Fourth Edition

HEART DISEASE

A Textbook of Cardiovascular Medicine

Edited by

EUGENE BRAUNWALD,
A.B., M.D., M.A. (hon.), M.D. (hon.), Sc.D. (hon.), F.R.C.P.
Hersey Professor of the Theory and Practice of Medicine,
Harvard Medical School;
Chairman, Department of Medicine,
Brigham and Women's Hospital, Boston

VOLUME 2

W. B. SAUNDERS COMPANY
A Division of Harcourt Brace & Company

Philadelphia, London, Toronto, Montreal, Sydney, Tokyo

W. B. SAUNDERS COMPANY
A Division of
Harcourt Brace & Company

The Curtis Center
Independence Square West
Philadelphia, PA 19106

Library of Congress Cataloging-in-Publication Data

Heart disease : a textbook of cardiovascular medicine / edited by
Eugene Braunwald. — 4th ed.
    p.   cm.
  Includes bibliographical references and index.
  ISBN 0-7216-3097-9 (single volume). — ISBN
0-7216-3096-0 (set). — ISBN 0-7216-2943-1 (v. 1). — ISBN
0-7216-3094-4 (v. 2)
    1. Heart— Diseases. 2. Cardiovascular system—Diseases.
I. Braunwald, Eugene
    [DNLM: 1. Heart Diseases.   WG 200 H4364]
RC681.H362   1992
616.1′2—dc20
DNLM/DLC   91-27954

Manuscript Editor: Edna Dick
Production Manager: Frank Polizzano
Illustration Coordinator: Joan Sinclair
Indexer: Mark Coyle

ISBN	Single Volume	0-7216-3097-9
ISBN	Set	0-7216-3096-0
ISBN	Volume 1	0-7216-2943-1
ISBN	Volume 2	0-7216-3094-4

HEART DISEASE

Printed in the United States of America.

Last digit is the print number: 9   8   7   6   5   4   3

CONTRIBUTORS

ELLIOTT M. ANTMAN, M.D.

Associate Professor of Medicine, Harvard Medical School. Director, Samuel A. Levine Cardiac Unit, Cardiovascular Division, Department of Medicine, Brigham and Women's Hospital, Boston, Massachusetts

Medical Management of the Patient Undergoing Cardiac Surgery

DONALD S. BAIM, M.D.

Associate Professor of Medicine, Harvard Medical School. Director of Invasive Cardiology, Beth Israel Hospital, Boston, Massachusetts

Interventional Catheterization Techniques: Percutaneous Transluminal Balloon Angioplasty, Valvuloplasty, and Related Procedures

S. SERGE BAROLD, M.D.

Professor of Medicine, University of Rochester School of Medicine and Dentistry. Chief, Cardiology Division, Department of Medicine, The Genesee Hospital, Rochester, New York

Cardiac Pacemakers and Antiarrhythmic Devices

WILLIAM H. BARRY, M.D.

Nora Eccles Harrison Professor of Cardiology, University of Utah School of Medicine. Attending Physician, University of Utah Medical Center, Salt Lake City, Utah

Cardiac Catheterization

EUGENE BRAUNWALD, A.B., M.D., M.A.(hon.), M.D.(hon.), Sc.D.(hon.), F.R.C.P.

Hersey Professor of the Theory and Practice of Medicine, Harvard Medical School. Chairman, Department of Medicine, Brigham and Women's Hospital, Boston, Massachusetts.

The History; The Physical Examination; Mechanisms of Cardiac Contraction and Relaxation; Pathophysiology of Heart Failure; Assessment of Cardiac Function; Clinical Aspects of Heart Failure; The Management of Heart Failure; Pulmonary Edema: Cardiogenic and Noncardiogenic; Pulmonary Hypertension; Valvular Heart Disease; Coronary Blood Flow and Myocardial Ischemia; Acute Myocardial Infarction; Chronic Ischemic Heart Disease; The Cardiomyopathies and Myocarditides: Toxic, Chemical, and Physical Damage to the Heart; Primary Tumors of the Heart; Pericardial Disease; Traumatic Heart Disease; Pulmonary Embolism; Cor Pulmonale; General Anesthesia and Noncardiac Surgery in Patients with Heart Disease; Hematological-Oncological Disorders and Heart Disease; Endocrine and Nutritional Disorders and Heart Disease; Renal Disorders and Heart Disease

AGUSTIN CASTELLANOS, M.D.

Professor of Medicine, University of Miami School of Medicine. Director, Clinical Electrophysiology, Jackson Memorial Medical Center, Miami, Florida

Cardiac Arrest and Sudden Cardiac Death

BERNARD R. CHAITMAN, M.D.

Professor of Medicine, St. Louis University School of Medicine. Director, Division of Cardiology, St. Louis University Medical Center, St. Louis, Missouri

Exercise Stress Testing

PETER F. COHN, M.D.

Professor of Medicine and Chief, Cardiology Division, State University of New York Health Sciences Center, Stony Brook, New York

Traumatic Heart Disease

WILSON S. COLUCCI, M.D.

Associate Professor of Medicine, Harvard Medical School. Associate Physician, Cardiovascular Division, Brigham and Women's Hospital, Boston, Massachusetts

Primary Tumors of the Heart

CHARLES A. DENNIS, M.D.

Director, Comprehensive Cardiac Therapy, Scripps Clinic and Research Foundation, La Jolla, California

Rehabilitation of Patients with Coronary Artery Disease

ROMAN W. DeSANCTIS, M.D.

Professor of Medicine, Harvard Medical School. Physician, Director of Clinical Cardiology, Massachusetts General Hospital, Boston, Massachusetts

Diseases of the Aorta

KIM A. EAGLE, M.D.

Assistant Professor of Medicine, Harvard Medical School. Assistant Chief of Medicine-Residency Training, and Co-Director of Cardiology Fellowship Training, Massachusetts General Hospital, Boston, Massachusetts

Diseases of The Aorta

URI ELKAYAM, M.D.

Professor of Medicine, University of Southern California School of Medicine. Chief of Cardiology, USC University Hospital, Los Angeles, California

Pregnancy and Cardiovascular Disease

JOHN A. FARMER, M.D.

Associate Professor, Department of Medicine, Baylor College of Medicine. Associate Physician, Internal Medicine and Cardiology Service, The Methodist Hospital; Associate Physician, Ben Taub General Hospital, Houston, Texas

Risk Factors for Coronary Artery Disease

HARVEY FEIGENBAUM, M.D.

Distinguished Professor of Medicine, and Director, Hemodynamic Laboratory, Indiana University School of Medicine. Senior Research Associate, Krannert Institute of Cardiology, Indianapolis, Indiana

Echocardiography

CHARLES FISCH, M.D.

Distinguished Professor of Medicine, Indiana University School of Medicine, Indianapolis, Indiana

Electrocardiography and Vectorcardiography

WILLIAM F. FRIEDMAN, M.D.

J. H. Nicholson Professor of Pediatrics and Executive Chairman, Department of Pediatrics, University of California, Los Angeles, School of Medicine. Pediatrician-in-Chief, University of California at Los Angeles Medical Center, Los Angeles, California

Congenital Heart Disease in Infancy and Childhood; Acquired Heart Disease in Infancy and Childhood

GEOFFREY A. GARDINER, Jr., M.D.

Associate Professor of Radiology, Jefferson Medical College of Thomas Jefferson University. Director of Cardiovascular and Interventional Radiology, Thomas Jefferson University Hospital, Philadelphia, Pennsylvania

Coronary Arteriography

GARY GERSTENBLITH, M.D.

Associate Professor of Medicine, Johns Hopkins Hospital and Francis Scott Key Medical Center, Baltimore, Maryland

Aging and The Heart

SAMUEL Z. GOLDHABER, M.D.

Associate Professor of Medicine, Harvard Medical School. Associate Physician, Brigham and Women's Hospital, Boston, Massachusetts

Pulmonary Embolism

LEE GOLDMAN, M.D.

Professor of Medicine, Harvard Medical School. Vice-Chairman, Department of Medicine, Brigham and Women's Hospital, and Chief, Division of Clinical Epidemiology, Brigham and Women's Hospital and Beth Israel Hospital, Boston, Massachusetts

Cost-Effective Strategies in Cardiology; General Anesthesia and Noncardiac Surgery in Patients with Heart Disease

ANTONIO M. GOTTO, Jr., M.D., D.Phil.

Professor of Medicine, and Chairman, Department of Medicine, Baylor College of Medicine. Chief, Internal Medicine Service, The Methodist Hospital, Houston, Texas

Risk Factors for Coronary Artery Disease

WILLIAM GROSSMAN, M.D.

Herman Dana Professor of Medicine, Harvard Medical School. Chief, Cardiovascular Division, Beth Israel Hospital, Boston, Massachusetts

Cardiac Catheterization; Clinical Aspects of Heart Failure; Pulmonary Hypertension

ROBERT I. HANDIN, M.D.

Associate Professor of Medicine, Harvard Medical School. Chief, Hematology Division, Brigham and Women's Hospital, Boston, Massachusetts

Hemostasis, Thrombosis, Fibrinolysis, and Cardiovascular Disease

CHARLES B. HIGGINS, M.D.

Professor of Radiology, University of California at San Francisco School of Medicine. Chief, Magnetic Resonance Imaging, University of California at San Francisco Medical Center, San Francisco, California

Newer Cardiac Imaging Techniques (CT, MRI)

ROLAND H. INGRAM, Jr., M.D.

Professor and Vice Chairman of Medicine, University of Minnesota Medical School. Chief of Internal Medicine, Hennepin County Medical Center, Minneapolis, Minnesota

Pulmonary Edema: Cardiogenic and Noncardiogenic

NORMAN M. KAPLAN, M.D.

Professor of Internal Medicine, University of Texas Southwestern Medical School, Dallas, Texas

Systemic Hypertension: Mechanisms and Diagnosis; Systemic Hypertension: Therapy

WISHWA N. KAPOOR, M.D.

Professor of Medicine, University of Pittsburgh. Attending Physician, Presbyterian-University Hospital, Pittsburgh, Pennsylvania

Hypotension and Syncope

DONALD KAYE, M.D.

Professor and Chairman, Department of Medicine, Medical College of Pennsylvania. Chief of Medicine, Hospital of Medical College of Pennsylvania; Consultant, Philadelphia Veterans Administration Medical Center, Philadelphia, Pennsylvania

Infective Endocarditis

vi

RALPH A. KELLY, M.D.

Assistant Professor of Medicine, Harvard Medical School. Associate Physician, Division of Cardiology, Department of Medicine, Brigham and Women's Hospital, Boston, Massachusetts

The Management of Heart Failure

OKSANA M. KORZENIOWSKI, M.D.

Associate Professor, Medical College of Pennsylvania, Philadelphia, Pennsylvania

Infective Endocarditis

EDWARD G. LAKATTA, M.D.

Professor of Medicine, Johns Hopkins University School of Medicine, and Professor of Physiology, University of Maryland School of Medicine. Visiting Physician, Francis Scott Key Medical Center, Baltimore, Maryland

Aging and The Heart

DAVID C. LEVIN, M.D.

Professor of Radiology, Jefferson Medical College of Thomas Jefferson University. Chairman, Department of Radiology, Thomas Jefferson University Hospital, Philadelphia, Pennsylvania

Radiology of the Heart; Coronary Arteriography

BEVERLY H. LORELL, M.D.

Associate Professor of Medicine, Harvard Medical School. Co-Director, Hemodynamic Research Laboratory, Beth Israel Hospital, Boston, Massachusetts

Pericardial Disease

JOSEPH LOSCALZO, M.D., Ph.D.

Associate Professor of Medicine, Harvard Medical School. Director, Center for Research in Thrombolysis, Brigham and Women's Hospital; Chief, Cardiology Section, Brockton/West Roxbury Veteran's Administration Medical Center, Boston, Massachusetts

Hemostasis, Thrombosis, Fibrinolysis, and Cardiovascular Disease

VIJAK MAHDAVI, Ph.D.

Associate Professor, Department of Pediatrics (Genetics), Harvard Medical School. Associate in Cardiology, Children's Hospital, Boston, Massachusetts

General Principles of Cardiovascular Cellular and Molecular Biology

MELVIN L. MARCUS, M.D. (Deceased)

Professor, Department of Internal Medicine, College of Medicine, The University of Iowa. Director, Coronary Physiology Laboratory, and Director, Specialized Center of Research in Ischemic Heart Disease, The University of Iowa College of Medicine; Consultant Physician, Department of Veterans Affairs Medical Center, Iowa City, Iowa

Relative Merits of Imaging Techniques

E. REGIS McFADDEN, Jr., M.D.

Argyle J. Beams Professor of Medicine, Case Western Reserve University School of Medicine. Director, Airway Disease Center, University Hospitals of Cleveland, Cleveland, Ohio

Cor Pulmonale

ROBERT J. MYERBURG, M.D.

Professor of Medicine and Physiology, and Director of the Division of Cardiology, University of Miami School of Medicine. Chief of Cardiology Services, Jackson Memorial Hospital, Miami, Florida

Cardiac Arrest and Sudden Cardiac Death

BERNARDO NADAL-GINARD, M.D., PH.D.

Alexander S. Nadas Professor of Pediatrics and Cellular and Molecular Physiology, Harvard Medical School. Chairman, Department of Cardiology, Children's Hospital, Boston, Massachusetts

General Principles of Cardiovascular Cellular and Molecular Biology

STEPHEN O. PASTAN, M.D.

Assistant Professor of Medicine, Indiana University School of Medicine. Attending Physician, Indiana University Hospitals, Indianapolis, Indiana

Renal Disorders and Heart Disease

RICHARD C. PASTERNAK, M.D.

Assistant Professor of Medicine, Harvard Medical School. Director, Coronary Care Unit, Beth Israel Hospital, Boston, Massachusetts

Acute Myocardial Infarction

D. GLENN PENNINGTON, M.D.

Professor of Surgery, and Director of Heart Replacement Services, St. Louis University Medical Center. Director of Cardiac Surgery, Cardinal Glennon Children's Hospital, St. Louis, Missouri

Assisted Circulation and the Mechanical Heart

JOSEPH K. PERLOFF, M.D.

Streisand/American Heart Association Professor of Medicine and Pediatrics, University of California, Los Angeles, School of Medicine. Division of Cardiology, Departments of Medicine and Pediatrics, UCLA Center for the Health Sciences, Los Angeles, California

Heart Sounds and Murmurs; Congenital Heart Disease in Adults; Neurological Disorders and Heart Disease

REED E. PYERITZ, M.D., PH.D.

Professor of Medicine and Pediatrics, Johns Hopkins University School of Medicine. Clinical Director, Center for Medical Genetics, Johns Hopkins Hospital, Baltimore, Maryland

Genetics and Cardiovascular Disease

ERIC C. RACKOW, M.D.

Professor and Chairman, Department of Medicine, St. Vincent's Hospital and Medical Center of New York Medical College, New York, New York

Acute Circulatory Failure

BRUCE A. REITZ, M.D.

Professor of Surgery, Johns Hopkins University School of Medicine. Cardiac Surgeon-in-Charge of New York Medical College, Johns Hopkins Hospital; Attending Cardiac Surgeon, Sinai Hospital, Baltimore, Maryland

Heart and Heart-Lung Transplantation

DAVID S. ROSENTHAL, M.D.

Associate Professor of Medicine, Harvard Medical School; Henry K. Oliver Professor of Hygiene, Harvard University. Physician and Hematologist, Brigham and Women's Hospital; Director and Physician, University Health Services, Harvard University, Boston, Massachusetts

Hematological-Oncological Disorders and Heart Disease

JOHN ROSS, JR., M.D.

Professor of Medicine, and Co-Director, Scientific Affairs, Department of Medicine, Division of Cardiology, University of California at San Diego. Attending Physician, University of California at San Diego Medical Center, San Diego, California; Editor-in-Chief, *Circulation*

Mechanisms of Cardiac Contraction and Relaxation

viii **RUSSELL ROSS, Ph.D., D.D.S.**

Professor and Chairman of Pathology, University of Washington, Seattle, Washington
The Pathogenesis of Atherosclerosis

JOHN D. RUTHERFORD, M.B., Ch.B., F.R.A.C.P.

Assistant Professor of Medicine, Harvard Medical School. Co-Director, Clinical Cardiology Service, Brigham and Women's Hospital, Boston, Massachusetts
Chronic Ischemic Heart Disease

HEINRICH R. SCHELBERT, M.D.

Professor of Radiological Sciences, Division of Nuclear Medicine and Biophysics, Department of Radiological Sciences, University of California at Los Angeles School of Medicine. Principal Investigator, The Laboratory of Nuclear Medicine and The Laboratory of Biomedical and Environmental Sciences, University of California at Los Angeles, Los Angeles, California
Relative Merits of Imaging Techniques

DAVID J. SKORTON, M.D.

Professor and Associate Chair for Clinical Programs, Department of Internal Medicine, College of Medicine, and Professor, Department of Electrical and Computer Engineering, College of Engineering, University of Iowa. Consultant Physician, Department of Veterans Affairs Medical Center, Iowa City, Iowa
Relative Merits of Imaging Techniques

THOMAS W. SMITH, A.B., M.D.

Professor of Medicine, Harvard Medical School. Chief, Cardiovascular Division, and Senior Physician, Brigham and Women's Hospital, Boston, Massachusetts
The Management of Heart Failure

BURTON E. SOBEL, M.D.

Lewin Professor of Medicine, and Director, Cardiovascular Division, Washington University School of Medicine; Cardiologist-in-Chief, Barnes Hospital, St. Louis, Missouri
Coronary Blood Flow and Myocardial Ischemia; Acute Myocardial Infarction

EDMUND H. SONNENBLICK, M.D.

Olson Professor of Medicine, The Albert Einstein College of Medicine. Chief, Division of Cardiology, Hospital of The Albert Einstein College of Medicine and The Bronx Municipal Hospital Center, Bronx, New York
Mechanisms of Cardiac Contraction and Relaxation

ROBERT SOUFER, M.D.

Associate Professor of Diagnostic Radiology and Medicine (Cardiovascular Medicine), and Director, Positron Emission Tomography Center, Yale University. Attending Physician, Internal Medicine, Yale–New Haven Hospital; Director, Nuclear Medicine Service, West Haven VA Hospital, West Haven, Connecticut
Nuclear Cardiology

ROBERT M. STEINER, M.D.

Professor of Radiology and Associate Professor of Medicine, Jefferson Medical College of Thomas Jefferson University. Chief, Section of Thoracic Radiology and Director, Division of General Diagnostic Radiology, Thomas Jefferson University Hospital, Philadelphia, Pennsylvania
Radiology of the Heart

GENE H. STOLLERMAN, M.D.

Professor of Medicine, Boston University School of Medicine. VA Distinguished Physician, Edith Nourse Rogers Memorial Veterans Hospital, Bedford, Massachusetts
Rheumatic Fever and Other Rheumatic Diseases of the Heart

MARC T. SWARTZ

Director of Circulatory Support, St. Louis University Medical Center, St. Louis, Missouri

Assisted Circulation and the Mechanical Heart

MARTIN VON PLANTA, M.D.

Chief Resident, Department of Medicine, University Hospital Basle, Basle, Switzerland

Acute Circulatory Failure

FRANS J. TH. WACKERS, M.D.

Professor of Diagnostic Radiology and Medicine, and Director, Cardiovascular Nuclear Imaging and Exercise Laboratories, Yale University School of Medicine and Yale–New Haven Hospital, New Haven, Connecticut

Nuclear Cardiology

MYRON L. WEISFELDT, M.D.

Professor of Medicine, Johns Hopkins University School of Medicine and Francis Scott Key Medical Center, Baltimore, Maryland

Aging and the Heart

MAX HARRY WEIL, M.D., PH.D.

Distinguished Professor and Chairman, Department of Medicine, The Chicago Medical School, North Chicago, Illinois

Acute Circulatory Failure

GORDON H. WILLIAMS, M.D.

Professor of Medicine, Harvard Medical School. Chief, Endocrine-Hypertension Division, Department of Medicine, Brigham and Women's Hospital, Boston, Massachusetts

Endocrine and Nutritional Disorders and Heart Disease

GERALD L. WOLF, PH.D., M.D.

Professor of Radiology, Harvard Medical School. Director, Center for Imaging and Pharmaceutical Research, Massachusetts General Hospital, Boston, Massachusetts

Relative Merits of Imaging Techniques

JOSHUA WYNNE, M.D.

Professor of Medicine, Wayne State University. Chief of Cardiology, Harper Hospital, Detroit, Michigan

The Cardiomyopathies and Myocarditides: Toxic, Chemical, and Physical Damage to the Heart

BARRY L. ZARET, M.D.

Robert W. Berliner Professor of Medicine, Professor of Diagnostic Radiology, and Chief, Section of Cardiovascular Medicine, Yale University School of Medicine. Chief of Cardiology, Yale–New Haven Medical Center, New Haven, Connecticut

Nuclear Cardiology

DOUGLAS P. ZIPES, M.D.

Professor of Medicine, Indiana University School of Medicine. Attending Physician, University Hospital, Wishard Memorial Hospital, and Roudebush Veterans Administration Hospital, Indianapolis, Indiana

Genesis of Cardiac Arrhythmias: Electrophysiological Considerations; Management of Cardiac Arrhythmias: Pharmacological, Electrical, and Surgical Techniques; Specific Arrhythmias: Diagnosis and Treatment; Cardiac Pacemakers and Antiarrhythmic Devices

CONTENTS

PART IV
BROADER PERSPECTIVES ON HEART DISEASE AND CARDIOLOGIC PRACTICE

PART V
HEART DISEASE AND DISORDERS OF OTHER ORGAN SYSTEMS

PART III

DISEASES OF THE HEART, PERICARDIUM, AORTA, AND PULMONARY VASCULAR BED

31

Congenital Heart Disease in Infancy and Childhood
by WILLIAM F. FRIEDMAN, M.D.

General Considerations

DEFINITION

Congenital cardiovascular disease is defined as an *abnormality in cardiocirculatory structure or function that is present at birth, even if it is discovered much later.* Congenital cardiovascular malformations usually result from altered embryonic development of a normal structure or failure of such a structure to progress beyond an early stage of embryonic or fetal development. The aberrant patterns of flow created by an anatomical defect may, in turn, significantly influence the structural and functional development of the remainder of the circulation. For instance, the presence in utero of mitral atresia may prohibit normal development of the left ventricle, aortic valve, and ascending aorta. Similarly, constriction of the fetal ductus arteriosus may result directly in right ventricular dilatation and tricuspid regurgitation in the fetus and newborn, contribute importantly to the development of pulmonary arterial aneurysms in the presence of ventricular septal defect and absent pulmonic valve, or, further, result in an alteration in the number and caliber of fetal and newborn pulmonary vascular resistance vessels. In this same regard, postnatal events may markedly influence the clinical presentation of a specific "isolated" malformation. The infant with Ebstein's malformation of the tricuspid valve may improve dramatically as the magnitude of tricuspid regurgitation diminishes with normal fall in pulmonary vascular resistance after birth; the infant with hypoplastic left heart syndrome or interrupted aortic arch may not exhibit circulatory collapse, and the baby with pulmonic atresia or severe stenosis may not become cyanotic until normal spontaneous closure of a patent ductus arteriosus occurs. Ductal constriction many days after birth also may be a central factor in some infants in the development of coarctation of the aorta. Still later in life the patient with a ventricular septal defect may experience spontaneous closure of the abnormal communication, or develop right ventricular outflow tract obstruction and/or aortic regurgitation, or pulmonary vascular obstructive disease. These selected examples serve to emphasize that anatomical and physiological changes in the heart and circulation may continue indefinitely from prenatal life in association with any specific congenital cardiocirculatory lesion.

Certain congenital defects are not apparent on gross inspection of the heart or circulation. Examples include the electrophysiological pathways for ventricular preexcitation or interruptions in the cardiac conduction system giving rise to paroxysmal supraventricular tachycardia or congenital complete heart block, respectively. Similarly, abnormalities in the development of myocardial autonomic innervation or in the ultrastructure of myocardial cells may ultimately prove to contribute to asymmetrical septal hypertrophy and left ventricular outflow tract obstruction. These examples make clear that occasional difficulties arise in distinguishing between congenital anomalies that are readily apparent at or shortly after birth and lesions that may have as their basis a subtle or undetectable abnormality that is present at birth.

INCIDENCE. The true incidence of congenital cardiovascular malformations is difficult to determine accurately, partly because of the difficulties in definition discussed above. About 0.8 per cent of live births are complicated by a cardiovascular malformation.[1] This figure does not take into account what may be the two most common cardiac anomalies: the congenital, nonstenotic bicuspid aortic valve[2] and the leaflet abnormality associated with mitral valve prolapse.[3] Moreover, the widely quoted 0.8 per cent incidence figure fails to include small preterm infants, almost all of whom have persistent patent ductus arteriosus. Further, if the calculations were to include stillbirths and abortuses, the incidence would be greatly increased. Cardiac malformations occur 10 times more often in stillborn than in liveborn babies, and many early spontaneous abortions are associated with chromosomal defects (see Chap. 51).[1] Thus, it is clear that past statistical analyses have seriously underestimated the incidence of congenital heart disease.

Precise data concerning frequency of individual congenital lesions also are lacking, and the results of many analyses differ, depending on the source (living or dead) and the selection of the study population. Table 31–1 is a compilation from both clinical and pathological studies that approximates the frequency of occurrence of specific cardiovascular malformations.[4,5]

Taken in toto, children with congenital heart disease are predominantly male. Moreover, specific defects may show a definite sex preponderance; patent ductus arteriosus and atrial septal defect are more common in females, whereas valvular aortic stenosis, congenital aneurysm of the sinus of Val-

salva, coarctation of the aorta, tetralogy of Fallot, and transposition of the great arteries are more common in males.

Extracardiac anomalies occur in about 25 per cent of infants with significant cardiac disease,[6] and their presence may significantly increase mortality. The extracardiac anomalies often are multiple, in part involving the musculoskeletal system; one third of infants with both cardiac and extracardiac anomalies have some established syndrome.

ETIOLOGY

Malformations appear to result from an interaction between multifactorial genetic and environmental systems too complex to allow a single specification of cause;[7,7a] in most instances, a causal factor cannot be identified. Maternal rubella, ingestion of thalidomide early during gestation, and chronic maternal alcohol abuse are environmental insults known to interfere with normal cardiogenesis in humans.[8–10] *Rubella syndrome* consists of cataracts, deafness, microcephaly, and, either singly or in combination, patent ductus arteriosus, pulmonic valvular and/or arterial stenosis, and atrial septal defect. *Thalidomide* exposure is associated with major limb deformities and, occasionally, with cardiac malformations without predilection for a specific lesion. Tricuspid valve anomalies are associated with the ingestion of *lithium* during pregnancy. The *fetal alcohol syndrome* consists of microcephaly, micrognathia, microphthalmia, prenatal growth retardation, developmental delay, and cardiac defects. The latter— often defects of the ventricular septum—occur in about 45 per cent of affected infants. *Maternal lupus erythematosus* during pregnancy has been linked to congenital complete heart block (p. 714). Animal experiments have incriminated hypoxia, deficiency or excess of several vitamins, intake of several categories of drugs, and ionizing irradiation as teratogens capable of causing cardiac malformations. The precise relation of these animal teratogens to human malformations is not clear.

The genetic aspects of congenital heart disease are discussed extensively in Chap. 51. A single gene mutation may be causative in the familial forms of atrial septal defect with prolonged AV conduction, mitral valve prolapse, ventricular septal defect, congenital heart block, situs inversus, pulmonary hypertension, the combination of supravalvular aortic stenosis and peripheral pulmonary arterial stenosis, and the syndromes of Noonan, LEOPARD, Holt-Oram, Ellis–van Creveld, and Kartagener. Table 31–2 provides a partial list of syndromes in which cardiovascular anomalies may be manifestations of the pleiotropic effects of single genes or examples of gross chromosomal defects.[10a] Less than 10 per cent of all cardiac malformations can be accounted for by chromosomal aberrations or genetic mutations or transmission.

The finding that, with some exceptions, only one of a pair of monozygotic twins is affected by congenital heart disease indicates that the vast majority of cardiovascular malformations are not inherited in a simple manner.[11] Family studies indicate a twofold to tenfold increase in the incidence of congenital heart disease in siblings of affected patients or in the offspring of an affected parent. Malformations often are concordant or partially concordant within families.[12] Because the incidence of congenital heart disease in the offspring or siblings of an index patient is only 2 to 10 per cent, it is seldom wise to discourage the parents of one affected child from having additional children if either parent is free of a cardiovascular anomaly.[1] Moreover, the low recurrence rate and the increasing possibilities for effective treatment for nearly all cardiac lesions usually justify a positive approach to family counseling. When two or more members of the family are affected, the recurrence risk may be quite high, and a pedigree should be obtained before further counseling. If a dominant or recessive mendelian pattern is established, the mendelian laws apply, and the risk of recurrence in each pregnancy is equal.

TABLE 31–1 FREQUENCY OF OCCURRENCE OF CARDIAC MALFORMATIONS AT BIRTH

DISEASE	PERCENTAGE
Ventricular septal defect	30.5
Atrial septal defect	9.8
Patent ductus arteriosus	9.7
Pulmonic stenosis	6.9
Coarctation of the aorta	6.8
Aortic stenosis	6.1
Tetralogy of Fallot	5.8
Complete transposition of the great arteries	4.2
Persistent truncus arteriosus	2.2
Tricuspid atresia	1.3
All others	16.5

Data based on 2310 cases.

SYNDROME	MAJOR CARDIOVASCULAR MANIFESTATIONS	MAJOR NONCARDIAC ABNORMALITIES
Heritable and Possibly Heritable		
Ellis–van Creveld	Single atrium or atrial septal defect	Chondrodystrophic dwarfism, nail dysplasia, polydactyly
TAR (thrombocytopenia–absent radius)	Atrial septal defect, tetralogy of Fallot	Radial aplasia or hypoplasia, thrombocytopenia
Holt-Oram	Atrial septal defect (other defects common)	Skeletal upper limb defect, hypoplasia of clavicles
Kartagener	Dextrocardia	Situs inversus, sinusitis, bronchiectasis
Laurence-Moon-Biedl-Bardet	Variable defects	Retinal pigmentation, obesity, polydactyly
Noonan	Pulmonic valve dysplasia, cardiomyopathy (usually hypertrophic)	Webbed neck, pectus excavatum, cryptorchidism
Tuberous sclerosis	Rhabdomyoma, cardiomyopathy	Phakomatosis, bone lesions, hamartomatous skin lesions
Multiple lentigines (LEOPARD)	Pulmonic stenosis	Basal cell nevi, broad facies, rib anomalies
Rubinstein-Taybi	Patent ductus arteriosus (others)	Broad thumbs and toes, hypoplastic maxilla, slanted palpebral fissures
Familial deafness	Arrhythmias, sudden death	Sensorineural deafness
Weber-Osler-Rendu	Arteriovenous fistulas (lung, liver, mucous membranes)	Multiple telangiectasias
Apert	Ventricular septal defect	Craniosynostosis, midfacial hypoplasia, syndactyly
Incontinentia pigmenti	Patent ductus arteriosus	Irregular pigmented skin lesions, patchy alopecia, hypodontia
Alagille (arteriohepatic dysplasia)	Peripheral pulmonic stenosis, pulmonic stenosis	Biliary hypoplasia, vertebral anomalies, prominent forehead, deep-set eyes
DiGeorge	Interrupted aortic arch, tetralogy of Fallot, truncus arteriosus	Thymic hypoplasia or aplasia, parathyroid aplasia or hypoplasia, ear anomalies
Friedreich's ataxia	Cardiomyopathy and conduction defects	Ataxia, speech defect, degeneration of spinal cord dorsal columns
Muscular dystrophy	Cardiomyopathy	Pseudohypertrophy of calf muscles, weakness of trunk and proximal limb muscles
Cystic fibrosis	Cor pulmonale	Pancreatic insufficiency, malabsorption, chronic lung disease
Sickle cell anemia	Cardiomyopathy, mitral regurgitation	Hemoglobin SS
Conradi-Hünermann	Ventricular septal defect, patent ductus arteriosus	Asymmetrical limb shortness, early punctate mineralization, large skin pores
Cockayne	Accelerated atherosclerosis	Cachectic dwarfism, retinal pigment abnormalities, photosensitivity dermatitis
Progeria	Accelerated atherosclerosis	Premature aging, alopecia, atrophy of subcutaneous fat, skeletal hypoplasia
Connective Tissue Disorders		
Cutis laxa	Peripheral pulmonic stenosis	Generalized disruption of elastic fibers, diminished skin resilience, hernias
Ehlers-Danlos	Arterial dilatation and rupture, mitral regurgitation	Hyperextensible joints, hyperelastic and friable skin
Marfan	Aortic dilatation, aortic and mitral incompetence	Gracile habitus, arachnodactyly with hyperextensibility, lens subluxation
Osteogenesis imperfecta	Aortic incompetence	Fragile bones, blue sclerae
Pseudoxanthoma elasticum	Peripheral and coronary arterial disease	Degeneration of elastic fibers in skin, retinal angioid streaks
Inborn Errors of Metabolism		
Pompe disease	Glycogen storage disease of heart	Acid maltase deficiency, muscular weakness
Homocystinuria	Aortic and pulmonary artery dilatation, intravascular thrombosis	Cystathionine synthetase deficiency, lens subluxation, osteoporosis
Mucopolysaccharidoses: Hurler; Hunter	Multivalvular and coronary and great artery disease, cardiomyopathy	Hurler: Deficiency of α-L-iduronidase, corneal clouding, coarse features, growth and mental retardation Hunter: Deficiency of L-idurano-sulfate sulfatase, coarse facies, clear cornea, growth and mental retardation

Table continued on following page

SYNDROME	MAJOR CARDIOVASCULAR MANIFESTATIONS	MAJOR NONCARDIAC ABNORMALITIES
Morquio; Scheie; Maroteaux-Lamy	Aortic regurgitation	Morquio: Deficiency of *N*-acetylhexosamine sulfate sulfatase, cloudy cornea, severe bone changes involving vertebrae and epiphyses Scheie: Deficiency of α-L-iduronidase, cloudy cornea, normal intelligence, peculiar facies Maroteaux-Lamy: Deficiency of arylsulfatase B, cloudy cornea, osseous changes
Chromosomal Abnormalities		
Trisomy 21 (Down syndrome)	Endocardial cushion defect, atrial or ventricular septal defect, tetralogy of Fallot	Hypotonia, hyperextensible joints, mongoloid facies, mental retardation
Trisomy 13 (D)	Ventricular septal defect, right ventricle patent ductus arteriosus, double-outlet right ventricle	Single midline intracerebral ventricle with midfacial defects, polydactyly, nail changes, mental retardation
Trisomy 18 (E)	Congenital polyvalvular dysplasia, ventricular septal defect, patent ductus	Clenched hand, short sternum, low arch dermal ridge pattern on fingertips, mental retardation
Cri du chat (short-arm deletion-5)	Ventricular septal defect	Cat cry, microcephaly, antimongoloid slant of palpebral fissures, mental retardation
XO (Turner)	Coarctation of aorta, biscuspid aortic valve, aortic dilatation	Short female, broad chest, lymphedema, webbed neck
XXXY and XXXXX	Patent ductus arteriosus	XXXY: Hypogenitalism, mental retardation, radial-ulnar synostosis XXXXX: Small hands, incurving of fifth fingers, mental retardation
Sporadic Disorders		
VATER association	Ventricular septal defect	Vertebral anomalies, anal atresia, tracheo-esophageal fistula, radial and renal anomalies
CHARGE association	Tetralogy of Fallot (other defects common)	Colobomas, choanal atresia, mental and growth deficiency, genital and ear anomalies
Williams	Supravalvular aortic stenosis, peripheral pulmonic stenosis	Mental deficiency, elfin facies, loquacious personality, hoarse voice
Cornelia de Lange	Ventricular septal defect	Micromelia, synophrys, mental and growth deficiency
Shprintzen (velocardiofacial)	Ventricular septal defect, tetralogy of Fallot, right aortic arch	Cleft palate, prominent nose, slender hands, learning disability
Teratogenic Disorders		
Rubella	Patent ductus arteriosus, pulmonic valvular and/or arterial stenosis, atrial septal defect	Cataracts, deafness, microcephaly
Alcohol	Ventricular septal defect (other defects)	Microcephaly, growth and mental deficiency, short palpebral fissures, smooth philtrum, thin upper lip
Dilantin	Pulmonic stenosis, aortic stenosis, coarctation, patent ductus arteriosus	Hypertelorism, growth and mental deficiency, short phalanges, bowed upper lip
Thalidomide	Variable	Phocomelia
Lithium	Ebstein's anomaly, tricuspid atresia	None

Modified from Friedman, W. F.: Congenital heart disease. *In* Wilson, J. D., et al. (eds): Harrison's Principles of Internal Medicine. 12th ed. New York, McGraw-Hill Book Co., 1991, p. 924.

PREVENTION

The feasibility of preventive programs depends on what is learned in the future about the 90 per cent or more of cardiovascular anomalies for which no cause currently is known. Strict testing in animals of new drugs that may be teratogenic when taken during pregnancy may be expected to reduce the chances of another thalidomide tragedy. In this regard, the dictum cannot be emphasized too strongly that no medication should be taken during pregnancy without prior consultation with a physician. Physicians who deal with pregnant women should be aware of known teratogens as well as drugs that may have a functional rather than a structural damaging influence on the fetal and newborn heart and circulation, and should recognize that drugs abound for which there is inadequate information concerning their teratogenic potential. Similarly, appropriate radiological equipment and techniques for reducing gonadal and fetal radiation exposure should always be used to reduce the potential hazards of this likely cause of birth defects.

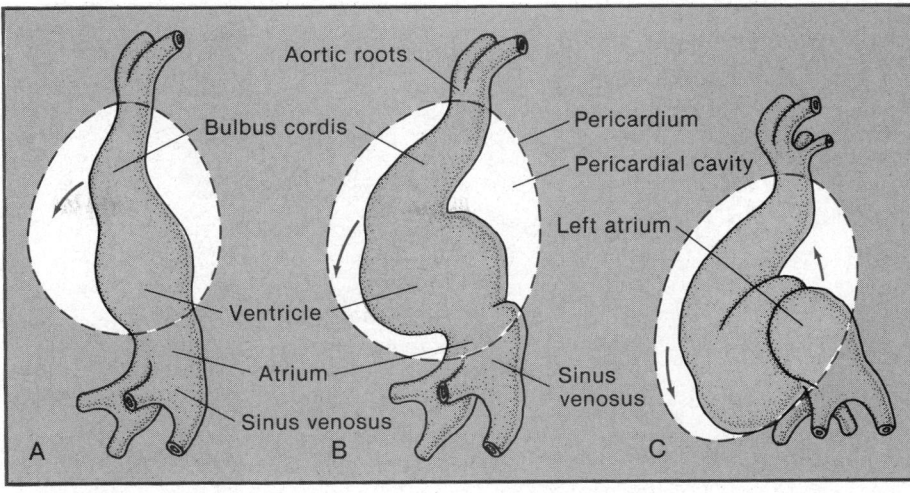

FIGURE 31-1. Formation of the cardiac loop as seen from the left side at *(A)* 32 days, *(B)* 34 days and *(C)* 38 days. Dashed line indicates parietal pericardium. The atrium gradually assumes an intrapericardial position. (From Clark, E. B., and Van Mierop, L. H. S.: Development of the cardiovascular system. *In Moss'* Heart Disease in Infants, Children, and Adolescents. Baltimore, Williams and Wilkins, 1989.)

Detection of abnormal chromosomes in fetal cells obtained from amniotic fluid or chorionic villus biopsy (Chap. 51) may predict cardiac malformation as one component of the multisystem involvement that may exist in such syndromes as Down, Turner, or trisomy 13–15 (D1) or 16–18 (E). Similarly, identification in such cells of the enzyme disorders observed in the mucopolysaccharidoses, homocystinuria, or type II glycogen storage disease may allow one to predict the ultimate presence of cardiac disease. Finally, immunization of children with rubella vaccine will avoid the effects of maternal rubella and its cardiac consequences.

EMBRYOLOGY

NORMAL CARDIAC DEVELOPMENT. Correlation of anatomical features of malformed hearts and embryonic cardiac morphology allows a developmental analysis of various anomalies. Detailed accounts of the normal development of the cardiovascular system are provided elsewhere.[13-15] In brief, during the first month of gestation the primitive, straight cardiac tube is formed, comprising the sinuatrium, the primitive ventricle, the bulbus cordis, and the truncus arteriosus in series (Fig. 31–1). In the second month of gestation this tube doubles over on itself to form two parallel pumping systems, each with two chambers and a great artery. The two atria develop from the sinuatrium; the atrioventricular canal is divided by the endocardial cushions into tricuspid and mitral orifices; and the right and left ventricles develop from the primitive ventricle and bulbus cordis. Differential growth of myocardial cells causes the straight cardiac tube to bear to the right, and the bulboventricular portion of the tube doubles over on itself, bringing the ventricles side by side (Fig. 31–2). Migration of the atrioventricular canal to the right and of the ventricular septum to the left serves to align each ventricle with its appropriate atrioventricular valve. At the distal end of the cardiac tube the bulbus cordis divides into a subaortic muscular conus and a subpulmonic muscular conus; the subpulmonic conus elongates and the subaortic conus resorbs, allowing the aorta to move posteriorly and connect with the left ventricle.

ABNORMAL DEVELOPMENT. A host of anomalies may result from defects in this basic developmental pattern. Thus, double-inlet left ventricle (p. 953) is observed if the tricuspid orifice does not align over the right ventricle. The various types of persistent truncus arteriosus (p. 915) result from failure of the truncus to divide into main pulmonary artery and aorta. Double-outlet anomalies of the right ventricle (p. 953) are produced by failure of either the subpulmonic or subaortic conus to resorb, whereas resorption of the subpulmonic instead of the subaortic conus may be central to transposition of the great arteries (p. 941).

THE ATRIA. The primitive sinuatrium is separated into right and left atria by the downgrowth from its roof of the septum primum toward the atrioventricular canal, thereby creating an inferior intraatrial ostium primum opening (Fig. 31–3). Multiple perforations form in the anterosuperior portion of the septum primum as the septum secundum begins to develop to the right of the former. The coalescence of these perforations forms the ostium secundum. The septum secundum completely separates the atrial chambers except for a central opening — the fossa ovalis — which is covered by tissue of the septum primum, forming the valve of the foramen ovale. Fusion of the endocardial cushions anteriorly and posteriorly divides the atrioventricular canal into tricuspid and mitral inlets (Fig. 31–4). The inferior portion of the atrial septum, the superior portion of the ventricular septum, and portions of the septal leaflets of both the tricuspid and mitral valves are formed from the endocardial cushions. The integrity of the atrial septum depends on growth of the septum primum and septum secundum and proper fusion of the endocardial cushions. Atrial septal defects (p. 906) and varying degrees of endocardial cushion defect (p. 92) are the result of developmental deficiencies of this process.

THE VENTRICLES. Partitioning of the ventricles occurs as cephalic growth of the main ventricular septum results in its fusion with the endocardial cushions and the infundibular or conus septum. Defects in the ventricular septum may occur owing to a deficiency of septal substance; malalignment of septal components in different planes, preventing their fusion; or an overly long conus, keeping the septal components apart. Isolated defects probably result from the first mechanism, whereas the latter two appear to generate the ventricular defects seen in tetralogy of Fallot (p. 935) and transposition complexes (p. 941).

THE LUNGS. These structures arise from the primitive foregut and are drained early in embryogenesis by channels from the splanchnic plexus to the cardinal and umbilicovitelline veins. An outpouching from the posterior left atrium forms the common pulmonary vein, which communicates with the splanchnic plexus, establishing pulmonary venous drainage to the left atrium. The umbilicovitelline and anterior cardinal vein communications atrophy as the common pulmonary vein is incorporated into the left atrium. Anomalous pulmonary venous connections (p. 951) to the umbilicovitelline (portal) venous system or to the cardinal system (superior vena cava) result from failure of the common pulmonary vein to develop or establish communications to the splanchnic plexus. Cor triatriatum (p. 929) results from a narrowing of the common pulmonary vein–left atrial junction.

THE GREAT ARTERIES. The truncus arteriosus is connected to the dorsal aorta in the embryo by six pairs of aortic arches. Partition of the truncus arteriosus into two great arteries is a result of the fusion of tissue arising from the back wall of the vessel and the truncus septum. Rotation of the truncus coils the aorticopulmonary septum and creates the normal

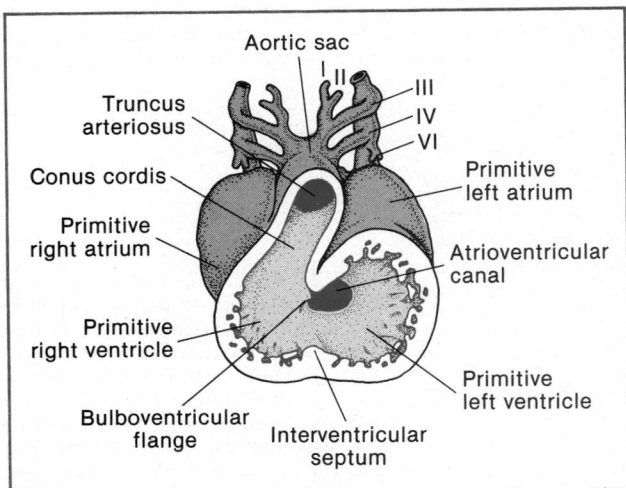

FIGURE 31-2. Frontal section through the heart of a 5-mm embryo showing the side-by-side primitive ventricles and the single opening of the atrium into the ventricles. (From Clark, E. B., and Van Mierop, L.H.S.: Development of the cardiovascular system. *In Moss'* Heart Disease in Infants, Children, and Adolescents. Baltimore, Williams and Wilkins, 1989.)

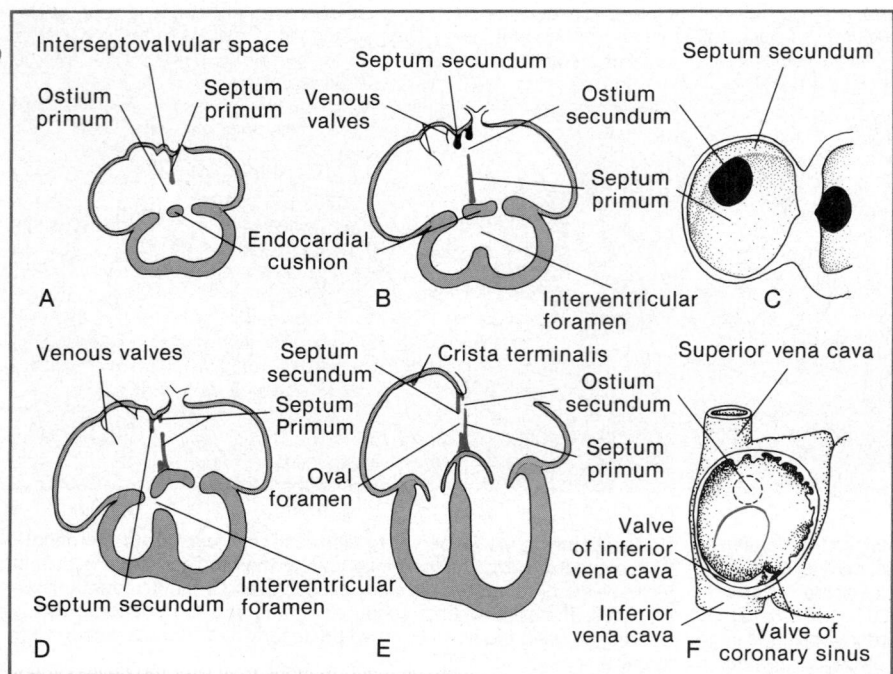

FIGURE 31–3. Diagrammatic representation of the atrial septa at 30 days (A), at 33 days (B), at 33 days (seen from the right side) (C), at 37 days (D), and in the newborn (E); the newborn atrial septum viewed from the right (F). (From Clark, E. B., and Van Mierop, L.H.S.: Development of the cardiovascular system. In Moss' Heart Disease in Infants, Children, and Adolescents. Baltimore, Williams and Wilkins, 1989.)

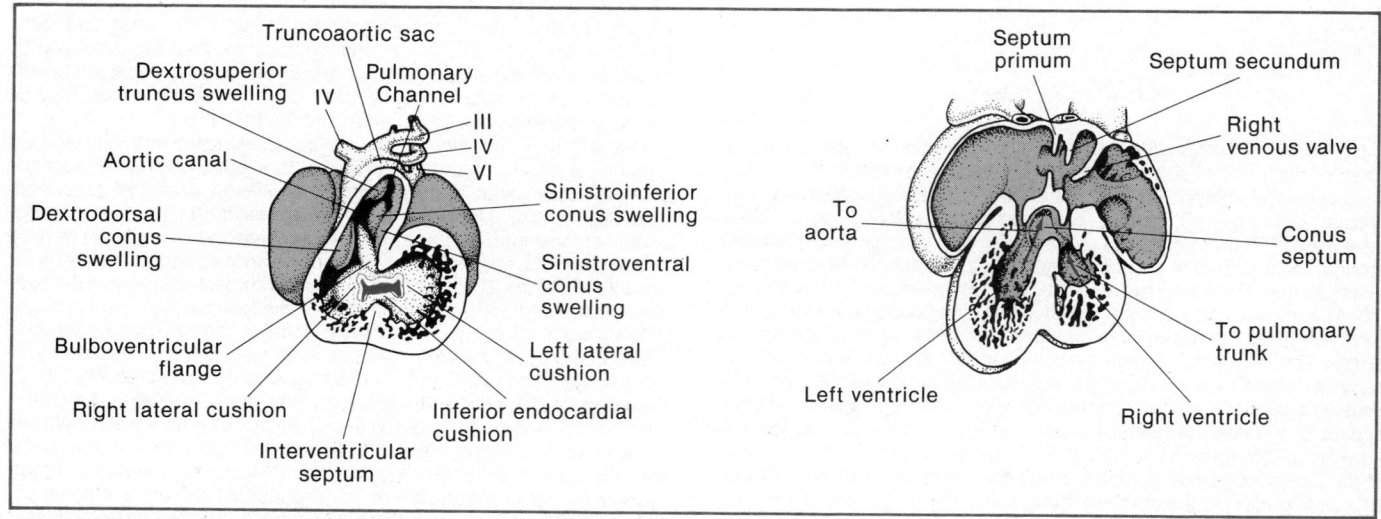

FIGURE 31–4. Frontal section through the heart of a 9-mm embryo (left panel) and 15-mm embryo (right panel). At 9 mm, development is noted of the cushions in the atrioventricular canal, and the truncus and conus swellings are visible. At 15 mm, the conus septum is completed; note the septation in the atrial region. (From Clark, E. B., and Van Mierop, L.H.S.: Development of the cardiovascular system. In Moss' Heart Disease in Infants, Children, and Adolescents. Baltimore, Williams and Wilkins, 1989.)

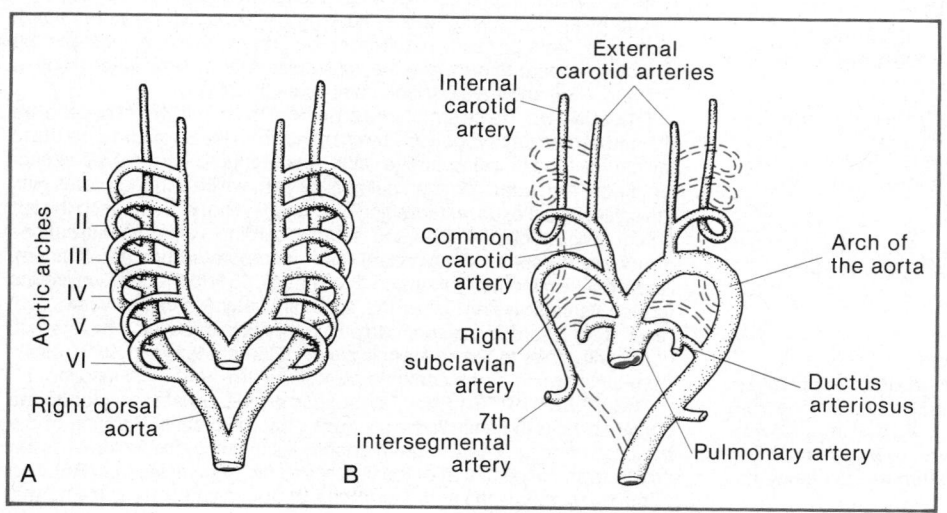

FIGURE 31–5. A, Aortic arches and dorsal aortas before transformation into the definitive vascular pattern. B, Aortic arches and dorsal aortas after transformation. The obliterated components are indicated by broken lines. (From Clark, E. B., and Van Mierop, L.H.S.: Development of the cardiovascular system. In Moss' Heart Disease in Infants, Children, and Adolescents. Baltimore, Williams and Wilkins, 1989.)

spiral relation between aorta and pulmonary artery. Semilunar valves and their related sinuses are created by absorption and hollowing out of tissue at the distal side of the truncus ridges. Aorticopulmonary septal defect (p. 915) and persistent truncus arteriosus (p. 915) represent varying degrees of partitioning failure.

Although the six aortic arches appear sequentially, portions of the arch system and dorsal aorta disappear at different times during embryogenesis (Fig. 31–5). The first, second, and fifth sets of paired arches regress completely. The proximal portions of the sixth arches become the right and left pulmonary arteries and the distal left sixth arch becomes the ductus arteriosus. The third aortic arch forms the connection between internal and external carotid arteries, while the left fourth arch becomes the arterial segment between left carotid and subclavian arteries; the proximal portion of the right subclavian artery forms from the right fourth arch. An abnormality in regression of the arch system in a number of sites can produce a wide variety of arch anomalies, whereas a failure of regression usually results in a double aortic arch malformation.

FETAL AND TRANSITIONAL CIRCULATIONS

Although the illness created by the presence of a cardiac malformation is almost always recognized only after an affected baby is born, important effects on the circulation have existed from early in pregnancy until the time of delivery. Thus knowledge of the changes in cardiocirculatory structure, function, and metabolism that accompany development is central to a systematic comprehension of congenital heart disease.

FETAL CIRCULATORY PATHWAYS. Dynamic alterations occur in the circulation during the transition from fetal to neonatal life when the lungs take over the function of gas exchange from the placenta. The single fetal circulation consists of parallel pulmonary and systemic pathways (Fig. 31–6) in contrast to the two-circuit system in the newborn and adult, in whom the pulmonary vasculature exists in series with the systemic circulation. Prenatal survival is not endangered by major cardiac anomalies as long as one side of the heart can drive blood from the great veins to the

aorta; in the fetus, blood can bypass the nonfunctioning lungs both proximal and distal to the heart. Oxygenated blood returns from the placenta through the umbilical vein and enters the portal venous system. A variable amount of this stream bypasses the hepatic microcirculation and enters the inferior vena cava by way of the ductus venosus. Inferior vena caval blood is composed of flow from the ductus venosus, hepatic vein, and lower body venous drainage, which is summarily deflected to a significant extent across the foramen ovale into the left atrium. Almost all superior vena caval blood passes directly through the tricuspid valve entering the right ventricle. Most of the blood that reaches the right ventricle bypasses the high-resistance, unexpanded lungs and passes through the ductus arteriosus into the descending aorta. The right ventricle contributes about 55 per cent and the left 45 per cent to the total fetal cardiac output. The major portion of blood ejected from the left ventricle supplies the brain and upper body, with lesser flow to the coronary arteries; the balance passes across the aortic isthmus to the descending aorta, where it joins with the large stream from the ductus arteriosus before flowing to the lower body and placenta.

FETAL PULMONARY CIRCULATION. In fetal life, pulmonary arteries and arterioles are surrounded by a fluid medium, have relatively thick walls and small lumina, and resemble comparable arteries in the systemic circulation. The low pulmonary blood flow in the fetus (7 to 10 per cent of the total cardiac output) is the result of high pulmonary vascular resistance. Fetal pulmonary vessels are highly reactive to changes in oxygen tension or in the pH of blood perfusing them as well as to a number of other physiological and pharmacological influences.

EFFECTS OF CARDIAC MALFORMATIONS ON THE FETUS. Although fetal somatic growth may be unimpaired, the hemodynamic effects in utero of many cardiac malformations may alter the development and structure of the fetal heart and circulation.[16] Thus, total anomalous pulmonary venous connection in utero may result in underdevelopment of the left atrium and left ventricle (p. 949), and premature closure of the foramen ovale may result in hypoplasia of the left ventricle. Moreover, postnatally, the caliber of the aortic isthmus may be reduced (p. 922) in the presence of lesions in utero that create left ventricular hypertrophy and impede filling because of reduced compliance of that chamber. It may also

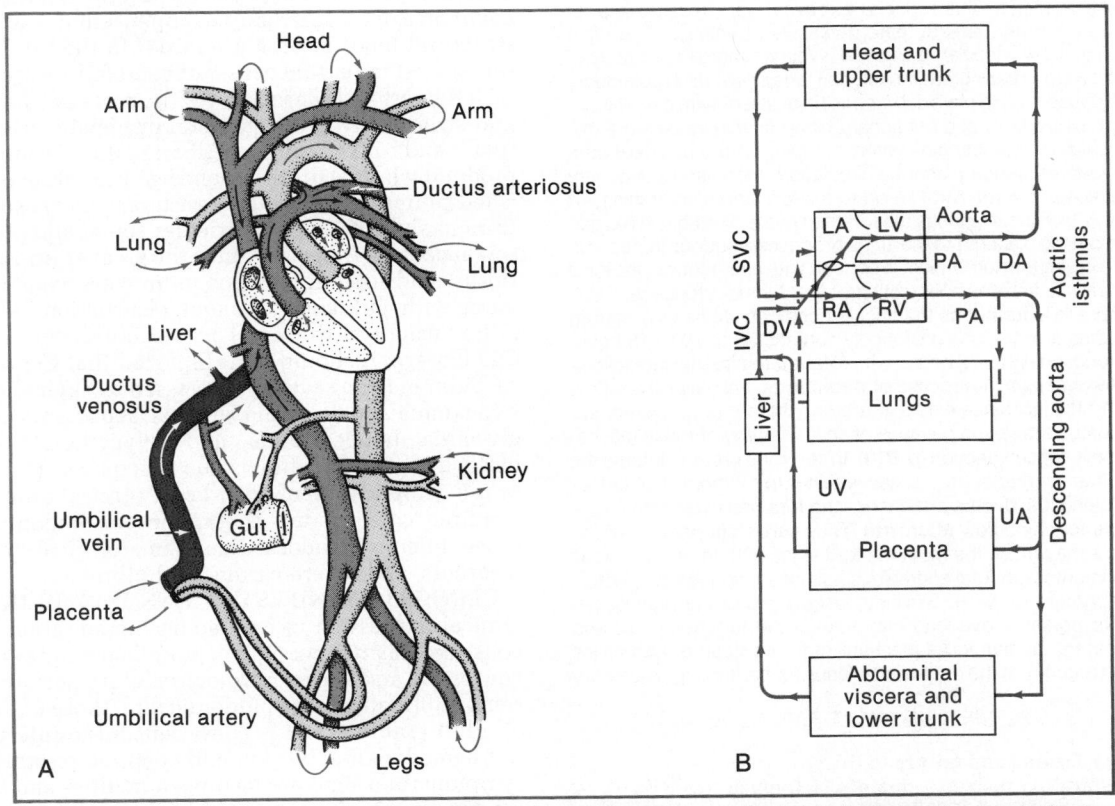

FIGURE 31–6. *A,* The fetal circulation. Shading shows the relative oxygenation of the blood, and arrows indicate its direction of flow. *B,* Prenatally, a fraction of umbilical venous (UV) blood enters the ductus venosus (DV) and bypasses the liver. This relatively well-oxygenated blood flows across the foramen ovale to the left heart, preferentially perfusing the coronary arteries, head, and upper trunk. Superior vena caval (SVC) blood is ejected by the right heart into the pulmonary artery (PA) and ductus arteriosus (DA). This stream circulates to the placenta as well as to the abdominal viscera and lower trunk. Dashed lines indicate diminished blood flow to and from the lungs and across the aortic isthmus. IVC = inferior vena cava, RA = right atrium, LA = left atrium, RV = right ventricle, LV = left ventricle, PA = pulmonary artery. (From Kaplan, S.: Congenital heart disease. *In* Vaughan, V. C., and McKay, R. J. [eds.]: Nelson Textbook of Pediatrics. 10th ed. Philadelphia, W. B. Saunders Company, 1975.)

be reduced in the presence of a lesion that interferes with left ventricular filling directly (e.g., mitral stenosis) or indirectly by diverting a proportion of left ventricular output away from the ascending aorta while increasing right ventricular output and ductus arteriosus flow (e.g., atrioventricular septal defect with left ventricular–right atrial shunt or aortic or subaortic stenosis with ventricular septal defect). Similarly, obstruction in utero to right ventricular outflow is associated with an increase in proximal aortic flow and diameter and almost never with aortic coarctation (p. 967). In these and other examples it is important to recognize that malformations compatible with fetal survival may nonetheless result in abnormal development of the circulation in utero and also affect circulatory adjustments after birth.

FUNCTION OF THE FETAL HEART. Compared with the adult heart, the fetal and newborn heart is unique with respect to its ultrastructural appearance,[17] its mechanical and biochemical properties,[17-20] and its autonomic innervation.[19-22] During late fetal and early neonatal development there is maturation of the excitation-contraction coupling process[23,24] and the biochemical composition of the heart's energy-utilizing myofibrillar proteins and of adenosine triphosphate and creatine phosphate energy-producing proteins.[20] Moreover, fetal and neonatal myocardial cells are small in diameter and reduced in density, so that the young heart contains relatively more noncontractile mass (primarily mitochondria, nuclei, and surface membranes) than later in postnatal life. As a result, force generation and the extent and velocity of shortening are decreased, and stiffness and water content of ventricular myocardium are increased in the fetal and early newborn periods. The diminished function of the young heart is reflected in its limited ability to increase cardiac output in the presence of either a volume load or a lesion that increases resistance to emptying.[25] Although functional integrity exists of efferent and afferent cardiac autonomic pathways early in life, fetal and newborn myocardium lacks the complete development of sympathetic but not cholinergic innervation. Thus, adaptation to cardiocirculatory stress in fetal or early newborn life may be less effective than in adulthood.

CHANGES AT BIRTH. The fundamental change that normally occurs at birth is a division of the single parallel fetal circulation into separate, independent circulations. Inflation of the lungs at the first inspiration produces a marked reduction in pulmonary vascular resistance owing partly to the sudden suspension in air of fetal pulmonary vessels previously supported by fluid media. The reduced extravascular pressure assists new vessels to open and already patent vessels to enlarge. The rapid decrease in pulmonary vascular resistance is related more importantly to vasodilatation owing to the increase in oxygen tension to which pulmonary vessels are exposed than to physical expansion of alveoli with gas. Pulmonary arterial pressure falls, and pulmonary blood flow increases greatly. Systemic vascular resistance rises when clamping of the umbilical cord removes the low-resistance placental circulation. Increased pulmonary blood flow increases the return of blood to the left atrium and raises left atrial pressure, which in turn closes the foramen ovale. The shift in oxygen dependence from the placenta to the lungs produces a sudden increase in arterial blood oxygen tension, which, in concert with alterations in the local prostaglandin milieu, initiates constriction of the ductus arteriosus.[26] Pulmonary pressure falls further as the ductus constricts. In healthy mature infants the ductus arteriosus is profoundly constricted at 10 to 15 hours and is closed functionally by 72 hours, with total anatomical closure following within a few weeks by a process of thrombosis, intimal proliferation, and fibrosis. A high incidence exists in preterm infants of persistent patency of the ductus arteriosus because of an immaturity of those mechanisms responsible for constriction (p. 913). In surviving preterm infants the ductus arteriosus spontaneously closes within 4 to 12 months of birth.

The ductus venosus, ductus arteriosus, and foramen ovale remain potential channels for blood flow after birth. Thus persistent patency of the ductus venosus may mask the most marked signs of pulmonary venous obstruction in infants with total anomalous pulmonary venous connection below the diaphragm (p. 949). Similarly, lesions producing right or left atrial volume or pressure overload may stretch the foramen ovale and render incompetent the flap valve mechanism for its closure. Anomalies that depend on patency of the ductus arteriosus for preserving pulmonary

or systemic blood flow remain latent until the ductus arteriosus constricts. A common example is the sudden intensification of cyanosis observed in the infant with tetralogy of Fallot when the magnitude of pulmonary hypoperfusion is unmasked by spontaneous closure of the ductus arteriosus. Moreover, there is increasing evidence that ductal constriction is a key factor in the postnatal development of coarctation of the aorta (p. 967). Lastly, it should be recognized that because the ductus arteriosus is potentially patent after birth and the pulmonary resistance vessels are hyperreactive, hypoxic pulmonary vasoconstriction of diverse causes may result in a right-to-left shunt through the ductus.

PATHOLOGICAL CONSEQUENCES OF CONGENITAL CARDIAC LESIONS

CONGESTIVE HEART FAILURE
(See also p. 446)

Although the basic mechanisms of cardiac failure, as outlined in Chap. 14, are similar for all ages, the pediatric cardiologist should clearly recognize that the common causes, time of onset, and often the approach to treatment vary with age.[27-29] The development of fetal echocardiography has allowed the diagnosis of intrauterine cardiac failure.[30,31] The cardinal findings of fetal heart failure are scalp edema, ascites, pericardial effusion, and decreased fetal movements. Although abnormalities in several organ systems may result in nonimmunological fetal hydrops, cardiac causes include a host of structural, functional, rhythm, and metabolic disturbances of the heart. Infants under 1 year of age with cardiac malformations account for 80 to 90 percent of pediatric patients who develop congestive failure. Moreover, cardiac decompensation in the infant is a medical emergency necessitating immediate treatment if the patient is to be saved.

In the preterm infant, especially under 1500 gm birthweight, persistent patency of the ductus arteriosus is the most common cause of cardiac decompensation, and other forms of structural heart disease are rare.[32] In the full-term newborn the earliest important causes of heart failure are the hypoplastic left heart and coarctation of the aorta syndromes, paroxysmal atrial tachycardia, cerebral or hepatic arteriovenous fistula, and myocarditis. Among the lesions commonly producing heart failure beyond age 1 to 2 weeks, when diminished pulmonary vascular resistance allows substantial left-to-right shunting, are ventricular septal and atrioventricular septal defects, transposition of the great arteries, truncus arteriosus, and total anomalous pulmonary venous connection, often with pulmonary venous obstruction. Although heart failure usually is the result of a structural defect or of myocardial disease, it should be recognized that the newborn myocardium may be severely depressed by such abnormalities as hypoxemia and acidemia, anemia, septicemia, marked hypoglycemia, hypocalcemia, and polycythemia. In the older child, heart failure often is due to acquired disease (Chap. 33) or is a complication of open-heart surgical procedures. In the acquired category are rheumatic and endomyocardial diseases, infective endocarditis, hematological and nutritional disorders, and severe cardiac arrhythmias.

CLINICAL MANIFESTATIONS IN THE INFANT. The clinical expression of cardiac decompensation in the infant consists of distinctive signs of pulmonary and systemic venous congestion and altered cardiocirculatory performance that resemble, but often are not identical to, those of the older child or adult (Table 31–3).[33] These reflect the interplay between the hemodynamic burden and adaptive responses. Common symptoms and signs are feeding difficulties and failure to gain weight and grow, tachypnea, tachycardia, pulmonary rales and rhonchi, liver enlargement, and cardiomegaly. Less frequent manifestations include peripheral edema, ascites, pulsus alternans, gallop rhythm, and inappropriate sweating. Pleural and pericardial effusions are exceedingly rare. The distinction between left and right heart failure is less obvious in the infant than in the older child or adult, since most lesions that create a left ventricular pressure or volume overload also

TABLE 31–3 FEATURES OF HEART FAILURE IN INFANTS

> Poor feeding and failure to thrive
> Respiratory distress—mainly tachypnea
> Rapid heart rate (160 to 180 beats/min)
> Pulmonary rales or wheezing
> Cardiomegaly and pulmonary edema on x-ray
> Hepatomegaly (peripheral edema unusual)
> Gallop sounds
> Color—ashen pale or faintly cyanotic
> Excessive perspiration
> Diminished urine output

result in left-to-right shunting of blood through the foramen ovale and/or patent ductus arteriosus as well as pulmonary hypertension owing to elevated pulmonary venous pressures. Conversely, augmented filling or elevated pressure of the right ventricle in the infant reduces left ventricular compliance disproportionately when compared with the older child or adult and gives rise to signs of both systemic and pulmonary venous congestion.[19]

Fatigue and dyspnea on exertion express themselves as a feeding problem in the infant. Characteristically, the respiratory rate in heart failure is rapid (50 to 100 breaths/min). In the presence of left ventricular failure, interstitial pulmonary edema reduces pulmonary compliance and results in tachypnea and retractions. Excessive pulmonary blood flow by way of significant left-to-right shunts may further decrease lung compliance. Moreover, upper airway obstruction may be produced by selective enlargement of cardiovascular structures. In patients with large left-to-right shunts and left atrial and main pulmonary artery enlargement, the left main stem bronchus may be compressed, resulting in emphysematous expansion of the left upper or lower lobe or left lower lobe collapse.[34] Respiratory distress with grunting, flaring of the alae nasi, and intercostal retractions is observed when failure is severe and especially when pulmonary infection precipitates cardiac decompensation, which often is the case. Under these circumstances pulmonary rales may be due to the infection or failure, or both. A resting heart rate with little variability is characteristic of heart failure. Hepatomegaly is regularly seen in infants in failure, although liver tenderness is uncommon. Cardiomegaly may be assessed roentgenographically, but it must be recognized that in the normal newborn infant, the cardiac diameter may be as much as 60 per cent of the thoracic diameter, and the large thymus gland in infants occasionally interferes with evaluation of heart size. Two-dimensional and Doppler echocardiography provide a good estimate of cardiac performance and chamber dimensions, and values may be compared with data derived from normal infants.[35-39]

Cardiac decompensation may progress with extreme rapidity in the first hours and days of life, producing a clinical picture of advanced cardiogenic shock and a profoundly obtunded infant. The presence of marked hepatomegaly and gross cardiomegaly usually allows distinction from noncardiac causes of diminished systemic perfusion.

CYANOSIS

(See also page 7)

Cyanosis is produced by reduced hemoglobin in cutaneous vessels in excess of approximately 3 gm/dl. Peripheral cyanosis usually reflects an abnormally great extraction of oxygen from normally saturated arterial blood, commonly the result of peripheral cutaneous vasoconstriction. Central cyanosis is a result of arterial blood oxygen unsaturation, most often in patients with congenital heart disease caused by shunting of systemic venous blood into the arterial circuit. Infants especially (as compared with adults) may appear cyanotic when in heart failure because of both peripheral and central factors; the latter may include severe impairment of pulmonary function that commonly exists with alveolar hypoventilation, ventilation-perfusion inequality, or impaired oxygen diffusion. In patients with central cyanosis owing to arterial oxygen unsaturation, the degree of cutaneous discoloration depends on the absolute amount of reduced hemoglobin, the magnitude of the right-to-left shunt relative to systemic flow, and the oxyhemoglobin saturation of venous blood. The last of these depends in turn on the tissue extraction of oxygen. Commonly, cyanosis appears or intensifies with physical activity or exercise as the saturation of systemic venous blood declines concurrent with an increase in right-to-left shunting across a defect as peripheral vascular resistance decreases. Oxygen transfer to the tissues is affected by shifts in the oxygen hemoglobin dissociation relation, which may be altered

by blood pH and levels of red blood cell 2,3-diphosphoglycerate concentration.

CLUBBING AND POLYCYTHEMIA. Prominent accompaniments of arterial hypoxemia are polycythemia and clubbing of the digits. The latter is associated with an increased number of capillaries with increased blood flow through extensive arteriovenous aneurysms and an increase of connective tissue in the terminal phalanges of the fingers and toes. Polycythemia is a physiological response to chronic hypoxemia that stimulates erythrocytosis. The extremely high hematocrits observed in patients with arterial oxygen unsaturation cause a progressive increase in blood viscosity, especially beyond packed red blood cell volumes of 60 per cent. Both the hematocrit and the circulating whole blood volume are increased in polycythemia accompanying cyanotic congenital heart disease; the hypervolemia is the result of an increase in red cell volume. The augmented red blood cell volume provoked by hypoxemia provides an increased oxygen-carrying capacity and enhanced oxygen supply to the tissues. The compensatory polycythemia often is of such severity that it becomes a liability and produces adverse physiological effects such as thrombotic lesions in diverse organs and a hemorrhagic diathesis.[41] In this regard, oral steroid contraceptives are contraindicated in the adolescent cyanotic female because of the enhanced risk of cerebral thrombosis.

MANAGEMENT. Red cell volume reduction and replacement with plasma or albumin (erythrophoresis) lowers blood viscosity and increases systemic blood flow and systemic oxygen transport, and thus may be helpful in the management of patients with severe hypoxic polycythemia (hematocrit $\geq$ 65 per cent). A final hematocrit of 55 to 63 per cent should be achieved; the higher level is necessary in patients with low initial oxygen saturation to avoid a severe reduction in arterial oxygen content. Acute phlebotomy without fluid replacement is contraindicated.

CEREBRAL AND PULMONARY COMPLICATIONS. Cerebrovascular accidents and brain abscesses occur particularly in cyanotic patients with substantial arterial desaturation.[42-44] *Cerebral thrombosis* is most common under age 2 years in severely cyanotic children, even in the presence of relatively low hematocrits, and occurs especially in a clinical setting in which oxygen requirements are raised by fever or, if blood viscosity is increased, dehydration.

Brain abscess is an important complication of cyanotic heart disease.[43,44] Such abscesses are rare under 18 months of age and commonly are of insidious onset marked by headache, low-grade fever, vomiting, and a change in personality. Seizures or paralysis less frequently heralds the onset of a brain abscess. Abscess must be suspected in any cyanotic child with focal neurological signs. Morbidity and mortality are related inversely to oxygen saturation levels. Brain abscess is thought to occur in about 2 per cent of the population with cyanotic congenital heart disease; a mortality rate of 30 to 40 per cent often is related to delay in diagnosis and treatment.

Paradoxical embolus is a rare complication of cyanotic heart disease, usually observed only at necropsy.[45] Emboli arising in systemic veins may pass directly to the systemic circulation, since right-to-left intracardiac shunts allow venous blood to bypass the normal filtering action of the lungs.

Retinopathy, consisting of dilated tortuous vessels progressing to papilledema, and retinal edema occasionally are observed in cyanotic patients, and appear to be related to decreased arterial oxygen saturation and/or to erythrocytosis but not to hypercapnia.

Hemoptysis is an uncommon but major complication in cyanotic patients with congenital heart disease, and occurs most often in the presence of pulmonary vascular obstructive disease or in patients with an extensive bronchial collateral circulation or pulmonary venous congestion.[46] Massive hemoptysis almost always represents rupture of a dilated bronchial artery.

SQUATTING. After exertion, patients with cyanotic heart disease, especially tetralogy of Fallot, typically assume a squatting posture to obtain relief from breathlessness.[47] Squatting appears to improve arterial oxygen saturation by increasing systemic vascular resistance, thereby diminishing the right-to-left shunt, and also by the pooling of markedly desaturated blood in the lower extremities. In addition, systemic venous return, and therefore pulmonary blood flow, may increase.

HYPOXIC SPELLS. Hypercyanotic or hypoxemic spells commonly complicate the clinical course in younger children with certain types of cyanotic heart disease, especially tetralogy of Fallot (p. 935).[47] The spells are characterized by anxiety, hyperpnea, and a sudden marked increase in cyanosis; they are the result of an abrupt reduction in pulmonary blood flow. Unless terminated, the hypercyanotic episodes may lead to convulsions and may even be fatal. The sudden reduction in pulmonary blood flow may be precipitated by fluctuations in arterial pCO_2 and pH, a sudden fall in systemic or increase in pulmonary vascular resistance, or an acute increase in the severity of right ventricular outflow tract obstruction either by augmented contraction of the hypertrophied muscle in the right ventricular outflow tract or by a decrease in right ventricular cavity volume owing to tachycardia.

Treatment. This consists of oxygen administration, placing the child in the knee-chest position, and administration of morphine sulfate. Additional medications that may prove of value include the intravenous administration of sodium bicarbonate to correct the accompanying acidemia, alpha-adrenoceptor stimulants such as phenylephrine hydrochloride (Neo-Synephrine) or methoxamine to raise peripheral resistance and diminish right-to-left shunting, and beta-adrenoceptor blocking agents, which reduce cardiac sympathetic tone and depress cardiac contractility directly, and which increase ventricular volume by reducing heart rate.

ACID-BASE IMBALANCE

Disturbances in blood gas and acid-base equilibrium are noted particularly in infants with either congestive heart failure or cyanosis.[48] Large-volume left-to-right shunts, especially with pulmonary edema, may be associated with moderate respiratory acidemia and a lowering of arterial oxygen tensions, reflecting an increase in the alveolar-arterial oxygen tension gradient and ventilation-perfusion imbalance. Interference with carbon dioxide transport implies moderate to severe failure in these infants. Lesions associated with a reduced systemic cardiac output, such as severe coarctation of the aorta or critical aortic stenosis in infancy, often present as cardiac failure complicated by a severe metabolic acidemia and relatively high values of arterial oxygen tension. The latter finding, even in the presence of right-to-left shunting across a patent ductus arteriosus, is a result of diminished systemic perfusion and an elevated pulmonary-systemic blood flow ratio. Respiratory acidemia and depressed levels of oxygen tension are observed in infants with obstruction to pulmonary venous return and right-to-left atrial shunting. Many infants with severe hypoxemia caused by lesions such as transposition of the great arteries or pulmonic atresia show metabolic acidemia and marked reductions in carbon dioxide tension secondary to hyperventilation, resulting from hypoxic stimulation of peripheral chemoreceptors.

IMPAIRED GROWTH

Impaired growth and physical development and delayed onset of adolescence are common features of many cyanotic and, to a lesser extent, acyanotic forms of congenital heart disease.[49] Mental development seldom is affected. The severity of growth disturbance depends on the anatomical lesion and its functional effect. Most children with mild defects grow normally. Weight gain is commonly slower than linear growth in acyanotic patients with large left-to-right shunts, whereas in cyanotic congenital heart disease, height and weight usually parallel each other. Boys appear to be more retarded in growth than girls, especially in the second decade. Skeletal maturity (i.e., bone age) is delayed in cyanotic children in relation to the severity of hypoxemia.

In some children, prenatal factors such as intrauterine infection and chromosomal or other hereditary and nonhereditary syndromes are responsible for growth retardation. In other patients, extracardiac malformations may contribute to poor weight gain and linear growth. Additional explanations for the mechanisms of growth interference have implicated malnutrition as a result of anorexia and inadequate nutrient and caloric intake, hypermetabolic state, acidemia and cation imbalance, tissue hypoxemia, diminished peripheral blood flow, chronic cardiac decompensation, malabsorption or protein loss, recurrent respiratory infections, and endocrine or genetic factors. In some instances, the underdevelopment is influenced little by operative correction of the underlying cardiac anomaly. Among factors that may be responsible for persistent growth retardation postoperatively are age at operation, hemodynamically significant residual lesions, and sequelae or complications of operation. As a general rule, it is unwise preoperatively to guarantee to the parents of a child with heart disease that surgery will result in accelerated growth and development.

PULMONARY HYPERTENSION

(See also Chap. 27)

Pulmonary hypertension is a common accompaniment of many congenital cardiac lesions, and the status of the pulmonary vascular bed often is the principal determinant of the clinical manifestations, the course, and whether surgical treatment is feasible.[50] Increases in pulmonary arterial pressure result from elevations of pulmonary blood flow and/or resistance, the latter sometimes caused by an increase in vascular tone, but usually the result of underdevelopment and/or obstructive, obliterative structural changes within the pulmonary vascular bed.[51-53]

Pulmonary vascular resistance normally falls rapidly im-

mediately after birth, owing to onset of ventilation and subsequent release of hypoxic pulmonary vasoconstriction. Subsequently the medial smooth muscle of pulmonary arterial resistance vessels thins gradually.[54] This latter process often is delayed by several months in infants with large aorticopulmonary or ventricular communications, at which time levels of pulmonary vascular resistance are still somewhat elevated. In patients with high pulmonary arterial pressure from birth, failure of normal growth of the pulmonary circulation may occur, and anatomical changes in the pulmonary vessels in the form of proliferation of intimal cells and intimal and medial thickening often progress, so that in the older child or adult vascular resistance ultimately may become fixed by obliterative changes in the pulmonary vascular bed. The causes of pulmonary vascular obstructive disease remain unknown, although increased pulmonary blood flow, increased pulmonary arterial blood pressure, elevated pulmonary venous pressure, polycythemia, systemic hypoxia, acidemia, and the nature of the bronchial circulation have all been implicated. There are many patients with pulmonary vascular obstruction whose cardiac anomaly places them at particular risk quite early in life, precluding survival to adulthood. Patients at particularly high risk for the development of significant pulmonary vascular obstruction are those with certain forms of cyanotic congenital heart disease, such as complete transposition of the great arteries with or without ventricular septal defect or patent ductus arteriosus, single ventricle without pulmonary stenosis, double-outlet right ventricle, and truncus arteriosus. Other conditions in which pulmonary vascular obstruction appears to progress rapidly include large ventricular septal defect, as well as the less common conditions of unilateral pulmonary artery absence, congenital left-to-right shunts in an environment of high altitude or in association with the Down syndrome of trisomy 21, and complete atrioventricular canal defects, even those unassociated with a chromosomal anomaly.

MECHANISMS OF DEVELOPMENT OF PULMONARY HYPERTENSION. Intimal damage appears to be related to shear stresses, since endothelial cell damage occurs at high-flow shear rates. A reduction in pulmonary arteriolar lumen size due to either thickened medial muscle or vasoconstriction increases the velocity of flow. Shear stress also increases as blood viscosity rises; therefore, infants with hypoxemia and high hematocrits as well as increased pulmonary blood flow are at increased risk of developing pulmonary vascular disease. In patients with left-to-right shunts, pulmonary arterial hypertension, if not present in infancy or childhood, may never occur or may not develop until the third or fourth decade or later. Once developed, intimal proliferative changes with hyalinization and fibrosis are not reversible by repair of the underlying cardiac defect. In severe pulmonary vascular obstructive disease, arteriovenous malformations may develop and predispose to massive hemoptysis.

Most vexing is the variability among patients with the same or similar cardiac lesions in both the time of appearance and rate of progression of their pulmonary vascular obstructive process. Although genetic influences may be operative (an example is the apparent acceleration of pulmonary vascular disease in patients with congenital heart disease and trisomy 21), evidence is now accumulating for important prenatal and postnatal modifiers of the pulmonary vascular bed that appear, at least in part, to be lesion-dependent. Thus a quantitative variability exists in the pulmonary vascular bed related to the *number,* not just the size and wall structure, of arterial vessels within the pulmonary circulation.[55,56] Modeling of the blood vessels occurs proximal to and within terminal bronchioles (preacinar and intraacinar vessels, respectively) continuously from before birth. The intraacinar vessels, in particular, increase in size and number from late fetal life throughout childhood with minimal muscularization of their walls. The ensuing increase in the cross-sectional area of the pulmonary arterial circulation allows the cardiac output to rise substantially without an increase in pulmonary arterial pressure. If, however, the presence of a cardiac lesion interferes with the normal growth and multiplication of these most peripheral arteries, the resulting elevation of pulmonary vascular resistance may first be related to failure of the intraacinar pulmonary circulation to develop fully, and then secondarily to the morphological changes of obliterative vascular disease—medial thickening, intimal proliferation, hyalinization and fibrosis, angiomatoid and plexiform lesions, and ultimately, arterial necrosis.[53]

In essence, the morphometric framework adds an important dimension, that of growth and development of the pulmonary circulation, to the traditional view of pulmonary vascular obstructive disease occurring primarily as a result of anatomical changes in the individual pulmonary arterioles. Research attention currently focuses on the cell biology of the vessel wall and abnormalities in endothelial cell–smooth muscle interactions in pulmonary hypertension.[51,56]

ASSESSMENT OF THE PATIENT WITH PULMONARY HYPERTENSION. It is important to understand the difficulties that exist with standard methods of assessing the severity of pulmonary vascular obstructive disease. Clinical, electrocardiographic, and echocardiographic observations do not distinguish between reversible and irreversible elevations in pulmonary vascular resistance. Hemodynamic measurements at cardiac catheterization are the mainstay in assessing the pulmonary vascular bed, especially its reactivity. The premium on accuracy is high because the presence, degree, and reactivity of pulmonary vascular obstruction determine the feasibility and long-term outcome of operation. Surgery must not be offered to patients with severe, fixed pulmonary vascular obstruction, even when the cardiac defect is anatomically correctable. Such patients either do not survive operation or, if they do, are not benefited and more often than not are harmed.

The aims of hemodynamic study are to quantify and compare the pulmonary and systemic flows and resistances and to determine the reactivity of the pulmonary vascular bed in patients with pulmonary hypertension. Because resistance to pulmonary blood flow cannot be measured directly, it is calculated from the ratio of pressure gradient to flow across the pulmonary bed according to Poiseuille's equation, which refers to steady flow of a newtonian fluid through straight, rigid tubes. There are potential errors in applying the equation and errors inherent in the methods of measurement. Furthermore, it is not possible in every patient to catheterize the pulmonary artery; when this is the case pulmonary venous wedge pressures may be used, but they are not always reliable indicators of pulmonary artery pressure, and the moment of hemodynamic evaluation may not be representative of potentially variable states of the pulmonary circulation. Nonetheless, a practical index of pulmonary vascular resistance can be established from measurements of pulmonary and systemic arterial pressures and calculated flows. One can then determine whether administration of drugs or oxygen reduces the pulmonary vascular resistance, implying that the resistance is not fixed and therefore may decrease or at least not progress after successful operation. A reduction in calculated pulmonary vascular resistance in response to oxygen inhalation or pharmacological intervention does not exclude coexisting anatomical pulmonary vascular disease, but does imply that there is a component of potentially reversible vasoconstriction contributing to the high resistance.

Other Diagnostic Methods. Because of the aforementioned shortcomings, additional methods have been developed to study the morphology of the small pulmonary arteries in patients with pulmonary hypertension. An example is the use of high-resolution magnification for *pulmonary wedge angiography* to determine the presence and extent of obstructive pulmonary vascular changes.[57] Pulmonary wedge angiograms, assessed quantitatively, appear to correlate well with both hemodynamic findings and histological observations of the structural state of the pulmonary vascular bed. Of additional interest is the current practical application of morphometric structural analyses that attempt to identify for operation patients whose postoperative pulmonary hemodynamics might be expected to improve, if not normalize.[58] Thus, *lung biopsy* at surgery has been proposed in patients with equivocal hemodynamic data to aid in determining whether to proceed with operation in reasonable anticipation of postoperative regression of elevated pulmonary vascular resistance.

THE MORPHOMETRIC APPROACH. Decisions on optimal timing of operations often are difficult because of the varying rates of development of pulmonary vascular disease in different patients with the same anomaly and because the evaluation of pulmonary vascular resistance and reactivity in the catheterization laboratory is a less than perfect science. Preoperative lung biopsy using the Heath-Edwards criteria has enjoyed little popularity, especially because sampling errors may result from the scatter of different grades of lesions in different parts of the lung. Accordingly, it is attractive to seek an alternative method that would obviate these problems. In this regard, application of a morphometric approach holds promise because the described changes in pulmonary vessel morphological characteristics are more uniformly distributed throughout the lung and, importantly, lend themselves to quantification.

Three abnormalities have been identified as anatomical markers of elevated pulmonary vascular resistance: (1) an excessive and premature extension of vascular smooth muscle into intraacinar pulmonary arteries, (2) failure of preacinar arterial wall thickness to regress normally, and (3) failure of pulmonary arteries to grow and proliferate normally during postnatal development. Frozen-section lung biopsy provides a firmer basis for judgment of whether reparative or palliative operation should proceed. The technique has proved useful in patients with univentricular hearts or tricuspid atresia in determining the feasibility of a Fontan procedure (p. 975) and in patients with lesions known to exhibit early and rapidly progressive pulmonary vascular disease, such as complete transposition of the great arteries, complete atrioventricular canal defect, and nonrestrictive ventricular septal defect.

CLINICAL MANIFESTATIONS OF PULMONARY HYPERTENSION. When this condition is associated with a large left-to-right shunt, the clinical manifestations reflect the specific malformation responsible. When pulmonary vascular resistance is elevated and a significant right-to-left shunt exists, the patient is cyanotic, and polycythemia and clubbing are noted. A dominant *a* wave in the jugular venous pulse may be seen, reflecting vigorous right atrial contraction caused by diminished compliance of the right ventricle. In some instances there are large systolic *c-v* waves, which suggest tricuspid regurgitation. A prominent right ventricular parasternal lift and palpable systolic expansion of the pulmonary artery are present. A soft pulmonary systolic ejection murmur preceded by an ejection sound and followed by a markedly accentuated pulmonic component of the second heart sound often is audible on auscultation; an early diastolic decrescendo blowing murmur of pulmonary regurgitation may be heard. If right ventricular failure and dilatation supervene, the systolic murmur of tricuspid regurgitation may be audible at the lower left sternal border. Right ventricular enlargement may be evident on the chest roentgenogram and electrocardiogram. The former examination also reveals a conspicuously enlarged pulmonary artery, prominent hilar pulmonary vascular markings, and attenuated peripheral vessels. The presence of pulmonary hypertension is suggested by analysis of Doppler waveforms of right and left ventricular ejection.[59,60] The site of the underlying defect may be localized by means of two-dimensional and Doppler echocardiography and/or cardiac catheterization and angiocardiography. Pressures in the right side of the heart are essentially identical to systemic pressures in cyanotic patients if the shunt is at the ventricular or aorticopulmonary levels, but they usually are lower than systemic pressures in patients with an intraatrial shunt. No specific treatment has proved beneficial for obstructive pulmonary vascular disease.

This fact underscores the importance of efforts to define the optimal age at operation to provide the highest probability of postoperative normalization of the pulmonary vascular bed. It is important to emphasize that almost all congenital cardiovascular defects are amenable to surgical repair in infancy, and it is likely that the surgical art will progress to the point that virtually all patients with lesions associated with pulmonary hypertension will be operated on within the first 3 to 18 months of life. When this goal is reached without increased operative mortality, the incidence of postoperative pulmonary vascular obstruction may well achieve the status of a bygone concern.

OTHER CONSEQUENCES OF CONGENITAL HEART DISEASE

INFECTIVE ENDOCARDITIS (see also Chap. 35). Infective endocarditis is uncommon under age 2 years, and thereafter most often affects children with tetralogy of Fallot (especially after systemic-pulmonary anastomosis), ventricular septal defect, aortic stenosis, and patent ductus arteriosus. Postsurgical patients with prosthetic heterograft or homograft valves or conduits are at particular risk. A causative organism can be isolated in about 90 per cent of children, usually either alpha-streptococci (usually *Streptococcus viridans*) or *Staphylococcus aureus*.[61,62] Fungal endocarditis is quite rare in the pediatric age group. Mortality appears to be highest when coagulase-positive *Staphylococcus* is the offending organism and when the endocarditis involves the left, rather than the right, side of the heart. Most recent data suggest 75 to 80 per cent overall survival.[61] Factors predisposing to endocarditis may be identified in about one-third of cases. These include cardiovascular surgery with infection during the perioperative period; respiratory tract infections; and ear, nose, throat, and dental procedures. Less often contamination during a surgical procedure or cardiac catheterization or an infection involving the skin, genitourinary tract, or other organ system has been the cause.

Although routine antimicrobial prophylaxis is recommended for all children with congenital heart disease and for the majority of patients after operative repair of the lesion, it should be recognized that many different microbes are responsible for the disease and that an effective preventive approach ultimately may center on active immunization rather than antibiotics. Antibiotic prophylaxis currently is recommended for all dental procedures known to induce gingival or mucosal bleeding, including cleaning, oral trauma, and other procedures such as tonsillectomy, gastrointestinal surgery, genitourinary surgery, and incision and drainage of infected tissue (Table 31–4). The risk of endocarditis is undoubtedly related both to the magnitude of bacteremia and to the type of underlying heart disease. Because infection on a prosthetic heart valve or conduit may be devastating, combinations of antibiotics given parenterally are advisable in these patients.

CHEST PAIN (see also pages 4 and 1295). *Angina pectoris* is an uncommon symptom of cardiac disease in infants and children, occurring in association with anomalous pulmonary origin of a coronary artery or, occasionally, in association with severe aortic stenosis, pulmonic stenosis, or pulmonary hypertension owing to pulmonary vascular obstruction. Cardiac pain in the infant with anomalous coronary artery (p. 918) usually takes the form of irritability and crying during feeding or straining at bowel movement. In children with severe left or right ventricular outflow tract obstruction chest pain commonly follows effort and is identical to angina observed in adults. Cardiac pain associated with *pulmonary vascular obstruction* may be anginal in nature but often is evanescent and pleuritic in type. Atypical forms of chest pain associated with the syndrome of *mitral valve prolapse* are much less usual in children than in adults. A sensation of chest discomfort or cardiac awareness frequently is interpreted as pain by the parents of children with cardiac arrhythmias. Careful questioning serves to identify palpitations rather than pain as the symptom and often elicits an additional history of anxiety, pallor, and sweating. Pain caused by *pericarditis* is commonly of acute onset and associated with fever, and can be identified by specific physical, roentgenographic, and echocardiographic findings.

Most commonly, chest pain in children is *musculoskeletal* in origin and may be reproduced on upper-extremity movement or by palpation; chest wall pain often is the result of *costochondritis*.[63] Finally, children, like adults, may suffer chest pain of nonspecific pattern owing to *anxiety*, with or without hyperventilation; a history often is elicited of a family member or friend who had recently died from or suffered myocardial infarction.

SYNCOPE (see also Chap. 30). Syncope is an unusual feature of heart disease in children; its presence suggests specific diagnoses, the most common being an arrhythmia. The symptom is observed in children with complete atrioventricular block that is less often of congenital origin than a

TABLE 31–4 PROPHYLACTIC ANTIBIOTICS FOR PROTECTION FROM BACTERIAL ENDOCARDITIS

I. STANDARD PROPHYLACTIC REGIMEN FOR DENTAL/ORAL/UPPER RESPIRATORY TRACT PROCEDURES

Amoxicillin 3.0 gm orally 1 hour before procedure, then 1.5 gm 6 hours after initial dose.

For amoxicillin/penicillin-allergic individuals:

Erythromycin ethylsuccinate 800 mg or erythromycin stearate 1 gm orally 2 hours before a procedure, then one-half the dose 6 hours after the initial administration.

-OR-

Clindamycin 300 mg 1 hour before a procedure, and 150 mg 6 hours after initial dose.

II. ALTERNATIVE PROPHYLACTIC REGIMENS FOR DENTAL/ORAL/UPPER RESPIRATORY TRACT PROCEDURES

For patients unable to take oral medications:

Ampicillin 2.0 gm IV (or IM) 30 minutes before procedure, then 1.0 gm ampicillin IV (or IM) or 1.5 gm amoxicillin orally 6 hours after initial dose.

For ampicillin/amoxicillin/penicillin-allergic patients unable to take oral medications:

Clindamycin 300 mg IV 1 hour before a procedure and 150 mg IV (or orally) 6 hours after initial dose.

Optional regimen for individuals considered to be at very high risk who are not candidates for the standard regimen:

Ampicillin 2.0 gm IV (or IM) plus gentamicin 1.5 mg/kg IV (or IM) (not to exceed 80 mg) one-half hour before procedure, followed by 1.5 gm oral amoxicillin 6 hours after the initial dose. Alternatively, the parenteral regimen may be repeated 8 hours after the initial dose.

Optional regimen for amoxicillin/ampicillin/penicillin-allergic patients:

Vancomycin 1.0 gm IV administered over 1 hour, starting 1 hour before the procedure. No repeat dose is necessary.

III. REGIMENS FOR GENITOURINARY/GASTROINTESTINAL PROCEDURES

Standard regimen:

Ampillicin 2.0 gm IV (or IM) plus gentamicin 1.5 mg/kg IV (or IM) (not to exceed 80 mg) one-half hour before procedure, followed by 1.5 gm oral amoxicillin 6 hours after the initial dose. Alternatively, the parenteral regimen may be repeated once 8 hours after the initial dose.

For amoxillin/ampicillin/penicillin-allergic patients:

Vancomycin 1.0 gm IV administered over 1 hour plus gentamicin 1.5 mg/kg IV (or IM) (not to exceed 80 mg) 1 hour before the procedure. May be repeated once 8 hours after initial dose.

Alternative oral regimen in low-risk patients:

Amoxicillin 3.0 gm orally 1 hour before the procedure, then 1.5 gm 6 hours after the initial dose.

Note: Initial pediatric dosages are listed below. Follow-up doses should be one-half the initial dose. Total pediatric dose should not exceed total adult dose.

Amoxicillin:	50 mg/kg
Ampicillin:	50 mg/kg
Clindamycin:	10 mg/kg
Gentamicin:	2.0 mg/kg
Vancomycin:	20 mg/kg
Erythromycin ethylsuccinate or stearate:	20 mg/kg

Adapted from Dijani, A.S., et al.: Prevention of bacterial endocarditis. Recommendations by the American Heart Association. JAMA *264*: 2919, 1990.

sequela of cardiac operation. Syncope caused by abrupt episodes of either bradycardia or tachycardia occurs in association with the sick sinus syndrome. The latter is most commonly produced in children after surgical procedures that involve the region of the sinoatrial node, e.g., atrial septal defect closure or Mustard's procedure for transposition of the great arteries (p. 941). Syncope is an occasional but ominous symptom if associated with severe aortic stenosis, pulmonary vascular obstruction, or a left atrial myxoma that transiently occludes left ventricular inflow.[64]

SUDDEN DEATH (see also Chap. 26). In contrast to adults, children seldom die suddenly and unexpectedly from cardiovascular disease. Arrhythmias, hypoxemia, and coronary insufficiency secondary to left ventricular outflow tract obstruction are the most frequent causes of death.[65,66] Sudden death most often is reported in patients with aortic stenosis or hypertrophic obstructive cardiomyopathy, primary pulmonary hypertension, the Eisenmenger syndrome of pulmonary vascular obstruction, myocarditis, congenital complete heart block, primary endocardial fibroelastosis, anomalies of the coronary arteries, and cyanotic congenital heart disease with pulmonic stenosis or atresia. A relation exists between strenuous exercise and sudden death in patients with aortic stenosis or obstructive cardiomyopathy, thus providing justification for restricting patients with these lesions from gymnastic activities and strenuous competitive sports.

APPROACH TO THE HIGH-RISK INFANT WITH CONGENITAL HEART DISEASE

Without prompt recognition, accurate diagnosis, and treatment about one-third of all infants born with congenital heart disease will die in the first months of life. Heart failure and cyanosis are the two cardinal signs in the high-risk infant with heart disease, and this section provides an approach for the management of each.

HEART FAILURE
(See also p. 446 and Chap. 17)

Care of the infant with heart failure must include careful consideration of the underlying structural or functional disturbance. The general aims of treatment are to achieve an increase in cardiac performance, augment peripheral perfusion, and decrease pulmonary and systemic venous congestion. It must be emphasized, however, that under many conditions medical management cannot control the effects of the abnormal loads imposed by a host of congenital cardiac lesions. Under these circumstances cardiac catheterization and operative intervention may be urgently required.[27,67] Thus initial therapy is aimed at stabilizing the infant's condition for diagnostic hemodynamic and angiocardiographic study as soon as possible. In almost all situations the decision to intervene surgically or to continue medical management requires a definitive anatomical diagnosis.

RESERVE MECHANISMS IN THE NEONATAL HEART

Pediatricians, in particular, should be aware of the important concept of cardiac reserve because it is in this regard that important differences exist between the young heart (of the preterm or newborn infant) and the fully developed heart of the older child, adolescent, and adult (Fig. 31-7).

Clinicians have long recognized the unique fragility and lability of the neonatal circulation in response to disease states and various physiological stimuli. Moreover, it often is apparent that newborns may exhibit suboptimal therapeutic responses to drugs such as digitalis, which directly stimulate cardiac contractility. The reasons for the age dependency of these observations have their basis in the reduced ability of the hearts of premature and full-term newborns, when compared with the hearts and circulation of older children or adults, to call on a functional reserve capacity to adapt to stress.[27,67,68]

Studies from the author's and other laboratories have shown that structural, functional, biochemical, and pharmacological properties of the young heart differ considerably from those of its older counterpart. The young heart contains fewer myofilaments to generate force with and to shorten during contraction. In addition, the chamber stiffness of the young heart's ventricles is greater than that seen later in life. This means that any increase in ventricular filling or volume in the small, young heart results in a disproportionately greater rise in ventricular wall tension or stress. Similarly, it takes a smaller increase in ventricular filling to reach the limits of

assistance given to cardiac pump and muscle function by stretching the myofilaments; that is, *preload or diastolic reserve is limited.* The young heart generates relatively less force and contracts less; it cannot generate the same ventricular systolic pressure or wall tensions, or obtain the same stroke volume augmentation from any initial stretch, as can the older heart. With these facts in mind, it must be remembered that the oxygen consumption of the normal newborn is considerably higher than later in life; accordingly, the newborn at rest has a much higher cardiac output/m^2 than the child or adult. Thus, even in the absence of stress, the young heart must function near peak performance just to satisfy the normal demands of the peripheral tissues. Because newborn cardiac performance at rest is so close to its ceiling, or limits of function, there is little *systolic reserve* that may be called on to adapt to an acute or chronic stress such as a pressure or volume load from an obstructive lesion or left-to-right circulatory shunt, respectively, or asphyxia.

In addition to *preload reserve* available to the heart from the Frank-Starling mechanism, and *systolic reserve* available through direct stimulation of cardiac contractility or through decreasing afterload to mechanically augment systolic emptying, there is a third, *heart rate reserve* mechanism. The latter consists of the ability of the heart to change its rate of pumping to raise the level of cardiac output. In this regard the newborn also is limited, since in this age group the intrinsic heart rate normally is quite high. In addition, heart failure per se will raise the frequency of contraction even further, primarily as a result of high circulating levels of catecholamines. In this sense, the newborn's heart rate also is closer than the child's or adult's to its ceiling, or upper limits of effectiveness. Furthermore, increases in heart rate occur largely at the expense of diastolic filling time. Thus, at very rapid heart rates, there is a disproportionately dimin-

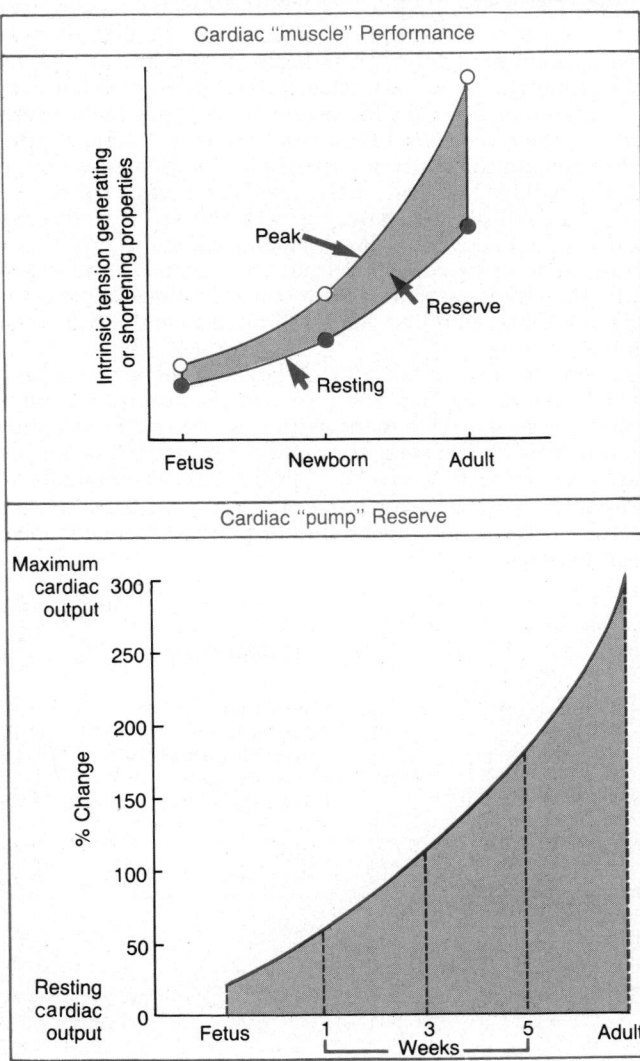

FIGURE 31-7. Schema of reduced cardiac reserve in fetal and newborn hearts compared with the adult's. In the newborn infant, resting cardiac muscle performance (top panel) is close to the peak of ventricular function because of limitations in diastolic, systolic, and heart rate reserve. Similarly, pump reserve (bottom panel) early in life is limited by these factors, as well as by a much higher resting cardiac output relative to body weight, compared with the adult.

ished diastolic time and therefore diminished time for perfusion of the myocardium by its own coronary arterial system. In addition, rapid heart rates result in elevated myocardial energy expenditure and increased myocardial demand for oxygen. The sum of these considerations indicates that newborn *heart rate reserve* is reduced.

TREATMENT OF HEART FAILURE (see also Chap. 17). Table 31–5 lists supportive and pharmacological measures in the treatment of the newborn with heart failure. The supportive measures are designed to increase tissue oxygen supply, decrease tissue oxygen consumption, and correct metabolic abnormalities. Digitalis glycosides and certain diuretic agents provide the most important elements of medical therapy, but it is important to recognize that the dosage regimen of drugs administered to young patients must be adjusted to take into account the age and size of the patient and the maturity-dependent pharmacological properties of cardioactive drugs.[67,69] Because this is especially true in early infancy, Table 31–6 provides the dosages of digoxin and diuretics commonly used for infants. Digoxin is the glycoside used exclusively to treat pediatric patients in most cardiac centers, since it is readily absorbed, available in convenient dosage form, and excreted rapidly from the body. Premature infants are more sensitive to digitalis than are full-term newborns, who, in turn, are more sensitive than older infants. Infants absorb and excrete digoxin as well as adults do, and their relative distribution of the glycoside to different body tissues also is similar. The prevailing dose schedules for digoxin produce higher serum concentrations in infants than would be considered optimal for adults.[70] The basis for the higher digitalis requirement in infancy is unclear, although it may relate to an age-dependent alteration in the sensitivity of the myocardium per se to the glycosides. In this regard, infants tolerate higher serum digoxin concentrations than adults without developing signs of toxicity. In the adult, the usual therapeutic concentrations of digoxin are less than 2 ng/ml blood, and toxicity commonly occurs above that level. In contrast, in infants, therapeutic levels of digoxin range from 1 to 5 ng/ml (mean = 3.5), while toxicity is associated with concentrations in excess of 3 ng/ml. Older children have therapeutic and toxic levels similar to those of adults.

A restricted fluid intake (65 ml/kg/day) and a low-sodium diet (1 to 2 mEq/kg/day) should accompany diuretic therapy in the most seriously ill infants with heart failure. Furosemide is the agent of choice when the rapid elimination of excess salt and water is needed. Hydrochlorothiazide, occasionally in conjunction with spironolactone or triamterene to reduce potassium loss and sodium retention, is convenient for long-term therapy.

TABLE 31–5 TREATMENT OF CONGESTIVE HEART FAILURE

I. GENERAL INTERVENTIONS
    Rest (occasional sedation)
    Semi-Fowler position
    Temperature and humidity control
    Oxygen
    Decrease sodium load
    Avoid aspiration
    Treat infection, if present

II. SPECIFIC INTERVENTIONS
    Preload manipulation
        Move ventricular function curve up by volume infusion to increase venous return
        Move ventricular function curve down with diuretics, venodilators
    Afterload reduction
        Facilitate ventricular emptying by reducing wall tension
        Reduce blood viscosity
        Drugs, arteriolar dilators, mechanical counterpulsation
    Inotropic stimulation
        Improve physical and metabolic milieu: pH, PaO_2, glucose, calcium, hemoglobin
        Inotropic drugs: digitalis, catecholamines, dobutamine, dopamine
    Heart rate
        Control rhythm disturbances with pacing, drugs
    Other
        Mechanical ventilation
        Prostaglandin manipulation
        Peritoneal dialysis

III. SURGERY (may include transplantation)

Other pharmacological approaches may prove to be of significant benefit in selected instances in which digitalis and diuretics are relatively ineffective. In situations in which cardiac decompensation is not the result of an obstructive lesion, catecholamines may be used temporarily to alleviate cardiac failure while the patient is awaiting more definitive operative treatment (Table 31–7).[67] In infants with the coarctation of the aorta syndrome, in whom ductal constriction unmasks the aortic branch point producing aortic narrowing (p. 967), or with aortic arch interruption, heart failure may be reversed dramatically by the intravenous infusion of prostaglandin E_1 (0.03–0.1 mg/kg/min), which results in dilatation of the ductus arteriosus and relief of the obstruction.[71,72] Conversely, in preterm infants in whom patent ductus arteriosus is responsible for profound cardiopulmonary deterioration, constric-

TABLE 31–6 DIURETIC AND DIGITALIS DOSAGES FOR INFANTS

PREPARATION	DOSAGE AND ROUTE OF ADMINISTRATION
Furosemide	IV, 1 mg/kg/dose; oral, 2 to 6 mg/kg/day
Ethacrynic acid	IV, 1 mg/kg/dose; oral, 2 to 3 mg/kg/day
Hydrochlorothiazide	Oral, 2 to 5 mg/kg/day
Spironolactone	Oral, 1 to 3 mg/kg/day
Triamterene	Oral, 2 to 4 mg/kg/day
Digoxin	
Elixir	0.05 mg/ml
Parenteral	0.10 mg/ml

| AGE AND WEIGHT | DOSE AND ROUTE* | |
	Acute Digitalization	Maintenance
Prematures <1.5 kg	10–20 µg/kg IV TDD: ½, ¼, ¼ of dose q 8h	4 µg/kg/day IV (may increase to 4 µg/kg q 12h at age 1 month)
1.5–2.5 kg	Same as above	4 µg/kg q 12h IV
Full-term newborns	30 µg/kg IV, TDD	4–5 µg/kg q 12h IV
Infants (1–12 months)	35 µg/kg IV, TDD	5–10 µg/kg q 12h IV
>12 months	40 µg/kg IV, TDD (maximum 1.0 mg)	5–10 µg/kg q 12h IV
Older children (over 20 kg)	1.0–2.0 mg IV, TDD over 48 hours	0.125–0.250 mg IV q day

* P.O. Oral dose approximately 20 per cent greater than IV dose except in "older children." In older children, IV = oral dose.
TDD = Total digitalizing dose.

TABLE 31-7   DOSAGE REGIMENS: INOTROPIC AGENTS

901

CHAP
31

DRUG	DOSE	COMMENTS
Epinephrine (Adrenalin)	0.05–1.0 μg/kg/min IV	May cause hypertension and cardiac arrhythmias; inactivated in alkaline solution
Isoproterenol (Isuprel)	0.05–0.5 μg/kg/min IV	May decrease coronary blood flow; results in peripheral and pulmonary vasodilation
Norepinephrine (Levophed)	0.05–0.5 μg/kg/min IV	Causes significant vasoconstriction
Dobutamine (Dobutrex)	2–10 μg/kg/min IV (Max 40 μg/kg/min)	No direct effect on renal perfusion, little or no peripheral vasodilatation or tachycardia
Dopamine (Intropin)	2–20 μg/kg/min IV (Max 50 μg/kg/min) 2–5 μg/kg/min 5–8 μg/kg/min >8 μg/kg/min >10 μg/kg/min 15–20 μg/kg/min	Significant renal vasodilatation Inotropic ± heart rate acceleration Significant heart rate acceleration ± Vasoconstriction Significant vasoconstriction
	(Above dose/effect relations speculative in neonates)	
Amrinone	Dose schedule not established for infants and children Adults: 40 μg/kg/min IV for 1 hr, then 6–10 μg/kg/min; 50–450 mg/day po divided TID	May cause thrombocytopenia, hepatic and GI disturbance, fever, and arrhythmias

From Friedman, W. F., and George, B. L.: New concepts and drugs in the treatment of congestive heart failure. Pediatr. Clin. North Am. 31:1197, 1984.

tion of the ductus arteriosus may be accomplished by inhibition of prostaglandin synthesis with the nonsteroidal anti-inflammatory agent indomethacin (0.2 mg/kg IV).[73,74] Vasodilator therapy also is used in infants or children with heart disease in whom preload or afterload alterations may be expected to improve cardiac performance (Table 31–8).[27,28,67,75] Moreover, treatment of severe cardiac failure often requires combining inotropic and afterload-reducing agents (p. 500). Combinations of dopamine, dobutamine, and nitroprusside have been used extensively and effectively in the pediatric population, primarily in the setting of low cardiac output after open-heart surgery.[67] Use of oral afterload-reducing agents, e.g., hydralazine or captopril, in association with digoxin is worthwhile in the long-term therapy of outpatients with congestive cardiomyopathy and/or significant mitral or aortic regurgitation.

CYANOSIS

(See also p. 895)

Cyanosis in the infant often presents as a diagnostic emergency, necessitating prompt detection of the underlying cause. The schema in Figure 31–8 outlines a general approach to diagnosis. The cardiologist must distinguish between three types of cyanosis—peripheral, differential, and central—while recognizing that cyanosis may accompany diseases of the central nervous, hematological, respiratory, and cardiac systems.

PERIPHERAL CYANOSIS. Peripheral cyanosis (normal arterial oxygen saturation and widened arteriovenous oxygen differences) usually indicates stasis of blood flow in the periphery. The level of reduced hemoglobin in the capillaries of the skin usually exceeds 3 gm/100 dl. The most prominent causes of peripheral cyanosis in the newborn are autonomically controlled alterations in the cutaneous distribution of capillary blood flow (acrocyanosis) and septicemia associated with evidence of a low cardiac output, i.e., hypotension, weak pulse, and cold extremities. In many instances peripheral cyanosis is clearly the result of a cold environment or high hemoglobin content. When cyanosis is caused by the former, vasodilatation produced by immersing the extremity in warm water for several minutes will reverse the cyanosis.

CENTRAL CYANOSIS. Oxygen unsaturation in central cyanosis may result from inadequately oxygenated pulmonary venous blood, in which case inhalation of 100 per cent oxygen may diminish or clear the discoloration (see below). Conversely, in instances in which cyanosis is due to an intracardiac or extracardiac right-to-left shunt, pulmonary venous blood is fully saturated, and inhalation of 100 per cent oxygen usually will not improve the infant's color. It is necessary to qualify the latter statement because oxygen may act directly in infants with elevated pulmonary vas-

TABLE 31-8   DOSAGE REGIMENS: VASODILATORS

DRUG	DOSE AND ROUTE OF ADMINISTRATION	COMMENTS
Nitroglycerin	0.5–20 μg/kg/min IV (Max 60 μg/kg/min IV)	Dosage schedule for IV and other routes of administration not well established for children
Hydralazine (Apresoline)	0.5 mg/kg/day po q 6-8h (Max 200 mg/day or 7 mg/kg/day) 1.5 μg/kg/min IV or 0.1–0.5 mg/kg/dose IV q 6h (Max 2 mg/kg-q 6h)	May cause tachycardia, GI symptoms, neutropenia, lupus-like syndrome
Captopril (Capoten)	0.1–0.4 mg/kg/dose po given q 6-24h as needed	May cause neutropenia/proteinuria
Nitroprusside (Nipride)	0.5–8 μg/kg/min IV	May result in thiocyanate or cyanide toxicity if used in high doses or for prolonged periods of time; light-sensitive
Prazosin (Minipress)	1st dose: 5 μg/kg/po (Max 25 μg/kg/dose q 6h)	Initial dose used to elevate hypotensive effects; orthostatic hypotension, attenuation of hemodynamic effects may occur.

From Friedman, W. F., and George, B. L.: New concepts and drugs in the treatment of congestive heart failure. Pediatr. Clin. North Am. 31:1197, 1984.

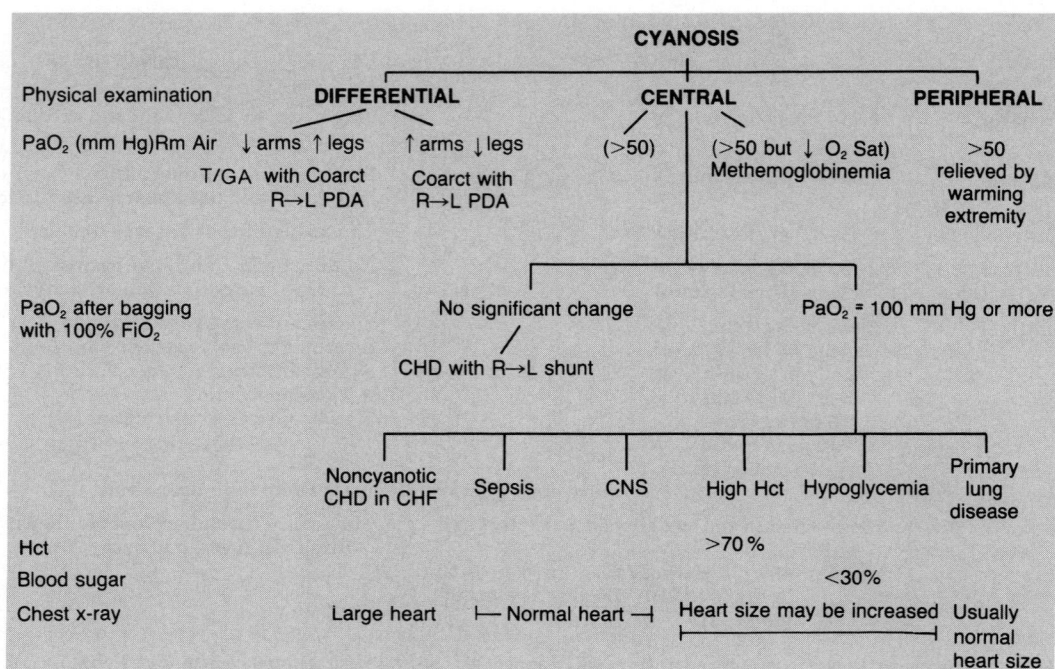

FIGURE 31–8. Flow chart for the evaluation of cyanotic infants. Tests to be done are listed at the left. The response to each of these tests leads along the line to the proper diagnostic category. CHD = congenital heart disease, CHF = congestive heart failure, CNS = central nervous system, Hct = hematocrit, PDA = patent ductus arteriosus, T/GA = transposition of great arteries. (From Kirkpatrick, S. E., et al.: Differential diagnosis of congenital heart disease in the newborn – University of California, San Diego, School of Medicine, and University Hospital, San Diego [Specialty Conference]. West. J. Med. *128*:127, 1978.)

cular resistance to dilate the pulmonary blood vessels and thus reduce the magnitude of the venoarterial shunt. Central cyanosis also may be due to the replacement of normal by abnormal hemoglobin, as in methemoglobinemia.

Several factors influence the oxygen saturation produced at any given arterial pO_2. These include temperature, pH, ratio of fetal to adult hemoglobin, and erythrocyte concentration of 2,3-diphosphoglycerate. For example, fetal hemoglobin has a higher affinity for oxygen than does adult hemoglobin and therefore would be more highly saturated at any given pO_2. Thus, determination of the systemic arterial oxygen tension may provide a more accurate picture of the underlying pathophysiology than simply measuring the oxygen saturation.[76]

DIFFERENTIAL CYANOSIS. Differential cyanosis virtually always indicates the presence of congenital heart disease, often with patency of the ductus arteriosus and coarctation of the aorta as components of the abnormal anatomical complex. If the upper part of the body is pink and the lower part of the body blue, coarctation of the aorta or interruption of the aortic arch is probable, with oxygenated blood supplying the upper body and desaturated blood supplying the lower body by way of right-to-left flow through the ductus arteriosus. The latter also occurs in patients with patent ductus arteriosus and markedly elevated pulmonary vascular resistance. A patient with transposition of the great arteries and coarctation of the aorta with retrograde flow through a patent ductus arteriosus demonstrates the reverse situation, i.e., the lower part of the body is pink and the upper part blue. Simultaneous determinations of oxygen saturation in the temporal or right brachial artery and the femoral artery are helpful in confirming the presence of differential cyanosis.

CENTRAL NERVOUS SYSTEM AND HEMATOLOGICAL CAUSES OF CYANOSIS. Irregular, shallow breathing secondary to central nervous system depression results in reduced alveolar ventilation and an abnormally low alveolar oxygen tension. Alveolar arterial pCO_2 becomes elevated, and arterial pO_2 is reduced. Sedatives and hypnotics administered to the mother during labor cause central nervous system depression in the newborn and intracranial hemorrhage secondary to birth trauma, accounting for most cases.

Methemoglobinemia, either congenital or acquired, is a rare cause of cyanosis in the newborn, with recognizable cyanosis occurring in affected babies when 15 per cent or more of the total hemoglobin is replaced by methemoglobin. Venous blood exposed to room air normally becomes pink but remains dark in infants with methemoglobinemia. Arterial blood with a normal partial pressure of oxygen but a low oxygen saturation should suggest the diagnosis, which may be established conclusively by spectrophotometry.

Differentiating Between Pulmonary and Cardiac Causes of Cyanosis

The distinction between respiratory signs and symptoms arising from cyanotic cardiac disease and those associated with a primary pulmonary disorder is an important challenge to the cardiologist.[33] Upper airway obstruction precipitates cyanosis by producing alveolar hypoventilation owing to reduced pulmonary ventilation. Mechanical obstruction may occur from the nares to the carina, and the important diagnostic possibilities among congenital abnormalities are choanal atresia, vascular ring, laryngeal web, and tracheomalacia. Acquired causes include vocal cord paresis, obstetrical injury to the cricothyroid cartilage, and foreign body. Structural abnormalities in the lungs resulting from intrapulmonary disease are more frequently a basis for cyanosis among newborns than is upper airway obstruction. Hyaline membrane disease, atelectasis, or pneumonitis causing inflammation, collapse, and fluid accumulation in the alveoli results in reduction of the oxygenation of blood reaching the systemic circulation.

Successfully distinguishing between these various causes of cyanosis depends on interpretation of the respiratory pattern, the cardiac physical examination, evaluation of arterial blood gases (Table 31–9), and interpretation of the electrocardiogram, chest x-ray, and echocardiogram.

RESPIRATORY PATTERNS. The key to differential diagnosis at the bedside commonly is the proper evaluation of the pattern of respiration. Term infants normally exhibit a progressive reduction in respiratory rate during the first day of life from 60 to 70 per minute to 35 to 55 per minute. Moreover, mild intercostal retractions and minimal expiratory grunting disappear within several hours of birth. An increased depth of respiration in the presence of cyanosis, but without other signs of respiratory distress, often is associated with congenital cardiac disease in which inadequate pulmonary blood flow is the most important functional component.

The most important variations from normal respiratory patterns are apnea and bradypnea, and tachypnea. Intermittent apneic episodes are common in premature infants with central nervous system immaturity or disease. In addition, higher

TABLE 31–9 ARTERIAL BLOOD GAS PATTERNS IN VARIOUS DISORDERS CAUSING CYANOSIS IN INFANTS

PATTERN	pH	pO_2	pCO_2	RESPONSE TO O_2	VENOUS pH	SUGGESTED CONDITION
1	↓	↓↓	↑	↑↑	↓	Hyaline membrane or other pulmonary parenchymal disease
2	↓	↓	↑↑↑	↑↑	↓	Hypoventilation
3	—	↓	↓	↑	—	Venous admixture
4	↓	↓↓	—	—	↓	Decreased or ineffective pulmonary blood flow
5	↓↓↓	↓	—↑	—↑	↓↓↓	Systemic hypoperfusion

— = no effect.

centers may be depressed as a result of severe hypoxemia, acidemia, or the administration of pharmacological agents to mother or baby. The association of apneic episodes, lethargy, hypotonicity, and a reduction in spontaneous movements most often points to intracranial disease as an underlying cause.

Diverse conditions result in tachypnea in the newborn period. Tachypnea in the presence of intrinsic pulmonary disease with upper or lower airway obstruction usually is accompanied by flaring of the alae nasi, chest-wall retractions, and grunting. In contrast, tachypnea associated with intense cyanosis in the absence of obvious respiratory distress suggests the presence of cyanotic congenital heart disease. In general, highest respiratory rates (80 to 110/min) are seen in association with primary lung, and not heart, disease. An initial chest x-ray frequently is diagnostic, especially if the problem is aspiration, mucous plug, adenomatoid malformation, lobar emphysema, diaphragmatic hernia, pneumothorax, lung agenesis, pulmonary hemorrhage, or an abnormal thoracic cage configuration. Choanal atresia may be excluded by passing a feeding tube through the nares, and the more common types of esophageal atresia and tracheoesophageal fistula may be excluded by passing the tube farther into the stomach.

CARDIAC EXAMINATION. Specific findings on cardiovascular examination may direct attention to a cardiac cause for cyanosis. Peripheral perfusion is poor in the presence of severe primary myocardial disease or the hypoplastic left heart syndrome. In contrast, peripheral pulses are bounding and the dorsalis pedis and palmar pulses are easily palpable in infants with patent ductus arteriosus, truncus arteriosus, or aorticopulmonary window. A marked discrepancy between upper- and lower-extremity blood pressures helps to identify the infant with coarctation of the aorta. Inspection and palpation of the precordium allow an overall estimate of cardiac activity. A suprasternal notch and precordial thrill occasionally may be felt in the infant with patent ductus arteriosus, critical aortic stenosis, or coarctation of the aorta. Characterization of the second heart sound may be of help, since it often is single in infants with a hypoplastic left heart complex, pulmonary atresia with or without an intact ventricular septum, or truncus arteriosus. Wide splitting of the second heart sound may occur in infants with total anomalous pulmonary venous return. Ejection sounds often are detectable in infants with persistent truncus arteriosus and occasionally with critical aortic or pulmonic stenosis. The presence of a third heart sound is normal, but a gallop rhythm may provide a clue to myocardial failure. Wide splitting of the first and second heart sounds and prominent third and fourth heart sounds may produce the characteristically rhythmic auscultatory cadence of Ebstein's anomaly of the tricuspid valve (p. 940). The presence of a cardiac murmur may point clearly to underlying cardiac disease, but the absence of a murmur does not exclude the presence of a cardiac malformation. Moreover, cardiac murmurs of specific anomalies often are atypical in the newborn period. However, certain cardiac murmurs such as the decrescendo holosystolic murmur of tricuspid regurgitation in Ebstein's anomaly or the transient tricuspid regurgitation of infancy may point clearly to an accurate diagnosis. Auscultation of the head and abdomen may detect the murmur of an arteriovenous malformation at those sites in infants who present with findings of severe heart failure.

BLOOD GAS AND pH PATTERNS. Arterial blood gas analysis may be a reliable method of evaluating cyanosis, suggesting the type of altered physiology, and assessing responses to therapeutic maneuvers.[48] Specimens for blood gas analysis should be obtained in room air and in 100 per cent oxygen. Stick capillary samples from the patient's warmed heel may be used, although determinations obtained by arterial puncture are preferable for evaluation of oxygenation, since they are less susceptible to alterations in regional blood flow in the critically ill infant. Sampling of right radial or temporal arterial blood is preferable, since these sites are proximal to flow through a ductus arteriosus and do not reflect right-to-left ductal shunting, as would a sample from the descending aorta obtained by means of an umbilical artery catheter. A trial of continuous positive airway pressure may improve oxygenation in infants with either hyaline membrane disease or pulmonary edema. Arterial blood gas patterns in various pathophysiological conditions are listed in Table 31–9. Pattern 1 typically is observed in infants with ventilation-perfusion abnormalities resulting from primary respiratory disease, often associated with elevated pulmonary vascular resistance and venoarterial shunting across a patent foramen ovale or patent ductus arteriosus. Pulmonary hypoventilation with CO_2 retention produces pattern 2. In the presence of a lesion causing obligatory venous admixture, such as total anomalous pulmonary venous connection (pattern 3), the response to oxygen may reflect an increase in pulmonary venous return secondary to a fall in pulmonary vascular resistance. Pattern 4 typically is seen in infants with a cardiac malformation that results in reduced pulmonary blood flow. Oxygen administration in these infants does not alter the arterial pO_2. The alterations of pattern 5 are observed when systemic hypoperfusion is the principal hemodynamic problem. In these babies the arteriovenous oxygen difference is high, and the acidemia may be progressive and unrelenting.

ELECTROCARDIOGRAM. This is less helpful in suggesting a diagnosis of heart disease in the premature and newborn infant than in the older child. Right ventricular hypertrophy is a normal finding in the neonate, and the range of normal voltages is wide. However, specific observations may offer major clues to the presence of a cardiovascular anomaly. A counterclockwise, superiorly oriented frontal QRS loop with absent or reduced right ventricular forces suggests the diagnosis of tricuspid atresia (p. 938). In contrast, when the QRS axis is normal but left ventricular forces predominate, the diagnosis of pulmonic atresia must be considered (p. 933). The counterclockwise, superior QRS orientation also is observed in infants with an endocardial cushion defect (p. 92) and in some with double-outlet right ventricle (p. 948); right ventricular forces in these babies are increased. The initial septal vector should be assessed from the electrocardiogram. Often Q waves are not clearly seen in the lateral precordial leads in the first 72 hours of life. A leftward, posteriorly directed septal vector giving rise to Q waves in the right precordial leads is abnormal, and suggests the presence of marked right ventricular hypertrophy, single ventricle (p. 953), or inversion of the ventricles. T-wave alterations may be seen in a normal neonatal electrocardiogram and may be of no particular consequence. However, by 72 hours of age the T waves should be inverted in V_3 and V_1 and upright in the lateral precordium; persistently upright T waves in the right precordial leads are a sign of right ventricular hypertrophy. Depressed or flattened T waves in the lateral precordium may suggest subendocardial ischemia and a left heart outflow tract obstructive lesion, electrolyte disturbance, acidosis, or hypoxemia. An electrocardiographic pattern of myocardial infarction suggests a diagnosis of anomalous pulmonary origin of the coronary artery (p. 918). Finally, rhythm disturbances such as complete heart block or supraventricular tachycardia can be detected readily by electrocardiography.

RADIOGRAPHIC EXAMINATION (see also p. 228). The chest x-ray often is the single most useful part of the examination in differentiating between respiratory and cardiac causes of cyanosis in the newborn period. Determination of a normal cardiac and abdominal situs aids in ruling out several kinds of complex cyanotic cardiac malformations associated with asplenia or polysplenia with abdominal heterotaxy and dextrocardia (p. 969). The distinct appearance of pulmonary parenchymal disease, such as the classic reticulogranular pattern of hyaline membrane disease, may allow a specific radiological diagnosis. In those premature infants with a large ductus arteriosus the x-ray appearance often evolves from the typical findings of hyaline membrane disease to increased pulmonary vascular markings and finally to perihilar and generalized pulmonary edema. Most important, the pediatric cardiologist depends heavily on the evaluation of pulmonary vascular markings to categorize congenital cardiac malformations in the newborn infant according to function. In the presence of cyanosis, diminished pulmonary vascular markings call attention to the group of anomalies that includes tetralogy of Fallot, pulmonic stenosis with intact ventricular septum, pulmonic atresia, tricuspid atresia, and Ebstein's malformation of the tricuspid valve. Reduced pulmonary blood flow is responsible for the systemic arterial desaturation in these babies. Increased pulmonary vascular markings in the cyanotic infant are associated with lesions in which an obligatory admixture of systemic venous and pulmonary venous blood occurs. The more common anomalies in this category include transposition of the great arteries, hypoplastic left heart syndrome, truncus arteriosus, and total anomalous pulmonary venous drainage.

As mentioned earlier, overall heart size in the normal newborn infant is greater than in the older child, and cardiothoracic ratios up to 0.60 are within normal limits. The thymus shadow occasionally obscures the cardiac silhouette and prohibits accurate estimation of heart size. An enlarged heart on x-ray examination suggests a cardiac disorder. However, in the presence of severe respiratory difficulties with an increase in carbon dioxide tension and a decrease in both pH and arterial oxygen tension, cardiomegaly may be only moderate. A right aortic arch suggests the presence of either tetralogy of Fallot or persistent truncus arteriosus. An ovoid heart with a narrow base associated with increased pulmonary vascular marking is typical of transposition of the great arteries. A boot-shaped heart with concavity of the pulmonary outflow tract suggests tetralogy of Fallot, pulmonic atresia, or tricuspid atresia.

FETAL ECHOCARDIOGRAPHY (see also pp. 89 to 92). Ultrasound technology now allows examination of human fetal cardiac development and function in utero.[30,31] Diagnostic-quality images of the fetal heart in utero can be obtained as early as 16 weeks of gestation. Cardiac structures are imaged primarily by cross-sectional echocardiography and augmented by a combination of rangegated pulse Doppler ultrasonography and M-mode echocardiography.[77–79] The analysis of the structure and function of the fetal heart during the second and third trimesters of pregnancy has allowed cardiologists to counsel prospective parents, and in a number of instances to formulate management plans for pregnancy, delivery, and the immediate postnatal period. Using fetal echocardiography, major forms of congenital heart disease have been diagnosed in utero, and cardiac rhythm abnormalities have been detected, permitting direct efforts at transplacental therapy. In particular, it has been established that a high incidence exists

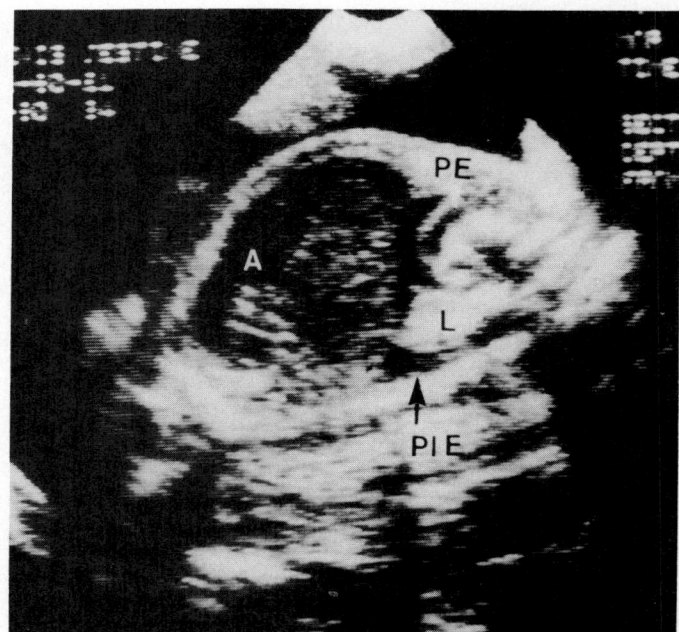

FIGURE 31–9. Abdominal ultrasound examination of a 28-week fetus with nonimmunological hydrops fetalis. A = ascites, PE = pericardial effusion, L = lung, PIE = pleural effusion. The fetal heart is to the right and inferior of the white arrow showing the pericardial effusion.

of cardiac pathology in the presence of nonimmune fetal hydrops. It appears clear that hydrops fetalis often represents end-stage fetal cardiac decompensation (Fig. 31–9). Atrioventricular valve insufficiency often causes fetal right ventricular volume overload and systemic venous hypertension leading to hydrops fetalis.

Pulsed Doppler ultrasound examination of the fetus importantly supplements the echocardiographic findings in identifying the responsible defects, such as Ebstein's malformation of the tricuspid valve, atrial isomerism with atrioventricular septal defects, and the absent pulmonary valve and hypoplastic left heart syndromes.

Fetal cardiac ultrasound is of especial importance in analyzing disturbances of fetal cardiac rhythm, which usually are first suspected on the basis of auscultatory findings. Transabdominal electrocardiography cannot identify atrial depolarization, and is of limited value in the analysis of cardiac arrhythmias in utero. However, M-mode recordings of cardiac motion versus time allow conclusions regarding electrical events in the fetal heart, as they are reflected by the mechanical responses that are recorded echocardiographically. Supraventricular tachyarrhythmias are a common cause of nonimmune fetal hydrops (Fig. 31–10). Detection is of practical use in the management of these patients because the arrhythmia is treatable with use of various antiarrhythmic drugs, such as digoxin, procainamide, propranolol, and verapamil, administered to the mother and reaching the fetus transplacentally or, rarely, under sonographic guidance, by means of injection of drugs, such as amiodarone, into the umbilical vein.[80]

ECHOCARDIOGRAPHY IN THE NEONATE. Echocardiography is of immense value in distinguishing heart disease from lung disease in the newborn.[81] Echocardiographic diagnoses that often can be made with certainty include hypoplastic left heart syndrome, aortic valve stenosis, membranous and fibromuscular subvalvular aortic stenosis, aortic coarctation, hypertrophic cardiomyopathy, cor triatriatum, atrial septal defect, tricuspid atresia, Ebstein's anomaly of the tricuspid valve, valvular pulmonic stenosis, atrioventricular septal defect, single ventricle, double-outlet right ventricle, transposition of the great arteries, and patent ductus arteriosus. The echocardiogram provides suggestive and occasionally conclusive evidence for tetralogy of Fallot, truncus

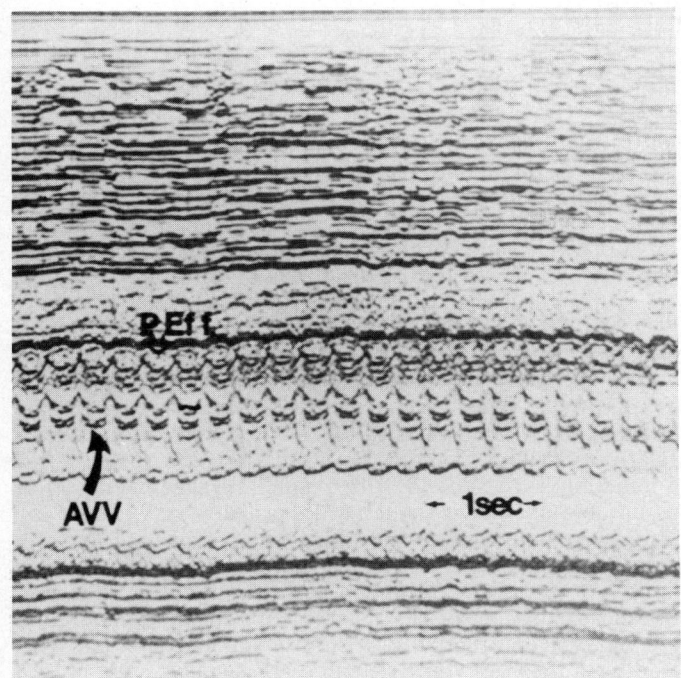

FIGURE 31–10. M-mode echocardiogram at 35 weeks' gestation, showing fetal supraventricular tachycardia and pericardial effusion (PEff). The tracing, taken at the midventricular level, allows the heart rate to be calculated from atrioventricular valve (AVV) motion (250 beats/min). (Courtesy of Charles Kleinman, M.D.)

arteriosus, total anomalous pulmonary venous connection, and pulmonary atresia with an intact ventricular septum.

Doppler ultrasonography (p. 67) has supplemented the two-dimensional echocardiographic examination by its ability to quantify valve gradients, cardiac output, blood flow patterns in the cardiac chambers and great arteries, and often shunt size.[81–84] For example, the pulmonary-systemic blood flow ratio can be calculated by multiplying the square of the ratio of the great vessel diameters by the ratio of the peak systolic flow velocities, the pulmonary variable being the numerator in each ratio.[82] The coupling of Doppler ultrasonographic techniques with the two-dimensional echocardiogram, and the representation in color of abnormalities in flow, volume, and direction (p. 68), greatly improves diagnostic accuracy.

CARDIAC CATHETERIZATION (see also Chap. 7). If a cardiac anomaly is identified by noninvasive studies or if a clear-cut differentiation cannot be made between cardiac and pulmonary disease, heart catheterization and angiocardiography often are necessary to define the underlying state precisely. However, fewer cardiac catheterizations are being performed in infants and children of all ages since the beginning of aggressive pursuit of preoperative diagnoses by noninvasive imaging modalities, particularly two-dimensional–Doppler flow echocardiography.[84] Hemodynamic study of the newborn infant carries a small but distinct risk.[85] As a general rule, cardiac catheterization is not performed unless the information sought is central to the management of the infant. Most infants with serious heart disease require therapeutic intervention, and thus catheterization should be performed only when surgical support is readily available. Cardiac catheterization usually is indicated in most newborns who experience congestive heart failure in the first days after birth if the cause is an anatomical abnormality rather than an arrhythmia or a metabolic disturbance. Preferably, medical measures will

have been instituted to stabilize the clinical state before a hemodynamic study is performed.

It is generally agreed that many newborns with cyanotic congenital heart disease require prompt cardiac catheterization, since there is considerable risk of rapid deterioration.[16] Under these circumstances hemodynamic and angiographic study may not only provide the anatomical diagnosis required before emergency operation but also allow the opportunity for therapeutic maneuvers such as balloon atrial septostomy to facilitate intercirculatory mixing in patients with complete transposition of the great arteries or to augment interatrial shunting in patients with a restrictive patent foramen ovale and either tricuspid, pulmonic, or mitral atresia, or total anomalous pulmonary venous connection. The selective infusion of low doses of prostaglandin E_1 (0.05–0.1 μg/kg/min) intravenously has been used before and at cardiac catheterization for the emergency palliation of ductus-dependent cardiac lesions such as pulmonary atresia, aortic coarctation, and interruption of the aortic arch.[71] Because a patent ductus arteriosus maintains pulmonary and systemic blood flow, respectively, in these infants, dilatation of the ductus with vasodilatory prostaglandins may retard their clinical deterioration. Thus, prostaglandin E_1 infusion has been shown to be an effective short-term measure to correct hypoxemia and acidemia and to improve the preoperative and intraoperative status of infants who require surgical relief of the congenital cardiac lesion that is causing pulmonary or systemic hypoperfusion.

Therapeutic Catheterization (see also Chap. 41). Balloon atrial septostomy was the first catheter intervention that proved useful to treat congenital heart disease, and remains the standard initial palliation in infants with complete transposition of the great arteries.[86] Recently, additional transcatheter techniques have been used successfully to treat congenital heart disease.[87–92] These include knife blade atrial septostomy, umbrella closure of patent ductus arteriosus and atrial septal defect, and balloon and coil embolization of large systemic pulmonary artery collateral vessels and arteriovenous fistulas. Other procedures that have expanded the role of the cardiac catheter from a diagnostic tool to a therapeutic instrument include transvenous or transarterial pacemaker insertion and retrieval of foreign bodies from the cardiovascular system. Transluminal balloon angioplasty currently is used principally in pediatrics for dilation of pulmonic valve stenosis, recoarctation of the aorta, and peripheral pulmonary artery stenosis. Unresolved questions exist about transluminal angioplasty in native coarctation and congenital aortic, subaortic, and mitral stenosis. Also investigational is the use of vascular stents, particularly after recurrence of vessel stenoses after balloon dilatation.

Electrophysiological Studies (see also Chap. 22). The cardiac catheterization laboratory also is being used with increasing frequency to define the anatomical and physiological diagnoses of arrhythmias, thus facilitating an accurate prognosis and providing a rational basis for pharmacological or surgical treatment.[93–96] The invasive electrophysiological approach provides unique information that cannot be obtained noninvasively. These include determination of conduction times of individual components of the conducting system and measurement of refractory periods for structures such as the atrioventricular node, His bundle, and bundle branches. In addition, one can determine the initiating features, sustaining mechanisms, and possible perturbations that terminate the arrhythmia. This last maneuver is particularly important, because it may enable the planning of effective drug treatment. It also may determine the advisability of catheter ablation, pacemaker control, or surgical treatment of the rhythm disturbance.

Many classifications of congenital cardiovascular lesions have been proposed on the basis of hemodynamic, anatomical, and radiographic factors. Although there is overlapping between groups, the following arrangement of cardiac anomalies is used in this chapter: (1) communications between the systemic and pulmonary circulations without cyanosis (left-to-right shunts), (2) obstructing valvular and vascular lesions with or without associated right-to-left shunt, (3) abnormalities in the origins of the great arteries and veins (the transposition complexes), (4) malpositions of the heart and cardiac apex, and (5) miscellaneous anomalies.

LEFT-TO-RIGHT SHUNTS

ATRIAL SEPTAL DEFECT
(See also p. 1632)

MORPHOLOGY. Atrial septal defect is one of the most commonly recognized congenital cardiac anomalies in adults but is very rarely diagnosed and even less commonly results in disability in infants.[97] The anatomical sites of interatrial defects are shown in Figure 31–11. Defects of the sinus venosus type are high in the atrial septum near the entry of the superior vena cava and are frequently associated with and may be a consequence of anomalous connection of pulmonary veins from the right lung to the junction of the superior vena cava and right atrium.[98] Most often the atrial septal defect involves the fossa ovalis, is midseptal in location, and is of the ostium secundum type. This type of defect is a true deficiency of the atrial septum and should not be confused with a patent foramen ovale. Embryologically the left side of the atrial septum is derived from the septum primum, which possesses an opening—the interatrial ostium secundum (Fig. 31–3). The ostium secundum lies forward and superior to the position of the foramen ovale. The latter is formed by the septum secundum and occupies the right side of the atrial septum. Tissue of the septum primum lying to the left of the foramen ovale serves as a flap valve that usually becomes fused postnatally with the side of the foramen ovale, yielding an anatomically closed or sealed foramen. "Probe patency," or an incomplete seal of the foramen ovale, occurs in about 25 per cent of adults. A widely patent foramen ovale may be considered an acquired form of atrial septal defect that occurs especially when a disproportion exists between the size of the foramen ovale and the effective length of its valve. Enlargement of the foramen ovale per se is commonly associated with obstructive lesions of the right side of the heart, whereas a short valve relative to the size of the foramen often is seen in large-volume left-to-right shunts in which left atrial dilatation is prominent.

Ostium primum atrial septal anomalies are a form of atrioventricular septal defect and will be dealt with in the next section. Lutembacher's syndrome is a designation applied to the rare combination of atrial septal defect and mitral stenosis, which is almost invariably the result of acquired rheumatic valvulitis.[99] Ten to 20 per cent of patients with ostium secundum atrial septal defect also have prolapse of the mitral valve as an associated anomaly.[100]

HEMODYNAMICS. The magnitude of the left-to-right shunt through an atrial septal defect depends on the size of the defect and the relative compliance of the ventricles, and the relative resistance in both the pulmonary and the systemic circulation.[101] In patients with a small atrial septal defect or patent foramen ovale, the left atrial pressure may exceed the right by several millimeters of mercury, whereas the mean pressures in both atria are nearly identical when the defect is large. Left-to-right shunting occurs predominantly in late ventricular systole and early diastole with some augmentation during atrial contraction. The shunt results in diastolic overloading of the right ventricle and increased pulmonary blood flow. During the first few days and weeks of life pulmonary resistance falls and systemic resistance rises, facilitating right ventricular emptying and impeding left ventricular emptying; the left-to-right shunt rises. Early in infancy left-to-right flow through even a large interatrial communication commonly is limited by both the reduced chamber compliance of the thick neonatal right ventricle and the elevated pulmonary and reduced systemic vascular resistance of the neonate. The pulmonary vascular resistance commonly is normal or low in the older infant or child with atrial septal defect, and the volume load usually is well tolerated, even though pulmonary blood flow may be two to five times greater than systemic. A transient and small right-to-left shunt occurring with the onset of left ventricular contraction and especially during respiratory periods of decreasing intrathoracic pressure is common in patients with ostium secundum defect, even in the absence of pulmonary hypertension.

CLINICAL FINDINGS. Patients with atrial septal defect usually are asymptomatic early in life, although occasional reports exist of congestive heart failure and recurrent pneumonia in infancy.[97] Children with atrial septal defect may experience easy fatigability and exertional dyspnea. They tend to be somewhat underdeveloped physically and prone to respiratory infection. Atrial arrhythmias, pulmonary arterial hypertension, development of pulmonary vascular obstruction, and heart failure are exceedingly uncommon in the pediatric age range, in contrast to their common appearance in adults with atrial septal defect. In the former group, diagnosis often is entertained after detection of a heart murmur on routine physical examination prompts a more extensive cardiac evaluation.

Common findings on *physical examination* include a prominent right ventricular cardiac impulse and palpable pulmonary artery pulsation. The first heart sound is normal or split, with accentuation of the tricuspid valve closure sound. Increased flow across the pulmonic valve is responsible for a midsystolic pulmonary ejection murmur. After the normal postnatal drop in pulmonary vascular resistance, the second heart sound is split widely and is relatively fixed in relation to respiration in patients with normal pulmonary pressures and low pulmonary vascular impedance because of a delay in pulmonic valve closure. With pulmonary hypertension the splitting interval is a function of the electromechanical intervals of each ventricle; wide splitting occurs with shortening of the left and/or lengthening of the right ventricular electromechanical interval.[102] If the shunt is large, increased blood flow across the tricuspid valve is responsible for a middiastolic

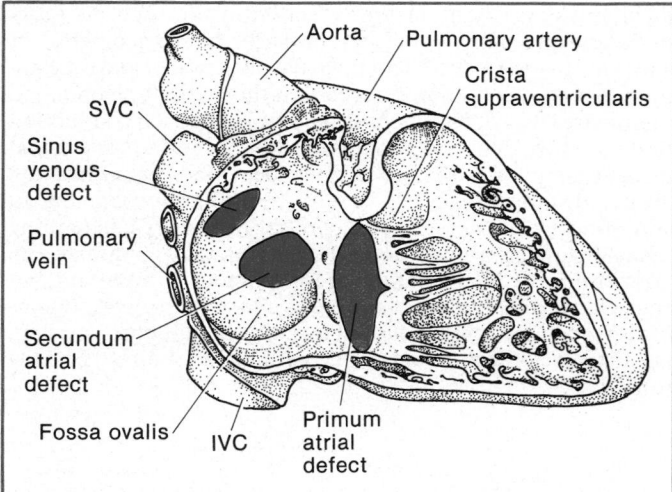

FIGURE 31–11. Composite locations of atrial defects. S.V.C. = superior vena cava, I.V.C. = inferior vena cava.

rumbling murmur at the lower left sternal border. In patients with associated prolapse of the mitral valve an apical holosystolic or late systolic murmur radiating to the axilla often is heard, but a midsystolic click may be difficult to discern. Moreover, left ventricular precordial overactivity usually is absent because mitral regurgitation is mild in most patients.

In the teenage patient, the physical findings may be altered when an increase in pulmonary vascular resistance results in diminution of the left-to-right shunt. Both the pulmonary and the tricuspid murmurs decrease in intensity, whereas the pulmonic component of the second heart sound becomes accentuated and the two components of the second heart sound may fuse; a diastolic murmur of pulmonic incompetence appears. Cyanosis and clubbing accompany development of a right-to-left shunt.

The *electrocardiogram* in patients with an ostium secundum defect usually shows right-axis deviation, right ventricular hypertrophy, and rSR' or rsR' pattern in the right precordial leads with a normal QRS duration (Fig. 31–12 and Fig. 30, p. 159). It is not clear whether the delay in right ventricular activation is a manifestation of right ventricular volume overload or a true conduction delay in the right bundle branch and peripheral Purkinje system.[103] Left-axis deviation of the P wave in the frontal plane (manifested by a negative P wave in lead III) suggests the presence of a sinus venosus rather than an ostium secundum type of atrial septal defect. Left-axis deviation and superior orientation and counterclockwise rotation of the QRS loop in the frontal plane suggests the presence of either an ostium primum defect or a secundum atrial septal defect in association with mitral valve prolapse. Prolongation of the P-R interval may be seen with all types of atrial septal defects; the prolonged internodal conduction time may be related to both the increased size of the atrium and the increased distance for internodal conduction produced by the defect itself.[103] *Chest roentgenograms* (Figs. 8–41A, p. 229, and 32–4, p. 969) reveal enlargement of the right atrium and ventricle, dilatation of the pulmonary artery and its branches, and increased pulmonary vascular markings. Dilatation of the proximal portion of the superior vena cava occasionally is noted in patients with a sinus venosus defect. Left atrial dilatation is

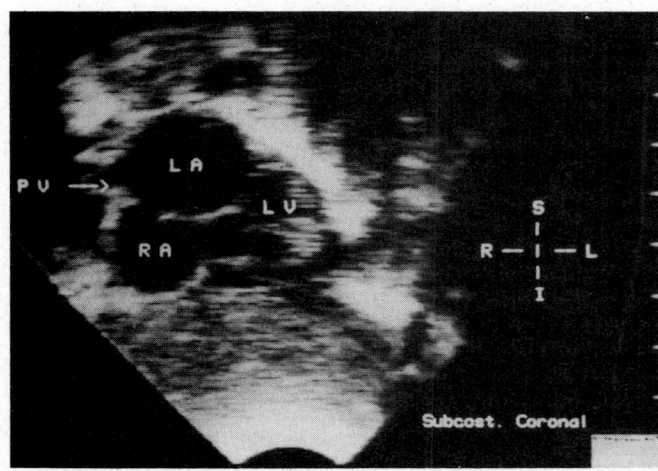

FIGURE 31–13. Subcostal coronal view showing a secundum atrial septal defect between the left atrium (LA) and the right atrium (RA). The right upper pulmonary vein (PV) is seen entering the left atrium. This view is posterior to the major portion of the ventricles; the left ventricle (LV) is seen, but only a small portion of the right ventricle (unlabeled) is apparent. I = inferior, L = left, R = right, S = superior. (Courtesy of Norman Silverman, M.D.)

extremely rare but may be observed when significant mitral regurgitation exists. Echocardiographic features include pulmonary arterial and right ventricular dilatation and anterior systolic (paradoxical) or "flat" interventricular septal motion if significant right ventricular volume overload is present.[81] The defect may be visualized directly by two-dimensional echo imaging, particularly from a subcostal view of the interatrial septum[36] (Fig. 31–13; also see Fig. 4–76, p. 93). Transesophageal color-coded Doppler echocardiography provides excellent visualization of defects of the atrial septum.[104] Associated mitral valve prolapse also may be identified by echocardiographic examination (Figs. 4–50 and 4–51, p. 84). Findings on ultrafast computed tomographic scanning are illustrated in Figure 11–12, p. 319.

In most institutions, two-dimensional echocardiography, supplemented by conventional or color-coded Doppler flow and/or contrast echocardiography, has supplanted cardiac catheterization as the confirmatory test for atrial septal defect.[105,106] Cardiac catheterization is then used if inconsistencies exist in the clinical data or if significant pulmonary hypertension is suspected.

Diagnosis may be readily confirmed at *cardiac catheterization* by passage of the catheter across the atrial defect. The site at which the catheter crosses, if high in the cardiac silhouette, may suggest a sinus venosus defect; if midseptal, a patent foramen ovale or ostium secundum defect; or, if low, a primum defect.[107] Serial determinations of the oxygen saturation or indicator dilution curve techniques may be used to estimate the magnitude of the shunt. In young patients, pressures on the right side of the heart often are normal, despite a large shunt. When a high oxygen saturation is found in the superior vena cava or when the catheter enters pulmonary veins directly from the right atrium, a sinus venosus defect is likely, and indicator dilution curves and selective angiography will aid in identifying the number and location of the anomalous veins. Partial anomalous pulmonary venous connection, although usually associated with sinus venosus defect, may accompany secundum defects. Selective left ventricular angiography will identify prolapse of the mitral valve and allow assessment of the magnitude of mitral regurgitation that may be present in such patients.

In contrast to adults, children with sinus venosus or secundum types of atrial septal defect seldom require treatment for heart failure or antiarrhythmic medications for atrial fibrillation or supraventricular tachycardia. Respiratory tract infections should be treated promptly. Although the risk of infective endocarditis is low, antibiotics should be administered prophylactically before dental procedures.

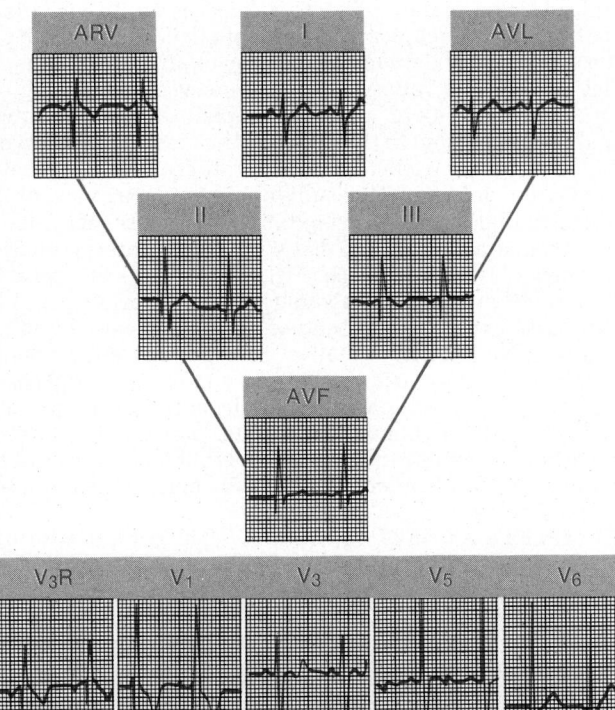

FIGURE 31–12. Typical electrocardiographic tracing in secundum atrial septal defect showing right axis deviation, rSR' in the right precordial leads, and right ventricular hypertrophy. (Courtesy of Delores A. Danilowicz, M.D.)

MANAGEMENT. *Operative repair* (ideally in those 2 to 4 years of age) should be advised for all patients with uncomplicated atrial septal defects in whom there is evidence of significant left-to-right shunting, i.e., with pulmonary-systemic flow ratios exceeding about 1.5:1.0. Rarely, an atrial septal aneurysm is seen in association with a secundum-type atrial septal defect.[108] Such patients may experience spontaneous closure, and may be followed more conservatively until an older age before advising operation. The defect is closed by suture or with a patch of prosthetic material with the patient on cardiopulmonary bypass. Earlier surgical repair is definitive treatment for the small number of infants and young children with significant symptoms or congestive failure. The surgical mortality rate is less than 1 per cent, and results usually are excellent. Although the mitral valve may be examined directly at operation, it seldom is necessary in childhood to attempt plication or replacement of a ballooning or prolapsing mitral valve. Operation should not be carried out in patients with small defects and trivial left-to-right shunts (pulmonary-systemic flow ratio ≤1.5:1.0) or in those with severe pulmonary vascular disease (pulmonary-systemic resistance ratio ≥0.7:1.0) without a significant left-to-right shunt.[109] Still investigational is the use of transcatheter closure by way of a clamshell-configuration double umbrella using fluoroscopic or transesophageal echocardiographic imaging guidance.[89]

Subtle evidence of left ventricular dysfunction may be observed preoperatively at cardiac catheterization in children with isolated large atrial septal defects but without overt left or right ventricular failure.[110] Thus decreased left ventricular stroke volume and cardiac output have been observed in children with both low and normal left ventricular end-diastolic volumes. In routine catheterization studies carried out on patients whose atrial septal defects were closed during preadolescence or later, a residual reduced cardiac output response to intense upright exercise in the absence of residual shunts, arrhythmias, or pulmonary arterial hypertension has been observed.[110,111] Normal myocardial function is preserved in patients in whom the defects were closed in early childhood.

Intracardiac electrophysiological studies reveal a high incidence of intrinsic dysfunction of the sinoatrial and atrioventricular nodes, which persists after surgical repair. These intrinsic nodal abnormalities are more common in sinus venosus than in ostium secundum defects,[112,113] but occur in both varieties. There also is evidence that the type of venous cannulation at the time of operative repair may contribute to the incidence and severity of arrhythmias observed at long-term follow-up.[114]

ATRIOVENTRICULAR (AV) SEPTAL DEFECT

AV septal defects comprise a range of malformations characterized by varying degrees of incomplete development of the inferior portion of the atrial septum, the inflow portion of the ventricular septum, and the AV valves (Fig. 31–3). These anomalies also have been called endocardial cushion defects and AV septal defects. The basic defect is a deficiency of the AV septum which separates the left ventricular inlet from the right atrium; it causes anomalies which range in severity from a small ostium primum atrial septal defect to a complete AV septum, which also involves defects in the interventricular septum and the mitral and tricuspid valves. The latter often are abnormal to varying degrees, with five or six leaflets present of variable size, and variability also in the completeness of their commissures. Often AV septal defects are encountered in association with other congenital abnormalities, such as asplenia or polysplenia syndromes, trisomy 21 (Down syndrome), and Ellis–van Creveld syndrome of ectodermal dysplasia and polydactyly.

OSTIUM PRIMUM DEFECT (PARTIAL AV CANAL). Ostium primum atrial septal defects lie immediately adjacent to the AV valves, either of which may be deformed and incompetent. Most often only the anterior or septal leaflet of the mitral valve is displaced, and it commonly is cleft; the tricuspid valve usually is not involved. A cleft often is considered to be present in the mitral valve, although it is likely that the valve is in fact a trileaflet structure, with the cleft representing an abnormal commissure. The interatrial defect often is large, and the size of the left-to-right interatrial shunt in these patients is controlled by the same factors that exist in patients with ostium secundum atrial septal defect. Moreover, the clinical features are quite similar, and principally consist of right ventricular precordial hyperactivity, a wide and persistently split second heart sound, a right ventricular outflow tract systolic ejection murmur, and a middiastolic tricuspid flow rumble. The murmurs of AV valve regurgitation may be audible if either valve is significantly abnormal; however, serious AV valve regurgitation usually is absent. In the occasional patient, mitral regurgitation is substantial and creates prominent signs of left ventricular overload.

Chest roentgenography usually reveals right atrial and ventricular cardiomegaly, prominence of the right ventricular outflow tract, and increased pulmonary vascular markings. The *electrocardiogram* is characteristic, and shows a right ventricular conduction defect accompanied by left anterior division block, left-axis deviation, and superior orientation and counterclockwise rotation of the QRS loop in the frontal plane (Fig. 5–21, p. 131).[115] Hemodynamic factors do not appear to be important in producing the characteristic electrocardiogram. Rather, the superior QRS vector in patients with a shortened H-V interval appears to be related to early activation of the posterobasal left ventricular wall; in other patients with a normal conduction time between the bundle of His and the ventricles, the counterclockwise superior inscription of the frontal plane vector appears to be related to late activation of the anterolateral left ventricular wall.[116,117] A prolonged P-R interval is observed in many patients with an ostium primum atrial septal defect; prolonged internodal conduction may be related to displacement of the AV node in a posteroinferior direction in some patients or to the enlarged right atrium, or both.[118]

Echocardiographic features (Fig. 4–77, p. 93) include enlargement of both the right ventricle and the pulmonary artery, systolic anterior ventricular septal motion, prolonged mitral-septal apposition in diastole, and various abnormalities in mitral valve motion.[119,120] The defect is easily visualized from the precordial apical and subxiphoid positions, with the latter views best demonstrating the relation between the atrial defect, AV valves, and the interventricular septum (Figs. 31–14 and 4–77, p. 93, color plate No. 4). Interatrial septal tissue is absent in the region of the crest of the interventricular septum; the trileaflet configuration of the mitral valve also may be identified. The subxiphoid long-axis view of the left ventricular outflow tract exhibits the "gooseneck" deformity in a manner similar to that with a right anterior oblique left ventricular angiogram (see Fig. 31–16). Echocardiography is particularly useful for detecting and characterizing double-orifice mitral valve, an association in about 3 per cent of patients with ostium primum atrial defect. It also allows detection of single left ventricular papillary muscle, hypoplasia of the left ventricle, and coarctation of the aorta, seen especially in symptomatic infants with an ostium primum atrial defect but without trisomy 21.[121] The *angiographic features* resemble those in the complete form of AV septal defect and are discussed below.

COMPLETE AV SEPTAL DEFECT. The complete form of the AV septal defect includes, in addition to the ostium primum atrial septal defect, a ventricular septal defect in the posterior basal inlet portion of the ventricular septum and a common AV orifice. The common AV valve usually has six leaflets: left superior and inferior, left and right lateral, and right superior and inferior. The left and right superior leaflets together often are referred to as the "anterior" bridging leaflet. No attachment exists between the left superior and inferior leaflets and the right superior and inferior leaflets. The left superior leaflet may cross the crest of the ventricular septum to reside partially on the right ventricular side. A classifica-

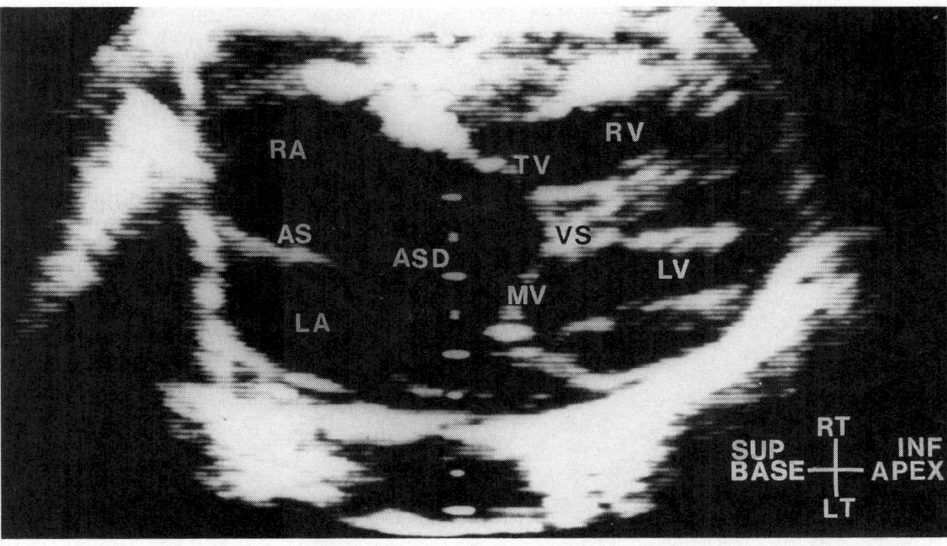

FIGURE 31–14. Subcostal four-chamber view showing an ostium primum atrial septal defect (ASD). There is echo dropout in the inferior portion of the atrial septum (AS). RA = right atrium, LA = left atrium, TV = tricuspid valve, MV = mitral valve, VS = ventricular septum, RV = right ventricle, LV = left ventricle. (Courtesy of Thomas DiSessa, M.D.)

tion of complete AV canal defect into types A, B, and C reflects the variability and the degree of left superior leaflet bridging of the ventricular septum. Thus in type A the left superior leaflet is entirely over the left ventricle, and together with the right superior leaflet is attached by chordae tendineae to the crest of the ventricular septum. In type C there is marked rightward displacement of the left superior leaflet, which floats freely over the crest of the ventricular septum and is not attached to it by chordae tendineae. In type B chordal attachments extend medially to an anomalous papillary muscle adjacent to the septum in the right ventricle.

A high incidence (about 35 per cent) of additional cardiovascular lesions exists in patients with common AV canal. Principal among these are tetralogy of Fallot, double-outlet right ventricle, transposition of the great arteries, total anomalous pulmonary venous connection, variable sites of left ventricular outflow tract obstruction, pulmonic stenosis, and persistent left superior vena cava. Moreover, the complete AV septal anomaly commonly is seen in patients with Down syndrome.

Diagnosis. Patients with common AV septal defects present clinically under age 1 year with a history of frequent respiratory infections and poor weight gain. Heart failure in infancy is extremely common. The *physical findings* are similar to those observed in patients with ostium primum atrial septal defect but may include as well the holosystolic, lower left sternal border murmur of an interventricular communication and/or the decrescendo, holosystolic apical murmur of mitral regurgitation. The *electrocardiographic features* of complete AV canal defects resemble those in the partial ostium primum variety of AV septal anomalies (Fig. 31–12, p. 907). *Radiographically,* the usual findings are generalized cardiomegaly and engorged pulmonary vessels. Two-dimensional echocardiography is diagnostic (Figs. 31–15 and 4–78, p. 94).[119,120] The atrial defect appears as a dropout of echoes from the leftmost portion of the interatrial septum immediately above the AV valves. AV leaflet morphology is best seen from the parasternal and subxiphoid short-axis views, with simultaneously visualized superior and inferior leaflets. The ventricular defect lies beneath the AV valve leaflets. On *hemodynamic study,* patients with persistent common AV canal invariably have elevated pulmonary arterial pressures; beyond age 2 years a significant number of these patients have progressively severe pulmonary vascular obstructive disease.

Diagnosis also is reliably established by selective left ventricular *angiocardiography* using rapid injection of relatively large quantities of contrast material. The findings include an absence of the AV septum and a deficiency of the inlet portion of the ventricular septum, with elongation of the left ventricular outflow tract in relation to the inflow tract. The leaflets of the left AV valve often may be visualized to determine the location and magnitude of valvar incompetence. The aortic

valve is elevated and displaced anteriorly relative to the AV valves, changing the relation between the anterior components of the left AV valve and the aorta, which produces a pathognomonic "gooseneck" deformity seen angiographically in diastole (Fig. 31–16). Additional findings include a jet of

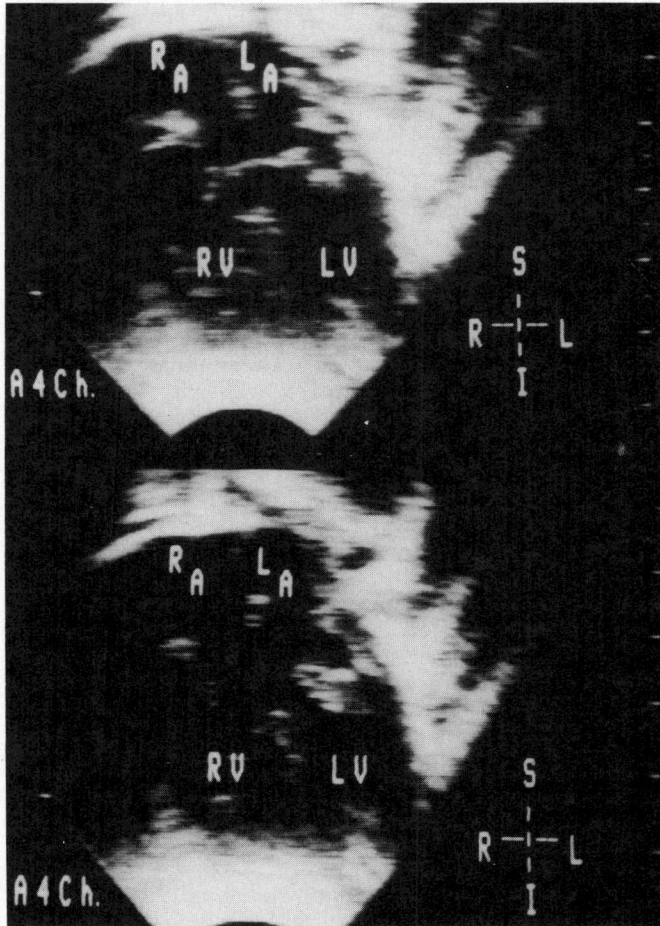

FIGURE 31–15. Apical four-chamber views of a common atrioventricular septal defect. The images are oriented anatomically. In systole, shown in the top panel, the atrioventricular valve leaflet is closed, with no apparent attachment of the atrioventricular valve to the ventricular septum. The interatrial and interventricular septal defects are represented by echo dropout above and below the common AV valve. In diastole, shown in the bottom panel, the AV valve is open, showing the valve resting on the crest of the ventricular septum and the entire defect allowing communication between all four cardiac chambers. RA = right atrium, LA = left atrium, RV = right ventricle, LV = left ventricle. (Courtesy of Norman Silverman, M.D.)

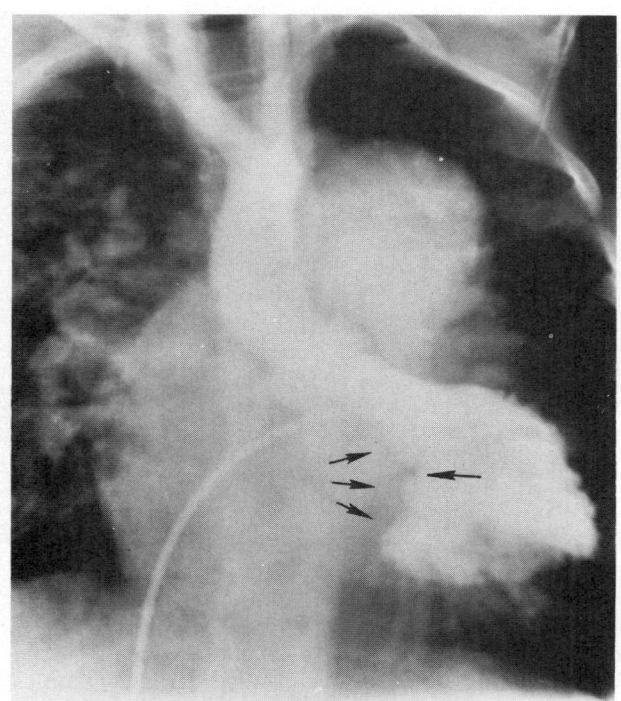

FIGURE 31–16. Left ventriculogram in systole in a patient with an endocardial cushion defect. The concavity of the right border of the left ventricle (left arrows) is caused by the abnormal position of the mitral orifice.

contrast material from left ventricle directly to right atrium or by way of mitral regurgitation and left-to-right atrial shunting. Conventional anteroposterior and lateral left ventricular angiographic views may not always differentiate between the partial and complete types of AV septal defects because all have the characteristic "gooseneck" left ventricular outflow tract deformity and because mitral regurgitation into the right atrium may obscure the presence or absence of a defect in the ventricular septum. Axial cine angiography, however, permits a more accurate distinction between types of AV septal defects, since the hepatoclavicular view helps greatly in separating a left ventricular–right atrial communication and shunt from left ventricular–left atrial regurgitation with subsequent left-to-right atrial shunt. In addition, the long axial oblique view portrays the AV portion of the ventricular septum.[122]

Management. In patients with complete AV canal, cardiac decompensation should be controlled initially. If an adequate response to medical therapy occurs early in life, hemodynamic study is indicated at about age 3 to 6 months to determine the level of pulmonary vascular resistance, since infants with the complete form of the AV septal defect are at high risk of obstructive pulmonary vascular disease. The level of major shunting should be determined during the initial hemodynamic and angiographic study, since if it is mainly at the ventricular level, pulmonary artery banding occasionally may be advised for intractable heart failure and failure to thrive. Often, however, there is a significant left ventricular–right atrial shunt either directly or indirectly by way of mitral regurgitation and left-to-right interatrial shunting, which will be unaffected by pulmonary artery banding and requires complete surgical correction. In most centers primary repair in patients who have intractable heart failure, growth failure, or severe pulmonary hypertension is the preferred approach at any age.[123-126] Mild to moderate regurgitation often persists after surgical repair, particularly if significant AV valve incompetence existed preoperatively.[127] Rarely, if left AV leaflet tissue is remarkably deficient or deformed, mitral valve replacement may be required. Recent advances in the surgical approach to complex forms of AV septal defects have greatly improved the outlook for patients born with this malforma-

tion.[127a] These include a more precise preoperative detection of such anatomical features as additional muscular ventricular septal defects, malalignment of the complete AV septum, and left ventricular hypoplasia.[126] Operative improvement is primarily related to a clearer understanding of the anatomy of this complex lesion and to the ability to reconstruct the left AV valve, often by splitting of papillary muscles and shortening of chordae tendineae, with or without annuloplasty. Many surgeons prefer to close the septal defects with a single patch rather than separating ventricular and atrial patches. Suture placement is avoided in the region of the AV node and the bundle of His.

VENTRICULAR SEPTAL DEFECT
(See also p. 944)

(See also p. 944)

Among the most prevalent of cardiac malformations, defects of the ventricular septum occur commonly, both as isolated anomalies and in combination with other anomalies. The ventricular septum is made up of four compartments: the membranous septum, the inlet septum, the trabecular septum, and the outlet, or infundibular, septum. Defects result from a deficiency of growth or a failure of alignment or fusion of component parts. Defects most commonly are classified as occurring in or adjacent to one or more of the septal components (Fig. 31–17).[127-130]

The most common defects occur in the region of the membranous septum, and are referred to as paramembranous or perimembranous defects because they are larger than the membranous septum itself, and are associated with a muscular defect at a portion of their perimeter. They also are known as infracristal, subaortic, or conoventricular defects. These perimembranous defects also can be defined by their adjacent

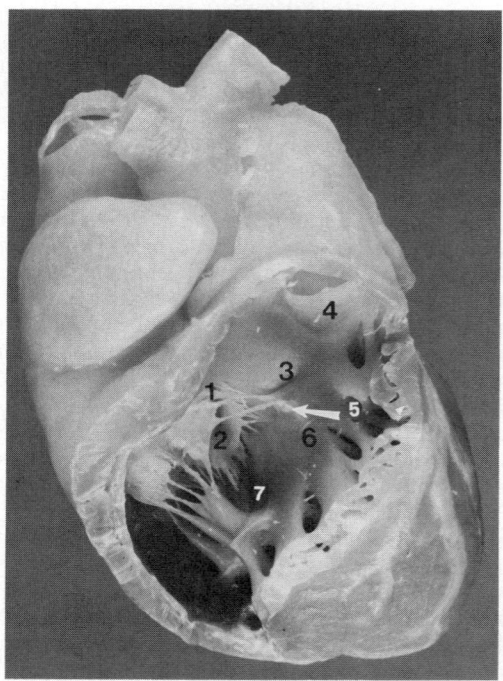

FIGURE 31–17. Heart specimen with right ventricular free wall removed to expose the locations of the various sites of ventricular septal defects. Perimembranous defects (1) lie at the right superior margin of the tricuspid valve. Inlet or atrioventricular septal defects (2) lie beneath the septal leaf of the tricuspid valve and may extend to the tricuspid annulus. Malalignment subaortic outflow or conoseptal defects (3) lie superior to the attachment of the septal tricuspid leaflet to the papillary muscle of the conus (arrow). The subpulmonary defect (4) is to the left of malalignment defects, and also is referred to as doubly committed subarterial. Muscular defects lie within the trabecular septum and may be located in the anterior (5), middle (6), or posterior (7) muscular septum. (Courtesy of Roberta G. Williams, M.D.)

areas as inlet, trabecular, or outlet. A second type of defect is one with an entirely muscular rim. Such muscular defects also can be defined as inlet, trabecular, outlet, or various combinations, and vary greatly in size, shape, and number. A third type of defect occurs when the outlet septum is deficient, and commonly is referred to as supracristal, subpulmonary, outlet, infundibular, or conoseptal. Because the aortic and pulmonary valves are in fibrous continuity, this type of defect also may be referred to as doubly committed subarterial. A septal deficiency of the site of the atrioventricular septum characterizes defects called atrioventricular septal, atrioventricular canal, or inlet septal defects.

The other feature of any defect may be a malalignment of the septal components. Either the inlet or the outlet septum can be malaligned. Malalignment of the inlet septum produces either mitral or tricuspid valve override and/or straddle. Malalignment of the outlet septum can be to the right or the left of the trabecular septum; when to the left of the trabecular septum, the ventricular septal defect is characteristic of tetralogy of Fallot, double-outlet ventricle, truncus arteriosus, and, in some cases, transposition of the great arteries.

TWO-DIMENSIONAL ECHOCARDIOGRAPHY. This technique identifies the type of defect in the ventricular septum.[131-134] Perimembranous ventricular septal defects are identified by septal dropout in the area behind the septal leaflet of the tricuspid valve and below the right border of the aortic annulus. The subaortic or anterior malalignment type of ventricular septal defect appears just below the posterior semilunar valve cusps, entirely superior to the tricuspid valve. The subpulmonary ventricular septal defect appears as echo dropout within the outflow septum, which extends to the pulmonary annulus. One or two of the aortic cusps may be visualized protruding through the defect into the right ventricular outflow tract. The inlet atrioventricular septal–type of ventricular septal defect extends from the fibrous annulus of the tricuspid valve into the muscular septum, and often is entirely beneath the septal tricuspid leaflet. Muscular defects may appear anywhere throughout the ventricular septum, and may be either single and large, or small and multiple. Anatomical localization of all ventricular septal defects is facilitated by coupling two-dimensional ultrasound images (Fig. 4–80, p. 94) with a Doppler system, and also by superimposing a color-coded direction and velocity of blood flow on the real-time images.[135-138]

PATHOPHYSIOLOGY. In general, the functional disturbance caused by a ventricular septal defect depends primarily on its size and the status of the pulmonary vascular bed rather than on the location of the defect. A small ventricular septal defect with high resistance to flow permits only a small left-to-right shunt. A large interventricular communication allows a large left-to-right shunt only if there is no pulmonic stenosis or high pulmonary vascular resistance, since these factors also determine shunt flow. Resistance to left ventricular emptying also affects shunt flow because it is an important factor in determining left ventricular pressure. Large defects allow both ventricles to function hemodynamically as a single pumping chamber with two outlets, equalizing the pressure in the systemic and pulmonary circulations. In such patients the magnitude of the left-to-right shunt varies inversely with pulmonary vascular resistance.

A wide spectrum exists in the natural history of ventricular septal defects, ranging from spontaneous closure to congestive cardiac failure and death in early infancy. Within this spectrum are possible development of pulmonary vascular obstruction, right ventricular outflow tract obstruction, aortic regurgitation, and infective endocarditis.[137-146]

INFANCY. It is unusual for a ventricular septal defect to cause difficulties in the immediate postnatal period, although congestive heart failure during the first 6 months of life is a frequent occurrence. Early diagnosis is helpful to insure more careful observation of the affected infant.[143] The examining physician usually suspects the diagnosis because of a harsh systolic murmur at the lower left sternal border. The electro-cardiogram and chest roentgenogram are within normal limits in the immediate neonatal period because appreciable left-to-right shunting occurs only after the pulmonary vascular resistance decreases as the pulmonary vessels lose their fetal characteristics. It is desirable to follow these infants closely. A ventricular septal defect that either decreases in size or closes completely during the first year of life presents no problems to the practicing physician. Spontaneous closure occurs by age 3 years in about 45 per cent of patients born with ventricular septal defect; occasional patients, however, do not experience spontaneous closure until age 8 to 10 years.[141] Closure is more common in patients born with a small ventricular septal defect; nonetheless, about 7 per cent of infants with a large defect and congestive heart failure early in life also may experience spontaneous closure. Partial rather than complete closure is common in patients with both large and small ventricular septal defects. Anatomically, reduction of the ventricular septal defect often is based on adherence of the tricuspid valve to the defect, hypertrophy of septal muscle, or ingrowth of fibrous tissue. Rarely, closure of the ventricular septal defect is the result of prolapse of an aortic cusp[145] or infective endocarditis.[144] Some defects close when an aneurysm forms in the ventricular septum.[142] On auscultation a click may be heard in early systole as the aneurysm tenses toward the right; the septal aneurysm may be detected by echocardiography as an anterior systolic bulge in the right ventricular outflow tract. A persistent minute ventricular septal defect is not life-threatening unless infective endocarditis develops. With proper precautions the incidence of this complication is less than 1 per cent.

If a moderate or large defect maintains its size after birth, the net left-to-right shunt increases during the first month of life as pulmonary vascular resistance falls. *Physical examination* during this time usually reveals a thrill along the lower left sternal border, and the holosystolic murmur of flow across the interventricular defect is accompanied by a low-pitched diastolic rumble at the apex, reflecting increased flow across the mitral valve. *Chest roentgenograms* reveal increased pulmonary vascular markings; evidence of left or biventricular hypertrophy may be observed on the electrocardiogram. Infants with a large left-to-right shunt tend to do poorly, with recurrent upper and lower respiratory tract infections, failure to gain weight, and congestive heart failure. Congestive heart failure may be severe and intractable despite intensive medical management.

Management. We currently recommend primary intracardiac repair of the ventricular septal defect rather than surgical banding of the pulmonary artery[147] to reduce pulmonary blood flow and alleviate heart failure. An exception is made for the rare infant with multiple ventricular septal defects and a sievelike septum, who is at higher risk for complications following operative repair. Operation usually is deferred, along with debanding of the pulmonary artery, until the child reaches 3 to 5 years. Primary closure of the ventricular septal defect, preferably through the right atrium, may be performed in infancy using cardiopulmonary bypass, profound hypothermia and cardiocirculatory arrest, or a combination of the two techniques. Mortality is less than 10 per cent if the defect is isolated and uncomplicated but approaches 25 per cent if multiple anomalies are present.[148]

Fortunately, medical treatment often is successful in controlling congestive heart failure. Nevertheless, these infants should be referred for cardiac catheterization to evaluate pulmonary vascular resistance and to detect associated defects that may require operation, such as patent ductus arteriosus and coarctation of the aorta.

It is of utmost importance to identify patients who may develop irreversible pulmonary vascular obstructive disease (the Eisenmenger reaction).[146,149,150] Retrospective analyses of children who develop this complication indicate that infants with systemic or near systemic pressures in the pulmonary artery at the time of initial hemodynamic study are most at risk. If early primary closure is not recommended, recatheterization before age 18 months and a second determination of pulmonary vascular resistance should be performed in these patients to decide whether surgical intervention is obligatory to prevent development of fixed obliterative changes in the pulmonary vessels. It is likely that multiple factors are involved in the development of pulmonary vascular disease (Chap. 27 and p. 896).[50-56] The anatomically large ventricular septal defect allows some or all of the systemic pressure to be transmitted to the pulmonary arteries, thereby retarding regression of their muscular media. Medial hypertrophy in the first months of life is responsible for higher pulmonary vascular resistance than would be anticipated for the amount of pulmonary blood flow. The shearing forces created by the high velocity of flow through narrowed pulmonary arterioles cause endothelial damage that is progressive. Although an elevation in left atrial pressure may contribute to the rise in pulmonary vascular resistance, it is not an essential factor, since pulmonary venous pressures can be low in patients who later develop pulmonary vascular disease. Nonetheless, pulmonary venous hypertension also may contribute to pulmonary arterial vasoconstriction and thus to increased shear forces. In this same regard, pulmonary vasoconstriction enhancing the risk of pulmonary vascular obstruction also may be caused by hypoxia caused by either high altitude or lung disease. At high altitudes, large ventricular septal defects have higher pulmonary vascular resistances and smaller shunts than at low altitudes.

CHILDHOOD. Beyond the first year of life a variable clinical picture emerges in children with ventricular septal defect.[139-147] If a small defect is present, the child usually is asymptomatic, the electrocardiogram usually is normal, and the chest roentgenogram shows normal or only a mild increase in pulmonary vascular markings. Effort intolerance and fatigue are associated with moderate left-to-right shunts. These children exhibit cardiomegaly with a forceful left ventricular impulse and a prominent systolic thrill along the lower left sternal border. The second heart sound normally is split, with moderate accentuation of the pulmonic component; a third heart sound and rumbling diastolic murmur that reflects increased flow across the mitral valve are audible at the cardiac apex. The characteristic murmur resulting from flow across the defect is harsh and holosystolic, is best heard along the third and fourth interspaces to the left of the sternum, and is widely transmitted over the precordium. A basal midsystolic ejection murmur due to increased flow across the pulmonic valve also may be heard. The electrocardiogram reveals left or combined ventricular hypertrophy (Fig. 31, p. 159), and the chest roentgenogram and CT scan (Fig. 8–41C, p. 229) show cardiomegaly, left atrial enlargement, and vascular engorgement (Fig. 11–13, p. 319).

RIGHT VENTRICULAR OUTFLOW TRACT OBSTRUCTION. With time, the clinical picture changes in 5 to 10 per cent of patients with ventricular septal defect and a moderate to large left-to-right shunt early in life. It begins to resemble more closely the tetralogy of Fallot (p. 935), i.e., subvalvular right ventricular outflow tract obstruction develops owing to progressive hypertrophy of the crista supraventricularis. Depending on the severity of the latter process, it ultimately may result in reduced blood flow and a right-to-left shunt across the ventricular septal defect. As right ventricular outflow tract obstruction develops, the holosystolic murmur is replaced by the crescendo-decrescendo ejection systolic murmur of pulmonic stenosis, and the pulmonary closure sound becomes softer. Right ventricular hypertrophy is evident on the electrocardiogram, and the chest roentgenogram shows a reduction in pulmonary vascular markings and a smaller heart size with a right ventricular configuration. Infundibular hypertrophy may progress quite rapidly within the first year of life, but the typical evolution to a clinical picture of cyanotic tetralogy of Fallot often takes 1 to 4 years. In those infants who develop right ventricular outflow obstruction the incidence of spontaneous closure or reduction in size of a ventricular septal defect is low.

AORTIC REGURGITATION. This well-described complication of ventricular septal defect occurs in about 5 per cent of patients.[151-153] It usually is noted after age 5 years when a physician detects the early diastolic blowing murmur and wide pulse pressure of aortic regurgitation while following a patient with a ventricular septal defect. The diagnosis is readily confirmed by Doppler echocardiography. In such patients aortic regurgita-

tion may become the predominant hemodynamic abnormality. It is of interest that ventricular septal defect with aortic regurgitation is rare in Europe and the United States, with an incidence of about 4 per cent of all cases of isolated ventricular septal defect, whereas in Japan the incidence is substantially higher (about 10 per cent). In the Japanese, in particular, aortic regurgitation is the result of herniation of an aortic leaflet (usually the right coronary) through a subpulmonic supracristal ventricular septal defect. In these patients, closure of the ventricular septal defect may be all that is required to relieve aortic regurgitation. In many patients, however, especially in the Western world, the ventricular septal defect is below the infundibular septum (crista supraventricularis). Although aortic leaflet herniation, especially of the right or noncoronary cusp, may occur in some of these patients, quite often aortic regurgitation results from a primary abnormality of the valve, usually one defective commissure. In the latter situation, plication of the elongated leaflet may lessen, but not abolish, the aortic regurgitation; in some patients prosthetic aortic valve replacement may be necessary to provide hemodynamic relief. In most patients with ventricular septal defect and aortic regurgitation, the ventricular septal defect is small to moderate in size, and mild right ventricular outflow tract obstruction exists. The latter is caused by either subpulmonic infundibular stenosis or projection of the herniated aortic cusp into the right ventricular outflow tract. The distinction between types of ventricular septal defect with aortic regurgitation usually can be made by two-dimensional and Doppler echocardiography and by selective left ventricular angiocardiography to define the site of the interventricular communication in combination with retrograde aortography to assess the anatomy and competence of the aortic valve (Fig. 31–18).[152,153]

Management. Treatment of the patient with ventricular septal defect and aortic regurgitation is controversial. In patients with a large, hemodynamically significant left-to-right shunt, repair of the ventricular septal defect is indicated, but aortic regurgitation is repaired only if at least moderate aortic regurgitation exists. If a supracristal ventricular septal defect without aortic regurgitation is identified at cardiac catheterization in early childhood, a sensible argument for prophylactic closure of the ventricular septal defect can be put forth to prevent the potential complication of aortic valve incompetence. In the presence of moderate or severe aortic regurgitation, valvuloplasty is preferred to valve replacement, in recognition of the fact that the severity of aortic regurgitation may increase in subsequent years and that reoperation with valve replacement may be necessary. Operation should probably be deferred in asymptomatic patients with a subcristal ventricular septal defect and an insignificant left-to-right shunt in whom aortic regurgitation is not severe. If the defect is

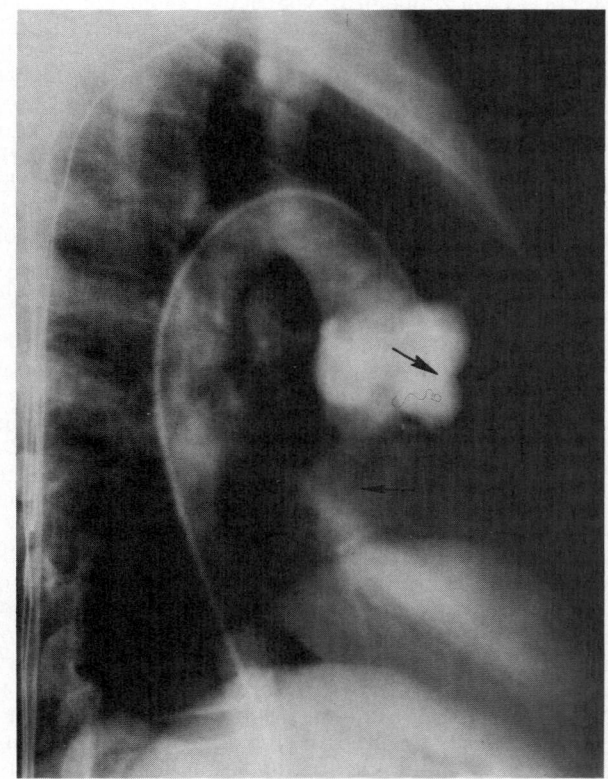

FIGURE 31–18. Retrograde aortogram showing herniation of the right coronary cusp through a supracristal ventricular septal defect (upper arrow) and the jet of aortic regurgitation (lower arrow). (Courtesy of Robert White, M.D.)

supracristal in the same clinical setting, its closure may not alleviate the mild degree of aortic incompetence but may retard its progression.

PULMONARY VASCULAR OBSTRUCTION. If a child who previously had a loud murmur and thrill associated with poor growth suddenly has a growth spurt, fewer respiratory infections, and a diminution of the intensity of the cardiac murmur and disappearance of the thrill, he or she may be developing severe obliterative changes in the pulmonary vascular bed. An increase in intensity of the pulmonic component of the second heart sound, a reduction in heart size on the chest roentgenogram (Fig. 32–9, p. 971), and more pronounced right ventricular hypertrophy on the electrocardiogram also are noted. These changes occur because the increased pulmonary vascular resistance causes a decrease in the left-to-right shunt. If these changes are suspected, cardiac catheterization should be repeated; if they are confirmed, prompt surgical repair is indicated before an inoperable predominant right-to-left shunt ensues. If operation is performed under age 2 years, pulmonary vascular resistance may be expected to fall to normal levels.[150] In older patients the degree to which pulmonary vascular resistance is elevated before operation is a critical factor determining prognosis. If the pulmonary vascular resistance is one-third or less of the systemic value, progressive pulmonary vascular disease after operation is unusual. However, if a moderate-to-severe increase in pulmonary vascular resistance exists preoperatively, either no change or progression of pulmonary vascular disease is common postoperatively. Moreover, the presence of increased pulmonary vascular resistance results in a higher immediate postoperative mortality rate for surgical closure of ventricular septal defect. These observations make it clear that a large ventricular septal defect should be approached surgically very early in life when pulmonary vascular disease is still reversible or has not yet developed.

OTHER FORMS OF VENTRICULAR DEFECT. Unusual forms of ventricular septal defect include multiple muscular defects and left ventricular–right atrial communications. Defects in the muscular ventricular septum frequently are multiple small fenestrations that produce a large net left-to-right shunt.[139] Their recognition is a necessary preliminary to successful operation, since incomplete repair may result in postoperative cardiac failure and death. A shunt from the left ventricle to right atrium may occur with a ventricular septal defect in the most superior portion of the ventricular septum, since the tricuspid valve is lower than the mitral valve. The clinical, electrocardiographic, and radiological findings in these patients do not differ appreciably from those in patients with a simple ventricular septal defect, although right atrial enlargement may provide a clue to correct diagnosis of left ventricular–right atrial communication.[155] The pathophysiology of single or common ventricle (p. 953) may resemble that of a large ventricular septal defect, although these defects are dissimilar embryologically. The single chamber frequently is the morphological left ventricle; malposition of the great arteries is quite common. There may be no detectable cyanosis if selective streaming and increased pulmonary blood flow rather than complete mixing occurs. Pulmonary hypertension invariably is present unless pulmonic stenosis exists. It is imperative to differentiate a single ventricle from a large ventricular septal defect by echocardiography[134] and angiography[122] because the operative approaches to the former malformation require a complex septation technique or the atriopulmonary Fontan connection.

MANAGEMENT OF VENTRICULAR SEPTAL DEFECT.
It is rarely necessary to restrict the activities of a child with an isolated ventricular septal defect. Infective bacterial endocarditis is always a threat, and antibiotic prophylaxis for dental procedures and minor surgery is indicated (Table 31–4).[156] Respiratory infections require prompt evaluation and treatment. These children should be seen at least once or twice yearly to detect changes in the clinical picture that suggest the development of pulmonary vascular obliterative changes.

When clinical findings suggest a moderate shunt but no pulmonary hypertension, elective hemodynamic evaluation should be advised between ages 3 and 6 years. Of prime importance in the hemodynamic evaluation is a determination of pressure and blood flow in the pulmonary artery.[157] Surgical treatment is not recommended for children who have normal pulmonary arterial pressures with small shunts (pulmonary-systemic flow ratios of less than 1.5 to 2.0 : 1). In such patients the remaining risk of infective endocarditis[156] does not exceed the risk of operation. Moreover, although the inherent risk of operation is small, the possibility of postoperative heart block, infection, or other complications of operation and cardiopulmonary bypass dictates a conservative approach when the cardiac defect may be well tolerated for life. With larger shunts, elective operation may be advised before the child enters school, thus minimizing any subsequent

distinction of these patients from their normal classmates. A total assessment of the psychosocial dynamics of the family and child is helpful in determining the proper age for elective operation in each patient.

Under investigation is transcatheter closure by umbrella or clamshell occluder devices (p. 915) inserted by crossing the ventricular defect by way of the left ventricle to guide a venous catheter through a long sheath, and, ultimately, placing the device across the ventricular septum from the right ventricular side.[158]

Complete heart block is the most significant surgically induced conduction system abnormality, occurring immediately after surgery in fewer than 1 per cent of patients. Late-onset complete heart block occasionally is a problem, especially in the 10 to 25 per cent of patients whose postoperative electrocardiographic findings show complete right bundle branch block with left anterior hemiblock.[159] When the latter electrocardiographic pattern is observed in patients with transient complete heart block in the early postoperative period, electrophysiological studies should be conducted at postoperative cardiac catheterization. It would appear that patients presenting postoperatively with right bundle block and left anterior hemiblock fall into two populations, defined by either peripheral damage to the conduction system or damage to the bundle of His or its proximal branches.[160] The former has not been associated with transient postoperative complete heart block, and these patients usually have a benign course. Trifascicular damage may be demonstrated in the latter population by a prolonged H-V interval, which implies a higher risk of complete heart block later in life. Although the prophylactic use of permanent pacemakers in asymptomatic patients with evidence of trifascicular damage is not currently recommended, this group certainly requires careful follow-up and continued study.

Treadmill exercise studies in patients who preoperatively had normal or only moderately elevated pulmonary vascular resistance and essentially normal postoperative cardiac catheterization data may uncover late abnormalities in circulatory function.[161,162] Despite normal cardiac output at rest, an impaired cardiac output response to exercise is noted in some. Moreover, despite a normal pulmonary arterial pressure at rest, markedly abnormal increases in pulmonary arterial pressure may be noted during exercise. These findings may be related to abnormal left ventricular function after closure of the ventricular septal defect and/or to persistent pathological changes in the pulmonary arterioles or to abnormal pulmonary vascular reactivity.[163] A direct relation exists between age at operation and the magnitude of the pulmonary arterial pressure response to intense exercise, suggesting that early operation may prevent permanent impairment of the functional capacity of the myocardium and pulmonary vascular bed.

Occasionally a child may come to medical attention who has already developed pulmonary vascular obstruction and a net right-to-left shunt across the ventricular septal defect. Symptoms may consist of exertional dyspnea, chest pain, syncope, and hemoptysis; the right-to-left shunt leads to cyanosis, clubbing, and polycythemia. There currently is little to offer this group of patients other than continuing support to the patient and family.

PATENT DUCTUS ARTERIOSUS
(See also p. 974)

The ductus arteriosus normally exists in the fetus as a widely patent vessel connecting the pulmonary trunk and the descending aorta just distal to the left subclavian artery (Fig. 31–5). In the fetus most of the output of the right ventricle bypasses the unexpanded lungs by way of the ductus arteriosus and enters the descending aorta, where it travels to the placenta, the fetal organ of oxygenation. Until recently it was assumed that during fetal life the ductus arteriosus was a passively open channel that constricted postnatally by means of undefined molecular mechanisms in response to the abrupt rise in arterial pO$_2$ accompanying the first breath of life.[164] Even in utero the lumen of the ductus arteriosus may be influenced by vasoactive substances, particularly prostaglandins.[73,74,165-167] Thus inhibition of prostaglandin synthesis causes profound constriction of the ductus arteriosus in the mammalian fetus that may be reversed by administration of vasodilatory E-type prostaglandins. Initial contraction and functional closure of the ductus arteriosus shortly after birth is related both to the sudden increase in arterial oxygen saturation that accompanies ventilation and to changes in the synthesis and metabolism of vasoactive eicosanoids. Intimal proliferation and fibrosis proceed more gradually, so that anatomical closure may take as long as several weeks for completion.[168]

The ductus arteriosus is a unique structure after birth, since its patency may, on the one hand, result in cardiac decompensation but may, on the other hand, provide the only life-sustaining conduit to preserve systemic or pulmonary arterial blood flow in the presence of certain cardiac malformations.[71] Appreciable left-to-right shunting across the patent ductus arteriosus frequently complicates the clinical course of infants born prematurely.[169] The ductal shunt has been implicated specifically in the deterioration of pulmonary function in infants with the respiratory distress syndrome in whom severe congestive heart failure often is unresponsive to digitalis and diuretics.[74]

A distinction should be made between patency of the ductus arteriosus in the *preterm* infant, who lacks the normal mechanisms for postnatal ductal closure because of immaturity, and the full-term newborn, in whom patency of the ductus is a true congenital malformation, probably related to a primary anatomical defect of the elastic tissue within the wall of the ductus.[168] In the former circumstance, delayed spontaneous closure of the ductus may be anticipated if the infant does not succumb to the cardiopulmonary difficulties caused by the ductus itself or to some lethal complication of prematurity, such as hyaline membrane disease, intraventricular hemorrhage, or necrotizing enterocolitis. In a similar manner, some full-term newborns have persistent patency of the ductus arteriosus for weeks or months because their relative hypoxemia contributes to vasodilatation of the channel. In the latter category are infants born at high altitude; those born with congenital malformations causing hypoxemia, such as pulmonic atresia with or without ventricular septal defect; or malformations in which ductal flow supplies the systemic circulation, such as hypoplastic left heart syndrome, interruption of the aortic arch, or some examples of coarctation of the aorta syndrome. In the clinical settings in which the ductus preserves pulmonary blood flow, the essentially inevitable spontaneous closure of the vessel is associated with profound clinical deterioration. The latter may be reversed medically within the first 4 to 5 days of life by infusion of prostaglandin E$_1$ intravenously. By dilating the constricted ductus arteriosus, this results in a temporary increase in arterial blood oxygen tension and oxygen saturation and correction of acidemia.[71] These infants can then undergo operative repair or a palliative systemic-pulmonary anastomosis, under more optimal circumstances. Pharmacological dilation of the ductus arteriosus also is effective in the preoperative restoration of systemic blood flow and the alleviation of heart failure, especially in infants with aortic coarctation or hypoplastic left heart syndrome, and in infants with complete transposition of the great arteries in whom intercirculatory mixing is augmented.[71]

PREMATURE INFANTS. In most, if not all, preterm infants under 1500 gm birthweight, persistence of a patent ductus arteriosus is prolonged, and in about one-third of these infants a large aorticopulmonary shunt is responsible for significant cardiopulmonary deterioration.[169,170] Radiographic, echocardiographic, and Doppler ultrasound signs of significant left-to-right shunting usually precede the appearance of physical findings suggesting ductal patency.[32,171-175] A significant increase in the cardiothoracic ratio is seen on sequential roentgenograms as well as increased pulmonary arterial markings progressing to perihilar and generalized pulmonary edema. Serial echocardiographic evaluations that demonstrate increases in left ventricular end-diastolic and left atrial dimensions, especially when correlated with the aforementioned radiographic signs, are highly suggestive of a large shunt.[171] Two-dimensional and Doppler echocardiography directly visualize and define the flow characteristics of the ductus arteriosus with great accuracy (Fig. 4-80, p. 94).[32,172,173] The clinical findings include bounding peripheral pulses, an infraclavicular and interscapular systolic murmur (occasionally a continuous murmur), precordial hyperactivity, hepatomegaly, and either multiple episodes of apnea and bradycardia or respirator dependency. Cardiac catheterization carries a high risk in the preterm infant and seldom is indicated unless the diagnosis is obscure.

Management of the preterm infant with a patent ductus arteriosus varies, depending on the magnitude of shunting and the severity of hyaline membrane disease, since the ductus may contribute importantly to mortality in the respiratory distress syndrome. Intervention in an asymptomatic infant with a small left-to-right shunt is unnecessary, since the patent ductus arteriosus will almost invariably undergo spontaneous closure and will not require late surgical ligation and division. Those infants who demonstrate unmistakable signs of a significant ductal left-to-right shunt during the course of the respiratory distress syndrome often are unresponsive to medical measures to control congestive heart failure, and require closure of the patent ductus arteriosus to survive. These infants are best managed within the first 2 to 7 days of life by pharmacological inhibition of prostaglandin synthesis with indomethacin to constrict and close the ductus[169,175-178]; surgical ligation is required in the estimated 10 per cent of infants who are unresponsive to indomethacin.[175,180] Early intervention is advised to reduce the likelihood of necrotizing enterocolitis and of bronchopulmonary dysplasia related to prolonged respirator and oxygen dependency.[179] Less often, indications for pharmacological or surgical closure of the ductus consist of life-threatening episodes of apnea and bradycardia or a prolonged failure to gain weight and grow.

FULL-TERM INFANTS AND CHILDREN. In full-term newborns and older infants and children, patency of the ductus arteriosus occurs particularly in females and in the offspring of pregnancies complicated by first-trimester rubella. Although most frequent in isolated form, the anomaly may coexist with other malformations, particularly coarctation of the aorta, ventricular septal defect, pulmonic stenosis, and aortic stenosis. Flow across the ductus is determined by the pressure relation between the aorta and the pulmonary artery and by the cross-sectional area and length of the ductus itself.[181] Pulmonary pressures most commonly are normal, and a persistent gradient and shunt from aorta to pulmonary artery exist throughout the cardiac cycle. Physical examination reveals a characteristic thrill and a continuous "machinery" murmur with a late systolic accentuation at the upper left sternal border. The left atrium and left ventricle enlarge to accommodate the increased pulmonary venous return, and flow murmurs across the mitral and aortic valves may be detected. With significant left-to-right shunting, the runoff of blood through the ductus causes a widened systemic pulse pressure and bounding peripheral pulses. The hemodynamic abnormality is reflected in the electrocardiogram by left ventricular and occasionally left atrial hypertrophy, and in the chest roentgenogram by left atrial and ventricular enlargement, prominent ascending aorta and pulmonary artery, and pulmonary vascular engorgement (Fig. 8-41B, p. 229 and Fig. 32-5, p. 969). The clinical diagnosis may be difficult when the findings do not conform to the classic presentation.[182] As mentioned above, disappearance of the diastolic component of the murmur is common in premature infants because higher pulmonary arterial diastolic pressures exist at that age.

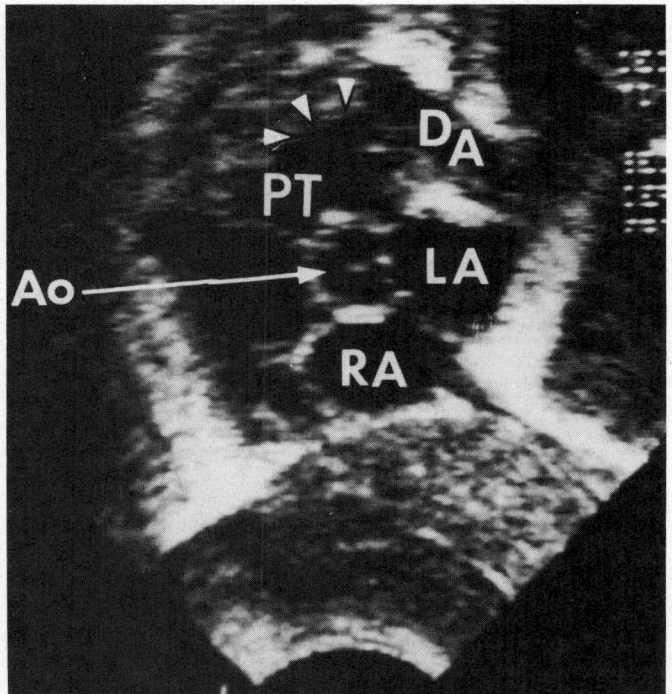

FIGURE 31-19. Parasternal short-axis view of a patent ductus arteriosus (arrowheads) in an infant. The pulmonic valve is the linear echo just beneath the pulmonary trunk (PT). AO = aortic valve, DA = descending aorta, RA = right atrium, LA = left atrium. (From Perloff, J.: The Clinical Recognition of Congenital Heart Disease. 3rd ed. Philadelphia, W. B. Saunders Company, 1986.)

In older patients both heart failure and pulmonary hypertension are associated with a reduction in the pressure gradient across the ductus arteriosus and result in atypical systolic murmurs. When severe pulmonary vascular obstructive disease results in reversal of flow through the ductus and preferential shunting of unoxygenated blood to the descending aorta, the toes, rather than the fingers, may show cyanosis and clubbing.

The full-term infant with patent ductus arteriosus may survive for a number of years, although occasionally a large defect results in heart failure and pulmonary edema early in life. The leading causes of death in older children are infective endocarditis and heart failure. Beyond the third decade severe pulmonary vascular obstruction has been known to cause aneurysmal dilatation, calcification, and rupture of the ductus.[182]

The patent ductus usually can be directly visualized by two-dimensional echocardiography (Figs. 31-19 and 4-81, p. 94); range-gated pulse Doppler echocardiography shows the characteristic flow abnormalities across the ductus, as well as a continuous flow disturbance in the pulmonary artery.[174] Cardiac catheterization may be indicated when additional lesions or pulmonary vascular obstruction is suspected. In the absence of severe pulmonary vascular disease with predominant right-to-left shunting the anatomical presence of a patent ductus usually is considered sufficient indication for operation. Ligation or division of the ductus carries a low risk, whether performed electively in the asymptomatic child or at any age if symptoms are present. The operative risk is reduced if heart failure can be compensated by medical measures before surgery. Operation should be deferred for several months in patients treated successfully for infective endarteritis because the ductus may remain somewhat edematous and friable. Rarely, when the infection will not subside with intensive antibiotic treatment, surgical ligation may be necessary to eradicate the infection. Although still investigational, substantial experience exists with transcatheter closure of the patent ductus using a spring-loaded, double-disk (clamshell configuration) umbrella occluder device introduced through

a relatively large-diameter sheath from the femoral vein. The approach is especially feasible in patients who weigh more than 10 kg, and with neither a long tubular ductus nor a ductus with a long, narrow aortic end.[183-187]

AORTICOPULMONARY SEPTAL DEFECT

Aorticopulmonary window or fenestration, partial truncus arteriosus, and aortic septal defect are other designations applied to this relatively uncommon anomaly. Septation of the aortopulmonary trunk occurs by fusion of the conotruncal ridges (Fig. 31-4). The right and left sixth aortic arches, destined to become the pulmonary arteries, join the pulmonary artery to complete great artery development (Fig. 31-5). Congenital defects between the ascending aorta and the pulmonary artery result from faulty development of this area during embryonic life. The typical aortopulmonary septal defect results because of incomplete fusion of the distal aortopulmonary septum.[188] Malalignment of the conotruncal ridges results in unequal partitioning of the aortopulmonary trunk, which may result in partial or complete fusion of the right pulmonary artery to the aorta. The usual defect consists of a communication between the aorta and pulmonary artery just above the semilunar valves. Persistent patency of the ductus arteriosus is an associated lesion in 10 to 15 per cent of cases. Less common accompanying cardiovascular lesions include ventricular septal defect, aortic origin of the right pulmonary artery, aortic arch interruption, coarctation of the aorta, and right aortic arch. Aorticopulmonary septal defects usually are large and are accompanied by severe pulmonary arterial hypertension and early-onset pulmonary vascular obstruction.

PHYSICAL EXAMINATION. The pulses typically are bounding, like those of a large patent ductus arteriosus. The murmur, however, seldom is continuous, and a basal systolic murmur is most common. Cardiomegaly is present, and pulmonary hypertension is reflected in a loud and palpable sound of pulmonary valve closure. Aorticopulmonary septal defect should be suspected whenever a large shunt into the pulmonary artery is demonstrated at catheterization. Diagnosis of the anomaly and its distinction from patent ductus and persistent truncus arteriosus usually can be done by two-dimensional echocardiography, but definitive identification of the aortopulmonary window and associated malformations requires hemodynamic study and selective angiocardiography with the injection of contrast material into the left ventricle and/or the root of the aorta (Fig. 31-20). Although some patients may survive to adulthood with uncorrected aorticopulmonary septal defect, most will die early in life unless surgical treatment is undertaken. Operative correction is indicated in all symptomatic infants when the diagnosis is made. Elective repair is advised at 3 to 6 months. Profound hypothermic total circulatory arrest or total cardiopulmonary bypass is required, and the defect is closed by way of a transaortic approach, usually with a prosthetic patch.[189,190]

PERSISTENT TRUNCUS ARTERIOSUS

Persistent truncus arteriosus is a rare but serious anomaly in which a single vessel forms the outlet of both ventricles and gives rise to the systemic, pulmonary, and coronary ar-

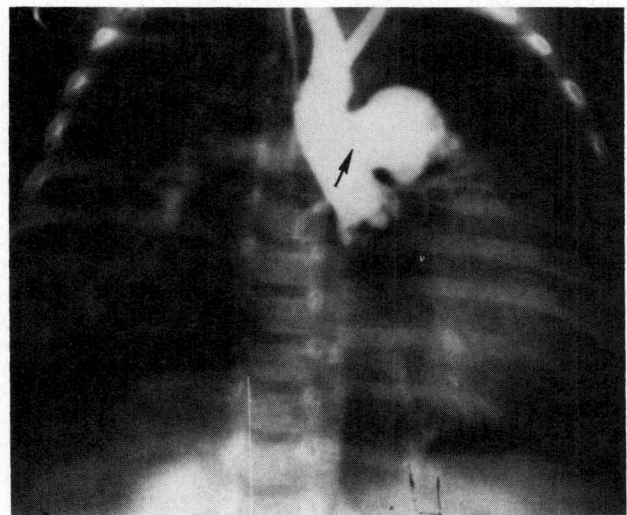

FIGURE 31-20. Aortic root injection of contrast material in the frontal view produces simultaneous opacification of aorta and pulmonary artery through a large aorticopulmonary septal defect (arrow). (Courtesy of Robert White, M.D.)

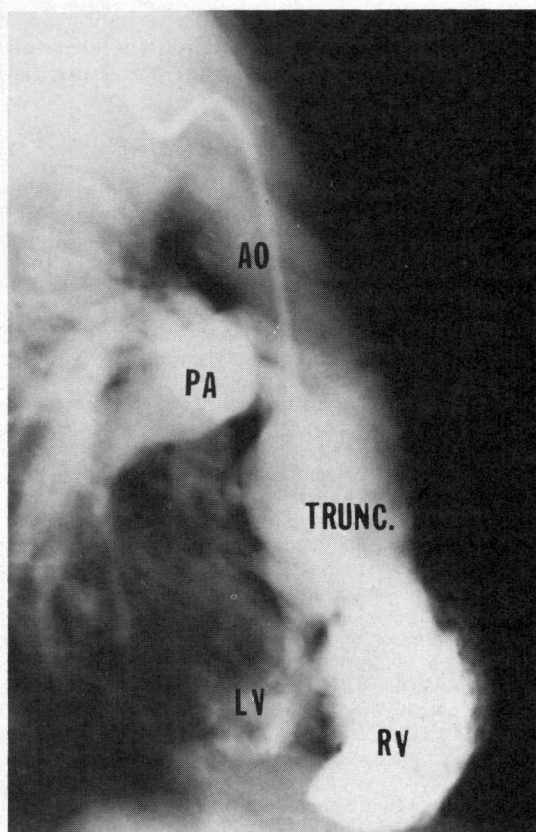

FIGURE 31–21. Right ventriculogram in the lateral view in a patient with type I truncus arteriosus. The contrast agent enters the left ventricle (LV) across a ventricular septal defect. The pulmonary artery (PA) arises directly from the persistent truncus arteriosus (TRUNC). AO = aorta, RV = right ventricle. (Courtesy of Robert White, M.D.)

teries.[191] The defect results from failure of septation of the embryonic truncus by the infundibular truncal ridges (Fig. 31–4). It is always accompanied by a ventricular septal defect, frequently with a right-sided aortic arch. The ventricular septal defect is due to the absence or underdevelopment of the distal portion of the pulmonary infundibulum. The truncal valve usually is tricuspid but is quadricuspid in about one-third of patients and rarely can be bicuspid. Truncal valve regurgitation and truncal valve stenosis are each seen in 10 to 15 per cent of patients. There may be a single coronary artery, displacement of the coronary ostia (usually the left ostium posteriorly), or a single posterior descending coronary artery arising from the right coronary or, less often, from the left circumflex artery, especially in patients with a single coronary artery.[192,193]

Truncus malformations may be classified either anatomically according to the mode of origin of pulmonary vessels from the common trunk or from a functional point of view, based on the magnitude of blood flow to the lungs.[194] In the common type (type I) of truncus arteriosus malformation a partially separate pulmonary trunk of variable length exists because of the presence of an incompletely formed aorticopulmonary septum (Fig. 31–21). The pulmonary trunk usually is very short and gives rise to left and right pulmonary arteries. When the aorticopulmonary septum is absent, there is no discrete main pulmonary artery component, and both pulmonary artery branches arise directly from the truncus. In type II, each pulmonary artery arises separately but close to the other from the posterior aspect of the truncus. In type III, each pulmonary artery arises from the lateral aspect of the truncus. Less commonly, one pulmonary artery branch may be absent, with collateral arteries supplying the lung that does not receive a pulmonary artery branch from the truncus. Truncus arteriosus malformation should not be confused with "pseudotruncus arteriosus," which is the severe form of tetralogy of

Fallot with pulmonary atresia in which the single aorta arises from the heart accompanied by a remnant of atretic pulmonary artery (p. 935).

Pulmonary blood flow is governed by the size of the pulmonary arteries and the pulmonary vascular resistance. In infancy, pulmonary blood flow is usually excessive, since pulmonary vascular resistance is not greatly increased. Thus, despite an obligatory admixture of systemic and pulmonary venous blood in the common trunk, only minimal cyanosis is present. Rarely, pulmonary blood flow is restricted by hypoplastic or stenotic pulmonary arteries arising from the truncus. Pulmonary vascular obstruction usually does not restrict pulmonary blood flow before 1 year of age.[195] Hence, the infant with truncus arteriosus usually presents with mild cyanosis coexisting with the cardiac findings of a large left-to-right shunt. Symptoms of heart failure and poor physical development usually appear in the first weeks or months of life. The most frequent physical findings include cardiomegaly, a systolic ejection sound accompanied by a thrill, a loud single second heart sound, a harsh systolic murmur, and a low-pitched middiastolic rumbling murmur and bounding pulses. Truncus arteriosus often is a feature of the *DiGeorge syndrome* (Table 31–2); thus facial dysmorphism, a high incidence of extracardiac malformations (particularly of the limbs, kidneys, and intestines), atrophy or absence of the thymus gland, T-lymphocyte deficiency, and predilection to infection also may be features of the clinical presentation.[196] Recent evidence suggests that embryonic abnormalities in the cardiac neural crest play a major role in the creation of the cardiovascular malformation as well as the other components of the syndrome.[196a]

Truncal valve incompetence is suggested by the presence of a diastolic decrescendo murmur at the base of the heart.[197] The physical findings are quite different if pulmonary blood flow is restricted by either high pulmonary vascular resistance or pulmonary arterial stenosis: cyanosis is prominent, congestive failure is rare, and only a short systolic ejection may be audible occasionally accompanied by continuous murmurs posteriorly of bronchial collateral flow. Left ventricular hypertrophy alone or in combination with right ventricular hypertrophy is present electrocardiographically when a prominent left-to-right shunt exists; right ventricular hypertrophy is observed in patients with restricted pulmonary blood flow. The radiographic findings depend on the hemodynamic circumstances. Gross cardiomegaly with left or combined ventricular enlargement, left atrial enlargement, and a small or absent main pulmonary artery segment with pulmonary vascular engorgement are the usual radiographic features. A right aortic arch is common (25 to 30 per cent of patients). When pulmonary blood flow is reduced, both heart size and pulmonary vascular markings are less prominent.

The *echocardiographic* features of truncus arteriosus (Fig. 31–22) include the detection of a large truncal root overriding the ventricular septum, truncal valve abnormalities, an in-

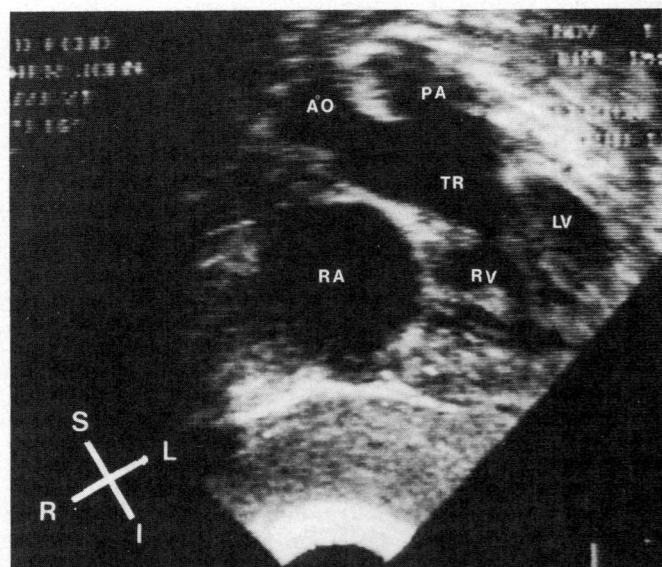

FIGURE 31–22. Truncus arteriosus, shown by a subcostal view with superior angulation of the transducer to image the truncal root (TR). The tricuspid valve is closed in ventricular systole. The truncal root sits above both the right ventricle (RV) and left ventricle (LV). The pulmonary artery (PA) arises directly from the truncus. AO = aorta, RA = right atrium.

crease in the right ventricular dimension, and mitral valve–truncal root continuity. The dimension of the left atrium determined echocardiographically provides a good index of pulmonary flow. Differentiation between truncus arteriosus and tetralogy of Fallot by ultrasound may be difficult unless either the separate origin of the pulmonary arteries or a single trunk from the ascending portion of a single arterial root can be identified. Diagnosis should be suspected at cardiac catheterization if the catheter fails to enter the central pulmonary arteries from the right ventricle. Selective angiocardiography and retrograde aortography are necessary to establish a precise diagnosis and to reveal the common trunk arising from the heart and the origin of the pulmonary arteries from the truncus.[198]

The early fatal course as well as early development of pulmonary vascular obstructive disease in patients surviving infancy is responsible for the poor prognosis associated with truncus arteriosus. In infants and young children with large left-to-right shunts, surgical banding of one or both pulmonary arteries to reduce pulmonary flow has been used with little success. Corrective operation is preferred before age 3 months to avoid the development of severe pulmonary vascular obstructive disease.[199]

SURGICAL TREATMENT. Operation consists of closure of the ventricular septal defect, leaving the aorta arising from the left ventricle; the pulmonary arteries are excised from their truncus origin and a valve-containing prosthetic conduit or aortic homograft valve conduit is used to establish continuity between the right ventricle and the pulmonary arteries (Fig. 31–23). Truncal valve regurgitation significantly enhances the risk of corrective surgery, since valve replacement is associated with significantly increased surgical mortality. Patients with only one pulmonary artery are especially prone to early development of severe pulmonary vascular disease but otherwise are not at increased risk from surgery. With truncus arteriosus defects, the possible inequalities of pressure and flow between the two pulmonary arteries often make precise calculation of pulmonary resistance difficult. Corrective operation may be performed in patients with at least one adequate pulmonary artery having low distal pressure or arteriolar resistance. Conversely, significant systemic arterial desaturation in a patient with two pulmonary arteries and with neither pulmonary artery stenosis nor a previous pulmonary artery band signifies that high pulmonary vascular resistance exists and that the condition is probably inoperable. It is not yet clear how often and at what age the conduit between the right ventricle and pulmonary artery must be replaced with a larger prosthesis because of either growth of the patient, in whom a small conduit causes eventual obstruction, heterograft valve degeneration, or obstruction created by neointimal proliferation within a prosthetic conduit. When operation is carried out with a conduit in the first year of life, conduit replacement often is required within 3 to 5 years.

CORONARY ARTERIOVENOUS FISTULA
(See also p. 970)

Coronary arteriovenous fistula is an unusual anomaly that consists of a communication between one of the coronary arteries and a cardiac chamber or vein. The right coronary artery, or its branches, is the site of the fistula in about 55 per cent of cases; the left coronary artery is involved in about 35 per cent, and both coronary arteries in 5 per cent. Connections between the coronary system and a cardiac chamber appear to represent persistence of embryonic intertrabecular spaces and sinusoids. Most of these fistulas drain into the right ventricle, right atrium, or coronary sinus; fistulous communication to the pulmonary artery, left atrium, or left ventricle is much less frequent. Most often the shunt through the fistula is of small magnitude, and myocardial blood flow is not compromised.[199] Potential complications include pulmonary hypertension and congestive heart failure if a large left-to-right shunt exists, bacterial endocarditis, rupture or thrombosis of the fistula or an associated arterial aneurysm, and myocardial ischemia distal to the fistula due to decreased coronary blood flow.

Most patients are asymptomatic and are referred because of a cardiac murmur that is loud, superficial, and continuous at the lower or midsternal border. The site of maximal intensity of the murmur is related to the site of drainage and usually is different from the second left intercostal space—the classic site of the continuous murmur of persistent ductus arteriosus —except when the fistula drains into the pulmonary artery or right ventricle. In the latter situation the murmur is louder in diastole than in systole because of compression of the fistula by contracting myocardium. The electrocardiogram and chest roentgenogram quite often are normal and seldom show selective chamber enlargement or myocardial ischemia. Significantly enlarged coronary arteries may be detected by two-dimensional echocardiography, and the actual diagnosis of an arteriovenous fistula occasionally can be made by combining two-dimensional echocardiography and Doppler techniques to detect the entrance site of the shunt, which is characterized by a continuous turbulent systolic and diastolic flow pattern.[200,201] (Fig. 32–7, p. 970)

Retrograde thoracic aortography or coronary arteriography can be used reliably to identify the size and anatomical features of the fistulous tract, which can be closed by suture obliteration in most cases.[202] In the presence of a large left-to-right shunt and symptoms of heart failure, the decision to

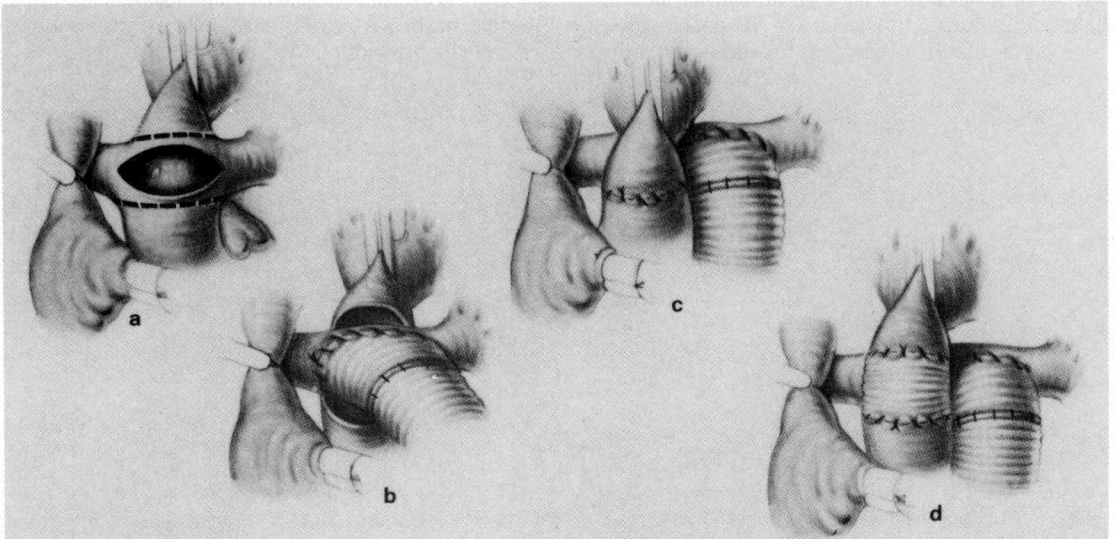

FIGURE 31–23. Operative correction of truncus arteriosus, type III. The pulmonary arteries arise separately from the truncus. An anterior incision is made and a segment of aorta containing the orifices of both pulmonary arteries is excised from the truncus (a). The cuff of tissue containing the two pulmonary arteries is anastomosed to an extracardiac valved conduit (b). Aortic continuity is restored by direct suture (c), or by interposing a preclotted graft (d). The diagram does not show closure of the ventricular septal defect. (From Stark, J., and DeLaval, M.: Surgery for Congenital Heart Defects. New York, Grune and Stratton, 1983, p. 420.)

operate is clearly justified. Most often the fistula is closed in asymptomatic patients to prevent future symptoms or complications, such as infective endocarditis. The prognosis after successful closure of a coronary artery–cardiac chamber fistula is excellent.

ANOMALOUS PULMONARY ORIGIN OF THE CORONARY ARTERY

This rare malformation occurs in about 0.4 per cent of patients with congenital cardiac anomalies. In almost all patients the left coronary artery originates from the posterior sinus of the pulmonary artery.[203]

Unusual cases have been reported in which the right coronary artery, or the entire coronary artery system, originates from the main pulmonary trunk. Embryologically the distal coronary artery system is formed by 9 weeks from solid angioblastic buds that extend throughout the epicardium to form the major coronary artery branches. Proximally the coronary network forms a ring around the truncus arteriosus, joining with coronary buds from the primitive aortic sinuses as the truncus partitions to form the great arteries. The varieties of anomalous pulmonary origin of the coronary artery are the result of displacement in this proximal process.

During fetal life pulmonary artery pressure is slightly greater than aortic pressure, and perfusion of the left coronary artery is antegrade. After birth, when pulmonary artery pressure falls below aortic pressure, perfusion of the left coronary artery from the pulmonary artery ceases, and the direction of flow in the anomalous vessel reverses. Blood flows from the aorta to the right coronary artery, then through collateral channels to the left coronary artery, and finally to the pulmonary artery. In effect, the left coronary artery behaves as a fistulous communication between the aorta and pulmonary artery. If adequate collateral channels exist or develop between the two coronary artery circulations, total myocardial perfusion through the right coronary artery increases. In 10 to 15 per cent of patients myocardial ischemia never develops because extensive intercoronary collaterals allow survival to adolescence or adulthood. In fact, if collateral blood flow is considerable, the patient may develop the clinical manifestations of a large arteriovenous shunt and a continuous or diastolic murmur. Older children or adults usually present with a continuous murmur or with mitral regurgitation resulting from dysfunction of ischemic or infarcted papillary muscles. In some instances the coronary anomaly is unsuspected until a previously well adolescent or adult experiences angina, heart failure, or sudden death.

By far the most common clinical presentation is that of the infant who suffers a myocardial infarction and develops congestive heart failure.[204,205] The infant syndrome usually becomes manifested at age 2 to 4 months with angina-like symptoms that may be misinterpreted as colic. Feeding and defecation often are accompanied by dyspnea, irritability and crying, pallor, diaphoresis, and occasional loss of consciousness. The diagnosis of anomalous origin of the coronary artery is supported by the electrocardiographic demonstration of deep Q waves in association with ST-segment alterations and T-wave inversions in leads I, aV_L, V_5, and V_6 (Fig. 31–24). Chest roentgenograms show moderate to severe enlargement of the left atrium and ventricle. The origin of the anomalous left coronary artery occasionally may be visualized echocardiographically from long- or short-axis views of the pulmonary artery.[206,207] Absence of the left coronary artery from its usual origin in the left sinus of Valsalva does not distinguish this lesion from single coronary artery. Color-flow Doppler examination reveals diastolic turbulent flow in the pulmonary artery near the coronary orifice, and also may disclose associated mitral regurgitation. Contrast echocardiography from a radial artery injection demonstrates even small left-to-right shunts from the right coronary artery system, through the anomalous left coronary artery, into the pulmonary artery.[207] Ischemia or infarction is suggested by the echocardiographic findings of segmental wall motion abnormalities, particularly involving the anterolateral free wall of the left ventricle. Stress thallium scintigraphy shows a characteristic defect of the anterolateral wall of the left ventricle.

Aortography or coronary angiography is the definitive diagnostic procedure, and demonstrates the retrograde drainage of the coronary vessel into the pulmonary artery (Fig. 31–25). It should be recognized that ventricular arrhythmias may complicate the course of hemodynamic study. Management of these infants depends, in part, on the magnitude of shunting into the pulmonary artery, which may be determined by oximetry, indicator dilution curves, or angiography.

MANAGEMENT. *Medical treatment* is indicated in infants with myocardial infarction for congestive heart failure, arrhythmias, and cardiogenic shock. In patients with a small left-to-right shunt or no shunt at all, the prognosis is exceedingly poor with conservative management, justifying an attempt to reestablish a two–coronary artery system. The *operations* that have been used include reimplanting the left coronary artery into the aortic root, surgically creating an aortopulmonary window and a tunnel to convey blood from the window across the back of the pulmonary trunk to the origin of the anomalous left coronary artery, with reconstruction of the anterior wall of the pulmonary trunk, or anastomosis of the left coronary artery with the subclavian artery or with the aorta by means of a graft.[208,209] If clinical deterioration occurs in infants in whom a sizable left-to-right shunt into the pulmonary artery exists, simple ligation of the left coronary artery at its origin prevents retrograde flow and allows perfusion of the left ventricle with blood supplied through anastomoses with the right coronary artery. If medical management stabilizes the infant with significant intercoronary collaterals, operation may be postponed to allow the patient to grow, since increased

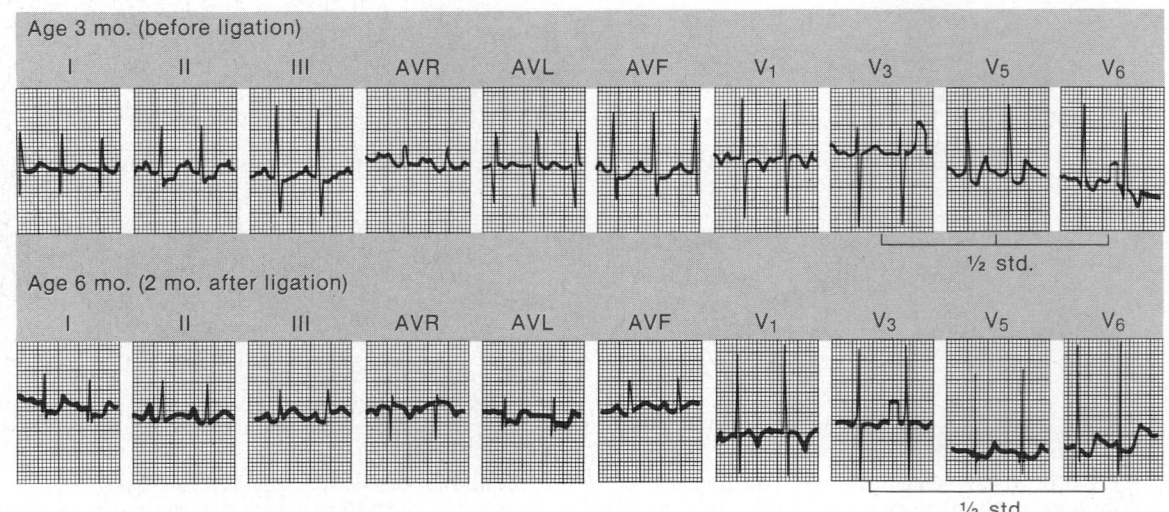

FIGURE 31–24. Typical electrocardiogram of an infant with anomalous left coronary artery before *(above)* and after *(below)* ligation of the anomalous left coronary artery. Arrows point to the abnormal Q waves. (Courtesy of Delores A. Danilowicz, M.D.)

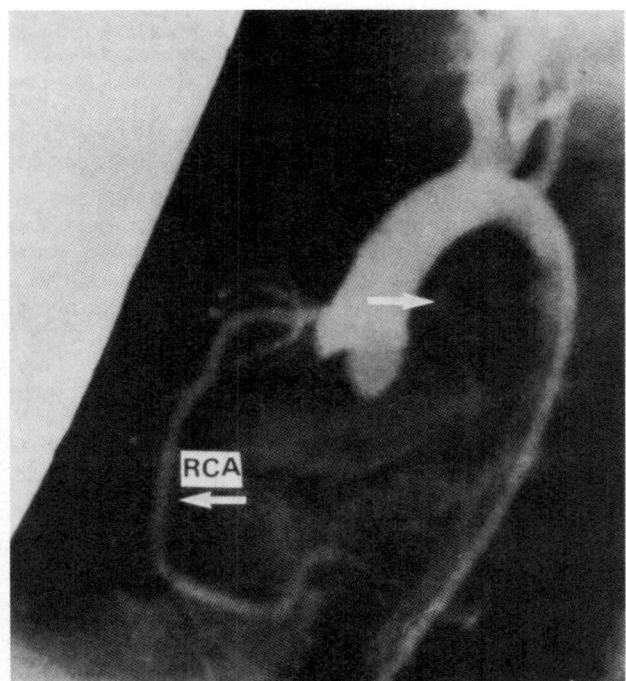

FIGURE 31–25. Lateral view of anomalous left coronary artery. Retrograde aortogram fills the right (RCA) and then the left coronary artery through collateral channels. The left coronary artery enters the main pulmonary artery (upper arrow). (Courtesy of Robert Freedom, M.D.)

size of the vessels enhances the likelihood of successful reimplantation or coronary arterial bypass surgery. The outcome of surgery and ultimate prognosis are significantly influenced by the degree of myocardial damage suffered preoperatively. Uncommonly, it is necessary to consider aneurysmectomy or mitral valve replacement.

AORTIC SINUS ANEURYSM AND FISTULA
(See also p. 970)

Congenital aneurysm of an aortic sinus of Valsalva, particularly the right coronary sinus, is an uncommon anomaly that occurs more often in males than in females. The malformation consists of a separation, or lack of fusion, between the media of the aorta and the annulus fibrosis of the aortic valve.[210] The receiving chamber of the aorticocardiac fistula usually is the right ventricle, but occasionally, when the noncoronary cusp is involved, the fistula drains into the right atrium.

Five to 15 per cent of aneurysms originate in the posterior or noncoronary sinus; seldom is the left aortic sinus involved. Associated anomalies are common and include bicuspid aortic valve, ventricular septal defect, and coarctation of the aorta.

It is not clear whether the aneurysm itself is present at birth, although the deficiency in the aortic media would appear to be congenital. Reports in children are infrequent, since progressive aneurysmal dilatation of the weakened area develops but may not be recognized until the third or fourth decade of life, when rupture into a cardiac chamber occurs.

The *unruptured aneurysm* usually does not produce a hemodynamic abnormality, although pressure on the intracardiac conduction system by an unruptured aneurysm may be a rare cause of complete atrioventricular block; rarely, myocardial ischemia may be caused by coronary arterial compression. Rupture often is of abrupt onset, causes chest pain, and creates continuous arteriovenous shunting and volume loading of both right and left heart chambers, which results in heart failure. An additional complication is bacterial endocarditis, which may originate either on the edges of the aneurysm or on those areas in the right side of the heart that are traumatized by the jet-like stream of blood flowing through the fistula.

The presence of this anomaly should be suspected in a patient with a history of chest pain or recent onset, symptoms of diminished cardiac reserve, bounding pulses, and a loud superficial continuous murmur accentuated in diastole when the fistula opens into the right ventricle, as well as a thrill

along the right or left lower parasternal border. The *physical findings* may be difficult to distinguish from those produced by a coronary arteriovenous fistula. *Electrocardiography* shows biventricular hypertrophy, and chest roentgenography demonstrates generalized cardiomegaly. Two-dimensional and pulsed Doppler *echocardiographic* studies may detect the walls of the aneurym and disturbed flow within the aneurysm or at the site of perforation, respectively.[211] *Cardiac catheterization* reveals a left-to-right shunt at the ventricular or, less commonly, the atrial level; the diagnosis may be established definitively by retrograde thoracic aortography (Fig. 31–26). Preoperative medical management consists of measures to relieve cardiac failure and to treat coexistent arrhythmias or endocarditis, if present. At operation the aneurysm is closed and amputated, and the aortic wall is reunited with the heart, either by direct suture or with a prosthesis.[212] Every effort should be made to preserve the aortic valve in children, since patch closure of the defect combined with prosthetic valve replacement greatly enhances the risk of operation in small patients.

VALVULAR AND VASCULAR LESIONS WITH OR WITHOUT RIGHT-TO-LEFT SHUNT

AORTIC ARCH OBSTRUCTION

The conventional anatomical and clinical divisions into preductal and postductal coarctation or infantile and adult types, respectively, is misleading, since the anatomical localization is inaccurate and the age-dependency of clinical presentation does not hold true (i.e., the adult type often is seen in the first weeks of life). A spectrum of anatomical lesions exists, causing obstruction of the aortic arch or proximal portion of the descending aorta. These range from a localized coarctation or constriction of the lumen, most commonly located just distal to the origin of the left subclavian artery and closely related to the attachment of the ductus arteriosus with the aorta, to diffuse narrowing or interruption of a portion of the aortic arch. In this chapter, aortic arch obstruction is divided into three types: (1) localized juxtaductal coarctation, (2) hypoplasia of the aortic isthmus, and (3) aortic arch interruption. *Pseudocoarctation* is used synonymously with "kinking," or

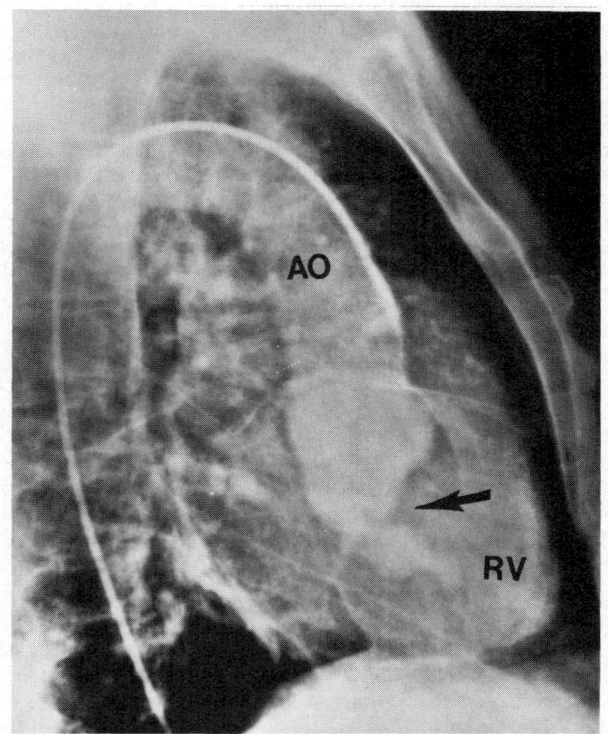

FIGURE 31–26. A retrograde aortogram shows the fistulous connection between the noncoronary sinus of Valsalva and the right ventricle (RV) (arrow). AO = aorta. (Courtesy of Robert White, M.D.)

"buckling," of the aorta, which is a subclinical form of localized juxtaductal coarctation of the aorta.[213]

LOCALIZED JUXTADUCTAL COARCTATION
(See also p. 967)

MORPHOLOGY. This lesion consists of a localized shelf-like thickening and infolding of the media of the posterolateral aortic wall opposite the ductus arteriosus; the wall of the aorta into which the ductus or ligamentum arteriosum inserts is not involved.[214] Juxtaductal coarctation occurs two to five times more commonly in males than in females, and there is a high degree of association with gonadal dysgenesis (Turner syndrome) and bicuspid aortic valve. Other common associated anomalies include ventricular septal defect and mitral stenosis or regurgitation. The most important extracardiac anomaly is aneurysm of the circle of Willis.

PATHOGENESIS. Juxtaductal coarctation is probably related to an abnormality in the pattern of ductus arteriosus blood flow in utero, which, in turn, may be the result of associated intracardiac anomalies.[214,215] Thus, in fetal life, blood flow through the aortic isthmus constitutes only 12 to 17 per cent of the total cardiac output, while blood flow through the ductus arteriosus exceeds that across the aortic valve. The dorsal aortic wall directly opposite the ductus arteriosus will resemble morphologically the apex of a normal branch point of the aorta if ductal flow pathways in utero diverge, with some flow directed cephalad into the aortic isthmus and the remainder proceeding into the descending aorta. The aortic branch point is identical histologically to the posterior shelf of juxtaductal aortic coarctation. A divergence of ductal flow is fostered by the presence of lesions in the fetus that create an imbalance between left and right ventricular outputs, with right-sided flow predominating (e.g., bicuspid aortic valve, mitral valve anomaly). In the absence of an anomaly fostering augmented ductal flow, a branch point may be created by an alteration in the angle at which the ductus arteriosus meets the aorta, pointing the ductal stream directly against the posterior aortic wall rather than obliquely down into the descending aorta. Cardiac anomalies that cause augmented ascending aortic blood flow (e.g., pulmonic atresia or stenosis, tetralogy of Fallot) prevent development of a branch point and indeed are almost never seen in association with juxtaductal coarctation of the aorta.

During fetal life the posterior aortic shelf is not obstructive, since blood may pass readily from the ascending aorta to the descending aorta by traversing the anterior aortic segment and the aortic end of the ductus arteriosus. Postnatally, however, when the ductus undergoes obliteration at its aortic end, the shelf-like projection of the posterior aortic wall unmasks the obstruction to aortic flow (Fig. 31–27). After pharmacological interventions that dilate the ductus arteriosus (prostaglandin E₁ infusion) the pressure difference may be obliterated across the site of coarctation, since the fetal flow pattern is reestablished.[71,216]

The pathogenesis of juxtaductal coarctation already described explains the prevalence of associated intracardiac anomalies that foster reduced ascending aortic flow and augmented ductus arteriosus flow in utero, and the absence of associated intracardiac anomalies in which the converse flow conditions exist in utero. The dependence of aortic obstruction on constriction of the ductus arteriosus postnatally explains the variable onset after birth of the clinical manifestations of coarctation, as well as the dramatic alleviation of obstruction produced pharmacologically by dilatation of the ductus arteriosus.

CLINICAL FINDINGS. The manifestations of juxtaductal coarctation of the aorta depend on the prominence of the posterolateral aortic shelf, which determines the intensity of obstruction, and on the rapidity with which obstruction develops. Rapid, severe obstruction in infancy is a prominent cause of left ventricular failure and systemic hypoperfusion. Substantial left-to-right shunting across a patent foramen ovale and pulmonary venous hypertension secondary to heart failure cause pulmonary arterial hypertension. Because little or no aortic obstruction existed during fetal life, the collateral circulation in the newborn period is often poorly developed. Characteristically in these infants, peripheral pulses are weak throughout the body until left ventricular function is improved with medical management; a significant pressure difference then develops between the arms and the legs, allowing detection of a pulse discrepancy. Cardiac murmurs are nonspecific in infancy and commonly are derived from associated lesions. The electrocardiogram shows right-axis devia-

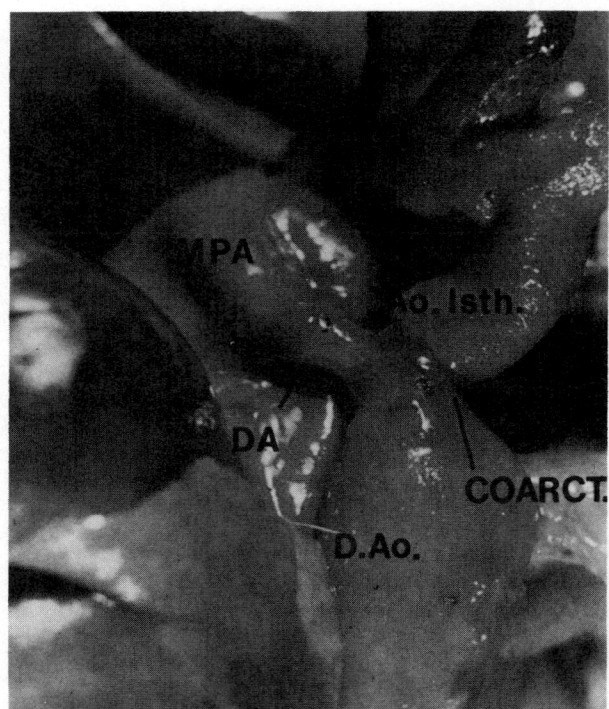

FIGURE 31–27. Juxtaductal coarctation (COARCT) unmasked by constriction of the ductus arteriosus (DA). MPA = main pulmonary artery, D.Ao. = descending aorta, Ao.Isth. = aortic isthmus. (Courtesy of Norman Talner, M.D.)

tion and right ventricular hypertrophy; the chest x-ray shows generalized cardiomegaly and pulmonary arterial and venous engorgement. Hemodynamic study allows delineation of the site and extent of aortic obstruction and the detection of associated cardiac malformations. Most infants with early-onset severe heart failure respond poorly to medical management, and balloon angioplasty,[217] surgical excision of the coarctation, or a subclavian flap angioplasty[218] often is required.

Aortic obstruction may develop slowly in infants in whom the posterolateral aortic shelf is not prominent at birth and in whom ductus arteriosus constriction is gradual. In these babies compensatory myocardial hypertrophy and an extensive collateral circulation have time to develop. If the obstruc-

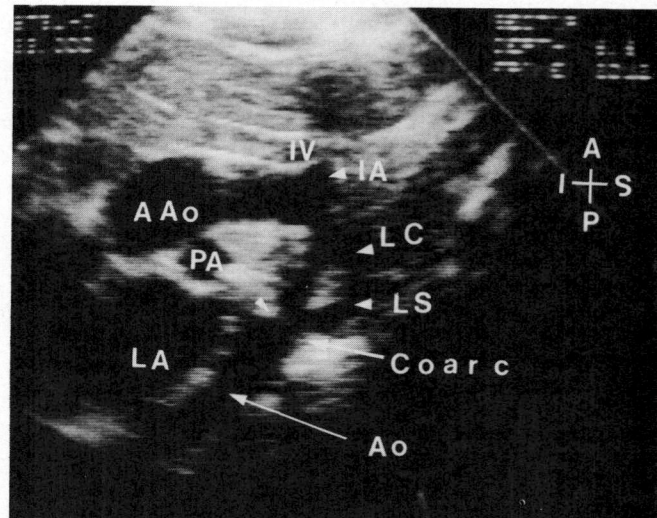

FIGURE 31–28. Aortic coarctation (Coarc) is visualized from the suprasternal notch. The aorta (Ao) can be traced from the ascending aorta (AAo). The aortic arch is somewhat narrowed and the relationship of the left subclavian artery (LS) to the coarctation is identified clearly. LA = left atrium, PA = pulmonary artery, IA = innominate artery, LC = left carotid artery. (Courtesy of Norman Silverman, M.D.)

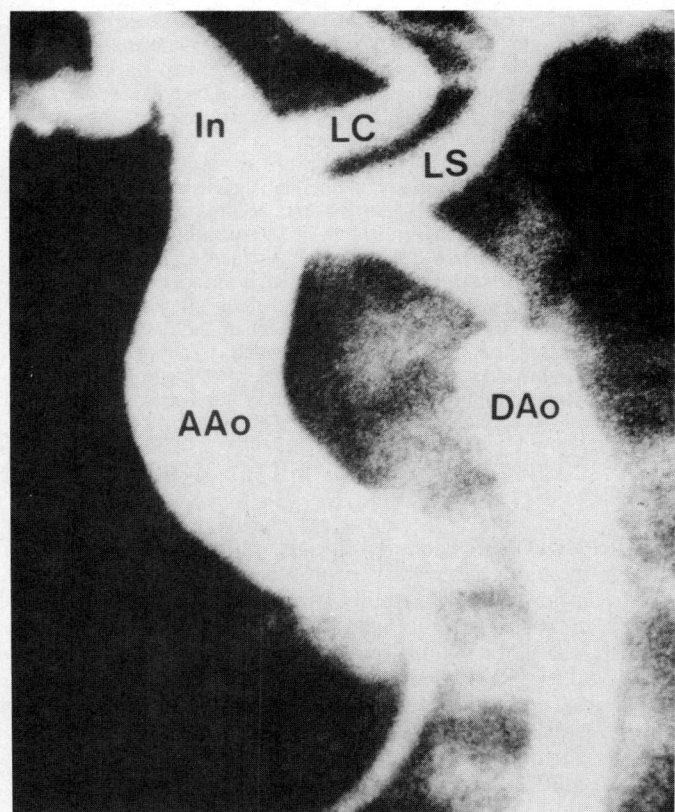

FIGURE 31–29. Retrograde aortogram demonstrates the discrete site of coarctation of the aorta, hypoplasia of the aortic isthmus, and poststenotic dilation of the descending aorta (DAo). AAo = ascending aorta, In = innominate artery, LC = left common carotid artery, LS = left subclavian artery.

ciently narrowed to result in a high-velocity jet across the lesion throughout the cardiac cycle. Additional systolic and continuous murmurs over the lateral thoracic wall may reflect increased flow through dilated and tortuous collateral vessels. *Electrocardiography* reveals left ventricular hypertrophy of varying degrees, depending on the height of arterial pressure above the obstruction and the patient's age. Combined with right ventricular hypertrophy, this usually implies a complicated lesion. *Chest roentgenograms* (Fig. 8–40, p. 229) may show a dilated left subclavian artery high on the left mediastinal border and a dilated ascending aorta. Indentation of the aorta at the site of coarctation and prestenotic and poststenotic dilatation (the "3" sign) along the left paramediastinal shadow is almost pathognomonic. Poststenotic dilation also may be detected by indentation of the barium-filled esophagus. Notching of the ribs, an important radiographic sign, is due to erosion by dilated collateral vessels, increases with age, and usually becomes apparent between the 4th and 12th years of life. The aortic coarctation may be visualized directly by two-dimensional echocardiography from high parasternal or suprasternal notch views with short focused transducers, and from the subxiphoid window with extended focal range transducers (Fig. 31–28). Doppler examination reveals a flow disturbance and high-velocity jet at the site of obstruction and provides a reasonable estimate of the transcoarctation pressure gradient.[220,221] Computed tomography,[222] magnetic resonance imaging (Fig. 11–39, p. 331), or cardiac catheterization and aortography (Fig. 31–29) are usually indicated to accurately localize the site of obstruction, determine the length of the coarctation, and, particularly, identify associated malformations.[223] Preoperative catheterization may be avoided for selected patients with typical clinical and two-dimensional and Doppler echocardiographic findings.[224]

MANAGEMENT. Controversy exists concerning the role of balloon angioplasty (p. 1365) in the treatment of native coarctation.[217] Concerns exist about residual pressure gradients and aneurysm formation, especially late after angioplasty. It is clear that angioplasty can effectively reduce obstruction in many patients, albeit with an unpredictable late outcome.

Subclavian flap aortoplasty (Fig. 31–30), particularly in neonates and infants, or surgical resection and end-to-end anastomosis of uncomplicated juxtaductal coarctation of the aorta can be accomplished with excellent results in most patients[218,225]; some surgeons prefer an on-lay patch across the site of obstruction.[226] In children who are asymptomatic it is preferable to delay surgery until age 4 to 6 years, at which time coarctation seldom recurs.[227] Paradoxical hypertension of short duration often is noted in the immediate postoperative period. A resetting of carotid baroreceptors and increased catecholamine secretion appear to be responsible for the initial phase of systemic hypertension with a later, second phase of prolonged elevation of systolic and particularly diastolic blood

tion does not intensify and cardiac failure does not occur by age 6 to 9 months, circulatory compensation is likely until adult life.

Most children with isolated juxtaductal coarctation are asymptomatic. Complaints of headache, cold extremities, and claudication with exercise may be noted, although attention usually is directed to the cardiovascular system by detection of a heart murmur or upper-extremity hypertension on routine physical examination. Mechanical factors rather than those of renal origin play the primary role in the production of hypertension. Absent, markedly diminished, or delayed pulsations in the femoral arteries and a low or unobtainable arterial pressure in the lower extremities with hypertension in the arms are the basic clues to the diagnosis.[219] A midsystolic murmur over the anterior chest, back, and spinous processes is most frequent, becoming continuous if the lumen is suffi-

FIGURE 31–30. Subclavian flap aortoplasty repair of aortic coarctation. *A*, The left subclavian artery has been ligated and divided; the aorta is incised from below the coarctation ridge of tissue, which is carefully excised. *B*, The distal end of the subclavian artery forms a flap, which is sutured to the aortotomy. (From Stark, J., and DeLaval, M.: Surgery for Congenital Heart Defects. New York, Grune and Stratton, 1983, p. 216.)

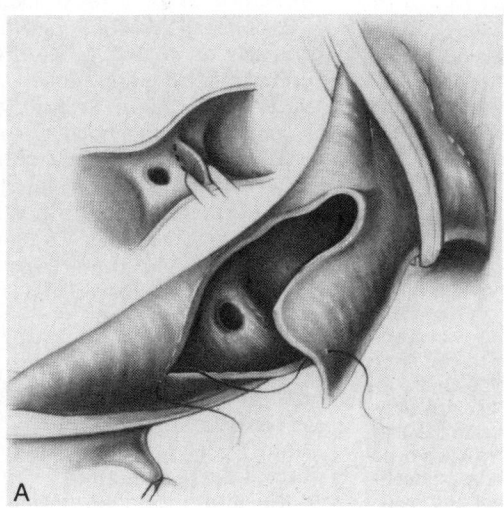

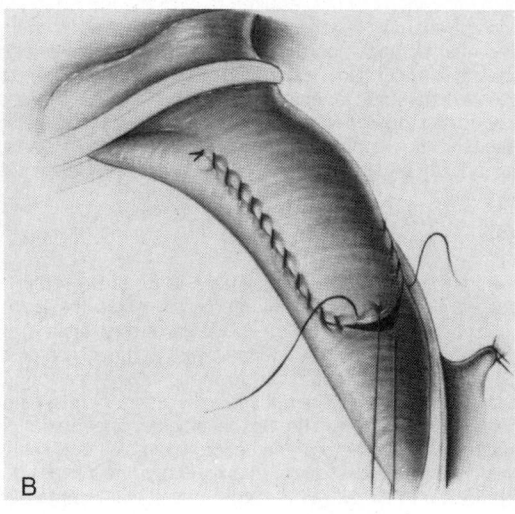

A

B

pressure related to activation of the renin-angiotensin system.[228,230] A necrotizing panarteritis of the small vessels of the gastrointestinal tract of uncertain cause occasionally complicates the course of recovery.

A 5 to 10 per cent risk of recurrent narrowing exists after repair of coarctation in infancy.[231] This problem is treated most effectively by transcutaneous balloon angioplasty,[232] which may be expected to markedly reduce, but not abolish entirely, the pressure differences across the site of recoarctation.

In those patients who survive the first 2 years of life, complications of juxtaductal coarctation are uncommon before the second or third decade. The chief hazards to patients with coarctation result from severe hypertension, and include the development of cerebral aneurysms and hemorrhage, hypertensive encephalopathy, rupture of the aorta, left ventricular failure, and infective endocarditis. Systemic hypertension in the absence of residual coarctation has been observed in resting or exercise-stressed patients postoperatively and appears to be related to the duration of preoperative hypertension.[233,234] Lifelong observation is desirable because of the late onset of hypertension in some postoperative patients.

HYPOPLASIA OF THE AORTIC ARCH

The aortic isthmus, the portion of aorta between the left subclavian artery and the ductus arteriosus, normally is narrowed in the fetus and newborn. The lumen of the aortic isthmus is about two-thirds that of the ascending and descending portions of the aorta until age 6 to 9 months, when the physiological narrowing disappears.[235] Pathological tubular hypoplasia of the aortic arch usually is noted in the aortic isthmus and often is referred to as preductal or infantile coarctation of the aorta.[236] Associated major cardiac malformations occur in virtually all such infants and include large ventricular septal defect, atrioventricular septal defect, transposition of the great arteries, the Taussig-Bing type of anomaly, and double-outlet right ventricle. The ventricular septal defect most often is subpulmonary, lying within the substance of the infundibular septum. Thus, muscle persists between the aortic and pulmonary valve leaflets, which, when displaced leftward, produces subaortic stenosis. Persistent patency of the ductus arteriosus commonly coexists, and right-to-left flow across the ductus arteriosus usually provides filling of the descending aorta. The adequacy of blood flow to the lower body depends on the degree of aortic hypoplasia, the caliber of the ductus arteriosus, and the relationship between pulmonary and systemic vascular resistance. Substantial right-to-left shunting through a wide-open ductus arteriosus minimizes the arterial blood pressure difference between the upper and lower body. Differential cyanosis of the toes and feet with normal color of the fingers and hands may be difficult to discern because intracardiac left-to-right shunting and pulmonary edema attenuate the differences in oxygen saturation in the ascending and descending aorta. Clinical deterioration is associated with ductal constriction or a fall in pulmonary vascular resistance. Moreover, the clinical presentation often is dictated by the hemodynamic effects of complex associated intracardiac malformations. Infants most often present with findings of a large left-to-right intracardiac shunt, pulmonary hypertension, and marked cardiac decompensation. Although tubular hypoplasia is detectable by two-dimensional echocardiography, cardiac catheterization often is required to evaluate the full extent of intracardiac and extracardiac lesions.[237] Surgical repair of aortic arch hypoplasia usually must be accompanied by operative palliation or correction of associated intracardiac lesions. Aortic angioplasty incorporating the subclavian–aortic anastomosis, and a tubular prosthetic conduit are among the operative approaches to correct long segment narrowing. Recoarctation is common and often necessitates transcatheter balloon aortoplasty and/or a second operation later in life to relieve anastomotic stenosis.

AORTIC ARCH INTERRUPTION

Aortic arch interruption is a rare and usually lethal anomaly; unless treated surgically almost all infants die within the first month of life.[238] Interruptions distal to the left subclavian artery (Type A) occur with almost equal frequency to interruptions distal to the left common carotid artery (Type B); interruptions distal to the innominate artery (Type C) are extremely uncommon. The right subclavian artery often is of variable origin, frequently arising from the descending aortic segment distal to the interruption.[239] The clinical presentation resembles that seen in tubular hypoplasia or severe juxtaductal coarctation of the aorta with a patent ductus arteriosus. In almost all patients a ventricular septal defect and patent

ductus arteriosus coexist with the arch interruption. Because the ductus arteriosus provides lower-body blood flow, its spontaneous constriction results in profound clinical deterioration. The latter may be temporarily ameliorated by prostaglandin E₁ infusion.[71,216] The ventricular septal defect most often is subpulmonary, lying within the substance of the infundibular septum. Thus, muscle persists between the aortic and pulmonary valve leaflets, which, when displaced leftward, produces subaortic stenosis. Other complex intracardiac malformations, such as transposition of the great arteries, aortopulmonary window, and truncus arteriosus, are common.[240] An association is frequent with DiGeorge syndrome of thymic hypoplasia or aplasia and the accompanying immunological and hypocalcemia problems.[241] The major clinical problem is severe congestive heart failure as a consequence of volume overload of the left ventricle resulting from an associated intracardiac left-to-right shunt and of pressure overload imposed by systemic hypertension. Operation by direct anastomosis seldom is possible, and reconstitution usually necessitates interposition of a tubular synthetic graft or a direct anastomosis between the aorta and one of its major brachiocephalic vessels.[238,239]

CONGENITAL VALVULAR AORTIC STENOSIS
(See also p. 1035)

MORPHOLOGY. Congenital valvular aortic stenosis is a relatively common anomaly, estimated to occur in 3 to 6 per cent of patients with congenital cardiovascular defects. However, it must be appreciated that the true incidence of the malformation is probably grossly underestimated because the congenital bicuspid aortic valve may be undetected in early life, and becomes stenotic and of clinical significance only in adult life, at a time when it may be indistinguishable from the acquired forms of aortic stenosis (Fig. 32–1, p. 967). Congenital valvular aortic stenosis occurs much more frequently in males than in females, with the sex ratio approximating 4 : 1. Associated cardiovascular anomalies have been noted in as many as 20 per cent of patients.[241] Patent ductus arteriosus and coarctation of the aorta occur most frequently with valvular aortic stenosis; all three of these lesions may coexist.

The basic malformation consists of thickening of valve tissue with varying degrees of commissural fusion. The valve most commonly is bicuspid with a single fused commissure and an eccentrically placed orifice. Sometimes a third commissure, incomplete or rudimentary, is apparent. Less commonly, the valve has three fused cusps with a stenotic central orifice. In some patients the stenotic aortic valve is unicuspid and dome-shaped with no or one lateral attachment to the aorta at the level of the orifice. In infants and young children with severe aortic stenosis the aortic valve ring may be relatively underdeveloped. This lesion forms a continuum with the hypoplastic left heart syndrome and the aortic atresia and hypoplasia complexes. Secondary calcification of the valve is extremely rare in childhood, but the dynamics of blood flow associated with the congenitally deformed aortic valve ultimately lead to thickening of the cusps and calcification in adult life. When the obstruction is hemodynamically significant, concentric hypertrophy of the left ventricular wall and dilatation of the ascending aorta occur.

HEMODYNAMICS (see also Figs. 4–55, p. 86; 7–9, p. 188; and 34–25, p. 1036). The hemodynamic abnormalities produced by obstruction to left ventricular outflow are discussed on p. 1036. A peak systolic gradient exceeding 75 mm Hg in association with a normal cardiac output or an effective aortic orifice less than 0.5 cm²/m² body surface area is considered to reflect critical obstruction to left ventricular outflow.[241,242] The normal outflow orifice approximates 2.0 cm²/m² body surface area; areas of 0.5 to 0.8 cm²/m² signify moderate obstruction. When the area is larger than 0.8 cm²/m², the obstruction is considered to be mild; when less than 0.4 cm²/m², it is severe.

The resting cardiac output and stroke volume usually are within normal limits. During exercise, most children with critical stenosis show an elevation of the cardiac output and an associated elevation in the transvalvular pressure gradient.[243,244] When left ventricular failure occurs, the cardiac output decreases, and the left atrial, left ventricular end-diastolic, and pulmonary vascular pressures increase.

The blood supply to the myocardium may be significantly compromised in infants and children with aortic stenosis, despite normal patency of the coronary arteries.[245] Coronary blood flow and arterial oxygen content are critical determinants of oxygen supply to the myocardium. Because intramyocardial compressive forces are greatest in the subendocardium, blood flow to that region of left ventricle is entirely diastolic in the presence of elevated left ventricular systolic pressure. In patients with left ventricular outflow tract obstruction, coronary vasodilatation may give an inadequate response to an increase in the demands of the myocardium for oxygen at rest or with exercise. When subendocardial vessels are maximally dilated, the coronary artery driving pressure and the duration of diastole determine the magnitude of subendocardial flow. When the duration of systolic ejection lengthens across the stenotic orifice, diastole is shortened, especially at high heart rates. Moreover, a reduction occurs in coronary driving pressure if left ventricular end-diastolic pressure is high or if aortic diastolic pressure is low, e.g., with aortic regurgitation or heart failure. In patients with severe aortic stenosis the redistribution of flow away from the subendocardium and the ischemia that results in that portion of ventricular muscle may be estimated by relating the diastolic pressure–time index (DPTI) (i.e., the area between the aortic and left ventricular pressures in diastole) to the systolic pressure–time index (SPTI) (a measure of myocardial oxygen demands). Inadequate subendocardial oxygen delivery has been shown to exist when the ratio [DPTI × arterial oxygen content/SPTI] falls below 10.[245]

INFANCY. Special comment concerning this malformation as it is seen in infants is warranted, in view of the unique problems presented by patients in this age group.[246–250] Fortunately isolated aortic valvular stenosis seldom causes symptoms in infancy. This lesion, however, occasionally may be responsible for profound and intractable heart failure. Despite normal coronary arterial anatomy, infarction of left ventricular papillary muscles may occur, resulting in an acquired form of mitral valvular regurgitation that intensifies the heart failure state. In addition, endocardial fibroelastosis may result from limited subendocardial oxygen delivery and myocardial degeneration may be significant.[250] The symptomatic infant with isolated valvular aortic stenosis is irritable, pale, and hypotensive, and presents with tachycardia, cardiomegaly, and pulmonary congestion manifested by dyspnea, tachypnea, subcostal retractions, and diffuse rales. Cyanosis may be observed secondary to pulmonary venous desaturation. The systolic murmur in infants often is atypical; it is best heard at the apex or along the lower left sternal border and may be confused with that caused by a ventricular septal defect. In infants with heart failure the murmur occasionally may be absent or extremely soft, becoming louder when myocardial contractility is improved with digitalis and other medical measures. The response to medical management of the infant with heart failure is frequently poor.

The electrocardiographic findings may not be characteristic; left ventricular hypertrophy and/or strain as well as right atrial enlargement and right ventricular hypertrophy may be detected shortly after birth.[246] The latter signs of right heart involvement result from both pulmonary hypertension secondary to elevated left ventricular diastolic and left atrial pressures and from volume loading of the right ventricle caused by left-to-right shunting across the foramen ovale. Survival past the early neonatal period does not preclude subsequent difficulties, and clinical deterioration may recur with the onset of physiological anemia.

Congenital aortic stenosis must be considered a medical emergency in the seriously ill newborn, and echocardiography, and sometimes cardiac catheterization and angiocardiography, may be indicated in the first 24 hours of life. Two-dimensional echocardiographic long-axis views of the left ventricular outflow tract demonstrate doming of the aortic valve. The parasternal short-axis view bisects the face of the valve, demonstrating the anatomy of the commissures.[251,252]

M-mode recordings best demonstrate wall thickness and motion. Doppler echocardiography provides an accurate estimate of the pressure gradient across the site of obstruction (Fig. 4–54, p. 85).[253–255] Hemodynamic findings commonly include left-to-right shunting at the atrial level, elevated left atrial and left ventricular end-diastolic pressures, and a small pressure drop across the aortic valve as a result of a markedly reduced cardiac output. Occasionally, right-to-left shunting across a patent ductus arteriosus is encountered. The presence of a normal or enlarged left ventricular cavity and normal or dilated ascending aorta allows distinction of aortic stenosis from the hypoplastic left heart syndrome angiographically. Because prolonged periods of stabilization are uncommon with medical therapy, early and definitive establishment of the diagnosis and prompt balloon valvuloplasty or valvulotomy usually are justified.[256–258] Poor myocardial performance resulting from endocardial fibroelastosis, subendocardial ischemia, or reduced left ventricular compliance, and inadequate relief of obstruction with or without significant aortic regurgitation are among the factors accounting for high operative mortality and morbidity. Open repair under direct vision is the preferred type of operation.[257,258,258a]

CHILDHOOD. Congenital aortic stenosis may be responsible for severe obstruction to left ventricular outflow in the absence of the clinical symptoms of diminished cardiac reserve that are so frequent in other forms of congenital heart disease. Most children with congenital aortic stenosis grow and develop normally and are asymptomatic. Attention usually is called to these children when a murmur is detected on routine examination. When symptoms occur, those noted most commonly are fatigability, exertional dyspnea, angina pectoris, and syncope. Less often described are abdominal pain, profuse sweating, and epistaxis. The symptomatic child usually has critical stenosis. There is a distinct threat of sudden death in patients with severe obstruction[242] (p. 899). Although the precise cause is poorly understood, ventricular arrhythmias, perhaps initiated by acute myocardial ischemia, are probably the most common inciting event. It has been speculated that an abrupt rise in intracavity left ventricular systolic pressure elicits a reflex hypotensive syncope that promotes acute ischemia and ventricular fibrillation.[260] Bacterial endocarditis occurs in about 4 per cent of patients with congenital valvular aortic stenosis.

DIAGNOSIS. Physical Findings. When the magnitude of obstruction is significant, a left ventricular lift usually is palpable, and a precordial systolic thrill often is palpated over the base of the heart with transmission to the jugular notch and along the carotid arteries; presystolic expansion often is palpable. The obstruction usually is mild if neither a left ventricular lift nor a thrill is present.

Opening of the aortic valve produces a systolic aortic ejection sound that typically is present at the cardiac apex when the valve is mobile, particularly in patients with mild to moderate stenosis. A delay in closure of the stenotic aortic valve leads to a single or a closely split second heart sound, and paradoxical splitting may be present. A fourth heart sound normally is associated with severe obstruction. A loud, harsh, rhomboid-shaped systolic murmur starts after completion of left ventricular isometric contraction and is best heard at the base of the heart. The murmur, like the thrill, radiates to the suprasternal notch and carotid vessels as well as to the apex. An early diastolic blowing murmur of aortic regurgitation is present in some patients, but unless the valve leaflets have been eroded by bacterial endocarditis, the regurgitation usually is not hemodynamically significant; uncommonly, in patients with a congenitally bicuspid valve, aortic regurgitation may be severe and may predominate.

Electrocardiography. There is a tendency for electrocardiographic signs of left ventricular hypertrophy to vary with the severity of obstruction, although a normal or near-normal electrocardiogram does not exclude severe aortic stenosis.[261] The presence of a left ventricular "strain pattern," consisting of left ventricular hypertrophy combined with ST-segment

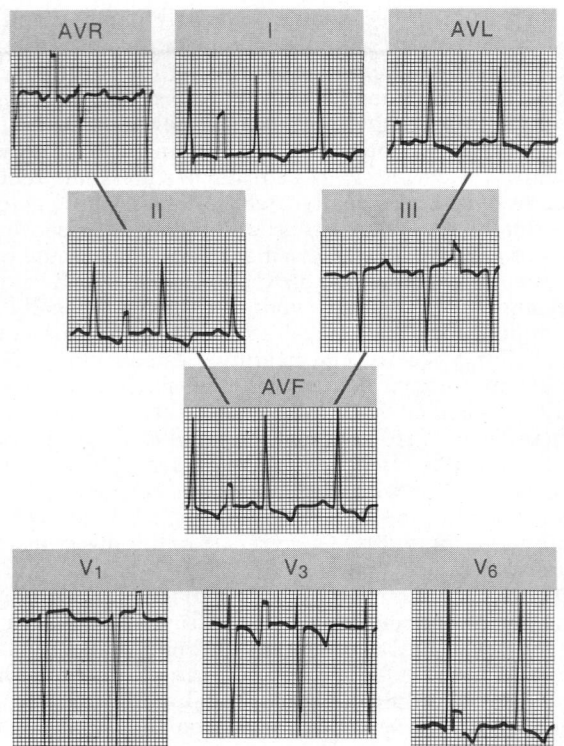

FIGURE 31–31. Electrocardiogram in congenital aortic stenosis. This tracing shows left ventricular hypertrophy and the typical left ventricular "strain" pattern (V_6, arrow). (Courtesy of Delores A. Danilowicz, M.D.)

depressions and T-wave inversion in the left precordial leads, usually indicates that severe aortic stenosis is present (Fig. 31–31).

In patients under 10 years of age the electrocardiogram is a more reliable guide in indicating the severity of the stenosis than it is in older patients.[259] Findings in the younger age group that often accompany severe obstruction are T-wave vectors in the frontal plane to the left of −40 degrees, widening of the angle between the mean QRS and T forces in the frontal plane in excess of 100 degrees, an S wave in V_1 greater than 16 mm, and an R wave in V_5 exceeding 20 mm. Nonetheless, it is important to recognize that these voltages may be excessive in patients who do not have severe stenosis. A good relation appears to exist between exercise-induced electrocardiographic changes and the severity of obstruction; ischemic ST-segment changes have been observed in patients with normal resting cardiac indices and transvalvular pressure differences in excess of 50 mm Hg or an abnormal left ventricular oxygen supply-demand ratio.[243]

Roentgenography. Overall heart size is normal or the degree of enlargement is slight in most children with congenital valvular aortic stenosis. Concentric left ventricular hypertrophy accompanies moderate or severe obstruction and is manifested by rounding of the cardiac apex in the frontal projection and posterior displacement in the lateral view.

Echocardiography. The M-mode echocardiographic findings that may suggest a diagnosis of aortic valve stenosis include multiple diastolic closure lines, or a single eccentrically placed diastolic closure line in the aortic lumen; left ventricular posterior wall and septal thickening; reduced separation of thickened aortic valve leaflets; and aortic root dilation. Two-dimensional echocardiography demonstrates a bicuspid aortic valve, impaired mobility of cusp tissue, altered phasic movement of the aortic valve with increased superior and reduced lateral excursions of valve echoes, and an increase in the internal aortic root dimension distal to the level of the valve annulus.[241] The parasternal short-axis view of the valve demonstrates the leaflet anatomy (Fig. 31–32).

The most accurate noninvasive approach to quantify the severity of obstruction combines continuous-wave Doppler flow analysis with the two-dimensional echocardiographic determination of the area of the orifice.[253–255] A simple estimate of the transvalvular gradient (in millimeters of mercury) may be calculated as four times the square of the peak Doppler velocity (meters per second).

The Doppler-derived aortic valve area, calculated by the continuity equation, correlates well with the catheterization-derived aortic valve area, calculated by the Gorlin equation, when either the time-velocity integral ratio or the peak flow velocity ratio between the left ventricular outflow tract and the aortic valve is used in the equation as follows:

$$AVA = (area)_{LVOT} \times \frac{(TVI)_{LVOT}}{(TVI)_{AV}}$$

where AV = aortic valve, AVA = aortic valve area, LVOT = left ventricular outflow tract, and TVI = time-velocity integral. The simplified continuity equation uses peak velocity ratio instead of time-velocity integral:

$$AVA = (area)_{LVOT} \times \frac{(V)_{LVOT}}{(V)_{AV}}$$

where V = peak flow velocity.[253]

Cardiac catheterization is more important for establishing the site and severity than for detecting the presence of aortic stenosis, since the malformation usually is readily diagnosed by clinical examination. Catheterization is indicated in any child with a clinical diagnosis of aortic stenosis in whom the clinical examination, roentgenogram, resting or exercise electrocardiogram, or echocardiogram suggests the possibility of severe obstruction.[242] Even in the absence of such findings, hemodynamic study should be performed if symptoms exist that might be related to aortic stenosis.

The site and severity of obstruction are established at car-

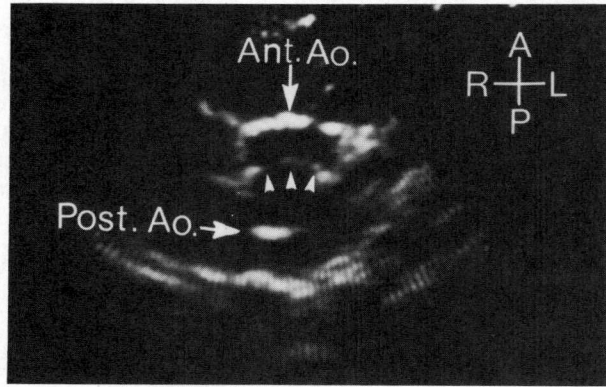
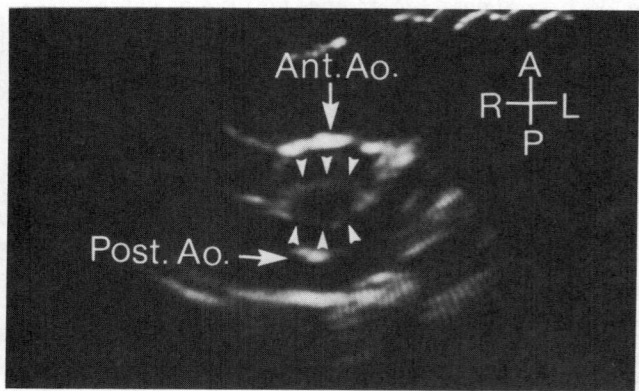

FIGURE 31–32. Short-axis view at the base of the heart of a bicuspid aortic valve. In the left panel the valve is imaged as a single diastolic echo (arrows) in the aortic root. In systole (right panel), the valve opens (arrows) with a typical fish-mouth appearance. Ant.Ao. = anterior aorta, Post.Ao. = posterior aorta. (From DiSessa, T. G., and Friedman, W. F.: Cardiovascular Clinics. Fowler, N. [ed.], Philadelphia, F. A. Davis Co., 1983.)

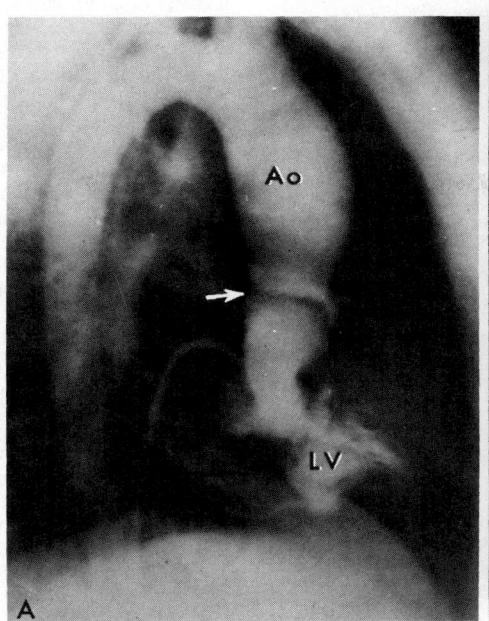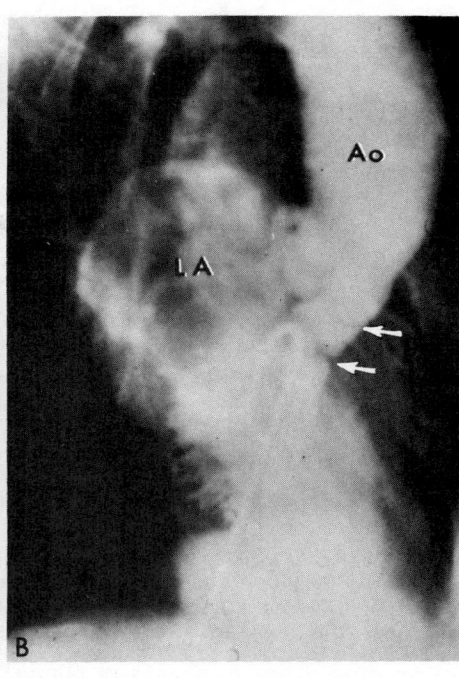

FIGURE 31-33. *A,* Left ventricular angiocardiogram obtained by the transseptal method in a patient with congenital valvular aortic stenosis. Ao = post-stenotic dilation of the aorta; LV = left ventricle. Arrow denotes the thickened valve cusp. *B,* Selective angiocardiogram in a patient with discrete subvalvular stenosis (bottom arrow). Associated mitral regurgitation is evident from the reflux of contrast into an enlarged left atrium (LA). The aortic valve (top arrow) is normal, and the right coronary artery is visualized. (From Friedman, W. F., and Kirkpatrick, S. E.: Congenital aortic stenosis. *In* Moss, A. J., Adams, F. H., and Emmanouilides, G. C. [eds.]: Heart Disease in Infants, Children and Adolescents. 2nd ed. Baltimore, Williams and Wilkins, 1977.)

diac catheterization, and associated malformations are identified. Typically, the angiocardiographic features of valvular stenosis are thickening of the aortic cusps and of the left ventricular wall with slight or no dilatation of the left ventricular cavity, poststenotic dilatation of the ascending aorta, and occasionally a jet of contrast material entering the ascending aorta through a narrowed valve orifice that is central or eccentric (Fig. 31-33). The leaflets of the bicuspid valve are domed in systole; a central jet corresponds to the orifice of the stenotic valve. In contrast, the stenotic orifice of the unicommissural valve may be visualized by the systolic jet in contact with the posterior wall of the aorta, with leaflet tissue and valve motion seen only anteriorly.

Congenital aortic stenosis frequently is a progressive disorder, even early in life, in a significant fraction of patients presenting initially with mild obstruction.[262-265] Thus, clinical deterioration may be anticipated because of an intensification in the severity of stenosis rather than the development of significant aortic regurgitation. Progression of obstruction usually is the result of the increase in cardiac output that occurs concurrent with increased body growth. Less often, a decrease in the area of the orifice is an added factor in the intensification of obstruction. The onset of symptoms or changes in the phonocardiogram or graphic pulse tracings, chest roentgenograms, electrocardiograms, or vectorcardiograms cannot be depended on to indicate progressive obstruction in the individual patient; Doppler echocardiography is most reliable.

MANAGEMENT. The malformed aortic valve is a potential site of bacterial infection; antibiotic prophylaxis is recommended for all patients, regardless of the severity of obstruction. Strict avoidance of strenuous physical activity is advised if severe aortic stenosis is present. Participation in competitive sports also should probably be restricted in patients with milder degrees of obstruction. Digitalis should be administered to patients who have symptoms of diminished cardiac reserve and also should be considered in patients with left ventricular hypertrophy, even if they are not in heart failure.

The most important decision concerns the advisability of *surgical treatment.* Among the factors influencing the indications, techniques, and results of operation are the patient's age, the nature of the valvular deformity, and the experience of the surgical team.[242] The recommendation that operation is indicated depends more often on the presence of severe obstruction than on the symptoms described by the patient. Operation currently is advised for any child with critical stenosis (i.e., a peak systolic pressure gradient exceeding 75 mm Hg, measured in the basal state when the cardiac output is

normal) or a calculated effective orifice less than 0.5 cm²/m² body surface area. In the presence of clinical symptoms, a left ventricular strain pattern on the electrocardiogram, or an abnormal exercise electrocardiogram, operation may be recommended with less rigid regard to the hemodynamic assessment of the severity of stenosis. After severe stenosis has been established hemodynamically, the potential hazard of sudden death dictates that surgical treatment not be postponed unnecessarily. Operation is carried out under direct vision after institution of cardiopulmonary bypass; judicious incision of the fused commissures enlarges the valve orifice and does not result in significant aortic regurgitation. A mortality rate less than 2 per cent can be expected when operation is performed by an experienced surgeon. Substantial relief of obstruction occurs in most patients unless the valve ring is hypoplastic. Balloon aortic valvuloplasty (p. 1043) currently is an experimental procedure for unoperated congenital valvular aortic stenosis. Preliminary data suggest that percutaneous valvuloplasty provides effective acute relief of valvular aortic stenosis. Significant complications have included death, aortic regurgitation, and femoral artery thrombosis or damage. Follow-up data are required before the percutaneous approach can be established as a treatment of choice for infants or children with this anomaly.[256,266]

Long-term follow-up studies have provided evidence that aortic valvulotomy is a safe and effective means of treatment with excellent relief of symptoms that were present preoperatively.[267-269] In some patients, aortic regurgitation may be progressive and require prosthetic valve replacement. Moreover, after commissurotomy the valve leaflets remain somewhat deformed, and it is quite possible that further degenerative changes, including calcification, will lead to significant stenosis later in life.[269-271] Thus, prosthetic valve replacement is required in about 35 per cent of patients within 15 to 20 years of the original operation. Because the valves are not rendered anatomically normal, antibiotic prophylaxis is indicated in all patients postoperatively, even if the systolic pressure gradient has been completely abolished.

DISCRETE SUBAORTIC STENOSIS

This malformation accounts for 8 to 10 per cent of all cases of congenital aortic stenosis and occurs twice as frequently in males as in females. The lesion consists of a membranous diaphragm or fibromuscular ring encircling the left ventricular outflow tract just beneath the base of the aortic valve.

Distinction of subvalvular from valvular aortic stenosis is

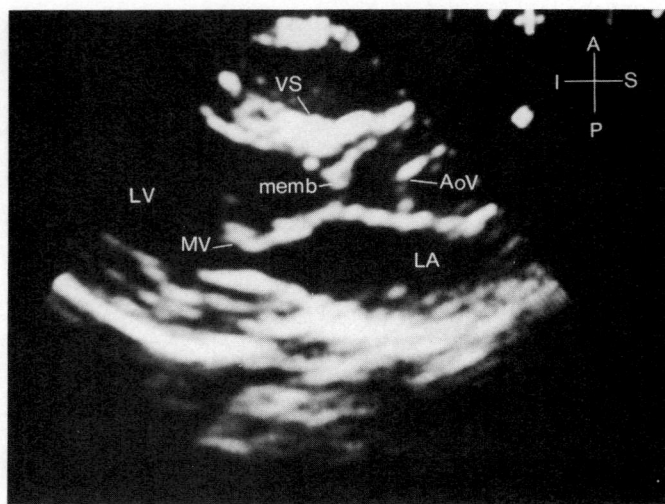

FIGURE 31–34. Long-axis view of discrete membranous subaortic stenosis. A discrete membrane (memb) is imaged in the left ventricular (LV) outflow tract beneath and parallel to the aortic valve (AoV), extending from the ventricular septum (VS) to the anterior leaflet of the mitral valve (MV). LA = left atrium.

extremely difficult by means of clinical findings alone.[241] Rarely, systolic ejection sound is heard, and the diastolic murmur of aortic regurgitation is more common than it is in valvular aortic stenosis. Dilatation of the ascending aorta is common, but valvular calcification is not observed.

Echocardiography is useful in the differentiation between valvular and subvalvular stenosis (Figs. 4–71 and 4–72, p. 92).[272,273] Two-dimensional echocardiographic studies from the apical two-chamber and left parasternal and subxiphoid long-axis views demonstrate persistent, prominent echoes in the subaortic left ventricle in both systole and diastole (Fig. 31–34). Doppler sampling proximal to the aortic valve shows increased flow velocity.[274] Most important, echocardiography also can identify hypertrophic subaortic stenosis when it coexists with fixed subaortic stenosis and can differentiate between the two forms of obstruction.

Definitive distinction between valvular and subvalvular obstruction is provided by transesophageal Doppler echocardiography[275] and by recording pressure tracings as a catheter is withdrawn across the outflow tract and valve, or by localizing the site of obstruction with selective left ventricular angiocardiography (Fig. 31–33).

Mild degrees of aortic valvular regurgitation commonly are observed in patients with discrete subaortic stenosis and appear to be caused by thickening of the valve and impaired mobility of the cusps secondary to the trauma created by the high-velocity jet passing through the subaortic diaphragm. Further deformation of these abnormal valve cusps by the vegetations of bacterial endocarditis often results in severe aortic regurgitation.

Because of the likelihood of both progressive obstruction and aortic regurgitation, the presence of even mild or moderate subaortic stenosis warrants consideration of elective operation.[276,277] The risks of operation in patients with discrete subaortic stenosis and valvular aortic stenosis are essentially the same. Surgical correction is accomplished by excising the membrane or fibrous ridge. Operation may be expected to improve the hemodynamic state substantially; it frequently is totally curative.[278–280] In a small number of patients, secondary muscular hypertrophy of the outflow tract and a pressure gradient may persist after the operative relief of valvular or discrete subvalvular aortic stenosis. Balloon dilatation also has been reported to be a successful mode of therapy, but is still considered experimental.[281]

UNCOMMON FORMS OF SUBAORTIC STENOSIS

In some patients, valvular and subvalvular aortic stenosis coexist, with hypoplasia of the aortic valve ring and thickened valve leaflets, producing a tunnel-like narrowing of the left ventricular outflow tract.[282] Additional findings often include a small ascending aorta. The subvalvular fibrous process usually extends onto the aortic valve cusps and almost always makes contact with the ventricular aspect of the anterior mitral leaflet at its base. The presence of "tunnel stenosis" may be suspected echocardiographically and angiographically from the appearance of the outflow tract and the aortic root. Operative treatment often is complicated by the necessity for prosthetic or homograft replacement of the aortic valve as well as for enlarging the aortic annulus, proximal aorta, and left ventricular outlet tract (the Konno operation). Operation is controversial, utilizing a prosthetic, valve-containing conduit between the left ventricular apex and descending aorta.[283]

Various anatomical lesions other than a discrete membrane or ridge may produce subaortic stenosis.[277,284] Among these are abnormal adherence of the anterior leaflet of the mitral valve to the left septal surface, and the presence in the left ventricular outflow tract of accessory endocardial cushion tissue. In some patients with atrioventricular canal, the part of the ventricular septum that contributes to the wall of the left ventricular outflow tract is deficient, and the ventricular aspect of the anterior leaflet of the common atrioventricular valve is adherent to the posterior edge of the deficient septum, resulting in a narrow left ventricular outflow tract. Malalignment of the conoventricular septum, resulting in an inferior ventricular septal defect, produces a leftward superior deviation and insertion of the conal septum, obstructing left ventricular outflow.[284] In patients with a single ventricle and an outflow chamber, the bulboventricular foramen serves as a potential site of aortic outflow obstruction. Additional, rarer causes of subaortic stenosis include redundant dysplastic left atrioventricular valve tissue in patients with congenitally corrected transposition of the great arteries and anomalous muscle bundles of the left ventricular outflow tract. A muscular type of subaortic stenosis may result from a convergence of all the mitral chordae into one or two fused papillary muscles; a "parachute" deformity of the mitral valve is produced that often is seen in association with supravalvular stenosis of the left atrium and coarctation of the aorta. In some of these patients, discrete membranous subvalvular aortic obstruction also has been noted.

In patients with ventricular septal defect, muscular subaortic stenosis has been shown to develop after surgical banding of the pulmonary artery, possibly as a result of hypertrophy of the conal septum or crista supraventricularis encroaching on the left ventricular outflow tract above the septal defect.

Subaortic muscular hypertrophy secondary to diffuse involvement of the myocardium by glycogen storage disease (Pompe's disease) is an extremely rare cause of obstruction to left ventricular outflow. A positive family history, symptoms of muscle weakness, heart failure in infancy, and the characteristic electrocardiographic findings of a short PR interval, high-voltage QRS and T waves, and left ventricular hypertrophy warrant skeletal muscle biopsy or fibroblast culture, permitting an antemortem diagnosis.

The last, relatively uncommon form of subaortic stenosis to be mentioned occurs infrequently in patients with congenitally corrected transposition of the great arteries in whom an anomalous muscle bundle in the subaortic area of the arterial ventricle obstructs outflow.

SUPRAVALVULAR AORTIC STENOSIS

Supravalvular aortic stenosis is a congenital narrowing of the ascending aorta that may be localized or diffuse, originating at the superior margin of the sinuses of Valsalva just above the levels of the coronary arteries.

The clinical picture of supravalvular obstruction usually differs in major respects from that observed in the other forms of aortic stenosis. Chief among these differences is the association of supravalvular aortic stenosis with idiopathic infantile hypercalcemia, a disease that may be related to deranged vitamin D metabolism.[285–288]

The designation supravalvular aortic stenosis syndrome, or Williams' syndrome, is applied to the distinctive clinical picture produced by coexistence of the cardiac and multisystem disorder. Additional manifestations of this syndrome include a peculiar elfin facies (Fig. 31–35), mental retardation, auditory hyperacusis, narrowing of peripheral systemic and pulmonary arteries, inguinal hernia, strabismus, and abnormalities of dental development.[289] In some patients, moderate thickening of the aortic cusps and valvular pulmonary stenosis may occur in association with peripheral pulmonary artery stenosis. Rarely, patients have mitral valve abnormalities with prolapse and mitral regurgitation.

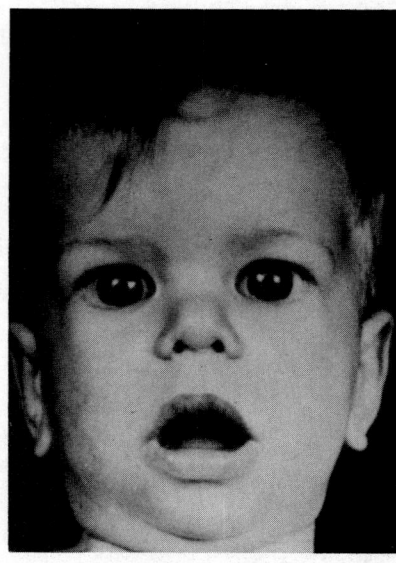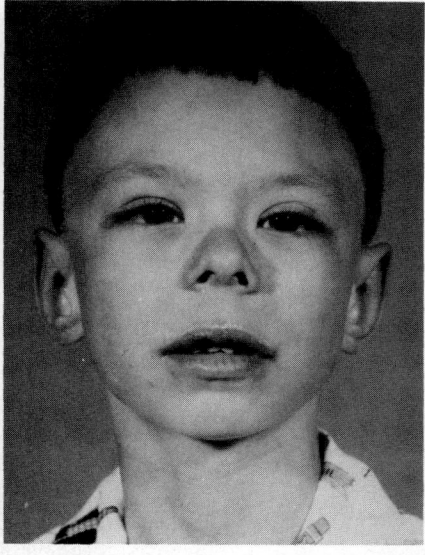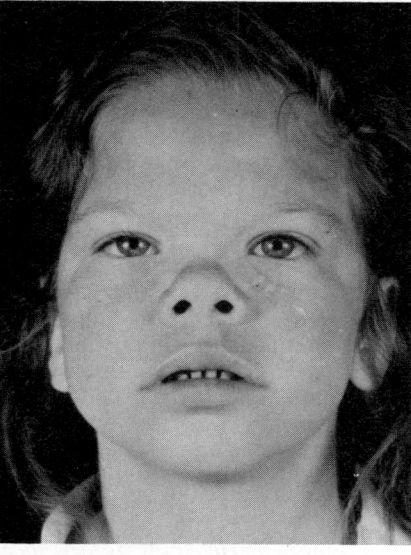

FIGURE 31–35. Typical elfin facies in three patients with supravalvular aortic stenosis. (From Friedman, W. F., and Kirkpatrick, S. E.: Congenital aortic stenosis. *In* Moss, A. J., Adams, F. H., and Emmanouilides, G. C. [eds.]: Heart Disease in Infants, Children and Adolescents. 2nd ed. Baltimore, Williams and Wilkins, 1977.)

Experimental hypervitaminosis D produced in the pregnant rabbit has caused craniofacial abnormalities and malformations resembling those of supravalvular aortic stenosis in the offspring.[285,286] In patients the metabolism of vitamin D is abnormal.[290] In humans, with one exception, chromosomal studies have consistently revealed normal karyotypes. Supravalvular aortic stenosis most often is a feature of the distinctive syndrome described above. Peripheral pulmonary artery stenosis and the aortic anomaly also are seen, however, in familial and sporadic forms unassociated with the other features of the syndrome.[291] Genetic studies suggest that the familial anomaly is transmitted as an autosomal dominant with variable expression. Some family members may have supravalvular pulmonic stenosis either as an isolated lesion or in combination with the supravalvular aortic anomaly. Unlike with the other forms of aortic stenosis, there appears to be no sex predilection.

Three anatomical types of supravalvular aortic stenosis are recognized, although some patients may have findings of more than one type. Most common is the hourglass type, in which marked thickening and disorganization of the aortic media produce a constricting annular ridge at the superior margin of the sinuses of Valsalva. The membranous type is the result of fibrous or fibromuscular semicircular diaphragm with a small central opening stretched across the lumen of the aorta. Uniform hypoplasia of the ascending aorta characterizes the hypoplastic type.

Because the coronary arteries arise proximal to the site of outflow obstruction in supravalvular aortic stenosis, they are subjected to the elevated pressure that exists within the left ventricle. These vessels often are dilated and tortuous, and premature coronary arteriosclerosis has been observed. Moreover, if the free edges of some or all of the aortic cusps adhere to the area of supravalvular stenosis, coronary artery inflow may be reduced. The formation of thoracic aortic aneurysms has been described in several patients.

Most patients with supravalvular aortic stenosis syndrome are mentally retarded and resemble one another in their facial features. The typical appearance is similar to that of the elfin facies observed in the severe form of idiopathic infantile hypercalcemia and is characterized by a high prominent forehead, epicanthal folds, underdeveloped bridge of the nose and mandible, overhanging upper lip, strabismus, and anomalies of dentition (Fig. 31–35). Recognition of this distinctive appearance, even in infancy, should alert the physician to the possibility of underlying multisystem disease. In addition, a positive family history in a patient with a normal appearance and clinical signs suggesting left ventricular outflow obstruction should lead to the suspicion of either supravalvular aortic stenosis or hypertrophic obstructive cardiomyopathy.[291] Patients with supravalvular aortic obstruction appear to be subject to the same risks of unexpected sudden death and infective endocarditis as those with valvular aortic stenosis.

With few exceptions, the major *physical findings* resemble those observed in patients with valvular aortic stenosis. Among these exceptions are accentuation of aortic valve clo-

sure due to elevated pressure in the aorta proximal to the stenosis, an infrequent systolic ejection sound, and the especially prominent transmission of a thrill and murmur into the jugular notch and along the carotid vessels. Uncommonly, there is an early diastolic, decrescendo, blowing murmur of aortic regurgitation caused by the fusion of one or more cusps to the area of stenosis. The narrowing of the peripheral pulmonary arteries that often coexists in these patients frequently produces a late systolic or continuous murmur that may help to distinguish this anomaly from valvular aortic stenosis. This differentiation is reinforced by the frequent finding of a significant disparity between the arterial pressures in the upper extremities in supravalvular aortic stenosis; the systolic pressure in the right arm tends to be the higher of the two and occasionally exceeds that in the femoral arteries. The disparity in pulses may relate to the tendency of a jet stream to adhere to a vessel wall (Coanda effect) and selective streaming of blood into the innominate artery.[292,293]

Electrocardiography usually reveals left ventricular hypertrophy when obstruction is severe. Biventricular, or even right ventricular, hypertrophy may be found if significant narrowing of peripheral pulmonary arteries coexists. Radiographically, in contrast to valvular and discrete subvalvular

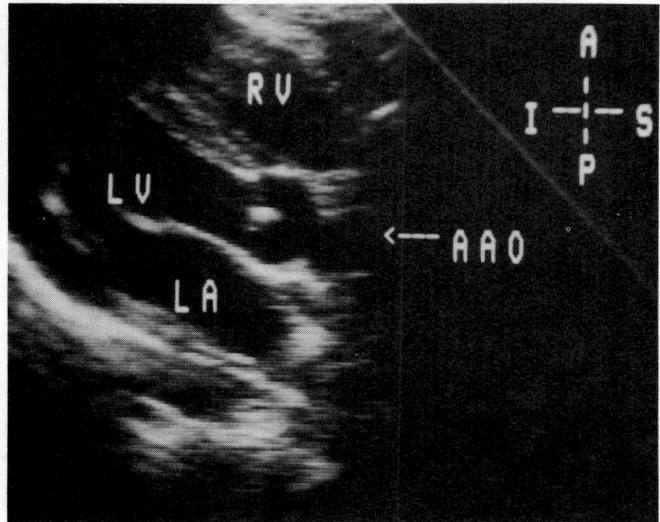

FIGURE 31–36. Supravalvar aortic stenosis is seen in a parasternal long-axis view. The constriction is distal to the sinuses of Valsalva in the ascending aorta (AAO). RV = right ventricle, LV = left ventricle, LA = left atrium. (Courtesy of Norman Silverman, M.D.)

aortic stenosis, poststenotic dilation of the ascending aorta seldom is seen. The sinuses of Valsalva usually are dilated, and the ascending aorta and aortic arch are of normal size or appear small.

Echocardiography is the most valuable technique for localizing the site of obstruction to the supravalvular area (Fig. 31–36), and Doppler examination and retrograde aortic catheterization can determine the degree of hemodynamic abnormality.[294]

The supravalvular aortic lumen may be widened by the insertion of an oval- or diamond-shaped fabric patch in those patients with a normal ascending aorta.[295,296] If the aorta is markedly hypoplastic, this operation merely displaces the pressure gradient distally without abolishing the obstruction. Under these circumstances, repair may require replacement or widening of the entire hypoplastic aorta with an appropriate prosthesis. Operation may be recommended when relatively little hypoplasia of the ascending aorta and arch exists and when the obstruction is discrete and significant, i.e., with a systolic gradient exceeding 50 mm Hg.

HYPOPLASTIC LEFT HEART SYNDROME

This designation is used to describe a group of closely related cardiac anomalies characterized by underdevelopment of the left cardiac chambers, atresia or stenosis of the aortic and/or the mitral orifices, and hypoplasia of the aorta.[297] These anomalies are an especially common cause of heart failure in the first week of life. The left atrium and ventricle often exhibit *endocardial fibroelastosis.* Pulmonary venous blood traverses a patent foramen ovale, and a dilated and hypertrophied right ventricle acts as the systemic, as well as the pulmonary, ventricle; the systemic circulation receives blood by way of a patent ductus arteriosus (Fig. 31–37). The diagnosis should be considered in infants, particularly males, with the sudden onset of heart failure, systemic hypoperfusion, and nonspecific murmur. Electrocardiography frequently reveals right axis deviation, right atrial and ventricular enlargement, and ST and T-wave abnormalities in the left precordial leads. Chest roentgenography may show only slight enlargement shortly after birth, but with clinical deterioration there are marked cardiomegaly and increased pulmonary venous and arterial vascular markings.

The *echocardiographic* findings usually are diagnostic (Fig.

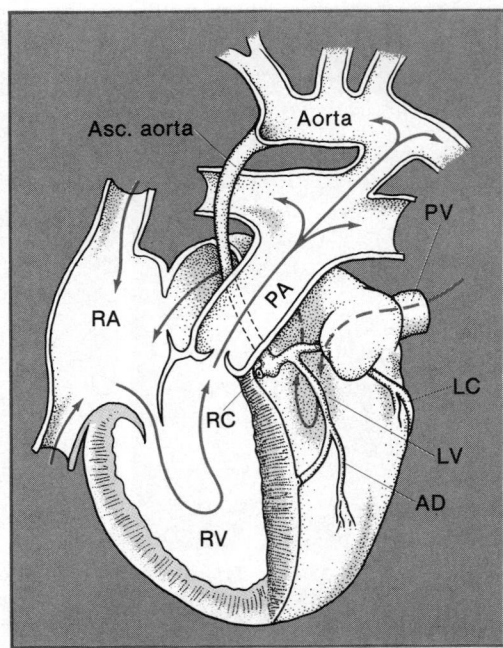

FIGURE 31–37. Hypoplastic left heart with aortic hypoplasia, aortic valve atresia, and a hypoplastic mitral valve and left ventricle. R.A. = right atrium, R.V. = right ventricle, R.C. = right coronary artery, P.A. = pulmonary artery, P.V. = pulmonary vein, L.C. = left coronary artery, L.V. = left ventricle, A.D. = anterior descending coronary artery. (From Neufeld, H. N., et al.: Diagnosis of aortic atresia by retrograde aortography. Circulation 25:278, 1962, by permission of the American Heart Association, Inc.)

31–38), and include a diminutive aortic root and left ventricular cavity and absence or poor visualization of aortic and mitral valve echoes, which, when seen, are of diminished amplitude and mobility.[298] Retrograde aortography shows hypoplasia of the ascending aorta (Fig. 31–39).

MANAGEMENT. Medical therapy directed at cardiac decompensation, hypoxemia, and metabolic acidemia seldom prolongs survival beyond the first days of life. Constriction of the patent ductus arteriosus and limited flow through a re-

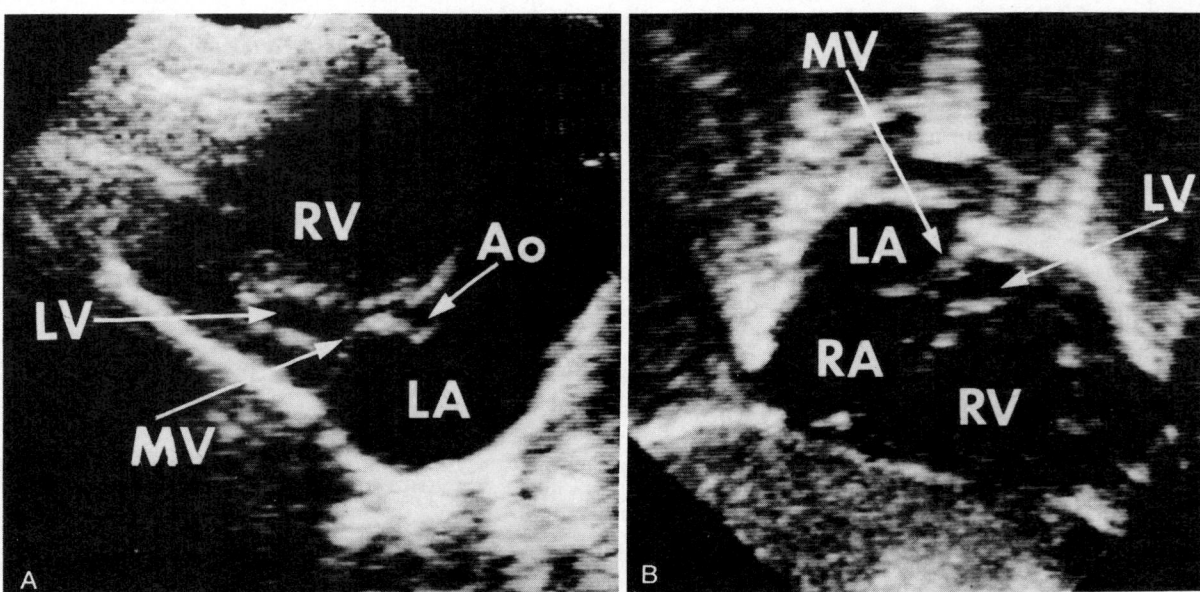

FIGURE 31–38. *A,* Hypoplastic left heart in a parasternal long-axis view in a newborn with aortic atresia, intact ventricular septum, and patent but hypoplastic mitral valve (MV). The left ventricular (LV) cavity is diminutive and the ascending aorta (Ao) is hypoplastic. Right ventricular (RV) dilation is noted. *B,* In the subcostal four-chamber view dilatation of the right atrium (RA) and right ventricle (RV) is noted. The endocardial echoes are very bright owing to fibroelastosis. (From Perloff, J.: The Clinical Recognition of Congenital Heart Disease. 3rd ed. Philadelphia, W. B. Saunders Company, 1986.)

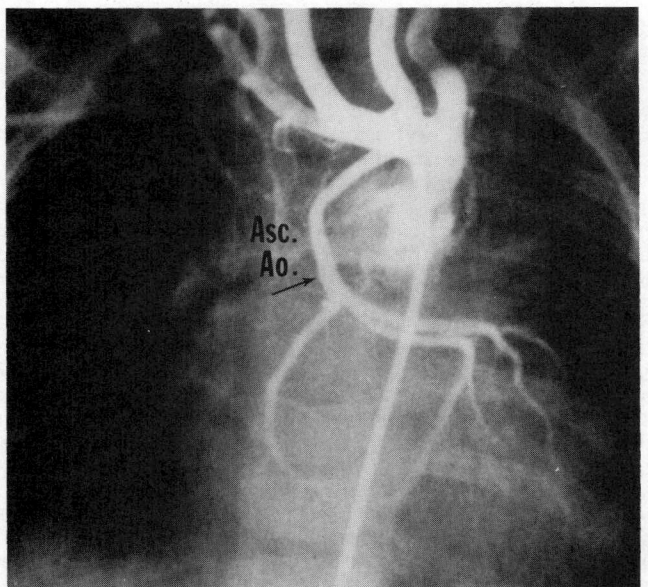

FIGURE 31–39. Retrograde aortogram showing marked hypoplasia of the ascending aorta (asc. Ao.) (arrow) in an infant with hypoplastic left heart syndrome. (From Freedom, R. M., et al.: Aortic atresia with normal left ventricle: Distinctive angiocardiographic findings. Cath. Cardiovasc. Diag. 3:283, 1977.)

consideration for prosthetic valve replacement. The aortico–left ventricular tunnel is an abnormal channel beginning in the ascending aorta above the right coronary orifice and ending in the left ventricle below the right aortic cusp. The channel usually passes behind the right ventricular infundibulum and through the ventricular septum.

Echocardiography, Doppler studies, and aortography combine to establish a precise diagnosis. Exercise testing is useful to assess the severity of the lesion.[307] In infants and children with congenital aortic regurgitation the severity of regurgitation increases with time, and valve replacement, rather than plication, is almost always necessary to correct the lesion. Operation should be deferred until symptoms, signs, and noninvasive assessment dictate its necessity. Conversely, closure of an aortic–left ventricular communication is advisable before progressive dilation of the aortic annulus creates secondary changes in the aortic valve itself which may necessitate aortic valve replacement.

PULMONARY VEIN ATRESIA AND STENOSIS

Pulmonary vein atresia is a rare anomaly in which the pulmonary veins do not connect with the heart or with a major systemic vein.[308] The lesion is incompatible with life, but infants may survive for days, probably because communications exist between the pulmonary veins and the bronchial or esophageal veins that allow limited egress for pulmonary venous blood. Pulmonary vein stenosis may occur as a focal stenosis at the atrial junction or generalized hypoplasia or one or more pulmonary veins. There is an extremely high incidence of associated cardiac malformations, including atrial septal defect, tetralogy of Fallot, tricuspid and mitral atresia, and endocardial cushion defect. The severe pulmonary vein obstruction imposed by pulmonary vein abnormalities causes severe cyanosis, congestive cardiac failure, and early death. Focal stenosis of one or more pulmonary veins at the atrial junction, recognized by two-dimensional echocardiography or angiography, may be relieved surgically.[309] Results of transcutaneous balloon angioplasty have been disappointing.

COR TRIATRIATUM

In this malformation failure of resorption of the common pulmonary vein results in a left atrium divided by an abnormal fibromuscular diaphragm into a posterosuperior chamber receiving the pulmonary veins and an anteroinferior chamber giving rise to the left atrial appendage and leading to the mitral orifice.[310] The communication between the divided atrial chambers may be large, small, or absent, depending on the size of the opening in the subdividing diaphragm, which determines the degree of obstruction to pulmonary venous return. Elevations of both pulmonary venous pressure and pulmonary vascular resistance result in severe pulmonary artery hypertension.

The diagnosis is established by two-dimensional echocardiography; cardiac catheterization and angiography are necessary only if major associated cardiac anomalies are suspected.[311,312] The obstructive membrane is visualized in the parasternal long- and short-axis and four-chamber (Fig. 31–40) views and can be distinguished from a supravalvular mitral ring by its position superior to the left atrial appendage, which forms part of the distal chamber. Also present are diastolic fluttering of the mitral leaflets and high-velocity flow detected by Doppler examination in the distal atrial chamber and at the mitral orifice.

The diagnosis should be suspected at cardiac catheterization if the pulmonary arterial wedge pressure is higher than a simultaneous left atrial pressure. The diagnosis also may be established by visualizing the obstructing lesion angiographically. Although rare, it is important to recognize the malformation because it may be easily correctable at operation.[313]

CONGENITAL MITRAL STENOSIS

Anatomical types of mitral stenosis include the parachute deformity of the valve, in which shortened chordae tendineae converge and insert into a single large papillary muscle; thickened leaflets with shortening and fusion of the chordae tendinae; an anomalous arcade of obstructing papillary muscles; accessory mitral valve tissue; and a supravalvular circumferential ridge of connective tissue arising at the base of the atrial

strictive patent foramen ovale are the principal factors responsible for early death. Prostaglandin E₁ infusion is effective in maintaining ductal patency. Some centers are attempting staged surgical management in an effort to provide long-term palliation.[297,299–302] The first stage, often referred to as the Norwood procedure, consists of creating an unobstructed communication between the right ventricle and aorta, and enlargement of the ascending aorta. The right ventricular–aortic connection has been accomplished with homograft or prosthetic conduits from the right ventricle or pulmonary trunk to the descending aorta, or by direct connection between the proximal pulmonary trunk and ascending aorta, which also enlarges the ascending aorta. Pulmonary blood flow and pressure are controlled by a tubed interposition systemic-pulmonary shunt to the distal pulmonary artery. The patent ductus arteriosus is ligated. A large interatrial communication also must be assured in stage 1 to allow free access of pulmonary venous blood to the tricuspid valve. In stage 2 an interatrial baffle is created to provide continuity between left atrium and tricuspid valve; the pulmonary arterial circulation is provided by direct anastomosis of the right atrium to the pulmonary arteries (the Fontan connection). Some surgeons prefer to perform a modified superior vena cava–pulmonary artery shunt (the Glenn operation) as an intermediate step before the Fontan procedure. In some centers, the preferred operation is human cardiac transplantation.[303]

CONGENITAL AORTIC REGURGITATION

Congenital aortic valve regurgitation is a rare isolated congenital cardiac lesion.[304] Aortic regurgitation most often occurs in association with congenital valvular aortic stenosis in which the valve commissures are fused, inhibiting cusp mobility, subvalvular aortic stenosis in which the aortic ring is dilated and the valve cusps are deformed, coarctation of the aorta when the aortic ring is dilated and the aortic valve is bicuspid, ventricular septal defect (p. 910), and endocardial fibroelastosis. Aortic valve regurgitation also may accompany aortic sinus aneurysm or be secondary to dilatation of the ascending aorta in patients with Marfan syndrome, Turner syndrome, cystic medial necrosis, or osteogenesis imperfecta, in which the aortic lesions are manifestations of the underlying connective tissue disorder.

Severe aortic regurgitation also may occur through channels other than the aortic valve.[305,306] Thus aortico–left ventricular tunnel is a rare anomaly that must be distinguished from congenital aortic valve regurgitation, since the approach to management of the former usually does not include

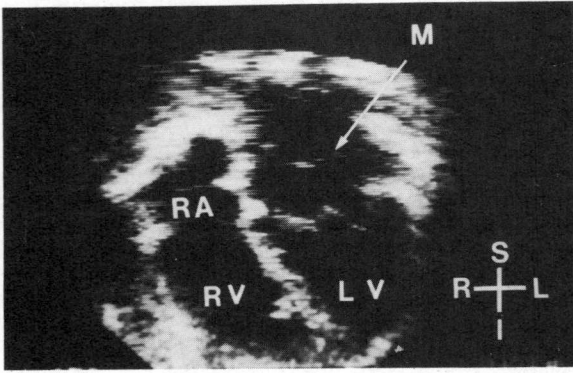

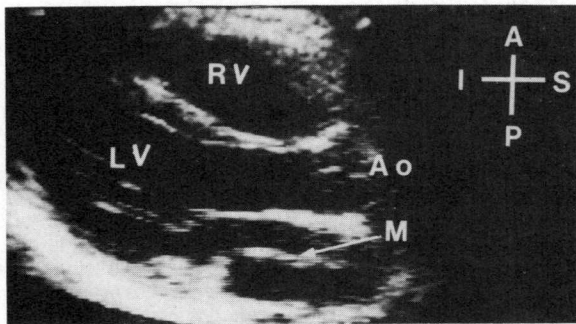

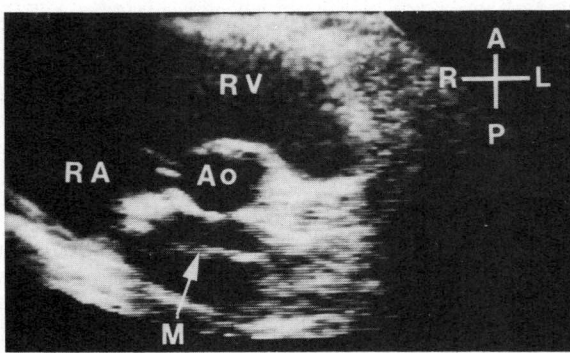

FIGURE 31-40. Echocardiograms demonstrating the membrane (M) of cor triatriatum. The apical four-chamber view (top panel) shows the membrane lying within the left atrial chamber. The atrial appendage is distal to the membrane and the pulmonary veins drain into the proximal portion. The parasternal long-axis view (center panel) shows the membrane posterior to the aortic root (AO) and mitral valve, dividing the left atrium into two chambers. In the parasternal short-axis view (bottom panel), the membrane is within the left atrium close to the posterior aortic root. RA = right atrium, RV = right ventricle, LV = left ventricle. (Courtesy of Norman Silverman, M.D.)

aspect of the mitral leaflets.[314,315] Associated cardiac defects are common, including endocardial fibroelastosis, coarctation of the aorta, patent ductus arteriosus, and left ventricular outflow tract obstruction. Two-dimensional echocardiography, combined with Doppler studies, often provides a complete analysis of the anatomy and function of congenital left ventricular inflow lesions.[316,317] The clinical and hemodynamic consequences of isolated congenital mitral stenosis are similar to those of acquired mitral obstruction with modifications imposed by coexisting anomalies.

The prognosis is poor; symptoms attributable to pulmonary vein obstruction begin usually in infancy and the majority of patients expire before age 1 year unless successfully operated upon. Conduit bypass of the mitral valve and prosthetic valve replacement are required if a reparative operation is not possible.[318-320] The use of a porcine bioprosthesis is contraindicated because of its rapid degeneration in the infant or young child. Transcatheter balloon valvuloplasty may prove to be an alternative to surgical mitral commissurotomy in selected patients beyond infancy.[321]

CONGENITAL MITRAL REGURGITATION
(See also p. 970)

The syndrome of *mitral valve prolapse* is discussed on pp. 1029 to 1035. This condition usually is quite benign in children. However, occasional difficulties exist with infective endocarditis, arrhythmias, atypical chest pain, and sudden death.

Isolated congenital mitral regurgitation of hemodynamic significance is an unusual lesion in infants and children. Congenital malformations of the mitral valve producing insufficiency most often are encountered in association with endocardial cushion defect, congenitally corrected transposition of the great arteries, endocardial fibroelastosis, anomalous pulmonary origin of the coronary artery, congenital subaortic stenosis, hypertrophic obstructive cardiomyopathy, and coarctation of the aorta. Mitral valve dysfunction also commonly is seen in various metabolic disorders (e.g., the mucopolysaccharidoses), primary and secondary cardiomyopathies, connective tissue disease (e.g., rheumatoid arthritis, Marfan syndrome, Ehlers-Danlos syndrome, pseudoxanthoma elasticum), and rheumatic and nonrheumatic inflammatory diseases of the myocardium.[322]

The various anatomical lesions that result in isolated congenital mitral regurgitation include prolapse of one or both mitral leaflets, cleft or perforated mitral leaflet, inadequate leaflet tissue, double orifice of the mitral valve, anomalous insertion of chordae tendineae (anomalous mitral arcade), redundant leaflet tissue, displacement inferiorly of the ring of the inferior leaflet into the left ventricle, and abnormal length of the chordae tendineae.[323] The clinical and henodynamic findings in patients with isolated congenital mitral incompetence resemble those observed in acquired mitral regurgitation. Mitral annuloplasty (which is preferred) and prosthetic valve replacement are procedures reserved for infants or children who are at least moderately symptomatic despite comprehensive medical management, often with repeated episodes of pulmonary infection, or cardiac failure with anorexia and retarded growth and development.[323,324] Operative condidates are shown by echocardiographic, Doppler, hemodynamic, and angiographic studies to have pulmonary hypertension, a regurgitant fraction in excess of 50 per cent, and a marked increase in left ventricular end-diastolic volume.[325]

PULMONARY ARTERIOVENOUS FISTULA
(See also p. 970)

Abnormal development of the pulmonary arteries and veins in a common vascular complex is responsible for this rare congenital anomaly. A variable number of pulmonary arteries communicate directly with branches of the pulmonary veins; in some cases the fistula receives systemic arterial branches.[326,327] Most patients have an associated Weber-Osler-Rendu syndrome; additional associated problems include bronchiectasis and other malformations of the bronchial tree, and absence of the right lower lobe. Venoarterial shunting depends on the extent of the fistulous communications and may result in cyanosis and secondary polycythemia. Patients with hereditary hemorrhagic telangiectasis often are anemic owing to repeated blood loss and may have less obvious cyanosis. Systolic and continuous murmurs are audible over areas of the fistula. Rounded opacities of variable size in one or both lungs on chest roentgenogram may suggest the presence of the lesion. Pulmonary angiography reveals the site and extent of the abnormal communication (Fig. 32-22, p. 984). Unless the lesions are widespread throughout both lungs, surgical treatment aimed at removing the lesions with preservation of healthy lung tissue commonly is indicated to avoid the complications of massive hemorrhage, bacterial endocarditis, and rupture of arteriovenous aneurysms.

Transcatheter balloon or plug or coil occlusion embolotherapy may prove to be the therapeutic procedure of choice.[328]

PERIPHERAL PULMONARY ARTERY STENOSIS

Stenosis of the pulmonary artery may occur as single or multiple lesions located anywhere from the main pulmonary trunk to the smaller peripheral arterial branches.[329] Associated defects are observed in most patients and include pulmonic valvular stenosis, ventricular septal defect, tetralogy of Fallot, and supravalvular aortic stenosis.

ETIOLOGY. The most important cause of significant pulmonary artery stenoses producing symptoms in the newborn is intrauterine rubella infection.[330] Diagnosis is facilitated in these infants by finding elevations of the IgM fraction and rubella antibody titer. Other cardiovascular malformations commonly seen in association with congenital rubella include patent ductus arteriosus, pulmonic valve stenosis, and atrial septal defect. Generalized systemic arterial stenotic lesions also may be a feature of the rubella embryopathy, often involving large and medium-sized vessels such as the aorta and coronary, cerebral, mesenteric, and renal arteries. Cardiovascular lesions are but one manifestation of intrauterine rubella infection, since cataracts, microphthalmia, deafness, thrombocytopenia, hepatitis, and blood dyscrasias also are common. Thus, the clinical picture in infants with rubella syndrome depends on the severity of the cardiovascular lesions and the associated abnormalities of other organs and system. Peripheral pulmonary stenosis also often is associated with supravalvular aortic stenosis in patients with the familial form of the latter anomaly or in patients with the Williams syndrome (see also p. 1633).

MORPHOLOGY. Obstruction within the pulmonary arterial tree may be classified into four types: (1) stenosis of the main pulmonary trunk or the main left or right branch; (2) narrowing at the bifurcation of the pulmonary artery, extending into both right and left branches; (3) multiple sites of peripheral branch stenosis; and (4) a combination of main and peripheral stenosis. Pulmonary artery obstruction may be produced by localized narrowing, diffuse constrictions, or, rarely, a membrane or diaphram. Poststenotic dilatation is usual when the stenosis is localized but may be absent or minimal with elongated constriction. It should be recognized that a physiological branch pulmonary artery stenosis often is present in the normal newborn in whom both right and left main pulmonary arteries are small and arise almost perpendicular from a large main pulmonary artery.[331] The branch vessels increase in size with growth and become less angulated in their take-off from the main pulmonary artery.

CLINICAL FINDINGS. The degree of obstruction is the principal determinant of clinical severity; the type of obstruction determines the feasibility of direct surgical relief. The clinical features vary; most infants and children are asymptomatic.[332] An ejection systolic murmur at the upper left sternal border that is well transmitted to the axillae and back is most common. The presence of an ejection sound suggests that pulmonic valve stenosis coexists. The pulmonic component of the second heart sound may be slightly accentuated, but occasionally is extremely loud if multiple peripheral stenoses exist. A continuous murmur is audible, especially in patients with main or branch stenosis, and particularly if an associated cardiovascular anomaly produces increased pulmonary blood flow. Electrocardiography shows right ventricular hypertrophy when obstruction is severe; left-axis deviation with counterclockwise orientation of the frontal QRS vector is common in the rubella syndrome and when the lesion coexists with supravalvular aortic stenosis. Mild or moderate stenosis usually produces a normal chest roentgenogram; detectable differences in vascularity between regions of the lungs or dilated pulmonary artery segments are uncommon. When obstruction is bilateral and severe, right atrial and ventricular enlargement may be observed.

Diagnosis is confirmed by observing pressure gradients within the pulmonary arterial system at cardiac catheteriza-

tion; digital subtraction and/or selective pulmonary angiography defines the exact location, extent, and distribution of the lesion (Fig. 31–41). Mild to moderate unilateral or bilateral stenosis does not require surgical relief; numerous stenotic areas are not amenable to correction, even with intraoperative balloon angioplasty. Well-localized obstruction of severe degree in the main pulmonary artery or its major branches may be alleviated by percutaneous transcatheter balloon angioplasty (p. 1316)[333] or with a patch graft or bypassed with a tubular conduit. The efficacy and safety of implantation of expandable mesh stents to dilate vessel stenoses await testing.[334] The natural history of peripheral pulmonary stenosis is not clear. Obstruction may increase by discrepant growth between a stenotic area and normal portions of the pulmonary artery tree, or as a result of an increase in cardiac output, especially during adolescence. Rarely, hypertrophy of right ventricular infundibular muscle is progressive and results in hypercyanotic spells.

PULMONIC STENOSIS WITH INTACT VENTRICULAR SEPTUM
(See also p. 1059)

Valvular pulmonic stenosis, resulting from fusion of the valve cusps during mid to late intrauterine development, is the most common form of isolated right ventricular obstruction and occurs in about 7 per cent of patients with congenital heart disease. Hypertrophy of the septal and parietal bands narrowing the right ventricular infundibulum often accompanies the pulmonic valve lesion, especially if it is severe. Fused cusps of varying thickness and rigidity form a fibrous dome in the severest forms. Pulmonic valve dysplasia, especially common in patients with Noonan syndrome (p. 1634), produces obstruction in the absence of adherent leaflets because leaflets are thickened, rigid, and myxomatous and are limited in their lateral movement because of the presence of tissue pads within the pulmonic valve sinuses.[335]

INFANCY. The clinical presentation and course of circulation in the newborn with pulmonic stenosis depends on the severity of obstruction and the degree of development of the right ventricle and its outflow tract, the tricuspid valve, and the pulmonary arterial tree. The greater the degree of pulmonic valve stenosis, the more closely the manifestations resemble those observed with pulmonary atresia and intact ventricular septum (see p. 933). Severe pulmonic stenosis is characterized by cyanosis caused by right-to-left shunting through the foramen ovale, cardiomegaly, and diminished pulmonary blood flow in the absence of persistent patency of the ductus arteriosus. Hypoxemia and metabolic acidemia, rather than right ventricular failure, are the main clinical disturbances in the symptomatic neonate and can be alleviated temporarily by infusion of prostaglandin E_1 to dilate the ductus arteriosus and increase pulmonary blood flow. Distinction of these babies from those with tetralogy of Fallot or tricuspid or pulmonary atresia usually is possible, since infants with tetralogy usually do not have roentgenographic evidence of cardiomegaly; infants with tricuspid and pulmonary atresia show a preponderance of left ventricular forces by electrocardiography in contrast to the right ventricular hypertrophy usually observed with critical pulmonic stenosis in the absence of right ventricular hypoplasia. Combined two-dimensional echocardiographic and continuous-wave Doppler examination (Figs. 4–67, p. 90, and 4–68, p. 90) characterizes the anatomical valve abnormality and its severity, and has importantly reduced the requirement for cardiac catheterization and angiographic studies to establish a precise diagnosis (Fig. 31–42).[336,337] Balloon dilatation of the pulmonary valve often is the therapeutic procedure of choice, but a pulmonary valvotomy and systemic-to-pulmonary arterial shunt may be necessary in infants with underdevelopment of the right ventricular cavity.[338] Transcatheter balloon valvuloplasty may be expected to reduce, but not abolish, the pressure difference in neonates with mobile doming valves. This

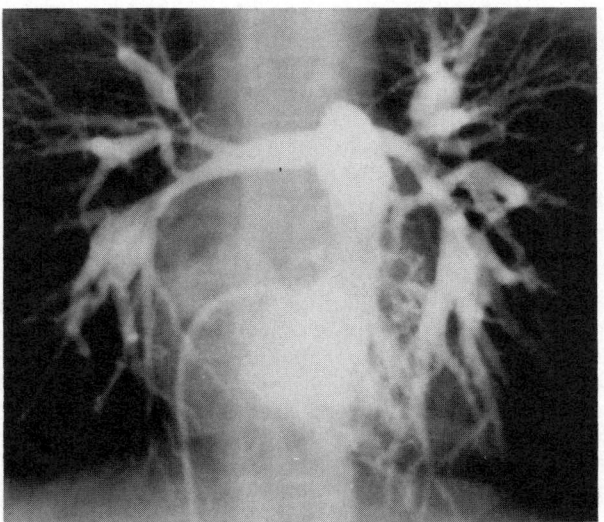

FIGURE 31–41. Right ventricular angiocardiogram showing multiple sites of peripheral pulmonic stenosis and poststenotic dilatation of the peripheral pulmonic arteries.

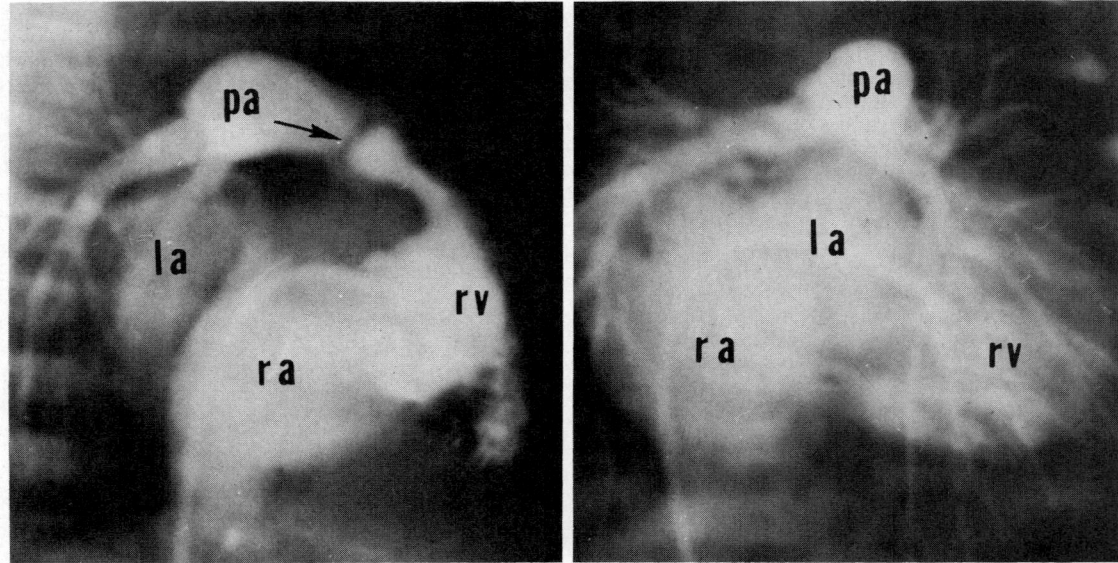

FIGURE 31–42. Right ventriculogram in an infant with critical pulmonic stenosis shows the thickened, nonmobile pulmonic valve (arrow) in the lateral projection *(left).* Both the lateral and frontal *(right)* projections show regurgitation of contrast material across the tricuspid valve into the right atrium (ra), with subsequent shunting across the foramen ovale to the left atrium (la). rv = right ventricle; pa = pulmonary artery. (Courtesy of Norman Talner, M.D.)

approach is of lesser efficacy in those patients with dysplastic valves, and is contraindicated if valve dysplasia is associated with annular hypoplasia.[339–342]

CHILDHOOD. The clinical profile of patients with valvular pulmonic stenosis beyond infancy usually is distinctive.[343,344] The severity of obstruction is the most important determinant of the clinical course. In the presence of a normal cardiac output a peak systolic transvalvular pressure gradient between 50 and 80 mm Hg or a peak systolic right ventricular pressure between 75 and 100 mm Hg is considered to be indicative of moderate stenosis; levels below and above that range are classified as mild and severe, respectively. Most patients with mild pulmonic stenosis are asymptomatic, and the condition is discovered during routine examination. In patients with more significant obstruction the severity of stenosis may increase with time. Progression may be relative and reflect disproportionate physical growth of the patient, infundibular narrowing due to progressive hypertrophy of the right ventricular outflow tract, or fibrosis of the valve cusps. Symptoms, when present, vary from mild exertional dyspnea and mild cyanosis to signs and symptoms of heart failure, depending on the degree of obstruction and the level of myocardial compensation. Exertional fatigue, syncope, and chest pain are related to an inability to augment pulmonary blood flow during exercise in some patients with moderate or severe obstruction.

The severity of obstruction often is suggested by the physical findings. Right ventricular hypertrophy reduces compliance of that chamber, and a forceful right atrial contraction is necessary to augment right ventricular filling. Prominent *a* waves in the jugular venous pulse, a fourth heart sound, and, occasionally, presystolic pulsations of the liver reflect a vigorous atrial contraction and suggest the presence of severe stenosis. Cardiomegaly and a right ventricular parasternal lift accompany moderate or severe obstruction. A systolic thrill is palpable along the upper left sternal border in all but the mildest forms of stenosis. The first heart sound is normal and is followed by a systolic ejection sound at the upper left sternal edge produced by sudden opening of the stenotic valve; an ejection sound is not heard in patients with pulmonic valve dysplasia. The ejection sound typically is louder during expiration; when it is inaudible or occurs less than 0.08 second from the onset of the Q wave on electrocardiogram, severe obstruction is suggested. Right ventricular ejection is prolonged in patients with moderate or severe stenosis, and the sound of pulmonic valve closure is delayed and soft. The characteristic feature of valvular pulmonic stenosis on ausculta-

tion is a harsh, diamond-shaped systolic ejection murmur heard best at the upper left sternal border. The systolic murmur becomes louder and its crescendo occurs later in systole, obscuring the aortic component of the second sound with more severe degrees of valvular obstruction, since these patients have a greater prolongation of right ventricular systole. The holosystolic decrescendo murmur of tricuspid regurgitation may accompany severe pulmonic stenosis, especially in the presence of congestive heart failure. Cyanosis, reflecting venoarterial shunting through a patent foramen ovale, is absent with mild stenosis and infrequent with moderate obstruction. Cyanosis may not be apparent in patients with severe obstruction if the atrial septum is intact.

Electrocardiography. (Fig. 7, p. 156 and Fig. 32–24, p. 987). This technique may be helpful in assessing the degree of obstruction to right ventricular output.[345] In mild cases the electrocardiogram often is normal, whereas moderate and severe stenoses are associated with right axis deviation and right ventricular hypertrophy. A tall QR wave in the right precordial leads with T-wave inversion and ST-segment suppression (right ventricular "strain") reflects severe stenosis. When an rSR′ pattern is observed in lead V_1 (20 per cent of patients) lower right ventricular pressures are found than in patients with a pure R wave of equal amplitude. High-amplitude P waves in leads II and V_1 indicating right atrial enlargement are associated with severe stenosis.

Chest Roentgenography. In patients with mild or moderate pulmonic stenosis chest roentgenography often shows a heart of normal size and normal pulmonary vascularity (Fig. 6–42A, p. 230). Poststenotic dilatation of the main and left pulmonary arteries often is evident. Right atrial and right ventricular enlargement are observed in patients with severe obstruction and resultant right ventricular failure. The pulmonary vascularity may be reduced in patients with severe stenosis, right ventricular failure, and/or a venoarterial shunt at the atrial level (p. 987).

Echocardiography. Reliable localization of the site of obstruction and assessment of its severity are obtained by combined continuous-wave Doppler and two-dimensional echocardiography[336,337] (Figs. 4–67, p. 90, and 32–3, p. 968). Parasternal and subcostal views are required to detect most accurately maximal pulmonary artery blood flow velocity, which is converted to a pressure difference across the valve utilizing a modified Bernoulli equation [pressure difference (mm Hg) = 4 × the squared peak Doppler velocity (m/s)].

Cardiac Catheterization and Angiocardiography. These

techniques also localize the site of obstruction, evaluate its severity, and document the coexistence of additional cardiac malformations (Fig. 31–43). The resting cardiac output usually is normal, even in cases of severe stenosis, and most children show the ability to increase cardiac output with exercise.[346] Right ventricular dysfunction occurs especially when venoarterial shunting is significant and produces systemic arterial desaturation. In patients with critical stenosis, care must be taken during hemodynamic study that the cardiac catheter does not dangerously occlude the stenotic valve opening. The angiographic appearance of a typical valvular pulmonic stenosis differs from that of a dysplastic valve. The former is thickened and domes during systole, returning to a normal configuration in diastole. Poststenotic dilatation of the main pulmonary trunk and sometimes of the left pulmonary artery often is observed. The leaflets of the dysplastic valve are not fused anatomically, but are thickened and immobile, creating little change in the angiographic picture during the cardiac cycle. Moreover, a small annulus and narrow sinuses of Valsalva are common accompaniments of valve dysplasia. With either type of valve, systolic narrowing of the right ventricular infundibulum usually is associated with moderate or severe obstruction.

Natural History. Mild and moderate pulmonic valve stenoses have a generally favorable course; uncommonly, progression occurs in the severity of obstruction.[347,348] Serial hemodynamic studies reveal unchanged pressure gradients over 4- to 8-year intervals in three-fourths of patients. Equal percentages of the remainder have an increase or a decrease in the severity of obstruction; significant increases in the pressure gradient occur especially in children with a gradient in excess of 50 mmHg at initial examination.[343]

Management. Percutaneous transluminal balloon valvuloplasty (p. 1316) is the initial procedure of choice in patients with typical pulmonary valve stenosis and moderate to severe degrees of obstruction.[339–342] This approach provides palliative improvement; it is not yet clear if improvement is permanent. In these same patients *surgical relief* also can be accomplished at extremely low risk.[349] The valve is approached through an incision in the pulmonary arterial trunk, and resection of infundibular muscle, if necessary, may be accomplished through the pulmonic valve. In patients with a dysplastic valve, in whom transcatheter valvuloplasty is ineffective, the thickened valve tissue is removed and a patch often is required to widen the annulus and proximal main pulmonary artery. In children with mild pulmonary valve ste-

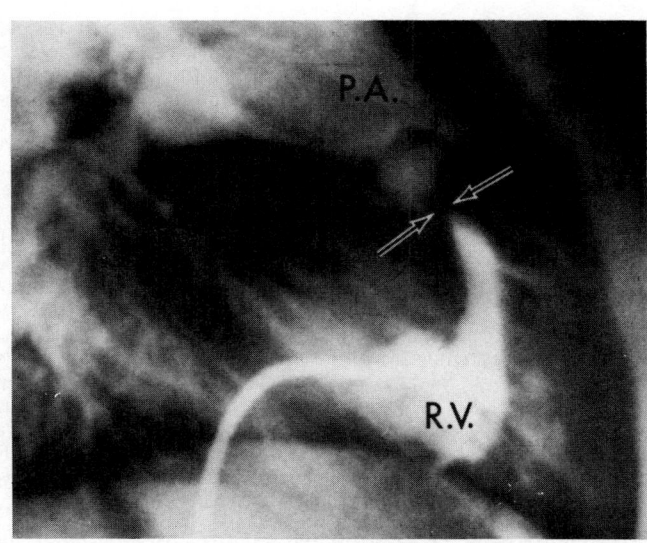

FIGURE 31–43. Lateral view of a right ventricular (R.V.) angiogram in a patient with severe pulmonic stenosis shows a thickened, domed pulmonic valve, below which exists marked hypertrophy of the right ventricular infundibulum (arrows). Poststenotic dilatation of the pulmonary artery (P.A.) is evident.

nosis prophylaxis against infective endocarditis is recommended; these patients need not restrict their physical activities.

PULMONIC ATRESIA WITH INTACT VENTRICULAR SEPTUM

MORPHOLOGY. This anomaly is an uncommon and serious cause of cyanosis in the neonatal period that may respond well to aggressive medical and surgical treatment.[349] In almost all infants the pulmonic valve is atretic; in the majority both the valve ring and the main pulmonary artery are hypoplastic. The right ventricular infundibulum occasionally may be atretic or extremely narrowed. A spectrum exists in right ventricular cavity size and configuration, from a diminutive right ventricular chamber, often with tricuspid stenosis, to a large right ventricle, frequently with tricuspid regurgitation (Fig. 31–44). In most infants the right ventricle is hypoplastic, and sinusoidal communications exist between the right ventricular cavity and the coronary circulation.[349a–352]

The intramyocardial sinusoids may end blindly or communicate with coronary arteries. Further, these communications may be multiple and

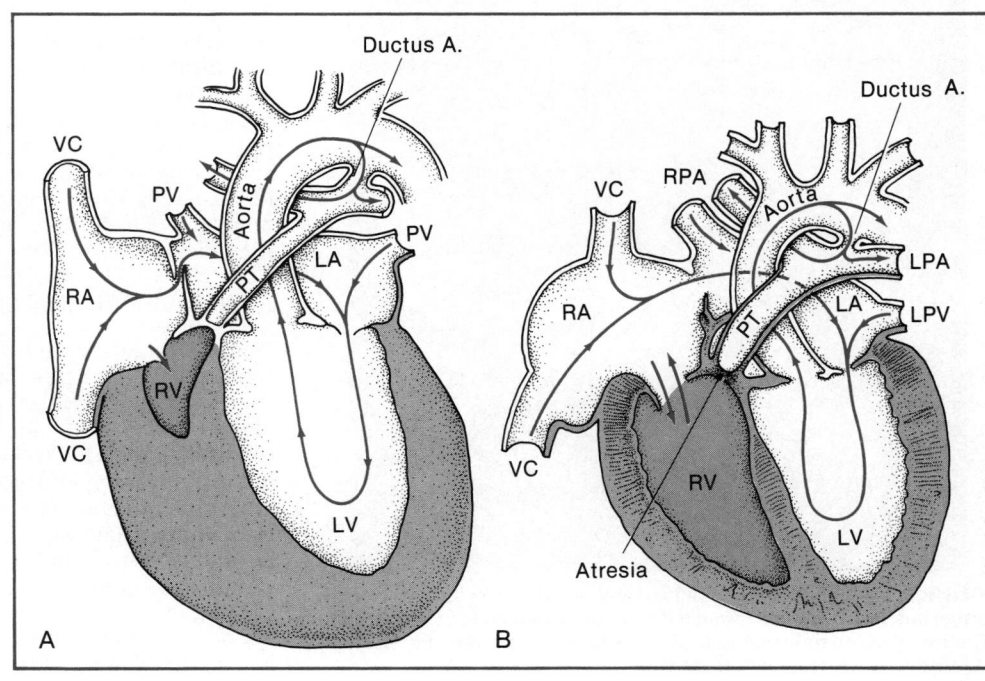

FIGURE 31–44. Pulmonic atresia with intact ventricular septum. With a competent tricuspid valve the right ventricular chamber is diminutive *(A)*; significant tricuspid regurgitation is associated with a normal or large right ventricular cavity *(B)*. V.C. = vena cava; R.A. = right atrium; R.V. = right ventricle; P.T. = pulmonary trunk; P.V. = pulmonary vein; L.A. = left atrium; L.V. = left ventricle; Ductus A. = ductus arteriosus; L.P.A. = left pulmonary artery; R.P.A. = right pulmonary artery; L.P.V. = left pulmonary vein. (From Edwards, J. E.: Congenital malformations of the heart and great vessels. *In* Gould, S. E. [ed.]: Pathology of the Heart. 2nd ed. Springfield, Ill., Charles C Thomas, 1960.)

feed both the left and right coronary systems, or they may be via a single, dilated vessel. The proximal coronary arteries in some patients may be atrophic, proximal to a communication between the sinusoids and the distal coronary artery, particularly in hearts with severe hypoplasia of the right ventricle. In these circumstances, the distal coronary vessels are supplied by communications with the right ventricle, and the coronary circulation is, therefore, right ventricule–dependent. In this group, decompression of the right ventricle by a surgical procedure would be associated with a high risk of myocardial ischemia and death.

Because the pulmonic valve is imperforate and completely obstructed, systemic venous blood returning to the heart bypasses the right ventricle through an interatrial communication. Right ventricular output does not contribute to the effective cardiac output and is proportional to the magnitude of tricuspid regurgitation and the size and extent of the sinusoidal communications with the coronary arterial tree. The blood supply to the lungs is derived from the bronchial circulation and from flow through a persistently patent ductus arteriosus. The size and patency of the ductus arteriosus are critical determinants in postnatal survival; ductus closure results in death. Reduced pulmonary blood flow by way of a partially constricted ductus arteriosus results in profound hypoxemia, tissue hypoxia, and metabolic acidemia.

CLINICAL FEATURES. The diagnosis is suggested by roentgenographic findings of pulmonary hypoperfusion and the electrocardiographic observation of a normal QRS axis, absent or diminished right ventricular forces, and/or dominant left ventricular forces. In the minority of infants with marked tricuspid regurgitation, the right ventricle and right atrium are massively enlarged. The echocardiogram in the usual infant shows a small right ventricular cavity and diminutive or absent pulmonic valve echoes.[353,354] Doppler examination shows continuous retrograde flow to the pulmonary artery and/or its branches through a patent ductus arteriosus which usually is narrow and tortuous. Only if tricuspid valve echoes are imaged by ultrasound examination can tricuspid atresia be distinguished from pulmonic atresia. Contrast echocardiography showing filling of the right ventricle across the tricuspid valve in diastole may clarify the latter distinction.

Cardiac catheterization usually is performed on an emergency basis. Because survival depends on patency of the ductus arteriosus, infusion of prostaglandin E$_1$ (0.05–0.1 μg/kg/min) intravenously may dramatically reverse clinical deterioration and improve arterial blood gases and pH.[71] The usual hemodynamic findings are right atrial and right ventricular hypertension, with right ventricular pressure often greater than systemic pressure, and a massive right-to-left interatrial shunt. Selective angiocardiography establishes the

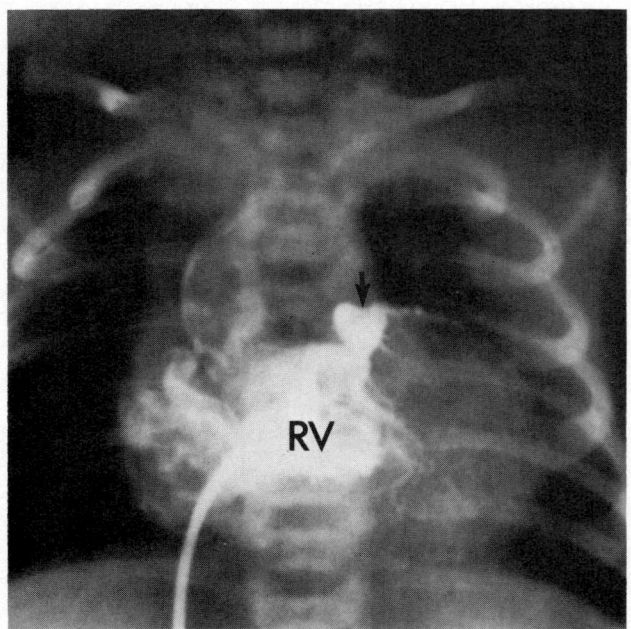

FIGURE 31–45. Right ventricular angiocardiogram in the frontal projection in a 1-day-old infant with an atretic pulmonic valve (arrow). The cavity of the right ventricle (RV) is small and eccentrically shaped. (Courtesy of Robert Freedom, M.D.)

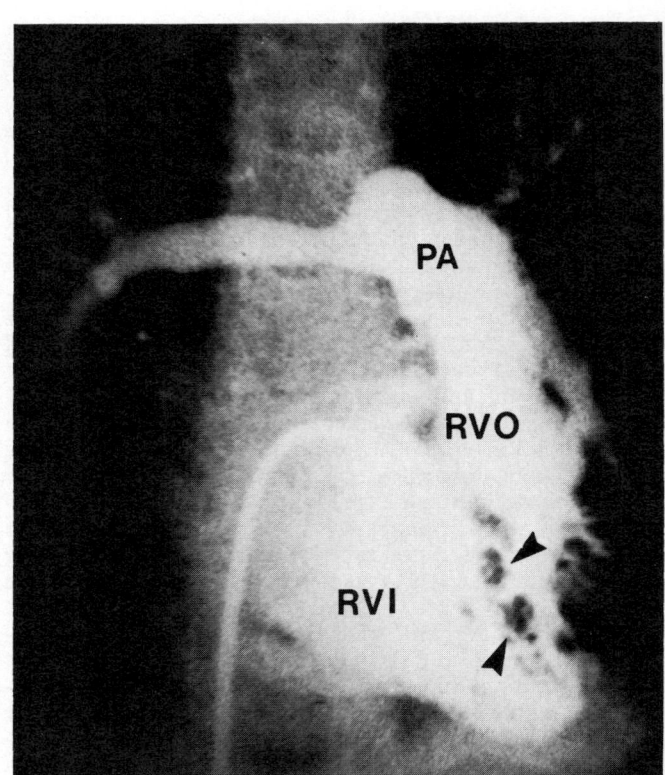

FIGURE 31–46. Intraventricular right ventricular obstruction. The right ventricular inflow (RVI) and outflow (RVO) tracts are separated by bands (arrows), creating intraventricular right ventricular obstruction. PA = pulmonary artery.

diagnosis and allows evaluation of the degree of separation between the right ventricular infundibular and pulmonary trunk, the size of the right ventricular cavity and of the pulmonary arteries (Fig. 31–45), the anatomy and function of the tricuspid valve, and the anatomical and functional details of the coronary circulation.

MANAGEMENT. In the majority of infants with a diminutive right ventricle, balloon atrial septostomy followed by a systemic-pulmonary artery shunt provides palliation. Infants with moderate right ventricular hypoplasia most often require a surgical pulmonary valvotomy and a systemic-pulmonary artery shunt, whereas in infants with only mild right ventricular hypoplasia, often valvotomy alone is necessary. The ultimate prognosis is poor unless continuity can be established between the right ventricle and the pulmonary arteries by pulmonary valvotomy or prosthetic conduit at initial or second operation.[349,355] Decompression of the right ventricle permits that chamber to grow and both the tricuspid and the pulmonary orifices to enlarge. In other patients who are unsuitable candidates for a one- or two-stage approach to biventricular repair, the Fontan right atrium–pulmonary anastomosis may be effective several years after shunt pallliation in the newborn period.[349]

INTRAVENTRICULAR RIGHT VENTRICULAR OBSTRUCTION

Infundibular pulmonic stenosis with an intact ventricular septum and the presence of anomalous muscle bundles are the two principal causes of intraventricular right ventricular obstruction (Fig. 31–46).[356]

SUBPULMONIC INFUNDIBULAR STENOSIS. This anomaly usually occurs at the proximal portion of the infundibulum and consists of a fibrous band at the junction of the right ventricular cavity and outflow tract. The clinical manifestations, course, and prognosis of patients with infundibular stenosis are similar to those of patients with valvular stenosis, although the former diagnosis is suggested by the absence of a systolic ejection sound and a systolic murmur lower along the left sternal border. Doppler echocardiography, withdrawal pressure tracings, and selective right ventricular angiocardiography permit localization of the site of obstruction and assessment of its extent and severity. Surgical treatment consists of resection of the fibrotic narrowed area and hypertrophied muscle. Occasionally it may be necessary to widen the outflow tract with a pericardial or prosthetic patch.

ANOMALOUS MUSCLE BUNDLES. A two-chambered right ventricle is formed by right ventricular obstruction due to anomalous muscle bundles; most of the patients have an associated malalignment or perimembranous ventricular septal defect, and about 5 per cent have subaortic stenosis.[356] Aberrant hypertrophied muscle bands traverse the right ventricular cavity, extending from its anterior wall to the crista supraventricularis and/or the portion of the adjacent interventricular septum. The anomalous pyramid-shaped muscle mass obstructs blood flow through the body of the right ventricle and produces a proximal high-pressure inflow chamber and a distal low-pressure chamber. Thus this type of obstruction is distinguishable from that in tetralogy of Fallot, in which hypertrophied infundibular muscle protrudes into but does not cross the cavity of the right ventricle.

The clinical, electrocardiographic, and chest roentgenographic findings resemble those observed in pulmonic valvular or subvalvular infundibular obstruction, although the systolic thrill and murmur may be displaced lower along the left sternal border. Progressive obstruction occurs in some patients. The diagnosis may be established by two-dimensional echocardiography. Selective right ventricular angiocardiography is necessary for most accurate diagnosis and reveals a filling defect in the midportion of the right ventricle which often does not change significantly with systole and diastole.

Management. The treatment for anomalous muscle bundles consists of surgical removal.[357,358] In the absence of preoperative recognition of the anomaly, the surgeon should be alerted to the correct diagnosis by the presence of a dimple on the ordinarily smooth anterior surface of the right ventricle and/or the inability to view the tricuspid valve through a longitudinal ventriculotomy because of the presence of the abnormal muscle mass.

TETRALOGY OF FALLOT

(See also p. 971)

DEFINITION. The overall incidence of this anomaly approaches 10 per cent of all forms of congenital heart disease, and it is the most common cardiac malformation responsible for cyanosis after 1 year of age.[359,360] The four components of this malformation are (1) ventricular septal defect, (2) obstruction to right ventricular outflow, (3) overriding of the aorta, and (4) right ventricular hypertrophy. The basic anomaly is the result of an anterior deviation of the septal insertion of the infundibular ventricular septum from its usual location in the normal heart between the limbs of the trabecular septum. The malalignment interventricular defect usually is large, approximating the aortic orifice in size, and is located high in the septum just below the right cusp of the aortic valve, separated from the pulmonic valve by the crista supraventricularis. The aortic root may be displaced anteriorly and straddle or override the septal defect, but, as in the normal heart, it lies to the right of the origin of the pulmonary artery. In most cases no dextroposition of the aorta exists; overriding of the aorta is a phenomenon secondary to the subaortic location of the ventricular septal defect.

HEMODYNAMICS. The degree of obstruction to pulmonary blood flow is the principal determinant of the clinical presentation. The site of obstruction is variable[361]; infundibular stenosis is the only major obstruction in about 50 per cent of patients and coexists with valvular obstruction in another 20 to 25 per cent (Fig. 31–47). Supravalvular and peripheral pulmonary arterial narrowing may be observed, and unilateral absence of a pulmonary artery (usually the left) is found in a small number of patients. Circulation to the abnormal lung is accomplished by bronchial and other collateral

arteries.[362-365] Atresia of the pulmonic valve, infundibulum, or main pulmonary artery occasionally is referred to as "pseudotruncus arteriosus." True truncus arteriosus with absent pulmonary arteries (Type 4) differs from Fallot's tetralogy, in which pulmonary artery branches are present but are fed by a patent ductus arteriosus and/or bronchial arteries (see Fig. 31–50).[363] A right-sided aortic knob, aortic arch, and descending aorta occur in about 25 per cent of patients with tetralogy of Fallot. The coronary arteries may have surgically important variations[366-368]: the anterior descending artery may originate from the right coronary artery; a single right coronary artery may give off a left branch that courses anterior to the pulmonary trunk; a single left coronary artery may give off a right branch that crosses the infundibulum of the right ventricle. Enlargement of the infundibular branch of the right coronary artery often presents a problem with respect to a right ventriculotomy. Associated cardiac anomalies exist in about 40 per cent of patients. Major associated cardiac anomalies include patent ductus arteriosus, multiple (usually muscular) ventricular septal defects, and complete atrioventricular septal defects. Localized single or multiple peripheral pulmonary arterial stenotic lesions are common; rarely, the right or left pulmonary artery may arise anomalously from the ascending aorta. Infrequently, aortic valve regurgitation results from aortic cusp prolapse. Associated extracardiac anomalies are present in 20 to 30 per cent of patients.

The relation between the resistance to blood flow from the ventricles into the aorta and into the pulmonary vessels plays a major role in determining the hemodynamic and clinical picture.[359] Thus, the severity of obstruction to right ventricular outflow is of fundamental significance. When right ventricular outflow tract obstruction is severe, the pulmonary blood flow is markedly reduced, and a large volume of unsaturated systemic venous blood is shunted from right to left across the ventricular septal defect. Severe cyanosis and polycythemia occur, and symptoms and sequelae of systemic hypoxemia are prominent. At the opposite end of the spectrum, the term "acyanotic" or "pink" tetralogy of Fallot often is used to describe an interventricular communication and a milder degree of obstruction to right ventricular outflow with little or no venoarterial shunting. In many infants and children the obstruction to right ventricular outflow is mild but progres-

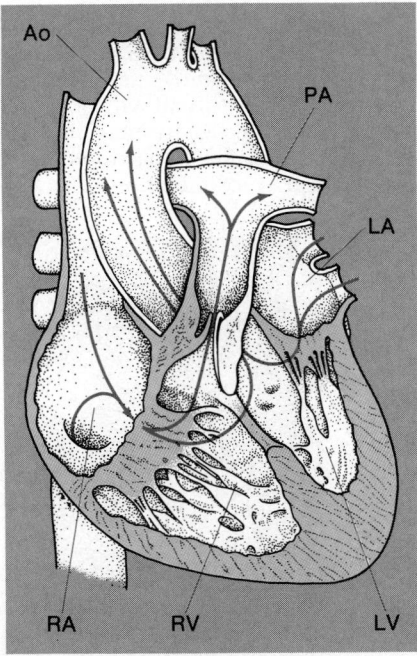

FIGURE 31–47. Tetralogy of Fallot with infundibular and valvular pulmonic stenosis. The arrows indicate direction of blood flow. A substantial right-to-left shunt exists across the ventricular septal defect. RA = right atrium; LA = left atrium; RV = right ventricle; LV = left ventricle; Ao = aorta; PA = pulmonary artery.

sive, so that early in life pulmonary exceeds systemic blood flow, and the symptoms resemble those produced by a simple ventricular septal defect.

CLINICAL MANIFESTATIONS. Few children with tetralogy of Fallot remain asymptomatic or acyanotic. Most are cyanotic from birth or develop cyanosis before age 1 year. In general, the earlier the onset of systemic hypoxemia, the more likely the possibility that severe pulmonary outflow tract stenosis or atresia exists. Dyspnea with exertion, clubbing, and polycythemia is common. When resting after exertion, children with tetralogy characteristically assume a squatting posture. The latter may be obvious even in infancy; many cyanotic infants prefer to lie in a knee-chest position. Spells of intense cyanosis related to a sudden increase in venoarterial shunting and a reduction in pulmonary blood flow most often have their onset between 2 and 9 months of age and constitute an important threat to survival.[369,370] The attacks are not restricted to patients with severe cyanosis; they are characterized by hyperpnea and increasing cyanosis that progresses to limpness and syncope and occasionally terminates in convulsions, a cerebrovascular accident, and death.

Physical Examination. This reveals variable degrees of underdevelopment and cyanosis. Clubbing of the terminal digits may be prominent after the first year of life. The heart is not hyperactive or enlarged; a right ventricular impulse and systolic thrill often are palpable along the left sternal border. An early systolic ejection sound that is aortic in origin may be heard at the lower left sternal border and apex; the second heart sound is single, the pulmonic component rarely being audible. A systolic ejection murmur is produced by flow across the narrowed right ventricular infundibulum or pulmonic valve. The intensity and duration of the murmur vary inversely with the severity of obstruction—the opposite of the relation that exists in patients with pulmonic stenosis and an intact ventricular septum. Polycythemia, decreased systemic vascular resistance, and increased obstruction to right ventricular outflow may all be responsible for a decrease in intensity of the murmur; with extreme outflow tract stenosis or pulmonic atresia and during an attack of paroxysmal hypoxemia, there may be no or only a very short, faint murmur. A continuous murmur faintly audible over the anterior or posterior chest reflects flow through enlarged bronchial collateral vessels. A loud continuous murmur of flow through a patent ductus arteriosus occasionally may be heard at the upper left sternal border.

LABORATORY EXAMINATIONS. The *electrocardiogram* ordinarily shows right ventricular and, less frequently, right atrial hypertrophy. In a patient with acyanotic tetralogy, combined ventricular hypertrophy may be noted initially, progressing to right ventricular hypertrophy as cyanosis develops. *Roentgenographic* examination (Fig. 32–14, p. 974)

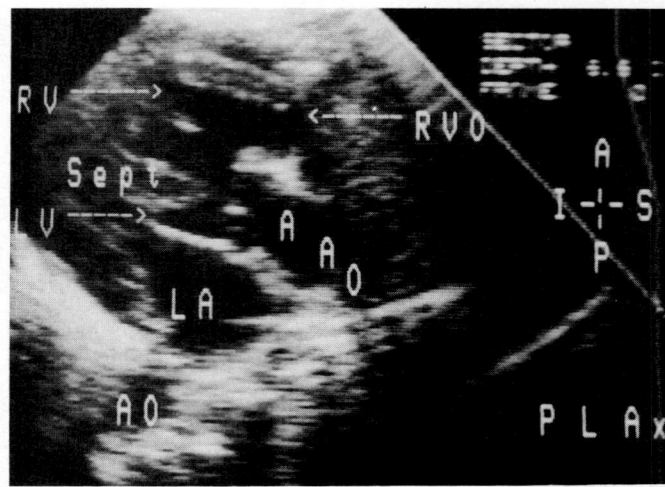

FIGURE 31–48. Tetralogy of Fallot in a parasternal long-axis (PLAx) view, which demonstrates the aorta overriding the ventricular septum (Sept). RV = right ventricle, RVO = right ventricular outflow tract, LV = left ventricle, LA = left atrium, AO = ascending aorta. (Courtesy of Norman Silverman, M.D.)

characteristically reveals a normal-sized, boot-shaped heart (coeur en sabot) with prominence of the right ventricle and a concavity in the region of the underdeveloped right ventricular outflow tract and main pulmonary artery. The pulmonary vascular markings typically are diminished, and the aortic arch and knob may be on the right side; the ascending aorta usually is large. A uniform, diffuse, fine reticular pattern of vascular markings is noted in the presence of prominent collateral vessels.

Echocardiographic findings include aortic enlargement, aortic–septal discontinuity, and aortic overriding of the ventricular septum.[371] Two-dimensional echocardiography (Fig. 4–82, p. 94) shows the right ventricular outflow tract to be narrowed and in a more horizontal orientation than normal. The main pulmonary artery and its branches are mildly to severely hypoplastic. The usual malalignment ventricular septal defect lies superior to the tricuspid valve and immediately below the aortic valve cusps. These findings are best displayed in views of the long axis of the right ventricular outflow tract, which are the subxiphoid short axis and the high transverse parasternal echo windows. Echo views which show the anteroposterior coordinates best indicate the overriding of the aorta; these are the parasternal long-axis, apical two-chamber, and subxiphoid views (Fig. 31–48). The echocardiographic examination also reveals the origin of the main pulmonary artery from the right ventricle, and continuity of the main pulmonary artery with its right and left branches,

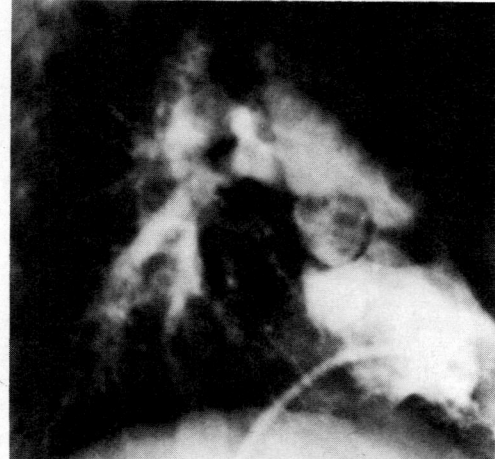

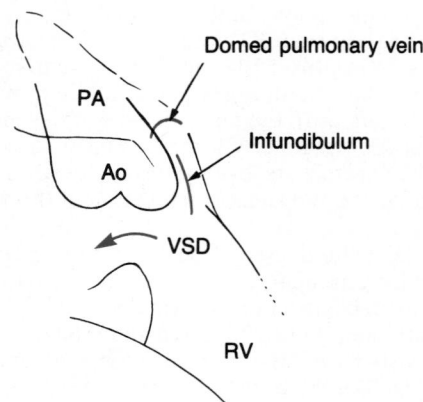

FIGURE 31–49. Lateral view of a right ventriculogram in a child with tetralogy of Fallot showing simultaneous opacification of the pulmonary artery (P.A.) and aorta (Ao.). P.V. = pulmonic valve; V.S.D. = ventricular septal defect; R.V. = right ventricle.

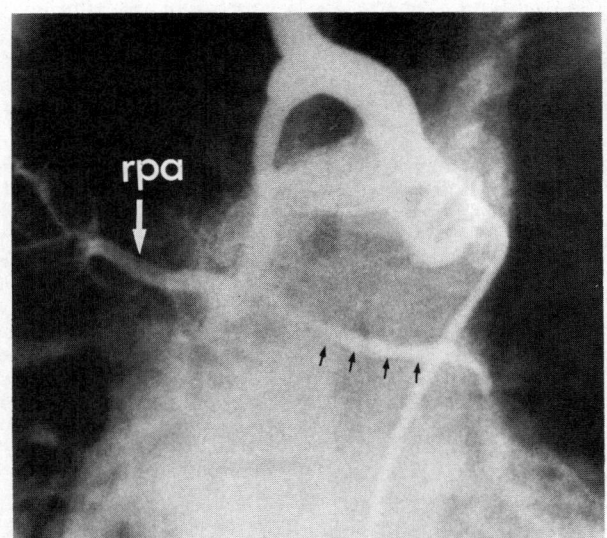

FIGURE 31–50. Selective systemic collateral bronchial arteriogram demonstrates "gull-wing" configuration of the hypoplastic right pulmonary artery (rpa) and left pulmonary artery (arrows) in a patient with tetralogy of Fallot and pulmonic atresia. (Courtesy of Robert Freedom, M.D.)

and is accurate for diagnosing coronary abnormalities.[367,368] The demonstration of mitral–semilunar valve continuity helps to distinguish tetralogy from double-outlet right ventricle with pulmonic stenosis, in which discontinuity of the mitral valve echo and the aortic cusp echo is a critical feature.

Cardiac Catheterization and Angiocardiography (Fig. 31–49). These are necessary to confirm the diagnosis; assess the magnitude of right-to-left shunting; provide details of additional muscular ventricular septal defects, if present; evaluate the architecture of the right ventricular outflow tract, pulmonic valve, and annulus and the morphology and caliber of the main branches of the pulmonary arteries; and analyze the anatomy of the coronary arteries. *Axial cineangiography*, utilizing the sitting-up projection, greatly facilitates evaluation of the pulmonary outflow tract and arteries.[122,361,365] The preoperative assessment of tetralogy with pulmonic atresia must include delineation of the arterial supply to both lungs by selective catheterization and visualization of bronchial collateral arteries with late serial filming; pulmonary arteries may be opacified only after the bronchial collateral arteries have cleared of contrast material (Fig. 31–50).[361,363] A patient with pulmonic atresia should not be ruled out as a candidate for surgical correction unless an inadequate pulmonary arterial supply to the lungs is clearly demonstrated.[362] Rarely, injection of contrast through a catheter in the pulmonary venous capillary wedge position is required to assess the possibility that anatomical pulmonary arteries are present.[364] Computer-assisted axial tomography may visualize central pulmonary arteries when conventional angiography cannot.

MANAGEMENT. Among the factors that may complicate the management of patients with tetralogy are iron deficiency anemia, infective endocarditis, paradoxical embolism, polycythemia, coagulation disorders, and cerebral infarction or abscess. Paroxysmal hypercyanotic spells may respond quickly to oxygen, placing the child in the knee-chest position, and morphine. If the spell persists, metabolic acidosis will develop from prolonged anaerobic metabolism, and infusion of sodium bicarbonate may be necessary to interrupt the attack. Vasopressors, beta-adrenoceptor redundant blockade, or general anesthesia occasionally may be necessary.[370]

Total Surgical Correction. This operation is advisable ultimately for almost all patients with tetralogy of Fallot.[367a–369a] Early definitive repair, even in infancy, currently is advocated in most centers that are experienced in intracardiac surgery in infants. Successful early correction appears to prevent the consequences of progressive infundibular obstruction and ac-

quired pulmonic atresia, delayed growth and development, and complications secondary to hypoxemia and polycythemia with bleeding tendencies. The size of the pulmonary arteries, rather than the age or size of the infant or child, is the most important determinant in assessing candidacy for primary repair; marked hypoplasia of the pulmonary arteries is a relative contraindication for early corrective operation.

Palliative Surgery. When marked hypoplasia of the pulmonary arteries exists, a palliative operation designed to increase pulmonary blood flow is recommended and usually consists in the smallest infants of a systemic-pulmonary arterial anastomosis.[370a] A transventricular infundibulectomy or valvulotomy is an alternative palliative procedure that may be considered. Balloon dilatation of the pulmonary valve may afford palliation in selected infants.[372] Total correction can then be carried out at a lower risk later in childhood or adolescence. The palliative procedures relieve hypoxemia caused by diminished pulmonary blood flow and reduce the stimulus to polycythemia. Because pulmonary venous return is augmented, the left atrium and ventricle are stimulated to enlarge their capacity in anticipation of total correction. In the most severe forms of tetralogy of Fallot with pulmonic atresia, the goals of operation include establishment of nonstenotic continuity between the right ventricle and pulmonary arteries, closure of the intracardiac shunt, and interruption of surgically created shunts or major collateral arteries to the lungs.[360,371a] When atresia is confined to the infundibulum or pulmonic valve, repair may be accomplished by infundibular resection and reconstruction of the outflow tract with a pericardial patch. If a long segment of pulmonary arterial atresia exists, a valve-containing conduit is inserted from the right ventricle to the distal pulmonary artery. The presence of a single pulmonary artery in the hilus of either lung is a prerequisite for repair of pulmonic atresia. A conduit also may be necessary in less severe forms of right ventricular outflow tract obstruction when an anomalous coronary artery crosses the right ventricular outflow tract.

A variety of complications are common in the postoperative period after palliative or corrective operation. Mild-to-moderate left ventricular decompensation may be secondary to the sudden increase in pulmonary venous return; varying degrees of pulmonic valvular regurgitation increase right ventricular cavity size further.[373] Bleeding problems frequently are seen, especially in older polycythemic patients. Complete right bundle branch block or the pattern of left anterior hemiblock often is seen, but disabling dysrhythmias are infrequent.[374,376] Restricted pulmonary arterial flow is the greatest cause for early and late mortality and poor late results.[359] After convalescence from intracardiac repair, symptoms of hypoxemia and severe exercise intolerance are relieved even in the presence of some residual right ventricular outflow tract obstruction, pulmonic valve incompetence, and/or cardiomegaly.[371,377] However, cardiovascular performance at rest or during exercise may remain below normal,[378,379] and major complications, such as trifascicular block, complete heart block, ventricular arrhythmias, and sudden death, may rarely occur many years after surgical treatment.

CONGENITAL ABSENCE OF THE PULMONIC VALVE

PATHOLOGY AND PATHOGENESIS. In the majority of cases of this rare malformation the lesion is associated with a ventricular septal defect, a narrowed obstructive annulus of the pulmonic valve, and marked aneurysmal dilatation of the pulmonary arteries. The combination of anomalies often is referred to as tetralogy of Fallot with absent pulmonic valve. The obstructing lesion principally consists of underdeveloped, primitive valve tissue within a hypoplastic annulus; infundibular obstruction and the ventricular septal defect do not differ from classic tetralogy of Fallot. The massively dilated pulmonary arteries often are the major determinant of the clinical course, since they frequently result in upper airway obstruction and severe respiratory distress in infancy.[380] Poststenotic pulmonary artery aneurysms develop in utero, and their size and location appear to be related to the magnitude of pulmonic regurgitation in fetal life, the orienta-

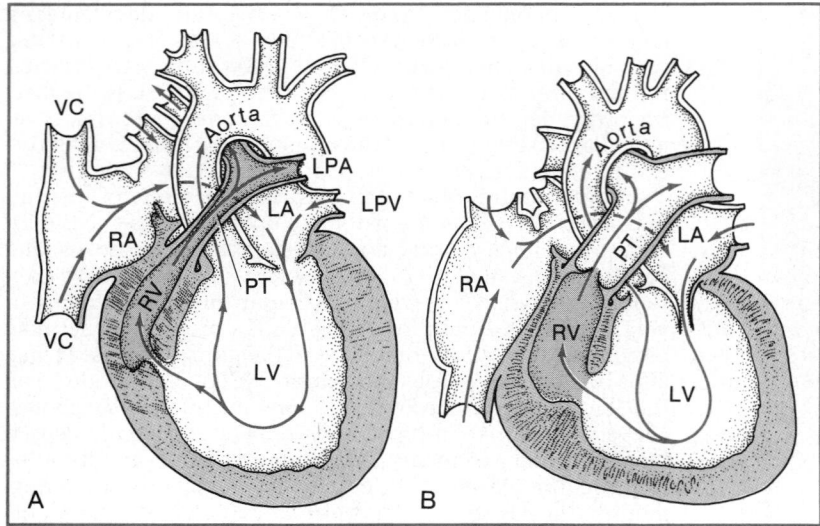

FIGURE 31–51. *A,* Tricuspid atresia with normally related great arteries, a small ventricular septal defect, diminutive right ventricular chamber, and narrowed outflow tract. *B,* An example of tricuspid atresia and complete transposition of the great arteries in which the left ventricular chamber is essentially a common ventricle, with the aorta arising from an infundibular component (R.V.) of the common ventricle. V.C. = vena cava; R.A. = right atrium; L.A. = left atrium; R.V. = right ventricle; L.V. = left ventricle; L.P.V. = left pulmonary vein; L.P.A. = left pulmonary artery. (Modified from Edwards, J. E., and Burchell, H. B.: Congenital tricuspid atresia: Classification. Med. Clin. North Am. 33:1177, 1949.)

tion of the right ventricular infundibulum to the right or left, and the size of the ductus arteriosus.[381] It has been suggested that the aneurysmal dilatation is related pathogenetically to agenesis of the ductus arteriosus.[382]

CLINICAL AND LABORATORY FINDINGS. The *clinical features* often are distinctive, with an early onset of severe respiratory distress caused by tracheobronchial compression accompanied by a systolic ejection and a widely transmitted low-pitched, decrescendo diastolic murmur at the upper left sternal border. In the absence of pulmonary complications cyanosis is commonly mild. *Roentgenographically* the heart is moderately enlarged; hyperinflated lung fields are observed with large hilar densities representing the aneurysmally dilated pulmonary arteries. The *echocardiographic* features are similar to those seen in classic tetralogy of Fallot, in addition to massive dilatation of the main pulmonary artery and branch pulmonary arteries. Remnants of pulmonary cusps may be visible. Right ventricular dilatation is produced by significant pulmonary regurgitation; the latter is identified by retrograde diastolic flow in the pulmonary arteries and right ventricle at Doppler examination. Definitive diagnosis is established by cardiac catheterization and selective angiocardiography.

Prognosis is related to the intensity of upper airway obstruction; pulmonary complications are the usual cause of death in infancy. If survival beyond infancy is accomplished, the respiratory symptoms usually diminish, probably because of maturational changes in the structure of the tracheobronchial tree. The surgical approach in infancy often is unsatisfactory; a variety of procedures have been attempted, ranging from aneurysmorrhaphy to pulmonary artery suspension to transection and reanastomosis of pulmonary artery segments to homograft insertion.[383,384] Also suggested are ligation of the main pulmonary artery and creation of a systemic-pulmonary shunt, and primary repair of the ventricular septal defect with pulmonary arterial plication. In older patients the stenotic annulus may be widened with a patch and the ventricular septal defect closed. It seldom is necessary to replace the pulmonic valve.

TRICUSPID ATRESIA

MORPHOLOGY. This anomaly is characterized by absence of the tricuspid orifice, an interatrial communication, hypoplasia of the right ventricle, and the presence of a communication between the systemic and pulmonary circulations, usually a ventricular septal defect.[385,386] Thus there is a univentricular atrioventricular connection, consisting of a left-sided mitral valve between the morphological left atrium and left ventricle. Unequal division of the atrioventricular canal by fusion of the right-sided endocardial cushions has been proposed as the embryological fault. Patients may be subdivided into those with normally related great arteries (60 to 70 per cent of cases) and those with D-transposition of the great arteries; further classification depends on the presence of pulmonic stenosis or atresia and the absence or size of the ventricular septal defect (Fig. 31–51). Additional cardiovascular malformations often are present, especially in patients with D-transposition of the great arteries, and include persistent left superior vena cava, patent ductus arteriosus, coarctation of the aorta, and juxtaposition of the atrial appendages.

PATHOPHYSIOLOGY. The association with other cardiac malformations determines whether or not pulmonary blood flow is decreased, normal, or increased and therefore the degree of systemic hypoxemia.[387] The clinical picture usually is dominated by symptoms resulting from greatly diminished pulmonary blood flow with severe cyanosis. Cyanosis results from an obligatory admixture of systemic and pulmonary venous blood in

the left atrium, and its intensity primarily depends on the magnitude of pulmonary blood flow. Heart failure, rather than cyanosis, is the predominant problem in infants with torrential pulmonary blood flow, which results when D-transposition of the great arteries, a ventricular septal defect, and an unobstructed pulmonary outflow tract coexist. If the latter patients survive infancy, they are candidates for pulmonary vascular obstructive disease; a favorable response to pulmonary arterial banding is common early in life.

CLINICAL FEATURES. The diagnosis is easily established in the vast majority of infants with tricuspid atresia and pulmonary hypoperfusion. The *electrocardiographic* findings of left-axis deviation, right atrial enlargement, and left ventricular hypertrophy in a cyanotic infant strongly suggest tricuspid atresia.[387] *Echocardiography* reveals a small or absent right ventricle, large left ventricle, and absent tricuspid valve echoes (Figs. 31–52 and 4–70, p. 91); further, it may demonstrate the relation of the great arteries unless pulmonic atresia is present. Contrast cross-sectional echocardiography reveals the abnormal flow patterns; apical and subxiphoid cross-sectional views best reveal the atretic tricuspid orifice. *Roentgenographically,* there are diminished pulmonary vascular markings and a concavity in the region of the cardiac silhouette usually occupied by the main pulmonary artery. The

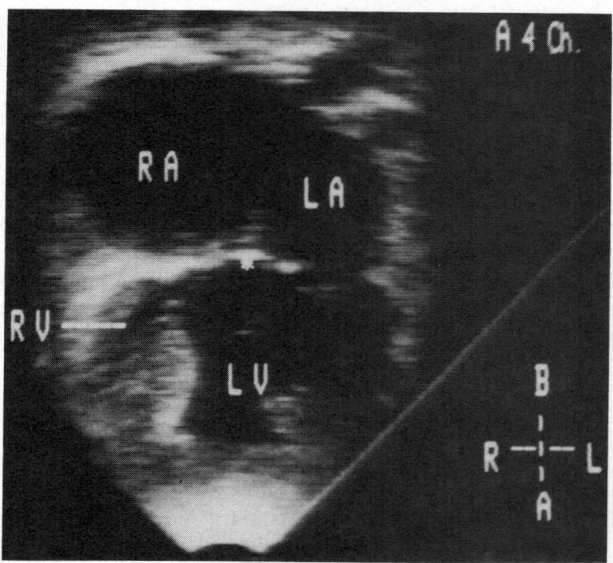

FIGURE 31–52. Tricuspid atresia is seen in an apical four-chamber view. The bright horizontal echoes arise from the AV sulcus tissue preventing communication between the right atrium (RA) and right ventricle (RV). The RV is small and communicates with the left ventricle (LV) via a small ventricular septal defect. (Courtesy of Norman Silverman, M.D.)

right atrial shadow may be prominent unless left-sided juxta-position of the atrial appendages exists, which produces a straight and flattened right heart border.

CARDIAC CATHETERIZATION AND ANGIOGRAPHY. The right ventricle cannot be entered directly from the right atrium. When the great arteries are related normally, pulmonary blood flow is found to be derived from shunting through a ventricular septal defect or by way of a patent ductus arteriosus; the latter and the bronchial collaterals are the source of pulmonary flow if the ventricular septum is intact. In complete transposition the pulmonary artery fills directly from the left ventricle and the aorta indirectly through a ventricular septal defect and the hypoplastic right ventricle. Because complete admixture exists in the left atrium of pulmonary and systemic venous return, the degree of systemic arterial hypoxemia depends on the pulmonary-systemic flow ratio. Right atrial angiography does not opacify the right ventricle unless by way of a ventricular septal defect (Fig. 31–53). Selective left ventricular *angiography* permits identification of the hypoplastic right ventricle, the size and location of the ventricular septal defect, the type of pulmonary obstruction, the relation between the great arteries, and the size of the distal pulmonary arterial tree.

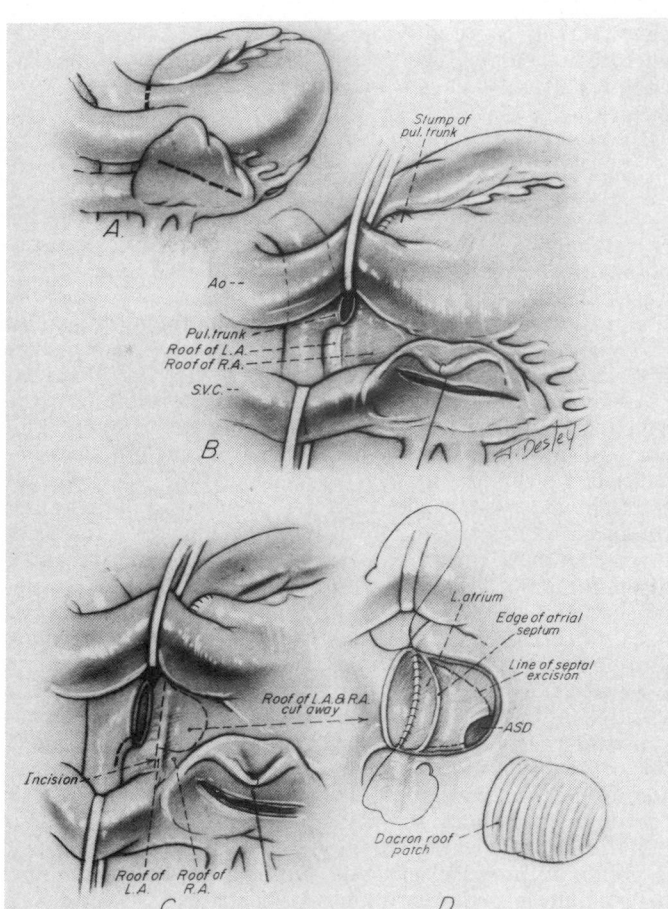

FIGURE 31–54. The Fontan operation with direct right atrial-pulmonary artery connection. *A,* The right atrium is opened through an oblique incision and the pulmonary artery transsected above the pulmonary valve. *B,* The proximal pulmonary trunk is closed and the distal end brought toward the right atrium beneath the aorta. *C,* The pulmonary artery is enlarged if a complex atrial septal baffle is required, the atrial septum is excised, and a circular button of atrial roof is removed. *D,* The posterior wall of the openings into the pulmonary artery and the atria are anastomosed; if the anterior wall of the right atrium and the pulmonary artery cannot easily be brought together for direct anastomoses, a convex Dacron roof patch is employed. AO = aorta, RA = right atrium, LA = left atrium, ASD = atrial septal defect. (From Kirklin, J. W., and Barratt-Boyes, B. G.: Cardiac Surgery. New York, John Wiley & Sons, 1986, p. 873.)

MANAGEMENT. *Balloon atrial septostomy* in those infants with a restrictive interatrial communication and palliative operations designed to increase pulmonary blood flow (systemic arterial– or venous–pulmonary artery anastomosis) are capable of producing clinical improvement of significant duration in patients with diminished blood flow.[387,388]

Functional correction of the anomaly has been accomplished by direct anastomosis or insertion of a nonvalved prosthetic conduit between the right atrium and pulmonary artery and closure of the interatrial communication (Fontan procedure) (Fig. 31–54).[389,390,390a,390b] If the right ventricle is not markedly hypoplastic, it may be utilized in the correction to generate forward flow into the pulmonary vascular bed. Also, if the right ventricle is not too hypoplastic, it may be used as a pumping chamber by anastomosis of the right atrial appendage to the right ventricle with the aid of a pericardial patch, leaving the outflow tract and pulmonic valve intact.[387] A previously existing systemic artery–to–pulmonary artery anastomosis must be closed, but a systemic vein–to–pulmonary artery anastomosis may be left in place. Candidates for these corrective procedures must have normal pulmonary vascular resistance and a mean pulmonary artery pressure less than 20 mm Hg, pulmonary arteries of adequate size, and good left ventricular function.[389,391] The postoperative period usually is

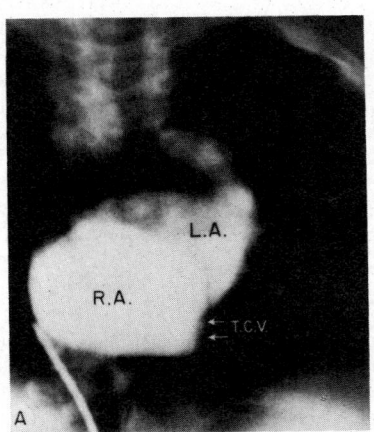
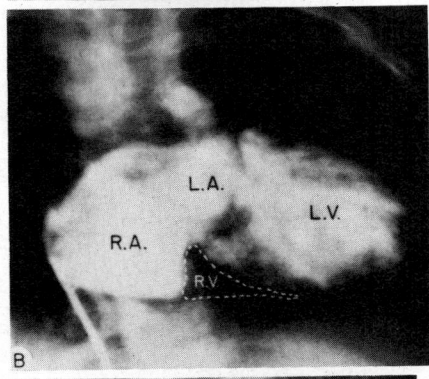
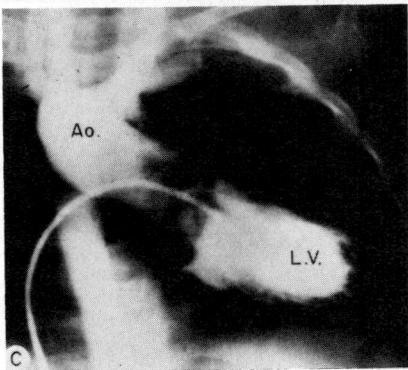

FIGURE 31–53. Right atrial angiogram in an infant with tricuspid atresia shows flow of contrast material from right atrium (R.A.) to left atrium *(A),* and then to left ventricle (L.V.) *(B)* and aorta (Ao.) *(C).* The tricuspid valve (T.C.V.) is atretic, and a radiolucency exists in the region of the right ventricle (R.V.).

characterized transiently by a superior vena cava syndrome with right heart failure, edema, ascites, and hepatomegaly. Long-term results have been good.[392-397]

EBSTEIN'S ANOMALY OF THE TRICUSPID VALVE
(See also p. 970)

This malformation is characterized by a downward displacement of the tricuspid valve into the right ventricle due to anomalous attachment of the tricuspid leaflets (Fig. 31–55).[398] Case-control studies suggest that maternal exposure in the first trimester to lithium carbonate, used in the management of manic-depressive psychosis, is associated with a greatly increased risk of this anomaly in exposed offspring.[399] Tricuspid valve tissue is dysplastic, and a variable portion of the septal and inferior cusps adhere to the right ventricular wall some distance away from the atrioventricular junction. Because of the abnormally situated tricuspid orifice, a portion of the right ventricle lies between the atrioventricular ring and the origin of the valve, which is continuous with the right atrial chamber. This proximal segment is "atrialized," and a distal, functionally small ventricular chamber exists. The degree of impairment of right ventricular function depends primarily on the extent to which the right ventricular inflow portion is atrialized and on the magnitude of tricuspid valve regurgitation.

CLINICAL MANIFESTATIONS. These are variable because the spectrum of pathology varies widely and because of the presence of associated malformations.[400] An interatrial communication consisting of a patent foramen ovale or an ostium secundum atrial septal defect is present in more than half the cases. The most common important associated defect is pulmonic stenosis or atresia. Other coexistent anomalies may include an ostium primum type of atrial septal defect and ventricular septal defect alone or in combination with other lesions. The Ebstein's lesion commonly is observed in associa-

tion with congenitally corrected transposition of the great arteries, in which the tricuspid valve is in the left atrioventricular orifice (p. 946). The usual manifestations in infancy are cyanosis, a cardiac murmur, and severe congestive heart failure. The magnitude of tricuspid regurgitation in the neonate is enhanced because the pulmonary vascular resistance is normally high early in life.[401] In this regard it may be difficult in some newborn infants with Ebstein's anomaly and massive tricuspid regurgitation to distinguish between organic pulmonic atresia and the presence of elevated perinatal pulmonary vascular resistance.[402] In such infants retrograde aortography is quite likely to fill the pulmonary root and allow visualization of the pulmonic valve by way of a patent ductus arteriosus, serving to differentiate a normal from an abnormal pulmonary outflow tract.[403] The tricuspid regurgitation in infants with Ebstein's anomaly may lessen substantially, and cyanosis may disappear early in life as pulmonary vascular resistance falls, only to recur at a later age when right ventricular dysfunction and/or paroxysmal arrhythmias develop. In some infants with Ebstein's malformation, cyanosis is suddenly intensified as the degree of pulmonary hypoperfusion is unmasked by spontaneous closure of a patent ductus arteriosus.

Beyond infancy the onset of symptoms is insidious; the most common complaints are exertional dyspnea, fatigue, and cyanosis. About 25 per cent of patients suffer episodes of paroxysmal atrial tachycardia. A prominent systolic pulsation of the liver and a large v wave in the jugular venous pulse accompany the systolic thrill and murmur of tricuspid regurgitation. Wide splitting of the first and second heart sounds and prominent third and fourth heart sounds may produce a characteristically rhythmic auscultatory cadence with a triple, quadruple, or quintuple combination of sounds.

LABORATORY FINDINGS. The *electrocardiographic abnormalities* commonly fall into two categories: those with a right bundle branch block pattern and those with the Wolff-Parkinson-White syndrome (Fig. 32–10, p. 972). The pattern in the latter is almost always type B, resembling left bundle branch block with predominant S waves in the right precordial leads. The presence of the Wolff-Parkinson-White pattern increases the risk of supraventricular paroxysmal tachycardia.[404] The electrocardiogram most often shows giant P waves, a prolonged P-R interval, and prolonged terminal QRS depolarization, producing variable degrees of right bundle branch block. These distinctive findings help to distinguish Ebstein's anomaly from other forms of right ventricular dysplasia whose presenting problem often is an arrhythmia. *Roentgenographic* (Figs. 8–42C, p. 230, and 32–6, p. 970) and fluoroscopic studies usually demonstrate an enlarged right atrium, a small right ventricle, and a pulmonary artery with reduced pulsations; the pulmonary vascularity may be reduced if a large right-to-left shunt is present.

The principal *echocardiographic findings* observed in patients with this anomaly, as well as in those with other forms of right ventricular volume overload, are an increase in right ventricular dimension, paradoxical ventricular septal motion, an increase in tricuspid valve excursion, and an abnormal closing velocity of the tricuspid valve. More specific findings for Ebstein's anomaly include a delay in tricuspid valve closure relative to mitral closure and a decrease in the E-F slope of the tricuspid valve, an abnormal anterior position of the tricuspid valve during diastole, and the detection of tricuspid valve echoes with more lateral placement of the transducer than usual.[405] Two-dimensional echocardiographic techniques are superior for observation of the inferior and leftward displacement of the tricuspid valve and simultaneously demonstrate the abnormal positional relation between the tricuspid and mitral valves (Figs. 31–56 and 4–69, p. 91).[402,405] Moreover, the boundaries of the atrialized right ventricle may be defined. Specific diagnosis requires identification, usually from an apical four-chamber view, of displacement of the septal tricuspid leaflet.[406] Tricuspid regurgitation, if present, is detected by Doppler examination.

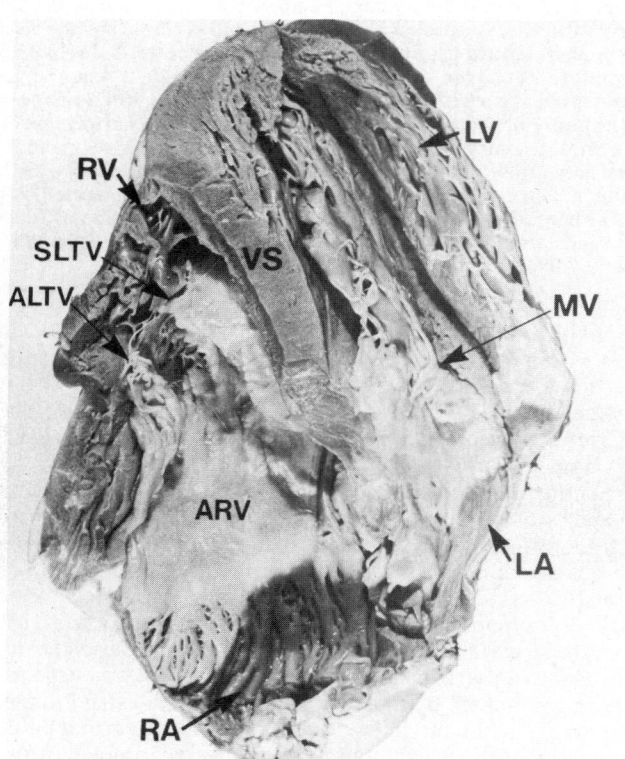

FIGURE 31–55. Anatomical specimen of Ebstein's anomaly of the tricuspid valve, cut in the same plane as an apical four-chamber echocardiographic view (Fig. 31–56). The septal and anterior leaflets of the tricuspid valve (SLTV, ALTV) are displaced into the right ventricle (RV), producing a large atrialized right ventricle (ARV). VS = ventricular septum, RA = right atrium, LA = left atrium, MV = mitral valve, LV = left ventricle. (Courtesy of Thomas DiSessa, M.D.)

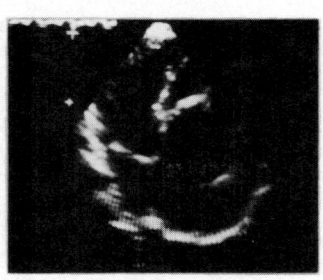

FIGURE 31–56. Apical four-chamber view of Ebstein's anomaly, corresponding to the anatomical specimen in Figure 31–55. RA = right atrium, LA = left atrium, MV = mitral valve, LV = left ventricle, TV = tricuspid valve, ARV = atrialized right ventricle, RV = right ventricle. (Courtesy of Thomas DiSessa, M.D.)

At *cardiac catheterization* the intracavitary electrocardiogram recorded just proximal to the tricuspid valve shows a right ventricular type of complex, while the pressure recorded is that of the right atrium (Fig. 31–57). A right-to-left atrial shunt normally is present. The hemodynamic findings depend on the degree of tricuspid regurgitation. The cardiac muscle is unusually irritable, and a high incidence of significant arrhythmias during catheterization has been noted. Selective right ventricular *angiocardiography* shows the position of the displaced tricuspid valve, the size of the right ventricle, and the configuration of the outflow portion of the right ventricle.

MANAGEMENT. Ebstein's anomaly may be compatible with a relatively long and active life, with most patients surviving into the third decade.[400,407] In some disabled patients moderate improvement has resulted from anastomosis of the superior vena cava to the right pulmonary artery (the Glenn procedure) to divert systemic venous return from the right atrium and to increase pulmonary blood flow. Benefit has resulted in older patients from replacement or repair of the tricuspid valve and closure of the atrial defect with or without ligation and marsupialization of the thin atrialized portion of the right ventricle.[408,409,409a] In patients with a preexcitation syndrome (p. 693) that is producing life-threatening rhythm disturbances the accessory conduction pathways should be divided. It should be recognized, however, that patients with Ebstein's anomaly are poor surgical risks at all ages.

The term *transposition* identifies a group of malformations that have in common abnormal relation between the cardiac chambers and great arteries. In this chapter the term is used to include both anomalous insertion of the pulmonary veins and cardiac malpositions.

COMPLETE TRANSPOSITION OF THE GREAT ARTERIES
(See also p. 946)

MORPHOLOGY. This is a common and potentially lethal form of heart disease in newborns and infants.[410] The malformation consists of the origin of the aorta arising from the morphological right ventricle and that of the pulmonary artery from the morphological left ventricle. With rare exceptions there is no fibrous continuity between the aortic and mitral valves. The origin of the aorta usually is to the right and anterior to, but may be lateral to, the main pulmonary artery. Thus, dextro- or D-transposition is a term often used interchangeably with complete transposition. The embryogenesis of complete transposition of the great arteries is controversial. There is consensus that the ventricular origins of the great arteries are reversed after development of a straight rather than a spiral infundibulotruncal septum. Transposition appears to result from a transfer of the pulmonary artery, instead of the aorta, from the heart tube's outlet zone to the left ventricle.[410a] The latter may result from maldevelopment of the infundibulum, or a combination of both infundibulum maldevelopment and truncal malseptation; the former results if the subpulmonary, rather than the subaortic, infundibulum is absorbed.

The anatomical arrangement results in two separate and parallel circulations. Some communication between the two circulations must exist after birth to sustain life; otherwise, unoxygenated systemic venous blood is directed inappropriately to the systemic circulation and oxygenated pulmonary venous blood is directed to the pulmonary circulation. Almost all patients have an interatrial communication (Fig. 31–58). Two-thirds have a patent ductus arteriosus, and about one-third have an associated ventricular septal defect. Complete transposition occurs more frequently in the offspring of diabetic mothers and more often in males than in females. Without treatment, about 30 per cent of these infants die within the first week of life, 50 per cent within the first month, 70 per cent within 6 months, and 90 per cent within the first year.[410] Those who live beyond infancy have, as a general rule, either

FIGURE 31–57. With a catheter in the "atrialized" portion of the right ventricle (RV), the intracardiac electrocardiogram in a patient with Ebstein's anomaly continues to show a ventricular complex, while right atrial pressure (RA) is recorded at the same site. (Courtesy of Delores A. Danilowicz, M.D.)

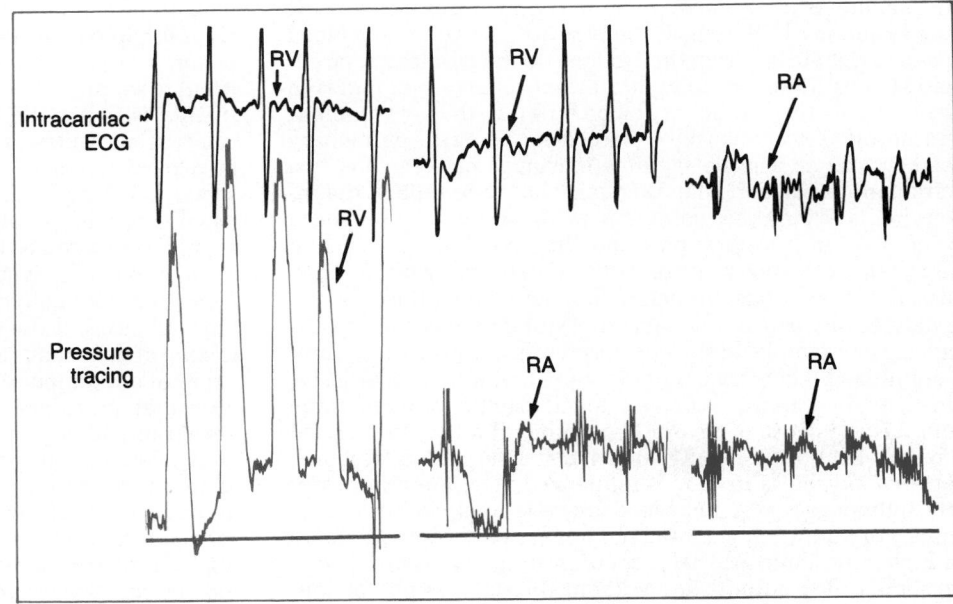

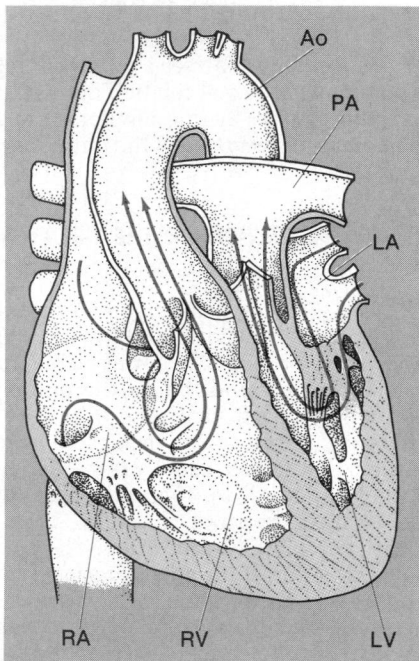

FIGURE 31-58. Complete transposition of the great arteries. Intercirculatory mixing occurs only at the atrial level. RA = right atrium; LA = left atrium; RV = right ventricle; LV = left ventricle; Ao = aorta; PA = pulmonary artery.

an isolated large atrial septal defect or a single ventricle, or ventricular septal defect and pulmonic stenosis. Current aggressive medical and surgical approaches to this group of patients have transformed the prognosis for an infant with this malformation from hopeless to hopeful.

The *clinical course* is determined by the degree of tissue hypoxia, the ability of each ventricle to sustain an increased workload in the presence of reduced coronary arterial oxygenation, the nature of the associated cardiovascular anomalies, and the anatomical and functional status of the pulmonary vascular bed.[411] A bidirectional shunt is always present because continuous unidirectional shunting would result in a progressive depletion of the circulating volume in either the pulmonary or the systemic vascular bed.

HEMODYNAMICS. A major determinant of the systemic arterial oxygen saturation is the amount of blood exchanged between the two circulations by intercirculatory shunts. The net volume of blood passing left to right from the pulmonary to the systemic circulation represents the anatomical left-to-right shunt and is in fact the effective systemic blood flow (i.e., the amount of oxygenated pulmonary venous return reaching the systemic capillary bed). Conversely, the volume of blood passing right to left from the systemic to the pulmonary circulation constitutes the anatomical right-to-left shunt and is in fact the effective pulmonary blood flow (i.e., the net volume of unsaturated systemic venous return perfusing the pulmonary capillary bed). The net volume exchange between the two circulations per unit time is equal. The magnitude of the intercirculatory mixing volume is modified by the number of intercirculatory communications that exist, the presence of associated obstructive intracardiac and extracardiac anomalies, the extent of the bronchopulmonary circulation, and the relation between pulmonary and systemic vascular resistance. For example, in the newborn with an intact ventricular septum and a constricted or closed patent ductus arteriosus, inadequate mixing through a small patent foramen ovale often is the cause of severe hypoxemia. If a large interatrial communication or a ventricular septal defect exists, systemic arterial oxygen saturation is influenced more importantly by the pulmonary–systemic blood flow relation than by the adequacy of mixing; augmented pulmonary blood flow produces a higher systemic arterial saturation if the left ventricle can sustain a high-output state without the intervention of con-

gestive heart failure and pulmonary edema. The systemic arterial oxygen saturation will be quite low, despite adequate intercirculatory mixing sites, if pulmonary blood flow is reduced by left ventricular outflow tract obstruction or increased pulmonary vascular resistance.

Infants with complete transposition of the great arteries are particularly susceptible to the early development of *pulmonary vascular obstructive disease.*[52,412] Severe morphological alterations develop in the pulmonary vascular bed by the age of 1 or 2 years in almost all patients with an associated large ventricular septal defect or large patent ductus arteriosus in the absence of obstruction to left ventricular outflow. Advanced pulmonary vascular disease also is seen within this same time frame in 5 to 10 per cent of patients without a patent ductus arteriosus and with an intact ventricular septum. Systemic arterial hypoxemia, increased pulmonary blood flow, and pulmonary hypertension contribute to the development of pulmonary vascular obstruction in these patients as they do in other forms of congenital heart disease. Among the additional factors implicated in the accelerated and more widespread pulmonary vascular obstruction found in patients with complete transposition is the presence of extensive bronchopulmonary anastomotic channels, which enter the pulmonary vascular bed proximal to the pulmonary capillary bed; thus, oxygen tension is reduced at the precapillary level, causing pulmonary vasoconstriction.[413] Beyond the early neonatal period many patients have an abnormal distribution pattern of pulmonary blood flow, with preferential flow to the right lung.[414] The asymmetrical distribution of pulmonary blood flow in these individuals results from an abnormal rightward inclination of the main pulmonary artery in the transposition malformation that favors flow from the main to the right pulmonary artery. Persistently increased pulmonary blood flow to the right lung would be expected to contribute to pulmonary vascular obstructive changes within the lung; in the left pulmonary vascular bed, thrombotic changes may occur because of the combination of reduced flow and polycythemia. Finally, it should be recognized that a prenatal alteration in pulmonary vascular smooth muscle may exist, since blood perfusing the fetal lungs in complete transposition of great arteries has a higher than normal pO_2 and may serve to dilate pulmonary vessels in utero. Postnatally such vessels may have an enhanced capacity to constrict in response to vasoactive stimuli and suffer anatomical, obliterative changes.

CLINICAL FINDINGS. Average birthweight and size of infants born with complete transposition of the great arteries are greater than normal. The usual clinical manifestations are dyspnea and cyanosis from birth, progressive hypoxemia, and congestive heart failure. Early in postnatal life the clinical manifestations and course are influenced principally by the magnitude of intercirculatory mixing. The most severe cyanosis and hypoxemia are observed in infants with only a small patent foramen ovale or ductus arteriosus and an intact ventricular septum in whom mixing is inadequate, or in those infants with relatively reduced pulmonary blood flow because of left ventricular outflow tract obstruction.[415,416] With a large persistent patent ductus arteriosus or a large ventricular septal defect, cyanosis may be minimal and heart failure is the usual dominant problem after the first few weeks of life.[410] It should be recognized that a patent ductus arteriosus is present in about half of newborn infants with transposition, although it closes functionally and anatomically soon after birth in almost all cases. If the ductus arteriosus remains open, better mixing of the venous and arterial circulations usually is at the expense of pulmonary artery hypertension.[417]

Cardiac murmurs are of little diagnostic significance and are absent or insignificant in about 30 to 50 per cent of infants with complete transposition of the great arteries and an intact ventricular septum. In infants with a large persistent patent ductus arteriosus, fewer than half exhibit physical signs typical of ductus arteriosus, such as continuous murmur, bounding pulses, or a prominent middiastolic rumble. Moreover, *differential cyanosis* caused by reversed pulmonary-to-sys-

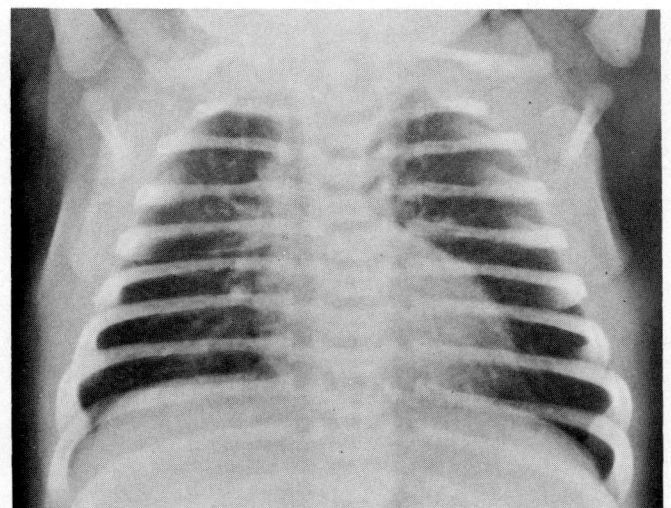

FIGURE 31-59. Chest roentgenogram in a 4-day-old infant with complete transposition of the great arteries showing an oval-shaped heart with a narrow base and increased pulmonary vascular markings.

anteriorly or posteriorly. A subaortic obstruction may be created by anterior shifting of the infundibular septum, whereas a posterior shift may narrow the subpulmonary area. The nature of left ventricular outflow tract obstruction may be further identified as a fixed obstruction caused by a fibromuscular ridge or as a dynamic obstruction caused by deviation of the interventricular septum toward the left ventricular cavity and the apposition between a thickened interventricular septum and systolic anterior motion of the mitral valve.[422,423]

CARDIAC CATHETERIZATION AND ANGIOCARDIOGRAPHY. Infants with simple, complete transposition of the great arteries who present in the first few weeks of life to a center prepared to correct the anomaly by the arterial switch operation (see below) often are taken to the operating room shortly after two-dimensional echocardiography and Doppler examination are performed.[422a] In these cases, transcatheter balloon atrial septostomy is not performed unless a delay is expected in taking the patient to the operating room. In essentially all other patients, cardiac catheterization and angiography are components of the initial evaluation of the patient.

The diagnostic portion of the cardiac catheterization allows confirmation of the anatomical derangement of the great ar-

temic shunting across the ductus arteriosus is difficult to detect because of generalized arterial desaturation. In those infants with a large ventricular septal defect, a pansystolic murmur usually emerges within the first 7 to 10 days of life. In newborns with transposition and severe pulmonic stenosis or atresia, the clinical findings are similar to those in the infant with tetralogy of Fallot.

The most usual *electrocardiographic findings* include right-axis deviation, right atrial enlargement, and right ventricular hypertrophy, reflecting that the right ventricle is the systemic pumping chamber. Combined ventricular hypertrophy may be present in those patients with a large ventricular septal defect and elevated pulmonary blood flow. Isolated left ventricular hypertrophy is encountered rarely in patients with a ventricular septal defect and a hypoplastic right ventricle, in many of whom the tricuspid valve is displaced abnormally and straddles a ventricular septal defect. In the first days of life the chest x-ray may appear normal, particularly in infants with an intact ventricular septum. Thereafter, roentgenographic findings often are highly suggestive of the diagnosis,[418] and consist of (1) progressive cardiac enlargement in early infancy; (2) a characteristic oval or egg-shaped cardiac configuration in the anteroposterior view, and a narrow vascular pedicle created by superimposition of the aortic and pulmonary artery segments; and (3) increased pulmonary vascular markings (Fig. 31-59). A right aortic arch is seen in about 4 per cent of infants with an intact ventricular septum and 11 per cent of infants with a ventricular septal defect.

CT scanning (Fig. 11-17, p. 321) and MR imaging (Fig. 11-38, p. 331) may be helpful in diagnosis as well.

ECHOCARDIOGRAPHY. Two-dimensional echocardiography is extremely useful in the diagnosis of complete transposition of the great arteries.[419-422,422a] In sagittal cross sections the aorta is observed to ascend retrosternally in contrast to the normal posterior sweep of the pulmonary artery. With transverse short-axis cross-sectional imaging, the diagnosis is confirmed by demonstrating that the anterior great artery (the aorta) is to the right of the posterior great artery (pulmonary) or that the two arteries are visualized side by side (Fig. 31-60). Moreover, from this plane the course of the two great arteries may be traced to delineate their ventricle of origin, demonstrating that the anterior rightward vessel (aorta) originates from the right ventricle and the posterior leftward vessel (pulmonary artery) originates from the left ventricle (Fig. 31-61). Echocardiography also may assist in identifying associated defects. Ventricular septal defects may be localized to the membranous, atrioventricular, and trabecular muscular septa, and malalignment types of ventricular septal defects may be identified if the infundibular septum is shifted either

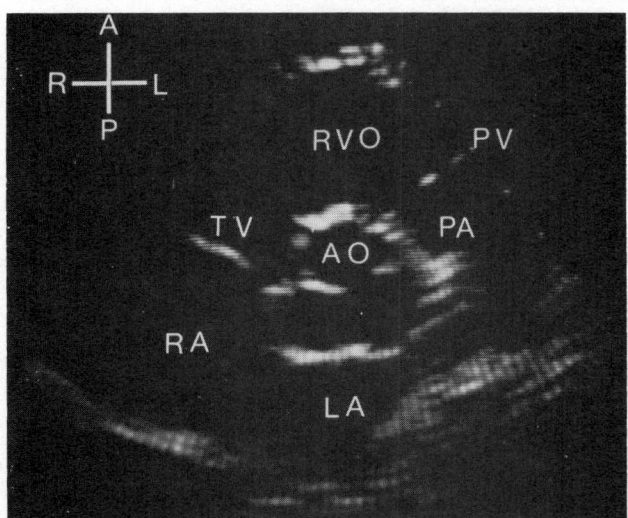

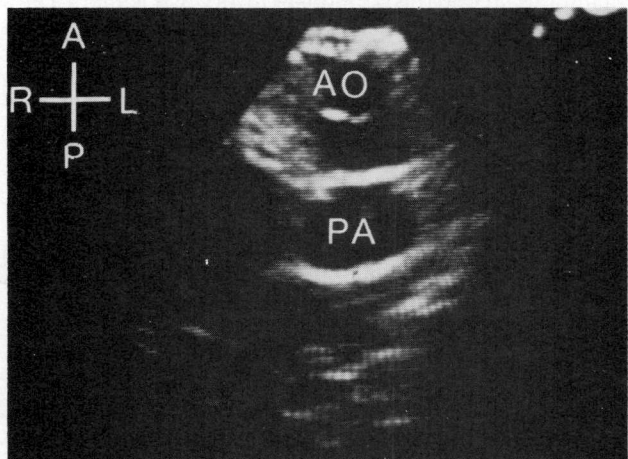

FIGURE 31-60. *Top*, A two-dimensional echocardiographic short-axis scan demonstrates normal great artery relations. The right ventricular outflow tract (RVO) wraps around the aorta (AO) in a clockwise manner. The pulmonic valve (PV) is to the left of the aortic valve. *Bottom*, Short-axis scan shows the abnormal great artery relations in an infant with transposition of the great arteries. The aorta (AO) is directly anterior and slightly to the right of the pulmonary artery (PA). The clockwise partial encirclement of the aorta by the right ventricular outflow tract is no longer observed. A = anterior, L = left, P = posterior, R = right, LA = left atrium, RA = right atrium, TV = tricuspid valve.

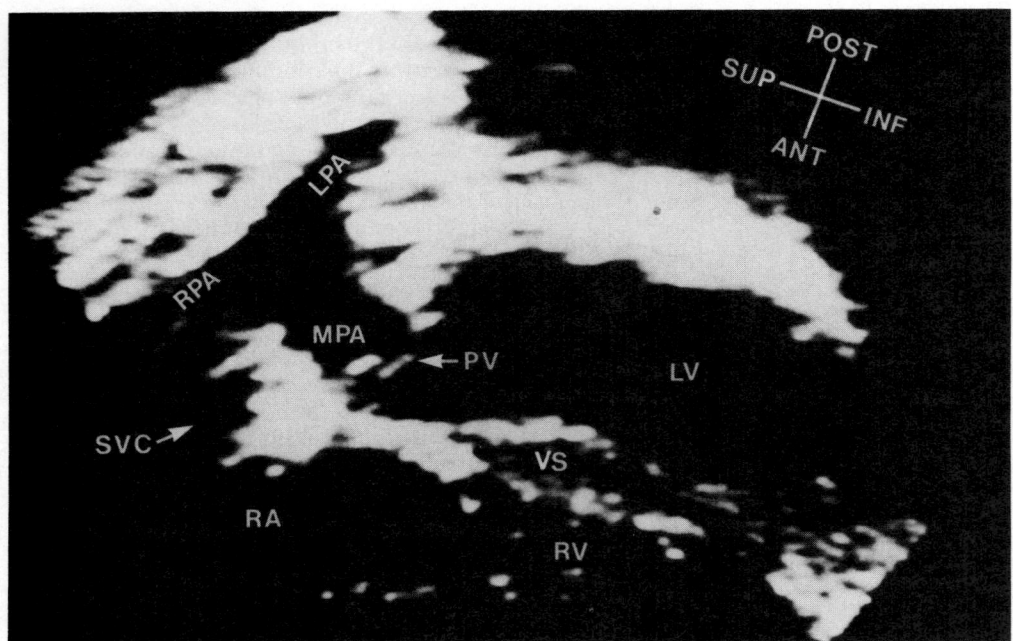

FIGURE 31–61. Complete transposition of the great arteries in a subcostal long-axis view with anterior transducer tilt. The main pulmonary artery (MPA) is seen exiting the left ventricle (LV) and bifurcating into its right and left branches (RPA, LPA). SVC = superior vena cava, RA = right atrium, RV = right ventricle, VS = ventricular septum, PV = pulmonary valve. (Courtesy of Thomas DiSessa, M.D.)

teries and establishes the presence of associated lesions; in the newborn, unless prompt arterial switch repair is planned, as discussed above, it should always be accompanied by a palliative balloon atrial septostomy, which serves to enlarge the interatrial communication and improve oxygenation. In the older neonate, usually beyond age 3 weeks, thickening of the atrial septum may preclude satisfactory balloon septostomy. In these instances, transcatheter blade septostomy is the preferred approach to palliation. Two-dimensional echocardiography, with or without fluoroscopy, may be used as the imaging mode for both balloon and blade creation of an atrial septal defect.[424] Subcostal four-chamber and sagittal views image cardiac anatomy and catheter position during the procedure, substantially reducing radiation dosage.

Both the diagnostic and the palliative procedures can be performed by percutaneous entry into the femoral vein, umbilical vein catheterization, or direct cutdown into the femoral or saphenous vein. The catheter passes easily across the foramen ovale into the left atrium and left ventricle and may be manipulated into the pulmonary artery by means of a flow-directed balloon-guided catheter or by manipulation of a standard catheter bent in the form of a J loop within the left ventricle, with the tip pointed posteriorly to the pulmonary artery. When a large ventricular septal defect is present, a catheter often can be manipulated directly across it from the right ventricle into the pulmonary artery.

The major abnormal hemodynamic findings include right ventricular pressure at systemic levels and either a high or low left ventricular pressure, depending on pulmonary blood flow, pulmonary vascular resistance, and the presence or absence of left ventricular outflow tract obstructive lesions. Oxygen saturation in the aorta is lower than that in the pulmonary artery. Application of the Fick principle to the calculation of pulmonary and systemic blood flow rates in these patients is an important source of error. Assumed values of oxygen consumption are unreliable in the severely hypoxemic infant. Moreover, because systemic and particularly pulmonary arteriovenous oxygen differences may be quite reduced, small errors in oxygen saturation values result in large errors in flow calculations. Furthermore, because bronchial collaterals enter the pulmonary circuit at the precapillary level, a true mixed pulmonary artery saturation cannot be sampled; pulmonary blood flow is therefore overestimated when one uses a sample from the central pulmonary artery, and pulmonary vascular resistance values often are underestimated.

Selective Ventricular Angiography. This is diagnostic and demonstrates that the anteriorly placed aorta arises from the right ventricle and that the posteriorly placed pulmonary artery in continuity with the mitral valve arises from the left ventricle. The status of the ductus arteriosus and the site and size of a ventricular septal defect can be well visualized by angiography (Fig. 31–62). Interventricular defects posterior and inferior to the crista supraventricularis occur in about

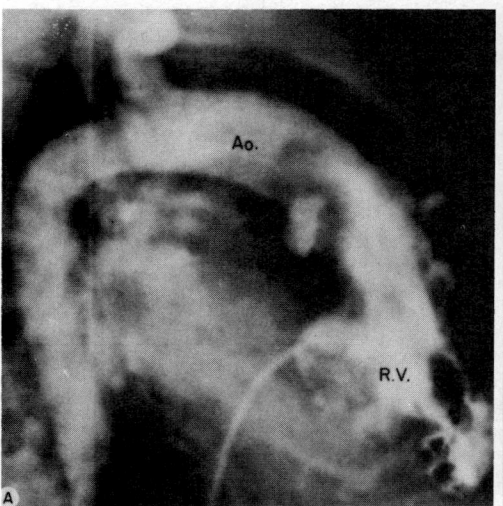

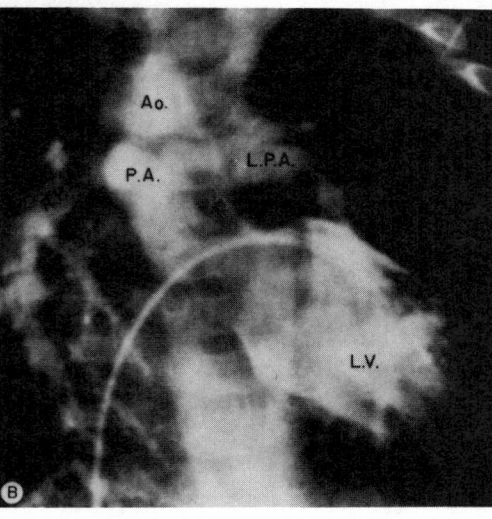

FIGURE 31–62. Lateral (A) and frontal (B) views of selective ventriculograms in a child with complete transposition of the great arteries and a ventricular septal defect (V.S.D.). Ao. = aorta, R.V. = right ventricle, P.A. = pulmonary artery, L.V. = left ventricle, R.P.A. = right pulmonary artery, L.P.A. = left pulmonary artery. (Courtesy of Delores A. Danilowicz, M.D.)

half of these patients; less often the defects are anterior and superior to the crista supraventricularis or are of the atrioventricular septal type.[425] A variety of lesions may be identified as the cause of left ventricular outflow tract obstruction, including ventricular septal hypertrophy with systolic anterior movement of the mitral valve, discrete or tunnel fibromuscular subpulmonic stenosis, valvular and supravalvular stenosis, and, rarely, an aneurysm of the membranous ventricular septum or redundant tricuspid valve tissue protruding through a ventricular septal defect.

A number of coronary arterial patterns are seen in patients with complete transposition of the great arteries.[426,427] In the majority, the left coronary artery originates in the left sinus and the right coronary artery originates in the posterior sinus, with single ostium above both the left and the posterior sinus. In almost 20 per cent of patients the left circumflex artery arises as a branch of the right coronary artery; a single coronary artery is present in about 6 per cent; in 3 to 4 per cent of patients either the right coronary and anterior descending arteries originate in the left sinus, with the left circumflex originating in the posterior sinus, or two ostia are present above one sinus, one giving rise to the right and the other to the left coronary artery.

MANAGEMENT. Medical treatment often is of limited help but should be vigorous since both functional and anatomical corrections of the malformation achieve good results. Conservative measures include the use of oxygen, digitalis, diuretics, iron (if an associated iron-deficiency anemia is present), and intravenous sodium bicarbonate for severe hypoxemic metabolic acidosis. Dilatation of the ductus arteriosus by prostaglandin E_1 in the early neonatal period both augments pulmonary blood flow and enhances intercirculatory mixing.[71] The creation or enlargement of an interatrial communication is the simplest procedure for providing increased intracardiac mixing of systemic and pulmonary venous blood; preferably this is achieved by rupturing the valve of the foramen ovale by balloon catheter during transseptal catheterization of the left side of the heart (Rashkind's procedure), or by blade septostomy. Surgical atrial septectomy seldom is required. The balloon should be inflated to a diameter of about 15 mm before pullback to the right atrium. Salutary results consist of a fall in left atrial pressure, equalization of mean left and right atrial pressures, and an increase in the systemic arterial oxygen saturation. When the foramen ovale is stretched by the balloon without accomplishing rupture of the septum primum valve of the fossa ovalis, the improvement in oxygenation is short-lived. Infusion or reinfusion intravenously of prostaglandin E_1 (0.05 to 0.1 mg/kg/min) has been shown to improve systemic oxygenation temporarily in the latter situation, by dilating the ductus arteriosus and thereby facilitating intercirculatory mixing.[71] Although balloon atrial septotomy usually is successful in stabilizing the infant's con-

dition and allowing survival in the neonatal period, the initial rise in systemic arterial oxygen saturation to 65 to 75 per cent often is not sustained beyond 6 to 9 months of age.

Surgical Treatment. The development of *corrective operations* for infants born with transposition of the great arteries has greatly improved prognosis.[428,428a] Intraatrial correction by the *Mustard* technique is accomplished by excision of the interatrial septum and creation of a new interatrial septum with a pericardial baffle diverting the systemic venous return into the left ventricle through the mitral valve and thence to the left ventricle and pulmonary artery, while the pulmonary venous blood is diverted through the tricuspid valve and right ventricle to the aorta.[428b] The *Senning* procedure is based on a similar principle and consists of diversion of left pulmonary venous blood by a coronary sinus flap and rerouting of caval flow by the use of an atrial wall flap.[428c] In medical centers in which the venous switch approach is preferred, the intraatrial corrective operation is performed at any age in patients with an intact ventricular septum who do not improve after balloon atrial septotomy. If palliative septotomy provides adequate relief of hypoxemia, the atrial rerouting operation is performed routinely in most infants with transposition of the great arteries and intact ventricular septum by 3 to 9 months of age, with a surgical mortality less than 5 per cent.[428] Clinical improvement usually is quite dramatic. In some patients postoperative complications are observed that are directly related to the intraatrial repair (shunts across the intraatrial patch and obstruction to either systemic or pulmonary venous return or both).[429] There is a high incidence of early and late postoperative dysrhythmias that are more likely to have their basis in injury to the sinoatrial node and/or its arterial supply than in disruption of internodal tracts or damage to the atrioventricular node.[430,431,431a] Tricuspid regurgitation is a less common complication of operation and may be related in some patients to a preexisting abnormality of the tricuspid valve, whereas in most it is related to right ventricular dysfunction.[432] Although the assessment of right ventricular contractility is difficult, it would appear that the right ventricular pump function is impaired before Mustard operation and does not return to normal after successful surgery.[433-438] It seems unlikely that the right ventricle can perform as a systemic pumping chamber for the duration of a normal life span.

A one-stage anatomical correction is now the approach of choice in major centers that care for infants with congenital heart disease.[428,439-443,443a] In this operation both coronary arteries are transposed to the posterior artery; the aorta and pulmonary arteries are transsected, contraposed, and anastomosed (Jatene operation) (Fig. 31-63). The arterial switch anatomical correction may be complicated by coronary ostial stenosis, acquired supravalvular aortic and/or pulmonary stenosis, and pulmonic and/or aortic incompetence. The major advantages of the arterial switch procedure, when com-

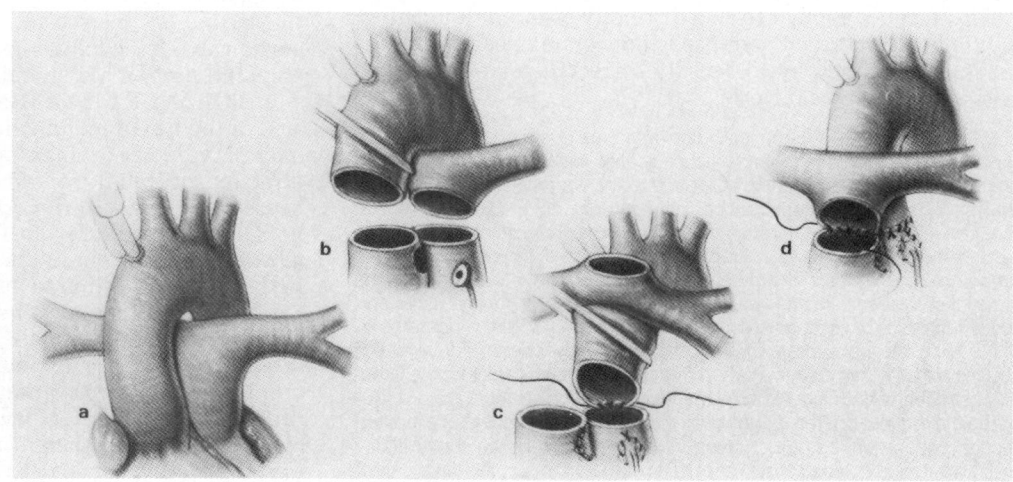

FIGURE 31–63. Complete transposition of the great arteries, corrected by a modified arterial switch operation. The aorta and pulmonary artery are transected and the orifices of the coronary arteries are excised with a rim of adjacent aortic wall (b). The aorta is brought under the bifurcation of the pulmonary artery, and the proximal pulmonary artery and the aorta are anastomosed without necessitating graft interposition. The coronary arteries are transferred to the pulmonary artery (c). The mobilized pulmonary artery is directly anastomosed to the proximal aortic stump (d). (From Stark, J., and DeLaval, M.: Surgery for Congenital Heart Defects. New York, Grune and Stratton, 1983, p. 379.)

pared with the atrial switch procedure, are the restoration of the left ventricle as the systemic pump and the potential for long-term maintenance of sinus rhythm.[444-450,450a]

Within the first month of life the arterial switch operation may be performed as a single-stage repair. In such patients, the origin and branching patterns of the coronary arteries are defined reliably preoperatively by two-dimensional echocardiography.[426] In older infants it appears necessary to prepare the left ventricle to withstand the systemic pressure which is produced after switching the great arteries, since, if the ventricular septum is intact, left ventricular pressure and left ventricular wall thickness diminish normally in relation to the postnatal reduction in pulmonary artery pressure. In these infants a two-stage approach is used, the first of which consists of banding the pulmonary artery; the arterial switch is performed soon thereafter, in some centers as early as 1 to 2 weeks later.[451]

In the unusual infant with an intact ventricular septum and a significant patent ductus arteriosus, an early intraatrial corrective operation with closure of the ductus is indicated at 4 to 6 months of age to prevent the likely progression of pulmonary vascular disease. Debate exists concerning the optimal management of patients with a large ventricular septal defect.[428] In some centers pulmonary artery banding is advocated early in life, followed by definitive intracardiac repair at 1 to 2 years of age. Others favor a one-stage intraatrial repair with patch closure of the ventricular septal defect before age 3 to 6 months. Still others perform an arterial switch anatomical correction within the first 3 to 4 months of age, unless the coronary arterial anatomy is considered unfavorable at operation.[440-442] Infants with transposition of the great arteries plus a ventricular septal defect and left ventricular outflow tract obstruction may require a systemic–pulmonary artery anastomosis when a pronounced diminution in pulmonary blood flow exists. A later corrective procedure for these patients bypasses the left ventricular outflow obstruction and uses an intracardiac ventricular baffle connecting the left ventricle to the aorta and an extracardiac prosthetic conduit between the right ventricle and the distal end of a divided pulmonary artery (Rastelli procedure).[440] In patients with significant pulmonary vascular obstructive disease the risk associated with definitive repair (anatomical correction or intraatrial baffle and closure of the ventricular septal defect) is great. In this group of patients a "palliative" Mustard or Senning procedure leaving the ventricular septal defect open often provides good, short-term, symptomatic improvement by increasing arterial oxygen tension and reducing the stimulus to progressive polycythemia.[452]

CONGENITALLY CORRECTED TRANSPOSITION OF THE GREAT ARTERIES
(See also p. 941)

This term is applied to two distinctly different anomalies: anatomically corrected transposition or malposition of the great arteries and physiologically corrected, levo- or L-transposition of the great arteries.

MORPHOLOGY. Anatomically corrected malposition of the great arteries is a rare form of congenital heart disease in which the great arteries are abnormally related to each other and to the ventricles but arise, nonetheless, above the anatomically correct ventricles.[453,454] Because of this, the term malposition, rather than transposition, is preferable. The anomaly results from either leftward looping of the ventricular segment of the embryonic heart tube in the situs solitus heart, or rightward looping in the situs inversus heart. In this unusual malformation the aorta is anterior and to the left (levo- or L-malposition) and the pulmonary artery is posteromedial and to the right, presumably because of a subaortic conus which causes mitral-aortic discontinuity. When no other defect exists, the circulation proceeds normally. When an associated lesion prompts echocardiographic examination, the diagnosis is indicated by the finding of atrioventricular concordance in association with wide mitral-aortic discontinuity with an anteriorly placed aorta. At cardiac catheterization, the diagnosis of the abnormal relation between the great arteries may be made by biplane angiocardiography. Anomalies commonly associated with anatomically corrected malposition of the great arteries include ventricular septal defect, left juxtaposition of the atrial appendages, tricuspid atresia or stenosis, and valvular and subvalvular pulmonic stenosis.

DEFINITION. Invariably, the term congenitally corrected transposition is applied to the heart in which a functional correction of the circulation exists by virtue of the relation between the ventricles and great arteries.[455,456] Corrected or L-transposition occurs when the primitive cardiac tube loops to the left, instead of to the right, during embryogenesis.[457] The anatomical right ventricle comes to lie on the left and receives oxygenated blood from the left atrium; this blood is ejected into an anteriorly placed, left-sided aorta. The anatomical left ventricle lies to the right and connects the right atrium to a posteriorly placed pulmonary artery. Thus, there are both ventriculoarterial and atrioventricular discordant connections, with ventricular inversion. This arrangement of the great arteries and ventricles (in contrast to the uncorrected, complete, or D-transposition) permits functional correction, so that systemic venous blood passes into the pulmonary trunk while arterialized pulmonary venous blood flows into the aorta. In the heart with congenitally corrected transposition, the venae cavae and coronary sinus drain into a right atrium that is normal in position and structure.

Venous blood flows from the right atrium, designated as the "venous atrium," across an atrioventricular valve that has the structure of a normal mitral valve and into the right-sided "venous ventricle." The venous ventricle, however, has the morphological characteristics of a normal left ventricle, i.e., its interior lining is trabeculated, it has no crista supraventricularis, and the atrioventricular valve is in continuity with the posteriorly placed semilunar valve. It ejects blood into the pulmonary trunk, which arises posterior to the ascending aorta. Oxygenated blood returns from the lungs to the left atrium, which is normal in position and structure; from here it flows into the left-sided "arterial ventricle" across an atrioventricular valve that has the structure of a normal tricuspid valve. The interior lining of the arterial ventricle has the morphological characteristics of a normal right ventricle (i.e., it has coarse trabeculations and a crista supraventricularis), and the tricuspid atrioventricular valve is not in continuity with the anteriorly placed semilunar valve. The arterial ventricle ejects blood into the aorta, which arises anterior to the pulmonary trunk. In addition to inversion of the cardiac ventricles, there is inversion of the conduction system and coronary arteries. Commonly associated anatomical lesions include atrial and ventricular septal defects, often accompanied by valvular or subvalvular pulmonary stenosis; single ventricle with an outlet chamber with or without pulmonic stenosis; left atrioventricular valve regurgitation, usually because of an Ebstein's malformation of the left-sided tricuspid valve; and abnormalities of visceral and atrial situs.[458]

CLINICAL MANIFESTATIONS. The clinical presentation, course, and prognosis of patients with congenital functionally corrected transposition vary, depending on the nature and severity of the complicating intracardiac anomalies.[458,459] Patients in whom corrected transposition exists as an isolated anomaly present no functional alterations and have no symptoms. Asymptomatic children with an increase in the size of the systemic ventricle, due to significant left-to-right shunting or tricuspid regurgitation, usually develop symptoms of systemic ventricular dysfunction by the third or fourth decade.[458-461]

The physical findings in congenitally corrected transposition are those of the associated lesions with two exceptions: (1) a single accentuated second heart sound usually is present in the second left intercostal space, representing closure of the aortic valve lying lateral and anterior to the pulmonic valve; and (2) there is a high incidence of cardiac dysrhythmias

LABORATORY EXAMINATION. Because of the inversion of the heart's conduction system, the electrocardiogram may provide important clues in the diagnosis. An abnormal direction of initial (septal) depolarization from right to left causes leftward, anterior, and superior orientation of the initial QRS forces and reversal of the precordial Q-wave pattern (Q waves are present in the right precordial leads and absent in the left). In addition to inversion of the conduction system, the His bundle is elongated because of the greater distance between the atrioventricular node and the base of the ventricular septum.[462] The His bundle is located beneath the pulmonic valve in the position of mitral pulmonary continuity; thus, it is subject to significant excursions during mitral valve closure. This arrangement may be a causal factor in the arrhythmias and atrioventricular conduction disturbances commonly observed in these patients. First-degree atrioventricular (AV) block occurs in about 50 per cent, and complete AV block occurs in 10 to 15 per cent of patients. Other degrees of AV dissociation may be observed as well as paroxysmal supraventricular tachycardia and ventricular extrasystoles. In some patients, Kent bundle connections provide the anatomical substrate for preexcitation.[463]

Roentgenographic examination characteristically reveals absence of the normal pulmonary artery segment and a smooth convexity of the left supracardiac border produced by the displaced ascending aorta (Fig. 8–42B, p. 230). The latter may be visualized by radionuclide scintillation scans of the central circulation. The main pulmonary trunk is medially displaced and absent from the cardiac silhouette; the right pulmonary hilus often is prominent and elevated compared with the left, producing a right-sided "waterfall" appearance.

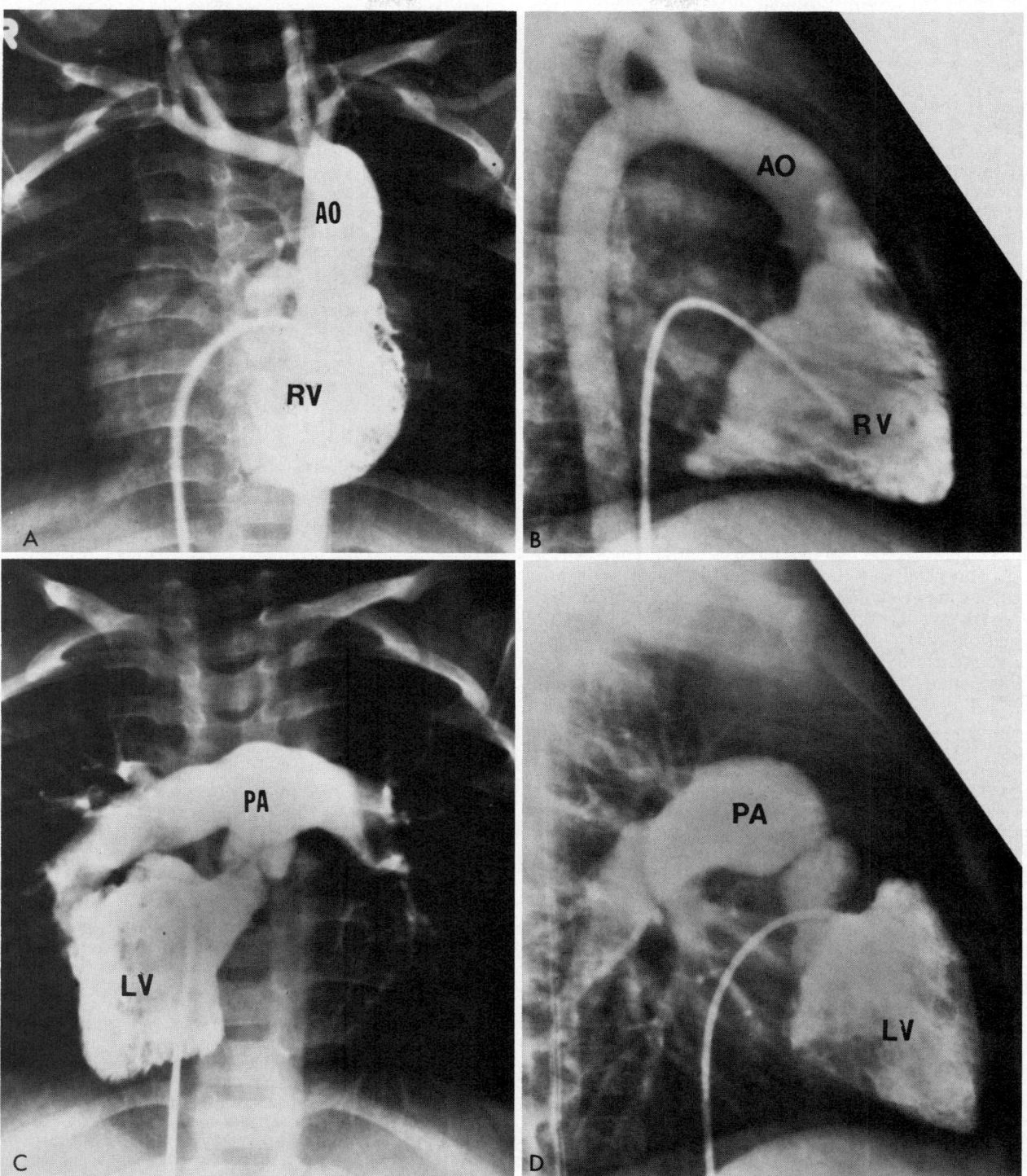

FIGURE 31–64. Congenitally corrected (levo-)transposition of the great arteries in a 4-year-old boy. *A*, Anteroposterior ventriculogram in left-sided ventricle with mesocardia. The morphological right ventricle (RV) is left-sided, indicating an L-ventricular loop (inverted ventricles in situs solitus). The aorta (AO) originates above the morphological right ventricle and is thus transposed and in the classic levo-transposition position. *B*, Lateral ventriculogram is left-sided ventricle (same frame as *A*). The aorta originates anteriorly above the morphological right ventricle (RV). *C*, Anteroposterior ventriculogram in right-sided morphological left ventricle (LV). The transposed pulmonary artery (PA) arises from this ventricle, and the ventricular septum appears intact. Pulmonic valve thickening is also evident. The aorta *(A)* is to the left of the pulmonary artery. Note that the ventricular septum in the L-ventricular loop is visualized best in the anteroposterior views. *D*, Lateral ventriculogram in right-sided ventricle (same frame as *C*). The pulmonary artery is posterior to the aorta, and supravalvular pulmonic narrowing is seen. (From Freedom, R. M., et al.: The differential diagnosis of levo-transposed or malposed aorta. An angiocardiographic study. Circulation 50:1040, 1974, by permission of the American Heart Association, Inc.)

Two-dimensional echocardiography seeks to identify the morphology of each ventricle by defining the characteristics of the inflow and outflow tracts and papillary and trabecular muscle morphology, ventricular shape, and great artery position.[464] By tracing the great arteries back to their ventricles of origin in subxiphoid and parasternal short-axis planes, one would find that the anterior leftward great artery (the aorta) arises from the left-sided ventricle and is not in continuity with the left-sided atrioventricular valve. The great arteries exit the heart in parallel fashion; the position, origin, and branching pattern of the great arteries are observed in subxiphoid and suprasternal views, while the anteroposterior and right-left positions of the great arteries can be seen from the parasternal short-axis view. Because the ventricular septum lies in the anteroposterior plane parallel to the echo beam, it may not be visualized from a left parasternal view. In apical-basal or subxiphoid, four-chamber echocardiographic views, the right and left ventricular morphology and the inverted position of the atrioventricular valves may be ascertained correctly. The latter views also demonstrate the level of attachment of the atrioventricular valves and allow detection of inferior displacement of the left-sided tricuspid valve when Ebstein's anomaly coexists.

At *cardiac catheterization* the diagnosis should be suspected when the venous catheter enters a posterior and midline main pulmonary trunk. Retrograde arterial catheter passage establishes the typical position of the ascending aorta at the upper left cardiac border. Hemodynamic abnormalities depend on the lesions associated with corrected transposition. Selective *angiocardiography* allows visualization of the transposed great arteries and morphological differentiation of the two ventricles (Fig. 31–64). The ventricles usually lie side by side, with the ventricular septum oriented in an anteroposterior direction. Selective aortography demonstrates the inverted coronary arterial pattern that is invariably present in corrected transposition. The competence of the left atrioventricular valve may be determined by injection of contrast material into the arterial ventricle.[465] When a left-sided Ebstein's malformation exists, the leaflets are displaced distal to the true valve annulus. The level of the annulus may be determined by visualization of the circumflex branch of the left coronary artery, which courses posteriorly in the AV groove.

Specific problems have attended operative repair of the lesions associated with congenitally corrected transposition, owing primarily to the course of the atrioventricular conduction system and the coronary arterial pattern.[466,467] Intraoperative electrophysiological mapping of the course of the conduction system has been proposed to reduce, but not abolish, the risk of surgically induced heart block. The AV bundle is located anteriorly and in relation to the anterolateral quadrant of the pulmonary outflow tract. Thus, when a ventricular septal defect is present, the bundle usually is related to the anterior and superior margins of the defect and lies beneath the pulmonic valve. In corrected transposition, the coronary arteries have a course appropriate to their ventricles, i.e., the anterior descending and circumflex arteries supply the morphological left ventricle, and the right coronary artery supplies the morphological right ventricle. However, because the great arteries are transposed, the noncoronary sinus is the anterior sinus of the aortic valve.

The inversion of the coronary arterial system occasionally may limit and preclude an incision into the venous ventricle, thereby interfering with exposure of intracardiac defects in the usual manner. The disadvantage in approaching intracardiac anomalies using an incision in the morphological right ventricle is that this is the systemic ventricle. When significant pulmonary stenosis exists with a ventricular septal defect, a valved extracardiac conduit often is a required part of the surgical repair. Surgical risks are especially high in patients in whom significant regurgitation exists from the arterial ventricle to the arterial atrium. In these patients, annuloplasty, or more usually valve replacement, is required. In all operative approaches, if complete heart block has been present intermittently or permanently preoperatively or intraoperatively, permanent epicardial atrial and ventricular pacemaker leads are implanted.

DOUBLE-OUTLET RIGHT VENTRICLE

MORPHOLOGY. Other designations applied to this lesion include origin of both great arteries from the right ventricle, partial transposition, complete transposition of the aorta and levo-position of the pulmonary

artery, complete dextroposition of the aorta, and the Taussig-Bing complex. This is an extremely heterogeneous category of malformations in which an abnormal relation exists between the aorta and the pulmonary trunk, which arise wholly or in large part from the right ventricle.[468,470]

A uniform definition or classification of double-outlet right ventricle does not exist.[469] To some, double-outlet right ventricle means origin of one great artery and at least 50 per cent of the other over the right ventricle; others require the presence of bilateral conus muscle between both great arteries and the atrioventricular annulus. One or both great arteries may arise from an infundibular chamber; there may be considerable variability in the amount of subarterial conus muscle. Thus, the semilunar valves may lie side by side, or with the pulmonary valve more anterior and superior, or with a more anterior and superior aortic valve. A malalignment type of ventricular septal defect is almost always present in double-outlet right ventricle because the infundibular septum is positioned abnormally. When the amount of conus muscle beneath the two great arteries varies, the ventricular septal defect commonly is positioned beneath the more posterior semilunar valve, which in fact usually overrides the interventricular septum through this ventricular septal defect. The amount of conus muscle underneath the valve determines the position of the semilunar root in relation to the ventricles below. Thus double-outlet right ventricle resides within the spectrum of conotruncal abnormalities ranging from tetralogy of Fallot to transposition of the great arteries. The ventricular septal defect occasionally extends beneath both great arteries and is referred to as doubly committed. In some instances, the ventricular septal defect is remote to both great arteries, or is considered uncommitted, in which case the defect often lies in the inlet or muscular portion of the interventricular septum.

More than half of patients with double-outlet right ventricle have associated anomalies of the atrioventricular valves.[471] Mitral atresia associated with a hypoplastic left ventricle is common; less often observed are tricuspid stenosis, Ebstein's anomaly of the tricuspid valve, complete atrioventricular septal defect, and overriding or straddling of either atrioventricular valve. Aortic coarctation may be associated with double-outlet right ventricle, particularly when the subaortic area is narrowed by malalignment of the infundibular septum. Double-outlet right ventricle also may be a component of the multiple cardiovascular anomalies of the splenic dysgenesis or heterotaxy syndromes. An increased incidence of the anomaly occurs in infants with the trisomy 18 syndrome.

The pathological features in most patients include side-by-side pulmonic and aortic valves and discontinuity between the mitral and aortic valves. The latter exists because muscular infundibulum is usual beneath both semilunar valves. The ventricular septal defect may be remote from or closely related to one or both semilunar valves (Fig. 31–65).[471] When the interventricular defect is subpulmonic, with or without a straddling pulmonary trunk, the complex is designated "Taussig-Bing." In most patients the interventricular septal defect is below the crista supraventricularis and is subaortic in location. Least often the defect either is remote from both semilunar valves ("uncommitted") or underlies both ("doubly committed").

CLINICAL MANIFESTATIONS. The clinical and physiological picture is determined by the size and location of the ventricular septal defect and the presence or absence of pulmonic stenosis. In the Taussig-Bing form of double-outlet right ventricle, the malformation resembles physiologically and clinically complete transposition with ventricular septal defect and pulmonary hypertension. When the ventricular septal defect is subaortic, the stream of blood from the left ventricle is directed preferentially to the aorta. Thus, there may be little or no detectable cyanosis, and these patients usually clinically resemble those with an isolated, large ventricular septal defect and pulmonary hypertension. The most important determinant of the natural history in both these types of double-outlet right ventricle is the progression of pulmonary vascular obstruction. In contrast, when there is pulmonary outflow tract obstruction, which often is severe and found commonly in those patients in whom the ventricular septal defect is subaortic, clinical findings are similar to those of cyanotic tetralogy of Fallot. In some patients, especially without pulmonic stenosis, the electrocardiogram shows a superiorly oriented counterclockwise frontal plane QRS loop in addition to right ventricular hypertrophy.[472] The pattern appears to result from relative hypoplasia of the anterosuperior left bundle and preferential activation of the posteroinferior left ventricular wall. The presence of the latter electrocardiographic pattern in patients with double-outlet right ventricle should raise the possibility of a coexistent atrioventricular septal defect or abnormality of the mitral valve.[471]

DIAGNOSIS. Two-dimensional *echocardiography* may reliably distinguish double-outlet right ventricle from other lesions causing cyanosis, such as tetralogy of Fallot and transposition of the great arteries.[469,473] The relative anteroposterior positions of the great arteries can be determined from the parasternal short-axis view. The parasternal long-axis view shows the position of the more posterior semilunar root relative to the interventricular septum and anterior mitral leaflet, and is the best view for demonstrating the presence of subarterial conus muscle. Subxiphoid

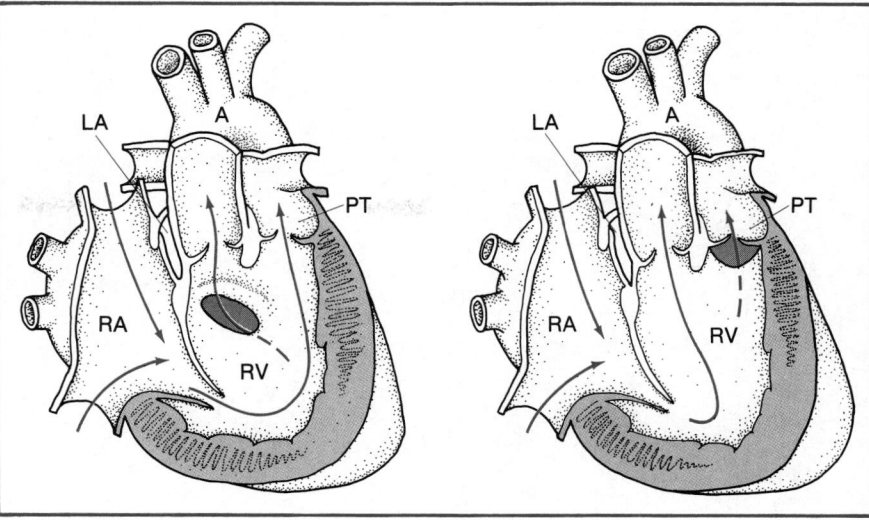

FIGURE 31–65. Double-outlet right ventricle (RV) with side-by-side relation of great arteries is illustrated in both panels. A subaortic ventricular septal defect (VSD) below the crista supraventricularis *(left)* favors delivery of left ventricular blood to the aorta (A). Location of the VSD above the crista *(right)* favors streaming to the pulmonary trunk (PT). LA = left atrium; RA = right atrium; PT = pulmonary trunk. (From Sridaromont, S., et al.: Double outlet right ventricle: Hemodynamic and anatomic correlations. Am. J. Cardiol. *38*:85, 1976.)

views best demonstrate the position of both great arteries over the ventricles. Each great artery is displayed on long- and short-axis subxiphoid sweeps. In reporting echocardiographic results, it is imperative to state each component anatomical feature, i.e., the position of both great arteries, the presence and amount of infundibulum under each semilunar valve, the anatomy of both subpulmonary and subaortic outflow tracts, the position and size of the associated ventricular septal defect, and the presence of all other associated lesions, particularly atrioventricular valve anomalies and coarctation of the aorta.

In each of the different types of double-outlet right ventricle, precise delineation of the malformation also depends on careful angiocardiographic analysis. The diagnosis can be established with confidence when the angiographic findings include simultaneous opacification of both great vessels from the right ventricle, aortic and pulmonic valves at the same transverse level, and separation of the aortic valve from the aortic leaflet of the mitral valve by the crista supraventricularis (Fig. 31–66).[474] The position of the ventricular septal defect and the relation between the great arteries must be defined to plan surgical procedures appropriately.

SURGICAL TREATMENT. In double-outlet right ventricle with subaortic ventricular septal defect, repair is accomplished by creating an intraventricular baffle that conducts left ventricular blood to the aorta.[475,476] When the ventricular septal defect is subpulmonic, repair is accomplished by use of one of three procedures: by creating an intraventricular conduit that conducts left ventricular blood to the pulmonary arteries and performing the Mustard or Senning procedure, by creating an intraventricular baffle directing left ventricular blood to the aorta and connecting the right ventricle to the pulmonary artery by use of a valve-containing conduit, or

by closure of the ventricular septal defect and arterial switch.[477–479] When the ventricular septal defect is doubly committed, i.e., both subaortic and subpulmonic, operation consists of creating an intraventricular baffle that conducts left ventricular blood to the aorta. The type of double-outlet right ventricle in which the ventricular septal defect is remote and uncommitted to either semilunar orifice may be approached by a venous switch operation, permitting the right ventricle to eject into the aorta, followed by placement of a conduit between the left ventricle and the pulmonary trunk. Alternatively, some patients may be candidates for a modified Fontan procedure (p. 939), particularly if additional findings include a common atrioventricular orifice, hypoplastic ventricles, a straddling tricuspid valve, or a straddling mitral valve.[477]

DOUBLE-OUTLET LEFT VENTRICLE

One of the rarest cardiac anomalies consists of the origin of both great arteries from the morphological left ventricle. Conal musculature or an infundibulum usually is absent or deficient beneath the orifices of both semilunar valves.[480] A broad spectrum of associated malformations exists. A ventricular septal defect and valvular or subvalvular pulmonic stenosis have been present in most patients. Angiocardiographic assessment of the spatial relations of the origins of the great arteries is essential to an accurate diagnosis and to evaluating the possibility of operative repair.[481]

TOTAL ANOMALOUS PULMONARY VENOUS CONNECTION

This anomaly has been estimated to account for 1 to 3 per cent of all cases of congenital heart disease and 2 per cent of deaths therefrom in the first year of life.[308,482] The anomaly is the result of persistence during embryogenesis of communications between the pulmonary portion of the foregut plexus and the cardinal or umbilicovitelline system of veins, resulting in the connection of all the pulmonary veins either to the right atrium directly or to the systemic veins and their tributaries. Because all venous blood returns to the right atrium, an interatrial communication is an integral part of this malformation. Additional major cardiac malformations occur in about 30 per cent of patients.[308] Among these are common atrium, single ventricle, truncus arteriosus, and anomalies of the systemic veins. Extracardiac malformations, particularly of the alimentary, endocrine, and genitourinary systems, are present in 25 to 30 per cent of cases.

MORPHOLOGY. The anatomical varieties of total anomalous pulmonary venous connection may be subdivided, depending on the level of the abnormal drainage (Fig. 31–67). Table 31–10 provides average figures of the distribution of the sites of anomalous connection.[308] The anomalous connection usually is supradiaphragmatic and to the left brachiocephalic vein, right atrium, coronary sinus, or superior vena cava. In about 13 per cent, particularly in males, the distal site of connection is below the diaphragm. In this situation a common trunk originates from the confluence of pulmonary veins and descends in front of the esophagus, penetrating the diaphragm through the esophageal hiatus. The anomalous trunk then connects into the portal vein or one of its tributaries, the ductus venosus, or, rarely, to one of the hepatic veins. In rare cases various combinations of anomalous connection occur in which drainage is to multiple levels.

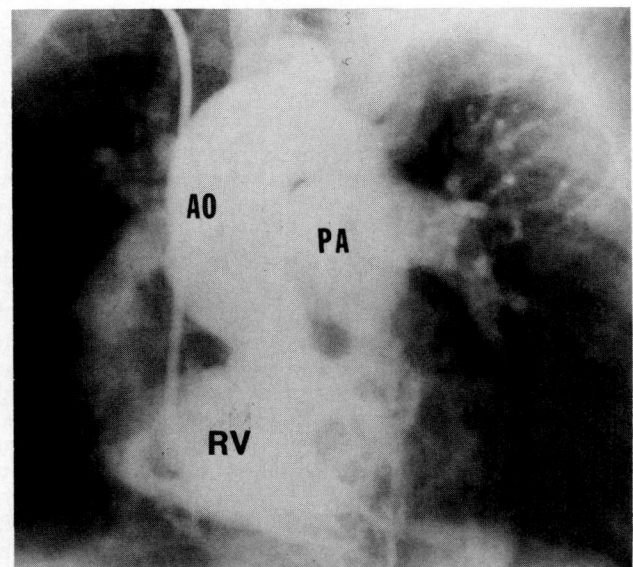

FIGURE 31–66. Simultaneous opacification of both great arteries from a right ventricular injection of contrast material in a patient with double-outlet right ventricle (RV). The aortic and pulmonic valves are at the same transverse level. AO = aorta, PA = pulmonary artery. (Courtesy of Robert White, M.D.)

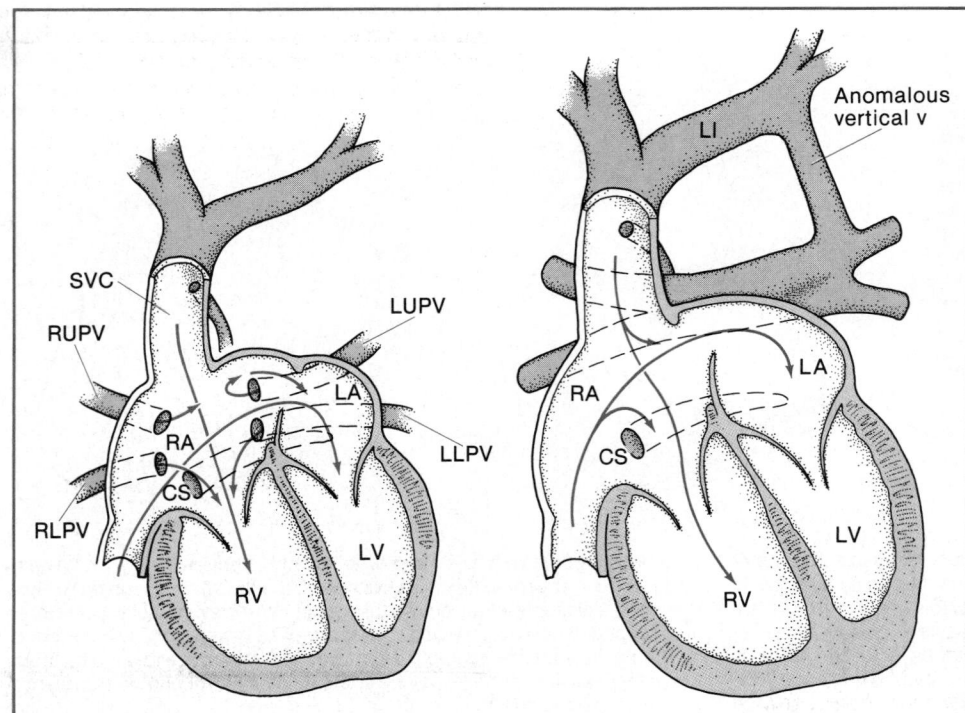

FIGURE 31–67. Two common types of total anomalous pulmonary venous connection are illustrated. These are connections to the right atrium *(left)* and to the left innominate vein *(right)*. S.V.C. = superior vena cava; I.V.C. = inferior vena cava; R.A. = right atrium; L.A. = left atrium; C.S. = coronary sinus; R.V. = right ventricle; L.V. = left ventricle; R.U.P.V. = right upper pulmonary veins; L.U.P.V. = left upper pulmonary veins; R.L.P.V. = right lower pulmonary veins; L.L.P.V. = left lower pulmonary veins; R.H. = right hepatic vein; L.H. = left hepatic vein; L.P.V. = left portal vein; R.P.V. = right portal vein; L.I. = left innominate vein. (From Wagenvoort, C. A., et al.: Pathology of the Pulmonary Vasculature. Springfield, Ill., Charles C Thomas, 1964.)

HEMODYNAMICS. The physiological consequences and, accordingly, the clinical picture depend on the size of the interatrial communication and on the magnitude of the pulmonary vascular resistance.[482] When the interatrial communication is small, systemic blood flow is markedly limited.[483] Right atrial and systemic venous pressures are elevated, and hepatic enlargement and peripheral edema are present. The size of the interatrial communication also is an important determinant in the development in utero and postnatally of the left atrium and left ventricle. Left atrial cavity size usually is somewhat reduced, whereas left ventricular volumes may be reduced or normal. The magnitude of pulmonary blood flow and therefore the ratio of oxygenated to unoxygenated blood that returns to the right atrium are a function of pulmonary vascular resistance. The arterial oxygen saturation, which ranges from markedly reduced to normal values, is inversely related to the pulmonary vascular resistance. In this regard, in most patients the principal determinant of pulmonary pressures and resistance is related less to augmented pulmonary blood flow and pulmonary arteriolar vascular obstruction than to the presence and intensity of pulmonary venous obstruction.[484–486] Obstruction to pulmonary venous return and pulmonary venous hypertension are invariably present in patients with infradiaphragmatic anomalous pulmonary

venous connection and in many with a supradiaphragmatic pathway. In the former type, pulmonary venous obstruction results from the length and narrowness of the common pulmonary venous trunk, compression at the esophageal hiatus of the diaphragm, constriction at the subdiaphragmatic site of insertion, or pulmonary venous return that must pass first through the portal-hepatic circulation before returning to the right atrium. When venous obstruction occurs in supradiaphragmatic types of drainage, constriction may exist at the entrance site of the anomalous veins into the systemic venous circulation, and/or the anomalous venous channel may be kinked or situated abnormally and compressed between the left pulmonary artery and left bronchus.[484,487] The presence of a small, restrictive patent foramen ovale occasionally results in pulmonary venous obstruction. Pulmonary vascular obstructive disease is rare during infancy, although exceptions have been reported.[488] In patients without pulmonary venous obstruction the risk of developing the Eisenmenger reaction is comparable to that in patients with an atrial septal defect.

CLINICAL MANIFESTATIONS. The majority of patients with total anomalous pulmonary venous connection have symptoms during the first year of life, and 80 per cent will die before age 1 year if left untreated.[482] The few who remain asymptomatic have a relatively good prognosis; once the condition is detected, operation may be elected later in childhood. Symptomatic infants with total anomalous pulmonary venous connection present with signs of heart failure and/or cyanosis. Infants with pulmonary venous obstruction present with the early onset of severe dyspnea, pulmonary edema, cyanosis, and right heart failure. Cardiac murmurs often are not prominent. In the unobstructed forms of total anomalous pulmonary venous connection the characteristic physical findings include right ventricular precordial overactivity and minimal cyanosis unless congestive heart failure intervenes. Multiple heart sounds often are audible, consisting of a first heart sound followed by an ejection sound; a fixed, widely split second heart sound with an accentuated pulmonic component; and a third and often a fourth heart sound. A soft systolic ejection murmur is usual along the left sternal border, and a middiastolic murmur of flow across the tricuspid valve commonly is audible at the lower left sternal border.

LABORATORY FINDINGS. The *electrocardiogram* shows right-axis deviation and right atrial and right ventricular hypertrophy. *Roentgenograms* of the chest reveal increased pul-

TABLE 31–10 SITE OF CONNECTION IN TOTAL ANOMALOUS PULMONARY VENOUS CONNECTION

1. Connection to right atrium	15%
2. Connection to common cardinal system	
a. (Right) superior vena cava	11%
b. Azygos vein	1%
3. Connection to left common cardinal system	
a. Left innominate vein	36%
b. Coronary sinus	16%
4. Connection to umbilicovitelline system	
a. Portal vein	6%
b. Ductus venosus	4%
c. Inferior vena cava	2%
d. Hepatic vein	1%
5. Multiple sites	7%
6. Unknown	1%

monary blood flow; the right atrium and ventricle are dilated and hypertrophied, and the pulmonary artery segment is enlarged (Fig. 31–68).[489] In addition, the specific site of anomalous connection may cause a characteristic appearance of the cardiac silhouette. Thus, in patients with total anomalous pulmonary venous connection to the left brachiocephalic vein, the superior vena cava on the right, left brachiocephalic vein superiorly, and vertical vein on the left produce a cardiac shadow that resembles a snowman or figure of eight. The upper right cardiac border may be prominent when the anomalous connection is to the right superior vena cava.

Echocardiography demonstrates marked enlargement of the right ventricle and a small left atrium.[490,491] An echo-free space representing the common pulmonary venous chamber occasionally may be seen to lie behind the left atrium on ultrasound examination. Diagnostic echocardiographic findings include an absence of pulmonary vein connections to a small left atrium in the presence of right to left bulging of the septum primum at the foramen ovale. Positive diagnosis is made by identifying pulmonary venous connection to the systemic veins, coronary sinus, or right atrium, rather than to the left atrium. All four pulmonary veins and their connections must be identified to diagnose mixed types accurately.[491] There is no standard echocardiographic method for tracing pulmonary venous pathways because of their diverse anatomical positions.

At *cardiac catheterization* those patients found to have systemic arterial saturations below 70 per cent and with pulmonary artery pressure at or above systemic levels are likely to have pulmonary venous obstruction. Variations in oxygen saturation in the systemic venous circulation may be helpful. In the subdiaphragmatic type, a step-up may not be apparent in inferior vena caval oxygen saturations obtained by way of femoral vein cannulation because of the contribution of highly oxygenated renal venous blood to the caval stream. In contrast, sampling of the hepatic or portal vein by way of a catheter inserted through the umbilical vein will yield diagnostically higher oxygen saturations, indicating anomalous return to those vessels. Selective pulmonary arteriography and *indicator dilution* studies at cardiac catheterization are especially helpful in determining the drainage pathways of the pulmonary veins. Indicator dye injected into the right ventricle or pulmonary artery takes longer to reach the peripheral arterial sampling site than does dye injected into the vena cava or right atrium. The contours of dilution curves obtained from a peripheral artery after injection into both the right atrium and a pulmonary vein are identical and show a large right-to-left shunt, while the left atrial curve is normal. If the cardiac catheter can be manipulated directly into the anomalous trunk through its site of connection, selective injection of contrast material into the common channel provides anatomical definition of the pulmonary venous tree. If the pulmonary veins cannot be entered directly, selective right and left main pulmonary artery injection of contrast material often is more helpful than is injection into a main pulmonary artery, since many infants have a persistent patent ductus arteriosus through which the contrast agent flows right to left. Moreover, the drainage from both lungs must be outlined clearly to exclude a mixed type of anomalous venous drainage. Pulmonary venous obstruction may be detected by noting a pressure difference between the pulmonary artery wedge pressure and the right atrium.

MANAGEMENT. Balloon atrial septotomy may provide dramatic palliation for the infant in whom the small size of an interatrial communication limits the amount of blood reaching the left side of the heart and systemic circulation.[483] Unless pulmonary vascular disease is present, results of operation for total anomalous pulmonary venous connection in patients beyond infancy are generally good.[491–493] The procedure consists of creating an anastomosis between the common pulmonary venous channel and left atrium and closing the atrial defect and the anomalous venous pathway. Improved results of operation in infancy require that postoperative pulmonary venous hypertension be averted by construction of a generally large anastomosis with or without enlargement of the left atrium. Normal hemodynamics and cardiac function have been demonstrated after surgical correction.[494]

PARTIAL ANOMALOUS PULMONARY VENOUS CONNECTION
(See also p. 949)

In this condition one or more of the pulmonary veins, but not all, are connected to the right atrium or to one or more of its venous tributaries. An atrial septal defect, particularly one of the sinus venosus type, commonly accompanies this anomaly; the usual connection involves the veins of the right upper and middle lobes and the superior vena cava.[308] Exclusive of atrial septal defects, major additional cardiac malformations occur in about 20 per cent of patients; these include ventricular septal defect, tetralogy of Fallot, and a variety of complex anomalies.

In the absence of associated anomalies the physiological disturbance is determined by the number of anomalous veins and their site of connection, the presence and size of an atrial septal defect, and the state of the pulmonary vascular bed.[495] In the usual patient with isolated partial pulmonary venous connection the hemodynamic state and physical findings are similar to those in atrial septal defect. Rarely, venous drainage of the right lung is into the inferior vena cava. This condition often is associated with hypoplasia of the right lung, dextroposition of the heart, pulmonary parenchymal abnormalities, and anomalous systemic supply to the lower lobe of the right lung from the abdominal aorta or its main branches.[496] This complex has been designated the "scimitar syndrome" because of the characteristic roentgenographic finding of a crescent-like shadow in the right lower lung field that is produced by the anomalous venous channel.

At *cardiac catheterization*, partial anomalous pulmonary venous connection to the coronary sinus, azygos vein, or superior vena cava may be identified by careful and frequent oximetry sampling. Oximetry is of limited value when the anomalous connection is to the inferior vena cava because of both reduced flow through the right lung and the contribution to the vena caval stream of highly oxygenated blood from the renal veins. Selective angiography is most helpful in cases in which the anomalous veins connect far away from the right atrium. Surgical repair offers definitive therapy at low risk if pulmonary vascular obliterative disease has not yet developed.

MALPOSITIONS OF THE HEART AND CARDIAC APEX

Positional anomalies of the heart are conditions in which the cardiac apex is located in the right side of the chest (dextrocardia) or is centrally located (mesocardia) or in which there is a normal location of the heart in the left side of the chest but abnormal position of the viscera (isolated levocardia). Such hearts commonly are abnormal with respect to chamber localization and great artery attachments; associated complex intracardiac and extracardiac lesions are common.

Problems of terminology abound in the literature describing these complex cardiac anomalies, although sensible and uniform systems of classification are available.[497,498]

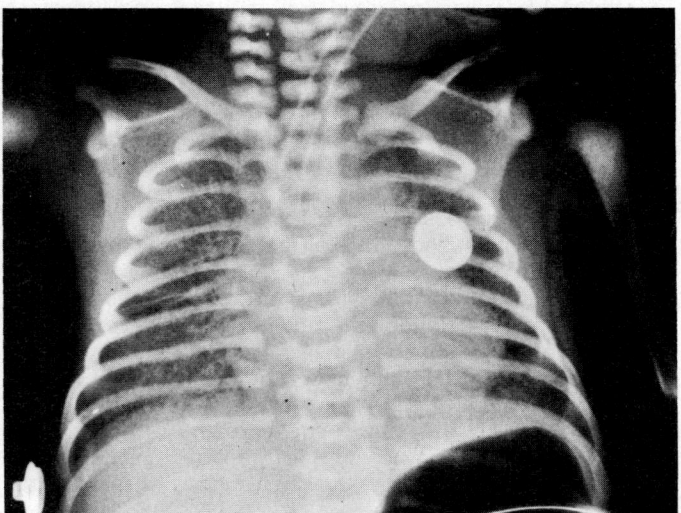

FIGURE 31–68. Chest roentgenogram in an infant with total anomalous pulmonary venous connection below the diaphragm shows normal overall heart size but diffuse pattern of pulmonary venous hypertension in both lung fields.

ANATOMICAL FEATURES. Defining the cardiac anatomy in instances of cardiac malposition requires a description of three cardiac segments — the visceroatrial situs, the ventricular loop, and the conotruncus (the atria, ventricles, and great arteries, respectively). In addition to defining positional interrelation, the description of the malposed heart also must include the connections of the ventricles to the atria and great arteries as well as chamber identification, both morphologically and functionally.

To accomplish accurate diagnosis often requires a synthesis of findings from noninvasive tests such as two-dimensional echocardiography, computed tomography, and magnetic resonance imaging (when available), as well as hemodynamic and cineangiographic findings obtained at cardiac catheterization.[499,500]

In general, the determination of the body situs indicates the position of the atria. The visceral situs usually can be determined by the location of the stomach bubble and liver on a routine roentgenogram and of the inferior vena cava by means of echocardiography or the position of a cardiac catheter, or by means of a computed axial tomogram or venous or radioisotope angiocardiography. Atrial anatomy is best investigated noninvasively by using subxiphoid long- and short-axis and apical four-chamber echocardiographic views. Venous contrast injections may be useful to define systemic venous connections.

Situs solitus is the normal arrangement of viscera and atria, with the right atrium right-sided and the left atrium left-sided. Situs solitus is further characterized by a trilobed right lung and eparterial bronchus (i.e., the right upper lobe bronchus passes above the right pulmonary artery), a bilobed left lung and hyparterial bronchus (i.e., the left bronchus passes below the left pulmonary artery), the major lobe of the liver on the right, a left-sided stomach and spleen, and right-sided venae cavae. Situs inversus is a mirror image of normal. Situs ambiguus or visceral heterotaxy refers to an anatomically uncertain or indeterminate body configuration. The latter often is seen in association with congenital asplenia, which resembles bilateral right-sidedness, and congenital polysplenia, which resembles bilateral left-sidedness.[501–503]

ASPLENIA. Cardiac anomalies associated commonly with asplenia include anomalous systemic venous connection, atrial septal or complete endocardial cushion defect, common ventricle, transposition of the great arteries, severe pulmonic stenosis or atresia, and anomalous pulmonary venous connection. Polysplenia commonly is associated with absence of the hepatic portion of the inferior vena cava with azygos continuation, bilateral superior venae cavae, anomalous pulmonary venous connection, and atrial septal defect (either ostium secundum or endocardial cushion). Pulmonic stenosis and double-outlet right ventricle are each observed in about 25 per cent of cases. It is important to recognize these complex syndromes to distinguish them from forms of cyanotic heart disease that may be more amenable to corrective surgical therapy. Diagnosis is suggested by a symmetrical liver shadow roentgenographically and, in asplenia, by the presence of Howell-Jolly and Heinz bodies in red blood cells demonstrated on blood smear, and it is confirmed by a negative or abnormal radioactive spleen scan.

Once the type of visceral situs is defined, it is necessary to describe the bulboventricular loop. The primitive cardiac tube normally bends to the right (D-loop), which brings the anatomical right ventricle to the right of the anatomical left ventricle. An L-loop brings the morphological right ventricle left-sided relative to the morphological left ventricle. The L-loop is normal in the presence of situs inversus, but in situs solitus it is synonymous with inverted ventricles.

VENTRICULAR MORPHOLOGY. The number, morphology, and size of the ventricle can be ascertained by using a variety of echocardiographic views. The morphological features of each ventricle also can be identified angiographically. The anatomical right ventricle is equipped with a tricuspid valve, is highly trabeculated, and contains the septal band of the single papillary muscle; its infundibulum lies anterior to and superiorly beyond the outlet of the left ventricle. The anatomical right ventricle usually connects with whichever of the two great arteries is the more anterior. The anatomical left ventricle is smooth-walled and contains an outlet that lies posterior to the right ventricular infundibulum; its entrance is guarded by a bicuspid mitral valve, the anterior leaflet of which is normally in continuity with elements of the semilunar valve at its outlet.

GREAT ARTERIES. The great arteries are described in terms of their positional interrelations and their ventricular connections. Each outflow tract and semilunar valve should be examined in both long- and short-axis echocardiographic views.[500] The ventriculoarterial alignments may be determined by direct visualization from the subxiphoid window. The relation between the great arteries can best be demonstrated noninvasively using parasternal short-axis echocardiographic views, which display the semilunar roots. The aortic arch and brachiocephalic arteries are seen well using suprasternal notch views. The pulmonary artery is seen from high parasternal or suprasternal notch short-axis sections. The ventricular attachments may be normal or may form the anomalies of double-outlet right or left ventricle or transposition. The arterial interrelations are described as D (dextro), in which the ascending aorta sweeps toward the right and lies

to the right of the main pulmonary artery; L (levo), in which the ascending aorta sweeps toward the left and lies to the left of the main pulmonary artery; or A (antero), which is the rare situation in which the aorta lies directly in front of the pulmonary artery. The D, L, and A descriptions of the aorticopulmonary artery interrelations should not be confused with the D- or L-loop designation of the ventricular interrelations.[498]

Using segmental sets composed of descriptive units of visceroatrial situs/ventricular loop/great artery relations greatly simplifies expression of the type of cardiac anatomy present in cardiac malposition. For example, the normal heart in a patient with situs inversus and dextrocardia is referred to as inversus/L loop/L normal; complete transposition of the great arteries in a patient with situs inversus is referred to as inversus/L loop/L transposition; functionally corrected transposition in a patient with situs solitus is referred to as solitus/L loop/L transposition; dextrocardia and functionally corrected transposition is designated solitus/D loop/D transposition with dextrocardia.

After the cardiac chambers are diagnosed functionally (arterial and venous), the positional and morphological relations are understood, and the presence of associated anomalies has been established, the principles of medical and surgical treatment apply to these cardiac malpositions as they do to normally located hearts.

OTHER CONDITIONS

Congenital Pericardial Defects

(See also p. 1506)

Isolated pericardial defects are rare. They most commonly occur in males and usually are left-sided, although they may be right-sided, diaphragmatic, or total.[504] The anomaly is produced by deficient formation of the pleuropericardial membrane, or, if diaphragmatic, defective formation of the septum transversum. Associated congenital anomalies of the heart and lungs occur in about 30 per cent of cases. Most patients with the isolated defect are asymptomatic. Nonspecific anterior chest pain may be the result of torsion of the great arteries due to absence of the stabilizing forces of the left pericardium.[505]

With complete absence of the left pericardium a conspicuous apical impulse may be noted shifted leftward to the anterior or midaxillary line. Electrocardiographic changes may be related to levo-position of the heart; a leftward displacement of the QRS transition in the precordial leads and vertical or right-axis deviation are usual. The diagnosis may be suggested by chest roentgenograms.[506] With complete left pericardial absence, the heart is levo-posed, and the aortic knob, pulmonary artery, and ventricles form three prominent left heart border convexities.

A partial left pericardial defect may be suspected on the basis of varying degrees of prominence of the pulmonary artery and/or the left atrial appendage. Echocardiographic findings often mimic those observed in patients with right ventricular volume overload (enlarged right ventricle and abnormal ventricular septal motion), probably owing to the altered cardiac position and motion within the thorax.[507,508] Other echocardiographic clues include lateral extension of the left atrial appendage as it herniates through the pericardial defect; this is best seen in short-axis views. The anomaly can be definitively diagnosed by computed tomography, magnetic resonance imaging, or angiocardiography, or by inducing a left pneumothorax and observing air under the right pericardium when the patient is placed in the right lateral decubitus position.[509]

Complete absence of the left pericardium requires no treatment. However, partial defects may impose serious risks, including herniation and strangulation of the ventricles or left atrial appendage with left-sided defects, or the possibility of a superior vena cava obstructive syndrome with right-sided defects.[510] In the diaphragmatic type, cardiac compression by abdominal contents requires surgical repair.[511] Partial left or right defects may be closed with a patch of mediastinal pleura.

Single Atrium

Single or common atrium is a rare, isolated defect. The anomaly consists of an absent atrial septum, usually with a cleft in the anteromedial leaflet of the mitral valve and, occasionally, with a cleft tricuspid valve as well. The lesion may be seen as one component of the Ellis–van Creveld syndrome (Table 31–2) or of the complex cardiac anomalies seen in patients with asplenia or polysplenia.

Single atrium may be suspected clinically by the presence of cardiac murmurs of an atrial septal defect and mitral regurgitation associated with mild cyanosis, roentgenographic evidence of cardiac enlargement and increased pulmonary blood flow, and electrocardiographic features of atrioventricular septal defect.[512] An absence of echoes from any part of the atrial septum is the essential feature of two-dimensional echocardiographic examination, which also may show a cleft anterior mitral leaflet, increased right ventricular end-diastolic dimension, paradoxical ventricular septal motion, and dilated, pulsatile pulmonary trunk. Angiographically, the absence of the atrial septum produces a large, globe-shaped single atrial structure. Selective left ventricular angiocardiography shows the characteristic gooseneck appearance seen in the various forms of atrioventricular septal defect. In the absence of pulmonary vascular obstructive disease surgical correction is indicated by means of a prosthetic patch.

Univentricular Atrioventricular Connection (Single Ventricle)

Hearts with univentricular atrioventricular connection constitute a family of complex lesions in which both atrioventricular valves, or a common atrioventricular valve, open into a single ventricular chamber.[513] Terminology is varied, and the anomaly often is referred to as single or common ventricle, which is imprecise but useful shorthand for the entity. The definition excludes examples of tricuspid or mitral atresia. Single ventricle is almost always accompanied by abnormal great artery positional relations; the incidence of L-malposition of the great arteries is about equal to that of D-malposition.[514] Associated anomalies are common, and include, in particular, pulmonic valvular or subvalvular stenosis, subaortic stenosis, total or partial anomalous pulmonary venous connection, and coarctation of the aorta.

MORPHOLOGY. In about 80 per cent of patients the single ventricle morphologically resembles a left ventricular chamber that is separated from an infundibular outlet chamber by a bulboventricular septum.[515] The opening is variously called the bulboventricular foramen and ventricular septal defect. The infundibular chamber is considered to represent developmentally the outflow tract of the right ventricle. When the great arteries are malposed the infundibulum lying anterior at the basal position of the single ventricle communicates with the aorta and may be in one of two positions: noninverted (D-malposition), when it is situated at the right basal aspect of the heart, or inverted (L-malposition), when it is located at the left base of the heart. In the unusual situation in which the great arteries normally are related, the infundibulum communicates with the pulmonary trunk.[514] *Double-inlet left ventricle* is a term used synonymously to describe the most frequently encountered single ventricular chamber that has the anatomical characteristics of the left ventricle. Less commonly the single ventricular chamber resembles a right ventricle (double-inlet right ventricle) or contains features suggestive of both ventricles or neither one; the latter two situations occasionally have been designated common ventricle and single ventricle of the primitive type, respectively.[514]

CLINICAL FINDINGS. Depending on the associated anomalies, the clinical presentation of single ventricle mimics other conditions in which cyanosis and decreased or increased pulmonary blood flow coexist, e.g., tetralogy of Fallot or tricuspid atresia in the former instance or complete transposition of the great arteries and double-outlet right ventricle in the latter. The *electrocardiogram in* double-inlet left ventricle without inversion of the infundibulum (D-malposition) usually shows features of left ventricular hypertrophy. With infundibular inversion (L-malposition) the electrical forces are directed anteriorly and rightward, as they are in ventricular inversion without associated defects. In patients with the more primitive types of common or single ventricle there is a repetitious rS pattern in all the precordial electrocardiographic leads. *Chest roentgenographic* findings resemble those observed in patients with complete (dextro-) transposition of the great arteries or functionally corrected (levo-) transposition of the great arteries without features distinctive for single ventricle.

In those patients in whom two separate atrioventricular valves communicate with the single ventricular chamber, *echocardiography* (Fig. 4–83,

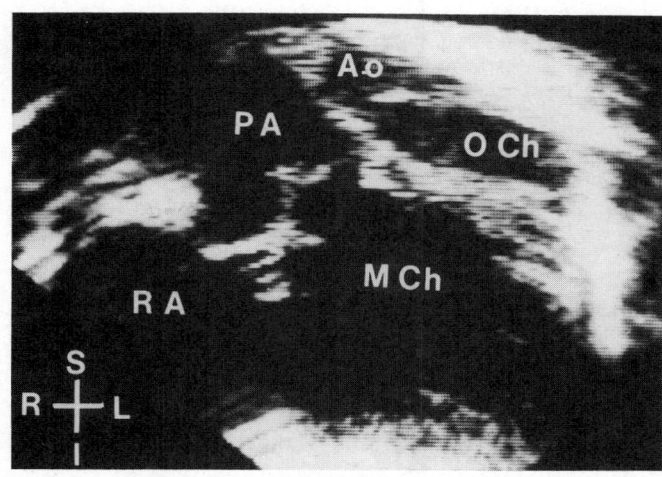

FIGURE 31–69. Single ventricle imaged in a subcostal coronal view. The pulmonary artery (PA) arises from a main chamber (MCh) of left ventricular type. The right atrioventricular valve is seen in part between the main chamber and the right atrium (RA). The ascending aorta (AO) arises anteriorly from a small outlet chamber (OCh). The bulboventricular foramen or ventricular septal defect is not identified in this plane. (Courtesy of Norman Silverman, M.D.)

p. 95) suggests the correct diagnosis when echoes are visualized from the two valves without an intervening interventricular septum.[515,516] In the absence of ventricular septal echoes when the two valves are not visualized simultaneously, they may be identified separately with a careful long-axis sweep of the ventricle. It is possible to detect the presence of a small outflow chamber anterior to the atrioventricular valves by using subxiphoid or parasternal short-axis views, and a plane orthogonal to the long-axis plane (Fig. 31–69). The single ventricle with a single atrioventricular valve is suspected when the excursion of echoes from the single valve located posteriorly in the ventricular chamber is of large amplitude. Enhanced assessment of the atrioventricular valve in patients with single

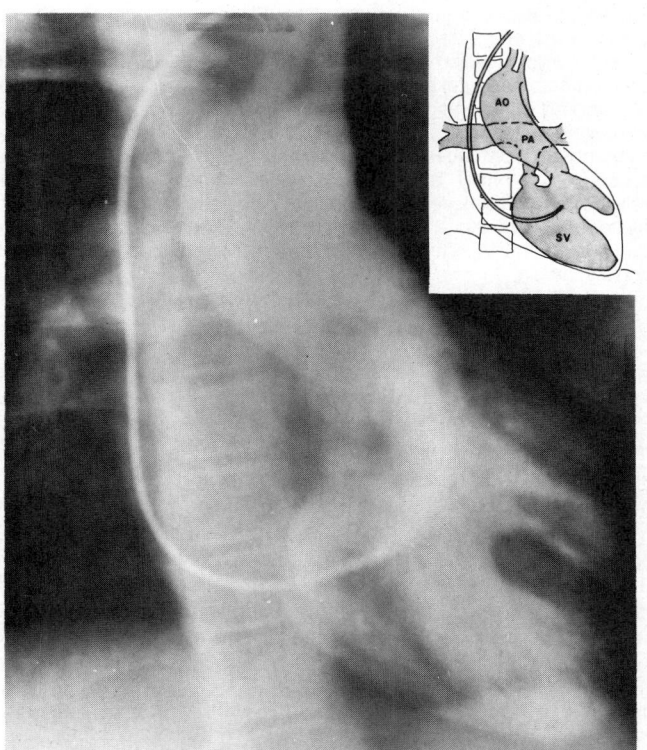

FIGURE 31–70. Selective ventriculogram in a child with single ventricle (SV). There is levo-malposition of the great arteries with the aorta (AO) communicating with a small outflow chamber. The pulmonary artery (PA) arises from a single ventricular chamber, which has the anatomical characteristics of a left ventricle. There is moderate pulmonic stenosis.

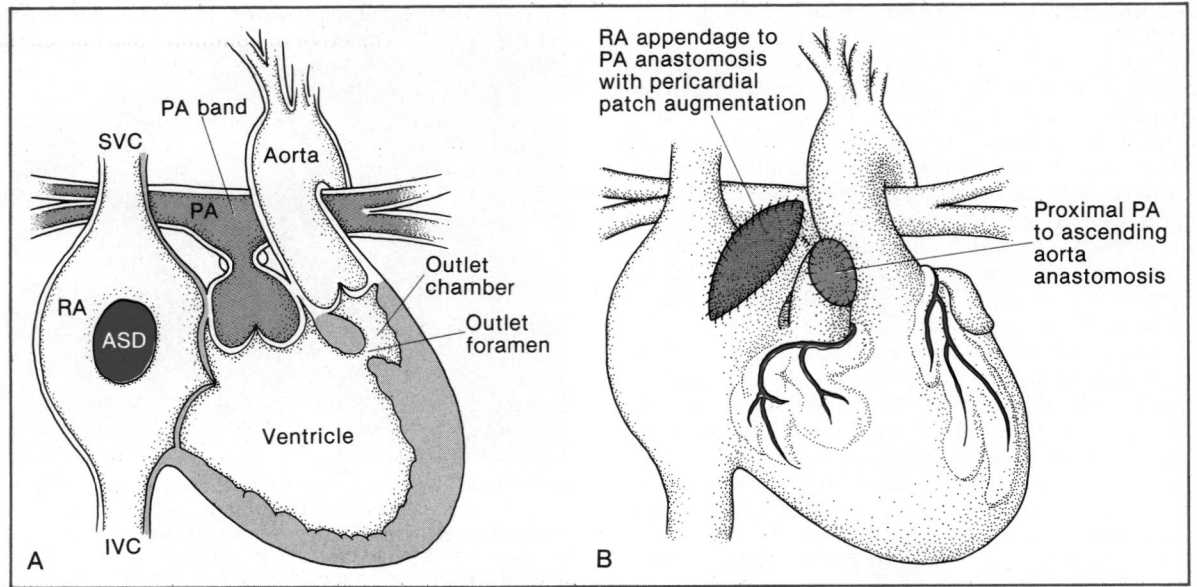

FIGURE 31-71. *A,* The preoperative anatomy of a univentricular heart of the left ventricular type with left anterior subaortic outlet chamber, ventricular arterial discordance, left atrioventricular valve atresia, atrial septal defect (ASD), and subaortic stenosis caused by a restrictive bulboventricular outlet foramen. *B,* The physiologic operative repair. The proximal pulmonary artery (PA) anastomosed to the ascending aorta (augmented by a prosthetic patch) and a modified Fontan procedure created (right atrial to the pulmonary artery anastomosis). Not shown is the interatrial baffle committing the pulmonary venous return to the right atrioventricular valve. (From Lin, A. E., et al.: Subaortic obstruction in complex heart disease. Reprinted with permission from the American College of Cardiology. J. Am. Coll. Cardiol. 7:617, 1986.)

ventricle is provided by Doppler echocardiography.[517] Selective ventriculography is necessary to delineate with certainty the anatomical type of single ventricle and to diagnose the associated great artery interrelations and the presence or absence of additional lesions (Fig. 31-70).[518,519]

SURGICAL TREATMENT. Attempts to partition the single ventricle with a Dacron or Teflon prosthetic patch have met with modest success as well as a high incidence of postoperative complete heart block.[520,521] The septation operation is best performed in patients with double-inlet left ventricle, a rudimentary right ventricular outflow chamber which is anterior and leftward, and a discordant ventriculoarterial connection, with either absent or mild pulmonary stenosis. Creation of an atriopulmonary conduit (the Fontan procedure) and closure of the tricuspid orifice is a technique best applied to patients with severe pulmonary stenosis or previous pulmonary artery banding procedure (Fig. 31-71).[522] In these patients, subaortic obstruction caused by a restricted bulboventricular foramen requires a pulmonary artery-to-ascending aorta anastomosis.[523,524] Palliative procedures designed to either increase pulmonary blood flow (systemic-pulmonary anastomosis) or limit pulmonary blood flow (pulmonary artery banding) often allow survival to adolescence in patients with a single ventricle.

VASCULAR RINGS

MORPHOLOGY. The normal development of the aortic arch system is described on page 1528 (Fig. 31-5). The term *vascular ring* is used for those aortic arch or pulmonary artery malformations that exhibit an abnormal relation with the esophagus and trachea, causing compression, dysphagia, and/or respiratory symptoms.[524a] The most common and serious vascular ring is produced by a double aortic arch in which both the right and left fourth embryonic aortic arches persist. In the most common type of double aortic arch there is a left ligamentum arteriosum or ductus arteriosus, and both arches are patent, the right being larger than the left. A right aortic arch with a left ductus or ligamentum arteriosum connecting the left pulmonary artery and the upper part of the descending aorta and with an anomalous right subclavian artery arising from the left descending aorta are additional important vascular ring arrangements.[525] The latter anomaly frequently exists in cases of tetralogy of Fallot and otherwise uncomplicated coarctation of the aorta. An unusual cause of tracheal compression is the "vascular sling" created by an anomalous left pulmonary artery that arises from a rightward, elongated pulmonary trunk and courses between the trachea and esopha-

gus before it branches normally within the left lung.[526] This arrangement commonly is associated with other cardiac and extracardiac anomalies.

CLINICAL FINDINGS. The symptoms produced by vascular rings depend on the tightness of anatomical constriction of the trachea and esophagus and consist principally of respiratory difficulties, cyanosis (associated especially with feeding), stridor, and dysphagia. The electrocardiogram is normal unless associated cardiovascular anomalies are present. The barium esophagogram is a useful screening procedure. Prominent posterior indentation of the esophagus is observed in the common vascular ring arrangements, although the pulmonary artery "vascular sling" produces an anterior indentation. Unusual and rare aortic arch anomalies may create rings that impinge on the trachea but do not compress the esophagus and that will be detected not by this simple radiographic procedure but rather by bronchoscopy. Computed tomography examination is helpful in the diagnosis of this malformation. Selective contrast angiography usually is required to delineate the anatomy of the aorta and its branches or the course of the main pulmonary arteries. Computed axial tomography and magnetic resonance imaging offer excellent imaging alternatives.[527,528]

MANAGEMENT. The severity of symptoms and the anatomy of the malformation are the most important factors in determining treatment. Patients, particularly infants, with respiratory obstruction require prompt surgical intervention. Operative repair of the double aortic arch requires division of the minor arch (usually the left).[529] A reported 20 to 30 per cent operative mortality is related, in part, to problems in postoperative respiratory care, especially when there is coexistent residual anatomical tracheal narrowing. Patients with a right aortic arch and a left ductus or ligamentum arteriosum require division of the ductus or ligamentum and/or ligation and division of the left subclavian artery, which is the posterior component of the ring. Operation seldom is indicated for patients with an aberrant right subclavian artery derived from a left aortic arch and left descending aorta. In patients with a pulmonary artery vascular sling, operation consists of detachment of the left pulmonary artery at its origin and anastomosis to the main pulmonary artery directly or by way of a conduit of its proximal end brought anterior to the trachea.[529]

CONGENITAL ARRHYTHMIAS

This classification refers to arrhythmias that are present in infancy, whose causes, when known, relate to a structural malformation or defect of the conduction system or to an acquired prenatal condition such as myocarditis, hypoxia, acidosis, or transplacental passage of a drug or substance from mother to fetus. In these latter examples, the substrate for the postnatal expression of the rhythm disturbance existed before birth and the arrhythmia is therefore designated "congenital." Complete heart block and supraventricular and ventricular tachycardias are the most common important congenital arrhythmias.[530] The electrophysiological and electrocardiographic features of these arrhythmias are discussed elsewhere in the text (Chaps. 24 and 25).

CONGENITAL COMPLETE HEART BLOCK
(See also p. 969)

The atrioventricular node and the His bundle originate during fetal development as separate structures and later join together. Anatomical studies have shown the basic lesion in congenital complete heart block to consist of discontinuity between the atrial musculature and the AV node or the His bundle, if the AV node is absent. The anatomical interruption occasionally may be situated between the AV node and the main His bundle, or within the bundle itself.[531,532] No known cause exists for the vast majority of cases of congenital heart block in infants, who usually have otherwise anatomically normal hearts. However, fetal myocarditis, idiopathic hemorrhage and necrosis involving conduction tissue, and degeneration and fibrosis related in some instances to the transplacental passage of anti–Ro antibody and other immune complexes from mothers with systemic lupus erythematosus are all entities capable of causing congenital heart block.[533-535] Less often, congenital heart block may be associated with various forms of congenital heart disease, the most common malformation being congenitally corrected transposition of the great arteries.

Detection of consistent fetal bradycardia (heart rate 40 to 80 beats/min) by auscultation, fetal echocardiography (Fig. 31–72), or electronic monitoring allows anticipation of the correct diagnosis.[536] The newborn, especially with a ventricular rate less than 50 beats/min and atrial rate in excess of 150 beats/min, is at highest risk; the presence of an associated cardiovascular anomaly greatly lessens the chances of survival. Treatment is not required for the asymptomatic infant.

Digitalization is recommended for the baby in congestive heart failure, irrespective of complete heart block. Isoproterenol and other sympathomimetic drugs and atropine do not have permanent or beneficial effects. Congestive heart failure and Stokes-Adams attacks require pacemaker treatment at any age.[530,537,540] Initial management of the child in whom permanent epicardial pacemaker insertion is indicated usually involves preoperative insertion of a transvenous intracardiac electrode into the right ventricle to protect the patient from serious arrhythmias during the induction of anesthesia.[538] A variety of problems may be anticipated after pacemaker implantation related to growth of the patient, which stresses the electrical lead system; the fragility of the lead system in a physically active young patient; and the limited life span of the pulse generator. Patients with congenital complete heart block who survive infancy usually remain asymptomatic until late in childhood or adolescence.[539]

SUPRAVENTRICULAR TACHYCARDIA

Paroxysmal tachycardia of supraventricular origin may have its origin in utero or in the immediate postnatal period.[30,541,542] The most frequent arrhythmias producing symptoms are paroxysmal atrial tachycardia with or without ventricular preexcitation, atrial flutter, and junctional tachycardia. The arrhythmia may cause intrauterine cardiac failure; its detection and persistence prenatally should prompt consideration of administration of digitalis, or if that fails, of propranolol or quinidine, to the mother if amniocentesis indicates surfactant deficiency and fetal lung immaturity, since early delivery is not indicated if the baby will have hyaline membrane disease. Cesarean delivery or induced labor may be indicated if the fetus is close to term. No recognizable cause exists for the disorder in the vast majority of infants. The transplacental passage of long-acting thyroid-stimulating (LATS) and immune gamma g globulin from hyperthyroid mothers, hypoglycemia, and Ebstein's anomaly of the tricuspid valve occasionally are causative.[543] Wolff-Parkinson-White syndrome (p. 693) is present in 10 to 50 per cent of infants with supraventricular tachycardia.[544] Symptoms produced by the tachyarrhythmia after birth are subtle and often go undetected until signs of heart failure have been present for 24 to 36 hours. Conversion to normal sinus rhythm usually is accomplished by administration of digitalis, direct-current cardioversion, transesophageal atrial pacing, or eliciting a diving reflex by covering the face with an ice-cold wet washcloth for 4 to 5 seconds.[545-548] Conversion should be fol-

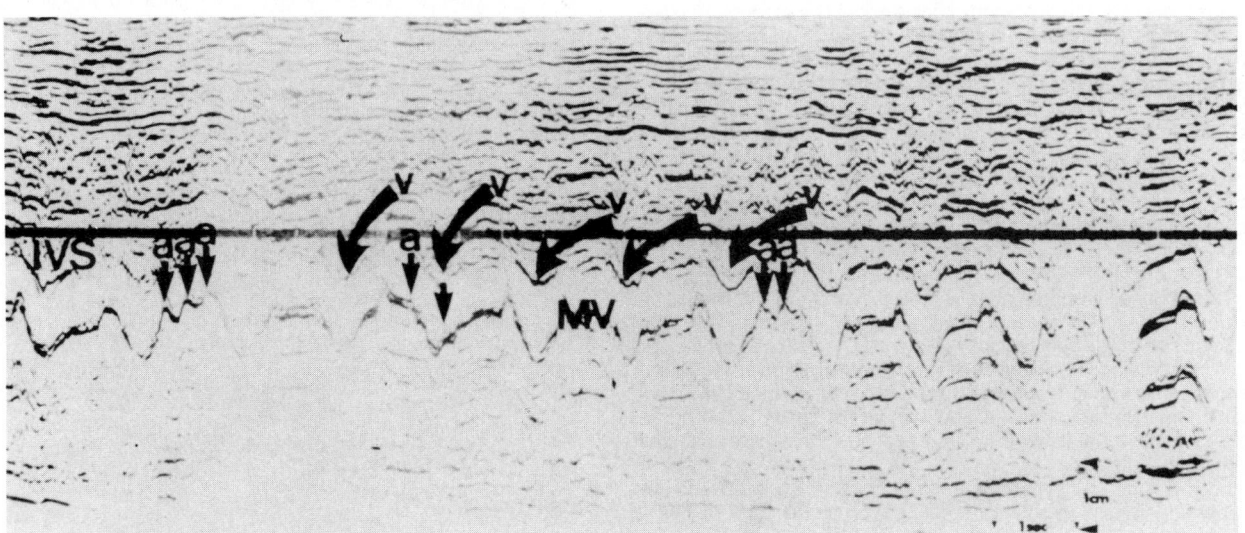

FIGURE 31–72. Fetal M-mode echocardiogram of complete heart block at 28 weeks' gestation. A slow ventricular rate of 45 to 50 beats/min is seen by the undulations (v, curved arrows) of the interventricular septum (IVS). Atrial contractions (a, straight vertical arrows) cause regular undulations of the mitral valve (MV) at a rate of 120–130 beats/min. The atrial activity has no fixed relationship to the idioventricular rhythm. (Courtesy of Charles Kleinman, M.D.)

lowed by digitalization on a prophylactic basis. Common practice consists of digitalis treatment for 9 to 12 recurrence-free months followed by its abrupt cessation. Recurrence of tachycardia, particularly in those infants with ventricular preexcitation, is not uncommon; maintenance of normal rhythm may require the administration, alone or in combination, of digitalis, phenytoin sodium, verapamil, and propranolol.[546a] The rate of recurrence falls substantially between ages 2 and 10 years, with a slight rise during adolescence. In general, the prognosis is excellent.[549]

ELECTROPHYSIOLOGICAL STUDIES. Beyond infancy, patients whose condition is refractory to medical treatment are candidates for electrophysiological catheter evaluation, which facilitates differentiation of a causative ectopic anatomical focus within the atria from accessory conduction pathways.[530,550] Endocardial mapping is performed to specifically localize the site of earliest activation in the atrium, or to identify multiple foci of ectopic impulses. Electrophysiological studies should include measurement of resting intervals and sinus and atrioventricular node function, including recovery times, effective refractory period, and Wenckebach conduction. Premature atrial stimulation may be used to interrupt tachycardia. Premature ventricular stimulation is used to measure retrograde conduction and localize the site of earliest atrial activation, and to assess the effective refractory period of the accessory pathway. Coronary sinus and right atrial catheters provide localization of the site of earliest atrial activation during tachycardia, and allow measurement of the antegrade effective refractory period of the accessory pathway.

If the tachyarrhythmia is refractory to pharmacological therapy or catheter ablative techniques, it may be treated definitively with intraoperative mapping and a variety of operative maneuvers, including cryoablation, surgical division of accessory conduction pathways, subendocardial excision of the ectopic focus, and atrial disconnection.[551,552]

ATRIAL FLUTTER. Uncommonly, atrial flutter is the cause of supraventricular tachycardia,[546] especially in the setting of newborn infants with hydrops fetalis, whose intrauterine tachyarrhythmia is an alternation between supraventricular tachycardia with Wolff-Parkinson-White syndrome and atrial flutter. Another common clinical setting for atrial flutter is in the infant under age 6 months with an otherwise normal heart, who shows frequent premature atrial contractions. In infants, classic flutter waves may not be present on a surface electrocardiogram or rhythm strip; detection may require recordings of transesophageal atrial electrograms. Acute treatment with electrical conversion or overdrive pacing, either through the esophagus or with an intracardiac atrial catheter, effectively terminates the rhythm disturbance.[546,547] If synchronized direct-current electrocardioversion is used, standby pacing should be available; if overdrive pacing is utilized, the same pacing catheter can be used to pace the heart in the event of a systole. Uncommonly, chronic drug treatment with digitalis, digitalis plus quinidine, or amiodarone may be required.

Junctional automatic tachycardia is characterized by a narrow QRS complex and AV dissociation, with the ventricular rate faster than the normal atrial rate. Ventricular dysfunction and congestive heart failure occur early, and the rhythm disturbance usually is not convertible to sinus rhythm by any medical treatment.[530] Because sudden death commonly occurs, pacemaker implantation is recommended with a subsequent effort at either catheter or surgical ablation.

VENTRICULAR TACHYCARDIA. Ventricular tachycardia is defined as three or more consecutive premature ventricular contractions. The definition, however, fails to identify a high-risk group. Infants or children who meet this criterion but seldom require treatment and seem to be at little risk have no symptoms and no evidence of anatomical heart disease. Potentially serious ventricular tachycardia in the newborn is associated with Q-T prolongation, mitral valve prolapse, and Marfan syndrome. In these settings the tachycardia is potentially life-threatening and always merits treatment.[530]

The cause of long Q-T syndrome (p. 708) is unknown; proposed are regional abnormalities of ventricular repolarization on the basis of an imbalance of right and left sympathetic innervation of the heart. The two most effective treatments are beta blockade and high thoracic left sympathectomy, which reduce the incidence of syncope and sudden death without affecting the Q-T interval.

The treatment of ventricular tachycardia (p. 651) consists of intravenous administration of lidocaine, followed by direct-current electrical cardioversion. In the absence of Q-T prolongation, but in the presence of mitral prolapse or other cardiac abnormalities, chronic treatment should be undertaken of multiform premature ventricular contractions, couplets, or ventricular tachycardia. In infants and children unresponsive to conventional or investigational antiarrhythmic drugs, surgical treatment — by either cryoablation or excision — may be lifesaving.[553]

REFERENCES

1. Hoffman, J.I.E.: Congenital heart disease. Ped. Clin. North Am. *37*:45, 1990.
2. Roberts, W. C.: Anatomically isolated aortic valvular disease: The case against its being of rheumatic etiology. Am. J. Cardiol. *49*:151, 1970.
3. Warth, D. C., King, M. E., Cohen, J. M., et al.: Prevalence of mitral valve prolapse in normal children. J. Am. Coll. Cardiol. *5*:1173, 1985.
4. Fontana, R. S., and Edwards, J. E.: Congenital Cardiac Disease: A Review of 357 Cases Studied Pathologically. Philadelphia, W. B. Saunders Company, 1962.
5. Bankl, H.: Congenital Malformations of the Heart and Great Vessels: Synopsis of Pathology, Embryology and Natural History. Baltimore-Munich, Urban and Schwarzenberg, 1977.
6. Greenwood, R. D.: Cardiovascular malformations associated with extracardiac anomalies and malformation syndromes. Clin. Pediatr. *23*:145, 1984.
7. Nora, J. J., and Nora, A. H.: Maternal transmission of congenital heart diseases: New recurrence risk figures and the questions of cytoplasmic inheritance and vulnerability to teratogens. Am. J. Cardiol. *59*:459, 1987.
7a. Kirby, M. L., and Waldo, K. L.: Role of neural crest in congenital heart disease. Circulation *82*:332, 1990.
8. de la Cruz, M. V., Munoz-Castellanos, L., and Nadal-Ginard, S.: Extrinsic factors in the genesis of congenital heart disease. Br. Heart J. *33*:203, 1971.
9. Ruttenberg, H. D.: Concerning the etiology of congenital cardiac disease. Am. Heart J. *84*:437, 1972.
10. Ouelette, E. M., Rossett, H. L., Rossman, M. P., and Wiener, L.: Adverse effects on offspring of maternal alcohol abuse during pregnancy. N. Engl. J. Med. *297*:528, 1977.
10a. Stevens, C. A., Carey, J. C., and Shigeoka, A. O.: DiGeorge anomaly and velocardiofacial syndrome. Pediatrics *85*:526, 1990.
11. Noonan, J.: Twins, conjoined twins, and cardiac defects. Am. J. Dis. Child. *132*:17, 1978.
12. Corone, P., Bonaiti, C., Feingold, J., et al.: Familial congenital heart disease: How are the various types related? Am. J. Cardiol. *51*:942, 1983.
13. Anderson, R. H., and Ashley, G. T.: Anatomic development of the cardiovascular system. In Davies, J., and Dobbing, J. (eds.): Scientific Foundations of Paediatrics. London, Heinemann, 1974, p. 165.
14. Langman, J., and van Mierop, L.H.S.: Development of the cardiovascular system. In Moss, A. J., and Adams, F. H. (eds.): Heart Disease in Infants, Children and Adolescents. Baltimore, Williams and Wilkins, 1968, p. 3.
15. Los, J. A.: Embryology. In Watson, H. (ed.): Paediatric Cardiology. London, Lloyd Luke Ltd., 1968, p. 1.
16. Rudolph, A. M.: Congenital Diseases of the Heart. Chicago, Year Book Medical Publishers, 1974.
17. Sheldon, C. A., Friedman, W. F., and Sybers, H. D.: Scanning electron microscopy of fetal and neonatal lamb cardiac cells. J. Molec. Cell. Cardiol. *8*:853, 1976.
18. McPherson, R. A., Kramer, M. F., Covell, J. W., and Friedman, W. F.: A comparison of the active stiffness of fetal and adult cardiac muscle. Pediatr. Res. *10*:660, 1976.
19. Friedman, W. F.: The intrinsic physiologic properties of the developing heart. Prog. Cardiovasc. Dis. *15*:87, 1972.
20. Ingwall, J. S., Kramer, M. F., Woodman, D., and Friedman, W. F.: Maturation of energy metabolism in the lamb: Changes in myosin ATPase and creatine kinase activities. Pediatr. Res. *15*:1128, 1981.
21. Friedman, W. F.: Physiological properties of the developing heart. Paediatric Cardiology. Vol. 6. New York, Churchill Livingstone, 1987, p. 3.
22. Geis, W. P., Tatooles, C. J., Priola, D. V., and Friedman, W. F.: Factors influencing neurohumoral control of the heart and newborn. Am. J. Physiol. *228*:1685, 1975.
23. Klitzner, T. S., and Friedman, W. F.: Excitation contraction coupling in developing mammalian myocardium. Pediatr. Res. *23*:428, 1988.
24. Klitzner, T. S., and Friedman, W. F.: A diminished role for the sarcoplasmic reticulum in newborn myocardial contraction. Pediatr. Res. *26*:98, 1989.
25. Romero, T. E., and Friedman, W. F.: Limited left ventricular response to volume overload in the neonatal period. Pediatr. Res. *13*:910, 1979.
26. Friedman, W. F., Printz, M. P., Kirkpatrick, S. E., and Hoskins, E. J.: The vasoactivity of the fetal lamb ductus arteriosus studied in utero. Pediatr. Res. *17*:331, 1983.

PATHOLOGICAL CONSEQUENCES

27. Friedman, W. F., and George, B. L.: Medical progress — Treatment of congestive heart failure by altering loading conditions of the heart. J. Pediatr. *106*:697, 1985.
28. Friedman, W. F., and George, B. L.: Treatment of cardiac failure in infants. Compr. Ther. *12*:8, 1986.

29. Artman, M., Parrish, M. D., and Graham, T. P., Jr.: Congestive heart failure in childhood and adolescence: Recognition and management. Am. Heart J. 105:471, 1983.

30. Schmidt, K. G., Araujo, L., and Silverman, N. H.: Evaluation of structural and functional abnormalities of the fetal heart by echocardiography. Am. J. Cardiol. Imag. 2:57, 1988.

31. Schmidt, K. G., Silverman, N. H., Van Hare, G. F., et al.: Two-dimensional echocardiographic determination of ventricular volumes in the fetal heart. Circulation 81:325, 1990.

32. Milne, M. J., Sung, R.Y.T., Fok, T. F., and Crozier, I. G.: Doppler echocardiographic assessment of shunting via the ductus arteriosus in newborn infants. Am. J. Cardiol. 64:102, 1989.

33. Sahn, D. J., and Friedman, W. F.: Difficulties in distinguishing cardiac from pulmonary disease in the neonate. Pediatr. Clin. North Am. 20:293, 1973.

34. Stanger, P., Lucas, R. V., Jr., and Edwards, J. E.: Anatomic factors causing respiratory distress in acyanotic congenital cardiac disease: Special reference to bronchial obstruction. Pediatrics 43:760, 1969.

35. DiSessa, T. G., and Friedman, W. F.: Echocardiographic evaluation of cardiac performance. Cardiol. Clin. 1:487, 1983.

36. DiSessa, T. G., and Friedman, W. F.: Echocardiographic evaluation of cardiac performance. In Friedman, W. F., and Higgins, C. B. (eds.): Pediatric Cardiac Imaging. Philadelphia, W. B. Saunders Company, 1984, p. 219.

37. Mercier, J. C., DiSessa, T. G., Jarmakani, J., and Friedman, W. F.: Two dimensional echocardiographic assessment of left ventricular volumes and ejection fraction. Circulation 65:962, 1982.

38. Hanseus, K., Bjorkhem, G., and Lundstrom, N. R.: Dimensions of cardiac chambers and great vessels by cross-sectional echocardiography in infants and children. Pediatr. Cardiol. 9:7, 1988.

39. Riggs, T. W., Rodriguez, R., Snider, A. R., and Batton, D.: Doppler echocardiographic evaluation of right and left diastolic function in normal neonates. J. Am. Coll. Cardiol. 13:700, 1989.

40. Teitel, D., and Rudolph, A. M.: Perinatal oxygen delivery and cardiac function. Adv. Pediatr. 32:321, 1985.

41. Rosenthal, A., Nathan, D. G., Marty, A. T., et al.: Acute hemodynamic effects of red cell volume reduction, polycythemia of cyanotic congenital heart disease. Circulation 42:297, 1970.

42. Voigt, G. C., and Wright, J. R.: Cyanotic congenital heart disease and sudden death. Am. Heart J. 87:771, 1974.

43. Fischbein, C. A., Rosenthal, A., Fischer, E. G., et al.: Risk factors for brain abscess in patients with congenital heart disease. Am. J. Cardiol. 34:97, 1974.

44. Shaher, R. M., and Deuchard, D. C.: Hematogenous brain abscess in cyanotic congenital heart disease. Am. J. Med. 52:349, 1972.

45. Corrin, C.: Paradoxical embolism. Br. Heart J. 26:549, 1964.

46. Haroutunian, L. M., and Neill, C. A.: Pulmonary complications of congenital heart disease: Hemoptysis. Am. Heart J. 84:540, 1972.

47. Guntheroth, W. G., Morgan, B. C., and Mullens, G. L.: Physiologic studies of paroxysmal hyperpnea in cyanotic congenital heart disease. Circulation 31:70, 1965.

48. Talmer, N. S.: Congestive heart failure in the infant. Pediatr. Clin. North Am. 18:1011, 1971.

49. Rosenthal, A., and Castaneda, A. R.: Growth and development after cardiovascular surgery in infants and children. In Rosenthal, A., Sonnenblick, E. H., and Lesch, M. (eds.): Postoperative Congenital Heart Disease. New York, Grune and Stratton, 1975, p. 110.

50. Friedman, W. F., Heiferman, M. F., and Perloff, J. K.: Late postoperative pulmonary vascular disease—Clinical concerns. In Engle, M. A., and Perloff, J. K. (eds.): Congenital Heart Disease After Surgery. New York, Yorke Medical Publishers, 1983, p. 151.

51. Rabinovitch, M.: Structure and function of the pulmonary vascular bed: An update. Cardiol. Clin. 7:227, 1989.

52. Rabinovitch, M., Keane, J. F., and Norwood, W. I.: Vascular structure and lung biopsy tissue correlated with pulmonary hemodynamic findings after repair of congenital heart defects. Circulation 69:655, 1984.

53. Heath, D., and Edwards, J. E.: The pathology of hypertensive pulmonary vascular disease. Circulation 18:533, 1958.

54. Levin, D. L., Rudolph, A. M., Heymann, M. A., and Phibbs, R. H.: Morphological development of the pulmonary vascular bed in the fetal lamb. Circulation 53:144, 1976.

55. Rabinovitch, M., and Reid, L. M.: Quantitative structural analysis of the pulmonary vascular bed in congenital heart defects. In Engle, M. A. (ed.): Pediatric Cardiovascular Disease. Philadelphia, F. A. Davis, 1981, p. 149.

56. Friedman, W. F.: Proceedings of the National Heart, Lung and Blood Institute Pediatric Cardiology Workshop: Pulmonary Hypertension. Pediatr. Res. 20:8, 1986.

57. Rabinovitch, M., Keane, J. F., Fellows, K. E., et al.: Quantitative analysis of the pulmonary wedge angiogram in congenital heart defects. Circulation 63:152, 1981.

58. Rabinovitch, M., Castaneda, A. R., and Reid, L.: Lung biopsy with frozen section as a diagnostic aid in patients with congenital heart defects. Am. J. Cardiol. 47:77, 1981.

59. Zeller, S. T., and Gutgesell, H. P.: Noninvasive estimation of pulmonary artery pressure. J. Pediatr. 114:735, 1989.

60. Morera, J., Hoadley, S. D., Roland, J. M., et al.: Estimation of the ratio of pulmonary to systemic pressures by pulsewave Doppler echocardiography for assessment of pulmonary artery pressures. Am. J. Cardiol. 63:862, 1989.

61. Van Hare, G. F., Ben-Shachar, G., Liebman, J., et al.: Infective endocarditis in infants and children during the past 10 years: A decade of change. Am. Heart J. 107:1235, 1984.

62. Dajani, A. S.: Prevention of bacterial endocarditis. Pediatr. Infect. Dis. 4:349, 1985.

62a. Dajani, A. S., Bisno, A. L., Chung, K. J., et al.: Prevention of bacterial endocarditis. Recommendations by the American Heart Association. JAMA 264:2919, 1990.

63. Selbst, S. M., Ruddy, R. M., Clark, B. J., et al.: Pediatric chest pain: A prospective study. Pediatrics 82:319, 1988.

64. Graham, T. P., Gessner, I. H., Friedman, W. F., et al.: Recommendations for use of laboratory studies for pediatric patients with suspected or proven heart disease: A statement of the Committee on Congenital Cardiac Defects of the Council on Cardiovascular Disease in the Young of the AHA. Circulation 74:443a, 1986.

65. Driscoll, D. J., and Edwards, W. D.: Sudden unexpected death in children and adolescents. J. Am. Coll. Cardiol. 5:118B, 1985.

66. Denfield, S. W., and Garson, A., Jr.: Sudden death in children and young adults. Ped. Clin. North Am. 37:215, 1990.

APPROACH TO THE HIGH-RISK INFANT

67. Friedman, W. F., and George, B. L.: New concepts and drugs in the treatment of congestive heart failure. Pediatr. Clin. North Am. 31:1197, 1984.

68. Anderson, P.A.W.: Maturation in cardiac contractility. Cardiol. Clin. 7:209, 1989.

69. Talner, N. S., and Lister, G.: Perioperative care of the infant with congenital heart disease. Cardiol. Clin. 7:419, 1989.

70. Park, M. K.: Use of digoxin in infants and children, with specific emphasis on dosage. J. Pediatr. 108:871, 1986.

71. Freed, M. D., Hegmann, M. A., Lewis, A. B., et al.: Prostaglandin E$_1$ in infants with ductus arteriosus dependent congenital heart disease. Circulation 64:899, 1981.

72. Lewis, A. B., Freed, M. D., Hegmann, M. A., et al.: Side effects of therapy with prostaglandin E$_1$ in infants with critical congenital heart disease. Circulation 64:893, 1981.

73. Friedman, W. F., Kurlinski, J., Jacob, J., et al.: Inhibition of prostaglandin and prostacyclin synthesis in clinical management of PDA. Semin. Perinatol. 4:125, 1980.

74. Friedman, W. F.: Patent ductus arteriosus in respiratory distress syndrome. Pediatr. Cardiol. 4(Suppl 2):3, 1983.

75. Montigny, M., Davignon, A., Fouron, J. C., et al.: Captopril in infants for congestive heart failure secondary to a large ventricular to right shunt. Am J. Cardiol. 63:631, 1989.

76. Snyder, J. V.: Assessment of systemic oxygen transport. In Snyder, J. V. (ed.): Oxygen Transport in the Clinically Ill. Chicago, Year Book Medical Publishing Co., 1987, p. 179.

77. Kleinman, C. S., and Donnerstein, R. L.: Ultrasonic assessment of cardiac function in the intact human fetus. J. Am. Coll. Cardiol. 5:84S, 1985.

78. Silverman, N. H., Kleinman, C. S., Rudolph, A. M., et al.: Fetal atrioventricular valve insufficiency associated with nonimmune hydrops: A two-dimensional echocardiographic and pulsed Doppler ultrasound study. Circulation 72:825, 1985.

79. Reed, K. L., Appelton, C. P., Anderson, C. F., et al.: Doppler studies of venacaval flows in human fetuses. Circulation 81:498, 1990.

80. Gembruch, U., Manz, M., Bald, R., et al.: Repeated intravascular treatment with amiodarone in a fetus with refractory supraventricular tachycardia and hydrops fetalis. Am. Heart J. 118:1335, 1989.

81. Silverman, N. H., and Schmidt, K. G.: The current role of Doppler echocardiography in the diagnosis of heart disease in children. Cardiol. Clin. 7:265, 1989.

82. Cloez, J. L., Schmidt, K. G., Birk, E., and Silverman, N. H.: Determination of pulmonary systemic blood flow ratio in children by simplified Doppler echocardiographic method. J. Am. Coll. Cardiol. 11:825, 1988.

83. Sahn, D. J.: Applications of color flow mapping in pediatric cardiology. Cardiol. Clin. 7:255, 1989.

84. Krabill, K. A., Ring, W. S., Foker, J. E., et al.: Echocardiographic versus cardiac catheterization diagnosis of infants with congenital heart disease requiring cardiac surgery. Am. J. Cardiol. 60:351, 1987.

85. Stanger, P., Heymann, M. A., Tarnoff, H., et al.: Complications of cardiac catheterization of neonates, infants and children. Circulation 50:595, 1974.

86. Rashkind, W. J., Tait, M.A.S., and Gibson, R. J., Jr.: Interventional cardiac catheterization in congenital heart disease. Int. J. Cardiol. 7:1, 1985.

87. Lock, J. E., Keane, J. F., and Fellows, K. E.: The use of catheter intervention procedures for congenital heart disease. J. Am. Coll. Cardiol. 7:1420, 1986.

88. Mullins, C. E., Latson, L. A., Neches, W. H. et al.: Balloon dilation of miscellaneous lesions: Results of valvuloplasty and angioplasty of congenital anomalies registry. Am. J. Cardiol. 65:802, 1990.

89. Mullins, C. E.: Pediatric and congenital therapeutic cardiac catheterization. Circulation 79:1153, 1989.

90. Beckman, R. H., Rocchini, A. P., and Rosenthal, A.: Therapeutic cardiac catheterization for pulmonary valve and pulmonary artery stenosis. Cardiol. Clin. 7:331, 1989.

91. Perry, S. B., Zeevi, B., Keane, J. F., and Lock, J. E.: Interventional catheterization of left heart lesions, including aortic and mitral valve stenosis and coarctation of the aorta. Cardiol. Clin. 7:341, 1989.

92. Hellenbrand, W. E., and Mullins, C. E.: Catheter closure of congenital heart defects. Cardiol. Clin. 7:351, 1989.

93. Zipes, D. P., Akthar, M., Denes, P., et al.: Guidelines for clinical intracar-

diac electrophysiologic studies. A report of the American College of Cardiology/AHA Task Force on assessment of diagnostic and therapeutic cardiovascular procedures. J. Am. Coll. Cardiol. 14:1827, 1989.

94. Perry, J. C., and Garson, A., Jr.: Diagnosis and treatment of arrhythmias. Adv. Pediatr. 36:177, 1989.

95. Case, C. L., Crawford, F. A., and Gillette, P. C.: Surgical treatment of dysrhythmias in infants and children. Ped. Clin. North Am. 37:79, 1990.

96. Kugler, J. D., Bansal, A. M., Cheatham, J. P., et al.: Drug-electrophysiology studies in infants, children and adolescents. Am. Heart J. 110:144, 1985.

SPECIFIC CARDIAC DEFECTS

97. Hunt, C. E., and Lucas, R. V., Jr.: Symptomatic atrial septal defect in infancy. Circulation 42:1042, 1973.

98. Davea, J. E., Cheitlin, M. D., and Bedynek, J. L.: Sinus venosus atrial septal defect. Am. Heart J. 85:177, 1973.

99. Bashi, V. V., Ravikumar, E., Jairaj, P. S., et al.: Coexistent mitral valve disease with left-to-right shunt at the atrial level: Clinical profile, hemodynamics, and surgical considerations in 67 consecutive patients. Am. Heart J. 114:1406, 1987.

100. Leachman, R. D., Cokkinos, D. V., and Cooley, D. A.: Association of ostium secundum atrial septal defects with mitral valve prolapse. Am. J. Cardiol. 38:167, 1976.

101. Levin, A. R., Spach, M. S., Boineau, J. P., et al.: Atrial pressure flow dynamics and atrial septal defects (secundum type). Circulation 37:476, 1968.

102. O'Toole, J. D., Reddy, I., Curtiss, E. I., and Shaver, J. A.: The mechanism of splitting of the second heart sound in atrial septal defect. Circulation 41:1047, 1977.

103. Clark, E. B., and Kugler, J. D.: Preoperative secundum atrial septal defect with coexisting sinus node and atrioventricular node dysfunction. Circulation 65:976, 1982.

104. Mugge, A., Daniel, W. G., Klopper, J. W., and Lichtlen, P. R.: Visualization of patent foramen ovale by transesophageal color-coded Doppler echocardiography. Am. J. Cardiol. 62:837, 1988.

105. Shub, C., Tajik, A. J., Seward, J. B., et al.: Surgical repair of uncomplicated atrial septal defect without "routine" preoperative cardiac catheterization. J. Am. Coll. Cardiol. 6:49, 1985.

106. Freed, M. D., Nadas, A. S., Norwood, W. I., and Castaneda, A. R.: Is routine preoperative cardiac catheterization necessary before repair of secundum and sinus venosus atrial septal defects? J. Am. Coll. Cardiol. 4:333, 1984.

107. Taketa, R. M., Sahn, D. J., Simon, A. L., et al.: Catheter positions in congenital cardiac malformations. Circulation 51:749, 1975.

108. Brand, A., Keren, A., Branski, D., et al.: Natural course of atrial septal aneurysm in children and the potential for spontaneous closure of associated septal defect. Am. J. Cardiol. 64:996, 1989.

109. Steele, P. M., Fuster, V., Cohen, M., et al.: Isolated atrial septal defect with pulmonary vascular obstructive disease—long term follow up and prediction of outcome after surgical correction. Circulation 76:1037, 1987.

110. Levin, A. R., Liebson, P. R., Ehlers, K. H., and Daimant, B.: Assessment of left ventricular function in atrial septal defect. Pediatr. Res. 9:894, 1975.

111. Epstein, S. E., Beiser, G. D., Goldstein, R. E., et al.: Hemodynamic abnormalities in response to mild and intense upright exercise following operative correction of an atrial septal defect or tetralogy of Fallot. Circulation 42:1065, 1973.

112. Karpawich, P. P., Antillon, J. R., Cappola, P. R., and Agarwal, K. C.: Pre- and postoperative electrophysiologic assessment of children with secundum atrial septal defect. Am. J. Cardiol. 55:519, 1985.

113. Bink-Boelkens, M.T.E., Bergstra, A., and Landsman, M.L.J.: Functional abnormalities of the conduction system in children with an atrial septal defect. Int. J. Cardiol. 20:263, 1988.

114. Bink-Boelkens, M.T.E., Meuzelaar, K. J., and Eygelaar, A.: Arrhythmias after repair of secundum atrial septal defect: The influence of surgical modification. Am. Heart J. 115:629, 1988.

115. Borkon, A. M., Pieroni, D. R., Varghese, P. J., et al.: The superior QRS axis in ostium primum ASD. Am. Heart J. 92:15, 1975.

116. Goodman, D. J., Harrison, D. C., and Cannom, D. S.: Atrioventricular conduction in patients with incomplete endocardial cushion defect. Circulation 49:630, 1974.

117. Jacobsen, J. R., Gillette, P. C., Corbett, B. N., et al.: Intracardiac electrography in endocardial cushion defects. Circulation 54:599, 1976.

118. Waldo, A. L., Kaiser, G. A., Bowman, F. O., Jr., and Malm, J. R.: Etiology of prolongation of the PR interval in patients with an endocardial cushion defect. Circulation 43:19, 1973.

119. Smallhorn, J. F., Tommasini, G., and Anderson, R. H.: Assessment of atrioventricular septal defects by two-dimensional echocardiography. Br. Heart J. 47:109, 1982.

120. Lipshultz, S. E., Sanders, S. P., Mayer, J. E., et al.: Are routine preoperative cardiac catheterization angiography necessary before repair of ostium primum atrial septal defect? J. Am. Coll. Cardiol. 11:373, 1988.

121. DeBia, S.E.L., DiCommo, V., Ballerini, L., et al.: Prevalence of left-sided obstructive lesions in patients with atrial ventricular canal without Down's syndrome. J. Thorac. Cardiovasc. Surg. 91:467, 1986.

122. Elliott, L. P., Bargeron, L. M., Jr., and Green, C. E.: Angled angiography: General approach and findings. In Friedman, W. F., and Higgins, C. B. (eds.): Pediatric Cardiac Imaging. Philadelphia, W. B. Saunders Company, 1984, p. 1.

123. Castaneda, A. R., Mayer, J. E., and Jonas, R. A.: Repair of complete atrioventricular canal in infancy. World J. Surg. 9:590, 1985.

124. Santos, A., Boucek, M., Ruttenberg, H., et al.: Repair of atrioventricular septal defects in infancy. J. Thorac. Cardiovasc. Surg. 91:505, 1986.

125. Clapp, S. K., Perry, B. L., Farooki, Z. Q., et al.: Surgical and medical results of complete atrioventricular canal: A ten-year review. Am. J. Cardiol. 59:454, 1987.

126. Pacifico, A. D.: Surgical treatment of complex atrial ventricular septal defects. Cardiol. Clin. 7:399, 1989.

127. Ceithaml, E. L., Midgley, F. M., and Perry, L. W.: Long term results after surgical repair of incomplete endocardial cushion defects. Am. Thorac. Surg. 48:413, 1989.

127a. Soto, B., Ceballos, R., and Kirklin, J. W.: Ventricular septal defects: A surgical viewpoint. J. Am. Coll. Cardiol. 14:1291, 1989.

128. Van Praagh, R., Geva, T., and Kreutzer, J.: Ventricular septal defects: How shall we describe, name and classify them? J. Am. Coll. Cardiol. 14:1298, 1989.

129. Hagler, D. J., Edwards, W. D., Seward, J. B., and Tajik, A. J.: Standardized nomenclature of the ventricular septum and ventricular septal defects, with applications for two-dimensional echocardiography. Mayo Clin. Proc. 60:741, 1985.

130. Baker, E. J., Leung, M. P., Anderson, R. H., et al.: The cross-sectional anatomy of ventricular septal defects: A reappraisal. Br. Heart J. 69:339, 1988.

131. Helmcke, F., Souza, A., Nanda, N. C., et al.: Two-dimensional and color Doppler assessment of ventricular septal defect of congenital origin. Am. J. Cardiol. 63:1112, 1989.

132. Sharif, D. S., Huhta, J. C., Marantz, P., et al.: Two-dimensional echocardiographic determination of ventricular septal defect size: Correlation of autopsy. Am. Heart J. 117:1333, 1989.

133. Beerman, L. B., Park, S. C., Fischer, D. R., et al.: Ventricular septal defect associated with aneurysm of the membranous septum. J. Am. Coll. Cardiol. 5:118, 1985.

134. Ortiz, E., Robinson, P. J., Deanfield, J. E., et al.: Localisation of ventricular septal defects by simultaneous display of superimposed colour Doppler and cross sectional echocardiographic images. Br. Heart J. 54:53, 1985.

135. Murphy, D. J., Ludomirsky, A., and Huhta, J. C.: Continuous-wave Doppler in children with ventricular septal defect: Noninvasive estimation of interventricular pressure gradient. Am. J. Cardiol. 57:428, 1986.

136. Kurokawa, S., Takahashi, M., Katoh, Y., et al.: Noninvasive evaluation of the ratio of pulmonary to systemic flow in ventricular septal defect by means of Doppler two-dimensional echocardiography. Am. Heart J. 116:1033, 1988.

137. Williams, R. G.: Doppler color-flow mapping and prediction of ventricular defect outcome. J. Am. Coll. Cardiol. 13:1119, 1989.

138. Hornberger, L. K., Sahn, D. J., Krabill, K. A., et al.: Elucidation of the natural history of ventricular septal defects by serial Doppler color-flow mapping studies. J. Am. Coll. Cardiol. 13:1111, 1989.

139. Friedman, W. F., Mehrizi, A., and Pusch, A. L.: Multiple muscular ventricular septal defects. Circulation 32:35, 1964.

140. Dickinson, D. F., Arnold, R., and Wilkinson, J. L.: Ventricular septal defects in children born in Liverpool. Evaluation of natural course and surgical implications in an unselected population. Br. Heart J. 46:47, 1981.

141. Weidman, W. H., Blount, S. G., Jr., DuShane, J. W., et al.: Clinical course in ventricular septal defect. Natural history study. Circulation 56(Suppl.):I-56, 1977.

142. Ramaciotti, C., Keren, A., and Silverman, N. H.: Importance of (perimembranous) ventricular septal aneurysm in the natural history of isolated perimembranous ventricular septal defect. Am. J. Cardiol. 57:268, 1986.

143. Friedman, W. F., and Pitlick, P. T.: Ventricular septal defect in infancy— University of California, San Diego (Specialty Conference). West. J. Med. 120:295, 1974.

144. Blumenthal, S., Griffiths, S. P., and Morgan, B. C.: Bacterial endocarditis in children with heart disease. (A review based on the literature and experience with 58 cases.) Pediatrics 26:993, 1960.

145. Moe, D. J., and Guntheroth, W. G.: Spontaneous closure of uncomplicated ventricular septal defect. Am. J. Cardiol. 60:674, 1987.

146. Neutze, J. M., Ishikawa, T., Clarkson, P. M., et al.: Assessment and follow up of patients with ventricular septal defect and elevated pulmonary vascular resistance. Am. J. Cardiol. 63:327, 1989.

147. Yeager, S. B., Freed, M. D., Keane, J. F., et al.: Primary surgical closure of ventricular septal defect in the first year of life: results in 128 infants. J. Am. Coll. Cardiol. 3:1269, 1984.

148. McDaniel, N., Gutgesell, H. P., Nolan, S. P., and Kron, I. L.: Repair of large muscular ventricular septal defects in infants employing left ventriculotomy. Ann. Thorac. Surg. 47:593, 1989.

149. Hislop, A., Haworth, S. G., Shinebourne, E. A., and Reid, L.: Quantitative structural analysis of pulmonary vessels in isolated ventricular septal defect in infancy. Br. Heart J. 37:1014, 1975.

150. DuShane, J. W., and Kirklin, J. W.: Late results of the repair of ventricular septal defect on pulmonary vascular disease. In Kirklin, J. W. (ed.): Advances in Cardiovascular Surgery. New York, Grune and Stratton, 1973, p. 9.

151. Rhodes, L. A., Keane, J. F., Keane, J. P., et al.: Long-term follow up (up to 43 years) of ventricular septal defect with audible aortic regurgitation. Am. J. Cardiol. 66:340, 1990.

152. Griffin, M. L., Sullivan, I. D., Anderson, R. H., and Macartney, F. J.: Doubly committed subarterial ventricular septal defect: New morphological criteria with echocardiographic and angiocardiographic correlation. Br. Heart J. 59:474, 1988.

153. Schmidt, K. G., Cassidy, S. C., Silverman, N. H., and Stanger, P.: Doubly

committed subarterial ventricular septal defects: Echocardiographic features and surgical implications. J. Am. Coll. Cardiol. *12*:1538, 1988.

154. Okita, Y., Miki, S., Kusuhara, K., et al.: Long-term results of aortic valvuloplasty for aortic regurgitation associated with ventricular septal defect. J. Thorac. Cardiovasc. Surg. *96*:769, 1988.

155. Leung, M. P., Mok, C. K., Lo, R.N.S., and Lau, K. C.: An echocardiographic study of perimembranous ventricular septal defect with left ventricular to right atrial shunting. Br. Heart J. *55*:45, 1986.

156. Gersony, W. M., and Hayes, C. J.: Bacterial endocarditis in patients with pulmonary stenosis, aortic stenosis, or ventricular septal defect. Natural history study. Circulation *56*(Suppl.):I-84, 1977.

157. deLeval, M.: Ventricular septal defects. In Stark, J., and deLeval, M. (eds.): Surgery for Congenital Heart Defects. New York, Grune and Stratton, Inc., 1983, p. 271.

158. Lock, J. E., Block, P. C., McKay, R. G., et al.: Transcatheter closure of ventricular septal defects. Circulation *78*:361, 1988.

159. Godman, M. J., Roberts, N. K., and Izukawa, T.: Late postoperative conduction disturbances after repair of ventricular septal defect in tetralogy of Fallot. Circulation *49*:214, 1974.

160. Okarama, E. O., Guller, B., Molony, J. D., and Weidman, W. H.: Etiology of right bundle-branch block pattern after surgical closure of ventricular-septal defects. Am. Heart J. *90*:14, 1975.

161. Otterstad, J. E., Simonsen, S., and Erikssen, J.: Hemodynamic findings at rest and during mild supine exercise in adults with isolated uncomplicated ventricular septal defects. Circulation *71*:650, 1985.

162. Maron, B. J., Redwood, D. R., Hirschfeld, J. W., Jr., et al.: Postoperative assessment of patients with ventricular septal defect and pulmonary hypertension. Response to intense upright exercise. Circulation *48*:864, 1973.

163. Graham, T. P., Jr., Atwood, G. F., Boucek, R. J., Jr., et al.: Right ventricular volume characteristics in ventricular septal defect. Circulation *54*:800, 1976.

164. Heymann, M. A., and Rudolph, A. M.: Control of the ductus arteriosus. Physiol. Rev. *55*:62, 1975.

165. Friedman, W. F., Printz, M. P., Kirkpatrick, S. E., and Hoskins, E. J.: The vasoactivity of the fetal lamb ductus arteriosus studied in utero. Pediatr. Res. *17*:331, 1983.

166. Skidgel, R. A., Friedman, W. F., and Printz, M. P.: Prostaglandin biosynthetic activities of the fetal lamb ductus arteriosus, other blood vessels and fetal lung. Pediatr. Res. *18*:12, 1984.

167. Printz, M. P., Skidgel, R. A., and Friedman, W. F.: Studies of pulmonary prostaglandin biosynthetic and catabolic enzymes as factors in ductus arteriosus patency and closure: Evidence for a shift in products with gestational age. Pediatr. Res. *18*:19, 1984.

168. Gittenberger-DeGroot, A. C.: Persistent ductus arteriosus: Most probably a primary congenital malformation. Br. Heart J. *39*:610, 1977.

169. Friedman, W. F., Hirschklau, M. J., Printz, M. P., et al.: Pharmacologic closure of patent ductus arteriosus in the premature infant. N. Engl. J. Med. *295*:526, 1976.

170. Douidar, S. M., Richardson, J., and Snodgrass, W. R.: Use of indomethacin in ductus closure: An update evaluation. Dev. Pharmacol. Ther. *11*:196, 1988.

171. Sahn, D. J., Vaucher, Y., Williams, D. E., et al.: Echocardiographic detection of large left to right shunts and cardiomyopathies in infants and children. Am. J. Cardiol. *38*:73, 1976.

172. Liao, P. K., Su, W. J., and Hung, J. S.: Doppler echocardiographic flow characteristics of isolated patent ductus arteriosus: Better delineation by Doppler color-flow mapping. J. Am. Coll. Cardiol. *12*:1285, 1988.

173. Hiraishi, S., Horiguchi, Y., Misawa, H., et al.: Noninvasive Doppler echocardiographic evaluation of shunt flow dynamics of the ductus arteriosus. Circulation *75*:1146, 1987.

174. Cloez, J. L., Issaz, K., and Pernot, C.: Pulsed Doppler flow characteristics of ductus arteriosus in infants with associated congenital anomalies of the heart or great arteries. Am. J. Cardiol. *57*:845, 1986.

175. Yeh, T. F., Achanti, B., Patel, H., and Pildes, R. S.: Indomethacin therapy in premature infants with patent ductus arteriosus — determination of therapeutic plasma levels. Dev. Pharmacol. Ther. *12*:169, 1989.

176. Jacob, J., Gluck, L., DiSessa, T. G., et al.: The contribution of PDA in the neonate with severe RDS. J. Pediatr. *96*:79, 1980.

177. Merritt, T. A., Harris, J. P., and Roghmann, K.: Early closure of the patent ductus arteriosus in very low birth weight infants: A controlled trial. J. Pediatr. *99*:281, 1981.

178. Gersony, W. M., Peckham, G. J., Ellison, R. C., et al.: Effects of indomethacin in premature infants with patent ductus arteriosus: Results of a national collaborative study. J. Pediatr. *102*:895, 1983.

179. Cassady, G., Crouse, D. T., Kirklin, J. W., et al.: A randomized control trial of very early prophylactic ligation of the ductus arteriosus in babies who weighed 1000 g or less at birth. N. Engl. J. Med. *320*:1511, 1989.

180. Wagner, H. R., Ellison, R. C., Zierler, S., et al.: Surgical closure of patent ductus arteriosus in 268 preterm infants. J. Thorac. Cardiovasc. Surg. *87*:870, 1984.

181. Jarmakani, M. M., Graham, T. P., Jr., Canent, R. V., Jr., et al.: Effect of site of shunt on left heart volume characteristics in children with ventricular septal defect and patent ductus arteriosus. Circulation *40*:411, 1969.

182. Bessenger, F. B., Jr., Blieden, L. C., and Edwards, J. E.: Hypertensive pulmonary vascular disease associated with patent ductus arteriosus. Circulation *52*:157, 1975.

183. Latson, L. A., Hofschire, P. J., Kugler, J. D., et al.: Transcatheter closure of patent ductus arteriosus in pediatric patients. J. Pediatr. *115*:549, 1989.

184. Krichenko, A., Benson, L. N., Burrows, P., et al.: Angiographic classifica-

tion of the isolated, persistently patent ductus arteriosus and implications for percutaneous catheter closure. Am. J. Cardiol. *63*:877, 1989.

185. Musewe, N. N., Benson, L. N., Smallhorn, J. F., and Freedom, R. M.: Two-dimensional echocardiographic and color-flow Dopper evaluation of ductal occlusion with the Rashkind prothesis. Circulation *80*:1706, 1989.

186. Ali Khan, M. A., Mullins, C. E., Nihill, M. R., et al.: Percutaneous catheter closure of the ductus arteriosus in children and young adults. Am. J. Cardiol. *64*:218, 1989.

187. Hellenbrand, W. E., and Mullins, C. E.: Catheter closure of congenital cardiac defects. Cardiol. Clin. *7*:351, 1989.

188. Kutsche, L. M., and Van Mierop, L.H.S.: Anatomy and pathogenesis of aorticopulmonary septal defect. Am. J. Cardiol. *59*:443, 1987.

189. Tiraboschi, R., Salomone, G., Crupi, G., et al.: Aorto-pulmonary window in the first year of life: Report on 11 surgical cases. Ann. Thorac. Surg. *46*:438, 1988.

190. Prasad, T. R., Valiathan, M. S., Chyamakrishnan, K. G., et al.: Surgical management of aortopulmonary septal defect. Ann. Thorac. Surg. *47*:877, 1989.

191. Crupi, G., Macartney, F. J., and Anderson, R. H.: Persistent truncus arteriosus: A study of 66 autopsy cases with special reference to definition and morphogenesis. Am. J. Cardiol. *40*:569, 1977.

192. Shrivastava, F., and Edwards, J. E.: Coronary arterial origin and persistent truncus arteriosus. Circulation *55*:551, 1977.

193. Suzuki, A., Ho, S. Y., Anderson, R. H., and Deanfield, J. E.: Coronary arterial and sinusal anatomy in hearts with a common arterial trunk. Ann. Thorac. Surg. *48*:792, 1989.

194. Calder, L., Van Praagh, R., Sears, W. P., et al.: Truncus arteriosus communis. Am. Heart J. *92*:23, 1976.

195. Juaneda, E., and Haworth, S. G.: Pulmonary vascular disease in children with truncus arteriosus. Am. J. Cardiol. *54*:1314, 1984.

196. Radford, D. J., Perkins, L., Lachman, R., and Thong, Y. H.: Spectrum of DiGeorge syndrome in patients with truncus arteriosus: Expanded DiGeorge syndrome. Pediatr. Cardiol. *9*:95, 1988.

196a. Kirby, M. L., and Waldo, K. L.: Role of neural crest in congenital heart disease. Circulation *82*:332, 1990.

197. Gelband, H., Van Meter, M., and Gersony, W. M.: Truncal valve abnormalities in infants with persistent truncus arteriosus. Circulation *45*:397, 1972.

198. Yoshizato, T., and Julsrud, P. R.: Truncus arteriosus revisited: An angiographic demonstration. Pediatr. Cardiol. *11*:36, 1990.

199. Bove, E. L., Beekman, R. H., Snider, A. R., et al.: Repair of truncus arteriosus in the neonate and young infant. Ann. Thorac. Surg. *47*:499, 1989.

200. Cooper, M. J., Bernstein, D., and Silverman, N. H.: Recognition of left coronary artery fistula to the left and right ventricles by contrast echocardiography. J. Am. Coll. Cardiol. *6*:923, 1985.

201. Miyatake, K., Okamoto, M., Kinoshita, N., et al.: Doppler echocardiographic features of coronary arteriovenous fistula. Complementary roles of cross sectional echocardiography and the Doppler technique. Br. Heart J. *51*:508, 1984.

202. Ruttenhouse, E. A., Doty, D. B., and Ehrenhaft, J. L.: Congenital coronary artery-cardiac chamber fistula. Review of operative management. Ann. Thorac. Surg. *20*:468, 1975.

203. Angelini, P.: Normal and anomalous coronary arteries: Definitions and classification. Am. Heart J. *117*:418, 1989.

204. Hurwitz, R. A., Caldwell, R. L., Girod, D. A., et al.: Clinical and hemodynamic course of infants and children with anomalous left coronary artery. Am. Heart J. *118*:1176, 1989.

205. Menahem, S., and Venables, A. W.: Anomalous left coronary artery from the pulmonary artery: A 15-year sample. Br. Heart J. *58*:378, 1987.

206. Vaksmann, G., Mauran, P., Ray, C., et al.: Visualization of anomalous origin of the left main coronary artery from the pulmonary trunk by pulsed and color Doppler echocardiography. Am. Heart J. *116*:181, 1988.

207. Schmidt, K. G., Cooper, M. J., Silverman, N. H., and Stanger, P.: Pulmonary artery origin of the left coronary artery: Diagnosis by two-dimensional echocardiography, pulsed Doppler ultrasound and color-flow mapping. J. Am. Coll. Cardiol. *11*:396, 1988.

208. Rein, A.J.J.T., Colan, S. D., Parness, I. A., and Sanders, S. P.: Regional and global left ventricular function in infants with anomalous origin of the left coronary artery from the pulmonary trunk: Preoperative and postoperative assessment. Circulation *75*:115, 1987.

209. Guikahue, M. K., Sidi, D., Kachaner, J., et al.: Anomalous left coronary artery arising from the pulmonary artery in infancy: Is early operation better? Br. Heart J. *60*:522, 1988.

210. Boutefeu, J. M., Morat, P. R., Hahn, C., and Hauf, E.: Aneurysms of the sinus of Valsalva. Report of seven cases in review of the literature. Am. J. Med. *65*:18, 1978.

211. Engle, P. J., Held, J. S., Bel-Kahn, J.V.D., and Spitz, H.: Echocardiographic diagnosis of congenital sinus of Valsalva aneurysm. Circulation *63*:705, 1981.

212. Barragry, T. P., Ring, W. S., Moller, J. H., and Lillehei, C. W.: 15 to 30 year follow up of patients undergoing repair of ruptured congenital aneurysms of the sinus of Valsalva. Ann. Thorac. Surg. *46*:515, 1988.

213. Smyth, P. T., and Edwards, J. E.: Pseudocoarctation, kinking or buckling of the aorta. Circulation *46*:1027, 1972.

214. Hutchins, G. M.: Coarctation of the aorta explained as a branch point of the ductus arteriosus. Am. J. Pathol. *63*:203, 1971.

215. Talner, N. S., and Berman, M. A.: Postnatal development of obstruction in coarctation of the aorta: Role of the ductus arteriosus. Pediatrics *56*:562, 1975.

216. Heymann, M. A., Berman, W., Jr., Rudolph, A. M., and Whitman, V.:

Dilatation of the ductus arteriosus by prostaglandin E₁ in aortic arch abnormalities. Circulation 59:169, 1979.

217. Tynan, M., Finley, J. P., Fontes, V., et al.: Balloon angioplasty for the treatment of native coarctation: Results of valvuloplasty and angioplasty of congenital anomalies registry. Am. J. Cardiol. 65:790, 1990.

218. Kopf, G. S., Hellenbrand, W., Kleinman, C., et al.: Repair of aortic coarctation in the first three months of life: Immediate and long-term results. Ann. Thorac. Surg. 41:425, 1986.

219. Van Son, J.A.M., Skotnicki, S. H., Van Asten, W. N., et al.: Quantitative assessment of coarctation in infancy by Doppler spectral analysis. Am. J. Cardiol. 63:1282, 1989.

220. Shaddy, R. E., Snider, A. R., Silverman, N. H., and Lutin, W.: Pulsed Doppler findings in patients with coarctation of the aorta. Circulation 73:82, 1986.

221. Rao, P. S., and Carey, P.: Doppler ultrasound in the prediction of pressure gradients across aortic coarctation. Am. Heart J. 118:299, 1989.

222. Godwin, G. D., Herfkens, R. L., Brundage, D. H., and Lipton, N. J.: Evaluation of coarctation of the aorta by computed tomography. J. Comput. Assist. Tomogr. 5:153, 1981.

223. Graham, T. P., Jr., Burger, J., Boucek, R. J., Jr., et al.: Absence of left ventricular volume loading in infants with coarctation of the aorta and a large ventricular septal defect. J. Am. Coll. Cardiol. 14:1545, 1989.

224. George, B., DiSessa, T. G., Williams, R. G., et al.: Coarctation repair without cardiac catheterization in infants. Am. Heart J. 114:1421, 1987.

225. Cohen, M., Fuster, V., Steele, P. M., et al.: Coarctation of the aorta: Long-term follow up and prediction of outcome after surgical correction. Circulation 80:840, 1989.

226. Bromberg, B. I., Beekman, R. H., Rocchini, A. P., et al.: Aortic aneurysm after patch aortoplasty repair of coarctation: A prospective analysis of prevalence, screening tests and risks. J. Am. Coll. Cardiol. 14:734, 1989.

227. Beekman, R. H., Rocchini, A. P., Behrendt, D. M., and Rosenthal, A.: Reoperation for coarctation of the aorta. Am. J. Cardiol. 48:1108, 1981.

228. Igler, F. O., Boerboom, L. E., Werner, P. H., et al.: Coarctation of the aorta and narrow receptor resetting. Circulation Res. 48:365, 1981.

229. Gidding, S. S., Rocchini, A. P., Beekman, R., et al.: Therapeutic effect of propranolol on paradoxical hypertension after repair of coarctation of the aorta. N. Engl. J. Med. 312:1224, 1985.

230. Choy, M., Rocchini, A. P., Beekman, R. H., et al.: Paradoxical hypertension after repair of coarctation of the aorta in children: Balloon angioplasty versus surgical repair. Circulation 75:1186, 1987.

231. Johnson, R. G., Williams, G. R., Razook, J. D., et al.: Reoperation in congenital aortic stenosis. Ann. Thorac. Surg. 40:156, 1985.

232. Hellenbrand, W. E., Allen, H. D., Golinko, R. J., et al.: Balloon angioplasty for aortic re-coarctation: Results of valvuloplasty and angioplasty of congenital anomalies registry. Am. J. Cardiol. 65:793, 1990.

233. Murphy, A. M., Blades, M., Daniels, S., and James, F. W.: Blood pressure in cardiac output during exercise: A longitudinal study of children undergoing repair of coarctation. Am. Heart J. 117:1327, 1989.

234. Maron, B. J., Humphries, J., Rowe, R. D., and Mellits, E. D.: Prognosis of surgically corrected coarctation of the aorta. Circulation 47:119, 1973.

235. Van Woezik, E.V.M., Kline, H. W., and Krediet, P.: Normal internal calibers of ostia, great arteries and aortic isthmus in children. Br. Heart J. 39:860, 1977.

236. Bharati, S., and Lev, M.: The surgical anatomy of the heart in tubular hypoplasia of the transverse aorta (preductal coarctation). J. Thorac. Cardiovasc. Surg. 91:79, 1986.

237. Graham, T. P., Jr., Atwood, G. F., Boerth, R. C., et al.: Right and left heart size and function in infants with symptomatic coarctation. Circulation 56:641, 1977.

238. Hammon, J. W., Jr., Merrill, W. H., Prager, R. L., et al.: Repair of interrupted aortic arch and associated malformations in infancy: Indications for complete or partial repair. Ann. Thorac. Surg. 42:17, 1986.

239. Sell, J. E., Jonas, R. A., Mayer, J. E., et al.: The results of a surgical program for interrupted aortic arch. J. Thorac. Cardiovasc. Surg. 96:864, 1988.

240. Dekker, A. O., Gittenberger-DeGroot, A. C., and Roozendaal, H.: The ductus arteriosus and associated cardiac anomalies in interruption of the aortic arch. Pediatr. Cardiol. 2:185, 1982.

241. Friedman, W. F.: Congenital aortic stenosis. In Adams, F. H., and Emmanouilides, G. C. (eds.): Moss' Heart Disease in Infants, Children and Adolescents. 4th ed. Baltimore, Williams and Wilkins, 1989.

241a. Stevens, C. A., Carey, J. C., and Shigeoka, A. O.: DiGeorge anomaly and velocardiofacial syndrome. Pediatrics 85:526, 1990.

242. Friedman, W. F., and Pappelbaum, S. J.: Indications for hemodynamic evaluation and surgery in congenital aortic stenosis. Pediatr. Clin. North Am. 18:1207, 1971.

243. Kveselis, D. A., Rocchini, A. P., Rosenthal, A., et al.: Hemodynamic determinants of exercise-induced ST-segment depression in children with valvar aortic stenosis. Am. J. Cardiol. 55:1133, 1985.

244. Cyran, S. E., James, F. W., Daniels, S., et al.: Comparison of the cardiac output and stroke volume response to upright exercise in children with valvular and subvalvular aortic stenosis. J. Am. Coll. Cardiol. 11:651, 1988.

245. Lewis, A. L., Heymann, M. A., Stanger, P., et al.: Evaluation of subendocardial ischemia in valvar aortic stenosis in children. Circulation 49:978, 1974.

246. Lakier, J. B., Lewis, A. B., Heymann, M. A., et al.: Isolated aortic stenosis of the neonate: Natural history and hemodynamic considerations. Circulation 50:801, 1974.

247. Balaji, S., Keeton, B. R., Sutherland, G., et al.: Aortic valvotomy for critical aortic stenosis in neonates and infants aged less than one year. Br. Heart J. 61:358, 1989.

248. Karl, T. R., Sano, S., Brawn, W. J., and Mee, R.B.B.: Critical aortic stenosis in the first month of life: Surgical results in 26 infants. Ann. Thorac. Surg. 50:105, 1990.

249. Sink, J. D., Smallhorn, J. F., Macartney, F. J.: Mangement of critical aortic stenosis in infancy. J. Thorac. Cardiovasc. Surg. 87:82, 1984.

250. Broderick, T. W., Higgins, C. B., and Friedman, W. F.: Critical aortic stenosis in neonates. Radiology 129:393, 1978.

251. Skjaerpe, T., Hegrenaes, L., and Hatle, L.: Noninvasive estimation of valve area in patients with arotic stenosis by Doppler ultrasound anad two-dimensional echocardiography. Circulation 72:810, 1985.

252. Ohlsson, J., and Wranne, B.: Noninvasive assessment of valve area in patients with aortic stenosis. J. Am. Coll. Cardiol. 7:501, 1986.

253. Oh, J. K., Taliercio, C. P., Holmes, D. R., et al.: Prediction of the severity of aortic stenosis by Doppler aortic valve area determination: Prospective Doppler-catheterization correlation in 100 patients. J. Am. Coll. Cardiol. 11:1227, 1988.

254. Bengur, A. R., Snider, A. R., Serwer, G. A., et al.: Usefulness of the Doppler mean gradient in evaluation of children with aortic valve stenosis in comparison to gradient at catheterization. Am. J. Cardiol. 64:756, 1989.

255. Meliones, J. N., Snider, R., Serwer, G. A., et al.: Pulsed Doppler assessment of left ventricular diastolic filling in children with left ventricular outflow obstruction before and after balloon angioplasty. Am. J. Cardiol. 63:231, 1989.

256. Kasten-Sportes, C. H., Piechaud, J. F., Sidi, D., and Kachaner, J.: Percutaneous balloon valvuloplasty in neonates with critical aortic stensis. J. Am. Coll. Cardiol. 13:1101, 1989.

257. Wheller, J. J., Hosier, D. M., Teske, D. W., et al.: Results of operation for aortic valve stenosis in infants, children and adolescents. J. Thorac. Cardiovasc. Surg. 96:474, 1988.

258. Karl, T. R., Sano, S., Brown, W. J., and Mee, R.B.B.: Critical aortic stenosis in the first month of life: Surgical results in 26 infants. Ann. Thorac. Surg. 50:105, 1990.

259. Braunwald, E., Goldblatt, A., Aygen, M. M., et al.: Congenital aortic stenosis. I. Clinical and hemodynamic findings in 100 patients. Circulation 27:426, 1963.

260. Johnson, A. M.: Aortic stenosis, sudden death, and the left ventricular baroreceptors. Br. Heart J. 33:1, 1971.

261. Wagner, H. R., Weidman, W. H., Ellison, R. C., and Miettinen, O. S.: Indirect assessment of severity in aortic stenosis. Natural history study. Circulation 56(Suppl.):I-20, 1977.

262. El-Said, G., Gallioto, F. J., Mullens, C. E., and McNamara, D. G.: Natural hemodynamic history of congenital aortic stenosis in childhood. Am. J. Cardiol. 30:6, 1972.

263. Hurwitz, R. A.: Aortic valve stenosis in childhood: Clinical and hemodynamic history. J. Pediatr. 82:228, 1973.

264. Friedman, W. F., Modlinger, J., and Morgan, J.: Serial hemodynamic observations in asymptomatic children with valvar aortic stenosis. Circulation 43:91, 1971.

265. Cohen, L. S., Friedman, W. F., and Braunwald, E.: Natural history of mild congenital aortic stenosis elucidated by serial hemodynamic studies. Am. J. Cardiol. 30:1, 1972.

266. Rocchini, A. P., Beekman, R. H., Ben Shachar, G., et al.: Balloon aortic valvuloplasty: Results of the valvuloplasty and angioplasty of congenital anomalies registry. Am. J. Cardiol. 65:784, 1990.

267. Bisset, G. S., III, Meyer, R. A., Hirschfeld, S. S., et al.: Aortic valve replacement in childhood: Evaluation of left ventricular function by electrocardiography, echocardiography and graded exercise testing. Am. J. Cardiol. 52:568, 1983.

268. Dorn, G. W., Donner, R., Assey, M. E., et al.: Alterations in left ventricular geometry, wall stress, and ejection performance after correction of congenital aortic stenosis. Circulation 78,:1358, 1988.

269. DeBoer, B. A., Robbins, R. C., Maron, B. J., et al.: Late results of aortic valvotomy for congenital valvular aortic stenosis. Ann. Thorac. Surg. 50:69, 1990.

270. DeBoer, B. A., Robbins, R. C., Maron, B. J., et al.: Late results of aortic valvotomy for congenital valvar aortic stenosis. Ann. Thorac. Surg. 50:69, 1990.

271. Friedman, W. F., Novak, V., and Johnson, A. D.: Congenital aortic stenosis in adults. In Roberts, W. C. (ed.): Congenital Heart Disease in Adults. Philadelphia, F. A. Davis, 1979, p. 235.

272. DiSessa, T. G., Hagan, A. D., Isabel-Jones, J. B., and Friedman, W. F.: Two-dimensional echocardiograpic evaluation of discrete subaortic stenosis from the apical long axis view. Am. Heart J. 101:774, 1981.

273. Pierli, C., Marino, B., Picardo, S., et al.: Discrete subaortic stenosis: Surgery in children based on two-dimensional and Doppler echocardiography. Chest 96:325, 1989.

274. Kinney, E. L., Machado, H., Cortada, X., and Galbut, D. L.: Diagnosis of discrete subaortic stenosis by pulsed and continuous wave echocardiography. Am. Heart J. 110:1069, 1985.

275. Mugge, A., Daniel, W. G., Wolpers, H. G., et al. Improved visualization of discrete subvalvular aortic stenosis by transesophageal color-coded Doppler echocardiography. Am. Heart J. 117:474, 1989.

276. Newfeld, E. A., Muster, A. J., Paul, M. H., et al.: Discrete subvalvular aortic stenosis in childhood. Am. J. Cardiol. 38:53, 1976.

277. Douville, E. C., Sade, R. M., Crawford, F. A., Jr., and Wiles, H. B.: Subvalvar aortic stenosis: timing of operation. Ann. Thorac. Surg. 50:29, 1990.

278. Brown, J., Stevens, L., Lynch, L., et al.: Surgery for discrete subvalvular aortic stenosis: Actuarial survival, hemodynamic results, and acquired aortic regurgitation. Ann. Thorac. Surg. 40:151, 1985.

279. Moses, R. D., Barnhart, G. R., and Jones, M.: The late prognosis after

localized resection for fixed (discrete and tunnel) left ventricular out-flow tract observation. J. Thorac. Cardiovasc. Surg. 87:410, 1984.

280. Ivert, T., Astudillo, R., Birdon, L., and Wranne, B.: Late results after a section of fixed subaortic stenosis. Scand. J. Thorac. Cardiovasc. Surg. 23:211, 1989.

281. Lababidi, Z., Weinhaus, L., Stoeckle, H., Jr., and Walls, J. T.: Transluminal balloon dilatation for discrete subaortic stenosis. Am. J. Cardiol. 59:423, 1987.

282. Maron, B. J., Redwood, D. R., Roberts, W. C., et al.: Tunnel subaortic stenosis. Circulation 54:404, 1976.

283. Ergin, M. A., Cooper, R., LaCourte, M., et al.: Experience with left ventricular apicoaortic conduits for complicated left ventricular outflow obstruction in children and young adults. Ann. Thorac. Surg. 32:369, 1981.

284. Waldman, J. D., Schneeweiss, A., Edwards, W. D., et al.: The obstructive subaortic conus. Circulation 70:339, 1984.

285. Friedman, W. G., and Roberts, W. C.: Vitamin D and the supravalvular aortic stenosis syndrome: The transplacental effects of vitamin D on the aorta of the rabbit. Circulation 34:77, 1966.

286. Friedman, W. F.: Vitamin D embryopathy. Adv. Teratol. 3:85, 1968.

287. Friedman, W. F., and Mills, L. F.: The relationship between vitamin D and the craniofacial and dental anomalies of the supraventricular aortic stenosis syndrome. Pediatrics 43:12, 1969.

288. Garcia, R. C., Friedman, W. F., Kaback, M. M., and Rowe, R. D.: Idiopathic hypercalcemia and supravalvular aortic stenosis: Documentation of a new syndrome. N. Engl. J. Med. 271:117, 1964.

289. Morris, C. A., Demsey, S. A., Leonard, C. O., et al.: Natural history of Williams syndrome: Physical characteristics. J. Pediatr. 113:318, 1988.

290. Taylor, A. B., Stern, P. H., and Bell, N. H.: Abnormal regulation of circulating 25-hydroxy vitamin D in the Williams syndrome. N. Engl. J. Med. 306:972, 1982.

291. Kahler, R. L., Braunwald, E., Plauth, W. H., Jr., and Morrow, A. G.: Familial congenital heart disease. Am. J. Med. 40:384, 1966.

292. French, J. W., and Guntheroth, W. G.: An explanation of asymmetric upper extremity blood pressure in supravalvular aortic stenosis: The Coanda effect. Circulation 42:31, 1970.

293. Goldstein, R. E., and Epstein, S. E.: Mechanism of elevated innominate artery pressures in supravalvular aortic stenosis. Circulation 42:23, 1970.

294. Brand, A., Keren, A., Reifen, R. M., et al.: Echocardiographic and Doppler findings in the Williams syndrome. Am. J. Cardiol. 63:633, 1989.

295. Stewart, S., Alexson, C., and Manning, J.: Extended aortoplasty to relieve supravalvular aortic stenosis. Ann. Thorac. Surg. 46:427, 1988.

296. Flaker, G., Teske, D., Kilman, J. et al.: Supravalvular aortic stenosis. A 20-year clinical perspective and experience with patch aortoplasty. Am. J. Cardiol. 15:256, 1983.

297. Sade, R. M., Crawford, F. A., Jr., and Fyfe, D. A.: Symposium on hypoplastic left heart syndrome. J. Thorac. Cardiovasc. Surg. 91:937, 1986.

298. Bash, S. E., Huhta, J. C., Vick, G. W., III, et al.: Hypoplastic left heart syndrome: Is echocardiography accurate enough to guide surgical palliation? J. Am. Coll. Cardiol. 7:610, 1986.

299. Norwood, W. I., Lang, P., and Hansen, D. D.: Physiologic repair of aortic atresia-hypoplastic left heart syndrome. N. Engl. J. Med. 308:23, 1983.

300. Norwood, W. I.: Hypoplastic left heart syndrome. Cardiol. Clin. 7:377, 1989.

301. Gustafson, R. A., Murray, G. F., Warden, H. E., et al.: Stage I palliation of hypoplastic left heart syndrome: The importance of neoaorta construction. Ann. Thorac. Surg. 48:43, 1989.

302. Pigott, J. D., Murphy, J. D., Barber, G., and Norwood, W. I.: Palliative reconstructive surgery for hypoplastic left heart syndrome. Ann. Thorac. Surg. 45:122, 1988.

303. Bailey, L. L., and Gundry, S. R.: Hypoplastic left heart syndrome. Pediatr. Clin. North Am. 37:137, 1990.

304. Frahm, C. J., Braunwald, E., and Morrow, A. G.: Congenital aortic regurgitation. Am. J. Med. 31:63, 1961.

305. Tuna, I. C., and Edwards, J. E.: Aortico-left ventricular tunnel and aortic insufficiency. Ann. Thorac. Surg. 45:5, 1988.

306. Hovaguimian, H., Cobanoglu, A., and Starr, A.: Aortico-left ventricular tunnel: A clinical review and new surgical classification. Ann. Thorac. Surg. 45:106, 1988.

307. Goforth, D., James, F. W., Kaplan, S., and Donner, R.: Maximal exercise in children with aortic regurgitation: An adjunct to noninvasive assessment of disease severity. Am. Heart J. 108:1306, 1984.

308. Lucas R. V., Jr.: Anomalous venous connection, pulmonary and systemic. In Adams, F. H., and Emmanouilides, G. C. (eds.): Moss' Heart Disease in Infants, Children and Adolescents. 4th ed. Baltimore, Williams and Wilkins, 1989, p. 580.

309. Pacifico, A. D., Mandke, N. V., McGrath, L. B., et al.: Repair of congenital pulmonary venous thrombosis with living autologous atrial tissue. J. Thorac. Cardiovasc. Surg. 89:604, 1985.

310. Marin-Garcia, J., Tandon, R., Lucas, R. V., Jr., and Edwards, J. E.: Cor triatriatum: Study of 20 cases. Am. J. Cardiol. 35:59, 1975.

311. Burton, D. A., Chin, A., Weinberg, P. M., Pigott, J. D.: Identification of cor triatriatum dexter by two-dimensional echocardiography. Am. J. Cardiol. 59:409, 1987.

312. Smith, I. O., Silverman, N. H., Oldershaw, P., et al.: Cor triatriatum sinistrum: Diagnostic features on cross-sectional echocardiography. Br. Heart J. 51:211, 1984.

313. Oglietti, J., Cooley, D. A., Izquierdo, J. P., et al.: Cor triatriatum: Operative results in 25 patients. Ann. Thorac. Surg. 35:415, 1983.

314. Ruckman, R. N., and Van Praagh, R.: Anatomic types of congenital mitral

stenosis: Report of 49 autopsy cases with consideration of diagnosis and surgical implications. Am. J. Cardiol. 42:592, 1978.

315. Parr, G. V. S., Fripp, R. A., Whitman, V., et al.: Anomalous mitral arcade: Echocardiographic and angiographic reception. Pediatr. Cardiol. 4:163, 1983.

316. Brandi-Pifano, S., Palacios, I. F., Block, P. C., et al.: Echophonocardiography in patients undergoing percutaneous mitral balloon valvotomy (PMV): The learning curve of PMV. Am. Heart J. 117:25, 1989.

317. Ortiz, E., and Somerville, J.: Assessment by cross-sectional echocardiography of surgical mitral valve disease in children and adolescents. Br. Heart J. 56:267, 1986.

318. Mazzera, E., Corno, A., Di Donato, R., et al.: Surgical bypass of the systemic atrioventricular valve in children by means of a valve conduit. J. Thorac. Cardiovasc. Surg. 96:321, 1988.

319. Stellin, G., Mazzucco, A., Bortolotti, U., et al.: Repair of congenital malformations of the mitral valve in children. Tex. Heart Inst. J. 16:102, 1989.

320. Zweng, T. N., Bluett, M. K., Mosca, R., et al.: Mitral valve replacement in the first 5 years of life. Ann. Thorac. Surg. 47:720, 1989.

321. Alday, L. E., and Juaneda, E.: Percutaneous balloon dilation in congenital mitral stenosis. Br. Heart J. 57:479, 1987.

322. Perloff, J. K.: Evolving concepts of mitral valve prolapse. N. Engl. J. Med. 307:369, 1982.

323. Carpentier, A.: Congenital malformations of the mitral valve. In Stark, J., and deLeval, M. (eds.): Surgery for Congenital Heart Defects. New York, Grune and Stratton, Inc., 1983, p. 467.

324. Carpentier, A., Branchini, B., Cour, J. C., et al.: Congenital malformations of the mitral valve in children: Pathology and surgical treatment. J. Thorac. Cardiovasc. Surg. 72:854, 1976.

325. Lamberti, J. J., Gensen, T. S., Grehl, T. M., et al.: Late reoperation for systemic atrioventricular valve regurgitation after repair of congenital heart defects. Ann. Thorac. Surg. 47:517, 1989.

326. White, R. I., Jr., Mitchell, S. E., Barth, K. H., et al.: Angioarchitecture of pulmonary arteriovenous malformations: An important consideration before embolotherapy. Am. J. Radiol. 140:681, 1983.

327. Gonzalez, V. R., Pieper, W. M., and Kap-herr, S. H.: Pulmonary arteriovenous fistula in childhood. Z. Kinderchir. 40:101, 1985.

328. Gomes, A. S., Busuttil, R. W., Baker, J. D., et al.: Congenital arteriovenous malformations: The role of transcatheter arterial embolization. Arch. Surg. 118:817, 1983.

329. D'Cruz, I. A., Agustssou, M. M., Bicoff, J. P., et al.: Stenotic lesions of the pulmonary arteries. Clinical hemodynamic findings in 84 cases. Am. J. Cardiol. 13:441, 1964.

330. Venables, A. W.: The syndrome of pulmonary stenosis complicating maternal rubella. Br. Heart J. 27:49, 1965.

331. Danilowicz, D. A., Rudolph, A. M., Hoffman, J. I. E., and Heymann, M. A.: Physiologic pressure differences between main and branch pulmonary arteries in infants. Circulation 45:410, 1972.

332. Eldredge, W. J., Tingelstad, J. B., Robertson, L. W., et al.: Observations on the natural history of pulmonary artery coarctation. Circulation 45:404, 1972.

333. Kan, J. S., Marvin, W. J., Jr., Bass, J. L., et al.: Balloon angioplasty-branch pulmonary artery stenosis: Results from the valvuloplasty and angioplasty of congenital anomalies registry. Am. J. Cardiol. 65:798, 1990.

334. Mullins, C. E., O'Laughlin, M. P., Vick, W., III, et al.: Implantation of balloon-expandable intravascular grafts by catheterization in pulmonary arteries and systemic veins. Circulation 77:188, 1988.

335. Koretzky, E., Moller, J. H., Korns, M. E., et al.: Congenital pulmonary stenosis resulting from dysplasia of valve. Circulation 40:43, 1969.

336. Aldousany, A. W., DiSessa, T. G., Dubois, R., et al.: Doppler estimation of pressure gradient in pulmonary stenosis: Maximal instantaneous vs peak-to-peak, vs mean catheter gradient. Pediatr. Cardiol. 10:145, 1989.

337. Frantz, E. G., and Silverman, N. H.: Doppler ultrasound evaluation of valvular pulmonary stenosis from multiple transducer positions in children requiring pulmonary valvuloplasty. Am. J. Cardiol. 61:844, 1988.

338. Srinivasan, V., Konyer, A., Broda, J. J., and Subramanian, S.: Critical pulmonary stenosis in infants less than three months of age: A reappraisal of closed transventricular pulmonary valvotomy. Ann. Thorac. Surg. 34:46, 1982.

339. Rao, P. S.: Balloon pulmonary valvuloplasty: A review. Clin. Cardiol. 12:55, 1989.

340. Radtke, W., and Lock, J.: Balloon dilation. Pediatr. Clin. North Am. 37:193, 1990.

341. Stanger, P., Cassidy, S. C., Girod, D. A., et al.: Balloon pulmonary valvuloplasty: Results of the valvuloplasty and angioplasty of congenital anomalies registry. Am. J. Cardiol. 65:775, 1990.

342. Marantz, P. M., Huhta, J. C., Mullins, C. E., et al.: Results of balloon valvuloplasty in typical and dysplastic pulmonary valve stenosis: Doppler echocardiographic follow up. J. Am. Coll. Cardiol. 12:476, 1988.

343. Lange, P. E., Onnasch, G. W., and Heintzen, P. H.: Valvular pulmonary stenosis. Natural history and right ventricular function in infants and children. Eur. Heart J. 6:706, 1985.

344. Mody, M. R.: The natural history of uncomplicated valvular pulmonary stenosis. Am. Heart J. 90:317, 1975.

345. Ellison, R. C., and Miettinen, O. S.: Interpretation of rSR' in pulmonic stenosis. Am. Heart J. 88:7, 1974.

346. Krabill, K. A., Wang, Y., Einzig, S., and Moller, J. H.: Rest and exercise hemodynamics in pulmonary stenosis: Comparison of children and adults. Am. J. Cardiol. 56:360, 1985.

347. Danilowicz, D., Hoffman, J. I. E., and Rudolph, A. M.: Serial studies of pulmonary stenosis in infancy and childhood. Br. Heart J. 37:808, 1975.

348. Wennevold, A., and Jacobsen, J. R.: Natural history of valvular pulmonary stenosis in children below the age of two years: Long-term follow-up with serial heart catheterizations. Eur. J. Cardiol. 8:371, 1978.

349. Kopecky, S. L., Gersh, B. J., McGoon, M. D., et al.: Long-term outcome of patients undergoing surgical repair of isolated pulmonary valve stenosis: Follow up at 20–30 years. Circulation 78:1150, 1988.

349a. Laks, H., and Billingsley, A. M.: Advances in the treatment of pulmonary atresia with intact ventricular septum: Palliative and definitive repair. Cardiol. Clin. 7:387, 1989.

350. Freedom, R. M., Wilson, G., Trusler, G., et al.: Pulmonary atresia and intact ventricular septum: A review of the anatomy, myocardium and factors influencing right ventricular growth and guidelines for surgical intervention. Scand. J. Thorac. Cardiovasc. Surg. 17:1, 1983.

351. Van de Wal, H.J.C.M., Smith, A., Becker, A. E., et al.: Morphology of pulmonary atresia with intact ventricular septum with patients dying after operation. Ann. Thorac. Surg. 50:98, 1990.

352. O'Connor, W. N., Stahr, B. J., Cottrill, C. M., et al.: Ventriculocoronary connections in hypoplastic right heart syndrome: Autopsy serial section study of six cases. J. Am. Coll. Cardiol. 11:1061, 1988.

353. Trowitzsch, E., Colan, S. D., and Sanders, S. P.: Two-dimensional echocardiographic evaluation of right ventricular size and function in newborns with severe right ventricular outflow tract obstruction. J. Am. Coll. Cardiol. 6:388, 1985.

354. Leung, M. P., Mok, C. K., and Hui, P. W.: Echocardiographic assessment of neonates with pulmonary atresia and intact ventricular septum. J. Am. Coll. Cardiol. 12:719, 1988.

355. Milliken, J. C., Laks, H., Hellenbrand, W., et al.: Early and late results in the treatment of patients with pulmonary atresia and intact ventricular septum. Circulation 72:II-61, 1985.

356. Danilowicz, D., and Ishmael, R.: Anomalous right ventricular muscle bundle: Clinical pitfalls and extracardiac anomalies. Clin. Cardiol. 4:146, 1981.

357. Kveselis, D., Rosenthal, A., Ferguson, P., et al.: Long-term prognosis after repair of double-chamber right ventricle with ventricular septal defect. Am. J. Cardiol. 54:1292, 1984.

358. Ford, D. K., Bollaboy, C. A., Derkac, W. M., et al.: Transatrial repair of double-chambered right ventricle. Ann. Thorac. Surg. 46:412, 1988.

359. Pinsky, W. W., and Arciniegas, E.: Tetralogy of Fallot. Pediatr. Clin. North Am. 37:179, 1990.

360. Perloff, J. K., Friedman, W. F., Laks, H., and Child, J. S.: From the cyanotic infant to the acyanotic adult—the odyssey of the blue baby. UCLA School of Medicine Interdisciplinary Conference. West. J. Med. 139:673, 1983.

361. Soto, B., and McConnell, M. E.: Tetralogy of Fallot: Angiographic and pathological correlation. Semin. Thorac. Cardiovasc. Surg. 2:12, 1990.

362. Barbero-Marcial, M., and Jatene, A. D.: Surgical management of the anomalies of the pulmonary arteries in the tetralogy of Fallot with pulmonary atresia. Semin. Thorac. Cardiovasc. Surg. 2:93, 1990.

363. Liao, P. K., Edwards, W. D., Julsrud, P. R., et al.: Pulmonary blood supply in patients with pulmonary atresia and ventricular septal defect. J. Am. Coll. Cardiol. 6:1343, 1985.

364. Johnson, R. J., Sauer, U., Buhlmeyer, K., and Haworth, S. G.: Hypoplasia of the intrapulmonary arteries in children with right ventricular overflow tract obstruction, ventricular septal defect, and major aortopulmonary collateral arteries. Pediatr. Cardiol. 6:137, 1985.

365. Smyllie, J. H., Sutherland, G. R., and Keeton, B. R.: The value of Doppler color-flow mapping in determining pulmonary blood supply in infants with pulmonary atresia with ventricular septal defect. J. Am. Coll. Cardiol. 14:1759, 1989.

366. Fellows, K. E., Freed, M. D., Keane, J. F., et al.: Results of routine preoperative coronary angiography and tetralogy of Fallot. Circulation 51:561, 1977.

366a. Kirklin, J. K., Kirklin, J. W., and Pacifico, A. D.: Transannular outflow tract patching for tetralogy: Indications and results. Semin. Thorac. Cardiovasc. Surg. 2:61, 1990.

367. Jureidini, S. B., Appleton, R. S., and Nouri, S.: Detection of coronary artery abnormalities in tetralogy of Fallot by two-dimensional echocardiography. J. Am. Coll. Cardiol. 14:960, 1989.

367a. Castaneda, A. R.: Classical repair of tetralogy of Fallot: Timing, technique, and results. Semin. Thorac. Cardiovasc. Surg. 2:70, 1990.

368. Pacifico, A. D., Kirklin, J. K., Colvin, E. V., et al.: Transatrial-transpulmonary repair of tetralogy of Fallot. Semin. Thorac. Cardiovasc. Surg. 2:76, 1990.

369. Morgan, B. C., Guntheroth, W. G., Blume, R. S., and Fyler, D. C.: A clinical profile of paroxysmal hyperpnea in cyanotic congenital heart disease. Circulation 31:66, 1965.

369a. Hammon, J. W., Jr., Henry, C. L., Jr., Merrill, W. H., et al.: Tetralogy of Fallot: Selective surgical management to minimize operative mortality. Ann. Thorac. Surg. 40:280, 1985.

370. Shaddy, R. E., Viney, J., Judd, V. E., and McGough, E. C.: Continuous intravenous phenylephrine infusion for treatment of hypoxemic spells in tetralogy of Fallot. J. Pediatr. 114:468, 1989.

370a. Rosankranz, E. R.: Modified Blalock-Taussig shunts in the treatment of tetralogy of Fallot. Semin. Thorac. Cardiovasc. Surg. 2:27, 1990.

371. McConnell, M. E.: Echocardiography in classical tetralogy of Fallot. Semin. Thorac. Cardiovasc. Surg. 2:2, 1990.

371a. Pacifico, A. D., Kirklin, J. K., Colvin, E. V., et al.: Tetralogy of Fallot: Late results and reoperations. Semin. Thorac. Cardiovasc. Surg. 2:108, 1990.

372. Qureshi, S. A., Kirk, C. R., Lamb, R. K., et al.: Balloon dilatation of the pulmonary valve in the first year of life in patients with tetralogy of Fallot: A preliminary study. Br. Heart J. 60:232, 1988.

373. Naito, Y., Fujita, T., Yagihara, T., et al.: Usefulness of left ventricular volume in assessing tetralogy of Fallot for total correction. Am. J. Cardiol. 56:356, 1985.

374. Garson, A., Jr., Randall, D. C., Gillette, P. C., et al.: Prevention of sudden death after repair of tetralogy of Fallot: Treatment of ventricular arrhythmias. J. Am. Coll. Cardiol. 6:221, 1985.

375. Zahka, K. G., Horneffer, P. J., Rowe, S. A., et al.: Long-term valvular function after total repair of tetralogy of Fallot: Relation to ventricular arrhythmias. Circulation 78(Suppl. III):14, 1988.

376. Chandar, J. S., Wolff, G. S., Garson, A., Jr., et al.: Ventricular arrhythmias in postoperative tetralogy of Fallot. Am. J. Cardiol. 65:655, 1990.

376a. Vaksmann, G., Fournier, A., Davignon, A., et al.: Frequency and prognosis of arrhythmias after operative "correction" of tetralogy of Fallot. Am. J. Cardiol. 66:346, 1990.

377. Oku, H., Shirotani, H., Sunakawa, A., and Yokoyama, T.: Postoperative long-term results in total correction of tetralogy of Fallot: Hemodynamics and cardiac function. Ann. Thorac. Surg. 41:413, 1986.

378. Rosenthal, A., Behrendt, D., Sloan, H., et al.: Long-term prognosis (15 to 26 years) after repair of tetralogy of Fallot: I. Survival and symptomatic status. Ann. Thorac. Surg. 38:151, 1984.

379. Sandor, G.G.S., Patterson, M.W.H., Tipple, M., et al.: Left ventricular systolic and diastolic function after total correction of tetralogy of Fallot. Am. J. Cardiol. 60:1148, 1987.

380. Ilbawi, M. N., Fedorchik, J., Muster, A. J., et al.: Surgical approach to severely symptomatic newborn infants with tetralogy of Fallot and absent pulmonary valve. J. Thorac. Cardiovasc. Surg. 91:584, 1986.

381. Fischer, D. R., Neches, W. H., Beerman, L. B., et al.: Tetralogy of Fallot with absent pulmonic valve: Analysis of 17 patients. Am. J. Cardiol. 53:1433, 1984.

382. Emmanouilides, G. C., Thanopoulos, B., Siassi, B., and Fishbein, M: Agenesis of ductus arteriosus associated with the syndrome of tetralogy of Fallot and absent pulmonary valve. Am. J. Cardiol. 37:403, 1976.

383. Dunnigan, A., Oldham, H. N., and Benson, D. W.: Absent pulmonary valve syndrome in infancy: Surgery reconsidered. Am. J. Cardiol. 48:117, 1981.

384. Kron, I. L., Johnson, A. M., Carpenter, M. A., et al.: Treatment of absent pulmonary valve syndrome with homograft. Ann. Thorac. Surg. 46:579, 1988.

385. Rigby, M. L., Carvalho, J. S., Anderson, R. H., and Redington, A.: The investigation and diagnosis of tricuspid atresia. Int. J. Cardiol. 27:1, 1990.

386. Wenink, A.C.J., and Ottenkamp, J.: Tricuspid atresia. Microscopic findings in relation to "absence" of the atrioventriculaar connection. Int. J. Cardiol. 16:57, 1987.

387. Sade, R. M., and Fyfe, D. A.: Tricuspid atresia: Current concepts in diagnosis and treatment. Pediatr. Clin. North Am. 7:151, 1990.

388. Fesslova, V., Hunter, S., Stark, J., and Taylor, J.F.N.: Long-term clinical outcome of patients with tricuspid atresia. I. "Natural history." J. Cardiovasc. Surg. 30:262, 1989.

389. Fontan, F., Deville, C., Quaegebeur, J., et al.: Repair of tricuspid atresia in 100 patients. J. Thorac. Cardiovasc. Surg. 85:647, 1983.

390. Fontan, F., Kirklin, J. W., Fernandez, G., et al.: Outcome after a "perfect" Fontan operation. Circulation 81:1520, 1990.

390a. Nakazawa, M., Katayama, H., Imai, Y., et al.: A quantitative analysis of hemodynamic effects of the right ventricle included in the circulation of the Fontan procedure. Circulation 83:822, 1991.

390b. Mayer, J. E., Jr., Bridges, N. D., Lock, J. E., et al.: Factors associated with improved survival after modified Fontan operations. J. Am. Coll. Cardiol. 17:33a, 1991.

391. Weber, H. S., Hellenbrand, W. E., Kleinman, C. S., et al.: Predictors of rhythm disturbances and subsequent morbidity after the Fontan operation. Am. J. Cardiol. 64:762, 1989.

392. Mair, D. D., Hagler, D. J., Puga, F. J., et al.: Fontan operation in 176 patients with tricuspid atresia. Circulation 82(Suppl. IV): 164, 1990.

393. Sampson, C., Martinez, J., Rees, S., et al.: Evaluation of Fontan's operation by magnetic resonance imaging. Am. J. Cardiol. 65:819, 1990.

394. Matsushita, T., Matsuda, H., Ogawa, M., and Yabuuchi, H.: Assessment of the intrapulmonary ventilation-perfusion distribution after the Fontan procedure for complex cardiac anomalies: Relation to pulmonary hemodynamics. J. Am. Coll. Cardiol. 15:842, 1990.

395. Fernandez, G., Costa, F., Fontan, F., et al.: Prevalence of reoperation for pathway obstruction after Fontan operation. Ann. Thorac. Surg. 48:654, 1989.

396. Zellers, T. M., Driscoll, D. J., Mottram, C. D., et al.: Exercise tolerance and cardiorespiratory response to exercise before and after the Fontan operation. Mayo Clin. Proc. 64:1489, 1989.

397. Rhodes, J., Garofano, R. P., Bowman, F. O., Jr., et al.: Effect of right ventricular anatomy on the cardiopulmonary response to exercise. Implications for the Fontan procedure. Circulation 81:1811, 1990.

398. Gussenhoven, E. J., Stewart, P. A., Becker, A. E., et al.: "Offsetting" of the septal tricuspid leaflet in normal hearts and in hearts with Ebstein's anomaly. Am. J. Cardiol. 53:172, 1984.

399. Zalzstein, E., Koran, G., Einarson, T., and Freedom, R. M.: A case control study on the association between first trimester exposure to lithium and Ebstein's anomaly. Am. J. Cardiol. 65:817, 1990.

400. Guiliani, E. R., Fuster, V., Brandenberg, R. O., and Mair, D. D.: Ebstein's anomaly; The clinical features and natural history of Ebstein's anomaly of the tricuspid valve. Mayo Clin. Proc. 54:163, 1979.

401. Boucek, R. J., Jr., Graham, T. P., Jr., Morgan J. P., et al.: Spontaneous resolution of massive congenital tricuspid insufficiency. Circulation 54:795, 1976.

402. Roberson, D. A., and Silverman, N. H.: Ebstein's anomaly: Echocardiographic and clinical features in the fetus and neonate. J. Am. Coll. Cardiol. 14:1300, 1989.

403. Freedom, R. M., Culham, J.A.G., Olley, P. M., et al.: The differentiation of functional from organic pulmonary atresia: The role of aortography. Am. J. Cardiol. 41:914, 1978.

404. Kastor, J. A., Goldreier, B. N., Josephson, M. E., et al.: Electrophysiologic characteristics of Ebstein's anomaly of the tricuspid valve. Circulation 52:987, 1975.

405. Gussenhoven, W. J., Spitaels, S.E.C., Bom, N., and Becker, A. E.: Echocardiographic criteria for Ebstein's anomaly of tricuspid valve. Br. Heart J. 43:31, 1980.

406. Hirschklau, M. J., Sahn, D. J., Hagan, A. D., et al.: Cross-sectional echocardiographic features of Ebstein's anomaly of the tricuspid valve. Am. J. Cardiol. 40:400, 1977.

407. Driscoll, D. J., Mottram, C. D., and Danielson, G. K.: Spectrum of exercise intolerance in 45 patients with Ebstein's anomaly and observations on exercise tolerance in 11 patients after surgical repair. J. Am. Coll. Cardiol. 11:831, 1988.

408. Pasque, M., Williams, W. G., Coles, G. J., et al.: Tricuspid valve replacement in children. Ann. Thorac. Surg. 44:164, 1987.

409. Carpentier, A., Chauvaud, S., Mace, L., et al.: A new reconstructive operation for Ebstein's anomaly of the tricuspid valve. J. Thorac. Cardiovasc. Surg. 96:92, 1988.

409a. Quaegebeur, J. M., Sreeram, N., Fraser, A. G., et al.: Surgery for Ebstein's Anomaly: The clinical and echocardiographic evaluation of a new technique. J. Am. Coll. Cardiol. 17:722, 1991.

410. Paul, M. H.: D-Transposition of great arteries. In Adams, F. H., and Emmanouilides, G. C. (eds.): Moss' Heart Disease in Infants, Children and Adolescents, 4th ed. Baltimore, Williams and Wilkins, 1989, p. 371.

410a. Anderson, R. H., Henry, G. W., and Becker, A. E.: Morphologic aspects of complete transposition. Cardiol. Young 1:41, 1991.

411. Mair, D. D., and Ritter, D. G.: Factors influencing systemic arterial oxygen saturation in complete transposition of the great arteries. Am. J. Cardiol. 31:742, 1973.

412. Lakier, J. B., Stanger, P., Heymann, M. A., et al.: Early onset of pulmonary vascular obstruction in patients with aortopulmonary transposition and intact ventricular septum. Circulation 51:875, 1975.

413. Aziz, K. U., Paul, M. H., and Rowe, R. D.: Bronchopulmonary circulation in D-transposition of the great arteries: Possible role and genesis of accelerated pulmonary vascular disease. Am. J. Cardiol. 39:432, 1977.

414. Muster, A. J., Paul, M. H., Van Grondell, E. A., and Conway, J. J.: Asymmetric distribution of the pulmonary blood flow between the right and left lungs in D-transposition of the great arteries. Am. J. Cardiol. 38:352, 1976.

415. Sansa, M., Tonkin, I. L., Bargeron, L. M., and Elliott, L. P.: Left ventricular outflow tract obstruction in transposition of the great arteries. Am. J. Cardiol. 44:88, 1979.

416. Chiu, I., Anderson, R. H., Macartney, F. J., et al.: Morphologic features of an intact ventricular septum susceptible to subpulmonary obstruction in complete transposition. Am. J. Cardiol. 53:1633, 1984.

417. Waldman, J. D., Paul, M. H., Newfeld, E. A., et al.: Transposition of the great arteries with intact ventricular septum and patent ductus arteriosus. Am. J. Cardiol. 39:232, 1977.

418. Tonkin, I. L., Kelley, M. J., Bream, P. R., and Elliott, L. P.: The frontal chest film as a method of suspecting transposition complexes. Circulation 53:1016, 1976.

419. Chin, A. J., Yeager, S. B., Sanders, S. P., et al.: Accuracy of prospective two-dimensional echocardiographic evaluation of left ventricular outflow tract in complete transposition of the great arteries. Am. J. Cardiol. 55:759, 1985.

420. Deal, B. J., Chin, A. J., Sanders, S. P., et al.: Subxiphoid two-dimensional echocardiographic identification of tricuspid valve abnormalities in transposition of the great arteries with ventricular septal defect. Am. J. Cardiol. 55:1146, 1985.

421. Marino, B., de Simone, G., Pasquini, L., et al.: Complete transposition of the great arteries: Visualization of left and right outflow tract obstruction by oblique subcostal two-dimensional echocardiography. Am. J. Cardiol. 55:1140, 1985.

422. Chin, A. J., Yeager, S. B., Sanders, S. P., et al.: Accuracy of prospective two-dimensional echocardiographic evaluation of left ventricular outflow tract in complete transposition of the great arteries. Am. J. Cardiol. 55:759, 1985.

422a. Rigby, M. L., and Chan, K-Y: The diagnostic evaluation of patients with complete transposition. Cardiol. Young 1:26, 1991.

423. DiSessa, T. G., Childs, W., Ti, C. C., and Friedman, W. F.: Systolic anterior motion of the mitral valve in a one day old infant with transposition of the great vessels. J. Clin. Ultrasound 6:186, 1978.

424. Lin, A. E., Di Sessa, T. G., Williams, R. G., et al.: Balloon and blade atrial septostomy facilitated by two-dimensional echocardiography. Am. J. Cardiol. 57:273, 1986.

425. Moene, R. J., Oppenheimer-Dekker, A., Wenink, A.C.G., et al.: Morphology of ventricular septal defect in complete transposition of the great arteries. Am. J. Cardiol. 55:1566, 1985.

426. Pasquini, L., Sanders, S. P., Parness, I. A., and Colan, S. D.: Diagnosis of coronary artery anatomy by two-dimensional echocardiography in patients with transposition of the great arteries. Circulation 75:557, 1987.

427. Oberhoffer, R. M., Ho, S. Y., and Anderson, R. H.: Coronary artery diameters in the heart with complete transposition of the great vessels. J. Am. Coll. Cardiol. 15:1433, 1990.

428. Kirklin, J. W., Colvin, E. V., McConnell, M. E., and Bargeron, L. M.: Complete transposition of the great arteries: Treatment in the current era. Pediatr. Clin. North Am. 37:171, 1990.

428a. Kirklin, J. W.: The surgical repair for complete transposition. Cardiol. Young 1:13, 1991.

428b. Oelert, H.: Modification of the Mustard operation for surgical treatment of complete transposition by creating a confluence of the caval veins. Cardiol. Young 1:71, 1991.

428c. Merrill, W. H., Stewart, J. R., Hammon, J. W., Jr., et al: The Senning operation for complete transposition: Mid-term physiologic, electrophysiologic, and functional results. Cardiol. Young 1:80, 1991.

429. Wong, K. Y., Venables, A. W., Kelly, M. J., and Kalff, V.: Longitudinal study of ventricular function after the Mustard operation for transposition of the great arteries: A long-term follow up. Br. Heart J. 60:316, 1988.

430. Vetter, V. L., Tanner, C. S., and Horowitz, L. N.: Inducible atrial flutter after the Mustard repair of complete transposition of the great arteries. Am. J. Cardiol. 61:428, 1988.

431. Duster, M. C., Bink-Boelkens, M.T.E., Wampler, D., et al.: Long-term follow-up of dysrhythmias following the Mustard procedure. Am. Heart J. 109:1323, 1985.

431a. Deanfield, J. E., Cullen, S., and Gewillig, M.: Arrhythmias after surgery for complete transposition: Do they matter? Cardiol. Young 1:91, 1991.

432. Kato, H., Nakano, S., Matsuda, H., et al.: Right ventricular myocardial function after atrial switch operation for transposition of the great arteries. Am. J. Cardiol. 63:226, 1989.

433. George, B. L., Laks, H., Klitzner, T. S., et al.: Results of the Senning procedure in infants with simple and complex transposition of the great arteries. Am. J. Cardiol. 59:426, 1987.

434. Reybrouck, T., Dumoulin, M., and Van Der Hauwaert, L. G.: Cardiorespiratory exercise testing after venous switch operation in children with complete transposition of great arteries. Am. J. Cardiol. 61:861, 1988.

435. Ensing, G. J., Heise, C. T., and Driscoll, D. J.: Cardiovascular response to exercise after the Mustard operation for simple and complex transposition of great arteries. Am. J. Cardiol. 62:617, 1988.

436. Musewe, N. N., Reisman, J., Benson, L. M., et al.: Cardiopulmonary adaptation at rest and during exercise 10 years after Mustard atrial repair for transposition of the great arteries. Circulation 77:1055, 1988.

437. Turina, M. I., Siebenmann, R., Von Segesser, L., et al.: Late functional deterioration after atrial correction for transposition of the great arteries. Circulation 80(Suppl. I):162, 1989.

438. Benson, L. N., Bonet, J., Olley, P. M., et al.: Assessment of right ventricular function during supine bicycle exercise after Mustard's operation. Circulation 65:1052, 1982.

439. Danford, D. A.: Factors influencing choice of procedure in transposition of the great arteries: A decision-analysis approach. J. Am. Coll. Cardiol. 16:471, 1990.

440. Corno, A., George, B., Pearl, J., and Laks, H.: Surgical options for complex transposition of the great arteries. J. Am. Coll. Cardiol. 14:742, 1989.

441. Bove, E. L., Beekman, R. H., Snider, A. R., et al.: Arterial repair for transposition of the great arteries and large ventricular septal defect in early infancy. Circulation 78(Suppl. III):26, 1988.

442. Di Donato, R. M., Wernofsky, G., Walsh, E. P., et al.: Results of the arterial switch operation for transposition of the great arteries with ventricular septal defect. Surgical considerations and mid-term follow up data. Circulation 80:1689, 1989.

443. Castaneda, A. R., Mayer, J. E., Jonas, R. A., et al.: Transposition of the great arteries: The arterial switch operation. Cardiol. Clin. 7:369, 1989.

443a. Planche, C., Serraf, A., Lacour-Gayet, F., et al.: Anatomic correction of complete transposition with ventricular septal defect in neonates: Experience with 42 consecutive cases. Cardiol Young 1:101, 1991.

444. Colan, S. D., Trowitz, S.C.H.E., Wernvosky, G., et al.: Myocardial performance after arterial switch operation for transposition of the great arteries with intact ventricular septum. Circulation 78:132, 1988.

445. Sandor, G.S.S., Freedom, R. M., Williams, W. G., et al.: Left ventricular systolic and diastolic function after two-stage anatomic correction of transposition of the great arteries. Am. Heart J. 115:1257, 1988.

446. Gleason, M. M., Chin, A., Andrews, B. A., et al.: Two-dimensional and Doppler echocardiographic assessment of neonatal arterial repair for transposition of the great arteries. J. Am. Coll. Cardiol. 13:1320, 1989.

447. Martin, M. M., Snider, R., Bove, E. L., et al.: Two-dimensional and Doppler echocardiographic evaluation after arterial switch repair in infancy for complete transposition of the great arteries. Am. J. Cardiol. 63:332, 1989.

448. Wernovsky, G., Hougen, T. J., Walsh, E. P., et al.: Mid-term results after the arterial switch operation for transposition of the great arteries with intact ventricular septum: Clinical, hemodynamic, echocardiographic, and electrophysiologic data. Circulation 77:1333, 1988.

449. Villafane, J., White, S., Elbl, F., et al.: An electrocardiographic mid-term follow up study after anatomic repair of transposition of the great arteries. Am. J. Cardiol. 66:350, 1990.

450. Martin, R. P., Ettedgui, J. A., Qureshi, S. A., et al.: A quantitative evaluation of aortic regurgitation after anatomic correction of transposition of the great arteries. J. Am. Coll. Cardiol. 12:1281, 1988.

450a. Redington, A. N.: Functional assessment of the heart after corrective surgery for complete transposition. Cardiol. Young 1:84, 1991.

451. Jonas, R. A., Gigliaa, T. M., Sanders, S. P., et al.: Rapid, two-stage arterial switch for transposition of the great arteries and intact ventricular septum beyond the neonatal period. Circulation 80(Suppl. I):203, 1989.

452. Corno, A. F., Parisi, F., Marino, B., et al.: Palliative Mustard operation: An expanded horizon. Eur. J. Cardiothorac. Surg. 1:144, 1987.

453. Colli, A. M., De Leval, M., and Somerville, J.: Anatomically corrected malposition of the great arteries. Am. J. Cardiol. 55:1367, 1985.

454. Kirklin, J. W., Pacifico, A. D., Bargeron, L. M., Jr., and Soto, B.: Cardiac repair and anatomically corrected malposition of the great arteries. Circulation 48:153, 1973.

455. Berry, W. B., Roberts, W. C., Morrow, A. G., and Braunwald, E.: Corrected transposition of the aorta and pulmonary trunk: Clinical, hemodynamic, and pathologic findings. Am. J. Med. 36:35, 1964.

456. Freedberg, D. Z., and Nadas, A. S.: Clinical profile of patients with congenital corrected transposition of the great arteries. N. Engl. J. Med. 282:1053, 1970.

457. Allwork, S. P., Bentall, H. H., Becker, A. E., et al.: Congenitally corrected transposition of the great arteries. Morphologic study of 32 cases. Am. J. Cardiol. 38:910, 1976.

458. Bjarke, B. B., and Kidd, B.S.L.: Congenitally corrected transposition of the great arteries: A clinical study of 101 cases. Acta Paediatr. Scand. 65:153, 1976.

459. Huhta, J. C., Danielson, G. K., Ritter, D. G., and Ilstrup, D. M.: Survival in atrioventricular discordance. Pediatr. Cardiol. 6:57, 1985.

459a. Dimas, A. P., Moodie, D. S., Strba, R., and Gill, C. C.: Long-term function of the morphologic right ventricle in adult patients with corrected transposition of the great arteries. Am. Heart J. 118:526, 1989.

460. Peterson, R. J., Franch, R. H., Fajman, W. A., and Jones, R. H.: Comparison of cardiac function in surgically corrected and congenitally corrected transposition of the great arteries. J. Thorac. Cardiovasc. Surg. 96:227, 1988.

461. Benson, L. N., Burns, R., Schwaiger, M., et al.: Radionuclide angiographic evaluation of ventricular function in isolated congenitally corrected transposition of the great arteries. Am. J. Cardiol. 58:319, 1986.

462. Waldo, A. L., Pacifico, A. D., Bargeron, L. M., Jr., et al.: Electrophysiological delineation of specialized AV conduction system in patients with corrected transposition of the great vessels and ventricular septal defect. Circulation 52:435, 1975.

463. Bharati, B., Rosen, K., Steinfield, L., et al.: The anatomic substrate for pre-excitation in corrected transposition. Circulation 62:831, 1980.

464. Meissner, M. D., Panidis, I. P., Eshaghpour, E., et al.: Corrected transposition of the great arteries: Evaluation by two-dimensional and Doppler echocardiography. Am. Heart J. 111:599, 1986.

465. Freedom, R. M., Harrington, D. P., and White, R. I., Jr.: The differential diagnosis of levotransposed or malposed aorta: An angiocardiographic study. Circulation 50:1040, 1974.

466. Russo, P., Danielson, G. K., and Driscoll, D. J.: Transaortic closure of ventricular septal defect in patients with corrected transposition with pulmonary stenosis or atresia. Circulation 76(Suppl. III):88, 1987.

467. McGrath, L. B., Kirklin, J. W., Blackstone, E. H., et al.: Death and other events after cardiac repair in discordant atrioventricular connection. J. Thorac. Cardiovasc. Surg. 90:711, 1985.

468. Piccoli, G., Pacifico, A. D., Kirklin, J. W., et al.: Changing results and concepts in the surgical treatment of double-outlet right ventricle: Analysis of 137 operations in 126 patients. Am. J. Cardiol. 52:549, 1983.

469. Hagler, D. J., Ritter, D. G., and Puga, F. J.: Double-outlet right ventricle. In Adams, F. H., and Emmanoulides, G. C. (eds.): Moss' Heart Disease in Infants, Children and Adolescents. 4th ed. Baltimore, Williams and Wilkins, 1989, p. 442.

470. Bostrom, M.P.G., and Hutchins, G. M.: Arrested rotation of the outflow tract may explain double-outlet right ventricle. Circulation 77:1258, 1988.

471. Sondheimer, H. M., Freedom, R. M., and Olley, P. M.: Double outlet right ventricle: Clinical spectrum and prognosis. Am. J. Cardiol. 39:709, 1977.

472. Goitein, K. J., Neches, W. H., Park, S. C., et al.: Electrocardiogram in double chamber right ventricle. Am. J. Cardiol. 45:604, 1980.

473. Macartney, F. J., Rigby, M. L., Anderson, R. H., et al.: Double outlet right ventricle. Cross-sectional echocardiographic findings, their anatomical explanation and surgical relevance. Br. Heart J. 52:164, 1984.

474. Sridaromont, S., Ritter, D. G., Feldt, R. H., et al.: Double outlet right ventricle: Anatomic and angiocardiographic correlations. Mayo Clin. Proc. 53:555, 1978.

475. Kirklin, J. W., Pacifico, A. D., Blackstone, E. H., et al.: Current risks and protocols for surgery for double outlet right ventricle: Derivation from an 18-year experience. J. Thorac. Cardiovasc. Surg. 92:913, 1986.

476. Musumeci, F., Shumway, S., Lincoln, C., and Anderson, R. H.: Surgical treatment for double-outlet right ventricle at the Brompton Hospital, 1973 to 1986. J. Thorac. Cardiovasc. Surg. 96:278, 1988.

477. Russo, P., Danielson, G. K., Puga, F. J., et al.: Modified Fontan procedure for biventricular hearts with complex forms of double-outlet right ventricle. Circulation 78(Suppl. III):20, 1988.

478. Shen, W. K., Holmes, D. R., Jr., Porter, C. J., et al.: Sudden death after repair of double-outlet right ventricle. Circulation 81:128, 1990.

479. Kanter, K., Anderson, R., Lincoln, C., et al.: Anatomic correction of double-outlet right ventricle and subpulmonary ventricular septal defect (the "Taussig-Bing" anomaly). Ann. Thorac. Surg. 41:287, 1986.

480. Van Praagh, R., and Weinberg, P. M.: Double outlet left ventricle. In Adams, F. H., and Emmanouilides, G. C. (eds.): Moss' Heart Disease in Infants, Children and Adolescents. 3rd ed. Baltimore, Williams and Wilkins, 1983, p. 370.

481. Murphy, E. A., Gillis, D. A., and Sridhara, K. S.: Intraventricular repair of double outlet left ventricle. Ann. Thorac. Surg. 31:364, 1981.

482. Gathman, G. E., and Nadas, A. S.: Total anomalous pulmonary venous connection: Clinical and physiologic observations in 75 pediatric patients. Circulation 42:143, 1970.

483. Ward, K. E., Mullins, C. E., Huhta, J. C., et al.: Restrictive interatrial communication in total anomalous pulmonary venous connection. Am. J. Cardiol. 57:1131, 1986.

484. Lucas, R. V., Jr., Lock, J. E., Tandon, R., and Edwards, J. E.: Gross and histologic anatomy of total anomalous pulmonary venous connections. Am. J. Cardiol. 62:292, 1988.

485. Jonas, R. A., Smolinsky, A., Mayer, J. E., and Castaneda, A. R.: Obstructed pulmonary venous drainage with total anomalous pulmonary venous connection to the coronary sinus. Am. J. Cardiol. 59:431, 1987.

486. Lincoln, C. R., Rigby, M. L., Marcanti, C., et al.: Surgical risk factors in total anomalous pulmonary venous connection. Am. J. Cardiol. 61:608, 1988.

487. Elliott, L. P., and Edwards, J. E.: The problem of pulmonary venous obstruction in total anomalous pulmonary venous connection to the left innominate vein. Circulation 25:913, 1962.

488. Newfeld, E. A., Wilson, A., Paul, M. H., and Reisch, J. S.: Pulmonary vascular disease in total anomalous pulmonary venous drainage. Circulation 61:103, 1980.

489. Haworth, S. G., Reid, L., and Simon, G.: Radiological features of the heart and lungs in total anomalous pulmonary venous return in early infancy. Clin. Radiol. 28:561, 1977.

490. Smallhorn, J. F., and Freedom, R. M.: Pulsed Doppler echocardiography in the preoperative evaluation of total anomalous pulmonary venous connection. J. Am. Coll. Cardiol. 8:1413, 1986.

491. Chin, A. J., Sanders, S. P., Sherman, F., et al.: Accuracy of subcostal two-dimensional echocardiography in prospective diagnosis of total anomalous pulmonary venous connection. Am. Heart J. 113:1153, 1987.

491a. Lamb, R. K., Qureshi, S. A., Wilkinson, J. L., et al.: Total anomalous pulmonary venous drainage. 17-year surgical experience. J. Thorac. Cardiovasc. Surg. 96:368, 1988.

492. Corno, A., Giamberti, A., Carotti, A., et al.: Total anomalous pulmonary venous connection: Surgical repair with a double-patch technique. Ann. Thorac. Surg. 49:492, 1990.

493. Phillips, S. J., Kongtahworn, C., Zeff, R. H., et al.: Correction of total anomalous pulmonary venous connection below the diaphragm. Ann. Thorac. Surg. 49:734, 1990.

494. Matthew, R., Thilenius, O. G., Replogle, R. L., and Arcilla, R. A.: Cardiac function in total anomalous pulmonary venous return before and after surgery. Circulation 55:361, 1977.

495. Van Meter, C., Jr., LeBlanc, J. G., Culpepper, W. S., III, and Ochsner, J. L.: Partial anomalous pulmonary venous return. Circulation 82(Suppl. IV):195, 1990.

496. Gikonyo, D. K., Tandon, R., Lucas, R. V., Jr., and Edwards, J. E.: Scimitar syndrome in neonates: Report of four cases and review of the literature. Pediatr. Cardiol. 6:193, 1986.

497. Stanger, P., Rudolph, A. M., and Edwards, J. E.: Cardiac malpositions: An overview based on a study of 65 necropsy specimens. Circulation 56:159, 1977.

498. Van Praagh, R.: Diagnosis of complex congenital heart disease: Morphologic-anatomic method and terminology. Cardiovasc. Intervent. Radiol. 7:115, 1984.

499. Tonkin, I.L.D.: The definition of cardiac malpositions with echocardiography and computed tomography. In Friedman, W. F., and Higgins, C. B. (eds.): Pediatric Cardiac Imaging. Philadelphia, W. B. Saunders Company, 1984, p. 157.

500. Silverman, N. H.: An ultrasonic approach to the diagnosis of cardiac situs, connections, and malposition. In Friedman, W. F., and Higgins, C. B. (eds.): Pediatric Cardiac Imaging. Philadelphia, W. B. Saunders Company, 1984, p. 188.

501. Anderson, C., Devine, W. A., Anderson, R. H., et al.: Abnormalities of the spleen in relation to congenital malformations of the heart: Survey of necropsy findings in children. Br. Heart J. 63:122, 1990.

502. Peoples, W. M., Moller, J. H., and Edwards, J. E.: Polysplenia: A review of 146 cases. Pediatr. Cardiol. 4:129, 1983.

503. Momma, K., Takao, A., and Shibata, T.: Characteristics and natural history of abnormal atrial rhythms in left isomerism. Am. J. Cardiol. 65:231, 1990.

504. Nasser, W. K.: Congenital absence of the left pericardium. Am. J. Cardiol. 26:466, 1970.

505. Morgan, J. R., Rogers, A. K., and Forker, A. D.: Congenital absence of the left pericardium: Clinical findings. Ann. Intern. Med. 74:370, 1971.

506. Pernot, C., Hoeffel, J. C., and Henry, M.: Radiologic patterns of congenital malformation of the pericardium. Radiol. Clin. (Basel) 44:505, 1975.

507. Nicolosi, G. L., Borgioni, L., Alberti, E., et al.: M-mode and two-dimensional echocardiography in congenital absence of the pericardium. Chest 81:610, 1982.

508. Rowland, T. W., Twible, E. A., Norwood, W. I., Jr., and Keane, J. F.: Partial absence of the left pericardium: Diagnosis by two-dimensional echocardiography. Am. J. Dis. Child. 136:628, 1982.

509. Schiavone, W. A., and O'Donnell, J. K.: Congenital absence of the left portion of parietal pericardium demonstrated by nuclear magnetic resonance imaging. Am. J. Cardiol. 55:1439, 1985.

510. Jones, J. W., and McManus, B. M.: Fatal cardiac strangulation by congenital partial pericardial defect. Am. Heart J. 107:183, 1984.

511. Rowland, T. W., Twible, E. A., Norwood, W. J., Jr., and Keane, J. F.: Partial absence of the left pericardium. Am. J. Dis. Child. 136:628, 1982.

512. Rastelli, G., Kirklin, J. W., and Titus, J. L.: Anatomic observations on complete form of persistent common atrioventricular canal with special reference to atrioventricular valves. Mayo Clin. Proc. 41:296, 1966.

513. Anderson, R. H., Macartney, F. J., Tynan, M., et al.: Univentricular atrioventricular connection: The single ventricle trap unsprung. Pediatr. Cardiol. 4:273, 1983.

514. Thies, W. R., Soto, B., Diethelm, E., et al.: Angiographic anatomy of hearts

with one ventricular chamber: The true single ventricle. Am. J. Cardiol. 55:1363, 1985.

515. Huhta, J. C., Seward, J. B., Tajik, A. J., et al.: Two-dimensional echocardiographic spectrum of univentricular atrioventricular connection. J. Am. Coll. Cardiol. 5:149, 1985.

516. DiSessa, T. G., Isabel-Jones, J. G., Heins, H., et al.: Two dimensional echocardiographic features of the univentricular heart. Cardiovasc. Ultrason. 3:89, 1984.

517. Moak, J. P., and Gersony, W. M.: Progressive atrioventricular valvular regurgitation in single ventricle. Am. J. Cardiol. 59:656, 1987.

518. Sano, T., Ogawa, M., Taniguchi, T., and Kawashima, Y.: Assessment of ventricular contractile state and function in patients with univentricular heart. Circulation 79:1247, 1989.

519. Sano, T., Ogawa, M., Yabuuchi, H., and Kawashima, Y.: Quantitative cineangiographic analysis of ventricular volume and mass in patients with single ventricle: Relation to ventricular morphologies. Circulation 77:62, 1988.

520. Stefanelli, G., Kirklin, J. W., Naftel, D. C., et al.: Early and intermediate-term (10-year) results of surgery for univentricular atrioventricular connection ("single ventricle"). Am. J. Cardiol. 54:811, 1984.

521. Pacifico, A. D., Kirklin, J. K., and Kirklin, J. W.: Surgical management of double inlet ventricle. World J. Surg. 9:579, 1985.

522. Laks, H., Milliken, J. C., Perloff, J. K., et al.: Experience with the Fontan procedure. J. Thorac. Cardiovasc. Surg. 88:939, 1984.

523. Rothman, A., Lang, P., Lock, J. E., et al.: Surgical management of subaortic obstruction in single left ventricle and tricuspid atresia. J. Am. Coll. Cardiol. 10:421, 1987.

524. Lin, A. E., Laks, H., Barber, G., et al.: Subaortic obstruction in complex congenital heart disease: Management by proximal pulmonary artery to ascending aorta end-to-side anastomosis. J. Am. Coll. Cardiol. 7:617, 1986.

524a. Stevenson, O., Soderlund, S., Thoren, C., and Wallgren, G.: Arterial anomalies causing compression of the trachea and/or the esophagus. Acta Paediatr. Scand. 60:81, 1971.

525. Park, C. D., Waldhausen, J. A., Friedman, S., et al.: Tracheal compression by the great arteries in the mediastinum: Report of 39 cases. Arch. Surg. 103:626, 1971.

526. Gikonyo, B. M., Jue, K. L., and Edwards, J. E.: Pulmonary vascular sling: Report of seven cases and review of the literature. Pediatr. Cardiol. 10:81, 1989.

527. Baron, R. L., Gutierrez, F. R., and McKnight, R. C.: Computed tomographic evaluation of the great arteries and aortic arch malformations. In Friedman, W. F., and Higgins, C. B. (eds.): Pediatric Cardiac Imaging. Philadelphia, W. B. Saunders Company, 1983, p. 135.

528. Biancaniello, T. M., and Heneghan, M. A.: Cardiac imaging with nuclear magnetic resonance: Technical considerations and potential clinical application. In Friedman, W. F., and Higgins, C. B. (eds): Pediatric Cardiac Imaging. Philadelphia, W. B. Saunders Company, 1983, p. 270.

529. deLeval, M.: Vascular rings. In Stark, J., and deLeval, M. (eds.): Surgery for Congenital Heart Defects. New York, Grune and Stratton, Inc., 1983, p. 227.

530. Perry, J. C., and Garson, A., Jr.: Diagnosis and treatment of arrhythmias. Adv. Pediatr. 36:177, 1989.

531. Anderson, R. H., Wenick, A.C.G., Losekoot, T. G., and Becker, A. E.: Congenitally complete heart block. Circulation 56:90, 1977.

532. Ho, S. Y., Esscher, E., Anderson, R. H., and Michaelsson, M.: Anatomy of congenital complete heart block and relation to maternal anti-ro antibodies. Am. J. Cardiol. 58:291, 1986.

533. Ross, B. A.: Congenital complete atrioventricular block. Pediatr. Clin. North Am. 37:69, 1990.

534. Sholler, G. F., and Walsh, E. P.: Congenital complete heart block in patients without anatomic cardiac defects. Am. Heart J. 118:1193, 1989.

535. Beyon, J. P., Ben-Chetrit, E., Karp, S., et al.: Acquired congenital heart block. Pattern of maternal antibody response to biochemically defined antigens in neonatal lupus. J. Clin. Invest. 84:627, 1989.

536. Steinfeld, L., Rappaport, H. L., Rossback, H. C., and Martinez, E.: Diagnosis of fetal arrhythmias using echocardiographic and Doppler techniques. J. Am. Coll. Cardiol. 8:1425, 1986.

537. Mahoney, L. T., Marvin, W. J., Jr., Atkins, D. L., et al.: Pacemaker management for acute onset of heart block in childhood. J. Pediatr. 107:207, 1985.

538. Epstein, M. L., Knauf, D. G., and Alexander, J. A.: Long-term follow-up of transvenous cardiac pacing in children. Am. J. Cardiol. 57:889, 1986.

539. Michaelsson, M., and Engle, M. A.: Congenital complete heart block: An international study of the natural history. Cardiovasc. Clin. 4:85, 1982.

540. Kugler, J. D., and Danford, D. A.: Pacemakers in children: An update. Am. Heart J. 117:665, 1989.

541. Zales, V. R., Dunnigan, A., and Benson, D. W., Jr.: Clinical and electrophysiologic features of fetal and neonatal paroxysmal atrial tachycardia resulting in congestive heart failure. Am. J. Cardiol. 62:225, 1988.

542. Kleinman, C. S., Donnerstein, R. L., DeVore, G. R., et al.: Fetal echocardiography for evaluation of in utero congestive heart failure. N. Engl. J. Med. 306:568, 1982.

543. Radford, D. J., Izukawa, T., and Rowe, R. D.: Congenital paroxysmal atrial tachycardia. Arch. Dis. Child. 51:613, 1976.

544. Deal, B. J., Keane, J. F., Gillette, P. C., and Gardon, A., Jr.: Wolff-Parkinson-White syndrome and supraventricular tachycardia during infancy: Management and follow-up. J. Am. Coll. Cardiol. 5:130, 1985.

545. Benson, D. W., Jr., Dunnigan, A., and Benditt, D. G., et al.: Prediction of digoxin treatment failure in infants with supraventricular tachycardia: Role of transesophageal pacing. Pediatrics 75:288, 1985.

546. Klitzner, T. S., and Friedman, W. F.: Cardiac arrhythmias: The role of pharmacologic intervention. Cardiol. Clin. 7:299, 1989.

546a. Garson, A., Jr., Bink-Boelkens, M., Hesslein, P. S., et al.: Atrial flutter in the young: A collaborative study of 380 cases. J. Am. Coll. Cardiol. 6:871, 1985.

547. Dunnigan, A., Benson, W., Jr., and Benditt, D. G.: Atrial flutter in infancy: Diagnosis, clinical features and treatment. Pediatrics 75:725, 1985.

547a. Trippel, D. L., and Gillette, P. C.: Atenolol in children with supraventricular tachycardia. Am. J. Cardiol. 64:233, 1989.

548. Dick, M., Scott, W. A., Serwer, G. S., et al.: Acute termination of supraventricular tachyarrhythmias in children by transesophageal atrial pacing. Am. J. Cardiol. 61:925, 1988.

549. Benson, D. W., Jr., Dunnigan, A., and Benditt, D. G.: Follow-up evaluation of infant paroxysmal atrial tachycardia: Transesophageal study. Circulation 75:542, 1987.

550. Zipes, D. P., et al.: Guidelines for clinical intracardiac electrophysiologic studies. A report of the American College of Cardiology/American Heart Association Task Force on Assessment of Diagnostic and Therapeutic Cardiovascular Procedures. J. Am. Coll. Cardiol. 14:1827, 1989.

551. Case, C. L., Crawford, F. A., and Gillette, P. C.: Surgical treatment of dysrhythmias. Pediatr. Clin. North Am. 37:79, 1990.

552. Garson, A., Jr., Moak, J. P., Friedman, R. A., et al.: Surgical treatment of arrhythmias in children. Cardiol. Clin. 7:319, 1989.

553. Garson, A., Jr., Gillette, P. C., Titus, J. L., et al.: Surgical treatment of ventricular tachycardia in infants. N. Engl. J. Med. 310:1443, 1984.

Congenital Heart Disease in Adults

by JOSEPH K. PERLOFF

Congenital heart disease in adults has emerged as a special area of cardiovascular interest.[1,1a] The patient population includes those who have never undergone cardiac surgery, those who have undergone cardiac surgery and require no further operation, those who have had palliation with or without anticipation of reparative surgery, and those who are inoperable apart from organ transplantation. The number of adults with congenital heart disease is steadily increasing, and the trend promises to continue. This chapter begins with a brief historical perspective and then focuses on the multidisciplinary facilities for comprehensive care, the survival patterns (natural and postoperative), medical considerations, surgical considerations, and postoperative residua and sequelae.

HISTORICAL PERSPECTIVES

Congenital heart disease is, by definition, present at birth, but survival patterns vary widely. In 1888, Etienne-Louis Arthur Fallot wrote: "We have seen from our observations that cyanosis, especially in the adult, is the result of a small number of cardiac malformations well determined."[2] Fallot was referring to the tetralogy that still bears his name.

In the first half of the twentieth century, the untiring work of Maude Abbott culminated in her remarkable *Atlas of Congenital Heart Disease,* which was based on 1000 pathology specimens personally studied.[3] The atlas was not only a landmark in the orderly classification of the anomalies but also provided invaluable information on natural survival patterns. The seminal contributions of Gross, Blalock, Taussig, and Crafoord materially modified those survival patterns, and the sense of despair that had surrounded congenital cardiac anomalies—those "hopeless futilities"—began to dissipate.

In 1939, Robert Gross, a pediatric surgeon at Harvard, ligated a patent ductus in a 7½-year-old girl.[4] A few years later, Helen Brooke Taussig, a pediatric cardiologist in Baltimore, conceived the idea of "creating" a patent ductus arteriosus in cyanotic children suffering from deficient pulmonary blood flow. In 1945, Alfred Blalock, a vascular surgeon at Johns Hopkins, sutured the end of a subclavian artery to the side of a pulmonary artery in a patient with Fallot's tetralogy, establishing the Blalock-Taussig anastomosis.[5] Previously, "a blue baby with a malformed heart was considered beyond the reach of surgical aid." In the early 1940s, Clarence Crafoord of the Karolinska Institute, while operating on patients with patent ductus arteriosus, "began to wonder whether it might not also be possible to treat coarctation of the aortic isthmus by surgical means."[6] The postwar introduction of cardiac catheterization, for which Andre F. Cournand, Dickinson W. Richards, and Werner Forssman received the Nobel prize in 1956, was a major step forward. The development of extra-corporeal circulation in the early to mid-1950's was destined to make virtually all congenital malformations of the heart accessible to the skills of cardiac surgeons. The stage was set for "accurate visualization of structures within the heart for a period sufficient to permit precise corrective measures."[7]

The culmination of these historical landmarks resulted in one of the most successful diagnostic and therapeutic programs that medicine has witnessed. Formidable technical resources are at our disposal, permitting remarkably accurate anatomical and physiological cardiac diagnoses and astonishing feats of reparative surgery. Survival patterns have been affected, often profoundly. Accordingly, congenital heart disease should be considered not only in terms of its age of onset but also in terms of the age range that survival now permits—an uninterrupted continuum from fetal life to senescence. Although long-term management remains concerned with natural survival, it is increasingly involved with the growing numbers of postoperative patients who continue to need medical surveillance. The quality of care provided by pediatric cardiologists to patients from birth to maturity must be matched with care of equal quality during adulthood.

Congenital heart disease in adults is represented by natural survival and postoperative survival patterns. *Unoperated* adults experience improved longevity and well-being owing to refinements in the medical management of hematological disorders, renal function, urate metabolism, pulmonary physiology, infective endocarditis, electrophysiological abnormalities, pregnancy, and noncardiac surgery. Proper care of patients *after* operation requires knowledge of the preoperative congenital cardiac malformation, the nature and effects of surgical intervention, and the presence, type, and extent of postoperative residua and sequelae. The ideal objective of complete cure is rarely achieved, so operations necessarily leave behind a broad range of residua and sequelae that require prolonged, if not indefinite, medical attention. Uninterrupted, long-term continuity care is essential if the concerns inherent in this new and increasing patient population are to be addressed.[8-10]

A MULTIDISCIPLINARY CENTER FOR CARE OF ADULTS WITH CONGENITAL HEART DISEASE

The UCLA Adult Congenital Heart Disease Center is a university hospital facility for congenital heart disease in adults.[1] The staff consists of a medical cardiologist, a pediatric cardiologist, a cardiologist with appointments in medicine and pediatrics, two cardiac surgeons, and a clinical cardiovascular nurse specialist. The cardiologists have a thorough understanding of the diagnostic modalities, the reparative and palliative surgical techniques, and the cardiovascular and general medical illnesses that adults with congenital heart disease may acquire during the course of aging. Dedication to task is a collaborative effort, especially in the setting of a university hospital in which intellectual interchange, teaching, and research are as paramount as optimal patient care.

Patients qualify for entry into the center when they reach age 18 years, or when they are judged to have achieved appropriate psychological and physical maturity. The transition from pediatric to adult care is simplest for 18-year-olds who consider themselves young adults. Conversely, patients in their 20's may be physically small, emotionally immature, and all too dependent on the familiar pediatric setting that has provided a sense of security for so many years. Every effort should be made to avoid reinforcing this dependency. Adult care is best provided in an adult setting, whether outpatient or inpatient. Referrals are from pediatric cardiology in the same institution, and from internists, family practitioners, pediatricians, or cardiologists within or outside the immediate geographical area. Patients are referred either directly to the Adult Congenital Heart Disease Center or to a colleague in the Division of Cardiothoracic Surgery.

The outpatient clinic is an important aspect of the center. Appointments are made through a single group of secretaries with whom the patients become familiar. The same outpatient rooms and the same nurses are used for each clinic session to provide the patients with a sense of familiarity. The outpatient laboratory serving the clinic gives priority to the processing of blood counts. The clinical nurse specialist arranges for phlebotomy during the outpatient visit as soon as its necessity is determined. Medical and pediatric cardiac fellows are assigned to the clinic together with medical and pediatric residents. Initial patient assessment is by a fellow or resident, who then confers with a staff cardiologist. When time permits, these presentations are made to the group as a whole, unless the problem is judged to be relatively routine. All follow-up and consultation reports are dictated by the staff cardiologists because the reports are designed to provide educational as well as practical information for referring physicians and to serve as reliable data sources. Inpatients include elective admissions for cardiac or noncardiac surgery, admissions for labor and delivery, admissions to the cardiac intensive care unit, usually for arrhythmias, and admissions for medical management. Other inpatients are referred directly to a cardiac surgeon and are routinely seen in hospital by a staff cardiologist. Before discharge, follow-up arrangements are made in collaboration with the surgeon and the referring physician. The clinical nurse specialist coordinates the inpatient-outpatient interface.

The noninvasive, catheterization, and angiographic laboratories must offer the same diagnostic quality for adults with congenital heart disease as that offered by the pediatric laboratories for infants and children. Adults with congenital heart disease are best studied in laboratories that are designed for adults, provided the quality of the investigations equals that achieved in pediatric laboratories. Results will be less than optimal unless the cardiologists and technologists in the adult laboratories have training, expertise, and experience in the complex problems of congenital heart disease, a goal that can be reached when there is a sufficient volume and variety of patients.

Noncardiac consultants formally incorporated into the Adult Congenital Heart Disease Center include those in hematology, renal function, urate metabolism, pulmonary medicine, cardiac surgery, electrophysiology, insurability and vocational counseling, genetics and epidemiology, gynecology and obstetrics, psychiatry, anesthesiology, and pathology. The objective is to have ready access to specialists who have gained experience in the specific problems associated with congenital heart disease in adults.

The center assumes a major role in the training and education of fellows, residents, and nurse specialists who will become the next generation of responsible professionals. Implicit in the educational mission is the idea that pediatric cardiologists should have an understanding of cardiovascular disease in adults, and medical cardiologists should have an understanding of heart disease in children.[11]

The center is a lively area of clinical research, which is prompted by a desire to address unresolved questions posed by the patient population under surveillance. Investigations usually require collaboration with colleagues in a number of other disciplines, thus stimulating valuable interdisciplinary interchange.

SURVIVAL PATTERNS

NATURAL SURVIVAL

Natural survival includes malformations that do not require operation, malformations that remain amenable to operation in adulthood, and malformations that are inoperable except for organ transplantation. Management of adults with congenital heart disease must take into account acquired disorders of the heart and circulation that may coexist and modify the physiological expressions of the basic congenital malformation. This discussion deals chiefly with common or uncommon defects in which survival to adulthood is expected, and with some common defects in which adult survival is exceptional, but does not deal with uncommon defects in which adult survival is exceptional.

Common Defects in Which Survival to Adulthood Is Expected

BICUSPID AORTIC VALVE (see also p. 922 and Figs. 4–66, p. 90; 31–31, p. 924; 31–32, p. 924; 31–33, p. 925). This disorder is the most frequent congenital anomaly to which that structure is subject and is one of the most common gross morphological congenital anomalies of the heart or great arteries.[12,13] Bicuspid aortic valves that are functionally normal at birth undergo one of several patterns of evolution.[12,13] The valve can remain functionally normal throughout a normal life span or can develop gradual obstruction caused by fibrocalcific thickening, a substrate that accounts for about one-half of surgical cases of calcific aortic stenosis in adults (Fig. 32–1).[14] The natural history of bicuspid aortic valves occasionally is punctuated by dissecting aortic aneurysms, which sometimes become manifested years after otherwise successful valve replacement. The relationship between aortic root disease and a congenitally bicuspid aortic valve is more than casual.[15] A bicuspid aortic valve may develop progressive regurgitation with or without the impetus of infective endocarditis and is an important cause of anatomically isolated valvular aortic regurgitation — mild to severe, chronic or acute — in adults.[16]

COARCTATION OF THE AORTA (see also p. 920 and Figs. 11–39, p. 331; 8–40, p. 229; 31–29, p. 921, 31–30, p. 921). This anomaly may not cause significant symptoms until after 20 to 30 years of age.[17] Most patients who survive infancy reach adulthood. Sporadic examples of exceptional longevity (Fig. 32–2) should not obscure the inherent risks that significantly shorten life span. On an average, death occurs in the mid-30's.[13] The oldest recorded survivor was Raynaud's patient (1828), a 92-year-old man.[18]

Longevity and morbidity in adults with coarctation of the aorta are influenced by coexisting congenital and acquired cardiac and vascular diseases. The most common associated congenital malformation is the bicuspid aortic valve,[13] the natural history of which was just described. Less common, but potentially lethal, is a congenital aneurysm of the circle of Willis, which typically announces itself by sudden rupture.[19] Aortic dissection or rupture is a dramatic complication, with peak incidence in the third and fourth decades.[20] Ruptures originate either in the proximal ascending aorta (the most common site) or in a post-coarctation aneurysm (distal compartment). Left ventricular failure in unoperated coarctation

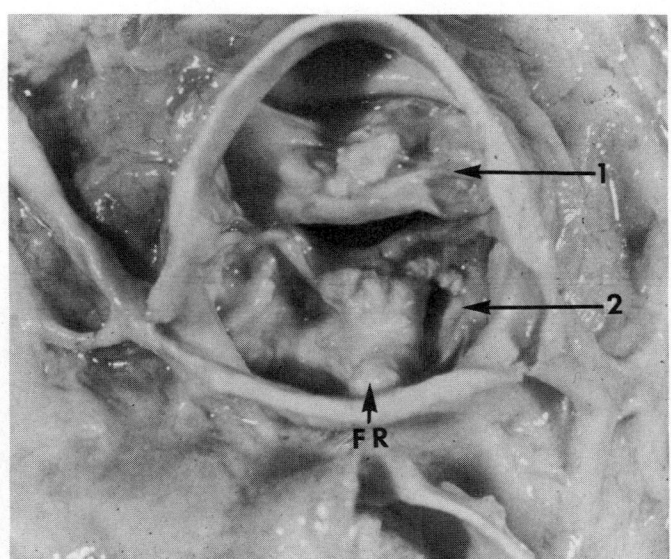

FIGURE 32–1. Necropsy specimen from an adult with bicuspid aortic stenosis. The first arrow points to one calcified leaflet, the second arrow points to a second calcified leaflet, and the vertical arrow points to calcium in the false raphe (FR). (Courtesy of Dr. William C. Roberts, National Heart Lung and Blood Institute, Bethesda, MD.)

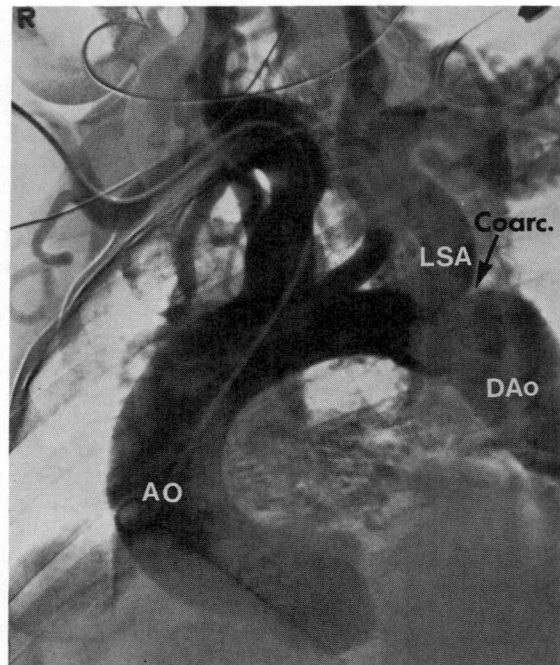

FIGURE 32-2. Lateral aortogram from a 62-year-old woman with coarctation (Coarc) of the aorta just distal to the left subclavian artery (LSA). There is poststenotic dilatation of the descending aorta (DAo). Arterial collaterals are conspicuous.

of the aorta occurs in patients who are either younger than 1 year of age or older than age 40 years, but seldom in between.[13] Hypertension predisposes to premature coronary artery disease.[21]

PULMONARY VALVE STENOSIS (see also p. 972, and Figs. 4-67 and 4-68, p. 90; 8-42A, p. 230; Fig. 7, p. 156; Fig. 31-42, p. 932; 31-43, p. 933). Represented by a pliant conical or dome-shaped valve with a narrow outlet at its apex, pulmonary valve stenosis typically occurs as an isolated congenital anomaly and is the most common variety of congenital obstruction to right ventricular outflow.[13] With the exception of pinpoint pulmonary valve stenosis in neonates, survival into adolescence and adulthood is the rule. Longevity depends chiefly on three variables: (1) the initial severity of obstruction, (2) whether a given degree of obstruction remains constant or progresses, and (3) the functional adequacy of the

pressure-overloaded right ventricle.[13] Patients with typical isolated pulmonary stenosis usually experience an increase in valve orifice with age, although the development of secondary hypertrophic subpulmonary stenosis (Fig. 32-3A) or fibrocalcific thickening may augment the degree of obstruction. While subjective complaints become more prevalent as years go by, equivalent degrees of stenosis may handicap one patient in childhood yet leave another relatively unencumbered as an adult. Right ventricular failure is the most common mode of death, usually occurring after the fourth decade.[22-25] Infective endocarditis is a risk (except perhaps in mild pulmonary valve stenosis), with a reported incidence of 2 to 7 per cent.

OSTIUM SECUNDUM ATRIAL SEPTAL DEFECT (see also p. 906 and Figs. 4-76, p. 92; 8-41A, p. 229; Fig. 30, p. 159; 31-11, p. 906; 31-12, p. 907; 31-13, p. 907). *This anomaly is among the most common congenital cardiac malformations in adults* (Fig. 32-4), accounting for 30 to 40 per cent in patients age 40 years or older.[13,26,27] The malformation often goes unrecognized for decades because symptoms may be absent and physical signs are subtle. Although life expectancy is not normal, survival into adulthood of patients who are not operated on is the rule, and many patients live to advanced ages.[26-31] Natural survival beyond age 40 to 50 years is, however, less than 50 per cent, with an attrition rate after age 40 years of about 6 per cent per annum.[13] One of the author's patients died at age 87 years with atrial fibrillation and right ventricular failure, and another lived relatively comfortably until 3 months before his 95th birthday.[32]

Virtually all patients with ostium secundum atrial septal defects who survive beyond the sixth decade are symptomatic. Older patients deteriorate chiefly on three counts. First, an age-related decrease in left ventricular distensibility augments the left-to-right shunt. Second, atrial arrhythmias, especially fibrillation but also atrial flutter or paroxysmal atrial tachycardia, increase in frequency after the fourth decade and precipitate right ventricular failure. Third, the majority of symptomatic adults older than age 40 have mild to moderate pulmonary hypertension in the presence of a persistent large left-to-right shunt, so the aging right ventricle is doubly beset by both pressure and volume overload.[13] If advanced pulmonary vascular disease occurs at all, it seldom does so before the third decade. Even so, the patient's life span often stretches into the fourth decade.[13,33]

The incidence, extent, and degree of mitral valve disease in patients with ostium secundum atrial septal defect increases with age, and significant mitral regurgitation occurs in about

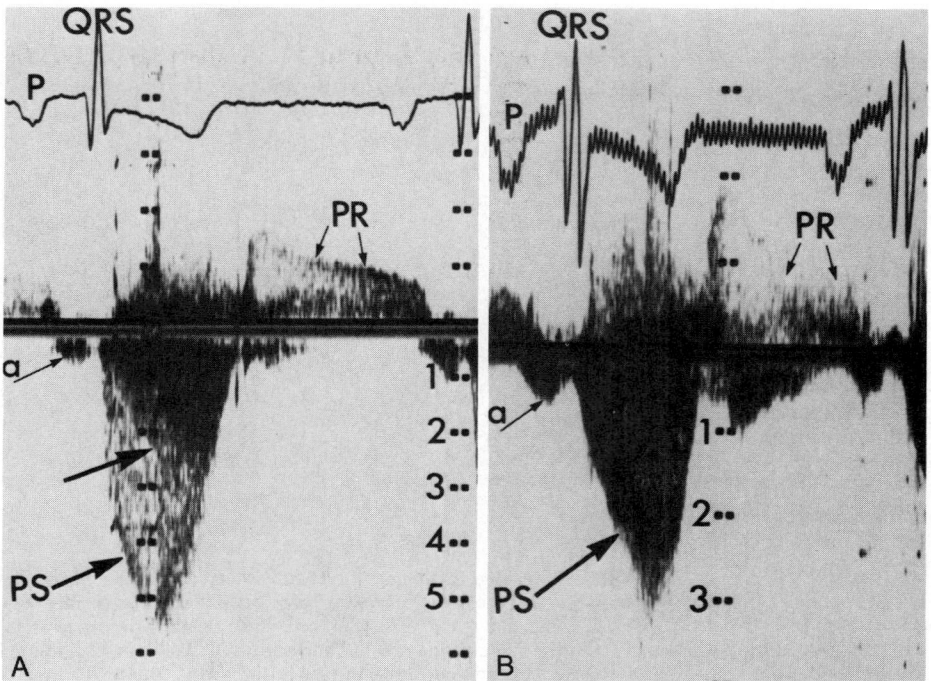

FIGURE 32-3. *A,* Continuous wave Doppler across the right ventricular outflow tract of a 33-year-old male with severe pulmonary valve stenosis (PS) and secondary hypertrophic subpulmonary stenosis. The peak instantaneous gradient across the valve was 120 mm Hg. Within the major symmetric flow disturbance envelope, there is an asymmetric, lower-velocity pattern (upper unmarked arrow) caused by the hypertrophic subpulmonary stenosis. a = presystolic flow in response to an increased force of right atrial contractions; PR = pulmonary regurgitation. *B,* After balloon dilatation, the gradient at valve level was virtually abolished, leaving only the subpulmonary (PS) gradient.

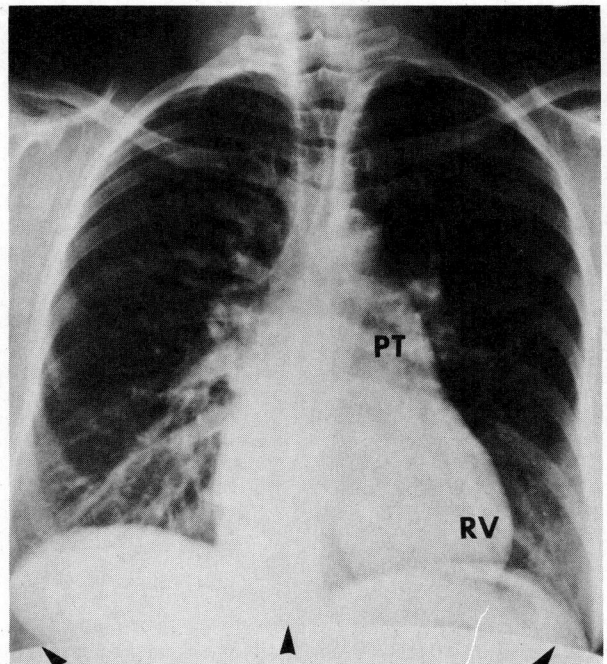

FIGURE 32–4. Chest radiograph from a 32-year-old woman with an uncomplicated ostium secundum atrial septal defect. She was in the third trimester of her ninth pregnancy. Note the lead shield (arrowheads) over the abdomen. The pulmonary trunk (PT) is dilated. An enlarged right ventricle (RV) occupies the apex.

15 per cent.[34-36] Mitral valve abnormalities have been attributed chiefly to the effects on the mitral apparatus of left ventricular cavity deformity (size as well as shape).[37,38] The female-male ratio is about two to one. Because the natural history of ostium secundum atrial septal defect extends into adulthood, it is the rule for women to reach childbearing age (Fig. 32–4) (see pp. 977 and 978).

PATENT DUCTUS ARTERIOSUS (see also p. 913 and Fig. 8–41B, p. 229). This congenital vascular anomaly permits asymptomatic survival in most patients, at least after the first year of life.[39-43] At the beginning of the second decade, the risk of infective endarteritis exceeds the risk of heart failure.[13] Beginning in the third decade (occasionally earlier), more and more patients with sizable left-to-right shunts develop cardiac failure, whereas those with small shunts (restrictive ductus) remain asymptomatic. One of the author's patients was an 84-year-old woman with a small patent ductus arteriosus of little or no physiological significance, and another 84-year-old

patient had a moderately restrictive ductus with atrial fibrillation and congestive heart failure (Fig. 32–5). There is a significant cumulative risk of infective endocarditis, especially if the patent ductus is restrictive (see later). Patients with patent ductus arteriosus and large shunts (nonrestrictive ductus) seldom reach adulthood unless a rise in pulmonary vascular resistance relieves the left ventricle of excessive volume overload.[42] Differential cyanosis is a distinctive feature of the reversed shunt.

Uncommon Defects in Which Survival to Adulthood Is Expected

SITUS INVERSUS WITH DEXTROCARDIA (p. 984). Patients with this anomaly, which usually occurs with a structurally normal heart,[13] experience normal longevity but are susceptible to *acquired* cardiac and noncardiac diseases. Symptoms so related may lead to the discovery of the hitherto unsuspected cardiac malposition. Angina pectoris or myocardial infarction in adults with complete situs inversus is associated with pain in the *right* anterior chest with radiation to the *right* shoulder and *right* arm. The pain of appendicitis is referred to the *left* lower quadrant, and biliary colic presents in the *left* upper quadrant, owing to the mirror image positions of the abdominal viscera. When situs inversus with dextrocardia coexists with congenital malformations of the heart, longevity is determined by the associated anomalies.

SITUS SOLITUS WITH DEXTROCARDIA. This malformation occasionally occurs with a structurally normal heart, which not only permits adult survival but usually delays clinical recognition.[13] A routine chest radiograph may provide the first evidence of the malposition. Coexisting congenital cardiac malformations, which normally are present, determine longevity.

CONGENITAL COMPLETE HEART BLOCK (see also pp. 955 and 984). This disorder usually permits survival into adulthood.[13,44-46] The key determinants of longevity are the ventricular rate, the presence of intrinsically normal ventricular myocardium, and the hemodynamic adjustments at rest and with exercise. Despite the frequency of asymptomatic survival into adulthood, optimism is dampened by the ultimate fate of large numbers of adolescents and adults with congenital complete heart block; nor is mortality in childhood negligible.[13,44]

UNCOMPLICATED CONGENITALLY CORRECTED TRANSPOSITION OF THE GREAT ARTERIES (see also p. 946 and Figs. 8–42A, p. 230; 31–65, p. 949). This malformation permits good but not normal longevity because of the functional inadequacy of a morphologic right ventricle in the systemic location.[47-50] More often than not the natural history is influenced by the presence and degree of the congenital cardiac malformations that commonly coexist.[13] Survival into the sixth decade is uncommon, with only a few patients reaching the seventh decade, and only one reaching age 73 years.[51] Incompetence of the inverted left atrioventricular valve (Ebstein-like anomaly) may go unrecognized until late childhood or early adulthood, prompting the mistaken diagnosis of acquired mitral regurgitation. The risk of complete atrioventricular block accrues at a rate of about 2 per cent per year.[13] Complete heart block may announce itself with a Stokes-Adams attack or sudden death.

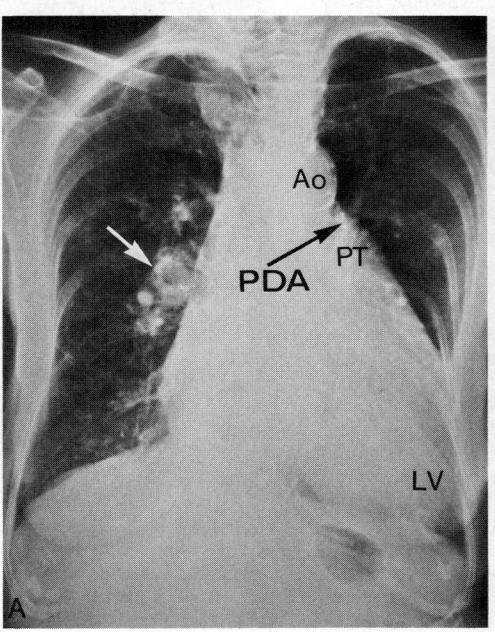
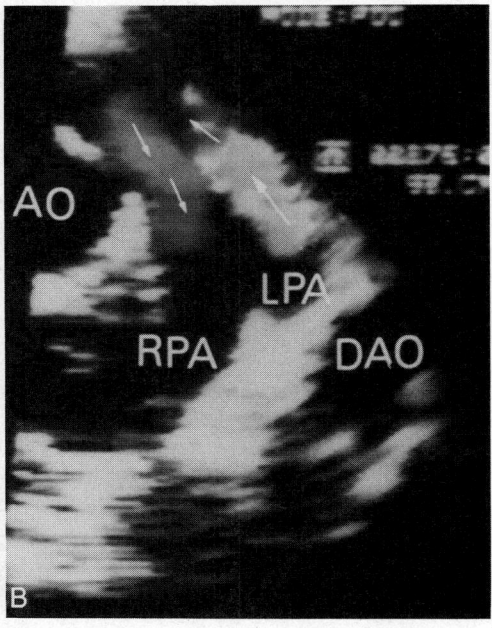

FIGURE 32–5. *A,* Radiograph from an 84-year-old woman with a moderately restrictive calcified patent ductus arteriosus (PDA). The pulmonary trunk (PT) and its right branch (unmarked white arrow) are dilated. Pulmonary arterial pressure was 90/40 mm Hg. The enlarged left ventricle (LV) occupies the apex. The aortic knuckle (Ao) is calcified. *B,* Black and white print of a color-flow image (parasternal short axis). Arrows trace the direction of ductal flow, moving first down the left lateral wall of the pulmonary trunk and then up the opposite wall. LPA = left pulmonary artery; RPA = right pulmonary artery; DAo = descending aorta.

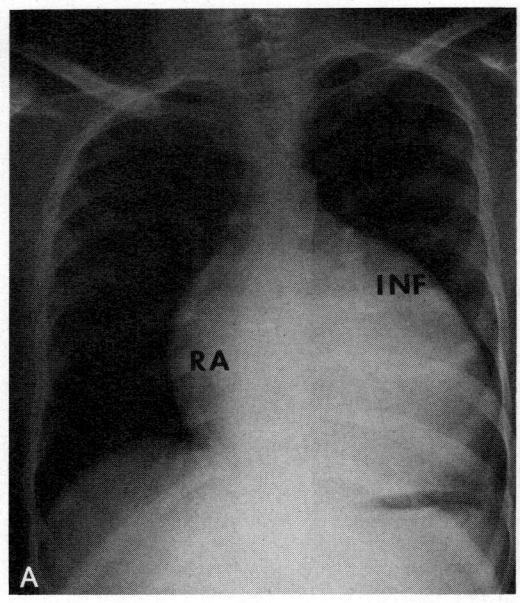
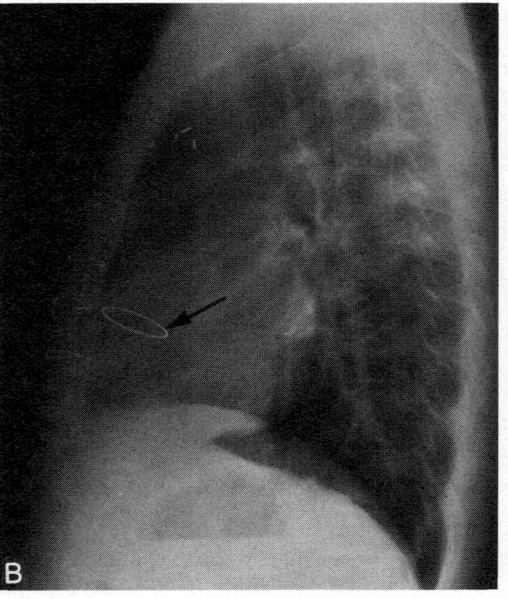

FIGURE 32-6. *A,* Preoperative chest radiograph from a 22-year-old man with cyanotic Ebstein's anomaly, Wolff-Parkinson-White bypass tracts, and syncope induced by atrial flutter with 1:1 antegrade conduction. There is a large right atrium (RA) and a hump-shaped infundibulum (INF). *B,* Lateral chest radiograph after tricuspid valve reconstruction and atrioventricular dissociation. Arrow identifies the Carpentier ring.

CONGENITAL MITRAL REGURGITATION (see also p. 930). Sometimes this lesion occurs as the only clinically overt component of an endocardial cushion defect.[13] Adult survival depends on the degree of regurgitation and the adaptive response of the volume-overloaded left ventricle. The mistaken diagnosis of acquired mitral regurgitation is not uncommon.

EBSTEIN'S ANOMALY OF THE TRICUSPID VALVE (see also p. 940 and Figs. 4-69, p. 91; 8-42C, p. 230). This lesion permits longevity into adulthood, depending on the physiological state of the malformed right ventricle, the presence of an interatrial communication (right-to-left shunt), and the presence and severity of atrial tachyarrhythmias, especially when accompanied by accelerated conduction through Wolff-Parkinson-White bypass tracts. The natural history ranges from neonatal death to relatively asymptomatic survival into adulthood, even to advanced age.[52-60,60a] For patients who survive the first year of life, a cumulative mortality of 12.4 per cent is distributed about evenly through childhood and adolescence.[13] Paroxysmal supraventricular tachycardia occurs in about 25 to 30 per cent of patients with Ebstein's anomaly.[13] Syncope heightens suspicion of accelerated bypass conduction (rapid atrial fibrillation or one-to-one atrial flutter). A rapid ventricular response by way of a bypass tract is held responsible for sudden death. Despite the aforementioned qualifications, there are accounts of astonishing longevity, with survivals into the eighth decade.[56,57] The oldest recorded patient with Ebstein's anomaly lived to age 85 years and had no cardiac symptoms until age 79.[13]

CONGENITAL PULMONARY VALVE REGURGITATION (see also p. 1059). This malformation typically permits adult survival. Longevity depends on the degree of regurgitant flow and on the adaptive response of the right ventricle to volume overload.[61,62] Because the regurgitation is seldom more than moderate, and because the right ventricle readily adapts to low pressure volume overload, most patients tolerate the anomaly through middle age and occasionally into the sixth or even eighth decade of life.[13,63] Right heart failure may occur in older adults after decades of stability because of the additive effects of a rise in pulmonary arterial pressure caused by acquired bronchopulmonary disease or because of the passive elevation of pulmonary arterial pressure that accompanies left ventricular failure.[13] The risk of infective endocarditis is relatively low.

LUTEMBACHER'S SYNDROME. This syndrome consists of an atrial septal defect that coexists with *acquired* mitral stenosis.[13] Longevity depends on the degree of mitral valve obstruction and the size of the interatrial communication. Mitral stenosis augments the left-to-right interatrial shunt, but the atrial septal defect decompresses the left atrium, reducing the gradient across the stenotic mitral valve. Lutembacher's original patient was a 61-year-old woman who had been pregnant 7 times,[68] and Firket's patient was a 74-year-old woman who had experienced 11 pregnancies.[69] The oldest reported patient was an 81-year-old woman who experienced no symptoms related to her heart until her 75th year.[70]

ANEURYSM OF A SINUS OF VALSALVA (see also p. 106). This defect typically begins as a blind pouch or diverticulum that takes origin from a localized site in one aortic sinus. The substantial majority of ruptures develop well after puberty but before age 30 years, usually in males ranging in age from 11 to 67 years.[71,72] The physiological consequences depend on the rapidity with which the rupture develops, the amount of blood flowing through the abnormal communication, and the chamber (site) that receives the shunt. Death usually is within a year after an unre-

lieved acute large perforation. A small perforation that progresses gradually may at first go unnoticed; small chronic perforations are susceptible to infective endocarditis. About 20 per cent of congenital sinus of Valsalva aneurysms are unperforated and are discovered at necropsy or cardiac surgery.[13] In one of our patients, an 85-year-old man, the diagnosis of a previously unsuspected aortic sinus aneurysm was made by echocardiography with Doppler interrogation and color-flow imaging.

CORONARY ARTERIOVENOUS FISTULAS (see also p. 917). This anomaly represents one of the most common major congenital malformations of the coronary circulation that permit adult survival.[13,73] Both coronary arteries arise from the aorta, but a fistulous branch of one or more arteries communicates directly with a cardiac chamber or with the pulmonary trunk, coronary sinus, vena cava, or a pulmonary vein (Fig. 32-7). Longevity depends on the amount of blood flowing through the communication, the chamber or vessel into which the fistula drains, and myocardial ischemia that may result from the fistulous bypass (coronary steal). Adult survival is expected, although life span is not normal. Survivals have been recorded in the seventh to the ninth decades, with the oldest patient living to age 85 years.[13]

CONGENITAL PULMONARY ARTERIOVENOUS FISTULAS (see also p. 930). These fistulas typically occur without coexisting congenital heart

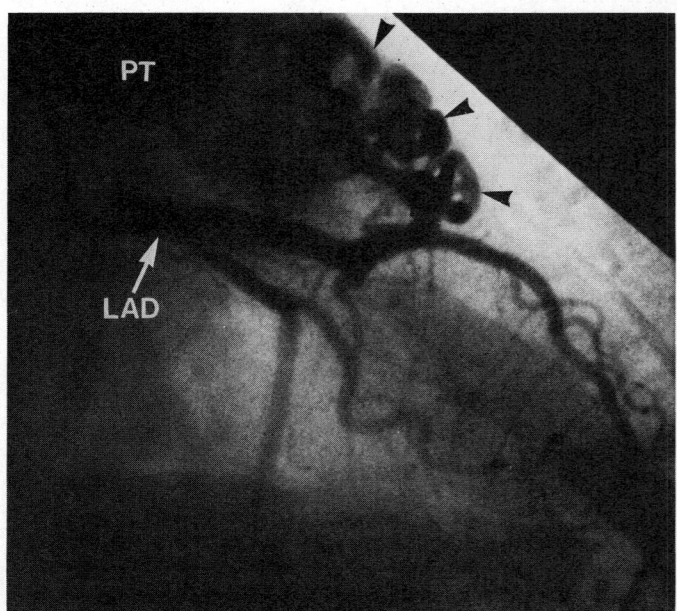

FIGURE 32-7. Selective left coronary arteriogram from an asymptomatic 63-year-old woman who had a continuous murmur beneath her left clavicle. Arrows at the right point to a congenital coronary arteriovenous fistula arising from a branch of the left anterior descending (LAD) coronary artery. PT = pulmonary trunk.

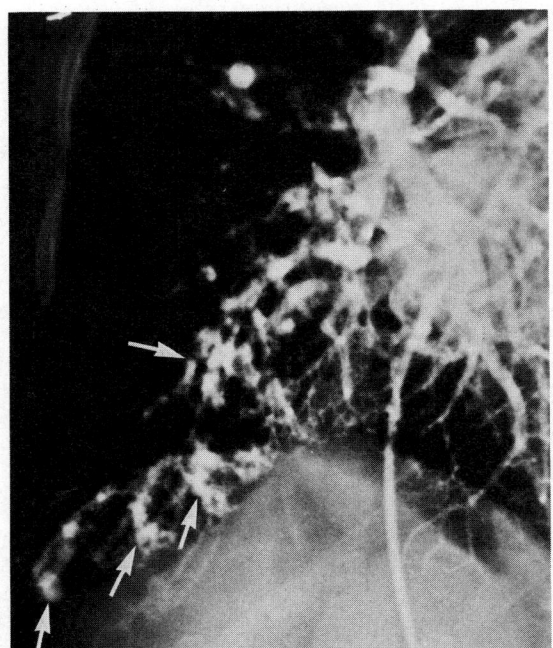

FIGURE 32–8. Selective right pulmonary arteriogram from a 71-year-old man with congenital bilateral pulmonary arteriovenous fistulae (arrows). His 73-year-old sister was similarly afflicted. Neither had telangiectasia.

disease but usually are associated with hereditary telangiectasia.[74] A substantial majority of the fistulas go unrecognized until adult life. In one large series, the mean patient age was 39 years (range 3 to 73 years), with the distinct minority younger than age 20 years.[13] Two of the author's patients without telangiectasia are siblings age 71 and 73 years (Fig. 32–8).[75]

Common Defects in Which Adult Survival Is Exceptional

VENTRICULAR SEPTAL DEFECT (see also p. 910, and Figs. 4–74, p. 93; Fig. 31, p. 159; 8–41C, p. 229; 11–13, p. 319). These are among the most common congenital cardiac malformations at birth but are seldom found in adults.[76–80] In his remarks on adult survival in congenital heart disease, Paul Wood asked, "Where's the maladie de Roger? Assuming it does not provide immortality, it must either close spontaneously in middle life or have long since run its mortal course."[81] Patients who survive into adulthood comprise two main groups: (1) those with small or moderately restrictive perimembranous or muscular defects that have closed spontaneously or that have decreased in size so that they are clinically inapparent, and (2) patients with nonrestrictive ventricular septal defects but with elevated pulmonary vascular resistance that relieves the left ventricle of excessive volume overload while imposing no increase in afterload on the right ventricle (Eisenmenger's complex).

The chief reason for adult survival of patients born with ventricular septal defects is spontaneous closure.[82] The long-term fate of perimembranous ventricular septal defects that have closed by aneurysm formation is unknown, but there is cautious optimism.[83] The occasional adult survivor with persistent patency of a small perimembranous ventricular septal defect confronts a cumulative risk of infective endocarditis.[84] It is not uncommon for patients with Eisenmenger's complex to reach adulthood (p. 763). The author's oldest patient died of noncardiac causes at age 69 years (Fig. 32–9). Longevity in Eisenmenger's complex has improved significantly because of meticulous hematological management (see later).

FALLOT'S TETRALOGY (see also p. 935 and Fig. 4–82, p. 94). This is the cyanotic malformation that most frequently permits survival to adulthood.[2,13] Individual reports describe survivals from the fifth to the seventh decades of life.[13,85,86] Nevertheless, survival patterns based on an analysis of more

than 500 necropsy cases disclosed that two-thirds of patients born with the tetralogy reached their first birthday, 50 per cent reached age 3 years, about 25 per cent completed the first decade of life, and thereafter the attrition rate was 6.4 per cent per year.[13] But differently, 11 per cent of patients are alive at age 20 years, 6 per cent at age 30 years, and 3 per cent at age 40. Systemic hypertension in adult survivors with the tetralogy is a special problem because the increased afterload is imposed on both the left *and* right ventricles (biventricular aorta).[13] The rise in right ventricular systolic pressure augments pulmonary blood flow and reduces cyanosis, but at the price of right ventricular (or biventricular) failure. Infective endocarditis on an incompetent biventricular aortic valve in Fallot's tetralogy may result in catastrophic acute severe regurgitation into both right and left ventricles.

SURVIVAL AFTER CARDIAC SURGERY OR INTERVENTIONAL CATHETERIZATION

An understanding of prognosis after cardiac surgery or interventional catheterization requires knowledge of the preoperative congenital malformation, the nature and effects of the therapeutic intervention, and the postoperative residua and sequelae.[1,87] Success is measured by the length of survival, the quality of life, and the need for reoperation. It is axiomatic that techniques have evolved and will continue to do so. Patients who underwent cardiac surgery two to three decades ago benefited from the anatomical repairs but often suffered from the deleterious effects of what would now be considered inadequate myocardial protection. Prosthetic materials—valves, patches, and conduits—that were state of the art at that time have been superseded by many generations of improved devices and materials. This discussion is concerned with late survival after surgery or interventional catheterization involving cardiac valves, intraatrial or intraventricular repairs, central arterial procedures, and creation of a complete or partial vena caval or atrial-dependent pulmonary circulation.

Congenitally Malformed Cardiac Valves

Congenitally stenotic or incompetent semilunar or atrioventricular valves are treated by cardiac surgery or, if ste-

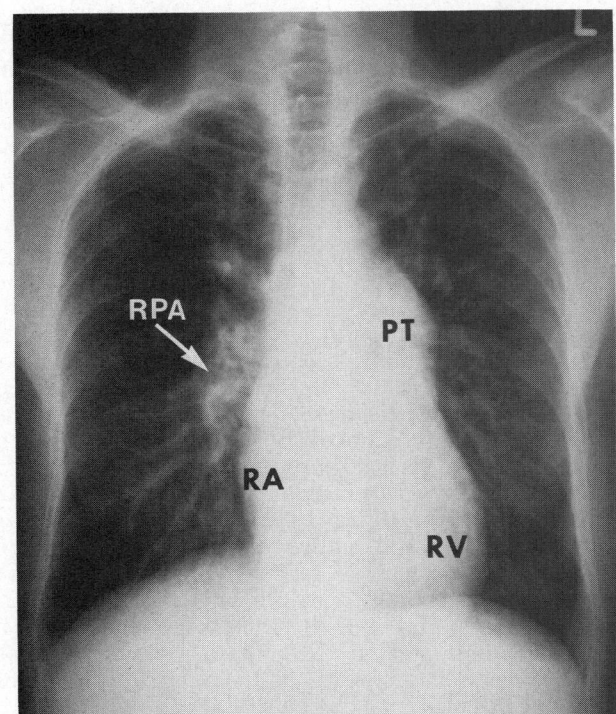

FIGURE 32–9. Radiograph from a 67-year-old man with Eisenmenger's complex; he died at age 69 of Legionnaire's disease. The pulmonary trunk (PT) and its branches (RPA = right pulmonary artery) are conspicuously dilated but the heart size is virtually normal.

notic, interventional catheterization. Surgery involves reconstruction or replacement of the malformed valve, either alone or with repair of coexisting defects. Long-term results are colored by these variables.

ISOLATED PULMONARY VALVE STENOSIS (see also p. 968). This anomaly lends itself to surgical repair with excellent results. Postoperative valvular residua are relatively minor, and residual poststenotic dilatation of the pulmonary arterial trunk is of no clinical significance, even when marked. These exemplary results are qualified by the age of the patient at operation and the severity of the preoperative gradient. If marked to severe pulmonary stenosis is relieved surgically during childhood, long-term survival patterns are similar to age- and sex-matched controls.[1] Adults who undergo surgical valvotomy after age 21 years also have excellent results, but the more severe the preoperative stenosis and the longer that the right ventricle has confronted the increased afterload, the less optimal are the long-term results, including late death from right ventricular failure. These conclusions support the current practice of relieving hemodynamically significant pulmonary stenosis during childhood and underscore the desirability of surveillance through adulthood.

Balloon dilatation has largely replaced surgical repair of typical isolated congenital pulmonary valve stenosis (Fig. 32–3).[88-91] Refinements in techniques have resulted in relief of gradients comparable to the results achieved at surgery. Long-term results are not yet available, but balloon valvuloplasty promises to be as effective as surgical valvotomy.

CONGENITAL AORTIC STENOSIS (see also p. 922). When caused by a bicuspid aortic valve, this malformation is amenable to direct repair in young patients or valve replacement in older patients.[92-95] Surgical valvotomy or balloon valvuloplasty presupposes that there is a pliant, noncalcified bicuspid valve with obstruction caused by congenital fusion (nonseparation) of the commissures. The best that valvotomy can achieve is a functionally normal bicuspid aortic valve with minor degrees of regurgitation. Valvotomy of a congenitally stenotic bicuspid aortic valve in childhood or adolescence provides temporary relief of obstruction, but the valve has the same, if not a greater, tendency than does a native, functionally normal bicuspid aortic valve to thicken, calcify, and become stenotic with the passage of time. Significant postvalvotomy aortic regurgitation tends to develop gradually, but infective endocarditis can cause sudden, severe incompetence that requires urgent valve replacement. The risk of infective endocarditis is not reduced by valvotomy, even if there is complete relief of bicuspid aortic stenosis. The longer the interval after operation, the greater the need for reoperation.[93-95]

Balloon dilatation in young patients with congenital bicuspid aortic stenosis is associated with considerable variability and unpredictability of results.[96,97] This procedure does not permit the meticulous relief of commissural fusion that is possible under direct vision. The best that can be achieved by ideal balloon separation of fused commissures is an outlook that approximates that just described for open operation.

Surgically important *congenital aortic regurgitation* may occur during the natural history of a bicuspid aortic valve or after valvotomy for bicuspid aortic stenosis. Prime objectives of operation (valve replacement) for aortic regurgitation are the removal of left ventricular volume overload and the preservation or restoration of satisfactory left ventricular function. Even if these objectives are achieved, a minority of patients succumb late after operation, not because of heart failure but because of what is presumed to be a disturbance in ventricular rhythm (sudden death). The fate of the aortic prosthesis and the need for anticoagulants are important determinants of late postoperative outcome.

EBSTEIN'S ANOMALY (see also pp. 940 and 970). This malformation is the most common cause of surgically important congenital tricuspid regurgitation. Operation relieves the right ventricular volume overload and improves right ventric-

ular function.[98-100] Closure of the interatrial communication removes the risk of paradoxical emboli, and interruption of right atrioventricular bypass tracts eliminates the risk of a rapid ventricular response to atrial flutter or fibrillation (Fig. 32–10). Supraventricular arrhythmias may recur postoperatively, but if the accessory pathways are divided, the ventricular response is not accelerated, and the arrhythmias respond to conventional pharmacological management.

Every attempt should be made to reconstruct rather than replace the tricuspid valve (Fig. 32–6), even though there are obligatory residual abnormalities following use of the large anterior leaflet to create a unicuspid valve. Replacement of the valve carries a late mortality of 10 to 15 per cent.[101] Tissue valves are preferred; a mechanical prosthesis poses the risk of pulmonary embolization even with anticoagulation. Abnormal left ventricular geometry and function have been identified in patients with Ebstein's anomaly,[53,60a] but the long-term postoperative effects are unknown.

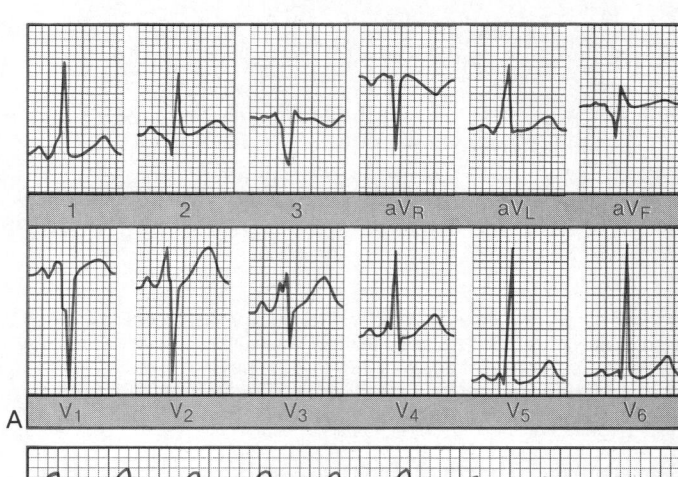
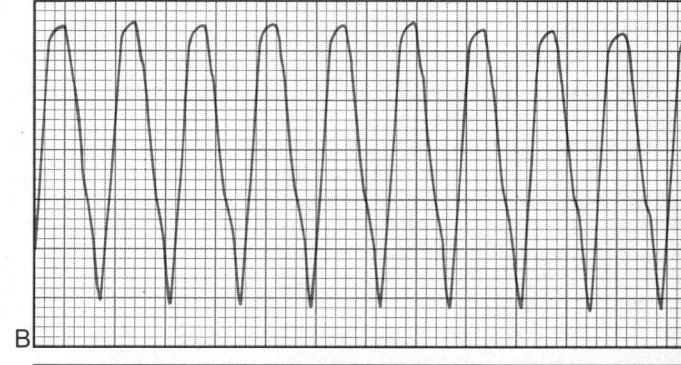
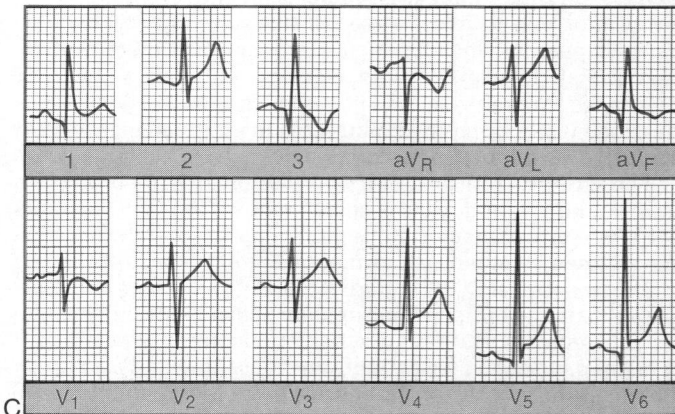

FIGURE 32–10. *A*, Twelve-lead electrocardiogram from a patient with Ebstein's anomaly of the tricuspid valve. There are typical fusion beats due to a right atrioventricular bypass tract. The delta wave is directed to the left, superior and posterior. *B*, Lead V₁ showing antegrade wide QRS tachycardia via the right bypass tract. *C*, Twelve-lead electrocardiogram after tricuspid valve reconstruction with interruption of the bypass tract by surgical dissociation between right atrium and right ventricle. The delta wave is absent.

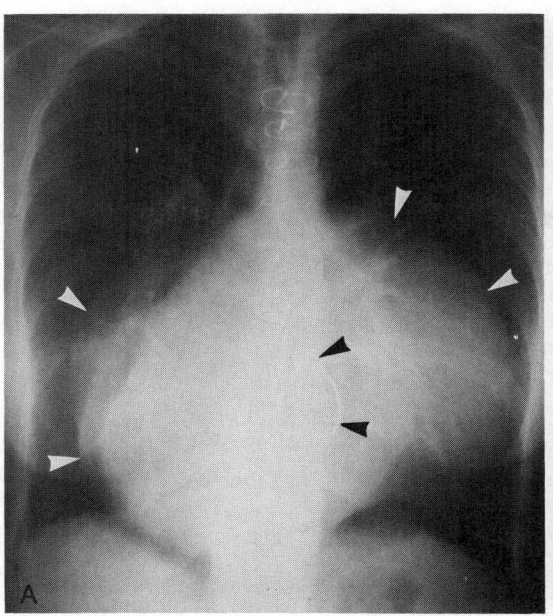
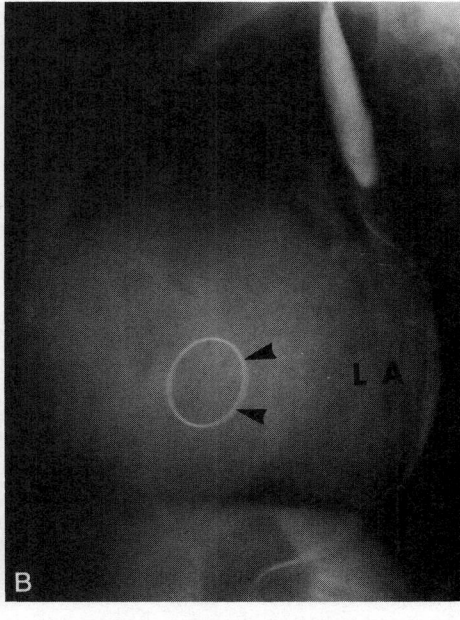

FIGURE 32–11. Chest radiographs from a 24-year-old woman with congenitally corrected transposition of the great arteries 5 years after replacement of an incompetent left atrioventricular valve with a tissue valve (arrowheads). *A,* The cardiac silhouette shown here is identical with the preoperative silhouette, resembling a huge ball consisting almost entirely of a massive left atrium (white arrowheads) that appears to be suspended from a narrow vascular pedicle. Neither great artery is border-forming. *B,* Lateral projection showing the prosthetic ring (black arrowheads) and the huge left atrium (LA).

ISOLATED INCOMPETENCE OF A LEFT-SIDED ATRIO-VENTRICULAR VALVE IN CONGENITALLY CORRECTED TRANSPOSITION OF THE GREAT ARTERIES. This lesion is caused by an Ebstein-like anomaly of a tricuspid valve in the systemic (inverted) position.[102] When surgical relief is indicated, the valve almost always requires replacement (Fig. 32–11). Long-term outcome is determined chiefly by the chronicity of preoperative regurgitation, by the functional adequacy (or inadequacy) of a morphological right ventricle in the systemic location, and by a 2 per cent per year accrued incidence of high-degree intranodal heart block.[13]

Intraatrial Surgery

ATRIAL SEPTAL DEFECT (OSTIUM SECUNDUM) (see also p. 906). This malformation lends itself to surgical closure with excellent long-term results. Operation before 24 years of age resulted in a 30-year actuarial survival that was the same as age- and sex-matched controls (98 per cent and 97 per cent).[103] When operation was performed on patients who were 24 to 40 years of age and whose preoperative pulmonary arterial pressures were normal, survival also approximated that of the control group. When pulmonary arterial systolic pressure exceeded 40 mm Hg, late survival was one-half of that of the control group, although life expectancy in the surgically treated older patients was better than with medical treatment. Even patients who were 60 years of age or older at the time of operation benefited, at least in the short term, regardless of pulmonary arterial pressure or functional class as long as the left-to-right shunt through the atrial septal defect remained large.[104]

After operation in childhood, right ventricular dimensions decrease, often strikingly,[105] but when adults undergo surgery, right ventricular dimensions remain abnormal in about 80 per cent of cases. If there is preoperative right ventricular failure and tricuspid regurgitation, late postoperative right atrial and right ventricular dilatation are the rule, and right ventricular ejection fraction seldom normalizes. These patients improve but usually remain symptomatic, and long-term outcome is influenced by preoperative pulmonary vascular resistance.[106]

A minority of patients who undergo surgical closure of an ostium secundum atrial septal defect during childhood experience the late onset of supraventricular arrhythmias believed to be related to patchy fibrosis of the right atrium secondary to dilatation, and perhaps to sinus node dysfunction.[107,108] In adults, chronic preoperative atrial fibrillation usually persists after surgical repair, but cardioversion followed by antiarrhythmic therapy may be efficacious. When operation is performed on patients older than age 40 years, about one-half of those in preoperative sinus rhythm experience late postoperative development of atrial fibrillation.

Intraatrial Surgery for Complex Cyanotic Congenital Heart Disease

COMPLETE TRANSPOSITION OF THE GREAT ARTERIES (p. 941). This malformation has been managed until recently by a Rashkind balloon atrial septostomy performed on the neonate followed by intraatrial redirection of venous return (Mustard or Senning venous switch operation) during the first 6 months of life.[1] These procedures have given way to the *arterial switch operation,* but there are large numbers of patients, including many young adults, who underwent intraatrial redirection of venous return 5 to 25 years ago.[109,110] Twenty-year survival after *atrial* switch operations has been reported at 80 to 90 per cent, but complications are the rule. Apart from postoperative electrophysiological sequelae (Fig. 32–12), an issue of fundamental importance is the long-term

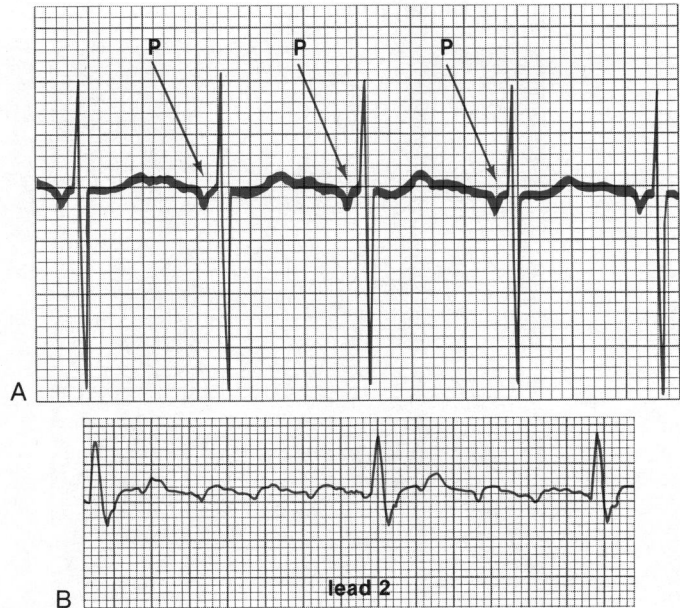

FIGURE 32–12. *A,* Junctional ectopic rhythm early after a Mustard repair for complete transposition of the great arteries. *B,* Late-onset atrial flutter with a slow ventricular response (impaired atrioventricular conduction) in a 25-year-old man who had a Mustard repair in infancy. The patient developed sinus node dysfunction in addition to atrial tachyarrhythmias.

adequacy of a morphological right ventricle in the systemic location.[111-113] The postoperative right ventricle normally does not increase its ejection fraction in response to exercise, and there is a high incidence of coexisting left ventricular dysfunction.

Intraventricular Surgery

Intraventricular surgery is performed through a right atrial incision or through a ventriculotomy in the morphological right ventricle. Long-term survival depends on a number of variables, including patient age at operation, the degree of relief of the loading conditions imposed on ventricular myocardium, myocardial protection during operation, electrophysiological sequelae, and the durability of prosthetic materials.

FALLOT'S TETRALOGY. This malformation is a case in point. When intraventricular repair is performed during infancy, long-term survival is good, but about 15 per cent of patients require reoperation.[114-117] The incidence of bifascicular block or high-degree heart block (Fig. 32–13) has decreased significantly with current operative techniques. Patients who had undergone early palliative shunts followed by intracardiac repair at about 2 years of age experienced 87 per cent survival 10 to 20 years after operation; all but a minority were free from significant cardiac or vascular symptoms and for all practical purposes were leading normal lives. Some patients who reach adulthood after having undergone Blalock-Taussig shunts in infancy or early childhood maintain symptomatic improvement for decades after operation, and benefit from intracardiac repair as adults (Fig. 32–14). However, patients who are 40 years or older at the time of intraventricular repair have a late mortality of about 15 per cent.[118,119] Late postoperative *left* ventricular function is related to age at the time of intracardiac repair and to previous shunt procedures (Fig. 32–14). Patients with severe cyanotic Fallot's tetralogy have reductions in left ventricular volume and ejection fraction related to decreased pulmonary arterial blood flow. If intracardiac repair is undertaken after 2 years of age, volumes of the left side of the heart increase but left ventricular function remains subnormal.[120,121]

Central Arterial Surgery

PATENT DUCTUS ARTERIOSUS (p. 913). Division of an isolated restrictive (small) patent ductus arteriosus in child-

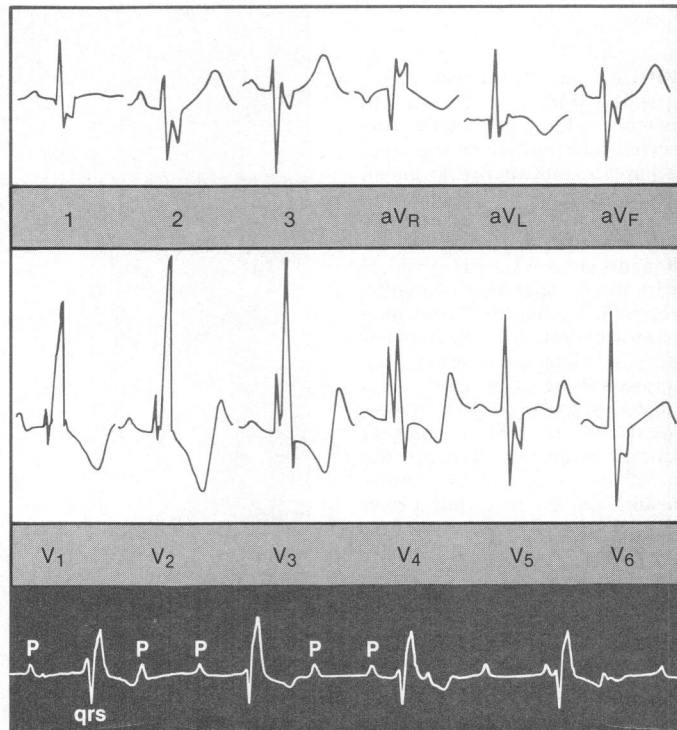

FIGURE 32–13. Twelve-lead electrocardiogram (top panel) and single channel electrocardiogram from a patient with Fallot's tetralogy after intracardiac repair. Bifascicular block (right bundle branch block with left anterior fascicular block) *(top)* progressed to complete atrioventricular block *(bottom)*.

hood represents one of the few categoric cures of congenital malformations of the heart and circulation. Transcatheter ductal occlusion must compete with this record, which is ideal except for the thoracotomy. After operation, patients are normal in the literal sense. When the ductus is moderately restrictive or nonrestrictive (large), division in childhood usually results in regression of left atrial and left ventricular enlargement, and in normalization of pulmonary arterial and right ventricular systolic pressures. If a relatively large (nonrestrictive) ductus remains undivided until after childhood, long-term outcome depends on the preoperative pulmonary

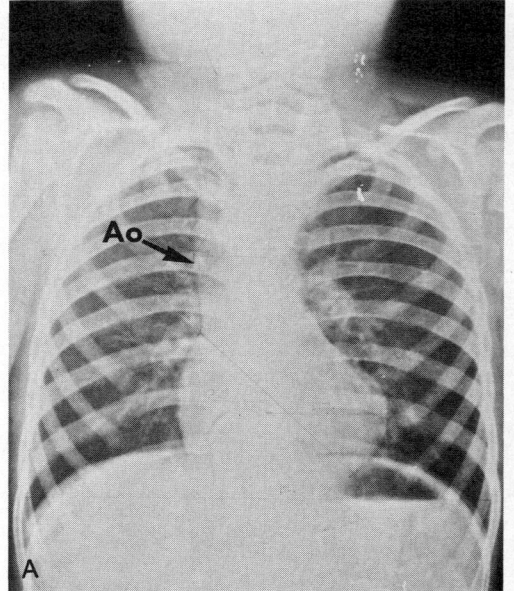

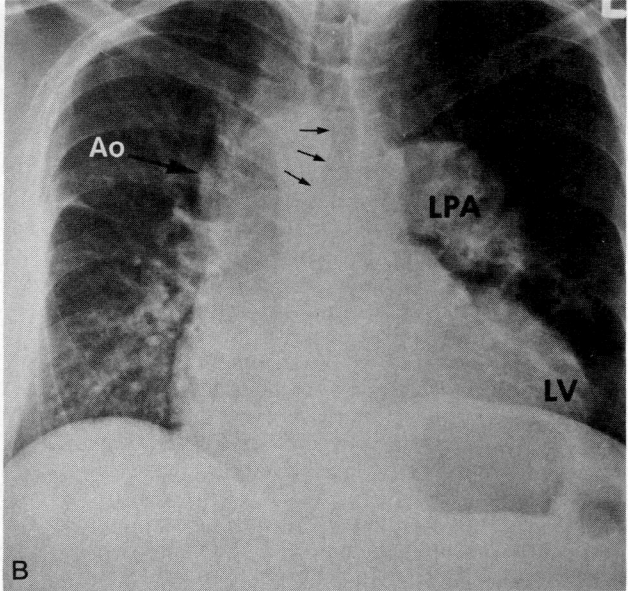

FIGURE 32–14. A, Radiograph before a left Blalock-Taussig shunt in a 4-year-old boy with cyanotic Fallot's tetralogy and a right aortic arch (Ao). B, Same patient at age 50 years. Pulmonary vascularity is increased. The left pulmonary artery (LPA) is aneurysmal. The large right ascending aorta (Ao) indents the trachea (small arrows), and an enlarged left ventricle (LV) occupies the apex. The patient underwent intracardiac repair with revision of the shunt.

vascular resistance and the effects of chronic left ventricular volume overload (Fig. 32–5).[122]

COARCTATION OF THE AORTA. After surgical repair, residual, sequelae, and complications are frequent and require indefinite follow-up.[123–127] There are three principal concerns: residual systolic hypertension despite absence of coarctation gradients, a bicuspid aortic valve, and recoarctation. The major predisposing factor for hypertension after coarctation repair is the duration of preoperative hypertension that results in baroreceptor abnormalities and changes in compliance of the walls of the major arteries.[124,128] The natural history of a coexisting functionally normal bicuspid aortic valve after coarctation repair is the same as that of an isolated congenitally bicuspid aortic valve, including the risk of infective endocarditis. Recurrence of coarctation after reparative surgery is related to the technique used for the initial operation.[129] After infancy, end-to-end anastomosis has the lowest incidence of recoarctation. Complications of premature coronary atherosclerosis, including myocardial infarction and congestive heart failure, were major causes of death in 12 per cent of patients 11 to 25 years after coarctectomy.[123] Cerebrovascular accidents owing to rupture of an aneurysm of the circle of Willis have been reported in normotensive patients long after successful coarctation repair.[126] Abnormalities of the mitral apparatus occur in 26 to 58 per cent of patients with coarctation of the aorta and vary from clinically occult and functionally benign to grossly overt stenosis or incompetence of the orifice.[130]

CONGENITAL SINUS OF VALSALVA ANEURYSMS. These typically rupture well after puberty but before age 30 years (see earlier discussion).[13] Surgical mortality is low, and when aortic regurgitation is not present preoperatively, late results of repair are excellent.

Caval to Pulmonary Arterial Circulations

THE FONTAN PROCEDURE[131] (see p. 954). This operation has undergone a number of modifications, the most recent of which is total caval–to–pulmonary arterial connection.[132] The Fontan and modified Fontan procedures are applied chiefly to tricuspid atresia or single ventricle with pulmonary stenosis but now include physiologically analogous complex cyanotic malformations in which biventricular repair is not feasible because of an underdeveloped ventricle. Late results depend principally on ventricular function and on maintenance of sinus rhythm.[133] Atrial fibrillation or flutter adversely elevates mean right atrial pressure chiefly because of the effect of the atrial arrhythmia on left ventricular filling pressure, a rise that results in an increase in right atrial and caval mean pressures. Ventricular function is better in the presence of a morphological *left* ventricle, as in tricuspid atresia or univentricular hearts of the left ventricular type.[134] Long-term function is, as a rule, not as good when a Fontan procedure is performed on patients with univentricular hearts of the *right* ventricular type.[134] Patients who are carefully selected for operation have fared well and often are New York Heart Association functional class I or II as late as 15 years after surgery. Operation in patients 18 years or older also has been successful, sometimes achieving remarkable degrees of rehabilitation. Ninety-three per cent of these adult patients are in New York Heart Association functional class I or II.[135–137]

MEDICAL MANAGEMENT OF CONGENITAL HEART DISEASE IN THE ADULT

CYANOTIC CONGENITAL HEART DISEASE: HEMATOLOGICAL MANAGEMENT, RENAL FUNCTION, AND URATE METABOLISM

In response to tissue hypoxia, erythropoietin is produced by specialized sensor cells in the kidneys, resulting in an increase in the number of circulating red blood cells and in an expanded blood volume.[138,139] If an increase in erythrocyte mass

is sufficient to raise the tissue oxygen concentration above the threshold for release of erythropoietin by the renal oxygen sensors, a new equilibrium is established at a higher hematocrit. However, erythrocytosis may exceed the range at which blood viscosity becomes a limiting factor in tissue oxygen delivery. An equilibrium is not achieved, and increased erythropoietin secretion and expansion of the erythrocyte mass proceed despite the detrimental effects of the further increase in hematocrit.[140] Iron deficiency significantly affects blood viscosity and shortens erythrocyte survival time.[141,142] Iron-deficient microcytic red cells are relatively rigid and resist deformation at high shear rates and in the microcirculation; accordingly, whole blood viscosity is increased. Phlebotomy-induced iron deficiency results in microcytosis, which leads to a reduction in the oxygen-carrying capacity of the erythrocytes and to an increase in viscosity that may offset potential benefits of hematocrit reduction. The erythrocytosis of cyanotic congenital heart disease is fundamentally different from polycythemia vera (primary polycythemia, p. 1749), an idiopathic clonal disorder of the bone marrow that results in an autonomous overproduction of red cells and is accompanied by thrombocytosis, leukocytosis, and basophilia.

Cyanotic patients with erythrocytosis fall into two categories: compensated and decompensated.[140,143] Those with *compensated* erythrocytosis establish equilibrium hematocrits in an iron replete state. Symptoms attributable to hyperviscosity usually are mild or absent when hematocrit levels are less than 65 per cent, and absent, mild, or moderate even at higher hematocrit levels, occasionally 70 per cent or more. Phlebotomy for relief of hyperviscosity symptoms is required rarely, if at all. Patients with *decompensated* erythrocytosis fail to establish equilibrium conditions and manifest unstable, rising hematocrit levels and recurrent, moderate to severe symptoms attributable to hyperviscosity. Erythrocyte production is not controlled, and negative feedback inhibition does not occur. Symptomatic hyperviscosity is common, prompting therapeutic phlebotomy that depletes iron stores. The pathophysiological mechanisms responsible for symptoms in patients with decompensated erythrocytosis are complex but are believed to be related to tissue hypoxia, iron deficiency, and hyperviscosity.

The risk of *cerebrovascular accidents* (stroke) in patients with cyanotic congenital heart disease is greatest in children younger than age 4 years with iron deficiency.[143,144] Dehydration is an important aggravating cause in these young patients in whom the cerebrovascular accidents are due to thromboses of intracranial veins and sinuses. By contrast, adults with cyanotic congenital heart disease do not appear to be at increased risk of stroke, even if the hematocrit level is above 65 per cent and the erythrocytosis is decompensated (iron deficient).[140,143] Cerebrovascular accidents in cyanotic adults usually are associated with excessive, injudicious phlebotomies or with use of aspirin or anticoagulants that reinforce the intrinsic hemostatic defects (see later) and cause intracranial bleeding.[143]

Phlebotomy is not recommended for adult patients with compensated erythrocytosis, including those with hematocrit levels in the range of 70 per cent, as long as symptoms attributed to hyperviscosity are mild or absent. Phlebotomy is recommended in patients with significant hyperviscosity symptoms and with hematocrit levels of 65 per cent or greater, provided dehydration is not the cause. Dehydration is treated by volume replacement, not phlebotomy. A comparatively simple, safe outpatient method for phlebotomy in adults involves the removal of 500 ml of blood over 30 to 45 minutes while quantitative volume replacement with isotonic saline or salt-free dextran is carried out.

Symptoms of iron deficiency usually are indistinguishable from those of hyperviscosity, but in adults with cyanotic heart disease, symptomatic hyperviscosity in an *iron replete state* seldom occurs with hematocrit levels of less than 65 per cent.[143] Symptoms in patients with hematocrit levels lower than 65 per cent are almost always due to iron deficiency, so phlebotomy aggravates rather than alleviates the symptoms.

Cyanotic congenital heart disease patients, especially those with decompensated erythrocytosis, should be cautioned to avoid over-the-counter preparations that contain iron. When iron is administered therapeutically in symptomatic iron-deficient patients with inappropriately low hematocrit levels, the dose should be small (325 mg of ferrous sulfate per day). Hematocrit levels rise quickly, so erythrocyte response should be closely monitored. Significant erythrocytosis can lead to inaccuracies in laboratory determinations. Hematocrits must be based on automated blood counts because microhematocrit centrifugation methods result in plasma trapping and falsely elevated hematocrit levels.[143]

Home oxygen therapy is sometimes advised, especially during sleep.[145] From both the hematological and respiratory points of view, there is little evidence that home oxygen is useful in adults with cyanotic congenital heart disease, and the drying effect on nasal mucous membranes tends to increase the risk of epistaxes.

HEMOSTASIS (see also p. 1767). Coagulation is abnormal in cyanotic congenital heart disease.[143,146–149] For the most part, bleeding tendencies are mild and characterized by easy bruising, petechial hemorrhages in the skin and mucous membranes, epistaxes, gingival bleeding, and hemoptysis.[143] Platelet counts usually are in the low range of normal, but when the increased blood volume is taken into account, the total circulating platelet mass is closer to normal than platelet concentrations indicate. Inherent abnormalities in platelet function[150] are reinforced by aspirin and other nonsteroidal antiinflammatory agents. Aspirin, oral anticoagulants, and heparin are ill-advised because the inherent risk of stroke is low and because these drugs have no demonstrated efficacy in reducing that negligible risk and instead may significantly aggravate the existing hemostatic defects and increase the risk of bleeding. Abnormalities of the intrinsic and extrinsic coagulation systems, with elevations of the prothrombin time and activated partial thromboplastin time, respectively, and specific deficiencies of several coagulation factors have been reported.[146] Failure to adjust the citrate concentration for the hematocrit level during blood collection may lead to spurious test results for the prothrombin time and activated partial thromboplastin time.

Serious bleeding may occur during surgery or accidental trauma.[151] Phlebotomy has been shown to temporarily improve hemostasis in some erythrocytotic patients, so preoperative phlebotomy is selectively used to reduce the hematocrit level to just below 65 per cent. The activated partial thromboplastin time is a useful estimate of the overall response of the intrinsic coagulation system to preoperative phlebotomy. Phlebotomized units are reserved for potential autologous transfusions.

RENAL FUNCTION AND URATE METABOLISM. These variables often are abnormal in adults with cyanotic congenital heart disease and erythrocytosis.[152,153] High plasma uric acid levels are secondary to inappropriately low fractional uric acid excretion by the kidney rather than to urate overproduction.[152] Enhanced urate reabsorption is believed to result from renal hypoperfusion reinforced by a high filtration fraction. Accordingly, hyperuricemia serves as a marker of abnormal intrauterine hemodynamics.[153] Renal histopathology is characterized by enlarged, hypercellular glomeruli, basement membrane thickening, focal interstitial fibrosis, tubular atrophy, and hyalinization of afferent and efferent arterioles.[154]

Arthralgias are relatively common in erythrocytotic adults with cyanotic congenital heart disease, but acute gouty arthritis is relatively uncommon, despite elevated uric acid levels, an observation similar to that in other forms of secondary hyperuricemia.[155] If colchicine is used to treat acute gouty arthritis, special care must be taken to avoid the dehydrating effects of vomiting and diarrhea. Nonsteroidal antiinflammatory agents may then be considered but should be used cautiously in patients with potential hemostatic defects. Whereas uricosuric agents are not routinely advised, they can be effica-

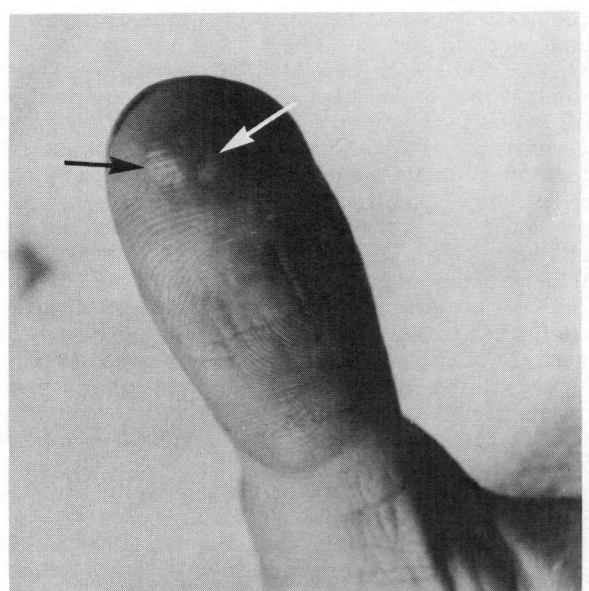

FIGURE 32–15. Urate deposit (arrows) on the pad of the thumb of a 24-year-old man with complex cyanotic congenital heart disease.

cious in patients with hyperuricemia and recurrences of gouty arthritis. Intraarticular steroid injections are sometimes required. Overt tophaceous deposits of urate are exceptional, even in patients with considerable chronic hyperuricemia (Fig. 32–15).[152]

CYANOTIC CONGENITAL HEART DISEASE: DYNAMICS OF OXYGEN UPTAKE AND CONTROL OF VENTILATION

Diversion of systemic venous blood from the pulmonary circulation into the systemic arterial circulation is a basic pathological fault in patients with cyanotic congenital heart disease. Exercise tends to increase significantly the degree of venoarterial shunting and materially influences the dynamics of oxygen uptake (VO_2) and ventilation. Patients with cyanotic congenital heart disease have markedly abnormal responses in achieving a new steady state for VO_2 after the onset of exercise.[156] The prolonged onset and recovery VO_2 kinetics result in large oxygen deficits and hypoxemia, even with low levels of exercise, and suggest that patients with significant right-to-left shunts may rely on an unusual degree of anaerobic metabolism to perform exercise. Patients with right-to-left

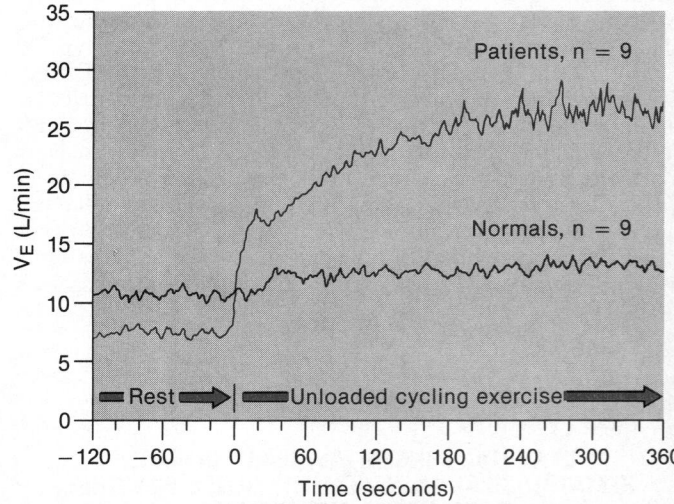

FIGURE 32–16. The increase in ventilation in response to unloaded cycle ergometric exercise in nine adults with right-to-left shunts, and in nine normal subjects. The patients had higher minute ventilation both at rest and in response to exercise. (From Sietsema, K. E., et al.: Control of ventilation during exercise in patients with central venous to systemic arterial shunts. J. Appl. Physiol. 64:234, 1988.)

shunts also have greater increases in ventilation during exercise than do normal subjects; dyspnea on exertion may be a prominent clinical complaint.[157] Unlike the prolonged kinetics of VO_2, cyanotic patients exhibit large increases in ventilation in phase I, and in contrast to normal subjects, ventilation increases more rapidly than VO_2 in phase II (Fig. 32–16).[157] Ventilatory stimuli that are potentially augmented by exercise in patients with right-to-left shunts include hypoxemia, metabolic acidosis, and shunting of carbon dioxide into the systemic arterial circulation.

INFECTIVE ENDOCARDITIS: RISKS AND PROPHYLAXIS

(See also Chap. 35)

With the advent of intracardiac surgery and of prosthetic devices, the clinical and bacteriological profile of infective endocarditis changed significantly.[1,158] Certain operations (ligation of a patent ductus arteriosus) eliminate the risk, whereas others (shunts, prosthetic valves, or conduits) materially increase the risk. However, certain general principles still prevail, namely, that there are two major predisposing causes of infective endocarditis: a susceptible cardiac or vascular substrate, and the presence of bacteremia. Susceptible lesions include those associated with high-velocity flow, jet impact, and focal increases in the rate of shear. Portals of entry include the oral cavity, the genitourinary tract in males, the upper and lower gastrointestinal tract, the airways and respiratory tract, obstetrical and gynecological procedures, and certain types of noncardiac surgery. Prophylaxis for infective endocarditis comprises nonchemotherapeutic and chemotherapeutic (antimicrobial) measures.

The risk of infective endocarditis in congenital heart disease has been classified as low-risk unoperated anomalies, low- or no-risk postoperative, intermediate-risk unoperated, intermediate-risk postoperative, and high-risk postoperative.[1] Examples of low-risk unoperated anomalies include ostium secundum atrial septal defect and mild pulmonary valve stenosis. A no-risk postoperative lesion is typified by division of a patent ductus arteriosus. Intermediate-risk unoperated lesions are represented by functionally normal bicuspid aortic valve, aortic regurgitation, restrictive ventricular septal defect, or patent ductus arteriosus. Intermediate-risk postoperative lesions are represented by bicuspid aortic stenosis, and residual left atrioventricular valve or aortic regurgitation. High-risk postoperative substrates include rigid prosthetic valves, especially left-sided, external valved conduits, and aortopulmonary shunts.

Chemotherapeutic prophylaxis is based on the cardiac lesion, the source of potential bacteremia, and the absence or presence of a history of antibiotic sensitivity. The American Heart Association recommendations (p. 1098) have been incorporated into convenient wallet-sized instructions that can be given to patients and referring physicians.

Nonchemotherapeutic prophylaxis includes day-to-day oral hygiene, skin care, nail care, and avoidance of certain female contraceptive devices.[1] The spongy, fragile gums of some patients with cyanotic congenital heart disease are of special concern, necessitating twice-yearly teeth and gum prophylaxis. Meticulous skin care is important, especially in adolescents and young adults with acne, which may be distributed beyond the face. Biting or picking of fingernails risks injury to contiguous skin and predisposes to paronychial infection with staphylococci. Intrauterine devices are best avoided because of the risk of bacteremia.

PREGNANCY AND CONGENITAL HEART DISEASE

(See p. 1793)

Central to this topic is the interplay between maternal circulatory and respiratory physiology and maternal congenital heart disease, and the effects of this interplay on the fetus, which is exposed to immediate risks that threaten its viability and to remote risks that express themselves as developmental defects or transmitted congenital anomalies.

In a practical sense, the most important category of unoperated patients are those with common congenital cardiac anomalies that are likely to be found in adult women.

OSTIUM SECUNDUM ATRIAL SEPTAL DEFECT (see also p. 1794). Because the natural history of this defect spans the reproductive years, and because the majority of affected patients are female, the malformation is of special importance. Young women with uncomplicated ostium secundum atrial septal defects usually tolerate pregnancy — even multiple pregnancies — with no tangible ill effects (Fig. 32–4). After the fourth decade, however, patients with otherwise uncomplicated secundum defects experience an increased incidence of supraventricular arrhythmia that may cause right ventricular failure and peripheral edema and, accordingly, serve to increase the probability of venous stasis and thrombophlebitis.

An important concern is the risk of paradoxical embolization from leg veins because emboli tend to course from the inferior vena cava through the atrial septal defect into the systemic circulation.[13,160,161] Meticulous leg care is advised to minimize venous stasis. Also important but less well known are potentially hazardous effects of acute blood loss in patients with unoperated ostium secundum atrial septal defects.[1] Hemorrhage during delivery results in a rise in systemic vascular resistance and a fall in systemic venous return, a combination that augments the left-to-right shunt, sometimes appreciably. Pulmonary hypertension is uncommon in young women with ostium secundum atrial septal defects, but its presence, even in the absence of a reversed shunt, increases the risk of pregnancy.

PATENT DUCTUS ARTERIOSUS (see also p. 1794). This anomaly occurs predominantly in females but is becoming less important as a complication of pregnancy because the clinical diagnosis is simple and surgical or bioprosthetic closure is routine and curative in childhood (see earlier). Asymptomatic young women with a small or moderate-sized ductus and normal pulmonary arterial pressure can anticipate an uncomplicated pregnancy, apart from the risk of infective endocarditis during delivery. One of the author's patients, a 57-year-old woman with a moderately restrictive patent ductus, endured 20 pregnancies with 12 live births (Fig. 32–17). The gestational fall in systemic vascular resistance tends to decrease ductal flow, but if the shunt is large, that benefit is not likely to compensate for the hemodynamic burden of pregnancy. At highest risk is the patient with a nonrestrictive patent ductus and a reversed shunt. The hazard of pulmonary vascular disease is again underscored, and the low oxygen saturation in the descending aorta puts the fetus at risk.

ISOLATED PULMONARY VALVE STENOSIS (see also p. 1795). Fifty per cent of patients are female[13]; survival to adulthood is usual, even if there is significant obstruction to right ventricular outflow. Mild to moderate pulmonary stenosis poses little or no threat to the mother, and occasionally even severe pulmonary stenosis is well tolerated despite the gestational volume overload imposed on an already pressure-overloaded

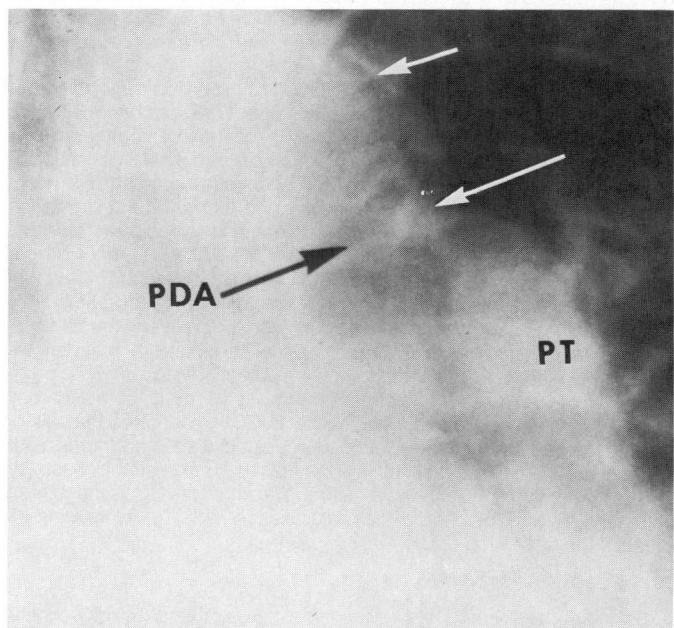

FIGURE 32–17. Chest radiograph (closeup) from a 57-year-old woman with a calcified patent ductus arteriosus (PDA, paired arrows) that was moderately restrictive. She had had 20 pregnancies with 12 live births. The pulmonary trunk (PT) is dilated. The aorta (Ao) also contains calcium (unmarked large white arrow).

right ventricle. Infective endocarditis prophylaxis is called for during delivery, although the risk in patients with mild pulmonary stenosis is negligible, if not absent.

COARCTATION OF THE AORTA

COARCTATION OF THE AORTA (see also p. 1794). This lesion occurs chiefly in males but is dealt with here because maternal morbidity is high.[13] Pregnancy increases the risk of aortic rupture or dissection and of cerebral hemorrhage from rupture of an aneurysm of the circle of Willis.[13,160] Blood pressure variations of pregnant women with aortic coarctation are similar in direction but occur from a higher initial level than in normal pregnancy. The incidence of toxemia is much less with the hypertension of coarctation than in pregnant women with other forms of hypertension. Left ventricular failure is exceptional despite the increased gestational blood volume that is added to the pressure-overloaded left ventricle. The risk of infective endocarditis is significantly higher on a coexisting bicuspid aortic valve than at the site of coarctation (see earlier).

BICUSPID AORTIC VALVE. An isolated functionally normal bicuspid aortic valve is likely to go unrecognized in young women. The clinical index of suspicion is low because the malformation occurs predominantly in males and the auscultatory signs are subtle. Because of the high susceptibility of the bicuspid aortic valve to infective endocarditis, the anomaly may become evident after delivery because of fever or the development of acute severe aortic regurgitation.[16]

CHRONIC BICUSPID AORTIC REGURGITATION. When moderate or even severe, this lesion usually is well tolerated during pregnancy, provided that the adaptive response of the left ventricle permits normal function, which normally is the case. The gestational fall in systemic vascular resistance coupled with a more rapid heart rate (shorter diastole) results in a decrease in regurgitant flow. The risk of infective endocarditis is high, and prophylaxis is required during delivery.

In the occasional young woman with congenital *bicuspid aortic stenosis,* the increased cardiac output of pregnancy is imposed on a pressure-overloaded left ventricle. Most asymptomatic women entering pregnancy with mild-to-moderate aortic stenosis do well, but if obstruction is marked to severe, circulatory reserve is limited. Dyspnea, angina pectoris, or cerebral symptoms that precede conception or that appear during early gestation predict serious sequelae. The stenotic valve is at risk of infective endocarditis.

FALLOT'S TETRALOGY (see also p. 1795). This is the most common cyanotic malformation that permits natural survival to reproductive age, and the sex distribution is nearly equal.[13] A paucity of symptoms and the presence of mild cyanosis before conception do not assure a smooth course. The gestational fall in systemic vascular resistance, coupled with the augmented cardiac output and increased venous return to an obstructed right ventricle, results in an augmentation of the right-to-left shunt and a fall in systemic arterial oxygen saturation. Cyanosis deepens, but the hematocrit level may rise less than anticipated because of the gestational increase in plasma volume. Labile hemodynamics during labor, delivery, and the puerperium incurs additional risks.[160] A sudden fall in systemic resistance may precipitate intense cyanosis, syncope, and death. Conversely, bearing down during labor may abruptly and dangerously reduce systemic blood flow. Infective endocarditis during delivery is an additional concern.

CONGENITAL COMPLETE HEART BLOCK. This uncommon disorder permits survival into childbearing age, and about one-half of patients are female. Asymptomatic young women with congenital complete heart block usually experience uneventful pregnancies, provided the duration of the QRS complex is not prolonged.[162-164] Stokes-Adams attacks occasionally occur during gestation, however, and the heart and circulation may not respond adequately to the volatile demands of labor and delivery.

EBSTEIN'S ANOMALY OF THE TRICUSPID VALVE. About 50 per cent of patients are female, and the majority reach adulthood.[13] The functionally inadequate right ventricle, already volume-overloaded by tricuspid regurgitation, copes poorly with the gestational increase in cardiac output.[165] Paroxysmal atrial arrhythmias occur in about one-third of nongravid patients with Ebstein's anomaly and are potential hazards during pregnancy. Wolff-Parkinson-White bypass tracts set the stage for excessively rapid ventricular rates in response to atrial fibrillation or flutter; the consequences can be catastrophic. Cyanosis in Ebstein's anomaly (right-to-left shunt at atrial level) may first become manifest during pregnancy because of a rise in right ventricular filling pressure. The right-to-left interatrial shunt increases the risk of paradoxical embolization, and the hypoxemia increases the risk to the fetus.

THE POSTOPERATIVE PATIENT

The postoperative woman with congenital heart disease now constitutes one of the most important categories of pregnancy and heart disease and represents a growing patient population. A prime objective of reparative surgery is to increase the safety and success of pregnancy and to preserve the subsequent health of mother and child. Operations should, therefore, be anticipatory. With few exceptions, cardiac surgery or interventional catheterization is not curative; the risk of pregnancy to the

mother is then determined chiefly by the presence, type, and degree of cardiac and vascular residua and sequelae. There is a consensus, however, that successful operation before gestation can be pivotal in reducing maternal risk. Operation has no bearing on genetic transmission of maternal congenital heart disease.

An asymptomatic woman of childbearing age who has undergone closure of an *ostium secundum atrial septal defect* as a child or young adult can anticipate pregnancy devoid of maternal risk.[160] Successful closure of the defect also eliminates the risk of paradoxical embolization. There are few or no significant postoperative residua or sequelae except for occasional atrial tachyarrhythmias years after successful repair. When a small *patent ductus arteriosus* has been closed in childhood, pregnancy is tolerated normally. More circumspect is the response to gestation after closure of a moderately restrictive or nonrestrictive ductus. Postoperative pulmonary vascular disease and depressed left ventricular function are important residua, depending on the degree. In any case, there is no risk of endocarditis. When surgical repair or balloon dilatation of *congenital pulmonary valve stenosis* leaves behind little or no gradient, the mother can anticipate a normal pregnancy except for a low, if not absent, risk of infective endocarditis. Mild-to-moderate low-pressure pulmonary regurgitation is not an important sequel.

Complete relief of *coarctation of the aorta,* especially in early childhood, materially increases the probability of long-term normalization of blood pressure and decreases the risk of gestational aortic dissection or rupture by removing the zone of aortic cystic medial necrosis.[166] Balloon dilatation of native (unoperated) coarctation may significantly reduce the intraaortic pressure gradient, but the risk of aortic rupture or dissection during pregnancy can be no less (and may be greater) than in mild native coarctation. Susceptibility to infective endocarditis at the site of successful coarctation repair is, for all practical purposes, absent, but the risk of infection on a coexisting bicuspid aortic valve is unaffected. To what extent successful correction of aortic coarctation diminishes the hazard of gestational rupture of an aneurysm of the circle of Willis is open to question, but the incidence of death resulting from intracranial hemorrhage is reassuringly low.[167]

In congenital *aortic valve stenosis,* surgical relief of gradients of 50 mm Hg or more appreciably lowers the risk of pregnancy except for susceptibility to infective endocarditis. Risk during pregnancy is lowest when postoperative left ventricular function is normal or nearly so. Aortic valve replacement should be avoided, especially with a rigid prosthesis that requires anticoagulants.

A woman with moderate to marked *aortic regurgitation* who wants to become pregnant is best advised to do so before aortic valve replacement. If a prosthetic valve is required in a female of reproductive age, there are persuasive arguments for the use of a tissue valve (no need for anticoagulants, with their adverse effects during pregnancy, p. 1797).

Pregnancy after successful intracardiac repair of *Fallot's tetralogy* is accompanied by justifiable optimism, especially in women with little or no outflow gradient and no more than mild postoperative low-pressure pulmonary regurgitation. Surgical relief of cyanosis increases the likelihood of successful conception and substantially improves the stability of the pregnancy and the prospect of normal growth and development of the fetus. However, electrophysiological sequelae of intracardiac repair—bifascicular block, high-degree heart block, or right ventricular electrical instability (Figs. 32–13 and 32–18)—cannot be ignored.

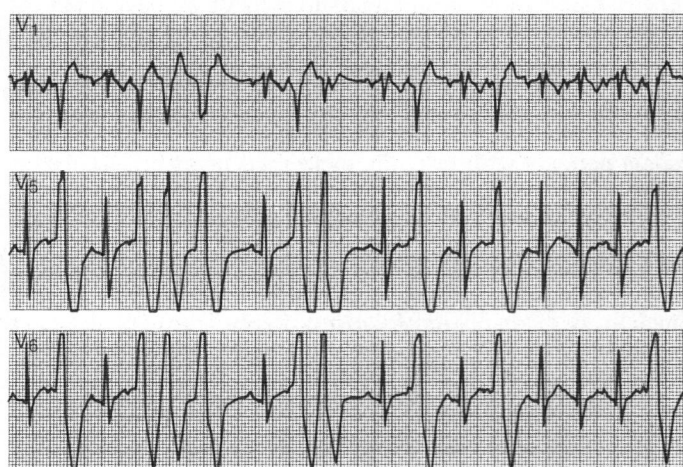

FIGURE 32–18. Rhythm response to isotonic exercise in a 41-year-old patient 5 years after intracardiac repair of Fallot's tetralogy. There are short runs of nonsustained ventricular tachycardia (From James, F. W., et al.: Response to exercise in patients after total correction of tetralogy of Fallot. *Circulation 54:*671, 1976.)

Congenital complete heart block in young women occasionally requires insertion of a pacemaker, but even so, relative confidence that pregnancy can proceed is justified. If ventricular function is normal, which usually is the case, an artificial fixed-rate pacemaker appears to provide satisfactory physiological support.

Surgical repair of *Ebstein's anomaly of the tricuspid valve* ideally takes the form of reconstruction into a relatively competent unicuspid atrioventricular valve. Dissociation of right atrium from right ventricle eliminates active or potential bypass tracts (Fig. 32–10). The risk of pregnancy to the mother, including susceptibility to infective endocarditis, is then appreciably reduced but not eliminated.

Pregnancy after repair of certain forms of *complex cyanotic congenital heart disease* is now a practical objective. After a Fontan operation for single ventricle or tricuspid atresia with pulmonary stenosis, patients can achieve a two-fold increment in cardiac index in response to isotonic exercise.[135] The implication is that women who have undergone successful Fontan repairs and have normal systemic ventricular function confront the physiological burden of pregnancy with circulations that potentially possess adequate hemodynamic reserve.[133]

MEDICAL MANAGEMENT OF THE PREGNANT WOMAN

The expectant mother's cardiac reserve is reduced by the hemodynamic burden of pregnancy, but the reduction can almost always be countered by addressing the factors that encroach on circulatory reserve. There is little or no convincing evidence that oxygen administration benefits cyanotic pregnant women.

Maternal mortality usually varies directly with functional class, but in the presence of certain congenital cardiac malformations, childbearing imposes such a formidable threat to maternal survival that pregnancy is proscribed or should be interrupted irrespective of functional class. The cardiac symptoms on which the New York Heart Association functional classes were originally based are more relevant to acquired than to congenital heart disease. In cyanotic patients, for example, what is subjectively reported as effort dyspnea is less likely to result from heart failure than from stimulation of the respiratory center by the changes in blood gas composition and pH in response to the increased right-to-left shunt induced by exercise. Effort fatigue may be due to the effect of iron deficiency on exercise performance (see p. 1791).

The two major maternal cardiac risks are pulmonary vascular disease and pulmonary edema. Pulmonary vascular disease limits or precludes appropriate adaptive responses to the circulatory changes of pregnancy and to the volatile changes during labor, delivery, and the puerperium. Primary pulmonary hypertension epitomizes this risk, and Eisenmenger's complex combines the maternal risk of pulmonary vascular disease with the fetal risk of cyanosis. A sudden fall in systemic vascular resistance in Eisenmenger's complex may precipitate intense cyanosis, and a sudden rise in systemic resistance associated with bearing down during labor may abruptly depress cardiac output and provoke fatal syncope. Pulmonary edema (p. 551) is less common in congenital heart disease than in acquired heart disease, but the functional adequacy of the ventricle that serves the systemic circulation—before or after operation—is central to this concern.

In women with functionally mild unoperated lesions and in patients after successful intracardiac repairs, management of labor and delivery is essentially the same as for normal women except for the selective risk of infective endocarditis (see Chap. 35). In high-risk patients, a flotation catheter offers the security of meticulous hemodynamic surveillance during labor and delivery and in the immediate postpartum period, but individual judgments are required. In Eisenmenger's complex, for example, the risks involved with use of a Swan-Ganz catheter outweigh the benefits.[168] Oxygen often is administered during labor, especially in cyanotic women, although the efficacy of so doing is unproved.

After expulsion of the placenta, bleeding can be reduced by uterine massage or intravenous oxytocin. Blood loss should be minimized, especially in patients with pulmonary vascular disease or Fallot's tetralogy. The risk of sudden hemorrhage in women with ostium secundum atrial septal defect was pointed out earlier.

The probability of thromboembolism increases during the postpartum period, and patients with lesions susceptible to paradoxical embolization are at particular risk (see earlier). Meticulous leg care, use of elastic support stockings, and early ambulation are important preventive measures.

Prophylaxis for infective endocarditis during labor and delivery is dealt with in Chapter 35.

MEDICAL MANAGEMENT OF THE FETUS

Maternal congenital heart disease exposes the fetus to immediate risks that threaten its intrauterine viability and to remote risks that are evidenced as congenital and developmental malformations. Immediate risks are determined chiefly by the functional class of the mother, maternal cyanosis, and anticoagulants. Extracorporeal circulation is associated with a high incidence of fetal wastage, but cardiac surgery seldom is required during pregnancy, especially in patients with congenital heart disease. The hypertension of coarctation of the aorta does not threaten the fetus as do other hypertensive disorders. Remote risks to the fetus take the form of genetic parental transmission, teratogenic effects of certain cardiac drugs, and the harmful effects of certain environmental toxins and environmental exposures.

Maternal cyanosis threatens the growth, development, and viability of the fetus, and materially increases fetal wastage.[160,169] Infants born to cyanotic mothers are typically dysmature (small for gestational age) or premature (gestation less than 37 weeks). There is little or no evidence that maternal oxygen administration favorably affects the growth-retarded fetus, despite the fact that high levels of inspired oxygen may raise arterial saturation even in the presence of a right-to-left shunt. The rate of spontaneous abortion is high and increases approximately in parallel to the mother's hypoxemia. Even when cyanosis is initially mild, the risk of fetal wastage is not low because a right-to-left shunt often increases during the course of pregnancy in response to the anticipated fall in systemic vascular resistance. Surgical correction of congenital heart disease eliminates cyanosis and improves maternal functional class, underscoring the desirability of anticipatory operative intervention.

The use of *anticoagulants* involves risks to the fetus that cannot be satisfactorily resolved. An attempt should be made to minimize the need for anticoagulants, and their use should be judicious. There is no consensus regarding the best method for administering anticoagulants to pregnant women. The options are discussed on pages 1805 and 1806.

GENETICS, EPIDEMIOLOGY, COUNSELING, AND PREVENTION

(See also Chap. 51)

There is substantial evidence that the presence of a congenital heart lesion in a first-degree relative is a risk factor to the fetus, even in the absence of a known genetic disorder.[170] There also is evidence that *maternal* congenital heart disease

TABLE 32–1 CHARACTERISTICS OF CYTOPLASMIC INHERITANCE

INHERITANCE OF MITOCHONDRIAL GENOMES			
Parental genotypes	Maternal Cc	Paternal × CC	Maternal CC Paternal × Cc
Offspring genotypes	Cc		CC

CC = normal mitochondrial genomes
Cc = some normal, some mutated mitochondrial genomes

CHARACTERISTICS OF INHERITANCE

Many mitochondrial gene copies are inherited. Inheritance is through the maternal lineage only. Offspring show variable phenotypes due to ratio of C:c mitochondrial DNAs caused by random segregation. Affected phenotypes are not manifested until a certain proportion of mutated mitochondrial DNAs is reached—a threshold effect.

is a greater fetal risk than congenital heart disease in other relatives, including the father. Possible reasons for this maternal effect include nonmendelian inheritance (cytoplasmic transmission [Table 32–1] and parental imprinting) and an effect of the maternal environment on the developing embryo.[170] If the mother has congenital heart disease, the recurrence risk in her offspring is 6.7 per cent (range 2.5 to 18 per cent), but if the father is affected, the risk is only 2.1 per cent (range 1.5 to 3 per cent). Potential parents with congenital heart disease — male or female — should be provided with genetic counseling regarding the recurrence risk in offspring.

Potential teratogenic or developmental fetal injury associated with cardiac or noncardiac drugs used during pregnancy is discussed on page 1803. In the first trimester, particularly before the 9th week, the risk of exposure is teratogenicity. In the second and third trimesters, the risks are represented by adverse effects on fetal growth and development, especially the central nervous system, which continues to develop throughout gestation.

In brief, congenital cardiovascular malformations cannot, as a rule, be assigned to specific antecedent causes, although malformations can result from heredity, from environmental exposures that require little or no apparent genetic predisposition, or from genetic-environmental interactions. Many cases of inherited malformations remain unexplained by classical genetics. Recent work has focused on cytoplasmic inheritance or parental imprinting to explain the observed risks.

EXERCISE AND ATHLETICS BEFORE AND AFTER SURGERY OR INTERVENTIONAL CATHETERIZATION

Patients with certain types of congenital disorders of the heart or circulation are at greater risk of complications or sudden death if they expose themselves to the stress of strenuous exercise or competitive sports.[171] Apart from the somewhat arbitrary distinction between competitive and recreational athletics, a number of other points are relevant. Consideration must be given to (1) the type, intensity, and duration of exercise; (2) the risk of body collision inherent in a given type of athletic activity, especially in patients receiving anticoagulants; (3) the training program (conditioning) required for a given sport; (4) the emotional response (stress) that the athlete experiences in anticipation of or during a particular sport event; and (5) the risk of injury either to the athlete or to spectators if the athletic activity induces loss of consciousness.[172]

Two general types of exercise are recognized: isotonic (dynamic) and isometric (static). *Isotonic exercise* is associated with changes in muscle length and with rhythmic muscle contractions that develop comparatively little force. A steady state can be achieved. *Isometric exercise* results in sudden development of a comparatively large force with little or no change in muscle length; a steady state cannot be achieved, even temporarily. There often is a continuum between the two types, with most physical activity incorporating both isotonic and isometric components. After certain types of reparative surgery, conditioning improves physical performance and permits activities at normal or near-normal levels. However, the risk entailed by conditioning (training) for a specific competitive athletic activity may exceed the risk of the competitive event itself. The heightened emotional response of an athlete before or during a sporting event may trigger a disturbance in cardiac rhythm and a loss of consciousness, putting the athlete, as well as participants and bystanders, at risk of injury. At issue in the following discussion are the type and severity of a given congenital malformation, whether surgery was undertaken and, if so, its type and success.

Sometimes patients with *congenital complete heart block* perform optimally,[13] but prolonged, high-intensity isotonic exercise is ill-advised, and strenuous isometric exercise is unwise, although often tolerated. If a pacemaker is required, patients are allowed isotonic or isometric exercise that falls within the limits of sensible moderation.

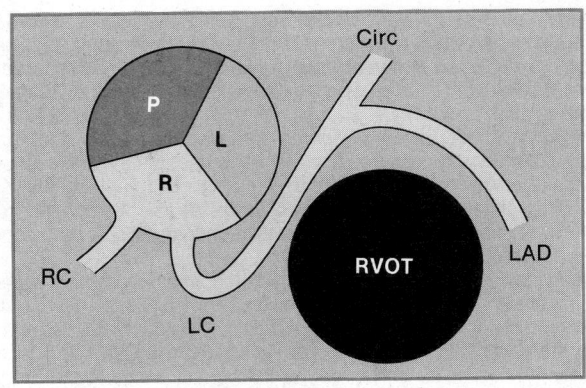

FIGURE 32–19. Illustration of the left coronary artery (LC) arising from a right aortic sinus (R) and coursing between the aorta and the right ventricular outflow tract (RVOT). P = posterior aortic sinus; L = left aortic sinus; RC = right coronary artery; Circ = circumflex coronary artery; and LAD = left anterior descending artery.

An aberrant coronary artery coursing between the aorta and right ventricular outflow tract can cause angina pectoris, myocardial infarction, and sudden death.[173] The risk is greatest when the *left* coronary artery arises from the right aortic sinus and passes between the aorta and the right ventricular outflow tract (Fig. 32–19), especially in males. Most cases of sudden death occur during or immediately after relatively strenuous physical effort. The mechanism is believed to be coronary arterial compression in response to exercise-induced dilatation of the great arteries in the setting of pre-existing acute angulation of the proximal course of the aberrant coronary, causing intrinsic narrowing of its lumen.[174,175] If the anomaly is identified and surgically corrected, subsequent athletic activity need not be restricted, provided that coronary flow is unobstructed and myocardial ischemia absent.

In *coarctation of the aorta*, the distensibility characteristics of the proximal aorta, the sensitivity or "set" of carotid sinus baroreceptors, and the efferent sympathetic activity play important roles in systemic hypertension (see earlier).[13] The aorta proximal to the coarctation is less distensible than is the postcoarctation aorta, accounting in part for the disproportionate rise in systolic blood pressure in the proximal compartment. The excessive rise in systolic blood pressure during isotonic exercise represents an exaggeration of the disproportionate systolic hypertension in the resting state. After successful repair of coarctation, the excessive rise in exercise-induced systolic hypertension is in large part related to the patient's age at the time of repair. Patients without recoarctation but with postoperative hypertension may experience abnormal increases in blood pressure (especially systolic) during exercise.

Unoperated patients with mild congenital *aortic valve stenosis* (resting gradient of 20 mm Hg or less) are not restricted in athletic activity, provided that the electrocardiogram is normal, the response to exercise stress testing is normal, left ventricular function is normal or supernormal, and there are no significant disturbances in rhythm as measured by 24-hour ambulatory electrocardiography. Patients with *moderate* congenital aortic stenosis (resting gradients higher than 20 but less than 50 mm Hg), especially those at the upper range, are advised to confine their athletics to low-intensity isotonic exercise. Isometric exercise, by increasing the aortic root systolic pressure, may reduce the gradient, but in so doing increases an already elevated left ventricular afterload. In patients with *marked* to *severe* aortic stenosis (peak systolic gradients in excess of 50 mm Hg), high-intensity isotonic or isometric exercise or competitive sports should be avoided.

A legitimate concern in advising exercise limitations in patients with aortic stenosis is the perceived risk of sudden death. The syncope that precedes sudden death is believed to be initiated by left ventricular baroreceptors activated by an exercise-induced increase in left ventricular pressure or stretch, which causes vasodilatation in skeletal muscle followed by systemic hypotension.[176] Malignant ventricular arrhythmias seldom *initiate* syncope but are believed to be the chief cause of death *after* a faint. Syncope-induced hypotension is much more likely to provoke electrical ventricular instability in adults with coexisting coronary artery disease than in younger patients with normal coronary arteries and no myocardial ischemia.

Recommendations based on the criteria above do not necessarily apply to exercise in patients after valvotomy or valvuloplasty for congenital aortic stenosis. Even if the postoperative pressure gradient is 20 mm Hg or less, athletic activity should be limited to low or moderate intensity when left ventricular internal dimensions at end-diastole are increased, when aortic regurgitation is more than mild, when the scalar electrocardiogram shows residual abnormalities of repolarization at rest or with exercise, or when important disturbances in ventricular rhythm are present at rest, with exercise, or on 24-hour ambulatory electrocardiogram. These recommendations are valid even if left ventricular systolic function is within normal range as measured by two-dimensional echocardiography or radionuclide imaging.

Patients with mild *pulmonary valve stenosis* (peak systolic gradient < 25 mm Hg) are allowed unrestricted athletic activity. When obstruction is moderate (gradient between 25 and 50 mm Hg) high-intensity competitive sports may be tolerated but are unwise because right ventricular systolic pressure rises appreciably in response to strenuous isotonic exercise. Most such patients have some degree of electrocardiographic evidence of right ventricular hypertrophy. When the resting peak systolic gradient exceeds 50 mm Hg, especially if there is echocardiographic or radionuclide evidence of impaired right ventricular function, isotonic exercise should be limited to mild intensity and short duration. After successful balloon dilatation or valvotomy, most patients need few restrictions and, as a rule, may participate in high-intensity competitive athletics. If residual obstruction to right ventricular outflow after surgery or balloon valvuloplasty is moderate or greater, athletic activity should be limited to noncompetitive low- to moderate-intensity exercise, especially if right ventricular internal dimensions are increased and systolic function is less than normal.

Most patients with uncomplicated *ostium secundum atrial septal defects* who escape early detection are asymptomatic and usually experience normal tolerance to high-intensity exercise. As long as the pulmonary vascular resistance is normal (which usually is the case), these young adults should not be restricted, although elective repair is advisable. When surgery abolishes the shunt in early childhood, long-term outlook is excellent and athletic activity is unrestricted, provided that the pulmonary vascular resistance is normal, the sinus node function and atrioventricular conduction are normal, and the right atrial and the right ventricular volumes are normal or nearly so.

A small *ventricular septal defect* with a functionally normal heart imposes no limitations on physical activity. Such patients can safely participate in competitive sports without restriction, but it is uncommon to find adult patients in this category. An important variation on the theme is the adult who had a moderately restrictive perimembranous ventricular septal defect that decreased in size or closed spontaneously in infancy. There is a consensus that such patients are physiologically normal and should be permitted unrestricted physical activity. Two-dimensional echocardiographic studies with Doppler interrogation and color-flow imaging should be performed to determine whether the defect closed by formation of a "septal aneurysm" and whether a trivial residual shunt persists. Although there is no evidence that strenuous athletic activity risks rupturing a septal aneurysm, it is prudent to be aware of the morphological substrate.

After surgical closure of a moderate to large ventricular septal defect, recommendations regarding levels of physical

activity and competitive sports depend on the postoperative pulmonary arterial pressure; the absence of significant disturbances in ventricular rhythm during maximal exercise stress testing and during 24-hour ambulatory electrocardiography; and two-dimensional echocardiographic evidence of an intact ventricular septum together with normalization of left ventricular and left atrial size and left ventricular function. It also is desirable for the 12-lead scalar electrocardiogram to exhibit little or no evidence of left ventricular volume overload or right ventricular pressure overload. If the aforementioned criteria are met, patients are permitted unrestricted isotonic or isometric exercise. Persistent postoperative elevation of pulmonary arterial pressure, especially if accompanied by exercise-induced right ventricular ectopic rhythms, requires that patients limit physical activity to low intensity and short duration.

A small *patent ductus arteriosus* is of little or no physiological significance, and patients are allowed normal physical activity. Similarly, there are no postoperative restrictions on athletic activity after division of an isolated restrictive patent ductus arteriosus in childhood. Recommendations for patients who have undergone division of a moderately restrictive or nonrestrictive patent ductus with large left-to-right shunt and variable elevations of pulmonary arterial pressure depend on the guidelines set forth earlier for postoperative moderately restrictive to nonrestrictive ventricular septal defect.

Pulmonary vascular disease is an important situation in which strenuous exercise should be avoided. In patients with suprasystemic pulmonary vascular resistance and right-to-left shunts (p. 919), even low levels of isotonic exercise tend to be accompanied by marked decrements in systemic arterial oxygen content and in the development of tissue lactic acidosis. The exercise-induced increase in right-to-left shunt poses a special problem in the elimination of metabolically produced carbon dioxide, resulting in high ventilatory requirements and subjective dyspnea (Fig. 32–16) and, occasionally, in respiratory acidosis. In nonrestrictive patent ductus arteriosus with suprasystemic pulmonary vascular resistance and reversed shunt, certain symptoms are related to selective flow of poorly oxygenated blood to the *lower* extremities (reversed shunt). Exercise may cause leg fatigue but comparatively little dyspnea because the ventilatory stimuli of hypoxemia, hypercapnia, and acidemia circumvent the respiratory center (venous blood is delivered to the lower body but not to the vital centers of the head and neck).[13]

In *Fallot's tetralogy*, isotonic exercise results in a fall in systemic resistance together with augmented venous return to a right ventricle with fixed obstruction to outflow, so the right-to-left shunt is increased. The subjective sensation of breathlessness is caused chiefly by the response of the respiratory center to the sudden change and blood gas composition and pH. The relief of effort-induced dyspnea by squatting, a time-honored hallmark of Fallot's tetralogy in children, is seldom witnessed in adults.[13] Squatting exerts its salutory effect by countering the exercise-induced fall in systemic vascular resistance and by decreasing the amount of low oxygen content inferior vena caval blood that is received by the right ventricle and shunted into the aorta during exercise. High-intensity *isometric* exercise in Fallot's tetralogy abruptly reduces flow from the right ventricle into the aorta in the face of fixed obstruction to right ventricular outflow, so systemic flow suddenly falls, precipitating syncope and, occasionally, sudden death. All but low-intensity isometric exercise is proscribed.

After intracardiac repair of Fallot's tetralogy, recommendations regarding the level of physical activity and participation in athletics depend on the patient's age at operation and the presence and degree of postoperative residua and sequelae.[177,178] Postoperative patients with Fallot's tetralogy should undergo two-dimensional echocardiography with Doppler interrogation and color-flow imaging, exercise stress testing, and 24-hour ambulatory electrocardiography. If obstruction to right ventricular outflow is mild or absent, if the shunt is absent or trivial, if low-pressure pulmonary valve regurgitation is no more than mild or moderate, if there are no detectable disturbances in ventricular rhythm, and if right ventricular size and function are normal, no limitations are imposed on athletic activity, either isotonic or isometric.[177,178] Of particular concern is a residual right ventricular outflow gradient that increases significantly with exercise and is accompanied by right ventricular electrical instability believed to originate at the site of the ventriculotomy scar (Fig. 32–18). Postoperative bifascicular block, uncommon with current operative techniques, is a potential electrophysiological risk (Fig. 32–13). Occurrence of bifascicular block in isolation (without the aforementioned residua or sequelae) does not in itself preclude unrestricted physical activity, provided the 24-hour ambulatory electrocardiogram records no additional evidence of impaired atrioventricular conduction.

In *complete transposition of the great arteries* (p. 944) data are derived chiefly from patients who have undergone atrial switch operations in early life. With few exceptions, obligatory and important postoperative residua and sequelae require that physical activity be restricted to mild or moderate intensity and limited duration. Recommendations regarding athletic activity for patients after undergoing the *arterial switch operation* cannot be made as of this writing. However, it is believed that uncomplicated arterial switch repairs may circumvent the electrophysiological sequelae after atrial switch operations (Fig. 32–12), while permitting the morphological left ventricle to serve as the systemic pump.

The *Fontan operation* (p. 975) permits study of the human circulation in which total right atrial or total caval flow is channeled directly into the pulmonary artery or into a small right ventricle that serves only as a conduit. The principal congenital malformations amenable to the Fontan repair are tricuspid atresia and single ventricle with pulmonary stenosis. Exercise performance improves but remains subnormal,[135,179] and cardiac index increases but seldom more than twofold. Patients with optimal repairs are permitted moderate-intensity isotonic and isometric exercise if the following criteria are met: (1) a satisfactory working capacity as judged by exercise stress testing; (2) stable sinus rhythm with no significant disturbances in atrial or ventricular rhythm in response to exercise or on 24-hour ambulatory electrocardiography; (3) normal ventricular function as determined by two-dimensional echocardiography or radionuclide imaging; and (4) normal systemic arterial oxygen saturation.

INSURABILITY, EMPLOYABILITY, AND PSYCHOSOCIAL CONSIDERATIONS

Most young adults who have undergone surgical repair of congenital heart lesions are eligible for *health insurance* and *life insurance*. As newer and more successful therapeutic modalities are applied, and as the long-term benefits of these therapeutic advances are realized, patients are likely to enjoy greater access to insurance. Life insurance ratings and premiums are based on known mortality rates over periods of 10 to 20 years, calculated from the age of the person at the time of application.[180,181] *Group life insurance* is a form of term life insurance that provides death benefits for applicants who are members of a specific group. The larger the group, the lower the premiums, as a rule. Comparatively less medical information is required for group term life insurance applications, so the probability of denial is significantly lower than for other types of life insurance. Term insurance is a relatively inexpensive solution for young parents who desire death benefits only, and policies are available to most young adults with congenital heart disease if purchased through a large group. Companies willing to consider applications for *whole life insurance* from patients with congenital heart disease may not insure a child, but might approve an adolescent (over age 15) with the same congenital malformation. These positions reflect the insurance companies' theory that by adolescence, a sufficient amount will be known about a patient's prognosis to provide a basis for judgment. *The Medical Information Bureau* pools medical information from life insurance applications. That information is available for review by referring physicians and patients.

The future of *health insurance* systems is uncertain, as reflected by major changes during the past 20 years. Options include fee-for-service insurance, health maintenance organizations, independent practice associations, Medicare, and Medicaid. An appreciable number of young adults who have had repair of congenital cardiac defects can anticipate a normal or near-normal life span and lifestyle, but the constraints imposed by fee-for-service health insurance plans (no coverage for preexisting conditions or for ambulatory services) make these plans least attractive. This is especially true for patients who anticipate further surgery or catheterization or for those who require frequent ambulatory evaluation or diagnostic testing.

EMPLOYABILITY. The opportunities for employment of adults with congenital cardiac defects are influenced by education, type of cardiac lesion, job discrimination, and cardiac surgery.[181] Legislation has been enacted to protect the rights of patients and to provide them with assistance in seeking employment. Overprotective attitudes by parents and teachers combined with absence of discipline may seriously reduce the patient's competitive spirit and curtail educational achievements. Job discrimination is one of the most important factors affecting employment opportunities for patients with congenital heart disease. The smaller the company to which the application is made, the greater the reluctance of employers to hire anyone with a thoracotomy scar or a preexisting cardiac disorder.

In selected occupations (bus drivers and airline pilots, for example), the safety of others is in the hands of a single person. To make rational recommendations about medical fitness for these occupations, the patient's risk of incapacity or sudden death must be clearly defined. The National Rehabilitation Act of 1973 prevents job discrimination against the disabled by almost all employers with 10 or more employees. The Vocational Rehabilitation Act of 1920, strengthened by amendments, offers a wide range of services, including medical evaluation and treatment, guidance and counseling, training for the right job, living expenses during rehabilitation, and follow-up to ascertain the satisfaction of the employee and employer. These services are significantly underutilized, especially by cardiac patients.

PSYCHOSOCIAL CONSIDERATIONS. There are special, if not unique, psychological problems of patients who have experienced dramatic and sometimes traumatic diagnostic and therapeutic interventions during key developmental phases of their lives. The trend toward earlier diagnosis and reparative surgery in congenital heart disease has made it difficult to generalize from results of studies done 10 to 20 years ago. Despite methodological difficulties and a number of constraints, some understanding has been achieved by critical assessment of available data combined with clinical experience. Most patients with congenital heart disease function psychologically within normal range, although sometimes low self-esteem, insecurity, and feelings of vulnerability are matters of concern.[182] Parental knowledge, understanding, and attitude largely determine patients' and parents' perceptions of the congenital heart disease and significantly affect psychological adjustments. Difficulty in accepting illness may be manifested by denial and potentially self-destructive behavior, especially in adolescents. The adult with congenital heart disease faces tangible problems in the workforce, in dating, in marriage, and in parenthood. Cyanosis impairs intellectual function, although the degree of impairment is usually mild and may be overestimated in IQ tests that depend on gross motor function at a young age.[183] Early surgery in patients with cyanotic congenital heart disease appears to improve intellectual and psychological development.[184,185] Circulatory arrest with profound hypothermia results in no major detrimental sequelae but may have subtle adverse effects on intellectual function, especially if the circulatory arrest and hypothermia are prolonged.[186] Longitudinal studies of the psychosocial aspects of congenital heart disease promise to improve our understanding of the expanding population of adolescents and adults with these disorders.

CARDIAC SURGICAL CONSIDERATIONS IN ADULTS WITH CONGENITAL HEART DISEASE

OPERATION AND REOPERATION

Operation or reoperation in adults with congenital heart disease often involves special surgical considerations peculiar to older patients.[1] These considerations must take into account the congenital cardiac malformation per se (previously operated or unoperated) together with acquired cardiac and noncardiac diseases of adulthood. Certain general considerations apply to adult congenital heart disease patients who have not had surgery and to those who have had palliative or reparative surgery. In cyanotic adults undergoing their initial operation, aortopulmonary collateral and hematological disorders are matters of concern. In patients who have had palliative procedures, the general concerns at the time of reoperation are shunts and bands. In adults who have undergone reparative surgery, the chief concerns at the time of reoperation are prosthetic materials such as conduits and valves. Concerns that apply to both unoperated patients and patients undergoing reoperation include pulmonary vascular disease, ventricular function, myocardial protection (cardioplegia), blood salvage techniques, the risk of infective endocarditis, the residua and sequelae of previous cardiac surgery, as well as coexisting acquired heart disease, the incidence of which varies with patient age.

Perioperative management of hemostatic defects in adult patients with cyanotic congenital heart disease is outlined on p. 1714. When preoperative phlebotomy is required to improve hemostasis, the blood should be stored for potential autologous transfusion. Reoperation after palliative procedures include revision of Blalock-Taussig shunts (Fig. 32–14), Glenn shunts, Potts or Waterston shunts, and pulmonary arterial bands. The most significant considerations regarding reoperation of patients who have had prior reparative surgery are related to native valve reconstruction and to prosthetic materials, either conduits or valves. Operative planning requires knowledge of the basic congenital malformation, knowledge of the initial surgical procedure, and knowledge of the postoperative residua, sequelae, and complications. Perhaps the most important variable that precludes reparative or palliative surgery or reoperation is pulmonary vascular disease. Ventricular function is the second major determinant of operability or reoperability. Volume and pressure overload, myocardial ischemia, and ventricular morphology are important variables that influence ventricular function and require meticulous preoperative assessment.

Certain general principles apply intraoperatively, such as myocardial protection and cardioplegia, and systemic hypothermia. Intraoperative salvage of red blood cells and platelet-rich plasma before cardiopulmonary bypass has greatly diminished the need for nonautologous blood and blood products. Minimizing blood and blood product usage is even more important at reoperation than at initial operation because of the greater risk of bleeding and the need for transfusions at reoperation. The sternotomy incision at reoperation is a technical concern. There is a significant risk of bleeding when an enlarged right ventricle is apposed to the sternum and when right ventricular outflow conduits adhere to the sternum. The risk of reopening the sternum can be materially reduced if reoperation is anticipated at the initial repair, with placement of an anterior patch of synthetic pericardium.

The selection, use, and long-term effects of prosthetic mate-

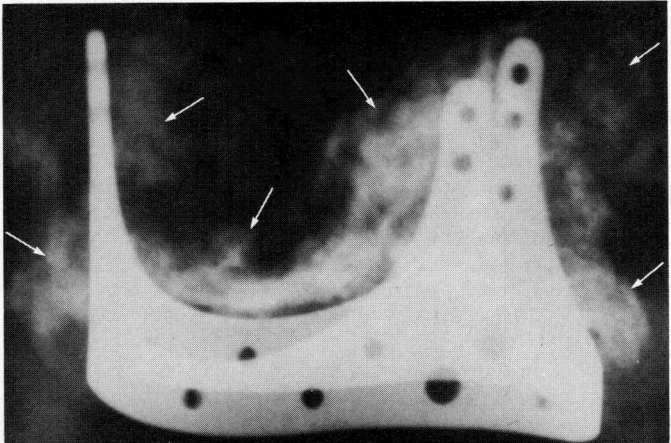

FIGURE 32–20. Lateral radiograph of an Ionescu-Shiley pericardial bioprosthetic valve removed from a 19-year-old male 4 years after insertion. The specimen shows extensive calcification (arrows).

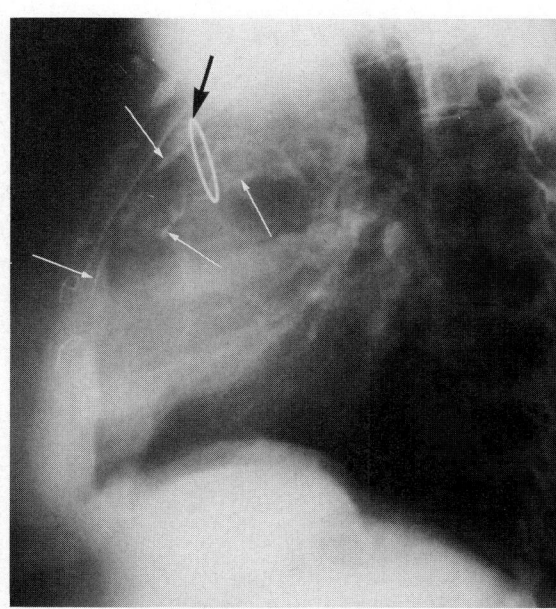

FIGURE 32–21. Lateral chest radiograph from a 19-year-old woman who, at age 8, underwent intracardiac repair for Fallot's tetralogy. An external valve conduit (porcine valve) was inserted because an anomalous coronary artery coursed across the right ventricular outflow tract. The radiograph shows calcification of the conduit (small arrows) above and below the porcine valve (large arrow).

rials are additional major considerations. There are three categories of prostheses: patches, valves, and conduits. The devices or materials selected must achieve an immediately successful technical result, while the long-term postoperative effects of the prosthetic materials on morbidity and mortality are taken into account (Figs. 32–20 and 32–21). The choice of materials is based on the patient's age and size, the nature of the congenital malformation, the type of repair undertaken, whether or not subsequent repairs are anticipated, the availability of various synthetic and biological materials and devices, complications of long-term anticoagulation, and the risk of infection.

CARDIAC CATHETERIZATION AS A THERAPEUTIC INTERVENTION

(See also Chap. 41)

Interventional cardiac catheterization is now the preferred primary treatment or an adjunct to the surgical treatment of increasing numbers of pediatric and adult patients with congenital malformations of the heart and circulation (see also p. 202).[90,91] Corrective or reparative interventional catheterization procedures apply to pulmonary valve stenosis, recoarctation of the aorta, patent ductus arteriosus, and potentially to selected patients with atrial septal defect or ventricular septal defect. Palliative interventions can be either instead of surgery or as adjuncts to surgery. Procedures performed in lieu of surgery are applied to lesions such as aortic valve stenosis, postoperative systemic or pulmonary venous obstruction, previously unoperated coarctation of the aorta, obstructed bioprosthetic valves, and congenital pulmonary arteriovenous fistulas (Fig. 32–22). Palliative procedures that are adjuncts to surgery apply to patients with systemic-to-pulmonary arterial collateral circulation, systemic-to-pulmonary arterial surgical shunts, pulmonary or systemic venous obstruction, certain intraatrial communications, and selected patients with peripheral pulmonary artery stenosis. Therapeutic cardiac catheterization, like cardiac surgery, has three principal objectives: (1) preservation of or improvement in cardiac function, (2) increase in longevity, and (3) maintenance of or improvement in quality of life. When the catheterization technique achieves these ends, surgical morbidity and mortality are circumvented.

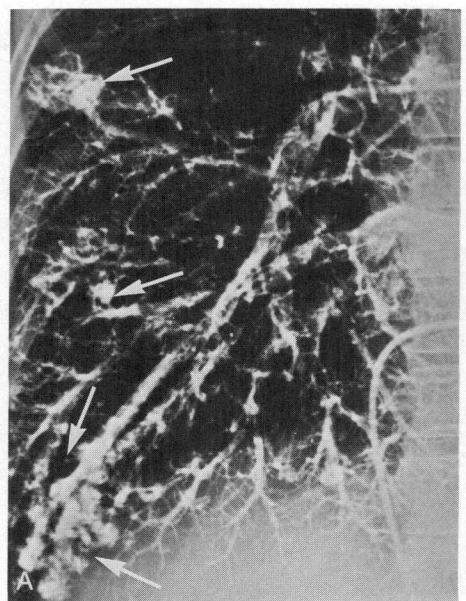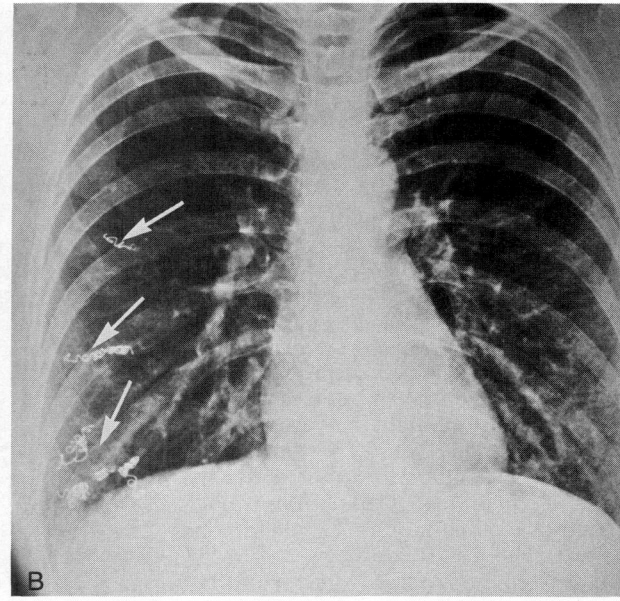

FIGURE 32–22. *A,* Pulmonary arteriogram showing congenital pulmonary arteriovenous fistulas in the right middle and lower lobes of a 50-year-old woman with hereditary hemorrhagic telangiectasia (Rendu-Osler-Weber syndrome). Arrows point to the larger fistula that was subjected to coil occlusion.

NONCARDIAC SURGERY IN ADULTS WITH CONGENITAL HEART DISEASE

(See also Chap. 55)

When adults with congenital heart disease require noncardiac surgery, perioperative risks can be reduced, often appreciably, when problems inherent in this patient population are anticipated. The author discusses patients with cyanotic or acyanotic congenital heart disease who have *not* undergone cardiac surgery and patients who have undergone reparative cardiac surgery.

SITUS INVERSUS WITH DEXTROCARDIA (p. 969). This arrangement usually occurs in people with structurally and functionally normal hearts and may go unrecognized until an illness that requires surgery brings an adult patient to attention. Accompanying symptoms are likely to be misconstrued and diagnostic conclusions incorrect unless the mirror image visceral positions are known. In acute appendicitis the abdominal pain is present in the *left* lower quadrant, and with biliary colic the pain is in the *left* upper quadrant. The risk of noncardiac surgery is the same in the presence of situs inversus as in patients with normal situs, provided no congenital malformations coexist in the mirror image heart.

CONGENITAL COMPLETE HEART BLOCK (p. 955). Patients with this condition who undergo noncardiac surgery should have electrocardiographic monitoring during and immediately after operation. Intraoperative vagotonic stimuli at ophthalmic or gastrointestinal surgery should be minimized and treated with intravenous atropine expectantly or if there is a sudden decrease in heart rate. If the preoperative scalar electrocardiogram shows wide QRS complexes and a relatively slow ventricular response, especially if the patient has a history of syncope or near syncope, a temporary right ventricular pacemaker should be inserted.

BICUSPID AORTIC VALVE. Noncardiac surgery in an adult with a functionally normal or mildly stenotic or incompetent bicuspid aortic valve imposes the risk of infective endocarditis. Fibrocalcific obstruction of a congenital bicuspid aortic valve accounts for about one-half the cases of surgically important pure aortic stenosis in adults.[14] The immediate risks of noncardiac surgery are determined by the degree of obstruction, the functional adequacy of the afterloaded left ventricle, and the presence of acquired coronary artery disease. When emergency noncardiac surgery is required in an adult with severe calcific bicuspid aortic stenosis and mar-

ginal left ventricular function, hemodynamic monitoring with a flotation catheter is obligatory. If surgery is elective, consideration should be given to aortic valve replacement. Balloon valvuloplasty in this setting is less successful if the stenosis is due to calcification of a congenitally *bicuspid* aortic valve than if the stenosis results from calcification of a previously normal *trileaflet* aortic valve. Coronary angiography helps to determine whether angina pectoris is caused by coexisting coronary artery disease or to augmented oxygen demands of the increased left ventricular mass. If the former is the case, the margin of safety during noncardiac surgery might be increased by preoperative coronary angioplasty. Intraoperative monitoring of systemic blood pressure is important because a sudden fall in systemic vascular resistance may not be compensated by an increase in stroke volume, owing to fixed obstruction to left ventricular outflow. An attempt to correct hypotension with rapid infusion of intravenous fluids may cause pulmonary edema. Pharmacological support of systemic resistance is safer than intravenous infusion and just as efficacious.

CONGENITAL BICUSPID AORTIC REGURGITATION. Patients with hemodynamically significant congenital bicuspid aortic regurgitation face noncardiac surgery with risks determined by left ventricular function and susceptibility to infective endocarditis. If left ventricular function is normal, noncardiac surgery is well tolerated. Moderate intraoperative anesthetic hypotension is not a hazard, serving instead to decrease regurgitant flow and reduce the volume overload on the left ventricle. If left ventricular function is depressed, elective noncardiac surgery raises the question of preemptive replacement of the aortic valve. A tissue valve is preferred to avoid anticoagulants in patients who anticipate subsequent noncardiac surgery. Emergency noncardiac operation in the presence of depressed left ventricular function calls for hemodynamic monitoring with a flotation catheter and postoperative pharmacological afterload reduction. Infective endocarditis is a risk; meticulous prophylaxis is mandatory.

EBSTEIN'S ANOMALY OF THE TRICUSPID VALVE (p. 940). Patients with acyanotic Ebstein's anomaly who require noncardiac surgery confront four risks: (1) the functionally inadequate right ventricle, (2) atrial tachyarrhythmias with or without accessory pathways, (3) paradoxical embolism through an intraatrial communication, and (4) infective endocarditis on the malformed tricuspid valve. Right ventricular failure is less a perioperative risk than the sudden occurrence of atrial flutter or fibrillation, especially with rapid antegrade conduction by way of right bypass tracts. Patients with histories of rapid heart action or with fusion beats (type B Wolff-Parkinson-White) on scalar electrocardiogram (Fig. 32–10A) require electrocardiographic monitoring. Postoperative thrombophlebitis and the attendant risk of paradoxical embolization are minimized by the use of support hose and early ambulation.

OSTIUM SECUNDUM ATRIAL SEPTAL DEFECT (p. 906). In asymptomatic young adults with this malformation normal pulmonary arterial pressure imposes comparatively little risk during noncardiac surgery, but there are two caveats. In response to hemorrhage, systemic resistance rises and venous return diminishes, a combination that augments the left-to-right intraatrial shunt, sometimes considerably. An additional concern is the risk of paradoxical emboli from leg veins because thrombi carried by the inferior vena cava tend to stream across the atrial septal defect into the systemic circulation. Meticulous leg care and early ambulation minimize venous stasis.

CYANOTIC CONGENITAL HEART DISEASE. In patients with these malformations both general and specific concerns apply. Cyanotic adults have an increased incidence of acute cholecystitis caused by *calcium bilirubinate stones* (Fig. 32–23). Accordingly, cholecystectomy is a surgical procedure that such patients may anticipate. Sometimes biliary colic becomes evident years after intracardiac surgery has eliminated the cyanosis. Perioperative improvement in *hemostasis* in cyanotic patients can be addressed if surgery is elective. Phlebotomized units are stored for potential autologous transfusion. *Oxygen inhalation* would seem to be desirable in cyanotic patients during and immediately after noncardiac surgery, and there are no ill effects from so doing. Administration of high levels of inspired oxygen may significantly raise arterial oxygen saturation even in the presence of right-to-left shunts, but there is little or no evidence that its routine perioperative use is beneficial. *Intravenous lines, infusions, and drugs* must be managed with special care in cyanotic patients. The introduction of air into peripheral veins risks delivery of the air into the systemic circulation because of the right-to-left shunt. Use of an air filter obviates the risk.

Fallot's tetralogy represents a large category of adults with uncorrected cyanotic congenital heart disease. Older patients with this malformation may, therefore, come to noncardiac surgery without intracardiac repair or with only a shunt created in infancy or childhood. Meticulous perioperative monitoring of oxygen saturation (pulse oximeter) and blood pressure is important because a sudden fall in systemic resistance may precipitate intense cyanosis and occasionally death, or a sudden rise in systemic resistance may abruptly and dangerously depress systemic blood flow. The risk of postoperative postural hypotension is mentioned later. Susceptibility to infective endocarditis requires prophylaxis.

Cyanotic patients with *elevated pulmonary vascular resistance* face noncardiac surgery with risks inherent in the cyanosis per se, in addition to the formidable risks of pulmonary vascular disease. Fixed pulmonary resistance precludes rapid adaptive responses to potentially labile intraoperative or postoperative hemodynamic changes. In Eisenmenger's complex or physiologically analogous lesions, a sudden fall or a sudden rise in systemic vascular resistance precipitates responses similar to those already described in Fallot's tetralogy. Every effort should be made to minimize the postural hypotension that tends to occur during early convalescence in patients having general anesthesia. Because the attendant drop in systemic vascular resistance suddenly augments the right-to-left shunt, convalescent cyanotic patients with pulmonary vascular disease should change positions slowly until the risk of postoperative postural hypotension has abated.

The Postoperative Patient

Adults with congenital heart disease who have undergone *reparative surgery* comprise an increasing percentage of patients who require subsequent noncardiac operations. If the cardiac surgery is curative, as it is after division of a small patent ductus arteriosus in childhood, there is no added risk of a noncardiac surgical procedure. Early uncomplicated correction of simple pulmonary valve stenosis also is close to a cure, and subsequent noncardiac surgery imposes little or no risk, including, in all probability, susceptibility to infective endocarditis. Closure of an ostium secundum atrial septal defect in childhood is close to a cure.

Valvular residua and sequelae after cardiac surgery or therapeutic catheterization are relevant to medical management when patients undergo noncardiac surgery in adulthood. Successful repair of coarctation of the aorta may leave behind a functionally normal bicuspid aortic valve susceptible to infective endocarditis. Direct repair of congenital bicuspid aortic stenosis at best creates a functionally normal bicuspid aortic valve that remains at risk of infective endocarditis. After complete relief of congenital pulmonary valve stenosis by direct repair or balloon dilatation, the risk of infective endocarditis is low, if not absent. The functional adequacy of the right ventricle is an important perioperative variable. In Fallot's tetralogy, reconstruction of the right ventricular outflow tract may largely or entirely abolish the pressure gradient, and if the functional adequacy of the right ventricle is satisfactory, the risk of noncardiac surgery is low. It is advisable to use prophylaxis for infective endocarditis, even though susceptibility is relatively low.

After surgical repair of *Ebstein's anomaly of the tricuspid valve* (tricuspid reconstruction and division of active or potential bypass tracts), atrial arrhythmias remain a consideration during medical management of noncardiac surgery, but without the fear of accelerated conduction (Fig. 32–10). Closure of the intraatrial communication eliminates cyanosis, so the hematological derangements are no longer concerns, and the risk of paradoxic embolization is eliminated. The postoperative right ventricle is not functionally normal, but the hemodynamic risk during subsequent noncardiac surgery is small. If residual tricuspid regurgitation is more than mild, prophylaxis for infective endocarditis is advisable.

PROSTHETIC MECHANICAL VALVES. These devices complicate the management of subsequent noncardiac surgery. The immediate intraoperative and perioperative concern is anticoagulation, in addition to and apart from the risk of infective endocarditis. If noncardiac surgery is elective, and if the prosthesis carries a high thromboembolic risk, warfarin should be replaced with an in-hospital continuous infusion of heparin, which is discontinued 4 to 6 hours before elective operation, restarted within 48 hours after operation, and then replaced by warfarin. For a lower-risk prosthetic valve in the aortic location, it is considered relatively safe to discontinue warfarin 2 to 3 days before noncardiac surgery and resume the drug 2 to 3 days postoperatively. Emergency noncardiac surgery in an anticoagulated patient with a mechanical prosthesis is managed differently. Cessation of warfarin and administration of vitamin K do not achieve immediate reversal of the anticoagulant effects, which persist for 24 hours or longer. Rapid reversal of the hemostatic defects before emergency noncardiac surgery requires infusion of fresh frozen plasma. If vitamin K is used preoperatively, the response to readministration of warfarin after operation is blunted.

ELECTROPHYSIOLOGICAL SEQUELAE. After reparative surgery for congenital heart disease, electrophysiological sequelae are important concerns in the management of subsequent noncardiac surgery. The most diverse and complex of these sequelae are after intraatrial repairs (Mustard or Senning operations) for complete transposition of the great

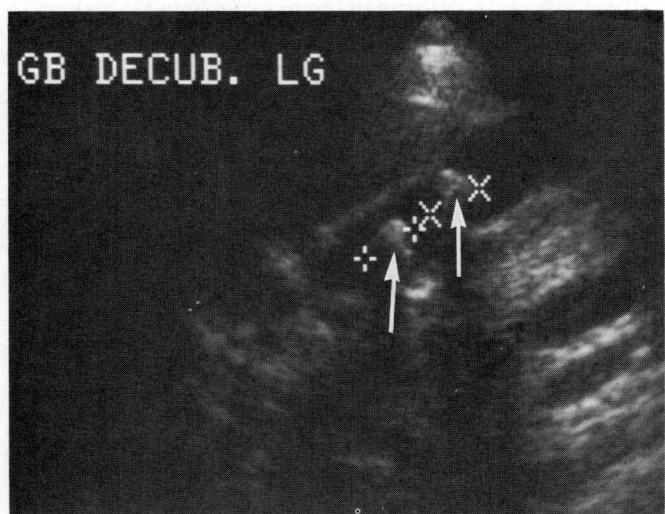

FIGURE 32–23. Abdominal ultrasound in a cyanotic 31-year-old woman with a univentricular heart and pulmonary vascular disease. She developed biliary colic due to calcium bilirubinate stones (arrows).

arteries (Fig. 32–12) and require monitoring during noncardiac surgery. Intraventricular surgery, as in Fallot's tetralogy, may result in electrophysiological sequelae that are potentially important concerns during noncardiac surgery (Figs. 32–13 and 32–18). Awareness of the presence or potential presence of these sequelae serves to decrease perioperative risk.

After repair of coarctation of the aorta, *systemic hypertension* may persist to some degree or recur even if the obstruction has been completely relieved, but the incidence is declining because of the success of early operation. Nevertheless, pharmacological control of perioperative systemic hypertension is sometimes necessary during noncardiac surgery. The longer the duration of systemic hypertension before repair of coarctation, the greater the incidence of premature coronary artery disease, a point to be considered in subsequent perioperative management.

VENTRICULAR FUNCTION. This is an important variable in the long-term management of patients after operation for congenital heart disease. The adequacy of ventricular function (left, right, or single ventricle) is a major determinant of risk during noncardiac surgery in adulthood. Excessive perioperative intravenous fluids should be avoided, and hemodynamic monitoring should be used when the morphological substrate permits.

Adults with congenital heart disease have not only the preoperative or postoperative malformation with which they were born but also *cardiovascular and noncardiac diseases that are acquired with age.* Medical management during noncardiac surgery must take into account acquired diseases of the heart and circulation, especially coronary artery disease and systemic hypertension, and noncardiac acquired medical disorders.

POSTOPERATIVE RESIDUA AND SEQUELAE

Residua

These are represented by cardiac, vascular, or noncardiovascular disorders that are intentionally left behind at the time of reparative heart surgery (Table 32–2). With few exceptions, the residua are obligatory, that is, do not result from the operation having fallen short of its goal, at least in a technical sense.[186] By contrast, *sequelae* are alterations or disorders that are intentionally incurred—occasionally or invariably—at the time of reparative surgery and are looked on as necessary and acceptable consequences of operation (Table 32–3). *Complications* are unintentional aftermaths of reparative surgery that range in severity from inconsequential to fatal; complications and sequelae may imperceptibly merge. Surgery is considered curative if no residua, sequelae, or complications of the heart or circulation are present after operation. This definition implies that normal cardiovascular function is achieved and maintained, life expectancy is normal, and further medical or surgical treatment for the congenital heart disease is unnecessary. These ideals seldom are realized, and even curative cardiac surgery does not preclude noncardiac residua.

Residua after reparative surgery for congenital heart disease are listed in Table 32–2. Electrophysiological abnormalities are, with some exceptions, inherent components of certain congenital cardiac malformations. These abnormalities often are evident in the standard preoperative 12-lead electrocardiogram, and they persist—sometimes harmlessly, sometimes not so harmlessly—after reparative surgery. Electrophysiological residua include: (1) axis deviation, especially left; (2) conduction defects, especially atrioventricular; (3) disorders of impulse formation, especially of the sinus node; and (4) arrhythmias, especially atrial.

RESIDUAL ABNORMALITIES OF CARDIAC VALVES. These abnormalities after reparative surgery for congenital heart disease fall into three general categories: (1) congenitally malformed cardiac valves that are functionally normal and do not require attention during reparative surgery; (2) intrinsically normal cardiac valves that are rendered incompetent because of the physiological stress imposed by the congenital malformation that prompted surgical repair; and (3) residually incompetent or stenotic congenitally malformed cardiac valves that do not lend themselves to complete repair. Aortic valve abnormalities that represent functionally unimportant residua include a bicuspid aortic valve with coarctation of the aorta, and mild aortic regurgitation that may accompany Fallot's tetralogy, perimembranous ventricular septal defect, or truncus arteriosus. Congenital mitral valve abnormalities that represent functionally unimportant residua include the "cleft" but competent anterior mitral leaflet of an endocardial cushion defect (p. 92) and a reduction in interpapillary muscle distance associated with coarctation of the aorta. Postoperative residual incompetence of intrinsically normal pulmonary or tricuspid valves usually is in response to pulmonary hypertension or right ventricular hypertension (obstruction to outflow) which is intrinsic to the basic congenital malformation that warranted surgery.

RESIDUAL VENTRICULAR ABNORMALITIES. After reparative surgery, certain ventricular abnormalities are permanent, such as the intrinsic morphology of a chamber, or may change with the passage of time, as in the case of alterations in chamber mass and function. In patients undergoing either atrial switch operations for complete transposition of the great arteries or operations for congenitally corrected transposition of the great arteries, an important postoperative residuum is the presence of a morphological right ventricle in the systemic location. A pivotal question is whether a morphological right ventricle that is perfused by a right coronary artery can, in the long run, perform as a systemic chamber as well as an anatomical left ventricle perfused by a left coronary artery.

The development of increased ventricular mass and its regression after reparative surgery are important properties of ventricular myocardium (Chap. 14).[187,188] An increase in ventricular mass in excess of the process of normal growth is determined by the nature of the inciting stimulus (hemodynamic or hypoxic), the duration and type of the hemodynamic stimulus (pressure or volume overload), myocardial age (ma-

---

TABLE 32–2 RESIDUA AFTER REPARATIVE SURGERY FOR CONGENITAL HEART DISEASE

1. **Electrophysiological**

2. **Valvular**

3. **Ventricular**
   a. **Chamber morphology**
   b. **Chamber mass**
   c. **Chamber function**
   d. **Myocardial connective tissue**

4. **Vascular**
   a. **Anatomical (morphological) vascular anomalies or defects**
   b. **Elevated resistance and/or pressure—systemic, pulmonic**

5. **Noncardiovascular residua**
   a. **Developmental abnormalities**
   b. **Somatic defects**
   c. **Medical disorders**

TABLE 32–3 SEQUELAE OF REPARATIVE SURGERY FOR CONGENITAL HEART DISEASE

A. **Electrophysiological**
   1. **Atriotomy**
      a. **Intraatrial repair**
      b. **Intraventricular repair**
   2. **Ventriculotomy**
      a. **The incision site**
      b. **The intracardiac repair**
B. **Native valves**
   1. **Left ventricular or right ventricular *outflow* repair**
   2. **Left ventricular or right ventricular *inflow* repair**
C. **Prosthetic materials**
   1. **Patches**
   2. **Valves**
   3. **Conduits**
D. **Myocardial and endocardial sequelae**

turity) at the time the stimulus is imposed, and the type of cell involved.[188-190] The response of a given cell type at the time of a hemodynamic or hypoxic stimulus depends chiefly on myocardial maturity. If overload or hypoxia is imposed on the immature heart, the cellular response is characterized by replication (hyperplasia) of myocytes and fibroblasts.[191] If the stimuli continue beyond immaturity, myocytes then respond by hypertrophy (enlargement) and fibroblasts by hyperplasia (replication).[189] Of concern is the cellular basis for the decrease in mass after surgical removal of ventricular overload or hypoxia[37,38] (Figs. 32–24 and 32–25). Regression of hypertrophy at the cellular level means a decrease in size of enlarged myocytes, but the fate of myocytes that had replicated in excess of their otherwise genetically regulated numbers is not clear.[192] A postoperative reduction in ventricular mass in the setting of hyperplasia implies, at least in part, that the numerically excessive myocytes become smaller in size, not fewer in number. If this contention is valid, its long-term functional significance is unknown. The response of preoperative hyperplasia of connective tissue cells to operative removal of the overload or hypoxic stimulus is also unknown, although there is evidence that connective tissue cells do not regress as readily as myocytes.[193]

VASCULAR RESIDUA. After primary repair of congenital cardiac malformations, vascular residua consist of anatomical anomalies or defects, or elevated resistance and/or pressure in the systemic or pulmonary circulation (Table 32–2). A more than casual relation exists between aortic root disease and bicuspid or unicuspid unicommissural aortic valves, and on rare occasions, bicuspid or unicuspid aortic stenosis is dramatically complicated by a dissecting aneurysm.[14] The aortic root defect—if present before operation—remains as a postoperative risk. Rupture of an aneurysm of the circle of Willis is a cerebral complication of coarctation of the aorta. The predisposition is likely to persist after surgery, and rupture may occur in normotensive patients long after successful coarctation repair.[194]

Congenital anomalies of the coronary arteries occur in a number of congenital malformations of the heart; an example is Fallot's tetralogy, in which a coronary arterial anomaly is

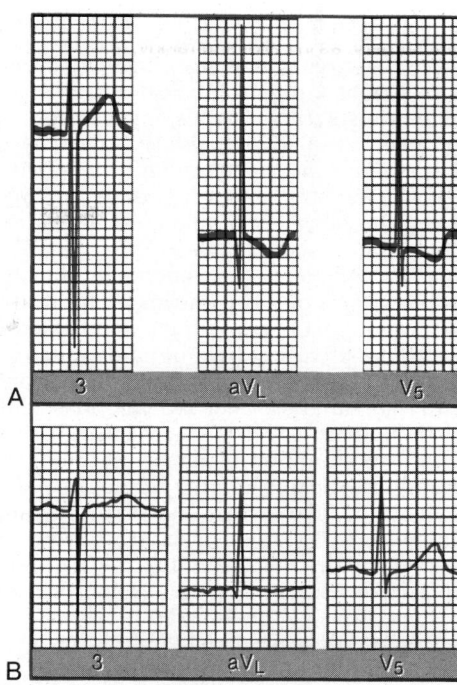

FIGURE 32–25. Electrocardiographic leads 3, aVl, and V₅ before and after ligation of an anomalous left coronary artery that arose from the pulmonary trunk. A, Before operation (age 4 months) there was left axis deviation with voltage and repolarization criteria for left ventricular hypertrophy in leads aVl and V₅. Lead aVl exhibits a deep but narrow Q wave. B, Five years after operation the left axis deviation persists, but left ventricular hypertrophy and the deep Q wave in lead aVl have disappeared.

present in 2 to 10 per cent of patients.[13] Although these anomalous arteries are functionally unimportant, they may be injured during operation. Not unimportant, however, is the residual coronary artery disease (intimal proliferation, medial thickening, premature atherosclerosis) initiated by the hypertension of coarctation of the aorta and that may become clinically overt after successful repair.

The younger the patient is at the time of successful coarctation repair, the more probable the long-term normalization of postoperative blood pressure.[195] Even if the resting blood pressure is normal after operation, systemic *systolic* pressure may rise disproportionately during exercise, implying a residual decrease in compliance of major proximal systemic arterial walls.

The preoperative status of the *pulmonary vascular bed*, especially the resistance vessels, is a major determinant of the presence and degree of residual postoperative pulmonary vascular disease. Early operation sets the stage for normal development of the pulmonary vascular bed, and reduces the probability that preoperative alterations will result in increased muscularity of small pulmonary arteries, intimal hyperplasia, and a reduction in the number of intraacinar vessels.[196] Refinements and safety of surgical repair within the first 6 to 12 months of life make it likely that postoperative pulmonary vascular disease will diminish in importance.

Noncardiac residua can be important long-term concerns after reparative surgery (Table 32–2). Developmental abnormalities such as the mental deficiency of Down syndrome or the physical deficiencies of Turner or the Ellis–van Creveld syndrome are examples. Specific residual somatic defects include dysmorphism and limb abnormalities. Spinal cord injuries during repair of coarctation of the aorta[197] are more properly considered complications rather than residua as defined earlier. Preoperative medical or psychosocial disorders may remain as important postoperative residua, and a healed brain abscess can serve as a focus of a seizure disorder. Cataracts and deafness persist as medical residua after division of the patent ductus in children with the rubella syndrome.[13]

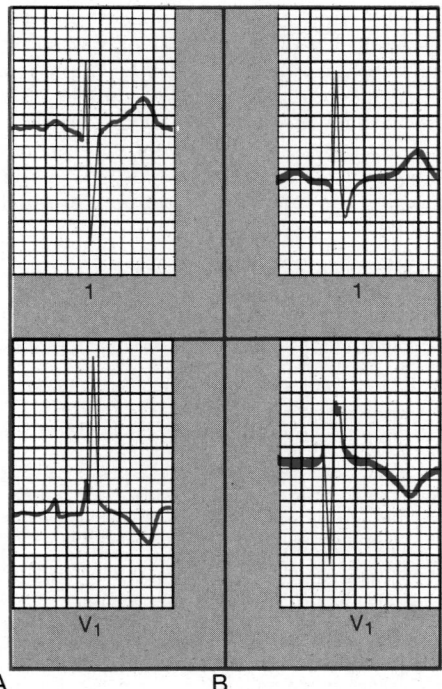

FIGURE 32–24. A, Leads 1 and V₁ from a 2-year-old boy with severe pulmonary valve stenosis. B, Leads 1 and V₁ 7 years after surgical pulmonary valvotomy. Right axis deviation has resolved and the rR' in lead V₁ has been replaced with an rSr'. These are electrocardiographic features of regression of right ventricular hypertrophy.

After reparative surgery for congenital heart disease, sequelae may involve electrophysiological mechanisms, native cardiac valves, prosthetic materials, myocardium, and endocardium (Table 32–3). *Electrophysiological sequelae* of intraatrial repair become overtly manifest as disturbances in rhythm and conduction, including sinoatrial dysfunction, junctional rhythm, atrial fibrillation, atrial flutter, and impaired atrioventricular conduction varying from P-R interval prolongation to complete atrioventricular block. Electrophysiological sequelae of intraventricular repair by way of a right atrial incision result from injury to internodal conduction pathways, the proximal right bundle branch alone or in combination with the left anterior fascicle (left anterior hemiblock with right bundle branch block or bifascicular block). A right ventriculotomy is responsible for two electrophysiological sequelae: an alteration in the sequence of ventricular activation, and electrical instability of the incised right ventricle (Fig. 32–18).[198] The surface electrocardiogram is useful in determining the site of origin of abnormal right ventricular activation when a right bundle branch block pattern coexists with left anterior fascicular block. Bifascicular block sets the stage for postoperative complete heart block, which is a hazardous electrophysiological sequel (Fig. 32–13).

Sequelae involving native cardiac valves occur after left ventricular or right ventricular outflow repairs, or left ventricular or right ventricular inflow repairs. Postoperative aortic regurgitation as a sequel of repair of congenital bicuspid aortic stenosis is an example. Direct repair or balloon dilation of simple congenital pulmonary valve stenosis is commonly followed by mild postinterventional pulmonary regurgitation (Fig. 32–26), a physiologically minor and therefore acceptable sequel. Repair of complex obstruction to right ventricular outflow, as in Fallot's tetralogy, usually induces pulmonary regurgitation. The importance of this sequel depends on the degree of regurgitant flow and the functional state of the recipient ventricle.

Sequelae associated with left ventricular inflow repair accompany operations for congenital mitral regurgitation or congenital obstruction to left ventricular inflow. Assuming complete relief of the mitral regurgitation of an endocardial cushion defect, the morphological abnormalities intrinsic to the congenitally malformed valve leave the left ventricular inflow guarded by an abnormal mitral apparatus. How these repaired valves will function decades after operation is not yet clear. Reconstruction of the tricuspid valve in Ebstein's anomaly is somewhat analogous. Repair is necessarily followed by sequelae intrinsic to the basic tricuspid valve malformation, even if competence is established.

PROSTHETIC MATERIALS. Insertion of these materials represents a special category of sequelae after reparative surgery for congenital heart disease. Patches often are devoid of sequelae, such as an endogenous pericardial patch for closure of an ostium secundum atrial septal defect. However, a patch can set the stage for undesirable sequelae, as when an ostium primum atrial septal defect is closed with synthetic material that is struck by a jet of mitral regurgitation, which causes hemolytic anemia. Valve replacement results in sequelae that vary in signficance according to the physical and hemodynamic characteristics of the prosthetic device (bioprosthetic or synthetic), the site of insertion, and patient age at the time of insertion. Sequelae and complications imperceptibly merge. Reoperation is required when an infant or child outgrows the original valve prosthesis. Bioprosthetic valves degenerate at rates determined chiefly by the patient's age at the time of insertion (p. 1065) and by the tissue characteristics of the device (endogenous or exogenous materials, homografts or xenografts) (Fig. 32–20). Susceptibility to infective endocarditis varies from negligible with aortic homografts to high with mechanical valvular prostheses. The incidence of thromboembolic complications is low with aortic homografts and high with rigid prostheses. Anticoagulants reduce but do not eliminate thromboembolic risks and carry inherent risks of anticoagulant-induced bleeding and the risks of teratogenicity during pregnancy (see earlier).

Conduits can be nonvalved (usually synthetic) or valved (bioprosthetic or mechanical valves). In addition to the risks of degeneration (Fig. 32–21), thrombogenicity, anticoagulation, and infective endocarditis, conduits—especially valved conduits—are subject to pseudointimal proliferation (peel). Conduit obstruction can therefore result from both nongrowth and pseudointimal proliferation.

MYOCARDIAL SEQUELAE. These originate at the site of the ventriculotomy or atriotomy incision. Morphological or mechanical sequelae at these sites usually are negligible or absent, unless there is aneurysm formation, which is more properly considered a complication. Electrophysiological sequelae were discussed earlier. *Endocardial sequelae* after intraventricular repair have been called "surgical fibroelastosis."[199,200] The cause and functional significance of these endocardial lesions, which are not necessarily confined to the chamber in which the intracardiac repair was done, have not been established.

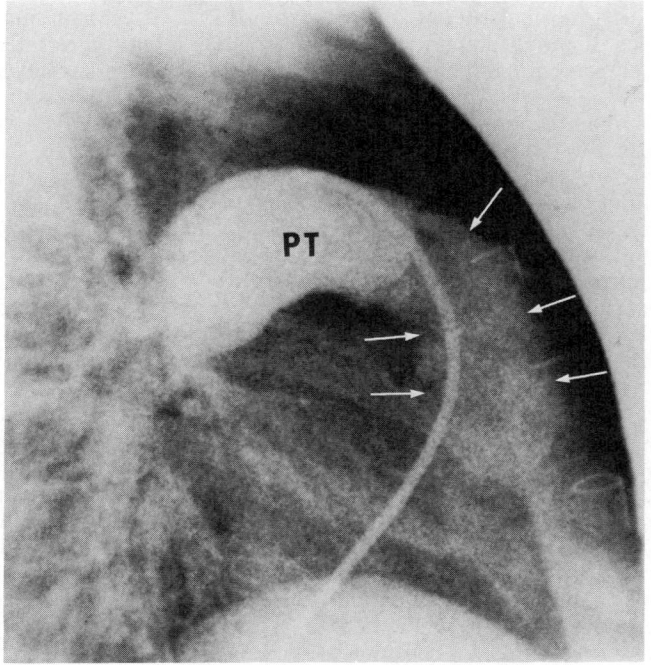

FIGURE 32–26. Pulmonary regurgitation (arrows) after open valvotomy for typical congenital pulmonary valve stenosis. PT = pulmonary trunk.

REFERENCES

1. Perloff, J. K., and Child, J. S.: Congenital Heart Disease in Adults. Philadelphia, W. B. Saunders Company, 1991.
2. Fallot, A.: Contribution a l'anatomie pathologique de la maladie bleue (cyanose cardiaque). Marseillemed. 25:418, 1888.
3. Abbott, M. E.: Atlas of Congenital Heart Disease. New York, American Heart Association, 1936.
4. Gross, R. E., and Hubbard, J. P.: Surgical ligation of a patent ductus arteriosus: Report of first successful case. JAMA 112:729, 1939.
5. Blalock, A., and Taussig, H. B.: Surgical treatment of malformations of the heart in which there is pulmonary stenosis or pulmonary atresia. JAMA 128:189, 1945.
6. Crafoord, C., and Nylin, G.: Congenital coarctation of the aorta and its surgical treatment. J. Thorac. Surg. 14:347, 1945.
7. Kirklin, J. W., DuShane, J. W., Patrick, R. T., et al.: Intracardiac surgery with the aid of a mechanical pump-oxygenator system (Gibbon type): Report of eight cases. Proc. Staff Meet. Mayo Clin. 30:201, 1955.
8. Perloff, J. K.: Pediatric congenital cardiac becomes a postoperative adult. The changing population of congenital heart disease. Circulation 47:606, 1973.
9. Somerville, J.: Congenital heart disease in adults and adolescents. Br. Heart J. 56:395, 1986.
10. Engle, M. A., Adams, F. H., Betson, C., et al.: Resources for long-term care of congenital heart disease. Circulation 44:A-205, 1971.

11. Garson, A.: The science and practice of pediatric cardiology in the next decade. Am. Heart J. *114*:462, 1987.

SURVIVAL PATTERNS

12. Roberts, W. C.: The congenitally bicuspid aortic valve: A study of 85 autopsy cases. Am. J. Cardiol. *26*:72, 1970.
13. Perloff, J. K.: The Clinical Recognition of Congenital Heart Disease. 3rd ed. Philadelphia, W. B. Saunders Company, 1987.
14. Subramanian, R., Olson, L. J., and Edwards, W. D.: Surgical pathology of pure aortic stenosis: A study of 374 cases. Mayo Clin. Proc. *59*:683, 1984.
15. Larson, E. W., and Edwards, W. D.: Risk factors for aortic dissection. A necropsy study of 161 cases. Am. J. Cardiol. *53*:849, 1984.
16. Morganroth, J., Perloff, J. K., Zeldes, S. M., and Dunkman, W. B.: Acute severe aortic regurgitation. Ann. Intern. Med. *87*:223, 1977.
17. Campbell, M.: Natural history of coarctation of the aorta. Br. Heart J. *32*:633, 1970.
18. Jarcho, S.: Coarctation of the aorta (Reynaud, 1828). Am. J. Cardiol. *9*:591, 1962.
19. Hodes, H. L., Steinfeld, L., and Blumenthal, S.: Congenital cerebral aneurysms and coarctation of the aorta. Arch. Pediatr. *76*:28, 1959.
20. Edwards, J. E.: Aneurysms of the thoracic aorta complicating coarctation. Circulation *48*:195, 1973.
21. Vladover, Z., and Neufeld, H. N.: Coronary arteries in coarctation of the aorta. Circulation *37*:449, 1968.
22. Campbell, M.: The natural history of congenital pulmonic stenosis. Br. Heart J. *31*:394, 1969.
23. Nugent, E. W., Freedom, R. M., Nora, J. J., et al.: Clinical course in pulmonary stenosis. Circulation *56*(Suppl I):38, 1977.
24. Moller, J. H., and Adams, P., Jr.: Natural history of pulmonary valvular stenosis: Serial cardiac catheterization in 21 children. Am. J. Cardiol. *16*:654, 1965.
25. Kaplan, S., and Adolph, R. J.: Pulmonic valve stenosis in adults. Cardiovasc. Clin. *10*:328, 1979.
26. Sanders, C., Bittner, V., Nath, P. H., et al.: Atrial septal defect in older adults: Atypical radiographic appearances. Radiology *167*:123, 1988.
27. Campbell, M.: Natural history of atrial septal defect. Br. Heart J. *32*:820, 1970.
28. Rodstein, M., Zeman, F. D., and Gerber, I. E.: Atrial septal defect in the aged. Circulation *23*:665, 1961.
29. Colmers, R. E.: Atrial septal defects in elderly patients: Report of three patients aged 68, 72, and 78. Am. J. Cardiol. *1*:768, 1958.
30. Craig, R. J., and Selzer, A.: Natural history and prognosis of atrial septal defect. Circulation *37*:805, 1968.
31. Markman, P. G., Horvitt, E. G., and Wade, E. G.: Atrial septal defect in the middle-aged and elderly. Q. J. Med. *34*:409, 1965.
32. Perloff, J. K.: Ostium secundum atrial septal defect—survival for 87 and 94 years. Am. J. Cardiol. *53*:388, 1984.
33. Wood, P.: The Eisenmenger syndrome or pulmonary hypertension with reversed central shunt. Br. Med. J. *2*:701, 1958.
34. Nagata, S., Yasuharu, N., Sakakibara, H., et al.: Mitral valve lesion associated with secundum atrial septal defect. Br. Heart J. *49*:51, 1983.
35. Davies, M. J.: Mitral valve in secundum atrial septal defect. Br. Heart J. *46*:126, 1981.
36. Boucher, C. A., Liberthson, R. R., and Buckley, M. J.: Secundum atrial septal defect and significant mitral regurgitation: Incidence, management and morphologic basis. Chest *75*:697, 1979.
37. Popio, K. A., Gorlin, R., Teichholz, L., et al.: Abnormalities of left ventricular function and geometry in adults with an atrial septal defect. Am. J. Cardiol. *36*:302, 1975.
38. Wanderman, K. L., Ovsyheer, I., and Gueron, M.: Left ventricular performance in patients with atrial septal defect: Evaluation with noninvasive methods. Am. J. Cardiol. *41*:487, 1978.
39. Campbell, M.: Natural history of persistent ductus arteriosus. Br. Heart J. *30*:4, 1968.
40. Marquis, R. M., Miller, H. C., McCormack, R.J.M., et al.: Persistence of ductus arteriosus with left to right shunt in the older patient. Br. Heart J. *48*:469, 1982.
41. White, P. D., Maxurkie, S. J., and Boschetti, A. E.: Patency of the ductus arteriosus at 90. N Engl. J. Med. *280*:146, 1969.
42. Fishman, L.: Patent ductus arteriosus in a patient surviving to seventy-four years. Am. J. Cardiol. *6*:685, 1960.
43. Bain, C.W.C.: Longevity in patent ductus arteriosus. Br. Heart J. *19*:574, 1957.

UNCOMMON DEFECTS WITH EXPECTED ADULT SURVIVAL

44. McHenry, M. M.: Factors influencing longevity in adults with congenital complete heart block. Am. J. Cardiol. *29*:416, 1972.
45. Reybrouck, T., Vanden Eynde, B. B., Dumoulin, M., and Van der Hauwaert, L. G.: Cardiorespiratory response to exercise in congenital complete atrioventricular block. Am. J. Cardiol. *64*:896, 1989.
46. Dewey, R. C., Capeless, M. A., and Levy, A. M.: Use of ambulatory electrocardiographic monitoring to identify high-risk patients with congenital complete heart block. N. Engl. J. Med. *316*:835, 1987.
47. Bjarke, B. B., and Kidd, B.S.L.: Congenitally corrected transposition of the great arteries: A clinical study of 101 cases. Acta Paediatr. Scand. *65*:153, 1976.

48. Cumming, G. R.: Congenital corrected transposition of the great vessels without associated intracardiac anomalies. Am. J. Cardiol. *10*:605, 1962.
49. Nagle, J. P., Cheitlin, M. D., and McCarty, R. J.: Corrected transposition of the great vessels without associated anomalies. Chest *60*:363, 1971.
50. Schiebler, G. L., Edwards, J. E., Burchell, H. B., et al.: Congenital corrected transposition of the great vessels. Pediatrics *27*:851, 1961.
51. Lieberson, A. D., Schumacker, R., and Childress, D.: Corrected transposition of the great vessels in a 73 year old man. Circulation *39*:96, 1969.
52. Anderson, K. R., Zuberbuhler, J. R., Anderson, R. H., et al.: Morphologic spectrum of Ebstein's anomaly of the heart. Mayo Clin. Proc. *54*:174, 1979.
53. Benson, L. N., Child, J. S., Schwaiger, M., et al.: Left ventricular geometry and function in adults with Ebstein's anomaly of the tricuspid valve. Circulation *75*:353, 1987.
54. Watson, H.: Natural history of Ebstein's anomaly of tricuspid valve in childhood and adolescence: An international cooperative study of 505 cases. Br. Heart J. *36*:417, 1974.
55. Radford, D. J., Graff, R. F., and Neilson, G. H.: Diagnosis and natural history of Ebstein's anomaly. Br. Heart J. *54*:517, 1985.
56. Makous, N., and Vander Veer, J. B.: Ebstein's anomaly and life expectancy: Report of a survival to over seventy-nine. Am. J. Cardiol. *18*:100, 1966.
57. Adams, J.C.L., and Hudson, R.: Case of Ebstein's anomaly surviving to age 79. Br. Heart J. *18*:129, 1956.
58. Giuliani, E. R., Fuster, V., Brandenburg, R. O., and Mair, D. D.: Ebstein's anomaly: The clinical features and natural history of Ebstein's anomaly of the tricuspid valve. Mayo Clin. Proc. *54*:163, 1979.
59. Seward, J. B., Tajik, A. J., Feist, D. J., and Smith, H. C.: Ebstein's anomaly in an 85 year old man. May Clin. Proc. *54*:193, 1979.
60. Leung, M. P., Baker, E. J., Anderson, R. H., and Zuberbuhler, J. R.: Cineangiographic spectrum of Ebstein's malformations: Its relevance to clinical presentation and outcome. J. Am. Coll. Cardiol. *11*:154, 1988.
60a. Saxena, A., Fong, L. V., and Tristam, M., et al: Left ventricular function in patients > 20 years of age with Ebstein's anomaly of the tricuspid valve. Am. J. Cardiol. *67*:217, 1991.
61. Collins, N. P., Braunwald, E., and Morrow, A. G.: Isolated congenital pulmonary valvular regurgitation. Am. J. Med. *28*:159, 1960.
62. Cortes, F. M., and Jacoby, W. J.: Isolated congenital pulmonary valvular insufficiency. Am. J. Cardiol. *10*:287, 1962.
63. Pouget, J. M., Kelly, C. E., and Pilz, C. G.: Congenital absence of the pulmonic valve: Report of a case in a 73 year old man. Am. J. Cardiol. *19*:732, 1967.
64. Rich, S., and Brundage, B. H.: Pulmonary hypertension: A cellular basis for understanding the pathophysiology and treatment. J. Am. Coll. Cardiol. *14*:545, 1989.
65. McGoon, M. D., and Edwards, W. D.: Primary pulmonary hypertension: Current status. Mod. Conc. Cardiovasc. Dis. *54*:29, 1985.
66. Fuster, V., Steele, P. M., Edwards, W. D., et al.: Primary pulmonary hypertension: Natural history and the importance of thrombosis. Circulation *70*:580, 1984.
67. Bjornsson, J., and Edwards, W. D.: Primary pulmonary hypertension: A histopathologic study of 80 cases. Mayo Clin. Proc. *60*:16, 1985.
68. Lutembacher, R.: De la stenose mitrale avec communication interauriculaire. Arch. Mal. Coeur *9*:237, 1916.
69. Firkett, C. H.: Examen anatomique d'un cas de persistence du trou ovale de botal, avec lésions valvulaires considérables du couer gauche, chez une femme de 74 ans. Ann. Soc. Med. Chir. Liege. *19*:188, 1880.
70. Rosenthal, L.: Atrial septal defect with mitral stenosis (Lutembacher's syndrome) in a woman of 81. Br. Med. J. *2*:1351, 1956.
71. Botefeu, J. M., Moret, P. R., Hahn, C., and Hauf, E.: Aneurysms of the sinus of Valsalva: Report of seven cases and review of the literature. Am. J. Med. *65*:18, 1983.
72. Mayer, E. D., Ruffman, K., Saggau, W., et al.: Ruptured aneurysms of the sinus of Valsalva. Ann. Thorac. Surg. *42*:81, 1986.
73. Liberthson, R. R., Sagar, K., Berkoben, J. P., et al.: Congenital coronary arteriovenous fistula: Report of 13 patients, review of the literature and delineation of management. Circulation *59*:849, 1979.
74. Dines, D. E., Seward, J. B., and Bernatz, P. E.: Pulmonary arteriovenous fistula. Mayo Clin. Proc. *58*:176, 1983.
75. Wong, L. B., and Perloff, J. K.: Familial occurrence of congenital pulmonary arteriovenous fistulae in octogenarian siblings. Am. J. Cardiol. *62*:1149, 1988.
76. Campbell, M.: Natural history of ventricular septal defect. Br Heart J. *33*:246, 1971.
77. Corone, P., Doyon, F., Gaudeau, S., et al.: Natural history of ventricular septal defect: A study involving 790 cases. Circulation *55*:908, 1977.
78. Weidman, W. H., DuShane, J. W., and Ellison, R. C.: Clinical course in adults with ventricular septal defect. Circulation *56*:I-78, 1977.
79. Ellis, J. H. IV, Moodie, D. S., Sterba, R., and Gill, C. C.: Ventricular septal defect in the adult: Natural and unnatural history. Am. Heart J. *114*:115, 1987.
80. Otterstad, J. E., Nitter-Hauge, S., and Myhre, E.: Isolated ventricular septal defect in adults: Clinical and haemodynamic findings. Br. Heart J. *50*:343, 1983.
81. Wood, P.: Foreword. In Bedford, E. D., and Caird, F. L.: Valvular Diseases of the Heart in Old Age. Boston, Little, Brown, and Company, 1960.
82. Moe, D. G., and Guntheroth, W. G.: Spontaneous closure of uncomplicated ventricular septal defect. Am. J. Cardiol. *60*:674, 1987.
83. Ramaciotti, C., Keren, A., and Silverman, N. H.: Importance of (perimembranous) ventricular septal aneurysm in the natural history of isolated perimembranous ventricular septal defect. Am. J. Cardiol. *57*:268, 1986.

84. Shah, P., Singh, W.S.A., Rose, V., and Keith, J. D.: Incidence of bacterial endocarditis in ventricular septal defects. Circulation 34:127, 1966.

85. Abraham, K. A., Cherian, G., Rao, V. D., et al.: Tetralogy of Fallot in adults: A report on 147 patients. Am. J. Med. 66:811, 1979.

86. Bertranou, E. G., Blackstone, E. H., Hazelrig, J. B., et al.: Life expectancy without surgery in tetralogy of Fallot. Am. J. Cardiol. 42:458, 1978.

87. Perloff, J. K.: Late postoperative concerns in adults with congenital heart disease. Cardiovasc. Clin. 11:431, 1980.

88. Kan, J. S., White, R. I., Jr., Mitchell, S. E., and Gardner, T. S.: Percutaneous balloon valvuloplasty: A new method for treating congenital pulmonary valve stenosis. N Engl. J. Med. 307:540, 1982.

89. Mullins, C. E.: Pediatric and congenital therapeutic cardiac catheterization. Circulation 79:1153, 1989.

90. Stanger, P., Cassidy, S. C., Girod, D. A., et al.: Balloon pulmonary angioplasty: Results of the valvuloplasty and angioplasty of congenital anomalies registry. Am. J. Cardiol. 65:775, 1990.

91. Nishimura, R. A., Holmes, D. R., and Reeder, G. S.: Percutaneous balloon valvuloplasty. Mayo Clin. Proc. 65:198, 1990.

92. Sandor, G.G.S., Olley, P. M., Trusler, G. A., et al.: Long-term follow-up of patients after valvotomy for congenital valvular aortic stenosis in children. J. Thorac. Cardiovasc. Surg. 80:171, 1980.

93. Presbitero, P., Sommerville, J., Revel-Chion, R., and Ross, D.: Open aortic valvulotomy for congenital aortic stenosis: Late results. Br. Heart J. 47:26, 1982.

94. Hsieh, K., Keane, J. F., Nadas, A. S., et al.: Long-term follow-up of valvulotomy before 1968 for congenital aortic stenosis. Am. J. Cardiol. 58:338, 1986.

95. Jones, M., Barnhart, G. R., and Morrow, A. G.: Late results after operation for left ventricular outflow tract obstruction. Am. J. Cardiol. 50:569, 1982.

96. Choy, M., Beekman, R. H., Rocchini, A. P., et al.: Percutaneous balloon valvuloplasty for valvar aortic stenosis in infants and children. Am. J. Cardiol. 59:1010, 1987.

97. Helgason, H., Keane, J. F., Fellow, K. E., et al.: Balloon dilatation of the aortic valve: Studies in normal lambs and in children with aortic stenoses. J. Am. Coll. Cardiol. 9:816, 1987.

98. Danielson, G. K., and Fuster, V.: Surgical repair of Ebstein's anomaly. Ann. Surg. 196:499, 1982.

99. Westaby, S., Karp, R. B., Kirklin, J. W., et al.: Surgical treatment in Ebstein's malformation. Ann. Thorac. Surg. 34:388, 1982.

100. Driscoll, D. J., Mottram, C. D., and Danielson, G. K.: Spectrum of exercise intolerance in 45 patients with Ebstein's anomaly and observations on exercise tolerance in 11 patients after surgical repair. J. Am. Coll. Cardiol. 11:831, 1988.

101. Behz, P. R., and Bleslovsky, A.: Ebstein's anomaly: Sixteen years' experience with valve replacement without plication of the right ventricle. Thorax 39:8, 1984.

102. Hwang, B., Bowman, F., Malm, J., and Krongrad, E.: Surgical repair of congenitally corrected transposition of the great arteries: Results and follow-up. Am. J. Cardiol. 50:781, 1982.

103. Murphy, J. G., Gersh, B. J., McGoon, M. D., et al.: Long-term outcome of patients undergoing surgical repair of isolated atrial septal defect: Follow-up at 28-32 years. (In press.)

104. St. John Sutton, M. G., Tajik, A. J., and McGoon, D. C.: Atrial septal defect in patients 60 years or older: operative results and long-term postoperative follow-up. Circulation 64:402, 1981.

105. Meyer, R. A., Korfhagen, J. C., Covitz, W., and Kaplan, S.: Long-term follow-up study after closure of secundum atrial septal defect in children: An echocardiography study. Am. J. Cardiol. 50:143, 1982.

106. Steele, P. M., Fuster, V., Cohen, M., et al.: Isolated atrial septal defect with pulmonary vascular obstructive disease—long-term follow-up and prediction of outcome after surgical correction. Circulation 76:1037, 1987.

107. Bink-Boelkens, M. T., Velvis, H., Van der Heide, J. J., et al.: Dysrhythmias after atrial surgery in children. Am. Heart J. 106:125, 1983.

108. Bolens, M., and Friedli, B.: Sinus node function and conduction system before and after surgery for secundum atrial septal defect: an electrophysiologic study. Am. J. Cardiol. 53:1415, 1984.

109. Williams, W. G., Trusler, G. A., Kirklin, J. W., et al.: Early and late results of a protocol for simple transposition leading to an atrial switch (Mustard) repair. J Thorac. Cardiovasc. Surg. 45:717, 1988.

110. Turina, M., Siebenmann, R., Nussbaumer, P., and Senning, A.: Long-term outlook after atrial correction of transposition of the great arteries. J. Thorac. Cardiovasc. Surg. 95:828, 1988.

111. Musewe, N. N., Reisman, J., Benson, L. N., et al.: Cardiopulmonary adaptation at rest and during exercise ten years after Mustard atrial repair for transposition of the great arteries. Circulation 77:1055, 1988.

112. Parrish, M. D., Graham, T. P., Bender, H. W., et al.: Radionuclide angiographic evaluation of right and left ventricular function during exercise after repair of transposition of the great arteries. Circulation 67:178, 1983.

113. Ramsay, J. M., Venables, A. W., Kelly, M. J., and Kalff, V.: Right and left ventricular function at rest and with exercise after the Mustard operation for transposition of the great arteries. Br. Heart J. 51:364, 1984.

114. Katz, N. M., Blackstone, E. H., Kirklin, J. W., et al.: Late survival and symptoms after repair of tetralogy of Fallot. Circulation 65:403, 1982.

115. Fuster, V., McGoon, D.C., Kennedy, M. A., et al.: Long-term evaluation (12 to 22 years) of open heart surgery for tetralogy of Fallot. Am. J. Cardiol. 46:635, 1980.

116. Abe, T., Asai, Y., Sugiki, K., and Komatsu, S.: Reoperation after initial correction of tetralogy of Fallot. J. Cardiovasc. Surg. 26:568, 1985.

117. Zhao, H., Miller, D. C., Reitz, B. A., and Shumway, N. E.: Surgical repair of tetralogy of Fallot: Long-term follow-up with particular emphasis on late death and reoperation. J. Thorac. Cardiovasc. Surg. 89:204, 1985.

118. Hu, D.C.K., Seward, J. B., Puga, F. J., et al.: Total correction of tetralogy of Fallot at age 40 years or older: long-term follow-up. J. Am. Coll. Cardiol. 5:40, 1985.

119. Hughes, C. F., Lim, Y. C., Cartmill, T. B., et al.: Total intracardiac repair for tetralogy of Fallot in adults. Ann. Thorac. Surg. 43:634, 1987.

120. Jarmakani, J. M., Graham, T. P., and Canent, R. V.: Left heart function in children with tetralogy of Fallot before and after palliative or corrective surgery. Circulation 46:478, 1972.

121. Borow, K. M., Green, L. H., Castenada, A. R., and Keane, J. F.: Left ventricular function after repair of tetralogy of Fallot and its relationship to age of surgery. Circulation 61:1150, 1980.

122. Fisher, R. G., Moodie, D. S., Sterba, R., and Gill, C. G.: Patent ductus arteriosus in adults—long-term follow-up: Nonsurgical versus surgical treatment. J. Am. Coll. Cardiol. 8:280, 1986.

123. Koller, M., Rothlin, M., and Senning, A.: Coarctation of the aorta: Review of 362 operated patients. Long-term follow-up and assessment of prognostic variables. Eur. Heart J. 8:670, 1987.

124. Daniels, S. R., James, F. W., Loggie, J.M.H., and Kaplan, S.: Correlates of resting and maximal exercise systolic blood pressure after repair of coarctation of the aorta: A multivariate analysis. Am. Heart J. 113:349, 1987.

125. Presbitero, P., Demarie, D., Villani, M., et al.: Long-term results (15 to 30 years) of surgical repair of aortic coarctation. Br. Heart J. 57:462, 1987.

126. Liberthson, R. L., Pennington, D. G., Jacobs, M. L., and Daggett, W. M.: Coarctation of the aorta: Review of 234 patients and clarification of management problems. Am. J. Cardiol. 43:835, 1979.

127. Cohen, M., Fuster, V., Steele, P. M., et al.: Coarctation of the aorta: Long-term follow-up and prediction of outcome after surgical correction. Circulation 80:840, 1989.

128. Clarkson, P. M., Nicholson, M. R., Barratt-Boyes, B. G., et al.: Results after repair of coarctation of the aorta beyond infancy: A 10 to 28 year follow-up with particular reference to late systemic hypertension. Am. J. Cardiol. 51:1481, 1983.

129. Hesslein, P. S., McNamara, D. G., Morriss, M.J.H., et al.: Comparison of resection versus patch aortoplasty for repair of coarctation in infants and children. Circulation 64:164, 1981.

130. Celano, V., Pieroni, D. R., Morera, J. A., et al.: Two-dimensional echocardiographic examination of mitral valve abnormalities associated with coarctation of the aorta. Circulation 69:924, 1984.

131. Fontan, F., and Baudet, E.: Surgical repair of tricuspid atresia. Thorax 26:240, 1971.

132. de Leval, M. R., Kilner, P., Gewillig, M., and Bull, C.: Total cavopulmonary connection: A logical alternative to atriopulmonary connection for complex Fontan operations. Experimental studies and early clinical experience. J. Thorac. Cardiovasc. Surg. 96:682, 1988.

133. Girod, D. A., Fontan, F., Deville, C., et al.: Long-term results after the Fontan operation for tricuspid atresia. Circulation 75:605, 1987.

134. Matsuda, H., Kawashima, Y., Kishimoto, H., et al.: Problems with the modified Fontan operation for univentricular heart of the right ventricular type. Circulation 76(suppl II):1, 1987.

135. Barber, G., DiSessa, T., Child, J. S., et al.: Hemodynamic responses to isolated increments in heart rate by atrial pacing after a Fontan procedure. Am. Heart J. 115:837, 1988.

136. Humes, R. A., Mair, D. D., Porter, C. J., et al.: Results of the modified Fontan operation in adults. Am. J. Cardiol. 61:602, 1988.

137. Laks, H., Milliken, J. C., Perloff, J. K., et al.: Experience with the Fontan procedure. J. Thorac. Cardiovasc. Surg. 88:939, 1984.

MEDICAL MANAGEMENT OF CONGENITAL HEART DISEASE IN THE ADULT

138. Berman, W., Jr., Wood, S. C., Yabek, S. M., et al.: Systemic oxygen transport in patients with congenital heart disease. Circulation 75:360, 1987.

139. Tyndall, M. R., Teitel, D. F., Lutin, W. A., et al.: Serum erythropoietin levels in patients with congenital heart disease. J. Pediatr. 110:538, 1987.

140. Rosove, M. H., Perloff, J. K., Hocking, W. G., et al.: Chronic hypoxaemia and decompensated erythrocytosis in cyanotic congenital heart disease. Lancet 2:313, 1986.

141. Linderkamp, O., Klose, H. J., Betke, K., et al.: Increased blood viscosity in patients with cyanotic congenital heart disease and iron deficiency. J. Pediatrics 95:567, 1979.

142. Giddings, S. S., and Stockman, J. A.: Effect of iron deficiency on tissue oxygen delivery in cyanotic congenital heart disease. Am. J. Cardiol. 61:605, 1988.

143. Perloff, J. K., Rosove, M. H., Child, J. S., and Wright, G. B.: Adults with cyanotic congenital heart disease: Hematologic management. Ann. Intern. Med. 109:406, 1988.

144. Cottrill, C. M., and Kaplan, S.: Cerebral vascular accidents in cyanotic congenital heart disease. Am. J. Dis. Child. 125:484, 1973.

145. Bowyer, J. J., Busst, C. M., Denison, D. M., and Shinebourne, E. A.: Effect of long term oxygen treatment at home in children with pulmonary vascular disease. Br. Heart J. 55:385, 1986.

146. Suarez, C. R., Menendez, C. E., Griffin, A. J., et al.: Cyanotic congenital heart disease in children: Hemostatic disorders and relevance of molecular markers of hemostasis. Semin. Thromb. Hemost. 10:285, 1984.

147. Rosove, M. H., Hocking, W. G., Harwig, S. S., and Perloff, J. K.: Studies of beta-thromboglobulin, platelet factor 4, and fibrinopeptide A in eryth-

rocytosis due to cyanotic congenital heart disease. Thromb. Res. 29:225, 1983.

148. Gill, J. C., Wilson, A. D., Endres-Brooks, J., and Montgomery, R. R.: Loss of the largest von Willebrand factor multimers from the plasma of patients with congenital cardiac defects. Blood 67:758, 1986.

149. Henriksson, P., Várendh, G., and Lundström, N. R.: Haemostatic defects in cyanotic congenital heart disease. Br. Heart J. 41:23, 1979.

150. Ware, J. A., Reaves, W. H., Horak, J. K., and Solis, R. T.: Defective platelet aggregation in patients undergoing surgical repair of cyanotic congenital heart disease. Ann. Thorac. Surg. 36:289, 1983.

151. Ekert, H., Gilchrist, G. S., Stanton, R., and Hammond, D.: Hemostasis in cyanotic congenital heart disease. J. Pediatr. 76:221, 1970.

152. Ross, E. A., Perloff, J. K., Danovitch, G. M., et al.: Renal function and urate metabolism in late survivors with cyanotic congenital heart disease. Circulation 73:396, 1986.

153. Young, D.: Hyperuricemia in cyanotic congenital heart disease. Am. J. Dis. Child. 134:902, 1980.

154. Spear, G. S.: The glomerular lesion of cyanotic congenital heart disease. Bull. Johns Hopkins Hosp. 140:185, 1977.

155. German, D. C., and Holmes, E. W.: Hyperuricemia and gout. Med. Clin. North Am. 70:419, 1986.

156. Sietsema, K. E., Cooper, D. M., Perloff, J. K., et al.: Dynamics of oxygen uptake during exercise in adults with cyanotic congenital heart disease. Circulation 73:1137, 1986.

157. Sietsema, K. E., Cooper, D. M., Perloff, J. K., et al.: Control of ventilation during exercise in patients with central venous-to-systemic arterial shunts. J. Appl. Physiol. 64:234, 1988.

158. Carvalho, J. S., Belcher, P., and Knight, W. B.: Infection of modified Blalock shunts. Br. Heart. J. 58:287, 1987.

159. Watanakunakorn, C.: Changing epidemiology and newer aspects of infective endocarditis. Adv. Intern. Med. 22:21, 1977.

160. Pitkin, R. M., Perloff, J. K., Koos, B. J., and Beall, M. H.: Pregnancy and congenital heart disease. Ann. Intern. Med. 112:445, 1990.

161. Loscalzo, J.: Paradoxical embolization: Clinical presentation, diagnostic strategies, and therapeutic options. Am. Heart J. 112:141, 1986.

162. Esscher, E. B.: Congenital complete heart block in adolescence and adult life: A follow-up study. Eur. Heart J. 2:281, 1981.

163. Esscher, E. B.: Congenital complete heart block (review). Acta Paediatr. Scand. 70:131, 1981.

164. Michaelson, M., and Engle, M. A.: Congenital complete heart block: An internal study of the natural history. Cardiovasc. Clin. 4:85, 1972.

165. Waickman, L. A., Skorton, D. J., Varner, M. W., et al.: Ebstein's anomaly and pregnancy. Am. J. Cardiol. 53:357, 1984.

166. Isner, J. M., Donaldson, R. F., Fulton, D., et al.: Cystic medial necrosis in coarctation of the aorta. Circulation 75:689, 1987.

167. Steele, P. M., Fuster, V., Ritter, D. G., and McGoon, D. C.: Isolated coarctation of the aorta—long term operative results. In Engle, M. A., and Perloff, J. K. (eds.): Congenital Heart Disease After Surgery. New York, Yorke Medical Books, 1983.

168. Devitt, J. H., Noble, W. H., and Byrick, R. J.: A Swan-Ganz catheter related complication in a patient with Eisenmenger's syndrome. Anesthesiology 57:335, 1982.

169. Shime, J., Mocarski, E. J., Hastings, D., et al.: Congenital heart disease in pregnancy: Short- and long-term implications. Am. J. Obstet. Gynecol. 156:313, 1987.

170. Nora, J. J., and Nora, A. H.: Maternal transmissions of congenital heart diseases: New recurrence risk figures and the questions of cytoplasmic inheritance and vulnerability to teratogens. Am. J. Cardiol. 59:459, 1987.

171. Maron, B. J., Epstein, S. E., and Mitchell, J. H.: Sixteenth Bethesda Conference: Cardiovascular abnormalities in the athlete: Recommendations regarding eligibility for competition. J. Am. Coll. Cardiol. 6:1189, 1985.

172. Mitchell, J. H., Blomqvist, G., Haskell, W. L., et al.: Classification of sports. Am. J. Coll. Cardiol. 6:1189, 1985.

173. Barth, C. W., and Roberts, W. C.: Left main coronary artery originating from the right sinus of Valsalva and coursing between the aorta and pulmonary trunk. J. Am. Coll. Cardiol. 7:366, 1986.

174. Cheitlin, M. D., De Castro, C. M., and McAllister, H. A.: Sudden death as a complication of anomalous left coronary origin from the anterior sinus of Valsalva, a not so minor congenital anomaly. Circulation 50:780, 1974.

175. Maron, B. J., Roberts, W. C., McAllister, H. A., et al.: Sudden death in young athletes. Circulation 62:218, 1980.

176. Mark, A. L., Abboud, F. M., Schmidt, P. G., and Heistad, D. D.: Reflex vascular responses to left ventricular outflow obstruction and activation of ventricular baroreceptors in dogs. J. Clin. Invest. 52:1147, 1982.

177. James, F. W., Kaplan, S., Schwartz, D. C., et al.: Response to exercise in patients after total correction of tetralogy of Fallot. Circulation 54:671, 1976.

178. Garson, A., Gillette, P. C., Gutgesell, H. P., and McNamara, D. G.: Stress-induced ventricular arrhythmias after repair of tetralogy of Fallot. Am. J. Cardiol. 46:1006, 1980.

179. Driscoll, D. J., Danielson, O. K., Puga, F. J., et al.: Exercise tolerance and cardiorespiratory response to exercise after the Fontan operation for tricuspid atresia or functional single ventricle. J. Am. Coll. Cardiol. 7:1087, 1986.

180. Truesdell, S. C., Skorton, D. J., and Lauer, R. M.: Life insurance for children with cardiovascular disease. Pediatrics 77:687, 1986.

181. Manning, J. A.: Insurability and employability of young cardiac patients. In Engle, M. A. (ed.): Pediatric Cardiovascular Disease. Philadelphia, F. A. Davis Co., 1981.

182. Sillanpaa, M.: Social adjustment and functioning of chronically ill and impaired children and adolescents. Acta Paediatr. Scand. [Suppl] 340:1, 1987.

183. Rasof, B., Linde, L. M., and Dunn, O. J.: Intellectual development in children with congenital heart disease. Child. Dev. 38:1043, 1967.

184. Finly, K. H., Buse, S. T., Popper, R. W., et al.: Intellectual functioning of children with tetralogy of Fallot: Influence of open heart surgery and earlier palliative operations. J. Pediatr. 85:318, 1974.

185. Baer, P. E., Freedman, D. A., and Garson, A.: Longterm psychological follow-up of patients after corrective surgery for tetralogy of Fallot. J. Am. Acad. Child. Psychiatry 5:622, 1984.

186. Dickinson, D. F., and Sambrooks, J. E.: Intellectual performance in children after circulatory arrest with profound hypothermia in infancy. Arch. Dis. Child. 54:1, 1979.

186. Stark, J.: Do we really correct congenital heart defects? J. Thorac. Cardiovasc. Surg. 97:1, 1989.

CARDIAC SURGICAL CONSIDERATIONS IN ADULTS WITH CONGENITAL HEART DISEASE

187. Grossman, W.: Cardiac hypertrophy: Useful adaptation or pathologic process? Am. J. Med. 69:576, 1980.

188. Zak, R., Kizu, A., and Bugaisay, L.: Cardiac hypertrophy: its characteristics as a growth process. Am. J. Cardiol. 44:941, 1979.

189. Zak, R.: Cell proliferation during cardiac growth. Am. J. Cardiol. 31:211, 1973.

190. Anversa, P., Ricci, R., and Olivetti, G.: Quantitative structural analysis of the myocardium during physiologic growth and induced cardiac hypertrophy: A review. J. Am. Coll. Cardiol. 7:1140, 1986.

191. Ghani, Q. P., and Hollenberg, M.: Poly-adenosine biphosphate ribose metabolism and regulation of myocardial cell growth by oxygen. Biochem. J. 170:378, 1978.

192. Hathaway, D. R., and March, K. L.: Molecular cardiology: New avenues for the diagnosis and treatment of cardiovascular disease. J. Am. Coll. Cardiol. 13:265, 1989.

193. Cutilleta, A. F., Bowell, R. T., Rudnik, M., et al.: Regression of myocardial hypertrophy: I. Experimental model, changes in heart weight, nucleic acids and collagen. J. Mol. Cell. Cardiol. 7:67, 1975.

194. Simon, A. B., and Zloto, A. E.: Coarctation of the aorta: Longitudinal assessment of operated patients. Circulation 50:456, 1974.

195. Nanton, M. A., and Olley, P. M.: Residual hypertension after coarctectomy in children. Am. J. Cardiol. 37:769, 1976.

196. Hislop, A., and Reid, L. M.: Intrapulmonary arterial development during fetal life—branching pattern and structure. J. Anat. 113:35, 1972.

197. Pollock, J. C., Jamieson, M. P., and McWilliams, R.: Somatosensory evoked potentials in the detection of spinal chord ischemia in aortic coarctation repair. Ann. Thorac. Surg. 41:251, 1986.

198. Horowitz, L. N., Alexander, J. A., and Edmunds, L. H.: Postoperative right bundle branch block: Identification of three levels of block. Circulation 62:319, 1980.

199. Bharati, S., and Lev, M.: Sequelae of atriotomy on the endocardium, conduction system and coronary arteries. In Engle, M. A., and Perloff, J. K. (eds.): Congenital Heart Disease After Surgery, New York, Yorke Medical Books, 1983.

200. Miller, A. J., Pick, R., and Katz, L. N.: Ventricular endomyocardial change after impairment of cardiac lymph flow in dogs. Br. Heart. J. 25:182, 1963.

Acquired Heart Disease in Infancy and Childhood

by WILLIAM F. FRIEDMAN, M.D.

Because many of the topics discussed in this chapter are given more substantial coverage elsewhere in this text, the emphasis herein is placed on features of acquired heart disease that are relatively unique to or common in infancy and childhood, although the disease processes per se may not recognize age-related boundaries. Acute rheumatic fever and rheumatic heart disease are discussed in Chapter 56. The hyperlipidemias are discussed in Chapter 37.

NONRHEUMATIC INFLAMMATORY DISEASE

INFECTIVE MYOCARDITIS
(See also Chap. 43)

Infectious processes that cause inflammatory disease of the heart may occur at any age, including fetal life. Causative agents include viruses, rickettsiae, bacteria, spirochetes, fungi, protozoa, and helminths. As a general rule, few of the generalized illnesses caused by these agents feature significant involvement of the heart. Myocardial involvement may be demonstrated histologically, but in most cases little or no expression of cardiac inflammation is detected clinically. Important exceptions are infections caused by certain viruses, diphtheria, and trypanosomes; these are discussed individually below.

VIRAL MYOCARDITIS. Coxsackie B and rubella viruses are the most common causative agents in infective myocarditis of the newborn. The rubella embryopathy and its associated cardiovascular malformations are discussed on page 888. Active *rubella myocarditis* occurs in utero, and may cause varying degrees of myocardial damage.[1] Invariably, however, other cardiovascular manifestations of the rubella syndrome dominate the clinical picture.

Coxsackie B typically causes outbreaks of epidemic myocarditis but may occur in the isolated infant in the newborn nursery, commonly with a fatal outcome.[2,3] The illness is of sudden onset, and is characterized by fever, tachycardia, signs of systemic hypoperfusion, cyanosis, and, occasionally, cardiac failure. In some infants signs and symptoms of encephalomyelitis and hepatitis predominate. The diagnosis is suggested by electrocardiographic findings of atrial and/or ventricular arrhythmias, generalized ST-segment and T-wave changes, and low-voltage QRS complexes, accompanied by the appearance of marked generalized cardiomegaly and pulmonary vascular congestion on the chest roentgenogram. Echocardiography reveals dilatation of both ventricles and depressed indices of cardiac performance. Echocardiography is especially helpful in excluding congenital cardiac struc-

tural anomalies. The diagnosis is strongly suggested or confirmed when the virus can be isolated from pericardial fluid, pharyngeal secretions, or feces, and when elevations occur in type-specific–neutralizing, hemagglutination-inhibiting, or complement-fixing antibody.[4] Digitalis, diuretics, and general supportive measures are of limited benefit. Although increased sensitivity to the toxic effects of the glycosides is common, digitalis should be administered cautiously and continued until heart size is normal, since cardiac failure may recur when the drug is discontinued.

Numerous viral agents have been identified as a cause of myocarditis in childhood beyond infancy.[5–7] The most common are Coxsackie A and B (Fig. 33–1), influenza, adenovirus, and ECHO virus. Moreover, myocarditis, usually of mild degree, may be associated with the common viral infectious diseases of childhood, including mumps, measles, infectious mononucleosis, varicella, and variola. Although the diagnosis usually is one of exclusion, it may be suggested by the presence of sustained tachycardia out of proportion to fever, cardiomegaly without significant murmurs, poor-quality heart sounds, a gallop rhythm, an unexplained arrhythmia, and the electrocardiographic findings already mentioned. Radionuclide gallium-67 scanning of the heart, showing a dense gallium uptake, provides suggestive evidence of active myocarditis.[8] Although endomyocardial biopsy is a reasonably safe procedure in infants, children, and adolescents, a poor correlation exists between clinical and endomyocardial biopsy diagnoses of acute myocarditis in these age-groups.[9–11a] Important differential diagnostic possibilities include endocardial fibroelastosis, glycogen storage disease with cardiac involvement, anomalous pulmonary origin of a coronary artery, critical aortic stenosis in infancy, and coarctation of the aorta or hypoplastic left heart syndromes.

The vast majority of these children recover from the acute episode of myocarditis with few or no sequelae. The results of treating patients with antiviral therapy or with immunosuppresants and antiinflammatory drugs have been disappointing.[11,12,12a] Some patients may retain a permanent conduction defect or mild cardiac enlargement as a result of the acute illness. Moreover, a child may progress from the acute episode to a chronic dilated cardiomyopathy, characterized by signs of left ventricular dysfunction and mitral valve insufficiency. Unfortunately there are no predictive criteria to identify the latter situation.[13] Cardiac transplantation has been successful in some of these children with cardiomyopathy and a chronic, relentless, and refractory course of heart failure. However, cardiac transplantation in children, especially in infants or very young children, is complicated by growth suppression related to the required corticosteriod doses, and the complex-

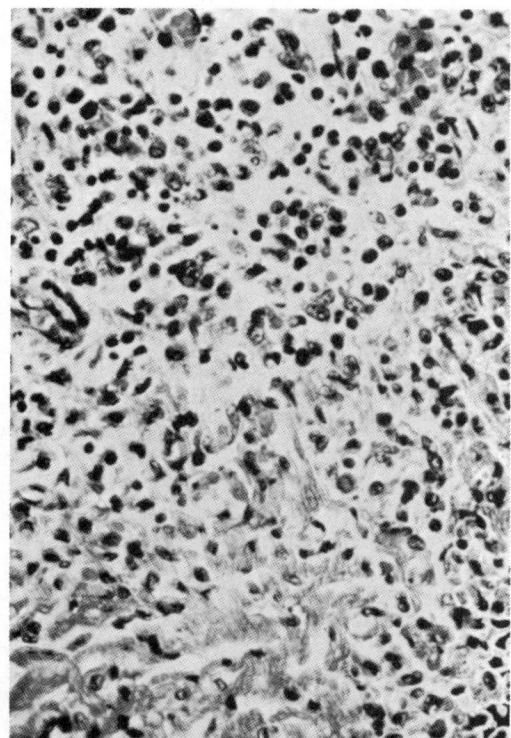

FIGURE 33-1. Photomicrograph of Coxsackie B₂ viral myocarditis. The major features are myocardial necrosis, edema, and heavy infiltrate of lymphocytes and large mononuclear cells. (×400.)(From Gore, I., and Kline, I. K.: Pericarditis and myocarditis. *In* Gould, S. E. (ed.): Pathology of the Heart and Blood Vessels. 3rd ed. Springfield, Ill., Charles C Thomas, 1968, p. 740.)

ity and severity of the immunosuppression in these infection-prone age groups.

DIPHTHERITIC CARDIOMYOPATHY. Diphtheria usually occurs in unimmunized children, especially in the western United States. Cardiac involvement is the result of the bacterial endotoxin rather than cardiac invasion by the bacillus.[14] Cardiac dysfunction appears to be related to abnormal fat metabolism, since diphtheria toxin causes marked depletion of myocardial carnitine, a cofactor required for the beta-oxidation of fats.[15] Thus, what was formerly designated a form of myocarditis is now considered an acute metabolic cardiomyopathy. The pathology includes extensive intracellular fat vacuolization and glycogen depletion. Plasma carnitine deficiencies have also been found in children with other forms of dilated cardiomyopathy.[16]

Cardiac involvement occurs in about 10 per cent of affected patients and is the most common cause of death from this disease. Heart disease is most reliably indicated by electrocardiographic changes, which range from ST-segment and T-wave changes to arrhythmias and conduction disturbances, including complete heart block.[17] Occasionally, the electrocardiographic pattern of myocardial infarction may emerge. The electrocardiogram is a fair indicator of the extent of myocardial involvement and of prognosis. The latter usually is favorable if only ST-segment and T-wave changes are observed in the absence of conduction system disturbances. Right or left bundle branch block and complete atrioventricular block are associated with mortality rates of 50 to 80 per cent. The electrocardiographic findings may be accompanied by evidence of myocardial dysfunction and ventricular chamber dilatation on cardiac ultrasound.

Treatment of diphtheritic cardiomyopathy usually is unsatisfactory. All patients should receive diphtheria antitoxin and intravenous penicillin after appropriate skin testing. Although corticosteroids have been used in the treatment of the myocardial problem, their value is debatable. Digitalis, diuretics, and antiarrhythmic medications usually are indicated. Parenteral adminstration of carnitine has been found to partially reverse diphtheritic cardiac dysfunction and reduce the risk of cardiac death.[18] This observation requires confirmation. If the child recovers from the acute episode of diphtheritic cardiomyopathy, the prognosis is quite good.

MYOCARDITIS CAUSED BY TRYPANOSOMAL INFECTION. Chagas' disease (p. 1432) is a chronic parasitosis caused by *Trypanosoma cruzi*, transmitted to humans by the bite of insects in the reduviid family. In the United States the disease is seen mostly in the southern states; endemic infection occurs in Latin America. Its most important clinical manifestation is a late-developing, chronic myocarditis and, much less frequently, an early acute myocarditis that is fatal in up to 10 per cent of cases.[19] In patients who survive the acute stage, cardiomyopathy may occur after an interval of 10 to 30 years.[20] Diagnosis of the acute illness is supported by findings of edema and adenitis in the region of the insect bite, associated with low-grade intermittent fever, sweating, muscle pain, and, at times, diarrhea and vomiting; weeks or months later cardiomegaly, gallop rhythm, and conduction disturbances may be noted. Xenodiagnosis (examination of the excreta of laboratory-bred insects fed on the patient) or complement-fixation tests provide confirmation. Endomyocardial biopsy reveals mitochondrial, nuclear, and cell membrane abnormalities early in the myocardial degenerative process. Late stages are characterized by severe myofibrillar lysis and variable amounts of fibrous tissue and cellular infiltrates.[21] There is no satisfactory treatment. Prophylaxis consists of control of the carrier of the parasites, reduviid bugs, by benzene hexachloride. A nitrofuran compound, nifurtinox, appears effective in the acute stage of infection, but not during the intracellular parasitic infection period.[22]

Trypanosoma rhodesiense, which causes African sleeping sickness, may also produce myocardial hemorrhage, interstitial edema, mononuclear infiltration, and myocardial degeneration.[23] Cardiac involvement is usually relatively mild, and the clinical picture is dominated by evidence of encephalitis.

MYOCARDITIS CAUSED BY HUMAN IMMUNODEFICIENCY VIRUS (see also p. 1427). In infants and children, the cardiac complications of the acquired immunodeficiency syndrome (AIDS) range from incidental microscopic inflammatory findings at necropsy to clinically significant, extensive, and chronic cardiac dysfunction.[24,25] In most patients infected with the human immunodeficiency virus (HIV), the virus appears to have been transmitted from mother to child; other routes of transmission include contaminated blood products. Older children or adolescents also can be infected by routes more commonly associated with adults, such as sharing needles used for the injection of drugs, and sexual activity.

Cardiovascular abnormalities have been observed in as many as 65 per cent of infants or children with AIDS, whether induced by opportunistic infection or by the HIV infection itself.[25] As the prevalence of AIDS escalates, it is predictable that the cardiac involvement in infants and children with this disease will become better defined. Ventricular dysfunction, pericardial effusion, dilated cardiomyopathy, and rhythm disturbances (including high-grade atrial and ventricular ectopy and sudden death) provide evidence that HIV infection may have multiple direct or indirect effects on the heart. The latter may be due to infection with a variety of opportunistic organisms as well as to toxins, drugs, and autoimmunity. Other possible contributors to the cardiomyopathy include the myocardial depressant action of overwhelming noncardiac infection, the hypoxic and ischemic influence of severe lung disease, renal failure, autonomic dysfunction, chronic anemia, malnutrition, elevated endogenous catecholamines, vasoactive substances related to stress, and therapeutic interventions, including the use of steroids. Serial noninvasive assessment of this patient population, particularly by echocardiography, will, it is hoped, enable early or even anticipatory medical therapy, improving the cardiovascular status of children with HIV infection.

Numerous infectious agents may be responsible for infective pericarditis. Viral and tuberculous inflammatory pericardial disease are discussed in detail in Chap. 45. Of special concern in infancy and childhood is disease caused by pyogenic bacteria.[26,27] Purulent pericarditis occurs most often in the first two decades of life, and is especially common in children under 6 years of age. Acute bacterial pericarditis usually is fatal if misdiagnosed or incorrectly treated. The most common pathogens are *Staphylococcus aureus, Streptococcus pneumoniae, Haemophilus influenzae,* and *Neisseria meningitides.* Unusual organisms that cause purulent pericarditis include *Escherichia coli, Pseudomonas, Salmonella, Klebisella, Proteus,* and *Bacteroides. H. influenzae,* in particular, affects infants and young children, usually in association either with upper respiratory tract infection and croup, with lower respiratory tract pneumonia, bronchitis, or, occasionally, with meningitis.

Presenting clinical signs and symptoms vary, depending on the age of the patient, the responsible organism, and the site(s) of associated infection. The latter two require identification if therapy is to be effective. Fever, tachycardia, dyspnea, and chest pain are invariably present. Pericardial exudate resulting from the acute suppurative process commonly produces signs of life-threatening cardiac tamponade. Physical findings suggestive of purulent pericarditis include neck vein distention and hepatomegaly, pulsus paradoxus, and/or systemic hypotension with a narrow pulse pressure, muffled and distant heart sounds, marked cardiomegaly, and a point of maximal cardiac impulse well within the area of percussed dullness. Although the presence of a pericardial friction rub clearly points to pericardial involvement, this sign occurs infrequently.

An enlarged, globular cardiac configuration on chest x-ray and electrocardiographic findings of diminished QRS amplitude and abnormalities of the ST segment (usually elevated) and T waves (often inverted) usually focus attention on the pericardium. Echocardiographic evaluation (p. 102) is reliable for establishing the diagnosis of significant pericardial effusion and for directing and guiding pericardiocentesis.[28] Culture and examination of pericardial fluid obtained by pericardiocentesis are essential for diagnosis and treatment. Unless effective surgical drainage is combined with antibiotic treatment, the mortality rate is high. Operation should consist of creation of a subxiphoid pericardial window with placement of a drainage tube, or anterior pericardiectomy with tube drainage.[29] Early aggressive diagnosis and treatment reduce the risk of death substantially (10 to 20 per cent). Pericardial constriction is uncommon, but all patients should be followed carefully for this complication.

POSTPERICARDIOTOMY SYNDROME (see also p. 1688)

In the first year after cardiac operation in which the pericardium is opened, and seldom in the second or third postoperative year, a febrile illness may occur, consisting of a pericardial and pleural inflammatory reaction with effusion and often with pulmonary parenchymal involvement. The illness occurs in about 35 per cent of children undergoing pericardiotomy and usually is self-limiting; infants undergoing open-heart surgery are seldom affected. It is characterized by fever; chest, neck, or shoulder pain that becomes worse with inspiration; anorexia; and laboratory findings of leukocytosis and an elevated erythrocyte sedimentation rate.[30] Recurrences are uncommon and usually mild. Physical, electrocardiographic, and roentgenographic signs of pericardial involvement vary with the magnitude of the effusion. Echocardiographic detection of the effusion is common between 4 and 10 days postoperatively.[31] Cardiac tamponade, although not usual, occurs with sufficient frequency to warrant careful observation of the patient.

Viral infection and an autoimmune reaction have been implicated in the pathogenesis. Serum antibodies and a rise in titer frequently are found against adenovirus, Coxsackie virus, and cytomegalovirus. Elevations in levels of heart-reactive antibody are common.

An association recently has been shown between antinuclear antibodies, which are immunoglobulins directed toward antigenic nuclear material, and postpericardiotomy syndrome.[32]

The syndrome must be distinguished from infective endocarditis and the postperfusion syndrome of atypical lymphocytosis and hepatosplenomegaly, which occurs about 3 to 6 weeks after extracorporeal circulation and is caused by cytomegalovirus infection.[33]

Treatment of the postpericardiotomy syndrome depends on the degree of patient discomfort and the magnitude of pericardial and/or pleural effusion. In some patients signs of cardiac tamponade will require pericardiocentesis. Bed rest and salicylates or indomethacin lessen patient discomfort and diminish the production of pleural or pericardial fluid. Corticosteroids are indicated for severe illness and promptly relieve fever and symptoms. Antibiotics are not useful in the treatment. Prolonged therapy is seldom necessary because of the self-limited nature of this postoperative complication. Late or recurrent tamponade, although rare, may require reinstitution of treatment.[34]

PRIMARY CARDIOMYOPATHIES
(See also Chap. 43)

The important *nonobstructive* cardiomyopathies, of special concern in infants and children, are the familial forms of endocardial fibroelastosis,[35-40] which afflict many of the patients also designated as having *dilated (congestive) cardiomyopathy.*[41-44] By definition, this diagnostic term excludes patients whose myocardial dysfunction is caused by infection, a congenital cardiac anomaly, or increased preload or afterload.[46] Dilated (congestive) cardiomyopathy often is a disease of infants, with most cases becoming manifested before the age of 1 year, with a history of respiratory or diarrheal illness preceding the onset of cardiac symptoms. Most severely ill patients probably have endocardial fibroelastosis, although the latter can be confirmed definitely only after myocardial biopsy or autopsy. Beyond age 2 years, dilated cardiomyopathy, like the condition in adults, is characterized by an unobstructed, dilated, and poorly contracting left ventricle. For this group of children, debate also exists as to whether endocardial fibroelastosis should be categorized as a separate entity under dilated or congestive cardiomyopathy, and whether it is an end stage of dilated cardiomyopathy of *any* cause.[45] In children with the clinical picture of dilated cardiomyopathy, a poor outcome is anticipated by a reduced left ventricular shortening fraction, a familial incidence of cardiomyopathy, and the presence of endocardial fibroelastosis. The overall mortality of dilated cardiomyopathy exceeds 30 per cent, the vast majority of fatal cases occurring during the first episode of cardiac failure.

ENDOCARDIAL FIBROELASTOSIS (EFE). Various designations have been applied to this condition, including endocardial sclerosis, fetal endocarditis, fetal endomyocardial fibrosis, and elastic tissue hyperplasia.[35] In recent years familial cases have been encountered more commonly than has the isolated form. The data provided by family studies fit neither an autosomal recessive nor a multifactorial mode of inheritance. Although the reasons are obscure, a marked reduction has been observed in the past decade of isolated, nonfamilial EFE. No definite cause for this condition has been established, although a host of theories have been proposed; inadequate subendocardial blood flow and/or prenatal or postnatal inflammation or infection currently are considered the most likely pathogenetic pathways.[37,45]

A distinction has been made between primary EFE, in which there is no cardiac malformation, and EFE secondary to congenital malformations of the heart.[38] In the *secondary* variety, focal areas of opaque fibroelastotic thickening of the mural endocardium or cardiac valves are observed in association with cardiac malformations. Underlying cardiovascular anomalies are almost always obstructive lesions, particularly of the left side of the heart, and these create cardiac hypertrophy and an imbalance in the myocardial oxygen supply-demand relation. Thus, secondary EFE quite commonly occurs in aortic stenosis, coarctation of the aorta, and hypoplastic left heart syndrome.

This discussion focuses on the *primary* form of EFE, which invariably involves the left ventricle and mitral and aortic valves without significant associated cardiac defects.

Although the use of the term "primary" implies that this form of EFE is a specific disease entity, most would agree that it is the end result of many different diseases.[45,46] Further, as already discussed, no clear separation exists clinically between primary EFE and dilated cardiomyopathy. Primary EFE commonly produces a marked dilatation of the left ventricle; rarely, a "contracted" type of primary EFE is observed, in which the left ventricle is relatively hypoplastic or normal in size. In the latter situation the right and left atria and the right ventricle are markedly enlarged and hypertrophied, with minimal or no endocardial sclerosis. In the common, dilated type of primary EFE, microthrombi may be found adherent to the endocardium. The diffuse endocardial hyperplasia may be several millimeters thick (Fig. 33–2). The aortic

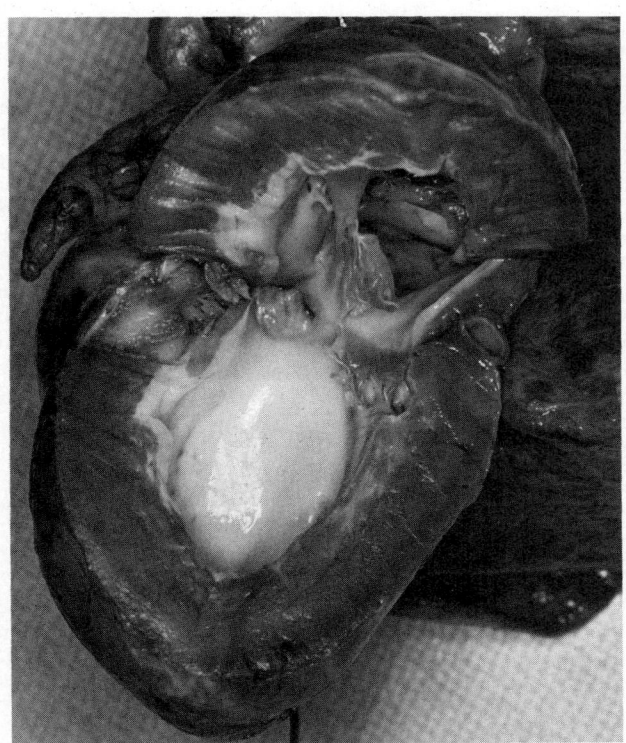

FIGURE 33-2. Diffuse left ventricular endocardial fibroelastosis. There is myocardial hypertrophy and obliteration of the papillary muscles as well as encroachment of the sclerotic subendocardial process onto the base of the aortic cusps. (From Tingelstaad, J. B., et al.: The electrocardiogram in the contracted type of primary endocardial fibroelastosis. Am. J. Cardiol. *27*:304, 1971.)

and mitral valve leaflets are thickened and distorted; mitral regurgitation is especially common. The papillary muscles and chordae tendineae are involved in the fibroelastic process and are shortened and distorted.

Primary EFE is a disease of infancy; symptoms usually develop between 2 and 12 months of age, although rarely they may be present shortly after birth. Clinical features reflect left ventricular dysfunction and congestive heart failure.[47,48] Noted initially are fatigue and breathlessness during feeding, failure to thrive, irritability, pallor, increased sweating, peripheral cyanosis, cough, wheezing, or grunting. Symptoms usually are rapidly progressive. Examination of the infant reveals tachycardia, cardiomegaly, a gallop rhythm, and hepatosplenomegaly. Cardiac murmurs may be absent; about 40 per cent of infants have the characteristic apical systolic murmur of mitral regurgitation.

Chest roentgenography reveals marked, generalized cardiomegaly with normal or congested pulmonary vascular markings. A typical electrocardiographic finding is left ventricular hypertrophy with inverted T waves in the left precordial leads; less common are tracings suggestive of myocardial infarction, varying degrees of atrioventricular block, and arrhythmias. Echocardiographic features include an increase in left atrial and left ventricular dimensions, reduced left ventricular septal and posterior wall motion, reduced ejection fraction, and abnormal mitral valve motion.[46,49] Dense echoes along the endocardium of the left ventricle are a diagnostic clue.

The *diagnosis* of primary EFE usually is made easily by the characteristic clinical findings but is, nonetheless, one of exclusion. Differential diagnosis includes anomalous pulmonary origin of the left coronary artery, myocarditis, hypertrophic obstructive cardiomyopathy, anomalies that cause left ventricular outflow tract obstruction, and glycogen storage disease of the heart. The first four of these entities differ appreciably from fibroelastosis in their electrocardiographic or echocardiographic features; the skeletal muscle biopsy in glycogen storage disease is diagnostic.

Hemodynamic studies reveal evidence of left ventricular dysfunction.[46a] This includes elevations in left ventricular end-diastolic and left atrial pressures, moderate pulmonary hypertension, widened arteriovenous oxygen differences, and reduced left ventricular stroke volume and cardiac output. Angiography usually demonstrates a markedly dilated left ventricle, a reduced ejection fraction, and varying degrees of mitral regurgitation. The configuration of the left ventricular chamber usually is globular or spherical; dyskinetic or akinetic patterns of contraction are uncommon. Endomyocardial biopsy shows a diagnostic invasion of the endocardium and subendocardium by fibroelastic tissue.[9-11,11a,50,51] The *contracted form* of primary EFE produces a clinical picture of left-sided obstructive disease, particularly if the mitral valve is small. Left atrial pressure is elevated, with pulmonary artery pressures at or near systemic arterial levels.

The optimal management of patients with primary EFE consists of early and prolonged treatment with digitalis. Glycoside therapy should be continued for many years after the disappearance of symptoms, since cessation of the drug may result in acute cardiac failure, even when the heart size has returned to normal. The results of pericardial poudrage and mitral valve replacement in seriously afflicted infants have been disappointing. Cardiac transplantation may be recommended, although the survival data for this approach have not been impressive for infants and children with cardiomyopathies.[44]

SECONDARY CARDIOMYOPATHIES

The designation "secondary" cardiomyopathy refers to intrinsic myocardial disease that is secondary to or associated with systemic disease or diseases of other organs or in other systems. Myocardial diseases coexisting with collagen vascular disorders (Chap. 56), neuromuscular disorders (Chap. 60), neoplasms (Chap. 57), acute glomerulonephritis (Chap. 62), and thalassemia (Chap. 57) are discussed elsewhere in this text. Additional secondary cardiomyopathies of special interest to those caring for infants and children are those seen in infants of diabetic mothers, and associated with glycogen storage disease, neonatal thyrotoxicosis, infantile beriberi, protein-calorie malnutrition, tropical endomyocardial fibrosis, anthracycline toxicity, and the mucocutaneous lymph node syndrome. Attention is directed to each of these latter disorders.

CARDIOMYOPATHY IN INFANTS OF DIABETIC MOTHERS

Infants born of diabetic mothers are exposed to chronic hyperinsulinism in utero and to reactive hypoglycemia after birth. Such infants occasionally display two basic forms of cardiomyopathy, both of which usually are transient.[52-55] Evidence exists that suboptimal metabolic control of maternal diabetes during pregnancy increases the incidence of these abnormalities.[55] In some of these infants, hypertrophy and hyperplasia of myocardial cells constitute a diffuse process, producing reversible signs and symptoms that resemble those of congestive cardiomyopathy. In other infants, the clinical findings are indistinguishable from those of hypertrophic obstructive cardiomyopathy.[56] The natural history in this latter group has been one of gradual spontaneous regression within 1 to 12 months of obstructive murmurs, cardiomegaly, and electrocardiographic and echocardiographic abnormalities typical of hypertrophic obstructive cardiomyopathy.

GLYCOGEN STORAGE DISEASE

Glycogen storage disease is the result of a deficiency of one or more of the enzymes involved in the biosynthesis and degradation of glycogen. The heart is importantly involved in type II (Pompe's disease), which results from a deficiency of alpha-1, 4-glucosidase (acid maltase), a lysosomal enzyme that hydrolyzes glycogen into glucose.[57] This disease is a heredi-

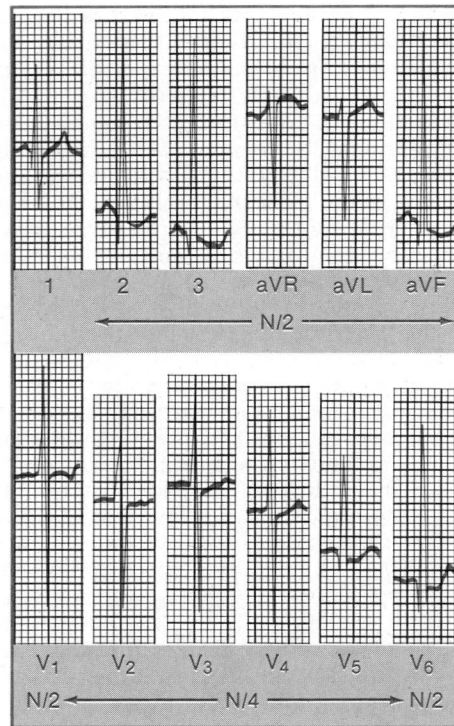

FIGURE 33-3. Electrocardiogram of an infant with glycogen storage disease showing a short PR interval and left ventricular hypertrophy.

tary error of metabolism transmitted through a single recessive gene. Generalized glycogenesis takes place, occurring especially in the heart, the skeletal muscles, and the liver. The glycogen within cardiac muscle cells is biochemically normal but is present in excessive amounts, both within lysosomes and free in the cytoplasm.[57] As a result, the heart enlarges, often to a marked degree, and congestive heart failure supervenes. Glycogen deposition within the myocardium usually is uniform, although occasionally the interventricular septum is especially involved, producing subpulmonic obstruction or a constellation of features indistinguishable from hypertrophic obstructive cardiomyopathy. Selective angiography has revealed a distinctive trabeculation of the left ventricle in some infants.[58]

Clinical signs of type II glycogen storage disease usually become prominent in the early neonatal period.[59,59a] Characteristic symptoms include failure to thrive, progressive hypotonia, lethargy, and a weak cry. Prominent early features include nonspecific cardiac murmurs, cardiomegaly, signs of congestive heart failure, macroglossia, poor skeletal muscle tone, and weakness. The electrocardiogram shows extremely tall, broad QRS complexes with a short P-R interval (commonly less than 0.09 sec) (Fig. 33-3).

The short P-R interval may be the result of facilitated atrioventricular conduction owing to myocardial glycogen deposition. Less often, deep Q waves are observed over the mid or left precordium as well as T-wave inversion and ST-segment elevation. Chest roentgenograms show an enlarged globular heart associated with pulmonary vascular congestion (Fig. 33-4). In rare patients with cardiac glycogenosis the cardiac murmur suggests left ventricular outflow tract obstruction and/or mitral regurgitation; the echocardiographic, hemodynamic, and angiographic features in this subgroup are indistinguishable from those in infants with hypertrophic obstructive cardiomyopathy. Diagnosis is confirmed by demonstrating the enzymatic deficiency in lymphocytes, skeletal muscle, or liver. Skeletal muscle biopsy reveals histological and histochemical evidence of glycogen deposition.

Cardiac glycogenosis may be confused with other entities that cause cardiac failure in the early months of life, including endocardial fibroelastosis, anomalous pulmonary origin of the left coronary artery, fixed and dynamic forms of left ventricu-

lar outflow tract obstruction, coarctation of the aorta, and myocarditis. The short P-R interval and the skeletal muscle hypotonia in glycogen storage disease help to distinguish this disorder from *endocardial fibroelastosis*. Infants with an anomalous pulmonary origin of the *left coronary artery* usually have a distinctive electrocardiographic pattern of anterolateral myocardial infarction. In infants with *coarctation of the aorta* the pulse and blood pressure discrepancies between the upper and lower extremities point to the proper diagnosis (p. 967). *Myocarditis* usually is of abrupt onset in a previously healthy child and is not associated with marked hypotonia; the generally low-voltage electrocardiogram does not show the short P-R interval. The skeletal muscle hypotonia and the macroglossia in infants with glycogen storage disease occasionally raise the possibilities of amyotonia congenita and cretinism or mongolism, respectively.

Cardiac glycogenosis leads to progressive impairment of myocardial function; Pompe's disease is uniformly fatal, usually within the first year of life. Death quite often is the result of either cardiac failure or complications of respiratory management such as pneumonia or aspiration.

NEONATAL THYROTOXICOSIS

Thyroid-stimulating immunoglobulin traverses the placental barrier and stimulates the fetal thyroid gland when maternal hyperthyroidism exists.[60] Many infants are born prematurely or are small for gestational age. Jitteriness and irritability are noted early. Cardiac findings include tachycardia, bounding pulses, systolic hypertension, and a precordial systolic murmur. Congestive heart failure frequently is present, and the presenting finding occasionally is an episode of paroxysmal atrial tachycardia. A neonatal goiter may be observed, especially if the mother received iodine therapy during pregnancy.

Diagnosis should be anticipated whenever a history of hyperthyroidism exists in the mother. Neonatal thyrotoxicosis occurs in the offspring of about 1 to 2 per cent of these women. A maternal level of thyroid-stimulating immunoglobulin should be obtained before delivery in anticipation of the problem arising in the newborn infant, since high levels often are observed in both mother and offspring. The serum levels of thyroxine are increased in the newborn.

The infant who has heart failure may be treated with digitalis and propylthiouracil or carbamizole. The latter two drugs will not be completely effective for many weeks; a beta blocker usually is helpful in addition to these agents. Supportive measures such as sedation and minimal stimulation may be helpful. Exchange transfusion or corticosteroid treatment is of no proven benefit.

Infants usually improve between the second and third month of life, although lack of attention to the problem or inadequate therapy may result in a fatal outcome.

INFANTILE BERIBERI (see also p. 461)

Thiamine (vitamin B_1) deficiency mainly occurs in regions of Southeast Asia, India, Brazil, and Africa, in which the dietary staple is polished rice or

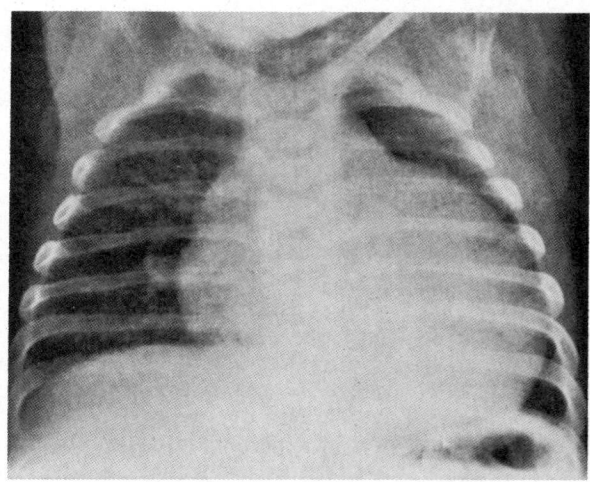

FIGURE 33-4. Chest roentgenogram of an infant with glycogen storage disease showing massive cardiomegaly and pulmonary edema. (From Taussig, H.: Congenital Malformations of the Heart. Vol. 2. 2nd ed. Boston, Commonwealth Fund, Harvard University, 1960, p. 901.)

cassava. Thiamine functions as a coenzyme in decarboxylation of alpha-keto acids and in the utilization of pentose in the hexose monophosphate shunt. A reduction in myocardial energy production causes symptoms in the infant, usually between 1 and 4 months of age, who is breastfed by a thiamine-deficient mother.[61] Such infants usually are edematous, irritable, pale, and anorectic. Hoarseness or aphonia is common, owing to involvement of the recurrent laryngeal nerve; blepharoptosis occurs in one-third of infants. Typically, cardiac involvement manifests as dilation of the right ventricle and prominent signs of systemic venous congestion. Electrocardiographic findings are nonspecific, and radiological findings principally consist of right ventricular dilatation. Infantile beriberi may be rapidly fatal but responds quickly and well to administration of thiamine (25 to 50 mg intravenously initially, with reduction of the dose to 10 mg/day for several days, and then orally for several weeks). Dramatic amelioration occurs within a few days of the cardiac findings. Cure is complete with no known sequelae.

PROTEIN-CALORIE MALNUTRITION (see also p. 1848)

This is a major public health problem in underdeveloped areas of the tropics.[62,63] In infants inadequate diet results in a state of emaciation termed "marasmus"; "kwashiorkor" is a designation applied to this syndrome in children beyond 1 year of age. The disease results from a deficiency of protein relative to calories, although the latter and other essential nutrients often are lacking as well. General muscle wasting, loss of subcutaneous fat, and atrophy of most organs, including the heart, are typical in marasmic infants. In both marasmus and kwashiorkor, thinning and atrophy of cardiac muscle fibers and interstitial edema or vacuolization of the myocardial fibers are noted.[64] As the condition progresses, listlessness becomes prominent. Cardiovascular collapse is easily precipitated in these infants by the stress of infection.

In both infancy and childhood the principal physical findings reflect systemic hypoperfusion and principally consist of hypothermia, hypotension, tachycardia, and low-amplitude peripheral arterial pulsations. Peripheral usually nonpitting edema is prominent, as are wasting of the skeletal musculature, exfoliative dermatitis, and gray or red discoloration of the hair. Changes seen on electrocardiogram and on radiographic examination are nonspecific.

Treatment should be directed at correction of fluid and electrolyte imbalance, eradication of infection, and management of such associated problems as anemia and parasitic infestation. Care is required in the correction of dehydration or severe anemia, since volume overload of the heart is easily produced. Supplements of potassium and magnesium often are required, and because of deficiencies in these elements, digitalis should probably be avoided or used with extreme caution. If the infant or child survives the initial phase, a well-balanced diet will effect an impressive recovery over several months' duration.

TROPICAL ENDOMYOCARDIAL FIBROSIS (see also p. 1422)

Endomyocardial fibrosis is a rare, acquired, progressive disease, usually involving children and young adults from Africa, Southeast Asia, and South America. This cardiomyopathy of unknown cause is characterized by focal endocardial fibrosis of one or, rarely, both ventricles.[65] Controversy exists as to whether or not endomyocardial fibrosis, which is not associated with eosinophilia, and Löffler's endocarditis with eosinophilia (Chap. 43) are the same disorder described from temperate climates.[66] Endocardial fibrosis is located almost exclusively in the inflow tracts of the ventricles, and commonly involves one or the other atrioventricular valve. Partial obliteration of either cardiac chamber results in reduced ventricular compliance with impairment of filling. The fibrotic process often involves the chordae tendineae, resulting in mitral and/or tricuspid regurgitation. Plaques of heaped-up fibrous tissue without elastic fibers are especially common within the left ventricle. Endomyocardial fibrosis involving the right ventricle may have to be differentiated from Ebstein's anomaly of the tricuspid valve (p. 940), and endomyocardial fibrosis involving the left ventricle may have to be differentiated from rheumatic mitral regurgitation.

When left ventricular disease predominates, the clinical findings often resemble those of mitral stenosis or regurgitation. When endocardial involvement of the right ventricle is more severe than that of the left ventricle, the patient usually presents with findings of markedly elevated systemic venous pressure and tricuspid regurgitation.

Treatment is supportive. Survival usually depends on the extent of endocardial and valvular involvement and is better when right ventricular disease predominates.[67] Mean survival after the onset of symptoms is about 24 months. Specific treatment does not exist, and corticosteroid therapy has not proved efficacious. Surgical excision (decortication) of affected tissue with prosthetic valve replacement has been associated with clinical improvement.[68] However, children most severely affected by this disease commonly reside in regions of the tropics and subtropics where cardiac surgery is not readily available.

The mucocutaneous lymph node syndrome in infancy (Kawasaki disease) was first described in Japan in 1967. Many thousands of cases from Japan have been reported, and the disorder is being recognized with increasing frequency in North America and Europe.[69]

The syndrome presents as a febrile illness in children that occurs before the age of 10 and usually before the age of 2 years. They commonly have fever and ocular and oral manifestations followed in 5 days by a rash and indurative edema of the hands and feet, with palmar and plantar erythema. Finally, after about 2 weeks, cutaneous desquamation occurs. Diagnostic criteria include (1) a fever lasting for 5 or more days that is unresponsive to antibiotics; (2) bilateral congestion of the ocular conjunctiva; (3) peripheral limb changes that include an indurative peripheral edema and erythema of the palms and feet, followed later in the course of the illness by a membranous desquamation of the fingertips; (4) changes in the lips and mouth, including dry, erythematous, and fissured lips, injected oropharyngeal mucosa, and a strawberry tongue; and (5) a polymorphous exanthema of the trunk without crusts or vesicles. Diagnosis is accepted when the first criterion and at least three of the remainder are present.

In addition to the mucous membrane and cutaneous effects, multiple organ system involvement has been noted. Noncardiovascular complications of the illness include arthritis, cerebrospinal fluid pleocytosis, pulmonary infiltrates, and hydrops of the gallbladder. The illness often is accompanied by cervical adenopathy, diarrhea, leukocytosis with a predominance of neutrophils, thrombocytosis, sterile pyuria and proteinuria, elevated liver transaminases, an elevation in the erythrocyte sedimentation rate and alpha$_2$-globulin, and a positive C-reactive protein.

An extensive search for the cause of Kawasaki disease has been unproductive. Multiple immunoregulatory abnormalities have been suggested to be involved in the pathogenesis of the illness.[70] Abnormalities include a T-cell lymphocytopenia, a decrease in CD8$^+$ T cells, increased numbers of activated CD4$^+$ lymphocytes, B-cell hyperactivity, and increased endothelial cell proliferation. Some hypothesize that a retrovirus with tropism for endothelial and lymphoid cells may be associated with the acute disease,[70] whereas others question the role of toxin-producing bacteria in pathogenesis, particularly streptococcal erythrogenic toxins.[71] Tumor necrosis factor, a polypeptide mediator secreted by activated macrophages and T lymphocytes, also has been viewed as a potential mediator of inflammation in this illness.[72]

On the basis of pathological data, progression of the disease may be divided into four stages.[73,74] In stage I, lasting for 1 to 9 days, acute perivasculitis of the small arteries is evident and involves the vasa vasorum of the major coronary arteries. Pericarditis, interstitial myocarditis, and endocardial inflammation also are seen; these changes chiefly consist of neutrophilic, eosinophilic, and lymphocytic infiltrations. In stage II, of 12 to 25 days' duration, panvasculitis involves the major coronary arteries. It affects the intima, media, and adventitia and results in aneurysm and thrombus formation. In stage III, of 28 to 31 days' duration, granulating thrombi and marked intimal thickening cause partial or total occlusion of the major coronary arteries. Stage IV follows and may be of many years' duration, during which healing occurs, consisting of scarring, calcification, and recanalization of occluded arteries.

The syndrome has an associated acute mortality of 1 to 3 per cent, secondary to complications from coronary artery involvement, myocarditis, or pericarditis, with a majority of deaths occurring in the third or fourth week of illness.[75] Other children may die later in life as a result of myocardial infarction.[76] Autopsy examination has almost uniformly demonstrated coronary arterial aneurysms, with occlusion caused by

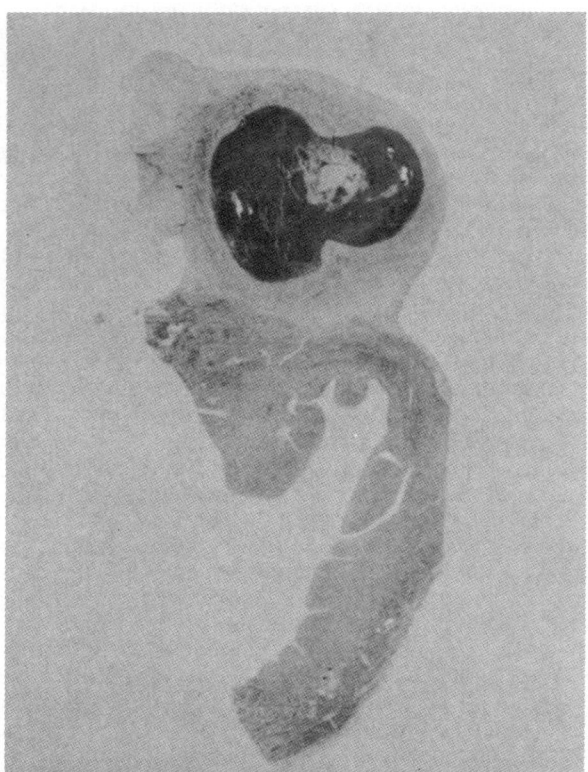

FIGURE 33–5. Low-power photomicrograph of a coronary artery aneurysm with recent occlusive thrombosis in a patient with mucocutaneous lymph node syndrome. (From Landing, B. H., and Larson, E. J.: Are infantile periarteritis nodosa with coronary artery involvement and fatal mucocutaneous lymph node syndrome the same? Comparison of 20 patients from North America with patients from Hawaii and Japan. Pediatrics 59:651, 1977. Copyright American Academy of Pediatrics, 1977.)

thromboendarteritis (Fig. 33–5). The spectrum of cardiovascular involvement is outlined in Table 33–1.

The disease often has been misdiagnosed in the United States as scarlet fever, Stevens-Johnson syndrome, Rocky Mountain spotted fever, rheumatoid arthritis, scleroderma, or lupus erythematosus.

TABLE 33–1   SPECTRUM OF CARDIOCIRCULATORY FINDINGS IN KAWASAKI DISEASE

CARDITIS (myocarditis, pericarditis)
  Congestive heart failure
  Arrhythmias
CORONARY ANGIITIS
  Thromboendarteritis—aneurysms
    Regression
    Thrombosis—recanalization
    Obstruction—stenosis
    Collaterals
    Rupture
  Myocardial ischemia or infarction
    Ventricular aneurysm
    Papillary muscle of dysfunction—mitral regurgitation
ARTERIAL INVOLVEMENT
  Pulmonary/renal angitis—pulmonary/renal hypertension
  Arteritis, aneurysms: femoral, iliac, brachial, cerebral, hepatic, etc.

Infants and children with this syndrome should be closely watched for signs of cardiac involvement. A significant number of patients show evidence of myocarditis or pericarditis, or both, in the early phases of the disease.[77] Electrocardiographic evidence of myocarditis with low voltage and nonspecific ST-T wave changes is seen in 45 per cent of patients, echocardiographic evidence of poor left ventricular function in 25 per cent, pericardial effusion in 9 per cent, cardiomegaly on chest radiographs in 25 per cent, pericardial effusion in 9 per cent, and a gallop rhythm in 12 per cent. Aneurysms of the coronary arteries with narrowing, tortuosity, and obstruction are almost invariably present on aortography and coronary angiography (Fig. 33–6).[78–82a] Success has been achieved in visualizing aneurysmal coronary lesions with two-dimensional cross-sectional echocardiography (Fig. 33–7).[83–85] About half of the children with coronary aneurysms diagnosed shortly after the acute phase of the disease subsides have normal-appearing vessels by angiography 1 or 2 years later.[86–89a] In those patients with residual cardiac abnormalities after recovery from the acute illness phase, a variety of findings have been described. These include impairment of left ventricular function secondary to the coronary arterial involvement, papillary muscle dysfunction with mitral regurgitation,[89b] impaired left

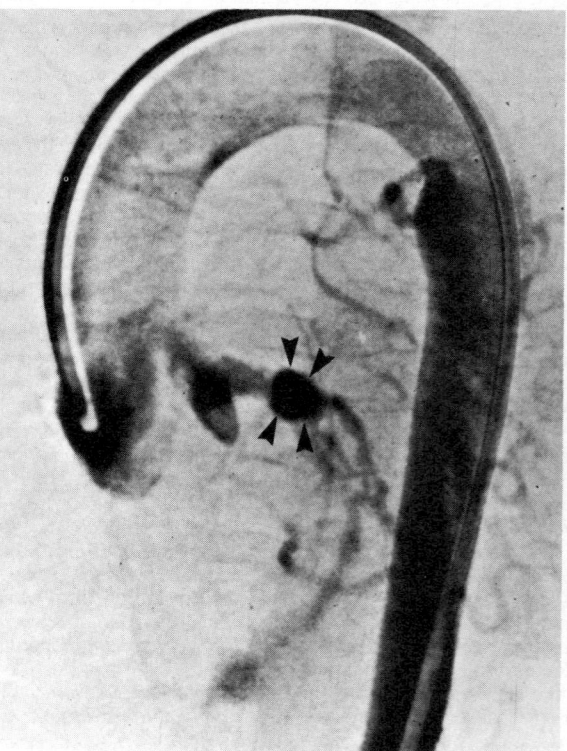

FIGURE 33–6. Aortic root cineangiograms from two patients with mucocutaneous lymph node syndrome. In the left panel, a dilated proximal left coronary artery is observed with collateral circulation and retrograde filling of the right coronary system, and three aneurysms of the right coronary artery. In the right panel, subtraction technique shows an aneurysm of the left coronary artery (arrowheads). (Courtesy of Thomas G. DiSessa, M. D.)

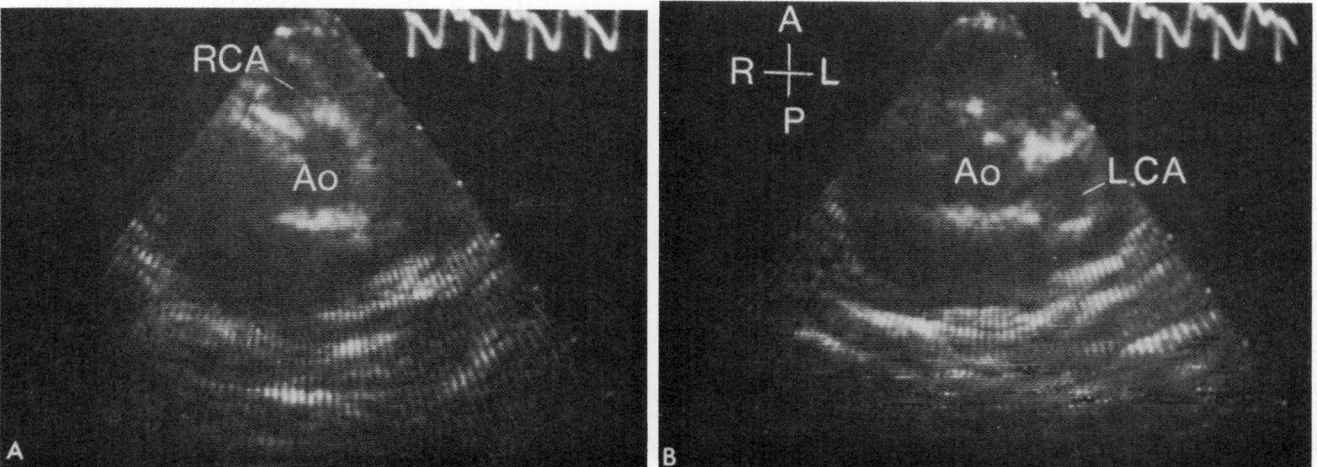

FIGURE 33–7. Short-axis cross-sectional echocardiographic views of aneurysms of the proximal right coronary artery (RCA) (A) and proximal left coronary artery (LCA) (B) in a 3-year-old boy with mucocutaneous lymph node syndrome. The right ventricular outflow tract is anterior (A) to the aorta (Ao) and the left atrium is posterior (P). R = right; L = left.

ventricular function,[89c] and abnormalities of the distensibility of the coronary arteries (even after aneurysms have disappeared and no morphological abnormalities are recognized by coronary arteriography).[90–94]

To date, no treatment has proved effective to prevent the formation of coronary artery aneurysms. It appears that corticosteroid therapy is *detrimental* during the acute illness. High-dose salicylate treatment (50 to 100 mg/kg/day) is advisable for all patients in the acute phase of the illness, and later in low doses (3–5 mg/kg/day) to inhibit platelet aggregation in the hope of preventing subsequent thrombus formation and occlusion of the coronary arteries. In many children with Kawasaki disease, there is failure to achieve therapeutic serum concentrations of salicylate despite high oral doses because of impaired gastrointestinal absorption of salicylate.[95] Therefore, regular monitoring of serum salicylate levels is advisable. In children who have no evidence of coronary artery disease and in whom the platelet count has returned to normal, the aspirin may be discontinued after 2 to 6 months. In patients who develop coronary arterial involvement, aspirin therapy should be maintained indefinitely (3 to 5 mg/kg/day). High-dose intravenous gamma globulin therapy has been demonstrated to be safe and effective in reducing the prevalence of coronary artery abnormalities when administered early in the course of Kawasaki disease.[96,97] The suggested dosage of intravenous gamma globulin has been 400 mg/kg/day for 4 days, although it is likely that a single large dose of intravenous gamma globulin (2 gm/kg), infused over 10 hours, is as safe and effective as the 4-day regimen.[98,99]

Two-dimensional echocardiography is indicated in all children with a diagnosis of Kawasaki disease, with or without evidence of significant cardiac involvement. Coronary angiography is recommended for those patients with severe symptoms of cardiovascular involvement, persistence of cardiomegaly or heart failure, ischemic ST-T wave changes or an electrocardiographic pattern of myocardial infarction, signs of mitral insufficiency, or cardiac calcification by chest x-ray. The prognosis for children with vascular involvement should be guarded;[100,101] some will be candidates for coronary arterial bypass surgery.[102]

Anthracycline Toxicity

(See also p. 1756)

Anthracycline drugs such as doxorubicin and daunomycin, used as cancer chemotherapeutic agents, cause a dose-related cardiomyopathy.[103] The risk of cardiac involvement increases significantly with doses in excess of 400 mg/m². [104] The onset

of cardiac symptoms often is delayed, occurring 2 to 3 months after the anthracycline dose. Cardiac dysfunction usually presents first as unexplained tachycardia, progressing to dyspnea, congestive heart failure, hepatomegaly, and, often, death. The cardiomyopathy most often is reversible only in its early stages. Later, it usually is poorly responsive to digitalis, diuretics, and afterload reducing agents. Quite often patients are in remission from their neoplasm when the drug's cardiotoxicity proves lethal. Long-term followup has disclosed elevated levels of left ventricular wall stress and impairment of diastolic function in children without overt cardiomyopathy.[105] Further, there are occasional reports of late-onset heart failure in previously asymptomatic children, many years after their cancer chemotherapy.[106]

SYSTEMIC HYPERTENSION

(See also p. 843)

Unfortunately, many physicians consider hypertension a disease of adults and not children. Thus, all too frequently, blood pressure is not recorded during the pediatric physical examination. It should be emphasized that elevations in systemic blood pressure may occur in as many as 2 per cent of children, and it has been well documented that undetected or untreated hypertension may lead to unfortunate consequences.[107] Three points in particular require recognition:[108]

1. Causes of hypertension in infants and children differ markedly from those in adults. Most children have secondary rather than essential forms of hypertension (Table 33–2); therefore, it is important to search for a remedial cause.
2. Offspring of hypertensive parents are known to have an increased susceptibility to blood pressure elevation.
3. Children with elevated blood pressure require the same surveillance and treatment as adults.

Accurate blood pressure measurements require cuffs of different sizes because of the variation in arm size from infancy through adolescence. To measure blood pressure correctly, the inner rubber bag should be wide enough to cover two-thirds of the length and three-fourths of the circumference of the upper arm or thigh while leaving the antecubital or popliteal fossa free. A cuff that is too small is likely to produce spuriously high readings. In infants under age 2 years the flush technique may be used, although a Doppler instrument is preferred.[109,110] Because disappearance of the Korotkoff sound may cause underestimation of the diastolic pressure, both muffling (the fourth phase of the Korotkoff sound) and disap-

TABLE 33-2 CONDITIONS AND DRUGS ASSOCIATED WITH HYPERTENSION IN INFANTS AND CHILDREN

CONGENITAL
Coarctation of the aorta
Gonadal dysgenesis (Turner syndrome)
Rubella syndrome
Pseudoxanthoma elasticum (Ehlers-Danlos syndrome)
Ask-Upmark syndrome (segmental renal artery dysplasia)
Renal arterial abnormalities
Multiple systemic and pulmonary artery stenoses
Solitary renal cyst
Hydronephrosis

GENETIC
Diabetes mellitus
Neurofibromatosis (von Recklinghausen's disease)
Adrenogenital syndrome
Pheochromocytoma
Polycystic kidney disease (infantile and adult forms)
Familial nephritis (Alport syndrome)
Little syndrome
Fabry's disease (angiokeratoma corporis diffusum)
Familial dysautonomia (Riley-Day syndrome)
Essential hypertension
Tuberous sclerosis with angiolipomas
Primary hyperparathyroidism
Porphyria

PHARMACOLOGICAL
Sympathomimetics: ephedrine, epinephrine, isoproterenol
Adrenal steroids
Heavy metals: mercury, lead
Licorice

ACQUIRED, RENAL
Unilateral hydronephrosis
Unilateral pyelonephritis
Renal trauma
Renal tumors
Unilateral multicystic kidney
Unilateral ureteral occlusion
Renal artery stenosis
Renal arteritis
Fibromuscular dysplasia of the renal artery
Renal fistula
Renal artery aneurysm
Chronic pyelonephritis superimposed on abnormal kidneys
Nephritis: shunt nephritis, acute poststreptococcal disease, anaphylactoid purpura, disseminated lupus erythematosus
Renal tuberculosis
Renal cortical necrosis: hemolytic uremic syndrome; sepsis
Renal vein thrombosis
Radiation nephritis
Postrenal transplantation

ACQUIRED, OTHER THAN RENAL
Hyperthyroidism
Retrosternal goiter
Guillain-Barré syndrome or poliomyelitis
Cerebral edema
Stevens-Johnson syndrome
Neuroblastoma
Hypercalcemia or hypernatremia
Adrenal adenoma or hyperplasia: primary aldosteronism or Cushing's syndrome
Hyperuricemic nephropathy
Burns

Modified from Lieberman, E.: Diagnostic evaluation of hypertensive children. Pediatr. Ann. 6:390, 1977.

pearance (fifth phase) should be recorded. The fourth phase is the more accurate measure of diastolic pressure in most prepubertal children; beyond adolescence the fifth phase sound more closely reflects diastolic pressure.[110,111]

The normal ranges of blood pressure relative to age are shown in Figures 33-8 through 33-13 and serve as a guide in judging unsafe levels. Because considerable variation exists in most children's pressures, it should be recognized that a single blood pressure recording at or higher than the 90th percentile at a single point in time may not be an abnormal finding. In an apparently healthy child measurements should be repeated serially; further investigation is warranted if the blood pressure persists at or above the 90th percentile.[112,113] In contrast, definite or severe hypertension (i.e., pressures repeatedly well beyond the broad limits of normal) requires prompt investigation and treatment.[114,115] Particularly urgent attention must be paid to those children whose systolic and diastolic pressures are remarkably high (i.e., equal to or greater than 180 and 110 mm Hg, respectively). Other findings identifying the patient at acute risk include localized neurological signs and/or generalized seizures; blurred vision or such eye ground changes as retinal hemorrhage, exudate, papilledema, or retinal arterial constriction; renal or abdominal pain; evidence of left ventricular hypertrophy or cardiac decompensation; renal

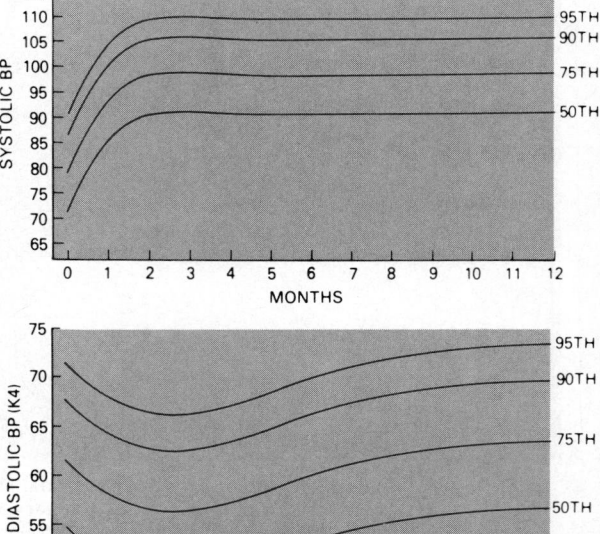

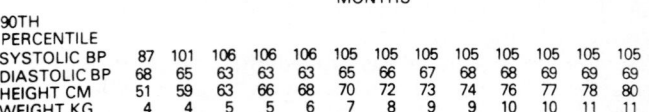

90TH PERCENTILE												
SYSTOLIC BP	87	101	106	106	106	105	105	105	105	105	105	105	105
DIASTOLIC BP	68	65	63	63	63	65	66	67	68	68	69	69	69
HEIGHT CM	51	59	63	66	68	70	72	73	74	76	77	78	80
WEIGHT KG	4	4	5	5	6	7	8	9	9	10	10	11	11

FIGURE 33-8. Age-specific percentiles of blood pressure measurements in boys — birth to 12 months of age. Korotkoff phase IV used for diastolic blood pressure. (From Horan, M. J., et al.: Report of the second task force on blood pressure control in children — 1987. Pediatrics 79:1, 1987. Copyright American Academy of Pediatrics, 1987.)

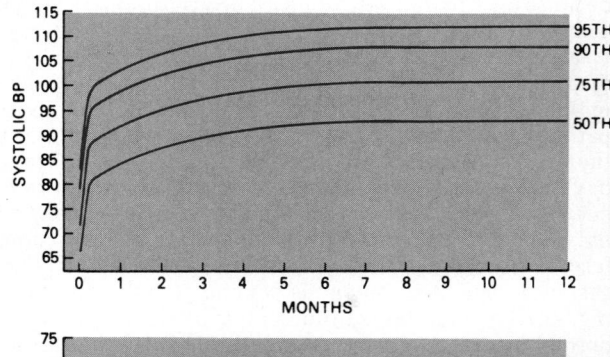

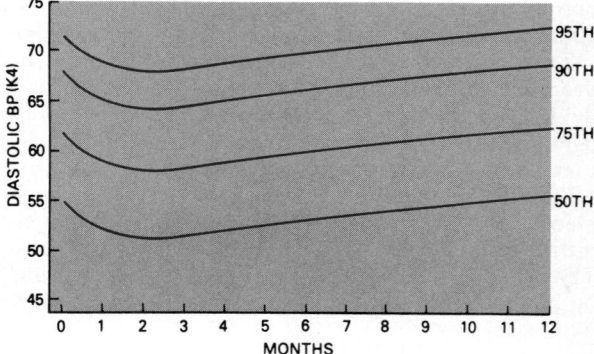

90TH PERCENTILE												
SYSTOLIC BP	76	98	101	104	105	106	106	106	106	106	106	105	105
DIASTOLIC BP	68	65	64	64	65	65	66	66	66	67	67	67	67
HEIGHT CM	54	55	56	58	61	63	66	68	70	72	74	75	77
WEIGHT KG	4	4	4	5	5	6	7	8	9	9	10	10	11

FIGURE 33-9. Age-specific percentiles of blood pressure measurements in girls — birth to 12 months of age. Korotkoff phase IV used for diastolic blood pressure. (From Horan, M. J., et al.: Report of the second task force on blood pressure control in children — 1987. Pediatrics 79:1, 1987. Copyright American Academy of Pediatrics, 1987.)

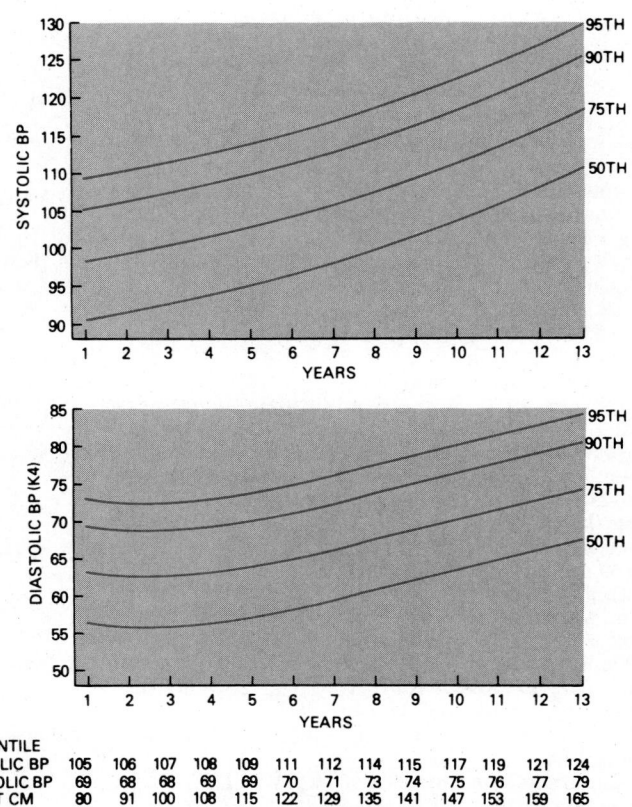

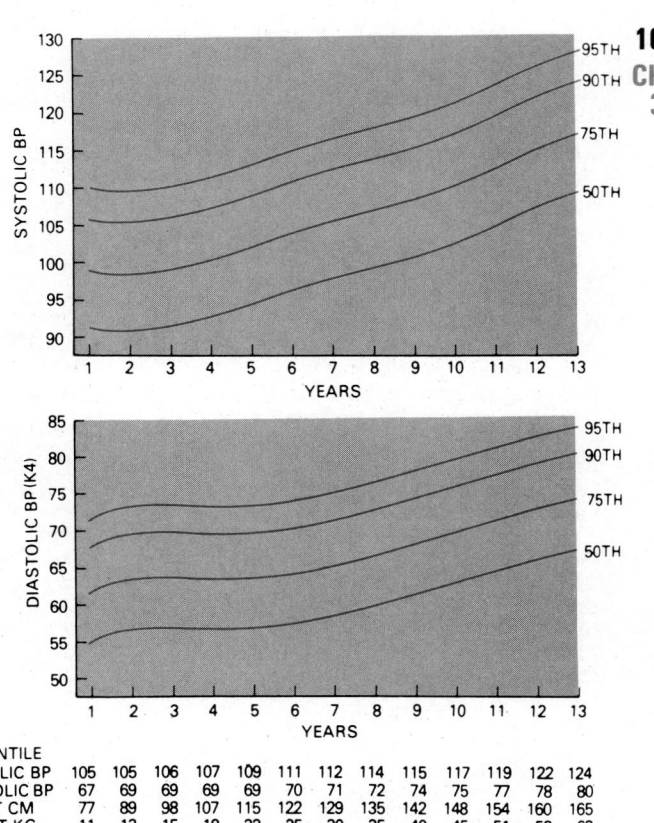

90TH PERCENTILE

SYSTOLIC BP	105	106	107	108	109	111	112	114	115	117	119	121	124
DIASTOLIC BP	69	68	68	69	69	70	71	73	74	75	76	77	79
HEIGHT CM	80	91	100	108	115	122	129	135	141	147	153	159	165
WEIGHT KG	11	14	16	18	22	25	29	34	39	44	50	55	62

FIGURE 33–10. Age-specific percentiles of blood pressure measurements in boys—1 to 13 years of age. Korotkoff phase IV used for diastolic blood pressure. (From Horan, M. J., et al.: Report of the second task force on blood pressure control in children—1987. Pediatrics 79:1, 1987. Copyright American Academy of Pediatrics, 1987.)

90TH PERCENTILE

SYSTOLIC BP	105	105	106	107	109	111	112	114	115	117	119	122	124
DIASTOLIC BP	67	69	69	69	69	70	71	72	74	75	77	78	80
HEIGHT CM	77	89	98	107	115	122	129	135	142	148	154	160	165
WEIGHT KG	11	13	15	18	22	25	30	35	40	45	51	58	63

FIGURE 33–11. Age-specific percentiles of blood pressure measurements in girls—1 to 13 years of age. Korotkoff phase IV used for diastolic blood pressure. (From Horan, M. J., et al.: Report of the second task force on blood pressure control in children—1987. Pediatrics 79:1, 1987. Copyright American Academy of Pediatrics, 1987.)

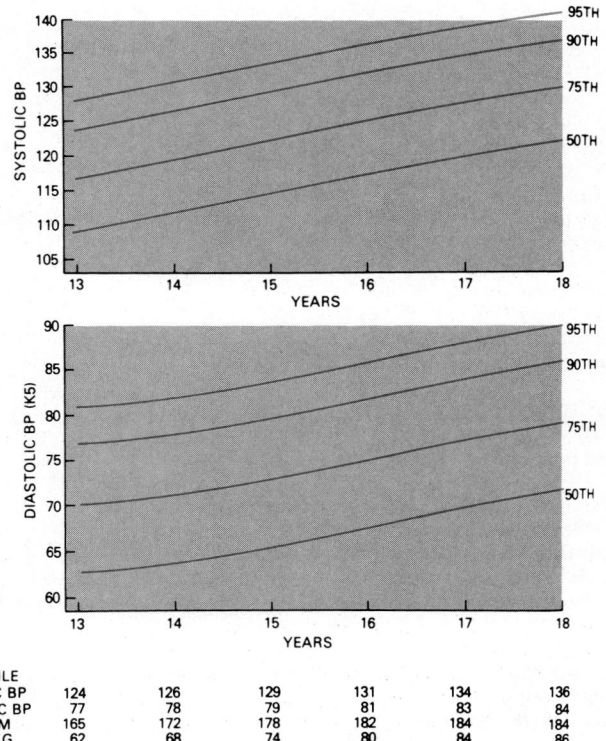

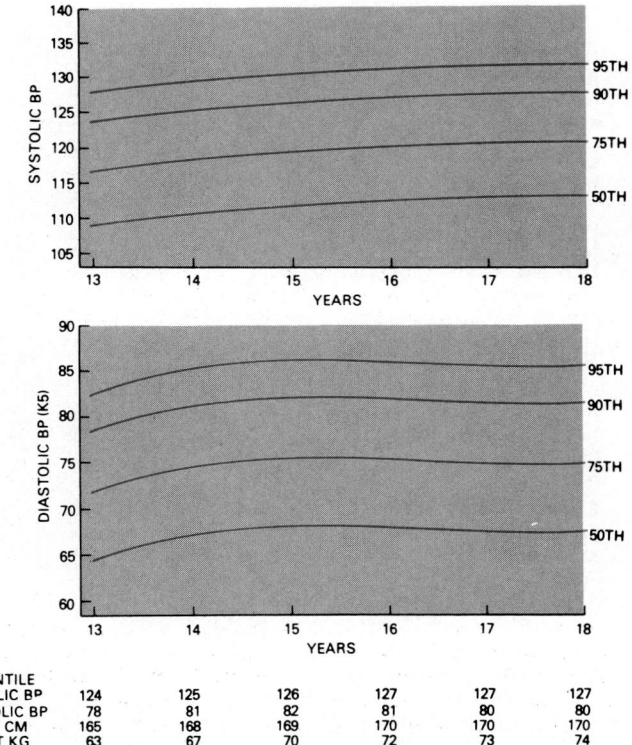

90TH PERCENTILE

SYSTOLIC BP	124	126	129	131	134	136
DIASTOLIC BP	77	78	79	81	83	84
HEIGHT CM	165	172	178	182	184	184
WEIGHT KG	62	68	74	80	84	86

FIGURE 33–12. Age-specific percentiles of blood pressure measurements in boys—13 to 18 years of age. Korotkoff phase V used for diastolic blood pressure. (From Horan, M. J., et al.: Report of the second task force on blood pressure control in children—1987. Pediatrics 79:1, 1987. Copyright American Academy of Pediatrics, 1987.)

90TH PERCENTILE

SYSTOLIC BP	124	125	126	127	127	127
DIASTOLIC BP	78	81	82	81	80	80
HEIGHT CM	165	168	169	170	170	170
WEIGHT KG	63	67	70	72	73	74

FIGURE 33–13. Age-specific percentiles of blood pressure measurements in girls—13 to 18 years of age. Korotkoff phase V used for diastolic blood pressure. (From Horan, M. J., et al.: Report of the second task force on blood pressure control in children—1987. Pediatrics 79:1, 1987. Copyright American Academy of Pediatrics, 1987.)

DRUG	ROUTE OF ADMINISTRATION	DOSAGE
Acetaminophen (Tylenol)	PO or PR	<1 year 60 mg (q4h); 1 to 3 years 120 mg (q4h); >3 years 120 to 240 mg (q4h)
Acetylsalicylic acid (Aspirin)	PO or PR	30 to 100 mg/kg/day (q4h)
ε-Aminocaproic acid (Amicar)	IV	Total 100 mg/kg; ¼ total dose (q1h)
Aminophylline	PO, PR, or IV	12 mg/kg/day (q6h)
Amiodarone	PO	10 mg/kg/day for 10 to 14 days, then 5 mg/kg/day for 1 to 2 mo, then 2.5 mg/kg/day
Ammonium chloride	PO	75 mg/kg/day (q6h)
Atropine	IV, SC, or PO	0.01 to 0.03 mg/kg (q4–6h)
Bicarbonate sodium	IV	1 to 2 mEq/kg/5 min
Bishydroxycoumarin (Dicumarol)	PO	Loading dose: 50 to 100 mg Maintenance: 10 to 50 mg/day (Regulate according to prothrombin times)
Bretylium	IV	5 mg/kg/dose over 10 minutes, then 50 to 100 μg/kg/min
Calcium chloride	IV	1 to 4 ml of 10% solution; for cardiac arrest, 10 mg/kg/dose
Calcium gluconate	IV	2 to 6 ml of 10% solution; for cardiac arrest, 10 mg/kg/dose
	PO	500 mg/kg/day (q6h)
Captopril	PO	0.1 to 0.4 mg/kg/dose (q6–24h)
Chlorothiazide (Diuril)	PO	20 to 40 mg/kg/day (q12h)
Chlorthalidone	PO	1 to 2 mg/kg/day (q12h)
Cholestyramine (Questran)	PO	250 to 1500 mg/kg/day (q6–12h)
Clofibrate (Atromid S)	PO	0.5 to 1.5 mg/day in divided doses
Clonidine (Catapres)	PO	0.002 to 0.008 mg/kg/day in divided doses
Codeine	PO	0.5 to 1.5 mg/kg/dose (q3h)
Dexamethasone (Decadron)	IV	0.2 to 0.4 mg/kg/dose (q6h) for cerebral edema
Diazoxide	IV	3 to 5 mg/kg/dose over 30 sec (q2–6h) (careful of severe hypotension)

Digitalis (Digoxin)		Loading dose:
		  Premature infants 0.01–0.02 mg/kg IV or IM
		  Term infants
		    Parenteral:
		      Up to 4 wk: 0.03 mg/kg; 4 wk to 12 mo: 0.035 mg/kg; Over 12 mo: 0.040 mg/kg; Beyond 2 yr: 0.03 mg/kg
		    Oral: approximately 20% greater than IV dose
		Maintenance: ⅓ to ¼ of loading dose, given in two divided doses/24 hr

Digoxin Specific Fab fragments (Ovine)	IV	0.6 mg digoxin bound by 40 mg Fab fragments
Dobutamine	IV	2 to 10 μg/kg/min
Dopamine	IV	1 gm in 250 ml D₅W; 2 to 20 μg/kg/min
Edrophonium chloride (Tensilon)	IV	0.05 to 0.2 mg/kg/dose
Ephedrine sulfate	IM or PO	0.8 to 1.6 mg/kg/day (q6h)
Epinephrine (Adrenalin)	IV	For cardiac arrest: single dose: 0.1 to 1.0 ml of 1:1000; 0.1 to 1.0 μg/min infusion
Ethacrynic acid (Edecrin)	IV	1.0 mg/kg/day
Ethylenediaminetetraacetic acid (EDTA) disodium salt	IV	20 mg/ml: 10 to 50 mg/kg (q12h)
Furosemide (Lasix)	IV or IM	1 to 2 mg/kg/dose
	PO	1 to 4 mg/kg/day
Glucagon	IV	0.05 to 0.10 mg/kg/hr
Glucose 50%	IV	1 mg/kg/dose
Glucose 50% + Insulin	IV	1 gm glucose/kg (50% solution) with insulin, 1 unit/3 gm glucose
Guanethidine sulfate (Ismelin)	PO	0.2 to 1.0 mg/kg/day (q6h)
Heparin	IV	100 units/kg (q4h)
Hydralazine hydrochloride (Apresoline)	IV	0.8 to 3.0 mg/kg/day (q4–6h)
	PO	0.75 to 7.5 mg/kg/day (q6–8h)
Hydrochlorothiazide	PO	1 to 3 mg/kg/day (q12h)
Hydrocortisone sodium succinate (Solu-Cortef)	IV	For shock: 50 to 75 mg/kg (q6h)
Indomethacin	IV	0.1 to 0.2 mg/kg/dose (premature, for ductal closure)
Innovar (fentanyl citrate & droperidol)	IV	0.01 to 0.02 ml/kg
Isoproterenol hydrochloride (Isuprel hydrochloride)	IV	0.05 to 0.25 μg/kg/min
Lidocaine (Xylocaine hydrochloride)	IV	Single dose: 1 mg/kg; 10 to 50 μg/kg/min infusion
Magnesium sulfate, 3%	IV	For neonatal seizure: single dose: 2 to 6 ml
Mannitol	IV	For cerebral edema: 1 to 2 gm/kg Repeated doses: 250 mg/kg (q4h) For hemoglobinuria: single dose: 0.5 gm/kg; 5% solution infusion if necessary
Meperidine hydrochloride (Demerol)	IM or IV	1 mg/kg/dose (q3h)
Meralluride (Mercuhydrin)	IM	<1 yr: single dose: 0.1 to 0.3 ml; 1 to 5 yr: single dose: 0.3 to 0.7 ml; >5 yr: single dose: 1 ml
Mercaptomerin sodium (Thiomerin sodium)	IM	Same as meralluride
Metaraminol (Aramine metaraminol bitartrate)	IV	Single dose: 0.1 mg/kg or 50 mg/500 ml; titrate to effect infusion
Methyldopa (Aldomet)	PO or IV	10 to 40 mg/kg/day (q6–8h)
Methylprednisolone (Solu-Medrol)	IV	For shock: 30 mg/kg/dose; for cerebral edema: 4 to 5 mg/kg/dose

DRUG	ROUTE OF ADMINISTRATION	DOSAGE
Mexiletine	PO	4 to 20 mg/kg/day (q8h)
Minoxidil	PO	0.05 to 2.0 mg/kg/day
Morphine sulfate	SC	0.1 to 0.2 mg/kg/dose (q3h)
Naloxone hydrochloride (Narcan)	IM or IV	0.01 mg/kg/dose
Nitroprusside, sodium	IV	0.5 to 8.0 μg/kg/min initial rate; titrate to effect
Norepinephrine (Levophed bitartrate)	IV	0.1 to 1.0 μg/kg/min
Pentobarbital (Nembutal)	PO or IM	2 to 3 mg/kg/dose
Phenobarbital	PO or IM	3 to 5 mg/kg/day (q8h)
Phenoxybenzamine	IV	0.5 to 1.0 mg/kg
Phentolamine	IV	0.05 to 0.10 mg/kg
Phenylephrine (Neo-Synephrine hydrochloride)	IV	10 mg/100 ml D_5W; 1 to 10 μg/kg/min, titrate to effect
Phenytoin (Dilantin)	PO or IV	For seizures: 5 to 10 mg/kg/day (q8h); for arrhythmias: 1 to 5 mg/kg/5 min
Potassium chloride	PO	1 to 2 mEq/kg/day
	IV	0.5 mEq/kg/hr not to exceed 2 mEq/kg, as 40 to 80 mEq/l solution
Potassium gluconate (Kaon) and Potassium triplex	PO	1 to 2 mEq/kg/day
Procainamide hydrochloride (Pronestyl)	PO	40 to 60 mg/kg/day (q4–6h)
	IM	5 to 8 mg/kg (q6h)
	IV	1 mg/kg/dose over 5 min
Propranolol hydrochloride (Inderal)	PO	1.0 to 6.0 mg/kg/day (divided q6h)
	IV	0.01 to 0.15 mg/kg (q6–8h)
	IM	0.5 to 1.0 mg/kg (q4–6h)
Promethazine	PO	1 to 2 mg/kg/day (q6–8h)
Prostaglandin E₁	IV	0.1 μg/kg/min, reduce to 0.01 μg/kg/min to maintain effect
Protamine sulfate	IV	3 mg for every 200 units of heparin
Quinidine gluconate	PO	10 to 30 mg/kg/day (q4–8h)
	IM or IV	2 to 10 mg/kg/dose (q3–6h)
Quinidine sulfate	PO	3 to 12 mg/kg/dose (q3h)
Reserpine (Serpasil)	PO	0.01 to 0.02 mg/kg/day (q12h)
	IM	0.07 mg/kg (q12h)
Sodium polystyrene sulfonate (Kayexalate)	PR	1 gm/kg mixed with 70% sorbitol
Spironolactone	PO	1 to 3 mg/kg/day (q6–12h)
Succinylcholine chloride (Anectine chloride)	IM	2 mg/kg/dose
	IV	1 mg/kg dose
Tolazoline (Priscoline)	IV	1 mg/kg/dose, then 1 to 3 mg/kg/hr
Triamterene	PO	2–4 mg/kg/day
Trimethaphan camsylate (Arfonad)	IV	50 mg in 100 ml D_5W, titrate to effect
Tris (hydroxymethyl) aminomethane (THAM)	IV	(0.3M) weight (kg) × base deficit = dose in ml
Tubocurarine chloride (curare)	IM or IV	Initial dose: 0.3 to 0.5 mg/kg; Subsequent dose: 0.1 mg/kg
Verapamil	IV	0.1 to 0.2 mg/kg/dose over 2 min
Vitamin K (AquaMEPHYTON)	IM or IV	Single dose (neonate): 1 mg
Warfarin sodium crystalline (Coumadin)	PO or IM	Initial dose: 0.5 mg/kg
		Maintenance: 1 to 5 mg/day (Regulate according to prothrombin times)

dysfunction; palpation of an abdominal mass or enlargement of the kidneys; or auscultation of an abdominal bruit.

Evaluation of the asymptomatic child or adolescent with a blood pressure level above the 90th percentile on three or more occasions includes a careful history focusing on conditions or drugs known to be associated with or to predispose to high blood pressure. These include oral contraceptives (p. 832), use of glucocorticoids, renal disease, and symptoms that suggest aldosteronism (p. 838) (i.e., spells, weakness, polyuria, muscle cramps) or pheochromocytoma (p. 1839) (i.e., excessive sweating, palpitations). The family history should be reviewed for eclampsia during the mother's pregnancy as well as any familial occurrence of hypertension, premature coronary artery disease, stroke, or renal failure.

Common *symptoms* in hypertensive children are headache, nausea and vomiting, loss of appetite, epistaxis, and palpitation. A dietary history should be obtained with an emphasis on sodium intake. The *physical examination* is directed at detecting conditions associated with secondary hypertension (Table 33–2) and finding evidence of target organ damage on funduscopic and cardiac examination. Typically, the physical findings in hypertensive disorders in children reflect the underlying cause of the elevated pressure; distinctive physical findings accompany many of the conditions listed in Table 33–1 (see also Chap. 28).

Laboratory studies are aimed primarily at identifying secondary causes of hypertension.[114,115] The minimal laboratory tests required are a urinalysis, complete blood count, serum electrolytes, blood urea nitrogen, serum creatinine, uric acid, echocardiogram, electrocardiogram, and chest roentgenogram. Because the most common cause of secondary hypertension in children is renal disease, evaluation often proceeds to include plasma renin activity with 24-hour urinary sodium excretion or plasma renin in response to captopril (p. 836), rapid-sequence intravenous pyelogram, ultrasound of the kidneys, and isotopic or angiographic analysis of the kidneys and/or their blood supply. Fortunately, most identifiable causes of correctable hypertension in children and adolescents are associated with clinical findings that direct attention to a particular organ system (renal, endocrine, central nervous, and cardiovascular). Less often, hypertension may result from tumors (ganglioneuroma, pheochromocytoma, Wilms', and neuroblastoma) or collagen vascular disease. Laboratory studies should be as specific as possible to avoid an unselected analysis of every organ system theoretically associated with hypertension. In general, the younger the child and the higher the blood pressure elevation, the more vigorous should be the laboratory evaluation. It should be recognized that although essential hypertension often is a diagnosis by exclusion in prepubertal children, it is a viable diagnosis, particularly in adolescents.[116,117] In the author's opinion the need for extensive laboratory investigations has been overemphasized in children or adolescents with mild sustained elevations in blood pressure.

Asymptomatic children and adolescents with borderline or only mildly elevated blood pressure (<5 to 10 mm Hg beyond the 90th percentile values for age) may not require antihypertensive pharmacological agents but should receive counseling regarding weight control, salt abuse, and avoidance of agents with pressor effects (e.g., caffeine, some bronchoconstrictors, nicotine). These patients should be encouraged to be physically active, especially in exercises improving cardiovascular fitness. Isometric or static exercise such as wrestling and weight lifting should be avoided, especially in children with evidence of left ventricular hypertrophy. If the latter exists or if these conservative measures do not result in normalization of blood pressure, treatment with antihypertensive drugs is indicated.

Drug therapy (Table 33–3) is aimed at prescribing the least complex regimen with the fewest side effects (see also Chap. 29). Pharmacological management is usually undertaken if diastolic blood pressure is greater than 85 mm Hg in children less than age 12 years, and greater than 90 mm Hg in children older than 12 years. If left ventricular hypertrophy is evident by echocardiogram, drug treatment is advisable at lower diastolic pressures. An oral thiazide diuretic usually is the initial drug of choice and may be combined with a potassium-sparing drug or with a dietary regimen that provides adequate potassium. If blood pressure control is not achieved, a beta-adrenergic blocking agent such as atenolol may be added to the regimen. Occasionally it is necessary to use an angiotensin enzyme blocker or a central sympathetic inhibitor such as clonidine. Of the calcium-antagonists, nifedipine has been used most often, but a broad experience in pediatric patients is lacking.

Acute, life-threatening episodes of hypertension occur rarely and in a variety of clinical situations.[118] Encephalopathy is the most severe complication of an acute hypertensive crisis; its presence demands immediate lowering of the systemic arterial blood pressure. Diazoxide is the agent of choice as a first drug for the patient with encephalopathy. If diazoxide is ineffective, catecholamine-producing tumors must be suspected and consideration given to using alpha-adrenergic blocking agents such as phentolamine or phenoxybenzamine. Sodium nitroprusside usually is considered the agent to be administered when all others have failed. If a cause for sustained hypertension has been detected, medical and/or surgical treatment should be directed at the underlying disease process.

HYPERLIPIDEMIAS

(See also Chap. 37)

The importance of prevention of arteriosclerosis in childhood is now generally accepted.[119-121] Hyperlipidemic children are at high risk of becoming hyperlipidemic adults and are therefore at greater risk of future atherosclerotic disease.[123-125] Although opinions vary about the feasibility of maintaining low serum lipid levels in normal children by dietary modification, a consensus exists that children whose serum cholesterol or triglyceride levels are beyond the 95th percentile for their age and sex should be treated. Guidelines for abnormal levels in the first two decades of life are provided in Table 33–4.

In the author's opinion, as part of routine pediatric practice, all children should have a random nonfasting cholesterol test performed. If the cholesterol level exceeds 200 mg/dl, a lipid profile should be obtained and, if the LDL cholesterol exceeds

TABLE 33–4   FASTING LIPID AND LIPOPROTEIN LEVELS (mg/dl) IN CHILDREN BY AGE

	MALES			FEMALES		
	5%	50%	95%	5%	50%	95%
Cholesterol						
0–4 yr	114	155	203	112	156	200
5–9 yr	121	160	203	126	164	205
10–14 yr	119	158	202	124	160	201
15–19 yr	113	150	197	120	158	203
Triglycerides						
0–4 yr	29	56	98	34	64	112
5–9 yr	30	56	101	32	60	105
10–14 yr	32	66	125	37	75	131
15–19 yr	37	78	148	39	75	132
HDL Cholesterol						
5–9 yr	38	56	74	36	53	73
10–14 yr	37	55	74	37	52	70
15–19 yr	30	46	63	35	52	74
LDL Cholesterol						
5–9 yr	63	93	129	68	100	140
10–14 yr	64	100	140	68	97	132
15–19 yr	62	94	130	59	96	137

Data from Lipid Research Clinics: Population Studies Data Book. Dept. of Health and Human Services (NIH) 80-1527, Vol. I: The Prevalence Study.

130 mg/dl, appropriate therapy should be instituted. Serum lipid levels should be analyzed at regular intervals in all children from families with hyperlipidemia or with histories that include hypertension, myocardial infarction, stroke, or peripheral vascular disease among parents or grandparents before age 50.[119,126-128] Differentiation is necessary between acquired hyperlipidemia and one of the familial, and presumably genetic, hyperlipidemias.[124]

Homozygous familial hypercholesterolemia causes severe atherosclerosis of the coronary arteries and myocardial infarction in childhood; rarely it causes atherosclerosis of the aortic valve, leading to critical aortic stenosis that requires surgical treatment.[128]

REFERENCES

NONRHEUMATIC INFLAMMATORY DISEASE

1. Ainger, L. E., Lawyer, N. G., and Fitch, C. W.: Neonatal rubella myocarditis. Br. Heart J. 28:691, 1966.
2. Ayuthya, T.S.N., Jayavasu, J., and Pongpanich, B.: Coxsackie group B virus in primary myocardial disease in infants and children. Am. Heart J. 88:311, 1974.
3. Suckling, P. V., and Vogelpoel, L.: Coxsackie myocarditis of the newborn. Lancet 2:421, 1970.
4. Lerner, A. M., and Wilson, F. M.: Virus myocardiopathy. Progr. Med. Virol. 15:63, 1973.
5. Oda, T., Hamamoto, K. and Morinaga, H.: Clinical aspects of non-rheumatic myocarditis in children. Jpn. Circ. J. 43:443, 1979.
6. Wink, K., and Schmitz, H.: Cytomegalovirus myocarditis. Am. Heart J. 100:667, 1980.
7. Arita, M., Ueno, Y., and Masuyama, Y.: Complete heart block in mumps myocarditis. Br. Heart J. 46:342, 1981.
8. O'Connell, J. B.: Gallium-67 imaging in patients with dilated cardiomyopathy and biopsy proven myocarditis. Circulation 70:58, 1984.
9. Leatherbury, L., Chandra, R. S., Shapiro, S. R., and Perry, L. W.: Value of endomyocardial biopsy of infants, children and adolescents with dilated or hypertrophic cardiomyopathy and myocarditis. J. Am. Coll. Cardiol. 12:1547, 1988.
10. Schmaltz, A. A., Apitz, J., Hort, W., and Maisch, B.: Endomyocardial biopsy in infants and children: Experience in 60 patients. Pediatr. Cardiol. 11:15, 1990.
11. Fisher, L. L., and Fisher, B. A.: Recognition and treatment of viral myocarditis. Primary Cardiol. 16:46, 1990.
11a. Yoshizato, T., Edwards, W. D., Alboliras, E. T., et al: Safety and utility of endomyocardial biopsy in infants, children and adolescents: Our view of 66 procedures in 53 patients. J. Am. Coll. Cardiol. 15:436, 1990.
12. Rezkalla, S. H., and Kolner, R. A.: Management strategies in viral myocarditis. Am. Heart J. 117:706, 1989.
12a. Chan, K. Y., Iwahara, M., Benson, L. N., et al.: Immunosuppressive therapy in the management of acute myocarditis in children: A clinical trial. J. Am. Coll. Cardiol. 17:458, 1991.

13. Taliercio, C. P., Seward, J. B., Driscoll, D. J., et al.: Idiopathic dilated cardiomyopathy in the young: Clinical profile and natural history. J. Am. Coll. Cardiol. 6:1126, 1985.

14. Wittels, B., and Bressler, R. J.: Biochemical lesions of diphtheria toxin in the heart. J. Clin. Invest. 43:630, 1964.

15. Challoner, D. R., and Prols, H. G.: Free fatty acid oxidation and carnitine levels in diphtheritic guinea pig myocardium. J. Clin. Invest. 51:2071, 1972.

16. Ino, T., Sherwood, W. G., Benson, L. N. et al.: Cardiac manifestations and disorders of fat and carnitine metabolism in infancy. J. Am. Coll. Cardiol. 11:1301, 1988.

17. Srivastava, S. C., Puri, D. S., and Lumba, S. T.: An electrocardiographic study of myocarditis and diphtheria. J. Assoc. Phys. India 14:365, 1966.

18. Ramos, A., Elias, P., Barrucand, L., and DaSilva, J.: The protective effect of carnitine in human diphtheritic myocarditis. Pediatr. Res. 18:815, 1984.

19. Prata, A.: Chagas' heart disease. Cardiologia 52:79, 1968.

20. Rosenbaum, M. B.: Chagasic myocardiopathy. Progr. Cardiovasc. Dis. 7:199, 1964.

21. Guerra, H. A. C., Palacios-Prue, E., Scorza, C. D., et al.: Clinical, histochemical, and ultrastructural correlation in septal endomyocardial biopsies from chronic chagasic patients: Detection of early myocardial damage. Am. Heart J. 113:716, 1987.

22. Drugs for parasitic infections. In Abramowicz, M. (ed.): The Medical Letter of Drugs and Therapeutics, Vol. 28 (Issue 706). The Medical Letter, Inc., New Rochelle, January 1986.

23. Koten, J. W., and DeRaadt, P.: Myocarditis and Trypanosoma rhodesiense infections. Trans. R. Soc. Trop. Med. Hyg. 63:485, 1969.

24. Stewart, J. M., Kaul, A., Gromisch, D. S., et al.: Symptomatic cardiac dysfunction in children with immunodeficiency virus infection. Am. Heart J. 117:140, 1989.

25. Lipshultz, S. E., Chanock, S., Sanders, S. P., et al.: Cardiovascular manifestations of human immunodeficiency virus infection in infants and children. Am. J. Cardiol. 63:1489, 1989.

26. Okoroma, E. O., Terry, L. W., and Scott, L. T.: Acute bacterial pericarditis in children: Report of 25 cases. Am. Heart J. 90:709, 1975.

27. VanReken, D., Strauss, A., Hernandez, A., and Feigin, R. D.: Infectious pericarditis in children. J. Pediatr. 85:165, 1974.

28. Callahan, J. A., Seward, J. B., Nishimura, R. A., et al.: Two dimensional echocardiographically guided pericardiocentesis: Experience in 117 consecutive patients. Am. J. Cardiol. 55:476, 1985.

29. Lajos, T. Z., Black, H. E., Cooper, R. G., and Wanka, J.: Pericardial decompression. Ann. Thorac. Surg. 19:47, 1975.

30. Engle, M. A., Ehlers, K. H., O'Laughlin, J. E., et al.: The post-pericardiotomy syndrome: Iatrogenic illness with immunologic and virologic components. In Engle, M. A. (ed.): Pediatric Cardiovascular Disease. Philadelphia, F. A. Davis Co., 1981, p. 381.

31. Clapp, S. K., Garson, J., Jr., Gutgesell, H. P., et al.: Postoperaive pericardial effusion and its relation to post-pericardiotomy syndrome. Pediatrics 66:585, 1980.

32. Mason, T. G., Neal, W. A., and DiBartolomeo, A. G.: Elevated antinuclear antibody titers and the postpericardiotomy syndrome. J. Pediatr. 116:403, 1990.

33. Paloheimo, J. A., Van Essen, R., Klemola, E., et al.: Sub-clinical cytomegalovirus infections and cytomegalovirus mononucleosis after open heart surgery. Am. J. Cardiol. 22:624, 1968.

34. Kron, I. L., Rheuban, K., and Nolan, S. P.: Late cardiac tamponade in children. Ann. Surg. 199:173, 1984.

PRIMARY CARDIOMYOPATHIES

35. Greenwood, R. D., Nadas, A. S., and Flyler, D. C.: The clinical course of primary myocardial disease in infants and children. Am. Heart J. 92:549, 1976.

36. Goodwin, J. F.: The frontiers of cardiomyopathy. Br. Heart J. 48:1, 1982.

37. Schryer, M. J. P., and Karnauchow, P. N.: Endocardial firboelastosis: Etiologic and pathogenic considerations in children. Am. Heart J. 88:557, 1974.

38. Moller, J. N., Lucas, R. V., Adams, P., et al.: Endocardial fibroelastosis. A clinical and anatomic study of 47 patients with emphasis on its relationship to mitral insufficiency. Circulation 30:759, 1964.

39. Taliercio, C. P., Seward, J. B., Driscoll, D. J., et al.: Idiopathic dilated cardiomyopathy in the young: Clinical profile and natural history. J. Am. Coll. Cardiol. 6:1126, 1985.

40. Hanukoglu, A., Fried, D., and Somekh, E.: Inheritance of familial primary endocardial fibroelastosis. Clin. Pediatr. 25:272, 1986.

41. Tripp, M. E.: Congestive cardiomyopathy of childhood. In Barness, L. A., (ed.): Advances in Pediatrics. Chicago, Year Book Medical Publishers, 1984, pp. 179–203.

42. Guntheroth, W. G.: Congestive cardiomyopathy in children. J. Am. Coll. Cardiol. 15:194, 1990.

43. Chen, S., Nouri, S., Balfour, I., et al.: Clinical profile of congestive cardiomyopathy in children. J. Am. Coll. Cardiol. 15:189, 1990.

44. Griffin, M. L., Hernandez, A., Martin, T. C., et al.: Dilated cardiomyopathy in infants and children. J. Am. Coll. Cardiol. 11:139, 1988.

45. Lurie, P. R.: Endocardial fibroeleastosis is not a disease. Am. J. Cardiol. 62:468, 1988.

46. Brandenburg, R. O.: Report of the WHO/ISFC Task Force on definition and classification of cardiomyopathy. Circulation 64:437a, 1971.

46a. Ino, T., Benson, L. N., Freedom, R. M., and Rowe, R. D.: Endocardial fibroelastosis: Natural history and prognostic risk factors. Am. J. Cardiol. 62:431, 1988.

47. Lambert, E. C., and Vlad, P.: Primary endomyocardial disease. Pediatr. Clin. North Am. 5:1057, 1958.

48. Sellers, F. J., Keith, J. D., and Manning, J. A.: The diagnosis of primary endocardial fibroelastosis. Circulation 29:49, 1964.

49. Akiba, T., Yoshikawa, M., Kinoda, M., et al.: Assessment of cardiac performance by first-pass radionuclide angiocardiography in infants and children with normal heart and endocardial fibroelastosis. Tohoku J. Exp. Med. 148:15, 1986.

50. Neustein, H. B., Lurie, P. R., and Fugita, M.: Endocardial fibroelastosis found on transvascular endomyocardial biopsy in children. Arch. Pathol. Lab. Med. 103:214, 1979.

51. Billingham, M. E.: The safety and utility of endomyocardial biopsy in infants, children and adolescents. J. Am. Coll. Cardiol. 15:443, 1990.

SECONDARY CARDIOMYOPATHIES

52. Gutgesell, H. P., Speer, M. E., and Rosenberg, H. S.: Characterization of the cardiomyopathy in infants with diabetic mothers. Circulation 51:441, 1980.

53. Trowitzsch, E, Bigalke, U., Gisbertz, R., and Kallfelz, H. C.: Echocardiographic profile of infants of diabetic mothers. Eur. J. Pediatr. 140:311, 1983.

54. Walther, F. J., Siassi, B., King, J., and Wu, P. Y-K.: Cardiac output in infants of insulin-dependent diabetic mothers. J. Pediatr. 107:109, 1985.

55. Miller, E., Hare, J. W., Cloherty, J. P., et al.: Elevated maternal hemoglobin A_{1C} in early pregnancy and major congenital anomalies in infants of diabetic mothers. N. Engl. J. Med. 304:1331, 1981.

56. Deorari, A. K., Saxena, A., Singh, M., and Shrivastava, S.: Echocardiographic assessment of infants born to diabetic mothers. Arch. Dis. Child 64:721, 1989.

57. Bordiuk, J. N., Logato, M. J., Lovelace, R. E., and Blumenthal, S: Pompe's disease: Electron myographic, electron microscopic and cardiovascular aspects. Arch. Neurol. (Chicago) 23:113, 1970,

58. Dickenson, E. F., Houlsby, W. T., and Wilkinson, J. L.: Unusual angiographic appearance of the left ventricle in two cases of Pompe's disease (glycogenosis type 2.) Br. Heart J. 41:238, 1979.

59. Hwang, G., Meng, C. C., Lin, C. Y., and Hsu, H. C.: Clinical analysis of five infants with glycogen storage disease of the heart—Pompe's disease. Jpn. Heart J. 27:25, 1986.

59a. DeDominicis, E., Finocchi, G., Vincenzi, M., et al.: Echocardiographic and pulsed Doppler features in glycogen storage disease type II of the heart (Pompe's disease). Acta Cardiologica XLVI:107, 1991.

60. Caddell, J. L.: Metabolic and nutritional disease. In Adams, F. H., and Emmanouilides, G. C. (eds.): Moss' Heart Disease in Infants, Children and Adolescents. 4th ed. Baltimore, Williams and Wilkins Co., 1989, pp. 750–777.

61. Sanstead, H. H.: Clinical manifestations of certain vitamin deficienceis. In Goodhart, M. S., and Shils, M. E. (eds.): Modern Nutrition in Health and Disease. 5th ed. Philadelphia, Lea and Febiger, 1973, p. 593.

62. Sanstead, H. H.: Mineral metabolism and protein malnutrition. In Olson, R. E. (ed.): Protein Calorie Malnutrition. New York, Academic Press, 1975, p. 213.

63. Cadell, J. L.: Diseases of the cardiovascular system. In Jelliffe, B. B. (ed.): Diseases of Children in the Subtropics and Tropics. London, Edward Arnold, Ltd., 1970, p. 398.

64. Nutter, D. O., Murray, T. G., Heymsfield, S. B., and Fuller, E. O.: The effect of chronic protein-calorie undernutrition in the rate on myocardial function and cardiac function. Circ. Res. 45:144, 1979.

65. Roberts, W. C., and Ferrans, V. J.: Pathological aspects of certain cardiomyopathies. Circ. Res. 34(Suppl. II):II–128, 1974.

66. Roberts, W. C., Buja, L. M., and Ferrans, V. J.: Löffler's fibroplastic parietal endocarditis, eosinophilic leukemia, and Davies' endomyocardial fibrosis: The same disease at different stages? Pathol. Microbiol. (Basel) 35:90, 1970.

67. Barretto, A. C. P., DaLuz, T. L., Oliveira, S. A, et al.: Determinants of survival in endomyocardial fibrosis. Circulation 80(Suppl. I):177, 1989.

68. Valithan, M. S., Balkrishnan, K. G., Sankarkumar, R., and Kartha, C. C.: Surgical treatment of endomyocardial fibrosis. Ann. Thorac. Surg. 43:68, 1987.

69. DiSessa, T. G., Klitzner, T., Hiraishi, S., et al.: Cardiovascular effects of Kawasaki's disease. J. Cardiovasc. Med. 6:1159, 1981.

70. Burns, J. C., Huang, A. S., Newburger, J. W., et al.: Characterization of the polymerase activity associated with cultured peripheral blood mononuclear cells from patients with Kawasaki disease. Pediatr. Res. 27:109, 1990.

71. Abe, Y., Nakano, S., Nakahara, T., et al.: Detection of serum antibody by the antimitogen assay against streptococcal erythrogenic toxins. Age distribution in children and the relation to Kawasaki disease. Pediatr. Res. 27:11, 1990.

72. Lang, B. A., Silverman, E. D., Laxer, R. M., and Lau, A. S.: Spontaneous tumor necrosis factor production in Kawasaki disease. J. Pediatr. 115:939, 1989.

73. Hiraishi, S., Yashiro, K., Oguchi, K., and Nakazawa, K.: Clinical course of cardiovascular involvement in the mucocutaneous lymph node syndrome. Am. J. Cardiol. 47:323, 1981.

74. Fujiwara, T., Fujiwara, H., and Hamashima, Y.: Frequency and size of coronary arterial aneurysm at necropsy in Kawasaki disease. Am. J. Cardiol. 59:808, 1987.

75. Nakano, H., Saito, A., Ueda, K., and Nojima, K.: Clinical characteristics of myocardial infarction following Kawasaki disease: Report of 11 cases. J. Pediatr. 108:198, 1986.

76. Kato, H., Ichinose, E., and Kawasaki, T.: Myocardial infarction in Kawasaki disease: Clinical analyses in 195 cases. J. Pediatr. *108*:923, 1986.

77. Meade, R. H., and Brandt, L.: Manifestation of Kawasaki disease in New England outbreak of 1980. J. Pediatr. *100*:558, 1982.

78. Onouchi, Z., Shimazu, S., Takamatsu, T., and Hamaoka, K.: Aneurysms of the coronary arteries in Kawasaki disease: An angiographic study of 30 cases. Circulation *66*:6,1982.

79. Nakanishi, T., Takao, A., Nakazawa, M., et al.: Mucocutaneous lymph node syndrome: Clinical, hemodynamic, and angiographic features of coronary obstructive disease. Am. J. Cardiol. *55*:6662, 1985.

80. Chung, K., Brandt, L., Fulton, D. R., and Kreidberg, M. B.: Cardiac and coronary arterial involvement in infants and children with mucocutaneous lymph node syndrome. Am. J. Cardiol. *50*:136, 1982.

81. Yoshida, H., Maeda, T., and Taniguchi, N.: Subcostal two-dimensional echocardiographic imaging of peripheral right coronary artery in Kawasaki disease. Circulation *65*:956, 1982.

82. Koren, G., Lavi, S., Rose, V., and Rowe, R.: Kawasaki disease. Review of risk factors for coronary aneurysms. J. Pediatr. *108*:388, 1986.

82a. Tatara, K., Kusakawa, S., Itoh, K., et al.: Collateral circulation in Kawasaki disease with coronary occlusion or severe stenosis. Am. Heart J. *121*:797, 1991.

83. Anderson, T. M., Meyer, R. A., and Kaplan, S.: Long-term echocardiographic evaluation of cardiac size and function in patients with Kawasaki's disease. Am. Heart J. *110*:107, 1985.

84. Ichida, F., Fatica, N. S., O'Loughlin, J. E., et al.: Correlation of electrocardiographic and echocardiographic changes in Kawasaki disease. Am. Heart J. *116*:812, 1988.

85. Fujiwara, T., Fujiwara, H., Ueda, T., et al.: Comparison of macroscopic, postmortem, angiographic and two-dimensional echocardiographic findings of coronary aneurysms in children with Kawasaki disease. Am. J. Cardiol. *6*:199, 1986.

86. Grenadier, E., Allen, H.D., Goldberg, S. J., et al.: Left ventricular wall motion abnormalities in Kawasaki's disease. J. Am. Coll. Cardiol. *1*:714, 1983.

87. Kato, H., Ichinose, E., Matsunaga, S., et al.: Fate of coronary aneurysms in Kawasaki disease: Serial coronary angiography and long-term follow-up study. Am. J. Cardiol. *49*:1758, 1982.

88. Anderson, T., Meyer, R. A., and Kaplan, S.: Long term evaluation of cardiac size and function in patients with Kawasaki disease. J. Am. Coll. Cardiol. *1*:714, 1983.

89. Suma, K., Takeuchi, Y., Shiroma, K., et al.: Early and late postoperative studies in coronary arterial lesions resulting from Kawasaki's disease in children. J. Thorac. Cardiovasc. Surg. *84*:224, 1982.

89a. Suzuki, A., Kamiya, T., Yasuo, O., and Kuroe, K.: Extended long-term follow-up study of coronary arterial lesions in Kawasaki disease. J. Am. Coll. Cardiol. *17*:33A, 1991.

89b. Akagi, T., Kato, H., Inoue, O., et al.: Valvular heart disease in Kawasaki syndrome: Incidence and natural history. Am. Heart J. *120*:366, 1990.

89c. Paridon, S. M., Ross, R. D., Kuhns, L. R., and Pinsky, W.W.: Myocardial performance and perfusion during exercise in patients with coronary artery disease caused by Kawasaki disease. J. Pediatr. *116*:52, 1990.

90. Takahashi, M., Mason, W., and Lewis, A. B.: Regression of coronary aneurysms in patients with Kawasaki syndrome. Circulation *75*:387, 1987.

91. Gidding, S. S., Shulman, S. T., Ilbawi, M., et al.: Mucocutaneous lymph node syndrome (Kawasaki's disease): delayed aortic and mitral insufficiency secondary to active valvulitis. J. Am. Coll. Cardiol. *7*:894, 1986.

92. Newburger, J. W., Sanders, S. P., Burns, J. C., et al.: Left ventricular contractility and function in Kawasaki syndrome: Effect of intravenous gamma globulin. Circulation *79*:1237, 1989.

93. Paridon, S. M., Ross, R. D., Kuhns, M. R., and Pinsky, W. W.: Myocardial performance and perfusion during exercise in patients with coronary-artery disease caused by Kawasaki disease. J. Pediatr. *116*:52, 1990.

94. Kurisu, Y., Azumi, T., Sugahara, T., et al.: Variation in coronary arterial dimension (distensible abnormality) after disappearing aneurysm in Kawasaki disease. Am. Heart J. *114*:532, 1987.

95. Koren, G., and MacLaod, S. M.: Difficulty in achieving therapeutic serum concentrations of salicylate in Kawasaki's disease. J. Pediatr. *105*:991, 1984.

96. Newburger, J. W., Takahasi, M., Burns, J. C., et al.: The treatment of Kawasaki syndrome with intravenous gamma globulin. N. Engl. J. Med. *315*:341, 1986.

97. Glode, M. P., Joffe, L. S., Wiggins, J., Jr., et al.: Effect of intravenous immune globulin on the coagulopathy of Kawasaki syndrome. J. Pediatr. *115*:469, 1989.

98. Engle, M. A., Fatica, N. S., Bussel, J. B., et al.: Clinical trial of single-dose intravenous gamma globulin in acute Kawasaki disease. Am. J. Dis. Child. *143*:1300, 1989.

99. Newburger, J. W., Takahashi, M., Beiser, A. S., et al.: A single intravenous infusion of gamma globulin as compared with four infusions in the treatment of acute Kawasaki syndrome. N. Engl. J. Med. *324*:1633, 1991.

99a. Shackelford, P. G., and Strauss, A. W.: Kawasaki syndrome. N. Engl. J. Med. *324*:1664, 1991.

100. Ohyagi, A., Hirose, K., Tsujimoto, S. et al.: Kawasaki's disease complicated by acute myocardial infarction nine years after onset. Am. Heart J. *110*:670, 1985.

101. Kohr, R. M.: Progressive asymptomatic coronary artery disease as a late fatal sequelae of Kawasaki's disease. J. Pediatr. *108*:256, 1986.

102. Suzuki, A., Kamiya, T., Ono, Y., et al.: Aorto-coronary bypass surgery for coronary arterial lesions resulting from Kawasaki disease. J. Pediatr. *116*:567, 1990.

103. Seraydarian, M. W., Artaza, L., and Yang, J. J.: Metablic involvement and adriamycin cardiotoxicity. *In* Tajaddin, M., Bhatrab, B., and Siddegue, H. H. (eds.): Advances in Myocardiology, Vol. 2. Baltimore, University Park Press, 1980.

104. Legha, S. S., Benjamin, R. S., and MacKay, H. J.: Reduction of doxorubicin cardiotoxicity by prolonged continuous intravenous infusion. Ann. Intern. Med. *96*:133, 1982.

105. Hausdorf, G., Morf, G., Beron, G., et al.: Long term doxorubicin cardiotoxicity in childhood: Noninvasive evaluation of the contractile state and diastolic filling. Br. Heart J. *60*:309, 1988.

106. Goorin, A. M., Chauvenet, A. R., Perez-Atayde, A. R., et al.: Initial congestive heart failure, six to 10 years after doxorubicin chemotherapy for childhood cancer. J. Pediatr. *116*:144, 1990.

SYSTEMIC HYPERTENSION

107. New, M. I., and Levine, L. S.: Hypertension in childhood and adolescence. Cardiovasc. Rev. *3*:115, 1982.

108. Lieberman, E.: Diagnostic evaluation of hypertensive children. Pediatr. Ann. *6*:390, 1977.

109. Colan, S. D., Fujii, A, Borow, K. M., et al.: Noninvasive determination of systolic, diastolic and end-systolic blood pressure in neonates, infants, and young children: Comparison with central aortic measurements. Am. J. Cardiol. *52*:867, 1983.

110. Horan, M. J., et al.: Report of the second task force on blood pressure control in children—1987. Pediatrics *79*:1, 1987.

111. Berenson, G. S., Webber, L. S., and Voors, A. W.: Diagnosing hypertension in children. J. Cardiovasc. Med. *6*:273, 1982.

112. Mehta, S. K.: Pediatric hypertension: A challenge for pediatrics. Am. J. Dis. Child. *141*:893, 1987.

113. Lauer, R. M., Burns, T. L., and Clarke, W. R.: Assessing children's blood pressure—considerations of age and body size: The Muscatine study. Pediatrics *75*:1081, 1985.

114. Rocchini, A. P.: Childhood hypertension: Etiology, diagnosis, and treatment. Pediatr. Clin. North Am. *31*:1259, 1984.

115. Balfe, J. W., Levin, L., Tsuru, N., and Chan, J. C. M.: Hypertension in childhood. Adv. Pediatr. *36*:201, 1989.

116. Lauer, R. M., and Clarke, W. R.: Childhood risk factors for high adult blood pressure: The Muscatine study. Pediatrics *84*:633, 1989.

117. Rocchini, A. P., Katch, V., Anderson, J. et al.: Blood pressure in obese adolescents: Effect of weight loss. Pediatrics *82*:16, 1988.

118. Fleischmann, L. E.: Management of hypertensive crises in children. Pediatr. Ann. *6*:410, 1977.

HYPERLIPIDEMIAS

119. Schieken, R. M.: The management of the family at high risk for coronary heart disease. *In* Friedman, W. F., and Talner, N. S. (eds.): Cardiology Clinics: Update in Pediatric Cardiology. Philadelphia, W. B. Saunders Company, Vol. 7, No. 2, 1989, pp. 467–477.

120. Garcia, R. E., and Moodie, D. S.: Routine cholesterol surveillance in childhood. Pediatrics *84*:751, 1989.

121. Jacobson, M. S., and Lillienfeld, D. E.: The pediatrician's role in atherosclerosis prevention. J. Pediatr. *112*:836, 1988.

122. Lauer, R. M., Lee, J., and Clarke, W. R.: Factors affecting the relationship between childhood and adult cholesterol levels: The Muscatine study. Pediatrics *82*:309, 1988.

123. Nader, P. R., Taras, H. L., Sallis, J. F., and Patterson, T. L.: Adult heart disease prevention in childhood: A national survey of pediatricians, practices and attitudes. Pediatrics *79*:843, 1987.

124. Breslow, J. L.: Genetic basis of lipoprotein disorders. J. Clin. Invest. *84*:373, 1989.

125. Leaf, A.: Management of hypercholesterolemia. Are preventive interventions advisable? N. Engl. J. Med. *321*:680, 1989.

126. Schaefer, E. J., and Levy, R. I.: Pathogenesis and management of lipoprotein disorders. N. Engl. J. Med. *312*:1300, 1985.

127. Neill, C. A., Ose, L., and Kwiterovich, P. O., Jr.: Hyperlipidemia: Clinical clues in the first two decades of life. Johns Hopkins Med. J. *140*:171, 1977.

128. Forman, M. B., Kinsley, R. M., DuPlessis, J. P., et al.: Surgical correction of combined supravalvular and valvular aotic stenosis in homozygous familial hypercholesterolemia. SA Med. J. *1*:579, 1982.

Valvular Heart Disease
by EUGENE BRAUNWALD, M.D.

Mitral Stenosis

ETIOLOGY AND PATHOLOGY

The predominant cause of mitral stenosis (MS) is rheumatic fever[1,2] (p. 1721). Far less frequently, MS is congenital in etiology,[3] and this form is observed almost exclusively in infants and young children (p. 929). Rarely, mitral stenosis is a complication of malignant carcinoid (p. 1424), systemic lupus erythematosus, rheumatoid arthritis,[4] and the mucopolysaccharidoses of the Hunter-Hurley phenotype.[5] Amyloid deposits may occur on rheumatic valves and contribute to the obstruction to left atrial emptying.[6] Methysergide therapy is an unusual but documented cause of MS.[7] MS, generally of rheumatic origin, may be associated with atrial septal defect in Lutembacher syndrome (p. 970). Left atrial tumor, particularly myxoma (p. 1454); ball-valve thrombus in the left atrium (usually associated with MS)[8]; and a congenital membrane in the left atrium, i.e., cor triatriatum (p. 929), may also obstruct left atrial outflow and therefore simulate MS. Although calcification of the mitral annulus usually causes mitral regurgitation (MR), when subvalvular or intravalvular extension is extensive, MS may result.[9] Approximately 25 per cent of all patients with rheumatic heart disease have pure MS, and an additional 40 per cent have combined MS and MR.[10] Two-thirds of all patients with rheumatic MS are female.

Rheumatic fever results in four forms of fusion of the mitral valve apparatus leading to stenosis: (1) commissural, (2) cuspal, (3) chordal, and (4) combined.[11] Thickening of the commissures alone occurs in 30 per cent, of the cusps alone in 15 per cent, and of the chordae alone in 10 per cent; in the remainder, thickening of more than one of these structures is involved. Characteristically, mitral valve cusps fuse at their edges, and fusion of the chordae results in thickening and shortening of these structures. The stenotic mitral valve is typically funnel-shaped, and the orifice is frequently shaped like a "fish mouth" or buttonhole, with calcium deposits in the valve leaflets sometimes extending to involve the valve ring, which may become quite thick[11] (Figs. 34–1 and 56–6, p. 1726). The thickened leaflets may be so adherent and rigid that they cannot open or shut, reducing or rarely even abolishing the first heart sound (S_1) and leading to combined MS and MR.[12] There is a rough correlation between the severity of calcification and the transvalvular gradient.[13] When rheumatic fever results exclusively or predominantly in contraction and fusion of the chordae tendineae, with little fusion of the valvular commissures, dominant MR results.[14]

It probably takes a minimum of 2 years after the onset of acute rheumatic fever for severe MS to develop, and most patients in temperate climates remain asymptomatic for at least a decade more.[1,15] Symptoms commence most commonly in the third or fourth decade, although mild MS in the aged is becoming a more frequent finding.[16,17] In the tropics, particularly in underdeveloped areas, the disease advances more rapidly, and severe MS may be present in early adolescence.[18] The debate continues about whether the anatomical changes in severe MS result from a smoldering rheumatic process or whether once the valve has been deformed by the initial episode, the constant trauma produced by the turbulent blood flow leads to progressive fibrosis, thickening, and calcification of the valve apparatus.[19]

Enlargement of the left atrium and resultant elevation of the left main stem bronchus, calcification of the left atrial wall, the development of mural thrombi, and obliterative changes in the pulmonary vascular bed (p. 796) may all result from chronic MS.

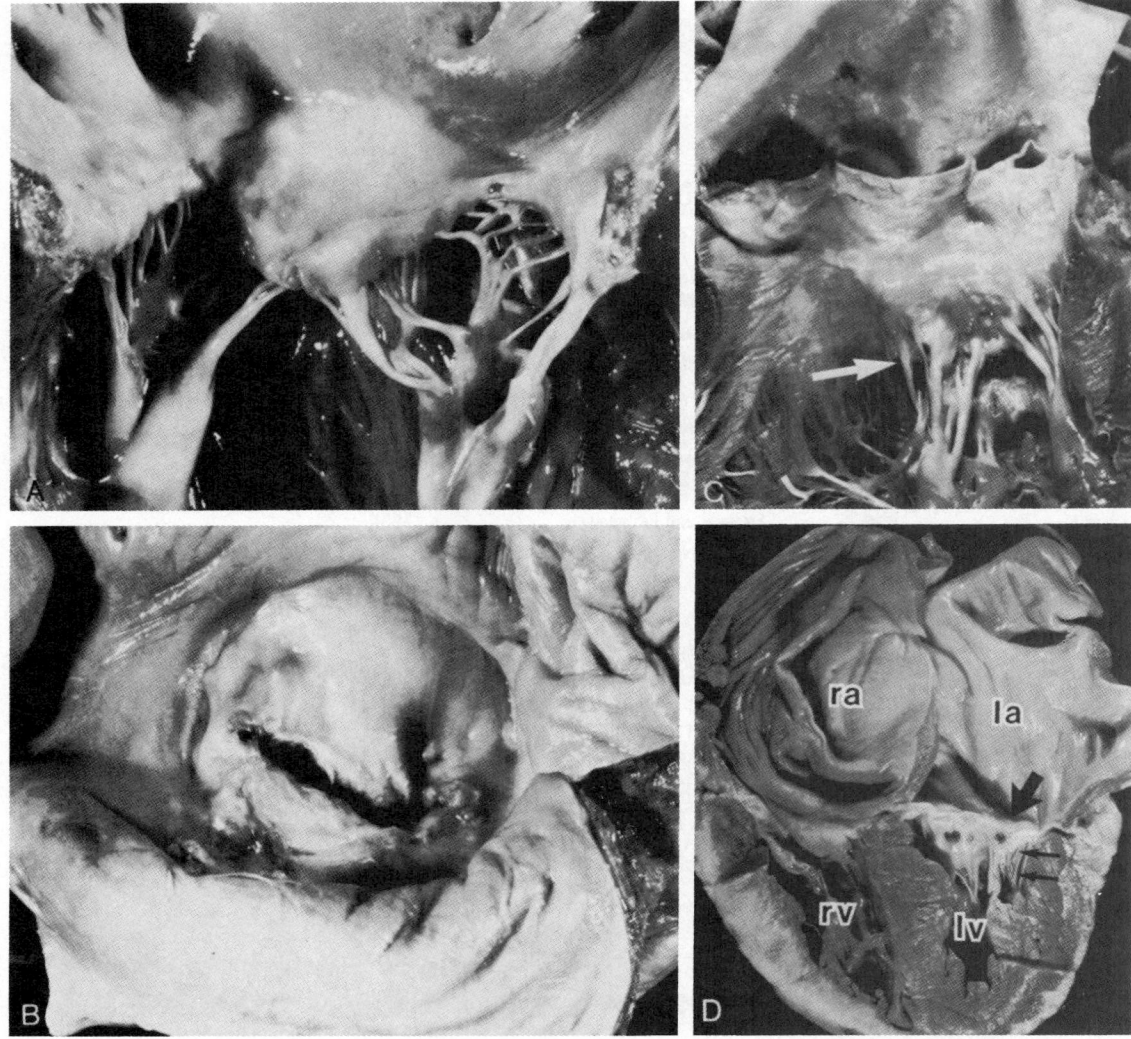

FIGURE 34–1. Rheumatic mitral stenosis. *A,* Moderate valvular changes including diffuse leaflet fibrosis, commissural fusion, and chordal thickening and fusion. In another case, atrial view (*B*) and subvalvular and aortic aspects (*C*) show prominent subvalvular involvement; severe subvalvular distortion is evident (arrow). *D,* Severe rheumatic mitral stenosis with specimen shown in apical four-chamber echocardiographic view, demonstrating small left ventricle (lv) and enlarged left atrium (la), right ventricle (rv), and right atrium (ra). Note the calcified stenotic valve (arrow) and prominent subvalvular changes (double arrows). (*A* and *D* from Schoen, F. J., and St. John Sutton, M.: Contemporary issues in the pathology of valvular heart disease. Hum. Pathol. *18:*568, 1987.)

PATHOPHYSIOLOGY

In normal adults the cross-sectional area of the mitral valve orifice is 4 to 6 cm². When the orifice is reduced to approximately 2 cm², which is considered to represent mild MS, blood can flow from the left atrium to the left ventricle only if propelled by an abnormal, though small, pressure gradient. When the mitral valve opening is reduced to 1 cm², which is considered to represent critical MS, a left atrioventricular pressure gradient of approximately 20 mm Hg (and therefore, in the presence of a normal left ventricular diastolic pressure, a mean left atrial pressure of approximately 25 mm Hg) is required to maintain normal cardiac output at rest (Figs. 34–2 and 34–3 and 7–10, p. 189). The elevated left atrial pressure in turn raises pulmonary venous and capillary pressures, resulting in exertional dyspnea (p. 449). The first bouts of dyspnea in patients with MS are usually precipitated by exercise, emotional stress, sexual intercourse, infection, or atrial fibrillation, all of which increase the rate of blood flow across the mitral orifice and result in further elevation of the left atrial pressure.[20,21]

In order to assess the severity of obstruction of the mitral valve (and, for that matter, of any valve), it is essential to measure both the transvalvular pressure gradient and the flow rate. The latter depends not only on cardiac output but on heart rate as well. An increase in heart rate shortens diastole proportionately more than systole and diminishes the time available for flow across the mitral valve. Therefore, at any given level of cardiac output, tachycardia augments the transmitral valvular pressure gradient and elevates left atrial pressures further.[22,23] This explains the sudden development of dyspnea and pulmonary edema in previously asymptomatic patients with MS who experience atrial fibrillation with a rapid ventricular rate[24]; it also accounts for the equally rapid improvement in these patients when the ventricular rate is slowed by means of cardiac glycosides and/or beta-adrenoceptor blocking agents, even when the cardiac output per minute remains constant. Hydraulic considerations dictate that at any given orifice size the transvalvular gradient is a function of the square of the transvalvular flow rate (p. 194 and Fig. 34–3).[25] Thus, a doubling of flow rate will quadruple the pressure gradient, so that a stress such as exercise in patients with moderate or severe MS will cause marked elevation of left atrial pressure.[26]

Atrial contraction augments the presystolic transmitral valvular gradient by approximately 30 per cent in patients with MS (Fig. 7–10, p. 189). Withdrawal of atrial transport when atrial fibrillation develops decreases cardiac output by about 20 per cent. The more rapid ventricular rate that occurs in atrial fibrillation until it is pharmacologically controlled raises the transvalvular pressure gradient. Thus, hemody-

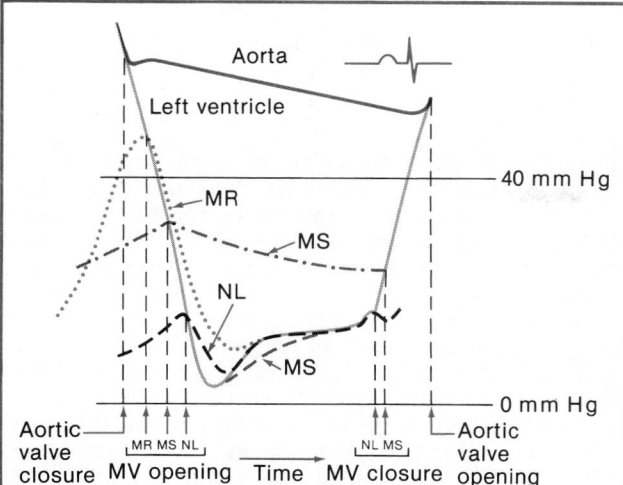

FIGURE 34–2. Schematic relationship of left ventricular (⎯⎯⎯⎯⎯), aortic (⎯⎯⎯⎯⎯), and pulmonary atrial wedge (PAW) pressures. Note that the higher the left atrial v wave, the earlier the pressure crossover, and the earlier the mitral valve (MV) opening. The higher left atrial end-diastolic pressure with severe mitral stenosis (MS) also results in later closure of the mitral valve. PAW pressures in severe mitral regurgitation (MR) (· · · · · · ·), mitral stenosis (⎯ · ⎯ · ⎯ ·), and normal (⎯ ⎯ ⎯ ⎯). The LV diastolic pressure in mitral stenosis (⎯ ⎯ ⎯ ⎯) rises slowly, denoting the absence of a rapid filling wave. (From Braunwald, E., and Turi, Z. G.: Pathophysiology of mitral valve disease. *In* Ionescu, M. I., and Cohn, L. H. [eds.]: Mitral Valve Disease. London, Butterworths, 1985, p. 3.)

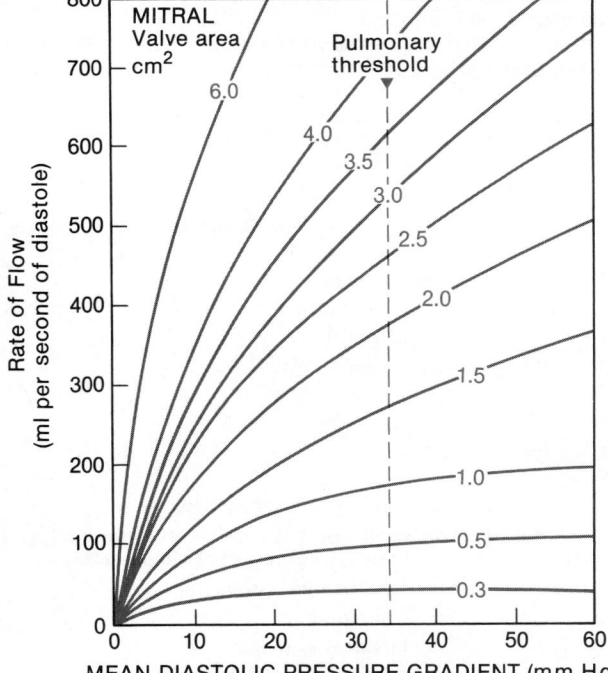

FIGURE 34–3. Graph illustrating the relation between mean diastolic gradient across the mitral valve and rate of flow across the mitral valve per second of diastole, as predicted by the Gorlin formula. Note that when the mitral valve area is 1.0 cm² or less, very little additional flow can be achieved by an increased pressure gradient. (From Wallace, A. G.: Pathophysiology of cardiovascular disease. *In* Smith, L. H., Jr., and Thier, S. O. [eds.]: Pathophysiology: The Biological Principles of Disease. The International Textbook of Medicine. Vol. 1. Philadelphia, W. B. Saunders Company, 1981, p. 1192.)

INTRACARDIAC AND INTRAVASCULAR PRESSURES

Left ventricular diastolic pressure is normal in patients with pure MS; coexisting MR, aortic valve lesions, systemic hypertension, ischemic heart disease, and cardiomyopathy may all be responsible for elevations of left ventricular diastolic pressure. In approximately 85 per cent of patients with pure MS, the end-diastolic volume is within the normal range, whereas it is reduced in the remainder.[28] In approximately one-fourth of patients with pure MS the ejection fraction and other ejection indices of systolic performance (p. 426) are below normal, most likely resulting from chronic reduction in preload and elevated afterload caused by reduced left ventricular thickness.[29] Regional hypokinesis is common,[30] perhaps caused by extension of the scarring process from the mitral valve into the adjacent posterior basal myocardium[31] or by associated ischemic heart disease. The left ventricular mass is normal or slightly reduced.[28] It has long been postulated that persistent myocardial dysfunction, perhaps caused by smoldering rheumatic myocarditis, may be responsible for the poor results following surgical treatment of some patients with pure MS.[32] The bulk of available evidence suggests that myocardial contractility (as opposed to systolic performance) is normal or slightly impaired in the majority of patients.[33,34] Associated ischemic heart disease may be responsible for myocardial dysfunction.[35] Most patients with MS show a normal elevation of ejection fraction and reduction of end-systolic volume during exercise.[36]

In MS and sinus rhythm, the *left atrial pressure pulse* generally exhibits a prominent atrial contraction (a) wave (Fig. 7–10, p. 189) and a gradual pressure decline after mitral valve opening (y descent); the mean left atrial pressure is elevated. In patients with mild to moderate MS without elevation of pulmonary vascular resistance, pulmonary arterial pressure may be normal or only slightly elevated at rest and may rise only during exercise. However, in patients with severe MS and/or those in whom the pulmonary vascular resistance is significantly increased, pulmonary arterial pressure is elevated when the patient is at rest, and in rare cases of extreme elevation of the pulmonary vascular resistance it may exceed the systemic arterial pressure. Further elevations of left atrial and pulmonary vascular pressures occur during exercise (Fig. 7–10, p. 189) or tachycardia or both. With moderate elevation of pulmonary artery pressure, right ventricular performance is maintained.[37] However, an elevation of pulmonary arterial systolic pressure exceeding 70 mm Hg represents a serious impedance to emptying of the right ventricle and causes right ventricular failure with elevations of the right ventricular end-diastolic and right atrial pressures. During exercise, patients with MS and pulmonary hypertension commonly fail to exhibit normal elevation of right ventricular ejection fraction.[36]

The *clinical and hemodynamic features* of MS of any given severity are dictated largely by the levels of cardiac output and pulmonary vascular resistance. The response to a given degree of mitral obstruction may be characterized at one end of the hemodynamic spectrum by a normal cardiac output and a high left atrioventricular pressure gradient or, at the opposite end of the spectrum, by a markedly reduced cardiac output and low transvalvular pressure gradient. In some patients with moderately severe stenosis (mitral valve area = 1.0 to 1.5 cm²) cardiac output at rest may be normal and it rises normally during exertion as well. In these patients, marked elevation of left atrial and pulmonary capillary pressures and the high transvalvular pressure gradient together lead to severe pulmonary congestion during exertion. However, in the majority of patients with severe MS, cardiac output rises subnormally during exertion, thus reducing the pulmonary venous pressure and the severity of symptoms of pulmonary congestion more than would be the case if the output rose normally. In patients with severe stenosis (mitral valve area < 1.0 cm^2), particularly when pulmonary vascular resistance is elevated, cardiac output is usually depressed at rest and may fail to rise at all during exertion. These patients frequently have prominent symptoms secondary to a low cardiac output, e.g., severe weakness and fatigue.

Pulmonary hypertension in patients with MS results from (1) passive backward transmission of the elevated left atrial pressure; (2) pulmonary arteriolar constriction, which presumably is triggered by left atrial and pulmonary venous hypertension (reactive pulmonary hypertension); (3) organic obliterative changes in the pulmonary vascular bed, which may be considered to be a complication of longstanding and severe MS[38] (Chap. 27); and (4) there is some evidence for reversible pulmonary vasoconstriction as well.[39-41] In time, severe pulmonary hypertension results in right-sided failure and tricuspid and sometimes pulmonic regurgitation. However, it has been suggested that these changes in the pulmonary vascular bed may also be considered to exert a protective effect; the elevated precapillary resistance makes the development of symptoms of pulmonary congestion less likely by tending to prevent blood from surging into the pulmonary capillary bed and damming up behind the stenotic mitral valve, although this protection occurs at the expense of a decreased cardiac output.[23] Patients with severe MS manifest a marked reduction in lung compliance, an increase in the work of breathing, and a redistribution of pulmonary blood flow from the bases to the apices.

The combination of mitral valve disease and atrial inflammation secondary to rheumatic carditis causes (1) left atrial dilatation, (2) fibrosis of the atrial wall, and (3) disorganization of the atrial muscle bundles. The third condition leads to disparate conduction velocities and inhomogeneous refractory periods. Premature atrial activation due either to an automatic focus or to reentry may stimulate the left atrium during the vulnerable period and may thus precipitate atrial fibrillation. Often this is episodic at first, but then it becomes more persistent. Atrial fibrillation per se causes diffuse atrophy of atrial muscle, further atrial enlargement,[42] and further inhomogeneity of refractoriness and conduction; these changes, in turn, lead to irreversible atrial fibrillation.[43]

CLINICAL MANIFESTATIONS

(Table 34–1)

HISTORY

The principal symptom of MS is dyspnea, largely the result of reduced compliance of the lungs. Vital capacity is reduced, presumably owing to the presence of engorged pulmonary vessels and interstitial edema. Patients with critical obstruction to left atrial emptying and dyspnea with ordinary activity (functional Class III) generally have orthopnea and are at risk of experiencing attacks of frank pulmonary edema. The latter may be precipitated by effort, emotional stress, respiratory infection, fever, sexual intercourse, pregnancy (p. 1796), or atrial fibrillation with a rapid ventricular rate or, indeed, by any condition that increases blood flow across the stenotic mitral valve, either by increasing total cardiac output or by reducing the time available for this flow of blood to occur. In patients with a markedly elevated pulmonary vascular resistance, right ventricular function is often impaired, and a rise in right ventricular output may be impossible. Therefore, they are less subject to sudden elevations of pulmonary capillary pressure and the accompanying attacks of pulmonary edema.[21,44]

HEMOPTYSIS. Wood has differentiated between several kinds of *hemoptysis* complicating MS.[21]

1. Sudden hemorrhage (sometimes called pulmonary apoplexy), while often profuse, is only rarely life-threatening.[45] It results from the rupture of thin-walled, dilated bronchial veins,[46] usually as a consequence of a sudden rise in left atrial pressure. After several years of pulmonary venous hypertension, the walls of these veins thicken appreciably, and this form of hemoptysis tends to disappear.

2. Blood-stained sputum associated with attacks of paroxysmal nocturnal dyspnea.

3. Pink, frothy sputum characteristic of acute pulmonary edema with rupture of alveolar capillaries.

4. Pulmonary infarction, a late complication of MS associated with heart failure.

5. Blood-stained sputum complicating chronic bronchitis; the edematous bronchial mucosa in patients with chronic MS

TABLE 34-1 DIAGNOSIS OF MITRAL VALVE DISEASE

	MITRAL STENOSIS	MITRAL REGURGITATION
Sex	Women > Men	Men > Women
Severity of rheumatic fever	Less severe	Often fulminating
Presystolic murmur	Present	Absent
First sound	Loud unless calcification	*Never loud*
Apical systolic murmur	Usually absent	Pansystolic or late
Mid-diastolic murmur	Long, not necessarily loud	*If present, short*
Opening snap of mitral valve	Present unless heavy calcification, pulmonary hypertension, or aortic regurgitation	
Third sound	*Never present*	Commonly present and loud
Cardiac impulse	Tapping ("closing snap"); right ventricular type if pulmonary vascular resistance raised	Left ventricular type; right ventricular type if pulmonary vascular resistance raised
Radial pulse	Small volume	Small volume but collapsing
Systemic emboli	Common	Less common
Left atrial size	Enlarged but rarely aneurysmal	May be aneurysmal; systolic
Left ventricle	*Normal or poor filling*, aorta hypoplastic	*Enlarged, rapidly filling*, and hyperdynamic
Electrocardiogram	RVH if pulmonary vascular resistance raised	LVH; RVH if pulmonary vascular resistance raised
	a. LAP may be greatly raised	a. Less severely raised as a rule
	b. Gradient across valve in diastole	b. No gradient usually
	c. PVR may be severely raised	c. PVR not commonly greatly raised

RVH = right ventricular hypertrophy, LVH = left ventricular hypertrophy, LAP = left atrial pressure, PVR = pulmonary vascular resistance.
Modified from Oram, S.: Clinical Heart Disease. London, William Heinemann Medical Books, 1981, p. 335.

increases the likelihood of chronic bronchitis, a common complication of MS, particularly in Great Britain.

CHEST PAIN. A small fraction, perhaps 15 per cent, of patients with MS experience chest discomfort that is indistinguishable from angina pectoris.[20,21] This symptom may be caused by right ventricular hypertension[47] or by coincidental coronary atherosclerosis,[35,48] or it may be secondary to coronary obstruction caused by coronary embolization.[49] In many such patients, however, a satisfactory explanation cannot be uncovered even after complete hemodynamic and angiographic studies.

THROMBOEMBOLISM. Prior to the advent of surgical treatment, this serious complication of MS[50] developed in at least 20 per cent of patients at some time during the course of their disease, and in the past as many as 10 to 15 per cent of this group died as a consequence. Before the era of anticoagulant therapy and surgical treatment, approximately one-fourth of all fatalities in patients with mitral valve disease were secondary to embolism. The tendency for embolization correlates inversely with cardiac output and directly with the patient's age and the size of the left atrial appendage; 80 per cent of patients with MS in whom systemic emboli develop are in atrial fibrillation. When embolization occurs in patients in sinus rhythm, the possibility of transient atrial fibrillation and underlying infective endocarditis should be considered. There is no simple correlation between the incidence of embolism on one hand and the size of the mitral orifice on the other. Indeed, embolism may be the first symptom of MS and may occur in patients with mild MS even before the development of dyspnea. Patients older than 35 with atrial fibrillation, especially with a low cardiac output and dilation of the left atrial appendage, are at the highest risk for emboli and therefore should receive prophylactic anticoagulant treatment.

Since thrombi are found in the left atrium at operation in only a minority of patients with a history of recent embolism, it is likely that only fresh clots are discharged. Approximately half of all clinically apparent emboli are found in the cerebral vessels. Coronary embolism may lead to myocardial infarction, angina pectoris, or both, and renal emboli may be responsible for the development of systemic hypertension. Emboli are recurrent and multiple in approximately 25 per cent of patients subject to this complication. Rarely, massive thrombosis develops in the left atrium, resulting in a pedunculated ball-valve thrombus, which may suddenly aggravate obstruction to left atrial outflow when a specific body position is assumed, or it may cause sudden death.[51] Similar consequences occur in patients with free-floating thrombi in the left atrium.[8]

INFECTIVE ENDOCARDITIS (see also Chap. 35). This complication tends to occur *less frequently* on rigid, thickened, calcified valves and is therefore more common in patients with mild than with severe MS.

OTHER SYMPTOMS. Compression of the left recurrent laryngeal nerve by a greatly dilated left atrium, enlarged tracheobronchial lymph nodes, and dilated pulmonary artery may cause hoarseness (Ortner syndrome).[52] A history of repeated hemoptysis is common in patients with pulmonary hemosiderosis, and longstanding elevation of pulmonary venous pressure is present in patients with pulmonary ossification. Systemic venous hypertension, hepatomegaly, edema, ascites, and hydrothorax are all signs of severe MS with elevated pulmonary vascular resistance and right heart failure.

PHYSICAL EXAMINATION[53,54]

Patients with severe MS, a low cardiac output, and systemic vasoconstriction often exhibit the so-called mitral facies, characterized by pinkish-purple patches on the cheeks.[21] The *arterial pulse* is usually normal, but in patients in whom the stroke volume is reduced, it may be small in volume. The *jugular venous pulse* usually exhibits a prominent *a* wave in patients with sinus rhythm and elevated pulmonary vascular

resistance. In atrial fibrillation, the x descent of the jugular pulse disappears, and there is only one crest, a prominent *v* or *c-v* wave, per cardiac cycle. *Palpation* of the cardiac apex usually reveals an inconspicuous left ventricle; the presence of either a palpable presystolic expansion wave or an early diastolic rapid filling wave speaks strongly against significant MS. A readily palpable, tapping first heart sound (S_1) suggests that the anterior mitral valve leaflet is pliable. When the patient is in the left lateral recumbent position, the low-pitched diastolic rumbling murmur of MS may be palpable as a thrill at the apex. Often a right ventricular lift is felt in the left parasternal region in patients with pulmonary hypertension (Fig. 2-19D, p. 29). A markedly enlarged right ventricle may displace the left ventricle posteriorly and produce a prominent apex beat that can be confused with a left ventricular lift. A loud pulmonic closure sound (P_2) may be palpable in the second left intercostal space in patients with MS and pulmonary hypertension.

AUSCULTATION. The auscultatory (and phonocardiographic) features of MS (some of which are illustrated in Fig. 3-28, p. 57) include an accentuated S_1 with prolongation of the Q-S_1 interval, correlating with the level of the left atrial pressure.[12] Accentuation of S_1 occurs when the mitral valve leaflets are flexible.[55,55a] It is caused, in part, by the rapidity with which left ventricular pressure rises at the time of mitral valve closure as well as by the wide closing excursion of the valve leaflets.[56] Marked calcification or thickening of the mitral valve leaflets or both reduce the amplitude of S_1, probably because of diminished motion of the leaflets. As pulmonary artery pressure rises, P_2 at first becomes accentuated and widely transmitted and can often be readily heard and recorded at both the mitral and the aortic areas. With further elevation of pulmonary artery pressure, splitting of S_2 narrows because of reduced compliance of the pulmonary vascular bed, which shortens the "hangout interval." Finally, S_2 becomes single and accentuated. Other signs of pulmonary hypertension include a nonvalvular pulmonic ejection sound that diminishes during inspiration, owing to dilation of the pulmonary artery; the systolic murmur of tricuspid regurgitation; a Graham Steell murmur of pulmonic regurgitation; and an S_4 originating from the right ventricle.[57] An S_3 originating from the left ventricle is absent, unless significant mitral or aortic regurgitation coexists.[58]

The *opening snap* (OS) of the mitral valve appears to be due to a sudden tensing of the valve leaflets after the valve cusps have completed their opening excursion. OS occurs when the movement of the mitral dome into the left ventricle suddenly stops.[56] It is best heard at the apex and with the diaphragm of the stethoscope and can usually be differentiated from P_2 because the OS occurs later, unless right bundle branch block is present. The mitral valve cannot be totally rigid if it produces an OS, which is usually accompanied by an accentuated S_1. These two sounds—the OS and the delayed S_1—are "reciprocal sounds," both caused by abrupt termination of movement of the fused mitral complex.[56] Calcification confined to the tip of the mitral valve leaflets does not preclude an OS, although calcification of the body and tip does.[59] In patients with combined MS and regurgitation, the OS may be followed by an S_3. The mitral OS follows A_2 by 0.04 to 0.12 sec, and the A_2-OS interval varies inversely with left atrial pressure.[60] Although a short A_2-OS interval is a reliable indicator of severe MS, the converse is not necessarily the case, since the time interval between the actual opening of the mitral valve and the OS can be prolonged in the presence of valvular calcification and tight stenosis. (Q-S_1)–(A_2-OS) correlates better with the height of the left atrial pressure than does either term alone.[61]

The diastolic murmur of MS is a low-pitched, rumbling murmur, best heard at the apex and with the bell of the stethoscope. When this murmur is soft, it is limited to the apex, but when louder, it may radiate to the axilla or the lower left sternal area. Although the intensity of the diastolic murmur is not closely related to the severity of stenosis, the *duration of* the murmur is a guide to the severity of mitral narrowing. In patients with combined MS and MR, a long diastolic murmur always signifies the presence of significant stenosis and, in general, persists for as long as the gradient across the mitral valve exceeds approximately 3 mm Hg. The murmur usually commences immediately after the mitral OS. In mild MS, the early diastolic murmur is brief but resumes in presystole. In severe stenosis, the murmur is holodiastolic, with presystolic accentuation in patients with sinus rhythm.

Although a *presystolic* murmur is usually present in patients with sinus rhythm in whom transvalvular blood flow is accelerated by atrial contraction, such a murmur may also occur in patients with atrial fibrillation, in whom it results from the increased velocity of blood flow across a mitral valve orifice that begins to narrow after the onset of left ventricular contraction.[62] Since, in patients with atrial fibrillation, this murmur results from motion of the mitral valve leaflets, a flexible mitral valve is required for its generation; its absence in a patient with moderate or severe obstruction suggests a rigid calcified valve or a markedly reduced cardiac output or both.

The *diastolic rumbling* murmur of MS may be masked by the presence of obesity, pulmonary emphysema, and a low cardiac output with a low flow rate across the mitral valve. The rumble may be sharply localized and thus missed unless palpation is used to detect the apex of the left ventricle and to pinpoint the area at which auscultation should be carried out. In so-called "silent" MS, there is usually marked right ventricular enlargement, so that the right ventricle occupies the cardiac apex, and cardiac output is reduced, so that the murmur either is not audible at all or can be heard only in the mid- or posterior axillary line.[63] Auscultation of the murmur is facilitated by placing the patient in the left lateral position and auscultating during expiration after a few sit-ups or other maneuvers described later.

Dynamic Auscultation. The diastolic murmur and OS of MS are often reduced during inspiration and augmented during expiration[53,54,64]—the opposite of what occurs when these findings are secondary to tricuspid stenosis (p. 1053). During inspiration the A_2-OS interval widens, and three sequential sounds (A_2, P_2, and OS) are frequently audible. Sudden standing and the resultant reduction of venous return lower left atrial pressure and widen the A_2-OS interval[65]; this maneuver is useful in distinguishing an A_2-OS combination from a split S_2, which narrows on standing. In contrast, A_2-OS is significantly narrowed during exercise as left atrial pressure rises. The diastolic rumbling murmur of MS is reduced during the strain of a Valsalva maneuver and in any condition in which transmitral valve flow rate declines. Amyl nitrite, coughing, isometric or isotonic exercise, and sudden squatting are all useful in accentuating a faint or equivocal murmur of MS. Progressive narrowing of A_2-OS on serial examinations suggests an increase in the severity of stenosis, whereas widening of A_2-OS after mitral commissurotomy indicates that the severity of stenosis has been reduced significantly.

DIFFERENTIAL DIAGNOSIS. It is important to recognize that a variety of conditions other than MS may exhibit auscultatory findings that can be confused with MS, and these are summarized in Table 34-2. In addition to the findings listed in the table, the *Carey-Coombs* murmur of acute rheumatic fever (p. 1727) is a sign of active mitral valvulitis and can be confused with the murmur of MS. It is a soft, early diastolic murmur, usually varies from day to day, and is higher pitched than the diastolic rumbling murmur of established MS. In pure, severe MR—indeed, in any condition in which there is increased flow across a nonstenotic mitral valve—there may also be a short, diastolic murmur following an S_3. *Left atrial myxoma* may produce auscultatory findings similar to those in rheumatic valvular MS (p. 1452). A high-frequency early systolic murmur is audible along the lower left sternal border in one-third of patients with MS.[66] This should be distinguished from the apical (often holosystolic or late systolic) murmur of MR. In addition, a *pansystolic murmur of tricuspid regurgitation* and an S_3 originating from the right ventricle may be audible in the fourth intercostal space in the left parasternal region in patients with severe mitral stenosis. These signs, secondary to pulmonary hypertension, may be confused with the findings of MR.[67] However, the inspiratory augmentation of the murmur and of the S_3 and the prominent v wave in the jugular venous pulse aid in establishing that the mur-

TABLE 34-2   CONDITIONS IN WHICH AUSCULTATORY FINDINGS MAY SIMULATE THOSE IN MITRAL STENOSIS

AUSCULTATORY EVENT	CONDITION OTHER THAN MITRAL STENOSIS	EXPLANATION OF EVENT
Loud and snapping first sound	Hyperkinetic states	High left ventricular dP/dt at time of mitral closure
Early diastolic opening snap	Myxoma of left atrium	Tumor movement into ventricle Abrupt checking of tumor (tumor plop)
	Constrictive pericarditis	Checking of ventricular filling by pericardium
	Tricuspid stenosis	Stenotic valve
Diastolic rumbling murmur	Aortic regurgitation (Austin Flint murmur)	Preclosure of mitral valve (?) Regurgitant stream (?) Fluttering of mitral valve

	Dilated ventricle
	  Myocarditis
	  Cardiomyopathy
		Preclosure of mitral valve
		(?) Centrifugal displacement of papillary muscles

	Hypertrophic, restrictive ventricle
	  Hypertrophic obstructive cardiomyopathy
	  Aortic valve disease
		Impaired filling of left ventricle
		(?) Impaired opening of mitral valve

	Tricuspid stenosis	Narrow orifice
	Myxoma of left atrium	Narrow orifice
	Augmented atrioventricular flow	Preclosure of valve
	Mitral regurgitation Left-to-right shunts	(?) Centrifugal displacement of papillary muscles
Crescendo presystolic murmur	Aortic regurgitation (Austin Flint murmur)	Preclosure of mitral valve opposing atrial systole
	Hypertrophic, restrictive ventricle	Summation of S_4 and S_1 may simulate presystolic murmur
	Tricuspid stenosis	Narrow orifice
	Myxoma of left atrium	Narrow orifice

Modified from Criley, J. M., et al.: Departures from the expected auscultatory events in mitral stenosis. In Likoff, W. (ed.): Cardiovascular Clinics, Vol. 5, No. 2, Valvular Heart Disease. Philadelphia, F. A. Davis, 1973, p. 213.

mur originates from the tricuspid valve. A decrescendo diastolic murmur along the left sternal border in patients with MS and pulmonary hypertension is usually due to aortic regurgitation and rarely represents a Graham Steell murmur of pulmonary regurgitation[68] (p. 56); the latter, when present, characteristically increases during inspiration.

LABORATORY EXAMINATION

ELECTROCARDIOGRAPHY. The ECG and vectorcardiogram are relatively insensitive techniques for the detection of mild MS, but they do show characteristic changes in moderate or severe obstruction[69,70] (Fig. 34-4). Left atrial enlargement (P-wave duration in lead II > 0.12 sec, terminal negative P force in lead V_1 > 0.003 mV/sec, P-wave axis between +45 and −30 degrees) is a principal electrocardiographic feature of MS (Fig. 5-10, p. 124) and is found in 90 per cent of patients with significant MS and sinus rhythm.[71] The ECG signs of left atrial enlargement correlate more closely with left atrial volume than with left atrial pressure[72] and often regress following successful valvulotomy.[21] When atrial fibrillation is present, the fibrillatory waves are coarse, i.e., greater than 0.1 mV in amplitude in V_1, also suggesting the presence of atrial enlargement.[73] The development of atrial fibrillation correlates with the preexistent ECG diagnosis of left atrial enlargement and is related to the size and the extent of fibrosis of the left atrial myocardium,[39-41] the duration of atriomegaly, and the age of the patient.[74]

Whether or not there is ECG evidence of right ventricular hypertrophy depends largely on the height of right ventricular systolic pressure; it is infrequent in patients with right ventricular systolic pressures less than 70 mm Hg.[71] However, approximately half of all patients with right ventricular systolic pressures between 70 and 100 mm Hg manifest the electrocardiographic criteria for right ventricular hypertrophy, including both a mean QRS axis that is greater than 80 degrees in the frontal plane and an R : S ratio greater than 1.0 in V_1.[75] In other patients with this degree of pulmonary hypertension there is no frank evidence of right ventricular hypertrophy, but the R : S ratio fails to increase from right to midprecordial leads. When right ventricular systolic pressures exceed 100 mm Hg, electrocardiographic evidence of right ventricular hypertrophy is found quite consistently. The mean QRS axis averages +150 degrees, and there is a Q-R morphology in the right precordial leads, accompanied by inverted or biphasic T waves.[76]

The *QRS axis in the frontal plane* often correlates with the severity of valve obstruction and with the level of pulmonary vascular resistance in pure MS; thus, a mean frontal axis between 0 and +60 degrees suggests that the mitral valve area exceeds 1.3 cm², whereas an axis greater than 60 degrees suggests that the valve area is less than 1.3 cm². In patients in whom pulmonary vascular resistance is greater than 650 dynes·sec·cm⁻⁵, the mean axis usually exceeds +110 degrees.[75]

VECTORCARDIOGRAPHY. The characteristic *vectorcardiographic finding* in MS is right ventricular hypertrophy Type C (Fig. 5-15, p. 128) characterized by counterclockwise rotation in the horizontal plane and a terminal deflection directed to the right, posteriorly, and superiorly.[71,75-77] In other patients with MS without frank right ventricular hypertrophy, QRS loops with posterior and rightward terminal appendages are evident without conduction delays.[71,75] There is vectorcardiographic evidence of right ventricular hypertrophy Type A (Fig. 5-15, p. 128) in only 10 per cent of patients with MS, but when present it indicates that both the hypertrophy and the stenosis are severe. Vectorcardiograms showing right ventricular hypertrophy Type B (Fig. 5-15) are infrequent in MS.

Rotation of the P loop in the frontal plane, with superior orientation of the terminal P forces and a wide angle between the initial and terminal P

vectors, occurs in about one-fourth of patients with pure mitral stenosis and may be the only evidence of left atrial enlargement.[78] The terminal portion of the P loop is usually directed posteriorly and inferiorly, and the T loop is often directed leftward and posterosuperiorly and is discordant with respect to the QRS loop, resulting in a diphasic T wave with initial negativity and terminal positivity in lead V_1.

RADIOLOGICAL FINDINGS (see also p. 223). Although the cardiac silhouette may be normal in the frontal projection, with the exception of an enlarged atrial appendage (Fig. 8-35, p. 224) in patients with hemodynamically significant MS, left atrial enlargement is almost invariably evident on the lateral and left anterior oblique views.[79,80] The size of the left atrium does *not* correlate with the severity of obstruction. However, extreme left atrial enlargement rarely occurs in pure MS; when it is present, MR is usually severe. Enlargement of the pulmonary artery, right ventricle, and right atrium (as well as the left atrium) is commonly seen in severe MS (Fig. 8-34, p. 224). Occasionally, calcification of the mitral valve is evident on the chest roentgenogram (Fig. 8-30, p. 221), but, more commonly, fluoroscopy is required to detect valvular calcification.

Radiological changes in the lung fields (Fig. 8-34, p. 224) are useful in estimating the height of pulmonary venous pressure and thereby the severity of MS. Interstitial edema, an indication of severe obstruction, is manifested as Kerley B lines (dense, short, horizontal lines most commonly seen in the costophrenic angles).[81] This finding is present in 30 per cent of patients with resting pulmonary artery wedge pressures below 20 mm Hg and in 70 per cent of patients with pressures exceeding 20 mm Hg. Severe, longstanding mitral obstruction often results in Kerley A lines (straight, dense lines up to 4 cm in length and running toward the hilum) as well as the findings of pulmonary hemosiderosis[82] (Fig. 8-34B, p. 224) and rarely of parenchymal ossification.

Angiography. Angiograms exposed in the right and left anterior oblique projections afford the best views of the mitral valve.[83] Although ideally contrast medium should be injected into the left atrium, it is often possible to achieve good visualization of the left side of the heart by injecting a large volume of contrast medium into the main pulmonary artery. Such angiograms provide an assessment of left atrial size, may demonstrate thickening and reduced motion of the valve leaflets, and may outline large intraluminal thrombi.[84] Left cine ventriculography is useful in the assessment of mitral valve motion. Although this technique allows visualization of only the ventricular aspect of the leaflet in patients with pure MS, it makes possible simultaneous assessment of left ventricular contractile function and of the subvalvular mitral apparatus.

ECHOCARDIOGRAPHY (see also p. 81). MS can ordinarily be readily diagnosed by M-mode echocardiography (Fig. 4-44, p. 82), but this technique does not allow a precise determination of its severity. Echocardiograms of a thickened, calcified stenotic rheumatic valve demonstrate increased acoustic impedance and fusion of the mitral valve leaflets and poor leaflet separation in diastole.[85,86] The leaflets fail to close in mid-diastole and may not reopen widely during atrial contraction. Normally, the posterior leaflet of the mitral valve moves posteriorly during early diastole, but in more than 90 per cent of patients with MS, both leaflets move anteriorly at this time (Fig. 34-5, *top*) and there is inadequate separation of the leaflets. The E−F slope is reduced,[87] but this finding is not

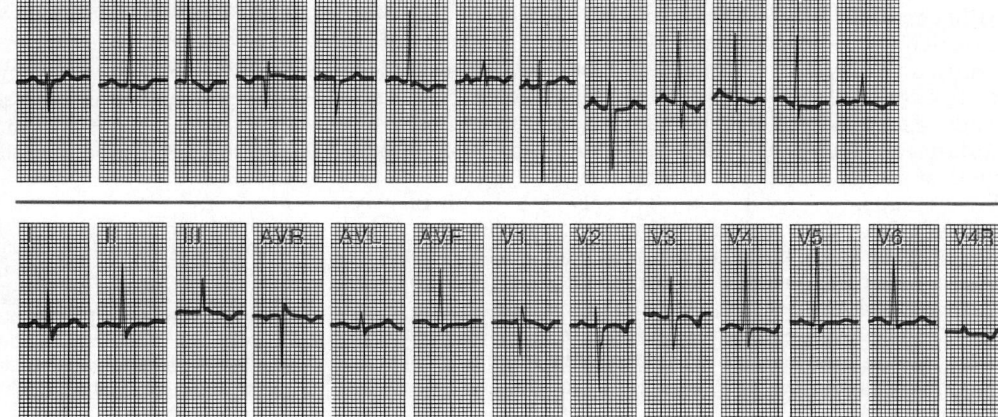

FIGURE 34-4. *Upper tracing,* ECG of a patient with tight mitral stenosis, pulmonary hypertension, right atrial enlargement, right axis deviation, and right ventricular hypertrophy. *Lower tracing,* Six months after commissurotomy, the signs of right ventricular hypertrophy have regressed. (From Barlow, J. B.: Perspectives on the Mitral Valve. Philadelphia, F. A. Davis, 1987, p. 169.)

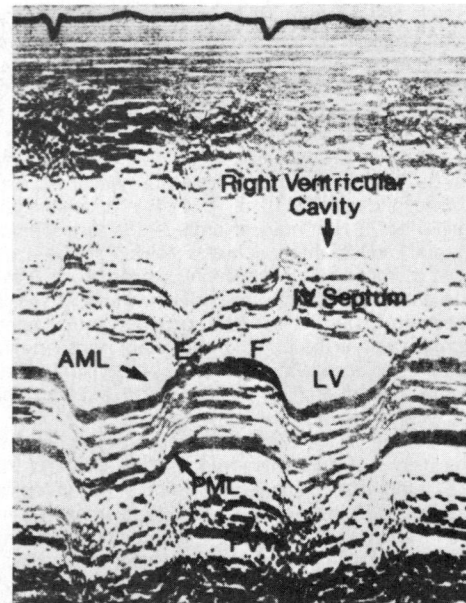

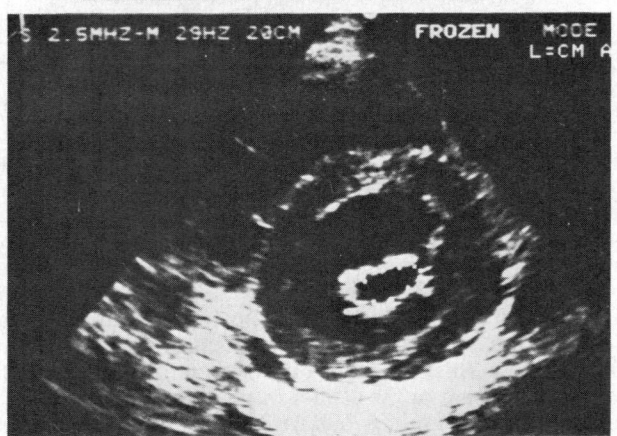

FIGURE 34–5. *Top,* M-mode echocardiogram of a patient with mitral stenosis. Note the decreased E-F slope, absence of the A wave, and thickened leaflets. The posterior mitral leaflet (PML) moves in an anterior direction with the anterior mitral leaflet (AML) during diastole. IV = interventricular septum, LV = left ventricle, PVW = posterior ventricular wall. (From Dalen, J. E.: Mitral stenosis. *In* Dalen, J. E., and Alpert, J. S. [eds.]: Valvular Heart Disease. 2nd ed. Boston, Little, Brown and Company, 1987, p. 73.) *Bottom,* Two-dimensional parasternal short-axis view of the mitral valve orifice during diastole, demonstrating the echocardiographic method of mitral valve area calculation. The innermost border of the mitral orifice was planimetered with the use of a light-pen system to obtain the area (in cm²). (From Smith, M. D., et al.: Comparative accuracy of two-dimensional echocardiography and Doppler pressure half-time methods in assessing severity of mitral stenosis in patients with and without prior commissurotomy. Circulation 73:100, 1986, by permission of the American Heart Association, Inc.)

pathognomonic of MS, since it may occur in other conditions in which left ventricular compliance and the velocity of left ventricular filling are reduced. However, in these other conditions the posterior leaflet of the mitral valve moves normally. The maximal diastolic separation of the anterior and posterior leaflets,[88] their rate of diastolic apposition, and the slope of motion of the left ventricular posterior wall during diastole appear to correlate more closely with the mitral valve area.[87,88] Two-dimensional echocardiography (Fig. 34–5, *bottom,* and Fig. 4–45, p. 82) is more accurate than M-mode echocardiography in determining mitral orifice size.[89–91] It reveals restricted motion and doming of the valve leaflets. The orifice can often be imaged directly and measured. This technique also provides information on the pliability and extent of calcification of the valve and its suitability for balloon mitral valvuloplasty (p. 1017).

Other important echocardiographic findings in patients with pulmonary hypertension and MS include a small or absent *a* wave in the pulmonic valve echogram (Fig. 4–42, p. 81). The left atrium is usually enlarged, and in isolated MS the left ventricular cavity is normal or reduced in size. Echocardiography is also useful in detecting mitral annular calcification, which may accompany MS and in which a band of dense echoes is present in the region of the mitral annulus, in contrast to the thin and delicate echoes recorded from the normal mitral annulus. The technique is helpful in the estimation of pulmonary artery pressure. Two-dimensional echocardiography may be helpful in the preoperative recognition of left atrial thrombus[92] in assessing mitral valve calcification and left ventricular contractility.

Doppler echocardiography is especially useful in quantifying the severity of MS[91,93] (Fig. 4–46, p. 82). The peak velocity of transmitral flow is increased, and the rate of decline of flow during early diastole is reduced. The time required for peak velocity to reach half its initial level correlates with the size of the mitral orifice. Doppler color flow imaging can be used to enhance the accuracy of the Doppler data by guiding the position of the beam[94] and to determine whether mitral regurgitation and other valvular abnormalities coexist. A detailed echocardiographic examination in a patient with MS can frequently provide sufficient information to allow development of a therapeutic plan without the need for invasive cardiac catheterization.

MANAGEMENT
MEDICAL TREATMENT

Patients with rheumatic heart disease should receive penicillin prophylaxis for beta-hemolytic streptococcal infections and prophylaxis for infective endocarditis (p. 1090). Anemia and infections should be treated promptly and aggressively in patients with valvular heart disease. Adolescents and young adults with serious valvular heart disease should be advised to avoid entering occupations requiring strenuous exertion.

In symptomatic patients with mitral valve disease, considerable improvement occurs with oral diuretics and the restriction of sodium intake. Digitalis glycosides do not alter the hemodynamics and usually do not benefit patients with MS and sinus rhythm[86,95] but are of great value in slowing the ventricular rate in patients with atrial fibrillation and in the treatment of right-sided heart failure. Measures designed to reduce pulmonary venous pressure, including sedation, assumption of the upright posture, and aggressive diuresis, are used to treat hemoptysis. Beta blockers may increase exercise capacity by reducing heart rate, even in patients with sinus rhythm.[96]

In patients with rheumatic heart disease and heart failure and/or atrial fibrillation, anticoagulant therapy is helpful in preventing venous thrombosis and pulmonary embolism in those who have experienced one or more previous embolic episodes, in those who are at high risk of embolization, i.e., with atrial fibrillation, and in those with mechanical prosthetic heart valves. However, no firm evidence exists that anticoagulant therapy reduces the incidence of pulmonary or systemic embolism in patients in sinus rhythm in whom such episodes have not previously occurred.

TREATMENT OF ARRHYTHMIAS. Frequent premature atrial contractions often presage atrial fibrillation, and the administration of antiarrhythmic drugs, as outlined on page 628, may be effective in preventing this complication. However, once atrial fibrillation has developed, these agents may be ineffective in restoring sinus rhythm or even in maintaining sinus rhythm following electrical cardioversion, because of the pathological changes that occur in the atrium secondary to the arrhythmia itself. After electrical cardioversion, sinus rhythm can often be maintained with antiarrhythmic drugs in young patients with mild MS without marked left atrial enlargement who have been in atrial fibrillation less than 6 months and who are maintained by adequate doses of quinidine. In any event, if elective cardioversion (pharmacological or electrical) is to be attempted in the patient with MS and atrial fibrillation, a preparatory three-week course of anticoagulation should be given to minimize the risk of systemic embolism when sinus rhythm resumes. Immediate treatment of atrial fibrillation should be directed toward reducing the ventricular rate by means of digitalis and, if possible, toward reestablishing sinus rhythm by a combination of pharmacological treatment and cardioversion. However, it must be appreciated that in 1 to 2 per cent of patients with MS, systemic embolism develops following electrical or pharmacological cardioversion. Paroxysmal atrial fibrillation and repeated conversions, spontaneous or induced, carry the risk of embolization.[97] In patients who cannot be converted or maintained in sinus rhythm, the ventricular rate at rest should be maintained at approximately 60 to 65 beats/min with digitalis. If this is not possible, small doses of a beta blocker, such as atenolol (25 mg daily), may be added. Multiple repeat cardioversions are not indicated if the patient has not sustained sinus rhythm while on adequate doses of quinidine.

NATURAL HISTORY

The development of effective surgical treatment has obscured our understanding of the natural history of MS (Fig. 34–6) and, for that matter, of all valvular lesions.[98] Although few meaningful data are available, it appears that in temperate zones such as the United States and Europe, after an asymptomatic period of 20 to 25 years following an attack of rheumatic fever, it takes approximately 5 years for most patients to progress from mild disability (i.e., early Class II) to severe disability (i.e., Class III or IV). The progression is much more rapid in patients in subtropical areas such as Pakistan, the Middle East, Central America, and the Philippines.[99] Polynesians, as well as Eskimos in Alaska and blacks in Alabama, also show an accelerated course. Economic conditions as well as genetic ones may play a role. In the presurgical era, Olesen found 62 per cent 5-year and 38 per cent 10-year survival rates among patients in New York Heart Association functional Class III but only 15 per cent 5-year survival rate in patients in Class IV.[100] Among asymptomatic patients (Class I) with MS treated medically, 40 per cent had a worsened course or had died within 10 years. Among mildly symptomatic patients (Class II), the comparable number was 80 per cent.[101] In medically treated patients with MS or with combined MS and MR, Munoz et al. found a 45 per cent 5-year survival rate.[44] In a comparable group of patients subjected to mitral commissurotomy, the 5-year survival rate was substantially better. In an unselected mix of patients with MS of varying severity, 80 per cent were alive after 5 years and 60 per cent after 10 years of medical treatment.[102]

SURGICAL TREATMENT

INDICATIONS FOR OPERATION. Patients with MS who are asymptomatic or minimally symptomatic frequently re-

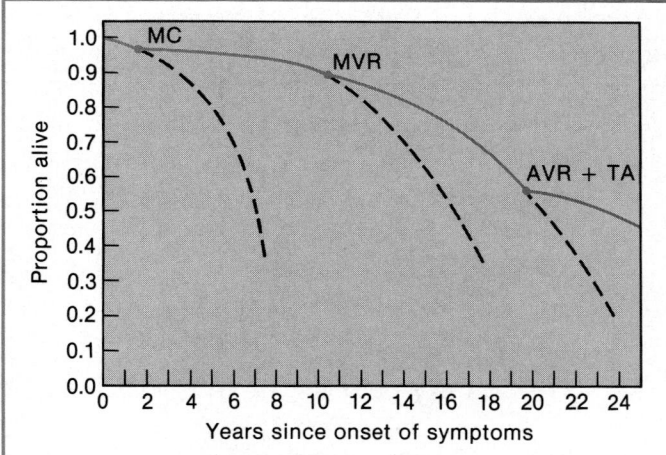

FIGURE 34–6. Schematic representation of the subsequent life history after the initial development of symptoms in a large group of patients with mitral stenosis. The red solid circles and red lines indicate a surgical procedure. The dashed lines represent estimated survival of patients not receiving the surgical procedure. MC = mitral commissurotomy, MVR = mitral valve replacement, TA = tricuspid annuloplasty, AVR = aortic valve replacement. (From Kirklin, J. W., and Barratt-Boyes, B. G.: Cardiac Surgery. New York, John Wiley and Sons, 1986, p. 328.)

main so for years. However, once severe symptoms develop, if the stenosis is not relieved mechanically, the disease may progress relatively rapidly, as already discussed. Operation (or balloon valvuloplasty) should therefore be carried out in symptomatic patients with moderate to severe MS (i.e., a mitral valve orifice size less than approximately 1.0 cm²/m² body surface area [BSA]).

There has been considerable debate concerning the need for routine cardiac catheterization in determining whether operation is indicated.[103–105] A careful clinical evaluation and noninvasive assessment, particularly using two-dimensional and Doppler echocardiography, can provide sufficient information to permit an informed decision in the majority of patients. However, the consequences of valvular surgery, particularly valve replacement, are so profound that I recommend preoperative catheterization and angiography in the following groups of patients with MS: (1) patients with heart murmurs and other findings suggesting the presence of valve lesions in addition to MS, (2) patients with associated chronic obstructive pulmonary disease, (3) patients in whom left atrial myxoma should be excluded, and (4) patients who have angina or angina-like chest pain or who have risk factors for coronary artery disease in whom associated coronary artery disease must be excluded. Critical narrowing of one or more coronary vessels occurs in approximately one-fourth of all adults with severe MS. It is more common in men over 45 years who have angina and risk factors for coronary artery disease.[35,106,107] I believe that preoperative catheterization can be omitted in the young (< 40 years) patient without angina who has typical symptoms and classic findings of pure, severe MS on physical examination and by noninvasive tests, including two-dimensional and Doppler echocardiography.

Care of mildly symptomatic patients (Class II) must be individualized. It is necessary to consider and balance three important factors: (1) the size of the mitral orifice, (2) the degree to which the patient's life style is impaired by the mitral obstruction, (3) the risk of the procedure (operation or balloon valvuloplasty), and (4) the history of complications, particularly systemic embolism. If there are no obvious contraindications to one of these procedures, left heart catheterization should be performed to determine the size of the valve orifice. In general, mechanical relief of obstruction can be deferred in patients with mild symptoms and mild stenosis (i.e., mitral valve orifice size > approximately 1.0 cm²/m² BSA), whereas it should be recommended for those with mild symptoms and more severe stenosis (i.e., mitral valve orifice size < approximately 1.0 cm²/m² BSA). However, this plan is subject to qualification. For instance, mechanical relief of obstruction might well be deferred in a retired, sedentary woman in her seventies and a mitral valve orifice of 0.8 cm²/m² BSA. On the other hand, a 25-year-old laborer whose family's economic well-being depends on his continued physical exertion might be an excellent candidate for mechanical relief of obstruction, although his mitral valve orifice size is 1.2 cm²/m² BSA.

Because of the high rate of recurrence, operation is also indicated in patients with MS in whom systemic embolism has previously occurred, even if they are otherwise asymptomatic and even though there is no definitive evidence that the incidence of recurrent emboli will be significantly reduced. Anticoagulants should be administered up to the time of operation. Although the risk of operation is higher in patients with advanced disease characterized by severe pulmonary hypertension and right-sided heart failure, surviving patients nearly always show striking clinical and hemodynamic improvement, with a marked reduction in pulmonary vascular pressures. In the pregnant patient with MS, operative treatment should be carried out only if serious pulmonary congestion occurs despite intensive medical treatment including bed rest (p. 1796).

There is no evidence that surgical treatment improves the prognosis of patients with no or only slight functional impairment. Therefore, valvulotomy is *not* indicated in patients who are entirely asymptomatic, except in unusual circumstances.

For example, some years ago I saw a 33-year-old woman with MS who had had hemoptysis and pulmonary edema during the second trimester of a pregnancy 2 years previously. She then became asymptomatic but wished to have another child. Hemodynamic study showed a pulmonary wedge pressure of 17 mm Hg and a mitral orifice area of 1.7 cm²/m² BSA. Prophylactic mitral commissurotomy was undertaken in this patient, since it was virtually certain that another pregnancy would have resulted in serious heart failure. At present I would recommend balloon mitral valvuloplasty (p. 1376) for such a patient.

SURGICAL TECHNIQUES. Three basically different operative approaches are available for the treatment of rheumatic MS (Fig. 34–7): (1) closed mitral valvotomy[108,109]; (2) open commissurotomy, i.e., commissurotomy carried out under direct vision with the aid of cardiopulmonary bypass; and (3) mitral valve replacement.[110] Closed mitral commissurotomy, performed with the aid of a transventricular dilator, is generally preferred to simple transatrial finger fracture.[108-110] It is an effective operation, provided that MR, atrial thrombosis, or valvular calcification is not serious and that chordal fusion and shortening are not severe. Unfortunately, few patients satisfy all these criteria, and they are difficult to identify preoperatively. In one large series,[108] hospital mortality was 1.5 per cent and 0.3 per cent of patients developed severe MR. Marked symptomatic improvement occurred in 86 per cent of survivors. Actuarial survival rate was 89.5 per cent after 18 years. Closed valvotomy for restenosis was carried out with a 6.7 per cent mortality. Long-term follow-up has shown that the results are best if the operation is carried out before chronic atrial fibrillation and/or heart failure have occurred.[109] Therefore, if possible, closed mitral commissurotomy should be carried out with "pump standby"; if the surgeon is unable to achieve a satisfactory result, the patient can be placed on cardiopulmonary bypass, and the commissurotomy carried out under direct vision. Closed mitral commissurotomy is rarely used in the United States today, but is more popular in developing nations, where the expense of open-heart surgery is a more important factor and where patients with mitral valve disease are younger. In any event, echocardiography is useful in selecting suitable candidates for closed mitral valvulotomy by identifying patients without valvular calcification or dense fibrosis.[111]

Most surgeons in the United States, Canada, and Western Europe now prefer to carry out *direct-vision* or *open commissurotomy*.[110-115] Cardiopulmonary bypass is established, and in order to obtain a dry, quiet heart, body temperature is usually lowered, the heart is arrested, and the aorta is occluded intermittently. Thrombi are removed from the left atrium and its appendage, and the latter is often amputated in order to remove a potential source of postoperative emboli. The commissures are incised, and when necessary fused chordae are separated, the underlying papillary muscle is split, and the valves are debrided of calcium; mild or even moderate mitral regurgitation may be corrected with suture plication or annuloplasty. Left atrial and ventricular pressures are measured after bypass has been discontinued to confirm that the commissurotomy has in fact been effective. In patients with atrial fibrillation, conversion to sinus rhythm is carried out at the completion of the operation. In a series of open mitral valve reconstructive procedures for MS at Brigham and Women's Hospital, the actuarial probability of survival at 10 years was 95 per cent; thromboemboli occurred in 9 of 120 patients. The annual reoperation rate was 1.7 per cent.[116]

The mortality rate after mitral commissurotomy, whether open or closed, ranges from 1 to 3 per cent, depending on the condition of the patient and the skill and experience of the surgical team.[113-116] In general, open commissurotomy provides better hemodynamic relief of mitral valve obstruction than does the closed procedure,[115,117] and the risk of dislodging thrombi from the atrium or calcium from the mitral valve is also less.[113,116] Left atrial size, the need for mitral or tricuspid

annuloplasty, and the presence of left atrial thrombus are all "risk factors" for a less than optimal outcome.[117] However, it must be recognized that mitral commissurotomy, whether open or closed, is a *palliative* rather than a curative operation, and even when successful, it merely "turns the clock back." (The generally more effective open valvulotomy turns the clock farther backward than does the closed valvulotomy or balloon mitral valvuloplasty.) Thus, valvulotomy does not result in a normal mitral valve but, at best, results in one resembling the valve as it existed perhaps a decade earlier. Since the valve is not normal postoperatively, turbulent flow usually persists in the paravalvular region, and the resultant trauma may well play a role in restenosis. These changes are analogous to the gradual development of obstruction in a congenitally bicuspid aortic valve (p. 967) and are not usually the result of recurrent rheumatic fever.

Mitral valve replacement is discussed on pages 1027 and 1042.

Although a contemporary control series of medically and surgically treated patients is not available (nor is it likely that it ever will be), appropriate surgical treatment appears to prolong survival substantially in patients with MS (Fig. 34–6).

Mitral Restenosis. This condition can be diagnosed with certainty only on the basis of three satisfactory hemodynamic or echocardiographic investigations: a preoperative study, a second study following a satisfactory operation in which an increase in the size of the valvular orifice can be demonstrated, and a third after the reappearance of symptoms, when a reduction in size relative to the earlier postoperative study is noted. On clinical grounds alone, the incidence of "restenosis" has been estimated to range widely, from 2 to 60 per cent[118]; approximately 10 per cent of patients who have undergone mitral commissurotomy require reoperation within 5

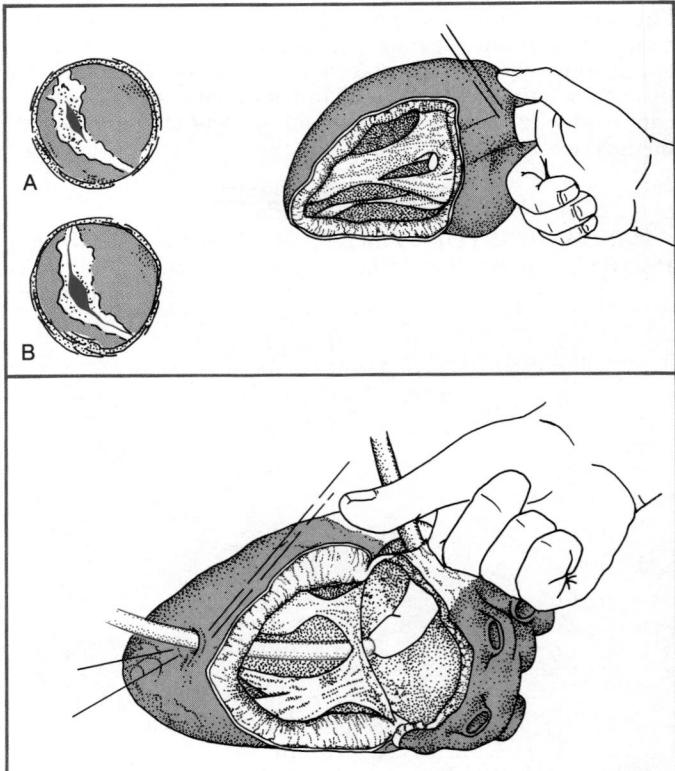

FIGURE 34–7. *Top,* Closed digital mitral commissurotomy. Mitral valve before (A) and after (B) valvotomy. *Bottom,* Transventricular closed mitral commissurotomy. Finger of the surgeon's right hand in the left atrium. Tubbs dilator through the apex of the left ventricle in the ostium of the mitral valve. (From deVivie, E. R., and Hellberg, K.: Closed transventricular mitral commissurotomy. *In* Ionescu, M. I., and Cohn, L. H. [eds.]: Mitral Valve Disease: Diagnosis and Treatment. London, Butterworths, 1985, pp. 140–141.)

years, but that fraction increases to 60 per cent by 10 years.[119] The recurrence of symptoms is *not necessarily* due to restenosis. Recurrent symptoms may be due to one of four other conditions: (1) an inadequate first operation with residual stenosis; (2) the presence or development of MR, either at operation or as a consequence of infective endocarditis; (3) the progression of aortic valve disease; and (4) the development of ischemic heart disease. In a study in which the size of the mitral valve orifice was estimated using two-dimensional echocardiography in 18 patients who had undergone successful mitral commissurotomy, no change in the mitral valve area occurred over a 10- to 14-year period in 13 patients, whereas in 5 (28 per cent) true restenosis developed.[119] Approximately 10 per cent of patients returning to the hospital with persistent or recurrent symptoms 6 years after operation have true restenosis.[120]

Thus, in properly selected patients, mitral commissurotomy results in a significant increase in the size of the mitral orifice and, at a low risk, favorably alters the clinical course of an otherwise progressive disease. Pulmonary artery pressure falls promptly and decisively when mitral obstruction is effectively relieved.[121-124] Some patients maintain clinical improvement for many (10 to 15) years of follow-up. When a second operation is required because of symptomatic deterioration, the valve is usually calcified and more seriously deformed than at the time of the first operation, and adequate reconstruction is not always possible. Accordingly, mitral valve replacement is often necessary.[125] Also, in patients with combined MS and MR, and in those with extensive calcification involving the commissures of the valve, mitral replacement rather than commissurotomy is often required. The operative mortality following mitral valve replacement ranges from 3 to 8 per cent in most hospitals. As described below (p. 1062), the long-term fate of the prosthetic valves is not yet clear; also, the hazards of lifelong anticoagulant treatment in patients with mechanical prostheses cannot be neglected. Therefore, in patients in whom preoperative evaluation suggests that valve replacement may be required, the threshold for operation should be higher than in patients believed to require commissurotomy alone. If possible, a second conservative procedure, i.e., open commissurotomy, should be performed; in some instances this has led to excellent outcome.[126]

BALLOON MITRAL VALVULOPLASTY

(See also Chap. 41)

This procedure represents an alternative to surgical treatment of MS. The technique consists of advancing a small balloon flotation catheter across the interatrial septum (after transseptal puncture), enlarging the opening and advancing one large (23 to 25 mm) or two smaller (12 to 18 mm) balloons across the mitral orifice, and inflating them within the orifice[86,127-133] (Fig. 41–19, p. 1376). Commissural separation and fracture of nodular calcium appear to be the mechanisms responsible for improvement in valvular function. In several series the hemodynamic results have been quite favorable (Fig. 34–8), with reduction of the gradient from an average of approximately 18 to 6 mm Hg, a small (average 20 per cent) increase in cardiac output, and, on the average, a 50 to 100 per cent increase in the calculated mitral valve area. The reported mortality ranges from 0 to 4 per cent. Complications include embolic events (despite absence of detectable thrombus on two-dimensional echocardiography), cardiac perforation in 0 to 4 per cent, and the development of mitral regurgitation severe enough to require operation in another 2 per cent (approximately one-third of patients develop milder degrees of regurgitation). Results are especially impressive in younger patients without valvular thickening or calcification.[133a] Improvement in exercise tolerance has paralleled the favorable hemodynamic changes (Fig. 34–9).

Approximately 35 per cent of patients are left with a small residual atrial septal defect, but this closes or decreases in size in the majority. Rarely, the defect is large enough to cause

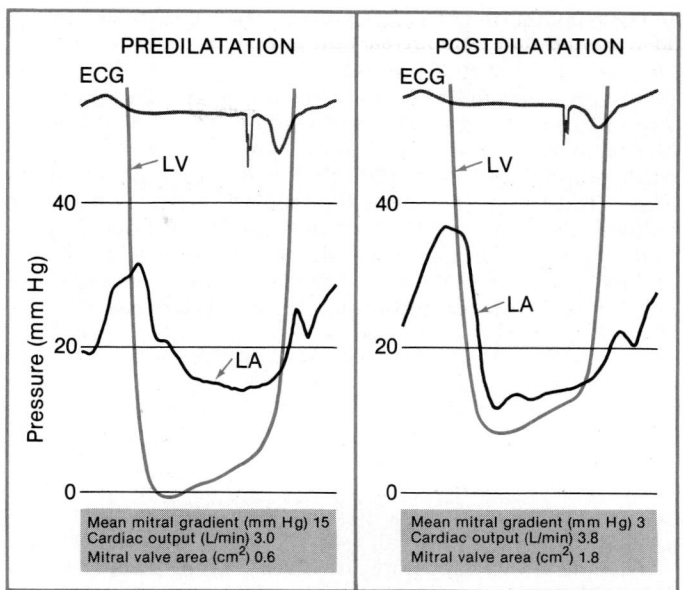

FIGURE 34–8. Simultaneous left atrial (LA) and left ventricular (LV) pressure before and after balloon valvuloplasty of the mitral valve in a patient with severe mitral stenosis. (Courtesy of Raymond G. McKay, M.D.)

right heart failure.[129,129a] Elevated pulmonary vascular resistance declines rapidly (but usually not completely) following mitral balloon valvuloplasty,[130,132] and pulmonary function improves as well.[131] In follow-up studies over 1 to 2 years, hemodynamic benefit has been maintained in the majority of patients, and they have not required surgical treatment, i.e., with commissurotomy or mitral valve replacement. Approximately 10 per cent have developed restenosis.

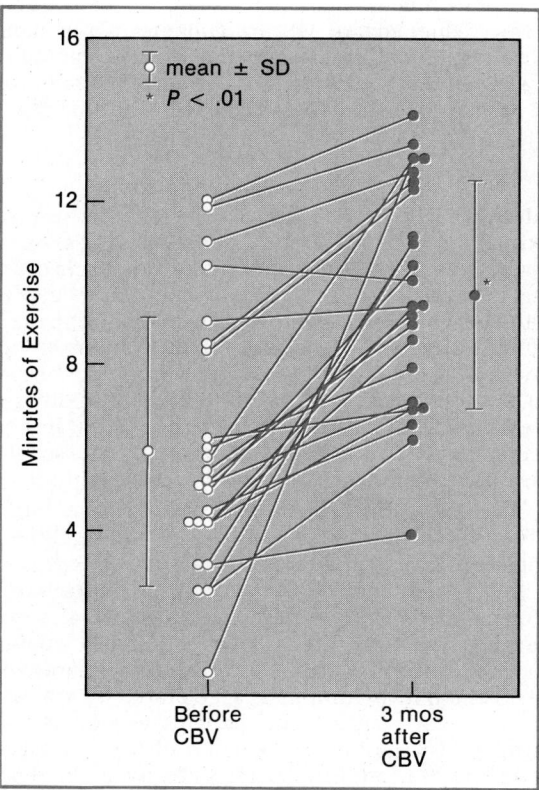

FIGURE 34–9. Exercise treadmill time (Bruce protocol) before and 3 months after catheter balloon valvuloplasty (CBV) in patients with mitral stenosis. (From McKay, C. R., et al.: Improvement in exercise capacity and exercise hemodynamics 3 months after double-balloon, catheter balloon valvuloplasty treatment of patients with symptomatic mitral stenosis. Circulation 77:1013, 1988, by permission of the American Heart Association, Inc.)

The combination of significant symptoms and documented MS generally serves as an indication for balloon valvulotomy. No hard and fast rules are possible as of this writing, when follow-up is limited to a relatively few years. The skill and experience of the operator (interventional cardiologist) must be considered. Detailed two-dimensional and Doppler echocardiographic studies are indicated before a decision is made. The mitral valves that show the greatest improvement with balloon mitral valvuloplasty are those that have mobility (particularly of the anterior cusp), little or no leaflet calcification, and little or no thickening and shortening of the subvalvular structures. An echocardiographic scoring system has been devised[133] that appears reasonably accurate in predicting the outcome of balloon mitral valvuloplasty.

While this technique is still in a developmental stage, it appears to be useful in patients who are unsuitable for surgery because of high risk.[130a] These may be very elderly patients with associated severe ischemic heart disease, as well as patients in whom MS is complicated by pulmonary, renal, or neoplastic disease. A second group consists of patients who refuse surgery. Also, it may be considered in women of childbearing age. The procedure may well be applicable for treating young patients with noncalcific MS in underdeveloped nations with limited facilities for open heart surgery.[131a]

Mitral Regurgitation

ETIOLOGY AND PATHOLOGY

The mitral valve apparatus involves the mitral annulus, the mitral leaflets per se, the chordae tendineae, and the papillary muscles. Abnormalities of any of these structures may cause mitral regurgitation (MR) (Table 34–3).[11] The mitral valve prolapse syndrome, an important cause of MR, is discussed in a separate section (p. 1029).

ABNORMALITIES OF VALVE LEAFLETS. MR due to involvement of the valve *leaflets* occurs most commonly in chronic rheumatic heart disease and is more frequent in men than in women. It is a consequence of shortening, rigidity, deformity, and retraction of one or both cusps of the mitral valve as well as shortening and fusion of the chordae tendineae and papillary muscles.[136] Destruction of the mitral valve leaflets can also be a consequence of systemic lupus erythematosus,[137] penetrating and nonpenetrating trauma (p. 1523), and infective endocarditis (Chap. 35). Retraction of the mitral valve cusps during the healing phase of endocarditis can also cause MR. When severe MR accompanies acute rheumatic fever, usually in children or in adolescents, regurgitation is due to a combination of prolapse of the anterior leaflet, elongation of the chordae, and dilatation of the annulus.[138]

ABNORMALITIES OF THE MITRAL ANNULUS

Dilatation. In a normal adult the mitral annulus measures approximately 10 cm in circumference. During systole, contraction of the surrounding left ventricular muscle causes the annulus to constrict, and this constriction contributes importantly to valve closure. MR secondary to dilatation of the mitral annulus can occur in any form of heart disease characterized by severe dilatation of the left ventricle,[139] especially dilated cardiomyopathy.[140] It is often difficult to differentiate this secondary from the primary forms of MR, but it is notable that primary valvular regurgitation is often more severe than is regurgitation secondary to dilatation of the annulus.

Calcification. Idiopathic calcification of the mitral annulus is one of the most common cardiac abnormalities found at autopsy; in most hearts this degenerative change is of little functional consequence.[141] However, when it is severe it may be an important cause of MR, and in contrast to MR secondary to rheumatic fever, this cause is more common in women than in men. In addition to the idiopathic form, degenerative calcification of the mitral annulus is accelerated by systemic hypertension, aortic stenosis, and diabetes, as well as by an intrinsic defect in the fibrous skeleton of the heart, such as occurs in the Marfan and Hurler syndromes. In these two conditions, the mitral annulus not only is calcified but also is dilated, further contributing to MR. The incidence of mitral annular calcification is also increased in patients with chronic renal failure with secondary hyperparathyroidism[142,143] (Fig. 62–11, p. 1867).

When annular calcification is severe, a rigid, curved bar or ring of calcium encircles the mitral orifice (Fig. 8–29, p. 221), and calcific spurs may project into the adjacent left ventricular myocardium[144,145]; the bulk of the calcium is located in the subvalvular region. The calcification may immobilize the basal portion of the mitral leaflets, preventing their normal excursion in diastole and coaptation in systole and aggravating the MR that results from loss of the normal sphincteric action of the mitral ring.[146,147] Rarely, when severe calcification encroaches on or protrudes into the mitral orifice, obstruction to left ventricular filling may occur. Calcification of the aortic valve cusps is an associated finding in approximately 50 per cent of patients with severe annular calcification, but this rarely causes aortic stenosis. In patients with severe calcification the conduction system may be invaded by calcium, leading to atrioventricular and/or intraventricular conduction defects.[148] Occasionally, calcific deposits extend into the coronary arteries. The annulus may also become thick and rigid as a consequence of rheumatic involvement, and when this process is severe, it also can interfere with valve closure.

ABNORMALITIES OF THE CHORDAE TENDINEAE. These are important causes of MR. The chordae may be congenitally abnormal; rupture may be spontaneous ("primary")[149] or may occur as a consequence of infective endocarditis, trauma, rheumatic fever, myxomatous proliferation, or rarely, osteogenesis imperfecta.[150-154] In most cases no cause for chordal rupture is apparent, other than increased mechanical strain.[153] Chordae to the posterior leaflet rupture more frequently than those to the anterior leaflet. Patients with idiopathic rupture of mitral chordae tendineae frequently exhibit pathological fibrosis of the papillary muscles. It is possible that the dysfunction of the papillary muscles may have caused stretching and ultimately rupture of the chordae. Chordal rupture may also result from acute left ventricular dilatation, regardless of etiology. Depending on the number of chordae involved in rupture and rate at which rupture occurs, the resultant MR may be mild, moderate, or severe and acute, subacute, or chronic, respectively.

INVOLVEMENT OF THE PAPILLARY MUSCLES. Diseases of the left ventricular papillary muscles frequently cause MR.[155] Since these muscles are perfused by the terminal portion of the coronary vascular bed, they are particularly vulnerable to ischemia, and any disturbance in coronary perfusion may result in papillary muscle dysfunction (Figs. 34–10 and 34–11). When ischemia is transient, it results in temporary papillary muscle dysfunction and may cause transient episodes of MR during attacks of angina pectoris (p. 1351). When ischemia of papillary muscles is severe and persistent, as in acute myocardial infarction, it produces papillary muscle scarring and chronic MR. The posterior papillary muscle, which is supplied by the posterior descending branch of the right coronary artery, becomes ischemic and infarcted more frequently than does the anterolateral papillary muscle, which is supplied by diagonal branches of the left anterior

TABLE 34-3 CAUSES OF ACUTE AND CHRONIC MITRAL REGURGITATION

TYPE	CONDITION
CHRONIC MITRAL REGURGITATION	
Inflammatory	Rheumatic heart disease
	Systemic lupus erythematosus
	Scleroderma
Degenerative	Myxomatous degeneration of mitral valve leaflets (Barlow's, click-murmur syndrome, prolapsing leaflet, mitral valve prolapse)
	Marfan syndrome
	Ehlers-Danlos syndrome
	Pseudoxanthoma elasticum
	Calcification of mitral valve annulus
Infective	Infective endocarditis affecting normal, abnormal, or prosthetic mitral valves
Structural	Ruptured chordae tendineae (spontaneous or secondary to myocardial infarction, trauma, mitral valve prolapse, endocarditis)
	Rupture or dysfunction of papillary muscle (ischemia or myocardial infarction)
	Dilatation of mitral valve annulus and left ventricular cavity (congestive cardiomyopathies, aneurysmal dilatation of the left ventricle)
	Hypertrophic cardiomyopathy
	Paravalvular prosthetic leak
Congenital	Mitral valve clefts or fenestrations
	Parachute mitral valve abnormality
	In association with
	Endocardial cushion defects
	Endocardial fibroelastosis
	Transposition of the great arteries
	Anomalous origin of the left coronary artery
ACUTE MITRAL REGURGITATION	
Inflammatory	Disorders of the mitral valve leaflets
	Infective endocarditis
	Trauma
	Left atrial myxoma
Degenerative	Disorders of the chordae tendineae
	Infective endocarditis
	Rheumatic valvulitis
	Trauma
	Acute rheumatic fever
	"Spontaneous" rupture
Infective	Disorders of the papillary muscles
	Dysfunction
	Ischemia
	Myocardial infarction
	Left ventricular dilatation
	Left ventricular aneurysm
	Rupture
	Trauma
	Acute myocardial infarct
	Myocardial abscess
Structural	Prosthetic valve malfunction
	Deterioration of Silastic disc
	Lodging of the ball or disc in the open position
	Dislodgement of the ball or disc
	Ring or strut fracture
	Paravalvular leak
	Suture or pledget dislodgement
	Deterioration of leaflets of tissue valve
	Prosthetic valve endocarditis

Data from Haffajee, C. I.: Chronic mitral regurgitation. *In* Dalen, J. E., and Alpert, J. S.: Valvular Heart Disease, 2nd ed. Boston, Little, Brown and Company, 1987, p. 112 (top portion); and from Rippe, J. M., and Howe, J. P., III: Acute mitral regurgitation. *In* Rippe, J. M., et al.: Intensive Care Medicine. Boston, Little, Brown and Company, 1985 (bottom portion).

descending coronary artery and often by marginal branches from the left circumflex artery as well. Ischemia of the papillary muscle is caused most commonly by coronary artery disease, but it may also occur in severe anemia, shock, coronary arteritis of any etiology, and anomalous left coronary artery. In patients with healed myocardial infarcts, MR is frequent and is caused by dyskinesis of the left ventricular myocardium at the base of a papillary muscle.[156,157]

Left ventricular dilatation of any cause, including ischemia, can alter the spatial relationships between the papillary muscles and the chordae tendineae and thereby result in MR.[158] Although *necrosis of a papillary muscle* is a frequent complication of myocardial infarction,[159] frank rupture of a papillary muscle is far less common; the latter is usually fatal because of the extremely severe MR that it produces.[160] However, rupture of one or two of the apical heads of a muscle, which results in a lesser degree of MR, makes survival possible, depending on the functional capacity of the left ventricle.

Some degree of MR is found in approximately 30 per cent of patients with coronary artery disease who are being considered for coronary bypass surgery,[156] and in them it is secondary to ischemic damage of the papillary muscles or dilatation of the mitral valve ring or both.[161] In most of these patients MR is mild, but in the small percentage in whom MR is severe (3 per cent in one large series of patients with coronary artery disease proved by coronary arteriography), it is associated with a poor prognosis.[157] The incidence and severity of regurgitation vary inversely with the left ventricular ejection fraction and directly with the left ventricular end-diastolic pressure.

A variety of other disorders of papillary muscles may also be responsible for the development of mitral regurgitation (Table 34–3). These include congenital malposition; absence of one papillary muscle, resulting in the so-called parachute mitral valve syndrome and involvement or infiltration of papillary muscles by a variety of processes, including abscesses, granulomas, neoplasms, amyloidosis, and sarcoidosis.

Other causes of MR, discussed in greater detail elsewhere, include obstructive cardiomyopathy (p. 1394), prolapse of the mitral valve (p. 1029), the hypereosinophilic syndrome,[162] en-

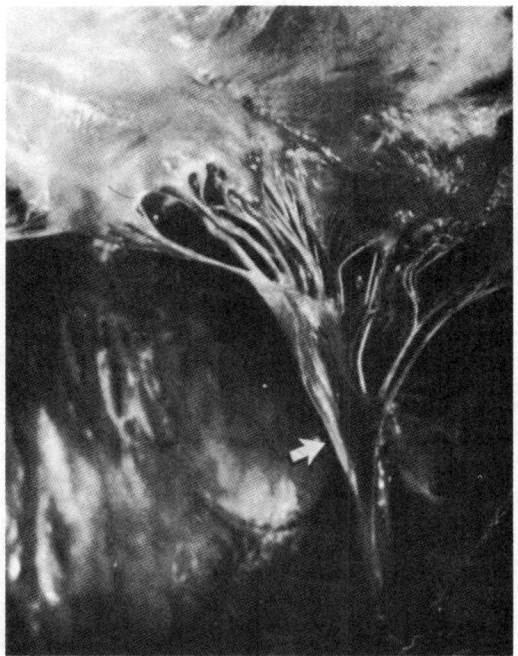

FIGURE 34–10. The posterior papillary muscle in a patient with chronic mitral regurgitation due to ischemic heart disease. The papillary muscle is thinned and replaced by fibrous tissue. The apical segment (arrows) is elongated and had undergone some calcification. (From Davies, M. J.: Aetiology and pathology of the diseased mitral valve. *In* Ionescu, M. I., and Cohn, L. H. [eds]: Mitral Valve Disease: Diagnosis and Treatment. London, Butterworths, 1985, p. 38.)

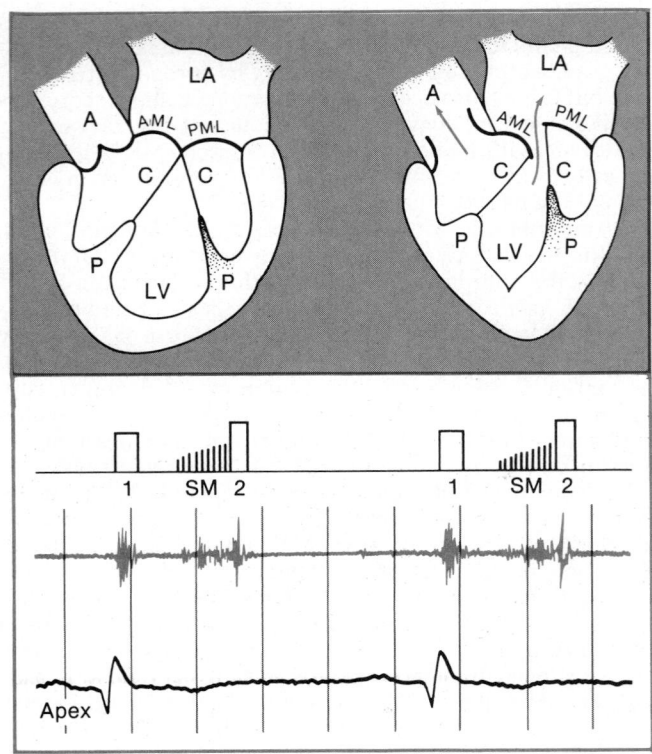

FIGURE 34–11. *Top,* Mitral regurgitation due to papillary muscle dysfunction. At the onset of systole (left), the anterior and posterior mitral valve leaflets (AML and PML) approximate. Later in systole (right), the anterior papillary muscle (P, nonhatched) contracts while the posterior papillary muscle (P, hatched) fails to contract because of ischemia or infarction. Part of the posterior leaflet is allowed to prolapse into the left atrium (LA) during systole, producing regurgitation. This process may involve either papillary muscle. C = chordae tendineae, LV = left ventricle, A = aorta. *Bottom,* Late systolic murmur (SM) that developed in a patient following an inferior myocardial infarction and is probably due to weakening of the posterior papillary muscle with prolapse of the mitral leaflet into the atrium during late systole. (From Ravin, A., et al.: Auscultation of the Heart. 3rd ed. Chicago, Year Book Medical Publishers, 1977, p. 99. Copyright © 1977 by Year Book Medical Publishers, Inc., Chicago.)

domyocardial fibrosis,[163] trauma affecting the leaflets[164] and/or papillary muscles[165] (p. 1523), Kawasaki disease (p. 997),[166] left atrial myxoma (p. 1454), a variety of congenital anomalies including cleft anterior leaflet,[167] and ostium secundum atrial septal defect.[168]

PATHOPHYSIOLOGY

Since the regurgitant mitral orifice is in parallel with the aortic valve, the impedance to ventricular emptying is reduced in MR. Consequently, as the left ventricle decompresses into the left atrium—both during isometric contraction and early during ejection—the left ventricular volume declines. Almost half of the regurgitant volume is ejected into the left atrium before the aortic valve opens.[169] The volume of MR is dependent on the impedance to left ventricular emptying and is increased by aortic stenosis.

The volume of mitral regurgitant flow depends on a combination of the instantaneous size of the regurgitant orifice and the pressure gradient between the left ventricle and left atrium[170-174]; both of these factors—orifice size and pressure

TABLE 34-4 HELPFUL POINTS IN DIFFERENTIAL DIAGNOSIS OF MITRAL REGURGITATION, VENTRICULAR SEPTAL DEFECT, TRICUSPID REGURGITATION, AND AORTIC STENOSIS

PHYSICAL, ROENTGENOGRAPHIC, OR ELECTROCARDIOGRAPHIC FEATURE	MITRAL REGURGITATION	VENTRICULAR SEPTAL DEFECT	TRICUSPID REGURGITATION	AORTIC STENOSIS
Systolic murmur	Harsh and pansystolic	Harsh and pansystolic	Pansystolic	Ejection, crescendo-decrescendo
Primary location of murmur	Apex	Left sternal border	Left sternal border	Base of heart; occasionally apical
Radiation of murmur	Axilla; occasionally base and neck	Left precordium	Little	Carotids
Thrill	Occasionally present at apex	Usually present at left sternal border	Rare	Occasionally present at base
Murmur with inspiration	No change	No change	Increases	No change
Valsalva maneuver	May increase	Increases or no change	No change	Decreases
Venous pressure	Often normal	Slightly elevated with prominent A and V waves	Elevated, with very prominent V waves	Usually normal
Pulsatile liver	No	No	Yes	No
Pulmonary component of S$_2$	Normal; occasionally increased	Normal or loud; usually delayed	Usually increased	Normal
Apical impulse	Hyperkinetic; occasional heaving	Hyperkinetic	Weak or normal	Forceful and sustained
ECG	Left ventricular hypertrophy; left atrial hypertrophy	Biventricular hypertrophy (Katz-Wachtel phenomenonon)	Right ventricular hypertrophy, occasional right atrial hypertrophy	Left ventricular hypertrophy with associated ST-T changes
Chest roentgenogram	Moderately enlarged heart, marked left atrial enlargement	Enlarged left and right ventricle	Enlarged right ventricle	Often normal heart size or left ventricular hypertrophy

From Haffajee, C. I.: Chronic mitral regurgitation. *In* Dalen, J. E., and Alpert, J. S.: Valvular Heart Disease. 2nd ed. Boston, Little, Brown and Company, 1987, p. 141.

gradient—are labile. Left ventricular systolic pressure and therefore the left ventricular–left atrial gradient are dependent on systemic vascular resistance and forward stroke volume,[170] and in patients in whom the mitral annulus is not calcific or rigid, the cross-sectional area of the mitral annulus may be altered by many interventions. Thus, increases of both preload and afterload and depressions of contractility increase left ventricular size and enlarge the mitral annulus and thereby the regurgitant orifice.[174] In MR caused by conditions in which the mitral valve apparatus is not rigid, such as ventricular dilatation due to ischemic heart disease, hypertensive heart disease or cardiomyopathy, dysfunction of papillary muscles, and rupture of chordae tendineae, the volume of regurgitant flow is influenced significantly by left ventricular dimensions, which in turn affect the regurgitant orifice. When ventricular size is reduced by treatment with positive inotropic agents, diuretics, and particularly vasodilators, the volume of regurgitant flow may become diminished, as reflected in the height of the v wave in the left atrial pressure pulse and in the intensity and duration of the systolic murmur. Conversely, left ventricular dilatation may increase MR.

In experiments in which the acute effects of equally severe MR and aortic regurgitation (AR) on the left ventricle were compared, left ventricular end-diastolic pressure, volume, and radius rose with both lesions, but far *less* so with MR.[175,176] Peak left ventricular wall tension rose markedly when AR was induced but either did not change greatly or actually declined with MR. According to Laplace's law (p. 377), myocardial wall tension is related to the product of intraventricular pressure and ventricular radius. Since acute MR reduces both late systolic ventricular pressure and radius, left ventricular wall tension declines markedly (and proportionately to a greater extent than left ventricular pressure), permitting the velocity of myocardial fiber shortening to increase. The ratio of wall thickness (h) to ventricular radius (r) is lower and the fractional shortening of myocardium greater in patients with MR than AR.[177,178]

At any given left ventricular end-diastolic and aortic systolic pressures, *acute* MR enhances early diastolic filling of the left ventricle[179] and reduces the tension developed by the left ventricular myocardium. The reduced load on the ventricle allows a greater proportion of the contractile energy of the myocardium to be expended in shortening than in tension development and explains how the left ventricle can adapt to the load imposed by MR. Thus, the reduction in left ventricular tension in *acute* MR may allow the left ventricle to increase its total output. Although the left ventricle initially compensates for the development of acute MR (in part by emptying more completely),[176,177] as regurgitation persists, the left ventricular end-diastolic volume increases. This may increase wall tension to normal or supranormal levels.[179,180] Then, an increase in left ventricular volume and mitral annulus diameter may create a vicious circle in which "MR begets more MR."[181]

A large volume of MR induced experimentally produces only slightly increased myocardial oxygen consumption,[182] because myocardial fiber shortening, which is elevated in MR, is not one of the principal determinants of myocardial oxygen consumption.[183] One of these, mean left ventricular wall tension, may actually be reduced in MR whereas the other two, contractility and heart rate, are little affected. In addition, the duration of left ventricular systolic tension is reduced in MR. These experimental observations correlate with the low incidence of clinical manifestations of myocardial ischemia in patients with severe MR compared with that occurring in aortic stenosis or aortic regurgitation, conditions in which myocardial oxygen demands are augmented.

In patients with chronic MR, both left ventricular end-diastolic volume and mass are increased; i.e., typical volume overload (eccentric) hypertrophy develops. The degree of hypertrophy is appropriate to the left ventricular dilatation, so that the ratio of left ventricular mass to end-diastolic volume is normal. In acute MR the left ventricle at first dilates rapidly. Before the myocardium becomes hypertrophied, the ratio of left ventricular mass to end-diastolic volume is reduced; i.e., the left ventricle is thin-walled. A shift to the right occurs in the left ventricular diastolic pressure-volume curve with chronic MR (Fig. 34–12).[183a]

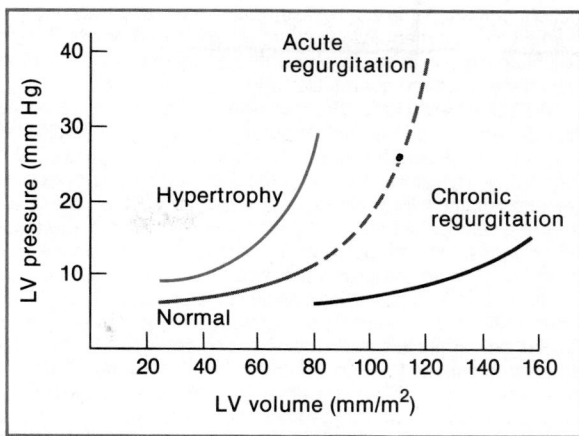

FIGURE 34–12. Diagrammatic representation of the changes in the diastolic pressure-volume relationship that occur in valve disease. Hypertrophy without significant ventricular dilatation (e.g., in aortic stenosis) produces a somewhat steeper curve than normal. Acute regurgitation produces a sudden volume load on the ventricle without time for other changes to occur and the ventricle operates at the upper (steep) end of the normal curve (broken line). Chronic aortic and mitral regurgitation with volume overload produces a flattened curve so that large volumes are accommodated without the large rise in end-diastolic pressure which occurs in acute regurgitation. (From Hall, R. J., and Julian, D. G.: Diseases of the Cardiac Valves. New York, Churchill Livingstone, 1989, p. 291.)

ASSESSMENT OF MYOCARDIAL CONTRACTILITY IN MITRAL REGURGITATION (see also p. 434)

Patients with severe MR often exhibit small elevations in ejection phase indices of myocardial contractility, such as ejection fraction (EF), fractional fiber shortening (FS), and velocity of circumferential fiber shortening (VCF) when they are in the compensated state as a consequence of reduced afterload.[184] However, by the time patients become seriously symptomatic, EF, FS, and mean VCF have usually declined to *normal* levels. As MR persists, the tendency for a low impedance leak, which usually increases myocardial shortening, is counteracted by the impairment of myocardial function characteristic of severe chronic diastolic overload. However, even in patients with overt heart failure secondary to MR, the EF and FS may be only slightly reduced.[179,180,184] Ejection phase indices of myocardial contractility are exquisitely sensitive to afterload, and wall tension (afterload) is dependent on preload (end-diastolic ventricular volume).[185,186] Therefore, *normal* values for the ejection phase indices of myocardial performance in patients with acute MR may actually reflect impaired myocardial function, whereas moderately reduced values (e.g., an ejection fraction of 40 to 50 per cent) generally signify severe, not moderate, impairment of contractility. An ejection fraction under 40 per cent in patients with severe MR usually represents advanced myocardial

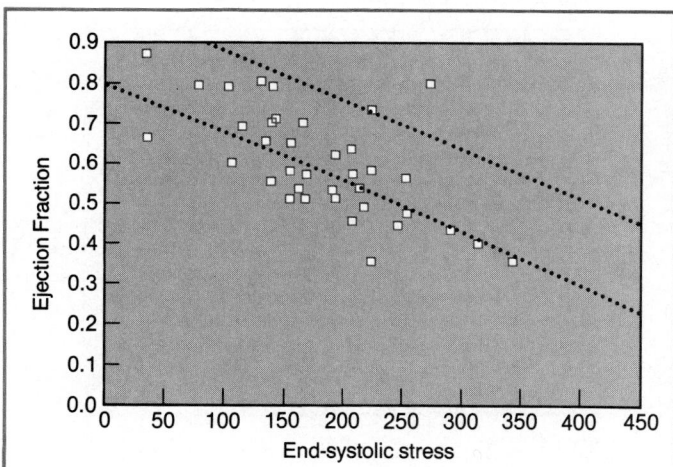

FIGURE 34–13. Ejection fraction–end-systolic stress (σ_{es}) relationships in 27 patients with MR (data points) versus the normal 95 per cent prediction (dashed lines). (From Wisenbach, T.: Does normal pump function belie muscle dysfunction in patients with chronic severe mitral regurgitation? Circulation 77:515, 1988, by permission of the American Heart Association, Inc.)

dysfunction; such patients are high operative risks and may not experience marked improvement following mitral valve replacement.[187] Reduction of ejection fraction at any level of end-systolic stress is often found in MR and reflects impaired contractility (Fig. 34–13).

END-SYSTOLIC VOLUME. Preoperative myocardial contractility is an important determinant of the risk of operative death and of cardiac failure in the perioperative period and of the level of left ventricular function postoperatively. Therefore, it is not surprising that the end-systolic pressure (or stress/dimension) relation has emerged as a useful index for evaluating left ventricular function in patients with valvular regurgitation (p. 428).[188–190] Indeed, the simple measurement of end-systolic volume has been found to be more useful as a predictor of outcome than the ejection fraction, end-diastolic volume, or end-diastolic pressure.[191–193] Patients with severe MR with a normal preoperative end-systolic volume (<30 ml/m^2) retained normal left ventricular function postoperatively, whereas marked enlargement of the end-systolic volume (>90 ml/m^2) signified a high perioperative mortality and residual left ventricular dysfunction. Patients with MR and modest enlargement of end-systolic volume (between 30 and 90 ml/m^2) usually tolerate operation satisfactorily but may have reduced left ventricular function postoperatively. For any level of end-systolic volume, patients with MR have more severe left ventricular dysfunction than do patients with aortic regurgitation.[189] This finding reflects the lower afterload in MR and correlates with the clinical observation that patients with MR have a less favorable response to surgical intervention than do those with aortic regurgitation.[191]

HEMODYNAMICS. Effective (forward) *cardiac output* is usually depressed in seriously symptomatic patients, whereas total left ventricular output (the sum of forward and regurgitant flow, which can be measured by radionuclide ventriculography)[192] is usually elevated until quite late in the patient's course. The atrial contraction (a) wave in the left atrial pressure pulse is usually not as prominent in MR as in MS, but the v wave is often much taller[173] (Figs. 7–15, p. 196 and 7–17A, p. 201), since it is inscribed during ventricular systole, when the left atrium is filled with blood from the pulmonary veins as well as from the left ventricle (Fig. 34–14). Indeed, backward transmission of the tall v wave into the pulmonary arterial bed may result in an early diastolic "pulmonary arterial v wave."[194] In patients with pure MR, during early diastole, as the distended left atrium suddenly empties, the y descent is

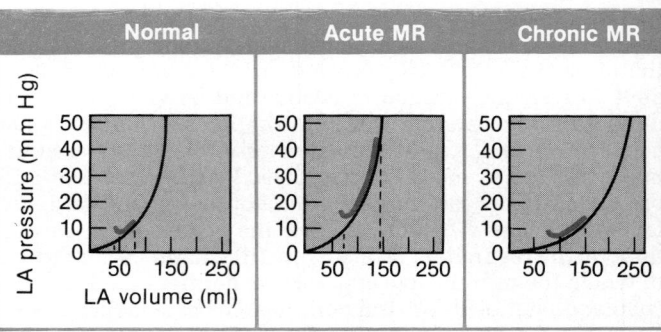

FIGURE 34–15. Schematic left atrial pressure-volume curves in a normal individual *(left)*, a patient with acute mitral regurgitation *(center)*, and a patient with chronic mitral regurgitation *(right)*. The phasic increase in left atrial pressure and volume during left ventricular systole is indicated by the heavy trace superimposed on the left atrial pressure-volume curve. In the normal subject, there is an LA volume increase of 40 ml, due to return of blood from the pulmonary veins, during the period of time when the mitral valve is closed. This causes a peak v wave of 10 mm Hg. This valve acutely becomes insufficient *(center)*, and the increase in LA volume during LV systole increases (in this example to 80 ml) because of the combination of the regurgitant volume and the pulmonary venous return, resulting in v waves to 45 mm Hg. In the same patient one year later *(right)* left atrial enlargement had occurred, so that the same degree of mitral regurgitation caused a much-reduced v wave because of increased left atrial compliance. (From Barry, W. H.: Invasive investigations for the diagnosis of mitral valve disease. *In* Ionescu, M. I., and Cohn, L. H. [eds.]: Mitral Valve Disease: Diagnosis and Treatment. London, Butterworths, 1985, p. 92.)

particularly rapid. However, in patients with combined MS and MR, the y descent is gradual. Although a left atrioventricular pressure gradient persisting throughout diastole signifies the presence of significant associated MS, a brief early diastolic gradient may occur in patients with pure severe regurgitation as a result of the torrential flow of blood across a normal-sized mitral orifice (Fig. 34–2).

LEFT ATRIAL COMPLIANCE. The compliance of the left atrium (and pulmonary venous bed) is an important determinant of the hemodynamic[193] and clinical picture in MR. Three major subgroups of patients with severe MR based on left atrial compliance have been identified[176,195,196] (Figs. 34–15 and 34–16) and are characterized as follows:

1. Normal or Reduced Compliance. There is little enlargement of the left atrium but marked elevation of the mean left atrial pressure, particularly of the v wave,[197–200] and pulmonary congestion is a prominent symptom. In most cases, severe MR has developed suddenly, as occurs with rupture of chordae tendineae, infarction of one of the heads of a papillary muscle, or perforation of a mitral leaflet as a consequence of trauma or endocarditis. Initially in acute MR the left atrium operates on the steep portion of the pressure-volume curve. Sinus rhythm is usually present; with the passage of weeks or a few months the left atrial wall frequently exhibits striking hypertrophy, is capable of contracting vigorously, and facilitates left ventricular filling.[193] Thickening of the walls of the pulmonary veins and proliferative changes in the pulmonary arteries as well as marked elevation of pulmonary vascular resistance usually develop over the course of 6 to 12 months.

2. Markedly Increased Compliance. At the opposite end of the spectrum from patients in the first group are those with severe, longstanding MR with massive enlargement of the left atrium and normal or only slightly elevated left atrial pressure. The atrial wall contains only a small remnant of muscle surrounded by a great deal of fibrous tissue. Longstanding MR in these patients has altered the physical properties of the left atrial wall and thereby displaced the atrial pressure-volume curve, allowing a normal or almost normal pressure to exist in a greatly enlarged left atrium. (This shift in the left atrial pressure-volume curve with persistent MR has been documented in animal experiments.[193]) Pulmonary artery pressure and

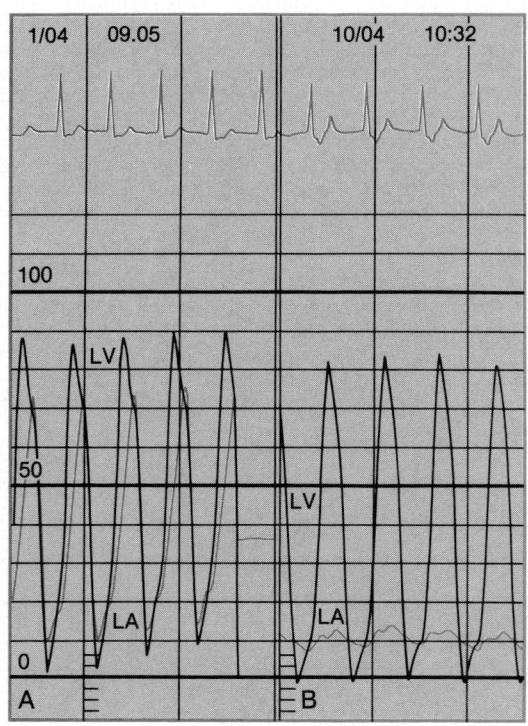

FIGURE 34–14. Intraoperative simultaneous left ventricular (LV) and left atrial (LA) pressures (mm Hg) before *(A)* and after *(B)* mitral valvuloplasty for correction of severe acute mitral regurgitation. Note the height of the v wave in the preoperative tracing. (From Barlow, J. B.: Perspectives on the Mitral Valve. Philadelphia, F. A. Davis, 1987, p. 257.)

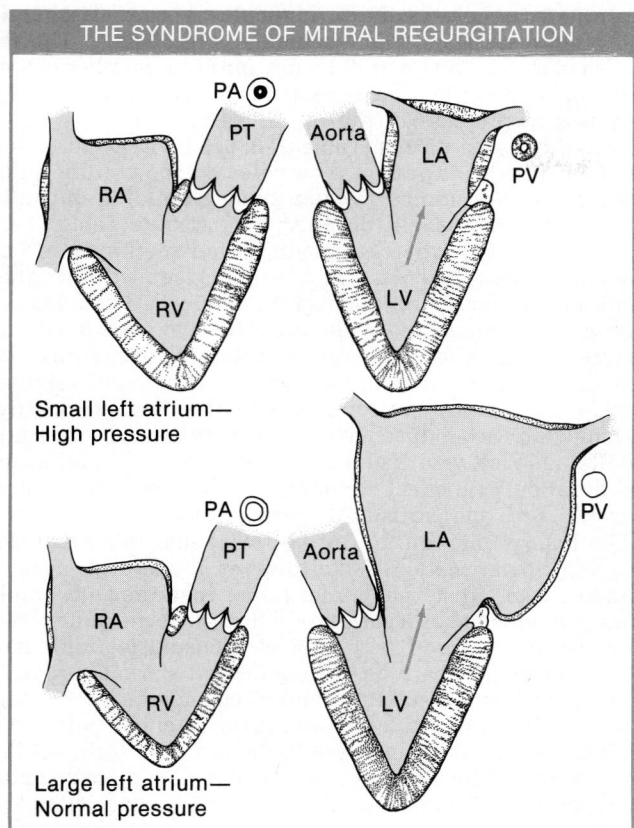

THE SYNDROME OF MITRAL REGURGITATION

Small left atrium—
High pressure

Large left atrium—
Normal pressure

FIGURE 34–16. Diagram depicting the two extremes of the spectrum in pure mitral regurgitation. When severe mitral regurgitation appears suddenly in individuals with previously normal or near-normal hearts (*top*), the left atrium (LA) is relatively small and the high pressure within it is reflected back into the pulmonary vessels and right ventricle (RV). The anatomical indicator of this latter physiological event is severe hypertrophy of the left atrial and right ventricular walls and marked intimal proliferation and medial hypertrophy of the pulmonary arteries (PA), arterioles, and veins (PV). At the other extreme with severe chronic mitral regurgitation (*bottom*), the left atrial cavity is of giant size and its wall is thin. It is thus able to "absorb" the left ventricular (LV) pressure without reflecting it back into the pulmonary vessels or right ventricle. As a consequence, pulmonary vessels remain normal, and the right ventricular wall does not thicken. PT = pulmonary trunk; RA = right atrium. (From Roberts, W. C., et al.: Nonrheumatic valvular cardiac disease. A clinicopathologic survey of 27 different conditions causing valvular dysfunction. *In* Likoff, W. [ed.]: Cardiovascular Clinics. Vol. 5, No. 2, Valvular Heart Disease. Philadelphia, F. A. Davis, 1973, p. 403.)

pulmonary vascular resistance are normal or only slightly elevated at rest. Atrial fibrillation and a low cardiac output are almost invariably present.[195]

3. Moderately Increased Compliance. This, the most common subgroup, consists of patients between the ends of the spectrum represented by groups 1 and 2; these patients have severe chronic MR and exhibit variable degrees of enlargement of the left atrium, associated with significant elevation of the left atrial pressure.

CLINICAL MANIFESTATIONS
(See Table 34–1, p. 1010)

HISTORY

The nature and severity of the symptoms of patients with chronic MR are a function of the severity of regurgitation, its rate of progression, the level of pulmonary artery pressure, and the presence of associated valvular, myocardial, or coronary artery disease. Since symptoms usually do not develop in patients with chronic MR until the left ventricle fails, the time interval between the initial attack of rheumatic fever (when one has occurred) and the development of symptoms tends to

be longer in MR than in MS and often exceeds 2 decades. Acute pulmonary edema occurs less frequently in chronic MR than in MS, presumably because sudden surges in left atrial pressure are less common.[20] Similarly, although hemoptysis and systemic embolization do occur in MR, they are less common than in MS. On the other hand, chronic weakness and fatigue secondary to a low cardiac output are more prominent features in MR.

Patients with mild MR may remain asymptomatic for their entire lives.[64] The majority of patients with MR of rheumatic origin have only mild disability, unless regurgitation progresses as a result of chronic rheumatic activity, infective endocarditis, or rupture of chordae tendineae.[196] The development of atrial fibrillation affects the course adversely but perhaps not as dramatically as it does in MS. The course in patients with chronic MR tends to be less dramatic and is punctuated with fewer acute complications than in patients with MS. However, this more indolent course may, in fact, be deceptive. By the time that symptoms secondary to a reduced cardiac output and/or pulmonary congestion become apparent, serious and sometimes even irreversible left ventricular dysfunction may have developed. In contrast, patients with MS have the benefit of an "early warning system," i.e., symptoms of pulmonary congestion with frequent, sudden elevations of left atrial pressure.

In patients with severe chronic MR with a greatly enlarged left atrium and with relatively mild left atrial hypertension (group 2 with increased left atrial compliance, already described), pulmonary vascular resistance does not usually rise appreciably. Instead, the major symptoms, fatigue and exhaustion, are related to a low cardiac output. However, right heart failure, characterized by congestive hepatomegaly, ankle edema, and ascites, is observed both in patients with longstanding severe MR and in patients with acute MR and elevated pulmonary vascular resistance. Angina pectoris is rare unless coronary artery disease coexists.

NATURAL HISTORY. This is variable and depends on a combination of the volume of regurgitation, the state of the myocardium, and the cause of the underlying disorder. The condition in asymptomatic patients with mild MR usually remains stable for many years[197]; severe regurgitation develops in only a small percentage of these, in some cases because of intervening infective endocarditis[196] or rupture of chordae tendineae or both. Regurgitation tends to progress more rapidly in patients with connective tissue diseases, such as Marfan syndrome, than in those with chronic MR on a rheumatic basis. Because the natural history of severe MR has been altered greatly by surgical intervention, it is difficult now to predict the course of patients on medical therapy alone. However, in an unselected group of patients with MR who were treated medically before surgical treatment of severe MR became commonplace, approximately 80 per cent survived 5 years after the diagnosis and almost 60 per cent survived 10 years.[102] Patients with combined MS and MR had a poorer prognosis, with only 67 per cent surviving 5 years and 30 per cent surviving 10 years after diagnosis. Munoz et al., in studying a group of patients with greater disability, found that medically treated patients with severe MR had a 5-year survival rate of only 45 per cent.[44] Among medically treated patients with MR, the arteriovenous oxygen difference and ventricular end-diastolic volume were significant (inverse) predictors of survival.[197]

PHYSICAL EXAMINATION

Palpation of the arterial pulse is helpful in differentiating aortic stenosis from MR; both may produce a prominent systolic murmur at the base of the heart. The carotid arterial upstroke is sharp in mitral regurgitation[201] and delayed in aortic stenosis; the volume of the pulse may be normal in both conditions or reduced in the presence of heart failure.

The cardiac impulse is brisk, hyperdynamic, and displaced to the left[20] (Table 2–1, p. 26; Fig. 2–18, p. 28), and a prominent left ventricular filling wave is frequently palpable in early diastole. Systolic expansion of the enlarged left atrium may result in a late systolic thrust in the parasternal region, which may be confused with right ventricular enlargement.[202]

AUSCULTATION.[203] With severe, chronic MR due to defective valve cusps, S_1, produced by valve closure, is usually diminished.[204] Wide splitting of S_2 is common and results from the shortening of left ventricular ejection and an earlier A_2 as a consequence of reduced resistance to left ventricular outflow. When pulmonary hypertension is present, P_2 is louder than A_2. The abnormal increase in the flow rate across the mitral orifice during the rapid filling phase is usually associated with an S_3, the auscultatory counterpart of a palpable rapid filling wave. A left ventricular S_3, i.e., one that is not augmented by inspiration, excludes predominant MS (unless aortic regurgitation, ischemic heart disease, or another cause of an S_3 is present).

The *systolic murmur* is the most prominent physical finding in MR; it must be differentiated from the systolic murmur heard in aortic stenosis, tricuspid regurgitation, ventricular septal defect, and sometimes MS (Table 34–4). In most cases of severe MR the systolic murmur commences immediately after the soft S_1 and continues beyond and may obscure A_2 because of the persistence of the pressure difference between the left ventricle and left atrium (Figs. 3–20 and 3–21, p. 53). The holosystolic murmur of chronic MR is usually constant in intensity, blowing, high-pitched, and loudest at the apex with radiation to the axilla and left infrascapular area; however, radiation toward the sternum or the aortic area may occur with abnormalities of the posterior leaflet. The murmur shows little change even in the presence of large beat-to-beat variations of left ventricular stroke volume, as occur in atrial fibrillation, in contrast to most midsystolic (ejection) murmurs, such as in aortic stenosis, which vary greatly in intensity with stroke volume and therefore with the duration of diastole.[205] There is little correlation between the intensity of the systolic murmur and the severity of MR. Indeed, in patients with severe MR due to left ventricular dilatation, acute myocardial infarction, or paraprosthetic valvular regurgitation or in those who have marked emphysema, obesity, chest deformity, or a prosthetic heart valve, the systolic murmur may be barely audible or even absent, a condition referred to as "silent MR."

Pansystolic and late systolic murmurs (and pansystolic murmurs with late systolic accentuation) are characteristic of MR. When the murmur is confined to late systole, the regurgitation is usually mild and may be secondary to prolapse of the mitral valve or papillary muscle dysfunction, conditions that cause late systolic regurgitation. These causes of MR are frequently associated with a normal S_1 because initial closure of the mitral valve cusps may be unimpaired. The systolic murmur is usually of no more than Grade 3/6 intensity and is a mid- to late diamond-shaped murmur, or exhibits late systolic accentuation and radiates more frequently to the lower left sternal border than to the axilla.[155] The murmur of papillary muscle dysfunction is particularly variable; it may become

accentuated or holosystolic during acute myocardial ischemia and often disappears when ischemia is relieved.[206] The response of a mid- to late-systolic murmur to a number of maneuvers, as described on page 1024, helps to establish the diagnosis of prolapse of the mitral valve.

Dynamic Auscultation (Table 2–8, p. 38; Fig. 2–20, p. 40). The holosystolic murmur of rheumatic MR shows little variation during respiration. However, sudden standing and amyl nitrite inhalation usually diminish the murmur (Table 34–5; Fig. 3–39, p. 62) whereas squatting and methoxamine or phenylephrine augment it. The murmur is reduced during the strain of the Valsalva maneuver and shows a left-sided response, i.e., a transient overshoot, six to eight beats following release. The murmur is usually intensified by isometric exercise, differentiating it from the systolic murmurs of valvular aortic stenosis and hypertrophic obstructive cardiomyopathy, both of which are reduced by this intervention. The murmur of MR due to left ventricular dilatation *decreases* in intensity and duration with effective therapy with cardiac glycosides, diuretics, rest, and particularly vasodilators.

The holosystolic murmur of MR resembles that produced by a ventricular septal defect. However, the latter is usually loudest at the left sternal border rather than the apex and is often accompanied by a parasternal thrill. The murmur of MR may also be confused with that of tricuspid regurgitation, which is usually heard best along the left sternal border, is augmented during inspiration, and is accompanied by a prominent v wave and y descent in the jugular venous pulse.

When the chordae tendineae to the posterior leaflet of the mitral valve rupture, the regurgitant jet is often directed anteriorly, so that it impinges on the atrial septum adjacent to the aortic root and causes a systolic murmur most prominent at the base of the heart, which can be confused with that of aortic stenosis. The acoustic energy derived from the mitral regurgitant jet may be transmitted to the aorta by the impact of the jet on the portion of the left atrial wall adjacent to the aortic root.[207] On the other hand, when the chordae to the anterior leaflet rupture, the jet is usually directed to the posterior wall of the left atrium, and the murmur may be transmitted to the spine or even to the top of the head.[208]

Differential Diagnosis. Patients with rheumatic disease of the mitral valve exhibit a spectrum of abnormalities, ranging from pure MS to pure MR. The presence of an S_3, a rapid left ventricular filling wave and left ventricular impulse on palpation, and a soft S_1 all favor predominant MR, whereas an accentuated S_1, a prominent OS with a short A_2-OS interval, and a soft short systolic murmur all point to predominant MS. Elucidation of the predominant valvular lesion may be complicated by the presence of a holosystolic murmur of tricuspid regurgitation in patients with pure MS and pulmonary hypertension; this murmur, as has already been noted, may sometimes be heard at the apex when the right ventricle is greatly enlarged and may therefore be mistaken for the murmur of MR. Many patients with severe tricuspid regurgitation have a low cardiac output and an inaudible or barely audible dia-

TABLE 34-5 EFFECT OF VARIOUS INTERVENTIONS ON SYSTOLIC MURMURS

INTERVENTION	HYPERTROPHIC OBSTRUCTIVE CARDIOMYOPATHY	AORTIC STENOSIS	MITRAL REGURGITATION	MITRAL PROLAPSE
Valsalva	↑	↓	↓	↑ or ↓
Standing	↑	↑ or unchanged	↓	↑
Handgrip or squatting	↓	↓ or unchanged	↑	↓
Supine position with legs elevated	↓	↑ or unchanged	Unchanged	↓
Exercise	↓	↑ or unchanged	↓	↓
Amyl nitrite	↑↑	↑	↓	↑
Isoproterenol	↑↑	↑	↓	↑

↑↑ = Markedly increased.

Modified from Paraskos, J. A.: Combined valvular disease. *In* Dalen, J. E., and Alpert, J. S. (eds.): Valvular Heart Disease. Boston, Little, Brown and Company, 1987, p. 365.

stolic murmur of MS, further complicating the clinical diagnosis. An S_3 originating from the right ventricle in patients with MS and pulmonary hypertension may falsely suggest the presence of MR. On the other hand, systolic expansion of the left atrium, as occurs in severe MR, often produces a late systolic parasternal expansion that may be confused with right ventricular hypertrophy and falsely attributed to mitral stenosis.

LABORATORY EXAMINATION
(Table 34–6)

ELECTROCARDIOGRAPHY. The principal *electrocardiographic* findings in patients with MR are left atrial enlargement and atrial fibrillation.[71,203,209] Electrocardiographic evidence of left ventricular enlargement occurs in about one-third of patients with severe MR. Approximately 15 per cent exhibit electrocardiographic evidence of right ventricular hypertrophy, a change which reflects the presence of pulmonary hypertension of sufficient severity to counterbalance even the hypertrophied left ventricle of MR.

RADIOLOGICAL FINDINGS (see also p. 224). Cardiomegaly with left ventricular and particularly with left atrial enlargement is a common finding in patients with chronic severe MR.[83,210] However, there is little correlation between left atrial size and pressure. Changes in the lung fields are less prominent in MR than in MS, but interstitial edema with Kerley B lines is frequently seen with acute regurgitation or with progressive left ventricular failure.

In patients with combined MS and MR, overall cardiac enlargement and particularly left atrial dilatation are prominent findings. However, it is often difficult to determine which lesion is predominant from the plain chest roentgenogram, since it may be difficult to distinguish between right and left ventricular enlargement. Predominant MS is suggested by relatively mild cardiomegaly, principally straightening of the left cardiac border with significant changes in the lung fields, whereas predominant MR is more likely when the heart is greatly enlarged and the changes in the lungs are relatively inconspicuous. When the left atrium is aneurysmally dilated chronic MR is almost always the dominant lesion. Calcification of the mitral valve occurs in patients with stenosis, regurgitation, or mixed lesions. *Calcification of the mitral annulus*, an important cause of MR in the elderly, is most prominent in the posterior third of the cardiac silhouette[83] and is best visualized on films exposed in the lateral or right anterior oblique projection, in which it appears as a dense, coarse, C-shaped opacity (Fig. 8–29, p. 221).

The diagnosis of MR can be established definitively by means of left ventricular angiocardiography:[211] the prompt appearance of contrast material in the left atrium following its injection into the left ventricle indicates the presence of MR. The injection should be rapid enough to permit left ventricular opacification but slow enough to avoid the development of premature ventricular contractions, which can induce spurious regurgitation.

The regurgitant volume can be determined from the difference between the total left ventricular stroke volume, estimated angiocardiographically, and the simultaneous measurement of the effective forward stroke volume by Fick's method (p. 189). The results of such studies suggest that in patients with severe regurgitation, the regurgitant volume may approach and in rare instances may even exceed the effective forward stroke volume.

Qualitative but clinically useful estimates of the severity of MR may be made by cineangiographic observation of the degree of opacification of the left atrium and pulmonary veins following the injection of contrast material into the left ventricle. MR secondary to rheumatic heart disease is characterized angiographically by a central regurgitant jet and by thickened leaflets that exhibit reduced motion, whereas in regurgitation due to other causes, particularly dilatation or calcification of the mitral annulus or ruptured chordae and papillary muscles, the systolic jet may be eccentric, and the valves consist of thin filaments that display excessive motion. The etiology of the regurgitation, e.g., prolapse of the mitral valve, and a flail leaflet are often distinguishable angiographically.

ECHOCARDIOGRAPHY (see also p. 83). Two-dimensional echocardiography is more useful in determining the etiology and hemodynamic consequences of than in estimating the severity of MR.[212] Severe MR results in enlargement of the left atrium and left ventricle, with increased systolic motion of both of these chambers. The underlying cause of the regurgitation—e.g., rupture of chordae tendineae,[213] mitral valve prolapse (Figs. 4–50 and 4–51, p. 84), a flail leaflet[213a] (Fig. 4–52, p. 84), and vegetation (Fig. 35–2, p. 1035)—can often be determined, and the echocardiogram may also show calcifi-

ACUTE MITRAL REGURGITATION	CHRONIC MITRAL REGURGITATION
ECG	
Commonly normal unless acute ischemia is the cause of regurgitation	Left atrial enlargement (P mitrale)
	Atrial fibrillation common
	Left ventricular hypertrophy common with severe regurgitation
Radiology and Fluoroscopy	
Heart size usually normal	Cardiomegaly common, mainly due to left ventricular enlargement
If regurgitation is severe there may be pulmonary congestion and interstitial edema	Left atrial enlargement, especially with rheumatic mitral disease
	Fluoroscopy may demonstrate calcium in rheumatic mitral disease
Phonocardiography and Pulse Tracings	
Systolic murmur frequently terminates before S_2	Systolic murmur usually holosystolic
S_3 common	S_3 occurs with more severe regurgitation
Apex cardiogram shows marked systolic impulse	Systolic impulse less marked than with acute severe mitral regurgitation
M-Mode Echocardiography	
Left atrium usually of normal size	Left atrium usually enlarged
Left ventricle usually of normal size, may be vigorously hypercontractile	Left ventricle frequently dilated, with signs of volume overload
Cause of acute regurgitation may be demonstrated; flail mitral leaflet, ruptured chordae or vegetations in infective endocarditis, etc.	Cause of chronic regurgitation may be defined; rheumatic disease, mitral valve prolapse, etc.

Two-Dimensional Echocardiography
In both acute and chronic regurgitation more clearly defines severity of left ventricular volume overload and enhances assessment of left ventricular function. In majority of cases can define etiology of regurgitation, and is especially useful in elucidating difficult diagnostic problems in M-mode echocardiography
Doppler Ultrasound
Facilitates detection of mitral regurgitation by identifying turbulent flow within left atrium in systole
Aids quantification of degree of mitral regurgitation
Nuclear Cardiology
Principal use is in quantitative assessment of ventricular performance, e.g., ejection fraction (EF). Quantification of the degree of mitral regurgitation can be achieved by comparing left and right ventricular stroke volumes. In acute regurgitation the EF is usually normal if increased. A decreased EF implies pre-existing regurgitation or severe ischemic damage to the left ventricle. In chronic regurgitation the EF is usually normal and may be decreased if long-standing volume overload leads to left ventricular dysfunction

From Bloomfield, P., et al.: Noninvasive investigations for the diagnosis of mitral valve disease. In Ionescu, M. I., and Cohn, L. H. (eds.): Mitral Valve Disease: Diagnosis and Treatment. London, Butterworths, 1985, p. 63.

cation of the mitral annulus as a band of dense echoes between the mitral apparatus and the posterior wall of the heart.[144,214] This technique is also useful for estimating the hemodynamic consequences of MR; with left ventricular dysfunction, end-diastolic and end-systolic volumes are increased.

Doppler echocardiography in MR reveals a high-velocity jet in the left atrium during systole. The severity of the regurgitation is a function of the distance from the valve that the jet can

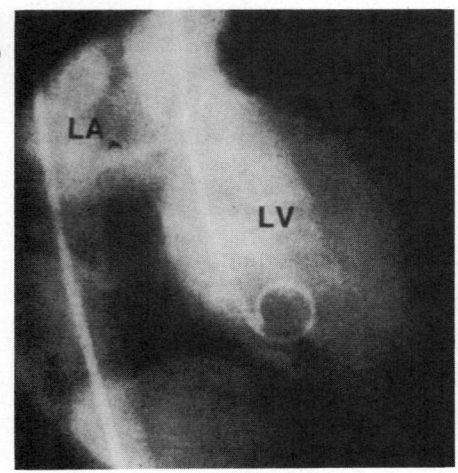 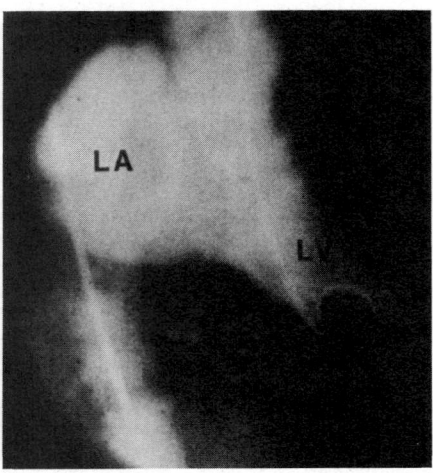

FIGURE 34–17. Diastolic *(left)* and systolic *(right)* frames of a left ventricular cineangiogram from a patient with severe mitral regurgitation. Dense opacification of the left atrium is seen in the first systolic frame. Left ventricular contraction is excellent. (From Hall, R. J., and Julian, D. G.: Diseases of the Cardiac Valves. New York, Churchill Livingstone, 1989, p. 66.)

be detected (Fig. 4–47, p. 83) and the size of the left atrium. Both color flow Doppler (Fig. 4–48, color plate No. 2, and Fig. 4–49, color plate No. 2) and pulsed techniques[215] have been found to correlate well with angiographic methods in estimating the severity of MR. Other methods of assessing the severity of MR include measurement of the absolute mitral jet (>8 cm^2 specifies severe MR[216]) and evaluation of the difference between left ventricular inflow and aortic outflow.[217]

ANGIOGRAPHY. Contrast left ventriculography shows systolic opacification of the left atrium (Fig. 34–17).

Gated pool imaging or first-pass angiography may reveal an increased end-diastolic volume; the regurgitant fraction can be estimated from the ratio of left ventricular to right ventricular stroke volume[192,218]; in patients with mitral regurgitation and impaired left ventricular function, ejection fraction fails to rise normally during exercise.[219] Radionuclide angiograms are useful for interval follow-up of patients. Progressive increases in ventricular end-diastolic or end-systolic volume often suggest that surgical treatment is necessary (discussed later).

ACUTE MITRAL REGURGITATION

The causes of acute MR are shown in Table 34–3 (*bottom*). They are diverse and represent acute manifestations of dis-

ease processes that may, under other circumstances, cause chronic MR. Especially important causes of acute MR are infective endocarditis with disruption of valve leaflets or rupture of chordae tendineae, ischemic dysfunction or rupture of a papillary muscle, and malfunction of a prosthetic valve.

One major hemodynamic difference between acute and chronic MR derives from the differences in the compliance of the left atrium, as discussed on page 1022 and as illustrated in Figures 34–15 and 34–16. As shown in Table 34–7 (*top*), acute severe MR causes a marked reduction of forward stroke volume, a slight reduction of end-systolic volume, a rise in end-diastolic volume. The differences in the clinical features between acute and chronic MR are summarized in Table 34–7 (*bottom*). In patients with acute MR with a normal-sized left atrium (group 1 with normal or reduced left atrial compliance, p. 1022) the left atrial pressure rises abruptly, possibly leading to pulmonary edema, marked elevation of pulmonary vascular resistance, and right-sided heart failure. Because the *v* wave is markedly elevated in acute MR, the pressure gradient between the left ventricle and atrium declines at the end of systole (Fig. 34–13A), and the murmur may not be holosystolic but decrescendo, ending well before A$_2$. It is usually lower-pitched and softer than the murmur of chronic MR. A left-sided S$_4$ is common.[197] Pulmonary hypertension, common in acute MR, may increase the intensity of P$_2$ and the mur-

TABLE 34-7   CHARACTERISTICS OF ACUTE AND CHRONIC REGURGITATION

	LV End Diastolic Volume	LV End Systolic Volume	Forward Stroke Volume	Ejection Fraction	Left Atrial Compliance	Left Atrial Pressure	LV Muscle Function
Acute MR	↑	↓	↓↓	↑	n	↑↑↑	n
Compensated chronic MR	↑↑↑	↓	n	↑	↑	n or ↑	n
Decompensated chronic MR	↑↑↑↑	↑↑	n or ↓	n or ↓	↑	↑↑	↓↓↓

CLINICAL FEATURE	CHRONIC MITRAL REGURGITATION	ACUTE MITRAL REGURGITATION
Systolic murmur	Harsh, pansystolic	Softer, low pitched, descrescendo, ends before A$_2$
Primary location of murmur	Apex	Base of heart
Radiation of murmur	Axilla	Neck, spine, top of head
Thrill	Apex	Absent
Venous pressure	Normal	Increased with large V waves
Apical impulse	Hyperkinetic, heaving	Hyperkinetic, heaving until LV failure occurs
ECG	LVH, LAE	Normal or infarct pattern
Chest x-ray	Cardiomegaly, marked LA enlargement, Kerley B lines	Normal size heart, may show pulmonary edema

n = normal, LA = left atrial, LAE = left atrial enlargement, LVH = left ventricular hypertrophy, MR = mitral regurgitation.
Data from Kusiak, V., and Brest, A. N.: Acute mitral regurgitation: Pathophysiology and management. *In* Frankl, W. S., and Brest, A. N. (eds.): Cardiovascular Clinics. Valvular Heart Disease: Comprehensive Evaluation and Management. Philadelphia, F. A. Davis, 1986, p. 273 (top portion); and from Carabello, B. A., and Grossman, W.: Effects of acute and chronic mitral regurgitation on left ventricular mechanics and contractile muscle function. *In* Duran, C., et al. (eds.): Recent Progress in Mitral Valve Disease. London, Butterworths, 1984, p. 188 (bottom portion).

murs of pulmonary and tricuspid regurgitation, and a right-sided S_4 may also develop. Rarely in patients with severe acute MR, a v wave (late systolic pressure rise) in the pulmonary artery pressure pulse may cause premature closure of the pulmonary valve, early P_2, and paradoxical splitting of S_2.[203] Acute MR, even if severe, often does not increase overall cardiac size on the chest roentgenogram and may produce only mild left atrial enlargement despite marked elevation of left atrial pressure. With acute MR, there may be little increase in the internal diameter of either of these chambers on the echocardiogram, but increased systolic motion of the ventricle is prominent.

ACUTE VS. CHRONIC MITRAL REGURGITATION

(See Table 34–7)

MANAGEMENT

MEDICAL TREATMENT

This includes all the measures used in the treatment of heart failure, as outlined in Chapter 17. Afterload reduction is of particular benefit in the management of MR—both the acute and the chronic forms.[220,221] By reducing the impedance to ejection into the aorta, the volume of blood regurgitating into the left atrium is reduced. In addition, decreasing left ventricular volume reduces the diameter of the mitral annulus and thereby the regurgitant orifice.[222] Mean left atrial pressure and, in particular, the elevated v wave, declines. Thus in the management of MR, vasodilator therapy is actually directed at relieving the physiological abnormality rather than simply dealing with its consequences. Afterload reduction with intravenous nitroprusside may be life-saving in acute MR due to rupture of the head of a papillary muscle occurring in the course of an acute myocardial infarction. It may permit stabilization of the patient's condition and thereby allow coronary arteriography and operation to be carred out with the patient in optimal condition. When surgical treatment is contraindicated, chronic afterload reduction with an angiotensin inhibitor or oral hydralazine may improve the clinical state for months or even years in patients with severe, chronic MR. Digitalis glycosides play a more important role in the management of MR than of MS. Like diuretics, they are indicated in patients with MR, cardiomegaly, and sinus rhythm. Cardiac glycosides are particularly helpful in patients with established atrial fibrillation.

Appropriate prophylaxis to prevent infective endocarditis (p. 1099) is indicated in MR as in all valvular lesions.

Left-sided cardiac catheterization, selective left ventricular angiocardiography, and coronary arteriography are indicated in patients with functional disability despite optimal medical management. The objectives of these studies are to (1) confirm the presence of regurgitation and estimate its severity; (2) aid in the identification of patients with primary myocardial disease and relatively mild, functional MR secondary to ventricular dilatation who are not likely to benefit greatly from operation and in whom the operative risk is relatively high; (3) detect and assess the severity of any associated valve lesions; and (4) determine the presence and assess the extent of coronary artery disease. Because of the additional risks when surgical treatment is carried out in patients with left ventricular dysfunction, definitive diagnosis and characterization of left ventricular function and consideration of surgical treatment should not be deferred until after the patient has developed severe heart failure.

SURGICAL TREATMENT

When operative treatment is under consideration, the chronic, often slowly progressive nature of MR must be weighed against the immediate risks and long-term uncertainties attendant upon surgery. Surgical mortality depends

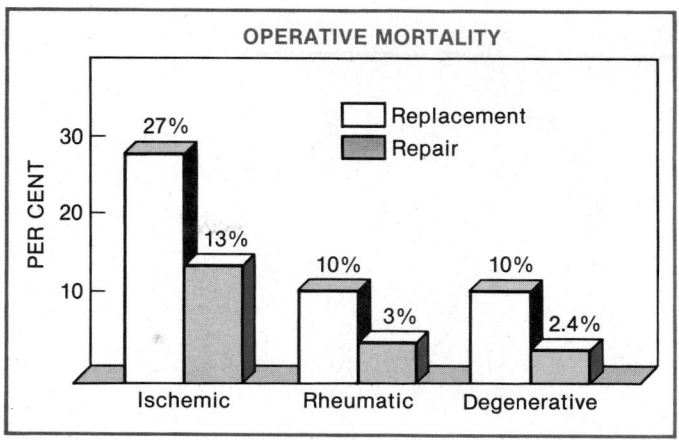

FIGURE 34–18. The operative mortality for mitral valve repair has been lower than for valve replacement regardless of the etiology. (From Cosgrove, D. M., and Stewart, W. J.: Mitral valvuloplasty. Curr. Prob. Cardiol. *14*:359, 1989.)

on the patient's hemodynamic and clinical state (particularly the function of the left ventricle) and on the presence of associated conditions such as renal, hepatic, or pulmonary disease, as well as on the skill and experience of the surgical team.[222a] The decision to replace or reconstruct the valve is of critical importance, since surgical mortality associated with mitral valve reconstruction appears to be lower than that associated with replacement (Fig. 34–18), although the patients selected for the two procedures differ. Surgical mortality does not depend significantly on *which* of the currently widely used tissue or mechanical valve prostheses is employed (pp. 1061 to 1062).

The reconstructive procedure consists of annuloplasty, often with use of a rigid prosthetic ring (Carpentier ring) or a flexible ring (Duran ring) (Fig. 34–19) or resection and repair of the valve (Fig. 34–20). Replacement,[223] reimplantation, elongation, or shortening of chordae tendineae has been successful in selected patients with pure or predominant MR. Reconstructive procedures have been useful in patients who have severe noncalcific MR with pliable valves, a dilated mitral annulus, MR secondary to ruptured chordae to the posterior leaflet, or perforation of a mitral leaflet due to infective endocarditis, in the absence of severe subvalvular chordal thickening and major loss of leaflet substance.[151,224–232] The results of these "plastic" operations have, in general, been more favorable in children and adolescents with pliable valves and in patients with MR secondary to mitral valve prolapse, annular dilatation, papillary muscle secondary to ischemia, dysfunction or rupture, or chordal rupture than they have been in older patients with the rigid, calcified deformed valves of rheumatic heart disease. Many of these patients still require mitral valve replacement, which is also usually the procedure of choice in patients with badly scarred mitral valves who have previously undergone mitral commissurotomy.

Although mitral valve replacement—with mechanical or bioprostheses—has been used successfully in the treatment of MR for 3 decades, there has been some dissatisfaction with the results of this operation. First, left ventricular function often deteriorates following this procedure, contributing to early and late mortality and late disability. The increase in afterload consequent to abolition of the low impedance leak was first believed to be responsible, but now it is clear that the loss of annular-chordal-papillary muscle continuity interferes with left ventricular function in patients who have undergone mitral valve replacement. This does not occur after mitral valve reconstruction.[233] Indeed, animal experiments have shown convincingly that the normal function of the mitral valve apparatus "primes" the left ventricle for normal contraction and that this is prevented when operation causes discontinuity of this apparatus.

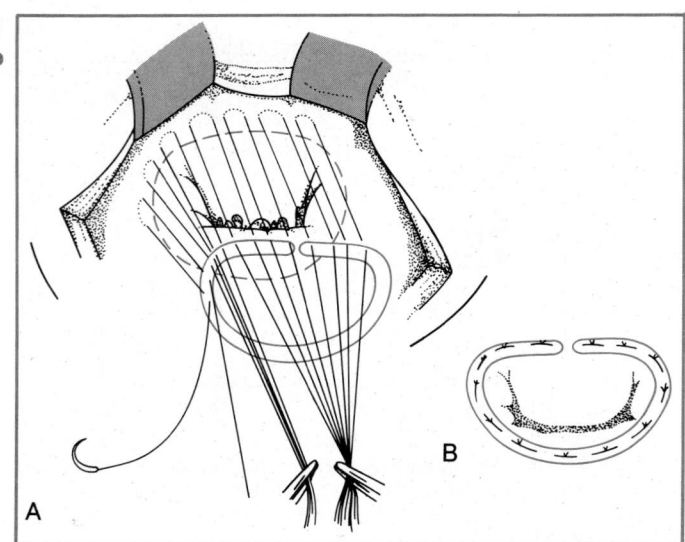

FIGURE 34–19. Illustration of insertion of annuloplasty ring. (From Galloway, A. C., Colvin, S. B., Baumann, F. G., et al.: Current concepts of mitral valve reconstruction for mitral insufficiency. Circulation 78:1087, 1988, by permission of the American Heart Association, Inc.)

A second disadvantage of prosthetic mitral valve replacement results from the prosthesis itself: thromboembolism or hemorrhage in the case of mechanical prostheses, late mechanical dysfunction of bioprostheses, and the hazard of infective endocarditis with all prostheses. For these reasons, increasing efforts are being made to reconstruct the mitral valve whenever possible, especially in patients with pure and predominant regurgitation. Indeed, these procedures, widely employed in Europe since the early 1960's, are now frequently used by U.S. surgeons as well. In many centers in the United States, approximately half of all patients requiring operation for pure or predominant MR receive reconstructive procedures and the other half valve replacement.

Intraoperative Doppler color flow mapping is extremely useful in assessing the adequacy of the reconstruction. In the minority of patients with persistent severe MR in whom the results are unsatisfactory, the problem can usually be corrected before the chest is closed.[234,235] Occasionally, the rigid Carpentier ring, placed in the mitral annulus with mitral valve reconstruction, causes serious left ventricular outflow tract obstruction.[236]

Progressive reduction in the prevalence of rheumatic heart disease — in which damaged valves often are not suitable for reconstructive surgery — with a simultaneous rise in degenerative causes of MR (including mitral valve prolapse and rupture of chordae tendineae) as well as in ischemic causes is producing an increase in the proportion of patients in whom reconstruction is carried out.

The potential advantages of repair of MR (as opposed to replacement with a prosthetic valve) are many; chronic anticoagulation and the hazards of bleeding and thromboembolism attendant upon implantation of a mechanical prosthesis are largely eliminated, as are the risks of late failure of a bioprosthesis. However, there is a distinct learning curve for mitral reconstructive procedures.[229] Furthermore, many regurgitant valves, particularly those which are thickened, severely deformed, calcified, and partly stenotic, do not lend themselves to reconstruction; mitral valve replacement is necessary. When severe MR is caused by myxomatous degeneration — especially when there is severe associated chordal disease — mitral valve replacement is usually required.[228]

RESULTS. Mortality rates of 1 to 4 per cent in patients with predominant MS and of 2 to 7 per cent in patients with pure or predominant MR in functional Class II or III who undergo elective isolated mitral valve replacement are now common in many centers.[151,237–239] Operative mortality tends to be

lower (1 to 4 per cent) in patients undergoing reconstructive surgery. Age per se is no barrier to successful surgery; mitral valve replacement can be carried out in patients older than 70 years with the same or only slightly higher risk as in younger patients, if their general health status is adequate. Surgical treatment substantially improves survival in patients with symptomatic MR. Factors such as an age of less than 60 years, a preoperative New York Heart Association functional Class of II, a cardiac index exceeding 2.0 liters/min/m², a left ventricular end-diastolic pressure less than 12 mm Hg, and a normal ejection fraction and end-systolic volume all correlate with improved immediate as well as long-term survival rates. Patients with moderate impairment of the ejection fraction (40 to 50 per cent) exhibit improved survival rates following surgical compared with medical treatment. In other series, only age and preoperative ejection fraction predicted long-term survival following mitral valve replacement.[240]

In most patients with MR, the clinical state and the quality of life improve following valve replacement. Severe pulmonary hypertension is relieved almost uniformly,[121,122] and left

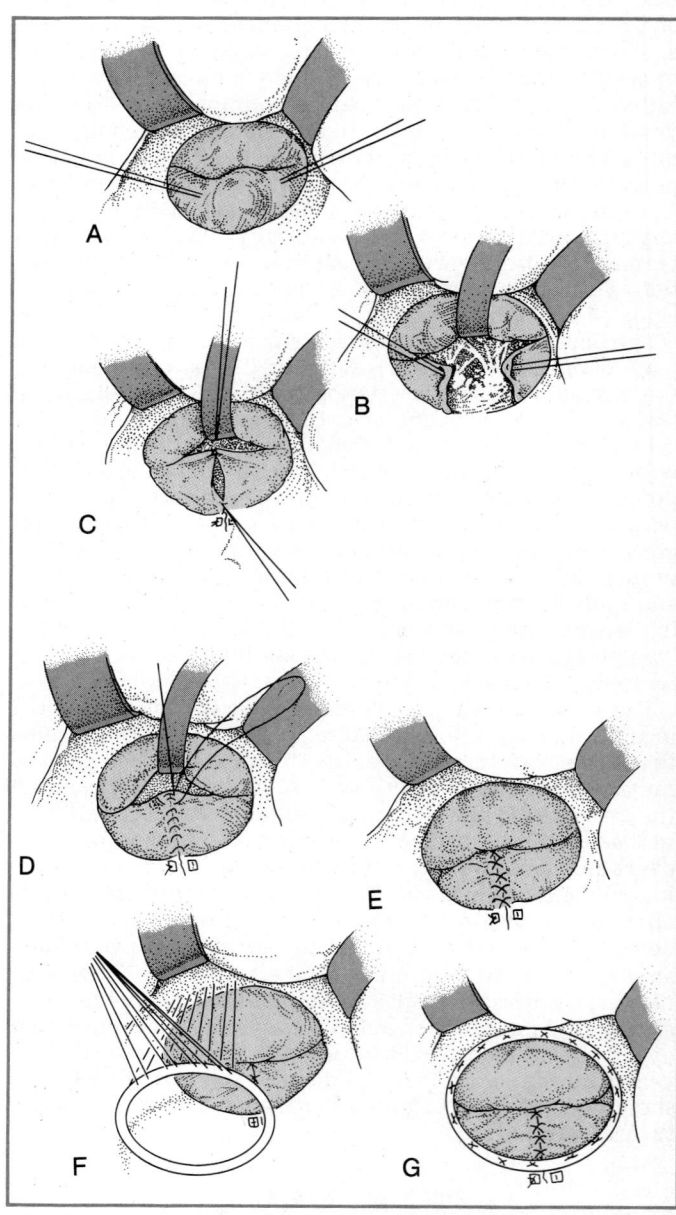

FIGURE 34–20. Valve repair techniques for quadrilateral resection of posterior leaflet of mitral valve. (From Cohn, L. H., DiSesa, V. J., Couper, G. S., et al.: Mitral valve repair for myxomatous degeneration and prolapse of the mitral valve. J. Thorac. Cardiovasc. Surg. 98:987, 1989.)

ventricular end-diastolic volume and mass are reduced. Depressed contractile function due to mitral regurgitation improves after mitral valve replacement.[240a] However, some patients with MR who had marked left ventricular dysfunction preoperatively sometimes remain symptomatic with a depressed ejection fraction[241] after a technically satisfactory operation, especially mitral valve replacement. Furthermore, long-term survival in patients with predominant MR who undergo mitral valve replacement may be poorer than in those with pure stenosis or mixed stenotic and regurgitant lesions, presumably because left ventricular dysfunction may be quite advanced and largely irreversible by the time patients with pure regurgitation become seriously symptomatic.[242-247] However, even though it is clearly desirable to operate on patients with MR before they develop marked left ventricular dysfunction, and despite these limitations of the results of surgical treatment in patients with severe left ventricular failure, operation is still indicated in the majority of these patients, since conservative therapy has little to offer.

The cause of the MR also plays an important role in the outcome following surgical treatment. In patients in whom mitral dysfunction is secondary to ischemic heart disease, the 5-year survival rate is about 30 per cent, whereas in rheumatic mitral regurgitation it is much better, approximately 70 per cent. Furthermore, occlusive coronary artery disease coexisting with, but not the primary cause of, mitral dysfunction is associated with decreased perioperative and long-term postoperative survival as well.[248] However, some improvement from mitral valve replacement can be expected even in patients with MR secondary to ischemic heart disease who are medically unresponsive and in congestive heart failure, as long as the cardiac index and ejection fraction exceed 1.5 liters/min/m² and 0.35, respectively. When left ventricular dysfunction is more severe, however, the risk of perioperative death becomes prohibitive.[249,250]

Surgical Treatment of Acute Mitral Regurgitation. Emergency surgical treatment of acute left ventricular failure caused by acute MR due to myocardial infarction and rupture of the head of a papillary muscle, by trauma to the mitral valve, or by endocarditis is associated with higher mortality rate than is the elective surgical treatment of chronic MR. However, unless such patients with acute, severe MR and heart failure are treated aggressively, a fatal outcome is almost certain. If the condition of patients with MR secondary to acute infarction can be stabilized by medical treatment, it is preferable to defer operation until 4 to 6 weeks after infarction. Vasodilator treatment may be useful during this period. However, medical management should not be prolonged if multisystem (renal or pulmonary or both) failure occurs. Surgical mortality is also higher in patients with refractory heart failure (functional Class IV), in those in whom a previously implanted prosthetic valve must be replaced because of

thromboembolism or valve dysfunction, and in those with active infective endocarditis (of a natural or prosthetic valve). Despite the higher surgical risks, the efficacy of early operation has been established in patients with infective endocarditis complicated by medically uncontrollable congestive heart failure, recurrent emboli, or both[244] (p. 1096). Since fungal endocarditis responds poorly to medical management, it is now the practice to recommend valve replacement in these cases *before* the onset of heart failure or embolization.

INDICATIONS FOR OPERATION. In view of advanced surgical techniques, reductions in operative mortality, and improvements in mitral reconstructive procedures and in artificial valves, as well as poor long-term results in many patients whose MR is corrected after a long history of heart failure, a more aggressive stance concerning the desirability of operation is in order. Only a few years ago I, along with many cardiologists, recommended operation for patients with chronic severe MR only if they were in functional Class III or IV,[251] i.e., with symptoms at rest or on ordinary activity despite intensive medical treatment. However, it is now my policy to recommend operation also for patients with severe MR who are in Class II, i.e., who become distinctly symptomatic only on heavy exertion, particularly if cardiomegaly and an elevated left ventricular end-systolic volume (> 30 ml/m² BSA) persist despite aggressive medical therapy.

The asymptomatic patient with severe MR presents a particularly challenging problem. Careful history and performance of an exercise test often reveal that these patients are not, in fact, truly asymptomatic. If that is the case, they may be considered for surgical treatment, as already discussed. However, patients with severe MR who are truly asymptomatic or only mildly symptomatic and have normal ventricular function (ejection fraction > 70 per cent) are followed. In asymptomatic patients with ejection fractions between 55 and 70 per cent it is useful to follow the end-systolic wall stress/end-systolic volume index ratio using noninvasive techniques and to time operation when these indices have begun to fall but before the patient becomes severely symptomatic. If valve replacement is likely to be necessary, a somewhat higher threshold for clinical and hemodynamic impairment is employed than if valvular reconstruction is contemplated.

The following preoperative hemodynamic indices are predictive of a favorable surgical outcome: EF > 0.70 and an end-systolic volume index < 50 ml/m², while predictors of poor outcome are an EF of < 0.55 and an end-systolic volume index of > 75 ml/m². Crawford et al. have reported that preoperative pulmonary hypertension (mean pulmonary artery pressure > 20 mm Hg) correlates with persistent postoperative left ventricular dilatation and that surgery should be considered in patients with MR before the ejection fraction decreases to 0.50 and before the end-systolic volume index exceeds 50 ml/m².[190]

The Mitral Valve Prolapse Syndrome

ETIOLOGY AND PATHOLOGY
(Fig. 34–21)

The mitral valve prolapse (MVP) syndrome has been given many names, including the systolic click–murmur syndrome, Barlow syndrome, billowing mitral valve syndrome, ballooning mitral cusp syndrome, floppy valve syndrome, and redundant cusp syndrome.[253-258] It is a common but variable clinical syndrome resulting from diverse pathogenic mechanisms of the mitral valve apparatus. The MVP syndrome has become recognized as one of the most prevalent cardiac valvular abnormalities, affecting as much as 5 to 10 per cent of the population.[256,259,260] It had been thought for many years that midsys-

tolic clicks and late systolic murmurs, the auscultatory hallmarks of this syndrome, were of extracardiac origin. However, in 1963 Barlow et al. demonstrated that these auscultatory findings are frequently associated with prolapse of the mitral valve, often with regurgitation.[261] Barlow and collaborators have distinguished between "billowing" and "prolapse" of the mitral valve.[261] Normally, the mitral valve billows slightly into the left atrium and an exaggeration should be termed "billowing mitral valve." A "floppy valve" is regarded as an extreme form of billowing. MVP occurs when the leaflet edges of the valve do not coapt, causing MR. With chordal rupture, the prolapsed mitral valve is "flail." Obviously, these conditions blend into one another, and it is often difficult to separate them sharply.

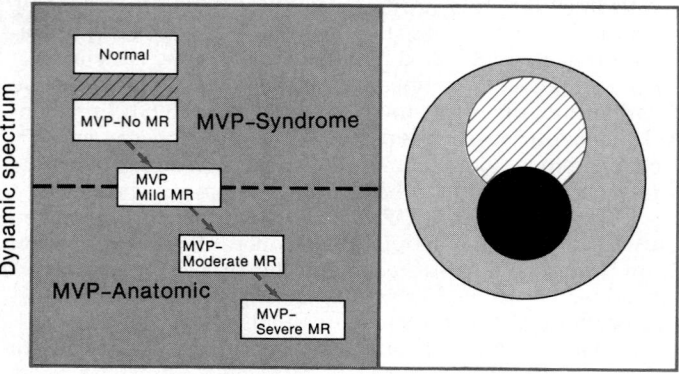

FIGURE 34–21. *Left panel,* The dynamic spectrum, time in years, and the progression of mitral valve prolapse (MVP) are shown. A subtle gradation (cross-hatched area) exists between the normal mitral valve and valves that produce mild MVP without mitral regurgitation (No MR). Progression from the level MVP–No MR to another level may or may not occur. Most of the MVP syndrome cases occupy the area above the dotted line, while progressive mitral valve dysfunction cases occupy the area below the dotted line. *Right panel,* The large circle represents the total number of patients with MVP. Patients with MVP may be symptomatic or asymptomatic. Symptoms may be directly related to mitral valve dysfunction (black circle), or to autonomic dysfunction (cross-hatched circle). Certain patients with symptoms directly related to mitral valve dysfunction may present with and continue to have symptoms secondary to autonomic dysfunction. (From Boudoulas, H., and Wooley, C. F.: Mitral Valve Prolapse and the Mitral Valve Prolapse Syndrome. Mount Kisco, NY, Futura Publishing Co., Inc., 1988.)

Perloff et al. have proposed specific clinical criteria for the diagnosis of MVP. They have divided the findings into three groups (Table 34–8): (1) major criteria, the presence of one or more of which establishes the diagnosis of MVP; (2) minor criteria, which cannot be discounted and which raise the suspicion of MVP but which by themselves are not sufficient to establish the diagnosis; and (3) nonspecific findings which, while often present in patients with MVP, are quite nonspecific. While they may alert the clinician, they do not aid in establishing the diagnosis. When rigorous two-dimensional echocardiography criteria (extension of leaflet tissue located cephalad to the plane of the mitral annulus) were employed, only two of 100 healthy young women displayed MVP.[262] In addition, Marks et al. have emphasized the importance of systolic displacement into the left atrium in the *parasternal view* in the diagnosis of MVP.[263,264] Such an approach may aid in avoiding overdiagnosis, which may occur with posterior bowing of the mitral valve on the M-mode echocardiogram and even in the four-chamber view on two-dimensional echocardiography.

The many causes of or conditions associated with prolapse of mitral valves into the left atrium during ventricular systole are shown in Table 34–9.[265-282] Prominent among these is myxomatous proliferation of the mitral valve, in which the spongiosa component of the valve, i.e., the middle layer of the leaflet composed of loose, myxomatous material, is unusually prominent[283,284] and the quantity of acid mucopolysaccharide is increased secondary to a fundamental but as yet undefined abnormality of collagen metabolism.[273,285] The concordance between inadequate production of type III collagen with echocardiographic findings of MVP in patients with type IV Ehlers-Danlos syndrome suggests that this abnormality of collagen is responsible in this subgroup.[286] Mucopolysaccharide infiltration and fragmentation of valvular collagen are common findings.[287] A reduction of type III and AB collagen has also been found in a patient with MVP without the Ehlers-Danlos syndrome.[288] While the majority of patients with MVP exhibit myxomatous degeneration of the valve, postinflammatory changes may also be responsible.[289]

Electron microscopy has shown haphazard arrangement, disruption, and fragmentation of collagen fibrils. In mild cases, the valvular myxoid stroma is enlarged on histological examination but the leaflets are grossly normal. However, with increasing quantities of myxoid stroma, the leaflets become grossly abnormal and redundant (Fig. 34–22) and prolapse. Regions of endothelial disruption, possible sites of endocarditis or thrombus formation, are common.[290] The severity of MR depends on the extent of the prolapse. The cusps of the mitral valve, the chordae tendineae, and the annulus may all be affected by myxomatous proliferation. Degeneration of collagen within the central core of the chordae tendineae is primarily responsible for chordal rupture, which occurs commonly in this syndrome and may intensify the severity of MR, although increased chordal tension resulting from the enlarged area of the valve cusps may play a contributory role.[291] Myxomatous changes in the annulus may result in annular dilatation and calcification—contributing to the severity of MR. Myxomatous proliferation, although most commonly affecting the mitral valve, is not limited to this

TABLE 34-8   DIAGNOSTIC CRITERIA AND NONSPECIFIC FINDINGS IN MITRAL VALVE PROLAPSE

MAJOR CRITERIA

Auscultation
  Mid- to late systolic clicks and late systolic murmur or whoop alone or in combination at the cardiac apex
Two-dimensional echocardiogram
  Marked superior systolic displacement of mitral leaflets with coaptation point at or superior to annular plane
  Mild to moderate superior systolic displacement of mitral leaflets with:
    Chordal rupture
    Doppler mitral regurgitation
    Annular dilatation
Echocardiogram plus auscultation
  Mild to moderate superior systolic displacement of mitral leaflets with:
    Prominent mid- to late systolic clicks at the cardiac apex
    Apical late systolic or holosystolic murmur in the young
    Late systolic "whoop"

MINOR CRITERIA

Auscultation
  Loud first heart sound with an apical holosystolic murmur
Two-dimensional echocardiogram
  Isolated mild to moderate superior systolic displacement of the posterior mitral leaflet
  Moderate superior systolic displacement of both mitral leaflets
Echocardiogram plus history
  Mild to moderate superior systolic displacement of mitral leaflets with:
    Focal neurologic attacks or amaurosis fugax in the young
    First-degree relatives with major criteria

NONSPECIFIC FINDINGS

Symptoms
  "Atypical" chest pain, dyspnea, fatigue, lassitude, giddiness, dizziness, syncope
  Psychological disturbances
Physical appearance
  Thoracic bony abnormalities
  Hypomastia
Electrocardiogram
  T-wave inversions in inferior limb leads or lateral precordial leads
  Premature ventricular beats at rest, during exercise, or on ambulatory ECG
  Supraventricular tachycardia
X-ray
  Scoliosis, pectus excavatum or carinatum, or loss of thoracic kyphosis
Two-dimensional echocardiogram
  Mild superior systolic displacement of anterior or anterior and posterior mitral leaflets

From Perloff, J. K., Child, J. S., and Edwards, J. E.: New guidelines for the clinical diagnosis of mitral valve prolapse. Am. J. Cardiol. 57:1124, 1986.

valve but has been described in the tricuspid,[281] aortic, and pulmonic valves, particularly in patients with Marfan syndrome, and may lead to regurgitation of these valves. It has been proposed that cellular proliferation in response to repeated minor stress applies to the mitral valve apparatus during the cardiac cycle results in increased production of type III collagen. This concept is supported by the observation of an increase in prevalence of MVP in late adolescence and an increase in severity with age.[292]

The MVP syndrome appears to exhibit a strong hereditary component,[293,294] transmitted as an autosomal dominant trait, and some cases of this syndrome appearing without any other obvious disorders may represent formes frustes of Marfan syndrome. However, genetic segregation analyses of familial MVP have shown no linkage to fibrillar collagen genes, providing evidence against the theory that the disease is a result of mutations of the genes encoding for the major collagens.[295] In an interesting report, MVP with transmission as an autosomal dominant was observed in 26 of a colony of 92 rhesus monkeys.[296] Although myxomatous proliferation of the mitral valve is idiopathic in most patients, it occurs in association with a variety of connective tissue disorders (Table 34–9) including Marfan syndrome, Ehlers-Danlos syndrome,[296] osteogenesis imperfecta, pseudoxanthoma elasticum,[297] and periarteritis nodosa, as well as with myotonic dystrophy,[272] Duchenne muscular dystrophy,[298] cardiomyopathy,[299] von Willebrand disease, keratoconus,[300] hyperthyroidism, and congenital malformations such as Ebstein's anomaly of the tricuspid valve, atrial septal defect of the ostium secundum variety,[265,301] and the Holt-Oram syndrome (p. 1633). There appears to be a high incidence of MVP in patients with asthenic habitus[302] and a variety of congenital thoracic deformities, including a straight back, a pectus excavatum, or a shallow chest.[276,279,280] The MVP syndrome may represent one manifestation of a number of systemic connective tissue disorders,[281] and thoracic abnormalities may represent another manifestation of the same disorders; frequently they coexist.

TABLE 34-9 CONDITIONS CAUSING OR ASSOCIATED WITH MITRAL VALVE PROLAPSE OR NONEJECTION CLICK/MITRAL REGURGITANT SYSTOLIC MURMUR

Primary mitral valve prolapse	von Willebrand syndrome
Marfan syndrome	Platelet abnormalities
Floppy valve syndrome	Migraine
Rheumatic endocarditis	Hypomagnesemia
Coronary artery disease	Osteogenesis imperfecta
Cardiomyopathy, congestive, hypertrophic	Inherited disorders of metabolism (Hunter-Hurler syndrome, Sanfilippo syndrome, Fabry disease, Sandhoff disease)
Myocarditis	
Trauma	
Left atrial myxoma	
Polyarteritis nodosa, systemic lupus erythematosus	Anxiety neurosis, neurocirculatory asthenia, autonomic dysfunction
Left ventricular aneurysm	
Ehlers-Danlos syndrome, pseudoxanthoma elasticum	Congenital prolonged QT syndrome
Pulmonary emphysema	Athelete's heart
Relapsing polychondritis	Turner syndrome
Muscular dystrophy	Noonan syndrome
Wolff-Parkinson-White syndrome	Congenital heart disease (atrial septal defect, ventricular septal defect, patent ductus arteriosus, aorticopulmonary window, complete-absence left pericardium, membranous subaortic stenosis, supravalvular aortic stenosis, Ebstein's anomaly, corrected transposition of great vessels, infundibular pulmonary stenosis, Uhl's anomaly)
Straight back syndrome	
Thoracic skeletal abnormalities	
Neuro-ecto-mesodermal histodysplasia	
Hyperthyroidism	

From Barlow, J. B.: Perspectives on the Mitral Valve. Philadelphia, F. A. Davis, 1987, p. 61.

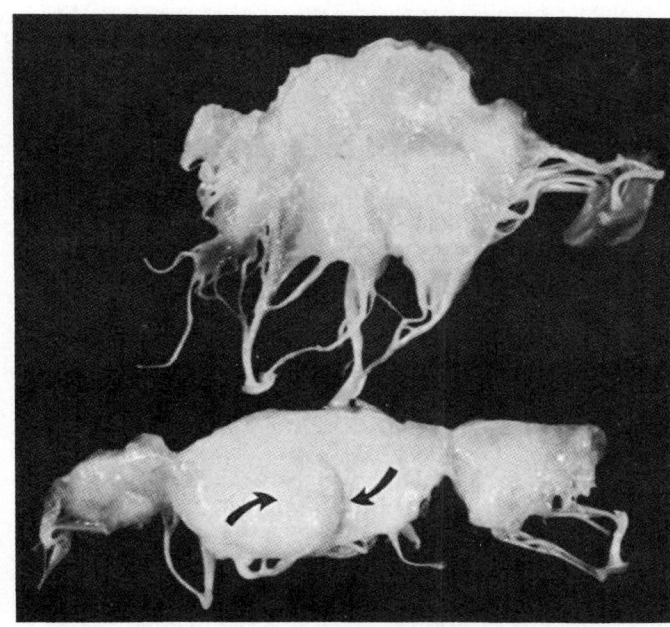

FIGURE 34–22. A resected floppy mitral valve from a 60-year-old man. Note the gelatinous appearance of the leaflets. The central scallop of the mural leaflet (arrows) shows a doming deformity. Some tendinous cords are ruptured in the vicinity of the dome. (From Turri, M., et al.: Surgical pathology of disease of the mitral valve, with special reference to lesions promoting valvular incompetence. Int. J. Cardiol. 22:213, 1989.)

It has been pointed out that the clinical phenotype of patients with MVP ranges from Marfan syndrome at one end to isolated MVP on the other. Many patients fall somewhere in between in what has been termed an "overlap heritable connective tissue disorder."[303]

The MVP syndrome can coexist with rheumatic MS, and it may develop following mitral commissurotomy for this lesion.[304] In hypertrophic obstructive cardiomyopathy, prolapse of the posterior leaflet of the mitral valve may accompany the usual anterior displacement of the anterior mitral valve leaflet.[305]

Ischemic heart disease and MVP are both common disorders and coexist not infrequently; MVP may also occur secondary to papillary muscle dysfunction. In some patients, MVP has been documented to develop for the first time *following* myocardial infarction.[306] Since MVP has also been reported in patients who have suffered acute myocardial infarction despite normal coronary arteriograms,[307] it is possible that coronary artery emboli are responsible for the infarction in this syndrome. MVP may cause myocardial ischemia by increasing tension on the base of the involved muscle.[305] It has also been proposed that coronary artery spasm occurs as a reflex response to prolapse of the posterior mitral leaflet and that the resultant ischemia may be responsible for angina or angina-like pain, myocardial infarction, arrhythmias, and sudden death in this syndrome.[308]

CLINICAL MANIFESTATIONS

The clinical presentations of the MVP syndrome are diverse.[309] The condition has been observed in patients of all ages and in both sexes. It is a common syndrome; indeed, prolapse of the mitral valve has been reported to occur in 6 per cent of healthy young women surveyed by echocardiography.[259] One series of 100 presumably healthy young women revealed that 17 had a midsystolic click or late systolic murmur or both and that 10 of these 17 had evidence of prolapse of the mitral valve on echocardiography.[260] However, as already noted, since billowing of the mitral valve is a normal variant and M-mode echocardiographic findings may be nonspecific, it is likely that more rigorous criteria for diagnosis based on two-dimensional echocardiography will indicate a much lower prevalence.[254] In one series, about 20 per cent of patients who underwent mitral valve replacement had myxomatous proliferation of the valve on histopathological examination.[310] Indeed, MVP is now the most common cause of isolated regurgitation requiring mitral valve replacement.[311] Echocardiographic evidence of MVP has been found in more than 90 per cent of patients with Marfan syndrome[312] and in many of their first-degree relatives.

HISTORY

The overwhelming majority of patients with MVP are asymptomatic[313] (Fig. 34–21). In many cases, otherwise asymptomatic patients with MVP suffer from undue anxiety, perhaps precipitated by their having been informed of the presence of heart disease. Boudoulas et al. have called attention to a "MVP syndrome" with a characteristic nonejection click and a variety of nonspecific symptoms, such as fatigability, palpitations, postural orthostasis, and neuropsychiatric symptoms, as well as symptoms of autonomic dysfunction.[313] Patients may complain of palpitations, chest discomfort, and, when MR is severe, symptoms of diminished cardiac reserve. Chest discomfort may be typical of angina but most often is atypical in that it is prolonged, not clearly related to exertion, and punctuated by brief attacks of severe stabbing pain at the apex. The discomfort may be secondary to tension on papillary muscles and may be associated with abnormalities of wall motion or indentations of the wall of the left ventricle at the base of these muscles on angiography. It may be difficult to differentiate this discomfort from angina because of the coexistence of the MVP syndrome and true angina pectoris secondary to coronary artery disease.

Since MVP is sometimes associated with another form of heart disease, e.g., atrial septal defect, symptoms produced by the latter may predominate. It has been suggested that many of the symptoms are related to dysfunction of the autonomic nervous system, which occurs frequently in the MVP syndrome.[314-316] Some patients with MVP exhibit increased excretion and circulating concentrations of epinephrine and norepinephrine, presumably secondary to increased adrenergic tone, which may be responsible for many of the symptoms of the syndrome. Some exhibit excessive vasoconstriction, others striking orthostatic tachycardia.[315] Although many of the symptoms of MVP resemble those of neurocirculatory asthenia, the two conditions appear to be distinct and unrelated.[317] Patients with MVP also have an unusually high incidence of migraine.[313]

PHYSICAL EXAMINATION

Palpation of the chest and of the carotid pulses confirms the presence of MR, which may range from nonexistent to severe. The physical findings unique to the MVP syndrome are detected by auscultation and can be corroborated by phonocardiography.[253,258] The most important is a systolic click at least 0.14 sec after S_1 (Figs. 3–7 and 3–8, p. 46). This can be differentiated from a systolic ejection click, since it occurs distinctly *after* the beginning of the upstroke of the carotid pulse. Occasionally multiple mid- and late-systolic clicks are audible most readily along the lower left sternal border and are believed to be produced by sudden tensing of the elongated chordae tendineae and of the prolapsing leaflets. The click is often, although not invariably, followed by a mid- to late-crescendo systolic murmur that continues to A_2. This murmur is similar to that produced by papillary muscle dysfunction (Fig. 2–20, p. 40), which is readily understandable, since both result from mid- to late-systolic MR. In general, the duration of the murmur is a function of the severity of the regurgitation, and when the murmur is confined to the latter portion of systole, regurgitation usually is not severe. However, as regurgitation becomes more severe, the murmur commences earlier and becomes holosystolic.

It is important to emphasize the variability of the physical findings in the MVP syndrome. Some patients exhibit both a midsystolic click and a mid- to late-systolic murmur; others present with one or the other of these two findings; still others have only a click on one occasion and only a murmur on another, both on a third examination, and no abnormality at all on a fourth. MVP may also cause an early diastolic sound or murmur, best heard at the apex or left sternal border 70 to 110 msec following A_2, at a time when the prolapsed posterior leaflet descends into the left ventricle.[318] Conditions other than MVP cause midsystolic clicks; these include tricuspid valve clicks, extracardiac causes, and atrial septal aneurysms.[319]

DYNAMIC AUSCULTATION. The auscultatory and phonocardiographic findings are exquisitely sensitive to physiological and pharmacological interventions, and recognition of the changes induced by these interventions is of great value in the diagnosis of the MVP syndrome (Fig. 2–20, p. 40) (Table 34–5).[253,258] The mitral valve begins to prolapse when the reduction of left ventricular volume during systole reaches a critical point at which the mitral valve leaflets no longer coapt; at that instant, the click occurs and the murmur commences. Any maneuver that decreases left ventricular volume, such as a reduction of impedance to left ventricular outflow, a reduction in venous return, or an augmentation of contractility, results in an earlier occurrence of prolapse during systole. As a consequence, the click and onset of the murmur move closer to S_1. When prolapse is severe or left ventricular size is markedly reduced or both, prolapse may begin with the onset of systole, and as a consequence, the click may not be audible and the murmur may be holosystolic. On the other hand, when left ventricular volume is augmented by an increase in venous return, a reduction of myocardial contractility, bradycardia, or an increase in the impedance to left ventricular emptying, both the click and the onset of the murmur will be delayed. Indeed, if the left ventricle becomes extremely large, prolapse may not occur at all, and the abnormal auscultatory features may disappear entirely.

During the straining phase of the Valsalva maneuver, upon sudden standing, and early during the inhalation of amyl nitrite, cardiac size decreases, and both the click and the onset of the murmur occur earlier in systole. In contrast, a sudden change from the standing to the prone position, leg-raising, squatting, maximal isometric exercise, and, to a lesser extent, expiration will delay the click and the onset of the murmur (Fig. 3–8, p. 46). During the overshoot phase of the Valsalva maneuver (i.e., six to eight cycles following release) and with prolongation of the R-R interval either following a premature contraction or in atrial fibrillation, the click and onset of the murmur are usually delayed, and the intensity of the murmur is reduced.

In general, when the onset of the murmur is delayed, both its duration and its intensity are diminished, reflecting a reduction in the severity of MR. With some maneuvers, however, there is a discrepancy between changes in the intensity and duration of the murmur. Following amyl nitrite inhalation, for example, the reduced left ventricular size results in an earlier click and longer murmur, but the lower left ventricular systolic pressure diminishes the severity of regurgitation and the intensity of the murmur. Conversely, phenylephrine and methoxamine delay the click and the onset of the murmur, but the larger volume of regurgitation consequent to the elevated left ventricular systolic pressure increases regurgitation and the intensity of the murmur. Emotional stress may increase the intensity of the click and exacerbate arrhythmias in MVP,[320] a finding that might explain the intermittency of the auscultatory findings and arrhythmias in these patients. In the diagnosis of the MVP syndrome, it is generally more helpful to determine the effect of interventions on the *timing of the click* and murmur than on the *intensity of the murmur.*

There may be confusion between the systolic murmurs of

hypertrophic cardiomyopathy (HCM) and of MVP, particularly because midsystolic clicks and a late systolic murmur have been reported in HCM and because the murmur may increase in intensity and duration with standing and decrease with squatting in both conditions (p. 1408). However, the response to several interventions may be helpful in differentiating these two conditions. During the strain of the Valsalva maneuver, the murmur of HCM increases in intensity[321] in contrast to that in the syndrome, which becomes longer but usually not louder. The murmur of HCM becomes louder after amyl nitrite inhalation, whereas that of MVP does not. Following a premature beat, the murmur of HCM increases in intensity and duration, whereas that due to MVP usually remains unchanged or decreases.

LABORATORY EXAMINATION

ELECTROCARDIOGRAPHY

Most commonly, the electrocardiogram is within normal limits in asymptomatic patients with typical auscultatory and echocardiographic findings. In a minority of asymptomatic patients and in many symptomatic patients, the electrocardiogram shows inverted or biphasic T waves and nonspecific ST-segment changes in leads II, III, and aV, and occasionally in the anterolateral leads as well.[253] The ST- and T-wave changes may become exaggerated during amyl nitrite inhalation and exercise. These electrocardiographic findings may be related to ischemia of the papillary muscles, or of the left ventricle at their bases, resulting from increased tension on these structures produced by the prolapsing valve. Alternatively, it is possible that the electrocardiographic abnormality reflects an underlying cardiomyopathy.

ARRHYTHMIAS. A spectrum of arrhythmias, including atrial and ventricular premature contractions and supraventricular and ventricular tachyarrhythmias[322-328] as well as bradyarrhythmias due to sinus node dysfunction or varying degrees of atrioventricular block,[329] have been observed in the MVP syndrome. Indeed, this syndrome should be considered patients with otherwise unexplained arrhythmias. The mechanism of the arrhythmias is not clear. Diastolic depolarization of muscle fibers in the anterior mitral leaflet in response to stretch has been demonstrated experimentally,[330] and the abnormal stretch of the prolapsed leaflet may be of pathogenetic significance. Wit et al. have shown that mitral valve leaflets contain atrium-like muscle fibers in continuity with left atrial myocardium. It is possible that mechanical stimulation of these fibers generates slow-response action potentials and sustained rhythmic action that penetrates the cardiac chambers.[331] Although most of these arrhythmias are of little clinical importance, recurrent ventricular tachycardia, refractory to the usual agents, and even ventricular fibrillation have been reported. These serious ventricular arrhythmias are significantly more frequent in patients with ST-segment and T-wave abnormalities on the resting electrocardiogram.[332]

Paroxysmal supraventricular tachycardia is the most common sustained tachyarrhythmia in patients with the MVP syndrome and may be related to the high incidence of atrioventricular bypass tracts in this condition.[322] These bypass tracts are always left-sided and may be associated with the mitral valve abnormality. In the general population only 20 per cent of patients with paroxysmal supraventricular tachycardia have such bypass tracts, whereas the incidence in patients with MVP is three times as great. Conversely, there is evidence that there is high incidence of MVP among patients with the Wolff-Parkinson-White syndrome.[333] However, the absence of electrocardiographic evidence of the Wolff-Parkinson-White syndrome should not be taken as evidence against the existence of bypass tracts in patients with the MVP syndrome who suffer attacks of supraventricular tachycardia. These considerations suggest that patients with the MVP syndrome who develop paroxysmal supraventricular tachycardia should be subjected to electrophysiological investigation. The outcome of such studies may be important, since digitalis or propranolol, which may be useful in reentry tachycardias, may be hazardous in the presence of antegrade conduction over an atrioventricular bypass tract. There is also an increased association between MVP and prolongation of the Q-T interval, and this association may play a role in the genesis of ventricular arrhythmias.[316,334]

MVP AND SUDDEN DEATH. The relation between the MVP syndrome and sudden death is not clear. Jeresaty collected 25 patients with MVP who died suddenly,[335] and Pocock et al. reviewed 17 patients.[336] But these are "numerators without denominators," and when the high incidence of both conditions is considered, it is difficult to interpret the coincidence. Considering the frequency of both conditions, these numbers are not very impressive. It is not clear how many, indeed if any, of these instances of sudden death were in fact caused by or related to the MVP syndrome. The immediate cause of the sudden, unexpected death is probably an episode of tachyarrhythmia,[337] although complete heart block with prolonged asystole has also been reported in this syndrome and cannot be excluded.[338]

Kligfield et al. have identified the following as potential risks for sudden death in MVP: the presence of significant MR, complex ventricular arrhythmias, prolongation of the Q-T interval, and a history of syncope and palpitations.[323,324] Boudoulas et al. identified nine patients with MVP who had experienced cardiac arrest. Ventricular fibrillation was documented in eight; seven were successfully resuscitated. Six living survivors have been followed for 3 to 14 years.[329]

ECHOCARDIOGRAPHY (see also p. 83). Echocardiography plays a key role in the diagnosis of MVP and has been most useful in the delineation of this syndrome[339] (Figs. 3–7, p. 46, 4–50 and 4–51, p. 84). The most common echocardiographic finding on M-mode echocardiography is abrupt posterior movement of the posterior leaflet or of both mitral leaflets in midsystole. A second finding is pansystolic posterior prolapse of one or both leaflets, giving rise to a U- or hammock-shaped configuration in the C-D segment (Fig. 4–50, p. 84) (the opposite of what is seen in hypertrophic obstructive cardiomyopathy, in which the anterior leaflet of the mitral valve moves toward the ventricular septum in midsystole). Holosystolic "hammocking" of less than 5 mm is not specific for MVP. Rarely, there is a sudden posterior collapse of the anterior mitral leaflet as it approaches the prolapsing posterior leaflet in early systole.[340] All three of these echocardiographic patterns have in common the motion of the mitral valve posterior to the C-point. Although the systolic click usually occurs at the time of the abrupt posterior movement, there is considerable variability in the relationship between the auscultatory and echocardiographic events.

In some patients, M-mode echocardiography has missed MVP that was detected by two-dimensional echocardiography.[341,342] The echocardiogram is helpful in the identification of patients at significant risk of developing severe MR or infective endocarditis; in addition to systolic displacement of one or both leaflets into the left atrium, the leaflets are distinctly thickened[263] or redundant[263] in these patients (Fig. 34–23). Doppler echocardiography frequently reveals mild MR that is not always associated with an audible murmur. Color flow Doppler is useful in identifying the location and severity of the regurgitant jets.[344] Moderate or severe MR is found in 10 per cent of patients, usually in men over the age of 50.[344]

The echocardiographic findings of MVP have been reported to occur in a large number of first-degree relatives of patients with established MVP,[345] but the variability in physical findings in this syndrome, already commented upon, extends to the echocardiogram.[346] Thus, some patients have a systolic click with or without a murmur and show no evidence of MVP on the echocardiogram. Conversely, the echocardiographic findings of MVP may be observed in patients without the click or murmur. Others have both the typical echocardiographic and auscultatory features.

Two-dimensional echocardiography has also revealed prolapse of the tricuspid and aortic valves in approximately one-fifth of patients with MVP.[347] Conversely, however, prolapse of the tricuspid and aortic valves[348] occurs uncommonly in patients without prolapse of the mitral valve; the latter echocardiographic finding is usually not associated with any aortic regurgitation.

STRESS SCINTIGRAPHY

The differential diagnosis between two common conditions—MVP associated with atypical chest pain and electrocardiographic abnormalities, and primary coronary artery disease associated with MVP—may be aided by exercise electrocardiography,[224] but myocardial scintigraphy using thallium-201 during exercise (p. 287) is probably more specific in this disorder. When findings are normal, i.e., when there is no evidence of exercise-induced regional myocardial ischemia, the diagnosis of MVP unrelated to ischemic heart disease is favored.[349] However, the reverse is not always the case, since patients having MVP with or without associated coronary artery disease may exhibit myocardial perfusion defects—

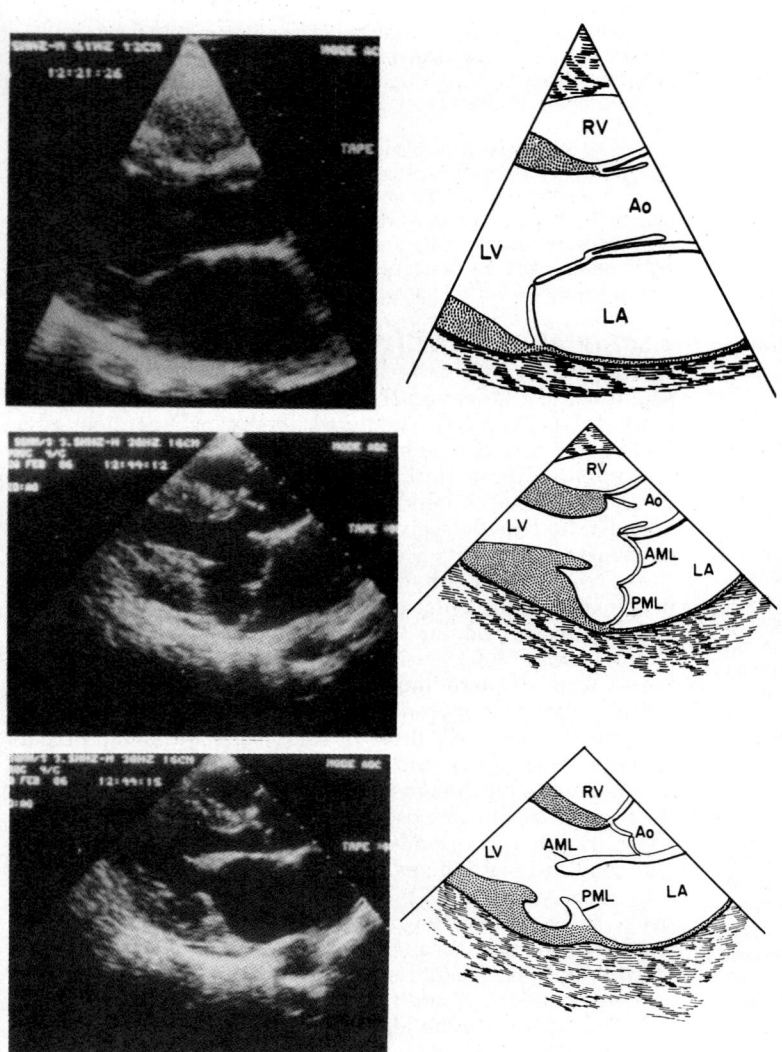

FIGURE 34–23. *Top,* Parasternal long-axis view of normal mitral valve leaflets during systole. RV = right ventricle, LV = left ventricle, Ao = aorta, and LA = left atrium. *Center,* Classic mitral-valve prolapse. The parasternal long-axis view shows the mitral leaflets prolapsing into the left atrium during systole. Note the relation of the mitral leaflets to the mitral annulus. RV denotes right ventricle; LV = left ventricle, Ao = aorta, LA = left atrium, AML = anterior mitral leaflet, and PML = posterior mitral leaflet. *Bottom,* Classic mitral-valve prolapse with leaflet thickening. The parasternal long-axis view of the same mitral valve as in center figure is shown during diastole. This view was used to measure the thickness of the leaflets. RV denotes right ventricle, LV = left ventricle, Ao = aorta, AML = anterior mitral leaflet, PML = posterior mitral leaflet, and LA = left atrium. (Reprinted by permission from Marks, A. R., Choong, C. Y., Sanfilippo, A. J., et al.: Identification of high-risk and low-risk subgroups of patients with mitral valve prolapse. N. Engl. J. Med. *320*:1031, 1989.)

exercise-induced or following redistribution or both.[350] Ejection fraction at rest determined by radionuclide angiography is normal in patients having MVP without associated MR. However, a subgroup of these patients do not exhibit a normal increase in ejection fraction during exercise, suggesting that a cardiomyopathic process may be responsible for the reduced cardiac reserve.[351]

ANGIOGRAPHY

The configuration of the left ventriculogram during systole is helpful in the diagnosis of MVP.[352] The right anterior oblique projection is most useful for defining the posterior leaflet of the mitral valve and the left anterior oblique projection for studying the anterior leaflet. The most helpful sign is extension of the mitral leaflet tissue inferiorly and posteriorly to the point of attachment of the mitral leaflets to the annulus fibrosis.[353] Angiography may also reveal scalloped edges of the leaflets, reflecting redundancy of tissue.

Other abnormalities noted on angiography of some patients with MVP include dilatation, decreased systolic contraction, and calcification of the mitral annulus and poor contraction of the basal portion of the left ventricle.[354] There may be an indentation at the base of the posteromedial papillary muscle associated with prolapse of the posterior leaflet and resulting from abnormal traction on this muscle. With involvement of both papillary muscles, there may be an indentation of the anterior as well as the inferior wall of the left ventricle, giving the cardiac silhouette an hourglass appearance. These left ventricular contraction abnormalities are secondary to redundancy of the mitral valve leaflets and transmission of the abnormal tension on these leaflets to the papillary muscles and underlying left ventricle. Patients with MVP and little or no MR have normal left ventricular hemodynamics. An increased rate of circumferential fiber shortening may be observed in the presence of significant MR, as in patients with regurgitation of other etiologies.[354]

NATURAL HISTORY

The outlook for MVP in children is excellent, a large majority remaining asymptomatic for many years without any change in clinical or laboratory manifestations.[355–357]

Progressive MR occurs in about 15 per cent of patients over a 10- to 15-year period; the incidence of this complication is significantly greater in patients with both murmurs and clicks than in those with an isolated click. In many patients, rupture of chordae tendineae or infective endocarditis is responsible for the intensification of the mitral regurgitation.[253] Severe MR occurs more frequently in men older than 50 years with MVP. Patients with the MVP syndrome are also at risk of developing infective endocarditis,[358–360] although the incidence appears to be extremely low in patients with a midsystolic click only; the incidence rises in patients with a systolic murmur.[361]

Acute hemiplegia, transient ischemic attacks, cerebellar infarcts, amaurosis fugax, and retinal arteriolar occlusions all appear to occur more frequently in patients with the MVP syndrome, suggesting that cerebral emboli are unusually common in this condition.[362–365] These neurological complications are often associated with shortened platelet survival. Loss of endothelial continuity and tearing of the endocardium overlying the myxomatous valve may initiate platelet aggregation and the formation of mural platelet-fibrin complexes.[362] The paroxysmal arrhythmias that occur in the MVP syndrome may contribute to the likelihood of embolization.

Indeed, it is possible that cerebral embolization secondary to MVP may be a significant cause for unexplained strokes and other cerebral and retinal complications in young people without cerebrovascular disease. Similarly, myocardial infarction in patients with MVP and normal coronary arteries may be secondary to embolization.[365]

MANAGEMENT

Asymptomatic patients (or those whose principal complaint is anxiety) with no arrhythmias evident on a routine extended electrocardiographic tracing and on prolonged auscultation, with normal ST segments and without evidence of serious MR, have an excellent prognosis. They should be reassured about the favorable prognosis but should have follow-up examinations every 2 to 4 years. This should include a two-dimensional echocardiogram and a Doppler study. Patients with a long systolic murmur may show progression of MR and should be examined more frequently, at intervals of approximately 12 months. Since infective endocarditis is a well-recognized complication of MVP,[358-360] *endocarditis prophylaxis* is advisable in patients, particularly men, with a typical systolic murmur and characteristic echocardiographic features. Although opinions on this point are not unanimous, prophylaxis is probably not necessary in patients, particularly women, with a midsystolic click without a systolic murmur.[358,359] Some, however, recommend prophylaxis when such patients are subjected to instrumentation of the upper respiratory or genitourinary tract.[360]

Patients with a history of palpitations, lightheadedness, dizziness, or syncope or those who have ventricular arrhythmias or Q-T prolongation on a routine electrocardiogram should undergo ambulatory (24-hour) electrocardiographic monitoring or treadmill exercise testing or both. A beta-adrenoceptor blocker is the drug of choice for many ventricular arrhythmias, and either propranolol or phenytoin is useful in patients

with prolongation of the Q-T interval. Beta-adrenoceptor blockade may also be useful in the treatment of chest discomfort, both in patients with associated coronary artery disease and in those with normal coronary vessels in whom the symptoms may be due to regional ischemia secondary to MVP.[366] Nitrates should be used with caution, since the reduction of cardiac size induced by these drugs may intensify the prolapse and the resultant ischemia of the base of the papillary muscles.

Patients with symptoms of reduced functional cardiac reserve attributable to MR should be treated like other patients with severe MR (p. 1027), and those with severe regurgitation who are not responsive to medical management may require mitral valve surgery. Often reconstructive surgery without valve replacement is possible (Fig. 34–20). Approximately half of all mitral valve reconstructions are carried out in patients with MVP. Among 62 such patients operated on at Brigham and Women's Hospital in Boston, resection of the posterior leaflet and insertion of an annuloplasty ring were the most commonly employed procedures.[367] In patients with angina on effort and/or ischemic electrocardiographic changes and abnormalities on a thallium perfusion scan during exercise, coronary arteriography should be performed, and treatment should take into account the responsiveness of symptoms to medical management and the coronary anatomy, as outlined in Chapter 40. In patients with MVP who have had any of the aforementioned cerebral events and in whom no other etiology is apparent, anticoagulant therapy and/or drugs that interfere with platelet function, such as aspirin, should be given.

Although this discussion has focused attention on complications of the MVP syndrome, it should not be forgotten that, on the whole, this is a benign condition and that the *vast majority* of patients with this syndrome remain asymptomatic for their entire lives and require, at most, observation every few years and reassurance.

Aortic Stenosis

ETIOLOGY AND PATHOLOGY

Obstruction to left ventricular outflow is localized most commonly at the aortic valve and is discussed in this section. However, obstruction may also occur above the valve (supravalvular stenosis [p. 926]) or below the valve (discrete subvalvular aortic stenosis [p. 925]) or may be caused by hypertrophic obstructive cardiomyopathy (p. 1404). In an analysis of the hearts of 543 patients with valvular disease, Roberts found isolated aortic stenosis (AS) to be the most common lesion.[368] Valvular AS *without accompanying mitral valve disease* is more common in men and very rarely occurs on a rheumatic basis but instead is usually either congenital or degenerative in origin[11,369,370] (Figs. 34–24 and 34–25).

CONGENITAL AORTIC STENOSIS (see also pp. 922 and 971). Congenital malformations of the aortic valve may be unicuspid, bicuspid, or tricuspid, or there may be a dome-shaped diaphragm.[11] *Unicuspid valves* produce severe obstruction in infancy and are the most frequent malformations found in fatal valvular aortic stenosis in children under the age of one year.[371] Congenitally *bicuspid valves* may be stenotic with commissural fusion at birth, but more commonly they are not responsible for serious narrowing of the aortic orifice during childhood; their abnormal architecture induces turbulent flow, which traumatizes the leaflets and ultimately leads to fibrosis, increased rigidity, and calcification of the leaflets and narrowing of the aortic orifice[372,373] (Fig. 34–26). Infective endocarditis may develop on a congenitally bicuspid valve, which then becomes regurgitant. Rarely, a congenitally bicuspid valve is purely regurgitant in the absence of antece-

ent infection. It should be emphasized that in a majority of cases, a bicuspid valve is not stenotic at birth and that the changes causing stenosis resemble those occurring in senile, degenerative calcific stenosis of a tricuspid aortic valve except that in the congenitally bicuspid valve these changes occur several decades earlier.

A third form of a congenitally malformed valve is tricuspid, with the cusps of unequal size and some commissural fusion. Although many of these valves retain normal function throughout life, it has been postulated that the turbulent flow produced by the mild congenital architectural abnormality may lead to fibrosis and ultimately to calcification and stenosis. Tricuspid stenotic aortic valves in adults may be congenital, rheumatic, or degenerative in origin.

ACQUIRED AORTIC STENOSIS. Rheumatic AS results from adhesions and fusions of the commissures and cusps and vascularization of the leaflets and the valve ring, leading to retraction and stiffening of the free borders of the cusps, with calcific nodules present on both surfaces and an orifice that is reduced to a small round or triangular opening. As a consequence, the rheumatic valve is often regurgitant as well as stenotic. The heart frequently exhibits other stigmata of rheumatic heart disease, especially mitral valve involvement. This form of AS appears to be decreasing in frequency.

In degenerative (senile) calcific AS, the cusps are immobilized by a deposit of calcium along their flexion lines at their bases. This common cause of AS in adults (which is now the most frequent in patients with AS requiring aortic valve replacement)[374] appears to result from years of normal mechanical stress on the valve. Although degenerative calcification

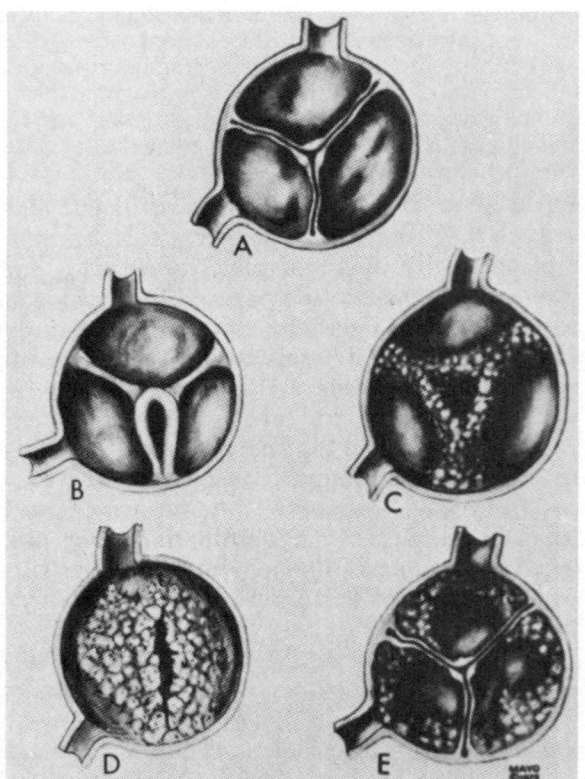

FIGURE 34-24. Types of aortic valve stenosis. *A,* Normal aortic valve. *B,* Congenital aortic stenosis. *C,* Rheumatic aortic stenosis. *D,* Calcific aortic stenosis. *E,* Calcific senile aortic stenosis. (From Brandenburg, R. O., et al.: Valvular heart disease — When should the patient be referred? Pract. Cardiol. *5:*50, 1979.)

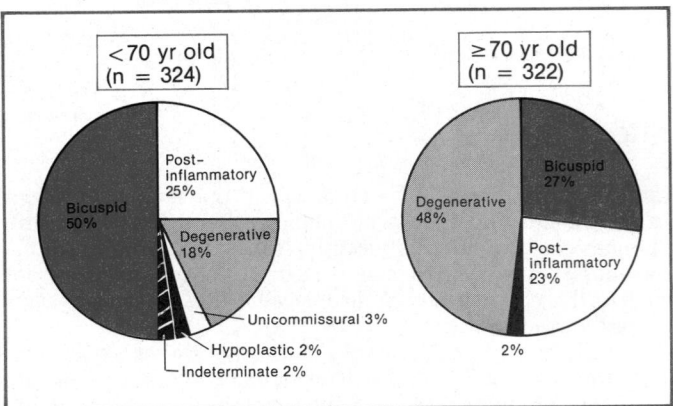

FIGURE 34-25. Causes of aortic stenosis, shown for two age groups. Among patients younger than 70 years (*left*), calcification of congenitally bicuspid valves accounted for half of the surgical cases. In contrast, in those 70 years of age or older (*right*), degenerative calcification accounted for almost half of the cases. (From Passik, C. S., et al.: Temporal changes in the causes of aortic stenosis: A surgical pathologic study of 646 cases. Mayo Clin. Proc. *62:*119, 1987.)

may extend in the direction of the cusps, no commissural fusion is present. Degenerative "wear and tear" appears to be the most likely cause of this form of AS, which is commonly accompanied by calcifications of the mitral annulus and coronary arteries but rarely by aortic regurgitation. Both diabetes mellitus and hypercholesterolemia are risk factors for the development of this lesion.[375,376] The stenosis is produced by the calcific deposits that prevent the cusps from opening normally during systole (Fig. 34-26).

In atherosclerotic aortic valvular stenosis, severe atherosclerosis involves the aorta and other major arteries; this form of AS occurs most frequently in patients with severe hyper-

cholesterolemia and is observed in children with homozygous type II hyperlipoproteinemia (p. 1137). Calcific aortic stenosis is observed in Paget's disease of bone[377] as well as in end-stage renal disease.[378,379] *Rheumatoid involvement* of the valve is a rare cause of AS and results in nodular thickening of the valve leaflets and involvement of the proximal part of the aorta (p. 1732). *Ochronosis* is another rare cause of aortic stenosis.[380]

Roberts studied hearts with AS obtained from patients between 15 and 65 years of age and found that almost 40 per cent were tricuspid. Since there were thickening of the mitral valve and a history of acute rheumatic fever in half of these cases, it is likely that the AS was rheumatic in etiology; in the remainder it was either congenital or degenerative in origin. In 90 per cent of hearts of patients with AS who were older than 65 years and who were examined at autopsy, the valves were tricuspid, with nodular calcific deposits on the aortic aspects of the cusps, but without commissural fusion.[368]

Hemodynamically significant AS leads to severe concentric left ventricular hypertrophy,[381] with heart weights as great as 1000 gm. The interventricular septum often bulges into and encroaches on the right ventricular cavity. When left ventricular failure supervenes, the left ventricle dilates,[381] the left atrium enlarges, and changes secondary to backward failure occur in the pulmonary vascular bed, right side of the heart, and systemic venous bed.

PATHOPHYSIOLOGY

The left ventricle responds to the *sudden* production of severe obstruction to outflow by dilatation and reduction of stroke volume. However, in adults with AS, the obstruction usually develops and increases gradually over a prolonged period. In infants and children with congenital AS, the valve orifice shows little change as the child grows, thereby also intensifying the relative obstruction quite gradually. Left ventricular function can be well maintained in experimentally produced, chronic, gradually developing subcoronary AS.[382] Left ventricular ouput is maintained by the presence of left ventricular hypertrophy, which may sustain a large pressure gradient across the aortic valve for many years without a reduction in cardiac output, left ventricular dilatation, or the development of symptoms. A peak systolic pressure gradient exceeding 50 mm Hg in the presence of a normal cardiac output or an effective aortic orifice less than about 0.75 cm² in an average-sized adult, i.e., 0.4 cm²/m² of body surface area (less than approximately one-fourth of the normal orifice) is generally considered to represent critical obstruction to left ventricular outflow.[383]

As contraction of the left ventricle becomes progressively more isometric, the left ventricular pressure pulse exhibits a rounded, rather than flattened, summit. The elevated left ventricular end-diastolic pressure, which is characteristic of severe AS, does not necessarily signify the presence of left ventricular dilatation or failure but often reflects diminished compliance of the hypertrophied left ventricular wall; usually it results from both processes.[384-386]

In patients with severe AS, large *a* waves usually appear in the left atrial pressure pulse because of the combination of enhanced contraction of a hypertrophied left atrium and diminished left ventricular compliance. Atrial contraction plays a particularly important role in filling of the left ventricle in AS.[27] It raises left ventricular end-diastolic pressure without producing a concomitant elevation of mean left atrial pressure.[387] This "booster pump" function of the left atrium prevents the pulmonary venous and capillary pressures from rising to levels that would produce pulmonary congestion, while at the same time maintaining left ventricular end-diastolic pressure at the elevated level necessary for effective left ventricular contraction. Loss of appropriately timed, vigorous atrial contraction, as occurs in atrial fibrillation or atrioventricular dissociation, may result in rapid clinical deterioration in patients with severe AS.

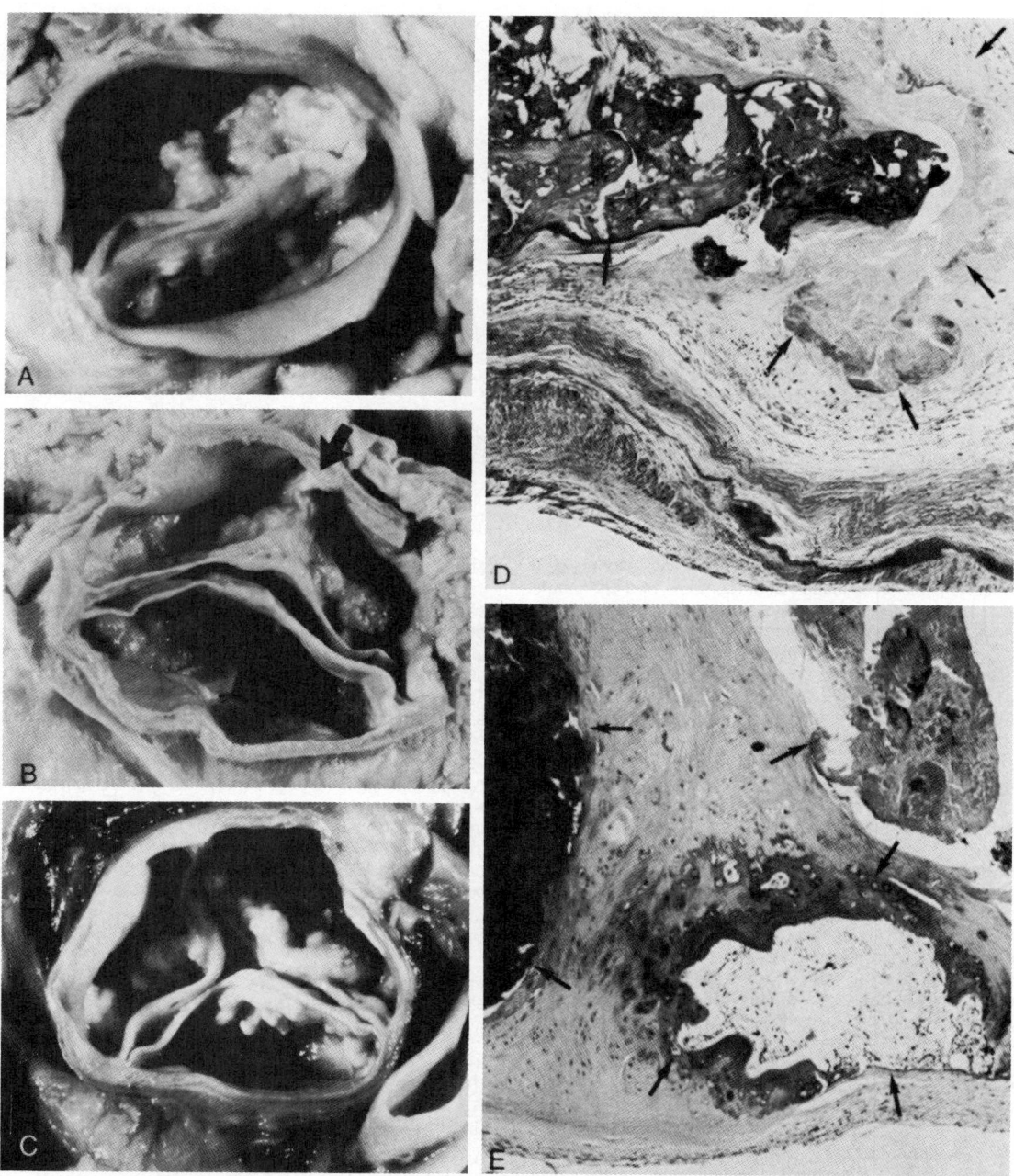

FIGURE 34–26. Calcific aortic stenosis. *A*, Congenitally bicuspid aortic valve, characterized by two equal cusps with basal mineralization. *B*, Congenitally bicuspid aortic valve having two unequal cusps, the larger with a central raphe (arrow). *C*, Otherwise anatomically normal tricuspid aortic valve in an elderly patient, characterized by isolated cusps with calcification localized to basilar aspect; cuspal free edges are not involved. *D* and *E*, Photomicrographs of calcific deposits in calcific aortic stenosis; deposits are rimmed by arrows (hematoxylin and eosin, 15×). *D*, Shows deposits with underlying cusp largely intact; transmural calcific deposits are shown in *E*. (*A* and *C*, from Schoen, F. J., St. John Sutton, M.: Contemporary issues in the pathology of valvular heart disease. Hum. Pathol. *18*:568, 1987.)

Although the *cardiac output* at rest is within normal limits in the majority of patients with severe AS,[383] it often fails to rise normally during exertion. Late in the course of the disease the cardiac output, stroke volume, and therefore the left ventricular–aortic pressure gradient all decline, whereas the mean left atrial, pulmonary capillary, pulmonary arterial, right ventricular systolic and diastolic, and right atrial pressures rise, often sequentially. AS intensifies the severity of any existing mitral regurgitation by increasing the pressure gradient responsible for driving blood from the left ventricle to the left atrium. In addition, the dilatation of the left ventricle, which occurs late in the course of some patients with aortic valve disease, may produce mitral regurgitation, superimposing the hemodynamic changes associated with this lesion on those produced by AS. Also, as a consequence of pulmonary

hypertension or bulging of the hypertrophied septum into the right ventricular cavity or both, the *a* wave in the right atrial pressure pulse becomes prominent.

Left ventricular end-diastolic volume usually remains normal until quite late in the course of the disease, but left ventricular mass increases in response to the chronic pressure overload, resulting in an increase in the mass/volume ratio. However, the increase in mass may not be as great as that seen with aortic regurgitation (AR) or combined AS and AR.

MYOCARDIAL FUNCTION IN AORTIC STENOSIS

In experimental animals, when the aorta is suddenly constricted, left ventricular pressure rises, and there is a large increase in wall stress, whereas both extent and velocity of shortening decline. As pointed out in Chapter 14, the development of ventricular hypertrophy is one of the principal mechanisms by which the heart adapts to such an increased

TABLE 34-10 EFFECT OF AORTIC VALVE DISEASE ON MYOCARDIAL OXYGEN SUPPLY AND DEMAND

$M\dot{V}O_2$

AS	AR	DETERMINANTS OF SUPPLY	DETERMINANTS OF DEMAND	AS	AR
−↑	↓↓↓	Diastolic BP	LV systolic pressure	↑↑↑	↑
↓	↓	Diastolic filling time	LV volume	—	↑↑↑
↓*	↓	Epicardial coronary arteries	Systolic ejection time	↑	↑
↓↓↓	↓	Coronary vascular resistance	Heart rate	—	—
		Humoral	Contractility	—	—
		Autonomic nervous system			
		Catecholamines	LV mass	↑↑↑	↑↑↑
		Compression by LV			
↓↓	↓↓	LV filling pressure (effect on intramural coronary veins)			
—	—	RV filling pressure			

AS, aortic stenosis; AR, aortic regurgitation; BP, blood pressure; LV, left ventricular; $M\dot{V}O_2$, myocardial oxygen consumption. Arrows refer to effect on supply or demand. Number of arrows indicates magnitude of effect. ↑ indicates increased demand; ↓, decreased demand; and —, no effect.

*If coronary disease present.

From Cheitlin, M. D.: The timing of surgery in mitral and aortic valve disease. Curr. Prob. Cardiol. 12:115, 1987.

hemodynamic burden.[388,389] The increased systolic wall stress induced by AS apparently leads to parallel replication of sarcomeres and concentric hypertrophy (Fig. 14–8, p. 400), and the increase in left ventricular wall thickness is often sufficient to counterbalance the increased pressure so that peak systolic wall tension returns to normal or remains so if the obstruction develops slowly[390–392] (Fig. 14–9, p. 401). An inverse correlation between wall stress and ejection fraction exists in patients with AS.[392] This suggests that the depressed ejection fraction and velocity of fiber shortening that occur in *some* patients are a consequence of inadequate wall thickening,[393] resulting in "afterload mismatch."[394] Patients having AS with compensated pressure overload as well as some with depressed left ventricular ejection fractions and overt congestive failure may have normal values for the rate of intraventricular stress (dσ/dt) and pressure (dP/dt) development.[395,396] In others, the lower ejection fraction is secondary to a depression of contractility; in the latter, the effectiveness of surgical treatment is reduced.[397] Thus, both altered contractility and increased afterload are operative in depressing left ventricular performance.[398]

From these considerations it is clear that in order to evaluate myocardial function in patients with AS, it is critical to relate the ejection phase indices to the existing wall tension (p. 422). Wall thickness is a critical determinant of ventricular performance in patients with AS; inadequate hypertrophy, an intrinsic depression of myocardial contractility, or a combination of these two defects may lead to a depression of ventricular performance.

DIASTOLIC STIFFNESS (see p. 402). Although ventricular hypertrophy is a key adaptive mechanism to the pressure load imposed by AS, it results in an adverse pathophysiological consequence, i.e., an increase in diastolic stiffness (Fig. 34–12, p. 1021). As a result, greater intracavitary pressure is required for ventricular filling. Some patients with AS manifest an increase in chamber stiffness due simply to an increase in muscle mass but with no alteration in muscle stiffness; others exhibit increases in muscle stiffness as well as in chamber stiffness, both of which contribute to the elevation of ventricular diastolic filling pressure at any level of ventricular diastolic volume.[384–386,399,400] Chamber stiffness may revert toward normal as hypertrophy regresses following relief of AS,[386] and at least in some patients muscle stiffness may also revert to normal. Whether this occurs in all patients is not clear. It is expected that this regression of stiffness would not occur in patients with extensive myocardial fibrosis. Indeed, in some patients stiffness increases postoperatively as ventricular hypertrophy regresses, while interstitial fibrosis remains unchanged.[385] The rate of ventricular thinning in diastole is slowed in AS (Fig. 15–25, p. 439).

STRUCTURE. A variety of changes in the myocardial ultrastructure have been documented in patients with severe AS. These include unusually large nuclei, loss of myofibrils, accumulation of mitochondria, large cytoplasmic areas devoid of contractile material, and proliferation of fibroblasts and collagen fibers in the interstitial space.[401] The depression of cardiac function that occurs late in the course of the disease may well be related to these morphological alterations. In adults with AS, both myocardial cellular hypertrophy and relative and absolute increases in connective tissue occur.[402–404] An inverse correlation between left ventricular ejection fraction and myocardial fiber diameter has been reported.[404]

ISCHEMIA (Table 34–10). In AS, coronary blood flow at rest is elevated in absolute terms but is normal when corrected for myocardial mass.[402] There may be inadequate myocardial oxygenation in severe AS, even in the absence of coronary artery disease. The hypertrophied left ventricular muscle mass, the increased systolic pressure, and the prolongation of ejection all elevate myocardial oxygen consumption,[405] and the

abnormally heightened pressure compressing the coronary arteries exceeds the coronary perfusion pressure, thereby interfering with coronary blood flow.[406,407] Myocardial perfusion is also impaired by the relative decrease in myocardial capillary density and by the elevation of left ventricular end-diastolic pressure, which lowers the aortic–left ventricular pressure gradient in diastole, i.e., the coronary perfusion pressure gradient. Therefore, the subendocardium in severe AS is susceptible to ischemia, and this underperfusion may be responsible for the development of myocardial ischemia.[406] Marcus et al. have demonstrated a reduction in the velocity of coronary blood flow during reactive hyperemia at the time of operation in patients with severe AS,[408] and this may be responsible for the angina commonly observed in these patients. Metabolic evidence of myocardial ischemia, i.e., lactate production, can be demonstrated when myocardial oxygen needs are stimulated by exercise or isoproterenol in patients with AS, in both the presence and the absence of coronary arterial narrowing.

CLINICAL MANIFESTATIONS

HISTORY

In the natural history of adults with AS, a long latent period exists during which there is gradually increasing obstruction and an increase in the pressure load on the myocardium while the patient remains asymptomatic. The cardinal manifestations of AS, which commence most commonly in the sixth decade of life, are angina pectoris, syncope, and heart failure.[409] In patients in whom the obstruction remains unrelieved, once these symptoms become manifested, the prognosis is poor; survival curves show that the interval from the onset of symptoms to the time of death is approximately 2 years in patients with heart failure, 3 years in those with syncope, and 5 years in those with angina.[410,411] *Dyspnea* is the most common initial complaint.[412] *Angina* occurs in approximately two-thirds of patients with critical AS (about half of whom have significant coronary artery obstruction)[413] and usually resembles that observed in patients with coronary artery disease, in that it is commonly precipitated by exertion and relieved by rest. It results from the combination of increased oxygen needs by the hypertrophied myocardium and reduction of oxygen delivery secondary to the excessive compression of coronary vessels[402,408,414] (see Ischemia, above). Rarely, it results from calcium emboli to the coronary vascular bed.[415] Angina may, of course, also result from coexisting coronary artery disease, but the absence of angina in a patient with severe AS does not exclude serious obstructive coronary artery disease.[416,417]

Syncope is often orthostatic and is most commonly due to the reduced cerebral perfusion that occurs during exertion when arterial pressure declines consequent to systemic vasodilatation in the presence of a fixed cardiac output. This may be related to an inappropriate left ventricular baroreceptor response.[418] It may also be caused by arrhythmias[419]; premonitory symptoms are common. Exertional hypotension may also be manifested as "graying out" spells or giddiness on effort.[420] Syncope at rest may be due to transient ventricular fibrillation, from which the patient recovers spontaneously; transient atrial fibrillation with loss of the "atrial kick" and a precipitous decline in cardiac output; or transient atrioventricular block due to extension of the calcification of the valve into the conduction system. Syncope has also been attributed to malfunction of the baroreceptor mechanism.[373] Exertional dyspnea with orthopnea, paroxysmal nocturnal dyspnea, and pulmonary edema reflect varying degrees of pulmonary venous hypertension. These are late symptoms in AS, and their presence for more than 5 years should suggest the possibility of associated mitral valvular disease. *Gastrointestinal bleeding*, idiopathic or due to angiodysplasia (most commonly of the right colon) or other vascular malformations, occurs more often than expected in patients with calcific AS; it may cease after aortic valve replacement.[421,422] Infective endocarditis is a greater risk in younger patients with milder valvular deformity than in older patients with rocklike calcific aortic deformities. Cerebral emboli resulting in stroke or transient ischemic attacks may result from microthrombi on thickened bicuspid valves.[423] Calcific AS may cause embolization of calcium to a variety of organs, including the heart, kidney, and brain. Abrupt loss of vision has been reported when calcific emboli occluded the central retinal artery.[424]

Since cardiac output is usually well maintained for many years in patients with severe AS, marked fatigability, debilitation, peripheral cyanosis, and other manifestations of a low cardiac output are usually not prominent until quite late in the natural history of the disease. Atrial fibrillation, pulmonary hypertension, and systemic venous hypertension in patients with isolated AS are often preterminal findings. Although AS may be responsible for sudden death (p. 763), this usually occurs in patients who had previously been symptomatic.

PHYSICAL EXAMINATION

The arterial pulse characteristically rises slowly and is small and sustained (pulsus parvus et tardus) (Fig. 2–12, p. 23).[425,426] In the advanced stage, systolic and pulse pressures are both reduced. However, in patients with mild stenosis with associated regurgitation and in older patients with an inelastic arterial bed, both systolic and pulse pressures may be normal or even increased. A systolic pressure exceeding 200 mm Hg is rare in patients with critical AS.[425] The anacrotic notch and coarse systolic vibrations are felt most readily in the carotid arterial pulse, producing the so-called carotid shudder. Simultaneous palpation of the apex and carotid arteries reveals a distinct lag in the latter in patients with severe AS.[427] Although pulsus alternans occurs commonly in AS with left ventricular dysfunction,[428] obstruction of the aortic valve may prevent its being recognized by examination of the peripheral arterial pulse. The jugular venous pulse usually shows prominent *a* waves, reflecting reduced right ventricular compliance consequent to hypertrophy of the ventricular septum.[429] With pulmonary hypertension and secondary right ventricular failure and tricuspid regurgitation, *v* or *c-v* waves may be prominent.

The cardiac impulse is sustained with left ventricular failure; it becomes displaced inferiorly and laterally (Table 2–1, p. 26). Presystolic distention of the left ventricle, i.e., a prominent precordial *a* wave, is often both visible and palpable. A hyperdynamic left ventricle suggests concomitant aortic or MR. A systolic thrill is usually best appreciated when the patient leans forward in full expiration. It is felt most readily in the second left intercostal space on either side of the sternum or in the suprasternal notch and is frequently transmitted along the carotid arteries.

Rarely, right ventricular failure with systemic venous congestion, hepatomegaly, and edema precedes left ventricular failure. Probably this is caused by the so-called Bernheim effect, which results from the hypertrophied ventricular septum's bulging into and encroaching on the right ventricular cavity and leads to impairment of right ventricular filling. In such cases, the jugular venous pressure is elevated and the *a* wave is prominent.

AUSCULTATION (Tables 34–4, p. 1020, and 34–11). S_1 is normal or soft and S_4 is prominent, presumably because atrial contraction is vigorous and the mitral valve is partially closed

TABLE 34-11 DIFFERENTIAL DIAGNOSIS OF AORTIC STENOSIS: PHYSICAL FINDINGS

TYPE OF STENOSIS	MAXIMUM MURMUR AND THRILL	AORTIC EJECTION SOUND	AORTIC COMPONENT OF SECOND SOUND	REGURGITANT DIASTOLIC MURMUR	ARTERIAL PULSE
Acquired nonrheumatic or rheumatic	Second right sternal border to neck; may be at apex in the aged	Uncommon	Decreased or absent	Common	Delayed upstroke; anacrotic notch; ± small amplitude
Hypertrophic subaortic	Fourth left sternal border to apex (± regurgitant systolic murmur at apex)	Rare	Normal or decreased	Very rare	Brisk upstroke, sometimes bisferiens
Congenital valvular	Second right sternal border to neck (along left sternal border in some infants)	Very common in children, disappearing with decrease in valve mobility with age	Normal or increased in childhood; decreased with decrease in valve mobility with age	Uncommon in child; not uncommon in adult	Delayed upstroke; anacrotic notch; ± small amplitude
Congenital subvalvular	Discrete: like valvular; tunnel: left sternal border	Rare	Not helpful (normal, increased, decreased or absent)	Almost all	
Congenital supravalvular	First right sternal border to neck and sometimes to medial aspect of right arm; occasionally greater in neck than in chest	Rare	Normal or decreased	Uncommon	Rapid upstroke in right carotid, delayed in left carotid; right arm pulse pressure greater than left

From Levinson, G. E.: Aortic stenosis. In Dalen, J. E., and Alpert, J. S.: Valvular Heart Disease. 2nd ed. Boston, Little, Brown and Company, 1987, p. 202.

during presystole.[430,431] S_2 may be single because calcification and immobility of the aortic valve make A_2 inaudible, because P_2 is buried in the prolonged aortic ejection murmur, or because prolongation of left ventricular systole makes A_2 coincide with P_2. Paradoxical splitting of S_2, which suggests associated left ventricular dysfunction, may also occur (Fig. 2–21, p. 31). With left ventricular failure and secondary pulmonary hypertension, P_2 may become accentuated. When the valve is rigid, A_2 may be inaudible, but when the valve is flexible, A_2 may be snapping and accentuated.

An aortic ejection sound (p. 44) occurs simultaneously with the halting upward movement of the aortic valve (Fig. 3–3, p. 45). It is dependent on mobility of the valve cusps and disappears when they become severely calcified. Thus, it is common in children with congenital AS but is rare in elderly adults with acquired calcific AS and rigid valves. This sound occurs approximately 0.06 sec after the onset of S_1, has a frequency similar to that of S_1, and is heard most readily with the diaphragm of the stethoscope along the left sternal border, although it is often well transmitted to the apex, where it may be confused with S_1 (and the S_1 may be mistaken for an S_4). In contrast to a pulmonic ejection sound, aortic ejection sounds usually do not vary with respiration.

The *systolic murmur* of AS is heard best at the base of the heart but is often well transmitted along the carotid vessels and to the apex (Fig. 3–16, p. 51). Cessation of the murmur before A_2 is usually helpful in differentiating it from a pansystolic mitral murmur, but it may be falsely considered to be a pansystolic murmur because it may end with S_2, which represents pulmonic valve closure, A_2 being soft or even inaudible. In patients with calcified aortic valves, the murmur is harsh and rasping at the base, but high-frequency components selectively radiate to the apex (the so-called Gallavardin phenomenon [Fig. 3–17, p. 51]), where it may actually be more prominent and where it may be mistaken for the murmur of MR. Frequently, there is a "quiet area" between the base and apex where the murmur is diminished in intensity, supporting the erroneous impression that the apical and basal murmurs have different origins. In general, the more severe the stenosis, the longer the duration of the murmur[432] and the more likely that it peaks in mid-systole.[433]

In patients with degenerative or atherosclerotic AS, there may be heavy valvular calcification, but obstruction may not be severe because the commissural fusion characteristic of congenital and rheumatic AS is absent. The nonfused calcified cusps vibrate freely, resulting in a softer, more musical murmur, more prominent at the apex than the murmur of congenital or rheumatic AS.[432] High-pitched decrescendo diastolic murmurs secondary to aortic regurgitation are common in many patients with dominant AS.

In hypertrophic cardiomyopathy (HCM), the murmur is delayed in onset and may continue up to A_2; the carotid artery characteristically rises sharply and is bisferiens. Palpation of the carotid pulse is also extremely helpful in differentiating between valvular AS on the one hand and HCM and MR on the other, because the arterial pulse generally rises slowly in AS but sharply in the other two conditions. However, confusion can arise in the young patient with congenital AS, in whom sudden upward displacement ("doming") of the pliant aortic leaflet or leaflets with ventricular systole may result in a brisk initial upstroke in the carotid pulse, coincident with the systolic ejection click.

When the left ventricle fails in AS and the cardiac output falls, the murmur becomes softer or disappears altogether, and the slowly rising pulse is more difficult to recognize. Stated simply, the clinical picture changes to that of severe left ventricular failure with a low cardiac output. Thus, occult AS may be a cause of intractable heart failure, and critical AS should be actively sought in patients with severe heart failure of unknown cause, since operative treatment may be life-saving and may result in substantial clinical improvement.[434,435]

Dynamic Auscultation (Table 34–5). The murmur of val-

vular AS is augmented by the inhalation of amyl nitrite and with squatting or lying flat and is reduced in intensity during the Valsalva strain, which increases the murmur of HCM or that produced with vasopressors, moderate isometric exercise, or standing.[436] It varies in intensity from beat to beat when the duration of diastolic filling varies, as in atrial fibrillation or following a premature contraction, and this characteristic is helpful in differentiating AS from MR, in which the murmur is usually unaffected. An aortic diastolic murmur is frequently present in patients with valvular AS.

LABORATORY EXAMINATION

ELECTROCARDIOGRAPHY

The principal electrocardiographic change is left ventricular hypertrophy, which is found in approximately 85 per cent of patients with severe AS. The absence of left ventricular hypertrophy does not exclude the presence of critical AS, and the correlation between the absolute voltages in precordial leads and the severity of obstruction, which is quite good in children with congenital AS, is not as good in adults. However, a good correlation has been reported between the sum of the QRS amplitudes in 12 leads and the height of the left ventricular systolic pressure.[437] T-wave inversion and ST-segment depressions in leads having upright QRS complexes are common. ST-segment depressions greater than 0.3 mV in patients with AS (left ventricular "strain") suggest that severe ventricular hypertrophy is present. The progressive development of ST-segment and T-wave abnormalities suggests that hypertrophy has progressed. Occasionally, a "pseudoinfarction" pattern is present, characterized by a loss of r waves in the right precordial leads and an early vector directed posteriorly in the horizontal plane of the vectorcardiogram, simulating anteroseptal infarction. There is evidence of left atrial enlargement in more than 80 per cent of patients with severe isolated AS[438]; the principal manifestation is prominent late negativity of the P wave in V_1 rather than an increased duration in lead II, suggesting that hypertrophy rather than dilatation is present. Atrial fibrillation is an uncommon and late sign of pure AS, and, when present in a patient who is not greatly disabled, should suggest the possibility of mitral valvular disease or ischemic heart disease.

The extension of calcific infiltrates from the aortic valve into the conduction system may cause various forms and degrees of atrioventricular and intraventricular block in 5 per cent of patients with calcific AS.[439–441] Conduction defects are more common in patients who also have mitral annular calcium.[441] Almost 10 per cent of all instances of left anterior hemiblock are secondary to aortic valvular disease.[442] Ambulatory electrocardiography frequently shows complex ventricular arrhythmias,[443] particularly in patients with myocardial dysfunction.[444]

VECTORCARDIOGRAPHY

In patients with severe AS, the vectorcardiogram usually shows an increase in the maximal spatial voltage and counterclock inscription of the loop in the transverse plane, with the major forces in the left posterior quadrant. In the left sagittal plane, the QRS loop is usually directed posteriorly and superiorly.[445]

GRAPHIC RECORDINGS

The indirect carotid, jugular, and apical pulse tracings and the phonocardiographic findings in AS are discussed in Chapters 2 and 3.

RADIOLOGICAL FINDINGS

Routine radiological examination may be entirely normal despite the presence of critical AS. The heart is usually of normal size or slightly enlarged, with a rounding of the left ventricular border and apex (Fig. 8–8A, p. 208), unless regurgitation or left ventricular failure is present and causes substantial cardiomegaly. Poststenotic dilatation of the ascending aorta is a common finding. Calcification of the aortic valve is found in almost all adults with hemodynamically significant AS[446,447] (Fig. 8–28, p. 220); it may have to be sought on fluoroscopy (or the echocardiogram) rather than on the roentgenogram. This is an important finding. Indeed, the *absence* of calcium in the region of the aortic valve on careful fluoroscopic examination in a patient older than 35 essentially rules out valvular AS. The converse is not true, however, and in patients over the age of 60, severe calcification of the aortic valve may occur with only mild obstruction. The left atrium may be slightly enlarged, and there may be radiological signs of pulmonary venous hypertension. However, when left atrial enlargement is marked, particularly if the atrial appendage is prominent, the presence of associated mitral valvular disease should be suspected.

Angiographic studies of the aortic valve are best performed by injecting contrast medium into the left ventricle and filming in the 30-degree right anterior oblique and 60-degree left anterior oblique projections. These examinations often make it possible to ascertain the number of cusps of the stenotic valve and to demonstrate doming of a thickened valve and a systolic jet. There is some hazard associated with the rapid injection of a large volume of contrast material into a high-pressure left ventricle, and this is ordinarily not indicated in patients with AS, critical obstruction, and/or left ventricular failure.

ECHOCARDIOGRAPHY (see also p. 85). The normal range of opening of the aortic valve is 1.6 to 2.6 cm, and normally the aortic valve leaflets are barely visible in systole. In patients with severe AS, thickened leaflets and a barely discernible aortic orifice in systole can often be recognized on the M-mode echocardiogram. However, a reduced aortic valve opening may also be seen in other conditions, such as heart failure, in which there is decreased blood flow across the aortic valve. In patients with a bicuspid aortic valve, the valve cusps are asymmetrical, resulting in their eccentric position within the aortic root. Dense, multiple echoes within the aortic root in the area of the aortic leaflets suggest valvular calcification and support the diagnosis of AS. Systolic vibrations of the interventricular septum are common in congenital AS.[448] Two-dimensional echocardiography may also be helpful in determining the severity of the stenosis, by imaging the orifice (Fig. 4–53, p. 85). Doppler echocardiography allows calculation of the left ventricular–aortic pressure gradient[449-452] using a modified Bernouilli equation (Fig. 4–54, p. 85). The noninvasively determined gradients correlate well with those determined by left heart catheterization.

MANAGEMENT

MEDICAL TREATMENT

Patients who are asymptomatic should be advised to report promptly to their physician the development of *any* symptoms possibly related to AS. Noninvasive assessment of the severity of obstruction by Doppler echocardiography should be carried out. In patients with mild obstruction, this measurement should be repeated every 2 years in asymptomatic patients because obstruction tends to become more severe over time.[453-456] There is a close correlation between the left ventricular–aortic systolic pressure gradient determined by echocardiography and left heart catheterization. Those with known or suspected critical obstruction should be cautioned to avoid vigorous athletic and physical activity. However, such restrictions do not apply to patients with mild obstruction. Because there is a tendency for the obstruction to become progressively more severe in patients with AS, asymptomatic patients with AS should be followed carefully; on follow-up examinations, it is essential to look for signs of possible progression.[457] Repeated clinical examinations and electrocardiographic and echocardiographic studies at intervals of 6 to 12 months are indicated in asymptomatic patients with severe AS. The necessity for endocarditis prophylaxis should be explained (p. 1097).

There is no need to use digitalis glycosides unless evidence exists of an increase in ventricular volume or a reduced ejection fraction. Although diuretics are beneficial when there is abnormal accumulation of fluid, they must be used with caution, because hypovolemia may reduce the elevated left ventricular end-diastolic pressure, lower cardiac output, and produce orthostatic hypotension. Beta-adrenoceptor blockers can depress myocardial function and induce left ventricular failure and should be used only with great caution, if at all, in patients with AS.

Atrial arrhythmias occur in fewer than 10 per cent of patients with severe AS, perhaps because of the late occurrence

of left atrial enlargement in this condition. When such an arrhythmia is observed in a patient with AS, the possibility of associated mitral valve disease should be considered. In light of the adverse hemodynamic effects of loss of atrial booster pump function with atrial fibrillation in patients with AS,[387] an effort should be made to prevent the development of this arrhythmia by prophylaxis with an antiarrhythmic agent when premature atrial contractions are frequent. When atrial fibrillation does occur, the rapid ventricular rate may cause angina or electrocardiographic evidence of myocardial ischemia or both; in some cases, loss of the "atrial kick" and a sudden fall in cardiac ouput may cause serious hypotension. Therefore, this arrhythmia should be treated promptly (p. 683), and a search for previously unrecognized mitral valve disease should be undertaken.

Adults considered to have severe AS should undergo catheterization if any symptoms develop. The purpose of catheterization in patients with AS is to localize the site and document the severity of the obstruction, to determine the state of left ventricular function, and to ascertain the presence or absence of associated valvular disease and coronary artery disease.

NATURAL HISTORY

In contrast to MS, which leads to symptoms almost immediately after its development, patients with severe AS may be asymptomatic for many years despite the presence of severe obstruction. The systolic pressure gradient can exceed 150 mm Hg, and the peak left ventricular systolic pressure can reach approximately 300 mm Hg with relatively little increase in overall heart size on radiographic examination and with normal left ventricular end-diastolic and end-systolic volumes. Patients with severe chronic AS tend to be free of cardiovascular symptoms until relatively late in the course of the disease. In Rapaport's series, 40 per cent of patients treated medically survived for 5 years and 20 per cent for 10 years after diagnosis.[102] In another series of patients with hemodynamically significant valvular AS treated medically, the 5-year survival rate was 64 per cent. However, once patients with AS become symptomatic with angina or syncope, the average survival is 2 to 3 years, whereas with congestive heart failure it is 1½ years[413] (Fig. 34–27). Sudden death, like syncope, in patients with severe AS may be due to cerebral hypoperfusion followed by arrhythmia. Among symptomatic patients with moderate or severe AS not subjected to operation, mortality rates from onset of symptoms were approximately 25 per cent at 1 year and 50 per cent at 2 years; more than half

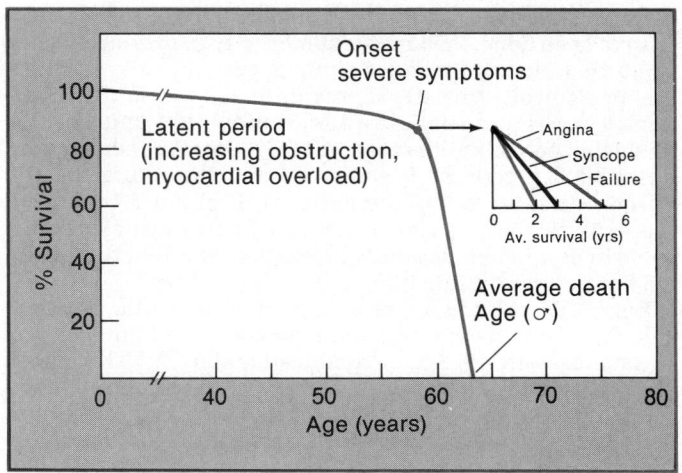

FIGURE 34–27. Natural history of aortic stenosis without operative treatment. (From Ross, J., Jr., and Braunwald, E.: Aortic stenosis. Circulation *38*[Suppl. V]:61, 1968, by permission of the American Heart Association, Inc.)

of the deaths were sudden. Asymptomatic patients have an excellent prognosis insofar as survival is concerned[458]; only about 4 per cent of the deaths in AS occur suddenly in asymptomatic patients. While severe AS is a potentially lethal disease, death, even when sudden, usually occurs in symptomatic patients. A number of authors have followed asymptomatic patients with critical AS,[459–462] and sudden death is extremely rare. Pellika et al. followed 113 asymptomatic patients; symptoms developed in 38 per cent within 2 years. No sudden deaths occurred during 118 patient-years of follow-up.[462] The obstruction tends to progress more rapidly in patients with degenerative calcific disease than in those with congenital or rheumatic disease.[463]

SURGICAL TREATMENT

INDICATIONS FOR OPERATION. The most critical decision in the management of patients with AS—indeed, of all patients with valvular heart disease—concerns the advisability and timing of surgical treatment.[464] The indications for surgery as well as the techniques and results of operation depend on the patient's age and the nature of the valvular deformity. In children and adolescents with noncalcific congenital AS, who most commonly have bicuspid aortic valves, simple commissural incision under direct vision usually leads to substantial hemodynamic improvement at a low risk, i.e., a mortality rate of less than 1 per cent (p. 925).[465] Therefore, this procedure (or aortic balloon valvuloplasty) is indicated not only in symptomatic patients but also in asymptomatic children and adolescents with critical aortic stenosis, i.e., a calculated effective orifice less than 0.75 cm²/m² BSA. Despite the salutary hemodynamic results following this procedure, the valve is not rendered entirely normal anatomically, and the turbulent blood flow through it may lead to further deformation, calcification, the development of regurgitation, and restenosis after 10 to 20 years, probably requiring reoperation and valve replacement later.

In most adults with calcific AS, satisfactory valvular function cannot be restored, even by deliberate sculpturing procedures carried out under direct vision, and valve replacement is the surgical treatment of choice.[466] Ultrasonic decalcification and other repairs may be effective immediately in a fraction of patients but even in them restenosis is a serious problem.[467–470] The aortic valve should, in general, be replaced in patients who have hemodynamic evidence of severe obstruction (aortic valve orifice < 0.75 cm² or < 0.4 cm²/m² BSA) as well as symptoms believed to result from AS. (Prosthetic valves are discussed on pp. 1061 to 1064.) Surgical treatment should also be carried out in asymptomatic patients with serious left ventricular dysfunction and progressive cardiomegaly. Although a prospective randomized controlled study has not been done, the long-term mortality in patients undergoing operation in the latter group appears to be lower than that in medically treated patients without operation.[471] As artificial valves and surgical skills continue to improve, it is likely that patients with severe AS will become candidates for operation at progressively earlier stages in the natural history of their disease. At the present time, I do not recommend prophylactic replacement of a critically narrow calcific aortic valve in *asymptomatic* adults unless they exhibit progressive left ventricular dysfunction.

RESULTS. Successful replacement of the aortic valve results in substantial clinical and hemodynamic improvement in patients with AS, AR, or combined lesions[466–475] including many patients in their 70's and 80's.[468,469] In patients without frank left ventricular failure, the operative risk ranges from 2 to 8 per cent in most centers. Risk factors for higher mortality include high New York Heart Association (NYHA) class, impairment of left ventricular function, age, and the presence of associated aortic regurgitation.[466] The 5-year actuarial survival rate of hospital survivors is approximately 85 per cent. Risk factors for late death include preoperative NYHA class, left ventricular function, preoperative ventricular arrhyth-

mias, associated significant aortic regurgitation, older age, and concomitant untreated coronary artery disease.[466] Symptoms secondary to elevations of left atrial pressure and myocardial ischemia are relieved in almost every patient. Hemodynamic results are equally impressive; elevated end-diastolic and end-systolic volumes show significant reductions. Ventricular performance often returns to normal more frequently in patients with AS than in those with AR.[476] However, the finding that the strongest predictor of postoperative left ventricular dysfunction is preoperative dysfunction[471,477] suggests that patients should, if possible, be operated on before left ventricular function becomes seriously impaired. The increased left ventricular mass is reduced toward (but not to) normal within 18 months after aortic valve replacement in patients with AS.[399,478] When restudied 5 years postoperatively, left ventricular mass had returned to normal.[479] Myocyte hypertrophy regresses before fibrous tissue is resorbed.

When operation is carried out in patients with frank left ventricular failure or a depressed ejection fraction, the operative risk is higher, and the mortality ranges from 10 to 25 per cent, depending on the skill of the surgical team and the severity of depression of left ventricular function.[480] A depressed relation between ejection fraction and wall stress is a poor prognostic index, as is a depressed level of dP/dt max at any given left ventricular end-diastolic pressure.[472] Obviously, it is desirable to perform surgery before the development of heart failure, but emergency operation is sometimes lifesaving even in the most desperate situations, such as cardiac arrest or pulmonary edema from AS. Certainly, in view of the extremely poor prognosis of such patients when they are treated medically, there is usually little choice but to advise immediate mechanical relief of obstruction, i.e., balloon angioplasty (see later discussion) or emergency surgery.[481] Many symptomatic patients with calcific AS are elderly, and particular attention must be directed to the adequacy of their hepatic, renal, and pulmonary function. However, the results of aortic valve replacement are satisfactory in patients older than 70[468] or even 80.[469] If the patient's general condition permits, age, per se, while adding to the risk, should not be considered a contraindication to operation.[482]

In patients with AS and obstructive coronary artery disease (a relatively common combination), aortic valve replacement and myocardial revascularization should be performed together.[417] Although the risk of aortic valve surgery is in-

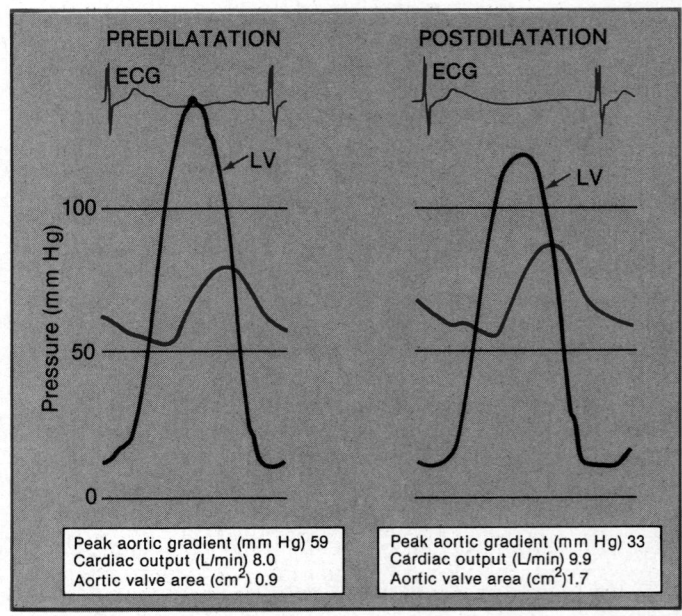

FIGURE 34–28. Simultaneous left ventricular (LV) and arterial pressure tracings recorded before and after balloon valvuloplasty in a patient with severe aortic stenosis. (Courtesy of Raymond G. McKay, M.D.)

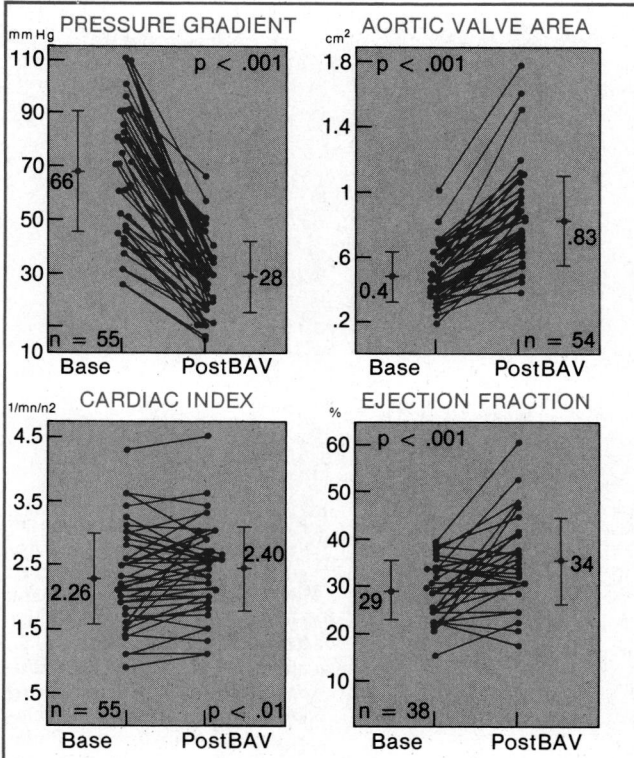

FIGURE 34-29. Plots of changes in pressure gradient, valve area, cardiac index, and ejection fraction at baseline (Base) after balloon aortic valvuloplasty (BAV). (From Berland, J., et al.: Percutaneous balloon valvuloplasty in patients with severe aortic stenosis and low ejection fraction. Circulation 79:1189, 1989, by permission of the American Heart Association, Inc.)

This technique (Fig. 41–20, p. 1377) represents an increasingly attractive alternative to aortic valvotomy in children and adolescents with congenital AS (p. 1035), but its value is limited in adults with calcific AS. A series of balloon dilatation catheters are advanced along a guidewire positioned at the left ventricular apex. In balloon dilatation of calcified stenotic aortic valves carried out on postmortem specimens and in the operating room, fracture of calcified nodules and/or separation of fused commissures were found to be responsible for the relief of obstruction[483]; stretching of the aortic valve ring is probably also involved.[484] There is considerable variation in patient response. However, this technique results initially in relief of obstruction in most patients[485,486,486a] (Fig. 34–28). On the average, valve area initially increases by about 60 per cent, from 0.50 to 0.80 cm,[2] and the mean gradient declines from approximately 60 to 30 mm Hg. Left ventricular ejection fraction tends to rise in patients with depressed left ventricular function. A major problem is restenosis, which occurs in about half of the patients within 6 months. Symptoms lessen in severity in the majority of patients but recur in approximately 30 per cent by 6 months. In most series, patients have been elderly, with heart failure, and were considered poor operative risks. One-year mortality is approximately 25 per cent. Independent correlates of event-free survival were a prevalvuloplasty left ventricular systolic pressure ≥130 mm Hg, a pulmonary capillary wedge pressure ≤15 mm Hg, an aortic valve area ≥0.8 cm[2], and a reduction in the transvalvular gradient >15 mm Hg.[487,487a]

In critically ill patients, the mortality from the procedure is 3 to 7 per cent, and another 6 per cent develop serious complications such as myocardial perforation, myocardial infarction, and severe aortic regurgitation.[484-490] While the overall intermediate-term (6 to 12 months) results of balloon aortic valvuloplasty have been disappointing, largely because of restenosis, the procedure does have a role in the management of severe calcific AS in patients who are not surgical candidates. This includes patients with cardiogenic shock due to critical AS,[484] patients with critical AS who require an urgent noncardiac operation, as a "bridge" to aortic valve replacement in patients with severe heart failure who are at extremely high operative risk, and in pregnant women with critical AS.[490a] In the adult, balloon aortic valvuloplasty is *not* a substitute for surgery (as balloon mitral valvuloplasty may be [p. 1017]).

Balloon aortic valvuloplasty appears to be useful in patients with critical AS who refuse surgical treatment or in whom surgical intervention is not advised because of an extremely high expected mortality. The procedure is also effective in young patients with noncalcific congenital AS.

creased by the association of coronary artery disease, the operative mortality in patients undergoing the combined procedure is not necessarily higher than that of isolated aortic valve replacement in this group.[466] Indeed, the surgical risk rises if severe coronary artery disease is left untreated. The ability to avoid serious myocardial ischemia in the perioperative period is a major factor that has served to reduce operative mortality. After the patient has been placed on cardiopulmonary bypass, the heart is protected by means of hypothermic cardiac arrest alone or combined with cardioplegia. The calcified valve must be removed with great care to avoid embolization of calcified fragments into the systemic circulation.

Aortic Regurgitation

ETIOLOGY AND PATHOLOGY

Aortic regurgitation (AR) may be caused by primary disease of either the aortic valve leaflets or the wall of the aortic root or both (Table 34–12 and Fig. 34–30). Among patients with pure AR coming to valve replacement, the percentage with aortic root disease has been increasing steadily during the past few decades and now accounts for more than one-third of the patients.[491]

VALVULAR DISEASE

Rheumatic fever is a common cause of primary disease of the valve leading to regurgitation.[11,491,492] The cusps become infiltrated with fibrous tissues and retract, a process that prevents cusp apposition during diastole and that usually leads to

regurgitation into the left ventricle through a defect in the center of the valve. Often the associated fusion of the commissures may also restrict the opening of the valve, resulting in combined AS and AR (Fig. 34–31B); some associated mitral valve involvement is common. Other primary valvular causes of AR include *infective endocarditis* (Chap. 35), in which the infection may destroy the valve or cause perforation of a leaflet, or the vegetations may interfere with proper coaptation of the cusps. *Trauma* (Fig. 46–8, p. 1524) resulting in a tear of the ascending aorta and loss of commissural support can cause prolapse of an aortic cusp. Although the most common complication of a congenitally *bicuspid valve* is stenosis in adult life, incomplete closure and/or prolapse of the larger of the two cusps of a *bicuspid valve* may cause regurgitation in childhood.[493] More commonly, progressive regurgitation of a

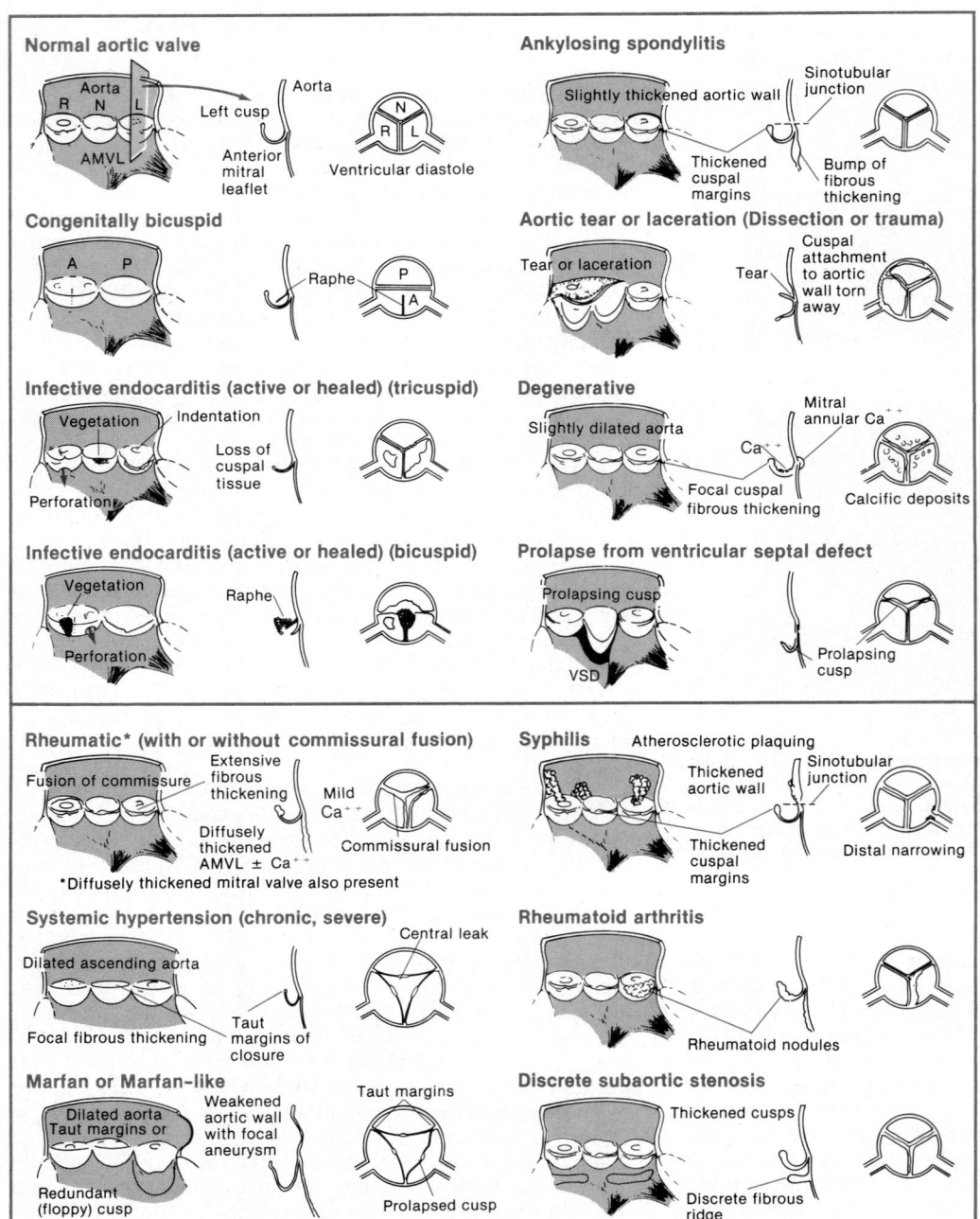

FIGURE 34–30. Diagram of various causes of pure aortic regurgitation. (From Waller, B. F.: Rheumatic and nonrheumatic conditions producing valvular heart disease. *In* Frankl, W. S., and Brest, A. N. [eds.]: Cardiovascular Clinics. Valvular Heart Disease: Comprehensive Evaluation and Management. Philadelphia, F. A. Davis, 1986, pp. 30–31.)

congenitally bicuspid valve develops in the third and fourth decades.[494,495] Progressive regurgitation may also occur in patients with Marfan syndrome, Ehlers-Danlos syndrome, cystic medionecrosis of the aorta, myxomatous proliferation of the aortic valve,[496] and related diseases of connective tissue. Less common causes of AR include a variety of forms of congenital AR; rupture of a congenitally fenestrated valve,[497] particularly in the presence of hypertension[498]; AR in association with systemic lupus erythematosus[499]; rheumatoid arthritis[500]; ankylosing spondylitis[501]; Jaccoud's arthropathy[502]; Whipple's disease[503]; and Crohn's disease in the absence of ankylosing spondylitis.[504] Isolated congenital AR is an uncommon lesion on necropsy studies, but when present, it is usually associated with a bicuspid valve.[505]

AORTIC ROOT DISEASE
(See also Chap. 47)

A variety of diseases produce aortic regurgitation by causing marked dilatation of the ascending aorta (Fig. 34–31C). These conditions include annuloaortic ectasia, cystic medionecrosis of the aorta (either isolated or associated with classic Marfan syndrome), osteogenesis imperfecta, syphilitic aor-

titis, ankylosing spondylitis, Behçet syndrome,[506] psoriatic arthritis, arthritis associated with ulcerative colitis, relapsing polychondritis, Reiter syndrome, giant cell arteritis, osteogenesis imperfecta, and systemic hypertension.[498,507–512]

Table 34–13 presents a comparison of the findings in four important conditions in which dilation of the aorta causes AR. In each of these, the aortic annulus may become greatly dilated, the aortic leaflets separate, and AR may ensue. Dissection of the diseased aortic wall may occur and may aggravate the AR. Dilatation of the aortic root may also have secondary effects on the aortic valve, since it results in tension and bowing of the individual cusps, which may thicken, retract, and become too short to close the aortic orifice. This leads to intensification of the AR, which increases left ventricular stroke volume, further dilating the ascending aorta and thus leading to a vicious circle in which "regurgitation begets regurgitation."

AR, regardless of its etiology, produces dilatation and hypertrophy of the left ventricle, dilatation of the mitral valve ring, and sometimes hypertrophy and dilatation of the left atrium. Endocardial pockets frequently develop in the left ventricular cavity at sites of impact of the regurgitant jet.

TABLE 34-12 MECHANISMS OF AORTIC REGURGITATION

1045

CHAP
34

1. Cusp abnormality	Perforation Reduction in area of cusps	Bacterial endocarditis Rheumatic disease Rheumatoid disease
2. Aortic root distortion (aortitis)		Ankylosing spondylitis Nonspecific urethritis Nonspecific aortitis Rheumatoid disease Syphilis Fallot-type VSD
3. Loss of commissural support		Dissection tears of aorta
4. Aortic root dilatation	Aortitis (inflammatory) "Aortopathy" (noninflammatory)	Syphilis All other aortitis Marfan syndrome Familial Idiopathic Ehlers-Danlos Pseudoxanthoma elasticum

From Davies, M. J.: Pathology of Cardiac Valves. London, Butterworths, 1980.

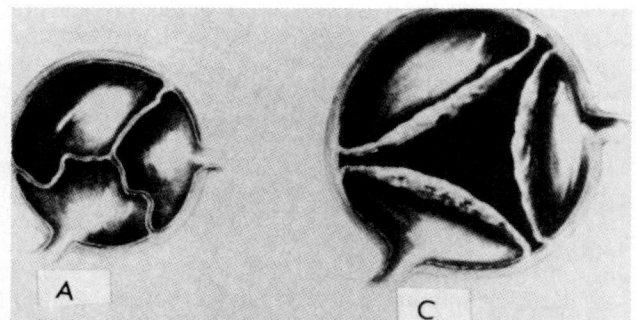

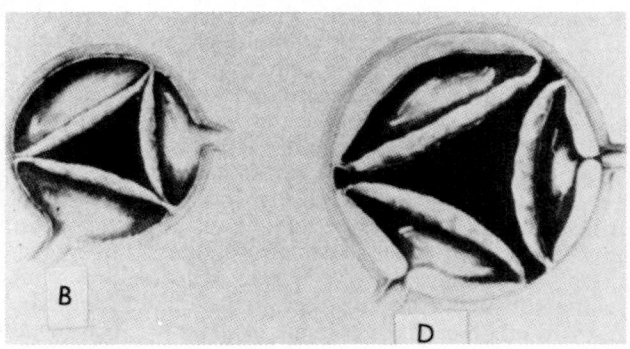

FIGURE 34–31. Variations in the aortic valve. *A,* The normal valve. *B,* Shortening of the cusps characteristic of rheumatic aortic regurgitation. The caliber of the aorta is normal. *C,* Dilatation of the aorta, as occurs in syphilitic aortitis and other conditions in which dilatation is responsible for aortic regurgitation. The main feature results from bowing of the leaflets. Commissural separation is illustrated and may also be present. *D,* In addition to the features shown in *C,* there is atherosclerosis of the aorta, as occurs in syphilitic aortitis, with consequent coronary ostial narrowing. (From Roberts, W. C.: Valvular, subvalvular and supravalvular aortic stenosis: Morphologic features. *In* Edwards, J. E. [ed.]: Clinical-Pathologic Correlations #2. Philadelphia, F. A. Davis, 1973, p. 133.)

PATHOPHYSIOLOGY

In contrast to MR, in which a fraction of the left ventricular stroke volume is ejected into the low-pressure left atrium, in AR the entire left ventricular stroke volume is ejected into a high-pressure chamber, i.e., the aorta (although the low aortic diastolic pressure does facilitate ventricular emptying during early systole). Whereas in MR the reduction of wall tension (i.e., reduced afterload) allows more complete systolic emptying, in AR the increase in left ventricular end-diastolic volume provides major hemodynamic compensation.[513-517]

Severe AR may occur with a normal effective forward stroke volume and a normal ejection fraction (total [forward plus regurgitant] stroke volume/end-diastolic volume), together with an elevated preload, i.e., left ventricular end-diastolic volume pressure and stress[518a] (Figs. 34–32 and 34–33). In accord with Laplace's law, left ventricular dilatation also increases the left ventricular systolic tension required to develop any level of systolic pressure. The increased end-diastolic wall stress leads to volume overload (eccentric) hypertrophy, with replication of sarcomeres in series, elongation of fibers, and sufficient wall thickening to maintain or return end-diastolic wall stress to normal levels the ratio of ventricular wall thickness to cavity radius (h/R) remains normal.[519]

TABLE 34-13 CARDIOVASCULAR MANIFESTATIONS OF CONDITIONS CAUSING AORTIC REGURGITATION

	SYPHILIS	AKYLOSING SPONDYLITIS	RHEUMATOID ARTHRITIS	MARFAN SYNDROME
Average age	50	45	70	30
Predominant sex	Men	Men	Women	Men
Aortic regurgitation	++++	++++	+	++++
Mitral regurgitation	0	++	+	+++
Conduction disturbances	+	++++	++	+
Serology (STS)	+	0	0	0
Morphology of aorta				
Thickened adventitia	++++	++++	+	+
Degenerated media	+++	+++	0	++++
Intimal proliferation	+++	+++	0	+
Vasa vasorum abnormal	++++	++++	0	0
Calcium	++	+	0	0
Aneurysms	+++	0	0	+++
Rupture	+	0	0	+
Dissection	0	0	0	+
Limited to sinuses	0	+	0	0
Morphology of aortic valve				
Cusp thickening				
Diffuse	0	+	0	0
Focal	+	0	+	+
Cusp calcification	0	0	0	0
Shortening	0	+	0	0
Commissural abnormality	+	+	0	0

From Roberts, W. C., et al.: Nonrheumatic valvular cardiac disease: A clinicopathologic survey of 27 different conditions causing valvular dysfunction. *In* Likoff, W. (ed.): Cardiovascular Clinics. Vol. 5, No. 2, Valvular Heart Disease. Philadelphia, F. A. Davis, 1973, p. 424.

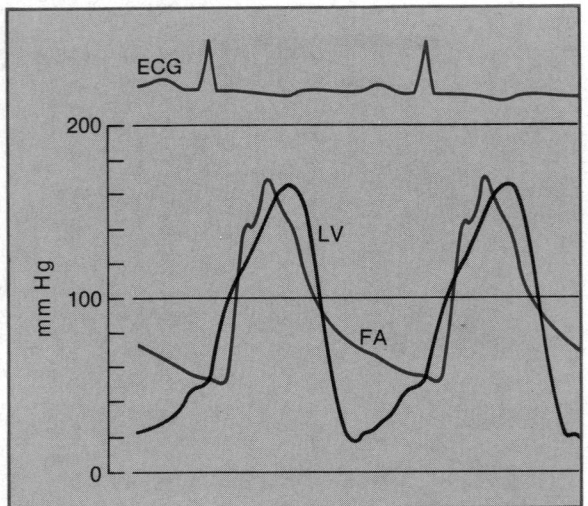

FIGURE 34–32. Pressure curves obtained from a 63-year-old man with symptoms of left ventricular failure and a loud decrescendo diastolic murmur. The femoral arterial (FA) pressure tracing demonstrates a widened pulse pressure of 115 mm Hg and equalization with left ventricular (LV) pressure late in diastole. The LV pressure curve exhibits a steady pressure increase throughout diastole, culminating in a markedly elevated end-diastolic pressure of 45 mm Hg. These findings are indicative of severe aortic regurgitation.

This contrasts with the events in AS, in which there is pressure overload (concentric) hypertrophy with replication of sarcomeres in parallel (p. 399) and an increased h/R (p. 402). In AR, left ventricular mass is usually greatly elevated, often to levels even higher than in isolated AS[381] and sometimes exceeding 1000 gm.

Patients with severe chronic AR have the largest end-diastolic volumes of those with any form of heart disease (resulting in so-called *cor bovinum*). However, end-diastolic pressure is not uniformly elevated (i.e., left ventricular compliance often becomes increased [Fig. 14–5, p. 398 and Fig. 34–12, p. 1021]), and there is a wide scatter in the relationship between end-diastolic volume and end-diastolic pressure.[381] In the more severe cases of AR, the regurgitant flow may exceed 20 liters/min, so that the total left ventricular output approaches 25 liters/min, a level that can be achieved only by a trained endurance runner during maximal exercise. Thus, the adaptive response to chronic and gradually increasing AR permits the ventricle to function as an effective high-compliance pump, handling large end-diastolic and stroke volumes, often with little increase in filling pressure (Fig. 34–33C). During exercise, peripheral vascular resistance declines, and with an increase in heart rate, diastole shortens and the regurgitation per beat decreases,[520–522] facilitating an increment in effective forward cardiac output without substantial increases in end-diastolic volume and pressure. The ejection fraction and related ejection phase indices (p. 426) are often within normal limits, both at rest and during exercise when

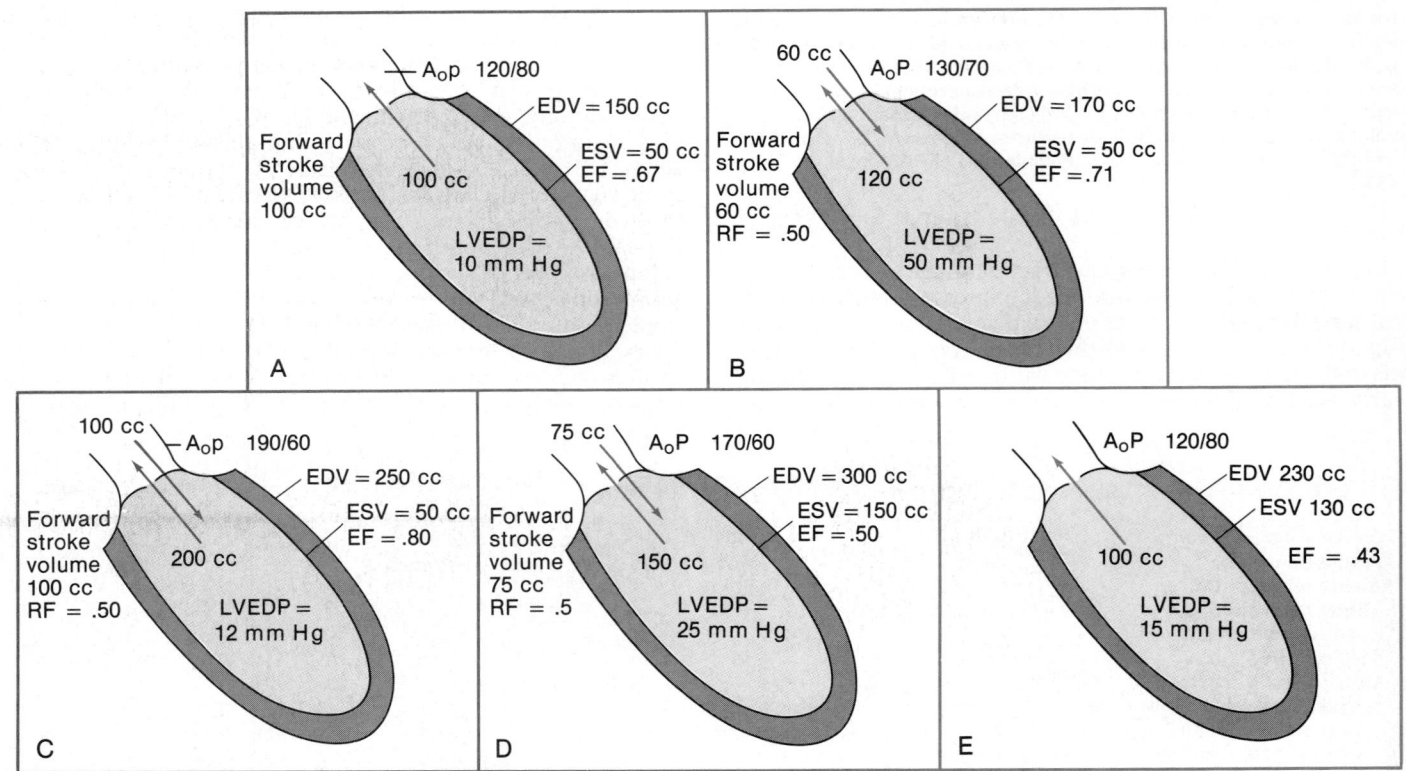

FIGURE 34–33. Hemodynamics of aortic regurgitation. *A,* Normal conditions. *B,* The hemodynamic changes that occur in severe acute aortic regurgitation. Although total stroke volume is increased, forward stroke volume is reduced. Left ventricular end-diastolic pressure rises dramatically. *C,* Hemodynamic changes occurring in chronic compensated aortic regurgitation are shown. Eccentric hypertrophy produces increased end-diastolic volume, which permits an increase in total as well as forward stroke volume. The volume overload is accommodated and left ventricular filling pressure is normalized. Ventricular emptying and end-systolic volume remain normal. *D,* In chronic decompensated aortic regurgitation, impaired left ventricular emptying produces an increase in end-systolic volume and a fall in ejection fraction, total stroke volume, and forward stroke volume. There is further cardiac dilatation and reelevation of left ventricular filling pressure. *E,* Immediately following valve replacement, preload estimated by end-diastolic volume decreases, as does filling pressure. End-systolic volume also is decreased but to a lesser extent. The result is an initial fall in ejection fraction. Despite these changes, elimination of regurgitation leads to an increase in forward stroke volume. AoP = aortic pressure; EDV = end-diastolic volume; ESV = end-systolic volume; EF = ejection fraction; LVEDP = left ventricular end-diastolic pressure; RF = regurgitant fraction. (From Carabello, B. A.: Aortic regurgitation: Hemodynamic determinants of prognosis. *In* Cohn, L. H., and DiSesa, V. J. [eds.]: Aortic Regurgitation: Medical and Surgical Management. New York, Marcel Dekker, Inc., 1986.)

myocardial function, as reflected in the slope of the end-systolic pressure-volume relation, is depressed.[523-525] Therefore, the latter is a more sensitive index of contractility than the former (p. 429).

As left ventricular function deteriorates, the left ventricle dilates (Fig. 34–33D). Ventricular end-diastolic volume increases without further elevation of the aortic regurgitant volume; left ventricular end-diastolic h/R declines,[526] systolic wall tension rises, and afterload mismatch occurs[527] so that ejection fraction declines with any additional stress.[528] Ultimately the ejection fraction and forward stroke volume decline at rest, and ventricular emptying is impaired; i.e., end-systolic volume increases. Many of these changes precede the development of symptoms. In advanced stages there may be considerable elevation of the left atrial, pulmonary artery wedge, pulmonary arterial, right ventricular, and right atrial pressures and lowering of the effective cardiac output, first during the stress of exercise[522] and then even at rest.

As is the case in MR (p. 1022), the end-systolic volume provides a useful overall index of myocardial function in patients with AR and correlates with operative mortality and postoperative left ventricular dysfunction.[191] Both the immediate and the long-term results are excellent in patients with normal left ventricular end-systolic volumes (<30 ml/m^2), poor in patients in whom this index is elevated (>90 ml/m^2), and variable in patients with intermediate values. In general, however, for any given preoperative level of impairment of left ventricular function, the outlook for left ventricular function in the postoperative period is somewhat better in patients with AR than with MR.

When *acute* AR is induced experimentally, preload, wall tension, and myocardial oxygen consumption all rise substantially,[182,514] a situation contrasting with that produced by *acutely* induced MR. In patients with chronic severe AR, total myocardial oxygen requirements are also augmented by the increase in left ventricular mass. Since the major portion of coronary blood flow occurs during diastole, when arterial pressure is lower than normal, coronary perfusion pressure is reduced.[529] The result—a combination of increased oxygen

demand and reduced supply—sets the stage for the development of myocardial ischemia, especially during exercise.[530] Indeed, patients with severe AR exhibit a reduction of coronary reserve,[531] which may be responsible for myocardial ischemia, which in turn may play a role in the deterioration of left ventricular function. The heightened activity of the adrenergic nervous system as a compensatory mechanism in patients with chronic AR is reflected in an abnormal increase in plasma catecholamine content during exercise, accompanied by a reduction in cardiac norepinephrine stores.[532]

Symptomatic patients with severe chronic AR generally exhibit a depression of the relations between end-systolic pressure (or wall stress) and end-systolic volume. This depression of myocardial function, combined with the increased demands placed on the left ventricle, augments left ventricular end-diastolic volume and ultimately pressure, causing symptoms of pulmonary congestion. These patients also demonstrate a failure of the normal decline in end-systolic volume or rise in ejection fraction during exercise, as determined by radionuclide angiography.[533] However, abnormal left ventricular function can be discerned even in subgroups of asymptomatic patients with normal ejection fractions; this dysfunction is reflected in failure of the normal increase in ejection fraction during exercise[534,535] or a depressed end-systolic pressure-volume relation.[535] Radionuclide ventriculography is of value in the identification of those patients with severe chronic AR, who, although asymptomatic or almost so, are at greater risk of developing left ventricular failure and therefore are candidates for consideration of surgical treatment.

ACUTE AORTIC REGURGITATION

In contrast to the pathophysiological events in chronic AR described above, in which the left ventricle has had the opportunity to adapt to the increased load, in *acute* regurgitation (caused most commonly by infective endocarditis, aortic dissection, and trauma) the regurgitant blood fills a ventricle of normal size that cannot accommodate the combined large regurgitant volume and inflow from the left atrium.[536,537] Since

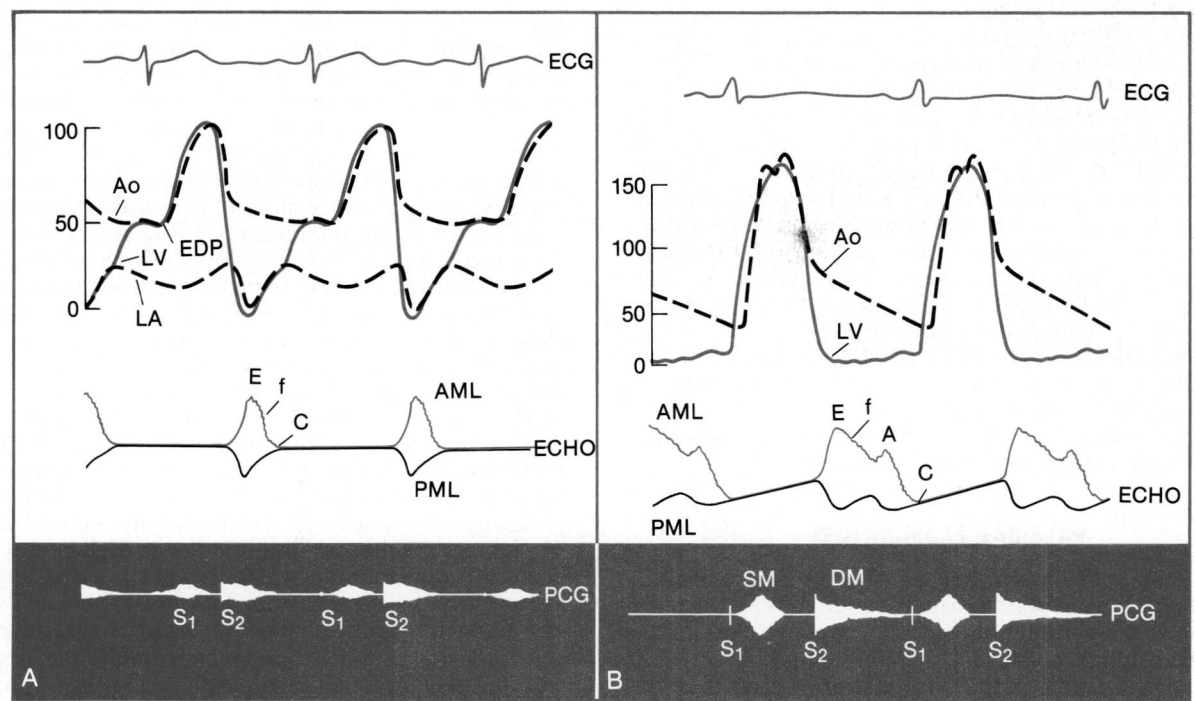

FIGURE 34–34. Schematic representations contrasting the hemodynamic, echocardiographic (ECHO), and phonocardiographic (PCG) manifestations of acute severe (A) and chronic severe (B) aortic regurgitation. Ao = aorta; LV = left ventricle; LA = left atrium; EDP = end-diastolic pressure; f = flutter of anterior mitral valve leaflet; AML = anterior mitral valve leaflet; PML = posterior mitral valve leaflet; SM = systolic murmur; DM = diastolic murmur; C = closure point of mitral valve. (From Morganroth, J., et al.: Acute severe aortic regurgitation. Ann. Intern. Med. 87:225, 1977.)

total stroke volume cannot rise a great deal acutely, *forward* stroke volume declines, left ventricular diastolic pressure rises rapidly to high levels,[513] and the left ventricle operates on a steep portion of its pressure-volume curve (Fig. 34–14).[514]

The hemodynamic findings in acute AR contrast with those in chronic AR.[538] For a similar severe degree of AR, the patient with acute regurgitation has a much smaller aortic pulse pressure and effective forward cardiac output, a smaller left ventricular volume throughout the cardiac cycle, and a higher heart rate than the patient with chronic AR. In addition, as left ventricular pressure rises rapidly above left atrial pressure during early diastole, the mitral valve closes prematurely in diastole (Fig. 34–34).[539] Preclosure of the mitral valve is accompanied by diastolic mitral regurgitation.[539] This protects the pulmonary venous bed from backward transmission of the greatly elevated end-diastolic pressure. Premature closure of the mitral valve, together with the tachycardia that shortens diastole, reduces the time interval during which the mitral valve is open. Left ventricular and aortic systolic pressures exhibit little change. Since aortic diastolic pressure cannot decline below the elevated left ventricular end-diastolic pressure, the systemic arterial pulse pressure widens relatively little.

CLINICAL MANIFESTATIONS

HISTORY

CHRONIC AORTIC REGURGITATION. In patients with chronic, severe AR, the left ventricle gradually undergoes enlargement while the patient remains asymptomatic or almost so.[492,540] Symptoms of reduced cardiac reserve or myocardial ischemia develop, most often in the fourth or fifth decade and usually only after considerable cardiomegaly and myocardial dysfunction have occurred. When symptoms do develop, exertional dyspnea, orthopnea, and paroxysmal nocturnal dyspnea are the principal complaints. Syncope is rare, and although angina pectoris is less frequent than it is in patients with AS, nocturnal angina, often accompanied by diaphoresis, which occurs when the heart rate slows and arterial diastolic pressure falls to extremely low levels, may be particularly troublesome. These episodes are occasionally accompanied by abdominal discomfort, presumably caused by splanchnic ischemia. Patients with severe AR often complain of an uncomfortable awareness of the heartbeat, especially on lying down, and disagreeable thoracic pain due to pounding of the heart against the chest wall. Tachycardia, occurring with emotional stress or exertion, may produce palpitations and head pounding; premature ventricular contractions are particularly distressing because of the great heave of the volume-loaded left ventricle during the postpremature beat. These complaints may be present for many years before symptoms of overt left ventricular dysfunction develop.

ACUTE AORTIC REGURGITATION. In light of the limited ability of the left ventricle to tolerate AR, patients with this valvular lesion often develop sudden clinical manifestations of cardiovascular collapse, with weakness, severe dyspnea, and hypotension; angina is uncommon.[538,541]

PHYSICAL EXAMINATION

In patients with chronic severe AR, the head frequently bobs with each heartbeat (*de Musset's sign*),[542] and the pulses are of the water-hammer or collapsing type with abrupt distention and quick collapse (*Corrigan's pulse*, p. 23). This pulse is readily visible in the carotid arteries and can be best appreciated by palpation of the radial artery with the patient's arm elevated. A *bisferiens pulse* may be present (Fig. 2–13, p. 24) and is more readily recognized in the brachial and femoral than in the carotid arteries. A variety of auscultatory findings provide confirmation of a wide pulse pressure. *Traube's sign* (also known as "pistol shot sounds"[542a]) refers to booming sys-

tolic and diastolic sounds heard over the femoral artery, *Müller's sign* consists of systolic pulsations of the uvula, and *Duroziez's sign* consists of a systolic murmur heard over the femoral artery when it is compressed proximally and a diastolic murmur when it is compressed distally. Capillary pulsations, i.e., *Quincke's sign*, can be detected by pressing a glass slide on the patient's lip or by transmitting a light through the patient's fingertips.

Systolic arterial pressure is elevated, and diastolic pressure is abnormally low. *Hill's sign* refers to popliteal cuff systolic pressure exceeding brachial cuff pressure by more than 60 mm Hg. Korotkoff sounds often persist to zero even though intraarterial pressure rarely falls below 30 mm Hg. The point of change in intensity of the Korotkoff sounds, i.e., the muffling of these sounds in phase IV, correlates with the diastolic pressure. As heart failure develops, peripheral vasoconstriction may occur and arterial diastolic pressure may rise. However, this finding should not be interpreted as a reduction in the severity of the AR.

The apical impulse is diffuse and hyperdynamic and is displaced laterally and inferiorly; there may be systolic retraction over the parasternal region. A rapid ventricular filling wave is often palpable at the apex, as is a systolic thrill at the base of the heart or suprasternal notch and over the carotid arteries, resulting from the augmented stroke volume. In many patients, a carotid shudder is palpable or may be recorded.[543]

AUSCULTATION. In *chronic* severe AR, a soft S_1 and prolongation of the P-R interval frequently are present. A_2 is soft or absent, and P_2 may be obscured by the early diastolic murmur.[544,544a] Thus, S_2 is variable; it may be absent or single or exhibit narrow or paradoxical splitting. A systolic ejection sound, presumably related to abrupt distention of the aorta by the augmented stroke volume, is frequently audible. An S_3 gallop correlates with an increased left ventricular end-systolic volume and has been suggested as a sign useful in considering patients with severe regurgitation for surgical treatment.[545]

The aortic regurgitant murmur is one of high frequency that begins immediately after A_2 (Figs. 2–24E, p. 35 and 3–31, p. 58). It may be distinguished from the murmur of pulmonic regurgitation (p. 1059) by its earlier onset, i.e., immediately after A_2 rather than after P_2, and often by the presence of a widened pulse pressure. The murmur is heard best through the diaphragm of the stethoscope while the patient is sitting up and leaning forward, with the breath held in deep expiration. In severe AR, the murmur reaches an early peak and then has a dominant decrescendo pattern throughout diastole.

The severity of the regurgitation correlates better with the *duration* than with the *intensity* of the murmur. In mild AR, the murmur may be limited to the early phase of diastole and is typically high-pitched; in moderately severe and severe regurgitation, the murmur is holodiastolic and may have a rough quality. When the murmur is musical ("cooing dove" murmur), it usually signifies eversion or perforation of an aortic cusp. In severe AR and left ventricular decompensation, equilibration of aortic and left ventricular pressures in late diastole (Fig. 34–32) abolishes this component of the regurgitant murmur. The diastolic murmur is best heard along the left sternal border in the third and fourth intercostal spaces when regurgitation is due to primary valvular disease, but it is often more readily audible along the right sternal border when it is due mainly to dilatation of the ascending aorta.[546] Murmurs in the latter position may be overlooked if auscultation along the right sternal border is not carried out routinely.

A mid- and late-diastolic apical rumble, the *Austin Flint murmur*, is common in severe AR and may occur in the presence of a normal mitral valve (Figs. 3–31 and 3–32, p. 58). This murmur appears to be created by rapid antegrade flow across a mitral orifice[520] that may be being narrowed by the rapidly rising left ventricular diastolic pressure caused by severe aortic reflux.[547] The Austin Flint murmur may be difficult to differentiate from that due to MS, but the presence of an opening snap and a loud S_1 in MS and the absence of these findings in AR are helpful clues (Table 34–14). As the left ventricular end-diastolic pressure rises, the Austin Flint murmur commences and terminates earlier, and in acute AR with premature diastolic closure of the mitral valve, the presystolic portion of the Austin Flint murmur is eliminated. A short, midsystolic murmur, grades 1 to 4/6, related to the increased ejection rate and stroke volume, may be audible at the base of the heart and transmitted to the carotid vessels. It may be higher pitched and less rasping than the murmur of aortic stenosis but is often accompanied by a systolic thrill.

Dynamic Auscultation. The diastolic murmur of AR may be accentuated when the patient sits up and leans forward or by any intervention that raises the arterial pressure, such as infusion of a vasopressor drug, squatting, or isometric exercise. It is reduced by interventions that lower the systolic pressure, such as amyl nitrite inhalation and the strain of the Valsalva maneuver.[548] The Austin Flint murmur, like that of AR, is augmented by isometric exercise and vasopressors and is reduced by amyl nitrite inhalation (Fig. 3–32, p. 58).[548]

ACUTE AORTIC REGURGITATION. These patients often appear gravely ill, with tachycardia, severe peripheral vasoconstriction and cyanosis, and sometimes pulmonary congestion and edema (Table 34–15).[536,538,541] The peripheral signs of AR are often not impressive and certainly not as dramatic as in patients with chronic AR.[539] Duroziez's murmur, pistol shot sounds over the peripheral arteries, and bisferiens pulses are usually absent in acute AR. The normal pulse pressure may lead to serious underestimation of the severity of the valvular lesion. The left ventricular impulse is normal or nearly so, and the rocking motion of the chest characteristic of chronic AR is not apparent. S_1 may be soft or absent because of premature closure of the mitral valve.[549] Instead, the sound of mitral valve closure is heard occasionally in mid-diastole. However, closure of the mitral valve may be incomplete, and diastolic mitral regurgitation may occur.[550] Evidence of pulmonary hypertension, with an accentuated P_2 and an S_3 and S_4, is frequently present. The early diastolic murmur of acute AR is lower pitched and shorter than that of chronic AR, because as left ventricular end-diastolic pressure rises, the pressure gradient between the aorta and the left ventricle is rapidly reduced. The Austin Flint murmur, if present, is brief and ceases when left ventricular pressure exceeds left atrial pressure in diastole.

TABLE 34-15 MANIFESTATIONS OF SEVERE AORTIC REGURGITATION

CLINICAL FINDING	ACUTE	CHRONIC
Congestive heart failure	Early and sudden	Late and insidious
Arterial pulse		
Rate per minute	Increased	Normal
Rate of rise	Not increased	Increased
Systolic pressure	Normal to decreased	Increased
Diastolic pressure	Normal to decreased	Decreased
Pulse pressure	Near-normal	Increased
Contour of peak	Single	Bisferiens
Pulsus alternans	Common	Uncommon
Left ventricular impulse	Near-normal to laterally displaced; not hyperdynamic	Laterally displaced, hyperdynamic
Auscultation		
First heart sound	Soft to absent	Normal
Aortic component of S_2	Soft	Normal or decreased
Pulmonic component of S_2	Normal or increased	Normal
Fourth heart sound	Consistently absent	Usually absent
Third heart sound	Common	Uncommon
Aortic systolic murmur	Grade 3 or less	Grade 3 or more
Aortic regurgitant murmur	Short, medium-pitched	Long, high-pitched
Austin Flint murmur	Mid-diastolic	Presystolic, mid-diastolic, or both
Peripheral arterial auscultatory signs	Absent	Present
LABORATORY FINDING		
ECG	Normal left ventricular voltage with minor repolarization abnormalities	Increased left ventricular voltage with major repolarization abnormalities
Chest roentgenogram		
Left ventricle	Normal to moderately increased	Markedly increased
Aortic root	Usually normal	Prominent
Pulmonary venous pattern	Redistributed to upper lobes	Normal
ECHOCARDIOGRAPHIC VARIABLE		
Mitral valve		
Closure	Early	Normal
Opening	Late	Normal
Anterior leaflet E-F slope	Reduced	Normal
Diastolic fluttering	Yes	Yes
Septal wall motion	Normal	Hyperkinetic
Posterior wall motion	Normal	Hyperkinetic
End-diastolic dimension	Normal	Increased
End-systolic dimension	Normal	Normal
Shortening fraction	Normal	Increased

Modified from Benotti, J. R.: Acute aortic insufficiency. In Dalen, J. E., and Alpert, J. S. (eds.): Valvular Heart Disease. 2nd ed. Boston, Little, Brown and Company, 1987, pp. 331 and 337.

TABLE 34-14 CHARACTERISTICS DISTINGUISHING THE MURMUR OF MITRAL STENOSIS FROM THE AUSTIN FLINT MURMUR

CLINICAL OR LABORATORY FINDING	MITRAL STENOSIS	AUSTIN FLINT MURMUR
Opening snap present	+	−
S_1 increased	+	−
S_3 present	−	+
Left ventricular enlargement and/or hypertrophy (physical examination, ECG, chest roentgenogram)	−	+
Right ventricular enlargement and/or hypertrophy (physical examination, ECG, chest roentgenogram)	+	−
Murmur decreases with amyl nitrite	−	+
Echocardiographic evidence of organic mitral stenosis	+	−
Presence of atrial fibrillation	+	−

From Alpert, J. S.: Chronic aortic regurgitation. In Dalen, J. E., and Alpert, J. S. (eds.): Valvular Heart Disease. 2nd ed. Boston, Little, Brown and Company, 1987, p. 291.

LABORATORY EXAMINATION

ELECTROCARDIOGRAM. *Chronic* AR results in left axis deviation and a pattern of left ventricular diastolic volume overload, characterized by an increase in initial forces (prominent Q waves in leads I, aV$_1$, and V$_3$ to V$_6$) and a relatively small *r* wave in V$_1$ (Fig. 34–35). With the passage of time, these initial forces diminish, but the total QRS amplitude increases. The T waves may be tall and upright in left precordial leads early in the course, but more commonly they are inverted, with ST-segment depressions.[551] Left intraventricular conduction defects occur late in the course and are usually associated with left ventricular dysfunction. When AR is caused by

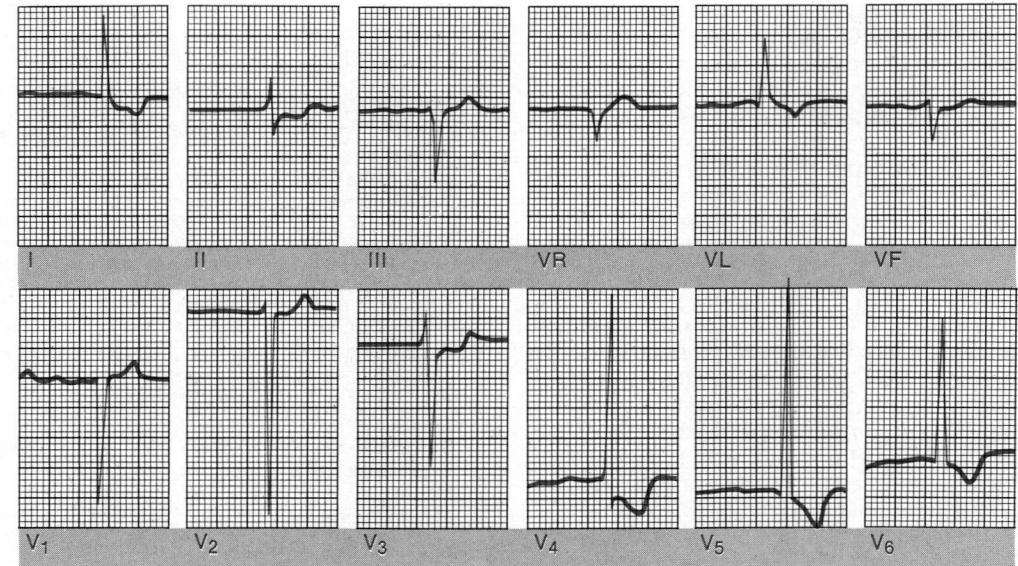

FIGURE 34–35. Atrial fibrillation and left ventricular hypertrophy. The most prominent features are the gross increase in precordial voltage (RV5 + SV2 = 70 mm) and the marked anterolateral ST/T wave changes (leads I, aVL, and V4-6). The patient had aortic regurgitation and normal coronary arteries and was not taking digitalis. (Normal standardization, i.e., 1 mV = 10 mm.) (From Hall, R. J., and Julian, D. G.: Diseases of the Cardiac Valves. New York, Churchill Livingstone, 1989, p. 39.)

an inflammatory process, P-R prolongation may result.[552] However, the electrocardiogram is not an accurate predictor of the severity of AR or cardiac weight.[552] In *acute* AR, the electrocardiogram may or may not show left ventricular hypertrophy, despite the presence of left ventricular failure, depending upon the severity and duration of the regurgitation. However, nonspecific ST-segment and T-wave changes are common.

RADIOLOGICAL FINDINGS (see also p. 223). Cardiac size is a function of the duration and severity of regurgitation and the state of left ventricular function. In acute AR, there may be little cardiac enlargement, but marked enlargement is a common finding in chronic AR. Typically, the left ventricle enlarges in an inferior and leftward direction, causing a significant increase in the long axis (Figs. 8–3, p. 207, 8–8B, p. 208, and 8–33, p. 223) but sometimes little or no increase in the transverse diameter of the heart. Calcification of the aortic valve is uncommon in patients with pure AR but is often present in patients with combined AS and AR. As in the case with AS, the presence of distinct left atrial enlargement in the absence of heart failure should suggest the possibility of mitral valve disease. Dilatation of the ascending aorta is usually more marked than in AS and may involve the entire aortic arch, including the aortic knob. Severe, aneurysmal dilatation of the aorta should suggest that aortic root disease (e.g., Marfan syndrome, cystic medionecrosis, or annuloaortic ectasia) is responsible for the AR. Linear calcifications in the wall of the ascending aorta are seen in syphilitic aortitis but are nonspecific and are observed in degenerative disease as well.

For angiographic assessment of AR, contrast material should be injected rapidly (i.e., 25 to 35 ml/sec) into the aortic root, and filming should be carried out in the right and left anterior oblique projections. Opacification may be improved by filming during a Valsalva maneuver. In acute AR, there is only a slight increase in ventricular end-diastolic volume, but with the passage of time both the end-diastolic volume and the thickness of the ventricular wall increase, usually in parallel.

ECHOCARDIOGRAPHY (p. 86). The severity of regurgitation is reflected in increased motion of the septum and posterior wall, as recorded by M-mode echocardiography. In chronic AR, the left ventricular end-diastolic diameter and extent of systolic shortening are both augmented (Fig. 34–36A). There is increased motion of the interventricular septum and posterior left ventricular wall in compensated patients, but shortening is normal or reduced in patients with left ventricular failure. Serial studies, particularly with two-dimensional echocardiography, may detect early changes in left ventricular function, as reflected in increased end-diastolic and end-systolic diameters and reduced fractional shortening, which may be of assistance in selecting the optimal time for surgical intervention. Echocardiography is helpful in identifying the cause of AR. It may show thickening of the valve cusps, prolapse of the valve, a flail leaflet (Fig. 34–

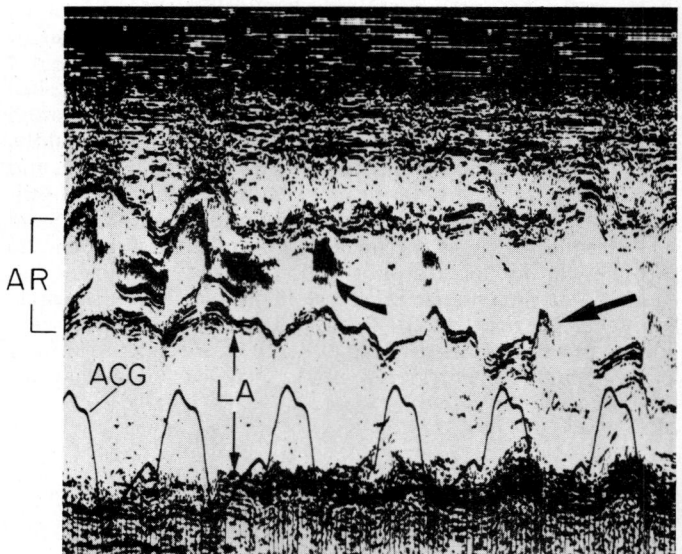

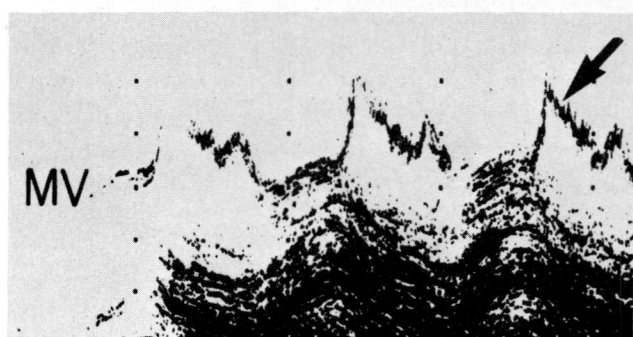

FIGURE 34–36. *Top*, M-mode electrocardiogram in severe aortic regurgitation. A markedly dilated aortic root (AR) is apparent on the left, appearing anterior to a slightly enlarged left atrium (LA). The left ventricle (at the right of the tracing) is dilated and demonstrates vigorous symmetrical contractile motion of the posterior wall and interventricular septum. Projecting anterior to the mitral valve is an abnormal diastolic echo (curved arrow) suggestive of a partially disrupted aortic valve cusp prolapsing into the left ventricular outflow tract. ACG = apexcardiogram. *Bottom*, Echocardiogram in aortic regurgitation. High-frequency diastolic vibrations (arrow) of the anterior mitral valve leaflet (MV) are typical of aortic regurgitation.

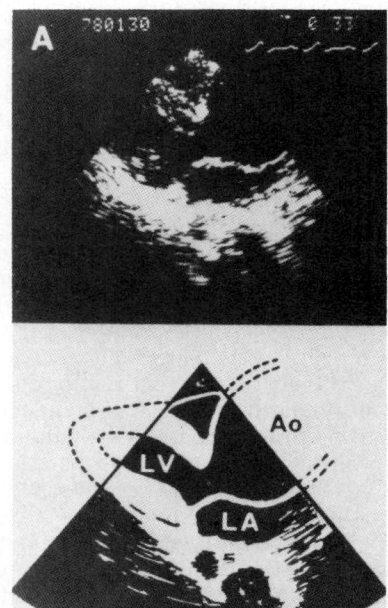

FIGURE 34–37. *A, B,* Long-axis view and schematic of the aortic root in end systole by two-dimensional echocardiography. The unusually dilated aortic root is visualized. (From Imaizumi, T., et al.: Utility of two-dimensional echocardiography in the differential diagnosis of the etiology of aortic regurgitation. Am. Heart J. *103:*887, 1982.)

are of value in the early detection of deterioration of left ventricular function.

MANAGEMENT

ACUTE AORTIC REGURGITATION. Since early death due to left ventricular failure is frequent in patients with *severe acute* AR despite intensive medical management, prompt surgical intervention is indicated. Even a normal ventricle cannot sustain the burden of acute severe volume overload; therefore, the risk of *acute* AR is much greater than that of chronic AR.[536,538,541] While the patient is being prepared for surgery, intravenous treatment with a positive inotropic agent (dopamine or dobutamine) and/or vasodilator (nitroprusside) may be necessary. The agent and dosage should be selected on the basis of arterial pressure (Chap. 17). In patients with acute AR secondary to active infective endocarditis who are stable hemodynamically, operation may be deferred to allow 7 to 10 days of intensive antibiotic therapy if the patient remains stable.[541] However, aortic valve replacement should be undertaken at the earliest sign of hemodynamic instability, if there is echocardiographic evidence of diastolic closure of the mitral valve,[562] or immediately upon completion of a 10-day course of antibiotics when acute, severe regurgitation has developed (p. 1091). The cautious use of vasodilators may be helpful in stabilizing the patient's condition but is no substitute for prompt surgery in the patients with pulmonary edema, severe pulmonary congestion, and/or an obvious low forward cardiac output state.

NATURAL HISTORY OF CHRONIC AORTIC REGURGITATION. Management must take into account the natural history of the lesion.[563] Moderately severe or even severe chronic AR is associated with a generally favorable prognosis for many years. Approximately 75 per cent of patients survive for 5 years and 50 per cent for 10 years after diagnosis.[102] However, as is the case for AS, once the patient becomes symptomatic, the condition often deteriorates rapidly, and sudden death may occur, usually in previously symptomatic patients. Without surgical treatment, death usually occurs within 4 years after the development of angina and within 2 years after the onset of heart failure. Even during the asymptomatic period gradual deterioration of left ventricular function may occur; it is important, therefore, to intervene surgically before these changes have become irreversible.

MEDICAL TREATMENT

Patients with mild or moderate AR who are asymptomatic with normal or only minimally increased cardiac size require no therapy but should be followed clinically and with echocardiography and with antibiotic prophylaxis for endocarditis. Patients with limitations of cardiac reserve and/or left ventricular dysfunction secondary to AR should not engage in vigorous sports or heavy exertion.[564] Cardiac glycosides should be employed in patients with severe AR, left ventricular dilatation, and sinus rhythm, even in the absence of symptoms. If present, systemic arterial diastolic hypertension should be treated, since it increases the regurgitant flow; however, drugs that impair left ventricular function, such as propranolol, should be avoided. Atrial fibrillation and bradyarrhythmias are poorly tolerated and should be prevented if possible. Since these and other cardiac arrhythmias and infections are poorly tolerated in patients with severe AR, such complications must be treated promptly and vigorously. Even though nitroglycerin and other nitrates are not as helpful in relieving anginal pain in patients with AR as they are in patients with coronary artery disease or AS, they are worth a trial. Patients with AR secondary to syphilitic aortitis (p. 1548) should receive a full course of penicillin therapy. Although patients with left ventricular failure secondary to AR require surgical treatment, they also respond, at least temporarily, to treatment with digitalis glycosides, salt restriction, and diuretics. The response to vasodilator therapy is often impres-

36A), vegetations, or dilatation of the aortic root[553] (Fig. 34–37).

In *acute* AR (Table 34–14 and Fig. 34–34) the echocardiogram reveals a reduction in amplitude of the opening movement of the mitral valve, premature closure and delayed opening of the mitral valve,[554] and a reduction in the E–F slope, indicating that the left ventricle is operating on the steep portion of its pressure-volume curve. Left ventricular end-diastolic dimensions are not markedly increased, and fractional shortening is normal. This contrasts with the findings in chronic AR, in which end-diastolic dimensions and wall motion are increased. Occasionally, with equilibration of aortic and left ventricular pressures in diastole, premature opening of the aortic valve may be detected.[555]

High-frequency, diastolic fluttering of the anterior leaflet of the mitral valve during diastole[556] (Fig. 34–36B) is an important echocardiographic finding in both acute and chronic AR; it does not occur, however, when the mitral valve is rigid. This sign, which, unlike the Austin Flint rumble, occurs even in mild AR, results from the movement imparted to the anterior leaflet of the mitral valve by the jet of blood regurgitating from the aorta.

Doppler echocardiography (Figs. 4–56, p. 86, 4–57, p. 87, and 4–58, p. 87) is the most sensitive and accurate noninvasive technique in the detection of AR and is superior to the M-mode and two-dimensional techniques in this regard.[557] It readily detects mild degrees of AR that may be inaudible. In addition, it provides an approach to the measurement of the regurgitation flow and the regurgitant orifice.[558,559]

RADIONUCLIDE TECHNIQUES. Radionuclide angiography, by allowing determination of the regurgitant fraction and of the left ventricular/right ventricular stroke volume ratio, provides an accurate noninvasive assessment of AR.[560,561] This technique is nonspecific, because the ratio will be increased by associated MR and reduced by tricuspid or pulmonary regurgitation. However, in the absence of these complicating lesions, a left ventricular/right ventricular stroke volume ratio of 2.5 or more denotes severe AR. As indicated earlier, these techniques are of value in the assessment of left ventricular function in patients with AR.[533–535] Serial measurements

sive. Hemodynamic studies have shown beneficial effects of intravenous hydralazine,[565,566] sublingual nifedipine,[567] and oral prazosin.[568] This form of therapy may be particularly helpful in stabilizing patients with acute lesions or those with decompensated chronic AR who are awaiting operation. Long-term administration of hydralazine[569-571] and nifedipine[572] appears to improve systolic function; either drug combined with digitalis glycosides[573] may be useful for the long-term management of the asymptomatic patient with severe AR.

Asymptomatic patients with severe *chronic* AR and normal left ventricular function should be examined at intervals of approximately 3 to 6 months. In addition to clinical examination, x-ray, and electrocardiogram, serial noninvasive assessments of left ventricular size and performance at rest and during exercise should be carried out using echocardiography or radionuclide angiography or both.

SURGICAL TREATMENT

INDICATIONS FOR OPERATION. There is general agreement that operative correction is *not* indicated in patients with severe chronic AR who are asymptomatic, have good exercise tolerance, and have normal left ventricular function. Similarly, there is a consensus that in the absence of contraindications surgical treatment is advisable in patients with severe AR who are symptomatic as a result of this lesion and who have impaired left ventricular function. Between these two ends of the clinical-hemodynamic spectrum are many patients in whom it may be quite difficult to balance the immediate risks of operation and the continuing risks of an implanted prosthetic valve on the one hand against the hazards of allowing a severe volume overload to damage the left ventricle on the other.[574-580]

Irreversible changes in left ventricular function can develop in some patients with AR so that even after successful correction of AR, this subset of patients may have persistent cardiomegaly and depressed left ventricular function.[581-585] Symptoms of impaired left ventricular function present preoperatively may persist and occasionally even get worse despite successful valve replacements. While it is best to operate on patients before irreversible left ventricular changes have occurred, most of the patients in the latter category are, in fact, also benefited, and do even worse with continued medical management. Patients whose ventricular function does not return to normal after aortic valve replacement often exhibit histological changes in the left ventricle, including massive fiber hypertrophy and increased interstitial fibrous tissue.[586] On the other hand, postoperative left ventricular function is usually excellent in patients who have normal systolic function preoperatively.[584]

In order to minimize the risk of postoperative left ventricular dysfunction, every effort should be made to operate on patients *before* serious left ventricular dysfunction occurs. Although quantitative biplane ventriculography is the most precise method for assessing left ventricular performance, it cannot be readily employed in serial fashion. Instead, serial echocardiograms or radionuclide ventriculograms should be obtained to detect changes in left ventricular size and function. These examinations can provide valuable information concerning progressive deterioration in left ventricular function at rest. Radionuclide angiography, in particular (p. 168), is a safe, simple, and noninvasive method that allows repeated evaluation of ejection fraction and end-systolic volume both at rest and during exercise. However, it is impaired ventricular function at *rest* that becomes the basis for selection of patients for operation; failure of a normal ejection fraction to respond normally to *exercise* portends impaired function at rest.

Since AR has complex effects on both preload and afterload, the selection of appropriate indices of ventricular contractility is a challenge.[587] Simple left ventricular end-diastolic volume

and the ejection phase indices such as ejection fraction and ventricular fraction shortening are too strongly influenced by loading to be accurate indicators of ventricular contractility but may be useful empirical predictors of postoperative function.[477] Preoperative left ventricular end-systolic volume and dimensions are largely preload dependent and are good predictors of postoperative left ventricular function.[588,589] The relationship between end-systolic wall stress and ejection fraction or per cent[590] fractional shortening may be even more useful. However, in the absence of such measurements *serial* changes in ventricular end-diastolic and/or ejection phase indices can be employed to detect *relative* deterioration of ventricular function.

Patients with severely impaired left ventricular systolic function preoperatively are at high risk of developing irreversible left ventricular dysfunction and, indeed, of dying of congestive heart failure postoperatively. Other patients with impaired left ventricular function preoperatively, improve postoperatively—both symptomatically and insofar as left ventricular function is concerned. Bonow et al. have reported that, after valve replacement, survival was excellent in patients with normal resting ejection fractions preoperatively. However, patients with subnormal ejection fraction and only a brief (<1 year) duration of left ventricular dysfunction also did well postoperatively and maintained their preoperative levels of exercise tolerance. On the other hand, patients with subnormal ejection fraction and impaired exercise tolerance and/or prolonged left ventricular dysfunction exhibited poor postoperative survival.[575,586]

In *conclusion*, the decision to recommend aortic valve replacement in some patients with severe AR remains difficult. Operation should be deferred in asymptomatic patients with normal left ventricular function and should be recommended in symptomatic patients regardless of the status of their left ventricular function. Asymptomatic patients with impaired left ventricular function must be treated individually, taking into account associated medical conditions and coronary artery disease that may add to the surgical risk, as well as the experience level of the surgical team. A decision should be based not on a single abnormal measurement of impaired left ventricular function but rather on several observations of depressed performance and impaired exercise tolerance, carried out at intervals of 4 to 6 months. If abnormalities are shown consistently and if any trend to deterioration is noted, operation should be carried out forthwith. If evidence of left ventricular dysfunction is borderline or is not consistent, the patient may be followed closely.

OPERATIVE PROCEDURES. The surgical treatment of AR and of combined AS and AR is valve replacement. (Prosthetic valves are discussed on pp. 1061–1064.) Since the aortic annulus in patients with severe AR is usually not as narrow as it is in patients with AS, a larger artificial valve can be inserted, and mild postoperative obstruction to left ventricular outflow is less of a problem than it is in some patients with AS. Occasionally, when a leaflet has been torn from its attachments to the aortic annulus by trauma, surgical repair without valve replacement may be possible. In patients in whom AR is due to aneurysmal dilatation of the aortic annulus (Chap. 47) and the ascending aorta, regurgitation may occasionally be reduced or eliminated by narrowing the annulus or by excising a portion of the aorta. More often, effective treatment in these patients requires replacement of the aortic valve and excision of the aneurysmal portion of the aorta and its replacement with a graft, sometimes with reimplantation of the coronary arteries. This more extensive procedure is associated with a higher operative risk than is aortic valve replacement alone.

Aortic valve replacement is discussed on page 1042. In general, results in patients with AR are similar to those in patients with AS, with a large percentage of patients exhibiting striking clinical improvement. Reductions in heart size and in left ventricular diastolic volume and mass occur in the majority of patients.[466,591] However, as already indicated, the extent of

FIGURE 34–38. Relation of preoperative ventricular function to postoperative survival. Data of Greves et al. *(left)* and those of Bonow et al. *(right)* show remarkable agreement: both groups incorporated limits clearly in abnormal range. Cunha et al *(center)* selected a limit that was well within normal range. These and other published data indicate that preoperative ventricular function is an important determinant of postoperative survival. SEF indicates systolic ejection fraction; ESD = echocardiographically measured dimension at end-systole; angio = angiography; echo = echocardiography. (From Errichetti, A., et al.: Is valve replacement indicated in asymptomatic patients with aortic stenosis or aortic regurgitation? *In* Cheitlin, M. [ed.]: Dilemmas in Clinical Cardiology. Philadelphia, F. A. Davis Co., 1990, p. 204.)

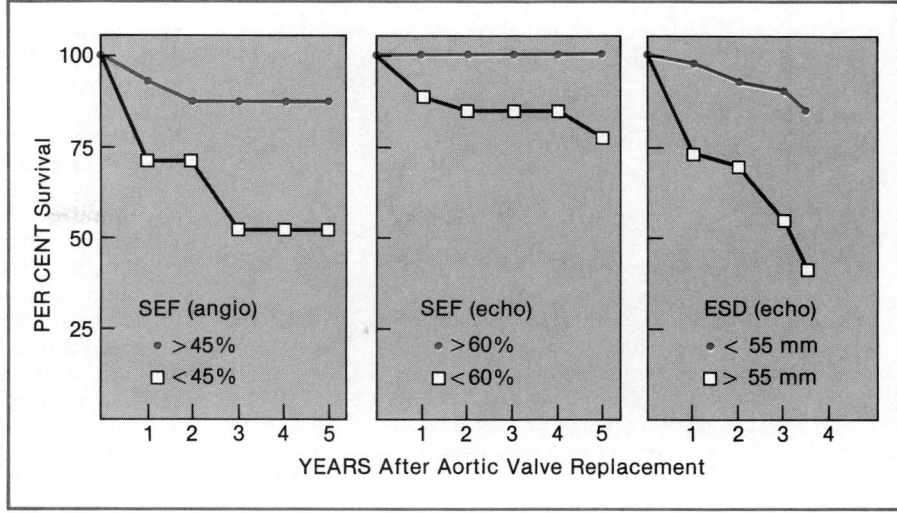

improvement in left ventricular function may not be as salutary as in patients with aortic stenosis, perhaps because the ventricular dysfunction is more advanced and less reversible in patients with volume overload by the time they become symptomatic and are referred for surgical treatment[592-593] than it is in patients with pressure overload. As is the case for AS, the operative risk of aortic valve replacement in patients with AR depends on the general condition of the patient, the state of left ventricular function, and the skill and experience of the surgical team; the mortality rate ranges from 3 to 8 per cent in most medical centers. A late mortality of approximately 5 to 10 per cent per year is observed in survivors in whom cardiac enlargement was marked and prolonged left ventricular dysfunction was present preoperatively (Fig. 34–38). Follow-up studies have shown both early rapid and then slower long-term reductions of ventricular mass, ejection fraction,[495] myocyte hypertrophy, and ventricular fibrous content.[404,479] By extending the indications for operation to symptomatic patients with normal left ventricular function as well as to asymptomatic patients with early left ventricular dysfunction, both early and late results are improving.[575,576,586] It is likely that with the continued improvement of surgical techniques and results, it will become possible to extend the recommendation for operative treatment to asymptomatic patients with severe regurgitation and normal or nearly normal cardiac function. However, given the risks of operation and the long-term complications of artificial valves, I believe that the time for such a policy has not yet arrived.

Tricuspid, Pulmonic, and Multivalvular Disease

TRICUSPID STENOSIS

ETIOLOGY AND PATHOLOGY

Tricuspid stenosis (TS) is almost always rheumatic in origin.[594] Other causes of obstruction to right atrial emptying are unusual and include congenital tricuspid atresia (p. 938), right atrial tumors (which may produce a clinical picture suggesting rapidly progressive TS [p. 1453]), and the carcinoid syndrome (which more frequently produces tricuspid regurgitation [TR] [p. 1056] but which may occasionally produce TS). Rarely, obstruction to right ventricular inflow can be due to pericardial constriction, extracardiac tumors, and vegetations.

Rheumatic TS *almost* never occurs as an isolated lesion but generally accompanies mitral valve disease[595-600]; in many patients the aortic valve is also involved. TS is present at autopsy in about 15 per cent of patients with rheumatic heart disease but is of clinical significance in only about 5 per cent.[601]

Organic tricuspid valve disease is more common in India than in North America or Western Europe; it has been reported to occur in the hearts of more than one-third of patients with rheumatic heart disease studied at autopsy on the subcontinent.[602] The anatomical changes of rheumatic TS resemble those of MS, with fusion and shortening of the chordae tendineae and fusion of the leaflets at their edges producing a diaphragm with a fixed central aperture.[11] As is the case for MS, TS is more common in women and, in the United States, TS is seen most commonly in persons between the ages of 20 and 60. Again, as in mitral valve disease, stenosis, regurgitation, or some combination of the two may exist.

The right atrium is often greatly dilated, and its walls are thickened. There may be evidence of severe passive congestion, with enlargement of the liver and spleen.

PATHOPHYSIOLOGY

A diastolic pressure gradient between the right atrium and ventricle—the hemodynamic expression of TS—is augmented when the transvalvular blood flow increases during exercise or inspiration and is reduced when flow declines during expiration. A mean diastolic pressure gradient exceeding 5 mm Hg is usually sufficient to elevate mean right atrial pressure to levels that result in systemic venous congestion and, unless sodium intake has been restricted or diuretics have been given, is associated with jugular venous distention, ascites, and edema.

In patients with sinus rhythm, the right atrial *a* wave may be extremely tall (Fig. 34–39) and may even approach the level of the right ventricular systolic pressure. Resting cardiac output is usually markedly reduced and fails to rise during exercise, accounting for the normal or only slightly elevated left atrial, pulmonary arterial, and right ventricular systolic pressures, despite the presence of accompanying mitral valve disease.

A *mean* diastolic pressure gradient across the tricuspid valve as low as 2 mm Hg is sufficient to establish the diagnosis

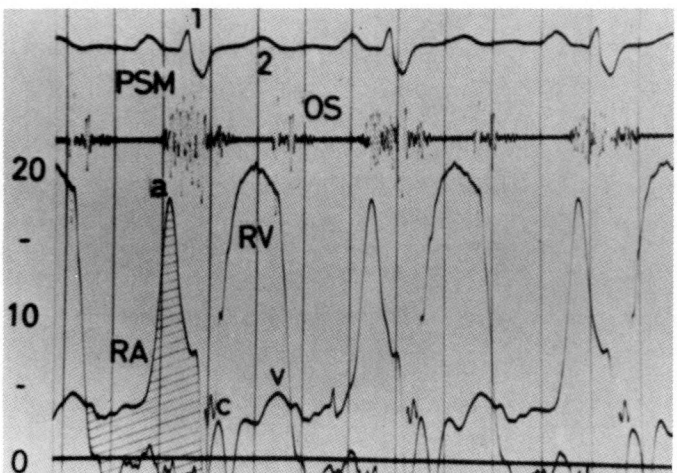

FIGURE 34–39. Phonocardiogram and right heart pressures in a patient with tricuspid stenosis. The giant right atrial *a* wave (a) nearly equals right ventricular (RV) systolic pressure and produces a large diastolic gradient (shaded area). A presystolic murmur (PSM), loud first heart sound (1), and early diastolic opening snap (OS) simulate the findings in mitral stenosis. (Time lines = 0.2 sec.) (From Criley, J. M., et al.: Departures from the expected auscultatory events in mitral stenosis. *In* Likoff, W. [ed.]: Valvular Heart Disease. Philadelphia, F. A. Davis, 1973, p. 214.)

of TS. However, exercise, deep inspiration, and the rapid infusion of fluid or the administration of atropine may enhance greatly a borderline gradient in the presence of TS.[596] Therefore, whenever this diagnosis is suspected, right atrial and ventricular pressures should be recorded simultaneously, using two catheters or a single catheter with a double lumen, with one lumen opening on either side of the tricuspid valve. The effects of respiration on any pressure difference should be examined.

CLINICAL MANIFESTATIONS
(Table 34–16)

HISTORY. The low cardiac output characteristic of TS causes fatigue, and patients often complain of discomfort due to hepatomegaly, swelling of the abdomen, and anasarca.[602a] The severity of these symptoms, which are secondary to an elevated systemic venous pressure, is out of proportion to the degree of dyspnea.[597] Some patients complain of a fluttering discomfort in the neck, caused by giant *a* waves in the jugular venous pulse. Despite the coexistence of MS, the symptoms characteristic of this valve lesion, i.e., hemoptysis, paroxysmal nocturnal dyspnea, and acute pulmonary edema, are usually absent in the presence of severe TS. Indeed, the *absence* of the symptoms of pulmonary congestion in a patient with obvious MS should suggest the possibility of TS.

PHYSICAL EXAMINATION. Because of the high frequency with which MS occurs in patients with TS, the diagnosis of the latter is commonly overlooked, since the physical findings are mistakenly attributed to MS, which is, of course, more common and may be more obvious. Therefore, a high index of suspicion is required to detect the tricuspid valve lesion. In the presence of sinus rhythm (which is surprisingly common), the *a* wave in the jugular venous pulse is tall, sharp, and flicking and on first impression may be confused with an arterial pulsation; a presystolic hepatic pulsation is often palpable. The *y* descent is slow and barely appreciable, indicating the absence of normal rapid, early right ventricular filling. The lung fields are clear, and despite engorgement of the neck veins and the presence of ascites and anasarca, the patient may be comfortable while lying flat. A parasternal (right ventricular) lift is inconspicuous, and pulmonic valve closure is not palpable, but occasionally the pulsations of a greatly enlarged right atrium may be felt to the right of the sternum.

Thus, on inspection and palpation the combination of a prominent *a* wave in the jugular venous pulse in a patient with MS without the clinical signs of pulmonary hypertension or right ventricular enlargement should suggest the diagnosis of TS. This suspicion is strengthened when a diastolic thrill is felt at the lower left sternal edge, particularly if it appears or becomes more prominent during inspiration.[20]

The auscultatory findings of the accompanying MS are usually prominent and often overshadow the more subtle signs of TS. A tricuspid valvular opening snap (OS) may be audible but is often difficult to distinguish from a mitral OS. However, the tricuspid OS usually follows the mitral OS, and is localized to the lower left sternal border, whereas the mitral OS is usually most prominent at the apex and radiates more widely. The diastolic murmur of TS is commonly heard best along the lower left parasternal border in the fourth intercostal space and is usually softer, higher pitched, and shorter in duration than the murmur of MS. The presystolic component has a scratchy quality, commences earlier (0.06 sec after the P wave in TS compared with 0.12 in MS), and has a crescendo-decrescendo configuration, diminishing before S_1.[598] The diastolic murmur and OS of TS are both augmented by inspiration (Fig. 3–34, p. 58), the Mueller maneuver, assumption of the right lateral decubitus position, leg-raising, inhalation of amyl nitrite, squatting, and both isotonic and isometric exercise. They are reduced during expiration or the strain of the Valsalva maneuver and return to control levels immediately (i.e., within two to three beats) after Valsalva release.

LABORATORY EXAMINATION

ELECTROCARDIOGRAM

In a patient with valvular heart disease in the absence of atrial fibrillation, TS is suggested by the presence of ECG evidence of right atrial enlargement disproportionate to the degree of right ventricular hypertrophy. The P-wave amplitude in leads II and V, exceeds 0.25 mV (p. 124), and there may be depression of the P-R segment resulting from increased magnitude of the atrial T wave. Since most patients with TS have mitral valve

---

TABLE 34-16   CLINICAL AND LABORATORY FEATURES OF RHEUMATIC TRICUSPID STENOSIS

HISTORY
Long history
Progressive fatigue, edema, anorexia
Minimal orthopnea, paroxysmal nocturnal dyspnea
Rheumatic fever in two-thirds of patients
Female preponderance
Orthopnea and paroxysmal nocturnal dyspnea are unusual
Pulmonary edema and hemoptysis are rare

PHYSICAL FINDINGS
Signs of multivalvular involvement
Wasting
Peripheral cyanosis
Neck vein distension, with prominent V waves
Right ventricular lift
Associated murmurs of mitral and aortic valve disease
Holosystolic murmur maximal at left lower sternal border, accentuating with inspiration
Hepatic pulsation
Ascites, peripheral edema

LABORATORY FINDINGS
Normal sinus rhythm is frequently present with large A waves in the neck veins
Absent right ventricular lift
Auscultation reveals a diastolic rumble at lower left sternal edge, increasing in intensity with inspiration
Electrocardiogram shows tall right atrial P waves and no right ventricular hypertrophy
Roentgenogram shows a dilated right atrium without an enlarged pulmonary artery segment

Modified from Ockene, I. S.: Tricuspid valve disease. *In* Dalen, J. E., and Alpert, J. S. (eds.): Valvular Heart Disease. 2nd ed. Boston, Little, Brown and Company, 1987, pp. 356 and 390.

disease, the ECG signs of biatrial enlargement (p. 125) with abnormally tall, broad P waves in leads II, III, and aV_f and prominent positive and negative deflections in V_f are commonly found. Right atrial dilatation may rotate the ventricular septum and affect QRS morphology in a manner so that the large volume of the right atrium between the exploring electrode and the ventricles reduces the amplitude of the QRS complex in lead V_1 (which often has a Q wave), whereas the QRS complex is much taller in V_2.

RADIOLOGICAL FINDINGS

The key radiological findings in TS are marked cardiomegaly, with conspicuous enlargement of the right atrium (i.e., prominence of the right heart border), which extends into a dilated superior vena cava and azygos vein, but without dilatation of the pulmonary artery. The vascular changes in the lungs characteristic of mitral valve disease may be masked, with little or no interstitial edema or vascular redistribution.

Angiography carried out following injection of contrast material into the right atrium and filming in the 30-degree right anterior oblique projection is useful for evaluating the appearance of the tricuspid valve. Thickening and decreased mobility of the leaflets, a jet through the constricted orifice, and thickening of the right atrial wall are characteristic findings.

ECHOCARDIOGRAM (see also p. 87). Although the motion of the normal tricuspid valve is similar to that of the normal mitral valve, it is more difficult to image. Not surprisingly, the changes in the echocardiogram of the tricuspid valve in TS resemble those observed in the mitral valve in MS (p. 1013). The M-mode echocardiogram usually shows thickening of the leaflets, a reduction in the E-F slope of the anterior leaflet, and paradoxical motion of the septal leaflet in diastole.[603,604] Calcification and thickening of the tricuspid valve often results in multiple and disorganized echoes. Two-dimensional echocardiography is more useful in the diagnosis of TS.[605] It characteristically shows diastolic doming of the leaflets, thickening and restriction of excision of the other leaflets, and reduced separation of the tips of the leaflets[606,607] (Fig. 34–40). Doppler echocardiography shows a prolonged slope of

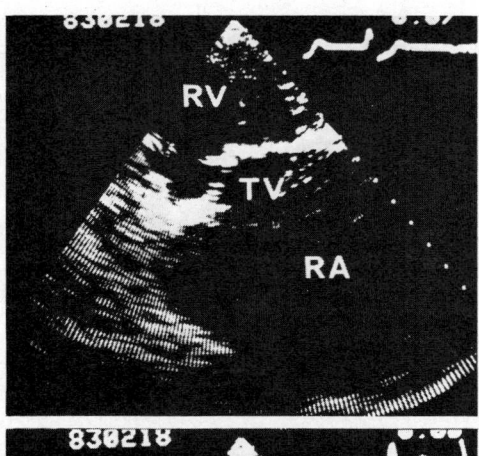
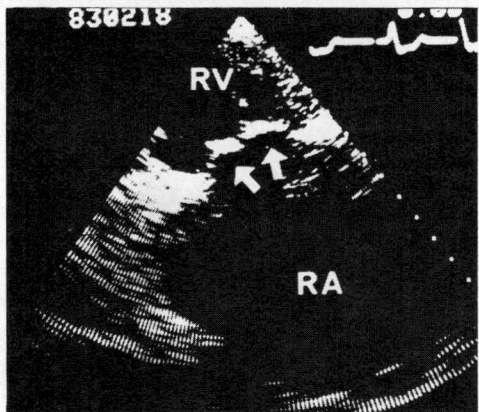

FIGURE 34–40. Two-dimensional echocardiograms in the long-axis view in a patient with tricuspid stenosis. *Top,* Systolic frame. *Bottom,* Diastolic frame that shows doming of both leaflets of the tricuspid valve (TV) (arrows). RA = right atrium; RV = right ventricle. (From Shimada, R., et al.: Diagnosis of tricuspid stenosis by M-mode and two-dimensional echocardiography. Am. J. Cardiol. *53*:164, 1984.)

antegrade flow[608] and compares well with cardiac catheterization in the quantification of TS and in the assessment of associated tricuspid regurgitation.[608]

MANAGEMENT

Although the fundamental approach to the management of severe TS is surgical treatment, intensive sodium restriction and diuretic therapy may diminish the symptoms secondary to the accumulation of excess salt and water. A prolonged preparatory period of diuresis may diminish hepatic congestive and thereby improve hepatic function sufficiently to diminish the risks of subsequent operation.

Surgical treatment of TS should be carried out at the time of mitral commissurotomy or valve replacement in patients with TS in whom mean diastolic pressure gradients exceed 5 mm Hg and tricuspid orifices are less than approximately 2.0 cm². Most patients with TS have coexisting valvular disease that requires surgery. The final decision concerning surgical treatment is made at the operating table. Since TS is almost always accompanied by some TR, simple finger fracture commissurotomy often does not result in significant hemodynamic improvement but may merely substitute severe regurgitation for stenosis. However, open valvulotomy in which the stenotic tricuspid valve is converted into a functionally bicuspid one may result in substantial improvement. The commissures between the anterior and septal leaflets and between the posterior and septal leaflets are opened; it is not advisable to open the commissure between the anterior and posterior leaflets for fear of producing severe regurgitation. If open commissurotomy does not restore reasonable normal valve function, the tricuspid valve may have to be replaced.[609,610] A tissue valve (p. 1062) is preferred to a mechanical prosthesis in the tricuspid position because of the high risk of thrombosis of the latter[611,612] (p. 1062) and the long-term durability of bioprostheses in the tricuspid position.[613] The feasibility of tricuspid balloon valvuloplasty has been demonstrated,[614] but it is not clear how this procedure will be used most effectively.

TRICUSPID REGURGITATION

ETIOLOGY AND PATHOLOGY
(Table 34–17)

The most common cause of tricuspid regurgitation (TR) is not intrinsic involvement of the valve itself but *dilatation of the right ventricle* and of the tricuspid annulus, which may be complications of right ventricular failure of any cause (Fig. 34–41). Functional TR is observed in patients with right ventricular hypertension secondary to any form of cardiac and pulmonary vascular disease, most commonly mitral valve disease,[613–617] right ventricular infarction[618] (p. 1205), congenital heart disease (e.g., pulmonic stenosis and pulmonary hypertension secondary to Eisenmenger syndrome), primary pulmonary hypertension, and rarely in cor pulmonale. Severe TR has been reported to be the presenting manifestation in thyrotoxicosis.[619] In infants, TR may complicate right ventricular failure secondary to neonatal pulmonary diseases and pulmonary hypertension with persistence of the fetal pulmonary circulation.[620] In all of these cases, TR reflects the presence of, and in turn aggravates, severe right ventricular failure. TR results from dilatation of the tricuspid annulus, reduction of the narrowing of the annulus during systole, and resultant failure of systolic valve coaptation of the tricuspid valve leaflets.[621–623] Functional regurgitation may diminish or disappear as the right ventricle decreases in size with the treatment of heart failure. TR can also occur as a consequence of dilatation of the annulus in Marfan syndrome, in which it is not associated with right ventricular dilatation secondary to pulmonary hypertension.

A variety of disease processes can affect the tricuspid valve

TABLE 34-17 CAUSES AND MECHANISMS OF PURE TRICUSPID REGURGITATION

CAUSES

I. Anatomically ABNORMAL valve
  A. Rheumatic
  B. Nonrheumatic
    1. Infective endocarditis
    2. Ebstein's anomaly
    3. Floppy (prolapse)
    4. Congenital (non-Ebstein's)
    5. Carcinoid
    6. Papillary muscle dysfunction
    7. Trauma
    8. Connective tissue disorders (Marfan)
    9. Rheumatoid arthritis
    10. Radiation injury
II. Anatomically NORMAL valve (functional)
  A. Elevated right ventricular systolic pressure (dilated annulus)

MECHANISMS

Condition	Leaflet Area	Annular Circumference	Leaflet Insertion
1. Floppy	↑	↑	Normal
2. Ebstein's anomaly	↑	↑	Abnormal
3. Pulmonary/right ventricular systolic hypertension	Normal	↑	Normal
4. Papillary muscle dysfunction	Normal	Normal	Normal
5. Carcinoid	↓/Normal	Normal	Normal
6. Rheumatic	↓/Normal	Normal	Normal
7. Infective endocarditis	↓/Normal	Normal	Normal

Modified from Waller, B. F.: Rheumatic and nonrheumatic conditions producing valvular heart disease. *In* Frankel, W. S., and Brest, A. N. (eds.): Cardiovascular Clinics. Valvular Heart Disease: Comprehensive Evaluation and Management. Philadelphia, F. A. Davis, 1986, pp. 35 and 95.

apparatus *directly* and lead to regurgitation. Thus, organic TR may occur on a congenital basis, as part of Ebstein's anomaly, (p. 940), in atrioventricular canal, and when the tricuspid valve is involved in the formation of an aneurysm of the ventricular septum,[624] or it may occur as an isolated congenital lesion.[625] Rheumatic fever may attack the tricuspid valve directly,[613] and when it does so, it usually leads to both regurgitation and stenosis (Fig. 34–41*B*). Infarction, rupture, or ischemia of the papillary muscles of the right ventricle in coronary artery disease[618] and in perinatal asphyxia is an important cause of TR. TR may result from prolapse of the tricuspid valve caused by myxomatous changes in the valve and chordae tendineae; this condition usually, but not always, accompanies prolapse of the mitral valve[626-628] and may be associated with atrial septal defect.[629] Other causes include trauma,[630] dilated cardiomyopathy[631] infective endocarditis,[632] particularly staphylococcal endocarditis in drug addicts, and surgical excision that has been necessary in patients with infective endocarditis unresponsive to medical management.[633]

TR can occur in the *carcinoid syndrome*[634] (Fig. 34–42, p. 1057), which leads to focal or diffuse deposits of fibrous tissue on the endocardium of the valvular cusps and cardiac chambers and on the intima of the great veins and coronary sinus. The white, fibrous carcinoid plaques are most extensive on the right side of the heart, where they are usually deposited on the ventricular surfaces of the tricuspid valve and cause the cusps to adhere to the underlying right ventricular wall, thereby producing tricuspid regurgitation.[635,636] Less common causes of tricuspid regurgitation include cardiac tumors, particularly right atrial myxoma; endomyocardial fibrosis; methysergide-induced valvular disease[637]; and systemic lupus erythematosus involving the tricuspid valve.[638]

CLINICAL MANIFESTATIONS

HISTORY. In the absence of pulmonary hypertension, TR is generally well tolerated. However, when pulmonary hypertension and TR coexist, cardiac output declines, and the manifestations of right-sided heart failure become intensified. Thus, the symptoms of TR result from a reduced cardiac output and from ascites, painful congestive hepatomegaly, and massive edema. Occasionally, patients complain of throbbing pulsations in the neck due to jugular venous distention, which intensify on effort,[20] and systolic pulsations of the eyeballs are sometimes noted.[639] In the many patients with TR who have mitral valve disease, the symptoms of the latter usually predominate. Symptoms of pulmonary congestion may abate as TR develops, but they are replaced by weakness, fatigue, and other manifestations of a depressed cardiac output.

PHYSICAL EXAMINATION (Figs. 2–7, p. 19, and 16–3, p. 453). Evidence of weight loss and cachexia, cyanosis, and jaundice is often present on inspection. Atrial fibrillation is common. There is jugular venous distention,[640] the normal *x* and *x'* descents disappear, and a prominent systolic ("*s*") wave, i.e., a *c-v* wave, is apparent. The descent of this wave, the *y* descent, is sharp and becomes the most prominent event in the venous pulse (unless there is coexisting TS, in which case it is slowed). The *s* waves and *y* descents become more prominent during inspiration.[641] A venous systolic thrill and murmur in the neck may be present in severe TR.[642] The right ventricular impulse is hyperdynamic and thrusting in quality. Rarely, a right atrial systolic impulse may be observed or palpated along the right lower sternal edge.[20] In patients with combined mitral valve disease and TR, a relatively quiet zone may be present between the apex and the left sternal edge.

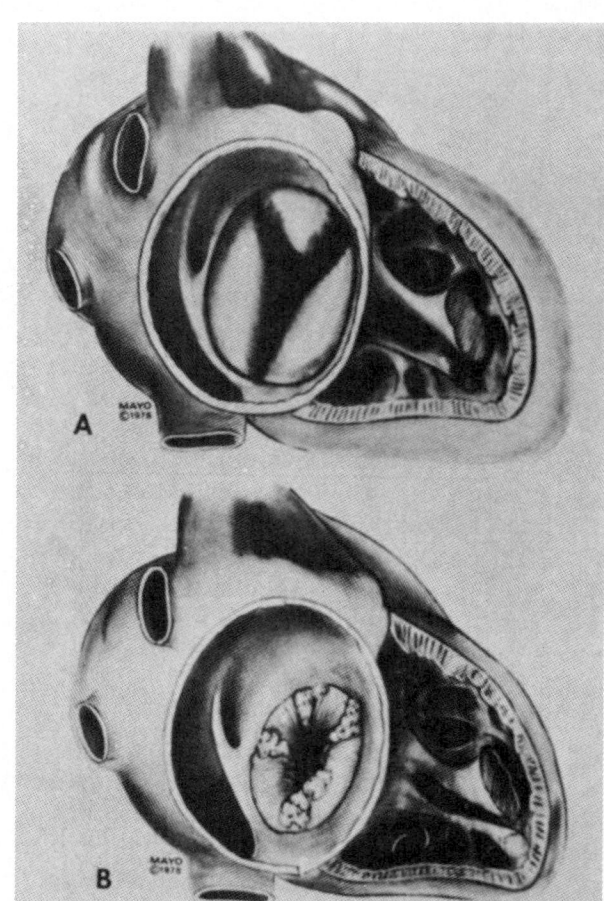

FIGURE 34-41. Types of tricuspid incompetence. *A*, Functional tricuspid incompetence secondary to dilatation of the right ventricle. *B*, Organic rheumatic tricuspid incompetence. (From Brandenburg, R. O., et al.: Valvular heart disease—When should the patient be referred? Pract. Cardiol. *5*:50, 1979.)

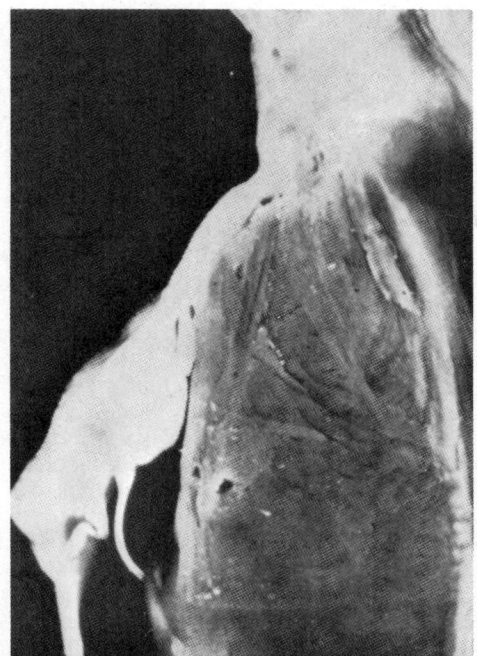

FIGURE 34–42. Septal tricuspid leaflet thickened by carcinoid plaques and fused to underlying ventricular septum. (From Callahan, J. A., et al.: Echocardiographic features of carcinoid heart disease. Am. J. Cardiol. 50:766, 1982.)

Systolic pulsations of an enlarged tender liver are commonly present initially, but in chronic TR with congestive cirrhosis, the liver may be firm and nontender. Ascites and edema are frequent.

Auscultation (Table 34–4, p. 1020). This usually reveals an S_3 originating from the right ventricle, i.e., one which is accentuated by inspiration; when TR is associated with pulmonary hypertension, P_2 is accentuated as well. The murmur of TR is usually high-pitched, pansystolic, and loudest in the fourth intercostal space in the parasternal region but occasionally in the subxiphoid area. When TR is mild, the murmur may be short. With acute TR due to infective endocarditis or trauma, the murmur is usually of low intensity and limited to the first half of systole. When the right ventricle is greatly dilated and occupies the anterior surface of the heart, the murmur may be most prominent at the apex and difficult to distinguish from that produced by MR.

The response of the murmur to respiration and other maneuvers is of considerable aid in establishing the diagnosis of tricuspid regurgitation (Table 2–8, p. 38). It is usually augmented during inspiration[20,643,644] (Rivero-Carvello's sign, p. 53). However, when the failing ventricle can no longer increase its stroke volume, the inspiratory augmentation is lost. Under these circumstances, respiratory variation may be elicited by standing and thereby reducing venous return. The murmur also increases during inspiration, the Mueller maneuver (forced inspiration against a closed glottis), exercise, leg-raising, hepatic compression, and amyl nitrite inhalation as well as after a prolonged diastole. It demonstrates an immediate overshoot after release of the Valsalva strain. It is reduced in intensity and duration in the standing position and during the strain of the Valsalva maneuver. Rarely, TR is silent except for the selective appearance of a soft systolic murmur during inspiration.[645]

Increased atrioventricular flow may cause a short early diastolic flow rumble in the left parasternal region following S_3.

LABORATORY EXAMINATION

ELECTROCARDIOGRAM. This is usually nonspecific and characteristic of the lesion causing TR. Incomplete right bun-

dle branch block, Q waves in lead V_1, and atrial fibrillation are commonly found.

RADIOLOGICAL FINDINGS. Marked cardiomegaly secondary to the condition responsible for the dilatation of the right ventricle is usually evident. The right atrium is prominent.[641] Evidence of elevated right atrial pressure may include distention of the azygos vein and the presence of pleural effusion. Ascites with upward displacement of the diaphragm may be present. Rarely, with prolonged elevation of right ventricular pressure, the tricuspid ring may calcify. The findings of pulmonary arterial and venous hypertension are common. Fluoroscopy may reveal systolic pulsations of the right atrium.

ECHOCARDIOGRAM (see also p. 87). In patients with TR secondary to dilation of the tricuspid annulus, the right atrium, right ventricle, and tricuspid annulus are usually dilated.[621–623] There is evidence of right ventricular diastolic overload, with paradoxical motion of the ventricular septum similar to that in atrial septal defect. Exaggerated motion and delayed closure of the tricuspid valve are evident in patients with Ebstein's anomaly. In patients with TR secondary to right ventricular dilatation and pulmonary hypertension, the pulmonic valve echogram shows a diminished or absent a deflection. *Prolapse of the tricuspid valve* due to myxomatous degeneration may be evident on M-mode and two-dimensional echocardiography[625,646] (Fig. 4–59, p. 87). Simultaneous echocardiographic studies of the tricuspid valve and phonocardiography may reveal a nonejection systolic click originating from the right side of the heart that occurs at the onset of prolapse. Echocardiographic indications of tricuspid valve abnormalities, especially TR by Doppler examination, can be detected in the majority of patients with carcinoid heart disease.[634]

Contrast echocardiography involving rapid injection of saline or indocyanine green dye into an antecubital vein made while a two-dimensional echocardiogram is being recorded (p. 69) is both sensitive and specific for TR.[647] The injection produces microcavities that are readily visible on echocardiography and normally travel as a bolus through the circulation. In TR, these microcavities can be seen to travel back and forth across the tricuspid orifice and to pass into the inferior vena cava and hepatic veins during systole.[648] TR secondary to carcinoid heart disease shows thickened, retracted valve leaflets, fixed in a semiopen position throughout the cardiac cycle[647,649] whereas that due to endocarditis may reveal vegetations on the valve, or a flail valve.

Pulsed Doppler echocardiography revealing systolic flow from right ventricle to right atrium is an exquisitely sensitive technique for detecting TR.[650] A semiquantitative assessment can be made by measuring reverse velocity in the inferior vena cava[651] and hepatic veins.[652] The peak velocity of TR flow is useful in the noninvasive estimation of right ventricular (and pulmonary artery) systolic pressure.[654] Real-time two-dimensional color-coded Doppler imaging is an extremely accurate, sensitive, and specific method for assessing TR[655] and is helpful in selecting patients for surgical treatment[656] and in assessing postoperative results.[657] The velocity of TR flow is useful in the noninvasive estimation of right ventricular (and pulmonary artery) systolic pressure.

HEMODYNAMIC AND ANGIOGRAPHIC FINDINGS. The right atrial and right ventricular end-diastolic pressures are characteristically elevated in TR, whether the condition is due to organic disease of the tricuspid valve or is secondary to right ventricular systolic overload (e.g., pulmonary hypertension and pulmonic stenosis). The right atrial pressure tracing reveals absence of the x descent and a prominent v or c-v wave ("ventricularization" of the atrial pressure). Therefore, as the severity of tricuspid regurgitation increases, the right atrial pressure pulse increasingly resembles the right ventricular pressure pulse (Fig. 34–43).[598] A rise or no change in right atrial pressure on deep inspiration, rather than the usual fall, is characteristic.[641,658] Pulmonary artery (or right ventricular) systolic pressure may offer a rough guide as to whether the TR

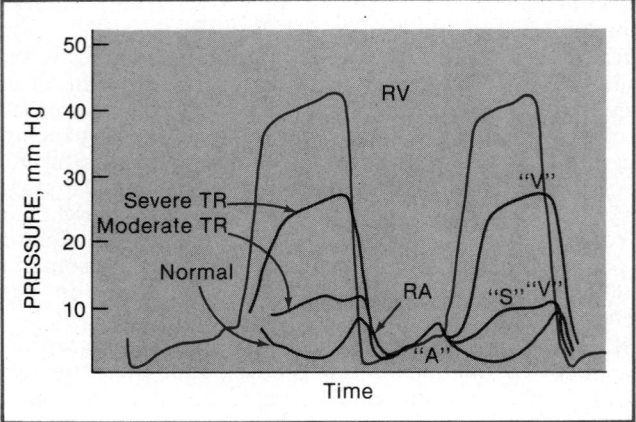

FIGURE 34–43. Appearance of right atrial (RA) pressure contour in patients with severe tricuspid regurgitation (TR), moderate TR, and no TR (normal). Note the regurgitant systolic ("S") wave that blends with the normal filling ("V") wave in severe TR. The resultant RA pressure waveform resembles a right ventricular (RV) pressure recording. (From Grossman, W. [ed.]: Cardiac Catheterization and Angiography. 3rd ed. Philadelphia, Lea and Febiger, 1986, p. 378.)

is primary (i.e., due to disease of the valve or its supporting structures) or secondary to right ventricular dilatation. A pulmonary artery or right ventricular systolic pressure less than 40 mm Hg favors a primary etiology, whereas a pressure greater than 60 mm Hg suggests that TR is secondary.

Diagnosis and quantitative assessment of TR can be aided in many instances by right ventriculography, but the fact that the catheter must be positioned across the tricuspid valve cannot exclude the possibility of a false-positive diagnosis of TR.[659] Modifications of previous angiographic techniques have been introduced in which a special, preformed catheter is positioned in the right ventricle, and angiography is carried out at low injection rates[660]; or a special balloon catheter is employed to minimize the induction of extrasystoles, which can also cause spurious regurgitation.[661]

MANAGEMENT

TR in the absence of pulmonary hypertension usually does not require surgical treatment. Indeed, both patients and experimental animals tolerate total excision of the tricuspid valve, as long as right ventricular systolic pressure is normal.[662] In some patients dilatation of the right side of the heart occurs months or years after tricuspid valvectomy (usually carried out for acute infective endocarditis), and insertion of a prosthetic valve can then be carried out after adequate sterilization of the valve ring.[662] *Surgical treatment* of acquired regurgitation secondary to annular dilatation was greatly improved when Carpentier introduced the concept of suturing the annulus to a right prosthetic ring of appropriate dimensions.[657,663] Annuloplasty without insertion of a prosthetic ring (so-called DeVega annuloplasty) has also been found to be effective in patients with annular dilatation. This technique is now widely employed.[664–666]

In patients with TR associated with mitral valve disease and pulmonary hypertension, the severity of the regurgitation should be assessed by palpation of the valve at the time of mitral commissurotomy or valve replacement. Patients with mild TR usually do not require surgical treatment[667]; pulmonary vascular pressures decline following successful mitral valve surgery, and the mild TR tends to disappear. Excellent results have been reported in patients with moderate TR with the use of tricuspid annuloplasty,[663] often utilizing a Carpentier ring[664,668,669] (Fig. 34–44). However, management of severe TR is more controversial. It is not clear whether severe TR should be treated by annuloplasty or valve replacement, but most surgeons prefer the former approach. If it does not pro-

vide a good functional result at the operating table, they resort to valve replacement.[670]

Organic disease of the tricuspid valve responsible for TR, as in Ebstein's anomaly[671,672] or carcinoid heart disease,[673] when severe enough to require surgery, usually requires valve replacement. The risk of thrombosis of valvular prostheses is greater in the tricuspid than in the mitral position, presumably because pressure and flow rates are lower in the right side of the heart. For this reason, the artificial valve of choice for the tricuspid position in adults at present is a large porcine heterograft. Anticoagulants are not required, and a durability of more than 10 years has been established.

In treating the difficult problem of tricuspid endocarditis in heroin addicts, it has been noted that total excision of the tricuspid valve *without immediate replacement* can be tolerated by these patients, who usually do not have associated pulmonary hypertension. However, surgery should be carried out in patients with resistant or relapsing infection after optimal antibiotic therapy.[661] When antibiotic therapy is unsuccessful, valvular replacement frequently results in reinfection or continued infection. Diseased valvular tissue should be excised to eradicate the endocarditis, and antibiotic treatment can be continued. Most patients tolerate loss of the tricuspid valve without great difficulty. However, if medical management does not control the tricuspid regurgitation and the infection has been controlled, an artificial valve can be inserted later.[662]

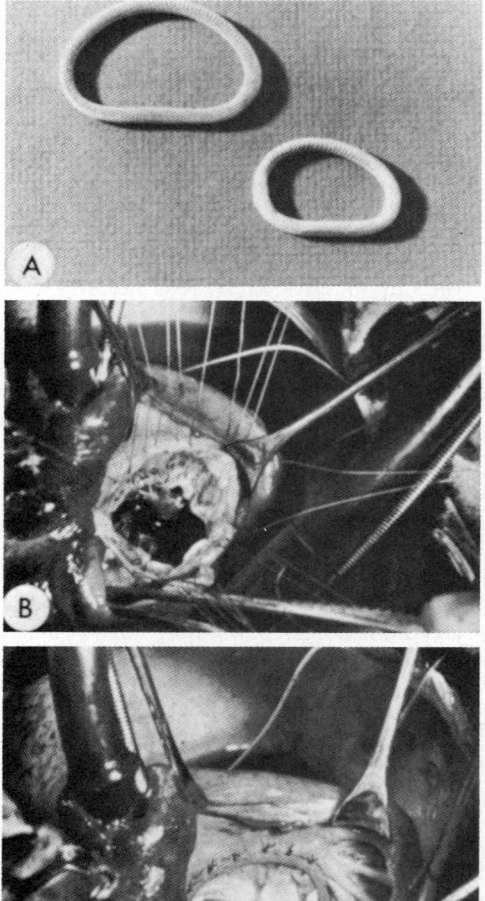

FIGURE 34–44. *A*, Carpentier rings. *B*, Ring being sutured into place. *C*, Completion of Carpentier ring annuloplasty. (From Starr, A.: Acquired disease of the tricuspid valve. *In* Sabiston, D. C., Jr., and Spencer, F. C. [eds.]: Gibbon's Surgery of the Chest. Philadelphia, W. B. Saunders Company, 1976, p. 1182.)

PULMONIC VALVE DISEASE

ETIOLOGY AND PATHOLOGY

The congenital form is the most common cause of *pulmonic stenosis* (PS).[674] Its manifestations in children are discussed on page 931 and in adults on page 968. *Rheumatic* inflammation of the pulmonic valve is very uncommon, is usually associated with involvement of other valves, and rarely leads to serious deformity. However, a high incidence of significant pulmonic valve involvement secondary to rheumatic fever has been reported in Mexico City, perhaps related to the pulmonary hypertension that occurs at high altitudes and the resultant greater stress on the pulmonic valve.[675] *Carcinoid* plaques, similar to those involving the tricuspid valve, are often present in the outflow tract of the right ventricle in patients with malignant carcinoid and result in constriction of the pulmonic valve ring, retraction and fusion of the valve cusps, and either PS or the combination of PS and pulmonic regurgitation (PR) (Fig. 34–45).[676] Obstruction in the region of the pulmonic valve may be extrinsic to the valve apparatus and may be produced by cardiac tumors or aneurysm of the sinus Valsalva.[677]

By far the most common cause of PR is dilatation of the valve ring secondary to pulmonary hypertension (of any etiology) or to dilatation of the pulmonary artery, either idiopathic[678,679] or consequent to a connective tissue disorder such as Marfan syndrome.[680] The second most common cause is infective endocarditis.[676,681–683] Less frequently, it is iatrogenic and is induced at the time of surgical treatment of congenital PS or tetralogy of Fallot. It may also result from a variety of lesions directly affecting the pulmonic valve. These include congenital malformations, such as absent, malformed, fenestrated, or supernumerary leaflets.[11] These anomalies may occur as isolated lesions[684] but more often are associated with other congenital anomalies, particularly tetralogy of Fallot, ventricular septal defect, and pulmonic valvular stenosis. Less common causes include carcinoid syndrome,[676] rheumatic involvement,[685] injury produced by a pulmonary artery flow-directed catheter,[686] syphilis,[629] and chest trauma.[683]

CLINICAL MANIFESTATIONS

Like TR, isolated PR causes right ventricular volume overload and may be tolerated for many years without difficulty unless it complicates or is complicated by pulmonary hypertension, in which case it is usually accompanied by and aggravates right ventricular failure. Patients with PR caused by infective endocarditis who develop septic pulmonary emboli and pulmonary hypertension often exhibit severe right ventricular failure.[683] In most patients the clinical manifestations of the primary disease are severe and usually overshadow the PR, which often results only in incidental auscultatory findings. *Physical examination* reveals a hyperdynamic right ventricle, producing palpable systolic pulsations in the left parasternal area and an enlarged pulmonary artery that often results in palpable systolic pulsations in the second left intercostal space; sometimes systolic and diastolic thrills are felt in the same area. A tap reflecting pulmonic valve closure is usually easily palpable in the second intercostal space in patients with pulmonary hypertension and secondary PR.

AUSCULTATION. In patients with congenital absence of the pulmonic valve, P_2 is not audible, but this sound is accentuated in patients with PR secondary to pulmonary hypertension, particularly when the dilated pulmonary artery is near the chest wall. There may be wide splitting of S_2 due to prolongation of right ventricular ejection accompanying the augmented stroke volume.[685] A nonvalvular systolic ejection click due to the sudden expansion of the pulmonary artery by the augmented right ventricular stroke volume frequently initiates a midsystolic ejection murmur, most prominent in the second left intercostal space. An S_3 and S_4 originating from the right ventricle are often audible, most readily in the fourth intercostal space at the left parasternal area, and are augmented by inspiration.

In the absence of pulmonary hypertension, the diastolic murmur of PR is low-pitched and is usually heard best at the third and fourth left intercostal spaces adjacent to the sternum (Fig. 3–32, p. 58). The murmur commences when pressures in the pulmonary artery and right ventricle diverge, approximately 0.04 sec after P_2. It is diamond-shaped in configuration and brief, reaching a peak intensity when the gradient between these pressures is maximal and ending with equilibration of the pressures.[687] The murmur becomes louder during inspiration[688] and following inhalation of amyl nitrite.

When pulmonary artery systolic pressure exceeds approximately 60 mm Hg, dilatation of the pulmonic annulus results in a regurgitant jet of high velocity that is responsible for the so-called Graham Steell murmur of PR. (Doppler ultrasound reveals pulmonary regurgitation at much lower pulmonary arterial pressures.[689]) The Graham Steell murmur is a high-pitched, blowing decrescendo murmur beginning immediately after P_2 and is most prominent in the left parasternal region in the second to fourth intercostal spaces. Thus, although it resembles the murmur of AR, it is usually accompanied by the findings of severe pulmonary hypertension, i.e., an accentuated P_2 or fused S_2, an ejection sound, and a systolic murmur of tricuspid regurgitation. Sometimes a low-frequency presystolic murmur is present, i.e., a right-sided Austin Flint murmur originating from the tricuspid valve that is analogous to the more common left-sided Austin Flint murmur originating from the mitral valve.[690]

The Graham Steell murmur of PR secondary to pulmonary hypertension usually increases in intensity with inspiration, exhibits little change after amyl nitrite inhalation or vasopressors, is diminished during the Valsalva strain, and returns to baseline intensity almost immediately after release of the Valsalva strain. This murmur resembles and may be confused with the diastolic blowing murmur of AR. However, indicator dilution studies[691] and aortography have established that a diastolic blowing murmur along the left sternal border in patients with rheumatic heart disease and pulmonary hypertension — even in the absence of peripheral signs of AR — is usually due to AR and not PR.

LABORATORY EXAMINATION

ELECTROCARDIOGRAM. In the absence of pulmonary hypertension, PR often results in an ECG that reflects right ventricular diastolic overload, i.e., an rSr' (or rsR') configuration in the right precordial leads. PR secondary to pulmonary hypertension is usually associated with ECG evidence of right ventricular hypertrophy.

RADIOLOGICAL FINDINGS. Both the pulmonary artery and the right ventricle are usually enlarged,[692] but these signs are nonspecific. Fluoros-

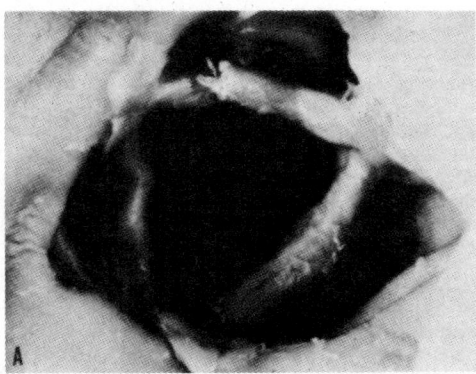

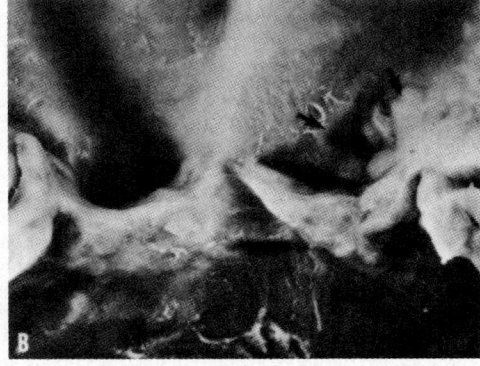

FIGURE 34–45. Carcinoid heart disease; pulmonary valve viewed from above (*A*) and opened (*B*). The thickened and retracted cusps result in valvular incompetence. The constricted annulus results in valvular stenosis. Carcinoid plaques (arrows) extend onto the pulmonary trunk. (From Callahan, J. A., et al.: Echocardiographic features of carcinoid heart disease. Am. J. Cardiol. *50*:767, 1982.)

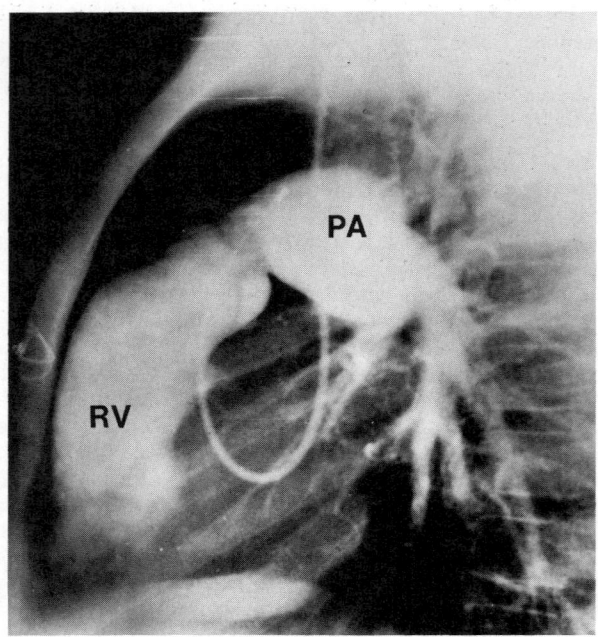

FIGURE 34–46. Pulmonic valvular regurgitation. Contrast medium has been injected into the main pulmonary artery (PA) and regurgitates back into an enlarged right ventricle (RV). (From Carlsson, E., et al.: The radiological diagnosis of cardiac valvular insufficiency. Circulation 55:921, 1977, by permission of the American Heart Association, Inc.)

copy may demonstrate pronounced pulsation of the main pulmonary artery. PR can be diagnosed by observing opacification of the right ventricle following injection of contrast material into the main pulmonary artery (Fig. 34–46). The diagnosis is supported by noting superimposition of the pulmonary artery and right ventricular pressure curves during mid and late diastole. Indicator dilution techniques with injections into the pulmonary artery and sampling from the right ventricle,[693] as well as intracardiac phonocardiography,[629] can also be helpful in establishing the diagnosis in mild cases.

ECHOCARDIOGRAM. This shows right ventricular dilatation and, in patients with pulmonary hypertension, right ventricular hypertrophy as well. Diastolic fluttering of the tricuspid valve leaflets, similar to that of the mitral valve leaflets in AR, is often noted. Abnormal motion of the septum characteristic of volume overload of the right ventricle in diastole and/or septal flutter[694] may be evident. The motion of the pulmonic valve may point to the etiology of the pulmonic regurgitation.[695] Absence of *a* waves and systolic notching of the posterior leaflet suggest pulmonary hypertension; large *a* waves indicate pulmonic stenosis. PR can be detected by contrast echocardiography.[696] The pulsed Doppler technique is extremely accurate in detecting PR. Abnormal Doppler signals in the right ventricular outflow tract whose velocity is sustained throughout diastole are generally observed in patients in whom dilatation of the valve ring (functional regurgitation) is the cause. When the velocity falls during diastole, the pulmonary artery pressure is usually normal, and the regurgitation is caused by an abnormality of the valve itself.[695]

MANAGEMENT. PR per se is seldom severe enough to require specific treatment. Cardiac glycosides are useful in the management of right ventricular dilatation or failure. Treatment of the primary condition such as infective endocarditis or of the lesion responsible for the pulmonary hypertension, such as surgical treatment of mitral valvular disease, often ameliorates the PR. Surgical treatment of primary PR directed specifically at the pulmonic valve is required only occasionally because of intractable right heart failure, and under such circumstances valve replacement may be carried out.[697]

MULTIVALVULAR DISEASE

Multivalvular involvement is common, particularly in patients with rheumatic heart disease, and a variety of clinical and hemodynamic syndromes can be produced by different combinations of valvular abnormalities. Development of PR and TR secondary to dilatation of the pulmonic valve ring and tricuspid annulus, respectively, as a consequence of pulmonary hypertension secondary to disease involving the mitral or aortic valve or both, has already been discussed (pp. 1055 and 1060), as has the combi-

nation of *organic* rheumatic tricuspid and mitral valvular disease. In patients with multivalvular disease, the clinical manifestations depend on the relative severities of each of the lesions.[698] When the valvular abnormalities are of approximately equal severity, as a general rule, clinical manifestations produced by the more proximal (upstream) of two valvular lesions, i.e., the mitral valve in patients with combined mitral and aortic valvular disease and the tricuspid valve in patients with combined tricuspid and mitral valvular disease, are more prominent than those produced by the distal lesion.

It is important to recognize multivalvular involvement preoperatively, since failure to correct all significant valvular disease at the time of operation increases mortality considerably. In patients with multivalvular disease, the relative severity of each lesion may be difficult to estimate by clinical examination and noninvasive techniques, because one lesion may mask the manifestations of the other. For this reason, patients suspected of multivalvular involvement and in whom surgical treatment is under consideration should undergo (in addition to careful clinical examination and noninvasive workup, with emphasis on two-dimensional and Doppler echocardiography), right- and left-sided cardiac catheterization and angiography. If there is any question concerning the presence of significant AS in patients undergoing an operation on the mitral valve, the aortic valve should be inspected, since overlooking this condition can lead to a high perioperative mortality. Similarly, it is useful to palpate the tricuspid valve at the time of operation on the mitral valve.

Mitral Stenosis and Aortic Regurgitation

Approximately two-thirds of patients with severe MS have an early blowing diastolic murmur along the left sternal border with a normal pulse pressure; in 90 per cent of these the murmur is due to AR and is usually of little clinical importance. However, approximately 10 per cent of patients with MS have severe rheumatic AR,[699] which can usually be recognized by the peripheral signs of a widened pulse pressure, left ventricular dilatation and increased wall motion on echocardiography, and signs of left ventricular enlargement on radiological and electrocardiographic examinations.

In keeping with the general observation that a proximal lesion may mask a distal lesion, significant AR may be missed in patients with severe MS. The widened pulse pressure, in particular, may be absent in the latter. On clinical examination of patients with obvious AR, errors may be made in that MS may be missed or, conversely, may be falsely diagnosed. An accentuated S_1 and an opening snap in a patient with AR should suggest the possibility of mitral valvular disease. On the other hand, an Austin Flint murmur is often inappropriately considered to be the diastolic rumbling murmur of MS (Table 34–14). These two murmurs may be distinguished at the bedside by means of amyl nitrite inhalation, which diminishes the Austin Flint murmur (Fig. 3–32, p. 58) but augments the murmur of MS; isometric handgrip and squatting augment both the diastolic murmur of AR and the Austin Flint murmur. Echocardiography, particularly pulsed Doppler echocardiography, is of decisive value in the detection of both lesions. Diastolic fluttering of the anterior leaflet of the mitral valve and of the ventricular spectrum is an important clue to the presence of AR in a patient with MS. Evidence of rapid left ventricular filling in diastole by echocardiography should suggest the presence of associated AR.

Hemodynamic analysis reveals that MS reduces the left ventricular volume overload characteristic of AR.[607] This combination is relatively uncommon.

Mitral Stenosis and Aortic Stenosis

When severe MS and AS coexist, the former masks many of the manifestations of the latter.[701] The cardiac output tends to be reduced further than in patients with isolated AS, and the atrial booster pump mechanism, so important in filling the ventricle in AS (p. 1035), has little impact when MS is present. The reduction in cardiac output lowers both the transaortic valvular pressure gradient and the left ventricular systolic pressure, diminishes the incidence of angina, and retards the development of aortic calcification and left ventricular hypertrophy.[702] On the other hand, clinical manifestations associated with MS, such as pulmonary congestion and hemoptysis, atrial fibrillation, and systemic embolization, occur more frequently than in patients with isolated AS. On physical examination, presystolic distention of the left ventricle and an S_4, common in pure AS, are usually not present. The midsystolic murmur characteristic of AS may be reduced in intensity and duration because of the reduced stroke volume. The *electrocardiogram* may fail to demonstrate left ventricular hypertrophy, but left atrial enlargement is common in patients in sinus rhythm. The *chest roentgenogram* is usually typical of MS except that calcium may be present in the region of the aortic valve. The two-dimensional and Doppler *echocardiograms* are of the greatest value because stenosis of both valves may be evident. However, the low cardiac output characteristic of the combination of lesions may reduce the transvalvular gradients estimated by Doppler echocardiography. The indirect *carotid pulse* tracing reveals a delayed upstroke.

It is vital to recognize the presence of hemodynamically significant aortic valvular disease (stenosis and/or regurgitation) preoperatively in patients who are to undergo surgical correction of MS, since isolated mitral valvulotomy may be hazardous in such patients; this operation can impose a sudden hemodynamic load on the left ventricle that may lead to acute pulmonary edema.

Aortic Stenosis and Mitral Regurgitation

The combination of severe AS and MR is a hazardous one, but fortunately it is relatively uncommon. Obstruction to left ventricular outflow augments the volume of MR flow,[170] whereas the presence of MR diminishes the ventricular preload necessary for maintenance of the left ventricular stroke volume in AS. The result is a reduced forward cardiac output and marked left atrial and pulmonary venous hypertension. The physical findings may be confusing because the delayed arterial pulse of AS may be counteracted by the sharp upstroke of MR, and it may be difficult to recognize two distinct systolic murmurs. Amyl nitrite tends to increase the intensity of the murmur of AS and to reduce that of MR. On echocardiography and roentgenography the left atrium and ventricle are usually larger than in isolated AS. Usually both valves must be treated surgically in patients with severe AS and MR.

Aortic Regurgitation and Mitral Regurgitation

This relatively frequent combination of lesions[703] may be caused by rheumatic heart disease or by prolapse of both valves due to myxomatous degeneration,[704] or dilatation of both annuli in connective tissue disorders. The clinical features of AR usually predominate, and it sometimes is difficult to determine whether the MR is due to organic involvement of this valve or dilatation of the mitral valve ring secondary to left ventricular enlargement. When both valvular leaks are severe, this combination of lesions is poorly tolerated. The normal mitral valve ordinarily serves as a "backup" to the aortic valve, and premature (diastolic) closure of the mitral valve limits the volume of reflux that occurs in patients with acute AR.[513] With combined regurgitant lesions, regardless of the etiology of the mitral lesion, blood may reflux from the aorta through both chambers of the left side of the heart into the pulmonary veins. Physical and laboratory examination will usually show evidence of both lesions. Both lesions are frequently associated with an S_3 and a brisk arterial pulse. The relative severity of each lesion can be assessed best by contrast angiography.

When MR occurs in patients with AR secondary to left ventricular dilatation, it often regresses following aortic valve replacement. If severe, it may be corrected by annuloplasty at the time of aortic valve replacement. Replacement of an intrinsically normal mitral valve that is regurgitant due to a dilated annulus is neither necessary nor advisable.

Surgical Treatment of Multivalvular Disease

Combined aortic and mitral valve replacement is usually associated with a higher risk and poorer survival than is replacement of either of the two valves alone.[705] Kirklin reported a 5-year survival rate of 70 per cent after double-valve replacement compared to 80 per cent for single-valve replacement.[706] The long-term survival is strongly dependent on the functional status preoperatively.[707] Also, patients operated on for the combination of AR and MR fared worse than did patients receiving double-valve replacement for any of the other combinations.[706] The operative risk of double valve replacement is about twice as high as it is for single valve replacement, and like the latter has been slowly but steadily declining.[708]

Hemodynamically significant disease involving the mitral, aortic, and tricuspid valves is uncommon. Patients with these lesions often present in advanced heart failure with marked cardiomegaly, and surgical correction of all three valvular lesions is imperative. Attempts to shorten the duration of operation by leaving one severely impaired valve in place after a double valve replacement are usually unsatisfactory. However, triple valve replacement is a long and complex operation. In one early series, the mortality rate was 18 per cent in patients in functional Class III and 40 per cent in Class IV.[709] In a more recent one it was only 5 per cent.[710,711] However, even this high risk must often be accepted because of the otherwise dismal prognosis in these patients. An alternative is to replace the mitral and aortic valves and carry out a tricuspid valvuloplasty.[710,711]

Patients who survive triple-valve replacement usually show substantial clinical improvement in the early postoperative period,[712-714] and postoperative catheterization studies show marked reductions in pulmonary arterial and capillary pressures.[715] However, some patients succumb to arrhythmias[714] or congestive heart failure in the late postoperative period despite normally functioning prostheses. The cause of cardiac failure in this situation is not known, but it may be related to intraoperative myocardial ischemia, microemboli from the multiple prostheses, or continued subclinical episodes of rheumatic myocarditis.

When multiple prosthetic valves must be inserted, it is logical to select either two (or three) bioprostheses or mechanical prostheses for the left side of the heart. If the patient is to be exposed to the hazards of anticoagulants for one mechanical prosthesis, it seems unreasonable to add the potential risks of early failure of a bioprosthesis. However, the use of a bioprosthesis in the tricuspid position is suggested.[710]

Prosthetic Cardiac Valves

The first successful replacements of cardiac valves in the human were accomplished by Nina Braunwald,[715] Harken et al.,[716] and Starr[717] in 1960. Two major groups of artificial (prosthetic) valves are currently available in models designed for both the atrioventricular (mitral and tricuspid) and the aortic positions: mechanical prostheses and bioprostheses (tissue valves).

MECHANICAL PROSTHESES
(Table 34–18)

Mechanical prosthetic valves are classified into two major groups: caged-ball and tilting-disc valves. The *Starr-Edwards* caged-ball valve (Figs. 34–47A and 34–48) is still widely used in both the aortic and mitral positions.[718,719] It has the longest record of predictable performance of any artificial valve. A disadvantage is its bulky cage design. It is therefore not suitable in patients with a small left ventricular cavity or a small aortic annulus or in a valve–aortic arch composite graft. In a small number of patients it induces hemolysis, which may be greatly exaggerated and become of clinical importance if a perivalvular leak develops.

Several types of tilting-disc valves are widely employed; these are less bulky and have a lower profile than the caged-ball valve. The *St. Jude* valve (Fig. 34–47E), constructed of pyrolytic carbon, has two semicircular discs that pivot between open and closed positions without the need for supporting struts (Fig. 34–48). It possesses favorable flow characteristics and causes a lower transvalvular gradient at any outer diameter and cardiac output than the caged-ball or tilting valves.[720,721] It is the most widely used mechanical prosthetic valve in the United States at the time of this writing. The St. Jude valve appears to have particularly favorable hemodynamic characteristics in the smaller sizes; therefore, it may be especially useful in children. Thrombogenicity in the mitral position *may* be less than for other prosthetic valves. As with other mechanical prostheses, permanent anticoagulation is needed—antiplatelet agents alone are not sufficient.[720] A variation of the St. Jude valve, the *Duromedics* prosthesis (Fig. 34–47F), is also a bileaflet valve with curved leaflets and a hinge design, which supposedly enhances central flow and hemodynamic performance. This valve appears to cause less regurgitation than other tilting-disc valves; the incidence of valve thrombosis and thromboembolism appears to be low.[722]

The *Lillehei-Kaster* pivoting-disc valve consists of a titanium valve housing with a Teflon fabric sewing ring in which a pyrolyte disc is suspended. In the open position, the disc swings to an angle of 80 degrees, providing a large central flow orifice. This is an excellent valve in larger sizes in the aortic position, but a relatively high incidence of thrombosis pre-

TABLE 34-18   RELATIVE RISK OF SPECIFIC PROSTHESIS-ASSOCIATED COMPLICATIONS WITH VARIOUS VALVE TYPES

COMPLICATIONS	GENERIC VALVE TYPE/MODELS USED						
	Caged-Ball (Bare-Cage)/ Starr-Edwards, Smerloff-Cutter	Caged-Ball (Cloth-Covered)/ Starr-Edwards, Braunwald-Cutter	Caged-Disc/ Beall	Tilting-Disc/ Björk-Shiley Hall-Medtronic Lillehei-Kaster	Bileaflet Tilting-Disc/ St. Jude/ Edwards-Duromedics	Porcine Bioprosthesis/ Hancock/ Carpentier-Edwards	Pericardial Bioprosthesis/ Ionescu-Shiley
Obstruction	++	++	+++	+	+	+	+
Hemolysis[a]	+	+	+	+	+	+	+
Paravalvular leak	++	++	++	++	++	++	++
Endocarditis	++	++	++	++	++	++	++
Thrombosis/thromboembolism	+++	+++	+++	+++	++	+	+
Extrinsic interference	+	++	++	++	+	+	+
Component fracture/ escape	+	++	+	+[b]	+	+	+
Ball (or disc) variance	+[c]	+	+	NA	+	NA	NA
Ball (or disc) abrasive wear	+	+[d]	+++[e]	+	+	NA	NA
Cloth wear	NA	++	NA	NA	NA	NA	NA
Leaflet tears	NA	NA	NA	NA	NA	+++	+++
Calcification	NA	NA	NA	NA	NA	+++	+++

NA = not applicable, + = rare, ++ = frequent, +++ = major problem; [a] = new onset or increasing hemolysis generally indicates dysfunctional valve; [b] = some Björk-Shiley valves are partially susceptible; [c] = lipid uptake unusual in valves fabricated since 1964; [d] = occurs only with cloth-covered valves with silicone ball; [e] = except in valves with pyrolytic carbon disc.

From Schoen, F. J.: Valvular heart disease. *In* Interventional and Surgical Cardiovascular Pathology. Philadelphia, W. B. Saunders Company, 1989, p. 156.

cludes its use in the mitral position.[723-725] Two adaptations of the Lillehei-Kaster tilting-disc valve, the *Omniscience*[724,726] (Fig. 34–47C) and the *Omnicarbon*[723] valves, have been introduced in an effort to improve hemodynamics and decrease thrombogenicity. Early reports suggest that both of these goals may have been achieved. A closely related valve is the *Medtronic-Hall* valve (Fig. 34–47D). Its pivoting disc has a central perforation that allows improved hemodynamics; thrombogenicity appears to be quite low, less than 1 episode per 100 patient-years in the aortic position and 1.5 per 100 patient-years in the mitral position[727,728]; mechanical performance is excellent over the long term. The *Björk-Shiley* valve[729-731] (Fig. 34–47B) consists of a low-profile cobalt base alloy covered with a Teflon fabric sewing ring; its design allows an excellent ratio between the diameter of the valve orifice and tissue annulus. It contains a suspended tilting-disc occluder made of pyrolytic carbon (pyrolyte). Two serious problems with this valve have been reported in a small number of patients: (1) sudden thrombosis and (2) strut fracture. Changes have been made to overcome the first of these problems, but in some models the incidence of strut fracture is prohibitive. Accordingly, this valve, previously very popular, is not being used in the United States at present.

DURABILITY AND THROMBOGENICITY. Most of these mechanical prosthetic valves have an excellent record of durability—up to 30 years in the case of the caged-ball valves. However, patients with any mechanical prosthesis, regardless of design or site of placement, require long-term anticoagulation because of the hazard of thromboembolism, which is greatest in the first postoperative year. Without anticoagulation, the incidence of thromboembolism is three- to sixfold higher than with proper doses.[731] Anticoagulation with sodium warfarin should begin about 2 days after operation, and a prothrombin time in the range of 1.5 times control should be achieved. This relatively conservative approach reduces the risk of anticoagulant hemorrhage yet does not appear to be associated with a greater frequency of thromboembolism than a prothrombin time of 2.0 to 2.5 times control. It must be recognized that (1) the administration of warfarin carries its own mortality and morbidity, estimated at 0.2 and 2.2 per 100 patient-years, respectively; and (2) despite treatment with anticoagulants, the incidence of thromboembolic complications with the best mechanical prostheses is still about 0.2 (fatal) and 1 to 2 (nonfatal) per 100 patient-years. This incidence tends to be slightly higher for prostheses in the mitral than in

the aortic position; thrombosis of mechanical prostheses in the tricuspid position is quite high, and for this reason bioprostheses are preferred at this site. The incidence of embolization in patients who have experienced repeated emboli from a prosthetic valve despite anticoagulants may be reduced by replacement with a tissue valve.

TISSUE VALVES

Largely to overcome the risk of thromboembolism that is inherent in all mechanical prosthetic valves and the attendant hazards and inconvenience of permanent anticoagulant therapy just discussed, considerable effort has been devoted to the development of nonthrombogenic tissue valves.[732,733] The first of these to be widely used were chemically sterilized homografts. These exhibited a high incidence of breakdown within 3 years. Fresh antibiotic-treated cryopreserved frozen-irradiated homografts were then developed. These are more durable[734-737]; while they have many desirable properties, their use has been restricted by the problems inherent in their procurement.

PORCINE HETEROGRAFTS. To overcome this difficulty, porcine heterografts were developed and have been used clinically since 1965. Two porcine heterografts are widely used today[725,726,738-742]: (1) The *Hancock* valve is fixed with 0.2 per cent glutaraldehyde and is mounted on a Dacron cloth–covered flexible polypropylene strut. In the smaller aortic models, the right coronary cusp is replaced by a posterior cusp from another valve to reduce obstruction resulting from the septal shelf of the valve. (2) The *Carpentier-Edwards* valve[738] (Fig. 34–47G) is pressure-fixed with 0.625 per cent glutaraldehyde and is mounted on a Teflon-covered Eljiloy strut in a manner as to minimize the septal shelf. The hemodynamic profiles of the porcine heterografts are similar to those of comparably sized low-profile mechanical prostheses.[743,744] In contrast to the latter, however, the valve orifice is blood flow–dependent, with greater orifice size as transvalvular flow increases. The Hancock valve has been reported to have slightly better hemodynamics than the Carpentier-Edwards valve.[734,735]

During the first 3 postoperative months, while the sewing ring becomes endothelialized, the thromboembolic rate is high enough that anticoagulation is extremely desirable. Thereafter, anticoagulants are not required for porcine valves in the aortic position, and the thromboembolic rate is approxi-

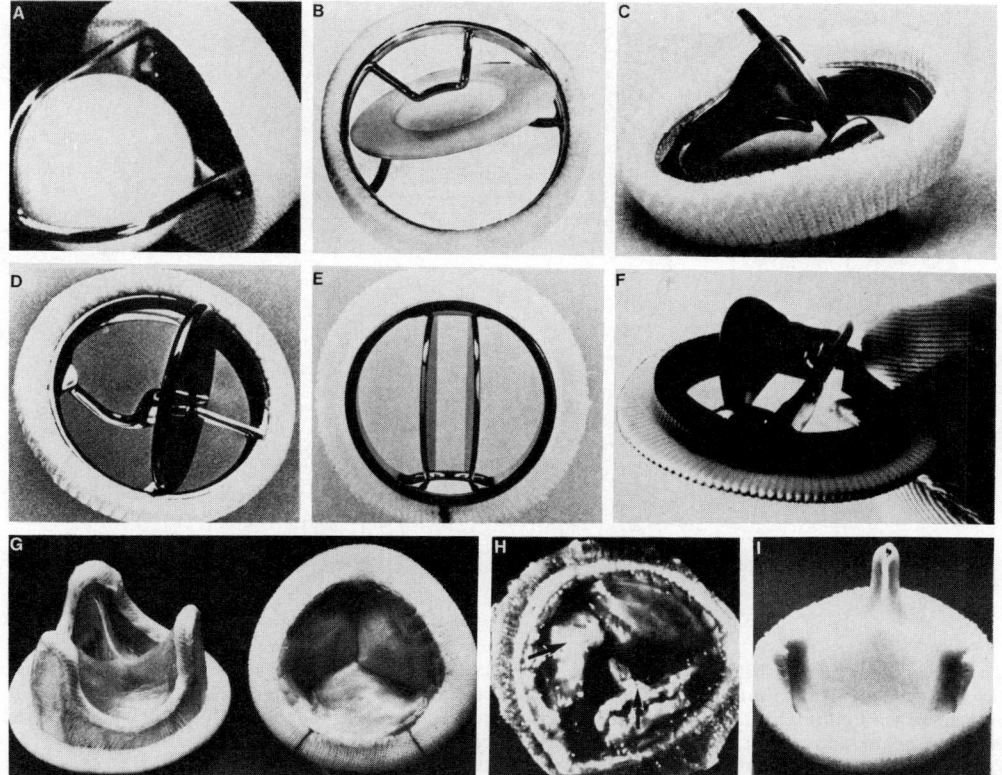

FIGURE 34–47. Prosthetic cardiac valves. *A*, Starr-Edwards caged-ball valve with cloth sewing ring and bare struts. *B*, Björk-Shiley tilting disc valve. *C*, Omniscience tilting disc valve. *D*, Medtronic-Hall tilting disc valve. *E*, St. Jude medical bileaflet valve as viewed end on. Note the large size of the effective orifice area compared with the potential orifice area and the minimal obstruction to flow by the leaflets. *F*, Duromedics bileaflet valve. *G*, Carpentier-Edwards prosthetic valve. *H*, Porcine valve removed several years following implantation because of primary valve failure; arrows point to areas of calcification and destruction of leaflets. *I*, Ionescu-Shiley pericardial valve. (*A* from Starek, P.J.K., and *F* from Clark, R. E., *in* Heart Valve Replacement and Reconstruction. Chicago, Year Book Medical Publishers, 1987, pp. 223 and 286. *B* from Björk, V.; C from Austin, E. H., III.; *E* and *I* from Crawford, F. A., Jr.; *G* and *H* from Magilligan, D. J., Jr., *in* Crawford, F. A. [ed.]: Cardiac Surgery: Current Heart Valve Prostheses, Vol. 1. Philadelphia, Hanley and Belfus, 1987, pp. 184, 204, 252, 270, 271, and 286. *D* from Cobanoglu, A., and Brockman, S. K., *in* Frankl, W. S., and Brest, A. N. [eds.]: Valvular Heart Disease: Comprehensive Evaluation and Management. Philadelphia, F. A. Davis, 1986, p. 404.)

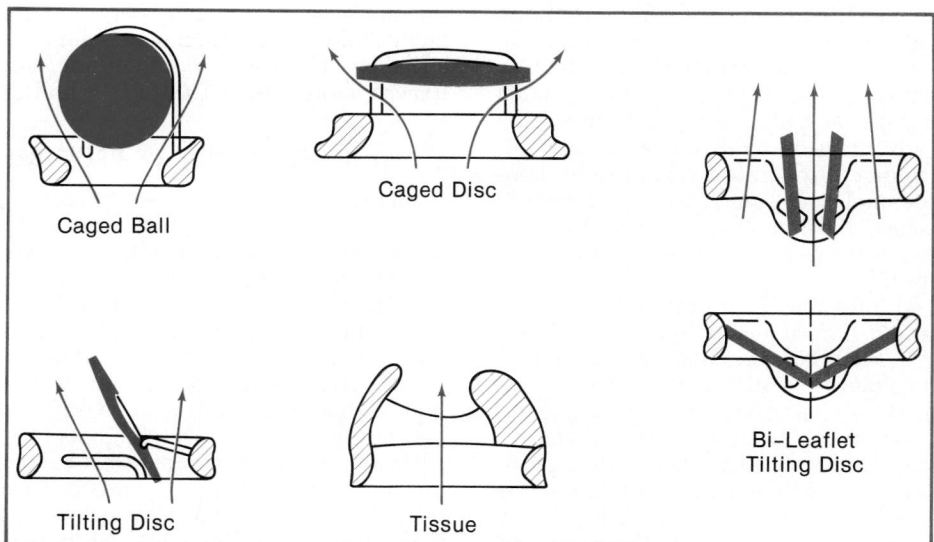

FIGURE 34–48. Designs and flow patterns of major categories of prosthetic heart valves: caged-ball, caged-disc, tilting-disc, bi-leaflet tilting-disc, and bioprosthetic (tissue) valves. While flow in mechanical valves must course along both sides of the occluder, bioprostheses have a central flow pattern. (Reproduced by permission from Schoen, F. J., et al.: Bioengineering aspects of heart valve replacement. Ann. Biomed. Eng. *10*:97, 1982. Copyright 1983, Pergamon Press Limited, 1983; and from Schoen, F. J.: Pathology of cardiac valve replacement. *In* Morse, D., Steiner, R. M., Fernandez, J. [eds.]: Guide to Prosthetic Cardiac Valves, p. 209. New York, Springer-Verlag, 1985. Copyright Springer-Verlag, Inc., 1985.)

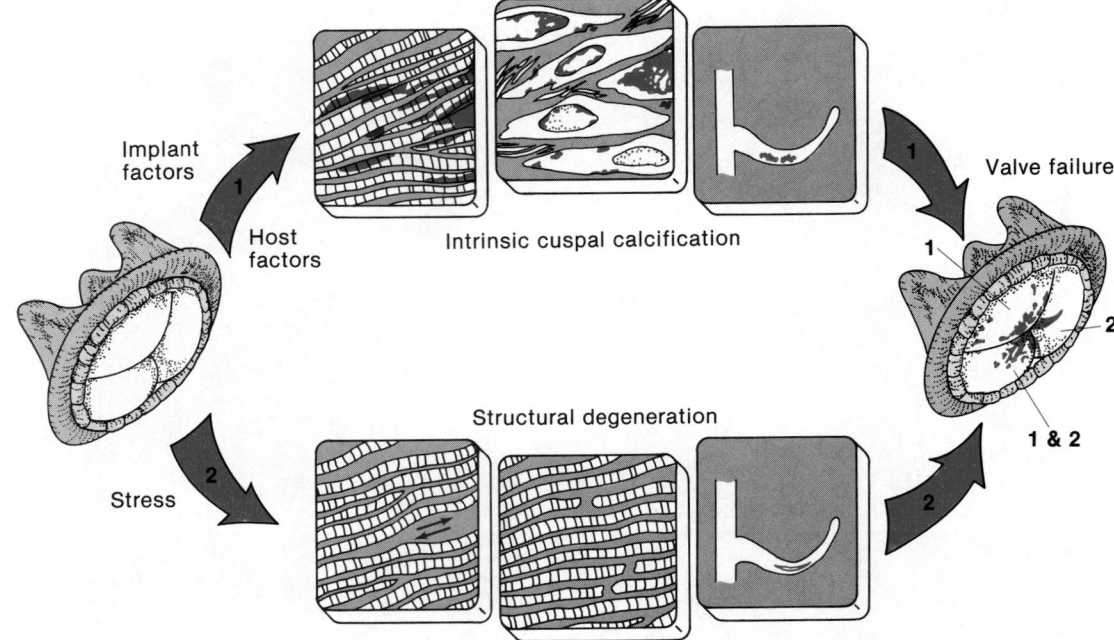

FIGURE 34–49. Unified model for bioprosthetic heart valve failure relating isolated tissue processes of mineralization (Pathway 1) and collagen degeneration (Pathway 2) to gross clinical failures. Such failures have calcification with cuspal stiffening (1), cuspal defects without calcific deposits (2), or cuspal tears associated with mineralization (1 and 2). These processes may occur independently or they may be synergistic. Specifically, implant and host factors interact to induce the collagen-oriented and cell-oriented calcific deposits noted ultrastructurally. The deposits predominate in the central portions of valve cusps, particularly at flexion points such as the commissures (Pathway 1). Stress causes shear between and fracture of collagen fibers, which may create gross cuspal defects (Pathway 2). Although dynamic mechanical activity is not a prerequisite for calcification, stress may promote (i.e., accelerate) this process through unknown mechanisms. (Amended from Schoen, F. J., and Levy, R. J.: Bioprosthetic heart valve failure: Pathology and pathogenesis. Cardiol. Clin. *2*:717, 1984.)

mately 1 to 2 episodes per 100 patient-years without these drugs.[733,739,742] When these valves have been placed in the mitral position in patients who are in sinus rhythm, anticoagulants are not needed (after the first 3 postoperative months), and the thromboembolic rate is also approximately 1 to 2 per 100 patient-years. This is comparable to that in patients with the St. Jude or other mechanical valves receiving anticoagulants and therefore subject to the risks of thrombosis. In patients undergoing mitral valve replacement who have experienced a previous embolus, in whom thrombus is found in the left atrium at operation or who remain in atrial fibrillation postoperatively (approximately one-third of all patients receiving mitral valve replacements), the hazard of thromboembolism persists. Indeed, in patients with atrial fibrillation the incidence of postoperative emboli following implantation of a porcine bioprosthesis into the mitral position is three times as high as in patients in sinus rhythm. Therefore, anticoagulants are required in those patients with these risk factors. This negates the principal advantage of the tissue valves. It is unlikely that any replacement of the mitral valve can be associated with a thromboembolic rate much below 0.5 per 100 patient-years, since some of the emboli in patients with long-standing mitral disease are derived from the left atrium rather than from the valve itself.[745]

The major problem with porcine bioprostheses is their limited durability (Fig. 34–49). Cuspal tears, degeneration, fibrin deposition, disruption of the fibrocollagenous structure, perforation, fibrosis, and calcification sufficiently severe to require reoperation (Fig. 34–47H) begin to appear in the fourth or fifth postoperative year, so that by 10 years the rate of primary tissue failure is approximately 20 per cent. It then accelerates,[733] and in one report in which a 15-year follow-up is described[734] the actuarial freedom from bioprosthetic primary tissue failure was only 45 per cent for valves in the mitral and 50 per cent for valves in the aortic position. It is likely that with the passage of time even more of these valves will fail, and essentially all valves implanted into patients aged less than 60 years will have to be replaced.[746] Fortunately, however, these valves usually do not fail suddenly (as is usually the case for failure of mechanical prostheses), and the second operation can often be carried out on an elective basis, with a

surgical mortality in the range of 10 to 15 per cent.[742] Color Doppler echocardiography with two-dimensional transthoracic[743,744] or transesophageal imaging is extremely helpful in the early detection of bioprosthetic malfunction. The time after implantation at which tissue valves fail varies inversely with age; it is prohibitively rapid in children and young adults. Valve degeneration is extremely rare in patients older than 70 years at the time of implantation.[733,739] Bioprostheses also have extremely limited durability in patients with chronic renal failure and hypercalcemia related to secondary hyperparathyroidism.

PERICARDIAL XENOGRAFT. A second major type of bioprosthetic valve is the *Ionescu-Shiley pericardial xenograft* (Fig. 34–47I),[747,748] which consists of glutaraldehyde-treated bovine pericardium from which three leaflets are mounted on a Dacron velour–covered titanium frame. This valve has an unacceptable rate of failure[747,748] and therefore is no longer widely used.

HEMODYNAMICS OF VALVE REPLACEMENTS

All valve replacements—mechanical prostheses as well as tissue valves—have an effective in vitro orifice size that is *smaller* than the normal valve at the same site.[732,733,749] After implantation, tissue ingrowth and endothelialization reduce the size of the in vivo effective orifice further. Therefore, all prosthetic valves currently available must be considered to be mildly stenotic. However, postoperative hemodynamic measurements of the rigid prostheses show reasonably good function, with effective mitral valve orifice areas averaging 1.7 to 2.0 cm^2 and mitral valve gradients of 4 to 8 mm Hg at rest. Although definitive comparisons have not been carried out, the cloth-covered Starr-Edwards valve appears to be intrinsically slightly more stenotic than the tilting-disc valves. The St. Jude valve, in turn, may be slightly superior to the latter. In hemodynamic studies, the porcine mitral valves behave in a manner similar to that of an artificial prosthetic valve of the same diameter.[645a,650a] Serious hemodynamic obstruction of an artificial valve in the mitral position is quite uncommon, unless the valve is placed in a small left ventricular cavity or an unusually small mitral annulus or unless the prosthesis chosen is inappropriate in size.

The problem of intrinsic stenosis may be more serious in patients who undergo aortic valve replacements for AS. The annulus into which the prosthesis is inserted in these patients is usually smaller than it is in patients with AR, and the surgeon may be forced to select an artificial valve of relatively small size. As a consequence, aortic valve replacement may not abolish obstruction in AS but may merely convert severe obstruction to a mild or moderate type. When the smaller models of the porcine xenograft or mechanical prosthesis are placed into the aortic position, effective orifice areas of about 1.1 to 1.3 cm^2 are common. In such patients, peak transvalvular gradients as high as 40 mm Hg during exercise have been recorded. It is possible that the poor late results observed in a minority of patients undergoing replacement of stenotic aortic valves may be the delayed effects of moderate stenosis of the prosthesis. In patients with AS who do not exhibit clinical improvement postoperatively, it is important to evaluate the function of both the prosthetic valve and the left ventricle. Rarely, reoperation to correct a malfunctioning prosthesis may be necessary.

SELECTION OF AN ARTIFICIAL VALVE

Most comparisons of mechanical and bioprostheses indicate similar overall results, in terms of early and late mortality, prosthetic valve endocarditis and other complications, and the need for reoperation, at least for the first 5 years postoperatively. As indicated, there appear to be no significant differences insofar as hemodynamics are concerned, except that in patients with an unusually small left ventricular cavity or mitral or aortic annulus, the low-profile (tilting-disc) St. Jude or Edwards-Duromedics prosthesis or a tissue valve may perform better than other valves.[749-751]

The major task in selection of an artificial valve is to weigh the advantage of durability and the disadvantage of the risk of thromboembolism and of anticoagulant treatment inherent in mechanical prostheses on the one hand with the advantages of low thrombogenicity and the serious disadvantage of abbreviated durability of the bioprostheses on the other. Tissue valves are preferred over mechanical prostheses in patients in whom anticoagulation is difficult to control or in whom it is especially hazardous because they are prone to hemorrhage or are noncompliant. Because of the problems with the long-term durability of bioprostheses, I believe that a mechanical prosthetic valve should be employed in patients under the age of approximately 65 to 70 years who do not have any of the aforementioned contraindications to anticoagulants.[752] Thus, the following groups of patients should receive bioprostheses: (1) those with coexisting disease who are prone to hemorrhage; (2) those who are noncompliant insofar as permanent anticoagulant treatment is concerned, (3) those who are unwilling to take anticoagulants on a regular basis; and (4) those over the age of 65 to 70 years, in whom bioprosthetic valves deteriorate very slowly and who by reason of their age may be at greater risk of hemorrhage while taking anticoagulants.

Special Situations

Pregnancy (see also p. 1802). Women with artificial valves can tolerate the hemodynamic burden of pregnancy well, but the hypercoagulable state of pregnancy increases the risk of thromboembolism in such patients. Anticoagulation must not be interrupted, although an increased risk of fatal fetal hemorrhage is seen in those in whom it is continued. There is also a risk of fetal malformation caused by the probable teratogenic effect of warfarin. Although these problems represent arguments for the use of tissue valves in all women of childbearing age,[753-756] their limited durability in young adults makes their use unacceptable. Therefore, every effort should be made to defer valve replacement until after childbirth. In pregnant women with critical mitral or aortic stenosis, balloon valvuloplasty should be considered. Women of childbearing potential with a mechanical prosthesis should be counseled against pregnancy. When a woman in whom a mechanical prosthetic valve is already in place becomes pregnant, the risk to the fetus if the mother receives oral anticoagulants appears to be lower than the risk to the mother if anticoagulants are discontinued.[757] Therefore, coumarin derivatives should be continued until 2 weeks before expected delivery, when the patient should probably be given prophylactic heparin.[753,754,756] This approach appears to be safe for the mother but is associated with increased fetal wastage.

Noncardiac Surgery. When this is required in patients with prosthetic valves who are receiving anticoagulants, the risk is minimal when the drug regimen is stopped 1 to 3 days preoperatively and for a similar period postoperatively. It may be desirable, however, to protect the patient with low molecular weight dextran during the perioperative period.

Patients Who Are Destined to Receive Anticoagulants. Patients with earlier implantation of a mechanical prosthesis, chronic atrial fibrillation in the presence of an enlarged left atrium, a history of thromboembolism, or the presence of a thrombus in the left atrium at operation (and who therefore are destined to receive anticoagulants) should receive a mechanical prosthesis because the potential advantage of a tissue valve is negated.

Children and Patients Receiving Chronic Hemodialysis. The high incidence of bioprosthetic valve failure in children and adolescents[752,758-760] and in patients on chronic hemodialysis virtually prohibits their use in these groups. In young adults between the ages of 25 and 35, the failure of bioprosthetic valves is somewhat higher than it is in older adults; this serves as a relative, but not an absolute, contraindication to their use in this age group.

In children, a mechanical prosthesis (generally the St. Jude valve) with its favorable hemodynamics is preferred despite the disadvantages inherent in anticoagulants in this age group.[761] Similarly, mechanical prostheses should be used in patients with chronic renal failure and/or hypercalcemia.

Tricuspid Position. The risk of thrombosis for all valves is highest in the tricuspid position because of the lower pressures and velocity of blood flow; this complication appears to be highest for tilting-disc valves, intermediate for caged-ball valves, and lowest for the bioprostheses, which are the valves of choice as tricuspid replacements. In the tricuspid position bioprostheses exhibit a much slower rate of mechanical deterioration than in the mitral or aortic position.

DETECTION OF PROSTHETIC VALVE DYSFUNCTION. Artificial valves have distinctive auscultatory and phonocardiographic characteristics.[762] Transthoracic and transesophageal echocardiography, phonocardiography, and cineradiography are extremely useful in the identification of artificial valve dysfunction.[762-765] Two-dimensional and Doppler echocardiography are particularly useful in the follow-up of patients who demonstrate clinical deterioration in the postoperative period following porcine heterograft implantation. These techniques may prove capable of distinguishing between failure of a bioprosthesis (abnormal valve motion) and left ventricular dysfunction.

REFERENCES
MITRAL STENOSIS

1. Kinare, S. G., and Kulkarni, H. L.: Quantitative study of the mitral valve in chronic rheumatic heart disease. Int. J. Cardiol. 16:271, 1987.
2. Olson, L. J., Subramanian, R., and Ackermann, D. M.: Surgical pathology of the mitral valve: A study of 712 cases spanning 21 years. Mayo Clin. Proc. 62:22, 1987.
3. Ruckman, R. N., and Van Praagh, R.: Anatomic types of congenital mitral stenosis: Report of 49 autopsy cases with consideration of diagnostic and surgical implications. Am. J. Cardiol. 42:592, 1978.
4. Bortolotti, U., Valente, M., Agozzino, L., et al.: Rheumatoid mitral stenosis requiring valve replacement. Am. Heart J. 107:1049, 1984.
5. Johnson, G. L., Vine, D. L., Cottrill, C. M., and Noonan, J. A.: Echocardiographic mitral valve deformity in the mucopolysaccharidoses. Pediatrics 67:401, 1981.
6. Ladefoged, C., and Rohr, N.: Amyloid deposits in aortic and mitral valves. Virchows Arch. (A) 404:301, 1984.
7. Misch, K. A.: Development of heart valve lesions during methysergide therapy. Br. Med. J. 2:365, 1974.
8. Matagliati, A., Pepi, M., and Fiorentini, C.: Doppler and echocardio-

graphic diagnosis of a free-floating left atrial thrombus. Int. J. Cardiol. 25:131, 1989.

9. Osterberger, L. E., Goldstein, S., Khaja, F., and Lakier, J. B.: Functional mitral stenosis in patients with massive annular calcification. Circulation 64:472, 1981.

10. Kumar, A., Sinha, M., and Sinha, D. N. P.: Chronic rheumatic heart diseases in Ranchi. Angiology 33:141, 1982.

11. Waller, B. F.: Rheumatic and nonrheumatic conditions producing valvular heart disease. In Frankl, W. S., and Brest, A. N. (eds.): Cardiovascular Clinics. Valvular Heart Disease: Comprehensive Evaluation and Management. Philadelphia, F. A. Davis, 1986, pp. 3–104.

12. Wells, B.: The assessment of mitral stenosis by phonocardiography. Br. Heart J. 16:261, 1954.

13. Lachman, A. S., and Roberts, W. C.: Calcific deposits in stenotic mitral valves. Circulation 57:808, 1978.

14. Ionescu, M. I., and Cohn, L. H. (eds.): Mitral Valve Disease: Diagnosis and Treatment. London, Butterworths, 1985, 367 pp.

15. Bowe, J. C., Bland, F., Sprague, H. B., and White, P. D.: Course of mitral stenosis without surgery: 10 and 20 year perspectives. Ann. Intern. Med. 52:741, 1960.

16. Somasundram, U., Euinton, H. A., and Williams, R. P.: Mitral valve stenosis in the elderly. Age Ageing 14:285, 1985.

17. Bell, M. H., and Mintz, G. S.: Mitral valve disease in the elderly. In Frankl, W. S., and Brest, A. N. (eds.): Cardiovascular Clinics. Valvular Heart Disease: Comprehensive Evaluation and Management. Philadelphia, F. A. Davis, 1986, pp. 313–324.

18. Chopra, P., Tandon, H. D., Raizada, V., et al.: Comparative studies in mitral valves in rheumatic heart disease. Arch. Intern. Med. 143:661, 1983.

19. Dalen, J. E., and Alpert, J. S. (eds.): Valvular Heart Disease. 2nd ed. Boston, Little, Brown and Company, 1987, 600 pp.

20. Reichek, N., Shelburne, J. D., and Perloff, J. R.: Clinical aspects of rheumatic valvular disease. Prog. Cardiovasc. Dis. 15:491, 1973.

21. Wood, P.: An appreciation of mitral stenosis. Br. Med. J. 1:1051 and 1113, 1954.

22. Leavitt, J. I., Coats, M. H., and Falk, R.H.: Effects of exercise on transmitral gradient and pulmonary artery pressure in patients with mitral stenosis or a prosthetic mitral valve: A Doppler echocardiographic study. J. Am. Coll. Cardiol. 17:1520, 1991.

23. Dalen, J. E.: Mitral stenosis. In Dalen, J. E., and Alpert, J. S. (eds.): Valvular Heart Disease. 2nd ed. Boston, Little, Brown and Company, 1987, pp. 49–110.

24. Selzer, A.: Effects of atrial fibrillation upon the circulation in patients with mitral stenosis. Am. Heart J. 59:518, 1960.

25. Gorlin, R., and Gorlin, S. G.: Hydraulic formula for calculation of the area of stenotic mitral valve, other cardiac valves and central circulatory shunts. Am. Heart J. 41:1, 1951.

26. Nakhjavan, F. K., Katz, M. R., Maranhao, V., and Goldberg, H.: Analysis of influence of catecholamine and tachycardia during supine exercise in patients with mitral stenosis and sinus rhythm. Br. Heart J. 31:753, 1969.

27. Stott, D. K., Marpole, D.G.F., Bristow, J. D., et al.: The role of left atrial transport in aortic and mitral stenosis. Circulation 41:1031, 1970.

28. Kennedy, J. W.: The use of quantitative angiocardiography in mitral valve disease. In Duran, C., Angell, W. W., Johnson, A. D., and Oury, J. H. (eds.): Recent Progress in Mitral Valve Disease. London, Butterworths, 1984, pp. 149–159.

29. Gash, A. K., Carabello, B. A., Cepin, D., and Spann, J. F.: Left ventricular ejection performance and systolic muscle function in patients with mitral stenosis. Circulation 67:148, 1983.

30. Colle, J. P., Rahal, S., Ohayon, J., et al.: Global left ventricular function and regional wall motion in pure mitral stenosis. Clin. Cardiol. 7:573, 1984.

31. Heller, S. J., and Carleton, R. A.: Abnormal left ventricular contraction in patients with mitral stenosis. Circulation 42:1099, 1970.

32. Harvey, R. M., Ferrer, M. I., Samet, P., et al.: Mechanical and myocardial factors in rheumatic heart disease in mitral stenosis. Circulation 11:531, 1955.

33. Bolen, J. L., Lopes, M. G., Harrison, D. C., and Alderman, E. L.: Analysis of left ventricular function in response to afterload changes in patients with mitral stenosis. Circulation 52:894, 1975.

34. Mohan, J. C., Khalilullah, M., and Arora, R.: Left ventricular intrinsic contractility in pure rheumatic mitral stenosis. Am. J. Cardiol. 64:240, 1989.

35. Reis, R. N., and Roberts, W. C.: Amounts of coronary arterial narrowing by atherosclerotic plaques in clinically isolated mitral valve stenosis: Analysis of 76 necropsy patients older than 30 years. Am. J. Cardiol. 57:1117, 1986.

36. Johnston, D. L., and Kostuk, W. J.: Left and right ventricular function during symptom-limited exercise in patients with isolated mitral stenosis. Chest 89:186, 1986.

37. Wroblewski, E., Spann, J. F., and Bove, A. A.: Right ventricular performance in mitral stenosis. Am. J. Cardiol. 47:51, 1981.

38. Haworth, S. G., Hall, S. M., and Patel, M.: Peripheral pulmonary vascular and airway abnormalities in adolescents with rheumatic mitral stenosis. Int. J. Cardiol. 18:405, 1988.

39. Halperin, J. L., Brooks, K. M., Rothlauf, E. B., et al.: Effect of nitroglycerin on the pulmonary venous gradient in patients after mitral valve replacement. J. Am. Coll. Cardiol. 5:34, 1985.

40. Kinare, S. G., and Kulkarni, H. L.: Quantitative study of the mitral valve in chronic rheumatic heart disease. Int. J. Cardiol. 16:271, 1987.

41. Olson, L. J., Subramanian, R., Ackerman, D. M., et al.: Surgical pathology of the mitral valve: A study of 712 cases spanning 21 years. Mayo Clin. Proc. 62:22, 1987.

42. Keren, G., Etzion, T., Sherez, J., et al.: Atrial fibrillation and atrial enlargement in patients with mitral stenosis. Am. Heart J. 114:1146, 1987.

43. Unverferth, D. V., Fertel, R. H., Unverferth, B. J., and Leier, C. V.: Atrial fibrillation in mitral stenosis: Histologic, hemodynamic, and metabolic factors. Int. J. Cardiol. 5:143, 1984.

44. Munoz S., Gallardo, J., Diaz-Gorrin, J. R., and Medina, O.: Influence of surgery on the natural history of rheumatic mitral and aortic valve disease. Am. J. Cardiol. 35:234, 1975.

45. Scarlat, A., Bodner, G., and Liron, M.: Massive haemoptysis as the presenting symptom in mitral stenosis. Thorax 41:413, 1986.

46. Ohmichi, M., Tagaki, S., Nomura, N., et al.: Endobronchial changes in chronic pulmonary venous hypertension. Chest 94:1127, 1988.

47. Ross, R. S.: Right ventricular hypertension as a cause of precordial pain. Am. Heart J. 61:134, 1961.

48. Saltups, A.: Coronary arteriography in isolated aortic and mitral valve disease. Aust. N.Z. J. Med. 12:494, 1982.

49. Baxter, R. H., Reid, J. M., McGuiness, J. B., and Stevenson, J. G.: Relation of angina to coronary artery disease in mitral and aortic valve disease. Br. Heart J. 40:918, 1978.

50. Nielson, G. H., Galea, E. G., and Houssack, K. F.: Thromboembolic complications of mitral valve disease. Aust. N.Z. J. Med. 8:372, 1978.

51. Lie, J. T., and Entman, M. L.: "Hole-in-one" sudden death: Mitral stenosis and left atrial thrombus. Am. Heart J. 91:798, 1976.

52. Sharma, N.G.K., Kapoor, C. P., Mahambre, L., and Borkar, M. P.: Ortner's syndrome. J. Indian Med. Assoc. 60:427, 1973.

53. Horwitz, L. D., and Groves, B. M. (eds.): Signs and Symptoms in Cardiology. Philadelphia, J. B. Lippincott, 1985, 506 pp.

54. Abrams, J.: Mitral stenosis. In Essentials of Cardiac Physical Diagnosis. Philadelphia, Lea and Febiger, 1987, pp. 275–306.

55. McCall, B. W., and Price, J. L.: Movement of mitral valve cusps in relation to first heart sound and opening snap in patients with mitral stenosis. Br. Heart J. 29:417, 1967.

55a. Longhini, C., Baracca, E., Aggio, S., et al.: The first heart sound in mitral stenosis. Acta Cardiol. (Brux.) XLVI:73, 1991.

56. Barrington, W. W., Boudoulas, H., Bashore, T., et al.: Mitral stenosis: Mitral dome excursion and M₁ and the mitral opening snap—the concept of reciprocal heart sounds. Am. Heart J. 115:1280, 1988.

57. Perloff, J. K.: Auscultatory and phonocardiographic manifestations of pulmonary hypertension. Prog. Cardiovasc. Dis. 9:303, 1967.

58. Nixon, P.G.F.: The genesis of the third heart sound. Am. Heart J. 65:712, 1963.

59. Chandraratna, P.A.N., Aronow, W. S., and Lurie, M.: Cross-sectional echocardiographic observations on the mechanism of preservation of the opening snap in calcific mitral stenosis. Chest 78:822, 1980.

60. Ebringer, R., Pitt, A., and Anderson, S. T.: Haemodynamic factors influencing opening snap interval in mitral stenosis. Br. Heart J. 32:350, 1970.

61. Craige, E.: Phonocardiographic studies in mitral stenosis. N. Engl. J. Med. 257:650, 1957.

62. Criley, J. M., Chambers, R. D., Blaufuss, A. H., and Friedman, N. J.: Mitral stenosis: Mechanico-acoustical events. In Leon, D. F., and Shaver, J. A. (eds.): Physiological Principles of Heart Sounds and Murmurs. New York, American Heart Association Monograph No. 46, 1975, pp. 149–159.

63. Harvey, W. P.: Silent valvular heart disease. In Likoff, W. (ed.): Cardiovascular Clinics. Vol. 5, No. 2, Valvular Heart Disease, Philadelphia, F. A. Davis, 1973, p. 77.

64. Stapleton, J. F.: Natural history of chronic valvular disease. In Frankl, W. S., and Brest, A. N. (eds.): Cardiovascular Clinics. Valvular Heart Disease: Comprehensive Evaluation and Management. Philadelphia, F. A. Davis, 1986, pp. 105–148.

65. Surawicz B.: Effect of respiration and upright position on the interval between the two components of the second heart sound and that between the second sound and mitral opening snap. Circulation 16:422, 1957.

66. Fuchs, R. M., Fisher, J., Schuster, E. H., and Fortuin, N. J.: The systolic murmur of mitral stenosis. Johns Hopkins Med. J. 151:220, 1982.

67. Aravanis, C., and Michaelides, G.: Tricuspid insufficiency masquerading as mitral insufficiency in patients with severe mitral stenosis. Am. J. Cardiol. 20:417, 1967.

68. McArthur, J. D., Sukumar, I. P., Munis, S. C., et al: Reassessment of Graham Steell murmur using platinum electrode technique. Br. Heart J. 36:1023, 1974.

69. Saunders, J. L., Calatayud, J. B., Schultz, K. J., et al.: Evaluation of ECG criteria for P-wave abnormalities. Am. Heart J. 74:757, 1967.

70. Walston, A., Harley, A., and Pipberger, H. V.: Computer analysis of the orthogonal electrocardiogram and vectorcardiogram in mitral stenosis. Circulation 50:472, 1974.

71. Cooksey, J. D., Dunn, M., and Massie, E.: Clinical Vectorcardiography and Electrocardiography. 2nd ed. Chicago, Year Book Medical Publishers, 1977, p. 272.

72. Kasser, I., and Kennedy, J. W.: The relationship of increased left atrial volume and pressure to abnormal P waves on the electrocardiogram. Circulation 39:339, 1969.

73. Mounsey, P.: The atrial electrocardiogram as a guide to prognosis after mitral valvulotomy. Br. Heart J. 21:617, 1961.

74. Probst, P., Goldschlager, N., and Selzer, A.: Left atrial size and atrial fibrillation in mitral stenosis: Factors influencing their relationship. Circulation 48:1281, 1973.

75. Cueto, J., Toshima, J., Armyo, G., et al.: Vectorcardiographic studies in acquired valvular disease with reference to the diagnosis of right ventricular hypertrophy. Circulation 33:588, 1967.

76. Taymor, R. C., Hoffman, I., and Henry, E.: The Frank vectorcardiogram in mitral stenosis. Circulation 30:865, 1964.

77. Donoso, E., Jick, S., Braunwald, E., et al.: The spatial vectorcardiogram in mitral valve disease. Am. Heart J. 53:760, 1957.

78. Gooch, A. S., Calatayud, J. B., Gorman, P. A., et al.: Leftward shift of the terminal P forces in the ECG associated with left atrial enlargement. Am. Heart J. 71:727, 1966.

79. Chen, J.T.T., Behar, V. S., Morris, J. J., Jr., et al.: Correlation of roentgen findings with hemodynamic data in pure mitral stenosis. Am. J. Roentgenol. Radium Ther. Nucl. Med. 102:280, 1968.

80. Amplatz, K.: The roentgenographic diagnosis of mitral and aortic valvular disease. Am. Heart J. 64:556, 1962.

81. Melhem, R. E., Dunbar, J. D., and Booth, R. W.: "B" lines of Kerley and left atrial size in mitral valve disease: Their correlation with mean left atrial pressure as measured by left atrial puncture. Radiology 76:65, 1961.

82. Fleischner, F. G., and Reiner, L.: Linear x-ray shadows in acquired pulmonary hemosiderosis and congestion. N. Engl. J. Med. 250:900, 1954.

83. Van Houten, F. X., Adams, D. F., and Abrams, H. C.: Radiology of valvular heart disease. In Sonnenblick, E. H., and Lesch, M. (eds.): Valvular Heart Disease. New York, Grune and Stratton, 1974, p. 1.

84. Parker, B. M., Friedenberg, M. J., Templeton, A. W. and Burford, T. H.: Preoperative angiocardiographic diagnosis of left atrial thrombi in mitral stenosis. N. Engl. J. Med. 273:136, 1965.

85. Come, P. C.: Echocardiographic evaluation of valvular heart disease. In Come, P. C. (ed.): Diagnostic Cardiology. Philadelphia, J. B. Lippincott, 1985, pp. 407–458.

86. Rahimtoola, S. H.: Perspective on valvular heart disease: An update. J. Am. Coll. Cardiol. 14:1, 1989.

87. Fisher, M. L., Parisi, A. F., Plotnick, G. D., et al.: Assessment of severity of mitral stenosis by echocardiographic leaflet separation. Arch. Intern. Med. 139:402, 1979.

88. Egeblad, H., Berning, J., Saunamaki, K., et al.: Assessment of rheumatic mitral valve disease: Value of echocardiography in patients clinically suspected of predominant stenosis. Br. Heart J. 49:38, 1983.

89. Thuillez, C., Theroux, P., Bourassa, M., et al.: Pulsed Doppler echocardiographic study of mitral stenosis. Circulation 61:381, 1980.

90. Glover, M. U., Warren, S. E., Vieweg, W.V.R., et al.: M-mode and two-dimensional echocardiographic correlation with findings at catheterization and surgery in patients with mitral stenosis. Am. Heart J. 105:98, 1983.

91. Smith, M. D., Handshoe, R., Handshoe, S., et al.: Comparative accuracy of two-dimensional echocardiography and Doppler pressure half-time methods in assessing severity of mitral stenosis in patients with and without prior commissurotomy. Circulation 73:100, 1986.

92. Schweizer, P., Bardos, P., Erbel, R., et al.: Detection of left atrial thrombi by echocardiography. Br. Heart J. 45:148, 1981.

93. Zoghbi, W. A., Farmer, K. L., Soto, J. G., et al.: Accurate noninvasive quantification of stenotic aortic valve area by Doppler echocardiography. Circulation 73:452, 1986.

94. Shandheria, B. K., Tajik, A. J., Reeder, G. S., et al.: Doppler color flow imaging: A new technique for visualization and characterization of the blood flow jet in mitral stenosis. Mayo Clin. Proc. 61:623, 1986.

95. Beiser, G. D., Epstein, S. E., Stampfer, M., et al.: Studies on digitalis. XVIII. Effects of ouabain on the hemodynamic response to exercise in patients with mitral stenosis in normal sinus rhythm. N. Engl. J. Med. 278:131, 1968.

96. Klein, H. O., Sareli, P., Schamroth, C. L., et al.: Effects of atenolol on exercise capacity in patients with mitral stenosis with sinus rhythm. Am. J. Cardiol. 56:598, 1985.

97. Levine, H. J.: Which atrial fibrillation patients should be on chronic anticoagulation? J. Cardiovasc. Med. 6:483, 1981.

98. Kloster, F. E., and Morris, C. D.: Natural history of valvular heart disease. Circulation 65:1283, 1982.

99. Joswig, B. C., Glover, M. U., Handler, J. B., et al.: Contrasting progression of mitral stenosis in Malayans versus American-born Caucasians. Am. Heart J. 104:1400, 1982.

100. Olesen, K. H.: The natural history of 271 patients with mitral stenosis under medical treatment. Br. Heart J. 24:349, 1962.

101. Rowe, J. C., Bland, E. F., Sprague, H. B., and White, P. D.: The course of mitral stenosis without surgery: Ten- and twenty-year perspectives. Ann. Intern. Med. 52:741, 1960.

102. Rapaport, E.: Natural history of aortic and mitral valve disease. Am. J. Cardiol. 35:221, 1975.

103. Sutton, M. J. St.J., Oldershaw, P., Sacchetti, R., et al.: Valve replacement without preoperative cardiac catheterization. N. Engl. J. Med. 305:1233, 1981.

104. Slater, J., Gindea, A. J., Freedberg, R. S., et al.: Comparison of cardiac catheterization and Doppler echocardiography in the decision to operate in aortic and mitral valve disease. J. Am. Coll. Cardiol. 17:1026, 1991.

105. O'Rourke, R. A.: Preoperative cardiac catheterization. Its need in most patients with valvular heart disease. JAMA 248:745, 1982.

106. Chun, P.K.C., Gertz, E., Davia, J. E., and Cheitlin, M. D.: Coronary atherosclerosis in mitral stenosis. Chest 81:36, 1982.

107. Ramsdale, D. R., Faragher, E. B., Bennett, D. H., et al.: Preoperative prediction of significant coronary artery disease in patients with valvular heart disease. Br. Med. J. 284:223, 1982.

108. John, S., Bashi, V. V., Jairaj, P. S., et al.: Closed mitral valvotomy: Early results and long-term follow-up of 3724 consecutive patients. Circulation 68:891, 1983.

109. Gautam, P. C., Coulshed, N., Epstein, E. J., et al.: Preoperative clinical predictors of long-term survival in mitral stenosis: Analysis of 200 cases

110. de Vivie, E. R., and Hellberg, K.: Closed transventricular mitral commissurotomy. In Ionescu, M. I., and Cohn, L. H. (eds.): Mitral Valve Disease: Diagnosis and Treatment. London, Butterworths, 1985, pp. 139–152.

111. Dernevik, L., Brorsson, L., Wallentin, I., and William-Olsson, G.: Improved results of closed commissurotomy for mitral stenosis using ultrasonocardiography as selection ground. Acta Med. Scand. 210:283, 1981.

112. Lower, R. R., and Ducey, K.: Open mitral valvotomy. In Ionescu, M. I., and Cohn, L. H. (eds.): Mitral Valve Disease: Diagnosis and Treatment. London, Butterworths, 1985, pp. 153–156.

113. Gross, R. I., Cunningham, J. N., Jr., Snively, S. L., et al.: Long-term results of open radical mitral commissurotomy: Ten year follow-up study of 202 patients. Am. J. Cardiol. 47:821, 1981.

114. Duran, C.: Mitral reconstruction in predominant mitral stenosis. In Duran, C., Angell, W. W., Johnson, A. D., and Oury, J. H. (eds.): Recent Progress in Mitral Valve Disease. London, Butterworths, 1984, pp. 255–264.

115. Farhat, M. B., Boussadia, H., Gandjbakhch, I., et al.: Closed versus open mitral commissurotomy in pure noncalcific mitral stenosis: Hemodynamic studies before and after operation. J. Thorac. Cardiovasc. Surg. 99:639, 1990.

116. Cohn, L. H., Allred, E. N., Cohn, L. A., et al.: Long-term results of open mitral valve reconstruction for mitral stenosis. Am. J. Cardiol. 55:731, 1985.

117. Eguaras, M. G., Luque, I., Montero, A., et al.: Conservative operation for mitral stenosis: Independent determinants of late results. J. Thorac. Cardiovasc. Surg. 95:1031, 1988.

118. Aora, R., Khalilullah, M., Gupta, M. P., and Padmavati, S.: Mitral restenosis. Incidence and epidemiology. Indian Heart J. 30:265, 1978.

119. Heger, J. J., Wann, L. S., Weyman, A. E., et al.: Long-term changes in mitral valve area after successful mitral commissurotomy. Circulation 59:443, 1979.

120. Higgs, L. M., Glancy, D. L., O'Brien, K. P., et al.: Mitral restenosis: An uncommon cause of recurrent symptoms following mitral commissurotomy. Am. J. Cardiol. 26:34, 1970.

121. Braunwald, E., Braunwald, N. S., Ross, J., Jr., and Morrow, A. G.: Effects of mitral valve replacement on the pulmonary vascular dynamics of patients with pulmonary hypertension. N. Engl. J. Med. 273:509, 1965.

122. Ward, C., and Hancock, B. W.: Extreme pulmonary hypertension caused by mitral valve disease. Natural history and results of surgery. Br. Heart J. 37:74, 1975.

123. Foltz, B. D., Hessel, E. A., and Ivey, T. D.: The early course of pulmonary artery hypertension in patients undergoing mitral valve replacement with cardioplegic arrest. J. Thorac. Cardiovasc. Surg. 88:238, 1984.

124. Dalen, J. E., Matloff, J. M., Evans, G. L., et al.: Early reduction of pulmonary vascular resistance after mitral valve replacement. N. Engl. J. Med. 277:387, 1967.

125. Scott, W. C., Miller, D. C., Haverich, A., et al.: Operative risk of mitral valve replacement: Discriminant analysis of 1329 procedures. Circulation 72(Suppl. II):108, 1985.

126. Peper, W. A., Lytle, B. W., Cosgrove, D. M., et al.: Repeat mitral commissurotomy: Long-term results. Circulation 76(Suppl. III):97, 1987.

127. Turi, Z. G., Reyes, V. P., Raju, B. S., et al.: Percutaneous balloon versus surgical closed commissurotomy for mitral stenosis. Circulation 83:1179, 1991.

128. Casale, P. N., Stewart, W. J., and Whitlow, P. L.: Percutaneous balloon valvotomy for patients with mitral stenosis: Initial and follow-up results. Am. Heart J. 121:476, 1991.

129. L'Epine, Y., Drobinski, G., Sotirov, Y., et al.: Right heart failure due to an inter-atrial shunt after percutaneous mitral balloon dilatation. Eur. Heart J. 10:285, 1989.

129a. Tuzcu, E. M., Block, P. C., and Palacios, I. F.: Comparison of early versus late experience with percutaneous mitral balloon valvuloplasty. J. Am. Coll. Cardiol. 17:1121, 1991.

130. Levine, M. J., Weinstein, J. S., Diver, D. J., et al.: Progressive improvement in pulmonary vascular resistance after percutaneous mitral valvuloplasty. Circulation 79:1061, 1989.

130a. Lefevre, T., Bonan, R., Serra, A., et al.: Percutaneous mitral valvuloplasty in surgical high risk patients. J. Am. Coll. Cardiol. 17:348, 1991.

131. Yoshioka, T., Nakanishi, N., Okubo, S., et al.: Improvement in pulmonary function in mitral stenosis after percutaneous transvenous mitral commissurotomy. Chest 98:290, 1990.

131a. Hung, J.-S., Chern, M.-S., Wu, J.-J., et al.: Short- and long-term results of catheter balloon percutaneous transvenous mitral commissurotomy. Am. J. Cardiol. 67:854, 1991.

132. Feldman, T., and Carroll, J. D.: Valve deformity and balloon mechanics in percutaneous transvenous mitral commissurotomy. Am Heart J. 121:1628, 1991.

133. Abascal, V. M., Wilkins, G. T., O'Shea, J. P., et al.: Prediction of successful outcome in 130 patients undergoing percutaneous balloon mitral valvotomy. Circulation 82:448, 1990.

133a. Kirklin, J. W.: Percutaneous balloon versus surgical closed commissurotomy for mitral stenosis. Circulation 83:1450, 1991.

134. Palacios, I. F., Block, P. C., Wilkins, G. T., et al.: Percutaneous mitral balloon valvotomy during pregnancy in a patient with severe mitral stenosis. Cathet. Cardiovasc. Diagn. 15:109, 1988.

135. Nobuyoshi, M., Hamasaki, N., Kimura, A., et al.: Indications, complications, and short-term clinical outcome of percutaneous transvenous mitral commissurotomy. Circulation 80:782, 1989.

136. Davies, M. J.: Aetiology and pathology of the diseased mitral valve. *In* Ionescu, M. I., and Cohn, L. H. (eds.): Mitral Valve Disease: Diagnosis and Treatment. London, Butterworths, 1985, pp. 27–42.

137. Dajee, H., Hurley, E. J., and Szarnicki, R. J.: Cardiac valve replacement in systemic lupus erythematosus. A review. J. Thorac. Cardiovasc. Surg. 85:718, 1983.

138. Marcus, R. H., Sareli, P., Pocock, W. A., et al.: Functional anatomy of severe mitral regurgitation in active rheumatic carditis. Am. J. Cardiol. 63:577, 1989.

139. Boltwood, C. M., Tei, C., Wong, M., and Shah, P. M.: Quantitative echocardiography of the mitral complex in dilated cardiomyopathy: The mechanism of functional mitral regurgitation. Circulation 68:498, 1983.

140. Keren, G., Sonnenblick, E. H., and LeJemtel, T. H.: Mitral annulus motion: Relation to pulmonary venous and transmitral flows in normal subjects and in patients with dilated cardiomyopathy. Circulation 78:621, 1988.

141. Bloor, C. M.: Valvular heart disease in the elderly. J. Am. Geriatr. Soc. 30:466, 1982.

142. Nestico, P. F., DePace, N. L., Kotler, M. N., et al.: Calcium phosphorus metabolism in dialysis patients with and without mitral anular calcium. Analysis of 30 patients. Am. J. Cardiol. 51:497, 1983.

143. Ritschard, T., Blumberg, A., and Jenzer, H. R.: Mitralanulusverkalkungen bei Dialyse-Patienten. Schweiz. Med. Wschr. 117:1363, 1987.

144. Zanolla, L., Marino, P., Nicolosi, G. L., et al.: Two-dimensional echocardiographic evaluation of mitral valve calcification. Sensitivity and specificity. Chest 82:154, 1982.

145. Mellino, M., Salcedo, E. E., Lever, H. M., et al.: Echographic-quantified severity of mitral annulus calcification: Prognostic correlation to related hemodynamic, valvular, rhythm, and conduction abnormalities. Am. Heart J. 103:222, 1982.

146. Labovitz, A. J., Nelson, J. G., Windhorst, D. M., et al.: Frequency of mitral valve dysfunction from mitral annular calcium as detected by Doppler echocardiography. Am. J. Cardiol. 55:133, 1985.

147. Kaul, S., Pearlman, J. D., Touchstone, D. A., and Esquival, L.: Prevalence and mechanisms of mitral regurgitation in the absence of intrinsic abnormalities of the mitral leaflets. Am. Heart J. 118:963, 1989.

148. Takamoto, T., and Popp, R. L.: Conduction disturbances related to the site and severity of mitral anular calcification: A two-dimensional echocardiographic and electrocardiographic correlative study. Am. J. Cardiol. 51:1644, 1983.

149. Scott-Jupp, W., Barnett, N. L., Gallagher, P. J., et al.: Ultrastructural changes in spontaneous rupture of mitral chordae tendineae. J. Pathol. 133:185, 1981.

150. Oliveira, D. B. G., Dawkins, K. D., Kay, P. H., and Paneth, M.: Chordal rupture I: Aetiology and natural history. Br. Heart J. 50:312, 1983.

151. Oliveira, D. B. G., Dawkins, K. D., Kay, P. H., and Paneth, M.: Chordal rupture II: Comparison between repair and replacement. Br. Heart J. 50:318, 1983.

152. Hickey, A. J., Wilcken, D. E. L., Wright, J. S., and Warren, B. A.: Primary (spontaneous) chordal rupture: Relation to myxomatous valve disease and mitral valve prolapse. J. Am. Coll. Cardiol. 5:1341, 1985.

153. Godley, R. W., Wann, L. S., Rogers, E. W., et al.: Incomplete mitral leaflet closure in patients with papillary muscle dysfunction. Circulation 63:565, 1981.

154. Gallagher, P. J., Caves, P. K., and Stinson, E. B.: Pathological changes in spontaneous rupture of chordae tendineae. Ann. Cir. Gynaecol. 66:135, 1977.

155. Burch, G. E., DePasquale, N. P., and Phillips, J. H.: The syndrome of papillary muscle dysfunction. Am. Heart J. 75:399, 1968.

156. Izumi, S., Miyatake, K., Beppu, S., et al.: Mechanism of mitral regurgitation in patients with myocardial infarction: A study using real-time two-dimensional Doppler flow imaging and echocardiography. Circulation 76:777, 1987.

157. Hickey, M. St.J., Smith, L. R., Muhlbaier, L. H., et al.: Current prognosis of ischemic mitral regurgitation: Implications for future management. Circulation 78(Suppl. I):I51, 1988.

158. Ballester, M., Jajoo, J., Rees, S., et al.: The mechanism of mitral regurgitation in dilated left ventricle. Clin. Cardiol. 6:333, 1983.

159. Becker, A. E., and Anderson, R. H.: Mitral insufficiency complicating acute myocardial infarction. Eur. J. Cardiol. 2:351, 1975.

160. Morrow, A. G., Cohen, L. S., Roberts, W. C., et al.: Severe mitral regurgitation following acute myocardial infarction and ruptured papillary muscle. Hemodynamic findings and results of operative treatment in four patients. Circulation 37(Suppl. II):124, 1968.

161. Balu, V., Hershowitz, S., Masud, A. R. Z., et al.: Mitral regurgitation in coronary artery disease. Chest 81:550, 1982.

162. Gottdiener, J. S., Maron, B. J., Schooley, R. T., et al.: Two-dimensional echocardiographic assessment of the idiopathic hypereosinophilic syndrome. Anatomic basis of mitral regurgitation and peripheral embolization. Circulation 67:572, 1983.

163. Metras, D., Ouezzin-Coulibaly, A., Ouattara, K., et al.: Endomyocardial fibrosis masquerading as rheumatic mitral incompetence. A report of six surgical cases. J. Thorac. Cardiovasc. Surg. 86:753, 1983.

164. Mazzucco, A., Rizzoli, G., Faggian, G., et al.: Acute mitral regurgitation after blunt chest trauma. Arch. Intern. Med. 143:2326, 1983.

165. Jolly, D. T.: Traumatic rupture of a papillary muscle of the mitral valve due to blunt thoracic trauma. Can. Fam. Phys. 29:1960, 1983.

166. Gidding, S. S., Shulman, S. T., Ibawi, M., et al.: Mucocutaneous lymph node syndrome (Kawasaki disease): Delayed aortic and mitral insufficiency secondary to active valvulitis. J. Am. Coll. Cardiol. 7:894, 1986.

167. DiSegni, E., and Edwards, J. E.: Cleft anterior leaflet of the mitral valve with intact septa. A study of 20 cases. Am. J. Cardiol. 51:919, 1983.

168. Nagata, S., Nimura, Y., Sakakibara, H., et al.: Mitral valve lesion associated with secundum atrial septal defect. Analysis of real-time two-dimensional echocardiography. Br. Heart J. 49:151, 1983.

169. Eckberg, D. L., Gault, J. H., Bouchard, R. L., et al.: Mechanics of left ventricular contraction in chronic severe mitral regurgitation. Circulation 47:1252, 1973.

170. Braunwald, E., Welch, G. H., Jr., and Sarnoff, S. J.: Hemodynamic effects of quantitatively varied experimental mitral regurgitation. Circ. Res. 5:539, 1957.

171. Pierpont, G. L., and Talley, R. C.: Pathophysiology of valvar heart disease. Arch. Intern. Med. 142:998, 1982.

172. Spratt, J. A., Olsen, C. O., Tyson, G. S., Jr., et al.: Experimental mitral regurgitation. Physiological effects of correction on left ventricular dynamics. J. Thorac. Cardiovasc. Surg. 86:479, 1983.

173. Braunwald, E., and Turi, Z. G.: Pathophysiology of mitral valve disease. *In* Ionescu, M. I., and Cohn, L. H. (eds.): Mitral Valve Disease: Diagnosis and Treatment. London, Butterworths, 1985, pp. 3–10.

174. Yellin, E. L., Yoran, C., Frater, R. W. M., and Sonnenblick, E. H.: Dynamics of acute experimental mitral regurgitation. *In* Ionescu, M. I., and Cohn, L. H. (eds.): Mitral Valve Disease: Diagnosis and Treatment. London, Butterworths, 1985, pp. 11–26.

175. Urschel, C. W., Covell, J. W., Sonnenblick, E. H., et al.: Myocardial mechanics in aortic and mitral valvular regurgitation: The concept of instantaneous impedance as a determinant of the performance of the intact heart. J. Clin. Invest. 47:867, 1968.

176. Braunwald, E.: Mitral regurgitation: Physiological, clinical and surgical considerations. N. Engl. J. Med. 281:425, 1969.

177. Corin, W. J., Monrad, E. S., Murakami, T., et al.: The relationship of afterload to ejection performance in chronic mitral regurgitation. Circulation 76:59, 1987.

178. Nwasokwa, O., Camesas, A., Weg, I., and Bodenheimer, M. M.: Differences in left ventricular adaptation to chronic mitral and aortic regurgitation. Chest 95:106, 1989.

179. Katayama, K., Tajimi, T., Guth, B. D., et al.: Early diastolic filling dynamics during experimental mitral regurgitation in the conscious dog. Circulation 78:390, 1988.

180. Knotos, G. J., Jr., Schaff, H. V., Gersh, B. J., and Bove, A. A.: Left ventricular function in subacute and chronic mitral regurgitation: Effect on function early postoperatively. J. Thorac. Cardiovasc. Surg. 98:163, 1989.

181. Keren, G., Katz, S., Strom, J., et al.: Dynamic mitral regurgitation: An important determinant of the hemodynamic response to load alterations and inotropic therapy in severe heart failure. Circulation 80:306, 1989.

182. Urschel, C. W., Covell, J. W., Graham, T. P., et al.: Effects of acute valvular regurgitation on the oxygen consumption of the canine heart. Circ. Res. 23:33, 1968.

183. Braunwald, E.: Control of myocardial oxygen consumption: Physiologic and clinical considerations. Am. J. Cardiol. 27:416, 1971.

183a. Corin, W. J., Murakami, T., Monrad, E. S., et al.: Left ventricular passive diastolic properties in chronic mitral regurgitation. Circulation 83:797, 1991.

184. Ross, J., Jr.: Left ventricular function and the timing of surgical treatment in valvular heart disease. Ann. Intern. Med. 94:498, 1981.

185. Mirsky, I., Corin, W. J., Murakami, T., et al.: Correction for preload in assessment of myocardial contractility in aortic and mitral valve disease: Application of the concept of systolic myocardial stiffness. Circulation 78:68, 1988.

186. Wisenbach, T.: Does normal pump function belie muscle dysfunction in patients with chronic severe mitral regurgitation? Circulation 77:515 1988.

187. Osbakken, M. D., Bove, A. A., and Spann, J. F.: Left ventricular regional wall motion and velocity of shortening in chronic mitral and aortic regurgitation. Am. J. Cardiol. 47:1055, 1981.

188. Ramanthan, K. B., Knowles, J., Connor, M. J., et al.: Natural history of chronic mitral insufficiency: Relation of peak systolic pressure/end-systolic volume ratio to morbidity and mortality. J. Am. Coll. Cardiol. 3:1412, 1984.

189. Wisenbaugh, T., Spann, J. F., and Carabello, B. A.: Differences in myocardial performance and load between patients with similar amounts of chronic aortic versus chronic mitral regurgitation. J. Am. Coll. Cardiol. 3:913, 1984.

190. Crawford, M. H., Souchek, J., Oprian, C. A., et al.: Determinants of survival and left ventricular performance after mitral valve replacement. Circulation 81:1173, 1990.

191. Borow, K., Green, L. H., Mann, T., et al.: End-systolic volume as a predictor of postoperative left ventricular performance in volume overload from valvular regurgitation. Am. J. Med. 68:655, 1980.

192. Boucher, C. A., Bingham, J. B., Osbakken, M. D., et al.: Early changes in left ventricular size and function after correction of left ventricular volume overload. Am. J. Cardiol. 47:991, 1981.

193. Kihara, Y., Sasayama, S., Miyazaki, S., et al.: Role of the left atrium in adaptation of the heart to chronic mitral regurgitation in conscious dogs. Circ. Res. 62:543, 1988.

194. Grose, R., Strain, J., and Cohen, M. V.: Pulmonary arterial V waves in mitral regurgitation. Clinical and experimental observations. Circulation 69:214, 1984.

195. Braunwald, E., and Awe, W. C.: The syndrome of severe mitral regurgitation with normal left atrial pressure. Circulation 27:29, 1963.

196. Roberts, W. C., Braunwald, E., and Morrow, A. G.: Acute severe mitral

regurgitation secondary to ruptured chordae tendineae. Clinical, hemodynamic and pathologic considerations. Circulation 33:58, 1966.

197. Cohen, L. S., Mason, D. T., and Braunwald, E.: Significance of an atrial gallop sound in mitral regurgitation: A clue to the diagnosis of ruptured chordae tendineae. Circulation 35:112, 1966.

198. Gorlin, R.: Natural history, medical therapy and indications for surgery in mitral valve disease. In Ionescu, M. I., and Cohen, L. H. (eds.): Mitral Valve Disease: Diagnosis and Treatment. London, Butterworths, 1985, pp. 105–126.

199. Kusiak, V., and Brest, A. N.: Acute mitral regurgitation: Pathophysiology and management. In Frankl, W. S., and Brest, A. N. (eds.): Cardiovascular Clinics. Valvular Heart Disease: Comprehensive Evaluation and Management. Philadelphia, F. A. Davis, 1986, pp. 257–280.

200. Rippe, J. M., and Howe, J. P., III: Acute mitral regurgitation. In Dalen, J. E., and Alpert, J. S. (eds.): Valvular Heart Disease. 2nd ed. Boston, Little, Brown and Company, 1987, pp. 151–176.

201. Elkins, R. C., Morrow, A. G., Vasko, J. S., and Braunwald, E.: The effects of mitral regurgitation on the pattern of instantaneous aortic blood flow. Clinical and experimental observations. Circulation 36:45, 1967.

202. Basta, L. L., Wolfson, P., Eckberg, D. L., and Abboud, F. M.: The value of left parasternal impulse recordings in the assessment of mitral regurgitation. Circulation 48:1055, 1973.

203. Barlow, J. B.: Mitral regurgitation. In Perspectives on the Mitral Valve. Philadelphia, F. A. Davis, 1987, pp. 113–141.

204. Haffajee, C. I.: Chronic mitral regurgitation. In Dalen, J. E., and Alpert, J. S. (eds.): Valvular Heart Disease. 2nd ed. Boston, Little, Brown and Company, 1987, pp. 111–150.

205. Karliner, J. S., O'Rourke, R. A., Kearney, D. J., and Shabetai, R.: Haemodynamic explanation of why the murmur of mitral regurgitation is independent of cycle length. Br. Heart J. 35:397, 1973.

206. Schreiber, T. L., Fisher, J., Mangla, A., and Miller, D.: Severe "silent" mitral regurgitation: A potentially reversible cause of refractory heart failure. Chest 96:242, 1989.

207. Antman, E. M., Angoff, G. H., and Sloss, J. J.: Demonstration of the mechanism by which mitral regurgitation mimics aortic stenosis. Am. J. Cardiol. 42:1044, 1978.

208. Merendino, K. A., and Hessel, E. A.: The murmur on top of the head in acquired mitral insufficiency. J.A.M.A. 199:392, 1967.

209. Morris, J. J., Estes, E. H., Whalen, R. E., et al.: P wave analysis in valvular heart disease. Circulation 29:242, 1964.

210. Priest, E. A., Finlayson, J. K., and Short, D. S.: The x-ray manifestations in the heart and lungs of mitral regurgitation. Prog. Cardiovasc. Dis. 5:219, 1962.

211. Wexler, L., Silverman, J. F., DeBusk, R. F., and Harrison, D. C.: Angiographic features of rheumatic and nonrheumatic mitral regurgitation. Circulation 44:1080, 1971.

212. Pizzarello, R. A., Turnier, J., Goldman, M. A., et al.: Clinical and echocardiographic features of isolated severe pure mitral regurgitation. Clin. Cardiol. 7:565, 1984.

213. Sweatman, T., Selzer, A., Kamageki, M., and Cohn, K.: Echocardiographic diagnosis of mitral regurgitation due to ruptured chordae tendineae. Circulation 46:580, 1972.

213a. Himelman, R. B., Kusumoto, F., Oken, K., et al.: The flail mitral valve: Echocardiographic findings by precordial and transesophageal imaging and Doppler color flow mapping. J. Am. Coll. Cardiol. 17:272, 1991.

214. Nair, C. K., Aronow, W. S., Sketch, M. H., et al.: Clinical and echocardiographic characteristics of patients with mitral annular calcification. Am. J. Cardiol. 51:992, 1983.

215. Helmcke, F., Nanda, N. C., Hsiung, M. C., et al.: Color doppler assessment of mitral regurgitation with orthogonal planes. Circulation 75:175, 1987.

216. Cujec, B., David, T., Wilansky, S., and Pollick, C.: Color flow imaging in severe mitral and aortic regurgitation. Can. J. Cardiol. 4:341, 1988.

217. Jenni, R., Ritter, M., Eberli, F., et al.: Quantification of mitral regurgitation with amplitude-weighted mean velocity from continuous wave Doppler spectra. Circulation 79:1294, 1989.

218. Thompson, R., Ross, I., and Elmes, R.: Quantification of valvular regurgitation by cardiac gated pool imaging. Br. Heart J. 46:629, 1981.

219. Boucher, C. A., Okada, R. D., and Pohost, G. M.: Current status of radionuclide imaging in valvular heart disease. Am. J. Cardiol. 46:1153, 1980.

220. Chatterjee, K.: Vasodilator therapy for mitral regurgitation. In Duran, C., Angell, W. W., Johnson, A. D., and Oury, J. H. (eds.): Recent Progress in Mitral Valve Disease. London, Butterworths, 1984, pp. 138–148.

221. Hoit, B. D.: Medical treatment of valvular heart disease. Curr. Opin. Cardiol. 6:207, 1991.

222. Yoran, C., Yellin, E. L., Becker, R. M., et al.: Mechanism of reduction of mitral regurgitation with vasodilator therapy. Am. J. Cardiol. 43:773, 1979.

222a. Cohn, L. H.: Valvular surgery. Curr. Opin. Cardiol. 6:235, 1991.

223. Frater, R.W.M., Vetter, O., Zussa, C., and Dahm, M.: Chordal replacement in mitral valve repair. Circulation 82(Suppl. IV):125, 1990.

224. Craver, J. M., Cohen, C., and Weintraub, W. S.: Case-matched comparison of mitral valve replacement and repair. Ann. Thorac. Surg. 49:964, 1990.

225. Tandon, A. P., Silverton, N. P., and Ionescu, M. I.: Mitral valve repair (the Woller annuloplasty). In Ionescu, M. I., and Cohn, L. H. (eds.): Mitral Valve Disease: Diagnosis and Treatment. London, Butterworths, 1985, pp. 171–178.

226. Rahko, P. S., and Berkoff, H. A.: Echocardiographic comparison of cardiac size and function before and after surgery for isolated MR: superiority of mitral valve repair vs replacement. Acta Cardiol. 45:189, 1990.

227. Duran, C. G., Revuelta, J. M., Gaite, L., et al.: Stability of mitral reconstructive surgery at 10–12 years for predominantly rheumatic valvular disease. Circulation 78(Suppl. I):I91, 1988.

228. Kirklin, J. W.: Mitral valve repair for mitral incompetence. Mod. Concepts Cardiovasc. Dis. 56:7, 1987.

229. Rankin, J. S., Feneley, M. P., Hickey, M. St.J., et al.: A clinical comparison of mitral valve repair versus valve replacement in ischemic mitral regurgitation. J. Thorac. Cardiovasc. Surg. 95:165, 1988.

230. Carpentier, A.: Mitral reconstruction in predominant mitral incompetence. In Duran, C., Angell, W. W., Johnson, A. D., and Oury, J. H. (eds.): Recent Progress in Mitral Valve Disease. London, Butterworths, 1984, pp. 265–276.

231. Galloway, A. C., Colvin, S. B., Baumann, F. G., et al.: Current concepts of mitral valve reconstruction for mitral insufficiency. Circulation 78:1087, 1988.

232. Cohn, L. H.: Surgery for mitral regurgitation. JAMA 260:2883, 1988.

233. Sarris, G. E., Cahill, P. D., Hansen, D. E., et al.: Restoration of left ventricular systolic performance after reattachment of the mitral chordae tendineae. J. Thorac. Cardiovasc. Surg. 95:969, 1988.

234. Stewart, W. J., Currie, P. J., Salcedo, E. E., et al.: Intraoperative Doppler color flow mapping for decision-making in valve repair for mitral regurgitation. Circulation 81:556, 1990.

235. Pitarys, C. J., III, Forman, M. B., Panayiotou, H., and Hansen, D. E.: Long-term effects of excision of the mitral apparatus on global and regional ventricular function in humans. J. Am. Coll. Cardiol. 15:557, 1990.

236. Shiavone, W. A., Cosgrove, D. M., Lever, H. M., et al.: Long-term follow-up of patients with left ventricular outflow tract obstruction after Carpentier ring mitral valvuloplasty. Circulation 78(Suppl. I):60, 1988.

237. Björk, V. O., Henze, A., and Lindblom, D.: The current status of prosthetic valves in the mitral position. In Duran, C., Angell, W. W., Johnson, A. D., and Oury, J. H. (eds.): Recent Progress in Mitral Valve Disease. London, Butterworths, 1984, pp. 201–210.

238. Gore, J. M.: Prosthetic heart valves. In Dalen, J. E., and Alpert, J. S. (eds.): Valvular Heart Disease. 2nd ed. Boston, Little, Brown and Company, 1987, pp. 509–528.

239. Lee, S.J.K., and Bay, K. S.: Mortality risk factors associated with mitral valve replacement: A survival analysis of 10 year follow-up data. Can. J. Cardiol. 7:11, 1991.

240. Phillips, H. R., Levine, F. H., Carter, J. E., et al.: Mitral valve replacement for isolated mitral regurgitation: Analysis of clinical course and late postoperative left ventricular ejection fraction. Am. J. Cardiol. 48:647, 1981.

240a. Nakano, K., Swindle, M. M., Spinale, F., et al.: Depressed contractile function due to canine mitral regurgitation improves after correction of the volume overload. J. Clin. Invest. 87:2153, 1991.

241. Huikuri, H.: Effect of mitral valve replacement on left ventricular function in mitral regurgitation. Br. Heart J. 49:328, 1983.

242. Schneider, R. M., and Helfant, R. H.: Timing of surgery in chronic mitral and aortic regurgitation. In Frankl, W. S., and Brest, A. N. (eds.): Cardiovascular Clinics. Valvular Heart Disease: Comprehensive Evaluation and Management. Philadelphia, F. A. Davis, 1986, pp. 361–374.

243. Carabello, B. A., and Grossman, W.: Effects of acute and chronic mitral regurgitation on left ventricular mechanics and contractile muscle function. In Duran, C., Angell, W. W., Johnson, A. D., and Oury, J. H. (eds.): Recent Progress in Mitral Valve Disease. London, Butterworths, 1984, pp. 181–192.

244. Smith, D. R.: Clinical diagnosis and evaluation of mitral valve disease. In Ionescu, M. I., and Cohn, L. H. (eds.): Mitral Valve Disease: Diagnosis and Treatment. London, Butterworths, 1985, pp. 43–52.

245. Cosgrove, D. M.: Valve reconstruction versus valve replacement. In Crawford, F. A. (ed.): Cardiac Surgery: Current Heart Valve Prostheses, Vol. 1. Hanley and Belfus, Philadelphia, 1987, pp. 143–158.

246. Peterson, K. L.: The timing of surgical intervention in chronic mitral regurgitation. Cathet. Cardiovasc. Diag. 9:433, 1983.

247. Peterson, K. L., and Tajimi, T.: The timing of surgical intervention in mitral regurgitation. In Duran, C., Angell, W. W., Johnson, A. D., and Oury, J. H. (eds.): Recent Progress in Mitral Valve Disease. London, Butterworths, 1984, pp. 171–180.

248. Bonchek, L. I.: Current status of cardiac valve replacement: Selection of a prosthesis and indications for operation. Am. Heart J. 101:96, 1981.

249. Pinson, C. W., Cobanoglu, A., Metzdorff, M. T., et al.: Late surgical results for ischemic mitral regurgitation. Role of wall motion score and severity of regurgitation. J. Thorac. Cardiovasc. Surg. 88:663, 1984.

250. Connolly, M. W., Gelbfish, J. S., Jacobowitz, I. J., et al.: Surgical results for mitral regurgitation from coronary artery disease. J. Thorac. Cardiovasc. Surg. 91:379, 1986.

251. Fowler, N. O., and van der Bel-Kahn, J. M.: Indications for surgical replacement of the mitral valve. With particular reference to common and uncommon causes of mitral regurgitation. Am. J. Cardiol. 44:148, 1979.

252. Cohn, L. H., Kowalker, W., Bhatia, S., et al.: Comparative morbidity of mitral valve repair versus replacement for mitral regurgitation with and without coronary artery disease. Ann. Thorac. Surg. 45:284, 1988.

THE MITRAL VALVE PROLAPSE SYNDROME

253. Pocock, W. A.: Mitral leaflet billowing and prolapse. In Barlow, J. B. (ed.): Perspectives on the Mitral Valve. Philadelphia, F. A. Davis, 1987, pp. 45–112.

254. Perloff, J. K., Child, J. S., and Edwards, J. E.: New guidelines for the clinical diagnosis of mitral valve prolapse. Am. J. Cardiol. 57:1124, 1986.

255. Krivokapich, J., Child, J. S., Dadourian, B. J., and Perloff, J. K.: Reassessment of echocardiographic criteria for diagnosis of mitral valve prolapse. Am. J. Cardiol. 61:131, 1988.

256. Savage, D. D., Garrison, R. J., Devereux, R. B., et al.: Mitral valve prolapse in the general population. I. Epidemiologic features: The Framingham Study. Am. Heart J. 106:571, 1983.

257. Fontana, M. E., Sparks, E. A., Boudoulas, H., and Wooley, C. F.: Mitral valve prolapse and the mitral valve prolapse syndrome. Curr. Prob. Cardiol. XVI:311–375, 1991.

258. Mitral valve prolapse. In Fowler, N. O.: Diagnosis of Heart Disease. New York, Springer-Verlag, 1991, pp. 171–180.

259. Procacci, P. M., Savran, S. V., Schreiter, S. L., and Bryson, A. L.: Prevalence of clinical mitral valve prolapse in 1,169 young women. N. Engl. J. Med. 294:1086, 1976.

260. Markiewicz, W., Stoner, J., London, E., et al.: Mitral valve prolapse in one hundred presumably healthy young females. Circulation 53:464, 1976.

261. Barlow, J. B., Pocock, W. A., Marchand, P., and Denny, M.: The significance of the late systolic murmurs. Am. Heart J. 66:443, 1963.

262. Wann, L. S., Grove, J. R., Hess, T. R., et al.: Prevalence of mitral prolapse by two-dimensional echocardiography in healthy young women. Br. Heart J. 49:334, 1983.

263. Marks, A. R., Choong, C. Y., Sanfilippo, A. J., et al.: Identification of high-risk and low-risk subgroups of patients with mitral valve prolapse. N. Engl. J. Med. 320:1031, 1989.

264. Levine, R. A., Handschumacher, M. D., Sanfilippo, A. J., et al.: Three-dimensional echocardiographic reconstruction of the mitral valve, with implications for the diagnosis of mitral valve prolapse. Circulation 80:589, 1989.

265. Ballester, M., Presbitero, P., Foale, R., et al.: Prolapse of the mitral valve in secundum atrial septal defect: A functional mechanism. Eur. Heart J. 4:472, 1983.

266. Goldhaber, S. Z., Rubin, I. L., Brown, W., et al.: Valvular heart disease (aortic regurgitation and mitral valve prolapse) among institutionalized adults with Down's syndrome. Am. J. Cardiol. 57:278, 1986.

267. Goldhaber, S. Z., Brown, W. D., and St. John Sutton, M. G.: High frequency of mitral valve prolapse and aortic regurgitation among asymptomatic adults with Down's syndrome. JAMA 258:1793, 1987.

268. Noah, M. S., Sulimani, R. A., Famuyiwa, F. O., et al.: Prolapse of the mitral valve in hyperthyroid patients in Saudi Arabia. Int. J. Cardiol. 19:217, 1988.

269. Froom, P., Margulis, T., Grenadier, E., et al.: Von Willebrand factor and mitral valve prolapse. Thromb. Haemost. 60:230, 1988.

270. Margaliot, S. Z., Barzilay, J., Bar-David, M., et al.: Spontaneous pneumothorax and mitral valve prolapse. Chest 89:93, 1986.

271. Jackson, A. C.: Neurologic disorders associated with mitral valve prolapse. Can. J. Neurol. Sci. 13:15, 1986.

272. Streib, E. W., Meyers, D. G., and Sun, S. F.: Mitral valve prolapse in myotonic dystrophy. Muscle Nerve 8:650, 1985.

273. Whittaker, P., Boughner, D. R., Perkins, D. G., and Canham, P. B.: Quantitative structural analysis of collagen in chordae tendineae and its relation to floppy mitral valves and proteoglycan infiltration. Br. Heart J. 57:264, 1987.

274. Johnson, G. L., Humphries, L. L., Shirley, P. B., et al.: Mitral valve prolapse in patients with anorexia nervosa and bulimia. Arch. Intern. Med. 146:1525, 1986.

275. Liberthson, R., Sheehan, D. V., King, M. E., and Weyman, A. E.: The prevalence of mitral valve prolapse in patients with panic disorders. Am. J. Psychiatry 143:511, 1986.

276. Waite, P., and McCallum, C. A.: Mitral valve prolapse in craniofacial skeletal deformities. Oral Surg. Oral Med. Oral Pathol. 61:15, 1986.

277. Sakuraba, H., Yanagawa, Y., Igarashi, T., et al.: Cardiovascular manifestations of Fabry's disease. Clin. Genet. 29:276, 1986.

278. Comens, S. M., Alpert, M. A., Sharp, G. C., et al.: Frequency of mitral valve prolapse in systemic lupus erythematosus, progressive systemic sclerosis and mixed connective tissue disease. Am. J. Cardiol. 63:59, 1989.

279. Chan, F. L., Chen, W. W., Wong, P.H.C., and Chow, J.S.F.: Skeletal abnormalities in mitral valve prolapse. Clin. Radiol. 34:207, 1983.

280. Chen, W. W., Chan, F. L., Wong, P.H.C., and Chow, J.S.F.: Familial occurrence of mitral valve prolapse: Is this related to the straight back syndrome? Br. Heart J. 50:97, 1983.

281. Kalter, S., Fuentes, F., and Price, E.: Mitral and tricuspid valve prolapse in a patient with mixed connective tissue disease. South. Med. J. 786:794, 1983.

282. Lu-Li, S., Guang-Gen, C., and Ru-Lian, L.: Valve prolapse in Behçet's disease. Br. Heart J. 54:100, 1985.

283. Olsen, E.G.J., and Al-Rufaie, H. K.: The floppy mitral valve. Study on pathogenesis. Br. Heart J. 44:674, 1980.

284. Pyeritz, R. E., and Wappel, M. A.: Mitral valve dysfunction in the Marfan syndrome. Am. J. Med. 74:797, 1983.

285. Davies, M. J., Moore, B. P., and Braimbridge, M. V.: The floppy mitral valve. Study of incidence, pathology and complications in surgical, necropsy and forensic material. Br. Heart J. 40:368, 1978.

286. Jaffe, A. S., Geltman, E. M., Rodey, G. E., and Uitto, J.: Mitral valve prolapse: A consistent manifestation of Type IV Ehlers-Danlos syndrome. The pathogenetic role of the abnormal production of Type III collagen. Circulation 64:121, 1981.

287. King, B. D., Clark, M. A., Baba, N., et al.: "Myxomatous" mitral valves: Collagen dissolution as the primary defect. Circulation 66:288, 1982.

288. Hammer, D., Leier, C. V., Baba, N., et al.: Altered collagen composition in a prolapsing mitral valve with ruptured chordae tendineae. Am. J. Med. 67:863, 1979.

289. Tomaru, T., Uchida, Y., Mohri, N., et al.: Postinflammatory mitral and aortic valve prolapse: A clinical and pathological study. Circulation 76:68, 1987.

290. Stein, P. D., Wang, C.-H, Riddle, J. M., et al.: Scanning electron microscopy of operatively excised severely regurgitant floppy mitral valves. Am. J. Cardiol. 64:392, 1989.

291. Baker, P. B., Bansal, G., Boudoulas, H., et al.: Floppy mitral valve chordae tendineae: Histopathologic alterations. Hum. Pathol. 19:507, 1988.

292. Hickey, A. J., and Wilcken, D.E.L.: Age and the clinical profile of idiopathic mitral valve prolapse. Br. Heart J. 55:582, 1986.

293. Malcolm, A. D.: Mitral valve prolapse associated with other disorders. Causal coincidence, common link, or fundamental genetic disturbance? Br. Heart J. 53:353, 1985.

294. Pader, E.: The familial incidence of mitral valve prolapse. A report of three generations in one family. N.Y. State J. Med. 84:395, 1984.

295. Wordsworth, P., Ogilvie, D., Akhras, F., et al.: Genetic segregation analysis of familial mitral valve prolapse shows no linkage to fibrillar collagen genes. Br. Heart J. 61:300, 1989.

296. Cabeen, W. R., Jr., Reza, M. J., Kovick, R. B., and Stern, M. S.: Mitral valve prolapse and conduction defects in Ehlers-Danlos syndrome. Arch. Intern. Med. 137:1227, 1977.

297. Lebwohl, M. G., Distefano, D., Prioleau, P. G., et al.: Pseudoxanthoma elasticum and mitral valve prolapse. N. Engl. J. Med. 307:228, 1982.

298. Sanyal, S. K., Johnson, W. W., Dische, M. R., et al.: Dystrophic degeneration of papillary muscle and ventricular myocardium. A basic for mitral valve prolapse in Duchenne's muscular dystrophy. Circulation 62:430, 1980.

299. Mason, J. W., Koch, F. H., Billingham, M. E., and Winkle, R. A.: Cardiac biopsy evidence for a cardiomyopathy associated with symptomatic mitral valve prolapse. Am. J. Cardiol. 42:557, 1978.

300. Beardsley, T. L., and Foulks, G. N.: An association of keratoconus and mitral valve prolapse. Ophthalmology 89:35, 1982.

301. Rippe, J. M., Sloss, J. J., Angoff, G., and Alpert, J. S.: Mitral valve prolapse in adults with congenital heart disease. Am. Heart J. 97:561, 1979.

302. Zema, M. J., Chiaramida, S., DeFilipp, G. J., et al.: Somatotype and idiopathic mitral valve prolapse. Cathet. Cardiovasc. Diagn. 8:105, 1982.

303. Giesby, M. J., and Pyeritz, R. E.: Association of mitral valve prolapse and systemic abnormalities of connective tissue: A phenotypic continuum. JAMA 262:523, 1989.

304. Gottdiener, J. S., Sherber, H. S., and Harvey, W. P.: Midsystolic click and mitral valve prolapse following mitral commissurotomy. Am. J. Med. 64:295, 1978.

305. Barlow, J. B., Pocock, W. A., and Obel, I.W.P.: Mitral valve prolapse: Primary, secondary, both or neither? Am. Heart J. 102:140, 1981.

306. Crawford, M. H.: Mitral valve prolapse due to coronary artery disease. Am. J. Med. 62:447, 1977.

307. Imaizumi, T., Chandraratna, P.A.N., Whayne, T. F., Jr., et al.: Transmural myocardial infarction. With the prolapsing mitral-leaflet syndrome and normal coronary arteries. Arch. Intern. Med. 138:1354, 1978.

308. Sakuma, T., Kakihana, M., Togo, T., et al.: Mitral valve prolapse syndrome with coronary artery spasm: A possible cause of recurrent ventricular tachyarrhythmia. Clin. Cardiol. 8:306, 1985.

309. Devereux, R. B., Kramer-Fox, R., and Kligfield, P.: Mitral valve prolapse: Causes, clinical manifestations, and management. Arch. Intern. Med. 111:305, 1989.

310. Tutassaura, H., Gerein, A. N., and Miyagishima, R. T.: Mucoid degeneration of the mitral valve. Clinical review, surgical management and results. Ann. J. Surg. 132:276, 1976.

311. Guy, F. C., MacDonald, R.P.R., Fraser, D. B., and Smith, E. R.: Mitral valve prolapse as a cause of hemodynamically important mitral regurgitation. Can. J. Surg. 23:166, 1980.

312. Pan, C. W., Chen, C. C., Wang, S. P., et al.: Echocardiographic study of cardiac abnormalities in families of patients with Marfan's syndrome. J. Am. Coll. Cardiol. 6:1016, 1985.

313. Boudoulas, H., Kolibash, A. J., Jr., Baker, P., et al.: Mitral valve prolapse and the mitral valve prolapse syndrome: A diagnostic classification and pathogenesis of symptoms. Am. Heart J. 118:796, 1989.

314. Davies, A. O., Mares, A., Pool, J. L., and Taylor, A. A.: Mitral valve prolapse with symptoms of beta-adrenergic hypersensitivity. Beta₂-adrenergic receptor supercoupling with desensitization on isoproterenol exposure. Am. J. Med. 82:193, 1987.

315. Gaffney, F. A., Bastian, B. C., Lane, L. B., et al.: Abnormal cardiovascular regulation in the mitral valve prolapse syndrome. Am. J. Cardiol. 52:316, 1983.

316. Puddu, P. E., Pasternac, A., Tubau, J. F., et al.: QT interval prolongation and increased plasma catecholamine levels in patients with mitral valve prolapse. Am. Heart J. 105:422, 1983.

317. Leor, R., and Markiewicz, W.: Neurocirculatory asthenia and mitral valve prolapse—Two unrelated entities? Isr. J. Med. Sci. 17:1137, 1981.

318. Wei, J. Y., and Fortuin, N. J.: Diastolic sounds and murmurs associated with mitral valve prolapse. Circulation 63:559, 1981.

319. Alexander, M. D., Bloom, K. R., Hart, P., et al.: Atrial septal aneurysm: A cause of midsystolic click. Report of a case and review of the literature. Circulation 63:1186, 1981.

320. Combs, R. L., Shah, P. M., Klorman, R. S., and Klorman, R.: Effects of induced psychological stress on click and rhythm in mitral valve prolapse. Am. Heart J. 99:714, 1980.

321. Braunwald, E., Oldham, H. N., Jr., Ross, J., Jr., et al.: The circulatory response of patients with idiopathic hypertrophic stenosis to nitroglycerin and to the Valsalva maneuver. Circulation 29:422, 1964.

322. Kligfield, P., Hochreiter, C., Kramer, H., et al.: Complex arrhythmias in mitral regurgitation with and without mitral valve prolapse: Contrast to

arrhythmias in mitral valve prolapse without mitral regurgitation. Am. J. Cardiol. 55:1545, 1985.

323. Kligfield, P., Levy, D., Devereux, R. B., and Savage, D. D.: Arrhythmias and sudden death in mitral valve prolapse. Am. Heart J. 113:1298, 1987.

324. Kligfield, P., and Devereux, R. B.: Is the mitral valve prolapse patient at high risk of sudden death identifiable? In Cheitlin, M. D. (ed.): Dilemmas in Clinical Cardiology. Philadelphia, F. A. Davis, 1991, pp. 143–157.

325. Bharati, S., Granston, A. S., Liebson, P. R., et al.: The conduction system in mitral valve prolapse syndrome with sudden death. Am. Heart J. 101:667, 1981.

326. Ware, J. A., Magro, S. A., Luck, J. C., et al.: Conduction system abnormalities in symptomatic mitral valve prolapse: An electrophysiologic analysis of 60 patients. Am. J. Cardiol. 53:1075, 1984.

327. Kavey, R.-E.W., Blackman, M. S., Sondheimer, H. M., and Byrum, C. J.: Ventricular arrhythmias and mitral valve prolapse in childhood. J. Pediatrics 105:885, 1984.

328. Kramer, H. M., Devereux, R. B., Savage, D. D., and Kramer-Fox, R.: Arrhythmias in mitral valve prolapse. Arch. Intern. Med. 144:2360, 1984.

329. Boudoulas, H., Schaal, S. F., Stang, J. M., et al.: Mitral valve prolapse: Cardiac arrest with long-term survival. Int. J. Cardiol. 26:37, 1990.

330. Wit, A. L., Fenoglio, J. J., Wagner, B. M., and Bassett, A. L.: Electrophysiological properties of cardiac muscle in the anterior mitral valve leaflet and the adjacent atrium in the dog. Possible implications for the genesis of atrial dysrhythmias. Circ. Res. 32:731, 1973.

331. Wit, A. L., Fenoglio, J. J., Hordof, A. J., and Reemtsma, K.: Ultrastructure and transmembrane potentials of cardiac muscle in the human anterior mitral valve leaflet. Circulation 59:1283, 1979.

332. Campbell, R.W.F., Godman, M. G., Fiddler, G. I., et al.: Ventricular arrhythmias in syndrome of balloon deformity of mitral valve. Definition of possible high risk group. Br. Heart J. 38:1053, 1976.

333. Gallagher, J. J., Gilbert, M., and Svenson, R. H.: Wolff-Parkinson-White syndrome. The problem, evaluation and surgical correction. Circulation 57:767, 1975.

334. Bekheit, S. G., Ali, A. A., Deglin, S. M., and Jain, A. C.: Analysis of QT interval in patients with idiopathic mitral valve prolapse. Chest 81:620, 1982.

335. Jeresaty, R. M.: Mitral Valve Prolapse. New York, Raven Press, 1979, 251 pp.

336. Pocock, W. A., Bosman, C. K., Chesler, E., et al.: Sudden death in primary mitral valve prolapse. Am. Heart J. 107:378, 1984.

337. Chesler, E., King. R. A., and Edwards, J. E.: The myxomatous mitral valve and sudden death. Circulation 67:632, 1983.

338. Leichtman, D., Nelson, R., Gobel, F. L., et al.: Bradycardia with mitral valve prolapse: A potential mechanism of sudden death. Ann. Intern. Med. 85:453, 1976.

339. Hershman, W. Y., Moskowitz, M. A., Marton, K. I., and Balady, G. J.: Utility of echocardiography in patients with suspected mitral valve prolapse. Am. J. Med. 87:371, 1989.

340. Waller, B. F., Maron, B. J., DelNegro, A. A., et al.: Frequency and significance of M-mode echocardiographic evidence of mitral valve prolapse in clinically isolated pure mitral regurgitation: Analysis of 65 patients having mitral valve replacement. Am. J. Cardiol. 53:139, 1984.

341. Abbasi, A. S., DeCristofaro, D., Anabtawi, J., and Irwin, L.: Mitral valve prolapse: Comparative value of M-mode, two-dimensional and Doppler echocardiography. J. Am. Coll. Cardiol. 2:1219, 1983.

342. Alpert, M. A., Carney, R. J., Flaker, G. C., et al.: Sensitivity and specificity of two-dimensional echocardiographic signs of mitral valve prolapse. Am. J. Cardiol. 54:792, 1984.

343. Morganroth, J., Mardelli, T. J., Naito, M., and Chen, C. C.: Apical cross-sectional echocardiography. Standard for the diagnosis of idiopathic mitral valve prolapse syndrome. Chest 79:23, 1981.

344. Panidis, I. P., McAllister, M., Ross, J., and Mintz, G. S.: Prevalence and severity of mitral regurgitation in the mitral valve prolapse syndrome: A Doppler echocardiographic study of 80 patients. J. Am. Coll. Cardiol. 7:975, 1986.

345. Sahn, D. J., Wood, J., Allen, H. D., et al.: Echocardiographic spectrum of mitral valve motion in children with and without mitral valve prolapse: The nature of false-positive diagnosis. Am. J. Cardiol. 39:422, 1977.

346. Arvan, S., and Tunick, S.: Relationship between auscultatory events and structural abnormalities in mitral valve prolapse: A two-dimensional echocardiographic evaluation. Am. Heart J. 108:1298, 1984.

347. Ogawa, S., Hayashi, J., Sasaki, H., et al.: Evaluation of combined valvular prolapse syndrome of two-dimensional echocardiography. Circulation 65:174, 1982.

348. Rodger, J. C., and Morley, P.: Abnormal aortic valve echoes in mitral prolapse. Echocardiographic features of floppy aortic valve. Br. Heart J. 47:337, 1982.

349. Klein, G. J., Kostuk, W. J., Boughner, D. R., and Chamberlain, M. J.: Stress myocardial imaging in mitral leaflet prolapse syndrome. Am. J. Cardiol. 42:746, 1978.

350. Butman, S., Chandraratna, P. A. N., Milne, N., et al.: Stress myocardial imaging in patients with mitral valve prolapse: Evidence of a perfusion abnormality. Cathet. Cardiovasc. Diagn. 8:243, 1982.

351. Gottdiener, J. S., Borer, J. S., Bacharach, S. L., et al.: Left ventricular function in mitral valve prolapse: Assessment with radionuclide cineangiography. Am. J. Cardiol. 47:7, 1981.

352. Ranganathan, N., Silver, M. D., Robinson, T. I., and Wilson, J. K.: Idiopathic prolapse mitral leaflet syndrome. Angiographic-clinical correlations. Circulation 54:707, 1976.

353. Cohen, M. V., Shah, P. K., and Spindola-Franco, H.: Angiographic-echo-

354. Cipriano, P. R., Kline, S. A., and Baltaxe, H. A.: An angiographic assessment of left ventricular function in isolated mitral valvular prolapse. Invest. Radiol. 15:293, 1980.

355. Mills, P., Rose, J., Hollingsworth, J., et al.: Long-term prognosis of mitral valve prolapse. N. Engl. J. Med. 297:13, 1977.

356. Greenwood, R. D.: Mitral valve prolapse: Incidence and clinical course in a pediatric population. Clin. Pediatr. 23:318, 1984.

357. Chesler, E., and Gornick, C. C.: Maladies attributed to myxomatous mitral valve. Circulation 83:328, 1991.

358. Devereux, R. B., Hawkins, I., Kramer-Fox, R., et al.: Complications of mitral valve prolapse: Disproportionate occurrence in men and older patients. Am. J. Med. 81:751, 1986.

359. Hickey, A. J., MacMahon, S. W., and Wilcken, D.E.L.: Mitral valve prolapse and bacterial endocarditis: When is antibiotic prophylaxis necessary? Am. Heart J. 109:431, 1985.

360. MacMahon, S. W., Hickey, A. J., Wilcken, D.E.L., et al.: Risk of infective endocarditis in mitral valve prolapse with and without systolic murmurs. Am. J. Cardiol. 59:105, 1987.

361. Danchin, N., Briancon, S., Mathieu, P., et al.: Mitral valve prolapse as a risk factor for infective endocarditis. Lancet 1:743, 1989.

362. Schnee, M. A., and Bucal, A. A.: Fatal embolism in mitral valve prolapse. Chest 83:285, 1983.

363. Vared, Z., Oren, S., Rabinowitz, B., et al.: Mitral valve prolapse. Quantitative analysis and long-term followup. Isr. J. Med. Sci. 21:644, 1985.

364. Barletta, G. A., Gagliardi, R., Benvenuti, L., and Fantini, F.: Cerebral ischemic attacks as a complication of aortic and mitral valve prolapse. Stroke 16:219, 1985.

365. Makino, H., and Al-Sadir, J.: Myocardial infarction in patients with mitral valve prolapse and normal coronary arteries. J. Am. Coll. Cardiol. 1:661, 1983.

366. Winkle, R. A., and Harrison, D.: Propranolol for patients with mitral valve prolapse. Am. Heart J. 93:422, 1977.

367. Cohn, L. H., DiSesa, V. J., Couper, G. S., et al.: Mitral valve repair for myxomatous degeneration and prolapse of the mitral valve. J. Thorac. Cardiovasc. Surg. 98:987, 1989.

AORTIC STENOSIS

368. Roberts, W. C.: Valvular, subvalvular and supravalvular aortic stenosis. Morphologic features. Cardiovasc. Clin. 5:97, 1973.

369. Panidis, I. P., and Segal, B. L.: Aortic valve disease in the elderly. In Frankl, W. S., and Brest, A. N. (eds.): Cardiovascular Clinics. Valvular Heart Disease: Comprehensive Evaluation and Management. Philadelphia, F. A. Davis, 1986, pp. 289–312.

370. Levinson, G. E.: Aortic stenosis. In Dalen, J. E., and Alpert, J. S. (eds.): Valvular Heart Disease. 2nd ed. Boston, Little, Brown and Company, 1987, pp. 197–282.

371. Moller, J. H., Nakib, A., Elliott, R. S., and Edwards, J. E.: Symptomatic congenital aortic stenosis in the first year of life. J. Pediatr. 67:728, 1966.

372. Braunwald, E., Goldblatt, A., Aygen, M. M., et al.: Congenital aortic stenosis: Clinical and hemodynamic findings in 100 patients. Circulation 27:426, 1963.

373. Selzer, A.: Changing aspects of the natural history of valvular aortic stenosis. N. Engl. J. Med. 317:91, 1987.

374. Passik, C. S., Ackermann, D. M., Pluth, J. R., and Edwards, W. D.: Temporal changes in the causes of aortic stenosis: A surgical pathologic study of 646 cases. Mayo Clin. Proc. 62:119, 1987.

375. Narang, N. K., Andrew, A.M.R., Chaudhury, H. R., and Gaba, B. S.: Aortic stenosis due to familial hypercholesterolemic xanthomatosis. A case report with brief review of literature. Indian Heart J. 30:189, 1978.

376. Deutscher, S., Rockette, H. E., and Krishnaswami, V.: Diabetes and hypercholesterolemia among patients with calcific aortic stenosis. J. Chron. Dis. 37:407, 1984.

377. Strickberger, S. A., Schulman, S. P., and Hutchins, G. M.: Association of Paget's disease of bone with calcific aortic valve disease. Am. J. Med. 82:953, 1987.

378. Maher, E. R., Pazianas, M., and Curtis, J. R.: Calcific aortic stenosis: A complication of chronic uraemia. Nephron 47:119, 1987.

379. Maher, E. R., Young, G., Smyth-Walsh, B., et al.: Aortic and mitral valve calcification in patients with end stage renal diseases. Lancet I:875, 1987.

380. Dereymacker, L., Van Parijs, G., Bayart, M., et al.: Ochronosis and alkaptonuria: Report of a new case with calcified aortic valve stenosis. Acta Cardiol. 45:98, 1990.

381. Kennedy, J. W., Twiss, R. D., and Blackmon, J. R.: Quantitative angiography. III. Relationships of left ventricular pressure volume and mass in aortic valve disease. Circulation 38:838, 1968.

382. Carabello, B. A., Mee, R., Collins, J. J., Jr., et al.: Contractile function in chronic gradually developing subcoronary aortic stenosis. Am. J. Physiol. 240:H80, 1981.

383. Grossman, W.: Profiles in valvular heart disease. In Grossman, W., and Baim, D. (eds.): Cardiac Catheterization and Angiography. 4th ed. Philadelphia, Lea and Febiger, 1991.

384. Diver, D. J., Royal, H. D., Aroesty, J. M., et al.: Influence of left ventricular load on abnormal diastolic function in patients with aortic stenosis. J. Am. Coll. Cardiol. (in press).

385. Hess, O. M., Ritter, M., Schneider, J., et al.: Diastolic stiffness and myocardial structure in aortic valve disease before and after replacement. Circulation 69:855, 1984.

386. Murakami, T., Hess, O. M., Gage, J. E., et al.: Diastolic filling dynamics in patients with aortic stenosis. Circulation 73:1162, 1986.

387. Braunwald, E., and Frahm, C. J.: Studies on Starling's law of the heart. IV. Observations on the hemodynamic functions of the left atrium in man. Circulation 24:633, 1961.

388. Donner, R., Carabello, B. A., Black, I., and Spann, J. F.: Left ventricular wall stress in compensated aortic stenosis in children. Ann. J. Cardiol. 51:946, 1983.

389. DePace, N. L., Ren, J-F., Iskandrian, A. S., et al.: Correlation of echocardiographic wall stress and left ventricular pressure and function in aortic stenosis. Circulation 67:854, 1983.

390. Sasayama, S., Ross, J., Jr., Franklin, D., et al.: Adaptations of the left ventricle to chronic pressure overload. Circ. Res. 38:172, 1976.

391. Spann, J. F., Bove, A. A., Natarajan, G., and Kreulens, T.: Ventricular performance, pump funcha, and compensatory mechanisms in patients with aortic stenosis. Circulation 62:576, 1980.

391a. Brouwer, C. B., Verwers, F. A., Alpert, J. S., and Goldberg, R. J.: Isolated aortic stenosis: Analysis of clinical and hemodynamic subsets. J. Appl. Cardiol. 4:565, 1989.

392. Krayenbuehl, H. P., Hess, O. M., Ritter, M., et al.: Left ventricular systolic function in aortic stenosis. Eur. Heart J. 9(Suppl. E):19, 1988.

393. Gunther, S., and Grossman, W.: Determinants of ventricular function in pressure overload hypertrophy in man. Circulation 59:679, 1979.

394. Ross, J., Jr.: Afterload mismatch and preload reserve: A conceptual framework for the analysis of ventricular function. Prog. Cardiovasc. Dis. 18:255, 1976.

395. Fifer, M. A., Gunther, S., Grossman, W., et al.: Myocardial contractile function in aortic stenosis as determined from the rate of stress development during isovolumic systole. Am. J. Cardiol. 44:1318, 1979.

396. Dineen, E., and Brent, B. N.: Aortic valve stenosis: Comparison of patients with to those without chronic congestive heart failure. Am. J. Cardiol. 57:419, 1986.

397. Carabello, B. A., Green, L. H., Grossman, W., et al.: Hemodynamic determinants of prognosis of aortic valve replacement in critical aortic stenosis and advanced congestive heart failure. Circulation 62:42, 1980.

398. Huber, D., Grimm, J., Koch, R., and Krayenbuehl, H. P.: Determinants of ejection performance in aortic stenosis. Circulation 64:126, 1981.

399. Dineen, E., and Brent, B. N.: Aortic valve stenosis: Comparison of patients to those without chronic congestive heart failure. Am. J. Cardiol. 57:419, 1986.

400. Fifer, M. A., Borow, K. M., Colan, S. D., and Lorell, B. H.: Early diastolic left ventricular function in children and adults with aortic stenosis. J. Am. Coll. Cardiol. 5:1147, 1985.

401. Schwarz, F., Flameng, W., Schaper, J., et al.: Myocardial structure and function in patients with aortic valve disease and their relation to postoperative results. Am. J. Cardiol. 41:661, 1978.

402. Bertrand, M. E., LaBlanche, J. M., Tilmant, P. Y., et al.: Coronary sinus blood flow at rest and during isometric exercise in patients with aortic valve disease. Mechanism of angina pectoris in presence of normal coronary arteries. Am. J. Cardiol. 47:199, 1981.

403. Bonow, R. O.: Left ventricular structure and function in aortic valve disease. Circulation 79:966, 1989.

404. Krayenbuehl, H. P., Hess, O. M., Monrad, E. S., et al.: Left ventricular myocardial structure in aortic valve disease before, intermediate, and later after aortic valve replacement. Circulation 79:744, 1989.

405. Smucker, M. L., Tedesco, C. L., and Manning, S. B.: Demonstration of an imbalance between coronary perfusion and excessive load as a mechanism of ischemia during stress in patients with aortic stenosis. Circulation 78:573, 1988.

406. Vinten-Johansen, J., and Weiss, H. R.: Oxygen consumption in subepicardial and subendocardial regions of the canine left ventricle—The effect of experimental acute aortic valve stenosis. Circ. Res. 46:139, 1980.

407. Matsuo, S., Tsuruta, M., Hayano, M., et al.: Phasic coronary artery flow velocity determined by Doppler flowmeter catheter in aortic stenosis and aortic regurgitation. Am. J. Cardiol. 62:917, 1988.

408. Marcus, M. L., Dot, D. B., Hiratzka, L. F., et al.: Decreased coronary reserve. A mechanism for angina pectoris in patients with aortic stenosis and normal coronary arteries. N. Engl. J. Med. 307:1362, 1982.

409. Kennedy, K. D., Nishimura, R. A., Holmes, D. R., et al.: Natural history of moderate aortic stenosis. J. Am. Coll. Cardiol. 17:313, 1991.

410. Ross, J., Jr., and Braunwald, E.: The influence of corrective operations on the natural history of aortic stenosis. Circulation 37(Suppl. V):61, 1968.

411. Frank, S., Johnson, A., and Ross, J., Jr.,: Natural history of valvular aortic stenosis. Br. Heart J. 35:41, 1973.

412. Kelly, T. A., Rothbart, R. M., Cooper, M., et al.: Comparison of outcome of asymptomatic to symptomatic patients older than 20 years of age with valvular aortic stenosis. Am. J. Cardiol. 61:123, 1988.

413. Hakki, A.-H., Kimbiris, D., Iskandrian, A. S., et al.: Angina pectoris and coronary artery disease in patients with severe aortic valvular disease. Am. Heart J. 100:441, 1980.

414. Lombard, J. T., and Selzer, A.: Valvular aortic stenosis: A clinical and hemodynamic profile of patients. Ann. Intern. Med. 106:292, 1987.

415. Holley, K. E., Bahn, R. C., McGoon, D. C., and Mankin, H. T.: Spontaneous calcific embolization associated with calcific aortic stenosis. Circulation 27:197, 1963.

416. Vandeplas, A., Willems, J. L., Piessens, J., and DeGeest, H.: Frequency of angina pectoris and coronary artery disease in severe isolated valvular aortic stenosis: Am. J. Cardiol. 62:117, 1988.

417. Mullany, C. J., Elveback, L. R., Frye, R. L., et al.: Coronary artery disease and its management: Influence on survival in patients undergoing aortic valve replacement. J. Am. Coll. Cardiol. 10:66, 1987.

418. Grech, E. D., and Ramsdale, D. R.: Exertional syncope in aortic stenosis: Evidence to support inappropriate left ventricular baroreceptor response. Am. Heart J. 121:603, 1991.

419. Schwartz, L. S., Goldfischer, J., Sprague, G. J., and Schwartz, S. P.: Syncope and sudden death in aortic stenosis. Am. J. Cardiol. 23:647, 1969.

420. Kulbertus, H. E.: Ventricular arrhythmias, syncope and sudden death in aortic stenosis. Eur. Heart J. 9(Suppl. E):51, 1988.

421. Shoenfeld, Y., Eldar, M., Bedazovsky, B., et al.: Aortic stenosis associated with gastrointestinal bleeding. A survey of 612 patients. Am. Heart J. 100:179, 1980.

422. Love, J. W.: The syndrome of calcific aortic stenosis and gastrointestinal bleeding: Resolution following aortic valve replacement. J. Thorac. Cardiovasc. Surg. 83:779, 1982.

423. Pleet, A. B., Massey, E. W., and Vengrow, M. E.: TIA, stroke, and the bicuspid aortic valve. Neurology 31:1540, 1981.

424. Brockmeier, L. B., Adolph, R. J., Gustin, B. W., et al.: Calcium emboli to the retinal artery in calcific aortic stenosis. Am. Heart J. 101:32, 1981.

425. Wood, P.: Aortic stenosis. Am. J. Cardiol. 1:553, 1958.

426. Aortic stenosis. In Fowler, N.O.: Diagnosis of Heart Disease. New York, Springer-Verlag, 1991, pp. 134–145

427. Abrams, J.: Aortic stenosis. In Essentials of Cardiac Physical Diagnosis. Philadelphia, Lea and Febiger, 1987, pp. 205–224.

428. Cooper, T., Braunwald, E., and Morrow, A. G.: Pulsus alternans in aortic stenosis: Hemodynamic observations in 50 patients studied by left heart catheterization. Circulation 18:64, 1958.

429. Perloff, J. K.: Clinical recognition of aortic stenosis. The physical signs and differential diagnosis of the various forms of obstruction to left ventricular outflow. Prog. Cardiovasc. Dis. 10:323, 1968.

430. Goldblatt, A., Aygen, M. M., and Braunwald, E.: Hemodynamic-phonocardiographic correlations of the fourth heart sound in aortic stenosis. Circulation 26:92, 1962.

431. Caulfield, W. H., deLeon, A. C., Perloff, J. K., and Steelman, R. B.: The clinical significance of the fourth heart sound in aortic stenosis. Am. J. Cardiol. 28:179, 1971.

432. Morton, B. C.: Natural history and management of chronic aortic valve disease. Can. Med. Assoc. J. 126:477, 1982.

433. Forssell, G., Jonasson, R., and Orinius, E.: Identifying severe aortic valvular stenosis by bedside examination. Acta Med. Scand. 218:397, 1985.

434. Morgan, D.J.R., and Hall, R.J.C.: Occult aortic stenosis as cause of intractable heart failure. Br. Med. J. 1:784, 1979.

435. Dymond, D. S., Wolf, F. G., and Schmidt, D. H.: Severe left ventricular dysfunction in critical aortic stenosis—reversal following aortic valve replacement. Postgrad. Med. J. 59:781, 1983.

436. Delman, A. J., and Stein, E.: Valvular aortic stenosis. In Dynamic Cardiac Auscultation and Phonocardiography. Philadelphia, W. B. Saunders Company, 1979, p. 795.

437. Siegel, R. J., and Roberts, W. C.: Electrocardiographic observations in severe aortic valve stenosis: Correlative necropsy study of clinical, hemodynamic, and ECG variables demonstrating relation of 12-lead QRS amplitude to peak systolic transaortic pressure gradient. Am. Heart J. 103:210, 1982.

438. Gooch, A. S., Calatayud, J. B., Rogers, P. A., and Garman, P. A.: Analysis of the P wave in severe aortic stenosis. Dis. Chest 49:459, 1966.

439. Thompson, R., Mitchell, A., Ahmed, M., et al.: Conduction defects in aortic valve disease. Am. Heart J. 98:3, 1979.

440. Rasmussen, K., Thomsen, P.E.B., and Bagger, J. P.: H-V interval in calcific aortic stenosis. Relation to left ventricular function and effect of valve replacement. Br. Heart J. 52:82, 1984.

441. Nair, C. K., Aronow, W. S., Stokke, K., et al.: Cardiac conduction defects in patients older than 60 years with aortic stenosis and without mitral annular calcium. Am. J. Cardiol. 53:169, 1984.

442. Rosenbaum, M., Elizari, M., and Lazari, J.: Los Hemibloques. Buenos Aires, Paidos, 1968, p. 363.

443. Klein, R. C.: Ventricular arrhythmias in aortic valve disease: Analysis of 102 patients. Am. J. Cardiol. 53:1079, 1984.

444. Olshausen, K. V., Schwarz, F., Apfelbach, J., et al.: Determinants of the incidence and severity of ventricular arrhythmias in aortic valve disease. Am. J. Cardiol. 51:1103, 1983.

445. Bell, H., Pugh, D., and Dunn, M.: Vectorcardiographic evolution of left ventricular hypertrophy. Br. Heart J. 30:70, 1968.

446. Siegel, R. J., Maurer, G., Navatpumin, T., and Shah, P. K.: Accurate noninvasive assessment of critical aortic valve stenosis in the elderly. J. Am. Coll. Cardiol. 1:639, 1983.

447. Szamosi, A., and Wassberg, B.: Radiologic detection of aortic stenosis. Acta Radiol. Diagn. 24:201, 1983.

448. Vukas, M., Wallentin, I., and Hjalmarson, A.: Analysis of systolic vibrations of interventricular septum in patients with aortic valvular stenosis. Acta Med. Scand. 210:397, 1981.

449. Galan, A., Zoghbi, W. A., and Quiñones, M. A.: Determination of severity of valvular aortic stenosis by Doppler echocardiography and relation of findings to clinical outcome and agreement with hemodynamic measurements determined at cardiac catheterization. Am. J. Cardiol. 67:1007, 1991.

450. Agatston, A. S., Chengot, M., Rao, A., et al.: Doppler diagnosis of valvular aortic stenosis in patients over 60 years of age. Am. J. Cardiol. 56:106, 1985.

451. Yeager, M., Yock, P. G., and Popp, R. L.: Comparison of Doppler-derived pressure gradient to that determined at cardiac catheterization in adults with aortic valve stenosis: Implications for management. Am. J. Cardiol. 57:644, 1986.

452. Currie, P. J., Hagler, D. J., Seward, J. B., et al.: Instantaneous pressure gradient: A simultaneous Doppler and dual catheter correlative study. J. Am. Coll. Cardiol. 7:800, 1986.

453. Jonasson, R., Jonsson, B., Nordlander, R., et al.: Rate of progression of severity of valvular aortic stenosis. Acta Med. Scand. 213:51, 1983.

454. Nestico, P. F., DePace, N. L., Kimbiris, D., et al.: Progression of isolated aortic stenosis. Analysis of 29 patients having more than one cardiac catheterization. Am. J. Cardiol. 52:1054, 1983.

455. Hoagland, P. M., Cook, E. F., Wynne, J., and Goldman, L.: Value of noninvasive testing in adults with suspected aortic stenosis. Am. J. Med. 80:1041, 1986.

456. Cohen, L. S., Friedman, W. F., and Braunwald, E.: Natural history of mild congenital aortic stenosis elucidated by serial hemodynamic studies. Am. J. Cardiol. 30:1, 1972.

457. Cheitlin, M. D., Gertz, E. W., Brundage, B. H., et al.: Rate of progression of severity of valvular aortic stenosis in the adult. Am. Heart J. 98:689, 1979.

458. Chizner, M. A., Pearle, D. L., and deLeon, A. C., Jr.: The natural history of aortic stenosis in adults. Am. Heart J. 99:419, 1980.

459. Braunwald, E.: On the natural history of severe aortic stenosis (editorial). J. Am. Coll. Cardiol. 15:1018, 1990.

460. Turina, J., Hess, O., Sepulchri, F., and Krayenbuehl, H. P.: Spontaneous course of aortic valve disease. Eur. Heart J. 8:471, 1987.

461. Kelly, T. A., Rothbart, R. M., Cooper, C. M., et al.: Comparison of outcome of asymptomatic patients older than 20 years with valvular aortic stenosis. Am. J. Cardiol. 61:123, 1988.

462. Pellikka, P. A., Nishimura, R. A., Bailey, K. R., and Tajik, A. J.: The natural history of adults with asymptomatic hemodynamically significant aortic stenosis. J. Am. Coll. Cardiol. 15:1012, 1990.

463. Wagner, S., and Selzer, A.: Patterns of progression of aortic stenosis: A longitudinal hemodynamic study. Circulation 65:709, 1982.

464. Usher, B. W.: Valve surgery: Indications and long-term results. Curr. Opin. Cardiol. 6:219, 1991.

465. Kirklin, J. W., and Barratt-Boyes, B. G.: Congenital valvular aortic stenosis. In Cardiac Surgery. New York, John Wiley and Sons, 1986, pp. 972–988.

466. Kirklin, J. W., and Barratt-Boyes, B. G.: Aortic valve disease. In Cardiac Surgery. New York, John Wiley and Sons, 1986, pp. 374–420.

467. McBride, L. R., Naunheim, K. S., Fiore, A. C., et al.: Aortic valve decalcification. J. Thorac. Cardiovasc. Surg. 100:36, 1990.

468. Culliford, A. T., Galloway, A. C., Colvin, S. B., et al.: Aortic valve replacement for aortic stenosis in persons aged 80 years and over. Am. J. Cardiol. 67:1256, 1991.

469. Shapira, N., Lemole, G. M., Fernandez, J., et al.: Aortic valve repair for aortic stenosis in adults. Ann. Thorac. Surg. 50:110, 1990.

470. Levinson, J. R., Akins, C. W., Buckley, M. J., et al.: Octagenarians with aortic stenosis: Outcome after aortic valve replacement. Circulation 80(Suppl. I):49, 1989.

471. Lund, O.: Preoperative risk evaluation and stratification of long-term survival after valve replacement for aortic stenosis. Circulation 82:124, 1990.

472. Mirsky, I., Henschke, C., Hess, O. M., and Krayenbuehl, H. P.: Prediction of postoperative performance in aortic valve disease. Ann. J. Cardiol. 48:295, 1981.

473. Acar, J., Ducimetiere, P., Cadilhac, M., et al.: Prognosis of surgically treated chronic aortic valve disease. Predictive indicators of early postoperative risk and long-term survival, based on 439 cases. J. Thorac. Cardiovasc. Surg. 82:114, 1981.

474. St. John Sutton, M., Plappert, T., Spiegel, A., et al.: Early postoperative changes in left ventricular chamber size, architecture, and function in aortic stenosis and aortic regurgitation and their relation to intraoperative changes in afterload: A prospective two-dimensional echocardiographic study. Circulation 76:77, 1987.

475. Monrad, E. S., Hess, O. M., Murakami, T., et al.: Abnormal exercise hemodynamics in patients with normal systolic function late after aortic valve replacement. Circulation 77:613, 1988.

476. Pantely, G., Morton, M., and Rahimtoola, S. H.: Effects of successful, uncomplicated valve replacement on ventricular hypertrophy, volume and performance in aortic stenosis and in aortic incompetence. J. Thorac. Cardiovasc. Surg. 75:383, 1978.

477. Hwang, M. H., Hammermeister, K. E., Oprian, C., et al.: Preoperative identification of patients likely to have left ventricular dysfunction after aortic valve replacement. Participants in the Veterans Administration Cooperative Study on Valvular Heart Disease. Circulation 80(Suppl. I):165, 1989.

478. Kennedy, J. W., Doces, J., and Stewart, D. K.: Left ventricular function before and following aortic valve replacement. Circulation 56:944, 1977.

479. Monrad, E. S., Hess, O. M., Murakami, T., et al.: Time course of regression of left ventricular hypertrophy after aortic valve replacement. Circulation 77:1345, 1988.

480. O'Tolle, J. D., Geiser, E. A., Reddy, S., et al.: Effect of preoperative ejection fraction on survival and hemodynamic improvement following aortic valve replacement. Circulation 58:1175, 1978.

481. Smith, N., McAnulty, J. H., and Rahimtoola, S. H.: Severe aortic stenosis with impaired left ventricular function and clinical heart failure: Results of valve replacement. Circulation 58:255, 1978.

482. Kay, P. H., and Paneth, M.: Aortic valve replacement in the over seventy age group. J. Cardiovasc. Surg. 22:312, 1981.

483. Safian, R. D., Mandell, V. S., Thurer, R. E., et al.: Postmortem and intraoperative balloon valvuloplasty of calcific aortic stenosis in elderly patients: Mechanisms of successful dilation. J. Am. Coll. Cardiol. 9:655, 1987.

484. Beatt, K. J.: Balloon dilatation of the aortic valve in adults: a physician's view. Br. Heart J. 63:207, 1990.

485. Kuntz, R. E., Tosteson, A. N. A., Berman, A. D., et al.: Predictors of event-free survival after balloon aortic valvuloplasty. N. Engl. J. Med. 325:17, 1991.

486. Bashore, T. M., Davidson, C. J., and the Mansfield Scientific Aortic Valvuloplasty Registry Investigators: Follow-up recatheterization after balloon aortic valvuloplasty. J. Am. Coll. Cardiol. 17:1188, 1991.

486a. Nishimura, R. A., Holmes, D. R., Jr., Michela, M. A., et al.: Follow-up of patients with low output, low gradient hemodynamics after percutaneous balloon aortic valvuloplasty: The Mansfield Scientific Aortic Valvuloplasty Registry. J. Am. Coll. Cardiol. 17:828, 1991.

487. McKay, R. G.: The Mansfield Scientific Aortic Valvuloplasty Registry: Overview of acute hemodynamic results and procedural complications. J. Am. Coll. Cardiol. 17:485, 1991.

488. Holmes, D. R., Jr., Nishimura, R. A., and Reeder, G. S.: In-hospital mortality after balloon aortic valvuloplasty: Frequency and associated factors. J. Am. Coll. Cardiol. 17:189, 1991.

489. Cribier, A., and Letac, B.: Percutaneous balloon aortic valvuloplasty in adults with calcific aortic stenosis. Curr. Opin. Cardiol. 6:212, 1991.

489a. Isner, J. A., and the Mansfield Scientific Aortic Valvuloplasty Registry Investigators: Acute catastrophic complications of balloon aortic valvuloplasty. J. Am. Coll. Cardiol. 17:1436, 1991.

490. Berland, J., Cribier, A., Savin, T., et al.: Percutaneous balloon valvuloplasty in patients with severe aortic stenosis and low ejection fraction. Circulation 79:1189, 1989.

490a. Angel, J. L., Chapman, C., and Knuppel, R. A.: Percutaneous balloon aortic valvuloplasty in pregnancy. Obstet. Gynecol. 72:438, 1988.

AORTIC REGURGITATION

491. Olson, L. J., Subramanian, R., and Edwards, W. D.: Surgical pathology of pure aortic insufficiency: A study of 225 cases. Mayo Clin. Proc. 59:835, 1984.

492. Alpert, J. S.: Chronic aortic regurgitation. In Dalen, J. E., and Alpert, J. S. (eds.): Valvular Heart Disease. 2nd ed. Boston, Little, Brown and Company, 1987, pp. 283–318.

493. Stewart, W. J., King, M. E., Gillam, L. D., et al.: Prevalence of aortic valve prolapse with bicuspid aortic valve and its relation to aortic regurgitation: A cross-sectional echocardiographic study. Am. J. Cardiol. 54:1277, 1984.

494. Frahm, C. J., Braunwald, E., and Morrow, A. G.: Congenital aortic regurgitation. Clinical and hemodynamic findings in four patients. Am. J. Med. 31:63, 1961.

495. Roberts, W. C., Morrow, A. G., McIntosh, C. L., et al.: Congenitally bicuspid aortic valve causing severe, pure aortic regurgitation without superimposed infective endocarditis. Am. J. Cardiol. 47:206, 1981.

496. Tonnemacher, D., Reid, C., Kawanishi, D., et al.: Frequency of myxomatous degeneration of the aortic valve as a cause of isolated aortic regurgitation severe enough to warrant aortic valve replacement. Am. J. Cardiol. 60:1194, 1987.

497. Morain, S. V., Casanegra, P., Maturana, G., and Dubernet, J.: Spontaneous rupture of a fenestrated aortic valve. Surgical treatment. J. Thorac. Cardiovasc. Surg. 73:716, 1977.

498. Waller, B. F., Kishel, J. C., and Roberts, W. C.: Severe aortic regurgitation from systemic hypertension. Chest 82:365, 1982.

499. Chartash, E. K., Lans, D. M., Paget, S. A., et al.: Aortic insufficiency and mitral regurgitation in patients with severe systemic lupus erythematosus and the antiphospholipid syndrome. Am. J. Med. 86:407, 1989.

500. Kramer, P. H., Imboden, J. B., Jr., Waldman, F. M., et al.: Severe aortic insufficiency in juvenile chronic arthritis. Am. J. Med. 74:1088, 1983.

501. Demoulin, J. C., Lespagnard, J., Bertholet, M., and Soumagne, D.: Acute fulminant aortic regurgitation in ankylosing spondylitis. Am. Heart J. 105:859, 1983.

502. Tahakur, R., Gupta, L. C., Misra, M., et al.: Jaccoud's arthropathy—diagnostic and therapeutic implications. Postgrad. Med. J. 64:809, 1988.

503. Bostwick, D. G., Bensch, K. G., Burke, J. S., et al.: Whipple's disease presenting as aortic insufficiency. N. Engl. J. Med. 305:995, 1981.

504. Burdick, S., Tresch, D. D., and Komokowski, R. A.: Cardiac valvular dysfunction associated with Crohn's disease in the absence of ankylosing spondylitis. Am. Heart J. 118:174, 1989.

505. Darvill, F. R., Jr.: Aortic insufficiency of unusual etiology. JAMA 184:753, 1963.

506. Chikamori, T., Doi, Y. L., Yonezawa, Y., et al.: Aortic regurgitation secondary to Behçet's disease. A case report and review of the literature. Eur. Heart J. 11:572, 1990.

507. Emanuel, R., Ng, R.A.L., Marcomichelakis, J., et al.: Formes frustes of Marfan's syndrome presenting with severe aortic regurgitation. Clinicogenetic study of 18 families. Br. Heart J. 39:190, 1977.

508. Reid, G. D., Patterson, M.W.H., Patterson, A. C., and Cooperberg, P. L.: Aortic insufficiency in association with juvenile ankylosing spondylitis. J. Pediatr. 95:78, 1979.

509. Paulus, H. E., Pearson, C. M., and Pitts, W., Jr.: Aortic insufficiency in five patients with Reiter's syndrome: A detailed clinical and pathologic study. Am. J. Med. 53:464, 1972.

510. Hollingsworth, P., Hall, P. J., Knight, S. C., and Newman, R.: Lone aortic regurgitation, sacroiliitis, and HLA B27: Case history and frequency of association. Br. Heart J. 42:229, 1979.

511. Heppner, R. L., Babitt, H. I., Blanchine, J. W., and Warbasse, J. R.: Aortic regurgitation and aneurysm of sinus of Valsalva associated with osteogenesis imperfecta. Am. J. Cardiol. 31:654, 1973.

512. Esdah, J., Hawkins, D., Gold, P., et al.: Vascular involvement in relapsing polychondritis. Can. Med. Assoc. J. 116:1019, 1977.

513. Welch, G. H., Jr., Braunwald, E., and Sarnoff, S. J.: Hemodynamic effects of quantitatively varied experimental aortic regurgitation. Circ. Res. 5:546, 1957.

514. Belenkie, I., and Rademaker, A.: Acute and chronic changes after aortic valve damage in the intact dog. Am. J. Physiol. 241:H95, 1981.

515. Iskandrian, A. S., Hakki, A-H., Manno, B., et al.: Left ventricular function in chronic aortic regurgitation. J. Am. Coll. Cardiol. 1:1374, 1983.

516. Boucher, C. A., Wilson, R. A., Kanarek, D. J., et al.: Exercise testing in asymptomatic or minimally symptomatic aortic regurgitation: Relationship of left ventricular ejection fraction to left ventricular filling pressure during exercise. Circulation 67:1091, 1983.

517. Johnson, L. L., Powers, E. R., Tzall, W. R., et al.: Left ventricular volume and ejection fraction response to exercise in aortic regurgitation. Am. J. Cardiol. 51:1379, 1983.

518. Florenzano, F., and Glantz, S. A.: Left ventricular mechanical adaptation to chronic aortic regurgitation in intact dogs. Am. J. Physiol. 252:H969, 1987.

518a. Borow, K. M., and Marcus, R. H.: Aortic regurgitation: The need for an integrated physiologic approach. J. Am. Coll. Cardiol. 17:898, 1991.

519. Grossman, W., Jones, D., and McLaurin, L. P.: Wall stress and patterns of hypertrophy in the human left ventricle. J. Clin. Invest. 56:56, 1975.

520. Laniado, S., Yellin, E. L., Yoran, C., et al.: Physiologic mechanism in aortic insufficiency. I. The effect of changing heart rate on flow dynamics. II. Determinants of Austin Flint murmur. Circulation 66:226, 1982.

521. Kawanishi, D. T., McKay, C. R., Chandraratna, A. N., et al.: Cardiovascular response to dynamic exercise in patients with chronic symptomatic mild-to-moderate and severe aortic regurgitation. Circulation 73:62, 1986.

522. Massie, B. M., Kramer, B. L., Loge, D., et al.: Ejection fraction response to supine exercise in asymptomatic aortic regurgitation: Relation to simultaneous hemodynamic measurements. J. Am. Coll. Cardiol. 5:847, 1985.

523. Mehmel, H. C., Olshausen, K. V., Schuler, G., et al.: Estimation of left ventricular myocardial function by the ejection fraction in isolated, chronic, pure aortic regurgitation. Am. J. Cardiol. 54:610, 1984.

524. Iskandrian, A. S., Hakki, A-H., and Kane-Marsch, S.: Left ventricular pressure/volume relationship in aortic regurgitation. Am. Heart J. 110:1026, 1985.

525. Shen, W. F., Roubin, G. S., Choong, C.Y.-P., et al.: Evaluation of relationship between myocardial contractile state and left ventricular function in patients with aortic regurgitation. Circulation 71:31, 1985.

526. Scognamiglio, R., Roelandt, J., Fasoli, G., et al.: Relation between myocardial contractility, hypertrophy and pump performance in patients with chronic aortic regurgitation: An echocardiographic study. Int. J. Cardiol. 6:473, 1984.

527. Ricci, D. R.: Afterload mismatch and preload reserve in chronic aortic regurgitation. Circulation 66:826, 1982.

528. Greenberg, B., Massie, B., Thomas, D., et al.: Association between the exercise ejection fraction response and systolic wall stress in patients with chronic aortic insufficiency. Circulation 57:1485, 1985.

529. Falsetti, H. L., Carroll, R. J., and Cramer, J. A.: Total and regional myocardial blood flow in aortic regurgitation. Am. Heart J. 97:485, 1979.

530. Uhl, G. S., Boucher, C. A., Oliveros, R. A., and Murgo, J. P.: Exercise-induced myocardial oxygen supply-demand imbalance in asymptomatic or mildly symptomatic aortic regurgitation. Chest 80:686, 1981.

531. Nitenberg, A., Foult, J-M., Antony, I., et al.: Coronary flow and resistance reserve in patients with chronic aortic regurgitation, angina pectoris, and normal coronary arteries. J. Am. Coll. Cardiol. 11:478, 1988.

532. Maurer, W., Ablasser, A., Tschada, R., et al.: Myocardial catecholamine metabolism in patients with chronic aortic regurgitation. Circulation 66(Suppl. I):139, 1982.

533. Dehmer, G. J., Firth, E. G., Hillis, L. D., et al.: Alterations in left ventricular volumes and ejection fraction at rest and during exercise in patients with aortic regurgitation. Am. J. Cardiol. 48:17, 1981.

534. Lewis, S. M., Riba, A. L., Berger, H. J., et al.: Radionuclide angiographic exercise left ventricular performance in chronic aortic regurgitation: Relationship to resting echographic ventricular dimensions and systolic wall stress index. Am. Heart J. 103:498, 1982.

535. Schuler, G., Olshausen, K. V., Schwarz, F., et al.: Noninvasive assessment of myocardial contractility in asymptomatic patients with severe aortic regurgitation and normal left ventricular ejection fraction at rest. Am. J. Cardiol. 50:45, 1982.

536. Benotti, J. R.: Acute aortic insufficiency. In Dalen, J. E., and Alpert, J. S. (eds.): Valvular Heart Disease. 2nd ed. Boston, Little, Brown and Company, 1987, pp. 319–352.

537. Dervan, J., and Goldberg, S.: Acute aortic regurgitation: Pathophysiology and management. In Frankl, W. S., and Brest, A. N. (eds.): Cardiovascular Clinics. Valvular Heart Disease: Comprehensive Evaluation and Management. Philadelphia, F. A. Davis, 1986, pp. 281–288.

538. Perloff, J. K.: Acute severe aortic regurgitation: Recognition and management. J. Cardiovasc. Med. 8:209, 1983.

539. Downes, T. R., Nomeir, A-M., Hackshaw, B. T., et al.: Diastolic mitral regurgitation in acute but not chronic aortic regurgitation: Implications regarding the mechanism of mitral closure. Am. Heart J. 117:1106, 1989.

540. Spagnuolo, M., Kloth, H., Taranta, A., et al.: Natural history of rheumatic aortic regurgitation: Criteria predictive of death, congestive heart failure and angina in young patients. Circulation 44:368, 1971.

541. Benotti, J. R., and Dalen, J. E.: Aortic valvular regurgitation: Natural history and medical treatment. In Cohn, L. H., and DiSesa, V. J. (eds.): Aortic Regurgitation: Medical and Surgical Management. New York, Marcel Dekker, 1986, pp. 1–14.

542. Sapira, J. D.: Quincke, DeMusset, Duroziez and Hill: Some aortic regurgitations. South. Med. J. 74:459, 1981.

542a. Boudoulas, H., Triposkiadis, F., Dervenagas, et al.: Mechanisms of pistol shot sounds in aortic regurgitation. Acta Cardiol. XLVI:139, 1991.

543. Alpert, J. S., Veiweg, W.V.R., and Hagan, A. D.: Incidence and morphology of carotid shudders in aortic valve disease. Am. Heart J. 92:435, 1976.

544. Sabbah, H. N., Khaja, F., Anbe, D. T., and Stein, P. D.: The aortic closure sound in pure aortic insufficiency. Circulation 56:859, 1977.

544a. Aortic Insufficiency, In Fowler, N. O.: Diagnosis of Heart Disease. New York, Springer-Verlag, 1991, pp. 123–133.

545. Abdulla, A. M., Frank, M. J., Erdin, R. A., Jr., and Canedo, M. I.: Clinical significance and hemodynamic correlates of the third heart sound gallop in aortic regurgitation. A guide to optimal timing of cardiac catheterization. Circulation 64:464, 1981.

546. Harvey, W., Corrado, M. A., and Perloff, J. K.: "Right-sided" murmurs of aortic insufficiency. Am. J. Med. Sci. 245:53, 1963.

547. Fortuin, N. J., and Craige, E.: On the mechanism of the Austin Flint murmur. Circulation 45:558, 1972.

548. Delman, A. J., and Stein, E.: Aortic regurgitation. In Dynamic Cardiac Auscultation and Phonocardiography. Philadelphia, W. B. Saunders Company, 1979, pp. 811–824.

549. Spring, D. A., Folts, J. D., Young, W. P., and Rowe, G. G.: Premature closure of the mitral and tricuspid valves. Circulation 45:663, 1972.

550. Wong, M.: Diastolic mitral regurgitation. Hemodynamic and angiographic correlation. Br. Heart J. 31:468, 1969.

551. Estes, E. H.: Left ventricular hypertrophy in acquired heart disease: A comparison of the vectorcardiogram in aortic stenosis and aortic insufficiency. In Hoffman, I. (ed.): Vectorcardiography. Amsterdam, North Holland Publishing Co., 1976.

552. Roberts, W. C., and Day, P. J.: Electrocardiographic observations in clinically isolated, pure, and chronic, severe aortic regurgitation: Analysis of 30 necropsy patients aged 19 to 65 years. Am. J. Cardiol. 55:431, 1985.

553. DePace, N. L., Nestico, P. F., Kotler, M. N., et al.: Comparison of echocardiography and angiography in determining the cause of severe aortic regurgitation. Br. Heart J. 51:36, 1984.

554. Meyer, T., Sareli, P., Pocock, W. A., et al.: Echocardiographic and hemodynamic correlates of diastolic closure of mitral valve and diastolic opening of aortic valve in severe aortic regurgitation. Am. J. Cardiol. 59:1144, 1987.

555. Weaver, W. F., Wilson, C. S., Rourke, T., and Caudill, C. C.: Mid-diastolic aortic valve opening in severe acute aortic regurgitation. Circulation 55:112, 1977.

556. Louie, E. K., Mason, T. J., Shah, R., et al.: Determinants of anterior mitral leaflet fluttering in pure aortic regurgitation from pulsed Doppler study of the early diastolic interaction between the regurgitant jet and mitral inflow. Am. J. Cardiol. 61:1085, 1988.

557. Grayburn, P. A., Smith, M. D., Handshoe, R., et al.: Detection of aortic insufficiency by standard echocardiography, pulsed Doppler echocardiography and auscultation. Ann. Intern. Med. 104:599, 1986.

558. Downes, T. R., Nomeir, A-D., Hackshaw, B. T., et al.: Diastolic mitral regurgitation in acute but not chronic aortic regurgitation: Implications regarding the mechanism of mitral closure. Am. Heart J. 117:1106, 1989.

559. Masuyama, T., Kodama, K., Kitabatake, A., et al.: Noninvasive evaluation of aortic regurgitation by continuous-wave Doppler echocardiography. Circulation 73:460, 1986.

560. Manyari, D. E., Nolewajka, A. J., and Kostuk, W. J.: Quantitative assessment of aortic valvular insufficiency by radionuclide angiography. Chest 81:170, 1982.

561. Steingart, R. M., Yee, C., Weinstein, L., and Scheuer, J.: Radio-nuclide ventriculographic study of adaptations to exercise in aortic regurgitation. Am. J. Cardiol. 51:483, 1983.

562. Sareli, P., Klein, H. O., Schamroth, C. L., et al.: Contribution of echocardiography and immediate surgery to the management of severe aortic regurgitation from active infective endocarditis. Am. J. Cardiol. 57:413, 1986.

563. Goldschlager, N., Pfeifer, J., Cohn, K., et al.: The natural history of aortic regurgitation. A clinical and hemodynamic study. Am. J. Med. 54:577, 1973.

564. Cheitlin, M. D., Bonow, R. O., Parmley, W. W., et al.: Task force II: Acquired valvular heart disease. J. Am. Coll. Cardiol. 6:1209, 1985.

565. Greenberg, B. H., DeMots, H., Murphy, E., and Rahimtoola, S. H.: Mechanism for improved cardiac performance with arteriolar dilators in aortic insufficiency. Circulation 63:263, 1981.

566. Elkayam, U., McKay, C. R., Weber, L., et al.: Favorable effects of hydralazine on the hemodynamic response to isometric exercise in chronic severe aortic regurgitation. Am. J. Cardiol. 54:1603, 1984.

567. Fioretti, P., Benussi, B., Scardi, S., et al.: Afterload reduction with nifedipine in aortic insufficiency. Am. J. Cardiol. 49:1728, 1982.

568. Jebavy, P., Koudelkova, E., and Henzlova, M.: Unloading effects of prazosin in patients with chronic aortic regurgitation. Am. Heart J. 105:567, 1983.

569. Kleaveland, J. P., Reichek, N., McCarthy, D. M., et al.: Effects of six-month afterload reduction therapy with hydralazine in chronic aortic regurgitation. Am. J. Cardiol. 57:1109, 1986.

570. Greenberg, B., Massie, B., Bristow, J. D., et al.: Long-term vasodilator therapy of chronic aortic insufficiency. Circulation 78:92, 1988.

571. Dumesnil, J. G., Tran, K., and Dagenais, G. R.: Beneficial long-term effects of hydralazine in aortic regurgitation. Arch. Intern. Med. 150:757, 1990.

572. Scognamiglio, R., Fasoli, G., Ponchia, A., and Dalla-Volta, S.: Long-term nifedipine unloading therapy in asymptomatic patients with chronic severe aortic regurgitation. J. Am. Coll. Cardiol. 16:424, 1990.

573. Crawford, M. H., Wilson, R. S., O'Rourke, R. A., and Vittitoe, J. A.: Effect of digoxin and vasodilators on left ventricular function in aortic regurgitation. Int. J. Cardiol. 23:385, 1989.

574. Hoshino, P. K., and Gaasch, W. H.: When to intervene in chronic aortic regurgitation. Arch. Intern. Med. 146:346, 1986.

575. Bonow, R. O., Picone, A. L., McIntosh, C. L., et al.: Survival and functional results after valve replacement for aortic regurgitation from 1976 to

1983: Impact of preoperative left ventricular function. Circulation 72:1244, 1985.

576. Turina, J., Turina, M., Rothlin, M., and Krayenbuehl, H. P.: Improved late survival in patients with chronic aortic regurgitation by earlier operation. Circulation 70(Suppl. I):147, 1984.

577. Gee, D. S., Juni, J. E., Santinga, J. T., and Buda, A. J.: Prognostic significance of exercise-induced left ventricular dysfunction in chronic aortic regurgitation. Am. J. Cardiol. 56:605, 1985.

578. Stone, P. H., Clark, R. D., Goldschlager, N., et al.: Determinants of prognosis of patients with aortic regurgitation who undergo aortic valve replacement. J. Am. Coll. Cardiol. 3:1118, 1984.

579. Nishimura, R., McGoon, M. D., Schaff, H. V., and Giuliani, E. R.: Chronic aortic regurgitation: Indications for operation — 1988. Mayo Clin. Proc. 63:270, 1988.

580. Louagie, Y., Brohet, C., Robert, A., et al.: Factors influencing postoperative survival in aortic regurgitation. J. Thorac. Cardiovasc. Surg. 88:225, 1984.

581. Borow, K. M., Surgical outcome in chronic aortic regurgitation: A physiologic framework for assessing preoperative predictors. J. Am. Coll. Cardiol. 10:1165, 1987.

582. Taniguchi, K., Nakano, S., Matsuda, H., et al.: Depressed myocardial contractility and normal ejection performance after aortic valve replacement in patients with aortic regurgitation. J. Thorac. Cardiovasc. Surg. 98:258, 1989.

583. Toussaint, C., Cribier, A., Cazor, J. L., et al.: Hemodynamic and angiographic evaluation of aortic regurgitation 8 and 27 months after aortic valve replacement. Circulation 64:456, 1981.

584. Bonow, R. O., Rosing, D. R., Kent, K. M., and Epstein, S. E.: Timing of operation for chronic aortic regurgitation. Am. J. Cardiol. 50:325, 1982.

585. Errichetti, A., Greenberg, J. M., and Gaasch, W. M.: Is valve replacement indicated in asymptomatic patients with aortic stenosis or aortic regurgitation? In Cheitlin, M. (ed.): Dilemmas in Clinical Cardiology. Philadelphia, F. A. Davis, 1991.

586. Bonow, R. O.: Noninvasive evaluation: Prognosis and timing of operation in symptomatic and asymptomatic patients with chronic aortic regurgitation. In Cohn, L. H., and DiSesa, V. J. (eds.): Aortic Regurgitation: Medical and Surgical Management. New York, Marcel Dekker, 1986, pp. 55–86.

587. Bonow, R. O., Dodd, J. T., Maron, B. J., et al.: Long-term serial changes in left ventricular function and reversal of ventricular dilatation after valve replacement for chronic aortic regurgitation. Circulation 78:1108, 1988.

588. Carabello, B. A., Usher, B. W., Hedrik, G. H., et al.: Predictors of outcome for aortic valve replacement in patients with aortic regurgitation and left ventricular dysfunction: A change in the measuring stick. J. Am. Coll. Cardiol. 10:991, 1987.

589. Taniguchi, K., Nakano, S., Hirose, H., et al.: Preoperative left ventricular function: Minimal requirement for successful late results of valve replacement for aortic regurgitation. J. Am. Coll. Cardiol. 10:510, 1987.

590. Wisenbaugh, T., Booth, D., DeMaria, A., et al.: Relationship of contractile state to ejection performance in patients with chronic aortic valve disease. Circulation 73:47, 1986.

591. Carroll, J. D., Gaasch, W. H., Naimi, S., and Levine, H. J.: Regression of myocardial hypertrophy: Electrocardiographic-echocardiographic correlations after aortic valve replacement in patients with chronic aortic regurgitation. Circulation 65:980, 1982.

592. Carroll, J. D., Gaasch, W. H., Zile, M. R., and Levine, H. J.: Serial changes in left ventricular function after correction of chronic aortic regurgitation. Dependence on early changes in preload and subsequent regression of hypertrophy. Am. J. Cardiol. 51:476, 1983.

593. Donaldson, R. M., Florio, R., Rickards, A. F., et al.: Irreversible morphological changes contributing to depressed cardiac function after surgery for chronic aortic regurgitation. Br. Heart J. 48:589, 1982.

TRICUSPID, PULMONIC, AND MULTIVALVULAR DISEASE

594. Hauck, A. J., Freeman, D. P., Ackermann, D. M., et al.: Surgical pathology of the tricuspid valve: A study of 363 cases spanning 25 years. Mayo Clin. Proc. 63:851, 1988.

595. Smith, J. A., and Levine, S. A.: Clinical features of tricuspid stenosis. Am. Heart J. 23:739, 1942.

596. Ribeiro, P. A., Al Zaibag, M., Al Kasab, S., et al.: Provocation and amplification of the transvalvular pressure gradient in rheumatic tricuspid stenosis. Am. J. Cardiol. 61:1307, 1988.

597. Perloff, J. K., and Harvey, W. P.: The clinical recognition of tricuspid stenosis. Circulation 22:346, 1960.

598. Morgan, J. R., Forker, A. D., Coates, J. R., and Myers, W. S.: Isolated tricuspid stenosis. Circulation 44:729, 1971.

599. Ockene, I. S.: Tricuspid valve disease. In Dalen, J. E., and Alpert, J. S. (eds.): Valvular Heart Disease. 2nd ed. Boston, Little, Brown and Company, 1987, pp. 353–402.

600. Wooley, C. F., Fontana, M. E., Kilman, J. W., and Ryan, J. M.: Tricuspid stenosis: Atrial systolic murmur, tricuspid opening snap and right atrial pressure pulse. Am. J. Med. 78:375, 1985.

601. Kitchin, A., and Turner, R.: Diagnosis and treatment of tricuspid stenosis. Br. Heart J. 26:354, 1964.

602. Mahapatra, R. K., Agarwal, J. B., and Wasir, H. S.: Rheumatic tricuspid stenosis. Indian Heart J. 30:138, 1978.

602a. Tricuspid valve disease. In Fowler, N. O.: Diagnosis of Heart Disease. New York, Springer-Verlag, 1991, pp. 181–186.

603. Daniels, S. J., Mintz, G. S., and Kotler, M. N.: Rheumatic tricuspid valve disease. Two-dimensional echocardiographic, hemodynamic, and angiographic correlations. Am. J. Cardiol. 51:492, 1983.

604. Pillai, M. G., Sharma, S., Munsi, S. C., Desai, A. G., and Panday, S. R.: Value of echocardiography in detecting rheumatic tricuspid stenosis. J. Cardiovasc. Ultrasonogr. 4:185, 1985.

605. Ribeiro, P. A., Al Zaibag, M., and Sawyer, W.: A prospective study comparing the haemodynamic with the cross-sectional echocardiographic diagnosis of rheumatic tricuspid stenosis. Eur. Heart J. 10:120, 1989.

606. Guyer, D. E., Gillam, L. D., Foale, R. A., et al.: Comparison of the echocardiographic and hemodynamic diagnosis of rheumatic tricuspid stenosis. J. Am. Coll. Cardiol. 3:1135, 1984.

607. Shimada, R., Takeshita, A., Nakamura, M., et al.: Diagnosis of tricuspid stenosis by M-mode and two-dimensional echocardiography. Am. J. Cardiol. 53:164, 1984.

608. Fawzy, M. E., Mercer, E. N., Dunn, B., et al.: Doppler echocardiography in the evaluation of tricuspid stenosis. Eur. Heart J. 10:985, 1989.

609. Péterffy, A., Jonasson, R., and Henze, A.: Haemodynamic changes after tricuspid valve surgery. Scand. J. Thorac. Cardiovasc. Surg. 15:161, 1981.

610. Throburn, C. W., Morgan, J. J., Shanahan, M. X., and Chang, V. P.: Long-term results of tricuspid valve replacement and the problem of prosthetic valve thrombosis. Am. J. Cardiol. 51:1128, 1983.

611. Boskovic, D., Elezovic, I., Boskovic, D., et al.: Late thrombosis of the Björk-Shiley tilting disc valve in the tricuspid position. J. Thorac. Cardiovasc. Surg. 91:1, 1986.

612. Cobanoglu, A., and Starr, A.: Tricuspid valve surgery: Indications, methods, and results. In Frankl, W. S., and Brest, A. N. (eds.): Cardiovascular Clinics. Valvular Heart Disease: Comprehensive Evaluation and Management. Philadelphia, F. A. Davis, 1986, pp. 375–388.

613. Guerra, F., Bortolotti, U., Thiene, G., et al.: Long-term performance of the Hancock porcine bioprosthesis in the tricuspid position. A review of 45 patients with 14-year follow-up. J. Thorac. Cardiovasc. Surg. 99:838, 1990.

614. Goldenberg, I. F., Pedersen, W., Olson, J., et al.: Percutaneous double balloon valvuloplasty for severe tricuspid stenosis. Am. Heart J. 118:417, 1989.

615. Shafie, M. Z., Hayat, N., and Majid, O. A.: Fate of tricuspid regurgitation after closed valvotomy for mitral stenosis. Chest 88:870, 1985.

616. Cohen, S. R., Sell, J. E., McIntosh, C. L., and Clark, R. E.: Tricuspid regurgitation in patients with acquired, chronic, pure mitral regurgitation. 1. Prevalence, diagnosis, and comparison of preoperative clinical and hemodynamic features in patients with and without tricuspid regurgitation. J. Thorac. Cardiovasc. Surg. 94:481, 1987.

617. Morrison, D. A., Ovitt, T., and Hammermeister, K. E.: Functional tricuspid regurgitation and right ventricular dysfunction in pulmonary hypertension. Am. J. Cardiol. 62:108, 1988.

618. Vatterott, P. J., Nishimura, R. A., Gersh, B. J., and Smith, H. C.: Severe isolated tricuspid insufficiency in coronary artery disease. Int. J. Cardiol. 14:295, 1987.

619. Dougherty, M. J., and Craige, E.: Apathetic hyperthyroidism presenting as tricuspid regurgitation. Chest 63:767, 1973.

620. Scheck-Krejca, H., Zulstra, F., Roelandt, J., and Vletter-McGhie, J.: Diagnosis of tricuspid regurgitation: Comparison of jugular venous and liver pulse tracings with combined two-dimensional and Doppler echocardiography. Eur. Heart J. 7:973, 1986.

621. Come, P. C., and Riley, M. F.: Tricuspid anular dilatation and failure of tricuspid leaflet coaptation in patients with tricuspid regurgitation. Am. J. Cardiol. 55:599, 1985.

622. Tei, C., Pilgrim, J. P., Shah, P. M., et al.: The tricuspid valve annulus: Study of size and motion in normal subjects and in patients with tricuspid regurgitation. Circulation 66:665, 1982.

623. Mikami, T., Kudo, T., Sakurai, N., et al.: Mechanisms for development of functional tricuspid regurgitation determined by pulsed Doppler and two-dimensional echocardiography. Am. J. Cardiol. 53:160, 1984.

624. Esaghpour, E., Kawai, N., and Linhart, J. W.: Tricuspid insufficiency associated with aneurysm of the ventricular septum. Pediatrics 61:586, 1978.

625. Sakai, K., Inoue, Y., and Osawa, M.: Congenital isolated tricuspid regurgitation in an adult. Am. Heart J. 110:680, 1985.

626. Schlamowitz, R. A., Gross, S., Keating, E., et al.: Tricuspid valve prolapse: A common occurrence in the click-murmur syndrome. J. Clin. Ultrasound 10:435, 1982.

627. Weinreich, D. J., Burke, J. F., Bharati, S., and Lev, M.: Isolated prolapse of the tricuspid valve. J. Am. Coll. Cardiol. 6:475, 1985.

628. Jackson, D., Gibbs, H. R., and Zee-Cheng, C. S.: Isolated tricuspid valve prolapse diagnosed by echocardiography. Am. J. Med. 80:281, 1986.

629. Chandraratna, P.A.N., Littman, B. B., and Wilson, D.: The association between atrial septal defect and prolapse of the tricuspid valve. An echocardiographic study. Chest 73:839, 1978.

630. Gayet, C., Pierre, B., Delahaye, J-P., et al.: Traumatic tricuspid insufficiency: An underdiagnosed disease. Chest 92:429, 1987.

631. Dickerman, S. A., and Rubler, S.: Mitral and tricuspid valve regurgitation in dilated cardiomyopathy. Am. J. Cardiol. 63:629, 1989.

632. Ginzton, L. E., Siegel, R. J., and Criley, J. M.: Natural history of tricuspid valve endocarditis: A two-dimensional echocardiographic study. Am. J. Cardiol. 49:1853, 1982.

633. Arbulu, A., and Asfaw, I.: Tricuspid valvulectomy without prosthetic replacement. Ten years of clinical experience. J. Thorac. Cardiovasc. Surg. 82:684, 1981.

634. Lundin, L., Norheim, I., Landelius, J., et al.: Carcinoid heart disease: Relationship of circulating vasoactive substances to ultrasound-detectable cardiac abnormalities. Circulation 77:264, 1988.

635. Callahan, J. A., Wroblewski, E. M., Reeder, G. S., et al.: Echocardiographic features of carcinoid heart disease. Am. J. Cardiol. 50:762, 1982.

636. Gutman, J. M., and Schiller, N. B.: Carcinoid heart disease: Diagnostic usefulness of echocardiography. Primary Cardiol. 9:130, 1983.

637. Mason, J. W., Billingham, M. E., and Friedman, J. P.: Methysergide-induced heart disease: A case of multivalvular and myocardial fibrosis. Circulation 56:889, 1977.

638. Laufer, J., Frand, M., and Milo, S.: Valve replacement for severe tricuspid regurgitation caused by Libman-Sacks endocarditis. Br. Heart J. 48:294, 1982.

639. Allen, S. J., and Naylor, D.: Pulsation of the eyeballs in tricuspid regurgitation. Can. Med. Assoc. J. 133:119, 1985.

640. Abrams, J.: Tricuspid regurgitation. In Essentials of Cardiac Physical Diagnosis. Philadelphia, Lea and Febiger, 1987, pp. 375–400.

641. Cha, S. D., and Gooch, A. S.: Diagnosis of tricuspid regurgitation: Current status. Arch. Intern. Med. 143:1763, 1983.

642. Amidi, M., Irwin, J. M., Salerni, R., et al.: Venous systolic thrill and murmur in the neck: A consequence of severe tricuspid insufficiency. J. Am. Coll. Cardiol. 7:942, 1986.

643. Cha, S. D., Gooch, A. S., and Maranhao, V.: Intracardiac phonocardiography in tricuspid regurgitation: Relation to clinical and angiographic findings. Am. J. Cardiol. 48:578, 1981.

644. Maisel, A. S., Atwood, J. E., and Goldberger, A. L.: Hepatojugular reflux: Useful in the bedside diagnosis of tricuspid regurgitation. Ann. Intern. Med. 101:781, 1984.

645. Sepulveda, G., and Lukas, D. S.: The diagnosis of tricuspid insufficiency: Clinical features in 60 cases with associated mitral valve disease. Circulation 11:552, 1955.

646. Hubbard, W. N., Westgate, C., Shapiro, L. M., and Donaldson, R. M.: Acquired abnormalities of the tricuspid valve—an ultrasonographic study. Int. J. Cardiol. 14:311, 1987.

647. Meltzer, R. S., van Hoogenhuyze, D., Serruys, P. W., et al.: Diagnosis of tricuspid regurgitation by contrast echocardiography. Circulation 63:1093, 1981.

648. Tei, C., Shah, P. M., and Ormiston, J. A.: Assessment of tricuspid regurgitation by directional analysis of right atrial systolic linear reflux echoes with contrast M-mode echocardiography. Am. Heart J. 103:1025, 1982.

649. Forman, M. B., Byrd, B. F., Oates, J. A., and Robertson, R. M.: Two-dimensional echocardiography in the diagnosis of carcinoid heart disease. Am. Heart J. 107:492, 1984.

650. Curtius, J. M., Thyssen, M., Breuer, H.W.M., and Loogen, F.: Doppler versus contrast echocardiography for diagnosis of tricuspid regurgitation. Am. J. Cardiol. 56:333, 1985.

651. Diebold, B., Touati, R., Blanchard, D., et al.: Quantitative assessment of tricuspid regurgitation using pulsed Doppler echocardiography. Br. Heart J. 50:443, 1983.

652. Pennestri, F., Loperfido, F., Salvatori, M. F., et al.: Assessment of tricuspid regurgitation by pulsed Doppler ultrasonography of the hepatic veins. Am. J. Cardiol. 54:363, 1984.

653. Yock, P. G., and Popp, R. L.: Noninvasive estimation of right ventricular systolic pressure by Doppler ultrasound in patients with tricuspid regurgitation. Circulation 70:657, 1984.

654. Skjaerpe, T., and Hatle, L.: Noninvasive estimation of systolic pressure in the right ventricle in patients with tricuspid regurgitation. Eur. Heart J. 7:704, 1986.

655. Suzuki, Y., Kambara, H., Kadota, K., et al.: Detection and evaluation of tricuspid regurgitation using a real-time, two-dimensional, color-coded, Doppler flow imaging system: Comparison with contrast two-dimensional echocardiography and right ventriculography. Am. J. Cardiol. 57:811, 1986.

656. Wong, M., Matsumara, M., Kutsuzawa, S., and Omoto, R.: The value of Doppler echocardiography in the treatment of tricuspid regurgitation in patients with mitral valve replacement. J. Thorac. Cardiovasc. Surg. 99:1003, 1990.

657. Lambertz, H., Minale, C., Flachskampf, F. A., et al.: Long-term follow-up after Carpentier tricuspid valvuloplasty. Am. Heart J. 117:615, 1989.

658. Lingameni, R., Cha, S. D., Maranhao, V., et al.: Tricuspid regurgitation: Clinical and angiographic assessment. Cathet. Cardiovasc. Diagn. 5:7, 1979.

659. Pepino, C. J., Nichols, W. W., and Selby, J. H.: Diagnostic tests for tricuspid insufficiency: How good? Cathet. Cardiovasc. Diagn. 5:1, 1979.

660. Lingameni, R., Cha, S. D., Maranhao, V., et al.: Tricuspid regurgitation: Clinical and angiographic assessment. Cathet. Cardiovasc. Diagn. 5:7, 1979.

661. Ubago, J. L., Figueroa, A., Colman, T., et al.: Right ventriculography as a valid method for the diagnosis of tricuspid insufficiency. Cathet. Cardiovasc. Diagn. 7:433, 1981.

662. Barbour, D. J., and Roberts, W. C.: Valve excision only versus valve excision plus replacement for active infective endocarditis involving the tricuspid valve. Am. J. Cardiol. 57:475, 1986.

663. Carpentier, A., Deloche, A., and Dauptain, J.: A new reconstructive operation for correction of mitral and tricuspid insufficiency. J. Thorac. Cardiovasc. Surg. 61:1, 1971.

664. Kirklin, J. W., and Barratt-Boyes, B. G.: Tricuspid valve disease. In Cardiac Surgery. New York, John Wiley and Sons, 1986, pp. 447–462.

665. Stolf, N.A.G., Moreira, L.F.P., Costa, R., et al.: The DeVega annuloplasty as surgical treatment for tricuspid incompetence. Int. J. Surg. 68:201, 1983.

666. Cohen, S. R., Sell, J. E., McIntosh, C. L., and Clark, R. E.: Tricuspid regurgitation in patients with acquired, chronic, pure mitral regurgitation. II. Nonoperative management, tricuspid valve annuloplasty, and tricuspid valve replacement. J. Thorac. Cardiovasc. Surg. 94:488, 1987.

667. Minale, C., Lambertz, H., Nikol, S., et al.: Selective annuloplasty of the tricuspid valve. Two years experience. J. Thorac. Cardiovasc. Surg. 99:846, 1990.

668. Duran, C.M.G., Pomar, J. L., Colman, T., et al.: Is tricuspid valve repair necessary? J. Thorac. Cardiovasc. Surg. 80:849, 1980.

669. Chidambaram, M., Abdulali, S. A., Baliga, B. G., and Ionescu, M. I.: Long-term results of DeVega tricuspid annuloplasty. Ann. Thorac. Surg. 43:185, 1987.

670. Kratz, J. M., Crawford, F. A., Stroud, M. R., et al.: Trends and results in tricuspid valve surgery. Chest 88:837, 1985.

671. Abe, T., and Komatsu, S.: Valve replacement for Ebstein's anomaly of the tricuspid valve. Chest 84:414, 1983.

672. Silver, M. A., Cohen, S. R., McIntosh, C. L., et al.: Late (5 to 132 months) clinical and hemodynamic results after either tricuspid valve replacement of annuloplasty for Ebstein's anomaly of the tricuspid valve. Am. J. Cardiol. 54:627, 1984.

673. Miller, B. R., Vohr, F. H., Christian, F. V., and Singh, A. K.: Cardiac valvular replacement in carcinoid heart disease. Am. J. Med. 75:896, 1983.

674. Kirshenbaum, H. D.: Pulmonary valve disease. In Dalen, J. E., and Alpert, J. S. (eds.): Valvular Heart Disease. 2nd ed. Boston, Little, Brown and Company, 1987, pp. 403–438.

675. Vela, J. E., Conteras, R., and Sosa, F. R.: Rheumatic pulmonary valve disease. Am. J. Cardiol. 23:12, 1969.

676. Altrichter, P. M., Olson, L. J., Edwards, W. D., et al.: Surgical pathology of the pulmonary valve: A study of 116 cases spanning 15 years. Mayo Clin. Proc. 64:1352, 1989.

677. Seymour, J., Emanuel, R., and Patterson, N.: Acquired pulmonary stenosis. Br. Heart J. 30:776, 1968.

678. Brayshaw, J. R., and Perloff, J. K.: Congenital pulmonary insufficiency complicating idiopathic dilatation of the pulmonary artery. Am. J. Cardiol. 10:282, 1962.

679. Runco, V., and Levin, H. S.: The spectrum of pulmonic regurgitation. In Physiologic Principles of Heart Sounds and Murmurs. American Heart Association Monograph No. 46, 1975, p. 175.

680. Childers, R. W., and McCrea, P. C.: Absence of the pulmonary valve. A case occurring in the Marfan's syndrome. Circulation 29:598, 1964.

681. Cassling, R. S., Rogler, W. C., and McManus, B. M.: Isolated pulmonic valve infective endocarditis: A diagnostically elusive entity. Am. Heart J. 109:558, 1985.

682. Cremieux, A. C., Witchitz, S., Malergue, M. C., et al.: Clinical and echocardiographic observations in pulmonary valve endocarditis. Am. J. Cardiol. 56:610, 1985.

683. DePace, N. L., Nestico, P. F., Iskandrian, A. S., and Morganroth, J.: Acute severe pulmonic valve regurgitation: Pathophysiology, diagnosis and treatment. Am. Heart J. 108:567, 1984.

684. Collins, N. P., Braunwald, E., and Morrow, A. G.: Isolated congenital pulmonic valvular regurgitation. Am. J. Med. 28:159, 1960.

685. Jacoby, W. J., Tucker, D. H., and Sumner, R. G.: The second heart sound in congenital pulmonary valvular insufficiency. Am. Heart J. 69:603, 1965.

686. O'Toole, J. D., Wurtzbacher, J. J., Wearner, N. E., and Jain, A. C.: Pulmonary valve injury and insufficiency during pulmonary-artery catheterization. N. Engl. J. Med. 301:1167, 1979.

687. Bousvaros, G. A., and Deuchar, D. C.: The murmur of pulmonary regurgitation which is not associated with pulmonary hypertension. Lancet 2:962, 1961.

688. Enomoto, D., Fenster, P. E., Ewy, G. A., and Salomon, N.: Effect of mitral regurgitation on the murmur of pulmonic regurgitation. Chest 83:822, 1983.

689. Masuyama, T., Kodama, K., Kitabatake, A., et al.: Continuous-wave Doppler echocardiographic detection of pulmonary regurgitation and its application to noninvasive estimation of pulmonary artery pressure. Circulation 74:484, 1986.

690. Green, E. W., Agruss, N. S., and Adolph, R. J.: Right-sided Austin Flint murmur. Documentation by intracardiac phonocardiography, echocardiography and postmortem findings. Am. J. Cardiol. 32:370, 1973.

691. Braunwald, E., and Morrow, A. G.: A method for detection and estimation of aortic regurgitant flow in man. Circulation 17:505, 1958.

692. Pernot, C., Hoeffel, J. C., Henry, M., et al.: Radiological patterns of congenital absence of the pulmonary valve in infants. Radiology 102:619, 1972.

693. Collins, N. P., Braunwald, E., and Morrow, A. G.: Detection of pulmonic and tricuspid valvular regurgitation by means of indicator solutions. Circulation 20:561, 1959.

694. Van Meurs-Van Woezik, H., McGhie, J., and Roelandt, J.: Septal flutter in pulmonary insufficiency. J. Cardiovasc. Ultrasonogr. 3:159, 1984.

695. Miyatake, K., Okamoto, M., Kinoshita, N., et al.: Pulmonary regurgitation studied with the ultrasonic pulsed Doppler technique. Circulation 65:969, 1982.

696. Meltzer, R. S., Vered, Z., Hegesh, T., et al.: Diagnosis of pulmonic regurgitation by contrast echocardiography. Am. Heart J. 107:102, 1984.

697. Emery, R. W., Landes, R. G., Moller, J. H., and Nicoloff, D. M.: Pulmonary valve replacement with a porcine aortic heterograft. Ann. Thorac. Surg. 27:148, 1979.

698. Paraskos, J. A.: Combined valvular disease. In Dalen, J. E., and Alpert, J. S. (eds.): Valvular Heart Disease. 2nd ed. Boston, Little, Brown and Company, 1987, pp. 439–508.

699. Segal, J., Harvey, W. P., and Hufnagel, C. A.: Clinical study of one hundred cases of severe aortic insufficiency. Am. J. Med. 21:200, 1956.

700. Gash, A. K., Carabello, B. A., Kent, R. L., et al.: Left ventricular performance in patients with coexistent mitral stenosis and aortic insufficiency. J. Am. Coll. Cardiol. 3:703, 1984.

701. Zitnik, R. S.: The masking of aortic stenosis by mitral stenosis. Am. Heart J. 69:22, 1965.

702. Schattenberg, T. T., Titus, J. L., and Parkin, T. W.: Clinical findings in

acquired aortic valve stenosis. Effect of disease of other valves. Am. Heart J. 73:322, 1967.

703. Melvin, D. B., Tecklenberg, P. L., Hollingsworth, J. F., et al.: Computer-based analysis of preoperative and postoperative prognostic factors in 100 patients with combined aortic and mitral valve replacement. Circulation 48(Suppl. III):58, 1973.

704. Rippe, J. M.: Multiple floppy valves. An echocardiographic syndrome. Am. J. Med. 66:817, 1979.

705. Baxley, W. A., and Soto, B.: Hemodynamic evaluation of patients with combined mitral and aortic prostheses. Am. J. Cardiol. 45:42, 1980.

706. Kirklin, J. W., and Barratt-Boyes, B. G.: Combined aortic and mitral valve disease with or without tricuspid valve disease. In Cardiac Surgery. New York, John Wiley and Sons, 1986, pp. 431–446.

707. Stephenson, L. W., Edie, R. N., Harken, A. H., and Edmunds, L. H.: Combined aortic and mitral valve replacement: Changes in practice and prognosis. Circulation 69:640, 1984.

708. Nitter-Hauge, S., and Horstkotte, D.: Management of multivalvular heart disease. Eur. Heart J. 8:643, 1987.

709. Stephenson, L. W., Kouchoukos, N. T., and Kirklin, J. W.: Triple valve replacement: An analysis of eight years' experience. Ann. Thorac. Surg. 23:327, 1977.

710. Coll-Mazzei, J. V., Jegaden, O., Janody, P., et al.: Results of triple valve replacement: Perioperative mortality and long-term results. J. Cardiovasc. Surg. 28:369, 1987.

711. Michel, P. L., Houdart, E., Ghanem, G., et al.: Combined aortic, mitral and tricuspid surgery: Results in 78 patients. Eur. Heart J. 8:457, 1987.

712. MacManus, Q., Grunkemeier, G., and Starr, A.: Late results of triple valve replacement: A 14-year review. Ann. Thorac. Surg. 25:402, 1978.

713. Péterffy, A., Jonasson, R., and Björk, V. O.: Ten years' experience of surgical management of triple valve disease. Early and late results in thirty-four consecutive cases. Scand. J. Thorac. Cardiovasc. Surg. 13:191, 1979.

714. Vatterott, P. J., Gersh, B. J., Fuster, V., et al.: Long-term followup (2–20 years) of patients with triple valve replacement (abstr.). J. Am. Coll. Cardiol. 1:586, 1983.

PROSTHETIC CARDIAC VALVES

715. Braunwald, N. S., Cooper, T. S., and Morrow, A. G.: Complete replacement of the mitral valve. J. Thorac. Cardiovasc. Surg. 40:1, 1960.

716. Harken, D. E., Soroff, M. S., and Taylor, M. C.: Partial and complete prostheses in aortic insufficiency. J. Thorac. Cardiovasc. Surg. 40:744, 1960.

717. Starr, A., and Edwards, M. L.: Mitral replacement: Clinical experience with a ball-valve prosthesis. Ann. Surg. 154:726, 1961.

718. Pilegaard, H. K., Lund, O., Nielsen, T. T., et al.: Twenty-two-year experience with aortic valve replacement: Starr-Edwards ball valves versus disc valves. Texas Heart Inst. J. 18:24, 1991.

719. Grunkemeier, G. L., and Starr, A.: Twenty-five year experience with Starr-Edwards heart valves: Follow-up methods and results. Can. J. Cardiol. 4:381, 1988.

720. Nair, C., Mohiuddin, S. M., Hilleman, D. E., et al.: Ten-year results with the St. Jude medical prosthesis. Am. J. Cardiol. 65:217, 1990.

721. Burckhardt, D., Streibel, D., Vogt, S., et al.: Heart valve replacement with St. Jude medical valve prosthesis: Long-term experience in 743 patients in Switzerland. Circulation 78(Suppl. I):I18, 1988.

722. Austin, E. H., III: Other mechanical prostheses. In Crawford, F. A. (ed.): Cardiac Surgery: Current Heart Valve Prostheses. Vol. 1. Hanley and Belfus, Philadelphia, 1987, pp. 237–268.

723. Damle, A., Gelfand, E., and Callaghan, J.: Six years clinical experience with the Omniscience cardiac valve. Can. J. Cardiol 4:372, 1988.

724. Stewart, S., Cianciotta, D., Hicks, G. L., and DeWeese, J. A.: The Lillehei-Kaster aortic valve prosthesis. J. Thorac. Cardiovasc. Surg. 95:1023, 1988.

725. Cobanoglu, A., and Brockman, S. K.: Selection of a prosthetic heart valve. In Frankl, W. S., and Brest, A. N. (eds.): Cardiovascular Clinics. Valvular Heart Disease: Comprehensive Evaluation and Management. Philadelphia, F. A. Davis, 1986, pp. 399–414.

726. Starek, P.J.K., Beaudet, R. L., and Hall, K.-V.: The Medtronic-Hall valve: Development and clinical experience. In Crawford, F. A. (ed.): Cardiac Surgery: Current Heart Valve Prostheses. Vol. 1. Hanley and Belfus, Philadelphia, 1987, pp. 223–236.

727. Beaudet, R. L., Nakhle, G., Beaulieu, C. R., et al.: Medtronic-Hall prosthesis: Valve related deaths and complications. Can. J. Cardiol. 4:376, 1988.

728. Lindblom, D., Rodriguez, L., and Björk, V. O.: Mechanical failure of the Björk-Shiley valve. J. Thorac. Cardiovasc. Surg. 97:95, 1989.

729. Lindblom, D.: Long-term clinical results after mitral valve replacement with the Björk-Shiley prosthesis. J. Thorac. Cardiovasc. Surg. 95:321, 1988.

730. Björk, V. O.: The Björk-Shiley tilting disc valve: Past, present, and future. In Crawford, F. A. (ed.): Cardiac Surgery: Current Heart Valve Prostheses. Vol. 1. Hanley and Belfus, Philadelphia, 1987, pp. 183–202.

731. Harker, L. A.: Antithrombotic therapy following mitral valve replacement. In Duran, C., et al. (eds.): Recent Progress in Mitral Valve Disease. London, Butterworths, 1984, pp. 340–348.

732. Alam, M., Rosman, H. S., Lakier, J. B., et al.: Doppler and echocardiographic features of normal and dysfunctioning bioprosthetic valves. J. Am. Coll. Cardiol. 10:851, 1987.

733. Akins, C. W., Carroll, D. L., Buckley, M. J., et al.: Late results with Carpentier-Edwards porcine bioprosthesis. Circulation 82(Suppl. IV):65, 1990.

734. Sugimoto, J. T., and Karp, R. B.: Homografts and cyropreserved valves. In Crawford, F. A. (ed.): Cardiac Surgery: Current Heart Valve Prostheses. Vol. 1. Hanley and Belfus, Philadelphia, 1987, pp. 295–316.

735. Khan, S. S., Mitchell, R. S., Derby, G. C., et al.: Differences in Hancock and

Carpentier-Edwards porcine xenograft aortic valve hemodynamics: Effect of valve size. Circulation 82(Suppl. IV):117, 1990.

736. Matsuki, O., Okita, Y., Almeida, R. S., et al.: Two decades experience with aortic valve replacement with pulmonary autograft. J. Thorac. Cardiovasc. Surg. 95:705, 1988.

737. O'Brien, M. F., Stafford, E. G., Gardner, M. A. H., et al.: A comparison of aortic valve replacement with viable cryopreserved and fresh allograft valves, with a note on chromosomal studies. J. Thorac. Cardiovasc. Surg. 94:812, 1987.

738. Carpentier, A., Lemaigre, G., and Robert, L.: Biological factors affecting long-term results of valvular heterografts. J. Thorac. Cardiovasc. Surg. 58:467, 1969.

739. Cohn, L. H., Collins, J. J., DiSesa, V. J., et al.: Fifteen-year experience with 1678 Hancock porcine bioprosthetic heart valve replacements. Ann. Surg. 210:435, 1989.

740. Bortolotti, U., Milano, A., Mazzucco, A., et al.: Results of reoperation for primary tissue failure of porcine bioprostheses. J. Thorac. Cardiovasc. Surg. 90:564, 1985.

741. Fawzy, M. E., Halim, M., Ziady, G., et al.: Hemodynamic evaluation of porcine bioprostheses in the mitral position by Doppler echocardiography. Am. J. Cardiol. 59:643, 1987.

742. Magilligan, D. J., Jr.: Porcine bioprostheses. In Crawford, F. A. (ed.): Cardiac Surgery: Current Heart Valve Prostheses. Vol. 1. Philadelphia, Hanley and Belfus, 1987, pp. 269–284.

743. Nellessen, U., Masuyama, T., Appleton, C. P., et al.: Mitral prosthesis malfunction: Comparative Doppler echocardiographic studies of mitral prostheses before and after replacement. Circulation 79:330, 1989.

744. Khuri, S. F., Folland, E. D., Sethi, G. K., et al.: Six month postoperative hemodynamics of the Hancock heterograft and the Björk-Shiley prosthesis: Results of a Veteran's Administration cooperative prospective randomized trial. J. Am. Coll. Cardiol. 12:8, 1988.

745. Janusz, M. T., Jamieson, W.R.E., Burr, L. H., et al.: Thromboembolism risks and role of anticoagulants in patients in chronic atrial fibrillation following mitral valve replacement with porcine bioprostheses. J. Am. Coll. Cardiol. 1:587, 1983.

746. Jamieson, W. R. E., Tyers, G. F. O., Janusz, M. T., et al.: Age as a determinant for selection of porcine bioprostheses for cardiac valve replacement: Experience with Carpentier-Edwards standard bioprosthesis. Can. J. Cardiol. 7:181, 1991.

747. Crawford, F. A.: The Ionescu-Shiley pericardial xenograft. In Crawford, F. A. (ed.): Cardiac Surgery: Current Heart Valve Prostheses. Vol. 1. Philadelphia, Hanley and Belfus, 1987, pp. 285–294.

748. Trowbridge, E. A., Lawford, P. V., Crofts, C. E., and Roberts, K. M.: Pericardiac heterografts: Why do these valves fail? J. Thorac. Cardiovasc. Surg. 95:577, 1988.

749. Bloomfield, P., Wheatley, D. J., Prescott, R. J., and Miller, H. C.: Twelve-year comparison of a Björk-Shiley mechanical heart valve with porcine bioprostheses. N. Engl. J. Med. 324:573, 1991.

750. Roberts, W. C.: Complications of cardiac valve replacement: Characteristic abnormalities of prostheses pertaining to any specific site. Am. Heart J. 103:113, 1982.

751. Nashof, S.A.M., Sethia, B., Turner, M. A., et al.: Björk-Shiley and Carpentier-Edwards valves: A comparative analysis. J. Thorac. Cardiovasc. Surg., 93:394, 1987.

752. Hammond, G. L., Geha, A. S., Klopf, G. S., and Hashim, S. W.: Biological versus mechanical valves. Analysis of 1116 valves inserted in 1012 adult patients with a 4818 patient-year and a 5327 valve-year followup. J. Thorac. Cardiovasc. Surg. 93:182, 1987.

753. Oakley, C.: Valve prostheses and pregnancy. Br. Heart J. 58:303, 1987.

754. Sareli, P., England, M. J., Berk, M. R., et al.: Maternal and fetal sequelae of anticoagulation during pregnancy in patients with mechanical heart valve prostheses. Am. J. Cardiol. 63:1462, 1989.

755. Salazar, E., Zajarias, A., Gutierrez, N., and Iturbe, I.: The problem of cardiac valve prostheses, anticoagulants, and pregnancy. Circulation 70(Suppl. I):169, 1984.

756. Iturbe-Alessio, I., Fonesca, M.D.C., Mutchinik, O., et al.: Risks of anticoagulant therapy in pregnant women with artificial heart valves. N. Engl. J. Med. 315:1390, 1986.

757. Limet, R., and Grondin, C. M.: Cardiac valve prostheses, anticoagulation and pregnancy. Ann. Thorac. Surg. 23:337, 1977.

758. John, S.: Valve replacement in the young patients with rheumatic heart disease: Review of a twenty year experience. J. Thorac. Cardiovasc. Surg. 99:631, 1990.

759. Ilbawi, M. N., Idriss, F. S., DeLeon, S. Y., et al.: Valve replacement in children: Guidelines for selection of prosthesis and timing of surgical intervention. Ann. Thorac. Surg. 44:398, 1987.

760. Selwyn, L., Rao, S., Mardin, M. K., et al.: Prosthetic valves in children and adolescents. Am. Heart J. 121:557, 1991.

761. Gardner, T. J.: Anticoagulants for children requiring heart valve replacement. In Dunn, J. M. (ed.): Cardiac Valve Disease in Children. New York, Elsevier, 1988, p. 359

762. Smith, N. D., Raizada, V., and Abrams, J.: Auscultation of the normally functioning prosthetic valve. Ann. Intern. Med. 95:594, 1981.

763. Radhakrishnan, S., Behl, V. K., Bajaj, R., et al.: Doppler echocardiographic evaluation of normal and thrombosed Björk-Shiley mitral prosthetic valves. Int. J. Cardiol 20:387, 1988.

764. Klein, H. O., Schamroth, C. L., Marcus, B. D., et al.: Echo-phonocardiographic assessment of the Medtronic-Hall mitral valve prosthesis: Observations on normal and abnormal function. J. Cardiovasc. Ultrasonogr. 5:115, 1986.

765. Alam, M., Serwin, J. B., Rosman, H. S., et al.: Transesophageal echocardiographic features of normal and dysfunctioning bioprosthetic valves. Am. Heart J. 121:1149, 1991.

Infective Endocarditis

by OKSANA M. KORZENIOWSKI, M.D., and DONALD KAYE, M.D.

DEFINITION AND CLASSIFICATION

Infective endocarditis (IE) usually refers to bacterial or fungal infection within the heart, although chlamydial and rickettsial infections also occur; the role of viruses is unknown. Extracardiac endothelium also can be colonized by microorganisms, and the infection (more properly called endarteritis) produces a clinical syndrome indistinguishable from that of IE.[1]

Endocarditis historically has been classified as *acute* or *subacute* on the basis of the clinical course as observed before availability of antimicrobial therapy. *Acute* endocarditis denoted infection on a normal valve by virulent organisms such as *Staphylococcus aureus*, *Streptococcus pneumoniae*, *Neisseria gonorrhoeae*, *Streptococcus pyogenes*, and *Haemophilus influenzae*, which rapidly destroyed the heart valve and caused widespread metastatic foci. Death occurred in less than 6 weeks. *Subacute* endocarditis referred to infection on abnormal valves (usually rheumatic) with relatively avirulent organisms such as viridans streptococci or *Staphylococcus epidermidis*. The course was indolent (up to 2 years), and metastatic foci were uncommon. Such classic presentations of IE are now encountered less frequently. Currently, patients with prosthetic cardiac valves, users of illicit parenteral drugs, and patients with mitral valve prolapse or other nonrheumatic abnormalities, rather than patients with rheumatic heart disease, account for the majority of cases of endocarditis. The bacteriology in each population differs, and correlations between organism and course are variable. Current useful classifications refer to underlying anatomy (i.e., native valve intravenous (IV) drug abuser or prosthetic valve) and infecting organism, and serve as a basis for therapy and prognosis (e.g., viridans streptococcal endocarditis on a native valve).

NATIVE VALVE ENDOCARDITIS

Most people (60 to 80 per cent) with native valve endocarditis who do not use parenteral drugs have an identifiable predisposing cardiac lesion.[2] The nature of the predisposing lesion and, to some extent, the bacteriology of the infection are determined by the patient's age.

Demographic Characteristics

CHILDREN (see also Chap. 33). The incidence of IE in infancy and childhood is low. It has been reported as 0.34 cases per 100,000 children per year and as ~1 in 4500 pediatric hospital admissions.[3]

Rheumatic Heart Disease. In children infected after the neonatal period, 75 to 100 per cent have identifiable predisposing lesions (Table 35–1).[5,6] Early series implicated rheumatic carditis as the underlying lesion in about one-third of cases of pediatric endocarditis.[7,8] Over the past 20 years the incidence of rheumatic fever has been decreasing and, consequently, rheumatic heart disease has been implicated in fewer cases of endocarditis. In several series from the 1970's and 1980's, only 1.5 to 10 per cent of endocarditis cases were on valves damaged by rheumatic fever.[3,9,10] Most infections involved the mitral and aortic valves. A resurgence in rheumatic fever recently was documented in several metropolitan areas in the United States (p. 1721), and carditis developed in 50 to 90 per cent of the affected children.[11,12] If the trend continues, an increase in the incidence of endocarditis on rheumatic valves can be anticipated.

Congenital Heart Disease. The association between congenital heart disease (CHD) and endocarditis was firmly established by autopsy series in the preantibiotic era. Of 181 children with CHD autopsied, 16.5 per cent had evidence of endocarditis.[13] Ventricular septal defect, patent ductus arteriosus, and tetralogy of Fallot were the most common underlying lesions, but patients with cyanotic heart disease associated with shunts and stenotic valves were noted to be at particular risk. Aortic valve disease accounted for 9 per cent of pediatric patients with IE. Infection of the pulmonary valve is uncommon but most often occurs in conjunction with infection at other structurally abnormal sites, such as uncorrected ventricular septal defect and tetralogy of Fallot.[14] Early series examining the impact of palliative or corrective surgery on the incidence of IE in CHD established cardiac surgery as a risk factor for endocarditis, both directly by way of postsurgical infections, especially in patients with synthetic material in the circulation, and indirectly as a consequence of prolongation of life in such patients.[15] Ostium secundum atrial septal defects seldom become infected because the lesion results in a low-pressure shunt with low turbulence; however, endocarditis that involves the mitral valve has been documented in patients with ostium primum defects.

Viridans streptococci and group D streptococci cause 40 to 50 per cent of pediatric cases (Table 35–1).[5,10,16] The beta-hemolytic streptococci seldom cause endocarditis. Enterococci are responsible for 4 per cent and pneumococci for less than 3 per cent of cases. *S. aureus* is responsible for 25 per cent of pediatric cases of endocarditis, but the incidence appears to be increasing.

ADULTS. The spectrum of recognized cardiac lesions underlying IE in adults has been changing as a result of the decline in the incidence of rheumatic heart disease and improvement in cardiac diagnostic techniques.[2] In a recent series, the major categories of underlying lesions, in descending frequency, were mitral valve prolapse, no underlying disease, degenerative lesions of the aortic and mitral valves, CHD, and rheumatic heart disease (Table 35–1).[2]

In most recent series evaluating nonaddict patients with native valve endocarditis, mitral valve prolapse (p. 1029) has gained prominence as the most common underlying predisposing cardiac lesion.[2,17,18] Mitral valve prolapse with redundancy of the mitral valve is an extremely common condition, with prevalence estimates ranging from 2.5 to 5.0 per cent in the general healthy population and up to 20 per cent in young women.[19] In two series prevalence rates of mitral valve prolapse in patients with IE were 32 per cent (18/56) and 54 per cent (19/35).[2,17] Male gender, the presence of a systolic murmur, and age above 45 years characterize patients at highest risk for IE. The risk for IE with mitral valve prolapse but no murmur is 0.0046 per cent per year; the risk for IE with mitral valve prolapse and a systolic murmur is 0.0520 per cent per year; the incidence of IE in the general population 15 years and older is 0.004 per cent per year.[18,20]

TABLE 35-1 INCIDENCE OF PREDISPOSING VALVULAR LESIONS AND MICROBIAL ISOLATES IN PATIENTS WITH ENDOCARDITIS ON NATIVE VALVES

	CHILDREN (%)		ADULTS %			
	Neonates	Older	< 60 yr.	> 65 yr.	Pregnant	Addict*
Predisposing Lesion						
RHD	–	1.5–10	25–30	8	74**	–
CHD	28	75–100	10–20	2		10
MVP	–	–	20–50	10	–	–
DHD	–	–	–	30		
Parenteral drug use	–	–	–	–	8	100*
Other	–	–	10–15	10	–	10
None	72	–	25–50	40	18	–
Organisms						
Streptococci	20	40–50	50–70	30	60	6–12
Enterococci	–	4	10	15	6	8
Staphylococci	60	30	25	45	18	60
S. aureus	(80)	(80)	(90)	(65)	(90)	(99)
S. epidermidis	(20)	(20)	(10)	(35)	(10)	(1)
GNB	10	5	<1	5	2	10
Fungi	10	1	<1	–	–	5
Diphtheroids	–	–	<1	–	–	2
Polymicrobial	4	–	–	–	4	5
Other	–	–	<1	–	6	–
Culture negative	4	0–15	5–10	5	4	4–10

RHD, rheumatic heart disease; CHD, congenital heart disease; MVP, mitral valve prolapse; DHD, degenerative heart disease; other, idiopathic hypertrophic subaortic stenosis, Marfan's syndrome, etc.; GNB, gram-negative bacilli.
* All patients are parenteral drug users.
** 74 percent includes RHD and CHD.

Rheumatic heart disease was the underlying lesion in 37 to 76 per cent of cases in the past.[2] It now accounts for about 30 per cent (21 to 42 per cent) of heart lesions in adults with endocarditis.[21] Most patients with rheumatic heart disease and endocarditis are middle-aged or older.[22] The mitral valve is the most commonly involved valve (>85 per cent), and women predominate (2:1) in series in which the mitral valve is solely involved. The aortic valve is the next most commonly affected site (50 per cent), and a male predominance (4:1) is seen with isolated lesions.[23] A tricuspid valve affected by rheumatic heart disease occasionally may be involved, but usually in association with involvement of either the mitral or aortic valve.

Congenital heart disease is the underlying lesion in 10 to 20 per cent of patients.[2] The most common predisposing lesions in adults include patent ductus arteriosus, ventricular septal defect, bicuspid aortic valve, coarctation of the aorta, and pulmonic stenosis. Isolated pulmonic valve endocarditis, in patients with CHD, in particular, atrial and ventricular septal defects, patent ductus arteriosus, and tetralogy of Fallot, is being increasingly recognized as improvements in echocardiographic technology have provided visual access to this site.[24] Bicuspid aortic valve is an important risk factor, especially in men over age 60. Hypertrophic obstructive cardiomyopathy (p. 1404) is a risk factor for endocarditis; about 5 per cent of patients with this condition develop IE.[25] Enhanced risk is conferred on people with a high peak systolic pressure gradient. Sites of involvement include the aortic valve, the mitral valve, and the subaortic endocardium, reflecting the hemodynamic abnormalities (i.e., mitral regurgitation caused by displacement of the anterior leaflet by the abnormal ventricular architecture and turbulence of the jet stream crossing the aortic valve distal to the intraventricular obstruction). Marfan syndrome, when associated with aortic insufficiency, has been involved in IE.[26] The vegetations are found primarily on the mitral valve. Luetic aortic valves are uncommon underlying lesions. Degenerative heart disease, particularly calcific aortic stenosis, is important in predisposing the elderly to endocarditis.

THE ELDERLY. There is a significant trend toward increased age among patients diagnosed with endocarditis.[27] In evaluating patients seen between 1976 and 1985, the percentage over age 60 ranged from 26 per cent of those treated in a veterans' hospital to 23 per cent treated in a university center to 60 per cent treated in a community hospital (the last institution having the lowest proportion of intravenous IV drug abusers).[28] The factors accounting for this shift in age distribution are a marked reduction in the frequency of rheumatic heart disease, longer survival as a result of modern medical and surgical therapy, of patients with CHD and those with valves damaged by rheumatic fever and aging of the population in general. The longer average life span is associated with an increased incidence of degenerative valve disease. The most common predisposing factor to endocarditis in those over age 65 is a prosthetic intravascular device. In elderly patients with native valve endocarditis, degenerative cardiac lesions (i.e., aortic sclerosis with or without a bicuspid aortic valve, calcified mitral annulus, postmyocardial infarction thrombi, atrial thrombi, and ventricular aneurysms) appear to be gaining prominence (Table 35-1).[29,30] Pomerance reported that of those with endocarditis, 33 per cent older than age 65 had no apparent underlying lesion at autopsy, compared with 22 per cent of those younger than 65 years.[31] It is likely that many of those older than 65 had minor degenerative cardiac lesions that were undetected at autopsy but were sufficient to serve as a nidus for initiation of endocarditis. Others may in fact have no structural defects but may have nosocomially acquired endocarditis related to intravenous catheters (23 per cent in one series) infected with a virulent organism such as S. aureus.[28] Overall, in the elderly, the mitral valve is involved more commonly than the aortic valve. However, gender difference exists—the aortic valve is involved in 61 per cent of male cases but in only 31 per cent of female cases.

DIABETES MELLITUS. Diabetes has been documented as an associated disease with IE in 15 per cent (8/53) of elderly patients.[28] Although not directly documented, metabolic, immunological, and vascular abnormalities in diabetes may have a significant impact on the susceptibility of patients to endocarditis.[32] Accelerated atherosclerosis results in a high incidence of calcific valvular nodular lesions.[33] Urinary tract infections and soft tissue infections are common in diabetes as a consequence of both poor perfusion and inhibition of leukocytic migration and phagocytosis by acidosis, and can serve as sources of bacteremia.[34] Furthermore, an increased incidence of colonization by S. aureus of the skin and nares has been documented in insulin-dependent diabetics.[35] A strong association of group B streptococcal infections with diabetes has been noted, and bacteremias and cases of endocarditis have been documented in diabetics.[36,37]

PREGNANCY (see also p. 1080). IE is an important but uncommon complication of pregnancy.[38] The calculated incidence of IE is 0.03 to 0.14 cases per 1000 deliveries and 5.5 to 9.0 cases per 1000 for patients with preexisting cardiac disease. These incidence rates, however, are based on earlier eras (1950's through 1970); the true incidence reflecting improved management of obstetric complications, legalization of abortion, falling incidence of rheumatic heart disease, and increasing use of IV drugs by women is unknown. Underlying cardiac disease was present in about 75 per cent of cases of IE in obstetric and gynecologic practice (Table 35–1).[39] Most cases were caused by streptococci—primarily viridans streptococci and S. aureus. In pregnancy, the most common portal of entry of bacteria was dental procedures. Puerperal endocarditis occurred after both vaginal delivery and cesarean delivery. Potential predisposing factors included premature labor, prolonged rupture of membranes, prolonged third stage of labor, and manual removal of the placenta.[39] Based on the number of abortions performed yearly in the United States, the incidence of endocarditis is believed to be below 1 per 1 million abortions.

MICROBIOLOGY

Streptococci (50 to 70 per cent), enterococci (10 per cent), and staphylococci (25 per cent) account for the majority of cases of endocarditis on native valves in nonintravenous drug abusers (Table 35–1).[2,18,27,28]

VIRIDANS STREPTOCOCCI. This organism is a normal inhabitant of the oropharynx, and accounts for more than half of all streptococcal infections.[40] These organisms usually are beta-hemolytic and nontypable by the Lancefield system. This group includes a variety of species, including *Streptococcus mitior* (25 per cent of cases of IE on native valves in non-drug abusers), *Streptococcus sanguis* (~20 per cent), *Streptococcus mutans* (~10%), *Streptococcus anginosus* (~5 per cent), and *Streptococcus salivarius* (~1 per cent).[40,41] Most are highly susceptible to penicillin and cause infections primarily on abnormal heart valves. The clinical course usually is indolent. *S. mutans* is fastidious on culture and frequently hydrolyzes bile-esculin; thus it may be confused with enterococci.[42] It grows best on horse blood agar in 5 to 10 per cent carbon dioxide on subculture, requires more than 3 days for primary isolation, and morphologically is quite pleomorphic. Nutritionally deficient variant streptococci, usually *S. mitior*, may be difficult to isolate.[43] Therapy for IE caused by nutritionally deficient variant streptococci tends to result in more frequent relapses than with other viridans species.[42]

ENTEROCOCCI. These organisms were classified as streptococci and recently reclassified as a separate genus. They include *Enterococcus faecalis, Enterococcus faecium,* and *Enterococcus durans.*[44] They are alpha-, beta-, or gamma-hemolytic, and normally inhabit the gastrointestinal tract and the anterior urethra. They grow well in sodium azide ("SF broth"), 40 per cent bile, 6.5 per cent sodium chloride, and 0.1 per cent methylene blue, and can survive at high temperatures (56°C) and high pH (9.6). Enterococci can attack normal or damaged heart valves.[45] Most patients are older men (60 years or older), many of whom give a recent history of genitourinary manipulation, trauma, or disease (cystoscopy, urethral catheterization, or prostatectomy), or, less commonly, young women (less than 40 years old) who have undergone abortion, pregnancy, or cesarean delivery.[46] Correct biochemical identification of enterococci is important because the organisms are relatively resistant to penicillin G and penicillin alone is not bactericidal. Thus, high doses of penicillin must be used and an aminoglycoside must be added to achieve a bactericidal effect on these organisms.[47] Recent identification of beta-lactamase–producing strains,[48] strains with high-level resistance to all aminoglycosides,[49] and vancomycin-resistant enterococci[50] has further increased the complexity of therapeutic regimens.

OTHER STREPTOCOCCI. *S. bovis* and *S. equinus* are group D streptococci. They differ biochemically from enterococci (which also type with group D typing serum) and can be separated from enterococci by determination of arginine or starch hydrolysis. They usually are readily killed by penicillin alone.[51] *S. bovis* endocarditis primarily occurs in the elderly (older than 60 years of age) and frequently is associated with the presence of colonic polyps (67 per cent versus 21 per cent of patients with enterococcal endocarditis) or colonic malignancy (18 per cent versus 2 per cent enterococcal endocarditis).[52,53]

Other Lancefield group streptococci account for less than 5 per cent of cases of endocarditis. Group A and group B streptococci can attack normal valves and produce distant metastases. Group B streptococci (*Streptococcus agalactiae*) are normal inhabitants of the mouth, vagina, anterior urethra, and gastrointestinal tract.[36] *S. agalactiae* has now been recognized as a significant pathogen in adults with diabetes mellitus, carcinoma, and hepatic failure as well as being a major pathogen in neonates and young pregnant women.[37] An association of *S. agalactiae* bacteremia with colonic villus adenomas recently has been noted.[54] More than 70 cases of *S. agalactiae* endocarditis have been reported since the 1940's. Most patients have fulminant disease with large, crumbling vegetations and systemic emboli, perhaps reflecting the absence of fibrinolysin production by the bacterium.[37] A similar clinical syndrome with high morbidity and mortality also has been reported as caused by group G streptococci.[55] Susceptibility to penicillin of the typable streptococci is variable, and an aminoglycoside may need to be added to achieve an adequate bactericidal effect.[55]

STREPTOCOCCUS PNEUMONIAE. This form of endocarditis occurred in 10 per cent of patients in series collected before the advent of penicillin. It now accounts for only 1 to 3 per cent of cases of IE, even though pneumococcal bacteremia remains common.[56–59] *S. pneumoniae* can infect normal valves, has a predilection for the aortic valve, and has an unusually high incidence of tricuspid valve involvement. Alcoholism is recognized as a risk factor for endocarditis (~40 per cent of patients), as are advanced age and diabetes. The course is fulminant with rapid valvular destruction, frequent perivalvular abscess formation, and purulent pericarditis. Sixty to 90 per cent of patients have concurrent meningitis. Most pneumococcal isolates remain sensitive to penicillin, but relatively resistant strains (minimal inhibitory concentration to penicillin ≥ 0.1 to ≤ 2.0 μg/ml) are being recognized with increasing frequency in the United States as well as in other countries.[60] Strains highly resistant to multiple antibiotics (but reliably susceptible to vancomycin), first recognized in South Africa, have been identified in Europe, the United States, and Canada.[61]

STAPHYLOCOCCI. These organisms cause 25 per cent of cases of native valve endocarditis.[62] Most are coagulase-positive (*S. aureus*). Coagulase-negative (*S. epidermidis*) species account for less than 10 per cent of isolates (1 to 3 per cent of cases of native valve endocarditis). The great majority of staphylococci, acquired either in the hospital or in the community, are highly resistant to penicillin G because of their ability to elaborate beta-lactamase.[63] *S. aureus* endocarditis usually is fulminant with multiple metastatic abscesses, and affected valves are rapidly destroyed.[64,65] *S. aureus* bacteremia commonly occurs in patients with soft tissue infections and as a nosocomial complication in patients with intravascular catheters. Because *S. aureus* can attack either normal or damaged valves, sometimes it is difficult to determine if a valve has been infected in patients with positive blood cultures for *S. aureus* but who have none of the characteristic clinical features of IE.

The percentage of patients with *S. aureus* bacteremia who have underlying IE is variable: 50 to 60 per cent of patients in populations with a high prevalence of underlying predisposing cardiac lesions, 15 to 25 per cent of patients in unselected populations, and 1 to 16 per cent of patients with a removable focus of infection (i.e., an IV catheter) but no underlying valvular disease.[66] Three clinical risk criteria—absent primary focus, community acquisition, and metastatic sequelae—that are strongly predictive (74 per cent) of IE in IV drug abusers (discussed below) are much less reliable (50 per cent predictive value) in non-addicts with *S. aureus* bacteremia.[66]

Community-acquired strains of *S. aureus* usually are susceptible to penicillinase-resistant beta-lactam antibiotics. The clinical significance of antibiotic tolerance (marked dissociation of minimal inhibitory concentration and minimal bactericidal concentration of cell wall–active antibiotics after 18 to 24 hours of incubation) has not been established.[67] Methicillin-resistant strains of *S. aureus* are becoming a major problem in nosocomially acquired infections.[62]

S. epidermidis. This organism causes an indolent infection on previously damaged valves.[62,68] Coagulase-negative staphylococci are common skin commensals, and the most common bacteria to contaminate blood cultures. A presumptive diagnosis of endocarditis caused by these organisms rests on repeated isolation of the same strain from multiple separate blood cultures. Determination of species, antibiogram analysis, phage typing, and plasmid profiles have been used with variable success to demonstrate strain identity.[62] Several reports have noted species other than *S. epidermidis* (*Staphylococcus warneri, Staphylococcus cohnii, Staphylococcus saprophyticus, Staphylococcus hemolyticus,* and *Staphylococcus hominis*) as causes of native valve endocarditis. In nosocomially acquired (i.e., catheter-related) coagulase-negative staphylococcal endocarditis, *S. epidermidis* predominated.[68] Most cases of coagulase-negative IE on native valves are community acquired, and the infecting strains are commonly susceptible to methicillin; nosocomial infections are caused by methicillin-resistant strains (frequently also gentamicin- and rifampin-resistant strains).[68] However, the association of antibiotic susceptibility and the location where endocarditis was acquired is not absolute. Thus, antibiotic susceptibility of isolates must be rigorously tested.[62]

OTHER ORGANISMS. Almost all species of bacteria occasionally are identified as causes of native valve endocarditis. Most commonly encountered are *N. gonorrhoeae*,[69,70] *Haemophilus* sp.,[71] and other closely related fastidious, slow-growing, gram-negative bacilli of the HACEK group (*Actinobacillus actinomycetemcomitans*, *Cardiobacterium hominis*, *Eikenella corrodens*, and *Kingella* sp.)[72-76]; *Pseudomonas*[77,77a]; *Listeria*[78]; and diphtheroids.[79] Clinical courses can be fulminant or indolent. Serum-susceptible gram-negative enteric organisms and anaerobic organisms are less capable of sustaining endocardial infection.[80,81] Spirochetes (e.g., *Spirillum minor*),[82] cell wall–deficient bacteria,[83] *Brucella*,[84] rickettsiae (*Coxiella burnetii*),[85] and chlamydiae[86] are rare causes of endocarditis.

Fungi. These organisms seldom cause native valve endocarditis in the absence of parenteral drug abuse. Factors that predispose to fungemia (i.e., severe underlying illness, corticosteroids, prolonged use of broad-spectrum antibiotics, and cytotoxic agents) can result in endocarditis in patients with IV catheters.[87] *Candida*, *Torulopsis*, and *Aspergillus* species usually are implicated. The course is indolent but grave; large vegetations frequently embolize to major vessels in the lower extremities.[87,88,88a]

ENDOCARDITIS IN INTRAVENOUS DRUG ABUSERS

The frequency of endocarditis in IV drug abusers is difficult to estimate.[89] There appear to be differences in relative risk for infection based on the drugs used (i.e., the risk with cocaine is lower than with heroin or amphetamines), the frequency of use, and the modes of drug preparation.[90] Such individuals with endocarditis usually are men (male-female ratio 3 : 1) and young (mean age 30 years).[64,91,92] Underlying cardiac disease is found in about 20 per cent, usually either congenital lesions or residua of previous endocarditis (Table 35–1).[93]

Recent echocardiographic studies have demonstrated mild degrees of tricuspid and pulmonic regurgitation in valves of IV drug abusers without a history of previous endocarditis (13/26 patients versus 1/13 controls).[94] This suggests that IV drug abuse is the human equivalent of stress-induced valvular abnormalities described in animals. These findings might explain the right-sided predilection of IE in drug users.[95] The sites of endocardial involvement based on clinical criteria are a tricuspid valve infected in about 54 per cent, aortic in 25 per cent, and mitral in 20 per cent.[64,91,93] The recent availability of Doppler echocardiography (p. 88) has led to the identification of vegetations that involve the pulmonic valve. In two series collectively describing 42 patients with isolated pulmonary valve endocarditis, 10 patients (24 per cent) were IV drug abusers.[14,96] Patients with pulmonic valve IE constitute 1.1 to 1.4 per cent of all patients with endocarditis. Mixed right- and left-sided endocarditis occurs in 6 per cent.

The sites of involvement as determined in a detailed autopsy series of 80 addicts dying during the first episode of endocarditis (59/80), recurrent endocarditis (10/80), or healed endocarditis (11/80) differ from clinically determined distributions, and reflect the increased mortality of IE in drug addicts when the left side of the heart is involved.[97] The first episode of IE involved a single right-sided cardiac valve in 30 per cent, both a right- and left-sided valve in 16 per cent, a single left-sided valve in 41 per cent, and both left-sided valves in 13 per cent—an average of 1.3 valves per patient. The tricuspid valve was infected in 44 per cent, the mitral in 43 per cent, aortic in 40 per cent, and pulmonic in 3 per cent. In 81 per cent of patients the infected valves were determined to have been anatomically normal before the onset of IE, and 71 per cent of patients had sufficient valvular damage to cause valvular dysfunction.

MICROBIOLOGY. The skin is the most frequent source of microorganisms responsible for endocarditis in IV drug abusers, although contamination of drugs and associated paraphernalia also contributes to bacteremias.[92,98] *S. aureus* is isolated from 60 per cent of cases of IE in these persons; various species of streptococci and enterococci from almost 20 per cent, gram-negative bacilli (predominantly *Pseudomonas* and *Serratia* sp.) from 10 per cent, and fungi (usually *Candida*) from 5 per cent. Anaerobic organisms are uncommon causes of IE, and diagnosis may be delayed because of difficulties in isolating such species from blood cultures.[99] Recent reports have identified *Streptococcus mitis* and group A streptococcus as causes of endocarditis among drug addicts.[100]

Five per cent of addict patients have more than a single microorganism isolated from the blood. In most cases of polymicrobial endocarditis, there are two or three isolates and rarely four or five pathogens.[101] Multiple organisms can either cause the primary infection or be acquired during the course of therapy. *S. aureus* is by far the most common organism isolated in tricuspid endocarditis, and accounts for 80 per cent of clinical isolates. Similarly, in 70 to 80 per cent of cases of *S. aureus* endocarditis in IV drug abusers only the tricuspid valve is involved.

The vast majority (70 to 100 per cent) of addicts with right-sided endocarditis are noted to have pneumonia or multiple septic emboli, but the murmur of tricuspid regurgitation frequently is not present, and that accompanying pulmonic valve endocarditis may be misinterpreted as a functional or flow murmur.[102] Moreover, patients with a syndrome compatible with tricuspid endocarditis may actually have an extracardiac site of endovascular infection (i.e., septic thrombophlebitis involving the subclavian or femoral venous system) rather than endocarditis.[103]

PROSTHETIC VALVE ENDOCARDITIS

Infections of prosthetic valves account for 5 to 15 per cent of all cases of endocarditis.[17,21] The overall incidence of endocarditis in patients with prosthetic valves is 1 to 4 per cent.[104-106,106a] Rutledge and coworkers retrospectively reviewed 1598 patients undergoing prosthetic valve replacement at the National Institutes of Health from 1961 to 1981, and performed an actuarial analysis of the risk of IE.[107] Overall, 43/1598 patients (2.7 per cent) developed endocarditis. The cumulative risk was 3 per cent at 5 years and 5 per cent at 10 years. The risk for prosthetic valve endocarditis (PVE) development peaked 15 days after operation at 45 episodes per 100,000 patient days; the risk then rapidly declined and from 150 days to 20 years remained stable at about 1 episode per 100,000 patient days. Using all patients and all episodes of PVE, the overall rate of infection was 5.9 episodes per 1000 patient years; if a patient survived 60 days without developing PVE, the subsequent rate was 3.7 episodes per 1000 patient years. These findings are consistent with results of others.[106,108]

By convention, PVE is termed "early" when symptoms appear within 60 days of valve insertion and "late" when symptoms occur after that time. The early and late groups differ in clinical features, microbial patterns, and mortality rates. Early PVE usually reflects contamination arising in the perioperative period. Most contamination probably occurs intraoperatively by way of direct wound inoculation or contamination of the bypass machine. Postoperative sources include IV catheters (particularly central lines), arterial lines, urethral catheters, cardiac pacing wires, and endotracheal tubes. The attack rate for early PVE before 1969 was 2.5 per cent of all patients undergoing valve replacement and subsequently has been 0.75 per cent of all such patients.[104-106]

Despite use of prophylactic antibiotics, staphylococcal infection accounts for 45 to 50 per cent of early PVE (Table 35–2). *S. epidermidis* is the most common organism isolated, with an average incidence of 25 to 30 per cent; *S. aureus* causes 20 to 25 per cent. The remainder of cases are caused by gram-negative aerobic organisms (about 20 per cent), fungi (particularly *Candida* and *Aspergillus*, 10 to 12 per cent), streptococci and enterococci (5 to 10 per cent), and diphtheroids (5 to 10 per cent). Occasional unusual causes of PVE include atypical mycobacteria,[109] *Legionella*,[110] mycoplasma,[111] unusual fungi,[112] and *Coxiella*.[113]

Late PVE occurs after valves have been endothelialized. The incidence depends on the length of follow-up. It has been estimated to occur at an overall incidence of 0.2 to 0.5 per cent per patient year. The source for infection is presumed to be seeding of the valve by transient bacteremia arising from dental, genitourinary, or gastrointestinal manipulation. Thus the bacteriology more closely resembles that of native valve endocarditis (Table 35–2). Viridans streptococci are the most

TABLE 35–2 INCIDENCE OF MICROBIAL ISOLATES IN PATIENTS WITH EARLY AND LATE PROSTHETIC VALVE ENDOCARDITIS

ORGANISMS	EARLY PVE (<2 mo) (%)	LATE PVE (>2 mo) (%)
Streptococci	5–10	25–30
Enterococci	<1	5–10
Staphylococci	45–50	30–40
S. aureus	(45–50)	(30)
S. epidermidis	(55–60)	(70)
GNB	20	10–12
Fungi	10–12	5–8
Diphtheroids	5–10	4–5
Polymicrobial	1–5	1–5
Other	8	8
Culture Negative	5–10	5–10

PVE, prosthetic valve endocarditis; GNB, gram-negative bacilli.

commonly isolated organisms (25 to 30 per cent) with a median time to onset of PVE of 24 months after valve implantation.[104] Other streptococci and enterococci account for 5 to 10 per cent. Staphylococci (*S. epidermidis*, 21 to 28 per cent; *S. aureus*, 9 to 12 per cent), gram-negative bacilli (10 to 12 per cent), fungi (5 to 8 per cent), and diphtheroids (4 to 5 per cent) occur more frequently in the first 18 months after implantation of the valve. Such infections probably reflect delayed clinical appearance of infection acquired perioperatively. Support of this hypothesis derives from the high frequency of methicillin resistance (84 to 87 per cent) among coagulase-negative staphylococci causing PVE throughout the initial 12 months after surgery as compared with the significantly lower frequency of methicillin resistance (23 to 30 per cent) of infections that occur later.[106,114]

RISK FACTORS. There appears to be no effect on the subsequent development of PVE of preoperative factors such as New York Heart Association functional class or hemodynamic measurements.[107] A higher risk for PVE was associated with the male sex in earlier series[108]; in the two most recent analyses, male sex was a risk factor only within 12 months of aortic valve replacement but not after mitral valve replacement.[106,107] Patients who develop PVE tend to be somewhat older (mean age 52) versus the population at risk (mean age 48 years); the risk appears to be associated with development of late PVE 12 or more months after surgery in recipients of multiple or mitral prostheses.[106] Black race and longer cardiopulmonary bypass time have been associated with higher incidence of PVE.[107]

In most series, infection more commonly involves the aortic prosthetic valve, but in Rutledge's series 2.6 per cent of aortic prostheses became infected versus 2.3 per cent of mitral prostheses; Calderwood and colleagues report no differences (4.2 versus 4.1 per cent). Most series also report a higher frequency of infection after multiple valve implantation than after replacement of either valve alone, but in Rutledge's series no significant difference in the frequency of PVE in patients with single-valve replacement (2.6 per cent) versus multiple valve replacement (3.0 per cent) was noted. In all series, right-sided PVE was negligible.

Currently there does not seem to be a significant difference in the cumulative risk of PVE by 5 years between mechanical and heterograft valves; however, the time course for development of infection appears to differ in Calderwood's series—recipients of mechanical valves had a higher risk of PVE within the first 3 months after surgery, but the risk for

PVE was higher for porcine valve recipients 12 or more months after surgery.[106] Valve make and model also do not appear to affect the frequency of PVE. The incidence of PVE after replacement of an infected, as opposed to a noninfected, native valve is increased (it is about 4 per cent) but usually is caused by an organism different from the original one.[104]

Early prosthetic valve endocarditis often is associated with valve dysfunction or dehiscence, a fulminant course, and a high mortality rate. Depending on the infecting organism, late PVE commonly is clinically indistinguishable from that occurring in patients without a prosthesis but also may be present with a fulminant course.

PATHOGENESIS

For endocarditis to develop, a complex interaction between the host vascular endothelium, the host hemostatic response, and adventitiously circulating bacteria must occur (Fig. 35–1). Normal endothelium is nonthrombogenic and poorly receptive to attachment by most bacteria.[115] When an endothelial surface (e.g., a valve) is denuded of cells, collagen (i.e., basement membrane or valve stroma), a potent stimulus to hemostasis, is exposed, and a clot of platelets and fibrin is deposited.[116] Such thrombi are believed to provide a more receptive surface to bacterial colonization during episodes of bacteremia.[117,118]

CONDITIONS PREDISPOSING TO ENDOCARDITIS. Three hemodynamic factors predispose patients to the development of IE by denuding endothelial surfaces: (1) a high-velocity abnormal jet stream; (2) flow from a high- to a low-pressure chamber; and (3) a comparatively narrow orifice separating the two chambers, creating a pressure gradient.[119] By injecting a bacterial aerosol into the air stream passing through an agar Venturi tube, Rodbard demonstrated that high pressure drives an infected fluid into a low-pressure sink and deposits the highest concentration of bacteria immediately below the obstructed orifice.[119] This model helps to explain the frequency of valvular involvement in IE and the distribution of lesions in various valvular defects.

In 1024 patients with IE studied at autopsy by Lepeschkin, the distribution of infected valves (i.e., mitral valves infected in 86 per cent, aortic valves in 55 per cent, tricuspid valves in 19.6 per cent, and pulmonic valves in 1.1 per cent) correlated with the degree of mechanical stress on such valves as reflected by resting pressures: mitral 116 mm Hg, aortic 72 mm Hg, tricuspid 24 mm Hg, and pulmonic 5 mm Hg.[120] Similarly, nonvalvular lesions with high degrees of turbulence (i.e., small ventricular septal defects with a jet lesion, arteriovenous fistula, coarctation of the aorta, and patent ductus arteriosus) readily create the Venturi effect and have a high incidence of endocarditis, whereas large defects (e.g., large ventricular septal defects), defects associated with low flow (e.g., secundum atrial septal defect), or conditions that result in attenuation of turbulence (e.g., congestive heart failure or atrial fibrillation) have a low incidence of endocarditis.

The lesions of IE tend to form just beyond the narrowed orifice through which the high-velocity jet stream passes (i.e., on the ventricular surfaces of the incompetent aortic valve, on the atrial surface of the incompetent mitral or tricuspid valve, and on the walls of the pulmonary artery at the orifice of the

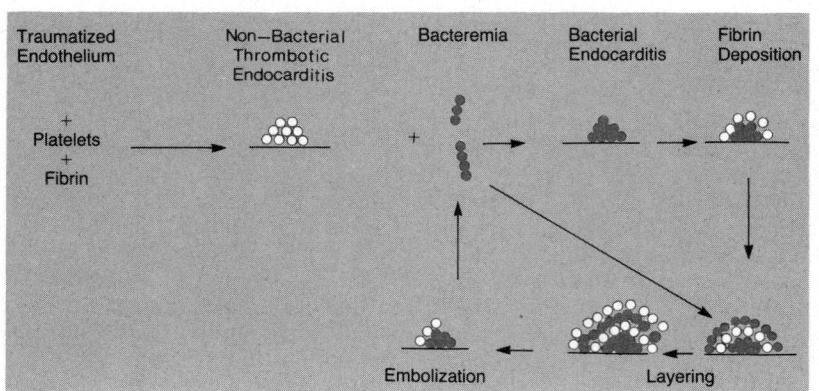

FIGURE 35–1. Evolution of an infected vegetation on a traumatized valve.

patent ductus arteriosus). Satellite lesions also can grow where the jet stream strikes the endocardium (e.g., the atrial wall opposite the mitral orifice in mitral regurgitation, the papillary muscle of the left ventricle in aortic regurgitation, and the surface of the pulmonary artery opposite the patent ductus areteriosus). The force of the jet stream presumably denudes the endothelium and promotes deposition of clumps of fibrin and platelets (Fig. 35-1), which form sterile vegetations termed nonbacterial thrombotic endocarditis (NBTE).[121]

Many forms of exogenous stress produce NBTE experimentally; these include systemic infection, hypersensitivity states, cold exposure, stress of captivity, simulated high altitude, high cardiac output states, cardiac lymphatic obstruction, and hormonal manipulations. Sterile vegetations also can occur in patients with wasting disease, particularly cancer (marantic endocarditis), in patients with uremia or connective tissue disorders, in areas surrounding foreign bodies such as intracardiac catheters, and at surgical sites, particularly vascular incisions and implants.[121]

IE occurs when microorganisms are deposited onto the sterile vegetation during the course of a bacteremia (Fig. 35-1).[122,123] In the absence of NBTE, it is nearly impossible to produce IE in laboratory animals with intravenously injected bacteria, even at high inocula.[124] Whether such sterile vegetations are essential for the development of endocarditis in humans is unknown. Organisms that adhere well to platelets, fibrin, or fibronectin (see below) and are resistant to host defense mechanisms, such as complement and other serum factors, are most likely to colonize sterile vegetations and at lower inocula. Subsequent deposition of platelets and fibrin over the bacteria forms a "protected site" into which phagocytic cells penetrate poorly, thus allowing survival and proliferation of the microorganisms.[117,118]

Fresh vegetations of IE are composed of clumps of microorganisms, fibrin, occasional red blood cells, and a few leukocytes, and are attached to the surface of a valve leaflet, chordae, or ventricular endocardium.[117,118,125] Underlying valve destruction occurs. The morphology of vegetations can vary, depending on the nature of the infecting organism and the activity of the disease, from small flat granular lesions to large pedunculated friable masses. Unimpaired bacterial growth results in extremely high colony counts of 10^9 to 10^{10} bacteria per gram of tissue.[126] As vegetations heal during the process of bacteriological cure, infiltration by polymorphonuclear leukocytes and fibroblasts occurs, leading to fibrosis, hyalinization, and, sometimes, calcification. Finally, the lesion is covered by endothelium.[127]

CONDITIONS PREDISPOSING TO BACTEREMIA. These have been extensively examined.[128-130] Transient bacteremia occurs whenever an area heavily colonized with bacteria is traumatized. The degree of bacteremia is proportional to the number of organisms inhabiting the area and the severity of trauma. The number of organisms in blood usually does not exceed 10 per milliliter, and intravascular residence is transient, lasting no more than 15 to 30 minutes.[128] Transient bacteremias most commonly are associated with dental extraction, periodontal surgery, and oropharyngeal, gastrointestinal, urological, or gynecological invasive diagnostic or surgical procedures (Table 35-3). Spontaneous bacteremia in the absence of trauma occurs with lung and skin infections and in patients with severe periodontal disease. Alone or mixed with other species, viridans streptococci are the most common bacteria isolated from blood, after trauma to tissues of the mouth.[131] A wide variety of trivial events (e.g., chewing and toothbrushing) induce streptococcal bacteremia. Most cases of streptococcal endocarditis (85 per cent) cannot be related to iatrogenic procedures.[132] Enterococcal and gram-negative bacillus bacteremia occur commonly after genitourinary or gastrointestinal surgery or instrumentation. Although about half of patients with enterococcal endocarditis report genitourinary tract manipulation before the onset of their disease, only six cases possibly related to gastrointestinal diagnostic procedures have been published.[132] In nonnosocomial staphylococ-

cal endocarditis, a portal of entry has been reported in 30 to 40 per cent of patients.[65]

Organisms that possess little inherent pathogenicity (e.g., viridans streptococci) usually implant only at sites with preexisting NBTE; more virulent organisms such as S. aureus and S. pneumoniae may be able to infect apparently normal valves. Factors that promote bacterial adherence to and propagation on susceptible valve surfaces have been studied extensively in vitro in systems utilizing fibrin-platelet matrices, endothelial cell cultures, and normal canine valve leaflets and in vivo in the rabbit and rat models of endocarditis.

Histopathological studies in animals established that initial bacterial colonization occurred on the endothelial surface of valves.[123,126] However, bacterial colonization of endothelial surfaces does not necessarily guarantee the establishment of endocarditis. To be pathogenic, organisms must be resistant to the complement-mediated bactericidal activity of serum (serum-resistant) and must circumvent clearance. Thus, although gram-negative aerobic bacilli are frequent causes of bacteremia, they are infrequent causes of IE. Susceptibility to bactericidal activity of serum is partially implicated in reduced virulence for IE, since only serum-resistant isolates of *Escherichia coli*, *Pseudomonas aeruginosa*, and *Serratia marcescens* have been isolated from human cases of gram-negative bacillus IE, and only such strains reliably produce experimental IE in rabbits. Experimental IE with "serum-sensitive" strains can be produced only in rabbits homozygous for C_6 deficiency or in rabbits with a permanent transaortic catheter; removal of the catheter results in prompt elimination of the organisms from the valve surface.[80]

Recent studies in laboratory animals indicate a protective role for humoral factors (preformed antibodies), although the results obtained vary with the species of bacteria studied. Protection may be conferred by more than one mechanism: preformed antibody inhibits adhesion of viridans streptococci and *Candida* to NBTE in vitro, whereas for pneumococci, immunization results in more rapid clearance of bacteria from blood.

Studies utilizing endothelial monolayers have demonstrated that vascular endothelial cells can phagocytize adherent *S. aureus* and *Candida*.[133,134] It is postulated that such ingested organisms may multiply intracellularly and kill the endothelial cell, thereby exposing the thrombogenic underlying extracellular matrix, and lead to the development and propagation of NBTE. It also is postulated that circulating organisms may become coated with fibronectin (a plasma glycoprotein that also is a major surface constituent of mammalian cells) and, as a consequence of its strong adhesive properties, become capable of adhering to intact endothelium.[135]

MECHANISMS OF BACTERIAL ADHERENCE TO NBTE. Numerous mechanisms that promote the adherence of bacteria to NBTE have been delineated.[136] The best characterized is the synthesis of extracellular polysaccharides, such as dextran, by viridans streptococci. Extracellular dextran production has been demonstrated in bacteria implicated in the production of dental caries, and is believed to promote attachment of such organisms to dental plaque.[137] In some series, dextran-producing strains are the most common viridans streptococci isolated from patients with IE, thus implicating dextran production as a possible virulence factor in human IE. In in vitro assays of adherence of streptococci to platelet-fibrin matrices and to traumatized canine aortic valves, adherence of dextran-producing strains has been shown to be superior to that of nonproducers. The degree of adherence is proportional to the amount of dextran produced. Dextran production also has been shown to correlate directly with the ability to produce IE in the rabbit model (71 per cent in dextran-positive strains versus 26 per cent in dextran-negative strains).[138]

Because dextran production can be implicated as a virulence factor in only a small number of bacterial species capable of causing IE, other mechanisms that mediate bacterial attachment to valve surfaces must exist. A central role has been postulated for fibronectin.[135] Cell-associated fibronectin is secreted by endothelial cells, fibroblasts, and platelets in response to a vascular injury. Soluble circulating fibronectin also binds to collagen exposed in such injury. Fibronectin receptors have been demonstrated on the surface of *S. aureus*, viridans streptococci, *S. pneumoniae*, streptococci of groups A, C, and G, as well as *Candida albicans* and *Candida tropicalis*. Binding of such organisms to analogs of traumatized valves is enhanced by the addition of fibronectin.[139-142] Lipoteichoic acid has been implicated as the fibronectin receptor on streptococci.[143] By virtue of the presence of multiple separate functional domains, fibronectin can simultaneously bind to fibrin, collagen, cells, and bacteria, and thus appears particularly well suited to act as a mediator of adherence during the pathogenesis of IE; for example, (1) circulating microorganisms may become coated with soluble fibronectin and thus adhere to either intact valves, exposed collagen, or fibrin; (2) circulating uncoated bacteria may bind to fibronectin-coated platelets or fibroblasts.[135]

Other bacterial-host interactions that may significantly affect the initia-

TABLE 35-3 INCIDENCE OF BACTEREMIA AND MOST LIKELY BACTERIAL ISOLATES (BY PROCEDURE GROUP) AFTER TISSUE TRAUMA IN DIAGNOSTIC PROCEDURES

PROCEDURES	BACTEREMIA (%)	REPORTED ISOLATES
DENTAL		
Tooth extraction		
No gingivitis	34	Streptococci, Diphtheroids, Anaerobes, and S. epidermidis
Gingivitis	70–75	
Chewing mint candy	20	
Brushing teeth	40	
Oral irrigation device	27–50	
Periodontal operations	31–88	
UPPER AIRWAY		
Massage of infected tonsils	23	Streptococci, diphtheroids, Haemophilus sp., S. pneumoniae, and S. epidermidis
Tonsillectomy	28–38	
Nasotracheal intubation	16	
Bronchoscopy—rigid	15	
—fiberoptic	0	
GASTROINTESTINAL—UPPER		
Upper GI endoscopy	4	Streptococci, S. epidermidis, S. aureus, and diphtheroids
Esophageal dilatation/sclerotherapy	50–53	
Endoscopic retrograde chlangiopancreatography	5	
GASTROINTESTINAL—LOWER		
Sigmoidoscopy—rigid	5	Enterococci, aerobic GNB
—flexible	0	
Proctoscopy	2	
Hemorrhoidectomy	8	
Barium enema	10	
Colonoscopy	5	
Liver biopsy	3–13	S. pneumoniae, GNB*
UROLOGICAL		
Urethral dilatation	28–33	Enterococci, GNB, and S. aureus
Urethral surgery	33–86	
Insertion/removal urethral catheter	8–26	
TU or retropubic prostatectomy		
—sterile urine	11–13	
—infected urine	58–82	
Suprapubic prostatectomy	7	
Massage of infected prostate	67	
Cystoscopy	0–17	
GYNECOLOGICAL		
Uncomplicated vaginal delivery	1–5	Streptococci (anaerobic and aerobic) and enterococci
IUD insertion/removal	0	
Punch biopsy cervix	0	
Endometrial biopsy	4	
OTHER		
Cardiac catheterization	0	
Manipulation of septic foci	39	S. aureus, others

TU, transurethral; IUD, intrauterine device; GNB, gram-negative bacilli.
* These isolates pertain to liver biopsy only.
Data from Everett, E. D., and Hirschmann, J. V.: Transient bacteremia and endocarditis prophylaxis. A review. Medicine (Baltimore) 56:61, 1977; Sipes, J. N., et al.: Prophylaxis of infective endocarditis: A re-evaluation. Ann. Rev. Med. 28:371, 1977; Baskin, G.: Prosthetic endocarditis after endoscopic variceal sclerotherapy: A failure of antibiotic prophylaxis. Am. J. Gastroenterol. 84:311, 1989; Rogosa, M., et al.: Blood sampling and cultural studies in the detection of post-operative bacteremia. J. Am. Dent. Assoc. 60:171, 1960; Durack, D. T.: Current issues in the prevention of infective endocarditis. Am. J. Med. 78(Suppl B):149, 1985.

tion or propagation of a vegetation include (1) the capacity of staphylococci and streptococci to aggregate platelets, thus enhancing their clearance from the circulation and reducing the probability of IE; (2) the capacity of these organisms to aggregate platelets and thus promote the growth of vegetations; and (3) the capacity of organisms to activate the clotting cascade either directly (staphylococci) or indirectly (enterococci) by stimulating local host cells (endothelial cells, stromal cells, or monocytes) to express tissue factor (i.e., tissue thromboplastin), thus increasing deposition of fibrin in the vegetation.[144-147]

PATHOPHYSIOLOGY

The signs and symptoms of IE are highly variable, and depend on the organ system involved. Clinical features result from (1) the local intracardiac infectious process and its attendant complications; (2) bland or septic embolization of

fragments of vegetations to virtually any organ; (3) constant bacteremia with seeding of distant foci; and (4) the development of immune complex–associated disease.

Intracardiac infection can lead to perforation of the valve leaflet or rupture of the chordae tendineae, interventricular septum, or papillary muscle (Fig. 35–2).[148] Infections, particularly with S. aureus, may result in valve ring abscesses, and extend into the myocardium to produce burrowing abscesses and purulent pericardial effusions.[149,150] Conduction abnormalities, fistulas between chambers of the heart and pericardium or major vessels, and aneurysms of the sinus of Valsalva may result.[151] Large vegetations, such as those caused by fungi or Haemophilus sp., can occlude a valve orifice.[152] Healing of the infection may cause scar formation with subsequent valvular stenosis or insufficiency.[153] Myocarditis and myocardial

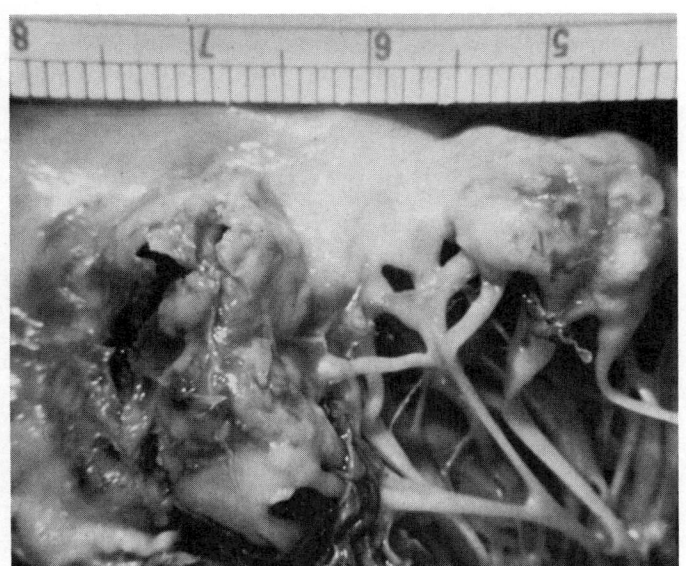

FIGURE 35-2. Large vegetations deforming the mitral valve leaflets in a patient with IE.

complexes are said to be detected in only 45 per cent of cases of IE in which cultures of blood are negative.[164] Serial quantitative determination of serum immune complex concentration (by Raji cell or Clq techniques) can be used to monitor response to therapy; decrease with eventual disappearance occurs with successful treatment. Rising titers or reappearance of complexes indicates therapeutic failure or relapse. Immune complex (containing IgG, IgA, IgM, and complement) deposition along the glomerular basement membrane results in the development of glomerulonephritis (Figs. 35-4 and 35-5). Histologically, the glomerulonephritis may be focal (48 to 88 per cent), diffuse (17 to 80 per cent) or membranoproliferative (rare).[165]

Arthritis and peripheral manifestations of IE such as Osler's nodes have been attributed to deposition of immune complexes in joints and mucocutaneous vessels.[166] Rheumatoid factor (IgM antibody directed against IgG) develops in about 50 per cent of patients with subacute IE.[167] The titers correlate with the level of hypergammaglobulinemia and decrease with therapy. Rheumatoid factor interacts with antigens located on the Fc portion of human IgG.[167] Immunofluorescent studies of valves removed at surgery from patients with streptococcal endocarditis have disclosed heavy deposits of IgG and bacterial antigen in vegetations and the underlying valve and diffuse endocardial and subendocardial deposits of C_2 and C_3 complement as well as rheumatoid factor.[168]

CLINICAL MANIFESTATIONS

Symptoms of endocarditis usually start within 2 weeks of the precipitating bacteremia. A study analyzing 76 patients with streptococcal endocarditis suggested that the median "incubation period" is about 1 week, and in this study 84 per cent of the patients developed symptoms within 2 weeks.[169] Nonspecific symptoms such as malaise, fatigue, night sweats, anorexia, and weight loss are common, particularly with organisms of low pathogenicity (e.g., viridans streptococci).[28] The onset of infection with organisms of high pathogenicity (e.g., S. aureus) usually is explosive.[64,65] Symptomatic predominance of extracardiac sites of infection may simulate other disorders, such as influenza, tuberculosis, collagen vascular diseases, congestive heart failure, stroke, subdiaphragmatic infection, or carcinoma. *Fever is present in almost all patients with IE* but may be absent in the elderly or those with severe debility, renal failure, or congestive heart failure or in those previously treated with antibiotics.[170] The fever usually is low grade (less than 39°C) except with acute disease, and usually is remittent. Shaking chills are infrequent except in patients with the acute form of IE or in patients receiving salicylates.

infarctions may be due to coronary artery emboli, myocardial abscesses, or immune complex vasculitis.[154] Coronary emboli with myocardial infarction are documented in 40 to 60 per cent of autopsies of patients with IE, although diagnostic antemortem electrocardiographic changes are infrequent. Sudden death caused by occlusion of a coronary ostium by a bulky vegetation has only rarely been reported.[155]

EMBOLIC PHENOMENA. These are common in IE.[155a] Although clinically apparent emboli occur in only 15 to 35 per cent of cases of IE, pathological evidence of emboli can be shown in 45 to 65 per cent of recent autopsy series.[156] Emboli originating from the left side of the heart are randomly distributed throughout the circulation; the resultant symptoms depend on the site of lodgment. The highest frequency of major emboli occurs in association with infections caused by organisms that produce large, mobile vegetations (e.g., fungi: group B and G streptococci; *Haemophilus parainfluenzae* and other slow-growing fastidious, gram-negative bacilli; S. aureus; and nutritionally deficient variant viridans streptococci.[37,43,55,71,88,90]) Infarcts and/or abscesses in major organs may result, depending on whether septic or bland embolization has occurred. Very large emboli, particularly to extremities, suggest fungal infection. *Pulmonary emboli* occur in right-sided endocarditis.[95-97]

Septic embolization to the vasa vasorum or direct bacterial invasion of the arterial wall produces *mycotic aneurysms*.[157-159] Sites of vessel branching favor the impaction of emboli and are the most common sites of lodgment. The most commonly involved vessels include the cerebral arteries, the aorta, the sinus of Valsalva, the ligated ductus arteriosus, and the superior mesenteric, splenic, coronary, and pulmonary arteries (Fig. 35-3). Although mycotic aneurysms usually appear during the active phase of endocarditis, they may remain silent at initial presentation, and rupture of the weakened vessel may occur during the episode of IE or years later.

STIMULATION OF IMMUNE SYSTEM. The persistent bacteremia of endocarditis stimulates both the humoral and the cell-mediated immune systems.[160] Cellular responses are characterized by the presence of activated circulating macrophages and splenomegaly.[161] Antibodies of the IgM, IgG, or IgA class of immunoglobulins, having opsonic, agglutinating, and complement-fixing properties for the infecting organisms, as well as cryoglobulins and macroglobulins have been described in IE. Nonspecific generalized hypergammaglobulinemia also develops, as in many other chronic infections.

Circulating Immune Complexes. These complexes are found in virtually all patients with IE and positive blood cultures.[162] Detection of high titers correlates with long duration of illness, the presence of extravascular sites of infection, hypocomplementemia, and right-sided IE.[163] Immune

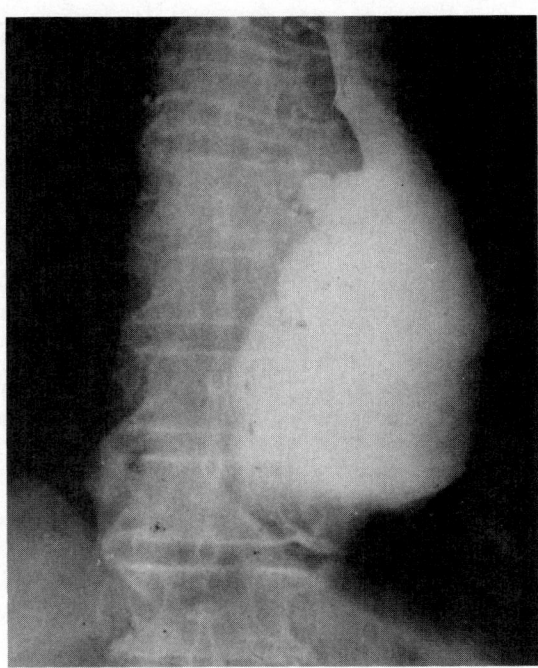

FIGURE 35-3. Angiographic demonstration of a mycotic aneurysm of the distal thoracic aorta in a patient with IE. (From Kaye, D.: Infective Endocarditis. Baltimore, University Park Press, 1976.)

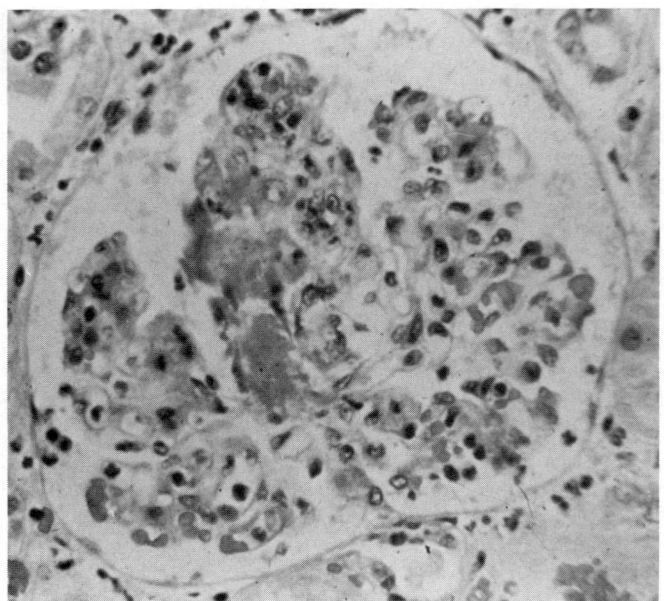

FIGURE 35–4. Microscopic section of glomerulus from patient with IE showing focal hypercellularity and focal necrosis (400×). (From Kaye, D.: Infective Endocarditis. Baltimore, University Park Press, 1976.)

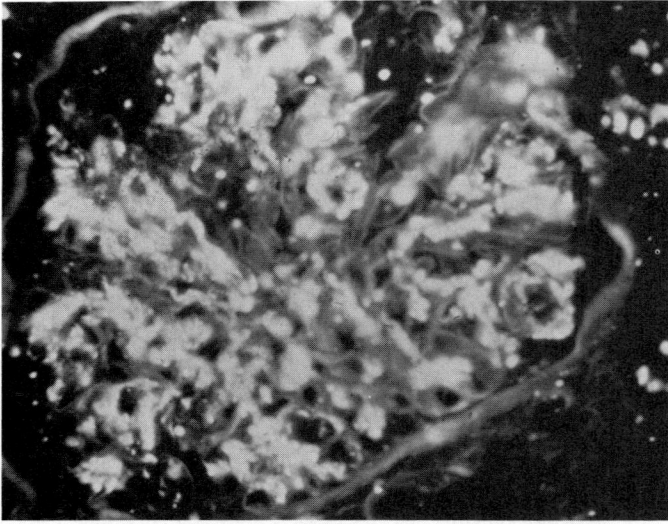

FIGURE 35–5. Microscopic section of glomerulus from patient with IE prepared with fluorescein-tagged antihuman globulin (bright areas). Granular immunoglobulin depositis are seen along the glomerular basement membrane and in the mesangium (400×). (From Kaye, D.: Infective Endocarditis. Baltimore, University Park Press, 1976.)

Heart murmurs are almost always present (> 99 per cent of cases) except in acute infections or with right-sided or mural infection. The appearance of a new regurgitant murmur or true changes in a preexisting murmur (not changes in intensity owing to differences in heart rate or cardiac output) have been reported as uncommon (only 16.7 per cent of subacute cases in earlier series[170]), but when present, they suggest acute staphylococcal disease and correlate with development of congestive heart failure. Of interest, in two recent series of patients with IE based on strict clinical criteria, new or changing murmurs were found in 36 to 52 per cent of patients.[28] New or changing murmurs are less common in the elderly. The possibility of endocarditis must always be considered in a febrile patient with a known heart murmur.[28]

Splenomegaly (present in about 30 per cent of cases), *petechiae* (20 to 40 per cent), and *clubbing* of the fingers tend to occur in disease of long duration (greater than 6 weeks).[170,171] *Splenic enlargement* occurred in 80 to 90 per cent of cases in the preantibiotic era; enlargement is still common except in acute cases but less pronounced. *Splenic infarctions*[155a] have been reported in 44 per cent of autopsy cases but are seldom detected clinically. *Clubbing*, formerly present in 25 to 30 per cent of patients with subacute forms of endocarditis, now occurs in only 10 to 20 per cent of patients with disease of long duration.

Petechiae (Fig. 35–6) are most frequently found on the conjunctivae, palate, buccal mucosa, and skin above the clavicles; they may be embolic or vasculitic. Petechiae are not specific to endocarditis, because lesions develop in patients with hematological disorders, vasculitis, scurvy, or renal insufficiency and as a consequence of fat or cholesterol emboli. *Splinter hemorrhages* (subungual, linear, dark red streaks) are nonspecific (Fig. 35–7). They often are related to trauma. Lesions located proximally in the nailbed are more suggestive of endocarditis than are distal lesions. The number of fingers involved is variable; in some cases the toes may be involved. *Osler nodes* (small, tender nodules, usually on the finger or toe pads, that persist for hours to days) occur in 10 to 25 per cent of patients, but also in other diseases.[172] They also may be present on the dorsal surfaces of toes, soles, forearms, and ears; on occasion they become necrotic[173] (p. 18). Immune complexes have been demonstrated in dermal vessels of Osler nodes, but occasional recovery of bacteria after aspiration suggests that they also may result from septic emboli.[174] *Janeway lesions* (1- to 4-mm, nontender, hemorrhagic areas on the palms and soles) are due to septic emboli.[175] They are most commonly seen in acute endocarditis (Fig. 35–8). *Roth spots* (oval, retinal hemorrhages with a pale center located near the optic disk) occur in less than 5 per cent of patients with endocarditis, and also are found in patients with connective tissue disease and hematological disorders (Fig. 35–9).

Musculoskeletal complaints (arthralgias or arthritis) may mimic rheumatological disorders.[166] *Systemic emboli* may occur during or after therapy, and are recognized in about a third of patients. *Pulmonary emboli* are common in addicts with tricuspid valve endocarditis (70 to 100 per cent are noted to have pneumonia or septic pulmonary emboli) and can be seen in left-sided endocarditis with left-to-right cardiac shunts.[64,65]

Neurological manifestations are present in about one-third of patients with endocarditis.[177] Major cerebral emboli to the middle cerebral artery system account for 25 per cent and mycotic aneurysms for 2 to 10 per cent, but brain abscesses and purulent meningitis, cerebral arteritis, cranial nerve palsy, intracerebral bleeding, and encephalomalacia have been documented. The most common complaint is *headache*, and most patients show improvement with supportive care and antimicrobial therapy. *Mycotic aneurysms* account for 2.5 to 6.2 per cent of all intracranial aneurysms (Fig. 35–10).[154] In a Mayo Clinic series of 628 patients with IE treated between 1963 and 1979, 8 (1.3 per cent) were found to have cerebral mycotic aneurysms; all 8 complained of severe, unremitting, localized headache, a complaint that should strongly suggest the possibility of a mycotic aneurysm.[154] Many other reports suggest that most patients with intracranial mycotic aneurysms are asymptomatic.[148] The true incidence of mycotic aneurysms is unknown. The diagnosis usually is made after a sudden catastrophic hemorrhage.[159]

Congestive heart failure (CHF) is the most common complication of IE.[178] Contributing factors include valve destruction, myocarditis, coronary artery emboli with myocardial infarction, and myocardial abscesses. CHF with aortic valve infective endocarditis is associated with a higher mortality than is CHF with mitral valve infection.[179] *Renal disease* is present in most patients with endocarditis, and is due to glomerulonephritis (up to 80 per cent), infarction (50 per cent), or abscesses (uncommon).[165] Renal insufficiency may result. Metastatic infection (i.e., pyogenic meningitis, splenic abscess, pyelonephritis, osteomyelitis, discitis) occurs most frequently in endocarditis caused by *S. aureus*.[148,154] Persistence of fever, localized pain, persistently abnormal results of liver function tests, and "breakthrough bacteremia" after institution of ap-

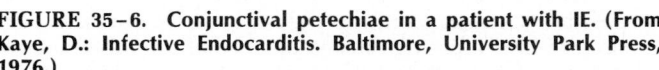

FIGURE 35–6. Conjunctival petechiae in a patient with IE. (From Kaye, D.: Infective Endocarditis. Baltimore, University Park Press, 1976.)

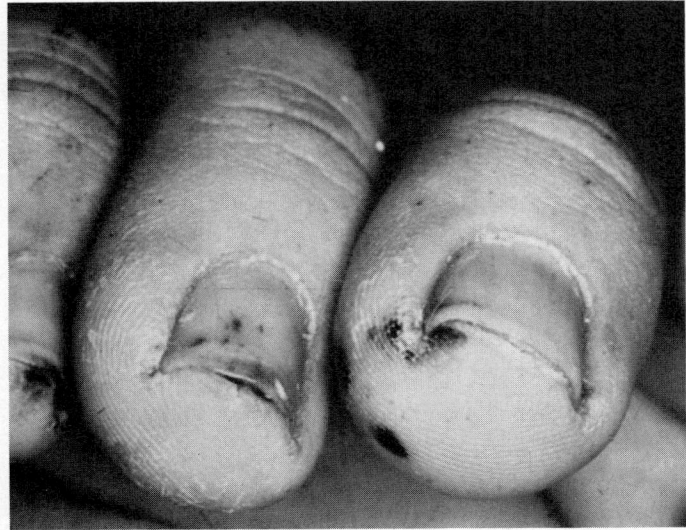

FIGURE 35–7. Subungual hemorrhages (splinter hemorrhages) and digital petechiae in a patient with IE.

FIGURE 35–8. Janeway lesions on the thumb in a patient with endocarditis.

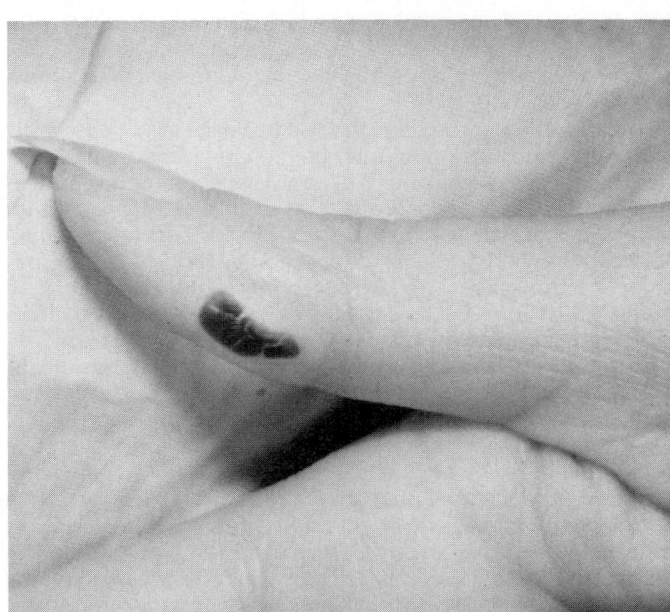

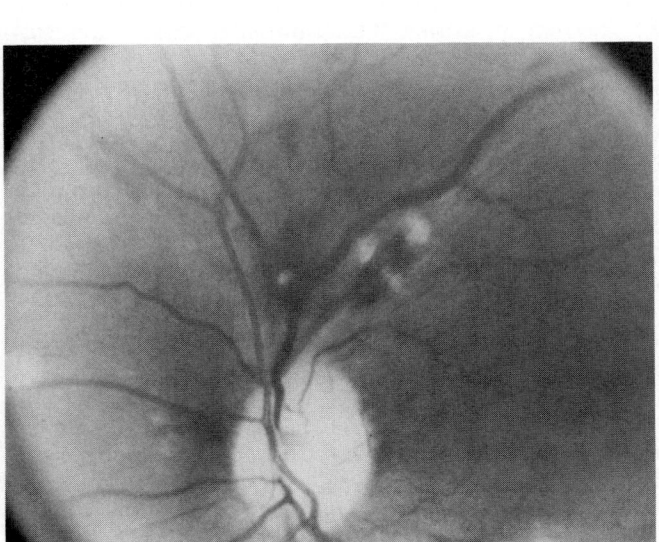

FIGURE 35–9. Roth spot (retinal hemorrhage with a clear center) in a patient with IE.

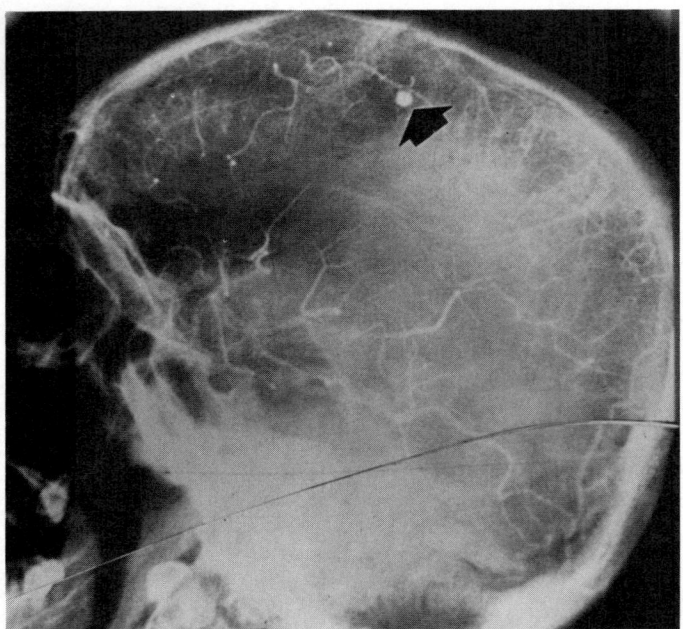

FIGURE 35-10. Angiographic demonstration of a large aneurysm (arrow) of cerebral artery in a patient with IE. (From Kaye, D.: Infective Endocarditis. Baltimore, University Park Press, 1976.)

propriate therapy suggest the diagnosis of metastatic abscess. Patients with metastatic infections are at high risk for relapse of IE.

DIFFERENTIAL DIAGNOSIS

The diagnosis of IE may be suspected either by clinical presentation or by results of blood cultures in the absence of a suggestive syndrome. Proof of endocarditis requires isolation of the infecting microorganism from blood, from an embolus, or from a vegetation or demonstration of infected vegetations at surgery or autopsy.[170]

Endocarditis should be suspected in a patient with a significant heart murmur when unexplained fever is present for at least 1 week or in a febrile IV drug abuser even in the absence of a murmur.[95,102] Endocarditis also should be suspected in a young person with a stroke[154,180] and in patients with a prosthetic valve who are febrile or who have valve dysfunction, such as a new murmur.[105,181] Even with a syndrome classic for endocarditis, a definitive diagnosis requires positive blood cultures or positive cultures of surgical or autopsy specimens (vegetation or emboli) because other diseases can duplicate the syndrome of endocarditis.[17,28a] For example, atrial myxoma, NBTE, acute rheumatic fever, systemic lupus erythematosus, other connective tissue diseases, thrombotic thrombocytopenic purpura, and sickle cell disease can produce a syndrome that is indistinguishable from that of IE.

After cardiac surgery, fever may be related to infection at other sites, to the postcardiotomy syndrome, or to a "postpump syndrome" (such as with cytomegalovirus infection) rather than to endocarditis (Chap. 53)[182] Furthermore, any patient with an existing heart murmur can develop fever related to another occult illness or to drugs. Therefore, in the absence of postive blood cultures, a search must be made for other causes of fever.

Another setting in which endocarditis should be suspected is in the patient who is treated with antimicrobial agents with response of symptoms (e.g., fever, malaise) only to relapse when therapy is stopped. Some patients have multiple episodes of symptoms, treatment, and then relapse. Furthermore, the therapy is likely to temporarily suppress positive blood cultures, confusing the diagnosis.

Although a murmur may not be present at the time of diagnosis, it may become detectable during therapy or even after therapy is completed.[28,169] Development of a murmur *during*

therapy is particularly prone to occur with acute endocarditis, most often caused by coagulase-positive staphylococci.[63-66] The appearance of a *new* murmur usually is related to perforation of the valve, rupture of chordae tendineae, or rupture of a papillary muscle. With prosthetic valve or tricuspid valve endocarditis, a murmur may never appear.[95,102,183]

Not uncommonly, febrile patients with or without a murmur have blood cultures performed as part of a diagnostic evaluation. When blood cultures are reported as positive, the possibility of endocarditis arises. Three factors must be considered in evaluating the significance of the microorganisms isolated from the blood. The first is whether the bacteremia is sustained or transient, as an intravascular infection such as endocarditis tends to produce sustained bacteremia[184]; in turn, sustained bacteremia must always raise the possibility of intravascular infection. We define sustained bacteremia as presence of the same microorganism in blood for at least 1 hour, as transient bacteremias are cleared in 30 minutes or less.[185] Isolation of an organism from blood cultures at only a single point in time may indicate contamination or transient bacteremia and does not constitute evidence for endocarditis.

The second major consideration is the identity of the microorganism. Certain bacteria, such as salmonellae, brucellae, meningococci, and enteric gram-negative bacilli, produce sustained bacteremia relatively frequently but are *rare causes of IE*. Other organisms, such as viridans streptococci and coagulase-negative staphylococci, seldom, if ever, produce sustained bacteremia without an intravascular focus. Coagulase-positive staphylococci and pneumococci often produce sustained bacteremia which may or may not be indicative of endocarditis.[66,186,187]

The third factor to consider is whether or not there is another explanation for the sustained bacteremia, such as infection at another site. Combinations of these factors often come into play. For example, sustained pneumococcal bacteremia in the absence of pneumonia strongly suggests endocarditis, but in the presence of pneumonia it may or may not indicate endocarditis. Sustained coagulase-negative staphylococcal bacteremia in the absence of an intravascular catheter is highly suggestive of endocarditis; in the presence of a catheter, endocarditis may or may not be present.

LABORATORY

BLOOD CULTURES

The critical diagnostic finding in IE is bacteremia or fungemia. In the absence of previous antimicrobial therapy, blood cultures are positive in more than 95 per cent of patients. The bacteremia is continuous; if any cultures are positive, all are likely to be positive.[184] For example, in one large series of 206 patients with blood culture-positive streptococcal endocarditis, 750 of 789 (95 per cent) blood cultures were positive for the causative organisms.[184] Intermittently positive and negative cultures were unusual. The first culture was positive in 95 per cent and the first or second in 98 per cent of the patients. Although constant, the bacteremia usually was low grade with less than 100 bacteria per milliliter of blood in more than 80 per cent of patients. Because the bacteremia of endocarditis is continuous, there is no advantage to obtaining cultures at any particular time or body temperature. Arterial blood offers *no* advantage over antecubital vein blood.[188]

In subacute disease, in the absence of previous therapy, three cultures should be obtained at least 1 hour apart. In those in whom the diagnosis seems likely, therapy should be started without waiting for a confirmatory positive culture. Blood cultures may be negative in as many as 25 per cent of patients who received recent outpatient antibiotic therapy,[189-191] and it is prudent, depending on the clinical status of the patient, to delay treatment to maximize the chance of obtaining positive blood cultures. In general, in acute disease, therapy should not be delayed for more than 2 to 3 hours while obtaining three blood cultures. Cultures should be spaced at least 30 minutes apart to allow proof that the bacteremia was continuous.

Only one culture should be obtained from each venipuncture site. At least 10 ml of blood should be obtained per culture and diluted tenfold in culture medium using both aerobic and anaerobic techniques. The yield of positive cultures is increased by observing them over 3 weeks and making periodic Gram stains and subcultures. Addition of pyridoxal hydrochloride to media will improve the chances of isolating nutritionally deficient variant streptococci.[43,192] Hypertonic media have been advocated to improve recovery of cell wall–deficient bacteria from previously treated patients. Their value, however, is controversial.[193]

Blood cultures may be negative in infections with fastidious organisms such as *H. parainfluenzae, Brucella* sp., or anaerobes. Prolonged incubation, up to 4 weeks, may increase recovery. Fifty per cent of patients with *Candida* endocarditis and almost all with *Aspergillus, Histoplasma, Coxiella burnetii,* or *Chlamydia psittaci* endocarditis have negative blood cultures.[85–88,194,195] With fungi, large peripheral emboli are common, necessitating embolectomy.[87,194] Histological examination and culture of the embolus may be diagnostic.

Although fastidious organisms are an occasional cause of negative blood cultures, administration of antimicrobial agents is a more common cause. The period of time required for the blood cultures to become positive again may be as short as 24 hours or as long as 2 weeks, depending on the activity of the antimicrobial agent against the infecting organism and the length of time the therapy was given. If therapy is given for only 2 to 3 days and then discontinued, cultures will probably rapidly revert to positive. With longer therapy, blood cultures will probably become positive by the time fever recurs.

Other obvious causes of negative blood cultures are incorrect diagnosis and improper blood culture techniques.

Other Laboratory Features[170,171,196]

In subacute IE a normochromic, normocytic *anemia* usually is present (70 to 90 per cent of cases) and worsens with duration of illness. The *white blood cell count* usually is normal, but the *differential count* may be slightly shifted to the left. In acute endocarditis (particularly staphylococcal), *leukocytosis* with a shift to the left often is present. *Thrombocytopenia* may occur. The *erythrocyte sedimentation rate* is almost always elevated except in patients with heart or kidney failure. A positive *rheumatoid factor* is present in 50 per cent of patients with endocarditis for 3 to 6 weeks.[167,197] Although circulating *immune complexes* are present in virtually all patients,[162,198] *hypergammaglobulinemia* is detected in only one-quarter. These tend to disappear with therapy.

High serum titers of *antibodies directed against teichoic acid* constituents of the cell wall of staphylococci suggest endocarditis or other deep-seated infection.[65,66,186] Unfortunately false-positive reactions and cross-reactions with other gram-positive bacteria limit their usefulness in diagnosis. Serologic tests for *C. burnetii, C. psittaci,* and *Brucella* are positive in endocarditis caused by these organisms but are not diagnostic of endocarditis.

Large mononuclear cells (earlobe histiocytes) occasionally can be seen on peripheral blood smears from patients with subacute endocarditis, but the yield is higher (25 per cent) if the first drop of blood obtained after earlobe massage and puncture is examined. These cells are not specific for endocarditis. *Intraleukocytic bacteria* can be seen in buffy coat preparations of blood in up to 50 per cent of patients.[199]

The urinalysis usually is abnormal, with *proteinuria, microscopic hematuria,* and/or *microscopic pyuria* in most patients. Reduction in *serum complement* parallels the incidence of abnormal renal function, especially that caused by diffuse glomerulonephritis.

IMAGING STUDIES

ECHOCARDIOGRAPHY (see also p. 88 and Figs. 4–60 to 4–62). This technique has assumed an increasingly important role in the assessment

and management of patients with suspected IE.[14,125,200–206,206a] Two-dimensional echocardiograms can demonstrate the vegetation in up to 80 per cent of patients with native valve endocarditis, but the usual sensitivity reported is about 60 per cent (Fig. 4–60, p. 88). In the absence of a prosthetic valve, vegetations larger than 5 mm in diameter are reliably detected and those under 3 mm usually are missed. Transesophageal echocardiography has been reported to be more sensitive than transthoracic echocardiography.[202–206,206b,206c] M-mode echocardiograms are less sensitive than two-dimensional studies in detecting vegetations. Knowledge of which valve is involved in endocarditis is important for surgical management and determination of prognosis. In addition, echocardiography can provide valuable information about the degree of valvular destruction and its hemodynamic effects and whether myocardial or valve ring abscess or aneurysm of the sinus of Valsalva is present. Doppler ultrasound can help to quantitate the degree of valvular insufficiency. Serial echocardiographic findings can contribute to decisions for surgical intervention.

In addition to the lack of sensitivity in terms of at least a 20 per cent false-negative rate, echocardiography lacks specificity. Thickened valves, noninfected thrombi, nodules, tumors, and flail leaflets can be misinterpreted as vegetations.[207,208]

Vegetations often are not visualized during the first 2 weeks of endocarditis. Once visualized, they usually remain unchanged in size during therapy and may remain the same size for months after successful therapy.[125,209]

Some have reported that patients with vegetations visualized on echocardiography have an increased risk of developing emboli and CHF, and require valve replacement.[200–202] Others have not found these relationships. It seems likely that vegetations greater than or equal to 10 mm in size are associated with a greater risk of emboli.[203,210]

Recent technological developments using digital image processing of two-dimensional echocardiograms may permit differentiation between active and healed vegetations.[209] Echocardiography usually is not useful in nontissue PVE because of the production of intense interfering echoes by the metal.[211]

Nontissue PVE more commonly is evaluated by serial phonocardiography, cineradiography, and Doppler echocardiography.[212] Changes in the timing or the intensity of the prosthetic sounds detected by phonocardiography may suggest obstruction by a vegetation. Disappearance of an opening click or the sound produced by a closing valve suggests presence of a vegetation. Cineradiography of the valve shows abnormal motion with valve dehiscence (Fig. 35–11). Doppler echocardiography is a sensitive detector of new valvular insufficiency, which indicates valvular dysfunction.

RADIOISOTOPIC SCANNING. This may be carried out with gallium-67 and with indium-111–labeled white blood cells, and has been used to localize vegetations and myocardial abscesses in endocarditis.[213–215] Although these techniques have been found to be useful in selected patients, because of their low sensitivity they add little to the usual diagnosis and management of endocarditis.

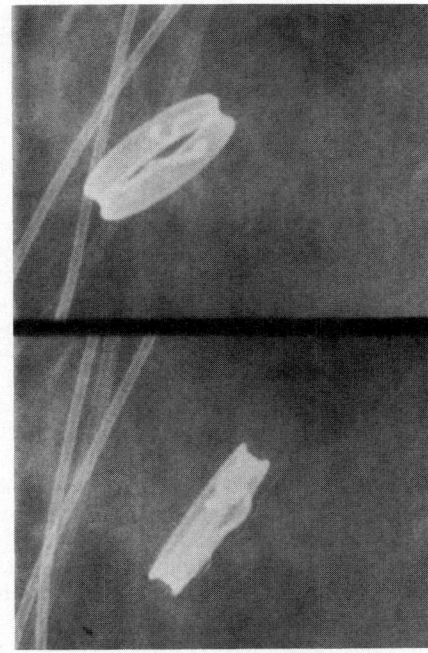

FIGURE 35–11. Fluoroscopic demonstration of the instability (rocking) of a prosthetic valve in a patient with IE.

MANAGEMENT

Before the availability of penicillin in the mid-1940's, IE was an almost uniformly fatal disease. Although a few cases had been cured with sulfonamides and there were rare reports of spontaneous cures, the advent of penicillin changed a disease with almost no chance of cure to one which usually could be cured. Even before the advent of antibiotic therapy, there were rare cases of IE endarteritis cured by surgical ligation of an infected patent ductus arteriosus. Since the 1970's cardiac surgery has evolved into an important adjunct for the management of endocarditis caused by organisms resistant to antimicrobial therapy as well as for drainage of intracardiac abscesses and repair of the damage done by endocarditis.

ANTIMICROBIAL THERAPY

Principles of Therapy

CHOICE, DOSE, DURATION, AND ROUTE OF ADMINISTRATION. Infecting organisms exist at extremely high densities inside the vegetation (e.g., 10^9 to 10^{10} per gram) in a state of reduced metabolic activity, protected from host defenses such as phagocytic cells.[185,216]

Cure of IE requires sterilization of the vegetation. If any microorganisms are viable after antimicrobial therapy is discontinued, multiplication and relapse will probably occur. Therefore, *bactericidal*, rather than bacteriostatic, agents must be used in high concentrations and must be given long enough to completely sterilize the vegetation. High doses of antimicrobial agents are required for two reasons. First, the bacteria are metabolizing slowly because of their extremely high density. Therefore, they are more resistant to many antibiotics, particularly the cell wall–active drugs such as the penicillins, cephalosporins, and vancomycin. Second, the bacteria are inside the vegetation and the therapeutic agents may not diffuse well into the vegetation.[217,218] The duration of therapy required to sterilize the vegetation varies with the microorganism, the valve involved, and the antimicrobial regimen used, but is a minimum of 2 weeks. Parenteral therapy is preferable to oral therapy, since higher and more predictable serum antibiotic levels are obtained. Deviation from these principles, such as use of bacteriostatic agents, unduly short courses, or oral therapy, tends to result in more relapses.

In evaluating the potential efficacy of an antibiotic, the minimal inhibitory concentration (MIC) and minimal bactericidal concentration (MBC) must be considered.[219] The MIC is the minimal concentration that inhibits growth of a bacterium in vitro, and the MBC is the minimal concentration that results in a 99.9 per cent decrease in titer (i.e., kill) within 24 hours. With most streptococci or staphylococci the MICs and MBCs of cell wall–active antibiotics (penicillins, cephalosporins, and vancomycin) do not differ or differ by only twofold to fourfold (i.e., they are bactericidal).[220] The MBCs of these antibiotics are much higher than the MIC's with a minority of strains of streptococci and staphylococci but with all strains of enterococci. When the difference is 10-fold or more, the strains are called *tolerant*.[221] Tolerance actually indicates a slower rate of kill than usually is observed. Tolerance can be overcome by addition of an aminoglycoside (e.g., gentamicin) to the cell wall–active agent, thereby resulting in more rapid bactericidal activity (i.e., a synergistic bactericidal effect).[222]

In therapy for enterococcal endocarditis an aminoglycoside must be added to a penicillin or vancomycin to develop an adequate bactericidal effect and result in cure (Fig. 35–12).[45,47,223,224] Studies in animal models of endocarditis have demonstrated that response to penicillin is slower with tolerant than with nontolerant strains of streptococci.[225] The presence of tolerance in streptococci and staphylococci, however, has not been shown to decrease cure rates in humans with penicillins, cephalosporins, or vancomycin used alone. Therefore, the presence of tolerance in streptococci and staphylococci has no implications for altering therapy from that used in nontolerant strains.[47]

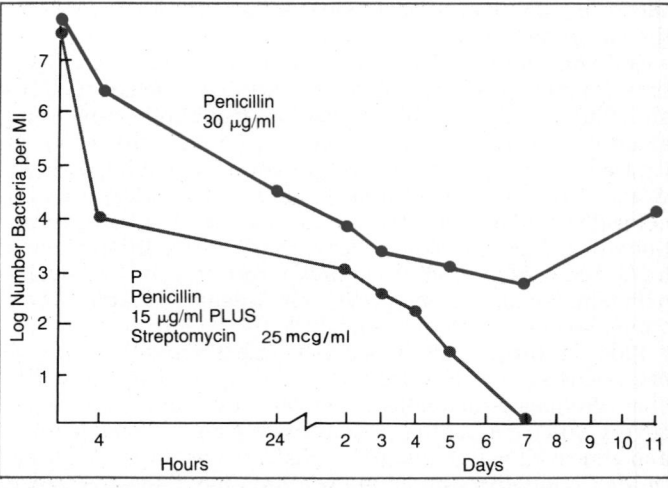

FIGURE 35–12. In vitro time/kill curves demonstrating synergistic activity of penicillin and streptomycin against *E. faecalis.*

FREQUENCY OF DOSING. The required frequency of dosing varies, depending on the microorganism and the therapeutic agent(s) being used. Administration should be frequent enough to guarantee that microbial multiplication does not occur between doses. Depending on the antimicrobial agent and the type of microorganism, after exposure to an antimicrobial agent, even in the absence of antimicrobial activity, there may be a "postantibiotic effect" during which organisms will not multiply.[226] In general, there is a postantibiotic effect of at least 2 hours with gram-positive cocci with penicillins, cephalosporins, and vancomycin. This means that even with an agent such as penicillin G that is rapidly cleared from the blood, administration over a period of 30 minutes, every 4 hours, will provide effective therapy. Penicillins and cephalosporins do not have a postantibiotic effect against gram-negative bacilli. Therefore, when treating gram-negative bacillary endocarditis with these agents, the next dose of antibiotic must be given before antibacterial levels in the vegetation are too low to be effective. In contrast to penicillins and cephalosporins, the quinolones (e.g., ciprofloxacin) and aminoglycosides do exert a postantibiotic effect against gram-negative bacilli.

The regimens recommended in this chapter take all of these factors into account and allow for appropriate doses, dosage intervals, and duration of therapy.

SERUM BACTERICIDAL TITER. The use of the Schlicter test, a determination of the serum bactericidal titer against the infecting organism, is controversial.[220,227–229] A peak serum bactericidal titer (the highest dilution of the patient's serum while receiving antibiotics that kills a standard inoculum of the patient's organism in vitro) of 1:8 or greater usually indicates an adequate therapeutic effect if these levels are achieved often enough each day. A peak bactericidal titer of 1/64 and a trough of 1/32 has been reported to represent optimal therapy.[227] The Schlicter test, however, may give false reassurance when highly protein-bound antibiotics are diluted in broth. As only free antibiotic is active, dilution in broth will result in more measured activity than exists in serum.[230] Furthermore, when combination therapy is required, the Schlicter test is likely to indicate infective serum bactericidal activity even with appropriate regimens. For example, in enterococcal endocarditis, for which an aminoglycoside is required in addition to penicillin or vancomycin to achieve a bactericidal effect, the aminoglycoside effect is likely to be diluted out at serum titers of 1/2 or 1/4.[47]

There is no need for the Schlicter test in the great majority of patients with endocarditis. Adequate therapeutic efficacy may be anticipated in streptococcal, enterococcal, and staphylococcal endocarditis with standard recommended regimens containing penicillins, cephalosporins, or vancomycin, provided the organisms are susceptible to these drugs.[47] Determination of the titer is valuable only when response to therapy with these regimens is suboptimal, when endocarditis is due to an unusual organism, or when an unconventional treatment regimen is used.[47]

ISOLATION OF THE INFECTING MICROORGANISM. Isolation of the infecting organism is extremely important, so that an appropriate antimicrobial regimen may be chosen.

The antimicrobial susceptibility of the infecting organism should be accurately determined.[219] Both MIC and MBC should be determined.[220] Disc diffusion sensitivities may be misleading, and are not a substitute for broth dilution techniques. The organism should be saved for future possible testing of serum bactericidal activity, further antimicrobial susceptibility testing if a change in therapy is indicated, determination of synergistic combinations of antibiotics, or comparison with a relapse strain.

TIMING OF INITIATION OF THERAPY. It is important to initiate antimicrobial therapy as soon as possible, and the dangers of delaying therapy must be weighed against the imperative of isolating the infecting organism. In general, in patients with suspected endocarditis, there is no advantage to delaying therapy beyond the 2 to 3 hours required for three blood cultures to be obtained. If antimicrobial agents have been given within the previous 2 weeks, treatment should be judiciously delayed in an attempt to isolate an organism. In patients with an acute course, even with recent therapy, it is unwise to delay therapy more than 2 to 3 hours, as valvular damage and abscess formation proceed rapidly. In patients with a subacute course and recent therapy it usually is safe to delay therapy for 2 to 3 days or even longer; during this time, two blood cultures are obtained each day. In the experience of the authors, patients in whom fever has recurred after discontinuing antimicrobials usually have positive blood cultures despite the recent administration of antimicrobial agents.

ROUTE OF ADMINISTRATION AND HOME THERAPY. With the advent of prospective payment for hospitalization, home therapy for endocarditis has become more common.[231] Home therapy should be considered only after response to treatment (i.e., afebrile with negative blood cultures), in the stable uncomplicated case (e.g., patients with no heart failure, emboli, or other manifestations of changing or complicating processes), and only in the patient who will receive medical follow-up daily. The preferred method of administration of antibiotics is intravenously or intramuscularly.

Although oral therapy has been used,[232] the risks of failure are clearly higher than with parenteral therapy. It is the authors' preference *not to use oral therapy, if at all possible,* in endocarditis. If oral therapy is to be considered, there must be repeated demonstration of adequate absorption of the agents used and the patient must be reliable enough not to omit any doses. If doses are missed, the organisms may regrow to their original density in the vegetation.

Specific Therapy

THERAPY BEFORE ISOLATION OF AN ORGANISM. The choice of antimicrobial therapy before isolation of the microorganism is based on the clinical setting. In the presence of an intracardiac prosthesis, therapy should be directed against S. epidermidis and S. aureus as well as gram-negative bacilli,[47,104,105,108,114,233] whereas in the absence of a prosthesis, with acute onset or drug abuse, therapy is directed against S. aureus.[47,65,91,92] With acute onset of endocarditis in a non-drug abuser with a native valve, an antistaphylococcal penicillin or cephalosporin can be used in the regimen (see Regimens A and B in Table 35–4). S. epidermidis strains that cause endocarditis in patients with prostheses and S. aureus strains isolated from intravenous drug abusers often are resistant to all beta-lactam antibiotics,[62,92,104,105,114,234–236] and therefore the regimen must include vancomycin (see Regimen C, Table 35–4, and Regimen D in Table 35–5).

With a subacute presentation in a non–intravenous drug abuser, therapy should be directed against the most resistant of the non-staphylococcal gram-positive cocci, the enterococcus.[47] This consists of high doses of intravenous penicillin G or ampicillin together with gentamicin (see Regimens F and G in Table 35–6).[45–47]

When the microorganism is isolated from the blood culture, antimicrobial susceptibility tests can indicate the most effective and least toxic therapy.

When blood cultures remain sterile but the clinical response is good, therapy is continued for the usual course of therapy for the suspected infecting organism. If blood cultures remain negative and there is no clinical response after 7 to 10 days, special cultures and serological studies should be performed for Brucella, Rickettsia, Legionella, and Chlamydia.[84–86,110] When, despite these measures, symptoms continue for more than 3 weeks of therapy with no blood isolates, consideration should be given to discontinuing the treatment and reevaluating the patient.

In the patient with fungal endocarditis (most prone to occur

TABLE 35–4   THERAPY FOR ENDOCARDITIS CAUSED BY STAPHYLOCOCCUS IN THE ABSENCE OF PROSTHETIC MATERIAL

REGIMEN	ANTIBIOTIC	ADULT DOSE AND ROUTE	DURATION
		METHICILLIN-SUSCEPTIBLE STAPHYLOCOCCI (NON-PENICILLIN ALLERGIC)	
A	Nafcillin	2 gm IV every 4 h	4–6 wk
	or		
	Oxacillin	2 gm IV every 4 h	4–6 wk
	plus optional		
	Gentamicin*	1 mg/kg IM or IV (not to exceed 80 mg) every 8 h	5 days
		METHICILLIN-SUSCEPTIBLE STAPHYLOCOCCI (PENICILLIN ALLERGIC)	
B	Cephalothin**	2 gm IV every 4 h	4–6 wk
	or		
	Cefazolin**	2 gm IV or IM every 8 h	4–6 wk
	plus optional		
	Gentamicin*	1 mg/kg IM or IV (not to exceed 80 mg) every 8 hr	First 3–5 days
	or		
	Vancomycin†	30 mg/kg/24 h IV in 2 or 4 equally divided doses, not to exceed 2 gm/24 h unless serum levels are monitored	4–6 wk
		METHICILLIN-RESISTANT STAPHYLOCOCCI	
C	Vancomycin†	30 mg/kg/24 h IV in 2 or 4 equally divided doses, not to exceed 2 gm/24 h unless serum levels are monitored	4–6 wk

* Benefit of additional aminoglycoside has not been established. Risk of toxic reactions caused by these agents is increased in patients who are older than age 65 years or who have renal or eighth nerve impairment.

** There is potential cross-allergenicity between penicillins and cephalosporins. Cephalosporins should be avoided in patients with immediate-type hypersensitivity to penicillin.

† Peak serum concentration of vancomycin should be obtained 1 hour after the termination of the infusion and should be in the range of 30 to 45 μg/ml for twice-daily dosing and 20 to 35 μg/ml for four-times-daily dosing. Each dose of vancomycin should be infused over 1 hour.

Modified from Bisno, A. L., et al.: Antimicrobial treatment of infective endocarditis due to viridans streptococci, enterococci and staphylococci, J.A.M.A. 261:1471, 1989.

TABLE 35-5 TREATMENT OF STAPHYLOCOCCAL ENDOCARDITIS IN THE PRESENCE OF A PROSTHETIC VALVE OR OTHER PROSTHETIC MATERIAL

REGIMEN	ANTIBIOTIC	ADULT DOSE AND ROUTE	DURATION
	METHICILLIN-RESISTANT STAPHYLOCOCCI		
D	Vancomycin*	30 mg/kg/24 h IV in 2 or 4 equally divided doses, not to exceed 2 gm/24 h unless serum levels are monitored	≥6 wk
	plus Rifampin** *and*	300 mg PO every 8 h	≥6 wk
	Gentamicin†	1 mg/kg IM or IV (not to exceed 80 mg) every 8 h	2 wk
	METHICILLIN-SUSCEPTIBLE STAPHYLOCOCCI		
E	Nafcillin *or* oxacillin‡	2 gm IV every 4 h	≥6 wk
	plus Rifampin** *and*	300 mg PO every 8 h	≥6 wk
	Gentamicin†	1 mg/kg IM or IV (not to exceed 80 mg) every 8 h	2 wk

* Peak serum concentrations of vancomycin should be obtained 1 hour after the termination of the infusion and should be in the range of 30 to 45 μg/ml for twice-daily dosing and 20 to 35 μg/ml for four-times-daily dosing. Each dose should be infused over 1 hour.

** Rifampin is recommended for therapy for infections caused by coagulase-negative staphylococci. Its use in coagulase-positive staphylococcal infections is controversial. Rifampin increases the amount of warfarin sodium required for antithrombotic therapy.

† Serum concentration of gentamicin should be monitored and dose should be adjusted to obtain a peak level of approximately 3 μg/ml.

‡ First-generation cephalosporins or vancomycin should be used in penicillin-allergic patients. Cephalosporins should be avoided in patients with immediate-type hypersensitivity to penicillin and in patients with methicillin-resistant staphylococci.

Modified from Bisno, A. L., et al.: Antimicrobial treatment of infective endocarditis due to viridans streptococci, enterococci and staphylococci. J.A.M.A. 261:1471, 1989.

TABLE 35-6 THERAPY FOR ENDOCARDITIS CAUSED BY ENTEROCOCCI (OR TO VIRIDANS STREPTOCOCCI WITH A MINIMUM INHIBITORY CONCENTRATION ≥0.5 μg/ml)

REGIMEN	ANTIBIOTIC	ADULT DOSE AND ROUTE	DURATION
	NONPENICILLIN-ALLERGIC PATIENTS		
F	Aqueous crystaline penicillin G	20-30 million U/24 h IV given continuously or in 6 equally divided doses	
	plus Gentamicin* ** *or*	1 mg/kg IM or IV (not to exceed 80 mg) every 8 h	4-6 wk
	Streptomycin* **	7.5 mg/kg IM (not to exceed 500 mg) every 12 h	
G	Ampicillin	12 gm/24 h IV given continuously or in 6 equally divided doses	
	plus Gentamicin* ** *or*	1 mg/kg IM or IV (not to exceed 80 mg) every 8 h	4-6 wk
	Streptomycin* **	7.5 mg/kg IM (not to exceed 500 mg) every 12 h	
	PENICILLIN-ALLERGIC PATIENTS (Desensitization Should Be Considered; Cephalosporins Are Not Satisfactory Alternatives)		
H	Vancomycin†	30 mg/kg/24 h IV in 2 or 4 equally divided doses, not to exceed 2 gm/24 h unless serum levels are monitored	
	plus Gentamicin* ** *or*	1 mg/kg IM or IV (not to exceed 80 mg) every 8 h	4-6 wk
	Streptomycin* **	7.5 mg/kg IM (not to exceed 500 mg) every 12 h	

* Choice of aminoglycosides depends on resistance level of infecting strain. Enterococci should be tested for high-level resistance (minimum inhibitory concentration, ≥2000 μg/ml).

** Serum concentration of gentamicin should be monitored and dose adjusted to obtain a peak level of about 3 μg/ml. Serum concentration of streptomycin should be monitored if possible and dose adjusted to obtain a peak level of about 20 μg/ml.

† Peak serum concentrations of vancomycin should be obtained 1 hour after the termination of infusion and should be in the range of 30 to 45 μg/ml for twice-daily dosing and 20 to 35 μg/ml for four-times-daily dosing. Each dose should be infused over 1 hour.

Modified from Bisno, A. L., et al.: Antimicrobial treatment of infective endocarditis due to viridans streptococci, enterococci and staphylococci. J.A.M.A. 261:1471, 1989.

on a prosthetic valve), blood cultures may remain sterile. The diagnosis may be suspected by the demonstration of very large vegetations or by the occurrence of large emboli.[87,194,237] Histological examination and culture of the extracted embolus may reveal the infecting fungus.[120,305]

STREPTOCOCCI. The ad hoc writing group of the Committee on Rheumatic Fever, Endocarditis, and Kawasaki Disease of the American Heart Association[47] has made recommendations for treatment of gram-positive coccal endocarditis for which the regimens in adults are outlined in this chapter. Regimens for streptococcal endocarditis are based primarily

on the MIC of the organism to penicillin G (i.e., MIC ≤ 0.1 μg/ml versus >0.1 μg/ml).

The great majority of streptococci, including the viridans group of streptococci, groups A and B streptococci, and S. bovis, are inhibited by 0.1 μg/ml penicillin G (highly susceptible). Endocarditis caused by these highly susceptible streptococci can be treated with one of the three regimens recommended by the American Heart Association shown in Table 35-7. Penicillin G alone for 4 weeks (Regimen I) gives bacteriological cure rates of 99 per cent. Addition of gentamicin or streptomycin (Regimen J) produces synergistic killing of the streptococci and sterilizes cardiac vegetations more rapidly. Equivalent cure rates are obtained in 2 weeks, which has obvious economic advantages over 4 weeks of treatment. Regimen J is appropriate only for uncomplicated infections (i.e., absence of shock, extracardiac foci of infection, or intracardiac abscess) and for disease of less than 3 months duration. Regimen I is preferred for patients likely to have side effects with aminoglycosides (i.e., those with renal insufficiency, eighth nerve disease, or age over 65 years).

Although not popular currently, procaine penicillin, 1.2 million units intramuscularly every 6 hours, has been used successfully instead of intravenous penicillin when there is difficulty with venous access. Penicillin for 4 weeks with an aminoglycoside for the first 2 weeks (Regimen K in Table 35–7) is used for nutritionally deficient variant strains of streptococci, a relapse, in the presence of complications such as shock and extracardiac foci of infection, and perhaps with endocarditis of more than 3 months' duration. Endocarditis caused by nutritionally deficient variant strains has a high relapse rate even when treated with this regimen.[40,43,224,238]

A 6-week regimen of penicillin with an aminoglycoside for at least the first 2 weeks is recommended for patients with prosthetic valve infections. Alternative regimens for penicillin-allergic patients (Table 35–8) include use of a cephalosporin, as in Regimen L, for those with a history of rash to penicillin, and use of vancomycin, as in Regimen M, for those with anaphylaxis when it is too risky to use a cephalosporin.

Endocarditis caused by relatively penicillin-resistant (MIC >0.1 μg/ml and <0.5 μg/ml) strains of streptococci is treated with penicillin in combination with an aminoglycoside (Table 35–9, Regimen N). The need to add an aminoglycoside has been questioned recently.[239] When penicillin cannot be used because of development of a rash, a cephalosporin can be substituted for the penicillin in Regimen N; in patients with immediate-type allergic reactions, vancomycin alone (Regimen M in Table 35–8) for 4 weeks is the substitute of choice. The approach to streptococci with an MIC greater than or equal to 0.5 μg/ml is identical to that used for enterococci (Regimens F, G, or H in Table 35–6).

ENTEROCOCCI. All enterococci are relatively resistant to penicillin G with an MIC greater than or equal to 0.5 μg/ml and a median MIC of 2 μg/ml. They are uniformly resistant to all cephalosporins. Although penicillin G, ampicillin, and vancomycin will inhibit the growth of enterococci, they are not bactericidal for most strains. For a bactericidal effect, it usually is

necessary to add an aminoglycoside (Fig. 35–12).[47,49,223,224,240] Furthermore, therapy with these agents alone results in high failure rates. Thus, treatment of enterococcal endocarditis requires the addition of an aminoglycoside to a penicillin, as in Regimen F or G, for routine therapy or to vancomycin (Regimen H) for penicillin-allergic patients (Table 35–6).[241] With Regimen H it is especially important to monitor antibiotic serum levels and observe patients for nephrotoxicity and ototoxity. With these regimens about 75 per cent of patients will be cured. Therapy usually is for 4 weeks but should be prolonged to 6 weeks when symptoms have been present for more than 3 months, the course is complicated, or the infection is on a prosthetic valve.[47,240]

It may be feasible to desensitize an patient allergic to penicillin G to avoid using vancomycin.[242] This involves a scratch test through a drop of penicillin G (100 U/ml). This is followed in 30 minutes by graded amounts of penicillin intradermally, beginning at .01 units in 0.1 ml of saline solution and continued in 10-fold increments every 30 minutes; with increasing amounts administration is changed to the subcutaneous, intramuscular, and, finally, intravenous route. Epinephrine and diphenhydramine should be on hand for emergency use during the procedure, if needed for an anaphylactic reaction, and preferably an intensive care unit should be used. If a reaction occurs, vancomycin therapy should be initiated.

The synergistic bactericidal effect of aminoglycosides on enterococci occurs only when in vitro growth is inhibited by 2000 μg/ml or less of the aminoglycoside. The degree of resistance as well as the susceptibility to individual aminoglycosides is highly variable; thus in vitro testing should be routine. Synergism is more likely with gentamicin than with streptomycin, and aminoglycosides other than gentamicin often lack activity against E. faecium. In some locales enterococci resistant to 2000 μg/ml of gentamicin have become common.[49,243,244] Although a minority of these strains are inhibited by streptomycin, most are resistant to all aminoglycosides. It is unlikely that the addition of an aminoglycoside would be of benefit with enterococci resistant to all aminoglycosides. Thus, with these organisms, aminoglycosides should probably be excluded from the regimen and the duration of therapy should be prolonged to 8 weeks. Unfortunately, with this approach, relapse is more likely.

In recent years, several additional complicating changes have been

TABLE 35–7 THERAPY FOR ENDOCARDITIS CAUSED BY PENICILLIN-SUSCEPTIBLE VIRIDANS STREPTOCOCCI AND *STREPTOCOCCUS BOVIS* (MINIMUM INHIBITORY CONCENTRATION ≤0.1 μg/ml)

REGIMEN	ANTIBIOTIC	ADULT DOSE AND ROUTE	DURATION
I	Aqueous crystalline penicillin G	10–20 million U/24 h IV either continuously or in 6 equally divided doses	4 wk
J	Aqueous crystalline penicillin G	10–20 million U/24 h IV either continuously or in 6 equally divided doses	
	plus Streptomycin*	7.5 mg/kg IM (not to exceed 500 mg) every 12 h	2 wk
	or Gentamicin*	1 mg/kg IM or IV (not to exceed 80 mg) every 8 hr	
K	Aqueous crystalline penicillin G	10–20 million U/24 h IV either continuously or in 6 equally divided doses	4 wk
	plus Streptomycin*	7.5 mg/kg IM (not to exceed 500 mg) every 12 h	First 2 wk
	or Gentamicin*	1 mg/kg IM or IV (not to exceed 80 mg) every 8 h	First 2 wk

* Peak streptomycin levels of about 20 μg/ml and peak gentamicin levels of about 3 μg/ml are desirable.
Modified from Bisno, A. L., et al.: Antimicrobial treatment of infective endocarditis due to viridans streptococci, enterococci and staphylococci. JAMA 261:1471, 1989.

TABLE 35–8 THERAPY FOR ENDOCARDITIS CAUSED BY PENICILLIN-SUSCEPTIBLE VIRIDANS STREPTOCOCCI AND *STREPTOCOCCUS BOVIS* (MINIMUM INHIBITORY CONCENTRATION ≤0.1 μg/ml) IN PATIENTS ALLERGIC TO PENICILLIN

REGIMEN	ANTIBIOTIC	ADULT DOSE AND ROUTE	DURATION
L	Cephalothin* *or*	2 gm IV every 4 h	4 wk
	Cefazolin*	1 gm IM or IV every 8 h	4 wk
M	Vancomycin**	30 mg/kg/24 h IV in 2 or 4 equally divided doses, not to exceed 2 gm/24 h unless serum levels are monitored	4 wk

* Streptomycin or gentamicin may be added to cephalothin or cefazolin for first 2 weeks in doses recommended in Table 35–4. There is potential cross-allergenicity between penicillins and cephalosporins. Cephalosporins should be avoided in patients with immediate-type hypersensitivity to penicillin.
** Peak serum concentrations of vancomycin should be obtained 1 hour after the termination of the infusion and should be in the range of 30 to 45 μg/ml for twice-daily dosing and 20 to 35 μg/ml for four-times-daily dosing. Each dose of vancomycin should be infused over 1 hour.
Modified from Bisno, A. L., et al.: Antimicrobial treatment of infective endocarditis due to viridans streptococci, enterococci and staphylococci. JAMA. 261:1471, 1989.

TABLE 35-9 THERAPY FOR ENDOCARDITIS CAUSED BY STRAINS OF VIRIDANS STREPTOCOCCI AND *STREPTOCOCCUS BOVIS* RELATIVELY RESISTANT TO PENICILLIN G (MINIMUM INHIBITORY CONCENTRATION >0.1 AND <0.5 μg/ml)*

REGIMEN	ANTIBIOTIC	ADULT DOSE AND ROUTE	DURATION
N	Aqueous crystalline penicillin G	20 million U/24 h IV either continuously or in 6 equally divided doses	4 wk
	plus Streptomycin**	7.5 mg/kg IM (not to exceed 500 mg) every 12 h	First 2 wk
	or Gentamicin**	1 mg/kg IM or IV (not to exceed 80 mg) every 8 h	First 2 wk

* Cephalothin or cefazolin (with aminoglycoside for the first 2 weeks) or vancomycin alone can be used in patients whose penicillin hypersensitivity is not of the immediate type. Vancomycin also can be used in patients with immediate penicillin allergy.

** Streptomycin or gentamicin should be given in addition to penicillin for the first 2 weeks. Peak streptomycin levels of about 20 μg/ml and peak gentamicin levels of about 3 μg/ml are desirable. For the rare viridans streptococcus with minimum inhibitory concentration greater than or equal to 0.5 μg/ml of penicillin G, aminoglycoside therapy should be continued for 4 weeks with appropriate monitoring of serum levels of streptomycin of gentamicin.

Modified from Bisno, A. L., et al.: Antimicrobial treatment of infective endocarditis due to viridans streptococci, enterococci and staphylococci. JAMA 261:1471, 1989.

noted. Beta-lactamase–producing enterococci have been isolated.[48,245] Patients infected with these organisms should receive vancomycin plus an aminoglycoside or ampicillin-sulbactam plus an aminoglycoside. A recent study found that most strains of *E. faecium* (14 per cent of enterococcal isolates) were highly resistant to penicillin by a mechanism other than beta-lactamase production.[246] Vancomycin would be required for therapy of patients infected with these strains. A few strains of enterococci resistant to vancomycin have been reported; some of these strains were sensitive to penicillin and ampicillin.[50,247,248]

Unlike in past years, the appropriate choice of therapy for enterococcal endocarditis cannot be determined without special in vitro sensitivity tests. Determination of the MIC of penicillin is required. If the enterococcus is resistant, it must be determined if the mechanism is beta-lactamase production. Susceptibility to 2000 μg/ml of aminoglycoside must be evaluated. It also is probably wise to determine the MIC of vancomycin if use of this agent is contemplated.

STAPHYLOCOCCI CAUSING NATIVE VALVE ENDOCARDITIS (Table 35–4). Most *S. aureus* and *S. epidermidis* that cause endocarditis produce a beta-lactamase and are therefore resistant to penicillin G. For the unusual strains that are inhibited by 0.1 μg/ml penicillin G, this agent can be used in a dose of 20 million units each day intravenously. The usual therapy for native valve endocarditis caused by *S. aureus* or *S. epidermidis* is with a penicillinase-resistant penicillin such as nafcillin or oxacillin, as in Regimen J. Although addition of gentamicin to nafcillin will increase the bactericidal rate both in broth cultures and in vegetations of laboratory animals infected by these organisms,[249] clinical trials have not demonstrated any advantage other than a small increase over the first few days in the rate at which fever and positive blood cultures normalize.[250–252] Furthermore, addition of gentamicin increases the risk of renal damage. Therefore, if gentamicin is added for the theoretical advantage of minimizing valvular damage, it should be continued for no more than 5 days, as in Regimen A.[67,251]

For penicillin-allergic patients, alternative regimens include substitution of a first-generation cephalosporin such as cephalothin or cefazolin for the penicillin in those with a history of a rash, or vancomycin for those with a history of anaphylaxis (Regimen B).

Staphylococci Resistant to Methicillin. These organisms also are resistant to all other penicillins and cephalosporins.[253] Methicillin-resistant *S. aureus* strains cause up to 50 per cent of cases of *S. aureus* endocarditis in drug abusers and may cause endocarditis acquired in hospitals where methicillin-resistant *S. aureus* are a cause of nosocomial infections.[234,253] Methicillin-resistant *S. epidermidis* strains are responsible for most cases of *S. epidermidis* endocarditis on prosthetic cardiac valves (discussed below) but uncommonly cause native valve endocarditis.[62,104,105,114,253] Treatment of suspected methicillin-resistant staphylococcal endocarditis in these settings or of proven methicillin-resistant staphylococcal endocarditis must be with vancomycin, as in Regimen C (Table 35–4).

Rifampin has been used as a supplement to therapy with a penicillin, cephalosporin, or vancomycin with or without aminoglycosides in patients who seemed to be responding poorly to these agents.[254,255] Most reports are of isolated cases, and indicate a positive clinical effect. However, they are difficult to interpret, as there are no controlled comparisons of regimens with and without rifampin. Furthermore, addition of rifampin to standard regimens in vitro has a variable effect (including antagonism) on the rate at which staphylococci are killed.[256] Therefore, rifampin should not be added routinely but should be considered in patients who responded poorly to conventional therapy.

The usual duration of therapy for staphylococcal endocarditis on native valves is 4 weeks. With evidence of metastatic infection or when response is poor (i.e., prolonged fever or bacteremia), therapy should be prolonged to 6 weeks.

S. aureus Endocarditis on the Tricuspid Valve. This form of IE is much easier to cure than left-sided *S. aureus* endocarditis. One series demonstrated that 2 weeks of nafcillin plus tobramycin resulted in a 94 per cent cure rate; 2 weeks of vancomycin plus tobramycin failed in two of three patients.[257] Until more series are available, such short courses cannot be recommended.

Vancomycin must be given intravenously, and this may be problematic in IV drug abusers with poor venous access. As a result, there has been an effort to find alternative therapies for endocarditis caused by methicillin-resistant *S. aureus*. Teicoplanin, an investigational agent, has activity similar to that of vancomycin (i.e., bactericidal against coagulase-positive and coagulase-negative methicillin-sensitive and methicillin-resistant *S. aureus* and *S. epidermidis*). It is being developed for intramuscular as well as intravenous use. It seems promising both in an animal model of endocarditis and in preliminary human studies.[258–260] Ciprofloxacin and other, newer fluoroquinolones have also been shown to be effective in staphylococcal endocarditis in animal models and in a small number of human cases.[261–263] Dworkin and coworkers[263] recently reported successful therapy of right-sided *S. aureus* endocarditis in a series of patients using 28 days of ciprofloxacin plus rifampin. Occasional emergence of resistance to the quinolones has occurred while therapy was being given, raising concerns about the reliability of these agents for staphylococcal endocarditis.[264]

STAPHYLOCOCCI CAUSING PROSTHETIC VALVE ENDOCARDITIS (Table 35–5). Most cases of staphylococcal endocarditis on prosthetic valves require both antibiotic and surgical management because of the frequent development of valve dysfunction or dehiscence or myocardial abscesses.[47,104,105,114] Staphylococcal endocarditis on prosthetic valves usually is caused by methicillin-susceptible *S. aureus* or methicillin-resistant *S. epidermidis*.[62,104,105,114,253] Data from an animal model and a relatively large clinical experience with methicillin-resistant *S. epidermidis* endocarditis on prosthetic valves have suggested that combination therapy with vancomycin plus gentamicin and rifampin gives better results than vancomycin alone.[62,114,253,265] Based on these data and the generally poor results of therapy for PVE in general, combination therapy is recommended for PVE.

Unless the infecting organism is demonstrated to be susceptible to methicillin, *S. epidermidis* infection on a prosthetic valve is treated with vancomycin and rifampin for at least 6 weeks with gentamicin (or an aminoglycoside to which it is sensitive) for the first 2 weeks (Regimen D).[47] If the organism is resistant to all aminoglycosides, they are omitted. If the *S. epidermidis* is susceptible to methicillin, a penicillinase-resistant penicillin is given instead of vancomycin with gentamicin and rifampin added (Regimen E).

S. aureus PVE also is treated with Regimen D or E but usually without rifampin, as there is no evidence of benefit from adding rifampin.

OTHER ORGANISMS.[266–268] Endocarditis caused by *Corynebacterium* sp., gram-negative bacilli, anaerobes, and other uncommon pathogens should be treated with the regimen of bactericidal drugs that demonstrates the best activity in vitro.[69–79,81–86] If in vitro efficacy can be demonstrated, the best results usually are obtained with combinations of penicillins (e.g., ampicillin or piperacillin), cephalosporins (e.g., cefazolin, cefotaxime, or ceftazidime), imipenem, aztreonam, or vancomycin with an aminoglycoside administered for at least 4 to 6 weeks. The use of the newer quinolone antibiotics, such as ciprofloxacin, may improve outcome in gram-negative bacillus endocarditis even further.[269] Serum bactericidal titers should be monitored. Valve replacement in addition to antimicrobial therapy often is necessary for cure. Most *Corynebacterium* strains are resistant to penicillin G.[79] Endocarditis caused by penicillin-susceptible strains can be treated with penicillin plus gentamicin, as in Regimen F in Table 35–6. For penicillin-resistant strains, vancomycin is used, as in Regimen C in Table 35–4.

TABLE 35-10 THERAPY FOR OTHER ORGANISMS

1095

CHAP
35

REGIMEN	ANTIBIOTIC	ADULT DOSE AND ROUTE	DURATION
	HACEK GROUP		
O	Ampicillin	12 gm/24 h IV in 6 divided doses	4 wk
	plus		
	Gentamicin	1.7 mg/kg IV every 8 h	4 wk
	ENTEROBACTERIACEAE		
P	Cefotaxime*	8 gm/24 h IV in 4 divided doses	4-6 wk
	or		
	Imipenem	2-4 gm/24 h IV in 4 divided doses	4-6 wk
	or		
	Aztreonam	8 gm/24 h IV in 4 divided doses	4-6 wk
	plus		
	Gentamicin	1.7 mg/kg IV every 8 h	4-6 wk
	PSEUDOMONAS AERUGINOSA		
Q	Piperacillin	18 gm/24 h IV in 6 divided doses	6 wk
	or		
	Ceftazidime	6 gm/24 h IV in 3 divided doses	6 wk
	or		
	Imipenem	2-4 gm/24 h IV in 4 divided doses	6 wk
	or		
	Aztreonam	8 gm/24 h IV in 4 divided doses	6 wk
	plus		
	Tobramycin	1.7 mg/kg IV every 8 h	6 wk
	FUNGI		
R	Amphotericin B	1 mg/kg/24 h IV	6-8 wk
	plus		
	Flucytosine	150 mg/kg/24 h orally in 4 divided doses	6-8 wk

* Or another third-generation cephalosporin.

The HACEK group of bacteria (*Haemophilus, Actinobacillus, Cardiobacterium, Eikenella,* and *Kingella*) usually are highly susceptible to ampicillin, and Regimen O in Table 35-10, consisting of ampicillin plus gentamicin, has been used most frequently.[71-76] If resistance to ampicillin is found, Regimen P in Table 35-10 should be used.

Enterobacteriaceae (*E. coli, Klebsiella, Enterobacter, Serratia, Proteus*) usually are highly susceptible to the third-generation cephalosporins, imipenem, and aztreonam,[270-275] and it seems most reasonable to use one of these agents plus gentamicin, as in Regimen P in Table 35-10. Emergence of resistance to the third-generation cephalosporins and aztreonam during therapy has been noted with *Enterobacter, Citrobacter,* and *Serratia* strains. This is less likely to occur with imipenem. *Pseudomonas aeruginosa* strains are likely to be susceptible to the ureidopenicillins (e.g., piperacillin), ceftazidime, imipenem, and aztreonam.[270-277] *P. aeruginosa* endocarditis is best treated with piperacillin, ceftazidime, imipenem, or aztreonam plus tobramycin, as in Regimen Q in Table 35-10. Emergence of resistance of the *Pseudomonas* has been noted on therapy. This is less likely to occur with imipenem. With availability of intravenous ciprofloxacin, fluoroquinolones may become the preferred therapy for endocarditis caused by Enterobacteriaceae and *P. aeruginosa*.

The current available antifungal agents usually will not cure fungal endocarditis[87,237] except in rare cases.[278] Thus, combined medical therapy (amphotericin B with flucytosine if the organism is susceptible), as in Regimen R in Table 35-10, and surgical therapy (excision of the vegetation or valve replacement) is advocated in the treatment of fungal endocarditis. After about a week of antifungal therapy the valve should be replaced. Outcome is poor at best. Even those cases of fungal endocarditis that are apparently cured may relapse after long, latent periods of time, such as 2 years.

The approach to both Q fever and chlamydial endocarditis usually has been valve replacement in association with prolonged antimicrobial therapy (i.e., months to years). The antimicrobial agents that seem to have been effective have been doxycycline (100 mg twice a day) and tetracycline (500 mg four times a day) with trimethoprim-sulfamethoxazole added in Q fever.[86,113,279-281] Valve cultures have yielded the infecting organism in many cases after months and even years of therapy.

LONG-TERM SUPPRESSIVE THERAPY. Occasionally, it is impossible to sterilize vegetations with antimicrobial therapy, and surgical excision is either refused or not feasible. This is most likely to occur with endocarditis on a prosthesis in a patient in whom the risk of cardiac surgery is excessive. In this situation long-term antimicrobial therapy can be tried in an attempt to suppress the manifestations of endocarditis.[282]

SURGICAL MANAGEMENT

Valve replacement is not without its problems (e.g., emboli, bleeding from anticoagulation, valve degeneration, prosthetic valve endocarditis), and therefore should be undertaken only in patients with IE when definite indications exist.[283-285,285a]

INDICATIONS. The major indications for surgical intervention in endocarditis are CHF secondary to valvular dysfunction, myocardial or valve ring abscess which requires drainage, uncontrolled infection, and prosthetic valve dysfunction or dehiscence (Table 35-11).[286-288] Mortality in patients with aortic regurgitation from endocarditis with moderate to severe CHF is extremely high.[289] Immediate valve replacement is essential. Valve replacement also is indicated in patients (1) with persistently positive blood cultures despite appropriate antimicrobial therapy; (2) when appropriate microbicidal therapy is not available (infections caused by organisms such as fungi or certain gram-negative bacilli); and (3) when recurrent relapse (i.e., two or more relapses) occurs despite appropriate antimicrobial therapy. In patients with early PVE (usually caused by organisms other than streptococci) surgery often becomes necessary either because of development of valve dysfunction or dehiscence or because of inability to eradicate the infection.[104,105,288] Late PVE (frequently caused by a streptococcus) often does not cause valve dys-

TABLE 35-11 INDICATIONS FOR CARDIAC SURGERY

ABSOLUTE INDICATIONS
Refractory heart failure related to valvular dysfunction*
Myocardial or perivalvular abscess*
Ineffective therapy such as persistent bacteremia or fungal
  infection*
Repeated relapses*
Unstable prosthesis

RELATIVE INDICATION
Multiple embolic episodes*

* Native or prosthetic valve endocarditis.

function.[104,105,288] Patients with delayed-onset streptococcal PVE are most likely to be cured with antibiotics alone.

Although it is ideal to treat with optimal antimicrobial therapy long enough to sterilize blood cultures before surgery, when a definite indication for surgery is present, the procedure should not be delayed. Delay of surgery, especially in the presence of heart failure, may convert an elective procedure with a relatively low mortality rate to an emergency procedure with a high mortality rate. Persistence of infection with the same organism has been uncommon (probably <5 per cent) after valve replacement, even when only short courses of antimicrobial therapy have been given before surgery.[286,290-293a] Postoperative antimicrobial therapy should be continued long enough to eradicate metastatic foci of infection.

Myocardial or valve ring abscesses must be drained surgically. Myocardial invasion extending from the valve annulus is common in PVE. Prompt surgical intervention may be lifesaving. Surgery should be considered in patients with large vegetations demonstrated by echocardiography and recurrent major arterial emboli. Many consider emboli a major indication for surgery. However, it is difficult to decide when to operate in patients with recurrent emboli, as there are no data to indicate the likelihood of additional emboli.[148,294] Our approach is not to routinely recommend surgery after one major embolus. With two or more emboli, and perhaps even after one embolus in the presence of very large vegetations on echocardiography (i.e., ≥10 mm), surgery often is recommended. We do not use size of the vegetation alone as an indication for cardiac surgery.

Some have considered infection caused by S. aureus to be an indication for cardiac surgery.[295] The authors do not advocate cardiac surgery for S. aureus infection unless other indications also are present.

A recent approach to the surgical management of IE has been valvuloplasty with resection of the vegetation. This procedure is applicable only to patients in whom the valve is relatively intact.[296-299] In future years this may become the preferred approach for patients with endocarditis refractory to therapy or with emboli.

Endocarditis restricted to the tricuspid valve is most often seen in IV drug abusers. When it is caused by fungi or antibiotic-resistant gram-negative bacilli, one approach has been resection of the valve without replacement.[299,300] This approach is of particular potential importance in those persons who are likely to return to use of intravenous drugs after surgery and in whom valvuloplasty with resection of the vegetatin is not possible. Presence of a prosthetic valve in an active IV drug abuser would provide an extremely susceptible focus for subsequent episodes of endocarditis. Many patients tolerate absence of the tricuspid valve for long periods of time. If pulmonary artery hypertension begins to develop, a tricuspid prosthetic valve can be implanted.

Recently, a patient with *Mycoplasma hominis* endocarditis involving mitral and aortic valve prostheses was cured with heart transplantation.[301] Noncardiac surgical intervention may be required for drainage of abscesses. Large emboli often require vascular procedures to reopen major arteries.

ANTICOAGULATION

Anticoagulants are of no value in treatment of IE. They do not prevent embolization of parts of the vegetation and do not add to the effectiveness of appropriate antimicrobial agents in preventing growth of the vegetation. Anticoagulation also increases the potential hazard of bleeding from a mycotic aneurysm or from a cerebral embolus and infarction. However, anticoagulation may have to be used if indications for anticoagulation exist, such as presence of a prosthetic valve or pulmonary emboli from a source other than from a cardiac vegetation.[148,302] Careful control is important to keep the parameters of anticoagulation (e.g., prothrombin time) in low therapeutic ranges.

RESPONSE TO THERAPY

Most patients defervesce by 3 to 7 days after effective antimicrobial therapy has been started.[251,303] *Persistence or recurrence of fever* may be due to associated myocardial or metastatic abscesses, recurrent emboli, superinfection of the vegetation, or (most commonly with recurrence of fever) febrile reactions to antimicrobial agents.[154,304,305] Blood cultures should be obtained periodically during treatment, and they usually become negative after several days of therapy. Lack of response of bacteremia may be associated with myocardial or metastatic abscess formation (especially with S. aureus)[148,154,251] Some patients may have positive blood cultures for as long as 1 or occasionally 2 weeks while receiving curative therapy. This is most likely to occur with enterococcal and especially S. aureus endocarditis.

If a *rash* develops, therapy can be continued and antihistamines or even corticosteroids given to suppress the reaction. If the rash is severe, therapy should be altered. Weight gain, improvement in appetite, and a rise in hemoglobin may not be seen until weeks after therapy has been completed. Petechiae, Osler nodes, and emboli may occur during and for weeks after successful antimicrobial therapy.[148] Splenomegaly may take months to resolve. Changes in murmurs from destruction of the valve or from shrinkage or rupture may occur during or after therapy. Heart failure may result, and is the principal cause of death, particularly in patients with aortic valve endocarditis.[154]

Mycotic aneurysms may regress on drug therapy or may rupture on therapy weeks to years later.[148,306] Despite the fact that cerebral aneurysms may rupture without warning, with present knowledge it is not reasonable to submit all patients with endocarditis for evaluation for cerebral aneurysm. Symptoms of headache and/or transient or permanent neurological abnormalities (e.g., visual field defects) in a patient with endocarditis must raise the question of cerebral aneurysm[148,154,157,306] and suggests leakage or enlargement of an aneurysm. Although computed tomographic scans may be suggestive, cerebral angiography is necessary for diagnosis and should be pursued in patients with central nervous system symptoms.[154,306] When aneurysms are found in symptomatic patients, surgical intervention must be seriously considered.

Aneurysms in the chest or abdomen often are asymptomatic and unsuspected until they rupture, requiring emergency surgery.[159] In an extremity a pulsatile mass suggests an aneurysm and the need for surgery.[154,158]

Renal insufficiency from glomerulonephritis usually improves with therapy for the endocarditis.[154,165,307] Occasional patients do not improve with control of the endocarditis, and in some of these patients corticosteroids, plasma exchange, and/or cytotoxic chemotherapy has been reported to be effective.[307-309]

RELAPSES AND NEW EPISODES

The great majority of relapses of endocarditis occur within 2 months of stopping antimicrobial therapy, and most occur within 4 weeks.[310,311] Blood cultures 2 to 4 weeks after completion of therapy detect the majority of relapses. Although delayed relapses are unusual with bacterial endocarditis, they are not uncommon with fungal endocarditis and Q fever endocarditis.[312] Relapses caused by the same fungus have been reported as long as 2 years after replacement of a prosthetic valve for fungal endocarditis. In fact, a case of ours reported as a cure subsequently relapsed after 2 years.[194]

New episodes of endocarditis commonly occur in patients who have had IE. At least 6 per cent of patients with native valve endocarditis and who are not drug abusers will have one or more additional episodes of endocarditis.[313] We saw one patient who had seven distinct episodes over a period of 20 years. IV drug abusers are at particularly high risk for additional episodes.[93,97] The results of treatment of those with subsequent episodes of endocarditis on native valves are no worse than results of therapy for first episodes of endocarditis.[313]

PROGNOSIS

The prognosis of IE varies according to the infecting microorganisms, the type of cardiac valve (native versus prosthetic and aortic versus mitral versus tricuspid), the age of the patient, and the presence or absence of complications.

NATIVE VALVE ENDOCARDITIS

The cure rates for native valve endocarditis are greater than or equal to 90 per cent for streptococcal endocarditis, 75 to 90 per cent for enterococcal endocarditis, and 60 to 75 per cent for *S. aureus* endocarditis (some series report mortality rates as high as 70 per cent in *S. aureus* endocarditis).[47,224,252,253,314] Mortality from streptococcal or enterococcal endocarditis is seldom related to failure of antibiotic therapy. (This may change with the emergence of antibiotic-resistant enterococci.) The usual causes of death are heart failure, emboli, rupture of mycotic aneurysms, complications of cardiac surgery, and renal failure. Death from *S. aureus* endocarditis may be caused by overwhelming infection or by the complications listed above. Results have been poor in endocarditis caused by fungi, gram-negative enteric organisms, and *Pseudomonas* sp. because of resistance to antimicrobial agents.

In addition to the effect of the microorganism on prognosis, a *poorer prognosis* has been associated with the old and the very young, aortic versus mitral valve involvement, left-sided versus right-sided endocarditis, myocardial abscess, rupture of a mycotic aneurysm, emboli (especially coronary artery emboli), heart failure, renal insufficiency, and cardiac surgery in the presence of active versus inactive endocarditis.[47,224,252,253,314,315]

Other underlying diseases also increase the chance of mortality. Delay of diagnosis results in more complications and a worse prognosis. The striking effect of right-sided versus left-sided endocariditis can be illustrated by the fact that more than 90 per cent of IV drug abusers with *S. aureus* endocarditis localized to the tricuspid valve can be cured with antibiotic therapy alone, as contrasted with at least a 25 to 40 per cent mortality with left-sided *S. aureus* endocarditis.[62] The presence of large vegetations on echocardiogram may indicate a poorer prognosis than small or absent vegetations.[200-203,210]

After cure of endocarditis the risk of increased mortality remains. Most of the deaths that occur during therapy or after cure of endocarditis are related to heart failure, a major embolus, or rupture of a mycotic aneurysm. Cardiac surgery with valve replacement may be required during therapy for the episode of endocarditis or after bacteriological cure. In a recent series of patents with IE,[314] 25 per cent died in the hospital, 30 per cent had died by 1 year after discharge, and about 40 per cent by 5 years.

PROSTHETIC VALVE ENDOCARDITIS

The prognosis is clearly worse in PVE than in native valve endocarditis. Late PVE (>60 days after surgery) has a better prognosis, with a mortality rate of 19 to 50 per cent, than early PVE (<60 days postoperatively), with a mortality rate of 41 to 80 per cent.[104,181,288,316,317] The valve dysfunction and dehiscence and intracardiac abscesses, which are much more common with early disease, and the antibiotic-resistant organisms associated with early disease contribute to the higher mortality. Streptococcal PVE has the best prognosis, whereas PVE caused by fungi, coagulase-positive and coagulase-negative staphylococci, *Corynebacterium* sp., enteric gram-negative bacilli, and *Pseudomonas* has a much worse prognosis.[104,181,288,316-318]

In addition to infecting organism and time of onset, increased mortality has been associated with the clinical observations of persistent fever on antibiotic therapy, changing murmurs, new conduction abnormalities, and increasing heart failure.[288,316,319] These poor prognostic clinical features are probably in turn related to uncontrolled infection, myo-

cardial abscesses, and/or valve dysfunction. It also has been observed that early valve replacement in PVE patients (who have indications for replacement) is associated with a lower mortality than when surgery is delayed.[288,320]

PREVENTION

In the pathogenesis of bacterial endocarditis the causative microorganisms usually gain access to the bloodstream from the oropharynx, but in IV drug abusers and occasionally others the portal of entry is the skin. The respiratory, genitourinary, or gastrointestinal tract or an intravascular catheter, suture, or infusion also can act as a portal of entry.

The optimal approach to prophylaxis of IE is prevention or correction of underlying cardiovascular defects which predispose to intravascular infection, and some progress toward this goal is being achieved through modern medicosurgical therapy. The other approach consists of use of antimicrobial agents to prevent bacterial invasion of the bloodstream and subsequent localization and multiplication at an intravascular site.

Antibiotic prophylaxis of IE can be applied only to events or procedures recognized as providing potential bacterial portals of entry and only in patients with a recognized predisposing cardiac lesion. Therefore, most cases of IE are not preventable, as only half of patients who develop endocarditis have a previously recognized predisposing cardiac lesion,[171,321] and an apparent portal of entry (other than in drug abusers) can be demonstrated in patients with IE in less than 25 per cent of cases.[169,321-326] In fact, it has been calculated that less than 10 per cent of cases of IE are theoretically preventable with prophylaxis.[322]

Viridans streptococci are the predominant organisms in the flora of the oral cavity, the most common bacterial species isolated from the blood after trauma to the tissues of the mouth, and the most common cause of IE. However, many other bacterial species can be detected in the mouth, are occasionally isolated from blood after dental trauma, and can cause IE (Table 35–3).[128] Prophylaxis of endocarditis after procedures in the mouth is aimed primarily at viridans streptococci. The frequency of bacteremia is related to the degree of disease of the gum and to the degree of trauma inflicted during the procedure (Table 35–3).[128] Procedures attended by bleeding are far more likely to cause bacteremia than those that are not.

Enterococci are responsible for a relatively large number of cases of IE that develop after urinary tract surgical procedures or delivery, abortion, pelvic inflammatory disease, and instrumentation of the female genitourinary tract.[45,46] Although *gram-negative enteric bacilli* are responsible for most of the cases of bacteremia after urinary tract manipulation, these organisms are unusual as causes of IE, and prophylaxis of endocarditis is directed at the enterococcus.

The *gastrointestinal tract* occasionally has been identified as a portal of entry for microorganisms in patients with IE. Although bacteremia occasionally occurs in association with instrumentation of the intestinal tract, such as sigmoidoscopy and colonoscopy, IE after these procedures is rare.[327,328] However, it appears advisable to administer antimicrobial agents to patients with valvular or congenital heart disease who undergo procedures on the lower gastrointestinal tract that are likely to be associated with considerable trauma to soft tissues (i.e., surgery).

Surgical procedures on the *gallbladder* also have occasionally been implicated as providing a portal of entry in IE; therefore, antimicrobial prophylaxis should be considered in connection with this type of surgery. Although the predominant bacterial flora of the gastrointestinal tract is anaerobic, anaerobes are rare causes of endocarditis. Gram-negative aerobic bacilli and enterococci also are found in large numbers in the intestinal tract, but, as the former organisms are rare causes of endocarditis, prophylaxis should be directed at the enterococcus. Endocarditis also may complicate localized infection at almost any site in the absence of demonstrable trauma. Obvious examples include endocarditis secondary to staphylococcal skin infections and pneumococcal pneumonia.

Finally, a clinically detectable portal of entry is absent in most patients with IE, and the source of infection in these patients is almost certainly asymptomatic transient bacteremia from the mouth, other mucous membranes, or sites of inapparent infection.[326,329,330] This is explained by the fact that although the risk of endocarditis after an episode of low-grade bacteremia caused by brushing the teeth or chewing a steak is undoubtedly much lower than that of the more intense bacteremia after tooth extraction, the cumulative risk of daily low-grade bacteremias is apparently higher than that from the occasional surgical procedure.[326] Cardiac catheterization has seldom been a predisposing event for endocarditis, and antibiotic prophylaxis is not recommended for routine cardiac catheterization.

The incidence of endocarditis is increased in two ways by prosthetic valve insertion: (1) the surgical maneuver itself, the use of intravascular catheters during the postoperative period, wound infection, and the occurrence of pneumonia all increase the possibility of bacteremia and subsequent endocarditis; and (2) the prosthetic valve is more susceptible to colonization by microorganisms immediately after insertion and probably permanently.

In one study,[331] which will undoubtedly never be repeated, when antibiotic medications were not used prophylactically, endocarditis occurred within 4 days after cardiac surgical intervention and was caused by S. pneumoniae and S. aureus. When prophylaxis is given, the frequency of early endocarditis seems to decrease. Although the evidence for or against antibiotic prophylaxis at the time of cardiac surgical procedures is inconclusive, all cardiac surgeons use prophylaxis. Because the staphylococcus is the most common cause of early PVE, it seems most reasonable to direct prophylaxis against this organism at time of operation.

General Methods

Patients with cardiovascular defects that predispose to endocarditis should be informed of the defect, the potential value of chemoprophylaxis, and the importance of sound routine dental care by a practitioner cognizant of their heart disease.[27,332,333] The highest level of oral health should be maintained. This will decrease daily bacteremias and is probably more important in preventing endocarditis than antibiotic prophylaxis before specific dental procedures.

There is a lack of awareness of the need for antibiotic prophylaxis among patients with cardiac lesions that predispose to IE and poor compliance with prophylactic regimens by physicians and dentists.[332-335] Therefore, it has been suggested that patients with predisposing heart disease carry a card indicating their cardiac lesion and recommendations for prophylaxis.

The incidence of bacteremia after trauma to contaminated epithelial surfaces or sites of local infection probably can be decreased by techniques that produce minimal damage to soft tissues.[336] There is no question that this is true in oral surgery. Furthermore, endodontic procedures are less likely to be associated with bacteremia than is tooth extraction or gingival surgery.[128] "De-germing" the mouth with antiseptic mouthwashes such as chlorhexidine just before a dental procedure can markedly decrease the intensity of subsequent bacteremia and, therefore, the risk of endocarditis.[332,336]

Use of an oral irrigation device should be *discouraged* in patients with cardiac lesions who are susceptible to endocarditis, because the appliance may produce bacteremia even in patients with normal-appearing gingiva (Table 35–3).[128]

To decrease the possibility of associated bacteremias and fungemias, central intravascular catheters should be avoided when possible. Infections (e.g., pneumonia, skin infections) should be promptly treated to decrease the possibility of duration of associated bacteremias. Urinary tract infection, prosta-

titis, and other deep infections should be treated before cystoscopy or prostatectomy, to eliminate infection and reduce the possibility of bacteremia from instrumentation of an infected bladder or from cutting into an infected prostate.

Chemoprophylaxis

Antibiotic agents may be effective in preventing IE by decreasing the incidence and magnitude of bacteremia associated with traumatic procedures, by decreasing adherence of microorganisms to endocardium and noninfected thrombi, and by eliminating bacteria in blood or, even more likely, on heart valves before an established vegetation is formed.

Despite the fact that antibiotic prophylaxis has been used for years, there is no definitive evidence that prophylaxis with antimicrobial agents is effective in preventing IE. Furthermore, there is a lack of information about risk-to-benefit or cost-to-benefit ratios for prophylaxis, and apparent failures of prophylaxis have occurred.[337] Nevertheless, it is important to apply prophylaxis to patients with high-risk lesions who are having procedures with a high risk of bacteremia. With low-risk lesions and low-risk procedures, the use of prophylaxis should clearly be optional or even discouraged.

Ideally, the antibiotic(s) used for prophylaxis should be the same as that used in the therapy for endocarditis caused by the organism against which the prophylaxis is aimed. The approach is to provide treatment sufficiently long to cure very early endocarditis (e.g., 10 bacteria on a valve rather than the 10^9 found in an established vegetation). Therapy usually is started about 1 hour before the procedure and continued for *less than 24 hours.* Starting prophylaxis earlier than 1 to 2 hours before the procedure has no advantages, and if started 1 or more days earlier, it increases the possibility of obtaining antibiotic-resistant strains of bacteria at the mucosal site.

Therapy with penicillin as well as with certain other antimicrobial agents produces only a moderate decrease in incidence of bacteremia after tooth extraction.[329] This is not necessarily a measure of effectiveness of an antibiotic in preventing IE; antimicrobial action in blood and on the valve is probably far more important in eradicating bacterial invaders. In addition, it has been demonstrated that antimicrobial agents, even at subinhibitory concentrations, may protect against development of endocarditis by interfering with adherence of bacteria to the cardiac lesion.[338,339]

The Committee on Rheumatic Fever and Infective Endocarditis of the American Heart Association has recently issued an update of guidelines on prevention of bacterial endocar-

TABLE 35–12 SELECTED CARDIAC CONDITIONS

ENDOCARDITIS PROPHYLAXIS RECOMMENDED
Prosthetic cardiac valves (bioprosthetic and homograft valves)
Previous bacterial endocarditis (even without heart disease)
Most congenital cardiac malformations
Rheumatic and other acquired valvular dysfunction (even after valvular surgery)
Hypertrophic cardiomyopathy (IHSS)
Mitral valve prolapse with valvular regurgitation

ENDOCARDITIS PROPHYLAXIS NOT RECOMMENDED
Isolated secundum atrial septal defect
Surgical repair without residua beyond 6 months of isolated secundum atrial septal defect, ventricular septal defect, patent ductus arteriosus
Previous coronary artery bypass graft surgery
Mitral valve prolapse without valvular regurgitation*
Physiological, functional, or innocent heart murmurs
Previous Kawasaki's disease without valvular dysfunction
Previous rheumatic fever without valvular dysfunction
Cardiac pacemakers and implanted defibrillators

* Patients with mitral valve prolapse associated with thickening and/or redundancy of the valve leaflets may be at increased risk for endocarditis, particularly in men over age 45 years.
Modified from Dajani, A. S., et al.: Prevention of bacterial endocarditis. JAMA 264:2919, 1990.

TABLE 35–13 SELECTED DENTAL AND SURGICAL PROCEDURES

ENDOCARDITIS PROPHYLAXIS RECOMMENDED

Dental procedures known to induce gingival or mucosal bleeding, including professional cleaning
Tonsillectomy and/or adenoidectomy
Surgical operations involving intestinal or respiratory mucosa
Bronchoscopy with a rigid bronchoscope
Sclerotherapy for esophageal varices
Esophageal dilatation
Gallbladder surgery
Cystoscopy
Urethral dilatation
Urethral catheterization if urinary tract infection is present*
Urinary tract surgery if urinary tract infection is present*
Prostatic surgery
Incision and drainage of infected tissue*
Vaginal hysterectomy
Vaginal delivery in the presence of infection*

ENDOCARDITIS PROPHYLAXIS NOT RECOMMENDED**

Dental procedures unlikely to induce gingival bleeding (e.g., simple adjustment of orthodontic appliances or fillings above gum line)
Injection of local intraoral anesthetic (except intraligamentary injections)
Shedding of primary teeth
Tympanostomy tube insertion
Endotracheal intubation
Bronchoscopy (flexible bronchoscope, with or without biopsy)
Cardiac catheterization
Endoscopy with or without gastrointestinal biopsy
Cesarean delivery
In the absence of infection: Urethral catheterization, dilatation and curettage, uncomplicated vaginal delivery, therapeutic abortion, sterilization procedure, insertion or removal of intrauterine devices

* In addition to prophylactic regimen for genitourinary procedures, antibiotic therapy should be directed against the most likely bacterial pathogen.
** In patients with prosthetic heart valves or a previous history of endocarditis, physicians may elect prophylaxis even for low-risk procedures that involve the lower respiratory, genitourinary, or GI tract.
Modified from Dajani, A. S., et al.: Prevention of bacterial endocarditis. JAMA 264:2919, 1990.

TABLE 35–14 STANDARD PROPHYLACTIC REGIMEN FOR DENTAL, ORAL, OR UPPER RESPIRATORY TRACT PROCEDURES IN PATIENTS AT RISK

Amoxicillin 3 gm orally 1 hour before procedure; then 1.5 gm 6 hours after initial dose.

FOR AMOXICILLIN/PENICILLIN-ALLERGIC PATIENTS:
Erythromycin ethylsuccinate 800 mg or erythromycin stearate 1 gm orally 2 hours before a procedure; then one-half the dose 6 hours after initial administration.
or
Clindamycin 300 mg orally 1 hour before a procedure and 150 mg 6 hours after initial dose.

Modified from Dajani, A. S., et al.: Prevention of bacterial endocarditis. JAMA 264:2919, 1990.

TABLE 35–15 ALTERNATE PROPHYLACTIC REGIMENS FOR DENTAL, ORAL, OR UPPER RESPIRATORY TRACT PROCEDURES IN PATIENTS AT RISK

FOR PATIENTS UNABLE TO TAKE ORAL MEDICATION:
Ampicillin 2 gm IV (or IM) 30 minutes before procedure; then ampicillin 1 gm IV (or IM) or amoxicillin 1.5 gm orally 6 hours after initial dose.

FOR AMPICILLIN/AMOXICILLIN/PENICILLIN-ALLERGIC PATIENTS UNABLE TO TAKE ORAL MEDICATIONS:
Clindamycin 300 mg IV 30 minutes before a procedure and 150 mg IV (or orally) 6 hours after initial dose.

FOR PATIENTS CONSIDERED TO BE AT VERY HIGH RISK:
Ampicillin 2 gm IV (or IM) plus gentamicin 1.5 mg/kg IV (or IM) (not to exceed 80 mg) 30 minutes before procedure, followed by amoxicillin 1.5 gm orally 6 hours after the initial dose.
Alternatively, parenteral regimen may be repeated 8 hours after initial dose.

AMOXICILLIN/AMPICILLIN/PENICILLIN-ALLERGIC PATIENTS CONSIDERED TO BE AT VERY HIGH RISK:
Vancomycin 1 gm IV administered over 1 hour, starting 1 hour before the procedure. No repeat dose is necessary.

Modified from Dajani, A. S., et al.: Prevention of bacterial endocarditis. JAMA 264:2919, 1990.

TABLE 35–16 REGIMENS FOR GENITOURINARY AND GASTROINTESTINAL PROCEDURES

STANDARD REGIMEN:
Ampicillin 2 gm IV (or IM) plus gentamicin 1.5 mg/kg IV (or IM) (not to exceed 80 mg) 30 minutes before procedure, followed by amoxicillin 1.5 gm orally 6 hours after the initial dose.
Alternatively, parenteral regimen may be repeated once 8 hours after initial dose.

FOR AMOXICILLIN/AMPICILLIN/PENICILLIN-ALLERGIC PATIENTS:
Vancomycin 1 gm IV administered over 1 hour plus gentamicin 1.5 mg/kg IV (or IM) (not to exceed 80 mg) 1 hour before procedure. May be repeated once 8 hours after initial dose.

ALTERNATE ORAL REGIMEN FOR LOW-RISK PATIENTS:
Amoxicillin 3 gm orally 1 hour before procedure; then 1.5 gm 6 hours after initial dose.

Modified from Dajani, A. S., et al.: Prevention of bacterial endocarditis. JAMA 264:2919, 190.

TABLE 35–17 PROPHYLACTIC REGIMENS FOR CARDIAC SURGERY WITH PLACEMENT OF FOREIGN MATERIAL

Cefazolin 2 gm IV immediately preoperatively and every 6 hours for 24–28 hours plus gentamicin 1.7 mg/kg IV immediately preoperatively and every 8 hours for 24 hours.

IN INSTITUTIONS WITH A HIGH INCIDENCE OF METHICILLIN-RESISTANT STAPHYLOCOCCI:
Vancomycin 15 mg/kg IV over 1 hour immediately preoperatively, followed by 10 mg/kg IV immediately after cardiopulmonary bypass surgery plus gentamicin as above.

---

ditis.[340] These are reviewed in Tables 35–12 through 35–17. Table 35–12 lists the cardiac conditions for which antibiotic prophylaxis is recommended (all of which have been associated with an increased frequency of IE). It also lists some of the conditions for which prophylaxis is not recommended.

Mitral valve prolapse is a particular problem because of its high frequency (estimated to occur in 2.5 to 5 per cent of the population and up to 20 per cent among young women[19]) and relatively low risk in predisposing to IE.[18,20] Controversy has raged over which patients with mitral valve prolapse should receive prophylaxis. Men with prolapse are at higher risk for IE than are women, and those with a murmur are at higher risk than those without a murmur, especially patients over age 45.[18,20,341,342] Without a murmur the risk is not much different from that in the population at large.[18] Several reports have suggested that the risk-to-benefit and cost-to-benefit ratios for prophylaxis with penicillin for all patients with mitral valve prolapse are unfavorable.[342–344] Restricting use of prophylaxis to prolapse with valvular regurgitation, as recommended by the American Heart Association committee, would be helpful, but the term regurgitation must be defined, especially with the advent of color Doppler ultrasound, which detects nonaudible regurgitation. We do not recommend prophylaxis in the absence of a murmur and make prophylaxis optional in cases with a late systolic murmur, either spontaneous or evoked with maneuvers.[345] Only with a holosystolic murmur do we mandate prophylaxis.

Antibiotic prophylaxis is to be used with procedures that are likely to cause bacteremia, as listed in Table 35–13, which also lists some procedures that infrequently cause bacteremia and for which prophylaxis is *not* recommended.

The regimens recommended for dental and other oral and upper respiratory tract procedures are aimed at viridans streptococci. The adult regimens are listed in Tables 35–14 and 35–15. The latter gives alternative regimens for patients who are unable to take oral medication. Although the oral regimen in Table 35–14 is appropriate for patients with all cardiovascular lesions, including those at high risk for IE (e.g., those with prosthetic valves), Table 35–15 outlines regimens for the physician who *elects* to use a parenteral regimen in high-risk patients.

When a series of dental procedures is anticipated, it is recommended to wait 7 days between procedures and to do multiple procedures at the same sitting. This may help to reduce the chances of emergence of antibiotic-resistant flora. If a patient is receiving continuous oral penicillin for prevention of rheumatic fever, mouth flora resistant to penicillin may develop. In such cases, erythromycin or another nonpenicillin regimen in Table 35–14 or 35–15 should be used.

Antibiotic prophylaxis is used with procedures that are likely to cause significant trauma to the large bowel, genitourinary tract, and the gallbladder and is directed at the enterococcus. Adult regimens are found in Table 35–16. Prophylaxis at the time of cardiac surgery with placement of foreign material (e.g., prosthetic valves) is directed primarily at staphylococci. An aminoglycoside often is added for activity against gram-negative bacilli in an attempt to prevent endocardial infection as well as infection at other sites, such as the sternum. Reasonable regimens are listed in Table 35–17.

REFERENCES

1. Johnson, F., Darling, R. C., Mundth, E. D., et al.: The management of infected arterial aneurysms. J. Cardiovasc. Surg. 18:361, 1977.
1a. Infective endocarditis. *In* Fowler, N. O.: Diagnosis of Heart Disease. New York, Springer-Verlag, 1991, pp. 410–416.

NATIVE VALVE ENDOCARDITIS

2. McKinsey, D. S., Ratts, T. E., and Bisno, A. L.: Underlying cardiac lesions in adults with infective endocarditis: The changing spectrum. Am. J. Med. 82:681, 1987.
3. Sholler, G. E., Hawker, R. E., and Celermajer, J. M.: Infective endocarditis in childhood. Pediatr. Cardiol. 6:183, 1986.
4. Millard, D. D., and Shulman, S. T.: The changing spectrum of neonatal endocarditis. Clin. Perinatol 15:587, 1988.
5. Saiman, L., and Prince, A.: Infections of the heart. Adv. Pediatr. Infect. Dis. 4:139, 1989.
6. Johnson, C. M., and Rhodes, K. H.: Pediatric endocarditis. Mayo Clin. Proc. 57:86, 1982.
7. Johnson, D. H., Rosenthal, A., and Nadas, A. S.: A forty-year review of bacterial endocarditis in infancy and childhood. Circulation 51:581, 1975.
8. Zakrzewski, T., and Keith, J. D.: Bacterial endocarditis in infants and children. J. Pediatr. 67:1179, 1965.
9. VanHare, G. F., Ben-Shachar, G., Liebman, J., et al.: Infective endocarditis in infants and children during the past 10 years: A decade of change. Am. Heart J. 107:1235, 1984.
10. Schollin, J., Bjarke, B., and Wesstrom, G.: Infective endocarditis in Swedish children. I. Incidence, etiology, underlying factors and port of entry of infection; II. Location, major complications, laboratory findings, delay of treatment, treatment and outcome. Acta Paediatr. Scand. 75:993, 1986; 75:999, 1986.
11. Wald, E. R., Dashefsky, B., Feidt, C., et al.: Acute rheumatic fever in western Pennsylvania and the tri-state area. Pediatrics 80:371, 1987.
12. Veasy, L. G., Weidmeier, S. E., Orsmond, G. S., et al.: Resurgence of acute rheumatic fever in the intermountain area of the United States. N. Engl. J. Med. 316:421, 1987.
13. Cutler, J. G., Ongley, P. A., Shwachman, H., et al.: Bacterial endocarditis in children with heart disease. Pediatrics 22:706, 1958.
14. Cremieux, A. C., Witchitz, S., Malergue, M. C., et al.: Clinical and echocardiographic observations in pulmonary valve endocarditis. Am. J. Cardiol. 56:610, 1985.
15. Blumenthal, S., Griffiths, S. P. and Morgan, B. C.: Bacterial endocarditis in children with congenital heart disease. Pediatrics 26:993, 1960.
16. Geva, T., and Frand, M.: Infective endocarditis in children with congenital heart disease: The changing spectrum 1965–1985. Eur. Heart J. 9:1244, 1988.
17. Nagger, C. Z., and Forgacs, P.: Infective endocarditis: A challenging disease. Med. Clin. North Am. 70:1279, 1986.
18. MacMahon, S. W., Roberts, J. K., Kramer-Fox, R., et al.: Mitral valve prolapse and infective endocarditis. Am. Heart J. 113:1291, 1987.
19. Lavie, C. J., Khandheria, B. K., Seward, J. B., et al.: Factors associated with the recommendation for endocarditis prophylaxis in mitral valve prolapse. JAMA 262:3308, 1989.
20. MacMahon, S. W., Hickey, A. J., Wilcken, D.E.L., et al.: Risk of infective endocarditis in mitral valve prolapse with and without precordial systolic murmurs. Am. J. Cardiol. 58:105, 1986.
21. Griffin, M. R., Wilson, W. R., Edwards, W. D., et al.: Infective endocarditis —Olmstead County, Minnesota, 1950 through 1981. JAMA 254:1199, 1985.
22. Weinberger, I., Rotenberg, Z., Zacharovitch, D., et al.: Native valve infective endocarditis in the 1970's versus the 1980's: Underlying cardiac lesions and infecting organisms. Clin. Cardiol. 13:94, 1990.
23. Kaye, D.: Definitions and demographic characteristics. In: Kaye, D. (ed.): Infective endocarditis. Baltimore, University Park Press, 1976, pp. 1–10.
24. Sharma, S., Desai, A. G., Pillai, M. G., et al.: Clinical and diagnostic features of pulmonary valve endocarditis in the setting of congenital cardiac malformations. Int. J. Cardiol. 9:457, 1985.
25. Stulz, P., Zimmerli, W., Mihatsch, J., and Gradel, E.: Recurrent infective endocarditis in idiopathic hypertrophic subaortic stenosis. Thorac. Cardiovasc. Surg. 37(2):99, 1989.
26. Soman, V. R., Breton, G., Hershkowitz, M., and Mark, H.: Bacterial endocarditis of mitral valve in Marfan syndrome. Br. Heart J. 36:1247, 1974.
27. Kaye, D.: Changing pattern of infective endocarditis. Am. J. Med. 78(Suppl 6B):157, 1985.
28. Terpenning, M. S., Buggy, B. P., and Kauffman, C. A.: Infective endocarditis: Clinical features in young and elderly patients. Am. J. Med. 83:626, 1987.
28a. von Reyn, C. E., Levy, B. S., Arbeit, N. O., et al.: Infective carditis: An analysis based on strict case definitions. Ann. Intern. Med. 94:505, 1981.
29. Stekilber, J. M., Melton, L. J., IV, Ilstrup, D. M., et al.: Influence of referral bias on the apparent clinical spectrum of infective endocarditis. Am. J. Med. 88:582, 1990.
30. Applefeld, M. M., and Hornick, R. B.: Infective endocarditis in patients over age 60. Am. Heart J. 88:90, 1974.
31. Pomerance, A.: Cardiac pathology in the elderly. Cardiovasc. Clin. 12:9, 1981.
32. Rayfield, E. J., Ault, M. J., Keusch, G. T., et al.: Infection and diabetes: The case for glucose control. Am. J. Med. 72:439, 1982.
33. Seltzer, A.: Changing aspects of the natural history of valvular aortic stenosis. N. Engl. J. Med. 317:91, 1987.
34. Cooper, G., and Platt, R.: Staphylococcus aureus bacteremia in diabetic patients. Endocarditis and mortality. Am. J. Med. 73:658, 1982.
35. Tuazon, C. U., Perez, A., Kishaba, T., et al.: Staphylococcus aureus among insulin-injecting diabetic patients; an increased carrier risk. J.A.M.A. 231:1272, 1975.
36. Casey, J. I., Maturlo, S., Albin, J., and Edberg, S. C.: Comparison of carriage rates of group B streptococcus in diabetic and non-diabetic persons. Am. J. Epidemiol. 116:704, 1982.
37. Gallagher, P. G., and Watanakunakorn, C.: Group B streptococcal endocarditis: Report on seven cases and review of the literature, 1962–1985. Rev. Infect. Dis. 8:175, 1986.
38. Seaworth, B. J., and Durack, D. T.: Infective endocarditis in obstetric and gynecologic practice. Am. J. Obstet. Gynecol. 54:180, 1986.
39. Cox, S. M., Hankins, G. D., Leveno, K. S., and Cunningham, F. G.: Bacterial endocarditis: A serious pregnancy complication. J. Reprod. Med. 33:671, 1988.
40. Roberts, R. B., Krieger, A. G., Schiller, N. L., et al.: Viridans streptococcal endocarditis: The role of various species including pyridoxal-dependent streptococci. Rev. Infect. Dis. 1:955, 1979.
41. Coykendale, A. L.: Classification and identification of the viridans streptococci. Clin. Microbiol. Rev. 2:315, 1989.
42. Harder, E. J., Wilkowske, C. J., Washington, J. A., et al.: Streptococcus mutans endocarditis. Ann. Intern. Med. 80:364, 1974.
43. Stein, D. S., and Nelson, K. E.: Endocarditis due to nutritionally deficient streptococci: Therapeutic dilemma. Rev. Infect. Dis. 9:908, 1987.
44. Facklam, R. R., and Carey, R. B.: Streptococci and aerococci. In: Lennete, E. H., Balows, A., Hausler, W. J., Jr., et al. (eds.): Manual of Clinical Microbiology. 4th ed. Washington, D.C., American Society of Microbiology, 1985, pp. 154–175.
45. Mandell, G. L., Kaye, D., Levison, M. E., et al.: Enterococcal endocarditis: An analysis of 38 patients observed at the New York Hospital—Cornell Medical Center. Arch. Intern. Med. 125:258, 1970.
46. Maki, D. G., and Agger, W. A.: Enterococcal bacteremia: Clinical features, the risk of endocarditis and management. Medicine (Baltimore) 67:248, 1988.
47. Bisno, A. L., Dismukes, W. E., Durack, D. T., et al.: Antimicrobial treatment of infective endocarditis due to viridans streptococci, enterococci and staphylococci. JAMA 261:1471, 1989.
48. Ingerman, M., Pitsakis, P. G., Rosenberg, A., et al.: Beta-lactamase production in experimental endocarditis due to aminoglycoside-resistant Streptococcus faecalis. J. Infect. Dis. 155:1226, 1987.
49. Zervos, M. J., Terpenning, M. S., Schaberg, D. R., et al.: High-level aminoglycoside-resistant enterococci colonization of nursing home and acute care hospital patients. Arch. Intern. Med. 147:1591, 1987.
50. Uttley, A.H.C., Collins, C. H., Naidoo, J., and George, R. C.: Vancomycin-resistant enterococci. Lancet 1:57, 1988.

51. Moellering, R. C., Watson, B. K., Kunz, L. J.: Endocarditis due to group D streptococci. Comparison of disease caused by *Streptococcus bovis* with that produced by enterococci. Am. J. Med. 57:239, 1974.

52. Leport, C., Bure, A., Leport, J., and Vilde, J. L.: Incidence of colonic lesions in *Streptococcus bovis* and enterococcal endocarditis. Lancet 1:748, 1987.

53. Emiliani, V. J., Chodos, J. E., Comer, G. M., et al.: *Streptococcus bovis* brain abscess associated with an occult colonic villous adenoma. Am. J. Gastroenterol. 85:78, 1990.

54. Wiseman, A., René, P., and Crelinsten, G. L.: *Streptococcus agalactiae* endocarditis: An association with villous adenomas of the large intestine. Ann. Intern. Med. 103:893, 1985.

55. Venezio, F. R., Gullberg, R. M., Westenfelder, G. O., et al.: Group G streptococcal endocarditis and bacteremia. Am. J. Med. 81:29, 1986.

56. Ugolini, V., Pacifico, A., Smitherman, T. C., and Mackowiak, P. A.: Pneumococcal endocarditis update: Analysis of 10 cases diagnosed between 1974 and 1984. Am. Heart J. 112:813, 1986.

57. Powderly, W. G., Stanley, S. L., Jr., and Medoff, G.: Pneumococcal endocarditis: Report of a series and review of the literature. Rev. Infect. Dis. 8:786, 1986.

58. Sands, M., Brown, R. B., Ryczak, M., and Hamilton, W.: *Streptococcus pneumoniae* endocarditis. South Med. J. 80:780, 1987.

59. Bruyn, G.A.W., Thompson, J., and van der Meer, J.W.M.: Pneumococcal endocarditis in adult patients. A report of five cases and review of the literature. Q. J. Med. 74:33, 1990.

60. Editorial: Penicillin-resistant pneumococci. Lancet 1:1142, 1988.

61. Klugman, K. P., and Koornof, H. J.: Drug resistance patterns and serogroups or serotypes of pneumococcal isolates from cerebrospinal fluid or blood, 1979–1986. J. Infect. Dis. 158:956, 1988.

62. Karchmer, A. W.: Staphylococcal endocarditis, laboratory and clinical basis for antibiotic therapy. Am. J. Med. 78:(Suppl 6B):116, 1985.

63. Eykyn, S. J.: Staphylococcal sepsis. The changing pattern of disease and therapy. Lancet 1:100, 1988.

64. Chambers, H. F., Korzeniowski, O. M., Sande, M. A., et al.: *Staphylococcus aureus* endocarditis: Clinical manifestations in addicts and non-addicts. Medicine 62:170, 1983.

65. Espersen, F., and Frimodt-Moller, N.: *Staphylococcus aureus* endocarditis. A review of 119 cases. Arch. Intern. Med. 146:1118, 1986.

66. Bayer, A. S., Lam, K., Ginzton, L., et al.: *Staphylococcus aureus* bacteremia clinical, serologic, and echocardiographic findings in patients with and without endocarditis. Arch. Intern. Med. 147:457, 1987.

67. Kaye, D.: The clinical significance of tolerance of *Staphylococcus aureus*. Ann. Intern. Med. 93:924, 1980.

68. Caputo, G. M., Archer, G. L., Calderwood, S. B., et al.: Native valve endocarditis due to coagulase-negative staphylococci, clinical and microbiologic features. Am. J. Med. 83:619, 1987.

69. Wall, T. C., Peyton, R. B., and Corey, G. R.: Gonococcal endocarditis: A new look at an old disease. Medicine (Baltimore) 68:375, 1989.

70. Owens, J. E., and Kelchak, J. A.: Gonococcal endocarditis: Report of a case and review of the literature. J.S.C. Med. Assoc. 86:93, 1990.

71. Lynn, D. J., Kane, J. G., and Parker, R. H.: *Haemophilus parainfluenzae* and influenzae endocarditis: A review of forty cases. Medicine (Baltimore) 56:115, 1977.

72. Ellner, J. J., Rosenthal, M. S., Lerner, P. I., et al.: Infective endocarditis caused by slow-growing, fastidious, gram-negative bacteria. Medicine (Baltimore) 58:145, 1979.

73. Schack, S. H., Smith, P. W., Penn, R. G., and Rapaport, J. M.: Endocarditis caused by *Actinobacillus actinomycetemcomitans*. J. Clin. Microbiol. 20:579, 1984.

74. Lane, T., MacGregor, R. R., Wright, D., et al.: *Cardiobacterium hominis*: An elusive cause of endocarditis. J. Infect. Dis. 6:75, 1983.

75. Decker, M. D., Graham, B. S., Hunter, E. R., et al.: Endocarditis and infections of intravascular devices due to *Eikenella corrodens*. Am. J. Med. Sci. 292:209, 1986.

76. Jenny, D. B., Letendre, P. W., and Iverson, G.: Endocarditis due to Kingella species. Rev. Infect. Dis. 10:1065, 1988.

77. Cohen, P. S., Maguire, J. H., and Weinstein, L.: Infective endocarditis caused by gram-negative bacteria: A review of the literature. Prog. Cardiovasc. Dis. 22:205, 1980.

77a. Komshian, S. V., Tablan, O. C., Palutke, W., and Reyes, M. P.: Characteristics of left-sided endocarditis due to *Pseudomonas aeruginosa* in the Detroit Medical Center. Rev. Infect. Dis. 12:693, 1990.

78. Carvajal, A., and Frederiksen, W.: Fatal endocarditis due to *Listeria monocytogenes*. Rev. Infect. Dis. 10:616, 1988.

79. Lindner, P. S., Hardy, D. J., and Murphy, T. E.: Endocarditis due to *Corynebacterium pseudodiphtheriticum*. N.Y. State J. Med. 86:102, 1986.

80. Yersin, B., Glauser, M. P., Guze, P. A., et al.: Experimental *Escherichia coli* endocarditis in rats. Roles of serum bactericidal activity and duration of catheter placement. Infect. Immunol. 56:1273, 1988.

81. Nord, C. E.: Anaerobic bacteria in septicemia and endocarditis. Scand. J. Infect. Dis. 31(Suppl):95, 1982.

82. McIntosh, C. S., Vickers, P. J., and Isaacs, A. J.: Spirillum endocarditis. Postgrad. Med. J. 51:645, 1975.

83. Popat, K., Barnardo, D., Webb-Peploe, M.: *Mycoplasma pneumoniae* endocarditis. Br. Heart J. 44:111, 1980.

84. Al-Kasab, S., Fagih, M. R., Al-Yousef, S., et al.: *Brucella* infective endocarditis: Successful combined medical and surgical therapy. J. Thorac. Cardiovasc. Surg. 95:862, 1988.

85. Shafer, R. W., and Braverman, E. R.: Q-fever endocarditis: Delay in diagnosis due to an apparent clinical response to corticosteroids. Am. J. Med. 86:729, 1989.

86. Jones, R. B., Priest, J. B., and Kuo, C. C.: Subacute chlamydial endocarditis. JAMA 247:655, 1982.

87. Rubinstein, E., Noriega, E. R., Simberkoff, M. S., et al.: Fungal endocarditis: Analysis of 24 cases and a review of the literature. Medicine 54:331, 1975.

88. Woods, G. L., Wood, R. P., and Shaw, B. W., Jr.: *Aspergillus* endocarditis in patients without prior cardiovascular surgery: Report of a case in a liver transplant recipient and review. Rev. Infect. Dis. 11:263, 1989.

88a. Johnston, P. G., Lee, J., Domanski, M., et al.: Late recurrent candida endocarditis. Chest 99:1531, 1991.

ENDOCARDITIS IN INTRAVENOUS DRUG ABUSERS

89. Scheidegger, C., and Zimmerli, W.: Infectious complications in drug addicts: Seven-year review of 269 hospitalized narcotics abusers in Switzerland. Rev. Infect. Dis. 11:486, 1989.

90. Chambers, H. F., Morris, D. L., Tauber, M. G., and Modin, G.: Cocaine use and the risk for endocarditis in intravenous drug users. Ann. Intern. Med. 106:833, 1987.

91. Julander, I.: Staphylococcal septicemia and endocarditis in 80 drug addicts. Aspects on epidemiology, clinical and laboratory findings and prognosis. Scand. J. Infect. Dis. 41(Suppl):49, 1983.

92. Levine, D. P., Crane, L. R., and Zervos, M. J.: Bacteremia in narcotic addicts at the Detroit Medical Center. II. Infectious endocarditis: A prospective comparative study. Rev. Infect. Dis. 8:374, 1986.

93. Baddour, L. M.: Twelve year review of recurrent native valve infective endocarditis: A disease of the modern antibiotic era. Rev. Infect. Dis. 10:1163, 1988.

94. Eichacker, P. Q., Miller, K., Robbins, M., et al.: Echocardiographic evaluation of heart valves in IV drug abusers without a previous history of endocarditis. Clin. Res. 32:670A, 1984.

95. Robbins, M. J., Sveiro, R., Fishman, W. H., and Strom, J. A.: Right-sided valvular endocarditis: Etiology, diagnosis, and approach to therapy. Am. Heart J. 111:128, 1986.

96. Cassling, R. S., Rogler, W. C., and McManus, B. M.: Isolated pulmonic valve infective endocarditis: A diagnostically elusive entity. Am. Heart J. 109:558, 1985.

97. Dressler, F. A., and Roberts, W. C.: Infective endocarditis in opiate addicts: Analysis of 80 cases studied at necropsy. Am. J. Cardiol. 63:1240, 1989.

98. Tuazon, C. W., and Sheagren, J. W.: Increased rate of carriage of *Staphylococcus aureus* among narcotic addicts. J. Infect. Dis. 129:725, 1974.

99. Kolander, S. A., Cosgrove, E. M., and Molavi, A.: Clostridial endocarditis. Report of a case caused by *Clostridium bifermentans* and review of the literature. Arch. Intern. Med. 149:455, 1989.

100. Rapeport, K. B., Girón, J. A., and Rosner, F.: *Streptococcus mitis* endocarditis. Report of 17 cases. Arch. Intern. Med. 146:2361, 1986.

101. Saravolatz, L. D., Burch, K. H., and Quinn, E. L.: Polymicrobial infective endocarditis: An increasing clinical entity. Am. Heart J. 95:163, 1978.

102. Burns, J.M.A., Hogg, K. J., Hillis, W. S., and Dunn, F. G.: Endocarditis in intravenous drug abusers with staphylococcal septicemia. Br. Heart J. 61:356, 1980.

103. Barg, W. L., Supena, R. B., and Fekety, R.: Persistent staphylococcal bacteremia in an intravenous drug abuser. Antimicrob. Agents Chemother. 29:209, 1986.

PROSTHETIC VALVE ENDOCARDITIS

104. Cowgill, L. D., Addonizio, V. P., Hopeman, A. R., and Harken, A. H.: Prosthetic valve endocarditis. Curr. Probl. Cardiol. 11:617, 1986.

105. Heimburger, T. S., and Duma, R. J.: Infections of prosthetic heart valves and cardiac pacemakers. Infect. Dis. Clin. North Am. 3:221, 1989.

106. Calderwood, S. B., Swinski, L. A., Waternaux, C. M., et al.: Risk factors for the development of prosthetic valve endocarditis. Circulation 72:31, 1985.

106a. Chen, S. C., Sorrell, T. C., Dwyer, D. E., et al.: Endocarditis associated with prosthetic cardiac valves. Med. J. Aust. 152:458, 1990.

107. Rutledge, R., Kim, J., and Applebaum, R. E.: Actuarial analysis of the risk of prosthetic valve endocarditis in 1,598 patients with mechanical and bioprosthetic valves. Arch. Surg. 120:469, 1985.

108. Ivert, I.S.A., Dismukes, W. E., Cobbs, G., et al.: Prosthetic valve endocarditis. Circulation 69:222, 1984.

109. Laskowski, L. F., Marr, J. J., Spernoga, J. F., et al.: Fastidious mycobacteria grown from porcine prosthetic heart valve cultures. N. Engl. J. Med. 297:101, 1977.

110. Thompkins, L. S., Roessler, B. J., Redd, S. C., et al.: *Legionella* prosthetic valve endocarditis. N. Engl. J. Med. 318:530, 1988.

111. Cohen, J. I., Sloss, L. J., Kundsin, R., and Golightly, L.: Prosthetic valve endocarditis caused by *Mycoplasma hominis*. Am. J. Med. 86:819, 1989.

112. Svirbely, J. R., Ayers, L. W., and Briesching, W. J.: Filamentous *Histoplasma capsulatum* endocarditis involving mitral and aortic valve porcine bioprostheses. Arch. Pathol. Lab. Med. 109:273, 1985.

113. Fernandez-Guerrero, M. L., Muelas, J. M., Aguado, J. M., et al.: Q-fever endocarditis on porcine bioprosthetic valves. Ann. Intern. Med. 108:209, 1988.

114. Karchmer, A. W., Archer, G. L., and Dismukes, W. E.: *Staphylococcus epidermidis* causing prosthetic valve endocarditis: Microbiologic and clinical observations as guides to therapy. Ann. Intern. Med. 98:447, 1983.

115. Rodgers, G. M., Greenberg, C. S., and Shuman, M. A.: Characterization of the effects of cultured vascular cells on the activation of blood coagulation. Blood 61:1155, 1983.

116. Richardson, M., Kinlough-Rathbone, R. L., Groves, H. M., et al.: Ultrastructural changes in re-endothelialized and non-endothelialized rabbit aorta neo-intima following reinjury with a balloon catheter. Br. J. Exp. Pathol. 65:597, 1984.

117. Ferguson, D.J.P., McColm, A. A., Savage, T. J., et al.: A morphologic study of experimental rabbit staphylococcal endocarditis and aortitis. I. Formation and effect of infected and uninfected vegetations on the aorta. Br. J. Exp. Pathol. 67:667, 1986.

118. Ferguson, D.J.P., McColm, A. A., Savage, T. J., et al.: A morphologic study of experimental rabbit staphylococcal endocarditis and aortitis. II. Inter-relationship of bacteria, vegetation and cardiovasculature in established infections. Br. J. Exp. Pathol. 67:679, 1986.

119. Rodbard, S.: Blood velocity and endocarditis. Circulation 27:18, 1963.

120. Lepeschkin, E.: On the relation between the site of valvular involvement in endocarditis and the blood pressure resting on the valve. Am. J. Med. Sci. 224:318, 1952.

121. Lopez, J. A., Ross, R. S., Fishbein, M. C., and Siegel, R. J.: Nonbacterial thrombotic endocarditis: A review. Am. Heart J. 113:773, 1987.

122. Durack, D. T., and Beeson, P. B.: Experimental bacterial endocarditis. I. Colonization of a sterile vegetation. Br. J. Exp. Pathol. 53:44, 1972.

123. Baddour, L. M., Christensen, G. D., Lowrance, J. H., and Simpson, W. A.: Pathogenesis of experimental endocarditis. Rev. Infect. Dis. 11:452, 1989.

124. Baddour, L. M. Production and progress of the disease in rabbits. Br. J. Exp. Pathol. 54:142, 1973.

125. Editorial: Vegetations, valves and echocardiography. Lancet 2:1118, 1988.

126. Durack, D. T.: Experimental bacterial endocarditis. IV. Structure and evolution of early lesions. J. Pathol. 115:81, 1975.

127. Roberts, W. C., and Buchbinder, N. A.: Healed left-sided infective endocarditis: A clinicopathologic study of 59 patients. Am. J. Cardiol. 40:876, 1977.

128. Everett, E. D., and Hirschmann, J. V.: Transient bacteremia and endocarditis prophylaxis. A review. Medicine (Baltimore) 56:61, 1977.

129. Sipes, J. N., Thompson, R. L., and Hook, E. W.: Prophylaxis of infective endocarditis: A re-evaluation. Ann. Rev. Med. 28:371, 1977.

130. Baskin, G.: Prosthetic endocarditis after endoscopic variceal sclerotherapy: A failure of antibiotic prophylaxis. Am. J. Gastroenterol. 84:311, 1989.

131. Rogosa, M., Hampp, E. G., Nevin, T. A., et al.: Blood sampling and cultural studies in the detection of post-operative bacteremia. J. Am. Dent. Assoc. 60:171, 1960.

132. Durack, D. T.: Current issues in the prevention of infective endocarditis. Am. J. Med. 78(Suppl B):149, 1985.

133. Hamill, R. J., Vann, J. M., and Proctor, R. A.: Phagocytosis of Staphylococcus aureus by cultured bovine aortic endothelial cells: Model for post-adherence events in endovascular infections. Infect. Immun. 54:833, 1986.

134. Rotrosen, D., Edwards, J. E., Jr., Gibson, T. R., et al.: Adherence of Candida to cultured vascular endothelial cells: Mechanisms of attachment and endothelial cell penetration. J. Infect. Dis. 152:1264, 1985.

135. Hamill, R. J.: Role of fibronectin in infective endocarditis. Rev. Infect. Dis. 9(Suppl 4):5360, 1987.

136. Sage, M. D., Koelmeyer, T. D., Smeeton, W.M.I., and Galler, L. L.: Evolution of Swan-Ganz catheter-related pulmonary valve nonbacterial endocarditis. Am. J. Forensic Med. Pathol. 9:112, 1988.

137. Gibbons, R. J., and Nygaard, M.: Synthesis of insoluble dextran and its significance in the formation of gelatinous deposits by plaque-forming streptococci. Arch. Oral Biol. 13:1249, 1968.

138. Scheld, W. M., Valone, J. A., and Sande, M. A.: Bacterial adherence in the pathogenesis of endocarditis. J. Clin. Invest. 61:1394, 1978.

139. Proctor, R. A., Mosher, D. F., and Olbrantz, P. J.: Fibronectin binding to Staphylococcus aureus. J. Biol. Chem. 257:14788, 1982.

140. Kuusela, P., Vartio, T., Vuento, M., and Myhre, E. B.: Attachment of staphylococci and streptococci on firbonectin, fibronectin fragments, and fibrinogen bound to a solid phase. Infect. Immun. 50:77, 1985.

141. Myhre, E. B., and Kuusela, P.: Binding of human fibronectin to groups A, C, and G streptococci. Infect. Immun. 40:29, 1983.

142. Skerl, K. G., Calderone, R. A., Segal, E., et al.: In vitro binding of Candida albicans yeast cells to human fibronectin. Can. J. Microbiol. 30:221, 1984.

143. Nealon, T. J., Beachey, E. H., Courtney, H. S., and Simpson, W. A.: Release of fibronectin-lipoteichoic acid complexes from group A streptococci with penicillin. Infect. Immun. 51:529, 1986.

144. Korzeniowski, O. M., Scheld, W. M., Bithell, T. C., et al.: Bacterial-platelet interaction in staphylococcal endocarditis (E). Abstr. 239. Presented at the 18th Interscience Conference on Antimicrobial Agents and Chemotherapy. American Society for Microbiology, October 1978.

145. Sullam, P. M., Valone, F. H., and Mills, J.: Mechanisms of platelet aggregation by viridans group streptococci. Infect. Immun. 55:1743, 1987.

146. Hendrix, H., Lindhou, T., Mertins, K., et al.: Activation of human prothrombin by stoichiometric levels of staphylocoagulase. J. Biol. Chem. 258:3637, 1983.

147. Drake, T. A., Rodgers, G. M., and Sande, M. A.: Tissue factor is a major stimulus for vegetation formation in enterococcal endocarditis in rabbits. J. Clin. Invest. 73:1750, 1984.

148. Weinstein, L.: Life-threatening complications of infective endocarditis and their management. Arch. Intern. Med. 146:953, 1986.

149. Arnett, E. N., and Roberts, W. C.: Valve ring abscess in active endocarditis: Frequency, location and clues to clinical diagnosis from the study of 95 necropsy patients. Circulation 54:140, 1976.

150. Sandler, M. A., Kotler, M. N., Bloom, R. D., and Jacobson, L.: Pericardial abscess extending from mitral vegetation: An unusual complication of infective endocarditis. Am. Heart J. 118:857, 1989.

151. DiNubile, M. J., Calderwood, S. B., Steinhaus, D. M., and Karchmer, A. W.: Cardiac conduction abnormalities complicating native valve active infective endocarditis. Am. J. Cardiol. 58:1213, 1986.

152. Bhatnagar, N. K., Dhasmana, J. P., Russell, G. A., and Jordan, S. C.: Aspergillus ball thrombus occluding a homograft conduit. Eur. J. Cardiothorac. Surg. 3:270, 1989.

153. Roberts, W. C., Ewy, G. A., Glancy, D. L., et al.: Valvular stenosis produced by active infective endocarditis. Circulation 36:449, 1967.

154. Wilson, W. R., Giulliani, E. R., Danielson, G. K., and Geraci, J. E.: Management of complications of infective endocarditis. Mayo Clin. Proc. 57:162, 1982.

155. Dowling, G. P., and Buja, M. L.: Sudden death due to left coronary artery occlusion in infective endocarditis. Arch. Pathol. Lab. Med. 112:932, 1988.

155a. Ting, W., Silverman, N. A., Arzouman, D. A., and Levitsky, S.: Splenic septic emboli in endocarditis. Circulation 82(Suppl. IV):IV–105, 1990.

156. Nakayama, D. K., O'Neill, J. A., Jr., Wagner, H., et al.: Management of vascular complications of bacterial endocarditis. J. Pediatr. Surg. 21:636, 1986.

157. Wilson, W. R., Lie, J. T., Houser, O. W., et al.: The management of patients with mycotic aneurysms. Curr. Clin. Top. Infect. Dis. 2:151, 1981.

158. Mansur, A. J., Grinberg, M., Leao, P. P., et al.: Extracranial mycotic aneurysms in infective endocarditis. Clin. Cardiol. 9:65, 1986.

159. Cosmo, L. Y., Risi, G., Nelson, S., et al.: Fatal hemoptysis in acute bacterial endocarditis. Am. Rev. Respir. Dis. 137:1223, 1988.

160. Bayer, A. S., and Theofilopoulos, A. N.: Immunopathogenetic aspects of infective endocarditis. Chest 97:204, 1990.

161. Maisch, B.: Autoreactive mechanisms in infective endocarditis. Springer Semin. Immunopathol. 11:439, 1989.

162. Bayer, A. S., Theofilopoulos, P. N., Eisenberg, R., et al.: Circulating immune complexes in infective endocarditis. N. Engl. J. Med. 295:1500, 1970.

163. McKenzie, P. E., Hawke, D., Woodroffe, A. J., et al.: Serum and tissue immune complexes in infective endocarditis. J. Clin. Lab. Immunol. 4:125, 1980.

164. Maisch, B., Mayer, E., Schubert, U., et al.: Immune reactions in infective endocarditis. II. Relevance of circulating immune complexes, serum inhibition factors, lymphocytotoxic reactions, and antibody dependent cellular cytotoxicity against cardiac target cells. Am. Heart J. 106:338, 1983.

165. Feinstein, E. I.: Renal complications of bacterial endocarditis. Am. J. Nephrol. 5:457, 1985.

166. Churchill, M. A., Geraci, J. E., and Hunder, G. G.: Musculoskeletal manifestations of bacterial endocarditis. Ann. Intern. Med. 87:754, 1977.

167. Williams, R. C.: Rheumatoid factors in subacute bacterial endocarditis and other infectious diseases. Scand. J. Rheumatol. Suppl 75:300, 1988.

168. Williams, R. C., Jr., and Kilpatrick, K.: Immunofluorescence studies of cardiac valves in infective endocarditis. Arch. Intern. Med. 145:297, 1985.

CLINICAL MANIFESTATIONS

169. Starkenbaum, M., Durack, D., and Beeson, P.: The "incubation period" of subacute bacterial endocarditis. Yale J. Biol. Med. 50:49, 1977.

170. Weinstein, L., and Schlesinger, J. J.: Pathoanatomic, pathophysiologic and clinical correlations in endocarditis. N. Engl. J. Med. 291:832, 1974.

171. Weinstein, L., and Rubin, R. H.: Infective endocarditis—1973. Prog. Cardiovasc. Dis. 16:239, 1973.

172. Yee, J., and McAllister, K.: The utility of Osler's nodes in the diagnosis of infective endocarditis. Chest 92:751, 1987.

173. Watanakunakorn, C.: Osler's nodes on the dorsum of the foot. Chest 94:1088, 1988.

174. Albeit, J. S., Krous, H. F., Dalen, J. E., et al.: Pathogenesis of Osler's nodes. Ann. Intern. Med. 85:471, 1976.

175. Kerr, A., Jr., and Tan, J. S.: Biopsies of the Janeway lesion of infective endocarditis. J. Cutan. Pathol. 6:124, 1979.

176. Silverberg, H. H.: Roth spots. Mt. Sinai J. Med. 37:77, 1970.

177. Salgado, A. V., Furlan, A. J., Keys, T. F., et al.: Neurologic complications of endocarditis: A 12 year experience. Neurology 39:173, 1989.

178. Varma, M.P.S., McCluskey, D. R., Khan, M. M., et al.: Heart failure associated with infective endocarditis. A review of 40 cases. Br. Heart J. 55:191, 1986.

179. Mills, J., Utley, J., and Abbott, J.: Heart failure in infective endocarditis: Predisposing factors, course and treatment. Chest 66:151, 1974.

180. Jones, H. R., and Siekert, R. G.: Neurological manifestations of infective endocarditis. Brain 112:1295, 1989.

181. Brottier, E., Gin, H., Brottier, L., et al.: Prosthetic valve endocarditis: Diagnosis and prognosis. Eur. Heart J. 5(Suppl C):123, 1984.

182. Armstrong, J. A., Tarr, G. C., Ho M., et al.: Cytomegalovirus infection in children undergoing open-heart surgery. Yale J. Biol. Med. 49:83, 1976.

183. Rouveix, E., Witchitz, S., Bouvet, E., et al.: Tricuspid infective endocarditis: 56 cases. Eur. Heart J. 5(Suppl C):111, 1984.

LABORATORY

184. Werner, A. S., Cobbs, C. G., Kaye, D., et al.: Studies on the bacteremia of bacterial endocarditis. JAMA 202:199, 1967.
185. Scheld, W. M.: Pathogenesis and pathophysiology of infective endocarditis. In: Sande, M. A., Kaye, D., and Root, R. K. (eds.): Endocarditis. New York, Churchill Livingstone, 1984, pp. 1–32.
186. Tuazon, C. U., Sheagren, J. N., Choa, M. S., et al.: Staphylococcus aureus bacteremia: Relationship between formation of antibodies to teichoic acid and development of metastatic abscesses. J. Infect. Dis. 137:57, 1978.
187. Ehni, W. F., and Reller, B.: Short-course therapy for catheter-associated Staphylococcus aureus bacteremia. Arch. Intern. Med. 149:533, 1989.
188. Hook, E. W.: Annotation. Yale J. Biol. Med. 38:521, 1966.
189. Pesanti, E. L., and Smith, I. M.: Infective endocarditis with negative blood cultures. An analysis of 52 cases. Am. J. Med. 66:43, 1979.
190. Van Scoy, R. E.: Culture-negative endocarditis. Mayo Clin. Proc. 57:149, 1982.
191. Pazin, G. J., Saul, S., and Thompson, M. E.: Blood culture positivity. Suppression by outpatient antibiotic therapy in patients with bacterial endocarditis. Arch. Intern. Med. 142:263, 1982.
192. Carey, R. B., Gross, K. C., and Roberts, R. B.: Vitamin-B_6-dependent Streptococcus mitior (mitis) isolated from patients with systemic infections. J. Infect. Dis. 131:722, 1975.
193. Auckenthaler, R. W.: Laboratory diagnosis of infective endocarditis. Eur. Heart J. 5(Suppl C):49, 1984.
194. Carrizosa, J., Levison, M. E., Lawrence, T., et al.: Cure of Aspergillus ustus endocarditis of prosthetic valve. Arch. Intern. Med. 133:486, 1974.
195. Pierce, M. A., Saag, M. S., Dismukes, W. E., et al.: Case report: Q fever endocarditis. Am. J. Med. Sci. 292:104, 1986.
196. Mandell, G. L.: The laboratory in diagnosis and management. In: Kaye, D. (ed.): Infective endocarditis. Baltimore, University Park Press, 1976, pp. 155–166.
197. Williams, R. C., Jr., and Kunkel, H. G.: Rheumatoid factor, complement and conglutinin aberrations in patients with subacute bacterial endocarditis. J. Clin. Invest. 41:666, 1962.
198. Mohammed, I., Ansell, B. M., Holborow, E. J., et al.: Circulating immune complexes in subacute endocarditis and poststreptococcal glomerulonephritis. J. Clin. Pathol. 30:308, 1977.
199. Powers, D. L., and Mandell, G. L.: Intraleukocytic bacteria in endocarditis patients. J.A.M.A. 227:312, 1974.
200. Buda, A. J., Zotz, R. J., Le Mire, M. S., et al.: Prognostic significance of vegetations detected by two-dimensional echocardiography in infective endocarditis. Am. Heart J. 112:1291, 1986.
201. Bayer, A. S., Blomquist, I. K., Bello, E., et al.: Tricuspid valve endocarditis due to Staphylococcus aureus. Chest 93:247, 1988.
202. Erbel, R., Rohmann, S., Drexler, M., et al.: Improved diagnostic value of echocardiography in patients with infective endocarditis by transoesophageal approach. A prospective study. Eur. Heart J. 9:43, 1988.
203. Mugge, A., Daniel, W. G., Frank, G., et al.: Echocardiography in infective endocarditis: Reassessment of prognostic implications of vegetation size determined by the transthoracic and the transesophageal approach. J. Am. Coll. Cardiol. 14:631, 1989.
204. Schwinger, M. E., Tunick, P. A., Freedberg, R. S., et al.: Vegetations on endocardial surface struck by regurgitant jets: Diagnosis by transesophageal echocardiography. Am. Heart J. 119:1212, 1990.
205. Taams, M. A., Gussenhoven, E. J., Bos, E., et al.: Enhanced morphological diagnosis in infective endocarditis by transoesophageal echocardiography. Br. Heart J. 63:109, 1990.
206. Klodas, E., Edwards, W. D., and Khandheria, B. K.: Use of echocardiography for improving detection of valvular vegetations in subacute bacterial endocarditis. J. Am. Soc. Echocardiogr. 2:386, 1989.
206a. Steckelberg, J. M., Murphy, J. G., Ballard, D., et al.: Emboli in infective endocarditis: The prognostic value of echocardiography. Ann. Intern. Med. 114:635, 1991.
206b. Tunick, P. A., Freedberg, R. S., Schrem, S. S., and Kronzon, I.: Unusual mitral annular vegetation diagnosed by transesophageal echocardiography. Am. Heart J. 120:444, 1990.
206c. Daniel, W. G., Mugge, A., Martin, R. P., et al.: Improvement in the diagnosis of abscesses associated with endocarditis by transesophageal echocardiography. N. Engl J. Med. 324:795, 1991.
207. Kinney, E. L., and Wright, R. J.: Aortic valve vegetations: Examples of overestimation and underestimation of disease by two-dimensional echocardiography. Am. Heart J. 113:1248, 1987.
208. Gross, C. M., Prisant, M., Paolini, D., et al.: Echocardiographic appearance of a flail bioprosthetic mitral valve leaflet mimicking vegetation. Am. Heart J. 117:953, 1989.
209. Tak, T., Rahimtoola, S. H., Kumar A., et al.: Value of digital image processing of two-dimensional echocardiograms in differentiating active from chronic vegetations of infective endocarditis. Circulation 78:116, 1988.
210. Jaffe, W. M., Morgan, D. E., and Pearlman, A. S.: Infective endocarditis, 1983–1988: Echocardiographic findings and factors influencing morbidity and mortality. J. Am. Coll. Cardiol. 15:1227, 1990.
211. Martin, R. P., French, J. W., and Popp, R. L.: Clinical utility of two-dimensional echocardiography in patients with bioprosthetic valves. Adv. Cardiol. 27:294, 1980.

212. Panidis, I. P., Ross, J., and Mintz, G. S.: Normal and abnormal prosthetic valve function as assessed by Doppler echocardiography. J. Am. Coll. Cardiol. 8:317, 1986.
213. Hardoff, R., Luder, A. S., and Lorber, A.: Early detection of infantile endocarditis by gallium-67 scintigraphy. Eur. J. Nucl. Med. 15:219, 1989.
214. Cerqueira, M. D., and Jacobson, A. F.: Indium-111 leukocyte scintigraphic detection of myocardial abscess formation in patients with endocarditis. J. Nucl. Med. 30:703, 1989.
215. Machac, J., Vallabhajosula, S., Goldman, M. E., et al.: Value of blood-pool subtraction in cardiac indium-111 labeled platelet imaging. J. Nucl. Med. 30:1445, 1989.

ANTIMICROBIAL THERAPY

216. Durack, D. T., and Beeson, P. B.: Experimental bacterial endocarditis. II. Survival of bacteria in endocardial vegetations. Br. J. Exp. Pathol. 53:50, 1972.
217. Cremieux, A. C., Maziere, B., and Vallois, J. M.: Evaluation of antibiotic diffusion into cardiac vegetations by quantitative autoradiography. J. Infect. Dis. 159:938, 1989.
218. Bayer, A. S., Crowell, D., and Nast, C. C.: Intravegetation antimicrobial distribution in aortic endocarditis analyzed by computer-generated model. Chest 97:611, 1990.
219. Washington, J. A.: In vitro testing of antimicrobial agents. Infect. Dis. Clin. North Am. 3:375, 1989.
220. Mulligan, M. J., and Cobbs, C. G.: Bacteriostatic versus bactericidal activity. Infect. Dis. Clin. North Am. 3:389, 1989.
221. Holloway, Y., Dankert, J., and Hess, J.: Penicillin tolerance and bacterial endocarditis. Lancet 1:589, 1980.
222. Eliopoulos, G. M.: Synergism and antagonism. Infect. Dis. Clin. North Am. 3:399, 1989.
223. Moellering, R. C.: Treatment of enterococcal endocarditis. In: Sande, M. A., Kaye, D., and Root, R. K. (eds.): Endocarditis. New York, Churchill Livingstone, 1984, pp. 113–133.
224. Wilson, W. R., and Geraci, J. E.: Treatment of streptococcal infective endocarditis. Am. J. Med. 78(Suppl 6B):128, 1985.
225. Meeson, J., McColm, A. A., and Acred, P.: Differential response to benzylpenicillin in vivo of tolerant and non-tolerant variants of Streptococcus sanguis. II. J. Antimicrob. Chemother. 25:103, 1990.
226. Levison, M. E., and Bush, L. M.: Pharmacodynamics of antimicrobial agents, bactericidal and post antibiotic effects. Infect. Dis. Clin. North Am. 3:415, 1989.
227. Weinstein, M. P., Stratton, C. W., Ackley, A., et al.: Multicenter collaborative evaluation of a standardized serum bactericidal test as a prognostic indicator in infective endocarditis. Am. J. Med. 78:262, 1985.
228. Wolfson, J. S., and Swartz, M. N.: Serum bactericidal activity as a monitor of antibiotic therapy. N. Engl. J. Med. 312:968, 1985.
229. Reller, L. B.: The serum bactericidal test. Rev. Infect. Dis. 8:803, 1986.
230. Craig, W. A., and Ebert, S. C.: Protein binding and its significance in antibacterial therapy. Infect. Dis. Clin. North Am. 3:407, 1989.
231. Poretz, D. M., Eron, L. J., Goldenberg, R. I., et al.: Intravenous antibiotic therapy in an outpatient setting. JAMA 248:336, 1982.
232. Guntheroth, W. G., Cammarano, A. A., and Kirby, W.M.M.: Home treatment of infective endocarditis with oral amoxicillin. Am. J. Cardiol. 55:1231, 1985.
233. Gayet, J. L., Etienne, J., Malquarti, V., et al.: Indices of effectiveness of medical and surgical treatment in 40 cases of prosthetic valve endocarditis. Eur. Heart J. 5:(Suppl C):133, 1984.
234. Myers, J. P., and Linnemann, C. C.: Bacteremia due to methicillin-resistant Staphylococcus aureus. J. Infect. Dis. 145:532, 1982.
235. Craven, D. E., Kollisch, N. R., Hsieh, C. R., et al.: Vancomycin treatment of bacteremia caused by oxacillin-resistant Staphylococcus aureus. J. Infect. Dis. 147:137, 1983.
236. King, K., and Harkness, J. L.: Infective endocarditis in the 1980s. Treatment and management. Med. J. Aust. 144:588, 1986.
237. Guzman, F., Gartmill, I., Holden, M. P., et al.: Candida endocarditis: Report of four cases. Int. J. Cardiol. 16:131, 1987.
238. Handrick, W., Kohler, W., Spencker, F. B., et al.: Endocarditis due to nutritionally variant streptococci. Infection 16:371, 1988.
239. DiNubile, M. J.: Treatment of endocarditis caused by relatively resistant nonenterococcal streptococci: Is penicillin enough? Rev. Infect. Dis. 12:112, 1990.
240. Wilson, W. R., Wilkowske, C. J., Wright, A. J., et al.: Treatment of streptomycin-susceptible and streptomycin-resistant enterococcal endocarditis. Ann. Intern. Med. 100:816, 1984.
241. Besnier, J. M., Leport, C., Bure, A., et al.: Vancomycin-aminoglycoside combinations in therapy of endocarditis caused by Enterococcus species and Streptococcus bovis. Eur. J. Clin. Microbiol. Infect. Dis. 9:130, 1990.
242. Green, G. R., Peters, G. A., and Geraci, J. E.: Treatment of bacterial endocarditis in patients with penicillin hypersensitivity. Ann. Intern. Med. 67:235, 1967.
243. Lipman, M. L., and Silva, J.: Endocarditis due to Streptococcus faecalis with high-level resistance to gentamicin. Rev. Infect. Dis. 11:325, 1989.
244. Eliopoulos, G. M., Eliopoulos, C. T.: Therapy of enterococcal infections. Eur. J. Clin. Microbiol. Infect. Dis. 9:118, 1990.
245. Patterson, J. E., Masecar, B. L., and Zervos, M. J.: Characterization and comparison of two penicillinase-producing strains of Streptococcus (Enterococcus) faecalis. Antimicrob. Ag. Chemother. 32:122, 1988.

246. Bush, L. M., Calmon, J., Cherney, C. L., et al.: High-level penicillin-resistance among isolates of enterococci. Ann. Intern. Med. 110:515, 1989.

247. Kaplan, A. H., Gilligan, P. H., and Facklam, R. R.: Recovery of resistant enterococci during vancomycin prophylaxis. J. Clin. Microbiol. 26:1216, 1988.

248. Leclerq, R., Derlot, E., Duval, J., et al.: Plasmid-mediated resistance to vancomycin and teicoplanin in Enterococcus faecium. N. Engl. J. Med. 319:157, 1988.

249. Sande, M. A., and Korzeniowski, O. M.: The antimicrobial therapy of infective endocarditis. New York, Grune & Stratton, 1981, pp. 113–122.

250. Watanakunakorn, C., and Baird, I. M.: Prognostic factors in Staphylococcus aureus endocarditis and results of therapy with a penicillin and gentamicin. Am. J. Med. Sci. 273:133, 1977.

251. Korzeniowski, O., and Sande, M. A.: The National Collaborative Endocarditis Study Group: Combination antimicrobial therapy for Staphylococcus aureus endocarditis in patients addicted to parenteral drugs and in nonaddicts. A prospective study. Ann. Intern. Med. 97:496, 1982.

252. Frimodt-Moller, N., Espersen, F., and Rosdahl, V. T.: Antibiotic treatment of Staphylococcus aureus endocarditis. A review of 119 cases. Acta Med. Scand. 222:175, 1987.

253. Karchmer, A. W.: Antibiotic therapy of nonenterococcal streptococcal and staphylococcal endocarditis: Current regimens and some future considerations. J. Antimicrob. Chemother. 21(Suppl C):91, 1988.

254. Faville, R. J., Zaske, D. E., Kaplan, E. L., et al.: Staphylococcus aureus endocarditis: Combined therapy with vancomycin and rifampin. JAMA 240:1963, 1978.

255. Acar, J. F., Goldstein, F. W., and Duval, J.: Use of rifampin for the treatment of serious staphylococcal and gram-negative bacillary infections. Rev. Infect. Dis. 5:S502, 1983.

256. Zak, O., Scheld, W. M., and Sande, M. A.: Rifampin in experimental endocarditis due to Staphylococcus aureus in rabbits. Rev. Infect. Dis. 5:S481, 1983.

257. Chambers, H. F., Miller, R. T., and Newman, M. D.: Right-sided Staphylococcus aureus endocarditis in intravenous drug abusers: Two-week combination therapy. Ann. Intern. Med. 109:619, 1988.

258. Chambers, H. F., and Sande, M. A.: Teicoplanin versus nafcillin and vancomycin in the treatment of experimental endocarditis caused by methicillin-susceptible or -resistant Staphylococcus aureus. Antimicrob. Ag. Chemother. 26:61, 1984.

259. Martino, P., Venditti, M., Micozzi, A., et al.: Teicoplanin in the treatment of gram-positive bacterial endocarditis. Antimicrob. Ag. Chemother. 33:1329, 1989.

260. Leport, C., Perronne, C., Massip, P., et al.: Evaluation of teicoplanin for treatment of endocarditis caused by gram-positive cocci in 20 patients. Antimicrob. Ag. Chemother. 33:871, 1989.

261. Kaatz, G. W., Barriere, S. L., Schaberg, D. R., et al.: Ciprofloxacin versus vancomycin in the therapy of experimental methicillin-resistant Staphylococcus aureus endocarditis. Antimicrob. Ag. Chemother. 31:527, 1987.

262. Rouse, M. S., Walcox, R. M., Henry, N. K., et al.: Ciprofloxacin therapy of experimental endocarditis caused by methicillin-resistant Staphylococcus epidermidis. Antimicrob. Ag. Chemother. 34:273, 1990.

263. Dworkin, R. J., Lee, B. L., Sande, M. A., et al.: Treatment of right-sided Staphylococcus aureus endocarditis in intravenous drug users with ciprofloxacin and rifampicin. Lancet 2:1071, 1989.

264. Humphreys, H., and Mulvihill, E.: Ciprofloxacin-resistant Staphylococcus aureus. Lancet 2:383, 1985.

265. Kobasa, W. D., Kaye, K. L., Shapiro, T., et al.: Therapy for experimental endocarditis due to Staphylococcus epidermidis. Rev. Infect. Dis. 5(Suppl 3):533, 1983.

266. Wilson, W. R., and Geraci, J. E.: Antibiotic treatment of infective endocarditis. Ann. Rev. Med. 34:413, 1983.

267. Levison, M. E.: Therapy of endocarditis due to gram-negative bacteria and fungi. In: Sande, M. A., Kaye, D., and Root, R. K. (eds.): Endocarditis. New York, Churchill Livingstone, 1984, pp. 151–161.

268. Geraci, J. E., and Wilson, W. R.: Endocarditis due to gram-negative bacteria. Report of 56 cases. Mayo Clin. Proc. 52:145, 1982.

269. Neu, H. C.: The quinolones. Infect. Dis. Clin. North Am. 3:625, 1989.

270. Donowitz, G. R., and Mandell, G. L.: Beta-lactam antibiotics. N. Engl. J. Med. 318:419, 1988.

271. Donowitz, G. R.: Third generation cephalosporins. Infect. Dis. Clin. North Am. 3:595, 1989.

272. Sobel, J. D.: Imipenem and aztreonam. Infect. Dis. Clin. North Am. 3:613, 1989.

273. Lipman, B., and Neu, H. C.: Imipenem: A new carbapenem antibiotic. Update on antibiotics. II. Med. Clin. North Am. 72:567, 1988.

274. Diekson, G., Rodriguez, K., and Arcey, S.: Efficacy of imipenem/cilastatin in endocarditis. Am. J. Med. 78:109, 1985.

275. Neu, H. C.: Aztreonam: The first monobactam. Med. Clin. North Am. 72:555, 1988.

276. Bush, L. M., Calmon, J., and Johnson, C. C.: Newer penicillins and beta-lactamase inhibitors. Infect. Dis. Clin. North Am. 3:571, 1989.

277. Reyes, M. P., and Lerner, A. M.: Current problems in the treatment of infective endocarditis due to Pseudomonas aeruginosa. Rev. Infect. Dis. 5:314, 1983.

278. Maderazo, E. G., Hickingbotham, N., and Cooper, B.: Aspergillus endocarditis: Cure without surgical valve replacement. South. Med. J. 83:351, 1990.

279. Haldane, E. V., Marrie, T. J., Faulkner, R. S., et al.: Endocarditis due to Q fever in Nova Scotia: Experience with five patients in 1981–1982. J. Infect. Dis. 148:978, 1983.

280. Street, A. C., and Durack, D. T.: Experience with trimethoprim-sulfamethoxazole in treatment of infective endocarditis. Rev. Infect. Dis. 10:915, 1988.

281. Brearley, B. F., and Hutchinson, D. N.: Endocarditis associated with Chlamydia trachomatis infection. Br. Heart J. 46:220, 1981.

282. Daikos, G. L., Kathpalia, S. B., Lolans, V. T., et al.: Long-term oral ciprofloxacin: Experience in the treatment of incurable infective endocarditis. Am. J. Med. 84:786, 1988.

SURGICAL MANAGEMENT

283. Abdelnoor, M., Nitter-Hauge, S., and Trettli, S.: Relative survival of patients after heart valve replacement. Eur. Heart J. 11:23, 1990.

284. Teoh, K. H., Ivanov, J., Weisel, R. D., et al.: Determinants of survival and valve failure after mitral valve replacement. Ann. Thorac. Surg. 49:643, 1990.

285. Jones, E. L., Weintraub, W. S., Craver, J. M., et al.: Ten-year experience with the porcine bioprosthetic valve: Interrelationship of valve survival and patient survival in 1,050 valve replacements. Ann. Thorac. Surg. 49:370, 1990.

286. Alsip, S. G., Blackstone, E. H., Kirklin, J. W., et al.: Indications for cardiac surgery in patients with active infective endocarditis. Am. J. Med. 78(Suppl 6B):138, 1985.

287. Karp, R. B.: Role of surgery in infective endocarditis. Cardiovasc. Clin. 17(3):141, 1987.

288. Cowgill, L. D., Addonizio, P. Hopeman, A. R., et al.: A practical approach to prosthetic valve endocarditis. Ann. Thorac. Surg. 43:450, 1987.

289. Griffin, F. M., Jr., Jones, G., and Cobbs, C. G.: Aortic insufficiency in bacterial endocarditis. Ann. Intern. Med. 76:23, 1972.

290. Sweeney, M. S., Ott, D. A., and Livesay, J. J.: Comparison of bioprosthetic and mechanical valve replacement for active endocarditis. J. Thorac. Cardiovasc. Surg. 90:676, 1985.

291. Mullany, C. J., McIsaacs, A. I., and Rowe, R. H.: The surgical treatment of infective endocarditis. World J. Surg. 13:132, 1989.

292. Aslamaci, S., Dimitri, W. R., and Williams, B. T.: Operative considerations in active native valve infective endocarditis. J. Cardiovasc. Surg. 30:328, 1989.

293. Tuna, I. C., Orszulak, T. A., Schaff, H. V., et al.: Results of homograft aortic valve replacement for active endocarditis. Ann. Thorac. Surg. 49:619, 1990.

293a. Dreyfus, G., Serraf, A., Jebara, V. A., et al.: Valve repair in acute endocarditis. Ann. Thorac. Surg. 49:706, 1990.

294. Cobbs, C. G., and Gnann, J. W.: Indications for surgery. In: Sande, M. A., Kaye, D., and Root, R. K. (eds.): Endocarditis. New York, Churchill Livingstone, 1984, pp. 201–212.

295. Richardson, J. V., Karp, R. B., Kirklin, J. W., et al.: Treatment of infective endocarditis: A 10-year comparative analysis. Circulation 58:589, 1978.

296. Fleisher, A. G., David, I., Mogtader, A., et al.: Mitral valvuloplasty and repair for infective endocarditis. J. Thorac. Cardiovasc. Surg. 93:311, 1987.

297. Evora, P.R.B., Brasil, J.C.F., and Elias, L. C.: Surgical excision of the vegetation: Treatment of tricuspid valve endocarditis. Cardiology 75:287, 1988.

298. Yee, E. S., and Ullyot, D. J.: Reparative approach for right-sided endocarditis. J. Thorac. Cardiovasc. Surg. 96:133, 1988.

299. Yee, E. S., and Khonsari, S.: Right-sided infective endocarditis: Valvuloplasty, valvectomy or replacement. J. Cardiovasc. Surg. 30:744, 1989.

300. Barbour, D. J., and Roberts, W. C.: Valve excision only versus valve excision plus replacement for active infective endocarditis involving the tricuspid valve. Am. J. Cardiol. 57:475, 1986.

301. DiSesa, V. J., Sloss, L. J., and Cohn, L. H.: Heart transplantation for intractable prosthetic valve endocarditis. J. Heart Transplant 9:142, 1990.

302. Wilson, W. R., Geraci, J. E., Danielson, G. K., et al.: Anticoagulant therapy and central nervous system complications in patients with prosthetic valve endocarditis. Circulation 57:1004, 1978.

RESPONSE TO THERAPY

303. Levison, M. E.: Response to therapy. In: Kaye, D. (ed.): Infective Endocarditis. Baltimore, University Park Press, 1976, pp. 185–199.

304. Douglas, A., Moore-Gillon, J. M., and Eykyn, S.: Fever during treatment of infective endocarditis. Lancet 1:1342, 1986.

305. Zabalgoitia-Reyes, M., Mehlman, D. J., and Talano, J. V.: Persistent fever with aortic valve endocarditis. Arch. Intern. Med. 145:327, 1985.

306. Brust, J.C.M., Dickinson, P.C.T., and Hughes, J.E.O.: The diagnosis and treatment of cerebral mycotic aneurysms. Ann. Neurol. 27:238, 1990.

307. Neugarten, J., and Baldwin, D. S.: Glomerulonephritis in bacterial endocarditis. Am. J. Med. 77:297, 1984.

308. Rovzar, M. A., Logan, J. L., Ogden, D. A., et al.: Immunosuppressive therapy and plasmapheresis in rapidly progressive glomerulonephritis associated with bacterial endocarditis. Am. J. Kidney Dis. 7:428, 1986.

309. McKinsey, D. S., McMurray, T. I., and Flynn, J. M.: Immune complex glomerulonephritis associated with Staphylococcus aureus bacteremia: Response to corticosteroid therapy. Rev. Infect. Dis 12:125, 1990.

310. Cates, J. E., and Christie, R. V.: Subacute bacterial endocarditis. Q. J. Med. 20:93, 1951.

311. Wilson, W. R., Giuliani, E. R., Danielson, G. K., et al.: Symposium on

infective endocarditis. II. General considerations in the diagnosis and treatment of infective endocarditis. Mayo Clin. Proc. 57:81, 1982.

312. Noseda, A., Liesnard, C., Goffin, Y., et al.: Q fever endocarditis: Relapse five years after successful valve replacement for a first unrecognized episode. J. Cardiovasc. Surg. 29:360, 1988.

313. Levison, M. E., Kaye, D., Mandell, G. L., and Hook, E.: Characteristics of patients with multiple episodes of bacterial endocarditis. JAMA 211:1355, 1970.

314. Malquarti, V., Saradarian, W., Etienne, J., et al.: Prognosis of native valve infective endocarditis: A review of 253 cases. Eur. Heart J. 5(Suppl C):11, 1984.

315. Julander, I.: Unfavorable prognostic factors in Staphylococcus aureus septicemia and endocarditis. Scand. J. Infect. Dis. 17:179, 1985.

316. Leport, C., Vilde, J. L., and Bricaire, F.: Fifty cases of late prosthetic valve endocarditis: Improvement in prognosis over a 15 year period. Br. Heart J. 58:66, 1987.

317. Dismukes, W. E.: Prosthetic valve endocarditis. Factors influencing outcome and recommendations for therapy. In: Bisno, A. L. (ed.) Treatment of Infective Endocarditis. New York, Grune & Stratton, 1981, pp. 167–191.

318. Wilson, W. R., Danielson, G. K., Giuliani, E. R., et al.: Prosthetic valve endocarditis. Mayo Clin. Proc. 57:155, 1982.

319. Calderwood, S. B., Swinski, L. A., Karchmer, A. W., et al.: Prosthetic valve endocarditis: Analysis of factors affecting outcome of therapy. J. Thorac. Cardiovasc. Surg. 92:776, 1986.

320. Cortina, J. M., Martinell, J., and Artiz, V.: Surgical treatment of active prosthetic valve endocarditis. J. Thorac. Cardiovasc. Surg. 35:209, 1987.

PREVENTION

321. Bayliss, R., Clarke, C., Oakley, C., et al.: The teeth and infective endocarditis. Br. Heart J. 50:506, 1983.

322. Kaye, D.: Prophylaxis against bacterial endocarditis: A dilemma. In: Kaplan, E. L., and Taranta, A. V. (eds.): Infective Endocarditis. Dallas, American Heart Association (AHA Monograph No. 52):67, 1977.

323. Pelletier, L. J., Jr., and Petersdorf, R. G.: Infective endocarditis: A review of 125 cases from the University of Washington hospitals, 1963–1972. Medicine (Baltimore) 56:282, 1977.

324. Lowes, J. A., Hamer, J., Williams, G., et al.: 10 years of infective endocarditis at St. Bartholomew's Hospital: Analysis of clinical features and treatment in relation to prognosis and mortality. Lancet 1:133, 1980.

325. Moulsdale, M. T., Eykyn, S. J., and Phillips, I.: Infective endocarditis, 1970–1979: A study of culture-positive cases in St. Thomas's Hospital. Q. J. Med. 49:315, 1980.

326. Guntheroth, W. G.: How important are dental procedures as a cause of infective endocarditis? Am. J. Cardiol. 54:797, 1984.

327. Meyer, G. W.: Endocarditis prophylaxis and gastrointestinal procedures. Am. J. Gastroenterol. 84(12):1492, 1989.

328. Fleischer, D: Recommendations for antibiotic prophylaxis before endoscopy. Am. J. Gastroenterol. 84(12):1489, 1989.

329. Kaye, D.: Prophylaxis of endocarditis. In Kaye, D. (ed.): Infective Endocarditis. Baltimore, University Park Press, 1976, pp. 245–265.

330. Lowy, F., and Steigbigel, N. H.: Infective endocarditis. Am. Heart J. 96:689, 1978.

331. Goodman, J. S., Schaffner, W., Collins, H. A., et al.: Infection after cardiovascular surgery: Clinical study including examination of antimicrobial prophylaxis. N. Engl. J. Med. 287:117, 1968.

332. Pallasch, T. J.: A critical appraisal of antibiotic prophylaxis. Int. Dent. J. 39:183, 1989.

333. Fekete, T.: Controversies in the prevention of infective endocarditis related to dental procedures. Dent. Clin. North Am. 34(1):79, 1990.

334. Lockhart, P. B., Crist, D., and Stone, P. H.: The reliability of the medical history in the identification of patients at risk for infective endocarditis. J. Am. Dent. Assoc. 119:417, 1989.

335. Sadowsky, D., and Kunzel, C.: Recommendations for prevention of bacterial endocarditis: Compliance by dental general practitioners. Circulation 77:1316, 1988.

336. Bender, I. B., Naidorf, I. J., and Garvey, G. J.: Bacterial endocarditis: A consideration for physician and dentist. J. Am. Dent. Assoc. 10:415, 1984.

337. Durack, D. T., Bisno, A. L., and Kaplan, E. L.: Apparent failure of endocarditis prophylaxis. Analysis of 52 cases submitted to a national registry. JAMA 250:2318, 1983.

338. Glauser, M. P., Bernard, J. P., Mareillon, P., and Francioli, P.: Successful single-dose amoxicillin prophylaxis against experimental streptococcal endocarditis: Evidence for two mechanisms of protection. J. Infect. Dis. 147:568, 1983.

339. Francioli, P., Mareillon, P., and Glauser, M. P.: Comparison of single-doses of amoxicillin or of amoxicillin-gentamicin for the prevention of endocarditis caused by Streptococcus faecalis and by viridans streptococci. J. Infect. Dis. 152:83, 1985.

340. Dajani, A. S., Bisno, A. L., Chung, K. J., et al.: Prevention of bacterial endocarditis. JAMA 264:2919, 1990.

341. Devereux, R. B., Hawkins, J., Kramer-Fox, R., et al.: Complications of mitral valve prolapse: Disproportionate occurrence in men and older patients. Am. J. Med. 81:751, 1986.

342. Hickey, A. J., MacMahon, S. W., and Wilcken, D.E.L.: Mitral valve prolapse and bacterial endocarditis: When is antibiotic prophylaxis necessary? Am. Heart J. 109(3 pt 1):431, 1985.

343. Bor, D. H., and Himmelstein, D. U.: Endocarditis prophylaxis for patients with mitral valve prolapse: A quantitative analysis. Am. J. Med. 76:711, 1984.

344. Clemens, J. D., and Ransohoff, D. F.: A quantitative assessment of predental antibiotic prophylaxis for patients with mitral valve prolapse. J. Chronic Dis. 37:531, 1984.

345. Kaye, D.: Prophylaxis for infective endocarditis: An update. Ann. Intern. Med. 104:419, 1986.

The Pathogenesis of Atherosclerosis
by RUSSELL ROSS, Ph.D., D.D.S.

Atherosclerosis, the principal cause of death in Western civilization,[1] is a progressive disease process that generally begins in childhood and has clinical manifestations in middle to late adulthood. Two decades ago, atherosclerosis was considered to be a degenerative process because of the accumulation of lipid and necrotic debris in the advanced lesions. We now recognize that it is a multifactorial process which, if it leads to clinical sequelae, requires extensive proliferation of smooth muscle cells within the intima of the affected artery. The form and content of the advanced lesions of atherosclerosis demonstrate the results of three fundamental biological processes. These are: (1) proliferation of intimal smooth muscle cells, together with variable numbers of accumulated macrophages and T-lymphocytes; (2) formation by the proliferated smooth muscle cells of large amounts of connective tissue matrix, including collagen, elastic fibers, and proteoglycans; and (3) accumulation of lipid, principally in the form of cholesteryl esters and free cholesterol within the cells as well as in the surrounding connective tissues.[2-5] Despite the fact that the term "atherosclerosis" is derived from the Greek "athero" (gruel or porridge) and "sclerosis" (hardening), it is important to note that there may be great variability in the relative amounts of tissue formed by each of these processes in the lesions. Consequently, many lesions of atherosclerosis are dense and fibrous, whereas others may contain large amounts of lipid and necrotic debris, with most demonstrating combinations and variations of each of these characteristics.

RISK FACTORS
(see also Chap. 37)

The development of the concept of "risk factors" and their relationships to the incidence of coronary artery disease evolved from prospective epidemiological studies in the United States and Europe.[6-9] These studies demonstrated a consistent association among characteristics observed at one point in time in apparently healthy individuals with the subsequent incidence of coronary artery disease in these individuals. These associations include an increase in the concentration of plasma cholesterol, the incidence of cigarette smoking, hypertension, clinical diabetes, obesity, age, or male sex, and the occurrence of coronary artery disease.[10-12] As a result of these associations, each characteristic has been termed a risk factor for coronary artery disease, and this terminology has been generally accepted and has become part of the scientific literature associated with this problem.

It is important to remember, however, that the presence of a risk factor does not necessarily imply a direct causal relationship. In most instances, a risk factor is the trait that predicts the risk of development of clinically significant disease within a population. In some cases, it may be involved in the causation of the disease; however, to achieve the latter requires a proved epidemiological association that is statistically valid. The risk factor concept has been extremely useful because it permits one to assess the importance not only of the aforementioned risk factors but also of genetic traits in given individuals, such as a family history of premature coronary artery disease. Using such information, it has become possible to determine whether modification of a given risk factor will result in modification of the risk of a particular disease.

Thus, a risk factor may be defined broadly as "any habit or trait that can be used to predict an individual's probability of developing that disease."[1] A risk factor so defined may be a causative agent but is not necessarily one. A more limited and specific definition is that a risk factor is a causative agent or condition that can be used to predict an individual's probability of developing disease. Used in this fashion, there are at least three independent predictors of risk for individuals within a population of the incidence of atherosclerosis. These are: plasma cholesterol concentration,[13-17] cigarette smoking,[18,19] and elevated blood pressure.[19-21]

THE NORMAL ARTERY

The normal artery (Fig. 36–1) consists of an intima lined by endothelium on the inner (luminal) aspect of the vessel and bounded by the internal elastic lamina on its outer aspect. The media is bounded by the internal elastic lamina and, in well-developed muscular and elastic arteries, by an external elastic lamina. The adventitia is bounded by the external elastic lamina and the exterior of the vessel itself.

THE INTIMA

At birth, the intima consists of a relatively thin layer of connective tissue which contains occasional solitary smooth muscle cells. Most of the connective tissue at birth consists of basement membrane. With increasing age, the amount of connective tissue increases, principally as a result of thickening of the basement membrane and formation of collagen fibrils and new elastic fibers. With increasing age, there appears to be a concentric increase in the numbers of intimal smooth muscle cells.

The intima is the site at which the lesions of atherosclerosis form. The lesions of atherosclerosis appear to be able to form

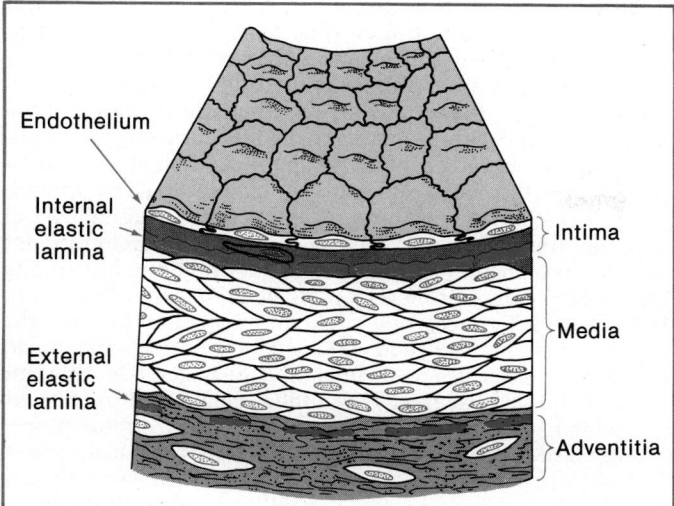

FIGURE 36–1. Structure of a normal muscular artery. (Reprinted by permission from Ross, R., and Glomset, J.: The pathogenesis of atherosclerosis. N. Engl. J. Med. 295:369, 1976.)

in two ways in different individuals. In those who develop clinical sequelae, the lesions form by a generally asymmetrical thickening of the intima which continually encroaches upon the lumen, resulting in a decrease in the flow of blood. The second form of intimal thickening is one in which the increase in the intima may be associated with continued dilation of the artery so that the actual lumen changes little, if at all, in diameter. In the latter case, although lesions of atherosclerosis may form, they are generally more symmetrical and concentric; few if any clinical sequelae appear to result.

THE MEDIA

The media is the muscular wall of the artery, bounded by the internal and external elastic laminae (Fig. 36–1). These laminae consist of fenestrated sheets of elastic fibers with numerous openings large enough to permit both substances and cells to pass in either direction. The media of muscular arteries consists of spiraling layers of smooth muscle cells attached to one another, each cell surrounded by a discontinuous basement membrane and by interspersed collagen fibrils and proteoglycan. Elastic arteries contain multiple lamellae of smooth muscle cells, each equivalent to a single media in a small muscular artery, or arteriole. Each lamella is bounded by an elastic lamina on its inner and outer aspects. The number of lamellar units present in elastic arteries has been shown to be highly predictable in relation to the size of the animal and to other factors, such as the anatomical position of the artery. Twenty-nine lamellar units have been suggested to represent the thickest amount of artery wall capable of transporting oxygenated metabolites from the lumen of the aorta to the outermost lamella. When more than 29 lamellar units are present, vasa vasorum that are derived from the adventitia appear to be necessary. These can provide nutrients to the remaining outer lamellar units.[22,23]

THE ADVENTITIA

The adventitia consists of a dense collagenous structure containing numerous bundles of collagen fibrils, elastic fibers, and many fibroblasts, together with some smooth muscle cells (Fig. 36–1). It is a highly vascular tissue and contains many nerve fibers as well. As indicated earlier, the adventitia provides the outermost portion of the media of large elastic arteries with much of their nutrition via vasa vasorum, as well as with lymphatic channels and innervation. Wolinsky and Glagov[23] have observed that the abdominal aorta in humans lacks vasa vasorum in its outermost aspects and have sug-

gested that this may be one of the reasons the abdominal aorta is particularly vulnerable to atherogenesis.

CELLS OF THE ARTERY AND FROM THE BLOOD POTENTIALLY INVOLVED IN ATHEROGENESIS

ENDOTHELIUM

The endothelial cells probably represent the largest and most extensive tissue in the body, since they line the entire vascular tree. In the arterial system, the endothelial cells form a continuous smooth, uninterrupted surface and represent the principal barrier between the elements of the blood and the artery wall (Fig. 36–2). In adulthood, the turnover of endothelial cells in those arteries that have been studied is relatively low; however, Schwartz and Benditt[24,25] have observed that there are "hot spots" where turnover of endothelium is high in the aorta, even in adults. These hot spots do not appear to be necessarily located at particular anatomical sites. The endothelium forms a highly selective permeability barrier,[26–28] is usually thought to be a nonthrombogenic surface,[29] is a highly active metabolic tissue,[30] and is capable of forming several vasoactive substances[29,31,32] and connective tissue macromolecules.[33] Endothelial cells examined in culture also have procoagulant properties[34]; however, it is probable that these procoagulant properties are manifested at times of "injury" to the endothelium and are probably not present in situ in the normal artery.

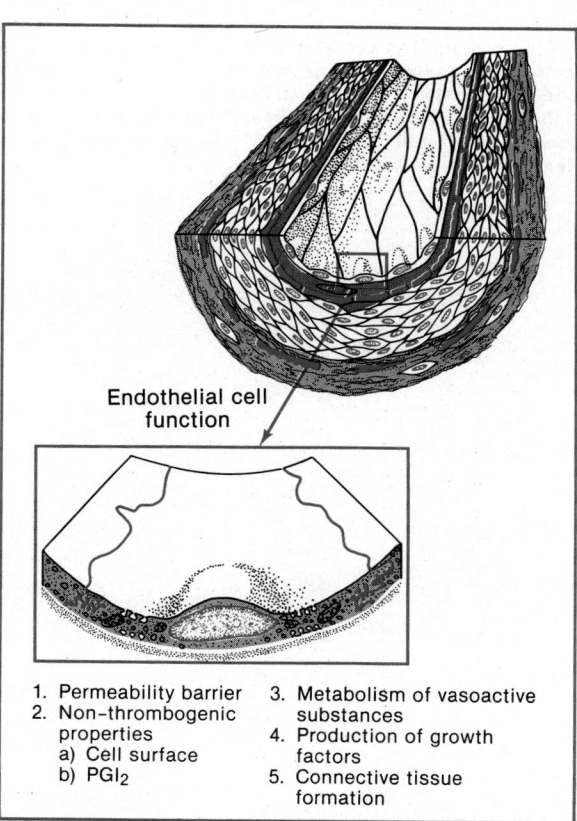

FIGURE 36–2. The endothelial barrier present in the normal artery wall. In the higher magnification insert, the borders between the endothelial cells are irregular, allowing the cells to interdigitate. Vesicles and infoldings at either cell surface permit the cells to transport materials from the lumen of the artery to the tissue by pinocytosis. Transport also occurs below the cell junctions, demonstrated by vesicles that fuse in these regions. In the artery, the cell rests on a connective-tissue matrix that consists of a basement membrane intermixed with collagen fibrils. (Reprinted by permission from Ross, R., and Glomset, J.: The pathogenesis of atherosclerosis. N. Engl. J. Med. 295:371, 1976.)

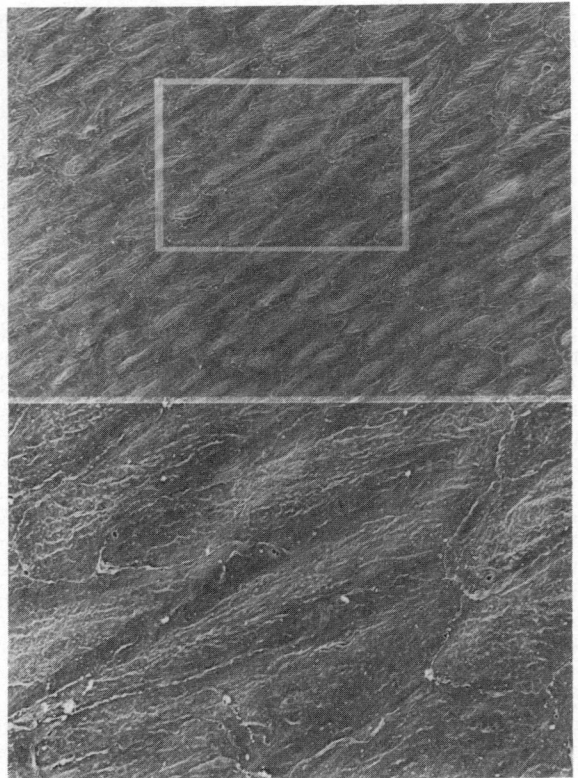

FIGURE 36–3. Scanning electron micrographs of the thoracic aorta endothelium from normal monkey *(Macaca nemestrina)*. ×540. At somewhat higher magnification, the overlapping folds of the endothelial cells can be clearly visualized. The elongated and elliptical appearance of the endothelium can also be seen. The long axes of the cells appear to be diagonal and are oriented in the main direction of the flow of blood in the artery. ×2100. (From Ross, R.: Atherosclerosis: A problem of the biology of arterial wall cells and their interactions with blood components. Arteriosclerosis *1*:297, 1981, by permission of the American Heart Association.)

Although the endothelial cells, as seen en face by light and scanning electron microscopy (Fig. 36–3) and in cross section by light and transmission electron microscopy (Fig. 36–4), appear to be highly similar morphologically in different parts of the arterial tree, there may be functional differences in these lining cells in different anatomical sites. For example, capillary endothelial cells contain receptors on their surfaces for a potent growth-regulatory peptide, platelet-derived growth factor (PDGF), whereas these receptors are absent on arterial endothelium.[35] Other differences are likely to be found, not only between capillary and arterial endothelium, but among endothelial cells in different parts of the arterial tree itself. With these differences, one might anticipate that there might be differences in the way in which endothelial cells respond to injury after exposure to various injurious agents in different parts of the arterial tree. Endothelial cells are normally attached to each other by tight junctions and by gap junctions. They transport substances in both directions via the process of endocytosis, sometimes called *transcytosis*. Transendothelial channels have been observed in capillary endothelium; however, it is not clear whether they play a role in macromolecular transport in arterial tissue. It has also been suggested that the junctions between endothelial cells may serve as potential sites of increased endothelial transport, particularly when the endothelium has been injured.

Endothelial cells rest on a basement membrane that consists of a particular form of collagen (type IV collagen) intermixed with particular types of proteoglycan molecules. The endothelial cells are undoubtedly responsible for the synthesis of these connective tissue molecules.[33] The basement membrane probably also serves as a crude form of filter.

Endothelial cells have receptors for many different molecules on their surface, including receptors for low-density lipoprotein (LDL),[36] for growth factors, and probably for a number of pharmacological agents. A special capacity of endothelium that may be particularly important in atherogenesis is its ability to modify lipoproteins. LDLs appear to be "modified" by a process of low-level oxidation when they are bound to LDL receptors, internalized, and transported through the

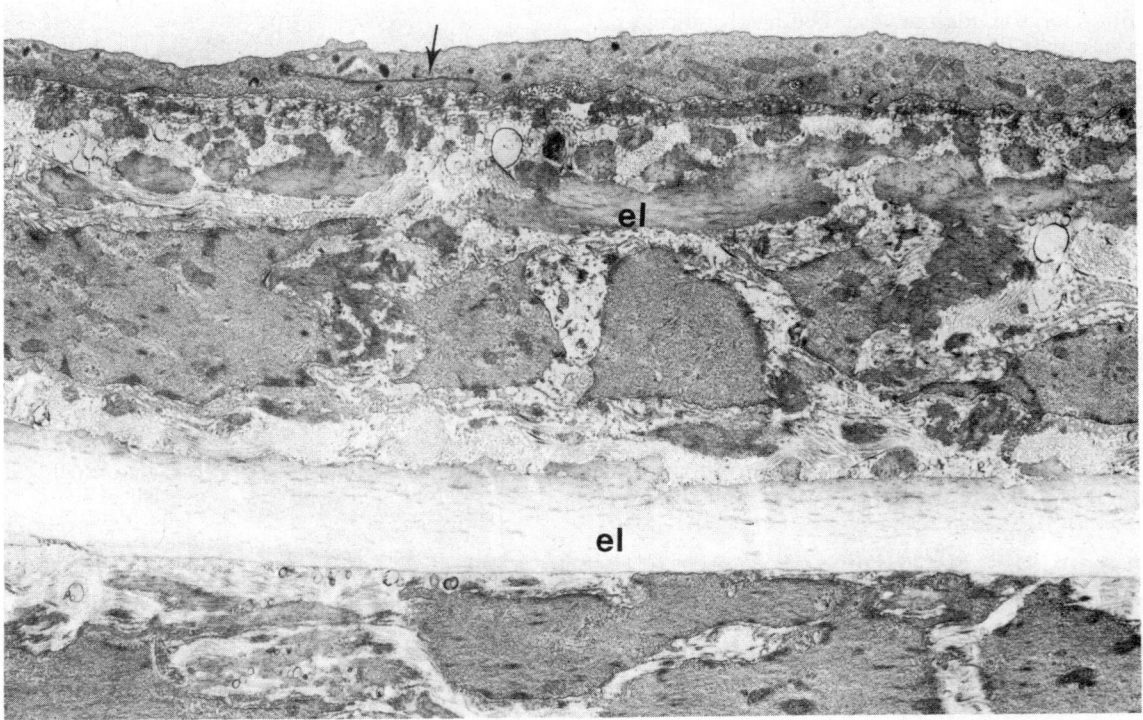

FIGURE 36–4. Transmission electron micrograph of a developing monkey aorta. Two endothelial cells can be seen at the lumen with a junction between them (arrow). Beneath the endothelial cells are newly forming elastic fibers (el) that are separated from the endothelium by basement membrane and collagen fibrils. Beneath the newly forming elastic fibers is a layer of smooth muscle cells separated from another layer by a well-formed elastica (el). No nuclei are apparent in the endothelial cells in this particular thin section.

endothelium. Such modified LDLs can bind to a specific type of receptor, termed a scavenger receptor, on the surface of macrophages, where they are ingested and contribute to the formation of foam cells. This activity is probably important in atherogenesis (see below). The endothelium normally provides a nonthrombogenic surface because of its capacity to form prostaglandin derivatives, particularly prostacyclin (PGI$_2$) (Chap. 59), a potent vasodilator that is an effective inhibitor of platelet aggregation,[29,32] and because of its surface coat of heparan sulfate. Endothelial cells also make the most potent vasodilator thus far discovered, endothelial-derived relaxing factor (EDRF), a thiolated form of nitric oxide. EDRF formation by endothelium may be critical in maintaining a balance between vasoconstriction and vasodilation in the process of arterial homeostasis.[37] Endothelial cells can also secrete agents that are effective in lysing fibrin clots, including plasminogen, as well as procoagulant materials such as von Willebrand factor.[34] They also secrete a number of vasoactive agents, such as endothelin,[38] angiotensin-converting enzyme, and platelet-derived growth factor, which may be important in vasoconstriction.

A particular characteristic of the endothelium that may be of great importance is the fact that endothelial cells grow in an obligate monolayer. Such growth is representative of cells that line most body surfaces, including epithelial surfaces, and is characterized by the fact that the endothelial cells cannot crawl over one another at sites of injury to facilitate repair of a surface that has been deendothelialized. In other words, only the cells at the margin of an injury can participate in the regenerative response. Thus if a particular anatomical site is repeatedly injured over a prolonged period, and if the endothelial cells that regenerate lose their replication capacity, cells distal to the site, capable of replicating, may not be able to participate simply because they cannot reach the site to do so.

Arterial endothelial cells are capable of synthesizing and secreting at least two mitogens, one of which is a form of PDGF.[39-41] PDGF is a growth factor for mesenchymally derived, connective tissue-forming cells such as fibroblasts and smooth muscle, but not for arterial endothelial cells. The capacity of endothelium, when it has been appropriately "activated," to form such growth factors may be important in atherogenesis. This will be discussed further in the section concerning the response-to-injury hypothesis of atherosclerosis (see p. 1113).

Thus, the endothelium forms an obligate monolayer that lines the entire arterial tree, is metabolically active, produces vasoactive substances, has a nonthrombogenic surface, and can form procoagulant materials. It also serves as the permeability barrier that controls the passage of molecules into the artery. All of these activities demonstrate the dynamic nature of the endothelial lining and how potentially important this cell layer is in the maintenance of arterial homeostasis.

SMOOTH MUSCLE

The cell that proliferates in the arterial intima to form the intermediate and advanced lesions of atherosclerosis, the smooth muscle cell, is originally derived from the media. In his early work, Wissler[42] described this cell as a "multifunctional medial mesenchymal cell." It is now widely accepted that proliferation of smooth muscle cells in the intima represents the sine qua non of the lesions of advanced atherosclerosis (Fig. 36-5).

Twenty years ago, the only functional capacity attributed to the smooth muscle cell was its ability to contract. In 1971, it became possible to maintain and propagate pure populations of smooth muscle cells in culture and to demonstrate that this cell, like the fibroblast, is one of the principal connective tissue-forming cells in the body.[43] It is capable of synthesizing and secreting several forms of collagen, both elastic fiber proteins and several different types of proteoglycans.[44] The prin-

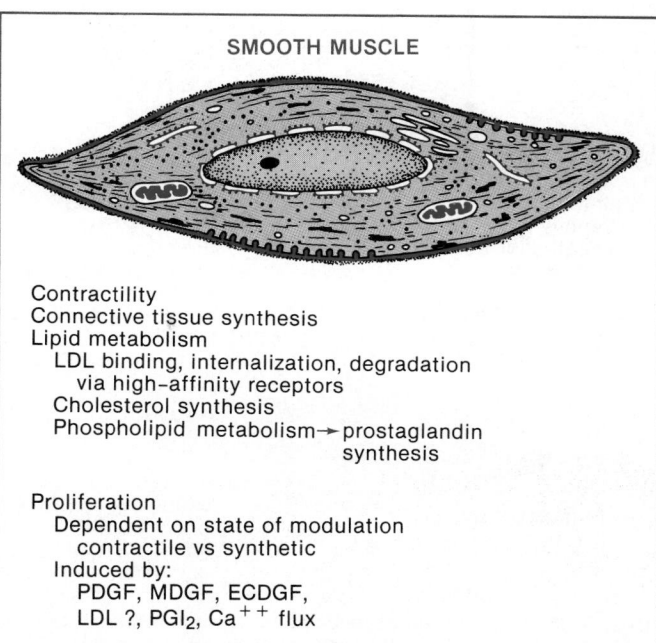

SMOOTH MUSCLE

Contractility
Connective tissue synthesis
Lipid metabolism
 LDL binding, internalization, degradation
  via high–affinity receptors
 Cholesterol synthesis
 Phospholipid metabolism → prostaglandin
  synthesis

Proliferation
 Dependent on state of modulation
  contractile vs synthetic
 Induced by:
  PDGF, MDGF, ECDGF,
  LDL ?, PGI$_2$, Ca^{++} flux

FIGURE 36-5. A smooth muscle cell showing many of the phenotypic characteristics of normal smooth muscle, as well as factors that can induce smooth muscle proliferation. (From Ross, R.: Atherosclerosis: A problem of the biology of arterial wall cells and their interactions with blood components. Arteriosclerosis 1:304, 1981, by permission of the American Heart Association.)

cipal role of the smooth muscle cell in the fully formed adult artery is presumably to maintain the tone of the arterial wall by its capacity to maintain the slow contractions peculiar to smooth muscle. The smooth muscle cell responds to numerous vasoactive agents, such as epinephrine and angiotensin, which induce contraction and vasoconstriction, and prostacyclin and EDRF, which can induce relaxation and vasodilation. Smooth muscle cells, like fibroblasts, contain specific high-affinity receptors for a number of ligands. These ligands include LDL[45] (see p. 1127) (which is the principal cholesterol-carrying plasma lipoprotein that participates in regulation of cholesterol metabolism), insulin (which is involved in glucose metabolism), and growth stimulators such as PDGF[46] and growth inhibitors such as transforming growth factor beta (TGF β) (which help to regulate cell multiplication). Arterial smooth muscle cells of the newborn rat, in contrast to adult rat smooth muscle, have been shown to be capable of synthesizing and secreting PDGF.[47] These observations suggest possible roles for smooth muscle in growth and development and possibly in atherosclerosis as well (to be discussed below).

Smooth muscle cells appear to be capable of presenting two different phenotypes in culture.[48,49] The first of these, the contractile phenotype, is generally thought to be associated with cell contractility because the cells contain extensive myofibrils throughout their cytoplasm consisting of actin and myosin filaments. These contractile filaments bind to one another and to the subplasmalemmal surface of the cell by dense bodies. Such cells do not appear to be capable of responding to mitogens such as PDGF. When a smooth muscle cell becomes appropriately stimulated, it loses its contractile phenotype and changes to a cell that has decreased content of myofilaments and that contains an extensively developed rough endoplasmic reticulum and Golgi complex. Such a cell has been described as being in a synthetic phenotype. Smooth muscle cells in the synthetic phenotype appear to be involved in the formation of numerous secretory proteins, including connective tissue matrix macromolecules. These two different smooth muscle phenotypes have been described in cell culture as well as in the artery wall.

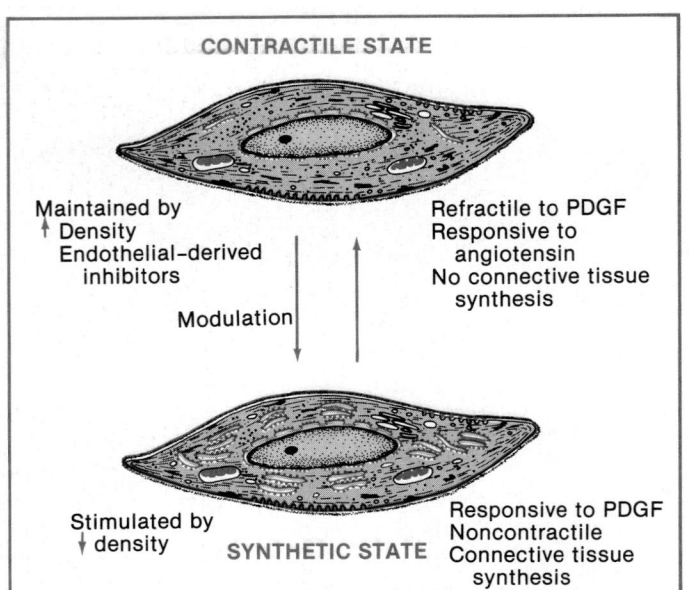

FIGURE 36-6. The state of modulation of smooth muscle cells in which the contractile versus the synthetic state is maintained by different sets of factors. (From Ross, R.: Atherosclerosis: A problem of the biology of arterial wall cells and their interactions with blood components. Arteriosclerosis 1:305, 1981, by permission of the American Heart Association.)

It has been suggested that the phenotypic differentiation of the smooth muscle cell may be important in terms of its capacity to respond to mitogens such as PDGF, and thus to form the proliferative lesions of atherosclerosis. Smooth muscle cells in the contractile phenotype have been described as nonresponsive to mitogens, whereas those in the synthetic phenotype have been described as responsive.[48,49] For the lesions of atherosclerosis to form, the smooth muscle cells must, in most cases, migrate from the media into the intima, where they can respond mitogenically. Consequently, control of the phenotypic state of smooth muscle cells could be important in understanding and preventing atherogenesis (Fig. 36-6).

One characteristic feature of the smooth muscle cells found in the lesions of atherosclerosis is the accumulation of lipid that results in formation of vacuolated cells, or foam cells. Most of the lipids that are deposited in these cells are in the form of cholesteryl esters that result from increase in cholesterol synthesis and esterification, and also a decrease in degradation of cholesteryl esters in the lysosomes of the cell.

Although smooth muscle cells were originally conceived of as only the receiver of signals such as those derived from mitogens, it has now been demonstrated that they not only can respond to mitogens such as PDGF but that they can synthesize and secrete substances such as PDGF and other growth-regulatory molecules so that they may stimulate themselves and their neighbors. Thus, smooth muscle cells may respond in autocrine fashion to molecules they themselves form. For example, it is well known that a marked intimal smooth muscle proliferative lesion can be induced by passing an intraarterial balloon embolectomy catheter through an artery. The pressure exerted by the balloon is sufficient to strip off the lining endothelium, expand the artery, and damage many of the smooth muscle cells in the wall of the artery. The exposed subendothelial connective tissue attracts platelets to adhere and degranulate, and many of the injured subendothelial smooth muscle cells undergo a change and migrate from the media into the intima, where they proliferate and form a myointimal hyperplastic fibrotic lesion. If the smooth muscle cells are cultured from such a lesion and are compared with those cultured from a contralateral uninjured artery, the cells from the proliferative lesion secrete a form of PDGF (see section on Growth Factors), and thus may participate in further enlargement of the lesion by autocrine stimula-

tion. Similarly, when smooth muscle cells derived from lesions of atherosclerosis are grown in culture, they secrete PDGF into the culture medium. Interestingly, there are data to suggest that smooth muscle cells derived from human occlusive fibrous plaques of the superficial femoral arteries have a limited capacity to divide in culture. When placed in culture, these cells respond less well to mitogens and act like senescent cells that have already undergone numerous cell doublings.[50] Although the cells may secrete mitogens in culture, it remains to be determined whether they are capable of secreting mitogens and responding to them in vivo.

Some data relevant to these observations have come from studies in nonhuman primates where Northern analyses of advanced lesions of atherosclerosis, using cDNA probes for different growth-regulatory peptides, have demonstrated increased messenger RNA for PDGF-B chain, and for both receptors of PDGF. Recent studies (see below), however, show that the principal source of the PDGF-B chain in these lesions is the macrophage. The smooth muscle cells appear to be the principal recipient of the growth regulatory peptides. Thus the regulation of smooth muscle cells via cellular interaction in the lesions of atherosclerosis needs to be further explored.

MACROPHAGES

Macrophages in all tissues, whether they are resident macrophages or cells that have entered the tissue during an inflammatory response, are derived at some point in their life span from circulating monocytes.[51] When the monocyte enters a tissue, it appears to take on characteristics peculiar to the host tissue. In most inflammatory sites, the macrophage acts as a scavenger cell to remove foreign substances by phagocytosis and intracellular hydrolysis and as a second line of defense after the neutrophil against microbial organisms.[52]

Macrophages are capable of secreting a large number of biologically important substances, including chemotactic agents such as leukotriene B4[53] and interleukin 1,[54] and oxygen metabolites such as superoxide anion,[55] which can be toxic to other cells. Macrophages have recently been shown to be capable of synthesizing and secreting at least six different growth factors.[56] These include (1) PDGF,[57] a growth factor for mesenchymal cells such as smooth muscle and fibroblasts; (2) interleukin 1, a cytokine that induces PDGF gene expression in fibroblasts[54,58]; (3) fibroblast growth factor (FGF),[59] a mitogen for endothelial cells and thus a potentially important angiogenic agent; (4) epidermal growth factor (EGF) and EGF-like molecules [e.g., transforming growth factor alpha (TGF α)], both of which bind to the same receptor and are capable of stimulating the growth of epithelial cells; (5) TGF β, a substance that participates in a synergistic way with some of the aforementioned growth factors in aiding the proliferation of many cells in different tissues and in many instances in inhibiting cell growth; and (6) M-CSF, a growth factor for monocyte macrophages[60] (Fig. 36-7).

As a result of its scavenging capacity and its ability to form and secrete growth factors, the macrophage is probably the key cell responsible for the promotion of connective tissue proliferation so commonly associated with chronic inflammatory responses. Macrophages, like smooth muscle, are a major source of foam cells in the lesions of atherosclerosis. In fact, they are the principal cells in the fatty streak, the initial lesion of atherosclerosis. They accumulate large amounts of lipid in the form of droplets that contain large amounts of cholesteryl ester. The role of the macrophage in atherogenesis will be discussed below.

PLATELETS

(see also Chap. 58)

Although they are probably uninvolved in the generation of many lesions, platelets are clearly implicated in the genesis of some of the lesions of atherosclerosis. (This will be discussed in greater detail below.) However, platelets are also important because they are regularly involved in one of the principal sequelae of atherosclerosis, thrombosis. It is usually a mural or occlusive thrombus or both that leads to infarction.

Platelets are amazing cells in that, although they are capable of little to no protein synthesis, they contain, sequestered in their granules, numerous prepacked extraordinarily potent molecules[61,62] (Fig. 36–8). Among these are a number of factors that participate in the coagulation cascade and, in addition, at least four extremely potent growth factors or mitogens. These are the same growth factors that can be formed by the activated macrophage, namely, PDGF,[63] FGF, EGF[64] or TGF α, and TGF β.[65] It appears that each of these growth factors is present in a class of granules, the alpha granules, which were originally thought to represent a single class on the basis of cell fractionation studies. They may, however, represent several different granules that are similar in morphological and flotation characteristics. Thus, when they are separated by cell fractionation and density gradient centrifugation, they appear to sequester into a single population.

When the platelet is exposed to substrates that induce platelet adherence, aggregation, and degranulation, each of these growth factors is potentially released and thus is capable of eliciting a proliferative response by essentially all of the resident cells in a particular tissue. In other words, platelets contain growth factors potentially stimulatory for each of the cell types present in any tissue in which platelet aggregation and release may occur. Thus, at sites of injury in which collagen exposure, thrombin and fibrin formation, or adenosine diphosphate release occur, platelet aggregation and thrombosis can occur, leading to release of the numerous vasoactive, stimulatory, and proliferative agents carried by the platelets. Each of these agents may play an important role in stimulating an early vasoconstrictive and proliferative response.[66] This

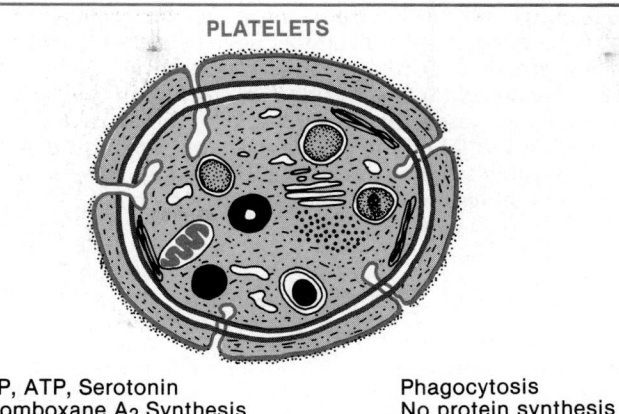

PLATELETS

ADP, ATP, Serotonin
Thromboxane A₂ Synthesis
β thromboglobulin
Platelet factor IV
Platelet–derived growth factor
Ca⁺⁺

Phagocytosis
No protein synthesis
Fibrinogen
Glycosidases
Proteinases
Cationic proteins

FIGURE 36–8. A platelet demonstrating the principal constituents of the platelet, which are listed beneath the figure. (From Ross, R.: Atherosclerosis: A problem of the biology of arterial wall cells and their interactions with blood components. Arteriosclerosis *1*:301, 1981, by permission of the American Heart Association.)

early reparative response to injury may be important in the initiation of the lesions of atherosclerosis as well.

T-LYMPHOCYTES

T-lymphocytes, both CD-8+ and CD-4+, have been observed in all phases of atherogenesis in humans and in nonhuman primates.[67–70] Their involvement in the lesions of atherosclerosis supports the notion that these lesions may develop, at least in part, as a result of an immune or possibly autoimmune response. Experimentally induced autoimmunity has been shown to induce rampant proliferative lesions of atherosclerosis in rabbits.[71] In humans, rejected cardiac transplants characteristically have extensive occlusive lesions of atherosclerosis in the coronary arteries. However, in contrast to the lesions observed in common atherosclerosis, the majority of which are eccentric lesions, those observed in the rejected hearts are concentric in appearance. The nature of the antigen(s) that may play a role in common atherosclerosis is unknown. However, interactions between T-lymphocytes and activated macrophages, both of which are prominent in the lesions, suggest that antigen presentation and the release of cytokines and growth factors between the activated macrophages and T cells may be important in this process.[72,73]

THE LESIONS OF ATHEROSCLEROSIS

Although atherosclerosis has been known for many centuries, its clinical effects are manifested principally in medium-sized muscular arteries, including the coronary, carotid, basilar, and vertebral arteries, as well as several arteries affecting the lower extremities, particularly the iliac and superficial femoral arteries. Larger arteries, such as the aorta and the iliac arteries, can also be involved, and the principal clinical sequelae in these large arteries is usually aneurysmal dilatation and its related effects.[74]

The earliest lesions of atherosclerosis can usually be found in young children and infants in the form of a lesion called the *fatty streak*, whereas the advanced lesion, the fibrous plaque, generally appears during early adulthood and progresses with age.[75–78] Until recently, most tissues that had been prepared for examination were derived from autopsy specimens and were sufficiently poorly preserved so that when the cells became laden with lipid and appeared as foam cells, it was vir-

MONOCYTE/MACROPHAGE

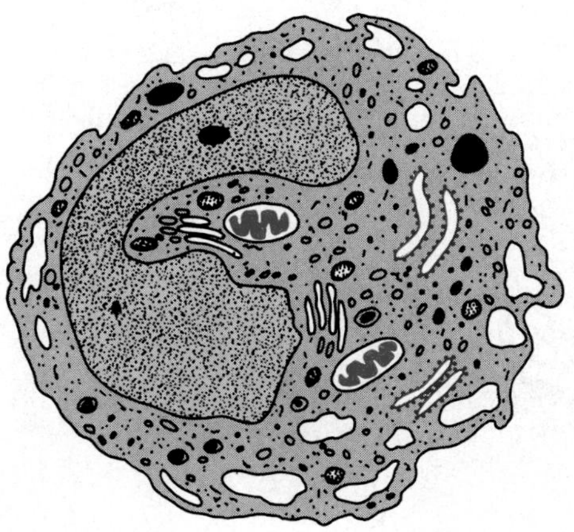

Neutral proteases
Acid hydrolases
Complement
Enzyme inhibitors
Reactive metabolites of O₂
Bioactive lipids
Chemotactic factors
Growth factors
Factors inhibitory to replication of lymphocytes,
    viruses, and tumor cells
Modified LDL receptors

FIGURE 36–7. A monocyte/macrophage cell containing a large number of substances, many of which are not present in the circulating monocyte but are formed after the monocyte leaves the blood and enters a specific tissue. A few of the components that can be found in macrophages are listed beneath the diagram. (From Ross, R.: Atherosclerosis: A problem of the biology of arterial wall cells and their interactions with blood components. Arteriosclerosis *1*:302, 1981, by permission of the American Heart Association.)

tually impossible to determine the origin of the cell. Advances in tissue fixation and embedding have permitted new modes of preservation. Furthermore, monoclonal antibodies have been developed that are specific for smooth muscle cells, for macrophages, and for lymphocytes. With the use of these antibodies and with improved preservation techniques, it has been possible to identify specifically the origin of the cells in the different lesions of atherosclerosis.

THE FATTY STREAK

Fatty streaks were observed by Stary[78] in his studies of a series of children and young adults. He demonstrated that by the age of 10 years, the fatty streaks consisted principally of lipid-laden macrophages, together with varying (but usually small) numbers of lipid-filled smooth muscle cells that accumulated beneath them as the lesions increased in size. Grossly, the fatty streak appears as an area of yellow discoloration due to the large amount of lipid deposited in the foam cells. The bulk of this lipid is in the form of cholesterol and cholesteryl ester, which probably enters the fatty streak by transport of lipoproteins from the plasma via the endothelial cells, after which it is taken up by macrophages and smooth muscle cells. The plasma lipids present in the intima are ingested by macrophages and are hydrolyzed and re-esterified once they have been taken up by these cells.

Stary also studied fatty streaks in the coronary arteries of a series of children and young adults and observed that they were localized at anatomical sites that were the same as the sites in other older individuals that were occupied by advanced fibromuscular lesions, or fibrous plaques. His data and that of others suggested that over a time, fatty streaks at particular sites are converted by a series of changes into the more advanced fibroproliferative lesions of atherosclerosis, whereas fatty streaks at other anatomical sites either remain the same or regress and disappear. McGill[79] has gone on to review data to demonstrate that with time, fatty streaks occupy increasing surface areas of the coronary arteries and that these sites also precede the formation of advanced lesions. Thus, although it is difficult to derive firm conclusions from these types of data, such observations suggest that the fatty streak in many instances, if not the large majority, is the precursor lesion that becomes converted into the advanced occlusive form of atherosclerosis.

Once foam cells have formed in fatty streaks and in advanced lesions, it may become extremely difficult to define the cell of origin. The cells become filled with lipid droplets that appear as empty vacuoles in paraffin-embedded tissues which are often surrounded by a very thin rim of cytoplasm (Fig. 36-9). Electron microscopic examination may permit identification of some of these cells; however, large numbers remain difficult if not impossible to identify using standard techniques of tissue staining.

Several monoclonal antibodies have been developed, at least two of which appear to be specific for cell type. Tsukada et al.[80] have developed monoclonal antibodies against smooth muscle–alpha actin and against a cytoplasmic antigen present in macrophages. Fortunately, these antigens resist some modes of fixation and embedding in paraffin. With these monoclonal antibodies, it has been possible to positively identify macrophages, T-lymphocytes, and smooth muscle cells in lesions of atherosclerosis. Thus it can be said definitively that the fatty streak consists principally of lipid-laden macrophages and T-lymphocytes, together with small and variable numbers of smooth muscle cells (Fig. 36-9).

DIFFUSE INTIMAL THICKENING

One form of lesion, described as a diffuse intimal thickening, consists of increased numbers of intimal smooth muscle cells surrounded by variable amounts of connective tissue. It is not entirely clear whether these sites of thickened intima represent developmental thickenings or whether such multi-layered cushions of intimal smooth muscle cells are sites that formed because of increased stress on the artery wall, but which do not progress to advanced lesions of atherosclerosis. This is a somewhat poorly understood and controversial subject.

THE FIBROUS PLAQUE

The advanced lesion of atherosclerosis is generally called a fibrous plaque. When the fibrous plaque becomes involved with thrombosis, hemorrhage, and/or calcification, it is often called a *complicated lesion*.

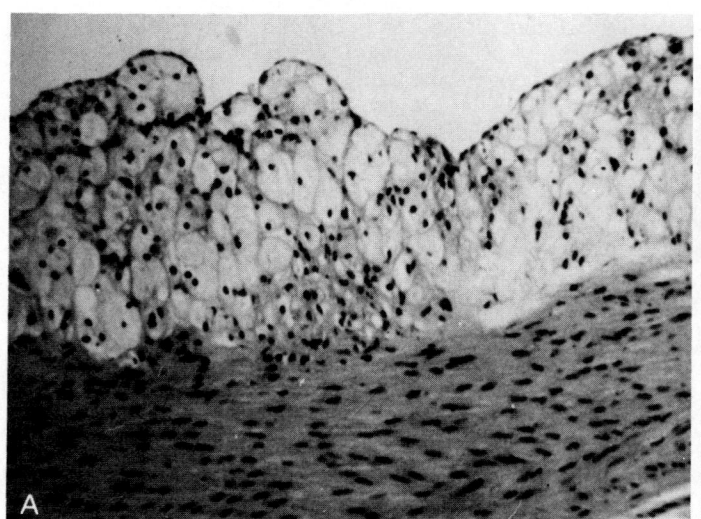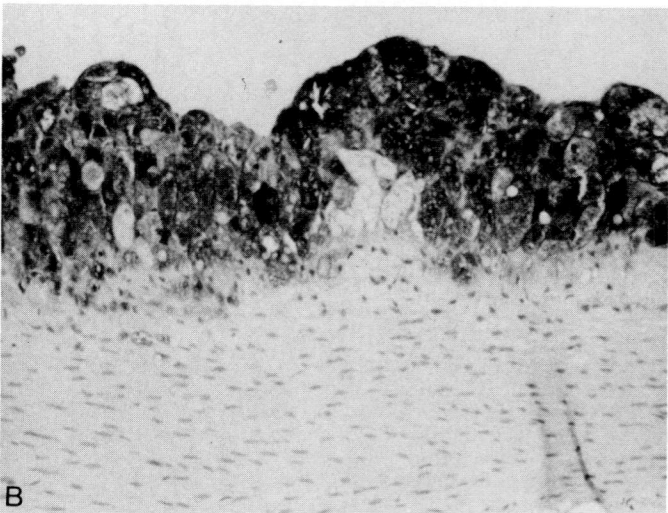

FIGURE 36-9. Light micrographs demonstrating portions of a fatty streak obtained from an aorta of a hypercholesterolemic monkey. This particular fatty streak contains several layers of macrophages. *A* is a routinely fixed and embedded paraffin section that has been stained with hematoxylin and eosin. The macrophage-rich areas are seen as clear, since they are lipid-containing and the lipid has been extracted during the process of dehydration and embedding. *B* demonstrates an adjacent section that has been stained with immunoperoxidase coupled to an antibody specific for a cytoplasmic antigen present within the macrophage. The macrophages stain densely black in this micrograph, demonstrating that the large majority of the lipid-rich cells in the fatty streak are macrophages. Such antibodies make it possible to recognize cell type, even after the cells have become distorted by inclusions.

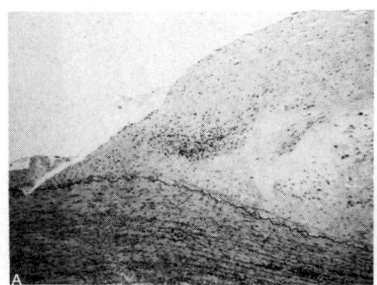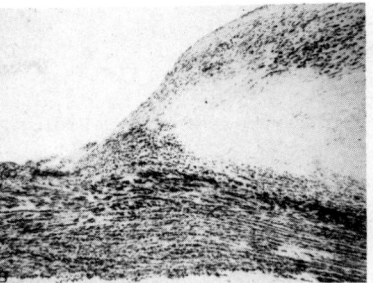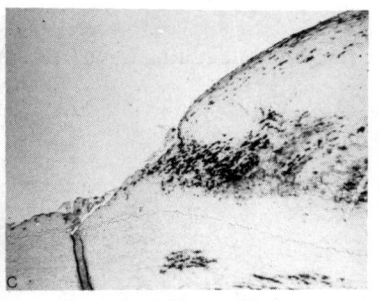

FIGURE 36-10. Three light micrographs demonstrating adjacent sections of a human fibrous plaque from a carotid endarterectomy specimen. *A* was stained with hematoxylin and eosin. In the elevated portion of the lesion, the area adjacent to the lumen consists of a fibrous cap of parallel layers of smooth muscle cells covering a mixture of cells. With H & E it is impossible to determine cell type. *B* is an adjacent section that has been stained using immunoperoxidase coupled to an anti–smooth muscle actin antibody. The smooth muscle cells in the fibrous cap, in the media underlying the lesion, and in patches and individual cells located throughout the lesion are stained black. *C* is an adjacent section stained with immunoperoxidase coupled to an anti-macrophage antibody. Individual macrophages can be seen dispersed among the smooth muscle cells in the fibrous cap, but are found principally in the area deep to the fibrous cap between the fibrous cap and the media, where most of the lipid-containing cells in this particular lesion can be found.

Fibrous plaques are grossly white in appearance and are usually elevated. In many cases they protrude into the lumen of the artery and, if sufficiently large, compromise the flow of blood. These lesions consist of large numbers of intimal smooth muscle cells, together with numerous macrophages and T-lymphocytes. When the macrophages and smooth muscle contain lipid, the lipid is primarily in the form of cholesterol and cholesteryl ester. The proliferated smooth muscle cells are surrounded by collagen and elastic fibers, by large amounts of proteoglycan, and, in individuals who are hypercholesterolemic, by varying amounts of lipid deposited in the cells and in the connective tissue. Fibrous plaques characteristically are covered by a fibrous cap.

In a study of a large series of male patients who had advanced occlusive lesions of the superficial femoral artery, we observed that the fibrous cap of each lesion consisted largely of a particular form of smooth muscle cell that is thin and pancake shaped and that is surrounded by numerous lamellae of basement membrane, proteoglycan, and large numbers of collagen fibrils. The connective tissue in the fibrous cap is exceedingly dense. Beneath the fibrous cap lies a mixture of smooth muscle cells, macrophages, and numerous lymphocytes, principally CD-8+ and some CD-4+ T cells. Using the monoclonal antibodies already described, as well as antibodies to lymphocytes, it has been possible to identify definitively each of these cell types in the advanced lesions of atherosclerosis. In this highly cellular portion of the fibrous plaque, there are also large amounts of connective tissue. Beneath the cell-rich region, there is often a zone of necrotic tissue and debris which may contain cholesterol crystals and regions of calcification as well as numerous enlarged foam cells (Fig. 36–10).

Some fibrous plaques are densely fibrous and contain relatively little lipid, whereas others are rich in lipid deposits. Such differences can be found in different arteries within a given individual but are often associated with different risk factors. For example, it is common that the fibrous plaques observed in the superficial femoral arteries of those who are heavy cigarette smokers are extremely fibrous and contain relatively little lipid. On the other hand, individuals who are hypercholesterolemic and have advanced lesions in the coronary arteries often have large amounts of lipid within the lesions.[50]

There appears to be a general pattern in the distribution of advanced lesions of atherosclerosis in humans. Generally, the abdominal aorta is more extensively involved than the thoracic aorta.[22] Lesions in the aorta are usually most prominent near the ostia of major branches that leave the aorta. Some arteries such as the renal arteries appear to be spared from atherosclerosis, except at their ostia.[81] The coronary arteries generally demonstrate the most intense involvement, with lesions of atherosclerosis located within the first 6 cm of the artery.[82] In hypertensive patients, lesions of the carotid, cerebral, and basilar arteries are more common. It has been suggested that the severity of lesion formation in a given artery may be related in part to the particular nature of the characteristics of the blood flow in the artery, and that rheological forces play a major role in determining the localization, extent, and severity of lesions in susceptible individuals.[83,84]

The principal clinical results of advanced lesions of atherosclerosis are derived either from the fact that they partially or totally occlude the lumen of the affected artery or because cracks and fissures develop in the lesions, leading to thrombosis and embolism or to aneurysmal dilatation (which usually occurs in large arteries such as the aorta).

HYPOTHESES OF ATHEROGENESIS

Current theories of the pathogenesis of the lesions of atherosclerosis relate back to early proposals made by Virchow,[85] Rokitansky,[86] and Duguid.[87] Virchow believed that a form of low-grade injury to the artery wall resulted in a type of inflammatory insudation, which in turn caused increased passage and accumulation of plasma constituents in the intima of the artery.[85] Rokitansky's belief, subsequently elaborated upon by Duguid, was that an encrustation of small mural thrombi existed at sites of arterial injury, that these thrombi went on to organize by the growth of smooth muscle cells into them, and they would become incorporated into the lesions and thus serve as sites where the lesions would progress.[86,87]

In 1973, these two notions about atherogenesis were combined with new knowledge of the cellular and molecular biology of the artery wall in a hypothesis termed the *response-to-injury hypothesis of atherosclerosis*.[2] This hypothesis has been modified as new data have come forth. It now takes into account many aspects of the behavior of arterial and blood cells described above, as well as the numerous risk factors that have been associated with atherogenesis, including hyperlipidemia, hormone dysfunction, altered rheological forces as may occur in hypertension, and alteration of the endothelial barrier by factors associated with cigarette smoking, diabetes, and so on.[3,6,88]

A second hypothesis that was also formulated in 1973, the *monoclonal hypothesis*, suggests that the lesions of atherosclerosis may represent some form of neoplasia.[14] Both of these are discussed below.

THE RESPONSE-TO-INJURY HYPOTHESIS

The response-to-injury hypothesis of atherosclerosis states that some form of "injury" may occur to the lining endothelial

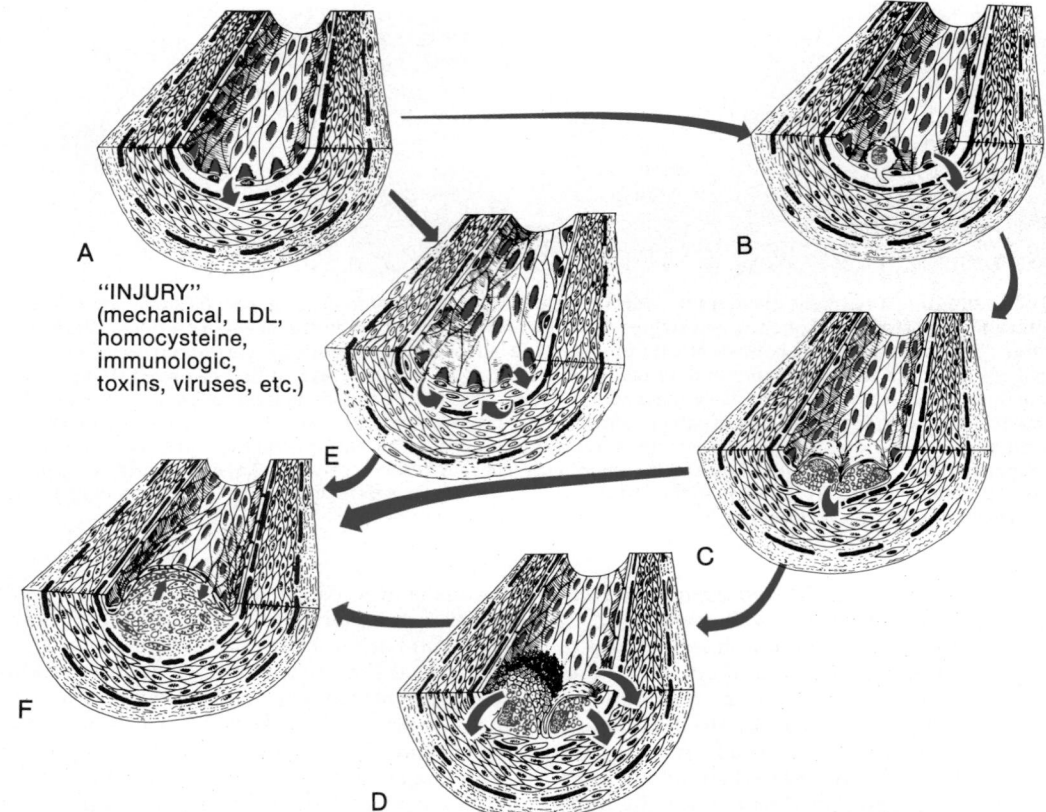

"INJURY"
(mechanical, LDL,
homocysteine,
immunologic,
toxins, viruses, etc.)

FIGURE 36–11. The response-to-injury hypothesis. Advanced intimal proliferative lesions of atherosclerosis may develop by at least two pathways. The pathway demonstrated by the clockwise (long) arrows to the right has been observed in experimentally induced hypercholesterolemia. Injury to the endothelium (A) may induce growth factor secretion (short arrow). Monocytes attach to endothelium (B), which may continue to secrete growth factors (short arrow). Subendothelial migration of monocytes (C) may lead to fatty streak formation and release of growth factors such as PDGF (short arrow). Fatty streaks may become directly converted to fibrous plaques (long arrow from C to F) through release of growth factors from macrophages or endothelial cells or both. Macrophages may also stimulate or injure the overlying endothelium. In some cases, macrophages may lose their endothelial cover, and platelet attachment may occur (D), providing three possible sources of growth factors—platelets, macrophages, and endothelium (short arrows). An alternative pathway for development of advanced lesions of atherosclerosis is shown by the arrows from A to E to F. In this case, the endothelium may be injured but remain intact. Increased endothelial turnover may result in growth factor formation by endothelial cells (A). This may stimulate migration of smooth muscle cells from the media into the intima, accompanied by endogenous production of PDGF by smooth muscle as well as growth factor secretion from the "injured" endothelial cells (E). These interactions could then lead to fibrous plaque formation and further lesion progression (F). (Reprinted by permission from Ross, R.: The pathogenesis of atherosclerosis—an update. N. Engl. J. Med. *314*:496, 1986.)

cells at particular anatomical sites in the artery wall. Injury to the endothelium is a key event in this hypothesis, and defining and understanding the subtleties of the nature of the various possible forms of injury is paramount in both testing the hypothesis and developing means of prevention and intervention.

Endothelial injury may be manifested as a number of forms of endothelial dysfunction. For example, interference with the permeability barrier role of the endothelium, alterations in the nonthrombogenic properties of the endothelial surface, promotion of the procoagulant properties of the endothelium, or increased release of vasoconstrictor or vasodilator molecules would all represent forms of dysfunction and injury that could result in some of the changes to be discussed below. Furthermore, maintenance of the continuity of the endothelial surface and maintenance of the normal low rates of turnover of the endothelial cells at most sites in the arterial tree are important in maintaining homeostasis. When turnover of the endothelium increases, it is possible that such turnover may be related to a series of changes in the endothelium, including the synthesis and secretion of vasoactive substances, of lipolytic enzymes, and of growth factors by the endothelial cells. Thus, endothelial injury could potentially lead to a host of changes in the functional activities of the lining endothelial cells which could then lead to a critical sequence of cellular

interactions, culminating in formation of lesions of atherosclerosis (Fig. 36–11).

In the case of chronic hyperlipidemia, the response-to-injury hypothesis proposes that an increase in plasma lipoproteins, principally oxidized LDL's and cholesterol, would result in toxic injury to the endothelium. It would also change the surface characteristics of both the endothelial cells and the circulating leukocytes, particularly circulating monocytes and possibly platelets as well. Hypercholesterolemia also somehow leads to increased adhesion of monocytes to endothelium at sites throughout the arterial tree.[89] When these monocytes adhere, they probe and are chemotactically attracted to migrate between endothelial cells and localize subendothelially, where they can become active as scavenger cells and are converted to macrophages. When they become macrophages, these cells take up lipid, principally modified, or oxidized LDL via receptors called scavenger receptors.[90] The lipid may enter the subendothelium in large quantities in the hypercholesterolemic state, resulting in the formation of foam cells and in the development of fatty streaks. The oxidized LDL may be toxic to the endothelium and to other cells in the microenvironment. The accumulation of macrophages in the intimal space would then establish conditions that could lead to further alterations in the endothelium. Macrophages are well known to be capable of synthesizing and secreting numerous injurious agents that normally could play a role in killing ingested microorganisms or in nullifying toxic substances.[52] In this instance, the macrophages could potentially secrete oxidative metabolites such as oxidized LDL and superoxide anion, which could further injure the overlying endothelial cells. It has been demonstrated that lipid-laden macrophages are capable of oxidizing LDL and of forming peroxide and superoxide anion in vitro,[55] suggesting that this may occur in vivo as well.

An additional and potentially important reaction of the macrophage is related to its capacity to form growth regulatory molecules. Activated macrophages can, as already noted, synthesize and secrete at least four potent growth factors: PDGF, FGF, an EGF-like factor, and TGF β. PDGF is a potent mitogen for smooth muscle cells, as is FGF under some circumstances. The combination of these growth factors, together with TGF β, has been shown in vivo to be extremely potent in stimulating the migration and proliferation of fibroblasts and potentially of smooth muscle cells, and in stimulating formation of new connective tissue by these cells.[91] TGF β is not only a potent stimulator of connective tissue synthesis but is also the most potent inhibitor of smooth muscle proliferation thus far discovered.[92] It is ubiquitous in the sense that most cells have the capacity to form it, and rich sources of this molecule are the platelet and the activated macrophage. Much of the TGF β that is secreted by these cells is in a latent form that requires decreased pH or proteolytic cleavage for activity. Nevertheless, the balance between inhibitors such as TGF β and stimulators of smooth muscle proliferation such as PDGF is probably critical in determining whether a net proliferative response of smooth muscle cells will occur, resulting in the formation of an atherosclerotic lesion. Thus, if the macrophage-derived foam cells are appropriately activated in the subendothelial space, they could potentially be involved in the secretion of growth factors that could chemotactically attract smooth muscle cells to migrate from the media into the intima, to proliferate within the intima, and to set up a series of conditions that could lead to the formation of an intimal, fibromuscular, proliferative lesion.

It has been demonstrated that PDGF-B-chain–containing protein is present in approximately 20 per cent of the macrophages in both human and nonhuman atherosclerotic lesions in all phases of development. PDGF is present in the non-foam-cell macrophages that are distributed throughout the lesion, as well as in macrophages present among the smooth muscle cells in the fibrous cap portion of the fibrous plaque[93] (Fig. 36–12). The presence of PDGF-B protein in the macrophages in these lesions provides the first convincing basis for assigning the macrophage a key role in the induction and maintenance of the smooth muscle proliferative response during atherogenesis, since PDGF-BB is one of the most potent growth factors, capable of stimulating smooth muscle migration, chemotaxis, and proliferation. Thus macrophage-derived PDGF-BB (Fig. 36–12) could be involved not only in the appearance of smooth muscle cells that migrate into macrophage-rich fatty streaks, but in the progression of these fatty streaks to intermediate or fibrofatty lesions, which may ultimately become advanced occlusive lesions, or fibrous plaques. If the cycle of "endothelial injury" and macrophage accumulation and stimulation is repeated, at least two cells capable of releasing growth factors into the intima — the activated endothelial cell and the activated macrophage — may continue to contribute to progression of the lesions.

The response-to-injury hypothesis also provides an opportunity for the interaction of a third cell, the platelet. The hypothesis suggests that if the flow properties of the blood at particular anatomical sites are such that these properties participate in the endothelial injury, endothelial cell-cell attachment may be affected and cell disjunction may occur, leading to retraction of endothelial cells and exposure of the underlying foam cells or connective tissue or both. In either case, this would permit opportunities for platelets to interact, adhere, aggregate, and form mural thrombi.[94-98] Should this occur, the platelet could provide a third potent source of growth factors, including the same four factors that can be released by the activated macrophage. Thus, there are numerous opportunities for mitogens to be deposited in the artery wall, which, under proper circumstances, could play critical roles in the genesis of proliferative smooth muscle lesions of atherosclerosis (Fig. 36–11).

It is important to point out that injury to the endothelium need not result in denudation of the endothelial cells. Endothelial injury may simply be manifested by relatively rapid replacement of individual endothelial cells that are lost, and is principally reflected in endothelial dysfunction such as alterations in endothelial permeability, and release of vasoactive substances and growth factors.

Finally, it has been shown that human arterial smooth muscle cells removed from lesions of atherosclerosis have the capacity to express one of the PDGF genes and secrete a form of PDGF when they are grown in cell culture.[99] If this were to occur in vivo, then as the smooth muscle cells proliferate in developing lesions, they could participate in inducing further progression of the lesions by release of PDGF. Thus a vicious circle might be established that would have to be stopped if one hoped to stop lesion progression and induce lesion regression.

THE MONOCLONAL HYPOTHESIS

The monoclonal hypothesis suggests that each lesion of atherosclerosis is derived from a single smooth muscle cell that serves as a source of all of the cells within the lesion. This hypothesis is based upon the Lyon, or inactive X chromosome, hypothesis, which states that each tissue is made of a small "patch" of related cells that have either an active maternal or an active paternal X chromosome, but not both. Such a fact would make little to no metabolic difference, since each X chromosome codes for similar enzymes. However, there is a special case that permits analysis of lesions by utilizing this fact. This is the case of some black females who are heterozygous for the enzyme glucose-6-phosphate dehydrogenase (G-6-PD). This enzyme is coded for by the X chromosome and occurs in two isozymic forms that can be separated by electrophoresis. When an individual is heterozygous for these two isozymes, one X chromosome codes for one and the second X chromosome for the other isoenzyme. Progenitor cells that have been committed to one or the other of the two X chromosomes therefore can replicate and form patches that will contain either one or the other isoenzyme.

This principle was taken advantage of by Lindner and Gartler,[100] who demonstrated that multiple samples of uterine leiomyomas are composed of cells that contain the same active X chromosome as denoted by G-6-PD, whereas when they examined samples of adjacent normal myometrium, they found both isozymes. More recently, studies of some tumors have also demonstrated similar phenomena, suggesting that in some tumors the tumor cells arose from a single cell, that is, they are monoclonal.

These observations were utilized in the proposal that some atherosclerotic plaques, which frequently appear as isolated nodules surrounded by areas of normal tissue, might be monoclonal. Benditt and Benditt[14] examined a series of plaques from a small number of black females that were obtained at autopsy. They dissected very small samples of each plaque

FIGURE 36–12. See color plate 9.

and examined the isozyme content of each sample and determined the number of lesions that contained one or the other isozyme or both isozymes. They interpreted their data to signify that each lesion of atherosclerosis represents a clone derived from a single smooth muscle cell, which they have termed monotypic rather than monoclonal. They have gone on to suggest, therefore, that each lesion of atherosclerosis is a benign neoplasm derived from a cell that has been transformed by viruses, by chemicals, or by other mutagens. More recently, investigators have looked for the presence of particular viruses, such as the herpes virus.[101] It is possible that some virally induced lesions could result in monoclonal lesions. It should be pointed out that contradictory data both supporting and refuting the monoclonal hypothesis have been published.

There are other possible interpretations of the data supporting the monoclonal hypothesis. Fialkow[102] has pointed out that the presence of a single-enzyme phenotype in a lesion does not necessarily mean that the lesion is clonal in origin. A single lesion could arise by the participation of more than one cell. If each cell that participated contained the same isozyme, and if some cells had a replicative advantage over others, it is possible that cells with a given isozyme type would replicate in preference to cells with the second isozyme type. The probability of such an origin would depend on the smooth muscle cell mosaic composition or patch size and distribution in the normal intima, which unfortunately is not known. If there were repeated cycles of cell death and cell proliferation in which a particular cell type had a selective advantage in proliferating, then repetitive sampling of these cells could lead to a single-enzyme phenotype, despite the fact that the lesions were multicellular in origin. In addition, clonal selection with evolution toward a single-enzyme phenotype has been shown to occur in several forms of focal hyperplasia. This makes it difficult if not impossible to determine whether the single-enzyme phenotype that has been observed is caused by monoclonality or by polyclonality based on selection as noted earlier.

LIPIDS AND LIPOPROTEINS IN ATHEROSCLEROSIS

Since hypercholesterolemia is the major risk factor associated with the increased incidence of atherosclerosis in the United States and Western Europe, it is important to understand the role that lipids play in this process. Although many lesions of atherosclerosis are fibrous and contain relatively little lipid, the effects of lipid on endothelium, monocytes, and smooth muscle, and the accumulation of lipid in the lesions of hypercholesterolemic individuals, are critical components of the process of atherogenesis. Consequently, it is important to understand specifically how elevated levels of cholesterol-bearing lipoproteins are related to the process of atherogenesis. These subjects are discussed in detail on pp. 1131 to 1139.

The Lipid Research Clinic Trials have provided data suggesting that it would be beneficial to lower plasma LDL levels.[16,17] Those studies showed that the decrease in plasma cholesterol can be correlated with a reduction in the incidence of myocardial infarction, and presumably atherosclerosis. The genetic basis for the increase in plasma LDL is not known for most individuals in the population who are hypercholesterolemic, although some may be heterozygous for the familial hypercholesterolemia (FH) trait. Nevertheless, our understanding of the LDL receptor control of HMG CoA reductase, and thus cholesterol synthesis, has been critical in permitting us to understand how cholesterol metabolism is regulated. As important as these studies are, however, they do not provide data that permit us to understand how the lesions of atherosclerosis form. In other words, although the LDL receptor pathway provides an understanding of the control of cholesterol metabolism, it yields no information concerning

the basis of the cellular changes and interactions that occur when elevated plasma cholesterol leads to atherosclerosis.

To answer this question, it has been necessary to devise experiments using appropriate animal models and appropriate cell culture systems. These tests provide opportunities to determine how smooth muscle cells proliferate and under what circumstances, what cellular interactions occur during the pathogenesis of this disease process, and what factors are elaborated by the cells that control not only smooth muscle multiplication but also connective tissue formation and lipid accumulation.

The response-to-injury hypothesis of atherosclerosis already discussed can be taken one step further in terms of asking how chronic hypercholesterolemia may "injure" endothelium. Jackson and Gotto[103] have suggested that one form of endothelial injury which may occur upon exposure to chronically elevated levels of LDL may result from the effects of an increase in the number of cholesterol molecules in the plasma membranes of cells, including the endothelial cells. When the cholesterol/phospholipid ratio of endothelial plasma membranes is elevated, this could theoretically lead to an increase in the viscosity of the membranes. Changes such as these would decrease the malleability of the endothelial cell surface and, should this occur, could have critical effects at particular anatomical sites such as branches of bifurcations in the arterial tree, where the endothelial cells are exposed to changes in the flow of blood. Such rheological changes could cause an otherwise normally malleable endothelial surface, if it becomes more viscous and this more rigid, to be incapable of dealing with the stresses caused by these changes in the flow characteristics. This could lead to endothelial cell–cell separation and endothelial retraction, particularly at sites where the blood flow has already been modified owing to the formation of fatty streaks, as has been found to occur in hypercholesterolemic monkeys, swine, and man. As already discussed, hypercholesterolemia also leads to changes in monocyte-endothelial adhesion properties and to the development of fatty streaks themselves.

It is also possible that hypercholesterolemia may alter the endothelial cells so that they are stimulated to produce increased amounts of growth factor. Recent studies with the Watanabe heritable hyperlipemic (WHHL) rabbit, an animal model of homozygous familial hypercholesterolemia, have demonstrated that probucol, a drug with mild lipid-lowering but powerful antioxidant properties, had a marked effect in significantly reducing the size and incidence of atherosclerotic lesions.[104,105] This led to studies suggesting that oxidized LDL might play a major role as an injurious agent responsible for many of the early events associated with atherogenesis, particularly since macrophages have scavenger receptors that can bind and permit phagocytosis of these oxidized lipid particles. The ingestion of oxidized LDL could lead to foam cell formation on the part of the macrophages, which can also engage in further oxidation of available molecules of LDL. Oxidized LDL is injurious to both endothelium and smooth muscle in vitro and has been found in both human and experimental lesions of atherosclerosis.[106] Thus the presence of this modified lipoprotein in the lesions suggests that it is the principal culprit in atherogenesis in hypercholesterolemic individuals and that interference with its formation could be an important step in lesion prevention. Studies are under way to examine further the capacity of antioxidants to prevent lesion formation in experimental atherosclerosis and in humans. All or any of these responses could lead to important changes that, step by step, lead to atherogenesis.

GROWTH FACTORS

As discussed earlier, growth factors can be elaborated by all four cells potentially involved in the lesions of atherosclerosis: endothelium, monocyte/macrophages, platelets, and smooth muscle. Although the first three of these cells can produce more than one growth factor, PDGF could play a critical role in the genesis of atherosclerosis because of its chemotactic and mitogenic effects on smooth muscle cells.

PDGF is a two-chain molecule of approximately 30,000 molecular weight that is highly cationic and highly disulfide bonded.[107-110] It is an extraordinarily potent mitogen that binds with very high affinity to responsive cells[111,112] and is chemotactic for the same cells for which it is mitogenic.[113,114] When it binds to its high-affinity cell-surface receptor, it induces a series of biological events, some of which are probably related to induction of DNA synthesis and cell division. These cellular responses include phosphorylation of the PDGF receptor through the activation of a tyrosine kinase on the receptor, and the activation of C-kinase in the subplasmalemmal cytoplasm resulting from phospholipase activation at the cell surface. C-kinase activation could ultimately lead to calcium transfer from intracellular compartments, which in itself may possibly be important in induction of the mitogenic signal.[56]

PDGF also induces increased binding of LDL to cells by increasing the numbers of LDL receptors,[45,115] increased cholesterol synthesis, increased endocytosis, increased flux of ions into the cell, reorganization of actin cables within the cells, and change in cell shape. It also has recently been found to be a potent vasoactive agent, even more potent than angiotensin II.[56] Thus, if PDGF is released from platelets when they adhere to the artery wall at sites of injury, from activated macrophages where it is now known to present in these cells[93] after they enter the artery wall (particularly during fatty streak formation), from activated endothelial cells if they are appropriately stimulated, and perhaps in some special instances from appropriately activated smooth muscle cells, then such responses would enhance lesion formation.

PDGF has an extremely short half-life when it is injected into the circulation.[116] This short half-life suggests that PDGF that is not bound locally to tissue would be cleared rapidly and thus would be unavailable at sites distant from its release. Furthermore, PDGF binds to a number of proteins in the plasma, including alpha$_2$-macroglobulin. These binding pro-

teins could serve to increase further the capacity of PDGF to act as a tissue mitogen at local sites where PDGF has been released and is bound to the tissue.[117]

There is a striking homology between the amino acid sequence of purified PDGF and that of a transforming protein derived from an oncogene of the simian sarcoma virus. This homology suggests that PDGF may be important in proliferation of cells transformed by the simian sarcoma virus.[118,119] Furthermore, numerous lines of transformed cells secrete a form of PDGF and have downregulated receptors for PDGF, suggesting that a form of PDGF may play a role in the proliferation of cells that are neoplastically transformed in other ways.[120] Both chains of PDGF and their receptors have been cloned. cDNA probes are available for each chain of PDGF and for both receptors. Investigations of these receptors have demonstrated a high degree of specificity of binding of the three different isomeric forms of PDGF (PDGF-AA, PDGF-AB, PDGF-BB) for the three different forms of the receptor (PDGF receptor $\alpha\alpha$, $\alpha\beta$, $\beta\beta$). For example, the A chain of PDGF can bind only to the α receptor subunit; thus PDGF-AA can bind only to PDGF receptor $\alpha\alpha$. In contrast, PDGF-BB can bind to any one of the three forms of the PDGF receptor.[121] It therefore becomes important to understand the relative numbers of receptors on the different smooth muscle cells in different regions of the artery wall if one is to determine how effective the specific form of PDGF will be on these cells in a given site in the arterial tree. Our increased understanding of these degrees of specificity and responsivity will increase opportunities to make effective agents that can either induce smooth muscle proliferation or, potentially, prevent such a proliferative response.

CELLULAR EVENTS THAT OCCUR DURING ATHEROGENESIS

Several animals form lesions of atherosclerosis similar to humans when they develop hypercholesterolemia from eat-

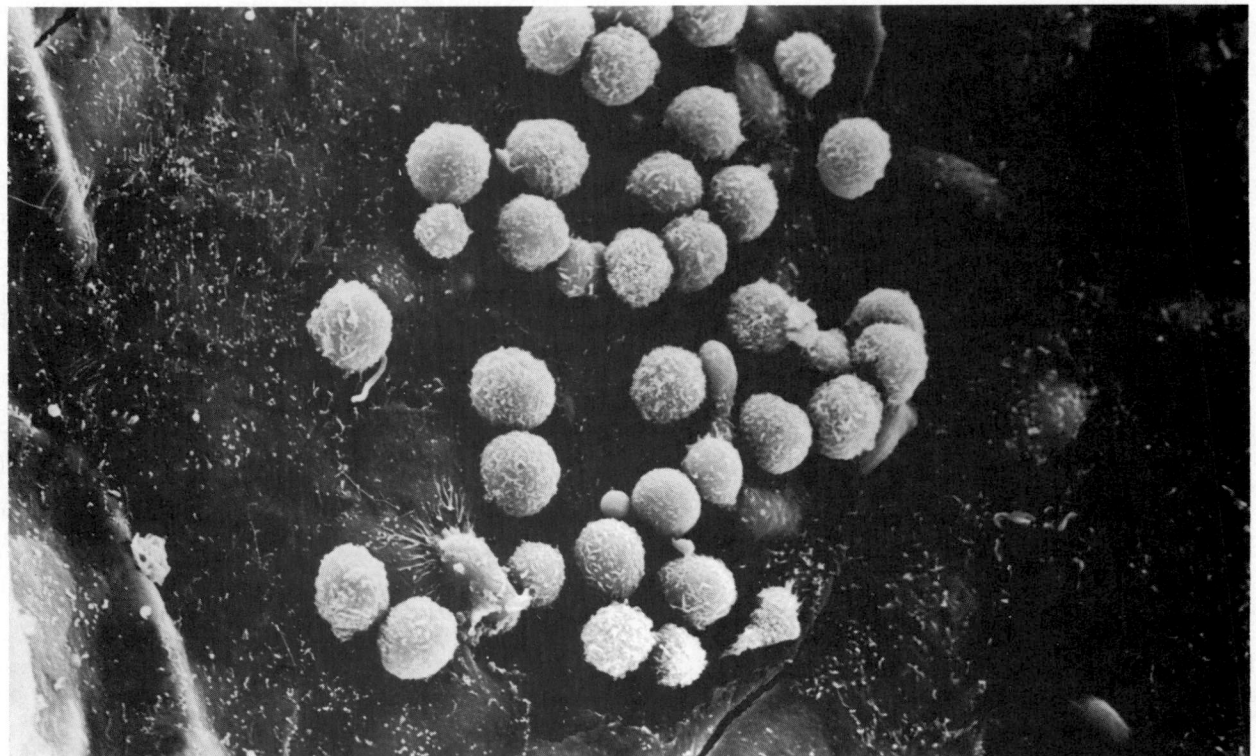

FIGURE 36-13. Electron micrograph demonstrating leukocytes adherent to the endothelium of the aorta of a hypercholesterolemic monkey after 14 days of an atherogenic diet. Adherent leukocytes (mostly monocytes) were found scattered in patches such as these randomly distributed at all levels of the aortic tree. Some of the cells appear spread on the surface, whereas others are rounded.

ing a fatty diet. This has made it possible to study the effects of hypercholesterolemia in terms of understanding the cellular interactions that occur that lead to the lesions of atherosclerosis. Such studies have been performed by Faggiotto et al.[122,123] and by Masuda and Ross[124,125] on nonhuman primates, by Gerrity[126-128] and his colleagues on swine, and by Rosenfeld et al.[129] on fat-fed rabbits and the WHHL rabbit. The latter studies have provided highly detailed observations concerning the sequence of cellular events that occur in endogenous hypercholesterolemia (the WHHL rabbit, a model of familial homozygous hypercholesterolemia) as compared with those that take place during diet-induced hypercholesterolemia.

EARLY CHANGES. The data of Faggiotto et al.[122,123] and Masuda and Ross[124,125] show that the first and most striking event occurs after 7 to 14 days of diet-induced hypercholesterolemia. This consists of the attachment of large numbers of leukocytes, principally monocytes, to the surface of the arterial endothelium (Fig. 36–13). The monocytes attach to the endothelial cells in clusters that appear to be randomly located throughout the arterial tree in all large and medium-sized arteries. The attached monocytes then migrate over the surface of the endothelium, where they probe, find a junction between the endothelial cells, and use this junctional site to slip between the cells and localize in the subendothelial space (Fig. 36–14). This process, as viewed in cell culture, appears to occur very rapidly and presumably does so in vivo as well. After finding their way into the subendothelial intimal space, the monocytes become converted into macrophages, so that within less than 1 month large numbers of foam cells, or lipid-

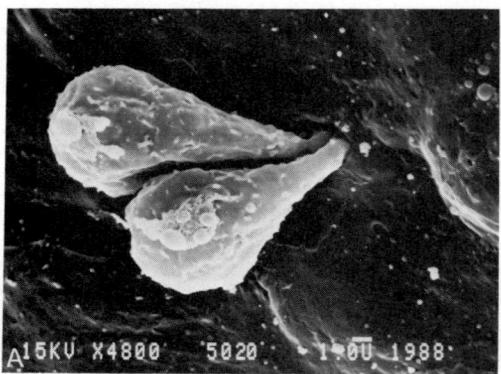

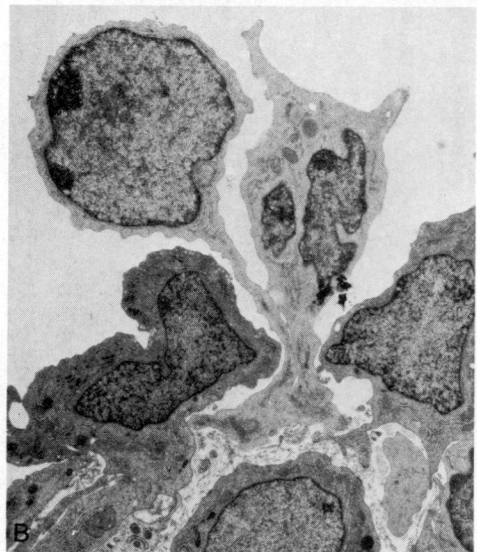

FIGURE 36–14. Scanning and transmission electron micrographs demonstrating leukocytes entering into the artery wall between endothelial junctions after 6 months and 1 year, respectively, of an atherogenic diet in nonhuman primates. *A*, Thoracic aorta, 6 months. ×4000. *B*, Thoracic aorta, 1 year. ×4700. (From Masuda, J., and Ross, R.: Atherogenesis during low level hypercholesterolemia in the nonhuman primate: I. Fatty streak formation. Arteriosclerosis 10:164, 1990, by permission of the American Heart Association.)

filled macrophages, are found beneath an intact endothelium. These cells continue to enlarge as they fill with lipid. Such accumulations of foam cells represent the establishment of the first and ubiquitous lesion of atherosclerosis, the fatty streak (Fig. 36–15).

The fatty streaks continue to expand in the hypercholesterolemic monkeys by continuing the process of monocyte adherence, subendothelial migration and localization, and lipid accumulation. As the fatty streaks expand, the surface of the artery becomes highly irregular and convoluted (Fig. 36–16). With increasing time, small numbers of smooth muscle cells begin to appear beneath the accumulated macrophages within the intima and also begin to accumulate deposits of lipid and take on the appearance of foam cells. As discussed earlier, monoclonal antibodies specific for smooth muscle and macrophages have made it possible to show that both types of cell become foam cells as the lesions expand. The cholesterol levels in the plasma of the fat-fed monkeys ranged between 500 and 1000 mg/dl, which are not dissimilar from the levels of plasma cholesterol found in humans with FH disease.

LATER CHANGES. After approximately 5 to 6 months at the very high cholesterol and LDL levels and after 1 year at levels closer to those observed in humans, a second series of changes occurred in the monkeys, initially at branches and bifurcations in the iliac arteries and subsequently at higher regions in the arterial tree. The changes that were found at branches and bifurcations suggest that they may be associated with the flow characteristics at these particular sites in the vessel. They consist of retraction of the endothelial cells covering some of the fatty streaks caused by endothelial cell-cell detachment. Endothelial retraction exposes the numerous lipid-filled macrophages to the circulation (Fig. 36–17) and permits them to remove the lipid they have ingested from the lesion by taking it with them into the circulation to the spleen and to lymph nodes. In this fashion, the macrophages play a role in the lesions of atherosclerosis similar to their role at sites of injury, where they are the principal scavenger cells. Thus, in a very real sense, the progressing lesions of atherosclerosis represent a special kind of inflammatory response in which macrophages (and perhaps T-lymphocytes) attempt initially to protect the tissues. With the continuing insult (hypercholesterolemia, diabetes, and so on), the response becomes excessive, and the resultant fibroproliferative events themselves become the disease process.

When the macrophages become exposed to the circulation they can serve as sites for platelet adherence and for microthrombi to form, demonstrating that the macrophages may represent a potent site for platelet interactions (Fig. 36–18). In these cases in which platelet interactions such as those just described occurred, similar anatomical sites were observed 1 to 2 months later to be occupied by space-filling lesions of advanced atherosclerosis, or fibrous plaques. These fibrous plaques had all of the characteristic appearances of fibrous plaques in humans, including a dense fibrous cap that overlay areas of extensive proliferation of smooth muscle cells intermixed with lipid-filled macrophages, beneath which were found areas of cell debris, lipid accumulation, and sometimes calcification (Fig. 36–19). The same changes occurred at the iliac bifurcation after approximately 7 months, in the abdominal aorta after 9 months, in the thoracic aorta by 11 months, and in the coronary arteries after a year to 13 months. By analyzing the distribution of these changes and correlating this distribution with the levels of cholesterol in the animals with time, Faggiotto et al.[122,123] and Masuda and Ross[124,125] were able to demonstrate that there was a correlation among three factors: the level of plasma cholesterol, the duration of the maintenance of this increased level of cholesterol, and the changes that occur at particular anatomical sites with time.

Another important observation was that there were many advanced lesions of atherosclerosis that also occurred at sites where fatty streaks were present but where there was no clear evidence of endothelial cell-cell separation and exposure of the subendothelium.[123] Thus, one has to conclude that proliferative lesions of atherosclerosis can occur at sites where the

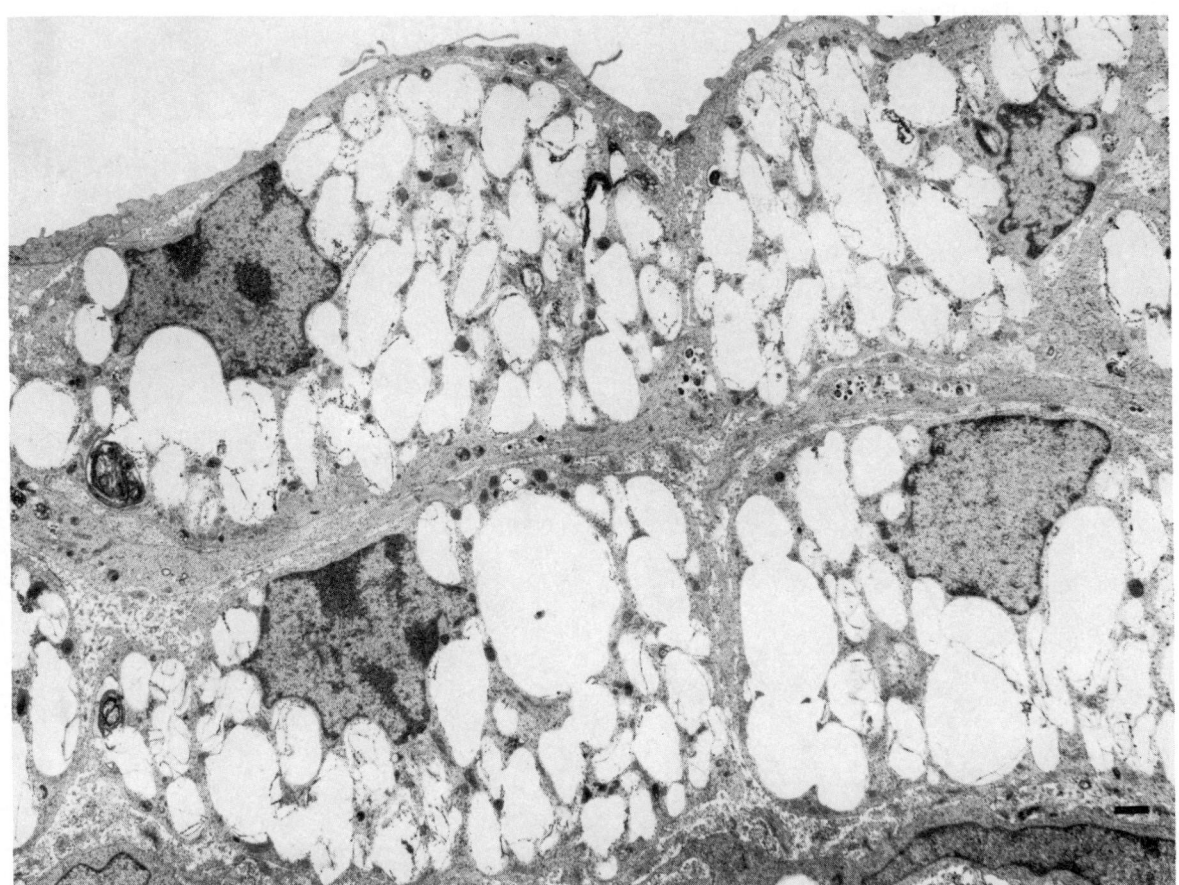

FIGURE 36–15. Transmission electron micrograph showing a fatty streak containing two layers of subendothelial foam cells after 2 months of hypercholesterolemia in a fat-fed nonhuman primate. The large lipid-filled macrophages are distributed focally in multilayers. The cells are four- to six-fold larger than lipid-laden macrophages observed in control animals. There is a small amount of intercellular matrix and some lipid debris. The macrophages maintain a close relationship to the intact endothelium. The endothelium is markedly stretched so that the endothelial cells have become very thin. (From Faggiotto, A., Ross, R., and Harker, L.: Studies of hypercholesterolemia in the nonhuman primate: I. Changes that lead to fatty streak formation. Arteriosclerosis 4:332, 1984, by permission of the American Heart Association.)

FIGURE 36–16. Scanning electron micrograph providing a surface view of a fatty streak from a fat-fed monkey after 2 months of hypercholesterolemia. The surface of the fatty streak has become highly irregular and has a striking nodular pattern with deep crevices between the nodules. Such a pattern forms by continuing adherence of monocytes to the endothelial cells that probe and migrate subendothelially between cells to continually expand the fatty streak. ⟶

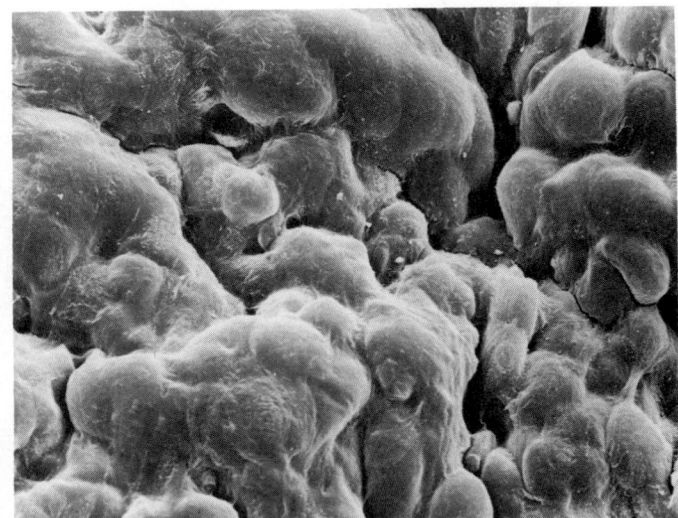

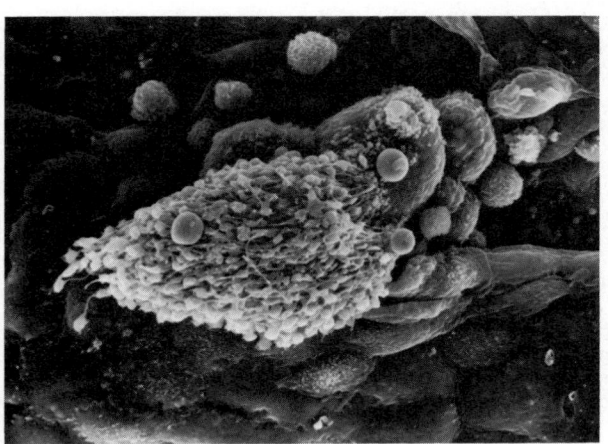

⟵
FIGURE 36–17. A scanning electron micrograph of the thoracic aorta of a nonhuman primate, showing the irregular surface of a fatty streak after 2 years of an atherogenic diet. Platelet microthrombi adherent to exposed macrophages are visible at a site of endothelial retraction. Many adherent leukocytes are also seen on the intact endothelial cells. ×720. (From Masuda, J., and Ross, R.: Atherogenesis during low level hypercholesterolemia in the nonhuman primate: II. Fatty streak conversion to fibrous plaque. Arteriosclerosis 10:178, 1990, by permission of the American Heart Association.)

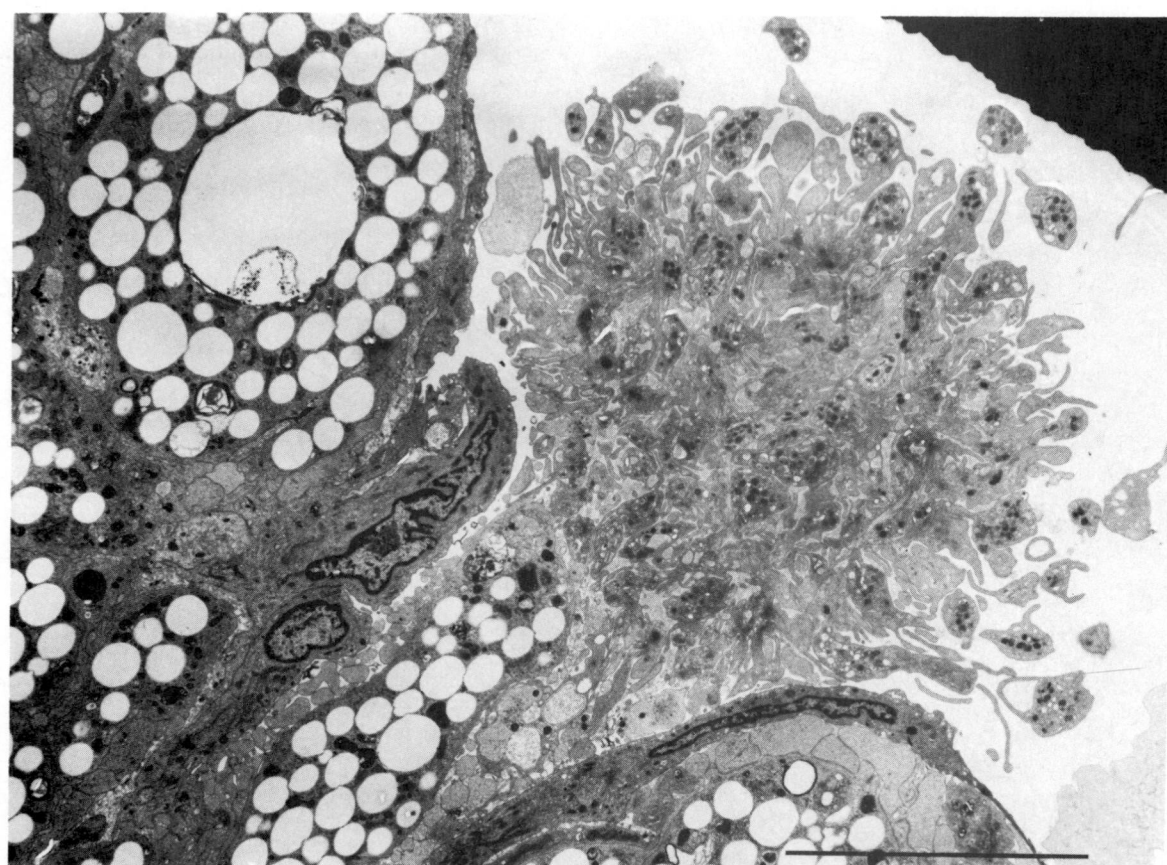

FIGURE 36–18. Transmission electron micrograph of platelets adherent to an exposed macrophage from a fatty streak in a fat-fed monkey that had been hypercholesterolemic for 6 months. The platelets in this thrombus are generally adherent to exposed foam cells and penetrate into the depth of a crevice in the fatty streak. Many of the platelets have undergone degranulation and have released their contents. Bar = 10 μ. (From Faggiotto, A., and Ross, R.: Studies of hypercholesterolemia in the nonhuman primate: II. Fatty streak conversion to fibrous plaque. Arteriosclerosis 4:349, 1984, by permission of the American Heart Association.)

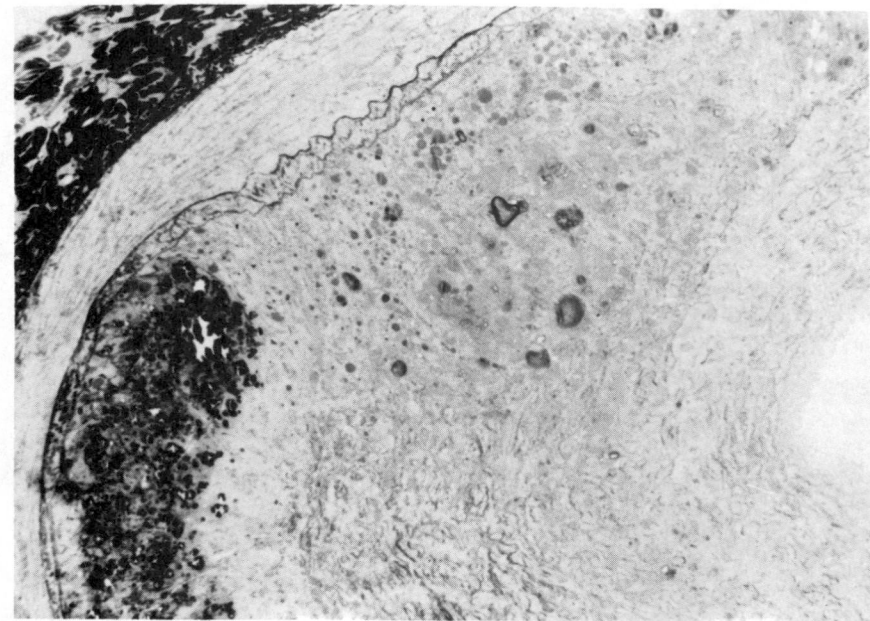

FIGURE 36–19. Light micrograph demonstrating an advanced fibrous plaque that formed in the internal iliac artery of a monkey that was hypercholesterolemic for 7 months. The lesion has occluded approximately 70 per cent of the arterial lumen and consists of numerous layers of smooth muscle cells surrounded by fibrous connective tissue. An area of lipid and necrotic tissue occupies the left side and upper portion of this lesion. (From Faggiotto, A., and Ross, R.: Studies of hypercholesterolemia in the nonhuman primate: II. Fatty streak conversion to fibrous plaque. Arteriosclerosis 4:345, 1984, by permission of the American Heart Association.)

endothelium remains intact over preexisting lesions such as fatty streaks. This can undoubtedly be explained by the fact that both activated macrophages and endothelium can serve as sources of growth factors so that platelet interactions are not required for smooth muscle proliferation to occur.

This leads to the need to determine what constitutes endothelial injury. It also suggests that nondenuding forms of injury or endothelial dysfunction are more important than the denuding forms described above. Reidy and Schwartz[130,131] have indicated that one of the most common results of endothelial injury may be detachment of individual endothelial cells, which are rapidly replaced by neighboring cells so that endothelial continuity is maintained. Several markers have been developed that can be used to identify sites of endothelial injury. Hansson et al.[132] demonstrated that injured endothelial cells take up IgG whereas normal endothelium will not, and that such IgG uptake can be correlated with increased replication of the endothelium. Furthermore, Reidy and Schwartz[133] showed that a linear correlation exists between the extent of endothelial injury (the number of denuded cells) and the localization of indium-111–labeled platelets at these sites. Platelets would adhere because injured endothelium appears to have lost its nonthrombogenic properties.

Thus, there may be several different forms of endothelial injury and more subtle techniques may be necessary to uncover them. This raises the interesting question, as suggested earlier, whether one subtle form of endothelial injury may be the stimulation of these cells to synthesize and secrete growth factors, including PDGF, that could then play a critical role in the genesis of the events previously described. If this were the case, then endothelial disjunction, retraction, and subendothelial exposure are clearly not necessary for lesions of atherosclerosis to develop, since both activated endothelium and macrophages could be sufficient in themselves to provide a mitogenic stimulus for smooth muscle cells to form lesions of atherosclerosis.

REGRESSION OF ATHEROSCLEROSIS

ANIMAL STUDIES. A number of studies have demonstrated that lesions of experimentally induced atherosclerosis can in fact regress. When hypercholesterolemic swine and nonhuman primates that have developed severe lesions are fed a normocholesterolemic diet, these lesions can regress. Fatty streaks formed in the monkeys receiving the high-fat, high-cholesterol diet of Faggiotto et al.[122] were found to regress completely within 1 month after the animals resumed a normal diet. Most of the studies of regression of the advanced lesions of atherosclerosis have been performed in nonhuman primates, principally in different strains of macaques and in squirrel monkeys. The studies were performed by providing the monkeys with atherogenic diets that took them through stages of fatty streak development and on to fibrous plaque formation. When cholesterol was removed from the diet and plasma cholesterol concentrations returned to normal, Faggiotto et al.[122] observed that reasonably rapid regression of fatty streaks occurred. Of greater potential interest, significant reduction in the size of the smooth muscle proliferative lesions has been observed by several different investigators. Some of the earliest studies were performed by Armstrong et al.,[134] who demonstrated that coronary atherosclerosis could regress. These studies were subsequently confirmed by Wissler and Vesselinovitch.[135] Perhaps the largest number of studies have been performed by Clarkson and his colleagues.[136] They demonstrated the clear therapeutic benefit of lowering plasma cholesterol concentrations after having induced fibrous plaques in animals on hypercholesterolemic regimens for periods of 12 months and longer. Regression occurred principally in lesions in the abdominal aorta and in the coronary arteries, in contrast to those that formed at the ca-

rotid bifurcation, which appeared, on some occasions, to develop lesions relatively independently of plasma lipid concentrations. When regression occurs and plasma cholesterol levels return to baseline, the lesions of atherosclerosis become smaller, contain less lipid, and demonstrate marked decreases in their content of cholesterol and cholesteryl esters. Remodeling of connective tissue proteins also appears to take place, as shown by decreases in both collagen and elastic fiber proteins in these lesions. Thus it seems that, over a sufficiently long period, advanced lesions can in some cases also regress.

HUMAN STUDIES. It has been demonstrated that advanced, semiocclusive lesions of human coronary atherosclerosis also can regress. In a quantitative image analysis study of coronary angiograms from a series of patients being aggressively treated with lipid-lowering regimens of either niacin and colestipol or lovastatin and colestipol, Brown and colleagues[137] have demonstrated statistically significant regression in association with decreases in plasma cholesterol and LDL. This provides clear evidence that the lesions of atherosclerosis are able to regress at apparently all stages of lesion development.

A number of investigators have probed the capacity of fish oils, which contain large amounts of omega-3 fatty acids, to decrease plasma cholesterol levels and potentially to induce lesion regression when added to the diet of hypercholesterolemic individuals.[138] Not only do these diets lead to decrease in plasma cholesterol levels, but they also change the balance of prostaglandins that are formed by the cells. It is well known that platelets have the capacity to use arachidonic acid to form the prostaglandin derivative thromboxane A_2, a proaggregating factor for platelets. On the other hand, endothelial cells and smooth muscle use the same fatty acid to form, via cyclooxygenase, the prostaglandin metabolite prostacyclin (PGI_2), an extraordinarily potent antiaggregant and vasodilator. When the omega-3 fatty acids are fed to animals (and if they are particularly rich in eicosapentaenoic acid), they shift the balance because thromboxane A_3 derived from this fatty acid is inactive as a platelet aggregant, whereas PGI_3 is as active as PGI_2, thus favoring antiaggregant, vasodilator effects over effects that might lead to platelet aggregation and thrombosis.

THROMBOSIS
(see also Chapter 58)

As described at the beginning of this chapter, thrombosis was originally considered to be an important component in the initiation and progression of the lesions of atherosclerosis. It now appears that thrombosis may play several roles. One prominent and potentially important clinical role is that of thrombi which become incorporated into existing advanced lesions of atherosclerosis, rapidly resulting in lumen narrowing and increase in lesion dimensions. Perhaps one of the most persistent and common complications of atherosclerosis is the formation of cracks and fissures in the advanced lesions of atherosclerosis that can act as sites for platelet attachment and formation of mural and potentially occlusive thrombi, which could lead to unstable angina or myocardial infarction.

As discussed earlier, there is good evidence in nonhuman primates and in rabbits that mural thrombi can contribute to the initiation and development of lesions of atherosclerosis.[94-98] This has also been demonstrated in humans at the perianastomotic site of coronary bypass surgery, where new lesions of atherosclerosis form in approximately 30 per cent of all bypass grafts.[139] In monkeys or rabbits receiving a hyperlipemic diet, intraarterial balloon catheter deendothelialization can lead to intimal smooth muscle proliferative lesions that appear very much like those found in hypercholesterolemic patients.

Thrombi have been observed in the coronary arteries of the vast majority of individuals who die from transmural myocardial infarction. However, thrombi are much less common in individuals who die from subendothelial infarction. Thrombosis is even less common in individuals who die of sudden cardiac death, although both thrombosis and embolism are well recognized as complications of cerebrovascular disease as well as peripheral vascular disease.

The role of the endothelium in the process of thrombosis is not entirely clear since, as discussed earlier, endothelial cells have both nonthrombogenic and procoagulant activities. Endothelial cells produce von Willebrand factor as well as plasminogen activator and prostacyclin. The development of agents that can alter thromboxane formation and thus prevent platelet interaction, or alter prostacyclin formation and thus promote platelet interactions, should make it possible to obtain a clearer idea of the role of these agents as compared with others that can be produced by the endothelial cells in the process of thrombosis in general.

CONCLUSIONS

It is clear that knowledge in the field of atherosclerosis has exploded and is changing rapidly. The opportunity to use the tools of cell and molecular biology, as well as new noninvasive methods for examining individuals at the clinical level, has broadened our understanding of the roles of the cells in atherogenesis. Cell and molecular biology have rapidly increased our understanding of the principal cells involved in atherosclerosis: endothelium, smooth muscle, platelets, and monocyte/macrophages and T-lymphocytes. How the risk factors that are commonly associated with an increased incidence of atherosclerosis are related to these cellular interactions is beginning to be understood, particularly in relation to hypercholesterolemia. Unfortunately, there are no good animal models that permit us to study the questions related to cigarette smoking, hypertension, diabetes, or some of the other risk factors that are epidemiologically associated with atherosclerosis. Without these, it is difficult to know the nature of the cellular interactions that occur during the genesis of the disease process as it is associated with each of these important risk factors.

Perhaps the most critical aspect of this problem is the need to understand the basis of the genetic susceptibility of individuals to these risk factors and thus to circumstances that can lead to these increased cellular interactions. Once the genetic loci for the various apoproteins are identified, and once it is possible to demonstrate altered genetic loci for these and other factors important in atherogenesis in individuals who are at increased risk for heart attack and/or stroke, it should be possible to begin to probe this question using these new tools.

Acknowledgments

This work was supported in part by U.S. Public Health Service Grant HL-18645 and NIH grant RR-00166 to the Northwest Regional Primate Center. The author is particularly indebted to Elaine Raines, Agostino Faggiotto, Junichi Masuda, Michael Rosenfeld, Toyohiro Tsukada, Masakiyo Sasahara, Shogo Katsuda, Allen Gown, and to Daniel Bowen-Pope, with whom work reported from his laboratory was performed.

REFERENCES

RISK FACTORS

1. Report of the Working Group on Arteriosclerosis of the National Heart, Lung, and Blood Institute. Vol. 2. DHEW Publication No. (NIH) 82-2035, Washington D.C., U.S. Government Printing Office, 1981.
2. Ross, R., and Glomset, J.: Atherosclerosis and the arterial smooth muscle cell. Science 180:1332, 1973.
3. Ross, R., and Glomset, J. A.: The pathogenesis of atherosclerosis. N. Engl. J. Med. 295:369, 1976.
4. Ross, R., and Harker, L.: Hyperlipidemia and atherosclerosis. Science 193:1094, 1976.
5. Wissler, R. W., Vesselinovitch, D., and Getz, G. J.: Abnormalities of the arterial wall and its metabolism in atherogenesis. Prog. Cardiovasc. Dis. 18:341, 1976.
6. Dawber, T. R., Moore, F. E., and Mann, G. V.: Measuring the risk of coronary heart disease in adult population groups: II. Coronary heart disease in the Framingham study. Am. J. Public Health 47:4, 1957.
7. Chapman, J. M., Goerke, L. S., Dixon, W., et al.: Measuring the risk of coronary heart disease in adult population groups: IV. The clinical status of a population group in Los Angeles under observation for two or three years. Am. J. Public Health 47:33, 1957.
8. Doyle, J. T., Heslin, A. S., Hillboe, H. E., et al.: Measuring the risk of coronary heart disease in adult population groups: III. A prospective study of degenerative cardiovascular disease in Albany: Report of three years' experience: I. Ischemic heart disease. Am. J. Public Health 47:25, 1957.
9. Drake, R. M., Buechley, R. W., and Breslow, L.: Measuring the risk of coronary heart disease in adult population groups: V. An epidemiological investigation of coronary heart disease in the California health survey population. Am J. Public Health 47:43, 1957.
10. Report of Inter-Society Commission for Heart Disease Resources. Primary prevention of the atherosclerotic disease. Circulation 42:55, 1970.
11. Stamler, J., Berkson, D. M., and Lindberg, H. A.: Risk factors: Their role in the etiology and pathogenesis of the atherosclerotic diseases. In Wissler, R. W., Geer, J. C., and Kaufman, N. (eds.): The Pathogenesis of Atherosclerosis. Baltimore, Williams and Wilkins, 1962, p. 41.
12. Kuller, L. H.: Epidemiology of cardiovascular disease: Current perspectives. Am. J. Epidemiol. 104:425, 1976.
13. Ross, R.: The pathogenesis of atherosclerosis—an update. N. Engl. J. Med. 314:488, 1986.
14. Benditt, E. P., and Benditt, J. M.: Evidence for a monoclonal origin of human atherosclerotic plaques. Proc. Natl. Acad. Sci. USA 70:1753, 1973.
15. Inkeles, S., and Eisenberg, D.: Hyperlipidemia and coronary atherosclerosis: A review. Medicine 70:110, 1981.
16. Lipid Research Clinics Program. The Lipid Research Clinics Coronary Primary Prevention Trial Results: I. Reduction in incidence of coronary heart disease. JAMA 251:351, 1984.
17. Lipid Research Clinics Program. The Lipid Research Clinics Coronary Primary Prevention Trial Results: II. The relationship of reduction in incidence of coronary heart disease to cholesterol lowering. JAMA 251:365, 1984.
18. Smoking and Health. Chap. 3. Criteria for Judgment. DHEW Publication No. (NIH) 1103, Washington, D.C., U.S. Government Printing Office, 1964.
19. The Pooling Project Research Group: Relationship of blood pressure, serum cholesterol, smoking habit, relative weight, and ECG abnormalities to incidence of major coronary events: Final report of the pooling project. J. Chronic Dis. 31:201, 1978.
20. Oberman, A., Harlan, W. R., Smith, M., and Graybiel, A.: The cardiovascular risk associated with different levels and types of elevated blood pressure. Minn. Med. 52:1283, 1969.

THE NORMAL ARTERY

21. Report of the Hypertension Task Force. Vol. 1. DHEW Publication No. (NIH) 79-1623, Washington, D.C., U.S. Government Printing Office, 1964.
22. Glagov, S.: Hemodynamic risk factors: Mechanical stress, mural architecture, medial nutrition and the vulnerability of arteries to atherosclerosis. In Wissler, R. W., and Geer, J. C. (eds.): The Pathogenesis of Atherosclerosis. Baltimore, Williams and Wilkins, 1972, p. 164.
23. Wolinsky, H., and Glagov, S.: Comparison of abdominal and thoracic aortic medial structure in mammals. Deviation of man from the usual pattern. Circ. Res. 25:677, 1969.

CELLS OF THE ARTERY AND FROM THE BLOOD POTENTIALLY INVOLVED IN ATHEROGENESIS

24. Schwartz, S. M., and Benditt, E. P.: Clustering of replicating cells in aortic endothelium. Proc. Natl. Acad. Sci. USA 73:651, 1976.
25. Schwartz, S. M., and Benditt, E. P.: Aortic endothelial cell replication. Effects of age and hypertension in the rat. Circ. Res. 41:248, 1977.
26. Simionescu, N., Simionescu, M., and Palade, G. E.: Permeability of muscle capillaries to small heme-peptides. Evidence for the existence of patent transendothelial channels. J. Cell Biol. 64:586, 1975.
27. Huttner, I., Boutet, M., and More, R. H.: Studies on protein passage through arterial endothelium. I. Structural correlates of permeability in rat arterial endothelium. Lab. Invest. 28:672, 1973.
28. Renkin, E. M.: Multiple pathways of capillary permeability. Circ. Res. 41:735, 1977.
29. Moncada, S., Herman, A. G., Higgs, E. A., and Vane, J. R.: Differential formation of prostacyclin (PGX or PGI$_2$) by layers of the arterial wall. An explanation for the antithrombotic properties of vascular endothelium. Thromb. Res. 11:323, 1977.
30. Fielding, C. J.: Metabolism of cholesterol-rich chylomicrons. Mechanism of binding and uptake of cholesteryl esters by the vascular bed of the perfused rat heart. J. Clin. Invest. 62:141, 1978.
31. Furchgott, R. F.: Role of endothelium in responses of vascular smooth muscle. Circ. Res. 53:557, 1983.
32. Gimbrone, M. A. Jr., and Alexander, R. W.: Angiotensin II stimulation of prostaglandin production in cultured human vascular endothelium. Science 189:219, 1975.

33. Jaffe, E. A., Minick, C. R., Adelman, B., et al.: Synthesis of basement membrane by cultured human endothelial cells. J. Exp. Med. 144:209, 1976.

34. Jaffe, E. A., Hoyer, L. W., and Nachman, R. L.: Synthesis of antihemophilic factor antigen by cultured human endothelial cells. J. Clin. Invest. 52:2757, 1973.

35. Rubin, K., Hansson, G. K. Ronnstrand, L. et al.: Induction of B-type receptors for platelet-derived growth factor in vascular inflammation: Possible implications for development of vascular proliferative lesions. Lancet 1:1353, 1988.

36. Steinberg, D.: Lipoproteins and atherosclerosis. A look back and a look ahead. Arteriosclerosis 3:283, 1983.

37. Yanagisawa, M., Kurihara, H., Kimura, S., et al.: A novel potent vasoconstrictor peptide produced by vascular endothelial cells. Nature 322:411, 1988.

38. Furchgott, R. F.: Role of endothelium in responses of vascular smooth muscle. Circ. Res. 53:557, 1983.

39. Gajdusek, C. M., DiCorleto, P. E., Ross, R., and Schwartz, S. M.: An endothelial cell-derived growth factor. J. Cell Biol. 85:467, 1980.

40. DiCorleto, P. E., Gajdusek, C. M., Schwartz, S. M., and Ross, R.: Biochemical properties of the endothelium-derived growth factor: Comparison to other growth factors. J. Cell. Physiol. 114:339, 1983.

41. DiCorleto, P. E., and Bowen-Pope, D. F.: Cultured endothelial cells produce a platelet-derived growth factor–like protein. Proc. Natl. Acad. Sci. USA 80:1919, 1983.

42. Wissler, R. W.: The arterial medial cell, smooth muscle, or multifunctional mesenchyme? J. Atheroscler. Res. 8:201, 1968.

43. Ross, R.: The smooth muscle cell: II. Growth of smooth muscle in culture and formation of elastic fibers. J. Cell Biol. 50:172, 1971.

44. Burke, J. M., and Ross, R.: Synthesis of connective tissue macromolecules by smooth muscle. Int. Rev. Connect. Tissue Res. 8:119, 1979.

45. Chait, A., Ross, R., Albers, J. J., and Bierman, E. L.: Platelet-derived growth factor stimulates activity of low density lipoprotein receptors. Proc. Natl. Acad. Sci. USA 77:4084, 1980.

46. Bowen-Pope, D. F., Seifert, R. A., and Ross, R.: The platelet-derived growth factor receptor. In Boynton, A. L., and Leffert, H. L. (eds): Control of Animal Cell Proliferation: Recent Advances. Vol. 1. New York, Academic Press, 1985, p. 281.

47. Seifert, R. A., Schwartz, S. M., and Bowen-Pope, D. F.: Developmentally regulated production of platelet-derived growth factor–like molecules. Nature 311:669, 1984.

48. Chamley-Campbell, J., Campbell, G., and Ross, R.: Phenotype-dependent response of cultured aortic smooth muscle to serum mitogens. J. Cell Biol. 89:379, 1981.

49. Thyberg, J., Palmberg, L., Nilsson, J., et al.: Phenotype modulations in primary cultures of arterial smooth muscle cells. On the role of platelet-derived growth factor. Differentiation 25:156, 1983.

50. Ross, R., Wight, T. N., Strandness, E., and Thiele, B.: Human atherosclerosis: I. Cell constitution and characteristics of advanced lesions of the superficial femoral artery. Am. J. Pathol. 114:79, 1984.

51. Van Furth, R.: Current view on the mononuclear phagocyte system. Immunobiology 161:178, 1982.

52. Nathan, C. F., Murray, H. W., and Cohn, Z. A.: Current concepts: The macrophage as an effector cell. N. Engl. J. Med. 303:622, 1980.

53. Martin, T. R., Altman, L. C., Albert, R. K., and Henderson, W. R.: Leukotriene B4 production by human alveolar macrophage: A potential mechanism for amplifying inflammation in the lung. Am. Rev. Respir. Dis. 129:106, 1984.

54. Bevilacqua, M. P., Pober, J. S., Cotran, R. S., and Gimbrone, M. A. Jr.: Interleukin 1 (IL1) acts upon vascular endothelium to stimulate procoagulant activity and leukocyte adhesion. J. Cell. Biochem. Suppl. 9A:148, 1985.

55. Cathcart, M. K., Morel, D. W., and Chisolm, G., III.: Monocytes and neutrophils oxidize low-density lipoprotein making it cytotoxic. J. Leuk. Biol. 38:341, 1985.

56. Ross, R., Raines, E. W., and Bowen-Pope, D. F.: The biology of platelet-derived growth factor. Cell 46:155, 1986.

57. Shimokado, K., Raines, E. W., Madtes, D. K., et al.: A significant part of macrophage-derived growth factor consists of at least two forms of PDGF. Cell 43:277, 1985.

58. Raines, E. W., Dower, S. K., and Ross, R.: IL-1 mitogenic activity for fibroblasts and smooth muscle cells is due to PDGF-AA. Science 243:393, 1989.

59. Baird, A., Mormede, P., and Bohlen, P.: Immunoreactive fibroblast growth factor in cells of peritoneal exudate suggests its identity with macrophage-derived growth factor. Biochem. Biophys. Res. Commun. 126:358, 1985.

60. Ralph, P.: Colony stimulating factors. In Zembala, M., and Asherson, G. (eds.): Human Monocytes. New York, Academic Press, 1989, p. 228.

61. Holmsen, H., and Weiss, H. J.: Secretable storage pools in platelets. Annu. Rev. Med. 30:119, 1979.

62. Pepper, D. S.: Macromolecules released from platelet storage organelles. Thromb. Haemost. 42:1667, 1980.

63. Ross, R., Glomset, J., Kariya, B., and Harker, L.: A platelet-dependent serum factor that stimulates the proliferation of arterial smooth muscle cells in vitro. Proc. Natl. Acad. Sci. USA 71:1207, 1974.

64. Oka, Y., and Orth, D. N.: Human plasma epidermal growth factor/beta-urogastrone is associated with blood platelets. J. Clin. Invest. 72:249, 1983.

65. Assoian, R. K., Komoriya, A., Meyers, C. A., et al.: Transforming growth factor-β in human platelets. Identification of a major storage site, purification, and characterization. J. Biol. Chem. 258:7155, 1983.

66. Baumgartner, H. R.: Platelet-interaction with vascular structures. Thromb. Diath. Haemorrh. 51(Suppl.):161, 1972.

67. Jonasson, L., Holm, J., Skalli, O., et al: Regional accumulations of T cells, macrophages, and smooth muscle cells in the human atherosclerotic plaque. Arteriosclerosis 6:131, 1986.

68. Gown, A. M., Tsukada, T., and Ross, R.: Human atherosclerosis: II. Immunocytochemical analysis of the cellular composition of human atherosclerotic lesions. Am. J. Pathol. 125:191, 1986.

69. Munro, J. M., van der Walt, J. D., Munro, C. S., et al.: An immunohistochemical analysis of human aortic fatty streaks. Hum. Pathol. 18:375, 1987.

70. Emeson, E. E., and Robertson, A. L.: T lymphocytes in aortic and coronary intimas. Their potential role in atherogenesis. Am. J. Pathol. 130:369, 1988.

71. Minick, C. R., and Murphy, G. E.: Experimental induction of atheroarteriosclerosis by the synergy of allergic injury to arteries and lipid-rich diet: II. Effect of repeated injections of horse serum in rabbits fed a lipid-rich, cholesterol-poor diet. Am. J. Pathol. 73:265, 1973.

72. Hansson, G. K., Holm, J., and Jonasson, L.: Detection of activated T lymphocytes in the human atherosclerotic plaque. Am. J. Pathol. 135:169, 1989.

73. Hansson, G. K., Jonasson, L., Holm, J., and Claesson-Welsh, L.: MHC antigen expression in the atherosclerotic plaque: Smooth muscle cells express HLA-DR, HLA-DQ, and the invariant gamma chain. Clin. Exp. Immunol. 64:261, 1986.

THE LESIONS OF ATHEROSCLEROSIS

74. McGill, H. C., Jr. (ed.): The Geographic Pathology of Atherosclerosis. Baltimore, Williams and Wilkins, 1968.

75. Geer, J. C., McGill, H. C., Jr., and Strong, J. P.: The fine structure of human atherosclerotic lesions. Am. J. Pathol. 38:263, 1961.

76. Geer, J. C.: Fine structure of human aortic intimal thickening and fatty streaks. Lab. Invest. 14:1764, 1965.

77. Ghidoni, J. J., and O'Neal, R. M.: Recent advances in molecular pathology. A review: Ultrastructure of human atheroma. Exp. Mol. Pathol. 7:378, 1967.

78. Stary, H. C.: Evolution of atherosclerotic plaques in the coronary arteries of young adults. Arteriosclerosis 3:471a, 1983.

79. McGill, H. C., Jr.: Persistent problems in the pathogenesis of atherosclerosis. Arteriosclerosis 4:443, 1984.

80. Tsukada, T., Rosenfeld, M., Ross, R., and Gown, A. M.: Immunocytochemical analysis of cellular components in atherosclerotic lesions. Use of monoclonal antibodies with the Watanabe and fat-fed rabbit. Arteriosclerosis 6:601, 1986.

81. Glagov, S., and Ozoa, A.: Significance of the relatively low incidence of atherosclerosis in the pulmonary, renal and mesenteric arteries. Ann. N.Y. Acad. Sci. 149:940, 1968.

82. Strong, J. P., Eggen, D. A., and Oalmann, M. C.: The natural history, geographic pathology, and epidemiology of atherosclerosis. In Wissler, R. W., and Geer, J. C. (eds.): The Pathogenesis of Atherosclerosis. Baltimore, Williams and Wilkins, 1972, p. 20.

83. Glagov, S., Rowley, D. A., Cramer, D. B., and Page, R. G.: Heart rate during 24 hours of usual activity in 100 normal men. J. Appl. Physiol. 29:799, 1970.

84. Wissler, R. W., and Vesselinovitch, D.: Atherosclerosis—relationship to coronary blood flow. Am. J. Cardiol. 52(2):2A, 1983.

THE HYPOTHESES OF ATHEROGENESIS

85. Virchow, R.: Phlogose und thrombose in gefassystem, gesammelte abhandlungen zur wissenschaftlichen medicin. Frankfurt-am-Main, Meidinger Sohn and Co., 1856, p. 458.

86. von Rokitansky, C.: A Manual of Pathological Anatomy, translated by Day, G. E. Vol. 4. London, The Sydenham Society, 1852.

87. Duguid, J. B.: Thrombosis as a factor in the pathogenesis of coronary atherosclerosis. J. Pathol. Bacteriol. 58:207, 1946.

88. Ross, R.: Atherosclerosis—a problem of the biology of arterial wall cells and their interaction with blood components. Arteriosclerosis 1:293, 1981.

89. Leary, T.: The genesis of atherosclerosis. Arch. Pathol. 32:507, 1941.

90. Parthasarathy, S., Quinn, M. T., Schwenke, D. C., et al.: Oxidative modification of beta-very low density lipoprotein. Potential role in monocyte recruitment and foam cell formation. Arteriosclerosis 9:398, 1989.

91. Assoian, R. K., Grotendorst, G. R., Miller, D. M., and Sporn, M. B.: Cellular transformation by coordinated action of three peptide growth factors from human platelets. Nature 309:804, 1984.

92. Sporn, M. B., Roberts, A. B., Wakefield, L. M., and de Crombrugghe, B.: Some recent advances in the chemistry and biology of transforming growth factor-beta. J. Cell Biol. 105:1039, 1987.

93. Ross, R., Masuda, J., Raines, E. W., et al.: Localization of PDGF-B protein in macrophages in all phases of atherogenesis. Science 248:1009, 1990.

94. Stemerman, M. B., and Ross, R.: Experimental arteriosclerosis: I. Fibrous plaque formation in primates, an electron microscope study. J. Exp. Med. 136:769, 1972.

95. Sheppard, B. L., and French, J. E.: Platelet adhesion in the rabbit abdominal aorta following the removal of the endothelium: A scanning and

transmission electron microscopical study. Proc. R. Soc. Lond. (Biol.) *176*:427, 1971.

96. More, S.: Thromboatherosclerosis in normolipemic rabbits: A result of continued endothelial damage. Lab. Invest. *29*:478, 1973.

97. Friedman, R. J., Moore, S., and Singal, D. P.: Repeated endothelial injury and induction of atherosclerosis in normolipemic rabbits by human serum. Lab. Invest. *32*:404, 1975.

98. Harker, L. A., Ross, R., Slichter, S. J., and Scott, C. R.: Homocystine-induced arteriosclerosis: The role of endothelial cell injury and platelet response in genesis. J. Clin. Invest. *58*:731, 1976.

99. Libby, P., Warner, S. J. C., Salomon, R. N., and Birinyi, L. K.: Production of platelet-derived growth factor-like mitogen by smooth-muscle cells from human atheroma. N. Engl. J. Med. *318*:1493, 1988.

100. Lindner, D., and Gartler, S. M.: Glucose-6-phosphate dehydrogenase mosaicism: Utilization as a cell marker in the study of leiomyomas. Science *150*:67, 1965.

101. Hajjar, D. P. Fabricant, C. G., Minick, C. R., and Fabricant, J.: Virus-induced artheriosclerosis: Herpesvirus infection alters aortic cholesterol metabolism and accumulation. Am. J. Pathol. *122*:62, 1986.

102. Fialkow, P. J.: Use of genetic markers to study cellular origin and development of tumor in human females. Adv. Cancer Res. *15*:191, 1972.

LIPIDS AND LIPOPROTEINS IN ATHEROSCLEROSIS

103. Jackson, R. L., and Gotto, A. M., Jr.: Hypothesis concerning membrane structure, cholesterol, and atherosclerosis. *In* Paoletti, R., and Gotto, A. M., Jr. (eds.): Atherosclerosis Reviews. Vol. 1. New York, Raven Press, 1976, p 1.

104. Carew, T., Schwenke, D. C., and Steinberg, D.: Antiatherogenic effect of probucol unrelated to its hypocholesterolemic effect: Evidence that the antioxidants in vivo can selectively inhibit low density lipoprotein degradation in macrophage-rich fatty streaks and slow the progression of atherosclerosis in the Watanabe heritable hyperlipidemic (WHHL) rabbit. Proc. Natl. Acad. Sci. USA *84*:7725, 1987.

105. Kita, T., Nagano, Y., Yokode, M., et al.: Probucol prevents the progression of atherosclerosis in Watanabe heritable hyperlipidemic rabbit, an animal model for familial hypercholestrolemia. Proc. Natl. Acad. Sci. USA *84*:5928, 1987.

106. Boyd, H. C., Gown, A. M., Wolfbauer, G., and Chait A.: Direct evidence for a protein recognized by a monoclonal antibody against oxidatively modified LDL in atherosclerotic lesions from a Watanabe heritable hyperlipidemic rabbit. Am. J. Pathol. *135*:815, 1989.

GROWTH FACTORS

107. Heldin, C.-H., Westermark, B., and Wasteson, A.: Platelet-derived growth factor: Purification and partial characterization. Proc. Natl. Acad. Sci. USA *76*:3722, 1979.

108. Antoniades, H. N.: Human platelet-derived growth factor (PDGF): Purification of PDGF-I and PDGF-II and separation of their reduced subunits. Proc. Natl. Acad. Sci. USA *78*:7314, 1981.

109. Raines, E. W., and Ross, R.: Platelet-derived growth factor: I. High yield purification and evidence for multiple forms. J. Biol. Chem. *257*:5154, 1982.

110. Huang, J. S., Huang, S. S., Kennedy, B., and Deuel, T. F.: Platelet-derived growth factor: Specific binding to target cells. J. Biol. Chem. *257*:8130, 1982.

111. Heldin, C.-H., Westermark, B., and Wasteson, A.: Specific receptors for platelet-derived growth factors on cells derived from connective tissue and glia. Proc. Natl. Acad. Sci. USA *78*:3664, 1981.

112. Bowen-Pope, D. F., and Ross, R.: Platelet-derived growth factor: II. Specific binding to cultured cells. J. Biol. Chem. *257*:5161, 1982.

113. Grotendorst, G., Seppa, H. E. J., Kleinman, H. K., and Martin, G.: Attachment of smooth muscle cells to collagen and their migration toward platelet-derived growth factor. Proc. Natl. Acad. Sci. USA *78*:3669, 1981.

114. Grotendorst, G. R., Chang, T., Seppa, H. E. J., et al.: Platelet-derived growth factor is a chemoattractant for vascular smooth muscle cells. J. Cell. Physiol. *113*:261, 1982.

115. Witte, L. D., and Cornicelli, J. A.: Platelet-derived growth factor stimulates low density lipoprotein receptor activity in cultured human fibroblasts. Proc. Natl. Acad. Sci. USA *77*:5962, 1980.

116. Bowen-Pope, D. F., Malpass, T. W., Foster, D. M., and Ross, R.: Platelet-derived growth factor in vivo: Levels, activity, and rate of clearance. Blood *46*:458, 1984.

117. Raines, E. W., Bowen-Pope, D. F., and Ross, R.: Plasma binding proteins for platelet-derived growth factor that inhibit its binding to cell-surface receptors. Proc. Natl. Acad. Sci. USA *81*:3424, 1984.

118. Doolittle, R. F., Hunkapiller, M. W., Hood, L. E., et al.: Simian sarcoma virus onc gene, v-sis, is derived from the gene (or genes) encoding a platelet-derived growth factor. Science *221*:275, 1983.

119. Waterfield, M. D., Scrace, G. T., Whittle, N., et al.: Platelet-derived growth factor is structurally related to the putative transforming protein P[28sis] of simian sarcoma virus. Nature *304*:35, 1983.

120. Bowen-Pope, D. F., Vogel, A., and Ross, R.: Production of platelet-derived growth factor-like molecules and reduced expression of platelet-derived growth factor receptors accompany transformation by a wide spectrum of agents. Proc. Natl. Acad. Sci. USA *81*:2396, 1984.

121. Seifert, R. A., Hart, C. E., Phillips, P. E., et al.: Two different subunits associate to create isoform-specific platelet-derived growth factor receptors. J. Biol. Chem. *264*:8771, 1989.

CELLULAR EVENTS THAT OCCUR DURING ATHEROSCLEROSIS

122. Faggiotto, A., Ross, R., and Harker, L.: Studies of hypercholesterolemia in the nonhuman primate: I. Changes that lead to fatty streak formation. Arteriosclerosis *4*:323, 1984.

123. Faggiotto, A., and Ross, R.: Studies of hypercholesterolemia in the nonhuman primate: II. Fatty streak conversion to fibrous plaque. Arteriosclerosis *4*:341, 1984.

124. Masuda, J., and Ross, R.: Atherogenesis during low-level hypercholesterolemia in the nonhuman primate: I. Fatty streak formation. Arteriosclerosis *10*:164, 1990.

125. Masuda, J., and Ross, R.: Atherogenesis during low-level hypercholesterolemia in the nonhuman primate: II. Fatty streak conversion to fibrous plaque. Arteriosclerosis *10*:178, 1990.

126. Gerrity, R. G., Naito, H. K., Richardson, M., and Schwartz, C. J.: Dietary induced atherogenesis in swine: Morphology of the intima in prelesion stages. Am. J. Pathol. *95*:775, 1979.

127. Gerrity, R. G.: The role of the monocyte in atherogenesis: I. Transition of blood-borne monocytes into foam cells in fatty lesions. Am. J. Pathol. *103*:181, 1981.

128. Gerrity, R. G., Goss, J. A., and Soby, L.: Control of monocyte recruitment by chemotactic factor(s) in lesion-prone areas of swine aorta. Arteriosclerosis *5*:55, 1985.

129. Rosenfeld, M. E., Faggiotto, A., and Ross, R.: The role of the mononuclear phagocyte in primate and rabbit models of atherosclerosis. *In* Van Furth, R. (ed.): Mononuclear Phagocytes: Characteristics, Physiology, and Function. The Hague, Netherlands, Martinus Nijhoff, 1985, p. 795.

130. Reidy, M. A., and Schwartz, S. M.: Endothelial regeneration: III. Time course of intimal changes after small defined injury to rat aortic endothelium. Lab. Invest. *44*:301, 1981.

131. Reidy, M. A., and Schwartz, S. M.: Endothelial injury and regeneration: IV. Endotoxin: A nondenuding injury to aortic endothelium. Lab. Invest. *48*:25, 1983.

132. Hansson, G. K., Bondjers, G., Bylock, A., and Hjalmarsson, L: Ultrastructural studies on nonatherosclerotic rabbits. Exp. Mol. Pathol. *33*:301, 1980.

133. Reidy, M. A., and Schwartz, S. M.: Recent advances in molecular pathology: Arterial endothelium—assessment of in vivo injury. Exp. Mol. Pathol. *41*:419, 1984.

REGRESSION OF ATHEROSCLEROSIS

134. Armstrong, M. L., Warner, E. D., and Conner, W. E.: Regression of coronary atheromatosis in rhesus monkeys. Circ. Res. *27*:59, 1970.

135. Wissler, R. W., and Vesselinovitch, D.: Studies of regression of advanced atherosclerosis in experimental animals and man. Ann. N.Y. Acad. Sci. *275*:363, 1976.

136. Clarkson, T. B., Bond, M. G., Bullock, B. C., et al.: A study of atherosclerosis regression in Macaca mulatta: V. Changes in abdominal aorta and carotid and coronary arteries from animals with atherosclerosis induced for 38 months and then regressed for 24 or 48 months at plasma cholesterol concentrations of 300 or 200 mg/dl. Exp. Mol. Pathol. *41*:96, 1984.

137. Brown, B. G., Albers, J. J., Fisher, L. D., et al.: Familial atherosclerosis treatment study: A randomized trial demonstrating coronary disease regression and clinical benefit from lipid-altering therapy among men with high apolipoprotein-B. N. Engl. J. Med. in press.

138. Cannon, P. J.: Eicosanoids and the blood vessel wall. Circulation *70*:00, 1984.

THROMBOSIS

139. Chesebro, J. H., Clements, L. P., Fuster, V., et al.: A platelet-inhibitor-drug trial in coronary-artery bypass operations. Benefit of perioperative dipyridamole and aspirin therapy on early postoperative vein-graft patency. N. Engl. J. Med. *307*:73, 1982.

Risk Factors for Coronary Artery Disease

by JOHN A. FARMER, M.D., and ANTONIO M. GOTTO, Jr., M.D., D.Phil.

DECLINING MORTALITY

Great progress against specific aspects of coronary artery disease (CAD) has been made over the past 40 years. For example, in 1950, the United States age-adjusted mortality rate from myocardial infarction was 226.4 per 100,000 people. By 1987 that rate had dropped to 124.1 per 100,000. Over the same period, the age-adjusted mortality rates from strokes and hypertension per 100,000 fell from 88.8 and 56.0, respectively, to 30.7 and 6.6.[1] These declining mortality rates mask the fact that CAD remains the major cause of death among Americans. In 1988, cardiovascular disease claimed 982,579 American lives (45.3 per cent of all deaths in the United States), and 511,050 of those deaths were due to CAD.[1] Moreover, the CAD mortality rate remains higher in the United States than in other industrialized nations. According to the World Health Organization, 55 of every 100,000 Americans die of CAD each year. That compares with CAD mortality rates of 33 and 15 per 100,000 people in Switzerland and Japan, respectively. Further progress against CAD in the United States may depend in part on whether we can precisely identify the factors behind the declining CAD mortality rates recorded since the 1950's and on whether we can continue to affect these factors positively.

Between 1968 and 1976, the age-adjusted mortality from CAD in the United States progressively declined by 20 per cent.[2] Goldman and Cook in 1984 estimated that more than half of that decline was related to lifestyle changes, specifically to decreases in serum cholesterol and cigarette smoking.[2a] They attributed as much as 24 per cent of the CAD reduction to smoking cessation. Dietary changes would also appear to be crucial. Since the 1950's, Americans have been eating less saturated fat and red meat and fewer dairy products while eating more polyunsaturated fats. Public concern about "heart-healthy" eating has grown stronger with each recent decade. The U.S. antihypertension campaign of the 1970's also is cited as a possible explanation for the declining CAD mortality rates during recent years. The declining rate of fatal cerebrovascular events, in particular, apparently reflects the growing awareness of hypertension as a cardiovascular risk factor, as well as the improved availability and effectiveness of well-tolerated antihypertensive agents. However, these advances against hypertension have not translated into fewer deaths from CAD. Indeed, clinical studies have indicated that some of the widely used antihypertensives, although they successfully lower blood pressure, tend to increase serum cholesterol levels, a result that negates the expected benefits of lower blood pressure on CAD mortality.

Other factors that have had a beneficial effect on CAD mortality rates in the United States include improvements in prehospital care, greater availability of coronary care units, the introduction of thrombolytic therapy and percutaneous transluminal angioplasty, and refinements in surgical techniques. Diagnostic advances such as thallium scintigraphy, gated wall-motion stress tests, and positron-emission tomography probably have not yet had an important impact on CAD mortality. But these imaging techniques are expected to cause further reductions in CAD mortality, especially among patients with subclinical or clinically manifest coronary atherosclerosis. That coronary artery bypass surgery has become part of common medical practice also should reduce these rates.

Because no single factor can be cited as the sole catalyst for the declining CAD mortality rates in the past, it is logical to assume that no one factor will be totally responsible for any mortality reductions in the future. Indeed, our ability to collectively identify and manage CAD risk factors will profoundly affect our efforts to maintain the trend of declining CAD mortality rates well into the 21st century. With this in mind, our goal here is to identify the risk factors for CAD and to review the current guidelines for their diagnosis and effective management.

DYSLIPIDEMIA

Dyslipidemia is one of three major modifiable risk factors for CAD. Hypertension and smoking, the other two such factors, are discussed in a later section.

Dyslipidemia has numerous forms, from hypercholesterolemia to hypoalphalipoproteinemia. The term itself simply refers to an abnormal metabolism of plasma lipids. This abnormal metabolism can be caused by genetic, dietary, or secondary disease factors. The various types of dyslipidemia, their probable causes, and the suggested treatment regimens for each are discussed later in this section. The traditional definition of hyperlipoproteinemia has been based on plasma cholesterol levels exceeding the 95th percentile value for age and sex, in comparison with measurements in a comparable nonrestricted population. The Lipid Research Clinics data provide the most complete sets available (Table 37–1).

TABLE 37-1 REFERENCE VALUES FOR PLASMA CHOLESTEROL AND LIPOPROTEIN CHOLESTEROL

	PLASMA CHOLESTEROL					LDL CHOLESTEROL				HDL CHOLESTEROL			
PERCENTILE	5	50	75	90	95	5	50	75	95	5	10	50	95
AGE (YR)													
Men													
5–19	115	155	170	185	200	65	95	105	130	35*	40*	55*	75*
20–24	125	165	185	205	220	65	105	120	145	30	30	45	65
25–29	135	180	200	225	245	70	115	140	165	30	30	45	65
30–34	140	190	215	240	255	80	125	145	185	30	30	45	60
35–39	145	200	225	250	270	80	135	155	190	30	30	45	60
40–44	150	205	230	250	270	85	135	155	185	25	30	45	65
45–69	160	215	235	260	275	90	145	165	205	30	30	50	70
70+	150	205	230	250	270	90	145	165	185	30	35	50	75
Women													
5–19	120	160	175	190	200	65	100	110	140	35	40	55	70
20–24	125	170	190	215	230	55	105	120	160	35	35	55	80
25–34	130	175	195	220	235	70	110	125	160	35	40	55	80
35–39	140	185	205	230	245	75	120	140	170	35	40	55	80
40–44	145	195	215	235	255	75	125	145	175	35	40	60	90
45–49	150	205	225	250	270	80	130	150	185	35	40	60	85
50–54	165	220	240	265	285	90	140	160	200	35	40	60	90
55+	170	230	250	295	295	95	150	170	215	35	40	60	95

From the Lipid Research Clinics Population Studies Data Book. Vol. 1: The Prevalence Study, Washington, D.C., U.S. Government Printing Office, 1988. USDHHS/NIH pub. no. 88-1927.
* For HDL values for men aged 15–19 yr use values for age group 20–24 yr.
HDL = high-density lipoprotein; LDL = low-density lipoprotein.

PLASMA LIPOPROTEINS

The major classes of plasma lipids are cholesterol, cholesteryl ester, triglyceride, and phospholipid. Although lipids are vital components of many of the body's tissues, they are insoluble in water. To reach those tissues, lipids must be transported in the bloodstream by complex, water-soluble molecules called *lipoproteins*. Structurally, lipoproteins consist of a core of nonpolar cholesteryl ester and triglyceride covered by a polar surface monolayer made up of phospholipids, free cholesterol, and the protein or polypeptide moieties called apolipoproteins, or apoproteins (apos) (Table 37–2). Each of the plasma lipids has one or more apoproteins that perform specific functions essential to lipid transport and cellular uptake (Figs. 37–1 and 37–2).

The five principal lipoprotein classes are defined according to their density on ultracentrifugation and by their mobility on agarose gel electrophoresis. In addition, they can be classified on the basis of size and relative concentrations of cholesterol or triglyceride and by their apoprotein content. The major lipoprotein classes are chylomicrons, very-low-density lipoproteins (VLDLs), intermediate-density lipoproteins (IDLs), low-density lipoproteins (LDLs), and high-density lipoproteins (HDLs).

CHYLOMICRONS. Chylomicrons are the largest of the lipoproteins. Their primary function is to transport dietary, or exogenous, triglyceride and cholesterol from the intestinal lumen to sites of metabolism or storage. The chylomicrons are formed in the gastrointestinal (GI) tract. In the lumen of the GI tract, dietary fat is degraded into free fatty acids and monoglycerides. These substances enter the intestinal villi, where they are reconstructed into a triglyceride particle. Dietary cholesterol absorbed into the intestinal wall is then esterified to cholesteryl esters, mainly cholesteryl oleate, by the enzymatic reaction catalyzed by acyl:cholesterol acyltransferase. The triglyceride and cholesteryl esters are then combined with apos B-48, A-I, and A-IV within the intestinal wall to form chylomicron particles.

The nascent chylomicrons enter the systemic circulation by way of the lymphatics. Apos E and C are then added to the

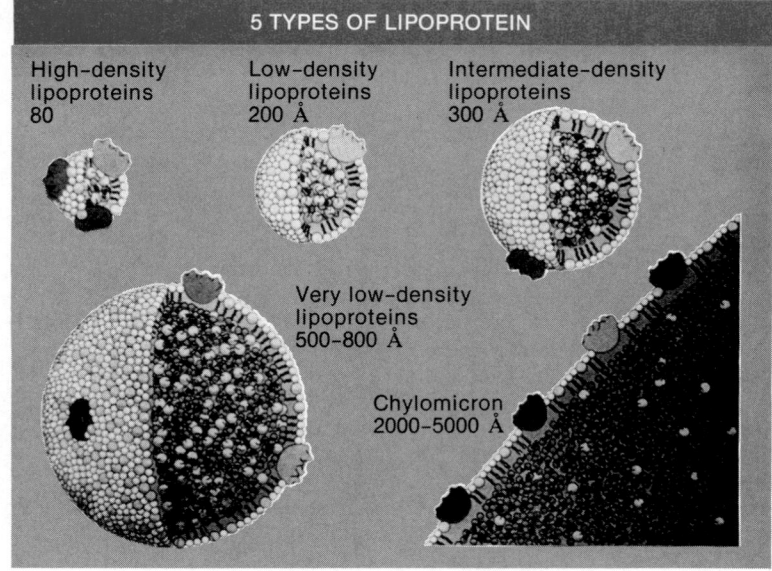

5 TYPES OF LIPOPROTEIN

High-density lipoproteins 80

Low-density lipoproteins 200 Å

Intermediate-density lipoproteins 300 Å

Very low-density lipoproteins 500–800 Å

Chylomicron 2000–5000 Å

FIGURE 37–1. The major categories of circulating lipoproteins differ as to size, relative lipid composition, electrophoretic mobility, and apoprotein content. Chylomicrons are large, triglyceride-rich particles that are formed in the wall of the intestine and carry dietary fat. Very low-density lipoproteins are smaller, triglyceride-rich particles of hepatic origin. Intermediate-density lipoproteins are formed from very low-density lipoprotein catabolism and are recognized by the apoprotein B/E receptor. The low-density lipoprotein particle has only apoprotein B-100 on its surface and is highly correlated with atherosclerosis risk. High-density lipoproteins are the smallest of the major lipoproteins and act in reverse cholesterol transport. (From Federman, D. D., and Rubenstein, E. (eds.): Scientific American Medicine, Section 9, Subsection II. © 1987 Scientific American, Inc., All rights reserved.)

TABLE 37-2 COMPOSITION AND PROPERTIES OF HUMAN PLASMA LIPOPROTEINS

PROPERTIES	CHYLOMICRONS	VLDL	IDL	LDL	HDL
Density (gm/ml)	0.95	0.95–1.006	1.006–1.019	1.019–1.063	1.061–1.210
Electrophoretic mobility	Origin	Pre-Beta	Beta	Beta	Alpha
Major lipid constituents	Triglyceride (exogenous)	Triglyceride (endogenous), phospholipid	Esterified cholesterol, phospholipid	Triglyceride, esterified cholesterol	Phospholipid, cholesterol
Apoprotein constituents	Apo A-I Apo II Apo IV Apo B-48	Apo B-100 Apo C-I Apo C-II Apo C-III Apo E	Apo B-100 Apo E	Apo B-100	Apo A-I Apo A-II Apo C-II Apo E

From Beigel, Y., and Gotto, A.: Lipoproteins in Health and Disease: Diagnosis and Management. The Baylor College of Medicine Cardiology Series 9:6, No. 1., 1986. Used with permission, Associates in Medical Marketing Co., Inc.

HDL = high-density lipoprotein; IDL = intermediate-density lipoprotein; LDL = low-density lipoprotein; VLDL = very low-density lipoprotein.

particles. Normally, the chylomicrons are cleared rapidly from the blood and are virtually absent in the fasting state. The clearing of the chylomicrons is modulated by the enzyme lipoprotein lipase (LPL). LPL catalyzes hydrolysis of the triglyceride core of the chylomicron, leaving a remnant particle rich in cholesterol, apo C, apo E, and apo B-48. During this process, apoproteins, phospholipids, and cholesterol from the surface of the chylomicron are transferred to HDL particles. The chylomicron remnants are cleared rapidly from the circulation by receptors present on the surface of liver cells. These receptors recognize the apo E component of the remnant particle. Remnants that contain the apo E_2 moiety bind less well, and are thus removed less quickly, than remnants that contain either the apo E_3 or E_4 moiety. The chylomicron remnant receptor, possibly identical to the LDL receptor–related entity, does not appear to be down-regulated as remnant particles are taken up.

Chylomicron remnants are thought to be atherogenic, and an abnormal delay in their clearance is therefore undesirable. Delays in chylomicron clearance may be secondary to a genetically inherited deficiency of LPL or its activator, apo C-II. Interestingly, in the most severe forms of these conditions,

which produce fasting hyperchylomicronemia syndromes, accelerated atherogenesis does not appear to be a clinical feature. Instead, it is partial degradation of the chylomicron to a remnant that renders the particle atherogenic. Delayed clearance of the remnant particles may damage the vascular endothelium, and thus predispose to atherosclerosis.

Hyperchylomicronemia also may be secondary to other acquired hypertriglyceridemic states, such as those seen with exogenous estrogen use, uncontrolled diabetes, and excessive alcohol intake. The presence of chylomicrons in the serum is necessary for the diagnosis of type I or V hyperlipoproteinemia in the Fredrickson and Lees classification system (see Typing of Hyperlipoproteinemia).

VERY LOW-DENSITY LIPOPROTEIN. VLDLs are intermediate in size between chylomicrons and IDLs. They are relatively large particles, with diameters ranging from 500 to 800 Å. VLDLs are produced in the liver. Their primary lipid component is triglyceride, but cholesterol, cholesteryl ester, and phospholipid are also present. Their surface components are apos B-100, C, and E and phospholipid. The synthesis of VLDL is increased by excess carbohydrate, alcohol, or caloric consumption. The function of VLDL is to transport endoge-

FIGURE 37-2. Model for plasma triglyceride and cholesterol transport in humans. VLDL, very low-density lipoprotein; IDL, intermediate-density lipoprotein; LDL, low-density lipoprotein; HDL, high-density lipoprotein; LCAT, lecithin:cholesterol acyltransferase; LP lipase, lipoprotein lipase; FFA, free fatty acids. The major apoprotein for each class of lipoproteins is shown. In HDL, apo E is a minor but crucial apoprotein. In chylomicrons, apo E and apo C-II are minor but crucial; they are added in the lymph or after the chylomicrons reach the circulation. (From Brown, M. S., and Goldstein, J. L.: The hyperlipoproteinemias and other disorders of lipid metabolism. In Wilson, J. E., et al. (eds.): Harrison's Principles of Internal Medicine. 12th ed. New York, McGraw-Hill, 1991, p. 1816.)

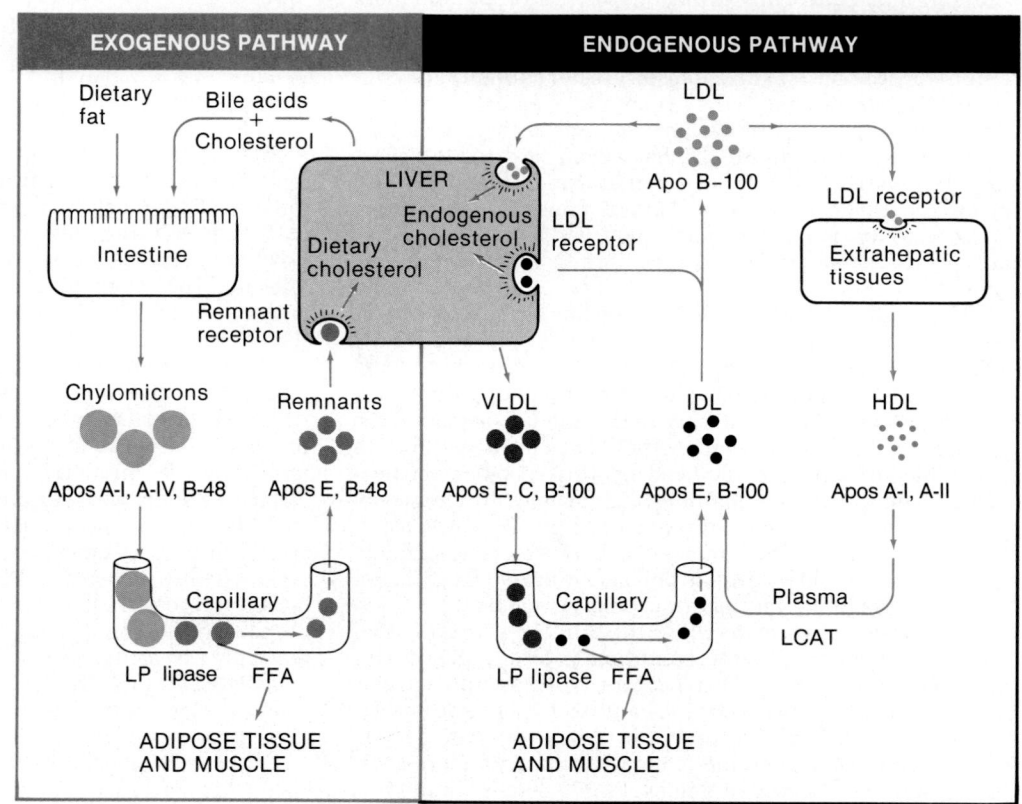

nously synthesized triglycerides and cholesterol into the peripheral tissues, where the lipids' fatty acids can be utilized for energy or stored as triglyceride.

When VLDL particles enter the systemic circulation, their triglyceride core is hydrolyzed by LPL. As the VLDL particle is degraded, most of its surface apoproteins, except for apo B-100, are transferred with other surface components to HDL. The remaining VLDL remnant is called IDL. Unlike the chylomicron remnant, IDL contains apo B-100 rather than apo B-48. The metabolism of VLDL is complex and not fully understood. Some of the larger particles appear to be directly removed from the circulation. The rest of the particles enter the cascade, in which they are converted to IDL and eventually to LDL, as discussed below.

INTERMEDIATE-DENSITY LIPOPROTEIN. IDLs, which carry both cholesterol and triglyceride, are the product of the enzymatic (LPL-mediated) breakdown of VLDL. After their formation, IDLs may be removed by the liver by means of the binding of apo E to the LDL, or B/E, receptor. The remainder are converted to LDL, a process thought to be mediated by hepatic triglyceride lipase. IDLs have a high cholesterol content and migrate in the beta region on electrophoresis. Elevations of IDLs are thought to predispose to premature CAD and peripheral artery disease. Accumulation of IDL is characteristic of dysbetalipoproteinemia, also called Fredrickson's type III hyperlipoproteinemia. This relatively uncommon form of hyperlipoproteinemia is associated with both triglyceride and cholesterol elevations (see Typing of Hyperlipoproteinemia, p. 1135).

LOW-DENSITY LIPOPROTEIN. LDL, which is 45 per cent cholesterol by weight, is the major carrier of cholesterol to the nerve tissues, cell membranes, and other cells that require the cholesterol for metabolic functions, including the synthesis of steroid hormones. LDLs have a density of 1.019 to 1.063 gm/ml, a diameter of 180 to 280 Å, and beta electrophoretic mobility. LDL usually is formed from VLDL breakdown. Direct synthesis has not been completely excluded. Increased LDL synthesis may occur by means of enhanced conversion of VLDL remnants or direct hepatic production of apo B–containing lipoproteins.

Apo B-100 is the only protein found in LDL, and makes up about 20 per cent of the LDL mass. Each particle is thought to contain 1 molecule of apo B-100, but the ratio of protein mass to total particle mass can vary from the large to the small particle range. LDL particles are heterogeneous, differing in their hydrated density and cholesteryl ester content. The content of cholesteryl ester in the LDL particle, for example, may vary up to 40 per cent by weight. Patients with greater concentrations of small, dense LDL have been reported to have a three-times greater risk for acute myocardial infarction (MI), regardless of weight or gender.[3] Small, dense LDL molecules are commonly associated with male gender, diabetes, depressed HDL levels, and familial combined hyperlipoproteinemia.

LDL particles are recognized by specific LDL, or apo B/E, receptors on the surfaces of hepatic and certain nonhepatic cells (Fig. 37–2). These receptors also recognize and bind some of the apo E–containing IDL particles, preventing their conversion into LDL. Bound LDL particles (and IDL particles) are then internalized into the cells.[4] About 75 per cent of the LDLs in the bloodstream are removed by this specific receptor-mediated binding. The remaining LDL particles are cleared by scavenger, or macrophage, receptors or by non-receptor-mediated mechanisms. The number of LDL receptors is not fixed, and can be modified by genetic defects, saturated fat and cholesterol intake, or certain pharmacological agents.

The prototype disease involving the LDL receptor is familial hypercholesterolemia. In this condition, heterozygotes have a 50 per cent reduction in LDL receptors, whereas homozygotes have little or no receptor activity. Familial hypercholesterolemia is fairly common, occurring in 1 in every 500 people. Familial combined hyperlipidemia (FCH) is even more common, possibly occurring in 1 in every 300 people. Clinically,

FCH patients may be difficult to differentiate from those with familial hypercholesterolemia. In FCH, most patients lack tendon xanthomas and the hyperlipidemia does not present in childhood; most family studies show varying Fredrickson's phenotypes.

The characteristic defect in FCH is thought to be an overproduction of apo B-100 by the liver.[5,6] Also, FCH patients have a lower ratio of apo A-I to apo B-100. About 80 per cent of patients with an elevated LDL value do not have only one gene defect; the dyslipidemia is secondary to polygenic factors. Hence, elevations of LDL due to primary receptor defects are relatively uncommon.

HIGH-DENSITY LIPOPROTEIN. HDLs are produced by the liver and the GI tract and by the peripheral catabolism of chylomicrons and VLDLs. HDL particles carry cholesteryl ester as their major lipid and apos A-I and A-II as their major proteins. Much of the apoprotein component of HDL is transferred in the systemic circulation to VLDLs or chylomicrons. Apo C-II, an obligatory activator of LPL, is one of the apoproteins transferred by HDL. By weight, HDL particles are about 30 per cent cholesterol, 45 per cent protein, and 25 per cent phospholipid (predominantly phosphatidylcholine). Small amounts of triglycerides are present.

HDL particles exist in several subtypes. For clinical purposes, HDL_2 and HDL_3 are the major circulating subfractions. HDL_2, which migrates with alpha mobility, is the subfraction most closely associated with statistical protection against premature atherosclerosis. It has a density of 1.061 to 1.25 gm/ml and a diameter of 90 to 120 Å. HDL_3 is a smaller particle, with a density of 1.125 to 1.210 gm/ml and a diameter of 50 to 90 Å. Alcohol consumption increases both HDL subfractions, with a greater impact on HDL_3. Lower levels of both subfractions are associated with male gender; hypertriglyceridemia; diabetes mellitus; obesity; uremia; the use of androgens, progestins, or tobacco products; and diets rich in polyunsaturated fat but low in total fat content.

Several epidemiological studies have addressed whether there is a varying clinical impact on CAD depending on the relative levels of HDL_2 and HDL_3.[7] In males with CAD who have an associated low level of circulating HDL, both fractions of HDL are depressed with more of a decline in HDL_2. The initial National Cholesterol Education Program (NCEP) guidelines (see below) do not recommend routine screening of HDL levels. In the authors' opinion, however, a complete lipoprotein profile, including determination of HDL levels, should be obtained in any patient with established CAD. In their own practice, they measure HDL cholesterol in anyone with a total cholesterol value exceeding 200 mg/dl.

HDL particles are thought to participate in the reverse transport of free cholesterol from peripheral tissues by way of a putative HDL receptor. Oram and coworkers[8] report that apos A-I and A-II interact with this receptor. This receptor-mediated reverse transport could explain why patients with elevated HDL concentrations are less prone to CAD.

Another explanation for the inverse relation between HDL levels and CAD incidence may be related to the observation that most patients with low levels of HDL have elevated levels of the more cholesterol- and triglyceride-rich lipoproteins. In this case, low HDL levels may serve only as a marker for other, concurrent lipid abnormalities. Hence, the independent clinical impact of low HDL concentrations is difficult to determine.[9] Patients with certain variant forms of apo A-I, such as A-I Milano, may have decreased levels of HDL without evidence of accelerated atherosclerosis.

Just as low levels of HDL are statistically associated with atherosclerosis, HDL is increased on a genetic basis in *familial hyperapolipoproteinemia*. This condition has been described as being associated with longevity.

LIPOPROTEIN (a) (see also p. 1780). Lipoprotein (a), or Lp(a), has been established as an independent CAD risk factor. The structure of Lp(a) is similar to that of an LDL molecule whose apo B-100 is linked by a disulfide bridge to apoprotein (a). It has a density of 1.05 to 1.12 gm/ml and a size of about

TABLE 37-3 SUMMARY OF APOPROTEINS

NAME	LIPOPROTEIN	MOLECULAR WEIGHT	FUNCTION
apo A-I	HDL, chylomicrons*	28,000	Structural; activator of LCAT enzyme
apo A-II	HDL, chylomicrons	16,000	Structural
apo A-IV	HDL, chylomicrons,* VLDL	46,000	Unknown
apo B-100	LDL, VLDL	550,000	Structural; synthesis and secretion of VLDL; binds to LDL receptor (B/E)
apo B-48	Chylomicrons	250,000	Structural; synthesis and secretion from intestine
apo C-I	HDL, chylomicrons, VLDL	6,000	Activator of LCAT
apo C-II	HDL, chylomicrons, VLDL	7,000	Activator of lipoprotein lipase
apo C-III	HDL, chylomicrons, VLDL	7,000	Stabilizes surface; provides negative charge
apo D	HDL, chylomicrons*	21,000	Cholesteryl ester exchange
apo E	HDL, VLDL, chylomicrons*	34,000	Binds to receptor on cell membrane of liver (E and B/E) and macrophage

From Cholesterol & Coronary Disease . . . Reducing the Risk. Lecture Guide. New York, Science & Medicine, 1986.
* Only in nascent chylomicrons.
HDL = high-density lipoprotein; LDL = low-density lipoprotein; LCAT = lecithin:cholesterol acyltransferase; VLDL = very low-density lipoprotein.

250Å, and it migrates in the pre-beta region. Lp(a) levels range from 1 mg/dl to 200 mg/dl, with the largest number of values below 20 mg/dl. Thus, this lipoprotein does not have the normal, bell-shaped distribution of population serum values seen in the other lipoproteins.

Although Lp(a) is structurally similar to LDL, the former appears to be regulated independently and carries an independent relation to overall coronary risk. If serum levels of both LDL and Lp(a) are elevated, the risk of CAD is markedly increased.[10] Recent angiographic studies have documented a positive correlation between Lp(a) levels and the severity of coronary atherosclerosis.[11,11a,11b]

The mechanism by which high levels of Lp(a) are related to coronary atherosclerosis is unclear. It has been suggested that because of the structural similarities of Lp(a) to plasminogen,[12] high levels of Lp(a) may inhibit the thrombolytic activity of naturally occurring tissue plasminogen activity. Plasminogen is composed of five sequences of amino acids rich in cysteine (Fig. 37–3). Each sequence is called a kringle. Lp(a) lacks the first three kringles, but has a sequence that is highly homologous to the fourth kringle of plasminogen. There is no serine protease activity in Lp(a) and no thrombolytic activity. An alternative explanation for the association between elevated Lp(a) levels and atherosclerosis is that Lp(a) may somehow alter the LDL-mediated delivery of cholesterol to the atherosclerotic plaque. Lp(a) is highly polymorphic and contains variable quantities of carbohydrate as well as having a heterogeneity of kringles.

The control mechanisms of Lp(a) are unknown. Dietary changes that increase LDL levels do not affect Lp(a) levels. The effects of pharmacological agents are unclear, although Lp(a) has been reported to be decreased by niacin, neomycin, and stanozolol.[13,14]

APOPROTEINS
(See Table 37–3)

Apoproteins are key lipoprotein components that serve both as enzymatic cofactors and as recognition elements that bind to specific receptors on peripheral tissues, including the vascular endothelial cells. It is the apo E component of the chylomicron remnant, for example, that is recognized by receptors on the hepatocyte. The apoproteins are distinguished alphabetically and numerically as apo A-I through apo E.

A great deal of research has been conducted in the use of apoproteins as CAD markers. Some investigators have found that the concentrations of apo A-I and apo B-100 are better predictors of CAD than are measurements of total plasma lipids or lipoproteins. In one study, apo A-I was the best predictor of atherosclerotic risk in patients undergoing coronary arteriography.[15] In this study, higher levels of apo A-I were associated with a decreased prevalence of obstructive coronary lesions. Indeed, apo A-I was found to be a better CAD predictor than either total cholesterol or HDL. These observations have not been generally reproduced.

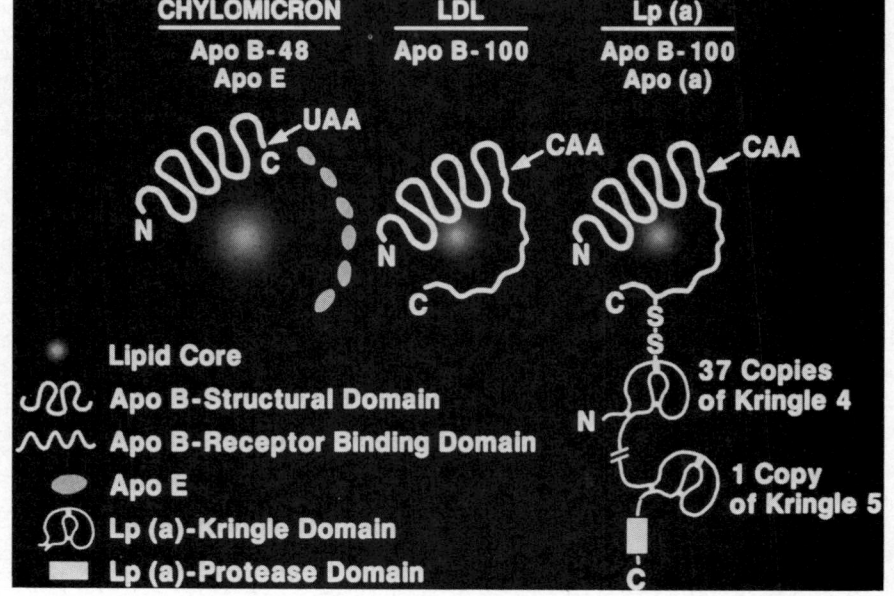

FIGURE 37–3. Chylomicrons are large, triglyceride-rich particles with several classes (A, B, C, E) of surface apoproteins. Apoprotein (apo) C-II activates lipoprotein lipase, which degrades the chylomicrons to remnant particles. The B class of apoproteins is apo B-48. Low-density lipoprotein (LDL) has only one apoprotein (B-100), which is recognized by the apo B/E receptor. Lipoprotein (a) [Lp(a)] has two major associated proteins—apo B-100 and apo(a), a unique protein. Lp(a) has structural similarity to plasminogen (one form has 7 repeating units of kringle 4) but lacks the serine protease activity. Arrow site at which codon 2,153 in the apo B gene is changed at the mRNA level from CAA (glutamine) to UAA (termination) in intestinal cells. (Adapted from Brown, M. S., and Goldstein, J. L.: Plasma lipoproteins: Teaching old dogmas new tricks. Nature 330:113, 1987.)

APOPROTEIN A. Apo A-I, the prototype of apo A, is a major protein in HDL and also is seen in chylomicrons. It has a molecular weight of 28,000 and is synthesized in the GI tract and liver. Its specific regions called amphipathic helices are enriched with charged amino acids that form areas of polar and nonpolar residues.[16] Apo A-I functions as the activator of lecithin:cholesterol acyltransferase (LCAT), and also has been found as a degradation product in amyloid fibrils.[17]

Apo A-II is a minor constituent of HDL and does not appear to be present in all species. Human apo A-II is of hepatic origin and consists of two identical chains attached by a single disulfide linkage. Apo A-II may be an activator of hepatic triglyceride lipase, which hydrolyzes triglyceride and phospholipid while utilizing HDL$_2$ as its preferred substrate. Apo A-IV is synthesized in the gut, and is present in HDL, chylomicrons, and as a free protein. Its molecular weight is 46,000, and its structure is helical. Although its function is not known, it also may be an activator of LCAT.

Although levels of apo A-I are inversely related to CAD risk, there are several genetic conditions in which the relationship of apo A-I to the subsequent development of coronary atherosclerosis is less clear. Genetic deficiencies of apo A-I are associated with extremely low HDL levels. The genetic codes for apos A-I, A-IV, and C-III are close together on the long arm of chromosome 11.[18] Combined A-I/C-III deficiency is associated with severe premature atherosclerosis.[19] A kindred with apo A-II deficiency has been reported with no significant reduction in either the level of circulating HDL or evidence of atherosclerosis.

APOPROTEIN B. Apo B occurs in two forms. Apo B-48 is synthesized by the small intestine, and apo B-100 is secreted by the liver. Apo B-48 is present on the surfaces of chylomicrons and chylomicron remnants. Apo B-100 is found in VLDL, IDL, and LDL. Apo B-100 is the primary apoprotein of LDL, and accounts for 25 per cent of its weight. It also is the recognition site for the LDL, or apo B/E, receptor on cell surfaces. It has recently been determined that a single gene regulates the synthesis of both apo B-48 and apo B-100. The gene for apo B-100 has been localized to chromosome 2 and exists as a 40-kilobase structure.[20] The structure in the amino acid sequence of human apo B-100 and the corresponding cDNA messenger have recently been determined.[21] A unique editing mechanism introduces a stop codon into the mRNA for apo B by means of a single base change. This allows the biosynthesis of two proteins from a single gene and mRNA, with either apo B-100 or apo B-48 being synthesized.[22,23]

APOPROTEIN D. Apo D is a relatively minor constituent found in HDL and the chylomicron. Its molecular weight is 21,000. It has been reported to be involved in cholesteryl ester exchange but does not appear to be the exchange site itself. Apo D is not in the family of the other soluble apoproteins.

APOPROTEIN E. Most apo E is synthesized in the liver. However, other tissues, including the small bowel, kidney, adrenals, and the cells of the reticuloendothelial system, have the ability to synthesize this apoprotein. Apo E accounts for about 15 per cent of the protein content of VLDL, 7 per cent of the protein content of chylomicron remnants, and 2 per cent of the protein content of HDL. It can be recognized by the LDL, or apo B/E, receptor and by specific apo E receptors in the liver whose function appears to be the removal of chylomicron remnants. The ability of apo E to interact with the LDL receptor is thought to be the result of ligand recognition sites between residues 140 and 150. Apo E is polymorphic and contains three major alleles: apos E$_2$, E$_3$, and E$_4$. These respective alleles are present in about 10 per cent, 76 per cent, and 13 per cent of whites. Their various combination results in homozygotes for apos E$_{2/2}$, E$_{3/3}$, and E$_{4/4}$. Also, apos E$_{2/3}$, E$_{2/4}$, and E$_{3/4}$ exist in the heterozygous state. The polymorphism of apo E has been determined on a molecular basis and results from the substitution of an amino acid at residues 112 and 158 in the protein.[23]

About 90 per cent of patients with type III hyperlipoproteinemia (HLP) are homozygous for the E$_{2/2}$ phenotype. This disorder is characterized by hypercholesterolemia, hypertriglyceridemia, and IDL or VLDL particles abnormally enriched in cholesterol. These particles have beta electrophoretic mobility and are termed beta-VLDLs. Premature coronary and peripheral vascular disease is characteristically associated with type III HLP. Type III HLP is also characterized by the delayed clearance of chylomicron remnants in the serum due to impaired binding of these remnants to the lipoprotein receptors in isolated cells. Because the E$_{2/2}$ genotype occurs in 1 per cent of the population, and type III HLP is rare, a second abnormality must be present.

Apo E isoforms may account for as much as 15 per cent of the variability of cholesterol and LDL levels in the population.[24] Also, recent Finnish studies suggest that E$_4$ may be associated with increased cholesterol absorption in the GI tract.[25] In the Prospective Cardiovascular Muenster (PROCAM) study, E$_2$ was associated with lower cholesterol levels and E$_3$ or E$_4$ with higher levels of total cholesterol and LDL in populations with and without CAD.[26,27]

GENETIC VARIATION OF APOPROTEINS

Restriction fragment length polymorphism (RFLP) analysis is a powerful tool for studying the genetic variation of apoproteins. When the genomic DNA molecules from different individuals are digested with enzymes called restriction endonucleases, the pattern of gene fragments varies. Each restriction endonuclease is specific for a defined DNA recognition sequence. A change in the digestion pattern could represent simply a point mutation, or it could be due to a deletion, insertion, or rearrangement of the DNA. RFLP analysis was initially used with the enzyme EcoRI to detect the abnormality in the DNA of patients with familial deficiency of apo A-I and apo C-III.

The genes for apos A-I, C-III, and A-IV have been localized to chromosome 11, and several kindreds have been described with abnormalities at this locus (see below). These genes have been isolated and shown clinically to be associated with abnormalities of HDL regulation. The most extensively evaluated RFLP for this locus used SacI.[28] This minor allele has been shown to be associated with elevated triglycerides and decreased HDL in certain racial groups. The RFLP may or may not be in the coding region of the protein. Association with elevations or decreases in serum lipid or lipoprotein levels could be due to a disequilibrium linkage with another gene.

Population screening has revealed at least 11 variants of apo A-I. The abnormal gene is associated with one normal gene in a heterozygous manner. It produces mutants that contain abnormal amino acid substitutions. Examples are apo A-I Milano and apo A-I Marburg. Both are associated with low HDL levels. Other apo A-I mutants (i.e., Giessen and Muenster) fail to activate LCAT. RFLP studies with apo A-II have revealed several alleles for the apo A-II gene.[29] A cDNA probe has revealed a minor allele of 3.7 kilobases. In patients homozygous for the minor allele, increased levels of apo A-II have been found.[29] Apo A-II has been reported to be an activator of hepatic triglyceride lipase.

RFLP analysis has been used to study the cluster of genes for apos A-I, C-III, and A-IV.[30] Two alleles have been identified in the apo C-III region: S1 and S2. They vary among racial groups; in addition, the S2 region has been associated with low HDL levels, MI survivors, and type V HLP. One of the most widely studied mutants is the XbaI polymorphism for apo B-100. Characteristic lipid changes are present in some populations but not in all. Unfortunately, this has been the case for most of the apoprotein polymorphism described, including that for apo A-I by Ordovas and associates.[31]

FAMILIAL APO C-II DEFICIENCY. The gene for apo C-II has been isolated, sequenced, and localized to chromosome 19.[32] The deficiency state involving apo C-II results in hyperchylomicronemia, but the disorder is highly complex and may involve a variety of potential defects. Several degradation steps occur before the final form of apo C-II is reached: pro-apo C-II and pre-pro-apo C-II isoforms undergo proteolysis and processing before the formation of the mature 73–amino acid sequence.[33] The deficiency of apo C-II on a familial basis has been well described. Its clinical presentation is similar to that of lipoprotein lipase deficiency. In one family, the apo C-II was nonfunctional and was characterized by an abnormal electrophoretic migration pattern due to an amino acid deletion.[34]

DEFECTS IN STRUCTURE AND SYNTHESIS OF APO B.[34a] The polymorphism of apo B has been observed in case-control studies of whites with and without CAD and in RFLP studies of the DNA coding sequence. So far, more than 60 variations have been reported.[35,36] The polymorphism is not associated with alterations in LDL content, although the X-2 allele with endonuclease XbaI and the B1 allele with EcoRI have been reported to occur with increased frequency in patients with CAD. There is great variability among populations.

Several genetic diseases have been described that result in decreased levels or the absence of apo B. Abetalipoproteinemia is characterized by the absence of LDL and by acanthocytosis. It appears to be transmitted as an autosomal recessive trait. On Southern blot analysis, the gene appears normal[37]; hence, the defect in abetalipoproteinemia appears to be a post-translational event. Homozygous hypobetalipoproteinemia has similar clinical manifestations; in this condition, however, the levels of apo B are reduced to one-half of normal. As a rule, CAD is not present, but the number of patients studied so far is small.

THE LIPID HYPOTHESIS OF ATHEROGENESIS

The lipid hypothesis states that dyslipidemia, as manifested by elevated LDL levels and/or decreased HDL levels, is central to the initiation and propagation of atherosclerotic plaque and CAD. It has been known since the nineteenth century that atherosclerotic plaques are laden with cholesterol. But the first scientific credence for the lipid hypothesis came in the early years of this century, when Anitschkow and his colleagues in czarist Russia experimentally induced atherosclerosis in rabbits by cholesterol feeding. Anitschkow reported that cholesterol was an essential ingredient in the development of atherosclerosis.

More recently, the lipid hypothesis has been supported by a large body of epidemiological studies that link the level of mean serum cholesterol to the incidence of coronary morbidity and mortality in many populations (Fig. 37–4). Indeed, virtually every major epidemiological study to date has shown a significant correlation between the level of serum cholesterol at the time of entry and the subsequent risk of CAD. The Seven Countries Study found that CAD was less common in Japan and Mediterranean countries (where the average diet is low in cholesterol and saturated fat) than in the United States, Finland, and The Netherlands (where the cholesterol and saturated fat content of the average diet is higher).[38] In the United States, the Framingham Heart Study and more recently the Multiple Risk Factor Intervention Trial (MRFIT) have shown that the incidence of CAD is positively associated with serum cholesterol levels in a continuous, graded, and progressive manner (Fig. 37–5).

Recent analyses of other epidemiological studies have also lent credence to the lipid hypothesis. Simons analyzed epidemiological data from 19 countries and found that in men, 45

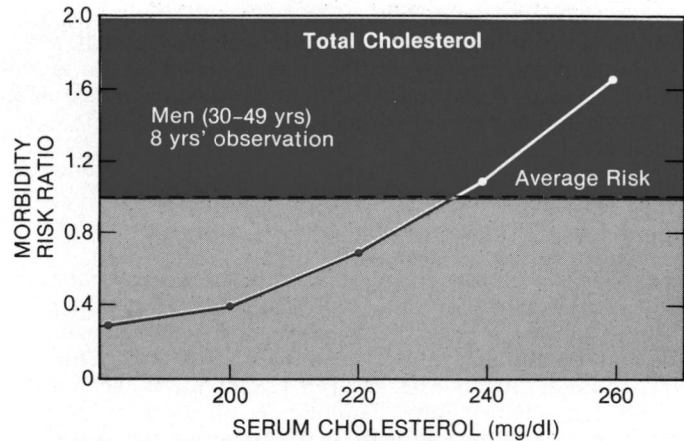

FIGURE 37–5. Various total cholesterol concentrations as related to coronary artery disease risk. Men in Framingham aged 30 to 49 were found to have significantly higher risk if their total cholesterol value exceeded 240 mg/dl.

per cent of the interpopulation differences in CAD mortality could be accounted for by the variation in serum cholesterol levels.[39] He noted that the variability in HDL levels could explain 32 per cent of the mortality differences, and the ratio of total serum cholesterol to HDL could account for 55 per cent. Meanwhile Peto, although unable to identify a level of cholesterol below which CAD is extremely rare, noted that in societies in which average cholesterol levels are under 150 mg/dl and low levels of total serum cholesterol are accompanied by low levels of LDL cholesterol, risks for atherosclerosis and CAD are greatly reduced (personal communication).

ATHEROSCLEROSIS PREVENTION STUDIES

Although the epidemiological data correlating the risk of CAD to levels of cholesterol are compelling, it does not necessarily follow that clinical benefits will accrue from dietary or pharmacological cholesterol lowering. Nonetheless, several controlled clinical trials of the lipid hypothesis have shown that reducing serum cholesterol will reduce overall CAD risk. This conclusion is substantiated by meta-analyses of the available trials. Yusuf and colleagues combined the results of 22 randomized trials involving more than 40,000 subjects.[40] In these trials, various means were used to alter serum cholesterol, including lowering total fat consumption, substituting polyunsaturated for saturated fat, and using pharmacological agents. The meta-analysis examined both primary prevention trials (for people with no clinical evidence of coronary atherosclerosis at the time of entry into the trial) and secondary prevention trials (for patients with documented atherosclerosis). The duration of these trials ranged from 1 to 7 years.

In the overall analysis, the treated subjects had 23 per cent fewer coronary events than the control subjects, a highly significant difference. It must be emphasized, however, that in the earlier trials, the degree of cholesterol lowering was relatively modest and the trials' durations were much shorter than the decades usually required for the buildup of atherosclerotic plaque. Nonetheless, in the 14 trials conducted for less than 4 years, a 10 per cent reduction in serum cholesterol level led to a 10 per cent reduction in coronary events. The reduction in CAD was double (lowering cholesterol 10 per cent leading to 20 per cent less CAD) in the eight trials that treated subjects for longer periods of time. Some of the more important prevention trials are summarized below.

Rossouw and colleagues performed a meta-analysis of the results of eight secondary prevention trials (post-MI, comprising 7837 participants) selected according to strict criteria. They found that across the eight trials, a 10 per cent mean

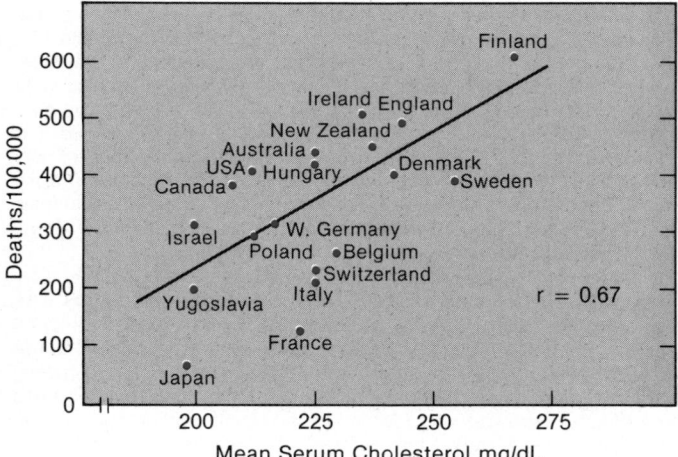

FIGURE 37–4. Coronary artery disease mortality rate versus serum cholesterol. (From Simons, L. A.: Interrelations of lipids and lipoproteins with coronary artery disease mortality in 19 countries. Am. J. Cardiol. 57:5G, 1986.)

reduction in serum cholesterol meant reductions of 19, 12, and 15 per cent in the number of nonfatal, fatal, and all MIs. Across four primary prevention trials selected by the same criteria, Rossouw and coworkers found respective reductions of 25, 12, and 22 per cent with a 10 per cent reduction in total cholesterol.[41]

SECONDARY PREVENTION TRIALS

Secondary prevention refers to the treatment of patients with established atherosclerotic disease in an attempt to prevent, postpone, or cause regression of the clinical or anatomical manifestations of atherosclerosis. The Veterans Administration Center in Los Angeles used a randomized trial design in 846 domiciled veterans. Patients with and without clinical evidence of coronary disease at the time of entry were included. The average patient age was 65 years. One group of patients was placed on a diet higher in unsaturated (versus saturated) fat content and somewhat lower in cholesterol content. By 8-year follow-up the group placed on the unsaturated fat diet had a 23 per cent reduced CAD incidence. Overall mortality was not different between the groups.[42]

The Coronary Drug Project was performed in post-MI patients and used high- or low-dose estrogens (allocation n = 2220) or clofibrate (n = 1103), niacin (n = 1119), dextrothyroxine (n = 1110), or placebo (n = 2789).[43] This trial was constituted as a randomized, double-blind clinical trial. The niacin, clofibrate, and placebo groups were on study for a mean 6.2 years; treatment in the other three arms was stopped early. No benefit was seen with clofibrate (1.8 gm per day), but niacin recipients (prescribed 3.0 mg/day) showed some improvement: average total serum cholesterol lowered from 253 to 227 mg/dl and average triglycerides lowered from 190 to 139 mg/dl at 1 year, with a 27 per cent lower incidence of nonfatal MI than placebo recipients at 5 years but without a significant difference in overall mortality. However, 9 years after the termination of the trial, total mortality was 11 per cent lower in the niacin group than in the placebo group, a highly significant difference.[44] The researchers estimated that nearly 30 per cent of the niacin recipients took less than 60 per cent of the protocol amount of drugs.[44]

The National Heart, Lung and Blood Institute (NHLBI) conducted a trial in patients with type II HLP and angiographic evidence of CAD.[45] Repeat angiography was performed in 116 of the 143 patients to determine CAD progression. Diet alone reduced the LDL cholesterol level 6 per cent in both the cholestyramine and placebo groups. After randomization, and averaged over the 5 years of treatment, LDL cholesterol was reduced another 26 per cent in the cholestyramine group (the drug allocated at 6 gm four times daily) and 5 per cent in the placebo group. HDL cholesterol increased 8 per cent in the drug group and 2 per cent in the placebo group over the 5 years. These lipid level modifications, in turn, greatly reduced the rate of progression of the angiographically demonstrated plaques.[45] Lack of progression correlated best with a favorable HDL–total cholesterol ratio.

The nonrandomized Leiden trial obtained similar results with a strict diet.[46] Other recent trials involving secondary prevention are discussed in the section on the progression of coronary atherosclerosis. These recent studies had adequate statistical power to analyze angiographic endpoints, in addition to the use of pharmacological agents, with a greater degree of lipid and lipoprotein modification.

PRIMARY PREVENTION STUDIES

The primary prevention studies reviewed in this section were designed to test whether modifying CAD risk factors, primarily hypercholesterolemia, would prevent the subsequent formation and progression of atherosclerotic plaque.

WORLD HEALTH ORGANIZATION TRIAL. In this trial, hypercholesterolemic European men were randomized in a double-blind manner and treated with a placebo or clofibrate (1.6 gm/daily). After 5 years of treatment,[47] the incidence of major ischemic heart disease was 20 per cent lower in the clofibrate group than in the control high-cholesterol group. Since the mortality from ischemic heart disease was essentially the same in the two groups, the difference lay in nonfatal MI (4.6 and 6.2 per thousand). Mean serum cholesterol was reduced 9 per cent from baseline levels in the clofibrate group. The overall mortality was increased in the group receiving the hypolipidemic agent; however, the excess mortality did not continue after the end of treatment.[48] This study had a number of flaws, but still raises a cautionary note about the risk of casual and relatively indiscriminate use of hypolipidemic drugs in a general population.

THE OSLO STUDY. This primary prevention trial used diet to lower cholesterol.[49] Because the study also incorporated programs to encourage smoking cessation, its results cannot be interpreted as a pure test of the lipid hypothesis. In the special-intervention group, 24 per cent of the control patients discontinued smoking, compared with 17 per cent in the placebo group. Also, the special-intervention group experienced a mean 13 per cent reduction in total cholesterol levels over the 5 years, compared with 3 per cent among controls. The smoking cessation and cholesterol lowering, in turn, resulted in 47 per cent fewer nonfatal and fatal MIs and sudden death for the special-intervention group and a 55 per cent reduction in CAD death. The statistical significance of this reduction could not be definitely determined because of the relatively small sample size. (N = 1232). More recent analysis of the Oslo Study, at a follow-up of 102 months, documented 19 deaths in the treated group versus 31 deaths in the control group, a difference approaching statistical significance.[50]

THE MULTIPLE RISK FACTOR INTERVENTION TRIAL. In the MRFIT, high-risk men either were referred to their own physicians for standard care or were enrolled in an intensive treatment program consisting of dietary treatment for lowering plasma cholesterol, counseling against cigarette smoking, and treatment of elevated blood pressure with diet and medication. This was not a placebo-controlled study; in fact, blood pressure and smoking cessation improved significantly in both groups. No significant difference in CAD or overall mortality was observed between the two groups after an average 7 years of follow-up.[51]

Special intervention led to a 49 per cent lower CAD mortality rate compared with usual care.[51] This was of particular interest because of the significant reductions in sudden coronary death and CAD incidence achieved by lipid-lowering dietary intervention and smoking cessation in the Oslo Study.[49] A negative aspect was the finding that patients with nonspecific ST-segment and T-wave changes on initial electrocardiograms who were treated with diuretics in the special-intervention group appeared to have a higher mortality rate. Whether these results were due to the lipid, insulin, or electrolyte effects of diuretic therapy is unclear.[51]

Recent MRFIT follow-up data have revealed a significant decrease in overall and CAD mortality in the special-intervention group at 10.5 years (an average 3.8 years after the end of intervention). The special-intervention patients had 11 per cent lower CAD mortality and 8 per cent lower all-causes mortality than the usual-care patients. The mortality differences were mainly due to a 24 per cent reduction in the death rate from acute MI in the special-intervention group compared with the usual-care groups.[52]

THE CORONARY PRIMARY PREVENTION TRIAL PERFORMED BY THE LIPID RESEARCH CLINICS (LRC-CPPT). This trial provided definitive proof of the lipid hypothesis.[53] This was a large-scale study carried out in 12 specialized lipid research clinics in North America. More than 3800 men were enrolled after meeting strict entry criteria: no clinical evidence of CAD, serum cholesterol in excess of 265 mg/dl and LDL elevation of 175 mg/dl or more even after dietary therapy, and without severe hypertension, hypertriglyceridemia, or diabetes. The men were randomized to receive either a placebo or the bile acid sequestrant cholestyramine. The prevalence of smoking was the same in both groups. The recommended dose of cholestyramine was 24 gm/day. Because of poor compliance, only a minority of patients took that much cholestyramine; the average actual dose was probably about 14 gm. Treatment was continued for 7 to 10 years (mean, 7.4 years), with definite endpoints of acute MI and CAD mortality tabulated.

Patients who received drug therapy lowered their total and LDL cholesterol levels 9 per cent and 13 per cent more than control patients. This degree of cholesterol lowering was associated with a graded effect on coronary endpoints (Fig. 37–6). The mean decrease in nonfatal MI and/or CAD death was 19 per cent. In patients who were randomized to cholestyramine but were unable to take the medication because of associated side effects, there was no reduction in cholesterol and no concomitant alteration in overall cardiac risk. However, those patients who daily took 20 gm or more of cholestyramine had a mean 19 per cent reduction in total cholesterol and a mean 28 per cent reduction in LDL cholesterol averaged over 7 years. Many cholestyramine recipients, especially those who took 20 gm or more daily, sustained total and LDL cholesterol levels at least 25

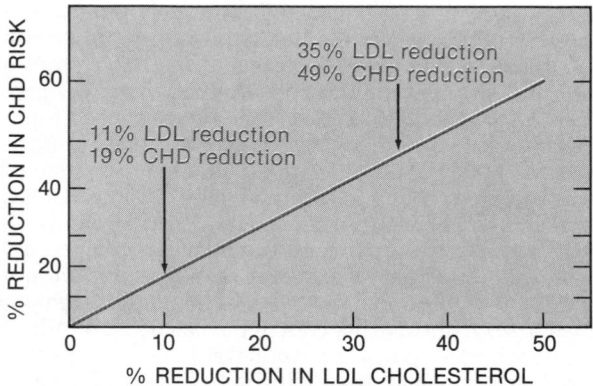

FIGURE 37-6. Relation of reduction in low-density lipoprotein (LDL) cholesterol to reduction in coronary heart disease (CHD) risk (Cox proportional hazards model) in the Lipid Research Clinics Coronary Primary Prevention Trial. When the cholestyramine-treated group was analyzed separately, a 19 per cent reduction in CHD was associated with each 11 per cent decrement in LDL cholesterol or 8 per cent decrement in total cholesterol.[44]

per cent and 35 per cent, respectively, below baseline. The proportional hazards model applied to the cholestyramine group predicted a 49 per cent reduction in CAD risk for a 35 per cent reduction in LDL cholesterol. As a rough rule of thumb, this study demonstrated that a 1 per cent reduction of total cholesterol results in a 2 per cent decrease in CAD risk.

Secondary cardiovascular endpoints were also lower in frequency in the cholestyramine-treatment group and on the order of the 19 per cent reduction of CAD risk. For example, there were reductions of 20, 25, and 21 per cent in the development of angina, new positive exercise test, and incidence of coronary bypass surgery, respectively, compared with those in the placebo group.

Total mortality was equivalent between the two groups, despite the decline in cardiovascular deaths. Apparently the treated group had a higher level of mortality from noncardiovascular causes, primarily motor vehicle accidents and other forms of violent death. These results have been extensively analyzed by the investigators, who perceive a statistical quirk unrelated to any pathological effect of cholestyramine or cholesterol lowering.

THE HELSINKI HEART STUDY. This primary prevention trial used gemfibrozil in the treatment of middle-aged men with dyslipidemia.[54] Like the LRC-CPPT, the Helsinki study was a randomized, double-blind trial of asymptomatic middle-aged men who ranged in age from 40 to 55 years and who had non-HDL cholesterol levels of 200 mg/dl or higher at entry. The total treatment group was 4081 men who were randomized to receive gemfibrozil 600 mg/twice daily or a placebo. Patients were followed for both cardiac death and MI for 5 years. By the end of the trial period, the treated group had experienced 34 per cent fewer coronary events. As in the LRC-CPPT, there was no decrease in overall mortality because of an increase in violent and other noncardiovascular deaths in the treatment group. There was no significant increase in serious drug-related side effects such as cholelithiasis, although GI side effects and the number of abdominal surgical procedures were increased in the gemfibrozil group.

Gemfibrozil has a powerful effect on hypertriglyceridemia, and when the effects on cardiovascular mortality in the Helsinki study were analyzed further, it became apparent that the largest benefit from the drug was seen in the patients with Fredrickson IIb HLP, a lipid disorder characterized by elevated cholesterol and triglycerides. The role of hypertriglyceridemia as a primary CAD risk factor remains controversial. However, there is an inverse relation between elevated triglycerides and low levels of HDL that may be reversed with gemfibrozil therapy. Although not definitely proved by the Helsinki Heart Study, it is attractive to speculate that the larger-than-expected improvement in mortality from a cholesterol lowering of 8 per cent was due to the combined effects on raising HDL and reducing LDL associated with gemfibrozil. On the basis of these findings, the Food and Drug Administration expanded its indication for gemfibrozil to subjects with elevated levels of LDL and triglycerides and low levels of HDL who have failed dietary therapy, resins, or nicotinic acid.

HYPERTRIGLYCERIDEMIA

Several genetic, epidemiological, and clinical studies have linked elevated triglycerides to an increased CAD risk. For

example, in the remnant lipoprotein disorder (type II), dysbetalipoproteinemia (which in part is characterized by elevated triglyceride levels), premature atherosclerosis, including CAD and peripheral arterial disease, frequently occurs. Also, a number of studies have shown that depressed lipoprotein lipase activity and the subsequent extended postprandial lipemia lead to a decreased clearance of triglyceride-rich lipoprotein remnants, an increased triglyceride exchange between LDL and HDL, a greater concentration of atherogenic small, dense LDL lipoproteins, and presumably an increased risk for CAD.[55]

At least two epidemiological or clinical studies lend credence to the positive correlation between elevated triglycerides and CAD risk. Recent analysis of the Framingham data indicates that triglyceride elevation constitutes a CAD risk, which for women is independent of other CAD risk factors. The triglyceride value was an independent risk factor in a Swedish study.[56]

As mentioned above, the Helsinki Heart Study patients in whom the greatest drop in CAD mortality was seen were those with type IIb HLP, a condition manifested by elevated LDL and triglyceride levels and depressed HDL levels. Gemfibrozil treatment in this study lowered the patients' LDL and triglyceride concentrations, while raising their HDL concentrations. The precise effect of the triglycerides modification cannot be determined at this point, and an independent effect of triglycerides could not be statistically validated.

In the *Cholesterol-Lowering Atherosclerosis Study* (CLAS) conducted by Blankenhorn et al. (see below), the proportion of apo C-III in HDL was correlated with decreased progression of disease. This suggests that a rapid rate of metabolism of the triglyceride-rich lipoproteins is anti-atherogenic. In addition, multivariate analysis of the placebo group in this study indicated that the concentration of triglyceride-rich lipoproteins was a significant predictor of atherosclerotic progression.[57] Despite this evidence, it is not clear whether elevated triglycerides are an independent and causal factor in the development of atherosclerosis. Multivariate analyses in many studies have failed to show the independent relation of hypertriglyceridemia and atherosclerosis.

The link between elevated triglycerides and CAD risk may be secondary to other disorders.[58] Various disease entities that are associated with hypertriglyceridemia, such as diabetes mellitus and chronic renal failure, have a definite association with atherosclerosis risk. Certain genetic disorders, such as FCH, which presents with several Fredrickson phenotypes within the same family, confer increased risk for atherosclerosis. In this situation, the triglycerides may represent the presence of other lipoprotein abnormalities that are associated with CAD, such as decreased levels of apo A-I and elevated levels of apo B-100 or remnant particles. However, the causal role of elevated triglycerides on CAD development cannot be ruled out for at least two reasons. First, it is not clear that multivariate analysis is a proper statistical tool to determine causal relations between lipoproteins, since the lipoproteins are highly interrelated metabolically and have rapid kinetic turnover rates. Second, cross-sectional studies have shown an inverse relation between hypertriglyceridemia and HDL, which is presumably due to the interrelated formation of HDL cholesterol with the efficient breakdown of the triglyceride core of VLDL particles.[59] Our ability to delineate further subfractions of the various lipoproteins may better determine the role of triglycerides in atherosclerosis. For example, it has been demonstrated that subforms of VLDL, particularly when associated with high levels of apo E, are readily taken up by residual macrophages with subsequent conversion into the foam cells that are precursors for advanced atherosclerosis.[60]

Current treatment guidelines for hypertriglyceridemia are based on the recommendations of a National Institutes of Health-sponsored consensus conference convened in 1983.[61] This conference classified triglyceride levels under 250 mg/dl as normal, levels between 250 and 500 mg/dl as borderline risk for CAD, and levels above 500 mg/dl as high risk. The guidelines of the European Atherosclerosis Society are quite different, and include triglyceride levels above 200 mg/dl in the treatment algorithm. Patients with borderline hypertriglyceridemia should be examined for possible secondary causes, such as obesity, diabetes, excess alcohol consumption, or the administration of certain drugs, such as noncardioselective beta blockers. Patients with elevated triglyceride levels are also at high risk for pancreatitis, and thus should be placed on a low-fat diet and treated with a fibric acid derivative, such as gemfibrozil, if diet therapy is ineffective.

CAN THE PROGRESS OF ATHEROSCLEROSIS BE HALTED?

Data from the *Bogalusa Heart Study* show a stepwise correlation between LDL concentrations and the extent of fatty streaks in the aorta (Fig. 37–7). It is believed, on the basis of the Bogalusa data, that the presence of fatty streaks in young people is the precursor of advanced atherosclerotic lesions. In the Bogalusa study, the aortic fatty streaks strongly correlated with antemortem levels of LDL and total serum cholesterol and were inversely related to the HDL-LDL ratio.[62]

Cabin and Roberts studied the relation between the autopsy extent of coronary artery narrowing by atherosclerotic plaques and fasting levels determined during life.[63] They quantitatively analyzed multiple 5-mm segments of 160 epicardial coronary arteries in 40 patients. Total cholesterol correlated positively with the number of severely narrowed coronary arteries per subject but not with the degree of severe narrowing. However, there was a significant relationship between triglyceride level and the (percentage) degree of severe narrowing.

Several studies have correlated aggressive control of dyslipidemia with angiographic regression of established CAD. As already mentioned, in the NHLBI's type II HLP trial, cholestyramine treatment lowered LDL levels. Also, cholestyramine improved the HDL–total cholesterol ratio. These changes, in turn, were associated with a decrease in the rate of progression of atherosclerosis.[64] Thirty-two per cent of the patients in the treatment group experienced atherosclerotic progression, compared with 49 per cent of the patients in the placebo group.

Blankenhorn and colleagues in CLAS studied the effects of combination hypolipidemic therapy on coronary atherosclerosis in patients who had angiographically documented CAD and who had undergone coronary artery bypass. Patients were enrolled in the study if they demonstrated that they

could tolerate full-dose niacin and colestipol therapy. Angiography was performed at the beginning of and post-study. A global coronary score was assigned to the angiograms after qualitative interpretation of both the native vessels and bypass grafts by a panel of experts. The scores ranged from -3, representing maximum regression, to $+3$, representing maximum progression. After 2 years,[65] patients in the pharmacologically treated group had experienced a 26 per cent decrease in total cholesterol, a 43 per cent decrease in LDL, and a 37 per cent increase in HDL concentrations, when compared with the placebo group. Moreover, a total of 16.2 per cent of patients in the treated group had evidence of anatomical regression, compared with only 3.6 per cent in the placebo group. In addition, no atherosclerotic progression was noted in 45 per cent of the treated group, compared with 36.6 per cent of the placebo group. A subgroup of patients continued on the study, and the results at 4 years[66] confirmed the 2-year findings.

Although only a minority of the general population with dyslipidemia is able to tolerate maximum colestipol plus niacin therapy, this study unequivocally demonstrated that modifying patient lipid profiles can delay progression of angiographically established atherosclerosis. Another interesting finding of the study was that among patients on placebo, those who did not develop new lesions had an average fat intake of 27 per cent of total calories, versus 34 per cent in those who formed new lesions.

The *Familial Atherosclerosis Treatment Study* (FATS) evaluated changes in angiographically demonstrable coronary disease on aggressive lipid lowering.[67] The men in this study had apo B-100 levels over 125 mg/dl and a family history of premature atherosclerosis. Participants were required to have at least 50 per cent stenosis in one vessel or 30 per cent or greater in three. Unlike the CLAS patients, the FATS patients had not had bypass grafts. Also, quantitative coronary angiography was used, viewing nine defined proximal segments of the major coronary arteries. Patients were divided into three comparably sized groups, two on treatment and one receiving placebo. All received dietary counseling. Treatment was daily, either colestipol 30 gm plus niacin 4 gm or colestipol 30 gm plus lovastatin 40 mg. Patients assigned to the placebo group whose baseline LDL cholesterol level exceeded the 90th percentile for age were given colestipol instead of placebo. A subgroup of patients in the niacin group received 6 gm of niacin a day when the LDL reduction was deemed inadequate. The patients were followed for 2.5 years and then underwent repeat angiography.

The colestipol-niacin group achieved a 32 per cent reduction in LDL and a 43 per cent increase in HDL. The colestipol-lovastatin group achieved a 46 per cent reduction in LDL and a 15 per cent increase in HDL. The control group achieved only a 7 per cent reduction in LDL and a 5 per cent increase in HDL. Moreover, in the colestipol-niacin group, only 25 per cent had definite lesion progression without regression, whereas 39 per cent had regression as the only change, comparable to figures of 21 per cent and 32 per cent in the colestipol-lovastatin group but quite different from values of 46 per cent for progression and 11 per cent for regression in the conventional-therapy group. Examples of regression in treated patients are shown in Figure 37–8. The negative anatomical changes correlated with a worsened clinical outcome. Three patients in the colestipol-lovastatin group experienced cardiovascular events, compared with two in the colestipol-niacin group and 10 in the control group. This well-designed study further supported the lipid hypothesis, and demonstrated that anatomical regression and decrease in clinical events can be achieved with lipid-lowering therapy. The role that HDL elevation played in these results is unclear. It has been suggested, however, that pharmacological elevations of HDL may also play a role in anatomical regression.

Quantitative angiography also showed atherosclerotic lesion regression with treatment (diet with niacin, colestipol, and/or lovastatin) versus lesion progression in a control group (diet, in some cases with low-dose colestipol) in the University

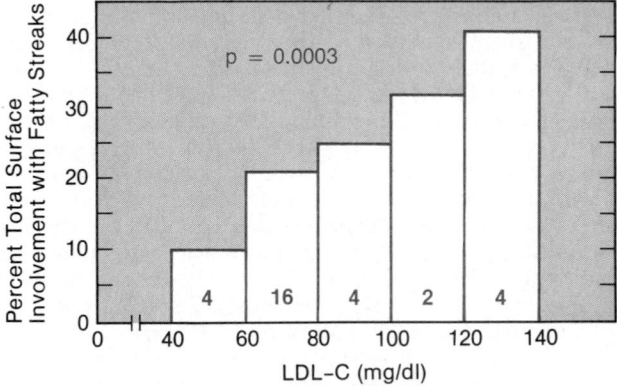

FIGURE 37–7. Atherosclerotic fatty streak involvement of the aorta related to levels of low-density lipoprotein cholesterol (LDL-C) in 30 young persons. Increasing LDL-C levels are significantly related to increasing amounts of aortic fatty streaks. (To convert values for cholesterol to millimoles per liter, multiply by 0.026.) (Reprinted by permission from Newman, W. P., Freedman, D. S., and Voors, A. W.: Relation of serum lipoprotein levels and systolic blood pressure to early atherosclerosis. The Bogalusa Heart Study. N. Engl. J. Med. *314*:138, 1986.)

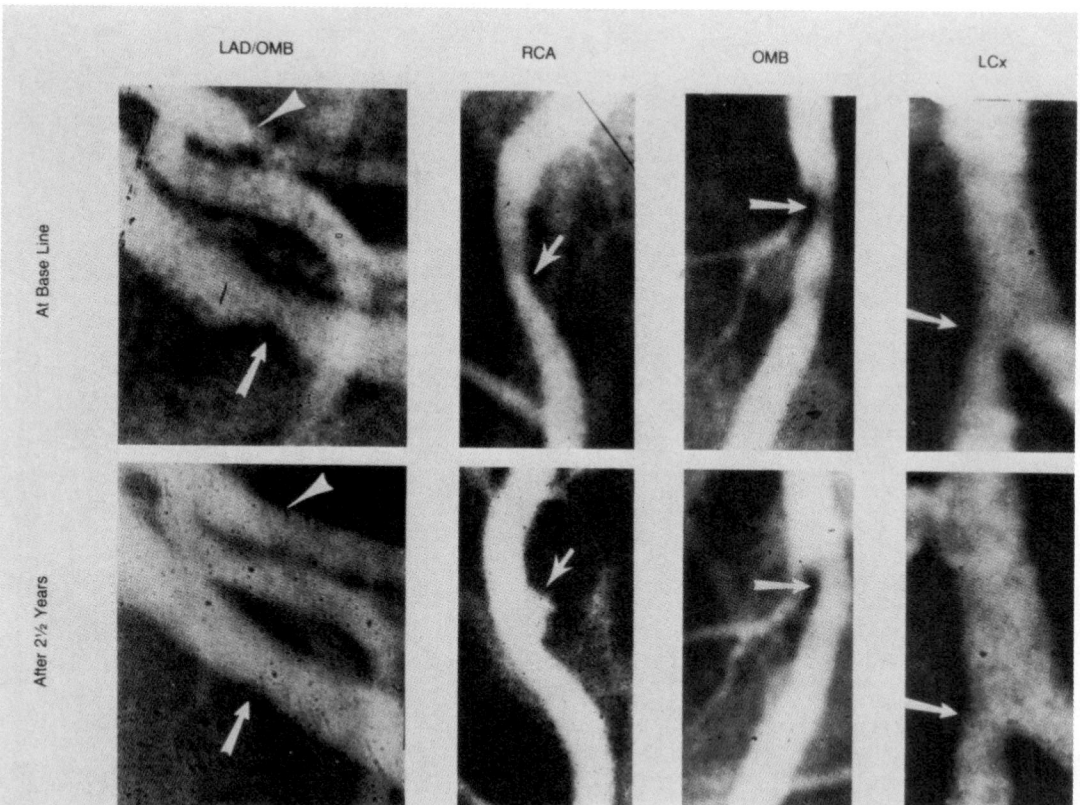

FIGURE 37–8. Examples of atherosclerotic lesion regression in patients treated intensively in the Familial Atherosclerosis Treatment Study. The top row shows images obtained at baseline; the bottom row, images obtained 2½
years later. LAD, left anterior descending artery; OMB, obtuse marginal branch; RCA, right coronary artery; LCx, left
circumflex artery. Stenosis caused by the lesions in these vessels decreased as follows: LAD, from 100 to 28 per cent;
OMB, from 39 to 18 per cent; RCA, from 48 to 30 per cent (note the plaque ulcer present at 2½ years); OMB, from 69
to 37 per cent; and LCx, from 44 to 30 per cent. (Reprinted by permission from Brown, G., Albers, J. J., Fisher, L. D.,
et al.: Regression of coronary artery disease as a result of intensive lipid-lowering therapy in men with high levels
of apolipoprotein B. N. Engl. J. Med. *323*:1289, 1990.)

of California, San Francisco Arteriosclerosis Specialized
Center of Research (SCOR) Intervention Trial.[68] All 72 patients in this randomized trial had heterozygous familial hypercholesterolemia, and the authors concluded that reduction of LDL cholesterol can induce lesion regression in CAD.

Gordon and associates in a meta-analysis of four major trials
found that a 1 mg/dl increment in HDL cholesterol was associated with significant reductions in CAD risk: 2 per cent in
men and 3 per cent in women.[69] They found HDL levels to be
essentially unrelated to noncardiovascular disease mortality.

DIAGNOSIS OF HYPERLIPIDEMIA

Because of the frequent lack of overt physical findings or
symptomatology in patients with dyslipidemia, the first step
when HLP is suspected is to determine accurate plasma lipoprotein levels. However, the basic screening test currently
recommended for all adults is that for serum cholesterol.

The traditional definition of HLP was levels of plasma cholesterol and triglycerides exceeding the 95th percentile for
adjusted age and gender. This approach used a statistical variation from the median and included patients who were 2 standard deviations above and below the mean cholesterol for that
group. In the United States and other countries where CAD
incidence is high, these statistically derived guidelines were
inadequate.

The National Cholesterol Education Program (NCEP) reported its findings after evaluating clinical risks from hypercholesterolemia and issued new screening recommendations
based on three categories of cholesterol levels (Fig. 37–9).[70–72]
According to the NCEP guidelines, less than 200 mg/dl cholesterol is desirable. Patients with these low cholesterol levels
should merely be given education concerning the risks in-

volved in the development of CAD, general dietary information, and instructions to repeat cholesterol testing within 5
years.

Borderline cholesterol levels in these guidelines are between 200 and 239 mg/dl in the absence of established CAD or
other CAD risk factors (hypertension, smoking, diabetes mellitus, body weight over 30 per cent of ideal, HDL under 35
mg/dl, family history of CAD, and male gender). Patients with
a cholesterol value in this range who do not have established
CAD or two other risk factors should be given dietary information and instructions to repeat cholesterol testing within 1
year. Patients with these borderline cholesterol levels who
have CAD or other CAD risk factors are considered at high
risk, as are patients with total cholesterol 240 mg/dl or higher.
High-risk patients should undergo a complete lipoprotein
analysis with further therapeutic intervention based on the
calculated LDL level.

From the fasting sample, total cholesterol, HDL, and triglycerides can be measured directly. LDL and its cholesterol content can be calculated mathematically. HDL is determined by
measuring the cholesterol that is in solution after precipitating the apo B–containing lipoproteins. LDL can then be
calculated by the following formula: LDL = total cholesterol − HDL − (triglycerides/5). The formula is not valid for triglyceride levels over 400 mg/dl or in type III HLP.

TYPING OF HYPERLIPOPROTEINEMIA

The Fredrickson and Lees classification of hyperlipoproteinemia (Table 37–4) remains a practical approach for the
clinician.[73] This system is based on laboratory definitions as
opposed to genetics and does not take into account underlying
pathophysiology or HDL measurements.

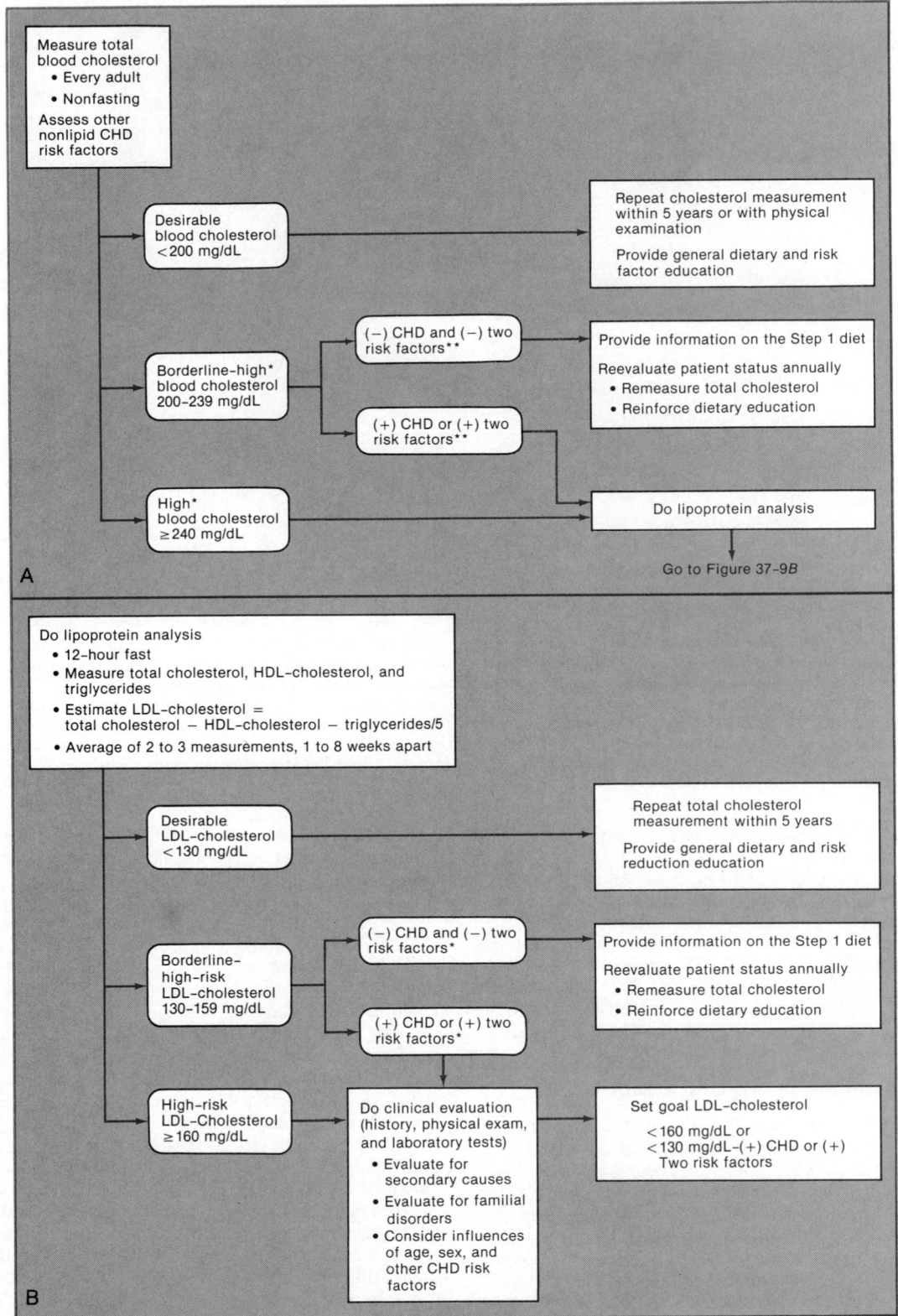

FIGURE 37–9. *A,* Initial classification based on total cholesterol. CHD indicates coronary heart disease; asterisk, must be confirmed by obtaining repeat measurements and then using the average value; double asterisks, one of which can be male sex. (From The Expert Panel: Report of the National Cholesterol Education Program Expert Panel on Detection, Evaluation and Treatment of High Blood Cholesterol in Adults. Arch. Intern. Med. *148*:36, 1988.) *B,* Classification based on low-density lipoprotein (LDL)-cholesterol. Asterisk, one of which can be male sex. CHD, coronary heart disease; HDL, high-density lipoprotein. (From The Expert Panel: Report of the National Cholesterol Education Program Expert Panel on Detection, Evaluation and Treatment of High Blood Cholesterol in Adults. Arch. Intern. Med. *148*:36, 1988.)

FREDRICKSON AND LEES PHENOTYPE	LABORATORY DEFINITION	ASSOCIATED WITH GENETIC DISORDERS	CONDITIONS ASSOCIATED WITH SECONDARY HYPERLIPOPROTEINEMIA
Type I	Hyperchylomicronemia and absolute deficiency of LPL Cholesterol normal Triglycerides greatly increased	Familial LPL deficiency Apo C-II deficiency	Dysglobulinemia, pancreatitis, poorly controlled diabetes mellitus
Type IIa	LDL increased Cholesterol increased Triglycerides normal VLDL normal	Familial hypercholesterolemia LDL receptor abnormal Familial combined hyperlipidemia Polygenic hypercholesterolemia	Hypothyroidism, acute intermittent porphyria, nephrosis, idiopathic hypercalcemia, dysglobulinemia, anorexia nervosa
Type IIb	LDL increased VLDL increased Cholesterol increased Triglycerides increased	Familial hypercholesterolemia Familial combined hyperlipidemia	
Type III	Floating beta lipoproteins VLDL cholesterol/VLDL triglyceride > 0.35 Apo E_2 homozygote on isoelectric focusing Cholesterol increased Triglycerides increased	Familial dysbetalipoproteinemia	Diabetes mellitus, hypothyroidism, dysglobulinemia (monoclonal gammopathy)
Type IV	VLDL increased Cholesterol normal or increased Triglycerides increased	Familial hypertriglyceridemia Familial combined hyperlipidemia	Glycogen storage disease, hypothyroidism, disseminated lupus erythematosus, diabetes mellitus, nephrotic syndrome, renal failure, ethanol abuse
Type V	Chylomicrons and VLDL increased LDL present but reduced Cholesterol increased Triglycerides greatly increased	Familial hypertriglyceridemia Familial multiple lipoprotein type hyperlipidemia	Poorly controlled diabetes mellitus, glycogen storage disease, hypothyroidism, nephrotic syndrome, dysglobulinemia, pregnancy, estrogen administration (either contraceptive or therapeutic) in women with familial hypertriglyceridemia

From Gotto, A. M.: Practical approach to phenotyping hyperlipoproteinemia. In Kligfield, P. D. (ed.): Cardiology Reference Book. New York, Co-Medica, Inc., 1984.
LDL = low-density lipoprotein; LPL = lipoprotein lipase; VLDL = very low density lipoprotein.

TYPE I HLP: FAMILIAL GENETIC DYSLIPIDEMIAS. The diagnosis of familial chylomicronemia, or type I HLP, requires the presence of chylomicrons in the fasting plasma above a clear supernatant. Type I HLP may be a primary genetic disorder, manifested chemically by the absence of apo C-II or lipoprotein lipase, or a condition secondary to poorly controlled diabetes mellitus, pancreatitis, or dysglobulinemia. The hyperchylomicronemic state of type I HLP is characterized by the appearance of extraordinarily large lipoprotein complexes. These macromolecular particles appear in normal people after consumption of a fatty meal. They usually are rapidly cleared from the plasma by means of activation of lipoprotein lipase by the apo C-II present on the surface of the chylomicrons. The diagnosis of type I HLP can be established by chemical determinations of the activity of lipoprotein lipase after heparin administration. The presence of an inhibitor to lipoprotein lipase can be determined by bioassay: there is a lack of activity when the patient's serum is added to a source that normally has enzyme activity. The primary genetic form of type I HLP—familial lipoprotein lipase deficiency—is not associated with complications of premature atherosclerosis, despite high levels of cholesterol and triglycerides. This disorder is clinically manifested in childhood by recurrent abdominal pain secondary to pancreatitis. The gene that governs the production of lipoprotein lipase has been mapped to chromosome 8.[74] The absence of lipoprotein lipase noted in some

forms of HLP may be secondary to mutations of this gene and to the subsequent accumulation of triglycerides localized to chylomicron particles because of impaired degradation. A clinically similar condition can occur when there is a deficiency of the apo C-II activator for lipoprotein lipase. This deficiency is less common than that of lipoprotein lipase enzyme. RFLP studies to determine genetic variation indicate that the genetic defect of apo C-II deficiency is heterogeneous.[75] The diagnosis of apo C-II deficiency depends on the determination of absent or defective apo C-II by electrophoretic techniques or assays.[76]

Dietary treatment is similar in both of these conditions. The infusion of fresh plasma with normal amounts of apo C-II may activate lipoprotein lipase if a deficiency state exists.

TYPE II HLP. Type II HLP is defined as an elevation of total plasma cholesterol, predominantly in the LDL fraction. It may represent a primary genetic disorder or be secondary to underlying disease such as hypothyroidism, nephrotic syndrome, or dysglobulinemia. In type IIa HLP, triglycerides and VLDL are normal. In type IIb, both these fractions are elevated.

GENETIC FORMS OF HYPERCHOLESTEROLEMIA

POLYGENIC HYPERCHOLESTEROLEMIA. The most common cause of an isolated elevation of total cholesterol and LDL cholesterol is polygenic hypercholesterolemia, which may be the underlying disorder in as many as 80 per cent of the people found to be hypercholesterolemic by routine screening. However, the exact incidence of polygenic hypercholesterolemia in patients with the type II phenotype has not been definitely determined. Polygenic hypercholesterolemia is not well understood from a genetic standpoint, and no single gene disorder has been implicated. Presumably, exogenous factors interact with a poorly understood genetic predisposition to result in increased LDL production or decreased LDL catabolism. Dietary treatment significantly reduces cholesterol levels in these patients.

FAMILIAL HYPERCHOLESTEROLEMIA. Familial hypercholesterolemia (FH) has a strong association with premature atherosclerosis. In the rare homozygous form of FH (which occurs in roughly 1 in 1 million Americans), clinical evidence of atherosclerosis—including acute MI, severe coronary atherosclerosis, and aortic stenosis—may occur in the first decade of life. The primary genetic defect in FH is an autosomal dominant disorder caused by a mutation in the LDL-receptor gene. The gene frequency in the United States is 1 per 500 people. Higher frequencies have been noted in Lebanon and among Afrikaners; this heterozygosity perhaps occurs in 1 per cent of these populations. In FH, LDL production is increased, whereas the cells' ability to recognize the apo B surface component of LDL is decreased. Also, the production of LDL may be increased because of a decrease in IDL removal by the liver and enhanced conversion to LDL.

The LDL receptor is located in coated pits on the surface of hepatic and extrahepatic tissues as a glycoprotein of 839 amino acids. The LDL receptor protrudes from the coated pit, and has a highly complex structure consisting of a ligand-binding domain of 292 amino acids that recognizes apos B and E. A subsequent domain is composed of about 400 amino acids with a homology to the precursors of the epidermal growth factor. This latter domain is followed by a series of O-linked sugars in a membrane-spanning domain of 222 amino acids. The carboxy-terminal portion of the LDL receptor is located within the cytoplasm and is composed of 50 amino acids.[77] Patients with homozygous FH typically have no functioning LDL receptors, although some homozygotes, called receptor defective, exhibit up to 10 per cent of normal receptor activity. Patients with the heterozygous state have about half of the normal-functioning LDL receptors. Goldstein and Brown have described four classes of LDL-receptor mutations that affect respectively the receptor's formation, transport, LDL binding, and clustering in the coated pit.[78]

In a class I mutation, a null allele results in a total failure to produce the LDL receptor. In a class II mutation, the LDL-receptor protein is formed, but with a transport defect that alters its migration between the endoplasmic reticulum and the Golgi complex. The class III mutation is associated with normal synthesis and transport of the LDL-receptor protein, but with LDL receptors that cannot recognize apoproteins on the LDL particle. With a class IV mutation, the LDL receptor fails to internalize and cluster properly in the coated pits. Many mutations of the LDL gene have been identified, each resulting in the phenotypic clinical manifestations of FH.

There is a mechanism for the clearance of LDL that is independent of the presence of the LDL receptor (Fig. 37-2, p. 1127). In receptor-absent homozygous patients, LDL clearance occurs by means of a non-receptor-mediated mechanism. This form of clearance is referred to as the "scavenger pathway" and presumably occurs in macrophages of the reticuloendothelial system or by other poorly defined non-receptor-mediated pathways. Patients with a normal complement of LDL receptors clear about one-third of their LDL by the scavenger pathway.

Monocytes and macrophages are able to express receptors for LDL that have been altered by oxidation or chemically. Contact with the endothelial cell can induce LDL oxidation. This uptake was attributed to the presence of a specific receptor—called the acetyl LDL receptor, or scavenger receptor—which is distinct from the LDL receptor. In fact, this specific receptor does not recognize native LDL.[79]

Most patients with a type IIa phenotype do not have FH. The clinical hallmarks of the FH patient are a positive family history and tendinous xanthomas. Quantification of the number and function of the LDL receptors can only be done by specialized medical centers.[80,81]

FAMILIAL COMBINED HYPERLIPIDEMIA. FCH is relatively common in the United States, occurring in about 1 in 300 people. It is an autosomal dominant disease. The presentation may vary within families, with several Fredrickson phenotypes seen (IIa, IIb, IV). FCH is associated with an increased risk for premature atherosclerosis. Although the disease may clinically mimic FH, patients with FCH lack tendinous xanthomas. FCH may be heterogeneous. The underlying mechanism is thought to be an overproduction of apo B-100 by the liver. Small, dense LDL particles with an increased content of apo B-100 are seen. It is possible the FCH could represent the heterozygous state of LPL deficiency.

TYPE III HLP: FAMILIAL DYSBETALIPOPROTEINEMIA. Type III HLP, or broad-beta-lipoproteinemia or dysbetalipoproteinemia, occurs in about 1 in 10,000 people. The expression of this genetic condition seldom occurs before adulthood, and the $E_{2/2}$ phenotype is seen in more than 90 per cent of patients. Atherosclerosis is clinically manifested as peripheral vascular disease or CAD.[3]

The lipid profile in patients with type III HLP is roughly equal elevations of both cholesterol and triglycerides, which are derived from incomplete catabolism of chylomicrons and VLDL particles. Lipoprotein electrophoresis reveals an increase in VLDL and a second band that encompasses both VLDL and LDL fractions. This broad band contains remnant intermediates termed beta-VLDLs. In normal subjects, the ratio of VLDL cholesterol to total triglycerides usually is less than 0.2, whereas in type III HLP, the ratio exceeds 0.37.

Delineation of apo E subtypes is a useful diagnostic tool for type III HLP, but it is not widely available. In patients with type III HLP, the presence of apo E_2 leads to defective binding of apo E–containing lipoproteins and the accumulation of remnant particles. Other factors must play a role, because approximately 1 per cent of the U.S. population carries the apo $E_{2/2}$ phenotype but without demonstrable lipoprotein abnormality or associated vascular disease. It has been suggested that some unknown environmental influence interacts with the underlying apo $E_{2/2}$ phenotype to alter the lipid profile. Type III HLP is associated in rare cases with another disease such as hypothyroidism. Although physical examination may be normal, a characteristic palmar lesion—xanthoma striatum palmare, which consists of yellow streaks in the palmar creases—frequently is present (Fig. 37-10). Tuberoeruptive xanthomas may be present on the tibial tuberosities and the

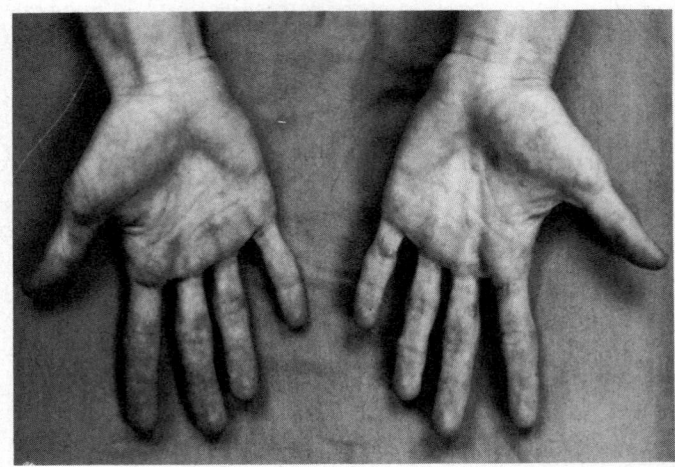

FIGURE 37-10. Palmar xanthomas.

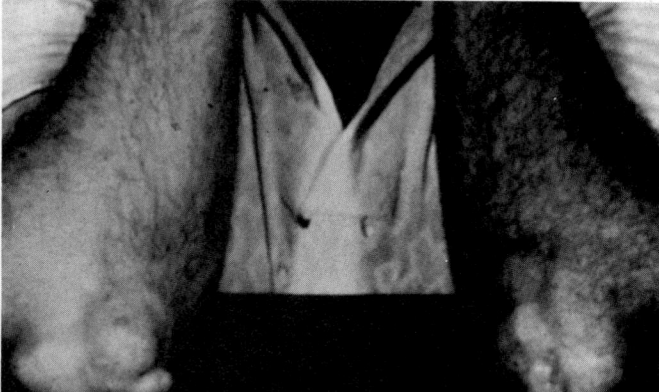

FIGURE 37-11. Tuberoeruptive xanthomas on the elbow.

elbows (Fig. 37-11). Tendinous xanthomas, which are common in type II, are rare in type III.[82]

GENETIC FORMS OF HYPERTRIGLYCERIDEMIA

Familial Combined Hyperlipoproteinemia

FAMILIAL DYSBETALIPOPROTEINEMIA. Hypertriglyceridemia's genetic forms have been described above.

TYPE IV HLP: FAMILIAL ENDOGENOUS HYPERTRIGLYCERIDEMIA. Type IV HLP is caused by an accumulation of VLDL in fasting plasma, which results in a cloudy or turbid appearance. Type IV HLP may be genetic in origin or secondary to another, underlying disease. Two main patterns with a genetic basis have been recognized. *Primary (familial) endogenous hypertriglyceridemia* is a relatively common autosomal dominant disorder. The incidence of its heterozygous form is 1 per cent in the general population. VLDL production is increased in this condition, whereas HDL levels are decreased.[83] The metabolic defect appears to be an oversynthesis of hepatic triglyceride and VLDL in which large triglyceride-rich particles are produced. Triglyceride levels usually are in the 200 to 500 mg/dl range.

FCH also may present as a type IV pattern. The physician should not be deterred by the overlap, since FCH patients also are predisposed to CAD. It should be noted, however, that the risk for patients with familial hypertriglyceridemia is less clearly delineated.[84] Premature CAD is common in some kindreds but not in others.

TYPE V HLP. Type V HLP is an uncommon dyslipidemia characterized by the presence of chylomicrons and VLDL in the fasting plasma. The phenotype occurs in about 2 of every 1000 men and is less frequent in women. Type V HLP usually is recognized in adults. Examination of fasting plasma reveals a creamy supernatant composed of chylomicrons overlying a turbid layer of VLDL-rich serum. The underlying causes are complex, and include genetic and secondary factors. Type V HLP does not have a clear pattern of inheritance, although elevations of chylomicrons usually are associated with a decreased activity of lipoprotein lipase. Type V HLP also can be associated with apo C-II deficiency. Other secondary causes include obesity (especially when associated with rapid weight gain), excessive alcohol intake, and administration of exogenous estrogens.[85,86]

A type V pattern may be seen in patients with genetic forms of hypertriglyceridemia. Effective treatment will decrease the chylomicron levels and cause the phenotype to revert to type IV or IIb. Type V HLP is difficult to differentiate from the frequently associated diabetes mellitus. The frequent presence of other risk factors for premature atherosclerosis, such as diabetes, hypertension, and obesity, clouds the primary contribution of type V HLP to CAD.[87,88]

Causes of secondary hypertriglyceridemia or of a type IV pattern are common and should be actively sought in any given patient. Diabetes mellitus frequently is associated with elevated triglycerides. There are several possible mechanisms for this association. For example, obese diabetics who are insensitive to the action of insulin require elevated levels of insulin to maintain a given level of plasma glucose. The increased insulin levels may, in turn, increase VLDL synthesis. In diabetics with insulin deficiency, the mechanism is more complex and relates to the prevention of triglyceride catabolism with lipoprotein lipase. The antilipolytic action of insulin prevents triglyceride breakdown and secondary free fatty acid release from adipocytes. The flux of unesterified fatty acids to the liver is thought to be a major factor driving VLDL synthesis. Insulin also is required to maintain adequate activity of lipoprotein lipase. As a result of absolute or relative insulin deficiency, remnant lipoproteins accumulate in the blood. Exogenous insulin restores lipoprotein lipase and prevents marked elevations of VLDL and chylomicrons.

Reduced lipoprotein lipase activity also occurs in myxedema and renal failure and may partially account for the commonly seen elevated triglyceride levels. If the nephrotic syndrome accompanies renal insufficiency, the associated hypoalbuminemia is thought to stimulate the VLDL production. Other causes of a type IV pattern are excessive alcohol intake and hepatocellular disease (glycogen or lipid storage abnormalities).

TREATMENT OF HYPERLIPOPROTEINEMIA

Before the initiation of therapy, a careful medical examination should be performed to determine if the hyperlipidemia is secondary to an underlying disease or has a genetic basis. Underlying conditions, such as diabetes, renal insufficiency, myxedema, biliary obstruction, nephrotic syndrome, and dysproteinemia, should be identified and treated. A careful dietary history also should be obtained to estimate caloric intake and the amounts of cholesterol, total fat, and saturated fat in the diet.

CONCURRENT MEDICATIONS. The concurrent use of medications should be documented and the need for continuation determined. Commonly used medications that alter lipid profiles include the diuretics and beta blockers. Estrogens tend to raise HDL, VLDL, and triglyceride levels while reducing LDL. Their effect on cardiac risk, especially in postmenopausal women, is the subject of current debate. Progesterone analogs decrease elevated levels of triglycerides but also decrease HDL.

The effect of antihypertensive agents on the blood lipids is complex. Noncardioselective beta blockers tend to increase VLDL levels, presumably because they also inhibit the adrenergic stimulation of lipoprotein lipase. It has been demonstrated that beta I and beta II agonists increase the lipase enzyme activity, whereas alpha agonists inhibit it. Despite their potential adverse effects on lipids, both cardioselective beta blockers (metoprolol) and nonselective beta blockers (propranolol, timolol) have been shown to reduce rates of MI and cardiac mortality.

Alpha-adrenergic blockers, such as prazosin, do not adversely affect lipids and may actually raise HDL. Whether this effect will translate into cardioprotection has not been determined. The calcium blockers, angiotensin-converting enzyme inhibitors, and centrally acting alpha$_2$ agonists tend to have a neutral effect on lipids. The role of the angiotensin-converting enzyme inhibitors is under investigation. There is increasing evidence that essential hypertension is associated with an insulin-resistant state. Captopril has been demonstrated to enhance, because of an increase in insulin sensitivity with its use, the insulin-mediated disposal of glucose when compared with hydrochlorothiazide.[89] The long-term clinical effects of this action have yet to be determined, but it may explain in part the lack of improvement in coronary mortality in hypertensive patients treated with thiazide derivatives.

LDL cholesterol below a level of 130 mg/dl is considered desirable (Fig. 37–9). LDL levels between 130 and 159 mg/dl are classified as borderline high risk if CAD or other CAD risk factors are absent. High-risk LDL elevations are values of 160 mg/dl or more, or between 130 and 159 mg/dl with existing CAD or two additional risk factors. The NCEP recommends dietary therapy for an LDL value of 160 mg/dl or higher if the patient is free of clinically evident coronary disease and does not have two of the established risk factors. The minimal goal is to lower the LDL cholesterol to under 160 mg/dl. If coronary disease is present or the patient has two or more of the established risk factors, the minimal goal for dietary therapy would be an LDL level below 130 mg/dl.

INDICATIONS FOR DRUG THERAPY. Drug therapy is recommended if a patient free of coronary disease and other risk factors has an LDL cholesterol value over 190 mg/dl after 3 to 6 months of dietary treatment. If the patient has coronary disease or the presence of two or more other risk factors, 160 mg/dl would be the threshold for the initiation of drug therapy after dietary therapy. Current NCEP treatment guidelines do not take into account for the LDL-HDL ratio.

As already stated, drug therapy should be considered only if patients still have high cholesterol levels despite at least 6 months of intensive dietary therapy. Drug therapy for patients who are at extreme risk for CAD or who have marked elevations of LDL might be considered at an earlier point. The treatment goal for LDL cholesterol should be to decrease the circulating LDL to less than 160 mg/dl if the patient is free of CAD and two of the established risk factors, or 130 mg/dl if these other factors are present. In the case of established atherosclerosis, the goal should not be limited to lowering the lipid value, but should include the anatomical regression of coronary disease. The threshold to achieve regression has not yet been determined but may be <100 mg/dl of LDL cholesterol. Drug therapy should be monitored by repeat cholesterol tests performed regularly every 4 to 6 weeks after the initiation of therapy. At the end of 12 weeks, the physician should check for any drug toxicity, altered liver function, or impairment of concomitant drug absorption due to binding in the GI tract.

DIETARY THERAPY

Dietary therapy should be the initial intervention in all forms of lipid disorders. Although there is considerable variability in individual response to a low-fat, low-cholesterol diet, alterations of diet can be expected to play a significant role in improving most lipid profiles.

Angiographic studies have demonstrated the benefit of dietary therapy in halting the progression of atherosclerosis. In the 2-year *Leiden Intervention Trial*, patients in whom angiography had shown at least one coronary vessel with 50 per cent obstruction were given a vegetarian diet that contained twice as much polyunsaturated as saturated fat. Less than 100 mg of cholesterol was consumed each day. By the end of the trial, body weight, systolic blood pressure, total cholesterol, and the

ratio of total cholesterol to HDL had all been lowered. There also was an increase in the linoleic acid content of cholesteryl esters. Angiograms performed after 24 months of dietary intervention indicated that about half of the patients showed no progression of coronary atherosclerosis. Progression of disease was seen in patients who had total cholesterol-HDL ratios greater than 6.9 throughout the trial period.[46]

The CLAS data (p. 1134) showed that the appearance of new coronary lesions can be influenced by diet.[90] This study's dietary therapy mainly involved the substitution of low-fat meats as a protein source. Similar findings on the benefits of dietary therapy were recently reported by Ornish and colleagues, whose study combined a vegetarian diet with relaxation therapy and exercise.[91]

Dietary goals should be established and a concerted effort made to ensure patient compliance. The diet should be nutritious, balanced, and of high culinary standard. These steps enhance adherence while achieving a reduction in circulating total and LDL cholesterol levels.

The minimal goals of dietary therapy should be to reduce LDL cholesterol to under 160 mg/dl and to lower the total cholesterol to under 240 mg/dl in patients without CAD or two additional risk factors and to less than 130 mg/dl if any of these conditions apply. Some clinicians would hold that the serum cholesterol should be more aggressively treated. The NCEP has described a two-step dietary program which parallels the dietary recommendations of the American Heart Association (AHA).[70,92] The NCEP specifically recommends a progressive initiation of dietary therapy designed to decrease dietary consumption of saturated fatty acids, promote weight loss, and lower total cholesterol. Although the AHA's Step One Diet can be initiated by the physician, implementation of the AHA's Step Two Diet should involve the aid of a registered dietitian. If a patient is overweight, total caloric intake should be decreased, as should the intake of saturated fat and cholesterol. In the average American diet, about 15 per cent of the total caloric intake consists of saturated fat, but in some people this may be considerably higher. A high consumption of saturated fat may decrease the activity of hepatic LDL receptors. In general, the diet should be aimed at balancing total calories and decreasing total fat, saturated fat, and cholesterol intake to the prescribed levels.

In the AHA's Step One Diet (Table 37–5), the recommended daily intake of total fat is less than 30 per cent of calories, with less than 10 per cent of total caloric intake coming from saturated fat. The daily consumption of total cholesterol should be less than 300 mg. The patient should have adequate instruction from the physician or staff, and a trial of 6 weeks should be implemented before lipids are rechecked. Not all saturated fatty acids elevate serum cholesterol. Recent studies by Bonanome and Grundy, for example, have shown that some saturated fatty acids have a neutral effect on cholesterol and that palmitic acid exerts a significant cholesterol-raising effect.[93] Saturated fatty acid intake can be replaced by the consumption of monounsaturated or polyunsaturated acids. Polyunsaturated fats can be increased to 10 per cent of calories, but the advisability of increasing their intake beyond this level is questioned by many authorities. The consumption of polyunsaturated fats has been shown to be associated with a better

TABLE 37-5 AMERICAN HEART ASSOCIATION DIETARY THERAPY OF HIGH BLOOD CHOLESTEROL IN ADULTS

NUTRIENT	RECOMMENDED INTAKE	
	Step One Diet	Step Two Diet
Total fat	Less than 30% of total calories	Less than 30% of total calories
Saturated fatty acids	Less than 10% of total calories	Less than 7% of total calories
Polyunsaturated fatty acids	Up to 10% of total calories	Up to 10% of total calories
Monounsaturated fatty acids	10% to 15% of total calories	10% to 15% of total calories
Carbohydrates	50% to 60% of total calories	50% to 60% of total calories
Protein	10% to 20% of total calories	10% to 20% of total calories
Cholesterol	Less than 300 mg/d	Less than 200 mg/d
Total calories	To achieve and maintain desirable weight	To achieve and maintain desirable weight

risk factor profile, including benefits in the lipid profile and alterations of glucose tolerance and blood pressure. The NCEP has recommended that monounsaturated fats, mainly oleic acid, make up 10 per cent to 15 per cent of total calories. These fats are found in olive oil and canola oil.

In Mediterranean countries, the intake of monounsaturated fats is high, primarily representing the consumption of olive oil. The incidence of CAD is considerably lower in these countries.[94]

A high dietary intake of cholesterol has been documented to induce the process of atherosclerosis in a variety of laboratory animals, including nonhuman primates. In humans, response of circulating cholesterol levels to alterations in diet is highly variable. However, an excess intake of cholesterol can elevate LDL in susceptible individuals and may add to the presence of cholesterol-rich atherogenic particles in the postprandial state. Hence, dietary restriction of cholesterol may be justifiable, even when other dietary measurements to minimize cholesterol have been successfully instituted.

Protein intake should be between 10 per cent and 20 per cent of the total caloric intake. The total amount of carbohydrates should be about 50 to 60 per cent of total calories. As dietary fat is reduced, it is considered prudent to replace it with complex carbohydrates, including vegetable fiber. The precise action of dietary fiber is not known. Although recent studies have shown that an increased consumption of oat bran may have a hypolipidemic effect, much of this effect may be due to the substitution of complex carbohydrates as fiber for fat in the diet rather than to a direct action.[95,96] There is a 4 to 5 per cent independent effect of soluble fiber in the reduction of serum cholesterol. Fiber in the diet may have other health benefits, including reduced risk from colon cancers.

If the patient is above ideal body weight, caloric restriction should be implemented to achieve weight reduction. Certain patients will respond to alterations in body weight with profound changes in circulating LDL levels. Ethanol is calorie dense, and its restriction can play a role in weight reduction; moderate use of ethanol can increase HDL cholesterol,[9] but the clinical significance of this effect is unknown.

After initiation of the Step One Diet, the serum cholesterol should be retested at 6 and 12 weeks. Serum cholesterol can serve as a surrogate measure of LDL in most patients. If specific goals are not achieved, and the patient can adhere to a more restricted diet, the patient should be referred to a registered dietitian for further instruction and for institution of the Step Two Diet. In the Step Two Diet (Table 37–5), saturated fats are decreased to less than 7 per cent of total calories and cholesterol to less than 200 mg/day. The polyunsaturated and monounsaturated fatty acid contents of the diet should remain at 10 per cent and in the 10 to 15 per cent range, respectively. Carbohydrate and protein intake should represent 50 to 60 per cent and 10 to 20 per cent of total calories, respectively, as in Step One.

An inadequate response to diet has several possible explanations. Some patients appear to be biologically resistant to an impact of diet on LDL lowering, despite good adherence. Adherence is a major problem and requires a concerted effort at guidance by physicians and dietitians. In some cases, a prolonged period of dietary therapy may be needed to alter the pattern of eating. Adequate time should be allowed for the patient to institute the recommended dietary changes and required adaptations of lifestyle. In patients with severe hyperlipidemia, it is not necessary to wait the 6 months before beginning pharmacological therapy.

The NCEP has also provided recommendations for dietary therapy in special groups. During pregnancy, elevated levels of triglycerides and cholesterol occur in the third trimester. As a general rule, these elevations are not clinically significant. The elevated lipids usually return to the baseline range about 4 to 6 weeks after delivery.

It is prudent to follow lipid values in hypertriglyceridemic patients and in those who have conditions that might predispose to this disorder. Dietary therapy in elderly patients should be individualized on physiological rather than chronological age, and the value of diet modification should be weighed against the possibility of an inadequate nutritional state. For the severe primary lipid disorders, such as FH, the lipid levels usually do not improve with dietary therapy alone. Dietary therapy should be implemented, however, to minimize the doses of pharmacological agents used.

For most patients with borderline elevations of lipids, intensive dietary therapy (i.e., the Step Two Diet) is not required. The NCEP states that population-based approaches to altering levels of lipids — in the entire community — will have a significant impact. Special attention should be given to younger people who are believed to be at increased risk for long-term development of CAD. The role of diet modification is pivotal in the treatment of the dyslipidemic patient and that dietary therapy must be continued, even after the decision has been made to use a pharmacological agent.

OMEGA-3 UNSATURATED FATTY ACIDS

The role of the consumption of oils from cold-water fish to protect against coronary disease remains controversial. The rationale for the use of these agents stems from the recognition that Greenland Eskimos have a low incidence of atherosclerotic cardiovascular disease, although this association has not been definitely established by extensive epidemiological data. Inhibition of atherosclerosis has been documented in several animal models on fish oil feeding.[97]

Fish oils are rich in eicosapentaenoic acid, an omega-3 unsaturated fatty acid that replaces an arachidonic acid in the platelet membrane. This replacement alters platelet aggregation and secondarily increases bleeding time. Eicosapentaenoic acid and docosahexaenoic acid appear to be the most important omega-3 fatty acids in the cold-water fish. Fish that contain omega-3 fatty acids include salmon, mackerel, rainbow trout, sardines, sablefish, and albacore tuna. In addition to the antiplatelet effect, the consumption of fish oil supplements has been shown to affect thrombosis. Experiments are under way to test the effects of fish oil supplements on patients undergoing angioplasty. The specific mechanisms are unknown, but it has been shown that fish oils will decrease fibrinogen levels.[98]

Fish oils may have beneficial effects on blood pressure as well. Human studies have documented that the intake of cold-water fish at a dose level of 280 gm/day can result in a 12 per cent decrease in systolic blood pressure.[99] Similar results were recorded in a number of epidemiological studies, in which fish consumption correlated with lower blood pressure.[100]

Although the consumption of fish oils does not greatly affect circulating LDL levels, it has been shown to decrease triglyceride levels markedly by inhibiting hepatic VLDL secretion. The benefit from fish oil supplements is rapid, and maximal lipid lowering can occur within 1 month of therapy. The use of fish oil supplements is more effective in the Fredrickson phenotypes associated with hypertriglyceridemia (IIb, IV, and V). Although usually this measure is effective in lowering lipids, there have been reports that a rebound phenomenon may occur later in the treatment phase, resulting in a decreased efficacy of therapy.[101] Moreover, fish oil supplements may have adverse effects in diabetic patients because of altered secretion of insulin and increased hepatic output of glucose.[102] Despite the apparent benefits of fish oil consumption in clinical and epidemiological studies, we do not recommend the intake of fish oil supplements as of this writing. It does seem prudent, however, to incorporate cold-water fish that are rich in omega-3 fatty acids into the diet at least twice a week.

DRUG TREATMENT
(See Tables 37–6 and 37–7)

Drug treatment of lipid disorders should not be used until a precise diagnosis is firmly established and the presence of

TABLE 37-6 SUMMARY OF LIPID-LOWERING AGENTS

AGENTS	MECHANISM OF ACTION	BIOCHEMICAL SIDE EFFECTS	SYSTEMIC SIDE EFFECTS	DOSAGE RANGE (DAILY)
Bile acid resins Cholestyramine; Colestipol	Increases excretion of bile acids in the stool, increases LDL-receptor activity	May prevent absorption of fat-soluble vitamins	Constipation, bloating	12–24 gm (cholestyramine) 15–30 gm (colestipol)
Nicotinic acid	Decreases plasma levels of free fatty acids, possibly inhibits cholesterol synthesis, decreases hepatic VLDL synthesis	Altered liver function tests, increased uric acid, increased glucose intolerance	Cutaneous flushing, pruritus, gastrointestinal upset	3–6 gm
Probucol	Enhances scavenger pathway removal of LDL	Decreased HDL	Diarrhea, nausea, flatulence	500–1000 mg
Fibric acid derivatives Gemfibrozil Clofibrate	Decreases hepatic VLDL synthesis, increases lipoprotein lipase activity	Altered liver function tests, increased CPK, potentiation of warfarin	Increased incidence of cholelithiasis and perhaps of GI cancer; myositis, diarrhea, nausea, rash (rare)	600–1200 mg (gemfibrozil) 1–2 gm (clofibrate)
HMG CoA reductase inhibitors Lovastatin Pravastatin	Inhibits HMG CoA reductase, increases LDL-receptor activity	Elevated transaminase levels, increased CPK	Mild GI symptoms; myositis syndrome	Starting dose 20 mg; range 40–80 mg

CPK = creatine phosphokinase; GI = gastrointestinal; HDL = high-density lipoprotein; HMG-CoA = 3-hydroxy-3-methylglutaryl coenzyme A; LDL = low-density lipoprotein; VLDL = very low-density lipoprotein.

treatable secondary causes has been ruled out. Before the institution of pharmacological hypolipidemic therapy, maximum dietary efforts should be instituted. As noted earlier, diet should be considered the mainstay of therapy, and a strenuous effort should be made to lower elevated lipids by nonpharmacological means. Drug therapy should be considered only when dietary treatment and other nonpharmacological interventions have failed to improve the lipid profile adequately.

The NCEP has provided risk-stratification guidelines for patients with hyperlipidemia. A number of factors—including the patient's age, associated illnesses, presence of documented atherosclerosis, and renal or hepatic dysfunction—play a role and must be considered before a patient is committed to pharmacological intervention.

The role of drugs in the treatment of hypertriglyceridemia is controversial. For example, Hoeg and coworkers recommend dietary therapy for patients in whom the triglyceride value is between 200 and 500 mg/dl.[103] If the value exceeds 500 mg/dl and the patient is at increased risk for pancreatitis or has a strong personal history of coronary disease, pharmacological therapy in addition to dietary measures is recommended.[103] If the triglyceride value exceeds 1000 mg/dl and this parameter

TABLE 37-7 DRUG TREATMENT FOR HYPERLIPIDEMIAS

PHENOTYPE	DRUG TREATMENT
Type I	None
Type IIa	LOV BAS NA and PRO BAS + NA BAS + LOV BAS + PRO
Type IIb	BAS + NA BAS + GEM
Type III	NA, GEM, Clo
Type IV	NA, GEM
Type V	NA (limited by glucose intolerance) GEM NA + GEM

BAS = bile-acid sequestrant (cholestyramine, colestipol); Clo = clofibrate; GEM = gemfibrozil; LOV = lovastatin; NA = nicotinic acid (niacin); Pro = probucol.

is uncontrolled, Hoeg and associates recommend referral to a specialized center for evaluation and treatment.[103] The NCEP recommends total and LDL cholesterol values as the keys to establishing treatment guidelines (see above). However, the importance of individualizing the therapy must be emphasized.

BILE ACID SEQUESTRANTS. Cholestyramine and colestipol are quaternary ammonium salts that act as anion-exchange resins and bind bile salts in the intestine. This binding leads to an interruption of the enterohepatic circulation of bile salts and causes an enhanced excretion of sterols in the stool. The number and function of LDL receptors also are increased, with a secondary rise in the plasma clearance of LDL.

Cholestyramine and colestipol are considered first-line agents by the NCEP for the treatment of type II HLP and are highly effective in decreasing LDL cholesterol.[104] They are efficacious if the cholesterol is moderately elevated, as in the sporadic, polygenic forms of hyperlipidemia, but usually are not sufficient as single agents if the cholesterol is severely elevated, as in heterozygous familial hypercholesterolemics. Cholestyramine and colestipol also are ineffective in the rare homozygous type II HLP.

The bile acid sequestrants are difficult to use because of their frequent side effects, which include nausea, abdominal discomfort, constipation, and indigestion, and their sandy, gritty texture and unpleasant taste. Systemic side effects are rare because of the drugs' lack of absorption. Sequestrants may interfere with the absorption of other agents, such as digitalis, phenobarbital, thiazides, Coumadin (warfarin), thyroxine, and tetracycline. GI side effects have been lessened with recent preparations that are less bulky and have decreased carbohydrate content.

The resins come as granulated preparations in 4- or 5-gm packets and should be mixed with fluids or taken with meals. Stool softeners and increased fluid intake also may minimize the side effects. The dose should be low initially (e.g., one packet per day before a meal) and gradually increased (by one packet per day). The drug should be given 1 hour before or 4 hours after other medications. For patients who tolerate these agents, the average dose is three to six packets per day, usually given in divided doses with meals. Although the maximum dose is difficult to attain because of poor compliance, a 20 to 25 per cent reduction in LDL levels may be attained.

The LRC-CPPT study used the bile acid sequestrant cholestyramine as a single agent.[53] As noted above, this study indicated that a 1 per cent drop in total cholesterol was associated with approximately a 2 per cent drop in CAD risk. However, only a 9 per cent reduction of cholesterol was achieved overall in this trial because of inadequate compliance in the use of the drug.

Colestipol was used in the recent CLAS[55,56] and FATS[67,105] studies in combination with nicotinic acid. This drug combination produced angiographic regression of coronary atherosclerosis among patients who had undergone coronary bypass surgery (CLAS) or who had elevated levels of apo B-100 (FATS).

NICOTINIC ACID. The B vitamin nicotinic acid (niacin) is applied pharmacologically in doses that far exceed the levels required for its action as a nutrient. At the maximum dose of 3 to 6 gm/day, nicotinic acid is effective in the pharmacological management of all types of HLP except type I. Nicotinic acid decreases LDL levels by about 25 per cent and VLDL levels by about 75 per cent. The mechanism of this agent is complex and involves a reduction in LDL production, secondary to a decreased hepatic VLDL synthesis.[106] Nicotinic acid also inhibits the release of fatty acids from adipose tissues and thus decreases the level of substrate available for synthesis of triglycerides. Nicotinic acid increases HDL levels by 20 to 40 per cent, also probably as a result of the decreased VLDL production. The subfraction of HDL increased with nicotinic acid therapy appears to be predominantly HDL_2.

Like bile acid resins, nicotinic acid has frequent side effects. Common problems include cutaneous flushing and GI symptoms. The flushing and pruritus usually occur within 1 hour of administration and can be minimized by taking the drug with meals along with aspirin prophylaxis. The flushing tends to decrease with time; its basis is a prostaglandin-mediated capillary dilation. The documented GI effects relate to the elevation of the liver enzymes and gastritis, which may predispose the patient to peptic ulcer disease. Increased pigmentation of the skin may occur as well. Liver function tests should be closely monitored. Because another potential side effect is impairment of glucose tolerance, the drug should be used with caution in diabetics. Hyperuricemia has been reported, particularly in patients with gout.

Initial doses of nicotinic acid should be low (e.g., 50 mg), given with each meal, and gradually advanced to 1 gm three times daily. Nicotinic acid can be used for aggressive LDL lowering when administered with bile acid sequestrants. In the Coronary Drug Project, nicotinic acid was shown to decrease coronary and total mortality 9 years after the trial was terminated.[44] An overall decrease in total mortality of 11 per cent was seen in the trial's long-term follow-up. In the CLAS study[65,66] nicotinic acid combined with colestipol markedly improved lipid profiles and produced angiographic coronary regression, when compared with dietary treatment. Entry into this study required that patients be able to tolerate full-dose niacin and colestipol. Anatomical coronary lesion regression was seen after 4 years in 18 per cent of the patients who underwent diet plus drug therapy, compared with 6 per cent of the group with dietary intervention alone.[66]

PROBUCOL. Probucol lowers both LDL and HDL fractions. LDL cholesterol reductions averaging about 20 per cent can be expected after a full therapeutic trial, although the magnitude of the effect varies considerably from patient to patient. Probucol's mechanism of action is complex, and does not require the presence of LDL receptors. Presumably, the effect on lipids is accomplished by a non-receptor–mediated or scavenger pathway–modulated removal of LDL. The decrease in HDL that occurs is of concern, but its clinical impact has not been determined. Probucol also may modify LDL in the Watanabe rabbit by protecting against LDL oxidation.[79,107] This effect has been correlated with an antiatherosclerotic effect in this animal. Native LDL is poorly taken up by the resident macrophages in foam cell genesis. However, oxidatively modified LDL is preferentially taken up by these scavenger receptors,

thus providing a mechanism for foam cell formation.[107a,107b] Apparently, antioxidants such as probucol can slow the progression of atherosclerosis in the Watanabe heritable hyperlipidemic (WHHL) rabbit. Probucol also may produce antiatherosclerotic activity, independent of its effect on lowering cholesterol.[108]

This pharmaceutical has been reported to increase the activity of the cholesteryl ester transfer protein, or lipid transfer protein. This effect would be expected to decrease HDL concentrations because of an alteration in lipoprotein kinetics. Probucol has been demonstrated to enhance a cholesterol efflux from human fibroblasts in vitro.[109] Its demonstrated stimulation of the production of apo E may further enhance the clearance of lipoproteins by way of their recognition and removal by the LDL receptor.[110] Probucol has little effect on VLDL; hence, it is most efficacious in the treatment of patients with type II HLP. Probucol has been combined with bile acid sequestrants for an additional effect on LDL lowering. The addition of probucol to lovastatin resulted in no further LDL decrease beyond that produced by lovastatin alone. There also appeared to be no added hypolipidemic benefit with the use of probucol as a third agent.[111]

The major side effects of probucol are gastrointestinal and usually are mild when the drug is used as a single agent. Prolongation of the QT and QT-C electrocardiogram intervals has been demonstrated experimentally and in humans. However, the relation of this alteration of repolarization to polymorphic ventricular tachycardia (torsades de pointes) has not been established.

As seen by a variety of imaging techniques, probucol yielded regression of tendinous xanthomas in FH patients; however, whether this effect correlates with coronary artery regression or has an impact on mortality has not been determined. A large-scale arterial regression study, the Probucol Quantitative Regression Swedish Trial, is investigating the development of atherosclerosis in hyperlipidemic patients through femoral quantitative angiographic techniques.[112,113]

FIBRIC ACID DERIVATIVES. Gemfibrozil and clofibrate are the fibric acid derivatives currently available in the United States. In Europe, fenofibrate, bezafibrate, and ciprofibrate are also used. The fibric-acid derivatives are effective in lowering VLDL, IDL, and triglycerides. Their mechanism of action is complex; one effect is to increase lipoprotein lipase activity and thereby increase the clearance of VLDL particles.[114,114a] Cholesterol secretion into the bile also is enhanced. These agents are effective in lowering triglycerides in patients with hypertriglyceridemia. In some cases, they can lower triglyceride levels by as much as 50 per cent, while increasing HDL levels by 10 per cent to 20 per cent.

Clofibrate was the agent used in the World Health Organization trial that showed a decrease in nonfatal MIs.[115] However, an increase in overall mortality was noted. In this trial, the MI incidence was directly related to serum cholesterol levels and blood pressure, and to the incidence of cigarette smoking. The decrease in MI was most evident in the patients who were hypertensive and heavy smokers. Clofibrate also appeared to lower fibrinogen levels, an effect that may have contributed to the lower MI incidence.

Gemfibrozil has been shown to be effective in all types of dyslipidemia with the exception of type I HLP.[114a] However, its main effect is the alteration of triglyceride-rich lipoproteins. Gemfibrozil reduces LDL cholesterol by about 10 per cent to 20 per cent, with a subsequent decrease in apo B in patients with type IIa HLP. Patients with type IIb experience minimal changes in LDL levels, whereas those with type IV HLP may experience an *increase* in LDL levels. VLDL and triglycerides may be decreased by up to 60 per cent, with a subsequent rise in the HDL fraction.

The efficacy of gemfibrozil in decreasing coronary death rates was demonstrated in the Helsinki Heart Study[54] (see p. 1133). This trial resulted in a 34 per cent reduction in coronary incidents with improvements seen in all of the Fredrickson

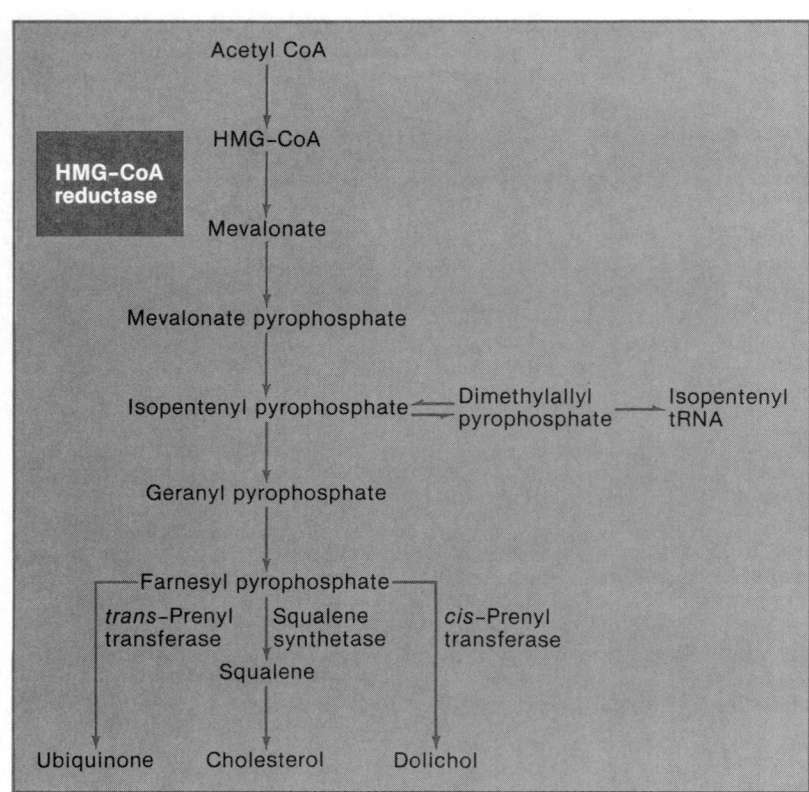

FIGURE 37–12. Cholesterol biosynthetic pathway. (From Alberts, A. W.: Effects of HMG CoA reductase inhibitors on cholesterol synthesis. Drug Invest. *2*(Suppl. 2):9, 1990.)

phenotypes in the study (IIa, IIb, and IV). The greatest benefit was experienced by patients with type IIb HLP.

Fibric-acid derivatives usually are well tolerated, with nausea and GI discomfort the major side effects. Myositis and glucose elevation have been reported but are relatively uncommon. Fibric acid derivatives may potentiate the effect of Coumadin.

HMG-CoA REDUCTASE INHIBITORS. Compactin, lovastatin, simvastatin, pravastatin, and fluvastatin are agents that inhibit 3-hydroxy-3-methylglutaryl coenzyme A HMG-CoA reductase, which is the rate-limiting enzyme in the cholesterol biosynthetic pathway (Fig. 37–12).[116] Their action is competition and partial blocking (Fig. 37–13), which occurs because the side chain in these agents has a structural resemblance to HMG-CoA. They decrease hepatic cholesterol synthesis and thus increase the number of LDL receptors expressed on the hepatic tissue surface. LDL-receptor activity can be determined by bioassay with culture of human fibroblasts, or by assay of the functional LDL-receptor activity on lymphocytes.[117,118]

The HMG-CoA reductase inhibitors represent a major advance in the treatment of hypercholesterolemic patients. Lovastatin and pravastatin are the only drugs of this class currently available in the United States. The prototype statin, compactin, was never marketed, presumably because of toxicity in animal experiments.

The main indication for the use of the HMG-CoA reductase inhibitors is in the treatment of patients with elevated levels of LDL cholesterol. In patients who also have mildly elevated triglycerides, lovastatin enhances clearance of postprandial lipoprotein levels, with a significant lowering of VLDL cholesterol and fasting triglycerides; hence its administration may benefit patients with type IIb HLP.[119] In patients with normal lipid profiles except for decreased levels of HDL, lovastatin has been shown to decrease LDL and apo B by about 25 per cent. In the large clinical trials in hypercholesterolemic subjects, reductase inhibitors have increased HDL cholesterol on average by 5 to 10 per cent.[120] The effects of reductase inhibitors on Lp(a) have not yet been well characterized. Lovastatin has reportedly decreased LDL cholesterol levels without a concomitant reduction in Lp(a). This suggests a different

mechanism of clearance of Lp(a) from the circulation. There are some reports of an increase in Lp(a) levels with lovastatin therapy, although the data are quite limited.[121]

In addition to lowering plasma lipids, the reductase inhibitor *simvastatin* has been reported to decrease platelet aggregation and thromboxane B_2 formation induced by collagen.[122]

The reductase inhibitors may be combined with bile-acid sequestrants (Fig. 37–14) to produce dramatic decreases in

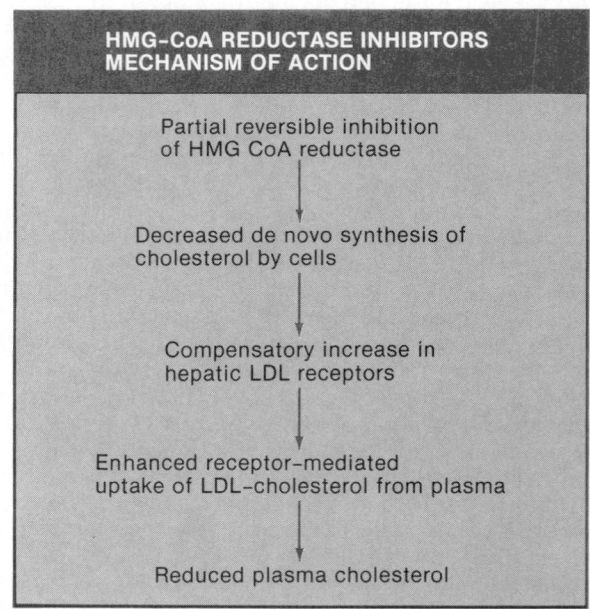

FIGURE 37–13. The mechanism of the 3-hydroxy-3-methylglutaryl–coenzyme A (HMG-CoA) reductase inhibitors involves partial inhibition of the rate-limiting enzyme in cholesterol synthesis that converts HMG-CoA to mevalonic acid. The subsequent decrease in intracellular cholesterol stimulates the synthesis of the low-density lipoprotein (LDL) or apoprotein B/E receptor, which allows increased recognition and plasma clearance of particles containing these apoproteins.

FIGURE 37–14. Rationale for the combination of a bile acid sequestrant and reductase inhibitor in the treatment of hypercholesterolemia. Bile acid sequestrants increase clearance of low-density lipoprotein (LDL) by increasing the number of apoprotein B/E receptors in addition to enhanced gastrointestinal loss via interception of the enterohepatic circulation. The compensatory increase in cholesterol synthesis may be blocked by addition of a reductase inhibitor that inhibits 3-hydroxy-3-methylglutaryl–coenzyme A (HMG-CoA) reductase–mediated cholesterol synthesis and further increases apoprotein B/E receptor activity. (From Brown, M. S., and Goldstein, J. L.: A receptor-mediated pathway for cholesterol homeostasis. Science *232:*34, 1986. Copyright 1986 by the American Association for the Advancement of Science.)

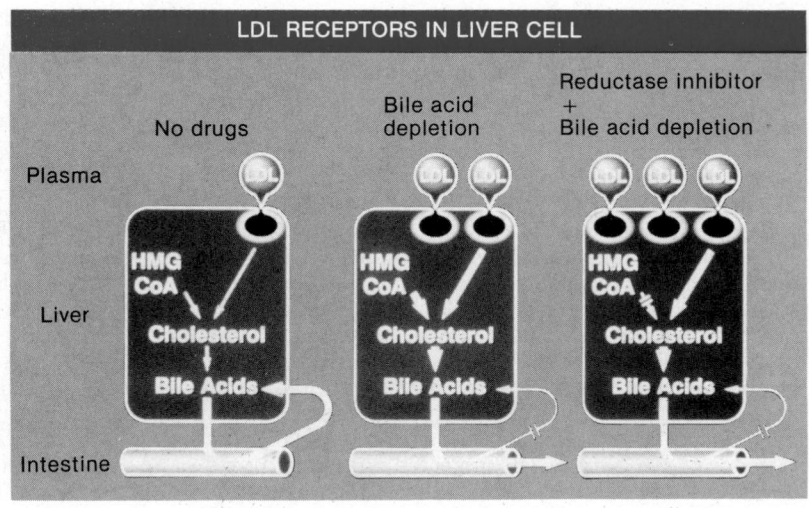

overall LDL levels. As already discussed, the bile-acid sequestrants increase LDL-receptor activity and sterol excretion in the GI tract. A compensatory increase in the activity of the HMG-CoA reductase enzyme system can be inhibited by the use of lovastatin, with reductions in LDL cholesterol of 50 per cent to 60 per cent reported.

The incidence of serious side effects with lovastatin is low. Nonetheless, the physician should be watchful for myositis, hepatocellular abnormalities, and lens opacities. Concerns about the potential for development of cataracts resulted from early experience with the drug MER-29, an agent that inhibited the penultimate step in the biosynthesis of cholesterol. This drug increased early cataract formation. Also, lovastatin at very high doses has been reported to cause cataracts in beagles, but this effect has not been encountered in other animals or in humans.

The inhibition of HMG-CoA reductase occurs early in the biosynthetic pathway of cholesterol (Fig. 37–12), and the fears concerning cataract formation have not been realized. Mild elevations of aspartate aminotransferase and alanine aminotransferase have been reported, requiring the discontinuation of therapy in about 0.6 per cent of outpatients. Myositis has been seen in transplant patients receiving concomitant cyclosporine therapy. The latter therapy raises blood levels of lovastatin and may result in marked elevation of creatinine phosphokinase and rhabdomyolysis. In patients not receiving cyclosporine, the incidence of myositis is probably 1 in 500. An increased incidence has been reported when the drug is given with gemfibrozil, nicotinic acid, or erythromycin. Available data on reductase inhibitors suggest that they are effectively removed in first-pass clearance by the liver and may be actively transported into hepatocytes. This highly effective first-pass clearance probably accounts for the relative efficacy and safety of the drugs as a class. Demonstrated differences in the uptake by nonhepatic tissues are potentially related to hydrophobicity and solubility in tissue. The clinical significance of these effects in humans is not established.

DEXTROTHYROXINE. Dextrothyroxine is the dextroisomer of the naturally occurring thyroid hormone levothyroxine and is used as a secondary drug in the treatment of type II HLP. Its mechanism of action is unclear, but it appears to increase the activity of LDL receptors in hypothyroid animals. Dextrothyroxine is approved by the Food and Drug Administration for use in patients with no evidence of CAD or cardiac arrhythmia. In the Coronary Drug Project, its use was associated with increased morbidity and mortality, leading to its early termination.[123] Dextrothyroxine should be reserved for selected young adults with primary hypercholesterolemia who are unable to take effective lipid-lowering drugs and who are free of CAD.

SPECIFIC TREATMENTS FOR HYPERLIPOPROTEINEMIA TYPES
(Table 37–7)

LIPOPROTEIN LIPASE AND APO C-II DEFICIENCY—TYPE I. Type I HLP is diagnosed in the pediatric age group as an autosomal recessive disorder of lipoprotein lipase.[124] A deficiency of apo C-II or a circulating inhibitor may cause a clinical presentation that is indistinguishable from other types of chylomicronemia. Therapy is initiated to decrease the risk of recurrent pancreatitis. Generally, if the triglyceride level can be kept under 1000 mg/dl, the development of pancreatitis is uncommon. Dietary fat should be restricted to 10 to 25 gm/day. Medium-chain triglycerides may be used to make the diet more palatable. These triglycerides are absorbed directly in the portal circulation and do not require lipoprotein lipase activation for metabolism. If there is documented apo C-II deficiency, the acute treatment of the abdominal pain associated with type I HLP can be specifically directed at replacement of the apoprotein. Apo C-II may be supplied by plasma infusions in a life-threatening situation. Drug therapy is ineffective in the three genetic defects that result in a type I phenotype. Hence, diet is the key to maintenance therapy of type I HLP.

POLYGENIC AND FAMILIAL HYPERCHOLESTEROLEMIA—TYPE II. Aggressive therapy is mandatory in patients with type II HLP because of the high incidence of premature coronary atherosclerosis and peripheral vascular disease. Therapy should be based on a careful genetic diagnosis, with secondary causes of elevated cholesterol diagnostically excluded. The patient should scrupulously follow the AHA Step One Diet and progress to the Step Two Diet before drug therapy is considered. Most patients with mild type II HLP have polygenic hypercholesterolemia and can be treated with diet alone. The NCEP recommends bile acid sequestrants (cholestyramine or colestipol) and niacin as primary therapeutic agents. Colestipol is given at 5 to 10 gm three times a day, cholestyramine at 4 to 8 gm three times a day. Nicotinic acid can be added in doses of 1.0 to 1.5 gm three times a day with meals and aspirin prophylaxis. The combination of colestipol and niacin has been shown to be associated with the regression of coronary atherosclerosis in both native circulation and coronary venous bypass grafts.[65] However, this combination often is hampered by poor compliance with therapy.

The advent of the HMG-CoA reductase inhibitors has markedly expanded the ability of the clinician to treat type II HLP successfully. These agents have been shown to be markedly effective in type II phenotypes, regardless of the underlying defect. Lovastatin in short-term use has been associated with a low incidence of serious side effects.[125] When it is combined with a bile acid sequestrant, dramatic reductions in LDL cholesterol (up to 60 per cent) can be achieved. Such a combination was shown in the FATS study to result in the regression of established atherosclerotic lesions as demonstrated by quantitative angiography (Fig. 37–8).[16] In that study, colestipol plus lovastatin resulted in a 46 per cent reduction in LDL levels and a 15 per cent increase in HDL levels over a treatment period of 2½ years.

Probucol can be used as a single agent to lower LDL levels. It stimulates LDL clearance by non-receptor–mediated mechanisms, and thus can be useful in the rare patient with homozygous familial hypercholesterolemia who has no functioning LDL receptors.[126] The clinical impact of probucol on the oxidative modification of the LDL molecule needs to be clarified by clinical trials. The fibric acid derivatives increase the clearance of VLDL by activating lipoprotein lipase and by increasing the secretion of cholesterol into the bile. An LDL reduction of about 15 per cent can be expected with gemfibrozil in patients with type IIa HLP. Plasma exchange or LDL-pheresis can be used for severe, refractory elevations of LDL. In rare cases of a familial hypercholesterolemic homozygote, liver transplantation may be required to supply functioning LDL receptors.

FAMILIAL DYSBETALIPOPROTEINEMIA—TYPE III. Patients with type III HLP respond to treatment of secondary factors such as metabolic abnormalities that result in IDL accumulation. Metabolic conditions that may unmask the underlying $E_{2/2}$ phenotype are excessive alcohol intake, hypothyroidism, and diabetes mellitus. Dietary modification should be aggressively attempted in type III HLP and frequently results in complete normalization of the lipid abnormality. Drugs that have been found to be useful for dietary failures are fibric acid derivatives and nicotinic acid. Gemfibrozil at 600 mg twice daily usually dramatically reduces VLDL, IDL, and triglycerides. Nicotinic acid can be expected to reduce VLDL cholesterol and plasma triglycerides by approximately 40 per cent. Simvastatin, a nonapproved drug, has recently been shown to be effective in treating type III HLP; it produced lipid profile improvements similar to those achieved with fibric acid derivatives.[127]

FAMILIAL COMBINED AND ENDOGENOUS HYPERTRIGLYCERIDEMIA—TYPE IV. The treatment of type IV HLP involves dietary management and weight control. Alcohol consumption should be minimized, and diabetes should be strictly regulated. The Step One Diet can be used as initial therapy for patients at risk for pancreatitis or other complications of hypertriglyceridemia. Pharmacological intervention should be individualized according to the cause of the elevated VLDL. The most commonly used medication is gemfibrozil, which increases VLDL clearance. Nicotinic acid can be used but may alter glucose tolerance in patients with diabetes. These drugs should be used when levels exceed 500 mg/dl and secondary causes have been excluded.

TYPE V. Treatment of type V HLP centers on the correction or control of the underlying cause, especially excessive alcohol use and diabetes. Estrogens should be avoided if possible. Dietary therapy should be directed toward the achievement of ideal body weight, and fats should not exceed 30 per cent of total caloric intake. Cholesterol consumption should be less than 300 mg/day. Polyunsaturated fats should be substituted for saturated fats in the diet. If drug therapy is required, gemfibrozil should be considered, since it has been shown to be well tolerated and effective in these patients.[128] Nicotinic acid in high doses is effective but may worsen glucose tolerance and hyperuricemia.

OTHER TYPES OF THERAPY FOR HYPERLIPOPROTEINEMIA

If diet and hypolipidemic agents are ineffective in lowering cholesterol to acceptable levels, more aggressive therapies are available. Bypassing the terminal 200 cm of the small intestine can be used to interrupt the anterohepatic circulation for

the reabsorption of bile salts and was evaluated in patients in the Program on the Surgical Control of the Hyperlipidemias (POSCH) trial.[129] Portacaval shunt appears to decrease LDL synthesis in familial hypercholesterolemia and will result in significant reductions in cholesterol. However, this treatment has been abandoned as a result of significant long-term side effects.[190-192] As mentioned, liver transplantation may be used in patients with total absence of LDL receptors.[299]

The serious problems attendant to these surgical approaches are obvious, and surgery should be considered only when diet and medications have failed to lower LDL cholesterol to acceptable levels. Plasma-exchange columns for LDL-pheresis and antibodies that extract LDL are available, but their current use is limited by expense and inconvenience. There have been reports of improved survival of patients with homozygous familial hypercholesterolemia who were treated with plasma exchange. The treatment interval was, on average, 2 weeks, and the treatment period was, on average, 8 years. The patients treated with plasma exchange had an average 37 per cent reduction in serum cholesterol and an average 5.5-year increase in survival.[134,135]

TOBACCO USE

The use of tobacco products remains a major remediable risk factor in patients prone to the development of CAD and may interact with a variety of the other CAD risk factors. Tobacco products may accelerate the process of atherosclerosis by a variety of mechanisms. Cigarette smoking has been demonstrated to have adverse effects on the lipid profile. Compared with nonsmokers, heavy smokers (more than 25 cigarettes per day) have lower levels of HDL and higher levels of LDL and triglycerides.[136,137] The precise mechanism by which smoking alters the lipid profile is unclear.

Use of tobacco products also has been correlated with alterations in blood pressure, although the effects are variable. In particular, the acute inhalation of tobacco smoke is associated with a rise in blood pressure.[138] However, a number of large-scale epidemiological studies have documented that chronic smokers tend to have lower blood pressure than nonsmokers, an effect that could be due to lower body weight.[139]

The use of tobacco products also may affect a patient's response to antihypertensive therapy. Smoking has worsened the outcome of patients with essential hypertension for all-causes cardiovascular mortality. This has been seen in many large-scale hypertension trials, including the Hypertension Detection and Follow-up Program, in which smokers had twice the rate of mortality of nonsmokers.[140]

Inhalation of cigarette smoke exerts many effects on clotting factors, platelet function, and other hematologic parameters that may play a role in atherosclerosis. In the Framingham Study, it was found that fibrinogen values are significantly higher in the smoking than in the nonsmoking population.[141] Fibrinogen levels have been reported to be an independent risk factor for CAD,[142] although the effects of secondary elevation of fibrinogen levels have not been studied. With smoking cessation, fibrinogen levels diminish to baseline, but this process may take as long as 5 years.[141] Alterations of the clotting mechanism also may attend to the effects of smoke inhalation on platelet function. Smokers have been found to have increased platelet aggregation and a prolongation in bleeding time.[143] Cigarette smoke may affect endothelial cell function directly by decreasing the ability to produce or release prostacyclin, thus changing platelet aggregation and vascular tone.[144]

Approximately 50 to 150 μg of nicotine is absorbed through the lung mucosa with each puff of tobacco. Nicotine is a potent agonist for the adrenergic nervous system and causes increased plasma norepinephrine release. Inhalation of tobacco smoke has been shown to induce increased coronary tone and enhance vasoconstriction in CAD patients.[145] The enhanced vasoconstriction may result in an imbalance between oxygen

TABLE 37-8 INCIDENCE OF CORONARY ARTERY DISEASE MORBIDITY RELATED TO CIGARETTE SMOKING

SMOKING PATTERN	INCIDENCE RATIO
Nonsmokers	58
Cigar and pipe smokers only	71
Cigarette smokers	
About 0.5 pack/day	104
About 1 pack/day	120
More than 1 pack/day	183

From Aronow, W. S., and Kaplan, N. M.: Smoking. *In* Kaplan, N. M., and Stamler, J. (eds.): Prevention of Coronary Heart Disease: Practical Management of the Risk Factors. Philadelphia, W. B. Saunders Company, 1983, p. 55.

Data from the Pooling Project Research Group: Relationship of blood pressure, serum cholesterol, smoking habit, relative weight and ECG abnormalities to incidence of major coronary events: Final report of the Pooling Project. J. Chron. Dis. 31:201, 1978.

supply and demand and has been associated with increased episodes of silent myocardial ischemia.[146] Many studies have shown that smokers have approximately twice the risk of CAD as nonsmokers (Table 37–8). In the Framingham Study, participants who discontinued smoking lowered their risk of MI within 2 years.[147] Other studies have found that men who have given up smoking for over 20 years still have an increased risk.[148] Kaufman and associates evaluated the components of cigarette smoke against the risk of MI in young men. These investigators compared 502 cases with 835 hospital controls between the ages of 30 and 54.[149] Overall, the relative-risk estimate for current smokers was 2.8, and risk showed a positive correlation with number of cigarettes smoked (2.1 for the lightest and 4.0 for the heaviest smokers). Risk did not vary with the quantity of nicotine or carbon monoxide in the cigarette. These results indicated that men who smoke cigarettes that contain less tar and less nicotine do *not* have a corresponding decrease in MI. In an animal model, inhalation of nicotine has been shown to increase markedly uptake of iodine-labeled fibrinogen by the arterial wall. This may be one mechanism by which cigarette smoking contributes to atherosclerosis.[150]

Despite the theoretical attractiveness of low-nicotine and low–carbon monoxide cigarettes, clinical studies have not shown that low-nicotine cigarettes reduce the incidence of MI. This may reflect a compensating factor, such as inhaling more deeply. In any case, patients who want to reduce their overall risk for CAD should not rely on any promised advantage of low-nicotine cigarettes.[151]

Even nonsmokers may be exposed to increased risk by passive smoking. In the MRFIT, subsets of patients were evaluated according to the smoking habits of their wives. The results indicate that passive exposure to cigarette smoke increased CAD risk.[152]

The incidence of MI is definitely diminished after patients quit smoking. The risk reduction occurs early, and may be demonstrated 12 months after the cessation of smoking. Major public health measures have been enacted to protect the nonsmoker from passive inhalation and to discourage consumption by reducing cigarette advertising and increasing excise taxes. The increase in cigarette smoking in young people, and particularly in young women, is of great concern for the future.

HYPERTENSION

(See also Chaps. 28 and 29)

Hypertension has been established as a major modifiable risk factor for the development of coronary atherosclerosis that extends across racial, gender, and age categories.[153,153a] It frequently coexists with other risk factors, and the impact may be synergistic, especially between hypertension and hyperlipidemia. The Framingham Study found an association between hyperlipidemia and increased hypertension.[147] Recent studies from Utah[154] have identified families with "dysli-

pidemic hypertension." This disorder may be related to "hyper-apo B," increased triglycerides, decreased HDL, small, dense LDL, hyperinsulinemia, and insulin resistance. Some antihypertensive agents, including diuretics and beta blockers, exacerbate dyslipidemia, although the clinical significance of these drug interactions is not known.[155] Pharmacological lowering of blood pressure has been reported to cause an increased risk for a cardiac event, especially in men with established coronary atherosclerosis.[156] This suggests that the relation between high blood pressure and CAD mortality follows a J-shaped curve, but the issue remains controversial.

Numerous prospective randomized clinical trials have addressed the impact of antihypertensive therapy on total and CAD morbidity and mortality. At least 14 trials have been completed, with a collective enrollment of over 37,000 patients and with long-term evaluation.[157] These intervention trials and epidemiological studies have described the prevalence rates and response to therapy of hypertension in the United States. The prevalence rates as defined by the Joint National Committee vary from 9.2 per cent among 18- to 24-year-olds to 64.3 per cent among 65- to 74-year-olds.[158]

Most of the hypertension trials used *stepped-care therapy*, with diuretics as the first-line agents. The efficacy of diuretic therapy in the prevention of CAD has been questioned, since a number of intervention trials did not show a decline in coronary mortality with these agents.

Beta blockers have a theoretical advantage in hypertension because of their multiplicity of effects and potential for cardioprotection. The Metoprolol Atherosclerosis Prevention in Hypertension (MAPHY) trial documented decreased total atherosclerotic death rates, including altered coronary heart disease mortality, in hypertensive patients who were smokers and receiving metoprolol therapy.[159] However, Kaplan[160] in a meta-analysis of antihypertensive trials attributed a lack of effect on CAD mortality (14 per cent reduction versus 42 per cent for stroke) in large part to the adverse effects of certain drugs on glucose tolerance, lipid levels, and insulin resistance. It was suggested that angiotensin-converting enzyme inhibitors through their favorable influence on CAD risk factors would reduce CAD mortality in patients treated for hypertension.[160]

SUCCESS OF DIETARY THERAPY FOR HYPERTENSION

There is no universal agreement on the optimal drug treatment goals in the management of hypertension. The recommendations of the British Hypertension Society are conservative. They suggest initial treatment at a diastolic level of 100 mm Hg, assuming the patient is less than 80 years old.[161] In the United States, the threshold generally recommended for treatment is 140/90 mm Hg. However, this threshold is not followed by all American physicians, especially when dealing with older patients.[162] Indeed, approximately half of American physicians use drug therapy in patients over age 60 whose systolic pressure is more than 160 mm Hg. Surveys also have shown that approximately 33 to 50 per cent of U.S. physicians begin to use drug therapy when an elderly patient's diastolic pressure exceeds 90 mm Hg.[163] Although Americans may be overly aggressive in using drugs to treat hypertension and the British too conservative, it is still useful to establish guidelines and goals.[164] These guidelines should include the identification of all curable forms of hypertension and stratify the remaining patients on the basis of underlying pathophysiology. The treatment should aim for minimum use of varied agents, lowest doses, and fewest side effects.

The 1988 recommendations of the U.S. Joint National Committee are a reasonable guide to the treatment of hypertension.[165] According to these recommendations, a diastolic pressure between 90 and 104 mm Hg constitutes "mild hypertension," a diastolic pressure between 105 and 114 mm Hg constitutes "moderate hypertension," and a diastolic pressure over 114 mm Hg defines "severe hypertension." With a diastolic pressure below 90 mm Hg, there is "borderline isolated systolic hypertension" when the systolic pressure is between 140 and 159 mm Hg and "isolated systolic hypertension" when the systolic pressure is 160 mm Hg or higher. These categorizations follow the documented clinical benefit of treating for diastolic pressures above 100 mm Hg and the suggested clinical benefit of treating for diastolic pressures between 90 and 99 mm Hg.

(see pp. 819 and 843)

A consensus report has been published to establish guidelines for the evaluation and treatment of pediatric patients as regards blood pressure.[166] This report stratifies blood pressure into three categories: (1) significant hypertension, in which the average confirmed systolic and diastolic pressures are above the 95th percentile for age and sex; (2) high normal, in which the average systolic and diastolic pressures are between the 90th and 95th percentiles for age and sex; and (3) normal, in which the average systolic and diastolic blood pressures are below the 90th percentile for age and sex.

The prevalence of significant hypertension is low in children. Markedly elevated blood pressure levels frequently are associated with a secondary cause (e.g., coarctation of the aorta, renal parenchymal anomalies, or reno-vascular disease), which should focus the investigation. A familial tendency for hypertension, hyperlipidemia, and increased insulin secretion, tentatively termed familial dyslipidemic hypertension, has been described in children and young adults, who often have truncal obesity. This may occur in 10 to 15 per cent of patients with presumed essential hypertension.[154,167] The urinary excretion of kallikrein has been reported to be inversely related to the level of high blood pressure and may be useful as a marker for some familial forms of hypertension.[168]

DIET AND HYPERTENSION

Although the exact relation of high sodium intake to hypertension has not been definitely established, an enormous amount of clinical evidence is available on this subject. The average U.S. consumption of salt is 10 to 15 gm/day, which exceeds the needs of the body. About two-thirds of the average dietary salt intake is obtained in processed food and one-third is added in cooking. NaCl has been shown to be more powerful in its pressor effect than other sodium salts.[169] Also, evaluation of 11 major clinical trials showed that an average decline in blood pressure of 6 mm Hg could be achieved by a 100-mmol/day decrease in sodium intake. A diet restricting sodium intake to a total of 2 gm, or 88 mmol, has been shown to be tolerable and efficacious.[170]

Although a vegetarian diet has been epidemiologically associated with lower blood pressure, these studies are fraught with potential methodological problems. Such a relation also is supported by experimental studies, although no precise mechanism has been described.[171,172] Daily consumption of more than 2 oz of alcohol is associated with an increased prevalence of hypertension.[173]

The role of dietary calcium in blood pressure remains controversial. Epidemiological studies suggest an inverse relationship.[174,175] The mechanism is unclear; the many explanations preferred include alteration of the vascular tone and the relationship of renin and angiotensin. Kaplan has hypothesized that volume expansion due to high dietary sodium intake will lead to hypercalciuria, secondary hyperparathyroidism, and subsequent hypertension. Increased dietary calcium intake would then restore parathormone levels to normal and thus reduce blood pressure.[176] Until the issue is clarified, dietary supplements of calcium for hypertension should not be routinely administered.

Decreased consumption of saturated fat has been correlated with lower blood pressure, as has increased intake of potassium.

EFFECTS OF TREATING HYPERTENSION

Meta-analysis of the major blood pressure–lowering trials has been performed by Yusuf and coworkers.[40] They reviewed the 14 major trials, which together involved 45,000 patients for an average of 5 years. In nine of the trials, a definite benefit was seen in stroke reduction. The impact on coronary disease was much less clear. The most important clinical trials are summarized below.

VETERANS ADMINISTRATION COOPERATIVE STUDY GROUP. The classic Veterans Administration trial demonstrated the efficacy of antihypertensive therapy in severe hypertension (> 114 mm Hg diastolic). The results in milder hypertension (90–104 mm Hg) were not statistically significant, although the numbers of patients were small.[177]

HYPERTENSION DETECTION AND FOLLOW-UP PROGRAM. More than 7800 patients with diastolic pressure between 90 and 104 mm Hg were enrolled in the Hypertension Detection and Follow-up Program (HDFP).[178] Half were referred to their usual source of medical care (referred care) and half received more intensive treatment under a stepped-care program (i.e., the study was not placebo controlled). The initial drug in the stepped-care approach was a diuretic, followed by addition of an adrenergic inhibitor and then hydralazine. After 5 years, the mean diastolic pressure was 83 mm Hg in the stepped-care group and 88 mm Hg in the referred-care group. The stepped-care group also had a 20 per cent lower overall mortality rate, including 45 per cent fewer deaths due to cerebrovascular disease, 46 per cent fewer deaths due to acute MI, and 20 per cent fewer deaths due to CAD. Across all the nearly 11,000 patients in the

trial (including the 4000 with higher blood pressure at entry), total mortality was reduced 17 per cent with stepped care compared with referred care. On the basis of these findings, the second U.S. Joint National Committee recommended that the initial goal of antihypertensive therapy be to maintain diastolic pressure under 90 mm Hg.

AUSTRALIAN THERAPEUTIC TRIAL. The Australian Therapeutic Trial enrolled patients with diastolic blood pressure between 95 and 109 mm Hg who were free of CAD. Patients were randomly assigned to placebo or stepped-care therapy similar to that in the HDFP. The trial was stopped after a statistically significant difference of 30 per cent between the two groups was attained. The patients were treated for an average of 4 years. Interestingly, the blood pressure in the group treated with placebo also fell, and, at the end of the trial, only 22 per cent of the patients whose initial pressure was between 100 and 104 mm Hg failed to lower their blood pressure. The treated group's average blood pressure fell 12.2 mm Hg, compared with 6.6 mm Hg in the placebo group. Improvement in total CAD outcome was noted. An excess in complications was noted in the placebo-treated patients whose pressure remained over 100 mm Hg.[179]

MULTIPLE RISK FACTOR INTERVENTION TRIAL. The MRFIT studied not only hypertension intervention, but also the impact of smoking cessation and cholesterol lowering on CAD mortality.[51] The MRFIT enrolled 12,866 men and assigned them to usual care by their private physicians or to a specialized center for aggressive intervention to reduce cardiac risk. Although the special-intervention patients were able to reduce their major risk factors, there were no significant differences between this group and the usual-care group in CAD or total mortality. The reason for this failure is unclear but may relate to the use of thiazide diuretic therapy in the special-care group.[180] Long-term follow-up (10.5 years) has revealed a beneficial impact on risk reduction in the special-intervention group, emphasizing the fact that risk-factor reduction should be considered a lifelong commitment.[181]

MEDICAL RESEARCH COUNCIL TRIAL. The Medical Research Council (MRC) Trial[182] was a large drug trial in mild hypertension carried out in the United Kingdom. Diuretics were used as the first step after nonpharmacological means were used. The MRC compared diuretics or beta blockers to placebo in patients who had no prior treatment for high blood pressure and no history of MI, diabetes, or angina pectoris. By the trial's end, the rate of strokes was decreased in the treated group. There was no decrease in coronary events.

INTERNATIONAL PROSPECTIVE PRIMARY PREVENTION STUDY IN HYPERTENSION. The International Prospective Primary Prevention Study in Hypertension (IPPPSH)[183] was a large-scale trial (6357 patients) that examined the impact of a noncardioselective beta blocker with partial agonist activity (oxprenolol) versus placebo plus other agents with a treatment goal of a diastolic pressure not to exceed 95 mm Hg. With 3 to 5 years of follow-up, there were no statistically significant differences between the groups in stroke, MI, or sudden cardiac death.

METOPROLOL ATHEROSCLEROSIS PREVENTION IN HYPERTENSION. The previously mentioned MAPHY trial was in a large subgroup (3234 men) of the original Heart Attack Primary Prevention in Hypertensives trial, and analyzed only the metoprolol versus diuretics results.[159] The drugs were administered in a nonblinded manner in this open trial. The metoprolol group had significant reductions in CAD, stroke, and overall mortality, as analyzed by the conservative intention-to-treat method. The benefit with metoprolol also was significant in the patients who used tobacco products. Despite some unanswered questions (e.g., study design, higher-than-expected mortality in the diuretics group), the MAPHY data suggest benefit from the use of a cardioselective beta blocker in hypertension.

REVIEW OF THE CLINICAL TRIALS. Diuretics and beta blockers are effective in reducing hypertension and subsequent morbidity and mortality from cardiovascular disease. Although they are well tolerated and effective in decreasing blood pressure, angiotensin-converting enzyme inhibitors and calcium antagonists have not been studied in placebo-controlled primary prevention trials. However, an impact on CAD is less clearly demonstrated. Care must be taken to correct induced metabolic abnormalities (e.g., hyperglycemia, hyperlipidemia, electrolyte abnormalities) and to avoid overzealous reduction of pressure to a point that jeopardizes coronary perfusion.

PHYSICAL ACTIVITY
(See also Chap. 42)

The role of physical activity in the prevention of CAD and in decreasing mortality after MI remains controversial. Recent epidemiological studies have shown an encouraging and beneficial trend in favor of this relatively low-cost and low-risk intervention (Fig. 37–15). Long-term physical activity is known to be important in maintaining ideal body weight and muscle mass. Exercise also may play an important role in

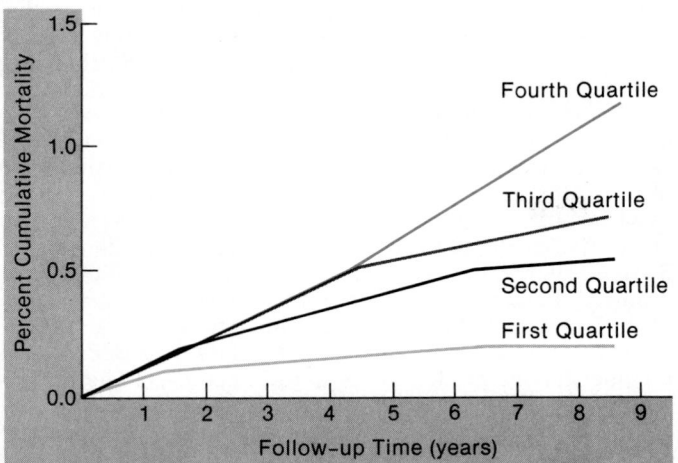

FIGURE 37–15. Life-table failure plots were computed from proportional hazards models that included age, smoking status, HDL level, LDL level, resting systolic blood pressure, and stage 2 exercise heart rate, with continuous variables set to mean values and smoking status to zero (yes = 1, no = 0). (Reprinted by permission from Ekelund, L.-G., Haskell, W. L., Johnson, J. L., et al.: Physical fitness as a predictor of cardiovascular mortality in asymptomatic North American men: The Lipid Research Clinics Mortality follow-up study. N. Engl. J. Med. 319:1379, 1988, p. 1383.)

maintaining normal blood pressure and optimizing lipid values. Patients who exercise regularly have been reported to show a decreased incidence of sudden cardiac death (Chap. 26). In contrast, some people who have been sedentary may be at increased risk for malignant ventricular arrhythmia or acute MI when they begin to exercise. Thus, patients over age 40 are urged to undergo a thorough physical examination and exercise stress test before undertaking a program of vigorous physical activity.

Several epidemiological studies have shown a consistent inverse relationship between caloric intake per kilogram of body mass and CAD, probably because of the protective effect of increased physical activity. Multivariate analyses have revealed that people with high levels of physical fitness have lower rates of CAD and cancer. Conversely, decreased levels of physical fitness are associated with increased risk of atherosclerosis.[184] Several studies have shown that the relative risk for cardiovascular disease conferred by physical inactivity appears to parallel in magnitude that conferred by hypertension, dyslipidemia, or the use of tobacco products.[185] This impact of physical inactivity was documented in well-designed prospective studies with large numbers of patients, superseding the lack of benefit described by small-scale and poorly designed studies.

In addition to its possible role as a primary risk factor for the development of coronary disease, physical inactivity may affect the secondary association of other cardiac risk factors.[185a] The Framingham Offspring Study found that patients who participated in at least 1 hour of conditioning activities per week had an improved cardiac risk profile when HDL, heart rate, body mass index, and tobacco use were analyzed.[186] Decreased presence of associated risk factors in physically active people would be predicted to translate into altered CAD mortality. The U.S. Railroad Study, with 17 to 20 years of mortality follow-up, confirmed that the age-adjusted risk estimate for CAD death was increased to 1.39 for sedentary men who expended less than 40 kcal/week. The relationship of physical activity was independent and statistically significant when controlled in multivariate analysis.[187]

MECHANISMS OF POSSIBLE BENEFIT

The exact mechanism of the apparent protection afforded against atherosclerosis by physical activity is doubtless multifactorial. Regular aerobic exercise decreases both systolic and diastolic blood pressure levels, although the precise mechanism is not clear. Regular aerobic physical training has been shown to increase cardiac output and decrease systemic vascular resistance.[188] Exercise also may alter the renin-angiotensin-aldosterone axis, with subsequent decreases in circulating renin levels, although the changes in renin have not been documented uniformly. It does appear that the decrease in plasma renin correlates significantly with the subsequent increase in physical activity.[189] Prostacyclin activity also is increased with exercise, although the role that this plays in the regulation of blood pressure is unclear.[190] Meta-analysis of studies that evaluated changes in blood pressure of normotensive patients with exercise has revealed a mild but significant decrease in both systolic and diastolic pressures of about 4 mm Hg. In patients with initial hypertension, the decrease may be more significant and has resulted in an average decline of 11 mm Hg for systolic pressure and 6 mm Hg for diastolic pressure. This has been corroborated by 24-hour ambulatory recordings.[191]

Additional benefit may accrue to patients who undergo exercise training, by means of an alteration in the lipid profile. Special interest has been directed to the effect of physical exertion on HDL levels. An inverse relation between HDL and obesity has been documented.[192] The role of exercise in the alteration of lipid profiles has been well studied. In most of these studies, intense exercise is associated with decreased total and LDL cholesterol values and with increased HDL levels.[193] In addition to the increases in total HDL induced by exercise, an associated increase in apo A-I levels has been shown to be produced by physical training.[194] The relation between exercise and alcohol consumption in runners and inactive men has been studied. Exercise has a more profound positive impact on HDL levels than does alcohol in people who run 12 or more miles per week.

Another benefit from regular exercise is improved glucose tolerance, although it is not clear that the reduction of blood glucose alters CAD mortality. However, meta-analyses of studies evaluating the impact of physical activity on cardiac mortality have been performed to circumvent the statistical limitations of smaller studies. Isolated clinical trials using samples of up to 750 patients usually have shown a trend of improvement in mortality (about a 20 per cent change). In general, these changes have not reached statistical significance when populations undergoing exercise training were compared with nonexercising controls. However, a meta-analysis involving the 12 major exercise trials has shown a statistically significant benefit to an endurance exercise program.[195]

EXERCISE LEVELS. The level of exercise required to provide CAD protection has not been established. Sedentary patients may produce alterations in other risk factors, such as blood pressure, weight, lipids, HDL, and glucose tolerance, by means of a moderate exercise program. Whether more sustained exercise will increase the benefit has not been shown. Exercise energy expenditures of about 2000 kcal/week, or the equivalent of jogging 20 miles per week, have correlated with protection from the development of CAD.[196,197] A practical exercise prescription depends on the clinical status of the patient and on the existence of CAD and peripheral arteriosclerosis. Patients at increased risk for atherosclerosis, such as those with hypertension, dyslipidemia, or diabetes, and patients in whom coronary disease is suspected should be evaluated by an exercise treadmill test, clinical history, and physical examination. Treadmill testing is recommended in sedentary patients over age 40 who plan to begin an exercise program. If the patient has no evidence or history of ischemic heart disease, exercise programs may not need close monitoring because of the low risk involved.

RECOMMENDATIONS

The best available evidence indicates that regular and moderate physical activity is beneficial in the primary and secondary prevention of CAD. This conclusion is endorsed by the World Health Organization, which predicts that increased physical activity should result in decreased health care costs and lower mortality rates.[198] Exercise programs can be inexpensive, and they seem a prudent way to improve the general health and well-being of the population. To bring about a significant improvement in aerobic capacity, at least three sessions per week are required, each lasting between 20 and 30 minutes. Five sessions produce the maximum result, which is achieved after 4 to 6 weeks of training. Adherence to exercise programs is a major problem, and half of those who begin a regular program drop out. All patients with known CAD should undergo treadmill testing before beginning an exercise program. Patients treated for MI may undergo a submaximal treadmill test before discharge from the hospital. Prognosis may be estimated by ST shifts, exercise time, ectopy, and inappropriate blood pressure responses.[199] The role of the physician is pivotal in helping the patient establish attainable goals for an exercise program. A regular routine should be advocated, with flexibility as to the type of calorie expenditure. The physician should encourage and support the patient to maximize benefits and to minimize dropout.

OBESITY

The precise role of obesity as an independent cardiac risk factor remains unclear. Analysis of the Framingham data reveals an independent contribution to the risk of coronary disease by elevated blood cholesterol, blood pressure, glucose, and uric acid. Although all are increased with increasing body mass index, obesity still makes an independent contribution to the overall risk of coronary disease on multivariate analysis. Mortality rates also are increased with overall obesity and central obesity. In people in the highest quintile by body mass index, increased waist circumference and subscapular skin folds were associated with increased risk of coronary and cerebrovascular disease. The definition of obesity is arbitrary; this condition frequently is defined as an increase of 20 per cent above ideal body weight. Actuarial studies have defined ideal weight as that weight associated with the lowest mortality rates in people applying for life insurance. Body mass index has been advocated as the best approach to estimating obesity. The prevalence of obesity averages about 20 per cent for men between ages 45 to 54 and 15 per cent for women in the same age range. About 16 per cent of men are at least 20 per cent overweight, and 28 per cent of women are 20 per cent or more overweight.

A National Institutes of Health consensus conference on obesity concluded that obesity adversely affects both health and longevity.[200] Obesity has a direct relationship with all the coronary risk factors except smoking.[201] The number of cigarettes smoked per day shows an inverse trend when compared with body weight, possibly because of appetite suppression by smoking.[202,203] The strongest correlations with obesity are with blood pressure, hypertriglyceridemia, hyperinsulinemia (all positive correlations), and the concentration of HDL cholesterol (an inverse relationship).

Body mass index correlates positively with total serum cholesterol and inversely with HDL level.[204] Although the epidemiological association of hypertension and obesity is well established, the precise mechanism involved in the genesis of elevated blood pressure is not known. Obesity may alter peripheral vascular resistance, dietary salt intake, and neuroendocrine homeostasis.

The role that dietary salt plays in elevating blood pressure in obese patients is controversial. Some obese patients who are salt sensitive lower their blood pressure when they reduce their sodium intake.[205] Certain obese patients increase renal sodium reabsorption, secondary to autonomic nervous system alterations, and have a low-renin or salt-sensitive hypertensive state.

In obese patients, hyperinsulinemia may play a role in ele-

vating blood pressure. Obese patients have resistance to the action of insulin because of decreased numbers of functioning receptors for insulin on the cell surface. Also, further decreases in insulin receptors occur when levels of circulating insulin are high. A relationship between insulin levels, diabetes, and hypertension has been determined epidemiologically.[206] Syndrome X has recently been defined as an underlying genetic disorder associated with insulin resistance, hyperinsulinemia, increased blood pressure, decreased HDL and HDL_2, increased VLDL triglyceride, and small, dense, apo B–rich LDL.[207] Postprandial lipemia may be part of this syndrome.[208] Familial dyslipidemic hypertension has been described as well.[209] Many of these characteristics are seen in familial combined hyperlipidemia. Possible suggested causes include the overproduction of hepatic apo B-100, heterozygous deficiency of lipoprotein lipase, and an increase in the activity of the cholesteryl ester transfer protein.[210]

FAT DISTRIBUTION

Studies carried out in several countries have shown the importance of the distribution of fat as a coronary risk factor. The difference in fat patterns between men and women implicates a hormonal basis for the variable degree of obesity in different anatomical areas. The waist–hip ratio (in women) has been positively correlated with the level of androgens.

The terms "overweight" and "obese" are not synonymous. Overweight refers to body mass index; obesity is estimated by the thickness of skin folds in various body regions. Upper values of body mass index and increased central obesity, as estimated by abdominal girth or waist–hip ratio, have been associated with increased relative risks of CAD.[211] Fat deposition in the abdomen has been associated both with hypertension and the risk of developing CAD complications (Fig. 37–16).[212] In men, CAD is correlated with the abdominal distribution of adiposity, which appears to be independent of obesity. The circumference of the waist compared with that of the hips has been associated with hypertension, hypercholesterolemia, elevated levels of fibrinogen, and hypertriglyceridemia. These variables have been epidemiologically correlated with CAD.[213]

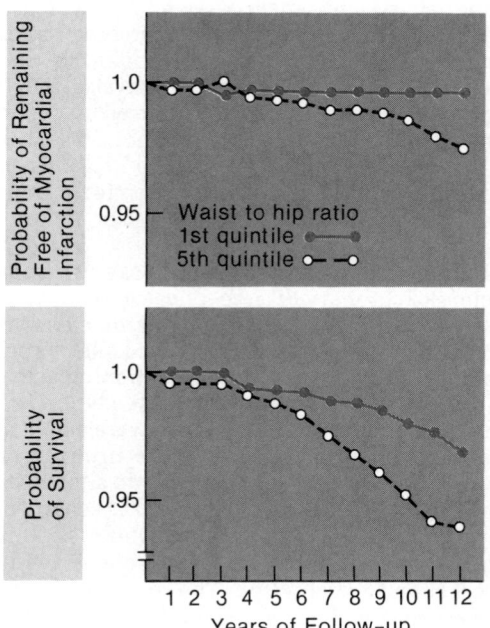

FIGURE 37–16. Probability of remaining free of myocardial infarction and dying of any cause for every year of a 12-year follow-up by highest and lowest quintiles of ratio of waist-to-hip circumference at entry. (From Lapidus, L., et al.: Distribution of adipose tissue and risk of cardiovascular disease and death: A 12-year follow-up of participants in the population study of women in Gothenburg, Sweden. Br. Med. J. **289**:1257, 1984.)

In women, the deposition of intraabdominal fat constitutes a greater risk for the development of CAD than obesity alone, when studied by a variety of anthropomorphic measurements: total body fat mass index, fat distribution (using waist–hip ratios), computed tomography, and subscapular-triceps skin fold ratios.[214] In women, body mass index and measurement of fasting levels of insulin are found to be strongly associated with CAD risk. The association is stronger for these variables than 2-hour postprandial glucose or insulin levels.[215] The positive association in women between the incidence of MI, angina, and stroke is linked to the waist–hip circumference ratio. This correlation is independent of age, smoking, serum cholesterol, systolic blood pressure, triglycerides, or body mass index.[211] Thus, a masculine distribution of adipose tissue increases CAD risk in both men and women. The waist–hip ratio appears to be a more significant predictor than the total degree of obesity. Although the role of obesity in the development of atherosclerotic complications is complex and remains controversial, obesity is associated with other cardiac risk factors and may increase the total risk in these patients. Hence, weight reduction should be encouraged in patients who have these additional risks. Dietary therapy should be aimed at weight reduction (to approach ideal body weight and to maintain the weight loss) as well as at any associated hyperlipidemia. Alteration of behavioral habits is a key element in the control of obesity. Exercise and other physical activities are adjuncts to weight control.

FAMILY HISTORY AND FAMILIAL AGGREGATION

A variety of studies, both case-control and prospective, point to familial aggregation of CAD. The aggregation of risk factors is well known and includes cholesterol, lipoproteins, blood pressure, diabetes, and obesity. Genetic and environmental influences on coronary risk may be difficult to distinguish.[216] A population predisposition to hypertension or hypercholesterolemia may be determined by its intake of salt, saturated fat, or calories overall. The family at high risk for the development of CAD usually has at least one member who has hyperlipidemia, low HDL, hypertension, a positive family history of coronary disease, or a positive family history of premature CAD. Familial-aggregation studies, genetic studies, and the tracking of blood pressure have yielded evidence that children born to families with a high prevalence of these risk factors also are at risk for development of CAD.[217] Preventive strategies are now available to the pediatrician.[218]

Familial-aggregation studies have included the evaluation of the siblings of patients with documented premature atherosclerosis. In the study by Becker and associates,[219] the siblings were apparently free of clinically evident coronary disease and were examined by questionnaire and interview. This wide-scale screening revealed that 48 per cent of the brothers and 41 per cent of the sisters were hypertensive, and that 45 per cent of the brothers and 22 per cent of the sisters had a lipid abnormality. There were high percentages of cigarette smoking and diabetes. Several risk factors frequently coexisted in the siblings; hence, there is a high degree of modifiable risk factors in first-degree relatives in families of a member affected by premature atherosclerosis. Despite the presence of classic risk factors in families, discriminant analyses evaluating the various risk factors have been unable to classify patients into exact risk groups. Hence, unknown risk variables must mediate the family history of coronary disease, and a positive family history for atherosclerosis should be considered an independent risk factor.[220]

Recent work by Austin and associates[221] has established a mendelian dominant inheritance for the atherogenic lipoprotein pattern associated with small, dense LDL. VLDL, IDL, and small, dense LDL are increased, whereas HDL and HDL$_2$ are decreased. Kindreds with this pattern may represent what has been called familial combined hyperlipidemia. This disorder

may be caused by partial lipase deficiency or by an increase in cholesteryl ester transfer protein.

DIABETES MELLITUS
(See also p. 1842)

Diabetes mellitus is a well-established risk factor for coronary disease.[222] However, problems have arisen in establishing standardized criteria for the diagnosis of diabetes and in comparing the risk inherent in diabetics with that of patients who have glucose intolerance. Also, diabetes frequently coexists with other cardiac risk factors; dyslipidemia and hypertension are increased in prevalence in the diabetic population compared with normals. The definition of diabetes mellitus of the National Diabetes Data Group is given in Table 37–9. The mechanism of coronary events for patients with overt diabetes is multifactorial and may include such factors as increased platelet aggregation. Strict control of glucose intolerance in type II diabetics has been shown to exert a favorable effect on the concentration of adenosine diphosphate and on collagen-induced platelet aggregation. Strict control of diabetes also has been shown to be associated with decreased thromboxane A$_2$ synthesis, which may play a further role in platelet aggregation in the diabetic patient.[223] Hyperinsulinemia may pose an additional risk in the development of atherosclerosis in patients with both diabetes and glucose intolerance. A number of epidemiological and clinical studies implicate hyperinsulinemia and insulin resistance in an increased frequency of CAD.[224]

Insulin is a growth factor and may stimulate smooth muscle cell proliferation. It has been found to enhance the local synthesis of lipids and the uptake of lipid by smooth muscle cells and fibroblasts,[225] which could enhance the transformation of these cells into foam cells. Epidemiological studies have documented that elevated fasting insulin levels are a predictor for the development of coronary atherosclerosis in nondiabetic patients, independent of other CAD risk factors.[226,226a] In addition, postprandial elevations of circulating insulin also play a role in increased coronary risk. Hypertension and obesity also have been found to be associated with diabetes and glucose intolerance. The frequency of hypertension is about doubled in patients with altered glucose tolerance.[226b]

The Framingham Study found diabetes to be a major risk for CAD, on the basis of a fasting glucose over 120 mg/dl or a blood glucose greater than 160 mg/dl at 1 hour and of more than 110 mg/dl at 2 hours after an oral glucose load.[227] This rather liberal definition of glucose intolerance probably contributed to inconsistencies in reports of various international studies relating hyperglycemia to CAD. Frank diabetes occurs in 2 per cent to 6 per cent of the general population, and

TABLE 37-9 CRITERIA FOR DIABETES AND GLUCOSE INTOLERANCE IN NONPREGNANT ADULTS

DIABETES MELLITUS
(Type I = Insulin-dependent; Type II = Non-insulin-dependent)
Fasting plasma glucose ≥ 140 mg/dl
Sustained elevated plasma glucose levels during the OGTT
  Two hour ≥ 200 mg/dl
  One other value between 0 and 2 hours ≥ 200 mg/dl
Classic symptoms of diabetes with unequivocal elevation of plasma glucose

IMPAIRED GLUCOSE TOLERANCE (OGTT)
Fasting plasma glucose <140 mg/dl
One value between 0 and 2 hours ≥ 200 mg/dl
Two hour = 140–199 mg/dl

From Kaplan, N. M.: Diabetes and glucose intolerance. In Kaplan, N. M., and Stamler, J. (eds.): Prevention of Coronary Heart Disease: Practical Management of the Risk Factors. Philadelphia, W. B. Saunders Company, 1983, p. 114. Reproduced from the National Diabetes Data Group: Classification and diagnosis of diabetes mellitus and other categories of glucose intolerance. Diabetes 28:1039, 1979.
OGTT = Oral glucose tolerance test.

impaired glucose tolerance may occur in up to 20 per cent, depending on the level of glucose used for the diagnosis.[228] However, overt diabetes develops in less than 5 per cent of patients with moderate glucose intolerance, defined by plasma glucose of 140 to 199 mg/dl 2 hours after an oral glucose load. Hence, the use of more conservative criteria to diagnose apparent glucose intolerance may alter epidemiological findings.

In overt diabetes, the mortality associated with coronary atherosclerosis is definitely increased. In the First National Health and Nutrition Examination Survey (NAHANES I), the age-adjusted death rates for diabetic men and women were twice those seen in nondiabetics.[229] Seventy-five per cent of the excess mortality among diabetic men was due to CAD. However, the risk of ischemic heart disease in patients with asymptomatic impairment of glucose tolerance is not clear. In a multivariate analysis of 15 studies, the International Collaborative Group raised the issue of absolute asymptomatic hyperglycemia, especially in combination with other risk factors such as hypertension, smoking, and hypercholesterolemia.[230] The relation between CAD risk and hyperinsulinemia is a consistent finding. As further studies implicating a role for hyperinsulinemia accumulate, more sophisticated analysis may further establish the relationship of glucose intolerance, insulin resistance, and hypertension.

Control of hypertension is particularly important in protecting against microvascular diabetic complications in the eye and kidney. Formation of glycosylated LDL has been suggested as a potential predisposing factor to macrovascular disease.[231] We do not yet know whether maintaining normal glucose levels will reduce the macrovascular or atherosclerotic complications in diabetics. In type II diabetes, weight control has been shown to improve glucose control, lipid abnormalities, and other CAD risk factors. Weight loss with normalization of glucose enhances the activity of lipoprotein lipase, with reduction of VLDL and an increase in HDL levels. Weight loss also augments control of the glucose level in patients with impaired glucose tolerance.[232]

Smoking should be discontinued and hypertension controlled in the diabetic. Drugs that adversely affect glucose tolerance, such as diuretics in high doses, should be avoided. Captopril, a sulfhydryl-containing angiotensin-converting enzyme inhibitor, has recently been shown to alter favorably the insulin and glucose relation in the treatment of hypertension.[233] The value of strict control of blood glucose as regards long-term vascular complications in diabetes has been controversial. However, a consensus exists that microangiopathy affecting the retina and kidney is reduced by maintaining more normal levels of glucose. Patients receiving a diuretic have increased insulin resistance.[233,234] Insulin resistance decreases lipoprotein lipase levels, which leads to an increase in remnant lipoproteins. It also may lead to increased lipolysis in adipose tissue, increased free fatty acid flux to the liver, and enhanced triglycerides and VLDL secretion.

OTHER INFLUENCES

PSYCHOSOCIAL AND BEHAVIORAL FACTORS

Many investigators have hypothesized that psychosocial factors play an important role in the incidence of CAD in Western society. The mechanisms of many psychosocial factors, such as stress, are not well delineated. Six prospective and many case-control studies have assessed for any correlation of depression, anxiety, and neuroticism with CAD.[235] These studies report consistently that emotional distress precedes the development of the symptoms of CAD. However, it has been difficult to define a statistical relation between MI and stress. The largest prospective study, involving Swedish construction workers, showed a statistically significant relation between emotional factors and acute MI.[235]

The means by which chronic emotional distress would ac-

celerate CAD have not been established, but mechanisms could include an imbalance between sympathetic- and parasympathetic-mediated release of catecholamines and acute increases in blood pressure. Several epidemiological studies have shown an inverse statistical relation of blood pressure and cigarette usage to educational level. There also appears to be, in general, an inverse correlation between educational level and both age-adjusted mortality from CAD and all-causes mortality, explained at least in part by shifts in exposure to (known) CAD risk factors as educational attainment increases.[236] Neither risk factor modification nor the decreases in the MI rates have been uniform across all socioeconomic groups. The higher the level of education and socioeconomic status, the greater the modification in life style, including adherence to a low-fat diet, and subsequent decline in the incidence of CAD.[237] Although such observations do not establish causality, the great challenge to the U.S. health care industry is to ensure that such changes are introduced in and adopted by all levels of society.

STRESS IN OCCUPATION. Job-related factors that appear to influence the induction or exacerbation of CAD include perceived job stress, role ambiguity, job autonomy, job change, unemployment, and retirement.[238] However, such causality is controversial, and several studies have revealed little statistical impact of occupational stress on cardiovascular morbidity and mortality. When stress was present, its demonstrable impact was believed to be weak.[239] The Honolulu Heart Study was unable to support the hypothesis that men in high-stress occupations have an enhanced risk of developing CAD. In this large-scale study involving more than 8000 men, there were no significant associations between the presence of CAD and individual job demands or low autonomy in the workplace.[240]

In a case-control study using death certificate verification derived from several geographical locations, the rates of acute MI and ischemic heart disease mortality were analyzed in police officers.[241] The authors proposed that the decreasing risk documented with increased age suggests that removal of stress at the time of retirement lowers the incidence of CAD. Various methodological problems exist in studies that attempt to correlate stress in the workplace and the development or exacerbation of CAD. This is especially pronounced in the assessment of the effect of blood pressure and its relation to job-induced stress. Random blood pressure measurements have a high potential for measurement error in addition to biological variability. This problem is compounded when a correlation is attempted with the assessment of stress. Blood pressure measurement has been improved with the availability of ambulatory monitoring, which increases the number of readings and minimizes interobserver variation. One study[242] weighed job-stimulated stress, as defined by high psychosocial demands associated with low decision latitude, against echocardiographically determined left ventricular mass and ambulatory blood pressure recordings. Multivariate analysis with control for age, race, body mass index, type A personality, 24-hour sodium excretion, education, alcohol consumption, and smoking showed a correlation between job strain and both hypertension and left ventricular mass index. Hence, job strain may predispose to left ventricular hypertrophy. Although not correlated with clinical events in this study, increased left ventricular mass has been linked in a number of epidemiological studies (e.g., Framingham Study[243]) to a variety of adverse cardiac outcomes, including stroke and CAD.

STRESS AND TYPE A PERSONALITY. The role of type A personality in the predisposition to CAD remains controversial. Type A people are characterized as highly competitive, ambitious, and in a constant struggle with their environment, in contradistinction to the type B personality, defined by greater passivity and less disturbance by environmental stress. The correlation of type A personality to CAD has been evaluated in several large studies, including the Framingham Study, in which type A behavior patterns were associated with a twofold increase in the development of angina pectoris.[244] However, there did not appear to be a translation into subsequent increases in fatal coronary events. The increased rate of stable angina among the subjects with type A personality traits could not be explained by the presence of other cardiac risk factors, such as diabetes, or by the presence of behavioral status, such as cigarette smoking or excessive alcohol intake. In addition, a high rate of silent MI occurs in type A subjects as assessed by exercise electrocardiography, with ST shifts as the basis for the diagnosis of total ischemic burden. Other studies have shown increased episodes of painful ischemia in type A people when compared with type B people with an equivalent ischemic burden.[245] More episodes of painful ischemia would seem to make seeking medical attention more likely, leading to treatment and thus introducing bias into a long-term study.

The Western Collaborative Group Study showed that type A men had more than twice the prevalence of CAD as type B men.[246] Interestingly, long-term survival data from this study revealed that the rate of sudden cardiac death did not relate to personality type (A versus B). However, among patients who survived at least 24 hours after a cardiac event, there appeared to be a protective benefit in the type A description: men with type A traits had a death rate of 19.1 per 1000 person-years (mean follow-up, 12.7 years), compared with 31.7 deaths per 1000 person-years in the type B group (mean follow-up, 11.5 years). This difference in mortality persisted after multivariate analysis for other cardiac risk factors.[247] Interpretation of the mortality data remains highly controversial, since other studies showed no effect or an inverse relation of type A personality to morbidity and mortality from CAD.[248,249]

The mechanism by which type A personality traits could influence atherogenesis is unclear. It is doubtless not a single mechanism. Stress may increase the risk imparted by traditional factors, and this process may be modulated by personal response. A rise in blood pressure might be expected to result from excess adrenergic output. Some studies have shown an increased adrenergic receptor density in the healthy offspring of parents with documented premature CAD and type A behavior. The pattern of receptor-density alteration was believed to be compatible with increased peripheral alpha-adrenergic receptor activity and potentially with increased coronary arterial vasoconstriction.[250] Lipid values are altered in people under stress, but this has not been conclusively shown to add to overall cardiac risk.[251] Type A people react differently even to nonstressful situations. Hence, although stress may play a role in the modification of risk factors, the effect of stress alone appears to be relatively minor and would not totally explain the epidemiologically documented risk.

Stress management has been advocated for primary and secondary prevention of CAD and has been shown to decrease reaction to anxiety-provoking situations. In particular, with an impetus from behavioral counseling, it may have a positive impact on the patient at risk for coronary disease.[252]

ESTROGENS AND GENDER

(See also p. 832)

The dictum that women have a lower incidence of CAD than men is a function of the age group examined. CAD is much less common in premenopausal women than in age-matched men, the difference most pronounced between ages 35 and 44. The purported protection of women from CAD becomes much less evident in their postmenopausal years, when the CAD rates for men and women begin to converge. The process of atherosclerosis does not appear to differ between men and women, and the risk factors correlated with the development of CAD appear to affect both sexes equally.

The presumption is that the differences in prevalence rates of coronary atherosclerosis between men and women are a function of the relative differences in estrogen and androgenic hormones. At puberty, circulating levels of testosterone increase in males and estrogen production increases in females.

HDL levels are approximately equivalent in males and females until puberty, when they drop in the male as a result of the androgenic effect of testosterone. The greatest effect is in the HDL_2 fraction. According to the Framingham Study, the total cholesterol–HDL ratio estimates the net effect of the "two-way traffic" of cholesterol in and out of the tissues. When this ratio exceeds 7.5 in women, they have the same CAD risk as men. The Framingham data also implicate the triglyceride concentration as an independent risk factor in older women.[253]

Determining the causes of the changes in CAD rates in postmenopausal women is difficult because of the complexity of factors. The Framingham Study did not show an effect of change in life style, thus implicating an alteration in reproductive physiology.

Natural menopause has not been documented to alter glucose tolerance, insulin levels, or blood pressure. In women who undergo natural menopause, serum levels of HDL gradually decline and total serum cholesterol and LDL levels gradually rise; that is, the lipid profile changes in a way that would predispose to atherosclerosis.[254] These lipid changes are favorably altered by hormone-replacement therapy (estrogens). Postmenopausal women also have been shown to have increased levels of circulating small, dense LDL particles, which may further increase their risk for the development of atherosclerosis.[255] Case-control studies revealed a significant benefit as regards severity of angiographically demonstrable coronary atherosclerosis in women receiving estrogen in the postmenopausal period. This protective effect was independent of other variables.[256] The roles that hormone-replacement therapy and gender play in the subsequent development of coronary atherosclerosis remain controversial[257]; the bulk of evidence favors hormone replacement therapy in the form of estrogen in postmenopausal women.

The effect of oral contraceptives is more complex, since these prescriptions contain both estrogen and progesterone in varying quantities. Progesterone analogs decrease both triglyceride and HDL levels. The progestational agents were added to the estrogen therapy, both in oral contraceptives and in replacement therapy, to decrease the risk of endometrial and breast cancer. The effect of this addition on the development of CAD needs further clarification.[258,259] The estrogen and progesterone doses in oral contraceptive pills are generally low, and the impact on cardiac risk depends on their relative concentrations. The nontestosterone agents are especially potent in reducing HDL levels. However, as mentioned, estrogen increases HDL and triglycerides and decreases LDL levels. The study by Mann and colleagues[260] was one of the first to demonstrate an increased associated risk of acute MI with the use of oral contraceptives. The relative risk in oral contraceptive users was estimated to be 4.5 compared with nonusers. The impact on risk of the use of oral contraceptives appears to be increased by the concomitant use of tobacco products. However, recent studies have provided conflicting data on the risk of oral contraceptive agents and subsequent development of atherosclerosis. In the Nurses' Health Study, about 120,000 women, ages 30 to 55, were prospectively evaluated for cardiovascular disease for 8 years. There appeared to be no increased risk for cardiovascular disease according to past use of oral contraceptives, despite prolonged use among a few participants. Past use also did not correlate on multivariate analysis with any material increase in risk for atherosclerosis.[261,262]

Estrogen and progesterone use should be addressed on an individual basis. For women at risk of thromboembolic disease who have associated risk factors such as hypertension or tobacco use, hormone replacement therapy should be addressed in light of the potential risk–benefit ratio.

ALCOHOL

Excessive ingestion of alcohol is an established preventable cause of morbidity and mortality. The effects of alcohol on the

TABLE 37-10 CASE-CONTROL STUDIES OF ALCOHOL CONSUMPTION AND CORONARY ARTERY DISEASE

STUDY	SIZE OF POPULATION	LEVEL OF CONSUMPTION	RELATIVE RISK DRINKERS : NONDRINKERS
Klatsky et al. 1974	661 cases* 661 controls	≤ 2 drinks/day 3-5 drinks/day 6+ drinks/day	0.7 0.7 0.4
Stason et al. 1976	399 cases† 2486 controls	< 6 drinks/day 6+ drinks/day	1.0 0.6
Hennekens et al. 1978	568 cases‡	≤ 2 oz alcohol/day > 2 oz alcohol/day	0.4 0.7
Petitti et al. 1979	Not given†	Any	0.3
Rosenberg et al. 1981	513 cases† 918 controls	Any	0.7

From Hennekens, C. H.: Alcohol. In Kaplan, N. M., and Stamler, J. (eds.): Prevention of Coronary Heart Disease: Practical Management of the Risk Factors. Philadelphia, W. B. Saunders Company, 1983, p. 132.
* Both fatal and nonfatal.
† Nonfatal.
‡ Fatal.

cardiovascular system are highly complex[262a]; alteration of cardiovascular function occurs by both primary and secondary mechanisms. Alcohol may be associated with a primary dilated cardiomyopathy in the absence of coronary atherosclerosis. The acute and chronic effects of ethanol on the cardiovascular system are variable, and epidemiological studies often are flawed by lack of control of other, coexisting risk factors. It is well established that excessive alcohol use is associated with high blood pressure.[263] However, it is not clear that alcohol intake of a moderate degree has a positive correlation with either total or CAD mortality. Multiple studies have demonstrated an inverse correlation between moderate alcohol consumption and subsequent cardiac events.[264]

The protective role that has been attributed to alcohol by some investigators has not been definitely established. Alcohol does raise HDL levels, although the specific subfraction (HDL$_2$, HDL$_3$, or a combined increase) involved has varied.[265] Low-dose alcohol (defined as one beverage per day) prospectively compared with abstention over an 8-week period increased apo A-I levels by 9 mg/dl and apo A-I–apo B ratios. But whether such lipid changes correlate with decreased prevalence or extent of CAD has not been established.

The epidemiological association between alcohol intake and CAD has been examined in a variety of large *case-control* studies (Table 37-10). There appears to be an inverse correlation between the daily consumption of small to moderate amounts of alcohol and coronary atherosclerosis. Of the five major *prospective* studies, four showed an inverse relationship to the incidence of CAD with mild to moderate alcohol use.[266] The Framingham Study assigned a relative risk of 0.7 to subjects consuming at least 30 oz of alcohol per month, the comparison with those drinking less.[267]

In other large epidemiological studies, light drinkers had a lower overall mortality rate than did heavy drinkers or nondrinkers. There remain many unanswered questions about the relationship of alcohol intake to coronary atherosclerosis. Overt CAD has been shown to be inversely related to moderate alcohol consumption, as has been the anatomical degree of atherosclerosis.[268-270] However, overt CAD correlated significantly with alcoholism. Also, heavy alcohol intake has been positively associated with prevalence of acute MI. This correlation was confirmed after control for tobacco usage and severity of underlying atherosclerosis, perhaps signifying a destabilizing effect by alcohol intake on the atherosclerotic plaque. Despite the inverse correlation of coronary mortality and moderate alcohol intake, other studies have shown associated problems of alcohol abuse to contribute to an increase in overall mortality. The authors currently do not recommend that patients consume alcohol as a preventive measure.

MINOR RISK FACTORS

A number of minor risk factors have also been implicated in the genesis of coronary atherosclerosis, notably certain trace elements, water hardness, hypercalcemia, hypercoagulability, vasectomy, coffee consumption, and hyperuricemia. In none of these categories is an effect fully documented or completely understood.

TRACE ELEMENTS. In the zinc/copper hypothesis, Klevay proposes that a deficiency of copper, or an excess of zinc, predisposes to secondary hypercholesterolemia, to result in coronary atherosclerosis.[271,272]

WATER HARDNESS. Both Leoni and coworkers[273] and Crawford and colleagues[274] in large studies found cardiovascular mortality to correlate inversely with water hardness. Unfortunately, in no such study has protection or risk clearly been linked to specific components in the water. Selenium and zinc have been described as protective, and lead and calcium as conferring increased risk, with magnesium variously placed in both categories. The inconsistency of the findings precludes any definite conclusions about CAD risk in relation to water hardness.

HYPERCALCEMIA. Calcium overload in the arterial wall may play a role in the pathogenesis of atherosclerosis. Intracellular calcium accumulation may increase vascular tone and enhance cholesterol accumulation and atherosclerotic plaque formation. The affinity of the arterial wall for calcium increases with age. Calcium antagonists such as verapamil, diltiazem, and nifedipine can inhibit experimental atherogenesis. Nifedipine has been reported in one clinical trial to decrease new coronary lesion formation.[275,276]

HYPERCOAGULABILITY[276a] (see also Chap. 58). Epidemiological studies, including the Framingham Study,[142] have shown a strong correlation between fibrinogen concentration and CAD risk.[277,277a] Indeed, this correlation is comparable in statistical strength to the classic CAD risk factors. Fibrinogen is positively associated with concentrations of cholesterol and triglycerides, and thus linked with hyperlipidemia. It correlates as well with smoking, obesity, and socioeconomic stress. Also, factor VII is positively correlated with hyperlipidemia, especially with elevated triglycerides. Because more than 90 per cent of patients with MI exhibit coronary thrombosis, one might expect high levels of fibrinogen to predispose to thrombotic events. But whether levels of fibrinogen and factor VII relate exclusively to the thrombotic process involved in coronary disease or play an accessory role in atherogenesis is not known. Fibrinogen has been statistically associated with the severity of angiographically determined CAD.[278] Fibrinogen remains significantly associated with the severity of coronary atherosclerosis in a progressive manner, even when adjustment is made for age, hypertension, dyslipidemia, cigarette smoking, and body mass index.[142,279]

Early on, researchers postulated that fibrin contributes to the growth of atherosclerotic plaque. The process may be by the incorporation of a mural thrombus into the intima of an artery. Fibrin can be diffusely or discretely deposited within an atherosclerotic plaque. Thus, it may be argued that the early proliferative plaque arises from a mural fibrin thrombus. All of the clotting factors are present in the intima. Prothrombin is present in the gelatinous atherosclerotic lesion, but the ratio of the antithrombin III inhibitor to prothrombin is 3 : 1.

Some studies have reported a reduction in the activity of antithrombin III with CAD, and many studies have described an apparent direct correlation between fibrinogen and cholesterol levels.[280] The relationship of the lipid profile to clotting mechanisms is complex. High levels of triglycerides have been shown to be associated with inhibitors of fibrinolysis, especially of alpha$_2$ antiplasmin.[281] With its close homology to plasminogen, Lp(a) at high concentrations might participate in the inhibition of thrombolysis, but this possibility remains to be explored. Split fibrin products have been demonstrated within the intima and exert potentially toxic effects, including chemotaxis and alteration of vascular permeability. Fibrin deposition in the vessel wall may be associated with the trapping of LDL. It has been shown that the intima contains not only extractable soluble LDL, but also an insoluble apo B–containing substance that remains in the tissues, some of which might be Lp(a).[282] This lighter substance can be released by pretreatment with plasminogen.

Platelet aggregation is believed to play a major role in atherogenesis. The role of antiplatelet therapy in the treatment of unstable angina and other acute ischemic syndromes has been well described (p. 1233).[283,284] Platelet aggregation is enhanced in patients with established coronary atherosclerosis.[285] The role of aspirin in the primary prevention of acute MI has recently been tested in the Physicians' Health Study,[286] in which the subjects were physicians. Aspirin prophylaxis (325 mg every other day) yielded a 44 per cent reduction in the risk of MI. The benefits of aspirin were significant for both fatal and nonfatal MI, and the MI benefit was apparent only in subjects 50 years of age or older. No reduction in overall mortality from cardiovasclar disease was established.

VASECTOMY. The subject of a correlation between vasectomy and nonfatal MI is controversial. In studies in nonhuman primates, vasectomy increased the severity of diet-induced atherosclerosis.[287] However, various investigators observed no excess risk for MI and no increase in the prevalence of hypertension or hypercholesterolemia in men who had undergone vasectomy. Moreover, epidemiological studies have shown no clear relation between vasectomy and coronary events. Finally, recent long-term studies have failed to indicate an association between the presence of sperm autoimmunization and the development of atherosclerosis.[288,289]

COFFEE CONSUMPTION. Epidemiological studies have not yet clarified whether coffee consumption is a risk factor for CAD. A recent Framingham multivariate analysis assessed survey data on coffee consumption in relation to age, systolic pressure, body mass index, and total cholesterol with regard to impact on CAD.[290] The analysis did not show an association between coffee consumption and the presence of atherosclerosis. Moreover, there was no demonstrable relationship between coffee intake and subsequent CAD events in patients with known CAD. The effects of coffee intake on lipids were gender dependent: an inverse correlation with total cholesterol and with LDL cholesterol in men, and a positive correlation with each of these lipid values in women.

HYPERURICEMIA. Several studies have shown a statistical association between elevated levels of uric acid and hypertriglyceridemia. The Framingham Study found that the concentration of uric acid also correlated with both systolic and diastolic blood pressure values.[291] Although uric acid was a predictor of MI in the Framingham cohort, on multivariate analysis—which included age, systolic blood pressure, relative weight, cigarette smoking, and serum cholesterol—serum uric acid was not an independent CAD predictor. Instead, hyperuricemia appeared to be a marker of metabolic disturbances that predispose to CAD.

ATHEROSCLEROSIS AFTER CARDIAC TRANSPLANTATION (see also p. 1352). For cardiac transplant patients, the advent of improved immunosuppressive agents has lowered the rates of morbidity and mortality due to acute rejection of the donor heart. However, accelerated atherosclerosis has emerged as a major problem affecting long-term post-transplant survival.[292] Chronic immune injury caused by the presence of cytotoxic B-cell antibodies and/or alterations of the lipid profile may play a role in transplant-associated atherosclerosis.[293] Cyclosporine has been shown to decrease LDL-receptor activity and thus to worsen the patient's lipid profile by increasing total and LDL cholesterol levels and by lowering HDL levels. Higher donor age and elevated plasma triglycerides also have been associated with atherosclerotic development in the donor heart.[294] Although logical on causative grounds, episodes of rejection or human leukocyte antigen mismatches have not been clearly shown to play a major role in transplant atherosclerosis. Moreover, several recent studies have shown no correlation of the level of maintenance steroids, the fasting blood sugar value, or the number of rejection episodes with the development of atherosclerosis in the donor heart.

REFERENCES

DECLINING MORTALITY OF CAD

1. American Heart Association. 1991 Heart and Stroke Facts. Dallas, American Heart Association, 1991.
2. Stern, M. P.: The recent decline in ischemic heart disease mortality. Ann. Intern. Med. 91:630, 1979.

2a. Goldman, L., and Cook, E. F.: The decline in ischemic heart disease mortality rates: An analysis of the comparative effects of medical interventions and changes in lifestyle. Ann. Intern. Med. 101:825, 1984.

DYSLIPIDEMIA

3. Austin, M. A., Breslow, J. L., Hennekens, C. H., et al.: Low-density lipoprotein subclass patterns and risk of myocardial infarction. JAMA 260:1917, 1988.
4. Goldstein, J. L., and Brown, M. S.: Atherosclerosis: The low-density lipoprotein receptor hypothesis. Metabolism 26:1257, 1977.
5. Teng, B., Sniderman, A. D., Soutar, A. K., and Thompson, G. R.: Metabolic basis of hyperapobetalipoproteinemia. Turnover of apolipoprotein B in low density lipoprotein and its precursors and subfractions compared with normal and familial hypercholesterolemia. J. Clin. Invest. 77:663, 1986.
6. Kwiterovich, P. O., Jr., White, S., Forte, T., et al.: Hyperapobetalipoproteinemia in a kindred with familial combined hyperlipidemia and familial hypercholesterolemia. Arteriosclerosis 7:211, 1987.
7. Miller, N. E.: Association of high density lipoprotein subclasses and apolipoprotein with ischemic heart disease and coronary atherosclerosis [Review]. Am. Heart J. 113:589, 1987.
8. Oram, J. F., Brinton, E. A., and Bierman, E. L.: Regulation of high-density lipoprotein receptor activity in cultured human skin fibroblasts and human arterial smooth muscle cells. J. Clin. Invest. 72:1611, 1983.
9. Gordon, D. J., and Rifkind, B. M.: High density lipoprotein. The clinical implication of recent studies [Review]. N. Engl. J. Med. 321:1311, 1989.
10. Armstrong, V. W., Cremer, P., Eberle, P., et al.: The association between serum Lp(a) concentrations and angiography assessed coronary atherosclerosis: Dependence on serum LDL levels. Atherosclerosis 62:249, 1986.
11. Dahlen, G. H., Guyton, J. R., Attar, M., et al.: Association of levels of Lp(a), plasma lipids, and other lipoproteins with coronary artery disease documented by angiography. Circulation 74:758, 1986.
11a. Genest, J., Jr., Jenner, J. L., McNamara, J. R., et al.: Prevalence of lipoprotein (a) [Lp(a)] excess in coronary artery disease. Am. J. Cardiol. 67:1039, 1991.
11b. Solymoss, B. C., Marcil, M., Lesperance, J., et al.: Lp(a) is related to complete obstruction of coronary arteries in men and to partial as well as complete obstruction in women. J. Am. Coll. Cardiol. 17:62A, 1991.
12. Eaton, D. L., Fless, G. M., and Kohn, W. J.: Partial amino acid sequence of apolipoprotein(a) shows that it is homologous to plasminogen. Proc. Natl. Acad. Sci. USA 84:3224, 1987.
13. Gurakar, A., Hoeg, J. M., Kostner, G., et al.: Levels of Lp(a) decline with neomycin and niacin treatment. Atherosclerosis 57:293, 1985.
14. Albers, J. J., Taggart, H. M., Applebaum-Bowden, D., et al.: Reduction of lecithin-cholesterol acyltransferase, apolipoprotein D, and the Lp(a) lipoprotein with the anabolic steroid stanozolol. Biochim. Biophys. Acta 795:293, 1984.
15. Kottke, B. A., Zinsmeister, A. R., Holmes, D. R., Jr., et al.: Apolipoproteins and coronary artery disease. Mayo Clin. Proc. 61:313, 1986.
16. Gotto, A. M., Pownall, H. R., and Havel, R. J.: Introduction to the plasma lipoproteins: Methods [Review]. Methods Enzymol. 128:3, 1986.
17. Michals, W. C., Duvulet, F. E., and Benson, M.: Apolipoprotein A-I in Iowa type hereditary amyloidosis. Clin. Res. 35:595A, 1987.
18. Karathanasis, S. K., Ferris, E., and Haddad, I. A.: DNA inversion within the apolipoprotein A-I/C-III/A-IV encoding gene cluster of certain patients with premature atherosclerosis. Proc. Natl. Acad. Sci. USA 89:7198, 1987.
19. Schaefer, E. J., Ordovas, J. M., Law, S. W., et al.: Familial apolipoprotein A-I and C-III deficiency, variant II. J. Lipid Res. 26:1089, 1985.
20. Higuchi, K., Monge, J. C., Lee, N., et al.: The human apo B-100 gene: Apo B-100 is encoded by a single copy gene in the human genome. Biochem. Biophys. Res. Commun. 144:1332, 1987.
21. Chen, S. H., Yang, C. Y., and Chen, P. F.: The completed cDNA and amino acid sequence of human apolipoprotein B-100. J. Biol. Chem. 261:12918, 1986.
22. Higuchi, K., Hospattankar, I. V., Law, S. W., et al.: Human (apolipoprotein B) mRNA: Identification of two distinct apo B mRNAs, an mRNA with the apoB-100 mRNA containing a premature w-frame translational stop codon in both liver and intestine. Proc. Natl. Acad. Sci. USA 85:1772, 1988.
23. Mahley, R. W.: Atherogenic lipoproteins and coronary artery disease: Concepts derived from recent advances in cellular and molecular biology. Circulation 72:943, 1985.
24. Lenzen, H. J., Assmann, G., Buchwalsky, R., and Schulte, H.: Association of apolipoprotein E polymorphism, low-density lipoprotein cholesterol, and coronary artery disease. Clin. Chem. 32:778, 1986.
25. Kesaniemi, Y. A., Ehnolm, C., and Miettinen, T. A.: Intestinal cholesterol absorption efficiency in man is related to apoprotein E phenotype. J. Clin. Invest. 80:578, 1987.
26. Assmann, G., and Schulte, H.: PROCAM-Studie. Zuerich, Panscientia Verlag, 1986.
27. Assmann, G., Schulte, H., Oberwittler, W., and Hauss, W. H.: New aspects in the prediction of coronary heart disease. In: Fidge, N. H., and Nestel, P. J. (eds). The Prospective Cardiovascular Müenster Study. Atherosclerosis VII. Proceedings of the 7th International Atherosclerosis Symposium. Amsterdam, Elsevier Science Publishers, 1986, p. 19.
28. Kessling, A. M., Berg, K., Mockelby, E., and Humphries, S. E.: DNA polymorphisms around the apo A-I gene in normal and hyperlipidemic individuals selected for a twin study. Clin. Genet. 29:485, 1986.

29. Scott, J., Knott, T. J., Priestley, L. M., et al.: High-density lipoprotein composition is altered by a common DNA polymorphism adjacent to apo A-II gene in man. Lancet 1:771, 1985.

30. Seilhamer, J. J., Protter, A. A., Frossard, P., and Levy-Wilson, B.: Isolation and DNA sequence of full-length cDNA and of the entire gene for human apolipoprotein AI—discovery of a new genetic polymorphism in the apo AI gene. DNA 3:309, 1984.

31. Ordovas, J. M., Schaefer, E. J., Salem, D., et al.: Apolipoprotein A-I gene polymorphism associated with premature coronary artery disease and familial hypoalphalipoproteinemia. N. Engl. J. Med. 314:671, 1986.

32. Fojo, S. S., Law, S. W., and Brewer, H. B., Jr.: The human preproapoprotein C-II gene. Complete nucleic acid sequence and genomic organization. FEBS Lett. 213:221, 1987.

33. Fojo, S. S., Taam, L., Fairwell, T., et al.: Human preproapolipoprotein C-II: Analysis of major plasma isoforms. J. Biol. Chem. 261:9591, 1986.

34. Connelly, P. W., Maguire, G. F., Hoffmann, T., and Little, J. A.: Structure of apolipoprotein CII Toronto, a nonfunctional human apolipoprotein. Proc. Natl. Acad. Sci. 84:270, 1987.

34a. Young, S. G., and Linton, M. F.: Genetic abnormalities in apolipoprotein B. Trends Cardiovasc. Med. 1:59, 1991.

35. Blackhart, B. D., Ludwig, E. M., Pierotti, V. R., et al.: Structure of the human apolipoprotein B gene. J. Biol. Chem. 261:15364, 1986.

36. Chan, L., Van Tuinen, P., and Gotto, A. M.: The human Apo B-100 gene: A highly polymorphic gene which maps to the short arm of chromosome 2. Biochem. Biophys. Res. Commun. 133:248, 1985.

37. Lackner, K. J., Monge, J. C., Gregg, R. E., et al.: Analysis of the apolipoprotein B gene and messenger ribonucleic acid in abetalipoproteinemia. J. Clin. Invest. 78:1707, 1986.

THE LIPID HYPOTHESIS OF ATHEROGENESIS

38. Keys, A. (ed.): Coronary heart disease in seven countries. Circulation 41(Suppl. 1), 1970.

39. Simons, L. A.: Interrelations of lipids and lipoproteins with coronary artery disease mortality in 19 countries. Am. J. Cardiol. 57:5G., 1986.

40. Yusuf, S., Wittes, J., and Friedman, L.: Overview of results of randomized clinical traits in heart disease. II. Unstable angina, heart failure, primary prevention with aspirin, and risk factor modification. JAMA 260:2259, 1988.

41. Rossouw, J. E., Lewis, B., and Rifkind, B. M.: The value of lowering cholesterol after myocardial infarction. N. Engl. J. Med. 323:1112, 1990.

42. Dayton, S., Pearce, M. L., Hashimoto, S., et al.: A controlled clinical trial of a diet high in unsaturated fat in preventing complications of atherosclerosis. Circulation 40(Suppl II):1, 1969.

43. Coronary Drug Project group: Clofibrate and niacin in coronary heart disease. JAMA 231:360, 1975.

44. Canner, P. L., Berge, K. G., Wenger, N. K., et al.: Fifteen year mortality in the Coronary Drug Project patients: Long-term benefit with niacin. J. Am. Coll. Cardiol. 8:1245, 1986.

45. Brensike, J. F., Levy, R. I., and Kelsey, S. F.: Effects of therapy with cholestyramine on progression of coronary arteriosclerosis: Results of the NHLBI Type II Coronary Intervention Study. Circulation 69:313, 1984.

46. Arntzenius, A. C., Kromhout, D., Barth, J. D., et al.: Diet, lipoproteins, and the progression of coronary atherosclerosis. The Leiden Intervention Trial. N. Engl. J. Med. 312:805, 1985.

47. Committee of Principal Investigators: A cooperative trial in the primary prevention of ischemic heart disease using clofibrate. Br. Heart J. 40:1069, 1978.

48. Committee of Principal Investigators: WHO cooperative trial on primary prevention of ischemic heart disease with clofibrate to lower serum cholesterol: Final mortality follow-up. Lancet 2:600, 1984.

49. Hjermann, I., Velve-Byre, K., Holme, I., and Leren, P.: Effect of diet and smoking on the incidence of coronary heart disease: Report from the Oslo Study Group of a randomized trial in healthy men. Lancet 2:1303, 1981.

50. Hjermann, I., Holme, I., and Leren, P.: Oslo Study, Diet and Antismoking Trial: Results after 102 months. Am. J. Med. 80(Suppl 2A):7, 1986.

51. Multiple Risk Factor Intervention Trial Research Group: Multiple Risk Factor Intervention Trial: Risk factor changes and mortality results. JAMA 248:1465, 1982.

52. Multiple Risk Factor Intervention Trial Research Group: Mortality rates after 10.5 years for participants in the Multiple Risk Factor Intervention Trial. Findings related to a priori hypotheses of the trial. JAMA 263:1795, 1990.

53. Lipid Research Clinics Program: The Lipid Research Clinics' Coronary Primary Prevention Trial results. I. Reduction in incidence of coronary heart disease. II. The relationship of reduction in incidence of coronary heart disease to cholesterol lowering. JAMA 251:351, 1984.

54. Manninen, V., Elo, M. O., and Frick, L.: Lipid alterations and decline in the incidence of coronary heart disease in the Helsinki Heart Study. JAMA 260:641, 1988.

55. Austin, M. A.: Epidemiologic association between hypertriglyceridemia and coronary heart disease. Semin. Thromb. Haemost. 14:137, 1988.

56. Carlson, L. A., and Bottiger, L. E.: Risk factors for ischemic heart disease in men and women. Results of the 19-year follow-up of the Stockholm Prospective Study. Acta Med. Scand. 218:207, 1985.

57. Blankenhorn, D. H., Alaupovic, P., Wickham, E., et al.: Prediction of angiographic change in native human coronary arteries and aortocoronary bypass grafts. Lipid and nonlipid factors. Circulation 81:470, 1990.

58. Kaplan, N. M.: The deadly quartet: upper body obesity, glucose intolerance, hypertriglyceridemia, and hypertension. Arch. Intern. Med. 149:1514, 1989.

59. Phillips, N. R., Havel, R. J., and Kane, J. P.: Levels and interrelationships of serum and lipoprotein cholesterol and triglycerides. Arteriosclerosis 1:13, 1981.

60. Havel, R. J.: Role of triglyceride-rich lipoproteins in progression of atherosclerosis. (comment). Circulation 81:694, 1990.

61. Consensus Conference: Treatment of hypertriglyceridemia. JAMA 251:1196, 1984.

62. Newman, W. P., III, Freedman, D. S., Voors, A. W., et al.: Relation of serum lipoprotein levels and systolic blood pressure to early atherosclerosis. The Bogalusa Heart Study. N. Engl. J. Med. 314:138, 1986.

63. Cabin, H. S., and Roberts, W. C.: Relation of serum total cholesterol and triglyceride levels to the amount and extent of coronary arterial narrowing by atherosclerotic plaque in coronary heart disease. Quantitative analysis of 2,037 five mm segments of 160 major epicardial coronary arteries in 40 necropsy patients. Am. J. Med. 73:227, 1982.

64. Levy, R. I., Brensike, J. F., Epstein, S. E., et al.: The influence of changes in lipid values induced by cholestyramine and diet on progression of coronary artery disease: Results of the NHLBI Type II Coronary Intervention Study. Circulation 69:325, 1984.

65. Blankenhorn, D. H., Nessim, S. A., Johnson, R. L., et al.: Beneficial effects of combined colestipol-niacin therapy on coronary atherosclerosis and coronary venous bypass grafts. JAMA 257:3233, 1987. (Published erratum appears in JAMA 259:2698, 1988.)

66. Cashin-Hemphill, L., Mack, W. J., Pogoda, J. M., et al.: Beneficial effects of colestipol-niacin on coronary atherosclerosis: A 4-year follow-up. JAMA 264:3013, 1990.

67. Brown, G., Albers, J. J., Fisher, L. D., et al.: Regression of coronary artery disease as a result of intensive lipid-lowering therapy in men with high levels of apolipoprotein B. N. Engl. J. Med. 323:1289, 1990.

68. Kane, J. P., Malloy, M. J., Ports, T. A., et al.: Regression of coronary atherosclerosis during treatment of familial hypercholesterolemia with combined drug regimens. JAMA 264:3007, 1990.

69. Gordon, D. J., Probstfield, J. L., Garrison, R. J., et al.: High-density lipoprotein cholesterol and cardiovascular disease: four prospective American studies. Circulation 79:8, 1989.

70. The Expert Panel: Report of the National Cholesterol Education Program Expert Panel on detection, evaluation and treatment of high blood cholesterol in adults. Arch. Intern. Med. 148:36, 1988.

71. National Cholesterol Education Program: Current status of blood cholesterol measurements in clinical laboratories in the U.S.: A report from the Laboratory Standardization Panel of the National Cholesterol Education Program. Clin. Chem. 80:193, 1988.

72. Goodman, D. S., Bradford, R. H., Brewer, H. B., Jr., et al.: AHA Conference Report on Cholesterol. Diagnosis, evaluation and treatment: Current status and issues [Review]. Circulation 80:735, 1989.

73. Fredrickson, D. S., and Lees, R. S.: System for phenotyping hyperlipoproteinemia. Circulation 31:321, 1965.

74. Sparks, R. S., Zollner, S., Klisak, I., et al.: Mapping of loci for lipoprotein lipase to 8p22 and hepatic lipase to 15q21. Genomics 1:138, 1987.

75. Hayden, M. R., Vergani, C., Humphries, S. E., et al.: The genetics and molecular biology of apolipoprotein C-II [Review]. Adv. Exp. Med. Biol. 201:241, 1986.

76. Brunzell, J. D., Miller, N. E., Alaupovic, P., et al.: Familial chylomicronemia due to a circulating inhibitor of lipoprotein in lipase activity. J. Lipid Res. 24:12, 1983.

77. Goldstein, J. L., Brown, M. S., Anderson, R. G., et al.: Receptor-mediated endocytosis: Concepts emerging from the LDL receptor system. Annu. Rev. Cell Biol. 1:1, 1985.

78. Goldstein, J. L., and Brown, M. S.: Progress in understanding the LDL receptor and HMG-CoA reductase, two membrane proteins that regulated the plasma cholesterol [Review]. J. Lipid Res. 25:1450, 1984.

79. Steinberg, D., Parthasarathy, S., Carew, T. E., et al.: Beyond cholesterol. Modifications of low-density lipoproteins that increase its atherogenicity [Review]. N. Engl. J. Med. 320:915, 1989.

80. Cuthbert, J. A., East, C. A., Bilheimer, D. W., and Lipsky, P. E.: Detection of familial hypercholesterolemia by assaying functional low-density lipoprotein receptors on lymphocytes. N. Engl. J. Med. 314:879, 1986.

81. Hobbs, H. H., Brown, M. S., Russel, D. W., et al.: Deletion in the gene for the low-density lipoprotein receptor in a majority of French Canadians with familial hypercholesterolemia. N. Engl. J. Med. 317:734, 1987.

82. Morganroth, J., Levy, R. I., and Fredrickson, D. S.: The biochemical, clinical and genetic features of Type III hyperlipoproteinemia. Ann. Intern. Med. 82:158, 1975.

83. Janus, E. D., Nicoll, A. M., Turner, P. R., et al.: Kinetic basis of the primary hyperlipidemias: Studies of apolipoprotein B turnover in genetically defined subjects. Eur. J. Clin. Invest. 10:161, 1980.

84. Sniderman, A. D., Wolfson, C., Teng, B., et al.: Association of hyperapobetalipoproteinemia with endogenous hypertriglyceridemia and atherosclerosis. Ann. Intern. Med. 97:833, 1982.

85. Chait, A., Mancini, M., February, A. W., and Lewis, B.: Clinical and metabolic study of alcoholic hyperlipidemia. Lancet 2:62, 1972.

86. Sadbank, V., Bechan, M., and Bonnstein, B.: Hyperlipidemia neuropathy. Acta Neuropathol. Berl. 19:290, 1971.

87. Fallat, R. W., and Glueck, C. J.: Familial and acquired Type V hyperlipoproteinemia. Atherosclerosis 23:41, 1976.

88. Zilversmit, D. B.: Atherogenesis: A postprandial phenomenon. Circulation 60:473, 1979.

89. Pollare, T., Lithell, H., and Berne, C.: A comparison of the effects of hydrochlorothiazide and captopril on glucose and lipid metabolism in patients with hypertension. N. Engl. J. Med. 321:868, 1989.

90. Blankenhorn, D. H., Johnson, R. L., Mack, W. J., et al.: The influence of diet on the appearance of new lesions in human coronary arteries. JAMA 263:1646, 1990.

91. Ornish, D., Brown, S. E., Scherwitz, L. W., et al.: Can lifestyle changes reverse coronary heart disease? The Lifestyle Heart Trial. Lancet 336:129, 1990.

92. Gotto, A. M., Jr., Bierman, E. L., Connor, E., et al.: Recommendations for treatment of hyperlipidemia in adults. A joint statement of the Nutrition Committee and the Council on Arteriosclerosis. Circulation 69:1065A, 1984.

93. Bonanome, A., and Grundy, S. M.: Effect of dietary stearic acid on plasma cholesterol and lipoprotein levels. N. Engl. J. Med. 318:1244, 1988.

94. Trevisan, M., Krogh, V., Freudenheim, J., et al.: Consumption of olive oil, butter, and vegetable oils and coronary heart disease risk factors. The Research Group ATS-RF2 of the Italian National Research Council. JAMA 263:688, 1990.

95. Swain, J. F., Rouse, I. L., Curley, C. B., and Sacks, F. M.: Comparison of the effects of oat bran and low-fiber wheat on serum lipoprotein levels and blood pressure. N. Engl. J. Med. 322:147, 1990.

96. Connor, W. E.: Dietary fiber—nostrum or critical nutrient? N. Engl. J. Med. 322:193, 1990.

97. Kim, D. N., Ho, H. T., Lawrence, D. A., et al.: Modification of lipoprotein patterns and retardation of atherogenesis by a fish oil supplement to a hyperlipidemic diet for swine. Atherosclerosis 76:35, 1989.

98. Rogers, S., James, K. S., Butland, B. K., et al.: Effects of a fish oil supplement on serum lipids, blood pressure, bleeding time, hemostatic and rheological variables. A double blind randomized controlled trial in healthy volunteers. Atherosclerosis 63:137, 1987.

99. Singer, P., Jaeger, W., Wirth, M., et al.: Lipid and blood pressure lowering effect of mackerel diet in man. Atherosclerosis 49:99, 1983.

100. Zhu, B. Q., and Parmley, W. W. Modification of experimental and clinical atherosclerosis by dietary fish oil. Am. Heart. J. 119:178, 1990.

101. Schectman, G., Kaul, S., Cherayil, G. D., et al.: Can the hypotriglyceridemic effect of fish oil concentrate be sustained? Ann. Intern. Med. 110:346, 1989.

102. Glauber, H., Wallace, P., Griver, K., et al.: Adverse metabolic effect of omega-3 fatty acids in non-insulin–dependent diabetes mellitus. Ann. Intern. Med. 108:663, 1988.

103. Hoeg, J. M., Gregg, R. E., and Brewer, H. B., Jr.: An approach to the management of hyperlipoproteinemia [Review]. JAMA 255:512, 1986.

104. Levy, R. I.: Drugs used in the treatment of hyperlipoproteinemia. In Goodman, A. S., Gilman, A. S., and Gilman, A. (eds.): The Pharmacologic Basis of Therapeutics. New York, Macmillan, 1980, pp. 834–877.

105. Brown, B. G., Lin, J. T., Schaefer, C. A., et al.: Niacin or lovastatin combined with colestipol regress coronary atherosclerosis and prevent clinical events in men with elevated apolipoprotein. Circulation 80(Suppl. II):II-266, 1989.

106. Grundy, S. M., Mok, H. Y., Zech, L., and Berman, M.: Influence of nicotinic acid on metabolism of cholesterol and triglycerides in man. J. Lipid Res. 22:24, 1981.

107. Steinberg, D., Parthasarathy, S., and Carew, T. E.: In vivo inhibition of foam cell development by probucol in Watanabe rabbits. Am. J. Cardiol. 62:6b, 1988.

107a. Tanner, F. C., Noll, G., Boulanger, C. M., and Luscher, T. F.: Oxidized low density lipoproteins inhibit relaxations of porcine coronary arteries. Role of scavenger receptor and endothelium-derived nitric oxide. Circulation 83:2012, 1991.

107b. Rosenfield, M. E.: Oxidized LDL affects multiple atherogenic cellular responses. Circulation 83:2137, 1991.

108. Carew, T., Schwenke, W., and Steinberg, D.: Antiatherogenic effect of probucol unrelated to its hypercholesterolemic effect: Evidence that antioxidants in vivo can selectively inhibit low density lipoprotein degradation in macrophage-rich fatty streaks and slow the progression of atherosclerosis in the Watanabe heritable hyperlipidemic rabbit. Proc. Natl. Acad. Sci. USA 84:7725, 1987.

109. Goldberg, R., and Mendez, A.: Probucol enhances cholesterol efflux from cultured skin fibroblasts. Am. J. Cardiol. 62:57B, 1988.

110. Aburatani, H., Matsumoto, A., Kodama, T., et al.: Increased levels of messenger ribonucleic acid for apolipoprotein E in the spleen of probucoltreated rabbits. Am. J. Cardiol. 62:60B, 1988.

111. Witztum, J. L., Simmons, D., Steinberg, D., et al.: Intensive combination drug therapy of familial hypercholesterolemia with lovastatin, probucol and colestipol hydrochloride. Circulation 79:16, 1989.

112. Erikson, U., Nilsson, S., and Stenport, G.: Probucol Quantitative Regression Swedish Trial: New angiographic technique to measure atheroma volume of the femoral artery. Am. J. Cardiol. 62:44B, 1988.

113. Walldius, G., Carlson, L. A., Erickson, U., et al.: Development of femoral atherosclerosis in hypercholesterolemic patients during treatment with cholestyramine and probucol/placebo. Probucol Quantitative Regression Swedish Trial (PQRST): A status report. Am. J. Cardiol. 62:37B, 1988.

114. Sitori, C. R., and Chiero, G.: Effects of lipid lowering agents and other treatment regimens on serum lipoprotein. Current Opinion in Lipidology 1:262, 1990.

114a. Lupien, P. J., Brun, D., Gagné, C., et al.: Gemfibrozil therapy in primary type II hyperlipoproteinemia: Effects on lipids, lipoproteins and apolipoproteins. Can. J. Cardiol. 7:27, 1991.

115. Committee of Principal Investigators: WHO cooperative trial of primary prevention of ischaemic heart disease with clofibrate to lower serum cholesterol: Final mortality follow-up. Lancet 2:600, 184.

116. Mabuchi, H., Sakai, T., Sakai, Y., et al.: Reduction of serum cholesterol in heterozygous patients with familial hypercholesterolemia. Additive effects of compactin and cholestyramine. N. Engl. J. Med. 308:609, 1983.

117. Bilheimer, D. W., Grundy, S. M., Brown, M. S., and Goldstein, J. L.: Mevinolin and colestipol stimulate receptor mediated clearance of low density lipoprotein from plasma in familial hypercholesterolemia heterozygotes. Proc. Natl. Acad. Sci. USA 80:4124, 1983.

118. Cuthbert, J. A., and Lipsky, P. E.: Assessment of functional LDL receptor activity on lymphocytes of normal subjects and patients with mild hypercholesterolemia. Trans. Assoc. Am. Physicians 101:1, 1988.

119. Weintraub, M. S., Eisenberg, S., and Breslow, J. L.: Lovastatin reduces postprandial lipoprotein levels in hypercholesterolemic patients with mild hypertriglycerides. Eur. J. Clin. Invest. 19:480, 1989.

120. Vega, G. L., and Grundy, S. M.: Comparison of lovastatin and gemfibrozil in normolipidemic patients with hypoalphalipoproteinemia. JAMA 262:3148, 1989.

121. Kostner, G. M., Gavish, D., Leopold, B., et al.: HMG-CoA reductase inhibitors lower LDL cholesterol without reducing Lp(a) levels. Circulation 80:1313, 1989.

122. Davi, G., Averna, M., Novo, S., et al.: Effects of synvinolin on platelet aggregation and thromboxane B2 synthesis in type IIa hypercholesterolemic patients. Atherosclerosis 79:79, 1989.

123. Coronary Drug Project Research Group: The Coronary Drug Project findings leading to further modifications of its protocol with respect to dextrothyroxine. JAMA 220:996, 1972.

124. Eckel, R. H.: Lipoprotein lipase. A multifunctional enzyme relevant to common metabolic diseases [Review]. N. Engl. J. Med. 320:1060, 1989.

125. Havel, R. J., Hunninghake, D. B., Illingworth, D. R., et al.: Lovastatin (mevinolin) in treatment of heterozygous familial hypercholesterolemia. Ann. Intern. Med. 107:609, 1987.

126. Blum, C. B., and Levy, R. I.: Current therapy for hypercholesterolemia [Review]. JAMA 261:3582, 1989.

127. Stuyt, P. M., Mol, M. J., Stalenhoef, A. F., et al.: Simvastatin in the effective reduction of plasma lipoprotein levels in familial dysbetalipoproteinemia (type III hyperlipoproteinemia). Am. J. Med. 88:42N, 1990.

128. Leaf, D. A., Connor, W. E., Illingworth, D. R., et al.: The hypolipidemic effects of gemfibrozil in type V hyperlipidemia. A double-blind, crossover study. JAMA 262:3154, 1989.

129. Buchwald, H., Varco, R. L., Matts, J. P., et al.: Effect of partial ileal bypass surgery on mortality and morbidity from coronary heart disease in patients with hypercholesterolemia. Report of the Program on the Surgical Control of the Hyperlipidemias (POSCH). N. Engl. J. Med. 323:946, 1990.

130. Miettinen, T. A., and Lempinen, M.: Cholestyramine and ileal bypass in the treatment of familial hypercholesterolemia. Eur. J. Clin. Invest. 7:509, 1977.

131. Starzl, T. E., Putnam, C. W., Chase, H. P., and Porter, K. A.: Portacaval shunt in hyperlipoproteinemia. Lancet 2:940, 1973.

132. Forman, M. B., Baker, S. G., Mieny, C. J., et al.: Treatment of homozygous familial hypercholesterolemia with portacaval shunt. Atherosclerosis 41:349, 1982.

133. Bilheimer, D. W., Goldstein, J. L., Grundy, S. C., et al.: Liver transplantation provides low density lipoprotein receptors and lowers plasma cholesterol in a child with homozygous familial hypercholesterolemia. N. Engl. J. Med. 311:1658, 1984.

134. Lupien, P. J., Moorjani, S., Lou, M., et al.: Removal of cholesterol from blood by affinity binding to heparin-agarose: Evaluation on treatment in homozygous familial hypercholesterolemia. Pediatr. Res. 14:113, 1980.

135. Thompson, G. R., Myant, N. B., Kilpatrick, D., et al.: Assessment of long-term plasma exchange for familial hypercholesterolemia. Br. Heart J. 43:680, 1980.

TOBACCO USE

136. Migas, O. D.: The lipid effects of smoking. Am. Heart J. 115:272, 1988.

137. Tiwari, A. K., Gode, J. D., and Dubey, G. P.: Effect of cigarette smoking on serum total cholesterol and HDL in normal subjects and coronary heart disease patients. Indian Heart J. 41:92, 1989.

138. Trap-Jensen, J.: Effects of smoking on the heart and peripheral circulation [Review]. Am. Heart J. 115:263, 1988.

139. Green, M. S., Jucha, E., and Luz, Y.: Blood pressure in smokers and nonsmokers: Epidemiologic findings. Am. Heart J. 111:932, 1986.

140. Langford, H. G., Stamler, J., Wassertheil-Smoller, S., and Prineas, R. J.: All-cause mortality in the Hypertension Detection and Follow-up Program. Findings for the whole cohort and for persons with less severe hypertension with and without other traits related to risk of mortality. Prog. Cardiovasc. Dis. 29:29, 1986.

141. Kannel, W. B., D'Agostino, R. B., and Belanger, A. J.: Fibrinogen, cigarette smoking, and the risk of cardiovascular disease: Insights from the Framingham Study. Am. Heart J. 113:1006, 1987.

142. Kannel, W. B., Wolf, P. A., Castelli, W. P., and D'Agostino, R. B.: Fibrinogen and risk of cardiovascular disease. The Framingham Study. JAMA 258:1183, 1987.

143. Meade, T. W., Imeson, J., and Stirling, Y.: Effects of changes in smoking and other characteristics on clotting factors and the risk of ischemic heart disease. Lancet 2:986, 1987.

144. Nowak, J., Murray, J. J., Oates, J. A., and FitzGerald, G. A.: Biochemical evidence of a chronic abnormality in platelet and vascular function in healthy individuals who smoke cigarettes. Circulation 76:6, 1987.

145. Winniford, M. D., Wheelan, K. R., Kremers, M. S., et al.: Smoking-induced coronary vasoconstriction in patients with atherosclerotic coronary artery disease: Evidence for adrenergically mediated alterations in coronary artery tone. Circulation 73:662, 1986.

146. Deanfield, J. E., Shea, M. J., Wilson, R. A., et al.: Direct effects of smoking on the heart: Silent ischemic disturbances of coronary flow. Am. J. Cardiol. 57:1005, 1986.

147. Kannel, W. B.: Hypertension, blood lipids, and cigarette smoking as co-risk factors for coronary heart disease. Ann. N.Y. Acad. Sci. 304:128, 1978.

148. Cook, D. G., Shaper, A. G., Pocock, S. J., and Kussick, S. J.: Giving up smoking and the risk of heart attacks: A report from the British Regional Heart Study. Lancet 2:1376, 1986.

149. Kaufman, D. W., Helmrich, S. P., Rosenberg, L., et al.: Nicotine and carbon monoxide content of cigarette smoke and the risk of myocardial infarction in young men. N. Engl. J. Med. 308:409, 1983.

150. Allen, D. R., Browse, N. L., and Rutt, D. L.: Effects of cigarette smoke, carbon monoxide and nicotine on the uptake of fibrinogen by the canine arterial wall. Atherosclerosis 77(1):83, 1989.

151. Palmer, J. R., Rosenberg, L., and Shapiro, S.: "Low yield" cigarettes and the risk of nonfatal myocardial infarction in women. N. Engl. J. Med. 320:1569, 1989.

152. Svendsen, K. H., Kuller, L. H., Martin, M. J., and Ockene, J. K.: Effects of passive smoking in the Multiple Risk Factor Intervention Trial. Am. J. Epidemiol. 126:783, 1987.

HYPERTENSION

153. Stamler, J., Stamler, R., and Liu, K.: High blood pressure. In Connor, W. E., and Bristow, J. D. (eds.): Coronary Heart Disease: Prevention, Complications, and Treatment. Philadelphia, J. B. Lippincott Company, 1985, pp. 85–109.

153a. Koren, M. J., Devereux, R. B., Casale, P. N., et al.: Relation of left ventricular mass and geometry to morbidity and mortality in uncomplicated essential hypertension. Ann. Intern. Med. 114:345, 1991.

154. Williams, R. R., Hunt, S. C., and Hopkins, P. H.: Familial dyslipidemic hypertension. Evidence of 58 Utah families for a syndrome present in approximately 12% of patients with essential hypertension. JAMA 259:3579, 1988.

155. Freis, E. D.: Critique of the clinical importance of diuretic induced hypokalemia and elevated cholesterol level. Arch. Intern. Med. 149:2640, 1989.

156. Safar, M.: Therapeutic trials and large arteries in hypertension [Review]. Am. Heart J. 115:702, 1988.

157. MacMahon, S. M., Cutler, J. A., Furburg, C. D., and Payne, G. H.: The effects of drug treatment for hypertension on morbidity and mortality from cardiovascular disease: A review of randomized controlled trials [Review]. Prog. Cardiovasc. Dis. 29(3 Suppl. 1):99, 1986.

158. Subcommittee on Definition and Prevalence of the 1984 Joint National Committee: Hypertension prevalence and the status of awareness, treatment, and control in the United States: Final report. Hypertension 7:457, 1985.

159. Wikstrand, J., Warnold, I., Olsson, G., et al.: Primary prevention with metoprolol in patients with hypertension. Mortality results from the MAPHY study. JAMA 259:1976, 1988.

160. Kaplan, N. M.: Cardiovascular risk reduction: The role of antihypertensive treatment. Am. J. Med. 90:19S, 1991.

161. Treating mild hypertension. Report of the British Hypertension Society Working Party. Recommendation for treatment of hypertension. Br. Med. J. [Clin. Res.] 298:694, 1989.

162. Breckenridge, M. B., and Kostis, J. B.: Isolated systolic hypertension in the elderly: Results of a statewide survey of clinical practice in New Jersey. Am. J. Med. 86:370, 1989.

163. Cloher, T. P., and Whelton, P. K.: Physician approach to the recognition and initial management of hypertension. Results of a statewide survey of Maryland physicians. Arch. Intern. Med. 146:529, 1986.

164. Laragh, J. H.: Issues, goals and guidelines in selecting first line drug therapy for hypertension. Hypertension 13:I103, 1989.

165. The 1988 Report of the Joint National Committee on Detection, Evaluation and Treatment of High Blood Pressure. Arch. Intern. Med. 148:1023, 1988.

166. Report of the Second Task Force on Blood Pressure in Children, 1987. Task Force on Blood Pressure Control in Children. National Heart, Lung, and Blood Institute, Bethesda, Maryland. Pediatrics 79:1, 1987.

167. Smoak, C. A., Burke, G. L., Webber, L. S., et al.: Relation of obesity to clustering of cardiovascular risk factors in children and young adults. The Bogalusa Heart Study. Am. J. Epidemiol. 125:364, 1987.

168. Williams, R. R., Hunt, S. C., Hasstedt, S., et al.: Biological markers of genetically predisposed hypertension. In Hofman, A., Grobbee, D. E., Schalekamp, M.A.D.H. (eds.): The Early Pathogenesis of Primary Hypertension. Amsterdam, Excerpta Medica, 187:208, 1987.

169. Weinberger, M. H.: Sodium chloride and blood pressure [Editorial]. N. Engl. J. Med. 317:1084, 1987.

170. Weinberger, M. H., Cohen, S. J., Miller, J. Z., et al.: Dietary sodium restriction as adjunctive treatment of hypertension. JAMA 259:2561, 1988.

171. Rouse, I. L., Beilin, L. J., and Mahoney, D. O.: Nutrient intake, blood pressure, serum and urinary prostaglandins and serum thromboxane B2 in a controlled trial with a lacto-ovo-vegetarian diet. J. Hypertens. 4:241, 1986.

172. Margetts, B. M., Beilin, L. J., Vandongen, R., et al.: Vegetarian diet in mild hypertension. A randomized controlled trial. Br. Med. J. [Clin. Res.] 293:1468, 1986.

173. Klatsky, A. L., Friedman, G. D., and Armstrong, M. A.: The relationships between alcoholic beverage use and other traits to blood pressure: A new Kaiser-Permanente study. Circulation 73:628, 1986.

174. Kok, F. J., Vandenbroucke, J. P., Wessel, C., and Van der Heide, R. M.: Dietary sodium, calcium potassium and blood pressure. Am. J. Epidemiol. 123:1043, 1986.

175. Trevisan, M., Krogh, V., Farinaro, E., et al.: Calcium-rich foods and blood pressure. Findings from the Italian National Research Council Study (the Nine Communities Study). Am. J. Epidemiol. 127:1155, 1988.

176. Kaplan, N. M.: Calcium and potassium in the treatment of essential hypertension [Review]. Semin. Nephrol. 8:176, 1988.

177. Veterans' Administration Co-operative Study Group on Antihypertensive Agents: Effects of treatment on morbidity in hypertension. JAMA 213:1143, 1970.

178. Hypertension Detection and Follow-up Program Cooperative Group: Five year findings of the Hypertension Detection and Follow-up Program. I. Reduction in mortality of persons with high blood pressure, including mild hypertension. JAMA 242:2562, 1979.

179. Management Committee: The Australian therapeutic trial in mild hypertension. Lancet 1:1261, 1980.

180. Multiple Risk Factor Intervention Trial Research Group: Coronary heart disease, death, non-fatal acute myocardial infarction and other clinical outcomes in the Multiple Risk Factor Intervention Trial. Am. J. Cardiol. 58:1, 1986.

181. Multiple Risk Factor Intervention Group: Mortality after 10.5 years for hypertensive patients in MRFIT. Circulation 82:1616, 1990.

182. Paul, O.: The Medical Research Council Trial. Hypertension 8:733, 1986.

183. The IPPPSH Collaborative Group: Cardiovascular risk and risk factors in a randomized trial of treatment based on the beta blocker oxprenolol: The International Prospective Primary Prevention Study in Hypertension (IPPPSH). J. Hypertens. 3:379, 1985.

PHYSICAL ACTIVITY AND OBESITY

184. Blair, S. N., Kohl, H. W., Paffenberger, R. S., Jr., et al.: Physical fitness and all-cause mortality. A prospective study of healthy men and women. JAMA 262:2395, 1989.

185. Powell, K. E., Thompson, P. D., Caspersen, C. J., and Kendrick, J. S.: Physical activity and the incidence of coronary heart disease [Review]. Annu. Rev. Public Health 8:253, 1987.

185a. Caspersen, C. J., Bloemberg, B. P. M., Saris, W. H. M., et al.: The prevalence of selected physical activities and their relation with coronary heart disease risk factors in elderly men: The Zutphen study, 1985. Am. J. Epidemiol. 133:1078, 1991.

186. Daneberg, A. L., Keller, J. B., Wilson, P. W., and Castelli, W. P.: Leisure time physical activity in the Framingham Offspring Study. Description, seasonal variation, and risk factor correlates. Am. J. Epidemiol. 129:76, 1989.

187. Slattery, M. L., Jacobs, D. R., Jr., and Nichaman, M. Z.: Leisure time physical activity and coronary heart disease death. The US Railroad Study. Circulation 79:304, 1989.

188. Jennings, G., Nelson, L., Nestel, P., et al.: The effects of changes in physical activity on major cardiovascular risk factors, hemodynamics, sympathetic function, and glucose utilization in man: A controlled study of four levels of activity. Circulation 73:30, 1986.

189. Hespel, P., Lijnen, P., Van Hoof, R., et al.: Effects of physical endurance training on the plasma renin-angiotensin-aldosterone system in normal man. J. Endocrinol. 116:443, 1988.

190. Fagard, R., Grauwels, R., Groeseneken, D., et al.: Plasma levels or renin, angiotensin II, and 6-keto-prostaglandin F1 alpha in endurance athletes. J. Appl. Physiol. 59:947, 1985.

191. Fagard, R., Bielen, D., Hespel, P., et al.: Physical exercise in hypertension. In Laragh, J. H., and Brenner, B. M. (eds.): Hypertension: Pathophysiology, Diagnosis, and Management. Vol. 2. New York, Raven Press, 1990, pp. 1985–1997.

192. Gordon, T., Castelli, W. P., Hjortland, M. C., et al.: High-density lipoprotein as a protective factor against coronary heart disease. The Framingham Study. Am. J. Med. 62:707, 1977.

193. Sellier, P., Corona, P., Audoin, P., et al.: Influence of training on blood lipids and coagulation. Eur. Heart J. 9:32, 1988.

194. Hamalainen, E., Tikkanen, H., Harkonen, M., et al.: Serum lipoproteins, sex hormones and sex hormone binding globulin in middle-aged men of different physical fitness and risk of coronary heart disease. Atherosclerosis 67:155, 1987.

195. Shepard, R. J.: Exercise in the tertiary prevention of ischemic heart disease: Experimental proof [Review]. Can. J. Sport Sci. 14:74, 1989.

196. Paffenbarger, R. S., Jr., Wing, A. L., and Hyde, R. T.: Physical activity as an index of heart attack risk in college alumni. Am. J. Epidemiol. 108:161, 1978.

197. Milvy, P., and Siegel, A. J.: Physical activity levels and altered mortality

from CHD with emphasis on marathon running: A critical review. Cardiovasc. Rev. Rep. 2:233, 1981.

198. Briazgounor, I. P.: The role of physical activity in the prevention and treatment of noncommunicable diseases. World Health Stat. Q. 41:242, 1988.

199. Froelicher, V. F., Perdue, S. T., Atwood, J. E., et al.: Exercise testing of patients recovering from myocardial infarction. Curr. Probl. Cardiol. 11:369, 1986.

200. Burton, B. T., Foster, W. R., Hirsch, J., and Van Itallie, T. B.: Health implications of obesity: An NIH consensus development conference. Int. J. Obes. 9:155, 1985 (Published erratum appears in Int. J. Obes. 10:79, 1986).

201. Kannel, W. B., and Gordon, T.: Physiological and medical concomitants of obesity: The Framingham Study. In Bray, G. A. (ed.): Obesity in America. Washington, D.C., U.S. Department of Health, Education and Welfare, 1979, pp. 125–163. NIH publication no. 79–359.

202. Higgins, M., Kannel, W., Garrison, R., et al.: Hazards of obesity–The Framingham experience. Acta Med. Scand. [Suppl] 723:23, 1988.

203. Jooste, P. L., Steenkamp, H. J., Benade, A. J., and Rossouw, J. E.: Prevalence of overweight and obesity and its relation to coronary heart disease in the CORIS Study. S. Afr. Med. J. 74:101, 1988.

204. Knuiman, J. T., West, C. E., and Burema, J.: Serum total and high density lipoprotein cholesterol concentrations and body mass index in adult men from 13 countries. Am. J. Epidemiol. 116:631, 1982.

205. Yamazi, I., Kobayakawa, H., and Komura, H.: Sympathetic nerve activity, plasma renin and water-sodium balance in obese patients with essential hypertension. Jpn. Circ. J. 50:1155, 1986.

206. Modan, M., Halkin, H., Almog, S., et al.: Hyperinsulinemia: A link between hypertension, obesity and glucose intolerance. J. Clin. Invest. 75:809, 1985.

207. Reaven, G. M., and Hoffman B. B.: Hypertension as a disease of carbohydrates and lipoprotein metabolism. Am. J. Med. 87(Suppl. 6A):2S, 1989.

208. Patsch, J. R., Prasad, S., Gotto, A. M., Jr., and Patsch, W.: High density lipoprotein. Relationship of the plasma levels of this lipoprotein species to its composition, to the magnitude of postprandial lipemia, and to the activities of lipoprotein lipase and hepatic lipase. J. Clin. Invest. 80:341, 1987.

209. Hunt, S. C., Wu, L. L., Hopkins, P. N., et al.: Apolipoprotein, low density lipoprotein subfraction, and insulin associations with familial combined hyperlipidemia. Study of Utah patients with familial dyslipidemic hypertension. Arteriosclerosis 9:335, 1989.

210. Bjorntorp, P.: The associations between obesity, adipose tissue distribution and disease. Acta Med. Scand. Suppl. 723:121, 1988.

211. Lapidus, L., Bentsson, C., and Larsson, B.: Distribution of adipose tissue and body fat and risk of cardiovascular disease. A 12-year follow-up of participants in the population study of women in Gothenburg, Sweden. Br. Med. J. [Clin. Res.] 289:1257, 1984.

212. Larsson, B., and Svardsudd, K.: Distribution and the risk of cardiovascular disease. Br. Med. J. [Clin. Res.] 288:1401, 1984.

213. Larsson, B., Seidell, J., Savardsudd, K., et al.: Obesity, adipose tissue distribution and health in men. The study of men born in 1913. Appetite 13:37, 1989.

214. Peiris, A. N., Sothmann, M. S., Hoffmann, R. G., et al.: Adiposity, fat distribution and cardiovascular risk. Ann. Intern. Med. 110:867, 1989.

215. Wing, R. R., Bunker, C. H., Kueller, L. H., et al.: Insulin, body mass index and cardiovascular risk factors in pre-menopausal women. Arteriosclerosis 9:479, 1989.

FAMILY HISTORY AND DIABETES MELLITUS

216. Feinleib, M.: Genetics. In Kaplan, N. M., and Stamler, J. (eds.): Prevention of Coronary Heart Disease: Practical Management of the Risk Factors. Philadelphia, W. B. Saunders Company, 1983, pp. 120–129.

217. Sinaiko, A. R., and Wells, T. G.: Childhood hypertension. In: Laragh J. H., and Brenner, B. M. (eds.): Hypertension, vol. 2. Raven Press, New York, 1990, pp. 1855–1868.

218. Schieken, R. M.: The management of the family at high risk for coronary heart disease. Cardiol. Clin. 7:467, 1989.

219. Becker, D. M., Becker, L. C., and Pearson, T. A.: Risk factors in siblings of people with premature coronary heart disease. J. Am. Coll. Cardiol. 12:1273, 1988.

220. Jorde, L. B., and Williams, R. R.: Relation between family history of coronary artery disease and coronary risk variables. Am. J. Cardiol. 62:708, 1988.

221. Austin, M. A., King, M. C., Vranizan, K. M., and Krauss, R. M.: Atherogenic lipoprotein phenotype. A proposed genetic marker for coronary heart disease risk. Circulation 82:495, 1990.

222. Garcia, M. J., McNamara, P. M., Gordon, T., and Kannel, W. B.: Sixteen year follow-up study. Morbidity and mortality in diabetics in the Framingham population. Diabetes 23:105, 1976.

223. Davi, G., Averna, M., Catalano, I., et al.: Platelet function in patients with Type II diabetes mellitus. The effect of glycemic control. Diabetes Res. 10:7, 1988.

224. Stolar, M. W.: Atherosclerosis in diabetes. The role of hyperinsulinemia. Metabolism. 37(Suppl. 1):J1, 1988.

225. Dzau, V. J.: Atherosclerosis and hypertension: Mechanisms and interrelationships. J. Cardiovasc. Pharmacol. 15(Suppl. 5):S59, 1990.

226. Black, H. R.: The coronary artery disease paradox: The role of hyperinsu-

linemia and insulin resistance and implications for therapy. J. Cardiovasc. Pharmacol. 15(Suppl. 5):S26, 1990.

226a. Kannel, W. B., and Ross, S. A.: States of insulin resistance: the interaction between hypertension, glucose intolerance, and coronary heart disease. Am. Heart J. 121:1267, 1990.

226b. Reaven, G. M.: Insulin resistance and compensatory hyperinsulinemia: Role in hypertension, dyslipidemia, and coronary heart disease. Am. Heart J. 121:1283, 1991.

227. Kannel, W. B., D'Agostino, R. B., Wilson, P. W., et al.: Diabetes, fibrinogen and risk of cardiovascular disease. The Framingham Experience. Am. Heart J. 120:672, 1990.

228. West, K. M.: Epidemiology of Diabetes and Its Vascular Lesions. New York, Elsevier, 1978.

229. Kleinman, J. C., Donahue, R. P., Harris, M. I., et al.: Mortality among diabetics in a national health sample. Am. J. Epidemiol. 128:389, 1988.

230. Joint Discussion: The International Collaborative Group. J. Chron. Dis. 32:829, 1979.

231. Ishii, H., Umeda, F., Kunisaki, M., et al.: Modification of prostaglandin synthesis in washed human platelets and cultured bovine aortic endothelial cells by glycosylated low density lipoprotein. Diabetes Res. 12:177, 1989.

232. Howard, B. V.: Lipoprotein metabolism in diabetes mellitus. J. Lipid Res. 28:613, 1987.

233. Pollare, T., Lithell, H., and Berne, C.: A comparison of the effects of captopril and hydrochlorothiazide on glucose and lipid metabolism in patients with hypertension. N. Engl. J. Med. 321:868, 1989.

234. Ferrannini, E., Buzzigoli, G., Bonadonna, R.: Insulin resistance in essential hypertension. N. Engl. J. Med. 317:350, 1987.

235. Jenkins, C. D.: Psychosocial and behavioral factors. In: Kaplan, N. M., and Stamler, J. (eds.): Prevention of Coronary Heart Disease: Practical Management of the Risk Factors. Philadelphia, W. B. Saunders Company, 1983, p. 99.

236. Liu, K., Cedres, L. B., and Stamler, J.: Relationship of education to major risk factors and death from coronary heart disease, cardiovascular diseases and all causes. Findings of three Chicago epidemiologic studies. Circulation 66:1308, 1982.

237. Colbourn, A. W.: The decline in coronary heart disease mortality: The DuPont experience. Part 2 (editorial). Del. Med. J. 58:351, 1986.

238. Davidson, D. M.: Cardiovascular disease and occupation. Cardiovasc. Rev. Rep. 5:503, 1984.

239. Aro, S., and Hasan, J.: Occupational class, psychosocial stress and morbidity. Ann. Clin. Dis. 19:62, 1987.

240. Reed, D. M., LaCroix, A. Z., Karasek, R. A., et al.: Occupational strain and the incidence of coronary heart disease. Am. J. Epidemiol. 129:495, 1989.

241. Dubrow, R., Burnett, C. A., Gute, D. M., and Brockert, J. E.: Ischemic heart disease and acute myocardial infarction among police officers. J. Occup. Med. 30:650, 1988.

242. Schnall, P. L., Pieper, C., Schwartz, J. E., et al.: The relationship between job strain, workplace diastolic blood pressure, and left ventricular mass index. Results of a case-control study. JAMA 263:1929, 1990.

243. Levy, D., Savage, D. D., Garrison, R. J., et al.: Echocardiographic criteria for left ventricular hypertrophy: The Framingham Heart Study. Am. J. Cardiol. 59:956, 1987.

244. Eaker, E. D., Abbott, R. D., and Kannel, W. B.: Frequency of uncomplicated angina pectoris in Type A compared with Type B persons. The Framingham Study. Am. J. Cardiol. 63:1042, 1989.

245. Siegel, W. C., Mark, D. B., Hlatky, M. A., et al.: Clinical correlates and prognostic significance of Type A behavior and silent myocardial ischemia on the treadmill. Am. J. Cardiol. 64:1280, 1989.

246. Rosenman, R. H., Friedman, M., Straus, R., et al.: A predictive study of coronary heart disease. The Western Collaborative Group Study. JAMA 189:15, 1964.

247. Ragland, D. R., and Brand, R. J.: Type A behavior and mortality from coronary heart disease. N. Engl. J. Med. 318:65, 1988.

248. Shekelle, R. B., Gale, M., and Norusis, M.: Type A score (Jenkins Activity Survey) and risk of recurrent heart disease in the Aspirin Myocardial Infarction Study. Am. J. Cardiol. 56:221, 1985.

249. Case, R. B., Heller, S. S., Case, N. B., et al.: Type A behavior and survival after acute myocardial infarction. N. Engl. J. Med. 312:737, 1985.

250. Kahn, J. P., Perumal, A. S., Gully, R. J., et al.: Correlates of Type A behaviour with adrenergic receptor density: Implications for coronary artery disease pathogenesis. Lancet 2:937, 1987.

251. Friedman, M., Rossenman, R. H., and Carroll, V.: Changes in serum cholesterol and blood clotting time in men subject to cycle variations of occupations stress. Circulation 17:852, 1980.

252. Friedman, M.: Type A behavior: Its diagnosis, cardiovascular relation and the effect of its modification or recurrence of coronary artery disease. Am. J. Cardiol. 64:12c, 1989.

253. Kannel, W. B.: Metabolic risk factors for coronary heart disease in women: Perspective from the Framingham Study. Am. Heart J. 114:413, 1987.

254. Matthews, K. A., Meilahn, E., Kuller, L. H., et al.: Menopause and risk factors for coronary artery disease. N. Engl. J. Med. 321:641, 1989.

255. Campos, H., McNamara, J. R., Wilson, P. W., et al.: Differences in low density lipoprotein subfractions and apolipoproteins in premenopausal and postmenopausal women. J. Clin. Endocrinol. Metab. 67:30, 1988.

256. Sullivan, J. M., Vander-Zwag, R., Lemp, G. F., et al.: Postmenopausal estrogen use and coronary atherosclerosis. Ann. Intern. Med. 108:358, 1988.

257. Godsland, I. F., Wynn, V., Crook, D., and Miller, N. E.: Sex, plasma, lipo-

proteins and atherosclerosis prevailing assumption and questions. Am. Heart J. *114*:1467, 1987.

258. Ernster, V. L., Bush, T. L., and Huggins, G. R.: Benefits and risks of menopausal estrogens and progestin hormone use. Prev. Med. *17*:201, 1988.

259. Stampfer, M. J., Willett, W. C., and Coldity, G. A.: A prospective study of this past use of oral contraceptive agents and risk of cardiovascular disease. N. Engl. J. Med. *319*:1313, 1988.

260. Mann, J. I., Vessey, M. P., Thorogood, M., and Doll, R.: Myocardial infarction in young women with special reference to oral contraceptive practice. Br. Med. J. [Clin. Res.] 2:241, 1975.

261. Stampfer, M. J., Willett, W. C., Colditz, G. A., et al.: A prospective study of past use of oral contraceptive agents and risk of cardiovascular disease. N. Engl. J. Med. *319*:1313, 1988.

262. Stampfer, M. J., Willett, W. C., Colditz, G. A., et al.: Past use of oral contraceptives and cardiovascular disease: A meta-analysis in the context of the Nurses' Health Study. Am. J. Obstet. Gynecol. *163*:285, 1990.

262a. Steinberg, D., Pearson, T. A., and Kuller, L. H.: Alcohol and atherosclerosis. Ann. Intern. Med. *114*:967, 1991.

263. Regan, T. J.: Alcohol and the cardiovascular system. JAMA *264*:377, 1990.

264. Handa, K., Sasaki, J., and Saku, K.: Alcohol consumption, serum lipids and severity of angiographically determined coronary artery disease. Am. J. Cardiol. *65*:287, 1990.

265. Hartung, G. H., Reeves, R. S., Krock, L. P., et al.: Effect of alcohol and exercise on plasma HDL cholesterol subfractions and apolipoprotein A-I(APOA-I) in middle-aged men. Circulation *72*(Suppl. III):452, 1985.

266. Hennekens, C. H.: Alcohol. *In* Kaplan, N. M., and Stamler, J. (eds.): Prevention of Coronary Heart Disease: Practical Management of the Risk Factors. Philadelphia, W. B. Saunders Company, 1983, pp. 130–138.

267. Stason, W. B., Neff, R. K., Miettinen, O. S., and Jick, H.: Alcohol consumption and nonfatal myocardial infarction. Am. J. Epidemiol. *104*:603, 1976.

268. Anderson, A. J., Barboriak, J. J., and Rimm, A. A.: Risk factors and angiographically determined coronary occlusion. Am. J. Epidemiol. *107*:8, 1978.

269. Barboriak, J. J., Rimm, A. A., and Anderson, A. J.: Coronary artery occlusion and alcohol intake. Br. Heart J. *39*:289, 1977.

270. Barboriak, J. J., Anderson, A. J., and Hoffman, R. G.: Interrelationships between coronary artery occlusion, high-density lipoprotein cholesterol and alcohol intake. J. Lab. Clin. Med. *94*:348, 1979.

271. Klevay, L. M.: The role of copper, zinc and other chemical elements in ischemic heart disease. *In*: Rennert, O. M., and Chan, W. Y. (eds.): Metabolism of Trace Metals in Man, vol. 1. Boca Raton, FL, CRC Press, 1984, pp. 129–158.

272. Klevay, L. M.: Copper and ischemic heart disease. Bio-Trace Element Res. *5*:245, 1983.

273. Leoni, V., Fabiani, L., and Ticchiarelli, L.: Water hardness and cardiovascular mortality rate in Abruzzo, Italy. Arch. Environ. Health *40*:274, 1985.

274. Crawford, M. D., Clayton, D. G., Stanley, F., and Shaper, A. G.: An epidemiological study of sudden death in hard and soft water areas. J. Chronic Dis. *30*:69, 1977.

275. Chobanian, A. V.: Effects of calcium channel antagonists and other antihypertensives on atherogenesis. J. Hypertens. *5*(Suppl. 4):S543, 1987.

276. Weinstein, D. B., and Heiden, J. G.: Antiatherogenic effects of calcium channel blockers. Am. J. Med. *84*:102, 1988.

276a. Broze, G. J., Jr.: Endothelial injury, coagulation, and atherosclerosis. Coronary Artery. Dis. *2*:131, 1991.

277. Meade, T. W., Mellows, S., Brozovic, M., et al.: Haemostatic function and ischemic heart diseases. Principal results of the Northwich Park Heart Study. Lancet *2*:533, 1986.

277a. Yarnell, J. W. G., Baker, I. A., Sweetnam, P. M., et al.: Fibrinogen, viscosity, and white blood cell count are major risk factors for ischemic heart disease. The Caerphilly and Speedwell collaborative heart disease studies. Circulation *83*:836, 1991.

278. Lipinska, I., Gurewich, V., and Meriam, C. M.: Lipids, lipoproteins, fibrinogen and fibrinolytic activity in angiographically assessed coronary heart disease. Artery *15*:44, 1987.

279. Handa, K., Kono, S., and Saku, K.: Plasma fibrinogen levels as an independent indicator of the severity of coronary atherosclerosis. Atherosclerosis *77*:209, 1989.

280. Lobo, R. A.: Lipids, clotting factors and diabetes. Endogenous risks for cardiovascular disease. Am. J. Obstet. Gynecol. *158*:1584, 1988.

281. Small, M., Lowe, G. D., Beattie, J. M., et al.: Severity of coronary artery disease and basal fibrinolysis. Haemostasis *17*:305, 1987.

282. Smith, E. B., Massie, I. B., and Alexander, K. M.: The release of an immobilized lipoprotein fraction from atherosclerotic lesions by incubation with plasmin. Atherosclerosis *25*:71, 1976.

283. Cairns, J. A., Gent, M., Singer, J., et al.: Aspirin, sulfinpyrazone or both to treat in unstable angina. N. Engl. J. Med. *313*:1369, 1985.

284. Theroux, P., Ouimet, H., McCans, J., et al.: Aspirin, heparin, or both treat acute unstable angina. N. Engl. J. Med. *319*:1105, 1988.

285. Jaschonek, K., Karsch, K. R., Weisenberger, H., et al.: Platelet prostacyclin binding in coronary artery disease. J. Am. Coll. Cardiol. *8*:259, 1986.

286. Steering Committee of the Physicians' Health Study Group: Final report on the aspirin component of the ongoing physicians' health study. N. Engl. J. Med. *321*:129, 1989.

287. Alexander, N. J., and Clarkson, T. B.: Vasectomy increases the severity of diet-induced atherosclerosis in *Macaca fascicularis*. Science *201*:538, 1978.

288. Walker, A. M., Jick, H., Hunter, J. R., and McEvoy, J.: Vasectomy and nonfatal myocardial infarction: Continued observations indicate no elevation of risk. J. Urol. *130*:936, 1983.

289. Liu, S. C., and Fang, G. H.: Serum autoimmunity in vasectomyed men and its relation to atherosclerotic coronary artery disease? Clin. Reprod. Fertil. *3*:343, 1985.

290. Wilson, P. W., Garrison, R. J., Kannel, W. B., et al.: Is coffee consumption a contribution to cardiovascular disease? Insights from the Framingham Study. Arch. Intern. Med. *149*:1169, 1989.

291. Brand, F. N., McGee, D. L., Kannel, W. B., et al.: Hyperuricemia as a risk factor of coronary heart disease: The Framingham Study. Am. J. Epidemiol. *121*:11, 1985.

292. Billingham, M. E.: Cardiac transplant atherosclerosis. Transplant Proc. *19*:19, 1987.

293. Hess, M. L., Hastillo, A., Mohanakumar, T., et al.: Accelerated atherosclerosis in cardiac transplantation: Role of cytoxic B-cell antibodies and hyperlipidemia. Circulation *68*(Suppl. 2):94, 1983.

294. Gao, S. Z., Schroeder, J. S., Alderman, E. L., and Hunt, S. A.: Clinical and laboratory correlates of accelerated coronary disease in the cardiac transplant patient. Circulation *76*(Suppl. 5):56, 1987.

Coronary Blood Flow and Myocardial Ischemia

by EUGENE BRAUNWALD, M.D., and BURTON E. SOBEL, M.D.

Hypoxia, or *hypoxemia*, is a state of reduced oxygen supply to tissue despite adequate perfusion; *anoxia* is the absence of oxygen supply despite adequate perfusion. These conditions should be distinguished from *ischemia*, which is a condition of oxygen deprivation accompanied by inadequate removal of metabolites consequent to reduced perfusion. Although clinical manifestations of coronary insufficiency generally reflect the effects of ischemia, under selected experimental and clinical conditions, deprivation of oxygen can be separated from reduced washout of metabolites.[1] For example, in isolated hearts perfused at high flow rates with media equilibrated with a gas mixture poor in oxygen, anoxia without ischemia results, since washout of metabolites is not hindered. An analogous situation occurs in patients with cyanotic congenital heart disease, as well as in those with cor pulmonale, severe anemia, asphyxiation, and carbon monoxide poisoning.

Neither ischemia nor hypoxia can be defined in absolute terms, since the blood flow and quantity of oxygen required to support myocardium under one set of conditions will not necessarily pertain under another. In humans, blood flow of 60 to 90 ml/min per 100 gm of myocardium is generally required under basal physiological conditions. On the other hand, when the mechanical activity of the heart and its metabolic requirements are markedly reduced, myocardial viability may be maintained by perfusion at much lower rates, approximately 10 to 20 ml/min per 100 gm, or even with complete interruption of perfusion for periods of up to 100 minutes. Examples of conditions that reduce oxygen needs markedly include hypothermia with ventricular fibrillation or asystole, techniques widely used in cardiovascular surgery. Other examples of lowered cardiac oxygen needs, though less drastic, occur following the administration of nitroglycerin and of other nitrates, which reduce the preload and afterload, and of beta-adrenoceptor blockers, which lower heart rate and contractility. This reduction of oxygen needs is perhaps the *principal* mechanism by which these agents relieve anginal pain (p. 1307).

The importance of defining ischemia in *relative* rather than absolute terms is underscored by the use of a variety of stress tests to detect or assess the severity of coronary artery disease. During relative ischemia an imbalance occurs between myocardial oxygen demands and supply (Fig. 38–1). Whether the ischemia is manifested as anginal discomfort, deviation of the ST segment on the electrocardiogram (Chap. 5), relative dimi-

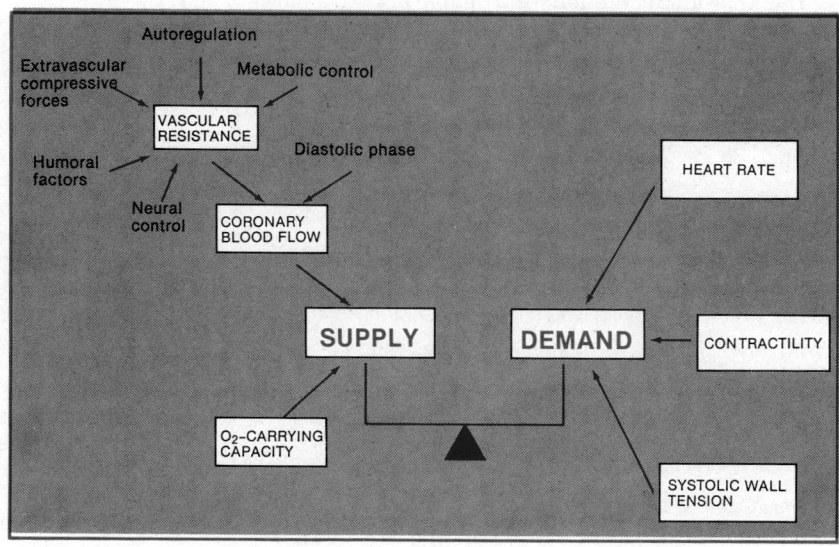

FIGURE 38–1. Factors influencing myocardial oxygen supply and demand. (From Ardehali, A., and Ports, T. A.: Myocardial oxygen supply and demand. Chest **98:**699, 1990.)

nution of accumulation of ^{201}Tl in myocardial "perfusion images," regional wall motion disorders, or diminution of ejection fraction detectable with gated blood pool images (Chap. 10), the underlying principle is the same. Induction of stress by isotonic exercise, atrial pacing, handgrip, or any other means leads to a transitory disparity in the balance between oxygen supply and demand. Although this balance may be adequate under conditions of rest, the disparity becomes apparent when the increased oxygen demands cannot be satisfied by an adequate augmentation of myocardial delivery. An additional cause of imbalance is a reduction of oxygen supply secondary to increased coronary vascular tone.

In this chapter we consider first the control of the balance between myocardial oxygen supply and demand and then the hemodynamic, biochemical, and electrophysiological consequences of ischemia.

DETERMINANTS OF MYOCARDIAL OXYGEN CONSUMPTION
(Table 38–1)

The heart is an aerobic organ; that is, it relies almost exclusively on the oxidation of substrates for the generation of energy, and it can develop only a small oxygen debt. Therefore, in a steady state, determination of the rate of myocardial oxygen consumption ($\dot{M}VO_2$) provides an accurate measure of its total metabolism. It has been known for many years that the total metabolism of the arrested, quiescent heart is only a small fraction of that of the working organ. The $\dot{M}VO_2$ of the beating canine heart ranges from 8 to 15 ml/min per 100 gm, while the oxygen of the noncontracting heart is approximately 1.5 ml/min per 100 gm.[2-4] This quantity of oxygen is required for those physiological processes not directly associated with contraction. Increases in the frequency of depolarization of the noncontracting heart are accompanied by only small increases of $\dot{M}VO_2$. Oxygen cost of electrical depolarization is trivial compared to the cost of contractile activity.[5]

MYOCARDIAL TENSION. As early as 1915 Evans and Matsuoka concluded from studies on the Starling heart-lung preparation that "there is a relation between the tension set up on contraction and the metabolism of the contractile tissue."[6] In 1955, in a systematic investigation of the relative effects of aortic pressure, stroke volume, and heart rate on $\dot{M}VO_2$, it became apparent that the energy needs of the myocardium do not correlate simply with the external work produced by the heart when work is calculated in the classic manner as the product of developed pressure and stroke volume. As a corollary, it was shown that myocardial efficiency, i.e., the ratio of the work performed to the oxygen consumed, varies widely according to the hemodynamic conditions.[7,8] These investigations suggested that the tension-time index, i.e. the area under the left ventricular pressure curve, is an important determinant of the $\dot{M}VO_2$. Subsequently, it was emphasized that the myocardial wall tension time integral is a

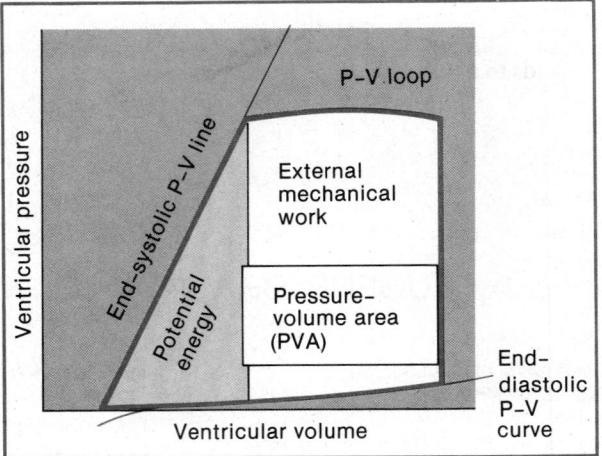

FIGURE 38–2. Schematic illustration of systolic pressure-volume area and its two components, external mechanical work (the P-V loop) and potential energy. End-systole is the time at which the P-V loop touches the end-systolic P-V relation line. The systolic segment of the P-V loop consists of the segments for the isovolumic contraction phase and the ejection phase. The diastolic segment of the P-V loop consists of the segments for the isovolumic relaxation phase and the filling phase. (From Suga, H., Goto, Y., Yamada, O., and Igarashi, Y.: Independence of myocardial oxygen consumption from pressure-volume trajectory during diastole in canine left ventricle. Circ. Res. *55*:735, 1984, by permission of the American Heart Association, Inc.)

more definitive determinant of myocardial energy utilization than is the developed pressure.[9,10] Later studies demonstrated that velocity of myocardial contraction—a reflection of the heart's contractility—is an additional important determinant of $\dot{M}VO_2$ (Fig. 38–1).[11]

Recent reexamination of the determinants of $\dot{M}VO_2$ has emphasized that they correlate closely with the left ventricular systolic pressure-volume area, which consists of the sum of the area within the systolic pressure-volume loop, i.e., the external mechanical work, and the end-systolic elastic potential energy in the ventricular wall, i.e., the area enclosed by the systolic pressure-volume trajectory and the E_{max} line[12-17a] (Fig. 38–2). The pressure-volume area varies linearly with $\dot{M}VO_2$ regardless of loading conditions. It has been demonstrated in isolated muscle as well as in the intact ventricle[18,19] that the pressure-volume area appears to be superior to the force-time integral as a correlate of $\dot{M}VO_2$.[13] Mechanical events during myocardial relaxation do *not* appear to affect $\dot{M}VO_2$ importantly.[4,12-15,20]

Rooke and Feigl have provided evidence that $\dot{M}VO_2$ is influenced by stroke volume, although less so than by pressure development.[3] They have also provided an experimental basis for the use of the systolic pressure–rate product (plus an estimate of the oxygen requirements of the noncontracting heart) as a clinically useful index of $\dot{M}VO_2$. These observations are consistent with Fenn's classic observations on skeletal muscle, which showed that the energy release (a variable related to oxygen consumption) is proportional to the sum of tension development and external work of the muscle.[21,22] Thus, both skeletal muscle and myocardium adjust their energy costs to external conditions imposed after stimulation (Fig. 38–3).[10]

MYOCARDIAL CONTRACTILITY. The net effect of positive inotropic stimuli (such as Ca^{++}, cardiac glycosides, and catecholamines) on $\dot{M}VO_2$ is the end result of their influence on two of its major determinants of that change in opposite directions in the intact heart. These are *wall tension*, which declines as a consequence of a reduction in heart size, and *myocardial contractility*, which, by definition, is augmented. In the failing, dilated ventricle, the increased contractility reduces the left ventricular end-diastolic pressure and volume. On the basis of the Laplace relation (p. 377), this reduction in ventricular volume leads to a decline in intramyocardial tension, which reduces $\dot{M}VO_2$. However, the decrease in $\dot{M}VO_2$

TABLE 38–1 MYOCARDIAL O_2 CONSUMPTION COMPONENTS

Total: 6–8 cc/min/100 gm			
Distribution			
Basal	20%	Volume work	15%
Electrical	1%	Pressure work	64%
Effects on $\dot{M}VO_2$ of 50% increases in			
Wall stress	25%	Heart rate	50%
Contractility	45%	Volume work	4%
Pressure work	50%		

The table demonstrates the dominant contribution to $\dot{M}VO_2$ made by pressure work and prominent effects of increasing pressure work and heart rate on $\dot{M}VO_2$.

From Gould, K. L.: Coronary Artery Stenosis. New York, Elsevier, 1991, p. 8.

that might be expected to result from falling tension in the ventricular wall is opposed by the increase in contractility, which tends to augment MVO_2. The net result of these opposing effects is to produce no change, a slight increase, or a small decrease in MVO_2. Thus, the change in MVO_2 that follows the stimulation of contractility depends on the extent to which intramyocardial tension is reduced in relation to the extent to which contractility is augmented.[10] In general, in the absence of heart failure, drugs that stimulate myocardial contractility elevate MVO_2, because heart size and therefore wall tension are not reduced substantially and do not offset the effect on metabolism of the stimulation of contractility. The importance of contractility as an independent predictor of MVO_2 is reflected in its displacement of the relation between the pressure-volume area and MVO_2.[15,23] The conclusion that myocardial contractility is an important determinant of MVO_2 is also supported by observations on the effects of reducing contractility. Thus, in animal experiments reductions in contractility and in the velocity of contraction produced by cardiac depressant drugs, including propranolol and procainamide, were shown to lower MVO_2 when wall tension was held constant or almost so.[24] Also, reductions of MVO_2 are sometimes seen in the presence of heart failure with its reduced contractility.

In experiments in which the relative effects on MVO_2 of changes in tension development and in myocardial contractility were assessed in the same heart, it was concluded that the quantitative effects on MVO_2 of changes in contractility and tension development are both substantial and of the same order of magnitude.[24] In these experiments heart rate was purposely held constant, since heart rate itself is an important determinant of MVO_2. An augmentation of heart rate elevates the MVO_2 by increasing the frequency of tension development per unit of time, as well as by increasing contractility.[7,25] Systolic wall tension, contractility, and heart rate thus have emerged as the three principal determinants of MVO_2[26] (Fig. 38–1).

Although the precise energy costs of the *maintenance* of the active state of the myocardium have not yet been clearly defined, they are likely to be relatively low. In studies on isolated papillary muscles, MVO_2 was found to be a function of the tension that is developed and the velocity of shortening of the unloaded muscle. Shortening against a load requires oxygen above and beyond that required for the development of tension. It has been suggested by Suga et al. that almost the entire increase in MVO_2 produced by the administration of positive inotropic agents such as Ca^{++} and epinephrine results from the energy costs of enhanced excitation-contraction coupling. Specifically the increased energy costs result from the greater and more rapid Ca^{++} uptake by the sarcoplasmic reticulum[27] as well as from the increased contractile activity, rather than from a direct stimulating effect of positive inotropic agents on basal myocardial metabolism. It has been suggested that when all other parameters affecting MVO_2 are held constant, severe valvular regurgitation does not increase MVO_2 significantly because of the relatively low O_2 cost of the additional myocardial shortening associated with valvular regurgitation[7,16,17,28] (Table 38–2).

MVO_2 is also influenced by the substrate utilized. Specifically, it varies directly with the fraction of energy derived

TABLE 38–2 DETERMINANTS OF MYOCARDIAL OXYGEN CONSUMPTION

1. **Tension development**
2. **Contractile state**
3. **Heart rate**
4. **Shortening against a load (Fenn effect)**
5. **Maintenance of cell viability in basal state**
6. **Depolarization**
7. **Activation**
8. **Maintenance of active state**
9. **Direct metabolic effect of catecholamines**
10. **Fatty acid uptake**

from the metabolism of fatty acids, which in turn varies directly with the arterial concentration of fatty acids and inversely with that of glucose and insulin.[29]

Alterations in contractile performance sometimes affect MVO_2 profoundly. For example, the spontaneously hypertensive rat exhibits reduced MVO_2 (per gm of myocardium) compared with the normal rat at comparable mechanical activity. This improved mechanical efficiency appears to be related to the shift from V_1 to V_3 myosin isoforms.[31] Similar changes have been described in nonischemic, nonworking hearts.[32] On the other hand, the acutely reduced mechanical activity of the postischemic (stunned) heart (p. 1329) is not associated with any reduction of MVO_2.[33] Presumably, abnormalities in energy utilization, in electromechanical coupling, or in the shunting of energy supplies to cellular repair processes might be responsible for the unexpectedly high MVO_2 (and the low efficiency) of stunned myocardium.[33]

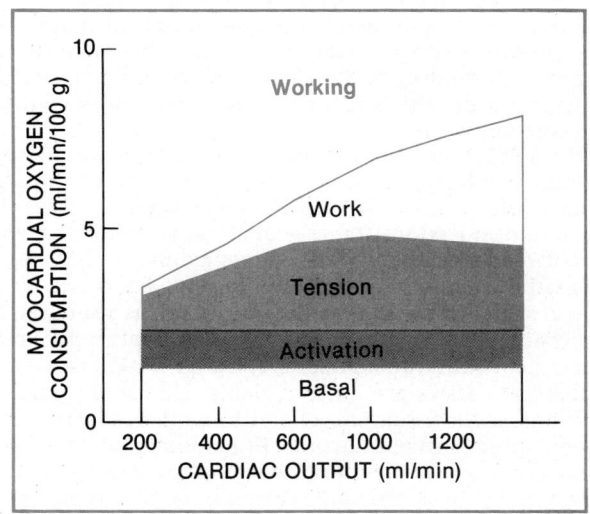

FIGURE 38–3. Basal metabolism, activation energy, tension-related energy, and energy for external work as components of myocardial oxygen consumption at various levels of cardiac output. (From Ando, H., Nakano, E., Ueno, Y., and Tokunaga, K.: New technique for analysis of cardiac energetics using a modified Fenn equation. J. Thorac. Cardiovasc. Surg. 97:565, 1989.)

Regulation of Coronary Blood Flow

ANATOMICAL FACTORS. Coronary blood flow is influenced by anatomical, hydraulic, mechanical, and metabolic factors.[34-37] During diastole, when the aortic valve is closed, aortic diastolic pressure is transmitted without impediment through the dilated sinuses of Valsalva to the coronary ostia. The aortic arch and sinuses then act as a miniature reservoir, facilitating maintenance of relatively uniform coronary inflow through diastole. Both the left and right coronary arteries course across the epicardial surface of the heart. The major vessels and their principal branches serve as conductance vessels and normally offer little resistance to coronary blood flow. The epicardial conductance vessels can constrict

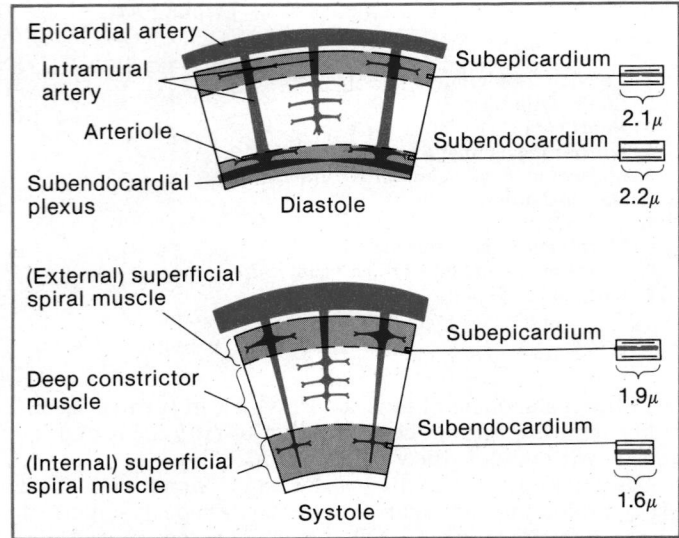

FIGURE 38–4. Cross-section of the left ventricular wall in diastole and systole. Factors involved in the susceptibility of the subendocardium to the development of ischemia include the greater dependence of this region on diastolic perfusion and the greater degree of shortening, and therefore of energy expenditure, of this region during systole. (From Bell, J. R., and Fox, A. C.: Pathogenesis of subendocardial ischemia. Am. J. Med. Sci. *268*:2, 1974.)

in response to alpha-adrenergic stimuli and dilate to nitroglycerin.[38] These vessels give rise to smaller penetrating vessels approximately at right angles (Fig. 38–4). A large pressure drop occurs in these intramural vessels and in the coronary arterioles, hence their designation as "resistance vessels." The dense capillary network of about 4000 capillaries/mm² cross-section of the normal heart is not uniformly patent, because precapillary sphincters appear to serve a regulatory function,[39] depending on the flow needs of the myocardium. This capillary density is reduced in the presence of ventricular hypertrophy.

COLLATERALS. Anastomotic connections without an intervening capillary bed exist between portions of the same coronary artery and between different coronary arteries. The distribution and extent of these collateral vessels differ markedly between species, as well as among different individuals of the same species. In canine or guinea pig hearts, an extensive epicardial network of collateral vessels is common, but epicardial collateral vessels are not prominent in porcine or primate hearts. In human hearts, the distribution and extent of collateral vessels are quite variable. Under physiological conditions, such vessels are generally less than 40 μ in diameter and appear to have little or no functional role. When myocardial perfusion is compromised by obstructions affecting major vessels, these collateral vessels enlarge and blood flow through them increases.[40] Exercise,[41,42] severe anemia,[43] and gradual (rather than abrupt) coronary occlusion[44] appear to enhance the development of collaterals. However, in experimental animals[44a] exercise does not reduce mortality resulting from subsequent coronary occlusion.[45] Perfusion via collaterals in the presence of total coronary occlusion may equal perfusion through a vessel with 90 per cent obstruction of the luminal diameter.[46] Positron emission tomographic imaging is a noninvasive technique for detecting coronary collaterals in humans.

Repeated brief (2 min) but not transient (15 sec) episodes of ischemia can serve as stimuli for collateral vessel formation.[47-49] With sustained coronary occlusion, collateral blood flow to salvaged tissue commences early, i.e., between 5 and 10 min following occlusion, and then rises progressively for 24 hours; this reflects the gradual recruitment of collateral vessels.[50]

Although debate continues concerning the functional significance of collaterals, two facts are clear: (1) collaterals become visible angiographically only when coronary occlusion is complete or virtually so, and (2) the presence of collaterals occasionally can prevent the development of a myocardial infarction in the presence of a total coronary occlusion. However, even when collaterals prevent myocardial infarction in the presence of coronary occlusion, they provide perfusion just sufficient to maintain myocardial viability; an increase in MVO₂ induced by electrical pacing results in a deterioration of myocardial function.[51] Some studies have shown that the presence of collaterals appears to reduce the frequency of wall motion disorders in the face of coronary obstruction,[46] while others have not confirmed this.[47-49] In any event, when cardiac muscle is supplied entirely or largely by collateral vessels, it often becomes ischemic if its oxygen demands increase above basal levels.

PERFUSION PRESSURE. As in any vascular bed, blood flow in the coronary bed depends on the driving pressure and the resistance offered by this bed. However, the coronary circulation differs from other circulations in that the resistance offered by the bed is influenced importantly by phasic systolic compression of the coronary vessels coursing through the myocardium. The perfusion or effective coronary driving pressure is the pressure gradient between the coronary arteries and the pressure in either the right atrium or the left ventricle in diastole, since coronary flow drains primarily into these two chambers. However, effective perfusion pressure is not constant throughout the cardiac cycle. When the aortic valve is open and ejected blood flows rapidly past the coronary ostia, perfusion pressure is reduced slightly below aortic pressure because of the Venturi effect. In addition, phasic changes in right atrial pressure occurring during the cardiac cycle and in the left ventricle during diastole modify the effective perfusion pressure gradient, albeit only slightly, except in the presence of a tall right atrial v wave, as in tricuspid regurgitation.

FACTORS EXTRINSIC TO THE VASCULAR BED. Coronary vascular resistance is influenced both by factors *extrinsic* to the bed, particularly compressive forces within the myocardium (intramyocardial forces acting on the intramyocardial vessels), and by metabolic, neural, and humoral factors *intrinsic* to the bed causing changes in the cross-sectional area of coronary resistance vessels. Intramyocardial wall tension varies throughout the cardiac cycle and is dependent on both load and contractility.[51,52] Because ventricular wall tension is much higher in systole than it is in diastole, forces compressing intramyocardial vessels are much greater during this phase of the cardiac cycle. Therefore, most of the coronary blood flow to the left ventricle occurs during diastole. Sometimes there is even some backflow in the major coronary arteries during systole. This "throttling" effect of systole on myocardial perfusion[34] is particularly important when systolic intraventricular pressure is elevated but coronary perfusion pressure is not, as is the case with obstruction to left ventricular outflow by valvular or subvalvular aortic stenosis, or with severe aortic regurgitation. Since an increase in heart rate diminishes the total amount of diastolic time per minute while myocardial oxygen demand is augmented, tachycardia may cause myocardial ischemia.

Extravascular Compressive Forces. The important resistance to coronary flow caused by left ventricular compression can be demonstrated experimentally in a beating heart perfused at constant pressure in which asystole is induced transiently by vagal stimulation. At this time, coronary blood flow suddenly increases by approximately 50 per cent because of relief of the compressive effect.[35] Because compressive forces exerted by the right ventricle are ordinarily far less than those of the left ventricle, perfusion of the right ventricle is not interrupted during systole.

The calculation of coronary vascular resistance is complicated by the observation that under normal conditions coronary blood flow ceases when coronary driving pressure reaches levels of approximately 40 mm Hg, the so-called P_{zf} (pressure at zero flow). Although there is no question concerning the existence of a P_{zf} substantially above coronary venous pressure, considerable debate continues about the responsible mechanism.[53,54] Extravascular compressive forces in humans are reflected in the phasic coronary artery flow velocity determined by Doppler flow meter catheters. Patients with aortic stenosis exhibit a reduction of the fraction of forward flow in systole.[55,56]

Susceptibility of the Subendocardium to Ischemia. Extravascular compressive forces during systole are greater in subendocardial zones of the heart than in subepicardial ones (Fig. 38–3). Therefore, systolic flow is greatly reduced in this area.

Under physiological conditions, marked transitory disparities exist between endocardial and epicardial wall stresses and, correspondingly, between endocardial and epicardial flow throughout the cardiac cycle. Nevertheless, under physiological conditions, in conscious dogs the ratio of endocardial to epicardial flow averaged throughout the cardiac cycle is approximately 1.25:1 as a consequence of preferential dilatation of the subendocardial vessel,[57] which appears to be secondary to the increased wall stress and oxygen consumption in this region. Interventions that reduce the perfusion pressure gradient during diastole (as occurs with coronary obstruction, elevation of ventricular diastolic pressure, and tachycardia) lower the ratio of subendocardial to subepicardial flow and may cause the subendocardium to become ischemic.

The combination of a greater wall stress, and hence greater resistance to flow, and higher metabolic demands results in lower coronary vascular tone in the subendocardium than in the subepicardium. As a consequence, the reserve for vasodilatation is also less in the subendocardium than in the subepicardium, and as perfusion is reduced the deeper layers of myocardium become ischemic before the more superficial ones. This phenomenon is manifested by reduced intracellular oxygen tension and contractility and increased production of lactate in the inner layers of the ventricular wall as the heart becomes ischemic[58,59] (see Fig. 38–31, p. 1182).

The preferential susceptibility of the subendocardium to ischemia by the combination of limited reserve for vasodilation, extrinsic compression from the higher wall stress to which it is subjected,[60] and the resultant high metabolic demands accounts for the electrocardiographic ST-segment depression characteristically associated with episodes of transient ischemia (Fig. 5–30, p. 137). Injury currents from the subendocardium, resulting in ST-segment depression, accompany the maldistribution of transmural flow and metabolic impairment of subendocardial tissue under these circumstances, even though net transmural flow may remain near normal[61] (Fig. 38–5). These considerations provide the basis for the recognition of myocardial ischemia by ST-segment depression during exercise stress testing (Chap. 6). When coronary flow is restricted, the adaptive changes in the subendocardium include its greater potential for glycolytic metabolism[62] due to higher glycolytic enzyme activity and, consequently, higher lactate production rates.[63] However, even though the glycogen content of subendocardium is higher than that of the subepicardium under aerobic conditions, concentrations of high-energy phosphate compounds are generally lower in the subendocardium than in other portions of the ventricular wall when coronary flow is restricted, because of the inability of the anaerobic metabolism of glucose to fulfill energy requirements completely.

PREDICTION OF SUBENDOCARDIAL ISCHEMIA. Griggs, Hoffman, Buckberg, Brazier and their collaborators have developed indexes for the evaluation of transmural blood flow and the prediction of subendocardial ischemia in the absence of coronary artery obstruction.[57,61–64] They reasoned that the delivery of oxygen to the subendocardium represents the product of arterial oxygen content and the driving force for subendocardial blood flow, which in turn depend on the integrated pressure difference between the aorta and left ventricle during diastole, termed the *diastolic*

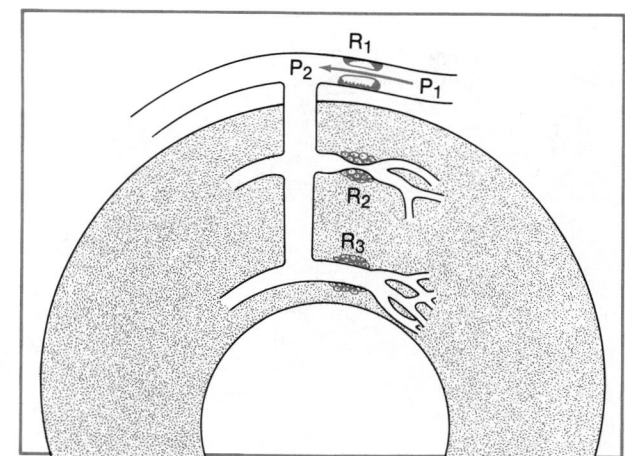

FIGURE 38–5. Effects of a stenosis in an epicardial vessel (R_1) on endocardial and epicardial flow. Endocardial vessels (R_3) are maximally dilated, whereas epicardial vessels (R_2) are not. A vasodilator stimulus resulting (for example, from an increase in heart rate) will augment transmural flow owing to dilation of subepicardial vessels. Increase in flow will cause a greater pressure drop across the stenosis (P_1-P_2) and the coronary driving pressure (P_2) will drop.

As long as the fall in resistance in subepicardial vessels (R_2) is greater than the resulting fall in driving pressure, flow will increase in the subepicardial region. However, because subendocardial vessels are already maximally dilated, the fall in coronary driving pressure will not be accompanied by a fall in resistance. Hence, flow to subendocardial vessels will fall. (From Epstein, S. E., Cannon, R. O., III, and Talbot, T. L.: Hemodynamic principles in the control of coronary blood flow. Am. J. Cardiol. 56:8E, 1985.)

pressure–time index (DPTI). The demand for blood flow, i.e., MVO_2, is closely related to the area beneath the systolic portion of the ventricular pressure curve, i.e., the *systolic pressure–time index* (SPTI). The ratio DPTI × oxygen content/SPTI has been used as an index of the relation between subendocardial oxygen supply and demand. This ratio can be reduced by (1) opening an arteriovenous fistula or patent ductus arteriosus or inducing aortic regurgitation to diminish aortic diastolic pressure and thereby reducing DPTI; (2) increasing preload or afterload, causing left ventricular dysfunction, or reducing left ventricular compliance; these maneuvers all raise left ventricular diastolic pressure and also reduce DPTI; (3) inducing tachycardia to shorten diastole[65]; and (4) causing severe anemia or hypoxemia to reduce arterial oxygen content. With reduction of the DPTI × oxygen content/SPTI below a critical value of approximately 10, the endocardial/epicardial blood flow ratio also decreased.

Although it is recognized that this index provides only an approximation of the oxygen supply-to-demand relationship,[51] it can explain a number of clinical findings, such as the development of angina and the electrocardiographic and biochemical evidence of ischemia caused by tachycardia in patients with aortic stenosis; in this situation DPTI falls and SPTI rises. Myocardial lactate production has been observed to occur during beta-adrenoceptor stimulation with isoproterenol in patients with aortic stenosis,[66] when left ventricular systolic pressure, contractility, heart rate, and therefore, MVO_2 rise while DPTI does not. When adrenergic stimulation was carried out in dogs with experimentally produced aortic stenosis, the myocardial lactate concentration and the lactate-pyruvate ratio rose while the reduction of ATP stores was more prominent in the inner than the outer half of the ventricle.[58,59] This indicates that the subendocardium is more vulnerable to ischemia and therefore becomes dependent on anaerobic metabolism more readily than does the subepicardium.

In experimentally produced aortic regurgitation, diastolic coronary blood flow falls but systolic flow rises, so that total coronary flow does not change.[67] However, with severe reductions in aortic diastolic pressure, DPTI declines and the subendocardial region exhibits biochemical evidence of anaerobic metabolism. As the DPTI × oxygen content/SPTI declines, the subendocardial lactate-pyruvate ratio rises, evidence of anaerobic metabolism in this region of myocardium. These observations are clinically relevant considering that angina pectoris occurs in a significant number of patients with severe aortic stenosis and/or regurgitation in the absence of coronary artery disease (Chap. 34). Other conditions in which subendocardial ischemia occurs include marked systemic hypotension, regardless of etiology (Chap. 21), and pulmonary embolism, particularly when complicated by fever, tachycardia, and anemia. In these conditions the ischemia results from a combination of lowered coronary perfusion

Normal
diastolic
perfusion
pressure

Spasm +
critical
stenosis

| NITRATES |

Vasodilation

Capillaries 3/5 open

NORMAL

Capillaries
4/5 open

ISCHEMIC

Fewer
capillaries
compressed

SUBENDO-
CARDIAL
ISCHEMIA
LESSENED

Less diastolic crunch

| NITRATES |

⬆LVEDP
in angina
(diastolic crunch)

LVEDP

Normal
LVEDP

FIGURE 38–6. Effects of a critical stenosis in an epicardial vessel and of nitrates on myocardial perfusion and function. When a patient with a critical stenosis exercises, subendocardial ischemia and an increase in left ventricular end-diastolic pressure (LVEDP) occur; this is accompanied by compression of subendocardial vessels. Alternatively, angina at rest can develop if there is superimposed coronary spasm. Nitrates bring relief by increasing the diameter of large coronary arteries, by relaxing spasm, by reducing LVEDP, and by decreasing diastolic compression. (Adapted from Parratt, J. R., Marshall, R. J., and Ledingham, M. C. A.: J. Physiol. [Paris] *76*:791, 1980.)

pressure, tachycardia, and increased subendocardial tension secondary to sympathetic stimulation of myocardial contractility. Since coronary blood flow ceases at a pressure higher than ventricular diastolic pressure (see discussion of P_{zf} above), as arterial pressure declines with systemic hypotension or aortic regurgitation, the coronary perfusion pressure declines to quite low levels.

In the presence of coronary obstruction the *effective* pressure perfusing the subendocardial region is determined by the gradient between the diastolic coronary pressure *distal* to the obstruction and the left ventricular end-diastolic pressure; hence the DPTI no longer reflects or even approximates the driving force for subendocardial blood flow. When left ventricular diastolic pressure is elevated in the ischemic ventricle, the endocardial/epicardial flow ratio declines, further reducing subendocardial blood flow.[68] The development of subendocardial ischemia can raise ventricular diastolic pressure further, largely by interfering with the ventricle's diastolic properties, thereby causing a vicious circle.

Since maldistribution of transmural blood flow compromises the subendocardial tissue, antianginal drugs may be effective if they improve the ratio of subendocardial to subepicardial flow even if they do not augment net transmural perfusion. Analysis of the washout of ^{86}Rb and fractional uptake of radioactive-labeled microspheres has shown that both nitroglycerin and beta-adrenoceptor blockers redistribute blood flow to the subendocardium.[69,70] This phenomenon may, in the case of nitroglycerin, reflect in part the direct effects of the drugs on the coronary vascular bed as well as the reduction of extravascular compressive forces induced by a lowering of ventricular diastolic pressure resulting from a reduction of preload (Fig. 38–6). Beta blockers reduce MVO$_2$ and thereby ischemia, which is most prominent in the subendocardium; the relief of ischemia in turn reduces diastolic wall tension (primarily in the subendocardium) and improves myocardial perfusion.

CONTROL OF CORONARY VASCULAR RESISTANCE

Coronary vascular resistance is influenced markedly by changes in the tone of the vascular bed, changes that are mediated by neural, metabolic, pharmacological, and myogenic factors, as well as by vasodilator and vasoconstrictor substances released by the endothelium.

NEURAL FACTORS. The coronary arteries are richly innervated by adrenergic and parasympathetic nerves,[35,38] and their activation can exert an important influence on coronary vasomotor tone. Both alpha$_1$ and alpha$_2$ adrenoceptors are present in the coronary arteries,[71] and when activated by neuronally released or circulating norepinephrine both cause

coronary vasoconstriction[72-74] (Fig. 38–7), which appears to be mediated ultimately by an increased concentration of calcium in coronary vascular smooth muscle.[73-76] When inotropic and chronotropic effects are blocked[77] (to prevent the development of metabolic vasodilator stimuli), stimulation of cardiac nerves causes coronary vasoconstriction. The activation of alpha$_1$ receptors induced by the infusion of methoxamine has been demonstrated to reduce the diameter of coronary arteries while increasing intraluminal pressure.[38,78] Activation of the carotid chemoreceptor reflex causes marked coronary constriction, which can be blocked by surgical denervation or by the alpha blocker phentolamine.[78] On the other hand, beta$_1$ and beta$_2$ adrenoceptors in the large and small coronary arteries mediate vasodilation.[38,79,80] Beta blockade induces coronary constriction, but this effect appears not to be a direct action on the coronary arteries. Rather it results from blockade of beta-adrenoreceptor–mediated increases in MVO$_2$.[81] The extent of cholinergic regulation of large coronary arteries is controversial,[82] although parasympathetic stimulation appears to dilate small coronary arteries.[38]

Intravenous administration of norepinephrine induces a brief fall, followed by a sustained rise, in coronary vascular resistance, accompanied by a decline in coronary sinus pO$_2$ (Fig. 38–7).[83] The early vasodilatation can be eliminated by beta-adrenoceptor blockade and presumably results from the augmented myocardial oxygen needs consequent to stimulation of myocardial beta receptors. The later increase in coronary vascular resistance can be prevented by alpha-adrenoceptor blockade and presumably results from stimulation by norepinephrine of alpha receptors in the coronary vascular bed. Blockade of alpha$_1$ receptors in patients with coronary artery disease attenuates the coronary vasoconstrictor response to the cold pressor test[84] and cigarette smoking,[85,86] indicating that both responses are mediated by stimulation of these receptors. Baroreceptor activity affects coronary vascular resistance reflexly. In the dog with sectioned vagal nerves, occlusion of the carotid arteries to produce baroreceptor hypotension induces an increase in heart rate and blood pressure, accompanied by a reduction in coronary vascular

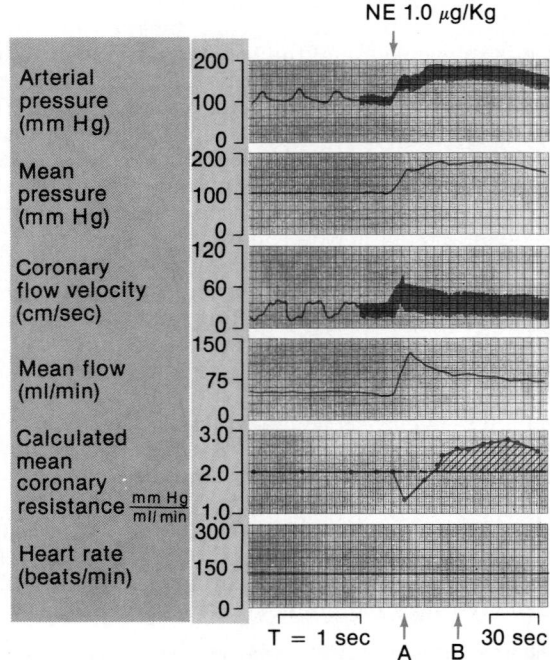

FIGURE 38–7. Effects of intravenously administered norepinephrine (NE) in the intact unanesthetized dog with heart rate held constant. Coronary vascular resistance fell initially (A) and then showed a sustained increase (B). (From Vatner, S. F., Higgins, C. B., and Braunwald, E.: Effects of norepinephrine on coronary circulation and left ventricular dynamics in the conscious dog. Circ. Res. *34*:812, 1974, by permission of the American Heart Association, Inc.)

resistance.[87] When the reflex tachycardia and myocardial contractility (which would be expected to increase MVO$_2$ and thereby lower coronary vascular resistance) are blocked with propranolol, an *increase* in coronary vascular resistance is observed, which can be prevented by cardiac sympathectomy. It may be concluded that with intact adrenergic nerves and beta receptors, the coronary dilatation consequent to carotid occlusion is due to heightened cardiac metabolic activity induced reflexly by baroreceptor hypotension. When this augmentation of myocardial beta-receptor–mediated activity is prevented by beta blockade, reflex coronary *vasoconstriction* secondary to carotid hypotension is unmasked.[88] Stimulation of the distal ends of the vagi produces coronary vasodilatation,[88,89] an effect that is mediated by the release of acetylcholine from vagal nerve endings and that can be blocked by atropine.[35]

Evidence also exists for *tonic* coronary constriction mediated by adrenergic nerves.[90] Acute surgical denervation of the heart produces a fall in coronary vascular resistance with a reduction in arteriovenous oxygen extraction and a rise in coronary venous O$_2$ content (primary vasodilatation).[91] Coronary vascular resistance in patients as well as in dogs[92] with innervated hearts declines by almost 25 per cent in response to alpha-adrenoceptor blockade, suggesting that basal coronary constrictor tone mediated by alpha receptors is released. However, coronary vascular resistance does *not* diminish when patients with cardiac transplants receive alpha-adrenoceptor blockade. This indicates that cardiac denervation had previously abolished the coronary constrictor tone.

In the conscious dog, stimulation of the carotid sinus nerves results in a substantial reduction in coronary vascular resistance.[90] This effect can be prevented by alpha-receptor blockade; therefore, it would appear that adrenergic coronary constrictor tone is present in the resting conscious dog and that coronary vasodilation attendant upon electrical stimulation of the carotid sinus nerves results from a reduction in this resting vasoconstrictor tone. Coronary vasodilation resulting from stimulation of the carotid sinus nerves occurs also during exercise. Apparently, alpha-receptor-mediated constrictor tone persists in the coronary vascular bed during exercise, despite the coexisting metabolic vasodilation. This conclusion is supported by studies using alpha-adrenoceptor blocking drugs which have shown that the increase in coronary blood flow and oxygen delivery to the myocardium during normal exercise is limited by alpha-adrenergic vasoconstriction.[93] Alpha$_1$ adrenoceptor stimulation of *ischemic* myocardium is capable of causing epicardial vasoconstriction and thereby influencing favorably the transmural distribution of blood flow[94-96] during exercise. Thus, alpha-adrenergic–mediated coronary constriction distal to the flow-limiting stenosis redistributes blood flow to the subendocardium.[97,98]

Efferent neural influences on the coronary vascular bed may also be activated reflexly by cardiopulmonary parasympathetic receptors. Stimulation of parasympathetic receptors leads to reflex systemic and coronary vasodilation,[99] while stimulation of somatic afferent fibers increases coronary resistance through alpha-adrenergically mediated vasoconstriction.[100] Chemoreceptor activation initially causes coronary dilation, a reflex that is mediated by the vagi and can be abolished by atropine.[35] As already noted, the late response is coronary vasoconstriction.[78] Intracoronary injection of veratrum alkaloids, as well as other metabolically active substances, induces reflex bradycardia and hypotension (the Bezold-Jarisch reflex),[101] the afferent limb of which involves the vagus nerves. The effects of efferent vagus nerve activity causing *coronary* vasodilation[102] have been documented, indicating that the Bezold-Jarisch reflex involves coronary efferent as well as afferent parasympathetic components.[99] Neurally controlled and alpha-adrenoceptor–mediated constriction of stenotic lesions of the coronary vascular bed in humans has been observed on coronary arteriograms[98] demonstrating the vasoconstrictor effects of handgrip.[103]

An increase in adrenergic outflow does *not* appear to be

responsible for the episodes of coronary spasm in patients with Prinzmetal's (variant) angina[104] (p. 1342) or in the genesis of ischemia in so-called syndrome X (p. 1346).[105,105a] However, it has been reported that alpha-adrenoceptor stimulation can induce coronary spasm that can be prevented by phenoxybenzamine or prazosin in some patients.[98] The finding that administration of alpha receptor blockers can reduce exercise-induced ST-segment depression and angina[98,106,106a,107] indicates that alpha receptor–mediated coronary vasoconstriction plays some role in angina on effort. It has also been shown that cocaine is a potent coronary vasoconstrictor in humans and dogs,[107a] and since this effect can be prevented by an alpha receptor blocker, phentolamine, it appears to be mediated through alpha-adrenergic stimulation.[108]

AUTOREGULATION OF CORONARY BLOOD FLOW

When sudden alterations in perfusion pressure are imposed in many vascular beds, the abrupt changes in blood flow are only transitory, with flow promptly returning toward the previous steady-state level.[109] This phenomenon, called *autoregulation* (Fig. 38–8), applies also to the coronary vascular bed and tends to maintain myocardial perfusion within a relatively narrow range, regardless of transitory changes in perfusion pressure between approximately 60 and 130 mm Hg.[52] Demonstration of autoregulation is difficult in intact animals because modification of coronary perfusion pressure also changes both MVO$_2$ and the extrinsic compression of the coronary vessels. However, under experimental conditions in which perfusion pressure is altered but ventricular pressure, cardiac contractility, and heart rate—the principal determinants of MVO$_2$—are maintained constant, autoregulation is clearly evident. Autoregulation is more prominent in the subepicardial than in the subendocardial layers of the left ventricle. Drugs that cause relaxation of coronary vascular smooth muscle diminish autoregulation.[51]

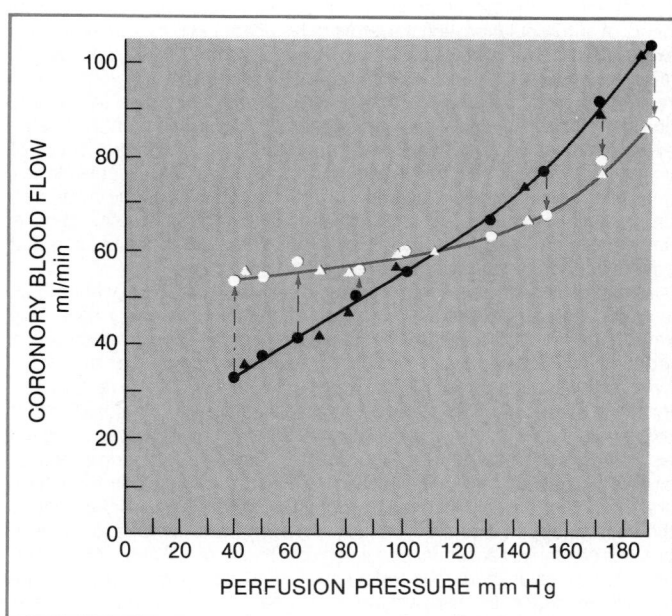

FIGURE 38–8. Autoregulation of coronary blood flow in the beating dog heart. The point where the curves cross represents the control steady-state pressure and flow. A sudden, sustained change in perfusion pressure caused an abrupt change in flow represented by the filled symbols and black line (transient flow). The open symbols and red line represent the steady-state flows obtained at each perfusion pressure. The points represented by triangles were obtained after blockade of cardiac prostaglandin synthesis with indomethacin. (Reproduced by permission from Rubio, K., and Berne, K. M.: Regulation of coronary blood flow. Prog. Cardiovasc. Dis. *18*:105, 1975.)

Autoregulation in the bed distal to a coronary obstruction may be compromised because the bed is already maximally dilated in the basal state. As a consequence, perfusion of this distal bed becomes dependent entirely on perfusion pressure (Fig. 38–5). Under these circumstances, augmentation of cardiac oxygen requirements, as occurs during exercise and *without* an increase in perfusion pressure, results in or intensifies ischemia. Since blood flow to regions supplied by normal vessels can be increased (because regional vasodilatation in these regions is possible), while blood flow to the compromised zone cannot (because its vessels are already maximally dilated), disparities in regional perfusion can become intensified. This explains exercise-induced regional dysfunction in the presence of subcritical coronary stenosis.[110] In addition, vasodilatation in the normal zones may reduce perfusion pressure to the ischemic area and deprive it further of blood flow, a phenomenon sometimes termed *coronary steal*. It has been observed that when coronary perfusion pressure falls to below the critical levels of 60 to 70 mm Hg, the coronary vessels become maximally dilated and flow becomes pressure-dependent, i.e., autoregulation is lost (Fig. 38–8). This observation underlines the importance of maintaining coronary perfusion pressure in patients with hypotension of any cause, including acute myocardial infarction.

When obstructive coronary artery disease is present, coronary perfusion pressure is lower than aortic pressure. A small reduction of the latter could then lower perfusion pressure below critical levels, thereby depressing myocardial perfusion, intensifying myocardial ischemia, and increasing left ventricular filling pressure, which decreases the perfusion pressure gradient further and may cause a vicious circle. In patients with cardiogenic shock, the reduction of perfusion pressure below the critical level at which autoregulation is lost lowers coronary blood flow even through nonobstructed vessels and may reduce collateral blood flow to the periinfarction zone, thereby enlarging the infarct (Fig. 39–11, p. 1210).

Several mechanisms have been implicated in the autoregulation of coronary blood flow, including myogenic and metabolic factors, vasoactive substances released by the endothelium, as well as extravascular compressive forces.[34,35]

MYOGENIC FACTORS. Stretch of vascular smooth muscle resulting from an increase in perfusion pressure stimulates the muscle to contract.[111] The consequent augmentation of resistance tends to return blood flow toward normal despite the higher perfusion pressure. Although this myogenic mechanism, sometimes called the *Bayliss effect* (after its discoverer, a collaborator of Ernest Starling), appears to be a general characteristic of vascular smooth muscle,[112] its role in the regulation of coronary blood flow has not been explicitly defined and is probably a modest one.[35]

METABOLIC CONTROL OF CORONARY BLOOD FLOW. It is likely that changes in regional myocardial metabolism are important determinants of autoregulation (and therefore coronary blood flow). Several mediators have been implicated, including oxygen, carbon dioxide, and vasodilator metabolites such as adenosine, that accumulate in hypoperfused regions of myocardium. There is a tight coupling between $M\dot{V}O_2$ and coronary blood flow.[52] It has been suggested that with increased energy expenditure by the heart there is a proportionally increased production of vasodilator metabolites, which in turn reduces coronary vascular resistance and raises coronary blood flow so that only small changes in myocardial oxygen extraction occur. This form of coronary vasodilatation is known as *secondary* dilatation, in contrast to the *primary* dilatation that occurs with denervation of the heart already described.

A marked reduction in coronary arterial perfusion pressure (while $M\dot{V}O_2$ is held constant) causes an immediate decrease in coronary flow. This would be expected to cause increased myocardial O_2 extraction and a reduced myocardial oxygen tension; the resultant hypoxia and accompanying accumulation of vasodilator metabolites then would be responsible for the ensuing (secondary) coronary vasodilatation.[113] It is possible that oxygen acts on vascular smooth muscle directly, possibly by altering the electrochemical potential of the muscle cells. Direct vasodilating effects of diminished oxygen tension have been demonstrated in the coronary, femoral, and other vessels.[114] Molecular oxygen diffusing across the walls of the vessels appears to be a primary determinant of constrictor tone of precapillary sphincters under physiological conditions.[115] Thus, diminution of oxygen tension increases the number of capillaries perfused within a predefined region of myocardium, presumably by relaxation of these sphincters.[116] In this manner, coronary blood flow would be expected to remain constant (or almost so) despite a reduction of coronary perfusion pressure. Transitory augmentation of the concentration of potassium in extracellular fluid, an early consequence of myocardial ischemia, may also modify the transmembrane potential of vascular smooth muscle cells, causing their relaxation and thus producing coronary vasodilatation.

Role of Adenosine (Fig. 38–9). Degradation of adenine nucleotides under conditions in which ATP utilization exceeds the capacity of myocardial cells to resynthesize high-energy phosphate compounds (a process dependent on oxidative phosphorylation in mitochondria) results in the production of adenosine monophosphate (AMP). The enzyme 5′-nucleotidase is responsible for the formation of adenosine.[117] Accordingly, adenosine and its metabolites, inosine and hypoxanthine, appear in interstitial fluid and in the coronary sinus venous effluent. *Adenosine* is a powerful vasodilator[118] that is considered to be an important, perhaps the critical, *mediator* linking metabolically induced vasodilatation to diminished coronary perfusion (Fig. 38–9). There is substantial evidence that an imbalance (a reduction) in the supply-to-demand ratio for oxygen is the primary determinant of adenosine formation.[117,119]

Concentrations of adenosine in the venous effluent are much lower than those in interstitial fluid, in part because capillary endothelium rapidly converts adenosine to inosine and hypoxanthine.[120] However, when the enzyme responsible for this conversion, adenosine deaminase, is inhibited by the administration of 8-azaguanine, marked increases in the concentration of adenosine in the effluent are unmasked.[121] If, at a constant level of myocardial metabolism, adenosine were being released at a constant rate, an elevation of coronary perfusion pressure and the resultant increase in coronary blood flow would augment the washout of adenosine, reduce its concentration, and thus increase coronary vascular resistance. Such a mechanism could provide a feedback to account for autoregulation of coronary blood flow. More important, it could also explain the close correlation between the energy expenditure of the heart and the level of coronary blood flow.[121,122] According to this concept, as the former rises, the ratio of oxygen supply to demand declines, and more ATP is degraded to AMP, which becomes available for and enhances adenosine formation. The latter causes coronary relaxation, thereby increasing coronary blood flow to a level appropriate to the $M\dot{V}O_2$.

It appears that adenosine acts on the surface of vascular smooth muscle cells, apparently on adenosine receptors on the cell membrane; presumably activation of these receptors blocks entry of Ca^{++} into these cells and thereby causes vasodilatation.[35] In addition to its potent vasodilating action, adenosine exerts a generally depressant activity on cardiac automaticity and atrioventricular conduction and attenuates the effects of adrenergic influences on myocardial contractility.[123]

Despite its importance, adenosine is almost certainly not the only metabolic factor involved, and its role in mediating the increase in coronary blood flow has been questioned. It is possible that adenosine does not act alone but interacts with other agents in response to hypoxia in causing coronary relaxation.[124] Prostaglandins, kinins, acetate, K^+, and a number of metabolites alter coronary vascular resistance profoundly and may play a role in mediating vasodilatation in response to hypoxia. The infusion of at least two prostaglandins synthesized in the heart (PGI_2 and PGE_2) can cause coronary vasodilatation,[125] and the inhibition of prostaglandin synthesis with indomethacin causes an increase in coronary vascular resistance in humans.[126]

ENDOTHELIAL CONTROL OF CORONARY VASCULAR TONE

The adult human possesses approximately 10^{12} vascular endothelial cells, which occupy an area exceeding 1000 m². It has long been appreciated that the endothelial cells serve as a nonthrombogenic diffusion barrier to the migration of substances out of and into the bloodstream and as a site for exchange of nutrients and metabolites between the capillaries and cells. However, during the past 15 years it has been appreciated that the endothelium is also the largest and most active paracrine organ in the body, producing potent vasoactive, anticoagulant, procoagulant, and fibrinolytic substances (Table 38–3).[126a] Abnormalities in the structure and function of the

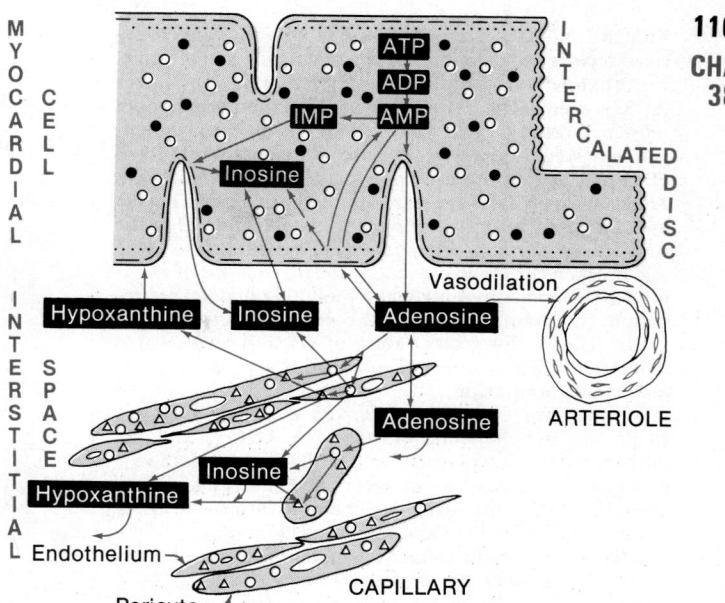

FIGURE 38-9. Schematic drawing depicting a myocardial interstitial space, an arteriole, and a capillary with the localization of enzymes involved in the formation and fate of adenosine. Adenosine formed by 5'-nucleotidase from AMP (which in turn arises from ATP) can enter the interstitial space. There it can induce arteriolar dilation and reenter the myocardial cell, where it is either phosphorylated to AMP by adenosine kinase or deaminated to inosine by adenosine deaminase, or it can enter the capillaries and leave the tissue. A large fraction of adenosine that crosses the capillary wall is deaminated to inosine, which in turn is split to hypoxanthine and ribose-1-PO₄ by nucleoside phosphorylase located in the endothelial cells, pericytes, and erythrocytes. Most of the adenosine is taken up by the myocardial cells, and that escaping into the circulation is largely in the form of inosine and hypoxanthine. Since adenylic acid deaminase (which deaminates AMP to IMP) is in low concentration in heart muscle, the major degradative pathway from AMP is via dephosphorylation to adenosine. ○, Adenosine deaminase; ●, adenylic acid deaminase; △, nucleoside phosphorylase; (---), 5'-nucleotidase; (···), adenosine kinase. (From Berne, R. M., and Rubio, R.: Coronary circulation. *In* Berne, R. M., Sperelakis, N., and Geiger, S. R. [eds.]: Handbook of Physiology, Section 2. The Cardiovascular System. Bethesda, Md., American Physiological Society, 1979, p. 924.)

endothelium are now believed to play important roles in the pathogenesis of many vascular (including coronary vascular) diseases.[127,128]

Among the many important vasoactive substances synthesized by endothelial cells is prostacyclin (PGI₂), an arachidonic acid metabolite whose release is stimulated by a variety of physiological stimuli (tissue hypoxia, hemodynamic stress, high-density lipoproteins, ATP, and leukotrienes) and pharmacological substances (calcium ionophores). Prostacyclin elevates intracellular concentrations of cyclic AMP and thereby serves as a potent relaxant of vascular smooth muscle and inhibitor of platelet aggregation.

ENDOTHELIUM-DERIVED RELAXING FACTOR. Endothelium also synthesizes *endothelium-derived relaxing factor* (EDRF),[129-131] which is, or acts like, nitric oxide (NO).[131a] It is derived from the amino acid L-arginine (through an as-yet unidentified biosynthetic pathway[132]) and is metabolized to

inactive nitrite; the synthesis of EDRF can be inhibited by the L-arginine analog N^G monomethyl L-arginine.[133] The principal target organs of EDRF are, on one side, the subadjacent vascular smooth muscle cells and on the other side, circulating platelets (Fig. 38-10).

EDRF is released from normal endothelial cells by a broad array of stimulants, including acetylcholine,[134] thrombin, bradykinin, thromboxane A₂, histamine, and aggregating platelets, and by catecholamines acting on alpha₂ receptors on endothelial cells.[129] Receptors on normal endothelium that cause the release of EDRF when stimulated include muscarinic receptors (for acetylcholine), thrombin receptors, histaminergic receptors, vasopressin(ergic) and oxytocin(ergic) receptors, alpha₂-adrenoceptors (for circulating catecholamines), purinergic and serotonergic receptors stimulated by aggregating platelets, ADP, and serotonin (Fig. 38-11). In contrast to prostacyclin (which acts by increasing intracellular

TABLE 38-3   IMPORTANT SUBSTANCES PRODUCED BY OR ACTING THROUGH VASCULAR ENDOTHELIUM

VASODILATOR	VASOCONSTRICTOR	ANTICOAGULANT/ ANTITHROMBOTIC/ ANTIPLATELET	PROCOAGULANT
Produced by endothelium			
Adenosine	? Endothelin	Adenosine	Collagen
EDRF	Peptidoleukotrienes	EDRF	FVIII-VWF complex
EDHF		Glycosaminoglycans	Fibronectin
Peptidoleukotrienes		Plasminogen activator	Plasminogen inhibitors
PGE₂		PGE₁, PGE₂	
PGF₁ₐ		PGI₂	
PGI₂		Thrombomodulin	
		Tissue factor	
Acts through endothelium			
Acetylcholine	Angiotensin	Heparin	
ADP	Vasopressin		
Bradykinin			
Catecholamines			
Histamine			
Peptidoleukotrienes			
Serotonin			

ADP = adenosine diphosphate; EDHF = endothelium-derived hyperpolarizing factor; EDRF = endothelium-derived relaxing factor; FVIII = coagulation factor VIII; PG = prostaglandin; VWF = von Willebrand factor.

From Dinerman, J. L., and Mehta, J. L.: Endothelial, platelet and leukocyte interactions in ischemic heart disease: Insights into potential mechanisms and their clinical relevance. Reprinted by permission of the American College of Cardiology. J. Am. Coll. Cardiol. *16*:207, 1990.

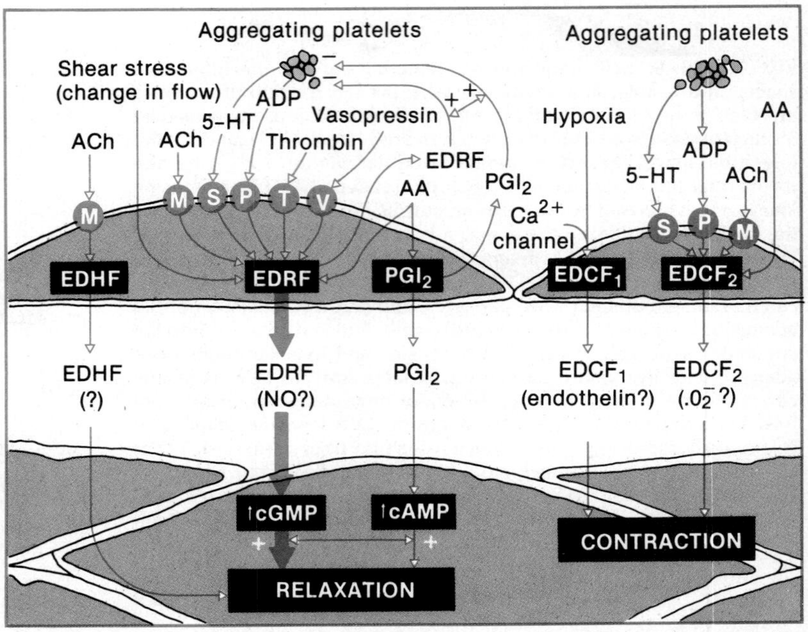

FIGURE 38–10. Current concepts of endothelium-derived factors and their modulation of vascular smooth muscle contraction. Endothelium-derived relaxing factor (EDRF), a powerful vasodilator of the underlying smooth muscle, increases cyclic GMP (cGMP) levels through activation of soluble guanylate cyclase. The chemical nature of EDRF may be simply nitric oxide or a complex containing it. Prostacyclin (PGI$_2$) is another vasodilator released from the endothelium whose effects depend on elevation of cyclic AMP (cAMP) through activation of adenylate cyclase. EDRF and prostacyclin could act synergistically in terms of relaxing vascular smooth muscle and inhibiting platelet aggregation. The endothelial cells also secrete a hyperpolarizing factor (EDHF). The exact nature of EDHF is unknown; is most likely is a metabolite of arachidonic acid, presumably an epoxide or lipoxide.

At least two endothelium-derived contracting factors exist; one is indomethacin-insensitive (EDCF$_1$) and the other is indomethacin-sensitive (EDCF$_2$). Recent data suggest that EDCF$_1$ may be endothelin, and EDCF$_2$ may be superoxide anions, although this remains to be proved. EDHF has a vasodilator effect and may contribute in part to the initial portion of endothelium-dependent relaxations. ACh, acetylcholine; 5-HT, 5-hydroxytryptamine, serotonin; ADP, adenosine diphosphate; AA, arachidonic acid; +, synergism or facilitation; −, inhibition; ?, exact nature unknown; M, muscarinic receptor; S, serotonergic receptor; P, purinergic receptor; T, thrombin receptor; V, vasopressinergic receptor. (From Vanhoutte, P. M., and Shimokawa, H.: Endothelium-derived relaxing factor and coronary vasospasm. Circulation *80*:1, 1989, by permission of the American Heart Association, Inc.)

cyclic AMP), EDRF acts on a receptor that is probably the heme moiety of soluble guanylate cyclase.[132] The resultant stimulation of guanylate cyclase increases vascular smooth muscle cell cyclic guanine monophosphate (GMP), which activates a cyclic GMP–dependent protein kinase. This in turn inhibits release of Ca^{++} from endoplasmic reticulum and other storage sites, causing relaxation of vascular smooth muscle. These biochemical actions of EDRF are shared by a number of nitrosodilators, such as nitroglycerin and nitroprusside, which act by generating NO. However, these substances do not require an intact endothelium for their vasodilator action, as do acetylcholine, thrombin, aggregating platelets, and the like. Thus, EDRF might be considered to be an "endogenous nitrate," while, conversely, nitroglycerin might be considered to be an "exogenous EDRF." N-Acetylcysteine, a reduced thiol, potentiates the inhibition of platelets by EDRF, an effect associated with increasing platelet cyclic GMP concentrations.[135]

The formation of EDRF in the basal state plays a significant role in setting resting arterial tone.[131] The endothelial response to shear stress plays an important physiological role in the control of vascular (including coronary vascular) tone. As blood flow through an artery increases, the shear stress on the endothelium rises. This in turn increases the release of EDRF and causes vasodilation, which enhances blood flow further. Absence of EDRF or damage to the endothelium abolishes this response to shear stress. Inflammatory mediators, such as bradykinin, histamine, and substance P, also augment local blood flow by increasing release of EDRF.

The two vasoactive and platelet-active products of normal endothelium, prostacyclin and EDRF, act in concert to inhibit platelet adhesion and aggregation and to relax vascular smooth muscle. Normal endothelium also opposes a variety of vasoconstrictor stimuli, including catecholamines, serotonin, and vasopressin, and enhances the vasorelaxant effects of dilators, such as histamine and adenosine nucleotides.[136] Vascular endothelium is normally the principal source of locally produced plasminogen activator, and by this action too it enhances the fluidity of the blood. Indeed, prostacyclin, EDRF, and t-PA act synergistically in this manner. In the absence of

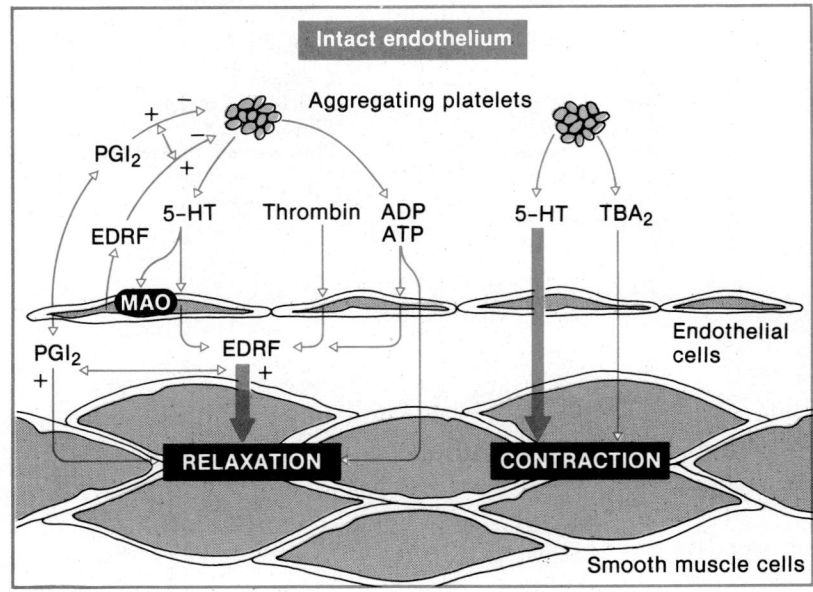

FIGURE 38–11. Illustration of several effects of endothelium-derived relaxing factor (EDRF) during platelet aggregation; inhibition of platelet adhesion and aggregation and of platelet-induced contraction. Endothelium-dependent relaxations to aggregating platelets are achieved mainly by adenine nucleotides (ADP and ATP) and serotonin (5-HT), whereas direct, endothelium-independent contractions are achieved mainly by serotonin (5-HT) and thromboxanes (TBA$_2$), depending on the species and vascular beds tested. Under normal conditions in the presence of intact endothelium, those relaxations and contractions may be well balanced. EDRF and prostacyclin could act synergistically (arrowheads) against platelet aggregation and platelet-induced contractions. +, facilitation; −, inhibition. MAO, monoamine oxidase; PGI$_2$, prostacyclin. (From Vanhoutte, P. M., and Shimokawa, H.: Endothelium-derived relaxing factor and coronary vasospasm. Circulation *80*:1, 1989, by permission of the American Heart Association, Inc.)

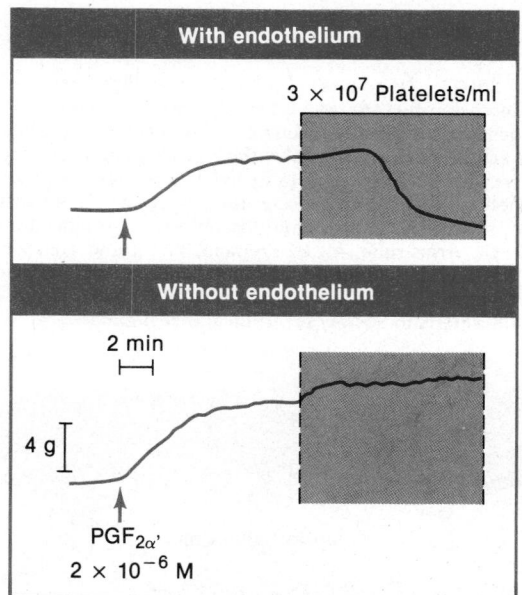

FIGURE 38-12. Example of the response of left circumflex artery rings with and without endothelium during contraction to prostaglandin $F_{2\alpha}$ ($PGF_{2\alpha}$) upon addition of platelet suspensions. The size of the contraction in response to $PGF_{2\alpha}$ was not significantly different in rings with or without endothelium. (From Cohen, R. A., Shepherd, J. T., and Vanhoutte, P. M.: Endothelial alpha receptors in canine pulmonary and systemic blood vessels. Eur. J. Pharmacol. *118*:123, 1985.)

an intact endothelium, platelets are potent vasoconstrictors, but in the presence of an intact endothelium, platelets actually exert an indirect vasodilating effect by effecting the release of EDRF (Fig. 38-12). Vascular endothelial cells also perform a variety of metabolic functions including the conversion of angiotensin I to II as well as the uptake of circulating norepinephrine and serotonin.[127]

In the face of thrombogenic vasoconstrictor stimuli, such as may be supplied by thrombin and platelets, the products of endothelial cells, i.e., prostacyclin and EDRF, oppose normal thrombogenesis and cause vascular dilatation. In contrast, in vessels with atherosclerotic plaques and in other conditions in which the endothelium has been damaged, the response to a thrombus is vascular contraction and further platelet aggregation, thereby resulting in interference with blood flow. A variety of disease processes interfere with the normal function of the endothelium. For example, disruption of the endothelium by atheromatous plaques can activate platelets and lead to thrombogenesis. Sites of endothelial damage in the coronary vascular bed can be responsible for localized regions of coronary spasm (Fig. 38-13). Indeed, the coronary spasm that frequently follows PTCA suggests that disruption of the endothelium may tip the balance of forces acting on the coronary artery diameter in favor of contraction.

There is experimental evidence that both hypertension and hypercholesterolemia also impair release of EDRF. Thus, endothelium-dependent relaxation in response to thrombin, ADP, and acetylcholine is reduced or absent in aortic rings from genetically hypertensive rats. Hypercholesterolemia in cynomolgus monkeys and swine[137a] impairs endothelium-dependent vascular relaxation.[137] Normal young adult human subjects exhibit coronary vasodilatation in response to the intracoronary artery infusion of acetylcholine, presumably as a consequence of the release of EDRF. In contrast, atherosclerotic coronary arteries, coronary vessels with minor irregularities, the apparently *uninvolved* vessels of patients with known coronary vascular disease,[138] vessels of patients after cardiac transplantation, and even apparently normal coronary arteries in older subjects all may display a constrictor effect to intracoronary acetylcholine, suggesting the presence of abnormally functioning endothelium.[139] The endothelial dysfunction characteristic of early atherosclerosis may, by impairing vasodilator function, cause abnormal coronary vasomotion during exercise.[140] In patients with ischemic heart disease, the combination of atherosclerotic plaques that encroach on the vascular lumen and the presence of vasoconstrictor stimuli, such as norepinephrine and angiotensin II, with the additional factor of endothelial dysfunction, may produce vascular obstruction.[141]

Oxygen-derived free radicals, frequently produced during postischemic reperfusion (p. 1239), inhibit endothelial dependent dilation and can thereby impede recovery of ischemically damaged myocardium.[142,143] In contrast, relaxation of coronary arteries to acetylcholine can be restored by dietary treatment of arteriosclerosis (Fig. 38-14). It is possible (through not proved) that the eicosapentaenoic acid in cod liver oil, by changing the fluidity of the membranes of endothelial cells, enhances synthesis and/or release of EDRF.[144]

ENDOTHELIN. Endothelial cells may also cause contraction of vascular smooth muscle cells (Fig. 38-15). Yanagisawa et al.[145] have cloned the precursor of a contractile factor produced by endothelial cells, a 21-residue vasoconstrictor polypeptide called *endothelin* (Fig. 38-16). Endothelin was ini-

FIGURE 38-13. Illustration of endothelium-dependent responses under pathological conditions. The endothelium is dysfunctional in a regenerated state, hypercholesterolemia and atherosclerosis, releasing less endothelium-derived relaxing factor (EDRF), whereas the ability of the smooth muscle to contract is unaltered. As a result, the contractions predominate. In atherosclerosis, the production of both EDRF and prostacyclin (PGI_2) is reduced, and their synergistic actions against aggregating platelets may not occur. 5-HT, 5-hydroxytryptamine, serotonin; ADP, adenosine diphosphate; ATP, adenosine triphosphate; TBA_2, thromboxane A_2; MAO, monoamine oxidase; −, inhibition; +, synergism. (From Vanhoutte, P. M., and Shimokawa, H.: Endothelium-derived relaxing factor and coronary vasospasm. Circulation *80*:6, 1989, by permission of the American Heart Association, Inc.)

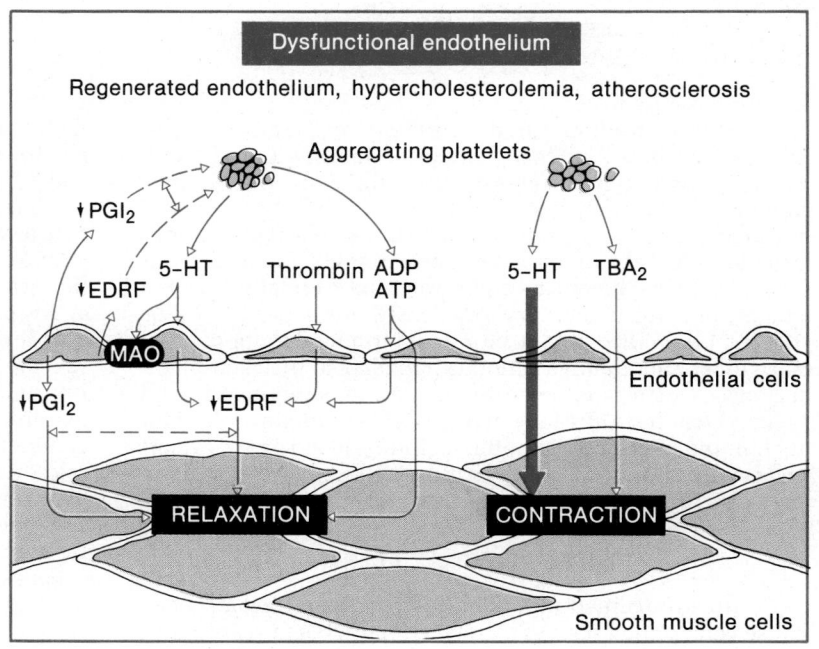

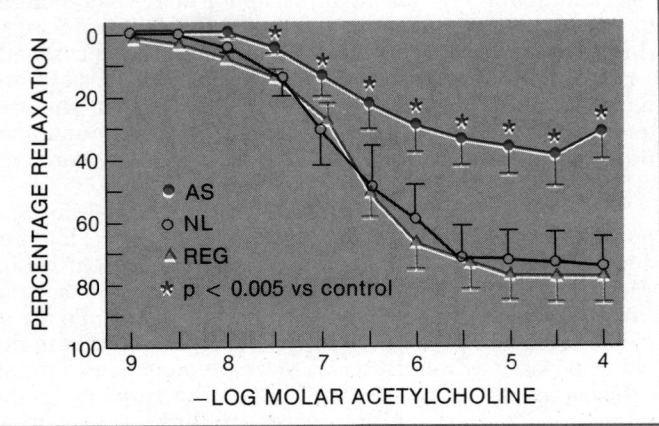

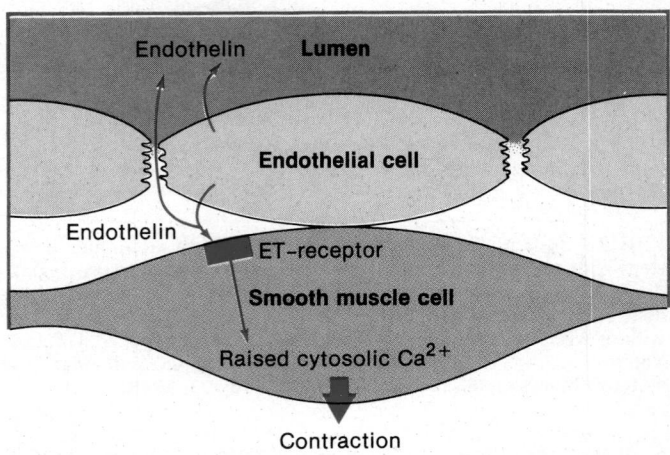

FIGURE 38–14. Responses to acetylcholine of iliac arteries of normal (NL), atherosclerotic (AS), and atherosclerosis regression (REG) monkeys. Atherosclerosis was induced by cholesterol feeding, while regression was achieved by withdrawal of the high cholesterol diet. *p < 0.05 vs. atherosclerotic. Responses to acetylcholine were reduced by approximately one-half in atherosclerotic vessels, and were restored to normal by dietary treatment of atherosclerosis. (Reproduced from Harrison, D. G., Armstrong, M. L., Freiman, P. C., and Heistad, D. D.: Restoration of endothelium-dependent relaxation by dietary treatment of atherosclerosis. J. Clin. Invest. *80*:1808, 1987, by copyright permission of the American Society for Clinical Investigation.)

FIGURE 38–15. Schematic representation of the "spill-over" *of* endothelin into the circulation. The target site for the released endothelin is the endothelin (ET) receptor on the smooth muscle cell. Activation of this receptor results in a sustained rise in cytosolic Ca++, and hence constriction. (From Naylor, W. G.: The Endothelins. Berlin, Springer-Verlag, 1990, p. 91.)

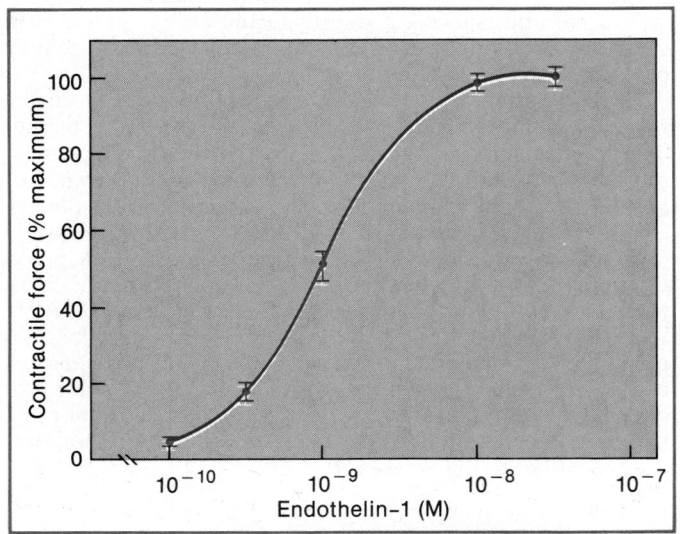

FIGURE 38–16. Dose-dependent constrictor effect of endothelin-1 on human left anterior descending coronary arteries. (From Naylor, W. G.: The Endothelins. Berlin, Springer-Verlag, 1990, p. 117, based on data from Chester, A. H., et al.: Influence of endothelin on human coronary arteries and localization of its binding sites. Am. J. Cardiol. *63*:1395, 1989.)

tially isolated from cultured endothelial cells, but it is also synthesized in a number of tissues, including the kidneys. Shear stress acting on endothelial cells apparently causes downregulation of the preendothelin gene, thereby contributing to flow-induced vasodilation.[146] Threshold concentrations of endothelin I also amplify the contractions of human arteries caused by norepinephrine and serotonin.[147] Endothelin has a potent, prolonged coronary vasoconstrictor action[148,149] (Fig. 38–16). Like EDRF, it may be a long-term modulator of coronary tone. Endothelin's action is not affected by calcium antagonists, but it is opposed by adenosine, substance P, and glyceryl trinitrate.[150] Many diverse tissues contain high-affinity binding sites for endothelin, including blood vessels, heart (especially the atria), lung, brain, and kidneys. Endothelin may also function as a neurotransmitter.[146]

PHARMACOLOGICAL AGENTS

As already pointed out, alpha₁-adrenoceptor agonists can cause constriction both of coronary conductance vessels, i.e.,

the large epicardial arteries, and coronary resistance vessels, i.e., the small intramural arteries and arterioles[38] (Figs. 38–7 and 38–8). This effect is opposed by the passive distention of these vessels consequent to an elevation of intravascular pressure as well as by the metabolically-induced coronary vasodilatation resulting from the increase in MVO₂ accompanying the arterial hypertension induced by these drugs. Directly acting coronary vasodilators, such as nitroglycerin and isosorbide dinitrate,[151–153] augment perfusion of ischemic zones, as reflected by the increased rate of clearance of ^{133}Xe injected into the coronary arteries of patients with coronary artery disease.[154] These drugs have been shown to dilate coronary conductance vessels, coronary collaterals, and even atherosclerotic stenoses[155–157] (Fig. 40–4, p. 1305) as well as to reduce ventricular diastolic tension, which tends to limit flow to the subendocardium. Nitrates have a lesser effect on coronary resistance vessels[158] (Fig. 38–6).

Papaverine and calcium antagonists exert a *direct* action on the large epicardial conductance vessels as well as on the resistance vessels.[157] These agents increase blood flow to normal as well as ischemic myocardium.[159] Dipyridamole dilates the distal (resistance) vessels.[151,160] Because these are acted upon also by the endogenous vasodilator (adenosine), dipyridamole is of little or no value in the treatment of acute myocardial ischemia. Prostacyclin, which is produced by endothelial cells and which inhibits platelet aggregation, also is a potent coronary vasodilator,[124] whereas thromboxane A_2, which is produced by and aggregates platelets, is a potent coronary vasoconstrictor. Dazoxiben, a thromboxane A_2 synthetase inhibitor, can prevent cyclic increases in coronary vascular resistance in stenotic coronary arteries.[161] Serotonin is an extremely potent coronary vasoconstrictor that acts on serotonergic receptors.[38,162] It can be blocked by serotonergic antagonists such as methysergide and ketanserin. Ergonovine and related ergot alkaloids are used diagnostically to provoke coronary spasm in patients suspected of having Prinzmetal's (variant) angina (p. 1342); these compounds cause coronary constriction by acting on both alpha-adrenergic and serotonergic receptors.[38] Atrial natriuretic peptide (p. 412) is a potent dilator of coronary arteries and collaterals in experimental animals and humans.[163,164]

REACTIVE HYPEREMIA AND CORONARY FLOW RESERVE

Ischemia caused by transient coronary arterial occlusion is followed by an increase in blood flow above control levels, a response called *reactive hyperemia* (Fig. 38–17). The flow debt (although not the oxygen debt) is overpaid by the marked vasodilation that characterizes reactive hyperemia; this overpayment is probably related to the accumulation of vasodilator metabolites, especially adenosine.[51,165] The difference between basal coronary blood flow and peak flow during reactive hyperemia represents the *coronary flow reserve*, which has been measured in experimental animals[166–168] and estimated in patients.[169] The coronary reserve is reduced, even absent, in patients with severe obstructive coronary artery disease, and it can be restored to normal by bypass grafting. The coronary flow reserve in the left ventricles of patients with severe left ventricular hypertrophy secondary to aortic stenosis is reduced,[170,171] perhaps because of failure of the coronary circulation to grow apace with the increase in ventricular mass[170] as well as by compression of the intramural coronary vascular bed by the hypertrophied myocardium. Regression of experimentally produced hypertrophy has been found to restore impaired coronary flow reserve toward normal.[172–174]

Coronary flow reserve can be estimated noninvasively by positron emission tomographic imaging (to measure cardiac perfusion) both in the basal state and under the influence of a powerful vasodilator stress—the combination of intravenous dipyridamole and handgrip stress. Patients with left ventricular hypertrophy exhibited a reduction of the stress-to-rest perfusion ratio to 1.06 from normal values of 1.41.[175] Good correlations also have been reported between the severity of

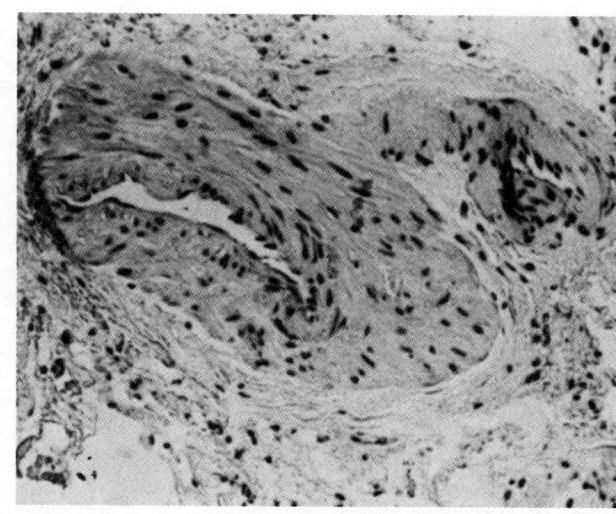

FIGURE 38–18. Light micrograph from patient 2, showing markedly thickened small coronary arteries (hematoxylin and eosin × 320). (From Mosseri, M., Yarom, R., Gotsman, M. S., and Hasin, Y.: Histologic evidence for small-vessel coronary artery disease in patients with angina pectoris and patent large coronary arteries. Circulation 74:964, 1986, by permission of the American Heart Association, Inc.)

coronary stenosis determined by quantitative coronary arteriography and myocardial perfusion determined by positron emission tomography.[176] Coronary flow reserve has been estimated in a wide variety of conditions. A reduction of the coronary blood flow response to the vasodilating actions of dipyridamole has been demonstrated in patients with essential hypertension.[177] Using electrical pacing of the heart to evoke a vasodilator response, Cannon and associates described an abnormally reduced coronary flow reserve in patients with hypertrophic cardiomyopathy, in whom elevation of left ventricular filling pressure, probably related to an ischemia-induced reduction in ventricular compliance during tachycardia, was associated with a decline in coronary blood flow.[178] Similar reductions in vasodilator reserve were demonstrated in patients undergoing rejection of the transplanted heart.[179]

Patients with dilated cardiomyopathy, anginal chest pain, and angiographically normal coronary arteries have exhibited impaired vasodilator response to a metabolic stimulus (cardiac pacing) and a pharmacological stimulus (dipyridamole) and increased sensitivity to a vasoconstrictor stimulus (ergonovine).[180]

An inadequate flow reserve secondary to a vascular or extravascular abnormality that prevents normal coronary arterial dilatation in the face of ischemia represents a cause of myocardial ischemia that is being recognized with increasing frequency. Indeed, among patients with angina pectoris and patent large coronary arteries, a reduced flow of angiographic contrast medium has been reported, and right ventricular endomyocardial biopsy specimens have shown fibromuscular hyperplasia, hypertrophy of the media, and endothelial degeneration[181] (Fig. 38–18). Many of these patients with so-called microvascular angina[181a] also demonstrate an abnormally reduced dilator capacity to dipyridamole with a paradoxical vasoconstrictor response to bicycle exercise.[182] At autopsy intramyocardial small arteries uniformly showed a reduction in the ratio of vessel lumen to wall thickness.[183]

FACTORS LIMITING CORONARY PERFUSION

The normal intramyocardial coronary vascular bed has the capacity to reduce its resistance to approximately 15 to 20 per cent of basal levels during the stress of maximal exercise, i.e., a five- to sixfold increase in coronary blood flow, which is

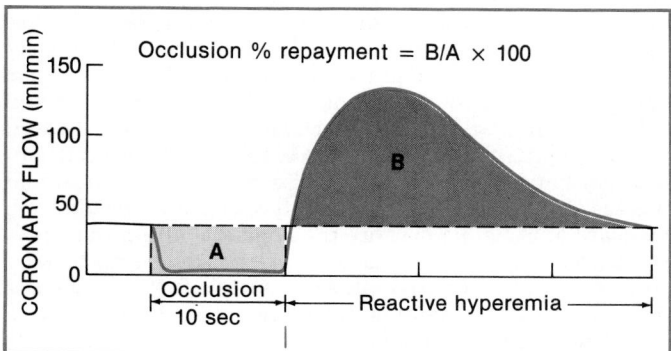

FIGURE 38–17. Mean coronary flow prior to, during, and following coronary occlusion. Arrow indicates the release of occlusion. Area A represents the flow debt, and area B its repayment. (From Gould, K. L.: Coronary Artery Stenosis. New York, Elsevier, 1991, p. 13.)

generally accompanied by an increase in arterial pressure and marked tachycardia, can occur during maximal exercise. It is then not surprising that when the diameter of a normal proximal coronary artery can be reduced by up to 80 per cent, sufficient dilatation of the intramyocardial coronary resistance vessels will occur so that the *total* coronary vascular resistance in series remains constant (Fig. 38–19).[184] However, when maximal dilatation of the resistance vessels has occurred in the presence of such a critical obstruction in a proximal artery, coronary blood flow cannot rise; any stimulus that increases MVO_2, such as exercise- or pacing-induced tachycardia, will of necessity elicit ischemia. When obstruction of a proximal coronary artery reduces the lumen by more than approximately 90 to 95 per cent of normal, ischemia will be present even in the basal state, despite maximal dilatation of the resistance vessels, unless the myocardium distal to the obstructed vessel is perfused by collateral vessels or unless mechanical activity of the myocardium is reduced. Transient severe obstruction, as may occur with coronary spasm, will result in brief periods of ischemia, chest pain, electrocardiographic changes, and myocardial dysfunction. When severe ischemia persists, myocardial necrosis usually ensues. With lesser degrees of obstruction of an epicardial artery (e.g., 40 to 80 per cent of the control diameter lumen) the distal bed is *not* maximally dilated in the basal state, and although the capacity for further dilatation exists, this capacity is subnormal and ischemia may develop if myocardial oxygen demands are sufficiently augmented. With less than 40 per cent diameter stenosis, maximum flow during exercise is usually normal.

Basic considerations of fluid mechanics indicate that the pressure drop across a stenosis varies directly with the length of the stenosis and inversely with the fourth power of the radius (Bernoulli's theorem), emphasizing the greater importance of changes in the latter compared with the former.[185,186] Stenosis resistance changes relatively little with mild degrees of vascular narrowing but rises progressively and precipitously with severe obstruction; indeed, resistance almost triples as stenosis severity increases from 80 to 90 per cent.[187] As a consequence, with even a slight increase in the severity of

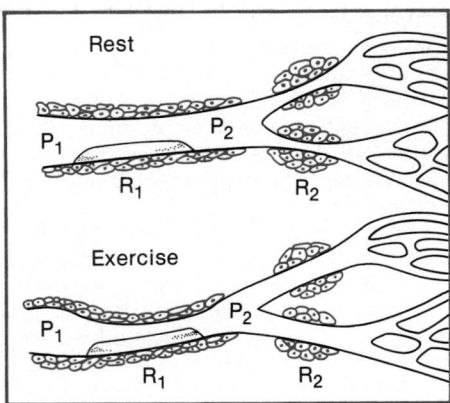

FIGURE 38–20. Diagrammatic representation of vessel collapse when myocardial flow increases. Under baseline conditions (Rest, *top*), flow across the stenosis (R_1) is modest and a large pressure gradient (P_1-P_2) does not develop. With a vasodilator intervention such as exercise *(bottom)*, the pressure gradient across the stenosis (P_1-P_2) increases. The resulting fall in intraluminal pressure may lead to collapse of the vessel at the level of the obstruction, thereby increasing the degree of stenosis. This leads to dilatation of the distal vessels (R_2). (From Epstein, S. E., Cannon, R. O., III, and Talbot, T. L.: Hemodynamic principles in the control of coronary blood flow. Am. J. Cardiol. *56:*9E, 1985.)

stenosis—as might occur when platelets aggregate on a critically narrowed plaque or when the pressure distending the narrowed coronary artery declines, as occurs with a rise in blood flow during exercise or following administration of dipyridamole—the perfusion pressure distal to the obstruction may become reduced and subendocardial perfusion impaired.[185] Vascular resistance is not fixed even in the presence of an atherosclerotic plaque. As flow across such a lesion rises, substantial energy losses due to turbulence occur that are proportional to the flow squared. As a result, there is an exponential rise in the pressure gradient across the stenosis. As the transstenotic pressure drop increases, the pressure distending the artery declines. This may result in passive collapse[188] (Fig. 38–20), causing further damage.

FIXED AND DYNAMIC OBSTRUCTION

Myocardial ischemia and its consequences may occur as a result of fixed atherosclerotic lesions or may be secondary to transitory reduction of myocardial blood flow caused by coronary spasm and/or platelet aggregation.[189,190] The clinical sequelae of myocardial ischemia, whether produced by an increase in MVO_2 in the face of fixed obstruction, by a reduction in myocardial oxygen supply, or by a combination of these factors, may be manifested clinically as angina pectoris, electrical instability, characteristic electrocardiographic changes, or depression of myocardial function, alone or in combination.

Maseri has clarified the interrelation between fixed and dynamic (variable) obstruction to blood flow.[189] Normal subjects can carry out maximal exercise, develop a 15- to 20-fold increase in body $\dot{V}O_2$ above resting levels, and yet not develop myocardial ischemia because they operate within their normal coronary reserve. Figure 38–21 shows the effects of fixed coronary obstruction that allows a fourfold increase in coronary blood flow. Ischemia occurs whenever $M\dot{V}O_2$ rises to a level that cannot be met by this coronary flow reserve. It is clear that transient reductions of coronary reserve below this level will occur in many patients with coronary atherosclerosis. In these patients, the anginal threshold will be quite variable (Fig. 38–21 II), a condition referred to as *mixed angina*.[191]

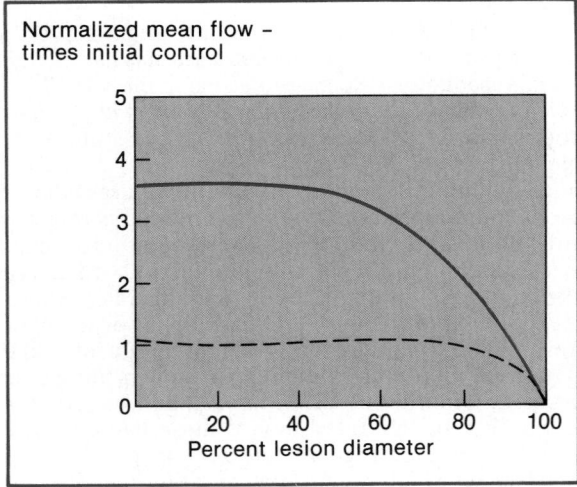

FIGURE 38–19. Relationship between resting *(dashed line)* and maximal coronary blood flow *(solid line)* and percentage of diameter stenosis in a dog. Progressive coronary stenosis was achieved by progressively narrowing a short segment of a proximal coronary artery. Resting coronary blood flow did not change until coronary diameter stenosis exceeded 80 percent. Maximal coronary blood flow began to decrease when percent diameter stenosis exceeded 50 percent. (From Marcus, M. L.: The Coronary Circulation in Health and Disease. New York, McGraw-Hill, 1983, and modified from Gould, K. L., Lipscomb, K.: Effects of coronary stenoses on coronary flow reserve and resistance. Am. J. Cardiol. *34:*50, 1974.)

PLATE 5

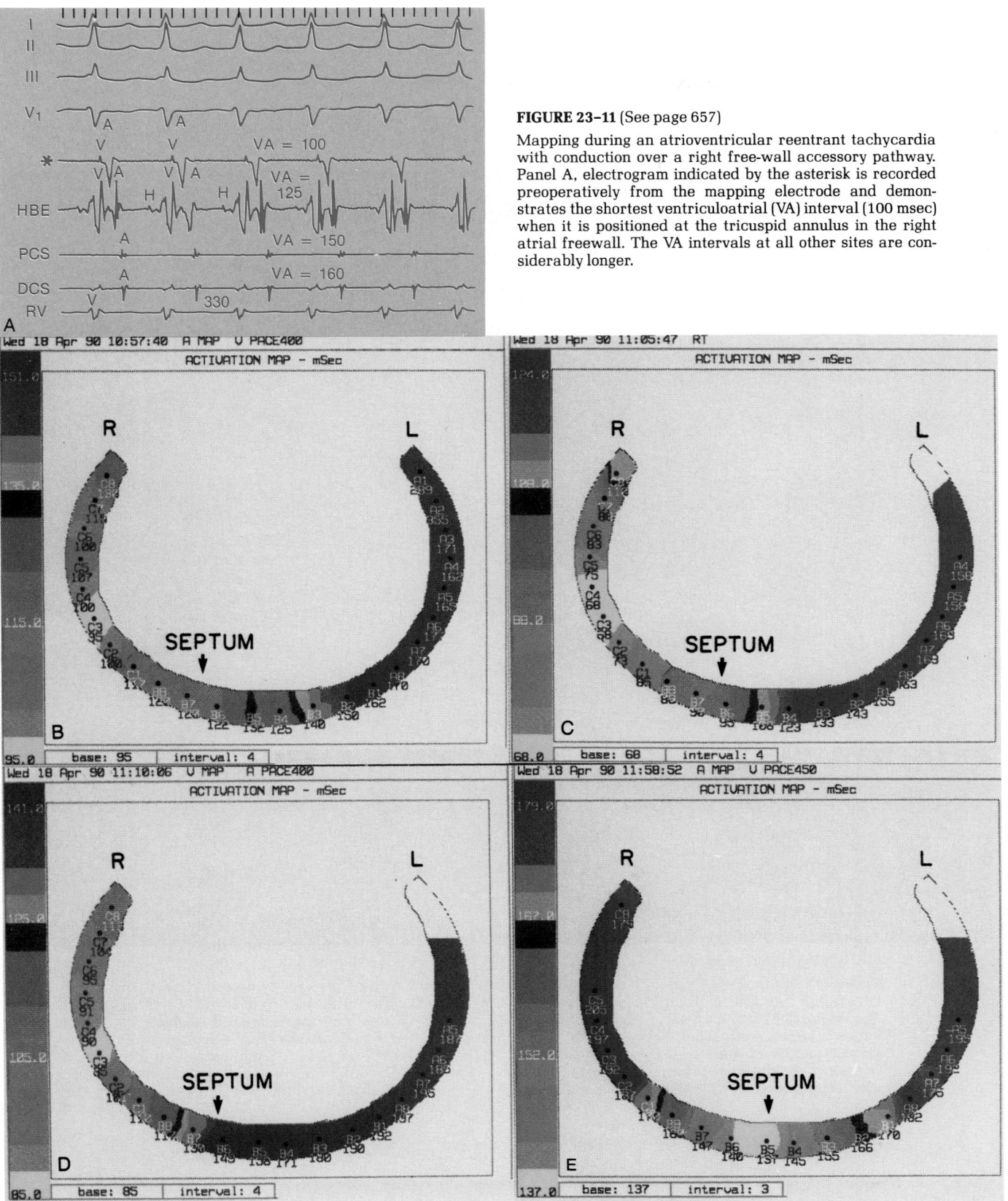

FIGURE 23–11 (See page 657)

Mapping during an atrioventricular reentrant tachycardia with conduction over a right free-wall accessory pathway. Panel A, electrogram indicated by the asterisk is recorded preoperatively from the mapping electrode and demonstrates the shortest ventriculoatrial (VA) interval (100 msec) when it is positioned at the tricuspid annulus in the right atrial freewall. The VA intervals at all other sites are considerably longer.

Panel B demonstrates the computerized isopotential map (Bard Systems) recorded at the atrial side of the annulus intraoperatively during ventricular pacing at a CL of 400 msec. The VA interval at site C3 is 95 msec (yellow). (The VA interval at site C6 registers 100 msec while at C5 it is 107 msec, probably due to slightly inappropriate electrode positioning.) The activation map during atrioventricular reentrant tachycardia confirms the location of the earliest atrial activation to be at C3 and C4 (panel C). During atrial pacing, the ventricle is similarly activated anterogradely early at the same site (panel D). Following surgical interruption of the accessory pathway, ventricular pacing results in earliest activation of the atrium concentrically, just to the right of the interventricular septum (panel E).

PLATE 6

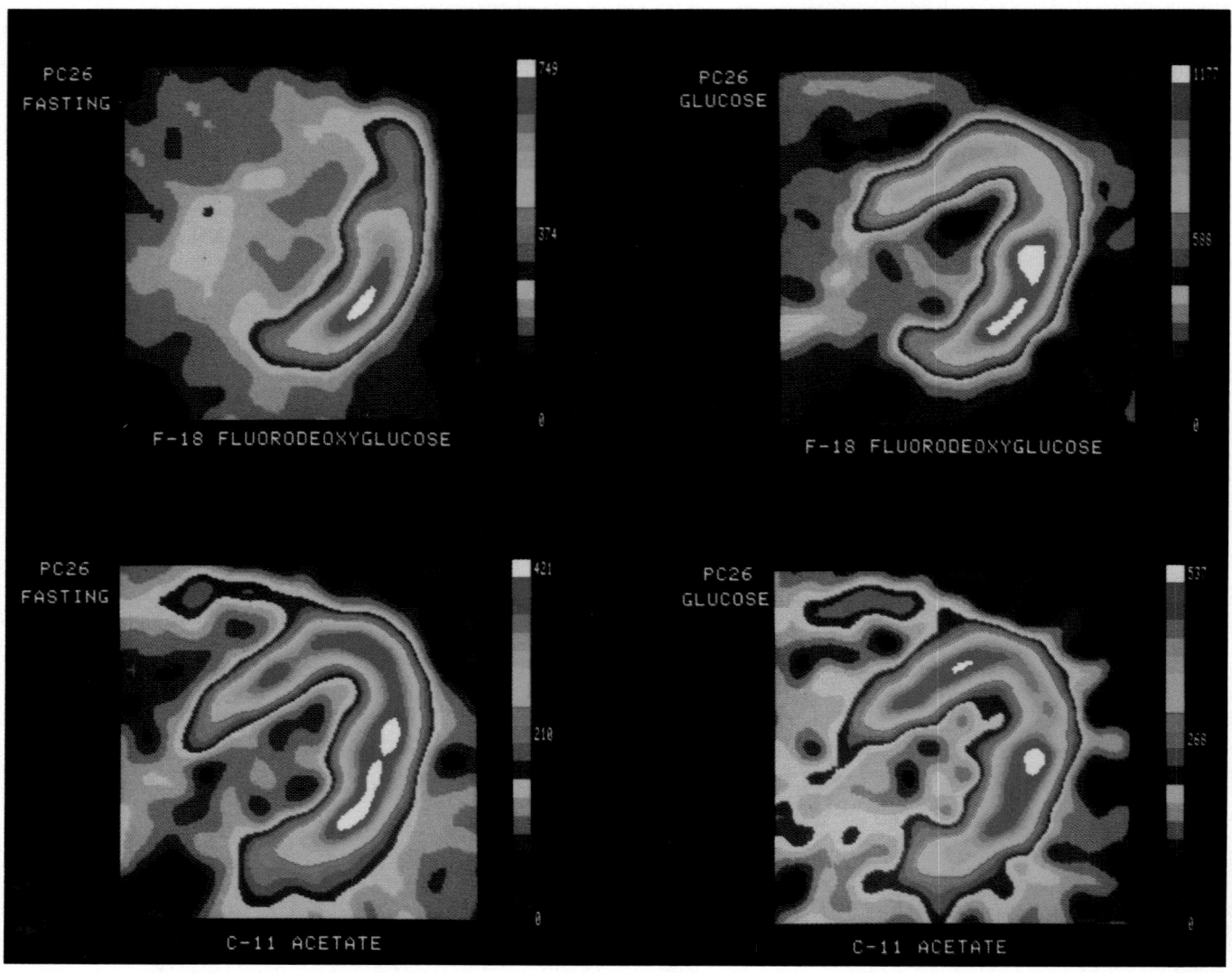

FIGURE 38–34 (See page 1184)

Midventricular positron-emission tomographic reconstructions are shown from a single normal subject. The tomograms depicted in the upper panels were performed after the intravenous administration of ^{18}F-fluorodeoxyglucose and those in the bottom panels after the intravenous administration of ^{11}C-acetate. The left-hand panels were acquired after a 5- to 8-hour fast; those in the right-hand panels were acquired after glucose administration. ^{11}C-acetate accumulation and clearance were homogenous during fasting and after feeding. (Reproduced, with permission, from Gropler, R., Siegel, B.A., Lee, K.J. et al.: Nonuniformity in myocardial accumulation of F-18 fluorodeoxyglucose in normal fasted humans. J. Nucl. Med. [in press].)

PLATE 7

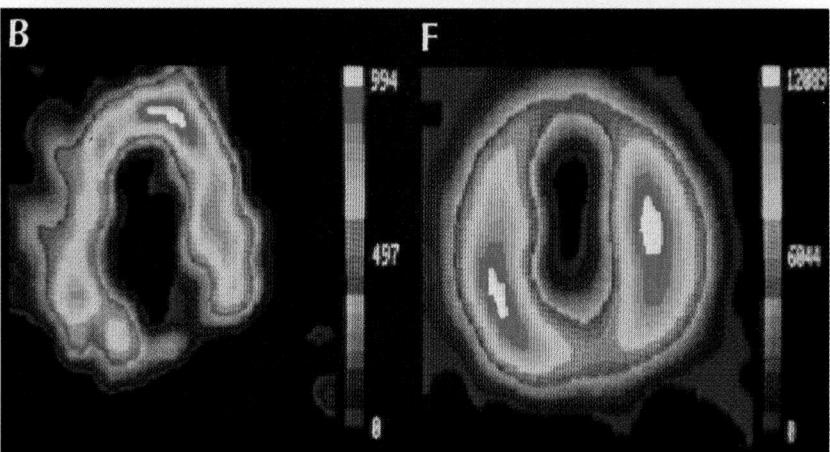

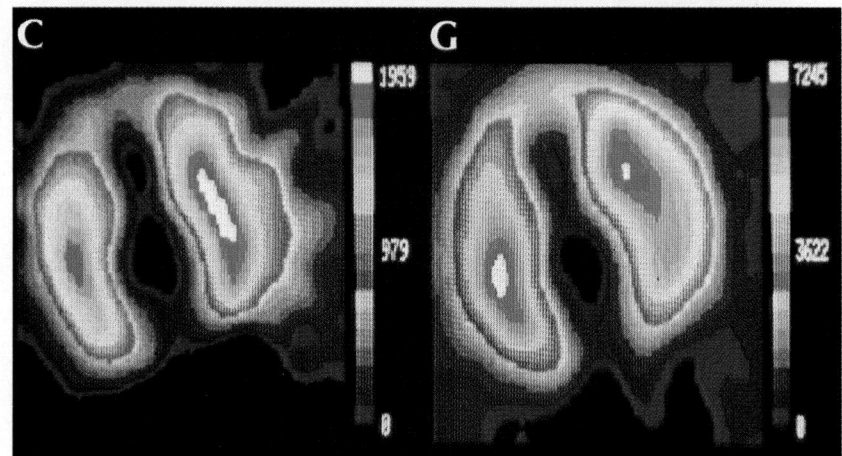

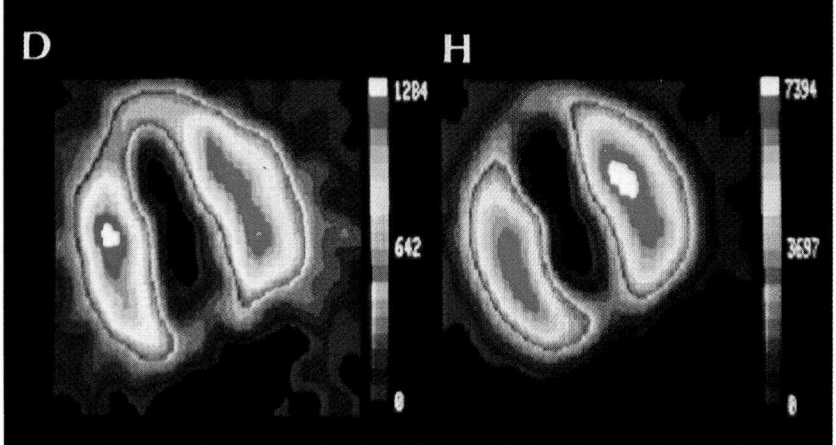

FIGURE 38–35 (See page 1184)

Transverse reconstructed tomograms from a single plane through the middle of the left ventricle of a dog given recombinant tissue-type plasminogen activator after 2 hours of coronary occlusion. Images have been corrected for vascular activity with the use of blood-pool images obtained prior to each flow determination after inhalation of ^{15}O-labeled carbon monoxide. Anterior myocardium is at the top of each image, with the lateral wall on the left, interventricular septum on the right, and the posterior region of the mitral valve at the bottom. Panels A through D represent myocardial perfusion and were obtained after intravenous injection of ^{15}O-labeled water. Panels E through H represent myocardial fatty acid uptake after intravenous injection of ^{11}C-labeled palmitate. Images A and E were obtained 90 minutes after occlusion of the left anterior descending coronary artery.

Note the large ischemic area in the anterior region, which partially resolves 1 hour after reperfusion (panels B and F). Panels C and G were obtained after 24 hours and show the late diminution in flow and metabolism in the reperfused zone. After 4 weeks of reperfusion, flow (panel D) has increased in the anterior region, but palmitate uptake (panel H) has recovered only minimally. (Reproduced, with permission, from Knabb, R.M., Bergmann, S.R., Fox, K.A.A., Sobel, B.E.: The temporal pattern of recovery of myocardial perfusion and metabolism delineated by positron emission tomography after coronary thrombolysis. J. Nucl. Med 28:1563, 1987.)

PLATE 8

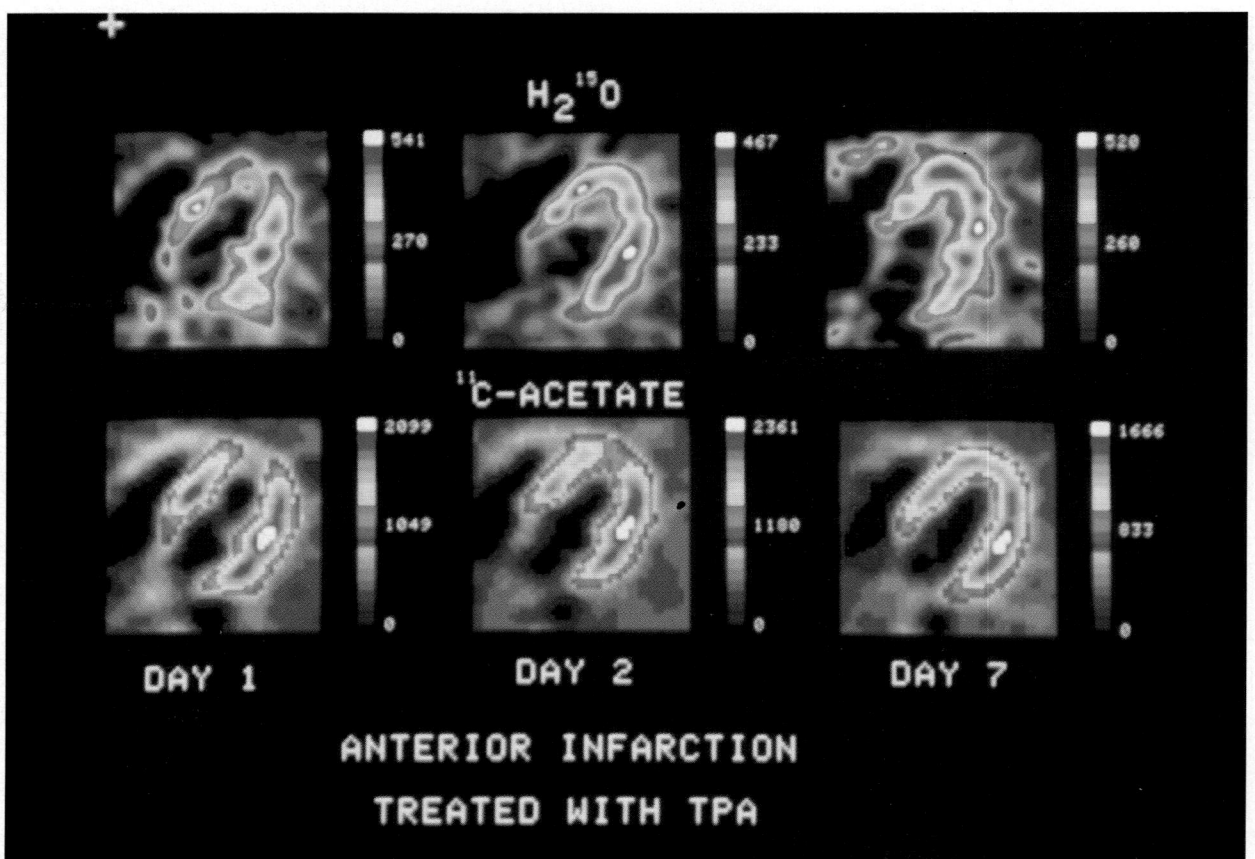

FIGURE 38-40 (See page 1190)

Midventricular positron-emission tomographic reconstructions from a patient with anterior myocardial infarction after treatment with t-PA are depicted at the intervals indicated. The top row of images represents relative perfusion. The bottom row of images illustrates the myocardial accumulation of ^{11}C-acetate reconstructed from data collected 3 to 8 minutes after administration of ^{11}C-acetate. The top of each image corresponds to the anterior and the left of each to the patient's right. Areas in white and red have the highest relative perfusion or content of tracer. Zones in blue and purple have the lowest. The discontinuity visible posteriorly is attributable to the mitral valve apparatus and atria, in which uptake is below the spatial resolution of the instrument.

A slight reduction in relative perfusion is observed in the anterior wall on the initial study, with normalization by 48 hours. A defect in accumulation of ^{11}C-acetate is evident in the initial study, with gradual improvement over the subsequent interval of observation. (Reproduced, with permission, from Henes, C.G., et al.: The time course of restoration of nutritive perfusion, myocardial oxygen consumption, and regional function after coronary thrombolysis. Coronary Artery Dis. 1:687,1990.)

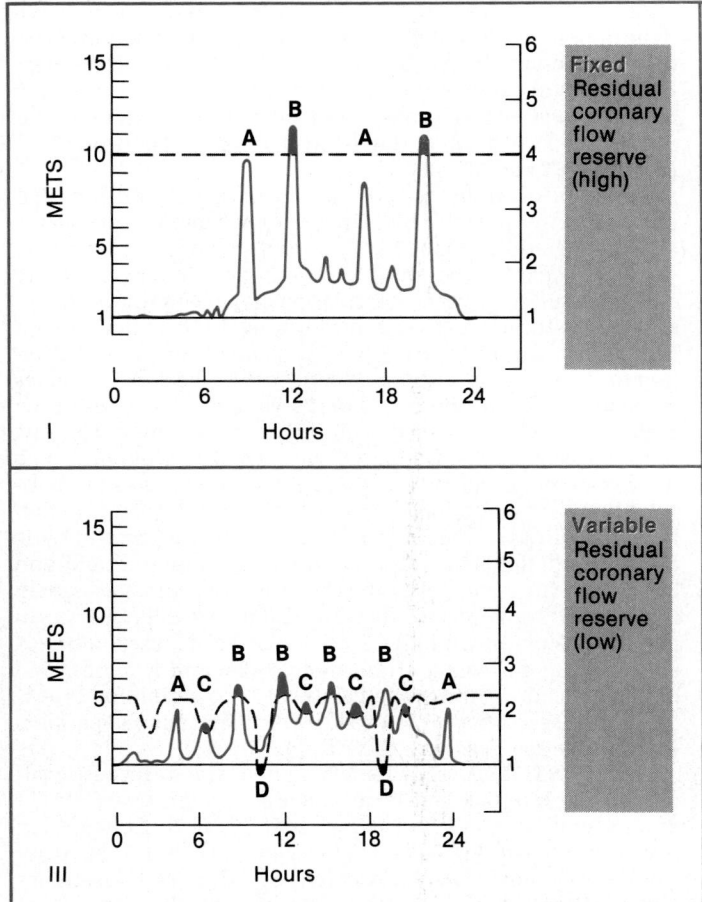

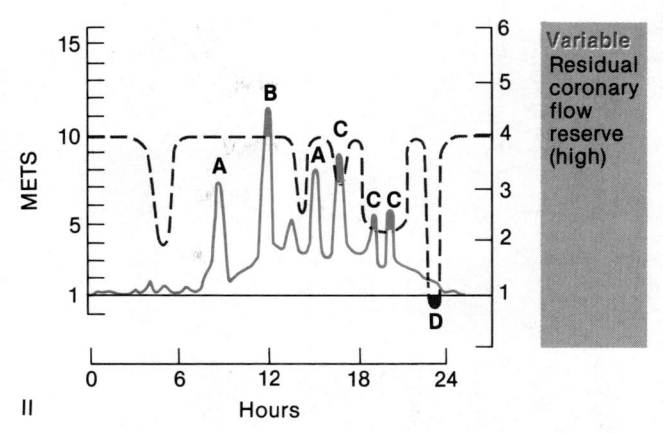

FIGURE 38–21. Schematic illustration of the relation between physical activity (during 24 hours) expressed as METS (multiple of basal metabolic oxygen consumption) and coronary flow reserve. Normally, during resting conditions, coronary flow reserve exactly matches the metabolic demand. However, when metabolic demands increase to a maximum of 16 METS, coronary flow reserve increases up to six times the resting value to match the increased demand for flow by the myocardium so that no ischemia occurs.

I. In this situation, a patient has a moderately severe fixed coronary artery obstruction that reduces coronary flow reserve to four times the resting value. *A,* the patient can exercise up to approximately 10 METS without developing ischemia; *B,* however, if he exercises above approximately 10 METS, he will consistently develop ischemia.

II. In this situation, the patient has a moderately severe stenosis that fixes the coronary reserve at four times resting levels as in I. In addition, he has a variable stenosis. Therefore, residual coronary flow reserve has an upper limit that is fixed but that can decrease because of the presence of the mechanisms that transiently interfere with coronary blood flow. Thus, the residual coronary flow reserve can vary throughout the day. Under these conditions, if the patient exercises beyond the maximal residual coronary flow reserve, he will always develop ischemia (*B*). However, he may also develop ischemia on other occasions after smaller degrees of exercise, when residual coronary flow reserve is decreased by these functional factors (*C*). Occasionally, coronary flow reserve decreases so that resting flow is impaired and ischemia occurs at rest (*D*). At other times of the day, this patient can exercise below the level of his maximal residual coronary flow reserve without experiencing ischemia (*A*).

III. In this situation, the patient has a very severe fixed stenosis and also variable stenosis. Maximal residual coronary flow reserve is reduced to little more than two times the resting value of coronary flow, thus allowing the patient to exercise up to a level of about 5 METS in the absence of any transient impairment of coronary flow. The combination of markedly reduced coronary flow reserve and of transient impairment of coronary flow results in frequent occurrences of ischemic episodes caused by excessive increase of demand above the maximal residual coronary flow (*B*) or by transient impairment of flow during exertion (*C*) or at rest (*D*). However, in the absence of transient impairment of flow, the patient can tolerate activities below 5 METS (*A*). (Modified from Maseri, A., Chierchia, S., and Kaski, J. C.: Mixed angina pectoris. Am. J. Cardiol., *56*:31E and 32E, 1985.)

Myocardial Ischemia and Ischemic Injury

EFFECTS OF ISCHEMIA ON MYOCARDIAL FUNCTION

In 1935 Tennant and Wiggers demonstrated that after ligation of a coronary artery the contraction of cardiac muscle supplied by this vessel ceases almost immediately and the affected area appears cyanotic, dilated, and bulging.[192] In the basal state there is no reserve in blood flow; any reduction in flow, even one as small as 10 to 20 per cent, results in an approximately similar percentage reduction of myocardial segment shortening.[193] Myocardial ischemia is generally associated with elimination of the normal contractile performance of a *localized area* of myocardium, resulting in an asynergic contraction.[194] Figure 38–22 shows the immediate regional myocardial functional responses to acute coronary occlusion: there is paradoxical motion (systolic bulging or dyskinesis) in the central ischemic zone, reduced contraction (akinesis or hypokinesis) in the adjacent area, and compensatory hyperfunction of the uninvolved normal myocardium, the latter mediated in part by adrenergic stimulation and the operation of the Frank-Starling mechanism.[195,196] A reduction of blood flow of 80 per cent below control results in akinesis, while a 95 per cent reduction causes dyskinesis. Animals and patients with a previous myocardial infarction exhibit impaired regional left ventricular function, although, if the damage is limited, hyperfunction of the residual myocardium will maintain global left ventricular function (Fig. 39–12, p. 1211). In the isolated heart, *global* ischemia causes a depression of myocardial contractility reflected in a decrease in the slope of the end-systolic pressure-volume relation (E_{max}) (p. 428). On the other hand, *regional* ischemia shifts the relationship

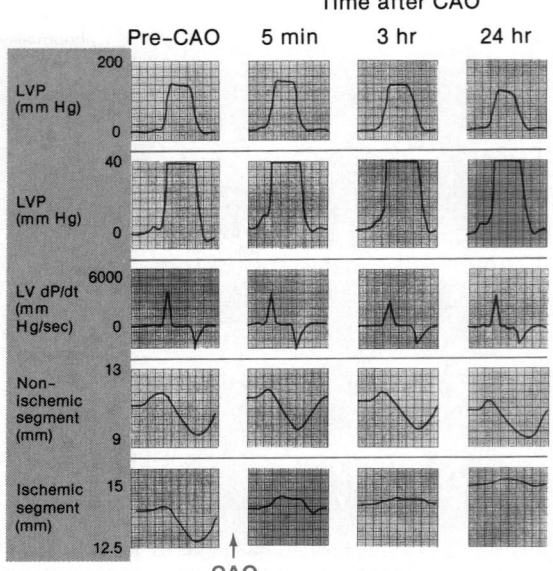

Time after CAO

FIGURE 38–22. Phasic recordings are shown for left ventricular (LV) systolic (1st trace) and end-diastolic (2nd trace) pressures, LV dP/dt, and segment shortening in nonischemic and ischemic zones in a normal dog, before coronary artery occlusion (CAO), at 5 minutes and 3 and 24 hours after CAO. (From Amano, J., Thomas, J. X., Jr., Lavallee, M., Mirsky, I., Glover, D., Manders, W. T., Randall, W. C., and Vatner, S. F.: Effects of myocardial ischemia on regional function and stiffness in conscious dogs. Am. J. Physiol. *252*:H113, 1987.)

rightward, without affecting E_{max}. The shift reflects the behavior of the noncontractile ischemic segment of the ventricle, while the normal slope results from the compensatory hyperfunction of the nonischemic segment.[197]

Myocardial Stunning and Hibernation

For approximately 4 decades following Tennant and Wiggers' classic observations on the effects of coronary occlusion on myocardial contraction,[192] it was thought that following severe ischemia myocardium either became irreversibly injured, i.e., infarction developed, or promptly recovered. However, in the 1970's it became clear that after a *brief* episode of *severe* ischemia, prolonged dysfunction with gradual return of contractile activity occurred, a condition termed *myocardial*

stunning[198–200] (Figs. 38–23 and 38–24). It then became evident in both experimental animals and patients that myocardial function could also be chronically depressed consequent to severe, chronic ischemia; this myocardial dysfunction could be ameliorated promptly by relief of the ischemia. This condition has been termed *myocardial hibernation*[201,202] (Figs. 38–25 and 38–26).

Those two conditions, myocardial stunning and hibernation, occur frequently, both in the experimental laboratory and in the clinic (Fig. 38–27). Since stunned myocardium occurs adjacent to necrotic tissue after prolonged coronary occlusion, many myocardial infarcts may be a mixture of necrotic and stunned tissue. Stunning may occur with demand-induced ischemia[203] with coronary spasm,[203a] and may be limited to the subendocardium.[204] It occurs in diastole as well as in systole[200,205] and can occur in the globally as well as in the regionally ischemic heart. Clinically, myocardial stunning probably occurs most frequently in the hearts of patients who have undergone ischemic cardiac arrest during cardiopulmonary bypass[206]; such hearts may not recover normal function for hours or days. Similarly, it occurs following thrombolytic therapy in patients having acute myocardial infarction[207] and in those with severe ischemia due to coronary vasospasm (Prinzmetal's angina) or unstable angina, or following coronary occlusion during balloon angioplasty. Myocardial hibernation is as common as stunning (p. 1329) and is manifested clinically as the improvement in ventricular function that is frequently seen after myocardial revascularization in patients with ischemic heart disease[208,209] (Fig. 38–25).

MECHANISM OF STUNNING. The mechanism responsible for stunning has not been elucidated definitively.[209a,209b] Studies with NMR spectroscopy demonstrate that changes in the ratio of phosphocreatine to inorganic phosphate correlate closely with reductions of nutritive perfusion and consequent changes in myocardial function.[210] Results implicate accumulation of inorganic phosphate or hydrogen ion or both as potential inhibitors of myocardial contractility. They are supported by studies with magnetic resonance imaging (MRI) in dogs subjected to coronary occlusion in which increased signal intensity with proton MRI was found to be a specific criterion of irreversible ischemic injury in contrast to stunning of myocardium.[211]

Stunned myocardium has been differentiated from irreversibly injured tissue by ultrasonic tissue characterization with

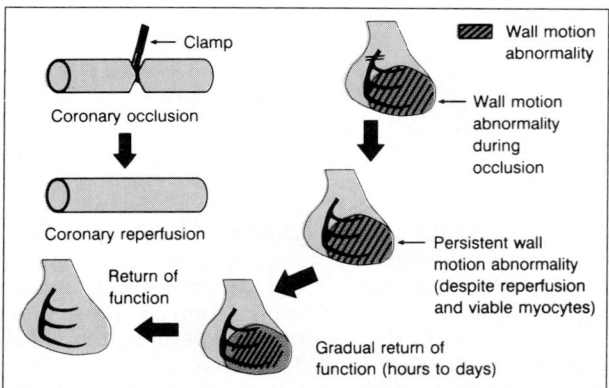

FIGURE 38–23. Schematic diagram of stunned myocardium. During coronary occlusion, a wall motion abnormality of the left ventricle is present in the region supplied by the occluded artery. With relief of ischemia and re-establishment of coronary blood flow, there is a persistent wall motion abnormality despite reperfusion and viable myocytes. There is then gradual improvement in function that requires hours to days for recovery. (From Kloner, R. A., Przyklenk, K., and Patel, B.: Altered myocardial states: The stunned and hibernating myocardium. Am. J. Med. *86*(Suppl. 1A):14, 1986.)

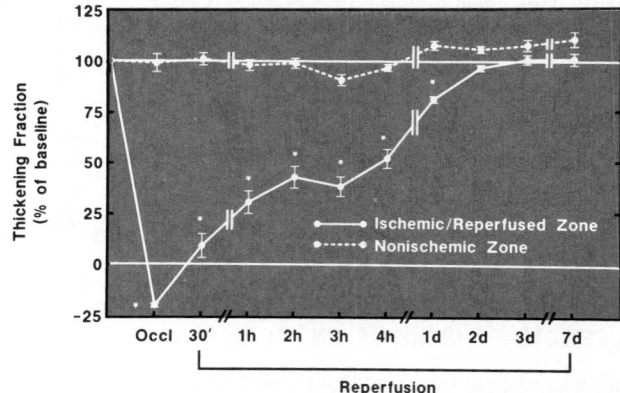

FIGURE 38–24. Changes in systolic thickening fraction during coronary occlusion (Occl) and at selected times after reperfusion in the nonischemic region and in the ischemic-reperfused region. Thickening fraction is expressed as percentage of preocclusion (baseline) values. It is an excellent indicator of local myocardial function. Data are mean values ± SEM (n = 10). Systolic function in the reperfused myocardium recovered slowly; on the average, thickening fraction was still significantly depressed at 24 hours, and returned to baseline at 48 hours after reflow. *p < 0.001 versus baseline. (From Charlat, M. L. et al.: Prolonged abnormalities of left ventricular diastolic wall thinning in the "stunned" myocardium in conscious dogs: Time course and relation to systolic function. Reprinted by permission of the American College of Cardiology. J. Am. Coll. Cardiol. *13*:185, 1989.)

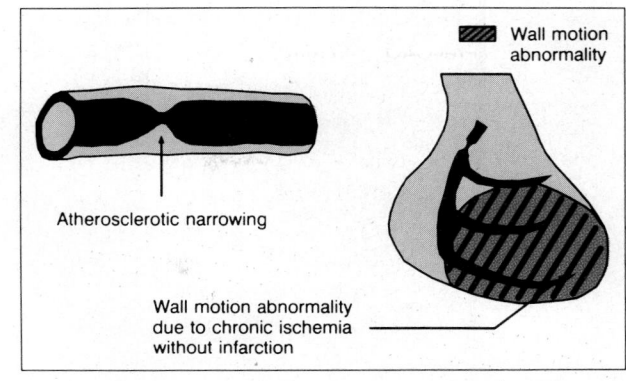

FIGURE 38–25. Schematic diagram of hibernating myocardium. Chronic ischemia without infarction results in a persistent regional wall motion abnormality. There is enough blood flow through the severe stenosis to allow for myocyte viability, but not enough to allow for normal contraction. The wall motion abnormality may be a protective mechanism whereby the left ventricle tries to reduce its oxygen demand in the setting of reduced oxygen supply. (From Kloner, R. A., Przyklenk, K., and Patel, B.: Altered myocardial states: The stunned and hibernating myocardium. Am. J. Med. **86**(Suppl. 1A):14, 1986.)

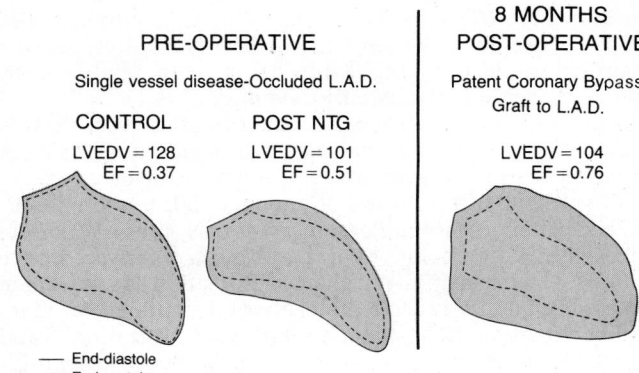

FIGURE 38–26. End-diastolic and end-systolic silhouettes of the left ventricle from the right anterior oblique contrast ventriculogram. In the preoperative studies, the ejection fraction (EF) in the control state was 0.37 and there was a large akinetic area involving the anteroapical wall. After nitroglycerin (NTG), there was an improvement of wall motion of the akinetic zone, and EF improved to 0.51. The patient had no history of myocardial infarction. Coronary arteriography showed one-vessel disease with a totally occluded left anterior descending coronary artery (LAD). The distal LAD was filled by collaterals from the circumflex coronary artery and the posterior descending coronary artery. Eight months postoperatively on routine study, the graft was fully patent and there was good filling of the LAD. The patient now shows normal left ventricular wall motion function and a normal ejection fraction of 0.76. LVEDV, Left ventricular end-diastolic volume. (From Rahimtoola, S. H.: Coronary bypass surgery for chronic angina—1981. Circulation **65**:225, 1982 by permission of the American Heart Association, Inc.)

integrated backscatter. Cardiac cycle–dependent variation of backscatter is depressed persistently in zones of infarction, whereas it is at least partially restored in stunned myocardium even before recovery of wall thickening is detectable echocardiographically.[212]

As judged from results of studies in patients with infarction treated with thrombolytic agents, in patients with angina, and in patients recovering from cardiopulmonary bypass, the duration of stunning is generally proportional to the duration of the preceding ischemia that is responsible.[213] In addition to local acidosis and accumulation of inorganic phosphate, increased intracellular sodium giving rise to excessive calcium uptake in myocardium subjected to ischemia has been impli-

cated.[214] As judged from studies of sarcoplasmic reticulum isolated from stunned tissue from hearts of dogs subjected to transitory coronary occlusion and reflow, impaired calcium uptake may contribute as well.[215] Inhibition of calcium influx into cells and competition for calcium binding sites appear to protect against stunning, as judged from results of laboratory studies with isolated perfused hearts.[216]

Metabolic abnormalities have been detected in stunned myocardium and implicated in its pathogenesis (Fig. 38–28). Although accumulation of oxygen-derived free radicals may occur through the xanthine-oxidase system in the hearts of experimental animals,[217] the absence of this system in human myocardium implicates other sources of free radicals in

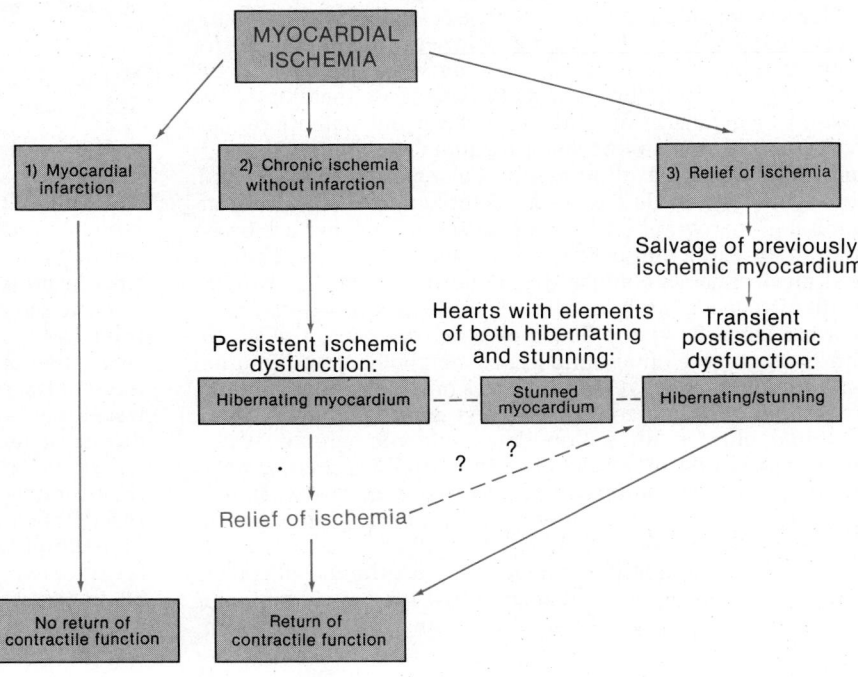

FIGURE 38–27. The three possible outcomes of myocardial ischemia. (From Kloner, R., et al.: Myocardial stunning and hibernation: Mechanisms and clinical implications. *In* Braunwald, E. (ed.): Heart Disease: A Textbook of Cardiovascular Medicine, 3rd ed. Philadelphia, W. B. Saunders Company. Update No. 11, p. 253, 1990.)

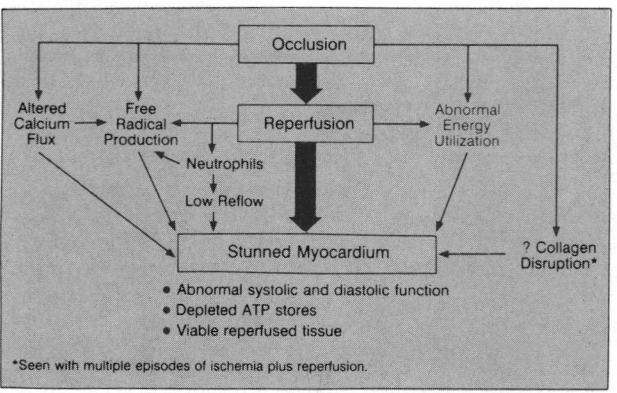

FIGURE 38–28. Potential mechanisms of stunned myocardium. (From Kloner, R. A., Przyklenk, K., and Patel, B.: Altered myocardial states: The stunned and hibernating myocardium. Am. J. Med. *86*(Suppl. 1A):14, 1986.)

human hearts. Infiltration of neutrophils into ischemic myocardium and consequent bombardment of the tissues with free radicals from activated white cells may be responsible for extending myocardial damage, in view of the diminution of apparent infarct size in dog hearts by prostacyclin analogs that inhibit neutrophil activation[218] and by free-radical scavengers.[219-223] Accumulating free radicals may contribute to stunning by direct attack on myocyte membranes resulting from lipid peroxidation, as judged from the protective effects of agents such as diltiazem that inhibit peroxidation without attenuating free-radical production in isolated perfused rabbit hearts.[224] Proarrhythmic effects that are manifested as reperfusion arrhythmias,[225] attenuation of vasodilator reserve,[226] and stunning may all be manifestations of free radical–induced injury accompanying ischemia. These effects may be attenuated by free-radical scavengers such as dimethylurea,[227] enzymes mediating catabolism of free radicals such as superoxide dismutase (SOD) and catalase,[228] and inhibitors of free-radical production.[229]

The contractility of stunned but viable myocardium can be stimulated by infused sympathomimetics.[230,231] However, it does not respond to sympathetic nerve stimulation.[232]

CLINICAL IMPLICATIONS OF STUNNING. The clinical importance of differentiating stunned from irreversibly injured myocardium cannot be overemphasized. If impaired ventricular performance is caused primarily by stunned myocardium, aggressive interventions designed to induce revascularization, including thrombolysis, angioplasty, and surgery, may be beneficial. Appropriate selection of patients for angiography and invasive intervention after attempted pharmacological thrombolysis rests in part on delineation of the extent of myocardium still in jeopardy but potentially salvageable. Several approaches are under development to facilitate differentiation of stunned from necrotic myocardium, including ultrasonic tissue characterization[212] and positron-emission tomography.[233-236] The latter approaches are based on the principle that persistent intermediary metabolism is a hallmark of persistent viability. Thus, in tomographic studies with nitrogen-13 ammonia ($^{13}NH_3$) (to estimate regional myocardial blood flow) and fluorine-18-deoxyglucose (^{18}FDG) (to measure glucose uptake and hence metabolism), wall motion abnormalities are reversible in areas in which glucose uptake is preserved before coronary bypass grafting.[233] In addition, residual glucose utilization detectable tomographically is often present despite fixed or only partially resolving stress thallium defects, underscoring the discordance between persistence of intermediary metabolism and apparent diminution of perfusion. Tomography is helpful in recognizing persistent aerobic oxidative metabolism with the use of tracers such as carbon-11–labeled acetate that may avoid ambiguities seen with tracers of aerobic and anaerobic metabolism combined, such as ^{18}FDG. In dogs with reperfusion after 15 minutes of myocardial ischemia, preservation of regional oxidative metabolism is detectable tomographically, as is oxidative metabolic reserve in stunned myocardium.

HEMODYNAMIC CONSEQUENCES OF ISCHEMIA

If sufficiently widespread, regional loss of myocardial contractile activity (whether sustained or transient) depresses overall left ventricular function, producing reductions of stroke volume, stroke work, cardiac output, and ejection fraction, while elevating ventricular of end-diastolic volume and pressure. Clinical evidence of heart failure occurs when regional asynergy is so severe and extensive that the uninvolved myocardium cannot sustain the excess load. Hemodynamic evidence of left ventricular failure develops when contraction ceases in 20 to 25 per cent of the left ventricle; with loss of 40 per cent or more of the left ventricular myocardium, severe pump failure ensues, and, if this loss is acute, fatal or near-fatal cardiogenic shock usually develops.

In patients with wall motion abnormalities secondary to coronary artery disease, maintenance of nearly normal regional myocardial oxygen consumption is a powerful predictor of subsequent resolution of regional wall motion abnormalities after revascularization, whereas preservation of glucose utilization before bypass grafting is of less predictive value.[235] The insensitivity of glucose utilization as a marker of persistent viability reflects the primary dependence of myocardial oxidative metabolism on fatty acid utilization[237] and the confounding effects of variable patterns of substrate utilization on the interpretation of tomographic images when labeled metabolites of carbohydrate utilization are used, as opposed to tracers of overall oxidative metabolism.[238-241]

Since the heart has virtually no stores of oxygen, its high rate of energy expenditure results in a sudden, striking decline of myocardial oxygen tension within seconds of coronary occlusion, coincident with the loss of contractility. During ischemia there is both a rightward shift and a reduction in the slope of the left ventricular end-diastolic pressure-volume relation.[242,243] The marginal zone contracts weakly, whereas the nonischemic myocardium exhibits a compensatory increase in its force of contraction. The rapid decline in contractility induced by ischemia cannot be attributed to alterations in excitability. Although the early stages of ischemia do not produce major changes in the amplitude and upstroke velocity of the action potential, the duration of the plateau phase of the action potential is shortened, which may signify a reduction in the slow inward current, carried largely by Ca^{++}.

Mechanism of Ischemic Impairment of Ventricular Contraction

The precise mechanism by which ischemia impairs left ventricular systolic function has not been defined. It is possible that ischemia reduces the release of Ca^{++} from the sarcolemma or the sarcoplasmic reticulum (SR)[244] or both and thereby interferes with the interaction of Ca^{++} with the contractile proteins. However, ischemic failure of cardiac contraction can occur despite normal or even elevated[245] intracellular Ca^{++} concentrations, and therefore ischemia must in some manner interfere with the ability of Ca^{++} to generate force in the myocardial cell.[246] During severe hypoxia the intracellular $[Ca^{++}]$ declines as contractility fails. In contrast, during ischemia $[Ca^{++}]$ usually rises, implying a reduced sensitivity to Ca^{++}.[247] One theory holds that the high intracellular $[H^+]$ induced by ischemia may compete with Ca^{++} for the receptors on the troponin molecules. Thus, the actin-myosin interaction is impaired, and it has been postulated that as a result of two processes, i.e., reduction of the sensitivity of the SR to any given concentration of Ca^{++} and competition between H^+ and Ca^{++} for the troponin receptor sites, contractility is reduced.[248] This idea is supported by the observations that the functional changes induced by primary acidosis in the face of adequate myocardial oxygenation are similar to those produced by ischemia[249] and that the reversal of acidosis by the administration of alkali improves contractile performance. In addition to the role played by intracellular [H+], minor reductions of ATP may be important. It is possible that the concentrations of high-energy phosphate compounds in critical locations—such as the SR or the sarcolemma (where ion fluxes and cell volume may be affected)—are reduced by ischemia even when the overall intracellular concentration of these compounds is still normal or near normal.

ISCHEMIA AND HIGH-ENERGY PHOSPHATE DEPLETION. Despite the fact that prolonged ischemia depletes ATP from myocardium, impairment of function after transitory ischemia is not closely correlated with depression of overall ATP content at the end of the ischemic interval. "Buffering" of ATP stores by phosphocreatine is one factor responsible for the disparity.[250] Results from studies of isolated perfused hearts with nuclear magnetic resonance (NMR) magnetization transfer indicate that despite reduction of the creatine kinase reaction velocity, high-energy phosphate transfer does not limit availability of high-energy phosphate for contraction.[251] In fact, impairment of mechanical function and diminution of the rate of oxidative metabolism are parallel even though tissue ATP content is sustained by dephosphorylation of phosphocreatine.[252] Thus, limitation of oxidative metabolic reserve is not responsible for depression of contractility in ischemic or stunned myocardium, as judged from the persistence of close coupling between contractile performance and oxidative metabolism.[252] However, when cells are subjected to profound or prolonged ischemia, or when profound ischemic injury is complicated by reperfusion and flooding of cellular organelles with calcium, postischemic oxidative capacity may be reduced and may limit the maximal postischemic mechanical performance obtainable.[253]

Effects of ischemia on myocardium lead within seconds to the loss of the capacity for development of tension. Phosphocreatine content also declines rapidly and may be marked within a few minutes; ATP content declines more slowly and is associated with progressive intracellular hypoxia and acidosis; and accumulation of intracellular sodium, calcium, and hydrogen ion is striking and associated with impaired compartmentalization of activator calcium available for initiation of contraction. Accumulation of amphipathic metabolites such as long-chain acyl carnitine and lysophospholipids, strongly implicated in the genesis of malignant arrhythmias, may impair mechanical performance as well. Excitation-contraction coupling can be affected adversely by oxygen-derived free radicals elaborated within myocardium or by neutrophils infiltrating ischemic zones.[254]

EFFECTS OF ISCHEMIA ON VENTRICULAR DIASTOLIC PROPERTIES. Myocardial ischemia and infarction alter not only the contractile properties of the heart but also the diastolic pressure-volume relations of the left ventricle. Myocardial ischemia impairs ventricular relaxation[255-256a] as evidenced by a decreased rate of left ventricular pressure decline (negative dP/dt) and ventricular wall thinning, and it prolongs the isovolumetric relaxation period.[255,256] The globally ischemic ventricle is less compliant than normal[255,257-258a] (Fig. 38-29). In the presence of regional ischemia, the reduction of compliance involves the ischemic region, while the behavior of the nonischemic region conforms to that described by a higher and steeper portion of the pressure-volume curve. These changes are exaggerated when ischemia is induced in hearts with pressure overload hypertrophy.[259] In turn, the ischemia-induced changes in diastolic properties increase the resistance to ventricular filling and together with the reduced systolic properties of the ventricle contribute to the elevation of left ventricular diastolic pressure during ischemia. The mechanism responsible for the ischemia-induced impairment of myocardial relaxation has not been fully

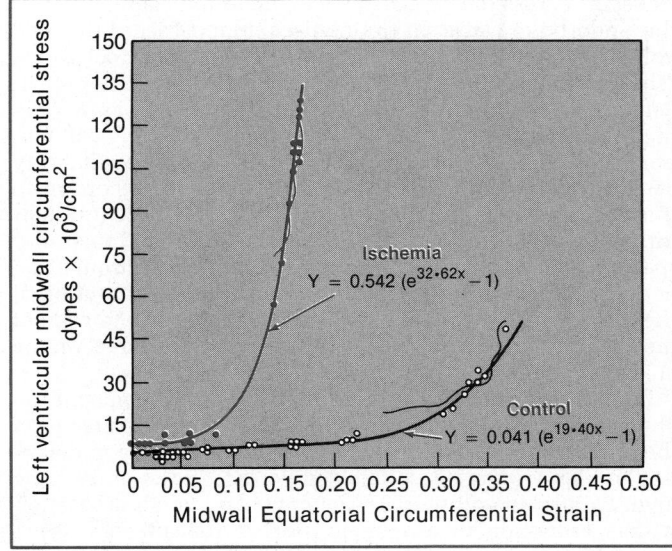

FIGURE 38-29. Diastolic pressure-strain and stress-strain relationships constructed from observations during control period and during ischemia. (From Visner, M. S., Arentzen, C. E., Parrish, D. G., Larson, E. V., O'Connor, M. J., Crumbley, A. J., III, Bache, R. J., and Anderson, R. W.: Effects of global ischemia on the diastolic properties of the left ventricle in the conscious dog. Circulation 71:616, 1985, by permission of the American Heart Association, Inc.)

elucidated, but it has been proposed that reductions of myocardial high-energy stores impair the rate of uptake of Ca^{++} from the vicinity of the myofilaments into the SR, thus prolonging contraction.[260] Ca^{++} channel blockade will antagonize this process and by diminishing Ca^{++} influx into the cell will lower cytosolic [Ca^{++}], restoring rapid relaxation. On the other hand, caffeine, an agent known to prolong Ca^{++} availability, potentiates the ischemia-induced impairment of ventricular relaxation. In addition to increases in myocardial stiffness induced by ischemia, alterations in ventricular diastolic properties may reflect protraction of systolic events locally with regionally delayed onset of relaxation (postsystolic contraction), passively decreased segmental lengthening corresponding to a decrease in segmental shortening preceding it, regionally nonuniform loading conditions, and changes in coronary vascular pressure and chamber geometry.[261-264]

Ischemia thus causes impairment of cardiac contraction and incomplete ventricular emptying (systolic failure). In addition, it impairs ventricular relaxation and shifts the diastolic pressure-volume curve upward (diastolic failure). The combination of systolic and diastolic failure leads to elevated ventricular filling pressures, ultimately causing symptoms of pulmonary congestion.

ELECTROPHYSIOLOGICAL CONSEQUENCES OF ISCHEMIA

ST-SEGMENT CHANGES IN THE DETECTION OF ISCHEMIA. It has been known for more than a half century that ST-segment elevation is an electrocardiographic sign of coronary artery occlusion. Within 30 to 60 seconds after occlusion in dogs with open chests, epicardial leads from within the area of cyanosis show ST-segment elevation, reaching a maximum 5 to 7 minutes after occlusion. ST-segment elevation in the central area of cyanosis is usually more marked than at the periphery. With the use of small intracavitary electrodes, simultaneous ST-segment elevation is also noted on the endocardial surface, although it is less marked than that recorded on the epicardium.

The electrophysiological basis of ST-segment changes in myocardial ischemia is discussed on page 137; altered ion transport across the myocardial cell membrane apparently is the underlying cause. In the nonischemic myocardium, cell volume is regulated within narrow limits by the sarcolemmal "sodium pump" (p. 592). This active, metabolically dependent pump maintains a high extracellular [Na$^+$] as well as high intracellular [K$^+$] and colloids, thus stabilizing cell volume. It has been postulated that with ischemia the availability of energy necessary for this pumping is reduced. According to this concept Na$^+$, accompanied by Cl$^-$ and H$_2$O, accumulates intracellularly and K$^+$ begins to leak into the extracellular space. The reduction in intracellular [K$^+$] or the accumulation of extracellular [K$^+$] or both are critical in the generation of the elevated ST segment, since small changes in the ratio of intracellular to extracellular [K$^+$] have a marked effect on the polarity of cellular membranes.

Interpretation of ST-Segment Elevations. The magnitude of epicardial ST-segment elevation generally correlates with the decrease in blood flow, lactate accumulation, and depletion of high-energy phosphate compounds in the underlying myocardium. In addition, ST-segment elevation is associated with a reduction in oxygen tension in the affected tissue below 65 per cent of control,[265] and the magnitude of the elevation correlates with intramyocardial oxygen tension. Measurements with a mass spectrometer have shown that intramyocardial ST-segment elevations are correlated with changes in myocardial gas tensions. Also, epicardial ST-segment elevations shortly after coronary artery occlusion correlate closely with subsequent depletion of myocardial creatine phosphokinase (CK) activity and with histological evidence of necrosis in the subjacent myocardium.[266] It is now clear that the distribution of *epicardial* ST-segment elevation provides an approximation of the extent of myocardial ischemia, but that the *intramyocardial* ST segment is a more sensitive index than the epicardial. However, it must be appreciated that ST-segment elevation, wherever measured, is not specific for myocardial ischemia, since the ST segment is also affected by changes in temperature, by drugs (including the digitalis glycosides and quinidine), by sympathetic stimulation of the heart, by epicardial injury due to pericarditis, and by localized intraventricular conduction defects.[267]

ALTERATIONS IN CELLULAR ELECTROPHYSIOLOGY INDUCED BY ISCHEMIA

The effects of ischemia on the electrophysiological properties of cardiac muscle are numerous and complex. Ischemia-induced ventricular tachyarrhythmias can be caused by increased automaticity (p. 603), triggered activity (p. 604), and reentry (p. 607). The early electrophysiological hallmarks of ischemia include a marked diminution in resting membrane potential, action potential amplitude, rate of upstroke of phase 0, and action potential duration. Activation of ATP-sensitive K$^+$ channels appears to be responsible for the latter. Within 10 minutes of ischemia, action potential alterations in amplitude and duration (2:1 alternans) become prominent, with subsequent diminution of excitability and conduction block. Although excitability may return transiently, it is generally persistently absent after 30 minutes of ischemia. Initially, the refractory period of cells in ischemic zones decreases, but with ischemia lasting for several minutes it lengthens and exceeds the duration of refractoriness in nonischemic tissue. Consequently, heterogeneity of refractoriness and postrepolarization refractoriness are prominent. These phenomena may account for continuous electrical activity spanning the interval between a normal sinus beat and a ventricular ectopic beat.[254] Although conduction velocity may increase transiently early after the onset of ischemia, it declines within 3 to 5 minutes as a result of hypoxia, acidosis, and increased intracellular calcium.[254] Initially, changes in passive membrane properties may contribute to the electrophysiologic effects induced first by ischemia increasing extracellular longitudinal resistance reflecting volume shifts and subsequently

by increased intracellular longitudinal resistance with irreversible uncoupling of cells.[269]

REENTRY ARRHYTHMIAS (see also p. 609). The development of conduction delay contributes to spatial inhomogeneity of electrophysiological alterations along with disparities in refractory period duration. These alterations predispose to development of arrhythmias reflecting reentry caused by slow conduction and unidirectional block combined with delayed activation and inhomogeneous recovery of excitability.

ABNORMAL AUTOMATICITY (see also p. 603). Ventricular arrhythmias associated with ischemia may reflect nonreentrant mechanisms as well,[270] such as abnormal automaticity favored by diminished negativity of resting membrane potentials and triggered activity precipitated by early or delayed afterdepolarizations. The rapid reversibility of both types of electrophysiological alterations by prompt restoration of perfusion and the lack of concomitant morphological manifestations of myocyte injury under such circumstances suggest that subtle biochemical derangements accompanying brief ischemia are responsible. Accumulation of specific metabolites and ions has been implicated. Thus, electrophysiological derangements underlying malignant arrhythmias induced by ischemia appear to depend on the accumulation of toxic metabolites as well as on lack of oxygen for energy production itself.[271]

EFFECTS OF ISCHEMIA ON THE SARCOLEMMA. The function of the sarcolemma is exquisitely dependent on its structural integrity. Disruption of sarcolemma secondary to ischemia appears to reflect altered lipid metabolism. The generation of amphipathic metabolites such as long-chain acyl carnitine and lysophosphatidyl choline (LPC) as a result of impairment of beta-oxidation of fatty acids, the activation of phospholipases, and the inhibition of enzymes that catalyze catabolism of LPC appear to be responsible.[271] Such metabolites are toxic because their combined hydrophobic and hydrophilic (amphiphilic) properties endow them with detergent-like properties. Their presence, in even minute concentrations in the sarcolemma, alters the behavior of ion channels, the activity of membrane-associated receptors, and thereby the electrophysiological properties of the sarcolemma.[270] Thus, exposure of normoxic myocytes to amphiphiles induces electrophysiological derangements comparable to those induced by ischemia. Induction of ventricular fibrillation early after the onset of ischemia can be prevented by pharmacological inhibition of accumulation of amphiphiles in hearts of experimental animals.[272]

Arrhythmias occur in three phases in dogs with coronary occlusion.[158,159]

THE EARLY PERIOD. This phase begins almost immediately after coronary ligation, frequently culminates in ventricular fibrillation within 3 to 6 minutes, and usually lasts less than 30 minutes. Within minutes after coronary occlusion, marked alterations occur in the electrophysiological properties of ventricular myocardial cells, with shortening of action potential duration and refractoriness, decreased amplitude, upstroke velocity, and resting potential. Extracellular recordings from the epicardial surface of the ischemic zone show marked loss of amplitude and delay and fractionation of recorded electrograms, suggesting that activation in the myocardium is irregular and that the effects of ischemia are heterogeneous.

Initially after coronary occlusion, conduction velocity increases presumably related to the increase in extracellular K$^+$ (which may also contribute to the abbreviation of the action potential). Subsequently, conduction velocity slows. Available evidence suggests that inhomogeneities in the conduction velocity and in the shortening of the refractory period create the conditions necessary for reentry, which in turn is responsible for ventricular tachycardia and ventricular fibrillation early during ischemia.[272a] The cause of ventricular premature beats is less clear but may be related to the triggering of automatic activity by the current of injury.

This early arrhythmic phase observed in experimental animals could be related to the "prehospital" phase of arrhythmias observed in patients, which is also marked by a high incidence of ventricular fibrillation and sudden death. The arrhythmias of the early phase are intimately rate-related. Thus, vagally induced cardiac slowing can avert or abort ectopic ventricular rhythms. Conversely, ectopic ventricular rhythm can be induced by cardiac pacing.

Regional myocardial sympathetic stimulation appears to contribute to early malignant ventricular arrhythmia. During ischemia, beta-adrenoceptors are redistributed from intracellular vesicles to the sarcolemma. This may enhance the response of the ischemic myocardium to sympathomimetics, causing arrhythmia, increase of MVO_2, and extension of the ischemic zone. Sympathectomy and beta-adrenoceptor blockade mitigate both the regional augmentation of cyclic AMP and the frequency and severity of the early phase of ventricular arrhythmias.[273] On the other hand, the effectiveness of antiarrhythmic drugs such as quinidine and lidocaine during the early phase has been questioned.

THE INTERMEDIATE PERIOD IN THE DOG. After a period of quiescence, a delayed arrhythmic phase begins at about 6 to 9 hours following coronary occlusion in the dog and lasts for 24 to 72 hours. During this period spontaneous polymorphic ventricular rhythms occur, but ventricular fibrillation is uncommon. Multiple electrophysiological mechanisms are probably involved in the delayed arrhythmic phase, particularly abnormal automaticity of subendocardial Purkinje fibers. This phase may correspond to ventricular tachycardia and "accelerated idioventricular rhythms" (p. 706) commonly seen on the second and third days following infarction in humans. Antiarrhythmic drugs such as quinidine, procainamide, lidocaine, and disopyramide suppress these arrhythmias by reducing automaticity.

THE LATE PHASE. By 72 hours after coronary ligation in the dog, the spontaneous polymorphic ventricular rhythms have nearly subsided, but the heart is still prone to ventricular tachyarrhythmias and, occasionally, ventricular fibrillation.[274] These arrhythmias may be easily induced by rapid cardiac pacing or programmed premature stimulation[275] and may be the result of reentrant circuits in the subepicardial layer of the infarction, including the boundary zone between the infarction and surrounding viable myocardium. This late phase of ventricular vulnerability may correspond to the "post-coronary care unit" ventricular arrhythmias and late in-hospital ventricular fibrillation. Antiarrhythmic drugs, such as lidocaine or procainamide, appear to abolish these late reentrant arrhythmias by further depression or block of the already slowed conduction in the reentrant circuit. Electrophysiological abnormalities persist for long periods after myocardial infarction. These may be responsible, in part, for the prolonged increased risk of sudden death in such patients.

REPERFUSION ARRHYTHMIAS. There has been considerable interest in the mechanism of ventricular arrhythmias that occur with release of coronary occlusion and reperfusion (whether induced or spontaneous). Ventricular fibrillation is likely to occur abruptly without warning following reperfusion, whereas it is often heralded by ventricular ectopic beats with increasing frequency after occlusion. Chemical and electrical gradients caused by washout of metabolites and electrolytes that have accumulated in the ischemic zone are probably responsible for the electrophysiological derangement responsible for reperfusion arrhythmias.[276] Reperfusion is accompanied by changes in regional concentrations of K^+, Ca^{++}, H^+, catecholamines, and lysophosphoglycerides; the last are derived from degradation of membrane phospholipids in cells undergoing infarction.[277] Since the free-radical scavenger superoxide dismutase can protect the heart from reperfusion arrhythmias, these substances may also be important in its generation.[278] Reperfusion arrhythmias are more common in experimental animals such as the dog and pig. However, while they are less common in patients, the occasional abrupt onset of ventricular fibrillation in those with coronary occlusion and myocardial infarction who are undergoing thrombolytic, mechanical, or spontaneous reperfusion and in those with Prinzmetal's angina at the termination of an episode of coronary spasm is a clinical example of reocclusion arrhythmia.

BIOCHEMICAL MECHANISMS OF ELECTROPHYSIOLOGICAL DERANGEMENTS INDUCED BY ISCHEMIA. Physiological changes have not been identified with certainty. Ischemia depresses the energy-dependent sarcolemmal Na pump, which leads to a gain in intracellular Na^+ and loss of intracellular K^+ with consequent elevation of extracellular K^+ concentration in the vicinity of the sarcolemma, and augmented intracellular Ca^{++} secondary to increased Na/Ca exchange.[279] As a result of anaerobic metabolism, intracellular pH declines. Ischemia also results in release of norepinephrine from adrenergic nerve endings and an increase of tissue levels of cyclic AMP. Although it has been postulated that in the ischemic zone high concentrations of extracellular K^+ may depolarize the cells to the extent that the rapid Na^+ channel is inactivated, and high concentrations of catecholamines may stimulate the slow current carried principally by Ca^{++}, resulting in slow response action potentials, slowed conduction and reentrant ventricular arrhythmias associated with ischemia are more likely to reflect depression of the rapid Na inward current.[254]

It is less likely that slow response action potentials are responsible for ischemia-induced electrophysiological disturbances in the later stage of myocardial infarction. The extracellular $[K^+]$ is probably not as high as in the early stage of ischemia. Besides, total catecholamines in the ischemic region decline to a very low level on the day after coronary occlusion. However, ischemic myocardium still shows markedly depressed action

potentials, slow conduction, and a high propensity for reentrant rhythms. In the later stage of ischemia, ischemic myocardial cells have been found to be exquisitely sensitive to the depressant effect of tetrodotoxin, a specific blocker of the fast Na^+ channel, and not to verapamil and D600, which are blockers of the slow Ca^{++} channel. These observations suggest that poor membrane responses of ischemic myocardial cells are related to depression of the fast Na^+ channel. The clinical relevance of studies of ischemia-induced ionic conductance changes relates to the choice of ideal antiarrhythmic therapy following ischemia. Thus, the antiarrhythmic effect of lidocaine on ischemia-induced reentrant ventricular arrhythmias (pp. 633 and 639) may be due to selective depression of ischemic myocardial cells forming part of the reentrant pathway. The finding that the effect of lidocaine on depressed ischemic cells is similar to that of tetrodotoxin suggests that lidocaine acts by further depressing the Na^+ channel in ischemic cells.

EFFECTS OF ISCHEMIA ON MYOCARDIAL METABOLISM

HIGH-ENERGY PHOSPHATE METABOLISM. During the first minutes of severe ischemia, the production of high-energy phosphates (the sum of ATP and creatine phosphate [CP]) declines and is greatly exceeded by their utilization (Figs. 38–30 and 38–31). Therefore, tissue stores decline progressively, with CP stores falling more rapidly than ATP stores. CP is depleted by transfer of high-energy phosphate to ADP as oxidative synthesis of ATP declines. In the absence of normal oxidative phosphorylation, ADP is converted to AMP (in the myokinase reaction), which in turn is broken down to adenosine and ultimately to inosine, hypoxanthine, and xanthine (Fig. 38–9, p. 1169).[280] When ATP content is reduced below 20 per cent of control values, cells become unable to regenerate high-energy phosphate, to maintain physiological ionic gradients, and to control their volume. The combination of reduced myocardial high-energy phosphate stores, cell swelling, and sarcolemmal damage (attributable potentially to oxygen-derived free radical attack with lipid peroxidation and the effects of accumulating amphipathic metabolites) appears to play a key role in cell death with ischemia or reperfusion (Fig. 38–32). When tissue is only *reversibly* injured by ischemia (i.e., when its viability can still be maintained by reperfusion), ATP stores are usually greater than 60 per cent of control and electronmicroscopy may reveal only glycogen loss, nuclear chromatin clumping, intermyofibrillar edema, and mitochondrial swelling but no sarcolemmal damage or accumulation of amorphous dense bodies in the mitochondria. Reduction of ATP below 30 per cent is usually associated with visible sarcolemmal damage and irreversible injury (i.e., the tissue is not viable despite reperfusion).

Phosphorus-31 NMR spectroscopy permits multiple sequential assessments of the same tissue and correlation of high-energy phosphate stores with mechanical activity. Both the magnitude of intracellular acidosis and associated increase in inorganic phosphate have been shown to correlate inversely with postischemic recovery of function; ATP but not CP content has been shown to correlate with return of contractile function after reperfusion.[281]

INTERMEDIARY METABOLISM IN ISCHEMIA (Fig. 38–33)

Under physiological conditions, myocardium derives most of its energy from oxidative phosphorylation, a process localized to the mitochondria. Oxidation of fatty acids predominates. When oxygen availability is limited, the rate of ATP synthesis declines, regeneration of ATP from ADP and phosphocreatine decreases, and ultimately, high-energy phosphate stores decline. Results of NMR spectroscopic studies indicate that the ratio of phosphocreatine to creatine is an index of energy reserve[282] and that energy production and consumption remain balanced when contractile reserve is taxed.[283] The diminution of contractility induced by ischemia reflects a limited turnover of high-energy phosphate stores[284,285] rather than reduction of total cellular content of ATP itself, until and unless ischemia is profound and sustained.[286] However, even intermittent ischemia depletes the mitochondria of adenine nucleotides[287] and may therefore limit oxidative metabolic reserve. After intense, transitory ischemia, the depletion of adenine nucleotides may persist for hours to days, in part

FIGURE 38-30. Principal reactions producing and utilizing high-energy phosphates (HEP) in ischemic tissue. The width of the arrows indicates the estimated quantitative importance of the various reactions. In severe ischemia, aerobic respiration is abolished. The preexisting stores of HEP, in the form of creatine phosphate (CP) or ATP, are relatively small. Thus, anaerobic glycolysis becomes the principal source of energy, producing 80 to 90 per cent of the HEP bonds that can be utilized by severely ischemic tissue. Substrate-level phosphorylation of α-ketoglutarate in the mitochondria does not require oxygen, but the tissue content of substrates that can be shuttled to α-ketoglutarate is small. Energy utilized also is markedly reduced during ischemia. Cardiac contraction, which is mediated by Ca++ activated myofibrillar ATPase, consumes much of the ATP produced in aerobic myocardium. However, contraction is abolished or severely depressed in areas of severe ischemia. Nevertheless, ATP continues to be required to remove Na+ from the cell, to keep Ca++ sequestered in the sarcoplasmic reticulum, and for a variety of other cellular processes that may continue to compete for the remaining ATP. (From Jennings, R. B., and Reimer, K. A.: Lethal myocardial ischemic injury. Am. J. Pathol. *102*:241, 1981.)

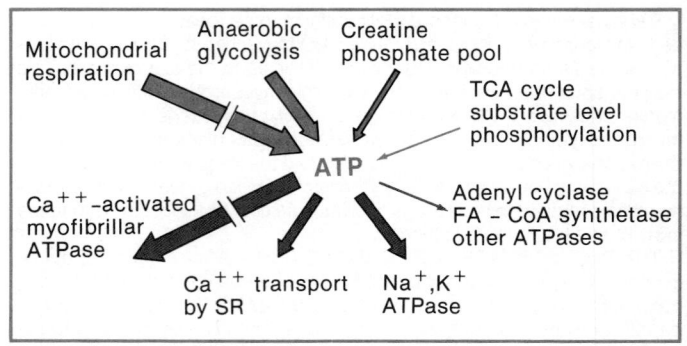

because of the limited capacity of myocardium for de novo purine synthesis. Depletion of adenine nucleotides may *contribute* to (but does not appear to be the cause of) stunning of myocardium, because recovery of segmental function with reperfusion is associated with restoration of high-energy phosphate stores.[287]

CARBOHYDRATE METABOLISM. During hypoxia, glycolytic flux increases, as does the uptake of glucose. There is evidence for functional compartmentalization of anaerobic glycolytic versus oxidative metabolism. Energy from glycolysis preferentially supports sarcolemmal function, whereas oxidative phosphorylation preferentially supports contractile function.[288] However, anaerobic glycolysis alone can meet myocardial energy requirements only transiently, even though augmentation of glycolytic flux by provision of glucose or prior augmentation of glycogen stores confers some resistance to the deterioration of function induced by anoxia or ischemia.[289] The persistence of anaerobic glycolytic flux may account for observations made with positron-emission tomography of patients in which metabolism/flow mismatches (persistence of uptake of [18]FDG despite diminished accumulation of [13]NH3 reflecting decreased perfusion) were seen in ischemic but presumably still viable myocardium[290,291,291a,291b] (p. 1301). However, tomographic documentation of viability may be provided more definitively by delineation of persistent oxidative metabolism, ascertainable by positron tomography with carbon-11-labeled acetate, which presages recovery of regional wall motion with reperfusion[235,238-241] (Fig. 38-34).

THE ROLE OF LACTATE. Lactate accumulates during ischemia, because oxidation of pyruvate is precluded by the inhibition of the tricarboxylic acid cycle, and washout of metabolites is reduced because of the limited perfusion. The initial burst of glycolytic activity accompanying hypoxia with or without ischemia appears to depend on allosteric effects of adenine nucleotides and other regulators of enzymes such as phosphorylase b, hexokinase, and phosphofructokinase.[292] However, under conditions of limited perfusion sufficient to induce hypoxia, the rapidly increasing concentration of lactic acid within the cell, the decline of pH, and the accumulation of other metabolites inhibit glycolytic flux at the phosphofructokinase and glyceraldehyde-3-phosphate dehydrogenase[292] steps, among others (Fig. 38-33).

In isolated perfused hearts, lactate exerts a deleterious effect on glycolytic flux independent of pH[190] by inhibiting the glyceraldehyde-phosphate dehydrogenase reaction, which is responsible for conversion of glyceraldehyde-3-phosphate to 1,2-diphosphoglyceric acid. On the other hand, acidosis itself inhibits glycolytic flux and the malate-aspartate cycle.[293] Persistent or prolonged ischemia results in inhibition of this and other shuttle reactions because of accumulation of reducing equivalents in the

FIGURE 38-31. Time course of metabolic changes during myocardial ischemia plotted by transmural layer (I = inner, subendocardial; M = middle; O = outer, subepicardial). Ischemia was induced by circumflex occlusion in anesthetized dogs. Data for different times are based on different groups of dogs; N = 4 to 6; brackets indicate plus or minus one standard error of the mean. *A*, More rapid depletion of ATP in the inner layer, highly significant after 5 min of ischemia ($p < 0.01$). *B*, Tissue lactate accumulation, with the most rapid accumulation in the subendocardium. For all layers there was a progressive increase in lactate content during the first 10 min of ischemia. Between 10 and 40 min there was continued lactate accumulation in the inner and middle layers, but not in the outer layer. *C*, Total adenine nucleotide content (ATP + ADP + AMP). Adenine nucleotide degradation was most rapid in the subendocardium. Note the time lag between ATP depletion (graph A) and adenine nucleotide breakdown. *D*, Total nucleosides and bases, which are the products of adenine nucleotide degradation. Accumulation was fastest in the subendocardium.

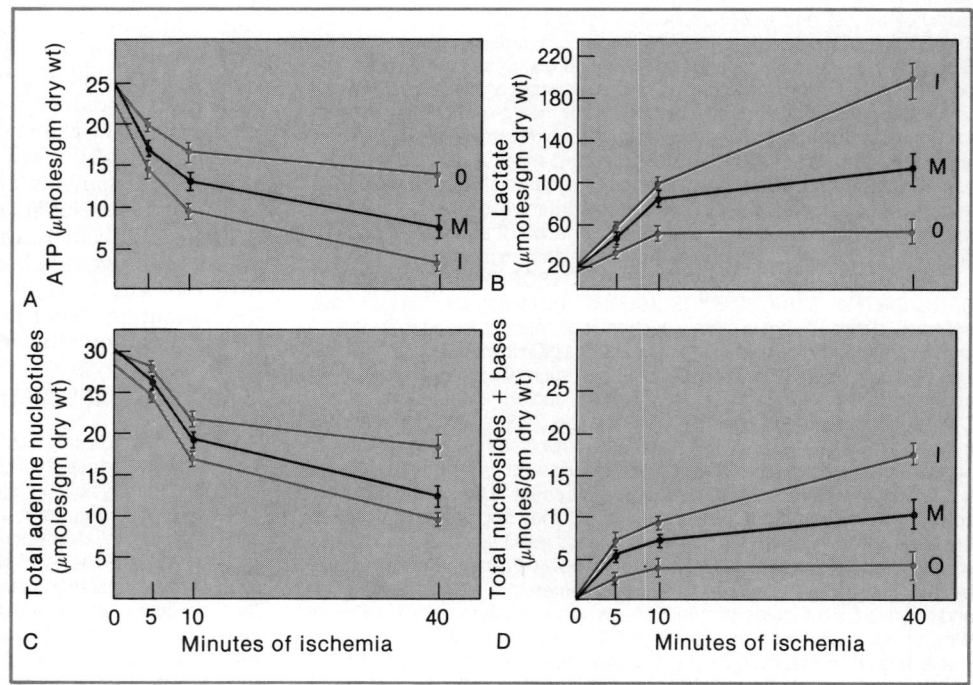

As with lactate (graph B), nucleoside and base content in the outer layer was maximal by 10 minutes and was not further increased at 40 minutes, even though adenine nucleotide breakdown in this layer continued (graph C). (From Reimer, K. A., and Jennings, R. B.: Myocardial ischemia, hypoxia and infarction. *In* Fozzard, H. A., Jennings, R. B., Haber, E., Katz, A. M., and Morgan, H. E. [eds.]: The Heart and Cardiovascular System. New York, Raven Press, 1986, p. 1144. From the studies of Murry, C. E. et al.: Collateral blood flow and transmural location: Independent determinants of ATP in ischemic canine myocardium. Fed. Proc. *44*:823, 1985.)

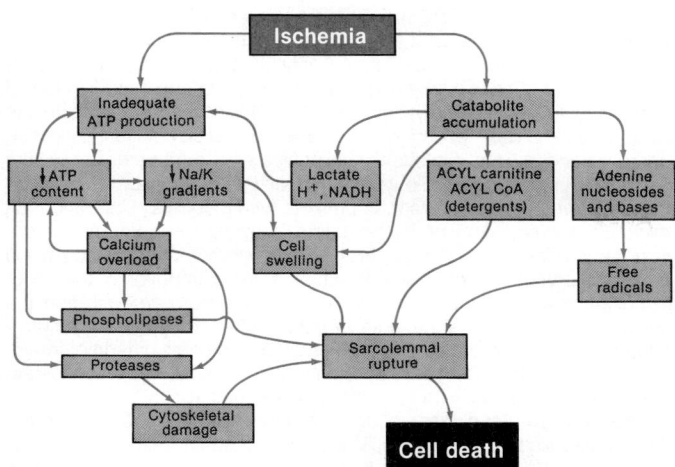

FIGURE 38-32. Some potential pathways leading to sarcolemmal damage, which form the basis for various hypotheses of events leading to irreversible ischemic cell injury. Two major facets of ischemia are the inadequate production of ATP and the accumulation of potentially noxious catabolites. Declining ATP content could have many adverse consequences including loss of sodium and potassium gradients, calcium overload, and activation of endogenous phospholipases or proteases. The latter could damage the sarcolemma and/or its cytoskeletal supports. Accumulation of catabolites such as lactate, H⁻, and NADH inhibits anaerobic glycolysis and thereby inhibits ATP production in ischemia. Products of lipid degradation may act as detergents and damage cell membranes. Adenine nucleosides and bases accumulate and might be a major source of free radicals via the xanthine oxidase reaction. In addition, accumulating catabolites are an intracellular osmotic load that may accentuate cell swelling and facilitate the rupture of already weakened membranes. The relative importance of these various pathways in the pathogenesis of ischemic cell death has not been established. Moreover, many reactions occur in ischemic myocardium which have been less well studied and are not included on this diagram; it is not even certain that the most important assays are illustrated. (From Reimer, K. A., and Jennings, R. B.: Myocardial ischemia, hypoxia and infarction. *In* Fozzard, H. A., Jennings, R. B., Haber, E., Katz, A. M., and Morgan, H. E. [eds.]: The Heart and Cardiovascular System. New York, Raven Press, 1986, p. 1163.)

mitochondria (due to the lack of oxygen as a terminal electron and hydrogen receptor), with consequent acidosis and accumulation of metabolites that inhibit glycolytic flux. When flux is sufficiently inhibited, ischemic contracture results.[289]

The relationship between lactate production and the severity of impaired perfusion can be exploited diagnostically. Under physiological aerobic conditions, myocardium extracts lactate from the arterial blood with extraction fractions in the range of 20 per cent. In normal subjects, extraction persists despite acceleration of ventricular rate by pacing. However, when myocardial ischemia is present at rest or develops in response to stress induced by pacing or other physiological stimuli, lactate extraction declines or is replaced by net lactate production. Dual carbon-labeled isotopic experiments have demonstrated that in patients with coronary artery disease simultaneous lactate production and extraction can occur. During a pacing stress test, significant lactate release occurs even in the presence of net lactate extraction. Unfortunately, relationships between the concentrations of lactate in coronary sinus blood and in extracellular fluid, cytosol, and mitochondrial compartments are complex and are influenced by nonspecific factors such as acid-base balance, adrenergic stimulation of the heart, substrate availability, permeability of cell membranes to lactate and pyruvate, concomitant disorders such as diabetes mellitus, and prevailing levels of plasma free fatty acids. Thus, net lactate extraction is a relatively insensitive index of changes occurring in localized regions of the heart.

DIFFERENCES BETWEEN ISCHEMIA AND ANOXIA

A number of important differences exist between anoxia and ischemia.[1] Not only is oxidative metabolism reduced during ischemia, as it is in anoxia, but the anaerobic production of ATP also proceeds at less than maximal capacity. In the ischemic working heart the concentration of lactic acid rises and the intracellular pH falls rapidly as the acid products of glycolysis accumulate. In contrast, in the anoxic heart perfusion results in the washout of the acid products of glycolysis, thereby retarding the rate of development of intracellular acidosis. The increased lactate production is not sustained by the ischemic heart, which has a glycolytic rate about one-fourth that of the anoxic heart in a steady state. This is unrelated to a reduction of substrate availability. Thus, the addition of insulin and glucose to the perfusion medium fails to stimulate glycolysis to the extent observed in anoxia or under normal aerobic conditions. While insulin and elevated glucose in the perfusate are able to increase glucose transport and augment the intracellular glucose concentration, they do not prevent ischemia from inhibiting glucose utilization.

FIGURE 38-33. Effects of ischemia on glycolysis and free fatty acid metabolism. Ischemia increases intracellular lactate concentration; this accumulation inhibits several enzymes in the glycolytic pathway: Phosphofructokinase (*A*); hexokinase (*B*); and phosphorylase kinase (*C*), which prevents activation of phosphorylase b to phosphorylase a and therefore suppresses conversion of glycogen to glucose-1-phosphate. Glyceraldehyde-3-phosphate dehydrogenase (*D*) is suppressed by an elevation of intracellular lactate. (* denotes that the glycolytic pathway has been condensed at this point.) Ischemia increases the intracellular concentration of acyl CoA esters, in part because the intracellular accumulation of lactate inhibits carnitine palmityl coenzyme A transferase (*E*), the enzyme that catalyzes the transfer of acyl CoA from the cell cytoplasm to the mitochondria. Acyl CoA esters inhibit the effective exchange of ADP and ATP between the cytoplasm of the cell and the mitochondria by suppressing the activity of adenine nucleotide translocase (*F*). The antilipolytic agents are effective because they prevent a build-up of acyl CoA esters within the cytoplasm, and 1-carnitine exerts a salutary effect on ischemic myocardium by reversing the inhibition of adenine nucleotide translocase, thus allowing continued movement of ADP and ATP between the cell cytoplasm and the mitochondria. (TCA = tricarboxylic acid.) (Reproduced with permission from Hillis, L. D., and Braunwald, E.: Myocardial ischemia. N. Engl. J. Med. *296*:971, 1034, and 1093; 1977.)

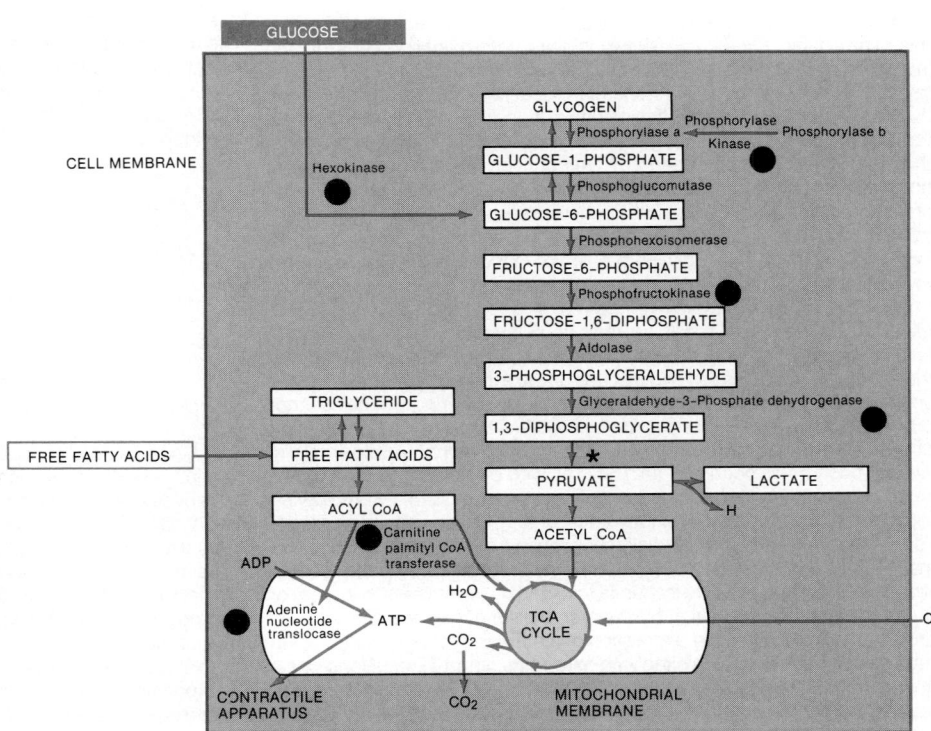

Figure 38-34. See color plate 6

The lower glycolytic flux in the ischemic as compared with the anoxic heart probably results in part from the inhibition by intracellular acidosis of PFK (Fig. 38-33), a key enzyme in the glycolytic chain. The importance of intracellular pH is further supported by the observation that pretreatment of rat myocardium to an alkaline pH of 7.9 maintains tension during a subsequent period of hypoxia.

In ischemic as opposed to anoxi perfused myocardium, accumulation of metabolites other than hydrogen ion, such as long-chain acyl carnitine (due to inhibition of β-oxidation of fatty acids) and lysophospholipids (due to activation of phospholipases and inhibition of enzymes responsible for lysophospholipid metabolism,[294-296] is likely to contribute not only to electrophysiological impairment and arrhythmogenesis but also to depression of mechanical performance and progression of injury in ischemic myocardium.

FATTY ACID METABOLISM IN ISCHEMIA

Under normal aerobic conditions, 60 to 90 per cent of myocardial energy requirements is met by oxidation of free fatty acids (FFA),[297] which are trapped in cells in the form of fatty (acyl) esters containing coenzyme A (acyl-CoA). The preferential utilization of FFA by myocardium appears to depend on the high activity of several enzyme systems, including the acyl-CoA-carnitine transferase systems that facilitate continuing transport of acyl-CoA from the cytosol to the mitochondria in a series of steps in which acyl-CoA and acyl-carnitine are interconverted.

After fatty acids are taken up by myocardial cells and undergo esterification with CoA, the acyl-CoA intermediates generally remain trapped in the cell. Acyl-CoA may be incorporated into triglycerides in the cytosol or oxidized after transport through the mitochondrial membrane. Under aerobic conditions, oxidation predominates since the products formed (two carbon moieties called acetyl groups) are readily incorporated as intermediates into the citric acid cycle and oxidized to carbon dioxide and water. Oxidation of fatty acids inhibits glucose uptake, glycolytic flux, and glycogenolysis. The increased production of acetyl-CoA accompanying fatty acid oxidation inhibits pyruvate dehydrogenase, thereby limiting the flow of carbohydrate metabolism through the citric acid cycle. Accumulation of glucose-6-phosphate inhibits hexokinase, decreasing phosphorylation of glucose. The decreased phosphorylation, coupled with direct inhibition of membrane transport of glucose mediated by fatty acids, contributes to the overall reduction of carbohydrate metabolism when fatty acid availability is high and oxygenation adequate.

Striking changes in fatty acid metabolism result from myocardial ischemia. The limited supply of oxygen inhibits beta-oxidation — as do the increased ratio of NADH/NAD and the reduced concentration of flavoproteins.[292] With more prolonged ischemia, oxidation of fatty acids is inhibited by another mechanism: inhibition or loss of long-chain acyl-carnitine transferase enzyme activity, necessary for transport of cytosolic acyl-CoA to the mitochondria before oxidation.[297] Accordingly, intracellular concentrations of acyl-CoA increase and acetyl-CoA content declines.[298] The increased acyl-CoA accompanied by increased production of glycerol, a byproduct of the enhanced glycolytic flux induced by ischemia, leads to increased synthesis of triglycerides, which accumulate in the ischemic myocardium.

INTRAMYOCARDIAL ACCUMULATION OF ACYL-CoA IN ISCHEMIA. Accumulation of acyl-CoA may be deleterious because it inhibits further formation of CoA esters of fatty acids. Thus, fatty acids entering the cell cannot be esterified and trapped and are therefore prone to egress promptly. Furthermore, oxidation of fatty acids entering the cell cannot proceed without initial esterification with CoA. Accordingly, accumulation of fatty acid labeled with carbon-11, which can be monitored externally in vivo by positron tomography (p. 1347) or with other tracers,[299] is diminished in ischemic or hypoxic zones. Restored metabolism accompanying reperfusion implemented promptly enough to maintain cell viability is reflected by a return of myocardial accumulation of fatty acid toward normal,[300] although the return of recovery may sometimes be prolonged. In working hearts subjected to ischemia followed by reperfusion, recovery of function cannot be sustained by the metabolism of glucose alone but, in fact, appears to depend on restoration of metabolism of fatty acids. When fatty acid metabolism is inhibited with oxfenicine, an inhibitor of long-chain acyl carnitine transferase activity,[301] ischemia followed by reperfusion results in profound stunning with concordant reduction of myocardial oxygen consumption despite increased oxidation of glucose. These results are consistent with the known coupling between diminished fatty acid oxidation and decreased function in ischemic myocardium.[299]

ISCHEMIA-INDUCED DEFECTS IN FATTY ACID METABOLISM. Detection of altered fatty acid metabolism is the basis for recognition of ischemic myocardium in experimental animals and patients after intravenous administration of cyclotron-produced, positron-emitting, ^{11}C-labeled fatty acids. In isolated perfused hearts, transitory diminution of perfusion leads to a reversible reduction of ^{11}C-palmitate accumulation, reflecting decreased uptake and oxidation of fatty acids in the perfusate. The uptake of tracer is independent of flow per se, as long as metabolic activity of the myocardium remains constant. In patients with myocardial infarction, diminished accumulation of ^{11}C-palmitate is evident in computer-reconstructed images obtained by positron emission tomography. Because this technique permits quantitative delineation of the distribution of the tracer in multiple cross-sections of the heart after intravenous administration, the diminution of ^{11}C-palmitate uptake detectable tomographically corresponds quantitatively to biochemical and morphometric criteria of infarction.[302] During physical exercise patients with ischemic heart disease exhibited reduced myocardial free fatty acid extraction.[303]

Reduced flow alone does not diminish uptake of a substrate if intermediary metabolism is not altered, since the extraction fraction increases. Thus, transitory ischemia without reduction of either myocardial oxygen consumption or fatty acid utilization would not be manifested tomographically by decreased ^{11}C-palmitate uptake.[304] However, prolonged ischemia, with impairment of oxidative metabolism but without necrosis, would give rise to a zone of decreased accumulation of the tracer evident by tomography. The two conditions (prolonged ischemia without necrosis and infarction per se) can be readily differentiated with the use of serial studies. Prolonged and persistent diminution of oxidative metabolism and hence persistently impaired regional uptake of ^{11}C-palmitate detectable tomographically are tantamount to necrosis in view of the well-established irreversibility of injury sustained by myocardium rendered ischemic for 2 hours or more.

In contrast to the regional variation of accumulation of [18]FDG in hearts of normal human subjects under conditions such as fasting,[305] accumulation of radiolabeled fatty acids is homogeneous.[306] Nevertheless, externally detectable clearance of radiolabeled tracers of fatty acid from myocardium does not provide a direct index of myocardial fatty acid metabolism because of sometimes pronounced and often variable efflux of nonmetabolized radiolabeled fatty acid.[307] Furthermore, variable contributions to overall energy production of diverse substrates, including glucose, palmitate, ketones, and lactate, preclude estimations of regional energy metabolism in ischemic or reperfused myocardium by analysis of uptake or clearance of a single tracer of any one metabolic pathway.[308,308a]

Uptake of Fatty Acids. Despite the limitations of estimation of fatty acid utilization (because of efflux) and the diversity of contributions of different pathways of intermediary metabolism to overall oxidative metabolism, uptake of palmitate quantifiable tomographically 1 hour after reperfusion is a powerful predictor of maintenance of myocardial viability evident 4 weeks later in the hearts of dogs subjected to coronary occlusion and reperfusion[240] (Fig. 38-35). Definitive assessments of overall myocardial oxygen utilization (and hence viability) can be made in normal, ischemic, and reperfused myocardium with the use of dynamic positron-emission tomography and radiolabeled acetate — a tracer entering essentially only one pathway of metabolism, namely mitochondrial oxidative phosphorylation.[239,241,254]

Figure 38-35. See color plate 7

PROTEIN AND NUCLEIC ACID METABOLISM IN ISCHEMIA

Characteristic changes in synthesis and degradation of myocardial proteins accompany ischemia. Synthesis decreases because of inhibition of peptide chain initiation and elongation. Efflux of alanine reflects not only its diminished utilization in protein synthesis but also augmented synthesis by transamination of pyruvate, a precursor accumulating because of impaired carbohydrate exudation. Thus, alanine release from the ischemic heart is analogous to lactate production, just as release of inosine (a product of degradation of adenine nucleotides) is analogous to lactate production.

Release of another amino acid, phenylalanine, has been employed in experimental preparations in which reincorporation into protein is prevented by pretreatment with cycloheximide (an inhibitor of protein synthesis) to provide an index of protein degradation under a variety of conditions, including normal oxygenation, anoxia, and simulated ischemia. The process of protein degradation requires energy derived from oxidative metabolism under physiological conditions based on observations with such preparations, since the rate of protein degradation declines by as much as 80 per cent in isolated hearts subjected to severe ischemia.[309] Although proteolysis mediated by lysosomal hydrolases has been implicated as a factor leading to irreversible injury in myocardium undergoing ischemic injury, increases in free and total lysosomal hydrolase activity do not occur until several hours after the onset of ischemia. Accordingly, it appears likely that the early loss of functional sarcolemmal integrity accompanied by electrophysiological manifestations, subsequent impairment of cell volume regulation, and leakage of cytoplasmic constituents reflects primary damage to the cell membrane itself. Only later during the evolution of ischemic injury do activation and liberation of lysosomal enzymes or activation of proteases appear to be prominent. It has been postulated that a Ca^{++}- activated neutral protease degrades subunits of troponin within the first few hours of severe ischemia. These and related observations suggest that the irreversible nature of injury sustained by ischemic myocardium is not due to proteolysis, even though activation of these enzymes may account for the release of relatively late markers of cell death and result in protein degradation late in the evolution of necrosis. Nevertheless, provision of branched chain amino acids along with glucose in oxygenated crystalloid solutions to energy-depleted ischemic rat hearts enhances protection of myocardium and recovery of function with reperfusion.[310]

Under physiological conditions, the myocardium extracts glutamic acid from arterial blood and produces ammonia and glutamine, which appear in the coronary venous effluent. When ischemia supervenes, ammonia derived from amino acids that cannot be incorporated into protein under these conditions is incorporated into alanine and glutamine with a consequent increase in their concentrations in the coronary sinus effluent. The increased production of alanine has been viewed as analogous to the increased production of lactate. Both are markers of ischemia. In the case of alanine, transamination of pyruvate serves as a sink for ammonia that would otherwise accumulate. In the case of lactate, the pyruvate serves as a sink for hydrogen ions.

EFFECTS OF ISCHEMIA ON GENETIC EXPRESSION OF SPECIFIC PROTEINS

As already outlined, the consequences of myocardial ischemia are prompt and are undoubtedly mediated initially by altered intermediary metabolism. Later or more sustained effects may reflect abnormalities in the synthesis of particular proteins mediated by changes in their genetic expression. In many tissues, "stress" such as hyperthermia or hypoxia induces the appearance of so-called heat shock or stress proteins with diverse effects. Recently, increased steady-state concentrations of a messenger RNA (mRNA) coding for one such protein in myocardium have been demonstrated after the induction of ischemia.[311] Proteins coded by the specific mRNA showed an increase in concentration despite a lack of overall change in the concentration of myosin and a decrease in the concentration of the predominant subunit of creatine kinase. Thus, myocardial ischemia induces specific alterations in steady-state concentrations of mRNAs coding for proteins with disparate functional properties in heart muscle cells.[311] These observations indicate that relatively long-term consequences of ischemia may reflect altered genetic expression leading to abnormal concentrations of specific intracellular proteins.[312]

Stimulation of hearts by heat shock, which induces expression of heat-shock proteins and acquisition of thermotolerance in other systems, can protect the stressed cells from injury induced by subsequent ischemia followed by reperfusion. Thus, when rats are rendered hyperthermic at 40°C for 15 minutes, hearts isolated and perfused later under conditions of low flow followed by reperfusion recover contractility within 5 minutes of reperfusion, in contrast to the case with hearts from control animals in which no recovery is evident at corresponding intervals. Release of creatine kinase induced by ischemia is markedly diminished, and ultrastructural integrity is better maintained as well.[312] The potential impact of altered genetic expression of specific proteins in mediating cardiac dysfunction is suggested by the relationship between slow relaxation and decreased relative expression of the calcium-ATPase gene with consequently diminished density of intracellular calcium pumps in rat hearts rendered hypertrophic.[313]

The importance of oxidative phosphorylation, i.e., the coupling of ATP synthesis to aerobic respiration, for the metabolic integrity of myocardium is underscored by some simple quantitative considerations. Complete oxidation of one mole of glucose gives rise to the net production of 36 moles of ATP. In contrast, only 2 moles of ATP are produced from complete anaerobic metabolism of 1 mole of glucose. Thus, even if the profound derangements in intermediary metabolism associated with increased production of reducing equivalents accompanying anaerobic glycolysis could be corrected, an 18-fold increase in glycolytic flux would be required for myocardium to synthesize comparable quantities of ATP via anaerobic compared to aerobic metabolism. The failure of energy production to keep pace with demand in ischemic cells is manifested by a prompt decline in the concentration of creatine phosphate, a major constituent of myocardial high-energy phosphate stores.

The dependence of myocardial viability on the availability of oxygen has stimulated careful assessment of the gradients of oxygen present within ischemic zones of the heart, based on analysis of the oxidation-reduction state of specific components of the electron transport chain and different spectra reflecting changes in the oxygenation of myoglobin.[314,315] Results obtained with optical techniques applied to the infarcted heart in vitro suggest that individual cells, and possibly individual mitochondria, are either fully aerobic or fully anaerobic in regions of myocardium subjected to ischemia. Thus, at any given instant, borders between anoxic and oxygenated tissue are very sharp. This phenomenon is in part a reflection of the very high affinity of mitochondria for oxygen. In response to ischemia, the mitochondria remain oxidized, despite very low levels of tissue oxygen tension, and become reduced only when virtually the last remaining oxygen has been utilized within a region. Thus, there appears to be a sharp, anatomically definable border between regions in which mitochondria are aerobic and anaerobic. However, this border is not static. As ischemia persists, there is expansion of the mass of severely ischemic tissue judging from morphological observations in canine hearts subjected to coronary occlusion. Early in the course of severe ischemia there is a potentially large mass of jeopardized but not yet irreversibly injured ischemic myocardium, susceptible to favorable influence by selected interventions.

THE "WAVEFRONT" OF ISCHEMIC NECROSIS. The percentage of transmural necrosis ultimately developing within a zone of myocardium rendered ischemic by coronary occlusion maintained for 40 minutes, 3 hours, 6 hours, and 24

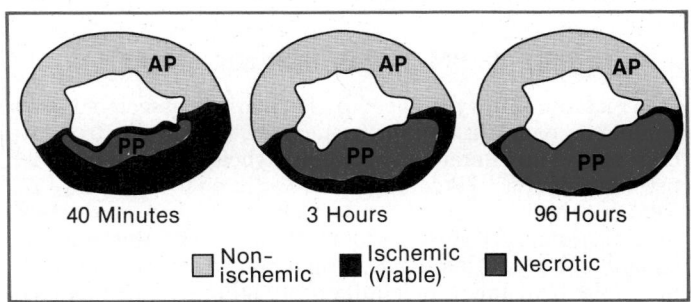

FIGURE 38–36. Progression of cell death versus time after circumflex coronary occlusion in dogs. Necrosis occurs first in the subendocardial myocardium. With longer occlusions, a wavefront of cell death moves from the subendocardial zone across the wall to involve progressively more of the transmural thickness of the ischemic zone. In contrast, the lateral margins in the subendocardial region of the infarct are established as early as 40 minutes after occlusion and are sharply defined by the anatomic boundaries of the ischemic bed. AP = anterior papillary muscle; PP = posterior papillary muscle. (From Reimer, K. A., Hill, M. L., and Jennings, R. B.: Prolonged depletion of ATP and of the adenine nucleotide pool due to delayed resynthesis of adenine nucleotides following reversible myocardial ischemic injury in dogs. J. Mol. Cell. Cardiol. *13*:229, 1981.)

hours, followed by reperfusion for 2 to 4 days, varies from 38 to 85 per cent with a "wavefront" of necrosis progressing from subendocardial to epicardial tissue,[1] presumably because the subendocardium has a greater oxygen demand and smaller oxygen supply than the epicardium (Fig. 38–36). Metabolic studies have shown greater and more rapid reductions of ATP and total adenosine nucleotides and greater and more rapid accumulation of lactate and nucleotides and bases, i.e., the products of degradation of adenine nucleotides in the subendocardium (Fig. 38–31). A cell in the subendocardium may be able to tolerate severe ischemia for a brief interval although it will become necrotic after 20 minutes. A cell with similar energy requirements in the subepicardium will be able to tolerate the milder degree of ischemia to which it is exposed following coronary occlusion for a longer period before becoming necrotic. As a consequence, when ischemic myocardium is reperfused 20 minutes to 5 hours after coronary occlusion, a progressively smaller epicardial zone of myocardium survives.[316]

ACTIVATION OF LYSOSOMAL ENZYMES AND COMPLEMENT

Most tissues contain latent lysosomal hydrolases capable of mediating proteolysis under certain conditions. Lysosomal hydrolases are activated by an acid pH, although mammalian cells contain neutral proteases as well. Relatively late reparative processes in myocardium undergoing infarction are accompanied by consistent increases in lysosomal hydrolase activity in tissue extracts as well as in the circulation, suggesting that activation of proteases with dissolution of cellular debris is a component to the response to irreversible injury. However, the extent to which activation of lysosomal hydrolase contributes to early manifestations of ischemia or irreversibility remains controversial. What is clear is that much of the lysosomal activity in the heart undergoing infarction comes from cells participating in the response to inflammation, such as polymorphonuclear leukocytes rather than myocardial cells per se.

In addition to degradation by activated lysosomal enzymes, ischemic injury may reflect the impact of activated complement either directly[317] or indirectly[318] by diminution of neutrophil activation. Complement may be activated by constituents of mitochondria released when heart muscle is subjected to ischemia.[317] Depletion of complement diminishes ischemic injury even when it is induced only after the onset of ischemia.[318] Salutary effects of depletion of complement appear to be greater than those seen with reduction of neutrophil activation and infiltration alone by nonsteroidal antiinflammatory agents such as ibuprofen.[318]

ROLE OF CALCIUM IN ISCHEMIC INJURY

Myocardial injury induced by ischemia is associated with complexes of calcium in the tissue detectable by electron microscopy.[1] The interaction between myocardial ischemia and myoplasmic [Ca^{++}] is complex, as illustrated in Figure 38–37. Ischemia, however produced, is characterized by a reduction of myocardial ATP stores, which interferes with the transsarcolemmal Na^+–K^+ exchange, which in turn elevates intracellular [Na^+], raising intracellular [Ca^{++}] through an enhanced Na^+–Ca^{++} exchange. Lowered ATP stores also reduce Ca^{++} uptake by the sarcoplasmic reticulum and reduce extrusion of Ca^{++} from cells. The resultant augmented intracellular [Ca^{++}][319,320] causes mitochondrial Ca^{++} overload, which depresses ATP production further. Activation of intracellular Ca^{++} ATPases augments ATP usage and activates sarcolemmal phospholipases, which release membrane phospholipid degradation products whose detergent properties impair the integrity of the cell membrane.[321,322] Calcium antagonists interfere with Ca^{++} influx through voltage-dependent channels. Beta-adrenoceptor agonists recruit additional receptor-operated channels, and beta-adrenoceptor blockers reduce Ca^{++}

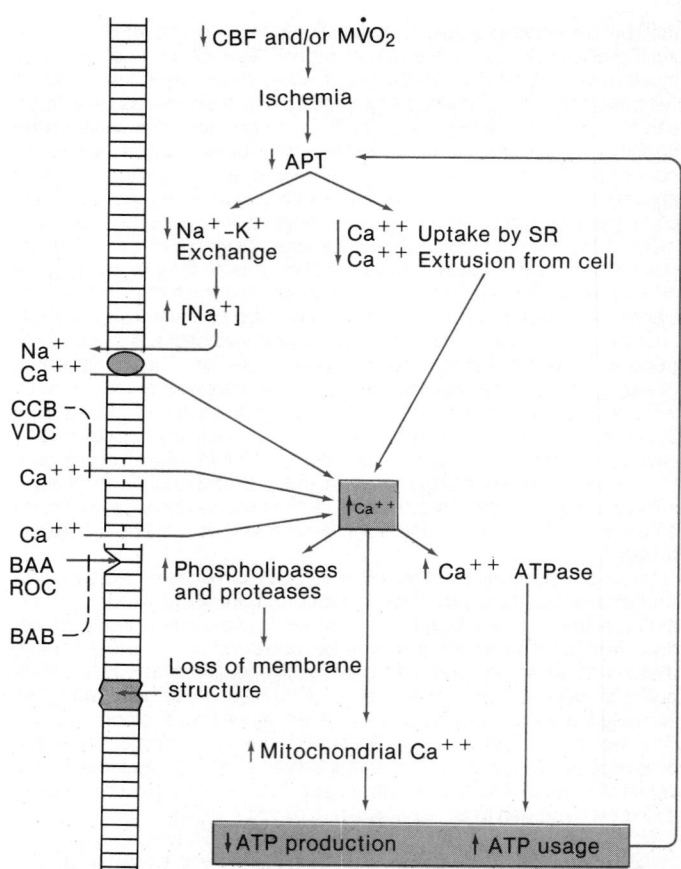

FIGURE 38–37. Interactions between myocardial ischemia and [Ca^{++}]. A reduction of coronary blood flow (CBF), sometimes accompanied by an increase in myocardial oxygen requirements (MVO₂), causes myocardial ischemia, which in turn reduces cellular ATP stores. This reduction interferes with the transsarcolemmal Na^+–K^+ exchange, which elevates intracellular [Na^+], raising intracellular [Ca^{++}] through an enhanced Na^+–Ca^{++} exchange. Lowered ATP stores also reduce Ca^{++} uptake by the sarcoplasmic reticulum (SR) and reduce extrusion of Ca^{++} from cells. The resultant augmented intracellular [Ca^{++}] causes mitochondrial Ca^{++} overload, which depresses ATP production further; activation of intracellular Ca^{++} ATPases, which augment ATP usage; and activation of sarcolemmal phospholipases and proteases, which impair the integrity of the cell membrane. Calcium-channel blockers (CCB) interfere with Ca^{++} influx through voltage-dependent channels (VDA). Beta-adrenoceptor agonists (BAA) recruit additional receptor-operated channels (ROC). Beta-adrenoceptor blockers (BAB) reduce Ca^{++} influx by interfering with the recruitment of ROC. (Reproduced with permission from Braunwald, E.: Mechanism of action of calcium channel blocking agents. N. Engl. J. Med. *307*:1618, 1982.)

influx by interfering with this recruitment of receptor-operated channels. Thus, one would expect beta blockers and Ca^{++} antagonists to have similar effects in the treatment of ischemia. Indeed, both groups of compounds delay ischemia-induced necrosis and, particularly when combined with reperfusion, reduce the extent of myocardial necrosis.[323–327]

The hypothesis that the entry of Ca^{++} into ischemic cells may be harmful is based on the observation that after a period of myocardial ischemia and subsequent reperfusion the accumulation of excess Ca^{++} in the mitochondria may interfere with their capacity to generate ATP. The destructive chain of metabolic events provoked by increased intracellular [Ca^{++}] appears to be responsible, at least in part, for the death of cells in the ischemic myocardium. Henry and associates[328] found that during one hour of severe ischemia, the left ventricle undergoes progressive ischemic contracture, with the development of an elevated ventricular diastolic pressure and a fourfold increase in mitochondrial Ca^{++}. With subsequent reperfusion, both myocardial systolic function and relaxation remain abnormal, and a further marked increase in Ca^{++} accumulation occurs. Administration of nifedipine prevents ischemic contracture and permits recovery of systolic contractile function and of myocardial relaxation. These favorable hemodynamic changes are accompanied by a marked reduction in the accumulation of Ca^{++} in the mitochondria.

Ca^{++} antagonists have also been shown to reduce ATP depletion and myocardial damage during coronary occlusion, and particularly during reperfusion,[327-331] and nifedipine preserved left ventricular function in dogs with cardiopulmonary bypass that were subjected to prolonged total ischemia. These experiments demonstrate that in a setting analogous to the clinical practice of cardiac surgery, Ca^{++} antagonists protect myocardium, which is at first ischemic and is then reperfused. Thus, Ca^{++} antagonists may be valuable in protecting the myocardium from the Ca^{++}-associated ischemic injury occurring during open heart surgery. However, Ca^{++} antagonists do not appear to inhibit Ca^{++} influx into irreversibly injured myocardium. Instead, their protective action depends on an antiischemic effect resulting from a reduction of $M\dot{V}O_2$.

The accumulation of Ca^{++} in myocardium undergoing ischemic injury has important diagnostic and therapeutic implications. Myocardial infarct scintigraphy with agents such as ^{99m}Tc-stannous pyrophosphate permits detection and localization of infarction after intravenous injection of tracer. The tissue's avidity for the tracer appears to depend on the accumulation of Ca^{++} (p. 291).

Reduction of accumulation of intracellular Ca^{++} in jeopardized ischemic myocardium that has not yet undergone necrosis appears to protect the tissue and enhance salvage induced by reperfusion, as judged from studies in dogs with induced thrombotic coronary occlusion followed by clot lysis with intravenous streptokinase.[332] Effects of intravenous diltiazem given 30 minutes before administration of steptokinase were evident on positron-emission tomograms with $H_2^{15}O$ (to characterize perfusion) and carbon-11–labeled palmitate (to characterize intermediary metabolism). The extent of infarction expressed as the percentage of risk region was reduced by reperfusion alone but was even more markedly reduced by reperfusion coupled with cardiac protection conferred by diltiazem. These results were confirmed by direct analysis of myocardial creatine kinase content, which demonstrated less depletion of the enzyme in hearts subjected to reperfusion and concomitant calcium blockage compared with depletion in hearts subjected to reperfusion alone.

PHOSPHOINOSITIDES AND CALCIUM. The effects of many agonists on diverse cells are transduced by their interactions with surface receptors that are coupled to specific intracellular second messengers. One familiar example is beta-adrenergic stimulation of cardiac myocytes (p. 363). Stimulation is transduced by activation of cell surface receptors coupled to specific G proteins (p. 363) (named because of their interaction with GTP) that modulate activity of adenylate cyclase, increased synthesis of cyclic AMP, and cyclic AMP–dependent phosphorylation of proteins, one of which alters calcium channel function and increases calcium influx. Another particularly important bifurcating signal pathway responds to activation of other surface receptors coupled to other G proteins in response to agonists such as alpha-adrenergic agents. Activation of this system in cardiac myocytes gives rise to inositol 1,4,5-triphosphate (IP_3) (or a cyclic compound, inositol 1:2-cyclic 4,5-triphosphate) and diacylglycerol—both of which are products of Ca^{++}-dependent phospholipase-catalyzed hydrolysis of phosphatidylinositol 4,5-biphosphate. IP_3 releases Ca^{++} from the sarcoplasmic reticulum, and diacylglycerol activates protein kinase C. Both components of this signaling pathway (IP_3 and diacylglycerol) influence intracellular Ca^{++}-dependent responses.[333]

Increases in intracellular concentrations of phosphoinositides may mediate the positive inotropic effects of alpha-adrenergic agonists and contribute to Ca^{++} overload and alpha-adrenergic receptor–mediated arrhythmogenesis in ischemic and reperfused myocardium.[334] Amphiphiles accumulating

with ischemia and reperfusion augment alpha-receptor density and Ca^{++} influx. Thus, it is not surprising that reperfusion appears to increase turnover of phosphoinositides.[335] Catecholamines increase intracellular Ca^{++} by beta-adrenergic cyclic AMP-mediated increased influx and by alpha-adrenergic IP_3-mediated effects on the sarcoplasmic reticulum, and increased adrenergic stimulation is a hallmark of ischemic and reperfused myocardium. Accordingly, attenuation of receptor-mediated activation of both the cyclic AMP and IP_3-diacylglycerol second messenger systems, inhibition of activation of phospholipase C, or inhibition of activated protein kinase C may retard the progression of ischemic injury and attenuate its manifestations, particularly when coupled with other measures designed to inhibit calcium overload secondary to ischemia or reperfusion.[336,337]

OXYGEN-DERIVED FREE RADICALS IN ISCHEMIC TISSUE INJURY

There is substantial evidence that ischemic tissue generates oxygen-derived free radicals (oxygen radicals), i.e., oxygen molecules containing an odd number of electrons, making them chemically reactive, and often leading to chain reactions.[338] There are three principal oxygen radicals: the superoxide anion ($\cdot O_2^-$), hydrogen peroxide (H_2O_2), and the hydroxyl radical ($\cdot OH$). Acute, severe ischemia appears to increase the production of oxygen radicals by several mechanisms: (1) dissociation of intramitochondrial electron transport; (2) ischemia-induced Ca^{++} influx activates phospholipase, which enhances arachidonic acid metabolism, which in turn may produce oxygen radicals; (3) ischemia converts the normal myocardial enzyme xanthine dehydrogenase to xanthine oxidase in some species, which in the presence of xanthine produces oxygen radicals; and/or (4) complement is activated in ischemic tissue and this enhances the accumulation of neutrophils, which in turn release oxygen radicals.[338]

The oxygen radicals, in turn, can contribute to ischemic damage or postischemic damage caused by reperfusion.[339] These moieties react with almost any biological molecule in their vicinity. It has been proposed that by causing perioxidation of cell membranes, oxygen radicals damage cell membranes and contribute to cell death. It has also been postulated that they can contribute to the development of irreversible injury by acting on the mitochondria and sarcoplasmic reticulum. This postulate is based largely on the observation that free radical scavengers such as superoxide dismutase and catalase prevent the ischemia-induced loss of Ca^{++} sequestration by the sarcoplasmic reticulum and preserve mitochondrial function.

Despite the demonstrable toxicity of oxygen-derived free radicals to cell membranes and the apparently protective effects of free radical scavengers in studies of experimental animals[225-228,340] and inhibitors of their production,[229,229a] salvage of myocardium by interventions attenuating free-radical production and persistence has not been observed consistently. High molecular weight "scavengers" such as catalase and superoxide dismutase may not penetrate the source of free radicals rapidly enough, and even brief exposure of vulnerable organelles to oxygen-derived free radicals may be sufficient to obviate their protective effects. Strategies focusing on attenuation of oxygen-derived free radical accumulation diminish stunning in ischemic myocardium subjected to reperfusion, and accordingly, these radicals have been implicated in its pathogenesis.[226,341-344] Neutrophil depletion during reperfusion reduces myocardial infarct size, presumably by reducing production of oxygen-derived free radicals.[345] Preservation of high concentrations of intracellular reducing agents such as glutathione that may attenuate otherwise increased concentrations of active oxygen radicals appears to confer protection as judged from preservation of both systolic and diastolic function in hearts subjected to ischemia and reperfusion.[346] In addition, agents such as diltiazem that inhibit lipid peroxidation inducible by oxygen-derived free radicals may be beneficial.[224]

RELEASE OF MYOCARDIAL ENZYMES IN DETECTION OF ACUTE MYOCARDIAL INFARCTION

(see also p. 1218)

Since biochemical markers of ischemic injury have become important clinical tools, some considerations required for their proper interpretation merit particular attention. Loss of functional integrity of the sarcolemma is a primary common denominator underlying liberation of cytoplasmic constituents into the circulation, such as transaminase (SGOT, AST), lactic dehydrogenase (LDH), and creatine kinase (CK).[347] Species of lower molecular weight, such as myoglobin, are liberated, but elevated concentrations persist in the circulation only briefly because of rapid renal clearance. Furthermore, myoglobin released from hypoperfused skeletal muscle may cloud interpretation of elevated values in plasma.

Accurate assessment of myocardial infarction based on analysis of plasma enzyme time-activity curves has been facilitated by the demonstration that one isoenzyme of creatine kinase, CK-MB, is localized primarily in the heart in humans.[347] Under carefully defined conditions in experimental animals, depletion of myocardial CK activity correlates with infarct size estimated independently by morphometric techniques or with the use of radioactively labeled microspheres. The corollary of these observations, namely, that increases in plasma enzyme activity reflect infarct size, has been recognized for many years.

On the basis of many clinical studies and observations in conscious experimental animals,[347,348] it has become clear that release of myocardial cytosolic enzymes into the circulation is tantamount to cell death when the cause of enzyme release is myocardial ischemia. Accordingly, infarct size has been estimated from analysis of plasma enzyme CK time-activity curves,[349-351] and from curves obtained by quantitative assay of plasma samples for CK-MB activity. Despite obvious imperfections, enzymatic estimates of infarct size have correlated with biochemical and morphological analyses of infarction in hearts of experimental animals, morbidity and mortality in patients, histochemical assessment of necrosis among patients who succumb to acute myocardial infarction,[352] early and late ventricular arrhythmia, and impairment of ventricular function. Time-activity curves are influenced by regional myocardial perfusion, local degradation of enzyme in the heart, the ratio of enzyme released compared with that destroyed,[353] inactivation of enzyme in lymph,[354] exchange of enzyme between vascular and extravascular compartments,[350] and potential variation in the rate of inactivation and removal of enzyme once it has reached the circulation.[354] Thus, the pattern of enzyme release and its overall magnitude may be influenced by interventions resulting in early reperfusion and accelerated washout. Nevertheless, analysis of plasma time-activity curves of CK-MB and other biochemical markers of ischemic injury has proved useful in quantitative assessment of the progress and extent of myocardial infarction in the clinical setting.

Because the rate of appearance of macromolecules such as CK in plasma is accelerated when myocardium is subjected to reperfusion (reflecting an increased rate of washout), the utility of enzymatic estimation of the extent of infarction in the setting of reperfusion has been questioned. However, recent studies in dogs in which estimates based on plasma enzyme time-activity curves were correlated with the actual extent of infarction as judged from direct measurements of infarct size in excised hearts demonstrated that enzymatic estimates remained valid when CK release was measured during the first 60 minutes after the onset of reperfusion. Analogous results were obtained in patients with myocardial infarction who had undergone early reperfusion and in whom enzymatic estimates were correlated with estimates of infarct size based on

positron-emission tomography 1 to 2 weeks after the index episode.[355]

Despite their usefulness, results of assays of plasma enzymes and other macromolecules must be interpreted cautiously. An apparent lack of elevation may occur in the setting of unequivocal acute myocardial infarction if the extent of injury sustained is minimal, the frequency of sampling insufficient, or the extent of the peak elevation modest and difficult to define in terms of the "normal" range reflecting a distribution of values in the population. The biological implications of severe myocardial ischemia without infarction may be as great for patients with unstable angina as they are for patients with incipient or early evolving infarction or infarction of minimal extent. Accordingly, it is inappropriate to deprive patients of continued medical surveillance if the index of suspicion of coronary insufficiency is high, even when statistically definable elevations of plasma enzymes and other macromolecular markers of ischemic injury are not present in initially obtained plasma samples.

CREATINE KINASE ISOFORMS. Subforms of individual isoenzymes of CK-MM (isoforms), which may be distinguished by differences in isoelectric points (PI), exist in the plasma soon after myocardial infarction (Fig. 38–38). When CK-MM is released into the bloodstream it is in the MM_3 isoform; this evolves in the plasma sequentially and in a time-dependent manner with cleavage of carboxyterminal lysines on each of the M subunits by carboxypeptidase N[356] into two other isoforms, MM_2 and MM_1, having lower isoelectric points. Both in experimental animals and in patients with coronary occlusion, within one hour after occlusion the percentage of total circulating MM comprised by the MM_3 isoform rises, with a reciprocal reduction of MM_2. No conversion of isoforms appears to occur in normal, ischemic, or necrotic myocardium.[357] It appears possible to use a single blood sample, available at the time of initial presentation, in which relative distribution of CK-MM isoforms is estimated both to diagnose (with a sensitivity of 94 per cent)[358] and to time the onset of myocardial infarction. The isoform profile may be distinctly abnormal in the face of normal total CK or CK-MB.[359] However, since the MM_3 isoform is present in tissues other than the

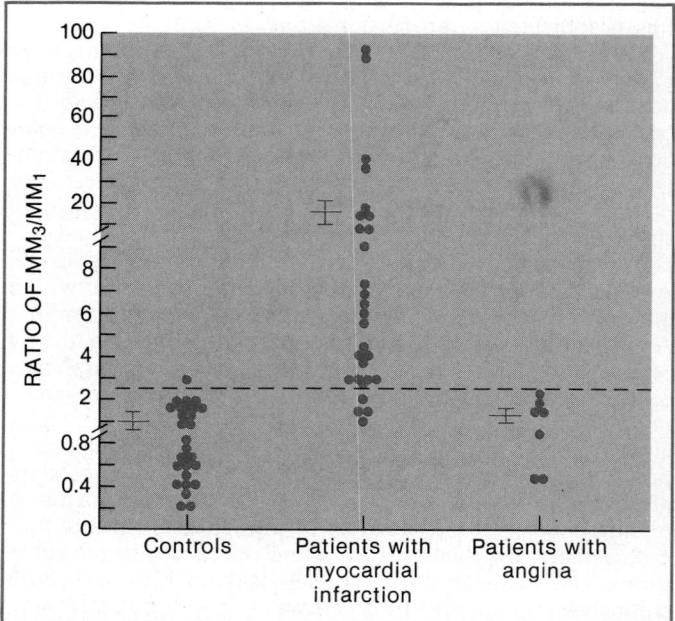

FIGURE 38–38. Comparison of the ratios of MM_3 to MM_1 in plasma from normal control subjects, patients with acute myocardial infarction, and patients with angina. (From Jaffe, A. S., Serota, H., Grace, A., and Sobel, B. E.: Diagnostic changes in plasma creatine kinase isoforms early after the onset of acute myocardial infarction. Circulation 74:105, 1986, by permission of the American Heart Association, Inc.)

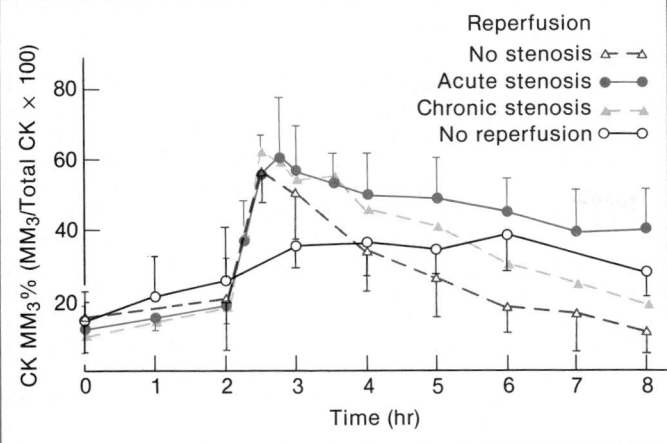

FIGURE 38-39. Plasma profiles of percent of creatine kinase activity composed of MM₃ in dogs subjected to coronary occlusion and release after 2 hours in the absence of coronary stenosis (n = 10) or with stenosis induced for 1 week (chronic, n = 5) or before occlusion (acute, n = 5), and in dogs subjected to persistent coronary occlusion (no reperfusion, n = 10). Data are presented as mean vaues ± 1 SD. (From Nohora, R., Myears, D. W., Sobel, B. E., and Abendschein, D. R.: Optimal criteria for rapid detection of myocardial reperfusion by creatine kinase MM isoforms in the presence of residual high grade coronary stenosis. Reprinted with permission from the American College of Cardiology. J. Am. Coll. Cardiol. *14*:1067, 1989.)

heart, the isoform profile in plasma is less specific for myocardial damage than is the CK-MB. The isoform profile (the percentage of concentrations of total CK activity in plasma comprised by MM₃) changes rapidly following myocardial reperfusion and appears to provide a prompt, reliable, and noninvasive index of the presence of myocardial reperfusion,[360,361] even in the presence of residual high-grade stenosis with the potential to attenuate washout of MM₃ into the circulation[362] (Fig. 38-39).

OTHER MACROMOLECULAR MARKERS. In addition to isoforms of CK-MM, isoforms of CK-MB have been recognized.[363] Three MB isoforms exist, but most assay systems detect only a tissue form and a second form that can comprise both converted products comigrating or copurifying under specific conditions. Alternatively, one of the two converted forms may be present only transiently in the circulation.[364,365] Despite the promise of analysis of CK-MB isoform profiles for early detection of reperfusion because of potentially greater specificity with MB- as opposed to MM-CK,[366] isoform analysis of MM is likely to afford more sensitivity and less ambiguity in view of the resolution of all three theoretically possible isoforms.

The pattern of release of many other macromolecular markers of ischemic injury into the circulation is qualitatively similar to that of individual isoenzymes of CK. Myoglobin has been used for early detection of reperfusion[367] because of its rapid clearance from the circulation as a result of glomerular filtration. In experimental animals, its pattern of release into the circulation with reperfusion is "staccato-like."[368] In patients, abrupt increases in the concentration of myoglobin in plasma are evident during the first 2 hours after coronary revascularization with myocardial infarction in progress.[369]

Myosin light chains have been assayed in plasma to detect irreversible ischemic injury. In dogs, the extent of infarction estimated from calculated myosin light-chain II release correlates closely with morphological estimates of infarct size whether or not reperfusion is induced within 3 or 6 hours after coronary occlusion.[370]

It appears likely that rapid, noninvasive estimation of the extent of infarction and accurate delineation of the time of occurrence of reperfusion based on assay of macromolecular markers will play an increasing role in decision making for

management of patients with evolving myocardial infarction treated with thrombolytic agents in whom angioplasty or emergency surgery may be required because of failure of initial recanalization or demonstrably successful recanalization with subsequent early reocclusion.

MODIFICATION OF ISCHEMIC INJURY

A variety of interventions have been shown in animal experiments to modify the severity of ischemic injury, and in some instances parallel changes in infarct size have been observed. The theoretical basis for these interventions and the experimental results are discussed below. The clinical application of these observations is discussed on page 1227. The potency of any intervention designed to limit ischemic injury is inversely related to the interval between the onset of the ischemic stimulus and the time the intervention is applied. In the normothermic working dog heart no intervention can be expected to exert a significant beneficial effect if it is initiated more than 4 to 6 hours after the onset of severe ischemia, because by this time all tissue in the distribution of the occluded vessel is likely to have become irreversibly injured.

INTERVENTIONS THAT INCREASE MYOCARDIAL INJURY AFTER CORONARY ARTERY OCCLUSION
(Table 38-4)

Certain interventions known to increase M$\dot{V}$O₂ also increase the severity and extent of myocardial injury in the presence of residual, albeit restricted coronary blood flow. In the dog without heart failure, isoproterenol, digitalis (in the absence of heart failure), and amrinone[371] have a deleterious effect on ischemic myocardium. Exercise can precipitate ischemia in the presence of obstruction not severe enough to cause ischemia at rest. Also, pacing-induced tachycardia increases ischemic damage,[372] and a similar observation in patients has been reported. Hypoxemia,[373] anemia, and hypotension, regardless of how produced,[374] increase myocardial ischemic injury after coronary occlusion, since in all of these conditions the delivery of oxygen to the ischemic tissue is reduced; similarly, hypoglycemia augments ischemic injury.[375] Hyperthermia impairs mechanical performance of the ischemic myocardium; through its direct stimulation of M$\dot{V}$O₂ and heart rate, it exerts an adverse effect on myocardial oxygen balance.

The positive inotropic and chronotropic effects of isoproterenol improve the function of normal myocardium and elevate M$\dot{V}$O₂. When isoproterenol is administered in the presence of global myocardial ischemia, however, myocardial function deteriorates rapidly because of the intensification of ischemia.[376] The effects of isoproterenol on myocardial function in

TABLE 38-4 INTERVENTIONS THAT INCREASE MYOCARDIAL INJURY AFTER CORONARY ARTERY OCCLUSION

Increase Myocardial Oxygen Requirements
  Isoproterenol
  Digitalis and amrinone (in the absence of heart failure)
  Tachycardia
  Hyperthermia

Decrease Myocardial Oxygen Supply
  Directly
    Hypoxemia
    Anemia
  Through collateral vessels, reducing coronary perfusion pressure
    Hemorrhage
    Sodium nitroprusside
    Other vasodilators (including isoproterenol)
    Coronary vasoconstriction (indomethacin)
  Decrease substrate availability
    Hypoglycemia

the presence of regional ischemia are more complex. In the conscious dog with regional myocardial ischemia, isoproterenol elicits a spectrum of reactions in areas with different degrees of ischemia.[377] Severely ischemic sites exhibit no increase in blood flow, and a deterioration of function occurs during infusion of isoproterenol, as a result of an increase in MVO_2, whereas normal or moderately ischemic areas show an improvement of both myocardial function and regional blood flow. The positive chronotropic and inotropic actions of isoproterenol cause an increase in infarct size in anesthetized dogs, and myocardial lactate production increases when isoproterenol is administered to patients with acute myocardial infarction.

An increase in the concentration of circulating fatty acids also aggravates ischemia following coronary occlusion. They augment MVO_2 in the presence of limited oxygen supply; this intensifies ischemia, depresses myocardial contractility, and probably precipitates arrhythmias.

INTERVENTIONS THAT REDUCE MYOCARDIAL INJURY AFTER CORONARY ARTERY OCCLUSION

(Table 38–5)

THE PRIMACY OF REPERFUSION FOR SALVAGE OF ISCHEMIC MYOCARDIUM. As discussed on page 1230, coronary thrombolysis has become a cornerstone of early treatment of acute myocardial infarction precipitated by coronary thrombosis. Results of numerous laboratory and clinical investigations[378] have demonstrated that (1) myocardial infarc-

TABLE 38–5 INTERVENTIONS THAT REDUCE EXPERIMENTAL MYOCARDIAL INJURY FOLLOWING CORONARY OCCLUSION

Increasing myocardial oxygen supply
  Directly
    Coronary artery reperfusion (surgery, PTCA, thrombolysis)
    Elevating arterial pO_2, hyperbaric oxygenation
    Fluorocarbons
  Through collateral vessels
    Elevation of coronary perfusion pressure (e.g., methoxamine, neosynephrine)
    Intraaortic balloon counterpulsation
  Coronary vasodilatation (calcium antagonists, nitroglycerin, prostacyclin)
  Coronary venous retroperfusion
Decreasing myocardial O_2 demand
  Beta-adrenoceptor blockers
  Cardiac glycoside in the failing heart
  Intraaortic balloon in counterpulsation
  Decreasing afterload in hypertensive individuals
  Decreasing preload (nitroglycerin)
  Inhibiting calcium influx (Ca^{++} antagonists)
  Hypothermia
Preventing myocardial edema
  Increasing plasma osmolality (mannitol, hypertonic glucose)
Augmenting anaerobic metabolism
  Glucose-insulin-potassium, fructose diphosphate, ribose hypertonic glucose
Enhancing transport to the ischemic zone of substrate utilized in energy production (presumed)
  Hyaluronidase
Prevention of injury by oxygen-free radicals (e.g., superoxide dismutase, allopurinol)
Reduction of catabolism
  Inhibition of adenine nucleotide catabolism (allopurinol)
  Inhibition of lipolysis (β-pyridilcarbinol)
Prevention of cell swelling
  Osmotic agents (mannitol), Ca^{++} antagonists
Reduction of inflammatory response
  Glucocorticosteroids
  Nonsteroidal antiinflammatory drugs (e.g., ibuprofen)
Reduction of microvascular damage
  Prevention of injury of vessels by free radicals
  Prevention of platelet aggregation
  Prevention of endothelial swelling (hypertonic agents)

tion is a dynamic process that can be interrupted by interventions restoring nutritive perfusion, limiting myocardial oxygen requirements, supporting myocardial metabolism, and inducing favorable ventricular loading conditions; (2) damage to ischemic myocardium can be limited by prompt and sustained recanalization of infarct-affected arteries; (3) most acute transmural infarcts and many non-Q-wave infarcts result from acute coronary thrombosis that can be documented biochemically, angiographically, or morphologically; (4) mortality attributable to acute myocardial infarction is directly related to the extent of damage sustained by heart muscle rendered ischemic, which is also reflected by impairment of regional ventricular function; and (5) preservation of myocardial viability, restoration of regional wall motion in jeopardized ischemic zones, and reduction of mortality are inversely related to the duration of ischemia preceding induction and persistence of reperfusion.

Myocardial ischemia in patients should be relieved by prompt and sustained recanalization of thrombotically occluded infarct-related arteries, generally accomplished with intravenous administration of activators of plasminogen.[379] The efficacy of coronary thrombolysis can be enhanced pharmacologically in two ways: with adjunctive agents and with conjunctive agents.[380]

Adjunctive Agents. Treatment with adjunctive agents is directed toward increasing the interval during which jeopardized ischemic myocardium remains salvageable as has been accomplished in experimental animals with calcium antagonists[332]; diminishing deleterious effects of neutrophil activation[381] or of oxygen-centered free radicals regardless of their origin[382-384]; diminishing calcium overload potentially exacerbated by reperfusion[385,386]; reducing oxygen requirements in jeopardized ischemic or reperfused myocardium with beta-adrenergic-blocking agents[387]; or preserving myocardial viability with combinations of protective measures.[388]

Treatment with conjunctive agents is directed toward accelerating thrombolysis or sustaining recanalization to prevent early thrombotic reocclusion or both on the basis of compelling evidence indicating that the efficacy of coronary thrombolysis depends on attenuation of ongoing thrombosis potentially exacerbated by procoagulant effects of plasminogen activators or plasmin[389-391] and by activation of platelets[392-395] as well as on fibrinolysis itself.[380,396] Conjunctive agents include PGE_1,[397,398] thromboxane receptor antagonists,[399] thromboxane synthetase inhibitors,[400] prostacyclin analogs,[401] alpha$_2$-antiplasmin,[402] heparin,[403] aspirin,[404] and hirudin.[405] Thus, even though protection of ischemic myocardium is best accomplished by prompt restoration of nutritive perfusion[406] and perfusion reserve[407] (as shown by positron-emission tomography with $H_2^{15}O$ before and after revascularization [Fig. 38–40]), the net impact of recanalization reflects the interplay of diverse factors that can affect myocardial viability.

Figure 38–40. See color plate 8

Several studies in animals have shown that early reperfusion results in smaller infarction than if the occlusion is sustained. As might be expected, the extent of salvage depends on the duration of occlusion.[1,315,408,409] Reperfusion after less than 15 to 20 minutes of coronary occlusion salvages essentially all of the ischemic tissue.[1] With longer periods of ischemia, a wavefront of necrosis beginning in the subendocardium and moving progressively outward, i.e., to the epicardium and laterally, occurs[410] (Fig. 38–36). When reperfusion is implemented after 6 hours of coronary occlusion, most of the jeopardized myocardium becomes necrotic and no tissue is salvaged.

OTHER INTERVENTIONS

The inhalation of an *oxygen-rich gas mixture* exerts a slight beneficial effect on the ischemic myocardium, presumably by enhancing delivery of oxygen to ischemic tissue through collaterals.[411] This may be greatly enhanced by combining inhalation of 100 per cent oxygen with fluorocarbon mixtures, i.e., so-called artificial blood, which greatly augments delivery.[412-415]

Intraaortic balloon counterpulsation (p. 580) reduces the severity of ischemic injury, presumably by reducing MVO_2, as a consequence of lowering systolic wall tension, while simultaneously augmenting oxygen delivery by increasing aortic diastolic (coronary perfusion) pressure. In experimental animals, *beta-adrenoceptor blockers* appear to prolong the survival of severely ischemic tissue, judging from changes in ST segments, QRS complexes, myocardial creatine kinase activity, and electron-microscopic, histochemical, and histological criteria.[416] In addition, these drugs appear to improve the ratio of subendocardial to subepicardial blood flow in both ischemic and normal areas of myocardium in dogs with coronary occlusion. Beta-adrenoceptor blockade appears to be more useful in *delaying* than preventing cell death and is especially effective in limiting infarct size in animals subjected to coronary occlusion and reperfusion.[325] Calcium antagonists have similar actions.[417] Ca^{++} antagonists may be beneficial when they are administered prophylactically, i.e., before the development of ischemia or early in its course.[323,326-331,418-420]

A number of *metabolic interventions* may also improve the energy balance of ischemic myocardium. As fatty acid oxidation is impaired by ischemia, glucose becomes the principal source of energy. In the ischemic dog heart, oxidative phosphorylation and cardiac function are enhanced by the infusion of glucose-insulin-potassium (GIK).[421] In the anoxic, isolated heart, both electrical and mechanical function improve and recovery occurs more rapidly when glucose is added to the perfusate,[422] and analogous effects have been observed in laboratory and some clinical studies in vivo.[423-425]

A number of agents that limit the inflammatory response reduce myocardial ischemic injury in the laboratory animal, and some have been tested in limited numbers of patients. *Cobra venom factor,* a protein that enzymatically cleaves C3 and prevents the effects of the complement system, reduces myocardial injury,[426] presumably by diminishing leukotaxis. The kallikrein system enhances leukotactic activity, capillary permeability, interstitial edema, and proteolytic activity, and *aprotinin,* an inhibitor of this system, diminishes ischemic injury.[427] Large doses of a *glucocorticosteroid* reduce myocardial infarct size in the dog with coronary occlusion.[428] However, they may inhibit healing of the infarct, increasing the risk of ventricular rupture or aneurysm formation.[429] Ibuprofen, a nonsteroidal antiinflammatory compound, reduces infarct size in experimental animals but interferes with infarct healing and scar formation.[430]

Mannitol reduces the extent of ischemic injury and improves the function of the ischemic myocardium, presumably by reducing cell swelling and improving collateral blood flow.[431]

Hyaluronidase, which depolymerizes mucopolysaccharides in extracellular matrix, has also been shown to reduce myocardial necrosis in the dog and rabbit, possibly by increasing the access of nutrients to myocytes or increasing washout of toxic metabolites. However, its clinical impact is modest, and it appears to be beneficial only to patients with infarction associated with early, spontaneous reperfusion.[432] In the dog, intravenous nitroglycerin, administered at a rate sufficient to cause a mild diminution in systemic arterial pressure, reduces the magnitude and extent of ischemic injury, particularly when reflex tachycardia secondary to hypertension is prevented. In addition, the administration of nitroglycerin shortly after coronary artery occlusion partially reverses the ventricular fibrillation threshold, whereas nitroglycerin and phenylephrine in combination restore this threshold to normal. Nitroglycerin is presumed to act by augmenting perfusion of the border of the ischemic zone by dilating collaterals and by reducing myocardial demands by lowering preload and afterload (Fig. 38-6).[433]

The idea that oxygen-derived free radicals may play a role in myocardial injury due to ischemia and reperfusion is discussed on page 1187. A variety of scavengers of oxygen radicals have been shown to reduce the size of myocardial infarction in some[338] but certainly not all experiments.[434,435] These agents include superoxide dismutase, catalase, their combination, N-2-mercaptopropionyl glycine, and allopurinol, an inhibitor of xanthine oxidase.[436] Neutrophils accumulate rapidly in ischemic tissue, and the injury they cause is mediated largely through release of oxygen radicals. Neutrophil depletion also limits infarct size[437]; however, beneficial effects of free radical scavengers have been seen even in animals depleted of neutrophils.

When myocardium is "preconditioned" by repeated brief episodes of ischemia, it appears to be protected from the deleterious effects of subsequent prolonged ischemia. It had been suggested that preconditioning reduces myocardial energy demand during subsequent ischemia.[438-440]

REPERFUSION INJURY

Despite the unequivocal utility of reperfusion in limiting cell death in the presence of severe ischemia, reperfusion can elicit a number of adverse reactions that may limit its beneficial actions[437a,437b].

ACCELERATION OF MYOCYTE NECROSIS. After reperfusion, ischemic cells often suddenly develop ultrastructural changes indicative of cell death, including "explosive swelling" and widespread architectural disruption. Nevertheless, it is likely that most—perhaps all—of the myocytes in which necrosis is accelerated by reperfusion were already irreversibly injured by the time reperfusion occurred and that reperfusion merely hastened the death of cells already destined not to recover. If reperfusion does cause necrosis of *reversibly* injured myocardium, the quantity of tissue so affected is likely to be small.

ISCHEMIC CELL SWELLING. This causes compression of myocardial capillaries interfering further with myocardial perfusion. Reperfusion intensifies this process and thereby contributes to necrosis of some reversibly injured cells.[441]

THE "NO-REFLOW" PHENOMENON. This refers to the failure to achieve sustained reperfusion after a prolonged period of ischemia. The areas of reduced or absent reflow often appear to result from ischemia-induced microvascular damage and myocardial contracture. The no-reflow phenomenon does *not* appear to augment myocyte death, because the zone of reflow is contained within areas in which myocytes were already necrotic at the time of the onset of reperfusion (Fig. 38-41).

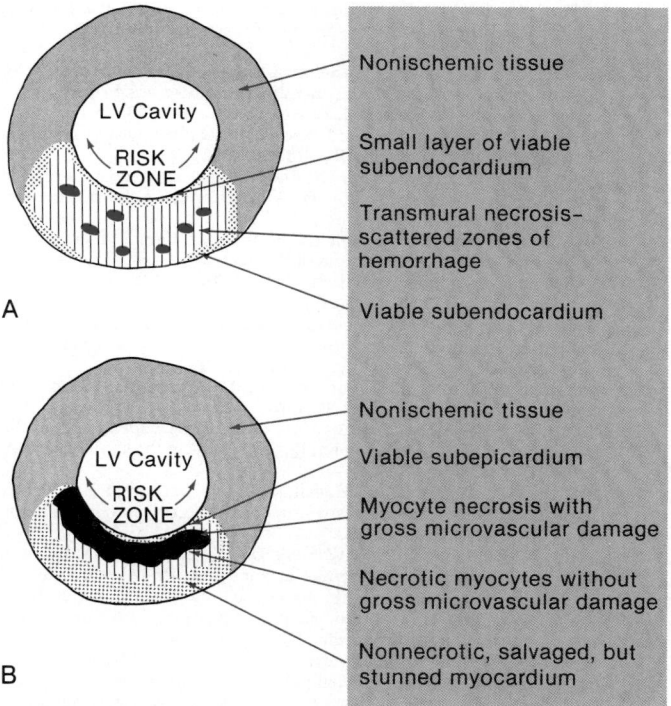

FIGURE 38-41. *A,* Schematic diagram showing a transverse section through a canine left ventricle subjected to a permanent coronary occlusion without reperfusion. The white area represents nonischemic myocardium supplied by the nonoccluded vessel. The infarct (hatched area) is transmural or near-transmural. There are scattered zones of hemorrhage (solid black). A small layer of viable subendocardium is present, which derives its oxygen directly from the ventricular cavity. Where collateral flow is high, there may be a small rim of surviving subepicardium (stippled areas). *B,* Schematic diagram showing a transverse section through a canine left ventricle subjected to coronary occlusion followed within 1 or 2 hours by coronary reperfusion. The hatched and solid black areas represent the infarct that is confined to the inner half of the myocardium. The solid black area represents the zone of gross microvascular damage including the zones of no-reflow and hemorrhage. It is smaller than and contained within the total infarct. The remainder of the infarct without severe microvascular damage is represented by the hatched area and is located in the midmyocardium. The epicardial portion of the ischemic zone (stippled area) has been salvaged by coronary reperfusion. It is nonnecrotic but stunned (postischemic ventricular dysfunction) for hours to days following coronary reperfusion. (From Braunwald, E., and Kloner, R. A.: Myocardial reperfusion: A double-edge sword? J. Clin. Invest. 76:1715, 1985.)

REPERFUSION-INDUCED HEMORRHAGE. Reperfused infarcts frequently contain hemorrhagic areas.[442] Reperfusion-induced hemorrhage, like the "no-reflow" phenomenon, is caused largely by microvascular damage. It is generally contained within areas of myocardium already necrotic at the time of reperfusion.[443]

THE CALCIUM PARADOX AND THE OXYGEN PARADOX. The reintroduction of Ca^{++} and/or of oxygen to hearts previously perfused with Ca^{++}-free hypoxic media causes marked damage to the sarcolemma and entry of large quantities of Ca^{++} into the ischemic cells. These phenomena have been termed the *calcium paradox* and the *oxygen paradox*, respectively. Perfusion of ischemic cells with Ca^{++}-free solution occurs clinically only in the special circumstances when cardioplegia is produced during cardiac surgery by means of a Ca^{++}-free solution. However, the oxygen paradox may have clinical relevance. It may be mediated by oxygen-derived free radicals and potentially can be limited by free-radical scavengers of these substances.

REFERENCES

CONTROL OF MYOCARDIAL OXYGEN CONSUMPTION

1. Reimer, K. A., and Jennings, R. B.: Myocardial ischemia, hypoxia and infarction. In Fozzard, H. A., Jennings, R. B., Haber, E., Katz, A. M., and Morgan, H. E. (eds.): The Heart and Cardiovascular System. New York, Raven Press, 1986, pp. 1133–1202.
2. McKeever, W. P., Gregg, D. E., and Canney, P. C.: Oxygen uptake of the nonworking left ventricle. Circ. Res. 6:612, 1958.
3. Rooke, G. A., and Feigl, E. O.: Work as a correlate of canine left ventricular oxygen consumption, and the problem of catecholamine oxygen wasting. Circ. Res. 50:273, 1982.
4. Suga, H., Goto, Y., Yamada, O., and Igarashi, Y.: Independence of myocardial oxygen consumption from pressure-volume trajectory during diastole in canine left ventricle. Circ. Res. 55:734, 1984
5. Klocke, F. J., Braunwald, E., and Ross, J., Jr.: Oxygen cost of electrical activation of the heart. Circ. Res. 18:357, 1966.
6. Evans, C. L., and Matsuoka, Y.: The effect of various mechanical conditions on the gaseous metabolism and efficiency of the mammalian heart. J. Physiol. 49:378, 1915.
7. Sarnoff, S. J., Braunwald, E., Welch, G. H. Jr., et al.: Hemodynamic determinants of oxygen consumption of the heart with special reference to the tension-time index. Am. J. Physiol. 192:148, 1958.
8. Braunwald, E., Sarnoff, S. J., Case, R. B., et al.: Hemodynamic determinants of coronary flow: Effect of changes in aortic pressure and cardiac output on the relationship between myocardial oxygen consumption and coronary flow. Am. J. Physiol. 192:157, 1958.
9. Rodbard, S., Williams, C. B., and Rodbard, D.: Myocardial tension and oxygen uptake. Circ. Res. 14:139, 1964.
10. Teplick, R., Haas, G. S., Trautman, E., et al.: Time dependence of the oxygen cost of force development during systole in the canine left ventricle. Circ. Res. 59:27, 1986.
11. Sonnenblick, E. H., Ross, J., Jr., Covell, J. W., and Braunwald, E.: Velocity of contraction as a determinant of myocardial oxygen consumption. Am. J. Physiol. 209:919, 1965.
12. Starling, M. R., Mancini, J., Montgomery, D. G., and Gross, M. D.: Relation between maximum time-varying elastance pressure-volume areas and myocardial oxygen consumption in dogs. Circulation 83:304, 1991.
13. Suga, H., Nozawa, T., Yasumura, Y., et al.: Force-time integral does not improve predictability of cardiac O_2 consumption from pressure-volume area (PVA) in dog left ventricle. Heart Vessels 5:152, 1990.
14. Suga, H., Goto, Y., Igarashi, Y., et al.: Cardiac cooling increases E_{max} without affecting relation between O_2 consumption and systolic pressure-volume area in dog left ventricle. Circ. Res. 63:61, 1988.
15. Schike, J. D., Burkhoff, D., Kass, D. A., et al.: Hemodynamic dependence of myocardial oxygen consumption indexes. Am. J. Physical. 258:H1281, 1990.
16. Yasumura, Y., Nozawa, T., Futaki, S., et al.: Time-invariant oxygen cost of mechanical energy in dog left ventricle: Consistency and inconsistency of time-varying elastance model with myocardial energetics. Circulation 64:764, 1989.
17. Ando, H., Nakano, E., Ueno, Y., and Tokunaga, K.: New technique for analysis of cardiac energetics using a modified Fenn equation. J. Thorac. Cardiovasc. Surg. 97:565, 1989.
17a. Hasenfuss, G., Mulieri, L. A., Blanchard, E. M., et al.: Energetics of isometric force development in control and volume-overloaded human myocardium: Comparison with animal species. Circ. Res. 68:836, 1991.
18. Hisano, R., and Cooper, G. IV: Correlation of force-length area with oxygen consumption in ferret papillary muscle. Circ. Res. 61:318, 1987.
19. Mast, F., and Elzinga, G.: Heat released during relaxation equals force-length area in isometric contractions of rabbit papillary muscle. Circ. Res. 67:893, 1990.
20. Duwel, C.M.B., and Westerhof, N.: Feline left ventricular oxygen consumption is not affected by volume expansion, ejection or redevelopment of pressure during relaxation. Pflugers Arch. 412:409, 1988.
21. Fenn, W. O.: A quantitative comparison between the energy liberated and the work performed by the isolated sartorius muscle of the frog. J. Physiol. (Lond.) 58:175, 1923.

22. Rall, J. A.: Sense and nonsense about the Fenn effect. Am. J. Physiol. 242(Heart Circ. Physiol. 11):H1, 1982.
23. Suga, H., Futaki, S., Tanaka, N., et al.: Paired pulse pacing increases cardiac O_2 consumption for activation without changing efficiency of contractile machinery in canine left ventricle. Heart Vessels 4:79, 1988.
24. Graham, T. P., Jr., Covell, J. W., Sonnenblick, E. H., et al.: Control of myocardial oxygen consumption: Relative influence of contractile state and tension development. J. Clin. Invest. 47:375, 1968.
25. Boerth, R. C., Covell, J. W., Pool, P. E., and Ross, J., Jr.: Increased myocardial oxygen consumption and contractile state associated with increased heart rate in dogs. Circ. Res. 24:725, 1969.
26. Ardehali, A., and Ports, T. A.: Myocardial oxygen supply and demand. Chest 98:699, 1990.
27. Suga, H., Hisano, R., Goto, Y., Yamada, O., and Igarashi, Y.: Effect of positive inotropic agents on the relation between oxygen consumption and systolic pressure volume area in canine left ventricle. Circ. Res. 53:306, 1983.
28. Urschel, C. W., Covell, J. W., Graham, T. P., et al.: Effects of acute valvular regurgitation on the oxygen consumption of the canine heart. Circ. Res. 23:33, 1968.
29. Vik-Mo, H., and Mjos, O. E.: Influence of free fatty acids on myocardial oxygen consumption and ischemic injury. Am. J. Cardiol. 48:361, 1981.
30. Loiselle, D. S.: Cardiac basal and activation metabolism. In Jacob, R., Just, H. J., and Holubarsch, C. H. (eds.): Cardiac Energetics: Basic Mechanisms and Clinical Implications. New York, Springer-Verlag, 1987, pp. 37–50.
31. Tubau, J. F., Wikman-Coffelt, J., Massie, B. M., et al.: Improved myocardial efficiency in the working perfused heart of the spontaneously hypertensive rat. Hypertension 10:396, 1987.
32. Hornby, L., Hamilton, N., Marshall, D., et al.: Role of cardiac work in regulating myocardial biochemical characteristics. Am. J. Physiol. 258:H1482, 1990.
33. Laxson, D. D., Homans, D. C., Dai, X., et al.: Oxygen consumption and coronary reactivity in postischemic myocardium. Circ. Res. 64:9, 1989.

REGULATION OF CORONARY BLOOD FLOW

34. Braunwald, E., Ross, J., Jr., and Sonnenblick, E. H.: Regulation of coronary blood flow. In Mechanisms of Contraction of the Normal and Failing Heart. 2nd ed. Boston, Little, Brown, 1976, p. 200.
35. Berne, R. M., and Rubio, R.: Coronary circulation. In Berne, R. M., Sperelakis, N., and Geiger, S. R. (eds.): Handbook of Physiology; Section 2, The Cardiovascular System. Bethesda, American Physiological Society, 1979, p. 897.
36. Feigl, E. O.: Coronary physiology. Physiol. Rev. 63:1, 1983.
37. Marcus, M. L., and Harrison, D. G.: Physiologic basis for myocardial perfusion imaging. In Marcus, M. L., et al. (eds.): Cardiac Imaging. Philadelphia, W. B. Saunders Company, 1991, pp. 8–23.
38. Young, M. A., and Vatner, S. F.: Regulation of large coronary arteries. Circ. Res. 59:579, 1986.
39. Provenza, D. V., and Scherlis, S.: Coronary circulation in dog's heart: Demonstration of muscle sphincters in capillaries. Circ. Res. 7:318, 1959.
40. Habib, G. B., Heibig, J., Forman, S. A., et al.: Influence of coronary collateral vessels on myocardial infarct size in humans: Results of Phase I thrombolysis in myocardial infarction (TIMI) trial. Circulation 83:739, 1991.
41. Cohen, M. V., Yipintsoi, T., and Scheuer, J.: Coronary collateral stimulation by exercise in dogs with stenotic coronary arteries. J. Appl. Physiol. 52:664, 1982.
42. Bloor, C. M., White, F. C., and Sanders, M.: Effects of exercise on collateral development in myocardial ischemia in pigs. J. Appl. Physiol. 56:656, 1984.
43. Scheel, K. W., and Williams, S. E.: Hypertrophy and coronary and collateral vascularity in dogs with severe chronic anemia. Am. J. Physiol. 249:H1031, 1985.
44. Patterson, R. E., Jones-Collins, B. A., Aamodt, R., and Ro, Y. M.: Differences in collateral myocardial blood flow following gradual vs. abrupt coronary occlusion. Cardiovasc. Res. 17:207, 1983.
44a. Sabri, M. N., DiSciascio, G., Cowley, M. J., et al.: Coronary collateral recruitment: Functional significance and relation to rate of vessel closure. Am. Heart J. 121:876, 1991.
45. Schaper, W.: Influence of physical exercise on coronary collateral blood flow in chronic experimental two-vessel occlusion. Circulation 65:905, 1982.
46. Verani, M. S.: The functional significance of coronary collateral vessels: Anecdote confronts science. Cathet. Cardiovasc. Diagn. 9:333, 1983.
47. Elayda, M. A., Mathur, V. S., Hall, R. J., et al.: Collateral circulation in coronary artery disease. Am. J. Cardiol. 55:58, 1985.
48. Demer, L. L., Gould, K. L., Goldstein, R. A., and Kirkeeide, R. L.: Noninvasive assessment of coronary collaterals in man by PET perfusion imaging. J. Nucl. Med. 31:259, 1990.
49. Mohri, M., Tomoike, H., Noma, M., et al.: Duration of ischemia is vital for collateral development: Repeated brief coronary artery occlusions in conscious dogs. Circ. Res. 64:287, 1989.
50. Shen, Y., Knight, D. R., Canfield, D. R., et al.: Progressive change in collateral blood flow after coronary occlusion in conscious dogs. Am. J. Physiol. 256:H478, 1989.
51. Marcus, M. L.: The Coronary Circulation in Health and Disease. New York, McGraw-Hill and Company, 1983, 465 pp.

52. Olsson, R. A., and Bugni, W. J.: Coronary circulation. *In* Fozzard, H. A., et al. (eds.): The Heart and Cardiovascular System. New York, Raven Press, 1986, pp. 987–1038.

53. Klocke, F. J., Mates, R. E., Canty, J. M., Jr., and Ellis, A. K.: Coronary pressure-flow relationships. Controversial issues and probable implications. Circ. Res. 56:311, 1985.

54. Spnan, J.A.E.: Coronary diastolic pressure-flow relation and zero flow pressure explained on the basis of intramyocardial compliance. Circ. Res. 56:293, 1985.

55. Matsuo, S., Tsuruta, M., Hayano, M., et al.: Phasic coronary artery flow velocity determined by Doppler flowmeter catheter in aortic stenosis and aortic regurgitation. Am. J. Cardiol. 62:917, 1988.

56. Cole, J. S., and Hartley, C. J.: The pulsed Doppler artery catheter. Circulation 56:18, 1977.

57. Klocke, F. J.: Coronary blood flow in man. Prog. Cardiovasc. Dis. 19:117, 1976.

58. Griggs, D. M., Jr., Chen, C. C., and Tchokoev, V. V.: Subendocardial metabolism in experimental aortic stenosis. Am. J. Physiol. 224:607, 1973.

59. Klocke, F. J.: Measurements of coronary flow reserve: Defining pathophysiology versus making decisions about patient care. Circulation 76:1183, 1987.

60. Sabbah, H. N., and Stein, P. D.: Effect of acute regional ischemia on pressure in the subepicardium and subendocardium. Am. J. Physiol. 242(Heart Circ. Physiol. 11):H240, 1982.

61. Brazier, J., Cooper, N., and Buckberg, G.: The adequacy of subendocardial oxygen delivery: The interaction of determinants of flow, arterial oxygen content and myocardial oxygen need. Circulation 49:968, 1974.

62. Lundsgaard-Hansen, P., Meyer, C., and Riedwyl, H.: Transmural gradients of glycolytic enzyme activities in left ventricular myocardium. I. The normal state. Pfluegers Arch. 297:89, 1967.

63. Buckberg, G. D., Fixler, D. E., Archie, J. P., and Hoffman, J.I.E.: Experimental subendocardial ischemia in dogs with normal coronary arteries. Circ. Res. 30:67, 1972.

64. Hoffman, J.I.E.: Determinants of prediction of transmural myocardial perfusion. Circulation 58:381, 1978.

65. Boudoulas, H.: Diastolic time: The forgotten dynamic factor. Implications for myocardial perfusion. Acta Cardiologica XLVI:61, 1991.

66. Fallen, E. L., Elliott, W. C., and Gorlin, R.: Mechanisms of angina in aortic stenosis. Circulation 36:480, 1967.

67. Griggs, D. M., Jr., and Chen, C. C.: Coronary hemodynamics and regional myocardial metabolism in experimental aortic insufficiency. J. Clin. Invest. 53:1599, 1974.

68. Dunn, R. B., and Griggs, D. M., Jr.: Ventricular filling pressure as a determinant of coronary blood flow during ischemia. Am. J. Physiol. 244:H429, 1983.

69. Becker, L. C., Fortuin, N. J., and Pitt, B.: Effect of ischemia and antianginal drugs on the distribution of radioactive microspheres in the canine left ventricle. Circ. Res. 28:263, 1971.

70. Mathes, P., and Rival, J.: Effect of nitroglycerin on total and regional coronary blood flow in the normal and ischaemic canine myocardium. Cardiovasc. Res. 5:54, 1971.

71. Vatner, S. F.: Alpha-adrenergic tone in the coronary circulation of the conscious dog. Fed. Proc. 43:2867, 1984.

72. Woodman, O. L., and Vatner, S. F.: Coronary vasoconstriction mediated by alpha$_1$ and alpha$_2$ adrenoceptors in the conscious dog. Am. J. Physiol. 253:H388, 1987.

73. Young, M. A., Vatner, D. E., Knight, D. R., et al.: Alpha-adrenergic vasoconstriction and receptor subtypes in large coronary arteries of calves. Am. J. Physiol. 255:H1452, 1988.

74. Morgan, K. G.: Role of calcium ion in maintenance of vascular smooth muscle tone. Am. J. Cardiol. 59:24A, 1987.

75. Johns, A., Leijten, P., Yamamoto, H., Hwang, K., and van Breemen, C.: Calcium regulation in vascular smooth muscle contractility. Am. J. Cardiol. 59:18A, 1987.

76. Adelstein, R. S., and Sellers, J. R.: Effects of calcium on vascular smooth muscle contraction. Am. J. Cardiol. 59:4B, 1987.

77. Rinkema, L. E., Thomas, J. X., Jr., and Randall, W. C.: Regional coronary vasoconstriction in response to stimulation of stellate ganglia. Am. J. Physiol. 243:H410, 1982.

78. Murray, P. A., Lavall, M., and Vatner, S. F.: Alpha-adrenergic-mediated reduction in coronary blood flow secondary to carotid chemoreceptor reflex activation in conscious dogs. Circ. Res. 54:96, 1984.

79. Vatner, D. E., Knight, D. R., Homcy, C. J., et al.: Subtypes of beta-adrenergic receptors in bovine coronary arteries. Circ. Res. 59:463, 1986.

80. Feldman, R. D., Christy, J. P., Paul, S. T., and Harrison, D. G.: Beta-adrenergic receptors on canine coronary collateral vessels: Characterization and function. Am. J. Physiol. 257:H1634, 1989.

81. Vatner, S. F., and Hintze, T. H.: Mechanism of constriction of large coronary arteries by beta-adrenergic receptor blockade. Circ. Res. 53:389, 1983.

82. Cox, D. A., Hintze, T. H., and Vatner, S. F.: Effects of acetylcholine on large and small coronary arteries in conscious dogs. J. Pharmacol. Exp. Ther. 225:764, 1983.

83. Vatner, S. F., Higgins, C. B., and Braunwald, E.: Effects of norepinephrine on coronary circulation and left ventricular dynamics in the conscious dog. Circ. Res. 34:812, 1974.

84. Kern, M. J., Horowitz, J. D., Ganz, P., et al.: Attenuation of coronary vascular resistance by selective alpha$_1$-adrenergic blockade in patients with coronary artery disease. J. Am. Coll. Cardiol. 5:840, 1985.

85. Winniford, M. D., Wheelan, K. R., Kremers, M. S., et al.: Smoking-induced coronary vasoconstriction in patients with atherosclerotic coronary ar-

tery disease: Evidence for adrenergically mediated alterations in coronary artery tone. Circulation 74:662, 1986.

86. Winniford, M. D., Jansen, D. E., Reynolds, G. A., et al.: Cigarette smoking-induced coronary vasoconstriction in atherosclerotic coronary artery disease and prevention by calcium antagonists and nitroglycerin. Am. J. Cardiol. 59:203, 1987.

87. Szentivanyi, M., and Juhasz-Nagy, N.: Physiological role of the coronary constrictor fibers. Q. J. Exp. Physiol. 48:93, 1963.

88. Hackett, J. G., Abboud, F. M., Mark, A. L., et al.: Coronary vascular responses to stimulation of chemoreceptors and baroreceptors. Circ. Res. 21:8, 1972.

89. Higgins, C. B., Vatner, S. F., and Braunwald, E.: Parasympathetic control of the heart. Pharmacol. Rev. 25:119, 1973.

90. Vatner, S. F., Franklin, D., VanCitters, R. L., and Braunwald, E.: Effects of carotid sinus nerve stimulation on the coronary circulation of the conscious dog. Circ. Res. 27:11, 1970.

91. Brachfeld, N., Monroe, R. G., and Gorlin, R.: Effects of pericoronary denervation on coronary hemodynamics. Am. J. Physiol. 199:174, 1960.

92. Macho, P., and Vatner, S. F.: Effects of prazosin on coronary and left ventricular dynamics in conscious dogs. Circulation 65:1186, 1982.

93. Heyndrickx, G. R., Muylaert, P., and Pannier, J. L.: Alpha-adrenergic control of oxygen delivery to myocardium during exercise in conscious dog. Am. J. Physiol. 242(Heart Circ. Physiol. 11):H805, 1982.

94. Laxson, D. D., Dai, X., Homans, D. C., and Bache, R. J.: The role of alpha$_1$- and alpha$_2$-adrenergic receptors in mediation of coronary vasoconstriction in hypoperfused ischemic myocardium during exercise. Circ. Res. 65:1688, 1989.

95. Feigl, E. O.: The paradox of adrenergic coronary vasoconstriction. Circulation 76:737, 1987.

96. Huang, A. H., and Feigl, E. O.: Adrenergic coronary vasoconstriction helps maintain uniform transmural blood flow distribution during exercise. Circ. Res. 62:286, 1988.

97. Chilian, W. M., and Ackell, P. H.: Transmural differences in sympathetic coronary constriction during exercise in the presence of coronary stenosis. Circ. Res. 62:216, 1988.

98. Heusch, G.: Alpha-adrenergic mechanisms in myocardial ischemia. Circulation 81:1, 1990.

99. Feigl, E. O.: Reflex parasympathetic coronary vasodilation elicited from cardiac receptors in the dog. Circ. Res. 37:175, 1975.

100. Pitetti, K. H., Iwamoto, G. A., Mitchell, J. H., and Ordway, G. A.: Stimulating somatic afferent fibers alters coronary arterial resistance. Am. J. Physiol. 256:R1331, 1989.

101. Jarisch, A., and Zotterman, Y.: Depressor reflexes from the heart. Acta Physiol. Scand. 16:31, 1948.

102. Feigl, E. O.: Parasympathetic control of coronary blood flow in dogs. Circ. Res. 25:509, 1969.

103. Brown, B. G., Lee, A. B., Bolson, E. L., and Dodge, H. T.: Reflex constriction of significant coronary stenosis as a mechanism contributing to ischemic left ventricular dysfunction during isometric exercise. Circulation 70:18, 1984.

104. Chierchia, S., Davies, G., Berkenboom, B., et al.: Alpha-adrenergic receptors and coronary spasm: An elusive link. Circulation 69:8, 1984.

105. Galassi, A. R., Kaski, J. C., Pupita, G., et al.: Lack of evidence for alpha-adrenergic receptor–mediated mechanisms in the genesis of ischemia in syndrome X. Am. J. Cardiol. 64:264, 1989.

105a. Cannon, R. O., III, Bonow, R. O., Bacharach, S. L., et al.: Left ventricular dysfunction in patients with angina pectoris, normal epicardial coronary arteries, and abnormal vasodilator reserve. Circulation 71:218, 1985.

106. Gould, L., Reddy, G. V., and Gombrecht, R. F.: Oral phentolamine in angina pectoris. Jpn. Heart J. 14:393, 1973.

106a. Cannon, R. O., III, Leon, M. B., Watson, R. M., et al.: Chest pain and "normal" coronary arteries—Role of small coronary arteries. Am. J. Cardiol. 55:50B, 1985.

107. Berkenboom, G. M., Abramowicz, M., Vandermoten, P., and Degre, S. G.: Role of alpha adrenergic coronary tone in exercise-induced angina pectoris. Am. J. Cardiol. 57:195, 1986.

107a. Hayes, S. N., Moyer, T. P., Morley, D., and Bove, A. A.: Intravenous cocaine causes epicardial coronary vasoconstriction in the intact dog. Am. Heart J. 121:1639, 1991.

108. Lange, R. A., Cigarra, R. G., Yancy, C. W., et al.: Cocaine-induced coronary-artery vasoconstriction. N. Engl. J. Med. 321:1557, 1989.

109. Johnson, P. C.: Autoregulation of blood flow. Circ. Res. 58:483, 1986.

110. Lee, J.-D., Tajimi, T., Guth, B., et al.: Exercise-induced regional dysfunction with subcritical coronary stenosis. Circulation 73:596, 1986.

111. Oien, A. H., and Aukland, K.: A mathematical analysis of the myogenic hypothesis with special reference to autoregulation of renal blood flow. Circ. Res. 52:241, 1983.

112. Bayliss, W. M.: On the local reaction of the arterial wall to changes in arterial pressure. J. Physiol. (Lond.) 28:220, 1902.

113. Coffman, J. D., and Gregg, D. E.: Oxygen metabolism and oxygen debt repayment after myocardial ischemia. Am. J. Physiol. 201:881, 1961.

114. Detar, R., and Bohr, D. F.: Oxygen and vascular smooth muscle contraction. Am. J. Physiol. 214:241, 1968.

115. Duling, B. R.: Microvascular responses to alterations in oxygen tension. Circ. Res. 31:481, 1972.

116. Martini, J., and Honig, C. R.: Direct measurement of intercapillary distance in beating rat heart in situ under various conditions of O_2 supply. Microvasc. Res. 1:244, 1969.

117. Sparks, H. V., Jr., and Bardenheuer, H.: Regulation of adenosine formation by the heart. Circ. Res. 58:193, 1986.

118. Rubio, R., and Berne, R. M.: Release of adenosine by the normal myocardium and its relationship to the regulation of coronary resistance. Circ. Res. 25:407, 1969.

119. Bardenheuer, H., and Schrader, J.: Supply-to-demand ratio for oxygen determines formation of adenosine by the heart. Am. J. Physiol. 250:H173, 1986.

120. Rubio, R., Berne, R. M., and Dobson, J. G., Jr.: Sites of adenosine production in cardiac and skeletal muscle. Am. J. Physiol. 225:938, 1973.

121. Rubio, R., Berne, R. M., and Katori, M.: Release of adenosine in reactive hyperemia of the dog heart. Am. J. Physiol. 216:56, 1969.

122. McKenzie, J. E., Steffen, R. P., and Haddy, F. J.: Relations between adenosine and coronary resistance in conscious exercising dogs. Am. J. Physiol. 242:H24, 1982.

123. Belardinelli, L., Vogel, S., Linden, J., and Berne, R. M.: Anti-adrenergic action of adenosine on ventricular myocardium in embryonic chick hearts. J. Mol. Cell. Cardiol. 14:291, 1982.

124. Gellai, M., Norton, J. M., and Detar, R.: Evidence for direct control of coronary vascular tone by oxygen. Circ. Res. 32:279, 1973.

125. Bergman, G., Atkinson, L., Richardson, P. J., et al.: Prostacyclin: Haemodynamic and metabolic effects in patients with coronary artery disease. Lancet 1:569, 1981.

126. Friedman, P. L., Brugada, P., Kuck, K. H., et al.: Coronary vasoconstrictor effect of indomethacin in patients with coronary artery disease. N. Engl. J. Med. 305:1171, 1981.

126a. Henderson, A.H.: Endothelium in control. Br. Heart J. 65:116, 1991.

127. Vanhoutte, P. M. (ed.): Vasodilatation: Vascular Smooth Muscle, Peptides, Autonomic Nerves, and Endothelium. New York, Raven Press, 1988, 572 pp.

128. Warren, J. B. (ed.): The Endothelium: An Introduction to Current Research. New York, Wiley-Liss, 1990, 317 pp.

129. Furchgott, R. F., and Vanhoutte, P. M.: Endothelium-derived relaxing and contracting factors. FASEB J. 3:2007, 1989.

130. Vanhoutte, P. M., and Shimokawa, H.: Endothelium-derived relaxing factor and coronary vasospasm. Circulation 80:1, 1989.

131. Kelm, M., and Schrader, J.: Control of coronary vascular tone by nitric oxide. Circ. Res. 66:1561, 1990.

131a. Ahlner, J., Ljusegren, M. E., Grundström, N., and Axelsson, K. L.: Role of nitric oxide and cyclic GMP as mediators of endothelium-independent neurogenic relaxation in bovine mesenteric artery. Circ. Res. 68:756, 1991.

131b. Schini, V.B.: Nitric oxide and vascular reactivity. Coronary Artery Dis. 2:293, 1991.

132. Ignarro, L. J.: Biological actions and properties of endothelium-derived nitric oxide formed and released from artery and vein. Circ. Res. 65:1, 1989.

133. Vallance, P., Collier, J., and Moncada, S.: Nitric oxide synthesised from L-arginine mediates endothelium dependent dilatation in human veins in vivo. Cardiovasc. Res. 23:1053, 1989.

134. Van Winkle, D. M., and Feigl, E. O.: Acetylcholine causes coronary vasodilation in dogs and baboons. Circ. Res. 65:1580, 1989.

135. Stamler, J., Mendelsohn, M. E., Amarante, P., et al.: N-acetylcysteine potentiates platelet inhibition by endothelium-derived relaxing factor. Circ. Res. 65:789, 1989.

136. Dinerman, J. L., and Mehta, J. L.: Endothelial, platelet and leukocyte interactions in ischemic heart disease: insights into potential mechanisms and their clinical relevance. J. Am. Coll. Cardiol. 16:207, 1990.

137. Sellke, F. W., Armstrong, M. L., and Harrison, D. G.: Endothelium-dependent vascular relaxation is abnormal in the coronary microcirculation of atherosclerotic primates. Circulation 81:1586, 1990.

137a. Shimokawa, H., and Vanhoutte, P. M.: Hypercholesterolemia causes generalized impairment of endothelium-dependent relaxation to aggregating platelets in porcine arteries. J. Am. Coll. Cardiol. 13:1402, 1989.

138. Werns, S. W., Walton, J. A., Hsia, H. H., et al.: Evidence of endothelial dysfunction in angiographically normal coronary arteries of patients with coronary artery disease. Circulation 79:287, 1989.

139. Yasue, H., Matsuyama, K., Matsuyama, K., et al: Responses of angiographically normal human coronary arteries to intracoronary injection of acetylcholine by age and segment: Possible role of early coronary atherosclerosis. Circulation 81:482, 1990.

140. Gordon, J. B., Ganz, P., Nabel, E. G., et al.: Atherosclerosis influences the vasomotor response of epicardial coronary arteries to exercise. J. Clin. Invest. 83:1946, 1989.

141. Tulenko, T. N., Constantinescu, D., Kikuchi, T., et al.: Mutual interaction of vasoconstriction and endothelial damage in stenotic arteries. Am. J. Physiol. 256:H881, 1989.

142. Stewart, D. J., Pohl, U., and Bassenge, E.: Free radicals inhibit endothelium-dependent dilation in the coronary resistance vessels. Am. J. Physiol. 255:H765, 1988.

143. Tsao, P. S., Aoki, N., Lefer, D. J., et al.: Time course of endothelial dysfunction and myocardial injury during myocardial ischemia and reperfusion in the cat. Circulation 82:1402, 1990.

144. Shimokawa, H., and Vanhoutte, P. M.: Dietary cod-liver oil improves endothelium-dependent responses in hypercholesterolemic and atherosclerotic porcine coronary arteries. Circulation 78:1421, 1988.

145. Yanagisawa, M., Kurihara, H., Kimura, S., et al.: A novel potent vasoconstrictor peptide produced by vascular endothelial cells. Nature 332:411, 1988.

146. Nayler, W. G.: Endothelin-1 and the cardiovascular system: A mini-review. J. Appl. Cardiol. 4:495, 1989.

147. Yang, Z., Richard, V., von Segesser, L., et al.: Threshold concentrations of endothelin-1 potentiate contractions to norepinephrine and serotonin in human arteries: A new mechanism of vasospasm? Circulation 82:188, 1990.

148. Clozel, J., and Clozel, M.: Effects of endothelin on the coronary vascular bed in open-chest dogs. Circ. Res. 65:1193, 1989.

149. Siegfried, M. R., Aoki, N., Mulloy, D., and Lefer, A. M.: Direct positive inotropic and vasoconstrictor effects of endothelin. Heart Vessels 5:146, 1990.

150. Prasad, K., Lee, P., and Kalra, J.: Influence of endothelin on cardiovascular function, oxygen-free radicals, and blood chemistry. Am. Heart J. 121:178, 1991.

151. Fam, W. M., and McGregor, M.: Effect of coronary vasodilator drugs on retrograde flow in areas of chronic myocardial ischemia. Circ. Res. 15:355, 1964.

152. Cohen, M. V., Downey, J. M., Sonnenblick, E. H., and Kirk, E. S.: The effects of nitroglycerin on coronary collaterals and myocardial contractility. J. Clin. Invest. 52:2836, 1973.

153. Schwartz, J. S., and Bache, R. J.: Pharmacologic vasodilators in the coronary circulation. Circulation 75:I–162, 1987.

154. Vatner, S. F., Pagani, M., Manders, T., and Pasipoularides, A. D.: Alpha-adrenergic vasoconstriction and nitroglycerin vasodilation of large coronary arteries in the conscious dog. J. Clin. Invest. 65:5, 1980.

155. Feldman, R. L., Marx, J. D., Pepine, C. J., and Conti, C. R.: Analysis of coronary responses to various doses of intracoronary nitroglycerin. Circulation 66:321, 1982.

156. Macho, P., and Vatner, S. F.: Effects of nitroglycerin and nitroprusside on large and small coronary vessels in conscious dogs. Circulation 64:1101, 1981.

157. Hinte, T. H., and Vatner, S. F.: Comparison of effects of nifedipine and nitroglycerin on large and small coronary arteries and cardiac function in conscious dogs. Circ. Res. 52(Suppl. I):139, 1983.

158. Ludmer, P. L., Selwyn, A. P., Shook, T. L., et al.: Paradoxical vasoconstriction induced by acetylcholine in atherosclerotic coronary arteries. N. Engl. J. Med. 315:1046, 1986.

159. Engle, H.-J., and Lichten, P. R.: Beneficial enhancement of coronary blood flow by nifedipine: Comparison with nitroglycerin and beta blocking agents. Am. J. Med. 71:658, 1981.

160. Cannon, R. O., III, Schenke, W. H., Leon, M. B., et al.: Limited coronary flow reserve after dipyridamole in patients with ergonovine-induced coronary vasoconstriction. Circulation 75:163, 1987.

161. Bush, L. R., Campbell, W. B., Buja, L. M., et al.: Effects of the selective thromboxane synthetase inhibitor dazoxiben on variations in cyclic blood flow in stenosed canine coronary arteries. Circulation 69:1161, 1984.

162. Bush, L. R., Campbell, W. B., Kern, K., et al.: The effects of alpha₂-adrenergic and serotonergic receptor antagonists on cyclic blood flow alterations in stenosed canine coronary arteries. Circ. Res. 55:642, 1984.

163. Foreman, B., Dai, X., Homans, D. C., et al.: Effect of atrial natriuretic peptide on coronary collateral blood flow. Circ. Res. 65:1671, 1989.

164. Chu, A., Morris, K. G., Kuehl, W. D., et al.: Effects of atrial natriuretic peptide on the coronary arterial vasculature in humans. Circulation 80:1627, 1989.

165. Wilson, R. F., Wyche, K., Christensen, B. V., et al: Effects of adenosine on human coronary arterial circulation. 82:1595, 1990.

166. Hoffman, J.I.E.: A critical review of coronary reserve. Circulation 75:I–6, 1987.

167. Klocke, F. J.: Measurements of coronary flow reserve: Defining pathophysiology versus making decisions about patient care. Circulation 76:1183, 1987.

168. Gould, K. L., Kirkeeide, R. L., and Buchi, M.: Coronary flow reserve as a physiologic measure of stenosis severity. J. Am. Coll. Cardiol. 15:459, 1990.

169. Marcus, M. L., Harrison, D. G., White, C. W., and Hiratzka, L. F.: Assessing the physiological significance of coronary obstruction in man. Can. J. Cardiol. Suppl. A:195A, 1986.

170. Marcus, M. L., Doty, D. B., Hiratzka, L. F., et al.: Decreased coronary reserve. A mechanism for angina pectoris in patients with aortic stenosis and normal coronary arteries. N. Engl. J. Med. 307:1362, 1982.

171. Marcus, M. L., Harrison, D. G., Chilian, W. M., et al.: Alterations in the coronary circulation in hypertrophied ventricles. Circulation 75:I–19, 1987.

172. Canby, C. A., and Tomanek, R. J.: Role of lowering arterial pressure on maximal coronary flow with and without regression of cardiac hypertrophy. Am. J. Physiol. 257:H1110, 1989.

173. Sato, F., Isoyama, S., and Takishima, T.: Normalization of impaired coronary circulation in hypertrophied rat hearts. Hypertension 16:26, 1990.

174. Tanaka, M., Fujiwara, H., Onodera, T., et al.: Quantitative analysis of narrowings of intramyocardial small arteries in normal hearts, hypertensive hearts, and hearts with hypertrophic cardiomyopathy. Circulation 75:1130, 1987.

175. Goldstein, R. A., and Haynie, M.: Limited myocardial perfusion reserve in patients with left ventricular hypertrophy. J. Nucl. Med. 31:255, 1990.

176. Goldstein, R. A., Kirkeeide, R. L., Demer, L. L., et al.: Relation between geometric dimensions of coronary artery stenoses and myocardial perfusion reserve in man. J. Clin. Invest. 79:1473, 1987.

177. Opherk, D., Mall, G., Zebe, H., et al.: Reduction of coronary reserve: A mechanism for angina pectoris in patients with arterial hypertension and normal coronary arteries. Circulation 69:1, 1984.

178. Cannon, R. O., III, Rosing, D. R., Maron, B. J., et al.: Myocardial ischemia in patients with hypertrophic cardiomyopathy: contribution of inade-

quate vasodilator reserve and elevated left ventricular filling pressures. Circulation 71:234, 1985.

179. Nitenberg, A., Tavolaro, O., Loisance, D., et al.: Maximal coronary vasodilator capacity of orthotopic heart transplants in patients with and without rejection. Am. J. Cardiol. 61:513, 1989.

180. Cannon, R. O., Cunnion, R. E., Parrillo, J. E., et al.: Dynamic limitation of coronary vasodilator reserve in patients with dilated cardiomyopathy and chest pain. J. Am. Coll. Cardiol. 10:1190, 1987.

181. Mosseri, M., Yarom, R., Gotsman, M. S., and Hasin, Y.: Histologic evidence for small-vessel coronary artery disease in patients with angina pectoris and patent large coronary arteries. Circulation 74:964, 1986.

181a. Cannon, R. O. III, Schenke, W. H., Quyyumi, A., et al.: Comparison of exercise testing with studies of coronary flow reserve in patients with microvascular angina. Circulation 83:(Suppl. III):77, 1991.

182. Bortone, A. S., Hess, O. M., Eberli, F. R., et al.: Abnormal coronary vasomotion during exercise in patients with normal coronary arteries and reduced coronary flow reserve. Circulation 79:516, 1989.

183. Tanaka, M., Fujiwara, H., Onodera, T., et al.: Quantitative analysis of narrowings of intramyocardial small arteries in normal hearts, hypertensive hearts, and hearts with hypertrophic cardiomyopathy Circulation 75:1130, 1987.

184. Gould, K. L.: Coronary Artery Stenosis. New York, Elsevier, 1991, 323 pp.

185. Gould, K. L.: Assessing coronary stenosis severity: A recurrent clinical need. J. Am. Coll. Cardiol. 8:91, 1986.

186. Epstein, S. E., and Talbot, T. L.: Dynamic coronary tone in precipitation, exacerbation, and relief of angina pectoris. Am. J. Cardiol. 48:797, 1981.

187. Klocke, F. J.: Measurements of coronary blood flow and degree of stenosis: Current clinical implications and continuing uncertainties. J. Am. Coll. Cardiol. 1:31, 1983.

188. Epstein, S. E., Cannon, R. O., III, and Talbot, T. L.: Hemodynamic principles in the control of coronary blood flow. Am. J. Cardiol. 56:4E, 1985.

189. Maseri, A.: Myocardial ischemia in man: Current concepts, changing views and future investigation. Can. J. Cardiol. Suppl. A:225A, 1986.

190. Ganz, P., Abben, R. P., and Barry, W. H.: Dynamic variations in resistance of coronary arterial narrowings in angina pectoris at rest. Am. J. Cardiol. 59:66, 1987.

191. Maseri, A., Chierchia, S., and Kaski, J. C.: Mixed angina pectoris. Am. J. Cardiol. 56:30E, 1985.

MYOCARDIAL ISCHEMIA AND ISCHEMIC INJURY

192. Tennant, R., and Wiggers, C. J.: The effect of coronary occlusion on myocardial contractions. Am. J. Physiol. 112:351, 1935.

193. Ross, J., Jr., Gallagher, K., Matzuski, M., et al.: Regional myocardial blood flow and function in experimental myocardial ischemia. Can. J. Cardiol. Suppl. A:9A, 1986.

194. Osakada, G., Hess, O. M., Gallather, K. P., et al.: End-systolic dimension-wall thickness relations during myocardial ischemia in conscious dogs. Am. J. Cardiol. 51:1750, 1983.

195. Amano, J., Thomas, J. X., Jr., Lavallee, M., et al.: Effects of myocardial ischemia on regional function and stiffness in conscious dogs. Am. J. Physiol. 252:H110, 1987.

196. Lew, W.Y.W., Chen, Z., Guth, B., and Covell, J. W.: Mechanisms of augmented segment shortening in nonischemic areas during acute ischemia of the canine left ventricle. Circ. Res. 56:351, 1985.

197. Sunagawa, K., Maughan, W. L., and Sagawa, K.: Effect of regional ischemia on the left ventricular end-systolic pressure-volume relationship of isolated canine hearts. Circ. Res 52:170, 1983.

198. Heyndrickx, G. R., Millard, R. W., McRitchie, R. J., et al.: Regional myocardial functional and electrophysiological alterations after brief coronary occlusion in conscious dog. J. Clin. Invest. 56:978, 1975.

199. Ellis, S. G., Henschke, C. I., Sandor, T., et al.: Time course of functional and biochemical recovery of myocardium salvaged by reperfusion. J. Am. Coll. Cardiol. 1:1047, 1983.

200. Braunwald, E., and Kloner, R. A.: The stunned myocardium: Prolonged, postischemic ventricular dysfunction. Circulation 66:1146, 1982.

200a. Braunwald, E., Rutherford, J. D.: Reversible ischemic left ventricular dysfunction: Evidence for the "hibernating myocardium." J. Am. Coll. Cardiol. 8:1467, 1986.

201. Rahimtoola, S. H.: A perspective on the three large multicenter randomized clinical trials of coronary bypass surgery for chronic stable angina. Circulation 72(Suppl. V):123, 1985.

202. Rahimtoola, S. H.: The hibernating myocardium. Am. Heart J. 117:211, 1989.

203. Thaulow, E., Guth, B. D., Heusch, G., et al.: Characteristics of regional myocardial stunning after exercise in dogs with chronic coronary stenosis. Am. J. Physiol. 257:H113, 1989.

203a. Fournier, C., Boujon, B., Hebert, J., et al.: Stunned myocardium following coronary spasm. Am. Heart J. 121:593, 1991.

204. Bolli, R., Patel, B. S., Hartley, C. J., et al.: Non-uniform transmural recovery of contractile function in stunned myocardium. Am. J. Physiol. 257:H375, 1989.

205. Charlat, M. L., O'Neill, P. G., Hartley, C. J., et al.: Prolonged abnormalities of left ventricular diastolic wall thinning in the "stunned" myocardium in conscious dogs: time course and relation to systolic function. J. Am. Coll. Cardiol. 13:185, 1989.

206. Braunwald, E.: The stunned myocardium: Newer insights into mechanisms and clinical applications. J. Thorac. Cardiovasc. Surg. 100:310, 1990.

207. Patel, B., Kloner, R. A., Przyklenk, K., and Braunwald, E.: Postischemic

208. Matsuzaki, M., Gallagher, K. P., Kemper, W. S., et al.: Sustained regional dysfunction produced by prolonged coronary stenosis: gradual recovery after reperfusion. Circulation 68:170, 1987.

209. Fedele, F. A., Gerwitz, H., Capone, R. J., et al.: Metabolic response to prolonged reduction of myocardial blood flow distal to a severe coronary artery stenosis. Circulation 78:729, 1988.

209a. Vandeplassche, G., Hermans, C., Thoné, F., and Borgers, M.: Stunned myocardium has increased mitochondrial NADH oxidase and ATPase activities. Cardioscience 2:47, 1991.

209b. Marban, E.: Myocardial stunning and hibernation: the physiology behind the colloquialisms. Circulation 83:681, 1991.

210. Schaefer, S., Schwartz, G. G., Gober, J. R., et al.: Relationship between myocardial metabolites and contractile abnormalities during graded regional ischemia: Phosphorus-31 nuclear magnetic resonance studies of porcine myocardium in vivo. J. Clin. Invest. 85:706, 1990.

211. Ryan, T., Tarver, R. D., Duerk, J. L., and Sawada, S. G.: Ability of magnetic resonance imaging to distinguish stunned from infarcted myocardium following transient experimental ischemia. J. Am. Coll. Cardiol. 15:162A, 1990.

212. Milunski, M. R., Mohr, G. A., Perez, J. E., et al.: Ultrasonic tissue characterization with integrated backscatter: Acute myocardial ischemia, reperfusion, and stunned myocardium in patients. Circulation 80:491, 1989.

213. Kloner, R. A., and Przyklenk, K.: Recent advances in stunned myocardium. Cardiovasc. Rev. Rep. 68, June 1990.

214. Tani, M., and Neely, J. R.: Role of intracellular Na$^+$ in Ca^{2+} overload and depressed recovery of ventricular function of reperfused ischemic rat hearts: Possible involvement of H$^+$-Na$^+$ and Na$^+$-Ca^{2+} exchange. Circ. Res. 65:1045, 1989.

215. Krause, S. M., Jacobus, W. E., and Becker, L. C.: Alterations in cardiac sarcoplasmic reticulum calcium transport in the postischemic "stunned" myocardium. Circ. Res. 65:526, 1989.

216. Kitakaze, M., Weisfeldt, M. L., and Marban, E.: Acidosis during early reperfusion prevents myocardial stunning in perfused ferret hearts. J. Clin. Invest. 82:920, 1988.

217. Thompson-Gorman, S. L., and Zweier, J. L.: Evaluation of the role of xanthine oxidase in myocardial reperfusion injury. J. Biol. Chem. 265:6656, 1990.

218. Simpson, P. J., Mickelson, J. Fantone, J. C., et al.: Iloprost inhibits neutrophil function in vitro and in vivo and limits experimental infarct size in canine heart. Circ. Res. 60:666, 1987.

219. Kuzuya, T., Hoshida, S., Nishida, M., et al.: Role of free radicals and neutrophils in canine myocardial reperfusion injury: Myocardial salvage by a novel free-radical scavenger, 2-octadecylascorbic acid. Cardiovasc. Res. 23:323, 1989.

220. Bolli, R., Jeroudi, M. O., Patel, B. S., et al.: Marked reduction of free radical generation and contractile dysfunction by antioxidant therapy begun at the time of reperfusion. Evidence that myocardial "stunning" is a manifestation of reperfusion injury. Circ. Res. 65:607, 1989.

221. Chi, L., Tamura, Y., Hoff, P. T., et al.: Effect of superoxide dismutase on myocardial infarct size in the canine heart after 6 hours of regional ischemia and reperfusion: a demonstration of myocardial salvage. Circ. Res. 64:665, 1989.

222. Naslund, U., Haggmark, S., Johansson, G., et al.: Limitation of myocardial infarct size by superoxide dismutase as an adjunct to reperfusion after different durations of coronary occlusion in the pig. Circ. Res. 66:1294, 1990.

223. Zweier, J. L., Kuppusamy, P., Williams, R., et al.: Measurement and characterization of postischemic free radical generation in the isolated perfused heart. J. Biol. Chem. 264:18890, 1989.

224. Koller, P. T., and Bergmann, S. R.: Reduction of lipid peroxidation in reperfused isolated rabbit hearts by diltiazem. Circ. Res. 65:838, 1989.

225. Pallandi, R. T., Perry, M. A., and Campbell, T. J.: Prearrhythmic effects of an oxygen-derived free radical generating system on action potentials recorded from guinea pig ventricular myocardium: A possible cause of reperfusion-induced arrhythmias. Circ. Res. 61:50, 1987.

226. Mehta, J. L., Nichols, W. W., Donnelly, W. H., et al.: Protection by superoxide dismutase from myocardial dysfunction and attenuation of vasodilator reserve after coronary occlusion and reperfusion in dog. Circ. Res. 65:1283, 1989.

227. Bolli, R., Zhu, W.-X., Hartley, C. J., et al.: Attenuation of dysfunction in the postischemic "stunned" myocardium by dimethylthiourea. Circulation 76:458, 1987.

228. Engler, R., and Gilpin, E.: Can superoxide dismutase alter myocardial infarct size? Circulation 79:1137, 1989.

229. Holzgrefe, H. H., and Gibson, J. K.: Beneficial effects of oxypurinol pretreatment in stunned, reperfused canine myocardium. Cardiovasc. Res. 23:340, 1989.

229a. Williams, R. E., Zweier, J. L., and Flaherty, J. T.: Treatment with deferoxamine during ischemia improves functional and metabolic recovery and reduces reperfusion-induced oxygen radical generation in rabbit hearts. Circulation 83:1006, 1991.

230. Ellis, S. G., Wynne, J., Braunwald, E., et al.: Response of reperfusion-salvaged stunned myocardium to inotropic stimulation. Am. Heart J. 107:13, 1984.

231. Arnold, J.M.O., Braunwald, E., Sando, T., and Kloner, R. A.: Inotropic stimulation of reperfused myocardium with dopamine: Effects on infarct size and myocardial function. J. Am. Coll. Cardiol. 6:1026, 1985.

232. Ekmekci, A., Toyoshima, H., Dowczynski, J. K., et al.: Angina pectoris. IV.

Clinical and experimental difference between ischemia with S-T elevation and ischemia with S-T depression, Am. J. Cardiol. 7:412, 1961.

233. Tillisch, J., Brunken, R., Marshall, R., et al.: Reversibility of cardiac wall-motion abnormalities predicted by positron tomography. N. Engl. J. Med. 314:884, 1986.

234. Brunken, R., Schwaiger, M., Grover-McKay, M., et al.: Positron emission tomography detects tissue metabolic activity in myocardial segments with persistent thallium perfusion defects. J. Am. Coll. Cardiol. 10:557, 1987.

235. Gropler, R. J., Siegel, B. A., Perez, J. E., et al.: Functional recovery after myocardial revascularization is characterized by improved glucose and oxidative metabolism. J. Nucl. Med. 31:773, 1990.

236. Bergmann, S. R., Shelton, M. E., Weinheimer, C. J., et al.: Persistence of perfusion, metabolic, and functional reserve capacity in stunned myocardium. J. Nucl. Med. 31:794, 1990.

237. Renstrom, B., Nellis, S. H., and Liedtke, A. J.: Metabolic oxidation of glucose during early myocardial reperfusion. Circ. Res. 65:1094, 1989.

238. Myears, D. W., Sobel, B. E., and Bergmann, S. R.: Substrate utilization in ischemic and reperfused canine myocardium: quantitative considerations. Am. J. Physiol. 253:H107, 1987.

239. Brown, M. A., Marshall, D. R., Sobel, B.E., and Bergmann, S. R.: Delineation of myocardial oxygen utilization with carbon-11-labeled acetate. Circulation. 76:687, 1987.

240. Knabb, R. M., Bergmann, S. R., Fox, K.A.A., and Sobel, B. E.: The temporal pattern of recovery of myocardial perfusion and metabolism delineated by positron emission tomography after coronary thrombolysis. J. Nucl. Med. 28:1563, 1987.

241. Walsh, M. N., Geltman, E. M., Brown, M. A., et al.: Noninvasive estimation of regional myocardial oxygen consumption by positron emission tomography with carbon-11 acetate in patients with myocardial infarction. J. Nucl. Med. 30:1798, 1989.

242. Kass, D. A., Marino, P., Maughan, W. L., and Sagawa, K.: Determinants of end-systolic pressure-volume relations during acute regional ischemia in situ. Circulation 80:1783, 1989.

243. Jennings, R. B., Murry, C. E., Steenbergen, C. Jr., and Reimer, K. A.: Development of cell injury in sustained acute ischemia. Circulation 82:(Suppl. II):2, 1990.

244. Stern, M. D., Silverman, H. S., Houser, S. R., et al.: Anoxic contractile failure in rat heart myocytes is caused by failure of intracellular calcium release due to alteration of the action potential. Proc. Natl. Acad. Sci. USA 85:6954, 1988.

245. Marban, E., Kitikaze, M., Kusuoka, H., et al.: Intracellular free calcium concentration measured with ^{19}F NMR spectroscopy in intact ferret hearts. Proc. Natl. Acad. Sci. USA 84:6005, 1987.

246. Barry, W. H.: Mechanical dysfunction of the heart during and after ischemia. Circulation 82:652, 1990.

247. Kihara, Y. Grossman, W., and Morgan, J. P.: Direct measurement of changes in intracellular calcium transients during hypoxia, ischemia, and reperfusion of the intact mammalian heart. Circ. Res. 65:1029, 1989.

248. Braunwald, E., Ross, J., Jr., and Sonnenblick, E. H.: Mechanisms of Contractions in the Normal and Failing Heart. 2nd Ed. Boston, Little, Brown and Company, 1976, p. 357.

249. Williamson, J. R., Schaffer, S. W., Ford, C., and Safer, B.: Contribution of tissue acidosis to ischemic injury in the perfused rat heart. Circulation 53(Suppl. I):3, 1976.

250. Gard, J. K., Kichura, G. M., Ackerman, J. J. H., et al.: Quantitative ^{31}P NMR analysis of metabolite concentrations in Langendorff-perfused rabbit hearts. Biophys. J. 48:803, 1985.

251. Neubauer, S., Hamman, B. L., Perry, S., B., et al. Velocity of the creatine kinase reaction decreases in postischemic myocardium: A^{31}P-NMR magnetization transfer study of the isolated ferret heart. Circ. Res. 63:1, 1988.

252. Marshall, R. C.: Correlation of contractile dysfunction with oxidative energy production and tissue high energy phosphate stores during partial coronary flow disruption in rabbit heart. J. Clin. Invest. 82:86, 1988.

253. Zimmer, S. D., Ugurbil, K., Michurski, S. P., et al.: Alterations in oxidative function and respiratory regulation in the post-ischemic myocardium. J. Biol. Chem. 264:12402, 1989.

254. Pogwizd, S. M., and Corr, P. B.: Electrophysiologic and biochemical mechanisms underlying malignant ventricular arrhythmias during early myocardial ischemia. In Heusch, G. (ed.): Pathophysiology and Rational Pharmacotherapy of Myocardial Ischemia. Darmstadt, Germany, Steinkopff Verlag Darmstadt, 1990, p. 137.

255. Visner, M. S., Arentzen, C. E., Parrish, G. D., et al.: Effects of global ischemia on the diastolic properties of the left ventricle in the conscious dog. Circulation 71:610, 1985.

256. Momomura, S-I, Ferguson, J. J., Miller, M. J., et al.: Regional myocardial blood flow and left ventricular diastolic properties in pacing-induced ischemia. J. Am. Coll. Cardiol. 17:781, 1991.

256a. Miyazaki, S., Guth, B. D., Miura, T., et al.: Changes of left ventricular diastolic function in exercising dogs without and with ischemia. Circulation 81:1058, 1990.

257. Kass, D. A., Midei, M., Brinker, J., and Maughan, W. L.: Influence of coronary occlusion during PTCA on end-systolic and end-diastolic pressure volume relations in humans. Circulation 81:447, 1990.

258. Wexler, L. F., Weinberg, E. O., Ingwall, J. S., and Apstein, C. S.: Acute alterations in diastolic left ventricular chamber distensibility: Mechanistic differences between hypoxia and ischemia in isolated perfused rabbit and rat hearts. Circ. Res. 59:515, 1986.

258a. Takahashi, T., Levine, M. J., and Grossman, W.: Regional diastolic mechanics of ischemic and nonischemic myocardium in the pig heart. J. Am. Coll. Cardiol. 17:1203, 1991.

259. Gaasch, W. H., Zile, M. R., Hoshino, P. K., et al.: Tolerance of the hypertrophic heart to ischemia: studies in compensated and failing dog hearts with pressure overload hypertrophy. Circulation 81:164, 1990.

260. Imai, K., Wang, T., Millard, R. W., et al.: Ischemia-induced changes in canine cardiac sarcoplasmic reticulum. Cardiovasc. Res. 17:696, 1983.

261. Krayenbuehl, H. P., Hess, O. M., and Nonogi, H.: On whether there is a true increase in myocardial stiffness during myocardial islchemia. Am. J. Cardiol. 63:78E, 1989.

262. Nakamura, Y., Sasayama, S., Nonogi, H., et al.: Alterations in left ventricular relaxation, early diastolic filling and passive viscoelastic properties during postpacing ischemia. Am. J. Cardiol. 63:72E, 1989.

263. Ross, J., Jr.: Is there a true increase in myocardial stiffness with acute ischemia? Am. J. Cardiol. 63:87E, 1989.

264. Sys, S. U., and Brutsaert, D. L.: Is stiffness increased during ischemia? Am. J. Cardiol. 63:83E, 1989.

ELECTROPHYSIOLOGICAL CONSEQUENCES OF ISCHEMIA

265. Sayen, J. J., Peirce, G., Katcher, A. H., and Sheldon, W. F.: Correlation of intramyocardial electrocardiograms with polarographic oxygen and contractility in the nonischemic and regional ischemic left ventricle. Circ. Res. 9:1268, 1961.

266. Maroko, P. R., Kjekshus, J. K., Sobel, B. E., et al.: Factors influencing infarct size following experimental coronary artery occlusions. Circulation 43:67, 1971.

266a. Carroll, J. D., Hess, O. M., Hirzel, H. O., and Krayenbuehl, H. P.: Exercise-induced ischemia: The influence of altered relaxation on early diastolic pressures. Circulation 67:521, 1983.

267. Muller, J. E., Maroko, P. R., and Braunwald, E.: Evaluation of precordial electrocardiographic mapping as a means of assessing changes in myocardial ischemic injury. Circulation 52:16, 1975.

268. Wilde, A.A.M., Escande, D., Schumacher, C. A., et al.: Potassium accumulation in the globally ischemic mammalian heart: A role for the ATP-sensitive potassium channel. Circ. Res. 67:835, 1990.

268a. Sasayama, S., Nonogi, H., Miyazaki, S., Sakurai, T., Kawai, C., Eiho, S., and Kuwahara, M.: Changes in diastolic properties of the regional myocardium during pacing-induced ischemia in human subjects. J. Am. Coll. Cardiol. 5:599, 1985.

269. Kleber, A. G., Riegger, C. B., and Janse, M. J.: Electrical uncoupling and increase of extracellular resistance after induction of ischemia in isolated, arterially perfused rabbit papillary muscle. Circ. Res. 61:271, 1987.

270. Creer, M. H., Dobmeyer, D. J., and Corr, P. B.: Amphipathic lipid metabolites and arrhythmias during myocardial ischemia. In Zipes, D., and Jalife, J. (eds.): Cardiac Electrophysiology. Philadelphia, W. B. Saunders, 1990, pp. 417–432.

271. Corr, P. B., Saffitz, J. E., and Sobel, B. E.: What is the contribution of altered lipid metabolism to arrhythmogenesis in the ischemic heart? In Hearse, D. J., Manning, A. S., and Janse M. (eds.): Life-Threatening Arrhythmias During Ischemia and Infarction. New York, Raven Press, 1987, pp. 91–114.

272. Corr, P. B., Creer, M. H., Yamada, K. A., et al.: Prophylaxis of early ventricular fibrillation by inhibition of acylcarnitine accumulation. J. Clin. Invest. 83:927, 1989.

272a. Mehra, R., Zeiler, R. H. Gough, W. B., and El-Sherif, N.: Reentrant ventricular arrhythmias in the late myocardial infarction period. 9. Electrophysiologic-anatomic correlation of reentrant circuits. Circulation 67:11, 1983.

273. Corr, P. B., Witkowski, F. X., and Sobel, B. E.: Mechanisms contributing to malignant dysrhythmias induced by ischemia in the cat. J. Clin. Invest. 61:109, 1978.

274. Kimura, S., Basset, A. L., Kohya, T., et al.: Automaticity, triggered activity, and responses to adrenergic stimulation in cat subendocardial Purkinje fibers after healing of myocardial infarction. Circulation 75:651, 1987.

275. El-Sherif, N., Hope, R. R., Scherlag, B. J., and Lazzara, R.: Re-entrant ventricular arrhythmias in the late myocardial infarction period. 2. Patterns of initiation and termination of reentry. Circulation 55:702, 1977.

276. Sobel, B. E., Corr, P. B., Robinson, A. K., et al.: Accumulation of lysophosphoglycerides with arrhythmogenic properties in ischemic myocardium. J. Clin. Invest. 61:109, 1978.

277. Corr, P. B., Cain, M. E., Witkowski, F. X., et al.: Potential arrhythmogenic electrophysiological derangements in canine Purkinje fibers induced by lysophosphoglycerides. Circ. Res. 44:822, 1979.

278. Bernier, M., Manning, A. S., and Hearse, D. J.: Reperfusion arrhythmias: Dose-related protection by anti-free radical interventions. Am. J. Physiol. 256:H1344, 1989.

279. Tani, M., and Neely, J. R.: Intermittent perfusion of ischemic myocardium. Possible mechanisms of protective effects on mechanical function in isolated rat heart. Circulation 82:536, 1990.

EFFECTS OF ISCHEMIA ON MYOCARDIAL METABOLISM

280. Jennings, R. B., Reimer, K. A., Hill, M. L., and Mayer, S. E.: Total ischemia in dog hearts in vitro. I. Comparison of high energy phosphate production, utilization and depletion, and of adenine nucleotide catabolism in total ischemia in vitro vs. severe ischemia in vivo. Circ. Res. 49:892, 1981.

281. Flaherty, J. T., Weisfeldt, M. L., Bulkley, B. H., et al.: Mechanisms of ischemic myocardial cell damage assessed by phosphorus-31 nuclear magnetic resonance. Circulation 65:561, 1982.

282. Schaefer, S., Camacho, S. A., Gober, J., et al.: Response of myocardial metabolites to graded regional ischemia: ^{31}P NMR spectroscopy of porcine myocardium in vivo. Circ. Res. 64:968, 1989.

283. Marshall, R. C., Nash, W. W., Bersohn, M. M., and Wong, G. A.: Myocardial energy production and consumption remain balanced during positive inotropic stimulation when coronary flow is restricted to basal rates in rabbit heart. J. Clin. Invest. 80:1165, 1987.

284. Bittl, J. A., Balschi, J. A., and Ingwall, J. S.: Effects of norepinephrine infusion on myocardial high-energy phosphate content and turnover in the living rat. J. Clin. Invest. 79:1852, 1987.

285. Bittl, J. A., Balschi, J. A., and Ingwall, J. S.: Contractile failure and high-energy phosphate turnover during hypoxia: ^{31}P-NMR surface coil studies in living rat. Circ. Res. 60:871, 1987.

286. Asimakis, G. K., Sandhu, G. S., Conti, V. R., et al.: Intermittent ischemia produces a cumulative depletion of mitochondrial adenine nucleotides in the isolated perfused rat heart. Circ. Res. 66:302, 1990.

287. Guth, B. D., Martin, J. F., Heusch, G., and Ross, J., Jr.: Regional myocardial blood flow, function and metabolism using phosphorus-31 nuclear magnetic resonance spectroscopy during ischemia and reperfusion in dogs. J. Am. Coll. Cardiol. 10:673, 1987.

288. Mazer, C. D., Stanley, W. C., Hickey, R. F., et al.: Myocardial metabolism during hypoxia: Maintained lactate oxidation during increased glycolysis. Metabolism 39:913, 1990.

289. Owen, P., Dennis, S., and Opie, L. H.: Glucose flux rate regulates onset of ischemic contracture in globally underperfused rat hearts. Circ. Res. 66:344, 1990.

290. Mody, F. V., Brunken, R. C., Stevenson, L. W., et al.: Differentiating cardiomyopathy of coronary artery disease from nonischemic dilated cardiomyopathy utilizing positron emission tomography. J. Am. Coll. Cardiol. 17:373, 1991.

291. Fudo, T., Kambara, H., Hashimoto, T., et al.: F-18 deoxyglucose and stress N-13 ammonia positron emission tomography in anterior wall healed myocardial infarction. Am. J. Cardiol. 61:1191, 1988.

291a. Bonow, R. O., Dilsizian, V., Cuocolo, A., and Bacharach, S. L.: Identification of viable myocardium in patients with chronic coronary artery disease and left ventricular dysfunction. Circulation 83:26, 1991.

291b. Bonow, R. O., Dilsizian, V., Cuocolo, A., and Bacharach, S. L.: Identification of viable myocardium in patients with chronic coronary artery disease and left ventricular function. Circulation 83:26, 1991.

292. Rovetto, M. J., Lamberton, W. F., and Neely, J. R.: Mechanisms of glycolytic inhibition in ischemic rat hearts. Circ. Res. 37:742, 1975.

293. Williamson, J. R., Schaffer, S. W., Ford, C., and Safer, B.: Contribution of tissue acidosis to ischemic injury in the perfused rat heart. Circulation 53(Suppl. I):3, 1976.

294. Corr, P. B., Saffitz, J. E., and Sobel, B. E.: Lysophospholipids, long chain acylcarnitines, and membrane dysfunction in the ischemic heart. In Lipid Metabolism in the Normoxic and Ischaemic Heart. New York, Springer-Verlag, 1987, p. 199.

295. Miyazaki, Y., Gross, R. W., Sobel, B. E., and Saffitz, J. E.: Selective turnover of sarcolemmal phospholipids with lethal injury. Am. J. Physiol., 259:C325, 1990.

296. Knabb, M. T., Saffitz, J. E., Corr, P. B., and Sobel, B. E.: The dependence of electrophysiologic derangements on accumulation of endogenous long-chain acyl carnitine in hypoxic neonatal rat myocytes. Circ. Res. 58:230, 1986.

297. Camici, P., Marraccini, P., Lorenzoni, R.: Metabolic markers of stress-induced myocardial ischemia. Circulation 83(Suppl. III)III8, 1991.

298. Neely, J. R., Rovetto, M. J., Whitmer, J. T., and Morgan, H. E.: Effects of ischemia on ventricular function and metabolism in the isolated working rat heart. Am. J. Physiol. 225:651, 1973.

299. Vyska, K., Machulla, H. J., Stremmel, W., et al.: Regional myocardial free fatty acid extraction in normal and ischemic myocardium. Circulation 78:1218, 1988.

300. Bergmann, S. R., Lerch, R. A., Fox, K. A. A., et al.: Temporal dependence of beneficial effects of coronary thrombolysis characterized by positron tomography. Am. J. Med. 73:573, 1982.

301. Renstrom, B., Nellis, S. H., and Liedtke, A. J.: Metabolic oxidation of glucose during early myocardial reperfusion. Circ. Res. 65:1094, 1989.

302. Weiss, E. S., Ahmed, S. A., Welch, M. J., et al.: Quantification of infarction in cross sections of canine myocardium in vivo with positron emission transaxial tomography and ^{11}C-palmitate. Circulation 55:66, 1977.

303. Kimihara, S., Yokota, M., Iwase, M., et al.: Early detection of myocardial ischemia by myocardial free fatty acid extraction in patients with exercise-induced angina pectoris. Am. J. Cardiol. 64:180–185, 1989.

304. Fox, K. A. A., Nomura, H., Sobel, B. E., and Bergmann, S. R.: Consistent substrate utilization despite reduced flow in hearts with maintained work. Am. J. Physiol. 244:H799, 1983.

305. Gropler, R. J., Siegel, B. A., Lee, K. J., et al.: Nonuniformity in myocardial accumulation of ^{18}F-fluorodeoxyglucose in normal fasted humans. J. Nucl. Med., 31:1749, 1990.

306. Eisenberg, J. D., Sobel, B. E., and Geltman, E. M.: Differentiation of ischemic from nonischemic cardiomyopathy with positron emission tomography. Am. J. Cardiol. 59:1410, 1987.

307. Rosamond, T. L., Abendschein, D. R., Sobel, B. E., et al.: Metabolic fate of radiolabeled palmitate in ischemic canine myocardium: Implications for positron emission tomography. J. Nucl. Med. 28:1322, 1987.

308. Myears, D. W., Sobel, B. E., and Bergmann, S. R.: Substrate use in ischemic and reperfused canine myocardium: Quantitative considerations. Am. J. Physiol. 253:H107, 1987.

308a. Henes, C. G., Bergmann, S. R., Walsh, M. N., et al.: Assessment of myocardial oxidative metabolic reserve with positron emission tomography and carbon-11 acetate. J. Nucl. Med. 30:1489, 1989.

309. Rannels, D. E., McKee, E. E., and Morgan, H. E.: Regulation of protein synthesis and degradation in heart and skeletal muscle. In Litwack, G. (ed.): Biochemical Actions of Hormones. New York, Academic Press, 1976.

310. Schwalb, H., Izhar, U., Yaroslavsky, E., et al.: The effect of amino acids on the ischemic heart: Improvement of oxygenated crystalloid cardioplegic solution by an enriched branched chain amino acid formulation. J. Thorac. Cardiovasc. Surg. 98:551, 1989.

311. Mehta, H. B., Popovich, B. K., and Dillmann, W. H.: Ischemia induces changes in the level of mRNAs coding for stress protein 71 and creatine kinase M. Circ. Res. 63:512, 1988.

312. Currie, R. W., Karmazyn, M., Kloc, M., and Mailer, K.: Heat-shock response is associated with enhanced postischemic ventricular recovery. Circ. Res. 63:543, 1988.

313. de la Bastie, D., Levitsky, D., Rappaport, L., et al.: Function of the sarcoplasmic reticulum and expression of its Ca$^+$-ATPase gene in pressure overload-induced cardiac hypertrophy in the rat. Circ. Res. 66:554, 1990.

314. Chance, B.: Discussion. Circ. Res. 38(Suppl. I):69, 1976.

315. Reimer, K. A., Lowe, J. E., Rasmussen, M. M., and Jennings, R. B.: The wavefront phenomenon of ischemic cell death. I. Myocardial infarct size vs duration of coronary occlusion in dogs. Circulation 56:786, 1977.

316. Lavellee, M., Cox, D., Patrick, T. A., and Vatner, S. F.: Salvage of myocardial function by coronary artery reperfusion 1, 2, and 3 hours after occlusion in conscious dogs. Circ. Res. 53:235, 1983.

317. Kagiyama, A., Savage, H. E., Michael, L. H., et al.: Molecular basis of complement activation in ischemic myocardium: Identification of specific molecules of mitochondrial origin that bind human C1q and fix complement. Circ. Res. 64:607, 1989.

318. Crawford, M. H., Grover, F. L., Kolb, W. P., et al.: Complement and neutrophil activation in the pathogenesis of ischemic myocardial injury. Circulation 78:1449, 1988.

319. Steenbergen, C., Murphy, E., Levy, L., and London, R. E.: Elevation of cytosolic free calcium concentration early in myocardial ischemia in perfused rat heart. Circ. Res. 60:700, 1987.

320. Marban, E., Koretsume, Y., Corretti, M., et al.: Calcium and its role in myocardial cell injury during ischemia and reperfusion. Circulation 80(Suppl. IV):4, 1989.

321. Corr, P. B., Gross, R. W., and Sobel, B. E.: Arrhythmogenic amphiphilic lipids and the myocardial cell membrane. J. Mol. Cell. Cardiol. 14:619, 1982.

322. Sedlis, S. P., Corr, P. B., Sobel, B. E., and Ahumada, G. G.: Lysophosphatidyl choline potentiates Ca^{++} accumulation in rat cardiac myocytes. Am. J. Physiol. 13:H32, 1983.

323. Kloner, R. A., DeBoer, L.W.V., Carlson, N., and Braunwald, E.: The effect of verapamil on myocardial ultrastructure during and following release of coronary artery occlusion. Exp. Mol. Pathol. 36:277, 1982.

324. Braunwald, E., Muller, J. E., Kloner, R. A., and Maroko, P. R.: Role of beta-adrenergic blockade in the therapy of patients with myocardial infarction. Am. J. Med. 784:113, 1983.

325. Hammerman, H., Kloner, R. A., Briggs, L. L., and Braunwald, E.: Enhancement of salvage of reperfused myocardium by early beta-adrenergic blockade. J. Am. Coll. Cardiol. 3:1438, 1984.

326. Lo, H. M., Kloner, R. A., and Braunwald, E.: Effect of intracoronary verapamil on infarct size in the ischemic, reperfused canine heart: Critical importance of the timing of treatment. Am. J. Cardiol. 56:672, 1985.

327. Campbell, C. A., Kloner, R. A., Alker, K. J., and Braunwald, E.: Effect of verapamil on infarct size in dogs subjected to coronary artery occlusion with transient reperfusion. J. Am. Coll. Cardiol. 8:1169, 1986.

328. Henry, P. D., Shuchleib, R., Davis, J., et al.: Myocardial contracture and accumulation of mitochondrial calcium in ischemic rabbit heart. Am. J. Physiol. (Heart Circ. Physiol.) 2:H677, 1977.

329. DeBoer, L.W.V., Strauss, H. W., Kloner, R. A., et al.: Autoradiographic method for measuring the ischemic myocardium at risk: Effects of verapamil on infarct size after experimental coronary artery occlusion. Proc. Natl. Acad. Sci. 77:6119, 1980.

330. Nayler, W. G., Panagiotopoulos, S., Elz, J. S., and Sturrock, W. J.: Fundamental mechanisms of action of calcium antagonist in myocardial ischemia. Am. J. Cardiol. 59:75B, 1987.

331. Kloner, R. A., and Braunwald, E.: Effects of calcium antagonists on infarcting myocardium. Am. J. Cardiol. 59:84B, 1987.

332. Knabb, R. M., Rosamond, T. L., Fox, K.A.A., and Geltman: Enhancement of salvage of reperfused ischemic myocardium by diltiazem. J. Am. Coll. Cardiol. 8:861, 1986.

333. Berridge, M. J.: Inositol trisphosphate and diacylglycerol: Two interacting second messengers. Annu. Rev. Biochem. 56:159, 1987.

334. Kohl, C., Schmitz, W., Scholz, H., and Scholz, J.: Evidence for the existence of inositol tetrakisphosphate in mammalian heart: Effect of α_1-adrenoceptor stimulation. Circ. Res. 66:580, 1990.

335. Otani, H., Prasad, R., Engelman, R. M., et al.: Enhanced phosphodiesteratic breakdown and turnover of phosphoinositides during reperfusion of ischemic rat heart. Circ. Res. 63:930, 1988.

336. Heathers, G. P., Yamada, K. A., Kanter, E. M., and Corr, P. B.: Long-chain acylcarnitines mediate the hypoxia-induced increase in α_1-adrenergic receptors on adult canine myocytes. Circ. Res. 61:735, 1987.

337. Heathers, G. P., Yamada, K. A., Pogwizd, S. M., and Corr, P. B.: The

contribution of α- and β-adrenergic mechanisms in the genesis of arrhythmias during myocardial ischemia and reperfusion. *In* Kulbertus, H. E., and Frank, G. (eds.): Neurocardiology. Mount Kisco, Futura, 1988, pp. 143–178.

338. Ambrosio, G., Weisfeldt, M. L., Jacobus, W. E., and Flaherty, J. T.: Evidence for a reversible oxygen radical-mediated component of reperfusion injury: reduction by recombinant human superoxide dismutase administered at the time of reflow. Circulation 75:282, 1987.

339. Rossen, R. D., Swain, J. L., Michael, L. H., et al.: Selective accumulation of the first component of complement and leukocytes in ischemic canine heart muscle. Circ. Res. 57:119, 1985.

340. Naslund, U., Haggmark, S., Johansson, G., et al.: Limitation of myocardial infarct size by superoxide dismutase as an adjunct to reperfusion after different durations of coronary occlusion in the pig. Circ. Res. 66:1294, 1990.

341. Kloner, R. A., Przyklenk, K., and Whittaker, P.: Deleterious effects of oxygen radicals in ischemia/reperfusion: Resolved and unresolved issues. Circulation 80:1115, 1989.

342. Cohen, M. V.: Free radicals in ischemic and reperfusion myocardial injury: It is the time for clinical trials? Ann. Intern. Med. 111:918, 1989.

343. Kaneko, M., Beamish, R. E., and Dhalla, N. S.: Depression of heart sarcolemmal Ca^{2+}-pump activity by oxygen free radicals. Am. J. Physiol. 256:H368, 1989.

344. van der Kraaij, A. M. M., van Eijk, H. G., and Koster, J. F.: Prevention of postischemic cardiac injury by the orally active iron chelator 1,2-dimethyl-3-hydroxy-4-pyridone (L1) and the antioxidant (+)-cyanidanol-3. Circulation 80:158, 1989.

345. Litt, M. R., Jeremy, R. W., Weisman, H. F., et al.: Neutrophil depletion limited to reperfusion reduces myocardial infarct size after 90 minutes of ischemia: Evidence for neutrophil-mediated reperfusion injury. Circulation 80:1816, 1989.

346. Blaustein, A., Deneke, S. M., Stolz, R. I., et al.: Myocardial glutathione depletion impairs recovery after short periods of ischemia. Circulation 80:1449, 1989.

347. Ahumada, G., Roberts, R., and Sobel, B. E.: Evaluation of myocardial infarction with enzymatic indices. Prog. Cardiovasc. Dis. 18:405, 1976.

348. Ahmed, S. A., Williamson, J. R., Roberts, R., et al.: The association of increased plasma MB CPK activity and irreversible ischemic myocardial injury in the dog. Circulation 54:187, 1976.

349. Shell, W. E., Kjekshus, J. K., and Sobel, B. E.: Quantitative assessment of the extent of myocardial infarction in the conscious dog by means of analysis of serial changes in serum creatine phosphokinase activity. J. Clin. Invest. 50:2614, 1971.

350. Sobel, B. E., Markam, J., Karlsberg, R. P., and Roberts, R.: The nature of disappearance of creatine kinase from the circulation and its influence on enzymatic estimation of infarct size. Circ. Res. 41:836, 1977.

351. Geltman, E. M., Ehsani, A. A., Campbell, M. K., et al.: The influence of location and extent of myocardial infarction on long-term ventricular dysrhythmia and mortality. Circulation 60:805, 1979.

352. Hackel, D. B., Reimer, K. A., Ideker, R. E., et al.: Comparison of enzymatic and anatomic estimates of myocardial infarct size in man. Circulation 70:824, 1984.

353. Vatner, S. F., Baig, H., Manders, W. T., and Maroko, P. R.: Effects of coronary artery reperfusion on myocardial infarct size calculated from creatine kinase. J. Clin. Invest. 61:1048, 1978.

354. Clark, G. L., Robison, A. K., Gnepp, D. R., et al.: Effects of lymphatic transport of enzyme on plasma CK time-activity curves after myocardial infarction. Circ. Res. 43:162, 1978.

355. Devries, S. R., Jaffe, A. S., Geltman, E. M., et al.: Enzymatic estimation of the extent of irreversible myocardial injury early after reperfusion. Am. Heart J. 117:31, 1989.

356. Abendschein, D. R., Serota, H., Plummer, T. H., Jr., et al.: Conversion of MM creatine kinase isoforms in human plasma by carboxypeptidase N. J. Lab. Clin. Med. 110:798, 1987.

357. Hashimoto, H., Abendschein, D. R., Strauss, A. W., and Sobel, B. E.: Early detection of myocardial infarction in conscious dogs by analysis of plasma MM creatine kinase isoforms. Circulation 71:363, 1985.

358. Abendschein, D., Seacord, L. M., Nohara, R., et al.: Prompt detection of myocardial injury by assay of creatine kinase isoforms in initial plasma samples. Clin. Cardiol. 11:661, 1988.

359. Jaffe, A. S., Serota, H., Grace, A., and Sobel, B. E.: Diagnostic changes in plasma creatine kinase isoforms early after the onset of acute myocardial infarction. Circulation 74:105, 1986.

360. Devries, S. R., Sobel, B. E., and Abendschein, D. R.: Early detection of myocardial reperfusion by assay of plasma MM-creatine kinase isoforms in dogs. Circulation 74:567, 1986.

361. Rude, R. E., Muller, J. E., and Braunwald, E.: Efforts to limit the size of myocardial infarcts. Ann. Intern. Med. 95:736, 1981.

362. Nohara, R., Myears, D. W., Sobel, B. E., and Abendschein, D. R.: Optimal criteria for rapid detection of myocardial reperfusion by creatine kinase MM isoforms in the presence of residual high-grade coronary stenosis. J. Am. Coll. Cardiol. 14:1067, 1989.

363. Wu, A.H.B.: Creatine kinase isoforms in ischemic heart disease. Clin. Chem. 35:7, 1989.

364. Puleo, P. R., Guadagno, P. A., Roberts, R., and Perryman, M. B.: Sensitive, rapid assay of subforms of creatine kinase MB in plasma. Clin. Chem. 35:1452, 1989.

365. Christenson, R. H., Ohman, E. M., Clemmensen, P., et al.: Characteristics of creatine kinase-MB and MB isoforms in serum after reperfusion in acute myocardial infarction. Clin Chem. 35:2179, 1989.

366. Garabedian, H. D., Gold, H. K., Yasuda, T., et al.: Detection of coronary artery reperfusion with creatine kinase-MB determinations during thrombolytic therapy: Correlation with acute angiography. J. Am. Coll. Cardiol. 11:729, 1988.

367. Katus, H. A., Diederich, K. W., Scheffold, T., et al.: Noninvasive assessment of infarct reperfusion: The predictive power of the time to peak value of myoglobin, CK MB, and CK in serum. Eur. Heart J. 9:619, 1988.

368. Ellis, A. K., and Saran, B. R.: Kinetics of myoglobin release and prediction of myocardial myoglobin depletion after coronary artery reperfusion. Circulation 80:676, 1989.

369. Ellis, A. K., Little, T., Zaki Masud, A. R., et al.: Early noninvasive detection of successful reperfusion in patients with acute myocardial infarction. Circulation 78:1352, 1988.

MODIFICATION OF ISCHEMIC INJURY

370. Isobe, M., Nagai, R., Yamaoki, K., et al.: Quantification of myocardial infarct size after coronary reperfusion by serum cardiac myosin light chain II in conscious dogs. Circ. Res. 65:684, 1989.

371. Maroko, P. R., Kjekshus, J. K., Sobel, B. E., et al: Factors influencing infarct size following experimental coronary artery occlusion. Circulation 43:67, 1971.

372. Shell, W. E., and Sobel, B. E.: Deleterious effects of increased heart rate on infarct size in the conscious dog. Am. J. Cardiol. 31:474, 1973.

373. Radvany, P., Maroko, P. R., and Braunwald, E.: Effect of hypoxemia on the extent of myocardial necrosis after experimental coronary occlusion. Am. J. Cardiol. 35:795, 1975.

374. DeBoer, L.W.V., Rude, R. E., Davis, R. F., et al.: Extension of myocardial necrosis into normal epicardium following hypotension during experimental coronary occlusion. Cardiovasc. Res. 16:423, 1984.

375. Libby, P., Maroko, P. R., and Braunwald, E.: The effect of hypoglycemia on myocardial ischemic injury during acute experiment coronary artery occlusion. Circulation 51:621, 1975.

376. Davidson, S., Maroko, P. R., and Braunwald, E.: Effects of isoproterenol on contractile function of the ischemic and anoxic heart. Am. J. Physiol. 227:439, 1974.

377. Vatner, S. F., Millard, R. W., Patrick, T. A., and Heyndrickx, G. R.: Effects of isoproterenol on regional myocardial function, electrogram, and blood flow in conscious dogs with myocardial ischemia. J. Clin. Invest. 57:1261, 1976.

378. Fry, E. T. A., and Sobel, B. E.: Coronary thrombolysis. *In* Zipes, D. P., and Rowlands, D. J. (eds.): Progress in Cardiology. Philadelphia, Lea and Febiger, 1990, p. 199.

379. Tiefenbrunn, A. J., and Sobel, B. E.: Thrombolysis and myocardial infarction. Fibrinolysis, 5:1, 1991.

380. Sobel, B. E.: Coronary thrombolysis. Coronary Artery Dis. 1:3, 1990.

381. Simpson, P. J., Fantone, J. C., Mickelson, J. K., et al.: Identification of a time window for therapy to reduce experimental canine myocardial injury: Suppression of neutrophil activation during 72 hours of reperfusion. Circ. Res. 63:1070, 1988.

382. Przyklenk, K., and Kloner, R. A.: "Reperfusion injury" by oxygen-derived free radicals? Effect of superoxide dismutase plus catalase, given at the time of reperfusion, on myocardial infarct size, contractile function, coronary microvasculature, and regional myocardial blood flow. Circ. Res. 64:86, 1989.

383. Engler, R. L.: Free radical and granulocyte-mediated injury during myocardial ischemia and reperfusion. Am. J. Cardiol. 63:19E, 1989.

384. Engler, R., and Covell, J. W.: Granulocytes cause reperfusion ventricular dysfunction after 15-minute ischemia in the dog. Circ. Res. 61:20, 1987.

385. Opie, L. H.: Reperfusion injury and its pharmacologic modification. Circulation 80:1049, 1989.

386. Klein, H. H., Pich, S., Lindert, S., et al.: Treatment of reperfusion injury with intracoronary calcium channel antagonists and reduced coronary free calcium concentration in regionally ischemic, reperfused porcine hearts. J. Am. Coll. Cardiol. 13:1395, 1989.

387. Jang, I.-K., Van de Werf, F., Vanhaecke, J., and De Geest, H.: Coronary reperfusion by thrombolysis and early beta-adrenergic blockade in acute experimental myocardial infarction. J. Am. Coll. Cardiol. 14:1816, 1989.

388. Torr, S., Drake-Holland, A. J., Main, M., et al.: Effects on infarct size of reperfusion and pretreatment with β-blockade and calcium antagonists. Basic Res. Cardiol. 84:564, 1989.

389. Eisenberg, P. R., Sherman, L., Rich, M., et al.: Importance of continued activation of thrombin reflected by fibrinopeptide A to the efficacy of thrombolysis. J. Am. Coll. Cardiol. 7:1255, 1986.

390. Eisenberg, P. R., Miletich, J. P., Sobel, B. E., and Jaffe, A. S.: Differential effects of activation of prothrombin by streptokinase compared with urokinase and tissue-type plasminogen activator (t-PA). Thromb. Res. 50:707, 1988.

391. Eisenberg, P. R., and Miletich, J. P.: Induction of marked thrombin activity by pharmacologic concentrations of plasminogen activators in nonanticoagulated whole blood. Thromb. Res. 55:635, 1989.

392. Sobel, B. E.: Coronary thrombolysis and the new biology. J. Am. Coll. Cardiol. 14:850, 1989.

393. Fry, E.T.A., Grace, A., and Sobel, B. E.: Interactions between pharmacologic concentrations of plasminogen activators and platelets. Fibrinolysis 3:127, 1989.

394. Fujii, S., and Sobel, B. E.: Induction of plasminogen activator inhibitor by products released from platelets. Circulation, 82:1485, 1990.

395. Torr, S. R., Winters, K. J., Santoro, S. A., and Sobel, B. E.: The nature of interactions between tissue-type plasminogen activator and platelets. Thromb. Res., 59:279, 1990.

396. Eisenberg, P. R., Miletich, J. P., and Sobel, B. E.: Factors responsible for differential procoagulation effects of diverse plasminogen activators in plasma. Blood, in press.

397. Terres, W., Beythien, C., Kupper, W., and Bleifeld, W.: Effects of aspirin and prostaglandin E₁ on in vitro thrombolysis with urokinase: Evidence for a possible role of inhibiting platelet activity in thrombolysis. Circulation 79:1309, 1989.

398. Vaughan, D. E., Plavin, S. R., Schafer, A. I., and Loscalzo, J.: PGE₁ accelerates thrombolysis by tissue plasminogen activator. Blood 73:1213, 1989.

399. Schumacher, W. A., and Grover, G. J.: The thromboxane receptor antagonist SQ 30,741 reduces myocardial infarct size in monkeys when given during reperfusion at a threshold dose for improving reflow during thrombolysis. J. Am. Coll. Cardiol. 15:883, 1990.

400. Lefer, A. M., Mentley, R., and Sun, J-Z.: Potentiation of myocardial salvage by tissue type plasminogen activator in combination with a thromboxane synthetase inhibitor in ischemic cat myocardium. Circ. Res. 63:621, 1988.

401. Nicolini, F. A., Mehta, J. L., Nichols, W. W., et al.: Prostacyclin analogue iloprost decreases thrombolytic potential of tissue-type plasminogen activator in canine coronary thrombosis. Circulation 81:1115, 1990.

402. Reed, G. L., III, Matsueda, G. R., and Haber, E.: Inhibition of clot-bound α₂-antiplasmin enhances in vivo thrombolysis. Circulation 82:164, 1990.

403. Hsia, J., Hamilton, W. P., Kleiman, N., et al.: The Heparin-Aspirin Reperfusion Trial (HART): A randomized trial of heparin versus aspirin adjunctive to tissue plasminogen activator-induced thrombolysis in acute myocardial infarction. N. Engl. J. Med., in press.

404. Thompson, P. L., Aylward, P. E., Federman, J., et al.: A randomized comparison of intravenous heparin versus oral aspirin and dipyridamole commenced at 24 hours after recombinant tissue plasminogen activator for acute myocardial infarction. Circulation, in press.

405. Haskel, E. J., Sobel, B. E., and Abendschein, D. R.: The relative efficacy of antithrombin compared with antiplatelet agents in accelerating coronary thrombolysis and preventing early reocclusion. Circulation, 83:1048, 1991.

406. Walsh, M. N., Geltman, E. M., Steele, R. L., et al.: Augmented myocardial perfusion reserve after coronary angioplasty quantified by positron emission tomography with H₂¹⁵O. J. Am. Coll. Cardiol. 15:119, 1990.

407. Geltman, E. M., Henes, C. G., Senneff, M. J., et al.: Increased myocardial perfusion at rest and diminished perfusion reserve in patients with angina and angiographically normal coronary arteries. J. Am. Coll. Cardiol., 16:586, 1990.

408. Schaper, J., and Schaper, W.: Reperfusion of ischemic myocardium: Ultrastructural and histochemical aspects. J. Am. Coll. Cardiol. 1:1037, 1983.

409. Ellis, S. G., Henschke, C. I., Sandor, T., et al.: Time course of functional and biochemical recovery of myocardium salvaged by reperfusion. J. Am. Coll. Cardiol. 1:1047, 1983.

410. Lavallee, M., Cox, D. A., and Vatner, S. F.: Effects of coronary artery reperfusion on recovery of regional myocardial function in conscious dogs. Eur. Heart J. 6:109, 1985.

411. Maroko, P. R., Radvany, P., Braunwald, E., and Hale, S. L.: Reduction of infarct size by oxygen inhalation following acute coronary occlusion. Circulation 52:360, 1975.

412. Glogar, D. H., Kloner, R. A., Muller, J., et al.: Fluorocarbons reduce myocardial ischemic damage after coronary occlusion. Science 211:1439, 1981.

413. Tokioka, H., Miyazaki, A., Fung, P., et al.: Effects of intracoronary infusion of arterial blood or Fluosol-DA 20% on regional myocardial metabolism and function during brief coronary artery occlusions. Circulation 75:473, 1987.

414. Schaer, G. L., Karas, S. P., Santoian, E. C., et al.: Reduction in reperfusion injury by blood-free reperfusion after experimental myocardial infarction. J. Am. Coll. Cardiol. 15:1385, 1990.

415. Bajaj, A. K., Cobb, M. A., Virmani, R., et al.: Limitation of myocardial reperfusion injury by intravenous perfluorochemicals. Role of neutrophil activation. Circulation 79:645, 1989.

416. Braunwald, E., Muller, J. E., Kloner, R. A., and Maroko, P. R.: Role of beta-adrenergic blockade in the therapy of patients with myocardial infarction. Am. J. Med. 74:113, 1983.

417. Nayler, W. G., Panagiotopoulos, S., Elz, J. S., and Sturrock, W. J.: Fundamental mechanisms of action of calcium antagonists in myocardial ischemia. Am. J. Cardiol. 59:75B, 1987.

418. Kloner, R. A., and Braunwald, E.: Effects of calcium antagonists on infarcting myocardium. Am. J. Cardiol. 59:84B, 1987.

419. Henry, P. R., Shuchleib, R., Borda, L. J., et al.: Effects of nifedipine on myocardial perfusion and ischemic injury in dogs. Circ. Res. 43:372, 1978.

420. Drury, J. K., Haendchen, R. V., Meerbaum, S., et al.: Diltiazem improves function and reduces infarct size after acute coronary occlusion. J. Am. Coll. Cardiol. 1:692, 1983.

421. Calva, E., Mujica, A., Bisteni, A., and Sodi-Pallares, D.: Oxidative phosphorylation in cardiac infarct: Effect of glucose-KCl-insulin solution. Am. J. Physiol. 209:371, 1965.

422. Henry, P. D., Sobel, B. E., and Braunwald, E.: Protection of hypoxic guinea pig hearts with glucose and insulin. Am. J. Physiol. 226:390, 1974.

423. Maroko, P. R., Libby, P., Sobel, B. E., et al.: Effect of glucose-insulin-potassium infusion on myocardial infarction following experimental coronary artery occlusion. Circulation 45:1160, 1972.

424. Mjøs, O. D.: Effect of reduction of myocardial free fatty acid metabolism relative to that of glucose on the ischemic injury during experimental coronary artery occlusion in dogs. In Hjalmarson, A., and Werko, L. (eds.): Experimental and Clinical Aspects on Preservation of the Ischemic Myocardium. Sweden, Molndal, 1976, p. 29.

425. Coleman, G. M., Gradinac, S., Taegtmeyer, H., et al.: Efficacy of metabolic support with glucose-insulin-potassium for left ventricular pump failure after aortocoronary bypass surgery. Circulation 80(Suppl. I):91, 1989.

426. Maroko, P. R., Carpenter, C. B., Chiariello, M., et al.: Reduction by cobra venom factor of myocardial necrosis following coronary artery occlusion. J. Clin. Invest. 61:661, 1978.

427. Diaz, P. E., Fishbein, M. C., Davis, M. A., et al.: Effect of kallikrein inhibitor aprotinin on myocardial ischemic injury following coronary artery occlusion in the dog. Am. J. Cardiol. 40:541, 1977.

428. Libby, P., Maroko, P. R., Bloor, C. M., et al.: Reduction of experimental myocardial infarct size by corticosteroid administration. J. Clin. Invest. 52:599, 1973.

429. Hammerman, H., Kloner, R. A., Hale, S., et al.: Dose-dependent effects of short-term methylprednisolone on myocardial infarct extent, scar formation, and ventricular function. Circulation 68:446, 1983.

430. Brown, E. J., Kloner, R. A., Schoen, F. J., et al.: Scar thinning due to ibuprofen administration following experimental myocardial infarction. Am. J. Cardiol. 51:877, 1983.

431. Willerson, J. T., Watson, J. T., and Platt, M. R.: Effect of hypertonic mannitol and intraaortic counterpulsation on regional myocardial blood flow and ventricular performance in dogs during myocardial ischemia. Am. J. Cardiol. 37:514, 1976.

432. Roberts, R., Braunwald, E., Muller, J. E., et al.: Effect of hyaluronidase on mortality and morbidity in patients with early peaking of plasma creatine kinase MB and non-transmural ischaemia. Br. Heart J. 60:290, 1988.

433. Flaherty, J. T.: Intravenous nitroglycerin in acute myocardial infarction. Cardiovasc. Rev. Rep. 46, June 1990.

434. Gallagher, K. P., Buda, A. J., Pace, D., et al.: Failure of superoxide dismutase and catalase to alter size of infarction in conscious dogs after three hours of occlusion followed by reperfusion. Circulation 73:1065, 1986.

435. Uraizee, A., Reiner, K. A., Murry, C. E., and Jennings, R. B.: Failure of superoxide dismutase to limit size of myocardial infarction after 40 minutes of ischemia and four days of reperfusion in dogs. Circulation 75:1237, 1987.

436. Werns, S. W., Shea, M. J., Mitsos, S. E., et al.: Reduction of the size of infarction by allopurinol in the ischemic-reperfused canine heart. Circulation 73:518, 1986.

437. Braunwald, E., and Kloner, R. A.: Myocardial reperfusion: A double-edged sword? J. Clin. Invest. 76:1713, 1985.

437a. Forman, M. B., Virmani, R., and Puett, D. W.: Mechanisms and therapy of myocardial reperfusion injury. Circulation 81(Suppl. IV)69, 1990.

437b. Lefer, A. M., Tsao, P. S., Lefer, D. J., and Ma, X-L.: Role of endothelial dysfunction in the pathogenesis of reperfusion injury after myocardial ischemia. FASEB J 5:2029, 1991.

438. Murry, C. E., Richard, V. J., Reimer, K. A., and Jennings, R. B.: Ischemic preconditioning slows energy metabolism and delays ultrastructural damage during a sustained ischemic episode. Circ. Res. 66:913, 1990.

439. Li, G. C., Vasquez, J. A., Gallagher, K. P., and Lucchesi, B. R.: Myocardial protection with preconditioning. Circulation 82:609, 1990.

440. Schott, R. J., Rohmann, S., Braun, E. R., and Schaper, W.: Ischemic preconditioning reduces infarct size in swine myocardium. Circ. Res. 66:1133, 1990.

441. Jennings, R. B., Schaper, J., Hill, M. L., et al.: Effect of reperfusion late in the phase of reversible ischemic injury: Changes in cell volume, electrolytes, metabolites, and ultrastructure. Circ. Res. 56:262, 1985.

442. Kloner, R. A., Ellis, S. G., Lange, R., and Braunwald, E.: Studies of experimental coronary artery reperfusion: Effects on infarct size, myocardial function, biochemistry, ultrastructure, and microvascular damage. Circulation 68(Suppl. I):8, 1983.

443. Kloner, R. A., Ellis, S. G., Carlson, N. V., and Braunwald, E.: Coronary reperfusion for the treatment of acute myocardial infarction. Postischemic ventricular dysfunction. Cardiology 70:233, 1983.

Acute Myocardial Infarction

by RICHARD C. PASTERNAK, M.D., EUGENE BRAUNWALD, M.D., and BURTON E. SOBEL, M.D.

In the United States nearly 1,500,000 patients suffer from acute myocardial infarction (AMI) annually and approximately one-fourth of all deaths are due to AMI.[1] More than 60 per cent of the deaths associated with AMI occur within one hour of the event and are attributable to arrhythmias, most often ventricular fibrillation (Chap. 26). Approximately 1.7 million patients with suspected AMI are admitted yearly to coronary care units in the United States; in about one-third of the patients, the diagnosis of MI is confirmed.[2]

In 1980, before the introduction of thrombolytic therapy, the mortality rates during hospitalization and the year following infarction were approximately 10 per cent each. However, there is considerable variation in prognosis depending on a wide variety of clinical factors, as discussed later, and several recent large-scale trials have suggested a far lower mortality when newer therapeutic modalities are used.[3,4] In the United States, the yearly economic burden of coronary artery disease is in excess of $100 billion.[5] Perhaps as much as half of this cost is related to myocardial infarction (MI) and its prevention and treatment. The average 5-year cost of an AMI has recently been estimated at over $50,000 per patient[6]; these costs appear to be increasing despite shorter average lengths of hospital stay.[7]

DIMINISHING MORTALITY IN MYOCARDIAL INFARCTION. In the United States, the decline in death rate from coronary artery disease (p. 1292) has been accompanied by diminished mortality from AMI. This fall in the mortality appears to be caused by two factors: a fall in the incidence of AMI by 25 per cent or more[8] and a similarly marked fall in the case fatality rate once a myocardial infarction has occurred.[8-11] The reasons for this decline in mortality undoubtedly are multifactorial. According to some estimates,[12,13] about 40 per cent of the fall in mortality is caused by such medical interventions as coronary care units, prehospital resuscitation, and newer mechanical and medical treatments of coronary artery

disease. A marked overall decline in the incidence of sudden cardiac death suggests the effectiveness of both preventive measures and early treatment.[14]

There is no doubt that careful monitoring of cardiac rhythm and prompt treatment of *primary* arrhythmias have reduced sharply the incidence of in-hospital deaths from AMI. Accordingly, most deaths among patients with this condition who reach the hospital are now attributable to left ventricular failure and shock, and occur within the 3 or 4 days after the onset of infarction.[15,16] Only a minority of in-hospital deaths now result from *primary* arrhythmias and most of these occur in

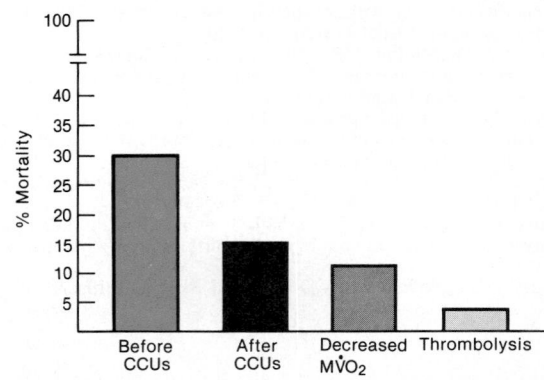

FIGURE 39–1. The mortality rates for patients with AMI managed in the era before use of defibrillation in coronary care units, after widespread utilization of defibrillation, and during the period in which reduction of myocardial oxygen requirements (MVO_2) was a major focus of cardiovascular care, and presently for patients treated with thrombolysis. (From Sobel, B. E.: Coronary thrombolysis and the new biology. Reprinted with permission of the American College of Cardiology. J. Am. Coll. Cardiol. *14*:858, 1989.)

settings in which monitoring and/or treatment is inadequate. Nevertheless, arrhythmias occurring in the setting of extensive infarction and left ventricular failure (*secondary* arrhythmias) represent a relatively common cause of death.[17]

Before the advent of coronary care units, treatment of AMI was directed almost exclusively toward allowing healing of the infarct, preventing cardiac rupture and other complications such as pulmonary and systemic embolism, and sustaining arterial pressure and urine output. Subsequently, the major emphasis was on the prevention and aggressive treatment of arrhythmias. The concept that infarct size is an important determinant of prognosis and that its ultimate extent might be modified favorably by early implementation of selected physiological and pharmacological interventions has directed attention to the protection of jeopardized myocardium by attempts to decrease myocardial oxygen demand as well as by restoration of perfusion to ischemic tissue.[17,18] There have been recent dramatic strides, particularly in the area of thrombolytic therapy for AMI.[16,19,20] These developments are responsible for an ever-decreasing mortality from AMI, a decrease of over 80 per cent in the past 3 decades (Fig. 39–1).

For several years now we have been in an era in which the management of AMI may be characterized as "aggressive,"[21] in which there is wide recognition of the dynamic nature of the infarction process, and in which technological advances are occurring rapidly. This chapter addresses the underlying pathophysiology of AMI and the resulting clinical manifestations. Rapidly evolving management strategies are discussed in this pathophysiological context.

Pathology of Acute Myocardial Infarction

Almost all myocardial infarctions result from atherosclerosis of the coronary arteries, generally with superimposed coronary thrombosis. Nonatherogenic forms of coronary artery disease are discussed on p. 1352. The genesis of the coronary atherosclerotic lesion is a complex and controversial issue (see Chap. 36), and a number of risk factors have been associated with the development of atherosclerosis (see Chap. 37). However, regardless of the etiology and pathogenesis of the atherosclerotic process, the end result is plaques that cause luminal narrowing of the coronary arterial tree and, in many instances, a thrombus that causes further narrowing and often total occlusion. Below a certain critical level of blood flow, myocardial cells develop ischemic injury, a process described in detail in Chapter 38. When severe ischemia is prolonged, irreversible damage, i.e., MI, occurs.

Since the coronary luminal narrowing affects the major coronary arteries and their various branches to a different extent, MI usually occurs focally in specific regions of the heart. The location and size of a particular infarction depend on a number of different factors including (1) the location and severity of the atherosclerotic narrowings in the coronary arterial tree; (2) the size of the vascular bed perfused by the narrowed vessel(s); (3) the oxygen needs of the poorly perfused myocardium; (4) the extent of development of collateral blood vessels; (5) the presence, site, and severity of coronary arterial spasm; (6) the presence of tissue factors capable of modifying the necrotic process; and (7) the activity and effect of endogenously released thrombotic and thrombolytic substances.

GROSS PATHOLOGICAL CHANGES

Myocardial infarctions may be divided into two major types: *transmural infarcts,* in which myocardial necrosis involves the full thickness of the ventricular wall, and *subendocardial (nontransmural) infarcts,* in which the necrosis involves the subendocardium, the intramural myocardium, or both without extending all the way through the ventricular wall to the epicardium (Fig. 39–2).

Acute coronary thrombosis appears to be far more common when the infarction is transmural.[21a,22] Furthermore, the histological pattern of necrosis may differ, with contraction band injury (see below) occurring almost twice as often in nontransmural as in transmural infarction.[21a] Transmural infarcts are more frequently localized to the zone of distribution of a single coronary artery. Nontransmural infarctions, however, frequently occur in the setting of severely narrowed but still patent coronary arteries,[23] often in patients with pulmonary embolism, hypertension, hypotension, anemia, aortic stenosis, operative procedures, or cerebrovascular accidents. In the presence of severe atherosclerotic narrowing of the coronary arteries, these and other conditions associated with increased myocardial metabolic demands or decreased myocardial oxygen delivery or both are capable of producing patchy nontransmural myocardial necrosis, which tends to involve the subendocardium. In other instances, nontransmural infarcts appear to result from a total thrombotic occlusion that undergoes early spontaneous thrombolysis. Paradoxically, before their infarction, patients with nontransmural infarcts have, on average, a more severe stenosis in the infarct-related coronary artery than do patients suffering from transmural infarcts.[24] This finding suggests that a more severe lesion occurring before infarction protects against the development of transmural infarction, perhaps by fostering the development of supportive collateral circulation.

Myocardial infarction most commonly involves the left ventricle and interventricular septum; however, depending upon the criteria used, approximately one-third to two-thirds of patients with inferior infarction have some involvement of the right ventricle.[25,26] Among these patients, right ventricular infarction occurs exclusively in those with transmural infarction of the inferior posterior wall and the posterior portion of the septum. Patients with preexisting right ventricular hypertrophy are predisposed to develop right ventricular infarction with acute inferior MI.[27] Although right ventricular infarction almost invariably develops in association with infarction of the adjacent septum and left ventricular myocardium, *isolated* infarction of the right ventricle is seen in 3 to 5 per cent of autopsy-proven cases of myocardial infarction, usually in patients with chronic lung disease and right ventricular hypertrophy.[28]

ATRIAL INFARCTION. This occurs in 7 to 17 per cent of autopsy-proven cases of MI,[29] is often seen in conjunction with left ventricular infarction, and can result in rupture of the atrial wall. This type of infarct is more common on the right than the left side and occurs more frequently in the atrial appendages than in the lateral or posterior walls of the atrium. These differences in incidence might be explained by the considerably higher oxygen content of left atrial blood. Since right atrial infarction is usually associated with obstructive disease of the sinus node artery, it is accompanied frequently by atrial arrhythmias.

Gross changes (Fig. 39–3) do not appear in the myocardium until 6 hours after the onset of MI.[30] Initially, the myocardium in the affected region appears pale, bluish, and slightly swollen. Eighteen to 36 hours after the onset of the infarct, the

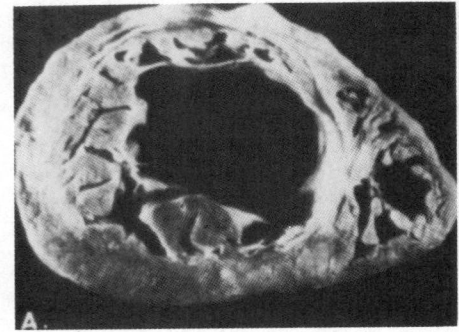
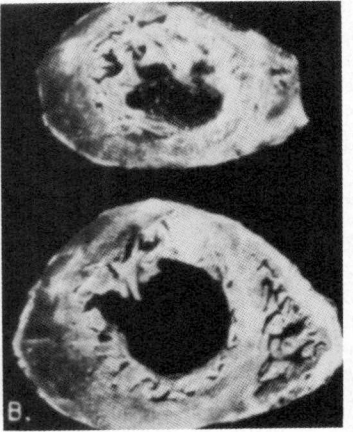
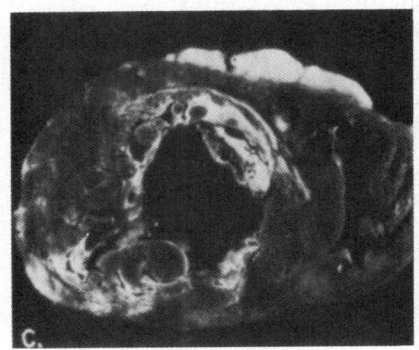
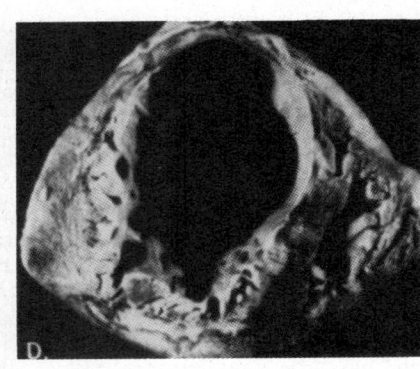

FIGURE 39–2. Examples of gross appearance of heart with healed myocardial infarct. *A,* Healed extensive anteroseptal infarction. The involved part of the wall is thin. *B,* Two levels of section showing healed anterior infarction with mural thrombosis at the apex. *C,* Healed subendocardial anterior infarction with endocardial fibrosis. In the inferolateral aspect there is scarring of healed infarction. *D,* Healed extensive anterior infarction and recent healing inferior infarction. The thin wall and endocardial fibrosis are characteristic of a healed extensive anterior infarct. In the inferior wall there is an infarct that is undergoing healing. (From Edwards, B. S., and Edwards, J. E.: Pathology of acute myocardial infarction. *In* Francis, G. S., and Alpert, J. S. [eds.]: Modern Coronary Care. Boston, Little, Brown and Co., 1990, p. 56.)

myocardium appears tan or reddish-purple, with a serofibrinous exudate evident on the epicardium in transmural infarcts. These changes persist for approximately 48 hours; the infarct then turns gray, and fine yellow lines, secondary to neutrophilic infiltration, appear at its periphery. This zone gradually widens and during the next few days extends throughout the infarct.

Eight to 10 days following infarction, the thickness of the cardiac wall in the area of the infarct is reduced as necrotic muscle is removed by mononuclear cells. The cut surface of an infarct of this age is yellow, surrounded by a reddish-purple band of granulation tissue that extends through the necrotic tissue by 3 to 4 weeks. Commencing at this time and extending over the next 2 to 3 months, the infarcted area gradually acquires a gelatinous, ground-glass, gray appearance, eventually converting into a shrunken, thin, firm scar,

which whitens and firms progressively with time.[31,32] This process begins at the periphery of the infarct and gradually moves centrally. The endocardium below the infarct increases in thickness and becomes gray and opaque.

HISTOLOGICAL AND ULTRASTRUCTURAL CHANGES

LIGHT MICROSCOPY. Severe ischemia, which is potentially reversible, causes cloudy swelling, as well as hydropic, vascular, and fatty degeneration.[33] For many years it was believed that no light microscopic changes could be seen in infarcted myocardium until 8 hours after interruption of blood flow. Bouchardy and Majno, however, have called attention to a wavy pattern of myocardial cells that occurs shortly after the onset of infarction (Fig. 39–4), a pattern that is probably the result of agonal contraction of myocardial cells.[34] With careful light microscopy,

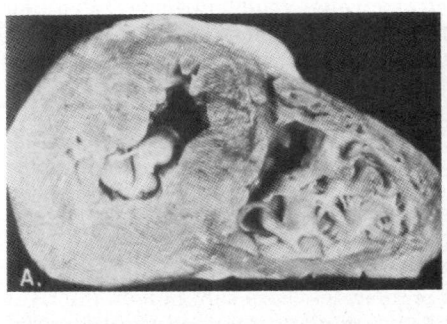
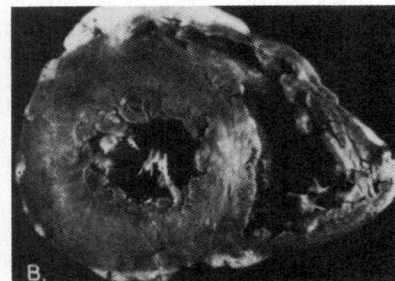
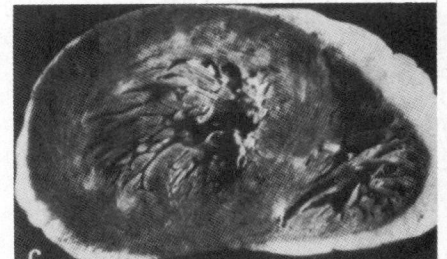
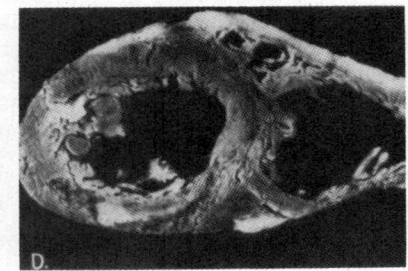

FIGURE 39–3. Gross pathology of AMI. *A,* Early anteroseptal infarction. The different texture of the anterior part of the septum and nearby anterior wall reflects a zone that in the fresh state yielded a cyanotic hue. *B,* Anterior infarction of about 4 days' duration. The pale area in the subendocardial half of the anterior wall and the nearby ventricular septum represents acute infarction. *C,* Healing infarction in midportion of the ventricular septum. The dark, depressed area represents a zone of necrotic muscle. *D,* Transmural acute inferior infarction. The pale area in the inferior wall represents necrotic muscle. Peripheral to this zone is a dark area characteristic of a 2- to 3-week-old infarct. (From Edwards, B. S., and Edwards, J. E.: Pathology of acute myocardial infarction. *In* Francis, G. S., and Alpert, J. S. [eds.]: Modern Coronary Care. Boston, Little, Brown and Co., 1990, p. 55.)

cell nuclei become pyknotic and then undergo karyolysis, and small blood vessels undergo necrosis.

By 24 hours there are clumping of the cytoplasm and loss of cross striations, with appearance of focal hyalinization and irregular cross bands in the involved myocardial fibers. The nuclei become pyknotic and sometimes even disappear. The myocardial capillaries in the involved region dilate, and polymorphonuclear leukocytes accumulate, first at the periphery and then in the center of the infarct. During the first 3 days, the interstitial tissue becomes edematous and red blood cells may extravasate (Fig. 39–5). Generally, on about the fourth day after infarction, removal of necrotic fibers begins, again commencing at the periphery. Later, lymphocytes, macrophages, and fibroblasts infiltrate between myocytes, which become fragmented. At 8 days the necrotic muscle fibers have become dissolved; by about 10 days the number of polymorphonuclear leukocytes is reduced, and granulation tissue first appears at the periphery. Ingrowth of blood vessels and fibroblasts continues, along with removal of necrotic muscle cells, until the fourth to sixth week following infarction, by which time much of the necrotic myocardium has been removed. This process continues along with increasing collagenization of the infarcted area. By the sixth week, the infarcted area has usually been converted into a firm connective tissue scar with interspersed intact muscle fibers (Fig. 39–5).

HISTOCHEMISTRY. A variety of *histochemical* approaches have been used to detect myocardial changes compatible with infarction before routine microscopic changes become evident at 6 hours. These include estimation of glycogen, using a periodic acid–Schiff stain (PAS) and succinic dehydrogenase activity. Glycogen stores may become depleted within 3 to 4 hours after the onset of severe myocardial ischemia. However, the reliability of these procedures diminishes with lengthening of the interval between death and the examination of the myocardium.[30]

The nitro–blue tetrazolium staining technique can distinguish viable zones of myocardium, which stain dark blue, from necrotic areas of myocardium, which therefore remain uncolored and identifiable. This reaction can distinguish infarcted myocardium 6 to 8 hours after the start of infarction.[35]

ELECTRONMICROSCOPY. In experimental infarction, the earliest ultrastructural changes in cardiac muscle following ligation of a coronary artery, noted within 20 minutes, consist of reduction in the size and number of glycogen granules, development of intracellular edema, and swell-

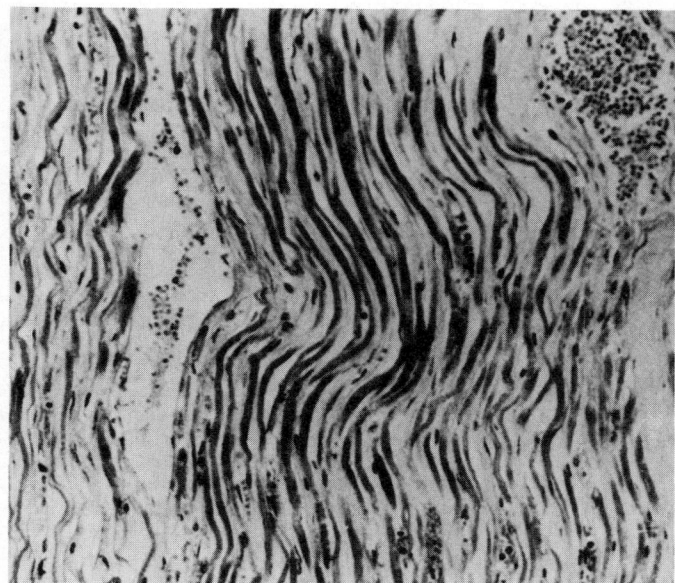

FIGURE 39–4. Wavy and stretched appearance of necrotic muscle cells in an acute myocardial infarct. The wavy myocardial fibers have pyknotic nuclei and hypereosinophilic cytoplasm. (Hematoxylin and eosin, × 128). (From Willerson J. T., Hillis, L. D., and Buja, L. M. [eds.]: Pathogenesis and pathology of ischemic heart disease. *In* Ischemic Heart Disease. Clinical and Pathophysiologic Aspects. New York, Raven Press, 1982, p. 46.)

contraction bands and small spaces between myocardial cells are also revealed. After 8 hours, edema of the interstitium becomes evident, as do increased fatty deposits in the muscle fibers, along with infiltration of neutrophilic polymorphonuclear leukocytes and red blood cells. Muscle

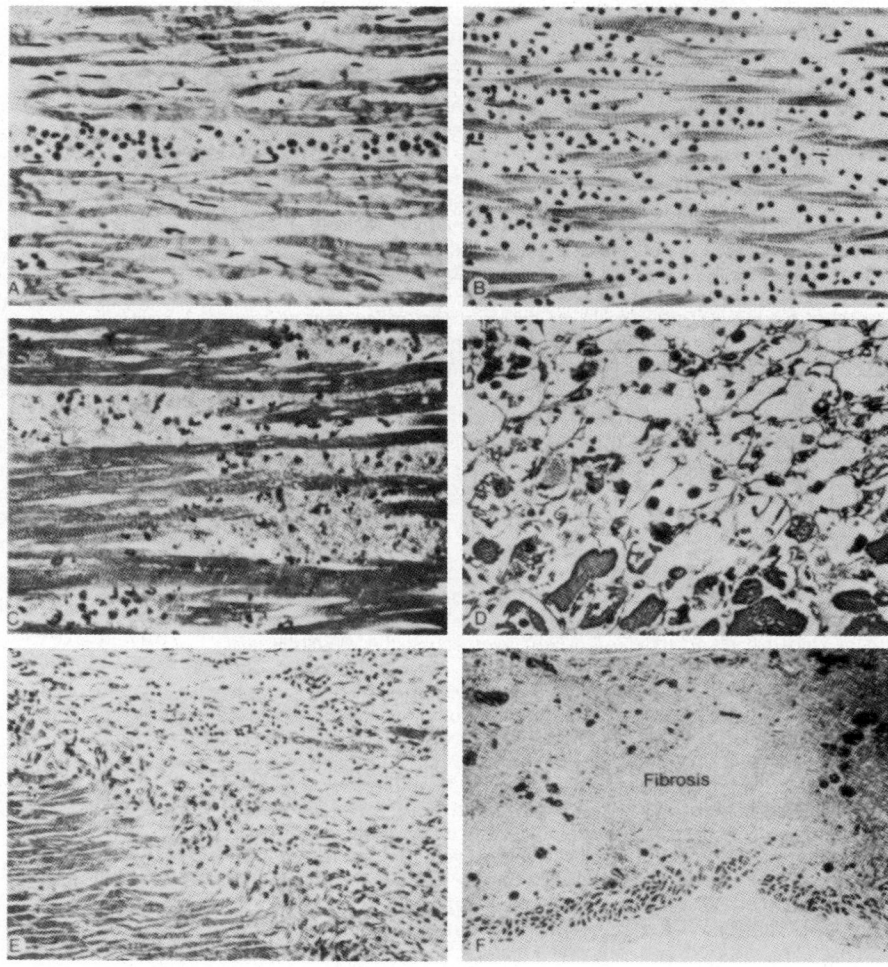

FIGURE 39–5. Histopathology of myocardial infarction. *A*, Acute myocyte ischemic injury with interstitial edema and early neutrophilic infiltration (1 day old). *B*, Necrotic myocytes and extensive neutrophilic infiltrate (2 to 4 days). *C*, Necrotic myocytes and basophilic interstitial debris (5 to 7 days). *D*, Extensive accumulation of macrophages within infarcted myocardium (8 to 11 days). *E*, Fibrovascular granulation tissue at border of infarct (12 to 16 days). *F*, Dense fibrosis, at low power (older than 16 days). (From Edwards, W. D.: Pathology of myocardial infarction and reperfusion. Reprinted by permission of the publisher. *In* Gersh, B. J., and Rahimtoola, S. H. [eds.]: Acute Myocardial Infarction. New York, Elsevier, 1991, p. 24.)

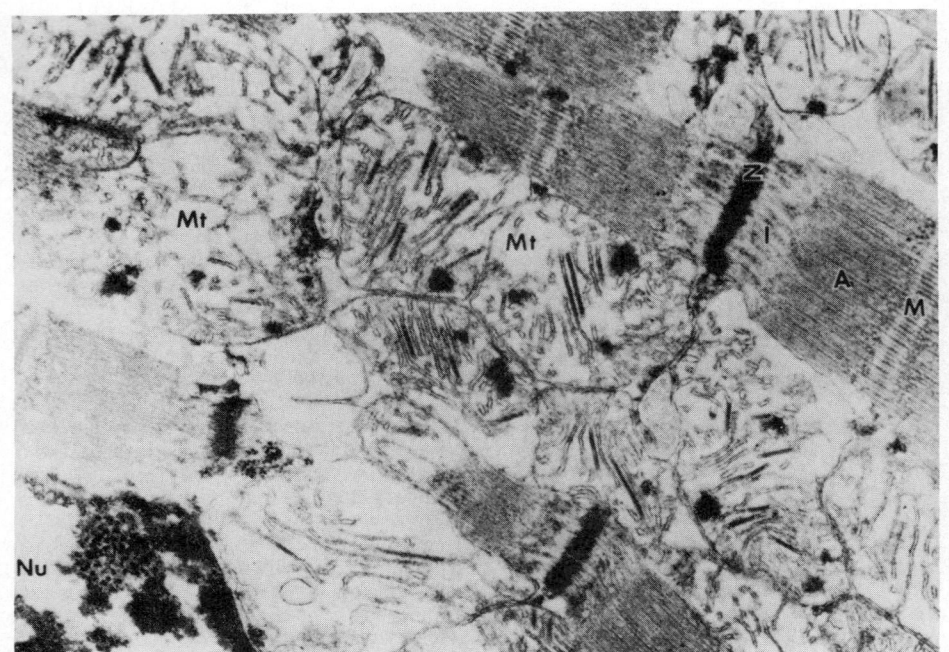

FIGURE 39-6. Electron micrograph of a muscle cell from the center of an infarct produced by permanent coronary occlusion in the dog. The myofibrils are fixed in a relaxed state and exhibit I, A, M, and Z bands. There is slight edema and no glycogen. (The clusters of granules resembling glycogen probably are ribosomes.) The mitochondria (Mt) are swollen and have linear densities and amorphous matrix (flocculent) densities. The nucleus (Nu) has clumped chromatin along the nuclear membrane and large lucent areas. (Tissue fixed with glutaraldehyde and osmium. Epoxy section stained with uranyl acetate and lead citrate, × 19,500.) (From Willerson, J. T., Hillis, L. D., and Buja, L. M. [eds.]: Pathogenesis and pathology of ischemic heart disease. *In* Ischemic Heart Disease. Clinical and Pathophysiological Aspects. New York, Raven Press, 1982, p. 47.)

ing and distortion of the transverse tubular system, the sarcoplasmic reticulum, and the mitochondria (Fig. 39-6).[36-38] When these changes are relatively mild, they are compatible with reversible ischemic injury. Changes after 60 minutes of occlusion include myocardial cell swelling, mitochondrial abnormalities such as swelling and internal disruption, aggregation and margination of nuclear chromatin, and relaxation of myofibrils. After 20 minutes to 2 hours of ischemia, changes in some cells become irreversible, and there is progression of these alterations; additional changes include indistinct, tight junctions at the intercalated discs, swollen sacs of the sarcoplasmic reticulum at the level of the A band, greatly enlarged mitochondria with few cristae, thinning and fractionation of myofilaments, disappearance of the heterochromatin, rarefaction of the euchromatin and peripheral aggregation of chromatin in the nucleus, disorientation of myofibrils, and clumping of mitochondria. Cells irreversibly damaged by ischemia are usually swollen, with an enlarged sarcoplasmic space; the sarcolemma may peel off the cells, defects in the plasma membrane may appear, and the mitochondria are fragmented.

The swollen mitochondria obtained from ischemic myocardium contain deposits of calcium phosphate and amorphous matrix densities[39]; many of these changes become more intense when blood flow is restored.[40] However, it appears unlikely that the structural and functional deterioration of mitochondria—the hallmark of ischemic injury—is the primary mediator of myocardial cell death. In experimental infarction, reflow into an area rendered ischemic for 40 to 60 minutes results in violent cell swelling with vacuolization of myocardial cell cytoplasm and marked swelling of mitochondria. Cell membranes are lifted off the myofibrils, and subsarcolemmal blebs appear. The speed with which these morphological changes occur early after ischemic reflow suggests that ischemia produces a defect of volume regulation in myocardial cells.

PATTERNS OF MYOCARDIAL NECROSIS

COAGULATION NECROSIS. This results from severe, persistent ischemia and is usually present in the central region of infarcts, which results in the arrest of muscle cells[44] in the relaxed state and the passive stretching of ischemic muscle cells. On light microscopy the myofibrils are stretched, many with unclear pyknosis, with vascular congestion and healing by phagocytosis of necrotic muscle cells. There is evidence of mitochondrial damage with prominent amorphous (flocculent) densities but no calcification.

COAGULATIVE MYOCYTOLYSIS.[34,42] This form of myocardial necrosis, also termed *contraction band necrosis*,[43] results primarily from severe ischemia followed by reflow.[36] It is caused by increased Ca^{++} influx into dying cells, resulting in the arrest of cells in the contracted state. It is seen in the periphery of large infarcts and is present to a greater extent in nontransmural infarcts than in transmural ones.[21a] The entire infarct may show this form of necrosis when reperfusion occurs experimentally[44] or by surgery.[43] While patches of contraction band necrosis are found after successful reperfusion by thrombolytic therapy,[45] its presence in a large

segment of some infarcts suggests that reperfusion through spontaneous thrombolysis or the release of spasm or both have occurred. It is characterized by hypercontracted myofibrils with contraction bands and mitochondrial damage, frequently with calcification, marked vascular congestion, and healing by lysis of muscle cells.

MYOCYTOLYSIS. This results from prolonged moderate ischemia and, like coagulative myocytolysis, is also frequently seen at the borders of an infarct as well as in patchy areas of infarction in patients with chronic ischemic heart disease. It is characterized by edema and cell swelling, early lysis of myofibrils, late lysis of nuclei, no neutrophilic response, and healing by lysis and phagocytosis of necrotic myocytes.[32,42]

CORONARY ARTERY ANATOMY AND PATHOLOGICAL ANATOMY

HISTORY. The importance of coronary artery obstruction has been the subject of much controversy since 1912, when Herrick proposed that AMI was due to occlusion of an epicardial coronary artery.[46] In the 3 decades following Herrick's description of the condition, the clinical manifestations of myocardial infarction were believed to stem from sudden coronary arterial occlusion, usually due to thrombosis; hence the terms *coronary thrombosis* and *acute myocardial infarction* became almost synonymous. One weakness of this concept was shown by Blumgart and colleagues, who demonstrated that *coronary occlusion could occur in the absence of infarction,* when the collateral circulation was adequate to maintain myocardial nutrition.[47] Equally important, Friedberg and Horn observed that *infarction could occur in the absence of coronary occlusion.*[48] The patients whom they described had severe coronary arterial narrowing. The areas of patchy, subendocardial infarction that occurred were thought to have developed secondary to relative insufficiency of coronary blood flow. Miller et al. then expanded on these observations, demonstrating that predominantly subendocardial infarcts were rarely associated with coronary occlusion, whereas transmural infarctions were frequently so.[23]

In over 75 per cent of patients with MI who come to autopsy, more than one coronary artery is severely narrowed.[32,49] One-third to two-thirds of patients with AMI have critical obstruction (to less than 25 per cent of luminal area) of all three coronary arteries, whereas the remainder are equally divided between those having one-vessel disease and those having two-vessel disease.[49,50] (Coronary arteriographic studies in surviving patients show that a higher percentage have one-vessel disease.) Most transmural infarcts occur distal to a totally occluded coronary artery. However, the converse is not the case, in that total occlusion of a coronary artery is not always associated with myocardial infarction. Collateral blood flow and other factors—such as the level of myocardial metabolism, the presence and location of stenoses in other coronary arteries, the rate of development of the obstruction, and the quantity of myocardium supplied by the obstructed vessel—all influence the viability of myocardial cells distal to the occlusion. In many series of patients studied at necropsy or by coronary arteriography, a small number (<5 per cent) of patients with MI are found to have normal coronary vessels.[32,50] In these patients, an embolus that has lysed or a prolonged episode of severe coronary spasm may have been responsible for the reduction in coronary flow.

Obstruction of the left anterior descending coronary artery usually causes infarction or threatens the viability of the anterior and apical regions of the left ventricle; portions of the septum, anterolateral wall, papillary muscles, and inferoapical wall of the left ventricle may also be involved. Obstruction of the left circumflex artery can cause infarction of the lateral or inferoposterior wall of the left ventricle. Occlusion of the right coronary artery usually results in infarction of the inferoposterior wall of the left ventricle, the inferior portions of the septum, posteromedial papillary muscle, and portions of the right ventricle. The size of the infarction and its location depend in part on the distribution of the obstructed coronary vessels. Thus, with occlusion of a dominant right coronary artery that supplies the posterior descending artery and posterior left ventricular wall, the inferoposterior wall of the left ventricle becomes infarcted, whereas the same region of the myocardium becomes involved with occlusion of the left circumflex coronary artery in the presence of a dominant left coronary artery.

Studies of patients who ultimately develop MI after having undergone coronary angiography at some time before its occurrence have been helpful in clarifying coronary anatomy before infarction. While high-grade stenoses, when present,[51,52] more frequently lead to MI than do less severe lesions, the majority of infarctions actually occur in areas supplied by a coronary artery with a previously identified stenosis of less than 50 per cent on angiograms performed months to years earlier.[53] This supports the concept (see below) that MI ultimately occurs secondary to recent destabilization of an atherosclerotic plaque. Certain angiographic characteristics, such as roughness of the luminal surface and lesion length, correlate with the risk of future infarction, further supporting this idea.[52]

RIGHT VENTRICULAR INFARCTION. Regardless of whether or not it is combined with involvement of the left ventricle, right ventricular infarction is generally associated with obstructive lesions of the right coronary artery. However, right ventricular infarction occurs less commonly than would be anticipated from the frequency of atherosclerotic lesions involving the right coronary artery.[54] This discrepancy probably can be explained by the lower oxygen demands of the right ventricle, since right ventricular infarcts occur more commonly in conditions such as pulmonary hypertension and right ventricular hypertrophy that are associated with increased right ventricular oxygen needs.[27,28] Moreover, the intercoronary collateral system of the right ventricle is richer than that of the left, and the thinness of the right ventricular wall allows the chamber to derive some nutrition from the blood within the right ventricular cavity.

Rather frequently, when an area of the ventricle is perfused by collateral vessels, an infarct occurs at a distance from a coronary occlusion. For example, following the gradual obliteration of the lumen of the right coronary artery, the inferior wall of the left ventricle may be maintained viable by collateral vessels arising from the left anterior descending coronary artery. In this circumstance, an occlusion of the left anterior descending artery may cause an infarct of the diaphragmatic wall.

CORONARY ARTERY THROMBOSIS

Conclusions drawn from autopsy studies of the coronary arteries following AMI are limited both by the selection bias (obviously only patients who die can be studied), and by post-

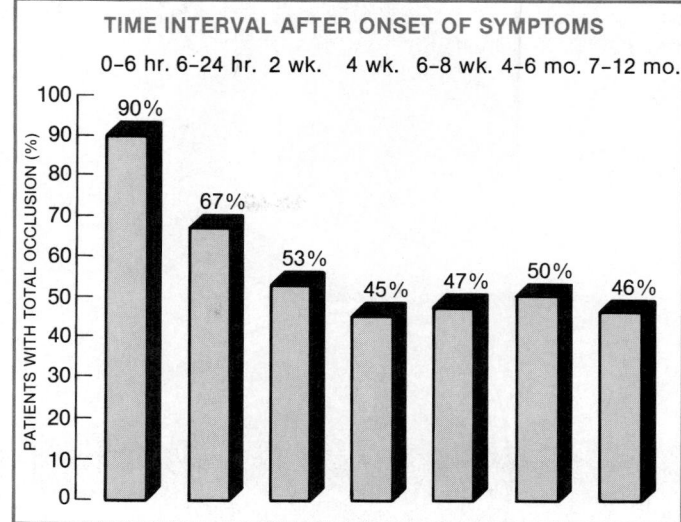

FIGURE 39–7. Percentage of patients with total coronary occlusion at different time intervals after the onset of symptoms of AMI. (Adapted from deFeyter, P. J., van den Brand, M., Serruys, P. W., and Wijns, W.: Early angiography after myocardial infarction: What have we learned? Am. Heart J. *109*:194, 1985.)

mortem events, including lysis of clots that were present premortem. For many years coronary angiography was avoided in the acute phases of MI because of potential complications.[55] Experience of the last decade, however, has shown that angiography is safe even during the acute phase of MI.[55,56] Angiographic studies performed in the earliest hours of transmural MI have revealed an approximate 90 per cent incidence of total occlusion in the infarct-related vessel.[56-58] Recanalization from spontaneous thrombolysis[58,59] as well as attrition due to some mortality among those patients with total occlusion results in a diminishing incidence of totally occluded vessels found in the period following myocardial infarction (Fig. 39–7).[50,56,59a]

Occlusion of a coronary artery leading to MI appears to be the final common pathway resulting from a complex and dynamic interaction among coronary atherosclerosis, vasospasm, plaque rupture, and platelet activation, ultimately leading to coronary artery thrombosis.[60-62]

CORONARY ATHEROSCLEROSIS IN MYOCARDIAL INFARCTION

At autopsy, the atherosclerotic plaque of patients who died of MI is primarily composed of fibrous tissue of varying density and cellularity.[63] Calcium, lipid-laden foam cells, and extracellular lipid each constitutes 5 to 10 per cent of the remaining area.[63] Roberts et al. have quantified the extent and severity of atherosclerosis in autopsied patients with a history of MI.[49,64] The entire length of the epicardial coronary tree was examined by dividing each coronary artery into 5-mm segments and assessing a cross-sectional area of each segment. The extent of severe narrowing (76 to 100 per cent) was largely unpredictable from clinical factors and varied between approximately 20 and 45 per cent of all coronary artery segments. Of the remaining segments without severe stenosis, about two-thirds showed moderate stenoses (51 to 75 per cent) and one-third, mild stenoses (26 to 50 per cent). Fewer than 6 per cent of segments examined were 25 per cent narrowed or less. Thus, the atherosclerotic processes were almost ubiquitous in most patients with MI. At autopsy, however, less advanced atherosclerosis may be present in survivors of MI.

The atherosclerotic plaques that are associated with thrombosis and a total occlusion, located in infarct-related vessels, are generally more complex and irregular than those in vessels not associated with MI.[65] Histological studies of these lesions often reveal plaque rupture or fissuring[66-69] (Fig. 39–8). Angiographic morphology suggestive of plaque rupture has been identified in the majority of stenoses associated with AMI or abrupt onset of unstable angina.[70] This finding is rare in the noninfarct-related vessels of AMI patients and in the vessels of patients with chronic stable angina pectoris.[70] While controversy exists regarding the exact role that plaque rupture plays in the sequence of events leading to coronary artery occlusion, it is probable that hemorrhage into an atherosclerotic plaque

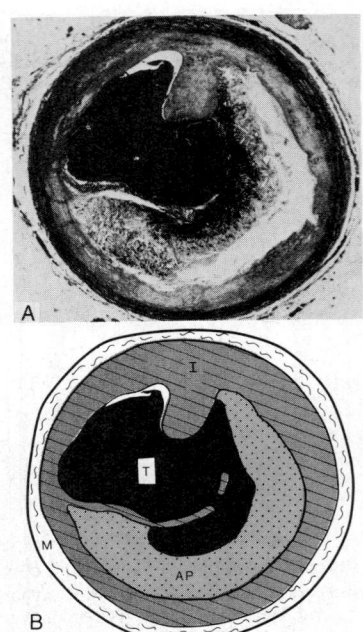

FIGURE 39-8. Histological cross section of a major plaque rupture (A) and accompanying diagram (B). The plaque (AP) has a large defect in the fibrous cap, through which a dumb-bell mass of thrombus (T) has formed, part being within the plaque and part virtually occluding the lumen. AP = atherosclerotic plaque; I = intima; M = media. (From Davies, M. J., and Thomas, A. C.: Plaque fissuring—the cause of acute myocardial infarction, sudden ischemic death, and crescendo angina. Br. Heart J. 53:363, 1985.)

can initiate a chain of events leading to coronary artery thrombus in MI.[61,62,66,68,69]

Platelet-rich thrombi are often associated with the surface of the most advanced atherosclerotic lesions, called *complicated plaques,* which are characterized by fibrocalcific degeneration, deposition of lipid, calcium, fibrous tissue, necrotic debris, extravasated blood, and a fibrous cap (Fig. 39-9). Impaired endothelial cell function associated with atherogenesis may predispose to platelet adhesion and activation. Conversely, platelet activation in association with such lesions may contribute to atherogenesis through release of growth factors. Luminal narrowing may potentiate platelet activation through augmentation of shear forces.

While it is now clear that transmural MI usually is caused by coronary thrombosis, the incidence of coronary thrombosis in subendocardial infarction is less clear, because angiographic studies provide only indirect evidence of thrombosis. The results of postmortem studies are difficult to interpret because thrombi can undergo organization or recanalization, which makes their pathological characteristics indistinguishable from nonocclusive atherosclerotic plaques.[66] Angiographic studies have suggested a wide variability in the frequency of coronary thrombosis with nontransmural infarction ranging from 20 to nearly 90 per cent.[22,71] The increasingly persuasive evidence that thrombosis plays a major role in patients with unstable ischemic syndromes[69-71] suggests that previous estimates of the incidence of thrombosis in nontransmural MI may have been less than the true frequency.

Rarely, coronary thrombosis may cause multifocal or circumferential infarction. However, the latter is more often the consequence of a severe imbalance between myocardial oxygen supply and demand when multiple high-grade fixed atherosclerotic lesions exist and myocardial oxygen demand is increased by such causes as tachycardia, increased ventricular wall tension, or increased myocardial contractility.

The rapidity with which thrombosis develops and the extent of coronary collaterals can determine whether acute coronary occlusion causes a transmural infarct, a subendocardial infarct, or no infarct.[36]

COMPOSITION OF THROMBI. At autopsy, coronary arterial thrombi, which are approximately 1 cm in length in most cases,[23] adhere to the luminal surface of an artery and are composed of platelets, fibrin, erythrocytes, and leukocytes. The composition of the thrombus may vary at different levels: A white thrombus is composed of platelets, fibrin, or both distally, and a red thrombus is composed of erythrocytes, fibrin, platelets, and leukocytes proximally. Early thrombi are usually small and nonocclusive and are composed almost exclusively of platelets.

In patients with MI, coronary thrombi are usually superimposed on or adjacent to atherosclerotic plaques (Fig. 39-8).[69] As already pointed out, the culprit plaques are often less than nearly occlusive. It has been suggested that degenerative changes in the atherosclerotic intima damage supportive perivascular tissue with resultant rupture of a plaque, sometimes accompanied by intramural hemorrhage.[36] This process may enlarge the volume of the plaque so that it occludes the arterial lumen without the occurrence of thrombosis, or the fissuring may disrupt the intima covering the plaque, thereby exposing collagen to flowing blood, a strong stimulus for thrombus formation.[67,68,72]

THE UNSTABLE PLAQUE. Pre- and postmortem angiographic studies have suggested that ulceration and plaque fissuring can be characterized radiographically as stenoses showing irregular borders (Fig. 8-35, p. 224) and intraluminal lucencies.[65,69] (The latter may be due to thrombus associated with the atherosclerotic lesion.) It has also been theorized that an angiographic pattern suggesting disruption of the atherosclerotic plaque is associated with histopathological evidence of coronary thrombosis as well as with the clinical syndromes of unstable angina (p. 1334) and AMI.[65,68-70]

ROLES OF PLATELETS AND COAGULATION FACTORS. While it is clear that platelets play an important role in the pathogenesis of atherosclerosis (Chap. 36), their precise *causal* role in MI remains controversial (p. 1110). It is quite likely that they are involved in the pathogenesis of coronary thrombosis.[60,62] Radiolabeled platelets incorporated into coronary thrombi have been identified scintigraphically in patients with AMI.[73] When atherosclerotic plaques undergo the changes noted earlier, exposed collagen leads to prompt platelet adhesion followed by formation of platelet aggregates, release of platelet granular constituents, and possible microembolization. The platelet in AMI has been characterized as hyperaggregable, and the degree of platelet hyperreactivity even appears to be a useful marker for future coronary events.[74] The phenomenon of hyperreactivity is probably related to the production, by aggregating platelets, of increased

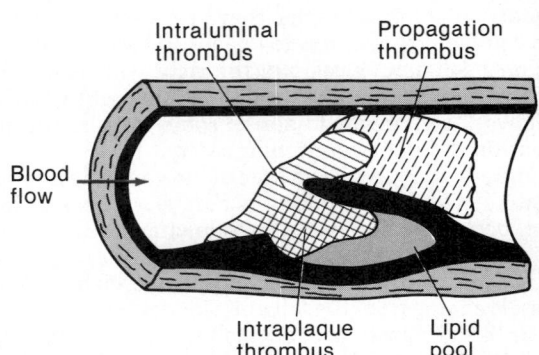

FIGURE 39-9. Representation of a longitudinal reconstruction of a coronary artery showing the histological components of an occluding thrombus. Much of the thrombus at the site of occlusion is contained within the plaque and compresses the lumen from outside. Intraluminal thrombus develops adjacent to a plaque fissure that propagates downstream. A plug of lipid has extruded into the lumen. (From Davies, M. J.: A macro and micro view of coronary vascular insult in ischemic heart disease. Circulation 82[Suppl. II]:38, 1990, by permission of the American Heart Association, Inc.)

amounts of thromboxane A_2 (a potent platelet-aggregating prostaglandin that is also a powerful vasoconstrictor).[60,75,76]

An imbalance in the clotting system between prothrombotic activity and the fibrinolytic system may also be related to the development of AMI. A hypercoagulable state may lead to MI in some patients who do not have atherosclerotic lesions (see below). A reduced fibrinolytic capacity due to the presence of a plasma inhibitor of tissue plasminogen activator (PAI-1) may be important in the pathogenesis of AMI in certain patients.[77] Elevated levels of urinary fibrinopeptide A in AMI patients provide evidence of activation of the clotting system, specifically of recent production of fibrin by the action of thrombin on fibrinogen.[78]

TEMPORAL CORRELATIONS. In order to define the precise relationship between coronary thrombosis and AMI, it is important to understand the time course of thrombus formation in relation to the onset of infarction. Unfortunately, estimates of the age of coronary thrombi and myocardial infarction by histological criteria may be quite imprecise,[79] but several lines of evidence suggest that a thrombus is present acutely. The findings of elevated levels of markers that indicate active coagulation[76,78,80] is considered circumstantial evidence. As already noted, studies in which coronary arteriography performed on patients within the first few hours after the onset of AMI have demonstrated that the coronary artery supplying the area of evolving infarction is totally occluded in the majority of these patients.[56,57,81,82] If fibrinolytic agents are infused into the occluded artery (or intravenously in large doses) patency is achieved in a high percentage of cases. Angiography performed after fibrinolytic therapy usually demonstrates residual stenotic lesions at the site where coronary arterial occlusion had existed. Fresh thrombi have been recovered from the majority of patients with acute myocardial infarction undergoing emergency coronary bypass surgery,[56] and have been directly visualized through coronary angioscopy in the setting of unstable angina, a condition that frequently precedes the development of AMI.[83]

CORONARY ARTERY SPASM

(See also p. 1338)

In addition to causing AMI in rare patients with normal coronary arteries (see below), coronary artery spasm may also play a broader role in patients with atherosclerotic coronary artery disease.[84] It has been postulated that spasm may cause intimal damage that can initiate formation of an atherosclerotic plaque.[85,86] Epicardial coronary artery spasm has been identified in patients with fixed atherosclerotic coronary artery stenosis before, during, and after AMI.[86-88] An association between coronary artery spasm and coronary artery thrombosis has also been documented clinically.[89]

In the setting of AMI, there is evidence of increased production of vasodilating and vasoconstricting prostaglandins,[75,90] but it appears that the vasoconstricting activity of thromboxane A_2 predominates.[60,75] Thus, the presence of thromboxane A_2 and other vasoconstricting substances released by the aggregating platelets at the site of a coronary artery stenosis has the potential to initiate or maintain coronary artery constriction. It may be responsible for some observed cases of coronary artery spasm occurring with and perhaps contributing to the pathogenesis of AMI.

COLLATERAL CIRCULATION

(See also p. 1164)

Normal hearts contain an extensive network of interarterial anastomotic blood vessels, greater than 60 μm in diameter, involving epicardial, intramyocardial, and subendocardial connections. This collateral circulation exists at birth and ap-

parently grows in size along with the rest of the coronary circulation but is beyond the limit of resolution of coronary arteriographic techniques and is not seen in living subjects without disease. In patients with coronary artery disease, these preexisting channels progressively enlarge, presumably as a consequence of the release of local vasodilators; flow through the collaterals will occur when pressure differences exist across these channels.[91] The coronary collateral circulation is particularly well developed in patients with (1) coronary occlusive disease, especially when it is severe, with the reduction of the luminal cross-sectional area by more than 75 per cent in one or more major vessels; (2) chronic hypoxia, as occurs in severe anemia, chronic obstructive pulmonary disease, and cyanotic congenital heart disease; and (3) left ventricular hypertrophy, which intensifies coronary collaterals. There is considerable variability in the development of collateral channels in patients with comparable degrees of obstructive coronary artery disease.

CORONARY COLLATERALS IN ACUTE MYOCARDIAL INFARCTION

Early angiography in patients with AMI and the performance of serial catheterizations for trials on the effects of reperfusion in these patients have allowed the careful study of the angiographic appearance of collaterals. Although well-developed collaterals are not the rule at the time of infarction, some collaterals are seen in nearly 40 per cent of patients with an acute total occlusion,[92] and more begin to appear soon after the total occlusion occurs.[22,93] The incidence of collaterals 1 to 2 weeks following AMI varies considerably and may be as high as 75 to 100 per cent in patients with persistent total occlusion of the infarct vessel, or as low as 17 to 42 per cent in patients with subtotal occlusion.[22,93-95,99a]

That the appearance of collaterals is closely related to the presence of a totally occluded vessel has been shown by studies at the time of coronary angioplasty. These studies have allowed for the demonstration that filling of collaterals improves within 1 to 2 minutes of a sudden temporary coronary artery occlusion induced by an angioplasty balloon.[96] Likewise, a total occlusion induced by transient coronary artery spasm may allow for the visualization of collaterals not seen before the spasm.[97] It is likely that the presence of a high-grade stenosis (> 90 per cent), possibly with periods of intermittent total occlusion, permits the development of collaterals that remain only as *potential* conduits until a total occlusion occurs or recurs. The latter event then brings these channels into full operation.

Supporting the argument in favor of a functional role for coronary collateral vessels is the finding that in patients with coronary occlusion and collaterals the area of myocardial necrosis is frequently smaller than the area supplied by an occluded coronary artery when collaterals are not present.[94,95,98,98a] Indeed, it is rather common for patients with abundant collaterals to have totally occluded coronary arteries without evidence of infarction in the distribution of that coronary vessel; thus, the survival of the myocardium distal to such occlusions must be dependent on collateral blood flow.

NONATHEROSCLEROTIC CAUSES OF ACUTE MYOCARDIAL INFARCTION

Numerous pathological processes other than atherosclerosis can, on occasion, involve the coronary arteries (p. 1213) and result in myocardial infarction (Table 39–1).[99,100] For example, coronary arterial occlusions can be the result of embolization of a coronary artery. Emboli most frequently lodge in the distribution of the left anterior descending coronary artery, commonly in the distal epicardial and intramural branches.[23] The causes of coronary embolism are numerous: infective and marantic endocarditis (Chap. 35), mural thrombi, prosthetic valves,[101] neoplasms,[102] air that is introduced at the time of cardiac surgery,[103] and calcium deposits from manipulation of calcified valves at operation. In situ thrombosis of coronary arteries can occur secondary to chest-wall trauma (Chap. 46). Oral contraceptive use probably is associated with AMI in healthy women,[104] although this point remains controversial.[105] The mechanism of this association may operate through an increased tendency for thrombosis.

A variety of inflammatory processes can be responsible for coronary artery abnormalities, some of which mimic athero-

TABLE 39–1   CAUSES OF MYOCARDIAL INFARCTION WITHOUT CORONARY ATHEROSCLEROSIS

CORONARY ARTERY DISEASE OTHER THAN ATHEROSCLEROSIS

Arteritis
  Luetic
  Granulomatous (Takayasu disease)
  Polyarteritis nodosa
  Mucocutaneous lymph node (Kawasaki) syndrome
  Disseminated lupus erythematosus
  Rheumatoid arthritis
  Ankylosing spondylitis
Trauma to coronary arteries
  Laceration
  Thrombosis
  Iatrogenic
  Radiation (radiotherapy for neoplasia)
Coronary mural thickening with metabolic disease or intimal
    proliferative disease
  Mucopolysaccharidoses (Hurler disease)
  Homocystinuria
  Fabry disease
  Amyloidosis
  Juvenile intimal sclerosis (idiopathic arterial calcification of
    infancy)
  Intimal hyperplasia associated with contraceptive steroids or
    with the postpartum period
  Pseudoxanthoma elasticum
  Coronary fibrosis caused by radiation therapy
Luminal narrowing by other mechanisms
  Spasm of coronary arteries (Prinzmetal's angina with normal
    coronary arteries)
  Spasm after nitroglycerin withdrawal
  Dissection of the aorta
  Dissection of the coronary artery

EMBOLI TO CORONARY ARTERIES

Infective endocarditis
Nonbacterial thrombotic endocarditis
Prolapse of mitral valve
Mural thrombus from left atrium, left ventricle, or pulmonary
    veins
Prosthetic valve emboli
Cardiac myxoma
Associated with cardiopulmonary bypass surgery and coronary
    arteriography
Paradoxical emboli
Papillary fibroelastoma of the aortic valve ("fixed embolus")
Thrombi from intracardiac catheters or guide wires

CONGENITAL CORONARY ARTERY ANOMALIES

Anomalous origin of left coronary from pulmonary artery
Left coronary artery from anterior sinus of Valsalva
Coronary arteriovenous and arteriocameral fistulas
Coronary artery aneurysms

MYOCARDIAL OXYGEN DEMAND-SUPPLY DISPROPORTION

Aortic stenosis, all forms
Incomplete differentiation of the aortic valve
Aortic insufficiency
Carbon monoxide poisoning
Thyrotoxicosis
Prolonged hypotension

HEMATOLOGICAL (IN SITU THROMBOSIS)

Polycythemia vera
Thrombocytosis
Disseminated intravascular coagulation
Hypercoagulability, thrombosis, thrombocytopenic purpura

MISCELLANEOUS

Cocaine abuse
Myocardial contusion
Myocardial infarction with normal coronary arteries
Complication of cardiac catheterization

Modified from Cheitlin, M., et al.: Myocardial infarction without athero-sclerosis. J.A.M.A. 231:951, 1975. Copyright 1975, American Medical Association.

sclerotic disease and may predispose to true atherosclerosis.[106] There is suggestive epidemiological evidence that viral infections, particularly with coxsackie B, may be an uncommon cause of MI.[107] Viral illnesses precede AMI occasionally in young persons who are later shown to have normal coronary arteries.[107,108]

Syphilitic aortitis may produce marked narrowing or occlusion of one or both coronary ostia,[109] whereas Takayasu's arteritis may result in obstruction of the coronary arteries (Chap. 47).[110] Necrotizing arteritis, polyarteritis nodosa,[111] mucocutaneous lymph node syndrome (Kawasaki disease) (p. 997),[112] systemic lupus erythematosus (p. 1234) and giant cell arteritis[114] (Chap. 56) can cause coronary occlusion. Therapeutic levels of mediastinal radiation can cause thickening and hyalinization of the walls of coronary arteries, with subsequent infarction.[115,116] MI may also be the result of coronary arterial involvement in amyloidosis (p. 1753), Hurler syndrome, pseudoxanthoma elasticum,[117] and homocystinuria (Chap. 51).

Involvement of the small coronary arteries (0.1 to 1.0 mm in diameter) by a number of disease processes may produce intimal and medial hyperplasia, necrosis, dissection, and thrombosis,[118] resulting in occlusions that produce *focal* areas of infarction and ultimately of fibrosis. Depending on the location and extent of the fibrotic reaction, arrhythmias, conduction defects, heart block, and heart failure can occur.

As *cocaine abuse* has become more common, reports of AMI following the use of cocaine have appeared with increasing frequency. Cocaine may cause AMI in patients with normal coronary arteries,[119-121] preexisting MI,[122] documented coronary artery disease,[121-123] or known coronary artery spasm.[125] Recurrent MI after further cocaine abuse has been reported as well.[119,124] Cocaine may cause MI by at least three mechanisms: (1) increasing myocardial oxygen demand via increases in heart rate and blood pressure, (2) diminishing coronary artery flow resulting from either coronary vasospasm and/or thrombosis,[119,121] and (3) active myocarditis (either hypersensitivity or toxic). Contraction band necrosis is the rule, and its extent appears to be related to the level of cocaine found in the blood or urine at autopsy.[126,128] In very high doses, cocaine appears to have a direct toxic effect on heart muscle that may produce cardiac failure and sudden death[127,129] with extensive myocyte necrosis.[126,127]

MYOCARDIAL INFARCTION WITH ANGIOGRAPHICALLY NORMAL CORONARY VESSELS

Approximately 6 per cent of all patients with AMI and perhaps four times that percentage of patients with this diagnosis under the age of 35 years do not have coronary atherosclerosis demonstrated by coronary arteriography or at autopsy.[50,59] Perhaps half the patients of this group, in turn, have a variety of other lesions involving the coronary vessels or myocardium (Table 39–1), whereas the others have no detectable coronary obstructive lesions.[130,131] Patients with AMI and normal coronary arteries tend to be young and to have relatively few coronary risk factors, except that they often have a history of cigarette smoking.[132-135] Usually they have no history of angina pectoris prior to the infarction.[136] The infarction in these patients is usually not preceded by any prodrome, but the clinical, laboratory, and electrocardiographic features of AMI are otherwise distinguishable from those present in the overwhelming majority of patients with AMI who have classic obstructive atherosclerotic coronary artery disease. In patients without coronary obstruction, the prognosis for survival of the acute event is usually excellent, but a few fatalities have occurred; therefore, it has been possible to document the presence of this syndrome at autopsy.[137] In 10 such patients, infarcts ranged from 5 to 33 per cent (mean of 18 per cent) of the left ventricle.[137] No thromboembolic material was seen in the coronary arterial tree despite the fact that the infarcts were only 2 days old in five patients and 3 or 4 days old in three others.

In patients who recover, areas of localized dyskinesis and hypokinesis can often be demonstrated by left ventricular angiography. Patients have been described as having both occlusion of the infarct-related artery during the acute phase of MI and normal coronary arteries during the convalescent phase.[138] In most cases, the initial total occlusion appears to have been due to thrombosis as thrombolytic therapy was used to produce complete recanalization.

POSSIBLE MECHANISMS

CORONARY SPASM. Numerous theories have been proposed to explain the occurrence of AMI in patients with normal coronary arteriograms. Patients with vasospastic angina are clearly at risk for MI: coronary spasm has been shown to cause MI in some patients with normal coronary arteries.[88,89] The administration of agents that provoke coronary artery spasm has been reported to cause MI in patients with normal coronary arteries,[139,140] and withdrawal of chronic nitrate vasodilation is presumably responsible for MI in others.[141] However, spasm may be induced in only a minority of patients with MI and normal coronary arteries.[132,133,138,142] Intracoronary vasodilators often have no effect when administered acutely

in MI, even when patients are later (after thrombolysis) shown to have normal coronary arteries. It is attractive to hypothesize that many of these cases are caused by combined coronary artery spasm and thrombosis, perhaps with underlying endothelial irregularities or small plaques that are not apparent on coronary angiography.[89,138,143]

OTHER CAUSES. Additional suggested causes include (1) coronary emboli (perhaps from a small mural thrombus, a prolapsed mitral valve,[144] or a myxoma); (2) coronary artery disease in vessels too small to be visualized by coronary arteriography or coronary arterial thrombosis with subsequent recanalization (Table 39–1); (3) a variety of hematological disorders causing in situ thrombosis in the presence of normal coronary arteries (polycythemia vera, cyanotic heart disease with polycythemia,[145] sickle cell anemia,[146] disseminated intravascular coagulation, thrombocytosis, and thrombotic thrombocytopenic purpura); (4) augmented oxygen needs (thyrotoxicosis,[147] amphetamine use[148]); (5) hypotension secondary to sepsis, blood loss, or pharmacological agents, and (6) anatomical variations such as anomalous origin of a coronary artery (p. 254), coronary arteriovenous fistula (p. 970), or a myocardial bridge.[149]

PROGNOSIS. The long-term outlook for patients who have survived an AMI with normal coronary vessels on arteriography appears to be substantially better than for patients with MI and obstructive coronary artery disease.[130–134,137] Following recovery from the initial infarct, recurrent infarction, heart failure, and death are unusual in patients with normal coronary arteries.[134,135] Indeed, most of these patients have normal exercise electrocardiograms[150] and only a minority develop angina pectoris.

Pathophysiology of Acute Myocardial Infarction

SYSTOLIC FUNCTION

The fundamental pathological alteration underlying left ventricular dysfunction in AMI is loss of functioning myocardium. Depression of cardiac function in myocardial infarction is directly related to the extent of left ventricular damage.[151] Cessation of blood flow to a region of myocardium produces four sequential abnormal contraction patterns[152]: (1) *dyssynchrony*, dissociation in the time course of contraction of adjacent segments of myocardial segments; (2) *hypokinesis*, reduction in the extent of shortening; (3) *akinesis*, cessation of shortening; and (4) *dyskinesis*, paradoxical expansion, systolic bulging.[153,154] Accompanying dysfunction of the infarcting segment is initial *hyperkinesis* of the remaining normal myocardium in the intact ventricle.[155] This increased motion of the noninfarcted region subsides within 2 weeks of infarction, during which time some degree of recovery can be seen in the infarct region as well, particularly if reperfusion (p. 1229) of the infarcted area occurs.[156] It is thought to be the result of acute compensatory mechanisms including the Frank-Starling mechanism and increased levels of circulating catecholamines.[155] If a sufficient amount of myocardium undergoes ischemic injury, left ventricular pump function becomes depressed, and cardiac output, stroke volume, blood pressure, and peak dP/dt are reduced,[151,154] and end-systolic volume is increased. In fact, the degree to which end-systolic volume increases is perhaps the most powerful predictor of mortality following AMI.[157] The paradoxical systolic expansion of an area of ventricular myocardium decreases the stroke output of the left ventricle. With the passage of time, edema and cellular infiltration and ultimately fibrosis increase the stiffness of the infarcted myocardium back to and beyond control values.[158] Increasing stiffness in the infarcted zone of myocardium improves left ventricular function, since it prevents systolic paradoxical wall motion.

Areas with reduced and absent wall motion are universally seen in patients with transmural AMI. Rackley and collaborators have demonstrated a linear relationship between specific parameters of left ventricular function and clinical symptoms.[159] The earliest abnormality is a reduction in diastolic compliance, which can be observed with infarcts that involve only 8 per cent of the total left ventricle on angiographic ex-

amination. When the abnormally contracting segment exceeds 15 per cent, the ejection fraction may be reduced and elevations of left ventricular end-diastolic pressure and volume occur. Clinical heart failure accompanies areas of abnormal contraction exceeding 25 per cent, and cardiogenic shock, often fatal, accompanies loss of more than 40 per cent of the left ventricular myocardium.[159]

Unless extension of the infarct occurs, some improvement in wall motion takes place during the healing phase, as recovery of function occurs in initially reversibly injured myocardium. Regardless of the age of the infarct, patients who continue to demonstrate abnormal wall motion of 20 to 25 per cent of the left ventricle manifest hemodynamic signs of left ventricular failure.[160] Physical signs and symptoms of left ventricular failure also increase proportionally to increasing areas of abnormal left ventricular wall motion.[154] These findings are of interest in view of the experimental work of Pfeffer et al., who produced infarcts of varying sizes and studied left ventricular performance 3 weeks later.[151] Rats with relatively small infarcts (< 30 per cent of the left ventricle) had no detectable impairment of function; those with moderate-sized infarcts (31 to 46 per cent) exhibited normal baseline measurements but inadequate responses to hemodynamic stresses; rats with large infarcts (> 46 per cent) uniformly exhibited left ventricular failure.

Patients with AMI often also show reduced myocardial contractile function in noninfarcted zones of myocardium.[161] This may result from obstruction of the coronary artery supplying this region of the ventricle, which is perfused by collaterals from the vessel that becomes occluded, a condition that has been termed *ischemia at a distance*.[162] Conversely, the presence of collaterals developing before MI may allow for greater preservation of regional systolic function in an area of distribution of the occluded artery and improvement in left ventricular ejection fraction early after infarction.[94,163]

DIASTOLIC FUNCTION

As pointed out on page 1178, myocardial ischemia alters not only the systolic performance but also the diastolic characteristics of the left ventricle, ultimately raising its diastolic pressure at any given volume.[158,164,165] Left ventricular diastolic properties are altered in infarcted and ischemic myocardium, leading initially to an increase but later to a reduction in left ventricular compliance. These changes are associated with an initial rise in left ventricular end-diastolic pressure. Over a period of 2 weeks, this pressure begins to fall toward normal, as there is a compensatory increase in end-diastolic volume.[166] As with impairment of systolic function, the magnitude of the diastolic abnormality appears to be related to the size of the initial infarct. Patients who have recovered from AMI frequently continue to manifest decreased left ventricular compliance secondary to the fibrous scar that remains in the left ventricle.

CIRCULATORY REGULATION IN ACUTE MYOCARDIAL INFARCTION

The abnormality in circulatory regulation that is present in AMI is diagrammed in Figure 39–10. The process begins with an anatomical or functional obstruction in the coronary vascular bed, which results in regional myocardial ischemia and, if the ischemia persists, in infarction. If the infarct is of sufficient size, it depresses overall left ventricular function so that left ventricular stroke volume falls and filling pressures rise. The hemodynamic deterioration is more severe if an atrioventricular conduction disturbance develops or if a mechanical complication such as mitral regurgitation or ventricular septal rupture occurs. A marked depression of left ventricular stroke volume ultimately lowers aortic pressure and reduces coronary perfusion pressure; this condition may intensify myocardial ischemia and thereby initiate a vicious circle (Fig. 39–11). The inability of the left ventricle to empty also leads to an increased preload—that is, it dilates the well-perfused, normally functioning portion of the left ventricle. This compensatory mechanism tends to restore stroke volume to normal levels, but at the expense of a reduced ejection fraction. However, the dilatation of the left ventricle also elevates ventricular afterload, because Laplace's law (p. 377) dictates that at any given arterial pressure the dilated ventricle must develop a higher wall tension. This increased afterload not only depresses left ventricular stroke volume but also elevates myocardial oxygen consumption, which in turn intensifies regional myocardial ischemia. When regional myocardial dysfunction is limited and the function of the remainder of the left ventricle is normal, compensatory mechanisms will sustain overall left ventricular function. If a large portion of the left ventricle becomes necrotic, pump failure occurs; i.e., overall left ventricular function becomes so depressed that the circulation cannot be sustained despite the dilatation of the remaining viable portion of the ventricle.

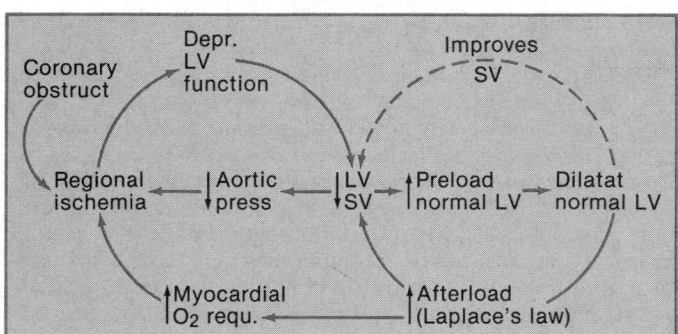

FIGURE 39–10. Changes in circulatory regulation in ischemic heart disease. DEPR. LV FUNCT., depressed left ventricular function; SV, stroke volume; DILATAT., dilatation; O₂ REQU., oxygen requirements. Solid lines indicate that the effect is produced or intensified; broken lines indicate that it is diminished. (Reprinted by permission from Braunwald, E.: Regulation of the circulation. N. Engl. J. Med. 290:1420, 1974.)

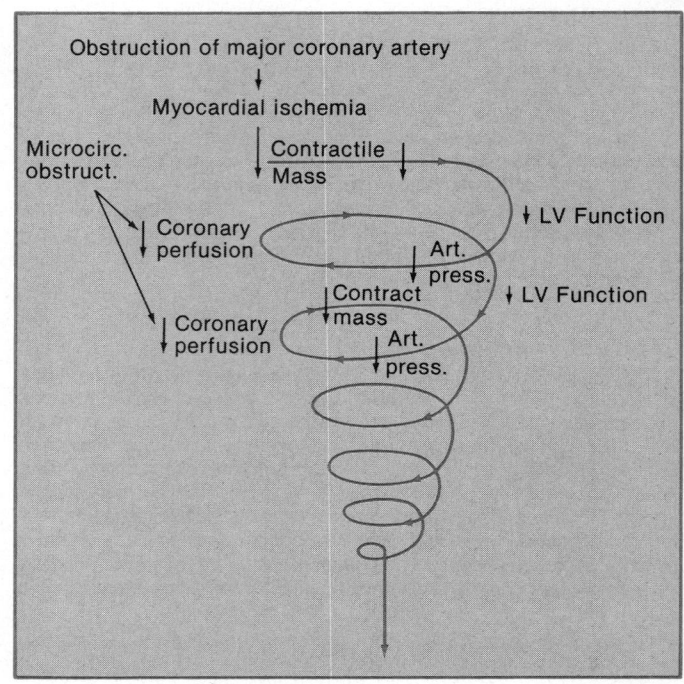

FIGURE 39–11. The sequence of events in the vicious circle in which coronary artery obstruction leads to cardiogenic shock and progressive circulatory deterioration. (From Pasternak, R. C., and Braunwald, E.: Acute myocardial infarction. *In* Wilson, J. D., et al. [eds.]: Harrison's Principles of Internal Medicine. New York, McGraw-Hill Book Co., 1991.)

EFFECTS OF TREATMENT. Some of the consequences of treating pump failure, discussed on page 1252, should be considered. The favorable effect of raising a depressed arterial pressure results from the increased coronary perfusion pressure and the subsequent augmented blood flow across the stenotic areas and through the collateral vessels. This improvement of coronary blood flow may limit the size of the infarction by improving oxygen delivery to the periinfarction zone. In this manner, myocardial fiber shortening may be augmented, thereby increasing stroke volume and cardiac output and elevating arterial pressure.

However, there are also some unfavorable effects of increasing arterial pressure because this intervention usually necessitates an elevation of left ventricular intracavitary pressure (unless it is achieved by a circulatory assist device, such as an intraaortic balloon). The increased afterload causes cardiac dilatation; intramyocardial tension rises, not only because of the higher intraventricular pressure but also because of the cardiac dilatation (p. 376). The increased wall tension augments myocardial oxygen needs and reduces myocardial fiber shortening (p. 425). These changes can cause further ischemia of the marginally viable myocardium adjacent to that supplied exclusively by the occluded vessel, and the area of infarction may be enlarged. Thus, cardiac function may deteriorate further.

It is obvious that the circulation is delicately balanced in patients with AMI. Unless the loss of viable myocardium is so extensive that it precludes survival, or is so small that the patient's survival is not threatened, the outcome may well depend on the clinician's appreciation of the interaction of the many factors that influence circulatory performance and their judicious manipulation.

VENTRICULAR REMODELING

As a consequence of MI, changes in left ventricular size, shape, and thickness involving both the infarcted and the noninfarcted segments of the ventricle often occur. These

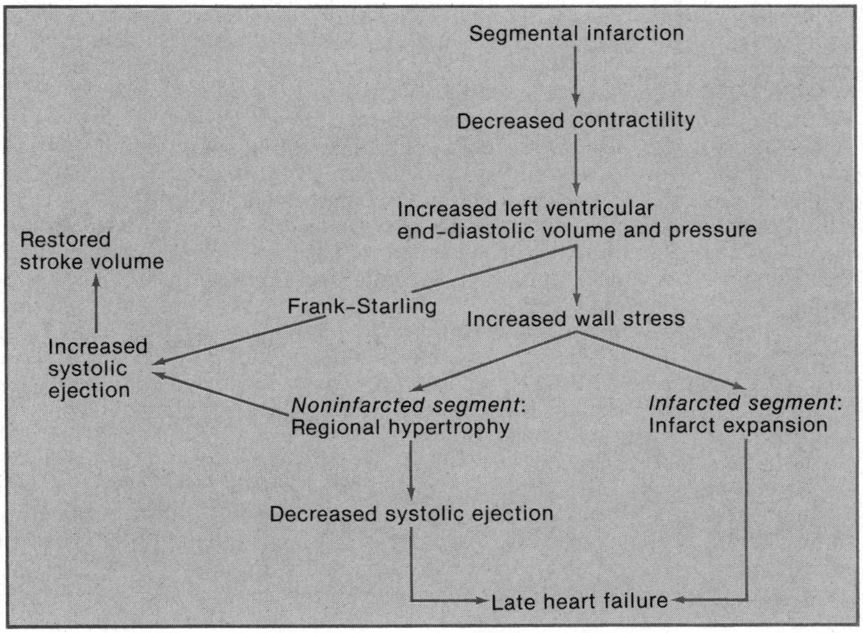

FIGURE 39-12. Hypothesis proposed to account for the mechanisms of left ventricular remodeling. (From McKay, R. G., et al.: Left ventricular remodeling after myocardial infarction: A corollary to infarct expansion. Circulation 74:693, 1986, by permission of the American Heart Association, Inc.)

changes are referred to as "ventricular remodeling," a process that in turn can influence ventricular function and prognosis.[167]

INFARCT EXPANSION. An increase in the size of the infarcted segment, known as *infarct expansion*, is defined as "acute dilatation and thinning of the area of infarction not explained by additional myocardial necrosis."[168] Infarct expansion appears to be caused by (1) a combination of slippage between muscle bundles, reducing the number of myocytes across the infarct wall; (2) disruption of the normal myocardial cells; and (3) tissue loss within the necrotic zone.[163,169,170] At autopsy, more than one-fourth of hearts of patients succumbing to AMI have severe infarct expansion and wall thinning.[168,171] Infarct expansion occurs almost exclusively in transmural infarcts, is far more common with anterior-apical than with other infarcts, and correlates directly with infarct size.[168,171] The degree of infarct expansion also appears to be related to the preinfarction wall thickness, with existing hypertrophy possibly protecting against infarct thinning.[171] Infarct expansion is associated with both a higher mortality and a higher incidence of nonfatal complications such as heart failure and ventricular aneurysm.[172] Rupture of the ventricle may be considered to be a consequence of extreme infarct expansion.[171,173] Infarct expansion can be recognized echocardiographically as elongation of the noncontractile region of the ventricle.[174]

VENTRICULAR DILATATION. While infarct expansion plays an important role in the ventricular remodeling that occurs in the early weeks following myocardial infarction, remodeling is also caused by dilatation of the viable portion of the ventricle, which commences immediately following AMI, but may progress for months thereafter.[166,175,176,176a] This dilatation may be accompanied by a shift to the right of the pressure-volume curve of the left ventricle, resulting in a larger left ventricular volume at any given diastolic pressure. This dilatation of the noninfarct zone may be viewed as a compensatory mechanism that maintains stroke volume in the face of a large infarction (Fig. 39-12). Following AMI, an extra burden is placed on the residual functioning myocardium,[160] a burden that presumably is responsible for the hypertrophy.[177] This adaptive hypertrophy could help to compensate for the functional impairment caused by the infarct and may be responsible for some of the initial hemodynamic improvement seen in the weeks after infarction in some patients.[178] However, as illustrated in Figure 39-12, adaptive hypertrophy may undergo a transition, with ultimate impairment of con-

tractile function of the viable myocardium in the presence of a large infarction, leading to further cardiac dilatation, loss of global function, and ultimately heart failure.[166]

In *summary*, ventricular remodeling occurs to an increasing extent with larger infarcts. It is a complex process that is not limited to areas of infarction. It begins at the time of AMI and probably continues for months to years, until either a stable hemodynamic state is achieved or progressively severe cardiac decompensation occurs, leading to death from congestive heart failure.

Ventricular remodeling after AMI can be affected by three independent factors, the first of which is infarct size. Acute reperfusion and other measures to restrict the extent of myocardial necrosis limit the increase in ventricular volume following AMI,[178a-180] and there is suggestive evidence that an open infarct artery per se also attenuates ventricular enlargement.[181,182,182a] The second factor is scar formation in the infarct. Glucocorticosteroids and nonsteroidal anti-inflammatory agents given early after MI can cause scar thinning and greater infarct expansion.[183,184] Third is the left ventricular distending pressures in the early post MI period; reduction of this pressure with nitroglycerin[185,186] or an angiotensin-converting enzyme inhibitor[187,187a] attenuates ventricular enlargement (p. 496).

PATHOPHYSIOLOGY OF OTHER ORGAN SYSTEMS IN ACUTE MYOCARDIAL INFARCTION

Alterations in Pulmonary Function

Changes in pulmonary gas exchange, ventilation, and distribution of perfusion all occur with AMI. Hypoxemia is a frequent consequence, with a severity, in general, proportional to that of left ventricular failure. Thus, there is an inverse relation between arterial oxygen tension and pulmonary artery diastolic pressure in patients with AMI. This suggests that increased pulmonary capillary hydrostatic pressure leads to interstitial edema, which results in arteriolar and bronchiolar compression that ultimately causes perfusion of poorly ventilated alveoli with resultant hypoxemia.[188] In addition to hypoxemia, there is a fall in diffusing capacity of carbon monoxide.[189] Hyperventilation often occurs in patients with AMI and may cause hypocapnia and respiratory alkalosis, particularly in restless, anxious patients with pain. Intrapulmonary shunting of blood has been noted in patients in whom left ventricular failure complicates AMI. With reversal of heart failure, hypoxemia and intrapulmonary shunting diminish.

INCREASE IN INTERSTITIAL WATER. A positive correlation has been demonstrated between pulmonary extravascular (interstitial) water content, left ventricular filling pressure, and the clinical signs and symptoms of left ventricular failure.[188] Over a period of 2 to 4 days following AMI, both the pulmonary extravascular water content and the wedge pressure decline. Presumably the increased pulmonary extravascular water represents a transudate secondary to increased pulmonary capillary pressure.

The increase in pulmonary extravascular water may also be responsible for the alterations in pulmonary mechanics observed in patients with AMI, i.e., reduction of airway conductance, pulmonary compliance, forced expiratory volume and midexpiratory flow rate, and an increase in closing volume — the last presumably related to the widespread closure of small, dependent airways during the first 3 days following AMI.[190] Ultimately, severe increases in extravascular water may lead to pulmonary edema (Chap. 20). Recovery of left ventricular function or diuresis reduces abnormally elevated values for closing volumes to normal. Presumably, competition for space between arteries and small airways in the bronchovascular sheath accounts for some of the elevation in airway resistance, particularly at left atrial pressures under 15 mm Hg. Higher left atrial pressures produce increases in airway resistance secondary to interstitial, alveolar, and peribronchial edema.

The "closing volume," i.e., the lung volume at which airway closure commences, can encroach on and sometimes exceed functional residual volume. This can lead to arterial hypoxemia by the shunting of blood through alveoli that are not well ventilated.

REDUCTION OF VITAL CAPACITY. For over 70 years it has been recognized that a fall in vital capacity is related to shortened life expectancy for the cardiac patient. It is now clear that virtually all indices of lung volume — total lung capacity, functional residual capacity, and residual volume, as well as vital capacity — fall in the setting of AMI.[191] These reductions correlate with the elevations of left-sided filling pressure and are most probably due to increases in pulmonary extravascular water. Lung volumes, oxygenation, and airway resistance all return toward normal by the time of discharge for most patients.[191]

Increased pulmonary venous pressure also results in redistribution of pulmonary blood flow from the bases to the apices of the lung in patients with AMI,[192] altering the relationship between ventilation and perfusion. However, at follow-up examination 3 to 25 weeks after MI, the ventilation/perfusion relationship has usually returned to normal or almost so.

REDUCTION OF AFFINITY OF HEMOGLOBIN FOR OXYGEN. In patients with MI, particularly when complicated by left ventricular failure or cardiogenic shock, the affinity of hemoglobin for oxygen is reduced, i.e., the P_{50} is increased.[193] The increase in P_{50} results from increased levels of erythrocyte 2,3-diphosphoglycerate (2,3-DPG), is maximal after 24 hours, and constitutes an important compensatory mechanism, responsible for an estimated 18 per cent increase in oxygen release from oxyhemoglobin in patients with cardiogenic shock.[193]

Alterations in Endocrine Function

PANCREAS. Hyperglycemia and impaired glucose tolerance are common in patients with AMI. Although the absolute levels of blood insulin are often in the normal range in patients with uncomplicated AMI, they are usually inappropriately low for the level of blood sugar elevation, and there may be relative insulin resistance as well.[194] Patients with cardiogenic shock often demonstrate marked hyperglycemia and depressed levels of circulating insulin, often with complete suppression of insulin secretion in response to tolbutamide.[195] These abnormalities in insulin secretion and the resultant

impaired glucose tolerance appear to be secondary to a reduction in pancreatic blood flow as a consequence of splanchnic vasoconstriction, which accompanies severe left ventricular failure. In addition, increased activity of the sympathetic nervous system with augmented circulating catecholamines[196] inhibits insulin secretion[197] and augments glycogenolysis, also contributing to the elevation of blood sugar.[198] In fact, hyperglycemia, even without prior diabetes mellitus, is associated with an increased incidence of heart failure following AMI and a high mortality.[199]

Since hypoxic heart muscle derives a considerable portion of its energy from the metabolism of glucose (Chap. 38), and since insulin is essential for the uptake of glucose by the myocardium as well as for myocardial protein synthesis and inhibition of lysosomal activity, the deleterious effects of insulin deficiency are clear.[200]

ADRENAL MEDULLA. Excessive secretion of catecholamines produces many of the characteristic signs and symptoms of AMI. The plasma and urinary catecholamine levels are highest during the first 24 hours after the onset of chest pain,[198] with the greatest rise in plasma catecholamine secretion occurring during the first hour after the onset of MI.[201,201a] These high levels of circulating catecholamines in patients with AMI correlate with the occurrence of serious arrhythmias[197] and result in an increase in myocardial oxygen consumption, both directly and indirectly, as a consequence of catecholamine-induced elevation of circulating free fatty acids.[201] As might be anticipated, the concentration of circulating catecholamines correlates with extent of myocardial damage, incidence of cardiogenic shock, as well as both early and late mortality rates.[197,202]

It is not clear, however, whether the elevation in plasma catecholamines plays some role in determining the amount of myocardium that becomes necrotic or whether this elevation is a consequence of the myocardial damage, i.e., whether it is cause or effect or both. The time course of sympathetic activation, which begins extremely early before extensive myocardial necrosis is present, suggests at least a potential role for these circulating hormones in extending myocardial damage and certainly in the genesis of arrhythmias.[202] Circulating catecholamines enhance platelet aggregation; when this occurs in the coronary microcirculation, the release of the potent vasoconstrictor thromboxane A_2 may further impair cardiac perfusion.[75]

ADRENAL CORTEX. Plasma and urinary 17-hydroxycorticosteroids and ketosteroids, as well as aldosterone, are also markedly elevated in patients with AMI.[198] Their concentrations correlate directly with the peak level of serum glutamic oxaloacetic transaminase and serum creatine kinase,[202] implying that the stress imposed by larger infarcts is associated with greater secretion of adrenal steroids. Glucocorticosteroids also contribute to the impairment of glucose tolerance. Although it has been suggested that the secretion of glucocorticoids is increased, it is inadequate to meet the demands for the stress imposed by a massive AMI, particularly if it is accompanied by cardiogenic shock.[198]

THYROID GLAND. Although patients with AMI are generally euthyroid, there is evidence for a significant transient decrease in serum T_3 levels, a fall that is most marked on about the third day after the infarct.[203,204] This fall in T_3 is usually accompanied by a rise in reverse T_3 with variable changes or no change in T_4 and TSH levels. The alteration in peripheral thyroxin metabolism appears to correlate with infarct size[203] and may be mediated by the rise in endogenous levels of cortisol that accompanies AMI.[204]

Hematological Function

ALTERATIONS IN PLATELETS. AMI generally occurs in the presence of extensive coronary and systemic atherosclerotic plaques, which may serve as the site for the formation of platelet aggregates, a sequence that has been suggested as the initial step in the process of coronary thrombosis, coronary occlusion, and subsequent MI. Circulating platelets are hyperaggregable in patients with AMI.[76] Approximately one-third of these patients demonstrate shortened platelet survival times.[205] Types III and IV hyperlipoproteinemia, frequently present in patients with AMI, can also be responsible for shortening platelet survival. Findings suggestive of a hypercoagulable state as a risk factor for AMI are discussed on page 1779, and the role of platelets in AMI is discussed on page 1206. A wide variety of platelet abnormalities have been described, including, most recently, an increase in thromboxane A$_2$ receptors on platelets from AMI patients.[206]

COAGULATION TESTS. Elevated levels of serum fibrinogen degradation products, an end product of thrombosis[207]—as well as release of distinctive proteins when platelets are activated, i.e., platelet factor 4[208] and beta thromboglobulin[209]—have been reported in some patients with AMI. Fibrinopeptide A, a protein released from fibrin by thrombin, is a marker of ongoing thrombosis and is elevated during the early hours of AMI.[210,211] In fact, markedly elevated levels of fibrinopeptide A may be a marker for coronary reocclusion after initially successful thrombolytic therapy.[211-213] The interpretation of the coagulation tests in patients with AMI may be complicated by elevated blood levels of catecholamines, concomitant shock, and/or pulmonary embolism, conditions which are all capable of altering various tests of platelet and coagulation function.[214] Thus, it is not yet clear whether the aforementioned changes are the causes or consequences of AMI.

LEUKOCYTES. AMI is usually accompanied by leukocytosis that is thought to be related both to the necrotic process and its magnitude, in which leukocytes play an active role, and to their stimulation by elevated glucocorticoids that occur with infarction. It is now recognized that leukocytes also participate in the thrombotic process.[215] Activation of neutrophils may produce important intermediates, such as leukotriene B$_4$ and oxygen free radicals,[216,217] that have important microcirculatory effects.[215]

BLOOD VISCOSITY. An increase in blood viscosity also occurs in patients with AMI. During the first few days after infarction, this is mainly attributable to hemoconcentration, but later the increases in plasma viscosity and red cell aggregation correlate with elevated serum concentrations of alpha$_2$ globulin and fibrinogen, which are nonspecific reactions to tissue necrosis and which are also responsible for the elevated sedimentation rate characteristic of AMI.[218] The high values of blood viscosity indices are observed most frequently in patients with complications such as left ventricular failure, cardiogenic shock, and thromboembolism.

OTHER BIOCHEMICAL TESTS. Over the years, many isolated abnormal blood chemistries have been reported in patients with AMI. Many have not led to further understanding of the pathophysiology of AMI or have not been confirmed in subsequent studies. New abnormalities are regularly reported—recent examples include decreased selenium[219] and pyridoxal 5'-phosphate (a metabolite of vitamin B6) levels.[220] The importance of both is unknown at present.

ALTERATIONS IN RENAL FUNCTION

Both prerenal azotemia and acute renal failure can complicate the marked reduction of cardiac output that occurs in cardiogenic shock. A physiological compensation for this occurs with the increase in atrial natriuretic peptide seen following AMI, an increase that is correlated with the degree of left ventricular failure present.[221] An increase in atrial natriuretic peptide is also found when right ventricular infarction accompanies inferior wall infarction, suggesting that this neurohumoral abnormality may play a role in the hemodynamic disturbances of the right ventricular infarction syndrome (p. 412).[222]

Clinical Features of Acute Myocardial Infarction

PRECIPITATING FACTORS

In about one-half of patients with AMI, no precipitating factor can be identified.[217a] An early study noted the following patient activities at the onset of AMI: heavy physical exertion, 13 per cent; modest or usual exertion, 18 per cent; surgical procedure, 6 per cent; rest, 51 per cent; and sleep, 8 per cent.[223] A more recent study has confirmed the importance of physical activity and pointed to emotional stress (in about 18 per cent of patients) as another important trigger of AMI.[224] Others, too, have reported that a significant number of AMIs occur within a few hours of severe physical exertion.[225,226] It has been pointed out that the *severe exertion* that preceded an infarction was often performed at times when the patient was unduly fatigued or emotionally stressed.[227] Exertion before infarction is somewhat more common among patients without preexisting angina than in patients who have had a history of angina.[228] Thus, although adequate control studies have not been carried out, there is *suggestive* evidence that heavy exercise may play a precipitating role in some patients. Such infarctions could be the result of marked increases in myocardial oxygen consumption in the presence of severe coronary arterial narrowing. Alternatively, exertion or mental stress may trigger plaque disruption, initiating a cascade of events leading to AMI. Such a scenario has been proposed by Muller[62] and is illustrated in Figure 39–13.

Surgical procedures associated with acute blood loss have also been noted as precursors of AMI (p. 1711). Reduced myocardial perfusion secondary to hypotension and increased myocardial oxygen demands secondary to fever, tachycardia, and agitation are presumably responsible for the myocardial necrosis. Other factors reported as predisposing to AMI include respiratory infections, hypoxemia of any cause, pulmonary embolism, hypoglycemia, administration of ergot preparations, serum sickness, allergy, and wasp stings.[229,230] In patients with Prinzmetal's angina (p. 1342), AMI may develop in the territory of the coronary artery, which repeatedly un-

dergoes spasm.[231] Rarely, munition workers exposed to high concentrations of nitroglycerin may develop myocardial infarction when they are withdrawn from this exposure, suggesting that it is caused by vasospasm.[141] Accelerating angina and rest angina, two forms of unstable angina, may culminate as infarction of the myocardium, again in the distribution of the affected vessel.[231]

Considerable evidence has accumulated that *emotional stresses* may be a precipitating factor in the initiation of AMI.[224,232] A number of reports have documented that upsetting life events occur commonly in patients who subsequently suffer an MI.[233] Such events have been quantified and scored as *Life Change Units*. Rahe and coworkers noted, on retrospective analysis, a significant buildup of Life Change Units in patients who subsequently suffered myocardial infarction or died suddenly.[233]

Trauma may precipitate an AMI in one of two ways. Myocardial contusion and hemorrhage into the myocardium may actually cause cell necrosis, or the injury may involve a coronary artery, causing occlusion of that vessel with resultant MI (Chap. 46). *Neurological disturbances* (transient ischemic attacks or strokes) may also precipitate AMI.[234]

CIRCADIAN PERIODICITY. An analysis of a large number of patients hospitalized with myocardial infarction, studied as part of the Multicenter Investigation of Limitation of Infarct Size (MILIS), has revealed a pronounced circadian periodicity for the time of onset of AMI.[235] In this retrospective review, a peak incidence of onset at about 9 AM was found when timing was estimated from either the occurrence of symptoms or from the first elevation of plasma creatine kinase MB (Fig. 39–14, *top*). This has been confirmed by other studies[236,237] such as a large World Health Organization report.[238] This early morning peak in MI parallels the onset of other related phenomena including sudden cardiac death,[239] thrombotic stroke,[240] and transient myocardial ischemia[241,242] (p. 1294) (Fig. 39–14, *bottom 3 panels*). Circadian rhythms affect many physiological and biochemical parameters; the

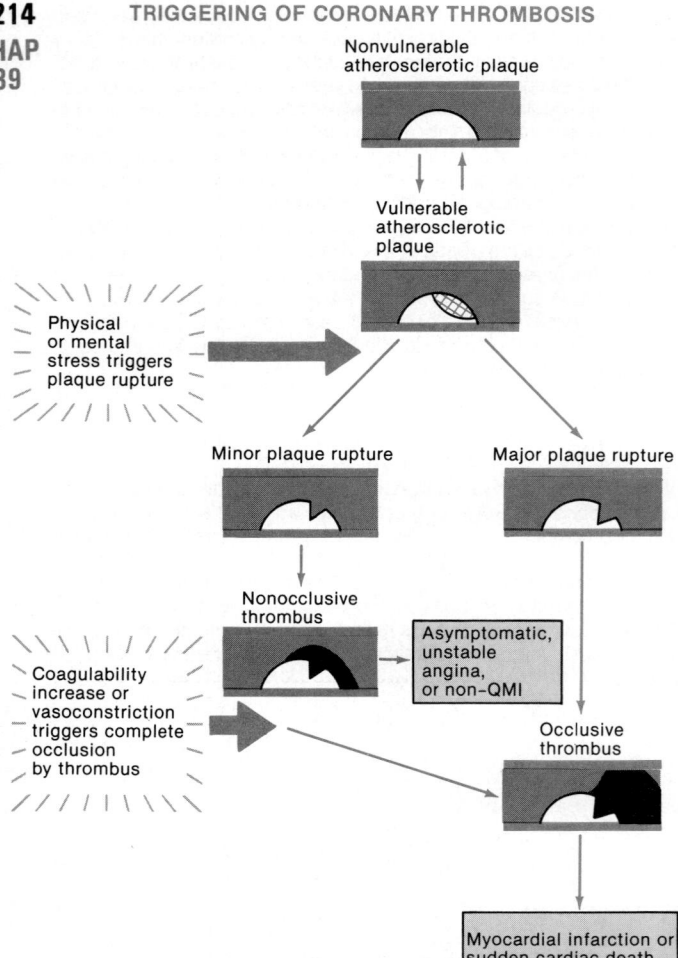

FIGURE 39–13. Schematic illustration of a hypothetical method by which daily activities may *trigger* coronary thrombosis. Three triggering mechanisms, (1) physical or mental stress producing hemodynamic changes leading to plaque rupture, (2) activities causing a coagulability increase, and (3) stimuli leading to vasoconstriction, have been added to the scheme depicting the role of coronary thrombosis in unstable angina, myocardial infarction, and sudden cardiac death. (From Muller, J. E., et al.: Circadian variation and triggers of onset of acute cardiovascular disease. Circulation *79*:733, 1989, by permission of the American Heart Association, Inc.)

resembling classic angina pectoris (described on pp. 4 and 1215), but it occurs at rest or with less activity than usual and can therefore be classified as unstable angina. However, the latter is often not disturbing enough to induce patients to seek medical attention, and if they do, they may not be hospitalized. Among patients who are hospitalized for unstable an-

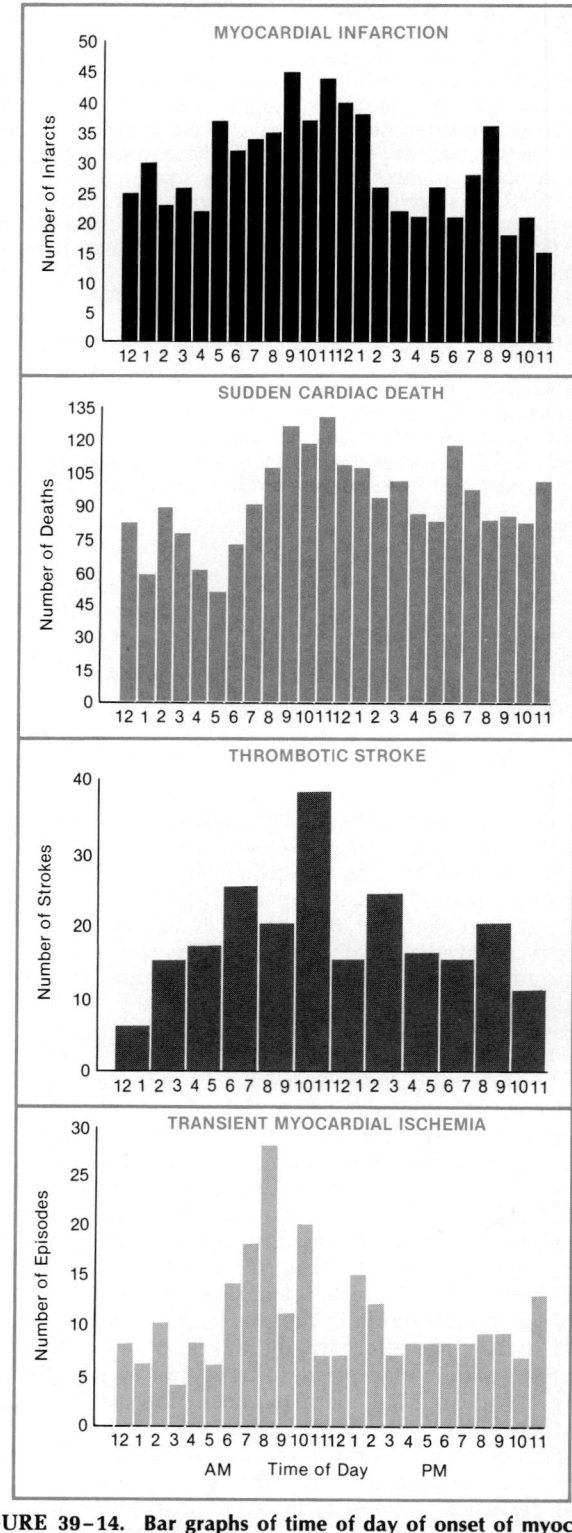

FIGURE 39–14. Bar graphs of time of day of onset of myocardial infarction, sudden cardiac death, stroke, and transient myocardial ischemia in four different groups of patients. The number of events is shown on the y axis and the hour of the day on the x axis. Note that each of the disorders exhibits a prominent increase in frequency of onset in the period from 6 AM to noon. (From Muller, J. E., et al.: Circadian variation and triggers of onset of acute cardiovascular disease. Circulation *79*:733, 1989, by permission of the American Heart Association, Inc.)

early morning hours are associated with rises in plasma catecholamines and cortisol and increases in platelet aggregability. Interestingly, the characteristic circadian peak was *absent* in patients receiving beta blocker or aspirin therapy before their presentation with AMI.[243,244] In addition to beta blockade and aspirin, previous heart failure or MI, history of smoking or diabetes, and non-Q-wave infarction have all been identified as blunting this circadian variability in AMI.[245] Nevertheless, it appears possible that some cyclical aspects of combined vasospastic and prothrombotic factors, in the setting of preexisting atherosclerosis, can lead to AMI. The apparent relationship between a patient's biological rhythm and the onset of AMI appears to be of both pathophysiological and clinical importance.

CLINICAL HISTORY

PRODROMAL SYMPTOMS. Despite recent advances in the laboratory detection of AMI, the history remains of substantial value in establishing a diagnosis. A prodromal history can be elicited in 20 to 60 per cent of patients with AMI.[246,247] The prodrome is usually characterized by chest discomfort,

gina, fewer than 15 per cent develop AMI (p. 1341). Of the patients with AMI presenting with prodromal symptoms of unstable angina, approximately one-third have had symptoms from 1 to 4 weeks before hospitalization; in the remaining two-thirds, symptoms predated admission by a week or less, with one-third of these patients (20 per cent of all with prodromes) having had symptoms for 24 hours or less.[248]

NATURE OF THE PAIN. The pain of AMI is variable in intensity; in most patients it is severe and, in some instances, intolerable. The pain is prolonged, usually lasting for more than 30 minutes and frequently for a number of hours. The discomfort is described as constricting, crushing, oppressing, or compressing; often the patient complains of something sitting on or squeezing the chest. Although usually described as a squeezing, choking, viselike, or heavy pain, it may also be characterized as a stabbing, knifelike, boring, or burning discomfort. The pain is usually retrosternal in location, spreading frequently to both sides of the anterior chest, with predilection for the left side. Often the pain radiates down the ulnar aspect of the left arm, producing a tingling sensation in the left wrist, hand, and even fingers. Some patients note only a dull ache or numbness of the wrists in association with severe substernal or precordial discomfort. In some instances, the pain of AMI may begin in the epigastrium and simulate a variety of abdominal disorders, a fact which often causes MI to be misdiagnosed as "indigestion." In other patients the discomfort of AMI radiates to the shoulders, upper extremities, neck, jaw, and interscapular region, again usually favoring the left side. In patients with preexisting angina pectoris, the pain of infarction usually resembles that of angina with respect to quality and location. However, it is generally much more severe, lasts longer, and is not relieved by rest and nitroglycerin.

What follows is a lucid, personal, published description of the pain of AMI, provided by a distinguished, experienced physician:

During the first 15 to 20 minutes when the pain was waxing and waning, I was pretending it was esophageal and popping a few Tums and drinking a glass of milk. After this, the pain certainly told me just what it seems to have told other patients. I felt I must sit down very, very quietly. Although I did so, the pain became a steadily expanding, deep, penetrating ache spreading from beneath mid-breast bone, around the sides of my chest, up my neck into my lower jaw, and down the inner aspect of my left arm into my fourth and fifth fingers. It cycled a bit. Sometimes it seemed most dreadful in my chest—then in my jaw and lower teeth—then in my left arm. But it conveyed one clear message. What I thought from the outset and continued to think through about 2 hours of what seemed absolutely intolerable pain was that if I remained *absolutely* immobile, not moving even an eyelash, perhaps it would let go of me. I would guess it took about 10 to 12 minutes to build to maximal intensity and there it stayed. During the entire period I sat absolutely still with my eyes closed, conscious of the fact that I was sweating profusely and that I probably looked very pale and lousy. Although my wife was bustling cheerfully about in the kitchen not 15 feet away, I said absolutely nothing, feeling that even moving my tongue or vocal chords was simply too much. There was no inclination to groan or cry out.

There was another aspect of the pain frequently alluded to by others. There was absolutely no doubt in my mind that I was about to die. As the pain remained, I simply wished exodus would go ahead and happen. . . . The quality of the pain is as difficult for me to describe as it seems to have been for other observers over the last 70 plus years. It was not the bright or burning or well-localized pain one feels with a cut, a puncture, or a burn, from which one instinctively and swiftly retreats. A very difficult set of nerve endings is involved. It was a dreadful, deep, nauseating ache. If you would try multiplying a hundred-fold the kind of ache you experience after working too long trying to screw a recalcitrant light bulb into a ceiling socket that's a little too high over your head to reach decently, you would be close. . . .

As to intensity, I keep wanting to use the word *unbearable*. Obviously, this word is not really appropriate, as I did manage somehow to bear the pain. But it was an absolutely monstrous,

awful sensation, and it was totally untouched by 20 or 30 or 40 milligrams of morphine administered to me over the next 2 hours. That morphine gave so little relief has made me empathize deeply with the hundreds of patients with the same disease I've treated with this drug over the years.[249]

In some patients, particularly the elderly, AMI is manifested clinically not by chest pain but rather by symptoms of acute left ventricular failure and chest tightness or by overwhelming weakness, accompanied by diaphoresis, nausea, vomiting, and diarrhea.[234] The pain of AMI may have disappeared by the time the physician first encounters the patient (or the patient reaches the hospital), or it may persist for many hours. Opiates—in particular, morphine—usually relieve the pain, although a persistent soreness, pressure, or dull ache may remain for several hours or more despite intensive treatment with analgesics. The longer a patient requires analgesic administration after hospital admission for ischemic pain, the more likely that MI will be confirmed in that patient.[250] Both angina pectoris and the pain of AMI are thought to arise from nerve endings in ischemic or injured, but not necrotic, myocardium.[251] Thus, in MI, stimulation of nerve fibers in an ischemic zone of myocardium surrounding the necrotic central area of infarction probably gives rise to the pain.

It has been suggested that the phenomenon of referred pain is modulated by the spatial and temporal patterns of excitation of these afferent sympathetic fibers as well as a variable contribution of vagal afferent fibers.[252] Experience with patients undergoing procedures to reperfuse myocardium in the setting of AMI suggests that pain often disappears suddenly and completely once blood flow to the infarct territory is restored.[253] In patients in whom reocclusion occurs after thrombolysis, pain recurs if the initial reperfusion has left viable myocardium. Thus, what has previously been thought of as the "pain of infarction," sometimes lasting for many hours, probably represents pain caused by ongoing ischemia. The recognition that pain implies ischemia and not inevitable infarction has important clinical ramifications and heightens the importance of seeking ways to relieve the ischemia, for which the pain is a marker. This finding suggests that the clinician should not be complacent about ongoing cardiac pain under any circumstances.

OTHER SYMPTOMS. Nausea and vomiting occur in more than 50 per cent of patients with transmural MI and severe chest pain,[254] presumably owing to activation of vagal reflex or to stimulation of left ventricular receptors as part of the Bezold-Jarisch reflex (p. 1167).[255] These symptoms occur more commonly in patients with inferior MI than in those with anterior MI. Occasionally a patient complains of diarrhea or a violent urge to evacuate the bowels during the acute phase of MI. Moreover, nausea and vomiting are common side effects of opiates. When the pain of AMI is epigastric in location and is associated with nausea and vomiting, the clinical picture may easily be confused with that of acute cholecystitis, gastritis, or peptic ulcer. Other symptoms include feelings of profound weakness, dizziness, palpitations, cold perspiration, and a sense of impending doom. On occasion, symptoms arising from an episode of cerebral embolism or other systemic arterial embolism are the first signs of an AMI. Rarely, patients with inferior infarction report intractable hiccupping, a finding which has been attributed to diaphragmatic irritation by the infarct. The aforementioned symptoms may or may not be accompanied by chest pain.[256] Finally, the feeling of general malaise or frank exhaustion often accompanies other symptoms preceding AMI.[257]

DIFFERENTIAL DIAGNOSIS. The pain of AMI may simulate the pain of *acute pericarditis* (p. 1469), which is usually associated with some pleuritic features, i.e., it is aggravated by respiratory movements and coughing and often involves the shoulder, ridge of the trapezius, and neck. *Pleural pain* is usually sharp, knifelike, and aggravated by each breath, which distinguishes it from the deep, dull, steady pain of AMI. *Pulmonary embolism* (Chap. 48) generally produces pain laterally in the chest, is often pleuritic in nature, and may be associated with hemoptysis. The pain due to *acute dissection of the aorta* (p. 1535) is usually localized in the center of the chest, is extremely severe, persists for many hours, and often radiates to the back and sometimes into the legs. Often one or more major arterial pulses are absent. Pain arising from the *costochondral and chondrosternal articulations* may be associated with localized swelling and redness; it is usually sharp and "darting" and is characterized by marked localized tenderness.

SILENT MI AND ATYPICAL PRESENTATION. Population studies suggest that between 20 and 60 per cent of nonfatal MIs are unrecognized by the patient and are discovered only on subsequent routine electrocardiographic[258,259] or postmortem examinations. Of these unrecognized infarctions, approximately half are truly silent, with the patients unable to recall any symptoms whatsoever referable to the infarction. The other half of patients with so-called silent infarction can recall an event characterized by symptoms compatible with acute infarction when leading questions are posed after the electrocardiographic abnormalities are discovered. Unrecognized or silent infarction occurs more commonly in patients without antecedent angina pectoris and is more common in patients with diabetes and hypertension,[258] although the association with diabetes is controversial. Silent MI is often followed by silent ischemia (p. 1347).

In an analysis of atypical presentations of AMI, Bean[260] lists the following: (1) congestive heart failure — beginning de novo or worsening of established failure; (2) classic angina pectoris without a particularly severe or prolonged attack; (3) atypical location of the pain; (4) central nervous system manifestations, resembling those of stroke, secondary to a sharp reduction in cardiac output in a patient with cerebral arteriosclerosis; (5) apprehension and nervousness; (6) sudden mania or psychosis; (7) syncope; (8) overwhelming weakness; (9) acute indigestion; and (10) peripheral embolism.

PHYSICAL EXAMINATION

GENERAL APPEARANCE. Patients suffering an AMI often appear anxious and in considerable distress. An anguished facial expression is common, and — in contrast to patients with angina pectoris, who often lie, sit, or stand quite still, realizing that all forms of activity increase the discomfort — patients suffering an AMI may be restless and move about in an effort to find a comfortable position. Others, like the physician who described his own symptoms (p. 1215), prefer to sit still. They often massage or clutch their chests and frequently describe their pain with a clenched fist held against the sternum. In patients with left ventricular failure and sympathetic stimulation, cold perspiration and skin pallor may be evident; they usually sit or are propped up in bed, gasping for breath. Between breaths, they may complain of chest discomfort or a feeling of suffocation. Cough production of frothy, pink, or blood-streaked sputum is common.

Patients in cardiogenic shock often lie listlessly, making few if any spontaneous movements. The skin is cool and clammy, with a bluish or mottled color over the extremities, and there is marked facial pallor with severe cyanosis of the lips and nailbeds. Depending on the degree of cerebral perfusion, the patient in shock may converse normally or may evidence confusion and disorientation. The patient is often anxious and frightened but may profess interest in only minimal communication.

VITAL SIGNS. The heart rate may vary from a marked bradycardia to rapid regular or irregular tachycardia, depending on the underlying rhythm and the degree of left ventricular failure. Most commonly, the pulse is rapid and regular initially (sinus tachycardia at 100 to 110 beats/min), slowing as the patient's pain and anxiety are relieved; premature ventricular beats are common, occurring in more than 95 per cent of patients evaluated early after the onset of symptoms.

Blood Pressure. The majority of patients with uncomplicated AMI are normotensive, although the reduced stroke volume accompanying the tachycardia may cause declines in systolic and pulse pressures and elevation of diastolic pressure. Among previously normotensive patients, a hypertensive response occasionally is seen, with the arterial pressure exceeding 160/90 mm Hg, presumably as a consequence of adrenergic discharge secondary to pain and agitation. It is rather common for previously hypertensive patients to become normotensive without treatment following AMI, although approximately two-thirds of these previously hypertensive patients eventually regain their elevated levels of blood pressure, generally 3 to 6 months after infarction. In patients with massive infarcts, arterial pressure falls acutely, owing to left ventricular dysfunction and venous pooling secondary to administration of morphine or nitrates or both; as recovery occurs, the arterial pressure tends to return to preinfarction levels. Patients in cardiogenic shock (p. 579), by definition, have systolic pressures below 90 mm Hg. However, hypotension does not necessarily signify cardiogenic shock, since some patients with inferior infarction, in whom the Bezold-Jarisch reflex is activated, may also have systolic blood pressure below 90 mm Hg.[261] Their prognosis is generally good and their hypotension eventually resolves spontaneously, although this resolution can be accelerated by atropine and assumption of the reverse Trendelenburg position. Other patients who are initially only slightly hypotensive may demonstrate gradually falling blood pressures with progressive reduction in cardiac output over several hours or days as they gradually develop cardiogenic shock as a consequence of increasing ischemia and extension of infarction (Fig. 38–11). Evidence of autonomic hyperactivity is common, varying in type with the location of the infarction. At some time in their initial presentation, more than half of patients with inferior MI have evidence of excess parasympathetic stimulation, with hypotension, bradycardia, or both, while about half of patients with anterior MI show signs of sympathetic excess, having hypertension, tachycardia, or both.[262]

Temperature and Respiration. Most patients with AMI develop *fever*, a nonspecific response to tissue necrosis, within 24 to 48 hours of the onset of infarction. Body temperature often begins to rise within 4 to 8 hours after the onset of infarction, and rectal temperature often reaches 101 to 102°F. Fever usually resolves by the seventh or eighth day following infarction.

The *respiratory rate* may be slightly elevated soon after the development of an AMI; in patients without heart failure, it results from anxiety and pain, since it returns to normal with treatment of physical and psychological discomfort. In patients with left ventricular failure, the respiratory rate correlates with the severity of failure; patients with pulmonary edema may have respiratory rates exceeding 40 per minute. However, the respiratory rate is not necessarily elevated in patients with cardiogenic shock. Cheyne-Stokes (periodic) respiration (p. 454) may occur in elderly individuals with cardiogenic shock and heart failure, particularly after opiate therapy and in the presence of cerebrovascular disease.

JUGULAR VENOUS PULSE. The height and contour of the jugular venous pulse reflect right atrial and right ventricular diastolic pressures (p. 18). Since these pressures are usually normal or only slightly elevated in patients with AMI (even in the presence of mild to moderate left ventricular failure), it is not surprising that usually the jugular venous pulse does not appear to be abnormal. The *a* wave may be prominent in patients with pulmonary hypertension secondary to left ventricular failure or reduced compliance. In contrast, right ventricular infarction (whether or not it accompanies left ventricular infarction) often results in marked jugular venous distention and, when it is complicated by necrosis or ischemia of right ventricular papillary muscles, tall *v* waves of tricuspid regurgitation are evident. In patients with AMI and cardiogenic shock, the jugular venous pressure is usually elevated. In patients with AMI, hypotension, and hypoperfusion, whose signs may specifically resemble those of patients with cardiogenic shock but who have flat neck veins, it is likely that the depression of left ventricular performance may be related, at least in part, to hypovolemia, but the differentiation can be made only by assessing left ventricular performance.

CAROTID PULSE. Palpation of the carotid arterial pulse provides a clue to the left ventricular stroke volume; a small pulse suggests a reduced stroke volume, whereas a sharp, brief upstroke is often observed in patients with mitral regurgitation or ruptured ventricular septum with a left-to-right shunt. Pulsus alternans reflects severe left ventricular dysfunction.

THE CHEST. Moist rales are audible in patients who develop left ventricular failure and/or a reduction of left ventricular compliance with AMI. Diffuse wheezing may be present in patients with severe left ventricular failure. Cough with hemoptysis, suggesting pulmonary embolism with infarction, may also occur. In 1967 Killip proposed a prognostic classification scheme based on the presence and severity of rales detected in patients presenting with AMI. Class I patients are free of rales and a third heart sound. Class II patients have rales but to only a mild-moderate degree (<50 per cent of lung fields) and may or may not have an S₃. Patients in Class III have rales in more than half of each lung field and frequently have pulmonary edema. Finally, Class IV patients are in cardiogenic shock. Despite overall improvement in mortality in each class, this classification remains useful today as evidenced by data from a recent large MI trial.[263]

CARDIAC EXAMINATION. Despite severe symptoms and extensive myocardial damage, the findings on examination of the heart may be surprisingly unremarkable in patients with AMI.[264] Palpation of the precordium may yield normal findings but more commonly reveals (in patients with sinus rhythm) a presystolic pulsation, synchronous with an audible fourth heart sound, reflecting a vigorous left atrial contraction filling a ventricle with reduced compliance. In the presence of left ventricular systolic dysfunction, an outward movement of the left ventricle may be palpated in early diastole, coincident with a third heart sound. When the anterior or lateral portion of the ventricle is dyskinetic, an abnormal systolic pulsation is present in the third, fourth, or fifth interspace to the left of the sternum. In some patients, this abnormal paradoxical precordial impulse is clearly separable from the point of maximal impulse, which is more lateral and to the left. In other patients, the abnormal impulse is a diffuse, rippling, precordial movement, approximately 5 to 10 cm in diameter, not clearly separable from the point of maximal impulse. Patients with longstanding hypertension or previous infarction with left ventricular hypertrophy often demonstrate a laterally displaced, sustained apical impulse.

Auscultation. The heart sounds, particularly the first sound, are frequently muffled and occasionally inaudible immediately after the infarct, and their intensity increases as healing occurs. A soft first sound may also reflect prolongation of the P-R interval. Patients with marked ventricular dysfunction and/or left bundle branch block may have paradoxical splitting of the second heart sound (p. 47). Individuals with postinfarction angina also may develop transient, paradoxically split second heart sounds during anginal episodes because of prolongation of the left ventricular preejection period.

A *fourth heart sound* is almost universally present in patients in sinus rhythm with AMI and is usually best heard between the left sternal border and the apex. This sound reflects atrial contraction and a reduction in left ventricular compliance (p. 50) and is associated with an elevation of left ventricular end-diastolic pressure, even in the absence of left ventricular systolic dysfunction. It is of little diagnostic value, since it is commonly audible in most patients with chronic ischemic heart disease and is recordable, although not often audible, in many normal subjects older than 45 years.

A *third heart sound* in AMI usually reflects extensive left ventricular dysfunction. It is usually heard in patients with large infarctions. This sound is heard best at the apex, with the patient in the left lateral recumbent position, and is more common in patients with transmural anterior infarctions than in those with inferior or nontransmural infarctions.[265] Patients with a third heart sound often have elevated left ventricular filling pressure. The mortality of patients who manifest a third heart sound during the acute phase of MI is higher than that of patients without such a sound.[265] A third sound may be caused not only by left ventricular failure but also by increased inflow into the left ventricle, as occurs when mitral regurgitation or ventricular septal defect complicates AMI. Third and fourth heart sounds emanating from the left ventricle are heard best at the apex; in patients with right ventricular infarcts, these sounds may be heard along the left sternal border and are intensified by inspiration.

Systolic murmurs, transient or persistent, are commonly audible in patients with AMI and generally result from mitral regurgitation secondary to papillary muscle dysfunction or left ventricular dilatation. A new, prominent holosystolic murmur at the apex, accompanied by a thrill, may represent rupture of a head of a papillary muscle (p. 1259). The findings in rupture of the interventricular septum are similar, although the murmur and thrill are usually most prominent along the left sternal border while being audible at the right sternal border as well. The systolic murmur of tricuspid regurgitation (caused by right ventricular failure due to pulmonary hypertension and/or right ventricular infarction or by infarction of a right ventricular papillary muscle) is also heard along the left sternal border but is characteristically intensified by inspiration and is accompanied by a prominent v wave in the jugular venous pulse. A *continuous murmur* is an unusual finding in AMI that may occur as a result of a variety of congenital abnormalities including a coronary artery arteriovenous fistula, an extremely rare cause of myocardial ischemia or infarction.[266]

Pericardial friction rubs are audible in 7 to 20 per cent of all patients with AMI and in a higher percentage of patients with transmural infarcts.[267] Rubs are notorious for their evanescence and, hence, are probably even more common than reported; frequent auscultation in patients with transmural infarction often results in the discovery of a rub which might otherwise have gone unnoticed. Although friction rubs may be heard by 24 hours or as late as 2 weeks after the onset of infarction, most commonly they are noted on the second or third day.[267] Occasionally, in patients with extensive infarction, a loud rub may be heard for many days. About 40 per cent of patients with a friction rub in the setting of AMI have a pericardial effusion on echocardiographic study[268] but only rarely are the classic electrocardiographic changes of pericarditis (p. 158) seen.[267] Delayed onset of the rub and the associated discomfort of pericarditis (as late as 3 months postinfarction) are characteristic of the postmyocardial infarction (Dressler) syndrome (p. 1263).[268–270]

Pericardial rubs are most readily audible along the left sternal border or just inside the point of maximal impulse and occur after either anterior or inferoposterior transmural infarction. Loud rubs may be audible over the entire precordium and even over the back. Occasionally, only the systolic portion of a rub is heard; it may be confused with a systolic murmur, and the diagnosis of rupture of the ventricular septum or mitral regurgitation may be considered. The presence of a pericardial friction rub does not exclude the presence of a significant pericardial effusion.

THE FUNDI. Hypertension, diabetes, and generalized atherosclerosis commonly accompany AMI, and since these conditions may produce characteristic changes in the fundus, a careful funduscopic examination may provide information concerning the underlying vascular status; this is particularly useful in patients unable to provide a detailed history.

THE ABDOMEN. As already noted, in patients with AMI (particularly inferior infarcts) with diaphragmatic irritation, the pain may localize in the epigastrium or the right upper quadrant. Pain in the abdomen associated with nausea, vomiting, restlessness, and even abdominal distention is often interpreted by patients as a sign of "indigestion,"[260] resulting in self-medication with antacids, and it may suggest an acute abdominal process to the physician. A normal abdominal examination aids in ruling this out and in pointing to the correct diagnosis. Right heart failure, characterized by hepatomegaly and a positive abdomino-jugular reflux, is unusual in patients with acute left ventricular infarction but does occur in patients with severe and usually prolonged left ventricular failure or right ventricular infarction.

THE EXTREMITIES. Coronary atherosclerosis is often associated with systemic atherosclerosis, and it is therefore common for patients with AMI to have a history of intermittent claudication and to demonstrate physical findings of peripheral vascular disease. Thus, diminished peripheral arterial pulses, loss of hair, and atrophic skin in the lower extremities are noted frequently in patients with coronary artery disease. Peripheral edema is a manifestation of right ventricular failure and, like congestive hepatomegaly, is unusual in patients with acute left ventricular infarction. Cyanosis of the nailbeds is common in patients with severe left ventricular failure and is particularly striking in patients with cardiogenic shock.

NEUROPSYCHIATRIC FINDINGS. Except for the altered mental status that occurs in patients with AMI who have a markedly reduced cardiac output and cerebral hypoperfusion, the neurological examination is normal unless the patient has suffered cerebral embolism secondary to a mural thrombus. Indeed, an underlying MI is common in patients with cerebral embolic stroke. There is an increased coincidence of cerebrovascular accidents and AMI. In a prospective study of patients with cerebrovascular accidents admitted to the hospital within 72 hours of the onset, 12.7 per cent have an associated AMI; in contrast, in a series of patients with AMI, only 1.7 per cent suffered a stroke. The coincidence was confined to patients with large myocardial infarcts as reflected in markedly elevated serum creatine kinase concentrations.[271] The coincidence between these two conditions may be explained by systemic hypotension due to MI precipitating a cerebral infarction and the converse, as well as by mural emboli from the heart causing cerebral emboli.

Patients with AMI often exhibit alterations of the emotional state, including intense anxiety, denial, and depression.

LABORATORY EXAMINATIONS

ENZYMES

Irreversibly injured myocardial cells release a number of enzymes into the circulation (Fig. 39–15), where they can be measured by specific chemical reactions (p. 1188).[272] Increased activities of many enzymes have been found in the serum or plasma of patients with AMI.[273] Following experimental MI, a small but significant myocardial venoarterial difference of enzyme activity can be measured, and elevated plasma levels of enzymes correlate with corresponding depletion of these same enzymes from infarcted tissue.[274] Determinations of serum activity of creatine kinase (CK), preferably its MB isoenzyme, and of lactic dehydrogenase (LDH) are frequently used in the laboratory diagnosis of AMI.

LACTIC DEHYDROGENASE (LDH). The activity of this

enzyme exceeds the normal range by 24 to 48 hours after the onset of AMI, reaches a peak 3 to 6 days after the onset of pain, and returns to normal levels 8 to 14 days after the infarction. The total LDH, while sensitive, is not specific; false-positive elevations occur in patients with hemolysis, megaloblastic anemia, leukemia, liver disease, hepatic congestion, renal disease, a variety of neoplasms, pulmonary embolism, myocarditis, skeletal muscle disease, and shock.[272,273]

LDH comprises five isoenzymes, which are numbered in the order of the rapidity of their migration toward the anode of an electrophoretic field. LDH_1 moves most rapidly, whereas LDH_5 is the slowest. Fractionation of serum LDH into its five isoenzymes increases diagnostic accuracy, since the heart contains principally LDH_1, whereas liver and skeletal muscle contain primarily LDH_4 and LDH_5. Thus, LDH_5 is commonly elevated in patients with congestive hepatomegaly. Most conditions causing elevated serum total LDH activity, such as liver or skeletal muscle disease or injury, are readily distinguished from AMI by analysis of LDH isoenzymes. Increased serum LDH_1 activity precedes elevation of serum total LDH and usually occurs within 8 to 24 hours after infarction.[275] Elevations of LDH and in the ratio of LDH_1 to total LDH occur in more than 95 per cent of patients with AMI.[272,276] Since hemolysis also raises serum LDH_1 activity, particular care must be taken in the withdrawal and handling of the blood specimens.

Many laboratories report the ratio of LDH_1 to LDH_2, which is elevated in MI. An LDH_1/LDH_2 ratio greater than 1.0 is commonly used as a cutoff defining abnormality in most series[273]; however, even a ratio as low as 0.76 has been reported to be more than 90 per cent sensitive and specific for the diagnosis of AMI.[275] LDH or LDH isoenzyme analysis for the diagnosis of AMI should be reserved for cases in which the CK has already fallen to normal—that is, when infarction is suspected to have occurred 2 to 4 days earlier. Although LDH isoenzyme testing may be useful, as already indicated, like aspartate aminotransferase (AST), the routine use of LDH and LDH isoenzyme determination is not justified and accounts for a considerable waste of resources.[277,278]

ASPARTATE AMINOTRANSFERASE (AST). For many years the activity of serum glutamic oxaloacetic acid transferase (SGOT)—now generally referred to as aspartate aminotransferase (AST)—was monitored for the diagnosis of AMI. Levels rise above normal 8 to 12 hours after the onset of chest pain, peak at 18 to 36 hours, and generally fall to normal within 3 to 4 days. However, because false-positive elevations occur frequently (with most hepatic or skeletal muscle diseases, following intramuscular injections or pulmonary embolism, and with shock), and because the time course of elevation and fall of AST is intermediate between that of CK and LDH, its incremental benefit for the diagnosis of AMI is negligible, and it is no longer routinely used.[277]

CREATINE KINASE (CK). Serum CK activity exceeds the normal range within 4 to 8 hours following the onset of AMI and declines to normal within 3 to 4 days after the onset of chest pain. The time of peak serum CK activity varies considerably, occurring as early as 8 hours after the onset of pain to as long as 58 hours later.[279] While the mean peak CK for AMI occurs at about 24 hours, peak levels occur earlier in patients who have had reperfusion as a result of the administration of thrombolytic therapy or mechanical recanalization (as well as in patients with early spontaneous thrombolysis), with peak CK occurring at about 12 hours after infarction in such cases.[273,280] With reperfusion, enzyme is released into the circulation more rapidly than for an infarct of comparable size without reperfusion.[281] Thus, reperfusion renders estimation of infarct size by enzyme analysis less accurate. Because the time-activity curve of serum CK is influenced by reperfusion, and because reperfusion itself influences infarct size, it has been suggested that the time to peak CK activity should be incorporated into enzymatic estimates of infarct size.[282]

Although elevation of the serum CK is the most sensitive enzymatic detector of AMI that can be used routinely,[272,273,283]

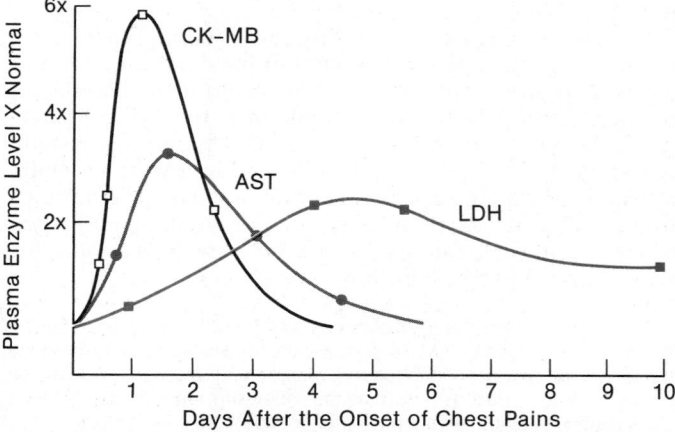

FIGURE 39–15. Typical plasma profiles for the MB isoenzyme of creatine kinase (CK-MB), aspartate amino transferase (AST), and lactate dehydrogenase (LDH) activities following onset of acute myocardial infarction. (Adapted from Hearse, D. J.: Myocardial enzyme leakage. J. Molec. Med. 2:185, 1977.)

15 per cent false-positive results will occur in patients with muscle disease, alcohol intoxication, diabetes mellitus, skeletal muscle trauma, vigorous exercise, convulsions, intramuscular injections, thoracic outlet syndrome, and pulmonary embolism.[272,284] However, serum CK activity is normal in patients with heart failure and hepatic disease. CK values in women are normally about two-thirds of those in men.

CK ISOENZYMES. Three isoenzymes of CK (MM, BB, and MB) have been identified by electrophoresis. Extracts of brain and kidney contain predominantly the BB isoenzyme, skeletal muscle contains principally MM, and both MM and MB isoenzymes are present in cardiac muscle. The MB isoenzymes of CK may also be present in minor quantities in the small intestine, tongue, diaphragm, uterus, and prostate.[283,285] Strenuous exercise, particularly in trained long-distance runners or professional athletes, may cause elevation of both total CK and CK-MB.[286,287] For some athletes, both the percentage of MB released and the characteristic rise and fall of CK-MB may be similar to the changes seen after MI. The possibility has been raised that isoenzyme production is at least partially dynamic, with the relative portion of MB isoenzyme in cardiac muscle perhaps depending on maturation, preexisting coronary artery disease, or left ventricular hypertrophy.[288] Despite these issues and the fact that small amounts of CK-MB isoenzyme are found in tissues other than heart, elevated serum activity of CK-MB may be considered, for practical purposes, to be the result of AMI (except in the case of trauma or surgery on the aforementioned organs, which contain small quantities of the enzyme).

Isoforms of the MM and MB *isoenzymes* have been identified[289-291] (p. 1188). Certain isoforms appear to be released into the blood quite rapidly—perhaps as soon as 1 hour—after the onset of infarction. An assay of these isoforms may permit early identification of patients with AMI and early detection of successful reperfusion with AMI,[292] with or without residual high-grade stenosis[293,294] (Fig. 38–38, p. 1188).

Nevertheless, measurement of serum CK-MB isoenzyme continues to be the most useful and widely available test for myocardial necrosis.[273,295,296] The development of radioimmunoassay for the measurement of serum CK-MB has been helpful in increasing the accuracy, sensitivity, and specificity of this test,[297] although agarose gel electrophoresis is used routinely in most laboratories. A newer solid-phase immunoradiometric assay may further improve sensitivity.[298] In addition to AMI secondary to coronary obstruction, other forms of injury to cardiac muscle—such as those resulting from myocarditis, trauma, cardiac catheterization, shock,[299] and cardiac surgery—may also produce elevated serum CK-MB activity.[299-301] These latter causes of elevation of serum CK-MB values can usually be readily distinguished from AMI by the clinical setting. In approximately 15 per cent of patients with apparent AMI, the CK-MB may be elevated despite a normal total CK.[302,303] The importance of this finding is unclear. In an animal model, it has been shown that CK-MB may be released into the blood by transient severe ischemia without myocardial necrosis[304]; thus, minor elevation of CK-MB may not be diagnostic of AMI. Patients with minimally elevated CK-MB and normal CK, however, do have a prognosis that is generally worse than patients with suspected MI and no CK-MB elevation.[298,303,305] Thus, whether or not such elevations represent true "microinfarctions" may be less important than the prognostic connotations of this isolated elevation. Therefore, total CK is not a sensitive adequate screening test. On the basis of a careful analysis of factors affecting serum enzyme assays and a rational approach to minimizing resource consumption without adversely affecting diagnostic accuracy, Lee and Goldman[273] have proposed the series of recommendations on the use of serum enzyme assays for the diagnosis of AMI, shown in Table 39–2.

Serial measurement of CK-MB and application of the methods devised by Sobel and Shell (p. 1189)[272] allow prediction of infarct size determined at necropsy[306]; infarct size estimated by this method varies inversely with ejection frac-

TABLE 39–2 RECOMMENDATIONS ON THE USE OF SERUM ENZYME ASSAYS IN THE DIAGNOSIS OF ACUTE MYOCARDIAL INFARCTION

1. A single set of cardiac enzyme values in the emergency room is not sufficiently sensitive to exclude myocardial infarction. Although a single, markedly positive CK-MB value will greatly increase the probability of acute infarction, data are insufficient to support or reject a policy whereby low-risk patients, who otherwise would be sent home, would be observed until one or more CK-MB values are obtained.

2. If myocardial infarction is suspected, then samples of total CK and CK-MB levels should be measured on admission and about 12 and 24 hours later, although condensed versions of this strategy may ultimately prove to be equally efficacious and more cost effective. If myocardial infarction may have occurred more than 24 hours before admission, and if CK and CK-MB levels are not diagnostic, a total LDH level should be ordered. If the total LDH level is elevated, an assay of LDH isoenzymes should be obtained. If the first LDH1/LDH2 ratio is only slightly less than 1.0, a second assay is probably indicated.

3. If chest pain recurs after admission, CK and CK-MB assays should be done at 0, 12, and 24 hours. "Surveillance" enzyme assays are not recommended in asymptomatic patients without electrocardiographic changes.

4. Routine use of enzyme assays other than those for CK, CK-MB, and LDH isoenzymes is not recommended.

5. If more than 2 hours may pass before CK isoenzymes will be assayed, the serum sample should be preserved on ice.

6. Strategies including CK-MB assays can be used to diagnose myocardial infarction in the setting of noncardiac surgery and cardiac catheterization and after electrical countershock.

7. In the setting of cardiac surgery, myocardial infarction should be diagnosed if any two of the following are present: CK-MB elevation persisting more than 12 hours; new Q waves on an electrocardiogram; or regional defects on technetium pyrophosphate scintigraphy.

8. False-positive elevations of CK-MB can be minimized by diluting samples with marked elevations of total CK; detecting isoenzyme variants that masquerade as CK-MB on column chromatography assays by retesting the sample on an electrophoretic assay if the clinical presentation is atypical for myocardial infarction; or consideration of other sources of CK-MB (for example, myocarditis, renal failure, neuromuscular diseases, trauma) if a true elevation of CK-MB levels is found in the absence of a typical rise and fall of CK and CK-MB levels and other evidence for myocardial infarction.

From Lee, T., and Goldman, L.: Serum enzyme assays in the diagnosis of acute myocardial infarction. Recommendations based on a quantitative analysis. Ann. Intern. Med. *102*:221, 1986.

tion[307] and with survival.[308] Coronary artery reperfusion influences infarct size estimates by CK-MB as it does total CK-derived estimates. Thus, further refinements in the estimation of infarct size from CK-MB will depend on the incorporation of the effect of acute reperfusion into such estimates.[309]

Other Laboratory Measurements

Numerous nonspecific manifestations may be recognized in patients with AMI. Although they are not generally employed in establishing the diagnosis, awareness of their coexistence with infarction is important in order to avoid misinterpretation or erroneous diagnosis of other disorders.

BLOOD SUGAR. Hyperglycemia occurs frequently following AMI, not only in diabetic patients, in whom ketoacidosis may be precipitated, but also (with a lower frequency) in nondiabetics, in whom several weeks may elapse before carbohydrate tolerance returns to normal[198,310] (p. 1212). The plasma urea and creatinine concentrations are normal, except in patients with severe left ventricular failure, in whom reduced renal perfusion and glomerular filtration may result in azotemia.

Hypokalemic alkalosis may be present in patients who develop an AMI while receiving thiazide or loop diuretics for antecedent hypertension or heart failure.

SERUM LIPIDS. These are often determined in patients with AMI.

However, the results may be misleading, since numerous factors that can alter the values are operating at the time of the patient's admission to the hospital; for example, stress increases serum cholesterol, whereas recumbency decreases it.[311] Serum triglycerides are affected by caloric intake, intravenous glucose, and recumbency.[311]

During the first 24 to 48 hours after admission, total cholesterol and HDL cholesterol remain at or near baseline values but generally fall precipitously after that.[312,313] The fall in HDL cholesterol after AMI is greater than the fall in total cholesterol; thus, the ratio of total cholesterol to HDL cholesterol is no longer useful for risk assessment early after MI.[314] Therefore, unless values are obtained very early in patients admitted for AMI, it is best to defer determinations of serum lipid levels until at least 8 weeks after the infarction has occurred.

MYOGLOBIN. This protein is released into the circulation from injured myocardial cells and can be demonstrated within a few hours after the onset of infarction; myoglobinemia is common in patients with AMI.[315] Peak levels of serum myoglobin are reached considerably earlier (3 to 20 hours) than peak values of serum CK.[316] However, the time of earlier appearance of myoglobin in the serum, its peak level, and the duration of detectable myoglobin release do *not* correlate well with these same parameters for serum CK and with clinical estimates of the severity of infarction. In contrast to CK, myoglobin (which has a molecular weight of only 17,000) is readily excreted into the urine. A more rapid rise in serum myoglobin has been observed following reperfusion, and its measurement has even been suggested as a useful index of successful reperfusion.[317] However, the clinical value of serial determinations of myoglobin in AMI is limited because of the brief duration of its elevation and the lack of specificity resulting from the fact that myoglobin is a constituent of skeletal muscle and is readily detected in the serum following damage to skeletal muscle.

HEMATOLOGICAL MANIFESTATIONS. An increase in the *white blood count* occurs frequently following AMI; it may be a response to tissue necrosis or increased secretion of adrenal glucocorticoids or both. The elevation of the white count usually develops within 2 hours after the onset of chest pain, reaches a peak 2 to 4 days following infarction, and returns to normal in 1 week; the peak white blood cell count usually ranges between 12 and 15 × 10³ per cubic millimeter but occasionally rises to as high as 20 × 10³ per cubic millimeter. Often there is an increase in the percentage of polymorphonuclear leukocytes and a shift of the differential count to band forms. The *erythrocyte sedimentation rate* (ESR) is usually normal during the first day or two after infarction, even though fever and leukocytosis may be present. It then rises to a peak on the fourth or fifth day and may remain elevated for several weeks. The increase in the ESR is secondary to elevated plasma alpha₂ globulin and fibrinogen,[318] but the peak does not correlate well with the size of the infarction or with the prognosis. The *hematocrit* often increases during the first few days following infarction as a consequence of hemoconcentration.[218]

ELECTROCARDIOGRAPHIC FINDINGS
(See also p. 136)

In the majority of patients with AMI, some change can be documented when serial electrocardiograms (ECGs) are compared. However, many factors limit the ability of the ECG to diagnose and localize MI: the extent of myocardial injury, the age of the infarct, its location, the presence of conduction defects, the presence of previous infarcts or acute pericarditis, changes in electrolyte concentrations, and the administration of cardioactive drugs. Nevertheless, serial standard 12-lead ECGs remain a clinically useful method for the detection and localization of MI.[296,319]

Although there is general agreement of electrocardiographic and vectorcardiographic criteria for the recognition of infarction of the anterior and inferior myocardial walls (Table 5–5, p. 144), there is less agreement on criteria for lateral and posterior infarcts[320]; here even the terminology may be confusing.[321] Although most patients continue to demonstrate the ECG changes from an infarction, particularly if they evolve Q waves for the rest of their lives, in a substantial minority the typical changes disappear, Q waves can regress,[322,323] and the ECG can even return to normal after a number of months or, more commonly, years.[324] Under many circumstances Q wave patterns may simulate MI.[325] Conditions that may mimic the electrocardiographic features of MI by producing a pattern of "pseudoinfarction" are listed in Table 39–3.

TABLE 39–3 CONDITIONS SIMULATING INFARCTION ON ECG

Ventricular hypertrophy
    Right ventricular (cor pulmonale)
    Left ventricular

Conduction disturbances
    Left bundle branch block
    Left anterior fascicular block

Wolff-Parkinson-White syndrome
Primary myocardial disease
    Myocarditis
    Dilated cardiomyopathy
    Hypertrophic cardiomyopathy (both obstructive and nonobstructive)
    Friedreich's ataxia
    Muscular dystrophy

Pneumothorax
Pulmonary embolus
Amyloid heart disease
Primary and metastatic tumors of the heart
Traumatic heart disease
Intracranial hemorrhage
Hyperkalemia
Pericarditis
Early repolarization
Sarcoidosis involving the heart

From Taussig, A. S., et al.: Misleading ECGs: Patterns of infarction. J. Cardiovasc. Med. 9:1147, 1983.

Q-WAVE AND NON-Q-WAVE INFARCTION. In the past an AMI (by enzyme or other clinical criteria) in which Q waves failed to develop on the ECG was referred to as a "subendocardial" or "nontransmural" MI. However, the presence or absence of Q waves on the surface ECG does not reliably predict the distinction between transmural and nontransmural or subendocardial MI.[326] True pathological subendocardial MI, as recognized at autopsy, is seen with ST-segment depression and/or T wave changes only about 50 per cent of the time.[327] Nevertheless, for the prognostic importance of identifying two different populations, a distinction should be made between AMI with and without Q waves.[328,329] Changes in the ST segment and T wave are quite nonspecific and may occur in a variety of conditions, including stable and unstable angina pectoris, ventricular hypertrophy, acute and chronic pericarditis, myocarditis, early repolarization, electrolyte imbalance, shock, metabolic disorders, and following the administration of digitalis (Ch. 17).[320] Serial ECGs may be of considerable aid in differentiating these conditions from non-Q-wave infarction.[330] Transient changes favor angina or electrolyte disturbances, whereas persistent changes argue for infarction if other causes such as shock, administration of glycoside, and persistent metabolic disorders can be eliminated. In the final analysis, the diagnosis of nontransmural infarction rests more on the combination of clinical findings and the elevation of serum enzymes than on the ECG.

ISCHEMIA AT A DISTANCE. Patients with new Q waves and ST-segment elevation diagnostic for MI in one territory often have ST-segment depression in other territories. These additional ST-segment changes may be caused by ischemia in a territory other than the area of infarction, termed "ischemia at a distance,"[162,331] or by reciprocal electrical phenomena.[332] A good deal of attention has been directed to associated ST-segment depression in the anterior leads, which occurs in the majority of patients with acute inferior MI.[333,334] However, despite the clinical importance of differentiation among causes of anterior ST-segment depression in such patients—including anterior ischemia, posterior wall infarction, and true reciprocal changes—such a differentiation cannot be made reliably by electrocardiographic or even vectorcardiographic[334] techniques. Although precordial ST-segment depression is more commonly associated with extensive infarction of the posterior, lateral, or inferior septal segments—rather than anterior wall subendocardial ischemia[335,336]—ancillary scintigraphic or angiographic techniques are necessary to document this. Regardless of whether the anterior ST-segment changes reflect anterior wall ischemia or are reciprocal to changes

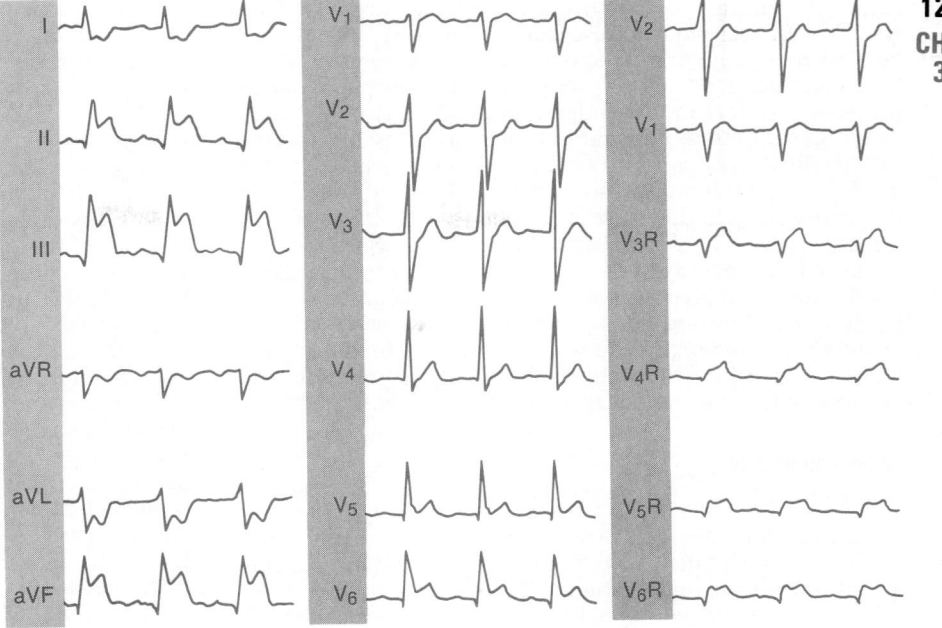

FIGURE 39–16. Leads I, II, III, aVR, aVL, aVF, leads V_1, V_2, V_3, V_4, V_5, and V_6, and right precordial leads V_2, V_1, V_3R, V_4R, V_5R, and V_6R recorded simultaneously. The ECG shows acute inferoposterior wall myocardial infarction. The right precordial leads show ST-segment elevation in leads V_3R, V_4R, V_5R, and V_6R, indicating right ventricular infarction as well. (From Brant, S. H.: Value of electrocardiography in diagnosing right ventricular involvement patients with an acute inferior wall myocardial infarction. Br. Heart J. 49:368, 1983.)

elsewhere, this finding, as with ischemia at a distance, implies a poorer prognosis than is the case if such changes are not present.[331,334]

RIGHT VENTRICULAR INFARCTION. This is difficult to diagnose by the electrocardiogram, presumably because the right ventricular myocardial mass is small in comparison with the left. However, ST-segment elevation in right precordial leads (V_1, V_3R-V_6R) has been noted to be a relatively sensitive and specific sign of right ventricular infarction[337–340] (Fig. 39–16). Occasionally ST-segment elevation in the usual precordial leads (particularly V_2 and V_3) may be due to acute right ventricular infarction; this appears to occur only when the injury to the left ventricular inferior wall is minimal.[341] Usually, the concurrent inferior wall injury suppresses this anterior ST-segment elevation resulting from right ventricular injury. Likewise, right ventricular infarction itself appears to reduce the anterior ST-segment depression often seen with inferior wall myocardial infarction.[342] A QS or QR pattern in leads V_3R and/or V_4R also suggest right ventricular myocardial necrosis but have less predictive accuracy than ST-segment elevation in these leads.[339,340]

ATRIAL INFARCTION. This can be suspected occasionally from the ECG[343,344]; the most common electrocardiographic patterns are depression or elevation of the PQ segment, alterations in the contour of the P wave, and abnormal atrial rhythms, including atrial flutter, atrial fibrillation, wandering atrial pacemaker, and AV nodal rhythm.[322]

IMAGING IN ACUTE MYOCARDIAL INFARCTION

ROENTGENOGRAPHY

(See also p. 224)

The initial chest roentgenogram in patients with AMI is almost invariably a portable film obtained in the emergency room or the coronary care unit. Two findings are common: signs of left ventricular failure and cardiomegaly. Although the pulmonary vascular markings on the roentgenogram generally reflect the left ventricular end-diastolic pressure, significant discrepancies may occur because of what have been termed *diagnostic lags* and *post-therapeutic lags*. In the former, patients may have elevated left ventricular filling pressure and normal chest roentgenogram, and, because of the time required for pulmonary edema to accumulate after left ventricular filling pressure has become elevated, 12 hours may elapse before the radiographic findings reflect the hemodynamic status. The post-therapeutic phase lag represents the longer time interval, generally 1 or 2 days, required for pulmonary edema to resorb and the radiographic signs of pulmonary congestion to clear after left ventricular filling pressure has returned toward normal.[345]

Cardiomegaly in a patient with AMI usually signifies prior infarction or another form of antecedent cardiovascular disease such as chronic hypertension with subsequent left ventricular dilatation, and it is usually associated with impaired left ventricular function.[346] Since the chest film (especially the portable film in the A-P projection) is not a sensitive indicator of ventricular size, the converse is not true, in that patients may have increased end-diastolic volume and still demonstrate a normal-sized heart on roentgenographic examination. The degree of congestion and the size of the left side of the heart on the chest film are highly useful predictors for defining groups of patients with AMI who are at increased risk of dying after the acute event.[347]

Computed tomography (CT) (p. 315) can provide useful cross-sectional information in patients with MI. In addition to the assessment of cavity dimensions and wall thickness, left ventricular aneurysms may be detected, and, of particular importance in AMI, intracardiac thrombi can be identified. Although cardiac CT is a less convenient technique, it probably is more sensitive for thrombus detection than echocardiography.[348] Infarct sizing is possible with CT scanning but for this purpose remains a research tool rather than a clinical one[349] (Fig. 11–4, p. 314).

Radioisotopic Studies

(See Chap. 10)

All major forms of nuclear cardiac imaging—radionuclide angiography, perfusion scintigraphy, infarct-avid scintigraphy, and positron-emission tomography—are useful in detecting AMI, in assessing infarct size and jeopardized myocardium, in determining the effects of the infarct on ventricular function, and in establishing prognosis. The application of these techniques is discussed in Chapter 11.[296,350–353]

A new radiopharmaceutical agent, ^{99m}Tc hexakis 2-methyoxy-2-isobutyl isonitrile ([99m] Sesta MIBI), has been developed for myocardial perfusion imaging[354] (p. 277). This agent has already proved useful for the measurement of the area of myocardium at risk in AMI[355] and the recognition of salvaged myocardium following thrombolytic therapy.[356] Its use is likely to increase in the next several years.

Magnetic Resonance Imaging

(See Figs. 11–22, 11–23, and 11–25, pp. 325–326)

Cardiac imaging with magnetic resonance imaging (MRI) has been employed in experimental and clinical studies of

AMI.[357] In addition to localizing and sizing the area of infarction,[358] MRI techniques are capable of early recognition of MI[359] and of providing an assessment of the severity of the ischemic insult.[360] While imaging with this technique presents practical problems for routine studies in coronary care unit patients because patients must be transported to the MRI facility, this safe, noninvasive modality holds much promise. Potential capabilities of MRI are likely to include not only the ability to detect, localize, and size AMI but also to assess perfusion of infarcted and noninfarcted tissue as well as of reperfused myocardium; to identify areas of jeopardized but not infarcted myocardium; to identify myocardial edema, fibrosis, wall thinning, and hypertrophy; to assess ventricular chamber size and segmental wall motion; and to identify the temporal transition between ischemia and infarction and eventually to assess coronary anatomy and flow.[359,361,362]

Echocardiography
(See also p. 97)

As major technical improvements have been made, echocardiography has emerged as an extremely important imaging modality in all cardiac patients. The relative portability of echocardiographic equipment makes this technique ideal for the assessment of patients with AMI hospitalized in the critical care setting[363] or even in the emergency department before admission. In patients with chest pain compatible with AMI, but with a nondiagnostic ECG, the finding on echocardiography of a distinct region of disordered contraction can be helpful diagnostically.

M-MODE ECHOCARDIOGRAPHY. This sensitive technique for examining regional left ventricular wall motion[364] is limited to the imaging of small segments of the interventricular septum and posterior and anterior left ventricular walls. Abnormalities of left ventricular wall motion, usually corresponding to the electrocardiographic site of infarction, may be recognized in the majority of patients with transmural infarction, and hyperkinetic motion can be found in noninfarcted areas in approximately one-third of patients.[365] M-mode echocardiography is also useful in detecting small pericardial effusions in patients with postinfarction pericarditis.[366]

TWO-DIMENSIONAL ECHOCARDIOGRAPHY (see Figs. 4–90, p. 98; 4–93, 4–94, p. 99). This technique can provide both longitudinal and transverse views of the left ventricle. Also, a much larger fraction of the ventricular wall—including significant portions of the left ventricular apical, anterior, septal, inferior, and posterior walls—can be imaged[363] by this method than by the M-mode technique. Areas of abnormal regional wall motion are observed almost universally in patients with AMI.[367] Abnormal wall motion is less often noted echocardiographically when the infarction is nontransmural; however, abnormalities are still present in more than two-thirds of patients.[368] Left ventricular function, estimated from two-dimensional echocardiograms,[368] correlates well with estimates for angiographic studies and may be useful in establishing prognosis.[369,370]

It has recently been shown that two-dimensional echocardiography is diagnostically useful and cost-effective in the emergency department setting.[367,370,371] In patients who arrive with chest pain, echocardiography may be utilized rapidly to identify regional wall motion abnormalities, which are nearly universally present in patients with AMI. The rapid application of this technique can then aid in admission decisions and in selecting among other important therapeutic options such as whether or not to use thrombolytic therapy (p. 1230). Furthermore, the *early* use of echocardiography can aid in the early detection of mechanical complications of AMI and in the early assessment of right and left ventricular function, as already noted.

In addition to the abnormal wall motion seen following AMI, myocardium in the area of infarction is usually much thinner than noninfarcted myocardium. Ultrasonic tissue characterization techniques, which take advantage of the known increase in echo intensity from myocardial scar, appear to aid in the differentiation between ischemic and infarcted myocardium.[372] Motion within the originally defined area of dyssynergy may improve during the recovery phase of AMI, suggesting a beneficial effect of reperfusion therapy.[373] While reliably detecting and localizing an AMI, two-dimensional echocardiography has been less useful for quantifying the area of infarction because of difficulties in distinguishing between ischemic and infarcted tissue. Both fail to contract normally; in such assessments the area of actual tissue necrosis usually is overestimated.[374]

Two-dimensional echocardiography is extremely useful for the detection of most mechanical complications of AMI. Left ventricular aneurysms[375] and pseudoaneurysms[376] usually are easily and reliably identified. In addition, in patients with AMI who develop a loud systolic murmur, this type of echocardiography can be used to detect and localize a ventricular septal defect, as well as detect mitral regurgitation, and elucidate its cause.[377] Myocardial rupture, pericardial effusion, and left ventricular thrombus formation, all of which occur with AMI, may also be detected by this method.[363,378]

DOPPLER ECHOCARDIOGRAPHY. This technique (p. 97) allows for assessment of blood flow in the cardiac chambers and across cardiac valves.[379] Used in conjunction with two-dimensional echocardiography, it is of benefit in detecting and assessing the severity of mitral[380] or tricuspid regurgitation following AMI. Identification of the site of acute ventricular septal rupture, as well as quantification of shunt flow across the resulting defect, is also possible.[380,381] Reliable estimation of cardiac output has been made by combining Doppler echocardiographic measurements of flow with two-dimensional echocardiographic measurements of ascending aortic cross-sectional area through which blood flows.[382]

Estimation of Infarct Size

ELECTROCARDIOGRAPHY. Interest in limiting infarct size, in large part because of the recognition that the quantity of myocardium infarcted has important prognostic implications, has focused attention on the accurate determination of MI size. The ECG initially received greatest attention. Early studies by Maroko and others demonstrated that the sum of ST-segment elevations measured from many precordial leads was useful for assessing the extent of myocardial injury in patients with anterior MI.[383] While this technique is practical and easily utilized, it is applicable only to anterior infarctions. It is limited by the inability to distinguish between reversibly and irreversibly ischemic tissue, and it depends on the influence of myocardial geometry.[384] QRS scoring systems with planar[385,386] or vectorcardiographic[387] techniques to estimate infarct size have been developed. While demonstrating good correlations with infarct size at autopsy and with enzymatic estimates, these ECG techniques are also subject to many limitations. These include the effects of ventricular geometry[384] as well as the inability to size infarcts in patients with conduction defects, nontransmural MI, and multiple infarctions.

ENZYMATIC METHODS. Serial measurements of enzymes released by necrotic myocardium, particularly creatine kinase (CK) and its MB isoenzyme, are helpful in determining AMI size. Clinically, the peak CK or CK-MB is useful for a rough estimate of infarct size and is widely used prognostically. However, coronary artery recanalization—spontaneous or pharmacologically or mechanically achieved—dramatically changes the wash-out kinetics of CK from myocardium, resulting in early and exaggerated peak enzyme levels.[280,281] Nevertheless, accuracy can be attained with appropriate modification of enzymatic estimates of impact size.[388] Quantification of the cumulative release of CK[399] or CK-MB[306,389,390] has been closely correlated with other techniques for estimating infarct size and with the area of necrosis at autopsy. This quantitative approach has proved useful for determining, in clinical trials on groups of patients, the effects (if any) of different forms of therapy for AMI and for prognostic assessment. However, accurate quantitation by this method is not available early enough to be useful for the clinician caring for patients with AMI.

NONINVASIVE IMAGING TECHNIQUES. Echocardiography (Chap. 4, p. 97), radionuclide scintigraphy (Chap. 10, p. 277), CT scanning (Chap. 11, p. 315), and magnetic resonance imaging (Chap. 11, p. 337) have all been utilized for the clinical and experimental assessment of infarct size. Contrast enhancement[391] may improve upon the tendency of two-dimensional echocardiography to overestimate infarct size.[392] Infarct-avid scintigraphy and the myocardial perfusion and wall motion types all have been used experimentally to quantify infarct size, but are limited by the inability to detect small infarcts, by ventricular geometry, and again by difficulty in distinguishing ischemic from infarcted myocardium. Tomography has improved on techniques employing technetium-99m pyrophosphate to image AMI.[393] Imaging of radiolabeled myosin-specific antibodies, which bind to myosin exposed by the loss of plasma membrane in early myocardial necrosis, is the newest scintigraphic technique and holds promise for highly accurate quantification of infarct size.[351,394]

A comprehensive method of infarct size estimation has been proposed incorporating enzymatic (CK-MB) and electrocardiographic indices and two-dimensional echocardiography.[395] While proving accurate in one prospective study, the proposed formula requires further validation.

Management of Acute Myocardial Infarction

Many options are available for the treatment of AMI. These include the use of pharmacological agents to dissolve occlusive thrombi and to prevent or delay necrosis of jeopardized myocardium and mechanical procedures to recanalize occluded coronary arteries. While such approaches have been termed "aggressive,"[21] they are clearly warranted in increasing numbers of patients. Nevertheless, the sound management of patients with AMI still depends on a variety of conventional management measures that have come into use in the decades since Herrick's original description of the condition at the beginning of this century. These measures, which consist of bed rest, oxygen, treatment of arrhythmias, and prevention of complications, will be considered in this section before the more aggressive therapies are discussed.

Physician practices have changed dramatically as newer approaches to the care of the AMI patient have become available.[395a,396] Virtually all physicians in the U.S. have intensive care facilities available for their patients with AMI. In 1970, such facilities were *unavailable* to almost 20 per cent of family physicians and general practitioners. The use of antiarrhythmic agents has increased markedly, while the regular prescription of long-term anticoagulant therapy and cardiac glycosides has fallen by 50 per cent or more. Nitrates and/or beta blockers, rarely prescribed in 1970, are now given to the majority of patients. Average hospital stay is less than one-half of what it was in 1970. Invasive and/or noninvasive procedures to evaluate prognosis and the need for further therapy are now used in most post-MI patients, whereas only a small percentage of patients had such procedures performed in the early 1970's.[397] Finally, thrombolytic therapy, available but unused in 1970, is now standard care in suitable patients.

PREHOSPITAL CARE

Most deaths associated with AMI occur within the first hour after its onset, and death usually is due to ventricular fibrillation (Chap. 26).[398] Accordingly, the importance of the immediate implementation of definitive resuscitative efforts and of rapidly transporting the patient to a hospital cannot be overemphasized.[398a] First and foremost, patients must be educated to seek immediate medical attention should they develop manifestations of MI. In patients with previous infarcts or in those with chronic stable angina, these manifestations are not difficult to describe—severe chest pain resembling that with the first infarct or more severe and prolonged than with ordinary angina. The task is more difficult in patients in whom the AMI is the first clinical manifestation of coronary artery disease.

Public campaigns must inform the susceptible population (most adults) about the clinical manifestations of AMI. In fact, it has been shown that a media campaign in Göteborg, Sweden, shortened significantly (from 3 to 2 hours) the median delay time for the onset of symptoms to hospital arrival.[399] People must be educated concerning the benefits of seeking immediate medical help if they are suffering an AMI, both in terms of prevention and treatment of potentially fatal arrhythmias as well as salvage of jeopardized myocardium by reper-

fusion, for which time is particularly crucial. In fact, when thrombolytic therapy is employed, prompt hospital arrival following the onset of symptoms (within 2 hours) is associated with a lower mortality rate.[263,400] It has been suggested that primary care physicians need to become familiar with newer strategies to help facilitate early treatment.[401] Well-equipped ambulances and helicopters staffed by personnel trained in the acute care of the infarction victim allow definitive therapy to commence while the patient is being transported to the hospital.[402,403] These specially equipped and staffed ambulances have been termed *mobile coronary care units*; to be used effectively, they must be placed strategically within a community and excellent radio communication systems must be available. They should be equipped with battery-operated monitoring equipment and direct writing electrocardiograph, a battery-operated DC defibrillator, oxygen, endotracheal tubes and suction apparatus, and commonly used cardiovascular drugs. A radiotelemetry system that allows transmission of the ECG to the hospital is desirable but not essential. The effectiveness of such a system depends upon the competency of paramedics, transmission distances, and the availability of expert consultation on the receiving end.[404]

The effectiveness of these systems in Belfast, Ireland,[402] Seattle, Washington,[405] and Columbus, Ohio[406] has been amply documented. The rapid initiation of prehospital cardiopulmonary resuscitation facilitated by mobile coronary care units and trained paramedical personnel results in initially successful resuscitation in approximately two-thirds of patients. It has been demonstrated that the frequency of death *during* transportation can be diminished from 22 to 9 per cent when defibrillation equipment and trained paramedical personnel are available,[407] although reduced overall mortality has not been shown.[403] In addition to prompt defibrillation, the efficacy of prehospital care appears to depend on several factors, including early relief of pain with its deleterious physiological sequelae, reduction of excessive activity of the autonomic nervous system, and abolition of prelethal arrhythmias, such as ventricular tachycardia. However, these efforts must not inhibit rapid transfer to the hospital, as recently the application of such therapies has been found actually to delay hospital arrival, possibly diminishing the benefit of such an approach.[403]

Communication systems capable of transmitting the ECG over regular telephone lines are now available for the home. The prehospital use of such a system has been shown to reduce morbidity and mortality in a high-risk subset of patients supplied with the device.[408] Mobile intensive care and prehospital monitoring systems have also facilitated the acquisition of data about the earliest signs and symptoms of AMI, both for the understanding of early complications of AMI and for identifying patient subgroups with differing risks.[409] Observations of simple variables such as heart rate and blood pressure permit initial classification to high- or low-risk subgroups because patients initially presenting with hypotension have a mortality in excess of 50 per cent, whereas patients with isolated sinus bradycardia (and a normal or elevated blood pressure) appear to have a mortality that approaches zero.[409]

Recently the possibility that the prehospital use of thrombolytic therapy might be of benefit has been addressed,[410,411] and several pilot studies have been carried out.[412-415] It is estimated that approximately one-quarter of patients presenting with AMI would be candidates for such early treatment[416] and that an organized paramedic-based treatment system could allow for thrombolytic therapy to be given, on average, about 70 minutes earlier.[416]

CORONARY CARE UNITS

During the past two and a half decades the mortality of patients with AMI treated in coronary care units has declined significantly from what it had been before the introduction of these units.[8,10,417] Reduction in mortality has resulted in large part from the elimination of *primary* arrhythmias as a cause of death. Actually, most instances of primary arrhythmias occur *before* the patient reaches the hospital, and only about 5 per cent of patients develop a primary ventricular arrhythmia *after* they reach the hospital, an average of 5 to 6 hours after the onset of the attack in most series. Deaths from primary ventricular fibrillation have been prevented because the coronary care unit allows continuous monitoring of cardiac rhythm by highly trained nurses with the authority to administer immediate treatment and prophylaxis of arrhythmias in the absence of physicians, and because of the specialized equipment (defibrillators, pacemakers) and drugs available for instantaneous use.[417] Although all of these benefits can certainly be achieved for patients scattered throughout the hospital, the clustering of patients with AMI in the coronary (or cardiac) care unit has greatly improved the efficient use of the trained personnel, facilities, and equipment. In recent years, with increasing emphasis on hemodynamic monitoring and treatment of the serious complications of AMI with such modalities as thrombolytic therapy, afterload reduction, and intraaortic balloon counter pulsation, the coronary care unit has assumed even greater importance.[417] As interventional strategies including thrombolytic therapy and acute coronary angioplasty are used more routinely in AMI patients, facilities in which patients may undergo diagnostic and therapeutic angiographic procedures are being integrated into the coronary care unit structure.

ROLE OF THE CORONARY CARE UNIT IN UNCOMPLICATED AMI PATIENTS. At the same time, the value of coronary care units for patients with *uncomplicated AMI* has been questioned and restudied.[418] In one widely publicized randomized trial, carried out in England, patients with suspected infarction were evaluated initially at home; after a 2-hour observation interval they were divided at random into home-management and hospital-management groups.[419] Although the 6-week mortality rates among patients with infarction in the two groups were similar (13 per cent and 11 per cent, respectively), such relatively low overall mortality rates make detection of small although real differences difficult (i.e., a high Type II error). Furthermore, hospital care was provided for all high-risk patients. Under the general conditions of medical practice in the United States, it is difficult to provide the same immediate intensive care at home for all patients with suspected infarction that was made available in this study. Since prediction of the occurrence of early complications is imperfect, it appears that the observation and prompt treatment possible in a well-staffed coronary care unit continue to justify the reliance placed upon this setting as the primary one for early management of patients with suspected or confirmed AMI. Unfortunately, patient delay in seeking medical attention and the medical system's delay in responding reduce the potential impact of the coronary care unit because the patients do not reach the unit until the maximum danger has passed. Therefore, education of the public, of patients at high risk of AMI, and of those members of the medical profession involved in responding to the initial complaints of these patients is likely to be rewarded by further reductions of mortality.[401]

SELECTION OF PATIENTS FOR THE CCU. With increasing attention directed to the limitation of resources and to the economic impact of intensive care, there have been efforts to identify patients for whom hospitalization in a coronary care unit would likely be of benefit (p. 1702).[417] A single set of cardiac enzyme measurements obtained in the emergency department is not of sufficient sensitivity to rule out an AMI. On the other hand, the ECG, particularly in conjunction with a general clinical assess-

ment, can be useful both for predicting which patients will have the diagnosis of AMI confirmed and identifying low-risk patients who may require less intensive care.[420] Of patients with a classic history of chest pain but with a normal ECG in the emergency department, less than 20 per cent will ultimately have an AMI on that admission, and less than 1 per cent will develop any significant complication.[421] Thus, a patient with a normal ECG may not require admission to a full-fledged coronary care unit. Careful analysis of the quality of pain may help identify such low-risk patients as well. Patients without a history of angina pectoris or MI presenting with pain that is sharp or stabbing and pleuritic, positional, or reproduced by palpation of the chest wall are extremely unlikely to have an AMI.[422]

More complex decision protocols, which have been utilized with the aid of simple computer programs accessible to the emergency department staff, have been successfully tested and found capable of accurately predicting which patients with acute chest pain are having an MI[423] and which have acute ischemic heart disease (including unstable angina).[424] These instruments, which incorporate clinical variables including ECG changes, the quality of pain and other symptoms, and the patient's age, have not yet achieved widespread use. As pressures increase to eliminate inappropriate coronary care unit admissions, emergency department clinicians may find it important to take advantage of such tools.

For patients with a low probability of MI, the clinician should consider admission to an intermediate care facility equipped with simple ECG monitoring and resuscitation equipment. This strategy has been shown to be cost-effective.[425] It may be preferable for many such patients who stand to gain little benefit from the high staffing, intense activity, and elaborate technology available to current coronary care units (with their attendant high costs) and who may be disturbed by that activity and equipment. Use of a nonintensive care facility for low-risk patients may reduce coronary care unit utilization by one-third, shorten hospital stays, and have no deleterious effect on patients' recovery.

RECOMMENDATIONS. While there is both a lack of direct evidence, in terms of improved patient survival, for the value of coronary care units and a lack of consensus concerning general admission policies and therapeutic strategies for these units,[426] several common principles and guidelines may be proposed: (1) Most patients with clear-cut AMI should be admitted to an intensive (coronary) care unit. Patients with hemodynamic instability, other serious medical problems, or continuing symptoms also should be admitted, even if the diagnosis of AMI is uncertain. Most patients with unstable angina (p. 1334), particularly if episodes of chest pain are occurring at rest, should also be admitted to the coronary care unit. (2) Once an AMI is ruled out, which may be as early as 24 hours after admission,[417,427] and symptoms are controlled with oral or topical pharmacological agents, discharge from the coronary care unit should be considered.[428] (3) In AMI patients with *uncomplicated* status, stays in the unit need be no longer than 2 days. (4) In patients with complicated AMI, the duration of the coronary care unit stay should depend on the need for "intensive" care—that is, hemodynamic monitoring, close nursing supervision, intravenous vasoactive drugs, and frequent changes in the medical regimen.

GENERAL MEASURES

General care measures should include (1) a liquid diet for 24 hours, because of the risk of nausea and vomiting or cardiac arrest early after infarction and the need to reduce the risk of aspiration. This should be followed by a 1500 calorie soft diet, with no added salt, divided into multiple small feedings for several days. Then, in the absence of heart failure, a regular diet, low in cholesterol and saturated fats, is appropriate. Caffeine-rich beverages should be avoided because of their possible arrhythmogenic effects. (2) Dioctyl sodium sulfosuccinate, 100 mg daily, or another stool softener should be used to prevent constipation and straining. (3) The emotional impact of an AMI and of hospitalization in a coronary care unit should be offset by thoughtful explanations of the nature of the illness, the function of the equipment, and the purpose of the procedures. A deliberate effort should be made to maintain the atmosphere in the coronary care unit as quiet and restful as possible. Oxazepam, 15 to 30 mg orally four times a day, is useful to allay the anxiety that is so common in this setting. Temazepam, 15 to 30 mg, or an equivalent may be given for sleep. (4) Derangements potentially contributing to arrhythmias, such as hypoxemia, hypovolemia, disturbances of acid-base balance or of electrolytes, and drug toxicity, should be identified and corrected.

CONTROL OF CARDIAC PAIN

The alleviation or reduction of pain is a critical factor in the care of patients with AMI.[429] Since the pain associated with MI is related to ongoing ischemia (p. 1201), many interventions that act to improve the oxygen supply-demand relationship (by either increasing supply or decreasing demand) may lessen the pain associated with AMI.

NITRATES. As long as hypotension (systolic pressure <100 mm Hg or a decline of >25 mm Hg from the patient's normal pressure) is not present, careful administration of nitrates may lessen pain. Once it is ascertained that hypotension is not present, a sublingual nitroglycerin tablet should be administered and the patient observed carefully for improvement in symptoms or change in hemodynamics. If an initial dose is well tolerated and appears to be of benefit, further nitrates should be administered, with careful monitoring of the vital signs. However, long-acting nitrate preparations should be avoided in the very early course of AMI. In patients with a prolonged period of waxing and waning chest pain, intravenous nitroglycerin may be of benefit in controlling symptoms and correcting ischemia, but careful monitoring of blood pressure is required.[430] Nitrates should be used cautiously in patients with inferior wall infarction because even small doses may produce sudden hypotension and bradycardia; a reaction that can be life-threatening can usually be easily reversed with intravenous atropine if it is recognized quickly.[431] In patients with suspected right ventricular myocardial infarction, nitrates should be used with *extreme caution*, if at all, since these patients may be particularly sensitive to the venodilating effects of the drug, with sudden hypotension resulting from inadequate right ventricular filling.[432]

ANALGESICS. Although a wide variety of analgesic agents has been used to treat the pain associated with MI, including meperidine, pentazocine, and morphine,[429] the last-named agent remains the drug of choice except in patients with well-documented morphine hypersensitivity. Four to 8 mg should be administered intravenously and doses of 2 to 8 mg repeated at intervals of 5 to 15 minutes until the pain is relieved or evident toxicity—i.e., hypotension, depression of respiration, or severe vomiting—precludes further administration of the drug. In some patients, remarkably large cumulative doses of morphine (2 to 3 mg/kg) may be required and are usually tolerated.

The reduction of anxiety resulting from morphine diminishes the patient's restlessness and the activity of the autonomic nervous system, with a consequent reduction of the heart's metabolic demands. The beneficial effect of morphine in patients with pulmonary edema is unequivocal (p. 563) and may relate to several factors, including peripheral arterial and venous dilatation (particularly among patients with excessive sympathoadrenal activity), reduction of the work of breathing, and slowing of heart rate secondary to combined withdrawal of sympathetic tone and augmentation of vagal tone.[433]

Hypotension following the administration of morphine can be minimized by maintaining the patient in a supine position and elevating the lower extremities if systolic arterial pressure declines below 100 mm Hg. Obviously, such positioning is undesirable in the presence of pulmonary edema, but morphine rarely produces hypotension under these circumstances. The concomitant administration of atropine in doses of 0.5 to 1.5 mg intravenously may be helpful in reducing the excessive vagomimetic effects of morphine, particularly when hypotension and bradycardia are present before it is administered. Respiratory depression is an unusual complication of morphine in the presence of severe pain or pulmonary edema, but as the patient's cardiovascular status improves, impairment of ventilation may supervene and should be watched for. It can be treated with naloxone, in doses of 0.1 to 0.2 mg intravenously initially, repeated after 15 minutes if necessary. Nausea and vomiting may be troublesome side effects of large doses of morphine and may be treated with a phenothiazine to avoid marked stress on the circulation.

Other analgesics such as meperidine are less effective than is morphine but equally likely to produce side effects and prone to augment ventricular rate.

OXYGEN. Hypoxemia is common in patients with AMI and is usually secondary to ventilation-perfusion abnormalities[434] that are sequelae of left ventricular failure; pneumonia and intrinsic pulmonary disease are additional causes of hypoxemia. It is common practice to treat all patients hospitalized with AMI with oxygen for 24 to 48 hours, based on the common occurrence of arterial hypoxemia and clinical[435] evidence that increased oxygen in the inspired air may protect ischemic myocardium. However, augmentation of the fraction of oxygen in the inspired air does not elevate oxygen delivery significantly in patients who are not hypoxemic. Furthermore, it may increase systemic vascular resistance and arterial pressure and thereby lower cardiac output slightly.

In view of these considerations, arterial oxygen tension may be estimated or measured at the time of the patient's admission to the coronary care unit; oxygen therapy may be omitted if it is normal. On the other hand, oxygen should be administered to patients with AMI when arterial hypoxemia is clinically evident or can be documented by measurement. In these patients, serial arterial blood gas measurements may be employed to follow the efficacy of oxygen therapy. Although patients with AMI may exhibit a reduction in precordial ST-segment elevation during 100 per cent oxygen breathing, no long-term effect on survival or on the development of complications has been documented.[435]

In general, the delivery of 2 to 4 liters/min of 100 per cent oxygen by mask or nasal prongs for 2 to 3 days is satisfactory for most patients with mild hypoxemia. If arterial oxygenation is still depressed on this regimen, the flow rate may have to be increased, and other causes for hypoxemia should be sought. In patients with pulmonary edema, endotracheal intubation and positive-pressure controlled ventilation may be necessary.

BETA-ADRENOCEPTOR BLOCKERS. Beta blocking agents have been used in the early hours of AMI in attempts to limit the size of the infarct (p. 1236). In the course of these studies, it has been recognized that beta blockers relieve pain and reduce the need for analgesics in many patients, presumably by reducing ischemia.[436] Patients most suited for the use of beta blockers early in the course of AMI are those who also have sinus tachycardia and hypertension, since beta blockers will improve the heart rate and blood pressure, thereby lowering myocardial oxygen demand. A popular and relatively safe protocol for the use of a beta blocker in this situation is as follows: (1) Patients with heart failure, hypotension, bradycardia, or heart block are first excluded. (2) Metoprolol is given in three 5-mg boluses. (3) Patients are observed for *2 to 5 minutes* after each bolus and if heart rate falls below 60 beats per minute, or systolic blood pressure falls below 100 mm Hg, no further drug is given; a total of three intravenous doses (15 mg) are administered. (4) If hemodynamic stability continues, 6 to 8 hours later the patient is begun on oral metoprolol 50 mg for one day, then advanced to 100 mg twice daily if the lower dose is well tolerated. An extremely short-acting beta blocker, esmolol, may also be useful and even safer than other currently available drugs.[436]

Unlike beta blockers, calcium antagonists are of little if any value in AMI and may be hazardous.[436a]

PHYSICAL ACTIVITY. In the absence of all complications, patients with AMI need not be confined to bed for more than 24 to 36 hours and, unless they are hemodynamically compromised, they may use a bedside commode from the time of admission. Progression of activity regimens should be individualized depending upon patients' clinical status, age, and physical capacity. A typical patient may sit in a chair for two half-hour periods on the second and for two one-hour periods or more on the third day. If arrhythmia, heart failure, and other significant complications have not occurred or if they are controlled, the patient may be transferred out of the coronary care unit after 2 to 3 days. Monitoring for at least an additional two days, and usually more, in an intermediate care unit is desirable.

In patients without hemodynamic compromise, early ambulation—including dangling feet on the side of the bed, sitting in a chair, standing, and walking around the bed—does not cause important changes in heart rate, blood pressure, or pulmonary wedge pressure.[437] While heart rate increases slightly (usually by less than 10 per cent), pulmonary wedge pressures fall slightly as the patient assumes the upright posture for activities. Early ambulatory activities are only rarely associated with any symptoms, and when symptoms do occur, they generally are related to hypotension. Thus, when Levine and Lown proposed the "armchair" treatment of AMI in the 1950's, they were undoubtedly correct that stress to the myocardium is less in the upright position.[438] As long as blood pressure and heart rate are monitored carefully, early ambulation offers considerable psychological and physical benefit without any clear medical risk.

HEMODYNAMIC ASSESSMENT

Major advances in the management of AMI have resulted from the hemodynamic monitoring that has become widespread in coronary care units.[439,440] This often consists of both an intraarterial catheter and a pulmonary artery catheter. The former is usually inserted into the radial artery for continuous monitoring of systemic pressure and for sampling for blood gas determination. Pulmonary artery catheterization is accomplished with a balloon-tipped flotation catheter, often advanced, with fluoroscopic guidance, from a peripheral or internal jugular vein through the right heart and into the pulmonary artery. Judicious positioning of the catheter allows recording of the pulmonary capillary wedge pressure when the balloon is inflated.[439] Blood may be sampled from the tip of the catheter in the pulmonary artery and, in some catheters, from a second lumen opening into the right atrium. Pulmonary artery balloon catheters with a thermistor near the tip for recording thermodilution measurements of cardiac output are used frequently.[441] Thus, a single catheter in the right heart can yield the following information: saturation of blood in the pulmonary artery and right atrium, pressures in the pulmonary artery, pulmonary wedge position, and right atrium and cardiac output. A good correlation exists between pulmonary artery wedge pressure (which is equal to pulmonary capillary pressure) and left ventricular diastolic pressure in patients with AMI.

Balloon-tipped catheters are now available with a fiberoptic bundle for transmission of light. By connecting this catheter to an oximeter, continuous pulmonary artery venous blood oxygen saturation can be monitored.[442]

In the past, central venous or right atrial pressure was used to gauge the degree of *left* ventricular failure in patients with AMI. However, this technique is fraught with error, since central venous pressure actually reflects *right* rather than left ventricular function. Right ventricular function, and therefore systemic venous pressure, may be normal or nearly so in patients with significant left ventricular failure.[440] Conversely, patients with right ventricular failure due to right ventricular infarction or pulmonary embolism may exhibit elevated right atrial and central venous pressures despite normal left ventricular function.[443] Low values for right atrial and central venous pressures imply hypovolemia, whereas elevated right atrial pressures usually result from right ventricular failure secondary to left ventricular failure, pulmonary hypertension, or right ventricular infarction, or less commonly from tricuspid regurgitation or pericardial tamponade.

The prognosis and the clinical status are related to both the cardiac output and the pulmonary artery wedge pressure. Patients with normal cardiac output after AMI have an extremely low expected mortality; prognosis worsens as cardiac output declines. Patients with cardiac indices in the range of 2.7 to 4.3 liters/min/sq meter usually have no clinical signs of impaired perfusion, whereas patients with cardiac indices ranging from 1.8 to 2.2 liters/min/sq meter demonstrate early signs of hypoperfusion (cool skin and decreasing urine output and mental acuity). Patients whose cardiac index is less than 1.8 liters/min/sq meter are usually in shock. The pulmonary artery wedge pressure reflects the state of left ventricular filling, its compliance, and its ability to empty. As pulmonary pressure rises, progressive increases in pulmonary congestion occur. Mortality is greater for patients with elevated pulmonary wedge pressures.[444]

Patients with intraventricular conduction defects or AV block or both after *anterior* infarction have lower cardiac indices and higher pulmonary capillary wedge pressures than do patients without these conduction disturbances. On the other hand, patients with these conduction defects and *inferior* myocardial infarction usually do not demonstrate such hemodynamic abnormalities.

PULMONARY ARTERY CATHETERIZATION (Table 39–4). Before inserting a pulmonary artery catheter into a patient with an AMI, the physician must decide that the potential benefit of the information to be obtained outweighs any potential risks. Complications from pulmonary artery catheters are relatively rare, but severe problems can occur, including sepsis, pulmonary infarction, and pulmonary artery rupture. By minimization of the duration of catheterization and by adherence to careful sterile techniques, risk can be diminished.[445] Accurate determination of hemodynamics by clinical assessment is difficult in critically ill patients. The use of a pulmonary artery catheter often leads to important changes in therapy that would not have occurred if the hemodynamic information had not been available.[446] Some believe, however, that the pulmonary artery catheter is often overused. It has been suggested that until clinical trials assessing its benefit are performed, the use of this technique should be curbed.[447,448] (At least one such trial has suggested that complications and mortality are actually higher in patients who received pulmonary artery catheterization,[449] although such patients might have been at higher risk initially.) This view emphasizes the importance of careful patient selection, meticulous technique, and correct interpretation of the data obtained.

TABLE 39–4 INDICATIONS FOR HEMODYNAMIC MONITORING OF AMI

Management of complicated AMI
  Hypovolemia vs. cardiogenic shock
  Ventricular septal rupture vs. acute mitral regurgitation
  Severe left ventricular failure
  Right ventricular failure
Refractory ventricular tachycardia
Differentiating severe pulmonary disease from left ventricular failure
Assessment of cardiac tamponade
Assessment of therapy in *selected* individuals
  Afterload reduction in patients with severe left ventricular failure
  Inotropic agents
  Beta blockers
  Temporary pacing (ventricular vs. atrioventricular)
  Intraaortic balloon counterpulsation
  Mechanical ventilation

From Gore, J. M., and Zwernet, P. L.: Hemodynamic monitoring of acute myocardial infarction. In Francis, G. S., and Alpert, J. S. (eds.): Modern Coronary Care. Boston, Little, Brown & Co., 1990, p. 138.

Patients most likely to benefit from pulmonary artery catheter monitoring include those whose AMI is complicated by: (1) hypotension that is not easily corrected by fluid administration; (2) hypotension in the presence of congestive heart failure; (3) hemodynamic compromise severe enough to require intravenous vasopressors or vasodilators or intraaortic balloon counterpulsation; and (4) mechanical lesions (or suspected ones) such as cardiac tamponade, severe mitral regurgitation, and a ruptured ventricular septum.[445]

THE INTERMEDIATE CORONARY CARE UNIT

Since the hazard of *primary* ventricular fibrillation is essentially over in 24 to 36 hours, there is little need for patients with entirely *uncomplicated* infarction to remain in a coronary care unit for more than 1 to 2 days. Obviously, patients with complicated infarction, particularly those with arrhythmias, pump failure, and recurrent ischemia, require continued care in such a unit. Patients who have undergone reperfusion and may be at risk of recurrent infarction also may require an extra day or so in the intensive cardiac care unit. There is an increased risk of ventricular tachycardia and ventricular fibrillation in the late MI period, particularly among patients with impaired left ventricular function or anterior infarction, accounting for between 10 and 30 per cent of total hospital deaths.[450] Recurrent ischemia or infarction also places such patients at increased risk.[451] In view of this significant in-hospital mortality after discharge from the coronary care unit, continued surveillance in intermediate coronary care units (also called step-down units) is justifiable. In fact, patients at an extremely low risk for complications should be considered as candidates for initial direct admission to such a facility.[425]

Risk factors for mortality in the hospital *after* discharge from the coronary care unit include intraventricular conduction defects,[452] sinus tachycardia persisting for more than 2 days, extensive anterior infarction, episodes of ventricular fibrillation and of atrial flutter or fibrillation occurring while the patient is in the coronary care unit, early recurrent angina and marked electrocardiographic ST-segment abnormalities induced by low levels of activity.[453,454] It is possible that a reduction in late hospital mortality can be achieved with the use of intermediate coronary care units, which permit prolonged continuous monitoring of the electrocardiogram and prompt, effective treatment of ventricular fibrillation and other serious arrhythmias. The availability of these units may be useful also in helping to identify those patients who remain free from complications for a minimum of one week, since early discharge from the hospital appears to be feasible for this subset.[455]

EARLY REHABILITATION (see p. 1263 and Chap. 42). Following myocardial infarction, patients are often eager for information, in need of reassurance, confused by misinformation and prior impressions, capable of counterproductive denial, and simply frightened. Cardiac rehabilitation should be carefully structured and often requires a considerable period of time, optimally beginning as early as possible once the patient is no longer in extreme danger. Intermediate care facilities provide ideal settings and ample opportunities to begin the rehabilitation process. Although intermediate care units were introduced for the purpose of decreasing mortality after coronary care unit discharge, studies have not shown any conclusive benefit in that regard.[456,457] Nevertheless, the capacity for the early detection of problems following AMI and the social and educational benefits of grouping such patients together strongly argue for continued utilization of the concept of intermediate coronary care. Furthermore, the economic advantage of grouping such patients together for sharing of resources, in terms of improving utilization of coronary care units and possibly for facilitating early discharge, outweighs any questions raised by the lack of a clear consensus regarding reduced mortality. An additional potential advantage that should not be underestimated is facilitation of patient education in a group setting with formal lectures and various types of audiovisual programs.

LIMITATION OF INFARCT SIZE

Infarct size is an important determinant of prognosis in patients with AMI.[458] Patients who succumb from cardiogenic shock generally exhibit massive infarcts.[459,460] Early impairment of ventricular function, presaging a poor prognosis, is correlated with extensive infarcts.[460,461] Survivors with large infarcts frequently exhibit late impairment of ventricular function, and the long-term mortality rate is higher than that for survivors with small infarcts (Fig. 39–17), who tend not to develop cardiac decompensation.[461-463] The occurrence of various manifestations and complications of AMI as well as the need for special treatments is also related to infarct size.[458] The influence of infarct size on mortality is most apparent during the patient's hospital course and in the first few months after infarction. The hospital mortality in patients with large infarcts, as estimated by technetium pyrophosphate scanning, is several times greater than it is in patients with small infarcts.[462] However, the importance of infarct size declines somewhat with time after the initial episode[463]; after recovery from an AMI it is the quantity of remaining myocardium whose viability is threatened because it is perfused by obstructed coronary vessels that becomes crucial to the prognosis.

In view of the prognostic importance of infarct size, the concept that modification of infarct size is possible has attracted a great deal of experimental and clinical attention over the past 2 decades.[17,18,464-466] Efforts to limit the size of the infarct have been divided among three different (sometimes overlapping) approaches: early reperfusion, reduction of myocardial energy demands, and stimulation of anaerobic energy production.[467] Before these areas are considered in more detail, issues concerning the infarction process and general clinical measures are discussed.

THE DYNAMIC NATURE OF INFARCTION. AMI is a dynamic process that often does not occur instantaneously but sometimes evolves relatively slowly, i.e., over a matter of hours (Fig. 39–18). As has been pointed out (p. 1190), in experimental animals the fate of jeopardized, ischemic tissue may be affected favorably by interventions that restore perfusion, reduce myocardial oxygen requirements, inhibit accumula-

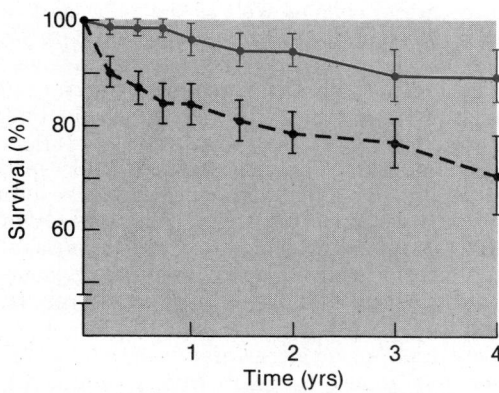

FIGURE 39–17. The influence of the extent of initial myocardial infarction on survival. Survival is shown after initial myocardial infarction in a total of 173 patients with infarct size index (expressed in terms of CK-gram-equivalents/m²) of < 15 (solid line) vs. ≥ 15 (interrupted line). Brackets indicate standard errors. The graph depicts survival curves for all patients who survived for at least 24 hours after the onset of an initial myocardial infarction. Survival was significantly greater for patients with small compared with large infarcts (P < 0.05). (From Geltman, E. M., et al.: The influence of location and extent of myocardial infarction on long-term ventricular dysrhythmia and mortality. Circulation 60:805, 1979, by permission of the American Heart Association, Inc.)

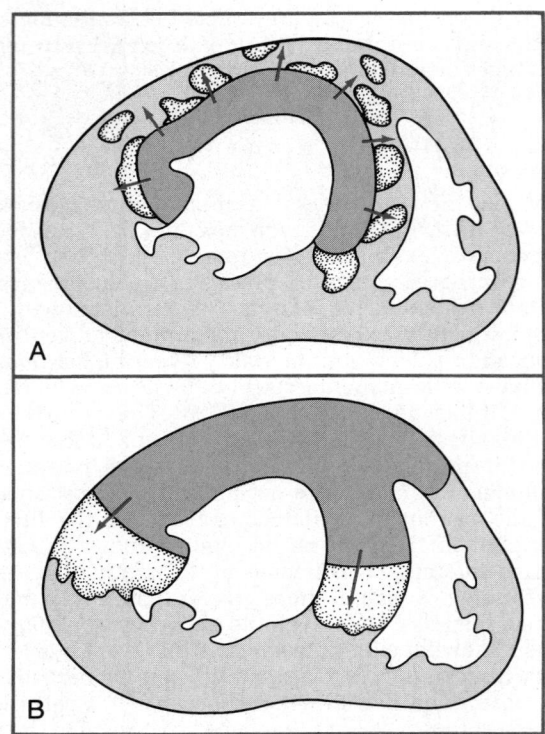

FIGURE 39–18. Two types of extension of myocardial infarction. Type A (*A*) was observed at the edges of an infarct, usually subepicardially. Type B (*B*) occurred at the lateral margins. (From Alonso, D. R., et al.: Pathophysiology of cardiogenic shock: Quantification of myocardial necrosis, clinical, pathological and electrocardiographic correlation. Circulation 48:588, 1973, by permission of the American Heart Association, Inc.)

tion or facilitate washout of noxious metabolites, augment the availability of substrate for anaerobic metabolism,[17,18,464,465,467] or blunt the effects of mediators of injury such as calcium or oxygen free radicals,[468–470,470a] metabolites, and constituents of cell membranes.[471,472]

The perfusion of the myocardium associated with AMI appears to be reduced maximally immediately following coronary occlusion. In experimental animals, increases in blood flow to the peripheral portions of the ischemic zones become evident within 24 hours of acute coronary occlusion,[472] suggesting that dynamic factors contribute to the early limitation of perfusion. These may include the efflux of potassium from injured myocardial cells as well as the release of catecholamines as a consequence of ischemia of adrenergic neurons (and the resultant vasospasm). Spasm of coronary vessels has been implicated not only in Prinzmetal's variant angina (p. 1342) but also in association with the more common forms of MI involving atherosclerosis,[473,474] as well as in patients experiencing postinfarction angina at rest.[475] While spasm may play a contributory role in enhancing infarct size, other than in patients with Prinzmetal's angina it is unlikely to be the *principal* cause. While coronary spasm might play a role at the inception of coronary occlusion, by the time an angiogram is performed intracoronary nitroglycerin very rarely results in reperfusion.

Relatively prompt, *partial* restoration of reduced blood flow to the ischemic zone may result from spontaneous thrombolysis, from relief of coronary spasm (see above), or from improved systemic hemodynamics; the last factor includes augmented coronary perfusion pressure and reduced left ventricular end-diastolic pressure. Subsequently, perfusion of the jeopardized zone may be enhanced by the development of collateral circulation.[476] The prompt implementation of measures designed to protect ischemic myocardium and support myocardial perfusion may provide sufficient time for the development of anatomical and physiological compensatory mechanisms that limit the ultimate extent of infarction.

AMI in hospitalized patients may be complicated by extension of infarction or early reinfarction (p. 1262). Depending on the criteria utilized for detection, the incidence of these complications ranges from 8 to 30 per cent.[477] It is possible that interventions designed to protect ischemic myocardium during the initial event may also reduce the incidence of extension of infarction or early reinfarction. On the other hand, it has been suggested that preservation of ischemic myocardium could lead to persistent survival of cells in regions subjected to repetitive episodes of severe ischemia, leading to the development of arrhythmias. The relatively poor *late* prognosis of patients with non-Q-wave infarction[478,479] is consistent with this possibility. However, despite these hazards, there is no evidence that the implementation of interventions designed to protect ischemic myocardium results in any late deleterious effects. Furthermore, it has been reported that preservation of ischemic myocardium by trimethaphan in hypertensive patients with evolving infarction,[480] by intravenous nitroglycerin in normotensive patients,[481] and by the early administration of beta-adrenoceptor blocking agents[482–484] is actually associated with a reduced rather than an increased mortality.

Proof of the clinical efficacy of specific interventions has been difficult to acquire, in part because of the wide variations in the size of infarcts and their rate of evolution, in part because of the difficulties involved in measuring infarct size, and in part because it is difficult to predict what size any given infarct would have attained had the intervention under study not taken place.

ROUTINE MEASURES FOR INFARCT SIZE LIMITATION

Recognition that the ultimate size of a myocardial infarct does not depend solely on the pathological anatomy of the coronary vascular bed (which supplies oxygen) but is also affected by a variety of physiological variables (which determine the heart's demands for oxygen) suggests emphasis on a number of principles to be considered in the routine care of AMI. It is mandatory to maintain an optimal balance between myocardial oxygen supply and demand so that as much of the jeopardized zone of the myocardium surrounding the most profoundly ischemic zones of the infarct can be salvaged. During the period before irreversible injury has occurred, myocardial oxygen consumption should be minimized by maintaining the patient at rest, physically and emotionally, and by utilizing mild sedation and a quiet atmosphere that may lower heart rate, a major determinant of myocardial oxygen consumption. If the patient was receiving a beta-adrenoceptor blocking agent at the time the clinical manifestations of the infarction commenced, the drug should not be discontinued unless a specific contraindication develops, such as left ventricular systolic failure or bradyarrhythmia. Marked sinus bradycardia (heart rate less than approximately 50 beats/min) and the frequently coexisting hypotension should be treated with postural maneuvers (the reverse Trendelenburg position) to increase central blood volume and atropine or electrical pacing, but *not* with isoproterenol. On the other hand, the *routine* administration of atropine, with the resultant increase in heart rate, to patients without serious bradycardia is contraindicated. All forms of tachyarrhythmias require prompt and direct treatment, since they increase myocardial oxygen needs.

Diuretics are the first line of drugs indicated in the treatment of congestive heart failure. If they prove insufficient, vasodilators should be added,[485] unless the patient is already hypotensive. Inotropic agents such as cardioactive sympathomimetics or the phosphodiesterase inhibitor amrinone (p. 503) should be added only if there is evidence of persistent and severe ventricular failure despite diuretics and vasodilators; these agents should *not* be given prophylactically. Of the various sympathomimetic amines available, isoproterenol with its chronotropic and vasodilator effects is the most hazardous.

Dobutamine (or small doses of dopamine) (p. 502), which has less effect on heart rate and systemic vascular resistance than does norepinephrine, epinephrine, or isoproterenol, is the drug of choice when cardiac contractility *must* be augmented.

Particular attention must be paid to preserving arterial oxygenation in patients with hypoxemia, such as occurs in patients with chronic pulmonary disease, pneumonia, or left ventricular failure. Oxygen-enriched air should be administered to patients with hypoxemia, and bronchodilators and expectorants should be used when indicated. Severe anemia, which can also extend the area of ischemic injury, should be corrected by the cautious administration of packed red cells, accompanied by a diuretic if there is any evidence of left ventricular failure. Associated conditions, particularly infections and the accompanying tachycardia, fever, and elevated myocardial oxygen needs, require immediate attention.

Systolic arterial pressure should not be allowed to deviate by more than approximately 25 to 30 mm Hg from the patient's usual level, unless marked hypertension had been present before the AMI. It is likely that each patient has an optimum level of arterial pressure; as coronary perfusion pressure deviates from this level, the unfavorable balance between oxygen supply (which is related to coronary perfusion pressure) and myocardial oxygen demand (which is related to ventricular wall tension) that ensues will increase the extent of ischemic injury.

Rather than simply maintaining the patient's vital signs, the physician's attention should be directed toward controlling ischemia and preserving the myocardium as well as maintaining perfusion of peripheral organs. However, these two objects may sometimes conflict. In the first 4 hours after the onset of the clinical event, when the ultimate size of the infarct may not yet have been established definitively, myocardial preservation should ordinarily be given the highest priority. This may mean foregoing the stimulation of cardiac contractility by inotropic agents. Later, once the size of the infarct is fixed and if heart failure supervenes, it may be appropriate to stimulate the heart with positive inotropic agents, i.e., to employ an intervention that might have increased infarct size if given at an earlier time.

In some patients, particularly those with cardiogenic shock, tissue damage occurs in a "stuttering" manner with persistent release of CK into the bloodstream rather than abruptly, a condition that might more properly be termed *subacute infarction*.[460] This concept of the dynamic nature of the infarction process as well as the observation that the incidence of complications of AMI in both the early and late postinfarction periods is a function of infarct size[458,463] greatly expands the horizon for what can *potentially* be accomplished by techniques to limit myocardial necrosis.

REPERFUSION OF MYOCARDIAL INFARCTION

One of the two most important developments in the treatment of patients with AMI since Herrick's description of the syndrome 80 years ago[46] consists of establishing reperfusion of ischemic heart muscle in the early hours of myocardial infarction.[486] (The second is the prevention and treatment of life-threatening arrhythmias.) While reperfusion occurs spontaneously in some patients,[280] this may not occur early enough to salvage ischemic myocardium, and in any event it is now well recognized that a persistent thrombotic occlusion is present in the majority of patients with AMI while the myocardium is undergoing necrosis.[56] Efforts to recanalize an occluded coronary artery by pharmacological and/or mechanical means have been increasingly successful. Timely reperfusion of jeopardized myocardium clearly represents the most effective way of restoring the balance between myocardial oxygen supply and demand. When carried out within the first several hours after coronary occlusion in several species of experimental animals, reperfusion improves hemodynamics and decreases infarct size, as assessed by both indirect

techniques (epicardial ST-segment recordings, precordial QRS maps, myocardial CK depletion, and positron-emission tomography) and direct techniques (morphology).[487-490] The extent of protection appears to be directly related to the rapidity with which reperfusion is implemented after the onset of coronary occlusion.[491]

While surgical reperfusion by coronary artery bypass grafting has been undertaken with variable success since the early 1970's,[492] the current era of nonsurgical reperfusion was launched by the pioneering effects of Chazov[493] and Rentrop[494] and their collaborators. These investigators demonstrated successful reperfusion of an occluded coronary artery by the intracoronary infusion of a thrombolytic agent, sometimes in conjunction with recanalization by means of a guidewire. Many different therapeutic approaches are now available to the clinician.[21] Much clinical research is currently directed at deciding on optimal reperfusion strategies and at understanding ancillary clinical issues such as patient selection, follow-up noninvasive testing, and the need for additional secondary preventive measures involving anticoagulants, antiplatelet agents, and revascularization.[495]

PATHOPHYSIOLOGY OF MYOCARDIAL REPERFUSION

By delivering oxygen to ischemic muscle, reperfusion has the potential to relieve ischemia. Prevention of cell death by the restoration of blood flow depends on the severity and duration of preexisting ischemia. Substantial experimental evidence for this concept[496] is supported by clinical studies showing that recovery of left ventricular systolic function,[497-499] improvement in diastolic function,[500] and reduction in overall mortality[466,501,502] are more favorably influenced, the earlier that blood flow is restored. Collateral coronary vessels also appear to play a role in the successful restoration of left ventricular function following reperfusion.[503] Collaterals are probably of greater importance in patients having reperfusion later than with reperfusion 1 to 2 hours after coronary artery occlusion; they provide sufficient perfusion of the myocardium to retard cell death.

REPERFUSION INJURY (see p. 1191). A specific form of reperfusion injury has been described as cell death that occurs following reperfusion in tissue that previously had been ischemic but not necessarily irreversibly damaged.[469,504,504a] Thus reperfusion may be a "double-edged sword."[505] On the one hand, blood flow must be restored to salvage ischemic myocardium, but it is possible, although not yet unequivocally established, that the process of restoring flow may damage cells not yet irreversibly injured. Reperfusion does increase the cell swelling that occurs with ischemia,[469,506] and this alone or with the condition known as the "no-reflow" phenomenon (impingement of swollen cells on the restoring of flow at the microvascular level[506]) could potentially lead to cellular injury. Available evidence indicates that, while reperfusion may accelerate necrosis of irreversibly injured myocytes, it does not add substantially to the area of myocardium ultimately damaged, for such cells are already destined to die.[507] Reperfusion of myocardium in which the microvasculature is damaged leads to the creation of a hemorrhagic infarct.[496,508] Reperfusion by means of thrombolytic therapy appears more likely to produce hemorrhagic infarction than reperfusion by mechanical means.[508] While concern has been raised that this hemorrhage may lead to extension of the infarct, this does not appear to be the case.[505,509] Histological study of patients not surviving in spite of successful reperfusion has revealed hemorrhagic infarcts, but this hemorrhage usually does *not* extend beyond the area of necrosis.[508-510] Necrosis in reperfused myocardium generally is of the contraction band type rather than the coagulation necrosis type seen after AMI.[510]

The sudden exposure of severely ischemic cells to both calcium and oxygen with the restoration of flow has been observed to affect the severity of ischemic damage.[504,505,510a] Toxicity from oxygen-derived free radicals, mediated at least in part by stimulated leukocytes, has attracted considerable attention[469,505,511] for its possible role in extending myocardial injury. Although unsupported by clinical evidence as of this writing, future therapy, likely to be carried out with reperfusion, may well include administration of agents that reduce leukocyte activation and scavenge oxygen free radicals. In addition, drugs such as beta-adrenoceptor blockers and verapamil, which *delay* the death of ischemic cells, may, if administered prophylactically to patients at high risk of occlusion (or reocclusion) or in the earliest phases of the development of an AMI, enhance the quantity of myocardium salvaged by early reperfusion.[512,513]

Reperfusion frequently causes changes in the cardiac rhythm. Transient sinus bradycardia occurs in many patients with inferior infarcts at the time of acute reperfusion; it is most often accompanied by some degree of hypotension. This combination of hypotension and bradycardia with a sudden increase in coronary flow has been ascribed to the Bezold-Jarisch reflex.[514] Premature ventricular contractions are the most common arrhythmia noted at the time of reperfusion, but these are frequent in all patients with AMI and it is not clear whether or not reperfusion actually increases their incidence. An accelerated idioventricular rhythm and ventricular tachycardia are more common acutely after successful reperfusion than after failed therapy.[515] When present, these rhythm disturbances may actually be a marker of successful restoration of coronary flow.[516] In general, clinical features are poor markers of reperfusion, with no single clinical finding or constellation of findings being reliably predictive of angiographically demonstrated coronary artery patency.[517] Nevertheless, the need for treatment of arrhythmias should be anticipated in any patient receiving therapy designed to recanalize a totally occluded coronary artery in the setting of AMI. Occasionally, reperfusion may actually lessen the severity of ventricular arrhythmias due to ongoing ischemia, or of heart block associated with an AMI.[518]

It has been suggested that improved survival and ventricular function after successful reperfusion are not due to limitation of infarct size alone.[181,495,519-521,521a] In addition to the possibility that early reperfusion may actually *prevent* AMI[519] and probably improves the electrical stability of the heart as noted earlier,[521b] the benefit of a patent artery may include a favorable effect on ventricular remodeling (p. 1210), improved diastolic function,[500] a lower incidence of cardiac rupture,[486,509] provision of collateral flow,[486,520] and later improvement in systolic left ventricular function.[521,522] Further support of this theory comes from information suggesting improved survival even when reperfusion occurs *after* the time period in which myocardial salvage could be anticipated. Therefore, it is reasonable to reexamine the width of the "time window"[490,491] previously thought to limit the benefit of reperfusion, but it is inappropriate to conclude that anything but maximum efforts should be applied to reducing the time interval between onset of clinical manifestations of AMI and institution of reperfusion therapy.[520]

CORONARY THROMBOLYSIS

Many years elapsed between the first report of intracoronary clot lysis in an experimental animal[524] and the widespread use of thrombolytic agents in AMI, even though the feasibility of such an approach was demonstrated as early as 1958.[525] It was not until relatively recently that the knowledge that coronary thrombosis is responsible for the initiation and/or the perpetuation of myocardial infarction (p. 1780) *and* the discovery that in most cases administration of thrombolytic agents restores angiographic patency to coronary vessels[57,81,493,526-528] sparked interest in the potential value of clot lysis in salvaging jeopardized tissue and limiting the extent of injury sustained in patients with evolving myocardial infarction. A large European trial in the late 1970's demonstrated that intravenous streptokinase reduced mortality at 6 months if given within 12 hours of AMI.[529] By the early 1980's reports of the use of thrombolytic agents in AMI became frequent. With publication of the first GISSI trial of over 11,000 patients in 1986,[512] in which intravenous streptokinase resulted in a significant reduction in mortality in patients treated within 6 hours of the onset of symptoms, the routine use of thrombolytic therapy in AMI was established. It is now clear that thrombolysis recanalizes thrombotic occlusion associated with the majority of cases, restoration of coronary flow improves myocardial function, and mortality is reduced.[530]

INTRACORONARY THROMBOLYSIS

Clinical investigation in the area of pharmacological reperfusion of ischemic myocardium initially focused on the use of *intracoronary* thrombolysis in the early hours of AMI (Fig. 39-19).[57,81,526,527] The fact that viability could be maintained in a portion of the successfully reperfused myocardium was reflected in studies showing the restoration of contractile activity.[155,498,507,528] On the basis of results of several successful trials, the Food and Drug Administration initially approved the use of *intracoronary* streptokinase and urokinase for the treatment of myocardial infarction.[507] Many factors affect the usefulness of this technique, which is dependent on the availability of a skilled catheterization team and well-equipped catheterization facility. Most reported experience with intracoronary thrombolysis has not been in both randomized and controlled trials, largely because it has been thought difficult to withhold thrombolytic therapy once a thrombotic coronary artery occlusion has been visualized angiographically, and it has not been considered ethical to catheterize patients if randomization to no thrombolytic therapy were possible for a portion of the patients. Because of the delay involved in catheterizing patients with AMI, current consensus is that intracoronary administration

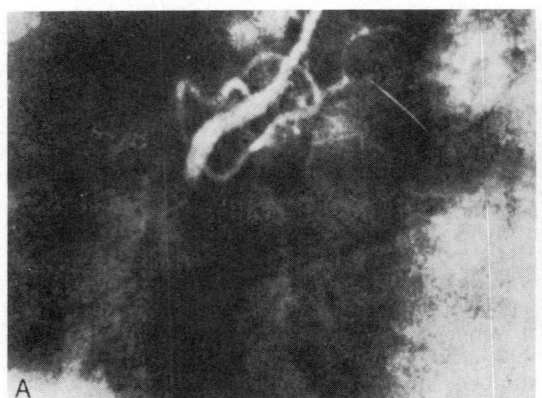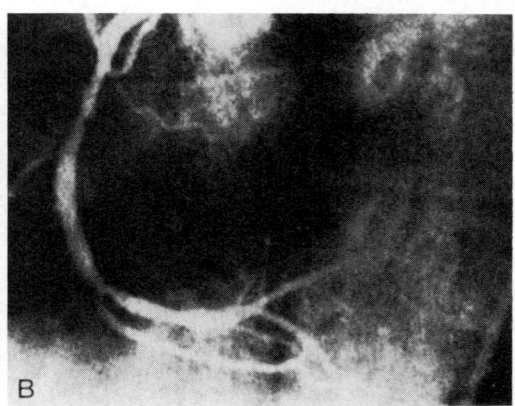

FIGURE 39-19. *A,* Complete occlusion of the right coronary artery in a 38-year-old man with evolving inferoposterolateral myocardial infarction. *B,* The artery was patent after 20 minutes of intracoronary streptokinase infusion. This arteriogram was taken after an additional infusion of streptokinase for 60 minutes, which further improved patency. (From Ganz, W., et al.: Intracoronary thrombolysis in evolving myocardial infarction. Am. Heart J. *101:*4, 1981.)

TABLE 39-5   OVERALL COMPARISON OF INTRAVENOUSLY ADMINISTERED STREPTOKINASE, RECOMBINANT TISSUE-TYPE PLASMINOGEN ACTIVATOR (rt-PA), AND ANISOYLATED PLASMINOGEN ACTIVATOR COMPLEX (APSAC)

1231

CHAP 39

FACTOR	STREPTOKINASE	rt-PA	APSAC
Usual dose	1.5 million U in 30–60 min	60 mg for first hour, 40 mg during hrs 2–3	30 mg in 5 min
Clot selectivity	None	Relative	Minor
Patency of infarct-related artery	50–60%	75–85%	60%
Time dependency	High; <30% after 4 h	None	?
Reocclusion	5–20%	10–20%	10–20%
Improvement of left ventricular function	Yes	Yes	Yes
Improvement of survival	Yes, in numerous trials	Yes, in two small trials	Yes
Hypotension	Severe in <5%	None	None
Half-life	Long	Short	Long
Allergic reactions	Yes	No	Yes
Fibrinogenolysis	Severe	Moderate	Severe
Periaccess bleeding	Common	Common	Common
Intracranial bleeding	<0.5%	<0.5%	<0.5%
Repeat dosing possible	No, because of antibodies	Yes	No
Patient cost/dose	$125	$2,800	$1,800

Data from references 486, 540, 573.
APSAC = anisoylated plasminogen streptokinase activator complex (Eminase).

of thrombolytic therapy should be reserved for patients who develop coronary thrombosis during the course of an angiographic procedure and in whom either a coronary catheter is already in place or such placement is easily and rapidly achieved.

Intravenous Thrombolysis

This form of thrombolytic therapy has several important advantages over intracoronary use. Since only the placement of a peripheral intravenous line is required, therapy may be initiated early, in a variety of locations (emergency room, ambulance, helicopter, or home[411,413]) and at relatively low cost. In fact, as already noted, intravenous streptokinase has been used in the treatment of AMI for decades, preceding our recent definitive knowledge that thrombosis is the focal event in initiating AMI. This subject has perhaps been one of the most rapidly evolving in the management of patients with AMI.

CHOICE OF AGENTS. Three thrombolytic agents, streptokinase, recombinant tissue-type plasminogen activator (rt-PA), and anisoylated plasminogen streptokinase activator complex (APSAC), are currently approved by the Food and Drug Administration for intravenous use in patients with AMI (Chap. 58) (Table 39–5). By far the greatest international experience has been accumulated with streptokinase, in part owing to its low cost and demonstrated efficacy in reducing mortality in very large trials.[466,502] The usual dose is 1.5 million units given over 1 hour. APSAC was developed in part to provide an agent with kinetics more favorable to sustain a thrombolytic effect, as the approved dose of 30 mg can be given over 2 to 5 minutes.[531] The initial hope that APSAC would be more fibrin clot–selective than streptokinase has not been borne out.[486,532] It appears to induce recanalization at a rate approaching that seen with *intracoronary* streptokinase.[531,533] It possesses the distinct advantage of allowing administration as a single bolus injection compared with continued intravenous infusion (for streptokinase or rt-PA).

Tissue plasminogen activator is an endogenously produced enzyme released from vascular endothelium as part of the body's defense against in vivo thrombosis (p. 1571).[533a,533b] Its isolation from a melanoma cell line led to later production by recombinant DNA techniques. Although the agent is expensive, it has received much attention as an "elegant product of the molecular biology revolution."[534] The currently approved dose is 100 mg, given as 60 mg in the first hour (of this, 6 to 10 mg is given as an initial bolus), followed by 20 mg per hour for the next 2 hours. Currently, different dosing strategies are being explored for improved efficacy and safety, as discussed below. Four relatively small trials have compared intrave-

nous streptokinase with rt-PA.[535–538] In the three trials employing early angiography, patency rate of the infarct-related artery was higher with rt-PA.[536–539] Although none of these studies showed reduced mortality with rt-PA, an analysis of pooled results suggests that mortality with streptokinase was 50 per cent greater than with rt-PA.[528,534] Additionally, pooled data from angiographic trials (of which there have been many) of streptokinase and rt-PA alone suggest a higher early patency rate with rt-PA.[540] However, the ultimate proof of superior efficacy depends on mortality trials that necessarily require many more patients. The results of one such trial (the International t-PA/SK Mortality Trial/GISSI 2) have recently been published.[263] Another (ISIS 3) has been presented[540a]; and one other large comparative trial (GUSTO) is under way. Both ISIS 3 and the International t-PA/SK Mortality Trial showed no significant difference in mortaity rates between the two agents.[263] However, in these trials, intravenous heparin was not administered early as it has been in most other trials with rt-PA, and this might have led to a lower early patency rate (as discussed below), thus diminishing its efficacy.

EFFECT ON MORTALITY. There is no doubt that early intravenous therapy with thrombolytic drugs improves survival in patients with AMI (Fig. 39–20). In fact, 30-day and 1-year mortality rates in some of the controlled trials are impressive, with survival in one treated group as high as 93.1 per cent at 12 months.[541] Mortality varies considerably depending on patients included for study and adjunctive therapies employed.[528] The benefit of thrombolytic therapy appears to be greatest when agents are administered as early as possible, with incremental benefit demonstrated if drug is administered less than 4 to 6 hours after the onset of pain, and even better results are seen when drug is given less than 1 to 2 hours after symptoms begin.[486,528] The impact of early treatment was first clearly shown in the initial GISSI trial[501] and confirmed in ISIS 2.[502] Although an analysis of patients treated 7 to 24 hours after symptom onset suggests a therapeutic benefit of thrombolysis as well, firm conclusions about the efficacy of such late therapy await the results of several ongoing placebo-controlled trials addressing this issue.

There has been debate about the relative benefit of thrombolytic therapy in inferior versus anterior myocardial infarction,[542] because, for example, initial results from the first GISSI trial showed no improvement in survival for inferior MI.[501] However, more careful analysis of data has subsequently shown that infarct *size* rather than *location* is the key variable, with no significant benefit in the smallest of infarcts, while the benefit (in terms of survival) increases with progressively larger infarcts.[501,543]

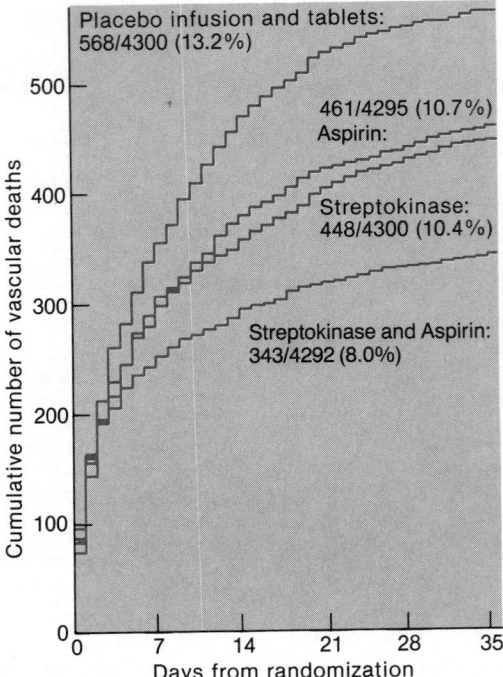

FIGURE 39–20. Cumulative vascular mortality (deaths from cardiac, cerebral, hemorrhagic, or other known vascular disease) in days 0–35 of the Second International Study of Infarct Survival (ISIS-2). The four curves describe mortality for patients allocated (i) active streptokinase only, (ii) active aspirin only, (iii) both active treatments, and (iv) neither. Note that individually, aspirin and streptokinase have a favorable effect of similar magnitudes, and that together the benefits appear additive. (From ISIS-2 [Second International Study of Infarct Survival] Collaborative Group: Randomized trial of intravenous streptokinase, oral aspirin, both, or neither among 17,187 cases of suspected acute myocardial infarction: ISIS-2. Lancet 2:349, 1988.)

A wide variety of other clinical benefits appear to accrue to patients treated with thrombolytic agents, including a reduction in ventricular arrhythmias,[486] asystole,[544] and cardiac arrest,[502] as well as a significantly lower incidence of cardiogenic shock.[544] Longer-term follow-up is now available from early trials.[545,546] Results indicate that the early favorable results of thrombolytic therapy are sustained over time, with one study showing that the benefit of a lower mortality is maintained over the 5-year follow-up.[546]

EFFECT ON LEFT VENTRICULAR FUNCTION. While precise measurements of infarct size would be an ideal endpoint for clinical reperfusion studies, such measures have been found to be impracticable. Trials have used the myocardial sparing as indirectly reflected in the preservation of left ventricular function as an important endpoint—one that is also well known to be prognostically important as well. As with survival, improvement in global left ventricular function is related to the time of thrombolytic treatment, with greatest improvement occurring with earliest therapy.[486,528,547] Improvement in left ventricular function is apparently greater with anterior than with inferior infarcts.[486] Trials have failed to demonstrate any difference in global left ventricular function when streptokinase and rt-PA were compared.[538,548,549] However, global ejection fraction is an imprecise measurement of ventricular function because hyperkinesis of noninvolved myocardium may prevent the reduction that would result from akinesis of the involved muscle. Regional left ventricular function of the ischemic myocardium has been shown to improve with streptokinase,[550] with APSAC,[551] and with rt-PA.[552] When regional wall motion was analyzed in a streptokinase versus rt-PA study, the latter appeared to be of greater benefit.[548] Reperfusion with either streptokinase or rt-PA appears to prevent some degree of late ventricular dilatation following AMI.[175,553] In many studies, the survival benefit appears to exceed measured improvements in ventricular

function.[547] This may reflect the impact on group data of survivors with markedly improved left ventricular function who would have died had they not been treated with a thrombolytic drug. In general, studies employing ventricular function as an endpoint have been much smaller than the survival trials and have at times included patients without Q-wave infarction in whom the benefit of thrombolytic therapy may well be produced by different mechanisms. Furthermore, as discussed on page 1267, long-term survival may be enhanced by long-term patency of the coronary artery as well as by diminished infarct size.

PATIENT SELECTION FOR THROMBOLYTIC THERAPY. In view of the established benefit of thrombolytic therapy, it is unfortunate that not more patients with AMI are being treated. Among patients presenting to emergency departments with MI, it has been estimated that 15 to 37 per cent are appropriate candidates for thrombolysis.[554-557] Firm recommendations cannot be made for the selection of patients in some instances. Most studies have excluded patients older than 70 to 75 years, yet among those that have included more elderly patients, thrombolytic therapy appears to be of benefit as judged from subgroup analysis.[501,502,558,559] In careful reviews of this subject, it was concluded that it is the elderly patient who may actually benefit most from thrombolytic therapy.[560,561] Patients with inferior, small, or prior infarcts have not been shown conclusively to benefit from thrombolytic therapy. Therapy should probably be reserved for those with at least a moderate amount of myocardium in jeopardy or otherwise at high risk (Table 39–6). The potential benefit of thrombolytic therapy in non-Q-wave MI is not yet clear but is currently under investigation. Finally, as already noted, the outside time limit for benefit is incompletely defined, and late therapy, while likely not to be universally helpful, should be considered for patients with clear evidence of ongoing ischemia.[561]

ADJUNCTIVE TREATMENT. Anticoagulants and antiplatelet therapy may play an important role in establishing and maintaining the success achieved by the use of thrombolytic drugs.[562a] The Second International Trial of Intravenous

TABLE 39–6
A) MORTALITY 6 WEEKS FOLLOWING THROMBOLYTIC THERAPY FOR EACH OF EIGHT RISK FACTORS IN 3261 PATIENTS*

RISK FACTOR	NO. OF PATIENTS WITH RISK FACTOR (%)	NO. OF DEATHS IN 6 WEEKS (%)
Age ≥70 years	374 (11.5)	42 (11.2)
Previous infarction	456 (13.7)	36 (7.9)
Anterior infarction	1681 (51.5)	94 (5.6)
Atrial fibrillation	66 (2.0)	7 (10.6)
Rales in more than one third of lung fields	105 (3.2)	13 (12.4)
Hypotension and sinus tachycardia	158 (4.8)	16 (10.1)
Female gender	577 (17.7)	41 (7.1)
Diabetes mellitus	425 (13.0)	36 (8.5)

B) MORTALITY 6 WEEKS FOLLOWING THROMBOLYTIC THERAPY ACCORDING TO NUMBER OF RISK FACTORS† PRESENT INITIALLY

NO. OF RISK FACTORS	NO. OF PATIENTS	NO. OF DEATHS WITHIN 6 WEEKS	MORTALITY RATE (%)
0	864	13	1.5
1	1384	32	2.3
2	689	48	7.0
3	231	30	13.0
≥4	93	16	17.2

* Seventy-eight patients with cardiogenic shock or pulmonary edema were excluded.

† Possible risk factors listed in A.

Data from analysis of patients enrolled in Phase II of the Thrombolysis in Myocardial Infarction (TIMI) trial. Hillis, L. D., Foreman, S., and Braunwald, E.: Risk stratification before thrombolytic therapy in patients with acute myocardial infarction. Reprinted by permission of the American College of Cardiology. J. Am. Coll. Cardiol. 16:313, 1990.

TABLE 39-7 EARLY MORTALITY (≤42 DAYS) IN PATIENTS TREATED WITH INTRAVENOUS THROMBOLYTIC DRUGS WITH AND WITHOUT HEPARIN

RESULTS*	PLACEBO GROUPS			TREATMENT GROUPS		
	No. of Patients	MORTALITY %	No.	No. of Patients	MORTALITY %	No.
With intravenous heparin	3025	9.3	280	8716	5.6	491
Without intravenous heparin	16,331	13.1	2144	34,581	9.3	3226

From Tiefenbrunn, A. J., and Sobel, B. E.: Thrombolysis and myocardial infarction. Fibrinolysis 5:1, 1991
* Trials included are:
With heparin: ASSET, initial European Cooperative Study Group Trial (ECSG), ECSG IV, ECSG V, HART, ISIS II patients treated with streptokinase for whom intention to treat with intravenous heparin was noted, New Zealand I, New Zealand II, SCATI, TIMI II, TIMI IIB.
Without heparin: GISSI I, GISSI II, ISIS II, HART (patients from the nonheparin arm of the trial), SCATI (patients from the nonheparin arm of the trial). (See references for further details of individual studies.)

Streptokinase[502,562a] demonstrated a clear benefit when aspirin was added to streptokinase (Fig. 39-20). Concurrent therapy with aspirin is now widely recommended with use of all thrombolytic agents, although optimal initial dose (80 to 325 mg) and ideal starting time (0 to 24 hours) have not been firmly established. Newer and potentially more potent antiplatelet drugs (p. 1266) are being actively studied and may well be of benefit in the future.[542]

The importance of interactions between heparin (and antiplatelet and other antithrombotic agents) and fibrinolytic drugs cannot be overemphasized. The clinical efficacy of thrombolysis appears to depend on a favorable balance between dissolution of clot and retardation or prevention of concomitant continuing thrombosis.[562,563] Unopposed, persistent thrombosis reflected by elevation of concentrations in plasma of fibrinopeptide A may compromise coronary thrombolysis by delaying recanalization or predisposing to early reocclusion or both. Results of laboratory studies demonstrate the efficacy of antithrombin agents in potentiating thrombolysis,[564] and a favorable impact of heparin on outcome in trials of thrombolytic agents is strongly suggested by comparison of recent results (Table 39-7).

In the absence of adequate anticoagulation, early patency induced by thrombolytic drugs may not be sustained.[565,566] Accordingly, apparent failure of thrombolysis may occur more often. Impairment of a treatment effect may be more prominent with rt-PA than with streptokinase because of the relative lack of generation of high concentrations of fibrin degradation products with rt-PA.

From a pathophysiological point of view, it should be recognized that fibrinolytic agents appear to exert clinically occult procoagulant effects even when lysis is successful. The presence of such effects underscores the importance of adequate concomitant anticoagulation.[567] While the use of heparin has been well studied, important questions remain. With rt-PA, intravenous heparin does not appear to be necessary in the first 90 minutes[568] or after 24 to 48 hours.[569] Likewise, subcutaneous heparin at 12 hours does not reduce mortality.[263] However, in the period immediately following discontinuation of intravenous rt-PA, heparin may be crucial in maintaining the high early patency rate of this agent,[565,566] for, without it, angiographic patency rates at 1 to 3 days are compromised by as much as 50 per cent. While the role of early intravenous heparin with streptokinase and APSAC has not been well studied, theoretically it may be of less importance in view of the prolonged half-lives of these agents. However, the results of one small trial suggest a benefit of early intravenous heparin with streptokinase.[570]

Many other potential adjunctive therapies have been or are being considered. Beta-adrenoceptor blockers appear to be useful for preventing recurrent ischemic episodes and reinfarction,[3,513] while no such benefit has been demonstrated for calcium antagonists.[571] While the early use of nitrates may improve coronary patency in some patients,[572] such concurrent therapy has not been tested in controlled prospective trials. Finally, the possibility has been raised that agents which scavenge damaging oxygen-derived free radicals may

reduce ischemic injury when given with thrombolytic agents[542] (p. 1187), and studies are being carried out to test this hypothesis.

COMPLICATIONS OF THROMBOLYTIC THERAPY. Recent (<1 year) exposure to streptococci or streptokinase produces some degree of antibody-mediated resistance to streptokinase (and APSAC) in most patients, but this is of clinical consequence only rarely. In the International tPA/SK Mortality Trial, allergic reactions were seen in 1.7 per cent of patients given streptokinase. Hypotension can be expected in 4 to 10 per cent.[263,502] Bleeding complications are, of course, most common and potentially the most serious.[573] Most bleeding is relatively minor with all agents, with more serious episodes occurring in patients requiring invasive procedures. Overall, 70 per cent of bleeding episodes occur at the site of vascular punctures.[573] Intracranial hemorrhage is the most serious complication of thrombolytic therapy[573a]; its frequency of about 0.5 per cent (as judged from results of numerous trials[486]) appears to be only slightly increased over that seen with anticoagulants alone.[592] The incremental incidence of intracranial hemorrhage with thrombolysis appears to be at least partially offset by a lower frequency of thrombotic strokes, so that the overall incidence of stroke is usually not much higher in patients receiving thrombolytic therapy compared with control patients. (However, the more devastating nature of hemorrhagic strokes as compared with the thrombotic type must be considered.) In addition to the risks introduced by invasive procedures, the following all appear to confer an increased risk of bleeding: female gender, lesser body weight, hypertension, older age, fibrinogen depletion, and a prolonged bleeding time at baseline.[573-575] Reports of more unusual complications such as splenic rupture[576] or aortic dissection[577] and cholesterol embolization[578] are beginning to appear as well.

DOSES. Most trials employing intravenous streptokinase have used 1.5 million units over 1 hour as a standard dose. The clinical acceptance of this dose was not preceded by the usual dose-response trials, however. Surprisingly, few studies have tried different doses until very recently. Although smaller doses have been found to be nearly as effective as the standard dose, trials testing these doses have not been of sufficient power to confirm this with a high degree of certainty.[579,580] One recent multicenter trial compared two smaller doses (200,000 units and 500,000 units) with the standard dose (1.5 million units) and one larger dose (3 million units).[581] Patency rates of the infarct-related artery were 38, 75, 60, and 82 per cent, respectively, with the lowest and highest doses each differing significantly from the middle two doses. Complications were low and similar in all groups. The implications of this preliminary trial are important: namely, that at twice the standard dose streptokinase may achieve patency rates comparable with those routinely seen with rt-PA and intravenous heparin together.

Alternative dosing strategies has been more extensively studied with rt-PA. Of the various regimens differing from the standard recommended doses that have been studied, two important newer strategies have clinical relevance. The first is that of so-called "front-loading."[582] Various regimens employing a larger *initial* bolus have shown a high patency rate.[583,584] The specific scheme proposed and tested by Neuhaus[585] appears most promising as it has produced the highest recanalization rate—92 per cent—yet reported for rt-PA: 15 mg intravenous bolus, 50 mg intravenous over 30 minutes, followed by 35 mg over the following 60 minutes (total dose 100 mg over 90 minutes). The improved efficacy of this regimen does not appear to be associated with a higher reocclusion rate, and the regimen does not seem to produce more frequent side effects. If these results are confirmed, current dosing recommendations for rt-PA should be modified to conform to this approach. The second important consideration is that of selection of optimal *total* dosage. It is widely recognized that bleeding complications increase with higher dosages and lesser patient body weights.[574] Accordingly, dosing on the basis of weight has been considered.[552,586,587] There are not sufficient data on which to base recommendations at present, although a total dosage of 2.0 mg/kg does appear to produce a higher incidence of intracranial bleeding (as was already recognized when 150 mg rather than 100 mg total dosage was given in the early phase of the TIMI II study[3]). It seems probable that an ideal regimen will eventually incorporate both front loading and dosing based on body weight.

Repeat dosing with rt-PA has been successfully employed in patients with acute reinfarction after initially successful thrombolysis with either rt-PA or streptokinase.[588] There does not appear to be an increased risk of bleeding, even when a full dosage of rt-PA is employed.[588] Because of antigenicity, repeat infusion of streptokinase or APSAC should be avoided.

INVESTIGATIONAL AGENTS AND COMBINATIONS. Urokinase (p. 1773), a thrombolytic agent that has been available for many years but is not approved for *intravenous* use in AMI, remains investigational in the United States. While probably as effective as streptokinase,[589] given its high cost, it appears to offer no advantage when used as the sole agent. *Single-chain urokinase-type plasminogen activator* (p. 1572) (scuPA or prourokinase) has been studied alone[590,591] and in combination with urokinase[592] and rt-PA.[593] Synergism has been suggested for these combinations, allowing for lower drug doses with higher clot specificity and less frequent bleeding complications. Combinations of urokinase and rt-PA[594] and streptokinase and rt-PA[595,595a] have also been tried for similar reasons. As yet, none of the newer agents or combinations have proved clearly to be of additional benefit, however. In the future, "protein engineering" may lead to molecular alterations of plasminogen activators that will improve both efficacy and safety.[596-598]

CORONARY ANGIOPLASTY IN AMI

It is now established that reperfusion *can* be achieved by emergency percutaneous transluminal coronary angioplasty (PTCA).[599-602] Using a guidewire and balloon catheter, it is technically easier to cross a total occlusion consisting of a fresh thrombus than to cross a longstanding occlusion of a coronary artery. Thus, wire-guided balloon angioplasty can be useful to achieve prompt reperfusion in two quite different situations: (1) in lieu of thrombolytic therapy, or (2) when thrombolysis has failed or when a severe stenosis remains after successful thrombolysis.

PRIMARY ANGIOPLASTY IN AMI. Although PTCA can be performed quickly and relatively safely after the onset of ischemia,[602,602a] the majority of patients with AMI do not have ready access to facilities in which this procedure can be performed. Emergency PTCA requires the ready availability of considerable resources but, despite the difficulty in mustering such resources, several centers have reported relatively extensive experiences with primary PTCA in AMI.[603-606] In these centers, outcome is generally quite favorable, with high primary success rates (78 to 94 per cent successful angioplasties), reocclusion rates of 10 to 15 per cent, improvement in global ejection fraction, and in-hospital mortality as low as 1

per cent in patients with single-vessel coronary artery disease,[607] but considerably higher (12 per cent) in patients with multivessel disease.[608] Small trials comparing thrombolytic therapy with PTCA directly suggest that the latter may result in less subsequent ischemia,[609,610,611a] presumably based on significantly less severe residual coronary artery stenosis produced by PTCA. While in-hospital mortality has generally been higher in patients with cardiogenic shock,[604,605] emergency PTCA in this setting (with or without prior thrombolytic therapy) can often be life-saving.[607,611] Despite the impressive results, the strategy of primary PTCA has not achieved widespread acceptance both because of the tremendous effort and resources (human and physical) required on a continuous standby basis and because, on a comparative basis, it has not been shown to be superior to an initial attempt at reperfusion with thrombolytic therapy.[612]

ANGIOPLASTY AS AN ADJUNCT TO THROMBOLYSIS. Immediate PTCA following thrombolytic therapy has the theoretical benefit of further opening of a stenosed coronary artery to increase flow, perhaps enhancing myocardial recovery and diminishing the possibility of reocclusion. However, in three separate trials of early emergency PTCA, it has been shown that this strategy actually increases the possibility of abrupt reclosure of the coronary artery and increases complications, including the need for urgent coronary artery bypass surgery, while providing no benefit in terms of overall mortality or recovery of ventricular function.[613-615] In the TIMI II study, the strategy of elective catheterization and PTCA, if suitable anatomy was found, within the first 2 days was compared with a strategy of catheterization and PTCA *only* if ischemia developed later in the hospital course or at predischarge exercise stress testing.[3] Here again, the more invasive course with early catheterization failed to provide any benefit in terms of either survival (Fig. 39-21) or improved ventricular function. As a result of this large trial as well as earlier key trials,[613-615] PTCA can be considered elective in most patients receiving thrombolytic therapy after AMI, with "watchful waiting" for ischemia at rest or during a prehospital discharge exercise test and a careful decision based on the clinical picture rather than routine catheterization and angioplasty.[616,617] Patients in whom thrombolytic therapy fails to achieve reperfusion represent candidates for PTCA (rescue angioplasty), and in such patients PTCA can usually be safe and effective (greater than 75 per cent success rates).[618-620] Unfortunately, it is difficult to know in advance of administering thrombolytic therapy which patients will require angioplasty, as *early* PTCA (as already noted) is *not* a practical technique to be used

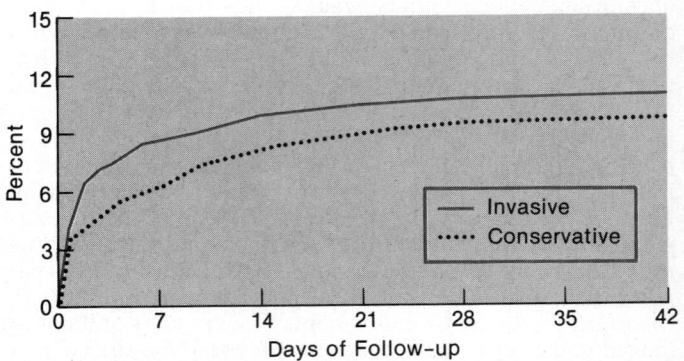

FIGURE 39-21. Cumulative percentage of patients in the invasive strategy and conservative strategy groups of the Thrombolysis in Myocardial Infarction (TIMI) Phase II trial who died or had confirmed nonfatal myocardial infarction (MI) during the 42 days after randomization. Invasive = coronary angiography and infarct-related artery coronary angioplasty (if vessel suitable) within 18–48 hours of thrombolytic therapy; Conservative = coronary angiography and angioplasty only if recurrent ischemia developed. (Reprinted by permission from the TIMI Study Group: Comparison of invasive and conservative strategies after treatment with intravenous tissue plasminogen activator in acute myocardial infarction. Results of the Thrombolysis in Myocardial Infarction [TIMI] Phase II Trial. N. Engl. J. Med. **320:**618, 1989.)

on a *routine* basis. Until there are better ways to recognize patients who might benefit from "rescue angioplasty," the question of optimal treatment of thrombolytic failure remains unresolved.[620] One approach employed in many centers is to perform emergency coronary arteriography on patients with AMI treated with thrombolytic therapy whose condition becomes or remains unstable followed by mechanical revascularization (PTCA or coronary bypass surgery) on those with persistently occluded infarct-related coronary arteries.

Either with or without previous thrombolytic therapy, certain clinical and angiographic features have been identified that can aid the clinician in selecting patients with AMI for PTCA. The most favorable outcome can be anticipated, not surprisingly, in younger patients with single-vessel disease and preserved ventricular function.[618,621] Emergency PTCA should probably be avoided in patients who have an open vessel if a clear-cut residual thrombus is present because abrupt closure appears to be relatively frequent in this situation. Emergency angioplasty also carries considerable more risk in patients with multilesion, multivessel disease and in those with severe hemodynamic compromise.[618,621] As already noted, however, in certain of the latter group, PTCA can be of substantial benefit albeit accompanied by high risk.[619]

Recommendations for Thrombolytic Therapy

On the basis of these considerations and of information from existing studies, as well as the authors' personal experience in the TIMI trials, and recognizing fully that this field is in rapid evolution, the following reperfusion strategy is recommended as of this writing.

1. Intravenous streptokinase (1.5 million units) administered over 1 hour, tissue plasminogen activator (t-PA) (a 6 mg bolus, a total of 60 mg during the first hour, 20 mg during the second hour and the third hour for a total of 100 mg), or Anistreplase (APSAC) (30 mg) given as a bolus should be given intravenously to all patients with impending or evolving transmural infarction (characteristic ischemic pain for ≥30 min, clear-cut new ST-segment elevation), if the drug can be administered within 4 to 6 hours of the onset of symptoms and if contraindications to the administration of this drug are not present (see below).

While as already stated there is still lively debate regarding the optimal thrombolytic agent(s), at this writing all three available thrombolytic agents appear to be effective in opening thrombolytically occluded coronary arteries and are approximately equally effective in reducing mortality. Cost considerations (SK is considerably less expensive than the other two agents) must sometimes influence the selection. This economic advantage must be considered in the light of the apparent greater effectiveness of rt-PA over SK in opening occluded coronary arteries SK and the concern that the large comparison trials of rt-PA and SK[263,540a] may not have used a heparin regimen optimal for rt-PA. This concern is being addressed in the ongoing GUSTO trial.

Patients who have received earlier treatment with either SK or APSAC should not receive these agents a second time because of the development of anti-SK antibodies. Finally, patients who are hypotensive or otherwise hemodynamically unstable should probably receive rt-PA because SK and APSAC may intensify the hypotension.

2. If symptoms have been present for more than 4 to 6 hours, thrombolytic therapy should be employed only if there is clinical evidence of ongoing ischemia, including continuing or recurrent chest pain and/or continuing elevation of electrocardiographic ST segments.

3. *Absolute* contraindications (Table 39-8) to thrombolytic therapy include active internal bleeding, recent prolonged or traumatic cardiopulmonary resuscitation, recent head trauma or known intracranial neoplasm, suspected or possible aortic dissection, suspected pregnancy, recorded blood pressure of greater than 200/110, previous allergic reaction to a thrombolytic agent (with streptokinase or APSAC only), and

TABLE 39-8 CONTRAINDICATIONS TO THROMBOLYTIC TREATMENT (GUIDELINES)

RISK OF BLEEDING
Recent trauma, major surgery, or head injury (within 6 weeks)
Gastrointestinal hemorrhage
Symptoms of proven peptic ulceration (within 3 months)
Bleeding diathesis or chronic liver disease with portal hypertension
Allergy (streptokinase or anistreplase)
Previous treatment with streptokinase or anistreplase
Stroke (residual disability), transient ischemic attack within 6 months, cerebrovascular hemorrhage (ever)
Pregnancy

RELATIVE CONTRAINDICATIONS
Serious organic disease associated with increased risk of bleeding or embolization
Uncontrolled hypertension
Systolic pressure >200 mm Hg or diastolic pressure >110 mm Hg
Noncompressible arterial puncture within 14 days
Dental extraction within 14 days
Active menstruation or lactation
Prolonged cardiopulmonary resuscitation
Diabetic proliferative retinopathy

From Verstraete, M.: Thrombolytic treatment in acute myocardial infarction. Circulation 82(Suppl.II):96, 1990, by permission of the American Heart Association.

presence of any condition that readily leads to hemorrhage (e.g., diabetic hemorrhagic retinopathy). *Relative* contraindications include history of a cerebrovascular accident, known bleeding diathesis, recent trauma or major surgery (within 6 weeks), history of severe recently uncontrolled hypertension, significant liver dysfunction, and prior exposure to streptokinase or APSAC (if either of those agents is to be given). Either rt-PA or urokinase can be used repeatedly or after streptokinase. Finally, thrombolytic therapy should be used with great caution in the elderly (over 80 years), and in any patient who is agitated, lethargic, or confused.

4. Before the institution of thrombolytic therapy, consideration should be given to the patient's need for intravascular catheterization, as would be required for the placement of an arterial pressure monitoring line, a pulmonary artery catheter for hemodynamic monitoring, or a temporary transvenous pacemaker. If any of these are required, ideally they should be placed, as expeditiously as possible, *before* infusion of the thrombolytic agent is begun. If such procedures will require an additional delay of more than 30 minutes, they should be deferred for as long as possible after thrombolytic therapy is begun. In the early hours *after* institution of thrombolytic therapy, such catheterization should be performed only if crucial to survival, and then sites where excessive bleeding can be controlled should be chosen (e.g., subclavian vein catheterization should be avoided).

5. With infusion of rt-PA, intravenous heparin should be employed initially given as a bolus of 5000 units intravenously, followed by a continuous infusion. It should be begun at the rate of 1000 units/hr and adjusted to keep the activated partial thromboplastin time at 1½ to 2 times control value. Aspirin (160 to 325 mg) should be administered within 24 hours of thrombolytic therapy regardless of the agent chosen. It should be continued indefinitely.

6. Emergency PTCA should be reserved for those patients who have access to a skilled cardiac catheterization team that is highly experienced in the performance of coronary angioplasty and readily available. Angioplasty should be employed on an emergency basis if thrombolytic therapy is contraindicated or if attempts at myocardial salvage have apparently failed after thrombolytic therapy, particularly if cardiac function is severely impaired and/or if there is clinical evidence of widespread ongoing ischemia. Primary PTCA may also be employed (without antecedent thrombolytic treatment or contraindications thereto) in the earliest (4) hours of an infarct in

patients with extensive ischemia and with the immediate availability of a skilled team and laboratory.

7. Elective PTCA should be reserved for patients who develop recurrent ischemia at any point during hospitalization, including during the predischarge exercise stress test. When a patient develops one of these indications and if a qualified catheterization team and well-equipped laboratory are not available in the facility in which the patient is located, the patient should be transferred promptly to a tertiary care center.

8. If recurrent ischemia develops and does not readily resolve, and if immediate catheterization with angioplasty backup is unavailable, retreatment with rt-PA should be considered. If prior therapy was within 12 hours (for rt-PA) or 24 hours (for streptokinase), the dose should be reduced by 25 to 50 per cent; otherwise a full dose can be administered, albeit cautiously.

9. Additional medical therapy with beta blockers, nitrates, and/or calcium antagonists should be routinely employed, as required, just as they are for other patients with AMI or for those undergoing coronary angioplasty.

SURGICAL REPERFUSION IN ACUTE MYOCARDIAL INFARCTION

There have been extensive improvements in intraoperative myocardial preservation with cardioplegia and hypothermia and in surgical techniques. These have allowed surgical reperfusion in coronary patients with AMI to be carried out at quite low short- and long-term mortality rates— approximately 2 per cent in-hospital and 25 per cent 10-year mortality rates in selected centers. This has kept alive the concept of emergency coronary revascularization as a possible measure to protect jeopardized myocardium in patients suffering AMI.[622-625] As appears to be the case for all methods designed to limit infarct size, this therapy can be successful only if it is applied within the first 4 to 6 hours (preferably the first 2 hours) of the onset of the acute event. In the usual patient who develops an AMI outside of the hospital, it is logistically difficult to bring the patient to the hospital, carry out a clinical evaluation, outline the coronary anatomy by arteriography, assemble the surgical team, commence operation, and place the patient on cardiopulmonary bypass in less than 4 hours after the onset of the event. It is therefore unlikely that surgical reperfusion can or will be widely applied on a regular basis in the routine treatment of AMI. Indeed, the operation is contraindicated in patients with uncomplicated transmural infarcts more than 6 hours after the onset of the event. When carried out at this time, surgical reperfusion appears to produce marked hemorrhage into the area of infarction.[626]

However, in some patients with AMI, including some with cardiogenic shock, infarction appears to occur in a stuttering manner over an interval of several days.[627] Theoretically, revascularization carried out more than 6 hours after the onset of the event might be of benefit in this group, but this has yet to be established firmly. Also, coronary bypass surgery can be carried out promptly in patients who develop coronary occlusion during cardiac catheterization, coronary arteriography, and PTCA, as well as in patients whose coronary anatomy has been assessed recently by coronary arteriography and who develop an infarction in the hospital while awaiting operation.

Patients undergoing successful thrombolysis but with important residual stenoses, who on anatomical grounds are more suitable for surgical revascularization than for PTCA, have undergone coronary artery bypass surgery with quite low mortality and morbidity.[628-630] Although postoperative chest tube drainage with relatively minor bleeding occurs more commonly than after elective bypass surgery, this problem is not of major concern.[628] PTCA is preferable in patients suitable for this procedure, whereas surgery should be reserved for those in whom PTCA has not been successful or could not be performed, or for patients with left main or extensive multivessel coronary artery disease for whom coronary

artery bypass graft surgery would be recommended even in the absence of AMI. Thus, it is in this group of patients with AMI, i.e., those who have undergone or who are undergoing thrombolytic therapy with continued severe ischemic and hemodynamic instability, that a small subgroup can be identified who are likely to benefit from emergency revascularization. In this group, bypass of noninfarct-related coronary artery obstructions can be expected to produce additional benefit.

Elective coronary artery bypass surgery has been carried out soon after AMI for much the same reasons as just outlined (see #6 above). If recurrent ischemia occurs in multivessel or left main coronary disease, that is, if the patient has coronary anatomy unsuitable for PTCA, coronary artery bypass grafting is a reasonable alternative and should be used—particularly in patients with easily provoked ischemia or impaired left ventricular function. Large series of patients operated on within 30 days of AMI have been reported with excellent long-term survival.[631,632] However, when surgery is performed under urgent conditions with active and ongoing ischemia or cardiogenic shock, operative mortality rises steeply.[631,632] At autopsy, such patients have extensive myocardial necrosis that is often hemorrhagic.[633]

PHARMACOLOGICAL THERAPY OF ACUTE MYOCARDIAL INFARCTION

BETA-ADRENOCEPTOR BLOCKADE
(See also p. 1225)

The immediate administration of beta-adrenoceptor blockers reduces cardiac index, heart rate, blood pressure, and tension-time index levels. The next effect of these drugs is a reduction in myocardial oxygen consumption per minute and per beat. Favorable effects of beta-adrenoceptor blockade on the balance of myocardial oxygen supply and demand are reflected in the reduction of myocardial lactate production and diminution of ventricular arrhythmias.[634] Since beta-adrenoceptor blockade diminishes circulating levels of free fatty acids by antagonizing the lipolytic effects of catecholamines, and since elevated levels of fatty acids augment myocardial oxygen consumption and probably increase the incidence of arrhythmias, these metabolic actions of beta-blocking agents may also be beneficial to the ischemic heart.[634] The effects of beta blockers on AMI can be divided into those that are immediate (when the drug is given very early in the course of infarction) and long-term (secondary prevention), when the drug is initiated sometime after infarction. The former type, which is part of the acute management of AMI, is considered this section; the latter, on p. 1254.

Objective evidence of beneficial effects of beta blockers in acute myocardial ischemia has been reported by several investigators using various modifications of the precordial ST-segment mapping technique.[635,636] For example, Gold et al.[635] found that the likelihood of a beneficial clinical and electrocardiographic response increased in the presence of residual antegrade or collateral blood flow to the infarct zone, as determined by coronary arteriography. Peter et al.[637] found that patients treated within 4 hours of onset of symptoms of uncomplicated MI had significantly lower peak serum creatine kinase levels and less cumulative creatine kinase release into plasma than did patients without specific therapy. The same group[638] also found that patients with suspected MI, treated with propranolol within 4 hours of the onset of symptoms, had a significantly lower incidence of infarction. This suggests that threatened infarction might actually be prevented by early beta blockade. Similarly, Yusuf et al. have reported that intravenous atenolol, given a median of 4 hours following onset of symptoms of AMI, decreased the incidence of AMI, CK-MB release, the electrocardiographic evolution of infarction, and the severity of ischemic pain.[639] Alprenolol[640] and metoprolol[641] begun early in the course of infarction have been shown to limit enzymatically estimated infarct size.

RESULTS OF MULTICENTER TRIALS. At least 27 randomized beta blocker trials involving over 27,000 patients have been undertaken.[16] Of these, there have been four large trials designed to test the effects of early beta blockade in myocardial infarction. In the *Multicenter Investigation for the Limitation of Infarct Size* (MILIS) study, propranolol adminis-

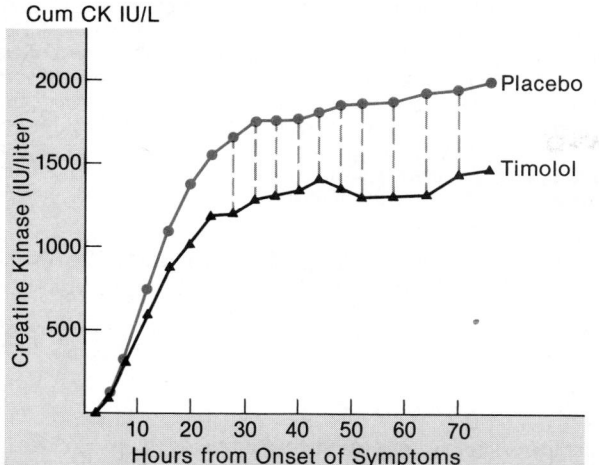

FIGURE 39-22. Mean cumulative release of creatine kinase during the evolution of acute myocardial infarction. Time zero denotes onset of symptoms. Significant differences between the two groups are indicated by vertical dashed lines. (Reprinted by permission from The International Collaborative Study Group: Reduction of infarct size with the early use of timolol in acute myocardial infarction. *N. Engl. J. Med. 310*:9, 1984.)

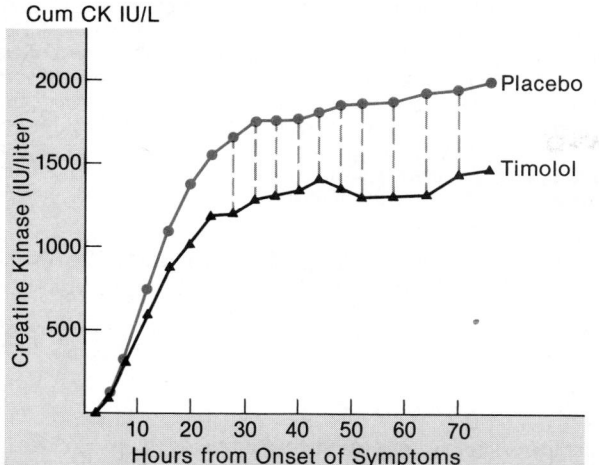

tered an average of 8.5 hours after the onset of symptoms, when compared to control, failed to reduce infarct size.[642] More favorable results were reported by the *International Collaborative Study Group*, which reported on the use of intravenous timolol in the early phase of AMI.[643] In this study, patients were treated a mean of 3.4 hours after the onset of symptoms, and infarct size was smaller in timolol-treated patients as assessed by cumulative release of CK (Fig. 39–22) and by electrocardiographic indices.

In a large randomized trial using intravenous metoprolol (the *MIAMI Trial*),[644] infarct size was found to be smaller by enzymatic criteria (maximum serum activity of aspartate aminotransferase [AST]) in the metoprolol group but only in patients treated within 7 hours. All these studies are consistent with experimental and other clinical evidence that ischemic myocardium can be spared from irreversible injury only if treated early enough in the infarction process. For most patients, the outside time limit for salvaging viable myocardium is probably in the range of 4 to 6 hours. Benefit is highly variable if treatment is begun between 6 and 12 hours.

In an additional large multicenter trial (*ISIS 1*) involving over 16,000 patients, investigators reported a significant reduction in mortality among the patients randomized to intravenous atenolol when compared to placebo-treated patients.[645] Patients were treated at a mean of 5 hours after the onset of suspected AMI. Mortality was reduced by 15 per cent at one week and this difference was maintained for the first year of follow-up. The study further suggests that treatment of approximately 200 patients would result in avoidance of one reinfarction, one cardiac arrest, and one death in the first week after onset of an AMI.[645]

In the TIMI II trial the addition of a beta blocker (metoprolol) to thrombolytic therapy was studied.[3] While recurrent ischemia and reinfarction were reduced by metoprolol, mortality was not reduced nor was ventricular function improved. Thus, beta blockade may not enhance salvage of myocardium in the setting of early reperfusion but may confer clinical benefit by means of its antiischemic effect.[513]

Given the overall favorable effects of beta blockade in the aforementioned clinical trials, patients in a hyperdynamic state (sinus tachycardia, hypertension, no evidence of heart failure or bronchospasm) as well as patients seen in the first 4 hours would appear to be good candidates for this therapy, regardless of whether thrombolytic therapy is employed. Unless there are contraindications, beta blockade probably should be continued in patients who develop AMI. In addition, beta blockers are indicated in patients in whom infarc-

tion is complicated by persistent or recurrent ischemic pain, progressive or repetitive serum enzyme elevations suggestive of infarct extension, or tachyarrhythmias refractory to lidocaine and procainamide early after the onset of infarction. If adverse effects of beta blockers develop, or if patients present with complications of infarction that are contraindications to beta blockade such as heart failure or heart block, the beta blocker should be withheld or can be discontinued safely.[646]

RECOMMENDATIONS. In patients with AMI who have not received beta blockers in the preceding 24 hours, this therapy may be administered as metoprolol 15 mg intravenously, divided into three equal doses given at 2- to 5-minute intervals. During this period, heart rate and arterial pressure should be determined, and an electrocardiographic strip should be recorded after each injection. Intravenous beta blockade should not be administered in patients with a history of bronchial asthma, and administration should be halted if any of the following events are present or develop:

1. Second- or third-degree AV block or lengthening of the P-R interval beyond 0.24 sec.
2. Rales extending more than one-third of the way up the lung fields, or wheezes detected on auscultation.
3. Heart rate below 50 per minute.
4. Systolic arterial pressure below 90 to 95 mm Hg.
5. Pulmonary artery wedge pressure above 20 to 24 mm Hg. (While it is useful to monitor this pressure in patients in whom a beta blocker will be administered, it is by no means essential.)

The intravenous administration of metoprolol is followed 6 to 8 hours later by oral metoprolol given first as 50 mg twice daily for the first day and then advanced to 100 mg twice daily, if the lower dose is tolerated. Ideally, the dose should keep the heart rate between 50 to 65 beats/min and the systolic pressure above 95 mm Hg in the absence of heart failure, wheezing, or advanced AV block.

Selection of Beta Blocker. At the time of this writing, only metoprolol has been approved for intravenous use in AMI by the Food and Drug Administration. However, favorable effects have also been reported with atenolol, timolol, and alprenolol; these benefits probably occur with propranolol and esmolol, an ultrashort-acting agent, as well.

In the absence of any favorable evidence supporting the benefit of agents with intrinsic sympathomimetic activity (ISA) such as pindolol and oxprenolol, and with some unfavorable evidence for any benefit of these agents in secondary prevention,[647] beta blockers with ISA probably should not be chosen for treatment of AMI. Occasionally the clinician may wish to proceed with beta blocker therapy even in the presence of *relative* contraindications, such as a history of mild asthma, mild bradycardia, mild heart failure, or first-degree heart block. In this situation, a trial of the very short-acting beta blocker esmolol (p. 1304) may help determine whether the patient can tolerate beta blockade.[648,649] Since the hemodynamic effects of this drug, with a half-life of 9 minutes, disappear in less than 30 minutes, it offers considerable advantage over longer-acting agents when the risk of a beta blocker complication is relatively high.

Although antagonism of sympathetic stimulation to the heart might be expected to exacerbate pulmonary edema in patients with occult heart failure, usually only small changes in pulmonary capillary wedge pressure occur when the drug is used in patients with AMI.[634]

NITRATES

(See also p. 1304)

Intravenous nitroglycerin has been reported to reduce infarct size in AMI patients.[650,651] The early use of intravenous nitroglycerin appears to diminish the frequency of mechanical complications of AMI and improves postinfarction ventricular remodeling.[651] Furthermore, in patients with heart failure, mortality and serious ventricular arrhythmias appeared to be reduced in the nitroglycerin-treated group.[650,651] Bussmann and associates[652] found significantly lower values of peak serum CK, lower rates of CK release, and smaller calculated infarct sizes in nitroglycerin-treated patients. Flaherty and colleagues[653] have shown in a prospective, randomized trial that treatment with intravenous nitroglycerin for 48 hours followed by nitroglycerin ointment therapy for 72 hours enhanced postinfarction improvement of myocardial perfusion measured with ^{201}Tl scintigraphy.

As with other interventions to spare ischemic myocardium in AMI, intravenous nitroglycerin appears to be of greatest benefit in patients treated earliest.[651,653] Patients with inferior wall infarction are particularly sensitive to an excessive fall in preload, particularly if concurrent right ventricular infarction is present.[432] In such cases nitrate-induced venodilatation could impair cardiac output and reduce coronary blood flow, thus worsening myocardial oxygenation rather than improving it.[654]

HEMODYNAMIC EFFECTS. In patients with AMI, the administration of nitroglycerin and other nitrates such as isosorbide dinitrate diminishes pulmonary capillary wedge pressure and systemic arterial pressure as well as left ventricular end-systolic and end-diastolic volumes. It also reduces ventricular asynergy, to the extent that the local impairment of left ventricular function is due to reversibly injured, depressed myocardium rather than to zones of completed infarction or scar.[655] When systemic arterial and pulmonary capillary wedge pressures are normal or low prior to the administration of nitroglycerin, reflex tachycardia may result from the further reduction of ventricular filling and arterial pressures.

MODE OF ADMINISTRATION. Intravenous nitroglycerin can be administered safely to patients with evolving MI as long as the dose is titrated carefully to avoid induction of reflex tachycardia or systemic arterial hypotension (systolic blood pressure ≤ 95 mm Hg).[485] One useful regimen employs an initial infusion rate of 10 µg/min with stepwise increases of 10 µg/min until the mean arterial blood pressure is reduced by 10 per cent of its baseline level. Alternatively, it may be administered sublingually at doses of 0.3 to 0.6 mg. This route may be more hazardous, since the rate of absorption is difficult to control and arterial pressure may decline precipitously. Nitroglycerin is often useful for the relief of persistent pain and as a vasodilator in patients with infarction associated with left ventricular failure.

When continuous infusion of intravenous nitroglycerin is used, two important potential complications must be considered. First, most commercially available nitroglycerin for intravenous use is prepared in a solution with ethanol as a diluent. When high infusion rates are continued for several days, signs and symptoms of alcohol intoxication may occur.[656] Second, clinically significant methemoglobinemia has been reported to occur during administration of intravenous nitroglycerin.[657] Although uncommon, this problem is seen when unusually large doses of nitrates are administered. It is important not only for its potential to cause symptoms of lethargy and headache but also because elevated methemoglobin levels can impair the oxygen-carrying capacity of blood, potentially exacerbating ischemia.

Tolerance to intravenous nitroglycerin (as manifested by increasing nitrate requirements) develops in many patients, often as soon as 12 hours after the infusion is started.[658] Despite the theoretical and demonstrated benefit of sulfhydryl agents in diminishing tolerance, their use has not become widespread.[659,660]

ACTIONS. According to all of the available evidence, nitroglycerin very rarely opens previously occluded coronary arteries. Nevertheless, one or two 0.3 mg tablets of nitroglycerin should be given when a patient presents with acute chest pain, particularly if the diagnosis of AMI is not clear. Patients in whom the pain is caused by unstable angina often respond with prompt relief of chest pain. Despite the evidence of a favorable effect of nitroglycerin on infarct size as already discussed, *routine* use of this drug is not recommended in patients with established AMI. However, in patients with pump failure, pulmonary edema, or continuing ischemia, intravenous nitroglycerin may be useful for lowering preload and afterload, and for improving flow to ischemic myocardium. It is contraindicated in the presence of hypotension.

OTHER POTENTIALLY USEFUL APPROACHES TO PROTECTION OF ISCHEMIC MYOCARDIUM

The experimental observations indicating the potential usefulness of the interventions described below are summarized on pages 1190 to 1192.

CALCIUM ANTAGONISTS

Nifedipine. In multiple trials involving a total of over 5000 patients, nifedipine has not shown any benefit in infarct size reduction, prevention of progression to infarction, control of recurrent ischemia, or lowering of mortality.[661] Furthermore, several trials suggest a detrimental effect of early nifedipine.[662-665] Nifedipine does not appear to be helpful in conjunction with either thrombolytic therapy[664] or beta blockade.[662,665]

VERAPAMIL AND DILTIAZEM. Verapamil, although less well studied, has not had any demonstrated favorable effect on infarct size or other important endpoints in patients with AMI, with the exception of control of supraventricular arrhythmias.[661] Both verapamil and diltiazem have apparently reduced mortality in subgroups of patients free of heart failure.[666,667] While diltiazem has been shown to diminish myocardial oxygen requirements,[668] it has failed convincingly to reduce infarct size, improve ventricular function, and reduce ischemia.[661] Thus far, the promising effects of calcium antagonists in studies of animals with infarction[669] have not been widely translated to clinical benefit in patients with AMI.[436a,670]

GLUCOSE-INSULIN-POTASSIUM. Administration of a solution of glucose-insulin-potassium (300 gm of glucose, 50 units of insulin, and 80 mEq of KCl in 1000 ml of water administered at a rate of 1.5 ml/kg/hr) lowers the concentration of plasma free fatty acids and improves ventricular performance, as reflected in systolic arterial pressure, cardiac output, and stroke work at any level of left ventricular filling pressure[671]; also the frequency of ventricular premature beats decreases.[672] In a nonrandomized study, mortality appeared to be reduced,[673] hemodynamics improved, global ejection fraction increased, and both asynergy in the ischemic zone and pulmonary artery diastolic pressure reduced.[672] However, no definitive effect on enzymatically estimated infarct size or long-term mortality has been described in a prospective, controlled, randomized trial.

INTRAAORTIC BALLOON COUNTERPULSATION. From a theoretical standpoint, intraaortic balloon counterpulsation might be expected to limit infarct size for several reasons. In experimental animals, intraaortic balloon counterpulsation decreases afterload and myocardial oxygen consumption,[630] decreases preload, increases coronary blood flow, and improves cardiac performance.[674] No definitive information is available indicating that intraaortic balloon counterpulsation alters the prognosis in patients with relatively uncomplicated infarction. Leinbach et al., however, have reported an immediate, persistent fall in ST-segment elevation. This occurred in patients with anterior MI who had preservation of precordial R waves and good ventricular function,[675] in whom the left anterior descend-

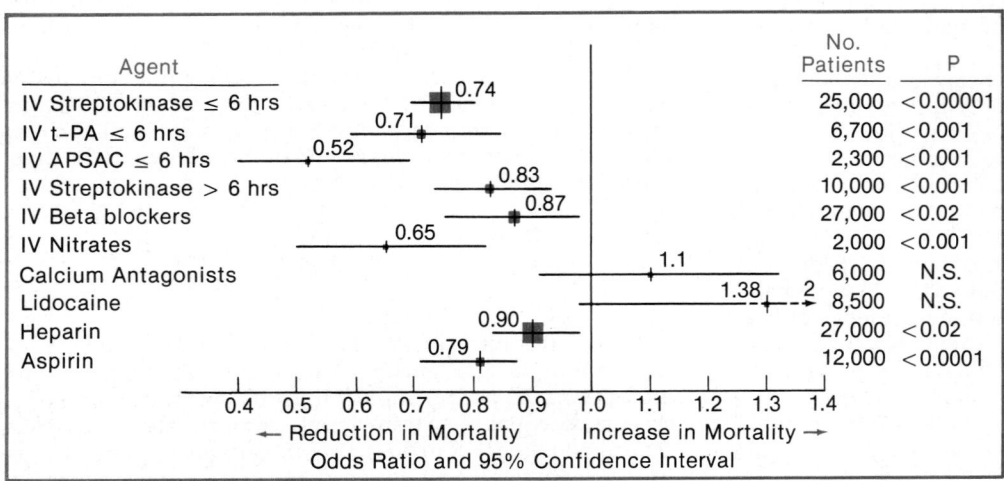

FIGURE 39–23. Summary of effects of various treatments on mortality in AMI. Odds ratios and their 95 per cent confidence intervals are plotted. The size of each square is related to the variance of the data. Larger squares reflect more data, and a narrower confidence interval indicates more precise estimates of treatment effect. IV, intravenous; t-PA, tissue plasminogen activator; APSAC, anisoylated plasminogen-streptokinase activator complex; NS, not significant. (From Yusuf, S., et al.: Routine medical management of acute myocardial infarction. Lessons from overviews of recent randomized controlled trials. *Circulation* 82[Suppl II]:117, 1990, by permission of the American Heart Association, Inc.)

Agent	Odds Ratio	No. Patients	P
IV Streptokinase ≤ 6 hrs	0.74	25,000	<0.00001
IV t-PA ≤ 6 hrs	0.71	6,700	<0.001
IV APSAC ≤ 6 hrs	0.52	2,300	<0.001
IV Streptokinase > 6 hrs	0.83	10,000	<0.001
IV Beta blockers	0.87	27,000	<0.02
IV Nitrates	0.65	2,000	<0.001
Calcium Antagonists	1.1	6,000	N.S.
Lidocaine	1.38	8,500	N.S.
Heparin	0.90	27,000	<0.02
Aspirin	0.79	12,000	<0.0001

0.4 0.5 0.6 0.7 0.8 0.9 1.0 1.1 1.2 1.3 1.4
← Reduction in Mortality   Increase in Mortality →
Odds Ratio and 95% Confidence Interval

ing coronary artery was not totally occluded and who underwent intraaortic balloon pumping within 6 hours.

In a relatively small prospective trial intraaortic balloon pumping with intravenous nitroglycerin appeared to preserve function only in noninfarcted segments.[676] Given the relatively frequent rate of complications[677] after intraaortic balloon insertion and the absence of convincing data for infarct size reduction, intraaortic balloon pumping should be reserved for hemodynamically compromised patients and for those with refractory ischemia, for whom the benefit of this approach has been demonstrated.

OTHER AGENTS. Oxygen-derived free radicals are abundant in ischemic tissue and may contribute to myocardial injury, particularly following reperfusion (p. 1187). Evidence from studies in animals suggests that the extent of myocardial necrosis can be affected favorably by treatment with oxygen free radical scavengers such as superoxide dismutase.[678]

Additionally, myocardial function is improved by the enhanced recovery induced by oxygen free radical scavengers after severe ischemia.[679] Studies in humans are under way to test the efficacy of this type of therapy for sparing injured myocardium.

The suggestion that magnesium metabolism is disturbed in AMI has led to several recent trials with intravenous magnesium. One such trial suggests that in-hospital mortality is reduced following a 48-hour magnesium infusion.[680] This improvement does not appear to be based solely on an antiarrhythmic effect.

Dozens of careful clinical trials carried out around the world by hundreds of collaborating investigators have made it possible to summarize and compare the results of different pharmacological therapies by the technique of meta-analysis. Such a comparison is shown in Figure 39–23.

Arrhythmias in Acute Myocardial Infarction

The genesis and diagnosis of arrhythmias are presented in Chapters 22 and 24 and their treatment in Chapters 23 and 25. The role of arrhythmias in complicating the course of patients with AMI and the prevention and treatment of these arrhythmias in this setting are discussed here and summarized in Table 39–9.

Some abnormality of cardiac rhythm has been noted in 72 to 96 per cent of patients with AMI treated in coronary care units.[234,681] The incidence of arrhythmias is higher in those patients seen earlier after the onset of symptoms. Moreover, many arrhythmias occur before hospitalization, before the pa-

tient is monitored.[682] Thus, the overall incidence of rhythm disturbance in AMI may actually be as high as 100 per cent. However, these data are difficult to interpret, since ambulatory electrocardiographic monitoring has also disclosed arrhythmias in a high percentage of asymptomatic, apparently healthy middle-aged men.[683]

Arrhythmias occurring in patients with AMI require vigorous treatment when they (1) impair hemodynamics; (2) compromise myocardial viability by augmenting myocardial oxygen requirements; or (3) predispose to malignant ventricular arrhythmias, i.e., ventricular tachycardia, ventricular fibril-

TABLE 39–9   CARDIAC ARRHYTHMIAS AND THEIR MANAGEMENT DURING ACUTE MYOCARDIAL INFARCTION

CATEGORY	ARRHYTHMIA	OBJECTIVE OF TREATMENT	THERAPEUTIC OPTIONS
I. *Electrical instability*	Ventricular premature beats	Prophylaxis against ventricular fibrillation	Antiarrhythmic agents (lidocaine, procainamide, beta blocker)
	Ventricular tachycardia	Prophylaxis against ventricular fibrillation, restoration of hemodynamic stability	Antiarrhythmic agents; cardioversion/defibrillation
	Ventricular fibrillation	Urgent reversion to sinus rhythm	Defibrillation; bretylium tosylate
	Accelerated idioventricular rhythm	Observation unless hemodynamic function is compromised	Increase sinus rate (atropine, atrial pacing); antiarrhythmic agents
	Nonparoxysmal AV junctional tachycardia	Search for precipitating causes (e.g., digitalis intoxication); suppress arrhythmia only if hemodynamic function is compromised	Atrial overdrive pacing; antiarrhythmic agents; cardioversion relatively contraindicated if digitalis intoxication present
II. *Pump failure/ Excessive sympathetic stimulation*	Sinus tachycardia	Reduce heart rate to diminish myocardial oxygen demands	Antipyretics; analgesics; consider beta blocker unless CHF present; treat latter if present with anticongestive measures (diuretics, afterload reduction)
	Atrial fibrillation and/or atrial flutter	Reduce ventricular rate; restore sinus rhythm	Verapamil, digitalis glycosides; anticongestive measures (diuretics, afterload reduction); cardioversion; rapid atrial pacing (for atrial flutter)
	Paroxysmal supraventricular tachycardia	Reduce ventricular rate; restore sinus rhythm	Vagal maneuvers; verapamil, cardiac glycosides, beta-adrenergic blockers; cardioversion; rapid atrial pacing
III. *Bradyarrhythmias and conduction disturbances*	Sinus bradycardia	Acceleration of heart rate only if hemodynamic function is compromised	Atropine; atrial pacing
	Junctional escape rhythm	Acceleration of sinus rate only if loss of atrial "kick" causes hemodynamic compromise	Atropine; atrial pacing
	Atrioventricular block and intraventricular block		Insertion of pacemaker

Modified from Antman, E. M., and Rutherford, J. D. (eds.): Coronary Care Medicine: A Practical Approach. Boston, Martinus Nijhoff Publishing, 1986, p. 78.

lation, or asystole. There is evidence that both the diminished threshold to ventricular fibrillation[684] and the incidence of malignant ventricular arrhythmias associated with infarction[463] are affected by the extent of the underlying infarction.[685]

When patients are seen *very early* during the course of MI they almost invariably exhibit evidence of increased activity of the autonomic nervous system. Thus sinus bradycardia, sometimes associated with AV block, and hypotension reflect the augmented vagal activity. Hypotension, regardless of cause, is hazardous in patients with AMI, since it impairs perfusion of marginally ischemic zones, intensifies ischemia, and may initiate or perpetuate the vicious circle illustrated in Figure 39–11 (p. 1210).

Activation of receptors within atrial and ventricular myocardium by necrotic tissue may cause enhanced efferent sympathetic activity, increased concentrations of circulating catecholamines, and local release of catecholamines from nerve endings within the heart. The last phenomenon may also result from direct ischemic damage of adrenergic neurons. In addition, ischemic myocardium may be hyperreactive to the arrhythmogenic effects of norepinephrine,[686] which may vary strikingly in concentration in different portions of the ischemic heart.[687] Sympathetic stimulation of the heart may also enhance the automaticity of ischemic Purkinje fibers. Furthermore, catecholamines facilitate propagation of slow current responses mediated by calcium, and stimulation of ischemic myocardium by catecholamines may exacerbate arrhythmias dependent on such currents.[686] Finally, it has been demonstrated that transmural infarction can interrupt both afferent and efferent limbs of the sympathetic nervous system innervating myocardium distal to the area of infarction (but still viable).[687] In addition to the potential for modifying a variety of cardiovascular reflexes, this creation of autonomic imbalance may promote the development of arrhythmias.[687] This explains why beta-adrenoceptor blocking agents may also be helpful in the treatment of ventricular arrhythmias, particularly when the latter are associated with other signs of heightened adrenergic activity.

The treatment of tachyarrhythmias involves not only the use of antiarrhythmic drugs but also correction of abnormalities of plasma electrolyte concentrations, acid-base balance disturbances, hypoxemia, anemia, and digitalis intoxication. In addition, it is essential to treat pericarditis, pulmonary emboli, and pneumonia or other infections, which may give rise to sinus tachycardia or other supraventricular tachyarrhythmias.

HEMODYNAMIC CONSEQUENCES OF CARDIAC ARRHYTHMIAS. Patients with significant left ventricular dysfunction have a relatively fixed stroke volume and depend on changes in heart rate to alter cardiac output. However, there is a narrow range over which the cardiac output is maximal, with significant reductions occurring at both faster and slower rates. Thus, all forms of bradycardia and tachycardia may depress the cardiac output in patients with AMI. Although the optimal rate insofar as cardiac output is concerned may exceed 100 per minute, it is important to consider that heart rate is one of the major determinants of myocardial oxygen consumption and that at more rapid heart rates myocardial energy needs can be elevated to levels that adversely affect ischemic myocardium. Therefore, in patients with AMI, the optimal rate is usually somewhat lower, in the range of 80 beats/min.

A second factor to consider in assessing the hemodynamic consequences of a particular arrhythmia is the loss of atrial transport function, i.e., the atrial "kick."[688] Studies in patients without AMI have demonstrated that loss of atrial transport decreases left ventricular output by 15 to 20 per cent.[689] However, in patients with reduced diastolic left ventricular compliance of any cause (including AMI), atrial systole is of greater importance for left ventricular filling. In patients with AMI, atrial systole boosts end-diastolic volume by 15 per cent,

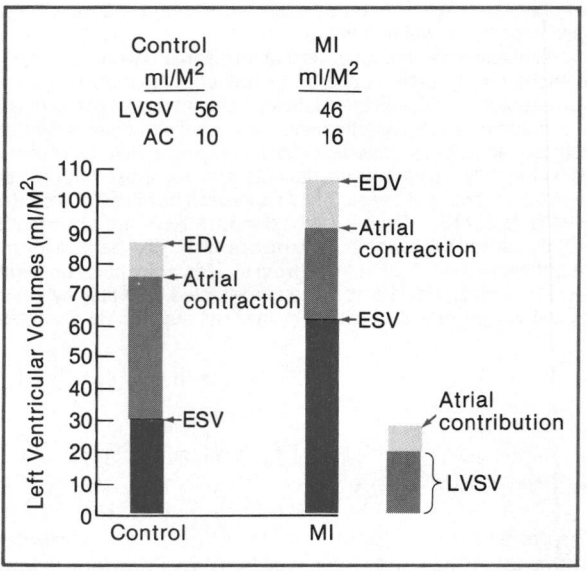

FIGURE 39–24. Average end-diastolic volumes (EDV), end-systolic volumes (ESV), left ventricular stroke volumes (LVSV), and atrial contribution (AC) in a control group of patients and in patients after myocardial infarction (MI). (From Rahimtoola, S. H., et al.: Left atrial transport function in myocardial infarction. *Am. J. Med. 59:686, 1975.*)

end-diastolic pressure by 29 per cent, and stroke volume by 35 per cent (Fig. 39–24).[690]

BRADYARRHYTHMIAS

SINUS BRADYCARDIA
(See also p. 674)

Sinus bradycardia is the most common arrhythmia occurring during the early phases of AMI, and it is particularly frequent in patients with inferior and posterior infarction.[691,692] Observations in mobile coronary care units indicate that 25 to 40 per cent of patients with AMI have electrocardiographic evidence of sinus bradycardia within the first hour after the onset of symptoms; however, 4 hours after infarction commences, the incidence of sinus bradycardia has declined to 15 to 20 per cent.[682] The cause of the vagotonia and resultant bradycardia and hypotension accompanying AMI is not entirely clear. One factor appears to be stimulation of cardiac vagal afferent receptors (which are more common in the inferoposterior than the anterior or lateral portions of the left ventricle) with resulting efferent cholinergic stimulation of the heart. The phenomenon is a manifestation of the Bezold-Jarisch reflex.[693] This reflex is mediated by the vagus nerves and occurs during thrombolytic reperfusion, particularly of the right coronary artery.[514] Often sinus bradycardia is a component of a vasovagal or vasodepressor response, which may be intensified by severe pain as well as by morphine, and may be related to vasovagal syncope (p. 875).

The clinical significance of sinus bradycardia is debated. On the one hand, this arrhythmia is a risk factor during the very early phase of AMI and predisposes the patient to the development of repetitive ventricular arrhythmias and hypotension. On the other hand, it has been suggested on the basis of data obtained in experimental infarction and from some clinical observations that the increased vagal tone that produces sinus bradycardia during the early phase of AMI may actually be protective, perhaps because it reduces myocardial oxygen demands.[692] Thus the acute mortality rate appears to be as low in patients with sinus bradycardia as in patients without this arrhythmia.

MANAGEMENT. This depends upon the timing and severity, and on other clinical manifestations. Isolated sinus bradycardia, unaccompanied by hypotension or ventricular ectopy, should be observed rather than treated initially. In the first 4 to 6 hours following infarction, if the sinus rate is extremely slow (under 40/min), administration of intravenous atropine in aliquots of 0.3 to 0.6 mg every 3 to 10 minutes (with a total dose not exceeding 2 mg) to bring heart rate up to approximately 60/min often abolishes the premature ventricular beats commonly associated with this degree of sinus bradycardia. Atropine often contributes to restoration of arterial pressure and hence coronary perfusion, and should be employed if hypotension accompanying any degree of sinus bradycardia is present. The favorable effects of atropine may be accompanied by regression of ST-segment elevation. Elevation of the lower extremities will also often elevate arterial pressure by redistributing blood from the systemic venous bed to the thorax, thereby augmenting ventricular preload, cardiac output, and arterial pressure.

Sinus bradycardia occurring more than 6 hours after the onset of the AMI is often transitory, is caused by sinus node dysfunction or atrial ischemia rather than vagal hyperactivity, is usually not accompanied by hypotension, and does not usually predispose to ventricular arrhythmias. Treatment is not required unless ventricular performance is compromised or the administration of a beta-adrenoceptor blocker or high doses of antiarrhythmic drugs (which may slow the sinus rate further) is planned. When atropine is ineffective and the patient is symptomatic and/or hypotensive, electrical pacing is indicated (Chap. 25). In patients with depressed ventricular performance, who require the "atrial kick," atrial pacing or atrioventricular sequential pacing is superior to simple ventricular pacing.[694]

CONDUCTION DISTURBANCES: ATRIOVENTRICULAR AND INTRAVENTRICULAR BLOCK

Ischemic injury can produce blocks at any level of the atrioventricular or intraventricular conduction system. Such blocks may occur in the atrioventricular node, producing various grades of AV block; in either main bundle branch, producing right or left bundle branch block; and in the anterior and posterior divisions of the left bundle, producing left anterior or left posterior (fascicular) divisional blocks. Disturbances of conduction can, of course, occur in various combinations. The mechanisms and recognition of intraventricular conduction disturbances are discussed in Chapter 5 and of atrioventricular conduction disturbances in Chapter 24.

FIRST-DEGREE AV BLOCK (see also p. 711). First-degree AV block (Fig. 24–40, p. 711) occurs in 4 to 14 per cent of patients with AMI admitted to coronary care units. His bundle electrocardiographic studies have shown that almost all patients with first-degree AV block have disturbances in conduction *above* the bundle of His, i.e., intranodal. The localization of the site of block is important, since development of complete heart block and ventricular asystole is restricted almost exclusively to those patients with first-degree block in whom the conduction disturbance is *below* the bundle of His[695]; this occurs more commonly in patients with anterior infarction and in those with associated bifascicular block.[696]

First-degree AV block generally does not require specific treatment. However, if digitalis intoxication is suspected as the cause, this drug should be discontinued. Beta blockers and calcium antagonists (other than nifedipine) prolong AV conduction and may be responsible for first-degree AV block as well. However, discontinuation of these drugs in the setting of AMI has the potential of increasing ischemia and ischemic injury. Therefore, in the presence of first-degree block alone, the clinician may consider decreasing the dosage of these drugs but for this reason alone should not discontinue them. Only if higher-degree block or hemodynamic impairment occurs should these agents be stopped. If the block is a manifestation of excessive vagotonia and is associated with sinus bradycardia and hypotension, administration of atropine, as

already outlined, may be helpful. In all circumstances, careful surveillance is important in view of the possibility of progression to higher degrees of block.[697]

SECOND-DEGREE AV BLOCK (see also p. 712). **Mobitz Type I, or Wenckebach.** Mobitz type I block (Fig. 24–43, p. 712) occurs in 4 to 10 per cent of patients with AMI admitted to coronary care units and accounts for about 90 per cent of all patients with AMI and second-degree AV block. This type of block (1) generally occurs within the AV node, (2) is usually associated with narrow QRS complexes, (3) is presumably secondary to ischemic injury, (4) occurs more commonly in patients with inferior than anterior myocardial infarction, (5) is usually transient and does not persist for more than 72 hours after infarction, (6) may be intermittent, and (7) rarely progresses to complete AV block. First-degree and type I second-degree AV block do not appear to affect survival, are most commonly associated with occlusion of the right coronary artery, and are caused by ischemia of the AV node.

Specific therapy also is not required in patients with second-degree AV block of the Mobitz type I variety when the ventricular rate is adequate and ventricular irritability, heart failure, and bundle branch block are absent. However, if these complications develop or if the heart rate falls below approximately 50 beats/min, immediate treatment with a temporary pacemaker is indicated.

Mobitz Type II. This is a rare conduction defect (Fig. 24–44, p. 712) following AMI, occurring in only 10 per cent of all cases of second-degree block[681]; thus, the overall incidence of Mobitz type II block after infarction is less than 1 per cent. In contrast to Mobitz type I block, type II second-degree block (1) usually originates from a lesion in the conduction system below the bundle of His, (2) is associated with a wide QRS complex, (3) often but not invariably reflects trifascicular block with impaired conduction distal to the bundle of His, (4) often progresses suddenly to complete AV block, and (5) is almost always associated with anterior rather than inferior infarction.

Because of its potential for progression to complete heart block, Mobitz type II second-degree AV block should be treated with a temporary demand pacemaker with the rate set at approximately 60 beats/min.

COMPLETE (THIRD-DEGREE) AV BLOCK (see also p. 714). The atrioventricular conduction system has a dual blood supply, the AV branch of the right coronary artery and the septal perforating branch from the left anterior descending coronary artery.[698] Therefore, complete AV block can occur in patients with either anterior or inferior infarction. Complete AV block develops in 5 to 8 per cent of patients with AMI. As with other forms of AV block, the prognosis depends on the anatomical location of the block in the conduction system and the size of the infarction.

In general, complete heart block in patients with inferior infarction results from an intranodal or prenodal lesion[699] and develops gradually, often progressing from first-degree or type I second-degree block. The escape rhythm is usually stable without asystole and often junctional, with a rate exceeding 40/min and a narrow QRS complex in 70 per cent of cases and a slower rate and wide QRS in the others. This form of complete AV block is often transient and resolves in a week.[696] The mortality is approximately 15 per cent unless right ventricular infarction is present, in which case the mortality associated with complete AV block may be more than doubled.[700]

In patients with anterior infarction, third-degree AV block often occurs suddenly, 12 to 24 hours after the onset of infarction, although it is usually preceded by intraventricular block and often a Mobitz type II pattern (not first-degree or Mobitz type I) AV block. Such patients have unstable escape rhythms with wide QRS complexes and rates less than 40 beats/min; ventricular asystole may occur quite suddenly. The mortality in this group of patients is extremely high, approximately 70 to 80 per cent.[701]

Prognosis. The prognosis for patients with AV block complicating AMI depends on the extent and secondarily on the anatomical site of the myocardial injury.[698] Thus, patients with inferior infarction often have concomitant ischemia or infarction of the AV node secondary to hypoperfusion of the AV node artery. However, the His-Purkinje system usually escapes injury in such individuals. Patients with inferior MI who develop AV block usually have lesions in both the right and left anterior descending arteries.[702] Likewise, patients with inferior MI and AV block have larger infarcts and more depressed right ventricular and left ventricular function than do patients with inferior infarct and no AV block. As already noted, junctional escape rhythms with narrow QRS complexes occur commonly in this setting. Hemodynamic derangements are often mild in these patients, and mortality is only slightly increased. In patients with anterior infarction, AV block usually develops as a result of extensive septal necrosis that involves the bundle branches. The high mortality in this group of patients with slow idioventricular rhythm and wide QRS complexes is the consequence of extensive myocardial necrosis resulting in severe left ventricular failure and often shock.

While data suggest that *complete* AV block is not an *independent* risk factor for mortality,[705] whether temporary transvenous pacing per se improves survival of patients with AMI remains controversial. Some investigators contend that ventricular pacing is useless when employed to correct complete AV block in patients with *anterior* infarction in view of the poor prognosis in this group regardless of therapy. We agree with others,[698,706] however, that ventricular or atrioventricular sequential pacing is indicated in essentially *all* patients with AMI with complete AV block. Pacing is likely to protect against transient hypotension with its attendant risks of extending infarction and precipitating malignant ventricular arrhythmias. Also, pacing protects against asystole, a particular hazard in patients with anterior infarction and infranodal block. Improved survival with pacing probably occurs in only a small fraction of patients with complete AV block and anterior wall infarcts, since the extensive destruction of the myocardium that almost invariably accompanies this condition results in a very high mortality rate, even in paced patients.

Given these considerations, an extremely large series of patients would be required to demonstrate the small reduction of mortality that might be achieved by pacing. The absence of data supporting such an effect, however, by no means excludes the possibility that it may be present. While it is generally agreed that pacing is indicated in patients with *inferior* wall infarction and complete AV block, it is of particular importance if the ventricular rate is very slow (<45 beats/min), if ventricular irritability or hypotension is present, or if pump failure develops; atropine is only rarely of value in these patients. Only when complete heart block develops in less than 6 hours after the onset of symptoms is atropine likely to abolish the AV block or cause acceleration of the escape rhythm.[707] In such cases the AV block is more likely to be transient and related to increases in vagal tone rather than the more persistent block seen later in the course of MI, which generally requires cardiac pacing.

INTRAVENTRICULAR BLOCK. Intraventricular conduction disturbances, i.e., block within one or more of the three subdivisions (fascicles) of the His-Purkinje system (the anterior and posterior divisions of the left bundle and the right bundle, p. 131), occur in 10 to 20 per cent of patients with AMI. The right bundle branch and the left posterior division have a dual blood supply from the left anterior descending and right coronary arteries, whereas the left anterior division is supplied by septal perforators originating from the left anterior descending coronary artery. Not all conduction blocks observed in patients with AMI can be considered to be complications of infarcts, since almost half are already present at the time the first ECG is recorded, and they may represent antecedent disease of the conduction system.

Isolated Left Anterior Divisional Block (Fig. 5–18, p. 130). This occurs in 3 to 5 per cent of patients with AMI,[708,709] and in an additional 5 per cent of patients with associated right bundle branch block and AMI.[708] Mortality is increased in these patients, although not as much as in patients with other forms of conduction block.

Left Posterior Divisional Block. This occurs in only 1 to 2 per cent of patients with AMI admitted to coronary care units. The posterior fascicle is larger than the anterior fascicle, and, in general, a larger infarct is required to block it. As a consequence, mortality is markedly increased.[708] Complete AV block is not a frequent complication of *either* form of isolated divisional block.

Right Bundle Branch Block. This defect alone occurs in approximately 2 per cent of patients with AMI and frequently leads to AV block because it is often a new lesion, associated with anteroseptal infarction. The mortality is high even if complete AV block does not occur.[681,708–711]

Bifascicular Block. The combination of right bundle branch block with either left anterior or posterior divisional block or the combination of left anterior and posterior divisional blocks (i.e., left bundle branch block) is known as bidivisional or bifascicular block (p. 132). If new block occurs in two of the three divisions of the conduction system, the risk of developing complete AV block is quite high.[681,708] Mortality is also high because of the occurrence of severe pump failure secondary to the extensive myocardial necrosis required to produce such an extensive intraventricular block.[712] Left bundle branch block occurs in approximately 5 per cent of patients with AMI. Although the latter defect progresses to complete AV block only half as frequently as does right bundle branch block, it is associated with as high a mortality as right bundle branch block and the other two forms of bifascicular block,[681,708,710,711] and with a high late mortality. Patients with intraventricular conduction defects, particularly right bundle branch block, account for the majority of patients who develop ventricular fibrillation late in their hospital stay. However, the high mortality in these patients occurs even in the absence of AV block and appears to be related to cardiac failure and massive infarction rather than to the conduction disturbance. Preexisting bundle branch block or divisional block is less often associated with the development of complete heart block in patients with AMI than are conduction defects acquired during the course of the infarct.[710] Bidivisional block in the presence of prolongation of the P-R interval (first-degree AV block) may indicate disease of the third subdivision rather than disease of the AV node. In such cases, termed trifascicular block, nearly 40 per cent will progress to complete heart block, a risk that is considerably greater than the risk of complete heart block without first-degree AV block.[706]

Complete bundle branch block (either left or right), the combination of right bundle branch block and left anterior divisional (fascicular) block, and any of the various forms of trifascicular block are all more often associated with anterior than inferoposterior infarction. All these forms are more frequent with large infarcts and in older patients and have a higher incidence of other accompanying arrhythmias than is seen in patients without bundle branch block.[711]

Use of Pacemakers in Acute Myocardial Infarction
(See also p. 728)

TEMPORARY PACING. Just as is the case for complete AV block, transvenous ventricular pacing has not resulted in statistically demonstrable improvement in prognosis among patients with AMI who develop intraventricular conduction defects. However, temporary pacing is advisable in certain of these patients because of the high risk of developing complete AV block. This includes patients with *new* bilateral (bifascicular) bundle branch block, i.e., right bundle branch block with left anterior or posterior divisional block and alternating right and left bundle branch block; first-degree AV block adds to this risk. Isolated new block in only one of the three fascicles even with P-R prolongation and preexisting bifascicular block and normal P-R interval poses somewhat less risk; these patients should be monitored closely, with insertion of a temporary pacemaker deferred unless higher-degree AV block occurs.

The risk of developing complete heart block following AMI can be predicted on the basis of results of an analysis of several large series of well-characterized patients with AMI.[712] The presence (new or preexisting) of any of the following conduction disturbances was considered a risk factor: first-degree AV block, Mobitz type I second-degree AV block, Mobitz type II second-degree AV block, left anterior hemiblock, left posterior hemiblock, right bundle branch block, and left bundle branch block. Each risk factor was assigned a score of 1, and the risk score was calculated as the sum of these electrocardiographic risk factors. The incidence of *complete heart block* occurred as follows: risk score 0, 1.2 to 6.8 per cent incidence; risk score 1, 7.8 to 10.4 per cent incidence; risk score 2, 25.0 to 30.1 per cent incidence; and risk score 3, 36 or greater per cent incidence.[712]

We believe that failure to demonstrate improved prognosis statistically does not belie the potential value of pacemaker therapy; it probably reflects the overriding impact on mortality of the extensive infarction responsible for the development of the conduction abnormality and the large number of patients required to permit statistical documentation of reduction of mortality.

Temporary pacing in AMI has been successfully employed for the last 2 decades. In assessing the need for temporary pacing (Table 39–10), the clinician must keep in mind that

TABLE 39-10   SUGGESTED USE OF TEMPORARY PACING WITH AMI

	STRENGTH OF INDICATION
Rate Disturbances	
Sinus bradycardia without hypotension, VEA, angina, left ventricular failure, or syncope	−
Sinus bradycardia with any of the above despite atropine	+
Accelerated idioventricular rhythm	−
Idioventricular rhythm with bradycardia, and hypotension or rate <45	+
Recurrent sick sinus syndrome, prolonged sinus pauses	+
Ventricular tachycardia (especially overdrive pacing for torsades de pointes)	+
Conduction Disturbances	
First-degree AV block	−
Second-degree AV block	
Mobitz I without bradycardia or hypotension	−
Mobitz I with bradycardia and hypotension	+
Mobitz II	+ +
Complete (third-degree) AV block	+ +
Isolated new or preexisting LAH, LPH, *or* RBBB	−
New LBBB	+
New bifascicular block*	+ +
Preexisting bifascicular block	−†
Asystole	+ +

Indications are graded as −, temporary pacing not indicated; +, temporary pacing should be considered, particularly if other therapeutic maneuvers have failed or if emergency pacer insertion would be difficult or logistically impossible at some other time (e.g., skilled personnel not always available); + +, temporary pacing should be instituted.

VEA = ventricular ectopic activity, AV = atrioventricular, LAH = left anterior hemiblock, LPH = left posterior hemiblock, RBBB = right bundle branch block, LBBB = left bundle branch block.

*Bifascicular block includes alternating right and left bundle branch block, right bundle branch block with left axis deviation, right bundle branch block with right axis deviation, and left bundle branch block with P-R interval prolongation.

†If duration of block is uncertain or if preexisting block occurs with new first-degree AV block, stronger consideration should be given.

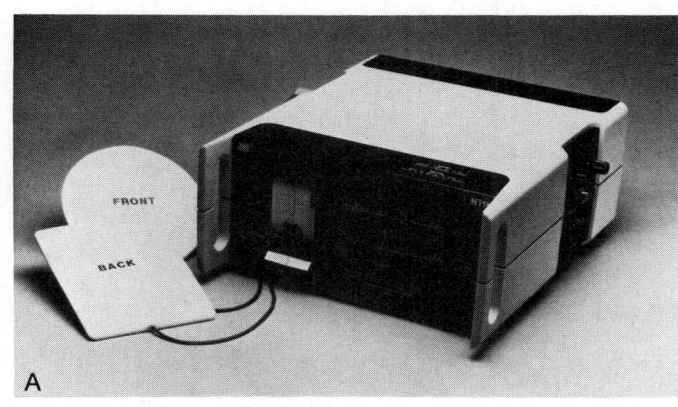
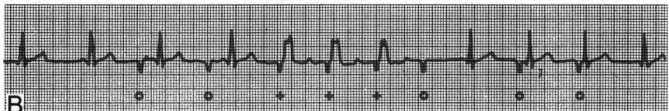

FIGURE 39-25. *A*, Noninvasive temporary pacing device shown with patient electrodes. The electrodes are self-adhering and applied to the left precordium (front) and posteriorly (back). The pacemaker includes an oscilloscopic monitor and strip recorder. Sensitivity, output, and rate adjustments can be made from the controls on the side of the device. *B*, Electrocardiographic strip during pacing with capture (+); also shown is the pacing artifact (0) when output of the pacer is lowered so as not to capture. The pacer rate is approximately 80 beats/min; the patient's intrinsic rate is approximately 60 beats/min. (Courtesy of P. Zoll, M.D.)

between 10 and 20 per cent of patients develop pacemaker-related complications.[713] A pericardial friction rub is heard in approximately 5 per cent of patients but does not necessarily indicate cardiac perforation, nor is such a finding an indication for withdrawal of the pacemaker electrode. Arrhythmias requiring cardioversion, right ventricular perforation, and local infectious complications occur in 1 to 3 per cent of cases.[713] Pacemaker malfunction also occurs rather frequently and is, in part, related to the experience of the clinical team in managing the device and its insertion.

Although external temporary cardiac pacing was introduced in 1952,[714] its widespread clinical use has not occurred until relatively recently, due to technical refinements making the technique safe, quickly applicable, and relatively well tolerated. Noninvasive external temporary cardiac pacing is now possible routinely in conscious patients and is acceptable to many but not all patients because of the discomfort[715] (Fig. 39–25). Used in a standby mode, it is virtually free of complications and contraindications and provides an important alternative to transvenous endocardial pacing. However, until its effectiveness has been more clearly documented, its routine use should be reserved for patients with moderate (or less) risk of complete heart block. Furthermore, once continuous pacing is required, external pacing is generally not well tolerated for more than minutes to hours. In such situations, it should be replaced by a temporary transvenous pacemaker.

PERMANENT PACING. The question of permanent pacing in survivors of AMI associated with conduction defects is still controversial[710,716,717] (Table 39–11). Patients with inferior infarction with *transient* type II second-degree block or complete AV block without an associated intraventricular conduction defect do not appear to require permanent pacing. Some contend that prophylactic pacing makes little difference in the long-term survival of patients with AMI and bundle branch block complicated by transient high-degree block.[718] On the other hand, in a retrospective multicenter study, survivors of AMI and bundle branch block who experienced transient high-degree (Mobitz type II second-degree, or third-degree) block had a high incidence of recurrent high-degree AV block and sudden death, and this incidence was reduced by insertion of a permanent demand pacemaker.[706,710] Thus, these findings suggest a role for prophylactic permanent pac-

**TABLE 39-11   SUGGESTED USE OF PERMANENT PACING
FOLLOWING AMI**

	STRENGTH OF INDICATION
Transient AV conduction disturbances in the absence of intraventricular conduction defects	−
Transient advanced* AV block and associated bundle branch block	+
Persistent first degree AV block with new bundle branch block	+
Persistent advanced* AV block	+ +

Indications are graded as −, permanent pacing not indicated; +, permanent pacing frequently used but opinion is divided (certain patients in this category warrant further testing, such as Holter monitoring or measurement of H-V conduction time before decision can be made); + +, permanent pacing indicated (insertion of pacemaker should take place before hospital discharge).

* Advanced heart block is defined as Mobitz II second-degree AV block or third-degree (complete) AV block.

ing in patients with AMI and bundle branch block with transient high-degree atrioventricular block.

The question of the advisability of permanent pacemaker insertion is complicated by the fact that not all sudden deaths in this population are due to recurrent high-degree block. A high incidence of late in-hospital ventricular fibrillation occurs in coronary care unit survivors with anteroseptal myocardial infarction complicated by either right or left bundle branch block.[719] If the propensity for this arrhythmia continued, ventricular fibrillation rather than asystole due to failure of atrioventricular conduction and of the infranodal pacemaker could be responsible for late sudden death.

Long-term pacing is often helpful when complete heart block persists throughout the hospital phase in a patient with acute myocardial infarction, or when sinus node function is impaired markedly, or when Mobitz II second- or third-degree block occurs intermittently. When block is associated with newly acquired bundle branch block or other criteria of impairment of conduction system function, prophylactic long-term pacing may be justified as well. Thus, despite the difficulty of proving that long-term pacing improves survival after MI because of the high mortality associated with extensive infarction frequently responsible for high degrees of heart block, prophylactic long-term pacing is prudent.

ASYSTOLE. This arrhythmia has been reported to occur in 1 to 14 per cent of patients with AMI admitted to coronary care units.[681] This wide variation in incidence reflects differences in the definition of this event. The lower incidence rates include only patients who develop asystole either as a primary event or following abnormalities of atrioventricular or intraventricular conduction, whereas the higher rates include patients who develop asystole as a terminal complication. In either event, the mortality is very high, ranging upward from 90 per cent.[681]

The presence of apparent ventricular asystole on monitor displays of continuously recorded electrocardiograms may be misleading, since the mechanism may in fact be fine ventricular fibrillation. Because of the predominance of ventricular fibrillation as the cause of cardiac arrest in this setting, initial therapy should include electrical countershock, even if definitive electrocardiographic documentation of this arrhythmia is not available. In the rare instance in which asystole can be documented to be the responsible electrophysiological disturbance, immediate transthoracic pacing (or stimulation with a transvenous pacemaker if one is already in place) is indicated. In this situation temporary noninvasive pacing with an external stimulating device may be life-saving.[715]

SUPRAVENTRICULAR TACHYARRHYTHMIAS

SINUS TACHYCARDIA (see also p. 673). Almost one-third of patients with an AMI will develop sinus tachycardia at some time during the first few days after the infarction,[681] an arrhythmia that may be associated with transient hypertension or hypotension and augmented sympathetic activity. The most common causes of sinus tachycardia are anxiety, persistent pain, and left ventricular failure. Other causes include fever, pericarditis, hypovolemia, atrial infarction, pulmonary embolism, and the administration of cardioaccelerator drugs such as atropine, epinephrine, or dopamine. Sinus tachycardia is particularly common in patients with anterior infarction. It is an undesirable rhythm in patients with AMI, since it results in an augmentation of myocardial oxygen consumption, as well as a reduction in the time available for coronary perfusion. Persistent sinus tachycardia may signify persistent heart failure and under these circumstances is a poor prognostic sign associated with an excess mortality. An underlying cause should be sought and appropriate treatment instituted, e.g., analgesics for pain, diuretics for heart failure, oxygen, beta blockers and nitroglycerin for ischemia, and aspirin for fever or pericarditis.

Administration of beta-adrenoceptor blocking agents, in the dosage and manner described on page 645, may be helpful in the treatment of sinus tachycardia, particularly when this arrhythmia is a manifestation of a hyperdynamic circulation, which is seen particularly in young patients with an initial MI without extensive cardiac damage. However, beta blockade is contraindicated in patients in whom the sinus tachycardia is a manifestation of hypovolemia or pump failure, the latter reflected by a systolic arterial pressure below 100 mm Hg, rales involving more than one-third of the lung fields, a pulmonary capillary wedge pressure exceeding 20 to 25 mm Hg, or a cardiac index below approximately 2.3 liters/min/m².

ATRIAL PREMATURE CONTRACTIONS (see also p. 377). Atrial premature contractions are relatively common after MI, occurring in up to half of all patients.[681,720,721] Atrial premature contractions, and the atrial tachyarrhythmias (paroxysmal supraventricular tachycardia, atrial flutter, and atrial fibrillation) that they often herald, may be caused by atrial distention secondary to increases in left ventricular diastolic pressure, by pericarditis with its associated atrial epicarditis, or, less commonly, by ischemic injury to the atria[722] and sinus node. Atrial premature beats per se are not associated with an increase in mortality,[721] and cardiac output is unaffected. Occasionally an atrial premature beat may initiate ventricular tachycardia or even ventricular fibrillation in the presence of AMI.

Premature atrial contractions require no specific therapy and may indicate atrial dilatation, excessive autonomic stimulation, or the presence of overt or occult heart failure. If they are related to heart failure, they often respond to treatment of this condition.

PAROXYSMAL SUPRAVENTRICULAR TACHYCARDIA (see also pp. 487 and 1684). This arrhythmia occurs in 2 to 11 per cent of patients with AMI.[721,723] It tends to be both transient and recurrent.[720] Its deleterious effects result from the elevation of myocardial oxygen consumption and the impairment of ventricular performance consequent to the rapid ventricular rate; it is associated with an increase in mortality.

Aggressive management is indicated for paroxysmal supraventricular tachycardia because of the rapid rate. Augmentation of vagal tone by manual carotid sinus stimulation may restore sinus rhythm. Intravenous verapamil is preferable to the use of alpha-adrenoceptor agonists to increase arterial pressure and activate carotid sinus baroreceptors. Although the latter is an acceptable form of therapy for paroxysmal supraventricular tachycardia under other circumstances, it can be hazardous in patients with AMI. Although digitalis glycosides may be useful in augmenting vagal tone, thereby terminating the arrhythmia, their effect is often delayed. Most rapidly acting is intravenous adenosine, which has recently been released for the treatment of supraventricular tachycardia. This agent should be *avoided* in MI patients with a low blood pressure because it is prone to cause hypotension. Accordingly, low-energy DC countershock or rapid atrial stimulation via a transvenous intraatrial electrode should be utilized if hemodynamic decompensation occurs or if the rhythm is refractory to conventional measures. *Paroxysmal atrial tachycardia with AV block* may be a manifestation of digitalis intoxication and should be treated by withholding this drug and instituting potassium therapy, when it is accompanied by hypokalemia.

ATRIAL FLUTTER AND FIBRILLATION (see also pp. 679 and 682). Atrial flutter is the least common major atrial arrhythmia associated with AMI, occurring in only 1 to 3 per cent of all patients.[721] As in patients who develop this arrhythmia in the absence of infarction, atrial flutter is usually associated with 2:1 atrioventricular block. Since the atrial rate ranges from 250 to 350 beats/min, the ventricular rate is usually 125 to 175 beats/min. Atrial flutter is usually transient and is a consequence of augmented sympathetic stimulation of the atria, often occurring in patients with left ventricular failure or pulmonary emboli. Atrial flutter often intensifies hemodynamic deterioration.[681,682,720]

Atrial fibrillation is far more common than flutter, occurring in 10 to 15 per cent of patients with AMI.[682,720,723] As with atrial premature contractions and atrial flutter, fibrillation is usually transient and tends to occur in patients with left ventricular failure but is also observed in patients with pericarditis and ischemic injury to the atria; it occurs more frequently following anterior than inferior infarction and appears to be a consequence of left atrial ischemia in the majority of cases.[724] The increased ventricular rate and the loss of the atrial contribution to left ventricular filling—i.e., the atrial kick—result in a significant reduction in cardiac output. Both atrial flutter and fibrillation are more common during the first 24 hours after infarction than later and are associated with increased mortality, particularly in patients with anterior wall infarction. However, because they are more common in patients with clinical and hemodynamic manifestations of extensive infarction and a poor prognosis, their *independent* contributions to increased mortality appear to be minor.[721,725] Unfortunately, their management is complicated by frequent recurrence, particularly when they result from left atrial dilatation secondary to left ventricular failure.

Management. Atrial flutter and fibrillation in patients with AMI are treated in a manner similar to that in other settings (pp. 681 and 683). However, because of the possibility that a rapid ventricular rate can increase infarct size and because of the important role played by atrial contraction in the support of cardiac output in patients with AMI (Fig. 39–24), treatment must be prompt, especially when the ventricular rate exceeds 100/min. *Digitalis glycosides* are the principal agents used to slow the ventricular response. Digitalis may be supplemented by small intravenous doses of a beta blocker, which also prolongs the AV nodal refractory period: 1 to 4 mg of propranolol in divided doses is often quite effective in reducing the ventricular rate and is well tolerated even in patients with mild heart failure and a rapid ventricular rate. Reduction of the rate of ventricular response to atrial fibrillation may be achieved also with verapamil administered intravenously via bolus injections of 60 to 120 μg/kg, followed by a continuous infusion of 2.5 to 5.0 μg/kg/min, although caution must be exercised to avoid systemic arterial hypotension. On the other hand, when hemodynamic decompensation is prominent, electrical cardioversion is indicated with anterior and laterally placed paddles,[726] beginning with 25 watt-seconds for atrial flutter and 50 watt-seconds for atrial fibrillation, with gradual increase if the initial shock is not successful.

An additional important option for the treatment of atrial flutter is the use of rapid atrial stimulation via a transvenous intraatrial electrode (p. 682); in contrast to DC cardioversion, this technique can be employed in the presence of possible digitalis intoxication, is less prone than DC countershock to elicit bradycardia after conversion to sinus rhythm, provides control of ventricular rate via atrial or ventricular pacing should this be necessary, and can be reapplied with less difficulty than cardioversion, should the patient experience recurrent atrial flutter. Following restoration of sinus rhythm, attention should be directed to the management of the underlying cause, usually heart failure, and to the prevention of recurrences, with antiarrhythmic agents such as quinidine. Patients with recurrent episodes should be treated with oral anticoagulants.

JUNCTIONAL RHYTHMS (see also p. 685). Sustained junctional rhythms fall into three categories:

1. *AV junctional rhythm* at a rate of 35 to 60 beats/min in which the AV junctional tissue simply assumes the role of the dominant pacemaker when the sinus node is depressed.

2. *Accelerated junctional rhythm* in which increased rhythmicity of the junctional tissue usurps the role of pacemaker, usually at a rate of 70 to 130 beats/min.

These two arrhythmias are often transient, occur during the first 48 hours of the infarction, usually develop and terminate gradually, and are characterized by QRS complexes that resemble those of normally conducted beats. Retrograde P waves may be evident, or atrioventricular dissociation may occur, with the junctional rate slightly in excess of the underlying sinus rate. Disagreement exists concerning the prognostic implications of these arrhythmias; some observers attach a poor prognosis to these arrhythmias, whereas others believe that they are benign.[720,727] However, in patients with relatively slow junctional rhythm, the process is generally a benign protective escape rhythm and is commonly seen among patients with a slow sinus rate in the presence of inferior myocardial infarction.

3. *Paroxysmal junctional tachycardia* usually produces rates between 160 and 220 beats/min.[720] This arrhythmia is uncommon in AMI, occurring in only 1 to 2 per cent of patients. In contrast to accelerated junctional rhythms, episodes of paroxysmal junctional tachycardia commence and terminate abruptly, thereby resembling other forms of paroxysmal supraventricular tachycardia, and they often occur in the presence of left ventricular failure, ischemia of the conduction system, or digitalis excess. When intraventricular conduction defects are present, it may be difficult to distinguish paroxysmal atrial or junctional tachycardia from ventricular tachycardia. The hemodynamic and prognostic significance of paroxysmal junctional tachycardia is similar to that for paroxysmal atrial tachycardia except that the atrial kick is lost with the junctional rhythm. As indicated above, the loss of atrial transport function may be tolerated poorly. When a junctional rhythm is present and there is hemodynamic impairment, transvenous sequential atrioventricular pacing may be required to facilitate ventricular performance and maintain adequate peripheral perfusion.

VENTRICULAR ARRHYTHMIAS

VENTRICULAR PREMATURE BEATS (VPBs) (see also p. 701). Although VPBs are very frequent, indeed almost universal[728] in the presence of AMI, the value of the so-called warning arrhythmias in the prediction of ventricular fibrillation is not clear. It was believed that warning arrhythmias—defined as frequent VPBs (more than five per minute), VPB's with multiform configuration, early coupling (the "R-on-T" phenomenon), and repetitive patterns in the form of couplets or salvos—presage ventricular fibrillation. However, it is now clear that they are present in as many patients who develop fibrillation as those who do not.[234] Several reports have shown that primary ventricular fibrillation (see below) occurs without antecedent warning arrhythmias in 40 to 83 per cent of cases.[728,729] On the other hand, frequent and complex VPBs are commonly observed in patients with AMI who never develop ventricular fibrillation.[728a,729]

Prognosis. The significance of early coupling ("R-on-T" phenomenon) has been reassessed in experimental[730] and clinical[729] studies. These have shown that ventricular tachyarrhythmias in patients with AMI are often initiated by a VPB that does *not* fall on an antecedent T wave. In fact, a majority of ventricular tachycardias in patients with AMI appear to be initiated by a *late*-coupled VPB.[731] In two clinical reports on electrocardiographic antecedents of primary ventricular fibrillation, 45 per cent[728] and 41 per cent[729] of episodes of ventricular fibrillation, respectively, were initiated by a late-coupled VPB. However, in one study[732] frequent VPBs showing the R-on-T phenomenon did appear to herald the development of ventricular fibrillation but not of ventricular tachycardia. Thus, the prognostic value, if any, of various forms of VPBs in AMI remains unclear.

Management. Historically, a large number of randomized trials have compared the routine (including prehospital[733]) administration of several potent antiarrhythmic drugs— lidocaine, quinidine, procainamide, and disopyramide, as well as beta-adrenoceptor blocking agents—against placebo.[734] All of these agents reduced the frequency of ventricular premature contractions, and in the case of lidocaine, routine administration lowered the incidence of ventricular fibrillation in some studies,[733,735,736] but not in all.[737] None of the agents administered in this fashion, however, conclusively reduced mortality.[738–740]

Frequent ventricular premature contractions occurring very soon after the onset of MI, particularly during the first hour, may depend primarily on reentry rather than on increased automaticity.[741] At this time, lidocaine, which impairs conduction in ventricular myocardium and diminishes automaticity, may be somewhat less effective than it is later.[738] When, at the very inception of an infarction, ventricular premature contractions are encountered in the presence of sinus tachycardia, augmented sympathoadrenal stimulation is often a contributing factor, and may be improved by beta-adrenoceptor blockade. In fact, early administration of an intravenous beta blocker is effective in reducing the incidence of ventricular fibrillation in evolving MI.[639,641] The effectiveness of beta-adrenoceptor blocking drugs under these circumstances may, in fact, play a role in the reduction in sudden deaths reported in patients who have recovered from AMI and are at high risk of recurrence.[645,647] The dosages and modes of administration as well as contraindications to beta blockade are discussed on pp. 645–646.

Lidocaine (see also p. 639). In the past, lidocaine was administered routinely to patients with AMI and "warning arrhythmias" including frequent ventricular premature contractions (>6/min), multiform premature contractions, extrasystoles occurring in pairs or salvos, and early premature contractions (R-on-T). On the basis of results of a recent trial[739] and pooled data from over 9000 patients,[740] this strategy can no longer be recommended. Furthermore, the complications of lidocaine prophylaxis might actually outweigh any small potential benefit, so that universal prophylaxis may actually be detrimental (Fig. 39–26). Lidocaine should be reserved for patients in whom sustained and/or symptomatic ventricular arrhythmias have occurred, for patients who cannot be managed with electrocardiographic monitoring, and possibly also for patients given thrombolytic agents because of the high incidence of "reperfusion" arrhythmias.

The pharmacology and pharmacokinetics of lidocaine are discussed on page 777. With regimens depending on continuous infusion alone, therapeutic blood levels (1.5 to 5 μg/ml) are reached only after several hours because of the short half-life of the drug. Therefore, a loading dose of 100 mg or 1.5 mg/kg should be given intravenously as a bolus injection at the time of admission or during the patient's transportation to the hospital, followed in 5 to 10 minutes by an injection of 0.5 mg/kg. An intravenous infusion should be started concomitantly; a dose of 50 μg/kg/min in patients without heart failure, hypotension, or primary hepatic dysfunction and of 20 μg/kg/min in patients with any of these problems is advised.[742] Intramuscular injections into the deltoid or gluteal muscles with conventional syringes and needles do not achieve therapeutic concentrations as promptly as do intravenous injections.

The maintenance dose of lidocaine should be adjusted within the range of 1 to 4 mg/min to reduce sharply or abolish premature ventricular contractions. It should be recognized that the metabolism of lidocaine is slowed not only in patients with heart failure or hypotension but also in those with diminution of hepatic blood flow due to effects of pharmacological agents such as propranolol.[743] The rate of infusion should be lower in patients taking cimetidine and in patients with renal failure. Therefore, careful titration is needed to avoid toxicity, manifested primarily by central nervous system hyperactivity, as well as by depression of intraventricular and atrioventricular conduction and cardiac contractility. Saturation of an extravascular pool normally occurs after a continuous infusion of approximately 3 hours, at which time blood levels will increase despite maintenance of a constant infusion rate.[744] At this time, it may be desirable to reduce the rate of administration by about 25 per cent.

Procainamide (see also p. 777). When ventricular premature contractions compromise hemodynamics and persist despite administration of lidocaine, or when lidocaine is contraindi-

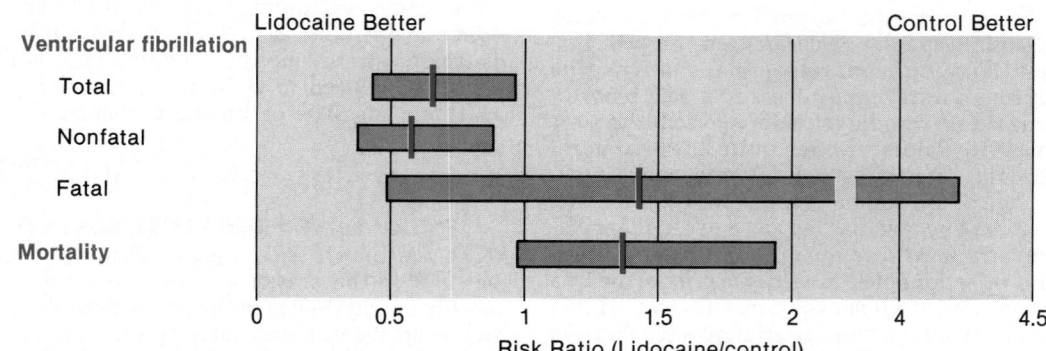

FIGURE 39–26. Pooled results of 14 randomized controlled trials of lidocaine in patients with suspected acute myocardial infarction suggest that the drug increases mortality despite reducing the risk of ventricular fibrillation. Patients received the drug intravenously (nine trials) or by intramuscular injection (five trials) and were followed for roughly the length of treatment (24 to 48 hours of IV administration, a few hours for IM). The narrow vertical bars represent the risk ratio derived from the pooled data and the broad horizontal bars show the 95% confidence limits for these ratios. (Adapted from Antman, E. M., and Braunwald, E.: Acute MI: Management in the 1990s. Hosp. Pract. July 15, 1990, p. 73.)

cated for other reasons (e.g., allergy), administration of procainamide intravenously in bolus doses of approximately 1 to 2 mg/kg intravenously over intervals of 5 minutes to a cumulative dose of approximately 1000 mg, followed by maintenance therapy with an intravenous infusion (20 to 80 μg/kg/min), may be effective. In patients with AMI, suppression of premature ventricular beats occurs at lower plasma concentrations of procainamide than are required in patients with chronic heart disease. This difference appears to reflect an electrophysiological difference, with the myocardium being more sensitive to the drug, rather than a change in procainamide pharmacokinetics, which is apparently normal in patients with AMI.[745]

Other Drugs. Other drugs such as tocainide[746] and propafenone[747] appear to be as effective as lidocaine for suppressing premature ventricular beats. Ventricular premature contractions that are unresponsive to lidocaine, procainamide, or tocainide in approximately the first 6 hours following AMI, particularly in the presence of sinus tachycardia, may be responsive to beta-adrenoceptor blocking agents.

Although phenytoin (Dilantin) (p. 641) (50 to 100 mg intravenously at 5 to 10 minute intervals to a total of 1000 mg) may diminish ventricular arrhythmia, it does not confer protection against ventricular fibrillation either in the first few hours[748] or later in the course of AMI.

The prognostic significance of VPBs in the postmyocardial infarction period continues to be controversial. Although there is little correlation between ventricular arrhythmias occurring in the early hours or days of AMI and those observed in the late postinfarction period,[749] frequent VPBs or ventricular tachycardia after hospital discharge are an independent risk factor for sudden death (p. 771).[750,751]

Because frequent and repetitive ventricular premature contractions are an independent risk factor for sudden cardiac death following AMI,[750,751] and because previous trials of antiarrhythmic agents to suppress ventricular ectopy in such patients have been flawed or inconclusive, a large placebo-controlled, double-blinded, multicenter study was initiated in 1987. This trial, known as the Cardiac Arrhythmia Suppression Trial (CAST), used the drugs flecainide, encainide, and moricizine to suppress ventricular arrhythmias in MI patients who were asymptomatic or mildly symptomatic. With over 1400 patients randomized and an average follow-up of 10 months, the flecanide and encainide arms of the trial were terminated prematurely because of a marked and unexpected increase (3.6 fold) in sudden cardiac death or arrest, and an increase in total mortality (2.5 fold) in the *treatment* groups[752] (Fig. 39–27). The important implications of this study have been much discussed.[753-755] They suggest that chronic prophylactic antiarrhythmic treatment of asymptomatic ventricular ectopy is *not* indicated after AMI, and specifically that type IC agents have powerful proarrhythmic effects that may entail risk with such drugs, particularly in patients who have recovered from AMI.

ACCELERATED IDIOVENTRICULAR RHYTHM (Fig. 24–35, p. 707). Commonly defined as a ventricular rhythm with a rate of 60 to 110 (or 125) beats/min,[756] and frequently called "slow ventricular tachycardia," this arrhythmia is seen in 8 to 20 per cent of patients with AMI, usually in the first 2 days, and seems to be equally common in anterior and inferior infarctions. About half of all episodes of accelerated idioventricular rhythm are manifested as an escape rhythm occurring during slowing of the sinus rhythm or gradual speeding of the ventricular pacemaker; the other half of accelerated idioventricular rhythms are initiated by a premature beat. Most episodes are of short duration, and the arrhythmia may terminate abruptly, slow gradually before termination, or be overdriven by acceleration of the basic cardiac rhythm. Variation of the rate is common. Accelerated idioventricular rhythms in patients with AMI probably result from enhanced automaticity of Purkinje fibers. In contrast to rapid ventricular tachycardia, accelerated idioventricular rhythms are thought not to affect prognosis.[234,756] However, accelerated idioventricular

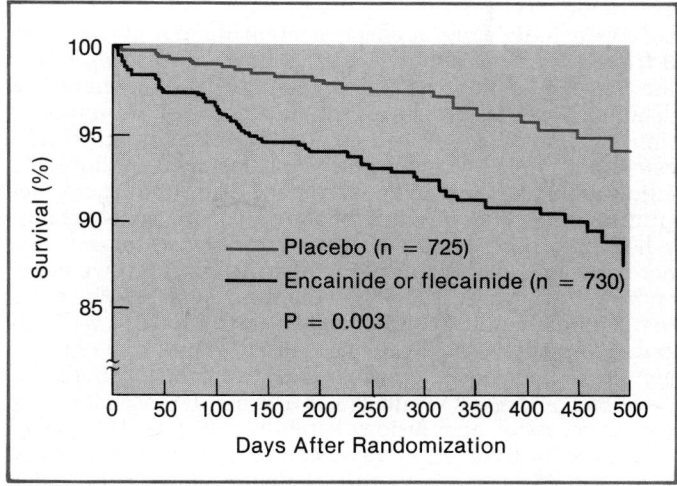

FIGURE 39–27. Survival among 1455 patients randomly assigned to receive encainide or flecainide, or matching placebo, from the Cardiac Arrhythmia Suppression Trial (CAST). The calculations were based on all causes of death. The nominal *p* value was based on a traditional two-sided log-rank test adjusted for multiple groups. A similarly significant difference in survival between groups was seen when only cardiac deaths were considered. (Reprinted by permission from the Cardiac Arrhythmias Suppression Trial [CAST] Investigators: Preliminary report: Effect of encainide and flecainide on mortality in a randomized trial of arrhythmia suppression after myocardial infarction. N. Engl. J. Med. *321*:406, 1989.)

rhythms are frequently associated with episodes of rapid ventricular tachycardia, and in many patients increased automaticity is manifested at times as accelerated idioventricular rhythms and at other times as ventricular tachycardia.

The need for treatment of this arrhythmia is controversial. Since these rhythms may deteriorate into ventricular tachycardia and since they may compromise cardiac function because of impairment of the physiological sequential relationship between atrial and ventricular contraction, it may be prudent to treat them by accelerating the sinus rate with atropine or atrial pacing or by suppressing the ventricular pacemaker with the administration of lidocaine intravenously. However, there is no definitive evidence that this arrhythmia, when left untreated, increases the incidence of either ventricular fibrillation or death.[757]

VENTRICULAR TACHYCARDIA (see also p. 658). This arrhythmia is generally defined as three or more consecutive ventricular ectopic beats occurring at a frequency exceeding 120 beats/min. It appears with a circadian variability similar to that seen with other phenomena associated with AMI, namely an increased incidence during the awake hours (Fig. 39–14, p. 1214).[758] The reported incidence of ventricular tachycardia in AMI is in the range of 10 to 40 per cent.[234,681] When this arrhythmia occurs within the first 24 hours, it is often precipitated by a late VPB and is generally transient and benign. Ventricular tachycardia occurring late in the course of AMI is more common in patients with transmural infarction and left ventricular dysfunction, is sustained, usually induces marked hemodynamic deterioration, and is associated with a relatively high hospital mortality rate—40 to 50 per cent.[681,759] However, the relative contribution to the high mortality rate of this arrhythmia per se, compared with that of the underlying impairment of left ventricular performance due to extensive infarction, is not clear.[759a] In addition, the long-term mortality in patients who exhibit ventricular tachycardia in the late hospital phase of AMI is greatly increased.[760]

Hypokalemia increases the risk of all ventricular tachycardia.[761] Low serum potassium should be identified quickly after a patient's admission for AMI and should be treated promptly. During the course of the patient's hospitalization, care should be taken to insure that the serum potassium level remains consistently above 4.0 mEq/liter. Care should be taken to identify and treat hypomagnesemia as well. Rapid abolition of ventricular tachycardia in patients with AMI is mandatory because of its deleterious effect on pump function and because it frequently deteriorates into ventricular fibrillation. When the ventricular rate is rapid (>150/min) and/or there is a decline in arterial pressure, a single attempt at "thump-version," i.e., striking a sharp blow to the precordium, is indicated (p. 775). If this maneuver is unsuccessful, it should be followed immediately by synchronized DC countershock, beginning with relatively low energies, i.e., 10 watt-seconds. When the ventricular rate is very rapid and synchronization is not possible, a defibrillatory impulse of 100 to 200 watt-seconds should be delivered. When the ventricular rate is slower than approximately 150/min and the arrhythmia is well tolerated hemodynamically, a brief (15 to 20 min) trial of treatment with lidocaine or procainamide, using the loading doses described on pages 636 and 639, is in order. If these measures are unsuccessful, an infusion of bretylium tosylate (1 to 2 mg/min) may be tried. After reversion to sinus rhythm, every effort should be made to correct underlying abnormalities such as hypoxia, hypotension, acid-base or electrolyte disturbances, and digitalis excess. Recurrent or refractory ventricular tachycardia may respond to aneurysm resection, encircling endocardial ventriculotomy, or endocardial resection with or without coronary artery bypass grafting (p. 1236); these surgical procedures are generally reserved for use until after the acute phase.[762-764]

VENTRICULAR FIBRILLATION (see also p. 709). This arrhythmia occurs in 4 to 18 per cent of patients with AMI treated in coronary care units.[728,729] It occurs with equal incidence in patients with anterior and with inferior Q-wave infarctions[234] and is rare in patients with non-Q-wave infarction. This arrhythmia may occur in three settings in hospitalized patients with AMI. (Its occurrence as a mechanism of sudden death is discussed in Chapter 26.) *Primary* ventricular fibrillation, responsible for more than 80 per cent of all instances of this arrhythmia, occurs suddenly and unexpectedly in patients with no or few signs or symptoms of left ventricular failure. Approximately 60 per cent of episodes occur within 4 hours and 80 per cent within 12 hours of the onset of symptoms. *Secondary* ventricular fibrillation, on the other hand, is the final phase of a progressive downhill course with left ventricular failure and cardiogenic shock.[681] So-called *late* ventricular fibrillation usually occurs 1 to 6 weeks following AMI. Patients with intraventricular conduction defects and anterior wall infarction, patients with persistent sinus tachycardia, atrial flutter, or fibrillation early in the clinical course, and those with right ventricular infarction who require ventricular pacing[765] all are at higher risk for suffering late *in-hospital* ventricular fibrillation than patients without these features. A recent large study has confirmed that the increase in mortality associated with late ventricular fibrillation (Fig. 39–28) is fully explained by the presence of heart failure in this group.[766]

Coronary care unit survivors with anteroseptal infarction complicated by right or left bundle branch block are particularly vulnerable to this late complication.[767] Those patients discharged alive with an anterior MI complicated by ventricular fibrillation face a much worse prognosis than those with inferior MI and ventricular fibrillation. In a case-controlled study, cumulative mortality at 5-year follow-up for the anterior MI group (54 per cent) was twice that for the inferior MI group (26 per cent).[768]

The effect of *primary* ventricular fibrillation on prognosis continues to be debated.[765,769] The MILIS study showed that it does not have an adverse effect,[769] while the first GISSI trial suggested that excess mortality due to primary ventricular fibrillation occurred only during the hospital phase but not thereafter.[770] On the other hand, *secondary* ventricular fibrillation occurring in association with marked left ventricular failure or hypotension clearly entails a dire prognosis, with only 20 to 25 per cent of patients surviving hospitalization.[757] The prognosis is intermediate in so-called late in-hospital ventricular fibrillation.[234] In the latter two forms it is the impair-

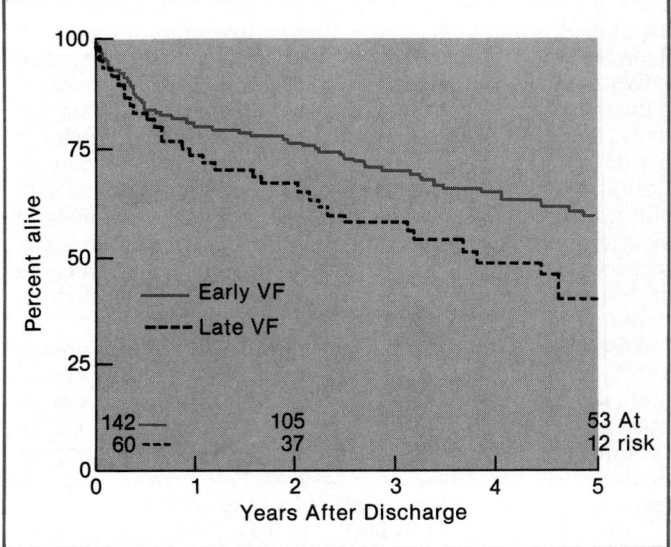

FIGURE 39–28. Kaplan-Meier survival curves from study of 422 consecutive patients discharged alive after acute myocardial infarction complicated by ventricular fibrillation (VF). (From Jeusen G.V.H., et al.: Prognosis of late versus early ventricular fibrillation in acute myocardial infarction. Am. J. Cardiol. 66:10, 1990.)

ment of cardiac function consequent to the loss of contracting myocardium rather than the arrhythmia per se that is responsible for the poor prognosis.

Procainamide, lidocaine,[733,735] and the beta-adrenoceptor blockers propranolol[639] and metoprolol[771] administered prophylactically have all been reported to reduce the incidence of primary ventricular fibrillation in hospitalized patients. However, they may not reduce overall mortality substantially because treatment of this arrhythmia is so successful in an efficient coronary care unit.

Management. The treatment of ventricular fibrillation is *electrical countershock*, implemented as rapidly as possible. The likelihood of successful restoration of an effective cardiac rhythm declines rapidly with time after the onset of uncorrected ventricular fibrillation. Irreversible brain damage may occur within 1 to 2 minutes, particularly in elderly patients. Despite the superficial appeal of "thump-version," which may sometimes terminate ventricular tachycardia (as opposed to fibrillation), no time should be lost before treating patients with ventricular fibrillation by means of electrical countershock.

Prompt electrical countershock generally interrupts fibrillation and restores an effective cardiac rhythm in patients under direct medical observation in the coronary care unit. When ventricular fibrillation occurs outside of an intensive care unit, resuscitative efforts are much less likely to be successful, primarily because the time interval between the onset of the episode and institution of definitive therapy tends to be prolonged. Since closed-chest cardiopulmonary resuscitation with external cardiac compression provides only a marginal cardiac output even under optimal circumstances, countershock should be implemented as soon as possible after the detection of ventricular fibrillation rather than deferred under the mistaken impression that adequate circulatory and respiratory support can be maintained in the interim. Failure of electrical countershock to restore an effective cardiac rhythm is due almost always to rapidly recurrent ventricular tachycardia or ventricular fibrillation, to electromechanical dissociation, or, very rarely, to electrical asystole.

Ventricular fibrillation often recurs rapidly and repeatedly when the metabolic milieu of the heart has been compromised by severe or prolonged hypoxemia, acidosis, electrolyte abnormalities, or digitalis intoxication. Under these conditions, continued cardiopulmonary resuscitation, prompt implementation of pharmacological and ventilatory maneuvers designed to correct these abnormalities, treatment with antiarrhythmic agents such as lidocaine, and rapidly repeated attempts with electrical countershock may be effective. Even though repeated shocks with excessive energy may damage the myocardium[772] and elicit arrhythmias,[773] speed is essential and prompt efforts with high-intensity shocks (generally 300 to 400 watt-seconds initially) are justified. When ventricular fibrillation persists without documented interruption by electrical countershock, the intracardiac administration of epinephrine (up to 10 ml of a 1 : 10,000 concentration) or calcium gluconate (up to 15 ml of 10 per cent calcium gluconate) may facilitate success in a subsequent attempt. Conversion of fine to coarse ventricular fibrillation by either or both of these drugs may augur well for subsequent successful defibrillation.

Successful interruption of ventricular fibrillation or prevention of refractory recurrent episodes may be facilitated by administration of *bretylium tosylate*, 5 mg/kg intravenously, repeated 20 minutes later if necessary (p. 648).[774] When synchronous cardiac electrical activity is restored by countershock, but contraction is ineffective—i.e., during electromechanical dissociation, the usual underlying cause is very extensive myocardial ischemia or necrosis or rupture of the ventricular free wall or septum.[775,776] If rupture has not occurred, intracardiac administration of calcium gluconate or epinephrine may facilitate restoration of an effective heartbeat. Another antifibrillatory agent is amiodarone (p. 646). It has a slow onset of action; therefore, its principal role may prove to be in the *prevention* rather than treatment of ventricular fibrillation.

Hemodynamic Disturbances in Acute Myocardial Infarction

More than one and a half decades ago Swan, Forrester, and their associates measured the cardiac output and wedge pressure simultaneously in a large series of patients with AMI and identified four major hemodynamic subsets of patients (Table 39–12): (1) patients with normal perfusion and without pulmonary congestion (normal cardiac output and normal wedge pressure); (2) patients with normal perfusion and pulmonary congestion (normal cardiac output and elevated wedge pressure); (3) patients with decreased perfusion but without pulmonary congestion (reduced cardiac output and normal wedge pressure); and (4) patients with decreased perfusion and pulmonary congestion (reduced cardiac output and elevated wedge pressure).[777] Although this classification has proved to be quite useful, patients frequently pass from one category to another with therapy and, sometimes, even apparently spontaneously.

HEMODYNAMIC SUBSETS. These are usually reflected in the patient's clinical status. Hypoperfusion usually becomes evident clinically when the cardiac index falls below approximately 2.2 liters/min/sq meter, whereas pulmonary congestion is noted when the wedge pressure exceeds approximately 20 mm Hg. However, approximately 25 per cent of patients with cardiac indices less than 2.2 liters/min/sq meter and 15 per cent of patients with elevated pulmonary capillary wedge pressures are not recognized clinically. Discrepancies in hemodynamic and clinical classification of patients with AMI arise for a variety of reasons. Patients may exhibit "phase lags" as clinical pulmonary congestion develops or resolves, symptoms secondary to chronic obstructive pulmonary disease may be confused with those resulting from pulmonary congestion, or longstanding left ventricular dysfunction may mask signs of hypoperfusion secondary to compensatory vasoconstriction.[777]

The hemodynamic subsets shown in Table 39–12 allow for rational approaches to therapy as indicated in Table 39–13.

The goals of hemodynamic therapy are to maintain ventricular performance, support blood pressure, and protect jeopardized myocardium. Since these goals occasionally may be at cross purposes, careful recognition of the hemodynamic profile, as assessed clinically or as available from hemodynamic monitoring, is required before optimal therapeutic interventions can be chosen.

INVASIVE HEMODYNAMIC MONITORING (see also p. 617 and Table 39–4 p. 1226). Hemodynamic assessment becomes possible once the patient reaches the hospital. An estimation of the presence or absence of gross abnormalities in cardiac index and left ventricular filling pressure can be made on the basis of clinical examination in approximately 80 per cent of patients. However, as noted above, severe depression of cardiac index and/or elevation of left ventricular filling pressure may be unsuspected in as many as 15 per cent of patients when estimates are based exclusively on clinical criteria.[440]

In patients with *clinically uncomplicated AMI*, invasive hemodynamic monitoring is not necessary, since the status of the circulation can be assessed by careful clinical evaluation. This ordinarily consists of monitoring of heart rate and rhythm, measurement of systemic arterial pressure by cuff, obtaining chest roentgenograms to detect heart failure, careful and repeated auscultation of the lung fields for pulmonary congestion, measurement of urine flow, examination of the skin and mucous membranes for evidence of the adequacy of perfusion, and arterial sampling for pO_2, pCO_2, and pH when hypoxemia or metabolic acidosis is suspected.

Invasive monitoring ordinarily consists of inserting an arterial line for the continuous measurement of arterial pressure and a balloon flotation catheter for measurement of pulmonary artery, pulmonary artery occlusive (equivalent to pulmonary wedge), and right atrial pressures, and cardiac output by thermodilution. In patients with hypotension, a Foley

TABLE 39–12 HEMODYNAMIC SUBSETS IN ACUTE MYOCARDIAL INFARCTION

CLINICAL SUBSET	CARDIAC INDEX (liter/min/sq meter)	PULMONARY CAPILLARY WEDGE PRESSURE (mm Hg)	MORTALITY (%)
I. No pulmonary congestion or peripheral hypoperfusion	2.7 ± 0.5	12 ± 7	2.2
II. Isolated pulmonary congestion	2.3 ± 0.4	23 ± 5	10.1
III. Isolated peripheral hypoperfusion	1.9 ± 0.4	12 ± 5	22.4
IV. Both pulmonary congestion and hypoperfusion	1.6 ± 0.6	27 ± 8	55.5

From Forrester, J. S., et al.: Medical therapy of acute myocardial infarction by application of hemodynamic subsets. N. Engl. J. Med. *295*:1404, 1976. Reprinted by permission of the New England Journal of Medicine.

TABLE 39–13 POTENTIALLY USEFUL THERAPEUTIC INTERVENTIONS IN HEMODYNAMIC CATEGORIES OF PATIENTS WITH ACUTE MYOCARDIAL INFARCTION

HEMODYNAMIC CATEGORY	P_a*	$\overline{PA}_o$†	CI‡	SUGGESTED INTERVENTION	REMARKS
Normal	≤15	≤12	2.7–3.5‡	None	β-Blockade may be beneficial
Hyperdynamic state	≤15	≤12	≥3.0	β-Adrenoceptor blockage	Tachycardia is a hallmark of subset
Hypotension or shock secondary to hypovolemia	≤15	≤9	≤2.7	Repletion of vascular volume	Reclassification may be necessary after PA_o is increased to range of 14 to 18 mm Hg
LV failure					
Mild	≥22	≥18 – ≤22	≤2.5	Diuretics	Dyspnea, hypoxemia, or mild pulmonary vascular congestion
Severe	≥25	≥22	≤1.8	Vasodilators + diuretics	Pulmonary vascular congestion and pulmonary edema; cardiac glycosides; positive pressure ventilation and/or circulatory assist may be useful
Cardiogenic hypotension or shock	≥22	≥18	≤1.8	Circulatory assist	Sympathomimetic agents with positive inotropic effects such as dopamine or dobutamine may be useful

* $\underline{P_a}$, mean pulmonary artery pressure in mm Hg.
† $\overline{PA}_o$, mean pulmonary artery occlusive pressure in mm Hg.
‡ CI, cardiac index in liter/min/sq mm.

catheter provides accurate and continuous measurement of urine output.

The importance of invasive hemodynamic monitoring[440] is based on the following principal factors:

1. Difficulty of interpreting clinical and radiographic findings of pulmonary congestion because of phase lags, such as those occurring after diuretic therapy.

2. Need for identifying noncardiac causes of arterial hypotension, particularly hypovolemia.

3. Possible contributions of reduced ventricular compliance to impaired hemodynamics, requiring judicious adjustment of intravascular volume to optimize left ventricular filling pressure.

4. Difficulty in assessing the severity and sometimes even determining the presence of lesions such as mitral regurgitation and ventricular septal defect when the cardiac output or the systemic pressures are depressed.

5. Establishing a baseline of hemodynamic measurements and guiding therapy in patients with clinically apparent pulmonary edema or cardiogenic shock.

6. Underestimation of systemic arterial pressure by the cuff method in patients with intense vasoconstriction.

HYPOTENSION IN THE PREHOSPITAL PHASE

During the *prehospital phase of AMI*, invasive hemodynamic monitoring is usually not practical, and during this period, therapy should be guided by frequent clinical assessment and measurement of arterial pressure by the cuff method, with the recognition that intense vasoconstriction can provide a falsely low pressure measured by this method. Hypotension associated with bradycardia often reflects excessive vagotonia, which may be responsive to atropine and elevation of the lower extremities. Relative or absolute hypovolemia is often present when hypotension occurs with a normal or rapid heart rate, particularly among patients receiving diuretics just prior to the occurrence of infarction. Marked diaphoresis, reduction of fluid intake, or vomiting during the period preceding and accompanying the onset of AMI may all contribute to the development of hypovolemia. Even if the effective vascular volume is normal, *relative* hypovolemia may be present, since ventricular compliance is reduced in AMI and a left ventricular filling pressure as high as 20 mm Hg may be needed to provide an optimal preload.

MANAGEMENT. In the absence of rales involving more than one-third of the lung fields, the patient should be put in the reverse Trendelenburg position and in those with sinus

bradycardia and hypotension, atropine should be administered (0.3 to 0.6 mg intravenously repeated at 3 to 10-min intervals up to 2.0 mg). If these measures do not correct the hypotension, crystalloid solutions should be administered intravenously, beginning with a bolus of 100 ml followed by 50-ml increments every 5 minutes. The patient should be carefully observed and the infusion stopped when the systolic pressure returns to approximately 100 mm Hg, if the patient becomes dyspneic, or if pulmonary rales develop or increase. Because of the poor correlation between left ventricular filling pressure and mean right atrial pressure, assessment of systemic (even central) venous pressure is of limited value as a guide to fluid therapy.

Administration of cardiotonic agents (see below) is indicated during the prehospital phase if systemic hypotension persists despite correction of hypovolemia and excessive vagotonia. In the absence of invasive hemodynamic monitoring, assessment of peripheral vascular resistance must be based on clinical observations. If cutaneous vasoconstriction is present, therapy with dobutamine, which stimulates cardiac contractility without unduly accelerating heart rate and which does not increase the impedance to ventricular outflow, may be helpful (p. 502). In hypotensive patients with AMI, when there is clinical evidence of vasodilatation, an uncommon circumstance, phenylephrine hydrochloride is preferable, although this agent, which increases coronary as well as peripheral vascular tone, should be used with caution.

HYPOVOLEMIC HYPOTENSION

Recognition of hypovolemia is of particular importance in hypotensive patients with AMI, because of the hazard it poses and because of the improvement in circulatory dynamics that can be achieved so readily and safely by augmentation of vascular volume. Since hypovolemia is often occult, it is frequently overlooked in the absence of invasive hemodynamic monitoring. It may be absolute, with low left ventricular filling pressure (<8 mm Hg), or relative, with normal (8 to 12 mm Hg) or even modestly increased (13 to 18 mm Hg) left ventricular filling pressures. Because of the reduction of left ventricular compliance that occurs with acute ischemia and infarction (p. 1178), left ventricular filling pressures between 13 and 18 mm Hg, while above the upper limits of normal, may actually be suboptimal.

Exclusion of hypovolemia as the cause of hypotension requires documentation of a reduced cardiac output despite left ventricular filling pressure *exceeding* 18 mm Hg. If, in a hypotensive patient, the pulmonary capillary wedge pressure (ordinarily measured as the pulmonary artery occlusive pressure) is below this level, fluid challenge should be carried out with sequential 50 ml intravenous bolus infusions, and serial assessments should be made of pulmonary capillary wedge pressure and cardiac output. Elevation of pulmonary capillary wedge pressure to between 18 and 24 mm Hg in patients with AMI reflects the achievement of a left ventricular filling pressure associated with an optimal cardiac output. If hypovolemia is documented or suspected, the fluid replaced should resemble the fluid lost. Thus, when a low hematocrit complicates AMI, infusion of packed red blood cells or whole blood is the treatment of choice. On the other hand, crystalloid or colloid solutions should be administered when the hematocrit is normal or elevated.

Hypotension caused by *right ventricular infarction* may be confused with that caused by hypovolemia, because both are associated with a low, normal, or minimally elevated left ventricular filling pressure. The findings in and management of right ventricular infarction are discussed on page 1205.

THE HYPERDYNAMIC STATE

When infarction is not complicated by hemodynamic impairment, no therapy other than general supportive measures and treatment of arrhythmias is necessary. However, if the hemodynamic profile is of the hyperdynamic state, i.e., elevation of sinus rate, arterial pressure, and cardiac index, occurring singly or together in the presence of a normal or low left ventricular filling pressure, and if other causes of tachycardia such as fever, infection, and pericarditis can be excluded, treatment with beta-adrenoceptor blockers is indicated. The rationale, dose, and mode of administration are discussed on pp. 1236–1237. Presumably, the increased heart rate and blood pressure are the result of inappropriate activation of the sympathetic nervous system, possibly secondary to augmented release of catecholamines or anxiety or both.

LEFT VENTRICULAR FAILURE AND CARDIOGENIC SHOCK

In patients with AMI, heart failure is characterized either by diastolic dysfunction alone or by both systolic and diastolic dysfunction.[777a] Left ventricular diastolic dysfunction leads to pulmonary venous hypertension and pulmonary congestion, while systolic dysfunction is principally responsible for a depression of cardiac output, and of the ejection fraction. Clinical manifestations of left ventricular failure become more common as the extent of the injury to the left ventricle increases. More than 75 per cent of patients with pulmonary congestion and AMI have an ejection fraction of less than 40 per cent and more than a third have an ejection fraction of less than 30 per cent.[778]

Clinical application of the Frank-Starling principle is useful for characterizing myocardial function in the AMI patient. If the cardiac index is plotted as a function of the pulmonary capillary wedge pressure (a modified Starling relationship) in patients with AMI, a wide range of left ventricular performances is apparent (Fig. 39–29). It is clear from this figure that one-third of patients with AMI have normal resting left ventricular hemodynamics and that mortality in AMI increases in association with the severity of the hemodynamic deficit.[777]

Physiological assessment of left ventricular function refines the information obtained by clinical means.[440] Among patients with AMI that is clinically uncomplicated (Killip Class I), approximately 50 per cent have a reduced cardiac output and 75 per cent have an elevated ventricular filling pressure. Patients with one or both of these hemodynamic abnormalities have a worse prognosis than those without any hemodynamic disturbance, even though their infarction may be clinically uncomplicated.[440] Similarly, the prognosis of patients in Killip Class IV (cardiogenic shock) is a function of the hemodynamic status. Rackley et al. reported that in such patients a filling pressure greater than 29 mm Hg was associated

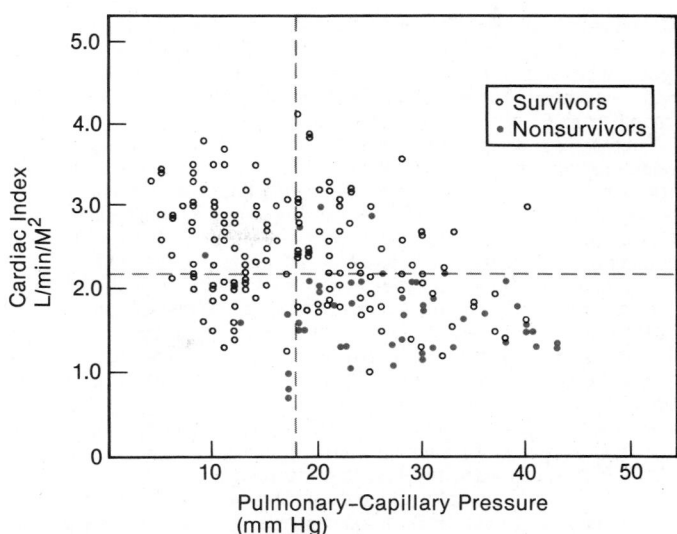

FIGURE 39–29. Relation between pulmonary-capillary pressure and cardiac index in 200 patients with acute myocardial infarction. The dotted lines are placed at the levels of 18 mm Hg for pulmonary-capillary pressure and 2.1 liters per minute per square meter for cardiac index. There is a wide degree of variability in left ventricular performance in patients with acute myocardial infarction, and mortality rate increases as cardiac performance deteriorates. (Reprinted by permission from Forrester, J. S., et al.: Medical therapy of acute myocardial infarction by application of hemodynamic subsets. N. Engl. J. Med. **295**:1356, 1976.)

with a mortality of 100 per cent, a filling pressure greater than 15 mm Hg and a cardiac index less than 2 liters/min/sq meter with a mortality of 93 per cent, and a filling pressure less than 15 mm Hg and a cardiac index less than 2 liters/min/sq meter with a mortality of 63 per cent.[440] Thus, hemodynamics and prognosis vary widely among patients with AMI with similar clinical presentations. Therefore, measurement of pertinent hemodynamic variables may be of great value in patients with complications.

THERAPEUTIC IMPLICATIONS. Classification of patients with AMI by hemodynamic subsets has therapeutic relevance. As already noted, patients with normal wedge pressures and hypoperfusion often benefit from infusion of fluids, since the peak value of stroke volume is usually not attained until left ventricular filling pressure reaches 18 to 24 mm Hg.[440] However, a low level of left ventricular filling pressure does not imply that left ventricular damage is necessarily slight. Such patients may be relatively hypovolemic and/or may have suffered a right ventricular infarct with or without severe left ventricular damage.[779]

The relation between ventricular filling pressure and cardiac index when preload is increased by an infusion of saline or dextran can provide valuable hemodynamic information, in addition to that obtained from baseline measurements. For example, the ventricular function curve rises steeply (marked increase in cardiac index, small increase in filling pressure) in patients with normal left ventricular function and hypovolemia, whereas the curve rises gradually or remains flat in those patients with a combination of hypovolemia and depressed cardiac function.

Cardiogenic Shock

(See also p. 576)

PATHOLOGICAL FINDINGS. The severest clinical expression of left ventricular failure, cardiogenic shock, is associated with extensive damage to the left ventricular myocardium. Page et al., who studied 20 such patients at autopsy, found that all exhibited necrosis of at least 40 per cent of the left ventricle. In contrast, 35 per cent or less of the left ventricle had been destroyed in all but 1 of 14 patients who succumbed without having been in cardiogenic shock.[780] Similar findings were reported by Alonso et al.: Patients with cardiogenic shock had lost an average of 51 per cent of the left ventricular myocardium (range: 35 to 68 per cent), whereas in a group of patients with AMI who died suddenly from arrhythmias and who had never been in cardiogenic shock, necrosis averaged 23 per cent (range: 14 to 31 per cent) of the left ventricle.[781]

Patients who die as a consequence of cardiogenic shock usually develop this complication while in the hospital. These individuals often have "piecemeal" necrosis, progressive myocardial necrosis from marginal extension of their infarct into an ischemic zone bordering on the infarction. This is generally associated with persistent elevation of CK-MB. Early deterioration in left ventricular function secondary to apparent extension of infarction may, in some cases, result from *expansion* of the necrotic zone of myocardium without actual *extension* of the necrotic process (p. 1219). Shearing forces that develop during ventricular systole can disrupt necrotic myocardial muscle bundles, with resultant expansion and thinning of the akinetic zone of myocardium, which in turn results in deterioration of overall left ventricular function.

At autopsy, patients with cardiogenic shock consistently demonstrate marginal extension of recent areas of infarction (Fig. 39–18) (p. 1228).[780,781] Additionally, focal areas of necrosis are frequently found in regions of the left and right ventricles that are not adjacent to the major area of recent infarction.[780] Such extensions and focal lesions are probably in part the result of the shock state itself, since they can also be found in the hearts of patients dying of noncardiogenic shock. Infarction of the ischemic periinfarction zone can be precipitated by a number of factors that adversely affect the supply of oxygen or the metabolic demand in this zone of myocardium. These adverse factors include a reduction of coronary perfusion pressure and an augmentation of myocardial oxygen demand resulting from the local release of catecholamines from ischemic adrenergic nerve endings in the heart as well as from circulating endogenous or infused catecholamines. Patients with rupture of the ventricular septum or of a papillary muscle can also exhibit cardiogenic shock. These patients often have smaller infarcts than do those with cardiogenic shock secondary to ventricular failure without a mechanical lesion. The prognosis is better in such patients, since the smaller infarct allows their left ventricle to support the circulation once the mechanical defect has been corrected surgically.

PATHOPHYSIOLOGY. The shock state in patients with AMI appears to be the result of a vicious circle, demonstrated in Figure 39–11, p. 1210. According to this formulation, coronary obstruction leads to myocardial ischemia, which impairs myocardial contractility and ventricular performance. This, in turn, reduces arterial pressure and therefore coronary perfusion pressure, leading to further ischemia and extension of necrosis until the left ventricle has insufficient contracting myocardium to sustain life. The progressive nature of the myocardial insult in this syndrome is reflected in the stuttering and progressive evolution of elevations in the plasma enzyme–time activity curves of markers specific for myocardial injury. Consideration of this vicious circle also points to the hazard of hypovolemic hypotension in patients with AMI but without cardiogenic shock; hypotension reduces coronary perfusion and thereby may enhance necrosis.

At autopsy, more than two-thirds of patients with cardiogenic shock demonstrate stenosis of 75 per cent or more of the luminal diameter of all three major coronary vessels, usually including the left anterior descending coronary artery.[782] Almost all patients with cardiogenic shock are found to have thrombotic occlusion of the artery supplying the major region of recent infarction.[780,781]

For many years the incidence of cardiogenic shock following AMI was about 15 per cent. Recent series have suggested that its incidence has fallen to about 7 per cent.[783] While this is in part related to newer interventional techniques, such as intraaortic balloon pumps and coronary angioplasty,[784] it is probable that medical therapy with thrombolysis and early treatment of ongoing ischemia are also responsible for this improvement.[783,785] Although the onset of shock is generally early in the course of AMI, when shock does develop later, it usually is due to infarct extension.[783]

MANAGEMENT OF LEFT VENTRICULAR FAILURE

Invasive hemodynamic monitoring is essential to guide therapy of patients with severe left ventricular failure.

AVOIDANCE OF HYPOXEMIA. The treatment of left ventricular failure with AMI requires meticulous attention to ventilation, since hypoxemia can impair the function of ischemic tissue at the margin of the infarct and thereby contribute to establishing or perpetuating the vicious circle (Fig. 39–11,

p. 1210) The combination of pulmonary vascular congestion (or when it is severe, pulmonary edema), reduced pulmonary compliance, and the respiratory depression that may be associated with excessive doses of analgesics conspires to impair ventilatory function and arterial oxygenation. When in patients with left ventricular failure secondary to AMI arterial oxygen tension cannot be maintained above 60 mm Hg despite inhalation of 100 per cent oxygen delivered at 8 liters/min by mask and the adequate use of bronchodilators, endotracheal intubation, assisted ventilation, and positive pressure should be considered. The improvement of arterial oxygenation and hence myocardial oxygen supply may help to restore ventricular performance. Positive end-expiratory pressure may diminish systemic venous return and reduce effective left ventricular filling pressure. Once a patient is intubated and mechanically ventilated, withdrawal of the support during the recovery phase must be undertaken extremely carefully. Since myocardial ischemia frequently occurs during the return to unsupported spontaneous breathing,[786] the weaning process should be accompanied by careful observation for signs of ischemia and is potentially facilitated by a period of intermittent mandatory ventilation before extubation. Continuous ST-segment monitoring has been recommended for these patients.[786]

When wheezing complicates pulmonary congestion, bronchodilators that act primarily on beta₂-adrenoceptors, such as isoetharine or metaproterenol, given as aerosols, or terbutaline, which can be administered subcutaneously or orally, are more desirable than conventional bronchodilators, such as isoproterenol or epinephrine, whose primary effects are on beta₁-receptors.

Although positive inotropic agents may be useful, they do *not* represent the *initial* therapy of choice in patients with AMI. Instead, heart failure in this setting is managed most effectively first by reduction of blood volume and ventricular preload, and then, if possible, by lowering afterload. Arrhythmias may contribute to hemodynamic compromise as discussed on page 1240 and should be treated promptly in patients with left ventricular failure.

The use of rotating tourniquets, routine in past years for advanced degrees of pulmonary congestion, is probably ineffective and not recommended.[787]

DIURETICS (see also p. 472). Mild heart failure in patients with AMI frequently responds well to diuretics such as furosemide, administered intravenously in doses of 10 to 40 mg, repeated at 3 to 4 hour intervals if necessary. The resultant reduction of pulmonary capillary pressure reduces dyspnea, and the lowering of left ventricular wall tension that accompanies the reduction of left ventricular diastolic volume diminishes myocardial oxygen requirements and may lead to improvement of contractility and augmentation of the ejection fraction, stroke volume, and cardiac output. The reduction of elevated left ventricular filling pressure may also enhance myocardial oxygen delivery by diminishing the impedance to coronary perfusion attributable to elevated ventricular wall tension. It may also improve arterial oxygenation by reducing pulmonary vascular congestion.

The intravenous administration of furosemide reduces pulmonary vascular congestion and pulmonary venous pressure within 15 minutes, before renal excretion of sodium and water has occurred; presumably this action results from a direct dilating effect of this drug on the systemic arterial bed. It is important not to "overshoot the mark" by reducing left ventricular filling pressure much below 18 mm Hg, the lower range associated with optimal left ventricular performance in AMI, since this may reduce cardiac output further and cause arterial hypotension. Excessive diuresis may also result in hypokalemia, with its attendant risk of digitalis intoxication.

VASODILATORS (see also p. 491). Myocardial oxygen requirements depend on left ventricular wall stress, which in turn is proportional to the product of peak developed left ventricular pressure, volume, and wall thickness. Vasodilator therapy is not currently recommended in patients with uncomplicated AMI (although the results of ongoing trials may alter this) but is useful in patients whose MI is complicated by: (1) heart failure unresponsive to treatment with diuretics, (2) hypertension, (3) mitral regurgitation, or (4) ventricular septal defect. In these patients, treatment with vasodilator agents increases stroke volume and may reduce myocardial oxygen requirements and thereby lessen ischemia. Hemodynamic monitoring of systemic arterial and, in many cases, pulmonary capillary wedge (or at least pulmonary artery) pressure and cardiac output in patients treated with these agents is important. Improvement of cardiac performance and energetics requires three simultaneous effects: (1) reduction of left ventricular afterload, (2) avoidance of excessive systemic arterial hypotension in order to maintain effective coronary perfusion pressure, and (3) avoidance of excessive reduction of ventricular filling pressure with consequent diminution of cardiac output. In general, pulmonary capillary wedge pressure should be maintained at approximately 20 mm Hg and arterial diastolic blood pressure above 60 mm Hg in patients who were normotensive before developing the AMI.

Appropriate doses of vasodilators generally enhance stroke volume and cardiac output, and reduce left ventricular filling pressure and volume and calculated systemic vascular resistance, without causing serious reflex tachycardia. While available data are not conclusive and do not apply to all subsets of patients with AMI, at least one vasodilator, nitroglycerin, when given early in the course of AMI, has been reported also to protect ischemic myocardium and limit infarct size[651] (p. 1237). Excessive doses of vasodilators may decrease cardiac output by reducing preload and left ventricular filling pressure below optimal levels or may decrease coronary perfusion by excessive depression of systemic arterial pressure. Compromise of coronary perfusion, in turn, may impair ventricular performance further, extend infarction, and give rise to lethal arrhythmias.

Vasodilator therapy is particularly useful when AMI is complicated by mitral regurgitation or rupture of the ventricular septum. In such patients, vasodilators alone or in combination with intraaortic balloon counterpulsation can sometimes serve as a "holding maneuver" and provide hemodynamic stabilization to permit definitive catheterization and angiographic studies to be carried out and to prepare the patients for early surgical intervention. Because of the precarious state of patients with complicated infarction and the need for meticulous adjustment of dosage, therapy is best initiated with agents that can be administered intravenously and that have a short duration of action, such as nitroprusside,[788,789] nitroglycerin,[790,791] or isosorbide dinitrate.[792] After initial stabilization, medications that may be useful are long-acting nitrates given by mouth, sublingually, or by ointment,[793] and angiotensin-converting enzyme inhibitors[794] such as captopril, or enalapril, which is now available for intravenous use.

Nitroprusside. There has been more experience with the intravenous infusion of sodium nitroprusside in patients with AMI than with other vasodilators. It is generally given initially in doses of 0.5 μg/kg/min,[795] which may be gradually and progressively increased up to 50 μg/kg/min. While it increases stroke volume and cardiac output in patients with AMI and left ventricular failure, nitroprusside diminishes arteriolar resistance and impedance to left ventricular ejection, pulmonary capillary wedge pressure, myocardial oxygen requirements, and sometimes the frequency of ventricular premature contractions. Nitroprusside may augment cardiac output even in patients with cardiogenic shock, if arterial diastolic and coronary perfusion pressures are maintained by concomitant intraaortic balloon counterpulsation.

Nitroglycerin. This drug has been shown in animal experiments to be less likely than nitroprusside to produce a "coronary steal," i.e., to divert blood flow from the ischemic to the nonischemic zone.[790] Therefore, used intravenously, it (or isosorbide dinitrate, which has a similar action[792]) may be a particularly useful vasodilator in patients with AMI.[650-652] Ten to 15 μg/min is infused and the dose is increased by 10 μg/min every 5 minutes until (1) the desired effect (improvement of hemodynamics or relief of ischemic chest pain) is achieved or (2) a decline in systolic arterial pressure to 90 mm Hg, or by more than 15 mm Hg, has occurred. Although both nitroglycerin and nitroprusside lower systemic arterial pressure, systemic vascular resistance, and the heart rate–systolic blood pressure product, the reduction of left ventricular filling pressure is more prominent with nitroglycerin because of its relatively greater effect than nitroprusside on venous capacitance vessels. Nevertheless, in patients with severe left ventricular failure, cardiac output often increases despite the reduction in left ventricular filling pressure produced by nitroglycerin.

Oral Vasodilators. The use of oral vasodilators in the treatment of chronic congestive heart failure is discussed on page 491. In patients who have persistent heart failure, long-term treatment with a converting enzyme inhibitor should be carried out. Studies are under way to determine the efficacy of these agents in patients with left ventricular dysfunction without heart failure. It is hoped that this reduced ventricular load will decrease the remodeling of the left ventricle that occurs commonly in the period after MI and thereby defer the development of heart failure and death therefrom[167] (Fig. 39–12, p. 1211).

DIGITALIS (see also p. 486). Although digitalis increases the contractility and the oxygen consumption of normal hearts, when heart failure is present the diminution of heart size and wall tension frequently results in a net reduction of myocardial oxygen requirements.[796] In animal experiments it fails to improve ventricular performance immediately following experimental coronary occlusion, but salutary effects are elicited when it is administered several days later.[797] The absence of early beneficial effects may be due to the inability of ischemic tissue to respond to digitalis, the already maximal stimulation of contractility of the normal heart by circulating and neuronally released catecholamines, or the dissipation of the force of contraction of normal myocardium into dyskinetic areas.

Although the issue is still controversial, arrhythmias may be increased by digitalis glycosides when they are given to patients in the first few hours after the onset of MI, particularly in the presence of hypokalemia. Also, undesirable peripheral systemic and coronary vasoconstriction may result from the rapid intravenous administration of rapidly acting glycosides such as ouabain.[797]

Administration of digitalis to patients hospitalized with AMI should generally be reserved for the management of supraventricular tachyarrhythmias such as atrial flutter and fibrillation and of heart failure that persists despite treatment with diuretics and vasodilators. There is no indication for its use as an inotropic agent in patients without clinical evidence of left ventricular dysfunction (Killip Class I), and it is too weak an inotropic agent to be relied upon as the principal cardiac stimulant in patients with overt pulmonary edema or cardiogenic shock (Class III or IV). It may, however, be useful as a supplement to vasodilator agents and in the treatment of persistent or recurrent left ventricular failure.[798] Cardiac glycosides appear to become progressively more effective in the treatment of heart failure as the interval from the acute events lengthens; i.e., they are more effective in the treatment of chronic than of acute heart failure secondary to ischemic heart disease. However, the possibility that continued administration of digitalis might contribute to late mortality in the two years following AMI has been raised[799] and debated.[800,801] While it is clear that mortality is greater in patients treated with digoxin after AMI, it is not clear that this increase in mortality is due to digoxin itself or to confounding variables that correlate with use of digoxin.[801] At this time, digoxin would appear to be indicated only if there is overt heart failure and/or supraventricular tachyarrhythmias.

BETA-ADRENOCEPTOR AGONISTS. When left ventricular failure is severe, as manifested by marked reduction of cardiac index (< 2 liters/min/sq meter), and pulmonary capillary wedge pressure is at optimal (18 to 24 mm Hg) or excessive (> 24 mm Hg) levels despite therapy with diuretics, beta-adrenoceptor agonists are indicated. Although isoproterenol is a potent cardiac stimulant and improves ventricular performance, it should be avoided in the MI patient. It also causes tachycardia and augments myocardial oxygen consumption and lactate production[802]; in addition, it reduces coronary perfusion pressure by causing systemic vasodilation and in animal experiments increases the extent of experimentally induced infarction.[803] Norepinephrine also increases myocardial oxygen consumption because of its peripheral vasoconstrictor as well as positive inotropic actions.

Dopamine (p. 501) and *dobutamine* (p. 502), which is relatively cardioselective and stimulates beta$_1$ receptors, exert predominantly positive inotropic effects and may be particularly useful in patients with AMI and reduced cardiac output, increased left ventricular filling pressure, pulmonary vascular congestion, and hypotension.[804] Fortunately, the potentially deleterious alpha-adrenergic vasoconstrictor effects exerted by *dopamine* occur only at higher doses than those required to increase contractility. Its vasodilating actions on renal and splanchnic vessels and its positive inotropic effects generally improve hemodynamics and renal function.[805] In patients with AMI and severe left ventricular failure, this drug should be administered at a dose of 3 μg/kg/min, while monitoring pulmonary capillary wedge and systemic arterial pressures as well as cardiac output. The dose may be increased stepwise to 20 μg/kg/min, in order to reduce pulmonary capillary wedge pressure to approximately 20 mm Hg and elevate cardiac index to exceed 2 liters/min/sq meter. However, it must be recognized that doses exceeding 5 μg/kg/min activate peripheral alpha receptors and cause vasoconstriction. While concern has been raised that the positive inotropic effect of even low-dose dopamine could extend infarct size, experimental evidence suggests that the enhancement in contractility by dopamine does not increase infarct size or lead to late deterioration of cardiac function even when the drug is administered to acutely reperfused, severely ischemic myocardium.[806]

Dobutamine has a positive inotropic action comparable to that of dopamine but a slightly less positive chronotropic effect,[807] and less vasoconstrictor activity at higher doses. In patients with AMI dobutamine improves left ventricular performance without augmenting enzymatically estimated infarct size.[808] It may be administered in a starting dose of 2.5 μg/kg/min and increased stepwise to a maximum of 30 μg/kg/min. Both dopamine and dobutamine must be given carefully and with constant monitoring of the ECG, systemic arterial pressure, and pulmonary artery or pulmonary artery occlusive pressure and, if possible, with frequent measurements of cardiac output. The dose must be reduced if the heart rate exceeds 100 to 110 beats/min, if supraventricular or ventricular tachyarrhythmias are precipitated, or if ST-segment changes increase.

AMRINONE (p. 503). This is a noncatecholamine, nonglycoside, inotropic, and vasodilating agent that is approved for clinical use parenterally.[809] Experience with it in the setting of AMI is relatively limited, but it appears to be an ideal agent for selected patients with heart failure persisting despite treatment with diuretics, who are not hypotensive and who are likely to benefit from both an enhancement in contractility and afterload reduction. In patients with left ventricular failure following AMI amrinone increases cardiac output while reducing pulmonary wedge pressure and systemic vascular resistance.[810,811] Heart rate increases only at relatively high doses.[811] In MI patients studied, no exacerbation of an-

gina or increased incidence of arrhythmias has been reported.[810] The initial intravenous dosage of amrinone is 0.75 mg/kg infused slowly over several minutes. This is then followed by a continued maintenance infusion started at 5 to 10 μg/kg/min and titrated to the patient's hemodynamic response. The total daily dose should not be greater than 10 mg/kg.[812]

TREATMENT OF CARDIOGENIC SHOCK
(See also p. 579)

When a massive AMI produces profound global impairment of left ventricular function, cardiogenic shock supervenes. This condition is characterized by marked and persistent (> 30 min) hypotension with systolic arterial pressure less than 80 mm Hg and a marked reduction of cardiac index (generally < 1.8 liters/mm/sq meter) in the face of elevated left ventricular filling pressure (pulmonary capillary wedge pressure > 18 mm Hg). Spurious estimates of left ventricular filling pressure based on measurements of the pulmonary artery wedge pressure can occur in the presence of marked mitral regurgitation, in which the tall v wave in the left atrial (and pulmonary artery wedge) pressure tracing elevates the mean pressure above left ventricular end-diastolic pressure. Accordingly, mitral regurgitation and other mechanical lesions such as ventricular septal defect, ventricular aneurysm, and pseudoaneurysm must be excluded before the diagnosis of cardiogenic shock due to global impairment of left ventricular function can be established. These potentially catastrophic mechanical complications should be suspected in any patient with AMI in whom circulatory collapse occurs. Immediate hemodynamic and angiographic evaluations are necessary in patients with cardiogenic shock. It is important to exclude these complications because primary therapy of such lesions usually requires immediate operative treatment with intervening support of the circulation by intraaortic balloon counterpulsation.

When the aforementioned mechanical complications are not present, cardiogenic shock is due to global impairment of left ventricular function. While dopamine or dobutamine usually improves hemodynamics in these patients, unfortunately neither appears to improve hospital survival significantly. Similarly, vasodilators have been utilized in an effort to elevate cardiac output and to reduce left ventricular filling pressure. However, by lowering the already markedly reduced coronary perfusion pressure, myocardial perfusion can be compromised further, accelerating the vicious circle illustrated in Figure 39–11 (p. 1210). Vasodilators may nonetheless be employed in conjunction with intraaortic balloon counterpulsation and inotropic agents in an effort to increase cardiac output while sustaining or elevating coronary perfusion pressure.

The systemic vascular resistance is usually elevated in patients with cardiogenic shock, but occasionally resistance is normal, and in a few cases vasodilation actually predominates. When systemic vascular resistance is *not* elevated in patients with cardiogenic shock, norepinephrine (in doses ranging from 2 to 10 μg/min), which has both alpha- and beta-adrenoceptor agonist properties, may be employed to increase diastolic arterial pressure, maintain coronary perfusion, and improve contractility, but, again, there is no definitive evidence that ultimate outcome is affected by this drug.[813] Norepinephrine should be used only when other means, including balloon counterpulsation, fail to maintain arterial diastolic pressure above 50 to 60 mm Hg in a previously normotensive patient. The use of alpha-adrenoceptor agents such as phenylephrine or methoxamine is contraindicated in most patients with cardiogenic shock (unless systemic vascular resistance is inordinately low).

REPERFUSION. Reversal of cardiogenic shock by acute reperfusion has been reported, usually with thrombolytic therapy, emergency PTCA, or a combination of these measures.[599,600,814,815] In a relatively large series of patients, the mortality of cardiogenic shock appears to have been reduced by early angioplasty.[814] Although data from a controlled trial are not available, such therapy appears warranted when suitable coronary anatomy is identified.[784] In several reported cases, cardiogenic shock due to total occlusion of the left main coronary artery was reversed by intravenous thrombolysis with streptokinase.[816,817]

INTRAAORTIC BALLOON COUNTERPULSATION (see also p. 537). Cardiogenic shock due to mechanical defects following AMI (pp. 1256 to 1259) or to severe left ventricular dysfunction may be managed by means of the appropriate use of intraaortic balloon counterpulsation (IABP) when other medical measures fail.[818-821] In present practice, the balloon is inserted percutaneously[822] or, rarely, via an arterial cutdown in the femoral artery and advanced into the thoracic aorta via the femoral artery. Phased pulsations, electrocardiographically synchronized, allow for inflation at the time of closure of the aortic valve and deflation just before the onset of systole. The augmented coronary perfusion pressure during diastole enhances coronary blood flow because coronary vascular resistance is minimal during this portion of the cardiac cycle (Fig. 13–32, p. 375). Since the balloon is deflated throughout systole, the left ventricle ejects against a lower impedance. Hemodynamic changes generally include a 10 to 20 per cent increase in cardiac output, a reduction in systolic and increase in diastolic arterial pressure with little change in mean pressure, a diminution of heart rate, and an increase in urine output.[818,819] The reduction in left ventricular afterload reduces myocardial oxygen consumption, and, as a consequence, anaerobic metabolism and myocardial ischemia are diminished.[819] Favorable effects are sometimes reflected in prompt resolution of electrocardiographic signs of ischemia.

Indications. Intraaortic balloon counterpulsation is utilized in the treatment of AMI in three groups of patients: (1) those whose conditions are hemodynamically unstable and in whom support of the circulation is required for the performance of cardiac catheterization and angiography carried out to assess lesions that are potentially correctable surgically; (2) those with cardiogenic shock that is unresponsive to medical management; and (3) rarely, those with persistent ischemic pain that is unresponsive to treatment with inhalation of 100 per cent oxygen, beta-adrenoceptor blockade, nitrates, and calcium channel blocking agents during the postinfarction state. Unfortunately, among patients with cardiogenic shock, improvement is often only temporary, and "balloon dependence" is common.[818,820] Patients with cardiogenic shock treated with this modality can be successfully weaned from the supporting system only occasionally. Counterpulsation alone does not improve overall mortality, either in patients with or those without a surgically remediable mechanical lesion.[820,821] However, it may be life-saving in allowing the patient to tolerate catheterization and coronary arteriography and to undergo coronary angioplasty or to be brought to the operating room for definitive treatment. Surgical treatment in cardiogenic shock (aside from correcting mechanical abnormalities) may involve bypassing severely obstructed nonoccluded vessels. Occlusion of one major vessel may cause left ventricular dysfunction and hypotension, which can then lead to hypoperfusion and ischemia of myocardium subserved by the other diseased vessels. Left ventricular function may be improved by relief of this ischemia with revascularization. It is possible that left ventricular bypass, a technique that reduces left ventricular oxygen demands more drastically, may ultimately prove to be more effective in improving survival in patients with cardiogenic shock than intraaortic balloon counterpulsation[823]; however, it is still experimental. Emergency percutaneous cardiopulmonary bypass has been uti-

lized in a small series of patients before catheterization.[824] While relatively successful in pilot studies, this complex strategy cannot be widely recommended until tested further.

Noninvasive approaches to circulatory assistance have been developed, such as external devices that apply pressure to the lower extremities during diastole, thereby promoting increased runoff during systole. However, this form of therapy likewise does not alter outcome decisively; its hemodynamic effects are, in fact, less than those of intraaortic counterpulsation.[825]

Complications. These occur infrequently but include damage to or perforation of the aortic wall, ischemia distal to the site of insertion of the balloon in the femoral artery, thrombocytopenia, hemolysis, renal emboli, and mechanical failure such as rupture of the balloon.[677,826] Those at highest risk include patients with peripheral vascular disease, the elderly, and women, particularly if they are small. These factors should be taken into consideration before an attempt to institute intraaortic balloon counterpulsation. Because of the potential for vascular bleeding complications there has been reluctance to use intraaortic pumps in patients who have undergone thrombolytic therapy. However, because of the poor outcome among patients with shock following thrombolysis (usually ineffective thrombolysis), and because balloon counterpulsation can be utilized relatively safely in this group,[827] this modality should be considered in carefully selected patients.

HYPOTENSION SECONDARY TO RIGHT VENTRICULAR INFARCTION

A characteristic hemodynamic pattern (Table 39–14) has been observed in patients with right ventricular infarc-

TABLE 39–14 FEATURES OF RIGHT VENTRICULAR INFARCTION

1. **Inferior-posterior myocardial infarction**

2. **Clinical findings may include:**
   A. Normal or depressed right ventricular function
   B. Shock
   C. Tricuspid regurgitation
   D. Ruptured ventricular septum

3. **Hemodynamic measurements**
   A. Abnormally elevated right atrial pressure
   B. Normal right ventricular and pulmonary artery systolic pressures
   C. Increased ratio of right ventricular to left ventricular filling pressure
   D. Depressed right ventricular function curve

4. **Scintigraphy**
   A. Uptake in right ventricular free wall
   B. Increased right ventricular dimensions and decreased wall motion

5. **Echocardiography**
   A. Increased right ventricular dimension
   B. Absence of pericardial effusion

6. **Cardiac enzymes**
   A. Increased magnitude of enzyme values to left ventricular dysfunction

7. **Cardiac catheterization**
   A. Involvement of right (usually) or left (rarely) circumflex coronary arteries
   B. Right ventricular akinesis

8. **Differential diagnosis**
   A. Hypotension with acute myocardial infarction
   B. Pericardial tamponade
   C. Constrictive pericarditis
   D. Pulmonary embolus

Modified from Rackley, C. E., Russell, R. O., Jr., Mantle, J. A., Rogers, W. J., Papapietro, S. E., and Schwartz, K. M.: Right ventricular infarction and function. Am. Heart J. *101*:215, 1981.

tion,[26,828] which frequently accompanies inferior left ventricular infarction,[704] or rarely occurs in isolated form.[829,830] Right-heart filling pressures (central venous, right atrial, and right ventricular end-diastolic pressures) are elevated while left ventricular filling pressure is normal or only slightly raised[779]; right ventricular systolic and pulse pressures are decreased, and cardiac output is often markedly depressed. Rarely, this disproportionate elevation of right-sided filling pressure causes right-to-left shunting through a patent foramen ovale.[831] This possibility should be considered in patients with right ventricular infarction who have unexplained systemic hypoxemia. The finding of an elevation in atrial natriuretic factor in this condition has led to the suggestion that abnormally high levels of this peptide might be, in part, responsible for the hypotension seen with right ventricular infarction.[832]

DIAGNOSIS. Many patients with the combination of normal left ventricular filling pressure and depressed cardiac index in fact have right ventricular infarcts (with accompanying inferior left ventricular infarcts). The hemodynamic picture may superficially resemble that seen in patients with pericardial disease (Chap. 45).[779] In it are seen elevated right ventricular filling pressure; steep, right atrial y descent; and an early diastolic dip and plateau (square root sign) in the right ventricular pressure tracing. Moreover, Kussmaul's sign (page 1484) and pulsus paradoxus (page 1474) may be present in patients with right ventricular infarction. In fact, Kussmaul's sign in the setting of inferior wall AMI is highly predictive of right ventricular involvement. The ECG may provide the first clue that right ventricular involvement is present in the patient with inferior wall MI (Fig. 39–16, p. 1221). Most patients with right ventricular infarction have ST-segment elevation in lead V_4R (right precordial lead in V_4 position).[340,833] Transient elevation of the ST segment in any of the right precordial leads may occur with right ventricular MI and the presence of ST-segment elevation of 0.1 mV or more in any one or combination of leads V_4R, V_5R, or V_6R in patients with the clinical picture of acute MI is highly sensitive and specific for the diagnosis of acute right ventricular MI.[339,340]

Echocardiography. This technique is helpful in the differential diagnosis[834] because in right ventricular infarction—in contrast to pericardial tamponade—no significant quantities of pericardial fluid are seen. On two-dimensional echocardiography, abnormal wall motion of the right ventricle as well as right ventricular dilatation and depression of the right ventricular ejection fraction can be noted.[834,835] Gated equilibrium radionuclide angiography also is useful for recognizing right ventricular MI.[26,836] Serial scintigraphic studies have shown that some degree of recovery of an initially depressed right ventricular ejection fraction is the rule with right ventricular myocardial infarction,[26,837,838] whereas this is not necessarily true for left ventricular ejection fraction.

Hemodynamics. Loss of atrial transport in patients with right ventricular infarction can result in marked reductions in stroke volume and arterial blood pressure.[837] As already noted, disproportionate elevation of the right-sided filling pressure compared with the left side is the hemodynamic hallmark of right ventricular infarction. Therefore, ventricular pacing, when required, may fail to increase cardiac output, and atrioventricular sequential pacing may be required.[694,839] In general, the hemodynamic importance of right ventricular infarction in patients with inferior infarction is reflected in the observations of Marmor et al. They noted that although infarct sizes (reflected in CK release curves) were similar in patients with anterior and inferior infarcts, the former had severe depression of the left ventricular ejection fraction and the latter had more severe depression of the right ventricular ejection fraction.[840]

TREATMENT. In patients with hypotension due to right ventricular MI, hemodynamics may be improved by a combination of expanding plasma volume to augment right ventricular preload and cardiac output and, when left ventricular failure is present, arterial vasodilators. The initial therapy for hypotension in patients with right ventricular infarction

should almost always be volume expansion. However, if hypotension has not been corrected after one or more liters of fluid has been administered briskly, consideration should be given to hemodynamic monitoring with a pulmonary artery catheter, because further volume infusion may be of little use and may produce pulmonary congestion.[443] Vasodilators reduce the impedance to left ventricular outflow and in turn left ventricular diastolic, left atrial, and pulmonary (arterial) pressures, thereby lowering the impedance to right ventricular outflow and enhancing right ventricular output. A remarkably high survival rate of 60 per cent, albeit in a small series of patients with right ventricular infarction and serious and prolonged hypotension, emphasizes the importance of recognition and vigorous medical therapy of this cause of serious hypotension in MI.[841]

Right ventricular infarction is common among patients with inferior left ventricular infarction. Therefore, otherwise unexplained systemic arterial hypotension or diminished cardiac output, or marked hypotension in response to small doses of nitroglycerin,[432] in patients with inferior infarction should lead to the prompt consideration of this diagnosis. In view of the importance of atrial transport, patients requiring pacing should have atrial or atrioventricular sequential pacing.[694,839] Replacement of the tricuspid valve has been carried out in the treatment of severe tricuspid regurgitation secondary to right ventricular infarction.[842]

MECHANICAL CAUSES OF HEART FAILURE AND SHOCK FOLLOWING ACUTE MYOCARDIAL INFARCTION

MYOCARDIAL RUPTURE

The most dramatic complications of AMI are those that involve tearing or rupture of acutely infarcted tissue. The clinical characteristics of these lesions vary considerably and depend on the site of rupture, which may involve the papillary muscles, the interventricular septum, or the free wall of either ventricle. The overall incidence of these complications is hard to assess because clinical and autopsy series differ considerably.[843,844] However, as a group they are probably responsible for about 15 per cent of all deaths from AMI.[843,845,845a] A large autopsy study suggests that the incidence of myocardial rupture has increased since the late 1960's, with a current rate of 31 per cent among necropsied cases.[844] The prior use of corticosteroids or nonsteroidal antiinflammatory agents has been implicated as predisposing to rupture as a result of impaired healing. Controversy remains about the actual relationship between the use of such agents and the frequency of rupture, with several series suggesting a correlation of rupture with their use[846,847] and others not.[843,845] Conversely, the early use of thrombolytic therapy appears to reduce the incidence of cardiac rupture,[848,849] an effect that is responsible in part for improved survival with effective thrombolysis. A recent detailed analysis[849] of many trials has, however, raised the possibility that late thrombolytic therapy may actually increase the risk of cardiac rupture despite improving overall survival. The comparative clinical profile of these complications, as gathered from different studies, is shown in Table 39–15.

Rupture of the Free Wall

Rupture of the free wall of the infarcted ventricle (Fig. 39–30) occurs in up to 10 per cent of patients dying in the hospital of AMI. Thinness of the apical wall, marked intensity of necrosis at the terminal end of the blood supply, poor collateral flow, the shearing effect of muscular contraction against an inert and stiffened necrotic area, and aging of the myocardium with laceration of the myocardial microstructure have all been proposed as the local factors that lead to rupture.[850-852]

The following are some features that characterize this serious complication of AMI. Rupture of the free wall:

1. Occurs more frequently in the elderly and possibly more frequently in women than in men with infarction[845];

VARIABLE	VENTRICULAR SEPTAL DEFECT	FREE WALL RUPTURE	PAPILLARY MUSCLE RUPTURE
Age (mean, years)	63	69	65
Days post-MI	3–5	3–6	3–5
Anterior MI	66%	50%	25%
New murmur	90%	25%	50%
Palpable thrill	Yes	No	Rare
Previous MI	25%	25%	30%
Echocardiographic findings			
2D	Visualize defect	May have pericardial effusion	Flail or prolapsing leaflet
Doppler	Detect shunt	—	Regurgitant jet in LA
PA catheterization	Oxygen step-up in RV	Equalization of diastolic pressure	Prominent V wave in PCW tracing
Incidence	2–4%	Up to 10%	1%
Mortality			
Medical	90%	90%	90%
Surgical	50%	Case reports	40–90%

MI = myocardial infarction, VSD = ventricular septal defect, 2D = two-dimensional, LA = left atrium, PA = pulmonary artery, RV = right ventricle, PCW = pulmonary capillary wedge.
Modified from Labovitz, A. J., et al.: Mechanical complications of acute myocardial infarction. Cardiovasc. Rev. Rep. 5:948, 1984.

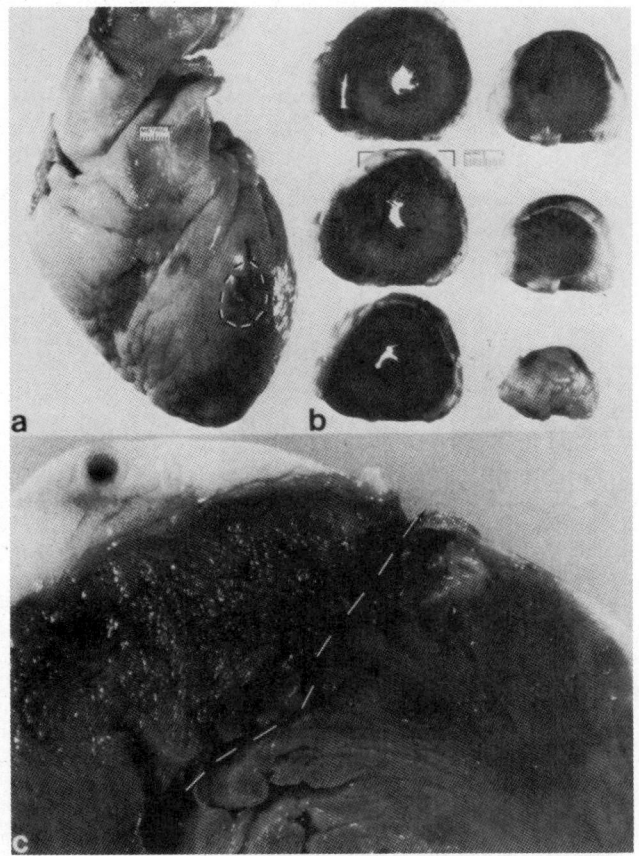

FIGURE 39-30. Heart of a 76-year-old woman who developed chest pain 14 hours before death. Her electrocardiogram showed changes of an anterior wall acute myocardial infarction. At necropsy, 300 ml of clotted blood was present in the pericardial sac. *A*, View of the anterior aspect of the heart showing the increased subepicardial adipose tissue and the rupture site (dotted circle). *B*, View of transverse cuts of the cardiac ventricles showing the acute myocardial infarct on the anterior left ventricular wall and the rupture site. *C*, Close-up view of the slice in brackets in *B* showing the acute myocardial infarct and the rupture site (arrow). (From Mann, J. M., and Roberts, W. C.: Rupture of the left ventricular free wall during acute myocardial infarction: Analysis of 138 necropsy patients and comparison with 50 necropsy patients with acute myocardial infarction without rupture. Am. J. Cardiol. 62:847, 1988.)

2. May be more common in hypertensive than normotensive patients[845,850];

3. Occurs approximately seven times more frequently in the left than the right ventricle and seldom occurs in the atria;

4. Usually involves the anterior or lateral walls[853] of the ventricle in the area of the terminal distribution of the left anterior descending coronary artery;

5. Is usually associated with a relatively large transmural infarction involving at least 20 per cent of the left ventricle[843];

6. Occurs between 1 day and 3 weeks, but most commonly 1 to 4 days, following infarction;

7. Is usually preceded by infarct expansion, i.e., thinning and a disproportionate dilatation within the softened necrotic zone[173];

8. Most commonly results from a distinct tear in the myocardial wall or a dissecting hematoma that perforates a necrotic area of myocardium (Fig. 39-31);

9. Usually occurs near the junction of the infarct and the normal muscle;

10. Occurs less frequently in the center of the infarct, but when rupture occurs here, it is usually during the second rather than the first week following the infarct;

11. Rarely occurs in a hypertrophied ventricle or in an area of extensive collateral vessels[851];

12. Most often occurs in patients without previous infarction.[843,853]

Rupture of the free wall of the left ventricle usually leads to hemopericardium and death from cardiac tamponade. Occasionally, rupture of the free wall of the ventricle occurs as the first clinical manifestation in patients with undetected or silent myocardial infarction, and then it may be considered a form of "sudden cardiac death" (Chap. 26).

The course of rupture varies from catastrophic, with an acute tear leading to immediate death, to slow and incomplete, leading to late rupture or formation of a false aneurysm.[854] In either case, survival depends on the recognition of this complication, hemodynamic stabilization of the patient —usually with inotropic agents and/or intraaortic balloon pump—and most importantly on immediate surgical repair.[855,856] Survival has occasionally been reported even in the most dire of circumstances, i.e., when the diagnosis is correctly made within moments of rupture, and through a well-coordinated operating room effort, the patients were placed on cardiopulmonary bypass within 1 hour and the defects then successfully repaired.[856,857]

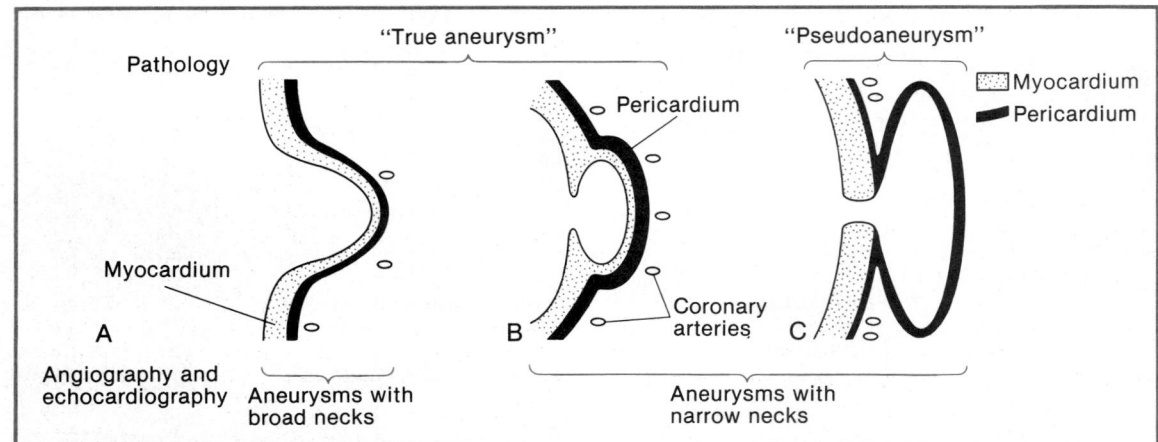

FIGURE 39–31. Pathological difference between true and pseudo-aneurysms. As can be seen in *B*, a narrow neck may occur with true aneurysms. A narrow neck may be a marker of higher risk for rupture, but it does not necessarily indicate that a pseudoaneurysm is present. (From Davies, M. J.: Ischemic ventricular aneurysm: True or false? Br. Heart J. *60*:95, 1990.)

Incomplete rupture of the heart may occur when organizing thrombus and hematoma, together with pericardium, seal a rupture of the left ventricle and thus prevent the development of hemopericardium (Fig. 39–31). With time, this area of organized thrombus and pericardium can become a small left ventricular diverticulum, or a large pseudoaneurysm that maintains communication with the cavity of the left ventricle.[858] In contrast to true aneurysms, which always contain some myocardial elements in their walls, the walls of false aneurysms are composed of organized hematoma and pericardium and lack any elements of the original myocardial wall. False aneurysms can become quite large, even equaling the true ventricular cavity in size, and they communicate with the left ventricular cavity through a narrow neck. Frequently, false aneurysms contain significant quantities of old and recent thrombus, superficial portions of which can cause arterial emboli. False aneurysms can drain off a portion of each ventricular stroke volume exactly as do true aneurysms. The diagnosis of pseudoaneurysm can usually be made by two-dimensional echocardiography (Fig. 4–88, p. 97) and contrast angiography, although at times differentiation between true and false aneurysms may be difficult by any imaging technique.[858a]

DIAGNOSIS. The recognition of rupture usually is first suggested by the development of sudden profound right heart failure associated with shock, often rapidly leading to electromechanical dissociation. Immediate pericardiocentesis will confirm the diagnosis and relieve the pericardial tamponade, at least momentarily. If the patient's condition is relatively stable, echocardiography may help in establishing the diagnosis of tamponade. Under the most favorable conditions, cardiac catheterization can be carried out, not necessarily to confirm the diagnosis of rupture but to delineate the coronary anatomy. This is helpful so that, in addition to ventricular repair, coronary artery bypass surgery can be performed in patients in whom high-grade lesions are seen. In situations in which hemodynamics are critically compromised, establishment of the diagnosis should be followed immediately by surgery for resection of the necrotic and ruptured myocardium with primary reconstruction. When rupture is subacute and a pseudoaneurysm is suspected or present, prompt elective surgery is indicated because rupture of the pseudoaneurysm occurs relatively frequently.[858,859]

Rupture of the Interventricular Septum

Although rupture of the interventricular septum appears to be less common than rupture of the free wall at autopsy,[850,860] our clinical experience is often otherwise,[843] perhaps because death usually is not immediate, and patients frequently can reach a referral center at which this complication is treated. The perforation usually is single (Fig. 39–32) and ranges in length from one to several centimeters. It may be a direct through-and-through hole or may be more irregular and serpiginous.[861,862] The size of the defect determines the magni-

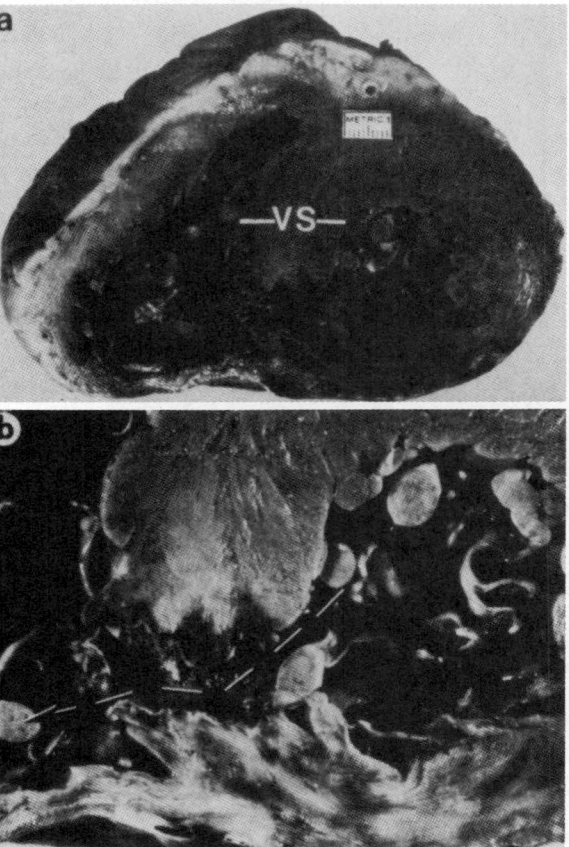

FIGURE 39–32. Heart of a 76-year-old woman who died 2 days after the onset of AMI. Her electrocardiogram had revealed an inferoposterior infarct and her course was complicated by complete heart block. *A*, View of the most basal transverse cut of the cardiac ventricles showing the posterior acute myocardial infarct and the posterior ventricular septal defect. VS = ventricular septum. *B*, Close-up view of the rupture site (arrow). (From Mann, J. M., and Roberts, W. C.: Acquired ventricular septal defect during acute myocardial infarction: Analysis of 38 unoperated necropsy patients and comparison with 50 unoperated necropsy patients without rupture. Am. J. Cardiol. *62*:8, 1988.)

tude of the left-to-right shunt and the extent of hemodynamic deterioration, which in turn affects the likelihood of survival. The development of shock and the likelihood of survival appear to depend critically on impairment of right ventricular function.[860,863,864] As in rupture of the free wall of the ventricle, transmural infarction underlies rupture of the ventricular septum. Rupture of the septum with an anterior infarction tends to be apical in location, whereas inferior infarctions are associated with perforation of the basal septum and with a worse prognosis.[663,864] Virtually all patients have multivessel coronary artery disease, with the majority exhibiting lesions in all of the major vessels.[860]

The development of ruptured interventricular septum is usually heralded by the appearance of a new harsh, loud holosystolic murmur that is heard best at the lower left and usually right sternal borders. A thrill may occur with the murmur. Biventricular failure generally ensues within hours to days. Confirmation of the diagnosis usually requires insertion of a pulmonary artery balloon catheter to document the left-to-right shunt. The defect can also be recognized by two-dimensional echocardiography with color flow Doppler imaging.[865,866,866a]

Catheter placement of an umbrella-shaped device within the ruptured septum has been reported to stabilize the conditions of critically ill patients with acute septal rupture following AMI.[867]

Rupture of a Papillary Muscle

Partial or total rupture of a papillary muscle is a rare but often fatal complication of transmural MI[868] (Fig. 39–33). Inferior wall infarction can lead to rupture of the posteromedial papillary muscle, which occurs more commonly than rupture of the anterolateral muscle, a consequence of anterolateral MI.[869,870] Rupture of a right ventricular papillary muscle is rare but can cause massive tricuspid regurgitation and right ventricular failure. Complete transection of a left ventricular papillary muscle is incompatible with life because the sudden massive mitral regurgitation that develops cannot be tolerated. Rupture of a portion of a papillary muscle, usually the tip or head of the muscle, resulting in severe, although not necessarily overwhelming, mitral regurgitation is much more fre-

quent. Unlike rupture of the ventricular septum, which occurs with large infarcts, papillary muscle rupture occurs with a relatively small infarction in approximately one-half of the cases seen.[868] The extent of coronary artery disease in these patients sometimes is modest as well.[869]

In a small number of patients, rupture of more than one cardiac structure is noted clinically[871] or at postmortem examination; all possible combinations of rupture of the free left ventricular wall, the interventricular septum, and papillary muscles have been described.[861]

As with patients who have a ruptured ventricular septal defect, those with papillary muscle rupture manifest a new holosystolic murmur followed by the development of increasingly severe heart failure. In both situations the murmur may become softer or disappear as arterial pressure falls. Mitral regurgitation due to partial or complete rupture of a papillary muscle may be promptly recognized echocardiographically.[872] Color flow Doppler imaging is particularly helpful in distinguishing acute mitral regurgitation from a ventricular septal defect in the setting of AMI.[873] Therefore, an echocardiogram should be obtained immediately on any patient in whom the diagnosis is suspected, because hemodynamic deterioration can ensue rapidly. Echocardiography also often permits differentiation of papillary muscle rupture from other, generally less severe forms of mitral regurgitation that occur with AMI.[874]

Hemodynamic Findings and Management in Ventricular Septal Rupture and Mitral Regurgitation

It may be difficult, on clinical grounds, to distinguish between acute mitral regurgitation and rupture of the ventricular septum in patients with AMI who suddenly develop a loud systolic murmur.[875] This differentiation can be made most readily by color flow Doppler echocardiography. In addition, a right-heart catheterization with a balloon-tipped catheter can readily distinguish between these two complications. As already noted, patients with ventricular septal rupture demonstrate a "step-up" in oxygen saturation in blood samples from the right ventricle and pulmonary artery compared with those from the right atrium. Patients with acute mitral regurgitation lack this step-up; they may demonstrate tall v waves in both

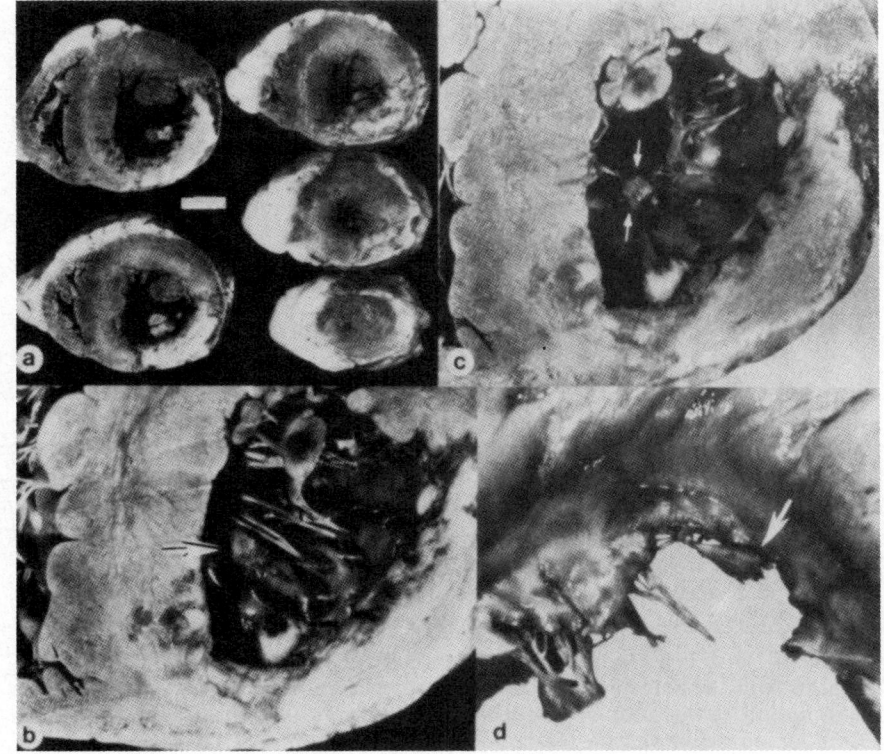

FIGURE 39–33. This 76-year-old woman had a large posterior wall acute myocardial infarction with incomplete rupture of the posteromedial papillary muscle. *A*, Ventricular transverse slices from base (top left) to apex (bottom left) demonstrating the extent of the infarction. *B* and *C*, Close-up of the basal portion of the left ventricle showing a portion of the ruptured posteromedial papillary muscle (arrows). *D*, Opened mitral valve showing the ruptured papillary muscle head (arrows) and the tangled chordae tendineae. (From Barbour, D. J., and Roberts, W. C.: Rupture of a left ventricular papillary muscle during acute myocardial infarction: Analysis of 22 necropsy patients. Reprinted with permission of the American College of Cardiology. J. Am. Coll. Cardiol. *8:*558, 1986.)

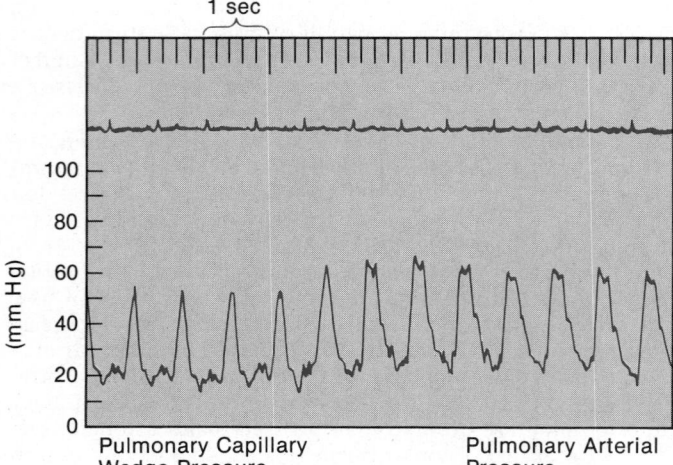

FIGURE 39-34. **Acute mitral regurgitation secondary to ruptured chord from infarcted papillary muscle in a 45-year-old man. Tracing shows mitral regurgitation, tall v waves in pulmonary capillary wedge and pulmonary artery tracings. (Courtesy of Ira S. Ockene, M.D.)**

A ventricular aneurysm, which is a circumscribed, noncontractile outpouching of the left ventricle, develops in 8 to 15 per cent of patients who survive a myocardial infarction.[880,881] The wall of the aneurysm is thin in comparison with the rest of the left ventricle (Figs. 39-31 and 39-36), and it is usually composed of fibrous tissue as well as necrotic muscle, occasionally mixed with viable myocardium.[882] Aneurysm formation presumably occurs when intraventricular tension stretches the noncontracting infarcted heart muscle, thus producing infarct expansion,[173] a relatively weak, thin layer of necrotic muscle, and fibrous tissue that bulges with each cardiac contraction. With the passage of time, the wall of the aneurysm becomes more densely fibrotic, but it continues to bulge with systole, thus "stealing" some of the left ventricular stroke volume during each systole.

When an aneurysm is present after anterior MI, there is generally a total occlusion of a poorly collateralized left anterior descending coronary artery.[883] An aneurysm is rarely seen with multivessel disease when there are either extensive collaterals or a nonoccluded left anterior descending artery.[883,884] Aneurysms usually range from 1 to 8 cm in diameter.[880] They occur approximately four times more often at the apex and in the anterior wall than in the inferoposterior wall.[880] The overlying pericardium is usually densely adherent to the wall of the aneurysm, which may even become partially calcified after several years. Rarely, a true left ventricular aneurysm ruptures soon after its development. In iso-

the pulmonary capillary and the pulmonary arterial pressure tracings (Fig. 39-34). However, patients with septal rupture may also develop large v waves and thus the presence of this finding is not necessarily useful in an individual patient. Cardiac output is usually significantly decreased in both conditions.

Invasive monitoring, which is essential in these patients, also allows for the critically important assessment of right ventricular function. Right and left ventricular filling pressures (right atrial pressure and pulmonary capillary wedge pressure) dictate fluid administration and the use of diuretics, while measurements of cardiac output and mean arterial pressure are obtained for calculation of systemic vascular resistance as a guide for vasodilator therapy. This therapy, generally using nitroprusside, should be instituted as early as possible once hemodynamic monitoring is available. This may be critically important for stabilizing the patient's condition in preparation for further diagnostic studies and surgical repair. If vasodilator therapy is not tolerated or if it fails to achieve hemodynamic stability, intraaortic balloon counterpulsation should be rapidly instituted.

Surgical Treatment of Hemodynamic Impairment

Operative intervention is most successful in patients with AMI and circulatory collapse when a surgically correctable mechanical lesion can be identified and repaired, such as ventricular septal defect.[876] In such patients the circulation should at first be supported by intraaortic balloon pulsation and a positive inotropic agent such as dopamine or dobutamine in combination with a vasodilator, unless the patient is hypotensive. Operation should not be delayed in patients with a correctable lesion who require pharmacological and/or mechanical (counterpulsation) support (Fig. 39-35).[876-879] Such patients frequently develop a serious complication—infection, adult respiratory distress syndrome, extension of the infarct, or renal failure—if operation is delayed. Surgical survival is predicted by early operation, short duration of shock, and mild degrees of right and left ventricular impairment.[876,878,879] When the hemodynamic status of a patient with one of these mechanical lesions complicating an AMI remains stable *after* the patient has been weaned from pharmacological and/or mechanical support, occasionally it may be desirable to postpone operation for 2 to 4 weeks to allow some healing of the infarct to occur. Surgical repair may involve either repair of a ventricular septal defect, correction of mitral regurgitation, or insertion of a prosthetic mitral valve, usually accompanied by coronary revascularization.

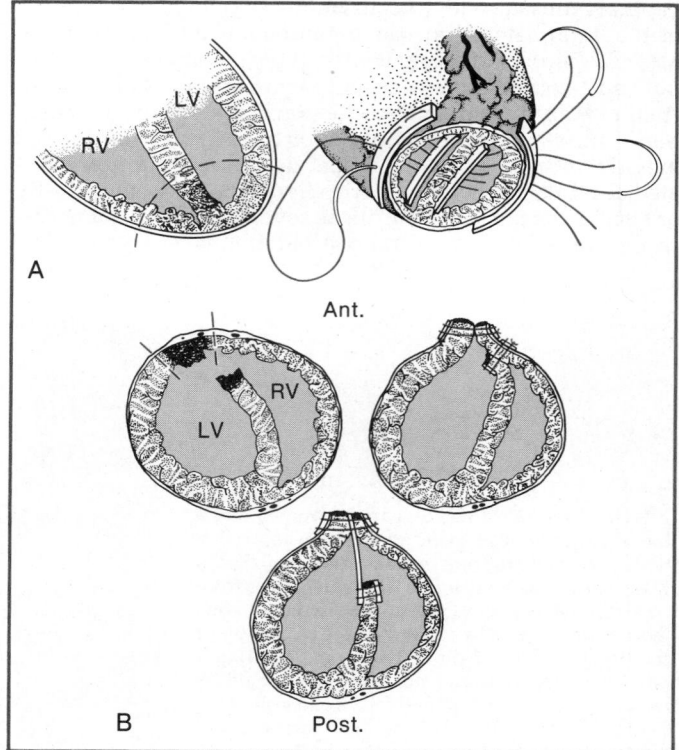

FIGURE 39-35. **A, Closure of apical ventricular septal rupture. The infarcted apex is resected, and the remaining viable myocardium of the septum and the left and right ventricular free walls are buttressed together using Teflon felt inside and outside the ventricle. B, Closure of a ventricular septal rupture with an extensive anterior infarct. The septum is reconstructed with a heavy Dacron patch that is sewn to the base of remaining septum using Teflon bolsters on both sides. The free edge of the patch is then brought out and the left and right ventricular free walls are attached to it. Ant. = anterior; LV = left ventricle; Post = posterior; RV = right ventricle. (Reproduced with permission from Kopf, G. S., Meshkov, A., Laks, H., Hammond, G. L., and Geha, A. S.: Changing patterns in the surgical management of ventricular septal rupture after myocardial infarction. Am. J. Surg. 143:465, 1982.)**

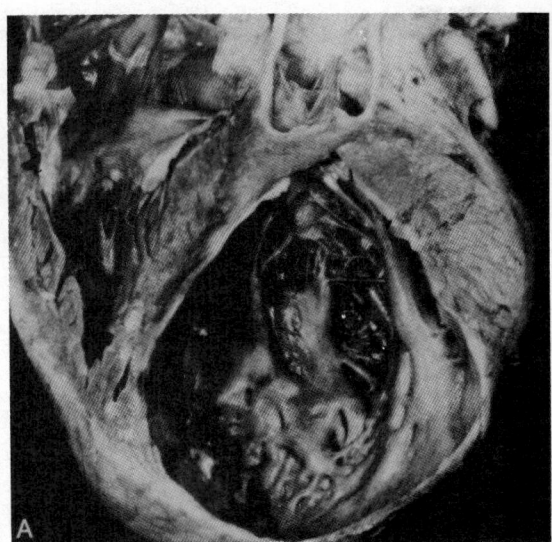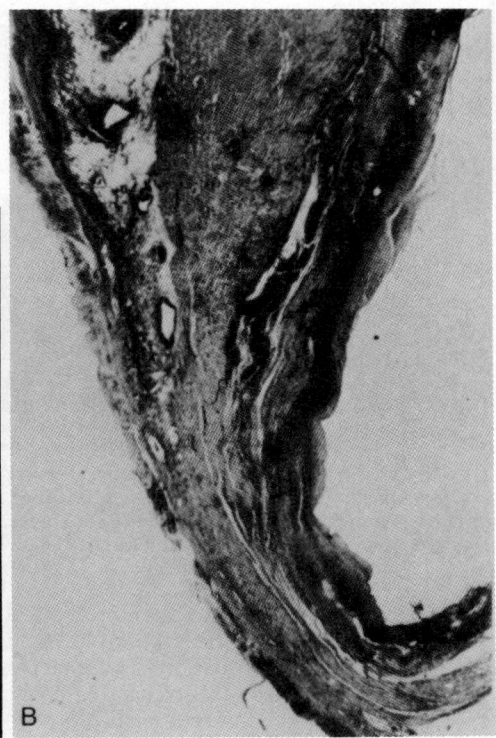

FIGURE 39–36. Example of true left ventricular aneurysm. *A,* Aneurysm complicating an anterior infarction. The ventricular portion of the heart, cut in frontal section and viewed from in front, shows the left ventricle to the left of the right ventricle. The aneurysm is thin-walled and has a fibroelastic lining. *B,* Photomicrograph of aneurysm. Epicardium is to the left. This low-power view shows virtual molding of the aneurysm at the edge of an infarct. The aneurysm displays endocardial fibrosis and some mural thrombosis. Elastic tissue stain, ×5. (From Edwards, B. S., and Edwards, J. E.: Pathology of acute myocardial infarction. *In* Francis, G. S., and Alpert, J. S. [eds.]: Modern Coronary Care. Boston, Little, Brown and Co., 1990, p. 64.)

lated cases this may be due to a degree of early myocardial rupture interrupted by subepicardial aneurysm formation, susceptible to later complete rupture. Late rupture, when the true aneurysm has become stabilized by the formation of dense fibrous tissue in its wall, almost never occurs.[858]

Mortality in patients with a left ventricular aneurysm is up to six times higher than in patients without aneurysms, even when compared to that in patients with comparable left ventricular ejection fraction.[885] Death in these patients is often sudden and presumably related to the high incidence of ventricular tachyarrhythmias that occur with aneurysms.

The presence of persistent ST-segment elevation in an electrocardiographic area of infarction, classically thought to suggest aneurysm formation, actually indicates a large infarct but does not necessarily imply an aneurysm.[886] The diagnosis of aneurysm is best made noninvasively by an echocardiographic study (Fig. 4–85, p. 95), by radionuclide ventriculography, or at the time of cardiac catheterization by left ventriculography. With the loss of shortening from the area of the aneurysm, the remainder of the ventricle is required to compensate. With relatively large aneurysms, complete compensation is impossible. The stroke volume falls, or if maintained, it is at the expense of an increase in end-diastolic volume, which in turn leads to increased wall tension and myocardial oxygen demand. Heart failure may ensue, and angina may appear or worsen.

TREATMENT. Aggressive management of AMI, including coronary thrombolysis, may diminish the incidence of ventricular aneurysms. Surgical aneurysmectomy generally is successful only if there is relative preservation of contractile performance in the nonaneurysmal portion of the left ventricle.[887] In such circumstances, when the operation is performed for worsening heart failure or angina, operative mortality is relatively low and clinical improvement can be expected.[887] Aneurysmectomy and special procedures carried out to control ventricular tachyarrhythmias occurring with left ventricular aneurysms are described on page 658.

OTHER COMPLICATIONS OF ACUTE MYOCARDIAL INFARCTION

LEFT VENTRICULAR THROMBUS AND ARTERIAL EMBOLISM

Mural thrombi (Fig. 39–37) are common in patients succumbing to AMI.[888] In one report, 44 per cent of 924 patients dying of AMI were found to have mural thrombi attached to the endocardium overlying the infarct[889]; thrombi are more common in patients with large than small infarcts and are more frequent in nonsurvivors than in survivors. They are almost universally located in the left ventricle, particularly at its apex. With extensive transmural infarction of the septum, however, mural thrombi may overlie infarcted myocardium in both ventricles. As noted earlier, mural thrombus is rather common in a ventricular aneurysm or pseudoaneurysm. Clinical series suggest that the incidence of left ventricular thrombi identified echocardiographically is 20 to 40 per cent, with the vast majority occurring in anterior MI[378,890–893] (Fig. 4–91, p. 98).[378,890–893] Computed tomography may be even more sensitive than echocardiography for the identification of intracardiac thrombi[348] (Fig. 11–37, p. 330). Mural thrombi have been found to be more frequent in patients treated with beta-adrenoceptor blockade after AMI.[894]

Although a mural thrombus adheres to the endocardium overlying the infarcted myocardium, superficial portions of it can become detached and produce systemic arterial emboli. Approximately half of patients with mural thrombi at autopsy also have evidence of systemic emboli.[881] Serial echocardiographic studies suggest that the incidence of emboli from documented mural thrombi in AMI is about 5 per cent,[895] but it is highly variable (0 to 25 per cent) even when a mural thrombus has been identified.[890–893] Occasionally, embolism from a mural thrombus is the presenting symptom with the underlying myocardial infarction either silent or overlooked. Prospec-

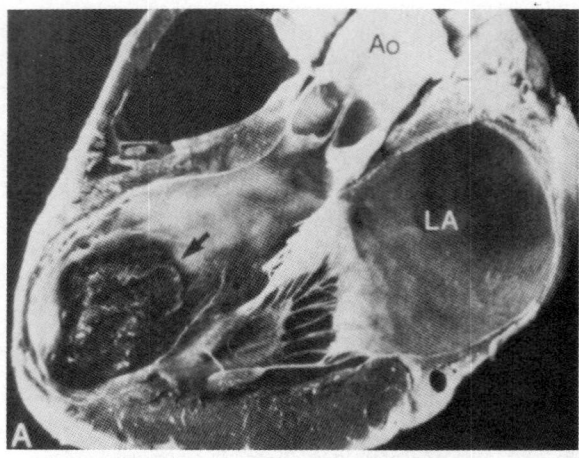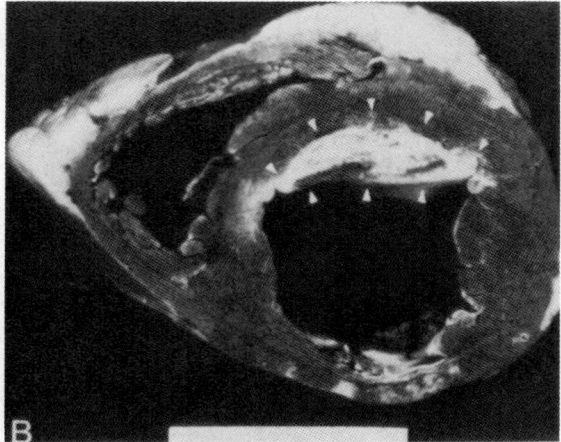

FIGURE 39–37. Postinfarction left ventricular mural thrombus. *A,* Recent thrombus (arrow) with central ulceration. Systemic embolization occurred in this patient. *B,* Old organized thrombus (arrowheads) adjacent to area of infarction. (From Edwards, W. D.: Pathology of myocardial infarction and reperfusion. *In* Gersh, B. J., and Rahimtoola, S. H. [eds.]: Acute Myocardial Infarction. New York, Elsevier, 1991, p. 29.)

tive studies have suggested that patients who develop a mural thrombus early (within 48 to 72 hours of infarction) have an extremely poor early prognosis.[878,892] In one series, over 90 per cent of the patients developing a thrombus within 48 hours died, all of causes related to the large infarction (shock, reinfarction, rupture, and ventricular tachyarrhythmia), while none had clinical evidence of emboli from the left ventricular thrombus.[378] Only 1 of the 24 patients with thrombus had a clinically apparent embolic episode. (None of the patients were receiving anticoagulation therapy.)

MANAGEMENT. It is not entirely clear whether heparinization or a combination of thrombolytic therapy with heparin prevents emboli from left ventricular thrombi,[890,895–897] although both heparin and thrombolytic therapy reduce the incidence or extent of mural thrombi.[898,899] Recommendations for anticoagulation vary considerably,[890,900–903] and thrombolysis has precipitated fatal embolization.[893] Nevertheless, prudent anticoagulation for 3 to 6 months with warfarin is advocated for many patients with demonstrable mural thrombi.[904,905] It is not our practice to recommend routine anticoagulation, even if a left ventricular thrombus is present, *unless:* (1) an embolic event has already occurred or (2) the thrombus appears highly mobile and/or markedly protuberant and shaggy on the echocardiogram.[891,893,906]

Antiplatelet therapy, while probably not capable of affecting thrombus size in most patients, may prevent further platelet deposition on existing thrombi.[907] Because it is generally so benign, antiplatelet therapy is therefore recommended for most patients with left ventricular thrombi in whom systemic anticoagulation is not undertaken. Independent of therapy, early spontaneous regression of a thrombus occurs in 20 per cent or more of patients,[378,891] while systemic thrombolytic therapy causes echocardiographic regression or disappearance of the thrombus in most patients so treated.[908]

VENOUS THROMBOSIS AND EMBOLISM

Almost all pulmonary emboli originate from thrombi in the veins of the lower extremities (Chap. 48); much less commonly, they originate from mural thrombi overlying an area of infarction in the right ventricle. Bed rest and heart failure predispose to venous thrombosis and subsequent pulmonary embolism, and both of these factors occur commonly in patients with AMI, particularly those with large infarcts. Several decades ago, at a time when patients with AMI were subjected to prolonged periods of bed rest, significant pulmonary embolism was found in more than 20 per cent of patients with MI at autopsy,[909] and massive pulmonary embolism accounted for 10 per cent of deaths from AMI.[889] In recent years, with early mobilization and the widespread use of low-dose anticoagu-lant prophylaxis, pulmonary embolism has become an uncommon cause of death in this condition.

POSTINFARCTION ISCHEMIA AND INFARCT EXTENSION

POSTINFARCTION ANGINA. *Angina* developing within the first 10 days following AMI is disconcerting to patients and physicians alike. In many patients, it responds to rest, nitroglycerin, beta-adrenoceptor blockade, and calcium channel antagonists,[904] just as does classic angina. In a minority of patients, postinfarction angina may be refractory to treatment and occurs at rest or is provoked by minimal activity, meals, or emotional upset. This represents a form of unstable angina (p. 1334). When accompanied by ST-T–wave changes in the same area where Q waves have appeared, it may be due to coronary spasm,[911] to occlusion of an initially patent vessel, or to reocclusion of a recanalized one.

Regardless of whether postinfarction angina is persistent or limited, its presence is important, for both short- and long-term mortality is higher among such patients.[331,912,913] For this reason we concur with the recommendation of others[914] that most patients who develop spontaneous angina early after AMI should undergo cardiac catheterization and coronary arteriography to assess their suitability for a revascularization procedure.

Exercise stress testing, particularly when used with stress-thallium scintigraphy, may be helpful in discerning whether chest pain following an AMI is due to ischemia. However, such tests should usually be avoided if symptoms have been persistent, accompanied by ECG changes, or have occurred at rest or with minimal activity. Positron-emission tomography has proved useful for recognizing hypoperfused but viable myocardium following AMI,[915] and its sensitivity is improved further when dual isotope imaging (with thallium and indium antimyosin) is utilized.[916] Early dipyridamole-thallium imaging performed within 4 days of AMI may be able to predict further in-hospital ischemia.[917]

INFARCT EXTENSION

Extension of the infarct occurs in approximately 7 to 10 per cent of patients with AMI during the first 10 days[912,918] and in closer to 20 per cent in patients who have undergone thrombolytic therapy.[919] In the latter group it is due to reocclusion. One study employing echocardiograms every 48 hours or less found extension in over 50 per cent of a selected group of patients with anterior MI.[920] While this incidence may be high, it is probable that many episodes of extension are unrecognized. It is frequently difficult to distinguish postinfarction angina from infarct extension. The latter is usually associated with more severe and prolonged discomfort, and *persistent* electrocardiographic changes (ST-T changes or QRS changes or both) may occur. It is generally defined as reelevation or reappearance of CK-MB in the serum after the initial peak. Neither chest pain nor the ECG provides accurate markers for recognizing infarct extension, as both occur in only about half of patients with extension. The majority of patients with cardiogenic shock have developed infarct extension.[781] In a prospective study of patients, it was found that mortality in those experiencing extension is more than double that noted in patients in whom extension did not occur.[921] Marmor reported that infarct extension occurred most frequently in obese females and was most common in patients with nontransmural infarction.[922] It is apparently more common in patients with diabetes mellitus, a previous MI, and in those with an early peaking CK-MB curve (<15 hours),[918] but it is not predictable from the angiographic appearance of the coronary artery early after infarction—at least when thrombolytic therapy has been given.[919] Presumably, the higher mortality associated with infarct extension is related to the larger mass of myocardium whose function becomes compromised.

PERICARDIAL EFFUSION AND PERICARDITIS
(See also p. 1495–1496)

PERICARDIAL EFFUSION. This is common after AMI. Effusions are generally detected echocardiographically, and their incidence varies with technique, criteria, and laboratory expertise. They occur in approximately 17 to 25 per cent of patients after MI.[923–925] Effusions are more common with anterior MI and with larger infarcts and when congestive failure is present.[923,925] This finding cannot be viewed as a complication because it does not necessarily lead to clinical problems. (When tamponade occurs, it is usually due to ventricular rupture or hemorrhagic pericarditis.)

The reabsorption rate of a postinfarction pericardial effusion is slow, with resolution often taking several months. The presence of an effusion does not indicate that pericarditis is present; although they may occur together, the majority of effusions occur without other evidence of pericarditis.[926]

PERICARDITIS. When secondary to transmural AMI, pericarditis may produce pain as early as the first day and as late as 6 weeks after MI. The pain of pericarditis may be confused with that resulting from persistent ischemia or extension of the infarct or both. Transmural myocardial infarction, by definition, extends to the epicardial surface and is responsible for causing local pericardial inflammation. Although transitory pericardial friction rubs are relatively common among patients with transmural infarction within the first 48 hours, the pain or electrocardiographic changes occur much less often. In one recent study of 423 consecutive patients with AMI, 31 (7.3 per cent) developed a pericardial friction rub, but only one patient had electrocardiographic changes diagnostic of acute pericarditis[267] (p. 1470). Pericarditis is more common in males, among patients with Q-wave infarction, and in those with congestive heart failure.[267,927] Fibrinous or serofibrinous pericarditis may be seen in up to 15 per cent of patients with AMI at autopsy, while clinical studies also suggest the presence of active pericarditis in 10 to 20 per cent of patients,[927,928] whereas pericardial effusion without evidence of pericarditis is far more common.[923] The discomfort of pericarditis usually becomes worse during a deep inspiration, but it may be somewhat relieved when the patient sits up and leans forward (Chap. 45).

Pericarditis generally occurs between the second and fourth days after the infarction. In some patients with diffuse pericarditis, an accompanying pericardial effusion may be large, but tamponade is rare, and as noted earlier no effusion is present in the majority of patients. Occasionally, hemorrhagic effusion with cardiac tamponade develops after myocardial infarction in patients who have been treated with anticoagulants.[929] Late pericardial constriction due to anticoagulant-induced hemopericardium has been reported.[930] While anticoagulation clearly increases the risk for hemorrhagic pericarditis early after MI, this complication has not been reported with sufficient frequency during heparinization or following thrombolytic therapy to warrant *absolute* prohibition of such agents when a rub is present. In cases in which continuation or initiation of anticoagulant therapy is *strongly* indicated (such as during cardiac catheterization or following coronary angioplasty), particularly careful attention is warranted to the clotting parameters and the duration of anticoagulation, and in observation for clinical signs of possible tamponade.

DRESSLER SYNDROME. Also known as the *postmyocardial infarction syndrome*,[269,270] this usually occurs 2 to 10 weeks after infarction. Its incidence is difficult to define because it often blends imperceptibly with the more common early postmyocardial infarction pericarditis. This incidence has decreased dramatically since the use of chronic anticoagulation has fallen out of favor and since antiinflammatory agents are used more vigorously. However, it has probably not disappeared completely as some have contended.[931,932] At autopsy, patients with this syndrome usually demonstrate localized fibrinous pericarditis[928] containing polymorphonuclear leukocytes.[269] The syndrome is treated with aspirin 650 mg, as often as every 4 hours. Other nonsteroidal antiinflammatory agents are best avoided in the AMI patient because of their potential to impair infarct healing,[933] to cause ventricular rupture,[934] and to increase coronary vascular resistance.[935] In occasional patients full-dose steroids are necessary to control what may be very severe symptoms.

Convalescence, Discharge, and Postmyocardial Infarction Care
(See also Chap. 42)

For the patient with an uncomplicated AMI, washing and personal care should be assisted by an attendant during the first 2 to 4 days. If the convalescence continues uneventfully, limited ambulation within the room can be begun on the third or fourth day. Once early ambulatory activities are begun, advancement in the activity should depend on the patient's condition. Activity can then increase progressively, and a shower may be allowed some time after the sixth day. In an era characterized by encouragement of earlier physical activity after AMI, investigators regularly have failed to identify any complication of early ambulation. One recent small study demonstrated that early "vigorous mobilization" (monitored brisk 10 to 15 minute walks from day 4 onward) produced no changes in ventricular volumes, heart rate, or cardiac output in a group of low-risk AMI patients compared with controls managed in a more conventional manner.[936] While concern has been raised from studies in animals[937,938] that such early activity might unfavorably influence ventricular remodeling, perhaps by causing infarct extension, there is no evidence to suggest that this concern is valid, and early mobilization does appear warranted in most stable AMI patients.

Prolonged hospitalization and enforced bed rest for any illness may lead to complications (particularly in elderly patients) such as constipation, decubitus ulcers, excessive resorption of bone with formation of renal calculi, atelectasis, thrombophlebitis, pulmonary emboli, urinary retention, mild anemia due to repetitive blood sampling for diagnostic tests, impaired oral intake of fluids, bleeding from the gastrointestinal tract due to stress ulcers, and deconditioning of cardiovascular reflex responses to postural changes. Because of the precarious status of the heart recovering from AMI, avoidance of such complications is of primary importance. For example, constipation may lead to straining, transitory reduction of venous return and diminution of cardiac output, impaired coronary perfusion, and ventricular arrhythmias, occasionally culminating in ventricular fibrillation. Early use of a bedside commode, stool softeners, and a bed-chair regimen appears to be useful in avoiding many of the difficulties encountered previously among patients confined to bed for several weeks.

TIMING OF HOSPITAL DISCHARGE

The time of discharge from the hospital is variable. It may be as early as 6 or 7 days after admission for patients who experience no complications, who can be followed readily at home, and for whom the family setting is conducive to convalescence.[939] Most complications that would preclude early discharge occur within the first day or so of admission; therefore, patients suitable for early discharge can be identified early during the hospitalization.[940] Ordinarily, discharge of patients without complications is deferred until approximately 7 to 8 days following infarction, at a time when the patient has become fully ambulatory. For patients who have experienced a complication, discharge is deferred until their condition has been stable for several days and it is clear that they are responding appropriately to necessary medications such as antiarrhythmic agents, vasodilators, or positive inotropic agents, or that they have undergone the appropriate work-up for recurrent ischemia.

TRIALS INVOLVING EARLY DISCHARGE. Several controlled trials and many uncontrolled trials of early discharge after AMI have been conducted.[940,940a] None have shown any increase in risk with early discharge, and some have actually shown significantly worse mortality and morbidity in the group discharged later,[941] although this may have been due to confounding variables. When considered together, the studies of early discharge are quite encouraging. Results involving 892 patients in 8 different trials of discharge between 7 and 14 days after admission for AMI suggest that there is no unfavorable effect on mortality and morbidity.[940] A multivariant statistical technique to determine risk of discharge for individual patients has been proposed.[942] Using 19 clinical variables, this technique was developed with the following assumptions: discharge would take place when the risk of a serious complication occurring in the 2 weeks following discharge was below 5 per cent, and when the risk of death in the first 30 days after admission for AMI was also less than 5 per cent. Tested retrospectively in over 1000 patients and prospectively in almost 200 patients, this statistical system confirmed that about 50 per cent of patients could be discharged safely after 5 days, and that up to a 20 per cent saving in hospitalization days could be obtained.[942] More recently, very early discharge (after *3 days*) has been reported without apparent clinical complications.[943] Furthermore, early discharge appeared to promote an earlier return to work and some degree of savings in hospital and professional costs. While conclusions from this study are intriguing, they are limited to a carefully selected group of patients, almost all of whom underwent cardiac catheterization with reperfusion by either thrombolytic therapy or coronary angioplasty. Whether the same savings would occur with the same degree of safety in patients not undergoing catheterization and reperfusion remains to be seen.[944]

While early discharge certainly is feasible for the majority of patients with uncomplicated MI, an attempt should be made before hospital discharge to identify patients at considerable risk of reinfarction or cardiac death. This usually involves noninvasive testing, which may lead to cardiac catheterization and coronary arteriography and, if indicated, to coronary revascularization. Much can be said for accomplishing such procedures, if necessary, before hospital discharge. Furthermore, since we do not yet know with certainty that vigorous exercise does not adversely affect scar formation or ventricular remodeling, an early increase in physical activity should be minimized by strict instructions to the patient and family concerning the gradual resumption of activity after discharge. In fact, patients with poor left ventricular function following relatively large anterior MI have

been shown to have infarct expansion and greater shape distortion of the left ventricle after a late exercise program (beginning 15 weeks after AMI).[945] Thus, in patients with extensive degrees of ventricular dysfunction, exercise should be undertaken with caution and monitoring.

COUNSELING. Before discharge from the hospital, all patients should receive detailed instruction concerning physical activity. Initially, this activity should consist of ambulation at home but avoidance of isometric exercise such as lifting; several rest periods should be taken daily. In addition, the patient should be given fresh nitroglycerin tablets and instructed in their use and should receive careful instructions about the use of any other medication prescribed. As convalescence progresses, graded resumption of activity should be encouraged. Many approaches have been utilized, ranging from formal rigid guidelines to general advice advocating moderation and avoidance of any activity that evokes symptoms. *Sexual counseling* is often overlooked during recovery from MI[946] and should also be included as part of the educational process. Such counseling should begin early after AMI and should include the recommendation that sexual activity be resumed after successful completion of either early submaximal or later symptom-limited exercise stress testing.[947]

There is some evidence that behavior alteration is possible after recovery from MI and that this may improve prognosis.[948,949] A cardiac rehabilitation program with supervised physical exercise and an educational component has been recommended for most MI patients following discharge.[950,951] While the overall clinical benefit of such programs continues to be debated,[952,953] there is little question that most people derive considerable knowledge and psychological security from such interventions. The physical and psychological aspects of rehabilitation of patients convalescing from AMI are discussed in Chapter 42.

SECONDARY PREVENTION OF MYOCARDIAL INFARCTION

The concept of secondary prevention of reinfarction and death after recovery from an AMI has been investigated actively during the past 2½ decades. Problems in proving the efficacy of various interventions have been related both to the ineffectiveness of certain strategies and to the difficulty in proving a benefit as mortality and morbidity have improved following AMI. Nevertheless, patients who survive the initial course of AMI are at increased risk due to coronary artery disease and its complications; therefore, it is imperative that efforts be made to reduce this risk.[954] While secondary prevention drug trials generally have tested one form of therapy against placebo in an attempt to demonstrate a benefit of that therapy, the physician must remember that disciplined clinical care of the individual patient is far more important than rote use of an agent found beneficial in the latest drug trial.[955]

In reviewing the results of any secondary prevention trial, the clinician must consider several issues before deciding on its relevance to a particular patient: (1) Was the intervention begun immediately (once AMI was identified) or was it applied later, and what is the relationship of its expected effectiveness to this timing? (2) Were patients in the trial similar to the patient for whom the intervention is contemplated, or would the specific patient under consideration have been excluded from the trial, thus rendering the trial's conclusion less meaningful for that particular patient? (3) Is there some reason to anticipate that the intervention being considered might be unusually risky in certain patients for whom it may be used (e.g., beta-adrenoceptor blockers in a patient with a history of obstructive lung disease)? (4) Once the intervention is started, how long should it be continued, or is this information unavailable because studies have not been ongoing for a sufficient time? (5) What is the underlying risk that the individual patient faces? As detailed on pages 1267 to 1270, patients with low risk can be separated from those with higher risk. In interventional strategies, the level of risk should be taken into consideration when any therapy, particularly if it is to be long term, is contemplated.

It is likely that secondary prevention efforts are, in fact, responsible in part for the remarkable decline in mortality and morbidity[12] in patients with coronary artery disease, although the magnitude of the impact is not clear.

RISK FACTOR REDUCTION. Efforts to improve survival and the quality of life after MI that relate to modification of known risk factors are considered in Chapter 37. Of the risk factors considered, cessation of smoking and control of hypertension are probably most important. It has been shown that within 2 years of quitting smoking, the risk of a nonfatal MI in these former smokers falls to a level compatible with that in never-smokers.[956] Being hospitalized for an AMI is a powerful motivation for patients to cease cigarette smoking, and this is an ideal time to encourage that clearly beneficial change. It is also an ideal time to begin to treat hypertension, to counsel patients to achieve optimal body weight, and to consider various strategies to improve the patient's lipid profile. Unfortunately, unless prior values of total cholesterol and HDL cholesterol are known, or unless measurements are obtained within the first 24 to 48 hours,[312–314] reliable values necessary to guide therapy will not be available until approximately 2 to 3 months after the MI. However, that is not too late to evaluate the lipid profile and to begin appropriate therapeutic measures as outlined in Chapter 37. Following a step I AHA diet (p. 1224) during the initial hospitalization and until the lipids have been evaluated is appropriate. As discussed in Chapter 42, cardiac rehabilitation efforts that include exercise programs and the teaching of stress reduction techniques are also likely to have an impact on secondary prevention.[952,953] However, despite the general desirability of these measures, for many patients with AMI, particularly the elderly, it is unlikely that much change in the underlying coronary atherosclerosis will take place with their institution.

Beta-Adrenoceptor Blockers

These drugs have been the most intensively investigated agents for secondary prevention following AMI. Numerous studies have now shown that beta blocker administration improves survival after AMI, and as a result, prescribing patterns for these agents have changed dramatically.[957] The first post-MI beta blocker trial was reported by Snow in 1965,[958] arousing a great deal of interest. Of the many beta blocking agents tested since then, propranolol,[642,959] metoprolol,[482,960] timolol,[961] and oxprenolol[962] have been tried in the greatest number of patients. Large trials with timolol, propranolol, and metoprolol have demonstrated that these drugs improve survival in a wide spectrum of postinfarction patients and also reduce the incidence of sudden death and reinfarction. Results with oxprenolol, a beta blocker with intrinsic sympathomimetic activity (ISA), are far less encouraging, with at least one trial of this agent appearing to show a slight adverse effect on mortality.[647] Structure in the various trials has varied considerably, making comparisons exceedingly difficult.[647] While increasingly rigorous trial design and analysis have allowed for more definitive conclusions, controversy continues regarding optimal selection of patients, variety of beta blocker, initial route (intravenous followed by oral vs. oral vs. intravenous), and timing of administration.[16]

Although differences in trials have made it statistically unsound to pool data from studies, one useful strategy, known as meta-analysis, has been to compare by graphs estimates of the mortality benefit (or lack of benefit) and the trial's 95 per cent confidence limits.[16,647,963] This form of analysis has been applied to beta blocker trials to demonstrate both the mode of benefit and the effect of ancillary properties of the beta blocker. It appears that improved mortality is related primarily to the prevention of sudden death and that, while there is no difference between cardioselective and noncardioselective beta blockers, agents with ISA are markedly less beneficial than those without ISA.[647]

ADVERSE EFFECTS. While adverse effects have required withdrawal of the beta blocker in approximately 10 per cent of patients, most of these effects can be ameliorated by varying the choice of beta blocker, reducing the dosage, or discontinuing the medication if necessary. There has been natural concern that, because of the beta blockers' negative inotropic effect, heart failure would complicate the administration of these agents to patients after AMI. Although a slight excess of clinical heart failure has been reported in some trials,[647] this difference appears to be at most trivial. Most studies have excluded patients with heart failure at entry, but even those including patients with mild failure do not show any increase

in either death or subsequent heart failure.[647] Subgroup analysis of patients from the Norwegian timolol study showed a more marked ability to prevent sudden death in patients with cardiac enlargement than in patients with normal heart size.[964] In the BHAT trial propranolol decreased the incidence of sudden death by 13 per cent in patients without heart failure and by 47 per cent in patients who had prior failure.[965] Early administration of beta blockers may reduce the incidence of heart failure by improving ischemia and by preventing reinfarction. At least one of the large trials suggests that this concept may be accurate. In the Göteborg metoprolol trial, a similar percentage of patients developed heart failure after AMI (27 per cent in the metoprolol group and 30 per cent in the control group), but significantly less diuretic was required among metoprolol-treated patients than among controls.[966] The results of the Beta-Blocker Pooling Project, in which data were examined from 9 separate studies involving more than 10,000 patients, suggest a highly significant reduction in overall mortality among treated patients *with* pump or mechanical failure compared with patients on placebo with such failure.[967] The relative benefit of beta blockers following thrombolytic therapy has been well studied in only one trial.[3] Early intravenous metoprolol reduced the incidence of recurrent ischemia and early reinfarction but did not affect 1-year survival or alter left ventricular function.

The mechanism by which beta blockers improve survival is not completely clear. It is likely that many factors are important, including control of hypertension and ischemia, an antiarrhythmic effect, perhaps an antiplatelet effect, an improvement in scar size, and possibly vascularity of the myocardium.[647] Blockade of the direct toxic effect of adrenergic stimulation on the myocardium may also be important. Since neither cardioselectivity or membrane-stabilizing activity appears to be requisite, the mechanism of beneficial effect appears to be due to a "class effect," i.e., it is secondary to beta blockade itself. The reduction in mortality is seen in all age groups and for all types of infarction.

RECOMMENDATIONS. On the basis of currently available evidence, patients without a contraindication to beta blockade (asthma, moderate or severe congestive heart failure, bradyarrhythmias) should have prophylactic treatment with beta blockers initiated after AMI. The dosage should be sufficient to blunt the heart rate response through stress or exercise. Since, in different trials, therapy has been initiated over a wide range of starting times (from hours to weeks) it is impossible to know which time is best from the available data. However, since the safety of early administration of beta blockers has been well documented,[958,960] it is reasonable to suggest that beta blocker administration should begin as early as possible, certainly before hospital discharge, as long as contraindications are not present. Since much of the impact in preventing mortality occurs in the first few weeks, not only is an excess degree of caution unwarranted, but delay may lead to failure to prevent a proportion of early deaths.[647] It is unclear how long patients should be treated. While it is reasonable to conclude that treatment need not extend beyond the period when mortality curves no longer diverge, this rationale is problematic: Will discontinuation of therapy lead to increasing mortality in some patients? Do mortality curves actually continue to diverge? Will continuing the drug lead to some degree of continued protection?

There are, in fact, conflicting data regarding the benefit of continuing therapy beyond 2 years. Late follow-up of a large metoprolol trial showed no significant difference in mortality at 5 years of treatment, even though a significant difference had existed at 2 years.[968] However, 6-year follow-up of the Norwegian timolol study showed lower cardiac mortality in the treated group, even 2 to 3 years after the study drug had been withdrawn.[961] Finally, in another trial, patients withdrawn from metoprolol demonstrated increased mortality following drug withdrawal.[969] Taken together, these studies suggest that therapy should be continued for at least 2 years.[16,970] At that time, if the beta blocker is well tolerated and if there is no reason to discontinue therapy, such therapy probably should be continued in most patients.

The 1 to 2 per cent overall reduction in mortality in postinfarction patients that would come from long-term use of beta blockers and secondary prevention may seem small, but it is comparable to the reduction in mortality achieved by long-term antihypertensive therapy, and would result in the saving of approximately 6000 lives per year in the United States.[647] While it should not be considered "ethically imperative" to treat all postinfarction patients, the fact that over 35,000 patients have been randomized into placebo-controlled beta blocker trials does make it important that the clinician be aware of the results of these trials, and at least consider beta blocker therapy in all patients, including the elderly, who survive MI.[647,971] The cost-effectiveness of such therapy in medium- or high-risk persons compares very favorably with many other accepted interventions such as coronary bypass surgery, angioplasty, and lipid-lowering therapy.[972] Beta blockers should not be given to patients who have clear contraindications, and *probably* need not be given to patients with an *extremely* good prognosis (first AMI, good ventricular function, no angina, negative stress test, and no complex ventricular ectopy) in whom a mortality rate of approximately 1 per cent per year can be anticipated.[973] Among such patients, long-term beta blockers do not appear to offer a benefit.[974]

Anticoagulants

(see also p. 1780)

There are at least three theoretical reasons for anticipating that anticoagulants might be beneficial in the management of AMI: (1) Since the coronary occlusion responsible for the AMI is often due to a thrombus (p. 1206), anticoagulants might be expected to halt or slow progression and to prevent the development of new thrombi elsewhere in the coronary arterial tree. (2) Anticoagulants might be expected to diminish the formation of mural thrombi and resultant systemic embolization. (3) Anticoagulants might be expected to reduce the incidence of venous thrombosis and pulmonary embolization.

After several decades of evaluation, the weight of evidence now suggests that anticoagulants appear to have a favorable effect on late mortality and reinfarction among patients hospitalized with AMI[975-978] (Fig. 39–38). While salutary effects on the underlying coronary disease and its progression have not been clearly demonstrated with conventional anticoagulant drugs, it is possible that they decrease the incidence of cerebral emboli resulting from mural thrombi (p. 1821).[969] In addition, the administration of heparin in doses sufficient to influence activation of factor X without affecting conventional laboratory tests of the coagulation system has in the past substantially diminished the incidence of deep vein thrombosis,[980] thereby reducing the incidence of pulmonary emboli. Whether anticoagulant therapy produces this benefit today, with earlier ambulation and discharge of patients, has not been retested. Nevertheless, it appears advisable to administer minidose heparin (5000 units subcutaneously) every 8 to 12 hours in the absence of specific contraindications.[981] The drug should be continued until 2 to 3 days before hospital discharge, although it is recognized that in patients with uncomplicated AMI there is no clear evidence that it reduces mortality. In any event, patients treated with thrombolytic agents require heparin therapy.

In patients at high risk of embolism (e.g., those with ventricular aneurysm, marked obesity, cardiogenic shock, low output state, present or past thrombophlebitis, arterial or pulmonary embolism), in the absence of contraindications, anticoagulant treatment does exert a favorable effect on survival, and full-dose anticoagulation with heparin is indicated (e.g., intravenous administration of 10,000 units, followed by continuous infusion of 1000 units per hour) to maintain the clotting time and partial thromboplastin time at 1.5 to 2.0 times normal. After 5 to 7 days of therapy, warfarin or continued administration of subcutaneous, adjusted doses of heparin may be employed if conditions exist that suggest that

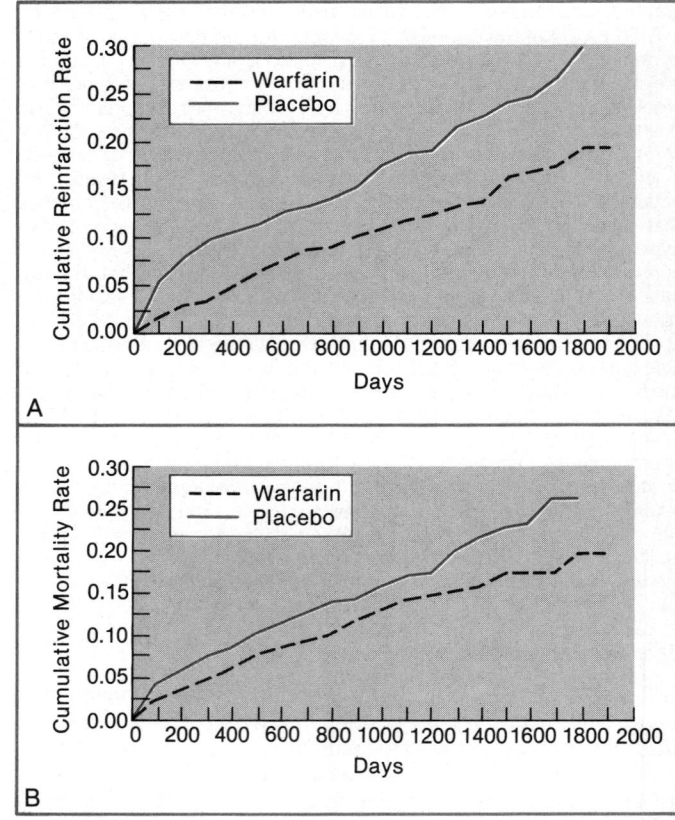

FIGURE 39–38. Cumulative rates of reinfarction (*A*) and death from all causes (*B*) according to original treatment assignment from randomized study of warfarin in 1214 patients with AMI. Treatment began a mean of 27 days after infarction. (Reprinted by permission from Smith, P., et al.: The effect of warfarin on mortality and reinfarction after myocardial infarction. N. Engl. J. Med. 323:147, 1990.)

venous thrombosis and embolism are likely to recur. These include continued or worsening heart failure, persistent thrombophlebitis, and the need for prolonged bed rest.

As anticoagulation does clearly reduce the occurrence of thromboembolic complications, it is reasonable to use chronic anticoagulants in patients in the posthospital phase with specific indications, including thrombophlebitis, a history of pulmonary or systemic embolism, evidence of a mural thrombus in the left ventricle on two-dimensional echocardiography (Fig. 4–91, p. 98), and severe heart failure.[982] As both warfarin and aspirin have now been shown to be of long-term benefit but have not been compared directly, the choice of one over the other must be based on individual physician preferences and patient characteristics.

Antiplatelet Agents

(See also p. 1340)

Secondary prevention trials with antiplatelet agents are based on the theory that platelets play a role in MI and sudden death. Thrombi may be composed of platelet aggregates at the site of an atherosclerotic coronary artery narrowing, and aggregates may obstruct the coronary microcirculation, inducing coronary vasospasm through the release of the vasoconstrictor thromboxane A_2. Platelets may also play a role in atherogenesis (p. 1337). In two different careful reviews of the major secondary prevention aspirin trials performed over the last 15 years, opposite conclusions were reached about the efficacy of aspirin after AMI.[983,984] Although seven of the eight trials reviewed showed a lower mean mortality with aspirin, the difference was statistically significant in only one (Table 58–3, p. 1785). However, pooling of the data suggests that aspirin prophylaxis could result in at least a 10 to 15 per cent reduction in total deaths and a 20 to 30 per cent reduction in reinfarction.[983,995] Accordingly, in the absence of contraindications to aspirin administration, particularly the history of peptic ulcer disease or gastrointestinal bleeding, we recommend 80 to 325 mg aspirin daily, which can be administered as an enteric-coated tablet. This dosage should minimize the risk of accompanying gastrointestinal side effects; the cost is low and inconvenience trivial. Despite the use of sulfinpyrazone in earlier trials,[986] there is no reason to anticipate that its antiplatelet effect is superior to aspirin's,[985] and it may, in fact, be less effective. Therefore, use of sulfinpyrazone in place of aspirin is not recommended. The addition of dipyridamole to aspirin for possible potentiation of antiplatelet effect has not convincingly improved on the effect of aspirin alone[987]; therefore, coadministration of dipyridamole also is not recommended.[985]

Other Measures

The effectiveness of secondary prevention with other agents, including calcium antagonists, nitrates, antiarrhythmics, lipid-lowering drugs, prostacyclin analogs, and thromboxane synthetase inhibitors, requires further investigation.

CALCIUM ANTAGONISTS. Studies of verapamil[670] and nifedipine[662,998] have failed to show any clear benefit with the *early* administration of these agents. In fact, three studies[663-665] have actually shown a higher early mortality when nifedipine was given early to patients with threatened or acute MI. Therefore, nifedipine cannot be recommended for secondary prevention following AMI, and, in fact, should probably be avoided in most patients.[989] Although diltiazem also showed no benefit in one large trial,[666] a subgroup analysis suggests that it may actually be harmful in patients with preexisting left ventricular dysfunction, while a parallel study showed potential benefit (reduction in reinfarction) in patients with non-Q wave infarction (Fig. 38–39).[990] This finding has led some to recommend diltiazem for patients with non-Q-wave MI.[991] Finally, verapamil also has produced mixed results, with one recent study showing a favorable long-term effect in patients free of heart failure.[667]

NITRATES. These agents are widely prescribed prophylactically to patients following AMI, usually for prevention of recurrent ischemia. However, controlled trials to test the long-term efficacy of this strategy have not been carried out; therefore, such an approach cannot be recommended on a routine basis. In one retrospective study, patients treated with long-acting nitrates had a significantly lower mortality (10 versus 26 per cent) than those not receiving this therapy.[992] This observational study cannot be used as justification for applying such therapy to all patients unless a specific indication such as continuing angina is present.

ANTIARRHYTHMICS. While it has been recognized for decades that antiarrhythmic therapy can control atrial and ventricular arrhythmias effectively in many patients, careful reviews of clinical trials have failed to suggest that routine use of these agents would be of any benefit.[993,994] Such agents have never been shown conclusively to reduce long-term mortality following AMI,[995] and certain agents (e.g., flecainide and encainide) appear to increase mortality,[752] as discussed on p. 643) (Fig. 39–27). Accordingly, the routine use of antiarrhythmic agents cannot be recommended. Whether subgroups with complex arrhythmias, particularly if they are symptomatic, should be treated remains unanswered by such studies, yet treatment of such patients with antiarrhythmic agents does seem reasonable in the absence of contraindications or newer data to the contrary.

Recently early treatment of AMI patients with intravenous magnesium (in patients with normal baseline magnesium levels) has been shown to reduce 1-year mortality, partly on the basis of a nearly 50 per cent reduction in arrhythmias.[996] This intriguing finding awaits confirmation before such therapy can be widely recommended.

RISK FACTOR MODIFICATION. This strategy applied universally after AMI has not been shown convincingly to affect long-term mortality and morbidity and is the subject of several large ongoing controlled studies. However, three trials are worthy of note. In the first, late follow-up (at a mean of 15 years) from the Coronary Drug Project, begun in 1966, has revealed lower mortality among patients treated with niacin to induce favorable effects on serum lipids.[997] Remarkably, this benefit was seen nearly 9 years after termination of the study, when patients were no longer taking niacin. The second, a recent trial from Sweden, demonstrated that clofibrate and nicotinic acid administered together reduced overt recurrent *ischemic* heart disease by 28 per cent at 5 years.[998] Third, it is known that type A behavior (an excessive sense of time urgency and easily aroused hostility, p. 1152) can be improved by training techniques, and it has been reported, although not yet confirmed, that the use of such techniques following AMI may reduce significantly the risk of recurrent AMI and sudden death.[999] It is clearly prudent to follow strategies known to improve

long-term cardiac risks such as encouraging smoking cessation, control of diabetes and hypertension if present, and treatment of elevated serum cholesterol or other prognostically unfavorable lipid profiles.[1000]

RISK STRATIFICATION FOLLOWING MYOCARDIAL INFARCTION

Both short-term and long-term survival after AMI depend on a number of factors,[1001,1002] (Table 39–16) the most important of which is the state of left ventricular function. Additional importance is ascribed to the severity and extent of the obstructive lesions in the coronary vascular bed perfusing residual viable myocardium.[1003,1004] In other words, survival relates to the quantity of myocardium that has become necrotic and the quantity at risk of becoming necrotic. At one extreme, the prognosis is best for the patient with normal intrinsic coronary vessels whose completed infarction constitutes a small fraction (less than 5 per cent) of the left ventricle as a consequence of a coronary embolus and who has no jeopardized myocardium. At the other extreme is the patient with a massive infarct who is in cardiogenic shock and whose residual viable myocardium is perfused by markedly obstructed vessels; obviously, progression of atherosclerosis or lowering of perfusion pressure in these vessels will impair the function and viability of the residual myocardium on which left ventricular function depends. The situation may not be hopeless even in such a patient, however, since revascularization may reduce the threat to the jeopardized myocardium.

CLINICAL FACTORS. Soon after coronary care units were instituted, it became apparent that left ventricular function is an important early determinant of survival. Thus, Killip divided patients into four groups on the basis of the clinical severity of left ventricular failure as assessed by physical examination at the time of admission to the coronary care unit. As noted in Table 39–12, hospital mortality from AMI depends directly on the severity of left ventricular dysfunction present at the time of admission.[1005] Similarly, Peel[1006] and Norris[1007] and their collaborators developed clinical prognos-

TABLE 39–16 ADVERSE RISK FACTORS AFTER ACUTE MYOCARDIAL INFARCTION

1. Congestive heart failure (clinical, hemodynamic, or radiographic)
2. Left ventricular ejection fraction less than 0.04
3. Large infarct size (estimated by enzymes, technetium-99m radionuclide scan, electrocardiographic QRS mapping, or echocardiographic techniques)
4. New bundle branch block (any type, including fascicular blocks)
5. Mobitz II second-degree or third-degree heart block
6. Anterior infarction
7. Reinfarction or infarct extension
8. Ventricular fibrillation or ventricular tachycardia
9. Ventricular premature beats (especially if frequent or complex)
10. Supraventricular arrhythmias (other than sinus bradycardia)
11. Abnormal signal-averaged electrocardiogram
12. Inducible sustained monomorphic ventricular tachycardia during electrophysiologic study
13. Postinfarction angina
14. Inability to perform exercise testing
15. Angina pectoris, ST-segment elevation or depression, abnormal blood pressure response, or ventricular ectopy induced by exercise testing
16. Diabetes mellitus
17. Hypertension or loss of preexisting hypertension
18. Age greater than 70 years
19. Female gender

Adapted from Hessen, S. E., and Brest, A. N.: Risk profiling the patient after acute myocardial infarction. In Pepine, C. J. (ed.): Acute myocardial infarction. Philadelphia, F. A. Davis, 1989, p. 284.

tic indices for patients with AMI. Although they used historical, electrocardiographic, and radiological data to predict hospital mortality, evidence of left ventricular failure heavily weigh these indices in the direction of poor prognosis.

Certain demographic and historical factors are associated with a poor prognosis after infarction, including female sex,[1008,1008a] age greater than 70 years,[1009,1010] a history of diabetes mellitus,[1011] hypertension, prior angina pectoris, and previous MI.[1012-1014] *Diabetes mellitus*, in particular, appears to confer a three- to fourfold increase in risk[1015,1016]; whether this is due to accelerated atherosclerosis or some other characteristic induced by the diabetic state (such as a larger infarct size[1017]) is unclear.[1018] Surviving diabetic patients also experience a more complicated postmyocardial infarction course than nondiabetic ones, including a greater incidence of postinfarction angina, infarct extension, and heart failure.[1011] Isolated elevation of systolic blood pressure and combined systolic and diastolic hypertension are also unfavorable prognostic factors.[1019] Interestingly, however, patients whose blood pressure falls after AMI seem to have a worse prognosis than those whose blood pressure increases or remains unchanged.[1019] There is also greater mortality after anterior wall MI than after inferior MI, even when corrected for infarct size.[1020,1021] As has already been discussed, infarct extension (p. 1262) influences prognosis adversely. Poor prognosis comes from the loss of viable myocardium with the resulting larger area of infarction creating a greater compromise in overall ventricular function. Postinfarction angina generally connotes a less favorable prognosis because it indicates the presence of jeopardized myocardium[1022]; however, if it is due to coronary artery spasm rather than critical organic obstruction, prognosis may be relatively good.[1023] In the current era of aggressive revascularization, early postinfarction angina often leads to early interventions that tend to improve outcome, diminishing the long-term impact and significance of angina early after AMI. Silent postinfarction ischemia detected by ambulatory monitoring is associated with the same unfavorable prognosis as symptomatic ischemia after AMI.[1024]

Although the incidence of unrecognized MI is less than that of clinically apparent MI,[258] the long-term prognosis from unrecognized infarction appears to be similar to, and as serious as, that following recognized infarction.[1025] Although the risk of angina recurring after an unrecognized MI is less than after a clinically apparent MI, the incidence of late stroke and heart failure may be even greater among patients with unrecognized MI.[1025]

Increasingly sophisticated statistical techniques have been applied to risk assessment following AMI. Madsen et al. have developed a discriminate function analysis score based on the presence or absence of four factors: heart failure, ventricular tachycardia, AV block, and previous infarction or extension of infarction.[1026] The accuracy of this score has been tested in several different populations and is useful for predicting both the risk of reinfarction and that of death following AMI.[1026] This group has also shown that reliable long-term prediction of outcome is possible using data from the first 24 hours of hospitalization,[1027] without a substantial increase in accuracy when further data from the rest of the hospitalization are added.[1028] Finally, they have applied these data to the development of a decision scheme for the selection of patients for coronary angiography after AMI,[1029] suggesting that the procedure be avoided in patients with a low 1-year mortality and recommending it for patients at higher risk.

As the widespread use of thrombolytic therapy is relatively recent, less is known about specific short- and long-term prognostic characteristics in patients having received such therapy. However, in studies carried out thus far, important risk factors appear to be no different in this group of patients from those in patients not undergoing thrombolysis.[1030,1031] The TIMI group has identified a series of clinical factors that can be detected at the time of presentation and used to help select patients at particularly high risk of death in the first 6 weeks following AMI[1031] (Table 39-6, p. 1232).

HEMODYNAMICS AND VENTRICULAR FUNCTION. Physiological evidence of compromised left ventricular function also correlates with hospital mortality in AMI, as already discussed. Thus, patients with hemodynamic (elevated pulmonary capillary wedge pressure and/or depressed cardiac index) or ventriculographic (depressed ejection fraction and elevated end-systolic volume by radionuclide angiography) evidence of left ventricular failure have a worse prognosis than patients without these findings.[1032,1033] Acute pulmonary edema with AMI, even if due to diastolic dysfunction and associated with a normal ejection fraction, can be used to identify a high-risk group.[1034]

Left ventricular ejection fraction may be the most easily assessed measurement of left ventricular function, and this measurement is extremely useful for risk stratification (Fig. 39-40). Further prognostic information can be obtained by the accurate assessment of end-systolic volume, which is an index superior even to ejection fraction for prediction of survival following AMI.[157] In patients with a low left ventricular ejection fraction, the measurement of exercise capacity is useful for further identifying those individuals at particularly high risk.[1035] Likewise, since a low ejection fraction per se is predictively highly variable, it is useful to know that patients with a *good* exercise capacity in this group fare far better than those who cannot perform more than modest exercise.[1036]

The presence or absence of concomitant right ventricular dysfunction with AMI (usually with inferior MI) does *not* appear to influence long-term outcome.[1037] The *chest roentgenogram* is of prognostic value because patients with cardiomegaly after infarction do not fare as well as individuals without this feature.

Because impaired ventricular function generally is a manifestation of the cumulative extent of myocardial damage sustained, one important determinant of prognosis is *infarct size*. This may be determined from an analysis of CK (or CK-MB) samples obtained at frequent intervals[273] or less accurately from the peak enzyme level. Thus, patients with markedly elevated plasma enzyme levels (CK > 2000 IU) often manifest left ventricular failure with concomitant poor prognosis. Furthermore, prognosis for as long as 4 years after an initial infarction is related to infarct size estimated from plasma CK time-activity curves at the time of the acute episode.[308] However, some patients with low peak CK levels may represent a higher-risk group with an increased incidence of late cardiac events, presumably due to jeopardized but noninfarcted myocardium.[1038] A large defect or multiple defects on a thallium-201 perfusion scintigram obtained early in the course of AMI, also presumably related to infarct size, is associated with a high incidence of mortality or subsequent cardiac events.[1032,1033] Similarly, patients with large infarcts on technetium-99m scintigrams have an adverse prognosis.[1039]

Experimental evidence suggests that an intervention aimed at improving ventricular function and ventricular remodeling after AMI (p. 1210), such as vasodilator therapy with captopril, may lessen ventricular dilatation and improve survival in the chronic phase of infarction.[167] A clinical trial is now under way to assess the possible benefit of this strategy in patients. Thus, in the future, ways may be found to improve upon the altered prognosis associated with large infarcts and compromised ventricular function.

Q-WAVE VERSUS NON-Q-WAVE INFARCTION (Table 39-17). Myocardial infarction occurring without the development of new Q waves has been called subendocardial, nontransmural, and non-Q-wave infarction. However, the correlation between the electrocardiographic findings of transmural or subendocardial myocardial infarction and the pathological counterparts is not good.[326] Indeed, many patients with pathological transmural infarctions have no Q waves or loss of R waves and vice versa. Consequently, it has been suggested that the description of MI based on electrocardiographic findings be confined to what is actually observed on the electrocardiogram—that is, "Q-wave" and "non-Q-wave" infarctions.

TABLE 39–17 DIFFERENCES IN PATIENTS WITH Q-WAVE AND NON-Q-WAVE MYOCARDIAL INFARCTION (MI)

CHARACTERISTIC	Q-WAVE MI	NON-Q-WAVE MI
Prevalence	60–70% of infarcts	30–40% of infarcts
Prior infarction	Rare	Frequent
Occluded infarct-related artery	75–80%	10–20%
Coronary collaterals	Less prominent	More prominent
ST-segment elevation	80%	40%
Peak creatine kinase	Higher	Lower
Ejection fraction	Lower	Higher
Wall motion	More dysfunction	Less dysfunction
Postinfarction ischemia	Less common	More common
Early infarction	~8%	~40%
In-hospital mortality	7–15%	5–10%
3-year mortality	10–30%	10–30%
Effect of medications		
Thrombolytic agents	Beneficial	Not established
β-Adrenergic blockers	Beneficial	Not established
Calcium channel blockers	Possibly detrimental	Possibly beneficial (diltiazem)

Adapted from Lavie, C. L., et al.: Acute myocardial infarction: Initial manifestations, management, prognosis. Mayo Clin. Proc. *65*:531, 1990.

The early (hospital) mortality in patients with Q-wave infarcts is approximately 1½ to 2 times that in patients with non-Q-wave infarcts,[451,1040,1041] unless early recurrent infarction or infarct extension occurs, in which case mortality is similar to that for both groups.[451] Patients with non-Q-wave infarction tend to have smaller infarcts initially and only infrequently have total occlusions of the infarct-related vessel when compared with patients with Q-wave infarction.[1041] Consistent with this finding are a lower incidence of heart failure early after infarction (as a consequence of a lesser degree of ventricular function impairment), and more frequent angina (related to the presence of preserved myocardium with marginal blood supply).[1040–1042] However, uncomplicated non-Q-wave infarctions are not benign conditions.[329,1040–1044] Thus, 60 per cent of these patients have critical obstruction in two or three of the major coronary arteries, and frequently go on to develop an acute Q-wave infarction within 12 months of the non-Q-wave infarct.[1040,1041] In one series almost half of the patients with non-Q-wave infarction developed unstable angina during a follow-up period averaging 11 months.[1045] In others, the incidence of infarct extension or early recurrent infarction was high.[1040,1041] In-hospital extension of a non-Q-wave infarction appears to increase long-term risk, with a doubling of 1-year mortality in one study.[1046]

Thus, it is clear that patients with non-Q-wave infarctions have a natural history different from that in patients with Q-wave infarction. The former may be considered a relatively unstable condition associated with a lower initial mortality rate but a higher risk of later infarction. The differing early and late risk patterns cancel each other out, to a certain extent, when overall long-term mortality is considered, because at late follow-up (1 to 3 years), both Q-wave and non-Q-wave MI patients have similar morbidities and mortalities.[1040,1044,1047,1048] The recognition of differences between the early natural histories of these two forms of infarction suggests the need for a more aggressive diagnostic approach including a careful noninvasive search for ischemia and often coronary arteriography perhaps followed by early coronary angioplasty[1049] or surgical treatment even in selected asymptomatic patients who have sustained an acute non-Q-wave infarction.[1044,1050]

Despite the logic inherent in this approach, there is no firm evidence that this strategy influences the course favorably, although it has been shown that the calcium antagonist diltiazem may be effective in preventing early recurrent MI and angina following non-Q-wave infarction. A multicenter study of this intervention in over 500 randomized patients showed a 50 per cent reduction in the cumulative incidence of such events after infarction (Fig. 39–39).[990] Patients with non-Q-wave infarction at greatest risk, who would appear likely to benefit most from the aforementioned interventions, include those with persistent ST-T–segment depression during hospitalization[1051] and those with spontaneous ischemia[1052] or ischemia provoked by stress testing.[1044,1053,1053a]

Patients with evidence of recurrent ischemia after infarction (regardless of location or ECG configuration) should receive medical therapy (bedrest, oxygen, nitrates, beta blockers, and calcium antagonists as tolerated) and should have coronary arteriography and be considered for revascularization (Chap. 40). However, it is particularly important to carefully follow symptomatic patients with non-Q-wave infarction because of the frequent presence of jeopardized but viable myocardium in such patients. Symptoms of recurrent angina or findings on noninvasive testing compatible with exercise-induced ischemia should be pursued vigorously and treated appropriately.[1050]

ELECTROCARDIOGRAM. Patients whose ECG demonstrates persistent advanced heart block (e.g., Mobitz type II, second-degree, or third-degree atrioventricular block) or new intraventricular conduction abnormalities (bifascicular or trifascicular) in the course of an AMI have a worse prognosis than do patients without these abnormalities. The influence of high degrees of heart block is particularly important in patients with right ventricular infarction, for such patients have a markedly increased mortality.[700] Other electrocardiographic findings that augur poorly for the postinfarction patient are repetitive ventricular ectopic activity (Table 39–9) (couplets, runs), persistent horizontal or downsloping ST-segment depression and Q waves in multiple leads, atrial arrhythmias (especially atrial fibrillation), voltage criteria for left ventricular hypertrophy, and an abnormal signal-averaged electrocardiogram (on a specially filtered and processed QRS complex).[1054–1057]

ST-segment depressions in leads other than those with acute Q waves are also a poor prognostic sign; for example, patients with acute inferior wall infarcts who demonstrate ST-segment depressions in precordial leads have a worse prognosis than do patients without this finding. There is con-

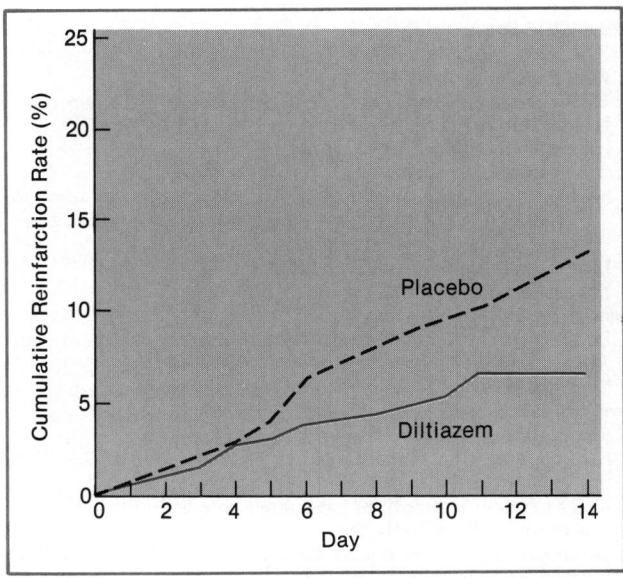

FIGURE 39–39. Life-table cumulative reinfarction rate, according to treatment group, from randomized study of 576 patients with non-Q-wave myocardial infarction. (Reprinted by permission from Gibson, R. S., et al.: Diltiazem and reinfarction in patients with non-Q-wave myocardial infarction. N. Engl. J. Med. *315*:423, 1986.)

troversy concerning whether these ST-segment depressions reflect reciprocal electrical changes, associated disease of the left anterior descending coronary artery, or, most likely, a larger inferior infarct.[332,333,335] Similarly, patients who develop angina during the first 10 days following infarction, with new electrocardiographic changes distant from the acute infarct, i.e., angina "at a distance," have a distinctly worse prognosis than do patients having postinfarct angina with ischemia in the infarct zone.[331]

LATE POSTINFARCT ASSESSMENT OF PROGNOSIS

Following recovery from AMI—i.e., by 10 days to 6 weeks after the event—long-term prognosis can be evaluated by ambulatory electrocardiographic monitoring and exercise testing,[1058,1059] with a recent survey suggesting that the vast majority employ at least the latter in most postinfarction patients.[1060] The development of ST-segment abnormalities, typical angina or exercise limitation by dyspnea at low levels of exercise (heart rate <120 beats/min or exercise duration <6 minutes on the Bruce protocol [p. 163]), and major (>2 mm) ST-segment depression and a stress-induced fall in blood pressure at any level of exercise all signify a poor prognosis.[1061–1063] A predischarge submaximal exercise test is useful for early risk stratification and can detect ischemia and arrhythmias among patients in whom these clinical features were not necessarily apparent during their hospital stay.[1059,1061,1064] A maximal stress test performed 4 to 6 weeks later may identify a greater number of patients with residual myocardial ischemia,[1066,1067] although this is controversial.[1063] Radionuclide angiography,[1067,1068] echocardiography,[1069] and thallium scintigraphy,[1066,1067] as well as coronary arteriography and left ventriculography, can provide additional important prognostic information.[1059] The high-risk variables which can be identified with noninvasive testing are shown in Table 39–18. Invasive tests are ordinarily carried out only if the patient is symptomatic or if the noninvasive tests suggest a poor prognosis and if the results of these examinations would alter the management (Chap. 40).[1029] A progressive increase in 1-year mortality is seen as ejection fraction, as measured by radionuclide angiography during hospitalization, falls below

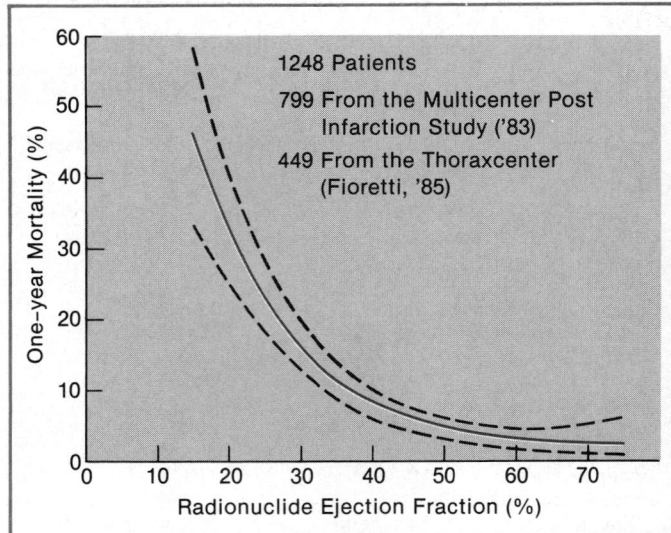

FIGURE 39–40. One-year mortality as a function of radionuclide ejection fraction (per cent) measured at hospital discharge after acute myocardial infarction. The solid line between the *dashed lines* indicates the corresponding 95 per cent confidence interval. The calculations are based on pooled data from the Multicenter Postinfarction Study and the Thoraxcenter. (From Serray, P. W., et al.: Preservation of global and regional left ventricular function after early thrombolysis in acute myocardial infarction. Reprinted with permission of the American College of Cardiology. J. Am. Coll. Cardiol. 7:729, 1986.)

0.40 (Fig. 39–40).[1070] Evidence indicates that electrical instability, as reflected in frequent, multiple, or complex ventricular extrasystoles, and left ventricular dysfunction, as reflected in a depressed left ventricular ejection fraction (<40 per cent) 10 days after the occurrence of an AMI, are independent risk factors[1071]; the presence of either risk factor was associated with an increased 15-month mortality.[1072]

Despite the clear prognostic importance of severe ventricular ectopy when detected during in-patient bedside or ambulatory monitoring, studies utilizing invasive programmed ventricular stimulation have provided conflicting evidence that ventricular arrhythmias provoked by this technique have any prognostic significance.[1073,1074] Patients who develop sustained ventricular tachycardia or fibrillation spontaneously in the early recovery period are at increased risk of sudden cardiac death following hospital discharge. Control of ventricular arrhythmias in such patients, by medical and (if necessary) surgical therapy, may improve long-term mortality but has not been shown definitely to do this.[1075] When considered together, the combination of clinical factors, radionuclide ejection fraction, and the results of ambulatory monitoring can provide an accurate assessment of prognosis—not surprisingly, the more risk factors present, the greater mortality at any time following AMI (Fig. 39–41).[15,1059,1070]

Use of readily available clinical variables[1076] and exercise electrocardiography is probably sufficient for risk stratification in most patients following AMI. The additional techniques of echocardiography, with or without dipyridamole[1076a] radionuclide angiography, thallium-201 scintigraphy (if necessary with dipyridamole[1077]), and ambulatory electrocardiography should probably be reserved for (1) patients who cannot undergo exercise electrocardiography, (2) those in whom it is not diagnostic, e.g. patients with left bundle branch block, and (3) those who are already thought to be at relatively high risk and in whom a search for specific risks (e.g. ventricular arrhythmia, myocardial dysfunction, or left ventricular thrombus) is appropriate and might lead to specific forms of therapy.[1059,1066,1078]

RECOMMENDATIONS. While there are many different strategies for the overall assessment of prognosis following

TABLE 39–18 HIGH-RISK EXERCISE TEST AND IMAGING VARIABLES AFTER ACUTE MYOCARDIAL INFARCTION

Exercise ECG Stress Testing
 Failure to reach target heart rate (120–130 beats per minute)
 Failure to achieve >3 METS
 Failure to increase systolic blood pressure by ≥10 mm Hg
 Exercise-induced ST-segment depression (>1.0 mm)
 Inducible angina
Exercise Thallium-201 Scintigraphy
 Multiple perfusion defects in more than one vascular region (for example, left anterior descending and circumflex zones)
 Presence of thallium-201 redistribution
 Increased lung thallium-201 uptake
 Exercise-induced LV cavity dilation
Exercise Radionuclide Angiography
 Decrease of >5% in LV ejection fraction from rest to exercise
 Absolute exercise LV ejection fraction <50%
 Exercise-induced increase in end-systolic volume
Rest Radionuclide Imaging
 Resting LV ejection fraction <45%
 Extensive resting thallium-201 or technetium-99m isonitrile persistent defects
 Large areas of technetium pyrophosphate or indium-111 antimyosin antibody uptake
 Large nitrogen-13 ammonia defect with no fluorine-18 2-deoxyglucose uptake

LV = left ventricular.
Adapted from Beller, G. A.: Radionuclide imaging in acute myocardial infarction. In Gersh, B. J., and Rahimtoola, S. H.: Acute myocardial infarction. New York, Elsevier, 1991, p. 192. By permission of the publisher.

results from left ventricular dysfunction, reflecting damaged myocardium as well as provokable ischemia, reflecting myocardium at risk.[1079] The strategy outlined is directed at identifying patients at more than low risk who can expect some benefit from anticipated interventions. Unfortunately, in patients at greatest risk—those with very severe left ventricular dysfunction—most currently available medical and surgical therapies are of little long-term benefit.

The general approach outlined in Figure 39–43 has been recommended by a combined American Heart Association and American College of Cardiology Task Force[1080] to help select patients for invasive investigations. Three different strategies can be employed depending upon physician preferences for an early symptom-limited stress test (Strategy I), combined early submaximal stress testing and later symptom-limited testing (Strategy II), or early discharge without stress testing followed by a relatively early (3-week) symptom-limited exercise test with or without thallium evaluation (Strategy III). Our own approach is as follows: In the first 5 days of hospitalization invasive or noninvasive testing generally is not performed in patients with uncomplicated AMI. However, if ischemia recurs after the first 24 hours, at any time before discharge, and if the patient is a suitable candidate for revascularization, consideration is given to proceeding with early cardiac catheterization and coronary arteriography to define the coronary anatomy and assess left ventricular function. Following AMI, symptoms secondary to left ventricular dysfunction are treated medically unless accompanied by evidence of reversible ischemia (angina, electrocardiographic changes, and/or reversible thallium-201 defects on imaging following an exercise stress test).

Before hospital discharge, patients without evidence of overt pump failure or ischemia and whose overall medical condition permits (e.g., excluding the very elderly or those with serious associated systemic diseases) undergo noninvasive testing. For most patients this means limited exercise stress (treadmill or bicycle) electrocardiography combined with thallium imaging for those with marked resting ECG abnormalities, or radionuclide ventriculography for those in whom an assessment of left ventricular function has not been obtained already (by echocardiography, for example).

Patients at high risk of recurrent MI or death should have cardiac catheterization and coronary arteriography. This includes patients with angina induced at a low level of exercise,

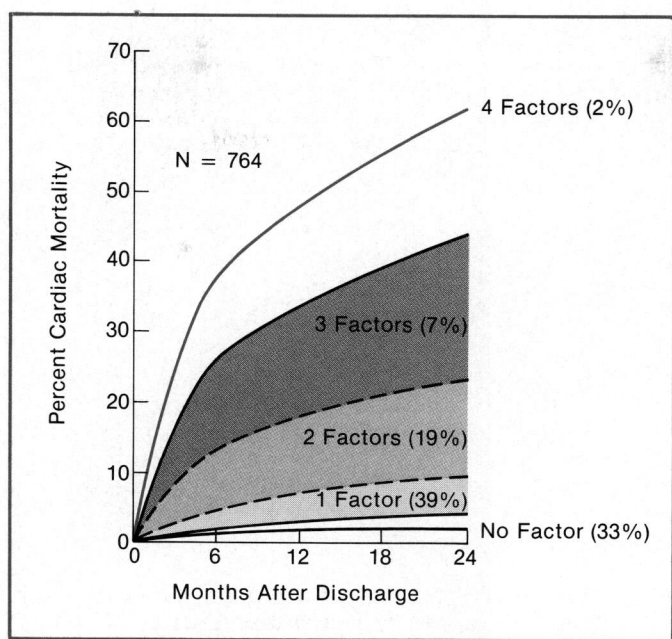

FIGURE 39–41. Mortality curves and zones of risk, according to number of risk factors. Individual risk factors included New York Heart Association functional classes II through IV (not class I) before admission, pulmonary rales, occurrence of 10 or more ventricular ectopic depolarizations per hour, and a radionuclide ejection fraction below 0.40. The variation of risk within each zone reflects the spectrum of relative risk for individual factors as well as the range of multiplicative risks for combinations of two and three factors. The numbers in the parentheses denote the percentage of the population with the specified number of factors. (Reprinted by permission from The Multicenter Post-infarction Research Group: Risk stratification and survival after myocardial infarction. N. Engl. J. Med. 309:331, 1983.)

particularly if associated with marked ECG changes (ST depressions >0.2 mV or serious electrical instability). Others in this category are those with a large reversible defect on thallium-201 imaging and those with an exercise-induced fall in left ventricular ejection fraction (more than 5 to 10 per cent)

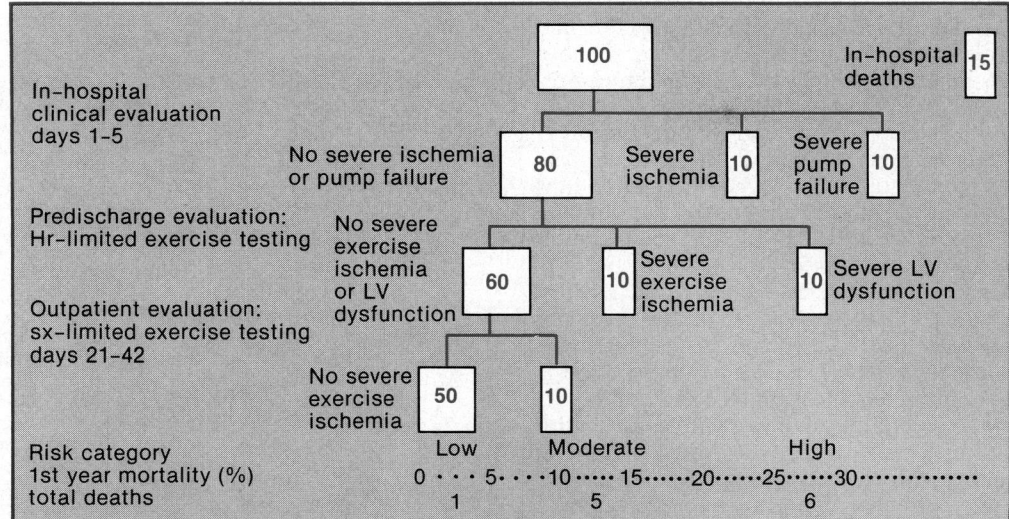

FIGURE 39–42. Prognostic stratification after acute myocardial infarction. The size of each patient subset (numbers in boxes) in the algorithm is approximate and will vary according to the patient population. Stratification of patients into the three main risk categories (low, moderate, and high) is based on the extent of myocardial ischemia (MI) and left ventricular (LV) dysfunction. A variety of clinical observations and tests may be used to detect these abnormalities at various times after acute myocardial infarction. Hr = heart rate, LV = left ventricle, SX = symptom. (Reprinted by permission from DeBusk, R. F., et al.: Identification and treatment of low-risk patients after acute myocardial infarction and coronary-artery bypass graft surgery. N. Engl. J. Med. 314:161, 1986.)

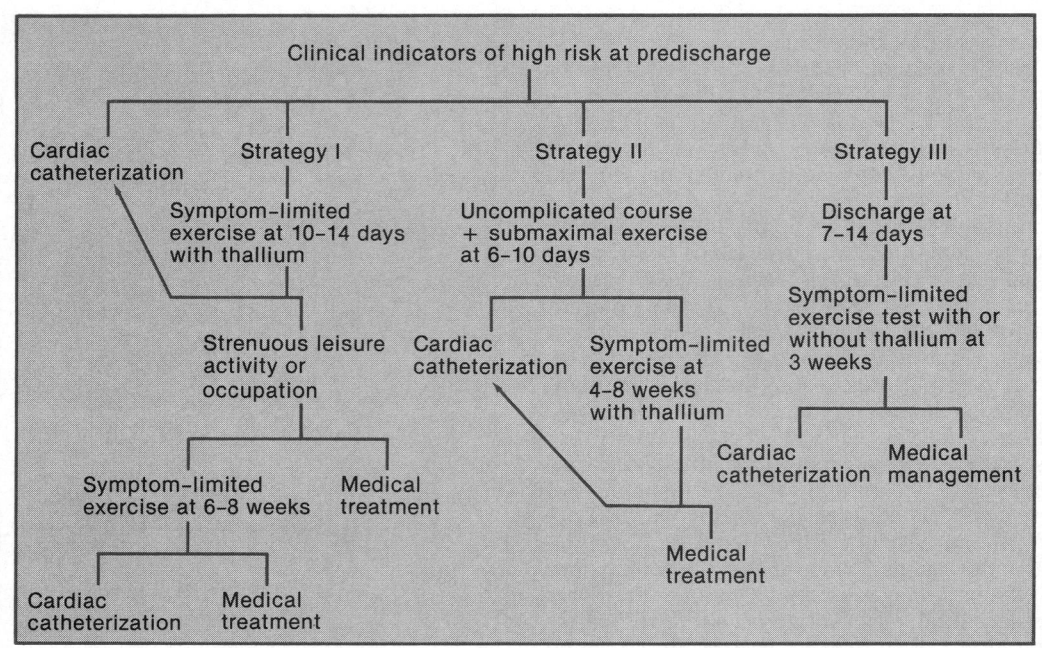

FIGURE 39-43. Strategies for predischarge or early postdischarge exercise evaluation. (From: A report of the American College of Cardiology/American Heart Association Task Force on Assessment, Diagnostic and Therapeutic Cardiovascular Procedures [Subcommittee to Develop Guidelines for the Early Management of Patients with Myocardial Infarction]: Guidelines for the early management of patients with acute myocardial infarction. Reprinted with permission of the American College of Cardiology. J. Am. Coll. Cardiol. 16:249, 1990.)

on radionuclide ventriculography. If exercise testing is negative or only mildly positive, the patient may be discharged.

The predischarge exercise test is useful not only for the detection of ischemia, arrhythmias, or symptoms of left ventricular dysfunction, but it also serves the patient and physician as a useful guide in developing activity recommendations and limitations for the early post-MI period. Patients with ventricular ectopy during hospitalization and those with severe left ventricular dysfunction should generally undergo ambulatory electrocardiographic monitoring before discharge as well. If symptomatic ventricular arrhythmias are detected, we recommend treatment with antiarrhythmic agents, recognizing that the value of this approach has not been established definitively. If high-grade ventricular ectopy occurs without symptoms, invasive electrophysiology evaluation may be indicated (p. 1351).

Four to six weeks after hospital discharge, further noninvasive testing, including maximal (symptom-limited) exercise stress testing, is appropriate for patients who are suitable candidates for revascularization (and have not already undergone such therapy). This would include those patients not already selected for invasive work-up by prior testing, those not suffering from associated debilitating diseases and those not very elderly — in other words, all patients for whom the results of noninvasive testing might lead to a change in the treatment program and for whom that change could affect the prognosis favorably. Catheterization and arteriography should be performed in patients whose noninvasive work-up suggests the presence of remaining jeopardized myocardium following AMI.[1081,1082a] Proceeding with an invasive work-up is therefore a consideration in any patient with a positive exercise stress test in the post-MI period. However, angiography is most strongly indicated in patients who have an exercise-induced fall in blood pressure, signs or symptoms of ischemia at a low workload, more than 0.2 mV of ST-segment depression on exercise electrocardiography, large (or multiple) reversible defects on thallium-201 imaging (or lung accumulation of thallium), or a marked fall in left ventricular ejection fraction with exercise radionuclide ventriculography.

REFERENCES

1. American Heart Association: 1990 Heart Facts. Dallas, American Heart Association National Center, p. 1.
2. National Center for Health Statistics. Utilization of short stay hospitals, United States, 1987. Vital Health Stat. 31:197, 1987.
3. The TIMI Study Group: Comparison of invasive and conservative strategies after treatment with intravenous tissue plasminogen activator in acute myocardial infarction. Results of the Thrombolysis in Myocardial Infarction (TIMI) Phase II Trial. N. Engl. J. Med. 320:618, 1989.
4. Califf, R. M., Topol, E. J., George, B. S., et al.: One-year outcome after therapy with tissue plasminogen activator: Report from the Thrombolysis and Angioplasty in Myocardial Infarction trial. Am. Heart J. 119:777, 1990.
5. Weinstein, M. C., and Stason, W. B.: Cost-effectiveness of interventions to prevent or treat coronary heart disease. Annu. Rev. Public Health 6:41, 1985.
6. Wittels, E. H., Hay, J. W., and Gotto, A. M.: Medical costs of coronary artery disease in the United States. Am. J. Cardiol. 65:432, 1990.
7. Sawitz, E., Showstack, J. A., Chow, J., et al.: The use of in-hospital physician services for acute myocardial infarction. Changes in volume and complexity over time. JAMA 259:2419, 1988.
8. Pell, S., and Fayerweather, W. E.: Trends in the incidence of myocardial infarction and in associated mortality and morbidity in a large employed population, 1957–1983. N. Eng. J. Med. 312:1005, 1985.
9. Pryor, D. B., Harrell, F. E. Jr., Lee, et al.: An improving prognosis over time in medically treated patients with coronary artery disease. Am. J. Cardiol. 52:444, 1983.
10. Elveback, L. R., and Connolly, D. C.: Coronary heart disease in residents of Rochester, Minnesota. V. Prognosis of patients with coronary heart disease based on initial manifestation. Mayo Clin. Proc. 60:305, 1985.
11. Gomez-Martin, O., Folsom, A. R., Kottke, T. E., et al.: Improvement in long-term survival among patients hospitalized with acute myocardial infarction, 1970 to 1980. N. Engl. J. Med. 316:1353, 1987.
12. Goldman, L., and Cook, E. F.: The decline in ischemic heart disease mortality rates. An analysis of the comparative effects of medical interventions and changes in lifestyle. Ann. Intern. Med. 101:825, 1984.
13. Beaglehole, R.: Medical management and the decline in mortality from coronary heart disease. Br. Med. J. 292:33, 1986.
14. Kuller, L. H., Traven, N. D., Rutan, G. H., et al.: Marked decline of coronary heart disease mortality in 35 44-year-old white men in Allegheny County, Pennsylvania. Circulation 80:261, 1989.
15. Ong, L., Green, S., Reiser, P., and Morrison, J.: Early prediction of mortality in patients with acute myocardial infarction: A prospective study of clinical and radionuclide risk factors. Am. J. Cardiol. 57:33, 1986.
16. Yusuf, S., Wittes, J., and Friedman, L.: Overview of results of randomized clinical trials in heart disease. 1. Treatments following myocardial infarction. JAMA 260:2088, 1988.

17. Rude, R. E., Muller, J. E., and Braunwald, E.: Efforts to limit the size of myocardial infarcts. Ann. Intern. Med. 95:736, 1981.
18. Lange, L. G., and Sobel, B. E.: Pharmacological salvage of myocardium. Annu. Rev. Pharmacol. Toxicol. 22:115, 1982.
19. Sobel, B.: Coronary thrombolysis and the new biology. J. Am. Coll. Cardiol. 14:850, 1989.
20. Califf, R. M., and Ohman, E. M.: Thrombolytic therapy: Overview of clinical trials. Coronary Artery Disease 1:23, 1990.

PATHOLOGY

21. Braunwald, E.: The aggressive treatment of acute myocardial infarction. Circulation 71:1087, 1985.
21a. Freifeld, A. G., Schuster, E. H., and Bulkley, B. H.: Nontransmural versus transmural myocardial infarction. Am. J. Med. 75:423, 1983.
22. DeWood, M. A., Stifter, W. F., Simpson, C. S., et al.: Coronary arteriographic findings soon after non-Q wave myocardial infarction. N. Engl. J. Med. 315:417, 1986.
23. Miller, R. D., Burchell, H. B., and Edwards, J. E.: Myocardial infarction with and without acute coronary occlusion: A pathologic study. Arch. Intern. Med. 88:597, 1951.
24. Ambrose, J. A., Tannenbaum, M. A., Alexopoulos, D., et al.: Angiographic progression of coronary artery disease and the development of myocardial infarction. J. Am. Coll. Cardiol. 12:56, 1988.
25. Haupt, H. M., Hutchins, G. M., and Moore, G. W.: Right ventricular infarction: Role of the moderator band artery in determining infarct size. Circulation 67:1268, 1983.
26. Shah, P. K., Maddahi, J., Berman, D. S., et al.: Scintigraphically detected predominant right ventricular dysfunction in acute myocardial infarction: Clinical and hemodynamic correlates and implications for therapy and prognosis. J. Am. Coll. Cardiol. 6:1264, 1985.
27. Forman, M. B., Wilson, B. H., Sheller, J. R., et al.: Right ventricular hypertrophy is an important determinant of right ventricular infarction complicating acute inferior left ventricular infarction. J. Am. Coll. Cardiol. 10:1180, 1987.
28. Kopelman, H. A., Forman, M. B., Wilson, B. H., et al.: Right ventricular myocardial infarction in patients with chronic lung disease: possible role of right ventricular hypertrophy. J. Am. Coll. Cardiol. 5:1302, 1985.
29. Lowe, T. E., and Wartman, W. B.: Myocardial infarction. Br. Heart J. 6:115, 1944.
30. Bloor, C. M.: Cardiac Pathology. Philadelphia, J. B. Lippincott Co., 1978, p. 176.
31. Mallory, G. K., White, P. D., and Salcedo-Salger, J.: The speed of healing of myocardial infarction: A study of the pathological anatomy in seventy-two cases. Am. Heart J. 18:647, 1939.
32. Buja, L. M., and Willerson, J. T.: Clinicopathologic correlates of acute ischemic heart disease syndromes. Am. J. Cardiol. 47:343, 1981.
33. Schlesinger, M. J., and Reiner, L.: Focal myocytolysis of the heart. Am. J. Pathol. 31:443, 1955.
34. Bouchardy, B., and Majno, G.: Histopathology of early myocardial infarcts. Am. J. Physiol. 74:301, 1974.
35. Kloner, R. A., Ganote, C. E., Whalen, D. A., Jr., and Jennings, R. B.: Effect of a transient period of ischemia on myocardial cells: Fine structure during the first few minutes of reflow. Am. J. Pathol. 74:399, 1974.
36. Willerson, J. T., Hillis, L. D., and Buja, L. M.: Ischemic Heart Disease. New York, Raven Press, 1982, 374 pp.
37. Kloner, R. A., Rude, R. E., Carlson, N., et al.: Ultrastructural evidence of microvascular damage and myocardial cell injury after coronary artery occlusion: Which comes first? Circulation 62:945, 1980.
38. Kloner, R. A., DeBoer, L. W. V., Carlson, N., and Braunwald, E.: The effect of verapamil on myocardial ultrastructure during and following release of coronary artery occlusion. Exp. Mol. Pathol. 36:277, 1982.
39. Caulfield, J., and Klionsky, B.: Myocardial ischemia and early infarction. An electron microscopic study. Am. J. Pathol. 35:489, 1959.
40. Jennings, R. B., and Ganote, C. E.: Structural change in myocardium during acute ischemia. Circ. Res. 35(Suppl. 3):156, 1974.
41. Kloner, R. A., Fishbein, M. C., Hare, C. M., and Maroko, P. R.: Early ischemic ultrastructural and histochemical alterations in the myocardium of the rat following coronary artery occlusion. Exp. Mol. Pathol. 30:129, 1979.
42. Baroldi, G.: Different types of myocardial necrosis in coronary heart disease: A pathophysiologic review of their functional significance. Am. Heart J. 89:742, 1975.
43. Hutchins, G. M., and Bulkley, B. H.: Correlation of myocardial contraction band necrosis and vascular patency: A study of coronary artery bypass graft anastomoses at branch points. Lab. Invest. 36:642, 1977.
44. Kloner, R. A., Ellis, S. G., Lange, R., and Braunwald, E.: Studies of experimental coronary artery reperfusion: effects on infarct size, myocardial function, biochemistry, ultrastructure and microvascular damage. Circulation 68(Suppl I):8, 1983.
45. Matsuda, M., Fujiwara, J., Onodera, T., et al.: Quantitative analysis of infarct size, contraction band necrosis, and coagulation necrosis in human autopsied hearts with acute myocardial infarction after treatment with selective intracoronary thrombolysis. Circulation 76:981, 1987.
46. Herrick, J. B.: Clinical features of sudden obstruction of the coronary arteries. JAMA 59:2015, 1912.
47. Blumgart, H. L., Schlesinger, M. J., and Davis, D.: Studies on the relation of the clinical manifestations of angina pectoris, coronary thrombosis, and myocardial infarction to the pathologic findings with particular reference to the significance of the collateral circulation. Am. Heart J. 19:1, 1940.
48. Friedberg, C. K., and Horn, H.: Acute myocardial infarction not due to coronary artery occlusion. JAMA 112:1675, 1939.
49. Roberts, W. C., Potkin, B. N., Solus, D. E., and Reddy, S. G.: Mode of death, frequency of healed and acute myocardial infarction, number of major epicardial coronary arteries severely narrowed by atherosclerotic plaque, and heart weight in fatal atherosclerotic coronary artery disease: analysis of 889 patients studied at necropsy. J. Am. Coll. Cardiol. 15:196, 1990.
50. Betriu, A., Castaner, A., Sanz, G. A., et al.: Angiographic finding 1 month after myocardial infarction: A prospective study of 259 survivors. Circulation 65:1099, 1982.
51. Ellis, S., Alderman E., Cain, K., et al.: Prediction of risk of anterior myocardial infarction by lesion severity and measurement method of stenoses in the left anterior descending coronary distribution: a CASS registry study. J. Am. Coll. Cardiol. 11:908, 1988.
52. Ellis, S., Alderman E. L., Cain, K., et al.: Morphology of left anterior descending coronary territory lesions as a predictor of anterior myocardial infarction: A CASS registry study. J. Am. Coll. Cardiol. 13:1481, 1989.
53. Little, W. C., Constantinescu, M., Applegate, R. J., et al.: Can coronary angiography predict the site of a subsequent myocardial infarction in patients with mild-to-moderate coronary artery disease? Circulation 78:1157, 1988.
54. Rackley, C. E., Russell, R. O., Jr., Mantle, J. A., et al.: Right ventricular infarction and function. Am. Heart J. 101:215, 1981.
55. deFeyter, P. J., van den Brand, M., Serruys, P. W., and Wijns, W.: Early angiography after myocardial infarction: What have we learned? Am. Heart J. 109:194, 1985.
56. DeWood, M. A., Spores, J., and Notske, R., Mouser, L. T., Burroughs, R., Golden, M. S., and Lang, H. T.: Prevalence of total coronary occlusion during the early hours of transmural myocardial infarction. N. Engl. J. Med. 303:897, 1980.
57. Ganz, W., Buchbinder, N., Marcus, H., et al.: Intracoronary thrombolysis in evolving myocardial infarction. Am. Heart J. 101:4, 1981.
58. Ong, L., Reiser, P., Coromilas, J., et al.: Left ventricular function and rapid release of creatine kinase MB in acute myocardial infarction: Evidence for spontaneous reperfusion. N. Engl. J. Med. 309:1, 1983.
59. DeWood, M. A., Notske, R. N., Simpson, C. S., et al.: Prevalence and significance of spontaneous thrombolysis in transmural myocardial infarction. Eur. Heart J. 6:33, 1985.
59a. Pichard, A. D., Ziff, C., Rentrop, P., et al.: Angiographic study of infarct-related coronary artery in the chronic stage of acute myocardial infarction. Am. Heart J. 106:687, 1983.
60. Willerson, J. T., Campbell, W. B., Winniford, M. D., et al.: Conversion from chronic to acute coronary artery disease: Speculation regarding mechanisms. Am. J. Cardiol. 54:1349, 1984.
61. Alpert, J. S.: Coronary vasomotion, coronary thrombosis, myocardial infarction and the camel's back. J. Am. Coll. Cardiol. 5:617, 1985.
62. Muller, J. E., Tofler, G. H., and Stone, P. H.: Circadian variation and triggers of onset of acute cardiovascular disease. Circulation 79:733, 1989.
63. Kragel, A. H., Reddy, S. G., Wittes, J. T., and Roberts, W. C.: Morphometric analysis of the composition of atherosclerotic plaques in the four major epicardial coronary arteries in acute myocardial infarction and in sudden coronary death. Circulation 80:1747, 1989.
64. Roberts, W. C.: Qualitative and quantitative comparison of amounts of narrowing by atherosclerotic plaques in the major epicardial coronary arteries at necropsy in sudden coronary death, transmural acute myocardial infarction, transmural healed myocardial infarction and unstable angina pectoris. Am. J. Cardiol. 64:324, 1989.
65. Levin, D. C., and Fallon, J. T.: Significance of the angiographic morphology of localized coronary stenoses: Histopathologic correlations. Circulation 66:316, 1982.
66. Ridolfi, R. L., and Hutchins, G. M.: Relationship between coronary artery lesions and myocardial infarcts: Ulceration of atherosclerotic plaques precipitating coronary thrombosis. Am. Heart J. 93:468, 1977.
67. Falk, E.: Plaque rupture with severe pre-existing stenosis precipitating thrombosis: Characteristics of coronary atherosclerotic plaque underlying fatal occlusion thrombi. Br. Heart J. 50:127, 1983.
68. Davies, M. J., and Thomas, A. C.: Plaque fissuring—the cause of acute myocardial infarction, sudden ischemic death, and crescendo angina. Br. Heart J. 53:363, 1985.
69. Falk, E.: Morphologic features of unstable atherothrombotic plaques underlying acute coronary syndrome. Am. J. Cardiol. 63:114E, 1989.
70. Wilson, R. F., Holida, M. D., and White, C. W.: Quantitative angiographic morphology of coronary stenoses leading to myocardial infarction or unstable angina. Circulation 73:286, 1986.
71. Mandelkorn, J. B., Wolf, N. M., Singh, S., et al.: Intracoronary thrombus in nontransmural myocardial infarction and in unstable angina pectoris. Am. J. Cardiol. 52:1, 1983.
72. Davies, M. J., and Thomas, A.: Thrombosis and acute coronary-artery lesions in sudden cardiac ischemic death. N. Engl. J. Med. 310:1137, 1984.
73. Fox, K. A. A., Bergmann, S. R., Mathias, C. J., et al.: Scintigraphic detection of coronary artery thrombi in patients with acute myocardial infarction. J. Am. Coll. Cardiol. 4:975, 1984.
74. Trip, M. D., Cats, V. M., Van Capelle, F. J. L., and Vreenken, J.: Platelet hyperactivity and prognosis in survivors of myocardial infarction. N. Engl. J. Med. 322:1549, 1990.

75. Hirsh, P., Campbell, W. B., Willerson, J. D., and Hillis, L. D.: Prostaglandins and ischemic heart disease. Am. J. Med. 71:1009, 1981.

76. Mueller, H. S., Rao, P. S., Greenberg, M. A., et al.: Systemic and transcardiac platelet activity in acute myocardial infarction in man: resistance to prostacyclin. Circulation 72:1336, 1985.

77. Hamstein, A., Wiman, B., De Faire, U., and Blomback, M.: Increased plasma levels of a rapid inhibitor of tissue plasminogen activator in young survivors of myocardial infarction. N. Engl. J. Med. 313:1557, 1985.

78. Wilensky, R. L., Zeller, J. A., Wish, M., and Tulchinsky, M.: Urinary fibrinopeptide A levels in ischemic heart disease. J. Am. Coll. Cardiol. 14:597, 1989.

79. Barold, G.: Pathological anatomy of myocardial infarction. In Wilhelmsen, L., and Hjalmarson, A. (eds.): Acute and Long-Term Medical Management of Myocardial Ischemia. Sweden, Mo Indal, 1978, p. 41.

80. Theroux, P., LaTour, J., Leger-Gautheir, C., and LeLara, J.: Fibrinopeptide A and platelet factor levels in unstable angina pectoris. Circulation 75:156, 1987.

81. Markis, J. E., Malagold, M., Parker, J. A., et al.: Myocardial salvage after intracoronary thrombolysis with streptokinase in acute myocardial infarction. N. Engl. J. Med. 305:777, 1981.

82. Gagnon, R. M., Morissette, M., Bensimon, H., et al.: The role of coronary thrombosis in myocardial infarction: Further evidence shown by intracoronary thrombolysis with streptokinase. Cathet. Cardiovasc. Diagn. 8:393, 1982.

83. Sherman, C. T., Litvack, F., Grundfest, W., et al.: Coronary angioscopy in patients with unstable angina pectoris. N. Engl. J. Med. 315:913, 1986.

84. Conti, C. R.: Myocardial infarction: thoughts about pathogenesis and the role of coronary artery spasm. Am. Heart J. 110:187, 1985.

85. Gertz, S. D., Merin, G., Pasternak, R. C., et al.: Endothelial damage and thrombosis following partial coronary artery constriction. Relevance to the pathogenesis of myocardial infarction. Israel J. Med. Sci. 14:384, 1978.

86. Marzilli, M., Goldstein, S., Trivella, M. G., et al.: Some clinical consideration regarding the relation of coronary vasospasm to coronary atherosclerosis: a hypothetical pathogenesis. Am. J. Cardiol. 45:882, 1980.

87. Cipriano, P. R., Koch, F. H., Rosenthal, S. M. K., et al.: Myocardial infarction in patients with coronary artery spasm demonstrated by angiography. Am. Heart J. 105:542, 1983.

88. Bertrand, M. E., Leblanche, J. M., Tilmant, P. Y., et al.: The provocation of coronary arterial spasm in patients with recent transmural myocardial infarction. Eur. Heart J. 4:532, 1983.

89. Vincent, G. M., Anderson, J. L., and Marshall, H. W.: Coronary spasm producing coronary thrombosis and myocardial infarction. N. Engl. J. Med. 309:220, 1983.

90. Friedrich, T., Lichey, J., Nigam, S., et al.: Follow-up of prostaglandin plasma levels after an acute myocardial infarction. Am. Heart J. 109:222, 1985.

91. Gorlin, R.: Coronary collaterals. In Coronary Artery Disease. Philadelphia, W. B. Saunders Co., 1976, p. 59.

92. Markis, J. E., Brewer, C. C., Alderman, J., et al.: Myocardial infarction without early coronary angiographic evidence of occlusion: The NHLBI thrombolysis in myocardial infarction trial (TIMI). Circulation 72(Suppl. III):56, 1985.

93. Schwartz, H., Leiboff, R. H., Bren, G. B., et al.: Temporal evolution of the human coronary collateral circulation after myocardial infarction. J. Am. Coll. Cardiol. 4:1088, 1984.

94. Freedman, S. B., Dunn, R. F., Bernstein, L., et al.: Influence of coronary collateral blood flow on the development of exertional ischemia and Q wave infarction in patients with severe single-vessel disease. Circulation 71:681, 1985.

95. Nakatsuka, M., Matsuda Y., Ozaki, M., et al.: Coronary collateral vessels in patients with previous myocardial infarction. Clin. Cardiol. 10:791, 1987.

95a. Habib, G. B., Heibig, J., Forman, S., et al.: Influence of coronary collateral vessels on myocardial infarct size in humans. Circulation 83:739, 1991.

96. Rentrop, K. P., Cohen, M., Blanke, H., and Phillips, R. A.: Changes in collateral channel filling immediately after controlled coronary artery occlusion by an angioplasty balloon in human subjects. J. Am. Coll. Cardiol. 5:587, 1985.

97. Tada, M., Yamagishi, M., Kodama, K., et al.: Transient collateral augmentation during coronary arterial spasm associated with ST-segment depression. Circulation 67:693, 1983.

98. Newman, P. E.: The coronary collateral circulation: determinants and functional significance in ischemic heart disease. Am. Heart J. 102:431, 1981.

98a. Topol, E. J., and Ellis, S. G.: Coronary collaterals revisited: Accessory pathway to myocardial preservation during infarction. Circulation 83:1084, 1991.

99. Cheitlin, M. D., McAllister, H. A., and deCastro, C. M.: Myocardial infarction without atherosclerosis. JAMA 231:951, 1975.

100. Forman, M., and Virmani, R. (eds.): Nonatherosclerotic ischemic heart disease. New York, Raven Press, 1989.

101. Dollar, A. L., Pierre-Louis, M.-L., McIntosh, C. L., and Roberts, W. C.: Extensive multifocal myocardial infarcts from cloth emboli after replacement of mitral and aortic valves with cloth-covered, caged-ball prostheses. Am. J. Cardiol. 64:410, 1989.

102. Ackermann, D. M., Hyma, B. A., and Edwards, W. D.: Malignant neoplastic emboli to the coronary arteries. Hum. Pathol. 18:955, 1987.

103. Obarski, T. P., Loop F. D., Cosgrove, D. M., et al.: Frequency of acute myocardial infarction in valve repairs versus valve replacement for pure mitral regurgitation. Am. J. Cardiol. 65:887, 1990.

104. Wei, J. Y., and Bulkley, B. H.: Myocardial infarction before age 36 years in women: predominance of apparent nonatherosclerotic events. Am. Heart J. 104:561, 1982.

105. Porter, J. B., Hunter, J. R., Jick, H., and Stergachis, A.: Oral contraceptives and nonfatal vascular disease. J. Am. Coll. Obstet. Gynecol. 66:1, 1985.

106. Parrillo, J. E., and Fauci, A. S.: Necrotizing vasculitis, coronary angiitis, and the cardiologist. Am. Heart J. 99:547, 1980.

107. Spodick, D. H.: Inflammation and the onset of myocardial infarction. Ann. Intern. Med. 102:699, 1985.

108. Miklozek, C. L., Crumpacker, C. S., Royal, H. D., et al.: Myocarditis presenting as acute myocardial infarction. Am. Heart J. 115:768, 1988.

109. Connolley, J. E., Eldridge, F. L., Calvin, J. W., and Stemmer, E. A.: Proximal coronary artery obstruction. N. Engl. J. Med. 271:213, 1964.

110. Roberts, W. C., MacGregor, R. R., DeBlanc, H. J., et al.: The prepulseless phase of pulseless disease, or pulseless disease with pulses. Am. J. Med. 46:313, 1969.

111. Pick, R. A., Glover, M. U., and Vieweg, W. V. R.: Myocardial infarction in a young woman with isolated coronary arteritis. Chest 82:378, 1982.

112. Kegel, S. M., Dorsey, T. J., Rowen, M., and Taylor, W. F.: Cardiac death in mucocutaneous lymph node syndrome. Am. J. Cardiol. 40:282, 1977.

113. Homcy, C. J., Liberthson, R. R., Fallon, J. T., et al.: Ischemic heart disease in systemic lupus erythematosus in the young patient: Report of six cases. Am. J. Cardiol. 49:481, 1982.

114. Lie, J. L., Failoni, D. D., and Davis, D. C., Jr.: Temporal arteritis with giant cell aortitis, coronary arteritis, and myocardial infarction. Arch. Pathol. Lab. Med. 110:857, 1986.

115. Taymor-Luria, H., Cohn, K., and Pasternak, R. C.: How to identify radiation heart disease. J. Cardiovasc. Med. 8:113, 1983.

116. Joensuu, H.: Acute myocardial infarction after heart irradiation in young patients with Hodgkin's disease. Chest 95:388, 1989.

117. Huang, S., Kumar, G., Steele, H. D., and Parker, J. O.: Cardiac involvement in pseudoxanthoma elasticum. Am. Heart J. 74:680, 1967.

118. James, T. N.: Small arteries of the heart. Circulation 56:2, 1977.

119. Wilkins, C. E., Mathur, V. S., Ty, R. C., and Hall, R. J.: Myocardial infarction associated with cocaine abuse. Texas Heart Inst. J. 12:385, 1985.

120. Rod, J. L., and Zucker, R. P.: Acute myocardial infarction shortly after cocaine inhalation. Am. J. Cardiol. 59:161, 1987.

121. Smith, H. W. B., III, Liberman, H. A., Brody, S. L., et al.: Acute myocardial infarction temporally related to cocaine use. Ann. Intern. Med. 107:13, 1987.

122. Coleman, D. L., Ross, T. F., and Naughton, J. L.: Myocardial ischemia and infarction related to recreational cocaine use. West. J. Med. 136:445, 1982.

123. Pasternack, P. F., Colvin, S. B., and Baumann, F. G.: Cocaine-induced angina pectoris and acute myocardial infarction in patients younger than 40 years. Am. J. Cardiol. 55:847, 1985.

124. Weiss, R. J.: Recurrent myocardial infarction caused by cocaine abuse. Am. Heart J. 111:793, 1986.

125. Schachne, J. S., Roberts, B. H., and Thompson, P. D.: Coronary artery spasm and myocardial infarction associated with cocaine use. N. Engl. J. Med. 310:1665, 1984.

126. Virmani, R., Robinowitz, M., Smialek, J. E., and Smyth, D. F.: Cardiovascular effects of cocaine: an autopsy study of 40 patients. Am. Heart J. 115:1068, 1988.

127. Karch, S. B., and Billingham, M. E.: The pathology and etiology of cocaine-induced heart disease. Arch. Pathol. Lab. Med. 112:225, 1988.

128. Tazelaar, H. D., Karch S. B., Stephens B. G., and Billingham, M. E.: Cocaine and the heart. Hum. Pathol. 18:195, 1987.

129. Ritchie, J. M., and Greene, N. M.: Local anesthetics. In Gilman, A. G. (ed.): The Pharmacologic Basis of Therapeutics. 8th ed. New York, Macmillan, 1990, pp. 311–331.

130. Glover, M. V., Kuber, M. T., Warren, S. E., and Vieweg, W. V. R.: Myocardial infarction before age 36: Risk factor and arteriographic analysis. Am. J. Cardiol. 49:1600, 1982.

131. Ciraulo, D. A., Bresnahan, G. F., Frankel, P. S., et al.: Transmural myocardial infarction with normal coronary angiograms and with single vessel coronary obstruction. Clinical-angiographic features and 5-year follow-up. Chest 83:196, 1983.

132. Pasternak, R. C., Thibault, G. E., Savola, M., et al.: Chest pain with angiographically insignificant coronary arterial obstruction. Clinical presentation and long term follow-up. Am. J. Med. 68:813, 1980.

133. Salem, B. I., Haikal, M., Zambrano, A., et al.: Acute myocardial infarction with "normal" coronary arteries: Clinical and angiographic profiles, with ergonovine testing. Texas Heart Inst. J. 12:1, 1985.

134. Pecora, M. J., Roubin, G. S., Cobbs, B. W., et al.: Presentation and late outcome of myocardial infarction in the absence of angiographically significant coronary artery disease. Am. J. Cardiol. 62:363, 1988.

135. Raymond, R., Lynch, J., Underwood, D., et al.: Myocardial infarction and normal coronary artiography: A 10 year clinical and risk analysis of 74 patients. J. Am. Coll. Cardiol. 11:471, 1988.

136. Rosenblatt, A., and Selzer, A.: The nature and clinical features of myocardial infarction with normal coronary arteriograms. Circulation 55:578, 1977.

137. Eliot, R. S., Baroldi, G., and Leone, A.: Necropsy studies in myocardial infarction with minimal or no coronary luminal reduction due to atherosclerosis. Circulation 49:1127, 1974.

138. Lindsay, J., and Pichard, A.: Acute myocardial infarction with normal coronary arteries. Am. J. Cardiol. 54:902, 1984.

139. Klein, L. S., Simpson, R. J., Stern, R., et al.: Myocardial infarction following administration of sublingual ergotamine. Chest 82:375, 1982.

140. Treasure, C. B., Vita, J. A., Cox, D. A., et al.: Acute myocardial infarction with normal coronary arteries associated with acetylcholine-induced vasoconstriction in the absence of a positive ergonovine test. Am. J. Cardiol. 65:255, 1990.

141. Lange, R. L., Reid, M. S., Tresch, D. D., Keelan, M. H., Bernhard, V. M., and Coolidge, G.: Nonatheromatous ischemic heart disease following withdrawal from chronic industrial nitroglycerin exposure. Circulation 46:666, 1972.

142. Heulpler, F. A., Proudfit, W. L., Razavi, M., et al.: Ergonovine maleate provocative test for coronary arterial spasm. Am. J. Cardiol. 41:631, 1978.

143. Braunwald, E.: Coronary spasm and acute myocardial infarction: New possibility for treatment and prevention. (editorial) N. Engl. J. Med. 299:1301, 1978.

144. Makino, H., and Al-Sadir, J.: Myocardial infarction in patients with mitral valve prolapse and normal coronary arteries. J. Am. Coll. Cardiol. 1:661, 1983.

145. Yeager, Sc. B., and Freed, M. D.: Myocardial infarction as a manifestation of polycythemia in cyanotic heart disease. Am. J. Cardiol. 53:952, 1984.

146. Martin, C. R., Cobb, C., Tatter, D., et al.: Acute myocardial infarction in sickle cell anemia. Arch. Intern. Med. 143:830, 1983.

147. Bergeron, G. A., Goldsmith, R., and Schiller, N. B.: Myocardial infarction, severe, reversible ischemia, and shock following excess thyroid administration in a woman with normal coronary arteries. Arch. Intern. Med. 148:1450, 1988.

148. Carson, P., Oldroyd, K., and Phadke, K.: Myocardial infarction due to amphetamine. Br. Med. J. 294:1525, 1987.

149. Vasan, R. S., Bahl, V. K., Rajani, M.: Myocardial infarction associated with a myocardial bridge. Int. J. Cardiol. 25:240, 1989.

150. Arnett, E. N., and Roberts, W. C.: Acute myocardial infarction and angiographically normal coronary arteries: An unproven combination. Circulation 53:395, 1976.

PATHOPHYSIOLOGY

151. Pfeffer, M. A., Pfeffer, J. M., Fishbein, M. C., et al.: Myocardial infarct size and ventricular function in rats. Circ. Res. 44:503, 1979.

152. Herman, M. V., Heinle, R. A., Klein, M. D., and Gorlin, R.: Localized disorders in myocardial contraction. N. Engl. J. Med. 227:222, 1967.

153. Swan, H. J. C., Forrester, J. S., Diamond, G., et al.: Hemodynamic spectrum of myocardial infarction and cardiogenic shock. Circulation 45:1097, 1972.

154. Forrester, J. S., Wyatt, H. L., Daluz, P. L., et al.: Functional significance of regional ischemic contraction abnormalities. Circulation 54:64, 1976.

155. Serruys, P. W., Simoons, M. L., Suryapranata, H., et al.: Preservation of global and regional left ventricular function after early thrombolysis in acute myocardial infarction. J. Am. Coll. Cardiol. 7:729, 1986.

156. Bourdillon, P. D. V., Broderick, T. M., Williams, E. S., et al.: Early recovery of regional left ventricular function after reperfusion in acute myocardial infarction assessed by serial two-dimensional echocardiography. Am. J. Cardiol. 63:641, 1989.

157. White, H. D., Norris, R. M., Brown, M. A., et al.: Left ventricular end-systolic volume as the major determinant of survival after recovery from myocardial infarction. Circulation 76:44, 1987.

158. Diamond, G., and Forrester, J. S.: Effect of coronary artery disease and acute myocardial infarction on left ventricular compliance in man. Circulation 45:11, 1972.

159. Rackley, C. E., Russell, R. O., Jr., Mantle, J. A., and Rogers, W. J.: Modern approach to the patient with acute myocardial infarction. Curr. Prob. Cardiol. 1:49, 1977.

160. Klein, M. D., Herman, M. V., and Gorlin, R. G.: A hemodynamic study of left ventricular aneurysm. Circulation 35:614, 1967.

161. Wynne, J., Sayres, M., Maddox, D. E., et al.: Regional left ventricular function in acute myocardial infarction: Evaluation with quantitative radionuclide ventriculography. Am. J. Cardiol. 45:203, 1980.

162. Schuster, H. E., and Bulkley, H. B.: Ischemia at a distance after acute myocardial infarction: A cause of early postinfarction angina. Circulation 62:3, 1980.

163. Cortina, A., Ambrose, J. A., Prieto-Granada, J., et al.: Left ventricular function after myocardial infarction: Clinical and angiographic correlations. J. Am. Coll. Cardiol. 5:619, 1985.

164. Paulus, W. J., Grossman, W., Serizawa, T., et al.: Different effects of two types of ischemia on myocardial systolic and diastolic function. Am. J. Physiol. 248:H719, 1985.

165. Aroesty, J. M., McKay, R. G., Heller, G. V., et al.: Simultaneous assessment of left ventricular systolic and diastolic function during pacing-induced ischemia. Circulation 71:889, 1985.

166. McKay, R. G., Pfeffer, M. A., and Pasternak, R. C.: Left ventricular remodeling following myocardial infarction: A corollary to infarct expansion. Circulation 74:693, 1986.

167. Pfeffer, M. A., and Braunwald, E.: Ventricular remodeling after myocardial infarction. Circulation 81:1161, 1990.

167a. Lamas, G. A., and Pfeffer, M. A.: Left ventricular remodeling after acute myocardial infarction: Clinical course and beneficial effects of angiotensin-converting enzyme inhibition. Am. Heart J. 121:1194, 1991.

168. Hutchins, G. M., and Bulkley, B. H.: Infarct expansion versus extension: two different complications of acute myocardial infarction. Am. J. Cardiol. 41:1127, 1978.

169. Roberts, C. S., Maclean D., Maroko, P., and Kloner, R. A.: Early and late remodeling of the left ventricle after acute myocardial infarction. Am. J. Cardiol. 54:407, 1984.

170. Weisman, H. F., Bush, D. E., Mannisi, J. A., et al.: Cellular mechanisms of myocardial infarct expansion. Circulation 78:186, 1988.

171. Pirolo, J. S., Hutchins, G. M., and Moore, G. W.: Infarct expansion: Pathologic analysis of 204 patients with a single myocardial infarct. J. Am. Coll. Cardiol. 7:349, 1986.

172. Meizlish, J. L., Berger, H. J., Plankey, M., et al.: Functional left ventricular aneurysm formation after acute anterior transmural myocardial infarction: Incidence, natural history, and prognostic implications. N. Engl. J. Med. 311:1001, 1984.

173. Schuster, E. H., and Bulkley, B. H.: Expansion of transmural myocardial infarction: a pathophysiologic factor in cardiac rupture. Circulation 60:1532, 1979.

174. Jugdutt, B. I., and Michorowski, B. L.: Role of infarct expansion in rupture of the ventricular septum after acute myocardial infarction. A two-dimensional echocardiographic study. Clin. Cardiol. 10:641, 1987.

175. Warren, S. E., Royal, H. D., Markis, J. E., et al.: Time course of left ventricular dilatation after myocardial infarction: Influence of infarct related artery and success of coronary thrombolysis. J. Am. Coll. Cardiol. 11:12, 1988.

176. Lamas, G. A., and Pfeffer, M. A.: Increased left ventricular volume following myocardial infarction in man. Am. Heart J. 111:30, 1986.

176a. Abernathy, M., Sharpe, N., Smith, H., and Gamble, G.: Echocardiographic prediction of left ventricular volume after myocardial infarction. J. Am. Coll. Cardiol. 17:1527, 1991.

177. Anversa, P., Loud, A. V., Levicky, V., and Guideri, G.: Left ventricular failure induced by myocardial infarction. I. Myocyte hypertrophy. Am. J. Physiol. 248:H876, 1985.

178. Ginzton, L. E., Conant, R., Rodrigues, D. M., and Laks, M. M.: Functional significance of hypertrophy of the noninfarcted myocardium after myocardial infarction in humans. Circulation 80:816, 1989.

178a. Touchstone, D. A., Beller, G. A., Nygaard, T. W., et al.: Effects of successful intravenous reperfusion therapy on regional myocardial function and geometry in humans: A tomographic assessment using two dimensional echocardiography. J. Am. Coll. Cardiol. 13:1506, 1989.

179. Marino, P., Zanolla, L., and Zardini, P: Effect of streptokinase on left ventricular modeling and function after myocardial infarction: The GISSI (Gruppo Italiano per lo Studio della Streptochinasi nell'Infarto Miocardico) Trial. J. Am. Coll. Cardiol. 14:1149, 1989.

180. Lavie, C. J., O'Keefe, J. H., Jr., Chesebro, J. H., et al.: Prevention of late ventricular dilatation after acute myocardial infarction by successful thrombolytic reperfusion. Am. J. Cardiol. 66:31, 1990.

181. Braunwald, E.: Myocardial reperfusion, limitation of infarct size, reduction of left ventricular dysfunction, and improved survival: Should the paradigm be expanded? Circulation 79:441, 1989.

182. Force, T., Kemper, A., Leavitt, M., and Parisi, A. F.: Acute reduction in functional infarct expansion with late coronary reperfusion: Assessment with quantitative two-dimensional echocardiography. J. Am. Coll. Cardiol. 11:192, 1988.

182a. Brown, E. J., Jr., Swinford, R. D., Gadde, P., and Lillis, O.: Acute effects of delayed reperfusion on myocardial infarct shape and left ventricular volume: A potential mechanism of additional benefits from thrombolytic therapy. J. Am. Coll. Cardiol. 17:1641, 1991.

183. Hammerman, H., Kloner, R. A., Hale, S., et al.: Dose-dependent effects of short-term methylprednisolone on myocardial infarct extent, scar formation, and ventricular function. Circulation 68:446, 1983.

184. Jugdutt, B. I., and Basualdo, C. A.: Myocardial infarct expansion during indomethacin or ibuprofen therapy for symptomatic post infarction pericarditis. Influence of other pharmacologic agents during remodeling. Can. J. Cardiol. 5:211, 1989.

185. Flaherty, J. T., Becker, L. C., Weiss, J. L., et al.: Results of a randomized prospective trial of intraaortic balloon counter pulsation and intravenous nitroglycerin in patients with acute myocardial infarction. J. Am. Coll. Cardiol. 6:434, 1985.

186. Jugdutt, B. I., and Warnica, J. W.: Intravenous nitroglycerin therapy to limit myocardial infarct size, expansion, and complications: Effect of timing, dosage, and infarct location. Circulation 78:906, 1988.

187. Pfeffer, J. M., Pfeffer, M. A., and Braunwald, E.: Influence of chronic captopril therapy on the infarcted left ventricle of the rat. Circ. Res. 57:84, 1985.

187a. Litwin, S. E., Litwin, C. M., Raya, T. E., et al.: Contractility and stiffness of noninfarcted myocardium after coronary ligation in rats. Circulation 83:1028, 1991.

188. Biddle, T. L., Yu, P. N., Hodges, M., et al.: Hypoxemia and lung water in acute myocardial infarction. Am. Heart J. 92:692, 1976.

189. Hales, C. A., and Kazemi, H.: Clinical significance of pulmonary function tests. Pulmonary function after uncomplicated myocardial infarction. Chest 72:350, 1977.

190. Hales, C. A., and Kazemi, H.: Small-airways function in myocardial infarction. N. Engl. J. Med. 290:761, 1974.

191. Gray, B. A., Hyde, R. W., Hodges, M., and Yu, P. N.: Alterations in lung volume and pulmonary function in relation to hemodynamic changes in acute myocardial infarction. Circulation 59:551, 1979.

192. Kazemi, H., Parsons, E. F., Valenca, L. M., and Strieder, D. J.: Distribution of pulmonary blood flow after myocardial ischemia and infarction. Circulation 41:1025, 1970.

193. DaLuz, P. L., Cavanilles, J. M., Michaels, S., et al.: Oxygen delivery, anoxic metabolism and hemoglobin-oxygen affinity (P50) in patients with acute myocardial infarction and shock. Am. J. Cardiol. 36:148, 1975.

194. Datey, K. K., and Nanda, N. C.: Hyperglycemia after acute myocardial infarction. N. Engl. J. Med. 276:262, 1976.

195. Vetter, N. J., Adams, W., Strange, R. C., and Oliver, M. F.: Initial metabolic and hormonal response to acute myocardial infarction. Lancet *1*:284, 1974.

196. Bertel, O., Buhler, F. R., Baitsch, G., et al.: Plasma adrenaline and noradrenaline in patients with acute myocardial infarction. Relationship to ventricular arrhythmias in varying severity. Chest *82*:64, 1982.

197. Taylor, S. H., Majid, P. A., Saxton, C., and Sharma, B.: Insulin secretion in heart failure. Am. Heart J. *83*:281, 1972.

198. Ceremuzynski, L.: Hormonal and metabolic reactions evoked by acute myocardial infarction. Circ. Res. *48*:767, 1981.

199. Bellodi, G., Manicardi, V., Malavasi, V., et al.: Hyperglycemia and prognosis of acute myocardial infarction in patients without diabetes mellitus. Am. J. Cardiol. *64*:885, 1989.

200. Jefferson, L. S., Rannels, D. E., Munger, B. L., and Morgan, H. E.: Insulin in the regulation of protein turnover in heart and skeletal muscle. Fed. Proc. *33*:1098, 1974.

201. Opie, L. H.: Metabolism of free fatty acids, glucose, and catecholamines in acute myocardial infarction: Relation to myocardial ischemia and infarct size. Am. J. Cardiol. *36*:938, 1975.

201a. Rouleau, J. L., Dagerais, G-R., Packer, M., et al.: Selective activation of neurohormonal systems in post-infarction left ventricular dysfunction. J. Am. Coll. Cardiol. *17*:21A, 1991.

202. Karlsberg, R. P., Cryer, P. E. and Roberts, R.: Serial plasma catecholamine response early in the course of clinical acute myocardial infarction: relationship to infarct extent and mortality. Am. Heart J. *102*:24, 1981.

203. Wiersinga, W. M., Lie, K. I., and Touber, J. L.: Thyroid hormones in acute myocardial infarction. Clin. Endocrinol. *14*:367, 1981.

204. Kahana, L., Keidar, S., Sheinfeld, M., and Palant, A.: Endogenous cortisol and thyroid hormone levels in patients with acute myocardial infarction. Clin. Endocrinol. *19*:131, 1983.

205. Steele, P., Rainwater, J., and Vogel, R.: Abnormal platelet survival time in men with myocardial infarction and normal coronary arteriogram. Am. J. Cardiol. *41*:60, 1978.

206. Dorn, G. W., II, Liel, N., Trask, J. L., et al.: Increased platelet thromboxane A₂/prostaglandin H₂ receptors in patients with acute myocardial infarction. Circulation *81*:212, 1990.

207. Laursen, B., and Gormsen, J.: Spontaneous fibrinolysis demonstrated by immunological technique. Thromb. Diath. Haemorrh. *17*:42, 1967.

208. Handin, R. I., McDonough, M., and Lesch, M.: Elevation of platelet factor 4 in acute myocardial infarction: Measurement by radioimmunoassay. J. Lab. Clin. Med. *91*:340, 1978.

209. Smitherman, T. C., Milam, M., Woo, J., et al.: Elevated beta thromboglobulin in peripheral venous blood of patients with acute myocardial ischemia: Direct evidence for enhanced platelet reactivity in vivo. Am. J. Cardiol. *48*:395, 1981.

210. Eisenberg, P., Sherman, L. A., Schechtman, K., et al.: Fibrinopeptide A: a marker for acute coronary thrombosis. Circulation *71*:912, 1985.

211. Rapold, H. J., Kuemmerli, H., Weiss, M., et al.: Monitoring of fibrin generation during thrombolytic therapy of acute myocardial infarction with recombinant tissue-type plasminogen activator. Circulation *79*:980, 1989.

212. Eisenberg, P. R., Sherman, L., Rich, M., et al.: Importance of continued activation of thrombin reflected by fibrinopeptide A to the efficacy of thrombolysis. J. Am. Coll. Cardiol. *7*:1255, 1986.

213. Eisenberg, P. R., Miletich, J. E., Sobel, B. E., and Jaffe, A. S.: Differential effects of activation of prothrombin by streptokinase compared with urokinase and tissue-type plasminogen activator (t-PA). Thromb. Res. *50*:707, 1988.

214. Cowan, D. H.: Acquired disorders of platelet function. *In* Colman, R. W., Hirsch, J., Marker, V. J., and Salzman, E. W. (eds.): Hemostasis and Thrombosis: Basic Principles and Clinical Practice. Philadelphia, J. B. Lippincott Co., 1982, pp. 516–524.

215. Marcus, A. J., Safier, L. B., Ullman, H. L., et al.: Inhibition of platelet function in thrombosis. Circulation *72*:698, 1985.

216. Fantone, J. C., and Ward, P. A.: Role of oxygen-derived free radicals and metabolites in leukocyte-dependent inflammatory reactions. Am. J. Physiol. *107*:397, 1982.

217. Engler, R. L., Dahlgren, M. D., Morris, D. D., et al.: Role of leukocytes in response to acute myocardial ischemia and reflow in dogs. Am. J. Physiol. *251*:H314, 1986.

217a. Acute Myocardial Infarction. *In* Fowler, N. O.: Diagnosis of Heart Disease. New York, Springer-Verlag, 1991, pp. 207–238.

218. Hershberg, P. I., Wells, R. E., and McGandy, R. B.: Hematocrit and prognosis in patients with acute myocardial infarction. JAMA *219*:855, 1972.

219. Kok, F. J., Hofman, A., Witteman, J.C.M., et al.: Decreased selenium levels in acute myocardial infarction. JAMA *261*:1161, 1989.

220. Kok, F. J., Schrijver, J., Hofman, A., et al.: Low vitamin B6 status in patients with acute myocardial infarction. Am. J. Cardiol. *63*:513, 1989.

221. Tomoda, H.: Atrial natriuretic peptide in acute myocardial infarction. Am. J. Cardiol. *62*:1122, 1988.

222. Robalino, B. D., Petrella, R. W., Jubran, F. Y., et al.: Atrial natriuretic factor in patients with right ventricular infarction. J. Am. Coll. Cardiol. *15*:546, 1990.

CLINICAL FEATURES

223. Phipps, C.: Contributory causes of coronary thrombosis. JAMA *106*:761, 1936.

224. Tofler, G. H., Stone, P. H., Maclure, M., et al.: Analysis of possible triggers of acute myocardial infarction (The MILIS Study). Am. J. Cardiol. *66*:22, 1990.

225. Smith, C., Sauls, H. C., and Ballew, J.: Coronary occlusion: A clinical study of 100 patients. Ann. Intern. Med. *17*:681, 1942.

226. French, A. J., and Dock, W.: Fatal coronary arteriosclerosis in young soldiers. JAMA *124*:1233, 1944.

227. Fitzhugh, G., and Hamilton, B. E.: Coronary occlusion and fatal angina pectoris: Study of the immediate causes and their prevention. JAMA *100*:475, 1933.

228. Matsuda, M., Matsuda, Y., Ogawa, H., et al.: Angina pectoris before and during acute myocardial infarction: Relation to degree of physical activity. Am. J. Cardiol. *55*:1255, 1985.

229. Knapp, R. B., Topkins, M. J., and Artusio, J. F., Jr.: The cerebrovascular accident and coronary occlusion in anesthesia. JAMA *182*:332, 1962.

230. Levine, H. D.: Acute myocardial infarction following wasp sting. Report of two cases and critical survey of the literature. Am. Heart J. *91*:365, 1976.

231. Maseri, A., L'Abbate, A., Baroldi, G., et al.: Coronary vasospasm as a possible cause of myocardial infarction. A conclusion derived from the study of "preinfarction" angina. N. Engl. J. Med. *299*:1271, 1978.

232. Jenkins, C. D.: Recent evidence supporting psychologic and social risk factors for coronary disease. N. Engl. J. Med. *294*:987, 1976.

233. Rahe, R. H., Romo, M., Bennett, L., and Siltanen, P.: Recent life changes, myocardial infarction, and abrupt coronary death. Arch. Intern. Med. *133*:221, 1974.

234. Norris, N. M.: Myocardial Infarction. New York, Churchill Livingstone, 1982, 322 pp.

235. Muller, J. E., Stone, P. H., Turi, Z. G., et al.: Circadian variation in the frequency of onset of acute myocardial infarction. N. Engl. J. Med. *313*:1315, 1985.

236. Mitler, M. M., and Kripke, D. F.: Circadian variation in myocardial infarction. N. Engl. J. Med. *314*:1187, 1986.

237. Goldberg, R. J., Brady, P., Muller, J. E., et al.: Time of onset of symptoms of acute myocardial infarction. Am. J. Cardiol. *66*:140, 1990.

238. Myocardial infarction community registers: Results of a WHO international collaborative study coordinated by the regional office for Europe. In: Public Health In Europe, No. 5. Copenhagen: Regional Office for Europe (World Health Organization), 1976, pp. 1–230.

239. Muller, J. E., Stone, P. H., Turi, Z. G., et al.: Circadian variation in the frequency of sudden cardiac death. Circulation *75*:131, 1987.

240. Tsementzis, S. A., Gill, J. S., Hitchcock, E. R., et al.: Diurnal variation of activity during the onset of stroke. Neurology *17*:901, 1985.

241. Quyyumi, A. A., Mockus, L., Wright, C., and Fox, K. M.: Morphology of ambulatory ST segment changes in patients with varying severity of coronary artery disease: investigation of the frequency of nocturnal ischemia and coronary spasm. Br. Heart J. *53*:186, 1985.

242. Rocco, M. B., Barry, J., Campbell, S., et al.: Circadian variation of transient myocardial ischemia in patients with coronary artery disease. Circulation *75*:395, 1987.

243. Willich, S. N., Linderer, T., Wegscheider, K., et al.: Increasing morning incidence of myocardial infarction in the ISAM study: absence with prior β-adrenergic blockade. Circulation *80*:853, 1989.

244. Ridker, P. M., Manson, J. E., Buring, J. E., et al.: Circadian variation of acute myocardial infarction and the effect of low-dose aspirin in a randomized trial of physicians. Circulation *82*:897, 1990.

245. Hjalmarson, A., Gilpin, E. A., Nicod, P., et al.: Differing circadian patterns of symptom onset in subgroups of patients with acute myocardial infarction. Circulation *80*:267, 1989.

246. Alonzo, A. M., Simon, A. B., and Feinleib, M.: Prodromata of myocardial infarction and sudden death. Circulation *52*:1056, 1975.

247. Muller, D. W. M., Topol, E. J., Califf, R. M., et al.: Relationship between antecedent angina pectoris and short-term prognosis after thrombolytic therapy for acute myocardial infarction. Am. Heart J. *119*:224, 1990.

248. Harper, R. W., Kennedy, G., DeSanctis, R. W., and Hutter, A. M., Jr.: The incidence and pattern of angina prior to acute myocardial infarction: a study of 577 cases. Am. Heart J. *97*:178, 1979.

249. Rogers, D. E.: Some observations on having a coronary. The Pharos of Alpha Omega Alpha *49*:12, 1986.

250. Baker, P.: Suspected myocardial infarction: Early diagnostic value of analgesic requirements. Br. Med. J. *290*:27, 1985.

251. Malliani, A., and Lombardi, F.: Consideration of the fundamental mechanisms eliciting cardiac pain. Am. Heart J. *103*:575, 1982.

252. Malliani, A.: The elusive link between transient myocardial ischemia and pain. Circulation *73*:201, 1986.

253. Ganz, W., Geft, I., Shah, P. K., et al.: Intravenous streptokinase in evolving acute myocardial infarction. Am. J. Cardiol. *53*:1209, 1984.

254. Ingram, D. A., Fulton, R. A., Portal, R. W., and Aber, C. P.: Vomiting as a diagnostic aid in acute ischemic cardiac pain. Br. Med. J. *281*:636, 1980.

255. Sleight, P.: Cardiac vomiting. Br. Heart J. *46*:5, 1981.

256. Uretsky, B. F., Farquhar, D. S., Borezin, A., and Hood, W. B.: Symptomatic myocardial infarction without chest pain: Prevalence and clinical course. Am. J. Cardiol. *40*:498, 1977.

257. Appels, A., Hoppener, P., and Mulder, P.: A questionnaire to assess premonitory symptoms of myocardial infarction. Int. J. Cardiol. *17*:15, 1987.

258. Margolis, J. R., Kannel, W. B., Feinleib, M., et al.: Clinical features of unrecognized myocardial infarction: Silent and symptomatic. Eighteen year follow-up: The Framingham Study. Am. J. Cardiol. *32*:1, 1973.

259. Yano, K., and MacLean, C. J.: The incidence and prognosis of unrecognized myocardial infarction in the Honolulu, Hawaii, Heart Program. Arch. Intern Med. 149:1528, 1989.

260. Bean, W. B.: Masquerade of myocardial infarction. Lancet 1:1044, 1977.

261. Chadda, K. D., Lichstein, E., Gupta, P. K., and Choy, R.: Bradycardia-hypotension syndrome in acute myocardial infarction. Reappraisal of the overdrive effects of atropine. Am. J. Med. 59:158, 1975.

262. Webb, S. W., Adgey, A. A., and Pantridge, J. F.: Autonomic disturbance at onset of acute myocardial infarction. Br. Med. J. 818:89, 1982.

263. The International Study Group: In-hospital mortality and clinical course of 20,891 patients with suspected acute myocardial infarction randomised between alteplase and streptokinase with or without heparin. Lancet 2:71, 1990.

264. Gadsboll, N., Hoilund-Carlsen, P. F., Nielsen, G. G., et al.: Symptoms and signs of heart failure in patients with myocardial infarction: Reproducibility and relationship to chest x-ray, radionuclide ventriculography and right heart catheterization. Eur. Heart J. 10:1017, 1989.

265. Riley, C. P., Russell, R. O., Jr., and Rackley, C. E.: Left ventricular gallop sound and acute myocardial infarction. Am. Heart J. 86:598, 1973.

266. Case Records of the Massachusetts General Hospital (Case 49-1986). N. Engl. J. Med. 315:1533, 1986.

267. Krainin, F. M., Flessas, A. P., and Spodick, D. H.: Infarction-associated pericarditis. Rarity of diagnostic electrocardiogram. N. Engl. J. Med. 311:1211, 1984.

268. Galve, E., Garcia-Del-Castillo, H., Evangelista, A., et al.: Pericardial effusion in the course of myocardial infarction: Incidence, natural history, and clinical relevance. Circulation 73:294, 1986.

269. Dressler, W.: The post-myocardial infarction syndrome: A report of 44 cases. Arch Intern. Med. 103:28, 1959.

270. Lichstein, E., Arsura, E., Hollander, G., Greengart, A., and Sanders, M.: Current incidence of postmyocardial infarction (Dressler's) syndrome. Am. J. Cardiol. 50:1269, 1982.

271. Thompson, P. L., and Robinson, J. S.: Stroke after acute myocardial infarction: Relation to infarct size. Br. Med. J. 2:457, 1978.

272. Sobel, B. E., and Shell, W. E.: Serum enzyme determinations in the diagnosis and assessment of myocardial infarction. Circulation 45:471, 1972.

273. Lee, T. H., and Goldman, L.: Serum enzyme assays in the diagnosis of acute myocardial infarction. Ann. Intern. Med. 105:221, 1986.

274. Shell, W. E., Kjekshus, J. K., and Sobel, B. E.: Quantitative assessment of the extent of myocardial infarction in the conscious dog by means of analysis of serial changes in serum creatine phosphokinase activity. J. Clin. Invest. 50:2614, 1971.

275. Vasudevan, G., Mercer, D. W., and Varat, M. A.: Lactic dehydrogenase isoenzyme determination in the diagnosis of acute myocardial infarction. Circulation 57:1055, 1978.

276. Weidner, N.: Laboratory diagnosis of acute myocardial infarct. Usefulness of determination of lactate dehydrogenase (LDH)-1 level and the ratio of LDH-1 to total LDH. Arch. Pathol. Lab. Med. 106:375, 1982.

277. Fisher, M. L., Kelemen, M. H., Collins, D., et al.: Routine serum enzyme tests in the diagnosis of acute myocardial infarction. Arch. Intern. Med. 143:1541, 1983.

278. Reis, G. J., Kaufman, H. W., Horowitz, G. L., and Pasternak, R. C.: Usefulness of lactate dehydrogenase and lactate dehydrogenase isoenzymes for diagnosis of acute myocardial infarction. Am. J. Cardiol. 61:754, 1988.

279. Herlitz, J.: Time lapse from estimated onset of acute myocardial infarction to peak serum enzyme activity. Clin. Cardiol. 7:433, 1984.

280. Ong, L., Reiser, P., Coromilas, J., et al.: Left ventricular function and rapid release of creatine kinase MB in acute myocardial infarction: Evidence for spontaneous reperfusion. N. Engl. J. Med. 309:1, 1983.

281. Blanke, H., von Hardenberg, D., Cohen, M., et al.: Patterns of creatine kinase release during acute myocardial infarction after nonsurgical reperfusion: Comparison with conventional treatment and correlation with infarct size. J. Am. Coll. Cardiol. 3:675, 1984.

282. Horie, M., Yasue, H., Omote, S., et al.: A new approach for the enzymatic estimation of infarct size: Serum peak creatine kinase and time to peak creatine kinase activity. Am. J. Cardiol. 57:76, 1986.

283. Roberts, R., and Sobel, B. E.: Isoenzymes of creatine phosphokinase and diagnosis of myocardial infarction. Ann. Intern. Med. 79:741, 1973.

284. Godfrey, N. F., Halter, D. G., Minna, D. A., et al.: Thoracic outlet syndrome mimicking angina pectoris with elevated creatine phosphokinase values. Chest 83:461, 1983.

285. Tsung, S. H.: Several conditions causing elevation of serum CK-BB. Am. J. Clin. Pathol. 75:711, 1981.

286. Apple, F. S., Rogers, M. A., Sherman, W. M., and Ivy, J. L.: Comparison of serum creatine kinase and creatine kinase MB activities post marathon race versus post myocardial infarction. Clin. Chim. Acta 138:111, 1984.

287. Jaffe, A. S., Garfinkel, B. T., Ritter, C. S., and Sobel, B. E.: Plasma MB creatine kinase after vigorous exercise in professional athletes. Am. J. Cardiol. 53:856, 1984.

288. Ingwall, J. S., Kramer, M. F., Fifer, M. A., et al.: The creatine kinase system in normal and diseased human myocardium. N. Engl. J. Med. 313:1050, 1985.

289. Morelli, R. L., Carlson, D. J., Emilson, B., et al.: Serum creatine kinase MM isoenzyme sub-bands after acute myocardial infarction in man. Circulation 67:1283, 1983.

290. Roberts, R.: Reperfusion and the plasma isoforms of creatine kinase isoenzymes: a clinical perspective. J. Am. Coll. Cardiol. 9:464, 1987.

291. Puleo, P. R., Guadagno, P. A., Roberts, R., et al.: Early diagnosis of acute myocardial infarction based on assay for subforms of creatine-kinase-MB. Circulation 82:759, 1990.

292. Puleo, P. R., Perryman, B., Bresser, M. A., et al.: Creatinine kinase isoform analysis in the detection and assessment of thrombolysis in man. Circulation 75:1162, 1987.

293. Abendschein, D., Seacord, L. M., Nohara, R., et al.: Prompt detection of myocardial injury by assay of creatine kinase isoforms in initial plasma samples. Clin. Cardiol. 11:661, 1988.

294. Nohara, R., Myears, D. W., Sobel, B. E., and Abendschein, D. R.: Optimal criteria for rapid detection of myocardial reperfusion by creatinine kinase MM isoforms in the presence of residual high-grade stenosis. J. Am. Coll. Cardiol. 14:1067, 1989.

295. Roberts, R., Gowda, K. S., Ludbrook, P. A., and Sobel, B. E.: Specificity of elevated serum MB creatine phosphokinase activity in the diagnosis of acute myocardial infarction. Am. J. Cardiol. 36:433, 1975.

296. Cooperating investigators from the MILIS study group: Electrocardiographic, enzymatic and scintigraphic criteria of acute myocardial infarction as determined from study of 726 patients (MILIS study). Am. J. Cardiol. 55:1463, 1985.

297. Roberts, R., Sobel, B. E., and Parker, C. W.: Radioimmunoassay for creatine kinase isoenzymes. Science 194:855, 1976.

298. Clyne, C. A., Medeiros, L. J., and Marton, K.: The prognostic significance of immunoradiometric CK-MB assay (IRMA) diagnosis of myocardial infarction in patients with low total CK and elevated MB isoenzymes. Am. Heart J. 118:901, 1989.

299. McGrath, R. B., and Revtyak, G.: Secondary myocardial injuries. Crit. Care Med. 12:1024, 1984.

300. Roberts, R., Sobel, B. E., and Ludbrook, P. A.: Determination of the origin of elevated plasma CPK after cardiac catheterization. Cathet. Cardiovasc. Diagn. 2:239, 1976.

301. Klein, M. S., Coleman, R. E., Weldon, C. S., et al.: Concordance of electrocardiographic and scintigraphic criteria of myocardial injury after cardiac surgery. J. Thorac. Cardiovasc. Surg. 71:934, 1976.

302. Smith, J. L., Ambos, D., Gold, H. K., et al.: Enzymatic estimation of myocardial infarct size when early creatinine kinase values are not available. Am. J. Cardiol. 51:1294, 1983.

303. Hong, R. A., Licht, J. D., Wei, J. Y., et al.: Elevated CK-MB with normal total creatine kinase in suspected myocardial infarction: Associated clinical findings and early prognosis. Am. Heart J. 111:1041, 1986.

304. Heyndrickx, G. R., Amano, J., Kenna, T., et al.: Creatine kinase release not associated with myocardial necrosis after short periods of coronary artery occlusion in conscious baboons. J. Am. Coll. Cardiol. 6:1299, 1985.

305. Yusuf, S., Collins, R., Lin, L., et al.: Significance of elevated MB isoenzyme with normal creatine kinase in acute myocardial infarction. Am. J. Cardiol. 59:245, 1987.

306. Grande, P., Hansen, B. F., Christiansen, C., and Naestoft, J.: Estimation of acute myocardial infarct size in man by serum CK-MB measurements. Circulation 65:756, 1982.

307. Hori, M., Inoue, M., Fukui, S., et al.: Correlation of ejection fraction and infarct size estimated from the total CK released in patients with acute myocardial infarction. Br. Heart J. 41:433, 1979.

308. Geltman, E. M., Ehsani, A. A., Campbell, M. K., et al.: The influence of location and extent of myocardial infarction on long-term ventricular dysrhythmia and mortality. Circulation 60:805, 1979.

309. Tamaki, S., Murakami, T., Kadota, K., et al.: Effects of coronary artery reperfusion on relation between creatine kinase-MB release and infarct size estimated by myocardial emission tomography with thallium-201 in man. J. Am. Coll. Cardiol. 2:1031, 1983.

310. Goldberger, E., Alesio, J., and Woll, F.: The significance of hyperglycemia in myocardial infarction. N.Y. State Med. J. 45:391, 1945.

311. Tan, M. H., Wilmshurst, E. G., Gleason, R. E., and Soeldner, J. S.: Effect of posture on serum lipids. N. Engl. J. Med. 289:416, 1973.

312. Gore, J. M., Goldberg, R. J., Matsumoto, A. S., et al.: Validity of serum total cholesterol level obtained within 24 hours of acute myocardial infarction. Am. J. Cardiol. 54:722, 1984.

313. Ryder, R.E.J., Hayes, T. M., Mulligan, I. P., et al.: How soon after myocardial infarction should plasma lipid values be assessed? Br. Med. J. 289:1651, 1984.

314. Ronnemaa, T., Viikari, J., Irjala, K., and Peltola, O.: Marked decrease in serum HDL cholesterol level during acute myocardial infarction. Acta Med. Scand. 207:161, 1980.

315. Isakov, A., Shapira, I., Burke, M., and Almog, C.: Serum myoglobin levels in patients with ischemic myocardial insult. Arch. Intern. Med. 148:1762, 1988.

316. Kagen, L., Scheidt, S., and Butt, A.: Serum myoglobin in myocardial infarction: The "staccato phenomenon." Is acute myocardial infarction in man an intermittent event? Am. J. Med. 62:86, 1977.

317. Ellis, A. K., Little, T., Masud, A.R.Z., et al.: Early noninvasive detection of successful reperfusion in patients with acute myocardial infarction. Circulation 77:1352, 1988.

318. Eastham, R. D., and Morgan, E. H.: Plasma-fibrinogen levels in coronary-artery disease. Lancet 2:1196, 1963.

319. Savage, R. M., Wagner, G. S., Ideker, R. E., et al.: Correlation of postmortem anatomic findings with electrocardiographic changes in patients with myocardial infarction. Circulation 55:279, 1977.

320. Cooksey, J. D., Dunn, M., and Massie, E.: Clinical Vectorcardiography and Electrocardiography. 2nd ed. Chicago, Year Book Medical Publishers, 1977, p. 361.

321. Seyal, M. S., and Swiryn, S.: True posterior myocardial infarction. Arch. Intern. Med. 143:983, 1983.

322. Jaarsma, W., Visser, C. A., Van Eenige, J., and Roos, J. P.: Left ventricular

wall motion with and without Q-wave disappearance after acute myocardial infarction. Am. J. Cardiol. 59:516, 1987.

323. Coll, S., Betriu, A., De Flores, T., et al.: Significance of Q-wave regression after transmural acute myocardial infarction. Am. J. Cardiol. 61:739, 1988.

324. Haiat, R., Worthington, F. X., Castellanos, A., and Lemberg, L.: Unusual normalization of the electrocardiogram on the 6th day of myocardial infarction. J. Electrocardiol. 4:363, 1971.

325. Goldberger, A. L.: Myocardial Infarction. St. Louis, C. V. Mosby, 1984, pp. 29–146.

326. Phibbs, B.: "Transmural" versus "subendocardial" myocardial infarction: An electrocardiographic myth. J. Am. Coll. Cardiol. 1:561, 1983.

327. Levine, H. D.: Subendocardial infarction in retrospect: Pathologic, cardiographic, and ancillary features. Circulation 72:790, 1985.

328. Spodick, D. H.: Q-wave infarction versus S-T infarction: Nonspecificity of electrocardiographic criteria for differentiating transmural and nontransmural lesions. Am. J. Cardiol. 51:913, 1983.

329. Zema, M. J.: Q wave, S-T segment, and T wave myocardial infarction. Am. J. Med. 78:391, 1985.

330. Goldberg, R. J., Gore, J. M., Alpert, J. S., and Dalen, J. E.: Non-Q wave myocardial infarction: Recent changes in occurrence and prognosis—a community-wide perspective. Am. Heart J. 113:273, 1987.

331. Schuster, E. H., and Bulkley, B. H.: Early postinfarction angina. Ischemia at a distance and ischemia in the infarct zone. N. Engl. J. Med. 305:1101, 1981.

332. Ferguson, D. W., Pandian, N., Kioschos, J. M., et al.: Angiographic evidence that reciprocal ST-segment depression during acute myocardial infarction does not indicate remote ischemia: Analysis of 23 patients. Am. J. Cardiol. 53:55, 1984.

333. Mukharji, J., Murray, S., Lewis, S. E., et al.: Is anterior ST depression with acute transmural inferior infarction due to posterior infarction? J. Am. Coll. Cardiol. 4:28, 1984.

334. Mirvis, D. M.: Physiologic bases for anterior ST segment depression in patients with acute inferior wall myocardial infarction. Am. Heart J. 116:1308, 1988.

335. Little, W. C., Rogers, E. W., and Sodums, M. T.: Mechanism of anterior ST segment depression during acute inferior myocardial infarction. Ann. Intern. Med. 100:26, 1984.

336. Lew, A. S., Weiss, A. T., Shah, P. K., et al.: Precordial ST segment depression during acute inferior myocardial infarction: Early thallium-201 scintigraphic evidence of adjacent posterolateral or inferoseptal involvement. J. Am. Coll. Cardiol. 5:203, 1985.

337. Chou, T., Van Der Bel-Kahn, J., Allen, J., et al.: Electrocardiographic diagnosis of right ventricular infarction. Am. J. Med. 70:1175, 1981.

338. Lopez-Sendon, J., Coma-Canella, I., Alcasena, S., et al.: Electrocardiographic findings in acute right ventricular infarction: Sensitivity and specificity of electrocardiographic alterations in right precordial leads V4R, V3R, V1, V2, and V3. J. Am. Coll. Cardiol. 6:1273, 1985.

339. Braat, S. H., Brugada, P., DeZwaan, C., et al.: Value of electrocardiogram in diagnosing right ventricular involvement in patients with an acute inferior wall myocardial infarction. Br. Heart J. 49:368, 1983.

340. Robalino, B. D., Whitlow, P. L., Underwood, D. A., and Salcedo, E. E.: Electrocardiographic manifestations of right ventricular infarction. Am. Heart J. 118:138, 1989.

341. Geft, I. L., Shah, P. K., Rodriguez, L., et al.: ST elevations in leads V1 to V5 may be caused by right coronary artery occlusion and acute right ventricular infarction. Am. J. Cardiol. 53:991, 1984.

342. Lew, A. S., Maddahi, J., Shah, P. K., et al.: Factors that determine the direction and magnitude of precordial ST-segment deviations during inferior wall acute myocardial infarction. Am. J. Cardiol. 55:883, 1985.

343. Lieu, C. K., Greenspan, G., and Piccirillo, R. T.: Atrial infarction of the heart. Circulation 23:331, 1961.

344. Silvertssen, E., Hoel, B., Bay, G., and Jorgensen, L.: Electrocardiographic atrial complex and acute atrial myocardial infarction. Am. J. Cardiol. 31:450, 1973.

345. Timmis, A. D., Fowler, M. D., Burwood, R. J., et al.: Pulmonary oedema without critical increase in left atrial pressure in acute myocardial infarction. Br. Med. J. 283:636, 1981.

346. Field, B. J., Russell, R. O., Jr., Moraski, R. E., et al.: Left ventricular size and function and heart size in the year following myocardial infarction. Circulation 50:331, 1974.

347. Brattler, A., Karliner, J. S., Higgins, C. B., et al.: The initial chest x-ray in acute myocardial infarction. Prediction of early and late mortality and survival. Circulation 61:1004, 1980.

348. Foster, C. J., Sekiya, T., Love, H. G., et al.: Identification of intracardiac thrombus: comparison of computed tomography and cross-sectional echocardiography. Br. J. Radiol. 60:327, 1987.

349. Rumberger, J. A., and Lipton, M. J.: Ultrafast cardiac CT scanning. Cardiol. Clin. 7:713, 1989.

350. Gibson, R. S., Taylor, G. J. Watson, D. D., et al.: Predicting the extent and location of coronary artery disease during the early postinfarction period by quantitative thallium-201 scintigraphy. Am. J. Cardiol. 47:1010, 1981.

351. Khaw, B. A., Gold, H. K., Yasuda, T., et al.: Scintigraphic quantification of myocardial necrosis in patients after intravenous injection of myosin-specific antibody. Circulation 74:501, 1986.

352. Hashimoto, T., Kambara, H., Fudo, T., et al.: Non-Q wave versus Q wave myocardial infarction: regional myocardial metabolism and blood flow assessed by positron emission tomography. J. Am. Coll. Cardiol. 12:88, 1988.

353. Johnson, L. L., Seldin, D. W., Becker, L. C., et al.: Antimyosin imaging in

354. Becker, L.: Technetium-99m isonitrile tomography in patients with acute myocardial infarction: measurement of myocardial salvage by thrombolysis. J. Am. Coll. Cardiol. 15:315, 1990.

355. Gibbons, R. J., Verani, M. S., Behrenbeck, T., et al.: Feasibility of tomographic 99mTc-hexakis-2-methoxy-2-methylopropyl, isonitrile imaging for the assessment of myocardial area at risk and the effect of treatment in acute myocardial infarction. Circulation 80:1277, 1989.

355a. Christian, T. F., Clements, I. P., and Gibbons, R. J.: Noninvasive identification of myocardium at risk in patients with acute myocardial infarction and nondiagnostic electrocardiograms with technetium-99m-Sestamibi. Circulation 83:1615, 1991.

356. Santoro, G. M., Bisi, G., Sciagra, R., et al.: Single photon emission computed tomography with technetium-99m hexakis 2-methoxyisobutyl isonitrile in acute myocardial infarction before and after thrombolytic treatment: Assessment of salvaged myocardium and prediction of late functional recovery. J. Am. Coll. Cardiol. 15:301, 1990.

357. Johnston, D. L., Thompson, R. C., Liu, P., et al.: Magnetic resonance imaging during acute myocardial infarction. Am. J. Cardiol. 57:1059, 1986.

358. Johns, J. A., Leavitt, M. B., Newell, J. B., et al.: Quantitation of acute myocardial infarct size by nuclear magnetic resonance imaging. J. Am. Coll. Cardiol. 15:143, 1990.

359. Johnston, D. L., Mulvagh, S. L., Cashion, R. W., et al.: Nuclear magnetic resonance imaging of acute myocardial infarction within 24 hours of chest pain onset. Am. J. Cardiol. 64:172, 1989.

360. Ratner, A. V., Okada, R. D., Newell, J. B., and Pohost, G. M.: The relationship between proton nuclear magnetic resonance relaxation parameters and myocardial perfusion with acute coronary arterial occlusion and reperfusion. Circulation 71:823, 1985.

361. Reeves, R. C., Evanochko, W. T., and Pohost, G. M.: Potential approaches to evaluating the cardiovascular system using NMR. Prog. Cardiovasc. Dis. 29:53, 1986.

362. Wisenberg, G., Finnie, K. J., Jablonsky, G., et al.: Nuclear magnetic resonance and radionuclide angiographic assessment of acute myocardial infarction in a randomized trial of intravenous streptokinase. Am. J. Cardiol. 62:1011, 1988.

363. Kloner, R. A., and Parisi, A. F.: Acute myocardial diagnostic and prognostic applications of two-dimensional echocardiography. Circulation 75:521, 1987.

364. Lindvall, K., Erhardt, L., and Sjögren, A.: Serial M-mode echocardiographic mapping in myocardial infarction: A quantitative evaluation of left ventricular wall motion abnormalities. Clin. Cardiol. 6:220, 1983.

365. Corya, B. C., Rasmussen, S., Knoebel, S. B., and Feigenbaum, H.: Echocardiography in acute myocardial infarction. Am. J. Cardiol. 36:1, 1975.

366. Feigenbaum, H., Corya, B. C., Dillon, J. C., et al.: Role of echocardiography in patients with coronary artery disease. Am. J. Cardiol. 37:775, 1976.

367. Peels, C. H., Visser, C. A., Funke Kupper, A. J., et al.: Usefulness of two-dimensional echocardiography for immediate detection of myocardial ischemia in the emergency room. Am. J. Cardiol. 65:687, 1990.

368. Mann, D. L., Gillam, L. D., and Weyman, A. E.: Cross-sectional echocardiographic assessment of regional left ventricular performance and myocardial perfusion. Prog. Cardiovasc. Dis. 23:1, 1986.

369. Oh, J. K., Miller, F. A., Shub, C., Reeder, G. S., and Tajik, A. J.: Evaluation of acute chest pain syndromes by two-dimensional echocardiography. Its potential application in the selection of patients for acute reperfusion therapy. May Clin. Proc. 62:59, 1987.

370. Berning, J., and Steensgaard-Hansen, F.: Early estimation of risk by echocardiographic determination of wall motion index in an unselected population with acute myocardial infarction. Am. J. Cardiol. 65:567, 1990.

371. Sabia, P., Afrookteh, A., Touchstone, D. A., et al.: Superiority of regional dyssynergy in the emergency room diagnosis of acute myocardial infarction: A prospective study utilizing two-dimensional echocardiography. Circulation (in press).

372. Parisi, A. F., Nieminen, M., O'Boyle, J. E., et al.: Enhanced detection of the evolution of tissue changes after acute myocardial infarction using color-coded two-dimensional echocardiography. Circulation 66:764, 1982.

373. Otto, C. M., Stratton, J. R., Maynard, C., et al.: Echocardiographic evaluation of segmental wall motion early and late after thrombolytic therapy in acute myocardial infarction: The Western Washington Tissue Plasminogen Activator Emergency Room Trial. Am. J. Cardiol. 65:132, 1990.

374. Weiss, J. L., Bulkley, B. H., Hutchins, G. M., and Mason, S. J.: Two-dimensional echocardiographic recognition of myocardial injury in man: Comparison with postmortem studies. Circulation 63:401, 1981.

375. Barrett, J. J., Charuzi, Y., and Corday, E.: Ventricular aneurysm: Cross sectional echocardiographic approach. Am. J. Cardiol. 46:1133, 1980.

376. Catherwood, E., Mintz, G. S., Kotler, M. N., et al.: Two-dimensional echocardiographic recognition of left ventricular pseudoaneurysm. Circulation 62:294, 1980.

377. Donaldson, R. M., and Ballester, M.: Echocardiographic visualization of the anatomic causes of mitral regurgitation resulting from myocardial infarction. Postgrad. Med. J. 58:257, 1982.

378. Spirito, P., Bellotti, P., Chiarella, F., et al.: Prognostic significance and natural history of left ventricular thrombi in patients with acute ante-

rior myocardial infarction: A two-dimensional echocardiographic study. Circulation 72:774, 1985.

379. Nishimura, R. A., Miller, F. A., Callahan, M. J., et al.: Doppler echocardiography: theory, instrumentation, technique, and application. Mayo Clin. Proc. 60:321, 1985.

380. Smyllie, J. H., Sutherland, G. R., Geuskens, R., et al.: Doppler color flow mapping in the diagnosis of ventricular septal rupture and acute mitral regurgitation after myocardial infarction. J. Am. Coll. Cardiol. 15:1449, 1990.

381. Harrison, M. R., MacPhail, B., Gurley, J. C., et al.: Usefulness of color Doppler flow imaging to distinguish ventricular septal defect from acute mitral regurgitation complicating acute myocardial infarction. Am. J. Cardiol. 64:697, 1989.

382. Chandrantna, P. A., Nanna, M., McKay, C., et al.: Determination of cardiac output by transcutaneous continuous-wave ultrasonic Doppler computer. Am. J. Cardiol. 53:234, 1984.

383. Maroko, P. R., Libby, P., Covell, J. W., et al.: Precordial ST-T segment elevation mapping: an atraumatic method for assessing alterations in the extent of myocardial ischemic injury. Am. J. Cardiol. 29:227, 1972.

384. Lekven, J., Chatterjee, K., Tyberg, J. V., and Parmley, W. W.: Influence of left ventricular dimensions on endocardial and epicardial QRS amplitude and ST segment elevations during acute myocardial ischemia. Circulation 61:679, 1980.

385. Ideker, R. E., Wagner, G. S., Ruth, W. K., et al.: Evaluation of a QRS scoring system for estimating myocardial infarct size. II. Correlation with quantitative anatomic findings for anterior infarcts. Am. J. Cardiol. 49:1604, 1982.

386. Roark, S. F., Ideker, R. E., Wagner, G. S., et al.: Evaluation of a QRS scoring system for estimating myocardial infarct size. III. Correlation with quantitative anatomic findings for inferior infarcts. Am. J. Cardiol. 51:382, 1983.

387. Cowan, M. J., Bruce, R. A., and Reichenbach, D. D.: Validation of a computerized QRS criterion for estimating myocardial infarction size and correlation with quantitative morphologic measurements. Am. J. Cardiol. 57:60, 1986.

388. Roberts, R.: Enzymatic estimation of infarct size. Thrombolysis induced its demise: will it now rekindle its renaissance? Circulation 81:707, 1990.

389. Morrison, J., Coromilas, J., Munsey, D., et al.: Correlation of radionuclide estimates of myocardial infarction size and release of creatine kinase-MB in man. Circulation 62:277, 1980.

390. Hackel, D. B., Reimer, K. A., Ideker, R. E., et al.: Comparison of enzymatic and anatomic estimates of myocardial infarct size in man. Circulation 70:824, 1984.

391. Armstrong, W. F., West, S. R., Dillon, J. C., and Feigenbaum, H.: Assessment of location and size of myocardial infarction with contrast-enhanced echocardiography. II. Application of digital imaging techniques. J. Am. Coll. Cardiol. 4:141, 1984.

392. Force, T., Kemper, A., Perkins, L., et al.: Overestimation of infarct size by quantitative two-dimensional echocardiography: The role of tethering and of analytic procedures. Circulation 63:1360, 1986.

393. Corbett, J. R., Lewis, S. E., Wolfe, C. L., et al.: Measurement of myocardial infarct size by technetium pyrophosphate single-photon tomography. Am. J. Cardiol. 54:1231, 1984.

394. Volpini, M., Giubbini, R., Gei, P., et al.: Diagnosis of acute myocardial infarction by indium-111 antimyosin antibodies and correlation with the traditional techniques for the evaluation of extent and localization. Am. J. Cardiol. 63:7, 1989.

395. Grande, P., Hindman, N. B., Saunamaki, K., et al.: A comprehensive estimation of acute myocardial infarct size using enzymatic, electrocardiographic and mechanical methods. Am. J. Cardiol. 59:1239, 1987.

MANAGEMENT

395a. Wenger, N. K., Hellerstein, H. K., Blackburn, H., and Castranova, S. J.: Physician practice in the management of patients with uncomplicated myocardial infarction: Changes in the past decade. Circulation 65:421, 1982.

396. Ericcson, C-G., Lindvall, B., Olsson, G., et al.: Trends in coronary care. A retrospective study of patients with myocardial infarction treated in coronary care units. Acta Med. Scand. 227:507, 1988.

397. Gore, J. M., Goldberg, R. J., and Alpert, J. S.: The increased use of diagnostic procedures in patients with acute myocardial infarction. A community-wide perspective. Arch. Intern. Med. 147:1729, 1987.

398. Antman, E. M., and Rutherford, J. D.: Coronary Care Medicine. Boston, Martinus Nijhoff, 1986, p. 20.

398a. Gibler, W. B., Kereiakes, D. J., Dean, E. N., et al.: Prehospital diagnosis and treatment of acute myocardial infarction: A North-South perspective. Am. Heart J. 121:1, 1991.

399. Herlitz, J., Hartford, M., Blohm, M., et al.: Effect of a median campaign on delay times and ambulance use in suspended acute myocardial infarction. Am. J. Cardiol. 64:90, 1989.

400. Maynard, C., Althouse, R., Olsufka, M., et al.: Early versus late hospital arrival for acute myocardial infarction in the Western Washington Thrombolytic Therapy Trials. Am. J. Cardiol. 63:1296, 1989.

401. British Heart Foundation Working Group: Role of the general practitioner in managing patients with myocardial infarction: impact of thrombolytic treatment. Br. Med. J. 299:555, 1989.

402. Pantridge, J. R., and Geddes, J. S.: Diseases of the cardiovascular system. Management of acute myocardial infarction. Br. Med. J. 2:168, 1976.

403. Dean, N. C., Haug, P. J., and Hawker, P. J.: Effect of mobile paramedic units on outcome in patients with myocardial infarction. Ann. Emerg. Med. 17:1034, 1988.

404. Dillon, J. C., Vasu, C. M., Berman, D. S., et al.: Thirteenth Bethesda Conference—Task Force III: Diagnostic Procedures. Am. J. Cardiol. 50:377, 1982.

405. Cobb, L. A., Baum, R. S., Alvarez, H., III, and Schaffer, W. A.: Resuscitation from out-of-hospital ventricular fibrillation: 4 years' follow-up. Circulation 51(Suppl. III):223, 1975.

406. Lewis, R. P., Lanese, R. R., Stang, J. M., et al.: Reduction of mortality from prehospital myocardial infarction by prudent patient activation of mobile coronary care system. Am. Heart J. 103:123, 1982.

407. Crampton, R. S., Aldrich, F. R., Gascho, J. A., et al.: Reduction of prehospital, ambulance and community coronary death rates by the community-wide emergency cardiac care system. Am. J. Med. 58:151, 1975.

408. Capone, R. J., Visco, J., Curwen, E., and VanEvery, S.: The effect of early prehospital transtelephonic coronary intervention on morbidity and mortality: experience with 284 postmyocardial infarction patients in a pilot program. Am. Heart J. 107:1153, 1984.

409. Pressley, J. C., Wilson, B. H., Severance, H. W., et al.: Basic emergency medical care of patients with acute myocardial infarction: Initial prehospital characteristics and in-hospital complications. J. Am. Coll. Cardiol. 4:487, 1984.

410. Gotsman, M. S.: Prehospital thrombolysis in acute myocardial infarction: is it feasible, practical and safe? Intensive Care World 5:9, 1988.

411. Califf, R. M., and Harrelson-Woodlief, S. L.: At home thrombolysis. J. Am. Coll. Cardiol. 15:937, 1990.

412. Weiss, A. T., Fine, D. G., Applebaum, D., et al.: Prehospital coronary thrombolysis. A new strategy in acute myocardial infarction. Chest 92:124, 1987.

413. The Thrombolysis Early in Acute Heart Attack Trial Study Group: Very early thrombolytic therapy in suspected acute myocardial infarction. Am. J. Cardiol. 65:401, 1990.

414. Roth, A., Barbash, G. I., Hod, H., et al.: Should thrombolytic therapy be administered in the mobile intensive care unit in patients with evolving myocardial infarction? A pilot study. J. Am. Coll. Cardiol. 15:932, 1990.

415. Castaigne, A. D., Herve, C., Duval-Moulin, A-M., et al.: Prehospital use of APSAC: results of a placebo-controlled study. Am. J. Cardiol. 64:30A, 1989.

416. Weaver, W. D., Eisenberg, M. S., Martin, J. S., et al.: Myocardial Infarction Triage and Intervention Project—Phase I: patient characteristics and feasibility of prehospital initiation of thrombolytic therapy. J. Am. Coll. Cardiol. 15:925, 1990.

417. Lee, T. H., and Goldman, L.: The coronary care unit turns 25: Historical trends and future directions. Ann. Intern. Med. 108:887, 1988.

418. Morris, A. L., Nernberg, V., Roos, N. P., et al.: Acute myocardial infarction: Survey of urban and rural hospital mortality. Am. Heart J. 105:44, 1983.

419. Hill, J. D., Hampton, J. R., and Mitchell, J.R.A.: A randomized trial of home-versus-hospital management for patients with suspected myocardial infarction. Lancet 1:837, 1978.

420. Fesmire, F. M., Percy, R. F., Wears, R. L., and MacMath, T. L.: Risk stratification according to the initial electrocardiogram in patients with suspected acute myocardial infarction. Arch. Intern. Med. 149:1294, 1989.

421. Brush, J. E., Brand, D. A., Acampora, D., et al.: Use of the initial electrocardiogram to predict in-hospital complications of acute myocardial infarction. N. Engl. J. Med. 312:1137, 1985.

422. Lee, T. L., Cook, E. F., Weisberg, M., et al.: Acute chest pain in the emergency ward: identification and evaluation of low risk patients. Arch. Intern. Med. 145:65, 1985.

423. Goldman, L., Weinberg, M., Weisberg, M., et al.: A computer-derived protocol to aid in the diagnosis of emergency room patients with acute chest pain. N. Engl. J. Med. 307:588, 1982.

424. Pozen, M. W., D'Agostino, R. B., Mitchell, J. B., et al.: The usefulness of a predictive instrument to reduce inappropriate admissions to the coronary care unit. Ann. Intern. Med. 92:238, 1980.

425. Fineberg, H., Scadden, D., and Goldman, L.: Management of patients with a low probability of acute myocardial infarction: Cost-effectiveness of alternatives to coronary care unit admission. N. Engl. J. Med. 310:1301, 1984.

426. McGregor, M.: The coronary care unit. A lack of consensus. Am. J. Med. 78:378, 1985.

427. Lee, T. H., Rouan, G. W., Weisberg, M. D., et al.: Sensitivity of routine clinical criteria for diagnosing myocardial infarction within 24 hours of hospitalization. Ann. Intern. Med. 106:181, 1987.

428. Weingarten, S., Ermann, B., Bolus, R., et al.: Early "step-down" transfer of low-risk patients with chest pain. A controlled interventional trial. Ann. Intern. Med. 113:283, 1990.

429. Herlitz, J., Hjalmarson, A., and Waagstein, F.: Treatment of pain in acute myocardial infarction. Br. Heart J. 61:9, 1989.

430. Mikolich, J. R., Nicoloff, N. B., Robinson, P. H., and Logue, H. B.: Relief of refractory angina with continuous intravenous infusion of nitroglycerin. Chest 77:375, 1980.

431. Come, P. C., and Pitt, B.: Nitroglycerin-induced severe hypotension and bradycardia in patients with acute myocardial infarction. Circulation 54:624, 1976.

432. Ferguson, J. J., Diver, D. J., Boldt, M., and Pasternak, R. C.: Significance of

nitroglycerin-induced hypotension with acute myocardial infarction. Am. J. Cardiol. 64:311, 1989.

433. Zelis, R., Mansour, E. J., Capone, R. J., and Mason, D. T.: The cardiovascular effects of morphine: The peripheral capacitance and resistance vessels in human subjects. J. Clin. Invest. 54:1247, 1974.

434. Fillmore, S. J., Shapiro, M., and Killip, T.: Arterial oxygen tension in acute myocardial infarction. Serial analysis of clinical state and blood gas changes. Am. Heart J. 79:620, 1970.

435. Madias, J. E., and Hood, W. B., Jr.: Reduction of precordial ST-segment elevation in patients with anterior myocardial infarction by oxygen breathing. Circulation 53(Suppl. I):198, 1976.

436. Richterova, A., Herlitz, J., Holmberg, S., et al.: Goteborg metoprolol trial: effects on chest pain. J. Cardiol. 53:32D, 1984.

436a. Yusuf, S., Held, P., and Furberg, C.: Update of effects of calcium antagonists in myocardial infarction or angina in light of the second Danish verapamil infarction trial (DAVIT-II) and other recent studies. Am. J. Cardiol. 67:1295, 1991.

437. Kirschenbaum, J. M., Koner, R. A., Antman, E., and Braunwald, E.: Use of an ultrashort acting β blocker in patients with acute myocardial ischemia. Circulation 72:873, 1985.

438. Levine, S. A., and Lown, B.: "Armchair" treatment of acute coronary thrombosis. JAMA 148:1365, 1952.

439. Swan, H.J.C., Ganz, W., Forrester, J. S., et al.: Catheterization of the heart in man with use of a flow-directed balloon-tipped catheter. N. Engl. J. Med. 283:447, 1970.

440. Rackley, C. E., Satler, L. F., Pearle, D. L., et al.: Use of hemodynamic measurements for management of acute myocardial infarction. In Rackley, C. E. (ed.): Advances in Critical Care Cardiology. Philadelphia, F. A. Davis Co., 1986, pp. 3–16.

441. Weisel, R. D., Berger, R. L., and Hechtman, H. B.: Measurement of cardiac output by thermodilution. N. Engl. J. Med. 292:682, 1975.

442. McMichan, J. C., Baele, P. L., and Wignes, M. W.: Insertion of pulmonary artery catheters—a comparison of fiberoptic and nonfiberoptic catheters. Crit. Care Med. 12:517, 1984.

443. Gewirtz, H., Gold, H. K., Fallon, J. T., et al.: Role of right ventricular infarction in cardiogenic shock associated with inferior myocardial infarction. Br. Heart J. 42:719, 1979.

444. Shell, W. E., DeWood, M. A., Peter, T., et al.: Comparison of clinical signs and hemodynamic state in the early hours of transmural myocardial infarction. Am. Heart J. 104:521, 1981.

445. Goldenheim, P. D., and Kazemi, H.: Cardiopulmonary monitoring of critically ill patients. N. Engl. J. Med. 311:776, 1984.

446. Eisenberg, P. R., Jaffe, A. S., and Schuster, D. P.: Clinical evaluation compared to pulmonary artery catheterization in the hemodynamic assessment of critically ill patients. Crit. Care Med. 12:549, 1984.

447. Robin, E. D.: The cult of the Swan-Ganz catheter. Ann. Intern. Med. 103:445, 1985.

448. Robin, E. D.: Death by pulmonary artery flow–directed catheter (editorial). Time for a moratorium? Chest 92:727, 1987.

449. Gore, J. M., Goldberg, R. J., Spodick, D. H., et al.: A community-wide assessment of the use of pulmonary artery catheters in patients with acute myocardial infarction. Chest 92:721, 1987.

450. Graboys, T. B.: In-hospital sudden death after coronary care unit discharge: A high risk profile. Arch. Intern. Med. 135:512, 1975.

451. Marmor, A., Geltman, E. M., Schechtman, K., et al.: Recurrent myocardial infarction: Clinical predictors and prognostic implications. Circulation 66:415, 1982.

452. Lie, K. I., Liem, K. L., Schuilenburg, R. M., et al.: Early identification of patients developing late in-hospital ventricular fibrillation after discharge from the Coronary Care Unit. Am. J. Cardiol. 41:674, 1978.

453. Starling, M. R., Crawford, M. H., Kennedy, G. T., and O'Rourke, R. A.: Treadmill exercise tests predischarge and 6-week postmyocardial infarction to detect abnormalities of known prognostic value. Ann. Intern. Med. 94:721, 1981.

454. Sellier, P., Plat, F., Corona, P., et al.: Prognostic significance of angina pectoris recurring soon after myocardial infarction. Eur. Heart J. 9:447, 1988.

455. Severance, H. W., Jr., Morris, K. G., and Wagner, G. S.: Criteria for early discharge after acute myocardial infarction. Validation in a community hospital. Arch. Intern. Med. 142:39, 1982.

456. Resnekov, L.: The intermediate care unit—a stage in continued coronary care. Br. Heart J. 39:357, 1977.

457. Weinberg, S. L.: Intermediate coronary care—observations on the validity of the concept. Chest 73:154, 1978.

458. van der Laarse, A., van Leeuwen, F. T., Krul, R., et al.: The size of infarction as judged enzymatically in 1974 patients with acute myocardial infarction. Relation with symptomatology, infarct localization and type of infarction. Int. J. Cardiol. 19:191, 1988.

459. Page, D. L., Caulfield, J. B., Kastor, J. A., et al.: Myocardial changes associated with cardiogenic shock. N. Engl. J. Med. 285:133, 1971.

460. Gutovitz, A. L., Sobel, B. E., and Roberts, R.: Progressive nature of myocardial injury in selected patients with cardiogenic shock. Am. J. Cardiol. 41:469, 1978.

461. Rogers, W. J., McDaniel, H. G., Smith, L. R., et al.: Correlation of angiographic estimates of myocardial infarct size and accumulated release of creatine kinase MB isoenzyme in man. Circulation 56:199, 1977.

462. Holman, B. L., Chisholm, R. J., and Braunwald, E.: The prognostic implications of acute myocardial infarct scintigraphy with 99m Tc-pyrophosphate. Circulation 57:320, 1978.

463. Geltman, E. M., Ehsani, A. A., Campbell, M. K., et al.: The influence of location and extent of myocardial infarction on long-term ventricular dysrhythmia and mortality. Circulation 60:805, 1979.

464. Sobel, B. E., and Shell, W. E.: Jeopardized, blighted and necrotic myocardium. Circulation 47:215, 1973.

465. Braunwald, E., and Maroko, P. R.: The reduction of infarct size—an idea whose time (for testing) has come. Circulation 50:206, 1974.

466. Yusuf, S., Collins, R., Peto, R., et al.: Intravenous and intracoronary fibrinolytic therapy in acute myocardial infarction: Overview of results on mortality, reinfarction and side effects from 33 randomized control trials. Eur. Heart J. 6:556, 1985.

467. Kubler, W., and Doorey, A.: Reduction of infarct size. An attractive concept: useful—or possible—in human? Br. Heart J. 53:5, 1985.

468. Christlieb, I. Y., Clark, R. E., and Sobel, B. E.: Three-hour preservation of the hypothermic globally ischemic heart with nifedipine. Surgery 90:947, 1981.

469. Weisfeldt, M. L.: Reperfusion and reperfusion injury. Clin. Res. 35:13, 1987.

470. Engler, R., and Gilpin, E.: Can superoxide dismutase alter myocardial infarct size? Circulation 79:1177, 1989.

470a. Murohara, Y., Yui, Y., Hattori, R., and Kawai, C.: Effects of superoxide dismutase on reperfusion arrhythmias and left ventricular function in patients undergoing thrombolysis for anterior wall acute myocardial infarction. Am. J. Cardiol. 67:765, 1991.

471. Corr, P. B., Snyder, D. W., Lee, B. I., et al.: Pathophysiological concentrations of lysophosphatides and the slow response. Am. J. Physiol. 12:187, 1982.

472. Schaper, W., and Pasyk, S.: Influence of collateral flow on the ischemic tolerance of the heart following acute and subacute coronary occlusion. Circulation 53(Suppl. I):57, 1976.

473. Braunwald, E.: Coronary artery spasm as a cause of myocardial ischemia. J. Lab. Clin. Med. 97:299, 1981.

474. Maseri, A., L'Abbate, A., Baroldi, G., et al.: Coronary vasospasm as a possible cause of myocardial infarction. N. Engl. J. Med. 299:1271, 1978.

475. Koiwaya, Y., Torii, S., Takeshita, A., et al.: Postinfarction angina caused by coronary arterial spasm. Circulation 65:275, 1982.

476. Williams, D. O., Amsterdam, E. A., Miller, R. R., and Mason, D. T.: Functional significance of coronary collateral vessels in patients with acute myocardial infarction: Relation to pump performance, cardiogenic shock and survival. Am. J. Cardiol. 37:345, 1976.

477. Baker, J. T., Bramlet, D. A., Lester, R. M., et al.: Myocardial infarction extension: Incidence and relationship to survival. Circulation 65:918, 1982.

478. Hutter, A. M., Jr., DeSanctis, R. W., Flynn, T., and Yeatman, L. A.: Nontransmural myocardial infarction. A comparison of hospital and late clinical course of patients with that of matched patients with transmural anterior and transmural inferior myocardial infarction. Am. J. Cardiol. 48:595, 1981.

479. Kao, W., Khaja, F., Goldstein, S., and Gheorghiade, M.: Cardiac event rate after non-Q-wave acute myocardial infarction and the significance of its anterior location. Am. J. Cardiol. 64:1236, 1989.

480. Shell, W. E., and Sobel, B. E.: Protection of jeopardized ischemic myocardium by reduction of ventricular afterload. N. Engl. J. Med. 291:481, 1974.

481. Derrida, J. P., Sal, R., and Chiche, P.: Nitroglycerin infusion in acute myocardial infarction. N. Engl. J. Med. 297:336, 1977.

482. Hjalmarson, A., Herlitz, J., Malek, I., et al.: Effect on mortality of metoprolol in acute myocardial infarction. Lancet 2:823, 1981.

483. Yusuf, S., Ramsdale, E., Peto, R., et al.: Early intravenous atentolol treatment in suspected acute myocardial infarction. Preliminary report of a randomized trial. Lancet 2:73, 1980.

484. Braunwald, E., Muller, J. E., Kloner, R. A., and Maroko, P. R.: Role of beta-adrenergic blockade in the therapy of patients with myocardial infarction. Am. J. Med. 74:113, 1983.

485. Chatterjee, K., and Parmley, W. W.: Vasodilator therapy for acute myocardial infarction and chronic congestive heart failure. J. Am. Coll. Cardiol. 1:133, 1983.

486. Lavie, C. J., Gersh, B. J., and Chesebro, J. H.: Reperfusion in acute myocardial infarction. Mayo Clin. Proc. 65:549, 1990.

487. Ginks, W. R., Sybers, H. D., Maroko, P. R., et al.: Coronary artery reperfusion: II. Reduction of myocardial infarct size at 1 week after the coronary occlusion. J. Clin. Invest. 51:2717, 1972.

488. Smith, G. T., Soeter, J. R., Haston, H. H., and McNamara, J. J.: Coronary reperfusion in primates: Serial electrocardiographic and histologic assessment. J. Clin. Invest. 54:1420, 1974.

489. Deloche, A., Fabiani, J. N., Camilleri, J. P., et al.: The effect of coronary artery reperfusion on the extent of myocardial infarction. Am. Heart J. 93:358, 1977.

490. Bergmann, S. R., Lerch, R. A., Fox, K.A.A., et al.: The temporal dependence of beneficial effects of coronary thrombolysis characterized by positron tomography. Am. J. Med. 73:573, 1982.

491. Reimer, K. A., and Jennings, R. B.: The wavefront phenomenon of myocardial ischemic cell death. II. Transmural progression of necrosis within the framework of ischemic bed size (myocardium at risk) and collateral flow. Lab. Invest. 40:633, 1979.

492. Cheauvechai, C., Effler, D. B., Loop, F. D., et al.: Emergency myocardial revascularization. Am. J. Cardiol. 32:901, 1973.

493. Chazov, E. I., Mateeva, L. S., Mazaev, A. V., et al.: Intracoronary administration of fibrinolysin in acute myocardial infarction. Ter. Arkh. 48:8, 1976.

494. Rentrop, P., DeVivie, E. R., Karsch, K. R., and Kreuzer, H.: Acute coronary occlusion with impending infarction as an angiographic complication relieved by a guide-wire recanalization. Clin. Cardiol. 1:101, 1978.

495. Califf, R. M., Topol, E., and Gersh, B. J.: From myocardial salvage to patient salvage in acute myocardial infarction: The role of reperfusion therapy. J. Am. Coll. Cardiol. *14*:1382, 1989.

496. Kloner, R. A., Ellis, S. G., Lange, R., and Braunwald, E.: Studies of experimental coronary artery reperfusion: Effects on infarct size, myocardial function, biochemistry, ultrastructure and microvascular damage. Circulation 68(Suppl I):8, 1983.

497. Schwartz, F., Schuler, G., Katus, H., et al.: Intracoronary thrombolysis in acute myocardial infarction: duration of ischemia as a major determinant of late results after recanalization. Am. J. Cardiol. *50*:933, 1982.

498. Sheehan, F. H., Mathey, D. G., Schofer, J., et al.: Factors that determine recovery of left ventricular function after thrombolysis in patients with acute myocardial infarction. Circulation *71*:1121, 1985.

499. Sheehan, F. H., Braunwald, E., Canner, P., et al.: The effect of intravenous thrombolytic therapy on left ventricular function: A report on tissue-type plasminogen activator and streptokinase from the thrombolysis in myocardial infarction (TIMI Phase I) trial. Circulation *75*:817, 1987.

500. Kurnik, P. B., Courtois, M. R., and Ludbrook, P. B.: Diastolic stiffening induced by acute myocardial infarction is reduced by early reperfusion. J. Am. Coll. Cardiol. *12*:1029, 1988.

501. Gruppo Italiano Per Lo Studio Della Streptochinasi Nell'infarcto Miocardico (GISSI): Effectiveness of intravenous thrombolytic treatment in acute myocardial infarction. Lancet *1*:397, 1986.

502. ISIS 2 Collaborative Group: Randomized trial of intravenous streptokinase, oral aspirin, both, or neither among 17,187 cases of suspected acute myocardial infarction: ISIS 2. Lancet *2*:349, 1988.

503. Saito, Y., Yasuno, M., Ishida, M., et al.: Importance of coronary collaterals for restoration of left ventricular function after intracoronary thrombolysis. Am. J. Cardiol. *55*:1259, 1985.

504. Nayler, W. G., and Elz, J. S.: Reperfusion injury: Laboratory artifact or clinical dilemma? Circulation *74*:215, 1986.

504a. Forman, M. B., Virmani, R., and Puett, D. W.: Mechanisms and therapy of myocardial reperfusion injury. Circulation *81*(Suppl. *IV*):IV–69, 1990.

505. Braunwald, E., and Kloner, R. A.: Myocardial reperfusion: A double-edged sword? J. Clin. Invest. *76*:1713, 1985.

506. Kloner, R. A., Ganote, C. E., and Jennings, R. B.: The "no-reflow" phenomenon after temporary coronary occlusion in the dog. J. Clin. Invest. *54*:1496, 1974.

507. Laffel, G. L., and Braunwald, E.: Thrombolytic therapy. A new strategy for treatment of acute myocardial infarction. N. Engl. J. Med. *311*:710, 1984.

508. Waller, B. F., Rothbaum, D. A., Pinkerton, C. A., et al.: Status of the myocardium and infarct-related coronary artery in 19 necropsy patients with acute recanalization using pharmacologic (streptokinase, r-tissue plasminogen activator), mechanical (percutaneous transluminal coronary angioplasty) or combined types of reperfusion therapy. J. Am. Coll. Cardiol. *9*:785, 1987.

509. Gertz, S. D., Kalan, J. M., Kragel, A. H., et al.: Cardiac morphologic findings in patients with acute myocardial infarction treated with recombinant tissue plasminogen activator. Am. J. Cardiol. *65*:953, 1990.

510. Mattfeldt, T., Schwarz, F., Schuler, G., et al.: Necropsy evaluation in seven patients with evolving acute myocardial infarction treated with thrombolytic therapy. Am. J. Cardiol. *54*:530, 1984.

510a. Carrea, F. P., and Lesnefsky, E. J., Repine, J. E., et al.: Reduction of canine myocardial infarct size by a diffusible reactive oxygen metabolite scavenger. Circ. Res. *68*:1652, 1991.

511. Werns, S. W., Shea, M. J., and Lucchesi, B. R.: Free radicals and myocardial injury: Pharmacologic implications. Circulation *74*:1, 1986.

512. TIMI Study Group: Comparison on invasive and conservative strategies following tissue plasminogen activator in acute myocardial infarction: Results of the Thrombolysis in Myocardial Infarction (TIMI-II) trial. N. Engl. J. Med. *320*:618, 1989.

513. Roberts, R., Rogers, W. J., Mueller, H. S., et al.: Immediate versus deferred β blockade following thrombolytic therapy in patients with acute myocardial infarction: Results of the Thrombolysis in Myocardial Infarction (TIMI) II-B Study. Circulation *83*:422, 1991.

514. Wei, J. Y., Markis, J. E., Malagold, M., and Braunwald, E.: Cardiovascular reflexes stimulated by reperfusion of ischemic myocardium in acute myocardial infarction. Circulation *67*:796, 1983.

515. Cercek, B., and Horvat, M.: Arrhythmias with brief, high-dose intravenous streptokinase infusion in acute myocardial infarction. Eur. Heart J. *6*:109, 1985.

516. Goldberg, S., Greenspan, A. J., Urban, P. L., et al.: Reperfusion arrhythmia: a marker of restoration of antegrade flow during intracoronary thrombolysis for acute myocardial infarction. Am. Heart J. *105*:26, 1983.

517. Califf, R. M., O'Neil, W., Stack, R. S., et al.: Failure of simple clinical measurements to predict perfusion status after intravenous thrombolysis. Ann. Intern. Med. *658*:108, 1988.

518. Wilber, D., Walton, J., O'Neill, W., et al.: Effects of reperfusion on complete heart block complicating anterior myocardial infarction. J. Am. Coll. Cardiol. *4*:1315, 1984.

519. Selzer, A.: Does thrombolytic therapy reduce infarct size? J. Am. Coll. Cardiol. *13*:1431, 1989.

519a. Deshmukh, P., Winters, S. L., and Gomes, J. A.: Frequency and significance of occult late potentials on the signal-averaged electrocardiogram in sustained ventricular tachycardia after healing of acute myocardial infarction. Am. J. Cardiol. *67*:806, 1991.

520. Braunwald, E.: Editorial Comment. Coronary artery patency in patients with myocardial infarction. J. Am. Coll. Cardiol. *16*:1550, 1990.

521. Fortin, D. F., and Califf, R. M.: Long-term survival from acute myocardial infarction: salutary effect of an open coronary vessel. Am. J. Med. *88*:1–9N, 1990.

521a. Bonaduce, D., Petretta, M., Villari, B., et al.: Effects of late administration of tissue-type plasminogen activator on left ventricular remodeling and function after myocardial infarction. J. Am. Coll. Cardiol. *16*:1561, 1990.

522. Grines, C. L., O'Neill, W. W., Anselmo, E. G., et al.: Comparison of left ventricular function and contractile reserve after successful recanalization by thrombolysis versus rescue percutaneous transluminal coronary angioplasty for acute myocardial infarction. Am. J. Cardiol. *62*:352, 1988.

523. Schroder, R., Neuhaus, K., Linderer, T., et al.: Impact of late coronary artery reperfusion on left ventricular function one month after acute myocardial infarction (results from the ISAM study). Am. J. Cardiol. *64*:878, 1989.

524. Agress, C. M., Jacobs, H. I., Clark, W. G., et al.: Intravenous trypsin in experimental acute myocardial infarction (abst). J. Pharmacol. Exp. Ther. *110*:1, 1952.

525. Fletcher, A. P., Alkjaersig, N., Smyriotis, F. E., and Sherry, S.: The treatment of patients suffering from early myocardial infarction with massive and prolonged streptokinase therapy. Trans. Assoc. Am. Phys. *71*:287, 1958.

526. Rentrop, P., Blanke, H., Marsch, K. R., et al.: Acute myocardial infarction: intracoronary application of nitroglycerin and streptokinase in combination with transluminal recanalization. Clin. Cardiol. *2*:354, 1979.

527. Khaja, F., Walton, J. A., Brymer, J. F., et al.: Intracoronary fibrinolytic therapy in acute myocardial infarction, report of a prospective randomized trial. N. Engl. J. Med. *308*:1305, 1983.

528. Tiefenbrunn, A. J., and Sobel, B. E.: The impact of coronary thrombolysis on myocardial infarction. Fibrinolysis *3*:1, 1989.

529. European Cooperative Study Group for Streptokinase Treatment in Acute Myocardial Infarction: Streptokinase in acute myocardial infarction. N. Engl. J. Med. *301*:797, 1979.

530. Fry, E.T.A., and Sobel, B. E.: Coronary thrombosis. *In* Zipes, D. P., and Rowlands, D. J. (eds.): Progress in Cardiology. Vol. II. Philadelphia, Lea & Febiger, 1990, pp. 199–239.

531. Anderson, J. L.: Reperfusion, patency, and reocclusion with anistreplase (APSAC) in acute myocardial infarction. Am. J. Cardiol. *64*:12A, 1989.

532. Sherry, S.: Unresolved clinical pharmacologic questions in thrombolytic therapy for acute myocardial infarction. J. Am. Coll. Cardiol. *12*:519, 1988.

533. Anderson, J. L., Rothbard, R. L., Hackworthy, R. A., et al.: Multicenter reperfusion trial of intravenous anisoylated plasminogen activator complex (APSAC) in acute myocardial infarction: controlled comparison with intracoronary streptokinase. J. Am. Coll. Cardiol. *11*:1153, 1988.

533a. Becker, R. C., Corrao, J. M., Harrington, R., et al.: Recombinant tissue-type plasminogen activator: Current concepts and guidelines for clinical use in acute myocardial infarction. Part 1. Am. Heart J. *121*:220, 1991.

533b. Becker, R. C., and Harrington, R.: Recombinant tissue-type plasminogen activator: Current concepts and guidelines for clinical use in acute myocardial infarction. Part II. Am. Heart J. *121*:627, 1991.

534. Topol, E. J., and Califf, R. M.: Tissue plasminogen activator: Why the backlash? J. Am. Coll. Cardiol. *13*:1477, 1989.

535. The TIMI Study Group: The thrombolysis in myocardial infarction (TIMI) trial. Phase I Findings. N. Engl. J. Med. *312*:932, 1985.

536. Verstraete, M., Bory, M., Collen, D., et al.: Randomised trial of intravenous recombinant tissue-type plasminogen activator versus intravenous streptokinase in acute myocardial infarction. Lancet *I*:842, 1985.

537. Chesebro, J. H., Knatterud, G., Roberts, R., et al.: Thrombolysis in myocardial infarction (TIMI) trial, phase I: a comparison between intravenous tissue plasminogen activator and intravenous streptokinase. Circulation *76*:142, 1987.

538. White, H. D., Rivers, J. T., Maslowski, A. H., et al.: Effect of intravenous streptokinase as compared with that of tissue plasminogen activator on left ventricular function after first myocardial infarction. N. Engl. J. Med. *320*:817, 1989.

539. Magnani, B., for the PAIMS Investigators: Plasminogen Activator Italian Multicenter Study (PAIMS): Comparison of intravenous recombinant single-chain human tissue-type plasminogen activator (rt-PA) with intravenous streptokinase in acute myocardial infarction. J. Am. Coll. Cardiol. *13*:19, 1989.

540. Collen, D.: Coronary thrombolysis: Streptokinase or recombinant tissue–type plasminogen activator? Ann. Intern. Med. *112*:529, 1990.

540a. Data presented at American College of Cardiology Annual Scientific Sessions, Atlanta, 1991.

541. Baim, D. S., Braunwald, E., Feit, F., et al.: The thrombolysis in myocardial infarction (TIMI) trial phase II: Additional information and perspectives. J. Am. Coll. Cardiol. *15*:1188, 1990.

542. Braunwald, E.: Thrombolytic reperfusion of acute myocardial infarction: resolved and unresolved issues. J. Am. Coll. Cardiol. *12*:85A, 1988.

543. Mauri, F., Gasparini, M., Barbonaglia, L., et al.: Prognostic significance of the extent of myocardial injury in acute myocardial infarction treated by streptokinase (the GISSI Trial). Am. J. Cardiol. *63*:1291, 1989.

544. Meinertz, T., Kasper, W., Schumacher, M., et al.: The German multicenter trial of anisoylated plasminogen activator complex versus heparin for acute myocardial infarction. Am. J. Cardiol. *62*:347, 1988.

545. Gruppo Italiano Per Lo Studio Della Streptochinasi Nell'Infarto Miocar-

dico (GISSI): Long-term effects of intravenous thrombolysis in acute myocardial infarction: Final report of the GISSI study. Lancet 2:871, 1987.

546. Simoons, M. L., Vos, J., Tijssen, J.G.P., et al.: Long-term benefit of early thrombolytic therapy in patients with acute myocardial infarction: 5-year follow-up of a trial conducted by the Interuniversity Cardiology Committee, University of the Netherlands. J. Am. Coll. Cardiol. 14:1609, 1989.

547. Sheehan, F. H.: Measurement of left ventricular function as an endpoint in trials of thrombolytic therapy. Coronary Artery Disease 1:13, 1990.

548. Wackers, F. J. Th., Terrin, M. L., Kayden, D. S., et al.: Quantitative radionuclide assessment of regional ventricular function after thrombolytic therapy for acute myocardial infarction: Results of phase I thrombolysis in myocardial infarction (TIMI) trial. J. Am. Coll. Cardiol. 13:998, 1989.

549. Gruppo Italiano Per Lo Studio Della Sopravvivenza Nell'Infarto Miocardico: GISSI-2: A factorial randomized trial of alteplase versus streptokinase and heparin versus no heparin among 12,490 patients with acute myocardial infarction. Lancet 336:65, 1990.

550. Touchstone, D. A., Beller, G. A., Nygaard, T. W., et al.: Effects of successful intravenous reperfusion therapy on regional myocardial function and geometry in humans: A tomographic assessment using two-dimensional echocardiography. J. Am. Coll. Cardiol. 13:1506, 1989.

551. Bassand, J.-P., Machecourt, J., Cassagnes, J., et al.: Multicenter trial of intravenous anisoylated plasminogen streptokinase activator complex (APSAC) in acute myocardial infarction: Effects on infarct size and left ventricular function. J. Am. Coll. Cardiol. 13:988, 1989.

552. Armstrong, P. W., Baigrie, R. S., Daly, P. A., et al.: Tissue plasminogen activator: Toronto (TPAT) placebo-controlled randomized trial in acute myocardial infarction. J. Am. Coll. Cardiol. 13:1469, 1989.

553. Lavie, C. J., O'Keefe, J. H., Chesebro, J. H., et al.: Prevention of late ventricular dilatation after myocardial infarction by successful thrombolytic reperfusion. Am. J. Cardiol. 66:31, 1990.

554. Lee, T. L., Weisberg, M. C., Brand, D. A., et al.: Candidates for thrombolysis among emergency room patients with acute chest pain. Ann. Intern. Med. 110:957, 1989.

555. Wasserman, A. G., and Ross, A. M.: Patient selection for thrombolytic therapy. Am. J. Cardiol. 64:17B, 1989.

556. Eisenberg, M. S., Ho, M. T., Schaeffer, S., et al.: A community survey of the potential use of thrombolytic agents for acute myocardial infarction. Ann. Emerg. Med. 18:838, 1989.

557. Karlson, B. W., Herlitz, J., Edvardsson, N., et al.: Eligibility for intravenous thrombolysis in suspected acute myocardial infarction. Circulation 82:1140, 1990.

558. Wilcox, R. G., Olsson, C. G., Skene, A. M., et al.: Trial of tissue plasminogen activator for mortality reduction in acute myocardial infarction. Anglo-Scandinavian Study of Early Thrombolysis (ASSET). Lancet 2:525, 1988.

559. AIMS Trial Study Group: Effect of intravenous APSAC on mortality after acute myocardial infarction: Preliminary report of a placebo-controlled clinical trial. Lancet 1:547, 1988.

560. Krumholz, H. M.: The clinical challenges of myocardial infarction in the elderly. West. J. Med. 151:304, 1989.

561. Grines, C. L., and DeMaria, A. N.: Optimal utilization of thrombolytic therapy for acute myocardial infarction: Concepts and controversies. J. Am. Coll. Cardiol. 16:223, 1990.

562. Eisenberg, P. R., Sherman, L., Rich, M., et al.: Importance of continued activation of thrombin reflected by fibrinopeptide A to the efficacy of thrombolysis. J. Am. Coll. Cardiol. 7:1255, 1986.

562a. Golino, P., and Willerson, J. T.: Is thrombolysis alone the best therapy for acute myocardial infarction? Current status and emerging strategies. Texas Heart Inst. J. 18:50, 1991.

563. Webster, M.W.I., Chesebro, J. H., and Mruk, J. S.: Antithrombotic therapy during and after thrombolysis for acute myocardial infarction. Coronary Artery Disease 1:190, 1990.

564. Haskel, E. J., Prager, N. A., Sobel, B. E., and Abendschein, D. R.: The relative efficacy of antithrombin compared with antiplatelet agents in accelerating coronary thrombolysis and preventing early reocclusion. Circulation 83:1048, 1991.

565. Hsia, J., Hamilton, W. P., Kleiman, N., et al.: The heparin-aspirin reperfusion trial (HART): A randomized trial of heparin versus aspirin adjunctive to tissue plasminogen activator–induced thrombolysis in acute myocardial infarction. N. Engl. J. Med. 323:1433, 1990.

566. Bleich, S. D., Nichols, T., Schumacher, R., et al.: The role of heparin following coronary thrombolysis with tissue plasminogen activator (t-PA). Circulation 80(Suppl. II):113, 1989.

567. Eisenberg, P. R., Miletich, J. P., and Sobel, B. E.: Factors responsible for differential procoagulant effects of diverse plasminogen activators in plasma. Fibrinolysis (in press).

568. Topol, E. J., George, B. S., Kereiakes, D. J., et al.: A randomized controlled trial of intravenous tissue plasminogen activator and early intravenous heparin in acute myocardial infarction. Circulation 79:281, 1989.

569. Kander, N. H., Holland, K. J., Pitt, B., and Topol, E. J.: A randomized pilot trial of brief versus prolonged heparin after successful reperfusion in acute myocardial infarction. Am. J. Cardiol. 65:139, 1990.

570. The SCATI (Studio Sulla Calciparina Nell' Angina E Nella Thrombosi Ventricolare Nell'Infarto) Group: Randomised controlled trial of subcutaneous calcium-heparin in acute myocardial infarction. Lancet 1:182, 1989.

571. Lavie, C. J., Murphy, J. G., and Gersh, B. J.: The role of beta-receptor and calcium-entry blocking agents in the treatment of acute myocardial infarction in the thrombolytic era: Can the results of thrombolytic therapy be enhanced? Cardiovasc. Drugs Ther. 2:601, 1988.

572. Hackett, D., Davies, G., Chierchia, S., and Maseri, A.: Intermittent coronary occlusion in acute myocardial infarction. Value of combined thrombolytic and vasodilator therapy. N. Engl. J. Med. 317:1055, 1987.

573. Sane, D. C., Califf, R. M., Topol, E. J., et al.: Bleeding during thrombolytic therapy for acute myocardial infarction: Mechanisms and management. Ann. Intern. Med. 111:1010, 1989.

573a. Gore, J. M., Sloan, M., Price, T. R., et al.: Intracerebral hemorrhage, cerebral infarction, and subdural hematoma after acute myocardial infarction and thrombolytic therapy in the Thrombolysis in Myocardial Infarction Study: TIMI Phase II Pilot and Clinical Trial. Circulation 83:448, 1991.

574. Califf, R. M., Topol, E. J., George, B. S., et al.: Hemorrhagic complications associated with the use of intravenous tissue plasminogen activator in treatment of acute myocardial infarction. Am. J. Med. 85:353, 1988.

575. Gimple, L. W., Gold, H. K., Leinbach, R. C., et al.: Correlation between template bleeding times and spontaneous bleeding during treatment of acute myocardial infarction with recombinant tissue-type plasminogen activator. Circulation 80:581, 1989.

576. Weiner, M. D., and Ong, L. S.: Streptokinase and splenic rupture. Am. J. Med. 86:249, 1989.

577. Blankenship, J. C., and Almquist, A. K.: Cardiovascular complications of thrombolytic therapy in patients with a mistaken diagnosis of acute myocardial infarction. J. Am. Coll. Cardiol. 14:1579, 1989.

578. Queen, M., Biem, J., Moe, G. W., and Suger, L.: Development of cholesterol embolization syndrome after intravenous streptokinase for acute myocardial infarction. Am. J. Cardiol. 65:1042, 1990.

579. Gottlich, M., Cooper, B., Schumacher, J. R., and Hillis, J. D.: Do different doses of intravenous streptokinase alter the frequency of coronary reperfusion in acute myocardial infarction? Am. J. Cardiol. 62:843, 1988.

580. Balnave, K., Moriarty, A. J., and Nelson, S. D.: Evaluation of optimum streptokinase dosage in systemic thrombolytic therapy for acute myocardial infarction: a randomized trial (abstr). Thromb. Haemost. 58:193, 1987.

581. Six, A. J., Louwerenburg, H. W., Braams, R., et al.: A double-blind randomized multicenter dose-ranging trial of intravenous streptokinase in acute myocardial infarction. Am. J. Cardiol. 65:119, 1990.

582. Braunwald, E.: Enhancing thrombolytic efficacy by means of "front-loaded" administration of tissue plasminogen activator. J. Am. Coll. Cardiol. 14:1570, 1989.

583. Tebbe, U., Tanswell, P., Seifried, E., et al.: Single-bolus injection of recombinant tissue–type plasminogen activator in acute myocardial infarction. Am. J. Cardiol. 64:448, 1989.

584. Tranchesi, B., Verstaete, M., Vanhove, Ph., et al.: Intravenous bolus administration of recombinant tissue plasminogen activator to patients with acute myocardial infarction. Coronary Artery Disease 1:83, 1990.

585. Neuhaus, K.-L., Feuerer, W., Jeep-Tebbe, S., et al.: Improved thrombolysis with a modified dose regimen of recombinant tissue-type plasminogen activator. J. Am. Coll. Cardiol. 14:1566, 1989.

586. Smalling, R. W., Schumacher, R., Morris, D., et al.: Improved infarct-related arterial patency after high dose, weight-adjusted, rapid infusion of tissue-type plasminogen activator in myocardial infarction: Results of a multicenter randomized trial of two dosage regimens. J. Am. Coll. Cardiol. 15:915, 1990.

587. Topol, E. J.: Ultrathrombolysis. J. Am. Coll. Cardiol. 15:922, 1990.

588. Barbash, G. I., Hod, H., Roth, A., et al.: Repeat infusions of recombinant tissue–type plasminogen activator in patients with acute myocardial infarction and early recurrent myocardial ischemia. J. Am. Coll. Cardiol. 16:779, 1990.

589. Wall, T. C., Phillips, H. R., Stack, R. S., et al.: Results of high dose intravenous urokinase for acute myocardial infarction. Am. J. Cardiol. 65:124, 1990.

590. PRIMI Trial Study Group: Randomized double-blind trial of recombinant pro-urokinase against streptokinase in acute myocardial infarction. Lancet 1:863, 1989.

591. Loscalzo, J., Wharton, T. P., Kirshenbaum, J. M., et al.: Clot-selective coronary thrombolysis with pro-urokinase. Circulation 79:776, 1989.

592. Bode, C., Schoenermark, S., Schuler, G., et al.: Efficacy of intravenous prourokinase and a combination of prourokinase and urokinase in acute myocardial infarction. Am. J. Cardiol. 61:971, 1988.

593. Bode, C., Schuler, G., Nordt, T., et al.: Intravenous thrombolytic therapy with a combination of single-chain urokinase-type plasminogen activator and recombinant tissue–type plasminogen activator in acute myocardial infarction. Circulation 81:907, 1990.

594. Neuhaus, K.-L., Tebbe, U., Gottwik, M., et al.: Intravenous recombinant tissue plasminogen activator (rt-PA) and urokinase in acute myocardial infarction: results of the German Activator Urokinase Study (GAUS). J. Am. Coll. Cardiol. 12:581, 1988.

595. Grines, C. L., Nissen, S. E., Booth, D. C., et al.: A new thrombolytic regimen for acute myocardial infarction using combination half dose tissue-type plasminogen activator with full dose streptokinase: A pilot study. J. Am. Coll. Cardiol. 14:573, 1989.

595a. Ott, P., and Fenster, P.: Combining thrombolytic agents to treat acute myocardial infarction. Am. Heart J. 121:1583, 1991.

596. Haber, E., Quertermous, T., Matsueda, G. R., and Runge, M. S.: Innovative approaches to plasminogen activator therapy. Science 243:51, 1989.

597. Sobel, B. E.: Coronary thrombolysis and the new biology. J. Am. Coll. Cardiol. *14*:850, 1989.

598. Tiefenbrunn, A. J., and Sobel, B. E.: Thrombolysis and myocardial infarction. Fibrinolysis *5*:1, 1991.

599. Meyer, J., Merx, W., Dorr, R., Lambertz, H., Bethge, C., and Effert, S.: Successful treatment of acute myocardial infarction shock by combined percutaneous transluminal coronary recanalization (PTCR) and percutaneous transluminal coronary angioplasty (PTCA). Am. Heart J. *103*:132, 1982.

599a. Kahn, J. K., Rutherford, B. D., McConahay, D. R., et al.: Catheterization laboratory events and hospital outcome with direct angioplasty for acute myocardial infarction. Circulation *82*:1910, 1990.

600. Holmes, D. R., Smith, H. C., Vliestra, R. D., et al.: Percutaneous transluminal coronary angioplasty alone or in a combination with streptokinase therapy, during acute myocardial infarction. Mayo Clin. Proc. *60*:449, 1985.

601. Hartzler, G. O., Rutherford, B. D., and McConahay, D. R.: Percutaneous transluminal coronary angioplasty: Application for acute myocardial infarction. Am. J. Cardiol. *53*:1176, 1984.

602. Sriram, R., Mullen, G. M., Foschi, A., and Bicoff, J. P.: Percutaneous transluminal coronary angioplasty in acute myocardial infarction without prior thrombolytic therapy. Am. J. Cardiol. *55*:842, 1985.

602a. Behrenbeck, T., Pellika, P. A., Huber, K. C., et al.: Primary angioplasty in myocardial infarction. Assessment of improved myocardial perfusion with technetium-99m isonitrile. J. Am. Coll. Cardiol. *17*:365, 1991.

603. Flaker, G. C., Webel, R. R., Meinhardt, S., et al.: Emergency angioplasty in acute anterior myocardial infarction. Am. Heart J. *118*:1154, 1989.

604. Ellis, S. G., O'Neill, W. W., Bates, E. R., et al.: Coronary angioplasty as primary therapy for acute myocardial infarction 6 to 48 hours after symptom onset: report of an initial experience. J. Am. Coll. Cardiol. *13*:1122, 1989.

605. O'Keefe, J. H., Rutherford, B. D., McConahay, D. R., et al.: Early and late results of coronary angioplasty without antecedent thrombolytic therapy for acute myocardial infarction. Am. J. Cardiol. *64*:1221, 1989.

606. Holmes, D. R., Smith, H. C., Vliestra, R. E., et al.: Percutaneous transluminal coronary angioplasty, alone or in combination with streptokinase therapy during acute myocardial infarction. Mayo Clin. Proc. *60*:449, 1985.

607. Stone, G. W., Rutherford, B. D., McConahay, D. R., et al.: Direct coronary angioplasty in acute myocardial infarction: Outcome in patients with single vessel disease. J. Am. Coll. Cardiol. *15*:534, 1990.

608. Kahn, J. K., Rutherford, B. D., McConahay, D. R., et al.: Results of primary angioplasty for acute myocardial infarction in patients with multivessel coronary artery disease. J. Am. Coll. Cardiol. *16*:1089, 1990.

609. O'Neill, W., Timmis, G. C., Bourdillon, P. D., et al.: A prospective randomized clinical trial of intracoronary streptokinase versus coronary angioplasty for acute myocardial infarction. N. Engl. J. Med. *314*:812, 1986.

610. Fung, A. Y., Lai, P., Juni, J. E., et al.: Prevention of subsequent exercise-induced periinfarct ischemia by emergency coronary angiplasty in acute myocardial infarction: Comparison with intracoronary streptokinase. J. Am. Coll. Cardiol. *8*:496, 1986.

611. Verna, E., Repetto, S., Boscarini, M., et al.: Emergency coronary angioplasty in patients with severe left ventricular dysfunction or cardiogenic shock after acute myocardial infarction. Eur. Heart J. *10*:958, 1989.

611a. Lee, L., Erbel, R., Brown, T. M., et al.: Multicenter registry of angioplasty therapy of cardiogenic shock: Initial and long-term survival. J. Am. Coll. Cardiol. *17*:599, 1991.

612. Brundage, B. H.: Because we can, should we? J. Am. Coll. Cardiol. *15*:544, 1990.

613. Topol, E. J., Califf, R. M., George, B. S., et al.: A randomized trial of immediate versus delayed elective angioplasty after intravenous tissue plasminogen activator in acute myocardial infarction. N. Engl. J. Med. *317*:581, 1987.

614. Simoons, M. L., Arnold, A.E.R., Betriu, A., et al.: Thrombolysis with tissue plasminogen activator in acute myocardial infarction: No additional benefit from immediate percutaneous coronary angioplasty. Lancet *1*:197, 1988.

615. Rogers, W. J., Baim, D. S., Gore, J. M., et al.: Comparison of immediate invasive, delayed invasive, and conservative strategies after tissue-type plasminogen activator. Results of the Thrombolysis in Myocardial Infarction (TIMI). Phase II—A trial. Circulation *81*:1457, 1990.

616. Guerci, A. D., and Ross, R. S.: TIMI II and the role of angioplasty in acute myocardial infarction. N. Engl. J. Med. *320*:663, 1989.

617. Holmes, D., and Topol, E. J.: Reperfusion momentum: Lessons from the randomization trials of immediate coronary angioplasty for myocardial infarction. J. Am. Coll. Cardiol. *14*:1572, 1989.

618. Stack, R. S., Califf, R. M., Hinohara, T., et al.: Survival and cardiac event rates in the first year after emergency coronary angioplasty for acute myocardial infarction. J. Am. Coll. Cardiol. *11*:1141, 1988.

619. Ellis, S. G., O'Neill, W. W., Bates, E. R., et al.: Implications for patient triage from survival and left ventricular functional recovery analyses in 500 patients treated with coronary angioplasty for acute myocardial infarction. J. Am. Coll. Cardiol. *13*:1251, 1989.

620. Erbel, R., Pop, T., Diefenbach, C., and Meyer, J.: Long-term results of thrombolytic therapy with and without percutaneous transluminal coronary angioplasty. J. Am. Coll. Cardiol. *14*:276, 1989.

621. Ellis, S. G., Topol, E. J., Gallison, L., et al.: Predictors of success for coronary angioplasty performed for acute myocardial infarction. J. Am. Coll. Cardiol. *12*:1407, 1988.

622. Phillips, S. J., Zeff, R. H., Skinner, J. R., et al.: Reperfusion protocol and results in 738 patients with evolving myocardial infarction. Ann. Thorac. Surg. *41*:119, 1986.

623. DeWood, M. A., Notske, R. N., Berg, R., et al.: Medical and surgical management of early Q wave myocardial infarction. I. Effects of surgical reperfusion on survival, recurrent myocardial infarction, sudden death and functional class at 10 or more years of follow-up. J. Am. Coll. Cardiol. *14*:65, 1989.

624. DeWood, M. A., Leonard, J., Grunwald, R. P., et al.: Medical and surgical management of early Q wave myocardial infarction. II. Effects on mortality and global and regional left ventricular function at 10 or more years of follow-up. J. Am. Coll. Cardiol. *14*:78, 1989.

625. Koshal, A., Beanlands, D. S., Davies, R. A., et al.: Urgent surgical reperfusion in acute evolving myocardial infarction. Circulation *78*(Suppl. I):171, 1988.

626. Montoya, A., Mulet, J., Pifarre, R., et al.: Hemorrhagic infarct following myocardial revascularization. J. Thorac. Cardiovasc. Surg. *75*:206, 1978.

627. Kagen, L., Scheidt, S., and Butt, A.: Serum myoglobin in myocardial infarction: The "staccato phenomenon": Is acute myocardial infarction in man an intermittent event? Am. J. Med. *62*:86, 1977.

628. Kay, P., Ahmad, A., Floten, S., and Starr, A.: Emergency coronary artery bypass surgery after intracoronary thrombolysis for evolving myocardial infarction. Int. J. Cardiol. *7*:281, 1985.

629. Meyer, J., Merx, W., Dorr, R., et al.: Sequential intervention procedures after intracoronary thrombolysis: balloon dilatation, bypass surgery, and medical treatment. Int. J. Cardiol. *7*:281, 1985.

630. Kereiakes, D. J., Topol, E. J., George, B. S., et al.: Favorable early and long-term prognosis following coronary bypass surgery therapy for myocardial infarction: results of a multicenter trial. Am. Heart J. *118*:199, 1989.

631. Naunheim, K. S., Kesler, K. A., Kanter, K. R., et al.: Coronary artery bypass for recent infarction. Predictors of mortality. Circulation *78*(Suppl. I):122, 1988.

632. Kennedy, J. W., Ivey, T. D., Misbach, G., et al.: Coronary artery bypass graft surgery early after acute myocardial infarction. Circulation *79*(Suppl. I):73, 1989.

633. Kalan, J. M., and Roberts, W. C.: Morphologic findings in patients undergoing coronary artery bypass grafting for acute myocardial infarction. Am. J. Cardiol. *62*:144, 1988.

634. Mueller, H. S., and Ayres, S. M.: The role of propranolol in the treatment of acute myocardial infarction. Prog. Cardiovasc. Dis. *19*:405, 1977.

635. Gold, H. K., Leinbach, C., and Maroko, P. R.: Propranolol-induced reduction of signs of ischemic injury during acute myocardial infarction. Am. J. Cardiol. *38*:689, 1976.

636. Pelides, L. J., Reid, D. S., Thomas, M., and Shillingford, J. P.: Inhibition by beta-blockade of the ST segment elevation after acute myocardial infarction in man. Cardiovasc. Res. *2*:295, 1972.

637. Peter, T., Norris, R. M., and Clarke, E. D.: Reduction of enzyme levels by propranolol after acute myocardial infarction. Circulation *57*:1091, 1978.

638. Norris, R. M., Clarke, E. D., Sammel, N. L., et al.: Protective effect of propranolol in threatened myocardial infarction. Lancet *2*:907, 1978.

639. Yusuf, S., Sleight, P., Rossi, P., et al.: Reduction in infarct size, arrhythmias and chest pain by early intravenous beta blockade in suspected acute myocardial infarction. Circulation *67*:12, 1983.

640. Jurgensen, H. J., Frederiksen, J., Hansen, D. A., and Pedersen-Bjorgaard, D.: Limitation of myocardial infarct size in patients less than 66 years treated with alprenolol. Br. Heart J. *45*:583, 1981.

641. Hjalmarson, A., Herlitz, J., Holmberg, S., et al.: The Goteborg metoprolol trial. Effects on mortality and morbidity in acute myocardial infarction. Circulation *67*:26, 1983.

642. Roberts, R., Croft, C., Gold, H. K., et al.: Effect of propranolol on myocardial infarct size in a randomized blinded multicenter trial. N. Engl. J. Med. *311*:218, 1984.

643. The International Collaborative Study Group: Reduction of infarct size with the early use of timolol in acute myocardial infarction. N. Engl. J. Med. *310*:9, 1984.

644. The MIAMI Trial Research Group: Metoprolol in acute myocardial infarction (MIAMI). A randomized placebo-controlled international trial. Eur. Heart J. *6*:199, 1985.

645. ISIS-1 (First International Study of Infarct Survival) Collaborative Group: Randomized trial of intravenous atenolol among 16,027 cases of suspected acute myocardial infarction. ISIS-I. Lancet *2*:57, 1986.

646. Croft, C. H., Rude, R. E., Gustafson, N., et al.: Abrupt withdrawal of β-blockade therapy in patients with myocardial infarction: Effects on infarct size, left ventricular function, and hospital course. Circulation *73*:1281, 1986.

647. Yusuf, S., Peto, R., Lewis, J., et al.: Beta blockade during and after myocardial infarction: an overview of the randomized trials. Prog. Cardiovasc. Dis. *27*:335, 1985.

648. Sung, R. J., Blanski, L., Kirschenbaum, J., et al.: Clinical experience with esmolol, a short-acting beta-adrenergic blocker in cardiac arrhythmias and myocardial ischemia. J. Clin. Pharmacol. *26*(Suppl. A):15, 1986.

649. Kirshenbaum, J. M., Kloner, R. F., McGowan, N., and Antman, E. M.: Use of an ultrashort-acting beta receptor blocker (esmolol) in patients with acute myocardial ischemia and relative contraindications to beta-blockade therapy. J. Am. Coll. Cardiol. *12*:773, 1988.

650. Derrida, J. P., Sal, R., and Chiche, P.: Favorable effects of prolonged nitroglycerin infusion in patients with acute myocardial infarction. Am. Heart J. 96:833, 1978.

651. Jugdutt, B. I., and Warnica, J. W.: Intravenous nitroglycerin therapy to limit myocardial infarct size, expansion, and complications. Effect of timing, dosage, and infarct location. Circulation 78:906, 1988.

652. Bussman, W. D., Passek, D., Seidel, W., and Kaltenbach, M.: Reduction of CK and CK-MB indexes of infarct size by intravenous nitroglycerin. Circulation 63:615, 1981.

653. Flaherty, J. T., Becker, L. C., Bulkley, B. H., et al.: A randomized prospective trial of intravenous nitroglycerin in patients with acute myocardial infarction. Circulation 68:576, 1983.

654. Osuna, P. B., Moreno, M. G., Jimenez, A. A., et al.: Isosorbide dinitrate sublingual therapy for inferior myocardial infarction: Randomized trial to assess infarct size limitation. Am. J. Cardiol. 55:330, 1985.

655. Shah, R., Bodenheimer, M. M., Banka, V. S., and Helfant, R. H.: Nitroglycerin and ventricular performance: Differential effect in the presence of reversible and irreversible asynergy. Chest 70:473, 1976.

656. Shook, T. L., Kirschenbaum, J. M., Hundley, R. F., et al.: Ethanol intoxication complicating intravenous nitroglycerin therapy. Ann. Intern. Med. 101:498, 1984.

657. Kaplan, K. J., Taber, M., Teagarden, J. R., et al.: Association of methemoglobinemia and intravenous nitroglycerin administration. Am. J. Cardiol. 55:181, 1985.

658. Jugdutt, B. I., and Warnica, J. W.: Tolerance with low dose intravenous nitroglycerin therapy in acute myocardial infarction. Am. J. Cardiol. 64:581, 1989.

659. Levy, W. E., Katz, R. J., Ruffalo, R. L., et al.: Potentiation of the hemodynamic effects of acutely administered nitroglycerin by methionine. Circulation 78:640, 1988.

660. Abrams, J.: Nitrates. Med. Clin. North Am. 72:1, 1988.

661. Skolnick, A. E., and Frishman, W. H.: Calcium channel blockers in myocardial infarction. Arch. Intern. Med. 149:1669, 1989.

662. Sirnes, P. A., Overskeid, K., Pederson, T. R., et al.: Evolution of infarct size during the early use of nifedipine in patients with acute myocardial infarction: The Norwegian Nifedipine Multicenter Trial. Circulation 70:738, 1984.

663. Muller, J. E., Morrison, J., Stone, P. H., et al.: Nifedipine therapy for patients with threatened and acute myocardial infarction: A randomized, double-blind, placebo-controlled comparison. Circulation 69:740, 1984.

664. Erbel, R., Pop, T., Meinertz, T., et al.: Combination of calcium channel blocker and thrombolytic therapy in acute myocardial infarction. Am. Heart J. 115:529, 1988.

665. Report of the Holland Interuniversity Nifedipine/Metoprolol Trial (HINT) Research Group: Early treatment of unstable angina in the coronary care unit: a randomised, double-blind, placebo-controlled comparison of recurrent ischaemia and thrombolytic therapy in patients treated with nifedipine or metoprolol or both. Br. Heart J. 56:400, 1986.

666. The Multicenter Diltiazem Postinfarction Trial Research Group: The effect of diltiazem on mortality and reinfarction after myocardial infarction. N. Engl. J. Med. 319:385, 1988.

667. The Danish Study Group on Verapamil in Myocardial Infarction: Effect of verapamil on mortality and major events after acute myocardial infarction (the Danish Verapamil Infarction Trial II — DAVIT II). Am. J. Cardiol. 66:779, 1990.

668. Renard, M., Sterling, I., Van Camp G., et al.: Comparison of the effect of intravenous diltiazem and a placebo on hemodynamics and blood gases in the acute phase of myocardial infarction. Ann. Cardiol. Angiol. 36:509, 1987.

669. Kloner, R. A., and Braunwald, E.: Effects of calcium antagonists on infarcting myocardium. Am. J. Cardiol. 59:84B, 1987.

670. Held, P. H., Yusuf, S., and Furberg, C. D.: Calcium channel blockers in acute myocardial infarction and unstable angina: an overview. Br. Med. J. 299:1187, 1989.

671. Mantle, J. A., Rogers, W. J., McDaniel, H. G., et al.: Metabolic support of mechanical performance in myocardial infarction in man — a randomized clinical trial of glucose-insulin-potassium. Am. J. Cardiol. 43:395, 1979.

672. Rogers, W. J., Segall, P. H., McDaniel, H. G., et al.: Prospective randomized trial of glucose-insulin-potassium in acute myocardial infarction. Am. J. Cardiol. 43:801, 1979.

673. Heng, M. K., Norris, R. M., Singh, B. N., and Barratt-Boyes, C.: Effects of glucose and glucose-insulin-potassium on haemodynamics and enzyme release after acute myocardial infarction. Br. Heart J. 39:748, 1977.

674. Powell, W. J., Jr., Daggett, W. M., Magro, A. E., et al.: Effects of intra-aortic balloon counterpulsation on cardiac performance, oxygen consumption, and coronary blood flow in dogs. Circ. Res. 26:753, 1970.

675. Leinbach, R. C., Gold, H. K., Harper, R. W., et al.: Early intraaortic balloon pumping for anterior myocardial infarction without shock. Circulation 58:204, 1978.

676. Flaherty, J. T., Becker, L. C., Weiss, J. L., et al.: Results of a randomized prospective trial of intraaortic balloon counterpulsation and intravenous nitroglycerin in patients with acute myocardial infarction. J. Am. Coll. Cardiol. 6:434, 1985.

677. Alderman, J. D., Gabliani, G. I., McCabe, C. H., et al.: Incidence and management of limp ischemia with percutaneous wire-guided intraaortic balloon catheters. J. Am. Coll. Cardiol. 9:524, 1987.

678. Werns, S. W., Shea, M. J., Driscoll, E. M., et al.: The independent effects of

679. oxygen radical scavengers on canine infarct size reduction by superoxide dismutase but not catalase. Circ. Res. 56:895, 1985.

679. Myers, M. L., Bolli, R., Lekich, R. F., et al.: Enhancement of recovery of myocardial function by oxygen free-radical scavengers after reversible regional ischemia. Circulation 72:915, 1985.

680. Shechter, M., Hod, H., Marks, N., et al.: Beneficial effects of magnesium sulfate in acute myocardial infarction. Am. J. Cardiol. 66:271, 1990.

ARRHYTHMIAS

681. Meltzer, L. E., and Cohen, H. E.: The incidence of arrhythmias associated with acute myocardial infarction. In Meltzer, L. E., and Dunning, A. J. (eds.): Textbook of Coronary Care. Philadelphia, Charles Press, 1972.

682. Pantridge, J. F., and Adgey, A.A.J.: Pre-hospital coronary care. The mobile coronary care unit. Am. J. Cardiol. 24:666, 1969.

683. Hinkel, L. E., Jr., Carver, S. T., and Stevens, M.: The frequency of asymptomatic disturbances of cardiac rhythm and conduction in middle-aged men. Am. J. Cardiol. 24:629, 1969.

684. Bloor, C. M., Ehsani, A., White, F. C., and Sobel, B. E.: Ventricular fibrillation threshold in acute myocardial infarction and its relation to myocardial infarct size. Cardiovasc. Res. 9:468, 1975.

685. Roque, F., Amuchastegui, L. M., Lopez Morillos, M. A., et al.: Beneficial effects of timolol on infarct size and late ventricular tachycardia in patients with myocardial infarction. Circulation 76:610, 1987.

686. Corr, P. B., and Gillis, R. A.: Autonomic neural influences on the dysrhythmias resulting from myocardial infarction. Circ. Res. 43:1, 1978.

687. Barber, M. J., Mueller, T. M., Davies, B. G., et al.: Interruption of sympathetic and vagal-mediated afferent responses by transmural myocardial infarction. Circulation 72:623, 1985.

688. Lassers, B. E., Anderton, J. L., George, M., et al.: Hemodynamic effects of artificial pacing in complete heart block complicating acute myocardial infarction. Circulation 38:308, 1968.

689. Ruskin, J., McHale, P. A., Harley, A., and Greenfield, J. C., Jr.: Pressure-flow studies in man; effects of atrial systole on left ventricular function. J. Clin. Invest. 49:472, 1970.

690. Rahimtoola, S. H., Ehsani, A., Sinno, M. Z., et al.: Left atrial transport function in myocardial infarction: Importance of its booster function. Am. J. Med. 59:686, 1975.

691. Adgey, A.A.J., Alley, J. D., Geddes, J. S., et al.: Acute phase of myocardial infarction. Lancet 2:501, 1971.

692. Graner, L. E., Gershen, B. J., Orlando, M. M., and Epstein, S. E.: Bradycardia and its complications in the pre-hospital phase of acute myocardial infarction. Am. J. Cardiol 32:607, 1973.

693. Mark, A. L.: The Bezold-Jarisch reflex revisited: Clinical implications of inhibitory reflexes originating in the heart. J. Am. Coll. Cardiol. 1:90, 1983.

694. Topol, E. J., Goldschlager, N., Ports, T. A., et al.: Hemodynamic benefit of atrial pacing in right ventricular myocardial infarction. Ann. Intern. Med. 96:594, 1982.

695. Damato, A. N., and Lau, S. H.: Clinical value of the electrogram of the conduction system. Prog. Cardiovasc. Dis. 13:119, 1970.

696. Rotman, M., Wagner, G. S., and Wallace, A.G.P.: Bradyarrhythmias in acute myocardial infarction. Circulation 45:703, 1972.

697. Norris, R. M., and Mercer, C. J.: Significance of idioventricular rhythms in acute myocardial infarction. Prog. Cardiovasc. Dis. 16:455, 1974.

698. Fisch, G. R., Zipes, D. P., and Fisch, C.: Bundle branch block and sudden death. Prog. Cardiovasc. Dis. 23:187, 1980.

699. Bilbao, F. J., Zabalza, I. E., Vilanova, J. R., and Froupe, J.: Atrioventricular block in posterior acute myocardial infarction. A clinicopathologic correlation. Circulation 75:733, 1987.

700. Mavric, Z., Zaputovic, L., Matana, A., et al.: Prognostic significance of complete atrioventricular block in patients with acute inferior myocardial infarction with and without right ventricular involvement. Am. Heart J. 119:823, 1990.

701. Kostuk, W. J., and Beanlands, D. S.: Complete heart block associated with acute myocardial infarction. Am. J. Cardiol. 26:380, 1970.

702. Bassan, R., Maia, I. G., Bozza, A., Amino, J.G.C., and Santos, M.: Atrioventricular block in acute inferior wall myocardial infarction: Harbinger of associated obstruction of the left anterior descending coronary artery. J. Am. Coll. Cardiol. 8:773, 1986.

703. Sagiura, T., Iwasaka, T., Takahashi, N., et al.: Factors associated with late onset of advanced atrioventricular block in acute Q wave inferior infarction. Am. Heart J. 119:1008, 1990.

704. Berger, P. B., and Ryan, T. J.: Inferior myocardial infarction. High-risk subgroups. Circulation 81:401, 1990.

705. Nicod, P., Gilpin, E., Dittrich, H., et al.: Long-term outcome in patients with inferior myocardial infarction and complete atrioventricular block. J. Am. Coll. Cardiol. 12:589, 1988.

706. Hindman, M. C., Wagner, G. S., JaRo, M., et al.: The clinical significance of bundle branch block complicating acute myocardial infarction. 2. Indications for temporary and permanent pacemaker insertion. Circulation 58:689, 1978.

707. Feigl, D., Ashkenazy, J., and Kishon, Y.: Early and late atrioventricular block in acute inferior myocardial infarction. J. Am. Coll. Cardiol. 4:35, 1984.

708. Mullins, C. B., and Atkins, J. M.: Prognoses and management of ventricular conduction blocks in acute myocardial infarction. Mod. Concepts Cardiovasc. Dis. 45:129, 1976.

709. Scheinman, M. M., and Gonzalez, R. P.: Fascicular block and acute myocardial infarction. JAMA 244:2646, 1980.

710. Hindman, M. C., Wagner, G. S., JaRo, M., et al.: The clinical significance of bundle branch block complicating acute myocardial infarction. I. Clinical characteristics, hospital mortality and one-year follow-up. Circulation 58:679, 1978.

711. Dubois, C., Pierard, L. A., Smeets, J.-P., et al.: Short- and long-term prognostic importance of complete bundle-branch block complicating acute myocardial infarction. Clin. Cardiol. 11:292, 1988.

712. Lamas, G. A., Muller, J. E., Turi, Z. G., et al.: A simplified method to predict occurrence of complete heart block during acute myocardial infarction. Am. J. Cardiol. 57:1213, 1986.

713. Hynes, J. K., Holmes, D. R., Jr., and Harrison, C. E.: Five-year experience with temporary pacemaker therapy in the coronary care unit. Mayo Clin. Proc. 58:122, 1983.

714. Zoll, P.: Resuscitation of the heart in ventricular standstill by external electrical stimulation. N. Engl. J. Med. 247:768, 1952.

715. Zoll, P. M., Zoll, R. H., Falk, R. H., et al.: External noninvasive temporary cardiac pacing: Clinical trials. Circulation 71:937, 1985.

716. Frye, R. L., Collins, J. J., DeSanctis, R. W., et al.: Guidelines for permanent cardiac pacemaker implantation. J. Am. Coll. Cardiol. 4:434, 1984.

717. ACC/AHA Task Force on Assessment of Diagnostic and Therapeutic Cardiovascular Procedures (Subcommittee on Pacemaker Implantation): Guidelines for permanent cardiac pacemaker implantation. J. Am. Coll. Cardiol. 4:434, 1984.

718. Ginks, W. R., Sutton, R., Oh, W., and Leatham, A.: Long-term prognosis after acute inferior infarction with atrioventricular block. Br. Heart J. 39:186, 1977.

719. Wilson, C., and Adgey, A.A.J.: Survival of patients with late ventricular fibrillation after acute myocardial infarction. Lancet 2:214, 1974.

720. DeSanctis, R. W., Block, P., and Hutter, A. M.: Tachyarrhythmias in myocardial infarction. Circulation 45:681, 1972.

721. Berisso, M. Z., Carratino, L., Ferroni, A., et al.: Frequency, characteristics and significance of supraventricular tachyarrhythmias detected by 24-hour electrocardiographic recording in the late hospital phase of acute myocardial infarction. Am. J. Cardiol. 65:1064, 1990.

722. Gordon, S., Finck, D. R., Perera, R. D., Levine, J., and Barnes, S. J.: Atrial infarction complicating an acute inferior myocardial infarction. Arch. Intern. Med. 144:193, 1984.

723. James, T. N.: Myocardial infarction and atrial arrhythmias. Circulation 24:761, 1961.

724. Hod, H., Lew, A. S., Keltai, M., et al.: Early atrial fibrillation during evolving myocardial infarction: A consequence of impaired left atrial perfusion. Circulation 75:146, 1987.

725. Goldberg, R. J., Seeley, D., Becker, R. C., et al.: Impact of atrial fibrillation on the in-hospital and long-term survival of patients with acute myocardial infarction: a community-wide perspective. Am. Heart J. 119:996, 1990.

726. Kerber, R. E., Jensen, S. R., Grayzel, J., et al.: Elective cardioversion: Influence of paddle-electrode location and size on success rates and energy requirements. N. Engl. J. Med. 305:658, 1981.

727. Konecke, L. L., and Knoebel, S. B.: Nonparoxysmal junctional tachycardia complicating acute myocardial infarction. Circulation 45:367, 1972.

728. Weinberg, B., and Zipes, D.: Strategies to manage the post-MI patient with ventricular arrhythmias. Clin. Cardiol. 12(Suppl. III):86, 1989.

728a. Lee, K. J., Wellens, H.J.J., Dorsnar, E., and Durrer, D.: Observations on patients with primary ventricular fibrillation complicating acute myocardial infarction. Circulation 52:755, 1975.

729. El-Sherif, N., Myerburg, R. J., Scherlag, B. J., et al.: Electrocardiographic antecedents of primary ventricular fibrillation. Value of the R-on-T phenomenon in myocardial infarction. Br. Heart J. 38:415, 1976.

730. El-Sherif, N., Scherlag, B. J., and Lazzara, R.: Electrode catheter recordings during malignant ventricular arrhythmias following experimental acute myocardial ischemia. Evidence for reentry due to conduction delay and block in ischemic myocardium. Circulation 51:1003, 1975.

731. DeSoyza, N., Meacham, D., Murphy, M. L., et al.: Evaluation of warning arrhythmias before paroxysmal ventricular tachycardia during acute myocardial infarction in man. Circulation 60:814, 1979.

732. Campbell, R.W.F., Murray, A., and Julian, D. G.: Relation of ventricular arrhythmias to ventricular fibrillation. Br. Heart J. 43:109, 1980.

733. Koster, R. W., and Dunning, J.: Intramuscular lidocaine for prevention of lethal arrhythmias in the prehospitalization phase of acute myocardial infarction. N. Engl. J. Med. 313:1105, 1985.

734. Josephson, M. E.: Treatment of ventricular arrhythmias after myocardial infarction. Circulation 74:653, 1986.

735. Lie, K. I., Wellens, H. J., and Van Capelli, F. J.: Lidocaine in the prevention of primary ventricular fibrillation. A double-blind randomized study of 212 consecutive patients. N. Engl. J. Med. 291:1324, 1974.

736. DeSilva, R. E., Hennekens, C. H., Lown, B., and Casscells, S. W.: Lidocaine prophylaxis in acute myocardial infarction: An evaluation of methodology. Lancet 1:855, 1981.

737. Dunn, H. M., McComb, J. M., Kinney, C. D., et al.: Prophylactic lidocaine in the early phase of suspected myocardial infarction. Am. Heart J. 110:353, 1985.

738. May, G. S., Furberg, C. D., Eberlein, K. A., and Geraci, B. J.: Secondary prevention after myocardial infarction. A review of short-term acute phase trials. Prog. Cardiovasc. Dis. 25:335, 1983.

739. Wyse, D. G., Kellen, J., and Rademaker, A. W.: Prophylactic versus selective lidocaine for early ventricular arrhythmias of myocardial infarction. J. Am. Coll. Cardiol. 12:507, 1988.

740. Hine, L. K., Laird, N., Hewitt, P., and Chalmers, T. C.: Meta-analytic evidence against prophylactic use of lidocaine in acute myocardial infarction. Arch. Intern. Med. 149:2694, 1989.

741. Mehra, R., Zeiler, R. H., Gough, W. B., and El-Sherif, N.: Reentrant ventricular arrhythmias in the later myocardial infarction period. 9. Electrophysiologic-anatomic correlation of reentrant circuits. Circulation 67:11, 1983.

742. Lopez, L. M., Mehta, J. L., Robinson, J. D., and Roberts, R. J.: Optimal lidocaine dosing in patients with myocardial infarction. Therap. Drug Monitoring 4:271, 1982.

743. Feely, J., Wade, D., McAllister, C. B., et al.: Effect of hypotension on liver blood flow and lidocaine disposition. N. Engl. J. Med. 307:866, 1982.

744. LeLorier, J., Grenon, D., Latour, Y., et al.: Pharmacokinetics of lidocaine after prolonged intravenous infusions in uncomplicated myocardial infarction. Ann. Intern. Med. 87:700, 1977.

745. Kessler, K. M., Kayden, D. S., Estes, D. M., et al.: Procainamide pharmacokinetics in patients with acute myocardial infarction or congestive heart failure. J. Am. Coll. Cardiol. 7:1131, 1986.

746. Keefe, D. L., Williams, S., Torres, V., et al.: Prophylactic tocainide or lidocaine in acute myocardial infarction. Am. J. Cardiol. 57:527, 1986.

747. Rehnqvist, N., Ericsson, G. G., Ericsson, S., et al.: Comparative investigation of the antiarrhythmic effect of propafenone and lidocaine in patients with ventricular arrhythmias during acute myocardial infarction. Acta Med. Scand. 216:525, 1984.

748. Lown, B., and Wolf, M.: Approaches to sudden death from coronary heart disease. Circulation 44:130, 1971.

749. Wenger, T. L., Bigger, J. T., Jr., and Merrill, G. S.: Ventricular arrhythmias in the late hospital phase of acute myocardial infarction. Circulation 52:110, 1975.

750. Moss, A. J., De Camilla, J. J., Davis, H. P., and Bayer, L.: Clinical significance of ventricular ectopic beats in the early post-hospital phase of myocardial infarction. Am. J. Cardiol. 39:635, 1977.

751. Mukharji, J., and MILIS Study Group: Risk factors for sudden death after acute myocardial infarction. Am. J. Cardiol. 54:31, 1984.

752. The Cardiac Arrhythmia Suppression Trial (CAST) Investigators: Preliminary report: effect on encainide and flecainide on mortality in a randomized trial of arrhythmia suppression after myocardial infarction. N. Engl. J. Med. 321:405, 1989.

753. Ruskin, J. N.: The cardiac arrhythmia suppression trial (CAST). N. Engl. J. Med. 321:386, 1989.

754. Pratt, C. M., and Moye, L. A.: The cardiac arrhythmia suppression trial: background, interim results and implications. Am. J. Cardiol. 65:20B, 1990.

755. Task Force of the Working Group on Arrhythmias of the European Society of Cardiology: CAST and beyond: implications of the cardiac arrhythmia suppression trial. Circulation 81:1123, 1990.

756. Sclarovsky, S., Strasberg, B., Martonovich, G., and Agmon, J.: Ventricular rhythms with intermediate rates in acute myocardial infarction. Chest 74:180, 1978.

757. Bigger, J. T., Jr., Dresdale, R. J., Heissenbuttel, R. H., et al.: Ventricular arrhythmias in ischemic heart disease: Mechanism, prevalence, significance, and management. Prog. Cardiovasc. Dis. 19:255, 1977.

758. Lucente, M., Rebuzzi, A. G., Lanza, G. A., et al.: Circadian variation of ventricular tachycardia in acute myocardial infarction. Am. J. Cardiol. 62:670, 1988.

759. Kleiman, R. B., Miller, J. M., Buxton, A. E., et al.: Prognosis following sustained ventricular tachycardia occurring early after myocardial infarction. Am. J. Cardiol. 62:528, 1988.

759a. El-Sherif, N., Gough, W. B., and Restivo, M.: Reentrant ventricular arrhythmias in the late myocardial infarction period: Mechanism by which a short-long-short cardiac sequence facilitates the induction of reentry. Circulation 83:268, 1991.

760. Bigger, J. T., Jr., Weld, F. M., and Rolnitzky, L. M.: Prevalence, characteristics and significance of ventricular tachycardia (three or more complexes) detected with ambulatory electrocardiographic recording in the late hospital phase of acute myocardial infarction. Am. J. Cardiol. 48:815, 1981.

761. Nordehaug, J. E., Johannessen, K. A., and von der Lippe, G.: Serum potassium concentration as a risk factor of ventricular arrhythmias early in acute myocardial infarction. Circulation 71:645, 1985.

762. Wald, R. W., Waxman, M. B., Corey, P. N., et al.: Management of intractable ventricular tachyarrhythmias after myocardial infarction. Am. J. Cardiol. 44:329, 1979.

763. Guiraudon, G., Fontaine, G., Frank, R., et al.: Encircling endocardial ventriculotomy: A new surgical treatment for life-threatening tachycardias resistant to medical treatment following myocardial infarction. Ann. Thorac. Surg. 26:438, 1978.

764. Bourke, J. P., Hilton, C. J., McComb, J. M., et al.: Surgery for control of recurrent life-threatening ventricular tachyarrhythmias within 2 months of myocardial infarction. J Am. Coll. Cardiol. 16:42, 1990.

765. Schwartz, P. J., Zaza, A., Grazi, S., et al.: Effect of ventricular fibrillation complicating acute myocardial infarction on long-term prognosis: importance of the site of infarction. Am. J. Cardiol. 56:384, 1985.

766. Jensen, G.V.H., Torp-Pedersen, C., Kober, L., et al: Prognosis of late versus early ventricular fibrillation in acute myocardial infarction. Am. J. Cardiol. 66:10, 1990.

767. Lie, K. I., Liem, K. L., Schuilenburg, R. M., et al.: Early identification of patients developing late in-hospital ventricular fibrillation after discharge from the coronary care unit. Am. J. Cardiol. 41:674, 1978.

768. Sclarovsky, S., Zafrir, N., Strasberg, B., et al.: Ventricular fibrillation complicating temporary ventricular pacing in acute myocardial in-

farction: significance of right ventricular infarction. Am. J. Cardiol. 48:1160, 1981.

769. Toffler, G. H., Stone, P. H., Muller, J. E., et al.: Prognosis after myocardial infarction complicated by ventricular fibrillation. Circulation 74(Suppl. II):304, 1986.

770. Volpi, A., Cavalli, A., Franzosi, M. G., et al.: One-year prognosis of primary ventricular fibrillation complicating acute myocardial infarction. Am. J. Cardiol. 63:1174, 1989.

771. Ryden, L., Ariniego, R., Arnman, K., et al.: A double-blind trial of metoprolol in acute myocardial infarction. Effects on ventricular tachyarrhythmias. N. Engl. J. Med. 308:614, 1983.

772. Ehsani, A., Ewy, G. A., and Sobel, B. E.: Effects of electrical countershock on serum creatine phosphokinase (CPK) isoenzyme activity. Am. J. Cardiol. 37:12, 1976.

773. Abboud, F. M., Pansegrau, D. G., and Mark, A. L.: Autonomic responses to ventricular defibrillation. In Proceedings, Cardiac Defibrillation Conference, Purdue University, West Lafayette, Ind., 1975.

774. Heissenbuttel, R. H., and Bigger, J. T., Jr.: Bretylium tosylate, a newly available antiarrhythmic drug for ventricular arrhythmias. Ann. Intern. Med. 91:229, 1979.

775. Bellotto, F., Forman, R., and Buja, G.: Electromechanical dissociation in the acute myocardial infarction. A review of the literature shows the need for a codified definition. J. Electrophys. 2:517, 1988.

776. Charlap, S., Kahlam, S., Lichstein, E., and Frishman, W.: Electromechanical dissociation: diagnosis, pathophysiology, and management. Am. Heart J. 118:355, 1989.

HEMODYNAMIC DISTURBANCES

777. Forrester, J. S., Diamond, G., Chatterjee, K., and Swan, H.J.C.: Medical therapy of acute myocardial infarction by application of hemodynamic subsets. N. Engl. J. Med. 295:1356, 1976.

777a. Noble, R. J.: Myocardial infarction with hypotension. Chest 99:1012, 1991.

778. Dwyer, E. M., Greenberg, H. M., Steinberg, G., and the Multicenter Postinfarction Research Group: Clinical characteristics and natural history of survivors of pulmonary congestion during acute myocardial infarction. Am. J. Cardiol. 63:1423, 1989.

779. Coma-Canella, I., Lopez-Sendon, J., and Gamallo, C.: Low output syndrome in right ventricular infarction. Am. Heart J. 98:613, 1979.

780. Page, D. L., Caulfield, J. B., Kastor, J. A., et al.: Myocardial changes associated with cardiogenic shock. N. Engl. J. Med. 285:133, 1971.

781. Alonso, D. R., Scheidt, S., Post, M., and Killip, T.: Pathophysiology of cardiogenic shock; quantification of myocardial necrosis, clinical, pathologic and electrocardiographic correlation. Circulation 48:588, 1973.

782. Wackers, F. J., Lie, K. I., Becker, A. E., et al.: Coronary artery disease in patients dying from cardiogenic shock or congestive heart failure in the setting of acute myocardial infarction. Br. Heart J. 38:906, 1976.

783. Hands, M. E., Rutherford, J. D., Muller, J. E., et al.: The in-hospital development of cardiogenic shock after myocardial infarction: Incidence, predictors of occurrence, outcome and prognostic factors. J. Am. Coll. Cardiol. 14:40, 1989.

784. Gunnar, R. M.: Cardiogenic shock complicating acute myocardial infarction. Circulation 78:1508, 1988.

785. Killip, T.: Cardiogenic shock complicating myocardial infarction. J. Am. Coll. Cardiol. 14:47, 1989.

786. Rasanen, J., Nikki, O. P., and Heikkila, J.: Acute myocardial infarction complicated by respiratory failure. The effects of mechanical ventilation. Chest 85:21, 1984.

787. Roth, A., Hochenberg, M., Keren, G., et al.: Are rotating tourniquets useful for left ventricular preload reduction in patients with acute myocardial infarction and heart failure? Ann. Emer. Med. 16:764, 1987.

788. Cohn, J. N., Franciosa, J. A., Francis, G. S., et al.: Effect of short-term infusion on sodium nitroprusside on mortality rate in acute myocardial infarction complicated by left ventricular failure. Results of a Veterans Administration Cooperative Study. N. Engl. J. Med. 306:1129, 1982.

789. Passamani, E. R.: Nitroprusside in myocardial infarction. N. Engl. J. Med. 306:1168, 1982.

790. Chiariello, M., Gold, H. K., Leinbach, R. C., et al.: Comparison between the effects of nitroprusside and nitroglycerin on ischemic injury during acute myocardial infarction. Circulation 54:766, 1976.

791. Flaherty, J. T.: Intravenous nitroglycerin. Johns Hopkins Med. J. 151:36, 1982.

792. Rabinowitz, B., Tamari, I., Elazar, E., and Neufeld, H. N.: Intravenous isosorbide dinitrate in patients with refractory pump failure and acute myocardial infarction. Circulation 65:771, 1982.

793. Franciosa, J. A., Mikulic, E., Cohn, J. N., et al.: Hemodynamic effects of orally administered isosorbide dinitrate in patients with congestive heart failure. Circulation 50:1020, 1974.

794. Cohn, J. N.: Editorial—Progress in vasodilator therapy for heart failure. N. Engl. J. Med. 302:1414, 1980.

795. Franciosa, J. A., Guiha, N. H., Limas, C. J., et al.: Improved left ventricular function during nitroprusside infusion in acute myocardial infarction. Lancet 1:650, 1972.

796. Covell, J. W., Braunwald, E., Ross, J., Jr., and Sonnenblick, E. H.: Studies on digitalis. XVI. Effects on myocardial oxygen consumption. J. Clin. Invest. 45:1535, 1966.

797. Ross, J., Jr., Waldhausen, J. S., and Braunwald, E.: Studies on digitalis. I. Direct effects on peripheral vascular resistance. J. Clin. Invest. 39:930, 1960.

798. Marchionni, N., Pini, R., Vannucci, A., et al.: Hemodynamic effects of digoxin in acute myocardial infarction in man: A randomized controlled trial. Am. Heart J. 109:63, 1985.

799. Moss, A. J., Davis, H. T., Conrad, D. L., et al.: Digitalis-associated cardiac mortality after myocardial infarction. Circulation 64:1150, 1981.

800. Muller, J. E., Turi, Z. G., Stone, P. H., et al.: Digoxin therapy and mortality after myocardial infarction. Experience in the MILIS study. N. Engl. J. Med. 314:265, 1986.

801. Bigger, J. T., Jr., Fleiss, J. L., Rolnitzky, L. M., et al.: Effects of digitalis treatment on survival after acute myocardial infarction. Am. J. Cardiol. 55:623, 1985.

802. Mueller, H., Ayres, S. M., Giannelli, S., Jr., et al.: Effect of isoproterenol, L-norepinephrine, and intra-aortic counterpulsation on hemodynamics and myocardial metabolism in shock following acute myocardial infarction. Circulation 45:335, 1972.

803. Shell, W. E., and Sobel B. E.: Deleterious effects of increased heart rate on infarct size in the conscious dog. Am. J. Cardiol. 31:474, 1973.

804. Ichard, C., Ricome, J. L., Rimailho, A., et al.: Combined hemodynamic effects of dopamine and dobutamine in cardiogenic shock. Circulation 67:620, 1983.

805. Holzer, J., Karliner, J. S., O'Rourke, R. A., et al.: Effectiveness of dopamine in patients with cardiogenic shock. Am. J. Cardiol. 32:79, 1973.

806. Arnold, J.M.O., Braunwald, E., Sandor, T., and Kloner, R. A.: Inotropic stimulation of reperfused myocardium with dopamine: Effects on infarct size and myocardial function. J. Am. Coll. Cardiol. 6:1026, 1985.

807. Tuttle, R. R., and Mills, J.: Development of a new catecholamine to selectively increase cardiac contractility. Circ. Res. 36:185, 1975.

808. Maekawa, K., Liang, C-S., and Hood, W. B., Jr.: Comparison of dobutamine and dopamine in acute myocardial infarction. Effects of systemic hemodynamics, plasma catecholamines, blood flows and infarct size. Circulation 67:750, 1983.

809. Mancini, D., LeJemtel, T., and Sonnenblick, E.: Intravenous use of amrinone for the treatment of the failing heart. Am. J. Cardiol. 56:8B, 1985.

810. Taylor, S. H., Verma, S. P., Hussain, M., et al.: Intravenous amrinone in left ventricular failure complicated by acute myocardial infarction. Am. J. Cardiol. 56:29B, 1985.

811. Verma, S. P., Silke, B., and Taylor, S. H.: Hemodynamic dose-response effects of amrinone in left ventricular failure complicating myocardial infarction. Br. J. Clin. Pharmacol. 19:540P, 1985.

812. Colucci, W. S., Wright, R. F., and Braunwald, E.: New positive inotropic agents in the treatment of congestive heart failure. N. Engl. J. Med. 314:349, 1986.

813. Mueller, H., Ayres, S. M., Gregory, J. J., et al.: Hemodynamics, coronary blood flow, and myocardial metabolism in coronary shock: Response to L-norepinephrine and isoproterenol. J. Clin. Invest. 49:1885, 1970.

814. Lee, L., Bates, E. R., Pitt, B., et al.: Percutaneous transluminal coronary angioplasty improves survival in acute myocardial infarction complicated by cardiogenic shock. Circulation 78:1345, 1988.

815. Sotolongo, R. P., Smith, M. L., and Margolis, W. S.: Coronary angioplasty in emergency treatment of myocardial infarction. Texas Heart Inst. J. 17:31, 1990.

816. Lew, A., Weiss, A. T., Shah, P. K., et al.: Extensive myocardial salvage and reversal of cardiogenic shock after reperfusion of the left main coronary artery by intravenous streptokinase. Am. J. Cardiol. 54:450, 1984.

817. Alosilla, C. E., Bell, W. W., Ferree, J., and De La Torre, A.: Thrombolytic therapy during acute myocardial infarction due to sudden occlusion of the left main coronary artery. J. Am. Coll. Cardiol. 5:1253, 1985.

818. Corral, C. H., and Vaughn, C. C.: Intraaortic balloon counterpulsation: An eleven-year review and analysis of determinants of survival. Texas Heart Inst. J. 13:39, 1986.

819. Mueller, H., Ayres, S. M., Conklin, E. F., et al.: The effects of intra-aortic counterpulsation on cardiac performance and metabolism in shock associated with acute myocardial infarction. J. Clin. Invest. 50:1885, 1971.

820. Johnson, S. A., Scanlon, P. J., Loeb, H. S., et al.: Treatment of cardiogenic shock in myocardial infarction by intraaortic balloon counterpulsation and surgery. Am. J. Med. 62:687, 1977.

821. O'Rourke, M. F., Norris, R. M., Campbell, T. J., et al.: Randomized controlled trial of intraaortic balloon counterpulsation in early myocardial infarction with acute heart failure. Am. J. Cardiol. 47:815, 1981.

822. Goldberg, M. J., Rubenfire, M., Kantrowitz, A., et al.: Intraaortic balloon pump insertion: A randomized study comparing percutaneous and surgical techniques. J. Am. Coll. Cardiol. 9:515, 1987.

823. Pae, W. E., Jr., and Pierce, W. S.: Temporary left ventricular assistance in acute myocardial infarction and cardiogenic shock. Rationale and criteria for utilization. Chest 79:692, 1981.

824. Shawl, F. A., Domanski, M. J., Hernandez, T. J., and Punja, S.: Emergency percutaneous cardiopulmonary bypass support in cardiogenic shock from acute myocardial infarction. Am. J. Cardiol. 64:967, 1989.

825. Gowda, S. K., Gillespie, T. A., Byrne, J. D., et al.: Effects of external counterpulsation on enzymatically estimated infarct size and ventricular arrhythmia. Br. Heart J. 40:308, 1978.

826. Isner, J. M., Cohen, S. J., Viruari, R., et al.: Complications of the intra-aortic balloon counterpulsation device: Clinical and morphologic observations in 45 necropsy patients. Am. J. Cardiol. 45:250, 1980.

827. Goodwin, M., Hartmann, J., McKeever, L., et al.: Safety of intraaortic balloon counterpulsation in patients with acute myocardial infarction receiving streptokinase intravenously. Am. J. Cardiol. 64:937, 1989.

828. Dell-Italia, L. J., Lembo, N. J., Starling, M. R., et al.: Hemodynamically important right ventricular infarction. Follow-up evaluation of right

ventricular systolic function at rest and during exercise with radionuclide ventriculography and respiratory gas exchange. Circulation 75:996, 1987.

829. Roberts, N., Harrision, D. G., Reimer, K. A., et al.: Right ventricular infarction with shock but without significant left ventricular infarction: A new clinical syndrome. Am. Heart J. *110*:1047, 1985.

830. Forman, M. B., Goodin, J., Phelan, B., et al.: Electrocardiographic changes associated with isolated right ventricular infarction. J. Am. Coll. Cardiol. *4*:640, 1984.

831. Bansal, R. C., Marsa, R. J., Holland, D., et al.: Severe hypoxemia due to shunting through a patent foramen ovale: A correctable complication of right ventricular infarction. J. Am. Coll. Cardiol. *5*:188, 1985.

832. Robalino, B. D., Petrella, R. W., Jubran, F. Y., et al.: Atrial natriuretic factor in patients with right ventricular infarction. J. Am. Coll. Cardiol. *15*:546, 1990.

833. Braat, S. H., Brugada, P., DeZwaan, C., et al.: Right and left ventricular ejection fraction in acute inferior wall infarction with or without ST segment elevation in lead V4R. J. Am. Coll. Cardiol. *4*:940, 1984.

834. Lopez-Sendon, J., Garcia-Fernandez, M. A., Coma-Canella, I., et al.: Segmental right ventricular function after acute myocardial infarction: Two-dimensional echocardiographic study in 63 patients. Am. J. Cardiol. *51*:390, 1983.

835. Arditti, A., Lewin, R. F., Hellman, C., et al.: Right ventricular dysfunction in acute inferoposterior myocardial infarction. An echocardiographic isotopic study. Chest *87*:307, 1985.

836. Starling, M. R., Dell'italia, L. J., Chaudhuri, T. K., et al.: First transit and equilibrium radionuclide angiography in patients with inferior transmural myocardial infarction: Criteria for the diagnosis of associated hemodynamically significant right ventricular infarction. J. Am. Coll. Cardiol. *4*:923, 1984.

837. Dell'italia, L. J., Starling, M. R., Crawford, M. H., et al.: Right ventricular infarction: Identification by hemodynamic measurements before and after volume loading and correlation with noninvasive techniques. J. Am. Coll. Cardiol. *4*:931, 1984.

838. Yasuda, T., Okada, R. D., Leinbach, R. C., et al.: Serial evaluation of right ventricular dysfunction associated with acute inferior myocardial infarction. Am. Heart J. *119*:816, 1990.

839. Matangi, M. F.: Temporary physiologic pacing in inferior wall acute myocardial infarction with right ventricular damage. Am. J. Cardiol. *59*:1207, 1987.

840. Marmor, A., Geltman, E. M., Biello, D. R., et al.: Functional response to the right ventricle to myocardial infarction: Dependence on the site of left ventricular infarction. Circulation *64*:1005, 1981.

841. Lorell, B., Leinbach, R. C., Pohost, G. M., et al.: Right ventricular infarction. Clinical diagnosis and differentiation from cardiac tamponade and pericardial constriction. Am. J. Cardiol. *43*:465, 1979.

842. Korr, K. S., Lewvinson, H., Bough, E. W., et al.: Tricuspid valve replacement for cardiogenic shock after acute right ventricular infarction. JAMA *244*:1958, 1980.

843. Pohjola-Sintonen, S., Muller, J. E., Stone, P. H., et al.: Ventricular septal and free wall rupture complicating acute myocardial infarction: Experience in the Multicenter Investigation of Limitation of Infarct Size. Am. Heart J. *117*:809, 1989.

844. Reddy, S. G., and Roberts, W. C.: Frequency of rupture of the left ventricular free wall or ventricular septum among necropsy cases of fatal acute myocardial infarction since introduction of coronary care units. Am. J. Cardiol. *63*:906, 1989.

845. Shapira, I., Isakov, A., Burke, M., and Almong, C. H.: Cardiac rupture in patients with acute myocardial infarction. Chest *92*:219, 1987.

845a. Pappas, P. J., Cernaianu, A. C., Baldino, W. A., et al.: Ventricular free-wall rupture after myocardial infarction. Chest *99*:892, 1991.

846. Silverman, H. S., and Pfeifer, M. P.: Relation between use of anti-inflammatory agents and left ventricular free wall rupture during acute myocardial infarction. Am. J. Cardiol. *59*:363, 1987.

847. Bulkley, B. H., and Roberts, W. C.: Steroid therapy during acute myocardial infarction: A cause of delayed healing and of ventricular aneurism. Am. J. Med. *56*:244, 1974.

848. Gertz, S. D., Kragel, A. H., Kalan, J. M., et al.: Comparison of coronary and myocardial morphologic findings in patients with and without thrombolytic therapy during fatal first acute myocardial infarction. Am. J. Cardiol. *66*:904, 1990.

849. Honan, M. B., Harrell, F. E., Reimer, K. A., et al.: Cardiac rupture, mortality and the timing of thrombolytic therapy: a meta-analysis. J. Am. Coll. Cardiol. *16*:359, 1990.

850. Edmondson, H. A., and Hoxie, H. J.: Hypertension and cardiac rupture: Clinical and pathological study of 72 cases, in 13 of which rupture of the interventricular septum occurred. Am. Heart J. *24*:719, 1942.

851. London, R. E., and London, S. B.: Rupture of the heart. A critical analysis of 47 consecutive autopsy cases. Circulation *31*:202, 1965.

852. Kassis, E., Vogelsang, M., and Lyngborg, K.: Cardiac rupture complicating myocardial infarction. A study concerning early diagnosis and possible management. Dan. Med. Bull. *48*:164, 1981.

853. Mann, J. M., and Roberts, W. C.: Rupture of the left ventricular free wall during acute myocardial infarction: Analysis of 138 necropsy patients and comparison with 50 necropsy patients with acute myocardial infarction without rupture. Am. J. Cardiol. *62*:847, 1988.

854. Balakumaran, K., Verbaan, C. J., Essed, C. E., et al.: Ventricular free wall rupture: sudden, subacute, slow, sealed and stabilized varieties. Eur. Heart J. *5*:282, 1984.

855. Coma-Canella, I., Lopez-Sendon, J., Gonzalez, L. N., and Ferrufino, O.: Subacute left ventricular free wall rupture following acute myocardial infarction: Bedside hemodynamics, differential diagnosis, and treatment. Am. Heart J. *106*:278, 1983.

856. Pifarre, R., Sullivan, H. J., Grieco, J., et al.: Management of left ventricular rupture complicating myocardial infarction. J. Thorac. Cardiovasc. Surg. *86*:441, 1983.

857. McMullan, M. H., Kilgore, T. L., Dear, H. D., and Hindman, S. H.: Sudden blowout rupture of the myocardium after infarction: Urgent management. J. Thorac. Cardiovasc. Surg. *89*:259, 1985.

858. Vlodaver, Z., Coe, J. L., and Edwards, J. E.: True and false left ventricular aneurysms. Circulation *51*:567, 1975.

858a. Lascault, G., Reeves, F., and Drobinski, G.: Evidence of the inaccuracy of standard echocardiographic and angiographic criteria used for the recognition of true and "false" left ventricular inferior aneurysms. Br. Heart J. *60*:125, 1988.

859. Shabbo, F. P., Dymond, D. S., Rees, G. M., and Hill, I. M.: Surgical treatment of false aneurysm of the left ventricle after myocardial infarction. Thorax *38*:25, 1983.

860. Radford, M. J., Johnson, R. A., Daggett, W. M., et al.: Ventricular septal rupture: A review of clinical and physiologic features and an analysis of survival. Circulation *64*:545, 1981.

861. Edwards, B. S., Edwards, W. D., and Edwards, J. E.: Ventricular septal rupture complicating acute myocardial infarction: Identification of simple and complex types in 53 autopsied hearts. Am. J. Cardiol. *54*:1201, 1984.

862. Mann, J. M., and Roberts, W. C.: Acquired ventricular septal defect during acute myocardial infarction: analysis of 38 unoperated necropsy patients and comparison with 50 unoperated necropsy patients without rupture. Am. J. Cardiol. *62*:8, 1988.

863. Moore, C. A., Nygaard, T. W., Kaiser, D. L., et al.: Postinfarction ventricular septal rupture: the importance of location of infarction and right ventricular function in determining survival. Circulation *74*:45, 1986.

864. Cummings, R. G., Reimer, K. A., Califf, R., et al.: Quantitative analysis of right and left ventricular infarction in the presence of postinfarction ventricular septal defect. Circulation *77*:33, 1988.

865. Bansal, R. C., Eng, A. K., and Shakudo, M.: Role of two-dimensional echocardiography, pulsed, continuous wave and color flow Doppler techniques in the assessment of ventricular septal rupture after myocardial infarction. Am. J. Cardiol. *65*:852, 1990.

866. Helmcke, F., Mahan, E. F., Nanda, N. C., et al.: Two-dimensional echocardiography and Doppler color flow mapping in the diagnosis and prognosis of ventricular septal rupture. Circulation *81*:1775, 1990.

866a. Fortin, D. F., Sheikh, K. H., and Kisslo, J.: The utility of echocardiography in the diagnostic strategy of postinfarction ventricular septal rupture: A comparison of two-dimensional echocardiography versus Doppler color flow imaging. Am. Heart J. *121*:25, 1991.

867. Lock, J. E., Block, P. C., McKay, R. G., et al.: Transcatheterization closure of ventricular septal defects. Circulation *78*:361, 1988.

868. Nishimura, R. A., Schaff, H. V., Shub, C., et al.: Papillary muscle rupture complicating acute myocardial infarction: Analysis of 17 patients. Am. J. Cardiol. *51*:373, 1983.

869. Barbour, D. J., and Roberts, W. C.: Rupture of a left ventricular papillary muscle during acute myocardial infarction: Analysis of 22 necropsy patients. J. Am. Coll. Cardiol. *8*:588, 1986.

870. Coma-Canella, I., Gamallo, C., Onsurbe, P. M., and Jadraque, L. M.: Anatomic findings in acute papillary muscle necrosis. Am. Heart J. *118*:1188, 1989.

871. Lader, E., Colvin, S., and Tunick, P.: Myocardial infarction complicated by rupture of both ventricular septum and right ventricular papillary muscle. Am. J. Cardiol. *52*:424, 1983.

872. Come, P. C., Riley, M. F., Weintraub, R., et al.: Echocardiographic detection of complete and partial papillary muscle rupture during acute myocardial infarction. Am. J. Cardiol. *56*:787, 1985.

873. Harrison, M. R., MacPhail, B., Gurley, J., et al.: Usefulness of color Doppler flow imaging to distinguish ventricular septal defect from acute mitral regurgitation complicating myocardial infarction. Am. J. Cardiol. *64*:697, 1989.

874. Ballester, M., Tasca, R., Marin, L., et al.: Different mechanisms of mitral regurgitation in acute and chronic forms of coronary heart disease. Eur. Heart J. *4*:557, 1983.

875. Meister, S. G., and Helfant, R. H.: Rapid bedside differentiation of ruptured interventricular septum from acute mitral insufficiency. N. Engl. J. Med. *287*:1024, 1972.

876. Jones, M. T., Schofield, P. M., Dark, J. F., et al.: Surgical repair of acquired ventricular septal defects: Determinants of early and late outcome. J. Thorac. Cardiovasc. Surg. *93*:680, 1987.

877. Miller, D. C., and Stinson, E. B.: Surgical management of acute mechanical defects secondary to myocardial infarction. Am. J. Surg. *141*:677, 1981.

878. Held, A. C., Cole, P. L., Lipton, B., et al.: Rupture of the interventricular septum complicating acute myocardial infarction: a multicenter analysis of clinical findings and outcome. Am. Heart J. *116*:1330, 1988.

879. Norell, M. S., Gershlick, A. H., Pillai, R., et al.: Ventricular septal rupture complicating myocardial infarction: Is earlier surgery justified? Eur. Heart J. *8*:1281, 1987.

880. Abrams, D. L., Edelist, A., Luria, M. H., and Miller, A. J.: Ventricular aneurysm: A reappraisal based on a study of 65 consecutive autopsied cases. Circulation *27*:164, 1963.

881. Faxon, D. P., Ryan, T. J., Davis, K. B., et al.: Prognostic significance of angiographically documented left ventricular aneurysm from the Coronary Artery Surgery Study (CASS). Am. J. Cardiol. *50*:157, 1982.

882. Schlichter, J., Hellerstein, H. K., and Katz, L. N.: Aneurysm of the heart: A correlative study of 102 proved cases. Medicine *33*:43, 1954.

883. Forman, M. D., Collins, H. W., Kipelman, H. A., et al.: Determinants of left ventricular aneurysm formation after anterior myocardial infarction: A clinical and angiographic study. J. Am. Coll. Cardiol. 8:1256, 1986.

884. Hirai, T., Fujita, M., Nakajima, H., et al.: Importance of collateral circulation for prevention of left ventricular aneurysm formation in acute myocardial infarction. Circulation 79:791, 1989.

885. Meizlish, J. L., Berger, H. J., Plankey, M., et al.: Functional left ventricular aneurysm formation after acute anterior transmural myocardial infarction: Incidence, natural history, and prognostic implications. N. Engl. J. Med. 311:1001, 1984.

886. Lindsay, J., Jr., Dewey, R. C., Talesnick, B. S., and Nolan, N. G.: Relation of ST-segment elevation after healing of acute myocardial infarction to the presence of left ventricular aneurysm. Am. J. Cardiol. 54:84, 1984.

887. Brawley, R. K., Magovern, G. J., Jr., Gott, V. L., et al.: Left ventricular aneurysmectomy. Factors influencing postoperative results. J. Thorac. Cardiovasc. Surg. 85:712, 1983.

888. Visser, C. A., Kan, G., Lie, K. I., and Durrer, D.: Incidence and one-year follow-up of left ventricular thrombus following acute myocardial infarction: An echocardiographic study of 96 patients. J. Am. Coll. Cardiol. 1:648, 1983.

889. Hellerstein, H. K., and Martin, J. W.: Incidence of thromboembolic lesions accompanying myocardial infarction. Am. Heart J. 33:443, 1947.

890. Nihoyannopoulos, P., Smith, G. C., Maseri, A., and Foale, R. A.: The natural history of left ventricular thrombus in myocardial infarction: a rationale in support of masterly inactivity. J. Am. Coll. Cardiol. 14:903, 1989.

891. Jugdutt, B. I., and Sivaram, C. A.: Prospective two-dimensional echocardiographic evaluation of left ventricular thrombus and embolism after acute myocardial infarction. J. Am. Coll. Cardiol. 13:554, 1989.

892. Funke Kupper, A. J., Verheugt, F.W.A., Peels, C. H., et al.: Left ventricular thrombus incidence and behavior studied by serial two-dimensional echocardiography in acute anterior myocardial infarction: left ventricular wall motion, systemic wall motion, systemic embolism and oral anticoagulation. J. Am. Coll. Cardiol. 13:1514, 1989.

893. Keren, A., Goldberg, S., Gottlieb, S., et al.: Natural history of left ventricular thrombi: their appearance and resolution in the posthospitalization period of acute myocardial infarction. J. Am. Coll. Cardiol. 15:790, 1990.

894. Johannessen, K. A., Nordehaug, J. E., and von der Lippe, G.: Increased occurrence of left ventricular thrombi during early treatment with timolol in patients with acute myocardial infarction. Circulation 75:151, 1987.

895. Gueret, P., Dubourg, O., Ferrier, A., et al.: Effects of full-dose heparin anticoagulation on the development of left ventricular thrombosis in acute transmural myocardial infarction. J. Am. Coll. Cardiol. 8:419, 1986.

896. Sharma, B., Carvalho, A., Wyeth, R., and Franciosa, J. A.: Left ventricular thrombi diagnosed by echocardiography in patients with acute myocardial infarction treated with intracoronary streptokinase followed by intravenous heparin. Am. J. Cardiol. 56:422, 1985.

897. Nordrehaug, J. E., Johannessen, K. A., and von der Lippe, G.: Usefulness of high-dose anticoagulants in preventing left ventricular thrombus in acute myocardial infarction. Am. J. Cardiol. 55:1941, 1985.

898. Turpie, A.G.G., Robinson, J. G., Doyle, D. J., et al.: Comparison of high-dose with low-dose subcutaneous heparin to prevent left ventricular mural thrombosis in patients with acute transmural anterior myocardial infarction. N. Engl. J. Med. 320:352, 1989.

899. Motro, M., Keren, G., Hod, H., et al.: Incidence of left ventricular thrombi formation after thrombolytic therapy with recombinant tissue plasminogen activator, heparin, and aspirin in patients with acute myocardial infarction. Am. J. Cardiol. (in press).

900. Halperin, J. L., and Fuster, V.: Left ventricular thrombus and stroke after myocardial infarction: toward prevention or perplexity? J. Am. Coll. Cardiol. 14:912, 1989.

901. Weintraub, W. S., and Ba'albaki, H. A.: Decision analysis concerning the application of echocardiography to the diagnosis and treatment of mural thrombi after anterior wall myocardial infarction. Am. J. Cardiol. 64:708, 1989.

902. Stein, B., Fuster, V., Halperin, J. L., and Chesebro, J. H.: Antithrombotic therapy in cardiac disease. An emerging approach based on pathogenesis and risk. Circulation 80:1501, 1989.

903. Kouvaras, G., Chronopoulos, G., Soufras, G., et al.: The effects of long-term antithrombotic treatment on left ventricular thrombi in patients after an acute myocardial infarction. Am. Heart J. 119:73, 1990.

904. Kouvaras, G., Chronopoulos, G., Soufras, G., et al.: The effect of long-term antithrombotic treatment on left ventricular thrombi in patients after an acute myocardial infarction. Am. Heart J. 119:73, 1990.

905. Halperin, J. L., and Fuster, V.: Left ventricular thrombi and cerebral embolism. N. Engl. J. Med. 320:392, 1989.

906. Visser, C. A., Kan, G., Meltzer, R. S., et al.: Embolic potential of left ventricular thrombus after myocardial infarction: A two-dimensional echocardiographic study of 119 patients. J. Am. Coll. Cardiol. 5:1276, 1985.

907. Stratton, J. R., and Ritchie, J. L.: The effects of antithrombotic drugs in patients with left ventricular thrombi: Assessment with indium-111 platelet imaging and two-dimensional echocardiography. Circulation 69:561, 1984.

908. Kremer, P., Fiebig, R., Tilsner, V., et al.: Lysis of left ventricular thrombi with urokinase. Circulation 72:112, 1985.

909. Eppinger, E. C., and Kennedy, J. A.: The cause of death in coronary thrombosis, with special reference to pulmonary embolism. Am. J. Med. Sci. 195:104, 1938.

910. Stone, P., and Muller, J. E.: Nifedipine therapy for recurrent ischemic pain following myocardial infarction. Clin. Cardiol. 5:223, 1982.

911. Koiwaya, Y., Torii, S., Takeshita, A., et al.: Postinfarction angina caused by coronary arterial spasm. Circulation 65:275, 1982.

912. Bosch, X., Theroux, P., Waters, D. D., et al.: Early postinfarction ischemia: Clinical, angiographic, and prognostic significance. Circulation 75:988, 1987.

913. Benhorin, J., Andrews, M. L., Carleen, E. D., et al.: Occurrence, characteristics, and prognostic significance of early postacute myocardial infarction angina pectoris. Am. J. Cardiol. 62:679, 1988.

914. Epstein, S. E., Palmeri, S. T., and Patterson, R. E.: Evaluation of patients after acute myocardial infarction. Indications for cardiac catheterization and surgical intervention. N. Engl. J. Med. 307:1467, 1982.

915. Brunken, R., Tillisch, J., Schwaiger, M., et al.: Regional perfusion, glucose metabolism, and wall motion in patients with chronic electrocardiographic Q wave infarctions: Evidence for persistence of viable tissue in some infarct regions by positron emission tomography. Circulation 73:951, 1986.

916. Johnson, L. L., Seldin, D. W., Keller, A. M., et al.: Dual isotope thallium and indium antimyosin SPECT imaging to identify acute infarct patients at further ischemic risk. Circulation 81:37, 1990.

917. Brown, K. A., O'Meara, J., Chambers, C. E., and Plante, D. A.: Ability of dipyridamole-thallium-201 imaging one to four days after acute myocardial infarction to predict in-hospital and late recurrent myocardial ischemic events. Am. J. Cardiol. 65:160, 1990.

918. Muller, J. E., Rude, R. E., Braunwald, E., et al.: Myocardial recurrence, outcome, and risk factors in the Multicenter Investigation of Infarct Size. Ann. Intern. Med. 108:1, 1988.

919. Ellis, S. G., Topol, E. J., George, B. S., et al.: Recurrent ischemia without warning. Analysis of risk factors for in-hospital ischemic events, following successful thrombolysis with intravenous tissue plasminogen activator. Circulation 80:1159, 1989.

920. Isaacsohn, J. L., Earle, M. G., Kemper, A. J., and Parisi, A. F.: Postmyocardial infarction pain and infarct extension in the coronary care unit: Role of two-dimensional echocardiography. J. Am. Coll. Cardiol. 11:246, 1988.

921. Baker, J. T., Bramlet, D. A., Lester, R. M., et al.: Myocardial infarct extension: Incidence and relationship to survival. Circulation 65:918, 1982.

922. Marmor, A., Sobel, B. E., and Roberts, E.: Factors presaging early recurrent myocardial infarction ("extension"). Am. J. Cardiol. 48:603, 1981.

923. Pierard, L. A., Albert, A., Henrard, L., et al.: Incidence and significance of pericardial effusion in acute myocardial infarction as determined by two-dimensional echocardiography. J. Am. Coll. Cardiol. 8:517, 1986.

924. Charlap, S., Greenberg, S., Greengart, A., et al.: Pericardial effusion early in acute myocardial infarction. Clin. Cardiol. 12:252, 1989.

925. Sugiura, T., Iwasaka, T., Takayama, Y., et al.: Factors associated with pericardial effusion in acute Q wave myocardial infarction. Circulation 81:477, 1990.

926. Somolinos, M., Violán, S., Sanz, R., and Marrero, P.: Early pericarditis after acute myocardial infarction: A clinical echocardiographic study. Crit. Care Med. 15:648, 1987.

927. Tofler, G. H., Muller, J. E., Stone, P. H., et al.: Pericarditis in acute myocardial infarction: Characterization and clinical significance. Am. Heart J. 117:86, 1989.

928. Lichstein, E., Liu, H.-M., and Gupta, P.: Pericarditis complicating acute myocardial infarction: incidence of complications and significance of electrocardiogram on admission. Am. Heart J. 87:246, 1974.

929. Blau, N., Shen, B. A., Pittman, D. E., and Joyner, C. E.: Massive hemopericardium in a patient with post-myocardial infarction syndrome. Chest 71:549, 1977.

930. Karim, A. H., and Salomon, J.: Constrictive pericarditis after myocardial infarction. Sequelae of anticoagulant-induced hemopericardium. Am. J. Med. 79:389, 1985.

931. Lichstein, E., Arsura, E., Hollander, G., et al.: Current incidence of postmyocardial infarction (Dressler's) syndrome. Am. J. Cardiol. 50:1269, 1982.

932. Northcote, R. J., Hutchinson, S. J., and McGuinness, J. B.: Evidence for the continued existence of the postmyocardial infarction (Dressler's) syndrome. Am. J. Cardiol. 53:1201, 1984.

933. Brown, E. J., Jr., Kloner, R. A., Schoen, F. J., et al.: Scar thinning due to ibuprofen administration following experimental myocardial infarction. Am. J. Cardiol. 51:877, 1983.

934. Silverman, H. S., and Pfeifer, M. P.: Relation between use of anti-inflammatory agents and left ventricular free wall rupture during acute myocardial infarction. Am. J. Cardiol. 59:363, 1987.

935. Friedman, P. L., Brown, E. J., Jr., Gunther, S., et al.: Coronary vasoconstrictor effect of indomethacin in patients with coronary artery disease. N. Engl. J. Med. 305:1171, 1981.

CONVALESCENCE, DISCHARGE, AND POST-MI CARE

936. Rowe, M. H., Jelinek, M. V., Liddell, N., and Hugens, M.: Effect of rapid mobilization on ejection fractions and ventricular volumes after acute myocardial infarction. Am. J. Cardiol. 63:1037, 1989.

937. Kloner, R. A., and Kloner, J. A.: The effect of early exercise on myocardial infarct scar formation. Am. Heart J. 106:1009, 1983.

938. Hammerman, H., Kloner, R. A., Alker, K. U., et al.: Effects of transient increased afterload during experimentally induced acute myocardial infarction in dogs. Am. J. Cardiol. 55:566, 1985.

939. Madsen, E. B.: Time of discharge for patients with acute myocardial infarction. Cardiovasc. Rev. Rep. 4:1301, 1983.

940. Pryor, D. B., Hindman, M. C., Wagner, G. S., et al.: Early discharge after acute myocardial infarction. Ann. Intern. Med. 99:528, 1983.

940a. Mark, D., Sigmon, K., Topol, E. J., et al.: Identification of acute myocardial infarction patients suitable for early hospital discharge after aggressive interventional therapy. Circulation 83:1186, 1991.

941. Abraham, A. S., Sever, Y., Weinstein, M., et al.: Value of early ambulation in patients with and without complications after acute myocardial infarction. N. Engl. J. Med. 292:719, 1975.

942. Madsen, E. B., Hougaard, P., Gilpin, E., and Pedersen, S.: The length of hospitalization after acute myocardial infarction determined by risk calculation. Circulation 68:9, 1983.

943. Topol, E. J., Burek, K., O'Neill, W. W., et al.: A randomized controlled trial of hospital discharge three days after myocardial infarction in the era of reperfusion. N. Engl. J. Med. 318:1083, 1988.

944. Bates, E. R., and Topol, E. J.: Early hospital discharge in the myocardial reperfusion era. Clin. Cardiol. 12(Suppl. III):65, 1989.

945. Jugdutt, B. I., Michorowski, B. L., and Kappagoda, C. T.: Exercise training after anterior Q wave myocardial infarction: Importance of regional left ventricular function and topography. J. Am. Coll. Cardiol. 12:362, 1988.

946. Papadopoulos, C.: A survey of sexual activity after myocardial infarction. Cardiovasc. Med. 3:821, 1978.

947. Tardif, G. S.: Sexual activity after a myocardial infarction. Arch. Phys. Med. Rehabil. 70:763, 1989.

948. Friedman, M., Thoresen, C. E., Gill, J. J., et al.: Feasibility of altering type A behavior pattern after myocardial infarction. Recurrent coronary prevention project study: Methods, baseline results and preliminary findings. Circulation 66:83, 1982.

949. Powell, L. H., and Thoresen, C. A.: Effects of type A behavioral counseling and severity of prior acute myocardial infarction on survival. Am. J. Cardiol. 62:1159, 1988.

950. Health and Public Policy Committee, American College of Physicians: Cardiac Rehabilitation Services. Ann. Intern. Med. 109:671, 1988.

951. Squires, R. W., Gau, G. T., Miller, T. D., et al.: Cardiovascular rehabilitation: Status, 1990. Mayo Clin. Proc. 65:731, 1990.

952. Greenland, P., and Chu, J. S.: Efficacy of cardiac rehabilitation services, with emphasis on patients after myocardial infarction. Ann. Intern. Med. 109:650, 1988.

953. O'Connor, G. T., Buring, J. E., Yusuf, S., et al.: An overview of randomized trials of rehabilitation with exercise after myocardial infarction. Circulation 80:234, 1989.

954. Moss, A. J., and Benhorin, J.: Prognosis and management after a first myocardial infarction. N. Engl. J. Med. 322:743, 1990.

955. Taylor, S. H.: Secondary prevention after myocardial infarction: Facts and fallacies. J. Cardiovasc. Pharmacol. 6:5914, 1984.

956. Rosenberg, L., Kaufman, D. W., Helmrich, S. P., and Shapiro, S.: The risk of myocardial infarction after quitting smoking in men under 55 years of age. N. Engl. J. Med. 313:1511, 1985.

957. Myers, M. G.: Changing patterns in drug therapy for ischemic heart disease. Can. Med. Assoc. J. 312:644, 1984.

958. Snow, P.J.D.: Effect of propranolol in myocardial infarction. Lancet 2:735, 1965.

959. Beta Blocker Heart Attack Study Group: The Beta-Blocker Heart Attack Trial. JAMA 246:2073, 1981.

960. Herlitz, J., Elmfeldt, D., Holmberg, S., et al.: Goteborg metoprolol trial: Mortality and causes of death. Am. J. Cardiol. 53:9D, 1984.

961. Pedersen, T. R., and the Norwegian Multicenter Study Group: Six-year follow-up of the Norwegian multicenter study on timolol after acute myocardial infarction. N. Engl. J. Med. 313:1055, 1985.

962. Taylor, S. H., Silke, B., Ebbutt, A., et al.: A long-term prevention study with oxprenolol in coronary heart disease. N. Engl. J. Med. 307:1293, 1982.

963. May, G. S.: A review of acute-phase beta-blocker trials in patients with myocardial infarction. Circulation 67(Suppl. I):21, 1983.

964. Gundersen, T.: Secondary prevention after myocardial infarction: subgroup analysis of patients at risk in the Norwegian timolol multicenter study. Clin. Cardiol. 8:253, 1985.

965. Chadda, K., Goldstein, S., Byington, R., and Curb, J. D.: Effect of propranolol after acute myocardial infarction in patients with congestive heart failure. Circulation 73:503, 1986.

966. Herlitz, J., Hjalmarson, A., Holmberg, S., et al.: Development of congestive heart failure after treatment with metoprolol in acute myocardial infarction. Br. Heart J. 51:539, 1984.

967. Beta-Blocker Pooling Project Research Group: The Beta-Blocker Pooling Project (BBPP): subgroup findings from randomized trials in post-infarction patients. Eur. Heart J. 9:8, 1988.

968. Herlitz, J., Hjalmarson, A., Swedberg, K., et al.: Effects on mortality during five years after early intervention with metoprolol in suspected acute myocardial infarction. Acta Med. Scand. 223:227, 1988.

969. Olsson, G., Oden, A., Johansson, L., et al.: Prognosis after withdrawal of chronic postinfarction metoprolol treatment: A 2–7 year follow-up. Eur. Heart J. 9:365, 1988.

970. Goldstein, S.: Review of beta blocker myocardial infarction trials. Clin. Cardiol. 12(Suppl. III):54, 1989.

971. Gundersen, T., Abrahamsen, A. M., Kjekshus, J., and Ronnevik, P. K.: Timolol-related reduction in mortality and reinfarction in patients ages 65–77 years surviving acute myocardial infarction. Circulation 66:1179, 1982.

972. Goldman, L., Sia, S.T.B., Cook, E. F., et al.: Costs and effectiveness of routine therapy with long-term beta-adrenergic antagonists after acute myocardial infarction. N. Engl. J. Med. 319:152, 1988.

973. Ahumada, G. G.: Identification of patients who do not require beta antagonists after myocardial infarction. Am. J. Med. 76:900, 1984.

974. Lopressor Intervention Trial Research Group: The Lopressor Intervention Trial: multicentre study of metoprolol in survivors of acute myocardial infarction. Eur. Heart J. 8:1056, 1987.

975. Modan, B., Shani, M., Schor, S., and Modan, M.: Reduction of hospital mortality from acute myocardial infarction by anticoagulant therapy. N. Engl. J. Med. 292:1359, 1975.

976. Horwitz, R. I., and Feinstein, A. R.: The application of therapeutic trial principles to improve the design of epidemiologic research: A case-control study suggesting that anticoagulants reduce mortality in patients with myocardial infarction. J. Chron. Dis. 34:575, 1981.

977. Turpie, A.G.G.: Anticoagulant therapy after acute myocardial infarction. Am. J. Cardiol. 65:20C, 1990.

978. Smith, P., Arnesen, H., and Holme, I.: The effect of warfarin on mortality and reinfarction after myocardial infarction. N. Engl. J. Med. 323:147, 1990.

979. Anticoagulants in acute myocardial infarction: Results of a cooperative clinical trial. JAMA 225:724, 1973.

980. Wray, R., Maurer, B., and Shillingford, J.: Prophylactic anticoagulant therapy in the prevention of calf-vein thrombosis after myocardial infarction. N. Engl. J. Med. 288:815, 1973.

981. Pitt, A., Anderson, S. T., Habersberger, P. G., and Rosengarten, D. S.: Low dose heparin in the prevention of deep thromboses in patients with acute myocardial infarction. Am. Heart J. 99:574, 1980.

982. Goldberg, R. J., Gore, J. J., Dalen, J. E., and Alpert, J. S.: Long-term anticoagulant therapy after acute myocardial infarction. Am. Heart J. 109:616, 1985.

983. Elwood, P. C.: Aspirin in the prevention of myocardial infarction: Current status. Drugs 28:1, 1984.

984. Friedewald, W. T., Furberg, C. D., and May, G. S.: Aspirin and myocardial infarction. Cardiovasc. Rev. Rep. 5:1285, 1984.

985. Antiplatelet Trialists' Collaboration: Secondary prevention of vascular disease by prolonged antiplatelet treatment. Br. Med. J. 296:320, 1988.

986. Anturane Reinfarction Trial Research Group: Sulfinpyrazone in the prevention of sudden death after myocardial infarction. N. Engl. J. Med. 302:250, 1980.

987. Klimt, C. R., Knatterud, G. L., Stamler, J., and Meier, P.: Persantine-aspirin reinfarction study. Part II. Secondary coronary prevention with persantine and aspirin. J. Am. Coll. Cardiol. 7:251, 1986.

988. Israeli Sprint Study Group: Secondary Prevention Reinfarction Israel Nifedipine Trial (SPRINT). A randomized intervention trial of nifedipine in patients with acute myocardial infarction. Eur. Heart J. 9:354, 1988.

989. Roberts, R.: Review of calcium antagonists trials in acute myocardial infarction. Clin. Cardiol. 12(Suppl. III):41, 1989.

990. Gibson, R. S., Boden, W. E., Theroux, P., et al.: Diltiazem and reinfarction in patients with non-Q wave infarction. N. Engl. J. Med. 315:423, 1986.

991. Gibson, R. S.: Management of acute non-Q-wave myocardial infarction: Role of prophylactic pharmacotherapy and indications for predischarge coronary arteriography. Clin. Cardiol. 12(Suppl. III):26, 1989.

992. Rapport, E.: Influence of long-acting nitrate therapy on the risk of reinfarction, sudden death, and total mortality in survivors of acute myocardial infarction. Am. Heart J. 110:276, 1985.

993. May, G. S., Furberg, C. D., Eberlein, K. A., and Geraci, B. J.: Secondary prevention after myocardial infarction: A review of short-term acute phase trials. Prog. Cardiovasc. Dis. 25:335, 1983.

994. May, G. S., Eberlein, K. A., Furberg, C. D., et al.: Secondary prevention after myocardial infarction: A review of long-term trials. Prog. Cardiovasc. Dis. 25:331, 1982.

995. Gottlieb, S. H., Achuff, S. C., Mellits, E. D., et al.: Prophylactic antiarrhythmic therapy of high-risk survivors of myocardial infarction: Lower mortality at 1 month but not at 1 year. Circulation 75:792, 1987.

996. Rasmussen, H. S., Gronbaek, M., Cintin, C., et al.: One-year death rate in 270 patients with suspected acute myocardial infarction, initially treated with intravenous magnesium or placebo. Clin. Cardiol. 11:377, 1988.

997. Canner, P. L., Berge, K. G., Weuger, N. K., et al.: Fifteen-year mortality in Coronary Drug Project patients: Long-term benefits with niacin. J. Am. Coll. Cardiol. 8:1245, 1986.

998. Carlson, L. A., and Rosenhaumer, G.: Reduction of mortality in the Stockholm ischaemic heart disease secondary prevention study by combined treatment with clofibrate and nicotinic acid. Acta Med. Scand. 223:405, 1988.

999. Freidman, M., Thoresen, C. E., Gill, J. J., et al.: Alteration of type A behavior and its effect on cardiac recurrences in post myocardial infarction patients: Summary results of the recurrent coronary prevention project. Am. Heart J. 112:653, 1986.

1000. Rossouw, J. E., Lewis, B., and Rifkind, B. M.: The value of lowering cholesterol after myocardial infarction. N. Engl. J. Med. 323:1112, 1990.

1001. Madsen, E. B., Hougaard, P., and Gilpin, E.: Dynamic evaluation of prognosis from time-dependent variables in acute myocardial infarction. Am. J. Cardiol. 51:1579, 1983.

1002. DeBusk, R. F., for the Health and Public Policy Committee of the Clinical Efficacy Assessment Subcommittee, American College of Physicians: Evaluation of patients after recent acute myocardial infarction. Ann. Intern. Med. 110:485, 1989.

1003. Taylor, G. J., Humphries, J. O., Mellits, E. D., et al.: Predictors of clinical course, coronary anatomy and left ventricular function after recovery from acute myocardial infarction. Circulation 62:960, 1980.

1004. Norris, R. M., Barnaby, P. F., Brandt, P.W.T., et al.: Prognosis after recovery from first acute myocardial infarction: Determinants of reinfarction and sudden death. Am. J. Cardiol. 53:408, 1984.

1005. Killip, T., and Kimball, J. I.: Treatment of myocardial infarction in a coronary care unit. A two year experience with 250 patients. Am. J. Cardiol. 20:457, 1967.

1006. Pell, A.A.F., Semple, T., Wang, I., et al.: A coronary prognostic index for garding the severity of infarction. Br. Heart J. 24:745, 1962.

1007. Norris, R. M., Brandt, P.W.T., Caughey, D. E., et al.: A new coronary prognostic index. Lancet 1:274, 1969.

1008. Tofler, G. H., Stone, P. H., Muller, J. E., et al.: Effects of gender and race on prognosis after myocardial infarction: Adverse prognosis for women, particularly black women. J. Am. Coll. Cardiol. 9:473, 1987.

1008a. Greenland, P., Reicher-Reiss, H., Goldbourt, U., et al.: In-hospital and 1-year mortality in 1524 women after myocardial infarction: comparison with 4315 men. Circulation 83:484, 1991.

1009. Tofler, G. H., Muller, J. E., Stone, P. H., et al.: Factors leading to shorter survival after acute myocardial infarction in patients aging 65 to 75 years compared with younger patients. Am. J. Cardiol. 62:860, 1988.

1010. Marcus, F. I., Friday, K., McCans, J., et al.: Age-related prognosis after acute myocardial infarction (The Multicenter Diltiazem Postinfarction Trial). Am. J. Cardiol. 65:559, 1990.

1011. Stone, P. H., Muller, J. E., Hartwell, T., et al.: The effect of diabetes mellitus on prognosis and serial left ventricular function after acute myocardial infarction: Contribution of both coronary disease and diastolic left ventricular dysfunction to the adverse prognosis. J. Am. Coll. Cardiol. 14:49, 1989.

1012. DeBusk, R. F., Kraemer, H. C., and Nash, E.: Stepwise risk stratification soon after acute myocardial infarction. Am. J. Cardiol. 52:1161, 1983.

1013. Merrilees, M. A., Scott, P. J., and Norris, R. M.: Prognosis after myocardial infarction: results of 15 year follow-up. Br. Med. J. 288:356, 1984.

1014. Benhorin, J., Moss, A. J., Oakes D., and the Multicenter Diltiazem Postinfarction Trial Research Group: Prognostic significance of nonfatal myocardial reinfarction. J. Am. Coll. Cardiol. 15:253, 1990.

1015. Smith, J. W., Marcus, F. I., and Serokman, R. with the Multicenter Postinfarction Research Group: Prognosis of patients with diabetes mellitus after acute myocardial infarction. Am. J. Cardiol. 54:718, 1984.

1016. Abbott, R. D., Donaue, R. P., Kannel, W. B., and Wilson, P. F.: The impact of diabetes on survival following myocardial infarction in men vs. women. The Framingham Study. JAMA 260:3456, 1988.

1017. Rennert, G., Saltz-Rennerts, H., Wanderman, K., and Weitzman, S.: Size of acute myocardial infarcts in patients with diabetes mellitus. Am. J. Cardiol. 55:1629, 1985.

1018. Gwilt, D.J.G., Petri, M., Lewis, P. W., et al.: Myocardial infarct size and mortality in diabetic patients. Br. Heart J. 54:466, 1985.

1019. The Coronary Drug Project Research Group: Blood pressure in survivors of myocardial infarction. J. Am. Coll. Cardiol. 4:1134, 1984.

1020. Maisel, A. S., Gilpin, E., Holt, B., et al.: Survival after hospital discharge in matched populations with inferior or anterior myocardial infarction. J. Am. Coll. Cardiol. 6:731, 1985.

1021. Hands, M. E., Lloyd, B. L., Robinson, J. S., et al.: Prognostic significance of electrocardiographic site of infarction after correction for enzymatic size and infarction. Circulation 73:885, 1986.

1022. Bosch, X., Theroux, P., Waters, D. D., et al.: Early postinfarction ischemia: Clinical, angiographic, and prognostic significance. Circulation 75:988, 1987.

1023. Koiwaya, Y., Nakagaki, O., Takeshita, A., and Nakamura, M.: Clinical characteristics and prognosis of patients with postinfarction angina caused by coronary artery spasm. Clin. Cardiol. 7:68, 1984.

1024. Tzivoni, D., Gavish, A., Zin, D., et al.: Prognostic significance of ischemic episodes in patients with previous myocardial infarction. Am. J. Cardiol. 62:661, 1988.

1025. Kannel, W. B., and Abbott, R. D.: Incidence and prognosis of unrecognized myocardial infarction. N. Engl. J. Med. 311:1144, 1984.

1026. Madsen, E. B., Gilpin, E., and Henning, H.: Evaluation and prognosis one year after myocardial infarction. J. Am. Coll. Cardiol. 4:985, 1983.

1027. Henning, H., Gilpin, E., Covell, J. W., et al.: Prognosis after acute myocardial infarction: A multivariate analysis of mortality and survival. Circulation 59:1124, 1979.

1028. Madsen, E. B., Gilpin, E., Henning, H., et al.: Prediction of late mortality after myocardial infarction from variables measured at different times during hospitalization. Am. J. Cardiol. 53:47, 1984.

1029. Ross, J., Gilpin, E. A., Madsen, E. B., et al.: A decision scheme for coronary angiography after acute myocardial infarction. Circulation 79:292, 1989.

1030. Chaitman, B. R., Thompson, B. W., Kern, M. J., et al.: Tissue plasminogen activator followed by percutaneous transluminal coronary angioplasty: one-year TIMI phase II pilot results. Am. Heart J. 119:213, 1990.

1031. Hillis, L. D., Forman, S., Braunwald, E., and The Thrombolysis in Myocardial Infarction (TIMI) Phase II Co-Investigators: Risk stratification before thrombolytic therapy in patients with acute myocardial infarction. J. Am. Coll. Cardiol. 16:313, 1990.

1032. Becker, L. C., Silverman, K. J., Bulkley, B. H., et al.: Comparison of early thallium-201 scintigraphy and gated blood pool imaging for predicting mortality in patients with acute myocardial infarction. Circulation 67:1272, 1983.

1033. Shiina, A., Tajik, A. J., Smith, H. C., et al.: Prognostic significance of regional wall motion abnormality in patients with prior myocardial infarction: A prospective correlative study of two-dimensional echocardiography and angiography. Mayo Clin. Proc. 61:254, 1986.

1034. Warnowicz, M. A., Parker, H., and Cheitlin, M. D.: Prognosis of patients with acute pulmonary edema and normal ejection fraction after acute myocardial infarction. Circulation 67:330, 1983.

1035. Work, J. W., Ferguson, J. G., and Diamond, G. A.: Limitations of a conventional logistic regression model based on left ventricular ejection fraction in predicting coronary events after myocardial infarction. Am. J. Cardiol. 64:702, 1989.

1036. Pilote, L., Silberberg, J., Lisbona, R., and Sniderman, A.: Prognosis in patients with low left ventricular ejection fraction after myocardial infarction. Circulation 80:1636, 1989.

1037. Haines, D. E., Beller, G. A., Watson, D. D., et al.: A prospective clinical, scintigraphic, angiographic and functional evaluation of patients after inferior myocardial infarction with and without right ventricular dysfunction. J. Am. Coll. Cardiol. 6:995, 1985.

1038. Piérard, L. A., Dubois, C., Albert, A., et al.: Prognostic significance of a low peak serum creatine kinase level in acute myocardial infarction. Am. J. Cardiol. 63:792, 1989.

1039. Holman, B. L., Chisholm, R. J., and Braunwald, E.: The prognostic implications of acute myocardial infarct scintigraphy with 99mTc-pyrophosphate. Circulation 57:320, 1978.

1040. Nicod, P., Gilpin, E., Dittrich, H., et al.: Short- and long-term clinical outcome after Q wave and non-Q wave myocardial infarction in a large patient population. Circulation 79:528, 1989.

1041. O'Brien, T. X., and Ross, J.: Non-Q-wave myocardial infarction: Incidence, pathophysiology, and clinical course compared with Q-wave infarction. Clin. Cardiol. 12(Suppl. III):3, 1989.

1042. Gibson, R. S., Beller, G. A., Gheorghiade, M., et al.: The prevalence and clinical significance of residual mycardial ischemia 2 weeks after uncomplicated non-Q wave infarction: A prospective natural history study. Circulation 73:1186, 1986.

1043. Connolly, D. C., and Elveback, L. R.: Coronary heart disease in residents of Rochester, Minnesota. VI. Hospital and posthospital course of patients with transmural and subendocardial myocardial infarction. Mayo Clin. Proc. 60:375, 1985.

1044. Gibson, R. S.: Clinical, functional, and angiographic distinctions between Q wave and non-Q wave myocardial infarction: Evidence of spontaneous reperfusion and implications for intervention trials. Circulation 75(Suppl. V):128, 1987.

1045. Madigan, N. P., Rutherford, B. D., and Frye, R. L.: The clinical course, early prognosis and coronary anatomy of subendocardial infarction. Am. J. Med. 60:634, 1976.

1046. Maisel, A. S., Ahnve, S., Gilpin, E., et al.: Prognosis after extension of myocardial infarct: The role of Q wave or non-Q wave infarction. Circulation 71:211, 1985.

1047. Benhorin, J., Moss, A. J., Oakes, D., et al.: The prognostic significance of first myocardial infarction type (Q wave versus non-Q wave) and Q wave location. J. Am. Coll. Cardiol. 15:1201, 1990.

1048. Fox, J. P., Beattie, J. M., Salih, M. S., et al.: Non Q wave infarction: Exercise test characteristics, coronary anatomy, and prognosis. Br. Heart J. 63:151, 1990.

1049. Safian, R. D., Snyder, L. D., Snyder, B. A., et al.: Usefulness of percutaneous transluminal coronary angioplasty for unstable angina pectoris after non-Q wave acute myocardial infarction. Am. J. Cardiol. 59:263, 1987.

1050. Ferlinz, J.: Acute myocardial infarction: Does the lack of Q waves help or hinder? J. Am. Coll. Cardiol. 15:1208, 1990.

1051. Schechtman, K. B., Capone, R. J., Kleiger, R. E., et al.: Differential risk patterns associated with 3 month as compared with 3 to 12 month mortality and reinfarction after non-Q wave myocardial infarction. J. Am. Coll. Cardiol. 15:940, 1990.

1052. Boden, W. E., Gibson, R. S., Kleiger, R. E., et al.: Importance of early recurrent ischemia on one-year survival after non-Q wave acute myocardial infarction. Am. J. Cardiol. 64:799, 1989.

1053. Krone, R. J., Dwyer, E. M., Greenberg, H., et al.: Risk stratification in patients with first non-Q wave infarction: Limited value of the early low level exercise test after uncomplicated infarcts. J. Am. Coll. Cardiol. 14:31, 1989.

1053a. Schechtman, K. B., Kleiger, R. E., Capone, R. J., et al.: In-hospital angina following non-Q wave myocardial infarction: the long-term prognostic significance. Coronary Artery Disease 2:67, 1991.

1054. Denniss, A. R., Richards, D. A., Cody, D. V., et al.: Prognostic significance of ventricular tachycardia and fibrillation induced at programmed stimulation and delayed potentials detected on the signal-averaged electrocardiograms of survivors of acute myocardial infarction. Circulation 74:731, 1986.

1055. Kostis, J. B., Byington, R., Friedman, L. M., et al.: Prognostic significance of ventricular ectopic activity in survivors of acute myocardial infarction. J. Am. Coll. Cardiol. 10:231, 1987.

1056. Cripps, T., Bennett, D., Camm, J., and Ward, D.: Prospective evaluation of clinical assessment, exercise testing and signal-averaged electrocardiogram in predicting outcome after myocardial infarction. Am. J. Cardiol. 62:995, 1988.

1057. Wong, N. D., Levy, D., and Kannel, W. B.: Prognostic significance of the electrocardiogram after Q wave myocardial infarction. Circulation 81:780, 1990.

1058. DeFeyter, P. J., van Eenige, M. J., Dighton, D. H., and Roos, J. P.: Exercise testing early after myocardial infarction. Chest 83:853, 1983.

1059. DeBusk, R. F.: Specialized testing after recent acute myocardial infarction. Ann. Intern. Med. 110:470, 1989.

1060. Hamm, L. F., Crow, R. S., Stull, G. A., and Hannan, P.: Safety and characteristics of exercise testing early after acute myocardial infarction. Am. J. Cardiol. 63:1193, 1989.

1061. Waters, D. W., Bosch, X., Bouchard, A., et al.: Comparison of clinical variables and variables derived from a limited predischarge exercise test—a predictor of early and later mortality after myocardial infarction. J. Am. Coll. Cardiol. 5:1, 1985.

1062. Madsen, E. B., Gilpin, E., Ahnve, S., Henning, H., et al.: Prediction of functional capacity and use of exercise testing for predicting risk after acute myocardial infarction. Am. J. Cardiol. 56:839, 1985.

1063. Senaratne, M.P.J., Hsu, L., Rossall, R. E., and Kappagoda, C. T.: Exercise testing after myocardial infarction: relative values of the low level predischarge and the postdischarge exercise trial. J. Am. Coll. Cardiol. 12:1416, 1988.

1064. Krone, R. J., Gillespie, J. A., Weld, F. M., et al.: Low-level exercise testing after myocardial infarction: Usefulness in enhancing clinical risk stratification. Circulation 71:80, 1985.

1065. Handler, C. E., and Sowton, E.: Stress testing predischarge and six weeks after myocardial infarction to compare submaximal and maximal exercise predischarge and to assess the reproducibility of induced abnormalities. Int. J. Cardiol. 9:173, 1985.

1066. Hakki, A., Nestico, P. F., Heo, J., et al.: Relative prognostic value of rest thallium-201 imaging, radionuclide ventriculography and 24-hour ambulatory electrocardiographic monitoring after acute myocardial infarction. J. Am. Coll. Cardiol. 10:25, 1987.

1067. Hung, J., Goris, M. L., Nash, E., et al.: The comparative prognostic value of standard treadmill testing, rest and exercise thallium myocardial perfusion scintigraphy and radionuclide ventriculography 3 weeks after myocardial infarction. J. Am. Coll. Cardiol. 1:654, 1983.

1068. Morris, K. G., Palmeri, S. T., Califf, R. M., et al.: Value of radionuclide angiography for predicting specific cardiac events after acute myocardial infarction. Am. J. Cardiol. 55:318, 1985.

1069. Berning, J., and Steensgaard-Hansen, F.: Early estimation of risk by echocardiographic determination of wall motion index in an unselected population with acute myocardial infarction. Am. J. Cardiol. 65:567, 1990.

1070. The Multicenter Postinfarction Research Group: Risk stratification and survival after myocardial infarction. N. Engl. J. Med. 309:331, 1983.

1071. Bigger, J. T., Jr., Fleiss, J. L., Kleiger, R., et al.: The relationships among ventricular arrhythmias, left ventricular dysfunction, and mortality in the 2 years after myocardial infarction. Circulation 69:250, 1984.

1072. Mukharji, J., Rude, R., Gustafson, N., et al.: Late sudden death following myocardial infarction: Interdependence of risk factors. J. Am. Coll. Cardiol. 1:585, 1983.

1073. Richards, D. A., Cody, D. V., Denniss, A. R., et al.: Ventricular electrical instability: A predictor of death after myocardial infarction. Am. J. Cardiol. 51:75, 1983.

1074. Roy, D., Marchand, E., Theroux, P., et al.: Long-term reproducibility and significance of provokable ventricular arrhythmias after myocardial infarction. J. Am. Coll. Cardiol. 8:32, 1986.

1075. DiMarco, J. P., Lerman, B. B., Kron, I. L., and Sellers, T. D.: Sustained ventricular tachyarrhythmias within 2 months of acute myocardial infarction: Results of medical and surgical therapy in patients resuscitated from the initial episode. J. Am. Coll. Cardiol. 6:759, 1985.

1076. Piérard, L. A., Dubois, C., Albert, A., et al.: Prediction of mortality after myocardial infarction by simple clinical variables recorded during hospitalization. Clin. Cardiol. 12:500, 1989.

1076a. Bolognese, L., Sarasso, G., Bongo, A. S., et al.: Stress testing in the period after infarction. Circulation 83(Suppl. III)32, 1991.

1077. Younis, L. T., Byers, S., Shaw, L., et al.: Prognostic value of intravenous dipyridamole thallium scintigraphy after an acute myocardial ischemic event. Am. J. Cardiol. 64:161, 1989.

1078. Fioretti, P., Brower, R. W., Simoons, M. L., et al.: Relative value of clinical variables, bicycle ergometry, rest radionuclide ventriculography and 24-hour ambulatory electrocardiographic monitoring at discharge to predict 1-year survival after myocardial infarction. J. Am. Coll. Cardiol. 8:40, 1986.

1079. DeBusk, R. F., Blomqvist, G., Kouchoukos, N. T., et al.: Identification and treatment of low-risk patients after acute myocardial infarction and coronary-artery bypass graft surgery. N. Engl. J. Med. 314:161, 1986.

1080. ACC/AHA Task Force on Early Management of Acute Myocardial Infarction: Guidelines for the early management of patients with acute myocardial infarction. J. Am. Coll. Cardiol. 16:249, 1990.

1081. Kulick, S. L., and Rahimtoola, S. H.: Risk stratification in survivors of acute myocardial infarction. Routine cardiac catheterization and angiography is a reasonable approach in most patients. Am. Heart J. 121:641, 1991.

1082. Topol, E. J., Holmes, D. R., and Rogers, W. J.: Coronary angiography after thrombolytic therapy for acute myocardial infarction. Ann. Intern. Med. 114:877, 1991.

40

Chronic Ischemic Heart Disease

by JOHN D. RUTHERFORD, M.B., Ch.B., and EUGENE BRAUNWALD, M.D.

Chronic ischemic heart disease is usually due to obstruction of the coronary arteries, which in turn most commonly results from atherosclerosis; the pathogenesis of atherosclerosis is described in Chapter 36 and factors that predispose to this condition in Chapter 37. The importance of ischemic heart disease in contemporary society is attested to by the almost epidemic number of persons afflicted—especially when this number is compared with the anecdotal reports of its occurrence in the medical literature before this century. Ischemic heart disease causes more deaths, disability, and economic loss in industrialized nations than any other group of diseases.

In this century a dramatic increase in coronary heart disease mortality has occurred, with a peak being reached in the late 1960's in most industrialized countries. Since then a continuing downward trend in coronary heart disease mortality has been noted in North America, Belgium, Finland, Israel, Japan, Australia, and New Zealand. In contrast, in most Eastern European countries and in the U.S.S.R. and Sweden, death rates from coronary heart disease are still increasing.[1] In the United States, coronary artery disease (CAD) is the leading cause of death, and in 1989 there were an estimated 27.7 million physician visits for this diagnosis.[2] In 1987, the total economic impact of coronary heart disease amounted to an estimated $43 billion.[2] Despite major declines in mortality, coronary heart disease still causes over half a million deaths annually. It is estimated that 3.1 per cent of Americans (about 7 million) have clinically active coronary heart disease.

Community-based studies carried out in Rochester, Minnesota showed that the incidence of CAD increased until 1959, fell to the level recorded in 1954 over the next 5 years, and thereafter slowly declined until 1969.[3,4] These observations applied to angina pectoris, myocardial infarction, and sudden unexpected death, with the greatest decline being noted in the incidence of sudden death. This fall in the incidence of CAD was followed a decade later by lowering of the overall annual mortality rate and probably was a contributing factor. The 5-year survival of patients with angina pectoris improved from 75 per cent in the years 1950 to 1970 to 87 per cent during 1970 to 1975. The Allegheny County Coronary Heart Disease Mortality Study, ongoing since 1970, showed a decline in coronary heart disease mortality from 91 to 40 deaths per 100,000 per year in the years 1970 to 1972 to 1985 to 1986, respectively.[5] Two-thirds of this decline was related to a decline in sudden deaths, and it was concluded that primary prevention had contributed substantially to this decline.[5] Mortality rate among diabetics did not decline during the 17 years of the study, and the proportion of diabetics with CAD deaths actually increased.

It remains to be seen whether the decline in CAD mortality (in the countries in which it has been observed) is due to a reduction in incidence, a change in case fatality rates, or both of these factors. Whereas changing incidence might suggest that preventive programs are having an impact, changing case fatality rates suggest improvements in medical and surgical management of patients known to have CAD.

The widespread decline in mortality secondary to CAD noted in different countries with different health systems and in all age groups appears to be real rather than the result of changes in methods of classifying patients. Studies in Rochester already mentioned[3] suggest that both the incidence and the case fatality rates may be falling. The fact that the population rates of CAD can change substantially over the course of several years provides a strong argument that efforts to prevent and/or treat the disease have the potential for success.[5,6]

There is no uniform presenting syndrome for chronic ischemic heart disease. Although chest discomfort is usually the predominant symptom in chronic (stable) or unstable angina and acute myocardial infarction, syndromes of ischemic heart disease also occur in which ischemic chest discomfort is absent or not prominent. These include asymptomatic (silent) myocardial ischemia, cardiac arrhythmias, and congestive heart failure. There are also nonatherosclerotic causes of obstructive coronary artery disease.[6a] Myocardial ischemia may also occur in the absence of CAD (as in aortic valve disease, hypertrophic cardiomyopathy, and syphilitic aortitis), and CAD may occur with these other forms of heart disease. Finally, the various syndromes characteristic of ischemic heart disease may complicate noncardiac disease, e.g., coronary atherosclerosis occurs commonly in patients with chronic renal failure requiring dialysis (p. 1863).

Chronic Stable Angina Pectoris

CLINICAL MANIFESTATIONS

CHARACTERISTICS OF ANGINA (see also p. 4). Angina pectoris is a discomfort in the chest or adjacent areas, which is caused by myocardial ischemia and is associated with a disturbance of myocardial function but without myocardial necrosis.[7] Heberden's initial description of the chest discomfort as conveying a sense of "strangling and anxiety" is still remarkably pertinent, although adjectives frequently used to describe this distress include "vise-like," "constricting," "suffocating," "crushing," "heavy," and "squeezing." In other patients, the quality of the sensation is more vague and may be described as a mild pressure-like discomfort or an uncomfortable numb sensation. The site of the discomfort is usually retrosternal, but radiation is common and usually occurs down the ulnar surface of the left arm; commonly the right arm and the outer surfaces of both arms are also involved[8,8a] (Fig. 1–1, p. 6). Sampson and Cheitlin have documented the large number of regions that can be sites of radiation, with neck, jaw, and throat pain observed most commonly.[9] The location of pain does not reliably identify the specific coronary artery involved.[10] Discomfort above the mandible or below the epigastrium due to angina is rare. Anginal "equivalents" (i.e., symptoms of myocardial ischemia other than angina) such as breathlessness, faintness, fatigue, and eructations have also been reported. A history of abnormal exertional dyspnea may be an early indicator of CAD even when angina is absent or there is no electrocardiographic evidence of ischemic heart disease.[11] Pain seldom occurs only in the left pectoral area, and a discomfort lasting all day is unlikely to be cardiac ischemia unless it is caused by myocardial infarction or an uncorrected arrhythmia. It is characteristic that patients with angina usually prefer to rest, sit, or stop walking during attacks.[7]

MECHANISM. The mechanism responsible for angina pectoris is complex and not fully understood. For example, the specific substance that actually stimulates sympathetic afferents and begins the series of interactions that culminate in chest discomfort has not been identified. Some evidence favors agents that are released from cells as a result of transient ischemia, such as adenosine,[12] bradykinin, histamine, or serotonin.[13] Acidosis or elevated potassium concentration in the involved tissues may trigger release of these substances to which the sensory end-plates of the intracardiac sympathetic nerves appear to be particularly sensitive. The end-plates are the receptors of a network of unmyelinated nerves that lie between cardiac muscle fibers and that are also found around coronary vessels, travel to a cardiac plexus, and then ascend to the sympathetic ganglia (C7–T4). Impulses are transmitted to corresponding spinal ganglia, then via the spinal cord to the thalamus, and finally to the cerebral cortex.

The discomfort of myocardial ischemia is perceived in various regions of the chest because it is "referred" to the corresponding peripheral dermatomes that supply afferent nerves to the same segment of the spinal cord as the heart. A plausible explanation is that a common pool of secondary neurons can be stimulated by somatic and visceral afferent impulses. If visceral stimuli are excessive, the nearby intermediate neurons that are receptors for somatic impulses may be excited, and the discomfort will then be perceived as being cutaneous in origin. Thus, pain impulses can be referred to the medial aspects of the arm via common connections to the brachial plexus and can be referred to the neck via connections with the cervical roots.

It is not clear why some patients with clear-cut evidence of ischemic heart disease experience no chest discomfort; diabetics appear to have a higher frequency of "silent" ischemia, perhaps because of autonomic denervation.[14] In some patients chest pain disappears after a myocardial infarction, even though other evidence of transient ischemia, such as ST-segment depression, may persist. It is postulated that in these patients the nerve endings may have been damaged as a result of the infarction. Patients with reproducible evidence of myocardial ischemia may or may not experience chest pain with each episode. Ambulatory electrocardiography has revealed that the majority of patients with angina also experience numerous episodes of silent ischemia, i.e., ST-segment and T-wave changes identical to those occurring during typical angina but unaccompanied by chest discomfort. These episodes are accompanied by reductions of myocardial perfusion, as measured by uptake of radioactive rubidium.[15] The frequency of episodes of silent ischemia is reduced by treatment with nitrates, beta blockers, and calcium antagonists, supporting the contention that they represent instances of myocardial ischemia (p. 1347). It has been suggested that patients with silent myocardial ischemia may have an altered central modulation of pain perception. This hypothesis is supported by the observations that, compared with patients who develop angina during myocardial ischemia, those who have silent ischemia have a higher dental pain threshold and, once the pain threshold is reached, feel it less intensely.[16] Other studies have suggested that the higher the endorphin level induced after exercise the less likely angina is to occur.[17]

FEATURES OF ANGINAL DISCOMFORT. The fact that the discomfort of angina is not uniform and that other entities can mimic it often makes the differential diagnosis of chest pain difficult[7,8] (see Table 1–1, p. 3). Constant[18] has suggested that physicians should ask specific questions to differentiate "nonanginal chest pain" from angina. He notes that some of the characteristics of *nonanginal* discomfort are episodes lasting less than 5 seconds or greater than 20 to 30 minutes; discomfort that is aggravated or precipitated by one deep breath; discomfort precipitated by a single movement of the trunk or arm; discomfort relieved within a few seconds of lying horizontally; discomfort relieved within a few seconds of one or two swallows of food or water; discomfort localized to a very small area, e.g., an area the size of the tip of a finger; pain associated with tenderness of the chest wall (unless the anginal pain is referred to a site of previous chest wall trauma). Differentiating the discomfort resulting from noncardiac disorders from angina pectoris is usually possible when the quality of the pain and its duration, precipitating factors, and associated symptoms are taken into consideration[9] (Table 1–3, p. 5). Thus, the typical anginal episode usually begins gradually and reaches maximum intensity over a period of minutes before dissipating—usually as a result of cessation of the activity that precipitated it. Noncoronary causes should be considered in patients with sharp, stabbing, or burning chest pain that comes and goes in a matter of seconds or with a dull, continuous ache in the chest that lasts for more than 30 minutes. Similarly, changes in posture do not usually affect immediately the discomfort of myocardial ischemia, and this maneuver helps to distinguish angina from pericardial disease or hiatus hernia.

Angina Due to Increased Oxygen Demand. In typical angina, the pain is related to an increase in myocardial oxygen demand, most commonly brought about by physical activity; the *rate* at which a task is carried out is also important. Hurrying is particularly likely to precipitate angina, as are efforts involving motion of the hands over the head. Emotion or eating, particularly when combined with physical activity, commonly causes angina, as do a variety of other factors, including the excessive metabolic demands imposed by chills and fever, thyrotoxicosis, tachycardia from any cause, severe anemia, and hypoglycemia. In all of these conditions, underlying fixed coronary artery obstruction is usually present, and the other factors (e.g., exercise, fever) increase the activity of the heart, stimulate myocardial oxygen needs in the presence of a fixed and limited oxygen supply, and thus precipitate ischemia and chest discomfort.

Angina Due to Transient Decreased Oxygen Supply. There is increasing evidence, however, that angina may also be caused by transient reductions of oxygen supply as a consequence of coronary vasoconstriction.[19,20] As pointed out on page 1164, the coronary arterial bed is well innervated, and a variety of stimuli alter coronary tone. There is a reciprocal relationship between the severity of dynamic and organic obstruction required to cause myocardial ischemia. Thus, in the occasional patient with no organic lesions, severe dynamic obstruction alone can cause myocardial ischemia and resultant angina. On the other hand, in patients with severe fixed obstruction to coronary flow, only a minor increase in dynamic obstruction is necessary for blood flow to fall below a critical level and cause myocardial ischemia (Fig. 38–21, p. 1175). Nonocclusive intracoronary thrombi are another cause of myocardial ischemia, although usually of angina at rest (unstable angina) rather than chronic stable angina.

FIXED COMPARED WITH VARIABLE-THRESHOLD ANGINA. The variability of the threshold for angina differs among patients. In patients with fixed-threshold angina precipitated by increased oxygen demands, with few if any dynamic (vasoconstrictive) components, the level of physical activity required to precipitate angina is relatively constant. Characteristically, these patients can predict with some precision the amount of physical activity that causes angina, e.g., walking up exactly two and a half flights of stairs. When these patients are tested on a treadmill or bicycle, the pressure-rate product that elicits angina and/or electrocardiographic evidence of ischemia is constant or almost so.

Patients with variable-threshold angina,[20a] the majority of whom have atherosclerotic coronary arterial narrowing, but in whom dynamic obstruction caused by vasoconstriction plays an important role in causing myocardial ischemia, typically have "good days," when they are capable of substantial physical activity, and "bad days," when even minimal activity can cause clinical and/or electrocardiographic evidence of myocardial ischemia or when angina occurs at rest. Often, even in the course of a single day, they may be capable of substantial physical activity at one time, while at another time minimal activity will result in angina. Patients with variable-threshold angina often complain of angina precipitated by cold temperatures, emotion, and meals and occasionally of angina occurring at rest or nocturnally. It is presumed that coronary vasoconstriction contributes to the development of angina under these circumstances. In many patients with stable angina, cold does not lower the ischemic threshold; however, others give a history that angina is more readily provoked by the cold and in them the ischemic threshold is lowered by cold.[21] Both beta blockers and calcium antagonists prolong the time to exercise-induced ischemia both at normal and cold temperatures.[21] The anginal threshold tends to be lower in the morning than in the afternoon, correlating with the angiographic finding of smaller coronary arterial lumina at that time of day. However, even in patients with angina at rest and nocturnal angina, an increase in myocardial oxygen demand may play a role.[22]

The term *mixed angina* has been suggested by Maseri to describe the many patients who fall between these two extremes of fixed threshold and variable threshold angina[23] (Fig. 38–21, p. 1175).

Changes in the blood pressure–heart rate product (the double product) provide an approximation of alterations of myocardial oxygen requirements (p. 1163). In patients with effort-induced, fixed-threshold angina, the specific threshold at which ischemia develops (as reflected in angina and/or ST-segment depression) is a function of the myocardial oxygen requirements. As the activity of the left ventricle (and therefore its oxygen consumption) increases, a point is reached at which perfusion distal to a critical coronary arterial obstruction cannot supply sufficient oxygen to the myocardium perfused by the obstructed artery; ischemia and angina ensue.

Observations in patients experiencing angina under circumstances other than exercise help to explain the pathophysiological bases of angina. For example, as already indicated, some patients with ischemic heart disease characteristically experience angina on exposure to cold weather or during or after meals. A cold environment has been shown to increase peripheral resistance at rest and during exercise.[24] The rise in arterial pressure, by augmenting myocardial oxygen requirements, lowers the threshold for the development of angina. An alternative, or additional, explanation is the development of cold-induced coronary vasoconstriction. The reduction in exercise capacity during or after meals has been explained by a more rapid rise in heart rate and blood pressure after meals as compared with before meals,[25] but the postprandial increase in myocardial oxygen needs may not be sufficient to explain the development of ischemia, and a dynamic component, i.e., coronary vasoconstriction, may also be involved.[26] Similarly, during angina induced by emotion, heart rate and blood pressure (and therefore myocardial oxygen needs) rise but usually not to the level required to produce angina during exercise. Therefore, a dynamic component probably plays a role here as well.[27]

Relief of anginal discomfort is usually afforded by rest and by sublingual use of nitroglycerin; indeed, the response to this drug is often a useful diagnostic tool.[28] A delay of more than 5 to 10 minutes before relief is obtained suggests that the pain is not ischemic in origin. As described by Levine, carotid sinus pressure can also often bring about rapid alleviation of discomfort.[29] Some patients experience loss of angina when they continue to exercise, a phenomenon described as "walk-through" angina.[30]

In atypical angina the precipitating factors may be similar to those of typical angina, but the quality of the discomfort is different (sharp and stabbing, for example); or, if the quality of the discomfort is angina-like, the precipitating causes are unusual, such as varying body positions; or the discomfort may be typical in quality and occur only at rest but may not be accompanied by characteristic ST-segment changes. Nonanginal chest pain has neither the quality of typical angina nor its usual precipitating causes.

GRADING OF ANGINA PECTORIS. A system of grading effort angina proposed by the Canadian Cardiovascular Society in 1972 has gained widespread acceptance.[31] This grading system is the New York Heart Association (NYHA) functional classification, modified to allow independent observers to categorize patients in more precise terms. The Specific Activity Scale described by Goldman et al.[32] is also useful in estimating symptomatic severity. These systems are described in Table 1–6 (p. 11). An anginal "score" describing the frequency, associated electrocardiographic or ST-segment changes, and whether or not the angina is stable or progressive or nocturnal can add significant, independent prognostic information over and above the patient's age, gender, and knowledge of left ventricular function and coronary anatomy.[33]

CLINICAL-PATHOLOGICAL CORRELATIONS. The incidence of CAD in subsets of patients with typical angina, atypical angina, and nonanginal chest pain has been estimated by Diamond and Forrester to be about 90 per cent, 50 per cent, and 16 per cent, respectively, while the incidence of CAD in asymptomatic middle-aged adults is estimated to be 3 to 4 per cent.[34] While the clinical manifestations of ischemia tend to be more severe in patients with multivessel than single-vessel disease,[35] in any individual patient the extent of the underlying disease cannot be predicted from the severity, nature, duration, or quality of the discomfort. Perhaps the best examples of this lack of clinical-pathological correlation are two subgroups of patients who have been well characterized: those with advanced obstructive CAD and so-called silent ischemia (p. 1347) and some with Prinzmetal's angina who may have episodes of excruciating angina yet have minimal or no coronary atherosclerosis (p. 1342).

For comparable degrees of obstructive CAD, as defined arteriographically, asymptomatic or minimally symptomatic patients have a better prognosis than do those with severe angina.[36] When infarction (without angina) is the first manifestation of ischemic heart disease, it is often associated with single-vessel disease; when infarction has been preceded by angina, two- or three-vessel disease is usually present. Gender also appears to influence the clinical expression of CAD. Among women, angina pectoris is by far the most frequent clinical expression, as compared with men, in whom fatal and nonfatal myocardial infarction are more common.[37]

DIFFERENTIAL DIAGNOSIS OF CHEST PAIN
(Table 1–1, p. 3 and Fig. 40–1)

The differentiation of various disorders from CAD is challenging because, as has already been noted, the severity of the chest pain and the seriousness of the underlying disorder are not necessarily related. Compounding the difficulty in differential diagnosis is the common myth that pain in the left arm or left side of the chest is an ominous sign signifying the presence of CAD. However, a host of disorders can cause these types of discomfort.

ESOPHAGEAL DISORDERS. These may produce symptoms that can mimic myocardial ischemia.[38,39] Abnormal regurgitation of acid from the stomach to the esophagus—esophageal reflux—is relatively common. This can cause inflammation of the esophageal mucosa and is often associated with retrosternal burning—"heartburn"—indigestion, and/or gaseous eructations. Esophageal spasm also may cause constant retrosternal discomfort of uniform intensity or severe spasmodic pain during or after swallowing. These symptoms are intermittent and often accompanied by

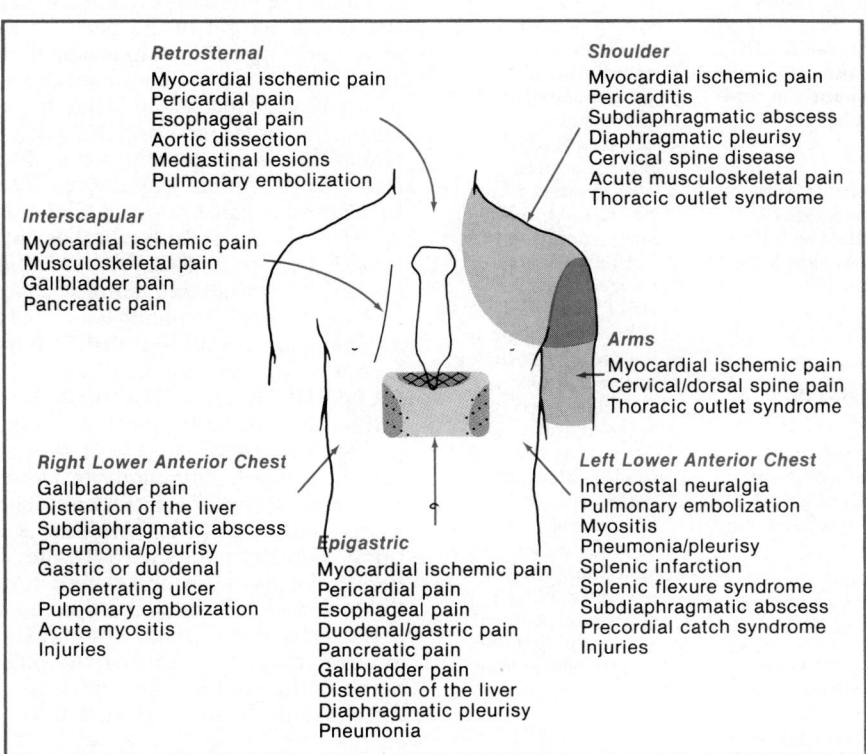

FIGURE 40–1. Differential diagnosis of chest pain according to location where pain starts. Serious intrathoracic or subdiaphragmatic diseases are usually associated with pains that begin in the left anterior chest, left shoulder or upper arm, the interscapular region, or the epigastrium. The scheme is not all-inclusive, e.g., intercostal neuralgia occurs in locations other than the left, lower anterior chest area. (From Miller, A. J.: Diagnosis of Chest Pain. New York, Raven Press, 1988, p. 175.)

difficulty in swallowing, although the pain may occur spontaneously at times. While esophageal disorders may produce substernal "burning," features more suggestive of esophageal than anginal pain include a background of continuous aching, discomfort that is not associated with exercise, and a pain disturbing sleep and occurring in association with other esophageal symptoms. Like angina, discomfort caused by esophageal spasm is often relieved by nitroglycerin (although not usually in less than 3 minutes). Unlike angina, esophageal pain is often also relieved by milk, antacids, foods, or occasionally warm liquids[18] (Table 40–1).

Acid regurgitation, or acid-induced esophageal spasm, as a cause of chest pain may be investigated by alternate infusions of dilute acid and normal saline via a nasogastric catheter with the tip at the level of the midesophagus (Bernstein test). In patients with subjective and objective evidence of gastroesophageal acid reflux, acid infusion readily produces pain within 2 to 4 minutes; however, pain may continue for more than 20 minutes in patients after the acid infusion is stopped despite the fact that the esophageal pH returns to normal much earlier.[40] Acid reflux into the esophagus can also be recognized by recording pH from an electrode at the tip of a catheter inserted into the distal esophagus.[41]

TABLE 40-1 SIMILARITIES AND DIFFERENCES BETWEEN ESOPHAGEAL AND CARDIAC PAIN

	SIMILARITIES OF CARDIAC AND ESOPHAGEAL PAIN	DISTINGUISHING FEATURES OF ESOPHAGEAL PAIN
Location	Mid or lower retrosternal. May be a severe epigastric pain with radiation up to neck.	High epigastric, behind xiphoid process or in low retrosternal area.
Nature	Heaviness, squeezing, tightness or burning. Can be associated with weakness, diaphoresis, and anxiety.	Often burning or perceived as spasm. Heartburn is frequent association. Can be associated with increased salivation. Dysphagia occurs.
Radiation	Upward toward throat. May radiate to left neck, shoulder, or arm.	Tends to ascend but not radiate to left side. Radiation to both shoulders and/or arms is less frequent. When pain begins in lower retrosternal area it often radiates down to epigastrium.
Precipitants	After eating. Angina is more likely with physical activity after eating.	After eating; certain foods—alcohol, coffee, spices. Less likely to be brought on by exertion. Can be precipitated by change in posture, e.g., by lying down.
Duration	Can last a short duration (2 to 10 min).	May last hours; may wax and wane.
Relieving factors	May be relieved or eased by nitroglycerin, standing, and relaxing.	

Modified from Miller, A. J.: Diagnosis of Chest Pain. New York, Raven Press, 1988, pp. 74–76.

Gastric reflux is often associated with hiatus hernia, which can be diagnosed radiographically. In patients with hiatus hernia, postprandial distress is most marked in the recumbent position, a feature that helps to differentiate it from angina pectoris. The differentiation between esophageal pain and angina is complicated by the observation that infusion of acid into the esophagus of patients with CAD can increase the rate-pressure product, can cause angina as well as electrocardiographic evidence of ischemia, and can cause pain indistinguishable from angina in patients with absence of or infrequent reflux symptoms.[42] Also, esophageal stimulation with acid will lower the threshold for exertional angina pectoris, especially in patients who have concurrent, regular esophageal symptoms.[43]

In patients with retrosternal chest pain of unclear cause, esophageal motility disorders are not uncommon[44,45] and should be specifically excluded or confirmed, if possible. In addition to chest pain, the majority of such patients have dysphagia. While barium studies may reveal motility problems, esophageal manometry may reveal diffuse esophageal spasm, increased pressure at the lower esophageal sphincter, and other disorders. Provocative pharmacological agents such as ergonovine[45] and methacholine[44] may provoke esophageal pain and manometric signs of spasm (in patients with normal coronary arteries). Surgical or medical therapy of esophageal reflux will improve symptoms in patients with normal coronary arteries whose experience of chest pain coincides with documented episodes of reflux (using esophageal pH monitoring).[41] While esophageal disease is frequent in patients with retrosternal chest pain of unclear cause, CAD occurs concomitantly in approximately 10 per cent of such patients. Thus, the diagnosis of CAD cannot be dismissed in such patients.[39]

BILIARY COLIC. This symptom is sometimes confused with angina pectoris. It is usually caused by a rapid rise in biliary pressure due to obstruction of the cystic or bile duct. The pain is steady, usually lasts 2 to 4 hours, and subsides spontaneously without any symptoms between attacks.[46] It is usually most intense in the right upper abdomen but may also be felt in the epigastrium, left abdomen, or precordium. This discomfort is often referred to the scapula, may radiate around the costal margin to the back, or rarely may be felt in the shoulder, suggesting diaphragmatic irritation. Although nausea and vomiting are common, the relationship of the pain to meals is variable. While a history of dyspepsia, flatulence, fatty food intolerance, and indigestion may be associated with cholelithiasis, these symptoms are also commonly experienced by the general population. Ultrasound is quite accurate in diagnosing gallstones and allows determination of gallbladder size, thickness, and whether or not the bile ducts are dilated.[46] Failure to opacify the gallbladder on oral cholecystography may indicate nonfunction due to disease.

Distention of the splenic flexure of the colon can also mimic anginal pain, but, unlike angina, relief of symptoms often follows a bowel movement.

COSTOSTERNAL SYNDROME. In 1921, Tietze first described a syndrome of local pain and tenderness, usually limited to the anterior chest wall, associated with swelling of the costal cartilages. This condition causes pain that can resemble angina pectoris. The full-blown Tietze syndrome, i.e., pain associated with tender swelling of the costochondral junctions, is uncommon, whereas costochondritis causing tenderness of the costochondral junctions (without swelling) is relatively common.[47] Pain on palpation of these joints is a useful clinical sign. Local pressure should be applied routinely to the anterior chest wall during the examination of the patient being evaluated for angina pectoris. Treatment of costochondritis usually consists of reassurance and antiinflammatory agents.

CERVICAL RADICULITIS. This may occur as a constant ache, sometimes resulting in a sensory deficit. The pain may be related to motion of the neck, just as motion of the shoulder triggers attacks of pain due to bursitis. A hyperalgesic area of skin, noted by running the finger down the back and exerting pressure, may lead to the suspicion of thoracic root pain.[18] Occasionally, pain mimicking angina can be due to compression of the brachial plexus via cervical ribs. Physical examination may also detect pain brought about by movement of an arthritic shoulder, a calcified shoulder tendon, and the like. The musculoskeletal disorders that can mimic angina include subacromial bursitis and costochondritis.

OTHER CAUSES OF ANGINA-LIKE PAIN. *Acute myocardial infarction* (Chap. 39) is usually associated with prolonged (> 30 minutes), severe pain that apart from duration and intensity may be similar to angina pectoris. It is associated with characteristic electrocardiographic and enzyme findings.

Severe pulmonary hypertension may be associated with exertional chest pain with the characteristics of angina pectoris (p. 806). Other associated symptoms include dyspnea on exertion, dizziness, and exertional syncope. Associated findings on physical examination, such as a parasternal lift, palpable and loud pulmonary component of the second sound, and right ventricular hypertrophy on the electrocardiogram usually are readily recognized.

Pulmonary embolism (Chap. 48) causes chest pain that is usually associated with dyspnea.[48] Associated pleuritic pain suggests pulmonary infarction, and a history of exacerbation of the pain with inspiration with findings of a pleural friction rub usually readily distinguish this from angina pectoris.

The pain of *acute pericarditis* (p. 1469) at times may be difficult to distinguish from angina pectoris. However, pericarditis tends to occur in younger patients than does angina, and the diagnosis depends on chest pain, a pericardial friction rub, and electrocardiographic changes. The chest pain usually is sudden in onset, severe and persistent, and is intensified by coughing, swallowing, and inspiration. Relief may be obtained by sitting up and leaning forward: palpation of the trapezius ridge often causes discomfort. A pericardial friction rub can be detected in most patients if listened for carefully, at different times, with the patient in different positions. Early widespread ST-segment elevation may be present.

In many of the disorders just mentioned, angina pectoris can usually be excluded by a careful history and physical examination. It must be emphasized, however, that chronic ischemic heart disease can and frequently does coexist with any of these other disorders and that noncardiac disease can trigger a true anginal attack in a patient with coronary artery disease.

PHYSICAL EXAMINATION

GENERAL EXAMINATION. In the patient with chronic ischemic heart disease and angina pectoris, the general examination may be entirely normal or may reveal the presence of risk factors for the development of coronary atherosclerosis. Inspection of the eyes, especially in men,[49] may reveal a *corneal arcus*, and examination of the skin may reveal xanthomas (Figs. 2–3, p. 17 and 37–10, p. 1138, and 37–11, p. 1139). In men, the size of the corneal arcus appears to correlate positively with age and levels of cholesterol and low-density lipoproteins.[50] The corneal arcus is not known to regress in humans and is unaffected by a reduction in the level of lipids.[51] *Xanthelasma*, in which lipid deposits are intracellular, appears to be promoted by increased levels of triglycerides and a relative deficiency of high-density lipoproteins. In the Lipid Research Clinic's study,[51] the incidence of both xanthelasma and corneal arcus increased with age and was highest in patients with Type II hyperlipoproteinemia and usually low in those with the Type IV phenotype (Ch. 37). In young persons, the presence of both xanthelasma and corneal arcus is closely correlated and identifies persons with plasma lipoprotein abnormalities. Adjusted-odds ratios for the presence of ischemic heart disease in individuals with xanthelasma and corneal arcus generally are increased.

There appears to be some correlation between CAD and *diagonal earlobe crease*, except in native American Indians,

Orientals, and children with Beckwith-Wiedemann syndrome (exomphalos, macroglossia, giantism).[52] It has been observed that there is often a unilateral diagonal earlobe crease in younger persons with CAD that becomes bilateral with advancing age.[53] Some believe that it develops along with CAD,[53] and pathological studies have linked diagonal earlobe creases and cardiovascular mortality.[54] Since the incidence of both diagonal earlobe creases and CAD increases with age,[55] it is not a very helpful clinical finding in persons over the age of 50 years.

The *blood pressure* may be chronically elevated or may rise acutely (along with the heart rate) during an anginal attack. Changes in blood pressure may precede (and precipitate) or follow (and be caused by) the anginal episode. Other features of the general physical examination that are important to seek are abnormalities of the arterial pulses and of the venous system. Major abnormalities of the carotid artery pulse, or bruits, associated with cerebral symptoms usually will lead to carotid ultrasonography and perhaps arteriography. Abnormality to palpation of the peripheral arterial pulses (femoral and popliteal) or the presence of bruits is not as accurate as are actual measurements of limb perfusion.[56] However, the positive correlation of CAD with carotid and peripheral arterial disease makes physical examination of these vessels, including palpation of the dorsalis pedis and posterior tibial pulses, an important part of the examination. Retinal arteriolar changes (p. 15) are common in patients with diabetes mellitus or hypertension and CAD. An abnormal light reflex is quite common, while abnormal vessel tortuosity and decreased caliber are less sensitive but more specific signs.

Evaluation of the patient's venous system, particularly in the legs, may have an important bearing on the type of grafting procedure employed in subsequent coronary artery surgery.

CARDIAC EXAMINATION. This may supply useful clues to both the diagnosis of ischemic heart disease and the functional state of the myocardium. First, the presence of murmurs of hypertrophic cardiomyopathy or aortic valve disease suggests that the ischemic chest pain may be due to conditions other than (or in addition to) CAD (Chaps. 2 and 3). Second, certain findings such as a third or loud fourth heart sound suggest ischemia as the basis for chest pain if other obvious cardiac diseases are absent. These sounds are common in patients with angina at rest, and their frequency is increased during handgrip exercise,[57] even if the latter does not precipitate angina pectoris. These sounds and pulsations are related to the functional state of the left ventricle, particularly its pressure and compliance during diastole (p. 370). In patients with moderate to severe left ventricular dysfunction, a sustained apical cardiac impulse is common. A palpable presystolic impulse may be more indicative of moderate than severe left ventricular dysfunction.[58] While a fourth heart sound may be recorded phonocardiographically in many apparently normal subjects over the age of 45, we agree with Tavel[59] that a clear, loud fourth heart sound accompanied by a palpable presystolic wave is an abnormal finding. It is not specific for ischemic heart disease but may be elicited in other conditions associated with left ventricular hypertrophy such as aortic stenosis, hypertrophic cardiomyopathy, and hypertension, in which left ventricular compliance is reduced (p. 50).

Paradoxical splitting of the second heart sound (p. 47) may occur transiently during an anginal attack and appears to be related to asynergy and prolongation of left ventricular contraction resulting in delayed closure of the aortic valve.

When patients with CAD lie in the left lateral recumbent position, dyskinetic bulges at the apex may be palpated or recorded by means of apexcardiography; these bulges correspond to dyskinetic areas and often complement the auscultatory findings of diastolic filling sounds. A transient apical systolic murmur is quite common in CAD and has been attributed to reversible papillary muscle dysfunction secondary to transient myocardial ischemia; when persistent, such murmurs may be due to fibrosis, often a manifestation of subendocardial infarction. These murmurs are more prevalent in patients with extensive coronary artery disease, especially those with prior myocardial infarction and left ventricular dysfunction. The systolic murmur may assume a variety of configurations (early, late, or holosystolic) and may be accentuated by exertion or during angina. A midsystolic click, often followed by a late systolic murmur characteristic of mitral regurgitation produced by mitral valve prolapse (Fig. 34–23, p. 1034), also occurs in patients with CAD. A diastolic murmur or a continuous murmur is an uncommon finding and has been attributed to turbulent flow across a proximal coronary artery stenosis.[60]

LABORATORY TESTS IN CHRONIC STABLE ANGINA

ELECTROCARDIOGRAM

(See also Chap. 5)

The resting electrocardiogram is normal in approximately one-third of patients with chronic stable angina pectoris. Patients with normal tracings at rest may have severe angina, but they usually have not previously suffered extensive infarction. When the electrocardiogram is abnormal, the most common findings are nonspecific ST-T changes with or without evidence of prior transmural infarction; however, a variety of conduction disturbances, most frequently left bundle branch block and left anterior fascicular block, have also been reported. When left bundle branch block is found in patients with chronic ischemic heart disease, it is often associated with marked impairment in left ventricular function,[61] presumably reflecting multivessel CAD and myocardial damage. The finding of incomplete right bundle branch block does not appear to be associated with an increased risk of death from CAD.[62] A variety of arrhythmias, especially ventricular premature beats, may be present, but they are not specific for identifying CAD. Abnormal Q waves are relatively specific but insensitive indicators of myocardial necrosis.

Interval electrocardiograms may reveal the development of Q-wave infarctions that are unrecognized clinically either by patients or their physicians. Such electrocardiographic abnormalities have as serious a prognosis as clinically recognized infarctions.[63] The increasing use of ambulatory electrocardiographic monitoring has shown that many patients with symptomatic myocardial ischemia also have episodes of silent ischemia that would otherwise go unrecognized during normal daily activities (p. 1347).

Exercise Electrocardiography

(See Chap. 6)

For appropriate application of noninvasive tests, it is important to consider Bayes' theorem (pp. 169 and 1697), which states that while the reliability of any test is defined by its sensitivity and specificity,* its predictability depends on the prevalence of the disease in the population under study (Table 54–2, p. 1697).

DIAGNOSIS OF CORONARY ARTERY DISEASE. Exercise electrocardiography is of limited value in predicting the *presence or absence* of CAD after other easily obtainable clinical data have been taken into account, e.g., the presence or absence of typical anginal symptoms, the presence or absence of Q waves, a clinical history of acute myocardial infarction, a history of cigarette smoking, elevated cholesterol level, and age.[64] However, the recording of an electrocardiogram during and after exercise—especially if angina is precipitated—is valuable in assessing the severity and prognosis of CAD.[65-67] Nonetheless, the exercise electrocardiogram may be of diagnostic value in several circumstances:

1. In patients with a chest pain syndrome and a normal resting electrocardiogram, we believe that a standard electro-

cardiographic exercise test is useful for detection of significant CAD.[67a]

2. Certain symptomatic and electrocardiographic responses during exercise testing suggest the presence of critical obstruction in one or more coronary arteries. The presence of *typical* anginal chest pain alone, in the absence of ST-segment changes, has a high predictive value for the detection of CAD.[67] However, the most useful exercise electrocardiographic variable for the detection of CAD is the ST-segment shift.[68] If typical chest discomfort occurs during the test associated with ≥ 1 mm ST-segment depression (of horizontal or downsloping nature) the predictive value for the detection of CAD is 90 per cent, and if > 2 mm ST-segment depressions coexist with typical chest discomfort, this is virtually diagnostic of significant CAD.[67] In the absence of typical angina pectoris, downsloping or horizontal ST-segment depressions ≥ 1 mm have a predictive value of 70 per cent, and ST depressions of ≥ 2 mm have a predictive value of 90 per cent for the detection of one or more significant coronary arterial narrowings.

3. An exercise test associated with a hypotensive response, i.e., a drop in systolic blood pressure during exercise below the preexercise value (in the absence of known major ventricular dysfunction), has an 80 per cent predictive value for the detection of significant CAD.[69]

4. Exercise-induced bundle branch block is relatively rare, is usually found in patients with significant CAD,[70-72] and is associated with a high incidence of critical obstruction of the proximal left anterior descending coronary artery.

5. The persistence of ST-segment changes at lower heart rates during the recovery period than the rate at which they develop represents additional evidence supporting the presence of significant CAD.[73]

6. Exercise test predictors of multivessel coronary artery disease include exercise-induced hypotension,[74,75] ST-segment changes ≥ 2 mm, a low work capacity or duration of exercise (which reflects the functional state of the left ventricle),[76] and persistent ST-segment depressions, especially beyond 5 minutes, in the recovery phase. Indeed, early onset of ST-segment depression, its long persistence following exercise, and, most importantly, its shape (downsloping or horizontal) are all strongly associated with multivessel CAD[77] (Fig. 40–2).

7. Failure to achieve a normal heart rate response to exer-

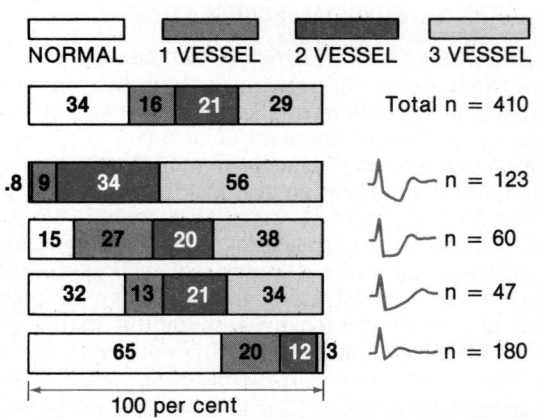

FIGURE 40–2. Relation between the type of ST-segment response in an exercise test and the extent of coronary artery disease. All numbers represent percentages. The total study population is represented at the top. Downsloping ST segments are highly specific for coronary disease, with only one false-positive response (0.8 per cent) encountered; most patients with this response (90 per cent) have double- and triple-vessel involvement. Neither the horizontal nor the slowly upsloping ST segments aid in identifying severe disease. A small percentage (15 per cent) of patients with entirely normal treadmill tests have double- and triple-vessel disease. (From Goldschlager, N., et al.: Treadmill stress tests as indicators of presence and severity of coronary artery disease. Ann. Intern. Med. **85:**277, 1976.)

---

*For definitions of these terms, see Table 6–2, p. 168.

cise (chronotropic incompetence) is also frequently observed in patients with multivessel or extensive CAD.[78,79] A low maximal heart rate associated with ST-segment depression increases the likelihood of the presence of CAD.[78]

8. Ventricular ectopic activity may be provoked during exercise testing, and if it is "high grade" (e.g., ventricular tachycardia, multiform ventricular ectopy) the likelihood that the patient has abnormal ventricular function or severe CAD is increased.[80]

ASSESSMENT OF PROGNOSIS. Several points should be considered in utilizing the electrocardiographic stress test to evaluate prognosis in patients *known* to have CAD.

1. One of the most important prognosticators derived from exercise electrocardiography is exercise duration or capacity. In symptom-limited exercise tests, *even in the presence of > 2 mm ST-segment depression*, patients who continue to exercise into stage 4 of a standard Bruce protocol have an excellent prognosis.[65,80a] In an 8-year follow-up of medically treated patients with angiographically confirmed CAD and a positive exercise test, the duration of exercise correlated significantly with survival—patients reaching stage 4 of a Bruce protocol had a survival rate of 93 per cent, compared with those terminating their exercise in stage 1 who had a survival rate of only 45 per cent.[66] This direct relationship between exercise duration and long-term survival held regardless whether the exercise test was terminated because of dyspnea, fatigue, or angina.[80b] Coronary artery revascularization appears to improve survival in comparison to medical treatment alone in patients with a positive exercise test and short exercise duration.[80c]

2. Exercise-induced hypotension not only correlates with left main CAD or multivessel disease[69,74,75] but also, in patients with evidence of ischemia during exercise testing who have a remote history of myocardial infarction, it indicates a three-fold increased risk for subsequent death or myocardial infarction.[69]

3. Early onset of angina with ST-segment depression is associated with a greater likelihood of myocardial infarction or coronary death.[81] In patients with known left ventricular dysfunction and multivessel coronary artery disease, the possibility of subsequent acute myocardial infarction or sudden death may be greater in patients who exhibit silent myocardial ischemia during exercise testing than in those who develop angina.[82] Therefore, in patients who exhibit substantial myocardial ischemia at levels of activity that they would normally exceed in daily living but *who do not have symptoms of angina, i.e., patients who have a defective anginal warning system*, an aggressive attitude should be adopted toward investigation and possible revascularization for prognostic reasons.

INFLUENCE OF ANTIANGINAL THERAPY. Antianginal pharmacological therapy reduces the sensitivity of exercise testing as a screening tool for left main coronary disease or three-vessel disease.[83] Beta blockade will increase the exercise duration and suppress, diminish, or delay the appearance of ST-segment depression and thus obscure the diagnostic interpretation of exercise testing.[84] In patients receiving antianginal medications, a positive exercise test will have the usual implications for management. However, a negative exercise test in patients receiving antianginal drugs does not exclude significant and possibly life-threatening myocardial ischemia. Therefore, if the purpose of the exercise test is to *diagnose* ischemia, it should be performed, if possible, in the absence of antianginal medications. The advisability of withdrawing medications in an individual patient before exercise testing is a matter of judgment. Unless the patient has severe angina, sublingual nitroglycerin for 1 or 2 days is likely to be sufficient to control symptoms if other therapy is withdrawn. For long-acting nitrates, calcium antagonists, and short-acting beta blockers, stopping the medications the day before testing usually will suffice. Two or three days are required for patients receiving long-acting beta blockers. However, if the purpose of the exercise test is to identify safe levels of daily activity, the test should be carried out while the patient is taking medications.

INCONCLUSIVE TESTS. In view of the relatively low sensitivity (approximately 75 per cent) of exercise stress electrocardiography in the diagnosis of CAD, a negative result does not exclude this diagnosis. However, it makes three-vessel or left main disease much less likely. Conversely, an adequate maximum exercise test—one achieving more than 85 per cent of predicted maximal heart rate—is unlikely to occur in patients with three-vessel or left main CAD.

A major limitation of the sensitivity of the exercise electrocardiogram is that it cannot be interpreted in many patients. This includes patients who are incapable of reaching the level of exercise required for near-maximal effort (85 per cent or more of maximal predicted heart rate), particularly those receiving beta-adrenoceptor blockers or those who develop fatigue, leg cramps, or dyspnea, and patients with abnormalities in the baseline electrocardiogram, including those taking digitalis. In patients with vascular, orthopedic, or neurological conditions who cannot perform leg exercise, the usual alternative tests considered include dipyridamole (or adenosine)-thallium imaging[85-87,87a] (p. 277), Holter monitoring to detect changes in ST segments (p. 1347), or, if appropriate, diagnostic coronary angiography.

RADIONUCLIDE IMAGING

STRESS THALLIUM-201 MYOCARDIAL PERFUSION IMAGING (see also p. 227). In this technique, the radionuclide is injected at peak exercise and the image is obtained several minutes later when the patient is at rest; it demonstrates the regional perfusion pattern that existed during the stress of exercise. Defects represent either areas of stress-induced impairment of blood flow or infarction. If a delayed image is obtained 2 to 3 hours later and the initial defect persists, it is probably due to an infarction. On the other hand, if it exhibits delayed uptake (i.e., redistribution), it probably represents an area of ischemic, transiently hypoperfused but viable myocardium. An electrocardiogram is ordinarily obtained at rest and during the various stages of exercise. Thus, stress thallium scintigraphy provides more information than exercise stress electrocardiography.[87b]

Since a stress thallium scan cannot ordinarily be performed in a physician's office and it is a relatively expensive test (three to four times the cost of a regular exercise electrocardiogram) requiring injection of a radionuclide, certain issues should be considered:

1. A regular exercise electrocardiogram should almost always be obtained first in patients with chest pain and a *normal resting electrocardiogram* for screening and detection of CAD. Stress thallium-201 scintigraphy should not be used as a screening test in populations in whom the prevalence of coronary disease is low or moderate since the sensitivity of exercise thallium imaging is approximately 70 to 85 per cent and the specificity is only 50 to 60 per cent.[88]

2. Thallium scanning is, in essence, either positive or negative and has little quantitative value in determining the number of vessels with significant coronary disease. However, in patients with an abnormal baseline electrocardiogram (e.g., left bundle branch block or right bundle branch block), a history of infarction, or a history of revascularization (by percutaneous transluminal coronary angioplasty or coronary bypass grafting) when the test is being used to assess whether significant stress-induced myocardial ischemia exists, thallium perfusion imaging may be the test of choice. In patients with single-vessel CAD, exercise thallium-201 perfusion imaging appears more sensitive in detecting CAD than an electrocardiographic exercise test[89] and will give information about the location and extent of the perfusion deficit. However, in most patients with single-vessel CAD (except those with a very proximal left anterior descending coronary artery stenosis) the prognosis is good.

3. Thallium scan results do not establish or exclude the

diagnosis of CAD with certainty. However, in patients with chest pain and normal findings during exercise thallium testing, the prognosis is excellent[90,91] even if angiography has demonstrated underlying CAD.[92]

4. If multiple thallium-201 redistribution defects are observed with exercise, especially if associated with abnormal lung uptake (reflecting a sudden rise in left ventricular diastolic pressure), multivessel or left main CAD causing significant ischemia is usually present.[93,93a] The finding of a larger left ventricle on the immediate post-stress image than on the delayed image, i.e., transient ischemic dilatation of the ventricle, is a highly specific marker of multivessel disease and left ventricular dysfunction.[94]

5. Single photon emission computed tomography (SPECT) offers an advantage over conventional planar thallium-201 imaging by providing a three-dimensional view of the myocardium and enhancement of lesion contrast.[95]

6. If a patient cannot perform a routine exercise test, dipyridamole-(or adenosine-[96]) induced maximal coronary vasodilation, when used in conjunction with thallium myocardial imaging (p. 277), offers sensitivity and specificity for the detection of CAD comparable to that of exercise thallium imaging and is relatively safe.[96a] Imaging 45 minutes after administration of oral dipyridamole is effective in unmasking regions of underperfused but viable myocardium.[97] A single high oral dose of dipyridamole (300 mg) followed by quantitative SPECT resulted in a sensitivity of approximately 92 per cent and specificity of 80 per cent in the diagnosis of CAD.[87]

Because thallium scintigraphy has certain disadvantages (unavailable in a physician's office, relatively costly, difficult to interpret), we generally proceed with exercise electrocardiography in the assessment of known or suspected chronic stable angina in patients with a normal resting electrocardiogram. In patients with major electrocardiographic conduction abnormalities at rest (left or right bundle branch block) and in patients with a history of infarction or revascularization in whom the significance of ST-segment changes may be difficult to assess and in whom we are primarily concerned with the consequences of CAD on regional perfusion during exercise, we would often proceed directly to stress thallium-201 myocardial perfusion imaging. In this situation, information concerning the location of ischemia, the extent of ischemia (presence or absence of multiple defects), irreversible ventricular damage (fixed defects), and ventricular dysfunction is useful clinically. In patients who cannot exercise we utilize dipyridamole-induced coronary vasodilation in conjunction with thallium myocardial imaging[85,86] or Holter monitoring of ST segments,[98] depending on the clinical circumstance.

EXERCISE RADIONUCLIDE ANGIOGRAPHY. Since two-dimensional (2-D) echocardiography at rest or during exercise (p. 96) may provide excellent information about ventricular function, radionuclide angiography has a somewhat diminished role in the assessment of patients with CAD than heretofore. It is unusual to use this test for the detection of CAD, but it can provide important information about the influence of known CAD on ventricular function at rest or the functional reserve of the ventricle. Normally, exercise should be associated with an increase in left ventricular ejection fraction of 5 per cent or more. The combination of failure of this normal rise in ejection fraction with exercise and development of new regional wall motion abnormalities is highly specific for CAD.[99]

It is important to realize that the failure of left ventricular ejection fraction to increase during exercise *unaccompanied* by regional wall motion abnormalities is a nonspecific finding that can occur in patients with conditions other than ischemic heart disease, including cardiomyopathy, valvular heart disease, and hypertension, and in some normal individuals receiving beta-adrenoceptor blocker. In patients unable to perform standard exercise testing, dipyridamole radionuclide ventriculography[100] may provide an alternative to ST-segment Holter monitoring, dipyridamole-thallium imaging, or coronary angiography in the detection of CAD.

Clinical Application of Noninvasive Tests
(See also p. 168)

In asymptomatic persons or in those with nonanginal chest pain who are being screened or examined for CAD, i.e., patients in whom the pretest likelihood of coronary disease is low (less than 15 per cent), a normal exercise electrocardiogram excludes, for practical purposes, ischemic heart disease. However, if in such a patient there is an abnormal exercise electrocardiographic test, several alternatives exist. If the patient demonstrates excellent exercise capacity (i.e., to stage IV of a Bruce protocol or the equivalent) then, since the likelihood of left main coronary disease or multivessel CAD is slight and the prognosis is excellent, the patient may be observed without further testing. If, on the other hand, the patient has an early abnormal exercise electrocardiogram, exercise-induced hypotension, or very poor work capacity, coronary angiography is generally indicated to determine whether or not left main CAD or severe multivessel disease with left ventricular dysfunction exists. If the patient falls into an intermediate category (a moderately positive exercise test) then a thallium scan may provide further information. If both the exercise electrocardiogram and thallium perfusion scan are abnormal, the likelihood of significant CAD exceeds 80 per cent. If there is a discrepancy in the results of the two tests, one may either proceed to coronary arteriography or follow up the patient medically, depending on the clinical circumstances.

In patients with atypical angina, if two noninvasive tests are abnormal, the likelihood of CAD exceeds 95 per cent; if both tests are normal, this likelihood falls below 5 per cent. When test results are discordant, they should be evaluated in the light of the level of exercise achieved as well as the degree of positivity (e.g., the presence of accompanying symptoms, the depth of the ST-segment response, the heart rate at which it occurred, and the persistence of the ST-segment response on the stress electrocardiogram; the size and number of perfusion defects on the stress perfusion scintigram; and the magnitude of the exercise-induced change in ejection fraction and regional wall-motion disorder on the exercise radionuclide angiogram). Thus, for example, a patient with a normal exercise electrocardiogram who develops multiple large perfusion defects on a thallium-201 scintigram (accompanied by chest pain at a heart rate of 130 beats/min) has a much greater likelihood of having ischemic heart disease than one who has a normal exercise electrocardiogram and develops a single small perfusion defect without chest pain at a heart rate of 185 beats/min.

In patients with typical angina (i.e., those with a high pretest likelihood of disease), noninvasive testing is most valuable for estimating the extent and severity of CAD and thereby the prognosis. The development of exertional hypotension, marked or prolonged ST-segment depression at low work levels and/or heart rate, striking decreases in ejection fraction and wall motion abnormalities, and large or multiple defects or lung uptake on the exercise thallium scintigram all point to severe multivessel disease in patients at high risk of subsequent coronary events, including sudden death.[101]

OTHER LABORATORY TESTS IN PATIENTS WITH KNOWN CORONARY ARTERY DISEASE

ECHOCARDIOGRAPHY (see also p. 95). Two-dimensional echocardiography allows visualization of large portions of the left ventricle, and serial recordings may detect wall-motion abnormalities due to transient myocardial ischemia. Echocardiography performed immediately after exercise (p. 96) is useful in the detection of wall-motion abnormalities and may enhance the diagnostic yield of a treadmill exercise test by providing information regarding functional reserve of the ventricles in addition to the usual information about exercise capacity, ST-segment changes, and the like.[102] Exercise echocardiography is moderately sensitive (75 to 90 per cent) and highly specific in detecting CAD in patients with normal ventricular wall motion at rest.[103] The test is also highly reproducible.[104] Adequate images can be obtained in more than 85 per cent of patients, and post-peak exercise imaging does not result in failure to detect significant CAD, because ventricular wall-motion abnormalities do not usually normalize immediately.[105] The development of wall-motion abnormalities detected by exercise echocardiography is closely related to the severity of coronary artery stenoses, measured by quantitative angiography.[106]

For patients who cannot exercise on a treadmill or bicycle, transesophageal atrial pacing combined with 2-D echocardiography[107] or dipyridamole–2-D echocardiographic testing may be utilized.[108,109] The development of wall-motion abnormalities and/or angina following the administration of intravenous dipyridamole predicts subsequent cardiac events.[108] During follow-up, cumulative survival rates free of cardiac events over 3 years were 92 per cent for patients with a normal dipyridamole–echocardiography test, 68 per cent for patients who had a positive test with a high dose of dipyridamole, and 50 per cent for patients with a positive test with a low dose of dipyridamole.[108]

It is unclear where exercise echocardiography will eventually fit into the overall scheme of available tests to evaluate CAD. Because, compared with radionuclide ventriculography, it is inexpensive, can be performed in a physician's office, and does not require injection of isotope, it is likely to be used widely. Two-dimensional echocardiography has also been used for defining obstructive lesions of the left main coronary artery[110] (Fig. 4–87, p. 96).

BIOCHEMICAL TESTS. Serum levels of cardiac enzymes (p. 1218) are normal in angina pectoris and serve to differentiate these patients from those with acute myocardial infarction. One of the striking features of chronic ischemic heart disease in relatively young persons is the frequency with which certain metabolic abnormalities are detected. Since hypercholesterolemia and carbohydrate intolerance are recognized as risk factors for the development of ischemic heart disease, the incidence of these abnormalities, particularly in patients under the age of 50 years, is impressive (Chap. 37). Over 90 per cent of patients under the age of 50 with angiographically proven ischemic heart disease have carbohydrate intolerance of either Type II or IV hyperlipoproteinemia.[111,112]

CHEST ROENTGENOGRAM. This is usually within normal limits in patients with chronic ischemic heart disease. However, coronary artery calcification detected fluoroscopically may be more diagnostic of CAD than was once thought, especially in young people. More than 90 per cent of patients with coronary artery calcification were found to have critical coronary artery obstruction; however, coronary calcification on fluoroscopy is not a very sensitive test, since it is found in only 40 per cent of patients with angiographically documented CAD.[113] When fluoroscopic evidence of coronary calcification is present in combination with a positive exercise test, the probability of finding CAD on coronary angiography is very high. Ultrafast computed tomography is more sensitive than fluoroscopy in detecting and quantifying coronary artery calcium.[114]

CATHETERIZATION, ANGIOGRAPHY, AND CORONARY ARTERIOGRAPHY

Although the clinical examination and noninvasive techniques described above are extremely valuable in establishing the diagnosis of ischemic heart disease and, in many instances, the prognosis as well, the definitive diagnosis of CAD and a precise assessment of its anatomical severity and its effects on cardiac performance require cardiac catheterization (Chap. 7), coronary arteriography (Chap. 9), and left ventricular angiography. Among patients with chronic stable angina pectoris referred to cardiologists, coronary arteriography usually reveals relatively equal distribution (approximately 25 per cent each) of critical (> 70 per cent luminal diameter) narrowing of one, two, and three of the major coronary ar-

teries. Five to 10 per cent of patients have obstruction of the left main coronary artery (these patients have a higher complication rate[115]), and in approximately 15 per cent no critical obstruction is detectable (Chap. 9). Total occlusion of at least one major coronary artery is more common in patients with chronic angina who have a history of prior infarction than in those without such a history.

Coronary artery ectasia, i.e., patulous, aneurysmal dilatation involving most of the length of a major epicardial coronary artery, is present in approximately 2 per cent of patients with obstructive CAD. This angiographic lesion does not appear to affect symptoms, survival, or the incidence of myocardial infarction.[116] Coronary ectasia should be distinguished from discrete *coronary artery aneurysms*, which are almost *never* found in arteries without severe stenoses, are most common in the left anterior descending coronary artery, and are usually associated with extensive CAD.[117] These discrete atherosclerotic coronary artery aneurysms do not appear to rupture, and their resection is not warranted.

The functional significance of *collateral vessels* (p. 1164) is unclear. They may protect against myocardial infarction when total occlusion occurs, provided they are of adequate size.[118] Thus, patients with a total occlusion of a major epicardial artery may have well-developed collateral vessels and normal ventricular function, i.e., no evidence of myocardial infarction. Thus, well-developed coronary collaterals may protect against resting ischemia even in the presence of total occlusion, but they may fail to meet the increased needs of exercise and therefore may not abolish exertion-induced angina. Patients with abundant collateral vessels appear to suffer smaller myocardial infarctions.[119,120]

Myocardial bridging of coronary arteries (Fig. 9–25, p. 253) is observed in angiographically normal coronary arteries and normally does not constitute a hazard for the patient. Occasionally, compression of a portion of a coronary artery by a myocardial bridge can be associated with clinical manifestations of myocardial ischemia during strenuous physical activity and may even initiate malignant ventricular arrhythmias.[121,121a]

Ventricular relaxation (p. 438), as reflected in the early diastolic ventricular filling rate, may be impaired at rest. Diastolic filling becomes even more abnormal (slowed) during exercise, when ischemia intensifies.

The frequency of abnormal left ventricular dynamics at rest, i.e., elevations of left ventricular end-diastolic pressure and reduced cardiac output, increases with the number of vessels exhibiting critical narrowing and with the number of prior infarctions,[122] but there is a great deal of overlap among individual patients so that the severity of coronary arterial disease cannot be predicted from these two measurements. The left ventricular end-diastolic pressure may be elevated because of reduced ventricular compliance, left ventricular systolic failure, or a combination of these two processes[123]; both impaired systolic and diastolic function may occur as a consequence of acute, reversible ischemia and chronic scar formation. The elevation of left ventricular diastolic pressure has its clinical correlate in the presence of diastolic (third and fourth) heart sounds. In many patients with normal hemodynamics in the basal state, abnormalities of left ventricular function can be elicited by dynamic or isometric exercise. Elevations of left ventricular end-diastolic pressure usually occur before the patient complains of chest discomfort and before there is electrocardiographic ST-segment depression.

Pacing-induced and post-pacing angina and/or ST-segment depression can also be observed in the catheterization laboratory. This form of stress testing is especially useful for combined hemodynamic-metabolic-ventriculographic studies[124] because quantitative left ventricular angiography and myocardial lactate metabolism can be obtained during or immediately after pacing, uncomplicated by an elevation of systemic arterial lactate levels, as occurs in dynamic exercise. When atrial pacing to induce ischemia is carried out in patients with chronic angina secondary to obstructive CAD, elevations in ventricular end-diastolic pressure occur frequently and usually in association with the development of angina and at a reproducible heart rate–blood pressure product.[124] Impaired ventricular relaxation and increased regional diastolic myocardial stiffness have also been demonstrated during pacing-induced ischemia[125] and represent one component of the altered diastolic properties of the ischemic ventricle (p. 1179).

LEFT VENTRICULAR FUNCTION. Left ventricular dysfunction can be detected with greatest accuracy by means of biplane contrast ventriculography. Global abnormalities of left ventricular function are expressed in elevations of left ventricular end-diastolic and end-systolic volumes and depression of the ejection fraction (p. 424). However, abnormalities of *regional* wall motion (hypokinesia, akinesia, or dyskinesia; Fig. 9–55, p. 272) are more sensitive, specific, and characteristic of CAD, since the latter is usually regional in distribution. Also, hyperkinetic contraction of nonischemic myocardium may compensate for hypokinetic or akinetic ischemic or necrotic myocardium, thereby maintaining normal or almost-normal *global* left ventricular function, despite marked depression of function in one region of the ventricle.[126]

Left ventricular function (global or regional) may be normal at rest in patients with chronic CAD without previous myocardial infarction but become abnormal during or after stress (exercise, pacing). While in most instances resting abnormalities of left ventricular function signify irreversible damage, i.e., prior infarction or acute ischemia, chronic hypoperfusion sufficient to maintain the viability but not the contractility of the myocardium can result in persistent ventricular dysfunction, a condition termed "myocardial hibernation"[127,128,128a] (p. 1176). This form of reversible left ventricular dysfunction may or may not be accompanied by angina pectoris or electrocardiographic changes of ischemia. The reversibility of this form of left ventricular dysfunction is reflected in long-term improvement after revascularization (by surgery or percutaneous transluminal coronary angioplasty) or transiently after an inotropic stimulus (postextrasystolic) potentiation[129] or the infusion of a sympathomimetic amine.[130]

Histopathological studies of myocardial biopsy specimens obtained at the time of coronary artery bypass operations have demonstrated that those segments that exhibit reversible asynergy at angiography are made up predominantly of histologically normal myocardium, while the segments that do not exhibit response to inotropic stimuli exhibit marked muscle loss and replacement by fibrous tissue.[131] The more responsive areas are usually better perfused, either by the native coronary artery or by collateral vessels, and are associated with a lower frequency of electrocardiographic Q waves.[132] The most severe aspect of left ventricular asynergy is the well-demarcated aneurysm, which not only exhibits contractile failure but also is unable to resist expansion during ventricular systole; in other words, it exhibits dyskinesis (paradoxical pulsation).

In addition to demonstrating areas of asynergy, left ventriculography may also show mitral valve prolapse, which occurs in 20 to 25 per cent of patients with obstructive CAD[133] and probably results from impaired contractility of the ventricular myocardium and papillary muscles.

Coronary Blood Flow and Myocardial Metabolism. Abnormal myocardial metabolism has also been documented by means of cardiac catheterization in patients with chronic stable angina. With a catheter in place in the coronary sinus, arterial and coronary venous lactate measurements are obtained at rest and after suitable stresses, such as the infusion of isoproterenol[134] or pacing.[135] Since lactate is a byproduct of anaerobic glycolysis, its production by the heart and subsequent appearance in coronary sinus blood is a reliable sign of myocardial ischemia (p. 1182). When combined with coronary arteriography, this technique may be helpful in localizing significant coronary obstructive lesions and myocardial ischemia.[136]

Coronary flow reserve (maximum flow divided by resting flow, p. 1173) has been measured in patients at cardiac catheterization with coronary sinus thermodilution, Doppler-tipped catheters, and digital subtraction angiography.[137] This invasive measurement is relatively imprecise. Another approach to obtain this variable is by means of quantitative coronary arteriography, which incorporates per cent narrowing with other measurements, including lumen area and vessel length derived by automated border recognition and densitometry. These dimensions can be integrated into a single number, stenosis flow reserve, which if it is below 2.0 to 2.5 is usually associated with clinical manifestations of ischemia, most commonly exertional angina.[137] If this technique is coupled with positron-emission tomography (p. 302), a complete description of the arterial narrowing and its metabolic consequences may be obtained.

Studies of endothelial function in the human coronary circulation (p. 1168) may reveal evidence of a diffuse abnormality of endothelial function even in the presence of angiographically normal coronary arteries.[138,139] An abnormal response, i.e., vasoconstriction, of coronary endothelium to a variety of vasoactive stimuli such as acetylcholine may precede the angiographic recognition of CAD.[139a]

RIGHT-HEART PRESSURE MEASUREMENTS. The value of right-heart catheterization in patients primarily undergoing routine evaluation for CAD has been questioned. It reveals previously unsuspected abnormalities such as right-sided pressure elevations or pulmonary hypertension in only 20 per cent of patients, and the data from right-sided catheterization alter management infrequently.[140] Therefore, routine right-sided catheterization is usually unnecessary in patients with a normal cardiac examination who are undergoing routine, diagnostic coronary angiography, if an echocardiogram has already been obtained and the clinician believes that CAD represents the patient's major cardiac problem.

MANAGEMENT

The management of chronic stable angina involves four aspects: (1) correction of specific coronary risk factors, discussed in Chapter 37; (2) general and nonpharmacological methods, with particular attention toward adjustment of the patient's life style; (3) various specific medications used to treat angina; and (4) revascularization by percutaneous transluminal angioplasty and coronary bypass surgery.

GENERAL MEASURES

General measures include the treatment of hypertension (Chap. 29), which not only is a risk factor for the development and progression of atherosclerosis but also causes cardiac hypertrophy, augments myocardial oxygen requirements, and thereby intensifies myocardial ischemia in patients with obstructive coronary disease. Attainment of an ideal body weight is particularly important in obese patients in whom weight reduction raises the threshold for and may even abolish angina pectoris.

It is imperative for patients with chronic CAD who are cigarette smokers to discontinue this practice. Among patients with angiographically documented CAD, cigarette smokers have a higher 5-year mortality and relative risk of infarction or sudden death than those who have quit smoking,[141] and smoking cessation lessens the risk of adverse coronary events in both older and younger persons with CAD.[142] Habitual smokers who survive out-of-hospital cardiac arrest have a lower incidence of recurrent arrest at 3 years if they stop smoking than do patients who continue to smoke.[143]

There appears to be a strong association between the risk of myocardial infarction and smoking,[144,145] and this risk appears related more to the number of cigarettes smoked per day than to the duration of smoking. Within a few years of stopping smoking this risk of infarction returns to a level similar to that in men who have never smoked.[146] These observations should

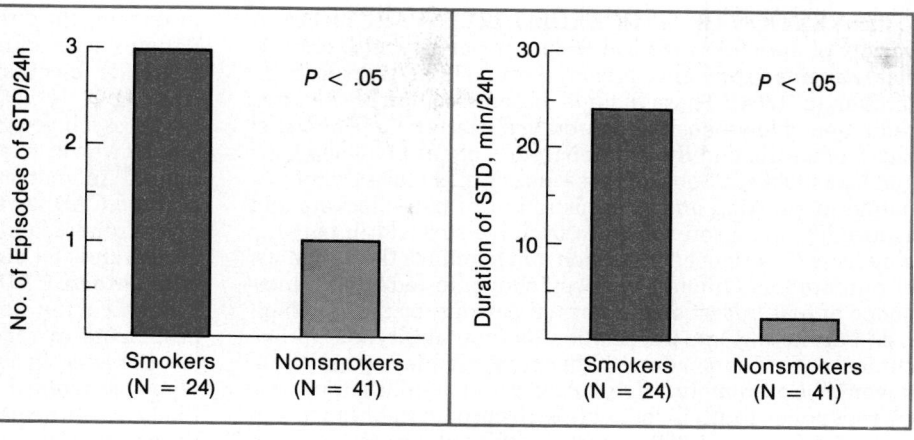

FIGURE 40-3. Influence of smoking on myocardial ischemia. Patients with chronic stable angina and a positive exercise test underwent continuous ambulatory monitoring to quantify the ischemic ST depression during daily life. The frequency of episodes of ischemia was 3 times greater and the duration of ischemia was 12 times longer in smokers than in nonsmokers. The histograms show the median number of episodes (left) and median duration of significant ST-segment depression (STD) (right) during 24 hours in 24 smokers and 41 nonsmokers. (From Barry, J., et al.: Effect of smoking on the activity of ischemic heart disease. JAMA *261*:398, 1989. Copyright 1989, American Medical Association.)

serve as a strong stimulus for discontinuing smoking. They suggest that cigarette smoking may be responsible for ischemic events other than through progression of atherosclerosis. Indeed, while cigarette smoking may increase myocardial oxygen demands and 24-hour energy expenditure (by approximately 10 per cent),[147] it can also cause reductions in coronary blood flow[148] due to an alpha-adrenergically mediated increase in coronary artery tone and increase myocardial ischemia (Fig. 40-3).[149,150]

Cigarette smoking also appears to interfere with the efficacy of antianginal drugs. Improvement in exercise tolerance and a reduction in angina pectoris were noted when cigarette smoking was discontinued while patients were receiving therapy with a beta blocker and nifedipine.[151] Active and passive cigarette smoking,[152] the inhalation of smog and carbon monoxide, and ascent to high altitude all lower the threshold for angina, and their avoidance represents an important aspect of therapy. Symptoms may be aggravated[153] or exercise performance impaired[153,154] in patients with chronic stable angina who encounter some specific environmental situations (traffic tunnels, houses with defective gas furnaces, and closed automobiles during heavy highway traffic).[154] The mechanism of symptom aggravation or exercise impairment is probably decreased oxygen delivery to the myocardium. Every effort must be made to avoid these aggravating stimuli.

In addition, fever, anemia, thyrotoxicosis, infection, tachycardia, hypoxemia (which occurs in acute and chronic pulmonary disease), and certain drugs used to treat noncardiac diseases (such as amphetamines and isoproterenol mists) all increase myocardial oxygen needs and may precipitate or intensify angina; cocaine can cause coronary spasm (p. 1167). These conditions and drugs must be eliminated. Congestive heart failure (by causing cardiac dilatation) and cardiac tachyarrhythmias can increase myocardial oxygen needs. Their treatment, as outlined in Chapters 17 and 24, will frequently diminish the frequency and severity of angina.

COUNSELING AND CHANGES IN LIFE STYLE. Effective communication with both the patient with angina pectoris and the family is essential. The psychosocial issues faced by the patient who develops chronic stable angina for the first time are similar to, although usually less intense than, those experienced by the patient with an acute myocardial infarction. Many patients have an unrealistically gloomy perception of their prognosis; they should be offered a realistic appraisal, together with an understandable explanation of the pertinent clinical features of the disease.

An important aspect of the physician's role is to counsel patients in the kind of work they can do, in their leisure activities, eating habits, vacation plans, and the like. It is desirable, if possible, to consult with the closest member(s) of the family, both to ensure an accurate and full assessment of the patient's activities and to inform the family of what can be expected in the course of the patient's illness.

Certain changes in life style may be helpful, such as modifying strenuous activities if they constantly and repeatedly produce angina. These changes may be minor in many instances. For example, golfing could be modified to include use of a golf cart instead of walking. Many activities, such as shopping or climbing stairs, need not be discontinued; often, it is merely necessary to perform them more slowly or to pause for brief periods of rest. The patient with chronic stable angina should avoid excessive fatigue and exhaustion; one or two regular rest periods during each day are often helpful. While it is desirable to minimize the number of bouts of angina, an occasional episode is not to be feared; indeed, unless patients occasionally reach their anginal threshold, they may not appreciate the extent of their exercise capacity. The vast majority of patients with chronic stable angina should not be treated as invalids. Often the propensity for angina actually declines, perhaps as a result of the development of collaterals or because of training effects, discussed later.

Eliminating or reducing the factors that precipitate anginal episodes is of obvious importance. Patients learn their usual threshold by trial and error. Since many anginal episodes are precipitated by increases in the mechanical activity of the heart (due to increases in myocardial oxygen consumption), the patient should avoid sudden bursts of activity, particularly after long periods of rest. Chronic angina exhibits a circadian rhythm (Fig. 39-14, p. 1214) characterized by a lower anginal threshold shortly after arising.[155] Therefore, morning activities such as showering, shaving, and dressing should be done at a slower pace, and if necessary with use of prophylactic nitroglycerin. The stress of sexual intercourse is ordinarily approximately equal to that of climbing one flight of stairs at a normal pace or of any activity that induces a heart rate of approximately 120 beats/min. With proper precautions, i.e., commencing more than 2 hours postprandially and taking an additional dose of a short-acting beta blocker 1 hour before and nitroglycerin 15 minutes before, the majority of patients with chronic stable angina are able to continue a satisfactory sexual life.

Just as there is a role for exercise in the management of CAD, so is there a role for rest, especially in situations in which angina has become frequent or severe. Marked restriction of activity or even complete bed rest, in addition to drug therapy, may be necessary to control symptoms. In less critical situations, merely reducing the amount of time spent working or increasing the rest periods will have a beneficial effect. For example, a long lunch break including a short nap may be beneficial. It may be helpful for the patient to use a face mask or scarf to cover the mouth or nose in cold weather. A hot, humid environment may also precipitate angina, and air conditioning may be a necessity rather than a luxury for patients with ischemic heart disease. Large meals can have a similar effect if they are followed by exertion. An effort should be made to minimize emotional outbursts, since they too increase myocardial oxygen requirements and sometimes induce coronary vasoconstriction. Occasionally antianxiety drugs or sedation may be useful.

PREVENTION OF MYOCARDIAL (RE)INFARCTION. A variety of measures are used widely in patients with chronic stable angina to prevent acute myocardial infarction and reinfarction (p. 1264). These include discontinuation of smoking, reduction of low-density lipoprotein cholesterol and elevated blood pressure, and the administration of antiplatelet agents and beta blockers. Some of these measures, such as discontinuation of smoking and administration of beta blockers and aspirin,[156] have been shown to improve survival in patients who have experienced infarction and to reduce the incidence of reinfarction. Others have been shown to reduce the incidence of first infarctions in normal persons, or those at high risk, but there is less information on their ability to improve clinical outcome in patients with chronic stable angina. While it would be extremely helpful to obtain such information, it is current policy to advise patients with chronic stable angina to cease smoking (p. 1303), assume an ideal body weight, and control blood pressure.

In men with chronic stable angina but no prior history of myocardial infarction who took aspirin, there was an 87-per cent reduction in the risk of myocardial infarction during 5 years of follow-up.[157] Therefore, in patients with chronic stable angina without contraindications to the drug, the administration of low-dose aspirin (160 mg/day or 325 mg every other day) may be beneficial in reducing the subsequent incidence of myocardial infarction. There is no evidence that long-term use of anticoagulants is indicated in these patients.

Whether beta blockers have any value in preventing infarction and sudden death in patients with chronic stable angina, as they do in patients after myocardial infarction, is not clear. However, since the beneficial effects observed in the post-myocardial infarction population (p. 1254) also possibly occur in the chronic stable angina group, it seems sensible to administer the drugs when angina or hypertension or both are present in these patients and when these drugs are well tolerated. Perhaps the antiarrhythmic and antiischemic effects exhibited by patients with recent myocardial infarction treated with beta blockers also occur in patients with chronic stable angina.

While strong effort should be made to bring total and LDL cholesterol to optimal levels in patients with chronic stable angina, it is not clear that intense dietary and pharmacological measures need be undertaken in the elderly (> 70 years). Men with CAD, thought to be at high risk for subsequent cardiovascular events, underwent intensive lipid-lowering therapy over a 2½-year period and demonstrated a reduced frequency of progression of coronary lesions, reduced incidence of adverse events (death, myocardial infarction, or revascularization), and increased frequency of regression of coronary lesions compared with patients assigned to conventional therapy.[158] This suggests that efforts to lower lipids in patients with a high-risk profile are justified and that this may influence favorably their long-term outcome.

EXERCISE (see also Chapter 42). The *conditioning effect of exercise* on skeletal muscles allows the patient to develop a greater workload at any level of total body oxygen consumption. The conditioning effect of exercise on the heart, by decreasing the heart rate at any level of exercise, allows a higher cardiac output to be achieved at any level of myocardial oxygen consumption. The combination of these two effects of exercise conditioning permits the patient with chronic stable angina to increase physical performance substantially following institution of a continuing exercise program. The reduced pressure-rate product lowers myocardial oxygen requirements during exertion and enables the patient with CAD to perform at higher workloads before reaching the ischemic threshold.[159] Therefore, physical conditioning reduces the amount of oxygen needed by the heart for any given amount of total body work. An example of this effect is seen in the study of Redwood et al. carried out in patients with chronic stable angina. They reported that a 6-week training program improved exercise performance by reducing the responses of heart rate and arterial pressure to bicycle exercise and by

prolonging the duration of exercise before angina occurred.[160] Patients with chronic ischemic heart disease may achieve a greater ejection fraction at equivalent workloads after training.

The psychological benefits of exercise are difficult to evaluate. However, exercise conditioning programs may be quite helpful in increasing the self-confidence of patients with chronic CAD (as they do in patients recovering from acute myocardial infarction). The question whether or not exercise accelerates the development of collateral vessels in patients with chronic CAD is unsettled.[161]

For all of the aforementioned reasons, patients are urged to participate in regular exercise programs — usually walking (see below) — in conjunction with their drug therapy. Patients who are involved in exercise programs usually are also more likely to be health conscious, to pay attention to diet and weight, and to discontinue cigarette smoking. Thus, in addition to a conditioning effect on skeletal and cardiac muscle, regular dynamic exercise provides the patient with a feeling of well-being, an important consideration in the management of any chronic disease.

The rationale and specific details for establishing an exercise program in patients with CAD are outlined in Chapter 42. Despite the many favorable effects of regular physical exercise in patients with chronic stable angina enumerated above, it must be acknowledged that there is no hard evidence that such programs improve survival or reduce the need for surgery in these patients.

NITRATES
(See also pp. 497 and 1172)

MECHANISM OF ACTION. Although the clinical effectiveness of amyl nitrite in angina pectoris was first described in 1867 by Brunton, organic nitrates are still the most common medications physicians employ to treat patients with this condition. The action of these agents is to relax vascular smooth muscle. The vasodilator effects of nitrates are evident in both systemic (including coronary) arteries and veins in normal subjects and in patients with ischemic heart disease, but they appear to be predominant in the venous circulation.[162] The decrease in venous tone reduces the return of blood to the heart and reduces preload and ventricular dimensions,[163] which in turn reduces wall tension and afterload. The actions of nitrates to reduce both preload and afterload make them useful in the treatment of heart failure as well as angina pectoris.

Posture is important in evaluating the hemodynamic effects of nitrates. In a patient in the supine position, venous return is normally greater while exercise tolerance and the anginal threshold are lower than in the upright position. The hemodynamic and angina-relieving effects of nitrates are most marked when patients are sitting or standing, i.e., when these drugs can reduce preload, and their hemodynamic effect resembles those of phlebotomy. By reducing the heart's mechanical activity, volume, and oxygen consumption, nitrates increase exercise capacity in patients with ischemic heart disease, i.e., a greater total body workload can be achieved before the anginal threshold is reached.

EFFECTS ON THE CORONARY CIRCULATION. A vasodilating effect of the nitrates on the larger (conductance) coronary arteries can be readily demonstrated, and there is evidence, obtained from quantitative, computer-assisted measurements of coronary arterial diameter, that nitroglycerin causes dilatation of epicardial stenoses. These are often eccentric lesions, and nitroglycerin causes relaxation of smooth muscle in the wall of the coronary artery that is not encompassed by the plaque. Even a small increase in the narrowed arterial lumen can produce a significant reduction in resistance to blood flow across the narrowed lesion (Fig. 40–4).[164]

Studies in experimental animals with coronary obstruction

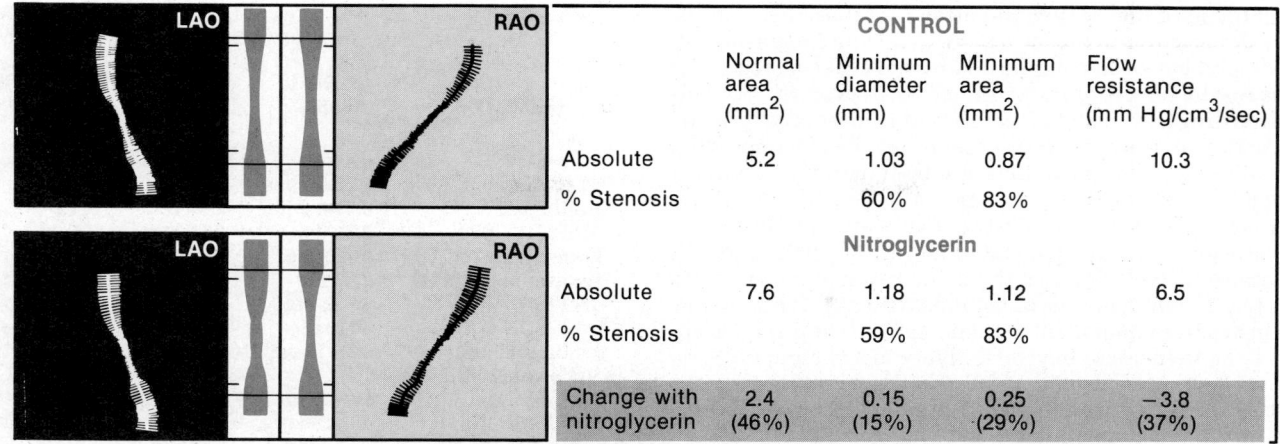

	CONTROL			
	Normal area (mm^2)	Minimum diameter (mm)	Minimum area (mm^2)	Flow resistance (mm Hg/cm^3/sec)
Absolute	5.2	1.03	0.87	10.3
% Stenosis		60%	83%	
	Nitroglycerin			
Absolute	7.6	1.18	1.12	6.5
% Stenosis		59%	83%	
Change with nitroglycerin	2.4 (46%)	0.15 (15%)	0.25 (29%)	−3.8 (37%)

FIGURE 40–4. A representative computer printout of segmental stenosis images and dimensional data for prenitroglycerin and postnitroglycerin (0.4 mg, sublingual) angiograms of this 60 per cent mid-right coronary artery stenosis. Each value is averaged from 8 estimates. LAO = left anterior oblique; RAO = right anterior oblique. (From Brown, B. G., et al.: The mechanisms of nitroglycerin action: Stenosis vasodilation as a major component of the drug response. Circulation 64:1089, 1981, by permission of the American Heart Association, Inc.)

have shown that nitroglycerin causes redistribution of blood flow from normally perfused to ischemic areas, particularly in the subendocardium,[165] perhaps mediated in part by an increase in collateral blood flow[166] and in part by a lowering of ventricular diastolic pressure, reducing subendocardial compression. The results of studies of nitroglycerin on coronary blood flow have been conflicting. Some studies in patients have reported increased blood flow after sublingual or intravenous nitroglycerin,[167] but most report no change or reduced flow.[168-170] However, since myocardial oxygen demands fell, the net effect on oxygen balance became favorable. In studies employing intracoronary injection of xenon-133[171] (as well as in retrograde perfusion studies performed during coronary bypass surgery), regional myocardial blood flow in areas perfused by stenotic coronary arteries rose after administration of nitroglycerin when well-developed collaterals supplying those regions were present. Atrial pacing studies indicate that after nitroglycerin the heart can be paced to higher rates before angina occurs. The nitrates have also been shown to improve ventricular wall motion in patients with ischemic heart disease, as demonstrated by contrast ventriculography,[172] echocardiography, and radionuclide ventriculography, at rest and during exercise.[173]

MECHANISM OF ANTIANGINAL ACTION. This action of the nitrates is complex (Fig. 40–5). Nitrates are not considered to exert a direct effect on the contractile state of the heart, although heart rate may rise reflexly as a consequence of the decline in blood pressure. When beta blockers are administered concurrently, the reflex tachycardia accompanying the nitrate-induced hypotension is blunted. Apparently, one action is to reduce the mechanical activity of the heart through the previously noted systemic effects, with subsequent reduction in left ventricular wall tension (which results from the simultaneous nitrate-induced reduction of arterial pressure and ventricular volume) and of myocardial oxygen consumption. Reduced left ventricular diastolic pressure may also decrease the resistance to coronary blood flow. It is probable that the cardiac actions of the nitrates—dilating epicardial stenoses, dilating coronary collateral vessels, and reducing ventricular diastolic pressure and thereby lowering extravascular resistance to endocardial perfusion—all act to increase oxygen delivery to ischemic myocardium. In the final analysis, some combination of a nitrate-induced reduction of myocardial oxygen requirements and increased oxygen delivery to the ischemic area relieves or prevents the development of myocardial ischemia in patients with chronic stable angina.

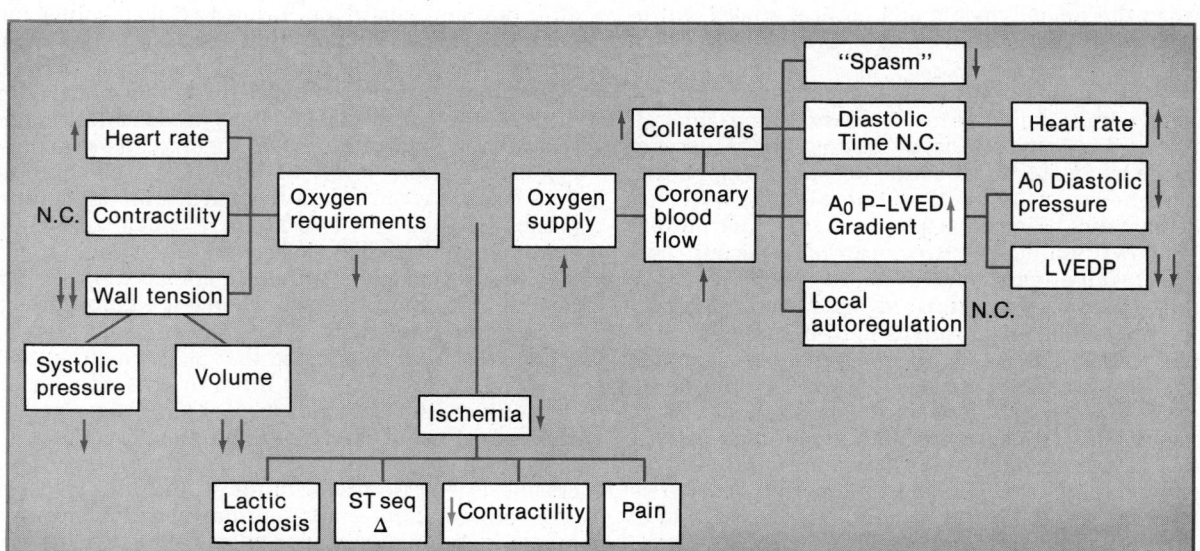

FIGURE 40–5. Factors influencing balance between myocardial oxygen requirements *(left)* and supply *(right)*. Arrows indicate effects of nitrates. In relieving angina pectoris, nitrates exert favorable effects by reducing oxygen requirements and increasing supply. Although a reflex increase in heart rate would tend to reduce the time for coronary flow, dilation of collaterals and enhancement of the pressure gradient for flow to occur as the LVEDP falls tend to increase coronary flow. AoP = aortic pressure; LVEDP = left ventricular end-diastolic pressure; NC = no change. (From Frishman, W. H.: Pharmacology of the nitrates in angina pectoris. Am. J. Cardiol. 56:81, 1985.)

Assessment of the relative importance of these two actions of nitroglycerin (reducing oxygen demand and increasing oxygen supply) has been complicated by the differing results of studies on the effects of intracoronary nitroglycerin. Any effect of the drug administered by this route must derive from its direct action on the coronary vascular bed, i.e., by improving myocardial oxygen supply; some studies have demonstrated a beneficial effect of intracoronary nitroglycerin,[164] while others have not. It is of interest that smoking-induced coronary vasoconstriction is prevented by nitroglycerin and calcium antagonists.[174] Perhaps the principal action of nitrates differs in different patients; in patients with a strong coronary vasoconstrictive component to their angina their principal action may be to increase oxygen delivery to ischemic myocardium, while in patients with relatively fixed lesions and constant-threshold angina their principal action may be to reduce myocardial oxygen demands.

Cellular Mechanism of Action. Nitrates have the ability to cause vasodilation whether or not endothelium is intact.[175] After entering the vascular smooth muscle cell, nitrates are converted to reactive nitric oxide–free radical (NO) or S-nitrosothiols, which activate intracellular guanylate cyclase to produce cyclic guanosine monophosphate (GMP),[162,175] which in turn triggers smooth muscle relaxation.[176] Sulfhydryl (SH) groups are required for both the formation of NO and the stimulation of guanylate cyclase, and nitroglycerin-induced vasodilation can be enhanced by prior administration of N-acetylcysteine, an agent that increases the availability of sulfhydryl groups.[177] This action of N-acetylcysteine potentiates the peripheral hemodynamic responses[177] and the coronary vasodilator effect of nitroglycerin[178] and reverses the partial tolerance to the coronary vasodilator effect of nitroglycerin.[179]

Types of Preparations and Routes of Administration

Nitroglycerin administered sublingually remains the drug of choice for treatment of acute anginal episodes. A transient but effective concentration of the drug rapidly appears in the circulation because sublingual administration avoids first-pass hepatic metabolism. The half-life of nitroglycerin itself is brief, and it is rapidly converted to two inactive metabolites, both of which are found in the urine after nitroglycerin administration. The liver possesses large amounts of hepatic glutathione organic nitrate reductase, but there is also evidence that blood vessels (veins and arteries) may metabolize nitrates directly. Thus, within 30 to 60 minutes hepatic breakdown has abolished the hemodynamic and clinical effects. Nitroglycerin is also available in a variety of other forms (Table 40–2).

The usual sublingual dosage is 0.3 to 0.6 mg, and most patients respond within 5 minutes to one or two 0.3-mg tablets. If symptoms are not relieved by a single dose, additional doses of 0.3 mg may be taken at 5-minute intervals, but no more than 1.2 mg should be used within a 15-minute period. The development of tolerance is rarely a problem with intermittent usage (see below). Sublingual nitroglycerin is especially useful when it is taken prophylactically shortly before activities are begun that are likely to cause angina. Used for this purpose, it may prevent angina for up to 30 to 40 minutes.

ADVERSE REACTIONS. These are common and include headache, flushing, and hypotension. The last is only rarely severe but can be potentially dangerous if the chest pain is due to a myocardial infarction rather than angina and arterial pressure has already declined because of pump failure and/or a vagal reaction or hypovolemia. In addition, the partial pressure of oxygen in arterial blood may fall after large doses of nitroglycerin because of a ventilation-perfusion imbalance due to inability of the pulmonary vascular bed to constrict in areas of alveolar hypoxia and thereby redirect perfusion to less hypoxic tissues.[180] Methemoglobinemia is a rare complication of very large doses of nitrates (p. 1761). Commonly used doses of nitrates cause small elevations of methemoglobin that probably are not of clinical significance.

TABLE 40-2   DOSAGE AND KINETICS OF NITROGLYCERIN AND LONG-ACTING NITRATES

MEDICATION	USUAL DOSAGE	ONSET OF ACTION	DURATION OF ACTION
Aerosol NTG	0.4 mg	2–5 min	10–30 min
NTG ointment (2%)	½–2 inches	20–60 min	3–8 hr
Sublingual NTG	0.3–0.6 mg	2–5 min	10–30 min
Oral NTG (SR)	2.5–9 mg	30–45 min	2–8 hr*
Transdermal NTG	5–15 mg	30–60 min	8–14 hr
Transmucosal NTG	1–3 mg	2–5 min	3–5 hr*
Oral ISDN	5–30 mg	15–30 min	3–6 hr
Oral ISDN (SR)	40 mg	30–60 min	6–10 hr
Sublingual and chewable ISDN	2.5–10 mg	3–15 min	1–2 hr
Oral ISMN	10–40 mg	30 min	6–8 hr
Oral ISMN (SR)	40–100 mg	30 min	6–10 hr
Sublingual and chewable ET	5–15 mg	3–15 min	2 hr
Oral ET	10 mg	30 min	Variable
Oral PET	10–40 mg	30 min	3–6 hr
Oral PET (SR)	30–80 mg	Slow	6–10 hr

* Duration of action lengthens with increasing dosage.

ET = erythrityl tetranitrate; ISDN = isosorbide dinitrate; ISMN = isosorbide-5-mononitrate (not available in the U.S.); NTG = nitroglycerin; PET = pentaerythrityl tetranitrate; SR = sustained release.

PREPARATIONS. Nitroglycerin tablets tend to lose their potency, especially if exposed to light, and should be kept in dark containers. Other nitrate preparations are available in sublingual, buccal, oral, spray, and ointment form (Table 40–2). Isosorbide dinitrate and other long-acting preparations are available in 2.5- and 5.0-mg sublingual tablets, 10-mg buccal (chewable) form, and 5-, 10-, and 20-mg tablets for oral use, as well as in 40-mg (sustained-release) capsules. An oral nitroglycerin spray that dispenses metered, aerosolized doses of 0.4 mg may be better absorbed than the sublingual form in patients with dry mucosal membranes. It can also be quickly sprayed onto, or under, the tongue with one hand and has a 3-year shelf life. For prophylaxis, the spray should be used 5 to 10 minutes before attack-provoking activities.[181]

Isosorbide Dinitrate. Isosorbide dinitrate is an effective antianginal agent but has low bioavailability after oral administration, because it undergoes rapid hepatic metabolism[182] and there are marked variations in plasma concentrations after oral administration. It has two metabolites (one has a potent vasodilator action) that are cleared less rapidly than the parent drug and are excreted unchanged in the urine.

Isosorbide-5-mononitrate,[183] an active metabolite of the dinitrate (not yet available in the United States), is completely bioavailable, since it does not undergo first-pass hepatic metabolism. Plasma levels of isosorbide-5-mononitrate reach their peak between 30 minutes and 2 hours, and the drug has a plasma half-life of 4 to 6 hours. A single 20-mg tablet still exhibits activity 8 hours after administration.

Partial or complete nitrate tolerance develops with regimens of isosorbide dinitrate when it is administered as 30 mg three or four times daily.[184,185] When this drug is used, a dosage schedule should be adopted that allows a 10- to 12-hour nitrate-free interval.[164,186-188] If the drug is administered on a three-times daily schedule (e.g., at 8 AM, 1 PM, and 6 PM), the antianginal benefit lasts for approximately 6 hours, and the magnitude of the antianginal benefit decreases with each successive dose.[185] Isosorbide dinitrate, like nitroglycerin, dilates both atherosclerotic and normal epicardial coronary segments, including diseased segments in small and medium-size arteries.[189] The drug has been shown to augment the increased exercise response observed with beta-adrenoceptor blockers.[190] While oral nitrates are not especially potent agents, they can reduce the incidence of anginal attacks and the need for sublingual nitroglycerin as well as raise the threshold of activity required for the development of angina.

TOLERANCE. Partial or complete nitrate tolerance develops with transdermal nitroglycerin patches,[191] once-daily applications of sustained-release isosorbide dinitrate ointment,[192] and regimens of isosorbide dinitrate administered 30 mg four times daily,[184] and 20 to 30 mg three times daily (at 8 AM, 1 PM, and 6 PM).[185] Thus, any regimen using frequent doses of long-acting nitrates (three or more times daily), continuous delivery systems (intravenous nitroglycerin or transdermal nitroglycerin patches) or long-acting (sustained-release) preparations *will result in tolerance unless there is a 10- to 12-hour nitrate-free interval.*[162,186-188,192a] Nitroglycerin administered by the buccal route does not result in tolerance and, even after 2 weeks of therapy, there is no diminished efficacy when buccal nitroglycerin is administered three times daily.[193] Even in patients who are already tolerant to long-acting oral nitrate therapy, intermittent doses of sublingual nitroglycerin will be effective.[194] Transdermal nitroglycerin patches will retain their efficacy provided patients have a 12-hour nitrate-free interval every 24 hours.[188]

The most commonly accepted hypothesis for the development of nitrate tolerance is that a depletion of intracellular sulfhydryl cofactors occurs in the metabolic conversion of nitroglycerin to nitric oxide or S-nitrosothiols, a conversion necessary for the activation of guanylate cyclase.[192,195,196] It is also possible that nitrate therapy is associated with increased catecholamine release and activation of the renin-angiotensin system, which might oppose the effect of nitrate-induced vasodilation.[195,196] It has been shown that if the sulfhydryl groups of the nitrate receptors are replenished by compounds such as N-acetylcysteine[177] or made more available by methionine,[197] then nitrate tolerance can be partially reversed[177] or the hemodynamic effects of intravenous nitroglycerin can be potentiated.[197]

Topical Nitroglycerin. Nitroglycerin ointment (15 mg/inch) is efficacious when applied (mostly commonly to the chest) in strips of 0.5 to 2.0 inches. Delay in the onset of action is approximately 30 minutes. Since it is effective for 4 to 6 hours, this form of the drug is particularly useful in patients with severe angina or unstable angina who are confined to bed and chair. Nitroglycerin ointment also may be used prophylactically after retiring by patients with nocturnal angina. Skin permeability increases with increased hydration, and absorption is also enhanced if the paste is covered with plastic whose edges are taped to the skin.

Transdermal Nitroglycerin Patches. A silicone gel or polymer matrix is impregnated with nitroglycerin, and absorption is then maintained for 24 to 48 hours at a rate determined by various methods of preparation, including a semipermeable membrane placed between the drug reservoir and the skin. The release rate of the patches varies from 2.5 to 15 mg/24 hours. Relatively low doses (2.5 mg to 5 mg/24 hours) may not produce sufficient plasma and tissue concentrations to sustain consistent, effective antianginal effects.[198]

A meta-analysis of randomized clinical trials of nitroglycerin patches suggested that in doses of 5 to 10 mg/24 hours exercise duration was improved early after administration, but by 24 hours the effect of nitroglycerin on exercise performance was attenuated by nitrate tolerance.[199] However, a regimen in which transdermal nitroglycerin was applied for 12 hours, and removed for 12 hours, improved exercise performance for 8 to 12 hours after application of the patch. After 1 month of such therapy, responsiveness to transdermal nitroglycerin remained virtually unchanged.[188] Therefore, after application of a transdermal nitroglycerin patch one can expect therapeutic efficacy (improved exercise performance) for 8 to 12 hours, and provided a substantial nitrate-free interval (of 10 to 12 hours) exists every 24-hour period, sustained improvement in exercise performance may be maintained. If a state of tolerance has been induced, a nitrate-free interval will restore responsiveness. If large, intermittent doses of transdermal or oral nitrates are employed (equivalent to 20 mg/24 hours of a transdermal patch), it is possible that rebound angina may occur during the nitrate-free period.[188,192]

WITHDRAWAL OF NITRATES. Because of the possibility of nitrate dependence, nitrate therapy should be withdrawn carefully. In individuals exposed to industrial doses of nitroglycerin, nitrate tolerance, nitrate dependence, and withdrawal symptoms may cause serious problems. During the manufacture of dynamite, substantial levels of nitrates are often present in the atmosphere and can be absorbed from the skin and lungs. After an acute response of headache, hypotension, palpitations, and gastrointestinal disturbance, adaptation occurs. Withdrawal from this environment may result in angina unrelated to exertion or emotion. In fact, spontaneous coronary vasospasm and acute myocardial infarction have been documented during a period of withdrawal.[200] A less dramatic, but far more common, form of nitrate withdrawal is observed in patients whose angina is intensified after discontinuation of large doses of long-acting nitrates.

BETA-ADRENOCEPTOR BLOCKING AGENTS
(See also p. 862)

These drugs constitute a cornerstone of therapy for effort-induced chronic stable angina. In the United States, four beta-adrenoceptor blocking drugs have been approved for the treatment of *angina*: atenolol, metoprolol, nadolol, and propranolol. A number of studies have shown that beta-adrenoceptor blockers, in doses that are generally well tolerated, reduce the frequency of anginal episodes and raise the anginal threshold, both when given alone and when added to other antianginal agents. The salutary action of these drugs, which have a chemical structure resembling that of isoproterenol and other beta-adrenoceptor agonists, depends on their ability to cause competitive inhibition of the effects of neuronally released and circulating catecholamines on beta-adrenoceptors.[201] In this manner, these drugs attenuate the cardiac responses to adrenergic stimulation (chiefly increases in heart rate and contractility). Thus, beta blockers reduce myocardial oxygen demands primarily during activity or excitement when surges of increased sympathetic activity occur. Effects on heart rate and myocardial contractility at rest are less prominent because of the lower adrenergic drive to the heart in the basal state. Beta-adrenoceptor blockers also lower myocardial oxygen needs by reducing arterial pressure, and they are extremely useful antihypertensive agents (p. 862).

Coronary vasoconstriction during the cold pressor test has been shown to be potentiated by beta-adrenergic receptor blockers in patients with coronary artery disease[202] but intracoronary administration of propranolol does not cause coronary vasoconstriction of epicardial vessels at rest or during exercise.[203] In clinical practice the potential adverse influence of unopposed increased alpha-receptor-mediated coronary artery tone associated with beta-blocker therapy is not a problem, except in some patients with variant angina (p. 1344).

Continuous ambulatory electrocardiographic and intraarterial blood pressure monitoring during normal daily activities of patients with chronic stable effort angina suggest that many ischemic events may be precipitated by transient impairment of regional myocardial perfusion rather than increases in myocardial oxygen demand.[20a] Beta blockers significantly reduce episodes of transient myocardial ischemia in these patients.[204]

CHARACTERISTICS OF DIFFERENT BETA BLOCKERS. The differing pharmacological properties of these agents affect their clinical effects (Table 40-3).

Selectivity. Two major subtypes of beta receptors, designated beta$_1$, and beta$_2$,[205] are present in different proportions in different tissues. Beta$_1$ receptors predominate in the heart, and their stimulation leads to an increase in heart rate and A-V conduction and contractility, whereas stimulation of these receptors leads to the release of renin in juxtaglomerular cells and lipolysis in adipocytes. Beta$_2$ stimulation results in bronchodilation, vasodilatation, and glycogenolysis.

The beta blockers have been classified according to their

TABLE 40-3 PHARMACOKINETICS AND PHARMACOLOGY OF SOME BETA-ADRENOCEPTOR BLOCKERS

	Atenolol	Metoprolol	Nadolol	Pindolol	Propranolol	Timolol	Propranolol HCl	Propranolol LA	Acebutolol	Labetalol
Extent of absorption (%)	≈50	>95	≈30	>90	90	>90	>90	>90	≈70	>90
Extent of bioavailability (% of dose)	≈40	≈50	≈30	≈90	≈30	75	≈30	≈20	≈50	≈25
Beta-blocking plasma concentration	0.2–0.5 μg/ml	50–100 ng/ml	50–100 ng/ml	50–100 ng/ml	50–100 ng/ml	5–10 ng/ml	50–100 ng/ml	20–100 ng/ml	0.2–2.0 μg/ml	0.7–3.0 μg/ml
Protein binding (%)	<5	12	≈30	57	93	≈10	93	93	30–40	≈50
Lipophilicity*	Low	Moderate	Low	Moderate	High	Low	High	High	Low	Low
Elimination half-life (hr)	6 to 9	3 to 4	14 to 25	3 to 4	3.5 to 6.0	3 to 4	3–4	10	3–4‡	≈6
Urinary recovery of unchanged drug (% of dose)	≈40	≈3	70	≈40	<1	≈20	<1	<1	≈40	<1
Total urinary recovery (% of dose)	>95	>95	70	>90	>90	65	>90	>90	>90	>90
Drug accumulation in renal disease	Yes	No	Yes	No	No	No	No	No	Yes§	No
Predominant route of elimination†	RE (mostly unchanged)	HM	RE	RE (≈40% unchanged) and HM	HM	RE (≈20% unchanged) and HM	HM	HM	HM§	HM
Active metabolites	No	No	No	No	Yes	No	Yes	Yes	Yes	No
β_1-blocker potency ratio (propranolol = 1)	1.0	1.0	1.0	6.0	1.0	6.0	1.0	1.0	0.3	0.3
Relative β_1 sensitivity	+	+	0	0	0	0	0	0	Yes	0
Intrinsic sympathetic activity	0	0	0	+	0	0	0	0	+	0
Membrane-stabilizing activity	0	0	0	+	++	0	++	++	+	0
Usual maintenance dose	50–100 mg/qd	50–100 mg/qid	40–80 mg/qd	5–20 mg/tid	60 mg/qid	20 mg/bid	60 mg/qid	80–160 mg/qd	200–600 mg/bid	100–600 mg/bid

*Determined by the distribution ratio between octanol and water.
†RE = renal excretion; HM = hepatic metabolism.
‡Half-life of the active metabolite, diacetolol, is 12 to 15 hours.
§Acebutolol is mainly eliminated by the liver, but its major metabolite, diacetolol, is excreted by the kidney.
Modified from Frishman, W. H., et al.: Antianginal agents, Part 2: β-Blockers. Hosp. Formul. 21:62, 1986.

relative cardioselectivity, i.e., beta₁-blocking properties. *Nonselective* beta-blocking drugs (propranolol, nadolol, oxprenolol, penbutolol, pindolol, sotalol, timolol, carteolol) block both beta₁ and beta₂ receptors, whereas *cardioselective* beta blockers (atenolol, betaxolol, bevantolol, esmolol, metoprolol) produce selective blockade of beta₁ receptors, while having lesser effects on beta₂ receptors. Thus, cardioselective beta blockers will reduce myocardial oxygen demands while tending not to block bronchodilation, vasodilatation, or glycogenolysis. As the dosages administered are increased, this cardioselectivity diminishes.[206] Since cardioselectivity is only relative, the use of cardioselective beta blockers in doses sufficient to prevent angina may still cause bronchoconstriction in some susceptible patients. Some drugs with beta-blocking properties also have the ability to cause vasodilatation. These include labetalol (an alpha-adrenergic blocking agent and a beta₂ agonist, p. 866), carvedilol (a direct vasodilator with beta₁- and beta₂-blocking activity), and dilevalol (the R,R isomer of labetalol that causes vasodilation due to beta₂-agonist activity and has beta₁- and beta₂-receptor competitive antagonist properties). Such agents are useful in the treatment of hypertension.

Membrane-Stabilizing Activity. This property refers to the "quinidine-like" effect of certain beta blockers that reduce the rate of rise of the cardiac action potential (p. 358). The clinical relevance of this effect is questionable because it is observed only at concentrations far exceeding therapeutic levels of the beta blockers that exhibit this action at all (propranolol, acebutolol).

Intrinsic Sympathomimetic Activity. Beta blockers with intrinsic sympathomimetic activity (acebutolol, carteolol, celiprolol, dilevalol, oxprenolol, penbutolol, pindolol) are "partial agonists" and produce blockade by shielding beta receptors from more potent beta agonists. Pindolol and acebutolol produce low-grade beta stimulation when sympathetic activity is low (at rest), while under conditions of stress and exercise, when sympathetic activity is high, partial agonists behave more like conventional beta blockers.

Pindolol causes little if any lowering of heart rate, depression of A-V conduction, or depression of contractility at rest but still blocks the effects of exercise on these variables. Its partial agonist activity also induces bronchodilation.[207] In patients with severe symptoms and nocturnal angina, agents with partial agonist activity may not be as effective at reducing heart rate or the frequency, duration, and magnitude of ambulatory ST-segment changes (monitored over 48 hours) or increasing the duration of exercise.[208]

Potency. This is the ability of beta blockers to inhibit the tachycardia produced by isoproterenol. All drugs are considered in reference to propranolol, which is given a value of 1.0 (Table 40–3). Timolol and pindolol are the most potent agents, while acebutolol and labetalol are the least.

Lipid Solubility. The hydrophilicity or lipid solubility of beta blockers is a major determinant of their absorption and metabolism. The lipid-soluble (lipophilic) beta blockers, propranolol, metoprolol, and pindolol (Table 40–3), are readily absorbed from the gastrointestinal tract. They are metabolized predominantly by the liver, have a relatively short half-life, and usually require administration twice or more daily to achieve continuing pharmacological effects. The water-soluble beta blockers (hydrophilic), atenolol, sotalol, and nadolol, are not as readily absorbed from the gastrointestinal tract, are not as extensively metabolized, have relatively long plasma half-lives, and can be administered once daily. Thus, in patients with renal or hepatic dysfunction the lipid-insoluble agents may be preferable.

Lipid-insoluble beta blockers are less likely to cross the blood-brain barrier; central nervous system side effects of beta blockers include depression, sleep disturbances, nightmares, fatigue, and weakness. While beta blockers with increased lipid solubility, such as pindolol and metoprolol, cross the blood-brain barrier more readily, there is no direct, consistent correlation between this property and central nervous system side effects.[209,210] For example, atenolol and metoprolol cause a similar degree of central nervous system effects despite large differences in lipid solubility[210] and, while the lipid-soluble agents propranolol, pindolol, and metoprolol cause more sleep interruptions and restlessness than either placebo or atenolol, other measures of mood and psychomotor and sexual function do not appear to correlate with lipid solubility.[211] Overall, atenolol (low lipid solubility) and metoprolol (moderate lipid solubility) may be useful if central nervous system side effects are a problem with other beta blockers.

Alpha-Adrenoceptor Blocking Activity. The alpha-blocking potency of labetalol is approximately 20 per cent of its beta-blocking potency, and it is also one of the weaker beta blockers compared with propranolol[212] (Table 40–3). Its combined alpha- and beta-blocking effects make it a particularly useful antihypertensive agent (p. 866), especially in patients with hypertension and angina. During exercise testing in normotensive patients with angina, labetalol prolonged exercise duration and blunted the exercise-induced tachycardia and increases in arterial pressure.[213]

Oxidation Phenotype. Metoprolol and propranolol are lipid-soluble beta blockers noted for the variability of their pharmacokinetics, drug metabolism, and pharmacodynamics. It has been found that the oxidative metabolism of metoprolol exhibits the debrisoquin type of genetic polymorphism (p. 630) and that poor hydroxylators, or metabolizers (up to 10 per cent of Caucasians), have significant prolongation of the elimination half-life of the drug as compared with extensive hydroxylators, or metabolizers. Thus, angina might be controlled by a single daily dose of metoprolol in poor metabolizers, whereas extensive metabolizers require the same dose two or three times a day.[214] Therefore, clinicians should be aware that if a patient exhibits an exaggerated clinical response (e.g., extreme bradycardia) following administration of metoprolol, propranolol, or other lipid-soluble beta blockers, it may be the result of prolongation of the elimination half-life due to slow oxidative metabolism of the drug.

First-Pass Effects. The lipid-soluble beta blockers are usually rapidly absorbed from the gastrointestinal tract and metabolized extensively by the liver (first-pass metabolism) before they reach the systemic circulation. Drugs such as propranolol and metoprolol have extensive first-pass metabolism, while timolol and pindolol have moderate first-pass metabolism. If either metoprolol or propranolol is administered intravenously, a much higher concentration reaches the bloodstream, and therefore intravenous dosing has much greater potency than oral dosing.

Effects on Serum Lipids. In general, beta blocker therapy (with agents without intrinsic sympathomimetic activity [ISA]) usually causes no significant changes in total or LDL cholesterol but increases triglycerides and decreases HDL.[215,216] The most commonly studied drug has been propranolol, which can increase plasma triglyceride concentrations by up to 50 per cent and reduce HDL cholesterol by approximately 15 per cent.[215] (Sotalol, a drug without ISA, increases total cholesterol, triglycerides, and LDL cholesterol and also decreases HDL cholesterol.) Two drugs possessing ISA, acebutolol and pindolol, do not significantly change total cholesterol, triglycerides, or LDL cholesterol, but pindolol *increases* serum HDL cholesterol. The clinical importance of these changes in serum lipids after long-term administration of beta blockers for either hypertension or angina is unknown, but obviously physicians should be aware that beta blockers may affect the serum lipid profile of their patients and should

take this into account when monitoring long-term therapy.[215,216]

DOSAGE. For optimal results, the dosage of beta blocker should be carefully titrated. In the case of propranolol, it is useful to start with 80 mg of propranolol daily (20 mg four times a day) or comparable doses of other blockers. It should be realized that with such a dosage regimen 24 to 48 hours will be required for the drug to reach levels of 100 ng/ml needed to achieve the physiological effect usually required to achieve an antianginal effect, i.e., to reduce resting heart rate to 50 to 60 beats/min and to cause increase of less than 20 beats/min with modest exercise (e.g., climbing one flight of stairs) and to produce 70 to 80 per cent reduction in the tachycardia induced by strenuous exercise on a treadmill.[217] The usual dosage of propranolol ranges from 80 to 320 mg/day, but some patients require (and tolerate) doses as high as 1000 mg daily.

ADVERSE EFFECTS AND CONTRAINDICATIONS. These drugs are well tolerated by the majority of patients with angina pectoris. Most of the adverse reactions are a consequence of their beta-blocking properties and include cardiac effects (severe sinus bradycardia, sinus arrest, AV block, reduced left ventricular contractility), bronchoconstriction, fatigue, mental depression, nightmares, gastrointestinal upset, sexual dysfunction, intensification of insulin-induced hypoglycemia, cutaneous reactions, and withdrawal syndrome.[218] Lethargy, weakness, and fatigue may be caused by reduced cardiac output or may arise from a direct effect on the central nervous system. Nightmares, depression, and very rarely even psychotic reactions may occur. Bronchoconstriction results from a blockade of beta₂ receptors in the tracheobronchial tree (Table 40-4). As a consequence, asthma and chronic obstructive lung disease are contraindications to the use of such agents. As already noted, cardioselectivity of beta blockers such as metoprolol and atenolol is only relative, and the use of such drugs in dosages sufficient to prevent angina may still cause bronchoconstriction in susceptible patients. In general, therefore, a history of asthma or wheezing probably constitutes a contraindication to the use of beta blockers. Other side effects include skin rash, fever, gastrointestinal symptoms (nausea, diarrhea, or constipation), and pharyngitis. In patients who already have impaired left ventricular function, congestive heart failure may be intensified, an effect that can be counteracted by the use of digitalis or diuretics.

Beta blockers should *not* be used in patients with bradyarrhythmias of any kind unless a pacemaker is in place. In patients with partial AV block, they may impair conduction further. Blockade of noncardiac beta₂ receptors inhibits

TABLE 40-4   CONTRAINDICATIONS TO USE OF NITRATES, CALCIUM CHANNEL ANTAGONISTS, AND BETA-ADRENOCEPTOR BLOCKING AGENTS

	NITRATES	VERAPAMIL	DILTIAZEM	NIFEDIPINE	BETA BLOCKER
Aortic stenosis (severe)	1	2	2	3	2
Asthma	0	0	0	0	3
A-V conduction defects	0	3	2	0	2
Congestive heart failure	0	3	3	2	3
Coronary spasm	0	0	0	0	1
Hypersensitivity or idiosyncrasy	3	3	3	3	3
Hypotension (BP < 90 mm Hg systolic)	3	3	3	3	3
Peripheral arterial disease and Raynaud's	0	0	0	0	2
Pregnancy	2(C)	2(C)	2(C)	2(C)	2(**)
Sick sinus syndrome	0	2	2	0	2
Sinus bradycardia	0	2	2	0	2
Unstable angina (in absence of beta blocker)	0	1	0	3	0

LEVEL OF CONTRAINDICATION: 3 = contraindication; 2 = relative contraindication; 1 = possible contraindication; 0 = no contraindication.
FDA CATEGORIES:
   (B) = FDA Category B. Either animal reproduction studies have not demonstrated a fetal risk but there are no controlled studies in women, or animal reproduction studies have shown an adverse effect that was not confirmed in controlled studies in women in the first trimester.
   (C) = FDA Category C. Either studies in animals have revealed adverse effects on the fetus and there are no controlled studies in women, or studies in women and animals are not available. Drugs should be given only if the potential benefit justifies the potential risk to the fetus.
   (D) = FDA Category D. There is positive evidence of human fetal risk, but the benefits from use in pregnant women may be acceptable despite the risk. There will be an appropriate statement in the "warnings" section of the label.
   (**). FDA Categories for Beta-Adrenergic Blocking Agents: FDA Category B = atenolol, metoprolol; FDA Category C = nadolol, timolol, pindolol, labetalol, and acebutolol; FDA Category D = propranolol.

catecholamine-induced glycogenolysis so that noncardioselective beta blockers can impair the defense to insulin-induced hypoglycemia. Blockage of vascular beta$_2$ receptors also inhibits the vasodilating effects of catecholamines in peripheral blood vessels and leaves the constrictive (alpha-adrenergic) receptors unopposed and thereby enhances vasoconstriction. Noncardioselective beta blockers may precipitate episodes of Raynaud's phenomenon in patients with this condition and may cause uncomfortable coldness of the distal extremities. In patients with peripheral vascular disease, reduced flow to the limbs may occur.[219]

In patients with chronic stable angina, abrupt withdrawal of

TABLE 40-5 INTERACTIONS OF BETA-ADRENOCEPTOR BLOCKING AGENTS WITH OTHER DRUGS

PHARMACOKINETIC INTERACTIONS

1. **Cimetidine:** Reduces hepatic metabolism of beta blockers; increased plasma levels of beta blockers and serum half-life prolonged. Bradycardia may be excessive.
   Management: Monitor heart rate and reduce dose of one or both drugs.
2. **Aluminum hydroxide gel:** Delay or reduction in GI absorption with reduced plasma levels of beta blocker.
   Management: Take drugs at different times or increase beta blocker dose.
3. **Barbiturates:** Induction of hepatic enzymes enhances metabolism of beta blockers and reduces plasma levels.
   Management: Avoid barbiturates or increase beta blocker dosage.
4. **Lidocaine:** Propranolol therapy reduces hepatic clearance of lidocaine; serum lidocaine levels may increase, and toxicity may ensue.
   Management: Monitor plasma lidocaine concentration and reduce dosage if appropriate.

PHARMACODYNAMIC INTERACTIONS

1. **Verapamil:** Hypotension, bradycardia, negative inotropic responses and abnormal A-V conduction are all additive with beta blockers. Avoid concurrent use (especially in patients with depressed left ventricular function). Monitor patients carefully if concurrent use unavoidable.
2. **Epinephrine:** Hypertension (and reflex bradycardia) result from unopposed alpha-vasoconstrictive effects of epinephrine.
3. **Aminophylline:** By phosphodiesterase inhibition, aminophylline increases cyclic AMP. Antagonism results from concurrent use with beta blockers.
4. **Antidiabetic agents:** Propranolol may induce hypoglycemia (reduced glycogenolysis), hyperglycemia (inhibition of insulin release); hypertension (release of endogenous epinephrine with hypoglycemia and unopposed alpha-vasoconstrictor effects ensue), absence of tachycardia with hypoglycemia. Avoid beta blockers in diabetics if possible. Cardioselective agents preferable.
5. **Clonidine:** Sudden withdrawal (and norepinephrine release) may result in severe hypertension if unopposed alpha-adrenergic tone exists because of beta-adrenergic blockade.
   Management: Withdraw beta blockers before clonidine.
6. **Cyclopropane:** Combined effects of cyclopropane and beta blockade may result in depression of LV function.

OTHER INTERACTIONS

1. **Indomethacin:** May reduce antihypertensive effect of beta blockers.
2. **Ergot alkaloids:** With beta blockers may cause excessive vasoconstriction.
3. **Tricyclic antidepressants:** May inhibit the bradycardia and negative inotropic effects of beta blockers.
4. **Monoamine oxidase inhibitors:** Enhance hypotensive effect of beta blockers.
5. **Tubocurarine, succinylcholine, and pancuronium:** Potentiate muscle relaxation when used with beta blockers.

beta-adrenoceptor blocking agents can result in increased total ischemic activity, as detected by ambulatory monitoring. This may be caused by a return to the previously high levels of myocardial oxygen demand while the underlying atherosclerotic process had progressed.[218] Occasionally this can precipitate unstable angina and rarely even provoke myocardial infarction. Although experimental evidence suggests that there may be increased myocardial sensitivity to catecholamines upon withdrawal of beta-adrenoreceptor blockade,[220] this may have limited biological and clinical importance; in patients without cardiac failure, it has never been proved that up-regulation of myocardial beta$_1$ receptors occurs during long-term beta blocker therapy. If abrupt withdrawal of beta blockers is required, patients should be instructed to reduce exertion, manage anginal episodes with sublingual nitroglycerin, and/or substitute a calcium antagonist.

Drug interactions involving beta blockers also occur. Most of the available information relates to propranolol, but detailed information regarding other beta blockers is available[221] (Table 40-5).

CALCIUM ANTAGONISTS
(See also p. 867)

The critical role played by calcium ions in the normal contraction of cardiac and vascular smooth muscle is discussed on page 357. Despite their chemical heterogeneity, the major action of these drugs is to interfere with the entry of calcium into myocytes and vascular smooth muscle cells.[222-224,224a] These agents are effective in the treatment of chronic stable angina, either alone or in combination with beta-adrenoceptor blockers and nitrates.[225-227] Calcium antagonists appear to be beneficial in controlling angina and improving exercise tolerance in patients with chronic stable angina due to coronary atherosclerosis as well as in patients with Prinzmetal's variant angina (p. 1344) and those in whom angina results from abnormal, small coronary arteries with limited vasodilator reserve.[228]

Five calcium antagonists—nifedipine, verapamil, diltiazem, nicardipine, and bepridil—are approved in the United States by the FDA for the treatment of angina pectoris (Table 40-6). All of these agents are effective in causing relaxation of vascular smooth muscle in both the systemic arterial and coronary arterial beds. In addition, the antagonism of entry of calcium into myocardium results in a negative inotropic effect. Peripheral vascular dilation is more prominent than the negative inotropic effects of the dihydropyridines—nifedipine and nicardipine—and to a lesser extent of diltiazem; verapamil's effects on the heart and vascular bed are approximately evenly balanced.

A large number of so-called second-generation calcium antagonists have been developed. They are mainly dihydropyridine derivatives and most have longer plasma half-lives and greater vascular selectivity than the prototypical agent, nifedipine (Table 40-7).[223] Several of these agents have potentially useful features. *Amlodipine*, which is less lipid soluble than nifedipine, has slow, smooth onset and ultralong duration of action (plasma half-life = 36 hours). It causes marked coronary and peripheral dilation and may be useful in the treatment of hypertension and angina. *Nicardipine* has a similar half-life to nifedipine (2 to 4 hours), but intravenous administration is easier because it is water soluble without associated light sensitivity. It also appears to have greater vascular selectivity.

Other compounds have interesting possibilities. *Bepridil* is a less specific calcium antagonist that interacts with the dihydropyridine binding site as well as having sodium channel blocking effects. This agent markedly prolongs the atrial refractory period and thus has some potential use in the treatment of atrial arrhythmias as well as angina, although it is also arrhythmogenic and causes Q-T prolongation and torsades de pointes.

TABLE 40-6 PHARMACOKINETICS OF CALCIUM ANTAGONISTS USED COMMONLY FOR ANGINA TREATMENT*

	DILTIAZEM	NICARDIPINE	NIFEDIPINE	NIFEDIPINE GITS	VERAPAMIL
Usual adult dose	IV: 0.075 to 0.15 mg/kg Oral: 30-90 mg tid or qid	IV: 10-15 mg/hr for 30 min then 3-5 mg/hr Oral: 20-30 mg tid	SL: 10-30 mg tid or qid Oral: 10-30 mg tid or qid	Oral: 30-90 mg daily	IV: 0.075 to 0.15 mg/kg Oral: 80-120 mg tid or qid
Per cent absorbed	80-90	~100	90	>90	90
Extent of bioavailability (% of dose)	40-70	30	65-75	45-70	20-35
Onset of action	Oral: <15 min	<20 min	SL: <3 min Oral: <20 min	Approximately 6 hr	IV: ~2 min Oral: 2 hr
Peak effect	Oral: 30 min	1 hr	Oral: 1-2 hr	After 6 hr	IV: 3-5 min Oral: 3-4 hr
Therapeutic serum levels (ng/ml)	50-200	30-50	25-100	25-100	80-300
Protein binding (%)	70-80	>95	95	95	80-90
Elimination half-life (hr)	3.5-6.0	2.0-4.0	2.0-5.0	2.0-5.0	3.0-7.0†
Elimination	60% metabolized by liver; remainder excreted by kidneys		High first-pass hepatic metabolism		85% eliminated by first-pass hepatic metabolism
Urinary recovery of unchanged drug (% of dose)	2-4	<1	1-2	1-2	3-4
Active metabolites	Yes‡	No	No	No	Yes§

*All agents approved by FDA for treatment of angina pectoris.
†4.5-12 hr with multiple dosing.
‡Desacetyl-diltiazem has 25-50% activity of parent compound.
§Norverapamil has 20% activity of parent compound.
GITS = gastrointestinal therapeutic system, IV = intravenous, SL = sublingual.

Perhexiline maleate is a less specific calcium antagonist that does not interact with the dihydropyridine binding site. It may be useful in refractory angina, but infrequently causes unpredictable serious hepatic and neurological toxicity.[228a] However, if plasma levels are maintained in the 150 to 600 ng/ml range, these toxicities are usually avoidable.

Studies in experimental animals, both in primates and nonprimates, have suggested that calcium antagonists might have an antiatherogenic effect, and recent human studies support this.[229,230] In a multicenter, randomized trial utilizing quantitative arteriography, patients showing mild coronary artery disease developed significantly fewer new lesions taking nifedipine than did patients taking placebo.[229] Preexisting lesions did not appear to be affected, however. Another study comparing the effects of nifedipine, propranolol, and isosorbide dinitrate on angiographic progression and regression of coronary arterial narrowing also showed that patients receiving nifedipine developed fewer new lesions than patients taking the other two agents over a 2-year period.[230] Prolonged follow-up in such studies will be required to determine whether these angiographic observations will be accompanied by clinical benefits.

NIFEDIPINE. This dihydropyridine is particularly effective in reducing the contractility of smooth muscle, especially vascular smooth muscle. The dose is 10 mg orally every 8 hours, increased stepwise to 20 mg every 6 hours, guided by the blood pressure response. The dosage of 160 mg daily is considered to be maximal. An extended-release formulation of nifedipine utilizes the gastrointestinal therapeutic system (GITS) of drug delivery (Table 40-6). The formulation is designed to deliver 30, 60, or 90 mg of nifedipine in a single daily dose at a relatively constant rate over a 24-hour period, and patients can be readily switched from nifedipine capsules to the nearest total daily dose of the extended-release preparation,[231] which is useful for the treatment of chronic stable angina, vasospastic angina, and hypertension.

Nifedipine is a more potent vasodilator than either diltiazem or verapamil. Although its in vitro actions on myocardium and specialized cardiac tissue, i.e., the sinoatrial and AV nodes, are similar to those of the other agents, the concentration required to reproduce effects on these tissues is not reached in vivo because of the early appearance of its powerful vasodilating effects. Thus, in clinical practice the potential negative chronotropic, inotropic, and dromotropic (on A-V conduction) effects of nifedipine are seldom a problem.

In patients with chronic stable angina, maximally tolerated doses of nifedipine result in a significant increase in heart rate at rest and at peak exercise and also in a reduced resting systolic blood pressure but have no effect on the blood pressure achieved at peak exercise. Compared with placebo the duration of a symptom-limited treadmill exercise is prolonged following nifedipine administration.[232] The beneficial effects of nifedipine in the treatment of angina result from its capacity to reduce myocardial oxygen needs consequent to afterload reduction, and to increase myocardial oxygen delivery consequent to its dilating action on the coronary vascular bed. In conscious animals, nifedipine has been shown to dilate both large coronary arteries and coronary resistance vessels.[233] Nifedipine decreases left ventricular afterload, while ejection fraction, velocity of circumferential fiber shortening, heart rate, and cardiac index all show slight reflex increases; these increases can be blocked by simultaneous administration of beta-adrenoceptor blockers. In patients with elevated left ventricular end-diastolic pressures and volumes, nifedipine reduces these variables and enhances ejection fraction more than it does in patients with normal baseline left ventricular function.[234]

Adverse Effects. These occur in 15 to 20 per cent of patients; they lead to discontinuation of medication in about 5 per cent (Table 40-8). Most adverse effects are related to the systemic vasodilation and include headache, dizziness, flushing, hypotension, and troublesome leg edema (not related to heart failure). Gastrointestinal side effects, including nausea, epigastric pressure, and vomiting, are noted in approximately 5 per cent of patients. Occasionally, nifedipine aggravates angina, presumably by lowering arterial pressure excessively with subsequent reflex tachycardia, in patients with extremely severe, fixed coronary obstructions. For this reason, combined therapy of nifedipine with a beta blocker is particularly effective in the treatment of chronic stable angina and is superior to nifedipine alone.[226,227] Most of the adverse effects are reduced by use of the extended-release preparations.

A comparison of the side effects of nifedipine with those of other calcium antagonists is shown in Table 40-8. Because of its potent vasodilator effects, nifedipine is *contraindicated* (Table 40-4) in patients who are hypotensive or who have severe aortic valve stenosis and also in patients with unstable angina who are not taking a beta blocker, in whom reflex-mediated increases in heart rate may be harmful. In patients with mild left ventricular dysfunction, sinus bradycardia, sick sinus syndrome, and AV block (particularly if a beta-adrenoceptor blocking agent is concurrently administered and additional drug therapy of angina is indicated), nifedipine is the calcium antagonist of choice.[226] This is because in the clinical dosage range tolerated it has fewer negative effects on myocardial contractility or on the specialized automatic and con-

TABLE 40-7 SECOND-GENERATION CALCIUM ANTAGONISTS AND RELATED COMPOUNDS

AGENTS	POSSIBLE USES	CHARACTERISTICS	AGENTS	POSSIBLE USES	CHARACTERISTICS
DIHYDROPYRIDINES			Nisoldipine	Hypertension, angina, ? CHF	Medium action duration, plasma half-life = 8–11 hr. Possibly more selective as a vasodilator than nifedipine. Highly specific for slow calcium channel.
Amlodipine	Hypertension, angina	Ultra long acting, plasma half-life = 36 hr. Marked coronary and peripheral dilator properties with minimal changes in inotropy, chronotropy, and cardiac conduction. Slow, smooth onset of action (less lipid soluble than nifedipine).			
			Nitrendipine	Hypertension, ? angina, ? CHF	Medium action duration, plasma half-life = 7–8 hr. Vascular selectivity without clinically significant negative inotropic effects and less reflex tachycardia. Pure calcium antagonist with some agonist properties. Increases serum digoxin levels.
Felodipine	Hypertension, ? angina, ? CHF	Medium action duration, plasma half-life = 8 hr. Vascular selectivity without negative chronotropic and inotropic effects clinically. Increases serum digoxin levels.			
Isradipine	Hypertension, angina, ? CHF	Medium action duration, plasma half-life = 8 hr. Vascular selectivity without negative chronotropic and inotropic effects clinically. No change in serum digoxin levels. Can cause arthralgia.	**OTHER COMPOUNDS**		
			Bepridil	Angina, ? atrial arrhythmias	Ultra long acting, plasma half-life = 40 hr. Combined sodium-calcium channel blockade. Marked prolongation of atrial refractory period. Arrhythmogenic, causing prolonged Q-T and torsades de pointes.
Nicardipine	Angina, hypertension	Short action duration, plasma half-life = 4–5 hr or less. Water soluble without light sensitivity (IV administration easier). Vascular selectivity, ? greater effect on coronaries, no clinically significant negative inotropic effects.	Perhexiline maleate	Refractory angina	Unclear mechanism of action, but current hypothesis is a drug-induced shift in myocardial metabolism. Hepatic and neurologic toxicity is usually avoidable by maintaining drug levels in 150–600 ng/ml range.
Nimodipine	Early stroke and subarachnoid hemorrhage	Short action duration, plasma half-life = 5 hr. Possibly more selective for cerebral than peripheral vessels.	**VERAPAMIL-LIKE AGENTS**		
			Anipamil	Hypertension	Long half-life, ? minimal effect on A-V conduction.

TABLE 40-8 SIDE EFFECTS OF ANTIANGINAL DRUGS*

	HYPOTENSION FLUSHING, HEADACHE	LEFT VENTRICULAR DYSFUNCTION	DECREASED HEART RATE ATRIOVENTRICULAR BLOCK†	GASTROINTESTINAL SYMPTOMS	BRONCHOCONSTRICTION‡
Beta blockers	0	++	+++	+	+++
Nitrates	+++	0	0	0	0
Diltiazem	+	+	+	0	0
Nifedipine	+++	0	0	0	0
Verapamil	+	+	++	++	0

*0 = absent; + = mild; ++ = moderate; +++ = sometimes severe.
†In patients with sick sinus node syndrome or conduction system disease.
‡In patients with obstructive lung disease.
Reprinted by permission from Braunwald, E.: Mechanism of action of calcium channel blocking agents. N. Engl. J. Med. 307:1618, 1982.

TABLE 40-9 DRUG INTERACTIONS WITH CALCIUM ANTAGONISTS

1313

CHAP
40

	VERAPAMIL	NIFEDIPINE	DILTIAZEM
Beta-adrenergic blockers (negative inotropic and chronotropic effects)	2(+)^A		2(+)
Carbamazepine (inhibition of hepatic metabolism)	3(+)		1(+)
Cimetidine (increased bioavailability of calcium antagonists)	3(+)	3(+)	3(+)
Cyclosporine (increased plasma levels of cyclosporine)	2(+)	1(−)?	2(+)
Digoxin (increased plasma digoxin levels)	3(+)	1(+)	1(+)
Disopyramide (sinus node depression)	1(+)		1(+)
Lithium carbonate (after plasma levels of lithium)	1(−)		2(+)
Neuromuscular blocking agents (verapamil potentiates action)	3(+)		
Phenobarbital (hepatic enzyme inducer)	3(−)		
Phenytoin (causes peak nifedipine levels to rise)		2(+)	
Prazosin (excessive hypotension)	2(+)	3(+)	
Quinidine (*hypotension and bradycardia,** decreased serum quinidine)	2(+)*	2(−)**	
Rifampin and sulfinpyrazone (hepatic enzyme inducers)	3(−)		
Theophylline (after pharmacological effects of theophylline)	1(+)	1(+/−)	1(+)

Modified from Pieho, R. W., et al.: Drug interactions with calcium-entry blockers. Circulation 75 (Suppl. V): 181, 1987, by permission of the American Heart Association, Inc.

(−) = decreased drug effect; (+) = increased drug effect (e.g., verapamil and beta blockers will interact so that the negative inotropic and chronotropic effects of verapamil will be increased significantly); 3 = significant, common interaction; 2 = significant, uncommon interaction; 1 = reported interaction of questioned significance; ? = debated response; A = the intravenous administration of a beta blocker while a patient is taking verapamil orally (or vice versa) may be hazardous.

duction systems than does verapamil or diltiazem. Nonetheless, in patients with left ventricular dysfunction all calcium antagonists—even nifedipine—can precipitate heart failure.[235] In patients already receiving maximal doses of nitrates and beta blocker therapy, the addition of nifedipine (80 to 100 mg/day) has been shown to improve diastolic function of the left ventricle at rest and during exercise.[236] However, in patients with severe left ventricular dysfunction, the addition of nifedipine may precipitate left ventricular failure. Nifedipine *interacts* significantly with prazosin (resulting in excessive hypotension), cimetidine, and phenytoin (resulting in increased bioavailability of nifedipine) and may result in reduced plasma quinidine levels (Table 40–9).

VERAPAMIL (see also p. 648).   The usual starting dose of verapamil for oral administration is 40 to 80 mg three times daily. It may later be increased to 80 to 120 mg three or four times daily to a maximum dose of 480 mg/day (Table 40–6). Sustained-release capsules of verapamil are available (60 mg, 90 mg, and 120 mg), and starting doses are 60 to 120 mg twice daily with a usual optimal dose range of 240 to 360 mg/day.

Parenteral verapamil dilates the systemic and coronary resistance vessels without clearly increasing myocardial metabolic demands. In addition, it has been shown to dilate large conductance vessels in both normal and diseased arterial segments, although this effect is not as potent as that of nitroglycerin. Verapamil appears to decrease myocardial oxygen demand without any change in the anginal threshold, i.e., in the rate-pressure product at the onset of angina. Trials comparing verapamil with a beta blocker (usually propranolol) in the treatment of effort-related angina have shown that the drugs are comparable in producing dose-dependent reductions in the frequency of anginal episodes. In a comparison of propranolol (480 mg/day) and verapamil (320 mg/day), the latter was found to be a more effective antianginal agent than the former, although the combination of both drugs resulted in better exercise capacity than did either alone.[237]

Verapamil accelerates left ventricular diastolic filling at rest and during exercise in patients with chronic stable angina (and hypertrophic cardiomyopathy [p. 1313]), whereas beta blockade does not have this effect.[237] Despite the marked negative inotropic effects of verapamil in isolated cardiac muscle preparations, changes in contractility are modest in patients with normal cardiac function. However, in patients with cardiac dysfunction, verapamil, like beta blockade, may reduce cardiac output and elevate left ventricular filling pressure.

In clinical doses, verapamil also inhibits calcium influx into specialized cardiac cells, sometimes causing slowing of heart rate and A-V conduction; it may cause slight P-R prolongation. Although the drug depresses sinus node automaticity, the systemic vasodilator effects of the drug activate reflexes that counteract or minimize this effect. Verapamil is therefore contraindicated in patients with sick sinus syndrome, A-V conduction abnormalities, or congestive heart failure and in patients with suspected digitalis toxicity.

Verapamil interacts significantly with a number of other drugs (Table 40–9). Intravenous verapamil should not be used together with an orally administered beta blocker nor should a beta blocker be administered intravenously in patients receiving oral verapamil, and certainly intravenous verapamil and intravenous beta blockade should not ordinarily be used together. The bioavailability of verapamil is increased by cimetidine and carbamazepine, while verapamil may increase plasma levels of cyclosporine and digoxin and may be associated with excessive hypotension with both quinidine and prazosin. Hepatic enzyme inducers such as phenobarbital may reduce the effects of verapamil.

Adverse effects of verapamil are noted in approximately 10 per cent of patients and relate to systemic dilation (hypotension and facial flushing), gastrointestinal symptoms (constipation and nausea), and central nervous system reactions such as headache and dizziness.

DILTIAZEM.   The dosage of diltiazem is 30 to 60 mg four times daily, although higher doses are sometimes needed.[238]

Diltiazem's actions are intermediate between those of nifedipine and verapamil. In clinically useful doses its vasodilator effects are somewhat less profound than nifedipine's, while its cardiac depressant action (on the sinoatrial and AV nodes and myocardium) may be less than those of verapamil. This profile may explain the remarkably low incidence of adverse effects of diltiazem. This drug is a systemic vasodilator, lowering arterial pressure at rest and during exertion and increasing the workload required to produce myocardial ischemia, but there is some evidence that the drug may also increase myocardial oxygen delivery.[239] Although diltiazem causes little vasodilation of epicardial coronary arteries under basal conditions, it may enhance perfusion of the subendocardium distal to a flow-limiting coronary stenosis[240]; it also blocks exercise-induced coronary vasoconstriction.[241,242] In patients with ischemic heart disease, diltiazem reduces afterload and depresses myocardial systolic function, although it improves left ventricular relaxation.[243] Studies in patients during tachycardia-induced angina pectoris suggest that the major benefit of diltiazem is related to reduction of myocardial oxygen demand rather than to enhancing myocardial oxygen delivery.[244] In patients with chronic stable angina receiving maximally tolerated doses of diltiazem there is a significant reduction in heart rate at rest, but there is no effect on peak blood pressure achieved during exercise, and the duration of symptom-limited treadmill exercise is prolonged.[232]

Diltiazem is a highly efficacious antianginal agent with minimal side effects when given to patients with angina pectoris that persists despite nitrate and beta blocker therapy.[245] High doses of diltiazem (mean dose 340 mg) have been shown to be a safe addition to maximally tolerated doses of isosorbide dinitrate and a beta blocker, causing increases in exercise tolerance and resting and exercise left ventricular ejection fraction without increasing side effects.[238] The combination of high doses of diltiazem with beta blockers is more effective in reducing symptoms and improving exercise capacity without increasing adverse effects than is the use of diltiazem alone.[244,246] The combination of diltiazem and nifedipine may be effective in patients who do not respond adequately to either agent alone.[247,248]

Like verapamil, diltiazem should be used with caution in patients with sick sinus syndrome and advanced degrees of AV block and left ventricular dysfunction. Diltiazem has *interactions* with other drugs, including beta-adrenergic blocking agents (with enhanced negative inotropic and chronotropic effects) and cimetidine (which increases the bioavailability of diltiazem), and diltiazem has been associated with increased plasma levels of cyclosporine, carbamazepine, and lithium carbonate. Diltiazem may cause excess sinus node depression if administered with disopyramide (Table 40–9).

SELECTION OF DRUGS FOR THE TREATMENT OF CHRONIC STABLE ANGINA

Verapamil (360 mg/day) and diltiazem (360 mg/day) appear to be equipotent antianginal agents and similar in efficacy to propranolol (320 mg/day). Nifedipine 60 mg/day appears to be equivalent to propranolol 160 to 240 mg/day. Diltiazem and verapamil, which reduce resting heart rate, appear to be more effective as single drugs for angina than is nifedipine, which causes reflex sympathetic stimulation; both diltiazem and verapamil appear to be safe and effective alternatives to beta blockers.[249]

RELATIVE ADVANTAGES OF BETA BLOCKERS AND CALCIUM ANTAGONISTS. There is some controversy whether a calcium antagonist or a beta blocker should be employed first in the treatment of chronic stable angina in patients in whom more than an occasional sublingual nitroglycerin tablet is required. Both classes of agents are effective. Long-term administration of beta-adrenoceptor blockers has been found to prolong life in patients after acute myocardial infarction.[249a] In general, however, agents without intrinsic sympathomimetic activity increase serum triglycerides[216] and decrease HDL cholesterol with uncertain long-term consequences. Long-term administration of calcium antagonists has not been shown definitively to improve long-term survival following acute myocardial infarction, although diltiazem apparently is effective in preventing severe angina and early reinfarction after non-Q-wave infarction,[250] and verapamil reduces reinfarction rates.[251] Nifedipine has been associated with the development of fewer new coronary artery lesions[229,230] in patients with coronary artery disease.

The choice of which agent to initiate therapy is influenced by a number of clinical factors:

1. Whether the patient's anginal threshold is fixed or variable, as discussed on page 1294. When there is a relatively fixed anginal threshold, it is presumed that myocardial ischemia is caused primarily by an increase in myocardial oxygen needs during exercise in the face of a fixed supply, and a beta blocker would usually be considered first (Table 40–10). Conversely, in patients with variable-threshold angina in whom reductions of myocardial blood supply may be caused by alterations in coronary vasomotor tone, a calcium antagonist may be preferable to a beta blocker.

2. If a patient is suspected of having variant angina (p. 1342) then calcium antagonists are clearly preferred, since occasionally beta blockers may aggravate angina under these circumstances.

3. The presence of moderate to severe left ventricular dysfunction in patients with angina limits the therapeutic options (Table 40–11). Obviously, cardiac failure may be controlled with diuretics, digitalis, and angiotensin-converting enzyme inhibitors, and nitrates can be used for angina. However, when cardiac failure is treated and angina persists, other agents may be required. Nifedipine and diltiazem are reasonable choices if the left ventricular ejection fraction is greater than 30 per cent and overt cardiac failure does not exist. Verapamil and beta blockers are more likely to be associated with adverse effects under these circumstances.

4. In patients with a history of asthma or chronic obstructive lung disease and/or with wheezing on clinical examination (in whom beta blockers, even relatively selective agents, are contraindicated), calcium antagonists and nitrates should be selected for the treatment of angina.

TABLE 40-10   EFFECTS OF ANTIANGINAL AGENTS ON INDICES OF MYOCARDIAL OXYGEN SUPPLY AND DEMAND*

INDEX	NITRATES	BETA-ADRENOCEPTOR BLOCKERS ISA† No	Yes	Cardio-Selective No	Yes	CALCIUM ANTAGONISTS Nifedipine	Verapamil	Diltiazem
Supply								
Coronary resistance								
Vascular tone	↓↓	↑	0	↑	0↑	↓↓↓	↓↓↓	↓↓↓
Intramyocardial diastolic tension	↓↓↓	↑	0	↑	↑	↓↓	0↑	0
Coronary collateral circulation	↑	0	0	0	0	↑	0	↑
Duration of diastole	0(↓)	↑↑↑	0↓	↑↑↑	↑↑↑	0↑(↓↓)	↑↑↑(↓)	↑↑(↓)
Demand								
Intramyocardial systolic tension								
Preload	↓↓↓	↑	0	↑	↑	↓0	↑0↓	0↓
Afterload (peripheral vascular resistance)	↓	↑	↑	↑↑	↑	↓↓	↓	↓
Contractility	0(↑)	↓↓↓	↓	↓↓↓	↓↓↓	↓(↑↑)‡	↓↓(↑)‡	↓(↑)‡
Heart rate	0(↑)	↓↓↓	0↓	↓↓↓	↓↓↓	0(↑↑)	↓↓(↑)	↓↓(↑)

*↑ = increase, ↓ = decrease, 0 = little or no definite effect. Number of arrows represents relative intensity of effect. Symbols in parentheses indicate reflex-mediated effects.

†ISA = intrinsic sympathomimetic activity.

‡Effect of calcium entry blockers on left ventricular *contractility*, as assessed in the intact animal model. The net effect on *left ventricular performance* is variable, being influenced by alterations in afterload, reflex cardiac stimulation, and the underlying state of the myocardium.

From Shub, C., et al.: Selection of optimal drug therapy for the patient with angina pectoris. Mayo Clin. Proc. 60:539, 1985.

TABLE 40-11 RECOMMENDED DRUG THERAPY (CALCIUM ANTAGONIST VS. BETA BLOCKER) IN PATIENTS WHO HAVE ANGINA IN CONJUNCTION WITH OTHER MEDICAL CONDITIONS*

CLINICAL CONDITION	RECOMMENDED DRUG (ALTERNATIVE DRUG)
Cardiac arrhythmias and conduction abnormalities	
Sinus bradycardia	Nifedipine
Sinus tachycardia (not due to cardiac failure)	Beta blocker
Supraventricular tachycardia	Verapamil or beta blocker
Atrioventricular block	Nifedipine
Rapid atrial fibrillation (with digitalis)	Verapamil or beta blocker
Ventricular arrhythmias	Beta blocker (± group 1 antiarrhythmic agent)
Left ventricular dysfunction	
Congestive heart failure	
Mild (LVEF ≥ 40%)	Nifedipine (verapamil, diltiazem, or beta blockers cautiously)
Moderate to severe (LVEF < 40%)	Nifedipine (cautiously, in combination with other therapy)
Left-sided valvular heart disease†	
Aortic stenosis (mild)‡	Beta blocker
Aortic insufficiency	Nifedipine
Mitral regurgitation	Nifedipine
Mitral stenosis§	Beta blocker
Miscellaneous medical conditions	
Systemic hypertension	Beta blocker (calcium antagonists)
Severe preexisting headaches	Beta blockers (verapamil or diltiazem)
COPD with bronchospasm or asthma	Nifedipine, verapamil, or diltiazem
Hyperthyroidism	Beta blocker
Raynaud's syndrome	Nifedipine
Claudication	Nifedipine, verapamil, or diltiazem (low-dose beta₁ blocker or beta-ISA)
Depression	Nifedipine, verapamil, or diltiazem
Neurasthenia or fatigue states	Nifedipine, verapamil, or diltiazem
Insulin-dependent diabetes mellitus	Nifedipine, verapamil, or diltiazem (low-dose beta₁ or beta-ISA)

From Shub, C., et al.: Selection of optimal drug therapy for the patient with angina pectoris. Mayo Clin. Proc. *60*:539, 1985.

* Beta-ISA = beta blocker with intrinsic sympathomimetic activity such as pindolol or acebutolol; COPD = chronic obstructive pulmonary disease; LVEF = left ventricular ejection fraction.

† Surgical therapy should be considered for patients with severe valvular heart disease; beta blockers are not routinely used in patients with valvular heart disease and left ventricular failure.

‡ Vasodilators may increase aortic valve gradient, and beta blockers can cause left ventricular failure. Any of these drugs should be used with extreme caution in patients with severe aortic stenosis.

§ If congestive heart failure (associated with normal left ventricular function) occurs in a patient with angina, severe mitral stenosis, and rapid atrial fibrillation, a beta blocker (in combination with digitalis) may be used to decrease the heart rate.

5. In patients with sick sinus syndrome, sinus bradycardia, or significant A-V conduction disturbances, nifedipine or nicardipine is the calcium antagonist of choice, and beta blockers and verapamil are often contraindicated and should be used only with great caution.

6. If patients have significant, symptomatic peripheral arterial disease, calcium antagonists are preferred over beta blockers.

7. In patients with new-onset or rapidly progressive angina or rest angina, i.e., unstable angina, nifedipine should not be used as the initial and only agent, but rather treatment should be initiated with nitrates, diltiazem, verapamil, or beta blockers to avoid the reflex-mediated tachycardia associated with nifedipine alone that may aggravate unstable angina. Nifedipine is, however, helpful when added to a beta blocker under this circumstance.

8. Beta blockers should usually be avoided in patients with significant depressive illness, a history of sexual dysfunction, or a history of sleep disturbance, nightmares, fatigue, or lethargy.

9. Hypertensive patients with angina pectoris do well with either beta blockers or calcium antagonists, since both agents have antihypertensive effects.

10. When treated with a beta blocker, patients with significant ambulatory asymptomatic ischemia appear to have a reduction in the number and duration of ischemic episodes as compared with results of calcium antagonist therapy.[252]

11. Verapamil is an effective alternative to beta-adrenergic blocking drugs for the treatment of chronic stable angina and may offer advantages over beta blockers in patients with fatigue, depression, impotence, memory loss, or bronchospasm.[237] Diltiazem is less likely than verapamil to exacerbate A-V conduction disturbances, is effective compared with nifedipine at reducing the frequency of angina attacks, and seems to be associated with fewer adverse reactions than nifedipine.[253]

COMBINATION THERAPY. A combination of a beta-adrenoceptor blocker, calcium antagonist, and long-acting nitrate may be employed. The hemodynamic spectrum of action of beta blockers, long-acting nitrates, and calcium antagonists is sufficiently different to suggest that combination therapy might be useful, and indeed it is, in patients with severe angina (Tables 40–4 and 40–8).

When adrenergic blockers and calcium antagonists are to be used together in the treatment of angina pectoris, a number of practical issues should be considered:

1. The combination of a beta blocker and calcium antagonist is not consistently better than the use of a beta blocker (or calcium antagonist) alone if the single agent is administered in a maximum tolerated dose.

2. However, if angina persists despite optimal doses of a beta blocker, then the addition of a calcium antagonist is likely to reduce angina and improve exercise performance.[254]

3. The addition of a beta blocker to either verapamil or diltiazem therapy does not appear to enhance antianginal efficacy,[227] although the addition of a beta blocker does seem to enhance the effects of nifedipine.

4. In patients with moderate or severe left ventricular dysfunction, sinus bradycardia, or A-V conduction disturbances, combination therapy with calcium antagonists and beta blockers either should be avoided or initiated with caution.[255,256] In patients with conduction system disease, the preferred combination is nifedipine and a beta blocker. The negative inotropic effects of calcium antagonists are not usually a problem in combined therapy with low doses of beta blockers but can become significant with high doses of beta blockers. Under these circumstances, nifedipine and nicardipine are the agents of choice. However, it should be noted that both nifedipine and diltiazem used alone can cause deterioration of left ventricular function in patients with treated cardiac failure.

5. The combination of nifedipine (or nicardipine) and long-acting nitrates is usually not optimal, since both are potent vasodilators.

Following (or simultaneously with) the general measures described on page 1302, we believe that it is usually advisable to initiate drug therapy of chronic stable angina with sublingual nitroglycerin (and aspirin). If the patient requires more than approximately three or four tablets per week either a beta blocker or calcium antagonist should be added, depending on the profile of the patient, as outlined above. The dosage of the drug selected is then raised progressively as efficacy and side effects are monitored and alternative agents added only if angina persists or side effects become a problem. With the recognition that all longer acting forms of oral or transdermal nitrate therapy provoke tolerance, regimens utilizing these agents are designed to allow a nitrate-free interval of about 10 hours. This is readily achieved with intermittent, transdermal nitrate therapy or careful dosage schedules of long-acting oral nitrates. At times, lower doses of triple-drug therapy (a long-acting nitrate, a beta blocker, and a calcium antagonist) are used early in the treatment plan if the patient can tolerate only low doses of the chosen agents. If symptoms persist despite these approaches and if there are no contraindications, myocardial revascularization is then considered.

In decisions about the management of individual patients with angina, the effects of the antianginal agents on indices of myocardial oxygen supply and demand should be considered.[257] When angina pectoris exists with other conditions that can complicate drug therapy, such as asthma and diabetes mellitus, the choice of therapy should be made especially carefully (Table 40–11).

GUIDELINES FOR MEDICAL TREATMENT OF CHRONIC STABLE ANGINA

Risk factor modification is most important in patients with chronic stable angina under the age of approximately 65 years. This is most easily accomplished by cessation of cigarette smoking and treatment of hypertension and low-density hyperlipoproteinemia. There is increasing evidence that *marked reduction* of elevated serum cholesterol levels will cause the regression of atheroma, but it is not yet clear that lowering a total cholesterol < 240 mg/dl and an LDL cholesterol < 175 mg/dl is of benefit in patients with chronic stable angina. At this time we recommend treatment above these thresholds but recognize that the results of ongoing trials may dictate an alteration of these limits. Perhaps currently available methods of diet and drug therapy may slow the progression of the disease. Similarly, the relationship between maintenance of blood sugar within the normal range in diabetics and preventing vascular disease is far from settled.

In mild chronic stable angina, drug therapy may be limited to sublingual nitroglycerin on an "as necessary" basis if pain episodes are relatively infrequent (once or twice a week). It should also be used prophylactically in situations known to precipitate angina. If nitroglycerin is required on a daily basis, either long-acting nitrate preparations or moderate doses of a beta blocker or a calcium antagonist may be employed. The doses of the drugs will depend on how well they are tolerated and on the clinical response. Resting heart rate should be lowered to 50 to 60 beats/min, and heart rate during ordinary activity should be below 100 beats/min. The clinical response can often be estimated by an improvement in exercise tolerance or the degree of ST-segment depression during a standard treadmill test. If the patient is still symptomatic at high doses of either a beta blocker or a calcium antagonist, then the other agent should be added. The relative advantages and disadvantages of the different agents have been discussed. Whichever is selected, a relatively low dose is given to begin and dosage is increased gradually.

There is no unanimity of opinion concerning when a patient with chronic angina pectoris should undergo cardiac catheterization, coronary arteriography, and left ventriculography. Some physicians take a more aggressive posture with patients under 50 years of age, with the hope of finding a lesion that demands revascularization; others prefer to wait for development of refractoriness to medical therapy, regardless of the patient's age. We believe that the use of noninvasive tests, as outlined on page 1298, can be extremely helpful in identifying patients with chronic stable angina at high risk of coronary events or early death; if there are no contraindications to coronary revascularization in such patients, they should undergo coronary arteriography, as should patients for whom medical therapy fails.

PERCUTANEOUS TRANSLUMINAL CORONARY ANGIOPLASTY

(See also Chap. 41)

With improved equipment and an increasing number of experienced operators, the primary success rate of coronary angioplasty (PTCA) has improved over the last 10 years, and the number of procedures performed has risen rapidly. Thus, PTCA is playing an increasingly important role in the treatment of chronic stable angina.[258,258a]

PATIENT SELECTION. PTCA should, in general, be carried out in patients with symptomatic angina, objective evidence of myocardial ischemia, and anatomical features on coronary arteriography that make them suitable for complete or nearly complete revascularization (Table 40–12). Ideally, such patients should also be suitable surgical candidates; however, selected patients with severe chronic angina who are not appropriate for surgical treatment (e.g., with advanced pulmonary or renal disease, and advanced age with infirmity) may be considered for PTCA. In such patients, PTCA may be undertaken as a palliative procedure and may, on occasion, be useful even in those with multivessel disease in whom all lesions are not suitable for dilatation.

The optimal lesion for PTCA in a patient with chronic stable angina pectoris involves a single, proximal coronary artery (but not at the coronary ostium) that is easily accessible. It is concentric, smooth, noncalcified, short (less than 0.5 cm), subtotal, and occupies a straight portion of the artery that has no side branches and that supplies an area of myocardium "protected" by distal collateral vessels.[258] PTCA of such lesions has a primary success rate of greater than 90 per cent.[259] If at the end of the procedure there is less than 30 per cent residual narrowing or a pressure gradient of less than 15 mm Hg at the site of the coronary lesion, there is a high chance of symptomatic relief.[259,260] However, PTCA is being carried out with increasing frequency in lesions that are eccentric, calcified, less accessible, and totally occluded.[261] Each of these factors reduces the chance of primary success and adds to the risk of the procedure.[261a]

RISKS. The NHLBI PTCA Registry, examining a cohort of 1801 patients treated in 1985 to 1986, compared with a cohort examined from 1977 to 1981, showed that in the latter period patients were older and had an increased incidence of multivessel coronary disease (double- or triplevessel disease in 51 per cent), and more patients had depressed left ventricular function or a history of prior infarction. Despite these differences in patient population, the risk of PTCA appeared to decrease. The most significant decreases in complication rates were a fall in the incidence of coronary spasm from 5.0 to 1.3 per cent and a decreased requirement for emergency coronary artery bypass grafting from 5.8 to 3.5 per cent. In-hospital mortality rates depended on the extent of coronary disease (0.2 per cent for single-vessel disease, 0.9 per cent for

TABLE 40-12   INDICATIONS FOR CORONARY ANGIOPLASTY

GENERALLY ACCEPTED INDICATIONS
Chronic stable angina unresponsive to medical therapy or unstable angina:
1. With objective evidence of myocardial ischemia
2. With normal or mildly reduced left ventricular function
3. With significant coronary artery stenoses involving one or two coronary arteries

EVOLVING INDICATIONS
1. Chronic stable angina unresponsive to medical therapy with multivessel disease
2. Acute myocardial infarction complicated by continuing unstable angina or cardiogenic shock
3. No angina, or mild angina, taking medical therapy, and with a strongly positive exercise test
4. Angina in patients with a recent coronary artery occlusion (less than 3 months)
5. Angina after coronary bypass surgery
6. Documented variant angina, taking medical therapy, with significant "fixed" coronary stenoses
7. Angina in inoperable/high-risk patients

RELATIVE CONTRAINDICATIONS
1. No angina or mild angina without evidence of myocardial ischemia
2. Significant left main coronary artery stenosis
3. Coronary artery stenoses with <50% diameter narrowing
4. Chronic, total coronary artery occlusions older than 3 months
5. Severe left ventricular dysfunction (ejection fraction <25%)

Adapted from Report of the ISFC/WHO Task Force on Coronary Angioplasty. Circulation *78*:780, 1988, by permission of the American Heart Association, Inc.

double-vessel disease, and 2.2 per cent for triple-vessel disease). The factors that showed an association with increased mortality included age greater than 64 years, female gender, new-onset angina, congestive heart failure, multivessel disease and left main coronary artery disease.[262] Even in patients with refractory angina and severe left ventricular dysfunction, both symptomatic and angiographic improvement can be accomplished in up to 90 per cent of patients, but major events (death, infarction, and emergency bypass surgery) may occur in about 8 per cent of patients.[263] Careful documentation of the risks of elective PTCA performed by experienced operators has shown that almost 90 per cent of procedures will be uneventful.

With steerable catheter systems, which are now used routinely, independent clinical predictors of *acute closure* are female gender, the presence of thrombus near the stenosis, stenosis occurring at a major bend or branch point, other stenoses in the same vessel, and the presence of multivessel disease.[264] At the time of the procedure the presence of an intimal tear or dissection, a post-PTCA stenosis of 35 per cent or more or a transtenotic gradient of 20 mm Hg or more, and the use of prolonged heparin infusion after PTCA were all associated with a higher incidence of acute closure.[264] Of particular importance is the observation that the presence of angiographic intimal dissection after PTCA substantially increases the immediate risk of a major complication.[264] The independent risk factors for in-hospital death following acute closure (<0.2 per cent in experienced centers) included female gender, the presence of multivessel disease, and collateral vessels *arising* from the vessel dilated.[265]

MULTIVESSEL PTCA. The overall clinical success rate of multivessel PTCA (angiographic success, clinical improvement, and absence of a major complication) initially is 83 to 95 per cent,[266-269,269a] with a mortality rate of 0.4 to 2.8 per cent.[266,267,270,270a] There is clinical recurrence or restenosis in approximately 30 per cent of patients during follow-up of 6 months or more,[266,268,270] even when initial technical success (at least a 35-per cent reduction in degree of stenosis and a decrease in the transstenotic gradient to 15 mm Hg or less) is seen in 89 per cent of vessels dilated.[266] The need for urgent revascularization surgery has been reported in 1 to 2.8 per cent,[266,268,270] and a major event (myocardial infarction, death, and need for emergency coronary artery surgery) occurred in 4 to 9 per cent of patients undergoing PTCA in two or more major epicardial vessels.[266,270] The acute occlusion rate of multivessel angioplasty has been reported as 2.9 per cent per patient and 1.7 per cent per vessel and is often linked to a hypotensive event occurring during dilation of the second vessel.[271]

Adverse procedural outcome is more likely in patients with high-grade (80 to 99 per cent) diameter stenoses, excessive tortuosity or a bend > 60 degrees, or in patients with chronic, total occlusion.[270a] Delayed closure (1 to 24 hours after PTCA) is usually related to intimal dissection.[271] Follow-up at 1 year reveals that approximately 80 per cent of patients who have undergone multivessel angioplasty exhibit continued improvement in symptoms[267] and may not experience death, myocardial infarction, or the need for revascularization surgery[267]; 5-year survival is nearly 90 per cent after initially successful PTCA.[269] Incomplete revascularization following multivessel PTCA may be associated with an increased restenosis rate, recurrence of angina, morbid events, and the need for coronary surgery.[272-274] Analyses of the degree of revascularization in patients with multivessel disease suggest that, while patients with one or more severe residual stenoses are more likely to require coronary artery revascularization surgery during follow-up, the risk of myocardial infarction or death is not different from that in patients who have no residual stenoses following successful angioplasty.[275,276]

RESTENOSIS. The risk of restenosis of a lesion is approximately 30 per cent[260,276a] within the first 6 months of the procedure, with angina recurring in the majority of patients with significant restenoses. Restenosis following successful PTCA appears to follow intimal hyperplasia in the dilated portion of the vessel.[277,277a] One factor that seems to increase the frequency of restenosis following PTCA is continued smoking.[266,278] While aspirin and dipyridamole do not appear to reduce the 6-month rate of restenosis after successful PTCA, they appear to reduce the incidence of transmural infarction during, or soon after, the procedure.[279]

Some factors suggestive of high risk for a second restenosis after a repeat PTCA include a lesion longer than 14 mm, the need to have an additional coronary artery dilated at the time of repeat PTCA, and a short interval between the initial and second angioplasty.[280,280a] Restenosis rates after third or fourth angioplasty procedures for recurrent restenosis are higher than those for initial procedures and approximate 50 per cent.[281] Emergency surgery will be required in 3 to 4 per cent[259,262] of patients undergoing elective PTCA (for severe coronary artery dissection, occlusion, or intractable angina) and is usually associated with higher morbidity and mortality[282] than routine coronary artery bypass grafting. An essential requirement for any institution performing PTCA is the immediate availability of surgical revascularization.

Left main coronary artery lesions are usually associated with significant

disease elsewhere in the coronary arteries and thus present major potential risks, both at the time of PTCA and later if restenosis occurs. In our view, attempts at PTCA of patients with left main coronary lesions are almost always contraindicated unless some protection is provided by a patent graft to the circumflex or anterior descending coronary arteries.

If left ventricular function is impaired, successful reperfusion by PTCA can improve both systolic[283] and diastolic[284] function, even though the risks of the procedure are increased. Indeed, significant long-term improvement in coronary artery dynamics (equivalent to the results of coronary artery surgery) is seen following successful PTCA.[285] This improvement is reflected in improved myocardial function during exercise[286] and long-term improvements in symptoms.[259,272-274,287,288]

PREVIOUS BYPASS SURGERY. Patients who have previously undergone coronary artery bypass surgery with recurrent angina can benefit from PTCA of the native coronary circulation and of the venous grafts to improve symptomatic status and avoid the need for reoperation.[289] Better long-term results are achieved with dilatation of distal graft lesions than of those located proximally or in the body of the graft. Angiographic success can approach 90 per cent at the distal site of the graft insertion, 70 per cent in the midportion, and 55 per cent proximally.[290] Cardiac complications occur in approximately 5 to 7 per cent,[289-291,291a] and the complication and recurrence rates of stenoses are significantly higher when PTCA is attempted in saphenous vein grafts failing 3 or more years after implantation than in those failing sooner after coronary artery surgery.[289,291,291a] Even totally occluded coronary arteries can be dilated,[292-294] especially if there is a short segment of occluded artery of known short duration.[293]

Invariably, a number of issues should be considered as the risks and benefits of PTCA are balanced against those of coronary artery surgery in individual patients. There are no absolute rules, but the following questions should be considered:

1. How experienced is the angioplasty team, and is there adequate surgical back-up?
2. How "favorable" is the lesion?
3. What are the potential consequences of abrupt total occlusion of the vessel to be dilated?
4. What are the chances of achieving adequate revascularization?

These factors involve judgment and discussion among cardiologists, surgeons, patients, and their families.

LASER ANGIOPLASTY (see also p. 1374). Successful vaporization of an atherosclerotic plaque (into its elementary components — water vapor, carbon dioxide, and other combustion byproducts) has been reported. Pulsed lasers[295] and excimer systems (which operate in the near-ultraviolet range) have the potential for minimizing adjacent thermal injury, and with the development of hydrophilic wires may become widely applicable with minimal risk of perforation of the vessel wall. Recent clinical reports of percutaneous excimer laser coronary angioplasty[296-298,298a] suggest that atheroma can be safely ablated, and with careful patient selection excimer laser angioplasty may become either a useful sole procedure or an adjunctive procedure to routine balloon coronary angioplasty.[296-298] This form of therapy is in a developmental phase, and issues remain, such as vessel restenosis and the development of flexible optical fibers or fiber bundles that can also achieve an adequate-sized lumen following the irradiation.[295]

CORONARY ATHERECTOMY (see also p. 1374). Directional, transluminal coronary atherectomy excises atherosclerotic plaque, whereas balloon angioplasty commonly disrupts plaque and separates it from the media. Early clinical studies suggest that the immediate angiographic results and incidence of serious complications are comparable to those of conventional balloon angioplasty.[299,300] As with balloon angioplasty, there is, however, a high incidence of early restenosis.[299] It remains to be established whether or not atherectomy provides long-term benefit relative to conventional PTCA.

CORONARY STENTS. These are discussed on page 1373.

CORONARY ARTERY BYPASS SURGERY

OPERATIVE PROCEDURE

When the decision has been reached to proceed with coronary artery bypass grafting (CABG), administration of beta-adrenoceptor blockers, nitrates, and calcium antagonists is continued until operation. Most surgeons perform coronary artery surgery using cardiopulmonary bypass at moderate hypothermia (24° to 32°C) with hemodilution. A motionless heart is achieved by continuous aortic cross-clamping with profound cardiac hypothermia and cardioplegia induced with cold potassium solution. Simultaneous topical and core myocardial hypothermia (such as achieved by direct injection of cold solutions into the coronary arteries) has been recommended to provide uniform myocardial cooling. Rapid diastolic cardiac arrest is the aim, and in the United States the most commonly used agent to achieve this is a highly concentrated solution of potassium chloride. Both crystalloid and blood cardioplegic solutions have been used with success.[301]

VENOUS CONDUITS. The saphenous vein is mainly used for distal branches of the right and circumflex coronary arteries and for sequential grafts to these vessels and diagonal branches[302] (Figs. 40–6 and 40–7). In emergency situations, many surgeons prefer the saphenous vein, which can be harvested and grafted more rapidly than the internal mammary artery. Arm vein grafts are not as effective as either saphenous veins or internal mammary artery grafts.[303,304] Since 8 to 12 per cent of saphenous vein grafts occlude in the early postoperative period, increasing attention has been directed to technical aspects of the procedure: avoidance of excessive distending pressures and atraumatic harvesting are employed to reduce intimal and medial injury of the graft.[302] When sequential vein grafts are used, the first side-to-side anastomosis has a higher patency rate than the more distal ones, and the terminal end-to-side anastomosis (end of saphenous vein to side of coronary artery) has the least favorable outcome. Indeed, the patency rate of such a distal anastomosis is lower than the patency rate of a single graft to the same vessel.[305]

INTERNAL MAMMARY ARTERY BYPASS GRAFTS. In patients under the age of 65 years, the internal mammary artery (also known as the internal thoracic artery) usually is remarkably free of atheroma. When it is grafted to a coronary artery, it appears to be virtually immune to the development of intimal hyperplasia, which is almost universally seen in aortocoronary vein grafts, and atherosclerotic changes in this vessel develop in only a small percentage of patients after coronary artery surgery. The internal mammary artery is delicate, and great care has to be taken to mobilize the vessel

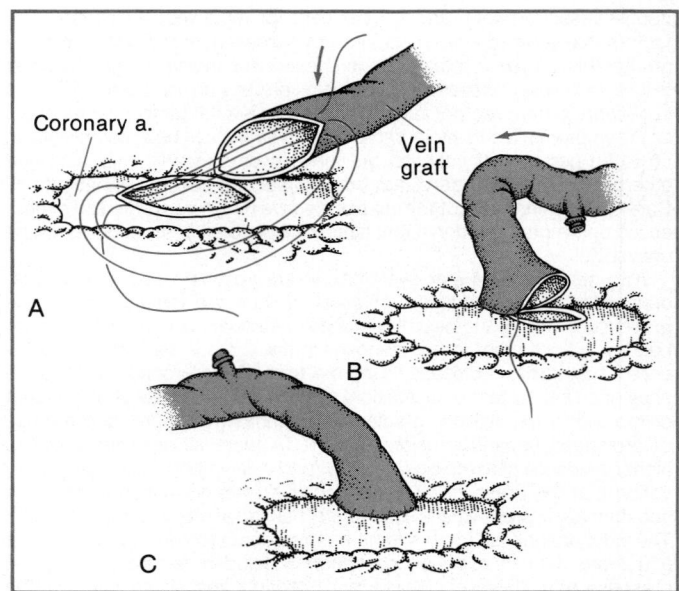

FIGURE 40–7. The venocoronary anastomosis to the proximal portion of the arteriotomy. (From Cohn, L. H.: Surgical techniques of emergency coronary revascularization. *In* Cohn, L. H. [ed.]: The Treatment of Acute Myocardial Ischemia: An integrated Medical-Surgical Approach. Mt. Kisco, N.Y., Futura Publishing Co., 1979, p. 87.)

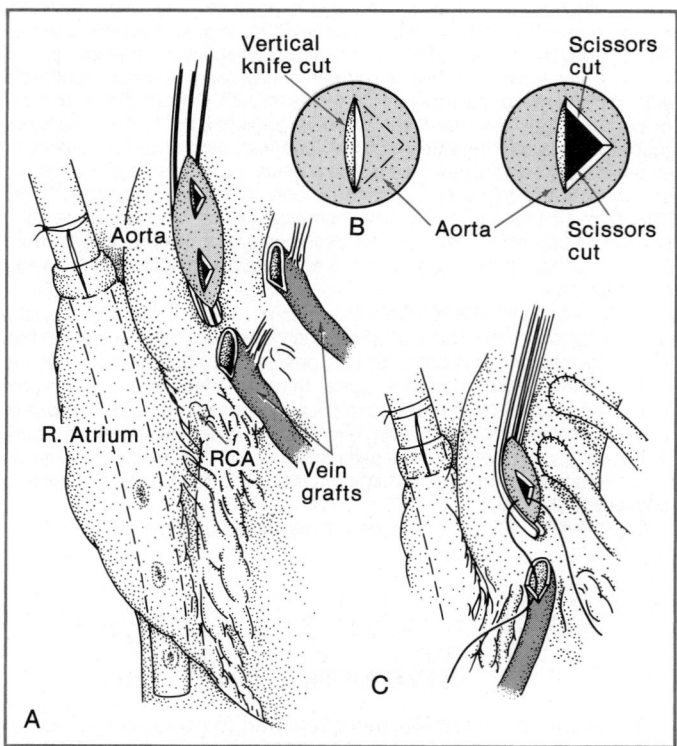

FIGURE 40–6. The aorticovenous anastomosis in a coronary arterial–saphenous vein bypass graft. *A* shows the direction of the anastomotic site for left-sided grafts; *B* shows details of aortic orifices; *C* shows the direction of right coronary artery (RCA) grafts. (From Cohn, L. H. [ed.]: The Treatment of Acute Myocardial Ischemia: An Integrated Medical-Surgical Approach. Mt. Kisco, N.Y., Futura Publishing Co., 1979, p. 87.)

without traumatizing it (Fig. 40–8).[306] This prolongs the operative time and often involves entry into the pleural space. Therefore, the internal mammary artery is not often used for emergency surgery. Comparative morphologic and angiographic studies of internal mammary arteries and saphenous vein bypass grafts that have been implanted long-term show that accelerated atherosclerosis occurs commonly in saphenous vein grafts but is extremely rare in internal mammary artery grafts. The media of the internal mammary artery may derive nourishment from the lumen rather than from vasa vasorum. Endothelium-dependent relaxation is more pronounced in the internal mammary artery than in vein grafts,[307] which may allow flow-dependent autoregulation to occur. The diameter of the internal mammary artery graft usually is a closer match to that of the recipient coronary artery than the diameter of a saphenous vein.

In contrast to the 40- to 60-per cent patency for vein grafts at 10 to 12 years following coronary surgery, that of internal mammary artery grafts exceeds 90 per cent.[308] However, fibrointimal proliferation may occasionally develop in internal mammary artery grafts and cause internal mammary artery narrowing and may be a factor in late graft closure.[309]

The improved 10-year survival described by Loop et al.[310] in patients who received an internal mammary artery graft to the anterior descending coronary artery alone, or combined with one or more saphenous vein grafts, compared with survival in patients who had only saphenous vein bypass grafts (Fig. 40–9) has been confirmed.[311,312] Indeed, in patients who receive an internal mammary artery graft to the left anterior descending coronary artery, the risk of dying is reduced by approximately 35 per cent compared to that in patients revascularized with vein grafts.[308] Most surgeons now believe that whenever it is technically feasible, internal mammary artery grafting is the preferable treatment (at least for lesions of the anterior descending coronary artery).

Multiple internal mammary artery grafts, which are technically more demanding and usually require more operative time compared with single internal mammary artery grafts (with or without concurrent vein grafts), do not appear to be associated with different operative mortality or morbidity than single internal mammary artery grafts, and intermediate (4-year) survival is similar (Fig. 40–10).[313]

OTHER CONDUITS. Other arterial conduits used for coro-

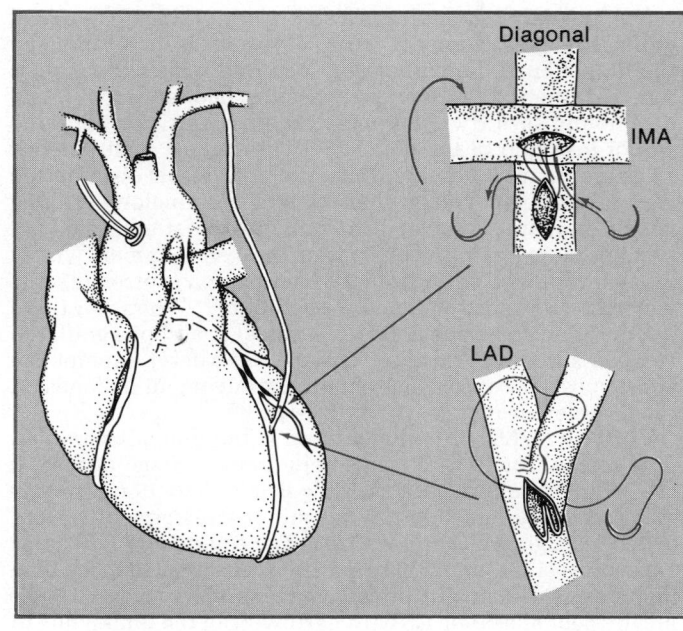

FIGURE 40–8. Internal mammary grafting: In situ left internal mammary artery (IMA) graft to the left anterior descending artery (end-to-side) and diagonal branch (side-to-side) employing the diamond anastomotic technique to the latter. The details show the IMA pedicle rolled up over the diagonal coronary artery to facilitate exposure and use of continuous suture. (From Jones, E. L.: Extended use of the internal mammary coronary artery bypass. J. Cardiac Surg. *1*:13, 1986.)

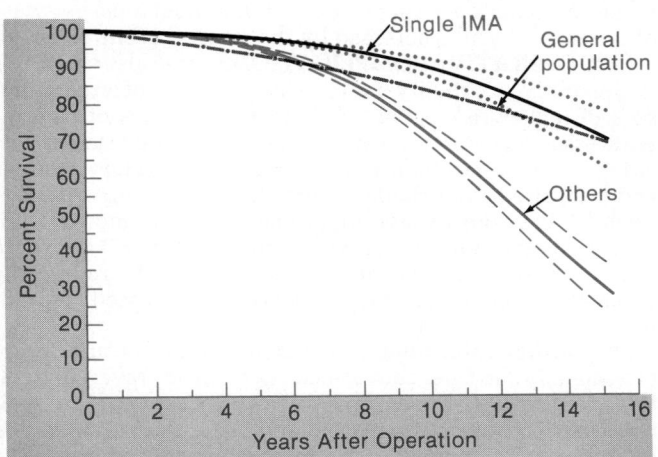

FIGURE 40–9. Survival of patients with extensive three-vessel disease according to whether or not a single internal mammary artery graft (IMA) to the left anterior descending coronary artery was used as a conduit in addition to whatever vein grafts were necessary. "General population" refers to an age, race, and gender-matched general population from government statistics and "Others" refers to patients revascularized without a single internal mammary artery graft applied to the left anterior descending coronary artery. These data strongly suggest that having a single IMA graft applied to the left anterior descending coronary artery is beneficial to survival in patients with extensive three-vessel coronary artery disease. (Modified from Kirklin J. W., et al.: Summary of a consensus concerning death and ischemic events after coronary artery bypass grafting. Circulation *79*[Suppl. I]:81, 1989, by permission of the American Heart Association, Inc.)

FIGURE 40–10. Different types of internal mammary artery grafts. A single attached internal mammary artery graft (either the right or left) remains attached proximally to the subclavian artery and is connected to the coronary arteries. Bilateral internal mammary artery grafts (right and left) are joined end to side to coronary arteries. Sequential internal mammary artery grafts consist of an attached or free internal mammary artery with one or more side-to-side anastomoses and one end-to-side anastomosis. The internal mammary artery Y graft has two terminal branches of either the attached or free internal mammary artery sutured to two coronary arteries. A free internal mammary artery graft is placed by transecting the right or left internal mammary artery near its origin in the subclavian artery, and the proximal artery is anastomosed to the aorta with the distal end to the coronary artery. (From Tector, A. J., et al.: Expanding the use of the internal mammary artery to improve patency in coronary artery bypass grafting. J. Thorac. Cardiovasc. Surg. *91*:9, 1986.)

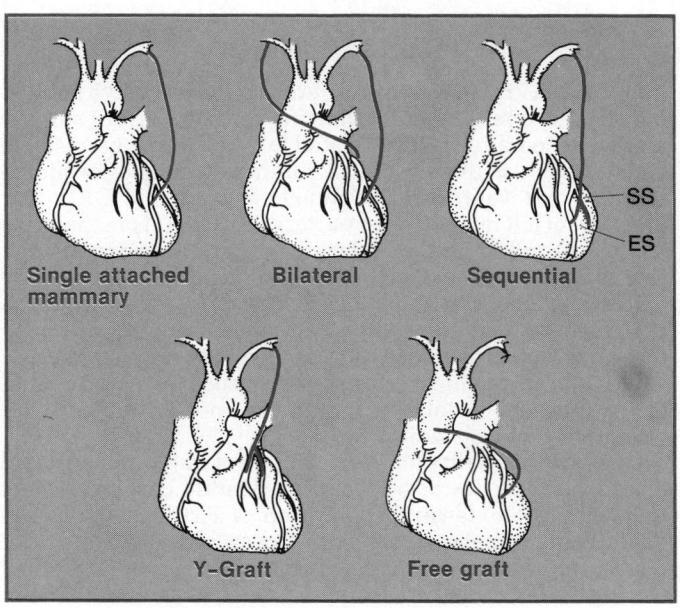

nary artery revascularization include the gastroepiploic artery,[314–316] which appears to be able to provide an adequate coronary artery supply even during exercise.[315] The radial artery is associated with poor patency rates,[314] and technical difficulty preparing the splenic artery for use as a graft has led to its disuse. The use of arm, allogeneic veins, and synthetic conduits have all been associated with relatively poor patency.[314]

MILD OBSTRUCTION. Intraoperative studies have shown that native arteries with less than 50 per cent luminal diameter obstruction often have minimal, if any, pressure gradients across the lesions and little difference in blood flow through the artery distal to the graft when the bypass graft is opened.[317] Patients with higher-grade obstructions usually have greater pressure gradients across the lesions, and flow through artery may increase significantly when the bypass graft is opened.

THE DISTAL VASCULATURE. The state of the distal coronary arterial vasculature is also important. Late patency of grafts is related to coronary arterial runoff, as determined by the diameter of the coronary artery into which the graft is inserted, the size of the distal vascular bed, and, to a lesser degree, the severity of coronary atherosclerosis distal to the site of insertion of the graft.[318,319] The highest graft patency rates are found when the lumina of the vessels distal to the graft insertion are greater than 1.5 mm in diameter, perfuse a large peripheral vascular bed, and are free of atheroma occluding more than 25 per cent of the vessel lumen. Vessel diameters measured at coronary arteriography correlate satisfactorily with those obtained at operation.[319] Whenever there is a question about the ability of a vessel to accept a graft, the surgeon should (consistent with patient safety) attempt the anastomosis because symptomatic improvement depends on the completeness of revascularization.[320]

FLOW RATES. When measured at the time of operation, flow rates through saphenous vein grafts average nearly 70 ml/min. Those in which the flow is less than 45 ml/min—and especially less than 25 ml/min—are frequently associated with graft closure, which is less common at flow rates exceeding 45 ml/min.[321] The possible causes for reduced flow include subcritical obstruction of the coronary artery; a technically poor anastomosis, with narrowing of the lumen due to kinking of the vessel or pinching at the site of the anastomosis; and a small myocardial mass perfused by the graft, which may in turn be due to diseased distal vasculature.

OTHER SURGICAL PROCEDURES FOR ISCHEMIC HEART DISEASE. Replacement of the aortic or mitral valve or both (Chap. 34) and left ventricular aneurysmectomy (p. 1350) may be performed with or without associated bypass grafting in patients with CAD. When valve replacement or aneurysmectomy is carried out as the sole procedure in such patients, it is usually because of the presence of heart failure refractory to medical management. These procedures add to the operative risk of bypass grafting, presumably because of the prolongation and greater technical complexity of the procedure, as well as because they are usually carried out on patients with left ventricular failure who are poor operative risks.

RESULTS OF SURGERY

OPERATIVE MORTALITY. As Kirklin et al. have pointed out, risk factors for death following coronary artery surgery are (1) preoperative factors related to CAD (severe or unstable angina, recent acute myocardial infarction, hemodynamic instability, left ventricular dysfunction, extent of CAD, and presence of left main coronary artery disease); (2) preoperative factors related to aggressiveness of the arteriosclerotic process, as reflected in associated carotid or peripheral vascular disease; (3) preoperative biological factors, (older age at operation, diabetes mellitus and perhaps female gender); (4) intraoperative factors (intraoperative ischemic damage and failure to use internal mammary artery grafts); and (5) environmental or institutional factors, including the specific surgeon and treatment protocols used.[311]

Operative mortality for the treatment of stable and unstable angina pectoris has been declining steadily despite the fact that with the extensive application of PTCD surgeons are operating on greater numbers of sicker, older patients with worse ventricular function and more extensive CAD.[322,323] During the last 10 years excellent operative results have been obtained even in patients with CAD and impaired ventricular function.[324-329] It is noteworthy that in patients of small stature (which probably correlates with small cardiac size and small coronary arteries), operative mortality is significantly increased and relief of angina is not as complete. In some series, operative mortality is 0.2 to 0.3 per cent.[330,331] However, *multi-institutional* results suggest hospital death rates of 6.5 per cent in community hospitals and 2.1 to 3.7 per cent in university hospitals.[311] Incremental risk factors for hospital death include increasing age, recent or previous myocardial

infarction, left ventricular dysfunction,[311] left main coronary artery disease (operative mortality 3.8 per cent compared with 2.6 per cent in patients with three-vessel disease),[332,332a] hemodynamic instability or cardiogenic shock, and the use of saphenous vein graft only.[311]

It has become increasingly clear that the use of internal mammary artery grafts (whether or not combined with vein grafts) is associated with reduced hospital and long-term mortality (Fig. 40–9).[311] The major areas of management that have been responsible for the currently low operative mortality of coronary artery surgery involve measures during both the intraoperative and perioperative periods. Improved anesthetic techniques, intraoperative protection of myocardium, conduit selection and preservation, blood conservation, perioperative hemodynamic monitoring, pharmacological left ventricular unloading, intraaortic balloon assistance, and arrhythmia control have all contributed.[301] In patients with active ischemia, cardiogenic shock, or extremely poor left ventricular function, operative mortality may be reduced when the intraaortic balloon is used to support the circulation during the perioperative period.[333]

There is still considerable variability in the results of various surgical groups, and the physician considering the referral of a particular patient for surgical treatment must be aware of the recent results obtained by the surgical group selected.

PERIOPERATIVE COMPLICATIONS (see also Chap. 53). Perioperative morbidity has increased because of larger numbers of higher-risk patients.[323] Greater numbers of patients with associated disease (hypertension, cerebrovascular disease), recent infarction, extensive coronary artery disease, and impaired ventricular function are being operated upon.[333a] Previous bypass surgery has become a more significant predictor of mortality with respect to time,[323] but there has also been a significant increase in patients undergoing emergency operation with associated increased mortality.[323,333a]

Myocardial Infarction. This complication occurs in approximately 2 to 5 per cent of elective coronary revascularizations.[330,331,334,335] In the Coronary Artery Surgery Study (CASS) trial, carried out between 1975 and 1979, the perioperative infarction rate, defined as the appearance of Q waves in the perioperative period, was reported as 6.4 per cent.[334] The incidence of perioperative infarction is usually related to the obstruction of a graft and correlates with the number of bypass grafts. Therefore, meticulous attention to anastomosis of the graft to the coronary artery is vital. Although the loss of any viable myocardium obviously is undesirable, in most patients the perioperative infarcts are small. In patients experiencing a perioperative myocardial infarction, perioperative mortality is higher, and in those with residual depressed left ventricular function (left ventricular ejection fraction < 40 per cent) and inadequate revascularization, the long-term prognosis is poorer.[336]

Intellectual Dysfunction. It is common for patients to show impaired cognitive function early following coronary artery bypass surgery. This occurs in the absence of evidence of a perioperative stroke.[337] It is important that the physician reassure the patient and family that this is usually a temporary phenomenon.[338]

Hypertension. This complication can occur in up to one-third of all patients after coronary artery surgery (p. 841). The mechanism is unclear, but it may be related to increased levels of circulating catecholamines and renin. With the use of agents such as calcium antagonists,[339] sodium nitroprusside,[339] or nitrates[340] in the perioperative period, it rarely presents a problem. Esmolol, a short-acting beta-blocking agent (p. 864) appears to be equally effective in reducing systolic and diastolic pressures and also slows heart rate.[341] It is important that hypertension be adequately controlled to prevent myocardial ischemia, cardiac failure, and excessive perioperative bleeding.

Intraventricular Conduction Disturbances. In general, patients with CAD who develop fascicular conduction disturbances have diffuse myocardial disease and an unfavorable prognosis. The subsequent causes of death are ventricular arrhythmias and cardiac failure. However, in one series of patients, the development of new perioperative ventricular conduction disturbances did not worsen the long-term survival rate.[342]

Complications in the Obese. Physicians, nurses, and physiotherapists involved in the perioperative care of obese patients are well aware of the need for aggressive chest physiotherapy and the potential problems with persistent immobilization. While obesity per se does not appear to increase significantly the operative mortality,[343] it is associated with a higher incidence of complications, including sternotomy dehiscence,[344] impaired leg wound healing following saphenous vein excision,[345] postoperative hypertension, and bronchoconstriction.[343]

SYMPTOMATIC RESULTS. Major relief of angina pectoris occurs in most appropriately selected patients after coronary artery surgery.[346-350] Approximately three-quarters of patients will be free from ischemic events (return of angina, occurrence of a myocardial infarction, or sudden death) for 5 years after coronary artery surgery, and nearly half of patients for at least 10 years (Fig. 40–11).[311] However, by 15 years only about 15 per cent of patients can be expected to remain free of an ischemic event.

Return to full employment has been disappointing in many series.[351] Factors that adversely affect the prospects of patients returning to work include increasing age,[352,353] postoperative angina,[352-354] and either unemployment or a period of disability before surgery.[352,353] Approximately half of patients will return to presurgery levels of household activity,[355] and most will experience improved physical and sexual functional status from presurgery levels.[356] However, with time there is a falloff in symptomatic benefit, and there is a suggestion that by 10 years after coronary vein graft surgery the relief of symptoms and improved exercise performance noted at 5 years have decreased to levels seen in medically treated patients.[357]

GRAFT PATENCY RATE AND CHANGES IN NATIVE CIRCULATION. Experimental studies and observations in patients suggest that there are several consecutive phases of disease development in venous aortocoronary artery bypass grafts (Fig. 40–12).

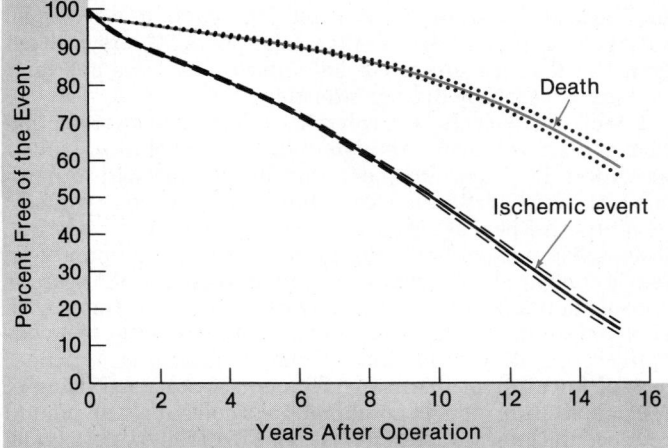

FIGURE 40–11. Freedom from the first ischemic event (angina, myocardial infarction, or sudden death) after coronary artery bypass grafting for ischemic heart disease. Freedom from death (the survivorship) is depicted, as is freedom from the first ischemic event after primary, isolated coronary artery bypass graft surgery for ischemic heart disease using any type of conduit (saphenous vein grafts and internal mammary grafts). In considering freedom from the first ischemic event, patients dying before the development of this event of causes other than sudden death (e.g., accidental death, cancer) have been censored at the time of death. (Modified from Kirklin J. W., et al.: Summary of a consensus concerning death and ischemic events after coronary artery bypass grafting. Circulation 79[Suppl. I]:81, 1989, by permission of the American Heart Association, Inc.)

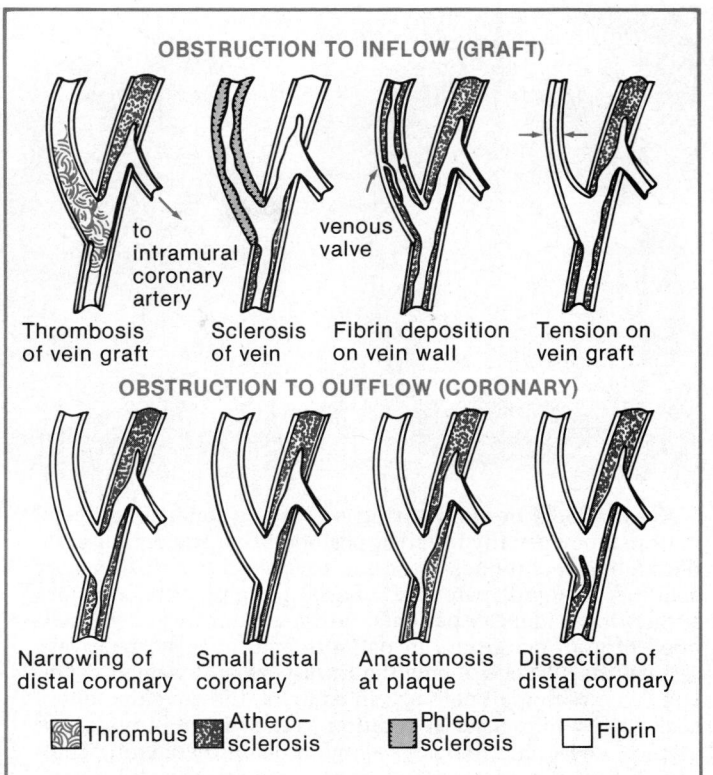

FIGURE 40–12. Anatomical and technical factors that can produce obstruction of a vein graft *(top)* and of arterial outflow *(bottom)*. (From Spray, T. L., and Roberts, W. C.: Morphologic observations in biologic conduits between aorta and coronary artery. *In* Rahimtoola, S. [ed.]: Coronary Bypass Surgery. Philadelphia, F. A. Davis, Co., 1977, p. 11.)

Early Occlusion. Early occlusion (prior to hospital discharge) occurs in 8 to 12 per cent of venous grafts, and by 1 year 12 to 20 per cent of vein grafts have become occluded.[302,305] Technical factors may cause closure at the proximal or distal anastomoses; both kinks due to excessive length and tension due to insufficient length may promote occlusion. Graft flow and distal vessel runoff are also important. Atheroma at the arteriotomy site may predispose to early occlusion. Perioperative platelet inhibitor therapy with both high-[358] and low-dose[359] aspirin and dipyridamole appears to diminish the rate of early occlusion.

Intermediate Phase. In vein grafts that have been implanted in the arterial circulation for 1 month to 1 year, there is substantial endothelial denudation and proliferation and migration of medial cells to the intima. These events are promoted by aggregation of platelets and growth factor secretion.[302] Intimal thickening and hyperplasia appear, but this process is not prevented by platelet inhibitor therapy. Histological studies of grafts that occlude within 1 year show either substantial thrombosis with minimal intima-medial changes or marked intimal hyperplasia and superimposed thrombus.[360] This accelerated process of intimal hyperplasia is an early stage of atherosclerotic plaque formation and is believed to occur because of an interaction between platelets and other circulating cells and chronic, mild endothelial damage. If the proliferation is severe and localized (as may occur at the site of the anastomosis between the grafts and the recipient artery), total occlusion can occur within 1 year.

Atherosclerosis in Venous Bypass Grafts. Beyond the first year, a histological picture occurs that is indistinguishable from that of arterial atherosclerotic disease (Fig. 40–13).[361] Some investigators believed that, as in native arteries, the development of atherosclerosis in vein grafts is a continuum starting from platelet deposition and advancing to smooth muscle cell proliferation and finally to lipid incorporation into the plaque. By 10 years, nearly one-half of venous grafts patent at 5 years have become occluded.[302,361a]

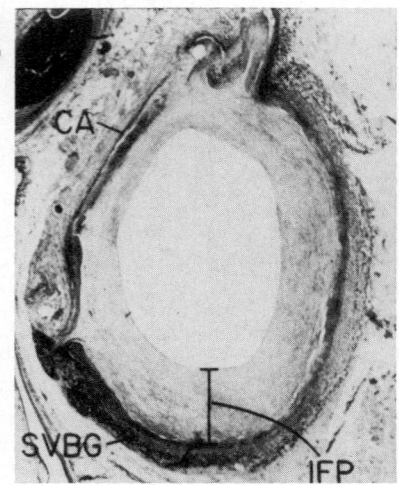 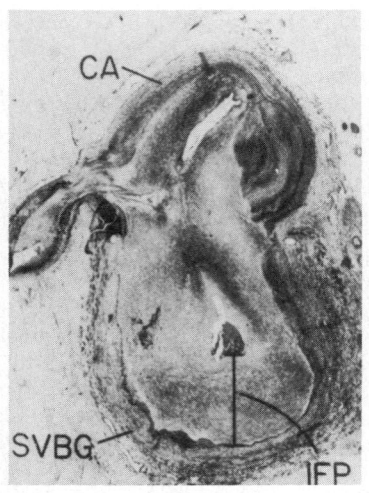

FIGURE 40–13. Postmortem histological sections through coronary artery (CA) anastomosis sites of saphenous vein bypass grafts (SVBG) show extensive fibrous tissue proliferation in the grafts' intimal layers. In the graft at *left,* the circumferential intimal fibrous plaque (IFP) developed in 5 months. In the graft at *right,* the process resulted in greater than 90 per cent stenosis 8 months after implantation. With time, such fibrous plaques may become infiltrated with lipids and calcium and increasingly resemble atherosclerotic plaques. (From Bulkley, B. H.: Why coronary bypass grafts fail: Early and late pathologic changes. J. Cardiovasc. Med. 5:1025, 1980.)

Nongrafted Coronary Arteries. While determination of graft patency usually involves postoperative angiography, radionuclide techniques assessing myocardial perfusion may also indicate graft patency.[362] Serial imaging after coronary surgery may identify patients with a greater or lesser likelihood of graft occlusion. In patients who have no recurrent angina, the absence of new thallium-perfusion defects correlates well with graft patency. In contrast, the development of new perfusion defects in addition to the return of typical or atypical chest pain indicates a high probability of graft occlusion.[362] Contrast-enhanced computer tomography also may be used to assess patency of saphenous vein grafts (Fig. 9–47, p. 267). Disease progression in nongrafted arteries (worsening of a preexisting lesion or appearance of a new diameter narrowing of greater than 49 per cent) can occur at a rate of 18 to 38 per cent over 5 to 10 years.[363–365] The rate of disease progression appears highest in arterial segments already showing evidence of disease.[364]

Late Occlusion. By the end of the first year, the overall occlusion rate per distal anastomosis is between 12 and 20 per cent (and the chance of one or more distal anastomoses being occluded in an individual patient with multiple venous grafts is approximately 45 per cent).[305,358,366] The occlusion rate decreases substantially beyond the first year to an annual rate of 2 per cent.[302] The attrition rate for grafts between 6 and 11 years after operation increases to 4 per cent per year.[305] Thus, the overall occlusion rate per distal anastomosis is 25 to 30 per cent at 5 to 7 years and 40 to 50 per cent at 10 years.

The risk of disease progression (appearance of a new lesion ≥50 per cent diameter stenosis or worsening of a preexisting lesion) is between three and six times higher in grafted native coronary arteries than in ungrafted native arteries,[363] and it is higher in arteries with patent grafts than in arteries with occluded grafts.[363] In the Veterans Administration Cooperative Study, the progression of disease in native grafted arteries was most often to total occlusion.[363] In general, progression usually occurs proximal to the site of graft insertion.[363,364] These data suggest that bypassing an artery with minimal disease, even if initially successful, may ultimately be harmful to the patient, who incurs both the risk of graft closure and the increased risk of accelerated obstruction of the native vessel.

Effects of Therapy on Vein Graft Occlusion and Native Vessel Progression. A meta-analysis of clinical trials suggests that antiplatelet or anticoagulant therapy after coronary artery bypass surgery may prevent graft occlusions.[367]

In a prospective randomized double-blind trial, dipyridamole (started 48 hours before operation) plus aspirin (started 7 hours after operation) was compared with placebo treatment. The daily maintenance therapy was dipyridamole 75 mg and aspirin 325 mg orally three times a day. Within 1 month of operation 3 per cent of vein-graft distal anastomoses were occluded in the treated patients compared to 10 per cent in the placebo group.[358] At angiography performed 1 year after operation, 11 per cent of vein-graft distal anastomoses were oc-

cluded in the treated group and 25 per cent in the placebo group.[366] It is possible, however, that dipyridamole is not an essential component of this treatment[368,368a] and that much lower doses of aspirin (40 to 80 mg/day) may be sufficient.

A Veterans Administration Cooperative Study Group has also examined the effect of specific antiplatelet therapy on vein graft[365,369] and internal mammary artery graft patency[370] after coronary artery bypass grafting. In this study, 772 patients were randomized to receive aspirin (325 mg once a day), aspirin (325 mg three times a day), aspirin plus dipyridamole (325 and 75 mg together three times a day), sulfinpyrazone (267 mg three times a day), or placebo.[369] In all aspirin subgroups, one 325-mg aspirin dose was given 12 hours before surgery and maintained thereafter according to the assigned regimen, but in other groups all therapy was started 48 hours before operation. Patients receiving aspirin required more reoperations for postoperative bleeding (6.6 per cent) compared with patients not receiving aspirin (1.7 per cent).[370a] All aspirin-containing therapeutic regimens improved vein graft patency compared with placebo.[369] Early graft patency rates were 94 per cent for aspirin daily, 92 per cent for aspirin three times daily, 92 per cent for aspirin and dipyridamole, and 90 per cent for dipyridamole alone compared with 85 per cent for placebo. At 1 year the graft occlusion rate in all the aspirin groups combined was 16 per cent compared with 23 per cent for the placebo group.[365] At 1 year the patency rate for all internal mammary artery grafts was 93 per cent (versus 90 per cent for all vein grafts to the left anterior descending artery) and aspirin therapy did not alter this.[370]

Effects of Hypercholesterolemia. It has been observed that LDL cholesterol levels are higher and HDL cholesterol levels are lower 11 years after operation in patients with atherosclerotic vein grafts than in patients with normal grafts.[371] Seventy-nine per cent of patients without new atherosclerotic lesions had normal lipid and normal plasma LDL apoprotein levels compared with only 8 per cent of patients whose grafts showed new atherosclerotic lesions. In addition, patients with elevated serum Lp(a) (p. 1129) have an increased risk of developing vein graft stenosis after coronary bypass surgery.[372] Successful lowering of total and LDL cholesterol and raising of HDL cholesterol (using a combination of colestipol and niacin) reduced the appearance of new lesions in coronary vein grafts as well as in the native coronary vessels.[373] Since late closure of venous grafts is invariably associated with atherosclerotic changes and is linked to continued smoking following surgery,[374] it is important for patients and physicians to work hard to maintain ideal body weight, reduce total and LDL cholesterol levels, and permanently cease smoking following coronary artery surgery.

LATE SURVIVAL. The large randomized trials of coronary artery surgery have provided detailed information of late survival (p. 1318). These studies predate the widespread use of the internal thoracic artery for revascularization, the use of PTCA, the use of aspirin, and an increasingly aggressive approach to the treatment of elevated levels of LDL cholesterol. Despite these improvements in medical and surgical management, preoperative left ventricular dysfunction continues to have a profound influence on both operative mortality and long-term survival. The beneficial influence of using the internal mammary artery as a conduit has been seen on early surgical mortality[311,330] and on later mortality.[308,311,312,330] Twelve-year follow-up in the European Coronary Surgery Study Group[375] suggests that the long-term benefits of surgery tend to be greater in patients at higher risk, i.e., patients over 50 years of age, with infarction on the preoperative electrocardiogram, a markedly ischemic response to exercise testing, and peripheral arterial disease. During short-term follow-up, there appears to be no significant difference with respect to relief of symptoms or survival between diabetics and nondiabetics,[376] although studies of patients with peripheral vascular disease show a cumulative 5-year survival of only 43 per cent for diabetics compared with 78 per cent for nondiabetics.[377] The results of coronary artery surgery in patients aged 35 or younger showed excellent actuarial survival rates of 94 per cent at 5 years and 85 per cent at 10 years despite the severity of the underlying disease and the rapidity of the atherosclerotic process in these patients.[378] However, during longer follow-up, atherosclerosis of the venous grafts becomes an increasingly important problem in these patients.[379]

COMPARISON OF MEDICAL AND SURGICAL THERAPY OF CHRONIC STABLE ANGINA PECTORIS

Prognostic Considerations

OBSERVATIONS WITHOUT ANGIOGRAPHIC ASSESSMENT. Prior to the widespread use of aspirin, beta blockers, and efforts to lower cholesterol in patients with CAD, the Framingham Study revealed that the average annual mortality of patients with chronic stable angina was 4 per cent.[380] Remission of angina may occur in up to one-third of patients with angina of recent onset. However, if the condition has been present for several years, remission is unusual. Survivors of myocardial infarction had a 5 per cent annual mortality after the first postinfarction year.[380] Others have reported similar,[381] higher,[382] and lower mortality rates.[383] In a long-term follow-up study of 586 men who had survived an attack of unstable angina or acute infarction and who were treated conservatively, the survival at 5 years was 80 per cent, at 10 years 61 per cent, and at 15 years 43 per cent.[383]

The severity of angina pectoris has some influence on the survival of patients with CAD. In a patient population with normal ventricular function and a similar extent of coronary disease, those with severe angina (perhaps reflecting, albeit indirectly, the severity of ischemia) have a worse prognosis.[384] Data from the Veterans Administration Study have shown that clinical factors such as the severity of symptoms, the presence of ST-segment depression on the resting electrocardiogram, and a history of either myocardial infarction or hypertension all adversely affect outcome in medically treated patients, particularly if two or more factors are present.[385] The European Coronary Study Group showed that an abnormal resting electrocardiogram and peripheral vascular disease also adversely affect survival in medically managed patients with chronic coronary artery disease.[347] Others have reported the adverse influence of hypertension on prognosis in patients with established CAD, and cigarette smoking appears to increase the incidence of sudden death. Cardiomegaly on a routine chest x-ray examination and the presence of a third sound on physical examination have adverse effects on prognosis because they reflect more extensive myocardial damage.[386]

PROGNOSIS BASED ON ANGIOGRAPHIC CRITERIA. In studies using angiographic criteria for prognostic evaluation, the two important variables are left ventricular function and the severity and extent of CAD. In general, the extent of left ventricular dysfunction is a more important determinant

of prognosis than the extent and severity of CAD.[387] The follow-up of patients in the CASS Registry has allowed accurate study of survival of medically treated patients with angiographically assessed CAD. Both the number of major coronary arteries with severe obstruction and the degree of depression of left ventricular ejection fraction were independent risk factors, the latter exerting the dominant influence.[388] These two risk factors are synergistic in that the adverse effects on prognosis of impaired ventricular function are more pronounced as the number of stenotic vessels increases (Fig. 40–14).

Studies in *symptomatic* patients have revealed that if only *one* of the three major coronary arteries has more than 50 per cent stenosis, the annual mortality rate will be approximately 2 per cent.[389] The importance to survival of the *quantity of* myocardium that is jeopardized is reflected in the observation that an obstructive lesion proximal to the first septal perforator of the left anterior descending coronary artery was associated with a 5-year survival of 90 per cent, compared with 98 per cent in patients with more distal lesions.[389] The survival rate of patients with isolated right CAD at 5 years appeared to be higher (96 per cent) than in patients with disease of the left anterior descending coronary artery (92 per cent). The overall survival of nonsurgically treated patients with left anterior descending and left circumflex CAD was not significantly different, but both were less than the survival of patients with isolated right CAD.[389] The risk of cardiac events does not appear to be related to the presence or absence of collateral vessels in patients with one-vessel coronary disease[390]; however, even in patients with single-vessel disease, left ventricular ejection fraction was the baseline descriptor most strongly associated with survival.

In symptomatic patients or survivors of infarction, if two of the major arteries exhibit severe stenosis, the 5-year mortality is approximately 9 per cent, and if all three vessels are stenotic it rises to approximately 15 per cent.[330,391] In an observational study of patients with obstructive coronary disease who initially were treated medically, 15-year survival rates were 48, 28, 18, and 9 per cent for patients with single-, double-, triple-, and left main vessel disease, respectively.[392] In addition to the number of vessels involved, the severity of obstruction is also important. Prognosis in patients with 50- to 75 per cent narrowing is better than in those with more than 75 per cent narrowing.[393]

High-grade lesions of the left main coronary artery are particularly life threatening.[394] Mortality among medically treated patients has been reported as 29 per cent at 18 months,[395] 39 per cent at 2 years,[396] and 43 per cent at 5 years.[397] Survival is better for patients having a 50 to 70 per cent stenosis (1- and 3-year survivals of 91 per cent and 66 per cent, respectively) than for patients with a greater than 70 per cent left main coronary artery stenosis (1- and 3-year survivals of 72 and 41 per cent)[394] (Fig. 40–15). Furthermore, a number of characteristics found at catheterization or noninvasive examination are predictors of an adverse prognosis in patients with 70 per cent or greater left main coronary artery stenosis; these include chest pain at rest, ST-T wave changes on the resting electrocardiogram, cardiomegaly on the chest roentgenogram, a history of congestive heart failure, findings of left ventricular dysfunction at catheterization, and elevation of the arterial-mixed venous oxygen difference.[394]

The severity of symptoms is a useful prognostic factor in conjunction with arteriographic findings. In asymptomatic or mildly symptomatic patients with one- or two-vessel disease, the prognosis is excellent, and the annual mortality is approximately 1.5 per cent. In patients with three-vessel disease with good exercise capacity (achievement of 85 per cent predicted heart rate or workload of 100 watts or more), the annual mortality rate also is only 4 per cent, but in those with poor exercise capacity it is much higher.[398] During exercise testing in the CASS randomized study (a group of patients with mild angina or history of infarction and a left ventricular ejection fraction of >35 per cent), the presence of exercise-induced angina identified patients who had a survival advantage over

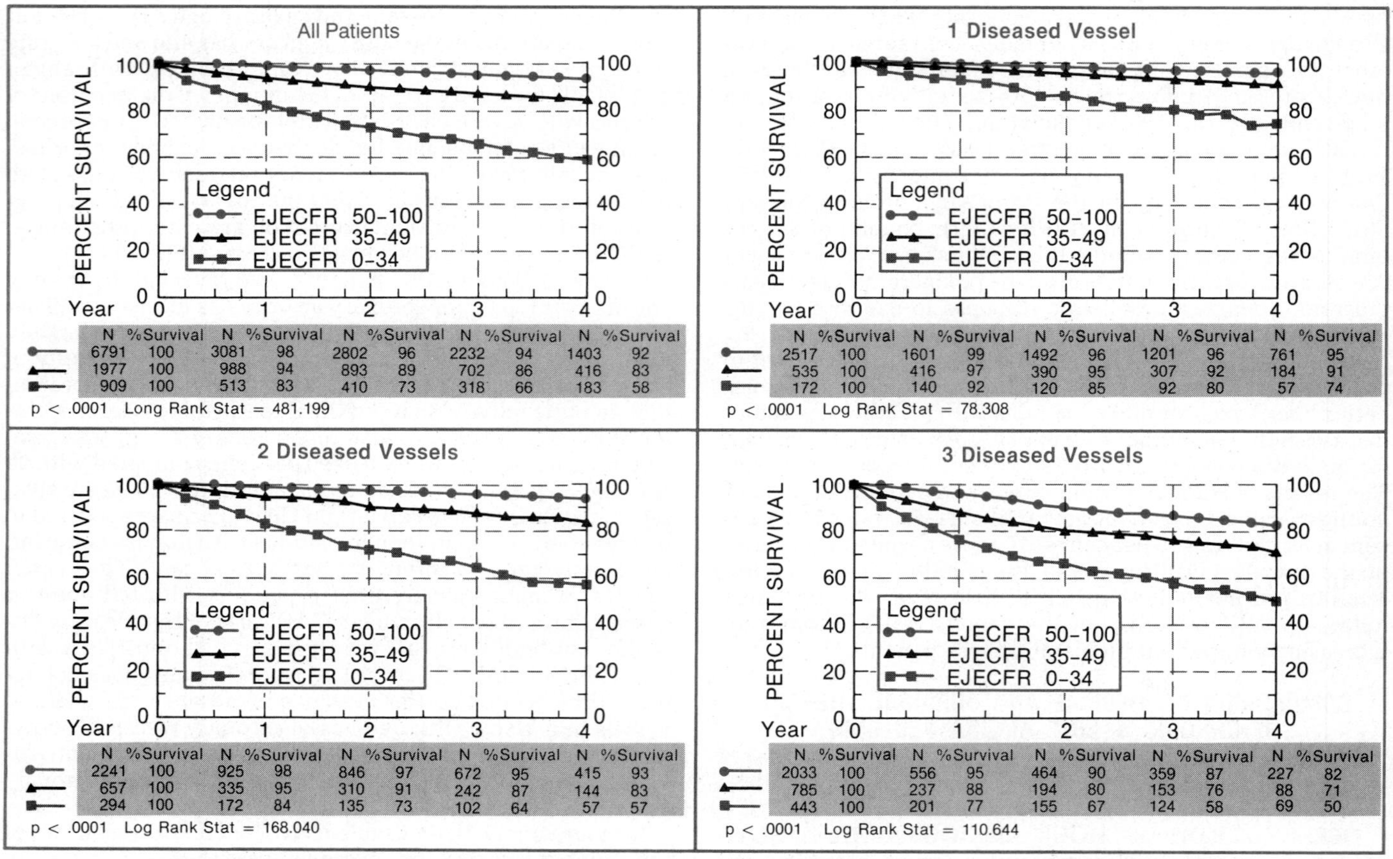

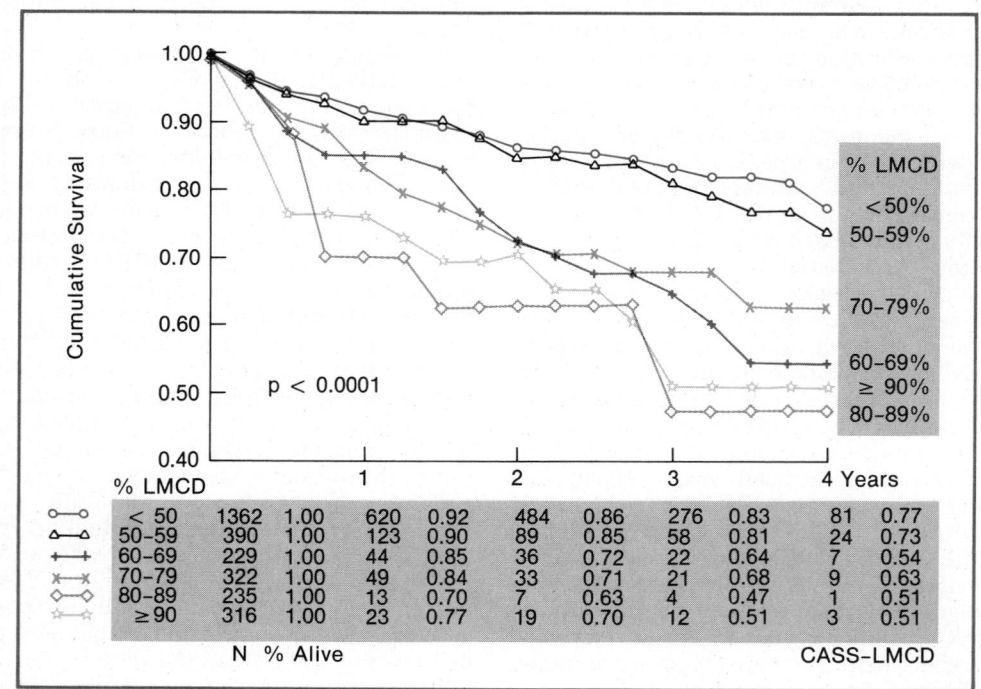

All Patients

	N	%Survival	N	%Survival	N	%Survival	N	%Survival	N	%Survival
●	6791	100	3081	98	2802	96	2232	94	1403	92
▲	1977	100	988	94	893	89	702	86	416	83
■	909	100	513	83	410	73	318	66	183	58

p < .0001   Long Rank Stat = 481.199

1 Diseased Vessel

	N	%Survival	N	%Survival	N	%Survival	N	%Survival	N	%Survival
●	2517	100	1601	99	1492	96	1201	96	761	95
▲	535	100	416	97	390	95	307	92	184	91
■	172	100	140	92	120	85	92	80	57	74

p < .0001   Log Rank Stat = 78.308

2 Diseased Vessels

	N	%Survival	N	%Survival	N	%Survival	N	%Survival	N	%Survival
●	2241	100	925	98	846	97	672	95	415	93
▲	657	100	335	95	310	91	242	87	144	83
■	294	100	172	84	135	73	102	64	57	57

p < .0001   Log Rank Stat = 168.040

3 Diseased Vessels

	N	%Survival	N	%Survival	N	%Survival	N	%Survival	N	%Survival
●	2033	100	556	95	464	90	359	87	227	82
▲	785	100	237	88	194	80	153	76	88	71
■	443	100	201	77	155	67	124	58	69	50

p < .0001   Log Rank Stat = 110.644

FIGURE 40–14. Effect of the anatomical extent of obstructive coronary artery disease and left ventricular function on survival in medically treated patients in the CASS Registry. Survival of medically treated patients with no significant obstructive disease was 97 per cent, in contrast to 92 per cent, 84 per cent, and 68 per cent of patients with one-, two-, and three-vessel disease, respectively. In patients with less than 50 per cent left main coronary artery obstruction and measured ejection fraction (EJEC FR), the effect of decreasing ejection fraction on survival is evident, even when the probability of survival is already high, as in patients with one or two obstructed arteries. As the severity of arterial disease increases, the impact of left ventricular dysfunction is even greater upon survival. (From Mock, M. B., et al.: Survival of medically treated patients in the Coronary Artery Surgery [CASS] Registry. Circulation 66:562, 1982, by permission of the American Heart Association, Inc.)

% LMCD

% LMCD	N	% Alive	N	% Alive	N	% Alive	N	% Alive	N	% Alive
< 50	1362	1.00	620	0.92	484	0.86	276	0.83	81	0.77
50–59	390	1.00	123	0.90	89	0.85	58	0.81	24	0.73
60–69	229	1.00	44	0.85	36	0.72	22	0.64	7	0.54
70–79	322	1.00	49	0.84	33	0.71	21	0.68	9	0.63
80–89	235	1.00	13	0.70	7	0.63	4	0.47	1	0.51
≥ 90	316	1.00	23	0.77	19	0.70	12	0.51	3	0.51

p < 0.0001

CASS–LMCD

FIGURE 40–15. Survival curves for medically treated patients with left main coronary artery disease. The cumulative survival rates of nonsurgically treated patients with left main coronary artery disease (LMCD) in the CASS Registry analyzed according to per cent intraluminal narrowing are demonstrated. The survival curves separate when the degree of angiographically assessed stenosis exceeds 60 per cent, so that patients with a lesser degree of narrowing have relatively favorable long-term prognosis. (From Chaitman, B. R., et al.: Effect of coronary bypass surgery on survival patterns in subsets of patients with left main coronary artery disease. Am. J. Cardiol. 48:765, 1981.)

7 years if assigned to surgical therapy (94 per cent), compared with medical therapy (87 per cent).[399]

The assessment of ventricular function and extent and severity of CAD have been major influences in determining our understanding of the natural history of CAD and have been of help in selecting patients for surgical therapy. Taken together, the available information suggests that the volume of myocardium perfused by critically narrowed vessels and the rate of progression of coronary atherosclerosis are the principal determinants of prognosis in patients with CAD. The likelihood that stable atherosclerotic plaque will develop into an ulcerated plaque leading to coronary thrombosis and development of electrical instability also affects prognosis.

EXERCISE ELECTROCARDIOGRAPHY AND OTHER NONINVASIVE TESTS FOR PROGNOSTIC EVALUATION. The aims of exercise electrocardiographic testing, thallium scintigraphy, and exercise radionuclide ventriculography are to provide data about ventricular function and the quantity of myocardium that becomes ischemic during stress. In this manner, an assessment of the patient's functional status and the quantity of "jeopardized" myocardium can be assessed. In patients in whom left ventricular function and coronary anatomy have also been defined, exercise stress testing can provide important additional prognostic information.

By means of the CASS Registry, 30 clinical and exercise variables were analyzed in 4083 patients with defined ventricular function and coronary anatomy to assess factors of prognostic importance.[400] The *duration* of exercise and the *ST-segment response* emerged as the most important exercise test variables. In a subgroup of 570 patients with three-vessel coronary disease and preserved left ventricular function, the probability of survival at 4 years ranged from 53 per cent for patients able to achieve only stage I of exercise to 100 per cent for patients able to exercise into stage V of the standard or modified Bruce protocol. Patients showing less than 0.1 mV of ST-segment depression who could exercise into stage III of the Bruce protocol or higher had an annual mortality of 1 per cent or less, while those with at least 0.1 mV ST-segment depression who could not complete stage I had an annual mortality of 5 per cent or more (Table 40–13).

STRESS THALLIUM-201 MYOCARDIAL PERFUSION IMAGING (see also p. 1270). Exercise thallium scintigraphy may be helpful in identifying areas of myocardium in which ischemia may be induced and that may benefit from revascularization. Predictors of adverse prognosis following thallium-201 scintigraphy performed during exercise, or after administration of dipyridamole, include a delayed tracer redistribution, multiple large perfusion defects, and abnormal lung uptake.[93] The disadvantages of thallium-201 scintigraphy include the high cost, the long time required for imaging, interpretation difficulties, and poor imaging in obese persons. The patient has to be able to attain a sufficient level of exercise before a normal perfusion pattern can be assumed confidently to indicate no significant underlying coronary artery disease, although dipyridamole can be employed in patients with severe exercise limitations.

EXERCISE RADIONUCLIDE ANGIOGRAPHY (see also p. 1300). A number of studies suggest that the exercise left ventricular ejection fraction is one of the best prognostic predictors of major future cardiac events or of high-risk CAD.[401] In patients with known CAD, if the left ventricular ejection fraction during exercise fails to rise appropriately or if it falls, it suggests that a substantial segment of myocardium has become ischemic, and correlates with multivessel disease, left main coronary artery disease, and a high mortality over the next 2 years.[401] During preoperative evaluation patients who had the most profound exercise-induced left ventricular dysfunction prior to myocardial revascularization had improved survival, compared to those treated medically,[402,403] while those with a normal ejection fraction response to exercise did not.

In patients whose left ventricular function and coronary anatomy have been defined, the demonstration of ischemia or jeopardized myocardium may have a profound bearing on management. In a study of minimally symptomatic patients with preserved resting left ventricular function and three-vessel disease, evidence of impaired exercise capacity combined with the demonstration of inducible myocardial ischemia (as manifested by a decrease in ejection fraction during exercise) identified those at high risk of death during medical therapy.[404] Patients who did not manifest ischemia during exercise by radionuclide angiography or exercise electrocardiography had an excellent prognosis compared with those with impaired exercise capacity, especially if it occurred at a low workload (Fig. 40–16).

Initial Results

RELIEF OF ANGINA PECTORIS. As early as 1972, a committee of the American Heart Association indicated that the most widely accepted indication for surgical revascularization was "significant disability from moderate to severe angina pectoris, unresponsive to optimal medical care."[404a] Two decades later angina pectoris remains the principal indication; however, coronary bypass surgery is now being carried out in increasing numbers of patients with multivessel coro-

TABLE 40-13   RISK STRATIFICATION BY EXERCISE TESTING

STUDY	PATIENTS (N)	RISK CLASSIFICATION		
		Low	Intermediate	High
McNeer et al. Circulation 57:64, 1978	1472	<1 mm ST ↓ FS ≥ IV Peak HR ≥ 160 beats/min		≥1 mm ST ↓ FS I or II
Bruce et al. (Seattle Heart Watch) Circulation 60:638, 1979	2001	<1 mm ST ↓ No LV dysfunction	≥1 mm ST ↓ No LV dysfunction	FS ≤ I Peak SBP <130 mm Hg, Cardiomegaly
Dagenais et al. Circulation 65:452, 1982	107	≤2 mm ST ↓ FS ≥ IV	≤2 mm ST ↓ FS ≥ III	≥2 mm ST ↓ FS ≤ I
Schneider et al. Am. J. Cardiol. 50:682, 1982	80			>1 mm ST ↓ FS I or II
Weiner et al. Am. Heart J. 105:749, 1983	292	≤2 mm ST ↓ No LV dysfunction		LV dysfunction or ≥2 mm ST ↓ beginning in stage I
Weiner et al. (CASS) J. Am. Coll. Cardiol. 3:772, 1984	4083	<1 mm ST ↓ FS ≥ III	≥1 mm ST ↓ FS ≥ III	≥1 mm ST ↓ FS I ≤ I

N = number; FS = final exercise stage (Bruce protocol); LV = left ventricular; SBP = systolic blood pressure; HR = heart rate; CASS = Coronary Artery Surgery Study.

From Deering, T. F., and Weiner, D. A.: Prognosis of patients with coronary artery disease. J. Cardiopulmon. Rehabil. 5:325, 1985.

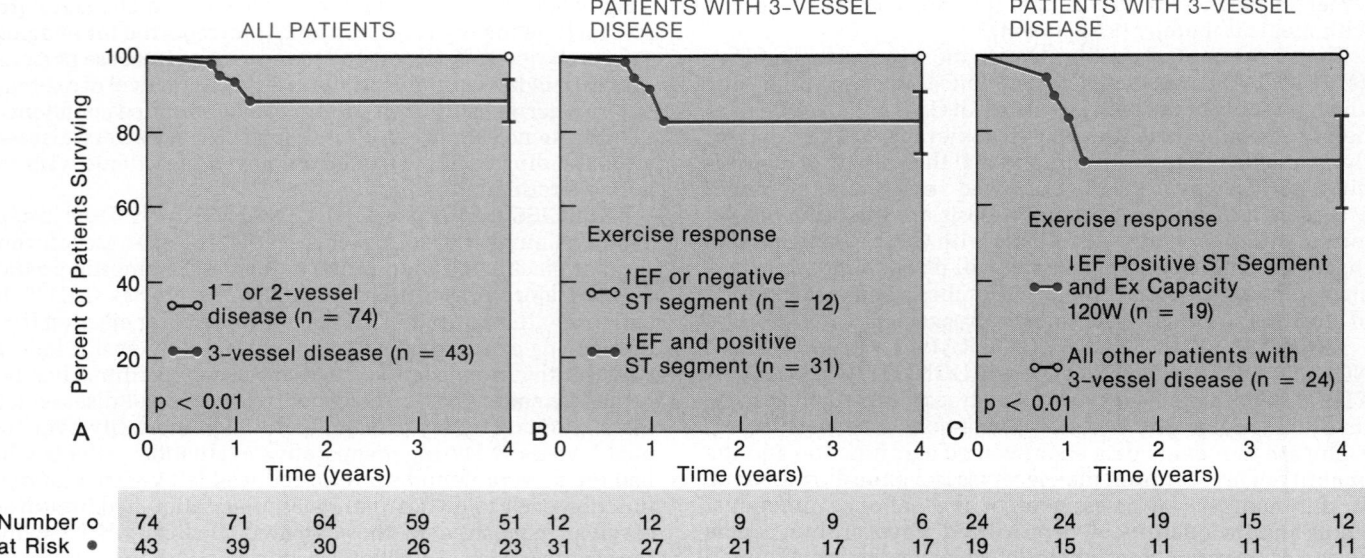

| Number ○ | 74 | 71 | 64 | 59 | 51 | 12 | 12 | 9 | 9 | 6 | 24 | 24 | 19 | 15 | 12 |
| at Risk ● | 43 | 39 | 30 | 26 | 23 | 31 | 27 | 21 | 17 | 17 | 19 | 15 | 11 | 11 | 11 |

FIGURE 40–16. Influence of anatomical severity of coronary artery disease, reversible ischemia, and exercise capacity on survival in mildly symptomatic patients with coronary artery disease and left ventricular ejection fractions greater than 40 per cent. Survival curves are shown for patients with three-vessel disease as compared with those with one- or two-vessel disease *(A)*; patients with three-vessel disease and an increase in ejection fraction (EF) or a negative ST-segment response to exercise as compared with those with three-vessel disease and both a decreased ejection fraction and a positive ST-segment response with exercise *(B)*; and patients with three-vessel disease and a decrease in ejection fraction during exercise, a positive ST-segment response, and exercise capacity of 120 watts or less as compared with all other patients with three-vessel disease *(C)*. The number of patients with potential follow-up at each time is shown for each group. Evidence of impaired exercise capacity associated with evidence of reversible myocardial ischemia defines a group of patients with three-vessel disease with an adverse prognosis long-term. (Reprinted with permission from Bonow, R. O., et al.: Exercise-induced ischemia in mildly symptomatic patients with coronary artery disease and preserved left ventricular function. N. Engl. J. Med. *311*:1339, 1984.)

nary disease and either mild to moderate symptoms, left ventricular dysfunction, or poor exercise tolerance, because of the apparent improval in survival in these groups. Patients with unstable angina[405] and left ventricular dysfunction as well as survivors of acute myocardial infarction[406] are also undergoing revascularization with increasing frequency.

Relief of angina pectoris occurs in up to 95 per cent of patients with chronic stable angina following coronary artery surgery. More than half of the patients become totally asymptomatic, at least initially. Most of the others exhibit substantial symptomatic relief.[346] The major randomized trials have all demonstrated greater relief of angina, better exercise performance, and a lower requirement for antianginal medications for surgically as opposed to medically treated patients 5 years postoperatively.[347-349] There is a reoperation rate of 6 to 8 per cent per year for recurrence of symptoms.[407] After 5 years, about three-quarters of patients can be predicted to be free from an ischemic event (return of angina, occurrence of myocardial infarction, or sudden death), about half remain free for approximately 10 years, and about 15 per cent for 15 or more years.[311] Compared with medical therapy, the overall advantages of angina relief, increased physical activity, and reduced use of antianginal medications are less apparent 10 years after coronary surgery[408]; symptomatic improvement is best maintained in those patients with the most complete revascularization.

For patients with persistent angina despite adequate medical therapy and for those who cannot tolerate the usual antianginal medications and who are not ideal candidates for PTCA, coronary artery surgery provides excellent symptomatic relief.[408a] With increasing use of internal mammary artery grafts, long-term relief of angina and freedom from subsequent cardiac events will improve, compared with previous patient populations who have received coronary artery vein grafts alone.

Long-Term Survival

Analyses from the Duke Database suggest changing survival benefits of coronary revascularization over time. In the present era, refinements in surgical care have improved survival after revascularization for patients with one-, two-, and three-vessel disease.[409] One important factor is the use of the internal mammary artery (IMA) graft to the left anterior descending coronary artery, in addition to other vein grafts as needed (Fig. 40–9, p. 1319).[311] Early[311,312] and later mortality[311,312,330] are both improved by the use of internal mammary grafting. By 10 years, the survival in typical patients with extensive three-vessel disease in whom the IMA graft is used to revascularize the left anterior descending artery is 89 per cent compared to 71 per cent when other conduits are used.[311] By 15 years, a further divergence in the survival curves is apparent. The lessons learned from the historical randomized trials of coronary artery surgery will be amended with time because of the known attenuation of survival advantage of surgical therapy (using only venous conduits) after 5 or 7 years in the subgroups of patients for whom it was shown initially to be beneficial (Fig. 40–17) and the slower attrition rate of internal mammary artery grafts over very long-term follow-up. Bilateral internal mammary artery grafts, sequential internal mammary artery anastomoses, and free internal mammary artery grafts have all been used since the large randomized trials were carried out[306,308] (Fig. 40–9). These latter studies also predated the widespread use of percutaneous transluminal coronary angioplasty and platelet inhibiting agents.

LEFT MAIN CORONARY ARTERY STENOSIS. There is general agreement that surgical treatment improves survival in patients with left main coronary artery obstruction[410,411] (Fig. 40–15). As already pointed out, the presence of left main coronary artery stenosis does not define a homogeneous population.[394] Coronary bypass surgery appears to confer the most benefit on patients with severe degrees of left main coronary

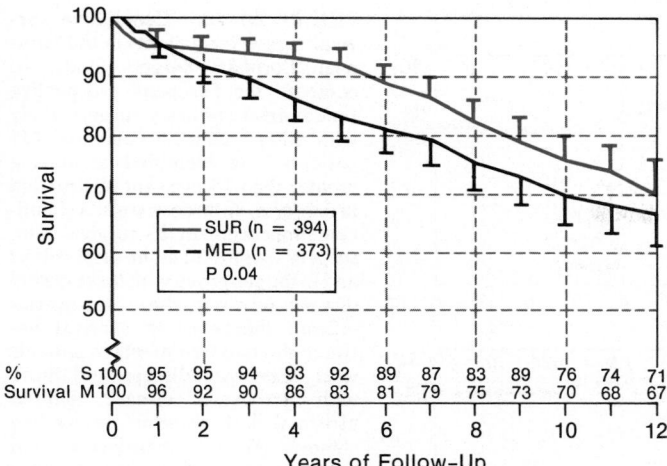

FIGURE 40–17. Cumulative survival curves for patients in the European Coronary Surgery Study. Twelve-year cumulative survival rates and 95 per cent confidence intervals for all patients randomly assigned to either surgical treatment (SUR,S), or medical therapy (MED,M). N denotes number of patients, and % survival denotes percentage surviving. The cumulative survival rate among patients who had early surgical treatment was significantly higher than those who had only medical treatment throughout the observation period. The significant difference in survival noted at 5 years between the two treatment groups (92 per cent medical treatment vs. 83 per cent surgical treatment) gradually decreased but remained significant at 10 years. After 5 years, the patients originally assigned to surgical treatment fared worse, and the benefit of early surgical treatment gradually decreased. The net result of these changes in the two treatment groups is a considerably smaller difference in survival rates at 10 and 12 years as compared with 5 years. (Reprinted with permission from Varnauskas E., and the ECSSG: Twelve-year follow-up of survival in the randomized European Coronary Surgery Study. N. Engl. J. Med. *319*:332, 1988.)

artery disease and/or those patients with impaired ventricular function. However, it is still beneficial in all patients with left main coronary stenoses greater than 50 per cent and for patients with normal left ventricular function.[411]

There is continuing debate whether there is a "left main equivalent," which has a natural history similar to that of left main coronary disease. The condition in question may consist of disease in the proximal portions of both the left anterior descending and left circumflex coronary arteries. We believe that the ominous nature of significant left main coronary disease exists because a single event (rupture of a single plaque) can cause infarction of a large quantity of myocardium. While combined disease of the proximal left anterior descending and circumflex coronary arteries does identify a subgroup of high-risk patients, the prognosis is not as poor as for those with left main coronary artery disease.[412] Nevertheless, patients with combined stenoses of 70 per cent or more in the left anterior descending coronary artery, before the first septal perforator, and in the proximal circumflex coronary artery before the first obtuse marginal branch who have impaired ventricular function appear to have improved longevity and less angina following revascularization surgery than if they are treated medically.[413] Not unexpectedly, the CASS Registry demonstrated that 96 per cent of patients with ≥50 per cent left main coronary artery stenoses were symptomatic and that the advantages of revascularization were equivalent in both symptomatic and asymptomatic patients with disease affecting this vessel.[397]

ONE-, TWO-, OR THREE-VESSEL CORONARY ARTERY DISEASE WITH OR WITHOUT IMPAIRED VENTRICULAR FUNCTION. Current clinical practice has been shaped by three major randomized trials in which patients were enrolled between 1972 and 1979, and follow-up has continued since then. In considering these studies today it is important to recognize that major improvements have taken place in both medical and surgical treatment, as well as in the postsurgical

medical treatment of patients with coronary artery disease in the 13 to 20 years since patients were entered into these trials. Nonetheless, some of the lessons they have taught us endure.

THE VETERANS ADMINISTRATION COOPERATIVE STUDY. This study prospectively examined the effects of coronary artery surgery as opposed to medical treatment in 686 adult males, randomly allocated to surgical or medical management in 1972 to 1974.[385,414–417] The patients were males who had stable angina pectoris of at least 6 months' duration, electrocardiographic evidence of either prior infarction or ischemia at rest or during exercise, significant coronary disease of at least one major coronary artery with a graftable distal segment, and a left ventricular ejection fraction greater than 25 to 30 per cent.

By 7 years after randomization, survival rates were 70 per cent with medical treatment and 77 per cent with surgical treatment (p = 0.043), but by 11 years the rates were 57 and 58 per cent, respectively, presumably because of later occlusion of the venous grafts.[417] Retrospective analyses have revealed that coronary artery surgery appears to confer an advantage in survival over medical therapy in patients at high clinical risk (having two or more of the following: NYHA Class III or IV, a history of hypertension, previous myocardial infarction, and ST-segment depression on the resting electrocardiogram). It also appeared to confer an advantage in a high angiographic risk group (impaired left ventricular function and three-vessel coronary artery disease).

The Veterans Administration Study investigators have summarized their long-term survival results as follows: coronary artery surgery did *not* significantly improve *overall* survival in patients without left main disease, while a significant survival benefit was seen with surgery at 5 to 7 years in subgroups of patients with multiple clinical and angiographic risk factors. This benefit diminished gradually when follow-up was extended to 11 years. The majority of patients who did not belong to high-risk subgroups derived no survival benefit from surgical treatment at any time.[416]

THE EUROPEAN CORONARY SURGERY STUDY GROUP. Men under the age of 65 with mild or moderately severe chronic stable angina (57 per cent were in Class I or II Canadian Cardiovascular Society and 42 per cent were in Class III), significant stenoses of at least two major coronary arteries, and good left ventricular function (ejection fraction greater than 50 per cent) were randomized to medical or surgical treatment between 1973 and 1976.[347,418] At 8 years of follow-up the policy of early surgery improved survival significantly compared with medical treatment in the total population (89 vs. 80 per cent), in the subgroup with three-vessel disease (92 vs. 77 per cent), and in the patients with two-vessel disease in which one of the diseased vessels was the proximal segment of the left anterior descending coronary artery (90 vs. 79 per cent) (Fig. 40–18).

There was no significant difference in survival between medical and surgical treatment in patients with one-vessel disease and in those with two-vessel disease without stenosis of the proximal left anterior descending coronary artery (Fig. 40–19). At 12 years of follow-up, it was apparent that the improvement in survival in patients treated surgically had become attenuated after 5 years and the percentage of patients surviving decreased more rapidly in the surgically treated patients (Fig. 40–17).[375] Nevertheless, the diminishing difference between the survival curves still favored surgical over medical treatment after 12 years (71 per cent vs. 67 per cent, respectively). The presence of proximal left anterior descending coronary artery stenosis as a component of two- or three-vessel disease was the outstanding predictor of poor prognosis with medical therapy and improved outcome with surgery.[375]

CORONARY ARTERY SURGERY STUDY (CASS). Patients age 65 or younger with mild angina or with a myocardial infarction more than 3 weeks previously were randomized to medical or surgical therapy between 1975 and 1979 if they had significant, operable coronary artery disease.[324,325,334] After 10 years, cumulative survival for CASS patients as a whole showed no significant difference in medical versus surgical 10-year survival (79 per cent vs. 82 per cent, respectively).[419] A significant advantage favoring initial surgical assignment was observed in patients with ejection fractions between 35 per cent and 50 per cent (medical, 61 per cent vs. surgical, 79 per cent; p = 0.01) (Fig. 40–20).[419] The CASS Registry observational studies have shown that in patients with mild[420] or severe[384,421] angina, surgery improves survival in patients with three-vessel disease regardless whether ventricular function is normal or depressed. However, in patients with more extensive disease and the worst ventricular function,[421] survival may be improved to an even greater extent by surgery. Other studies have also suggested that patients who demonstrate the most severe ischemia-induced ventricular dysfunction during exercise are most likely to benefit subsequently with respect to survival, relief of pain, and improvement in exercise capacity.[402,403,422]

TREATMENT OF PATIENTS WITH SEVERELY DEPRESSED LEFT VENTRICULAR FUNCTION. Studies have compared medical and surgical therapy in CAD patients with severely depressed left ventricular function.[326,327,329] In a

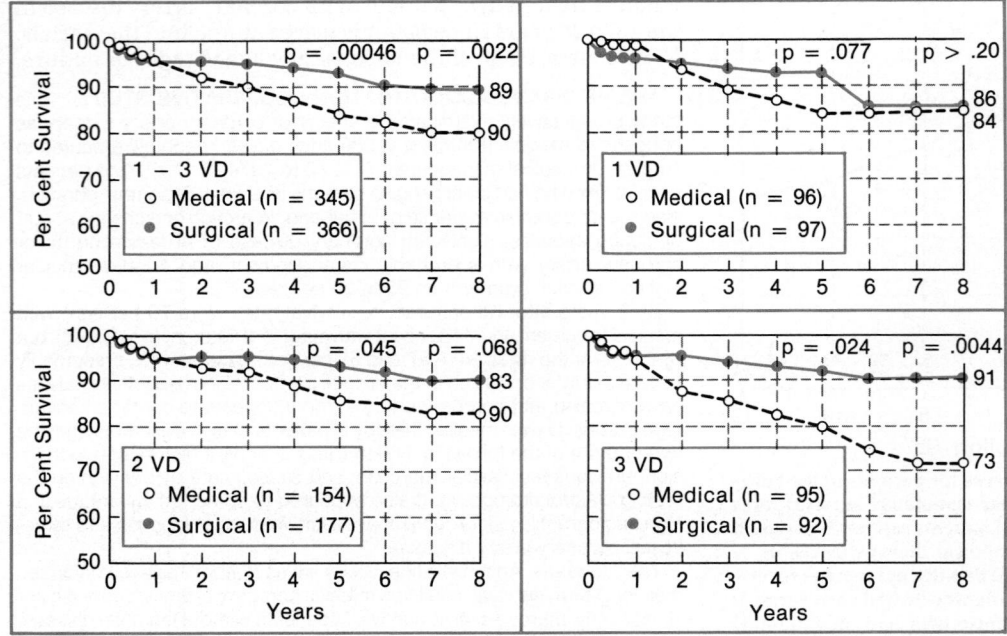

FIGURE 40–18. Cumulative survival curves for patients in the European Coronary Surgery Study. To compare the European prospective randomized coronary surgery study with other studies, a cohort of 711 patients was identified as having greater than 75 per cent obstruction in one, two, or three vessels. A significant improvement in survival with surgery was found in the total cohort and in the subgroup with three-vessel disease; however, there was no significant difference in survival between the two treatments in patients with one-vessel disease and those with two-vessel disease without proximal left anterior descending stenosis. (From Varnauskas, E., and the European Coronary Surgery Study Group: Survival, myocardial infarction, and employment status in a prospective, randomized study of coronary bypass surgery. Circulation 72[Suppl. V]:90, 1985, by permission of the American Heart Association, Inc.)

FIGURE 40–19. Cumulative survival for the subgroup of patients with double-vessel disease (2 VD group) in the European Coronary Study Group when disease is defined as 75 per cent or greater narrowing and is subdivided by the presence or absence of disease in the proximal segment of the left anterior descending coronary artery (LAD). This retrospective analysis suggests that surgery may confer an advantage over medical therapy in patients with two-vessel disease in whom both narrowings are greater than 75 per cent of luminal diameter, and one of them is the proximal segment of the left anterior descending coronary artery. (From Varnauskas, E., and European Coronary Surgery Study Group: Survival, myocardial infarction, and employment status in a prospective, randomized study of coronary bypass surgery. Circulation 72[Suppl. V]:90, 1985, by permission of the American Heart Association, Inc.)

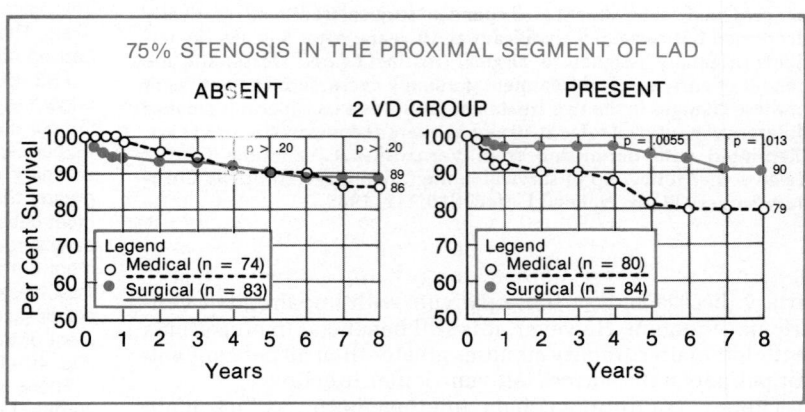

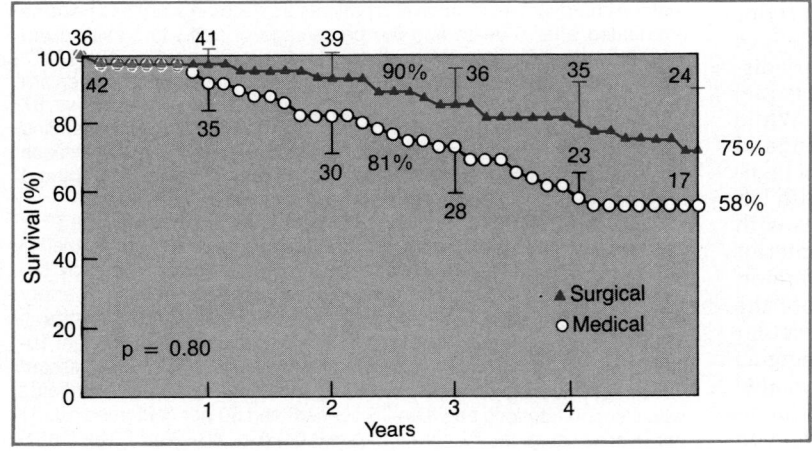

FIGURE 40–20. Survival of patients with three-vessel coronary disease and left ventricular dysfunction. Ten-year follow-up of survival in the Coronary Artery Surgery Study (CASS) in the subset of patients with an ejection fraction of less than 50 per cent and three-vessel coronary disease. Patients with left ventricular dysfunction exhibit long-term benefit from an initial strategy of surgical treatment, and this is particularly evident in patients with three-vessel coronary disease who show a survival benefit after 10 years with initial surgical treatment (75 per cent) vs. medical treatment (58 per cent). (From Alderman E. L., et al.: Ten-year follow-up of survival and myocardial infarction in the randomized Coronary Artery Surgery Study. Circulation 82:1629, 1990, by permission of the American Heart Association, Inc.)

CASS Registry study[423] surgical treatment was shown to prolong survival, particularly in patients with ejection fractions below 0.26 (Fig. 40–21). In another study examining the late results of surgical and medical therapy for patients with coronary artery disease and resting ejection fractions of less than 36 per cent, 7-year survival and freedom from nonfatal infarction were greater in the surgically than in the medically treated patients. Surgical treatment also was associated with improved survival in the patients with an ejection fraction of 25 per cent or less.[326] These studies, together with observa-

tions made by the Duke group (Fig. 40–22) suggest that if operative mortality is lower than approximately 7 per cent, surgery is likely to offer an advantage over medical therapy in terms of survival and relief of anginal symptoms in patients with ischemic myocardium and severely depressed left ventricular function.

Despite the advantage of surgical as opposed to medical therapy in patients with left ventricular dysfunction,[424] the relationship between poor surgical outcome and preoperative clinical evidence of congestive heart failure is well recog-

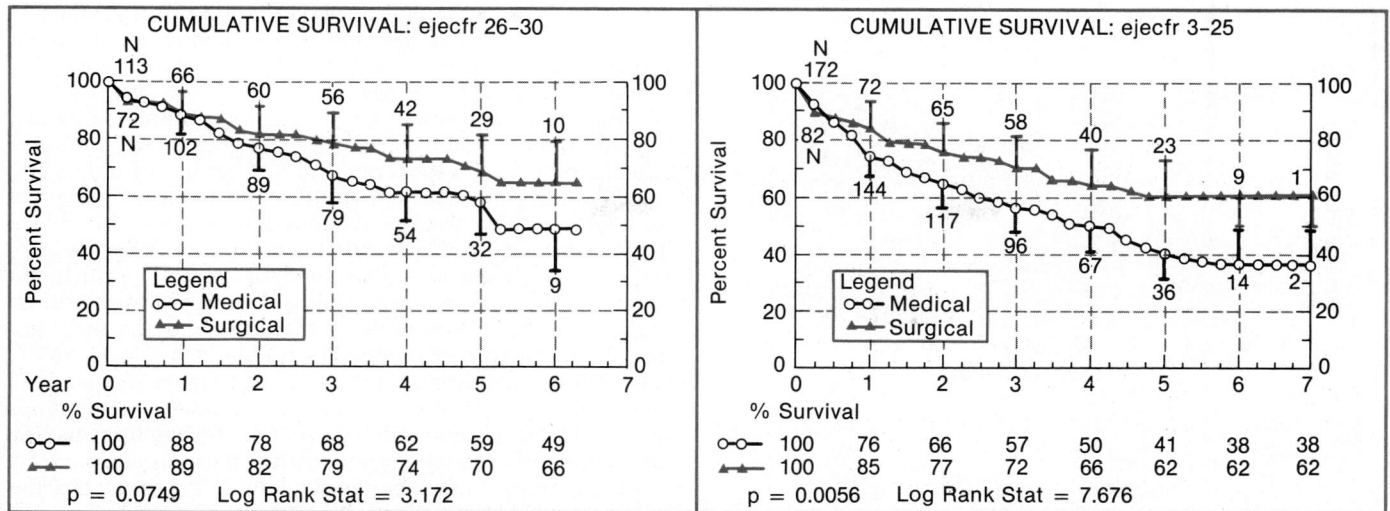

FIGURE 40–21. Life table cumulative survival curves for patients with severe left ventricular dysfunction. A CASS Registry study identified 420 medically treated and 231 surgically treated patients (coronary graft plus myocardial surgery in 30 per cent) who had severe left ventricular dysfunction manifested by an ejection fraction below 0.36 and markedly abnormal wall motion. Life table cumulative survivals for patients with an ejection fraction (ejecfr) of 0.26 to 0.30 *(left panel)*, and for patients with ejection fractions of 0.03 to 0.25 *(right panel)* are shown. The survival curves are adjusted for all other significant prognostic variables. The P values associated with each analysis are shown in the bottom left corner of the figures. Surgical benefit was most apparent for patients with ejection fractions below 0.26 who had a 43-per-cent 5-year survival with medical treatment vs. a 63-per-cent 5-year survival with surgery. Surgically treated patients experienced substantial symptomatic benefit compared with medically treated patients if their presenting symptoms were predominantly angina; however, there was no relief of symptoms caused primarily by heart failure. The operative mortality in this high-risk subset was 6.9 per cent. (From Alderman, E. L., et al.: Results of coronary artery surgery in patients with poor left ventricular function [CASS]. Circulation *68:*785, 1983, by permission of the American Heart Association, Inc.)

nized. Clinical descriptors, such as a history of heart failure (particularly if such a history predominates over a history of angina pectoris), pulmonary rales, previous need of a diuretic or digitalis, and a cardiothoracic ratio of 0.50 or more, are all associated with a significantly higher operative risk. In the CASS and the CASS Registry,[332] there was increasing operative mortality with increasing left ventricular dysfunction. Patients with normal or near-normal left ventricular function had an operative mortality rate of 2 per cent and a 5-year survival of 92 per cent. Patients with moderate impairment had an operative mortality of 4.2 per cent and a 5-year survival of 80 per cent, and in those with poor ventricular function the operative mortality was 6.2 per cent and 5-year survival 65 per cent. Thus, while left ventricular dysfunction indicates higher surgical risk than normal ventricular function, such patients also have more to gain from surgery.

ASSESSMENT OF CONTRACTILE RESERVE. In patients with impaired left ventricular function it may be useful to estimate ejection fraction and left ventricular wall motion in the basal state as well as after inotropic stimulation or afterload reduction to show enhancement of otherwise depressed wall motion.[128-130] The term *contractile reserve* is used to describe the ability of ventricular wall segments that contract abnormally in the basal state to exhibit augmented contractility, often with an increase in overall ejection fraction in response to a suitable stimulus. Zones of the myocardium responding to inotropic stimulation or to a decrease in afterload may improve functionally after revascularization[129] (Fig. 40–23). Methods for assessing the contractile reserve of potentially viable myocardium include use of postextrasystolic potentiation during left ventricular angiography[129]; the response of left ventricular ejection fraction to an inotropic stimulus such as an epinephrine infusion[130]; evidence of delayed uptake of thallium-201 after exercise testing in a dysfunctional region of myocardium, which suggests that it is viable[424a]; and, finally, positron emission tomography, which shows glucose utilization by the myocardium (p. 1182). Regions of myocardium with abnormal motion and preserved glucose uptake are likely to be viable, in contrast to regions with diminished uptake that are likely to be irreversibly damaged.[425] Nesto et al.

have reported that survival following revascularization is better among patients whose ejection fraction rose by more than 10 per cent when stimulated by either epinephrine or postextrasystolic potentiation than in those in whom this failed to occur.[130] The demonstration of augmentation of contractility acutely, and similar improvement after revascularization, is related to the finding that many hypokinetic (and even akinetic) areas of ventricular wall are composed either of ischemic, although viable, muscle or of a mixture of the latter and fibrous scar. The viable muscle is capable of responding to the inotropic stimulation, and its contraction may also respond to improved perfusion after operation.[131] In contrast, necrotic tissue obviously cannot be stimulated to contract by any pharmacological or hemodynamic intervention or by improved perfusion.

In patients with poor left ventricular function and poor contractile reserve (less than 10 per cent increase in ejection fraction with inotropic stimulation), perioperative mortality is high and long-term survival is poorer than in patients with equally depressed left ventricular function but with normal contractile reserve.[129-131] There are now a number of studies demonstrating that revascularization surgery will increase the ejection fraction at rest[426,427] and after exercise.[428] Regional wall-motion abnormalities have also shown improvement after revascularization surgery.[427,429,430] Percutaneous transluminal coronary angioplasty has also been shown to improve ischemic left ventricular dysfunction.[431,432]

MYOCARDIAL STUNNING AND HIBERNATION. Two related pathophysiological conditions termed myocardial stunning (prolonged but temporary postischemic ventricular dysfunction without myocardial necrosis) and myocardial hibernation (persistent left ventricular dysfunction when myocardial perfusion is chronically reduced but is still sufficient to maintain the viability of tissue) have been defined (pp. 1176 to 1178). In myocardial stunning there may be abnormalities of systolic and/or diastolic ventricular function. The stunned myocardium is viable and exhibits contractile reserve. There are a number of clinical situations in which myocardial stunning occurs, including delayed recovery of ventricular dysfunction after successful thrombolytic therapy administered

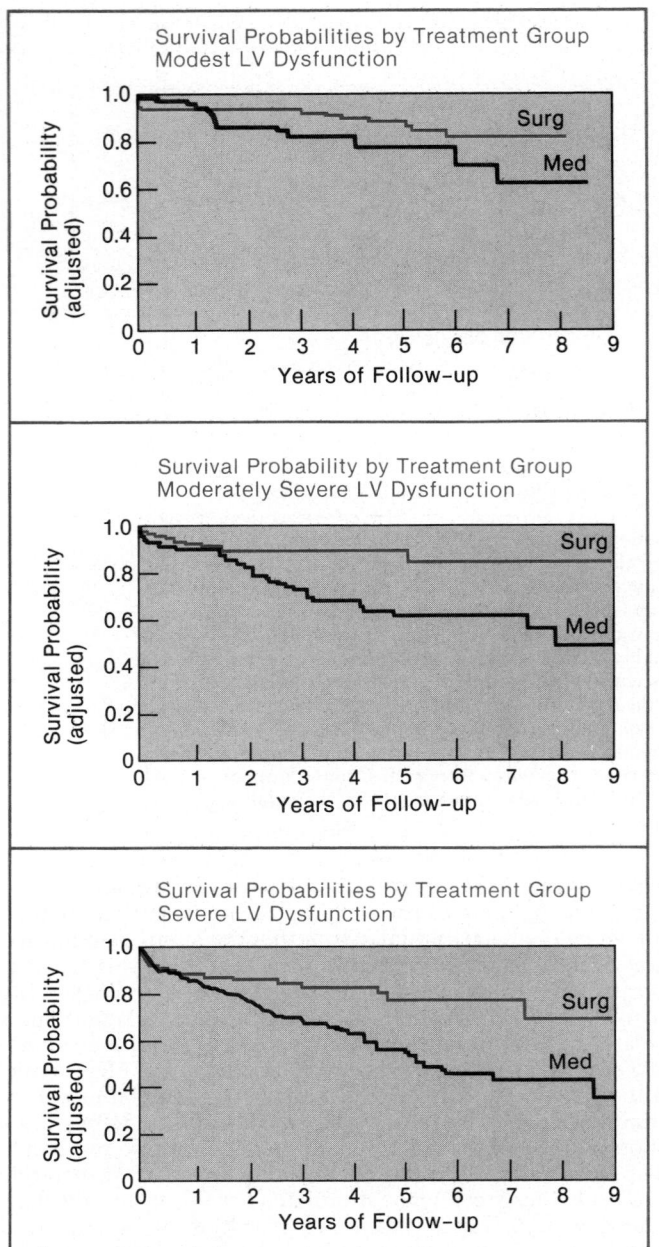

FIGURE 40–22. Survival of medically vs. surgically treated patients with left ventricular dysfunction. Patients undergoing first cardiac catheterization at Duke University Medical Center between 1976 and 1983 for any symptom of coronary artery disease with a 75 per cent or greater stenosis of at least one major coronary segment and a left ventricular ejection fraction of 40 per cent or less were reviewed. The survival curves were constructed from standard life table calculations after adjustment for differences in baseline prognostic factors, when appropriate, with the Cox proportional hazards model. Adjusted Kaplan-Meier survival estimates (survival probability) and time (years of follow-up) of the study population are divided according to baseline left ventricular ejection fraction. Med = medically treated; Surg = surgically treated. The upper panel shows upper tertile of ejection fraction (median ejection fraction 38 per cent). The middle panel shows mid tertile of ejection fraction (median ejection fraction 32 per cent). The lower panel shows lower tertile of ejection fraction (median ejection fraction 24 per cent). Surgical survival benefit was apparent in each third of the study group; however it appeared greater in those patients with moderate to severe left ventricular dysfunction than in those with only modest left ventricular dysfunction. (From Bounous E. P., et al.: Surgical survival benefits for coronary disease patients with left ventricular dysfunction. *Circulation 78*[Suppl. I]:151, 1988, by permission of the American Heart Association, Inc.)

during evolving acute myocardial infarction,[126] alterations in diastolic properties of the ventricle following percutaneous transluminal coronary angioplasty,[433] and following relief of ischemia caused by coronary vasospasm[434] or exercise.[435] In addition, delayed recovery of ventricular dysfunction following successful coronary artery bypass graft surgery may be explained by the disappearance of myocardial stunning.[436]

Hibernating myocardium results from months or years of ischemia, and ventricular dysfunction persists until blood flow is restored.[436a,436b] Hibernating myocardium can be associated with abnormal systolic and/or diastolic ventricular function; the dysfunction is reversible and the myocardium exhibits contractile reserve. In these patients the predominant clinical feature of myocardial ischemia may be elevation of left ventricular diastolic pressure and dyspnea secondary to ventricular systolic and/or diastolic dysfunction. Symptoms resulting from chronic left ventricular dysfunction may be inappropriately ascribed to myocardial necrosis and scarring when they may, in fact, be reversed when the chronic ischemia is relieved by coronary revascularization.[436c]

Surgical Results in Patients With Left-Ventricular Dysfunction. Surgical revascularization appears to confer the greatest advantage in those patients with the most severe anginal symptoms, the most severe left ventricular dysfunction (Fig. 40–22), and the most extensive coronary artery disease.[437] While the risk of operation is higher in patients with depressed left ventricular function, it has been found that patients with moderately impaired[324] and even severely impaired left ventricular function[326,423] may have improved long-term survival as compared with similar patients with CAD treated medically.[329,437,438] Indeed, patients with the worst ventricular function may show the most striking symptomatic and functional response to revascularization[423] and a greater survival advantage.[437] Since the prognosis with medical therapy is so poor in these patients, they have the most to gain from surgical treatment. Furthermore, in patients with a history of heart failure and three-vessel CAD, coronary artery surgery may reduce the incidence of sudden death, compared with those receiving medical therapy.[439]

It is helpful to evaluate heart failure secondary to CAD to determine whether the patient's myocardium exhibits contractile reserve. If it does, and the anatomy is appropriate, we recommend surgical treatment, recognizing that higher than usual risks are involved. When the myocardium fails to exhibit contractile reserve and when the patient has a history (and/or electrocardiographic findings) of extensive or multiple infarctions (and/or electrocardiographic findings) and no or little angina, it probably offers little benefit and is associated with substantial risk.

CONCLUSIONS. In considering which groups of patients are likely to achieve greater survival benefit from coronary artery surgery rather than medical therapy, the large randomized trials and CASS Registry studies all contribute important information. Clearly, coronary artery surgery is a procedure that prolongs survival in patients with significant left main coronary artery disease and those patients with multivessel disease associated with clinical or catheterization evidence of impaired ventricular function. In patients with moderately severe, stable angina pectoris and normal left ventricular function, the European study suggests that if several factors such as age greater than 50 years, an abnormal electrocardiogram at rest, ST-segment depression greater than 1.5 mm during exercise, and peripheral arterial disease are present (Table 40–14), coronary angiography should be performed. In such patients with three-vessel disease or coronary artery stenoses of greater than 75 per cent reduction in luminal diameter in the proximal left anterior descending coronary artery and one other major vessel, surgery appears superior to medical therapy.

Surgery also appears to have an advantage over medical therapy in patients with no or mild symptoms and three-vessel disease and impaired ventricular function. Other clinical risk factors in patients with three-vessel disease and either

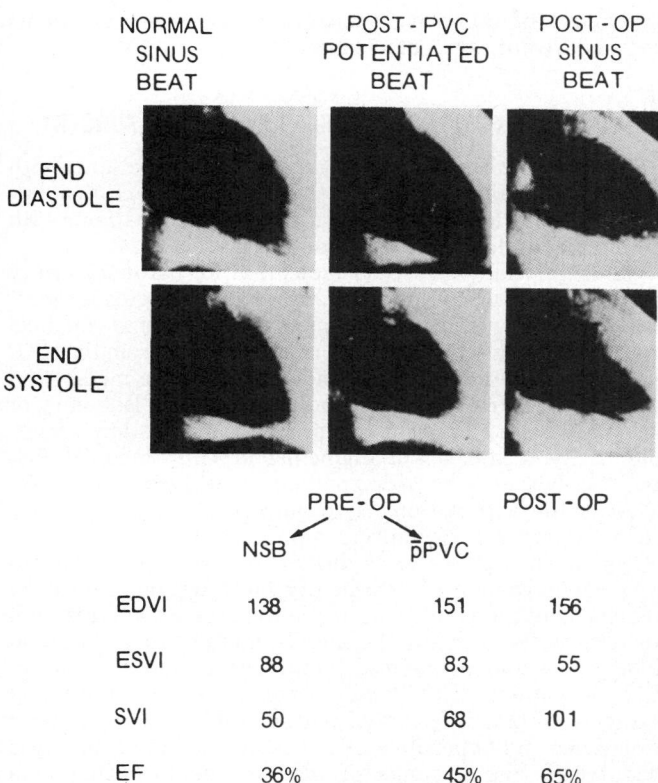

	PRE-OP		POST-OP
	NSB	p̄PVC	
EDVI	138	151	156
ESVI	88	83	55
SVI	50	68	101
EF	36%	45%	65%

FIGURE 40–23. Examples of the ventriculographic analysis performed to evaluate the effects of an inotropic stimulus, including some of the calculations made. p̄PVC = premature ventricular contraction; PRE-OP = preoperative; POST-OP = postoperative; NSB = normal sinus beat; p̄PVC = after premature ventricular contraction; EDVI = end-diastolic volume index (ml/m²); ESVI = end-systolic volume index (ml/m²); SVI = stroke volume index (ml/m²); EF = ejection fraction. (From Popio, K. A., et al.: Post extrasystolic potentiation as a predictor of potential myocardial viability. Am. J. Cardiol. 39:944, 1977.)

normal or impaired ventricular function that might lead to surgical rather than medical therapy include severe angina pectoris (Class III or IV NYHA), a history of myocardial infarction or hypertension, and resting ST-segment depression on the electrocardiogram. There is no evidence that surgical therapy confers any survival advantage over medical therapy in patients with two-vessel disease (which does not include severe proximal involvement of the left anterior descending coronary artery) and single-vessel disease. Patients in this latter category are being treated with increasing frequency by PTCA. As yet there is no evidence to suggest that the benefits of successful dilatation outweigh the risks of the procedure or whether any survival advantage is conferred upon such patients by PTCA. Patients with a left anterior descending stenosis of more than 50 per cent that is rough and long may have a greater risk of future myocardial infarction and therefore may be candidates for surgical revascularization.[440] There is some evidence that among patients with one- or two-vessel CAD and impaired left ventricular function, those who either have no change in their ejection fraction with exercise or a peak exercise ejection fraction less than 30 per cent have poor long-term survival.[441] If this subset of patients has angina and evidence of ischemia at a low or moderate level of exercise then they too may benefit from surgical revascularization.

The randomized trials of coronary bypass surgery have also suggested that both medical and surgical treatments have improved over time. In patients with angiographically confirmed three-vessel CAD treated medically, the annual mortality in the late 1960's was 11.4 per cent. Fifteen years later in the CASS it was only 2.1 per cent. (It is not clear how similar these two patient groups were.) For patients who have less than severe angina or who are free of angina after a recent infarc-

tion, if ventricular function is normal, surgical therapy does not appear to confer any benefits over medical therapy in terms of long-term survival for those with one-, two-, or three-vessel coronary disease. Surgical therapy may confer some survival advantage to patients with three-vessel and with two-vessel disease involving the proximal left anterior descending coronary artery if moderate angina pectoris exists, if the left ventricular ejection fraction decreases during exercise,[422] or if there is a positive symptom-limited exercise test in stage I or II of a standard Bruce protocol (or its equivalent) associated with 1.5 mm or greater ST-segment electrocardiographic depression (Table 40–15).

For patients with CAD whose dominant symptom is angina pectoris and who have severely depressed left ventricular function (ejection fraction ≤ 35 per cent), surgery appears to offer survival advantages if they can also be demonstrated to have critically narrowed vessels which perfuse viable myocardium. In patients whose dominant symptoms are heart failure without angina and diffuse poor contraction of the left ventricle without contractile reserve, revascularization is unlikely to be beneficial.

In patients with chronic stable angina who do not satisfy the indications for operation shown in Table 40–15, there is no evidence that survival is improved. Bypass grafting is usually associated with some small risk (< 1 per cent mortality, 5 per cent incidence of perioperative infarction), and progressive attrition of venous grafts occurs, particularly after 5 years.[305] Therefore it is suggested that in patients with normal ventricular function and mild to moderate symptoms with medical therapy, bypass surgery be postponed until the symptoms warrant consideration of this intervention.

OCCURRENCE OF MYOCARDIAL INFARCTION. The major randomized trials of patients with mild to moderate angina and absence of major left ventricular dysfunction suggested that the likelihood of occurrence of myocardial infarction after 5 to 10 years of follow-up was similar in medically and surgically treated patients.[418,419,442,443] In the CASS, in which the perioperative myocardial infarction rate was 6.4 per cent, surgery did not appear to prevent the occurrence of subsequent infarction. In the same study, the reported annual risk of nonfatal myocardial infarction (Q-wave) was 2.2 per cent per year with medical treatment compared with 2.8 per cent per year with surgical treatment.[443] In an attempt to ascertain whether the risk of subsequent myocardial infarction might be prevented by surgical revascularization in patients at higher risk for ischemic events (i.e., those with severe angina and three-vessel coronary artery disease), a CASS Registry study was performed.[444] During a 6-year follow-up period, 21 per cent of the medical patients and 13 per cent of the surgical patients had a new myocardial infarction, and the fatality rate of first new myocardial infarctions was 45 per cent for the medically treated patients and 16 per cent for the surgi-

TABLE 40–14 FIVE-YEAR SURVIVAL IN MEDICALLY MANAGED PATIENTS WITH TWO- OR THREE-VESSEL CORONARY ARTERY DISEASE

	RISK FACTORS			5-YEAR SURVIVAL (%)	
PROXIMAL LAD STENOSIS	ST Depression >1.5 mm With Exercise	Peripheral Vascular Disease	Abnormal Resting ECG	2-Vessel Disease	3-Vessel Disease
−	−	−	−	98	96
+	−	−	−	94	92
+	+	−	−	88	83
+	+	+	−	69	60
+	+	+	+	−	40

LAD = Left anterior descending coronary artery.
From Rutherford, J. D.: Coronary artery surgery, 1984. N. Z. Med. J. 97:813, 1984. Adapted from European Surgery Study Group: Long-term results of prospective, randomized study of coronary artery bypass surgery in stable angina pectoris. Lancet 2:1173, 1982.

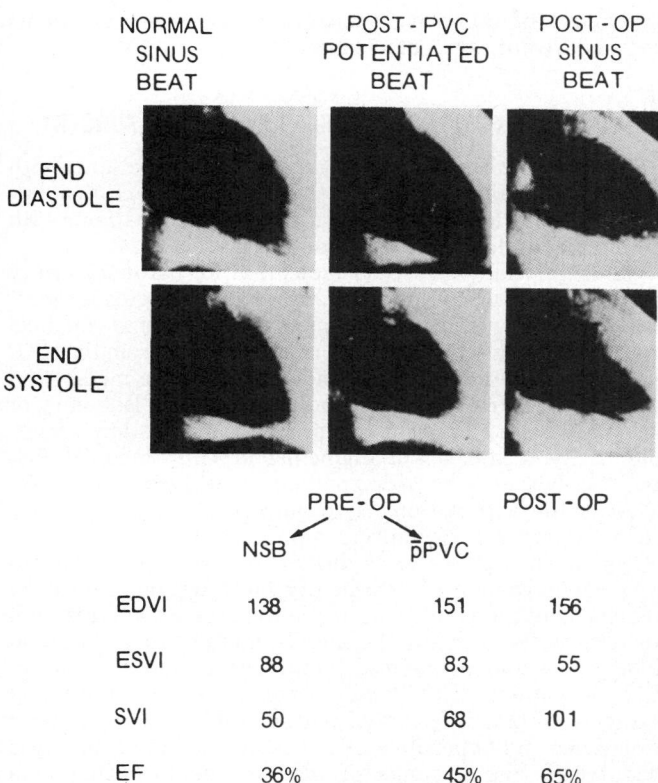

TABLE 40-15 INDICATIONS FOR CORONARY REVASCULARIZATION IN PATIENTS WITH CHRONIC STABLE ANGINA

1. Angina pectoris that is severe, disabling, or interfering with life style on maximally tolerated medical therapy.
2. Results of noninvasive stress testing indicate extensive inducible ischemia, poor functional capacity, associated with critical (>70%) obstruction in one or more vessels.
3. Left main coronary artery stenosis (>60%).
4. Critical obstruction (>70%) in three major coronary arteries with:
   a. Resting left ventricular dysfunction, or
   b. Normal resting left ventricular function + evidence of inducible ischemia or a poor exercise tolerance.
5. Critical obstruction of proximal left anterior descending artery with significant obstruction of one other major vessel + moderate angina pectoris and/or inducible ischemia.

cally treated patients (p < 0.0001). After adjustment for left ventricular dysfunction and the extent of CAD, 86 per cent of surgical and 73 per cent of medical patients were free of new myocardial infarction at 6 years (p < 0.0001). The advantage of surgical treatment was particularly evident in patients with stenoses of the left anterior descending coronary artery of 70 per cent or greater and moderate or severe impairment of left ventricular function, as well as those patients with two proximal coronary artery narrowings. This observational study suggests that coronary artery revascularization reduces the incidence of subsequent myocardial infarction in patients at high risk for subsequent ischemic events (those with severe angina, three-vessel CAD, or left anterior descending coronary artery stenoses). The risk of death following subsequent

myocardial infarction also appears to be lower in the patients who underwent revascularization.[444a]

PATIENT SELECTION FOR CORONARY ARTERY SURGERY

To undergo coronary artery bypass grafting, patients with chronic stable angina must usually meet certain clinical criteria.[444b] A plan for work-up and management of patients with mild to moderate angina is shown in Figure 40–24.

The most widely accepted indication for coronary artery bypass surgery in patients with chronic stable angina is significant disability from symptoms despite optimal medical care.[408a] Although this disability usually results from the CAD itself, it may be related to the side effects of the medication required to control the discomfort of myocardial ischemia, or patients may find taking large amounts of medication intolerable. Lastly, if the level of angina pectoris on a medical regimen clearly interferes with a patient's work, recreational activity, or life expectations, a recommendation for coronary artery surgery may be entirely appropriate.

Optimal medical care, as described earlier (p. 1302), involves achievement of satisfactory body weight, control of medical conditions such as thyrotoxicosis or anemia that might intensify myocardial ischemia, maintenance of normal blood pressure, assessment and control of arrhythmias (particularly in patients with impaired ventricular function), and treatment of metabolic abnormalities such as carbohydrate intolerance and hyperlipidemia. Abstinence from smoking is encouraged, and a range of medications including beta blockers, short- and long-acting nitrates, and calcium antagonists is used to control symptoms.

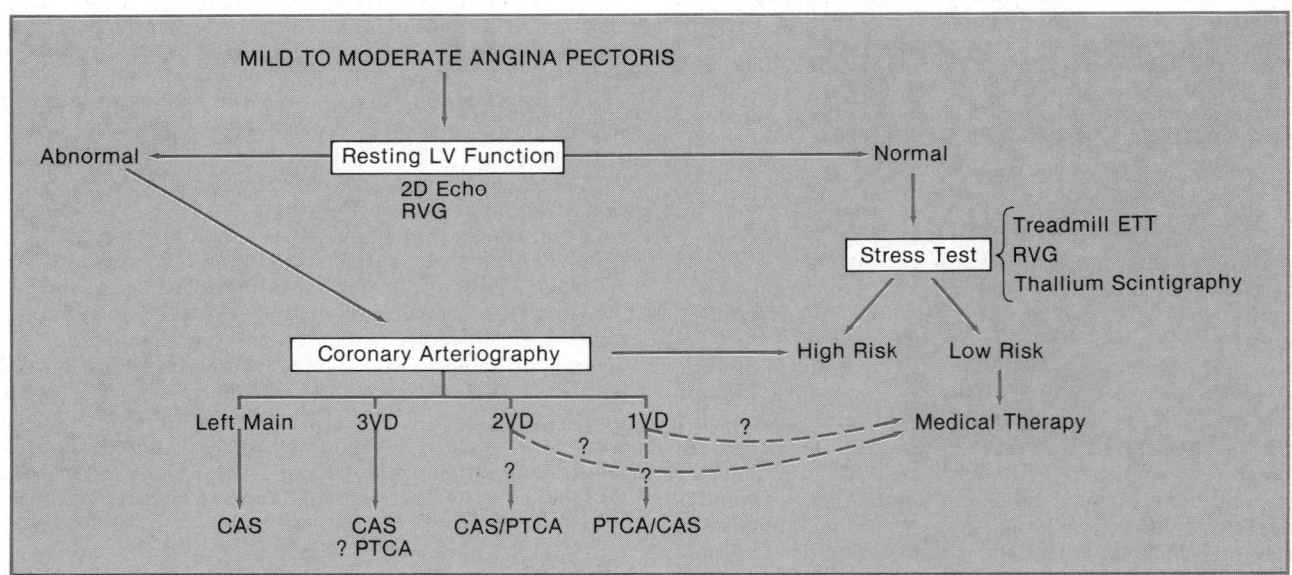

FIGURE 40–24. Management of patients with mild to moderate angina pectoris. Since coronary artery disease prognosis is worse in patients with left ventricular (LV) dysfunction, it is important to assess resting LV function (most readily accomplished noninvasively by either two-dimensional echocardiography [2D-echo] or radionuclide ventriculography [RVG].) If LV function is abnormal at rest, coronary angiography should be performed; if normal, some form of stress testing should be performed, e.g., treadmill exercise testing, radionuclide ventriculography at rest and during exercise, and thallium scintigraphy (with exercise or dipyridamole).

If there is evidence of significant exercise-induced ischemia or LV dysfunction, coronary arteriography should be performed. If stress is accomplished that is equivalent to or greater than completion of stage III of a Bruce protocol treadmill test without evidence of significant exercise-induced ischemia or LV dysfunction, a trial of medical therapy is reasonable. If this approach is used, the results of coronary arteriography will lead to logical management choices. For all patients with significant (>60 per cent) left main coronary artery disease and for most with significant (>70 per cent) three-vessel coronary artery disease (3VD), coronary artery surgery (CAS) is advised. With significant two- (2VD) and one-vessel disease (1VD), the options of CAS, percutaneous transluminal angioplasty (PTCA), or medical therapy will be considered.

In patients with critical obstruction of the proximal left anterior descending artery with significant obstruction of one other major vessel and moderate angina pectoris and/or inducible ischemia, either CAS or PTCA is usually advised. In patients with significant one-vessel coronary artery disease, the decision for CAS, PTCA, or medical therapy is made individually. Either PTCA or CAS is favored in those with results of noninvasive testing indicating extensive inducible ischemia, poor functional capacity, and a critical (>70 per cent) obstruction present. (Adapted from Corne, R. A.: Risk stratification in stable angina pectoris [editorial]. Am. J. Cardiol. 59:695, 1987.)

In the early 1970's most patients selected for operation were in functional Classes III and IV, but now patients with three-vessel disease and left ventricular dysfunction at rest or inducible by exercise, regardless of the severity or even the presence of symptoms, are appropriately undergoing coronary artery surgery.

WOMEN AS SURGICAL CANDIDATES. Symptomatic relief following revascularization surgery in women is not as good initially or as well sustained as it is in men.[323] In the CASS, 15 institutions carried out isolated coronary artery bypass grafting on 6258 men and 1153 women from 1975 to 1980. The operative mortality in men was 1.9 per cent, while the operative mortality for women undergoing coronary artery bypass grafting at the same institutions, during the same period, was 4.5 per cent. When matched for age, severity of angina, and the extent of coronary atherosclerosis, women appear to have twice the operative mortality of men.[445] Elderly women have a particularly high operative mortality.[323] After 2 years of follow-up, women were shown to have lower overall graft patency rates, and at 5 to 10 years postoperatively they had a higher incidence of recurrent angina than did men.[445] Women's smaller physical size and the smaller diameter of grafted coronary arteries may be responsible for this poorer response[446]; operative mortality increases in both men and women as physical size decreases.

CORONARY ARTERY BYPASS GRAFTING IN THE ELDERLY. During the past decade the hospital mortality of coronary artery surgery in the elderly (65 years or older) has declined to between 2.7 and 7.7 per cent.[447-450] In general, mortality is greater in patients over 75 years,[448,451] and women in this age group may be at even higher risk of hospital death than men. Variables predictive of perioperative mortality are the same as in younger patients and include rest angina,[451] the presence of 70 per cent or more severe stenosis of the left main coronary artery, severe left ventricular dysfunction,[447,448,451] and the presence of one or more associated medical diseases.[448,452] Compared with younger patients, the elderly spend more time in the hospital[449] and are more prone to complications,[449] which include cerebrovascular accidents, sternal dehiscence, and respiratory failure.[451] These complications, in turn, are associated with a higher perioperative mortality.[448,450,452a] However, angina is relieved or diminished in approximately 80 to 90 per cent of patients[451] more than 65 years of age, and the 5-year survival is generally excellent.[447,451] Thus, advanced age per se is not a contraindication to surgery.

REOPERATION. Six to 10 per cent of coronary artery surgery procedures are now reoperations.[407,453] Operative mortality rates for repeat coronary artery surgery are two to three times those of the initial procedure and range from 2 to 10 per cent[407,453-455,455a] for second operations and up to 15 per cent for third or more reoperations.[456] The reasons for reoperation include recurrence of angina due to primary graft failure (in approximately half of patients[407,455]), progression of disease with or without graft failure in 20 to 30 per cent,[407,455] and incomplete initial revascularization in the remainder.[407,455] At the time of reoperation, patients generally have more extensive CAD,[407,456] and the revascularization achieved at a second operation is less optimal,[455,456] which is reflected in an onset of recurrent angina at an earlier time than after initial cardiac revascularization surgery (Fig. 40–25).[407,455,456] The perioperative myocardial infarction rate in reoperations is approximately 10 per cent.[455] However, late survival is excellent, with 85 to 95 per cent of patients being alive at 5 years,[407,455,457] 89 per cent of patients being alive at 7 years[457] and 70 to 80 per cent at 10 years. Since long-term patency of internal mammary artery grafts is better than of vein grafts, if it is technically feasible this is the preferred conduit for both initial and repeat coronary artery surgery revascularization.

PATIENTS WITH ASSOCIATED CAROTID, ABDOMINAL AORTIC, AND PERIPHERAL VASCULAR DISEASE. The incidence of carotid arterial disease in patients undergoing coronary artery surgery varies from 2 to 12 per cent. Post-

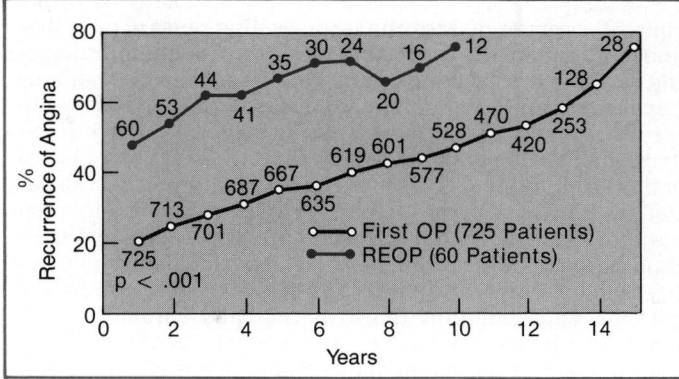

FIGURE 40–25. Recurrence of angina after initial operation and reoperation for coronary artery disease. Of 743 consecutive patients undergoing an initial coronary artery bypass procedure between 1970 and 1973, 64 patients required reoperation for angina recurrence and were followed up for 15 years or less (mean 6.2 years). Plot of annual recurrence of angina (%) and time (years) after initial operation (FIRST OP) and reoperation (REOP). The absolute numbers of patients at risk each year are indicated. There was less relief of angina in the first year after reoperation than after initial operation, but thereafter the annual increases in recurrence of angina were similar. Thus, less relief of angina after reoperation is predominantly attributable to early return of angina in the first postoperative year, rather than an accelerated return of angina in subsequent years, suggesting diffuse atherosclerosis is the cause of continuing angina rather than further progression of coronary artery lesions or occurrence of graft failure. (From Cameron A., et al.: Reoperation for coronary artery disease: 10 years of clinical follow-up. Circulation 78[Suppl. I]:158, 1988, by permission of the American Heart Association, Inc.)

operative strokes occur in 2 to 3 per cent of all patients following coronary revascularization, but in patients with known carotid disease it may occur in up to 20 per cent.[458] Conversely, myocardial infarction is responsible for a substantial number of late deaths following carotid endarterectomy. The risk factors for the development of stroke after coronary bypass grafting are increasing age, preexisting cerebrovascular disease, severe atheroma of the ascending aorta, prolonged cardiopulmonary bypass, and severe perioperative hypotension.[459]

When patients with asymptomatic carotid bruits have coronary artery bypass surgery the risk for stroke appears to be unaltered by prophylactic carotid endarterectomy.[460] Noninvasive diagnostic testing is recommended for patients with neurological symptoms and anterior-circulation transient ischemic attacks or previous minor strokes if coronary artery surgery is contemplated. For those patients who previously had minor strokes, selective carotid angiography can be performed directly, because they have a higher likelihood of a surgically approachable carotid lesion.[460] It is clear that the presence of carotid bruits increases the risk of stroke after coronary bypass surgery (2.9 per cent), but this risk is small and comparable to the reported risk of stroke from carotid endarterectomy.[461-463]

Simultaneous carotid-coronary operations should be considered in patients with symptomatic carotid disease with bilateral carotid arterial obstructions and concurrent unstable angina, left main coronary artery obstruction, or diffuse multivessel coronary artery disease. Combined coronary and carotid arterial[464] and coronary arterial and abdominal aortic[465] procedures can be performed with mortality and morbidity similar to that of isolated surgery on the carotid artery and abdominal aorta. Most patients with asymptomatic cervical bruits or mild to moderate carotid artery obstruction can undergo coronary artery surgery alone with a low incidence of perioperative stroke.[466] In patients with unstable angina and a prior stroke the perioperative risk of neurological injury may be increased, and decisions need to be made on a case-by-case basis. Asymptomatic, unilateral, internal carotid artery stenosis or occlusion does not appear to increase the stroke risk during coronary artery surgery.[467]

Coronary artery disease is commonly associated with peripheral vascular disease and is the leading cause of mortality and morbidity in the perioperative period of patients undergoing peripheral vascular surgery.[468] Commonly these patients have major exercise limitations because of peripheral vascular insufficiency, and they may have significant CAD. However, their angina is masked by the limitation in their physical activities. Routine exercise testing may be impossible. In patients admitted for nonemergency surgery on the abdominal aorta or vessels of the lower extremities, preoperative thallium imaging after administration of dipyridamole may identify ischemic myocardium. With this technique, one-half of patients with thallium redistribution had cardiac events, whereas there were no such events in patients whose thallium scan was either normal or showed only persistent defects.[469] These findings suggest that patients with redistribution following dipyridamole-thallium imaging should be considered for preoperative coronary angiography and possible myocardial revascularization to avoid perioperative myocardial infarction or ischemia and possibly to improve survival. Ambulatory electrocardiographic monitoring of patients undergoing peripheral vascular surgery has shown that the finding of preoperative ischemia (ST-segment deviations) is the most significant correlate of postoperative cardiac events and assessing cardiac risk in patients undergoing elective peripheral vascular surgery. The absence of ischemia during such monitoring indicates that the patient has a very low risk for cardiac events perioperatively.[98]

HEART FAILURE AND MYOCARDIAL INFARCTION. In the absence of severe angina, patients with overt heart failure secondary to myocardial infarctions are not good candidates for coronary revascularization. However, in patients in whom left ventricular failure is due to chronically ischemic but not irreversibly damaged tissue, regardless of the presence or absence of pain, surgical revascularization can improve left ventricular function. The most striking improvement in clinical manifestations of heart failure and survival in these patients is seen in those with the most severe ventricular dysfunction. Patients with overt heart failure should be studied carefully to exclude a mechanical lesion such as mitral regurgitation or a ventricular aneurysm, which is usually amenable to surgical treatment.

Elsewhere are discussed indications for coronary revascularization in patients with CAD and unstable angina (p. 1340, cardiogenic shock secondary to acute myocardial infarction (p. 1255), and intractable ventricular arrhythmias (p. 656).

Unstable Angina

Unstable angina (previously also known as preinfarction angina, crescendo angina, [acute] coronary insufficiency, and intermediate coronary syndrome) is important clinically because of its frightening and disabling nature and the distinct possibility that it heralds acute myocardial infarction.[469a] Pathological studies of patients with this syndrome who do not develop an acute fatal myocardial infarction are rare, but those that are available usually reveal multivessel disease but a low incidence of recent occlusive thrombi. These findings suggest that coronary vasospasm, transient platelet aggregation, and/or nonocclusive thrombi play a role in the development of the acute ischemic episodes occurring in the presence of severe obstructive organic disease.[470] Thus, ischemic heart disease may really represent a spectrum of severities, with acute transmural infarction at one end of the spectrum, ranging successively through acute subendocardial infarction, unstable angina, chronic stable angina, with occasional silent ischemia at the other end of the spectrum.

DEFINITION. In addition to the absence of clear-cut electrocardiographic and cardiac enzyme changes diagnostic of a myocardial infarction, the currently used definition of unstable angina pectoris depends on the presence of one or more of the following three historical features, accompanied by electrocardiographic changes: (1) crescendo angina (more severe, prolonged, or frequent) superimposed on a preexisting pattern of relatively stable, exertion-related angina pectoris; (2) angina pectoris at rest as well as with minimal exertion; or (3) angina pectoris of new onset (usually within 1 month), which is brought on by minimal exertion. The ischemic episodes of unstable angina pectoris can be related to obvious precipitating factors, such as anemia, infection, thyrotoxicosis, or cardiac arrhythmias and the condition is then called secondary unstable angina (Table 40–16). Prinzmetal's ("variant") angina is a different entity and is discussed on page 1342. The syndrome of unstable angina describes a heterogeneous population of patients. They may be patients with single- or multivessel coronary artery disease, they may or may not have a history of prior myocardial infarction, they may have unstable angina while receiving no medical therapy, or they may be suffering severe, transient episodes of ischemia despite a combination of medications including full doses of nitrates, calcium antagonists, beta blockers, and intravenous heparin.

To categorize the heterogeneous population of patients who get unstable angina, a classification has been suggested that focuses on three important issues: (1) the severity of the clinical manifestations, (2) the clinical circumstances in which the unstable angina occurs, and (3) whether or not the sympto-

TABLE 40-16 CLASSIFICATION OF UNSTABLE ANGINA

	SEVERITY
Class I	New-onset, severe, or accelerated angina.
	Patients with angina of less than 2 months' duration, severe or occurring three or more times per day, or angina that is distinctly more frequent and precipitated by distinctly less exertion. No rest pain in the last 2 months.
Class II	Angina at rest. Subacute.
	Patients with one or more episodes of angina at rest during the preceding month but not within the preceding 48 hr.
Class III	Angina at rest. Acute.
	Patients with one or more episodes at rest within the preceding 48 hr.

	CLINICAL CIRCUMSTANCES
Class A	Secondary unstable angina.
	A clearly identified condition extrinsic to the coronary vascular bed that has intensified myocardial ischemia, e.g., anemia, infection, fever, hypotension, tachyarrhythmia, thyrotoxicosis, hypoxemia secondary to respiratory failure.
Class B	Primary unstable angina.
Class C	Postinfarction unstable angina (within 2 weeks of documented myocardial infarction).

INTENSITY OF TREATMENT

1. Absence of treatment or minimal treatment.
2. Occurring in presence of standard therapy for chronic stable angina (conventional doses of oral beta blockers, nitrates, and calcium antagonists).
3. Occurring despite maximally tolerated doses of all three categories of oral therapy, including intravenous nitroglycerin.

Modified from Braunwald, E.: Unstable angina: A classification. Circulation 80:410, 1989, by permission of the American Heart Association, Inc.

matic ischemic episodes are accompanied by transient electrocardiographic changes[471] (Table 40-16). This classification notes whether or not rest pain is present, whether the episodes have occurred within the preceding 48 hours, and whether the unstable angina is provoked by conditions such as anemia, fever, infection, and tachyarrhythmias. It is also proposed that the amount of therapy administered be taken into account. Thus, a patient who experiences recurrent angina at rest, with transient ST-segment depression, several days after an acute myocardial infarction despite maximally tolerated doses of standard therapy (including intravenous nitroglycerin) would be Class III, C, 3. (Class III involves angina at rest, acute; C: postinfarction unstable angina; 3: occurring despite maximally tolerated doses of all three categories of oral therapy, including intravenous nitroglycerin.) While this is a clinical classification, it can be related to underlying disease. For example, Class III patients (with recent rest angina) are more likely to have intracoronary thrombus, and anticoagulants or perhaps thrombolytic therapy may be of greater value in such patients but of less value in patients in Classes I and II.

CLINICAL AND LABORATORY FINDINGS

SYMPTOMS. The chest discomfort in this syndrome is similar in quality to that of classic effort-induced angina, although it is often more intense, is usually described as pain, may persist for as long as 30 minutes, and occasionally awakens the patient from sleep. Longer episodes of ischemic pain are usually associated with acute myocardial infarction. The usual therapeutic regimen of bed rest and nitroglycerin administration often provides only temporary or incomplete relief. Several clues should alert the physician to a changing anginal pattern and the development of unstable angina; these include an abrupt and persistent reduction in the threshold of physical activity that provokes angina; an increase in the frequency, severity, and duration of angina; radiation of the discomfort to an additional or new site; and onset of new associated features such as diaphoresis, nausea, or palpitation.

The proportion of patients with unstable angina who have angina of new onset, a crescendo pattern superimposed on stable angina, or rest angina varies among different series and depends on how the observers defined the syndrome. Patients in whom unstable angina is superimposed on longstanding, stable angina often have multivessel disease, while patients with new onset of severe angina may have a strong dynamic (vasoconstrictive) component superimposed on fixed obstructive disease involving only a single coronary artery.

PHYSICAL EXAMINATION. This may reveal transient diastolic (third and fourth) heart sounds and a dyskinetic apical impulse suggesting left ventricular dysfunction, or a transient systolic murmur of mitral regurgitation during or immediately after an ischemic episode. These findings are nonspecific, since they may also be present in patients with chronic angina pectoris or acute myocardial infarction.

ELECTROCARDIOGRAM

Twelve-Lead Electrocardiogram. Transient deviations of the ST segment (depression or elevation) and/or T-wave inversions occur commonly but not universally in unstable angina. Usually these changes clear completely or partially with the relief of pain. Persistence of these electrocardiographic changes for more than 6 to 12 hours may suggest that a non-Q-wave infarction has occurred.

If patients have a typical history of chronic stable angina pectoris or established CAD (previous myocardial infarction, abnormal coronary arteriograms, or a history of a positive noninvasive stress test) before the development of symptoms of unstable angina, the diagnosis of unstable angina may be made with reliability if typical symptoms exist, even in the absence of electrocardiographic changes. It is in the subgroup of patients without evidence of previous CAD and no electrocardiographic change associated with pain that the diagnosis may be inaccurate. Also, in these patients no underlying CAD may be found at coronary arteriography.

Ischemic chest pain is not a reliable or sensitive marker of transient acute myocardial ischemia. Episodes of primary reduction in coronary blood flow may be associated with variable and minor electrocardiographic changes that precede symptoms of pain or discomfort.[472] In continuously monitored patients who demonstrated large falls in coronary sinus oxygen saturation, reflecting changes in myocardial blood flow, when the ischemic episodes were associated with chest pain (10 of 37) the pain always occurred 50 to 120 seconds after the onset of the ST-T changes.[472] Evaluation of the admission 12-lead electrocardiogram allows some risk stratification of patients admitted to the hospital with unstable angina. Patients with electrocardiographic ST-segment deviations (either depressions or elevations) are more likely to have a subsequent unfavorable hospital outcome (myocardial infarction, death, or the need for revascularization) than patients with no ST-segment deviations.[473]

Holter Monitoring. When continuous electrocardiographic monitoring is performed, many patients with unstable angina have a high incidence of ischemic electrocardiographic changes without accompanying symptoms, i.e., silent ischemia.[15,474-477] Recent studies suggest that more than 85 to 90 per cent of these ischemic episodes detected by Holter monitoring techniques are not associated with angina.[473,478] Furthermore, the presence of a significant degree of ischemia, detected by Holter monitoring, serves as a predictor of unfavorable outcome during hospital admission[473,479] and during follow-up (Fig. 40-26).[478,480] Holter monitoring appears to be more sensitive than ST-segment changes seen on the admission 12-lead electrocardiogram in predicting unfavorable outcome.[473] Ischemic electrocardiographic changes occurring without symptoms also correlate with transient reductions in myocardial perfusion and abnormalities of ventricular func-

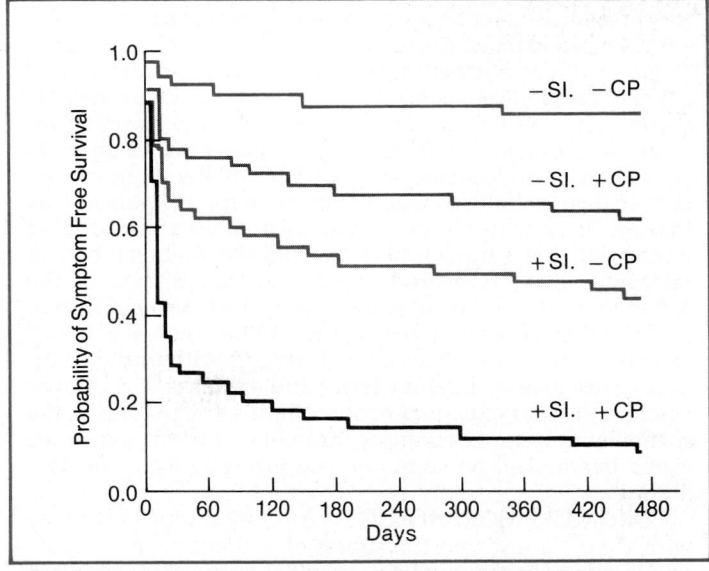

FIGURE 40-26. Symptom-free survival following unstable angina. Seventy patients with the clinical diagnosis of unstable angina treated with combination, triple-drug medical therapy were monitored electrocardiographically for silent ischemia for a 48-hour period, and the occurrence of chest pain during this period was documented. During follow-up, the influence of silent ischemia (SI) and recurrent chest pain (CP) on adverse outcome was assessed by Cox's hazard function analysis demonstrating the risk for death, myocardial infarction, or revascularization for recurrent symptoms. There was a five-fold relative risk for adverse outcomes associated with the presence of silent ischemia during the first 48 hours after the onset of unstable angina and a three-fold relative risk associated with the occurrence of chest pain during the initial 2 days of treatment for unstable angina. If both variables were present, the relative risk for experiencing an adverse outcome was increased by a factor of 15. (From Gottlieb S. O., et al.: Silent ischemia predicts infarction and death during 2 year follow-up of unstable angina. Reprinted with permission from the American College of Cardiology. J. Am. Coll. Cardiol. 10:756, 1987.)

tion.[15,475,476] Episodes of silent ischemia may persist and still be a sign of adverse prognosis in patients with unstable angina who are treated with conventional antianginal agents and whose symptoms are controlled.[478] Therefore, in patients with unstable angina, predischarge Holter monitoring may be helpful in detecting continuing ischemia and stratifying patients into groups who need early angiography and revascularization and groups who can continue on a conservative medical therapy regimen.[480] In the majority of patients adverse clinical outcomes are most likely within the first 2 to 4 months after hospitalization.[479,480]

STANDARD LABORATORY TESTS. Findings on chest roentgenogram, serum cholesterol level, and carbohydrate tolerance are similar to those observed in patients with chronic stable angina (p. 1298). Unlike acute myocardial infarction, nonspecific indicators of gross tissue necrosis, such as leukocytosis and fever, are usually absent. Cardiac enzymes are not abnormally elevated; when cardiac-specific enzymes are elevated, by definition the diagnosis is acute myocardial infarction and not unstable angina.

CARDIAC CATHETERIZATION AND CORONARY ARTERIOGRAPHY

Coronary arteriographic findings in patients with unstable angina vary according to the population being studied.[480a] In a population of male patients included in a randomized Veterans Administration study on unstable angina, 18 per cent had one-vessel coronary disease, 35 per cent had two-vessel coronary disease, and 46 per cent had three-vessel coronary disease. Similarly, in a population of patients from the CASS registry who received surgical therapy for unstable angina, 50 per cent had three-vessel coronary disease and 14 per cent had significant left main coronary artery stenoses.[481] However, in patients with new-onset unstable angina, and no previous history of myocardial infarction or chronic stable angina, there is a higher incidence of single-vessel disease (43 per cent versus 27 per cent) and a lower incidence of three-vessel disease (23 per cent versus 35 per cent) compared to patients with chronic stable angina.[482] The left anterior descending coronary artery is the most commonly affected vessel in patients with unstable (as well as chronic stable) angina. The collateral circulation appears less well developed in patients with unstable angina than in those with chronic stable angina, an arteriographic impression that is supported by findings at operation in which retrograde flow, measured directly by cannulation of the opened artery, was less in patients with unstable angina than in those with chronic stable angina.[483] The incidence of normal coronary arteriograms among patients with unstable angina varies among different series and averages 10 to 15 per cent. No obvious explanation other than coronary spasm, the spontaneous lysis of a coronary thrombus, or the presence of a lesion overlooked on coronary arteriography exists for this finding.

CORONARY MORPHOLOGY. Autopsy studies of patients with CAD suggest that the subset of patients with unstable angina can have the most severe and extensive CAD.[484] Such studies also have shown that about 70 per cent of specimens of diseased arterial segments with significant narrowings (greater than or equal to 50 per cent diameter loss) have an eccentric, residual arterial lumen that is partially circumscribed by an arc of at least 60 degrees of normal arterial wall.[485,486] The presence of this pliable, muscular elastic arc of normal wall provides a mechanism whereby variations in intraluminal pressure and/or vasomotor tone may alter lumen caliber and thus flow resistance. In patients with unstable angina, postmortem angiograms, histological examinations, and coronary arteriograms display eccentric stenoses with scalloped or overhanging edges more frequently than in patients with chronic stable angina (Fig. 9–64, p. 264).[487] In contrast, lesions with concentric, symmetrical narrowing, or asymmetrical narrowing with smooth borders and a broad neck are more common in patients with stable angina. In pa-

tients with known coronary artery anatomy and stable angina pectoris who were restudied after an episode of acute unstable angina, it appeared in most instances that acute progression had occurred from a previously insignificant lesion. Also, the eccentric lesion (type II lesion, that is, eccentrically placed convex stenosis with a narrow neck due to one or more overhanging edges or irregular, scalloped borders, or both [p. 263]) is the most common morphological feature of disease progression. This finding may represent either a disrupted atherosclerotic plaque or a partially lysed thrombus, or the combination.[487]

Plaque fissuring has been implicated in acute coronary syndromes, including acute myocardial infarction (p. 1205) and unstable angina.[488] The type of plaque most likely to undergo fissuring is one with an eccentrically situated pool of extracellular lipid (cholesterol) contained within the intima (Fig. 39–9, p. 1206). This pool is separated from the blood in the lumen of the artery by a cap of fibrous tissue covered by endothelium.[488] The cap seems most likely to tear at the lateral margin of the plaque where it is attached to more normal intima. Blood enters the lipid cavity from the lumen, and because of the thrombogenicity of the subendothelial tissues that are exposed a thrombus develops within the plaque itself. This thrombus can expand the volume of the plaque, but subsequently the tear may reseal, restabilize, and heal. Plaque fissures heal by smooth muscle proliferation that can contribute to an increase in the severity of chronic obstruction.[489] Some episodes of plaque fissuring are followed by the development of thrombus within the coronary arterial lumen. Pathological as well as coronary arteriographic studies have suggested the presence of subtotally occlusive coronary arterial thrombi in patients with unstable angina.[490-493]

Coronary angioscopy has revealed complex plaques or thrombi not detected by coronary angiography in such patients.[494] In patients presenting early after the onset of rest angina, coronary arteriography has shown a 40 per cent inci-

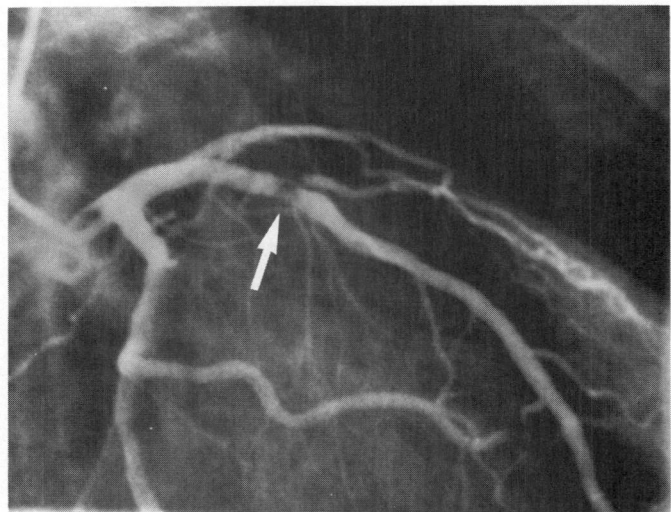

FIGURE 40–27. Coronary artery thrombus in a patient with unstable angina. A 60-year-old man was admitted to the hospital with a history of crescendo angina and prolonged rest pain. He had electrocardiographic T-wave inversions in leads V_2-V_5, I, aV_L and no abnormalities of serial cardiac enzymes. After 72 hours of hospital treatment with aspirin, heparin, and beta blocker therapy he had a further episode of rest pain associated with 5- to 8-mm anterior ST-segment elevations. Coronary angiography was performed, and the left coronary artery (right anterior oblique caudal projection) is shown. In the left anterior descending coronary artery, at the level of the second diagonal branch, an irregular hazy filling defect is present (arrow). It is surrounded by angiographic contrast medium and extends into the diagonal branch itself. After 4 further days of heparin and antianginal therapy, a repeat coronary angiogram was obtained, and the size of the intracoronary filling defect had decreased, confirming that it was a coronary thrombus.

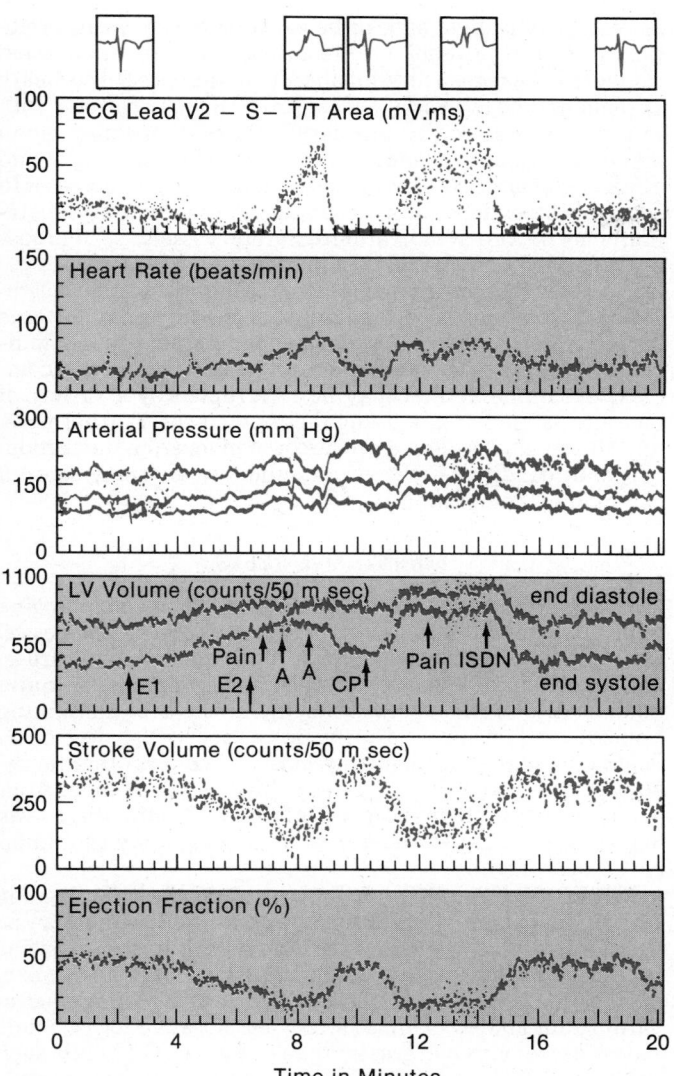

FIGURE 40-28. Changes in ventricular volume and function associated with myocardial ischemia. During spontaneous and ergometrine-induced ST-segment elevation, changes (from *top* to *bottom*) in ECG, heart rate, arterial pressure, left ventricular volume, stroke volume, and ejection fraction are parametrically displayed. E1 = ergometrine 0.025 mg IV; E2 = ergometrine 0.05 mg IV; A = amyl nitrite; CP = cold pressor test; ISDN = isosorbide dinitrate 2.5 mg IV. The small dose of ergometrine led to abrupt, severe left ventricular dilatation with reduction in stroke volume and ejection fraction. ST-segment elevation and pain were late events. Amyl nitrite administration led to resolution of all manifestations of the attack with left ventricular volume returning almost to the basal level. Cold pressor stimulation caused prompt recurrence of ST-segment elevation with extreme left ventricular dilatation and pain, and the episode was completely abolished by isosorbide dinitrate. (From Davies G. J., et al.: Sequence and magnitude of ventricular volume changes in painful and painless myocardial ischemia. Circulation *78*:310, 1988, by permission of the American Heart Association, Inc.)

dence of coronary thrombi (Fig. 40-27).[493] Cardiac events (death, myocardial infarction, and the need for urgent revascularization) were more frequent in patients with coronary thrombus (73 per cent), complex coronary morphology (55 per cent), or multivessel disease (58 per cent) than in patients without these angiographic features (17 per cent, 31 per cent, and 7 per cent, respectively). Similarly, intracoronary thrombi were present in 75 per cent of patients requiring urgent coronary arteriography for persistent angina later during admission.[493] Therefore, coronary thrombus is commonly present in patients with rest angina and appears to be an angiographic predictor of subsequent adverse cardiac events. It is not difficult to conceive that alterations in coronary artery tone at the site of irregular plaques may initiate and/or be exacerbated

by local formation of subtotally occlusive thrombi with resulting intensification of angina. In patients with well-formed coronary collaterals, total thrombotic occlusion of a coronary artery may lead to unstable angina without myocardial infarction.

Findings on left ventriculography are similar to those in patients with chronic stable angina and generally show good wall motion between episodes of acute ischemia, except of course in patients who have had prior myocardial infarction. During episodes of acute ischemia, localized areas of asynergy are present, and stroke volume and ejection fraction decline, while left ventricular end-systolic and end-diastolic volumes rise, as does left ventricular filling pressure; nitroglycerin restores both global and regional left ventricular function (Fig. 40-28).

PATHOPHYSIOLOGY

Most patients with unstable angina have severe obstructive CAD; episodes of myocardial ischemia can be precipitated by either an increase in myocardial oxygen demand and/or a reduction in supply.[473] Episodes of spontaneous (rest) angina can be preceded by arterial hypertension and/or tachycardia, which lead to increases in myocardial oxygen requirements. In patients with fixed atherosclerotic obstructive lesions, a primary reduction of myocardial oxygen supply (due to either coronary vasoconstriction, i.e., a further reduction in lumen diameter consequent to transient vasoconstrictor influences, or perhaps to platelet thrombi) may also be responsible for many cases of angina at rest and not merely those associated with Prinzmetal's angina (in which there is abnormal severe spasm of a proximal coronary artery [p. 1342]).

In many patients with unstable angina who are continuously monitored, an interesting sequence of events has been demonstrated (Fig. 40-28). First, there is a reduction of coronary sinus oxygen saturation (which, in the presence of constant myocardial oxygen needs, signifies a reduction of coronary blood flow). This is followed by the characteristic electrocardiographic changes discussed above, and only then does chest discomfort appear. Secondary to the latter, blood pressure and/or heart rate may rise.[472] Thus, in many patients with rest angina, ischemia appears to be precipitated by a reduction in oxygen supply rather than an increase in oxygen demand. It is also possible that in some instances an increase in myocardial oxygen demand and a reduction in supply occur simultaneously. Thus, in some patients with Prinzmetal's angina, coronary vasoconstriction has been observed to occur during exercise.[495] This is an example of simultaneous augmentation of myocardial oxygen needs with concurrent reduced availability. A similar mechanism may be operative in some patients with unstable angina.

Mechanisms contributing to the reduction of oxygen supply, and therefore to the precipitation of ischemic episodes in patients with unstable angina who have severe underlying obstructive CAD, include progression of atherosclerosis, platelet aggregation, thrombosis, and coronary vasoconstriction.

PROGRESSION OF ATHEROSCLEROSIS. Evidence exists that the development of unstable angina may be associated with more marked recent progression in the extent and severity of CAD than that seen in patients with chronic stable angina. Such progression appears to occur as commonly in areas that are minimally diseased as in segments that are initially severely narrowed.[496]

PLATELET AGGREGATION. There is substantial evidence to support the role of platelet aggregation in the precipitation of ischemic episodes in patients with unstable angina. Animal models have shown that spontaneous decreases in coronary blood flow through coronary artery stenoses may be due to episodic platelet aggregation (which may transiently occlude a partially constricted coronary artery) and that these cyclic reductions in coronary blood flow can be prevented by aspirin.[497] This suggests that platelet aggregation rather than fibrin deposition may cause the observed cyclic reductions of coronary flow. Platelets and the coronary vascular endothelium interact in a complex manner; platelets produce the proaggregatory and vasoconstrictive thromboxane A_2 (p. 1173), while the normal endothelium produces antiaggregatory prostacyclin (prostaglandin I_2), tissue plasminogen activator (t-PA), and endothelial-derived relaxing factor (p. 263). It is likely that other factors such as change in sympathetic vascular tone and the activation of platelet receptors (alpha$_2$-adrenergic and serotonergic) may promote platelet aggregation. It has been speculated that the abrupt conversion from chronic stable to unstable angina may result from the more intense myocardial ischemia initiated by platelet aggregation[498] and coronary vasoconstriction resulting from the local accumulation of thromboxane A_2 and serotonin, and also from reductions in the local concentrations of endothelially derived vasodilators and inhibitors of platelet aggregation.[499]

In patients with unstable angina who have had pain within 24 hours, the finding of elevated metabolites of thromboxane A_2 in plasma and urine suggests that local thromboxane release may be associated with the episodes of unstable angina.[498] The reductions in coronary blood flow in canine preparations with marked obstruction appear to be abolished by platelet inhibitors, including aspirin, sulfinpyrazone, prostacyclin, ibuprofen, and indomethacin but not by heparin, nitroglycerin, or papaverine.[500] Again this suggests that they are mediated by platelet aggregation rather than by vasospasm or fibrin deposition. Furthermore, four separate clinical trials have now shown that aspirin can protect against death and nonfatal acute myocardial infarction in patients with unstable angina.[501-504] Finally, in patients with unstable angina who suffer sudden death, aggregates of platelet emboli have been found in small intramyocardial vessels. These occur in segments of myocardium immediately downstream from a major epicardial coronary artery containing an atheromatous plaque that has undergone fissuring and on which mural thrombus had developed.[490]

THROMBOSIS. In addition to platelet aggregation, the presence of an active thrombotic process in patients with unstable angina is suggested by increased serum concentrations of fibrin-related antigen, and D-dimer (the principal breakdown fragment of fibrin) in patients with unstable angina, changes that do not occur in patients with chronic stable angina.[505] Several clinical studies have shown that when coronary angiography is performed in patients with unstable angina, intracoronary filling defects having the appearance of thrombi are commonly found[492,493,506]; coronary angioscopy has confirmed this interpretation.[494] Furthermore, when thrombolytic therapy is given to patients with unstable angina and recent pain, a reduction in the severity of coronary stenosis, dissolution of intracoronary filling defects, and opening of an occluded artery have all been observed.[506,507] The associations of persistent rest pain, intracoronary thrombus, and adverse outcome have also been noted.[493,506] Finally, postmortem observations in many patients with unstable angina have suggested an ongoing thrombotic process in a major coronary artery during the period of unstable angina. This process culminates in total vascular occlusion, which causes infarction and/or sudden death.[491]

CORONARY SPASM OR ALTERATIONS IN VASOMOTOR TONE. Quantitative angiography in patients with unstable angina has shown vasomotor hyperreactivity localized to regions of preexisting coronary atheroma.[508] Also, clinical studies have reported large-vessel coronary spasm as a cause of ST-segment elevation in such patients.[509] Postmortem studies have shown that in the majority of significantly diseased coronary arteries a portion of the circumference is circumscribed by normal arterial walls.[485,486] Because of this and because unstable angina pectoris is a dynamic, multifactorial process, it is likely that a normal pliable muscular elastic arc of vessel wall provides a mechanism whereby normal (vasoconstriction) or abnormally intense (vasospasm) increases in vasomotor tone may affect lumen caliber and thus flow resistance.[509a] Alterations in coronary artery tone at the site of

plaques may initiate and/or be exacerbated by local formation of platelet thrombi with resulting ischemia. Endothelial injury may be responsible for abnormal responses in coronary vasomotor tone to a variety of stimuli.[509] Even in patients with minimal disease of the coronary arteries, there may be an abnormal response to endothelium-dependent stimuli,[510] and dilatation of large coronary arteries in response to increases in coronary blood flow (flow-dependent coronary artery dilatation) may be impaired in atherosclerotic vessels,[511-514] probably reflecting endothelial dysfunction.

It is likely that progression of atherosclerosis, platelet aggregation, thrombus formation, and changes in vasomotor tone may operate either alone or together at different times in individual patients. The syndrome of unstable angina is a complex, dynamic one that may be interrupted by a variety of measures aimed at modifying these processes. Furthermore, unstable angina is often a precursor of myocardial infarction, and both conditions may occur suddenly and may share a common pathological link.

NONINVASIVE TESTS

Most patients who are hospitalized with unstable angina will, after initial therapy of bed rest, oxygen, analgesics, aspirin or heparin, nitrates, beta-adrenoceptor blocking drugs, and/or calcium antagonists, become asymptomatic quite quickly, and their electrocardiographic signs of continuing ischemia will disappear. During this period, serial electrocardiographic and enzyme evaluations will confirm that no infarction has taken place, thereby differentiating them from patients with acute myocardial infarction. Noninvasive tests may help determine whether or not angiography should be performed urgently.

EXERCISE TESTING. Exercise testing after stabilization of symptoms and before discharge from the hospital can be safely performed in patients admitted with unstable angina who have become asymptomatic.[515] When large numbers of such patients are studied, those with a normal resting electrocardiogram and an exercise stress test negative for ischemia have a 5-year survival greater than 95 per cent.[516] While such patients with chest pain but no changes on resting electrocardiograms or evidence of ischemia during exercise testing, are at very low risk for coronary events, the presence of chest pain at a low rate-pressure product associated with ST-segment changes during exercise testing identifies patients at high risk for subsequent morbid and fatal events.[515,516]

TWO-DIMENSIONAL ECHOCARDIOGRAPHY. This examination may reveal transient abnormalities of ventricular wall motion. Persistent abnormalities of wall motion are associated with an adverse prognosis.[517]

THALLIUM SCINTIGRAPHY. Abnormal thallium images indicating resting hypoperfusion of viable myocardium have been demonstrated to occur more commonly in patients with rapidly worsening exertional angina than in patients with chronic stable angina.[518,518a] In patients with rest angina, the combination of thallium defects and washout abnormalities has a sensitivity of 67 per cent for detecting coronary stenoses and a specificity of 59 per cent.[519] Detection of a reversible thallium defect by intravenous dipyridamole thallium scintigraphy can serve as a predictor of adverse cardiac events.[520] Exercise thallium testing performed when unstable angina had stabilized demonstrated that thallium defect size was a useful predictor of the extent of coronary artery disease[521] and of patients at higher risk for subsequent fatal and morbid events.[521a]

MANAGEMENT

INDICATIONS FOR CATHETERIZATION AND ANGIOGRAPHY. As is the case in patients with chronic stable angina, several questions need to be resolved: How will these tests aid in further management? In which patients should they be performed? What are the risks involved? Are any special precautions necessary? Although there is no unanimity of opinion regarding the answers, we believe that in most instances coronary arteriography is very helpful in the management of patients with unstable angina. For patients in whom medical therapy fails, i.e., who have continued episodes of ischemia at rest or with minimal exertion despite medical therapy described below, coronary arteriography should be carried out as soon as possible after the hemodynamic condition has been stabilized, unless there are obvious contraindications to possible angioplasty or coronary bypass surgery. On the other hand, in patients who respond to medical therapy, we recommend stress electrocardiography (and possibly a thallium scan). If these tests are strongly positive for myocardial ischemia, catheterization and coronary arteriography should be carried out.

Catheterization and arteriography are helpful in that they identify several subgroups of patients with unstable angina pectoris and can thus be used to dictate therapy: (1) Patients with left main coronary artery disease—the most life-threatening form of the disease—in whom urgent surgery is indicated. (2) Patients with multivessel obstructive disease without a clear "culprit" lesion and who are not suitable for angioplasty. Unless there are contraindications, we recommend that operation be planned on a semiurgent basis (within 10 days) after the patient's hemodynamic condition has stabilized. (3) Patients with left ventricular dysfunction and multivessel disease who should be revascularized to improve long-term survival. (4) A small number of patients (about 10 per cent of all patients with unstable angina) with no demonstrable CAD, in whom the prognosis appears to be excellent with medical management and in whom no further surgical consideration is necessary. In some of these patients, coronary spasm is responsible for the angina, and this can be established by provocative testing at the time of coronary arteriography (p. 1336); intensification of therapy with nitrates and calcium antagonists would then be indicated. (5) Patients with single-vessel or double-vessel disease with a discrete narrow proximal lesion (i.e., "culprit" lesion) amenable to percutaneous transluminal angioplasty (p. 1316). (6) Patients with diffuse distal CAD unsuitable for angioplasty or bypass grafting.

Which patients are unsuitable for cardiac catheterization and coronary arteriography? Obviously, patients who are suffering from another serious life-threatening illness with a poor prognosis do not require study. Advanced age per se is not considered a contraindication. The risks of coronary arteriography may be somewhat greater in patients with unstable angina than in those with chronic stable angina, but the addition of intraaortic balloon counterpulsation has reduced mortality to near zero. Maximal medical therapy, as described later, should be maintained up to and continued through the time of cardiac catheterization and arteriography.

Opinion is divided whether or not these procedures are necessary in patients in whom unstable angina has come under control and in whom severe ischemia cannot be provoked by a low level stress test. This question is currently being addressed in a large randomized clinical trial (TIMI III).

APPROACH TO MANAGEMENT. Unstable angina pectoris is a serious, potentially dangerous condition, and its management must be approached with this in mind. The patient should be admitted to the hospital and immediately placed at bed rest. Removal from an emotionally taxing situation, the presence of a quiet atmosphere, physical and emotional rest, the physician's reassurance, mild sedation, and antianxiety drugs are all helpful and will diminish or relieve episodes of rest pain in perhaps half of all patients. A vigorous effort must be undertaken immediately to diagnose and treat conditions that may be responsible for transient increases in myocardial oxygen demands, such as infection, fever, thyrotoxicosis, anemia, arrhythmias, exacerbation of preexisting heart failure, concurrent illnesses (particularly of the pulmonary tract, leading to coughing and hypoxemia, and acute gastrointestinal disturbances, causing vomiting, retching, or severe diarrhea), tachyarrhythmias (that increase myocardial oxygen

demand), and severe bradyarrhythmias that reduce myocardial perfusion. Control of these aggravating factors will be helpful in 10 to 15 per cent of patients. Placing the bed into the reverse Trendelenburg position (feet down) is a simple measure that may be helpful, as may the inhalation of 100 per cent oxygen during periods of pain.

The electrocardiogram should be monitored continuously; diagnostic tests to rule out a myocardial infarction should include serial CK-MB enzymes. Invasive monitoring is usually not necessary unless a serious hemodynamic disturbance is suspected. Frequent radionuclide angiograms, thallium perfusion scans, and two-dimensional echocardiograms, although useful in elucidating the mechanism and consequences of unstable angina, are not especially helpful in immediate management and may actually be harmful in that they disturb the patient's rest.

NITRATES. These are a mainstay of therapy. In addition to frequently relieving and preventing recurrence of pain, they have been shown to improve global and regional left ventricular function. Nitrates may be given sublingually, orally, topically, or intravenously, and they may be of the short- or long-acting variety. Intravenous nitroglycerin offers the advantage of more consistent control of ischemic episodes during the first 24 hours of treatment. An additional advantage of intravenous nitroglycerin in patients already receiving standard therapy of oral or topical nitrates and beta-blocking drugs is that it will reduce the number of anginal episodes, reduce the need for sublingual nitroglycerin and for analgesics. A dosage schedule designed to reduce mean arterial pressure by 10 per cent is a safe and effective way of treating unstable angina unresponsive to standard medical therapy.[522]

Nitroglycerin is relatively stable when stored in glass containers; however, plastic bags should be avoided because the drug is absorbed by the plastic. Polyvinylchloride tubing also has a great affinity for nitroglycerin.[523] Therefore, the quantity of nitroglycerin delivered to the patient may be much less than that ordered. Several companies offer a non-polyvinylchloride infusion set with preparations of intravenous nitroglycerin. Also, commercial preparations of intravenous nitroglycerin contain alcohol in quantities of 0.01 to 0.14 ml/mg of nitroglycerin, so that when large doses of the agent are administered the quantity of alcohol delivered may be substantial. Acute gout has been described in patients receiving intravenous nitroglycerin, and it has been postulated that the alcohol content of the preparation may have altered serum uric acid levels.[524] It has been demonstrated that platelets taken from patients treated with intravenous nitroglycerin exhibit attenuated aggregation responses ex vivo, and this effect depends on the adequacy of reduced intracellular thiol stores.[525] The combined administration of intravenous nitroglycerin and the sulfhydryl (SH) donor N-acetylcysteine (NAC) may augment the clinical efficacy of nitroglycerin but increase the risk of development of hypotension.[526] Pharmacological tolerance to continuous intravenous nitroglycerin therapy develops within 24 hours.[179,527]

BETA-ADRENOCEPTOR BLOCKERS. The role of beta-adrenoceptor blockade in the treatment of unstable angina pectoris is being reexamined because many episodes of myocardial ischemia in these patients are not preceded by increases in heart rate or blood pressure, which are the major determinants of myocardial oxygen consumption. However, immediately after the onset of ischemia, increases in heart rate and blood pressure commonly occur and may perpetuate the ischemia.[528]

Several randomized trials have placed the role of beta blockers in the treatment of unstable angina pectoris into better perspective. In unstable angina patients who have not previously been receiving beta blocker therapy, the addition of a beta blocker[529,530] or the combination of a beta blocker and nitrates[531] appears to reduce symptoms of recurrent ischemia[529-531] and the occurrence of myocardial infarction.[529,530] In patients already receiving nitrates and calcium antagonists, the addition of beta blockers reduces the frequency and duration of both symptomatic and silent ischemic episodes.[532] Propranolol and diltiazem may provide equivalent relief of symptoms, and the incidence of death, infarction, and the need for coronary artery surgery appears equal in patients treated with these.[533] In patients already taking a beta blocker with continuous episodes of angina at rest, the addition of nifedipine appears to provide additional symptomatic benefit.[529-531]

In conclusion, in patients not already receiving beta blockers who present with unstable angina, either a beta blocker alone,[529,530] a combination of a beta blocker and nitrates,[531] or a beta blocker with nifedipine would appear to be the preferred treatment regimen. Propranolol and diltiazem appear equivalent in providing symptomatic relief without any difference in adverse events.[533] When rapid beta blockade is desired to reduce angina by lowering heart rate and/or blood pressure, intravenous esmolol (p. 864) is efficacious and safe, even in patients with compromised left ventricular function.[534,535] Resolution of drug effect occurs within 20 to 30 minutes of discontinuing esmolol.

In patients who are already taking a beta blocker at the time unstable angina develops, the drug should be continued unless contraindications are present. The dosage of beta blockers should be adjusted so that the resting heart rate is reduced to between 50 and 60 beats/min. This usually requires 240 to 320 mg of propranolol per day (or the equivalent for other beta blockers). Beta blockade may improve pulmonary congestion if the elevated pulmonary venous pressure is due to an ischemia-induced reduction of left ventricular compliance or left ventricular systolic failure. Rarely, heart failure may be precipitated by beta blockade in patients with previous infarction. In this situation the drug should be discontinued or the dose reduced and treatment with diuretics instituted.

CALCIUM ANTAGONISTS. A systematic overview of all randomized trials of calcium antagonists in unstable angina suggests that they do not prevent the development of acute myocardial infarction or reduce mortality.[536] A large, randomized, double-blind, placebo-controlled comparison of recurrent ischemia in patients with unstable angina treated with nifedipine or metoprolol, or both, was terminated prematurely because it appeared that nifedipine therapy alone might have been associated with more nonfatal myocardial infarctions within the first 48 hours of treatment than therapy with metoprolol alone or a combination of nifedipine and metoprolol.[529,530] Studies of patients with unstable angina have suggested that the addition of nifedipine to beta blocker therapy[531] or to a combination of nitrates and beta blockers[537] is useful in relieving angina[531] and reducing the subsequent short-term risk of death, myocardial infarction, or the need for urgent coronary artery surgery.[537] We believe that unless contraindicated a calcium antagonist should be added to nitrates and a beta blocker in patients with continuing ischemia.

ANTICOAGULANTS AND ANTIPLATELET DRUGS. The potential importance of platelet activation and thrombus formation in the pathogenesis and the clinical outcome of unstable angina[488,492,493,506] has led to management strategies that include heparin[503,538] and aspirin.[501-504] Theroux et al.[503] have shown in a double-blind, placebo-controlled trial in patients with unstable angina that heparin alone (1000 units per hour), aspirin alone (325 mg twice daily), and their combination are effective in reducing subsequent in-hospital cardiac events. In patients receiving placebo therapy, myocardial infarction occurred in 12 per cent, compared with 0.8 per cent in patients receiving heparin, in 3 per cent of patients receiving aspirin, and in 1.6 per cent of patients receiving a combination of aspirin and heparin. Recurrent angina also occurred less frequently in the heparin-treated group. Thus, both heparin and aspirin appeared to reduce the incidence of myocardial infarction in patients presenting with unstable angina, but neither agent, taken as the sole therapy, appeared better than the other. The limited sample size precluded the evaluation of the effect of treatment on mortality. Long-term administration of

aspirin to patients with unstable angina reduces the incidence of nonfatal myocardial infarction and death.[501,502]

THROMBOLYTIC THERAPY. There is no agreement whether thrombolytic therapy plays a role in the clinical management of unstable angina. However, this question is currently being addressed by a large randomized trial (TIMI III).

INTRAAORTIC BALLOON COUNTERPULSATION (see also p. 580). This mode of therapy is considered when others have failed, and it is usually effective in stabilizing the patient's condition, both symptomatically and hemodynamically.[539] Intraaortic balloon counterpulsation is usually initiated either before or during coronary arteriography with a view to continuing it through revascularization.[540] This technique is useful primarily because it allows the safe performance of coronary arteriography and ensures that the patient goes to coronary artery surgery or PTCA under optimal conditions. Local complications related to intraaortic balloon placement are more common in the elderly, women, and diabetics.[541]

REVASCULARIZATION. PTCA. In patients with unstable angina, successful PTCA results in immediate abolition of ischemic episodes as well as improvement in both regional and global ischemic left ventricular dysfunction.[542] Patients with less than 50 per cent residual stenoses 6 months after PTCA often show sustained improvement in their functional status and myocardial perfusion 4 to 6 years later.[543] In large series of patients with unstable angina in whom PTCA is attempted, single-vessel CAD is present in 60 to 80 per cent.[544-546] The initial success rate of dilation of significant stenoses is 83 to 93 per cent.[544-549] Procedure-related myocardial infarction occurs in approximately 8 per cent of patients,[544-548] and in-hospital mortality is usually less than 1 per cent.[544,548] If PTCA is performed early after the *onset* of unstable angina, the complication rate is higher and the success rate is lower.[549a] Patients with unstable angina appear to be at higher risk of developing a myocardial infarction at the time of PTCA than do patients with chronic stable angina.[546,547] The risk factors for a procedure-related complication include severe degrees of stenosis,[548] the presence of thrombus and either ST-segment elevations, or persistent T-wave inversions on the electrocardiogram.[548]

The incidence of restenosis following PTCA appears to be similar in patients with unstable angina to those with chronic stable angina (approximately 30 per cent).[548-550] The risk factors for restenosis in patients with unstable angina appear to be multifactorial and include poor perfusion beyond the "culprit" lesion,[549] multiple irregularities in the vessel being dilated,[549] the presence of intraluminal thrombus,[549] involvement of the left anterior descending coronary artery,[548,549] and the presence of collateral vessels.[548] Urgent coronary artery surgery may be required in up to 10 per cent of patients.[548] Despite these problems, 18-month and 5-year survival are greater than 95 per cent[551] and approximately three-fourths of patients remain free of angina following successful angioplasty.[544,551] There is a myocardial infarction rate of 6 to 14 per cent during long-term follow-up,[546,551] which does not differ substantially from that following PTCA for chronic stable angina.[546]

Surgical Therapy. In patients with uncontrolled unstable angina (who have not suffered recent myocardial infarction) the operative mortality for coronary artery surgery is 3.7 per cent (approximately twice that observed in patients with chronic stable angina pectoris), the incidence of perioperative myocardial infarction is 10 per cent, and postoperative low cardiac output (patients requiring inotropic or intraaortic balloon support) is seen in 16 per cent of patients.[405] In patients observed for 7 to 10 years, either minimal angina or no angina is found in 80 per cent of patients, and survival at 5 years is approximately 90 per cent and at 10 years approximately 80 per cent.[405] It is estimated that the annualized rate of late nonfatal myocardial infarction is 3 to 4 per cent per year. In the Veterans Administration Cooperative Study that com-

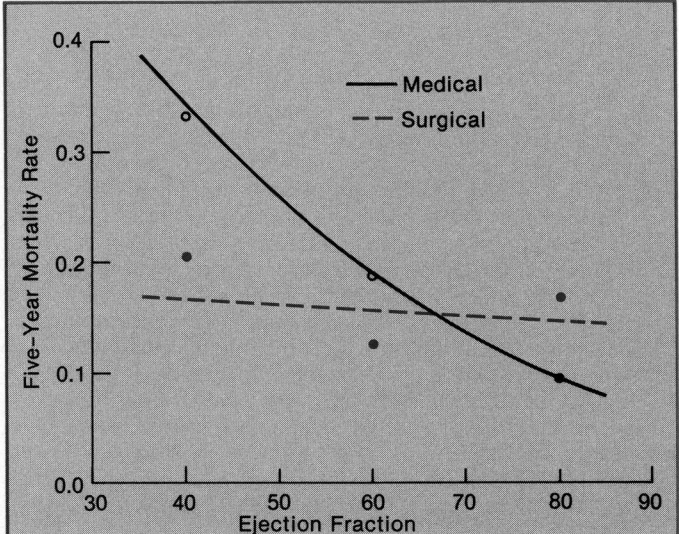

FIGURE 40–29. Mortality following medical and surgical treatment of unstable angina using ejection fraction as a continuous variable. Curves computed by logistic regression analysis based on 5-year mortality of 468 patients with unstable angina randomized to medical (open circles) and surgical (closed circles) therapy. The mean observed per cent mortality is illustrated for ejection fraction intervals 0.30–0.49, 0.50–0.69, and > 0.70. The worse the ejection fraction, the poorer the survival in medically treated patients; thus, surgery should be recommended for patients with unstable angina and reduced ejection fraction for three-vessel coronary artery disease suitable for surgical revascularization because it offers improved 5-year survival. (From Parisi A. F., et al.: Medical compared with surgical management of unstable angina: 5-year mortality and morbidity in the Veterans Administration Study. Circulation 80:1176, 1989, by permission of the American Heart Association, Inc.)

pared medical and surgical treatment for unstable angina pectoris,[552] no difference in 2-year mortality was seen in patients randomized to medical versus surgical therapy, although as is the case in patients with chronic stable angina, in patients with low ejection fractions surgical therapy conferred a survival advantage.[552] In patients with a left ventricular ejection fraction less than 50 per cent, the cumulative 3-year mortality for surgical patients was 6.1 per cent vs. 17.6 per cent for medical patients (p = 0.039), representing a 65-per-cent reduction in mortality with surgery.[553] Furthermore, at 5-year follow-up, patients with abnormal left ventricular function and three-vessel coronary disease had a survival of 75 per cent if treated medically and 89 per cent if treated surgically (Fig. 40–29).[554] The cumulative 5-year rate of repeat hospitalizations for cardiac reasons was lower in patients treated with surgery and the quality of their life appeared to be better.[554a] Interestingly, survival of patients whose ejection fractions were greater than 69 per cent was better with medical treatment.[553]

Thus, surgery appears to be the treatment of choice for patients with unstable angina pectoris, abnormal left ventricular function, and extensive CAD.[554] Risk factors for increased operative mortality in patients undergoing coronary artery bypass grafting for unstable angina include clinical and angiographic markers of left ventricular dysfunction[481,555] and the need for an intraaortic balloon for preoperative control of angina.[555] In patients who have postinfarction unstable angina, the independent predictors of perioperative mortality include the presence of an anterior transmural myocardial infarction and the need for preoperative intraaortic balloon pumping for either continuing angina or congestive heart failure.[539] In patients who have undergone coronary bypass grafting and later develop unstable angina, the risk of subsequent death and myocardial infarction is greater because they are less suitable candidates for further revascularization.[556]

The role of coronary arteriography and reperfusion and the timing of such therapy remain controversial. The choice of reperfusion technique depends on the findings in an individual patient, the local expertise, and experience. If a patient has received intensive medical therapy for a 48-hour period and there is persistent evidence of continuing ischemia, it is our policy to proceed with catheterization and coronary arteriography. Intraaortic balloon counterpulsation is often instituted either before or during cardiac catheterization if the patient exhibits any hemodynamic instability. If the patient has single-vessel disease and well-maintained left ventricular function, then PTCA is performed, if technically feasible. On the other hand, in patients in whom there is evidence of left main coronary disease, ventricular dysfunction, or multivessel disease and the anatomy is suitable for bypass grafting, operation is performed immediately.

Patients who respond to intensive medical therapy are gradually ambulated. If angina on mild effort recurs despite maximal medical therapy, coronary arteriography is performed, and PTCA or bypass grafting is carried out as in patients who did not respond to medical therapy initially. Patients who improve on medical management without recurrence of pain undergo exercise stress testing, often with [201]thallium, before hospital discharge. In many patients, the results of these tests will be positive and angiography is performed.[518] If the provocative tests are not indicative of high risk the patient may be discharged from the hospital.

PROGNOSIS

Unstable angina and acute myocardial infarction are closely related pathogenetically and clinically. While the majority of patients with acute myocardial infarction reported a prodrome of more intense or longer periods of angina, i.e., unstable angina shortly before infarction, the opposite is not the case, i.e., only a minority of patients with unstable angina pectoris develop early infarction. While patients with unstable angina may present difficult management problems, it is generally recognized that most *do not* in fact develop myocardial infarction over the short term. Documentation of all cardiac admissions to coronary and intensive care units in Hamilton, Ontario, over the 1-year period 1979–1980 revealed that in 811 patients admitted with unstable angina, hospital mortality was 1.5 per cent (compared with 17 per cent for acute myocardial infarction), 1-year mortality was 9.2 per cent (compared to 27 per cent for acute myocardial infarction), and only 16 per cent of the patients who died with unstable angina did so during the initial hospitalization. Repeat hospital admission occurred in 28 per cent of patients with unstable angina.[557] Patients with unstable angina who appear to have a worse prognosis and to be at high risk for adverse events while in the hospital include those of advanced age[518,557] with continuing rest pain and intracoronary thrombi,[493] and those with complex coronary morphology or multivessel disease.[493] Significant ischemia detected by Holter monitoring during hospitalization confers an immediate unfavorable outcome,[473,478,479] which extends to a follow-up of 2 years.[480]

Adverse events (death, myocardial infarction, or recurrent unstable angina) are most likely to occur in the first 2 to 4 months after discharge from the hospital.[479,480] Predischarge exercise testing shows that those patients whose exercise is limited by pain or who exhibit ST-segment depression or can achieve only a low rate-pressure product are likely to have a worse prognosis during 1 year of follow-up.[518] As already noted, revascularization is ordinarily the treatment of choice for patients presenting with unstable angina who are subsequently found to have abnormal ventricular function and extensive CAD[554]; 5-year survival is 75 per cent in such patients treated medically and 89 per cent if treated surgically.[554]

Variant Angina Pectoris (Prinzmetal's Angina)

In 1959, Prinzmetal et al. described an unusual syndrome of cardiac pain that occurs almost exclusively at rest, usually is *not* precipitated by physical exertion or emotional stress, and is associated with electrocardiographic ST-segment elevations.[558] This syndrome, now known as *Prinzmetal's*, or *variant*, *angina*, may be associated with acute myocardial infarction, severe cardiac arrhythmias, including ventricular tachycardia, and fibrillation, as well as sudden death.

MECHANISM

Variant angina pectoris has been demonstrated convincingly to be due to coronary artery spasm. The latter is a transient, abrupt, *marked* reduction in the diameter of an epicardial (or large septal) coronary artery resulting in myocardial ischemia in the absence of any preceding increases in myocardial oxygen demand (reflected in elevations of heart rate or blood pressure). This reduction in diameter can usually be reversed by nitroglycerin and can occur in either normal or diseased coronary arteries. The striking reduction in luminal diameter is usually focal and involves one or occasionally more than one site. The focal, severe vasospasm of Prinzmetal's angina should not be confused with vasoconstriction of both the large and small coronary resistance vessels, a normal response to stimuli such as cold exposure. The latter response is much less intense and occurs diffusely throughout the coronary vascular bed. In patients with Prinzmetal's angina, basal coronary artery tone may be increased. While responses to ergonovine and nitrates are greater in spastic segments of the coronary arteries, there is also hypersensitivity to vasoconstrictor stimuli throughout the entire coronary artery tree.[559] Sites of spasm in Prinzmetal's angina are often adjacent to atheromatous plaques. It has been suggested that in these patients the basic abnormality, i.e., coronary artery spasm, may be hypercontractility of the arterial wall associated with the atherosclerotic process itself.[560] Other mechanisms suggested include endothelial injury (which reverses the dilator response to a variety of stimuli, e.g., acetylcholine [p. 1169]), and hypercontractility of vascular smooth muscle due to vasoconstrictor mitogens, leukotrienes, serotonin,[560a] and higher local concentrations of blood-borne vasoconstrictors in areas of neovascularized atherosclerotic plaques.

During episodes of severe ischemia in patients with variant angina, coronary spasm associated with myocardial ischemia may induce stasis and result in fibrinogen-fibrin conversion in the coronary vessels with elevated levels of plasma fibrinopeptide A, an index of fibrin formation.[561] Furthermore, there appears to be a significant circadian variation in plasma levels of fibrinopeptide A, with the peak levels occurring from midnight to early morning in parallel with the frequency of the ischemic attacks in patients with variant angina.[562] Heparin suppressed the circadian variation and elevation of the plasma fibrinopeptide A levels but did *not* suppress the variant anginal attacks themselves. Therefore, increased plasma fibrinopeptide A levels, and thus, increased thrombin activity, appear to be the *result* rather than the *cause* of variant anginal attacks.[562] In support of the possibility that vasoactive substances may have a role in the pathogenesis of coronary spasm is the observation that an excessive number of mast cells have been noted in the adventitia of a vasospastic artery of a young patient succumbing to coronary artery spasm[563] and the occurrence of coronary artery spasm in carcinoid heart disease.[564]

Several studies suggest that magnesium ions play a role in the pathogenesis of attacks of variant angina. In patients with variant angina, magnesium sulfate has been shown to terminate cold-pressor–induced anginal attacks and prevent induction of further attacks.[565] Magnesium has also been shown to suppress variant anginal attacks induced by hyperventilation[566] and exercise.[567] Finally, in an anorexic patient with

intractable variant angina unresponsive to calcium antagonists and nitrates, intravenous magnesium sulfate prevented coronary spasm from being induced by ergonovine; subsequently, oral magnesium oxide stabilized the patient.[568]

Cocaine, which blocks the presynaptic uptake of the neurotransmitters norepinephrine and dopamine, not only causes alpha-adrenergically mediated coronary constriction when administered intranasally (near the dose used for topical anesthesia),[569] but there also appears to be a high incidence of spontaneous, silent myocardial ischemia in cocaine addicts (detected by Holter monitoring) during the early stages of withdrawal.[570] Obviously, clinicians must consider the possibility that coronary vasoconstriction may be mediated by therapeutic or illicit cocaine usage in patients with suspected coronary artery spasm.

CLINICAL MANIFESTATIONS

The history differs from that of typical angina; the principal finding is angina *at rest*. However, in contrast to the situation in many patients with unstable angina and the rest pain, the latter usually has not progressed from an earlier period in which pain occurred with decreasing levels of effort. Although exercise capacity is usually well preserved, some patients experience typical pain and ST-segment elevations not only at rest but during or after exertion as well. The anginal discomfort may be extremely severe, is generally referred to as "pain," and is accompanied by syncope, the latter presumably caused by arrhythmias. Attacks of variant angina tend to be clustered between midnight and 8 AM.[562] Patients studied with 48-hour Holter electrocardiograms, even those without clinically apparent angina pectoris, show more frequent abnormalities in the morning than in the afternoon.[571]

Clinical features do not reliably differentiate patients with Prinzmetal's angina with normal or mildly abnormal coronary arteriograms from those with fixed severe coronary obstruction. A large percentage of the latter are heavy smokers. This supports the observations that cigarette smoking may influence vasomotor tone.[572] These patients often have a combination of fixed-threshold exertion-induced angina with ST-segment depression and variant angina (rest angina with ST-segment elevation). Rarely, variant angina develops following coronary artery bypass grafting,[573] and coronary artery spasm has also been observed intraoperatively after the application of coronary vein grafts. In a few patients, variant angina appears to be a manifestation of a generalized vasospastic disorder associated with attacks of migraine and Raynaud's phenomenon and has been reported in association with aspirin-induced asthma.[574] Patients with Prinzmetal's angina tend to be younger than patients with chronic stable angina or unstable angina, and the male preponderance in the latter group is not evident.[575] In some patients there appears to be a distinct relationship between emotional distress and episodes of coronary vasospasm. Alcohol withdrawal may precipitate variant angina,[576] and alcohol administration may prevent coronary spasm.[577] Variant angina has been reported to be provoked by therapy with 5-fluorouracil[579,580] and by cyclophosphamide (p. 1759).[578]

Although patients with Prinzmetal's angina are often heavy cigarette smokers, on physical examination they do not usually exhibit the risk factors for coronary atherosclerosis. Cardiac examination is usually normal in the absence of ischemia (unless the patient has suffered a previous myocardial infarction) but often reveals signs of dyskinesis and impaired left ventricular function during episodes of myocardial ischemia.

ELECTROCARDIOGRAM. The key to the diagnosis of variant angina lies in the development of ST-segment elevations with pain (Fig. 40–30). In some patients, episodes of ST-segment depression follow episodes of ST-segment elevation and are associated with T-wave changes. The phenomenon of

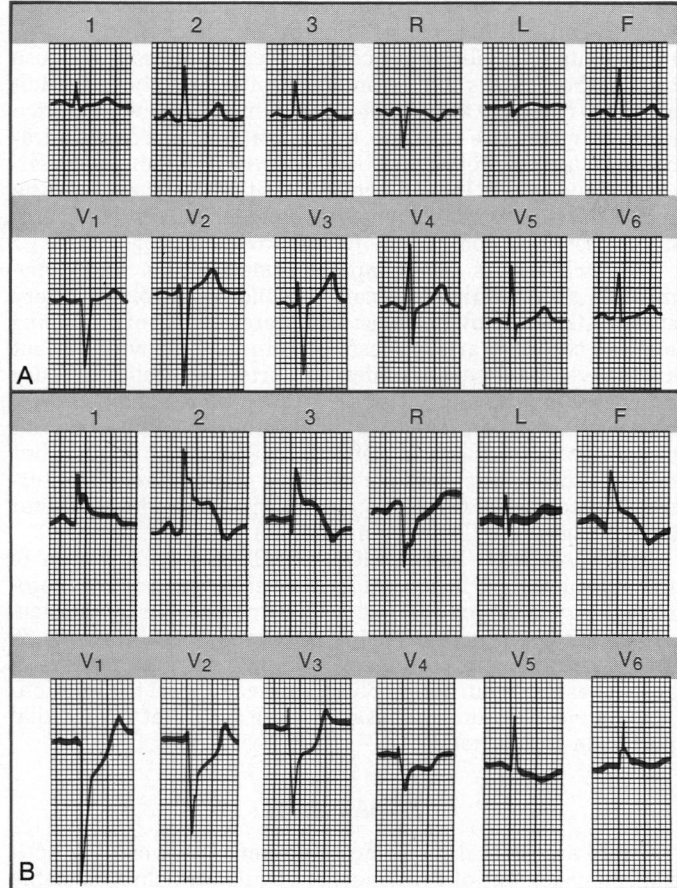

FIGURE 40–30. ECG **(A)** prior to an episode of Prinzmetal's angina and **(B)** during an episode of Prinzmetal's angina. ST segments are now markedly elevated in the inferior leads, with reciprocal depression in the anterior leads. After nitroglycerin was given, the electrocardiogram returned to baseline. (From Berman, N. D., et al.: Prinzmetal's angina with coronary artery spasm. Angiographic, pharmacologic, metabolic and radionuclide perfusion studies. Am. J. Med. 60:727, 1976.)

ST-segment and T-wave alternans[581] may be ominous (it is the result of ischemic conduction delay) and may be associated with potentially lethal ventricular arrhythmias.[582] The presence of R-wave "growth" may also be associated with the occurrence of ventricular arrhythmias.[583] Many patients exhibit multiple episodes of asymptomatic ST-segment deviation (silent ischemia). The ST-segment deviations may be present in any leads; however, the concurrent presence of ST-segment elevations in both the inferior and anterior leads (reflecting extensive ischemia) is associated with an increased risk of sudden death.[584]

Transient conduction disturbances may occur during episodes of ischemia.[585,586] The development of ventricular ectopic activity associated with episodes of spontaneous variant angina is always a serious clinical problem. Ventricular ectopic activity is more likely to be associated with ST-segment elevations,[587] is more frequent during longer episodes of ischemia, and is often associated with ST-segment and T-wave alternans.[583] Myocardial cell damage, as reflected by the release of small quantities of CK-MB, may occur in the absence of persistent electrocardiographic changes in patients with prolonged attacks of Prinzmetal's angina, and transient Q waves have been observed.[588]

Exercise testing in patients with variant angina is of limited value since the response is so variable. Approximately equal numbers of patients show ST-segment elevation, ST-segment depression, or no change in ST segments during exercise, reflecting the variability of the underlying fixed CAD in some patients, the absence of significant lesions in others, and the provocation of spasm by exercise in a few.

In contrast to the finding in patients with chronic stable (effort-induced) angina, episodes of Prinzmetal's angina often occur at rest or during mild exertion and are not usually preceded by increases in heart rate, arterial pressure, or myocardial contractility—all of which increase cardiac work or oxygen consumption. Spasm of a proximal coronary artery with resultant transmural ischemia, first postulated as the cause of variant angina, has been convincingly documented arteriographically (Fig. 9–62, p. 262). Exercise-induced ST-segment elevation can be associated with partial or total obstruction of large epicardial arteries in a manner similar to episodes observed during spontaneous or ergonovine-induced angina.[589,590] This suggests that coronary spasm may have a common mechanism despite being initiated by different stimuli. Echocardiographic studies performed during episodes of spontaneous variant angina have demonstrated abnormalities in ventricular function that precede the onset of symptoms of angina and electrocardiographic changes.[591]

The coronary anatomy in patients with Prinzmetal's angina has been defined both at autopsy and during coronary arteriography. Severe proximal coronary atherosclerosis of at least one major vessel occurs in approximately two-thirds of patients, and in them spasm usually occurs within 1 cm of the organic obstruction. The remainder have normal coronary arteries in the absence of ischemia. Spasm may occur at one or more sites in one artery or in multiple arteries simultaneously[592] and it is most common in the right coronary artery. Patients with variant angina with normal coronary arteriograms are more likely to have purely nonexertional angina and ST-segment elevations involving inferior leads. In contrast, patients with variant angina who have organic obstructive lesions with superimposed coronary artery spasm often have associated effort-induced angina and ischemia in anterolateral leads. Patients with no or mild fixed coronary obstruction tend to experience a more benign course than do patients with associated severe obstructive lesions.

THE ERGONOVINE TEST. A number of provocative tests for coronary spasm have been developed. Of these, the ergonovine test is the most sensitive and useful. Ergonovine maleate, an ergot alkaloid that stimulates both alpha-adrenergic and serotonergic receptors and therefore exerts a direct constrictive effect on vascular smooth muscle,[593] has been used to induce coronary artery spasm in patients with Prinzmetal's angina. Coronary arteries that constrict spontaneously appear to be abnormally sensitive to this agent. When administered intravenously in doses ranging from 0.05 to 0.40 mg, ergonovine provides a sensitive and specific test for provoking coronary artery spasm.[594] There is some correlation between the dose of ergonovine required to induce a positive test and the frequency of spontaneous attacks.[595] In low doses and in carefully controlled clinical situations, ergonovine is a relatively safe drug, but prolonged coronary artery spasm precipitated by ergonovine may cause myocardial infarction. Because of this hazard, it is recommended that ergonovine be administered only to patients in whom coronary arteriography has demonstrated normal or nearly normal coronary arteries and in gradually increasing doses, beginning with a very low dose.

The ergonovine test should be carried out only in a setting where appropriate resuscitative equipment, drugs, and personnel are readily available, usually in the cardiac catheterization laboratory, so that the angiographic diagnosis of spasm can be made and intracoronary nitroglycerin can be administered to abolish the spasm. Some investigators have also found that the ergonovine test can be carried out safely in the coronary care unit, with a positive test being reflected in the development of chest pain and ST-segment elevation; however, the safety of the test in this setting has not been firmly established. The normal response of the coronary arterial bed to larger doses (0.40 mg) of ergonovine is a diffuse reduction in arterial caliber by approximately 30 per cent.

In patients whose atypical chest pain is being evaluated (in

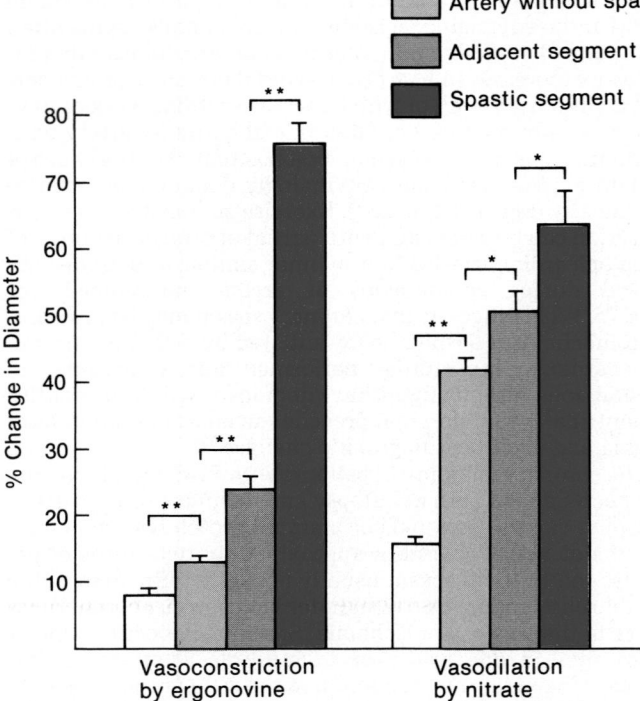

FIGURE 40-31. **Changes in coronary artery tone in patients with coronary spasm in response to ergonovine and nitrates.** A retrospective analysis was performed involving 159 patients who had undergone diagnostic coronary angiography with the ergonovine provocative test and who had normal coronary arteries or fixed lesions with < 40 per cent diameter reduction after nitrate administration. Per cent vasoconstriction after ergonovine (left panel) and vasodilation after nitrates (right panel) were compared among the spastic segments, adjacent segments, and segments of the coronary arteries without spasm in the vasospastic angina group, and the combined segments in the non-angina group. * P < 0.05; ** P < 0.01. Thus, in patients with vasospastic angina, coronary artery responses to both ergonovine and nitrate were greater in the spastic segments than in other segments. (From Hoshio, A., et al.: Significance of coronary artery tone in patients with vasospastic angina. Reprinted with permission of the American College of Cardiology. J. Am. Coll. Cardiol. *14*:604, 1989.)

Legend for figure:
- Non-angina group
- Artery without spasm
- Adjacent segment
- Spastic segment

the absence of a strongly positive exercise test and of evidence of organic coronary artery obstruction) who do *not* have Prinzmetal's angina, sequential intravenous bolus infusions of ergonovine maleate result in progressive nonspecific reductions in coronary dimensions. These vasoconstrictor responses appear to be accentuated in women and in patients with intimal coronary arteriographic irregularities suggesting the existence of minor atherosclerotic disease.[596] This dose-dependent phenomenon differs from the abnormal response in Prinzmetal's angina, which is characterized by severe focal spasm, usually at much lower doses of the agent (Fig. 40-31). The sensitivity of the ergonovine test is high in patients with active disease (who have at least one attack daily) and lower in patients with sporadic episodes of variant angina.[597]

HYPERVENTILATION. This stimulus has also been demonstrated to provoke some episodes of variant angina,[561,566,568,593,597,598] electrocardiographic ST-segment elevations,[561,568,597,598] angiographic evidence of coronary artery spasm,[593] and ventricular arrhythmias.[593,597,598] In patients with active disease who have at least one daily attack of variant angina, the sensitivity of hyperventilation was 95 per cent compared with 100 per cent for ergonovine. However, in patients with sporadic attacks of angina, hyperventilation has a lower sensitivity than ergonovine and, therefore, a limited diagnostic value.[597]

ACETYLCHOLINE. Intracoronary injections of acetylcholine have been shown to induce severe coronary spasm in patients with variant angina. (This should not be confused with the mild diffuse constriction that acetylcholine induces in patients with abnormal coronary endothelium.) Because this method allows induction of spasm separately in the left and right coronary arteries, it is useful in patients with known multivessel disease or spasm. In such patients, the use of intracoronary acetylcholine has been shown to be sensitive, reliable,[599] and safe.[600] Indeed, the sensitivity (90 per cent) and the specificity (99 per cent) of acetylcholine for induction of coronary spasm[599] is comparable to ergonovine testing.

Methacholine, a parasympathomimetic drug, and *dopamine*,[601] a catecholamine, can also induce coronary artery spasm. Like ergonovine, these agents are capable of producing marked coronary artery spasm both in patients with variant angina who have severe underlying arteriosclerotic coronary artery narrowing and in those without such fixed stenoses. Exercise, the cold pressor test, and induced alkalosis can all cause coronary spasm in patients with variant angina, but none of these tests is as sensitive as ergonovine. Catheter-induced coronary ostial spasm is nonspecific and not helpful in the diagnosis of Prinzmetal's angina.

MYOCARDIAL PERFUSION STUDIES. Localization of the myocardial perfusion defect to an area perfused by a coronary artery in which spasm can be demonstrated by arteriography has been reported using intravenous thallium-201,[602] and a reduction in coronary sinus flow during episodes of spasm has also been noted. These studies support the relationship between coronary spasm and the resultant myocardial perfusion and ischemia.

MANAGEMENT

There are several important differences between the optimal management of Prinzmetal's angina and chronic stable angina.

1. Patients with both forms of angina usually respond well to nitrates; sublingual or intravenous nitroglycerin often abolishes attacks of variant angina promptly, and long-acting nitrates are useful in preventing attacks.[603] However, the mechanism of action of the drugs may differ in the two types of angina. As already discussed (p. 1305), in chronic (effort-induced) stable angina, one important action of the nitrates appears to involve reducing myocardial oxygen needs. In Prinzmetal's angina, the nitrates abolish or prevent myocardial ischemia by exerting a direct vasodilating effect on the spastic coronary arteries.

2. In patients with chronic stable angina pectoris, beta-adrenoceptor blockade is usually beneficial, but the response in patients with Prinzmetal's angina is variable. Some, particularly those with associated fixed lesions, exhibit a reduction in the frequency of exertion-induced angina caused primarily by augmentation of myocardial oxygen requirements. In others, however, propranolol or any nonselective beta-adrenoceptor blocker may actually be detrimental, since blockade of the beta$_2$ receptors, which subserve coronary dilation, allows unopposed alpha-receptor–mediated coronary artery vasoconstriction to occur; the duration of episodes of vasotonic angina can be prolonged by propranolol.

3. In contrast to beta blockers, the calcium antagonists have been found to be extremely effective in preventing the coronary artery spasm of variant angina.[575,604] These drugs, along with long- and short-acting nitrates, are the mainstay of therapy in Prinzmetal's angina. Similar efficacy rates have been noted for nifedipine, diltiazem, and verapamil. Rarely, a patient will respond to only one of these three agents, and even less commonly simultaneous administration of two or even three antagonists is required.[605] A multicenter trial with nifedipine has shown dramatic reductions in the frequency of episodes and in the need for nitroglycerin. Because calcium antagonists act through a different mechanism than do nitrates, the vasodilatory actions of these classes of drugs may be additive. There have been reports suggesting a rebound of symptoms when nifedipine, verapamil, and diltiazem[606] are

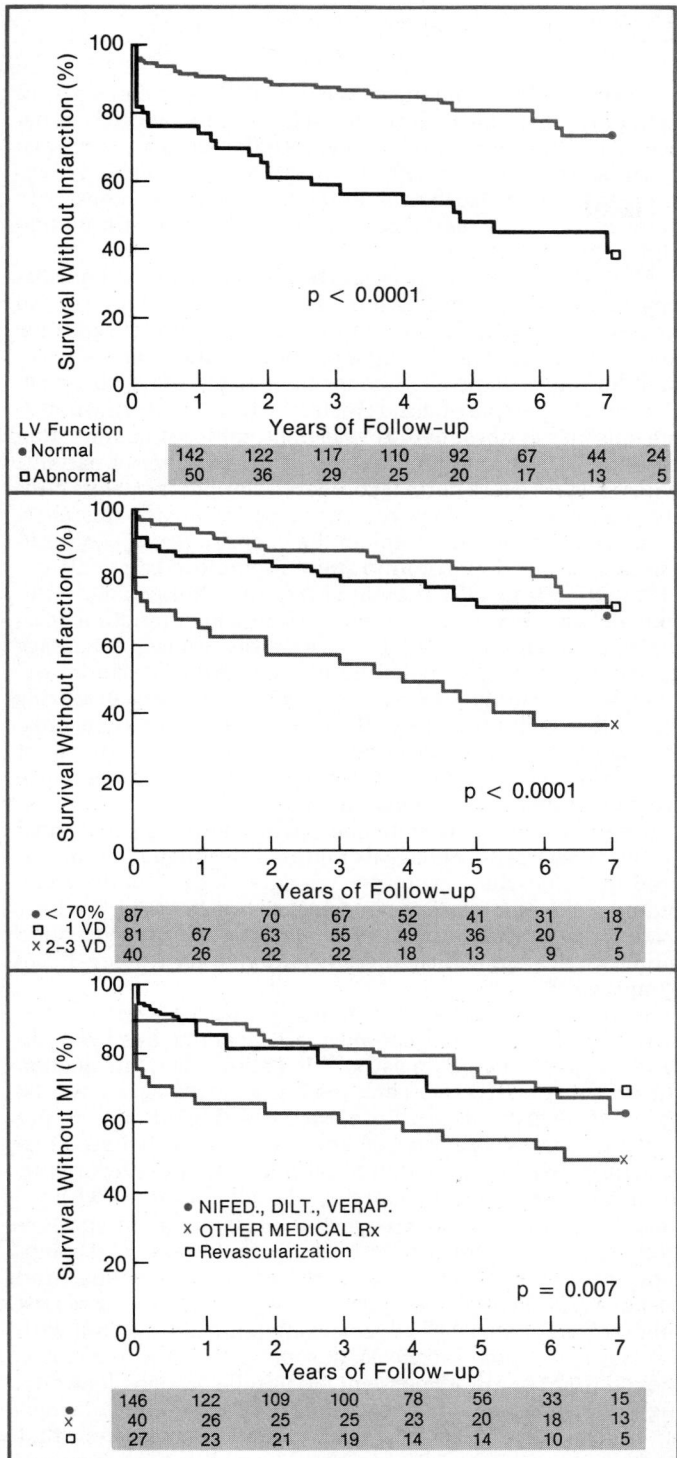

discontinued. Calcium antagonists ordinarily should be used in maximally tolerated doses.

The *natural history* of Prinzmetal's angina is characterized by cyclic periods of frequent spasm that alternate with asymptomatic periods. After 6 to 12 months of therapy, gradual tapering of the calcium antagonist with careful observation may be considered. Complete remission of variant angina, documented by both Holter recordings and ergonovine testing, has been demonstrated typically in patients who have had a shorter duration of symptoms and who have either shown normal or nonsignificantly diseased coronary arteries.[607]

4. *Prazosin*, a selective alpha-adrenoceptor blocker (p. 864), has also been found to be of value in patients with Prinzmetal's angina.[608] Aspirin, helpful in unstable angina (p. 1340), may actually increase the severity of ischemic episodes in patients with Prinzmetal's angina, because aspirin in high dosage inhibits biosynthesis of the naturally occurring coronary vasodilator prostaglandin I_2.[609] Provocation of asthma and variant angina by aspirin in the same patient has been reported.[574]

5. PTCA may be helpful in patients with variant angina[610] who have discrete proximal noncalcified obstructive lesions in a single major coronary artery. Calcium antagonists should be continued for at least 6 months following successful angioplasty. In patients with isolated coronary artery spasm without accompanying obstructive disease, PTCA and coronary artery bypass surgery are *not* indicated. In patients with Prinzmetal's angina who require coronary artery bypass surgery because of significant organic narrowings of the coronary arteries, the addition of verapamil to the priming solution for bypass appears to be effective in preventing perioperative coronary vasospasm.[611] Furthermore, internal mammary artery bypass grafts do not appear to show the hyperreactivity of the coronary arteries of patients with variant angina.[612]

PROGNOSIS

Many patients with Prinzmetal's angina go through an acute, active phase, with frequent episodes of angina and cardiac events during the first 6 months after their presentation. Over this period, nonfatal myocardial infarction occurs in up to 20 per cent of patients and death in up to 10 per cent.[613,614] Patients with variant angina who develop serious arrhythmias, ventricular tachycardia, ventricular fibrillation, high-degree atrioventricular block, or asystole during spontaneous episodes of pain have higher maximal ST-segment elevations and are at a higher risk for sudden death.[615] Patients with severe obstructive coronary artery lesions are at greater risk for persistent anginal symptoms, acute myocardial infarction, and death.[613,614] In most patients who survive an infarction or the initial 3- to 6-month period, the condition stabilizes and there is a tendency for symptoms and cardiac events to diminish with time. In patients who experience such remissions, cautious tapering or discontinuation of calcium antagonists may be attempted. For reasons that are not clear, some patients, after a relatively quiescent period of months or even years, experience a recrudescence of vasospastic activity with frequent and severe episodes of ischemia. Fortunately these patients respond to re-treatment with calcium antagonists.

Long-term survival at 5 years is excellent (89 to 97 per cent).[616,617] The extent and severity of CAD[614,616,617] and the activity of the disease[616,617] have an adverse influence on long-term survival free of myocardial infarction (Fig. 40–32). Calcium antagonist therapy improves long-term survival.[617] Overall patients without significant obstructive CAD have an excellent prognosis.[618]

FIGURE 40–32. Event-free 7-year survival of patients with variant angina; 217 consecutive patients with variant angina were observed for 7 years. Top panel: Survival without myocardial infarction is compared in patients with normal (closed circle) and abnormal (open squares) left ventricular function. The number of patients completing each year without an endpoint event are listed. Middle panel: Survival without infarction in patients with no stenoses of 70 per cent or greater (closed circles), those with one-vessel disease (open squares), and those with multivessel involvement (X 2-3 VD). Bottom panel: Influence of treatment on survival without infarction. Patients initially treated with nifedipine, diltiazem, or verapamil (closed circles) had a better outcome than patients receiving other medical treatment (X). Too few patients underwent bypass surgery or coronary angioplasty (open square, revascularization) to assess the value of these interventions. Thus, impaired ventricular function, the presence of multivessel coronary artery disease, and medical therapy not including calcium antagonists were all adverse factors for long-term survival in patients with variant angina. (From Walling, A., et al.: Long-term prognosis of patients with variant angina. Circulation 76:990, 1987, by permission of the American Heart Association, Inc.)

Chest Pain With Normal Coronary Arteriogram

The syndrome of angina or angina-like chest pain with a normal coronary arteriogram is an important clinical entity to be differentiated from classic ischemic heart disease caused by coronary atherosclerosis.[619] In this condition, sometimes referred to as *syndrome X*, the prognosis is usually excellent[620-621a]—contrasted with that in patients with coronary atherosclerosis—and its recognition is of clinical importance. Patients with chest pain who have normal coronary arteriograms may constitute as many as 10 to 20 per cent of those undergoing coronary arteriography because of the strong suspicion of angina. The cause of the syndrome is unknown. True myocardial ischemia, reflected in the production of lactate by the myocardium during exercise or pacing, is present in some of these patients.[622]

INADEQUATE VASODILATOR RESERVE (see also p. 1173). Several studies suggest that many patients with chest pain with angiographically normal coronary arteries and no evidence of large vessel spasm, even after an ergonovine challenge, demonstrate an abnormally reduced capacity to decrease coronary resistance and increase coronary flow in response to atrial pacing.[623] This abnormality appears to affect the smaller resistance vessels that are not visible angiographically, while the large proximal conductance vessels appear to be normal. This abnormal vasodilator reserve may be associated with exercise-induced regional wall-motion abnormalities and abnormalities of resting diastolic function.[624] Such patients, with low coronary flow reserve, may exhibit abnormalities of myocardial perfusion detectable noninvasively with positron emission tomography.[625] Some patients have an abnormally reduced dilator response of distal coronary arteries to the physiological dilator stimulus of exercise and also a reduced dilator capacity of the resistance vessels following administration of dipyridamole.[626] This same patient population also has an impairment of vasodilator reserve in forearm vessels[627] and airway hyperresponsiveness,[627a] suggesting that not only is their coronary circulation affected but also their peripheral arterial circulation.

In patients with hypertension and secondary left ventricular hypertrophy with angina pectoris and a normal coronary arteriogram, a reduced coronary blood flow response to dipyridamole has been observed. Similarly, patients with dilated cardiomyopathy and angiographically normal coronary arteries also exhibit impaired vasodilator responses to both rapid atrial pacing and pharmacological stimuli with an increased sensitivity to the vasoconstrictor effects of ergonovine.[628] Other patients with angina and normal coronary arteries are found on extensive investigation to have a cardiomyopathy—either hypertrophic[629] or dilated—and in these cases reduced perfusion, especially of the subendocardium, may be responsible for myocardial ischemia and angina. This finding correlates well with the autopsy observation of thickening of the walls of the coronary arterioles in hypertrophy obstructive cardiomyopathy.[630]

OTHER CAUSES. Patients with psychogenic chest pain, neurocirculatory asthenia, and DaCosta syndrome may also manifest chest pain and have normal coronary arteries.

CLINICAL FEATURES. The syndrome of angina or angina-like chest pain with normal large coronary arteries occurs more frequently in women, while obstructive CAD is found more commonly in men. Fewer than half of the patients with chest pain and normal coronary arteriograms have typical angina pectoris; the majority have a variety of forms of atypical chest pain.

In some patients with minimal or no coronary disease, an exaggerated preoccupation with personal health is associated with continued chest pain,[631] and panic disorder may account for a proportion of such patients.[632] Bass and Wade found that two-thirds of patients with chest pain and normal coronary arteries have predominantly psychiatric disorders.[633] Others

have reported that the incidence of CAD is extremely low in patients with atypical chest pain who are anxious and/or depressed.[634] At the time of cardiac catheterization, it has been observed that patients with syndrome X seem unusually sensitive to intracardiac instrumentation, with typical chest pain being consistently produced by direct right atrial stimulation and saline infusion.[635]

PHYSICAL AND LABORATORY FINDINGS. Abnormal physical findings indicative of ischemia, such as precordial bulges, gallop sounds, and murmurs of mitral regurgitation, are uncommon. The resting electrocardiogram may be normal, but nonspecific ST-T abnormalities are often observed. Commonly, perusal of serial electrocardiograms during multiple episodes of chest pain reveals no significant change from baseline. A minority, approximately 20 per cent of patients with chest pain and normal coronary arteriograms, have positive exercise tests. However, many patients with this chest pain syndrome fail to complete the exercise test, discontinuing because of fatigue or mild chest discomfort. Left ventricular function is usually normal at rest and after pacing,[622] unlike the situation in obstructive CAD in which function often becomes impaired during stress. However, a small percentage of patients with chest pain and normal coronary arteries exhibit lactate production and ST-segment depression during exercise (signifying ischemia). Some patients show abnormal myocardial perfusion reserve,[625] but there is no consistent pattern of abnormal myocardial blood flow, although coronary vasodilator reserve may be impaired.[623,624]

In patients with persistent chest pain syndrome and normal coronary arteries, esophageal abnormalities should be considered (p. 1295). Such patients may show either motility disorders of the esophagus or abnormal reflux. In patients whose experience of chest pain coincides with documented reflux, either surgical or medical therapy may give gratifying relief of symptoms.[636]

Important prognostic information on patients with either normal or near-normal coronary arteriograms has been obtained from the CASS Registry.[621] In patients with an ejection fraction of at least 50 per cent, the 7-year survival rate was 96 per cent for patients with a normal arteriogram and 92 per cent for those whose arteriographic study revealed mild disease (less than 50 per cent luminal stenosis). In such patients, an ischemic response to exercise was not associated with increased mortality although a history of smoking or hypertension was. Over follow-up periods of 4 to 6 years,[637,638] symptoms of angina, exercise test evidence of ischemia, and 24-hour ST-segment monitoring of ischemia can all persist relatively unchanged,[637] adversely affecting life style but with a seemingly benign prognosis. In some patients who have either constant or rate-dependent left bundle branch block during exercise there is significant deterioration of left ventricular function over a several-year follow-up, suggesting that they may comprise a subgroup of patients with a cardiomyopathy.[638] Inhibition of adenosine receptors by aminophylline appears to exert a beneficial effect on exercise-induced chest pain and ischemia-like electrocardiographic changes in patients with syndrome X.[639]

In *summary*, there are a number of possible explanations in patients having chest pain and normal coronary arteriograms. Sometimes review of angiography will reveal that significant CAD actually does exist (i.e., incorrect interpretation of angiograms with a false-negative result). When there is no evidence of coronary artery narrowing, even after ergonovine, other causes of pain may be defined (e.g., esophageal disease, mitral valve prolapse syndrome), although often other causes cannot be found even after exhaustive tests. However, a group of patients exists who have normal coronary arteries, symptoms of angina, evidence of ischemia, and abnormal coronary flow reserve with exercise.

MANAGEMENT. This should focus on the explanation of the relatively benign nature of the condition to the patient, psychological counseling, and analgesics to provide pain relief. Calcium antagonists appear to be effective in reducing the frequency and severity of angina and improving exercise tolerance in most patients with chest pain resulting from abnormal vasodilator reserve.[640] Aminophylline administration may be useful in some patients.[639] However, some patients continue to remain disabled with long-term chest discomfort. This can lead to multiple medical consultations and be responsible for a great deal of anxiety. Behavioral therapy may teach the patient with pain how to function more effectively, although unfortunately chronic symptoms may persist.

Ischemic Heart Disease in Which Discomfort Is Not The Dominant Symptom

SILENT MYOCARDIAL ISCHEMIA

There appear to be two forms of silent myocardial ischemia. The first and less common form, designated type I silent ischemia, occurs in patients with severe CAD who do not experience angina at any time; indeed, some of these patients do not even experience pain in the course of myocardial infarction. Epidemiological studies of sudden death (p. 756), clinical and postmortem studies of patients with silent myocardial infarction, and studies of patients with chronic angina pectoris suggest that many individuals with extensive coronary artery obstruction do not have angina pectoris in any of its recognized forms (stable, unstable, or variant).[641] These individuals, representative of type I silent ischemia, may be considered to have a defective anginal "warning system." Both the patient and physician may be unaware of the presence of ischemic heart disease until a fatal event ensues or an old infarction is detected on routine electrocardiogram. The second and much more frequent form, designated type II silent ischemia, occurs in patients with the usual forms of chronic stable angina, unstable angina, or Prinzmetal's angina. When carefully monitored, patients with type II are shown to have some episodes of ischemia that are associated with chest discomfort and other episodes that are not—i.e., episodes of silent ischemia. The term "total ischemic burden" refers to all episodes of myocardial ischemia, both symptomatic and asymptomatic.[642,642a]

During long-term follow-up in the Framingham Study, one-quarter of patients who developed myocardial infarction had unrecognized infarctions, detected only by pathological Q waves on routine 2-yearly electrocardiogram, and of these approximately half were truly silent.[63] In other patients, a myocardial infarction is the first clinical manifestation of ischemic heart disease, although postmortem or angiographic studies indicate that severe coronary atherosclerosis must have existed prior to the infarction yet the patient had never complained of angina. Such patients with silent ischemia may be identified prior to such an event because of cardiac arrhythmias or abnormal electrocardiograms (occasionally at rest, more commonly during exercise) or by means of coronary arteriography performed as a result of a positive exercise test.

AMBULATORY ELECTROCARDIOGRAPHY. The extensive use of ambulatory electrocardiographic monitoring has led to a greater appreciation of the frequency of "silent" ischemia.[642a] It has become apparent that anginal pain is a poor indicator of, and underestimator of, the frequency of significant cardiac ischemia.[642] Episodic hemodynamic changes indicative of myocardial ischemia (increasing left ventricular end-diastolic pressure and decreasing left ventricular ejection fraction with exercise) occur in patients with CAD, irrespective of the occurrence of angina pectoris.[643] Ambulatory studies in patients with chronic stable angina have also emphasized that, while increases in myocardial oxygen demand lead to ischemia, in many episodes of ischemia, both symptomatic and silent, heart rate is *not* accelerated and arterial pressure does *not* rise, suggesting that reductions in myocardial supply make an important contribution to the initiation of ischemia in such patients.[644] With the use of frequency-modulated ambulatory electrocardiographic recordings, it has been found that transient ST-segment depression of 0.1 mV or greater that lasts for more than 30 seconds is a very rare finding in normal subjects.[645] However, in patients known to have CAD there is a strong correlation between such transient ST-segment depression and independent measurements of regional myocardial perfusion and ischemia using rubidium-82 uptake measured by positron-emission tomography.[15] Perfusion defects occurred in the same myocardial segment during painful and silent episodes of ST-segment depression. These responses were significantly different from those observed in normal subjects studied similarly (Fig. 40–33).

Analyses of ambulatory electrocardiograms in patients with angina (exertion induced, and occurring at rest) suggest that the majority of ischemic episodes occurring during normal daily activities are asymptomatic (Fig. 40–34) (type II silent ischemia). Episodes of ST-segment depression, both symptomatic and silent, exhibit a circadian rhythm and are more common in the morning.[646] Nocturnal ST-segment changes are almost invariably an indicator of two- or three-vessel CAD or left main stem stenosis.[647]

MECHANISM OF SILENT ISCHEMIA. It is unclear why some episodes of myocardial ischemia are silent while others are symptomatic. It has been suggested that patients who have no episodes of symptomatic ischemia have a higher pain threshold.[16] Some, although not all, studies suggest that silent episodes may reflect less severe ischemia with less evidence of left ventricular dysfunction.[476] Among patients who experience both symptomatic and asymptomatic ischemia, the ST-segment changes recorded by ambulatory electrocardiographic monitoring are similar, although there is a tendency for symptomatic episodes to be accompanied by longer periods of ST-segment deviation and more marked ST depressions[647]; however, there is considerable overlap between symptomatic and asymptomatic episodes. In keeping with the increased incidence of silent myocardial infarction in patients with diabetes mellitus, there is a greater incidence of asymptomatic ischemia in patients with CAD and type II diabetes mellitus than in nondiabetic patients.[648]

Smokers with CAD may have profound asymptomatic disturbances of regional myocardial perfusion and ST-segment depressions during smoking.[649] Mental stress can also induce silent myocardial ischemia in patients with CAD.[650] Pharmacological agents that reduce or abolish episodes of symptomatic ischemia, i.e., nitrates, beta blockers[651] and calcium antagonists,[642] also reduce or abolish episodes of silent ischemia. It is not clear whether abolition of silent ischemia should be the endpoint of therapy and whether this will influence prognosis favorably, but patients with continuing ischemia despite treatment have a high risk of cardiac death.[652] Monitoring of patients with unstable angina pectoris also identifies a subset of patients with a worse long-term prognosis.[478–480] Elderly men frequently have asymptomatic silent ischemia, and if during these episodes they have ST-segment depressions greater than 0.1 mV, they have a higher relative risk of fatal or nonfatal myocardial infarction. When they also have a history

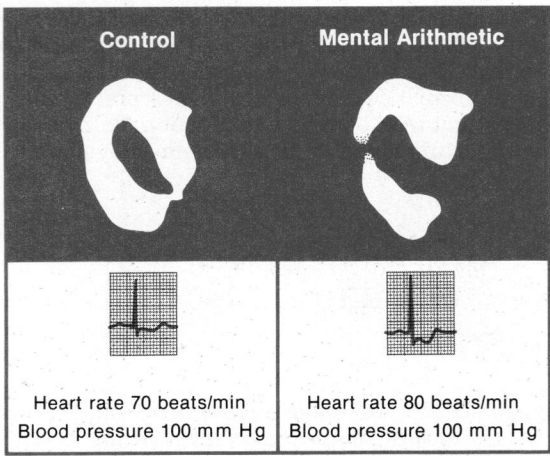

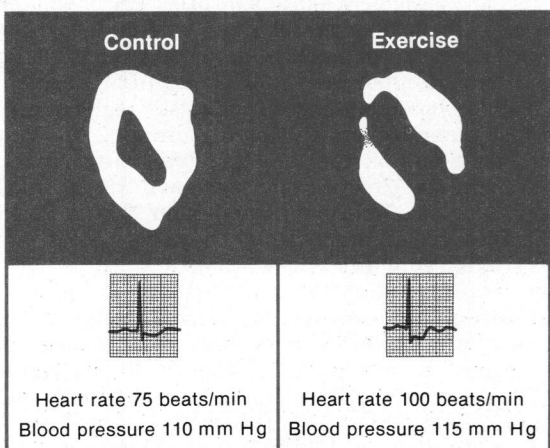

FIGURE 40–33. Tomographic slices of the myocardium recorded using positron-emission tomography in a patient with chronic stable angina, a positive exercise test, and proven coronary artery disease. The information from the heart is obtained from the short-lived tracer rubidium-82, which provides a measure of the distribution and changes in regional myocardial perfusion. The first image (control, *top left*) shows uniform perfusion to the posterior wall, free wall, anterior wall, and septum of the left ventricle. Regional myocardial perfusion during mental arithmetic *(top right)* shows a regional decrease in myocardial perfusion to the left ventricular free wall accompanied by ST-segment depression but not associated with chest pain. The second control image *(bottom left)* shows a return of myocardial perfusion to normal. During exercise *(bottom right)* there is recurrence of ischemia in the same area of the myocardium in which a perfusion abnormality occurred during the stress of mental arithmetic. With exercise, there were both ST-segment depression and symptoms of angina pectoris. Thus in this patient the ischemia provoked by mental arithmetic (asymptomatic) and exercise (symptomatic) showed similar ST-segment depression and myocardial perfusion abnormalities. (From Deanfield, J. E., et al.: Silent myocardial ischemia due to mental stress. Lancet 2:1001, 1984.)

of CAD, the risk is even greater.[653] In patients with stable CAD and positive exercise tests for myocardial ischemia, the presence of ischemia on ambulatory monitoring is a significant additional predictor of adverse outcome (Fig. 40–35).[654] Asymptomatic patients with positive thallium exercise tests have been treated in an uncontrolled manner with PTCA as the primary therapy for silent ischemia; whether this approach has any merit will be unknown until the results of controlled clinical trials become available.[655]

DETECTION. As of this writing, the detection of patients with CAD without angina (type I silent ischemia) is largely fortuitous. It is likely that screening of populations on a mass basis for silent ischemia would be extraordinarily costly. In Norway, an effort to detect such patients was carried out using a combination of screening techniques (questionnaires, resting and exercise electrocardiograms) in over 2000 asymptomatic and presumably healthy men aged 40 to 50 years.[656]

Overall, less than 4 per cent of this population had silent myocardial ischemia, with more than 75 per cent luminal stenosis of one or more coronary arteries. This figure is close to the 4 to 5 per cent of the population estimated by others to be the size of this subgroup.[641] Exercise testing appears to identify the majority of patients likely to have significant ischemia during their daily activities[657,657a] and remains the most important screening test for significant CAD (p. 167).

However, many patients with type I asymptomatic ischemia have been identified because of an asymptomatic positive exercise electrocardiogram obtained following myocardial infarction[658] or asymptomatic ST-segment deviation on an ambulatory (Holter) electrocardiogram.[659] In these patients with a defective anginal warning system it would appear to be useful to obtain coronary arteriograms. Consideration should be given to eliminating silent ischemia by antiischemic pharmacotherapy (nitrates, beta blockers, and Ca^{++} antagonists).[659a] If frequent episodes persist despite optimal drug therapy, critically obstructive lesions may be treated by revascularization (PTCA or surgery) so that severe asymptomatic ischemia is not induced repeatedly during normal life. Whether or not such an approach will improve survival has yet to be determined.

HEART FAILURE

Manifestations of congestive heart failure are common in patients with CAD, but it may be the dominant feature in some patients, especially those who have sustained prior myocardial infarctions and in whom the ischemic focus may have become replaced by fibrous scar, with disappearance or reduction of the angina. The three most common causes of congestive heart failure are (1) left ventricular aneurysm, (2) mitral regurgitation due to papillary muscle dysfunction, and (3) an inadequate quantity of normally contracting myocardium. The last may be secondary to extensive myocardial infarction, a large quantity of viable but "hibernating" myocardium, multiple scars and patchy fibrous replacement of myocardium, or a combination of these.

LEFT VENTRICULAR ANEURYSM

This is usually defined as a segment of the ventricular wall that exhibits paradoxical (dyskinetic) systolic expansion. It involves almost exclusively the left ventricle, most commonly

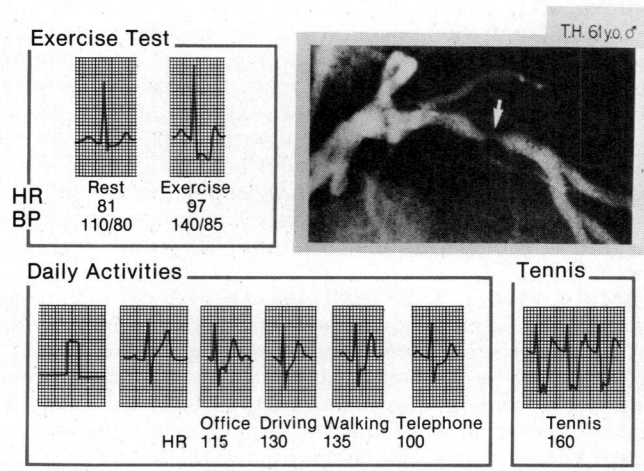

FIGURE 40–34. The ambulatory ECGs and coronary angiograms of a severe left anterior descending stenosis in a patient with fatigue (but not angina) during a tennis match. In stage II of a treadmill exercise test (Bruce protocol), 4 mm of ST-segment depression were seen in lead V_5. Ambulatory Holter monitoring of lead V_5 demonstrates ischemic ST-segment depressions during a number of ordinary activities, e.g., walking, telephoning. During a game of tennis, marked ST-segment depression was recorded when the patient was asymptomatic. (From Nabel, E. G., et al.: Characteristics and significance of ischemia detected by ambulatory electrocardiographic monitoring. Circulation 75[Suppl. II]:74, 1987, by permission of the American Heart Association, Inc.)

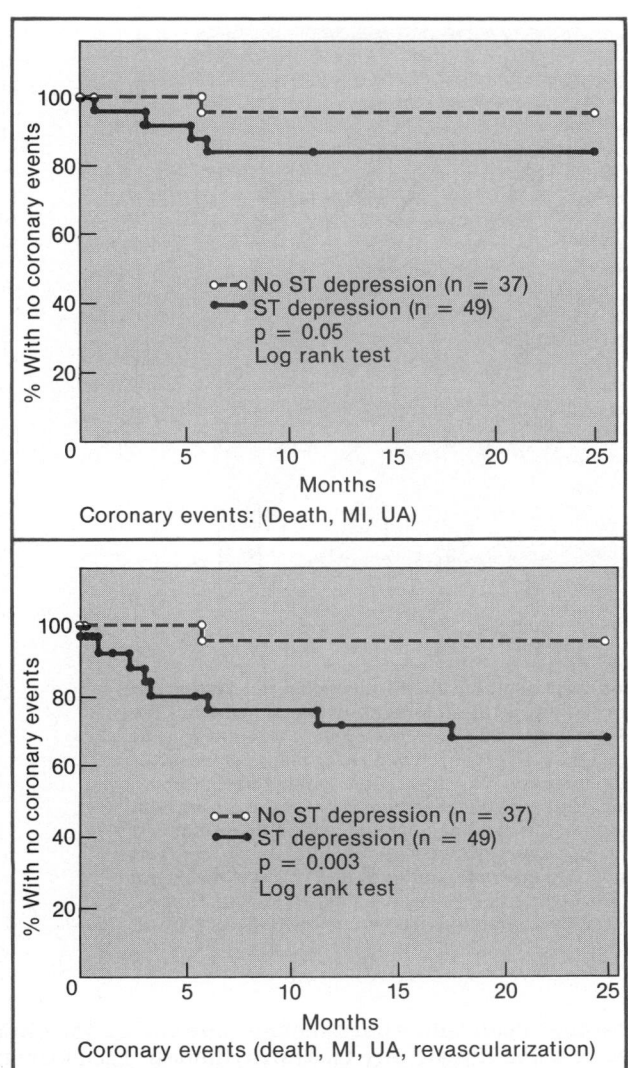

FIGURE 40–35. Prognostic importance of silent ischemia in patients with stable coronary artery disease. Ambulatory monitoring of the ECG was performed in 86 patients with stable coronary artery disease and positive exercise tests for myocardial ischemia. Monitoring was performed after withdrawal of antianginal medications. Prospective follow-up was obtained during routine medical care as prescribed by physicians who were unaware of the monitor results. Kaplan-Meier curves comparing the probability of not experiencing (top panel) an acute ischemic event (death, myocardial infarction, unstable angina), and (bottom panel) progressive ischemic events (acute events or revascularization for worsening symptoms) during follow-up for the 37 patients without ST-segment depression (open circles) and the 49 patients with ST-segment depression (closed circles) as detected by ambulatory monitoring. The presence of ischemia detected by ambulatory monitoring in patients with stable symptoms was common and identified a high-risk group for the development of subsequent unfavorable outcomes while receiving routine medical treatments. (From Rocco, M. B., et al.: Prognostic importance of myocardial ischemia detected by ambulatory monitoring in patients with stable coronary artery disease. Circulation 78:877, 1988, by permission of the American Heart Association, Inc.)

the anterior or apical segments. In vitro length-tension studies of tissue taken from human ventricular aneurysms have demonstrated that chronic fibrous aneurysms interfere with ventricular performance principally through loss of contractile tissue and that the extent of expansion and "lost work" by the normal left ventricle is minor. These might be considered to be anatomical aneurysms (Fig. 40–36). In contrast, aneurysms made up largely of a mixture of scar tissue and viable myocardium or of thin scar tissue produce a mechanical disadvantage by a combination of paradoxical expansion and loss of effective contraction; these might be considered to be functional

aneurysms. *False aneurysms* (pseudoaneurysms), which represent localized myocardial rupture, in which the hemorrhage is limited by pericardial adhesions (Fig. 39–31, p. 1258), have a mouth that is considerably smaller than the maximal diameter.

The frequency of ventricular aneurysm after myocardial infarction depends on the incidence of transmural myocardial infarction and congestive heart failure in the population studied. Left ventricular aneurysm can also result from myocardial infarction secondary to blunt chest trauma.[660] Anterior aneurysms are often associated with total occlusion of the left anterior descending coronary artery, and a poor collateral blood supply,[661] but are unusual in the presence of multivessel disease with a good collateral circulation or a patent anterior descending coronary artery.[662]

Over 80 per cent of left ventricular aneurysms are located anterolaterally near the apex, with approximately 5 to 10 per cent located posteriorly. Most anterior aneurysms are true aneurysms, whereas nearly half of the posterior aneurysms are false aneurysms. Three-quarters of patients with aneurysms have multivessel CAD.[663] Almost half of patients with moderate or large aneurysms have symptoms of heart failure, with or without associated angina. One-third have severe angina alone, and approximately 15 per cent have symptomatic ventricular arrhythmias. Mural thrombi are found in almost half of patients with chronic left ventricular aneurysms. Systemic embolic events in patients with thrombi in left ventricular aneurysms occur infrequently and tend to occur within the initial 4 to 6 months after infarction. Thrombi within the left ventricle can be detected by angiography and two-dimensional echocardiography (Figs. 4–91, p. 98 and 39–37, p. 1262). Available data are insufficient to suggest that long-term anticoagulant treatment is routinely indicated to prevent systemic embolization beyond the first 6 months after infarction.[664] Some patients with ventricular aneurysms have intractable life-threatening ventricular arrhythmias requiring operation (p. 656).[665]

DETECTION. Diagnostic clues to the presence of aneurysm include persistent ST-segment elevations on the electrocardiogram and a characteristic contour (bulge) of the silhouette of the left ventricle on a chest roentgenogram. These findings, when clear-cut, are relatively specific, but they have limited sensitivity. Radionuclide ventriculography and two-dimensional echocardiography can demonstrate ventricular aneurysm more readily. Color-flow echocardiographic imaging is useful in establishing the diagnosis of left ventricular pseudoaneurysm, since flow "in and out" of the aneurysm as well as abnormal flow within the aneurysm can be detected, and subsequent pulsed Doppler imaging can reveal a "to-and-fro" pattern with characteristic respiratory variation of the peak systolic velocity.[666] Computed tomography and magnetic resonance imaging are reliable noninvasive techniques for the identification of left ventricular aneurysms (Fig. 11–5, p. 314) and screening for resectability.[667] However, biplane left ventriculography remains the most precise method available for outlining a left ventricular aneurysm, assessing septal motion, and determining the quantity of functioning residual myocardium.

The motion of the interventricular septum, as assessed by echocardiography, is also of importance in evaluating the function of residual myocardium. Patients with akinesis of the interventricular septum tend to have less favorable outcomes following operation than patients who exhibit septal motion. On the other hand, patients who exhibit the most paradoxical systolic movement of the aneurysm tend to do better after operation than those showing akinesis.[668]

LEFT VENTRICULAR ANEURYSMECTOMY. Indications for this procedure include congestive heart failure, refractory ventricular tachycardia, recurrent thromboembolism, and refractory angina.[669] A large left ventricular aneurysm in a patient with symptoms of heart failure, particularly if angina pectoris is also present, is an indication for operation. The operative mortality rate for left ventricular

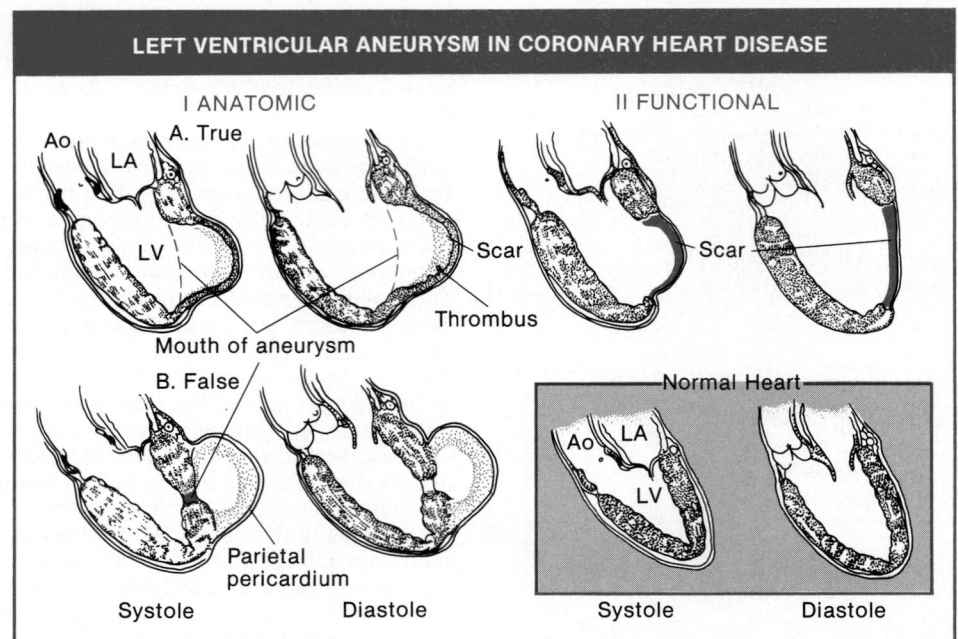

FIGURE 40-36. Hearts in systole and diastole with true and false anatomical and functional left ventricular aneurysms and healed myocardial infarction. A normal heart in systole and diastole is shown for comparison. The true anatomical left ventricular aneurysm protrudes during both systole and diastole, has a mouth that is as wide as or wider than the maximal diameter, has a wall that was formerly the wall of the left ventricle, and is composed of fibrous tissue with or without residual myocardial fibers. A true aneurysm may or may not contain thrombus and almost never ruptures once the wall is healed. The false anatomical left ventricular aneurysm protrudes during both systole and diastole, has a mouth that is considerably smaller than the maximal diameter of the aneurysm and represents a myocardial rupture site, has a wall made up of parietal pericardium, virtually always contains thrombus, and often ruptures. The functional left ventricular aneurysm protrudes during ventricular systole but not during diastole and consists of fibrous tissue with or without myocardial fibers. (From Cabin, H. S., and Roberts, W. C.: Left ventricular aneurysm, intraaneurysmal thrombus and systemic embolus in coronary heart disease. Chest **77**:586, 1980.)

aneurysmectomy is approximately 10 per cent (ranging from 2 to 19 per cent).[669,670] Risk factors for early death include poor left ventricular function,[663,670] resection of an akinetic rather than a dyskinetic aneurysm,[669] recent myocardial infarction,[671] the presence of mitral regurgitation,[672] and intractable ventricular arrhythmias.[670,671] Operation carries a particularly high risk in patients with symptoms of severe heart failure, a low-output state, a requirement for more than 80 mg of furosemide daily, and akinesis of the interventricular septum. Akinesia or dyskinesia of the posterior basal segment of the left ventricle and significant right coronary artery stenoses are additional risk factors.[663] Coronary revascularization is frequently carried out along with aneurysmectomy, especially in patients in whom angina accompanies heart failure.[663,669]

Risk factors for poor late survival following surgery include incomplete revascularization, impaired systolic function of the basal segments of the ventricle and of the septum not involved by the aneurysm, presence of a huge aneurysm with only an inadequate quantity of residual viable myocardium, and the presence of dominant symptoms of cardiac failure rather than angina pectoris (Fig. 40-37).[663] Improvement in left ventricular function has been reported in survivors 1[671] to 3[672] years following resection of left ventricular aneurysms complicated by cardiac failure. A concomitant improvement in exercise performance also occurs, particularly in patients who undergo complete revascularization.[671] After 5 years, 70 to 80 per cent of survivors are in NYHA Class I or Il, with a 10-year actuarial survival of 69 per cent in patients undergoing left ventricular aneurysmectomy and revascularization, compared with 57 per cent in those undergoing left ventricular aneurysmectomy alone.[673] Right ventricular dysfunction is relatively common in patients with left ventricular aneurysm and may not be improved by surgery.

True ventricular aneurysms do not rupture, and operative excision is carried out to improve the clinical manifestations

(most often heart failure but sometimes also angina, embolization, and life-threatening tachyarrhythmias). Pseudoaneurysms, on the other hand, do rupture frequently, and they should therefore be resected on an urgent basis as soon as the diagnosis is established.

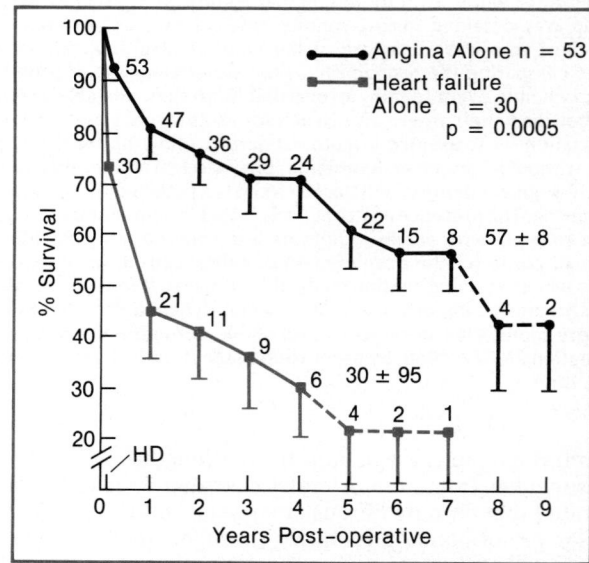

FIGURE 40-37. Survival curves for surgically treated patients with left ventricular aneurysm. Those patients complaining of angina rather than heart failure before operation have a more favorable long-term survival. The numbers of patients at risk are noted. (From Barratt-Boyes, B. G., et al.: The results of surgical treatment of left ventricular aneurysms: An assessment of risk factors affecting early and late mortality. J. Thorac. Cardiovasc. Surg. **87**:87, 1984.)

MITRAL REGURGITATION

Rupture of a papillary muscle, or of the head of a papillary muscle, usually causes severe acute mitral regurgitation in the course of an acute myocardial infarction (Fig. 39–33, p. 1259). Chronic mitral regurgitation in patients with ischemic heart disease is caused, most commonly, by papillary muscle dysfunction due to ischemia or fibrosis (Fig. 34–10, p. 1019) and/or by dilatation of the mitral annulus; many of the latter patients have ventricular aneurysms. Most patients with chronic CAD and mitral regurgitation have suffered a prior myocardial infarction, but the frequency of this syndrome (as with aneurysm) varies depending on the population studied. Clinical features that help to identify mitral regurgitation due to papillary muscle dysfunction as the cause of acute pulmonary edema or of milder symptoms of left-sided failure include a typical loud systolic heart murmur and demonstration of a flail mitral valve leaflet on echocardiography. The latter is the preferred diagnostic technique, since the timing and duration of the murmur are variable. Instead of being only mid to late systolic, as was originally thought, murmurs may be holosystolic or early systolic. Doppler echocardiography is helpful in assessing the severity of the regurgitation (p. 83).

The left atrium is usually not greatly enlarged unless severe mitral regurgitation has been present for more than 6 months. The electrocardiogram is nonspecific, and most patients have angiographic evidence of multivessel CAD. In patients with moderate to severe ischemic mitral regurgitation, variables influencing long-term survival include age, comorbid disorders (renal failure or pulmonary dysfunction), ventricular dysfunction, the need for intensive care management, and the extent of CAD.[674] In patients with posterior papillary muscle dysfunction resulting from acute myocardial infarction, reperfusion therapy with thrombolysis or PTCA may be attempted initially since urgent surgery often has a very high hospital mortality. In patients with rupture of a papillary muscle or, more frequently, one or more heads of a papillary muscle, immediate valve surgery is required provided the various descriptors of prognosis suggest a reasonable chance of satisfactory outcome.[675] Medical therapy is preferred in patients with generalized, severe ventricular dysfunction.

ISCHEMIC CARDIOMYOPATHY

Burch and colleagues used the term *ischemic cardiomyopathy* to describe the condition in which CAD results in severe myocardial dysfunction, with clinical manifestations often indistinguishable from those of primary dilated cardiomyopathy (p. 1398).[676] The fact that manifestations of cardiac dysfunction such as dyspnea or heart failure rather than anginal pain may be the predominant feature of ischemic myocardium is now well known. Observations have confirmed that in ambulatory patients with CAD the occurrence or frequency of angina pectoris is an inaccurate indicator of significant cardiac ischemia[474,645,651] and of ventricular dysfunction occurring during exertion.[643] Thus, symptoms of heart failure (caused by ischemic myocardial dysfunction, diffuse fibrosis, and multiple infarctions, alone or in combination) rather than a single discrete ventricular aneurysm may dominate the clinical picture. In some patients with chronic CAD, angina may be the principal clinical manifestation at one time but later diminishes or even disappears as heart failure becomes more prominent. Other patients have no history of angina or myocardial infarction (type I silent ischemia, p. 1347) and it is in this subgroup that ischemic cardiomyopathy may be confused with dilated cardiomyopathy.

The electrocardiogram may also be misleading. Myocardium with apparent electrocardiographic evidence of infarction, namely, pathological Q waves and diminished R wave height, can be successfully reperfused with improvement in myocardial function. Further evidence that electrocardiographic Q waves may overlie ischemic, rather than necrotic, myocardium is provided by the observation that Q waves may

be induced by exercise and subsequently disappear with rest.[677]

Long-term reduction of myocardial perfusion may cause persistent left ventricular dysfunction without tissue necrosis as long as myocardial flow is sufficient to maintain the myocardium viable but inadequate to sustain normal or even subnormal contractile function ("hibernating myocardium," pp. 1176 and 1329).[128] Thus, hibernating myocardium, which can be the basis of or play a role in the development of ischemic cardiomyopathy, can result from chronic ischemia and persist until blood flow is restored. The concept of myocardial hibernation is a useful one because symptoms resulting from chronic left ventricular dysfunction may be incorrectly thought to result from necrotic and scarred myocardium rather than from a reversible ischemic process. For this reason, attempts have been made to decide whether cardiac dysfunction is irreversible (due to necrosis) or potentially reversible (due to ischemia). If myocardial contractility can be improved by an inotropic stimulus such as postextrasystolic potentiation or the infusion of a sympathomimetic amine, it is said to exhibit contractile reserve (p. 1329). Hibernating myocardium may be present in patients with known or suspected CAD with a degree of cardiac dysfunction or heart failure not readily accounted for by other possible causes, e.g., cardiomyopathy of other etiology, longstanding hypertension, and prior myocardial infarctions.

In patients with heart failure in whom myocardial hibernation is suspected, cardiac catheterization and coronary arteriography should be carried out to assess hemodynamic parameters, ventricular function, and coronary anatomy. If myocardium exhibiting a contractile defect is supplied by stenotic coronary arteries or collateral vessels, it is helpful to determine whether it exhibits contractile reserve. If ventricular function improves with inotropic stimulation it is possible that revascularization carried out by surgery[128,130,429] or coronary angioplasty[263] may result in improved ventricular function and survival.[324,326,327,427]

The outlook for patients with ischemic cardiomyopathy treated medically is quite poor, and revascularization or cardiac transplantation may be considered.[679] Associated ventricular arrhythmias occurring in patients with ischemic cardiomyopathy usually are an ominous sign. Patients with diffuse disease have the worst outlook, with a slightly better clinical course being observed in patients with isolated wall-motion disorders.

CARDIAC ARRHYTHMIAS

Many patients with CAD and serious cardiac arrhythmias have other manifestations of active myocardial ischemia, such as acute myocardial infarction. Various degrees of ventricular ectopic activity are the most common arrhythmias. The frequency and severity of ventricular arrhythmias induced during exercise tests and ambulatory monitoring correlate, in general, with the degree of arteriographically documented CAD. Patients with severe left ventricular dysfunction associated with multivessel disease have more high-grade ectopic activity than do those with normal ventricular function and single-vessel disease. In some patients with CAD, cardiac arrhythmias are the predominant manifestation of their disease. That there is a substantial subgroup of patients with CAD and occult arrhythmias is suggested by the frequency with which sudden death is the first manifestation of ischemic heart disease (Ch. 26).

When arrhythmias are the predominant clinical manifestation, they are also the main focus of therapeutic interventions. This ordinarily involves pharmacological therapy, but in cases of drug failure, the implementation of an automatic cardiovascular defibrillator surgical therapy may be useful. Surgical revascularization in survivors of cardiac arrest can reduce the subsequent inducibility of ventricular arrhythmias in approximately one-half of patients, but advanced age and poor ventricular function are adverse prognostic indicators.[680]

Nonatheromatous CAD may also result from congenital abnormalities in the origin or distribution of the coronary arteries (p. 254). The most important of these are anomalous origin of a coronary artery (usually the left) from the pulmonary artery, origin of both coronary arteries from either the right or left sinus of Valsalva, and coronary arteriovenous fistula. Anomalous origin of either the left main coronary artery or right coronary artery from the aorta with subsequent coursing between the aorta and pulmonary trunk is a rare and sometimes fatal coronary arterial anomaly.[681]

Dissection of a coronary artery is often a postmortem finding. Two-thirds of the described cases have occurred in women, and one-half of these were associated with the postpartum state.[682] In patients who survive spontaneous coronary artery dissection, there is a 20-per cent mortality over the next 3 years. In general, coronary revascularization is recommended, particularly in patients who have ongoing ischemia.

A number of inherited connective tissue disorders are associated with myocardial ischemia.[6a] These include the Marfan syndrome (aortic dissection; p. 1641), Hurler syndrome (coronary obstruction; p. 1646), homocystinuria (coronary artery thrombosis; p. 1644), Ehlers-Danlos syndrome (coronary arterial dissection; p. 1643), and pseudo xanthoma elasticum (accelerated CAD; p. 1644). Kawasaki disease, the mucocutaneous lymph node syndrome, may cause coronary artery aneurysms and ischemic heart disease in children (p. 997). On rare occasions Takayasu disease (p. 1544) is associated with angina, myocardial infarction, and cardiac failure resulting from hypertension, aortic regurgitation, or annuloaortic ectasia in patients under the age of 40 years.[683] The average age of onset of symptoms is 24 years, and event-free survival at 10 years after diagnosis is approximately 60 per cent.[683]

Perhaps the most common cause of nonatheromatous CAD resulting in myocardial ischemia is the syndrome of angina-like pain despite normal coronary arteriograms, i.e., so-called syndrome X, which is discussed earlier in this chapter (p. 1346). Myocardial ischemia *not* caused by coronary atherosclerosis can also result from embolism, as in infective endocarditis (Chap. 35); implanted prosthetic heart valves (Ch. 34); primary tumors of the heart (Ch. 45); calcific emboli from calcified aortic valves; and emboli from mural thrombi. Luetic aortitis may also produce myocardial ischemia by causing obstruction of coronary ostia (p. 1548). Occasionally, a mass of amorphous, calcified material accumulates at the sinotubular ridge, i.e., the junction of the sinus and tubular portions of the ascending aorta, most commonly near the right aortic sinus. Complications can include coronary ostial stenosis or embolism to an epicardial coronary artery resulting from the lesion overhanging the ostium or invading the wall of the aorta at the site of the coronary artery takeoff.[684] Important CAD associated with systemic lupus erythematosus has been reported, but is rare.

Cardiac transplant–associated coronary arteriosclerosis (p. 528) is frequently observed in cardiac transplant survivors. It is a rapidly evolving, concentric, diffuse arteriosclerosis involving epicardial and intramural coronary vessels and appears to have an inconstant association with coronary risk factors. Suggested etiologic factors include opportunistic infection (cytomegalovirus infection), immunosuppressive therapy, and elevated lipid levels. Acute myocardial infarction can result and is usually not accompanied by chest pain or typical electrocardiographic changes. However infarction in these patients is associated with a high mortality rate, and, at anatomical examination, diffuse disease of the coronary arteries and multiple foci of nontransmural cardiac infarction.[685] It is likely that the initiating mechanism is in some way immunologically mediated, and intense research is continuing in this area.

An interesting nonatherosclerotic ischemic syndrome has been described in workers in the nitrate industry who apparently experience nitrate withdrawal symptoms on weekends, presumed to be secondary to coronary spasm when there is no counterstimulation to the vasoconstriction that they undergo as an adaptation to the vasodilating actions of the high concentrations of nitrates to which they are exposed.[686]

Acknowledgment

Dr. Peter Cohn was an author of this chapter in the first three editions of this book. He has had a lasting influence on its organization and contents. The authors gratefully acknowledge the secretarial help of Lisa McHale.

REFERENCES

INTRODUCTION

1. Marmot, M. G.: Interpretation of trends in coronary heart disease mortality. Acta Med. Scand. (Suppl.) 701:58, 1985.
2. National Heart, Lung, and Blood Institute: Morbidity from coronary heart disease in the United States. NHLBI Data Fact Sheet, June, 1990.
3. Connolly, D. C., Oxman, A. J., Nobrega, F. T., et al: Coronary heart disease in residents of Rochester, Minnesota, 1950–1975. I. Background in study design. Mayo Clinic Proc. 56:661, 1981.
4. Elveback, L. R., Connolly, D. C., and Kurland, L. T.: Coronary heart disease in residents of Rochester, Minnesota, 1950–1975. II. Mortality, incidence, and survival. Mayo Clin. Proc. 56:665, 1981.
5. Kuller, L. H., Traven, N. D., Rutan, G. H., et al.: Marked decline of coronary heart disease mortality in 35–44-year old white men in Allegheny County, Pennsylvania. Circulation 80:261, 1989.
6. WHO Expert Committee: Prevention of coronary heart disease. Tech. Rep. Ser. WHO No. 678, 1982.
6a. Virmani, R, and Forman, M. B.: Nonatherosclerotic ischemic heart disease. 1st ed. New York, Raven Press, 1989.

CHRONIC STABLE ANGINA PECTORIS

7. Matthews, M. B., and Julian, D. G.: Angina pectoris: Definition and description. In Julian, D. G. (ed.): Angina Pectoris. 2nd ed. New York, Churchill Livingstone, 1985, p. 2.
8. Christie, L. G., Jr., and Conti, C. R.: Systematic approach to evaluation of angina-like chest pain: Pathophysiology and clinical testing with emphasis on objective documentation of myocardial ischemia. Am. Heart J. 102:897, 1981.
8a. Angina pectoris. In Fowler, N.O.: Diagnosis of Heart Disease. New York, Springer-Verlag, 1991, pp. 187–206.
9. Sampson, J., and Cheitlin, M. D.: Pathophysiology and differential diagnosis of cardiac pain. Prog. Cardiovasc. Dis. 13:507, 1971.
10. Lichstein, E., Breitbart, S., Shani, J., et al.: Relationship between location of chest pain and site of coronary artery occlusion. Am. Heart J. 115:564, 1988.
11. Cook, D. G., and Shaper, A. G.: Breathlessness, angina pectoris and coronary artery disease. Am. J. Cardiol. 63:921, 1989.
12. Crea, F., Pupita, G., Galassi, A. R., et al: Role of adenosine in pathogenesis of anginal pain. Circulation 81:164, 1990.
13. Del Banco, P. L., Bel Bene, E., and Sicuteri, F.: Heart pain. In Bonica, J. J. (ed.): Advances in Neurology. Vol. 4. New York, Raven Press, 1974, p. 375.
14. Umachandran, V., Ranjadaylan, K., Ambepityia, G., et al.: The perception of angina in diabetes: Relation to somatic pain threshold and autonomic function. Am. Heart J. 121:1649, 1991.
15. Deanfield, J., Shea, M., Ribeiro, P., et al: Transient ST-segment depression as a marker of myocardial ischemia during daily life. Am. J. Cardiol. 54:1195,1984.
16. Falcone, C., Sconocchia, R., Guasti, L., et al: Dental pain threshold and angina pectoris in patients with coronary artery disease. J. Am. Coll. Cardiol. 12:348, 1988.
17. Sheps, D. S., Adams, K. F., Hindliter, A., et al.: Endorphins are related to pain perception in coronary artery disease. Am. J. Cardiol. 59:523, 1987.
18. Constant, J.: The clinical diagnosis of nonanginal chest pain: The differentiation of angina from nonanginal chest pain by history. Clin. Cardiol. 6:11, 1983.
19. Hillis, L. D., and Braunwald, E.: Coronary artery spasm. N. Engl. J. Med. 299:695, 1978.
20. Ganz, P., Abben, R. P., and Barry, W. H.: Dynamic variations in resistance of coronary arterial narrowings in angina pectoris at rest. Am. J. Cardiol. 59:66, 1987.
20a. Maseri, A.: Medical therapy of chronic stable angina pectoris. Circulation 82:2258, 1990.
21. Juneau, M., Johnstone, M., Dempsey, E., and Waters, D. D.: Exercise-induced myocardial ischemia in a cold environment. Effect of antianginal medications. Circulation 79:1015, 1989.
22. Quyyumi, A. A., Mockus, L. J., Wright, C. A., and Fox, K. M.: Mechanisms of nocturnal angina pectoris: Importance of increased myocardial oxygen demand in patients with severe coronary artery disease. Lancet 1:1207, 1984.
23. Maseri, A.: Mixed angina pectoris. Am. J. Cardiol. 56:30E, 1985.

24. Epstein, S. E., Stampfer, M., Beiser, G. D., et al: Effect of a reduction in environmental temperature on the circulatory response to exercise in man. Implications concerning angina pectoris. N. Engl. J. Med. 280:7, 1969.

25. Goldstein, R. E., Redwood, D. R., Beiser, G. D., and Epstein, S. E.: Alterations in the circulatory response to exercise following a meal and their relationship in postprandial angina pectoris. Circulation 44:90, 1971.

26. Figueras, J., Singh, B. N., Ganz, W., and Swan, H.J.C.: Hemodynamic and electrocardiographic accompaniments of resting postprandial angina. Br. Heart J. 42:402, 1979.

27. Schiffer, F., Hartley, L. H., Schulman, C. L., and Abelmann, W. H.: Evidence for emotionally induced coronary arterial spasm in patients with angina pectoris. Br. Heart J. 44:62, 1980.

28. Horowitz, L. D., Herman, M. V., and Gorlin, R.: Clinical response to nitroglycerin as a diagnostic test for coronary artery disease. Am. J. Cardiol. 29:149, 1972.

29. Levine, S. A.: Carotid sinus massage: A new diagnostic test for angina pectoris. JAMA 182:1332, 1962.

30. Joy, M., Cairns, A. W., and Sprigings, D.: Observations on the warm up phenomenon in angina pectoris. Br. Heart J. 58:116, 1987.

31. Campeau, L.: Grading of angina pectoris. Circulation 54:522, 1976.

32. Goldman, L., Hashimoto, B., and Cook. E. F.: Comparative reproducibility and validity of systems for assessing cardiovascular functional class: Advantages of a new specific activity scale. Circulation 64:1227, 1981.

33. Califf, R. M., Mark, D. B., Harrell, F. E., et al.: Importance of clinical measures of ischemia in the prognosis of patients with documented coronary artery disease. J. Am. Coll. Cardiol. 11:20, 1988.

34. Diamond, G. A., and Forrester, J. S.: Analysis of probability as an aid in the clinical diagnosis of coronary artery disease. N. Engl. J. Med. 300:1350, 1979.

35. Welch, C. C., Proudfit, W. L., and Sheldon, W. C.: Coronary arteriographic findings in 1000 women under age 50. Am. J. Cardiol. 35:211, 1975.

36. Cohn, P. F., Harris, P., Barry, W. H. et al.: Prognostic importance of anginal symptoms in angiographically defined coronary artery disease. Am. J. Cardiol. 47:233, 1981.

37. Reunanen, A., Suhonen, O., Aromaa, A., et al.: Incidence of different manifestations of coronary heart disease in middle-aged Finnish men and women. Acta Med. Scand. 218:19, 1985.

38. Davies, H. A., Jones, D. B., Rhodes, J., and Newcombe, R. G.: Anginal-like esophageal pain: Differentiation from cardiac pain by history. J. Clin. Gastroenterol. 7:477, 1985.

39. Conte, M. R., Orzan, F., Magnacca, M., et al.: Atypical chest pain: Coronary or esophageal disease? Int. J. Cardiol. 13:135, 1986.

40. Winnan, G. R., Meyer, C. T., and McCallum, R. W.: Interpretation of the Bernstein Test: A reappraisal of criteria. Ann. Intern. Med. 96:320, 1982.

41. DeMeester, T. R., O'Sullivan, G. C., Bermudez, G., et al.: Esophageal function in patients with angina-type chest pain and normal coronary angiograms. Ann. Surg. 196:488, 1982.

42. Mellow, M. H., Simpson, A. G., Watt, L., et al.: Esophageal acid perfusion in coronary artery disease. Gastroenterology 85:306, 1983.

43. Davies, H. A., Rush, E. M., Lewis, M. J., et al.: Oesophageal stimulation lowers exertional angina threshold. Lancet 1:1011, 1985.

44. Lee, M. G., Sullivan, S. N., Watson, W. C., and Melendez, L. J.: Chest pain—esophageal, cardiac, or both? Am. J. Gastroenterol. 80:320, 1985.

45. Eastwood, G. L., Weiner, B. H., Dickerson, W. J., et al.: Use of ergonovine to identify esophageal spasm in patients with chest pain. Ann. Intern. Med. 94:768, 1981.

46. Hargrove, M. D.: Gallbladder disease and chest pain. CV Dis & Chest Pain 2:3, 1987.

47. Epstein, S. E., Gerber, L. H., and Borer, J. S.: Chest wall syndrome. A common cause of unexpected cardiac pain. JAMA 241:2793, 1979.

48. Bettmann, M. A., and Salzman, E. W.: Current concepts in the diagnosis of pulmonary embolism. Mod. Concepts Cardiovasc. Dis. 53:1, 1984.

49. Pe'er J., Vidaurri, J., Halfon, S. T., et al.: Association between corneal arcus and some of the risk factors for coronary artery disease. Br. J. Ophthalmol. 67:795, 1983.

50. Winder, A. F.: Relationship between corneal arcus and hyperlipidaemia is clarified by studies in familial hypercholesterolaemia. Br. J. Ophthalmol. 67:789, 1983.

51. Segal, P., Insull, W., Chambless, L. E., et al.: The association of dyslipoproteinemia with corneal arcus and xanthelasma. The Lipid Research Clinic's Program Prevalence Study. Circulation 73:108, 1986.

52. Elliot, W. J.: Ear lobe crease and coronary artery disease. 1,000 patients and review of the literature. Am. J. Med. 75:1024, 1983.

53. Kaukola, S.: The diagonal ear-lobe crease, heredity and coronary heart disease. Acta Med. Scand. (Suppl.)668:60, 1982.

54. Kirkham, N., Murrells, T., Melcher, D. H., and Morrison, E. A.: Diagonal earlobe creases and fatal cardiovascular disease: A necropsy study. Br. Heart J. 61:361, 1989.

55. Brady, P. M., Zive, M. A., Goldberg, R. J., et al.: A new wrinkle to the earlobe crease. Arch. Intern. Med. 147:65, 1987.

56. Criqui, M. H., Coughlin, S. S., and Fronek, A.: Noninvasively diagnosed peripheral arterial disease as a predictor of mortality: Results from a prospective study. Circulation 72:768, 1985.

57. Cohn, P. F., Thompson, S., Strauss, W., et al.: Diastolic heart sounds during static (handgrip) exercise in patients with chest pain. Circulation 47:1217, 1973.

58. Ranganathan, N., Juma, Z., and Sivaciyan, V.: The apical impulse in coronary heart disease. Clin. Cardiol. 8:20, 1985.

59. Tavel, M. E.: the fourth heart sound—a premature requiem? Circulation 49:4, 1974.

60. Sangster, J. F., and Oakley, C. M.: Diastolic murmur of coronary artery stenosis. Br. Heart J. 35:840, 1973.

61. Hamby, R. I., Weissman, R. H., Prakash, M. N., and Hoffman, I.: Left bundle branch block: A predictor of poor left ventricular function in coronary artery disease. Am. Heart J. 106:471, 1983.

62. Liao, Y., Emidy, L. A., Dyer, A., et al.: Characteristics and prognosis of incomplete right bundle branch block: An epidemiologic study. J. Am. Coll. Cardiol. 7:492, 1986.

63. Kannel, W. B., and Abbott, R. D.: Incidence and prognosis of unrecognized myocardial infarction. N. Engl. J. Med. 311:1144, 1984.

64. Goldman, L., Cook, E. F., Mitchell, N., et al.: Incremental value of the exercise test for diagnosing the presence or absence of coronary artery disease. Circulation 66:945, 1982.

65. Dagenais, G. R., Rouleau, J. R., Christen, A., and Fabia, J.: Survival of patients with a strongly positive exercise electrocardiogram. Circulation 65:452, 1982.

66. Bogaty, P., Dagenais, G. R., Cantin, B., et al.: Prognosis in patients with a strongly positive exercise electrocardiogram. Am. J. Cardiol. 64:1284, 1989.

67. Weiner, D. A., McCabe, C., Hueter, D. C., et al.: The predictive value of anginal chest pain as an indicator of coronary disease during exercise testing. Am. Heart J. 96:458, 1978.

67a. Wilson, R. F., Marcus, M. L., Christensen, B. V., et al.: Accuracy of exercise electrocardiography in detecting physiologically significant coronary arterial lesions. Circulation 83:412, 1991.

68. Detrano, R., Gianrossi, R., Mulvihill, D., et al.: Exercise-induced ST segment depression in the diagnosis of multivessel coronary disease: A meta analysis. J. Am. Coll. Cardiol. 14:1501, 1989.

69. Dubach, P., Froelicher, V. F., Klein, J., et al.: Exercise-induced hypotension in a male population. Criteria, causes and prognosis. Circulation 78:1380, 1988.

70. Boran, K. G., Oliveros, R. A., Boucher, C. A., et al.: Ischemia-associated intraventricular conduction disturbances during exercise testing as a predictor of proximal left anterior descending coronary artery disease. Am. J. Cardiol. 51:1098, 1983.

71. Vasey, C., O'Donnell, J., Morris, S., and McHenry, P.: Exercise-induced left bundle branch block and its relation to coronary artery disease. Am. J. Cardiol. 56:892, 1985.

72. Williams, M. A., Esterbrooks, D. I., Nair, C. K., et al.: Clinical significance of exercise-induced bundle branch block. Am. J. Cardiol. 61:346, 1988.

73. Okin, P. M., Ameisen, O., and Kligfield, P.: Recovery-phase patterns of ST segment depression in the heart rate domain. Identification of coronary artery disease by the rate-recovery loop. Circulation 80:533, 1989.

74. Stone, P. H., LaFolette, E. L., and Cohn, K.: Patterns of exercise treadmill test performance in patients with left main coronary artery disease: Detection dependent on left coronary dominance or coexistent dominant right coronary disease. Am. Heart J. 104:13, 1982.

75. Nygaard, T. W., Gibson, R. S., Ryan, J. M., et al.: Prevalence of high-risk thallium-201 scintigraphic findings in left main coronary artery stenosis: Comparison of patients with multiple-and single-vessel coronary artery disease. Am. J. Cardiol. 53:462, 1984.

76. Bartel, A. L., Behar, V. S., Peter, R. H., et al.: Graded exercise stress tests in angiographically documented coronary artery disease. Circulation 49:348, 1974.

77. Goldschlager, N., Selzer, A., and Cohn, K.: Treadmill stress tests as indicators of presence and severity of coronary artery disease. Ann. Intern. Med. 85:282, 1976.

78. Hlatky, M. A., Pryor, D. B., Harrell, F. E., Jr., et al.: Factors affecting sensitivity and specificity of exercise electrocardiography. Am. J. Med. 77:64, 1984.

79. Weins, R. D., Lafia, P., Marder, C. M., et al.: Chronotropic incompetence in clinical exercise testing. Am. J. Cardiol. 54:74, 1984.

80. McHenry, P. L., Morris, S. N., Kavalier, M., and Jordan, J. W.: Comparative study of exercise-induced ventricular arrhythmias in normal subjects and patients with documented coronary artery disease. Am. J. Cardiol. 37:609, 1976.

80a. Podrid, P. J., Graboys, T. B., and Lown, B.: Prognosis of medically treated patients with coronary-artery disease with profound ST-segment depression during exercise testing. N. Engl. J. Med. 305:1111, 1981.

80b. Dagenais, G. R., Rouleau, J. R., Hochart, P., et al.: Survival with painless strongly positive exercise electrocardiogram. Am. J. Cardiol. 62:892, 1988.

80c. Weiner, D. A., Ryan, T. J., McCabe, C. H., et al.: The role of exercise testing in identifying patients with improved survival after coronary artery bypass surgery. J. Am. Coll. Cardiol. 8:741, 1986.

81. Cole, J. R., and Ellestad, M. H.: Significance of chest pain during treadmill exercise: Correlation with coronary events. Am. J. Cardiol. 41:227, 1978.

82. Weiner, D. A., Ryan, T. J., McCabe, C., et al.: Risk of developing an acute myocardial infarction or sudden coronary death in patients with exercise-induced silent myocardial ischemia. A report from the coronary artery surgery study (CASS) registry. Am. J. Cardiol. 62:1155, 1988.

83. Mukharji, J., Kremers, M., Lipscomb, K., and Blomqvist, C. G.: Early positive exercise test and extensive coronary disease: Effect of antianginal therapy. Am. J. Cardiol. 55:267, 1985.

84. Ho, S. W. -C., McComish, M. J., and Taylor, R. R.: Effect of beta-adrenergic blockade on the results of exercise testing related to the extent of coronary artery disease. Am. J. Cardiol. 55:258, 1985.

85. Severi, S., and Michelassi, C.: Prognostic impact of stress testing in coronary artery disease. Circulation 83:(Suppl. III):82, 1991.

86. Younis, L. T., Byers, S., Shaw, L., et al.: Prognostic importance of silent

myocardial ischemia detected by intravenous dipyridamole thallium myocardial imaging in asymptomatic patients with coronary artery disease. J. Am. Coll. Cardiol. 14:1635, 1989.

87. Borges-Neto, S., Mahmarian, J. J., Jain, A., et al.: Quantitative thallium-201 single photon emission computed tomography after oral dipyridamole for assessing the presence, anatomic location and severity of coronary artery disease. J. Am. Coll. Cardiol. 11:962, 1988.

87a. Coyne, E. P., Belvedere, D. A., Vande Streek, P. R., et al.: Thallium-201 scintigraphy after intravenous infusion of adenosine compared with exercise thallium testing in the diagnosis of coronary artery disease. J. Am. Coll. Cardiol. 17:1289, 1991.

87b. Brown, K. A.: Prognostic value of thallium-201 myocardial perfusion imaging: A diagnostic tool comes of age. Circulation 83:363, 1991.

88. Gould, K. L.: How accurate is thallium exercise testing for the diagnosis of coronary disease. J. Am. Coll. Cardiol. 14:1487, 1989.

89. Port, S. C., Oshima, M., Ray, G., et al.: Assessment of single-vessel coronary artery disease: Results of exercise electrocardiography, thallium-201 myocardial perfusion imaging and radionuclide angiography. J. Am. Coll. Cardiol. 6:75, 1985.

90. Wackers, F. J. T., Russo, D. J., Russo, D., and Clements, J. P.: Prognostic significance of normal quantitative planar thallium-201 stress scintigraphy in patients with chest pain. J. Am. Coll. Cardiol. 6:27, 1985.

91. Koss, J. H., Kobren, S. M., Grunwald, A. M., and Bodenheimer, M. M.: Role of exercise thallium-201 myocardial perfusion scintigraphy in predicting prognosis in suspected coronary artery disease. Am. J. Cardiol. 59:531, 1987.

92. Pamelia, F. X., Gibson, R. S., Watson, D. D., et al.: Prognosis with chest pain and normal thallium-201 exercise scintigrams. Am. J. Cardiol. 55:920, 1985.

93. Gill, J. B., Ruddy, T. D., Newell, J. B., et al.: Prognostic importance of thallium uptake by the lungs during exercise in coronary artery disease. N. Engl. J. Med. 317:1485, 1987.

93a. Pollock, S. G., Abbott, R. D., Boucher, C. A., et al.: A model to predict multivessel coronary artery disease from the exercise thallium-201 stress test. Am. J. Med. 90:345, 1991.

94. Weiss, A. T., Berman, D. S., Lew, A. S., et al.: Transient ischemic dilation of the left ventricle on stress thallium-201 scintigraphy: A marker of severe and extensive coronary artery disease. J. Am. Coll. Cardiol. 9:752, 1987.

95. Kiat, H., Berman, D. S., and Maddahi, J.: Comparison of planar and tomographic exercise thallium-201 imaging methods for the evaluation of coronary artery disease. J. Am. Coll. Cardiol. 13:613, 1989.

96. Coyne, E. P., Belvedere, D. A., Vande Streek, P. R., et al.: Thallium-201 scintigraphy after intravenous infusion of adenosine compared with exercise thallium testing in the diagnosis of coronary artery disease. J. Am. Coll. Cardiol. 17:1289, 1991.

96a. Ranhosky, A., Kempthorne-Rawson, J., and the Intravenous Dipyridamole Thallium Imaging Study Group: The safety of intravenous dipyridamole thallium myocardial perfusion imaging. Circulation 81:1205, 1990.

97. Kaul, S., Kiess, M., Liu, P., et al.: Comparison of exercise electrocardiography and quantitative thallium imaging for one-vessel coronary artery disease. Am. J. Cardiol. 56:257, 1985.

98. Raby, K. E., Goldman, L., Creager, M. A., et al.: Correlation between preoperative ischemia and major cardiac events after peripheral vascular surgery. N. Engl. J. Med. 321:1296, 1989.

99. Gibbons, R. J., Fyke, F. E., Clements, I. P., et al.: Noninvasive identification of severe coronary disease using exercise radionuclide angiography. J. Am. Coll. Cardiol. 11:28, 1988.

100. Cates, C. U., Kronenberg, M. W., Collins, H. W., and Sandler, M. P.: Dipyridamole radionuclide ventriculography: A test with high specificity for severe coronary artery disease. J. Am. Coll. Cardiol. 13:841, 1989.

101. Kaul, S., Lilly, D. R., Gascho, J. A., et al.: Prognostic utility of the exercise thallium-201 test in ambulatory patients with chest pain: Comparison with cardiac catheterization. Circulation 77:745, 1988.

102. Armstrong, W. F., O'Donnell, W. F., Dillon, J. C., et al.: Complementary value of two-dimensional exercise echocardiography to routine treadmill exercise testing. Ann. Intern. Med. 105:829, 1986.

103. Ryan, T., Vasey, C. G., Presti, C. F., et al.: Exercise echocardiography: Detection of coronary artery disease in patients with normal left ventricular wall motion at rest. J. Am. Coll. Cardiol. 11:993, 1988.

104. Oberman, A., Fan, P.-H., Nanda, N. C., et al.: Reproducibility of two-dimensional echocardiography. J. Am. Coll. Cardiol. 14:923, 1989.

105. Armstrong, W. F.: Exercise echocardiography: Ready, willing and able. J. Am. Coll. Card. 11:1359, 1988.

106. Sheikh, K. H., Bengtson, J. R., Helmy, S., et al.: Relation of quantitative coronary lesion measurements to the development of exercise-induced ischemia assessed by exercise echocardiography. J. Am. Coll. Cardiol. 15:1043, 1990.

107. Lim, T.-J., Nanto, S., Masuyama, T., et al.: Visualization of subendocardial myocardial ischemia with myocardial contrast echocardiography in humans. Circulation 79:233, 1989.

108. Picano, E., and Lattanzi, F.: Dipyridamole echocardiography. Circulation 83(Suppl. III):19, 1991.

109. Picano, E., Lattanzi, F., and L'Abbate, A.: Present application, practical aspects, and future issues on dipyridamole echocardiography Circulation 83(Suppl. III)111, 1991.

110. Ryan, T., Armstrong, W. F., and Feigenbaum, H.: Prospective evaluation of the left main coronary artery using digital two-dimensional echocardiography. J. Am. Coll. Cardiol. 7:807, 1986.

111. Neinle, R. A., Levy, R. I., Frederickson, D. S., and Gorlin, R.: Lipid and carbohydrate abnormalities in patients with angiographically documented coronary artery disease. Am. J. Cardiol. 24:178, 1969.

112. Falsetti, H. L., Schnatz, J. D., Greene, D. G., and Bunelli, I. L.: Lipid and carbohydrate studies in coronary artery disease. Circulation 37:184, 1968.

113. Margolis, J. R., Chan, J. T. T., Kong, Y., et al: The diagnostic and prognostic significance of coronary artery calcification. A report of 800 cases. Radiology 127:609, 1980.

114. Agatston, A. S., Janowitz, W. R., Hildner, F., et al.: Quantification of coronary artery calcium using ultrafast computed tomography. J. Am. Coll. Cardiol. 15:827, 1990.

115. Gordon, P. R., Abrams, C., Gash, A. K., and Carabello, B. A.: Pericatheterization risk factors in left main coronary artery stenosis. Am. J. Cardiol. 59:1080, 1987.

116. Hartnell, G. G., Parnell, B. M., and Pridie, R. B.: Coronary artery ectasia: Its prevalence and clinical significance in 4993 patients. Br. Heart J. 54:392, 1985.

117. Tunick, P. A., Slater, J., Kronzon, I., et al.: Discrete atherosclerotic coronary artery aneurysms: A study of 20 patients. J. Am. Coll. Cardiol. 15:279, 1990.

118. Agarwal, J. B., and Helfant, R. H.: Functional importance of coronary collateral circulation. Int. J. Cardiol. 4:94, 1983.

119. Newman, P. E.: The coronary collateral circulation: Determinants and functional significance in ischemic heart disease. Am. Heart J. 102:431, 1981.

120. Gregg, D. E., and Patterson, R. E.: Functional importance of the coronary collaterals. N. Engl. J. Med. 303:1404, 1980.

121. Kracoff, O. H., Ovsyshcher, I., and Gueron, M.: Malignant course of a benign anomaly: Myocardial bridging. Chest 92:1113, 1987.

121a. Bestetti, R. B., Costa, R. S., Kazava, D. K., and Oliveira, J. S. M.: Can isolated myocardial bridging of the left anterior descending coronary artery be associated with sudden death during exercise? Acta Cardiologica XLVI:27, 1991.

122. Moraski, R. E., Russell, R. O., Jr., Smith, M., and Rackley, C. E.: Left ventricular function in patients with and without myocardial infarction and one, two or three vessel coronary artery disease. Am. J. Cardiol. 35:1, 1975.

123. Mann, T., Brodie, B. R., Grossman, W., and McLaurin, L. P.: Effect of angina on the left ventricular diastolic pressure-volume relationship. Circulation 35:761, 1977.

124. Helfant, R. H., Forrester, J. S., Hampton, J. R., et al.: Coronary heart disease. Differential hemodynamic, metabolic, and electrocardiographic effects in subjects with and without angina pectoris during atrial pacing. Circulation 42:601, 1970.

125. Bourdillon, P. D., Lorell, B. H., Mirsky, I., et al.: Increased regional myocardial stiffness of the left ventricle during pacing-induced angina in man. Circulation 67:316, 1983.

126. Stack, R. S., Phillips, H. R., Grierson, D. S., et al.: Functional improvement of jeopardized myocardium following intracoronary streptokinase infusion in acute myocardial infarction. J. Clin. Invest. 72:84, 1983.

127. Rahimtoola, S. H.: A perspective on the three large multicenter randomized clinical trials of coronary bypass surgery for chronic stable angina. Circulation 72(Suppl. V):123, 1985.

128. Braunwald, E., and Rutherford, J. D.: Reversible ischemic left ventricular dysfunction: Evidence for the "hibernating myocardium." J. Am. Coll. Cardiol. 8:1467, 1986.

128a. Marban, E.: Myocardial stunning and hibernation. The physiology behind the colloquialisms. Circulation 83:681, 1991.

129. Popio, K. A., Gorlin, R., Bechtel, D., and Levine, J. A.: Postextrasystolic potentiation as a predictor of potential myocardial viability: Preoperative analyses compared with studies after coronary bypass surgery. Am. J. Cardiol. 39:944, 1977.

130. Nesto, R. W., Cohn, L. H., Collins, J. J., Jr, et al.: Inotropic contractile reserve: A useful predictor of increased 5-year survival and improved postoperative left ventricular function in patients with coronary artery disease and reduced ejection fraction. Am. J. Cardiol. 50:39, 1982.

131. Bodenheimer, M. M., Banka, V. S., Hermann, G. A., et al.: Reversible asynergy: Histopathologic and electrographic correlations in patients with coronary artery disease. Circulation 53:792, 1976.

132. Banka, V. S., Bodenheimer, M. M., and Helfant, R. H.: Determinants of reversible asynergy: The native coronary circulation. Circulation 52:810, 1975.

133. Verani, M. S., Carroll, R. J., and Falsetti, H. L.: Mitral valve prolapse in coronary artery disease. Am. J. Cardiol. 37:1, 1976.

134. Herman, M. V., Elliott, W. C., and Gorlin, R.: An electrocardiographic, anatomic, and metabolic study of zonal myocardial ischemia in coronary heart disease. Circulation 35:834, 1967.

135. Gertz, E. W., Wisneski, J. A., Neese, R., et al.: Myocardial lactate metabolism: Evidence of lactate release during net chemical extraction in man. Circulation 63:1273, 1981.

136. Cannon, P. J., Weiss, M. B., and Sciacca, R. R.: Myocardial blood flow in coronary artery disease: Studies at rest and during stress with inert gas washout techniques. Prog. Cardiovasc. Dis. 20:95, 1977.

137. Gould, K. L.: Identifying and measuring severity of coronary artery stenosis. Circulation 78:237, 1988.

138. Harrison, D. G.: From isolated vessels to the catheterization laboratory. Studies of endothelial function in the coronary circulation of humans. Circulation 80:703, 1989.

139. Werns, S. W., Walton, J. A., Hsia, H. H., et al.: Evidence of endothelial

dysfunction in angiographically normal coronary arteries of patients with coronary artery disease. Circulation 79:287, 1989.

139a. Zeiher, A. M., Drexler, H., Wollschläger, H., et al.: Modulation of coronary vasomotor tone in humans. Progressive endothelial dysfunction with different early stages of coronary atherosclerosis. Circulation 83:391, 1991.

140. Hill, J. A., Miranda, A. A., Keim, S. G., et al.: Value of right-sided cardiac catheterization in patients undergoing left-sided catheterization for evaluation of coronary artery disease. R_2 Management of Chronic Stable Angina Am. J. Cardiol. 65:590, 1990.

Management of Chronic Stable Angina

141. Kronmal, R. A., Oberman, A., Frye, R. L., and Killip, T., III: Effect of cigarette smoking on survival of patients with angiographically documented coronary artery disease. Report from CASS Registry. JAMA 255:1023, 1986.

142. Hermanson, B., Omenn, G. S., Kronmal, R. A., et al.: Beneficial six-year outcome of smoking cessation in older men and women with coronary artery disease. Results from the CASS Registry. N. Engl. J. Med. 319:1365, 1988.

143. Hallstom, A. P., Cobb, L. A., and Ray, R.: Smoking as a risk factor for recurrence of sudden cardiac arrest. N. Engl. J. Med. 314:271, 1986.

144. Rogot, E., and Murray, J. L.: Smoking and causes of death among U.S. veterans: 16 years of observation. Public Health Rep. 95:213, 1980.

145. Kannel, W. B., Castelli, W. P., and McNamara, P. M.: Cigarette smoking and risk of CHD: Epidemiologic clues to pathogenesis: The Framingham Study. N.C.I. Mongr. 28:9, 1968.

146. Kaufman, D. W., Helmich, S. P., and Shapiro, S.: The risk of myocardial infarction after quitting smoking in men under 55 years of age. N. Engl. J. Med. 313:1511, 1985.

147. Hofstetter, A., Schutz, Y., Jequier, E., and Wahren, J.: Increased 24-hour energy expenditure in cigarette smokers. N. Engl. J. Med. 314:79, 1986.

148. Nicod, P., Rehr, R., Winniford, M. D., et al.: Acute systemic and coronary hemodynamic and serologic responses to cigarette smoking in long-term smokers with atherosclerotic coronary artery disease. J. Am. Coll. Cardiol. 4:964, 1984.

149. Winniford, M. D., Wheelan, K. R., Kremers, M. S., et al.: Smoking-induced coronary vasoconstriction in patients with atherosclerotic coronary artery disease: Evidence for adrenergically mediated alterations in coronary artery tone. Circulation 73:662, 1986.

150. Winniford, M. D., Jansen, D. E., Reynolds, G. A., et al.: Cigarette smoking-induced coronary vasoconstriction in atherosclerotic coronary artery disease and prevention by calcium antagonists and nitroglycerin. Am. J. Cardiol. 59:203, 1987.

151. Deanfield, J., Wright, C., Kirkler, S., et al.: Cigarette smoking and the treatment of angina with propranolol, atenolol, and nifedipine. N. Engl. J. Med. 310:951, 1984.

152. Aronow, W. S.: Effect of passive smoking on angina pectoris. N. Engl. J. Med. 299:21, 1978.

153. Adams, K. F., Koch, G., Chatterjee, B., et al.: Acute elevation of blood carboxyhemoglobin to 6% impairs exercise performance and aggravates symptoms in patients with ischemic heart disease. J. Am. Coll. Cardiol. 12:900, 1988.

154. Alldred, E. N., Bleecker, E. R., Chaitman, B. R., et al.: Short-term effects of carbon monoxide exposure on the exercise performance of subjects with coronary artery disease. N. Engl. J. Med. 321:1426, 1989.

155. Rocco, M. B., Barry J., Campbell, S., et al.: Circadian variation of transient myocardial ischemia in patients with coronary artery disease. Circulation 75:395, 1987.

156. Hennekens, C. H., Buring, J. E., Sandercock, P., et al.: Aspirin and other antiplatelet agents in the secondary and primary prevention of cardiovascular disease. Circulation 80:749, 1989.

157. Ridker, P. M., Manson, J. E., Gaziano, J. M., et al.: Low-dose aspirin therapy for chronic stable angina. A randomized clinical trial. Ann. Intern. Med. 114:835, 1991.

158. Brown, G., Albers, J. J., Fisher, L. D., et al.: Regression of coronary artery disease as a result of intensive lipid-lowering therapy in men with high levels of apolipoprotein B. N. Engl. J. Med. 323:1289, 1990.

159. Ferguson, R. J., Taylor, A. W., Cote, P., et al.: Skeletal muscle and cardiac changes with training in patients with angina pectoris. Am. J. Physiol. 243:H830, 1982.

160. Redwood, D. R., Rosing, D. R., and Epstein, S. E.: Circulatory and symptomatic effects of physical training in patients with coronary artery disease and angina pectoris. N. Engl. J. Med. 286:959, 1972.

161. Ehsani, A. A., Biello, D. R., Schultz, J., et al.: Improvement of left ventricular contractile function by exercise training in patients with coronary artery disease. Circulation 74:350, 1986.

162. Parker, J. O.: Nitrate therapy in stable angina pectoris. N. Engl. J. Med. 316:1635, 1987.

163. Williams, J. F., Jr., Glick, G., and Braunwald, E.: Studies on cardiac dimensions in intact unanesthetized man. V. Effects of nitroglycerin. Circulation 32:76, 1965.

164. Brown, B. G., Bolson, E., Petersen, R. B., et al.: The mechanisms of nitroglycerin action: Stenosis vasodilation as a major component of the drug response. Circulation 64:1089, 1981.

165. Bache, R. J., Ball, R. M., Cobb, F. R., et al.: Effects of nitroglycerin on transmural myocardial blood flow in the unanesthetized dog. J. Clin. Invest. 55:1219, 1975.

166. Cohen, M. V., Downey, J. M., Sonnenblick, E. H., and Kirk, E. S.: The effects of nitroglycerin on coronary collaterals and myocardial contractility. J. Clin. Invest. 52:2836, 1973.

167. Cowan, C., Duran, P.V.M., Corsini, G., et al.: The effects of nitroglycerin on myocardial blood flow in man. Measured by coincidence counting and bolus injections of 84-rubidium. Am. J. Cardiol. 24:154, 1969.

168. Parker, J. O., West, R. O., and DiGiorgi, S.: The effect of nitroglycerin on coronary blood flow and the hemodynamic response to exercise in coronary artery disease. Am. J. Cardiol. 27:59, 1971.

169. Ganz, W., and Marcus, H. S.: Failure of intracoronary nitroglycerin to alleviate pacing-induced angina. Circulation 46:880, 1972.

170. Bernstein, L., Friesinger, G. C., Lichtlen, P. R., and Ross, R. S.: The effect of nitroglycerin on the systemic circulation in man and dog. Circulation 33:107, 1966.

171. Cohn, P. F., Maddox, D. E., Holman, B. L., et al.: Effect of sublingually administered nitroglycerin on regional myocardial blood flow in patients with coronary artery disease. Am. J. Cardiol. 39:672, 1977.

172. Dove, J. T., Shah, P. M., and Schreiner, B. F.: Effects of nitroglycerin on left ventricular wall motion in coronary artery disease. Circulation 49:682, 1974.

173. Borer, J. S., Bacharach, S. L., Green, M. V., et al.: Effect of nitroglycerin on exercise-induced abnormalities of left ventricular regional function and ejection fraction in coronary artery disease. Assessment by radionuclide cineangiography in symptomatic and asymptomatic patients. Circulation 57:314, 1978.

174. Winniford, M. D., Jansen, D. E., Reynolds, G. A., et al.: Cigarette smoking-induced coronary vasoconstriction in atherosclerotic coronary artery disease and prevention by calcium antagonists and nitroglycerin. Am. J. Cardiol. 59:203, 1987.

175. Murad, F.: Cyclic guanosine monophosphate as a mediator of vasodilation. J. Clin. Invest. 78:1, 1986.

176. Ignarro, L. J., Lippton, H., Edwards, J. C., et al.: Mechanism of vascular smooth muscle relaxation by organic nitrates, nitrites, nitroprusside, and nitric oxide: Evidence for the involvement of S-nitrosothiols as active intermediates. J. Pharmacol. Exp. Ther. 218:739, 1981.

177. Horowitz, J. D., Antman, E. M., Lorell, B. H., et al.: Potentiation of the cardiovascular effects of nitroglycerin by N-acetylcysteine. Circulation 68:1247, 1983.

178. Winniford, M. D., Kennedy, P. L., Wells, P. J., and Hillis, L. D.: Potentiation of nitroglycerin-induced coronary dilatation by N-acetylcysteine. Circulation 73:138, 1986.

179. May, D. C., Popma, J. J., Black, W. H., et al.: In vivo induction and reversal of nitroglycerin tolerance in human coronary arteries. N. Engl. J. Med. 317:805, 1987.

180. Hales, C. A., and Westphal. D.: Hypoxemia following the administration of sublingual nitroglycerin. Am. J. Med. 65:911, 1978.

181. Parker, J. O., Vankoughnett, K. A., and Farrell, B.: Nitroglycerin lingual spray: Clinical efficacy and dose response relation. Am. J. Cardiol. 57:1, 1986.

182. Needleman, P., Lang, S., and Johnson, E. M., Jr.: Organic nitrates: Relationship between biotransformation and rational angina pectoris therapy. J. Pharmacol. Exp. Ther. 181:489, 1972.

183. Belder, M. A., Schneeweiss, A., and Camm, A. J.: Evaluation of the efficacy and duration of action of isosorbide mononitrate in angina pectoris. Am. J. Cardiol. 65:6J, 1990.

184. Thadani, U., Fung, H. L., Darke, A. C., and Parker, J. O.: Oral isosorbide dinitrate in angina pectoris: Comparison of duration of action and dose-response relation during acute and sustained therapy. Am. J. Cardiol. 49:411, 1982.

185. Bassan, M. M.: The daylong pattern of the antianginal effect of long-term three times daily administered isosorbide dinitrate. J. Am. Coll. Cardiol. 16:936, 1990.

186. Abrams, J.: Interval therapy to avoid nitrate tolerance: Paradise regained? Am. J. Cardiol. 64:931, 1989.

187. Schaer, D. F., Buff, I. A., and Katz, R. J.: Sustained antianginal efficacy of transdermal nitroglycerin patches using an overnight 10-hour nitrate-free interval. Am. J. Cardiol. 61:46, 1988.

188. Demots, H., and Glasser, S. P.: Intermittent transdermal nitroglycerin therapy in the treatment of chronic stable angina. J. Am. Coll. Cardiol. 13:786, 1989.

189. Badger, R. S., Brown, B. G., Gallery, C. A., et al.: Coronary artery dilation and hemodynamic responses after isosorbide dinitrate therapy in patients with coronary artery disease. Am. J. Cardiol. 56:390, 1985.

190. Bassan, M. M., and Weiler-Ravell, D.: The additive antianginal action of oral isosorbide dinitrate in patients receiving propranolol. Magnitude and duration of effect. Chest 83:233, 1983.

191. Colditz, G. A., Halvorsen, K. T., and Goldhaber, S. Z.: Randomized clinical trials of transdermal nitroglycerin systems for the treatment of angina: A meta-analysis. Am. Heart J. 116:174, 1988.

192. Parker, J. O.: Intermittent transdermal nitroglycerin therapy in the treatment of chronic stable angina. J. Am. Coll. Cardiol. 13:794, 1989.

192a. Elkayam, U.: Tolerance to organic nitrates: evidence, mechanisms, clinical relevance, and strategies for prevention. Ann. Intern. Med. 114:667, 1991.

193. Parker, J. O., Vankoughnett, K. A., and Farrell, B.: Comparison of buccal nitroglycerin and oral isosorbide dinitrate for nitrate tolerance in stable angina pectoris. Am. J. Cardiol. 56:724, 1985.

194. Lee, G., Mason, D. T., and DeMaria, A. N.: Effects of long-term oral administration of isosorbide dinitrate on the antianginal response to nitroglycerin. Am. J. Cardiol. 41:82, 1978.

195. Marcus, F. I.: The rapid onset of nitrate tolerance. J. Am. Coll. Cardiol. 16:941, 1990.

196. Packer, M.: What causes tolerance to nitroglycerin? The 100 year old mystery continues. J. Am. Coll. Cardiol. 16:932, 1990.

197. Levy, W. S., Katz, R. J., and Wasserman, A. G.: Methionine restores the venodilative response to nitroglycerin after the development of tolerance. J. Am. Coll. Cardiol. 17:474, 1991.

198. Armstrong, P. W., Armstrong, J. A., and Marks, G. S.: Blood levels after sublingual nitroglycerin. Circulation 59:585, 1979.

199. Parker, J. O., Vankoughnett, K. A., and Fung, F.-L.: Transdermal isosorbide dinitrate in patients receiving propranolol. Magnitude and duration of effect. Chest 83:233, 1983.

200. Przybojewski, J. Z., and Heyns, M. H.: Acute coronary vasospasm secondary to industrial nitroglycerin withdrawal. S. Afr. Med. J. 63:158, 1983.

201. Watanabe, A. G.: Recent advances in knowledge about beta-adrenergic receptors: Application to clinical cardiology. J. Am. Coll. Cardiol. 1:82, 1983.

202. Kern, M. J., Ganz, P., Horowitz, J. D., et al.: Potentiation of coronary vasoconstriction by beta adrenergic blockade in patients with coronary artery disease. Circulation 67:1178, 1983.

203. Gaglione, A., Hess, O. M., Corin, W. J., et al.: Is there coronary vasoconstriction after intracoronary beta-adrenergic blockade in patients with coronary artery disease. J. Am. Coll. Cardiol. 10:299, 1987.

204. Chierchia, S., Muiesan, L., Davies, A., et al.: Role of the sympathetic nervous system in the pathogenesis of chronic stable angina. Implications for the mechanism of action of β-blockers. Circulation 82(Suppl. 11):71, 1990.

205. Lands, A. M., Arnold, A., McAuliff, J. P., et al.: Differentiation of receptor systems activated by sympathomimetic amines. Nature 214:597, 1967.

206. Conolly, M. E., Kersting, F., and Dollery, C. T.: The clinical pharmacology of beta-adrenoreceptor blocking drugs. Prog. Cardiovasc. Dis. 19:203, 1976.

207. Kostis, J. B., Frishman, W., Hosler, M. H., et al.: Treatment of angina pectoris with pindolol: The significance of intrinsic sympathomimetic activity of beta blockers. Am. Heart J. 104:496, 1982.

208. Quyyumi, A. A., Wright, C., Mockus, L., and Fox, K. M.: Effect of partial agonist activity in beta blockers in severe angina pectoris: A double-blind comparison of pindolol and atenolol. Br. Med. J. 289:951, 1984.

209. Drayer, D. E.: Lipophilicity, hydrophilicity and the central nervous system side effects of beta-blockers. Pharmacotherapy 7:87, 1987.

210. Gengo, F. M., Huntoon, L., and McHugh, W. B.: Lipid-soluble and water-soluble β-blockers. Comparison of the central nervous system depressant effect. Arch. Intern. Med. 147:39, 1987.

211. Kostis, J. B., and Rosen, R. C.: Central nervous system effects of the β-adrenergic-blocking drugs: The role of ancillary properties. Circulation 75:204, 1987.

212. Frishman, W., and Halprin, S.: Clinical pharmacology of the new beta-adrenergic blocking drugs. VII. New horizons in beta-adrenoceptor blocking therapy—labetalol. Am. Heart J. 98:660, 1979.

213. Prida, X.E., Hill, J. A., and Feldman, R. L.: Systemic and coronary hemodynamic effects of combined alpha- and beta-adrenergic blockade (Labetolol) in normotensive patients with stable angina pectoris and positive exercise test responses. Am. J. Cardiol. 59:1084, 1987.

214. Lennard, M. S.: The polymorphic oxidation of beta-adrenoceptor antagonists. Pharmacol. Ther. 41:461, 1989.

215. Lehtonen, A.: Effect of beta blockers on blood lipid profile. Am. Heart J. 109:1192, 1985.

216. Northcote, R. J., Todd, I. C., and Ballantyne, D.: Beta blockers and lipoproteins: A review of current knowledge. Scott Med. J. 31:220, 1986.

217. Rutherford, J. D., Singh, B. N., Ambler, P. K., and Norris, R. M.: Plasma propranolol concentration in patients with angina and acute myocardial infarction. Clin. Exp. Pharmacol. Physiol. 3:297, 1976.

218. Miller, R. R., Olson, H. G., Amsterdam, E. A., and Mason, D. T.: Propranolol withdrawal rebound phenomenon. Exacerbation of coronary events after abrupt cessation of antianginal therapy. N. Engl. J. Med. 293:416, 1975.

219. Hiatt, W. R., Stoll, S., and Nies, A. S.: Effect of beta-adrenergic blockers on the peripheral circulation in patients with peripheral vascular disease. Circulation 72:1226, 1985.

220. Cooper, G., Kent, R. L., McGonigle, P., and Watanabe, A.: Beta adrenergic receptor blockade of feline myocardium. Cardiac mechanics, energetics, and beta adrenoceptor regulation. J. Clin. Invest. 77:441, 1986.

221. Cardiology Drug Facts, 1989. 1st ed. St. Louis. C.V. Mosby.

222. Opie, L. H.: Calcium channel antagonists. A Review. Part 1. Fundamental properties: Mechanisms, classification, sites of action. Cardiovasc. Drugs Ther. I:411, 1987.

223. Opie, L. H.: Calcium channel antagonists. Part V. Second generation agents. Cardiovasc. Drugs Ther. 2:191, 1988.

224. Wood, A. J. J.: Calcium antagonists. Pharmacologic differences and similarities. Circulation 80(Suppl. IV):184, 1989.

224a. Hurwitz, L., Partridge, L. D., and Leach, J. K. (eds.): Calcium Channels: Their Properties, Functions, Regulation, and Clinical Relevance. Boca Raton, FL, CRC Press, 1991.

225. Stone, P. H., Turi, Z., Muller, J. E., et al.: Experience with nifedipine in 845 patients with refractory angina pectoris. J. Am. Coll. Cardiol. 1:596, 1983.

226. Strauss, W. E., and Parisi, S. F.: Combined use of calcium-channel and beta-adrenergic blockers for the treatment of chronic stable angina. Ann. Intern. Med. 109:570, 1988.

227. Packer, M.: Combined beta-adrenergic and calcium-entry blockade in angina pectoris. N. Engl. J. Med. 320:709, 1989.

228. Cannon, R. O., Watson, R. M., Rosing, D. R., and Epstein, S. E.: Efficacy of calcium channel blocker therapy for angina pectoris resulting from small-vessel coronary artery disease and abnormal vasodilator reserve. Am. J. Cardiol. 56:242, 1985.

228a. Cole, P. L., Beamer, A. D., McGowan, N., et al.: Efficacy and safety of perhexiline maleate in refractory angina. A double-blind placebo-controlled clinical trial of a novel antianginal agent. Circulation 81:1260, 1990.

229. Lichtlen, P. R., Hugenholtz, P. G., Raffenbleul, W. et al.: Retardation of angiographic progression of coronary artery disease by nifedipine. Results of the International Nifedipine Trial on Antiatherosclerotic Therapy (INTACT). Lancet 335:1109, 1990.

230. Loadi, A., Polese, A., Montorsi, P., et al.: Comparison of nifedipine, propranolol and isosorbide dinitrate on angiographic progression and regression of coronary arterial narrowings in angina pectoris. Am. J. Cardiol. 64:433, 1989.

231. Extended-release nifedipine: Effective 24-hour treatment for hypertension and angina. Hosp. Formul. (Suppl. A) 25:2, 1990.

232. Wallace, W. A., Wellington, K. L., Murphy, G. W., and Liang, C.-S.: Comparison of antianginal efficacies and exercise hemodynamic effects of Nifedipine and Diltiazem in stable angina pectoris. Am. J. Cardiol. 63:414, 1989.

233. Vatner, S. F., and Hintze, T. H.: Effects of a calcium-channel antagonist on large and small coronary arteries in conscious dogs. Circulation 66:579, 1982.

234. Ludbrook, P. A., Tiefenbrunn, A. J., Reed, F. R., and Sobel, B. E.: Acute hemodynamic responses to sublingual nifedipine: Dependence on left ventricular function. Circulation 65:489, 1982.

235. Elkayam, U., Amin, J., Mehra, A., et al.: A prospective, randomized, double-blind, crossover study to compare the efficacy and safety of chronic nifedipine therapy with that of isosorbide dinitrate and their combination in the treatment of chronic congestive heart failure. Circulation 82:1954, 1990.

236. White, H. D., Polak, J. F., Wynne, J., et al.: Addition of nifedipine to maximal nitrate and beta-adrenoreceptor blocker therapy in coronary artery disease. Am. J. Cardiol. 55:1303, 1985.

237. Leon, M. B., Rosing, D. R., Bonow, R. O., et al.: Clinical efficacy of verapamil alone and combined with propranolol in treating patients with chronic stable angina pectoris. Am. J. Cardiol. 48:131, 1981.

238. Boden, W. E., Bough, E. W., Reichman, M. J., et al.: Beneficial effects of high-dose diltiazem in patients with persistent effort angina on beta blockers and nitrates: A randomized, double-blind, placebo-controlled cross-over study. Circulation 71:1197, 1985.

239. Wagniart, P., Feguson, R. J., Chaitman, B. R., et al.: Increased exercise tolerance and reduced electrocardiographic ischemia with diltiazem in patients with stable angina pectoris. Circulation 66:23, 1984.

240. Bache, R. J.: Effects of calcium entry blockade on myocardial blood flow. Circulation 80(Suppl. IV):40, 1989.

241. Nonogi, H., Hess, O. M., Ritter, M., et al.: Prevention of coronary vasoconstriction during dynamic exercise in patients with coronary artery disease. J. Am. Coll. Cardiol. 12:892, 1988.

242. Rossen, J. D., Simonetti, I., Marcus, M. L., et al.: The effect of diltiazem on coronary flow reserve in humans. Circulation 80:1240, 1989.

243. Murakami, T., Hess, O. M., and Krayenbuehl, H. P.: Left ventricular function before and after diltiazem in patients with coronary artery disease. J. Am. Coll. Cardiol. 5:723, 1985.

244. DeServi, S., Ferrario, M., Ghio, S., et al.: Effects of diltiazem on regional coronary hemodynamics during atrial pacing in patients with stable exertional angina: Implications for mechanism of action. Circulation 73:1248, 1986.

245. O'Hara, M. J., Khurmi, N. S., Bowles, M. J., and Raftery, E. B.: Diltiazem and propranolol combination for the treatment of chronic stable angina pectoris. Clin. Cardiol. 10:115, 1987.

246. Strauss, W. E., and Parisi, A. F.: Superiority of combined diltiazem and propranolol therapy for angina pectoris. Circulation 71:951, 1985.

247. Frishman, W., Charlap, S., Kimmel, B., et al.: Diltiazem, nifedipine, and their combination in patients with stable angina pectoris: effects on angina, exercise tolerance, and the ambulatory electrocardiographic ST segment. Circulation 77:774, 1988.

248. Toyosaki, N., Toyo-Oka, T., Natsume, T., et al.: Combination therapy with diltiazem and nifedipine in patients with effort angina pectoris. Circulation 77:1370, 1988.

249. Van Dijk, R. B., Lie, K. I., and Crijns, H.J.G.M.: Diltiazem in comparison with metoprolol in stable angina pectoris. Eur. Heart J. 9:1194, 1988.

249a. Hampton, J. R.: Secondary prevention of acute myocardial infarction with beta-blocking agents and calcium antagonists. Am. J. Cardiol. 66:3c, 1990.

250. Gibson, R. S., Boden, W. E., Theroux, P., et al.: Diltiazem and reinfarction in patients with non-Q-wave myocardial infarction. Results of a double-blind, randomized, multicenter trial. N. Engl. J. Med. 315:423, 1986.

251. The Danish Study Group on Verapamil in Myocardial Infarction: Effect of Verapamil on mortality and major events after acute infarction (The Danish Verapamil Infarction Trial II-DAVIT II). Am. J. Cardiol. 66:779, 1990.

252. Stone, P. H., Gibson, R. S., Glasser, S. P., et al. (The ASIS Study Group): Comparison of propranolol, diltiazem, and nifedipine in the treatment of ambulatory ischemia in patients with stable angina. Differential effects on ambulatory ischemia, exercise performance, and anginal symptoms. Circulation 82:1962, 1990.

253. Klinke, W. P., Kvill, L., Dempsey, E. E., and Grace, M.: A randomized double-blind comparison of diltiazem and nifedipine in stable angina. J. Am. Coll. Cardiol. 12:1562, 1988.

254. Nesto, R. W., White, H. D., Wynne, J., et al.: Comparison of nifedipine and isosorbide dinitrate when added to maximum propranolol therapy in stable angina pectoris. Am. J. Cardiol. 60:256, 1987.

255. Packer, M., Meller, J., Medina, N., et al.: Hemodynamic consequences of combined beta-adrenergic and slow calcium channel blockade in man. Circulation 65:660, 1982.

256. Kieval, J., Kirsten, E. B., Kessler, K. M., et al.: The effects of intravenous verapamil on hemodynamic status of patients with coronary artery disease receiving propranolol. Circulation 65:653, 1982.

257. Shub, C.: Stable angina pectoris. 3. Medical treatment. Mayo Clin. Proc. 65:256, 1990.

258. Ellis, S. G., Cowley, M. J., DiSciascio, G., et al.: Determinants of 2-year outcome after coronary angioplasty in patients with multivessel disease on the basis of comprehensive preprocedural evaluation: Implications for patient selection. Circulation 83:1905, 1991.

258a. Wong, J. B., Sonnenberg, F. A., Salem, D. N., and Pauker, S. G. P.: Myocardial revascularization for chronic stable angina. Ann. Intern. Med. 113:852, 1990.

259. Cowley, M. J., Vetrovec, G. W., DiSciascio, G., et al.: Coronary angioplasty of multiple vessels: Short-term outcome and long-term results. Circulation 72:1314, 1985.

260. Leimgruber, P. P., Roubin, G. S., Hollman, J., et al.: Restenosis after successful coronary angioplasty in patients with single-vessel disease. Circulation 73:710, 1986.

261. Melchior, J. P., Meier, B., Urban, P., et al.: Percutaneous transluminal coronary angioplasty for chronic total coronary arterial occlusion. Am. J. Cardiol. 59:535, 1987.

261a. Savage, M. P., Goldberg, S., Hirshfeld, J. W., et al.: Clinical and angiographic determinants of primary coronary angioplasty success. J. Am. Coll. Cardiol. 17:22, 1991.

262. Holmes, D. R., Holubkov R., Vlietstra R. E., and the Coinvestigators of the NHLBI Transluminal Coronary Angioplasty Registry: Comparison of the complications during percutaneous transluminal coronary angioplasty from 1977 to 1981 and from 1985 to 1986. J. Am. Coll. Cardiol. 12:1149, 1988.

263. Kohli, R. S., DiSciascio, G., Cowley, M. J., et al.: Coronary angioplasty in patients with severe left ventricular dysfunction. J. Am. Coll. Cardiol. 16:807, 1990.

264. Ellis, S. G., Roubin, G. S., King, S. B., et al.: Angiographic and clinical predictors of acute closure after native vessel coronary angioplasty. Circulation 77:372, 1988.

265. Ellis, S. G., Roubin, G. S., King, S. B., et al.: In-hospital cardiac mortality after acute closure after coronary angioplasty: Analysis of risk factors from 8,207 procedures. J. Am. Coll. Cardiol. 11:211, 1988.

266. Stammen, F., Piessens, J., Vrolix, M., et al.: Immediate and short-term results of a 1988–1989 coronary angioplasty registry. Am. J. Cardiol. 67:253, 1991.

267. Deligonul, U., Vandormael, M. G., Kern, M. J., et al.: Coronary angioplasty: A therapeutic option for symptomatic patients with tow and three vessel coronary disease. J. Am. Coll. Cardiol. 11:1173, 1988.

268. DiSciascio, G., Cowley, M. J., Vetrovec, G. W., et al.: Triple vessel coronary angioplasty: Acute outcome and long-term results. J. Am. Coll. Cardiol. 12:42, 1988.

269. Vandormael, M., Deligonul, U., Taussig, S., and Kern, M. J.: Predictors of long-term cardiac survival in patients with multivessel coronary artery disease undergoing percutaneous transluminal coronary angioplasty. Am. J. Cardiol. 67:1, 1991.

269a. Thompson, R. C., Holmes, D. R., Gersh, B. J., et al.: Percutaneous transluminal coronary angioplasty in the elderly: Early and long-term results. J. Am. Coll. Cardiol. 17:1245, 1991.

270. O'Keefe, J. H., Rutherford, B. D., McConahay, D. R., et al.: Multivessel coronary angioplasty from 1980 to 1989: Procedural results and long-term outcome. J. Am. Coll. Cardiol. 16:1097, 1990.

270a. Ellis, S. G., Vandormael, M. G., Cowley, M. J., et al.: Coronary morphologic and clinical determinants of procedural outcome with angioplasty for multivessel coronary disease. Implications for patient selection. Circulation 82:1193, 1990.

271. Gaul, G., Hollman, J., Simpfendorfer, C., and Franco, I.: Acute occlusion in multiple lesion coronary angioplasty: Frequency and management. J. Am. Coll. Cardiol. 123:283, 1989.

272. Mabin, T. A., Holmes, D. R., Jr., Smith, H. E., et al.: Follow-up clinical results in patients undergoing percutaneous transluminal coronary angioplasty. Circulation 71:754, 1985.

273. Vandormael, M. G., Chaitman, B. R., Ischinger, T., et al.: Immediate and short-term benefit of multilesion coronary angioplasty: Influence of degree of revascularization. J. Am. Coll. Cardiol. 6:983, 1985.

274. Reeder, G. S., Vlietstra, R. E., Mock, M. B., et al.: Comparison of angioplasty and bypass surgery in multivessel coronary artery disease. Int. J. Cardiol. 10:213, 1986.

275. Reeder, G. S., Holmes, D. R., Detre, K., et al.: Degree of revascularization in patients with multivessel coronary disease: A report from the NHLBI Percutaneous Transluminal Coronary Angioplasty Registry. Circulation 77:638, 1988.

276. Bell, M. R., Bailer, K. R., Reeder, G. S., et al.: Percutaneous transluminal angioplasty in patients with multivessel coronary disease: How important is complete revascularization for cardiac event-free survival? J. Am. Coll. Cardiol. 16:553, 1990.

276a. Topol, E. J., and Faxon, D. P.: Symposium on restenosis: From basic studies to clinical trials. J. Am. Coll. Cardiol. 17:Suppl B, 1991, 199 pp.

277. Popma, J. J., and Topol, E. J.: Factors influencing restenosis after coronary angioplasty. Am. J. Med. 88:16N, 1990.

277a. Nobuyoshi, M., Kimura, T., Ohishi, H., et al.: Restenosis after percutaneous transluminal coronary angioplasty: Pathologic observations in 20 patients. J. Am. Coll. Cardiol. 17:433, 1991.

278. Galan, K. M., Deligonul, U., Kern, M. J., et al.: Increased frequency of restenosis in patients continuing to smoke cigarettes after percutaneous transluminal coronary angioplasty. Am. J. Cardiol. 61:260, 1988.

279. Schwartz, L., Bourassa, M. G., Lesperance, J., et al.: Aspirin and dipyridamole in the prevention of restenosis after transluminal coronary angioplasty. N. Engl. J. Med. 318:1714, 1988.

280. Black, A.J.R., Anderson, H. V., Roubin, G. S., et al.: Repeat coronary angioplasty: Correlates of a second restenosis. J. Am. Coll. Cardiol. 11:714, 1988.

280a. Hollman, J.: What does pathology teach us about recurrent stenosis after coronary angioplasty? J. Am. Coll. Cardiol. 17:440, 1991.

281. Teirstein, P. S., Hoover, C. A., Ligon, R. W., et al.: Repeat coronary angioplasty: Efficacy of a third angioplasty for a second restenosis. J. Am. Coll. Cardiol. 13:291, 1989.

282. Talley, J. D., Weintraub, W. S., Roubin, G. S., et al.: Failed elective percutaneous transluminal coronary angioplasty requiring coronary artery bypass surgery. Circulation 82:1203, 1990.

283. Bentivoglio, L. G., Van Raden, M. J., Kelsey, S. F., and Detre, K. M.: Percutaneous transluminal coronary angioplasty (PTCA) in patients with relative contraindications: Results of the National Heart, Lung, and Blood Institute PTCA Registry. Am. J. Cardiol. 53(Suppl. 1):82C, 1984.

284. Bonow, R. O., Kent, K. M., Rosing, D. R., et al.: Improved left ventricular diastolic filling in patients with coronary artery disease after percutaneous transluminal coronary angioplasty. Circulation 66:1159, 1982.

285. Bates, E. R., Aueron, F. M., Legrand, V., et al.: Comparative long-term effects of coronary artery bypass graft surgery and percutaneous transluminal coronary angioplasty on regional coronary flow reserve. Circulation 72:833, 1985.

286. Kent, K. M., Bonow, R. O., Rosing, D. R., et al.: Improved myocardial function during exercise after successful percutaneous transluminal coronary angioplasty. N. Engl. J. Med. 306:441, 1982.

287. Gruentzig, A. R., King, S. B., Schlumpf, M., and Siegenthaler, W.: Long-term follow-up after percutaneous transluminal coronary angioplasty. The early Zurich experience. N. Engl. J. Med. 316:1127, 1987.

288. Berger, E., Williams, D. O., Reinert, S., and Most, A. S.: Sustained efficacy of percutaneous transluminal coronary angioplasty. Am. Heart J. 111:233, 1986.

289. Webb, J. G., Myler, R. K., Shaw, R. E., et al.: Coronary angioplasty after coronary bypass surgery: Initial results and late outcome in 422 patients. J. Am. Coll. Cardiol. 16:812, 1990.

290. Cooper, I., Ineson, N., Demirtas, E., et al.: Role of angioplasty in patients with previous coronary artery bypass surgery. Cathet. Cardiovasc. Diagn. 16:81, 1989.

291. Platko, W. P., Hollman, J., Whitlow, P. L., and Franco, I.: Percutaneous transluminal angioplasty of saphenous graft stenosis: Long-term followup. J. Am. Coll. Cardiol. 14:1645, 1989.

291a. Plokker, H. W. T., Meester, B. H., and Serruys, P. W.: The Dutch experience in percutaneous transluminal angioplasty of narrowed saphenous veins used for aortocoronary arterial bypass. Am. J. Cardiol. 67:361, 1991.

292. Serruys, P. W., Umans, V., Heyndrickx, G. R., et al.: Elective PTCA of totally occluded coronary arteries not associated with acute myocardial infarction; short-term and long-term results. Eur. Heart J. 6:2, 1985.

293. Kereiakes, D. J., Selmon, M. R., McAuley, B. J., et al.: Angioplasty in total coronary artery occlusion: Experience in 76 consecutive patients. J. Am. Coll. Cardiol. 6:526, 1985.

294. DiSciascio, G., Vetrovec, G. W., Cowley, M. J., and Wolfgang, T. C.: Early and late outcome of percutaneous transluminal coronary angioplasty for subacute and chronic total coronary occlusion. Am. Heart J. 111:833, 1986.

295. Isner, J. M., Rosenfield, K., and Losordo, D. W.: Excimer laser atherectomy. The greening of Sisyphus. Circulation 81:2018, 1990.

296. Karsch, K. R., Haase, K. K., Voelker, W., et al.: Percutaneous coronary excimer laser angioplasty in patients with stable and unstable angina pectoris. Circulation 81:1849, 1990.

297. Veith, F. J., Bakal, C. W., Cynamon, J., et al.: Early experience with the smart laser in treatment of atherosclerotic occlusion. Am. Heart J. 121:1531, 1991.

298. Sanborn, T. A., Bittl, J. A., Hershman, R. A., and Siegel, R. M.: Percutaneous coronary excimer laser-assisted angioplasty: Initial multicenter experience in 141 patients. J. Am. Coll. Cardiol. (Suppl. B) 17:169B, 1991.

298a. Sanborn, T. A., Torre, S. R., Sharma, S. K., et al.: Percutaneous coronary excimer laser-assisted balloon angioplasty: Initial clinical and quantitative angiographic results in 50 patients. J. Am. Coll. Cardiol. 17:94, 1991.

299. Hillis, L. D.: Efficacy and safety of coronary balloon angioplasty and directional atherectomy. Circulation 82:305, 1990.

300. Safian, R. D., Gelbfish, J. S., Erny, R. E., et al.: Coronary atherectomy. Clinical, angiographic, and histological findings and observations regarding potential mechanisms. Circulation 82:69, 1990.

CORONARY ARTERY BYPASS SURGERY

301. Kaiser, G. C.: CABG 1984: technical aspects of bypass surgery. Circulation 72(Suppl. V):46, 1985.

302. Grondin, C. M., Campeau, L., Thornton, J. C., et al.: Coronary artery bypass grafting with saphenous vein. Circulation 79(Suppl. I):24, 1989.

303. Preito, I., Basil, E. F., and Abdulnou, R. E.: Upper extremity vein graft for aortocoronary bypass. Ann. Thorac. Surg. 37:218, 1984.

304. Stoney, W. S., Alford, W. C., Burrus, G. R., et al.: The fate of arm vein grafts used for coronary artery bypass grafts. J. Thorac. Cardiovasc. Surg. 88:522, 1984.

305. Campeau, L., Enjalbert, M., Lesperance, J., et al.: Atherosclerosis and late closure of aortocoronary saphenous vein grafts: Sequential angiographic studies at 2 weeks, 1 year, 5 to 7 years, and 10 to 12 years after surgery. Circulation 68(Suppl. II):1, 1983.

306. Green, G. E.: Use of internal thoracic artery for coronary artery grafting. Circulation 79(Suppl. I):30, 1989.

307. Luscher, T. F., Diederich, D., Siebenmann, R., et al.: Difference between endothelium-dependent relaxation in arterial and in venous coronary bypass grafts. N. Engl. J. Med. 319:462, 1988.

308. Loop, F. D., Lytle, B. W., and Cosgrove, D. M.: New arteries for old. Circulation 79(Suppl. I):40, 1989.

309. Shelton, M. E., Forman, M. B., Virmani, R., et al.: A comparison of morphologic and angiographic findings in long-term internal mammary artery and saphenous vein bypass grafts. J. Am. Coll. Cardiol. 11:297, 1988.

310. Loop, F. D., Lytle, B. W., Cosgrove, D. M., et al.: Influence of the internal mammary artery graft on 10-year survival and other cardiac events. N. Engl. J. Med. 314:1, 1986.

311. Kirklin, J. W., Naftel, D. C., Blackstone, E. H., and Pohost, G. M.: Summary of a consensus concerning death and ischemic events after coronary artery bypass grafting. Circulation 79(Suppl. I):81, 1989.

312. Cameron, A., Davis, K. B., Green, G. E., et al.: Clinical implications of internal mammary bypass grafts: The Coronary Artery Surgery Study experience. Circulation 77:815, 1988.

313. Morris, J. J., Smith, R., Glower, D. D., et al.: Clinical evaluation of single versus multiple mammary artery bypass. Circulation 82(Suppl. IV):214, 1990.

314. Foster, E. D., and Kranc, M. A.: Alternative conduits for aortocoronary bypass grafting. Circulation 79(Suppl. I):34, 1989.

315. Kusukawa, J., Hirota, Y., Kawamura, K., et al.: Efficacy of coronary artery bypass surgery with gastroepiploic artery. Assessment with thallium-201 myocardial scintigraphy. Circulation 79(Suppl. I):135, 1989.

316. Mills, N. L., and Everson, C. T.: Right gastroepiploic artery: A third arterial conduit for coronary artery bypass. Ann. Thorac. Surg. 47:706, 1989.

317. Smith, S. C., Jr., Gorlin, R., Herman, M. V., et al.: Myocardial blood flow in man. Effect of coronary collateral circulation and coronary artery bypass surgery. J. Clin. Invest. 51:2556, 1972.

318. Lesperance, J., Bourassa, M. G., Biron, P., et al.: Aorta to coronary artery saphenous vein grafts. Preoperative angiographic criteria for successful surgery. Am. J. Cardiol. 30:459, 1972.

319. Rosch, J., Dotter, C. T., Antonovic, R., et al.: Angiographic appraisal of distal vessel suitability for aortocoronary bypass graft surgery. Circulation 48:202, 1973.

320. Cukingnan, R. A., Carey, J. S., Wittig, J. H., and Brown, B. G.: Influence of complete coronary revascularization on relief of angina. J. Thorac. Cardiovasc. Surg. 79:188, 1980.

321. Grondin, C. M., Lapage, G., Castoguay, Y. R., et al.: Aortocoronary bypass graft. Initial blood flow through the graft, and early postoperative patency. Circulation 44:815, 1971.

322. Califf, R. M., Harrell, F. E., Lee, K. L., et al.: The evolution of medical and surgical therapy for coronary artery disease. A 15-year perspective. JAMA 261:2077, 1989.

323. Christakis, G. T., Ivanov, J., Weisel, R. D., et al.: The changing pattern of coronary artery bypass surgery. Circulation 80(Suppl. I):151, 1989.

324. Passamani, E., Davis, K. B., Gillespie, M. J., Killip, T., and the CASS principal investigators and their associates: A randomized trial of coronary artery bypass surgery. Survival of patients with a low ejection fraction. N. Engl. J. Med. 312:1665, 1985.

325. Killip, T., Passamani, E., Davis, K., and the CASS Principal Investigators and their Associates: Coronary artery surgery study (CASS): A randomized trial of coronary bypass surgery. Eight-year follow-up and survival in patients with reduced ejection fraction. Circulation 72(Suppl. V):102, 1985.

326. Pigott, J. D., Kouchoukos, N. T., Oberman, A., and Cutter, G. R.: Late results of surgical and medical therapy for patients with coronary artery disease and depressed left ventricular function. J. Am. Coll. Cardiol. 5:1036, 1985.

327. Vigilante, G. J., Weintraub, W. S., Klein, L. W., et al.: Improved survival with coronary bypass surgery in patients with three-vessel coronary disease and abnormal left ventricular function. Matched case-control study in patient with potentially operable disease. Am. J. Med. 82:697, 1987.

328. Mock, M. B., Fisher, L. D., Holmes, D. R., et al.: Comparison of effects of medical and surgical therapy on survival in severe angina pectoris and two-vessel coronary artery disease with and without left ventricular dysfunction. A coronary artery surgery study registry study. Am. J. Cardiol. 61:1198, 1988.

329. Bounous, E. P., Mark, D. B., Pollock, B. G., et al.: Surgical survival benefits for coronary disease patients with left ventricular dysfunction. Circulation 78(Suppl. I):151, 1988.

330. Proudfit, W. L., Kramer, J. R., Goormastic, M., and Loop, F. D.: Survival of patients with mild angina or myocardial infarction without angina; A comparison of medical and surgical treatment. Br. Heart J. 59:641, 1988.

331. Daily, P. O.: Early and 5-year results for coronary artery bypass grafting. A benchmark for percutaneous transluminal coronary angioplasty. J. Thorac. Cardiovasc. Surg. 96:67, 1989.

332. Myers, W. O., Davis, K., Foster, E. D., Maynard, C., and Kaiser, G. C.: Surgical survival in the Coronary Artery Surgery Study (CASS) Registry. Ann. Thorac. Surg. 40:245, 1985.

332a. Gomberg, J., Klein, L. W., Seelaus, P., et al.: Surgical revascularization of left main coronary artery stenosis: Determinants of perioperative and long-term outcome in the 1980s. Am. Heart J. 116:440, 1988.

333. Bolooki, H.: Emergency cardiac procedures in patients in cardiogenic shock due to complications of coronary artery disease. Circulation 79(Suppl. I):137, 1989.

333a. Naunheim, K. S., Fiore, A. C., Wadley, J. J., et al.: The changing profile of the patient undergoing coronary artery bypass surgery. J. Am. Coll. Cardiol. 11:494, 1988.

334. CASS Principal Investigators and their Associates: Coronary Artery Surgery Study (CASS): A randomized trial of coronary artery bypass surgery. Survival data. Circulation 68:939, 1983.

335. Chaitman, B. R., Alderman, E. L., Sheffield, L. T., et al.: Use of survival analysis to determine the clinical significance of new Q waves after coronary bypass surgery. Circulation 67:302, 1983.

336. Force, T., Hibberd, P., Weeks, G., et al.: Perioperative myocardial infarction after coronary artery bypass. Clinical significance and approach to risk stratification. Circulation 82:903, 1990.

337. Shaw, P. J., Bates, D., Cartlidge, N.E.F., et al.: Early intellectual dysfunction following coronary bypass surgery. Q. J. Med. 58:59, 1986.

338. Raymond, M., Conklin, C., Schaeffer, J., et al.: Coping with transient intellectual dysfunction after coronary bypass surgery. Heart Lung 13:531, 1984.

339. Mullen, J. C., Miller, D. R., Weisel, R. D., et al.: Postoperative hypertension: A comparison of diltiazem, nifedipine, and nitroprusside. J. Thorac. Cardiovasc. Surg. 96:122, 1988.

340. Durkin, M. A., Thys, D., Morris, R. B., et al.: Control of perioperative hypertension during coronary artery surgery. A randomized double-blind study comparing isosorbide dinitrare and nitroglycerin. Eur. Heart J. 9:A-181, 1988.

341. Gray, R. J., Bateman, T. M., Czer, L.S.C., et al.: Use of esmolol in hypertension after cardiac surgery. Am. J. Cardiol. 56:49F, 1985.

342. Tuzcu, E. M., Emre, A., Goormastic, M., et al.: Incidence and prognostic significance of intraventricular conduction abnormalities after coronary bypass surgery. J. Am. Coll. Cardiol. 16:607, 1990.

343. Koshal, A., Hendry, P., Roman, S. V., and Keon, W. J.: Should obese patients not undergo coronary artery surgery? Can. J. Surg. 28:331, 1985.

344. McDonald, W. S., Brame, M., Sharp, C., and Eggerstedt, J.: Risk factors for median sternotomy dehiscence in cardiac surgery. South. Med. J. 82:1361, 1989.

345. Utley, J. R., Thomason, M. E., Wallace, D. J., et al.: Preoperative correlates of impaired wound healing after saphenous vein excision. J. Thorac. Cardiovasc. Surg. 98:147, 1989.

346. Rutherford, J. D., Whitlock, R. M. L., McDonald, B. W., et al.: Multivariate analysis of the long-term results of coronary artery bypass grafting performed during 1976 and 1977. Am. J. Cardiol. 57:1264, 1986.

347. European Coronary Surgery Study Group: Long-term results of prospective randomized study of coronary artery bypass surgery in stable angina pectoris. Lancet 2:1173, 1982.

348. CASS Principal Investigators and their Associates: Coronary Artery Surgery Study (CASS): A randomized trial of coronary artery bypass surgery. Quality of life in patients randomly assigned to treatment groups. Circulation 68:951, 1983.

349. Hultgren, H. M., Peduzzi, P., Detre, K., Takaro, T., and the study participants: The 5-year effect of bypass surgery on relief of angina and exercise performance. Circulation 72(Suppl. V):79, 1985.

350. Johnson, W. D., Kayser, K. L., and Pedraza, P. M.: Angina pectoris and coronary bypass surgery: Patterns of prevalence and recurrence in 3105 consecutive patients followed up to 11 years. Am. Heart J. 108:1190, 1984.

351. Wenger, N. K.: Rehabilitation of the coronary patient: status 1986. Prog. Cardiovasc. Dis. 29:181, 1986.

352. Hymowitz, Z., Freiman, I., Borman, J., et al.: Work status before and after coronary artery bypass surgery. Publ. Health (Lond.) 99:367, 1985.

353. Misra, K. K., Kazanchi, B. N., Davies, G. J., et al.: Determinants of work capability and employment after coronary artery surgery. Eur. Heart J. 6:176, 1985.

354. Sergeant, P., Lesaffire, E., Flameng, W., and Suy, R.: How predictable is the postoperative work resumption after aortocoronary bypass surgery? Acta Cardiologica 41:41, 1986.

355. Hall, R.: Coronary artery bypass long-term follow-up on 22,284 consecutive patients. Circulation 68(Suppl. II):20, 1983.

356. Stanton, B., Jenkins, C. D., Savageau, J. A., and Thurer, R. L.: Functional benefits following coronary artery bypass graft surgery. Ann. Thorac. Surg. 37:286, 1984.

357. Peduzzi, P., Hultgren, H., Thomsen, J., and Detre, K.: Ten-year effect of medical and surgical therapy on quality of life: Veterans Administration Cooperative Study of Coronary Artery Surgery. Am. J. Cardiol. 59:1017, 1987.

358. Chesebro, J. H., Clements, I. P., Fuster, V., et al.: A platelet-inhibitor drug trial in coronary-artery bypass operations. Benefit of perioperative dipyridamole and aspirin therapy on early postoperative vein-graft patency. N. Engl. J. Med. 307:73, 1982.

359. Sanz, G., Pajaron, A., Alegria, E., et al.: Prevention of early aortocoronary bypass occlusion by low-dose aspirin and dipyridamole. Circulation 82:765, 1990.

360. Vlodaver, Z., and Edwards, J. E.: Pathologic changes in aortic-coronary arterial saphenous vein grafts. Circulation 44:719, 1971.

361. Lie, J. T., Lawrie, G. M., and Morris, G. C.: Aortocoronary bypass saphenous vein graft atherosclerosis. Am. J. Cardiol. 40:906, 1977.

361a. Fitzgibbon, G. M., Leach, A. J., Kafka, H. P., and Keon, W. J.: Coronary bypass graft fate: Long-term angiographic study. J. Am. Coll. Cardiol. 17:1075, 1991.

362. Rasmussen, S. L., Nielsen, S. L., Amtorp, O., et al.: 201-Thallium imaging as an indicator of graft patency after coronary artery bypass surgery. Eur. Heart J. 5:494, 1984.

363. Kroncke, G. M., Kosolcharoen, P., Clayman, J. A., et al.: Five-year changes in coronary arteries of medical and surgical patients of the Veterans Administration randomized study of bypass surgery. Circulation 78(Suppl. I):144, 1988.

364. Hwang, M. H., Meadows, W. R., Palac, R. T., et al.: Progression of native coronary artery disease at 10 years: Insights from a randomized study of medical versus surgical therapy for angina. J. Am. Coll. Cardiol. 16:1066, 1990.

365. Goldman, S., Copeland, J., Moritz, T., et al.: Saphenous vein graft patency 1 year after coronary artery bypass surgery and effects of antiplatelet therapy: Results of a Veterans Administration Cooperative Study. Circulation 80:1190, 1989.

366. Chesbro, J. H., Fuster, V., Elveback, L. R., et al.: Effect of dipyridamole and aspirin on late vein-graft patency after coronary bypass operations. N. Engl. J. Med. 310:209, 1984.

367. Henderson, W. G., Goldman, S., Copeland, J. G., et al.: Antiplatelet or anticoagulant therapy after coronary artery bypass surgery. A meta-analysis of clinical trials. Ann. Intern. Med. 111:743, 1989.

368. Fitzgerald, G. A.: Dipyridamole. N. Engl. J. Med. 316:1247, 1987.

368a. Gavaghan, T. P., Gebski, V., and Baron, D. W.: Immediate postoperative aspirin improves vein graft patency early and late after coronary artery bypass graft surgery. A placebo-controlled, randomized study. Circulation 83:1526, 1991.

369. Goldman, S., Copeland, J., Moritz, T., et al.: Improvement in early saphenous vein graft patency after coronary artery bypass surgery with antiplatelet therapy: Results of a Veterans Administration Cooperative Study. Circulation 77:1324, 1988.

370. Goldman, S., Copeland, J., Moritz, T., et al.: Internal mammary and saphenous vein graft patency. Circulation 82(Suppl. IV):237, 1990.

370a. Sethi, G. K., Copeland, J. G., Goldman, S., et al.: Implications of preoperative administration of aspirin in patients undergoing coronary artery bypass grafting. J. Am. Coll. Cardiol. 15:15, 1990.

371. Campeau, L., Enjalbert, M., Lesperance, J., et al.: The relation of risk factors to the development of atherosclerosis in saphenous-vein bypass grafts and the progression of disease in the native circulation. A study 10 years after aortocoronary bypass surgery. N. Engl. J. Med. 311:1329, 1984.

372. Hoff, H. F., Beck, G. J., Skibinski, C. I., et al.: Serum LP(A) level as a predictor of vein graft stenosis after coronary artery bypass surgery in patients. Circulation 77:1238, 1988.

373. Blankenhorn, D. H., Nessim, S. A., Johnson, R. L., et al.: Beneficial effects of combined colestipol-niacin therapy on coronary atherosclerosis and coronary vein bypass grafts. JAMA 257:3233, 1987.

374. Solymoss, B. C., Nadeau, P., Millette, D., and Campeau, L.: Late thrombosis of saphenous vein bypass grafts related to risk factors. Circulation 78(I):140–143, 1988.

375. Varnauskas, E., and The European Coronary Surgery Study Group: Twelve-year follow-up of survival in the randomized European Coronary Surgery Study. N. Engl. J. Med. 319:332, 1988.

376. Devineni, R., and McKenzie, F. N.: Surgery for coronary artery disease in patients with diabetes mellitus. Can. J. Surg. 28:367, 1985.

377. Hertzer, N. R., Young, J. R., Beven, E. G., et al.: Late results of coronary bypass in patients with peripheral vascular disease. II. Five-year survival according to sex, hypertension, and diabetes. Cleve. Clin. J. Med. 54:15, 1987.

378. Lytle, B. W., Kramer, J. R., Golding, L. R., et al.: Young adults with coronary atherosclerosis: 10-year results of surgical myocardial revascularization. J. Am. Coll. Cardiol. 4:445, 1984.

379. Fitzgibbon, G. M., Hamilton, M. G., Leach, A. J., et al.: Coronary artery disease and coronary bypass grafting in young men: Experience with 138 subjects 39 years of age and younger. J. Am. Coll. Cardiol. 9:977, 1987.

380. Kannel, W. B., and Feinleib, M.: Natural history of angina pectoris in the Framingham study: Progress and survival. Am. J. Cardiol. 29:154, 1972.

381. Frank, C. W., Weinblatt, W., and Shapiro, S.: Angina pectoris in men: Prognostic significance of related medical factors. Circulation 47:509, 1973.

382. Vedin, A., Wilhelmsson, C., Elmfeldt, D., et al.: Death and non-fatal reinfarctions during two years' follow-up after myocardial infarction. Acta Med. Scand. 198:353, 1975.

383. Graham, i., Mulcahy, R., Hickey, N., et al.: Natural history of coronary heart disease: A study of 586 men surviving an initial acute attack. Am. Heart J. 105:249, 1983.

384. Kaiser, G. C., Davis, K. B., Fisher, L. D., et al.: Survival following coronary artery bypass grafting in patients with severe angina pectoris (CASS). J. Thorac. Cardiovasc. Surg. 89:513, 1985.

385. Detre, K., Peduzzi, P., Murphy, M., et al.: Effect of bypass surgery on survival in patients with low- and high-risk groups delineated by the use of simple clinical variables. Circulation 63:1329, 1981.

386. Harlan, W. R., Oberman, A., Grimm, R., and Rosati, R. A.: Chronic congestive heart failure in coronary artery disease: Clinical criteria. Ann. Intern. Med. 86:133, 1977.

387. Sanz, G., Castaner, A., Betriu, A., et al.: Determinants of prognosis in survivors of myocardial infarction. A prospective clinical angiographic study. N. Engl. J. Med. 306:1065, 1982.

388. Mock, M. B., Ringqvist, I., Fisher, L. D., et al.: Survival of medically treated patients in the Coronary Artery Surgery Study (CASS) Registry. Circulation 66:562, 1982.

389. Califf, R. M., Tomabechi, Y., Lee, K. L., et al.: Outcome in one-vessel coronary artery disease. Circulation 67:283, 1983.

390. Nestico, P. F., Hakki, A. -H., Meissner, M. D., et al.: Effect of collateral vessels on prognosis in patients with one-vessel coronary artery disease. J. Am. Coll. Cardiol. 6:1257, 1985.

391. Humphries, J. O., Kuller, L., Ross, R. S., et al.: Natural history of ischemic heart disease in relation to angiographic findings. Circulation 49:489, 1974.

392. Proudfit, W. J., Bruschke, A. V. G., MacMillan, J. P., et al.: Fifteen-year survival study of patients with obstructive coronary artery disease. Circulation 68:986, 1983.

393. Harris, P. J., Behar, V. S., Conley, M. J., et al.: The prognostic significance of 50 per cent coronary stenosis in medically treated patients with coronary artery disease. Circulation 62:240, 1980.

394. Conley, M. J., Ely, R. L., Kisslo, J., et al.: The prognostic spectrum of left main stenosis. Circulation 57:947, 1978.

395. Conti, C. R., Selby, J. H., and Christie, L. G.: Left main coronary artery stenosis: Clinical spectrum, pathophysiology and management. Progr. Cardiovasc. Dis. 22:73, 1979.

396. Talano, J., Scanlon, P., Meadows, W., et al.: Influence of surgery on survival in 145 patients with left main coronary artery disease. Circulation 51, 52(Suppl. I):105, 1975.

397. Taylor, H. A., Deumite, N. J., Chaitman, B. R., et al.: Asymptomatic left main coronary artery disease in the coronary artery surgery study (CASS) registry. Circulation 79:1171, 1989.

398. Kent, K. M., Rosing, D. R., Ewels, C. J., et al.: Prognosis of asymptomatic or mildly symptomatic patients with coronary artery disease. Am. J. Cardiol. 49:1823, 1982.

399. Ryan, T. J., Weiner, D. A., McCabe, C. H., et al.: Exercise testing in the Coronary Artery Surgery Study randomized population. Circulation 72(Suppl. V):31, 1985.

400. Weiner, D. A., Ryan, T. J., McCabe, C. H., et al.: Prognostic importance of a clinical profile and exercise test in medically treated patients with coronary artery disease. J. Am. Coll. Cardiol. 3:772, 1984.

401. Lee, K. L., Pryor, D. B., Pieper, K. S., et al.: Prognostic value of radionuclide angiography in medically treated patients with coronary artery disease. A comparison with clinical and catheterization variables. Circulation 82:1705, 1990.

402. Jones, R. H., Floyd, R. D., Austin, E. H., and Sabiston, D. C.: The role of radionuclide angiography in the preoperative prediction of pain relief and prolonged survival following coronary artery bypass grafting. Ann. Surg. 197:743, 1983.

403. Kronenberg, M. W., Pederson, R. W., Harston, W. E., et al.: Left ventricular performance after coronary artery bypass surgery. Ann. Intern. Med. 99:305, 1983.

404. Bonow, R. O., Kent, K. M., Rosing, D. R., et al.: Exercise-induced ischemia in mildly symptomatic patients with coronary artery disease and preserved left ventricular function. N. Engl. J. Med. 311:1339, 1984.

404a. Report of Inter-Society Commission for Heart Disease Resources: Optimal resources for coronary artery surgery. Circulation 46:A–325, 1972.

405. Kaiser, G. C., Schaff, H. V., and Killip, T.: Myocardial revascularization for unstable angina pectoris. Circulation 79(Suppl. I):60, 1989.

406. Kouchoukos, N. T., Murphy, S., Philpott, T., et al.: Coronary artery bypass grafting for postinfarction angina pectoris. Circulation 79(Suppl. I):68, 1989.

407. Cameron, A., Kemp, H. G., and Green, G. E.: Reoperation of coronary artery disease. 10 years of clinical follow-up. Circulation 78(Suppl. I):158, 1988.

408. Rogers, W. J., Coggin, J., Gersh, B. J., et al.: Ten-year follow-up quality of life in patients randomized to receive medical therapy or coronary artery bypass graft surgery. The coronary artery surgery study (CASS). Circulation 82:1647, 1990.

408a. American College of Cardiology/American Heart Association Task Force on Assessment of Diagnostic and Therapeutic Cardiovascular Procedures (Subcommittee on Coronary Artery Bypass Graft Surgery): Guidelines and indications for coronary artery bypass graft surgery. J. Am. Coll. Cardiol. 17:543, 1991.

409. Pryor D. B., Harrell, F. E., Rankin, S. J., et al.: The changing survival benefits of coronary revascularization over time. Circulation 76(Suppl. V):13, 1987.

410. Takaro, T., Pifarre, R., and Fish, R.: Left main coronary artery disease. Progr. Cardiovasc. Dis. 28:229, 1985.

411. Chaitman, B. P., Fisher, L. D., and Bourassa, M. G.: Effect of coronary bypass surgery on survival patterns in subsets of patients with left main coronary artery disease. Report of the Collaborative Study in Coronary Artery Surgery (CASS). Am. J. Cardiol. 48:765, 1981.

412. Califf, R. M., Conley, M. J., Behar, V. S., et al.: "Left main equivalent" coronary artery disease: Its clinical presentation and prognostic significance with nonsurgical therapy. Am. J. Cardiol. 53:1489, 1984.

413. Chaitman, B. R., Davis, K. B., Kaiser, G. C., et al.: The role of coronary bypass surgery for "left main equivalent" coronary disease: The Coronary Artery Surgery Study Registry. Circulation 74(Suppl. III):17, 1986.

414. Detre, K. M., Takaro, T., Hultgren, H., Peduzzi, P., and the Study Participants: Long-term mortality and morbidity results of the Veterans Administration randomized trial of coronary artery bypass surgery. Circulation 72(Suppl. V):84, 1985.

415. Peduzzi, P., Detre, K., Murphy, M. L.: Ten-year incidence of myocardial infarction and prognosis after infarction: Department of Veterans Af-

fairs Cooperative study of coronary artery bypass surgery. Circulation 83:747, 1991.

416. Detre, K., Peduzzi, P., Scott, S. M., and Davies, B.: Long-term survival results in medically and surgically randomized patients. Progr. Cardiovasc. Dis. 28:235, 1985.

417. The Veterans Administration Coronary Artery Bypass Surgery Cooperative Study Group: Eleven-year survival in the Veterans Administration randomized trial of coronary bypass surgery for stable angina. N. Engl. J. Med. 311:1333, 1984.

418. Varnauskas, E., and the European Coronary Surgery Study Group: Survival, myocardial infarction, and employment status in a prospective randomized study of coronary bypass surgery. Circulation 72(Suppl. V):90, 1985.

419. Alderman, E. L., Bourassa, M. G., Cohen, L. S., et al.: Ten-year follow-up of survival and myocardial infarction in the randomized coronary artery surgery study. Circulation 82:1629, 1990.

420. Myers, W. O., Martshfield, W. I., Gersh, B. J., et al.: Medical versus early surgical therapy in patients with triple-vessel disease and mild angina pectoris: A CASS registry study of survival. Ann. Thorac. Surg. 44:471, 1987.

421. Myers, W. O., Schaff, H. V., Gersh, B. J., et al.: Improved survival of surgically treated patients with triple vessel coronary artery disease and severe angina pectoris. J. Thorac. Cardiovasc. Surg. 97:487, 1989.

422. Iskandrian, A. S., Hakki, A.-H., Goel, I. P., et al.: The use of rest and exercise radionuclide ventriculography in risk stratification in patients with suspected coronary artery disease. Am. Heart J. 110:864, 1985.

423. Alderman, E. L., Fisher, L. D., Litwin, P., et al.: Results of coronary artery surgery in patients with poor left ventricular function (CASS). Circulation 68:785, 1983.

424. Nwasokwa, O. N., Koss, J. H., Friedman, G. H., et al.: Bypass surgery for chronic stable angina: Predictors of survival benefit and strategy for patient selection. Ann. Intern. Med. 114:1035, 1991.

424a. Bonow, R. O., Dilsizian, V., Cucolo, A., and Bacharach, S. L.: Identification of viable myocardium in patients with chronic coronary artery disease and left ventricular dysfunction: Comparison of thallium scintigraphy with reinjection and PET imaging with 18F-fluorodeoxyglucose. Circulation 83:26, 1991.

425. Tillisch, J., Brunken, R., Marshall, R., et al.: Reversibility of cardiac wall-motion abnormalities predicted by positron tomography. N. Engl. J. Med. 314:884, 1986.

426. Shanes, J. G., Kondos, G. T., Levitsky, S., et al.: Coronary artery obstruction: A potentially reversible cause of dilated cardiomyopathy. Am. Heart J. 110:173, 1985.

427. Shearn, D. L., and Brent, B. N.: Coronary artery bypass surgery in patients with left ventricular dysfunction. Am. J. Med. 80:405, 1986.

428. Lim, Y. L., Kalff, V., Kelly, M. J., et al.: Radionuclide angiographic assessment of global and segmental left ventricular function at rest and during exercise after coronary artery bypass graft surgery. Circulation 66:972, 1982.

429. Kolibash, A. J., Goodenow, J. S., Bush, C. A., et al.: Improvement of myocardial perfusion and left ventricular function after coronary artery bypass grafting patients with unstable angina. Circulation 59:66, 1979.

430. Topol, E. J., Weiss, J. L., Guzman, P. A., et al.: Immediate improvement of dysfunctional myocardial segments after coronary revascularization: Detection by intraoperative transesophageal echocardiography. J. Am. Coll. Cardiol. 4:1123, 1984.

431. Cohen, M., Charney, R., Hershman, R., et al.: Reversal of chronic ischemic myocardial dysfunction after transluminal coronary angioplasty. J. Am. Coll. Cardiol. 12:1193, 1988.

432. Carlson, E. B., Cowley, M. J., Wolfgang, T. C., and Vetrovec, G. W.: Acute changes in global and regional rest left ventricular function after successful coronary angioplasty: Comparative results in stable and unstable angina. J. Am. Coll. Cardiol. 13:1262, 1989.

433. Wijns, W., Serruys, P. W., Slager, C. J., et al.: Effect of coronary occlusion during percutaneous transluminal angioplasty in humans on left ventricular chamber stiffness and regional diastolic pressure-radius relations. J. Am. Coll. Cardiol. 7:455, 1986.

434. Mathias, P., Kerin, N. Z., Blevins, R. D., et al.: Coronary vasospasm as a cause of stunned myocardium. Am. Heart J. 113:383, 1987.

435. Robertson, W. S., Feigenbaum, H., Armstrong, W. F., et al.: Exercise echocardiography: A clinically practical addition in the evaluation of coronary artery disease. J. Am. Coll. Cardiol. 6:1085, 1985.

436. Ballantyne, C. M., Verani, M. S., Short, H. D., et al.: Delayed recovery of severely "stunned" myocardium with the support of a left ventricular assist device after coronary artery bypass graft surgery. J. Am. Coll. Cardiol. 10:710, 1987.

436a. Ross, J., Jr.: Myocardial perfusion-contraction matching: Implications for coronary heart disease and hibernation. Circulation 83:1076, 1991.

436b. Lewis, S. J., Sawada, S. G., Ryan, T., et al.: Segmental wall motion abnormalities in the absence of clinically documented myocardial infarction: Clinical significance and evidence of hibernating myocardium. Am. Heart J. 121:1088, 1991.

436c. Bonow, R. O., Dilsizian, V., Cuocolo, A., and Bacharach, S. L.: Identification of viable myocardium in patients with chronic coronary artery disease and left ventricular dysfunction: Comparison of thallium scintigraphy with reinjection and PET imaging with ^{18}F-fluorodeoxyglucose. Circulation 83:26, 1991.

437. Gersh, B. J., Califf, R. M., Loop, F. D., et al.: Coronary bypass surgery in chronic stable angina. Circulation 79(Suppl. I):46, 1989.

438. Balu, V., Szmedra, L., Dean, D., and Bhayana, J.: Long-term survival of patients with low ejection fraction. Tex. Heart Inst. J. 15:44, 1988.

439. Holmes, D. R., Davis, K. B., Mock, M. B., et al.: The effect of medical and surgical treatment on subsequent sudden cardiac death in patients with coronary artery disease: A report from the Coronary Artery Surgery Study. Circulation 73:1254, 1986.

440. Ellis, S., Alderman, E. L., Cain, K., et al.: Morphology of left anterior descending coronary artery lesions as a predictor of anterior myocardial infarction. A CASS Registry Study. J. Am. Coll. Cardiol. 13:1481, 1989.

441. Mazzotta, G., Bonow, R. O., Pace, L., et al.: Relation between exertional ischemia and prognosis in mildly symptomatic patients with single or double vessel coronary artery disease and left ventricular dysfunction at rest. J. Am. Coll. Cardiol. 13:567, 1989.

442. Murphy, M. L., Meadows, W. R., Thomsen, J., et al.: The effect of coronary artery bypass surgery on the incidence of myocardial infarction and hospitalization. Progr. Cardiovasc. Dis. 28:309, 1986.

443. CASS principal investigators and their associates: Myocardial infarction and mortality in the Coronary Artery Surgery Study (CASS) randomized trial. N. Engl. J. Med. 310:750, 1984.

444. Myers, W. O., Schaff, H. V., Fisher, L. D., et al.: Time to first new myocardial infarction in patients with severe angina and three-vessel disease comparing medical and early surgical therapy: A CASS registry study of survival. J. Thorac. Cardiovasc. Surg. 95:382, 1988.

444a. Peduzzi, P., Detre, K., Murphy, M. L., et al.: Ten-year incidence of myocardial infarction and prognosis after infarction. Department of Veterans Affairs Cooperative Study of Coronary Artery Bypass Surgery. Circulation 83:747, 1991.

444b. Kirklin, J. W., Akins, C. W., Blackstone, E. H., et al.: ACC/AHA guidelines and indications for coronary artery bypass graft surgery. A report of the American College of Cardiology/American Heart Association Task Force on assessment of diagnostic and therapeutic cardiovascular procedures. Circulation 83:1125, 1991.

445. Loop, F. D., Golding, L. R., Macmillan, J. P., et al.: Coronary artery surgery in women compared with men: analyses or risks and long-term results. J. Am. Coll. Cardiol. 1:383, 1983.

446. Fisher, L. D., Kennedy, J. W., Davis, K. B., et al.: Association of sex, physical size, and operative mortality after coronary artery bypass in the Coronary Artery Surgery Study (CASS). J. Thorac. Cardiovasc. Surg. 84:334, 1982.

447. Gersh, B. J., Kronmal, R. A., Schaff, H. V., et al.: Comparison of coronary artery bypass surgery and medical therapy in patients 65 years of age or older. N. Engl. J. Med. 313:217, 1985.

448. Montague, N. T., Kouchoukos, N. T., Wilson, T.A.S., et al.: Morbidity and mortality of coronary bypass grafting in patients 70 years of age and older. Ann. Thorac. Surg. 39:552, 1985.

449. Roberts, A. J., Woodhall, D. D., Conti, C. R., et al.: Mortality, morbidity, and cost-accounting related to coronary artery bypass graft surgery in the elderly. Ann. Thorac. Surg. 39:426, 1985.

450. Rose, D. M., Gelbfish, J., Jacobowitz, I. J., et al.: Analysis of morbidity and mortality in patients 70 years of age and over undergoing isolated coronary artery bypass surgery. Am. Heart J. 110:361, 1985.

451. Ennabli, K., and Pelletier, L. C.: Morbidity and mortality of coronary artery surgery after the age of 70 years. Ann. Thorac. Surg. 42:197, 1986.

452. Rich, M. W., Keller, A. J., Schechtman, K. B., et al.: Increased complications and prolonged hospital stay in elderly cardiac surgical patients with low serum albumin. Am. J. Cardiol. 63:714, 1989.

452a. Hammermeister, K. E., Burchfiel, C., Johnson, R., and Grover, F. L.: Identification of patients at greatest risk for developing major complications at cardiac surgery. Circulation 82(Suppl. IV):380, 1990.

453. Foster, E. D., Fisher, L. D., Kaiser, G. C., et al.: Comparison of operative mortality and morbidity results for initial and repeat coronary artery bypass grafting: The Coronary Artery Surgery Study (CASS) Registry experience. Ann. Thorac. Surg. 38:563, 1984.

454. Lamas, G. A., Mudge, G. H., Collins, J. J., et al.: Clinical response to coronary reoperations. J. Am. Coll. Cardiol. 8:274, 1986.

455. Osaka, S., Barratt Boyes, B. G., Brandt, P. W., et al.: Early and late results of re-operation for coronary artery disease: A 13-year experience. Aust. N. Z. J. Surg. 58:537, 1988.

455a. Verheul, H. A., Moulijn, A. C., Hondema, S., et al.: Late results of 200 repeat coronary artery bypass operations. Am. J. Cardiol. 67:24, 1991.

456. Brenowitz, J. B., Johnson, D., Kayser, K. L., et al.: Coronary artery bypass grafting for the third time or more. Results of 150 consecutive cases. Circulation 78(Suppl. I):166, 1988.

457. Schaff, H. V., Orzulak, T. A., Gersh, B. J., et al.: The morbidity and mortality of reoperation for coronary artery disease and analysis of late results with use of actuarial estimate of event-free interval. J. Thorac. Cardiovasc. Surg. 85:508, 1983.

458. Brener, B. J., Brief, D. K., Alpert, J., et al.: A four-year experience with preoperative noninvasive carotid evaluation of 2,026 patients undergoing cardiac surgery. J. Vasc. Surg. 1:326, 1984.

459. Gardner, T. J., Horneffer, P. J., Manolio, T. A., et al.: Stroke following coronary artery bypass grafting: A ten-year study. Ann. Thorac. Surg. 40:574, 1985.

460. Feussner, J. R., and Matchar, D. B.: When and how to study the carotid arteries. Ann. Intern. Med. 109:805, 1988.

461. Reed, G. L., Singer, D. E., Picard, E. H., DeSanctis, R.: Stroke following coronary-artery bypass surgery. A case-control estimate of the risk from carotid bruits. N. Engl. J. Med. 319:1246, 1988.

462. Beebe, H. G., Clagett, G. P., DeWeese, J. A., et al.: Assessing risk associated with carotid endarterectomy. Circulation 79:472, 1989.

463. Grotta, J. C.: Current medical and surgical therapy for cerebrovascular disease. N. Engl. J. Med. 317:1505, 1987.

464. Babu, S. C., Shah, P. M., Singh, B. M., et al.: Coexisting carotid stenosis in patients undergoing cardiac surgery: Indications and guidelines for simultaneous operations. Am. J. Surg. 150:207, 1985.

465. David, T. E.: Combined cardiac and abdominal aortic surgery. Circulation 72(Suppl. II):18, 1985.

466. Jones, E. L., Craver, J. M., Michalik, R. A., et al.: Combined carotid and coronary operations: When are they necessary? J. Thorac. Cardiovasc. Surg. 87:7, 1984.

467. Furlan, A. J., and Craciun, A. R.: Risk of stroke during coronary artery bypass graft surgery in patients with internal carotid artery disease documented by angiography. Stroke 16:797, 1985.

468. Debakey, M. E., and Lawrie, G. M.: Combined coronary artery and peripheral vascular disease: Recognition and treatment. J. Vasc. Surg. 1:605, 1984.

469. Boucher, C. A., Brewster, D. C., Darling, R. C., et al.: Determination of cardiac risk by dipyridamole-thallium imaging before peripheral vascular surgery. N. Engl. J. Med. 312:389, 1985.

UNSTABLE ANGINA

469a. Bleifeld, W., Hamm, C. W., and Braunwald, E. (eds.): Unstable Angina. New York, Springer-Verlag, 1990, 270 pp.

470. Collins, P., and Fox, K. M.: Pathophysiology of angina. Lancet 1:94, 1990.

471. Braunwald, E.: Unstable angina. A classification. Circulation 80:410, 1989.

472. Chierchia, S., Brunelli, C., Simonetti, I., et al.: Sequence of events in angina at rest: Primary reduction in coronary blood flow. Circulation 61:759, 1980.

473. Langer, A., Freeman, M. R., and Armstrong, P. W.: ST segment shift in unstable angina: Pathophysiology and association with coronary anatomy and hospital outcome. J. Am. Coll. Cardiol. 13:1495, 1989.

474. Deanfield, J. E., Maseri, A., Selwyn, A. P., et al.: Myocardial ischaemia during daily life in patients with stable angina: Its relation to symptoms and heart rate changes. Lancet 2:753, 1983.

475. Cohn, P. F., Brown, A. J., Jr., Wynne, J., et al.: Global and regional left ventricular ejection fraction abnormalities during exercise in patients with silent myocardial ischemia. J. Am. Coll. Cardiol. 1:931, 1983.

476. Chierchia, S., Lazzari, M., Freedman, B., et al.: Impairment of myocardial perfusion and function during painless myocardial ischemia. J. Am. Coll. Cardiol. 1:924, 1983.

477. Campbell, S., Barry, J., Rocco, M. B., et al.: Features of the exercise test that reflect the activity of ischemic heart disease out of hospital. Circulation 74:72, 1986.

478. Nademanee, K., Intrachot, V., Josephson, M. A., et al.: Prognostic significance of silent myocardial ischemia in patients with unstable angina. J. Am. Coll. Cardiol. 10:1, 1987.

479. Gottlieb, S. O., Weisfeldt, M. L., Ouyang, P., et al.: Silent ischemia as a marker for early unfavorable outcomes in patients with unstable angina. N. Engl. J. Med. 314:1214, 1986.

480. Gottlieb, S. O., Weisfeldt, M. L., Ouyang, P., et al.: Silent ischemia predicts infarction and death during 2 years follow-up of unstable angina. J. Am. Coll. Cardiol. 10:756, 1987.

480a. Bugiardini, R., Pozzati, A., Borghi, A., et al.: Angiographic morphology in unstable angina and its relation to transient myocardial ischemia and hospital outcome. Am. J. Cardiol. 67:460, 1991.

481. McCormick, J. R., Schick, E. C., Jr., McCabe, C. H., et al.: Determinants of operative mortality and long-term survival in patients with unstable angina. The CASS experience. J. Thorac. Cardiovasc. Surg. 89:683, 1985.

482. Roberts, K. B., Califf, R. M., Harrell, F. E., Jr., et al.: The prognosis for patients with new-onset angina who have undergone cardiac catheterization. Circulation 68:970, 1983.

483. Parker, F. B., Jr., Neville, J. F., Jr., Hanson, E. C., and Webb, W. R.: Retrograde and antegrade pressures and flows in preinfarction syndrome. Circulation 50(Suppl. II):122, 1974.

484. Roberts, W. C.: Qualitative and quantitative comparison of amounts of narrowing by atherosclerotic plaques in the major epicardial coronary arteries at necropsy in sudden coronary death, transmural acute myocardial infarction, transmural healed myocardial infarction and unstable angina pectoris. Am. J. Cardiol. 64:324, 1989.

485. Freudenberg, H., and Lichtlen, P. R.: The normal segment in coronary stenosis—a postmortem study. Z. Kardiol. 70:863, 1981.

486. Saner, G. E., Gobel, F. L., Salomonowitz, E., et al.: The disease-free wall in coronary atherosclerosis: Its relation to degree of obstruction. J. Am. Coll. Cardiol. 6:1096, 1985.

487. Fuster, V., Stein, B., Ambrose, J. A., et al.: Atherosclerotic plaque rupture and thrombosis. Evolving concepts. Circulation 82(Suppl. II):47, 1990.

488. Davies, M. J., and Thomas, A. C.: Plaque fissuring—The cause of acute myocardial infarction, sudden ischaemic death, and crescendo angina. Br. Heart J. 53:363, 1985.

489. Moise, A., Theroux, P., Taeymans, Y., et al.: Unstable angina and progression of coronary atherosclerosis. N. Engl. J. Med. 309:685, 1983.

490. Davies, M. J., Thomas, A. C., Knapman, P. A., and Hangartner, J. R.: Intramyocardial platelet aggregation in patients with unstable angina suffering sudden ischemic cardiac death. Circulation 73:418, 1986.

491. Falk, E.: Unstable angina with fatal outcome: Dynamic coronary thrombosis leading to infarction and/or sudden death. Circulation 71:699, 1985.

492. Ambrose, J. A., Hjemdahl-Monsen, C., Borrico, S., et al.: Quantitative and qualitative effects of intracoronary streptokinase in unstable angina and non-Q infarction. J. Am. Coll. Cardiol. 9:1156, 1987.

493. Freeman, M. R., Williams, A. E., Chisholm, R. J., and Armstrong, P. W.: intracoronary thrombus and complex morphology in unstable angina. Relation to timing of angiography and in-hospital cardiac events. Circulation 80:17, 1989.

494. Sherman, C. T., Litvack, F., Grundfest, W., et al.: Coronary angioscopy in patients with unstable angina pectoris. N. Engl. J. Med. 315:913, 1986.

495. Speechia, G., De Servi, S., Falcon, C., et al.: Coronary arterial spasm as a cause of exercise-induced ST-segment elevation in patients with variant angina. Circulation 59:948, 1979.

496. Haft, J. I., Haik, B. J., Goldstein, J. E., and Brodyn, N. E.: Development of significant coronary artery lesions in areas of minimal disease. A common mechanism for coronary disease progression. Chest 94:731, 1988.

497. Folts, J. D., Crowell, E. B., and Rowe, G. G.: Platelet aggregation in partially obstructed vessels and its elimination with aspirin. Circulation 54:365, 1976.

498. Grande, P., Grauholt, A.-M., and Madsen, J. K.: Unstable angina pectoris. Platelet behaviour and prognosis in progressive angina and intermediate coronary syndrome. Circulation 81:(Suppl. I):16, 1990.

499. Willerson, J. T., Golino, P., Eidt, J., et al.: Specific platelet mediators and unstable coronary artery lesions. Experimental evidence and potential clinical implications. Circulation 80:198, 1989.

500. Folts, J. D., Gallagher, K., and Rowe, G. G.: Blood flow reductions in stenosed canine coronary arteries: Vasospasm or platelet aggregation. Circulation 65:248, 1982.

501. Lewis, H. D., Davis, J. W., Archibald, D. G., et al.: Protective effects of aspirin against acute myocardial infarction and death in men with unstable angina. N. Engl. J. Med. 309:396, 1983.

502. Cairns, J. A., Gent, M., Singer, J., et al.: Aspirin, sulfinpyrazone, or both in unstable angina. Results of a Canadian multicenter trial. N. Engl. J. Med. 313:1369, 1985.

503. Theroux, P., Ouimet, H., McCans, J., et al.: Aspirin, heparin, or both to treat unstable angina. N. Engl. J. Med. 319:1105, 1988.

504. The RISC Group: Risk of myocardial infarction and death during treatment with low-dose aspirin and intravenous heparin in men with unstable coronary artery disease. Lancet 336:827, 1990.

505. Kruskal, J. B., Commerford, P. J., Franks, J. J., et al.: Fibrin and fibrinogen related antigens in patients with stable and unstable coronary artery disease. N. Engl. J. Med. 317:1361, 1987.

506. Zalewski, A., Shi, Y., Nardone, D., et al.: Evidence for reduced fibrinolytic activity in unstable angina at rest: Clinical, biochemical, and angiographic correlates. Circulation 83:1685, 1991.

507. Gold, H. K., Johns, J. A., Leinbach, R. C., et al.: A randomized, blinded, placebo-controlled trial of recombinant human tissue-type plasminogen activator in patients with unstable angina pectoris. Circulation 75:1192, 1987.

508. Brown, B. G., Bolson, E. L., and Dodge, H. T.: Dynamic mechanisms in human coronary stenosis. Circulation 70:917, 1984.

509. Chesebro, J. H., Fuster, V., and Webster, M.W.I.: Endothelial injury and coronary vasomotion (editorial). J. Am. Coll. Cardiol. 14:1191, 1989.

509a. Kaski, J. C., Tousoulis, D., Heider, A. W., et al.: Reactivity of eccentric and concentric coronary stenoses in patients with chronic stable angina. J. Am. Coll. Cardiol. 17:627, 1991.

510. Zeiher, A. M., Drexler, H., Wollschlaeger, H., et al.: Coronary vasomotion in response to sympathetic stimulation in humans: Importance of the functional integrity of the endothelium. J. Am. Coll. Cardiol. 14:1181, 1989.

511. Drexler, H., Zeiher, A. M., Wollschlager, H., et al.: Flow-dependent coronary artery dilatation in humans. Circulation 80:466, 1989.

512. Cox, D. A., Vita, J. A., Treasure, C. B., et al.: Atherosclerosis impairs flow-mediated dilation of coronary arteries in humans. Circulation 80:458, 1989.

513. Hodgson, J.M.B, and Marshall, J. J.: Direct vasoconstriction and endothelium-dependent vasocilation. Mechanisms of acetylcholine effects on coronary flow and arterial diameter in patients with nonstenotic coronary arteries. Circulation 79:1043, 1989.

514. Vita, J. A., Treasure, C. B., Ganz, P., et al.: Control of shear stress in the epicardial coronary arteries of humans: Impairment by atherosclerosis. J. Am. Coll. Cardiol. 14:1193, 1989.

515. Swahn, E., Areskog, M., Berglund, U., et al.: Predictive importance of clinical findings and a predischarge exercise test in patients with suspected unstable coronary artery disease. Am. J. Cardiol. 59:208, 1987.

516. Severi, S., Orsini, E., Marraccini, P., et al.: The basal electrocardiogram and the exercise stress test in assessing prognosis in patients with unstable angina. Eur. Heart J. 4:441, 1988.

517. Nixon, J. V., Brown, C. N., and Smitherman, T. C.: Identification of transient and persistent segmental wall motion abnormalities in patients with unstable angina by two-dimensional echocardiography. Circulation 65:1497, 1982.

518. Brown, K. A., Okada, R. D., Boucher, C. A., et al.: Serial thallium-201 imaging at rest in patients with unstable and stable angina pectoris: Relationship of myocardial perfusion at rest to presenting clinical syndrome. Am. Heart J. 106:70, 1983.

518a. Zhu, Y. Y., Chung, W. S., Botvinick, E. H., et al.: Dipyridamole perfusion scintigraphy: the experience with its application in one hundred seventy patients with known or suspected unstable angina. Am. Heart J. 121:33, 1991.

519. Freeman, M. R., Williams, A. E., Chisholm, R. J., et al.: Role of resting thallium 201 perfusion in predicting coronary anatomy, left ventricular wall motion, and hospital outcome in unstable angina pectoris. Am. Heart J. 117:306, 1989.

520. Younis, L. T., Byers, S., Shaw, L., et al.: Prognostic value of intravenous

dipyridamole thallium scintigraphy after an acute myocardial ischemic event. Am. J. Cardiol. 64:161, 1989.

521. Freeman, M. R., Chisholm, R. J., and Armstrong, P. W.: Usefulness of exercise electrocardiography and thallium scintigraphy in unstable angina pectoris in predicting the extent and severity of coronary artery disease erratum published in Am. J. Cardiol. 63:392, 1989. Am. J. Cardiol. 62:1164, 1988.

521a. Brown, K. A.: Prognostic value of thallium-201 myocardial perfusion imaging in patients with unstable angina who respond to medical treatment. J. Am. Coll. Cardiol. 17:1053, 1991.

522. Lin, S.-G., and Flaherty, J. T.: Crossover from intravenous to transdermal nitroglycerin therapy in unstable angina pectoris. Am. J. Cardiol. 56:742, 1985.

523. Baaske, D. M., Amann, A. H., Wagenknecht, D. M., et al.: Nitroglycerin compatibility with intravenous fluid filters, containers, and administration sets. Am. J. Hosp. Pharm. 37:201, 1980.

524. Necoechea, A.J.C., Camacho, J. P., Gil, D., et al.: Acute gouty arthritis and intravenous nitroglycerin. Arch. Intern. Med. 148:2505, 1988.

525. Stamler, J., Cunningham, M., Loscalzo, J.: Reduced thiols and the effect of intravenous nitroglycerin on platelet aggregation. Am. J. Cardiol. 62:377, 1988.

526. Horowitz, J. D., Henry, C. A., Syrjanen, M. L., et al.: Combined use of nitroglycerin and N-acetylcysteine in the management of unstable angina pectoris. Circulation 77:787, 1988.

527. Jugdutt, B. I., and Warnica, J. W.: Tolerance with low dose intravenous nitroglycerin therapy in acute myocardial infarction. Am. J. Cardiol. 64:581, 1989.

528. Figueras, J., Singh, B. N., Ganz, W., et al.: Mechanism of rest and nocturnal angina: Observations during continuous hemodynamic and electrocardiographic monitoring. Circulation 59:955, 1979.

529. Hint Research Group: Early treatment of unstable angina in the coronary care unit: A randomized, double blind, placebo controlled comparison of recurrent ischaemia in patients treated with nifedipine or metoprolol or both. Br. Heart J. 56:400, 1986.

530. Tijssen, J. G., and Lubsen, J.: Early treatment of unstable angina with nifedipine and metoprolol—the HINT trial. J. Cardiovasc. Pharmacol. 12(Suppl. 71):1988.

531. Muller, J. E., Turi, Z. G., Pearle, D. L., et al.: Nifedipine and conventional therapy for unstable angina pectoris: A randomized, double-blind comparison. Circulation 69:728, 1984.

532. Gottlieb, S. O., Weisfeldt, M. L., Ouyang, P., et al.: Effect of the addition of propranolol therapy with nifedipine for unstable angina pectoris: A randomized, double-blind, placebo-controlled trial. Circulation 73:331, 1986.

533. Theroux, P., Taeymans, Y., Morissette, D., et al.: A randomized study comparing propranolol and diltiazem in the treatment of unstable angina. J. Am. Coll. Cardiol. 5:717, 1985.

534. Wallis, D. E., Pope, C., Littman, W. J., and Scanlon, P. J.: Safety and efficacy of esmolol for unstable angina pectoris. Am. J. Cardiol. 62:1033, 1988.

535. Kirshenbaum, J. M., Kloner, R. F., McGowan, N., and Antman, E. M.: Use of an ultrashort-acting beta-receptor blocker (esmolol) in patients with acute myocardial ischemia and relative contraindications to beta-blockade therapy. J. Am. Coll. Cardiol. 12:773, 1988.

536. Held, P. H., Yusuf, S., and Furberg, C. D.: Calcium channel blockers in acute myocardial infarction and unstable angina: An overview. Br. Med. J. 2:1187, 1989.

537. Gerstenblith, G., Ouyang, P., Achuff, S. C., et al.: Nifedipine in unstable angina: A double-blind, randomized trial. N. Engl. J. Med. 306:885, 1982.

538. Telford, A. M., and Wilson, C.: Trial of heparin versus atenolol in prevention of myocardial infarction in intermediate coronary syndrome. Lancet 1:1225, 1981.

539. Gardner, T. J., Stuart, R. S., Greene, P. S., and Baumgartner, W. A.: The risk of coronary bypass surgery for patients with postinfarction angina. Circulation 79(Suppl. I):79, 1989.

540. Szatmary, L. J., Marco, J., Fajadet, J., and Caster, L.: The combined use of diastolic counterpulsation and coronary dilation in unstable angina due to multivessel disease under unstable hemodynamic conditions. Int. J. Cardiol. 19:59, 1988.

541. Kantrowitz, A., Wasfie, T., Freed, P. S., et al.: Intraaortic balloon pumping 1967 through 1982: Analysis of complications in 733 patients. Am. J. Cardiol. 57:976, 1986.

542. de Feyter, P. J., Suryapranata, H., Serruys, P. W., et al.: Effects of successful percutaneous transluminal coronary angioplasty on global and regional left ventricular function in unstable angina pectoris. Am. J. Cardiol. 60:993, 1987.

543. Danchin, N., Haouzi, A., Amor, M., et al.: Sustained improvement in myocardial perfusion four to six years after PTCA in patients with a satisfactory angiographic result, six months after the procedure. Eur. Heart J. 9:454, 1988.

544. Leeman, D. E., McCabe, C. H., Faxon, D. P., et al.: Use of percutaneous transluminal coronary angioplasty and bypass surgery despite improved medical therapy for unstable angina pectoris. Am. J. Cardiol. 61:38G, 1988.

545. Timmis, A. D., Griffin, B., Crick, J. C., and Sowton, E.: Early percutaneous transluminal coronary angioplasty in the management of unstable angina. Int. J. Cardiol. 14:25, 1987.

546. Kamp, O., Beatt, K. J., De Feyter, P. J., et al.: Short-, medium-, and long-term follow-up after percutaneous transluminal coronary angioplasty for stable and unstable angina pectoris. Am. Heart J. 117:991, 1989.

547. Perry, R. A., Seth, A., Hunt, A., and Shiu, M. F.: Coronary angioplasty in

unstable angina and stable angina: A comparison of success and complications. Br. Heart J. 60:367, 1988.

548. De Feyter, P. J., Suryapranata, H., Serruys, P. W., et al.: Coronary angioplasty for unstable angina: immediate and late results in 200 consecutive patients with identification of risk factors for unfavorable early and late outcome. J. Am. Coll. Cardiol. 12:324, 1988.

549. Halon, D. A., Merdler, A., Shefer, A., et al.: Identifying patients at high risk for restenosis after percutaneous transluminal coronary angioplasty for unstable angina pectoris. Am. J. Cardiol. 64:289, 1989.

549a. Myler, R. K., Shaw, R. E., Stertzer, S. H., et al.: Unstable angina and coronary angioplasty. Circulation 82(Suppl. II):88, 1990.

550. Steffenino, G., Meier, B., Finci, L., and Ruitshauer, W.: Followup results of treatment of unstable angina by coronary angioplasty. Br. Heart J. 57:416, 1987.

551. Talley, J. D., Hurst, J. W., King, S., et al.: Clinical outcome 5 years after attempted percutaneous transluminal coronary angioplasty in 427 patients. Circulation 77:820, 1988.

552. Luchi, R. J., Scott, S. M., Deupree, R. H., and the principal investigators and their associates of Veterans Administration Cooperative Study No. 28: Comparison of medical and surgical treatment for unstable angina pectoris. N. Engl. J. Med. 316:977, 1987.

553. Scott, S. M., Luchi, R. J., Deupree, R. H., and the Veterans Administration Unstable Angina Cooperative Study Group: Veterans Administration Cooperative Study for treatment of patients with unstable angina. Results in patients with abnormal left ventricular function. Circulation 78(Suppl. I):113, 1988.

554. Parisi, A. F., Khuri, S., Deupree, R. H., et al.: Medical compared with surgical management of unstable angina. 5-Year mortality and morbidity in the Veterans Administration Study. Circulation 80:1176, 1989.

554a. Booth, D. C., Deupree, R. H., Hultgren, H. N., et al.: Quality of life after bypass surgery for unstable angina. 5-year follow-up results of a Veterans Affairs Cooperative Study. Circulation 83:87, 1991.

555. Naunheim, K. S., Fiore, A. C., Arango, D. C., et al.: Coronary artery bypass grafting for unstable angina pectoris: Risk analysis. Ann. Thorac. Surg. 47:569, 1989.

556. Waters, D., Walling, A., Roy, D., et al.: Previous coronary artery bypass grafting as an adverse prognostic factor in unstable angina pectoris. Am. J. Cardiol. 58:465, 1986.

557. Cairns, J. A., Singer, J., Gent, M., et al.: One year mortality outcomes of all coronary and intensive care unit patients with acute myocardial infarction, unstable angina or other chest pain in Hamilton, Ontario, a city of 375,000 people. Can. J. Cardiol. 5:239, 1989.

VARIANT ANGINA PECTORIS (PRINZMETAL'S ANGINA)

558. Prinzmetal, M., Kennamer, R., Merliss, R., et al.: A variant form of angina pectoris. Am. J. Med. 27:375, 1959.

559. Hoshio, A., Kotare, H., and Mashiba, H.: Significance of coronary artery tone in patients with vasospastic angina. J. Am. Coll. Cardiol. 14:604, 1989.

560. Ganz, P., and Alexander, R. W.: New insights into the cellular mechanisms of vasospasm. Am. J. Cardiol. 56:11E, 1985.

560a. McFadden, E. P., Clarke, J. G., Davies, G. J., et al.: Effect of intracoronary serotonin on coronary vessels in patients with stable angina and patients with variant angina. N. Engl. J. Med. 324:648, 1991.

561. Irie, T., Imaizumi, T., Matuguchi, T., et al.: Increased fibrinopeptide A during anginal attacks in patients with variant angina. J. Am. Coll. Cardiol. 14:589, 1989.

562. Ogawa, H., Yasue, H., Oshima, S., et al.: Circadian variation of plasma fibrinopeptide A level in patients with variant angina. Circulation 80:1617, 1989.

563. Forman, M. B., Oates, J. A., Robertson, D., et al.: Increased adventitial mast cells in a patient with coronary spasm. N. Engl. J. Med. 313:1138, 1985.

564. Topol, E. J., and Fortuin, N. J.: Coronary artery spasm and cardiac arrest in carcinoid heart disease. Am. J. Med. 77:950, 1984.

565. Cohen, L., and Kitzes, R.: Prompt termination and/or prevention of cold-pressor-stimulus-induced vasoconstriction of different vascular beds by magnesium sulfate in patients with Prinzmetal's angina. Magnesium 5:144, 1986.

566. Miyagi, H., Yasue, H., Okumura, K., et al.: Effect of magnesium on anginal attack induced by hyperventilation in patients with variant angina. Circulation 79:597, 1989.

567. Kugiyama, K., Yasue, H., Okumura, K., et al.: Suppression of exercise-induced angina by magnesium sulfate in patients with variant angina. J. Am. Coll. Cardiol. 12:1177, 1988.

568. Tanabe, K., Noda, K., Masaka, A., et al.: Variant angina due to deficiency of intracellular magnesium by anorexia nervosa. Kokyu To Junkan 37:467, 1989.

569. Lange, R. A., Cigarroa, R. G., Yancy, C. W., et al.: Cocaine-induced coronary-artery vasoconstriction. N. Engl. J. Med. 321:1557, 1989.

570. Nademanee, K., Gorelick, D. A., Josephson, M. A., et al.: Myocardial ischemia during cocaine withdrawal. Ann. Intern. Med. 111:876, 1989.

571. Waters, D. D., Muller, D., Bouchard, A., et al.: Circadian variation in variant angina. Am. J. Cardiol. 54:61, 1984.

572. Winniford, M. D., Jansen, D. E., Reynolds, G. A., et al.: Cigarette smoking-induced coronary vasoconstriction in atherosclerotic coronary artery disease and prevention by calcium antagonists and nitroglycerin. Am. J. Cardiol. 59:203, 1987.

573. Waters, D. D., Theroux, P., Crittin, J., et al.: Previously undiagnosed variant angina as a cause of chest pain after coronary artery bypass surgery. Circulation 61:1159, 1980.

574. Habbab, M. A., Szwed, S. A., and Haft, J. I.: Is coronary arterial spasm part of the aspirin-induced asthma syndrome? Chest 90:141, 1986.

575. Antman, E., Muller, J., Goldberg, S., et al.: Nifedipine therapy for coronary-artery spasm. Experience in 127 patients. N. Engl. J. Med. 302:12, 1980.

576. Pijls, N. J., and van der Werf, T.: Prinzmetal's angina associated with alcohol withdrawal. Cardiology 75:226, 1988.

577. Matsuguchi, T., Araki, H., Nakamura, N., et al.: Prevention of vasospastic angina by alcohol ingestion: Report of 2 cases. Angiology 39:394, 1988.

578. Stefenelli, T., Zielinski, C. C., Mayr, H., and Scoheithauer, W.: Prinzmetal's angina during cyclophosphamide therapy. Eur. Heart J. 9:1155, 1988.

579. Kleiman, N. S., Lehane, D. E., Geyer, C.E.J., et al.: Prinzmetal's angina during 5-flurouracil chemotherapy. Am. J. Med. 82:566, 1987.

580. Mancuso, L., Bondi, F., Marchi, S., et al.: Cardiac toxicity of 5-fluorouracil. Report of a case of spontaneous angina. Tumori 72:121, 1986.

581. Chockalingham, V., Jaganathan, V., Chandrasekar, P. V., et al.: A case of ST-segment and T-wave alternans. Arch. Intern. Med. 143:1792, 1983.

582. Salerno, J. A., Previtali, M., Panciroli, C., et al.: Ventricular arrhythmias during acute myocardial ischaemia in man. The role and significance of R-ST-T alternans and the prevention of ischaemic sudden death by medical treatment. Eur. Heart J. 7 (Suppl. A):63, 1986.

583. Bayes de Luna, A., Carreras, F., Cladellas, M., et al.: Holter ECG study of the electrocardiographic phenomena in Prinzmetal angina attacks with emphasis on the study of ventricular arrhythmias. J. Electrocardiol. 18:267, 1985.

584. Yasue, H., Takizawa, A., Nagao, M., et al.: Long-term prognosis for patients with variant angina and influential factors. Circulation 78:1, 1988.

585. Ortega, C. J., Garcia, N. F., Malillos, M., and Sanchez, F. A.: Transient left posterior hemiblock during Prinzmetal's angina culminating in acute myocardial infarction. Chest 84:638, 1983.

586. Ortega, C. J., and Paylos, J.: Transient right bundle branch block and left anterior hemiblock during Prinzmetal's angina. J. Electrocardiol. 16:419, 1983.

587. Gabliani, G. I., Winniford, M. D., Fulton, K. L., et al.: Ventricular ectopic activity with spontaneous variant angina: Frequency and relation to transient ST-segment deviation. Am. Heart J. 110:40, 1985.

588. Meller, J., Conde, C. A., Donoso, E., and Dack, S.: Transient Q waves in Prinzmetal's angina. Am. J. Cardiol. 35:691, 1975.

589. Matsuda, Y., Ozaki, M., Ogawa, H., et al.: Coronary arteriography and left ventriculography during spontaneous and exercise-induced ST-segment elevation in patients with variant angina. Am. Heart J. 106:509, 1983.

590. Crea, F., Davies, G., Romeo, F., et al.: Myocardial ischemia during ergonovine testing: Different susceptibility to coronary vasoconstriction in patients with exertional and variant angina. Circulation 69:690, 1984.

591. Distante, A., Rovai, D., Picano, E., et al.: Transient changes in left ventricular mechanics during attacks of Prinzmetal's angina: An M-mode echocardiographic study. Am. Heart J. 107:465, 1984.

592. Bell, M. R., Lapeyre, A. C., and Bove, A. A.: Angiographic demonstration of spontaneous diffuse three vessel coronary artery spasm. J. Am. Coll. Cardiol. 14:523, 1989.

593. Yokoyama, M., Akita, H., Hirata, K-I., et al.: Supersensitivity of isolated coronary artery to Ergonovine in a patient with variant angina. Am. J. Med. 89:507, 1990.

594. Winniford, M. D., Johnson, S. M., Mauritson, D. R., and Hillis, L. D.: Ergonovine provocation to assess efficacy of long-term therapy with calcium antagonists in Prinzmetal's variant angina. Am. J. Cardiol. 51:684, 1983.

595. Waters, D. D., Szlachcic, J., Theroux, P., et al.: Ergonovine testing to detect spontaneous remissions of variant angina during long-term treatment with calcium antagonists drugs. Am. J. Cardiol. 47:179, 1981.

596. Kimball, B. P., LiPreti, V., and Aldridge, H. E.: Quantitative arteriographic responses to ergonovine provocation in subjects with atypical chest pain. Am. J. Cardiol. 64:778, 1989.

597. Previtali, M., Ardissino, D., Barberis, P., et al.: Hyperventilation and ergonovine tests in Prinzmetal's variant angina pectoris in men. Am. J. Cardiol. 63:17, 1989.

598. Mortensen, S. A., Vilhelmsen, R., and Sande, E.: Nonpharmacological provocation of coronary vasospasm. Experience with prolonged hyperventilation in the coronary care unit. Eur. Heart J. 4:391, 1983.

599. Okumura, K., Yasue, H., Matsuyama, K., et al.: Sensitivity and specificity of intracoronary injection of acetylcholine for the induction of coronary artery spasm. J. Am. Coll. Cardiol. 12:883, 1988.

600. Okumura, K., Yasue, H., Horio, Y., et al.: Multivessel coronary spasm in patients with variant angina: A study with intracoronary injection of acetylcholine. Circulation 77:535, 1988.

601. Crea, F., Chierchia, S., Kaski, J. C., et al.: Provocation of coronary spasm by dopamine in patients with active variant angina pectoris. Circulation 74:262, 1986.

602. Maseri, A., Parodi, O., Severi, S., and Pesola, A.: Transient transmural reduction of myocardial blood flow, demonstrated by thallium-201 scintigraphy, as a cause of variant angina. Circulation 54:280, 1976.

603. Ginsburg, R., Lamb, I. H., Schroeder, J. S., et al.: Randomized double-blind comparison of nifedipine and isosorbide dinitrate therapy in variant angina pectoris due to coronary artery spasm. Am. Heart J. 103:44, 1982.

604. Beller, G.: Calcium antagonists in the treatment of Prinzmetal's angina and unstable angina pectoris. Circulation 80(Suppl. IV):78, 1989.

605. Prida, Z. E., Gelman, J. S., Feldman, R. L., et al.: Comparison of diltiazem

and nifedipine alone and in combination in patients with coronary artery spasm. J. Am. Coll. Cardiol. 9:412, 1987.

606. Pesola, A., Lauro, A., Gallo, R., et al.: Efficacy of diltiazem in variant angina. Results of a double-blind crossover study in CCU by Holter monitoring. The possible occurrence of a withdrawal syndrome. G. Ital. Cardiol. 17:329, 1987.

607. Previtali, M., Panciroli, C., Ardissino, D., et al.: Spontaneous remission of variant angina documented by Holter monitoring and ergonovine testing in patients treated with calcium antagonists. Am. J. Cardiol. 59:235, 1987.

608. Tzivoni, D., Keren, A., Benhorin, J., et al.: Prazosin therapy for refractory variant angina. Am. Heart J. 105:262, 1983.

609. Miwa, K., Kambara, H., and Kawai, C.: Effect of aspirin in large doses on attacks of variant angina. Am. Heart J. 105:351, 1983.

610. Corcos, T., David, P. R., Bourassa, M. G., et al.: Percutaneous transluminal coronary angioplasty for the treatment of variant angina. J. Am. Coll. Cardiol. 5:1046, 1985.

611. Katsumoto, K., and Niibori, T.: Prevention of coronary spasms during aorto-coronary (A-C) bypass surgery for variant angina and effort angina with ST elevation. J. Cardiovasc. Surg. 29:343, 1988.

612. Kitamura, S., Morita, R., Kawachi, K., et al.: Different responses of coronary artery and internal mammary artery bypass grafts to ergonovine and nitroglycerin in variant angina. Ann. Thorac. Surg. 47:756, 1989.

613. Waters, D. D., Miller, D., Szlachcic, J., et al.: Factors influencing the long-term prognosis of treated patients with variant angina. Circulation 68:258, 1983.

614. Mark, D. B., Califf, R. M., Morris, K. G., et al.: Clinical characteristics and long-term survival of patients with variant angina. Circulation 69:880, 1984.

615. Miller, D. D., Waters, D. D., Szlachcic, J., and Theroux, P.: Clinical characteristics associated with sudden death in patients with variant angina. Circulation 66:588, 1982.

616. Walling, A., Waters, D. D., Miller, D. D., et al.: Long-term prognosis of patients with variant angina. Circulation 76:990, 1987.

617. Yasue, H., Takizawa, D., Nagao, M., et al.: Long-term prognosis for patients with variant angina and influential factors. Circulation 78:1, 1988.

618. Shimokawa, H., Nagasawa, K., Irie, T., et al.: Clinical characteristics and long-term prognosis of patients with variant angina. A comparative study between western and Japanese populations. Int. J. Cardiol. 18:331, 1988.

CHEST PAIN WITH NORMAL CORONARY ARTERIOGRAM

619. Hutchison, S. J., Poole-Wilson, P. A., and Henderson, A. H.: Angina with normal coronary arteries: A review. Q. J. Med. 72:677, 1988.

620. Papanicolaou, M. N., Califf, R. M., Hlatky, M. A., et al.: Prognostic implications of angiographically normal and insignificantly narrowed coronary arteries. Am. J. Cardiol. 58:1181, 1986.

621. Kemp, H. G., Kronmal, R. A., Vlietstra, R. E., et al.: Seven-year survival of patients with normal or near normal coronary arteriograms: A CASS Registry study. J. Am. Coll. Cardiol. 7:479, 1986.

621a. Maseri, A., Crea, F., Kaski, C., and Crake, T.: Mechanisms of angina pectoris in syndrome X. J. Am. Coll. Cardiol. 17:499, 1991.

622. Camici, P., Marraccini, P., Lorenzoni, R., et al.: Coronary hemodynamics and myocardial metabolism in patients with syndrome X: Response to pacing stress. J. Am. Coll. Cardiol. 17:1461, 1991.

623. Cannon, R. O., III, Schenke, W. H., Quyyumi, A., et al.: Comparison of exercise testing with studies of coronary flow reserve in patients with microvascular angina. Circulation 83(Suppl. III):77, 1991.

624. Cannon, R. O., Bonow, R. O., Bacharach, S. L., et al.: Left ventricular dysfunction in patients with angina pectoris, normal epicardial coronary arteries, and abnormal vasodilator reserve. Circulation 71:218, 1985.

625. Geltman, E. M., Henes, C. G., Senneff, M. J., et al.: Increased myocardial perfusion at rest and diminished perfusion reserve in patients with angina and angiographically normal coronary arteries. J. Am. Coll. Cardiol. 16:586, 1990.

626. Bortone, A. S., Hess, O. M., Eberli, F. R., et al.: Abnormal coronary vasomotion during exercise in patients with normal coronary arteries and reduced coronary flow reserve. Circulation 79:516, 1989.

627. Sax, F. L., Cannon, R. O., Hanson, C., and Epstein, S. E.: Impaired forearm vasodilator reserve in patients with microvascular angina. N. Engl. J. Med. 317:1366, 1987.

627a. Cannon, R. O., III, Peden, D. B., Berkebile, C., et al.: Airway hyperresponsiveness in patients with microvascular angina: Evidence for a diffuse disorder of smooth muscle responsiveness. Circulation 82:2011, 1990.

628. Cannon, R. O., Cunnion, R. E., Parrillo, J. E., et al.: Dynamic limitation of coronary vasodilator reserve in patients with dilated cardiomyopathy and chest pain. J. Am. Coll. Cardiol. 10:1190, 1987.

629. Pasternac, A., Noble, J., Streulens, Y., et al.: Pathophysiology of chest pain in patients with cardiomyopathies and normal coronary arteries. Circulation 65:778, 1982.

630. Spray, T. L., Maron, B. J., Morrow, A. G., et al.: Clinical pathologic conference. A discussion on hypertrophic cardiomyopathy. Am. Heart J. 95:511, 1978.

631. Wielgosz, A. T., Fletcher, R. H., McCants, C. B., et al.: Unimproved chest pain in patients with minimal or no coronary disease: A behavioral phenomenon. Am. Heart J. 108:67, 1984.

632. Beitman, B. D., Mukerji, V., Lamberti, J. W., et al.: Panic disorder in

patients with chest pain and angiographically normal coronary arteries. Am. J. Cardiol. 63:1399, 1989.

633. Bass, C., and Wade, C.: Chest pain with normal coronary arteries. A comparative study of psychiatric and social morbidity. Psychol. Med. 14:51, 1984.

634. Channer, K. S., James, M. A., Papouchado, M., and Rees, J. R.: Anxiety and depression in patients with chest pain referred for exercise testing. Lancet 2:820, 1985.

635. Shapiro, L. M., Crake, T., and Poole-Wilson, P. A.: Is altered cardiac sensation responsible for chest pain in patients with normal coronary arteries? Clinical observation during cardiac catheterisation. Br. Med. J. 296:170, 1988.

636. DeMeester, T. R., O'Sullivan, G. C., Bermudez, G., et al.: Esophageal function in patients with angina-type chest pain and normal coronary angiograms. Ann. Surg. 196:488, 1982.

637. Pupita, G., Kaski, J. C., Galassi, A. R., et al.: Long-term variability of angina pectoris and electrocardiographic signs of ischemia in syndrome X. Am. J. Cardiol. 64:139, 1989.

638. Opherk, D., Schuler, G., Wetterauer, K., et al.: Four-year follow-up study in patients with angina pectoris and normal coronary arteriograms ("syndrome X"). Circulation 80:1610, 1989.

639. Emdin, M., Picano, E., Lattanzi, F., and L'Abbate, A.: Improved exercise capacity with acute aminophylline administration in patients with syndrome X. J. Am. Coll. Cardiol. 14:1450, 1989.

640. Cannon, R. O., Watson, R. M., Rosing, D. R., and Epstein, S. E.: Efficacy of calcium channel blocker therapy for angina pectoris resulting from small-vessel coronary artery disease and abnormal vasodilator reserve. Am. J. Cardiol. 56:242, 1985.

ISCHEMIC HEART DISEASE IN WHICH DISCOMFORT IS NOT THE DOMINANT SYMPTOM

641. Parmley, W. W.: Prevalence and clinical significance of silent myocardial ischemia. Circulation 80(Suppl. IV):68, 1989.

642. Mulcahy, D., Keegan, J., Crean, P., et al.: Silent ischemia in chronic stable angina: A study of its frequency and characteristics in 150 patients. Br. Heart J. 60:417, 1988.

642a. Kellermann, J. J., and Braunwald, E. (eds.): Silent Myocardial Ischemia: A Critical Appraisal. Basel, Karger, 1990, 358 pp.

643. Hirzel, H. O., Leutwyler, R., and Kralyenbuehl, H. P.: Silent myocardial ischemia: Hemodynamic changes during dynamic exercise in patients with proven coronary artery disease despite absence of angina pectoris. J. Am. Coll. Cardiol. 6:275, 1985.

644. Chierchia, S., Smith, G., Morgan, M., et al.: Role of heart rate in pathophysiology of chronic stable angina. Lancet 2:1353, 1984.

645. Deanfield, J. E., Ribiero, P., Oakley, K., et al.: Analysis of ST-segment changes in normal subjects: Implications for ambulatory monitoring in angina pectoris. Am. J. Cardiol. 54:1321, 1984.

646. Rocco, M. B., Barry, J., Campbell, S., et al.: Circadian variation of transient myocardial ischemia in patients with coronary artery disease. Circulation 75:395, 1987.

647. Quyyumi, A. A., Mockus, L., Wright, C., and Fox, K. M.: Morphology of ambulatory ST-segment changes in patients with varying severity of coronary artery disease. Investigation of the frequency of nocturnal ischaemia and coronary spasm. Br. Heart J. 53:186, 1985.

648. Langer, A., Freeman, M. R., Josse, R. G., et al.: Detection of silent myocardial ischemia in diabetes mellitus. Am. J. Cardiol. 67:1073, 1991.

649. Deanfield, J. E., Shea, M. J., Wilson, R. A., et al.: Direct effects of smoking on the heart: Silent ischemic disturbances of coronary flow. Am. J. Cardiol. 57:1005, 1986.

650. Rozanski, A., Bairy, C. N., Krantz, D. S., et al.: Mental stress and the induction of silent myocardial ischemia in patients with coronary artery disease. N. Engl. J. Med. 318:1005, 1988.

651. Deedwania, P. C., and Carbajal, E. V.: Prevalence and patterns of silent myocardial ischemia during daily life in stable angina patients receiving conventional antianginal drug therapy. Am. J. Cardiol. 65:1090, 1990.

652. Yeung, A. C., Barry, J., Orav, J., et al.: Effects of asymptomatic ischemia on long-term prognosis in chronic stable coronary disease. Circulation 83:1598, 1991.

653. Hedblad, B., Juul-Moller, S., Svensson, K., et al.: Increased mortality in men with ST segment depression during 24 h ambulatory long-term ECG recording. Eur. Heart J. 10:149, 1989.

654. Rocco, M. B., Nabel, E. G., Campbell, S., et al.: Prognostic importance of myocardial ischemia detected by ambulatory monitoring in patients with stable coronary artery disease. Circulation 78:877, 1988.

655. Bergin, P., Myler, R. K., Shaw, R. E., et al.: Transluminal coronary angioplasty in the treatment of silent ischemia. Cathet. Cardiovasc. Diagn. 15:223, 1988.

656. Erikssen, J., Enge, I., Forfang, K., and Storstein, O.: False-positive diagnostic tests and coronary angiographic findings in 105 presumably healthy males. Circulation 54:371, 1976.

657. Mulcahy, D., Keegan, J., Sparrow, J., et al.: Ischemia in the ambulatory setting—the total ischemic burden: Relation to' exercise testing and investigative and therapeutic implications. J. Am. Coll. Cardiol. 14:1166, 1989.

657a. Miranda, C. P., Lehmann, K. G., Lachterman, B., et al.: Comparison of silent and symptomatic ischemia during exercise testing in men. Ann. Intern. Med. 114:649, 1991.

658. Weiner, D. A.: The diagnostic and prognostic significance of an asymptomatic positive exercise test. Circulation 75(Suppl. II):20, 1987.

659. Yeung, A. C., Barry, J., and Selwyn, A. P.: Silent ischemia after myocardial infarction. Prognosis, mechanism and intervention. Circulation 82(Suppl. II):143, 1990.

659a. Hill, J. A., Gonzalez, J. I., Kolb, R., and Pepine, C. J.: Effects of atenolol alone, nifedipine alone and their combination on ambulant myocardial ischemia. Am. J. Cardiol. 67:671, 1991.

660. Grieco, J. G., Montoya, A., Sullivan, H. J., et al.: Ventricular aneurysm due to blunt chest injury. Ann. Thorac. Surg. 47:322, 1989.

661. Hirai, T., Fujita, M., Nakajima, H., et al.: Importance of collateral circulation for prevention of left ventricular aneurysm formation in acute myocardial infarction. Circulation 79:791, 1989.

662. Forman, M. B., Collins, H. W., Kopelman, H. A., et al.: Determinants of left ventricular aneurysm formation after anterior myocardial infarction: A clinical and angiographic study. J. Am. Coll. Cardiol. 8:1256, 1986.

663. Barratt-Boyes, B. G., White, H. D., Agnew, T. M., et al.: The results of surgical treatment of left ventricular aneurysms: An assessment of the risk factors affecting early and late mortality. J. Thorac. Cardiovasc. Surg. 87:87, 1984.

664. Meltzer, R. S., Visser, C. A., and Fuster, V.: Intracardiac thrombi and systemic embolization. Ann. Intern. Med. 104:689, 1986.

665. Stephenson, L. W., Hargrove, W. C., Ratcliffe, M. B., et al.: Surgery for left ventricular aneurysm. Early survival with and without endocardial resection. Circulation 79(Suppl. X):1, 1989.

666. Sutherland, G. R., Smyllie, J. H., and Roelandt, J. R.: Advantages of colour flow imaging in the diagnosis of left ventricular pseudoaneurysm. Br. Heart J. 61:59, 1989.

667. Marcus, M. L., Stanford, W., Hajduczok, Z. D., and Weiss, R. M.: Ultrafast computed tomography in the diagnosis of cardiac disease. Am. J. Cardiol. 64:54E, 1989.

668. Mangschau, A.: Akinetic versus dyskinetic left ventricular aneurysms diagnosed by gated scintigraphy: Difference in surgical outcome. Ann. Thorac. Surg. 47:746, 1989.

669. Couper, G. S., Bunton, R. W., Birjiniuk, V., et al.: Relative risks of left ventricular aneurysmectomy in patients with akinetic scars versus true dyskinetic aneurysms. Circulation 82(Suppl. IV):248, 1990.

670. Cosgrove, D. M., Lytle, B. W., Taylor, P. C., et al.: Ventricular aneurysm resection. Circulation 79(Suppl. I):97, 1989.

671. Mangschau, A., Forfang, K., Rootwelt, K., and Frysaker, T.: Improvement in cardiac performance and exercise tolerance after left ventricular aneurysm surgery: A prospective study. Thorac. Cardiovasc. Surg. 36:320, 1988.

672. Louagie, Y., Alouini, T., Lesperance, J., and Pelletier, L. C.: Left ventricular aneurysm complicated by congestive heart failure: An analysis of long-term results and risk factors of surgical treatment. J. Cardiovasc. Surg. 30:648, 1989.

673. Olearchyk, A. S., Lemole, G. M., and Spagna, P. M.: Left ventricular aneurysm. Ten years' experience in surgical treatment of 244 cases. Improved clinical status, hemodynamics, and long-term longevity. J. Thorac. Cardiovasc. Surg. 88:544, 1984.

674. Rankin, J. S., Hickey, M. S., Smith L. R., et al.: Ischemic mitral regurgitation. Circulation 79(Suppl. I):116, 1989.

675. Replogle, R. L., and Campbell, C. D.: Surgery for mitral regurgitation associated with ischemic heart disease. Circulation 79(Suppl. I):122, 1989.

676. Burch, G. E., Giles, T. D., and Colcolough, H. L.: Ischemic cardiomyopathy. Am. Heart J. 79:291, 1970.

677. Bateman, T. M., Czer, L.S.C., Gray, R. J., et al.: Transient pathologic Q waves during acute ischemic events: An electrocardiographic correlate of stunned but viable myocardium. Am. Heart J. 106:1421, 1983.

678. Shanes, J. G., Kondos, G. T., Levitsky, S., et al.: Coronary artery obstruction: A potentially reversible cause of dilated cardiomyopathy. Am. Heart J. 110:173, 1985.

679. Kron, I. L., Flanagan, T. L., Blackbourne, L. H., et al.: Coronary revascularization rather than cardiac transplantation for chronic ischemic cardiomyopathy. Ann. Surg. 210:348, 1989.

680. Kelly, P., Ruskin, J. N., Vlahakes, G. J., et al.: Surgical coronary revascularization in survivors of prehospital cardiac arrest: Its effect on inducible ventricular arrhythmias and long-term survival. J. Am. Coll. Cardiol. 15:267, 1990.

681. Kragel, A. H., and Roberts, W. C.: Anomalous origin of either the right or left main coronary artery from the aorta with subsequent coursing between aorta and pulmonary trunk: Analysis of 32 necropsy cases. Am. J. Cardiol. 62:771, 1988.

682. DeMaio, S. J., Kinsella, S. H., and Silverman, M. E.: Clinical course and long-term prognosis of spontaneous coronary artery dissection. Am. J. Cardiol. 64:471, 1989.

683. Subramanyan, R., Joy, J., and Balakrishnan, K. G.: Natural history of aortoarteritis (Takayasu's disease). Circulation 80:429, 1989.

684. Tveter, K. J., and Edwards, J. E.: Calcified aortic sinotubular ridge: A source of coronary ostial stenosis or embolism. J. Am. Coll. Cardiol. 12:1510, 1988.

685. Gao, S. Z., Schroeder, J. S., Hunt, S. A., et al.: Acute myocardial infarction in cardiac transplant recipients. Am. J. Cardiol. 64:1093, 1989.

686. Lange, R. L., Reid, M. S., Tresch, D. D., et al.: Nonatheromatous ischemic heart disease following withdrawal from chronic industrial nitroglycerin exposure. Circulation 46:666, 1972.

Interventional Catheterization Techniques: Percutaneous Transluminal Balloon Angioplasty, Valvuloplasty, and Related Procedures

by DONALD S. BAIM, M.D.

From 1950 through the 1970's essentially all cardiac catheterizations were performed to evaluate individual disease states, to guide medical therapy, or to provide a road map for cardiac surgical repair (see Chaps. 7 and 9). In the 1980's, however, cardiac catheterization began to play an increasingly important role in *treating* as well as *diagnosing* cardiovascular lesions. In the 1990's this new application of catheterization-based treatment has become known as "interventional" cardiology, which may involve delivery of mechanical, thermal, microsurgical, or light energy to cardiovascular lesions by means of specialized percutaneously inserted catheters. The end result may be to open stenotic blood vessels or cardiac valves, or to close undesired channels for blood flow, in an effort to achieve a physiological correction of the underlying cardiac pathology comparable to that obtained by traditional surgical techniques. If such a correction is possible (as it now is in one-half of the patients requiring coronary revascularization), it may be obtained frequently at a fraction of the expense, disability, and discomfort of surgery. The explosive growth of this area has already had a major impact on health care delivery and is likely to increase as these interventional techniques continue to mature. The delivery through catheters of electric currents to the heart and specialized conduction tissue for therapeutic purposes is another application of interventional catheterization and is described on pages 651 and 776.

Treatment of Vascular Stenosis

The development of vascular angiography made it possible to visualize atherosclerotic and fibromuscular stenoses in various arterial beds. In the course of such angiographic procedures, Dotter et al. noted that it was frequently possible to pass first a guidewire and then a catheter or rigid dilator through an area of stenosis in the iliac-femoral system, thereby enlarging the lumen and improving antegrade blood flow (Fig. 41–1).[1–3] While the so-called *Dotter technique* was used to some extent in Europe between 1964 and 1974,[4] its application was limited by the trauma to the artery which resulted from exertion of axial force on the stenosis, and the local complications which were related to the percutaneous introduction of the large-caliber rigid dilators. In 1974 Gruentzig and Kumpe modified the technique by substituting a balloon-tipped catheter for the rigid dilator.[5] This nonelastomeric balloon catheter could be introduced and passed across the stenosis in its smaller collapsed state and then inflated to a predetermined size with liquid contrast material in order to achieve the desired enlargement in luminal caliber (Fig. 41–2). Balloon angioplasty (the so-called *Gruentzig technique*) was applied first to peripheral[5] and then to renal arterial stenoses.[6] In 1977, after cadaver and intraoperative studies during bypass surgery, percutaneous balloon angioplasty was extended to stenoses of the epicardial coronary arteries.[7] Balloon angioplasty—albeit with many technical refinements—still constitutes the core of interventional cardiology and has provided major encouragement for the subsequent development of a variety of other interventional techniques for application in the heart and extracardiac vasculature.

PERCUTANEOUS TRANSLUMINAL CORONARY ANGIOPLASTY (PTCA)

EARLY EXPERIENCE. Between 1977 and 1980 coronary angioplasty used the original Gruentzig catheter,[7] a two-lumen device in which one

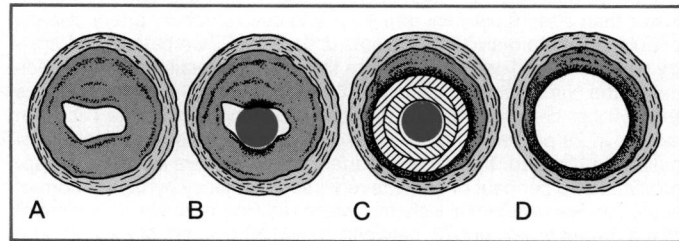

FIGURE 41–1. The Dotter technique. Cross sections of a stenotic arterial lumen are shown at baseline *(A)*, during the passage of the initial catheter *(B)*, during the passage of the coaxial dilators *(C)*, and after the procedure *(D)*. Note the improvement in luminal diameter without enlargement of the outer vessel caliber, suggesting compaction of the atheroma as the mechanism of dilatation. (From Dotter, C. T., Rosch, J., and Judkins, M. P.: Transluminal dilatation of atherosclerotic stenosis. Surg. Gynecol. Obstet. *127:*794, 1968.)

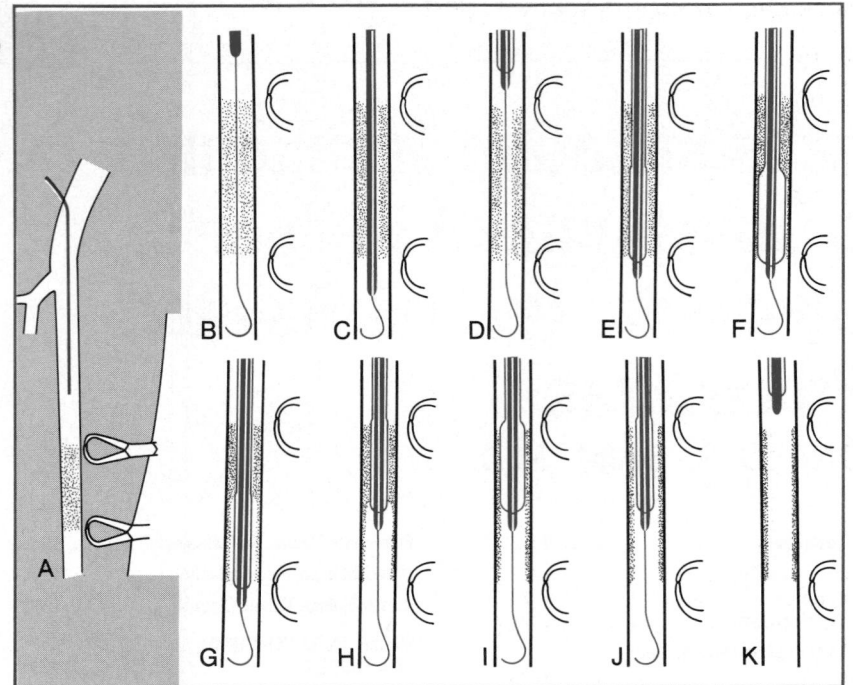

FIGURE 41-2. The Gruentzig technique. This series of diagrams depicts the application of balloon angioplasty to the treatment of a totally occluded peripheral artery (A). After diagnostic angiography a guidewire (B) and an angiographic catheter (C) are passed through the area of total occlusion. This creates a lumen for passage of the deflated dilatation catheter (D, E). The dilatation balloon is then inflated at several points throughout the stenotic lumen (F to I), resulting in improvement in vessel patency (J, K). Again note the absence of enlargement in the outer diameter, suggesting compaction of atherosclerotic material as the mechanism for luminal enhancement. (From Gruentzig, A., and Kumpe, D. A.: Technique of percutaneous transluminal angioplasty with the Gruentzig balloon catheter. Am. J. Radiol. *132*:547, 1979.)

lumen was used to inflate and deflate the polyvinylchloride (PVC) balloon, while the second lumen was used to monitor pressure or inject radiographic contrast material through a port near the catheter tip. A short segment of flexible guidewire was attached to the tip of the dilatation catheter. Although this guidewire reduced the chance of intimal dissection and subintimal passage, it could not be reshaped or manipulated once introduced into the patient, sharply limiting the ability to advance the dilatation catheter beyond all but the most proximal coronary stenoses. Moreover, the large diameter of these early balloon catheters in their deflated state (0.060 inch, or 1.5 mm) made it difficult to cross severe or inelastic stenoses, since the diameter of the deflated balloon was frequently larger than that of the stenotic lumen (i.e., 0.6 mm for an 80 per cent stenosis of a typical 3-mm diameter coronary artery). To deal with this problem, the dilatation catheter had to be advanced through a large (No. 8 or 9 French, 2.7 or 3.0 mm outer diameter), stiff "guiding catheter" positioned in the coronary ostium. The third limitation of the original Gruentzig catheter was its comparatively low balloon rupture pressure (6 atm, or 90 psi), which made it difficult to dilate rigid lesions adequately. In an effort to mitigate these problems, early angioplasty operators attempted to select patients considered to have "soft" rather than rigid lesions (as reflected by recent onset of anginal symptoms and absence of calcification of the lesion on fluoroscopy), and particularly those patients whose lesions were located in the proximal coronary segments.

To define better the results, complications, and long-term efficacy of this new technique, the National Heart, Lung, and Blood Institute (NHLBI) established a PTCA Registry in 1979.[8] Candidates for PTCA were selected to have severe enough angina to warrant consideration of bypass surgery, objective evidence of myocardial ischemia, and coronary anatomy (proximal, subtotal, discrete, concentric, noncalcified stenosis of a single coronary artery) thought to be approachable with the limited equipment then available. Although such patients were believed to represent fewer than 5 to 10 per cent of the symptomatic coronary artery disease population, more than 3,000 patients underwent PTCA before the Registry was closed in late 1981. Despite the careful selection of ideal candidates, the primary success rate of PTCA in the original Registry was less than 60 per cent, with failure to cross the stenosis with the dilatation system in 29 per cent and failure to dilate the stenosis in 12 per cent of patients attempted. Two other important problems were identified: (1) approximately 6 per cent of patients required emergency bypass to correct acute, severe myocardial ischemia which resulted from abrupt reclosure of the dilated artery, and (2) between 20 and 30 per cent of patients with an initially successful procedure experienced return of angina owing to angiographically evident renarrowing ("restenosis") of the dilated segment within 6 months after the procedure.

TECHNICAL ADVANCES. Shortly after the original NHLBI Registry was closed, a variety of technical improvements in PTCA equipment,[9,10] coupled with the availability of more experienced operators, facilitated major improvements

in the overall success of PTCA.[10a] The original dilatation catheter was redesigned so that the guidewire now extended the entire length of the dilatation catheter, allowing the wire to be advanced, withdrawn, reshaped, or steered during the procedure (Fig. 41-3).[11] Although these specialized guidewires are only 0.010 to 0.018 inch (0.3 to 0.5 mm) in diameter, sophisticated engineering has allowed the fabrication of devices with soft atraumatic tips, excellent torque control, and superb radiographic visibility. Current guidewires can be manipulated across stenoses located virtually anywhere in the coronary tree, and then serve as a "railroad track" over which advancement of the dilatation catheter can be performed. Special "exchange-length" guidewires (300 cm long) can be left positioned in the distal coronary artery as one balloon catheter is withdrawn and a second is inserted, or as contrast injection is

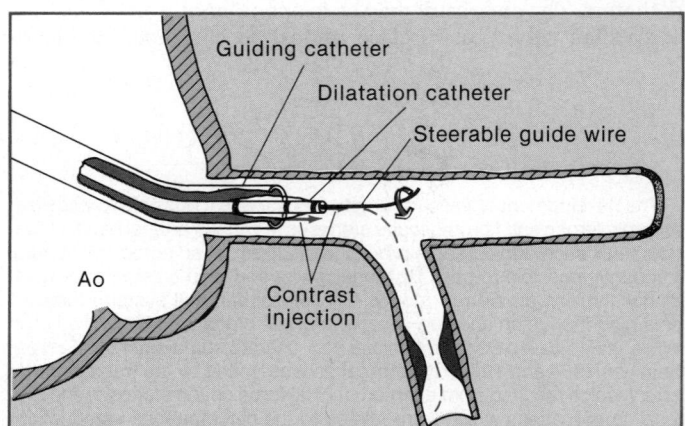

FIGURE 41-3. Movable guidewire dilatation system. The dilatation catheter is shown here at the end of a large (No. 8 or 9 French, 2.7- or 3.0-mm) guiding catheter, which is positioned at the ostium of the involved vessel. The soft, yet steerable guidewire is then advanced through the central lumen of the dilatation catheter and directed through and beyond the target lesion. The position of this guidewire relative to coronary branches and lesions can be revealed by contrast injection through the guiding catheter or through the central lumen of the dilatation catheter. Once the guidewire has been successfully positioned, it serves as a "track" over which the dilatation catheter itself can be advanced. (From Baim, D. S.: Coronary angioplasty. *In* Grossman, W., and Baim, D. S. [eds.]: Cardiac Catheterization, Angiography and Intervention. 4th ed. Philadelphia, Lea and Febiger, 1991.)

PLATE 9

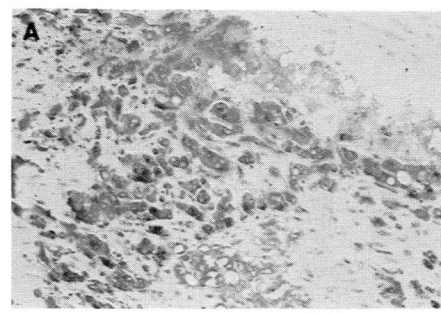 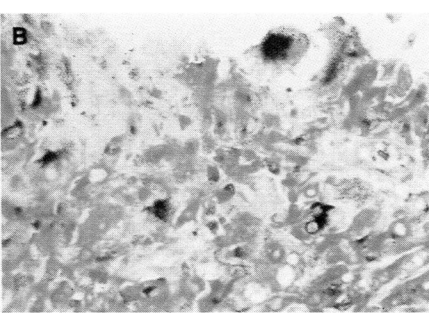 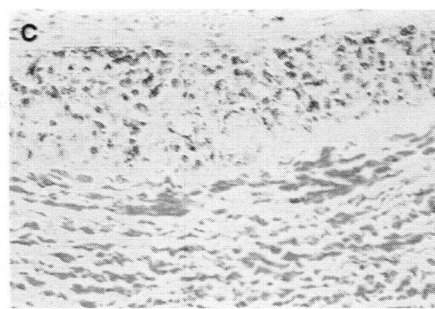

FIGURE 36–12 (See page 1115)

Double-immunostained preparations demonstrating the distribution of PDGF-B chain in methacarn-fixed, deparaffinized sections of advanced lesions of atherosclerosis from a high-level hypercholesterolemic nonhuman primate fed a hypercholesterolemic diet for one year. The sections were stained with a monoclonal antibody specific for PDGF-B-chain protein, and with cell-type-specific monoclonal antibodies for macrophages *(A, B)* or smooth muscle *(C)*, with IGSS and avidin-biotin immunoalkaline-phosphatase procedures.

A) PDGF-B chain (black, granular reaction product) is localized to HAM56-positive macrophages (red reaction product).
B) Positive cells at higher magnification.
C) PDGF-B chain (black, granular reaction product) and HHF35-positive smooth muscle cells (red reaction product) are identified in nonoverlapping cell populations. All sections were counterstained with methyl green. *A* and *C* original magnifications, X250; *B* original magnification, X400. (From Ross, R., Masuda, J., Raines, E.W., et al.: Localization of PDGF-B protein in macrophages in all phases of atherogenesis. Science 248:1009, 1990. © Copyright 1990 by the American Association for the Advancement of Science.

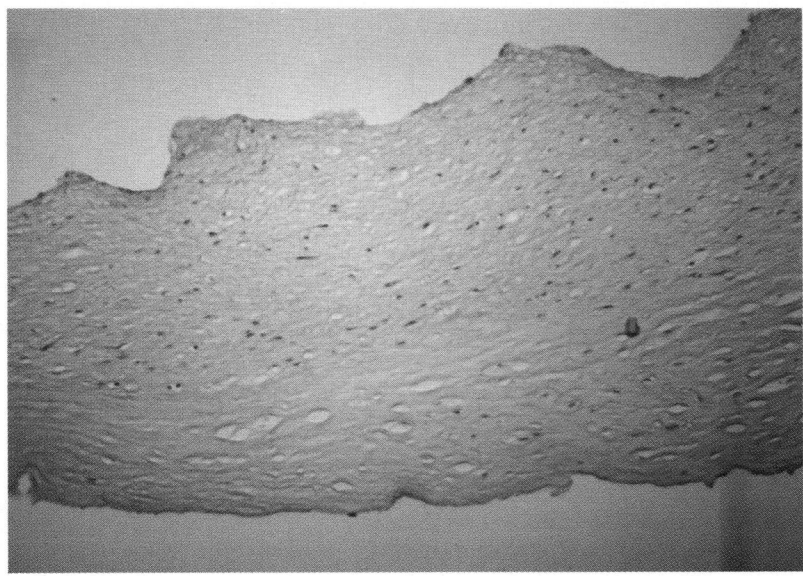

FIGURE 41–14 (See page 1372)

Histology of restenosis. This sample was obtained by directional coronary atherectomy from a patient who developed recurrent symptoms and angiographic restenosis 4 months after laser balloon angioplasty. There is a homogeneous population of smooth muscle cells showing a proliferative rather than contractile phenotype, wihch have grown within the initial treated lumen to renarrow the flow channel. Similar histological findings are apparent in postmortem specimens and atherectomy specimens in patients with restenosis after diverse coronary interventions. (From Safian, R. D., et al.: Coronary atherectomy: Clinical, angiographic and histologic findings and observations regarding mechanism. Circulation 82:69, 1990, by permission of the American Heart Association, Inc.)

PLATE 10

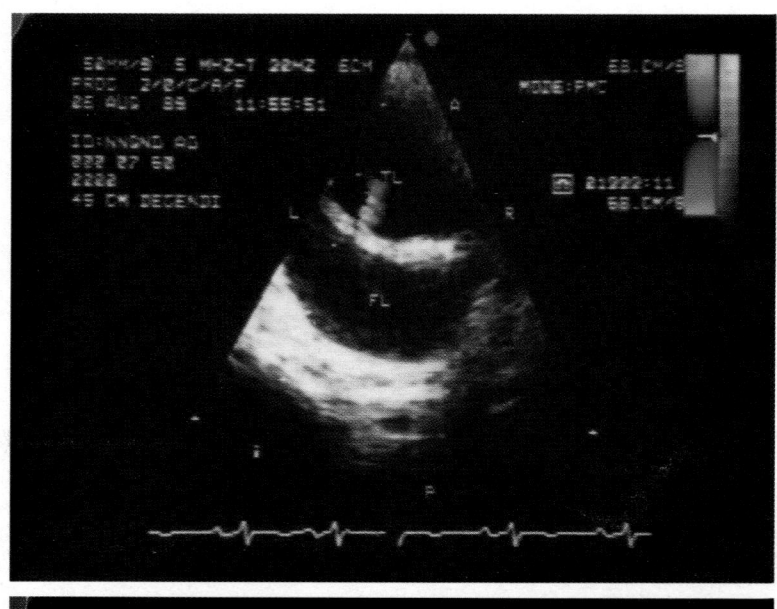

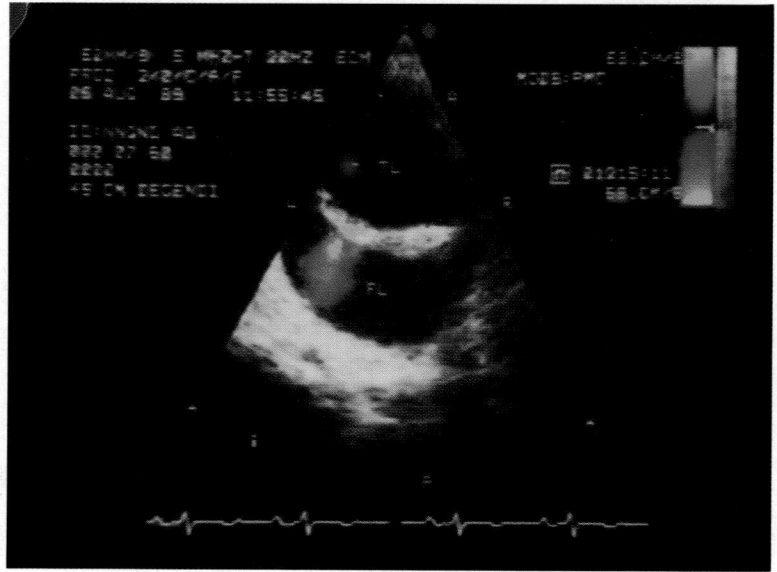

FIGURE 47–11 (See page 1538)

Transesophageal echocardiographic image of an aortic dissection, demonstrating a large false lumen posteriorly in the ascending aorta. Communication between the true lumen (TL) and false lumen (FL) is present. Bidirectional flow is demonstrated by transesophageal color Doppler echocardiography in these images of the descending aorta. The red jet indicates flow into true lumen from the false lumen; the blue jet indicates flow into the false lumen.

performed through the guiding catheter to assess adequacy of dilatation. Improvements in the design of dilatation catheters[10] have led to the development of devices with deflated diameters as small as 0.025 inch (0.60 mm), inflated diameters between 2.0 and 4.0 mm, and the ability to tolerate inflation pressures as high as 20 atm (300 psi). These devices can be used to cross and dilate even the most rigid stenoses. Specialized "balloon-on-a-wire" catheters are available with deflated profiles as small as 0.020 inch (0.5 mm) to allow dilatation of the most severe or most distal lesions.

The impact of these improvements in angioplasty catheters and guidewires was evident in PTCA Registry II,[12] which collected information on patients treated during 1985 and 1986 at 14 centers that had participated in the original Registry. Analysis demonstrated an improved success rate of 85 per cent, with concomitant reduction in the incidence of emergency bypass surgery to 3.5 per cent.[13] While the procedural mortality for patients with single-vessel disease had decreased compared to the original Registry (from 0.9 to 0.2 per cent), overall procedural mortality remained approximately 1 per cent because Registry II included more patients with multivessel disease (mortality 1.7 per cent). One-year follow-up of 838 patients with single-vessel disease showed a low incidence of death (1.6 per cent) and myocardial infarction (1.9 per cent), although repeat angioplasty (18.1 per cent) and bypass surgery (6.2 per cent) were required to treat restenosis or disease progression.[14] With the exception of a slight further increase in success (to 90 per cent) and reduction in emergency bypass surgery (to 2 per cent) as the result of further refinements in equipment and technique since 1986, the results of Registry II can be taken to reflect those obtainable by conventional balloon angioplasty at the time of this writing.

CURRENT TECHNIQUE

Patients undergoing coronary angioplasty are usually admitted to the hospital the day before or the morning of the procedure. Prior catheterization and exercise test data are reviewed, and a dilatation strategy is developed detailing the specific lesions, the sequence, and the equipment to be used for dilatation. The procedure—including the likelihood of successful dilatation, abrupt reclosure with emergency surgery, and late restenosis—is discussed with the patient and the family. Consent forms for both PTCA and possible emergency coronary artery bypass surgery are signed. Patients are proscribed from oral intake after midnight and asked to bathe with an antiseptic scrub. Aspirin (325 mg/day), dipyridamole (200 mg/day), and a calcium antagonist are added to existing medical therapy.

At the time of PTCA appropriate vascular access (by way of either brachial artery cutdown or femoral artery puncture) is obtained (Fig. 7–1, p. 182), and a guiding catheter is positioned at the ostium of the involved coronary artery. A venous catheter for monitoring right heart pressure and/or temporary ventricular pacing is usually placed, and full systemic anticoagulation is achieved using 10,000 units of intravenous heparin. Baseline angiography is performed to clarify any uncertainties (e.g., location of side branches relative to the target stenosis) and to document continued suitability of the lesion for dilatation. The guidewire is then passed across the target lesion and positioned in the distal segment of the involved vessel. A dilatation catheter comparable in size to the adjacent normal artery is advanced into the lesion and adequately pressurized to expand the balloon to its full diameter. Adequate dilatation is confirmed by repeat angiography and/or measurement of the translesional pressure gradient, after which the dilated segment is observed over 5 to 10 minutes to document the stability of the result. Additional lesions may then be dilated according to the predetermined dilatation strategy. The effect of heparin is allowed to wear off before removal of the vascular sheaths, although intravenous heparin infusion may be resumed for 24 to 48 hours if significant

intimal dissection is present at the dilatation site. After 8 to 24 hours of bed rest, the patient is ambulated and discharged.

Discharge medications typically include aspirin 325 mg/day and short-term (6 weeks) therapy with a calcium channel blocker.[15] The patient is scheduled for an exercise tolerance test during the following month but may typically return to work within 1 week of a successful and uncomplicated coronary angioplasty. A follow-up exercise tolerance test should be performed at 6 months (or sooner if anginal symptoms recur) to detect restenosis of the dilated segment(s). Annual exercise testing and continued attention to risk factor reduction are generally indicated in these coronary patients at high risk of additional coronary arterial lesions.

INDICATIONS
(See also pp. 1316–1317)

The indication for PTCA is myocardial ischemia (Table 41–1) owing to coronary stenosis(es) deemed suitable for this procedure.[16,17] With the advantage of improved guidewires, dilatation catheters, and guiding catheters, a high success rate is achieved despite the inclusion of patients with progressively more challenging anatomical and clinical disease.

ANATOMICAL INDICATIONS. Whereas PTCA was originally limited to proximal stenoses, more distal, eccentric, and calcified lesions are now approached on a routine basis.[9] Angioplasty of such lesions, however, is generally associated with less favorable results in terms of a lower success rate and/or a higher complication rate[18] than expected with an "ideal" lesion. This pattern is reflected in the ad hoc lesion grading system (Table 41–2) proposed by the AHA/ACC Task Force,[16] but also validated in a retrospective sample of multivessel angioplasty patients.[19] Lesions involving *coronary bifurcations*—previously avoided because of the 14 per cent incidence of "snowplow" occlusion of the side branch (Fig. 41–4)[20]—can now be dilated using the "kissing-balloon"[21] or double-wire (Fig. 41–5)[22] technique to preserve both the main and the side-branch lumina. *Totally occluded coronary arteries* are also approachable by PTCA, to revascularize areas of viable myocardium supplied by inadequate collateral flow (Fig. 41–6) or to provide collateral flow to other stenotic ves-

TABLE 41–1 INDICATIONS FOR AND CONTRAINDICATIONS TO PTCA

CLINICAL INDICATIONS FOR PTCA

Significant stenosis of one or more major epicardial arteries, which subtend at least a moderate-sized area of viable myocardium, in a patient who has:

1. Recurrent ischemic episodes after myocardial infarction or major ventricular arrhythmia,
2. Angina that has not responded adequately to medical therapy,
3. Clear evidence of myocardial ischemia on resting, ambulatory, or exercise electrocardiography, or
4. Objective evidence of myocardial ischemia that increases the overall risk of required noncardiac surgery.

ABSOLUTE OR RELATIVE CONTRAINDICATIONS TO PTCA

High-risk anatomy (including significant left main artery disease) in which vessel closure would likely result in hemodynamic collapse,

Severe, diffuse, and/or extensive coronary artery disease better treated surgically,

Target lesion morphology (type C) associated with an anticipated success <60%, unless PTCA is the only reasonable treatment option,

No coronary stenosis >50% diameter reduction,

No objective or compelling clinical evidence of myocardial ischemia, or

Absence of on-site surgical back-up, qualified PTCA operators, or adequate radiographic imaging equipment.

TABLE 41-2 ANTICIPATED SUCCESS IN VARIOUS LESIONS ACCORDING TO MORPHOLOGICAL TYPES

TYPE A LESION (HIGH [>85%] SUCCESS WITH LOW RISK)

Discrete (<10 mm long)	Little or no calcification
Concentric	Less than total occlusion
Readily accessible	Not ostial
Nonangulated segment	No major branch involvement
Smooth contour	Absence of thrombus

TYPE B LESION (MODERATE [60-85%] SUCCESS WITH MODERATE RISK)

Tubular (10-20 mm long)	Moderate calcification
Eccentric	Total occlusion <3 months
Moderate tortuosity	Ostial location
Moderate (45°-90°) angle	Treatable bifurcation lesion
Irregular contour	Some thrombus present

TYPE C LESION (LOW [<60%] SUCCESS WITH HIGH RISK)

Diffuse (>20 mm long)	Total occlusion >3 months
Excessive tortuosity or angulation	Bifurcation with nonprotect-able side branch
Degenerated vein graft	

(After Ryan, T. J., et al.[16])

sels undergoing dilatation (Fig. 41–7).[23] Although the primary success rate in dilatation of chronic total occlusions remains lower than that for other stenotic lesions (75 per cent for occlusions less than 3 months old and below 50 per cent for older occlusions), dilatation of total occlusions now accounts for 10 to 20 per cent of PTCA volume in large centers.[24]

An increasing number of patients with multivessel coronary artery disease are undergoing PTCA as an alternative to bypass surgery (Fig. 41–7). These patients account for more than half of those entered into the 1985–86 Registry, although fewer than two-thirds of patients identified as having multivessel *disease* actually underwent multivessel *dilatation*.[12] Preliminary data suggest that many patients with multivessel coronary artery disease may derive substantial clinical benefit from successful PTCA, but multivessel disease clearly imposes several additional difficulties to those of single-vessel disease. These include: (1) longer duration of the procedure and greater usage of radiographic contrast material, (2) more diffuse myocardial ischemia if abrupt reclosure should occur, (3) a greater chance that not all significant coronary lesions will be successfully dilated (incomplete revascularization), and (4) a greater chance that recurrent angina will develop owing to restenosis of a dilated segment or progression of disease in one or more undilated segments.[14] These difficulties affect both the selection of patients for and the performance of

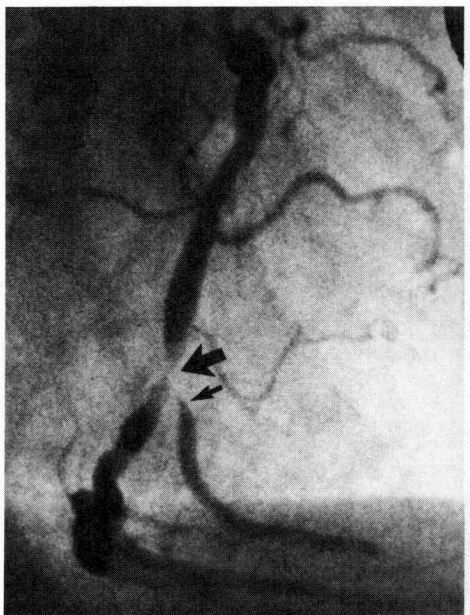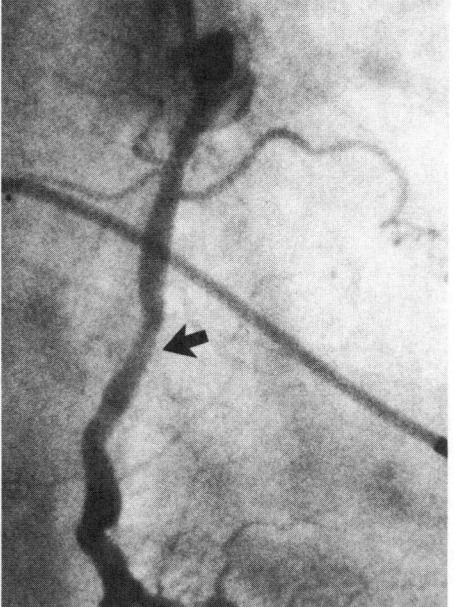

FIGURE 41–4. The "snowplow" effect. The left panel shows severe stenosis of the midportion of the right coronary artery (large arrow), from which a proximally diseased right ventricular branch (small arrow) originates. After PTCA (right panel), dilatation of the right coronary lesion has been achieved at the expense of occlusion of the right ventricular side branch. (From Baim, D. S.: Percutaneous transluminal angioplasty. *In* Petersdorf, R. G., et al. [eds.]: Harrison's Principles of Internal Medicine, Update VI. New York, McGraw-Hill Book Co., 1985.)

FIGURE 41–5. "Double-wire" and "kissing-balloon" techniques. To avoid occlusion of an involved branch, two guidewires are placed: one into the distal left anterior descending, and one into the involved diagonal. Repeated alternate balloon inflation in the two vessels resulted in alternating occlusion. With resort to a kissing-balloon approach, two balloons were inflated simultaneously to achieve patency of both vessels. (From Baim, D. S.: Coronary angioplasty. *In* Grossman, W., and Baim, D. S. [eds.]: Cardiac Catheterization, Angiography, and Intervention. 4th ed. Philadelphia, Lea and Febiger, 1991.)

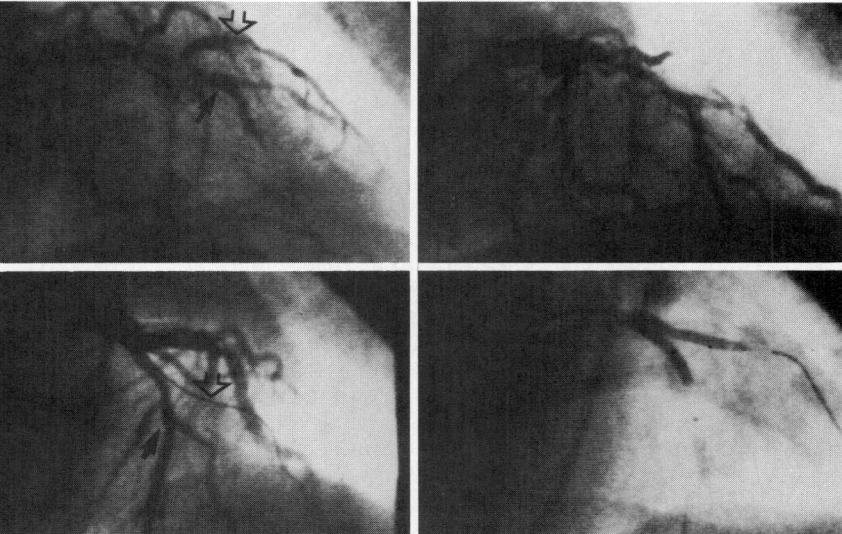

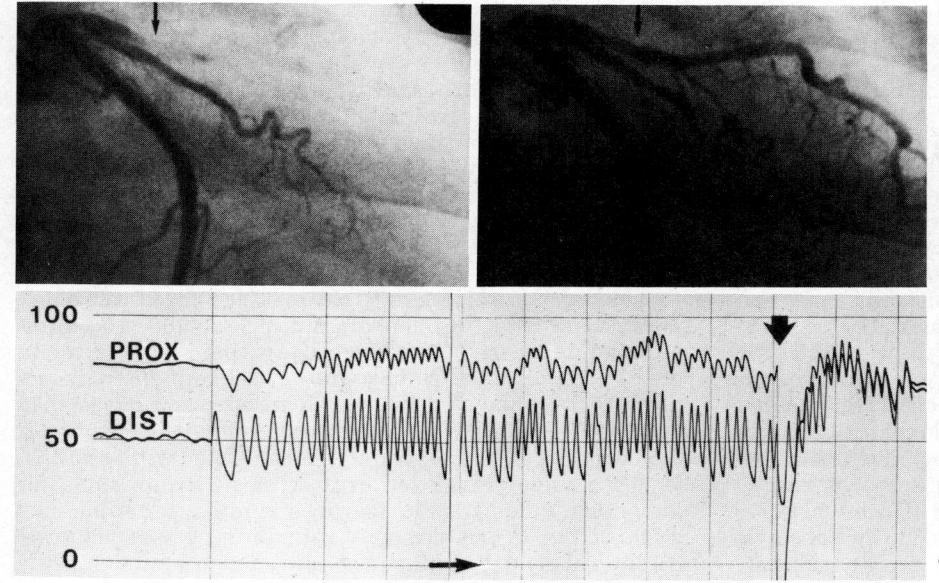

FIGURE 41-6. Angioplasty of a totally occluded coronary artery. Baseline angiography *(upper left)* shows total occlusion of the proximal left anterior descending. Prominent collateral filling of the distal vessel was evident during right coronary injection (not shown). Despite the presence of total occlusion of the involved vessel, this lesion was successfully crossed and dilated, with the result shown in the *upper right.* The *bottom panel* shows measurement of the "proximal" aortic and "distal" intracoronary pressure during inflation and after deflation (bold arrow) of the dilatation catheter. Note the presence of a high distal occluded coronary artery pressure (50 mm Hg), consistent with good collateral function, and the resolution of the pressure difference between the proximal and distal sampling sites after balloon deflation (residual transstenotic gradient 5 mm Hg). (From Dervan, J. P., Baim, D. S., Cherniles, J., and Grossman, W.: Transluminal angioplasty of occluded coronary arteries: Use of a movable guidewire system. Circulation *68:*776, 1983, by permission of the American Heart Association, Inc.)

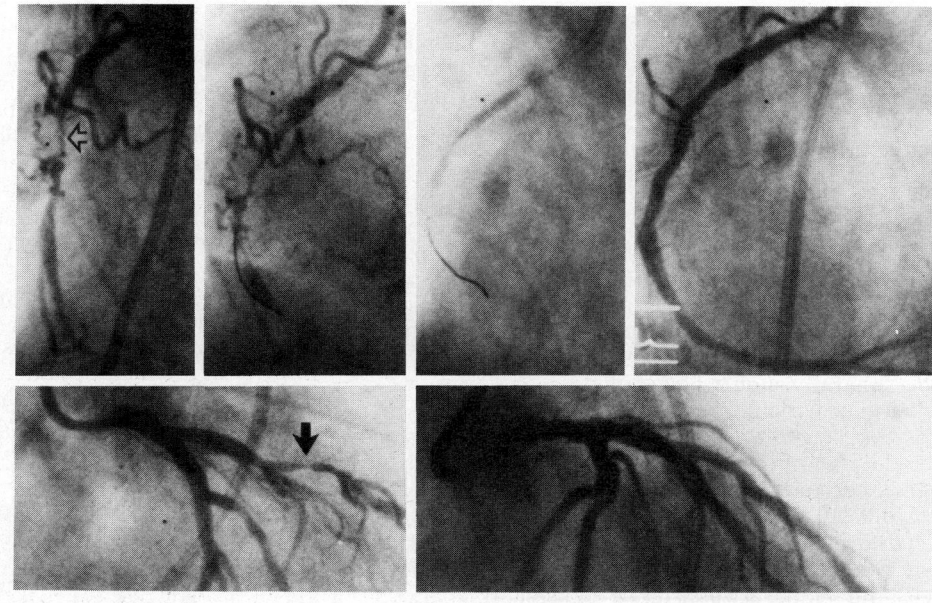

FIGURE 41-7. "Boot strap" two-vessel dilatation. *Upper panel* shows functionally occluded mid-right coronary artery, with filling of the distal vessel by way of bridging (right-to-right) and left-to-right collaterals. Successful dilatation of this lesion *(upper right)* restored antegrade flow in the right coronary artery and allowed reversal of the left-to-right collaterals to support the left anterior descending territory during dilatation of that vessel (bold arrow). (From Baim, D. S.: Coronary angioplasty. *In* Grossman, W. [ed.]: Cardiac Catheterization, Angiography, and Intervention. 4th ed. Philadelphia, Lea and Febiger, 1991.)

the actual PTCA procedure. The operator must decide which lesions are responsible for the patient's symptoms (the "culprit" lesions[25]) and therefore must be dilated, which lesions are mild enough to be left alone, what the sequence of dilatations should be, and whether a suboptimal result in one lesion necessitates deferral of other dilatations to a separate sitting (a "staged" multivessel PTCA procedure). These issues must be addressed on a case-by-case basis, but the general goal of PTCA in a patient with multivessel disease is to dilate all lesions which narrow the diameter of major coronary segments by more than 70 per cent. Milder lesions can be dilated easily, but such dilatation is not usually required to control symptoms and still entails some risk of abrupt reclosure or accelerated restenosis.[26] If natural progression of these mild lesions leads to recurrent ischemic symptoms, they can be addressed in a subsequent procedure. Given these uncertainties about PTCA in multivessel disease, an adequately controlled comparison of PTCA with bypass surgery—as in the Bypass Angioplasty Revascularization Intervention (BARI) Trial currently being conducted—will be required to establish the optimal application of PTCA in this important patient population.

CLINICAL INDICATIONS. At the same time PTCA has

been applied to progressively more difficult *anatomical* situations, it has also been applied to a broader spectrum of *clinical* disease states. Whereas PTCA was initially used largely in patients with chronic, stable angina, it is now used increasingly in patients with more unstable patterns, i.e., new onset, rest, or preinfarction angina (p. 1340).[27] Between one-half and three-quarters of such patients are anatomically suitable for PTCA, particularly if revascularization can be limited to dilatation of one or more severe "culprit" lesions responsible for the unstable clinical picture[28] without attempting revascularization of other milder lesions, small branches, or chronic total occlusions. In many instances PTCA can be performed in patients with unstable angina as an extension of the initial diagnostic catheterization procedure.[29] A tendency toward an increased incidence of ischemic complications initially reported for PTCA in the unstable angina population can be reduced by several days of intravenous heparin infusion prior to attempted dilatation.[30]

Acute Myocardial Infarction (see also p. 1316). The majority of patients with acute myocardial infarction have anatomical features that make them suitable for PTCA, either after or instead of thrombolytic therapy. While current thrombolytic regimens are capable of restoring patency to more than 75 per cent of infarct-related arteries within 90 minutes of initiation of therapy, patients typically are left with at least moderate stenosis of the infarct vessel, which makes them prone to reocclusion, reinfarction, or subsequent angina. Angioplasty can generally be performed safely in acute myocardial infarction, and it was initially thought that routine catheterization and angioplasty of such patients following thrombolytic therapy might reduce the incidence of subsequent adverse events. Several studies (including the Thrombolysis in Myocardial Infarction or TIMI IIA trial), however, have shown that routine *immediate* catheterization and angioplasty increase the risk of procedure-related complications (bleeding and emergency bypass surgery) without improving mortality, reinfarction, or left ventricular function.[31] Similarly, the overall TIMI II study has shown that even routine *delayed* (18 to 48 hours) catheterization and angioplasty fail to affect favorably either in-hospital or 1-year mortality or reinfarction rates compared to a *conservative* strategy (watchful waiting) in which catheterization and PTCA are reserved for patients who exhibit recurrent spontaneous or exercise-induced myocardial ischemia.[32] Although it has not yet been compared to the conservative TIMI strategy in a controlled trial, *primary* angioplasty (e.g., angioplasty without prior thrombolytic therapy) appears able to safely restore patency of the infarct artery.[33] It may be of particular value in patients with contraindications to thrombolytic therapy, who present within 4 to 6 hours of symptom onset to an institution with skilled angioplasty operators and in-house surgical standby.

Post Bypass. A rapidly growing indication for PTCA is seen in patients with *recurrent angina following bypass surgery*, who may undergo dilation of a lesion in a saphenous vein[34,35,35a] or internal mammary[36] graft or of a lesion in a previously grafted or ungrafted native coronary artery.[34] Saphenous vein graft lesions occurring within 1 year of surgery are typically due to local intimal hyperplasia and dilate quite nicely, albeit with a relatively high (50 per cent) restenosis rate. Atherosclerotic graft lesions occurring several years after surgery are more friable, and are prone to disruption with distal embolization during attempted angioplasty. Recently occluded grafts pose special problems with distal thromboembolization and long-term patency, so that PTCA of such vessels generally should be avoided.[37]

Patients with other factors increasing the risk of bypass surgery (advanced age[38] or other medical problems) may be offered PTCA of unprotected left main lesions or diffuse three-vessel coronary disease that would otherwise be rejected for angioplasty in favor of bypass surgery.[39] When it is necessary to perform angioplasty on patients at high risk because of poor left ventricular function, the procedure may be performed with the temporary assistance of intraaortic balloon counterpulsation[40] or percutaneous cardiopulmonary support.[41]

At the other end of the spectrum, some patients with *milder anginal symptoms* (Canadian Heart Class I or II) may be subjected to catheterization followed by dilatation of one or more severe underlying lesions, rather than continuing with medical antianginal therapy. Although such patients constitute less than 20 per cent of those currently subjected to PTCA,[42] it should be pointed out that there is no evidence that PTCA is superior to medical therapy for this patient group in terms of longevity, freedom from subsequent myocardial infarction, or reduced long-term health costs.

ECONOMIC AND REGULATORY IMPLICATIONS

The rapidly growing role of PTCA is reflected in current statistics. An estimated 250,000 PTCA procedures are being performed annually, compared with approximately the same number of coronary artery bypass operations. From another perspective, the current utilization of PTCA is reflected in the revascularization outcome of patients undergoing first-time diagnostic catheterizations for coronary artery disease. Approximately 60 per cent of such patients are referred for revascularization, which consists of nearly equal numbers of PTCA

and surgical bypass procedures.[42,43] Because PTCA can be performed for approximately one-half to one-third the in-hospital cost of bypass surgery, with a shorter length of stay and convalescent period, it is being increasingly favored by third-party payers. Most cost studies, however, do not factor in the hidden expenses of standby bypass surgery or the late expenses associated with treatment of restenosis, so that the magnitude of this cost savings may be somewhat less than expected.[44] Finally, both the success rate of PTCA and the resultant cost savings depend heavily on the experience and track record of the individual operator.

Standards for training in PTCA as a specialized part of fellowship are being developed[45] and include 150 procedures during training and 50 to 100 procedures per year to maintain the PTCA skills of individuals who have already entered practice. It is clear, however, that not all invasive cardiologists can or should perform PTCA, particularly complex procedures in which lack of ongoing experience is associated with less satisfactory results.[46] Moreover, because of the requirements for high-quality radiographic imaging and in-house cardiac surgical back-up to deal promptly with abrupt vessel reclosure, PTCA is likely to continue to be restricted to a fraction of the hospitals which currently perform diagnostic cardiac catheterization.

COMPLICATIONS

Like any cardiac catheterization procedure, PTCA is associated with risks relating to arrhythmia, arterial embolization, contrast agent toxicity, or vascular injury at the catheter entry site.[47,47a] One relatively unique complication, however, relates to the process by which angioplasty enlarges the stenotic coronary lumen. While angioplasty was initially thought to rely on compression of the atherosclerotic plaque[1,2,5] (Figs. 41–1 and 41–2), experimental studies disclose neither significant compression nor embolization of plaque elements.[48] Instead, the majority of improvement in vessel lumina appears to result from "cracking" and outward displacement of the plaque, associated with local plastic stretching of the media and adventitia (Fig. 41–8).[49,50] The use of a nonelastomeric balloon with an inflated diameter comparable to the diameter of the normal lumen adjacent to the stenotic segment is usually sufficient to achieve adequate dilatation. Use of a larger balloon increases the likelihood of excessive vessel trauma or

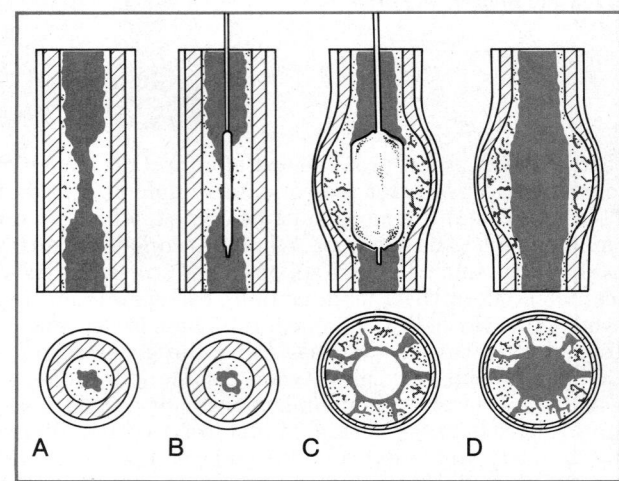

FIGURE 41–8. Current concept of the mechanism of balloon dilatation. Serial panels show the baseline stenosis (A), passage of the deflated balloon catheter (B), balloon inflation (C), and the postdilatation appearance (D), as drawn in longitudinal and transverse cross-sectional views. Balloon inflation (panel C) is associated with fracture and outward displacement of the atherosclerotic plaque, as well as plastic stretching of the media and adventitia. The result (panel D) is enlargement of the lumen owing to expansion of the entire vessel wall, rather than compaction of atherosclerotic material. (From Castaneda-Zuniga, W. R., et al.: The mechanism of balloon angioplasty. Radiology 135:565, 1980.)

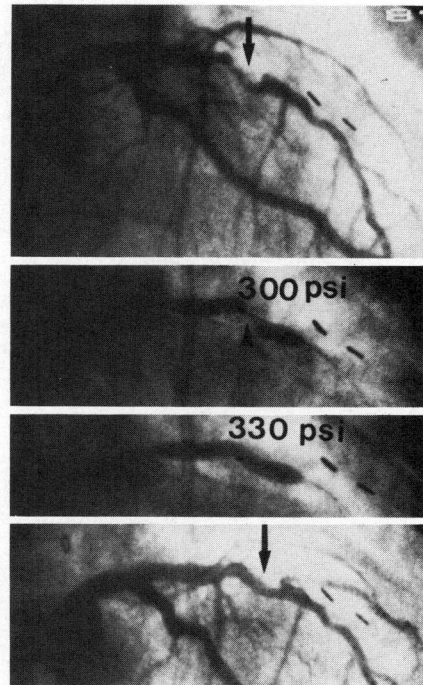

FIGURE 41–9. Angioplasty of a rigid lesion using a high-pressure balloon. This calcified stenosis in the midportion of the left anterior descending artery resisted dilatation at 300 psi (20 atm), but ultimately dilated at 330 psi with an acceptable result. Such rigid lesions are uncommon (<5 per cent) among angioplasty attempts. (From Baim, D. S.: Coronary angioplasty. In Grossman, W., and Baim D. S. [eds.]: Cardiac Catheterization, Angiography, and Intervention. 4th ed. Philadelphia, Lea and Febiger, 1991.)

vessel rupture precipitated by overdilatation.[51,52] Particularly rigid lesions may require inflation of the balloon to high pressure (10 to 20 atm, 150 to 300 psi) to achieve this result (Fig. 41–9), while eccentric lesions may require use of a slightly oversized balloon catheter, repeated inflations, or prolonged (1 minute) inflations to overcome the intrinsic elasticity of the normal arterial wall opposite the atherosclerotic plaque.[53] Although usually associated with transient left ventricular dysfunction,[54] these repeated transient coronary occlusions are usually well tolerated hemodynamically and do not cause serious arrhythmias. If limiting angina develops during balloon inflation in those patients who do not have good collateral flow to the dilated vessels, use of an autoperfusion balloon or distal Fluosol infusion through the inflated balloon[55] may help control temporary ischemia.

In the process of achieving adequate dilatation, neither too little nor too much "controlled injury" should be inflicted on the vessel wall. It is therefore important to monitor the adequacy of dilatation closely during the procedure, either by repeated angiographic examination of the dilated segment or by ongoing estimation of the residual translesional gradient,[56] i.e., the difference between mean aortic pressure and the mean coronary pressure distal to the dilated segment measured through the central lumen of the deflated balloon catheter (Fig. 41–6). Residual stenosis of less than 50 per cent and residual translesional gradients below 15 mm Hg are indicative of a successful procedure, although better results (30 per cent stenosis, or a 2-mm lumen in a 3-mm vessel) are commonly achieved.

Even when the dilatation has been successful, the vascular injury associated with PTCA is often evident in the radiographic appearance of intimal dissection at the dilatation site (Fig. 41–10). Patients with dissection may have some chest discomfort due to local vessel trauma, but limited dissection does not usually interfere with antegrade flow and goes on to heal by reendothelialization within 6 weeks of the dilatation procedure.

ABRUPT RECLOSURE. In approximately 4 per cent of

patients—particularly those undergoing dilatation of long (more than 2 cm), eccentric, or curved stenotic segments—local injury produces more extensive dissection.[57] This may (in conjunction with local vasospasm or thrombus formation) progress to abrupt vessel closure within 30 minutes of dilatation.[18,58] Half the vessels which manifest abrupt reclosure can be reopened by redilatation[59] (Fig. 41–11), but the other half (or approximately 2.5 per cent of the total PTCA attempts) currently require emergency surgery if vessel closure recurs and is associated with clinical and electrocardiographic evidence of myocardial ischemia.[60] Management of this complication necessitates prompt availability of an experienced cardiac surgical team and highlights the need for close cooperation between interventional cardiologists and their surgical colleagues. Although most patients requiring emergency surgery recover uneventfully,[61] up to half still sustain some degree of a myocardial infarction despite prompt revascularization, contributing heavily to the 0.4 per cent mortality associated with elective PTCA. Management of abrupt reclosure has been improved recently with the advent of special perfusion or "shunt" catheters[62] (Fig. 41–12), which can be placed across the occluded segment to permit perfusion of the distal bed while surgical control of the situation is being achieved. Better understanding of the dilatation process may allow more predictable responses and lower the incidence of significant dissection, while newer adjunctive techniques, e.g., the use of even more prolonged balloon inflations, thermal welding of the dissection plane, or placement of an intraluminal vascular stent (Fig. 41–12), may allow more consistent reversal of the reclosure phenomenon (see below). These advances may reduce further the incidence of emergency coronary bypass grafting and might even obviate the need for in-house surgical standby during PTCA procedures.

RESTENOSIS. Enhanced understanding of the biology of angioplasty will be required to prevent restenosis of the dilated segment. After successful PTCA there should be no clinical, electrocardiographic, or thallium perfusion evidence of myocardial ischemia,[63,64] but in approximately 20 per cent of patients, evidence of myocardial ischemia reappears within 6 months of the dilatation, coupled with angiographic evidence of restenosis of the dilated segment (Fig. 41–13). An additional 5 to 10 per cent of patients may remain free of recurrent symptoms but demonstrate partial angiographic renarrowing of the dilated segment. Some clinical parameters—severe baseline stenosis, incomplete dilatation, unstable angina with a brief duration of symptoms, male gender, stenosis of the left anterior descending coronary artery, ostial stenosis, uncontrolled vasospasm at the dilatation site,[65,66] a soft lesion which dilates without visible dissection, or early asymptomatic perfusion defects after PTCA[67]—are associated with a higher incidence of late restenosis.

Animal studies suggest that post-PTCA restenosis results from platelet adhesion to the area of endothelial damage at the

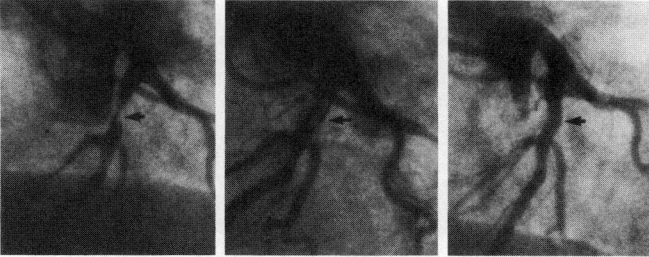

FIGURE 41–10. Intimal dissection during successful dilatation. Examination of the mid-left anterior descending artery (arrow) before *(left panel)* and immediately after (center panel) successful dilatation shows both enlargement of luminal caliber and the presence of two linear filling defects within the vessel lumen. This localized dissection did not impede antegrade flow and healed to leave an essentially normal vessel at 3-month restudy (right panel). (From Baim, D. S.: Percutaneous transluminal angioplasty. In Petersdorf, R. G., et al. [eds.]: Harrison's Principles of Internal Medicine, Update VI. New York, McGraw-Hill Book Co., 1985.)

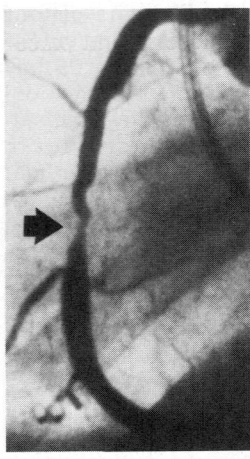
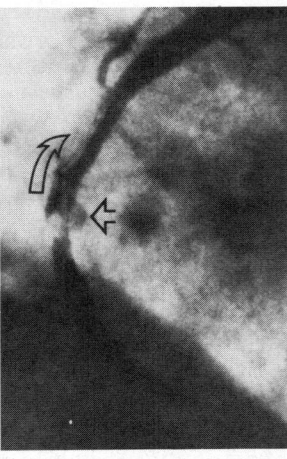
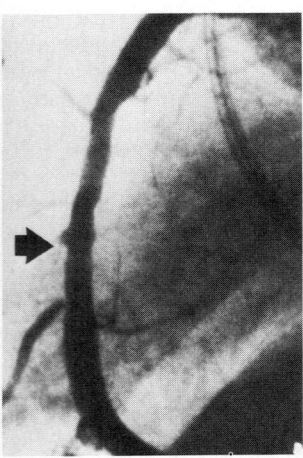

FIGURE 41–11. Dissection leading to abrupt closure. Baseline angiography (left panel) shows an eccentric lesion in the midportion of the right coronary artery. After dilatation with a 3.0-mm balloon (center panel) there is extensive dissection and imminent abrupt closure manifest as delayed propagation of distal contrast. Prolonged (10 minutes) inflation of a slightly larger 3.5-mm balloon catheter reestablished stable patency. (From Baim, D. S.: Coronary angioplasty. *In* Grossman, W., and Baim, D. S. [eds.]: Cardiac Catheterization, Angiography, and Intervention. 4th ed. Philadelphia, Lea and Febiger, 1991.)

FIGURE 41–12. Current alternatives for the management of abrupt reclosure. Abrupt reclosure owing to local dissection and accompanying thrombosis or spasm occurs in approximately 5 per cent of vessels treated with PTCA (left panel). Although such vessels were previously allowed to remain completely occluded during preparations for emergency bypass surgery (see color plate 9), four alternative management strategies have now been developed: *Redilatation* using multiple, prolonged inflations of the balloon catheter is successful in remolding the dissected vessel into a stable patent configuration in approximately one-half of the cases of abrupt reclosure. In the remaining cases a *shunt catheter* can be positioned within the occluded segment, over an exchange-length guidewire. Arterial blood can enter this catheter through side holes located proximal to the point of occlusion and exit through side

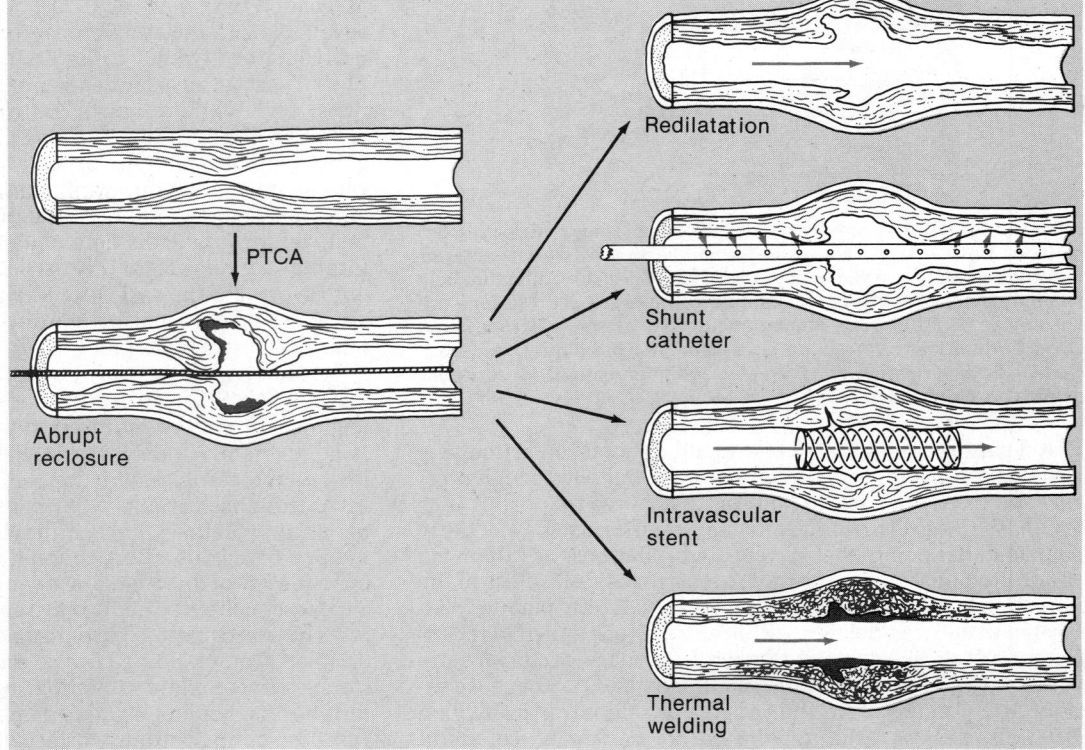

holes located distally, to maintain perfusion of the distal vessel as the patient is transported to the operating room. The catheter is then removed after the local delivery of cardioplegic solution and before placement of the aortic cross clamp. Two investigational approaches to abrupt reclosure include placement of an *intravascular stent* which can be delivered into the affected segment over a dilatation catheter and expanded to the caliber of the adjacent normal vessel by balloon inflation. This prevents the dissection flaps from acutely compromising lumen caliber and permits long-term patency and reendothialization in the presence of anticoagulant drugs. *Thermal welding* uses a laser-heated balloon catheter to coagulate and seal the local dissection and maintain vessel patency without placement of a prosthetic material.

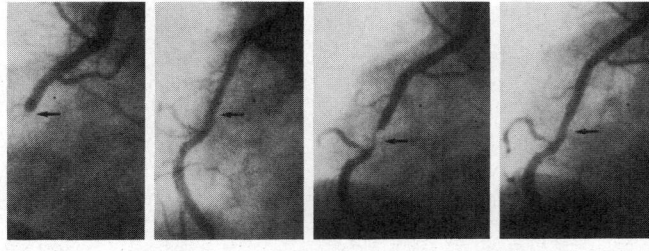

FIGURE 41–13. Restenosis of a dilated segment. The left panels show the appearance of a totally occluded mid-right coronary artery before and immediately after successful dilatation. Despite the absence of residual stenosis, this patient experienced recurrent symptoms 6 weeks after the procedure. Repeat catheterization (right panels) showed severe recurrence of the original lesion, which was successfully redilated. Restenosis developed again 6 weeks later (not shown), but this patient has now remained entirely asymptomatic for more than 4 years after a successful third dilatation. (From Baim, D. S.: Coronary angioplasty. In Grossman, W., and Baim, D. S. [eds.]: Cardiac Catheterization, Angiography, and Intervention. 4th ed. Philadelphia, Lea & Febiger, 1991.)

dilatation site, with subsequent release of potent smooth muscle vasoconstrictors and mitogens, such as platelet-derived growth factor (PDGF).[62] According to this hypothesis, restenosis represents a human correlate of the arterial injury technique used to create atherosclerotic plaques in experimental animals.[68a,68b] In support of this, postmortem and atherectomy[69] studies show that areas of restenosis tend to have a different, more proliferative histological appearance compared with the underlying primary plaque (color plate 9). This proliferative process (rather than simple recoil of the dilated vessel wall) is also favored by the angiographic finding of sta-

FIGURE 41–14. See color plate 9.

bility of the luminal diameter within the first month after PTCA, followed by subsequent progressive narrowing.[70,71]

On the other hand, adjunctive therapy with currently available antiplatelet agents (aspirin and dipyridamole) has failed to decrease the incidence of restenosis in PTCA patients, despite a favorable effect in some animal models. Clinical trials with other antiplatelet agents (prostacyclin analogs,[73] omega-3 fatty acids)[74] have similarly failed to show any consistent effect on restenosis. Other more potent antiplatelet agents[75-77] are currently being developed and may be at least partially effective if the platelet-triggered hypothesis is correct. A second avenue includes a search for pharmacological blockers of PDGF or techniques to leave behind a smoother and less platelet-attractive surface (thermal "smoothing" or mechanical plaque resection) in an effort to decrease the restenosis rate. Thus far, any favorable effects of new devices on restenosis appear to be the result of a larger initial lumen rather than reduction in intimal hyperplasia.[78] In the meantime, patients who have undergone successful PTCA should have their clinical symptoms and exercise test performance monitored closely over the 6 months following the procedure.

If clinical evidence of restenosis develops, repeat catheterization, including repeat PTCA, is the best management (Fig. 41–13). Repeat PTCA is almost always successful and is preferable to relying on intensified medical therapy alone, since the restenotic lesion may progress rapidly and produce escalating symptoms. Restenosis may develop in 30 to 40 per cent of patients after repeat PTCA, necessitating a third (or even a fourth) dilatation before long-term patency is secured.[79,80] If symptoms and signs of restenosis do not develop within 6 months of the dilatation procedure, they are unlikely to do so in future years, although anginal symptoms may develop because of progression of disease at other sites and require additional dilatation procedures.[64] Routine follow-up angiography is not clinically justified after PTCA, except in special situations (high-risk patients, commercial pilots). With the use of repeat PTCA for management of restenosis and progressive disease at other sites, fewer than 10 per cent of patients undergoing initially successful dilatation will require bypass surgery during the next several years.[8]

NEWER TECHNIQUES FOR TREATING VASCULAR STENOSIS

While essentially all experience in the treatment of coronary stenoses has involved the use of balloon dilatation, a number of other methods are under investigation.[81,81a] Given the advanced state and evident success of balloon dilatation, these methods must strive for the following goals: (1) to improve the crossing rate for difficult (e.g., totally occluded) lesions; (2) to dilate elastic, rigid, or diffusely diseased segments predictably; (3) to minimize or correct local injury responsible for abrupt vessel reclosure; and (4) to remove plaque and/or leave behind a smoother luminal surface in an effort to reduce the incidence of late restenosis.[82]

CORONARY STENTING. The concept of placing an intraluminal prosthesis to scaffold the treated vessel (stent) and maintain patency was advanced by Dotter more than 20 years ago[83] but has only recently become a therapeutic reality in the management of coronary artery disease.[83a] All current stents are made from polished metal wires or tubes and fall into two broad classes: (1) self-expanding stents (e.g., the Medinvent Wallstent), and (2) balloon-expandable stents (e.g., the Palmaz-Schatz or Gianturco-Roubin stent).[84,85] Regardless of design, use of all these devices presents difficulties in successful placement, prevention of thrombosis on the stent surface, and avoidance of excessive late intimal hyperplasia that can restrict the flow.[85a,85b]

Coronary stents remain investigational but have been implanted in more than 2,000 patients worldwide at the time of this writing. With suitable refinement of the delivery system, stent implantation can be accomplished in more than 97 per

cent of patients with relatively focal (<15 mm length) lesions. Because of the relative absence of elastic recoil, stent placement results in the creation of a large and smooth lumen whose diameter approximates or even slightly exceeds that of the adjacent reference segment, regardless of the underlying lesion morphology (eccentricity, ulceration, or friable plaque in an aged saphenous vein bypass graft)[86-89] (Fig. 41–15). Both mild intimal flaps and the more severe dissections responsible for post-PTCA abrupt vessel closure can be controlled by stent placement. Given the inherent thrombogenicity of current metallic stents, aggressive anticoagulation with heparin, aspirin, dipyridamole, and low molecular weight dextran (dextran 40) is generally required to prevent immediate thrombosis.[84] This is followed by continued heparin infusion until effective anticoagulation with oral warfarin is established, and given concurrently with aspirin and dipyridamole. Interruption of this regimen within the first 2 weeks after stent placement (i.e., to manage bleeding from the gastrointestinal system or the vascular puncture site) carries an incidence of subacute stent thrombosis as great as 15 per cent. On the other hand, removal of the vascular sheath on uninterrupted anticoagulation engenders a 5 to 10 per cent incidence of vascular complications requiring surgical correction under local anesthesia. Warfarin therapy may be discontinued in approximately 8 weeks, at which time the stent is fully endothelialized. Antibiotic prophylaxis for dental procedures is also imperative until the stent is fully endothelialized.

The fibrocellular layer that forms over the stent at the blood interface is typically 0.2 to 0.5 mm thick at 8 weeks, with some subsequent thinning as it matures further. By 6 months, this local intimal hyperplasia has caused the typical stented coronary lumen to lose 1 mm in luminal diameter, which is equivalent to a 30 per cent diameter stenosis in a 3-mm vessel. While the restenosis rate (defined as the fraction of patients with a stenosis > 60 per cent) may be as low as 15 to 20 per cent for stented vessels, it is important to emphasize that this appears to be because the larger stented lumen can tolerate more late loss due to intimal hyperplasia rather than because a stented vessel develops less local hyperplasia.[78]

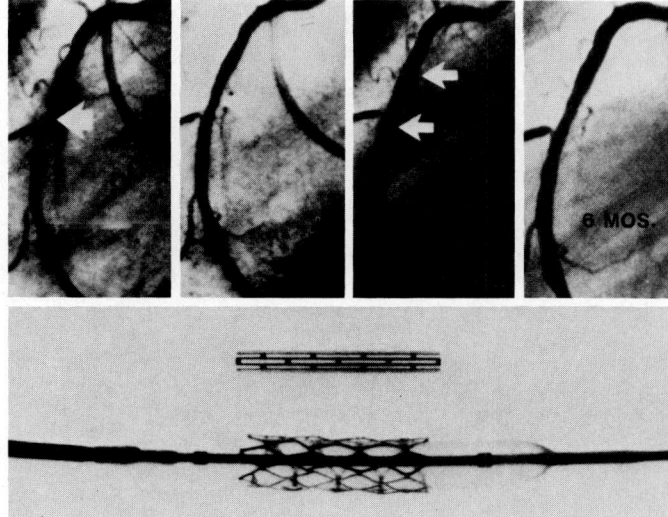

FIGURE 41–15. Placement of an intracoronary stent. This patient had an eccentric restenosis of the midportion of the right coronary artery *(left panel).* After predilation with a 3.0-mm balloon *(left center),* moderate (35 per cent) stenosis remained because of elastic recoil of the vessel wall. Placement of a single Palmaz-Schatz balloon-expandable stent *(right center)* allowed further enlargement of the vessel lumen. While there was some loss of luminal caliber due to intimal hyperplasia within the stent at 6-month routine follow-up angiography *(right panel),* the degree of stenosis was 32 per cent and the exercise test showed no evidence of ischemia. The stent itself is shown *(bottom panel)* in both its original and expanded configurations. (From Levine, M. J., et al.: Clinical and angiographic results of balloon-expandable intracoronary stents in right coronary artery stenoses. J. Am. Coll. Cardiol. *16:*332, 1990.)

ATHERECTOMY. While both conventional balloon angioplasty and coronary stenting work by outward displacement of plaque, several catheter designs have been developed to actually remove plaque mass. The first of these designs was the side-cutting directional atherectomy catheter designed by Simpson et al.[90,90a] It consists of a cylindrical metal chamber in which a 10 mm long window has been cut. On the outside of the chamber opposite the window, a small (1.8 mm) balloon is affixed. Low-pressure balloon inflation serves to press the window against the diseased vessel wall. Any plaque that prolapses into the cylinder is then cut free by a cup-shaped cutter and trapped in the tip of the catheter, allowing it to be removed from the body.

After trials of this concept in diseased peripheral arteries,[91] a coronary design entered clinical testing in 1988.[69] By mid 1990, more than 1,200 patients had been treated, with favorable rates of acute success (88 per cent) and emergency surgery (3 per cent). Perforation has been reported in 0.5 to 0.7 per cent of atherectomy-treated vessels, particularly when atherectomy is used in an effort to retrieve an extensive dissection that has developed following conventional PTCA. Treated vessels have a smoother surface and less residual stenosis than do vessels treated with conventional angioplasty,[92] and the technique appears to be particularly useful in larger (>3 mm diameter) noncalcified vessels with ostial, eccentric, or ulcerated lesions less than 20 mm in length (Fig. 41–16). Weighing shows a mean removed plaque sample weight of approximately 20 mg, suggesting that only part of the luminal improvement results from tissue removal per se.[69] The remainder of the improvement appears to result from "facilitated angioplasty" in which mechanical dilatation takes place within the bases of the initial atherectomy cuts. The restenosis rate for directional coronary atherectomy is currently 20 to 30 per cent, but has not yet been compared to that of conventional angioplasty in a randomized trial. The Simpson atherectomy system was approved by the Food and Drug Administration for general use in the coronary circulation in mid 1990.

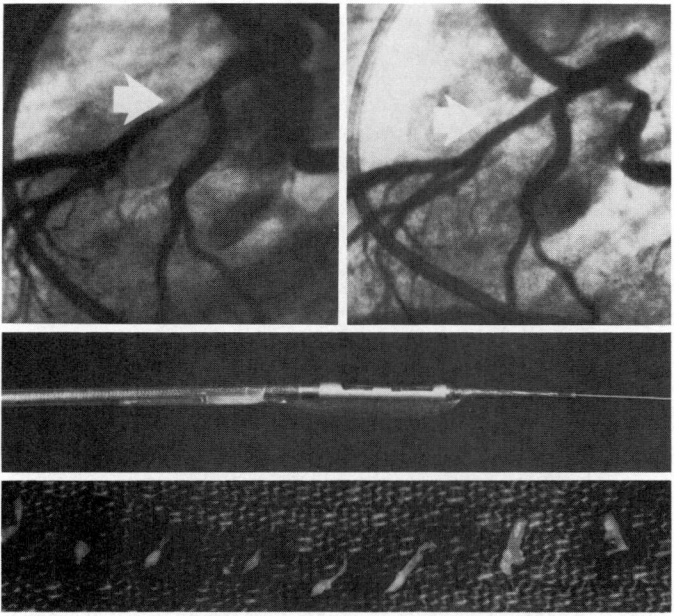

FIGURE 41–16. Directional coronary atherectomy. This patient had an eccentric restenosis lesion *(upper left)* **of the left anterior descending artery following conventional angioplasty. This lesion was treated by directional coronary atherectomy using a No. 6 French device** *(middle),* **with removal of the specimens shown** *(bottom),* **producing a smooth lumen without residual stenosis. There was slight stenosis evident at routine 6-month angiography** *(upper right)* **(presumably the result of local intimal hyperplasia), but no evidence of regional ischemia. (From Safian, R. D., et al.: Coronary atherectomy: Clinical, angiographic and histologic findings and observations regarding mechanism.** *Circulation* **82:69, 1990.)**

There has been less experience to date with two other atherectomy systems. The *end-cutting design* developed by Stack et al.[93] uses blades mounted on the tip of a rotating catheter to cut free fragments of plaque, which are then suctioned out of the body through the central lumen of the catheter. In the absence of mechanical advantage (i.e., a balloon catheter), this device typically cannot provide a larger lumen than the physical diameter of the cutter (2 mm), so that postatherectomy balloon angioplasty may be required to adequately treat larger vessels. The *Rotablator* developed by Auth et al. utilizes fine diamond chips mounted on the leading surface of a metal burr, which is rotated rapidly (100,000 rpm) as it is advanced down the diseased vessel over a guidewire.[94,95,95a] Plaque ground free from the lesion is pulverized into fragments averaging 25 μm in diameter. These fragments are generally well tolerated by the distal coronary circulation, although they may cause transient ischemia if generated in excessive size or number by aggressive cutting. Except in vessels of smaller diameter, subsequent PTCA is commonly required to achieve adequate lumen, and restenosis rates appear to be 30 to 40 per cent. Both devices seem to be particularly useful in smaller, diffusely diseased vessels.

LASER ANGIOPLASTY. Lasers emitting any of several wavelengths from the infrared to the ultraviolet bands can be used to deliver energy to the stenotic vessel by means of fiberoptic catheters. The fundamental goal of laser angioplasty is the direct ablation of plaque material.[96] This usually produces associated prothrombotic thermal charring and surrounding acoustic ("blast") injury of the adjacent vessel wall when the comparatively long wavelength lasers used in our medical applications (CO_2 = 10.6 μ, Nd:YAG = 1.06 μ, argon = 0.5 μ), are employed, but there is some evidence that the shorter wavelength excimer laser (less than 0.3 μ) achieves ablation of plaques with less surrounding thermal and acoustic injury.[96,97] Similar effects may be obtained by rapid-pulsing, high-energy lasers of longer wavelengths. Clinical trials with the excimer laser in the coronary circulation have utilized multifiber catheters that are advanced over a guidewire.[98,99] Because of the limited diameter of the catheter, these devices are most effective in smaller-diameter vessels or as pretreatment devices before conventional balloon dilatation. There is experimental evidence that the luminal surface present after excimer laser treatment is less thrombogenic than that seen after thermal injury as might be produced by a continuous-wave laser of longer wavelength.[100] Although the use of an over-the-wire system prevents use as a device to cross total occlusions, perforation appears to be much less frequent than was the case with earlier bare-fiber laser approaches. To date, a modified delivery system, plaque staining, or the use of fluorescence-guided ablation[101] has not overcome *that* limitation of laser ablation.

Another use of laser energy is as a thermal source to intentionally heat the diseased vessel segment. The so-called hot-tip design utilized a metal cap placed over the end of the laser fiber, which was heated to several hundred degrees during laser activation. Clinical trials, however, suggest that much of the ability of this device to cross chronic total occlusions in the peripheral circulation was the result of its mechanical properties rather than tip heating.[102] On the other hand, the "laser balloon" catheter developed by Spears et al.[103] uses a diffusing fiber wrapped around the central core of a balloon catheter to deliver Nd:YAG laser energy to the vessel wall during balloon inflation. It appears to be at least partially effective in overcoming vessel elasticity and providing a smooth luminal surface despite preexisting dissections or flaps (Fig. 41–17), but has thus far been associated with a restenosis rate of 35 to 50 per cent. If the restenosis limitation can be overcome, other thermal sources might be employed in a similar fashion.[104]

OTHER APPROACHES TO TOTAL OCCLUSIONS. Difficulty in crossing a chronically occluded segment constitutes one of the main remaining limitations of conventional angioplasty[24] and has thus been a driving force for device development. Modifications of mechanical force[105,106] appear to offer

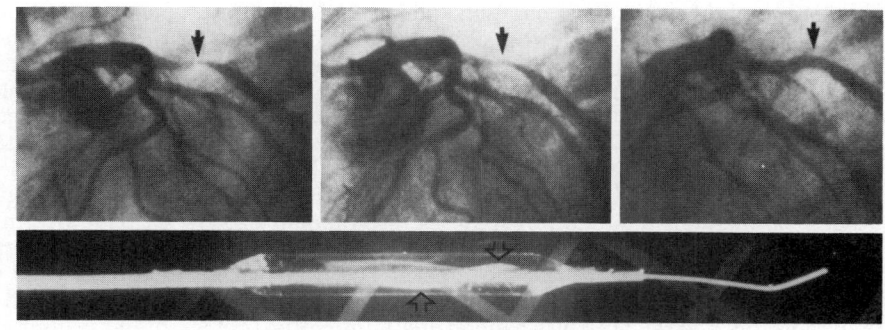

FIGURE 41–17. Laser balloon angioplasty. An eccentric lesion in the circumflex *(left)* responded elastically to conventional angioplasty using a 3.0-mm balloon *(center)*. Following treatment with an identical-size laser balloon with 20 sec of Nd:YAG delivery during balloon inflation, adequate to heat the vessel wall to 80 to 90°C, wide luminal patency was obtained *(right)*. The design of the Spears laser balloon is shown *(bottom)* with a diffusing fiber wrapped helically around the balloon central shaft.

some increase in crossing rate without a significant increase in vessel perforation. Because an ablative laser system usable in this situation is lacking, other alternatives utilizing ultrasonic energy are currently being explored.[107,108]

ANGIOPLASTY OF OTHER (NONCORONARY) ARTERIES

Most interventional techniques have been developed and tested in peripheral vessels (femoral or iliac arteries).[1,5,90,106,109] The number of peripheral angioplasty procedures, however, remains much smaller than the number of coronary angioplasties because of a lack of established referral pattern among the involved (medical, surgical, radiological) specialties, general lack of knowledge about interventional alternatives to vascular surgery, and lack of enthusiasm for angiography in patients with ischemic syndromes milder than rest pain.[110,111] In general, the results of peripheral angioplasty are similar to those described for PTCA. Primary success rates for peripheral arterial balloon dilatation exceed 95 per cent for the iliac and 87 per cent for the femoral arteries, with a 5-year restenosis rate which varies from 10 per cent for iliac vessels up to 40 per cent for smaller popliteal vessels.[112-114] Peripheral lesions, however, are more likely to be long (up to 10 cm) or totally occluded, in comparison to coronary arterial lesions. These technical challenges, coupled with better end-organ tolerance of ischemia and the absence of cardiac tamponade as a complication of vessel perforation or rupture, have fostered more aggressive trials of mechanical, thermal, or laser techniques in the peripheral circulation.

As in coronary angioplasty, peripheral angioplasty of technically suitable lesions may offer significant clinical and economic benefits over surgical repair, particularly since patients with peripheral vascular disease frequently have other cardiac or pulmonary disease that increases the risk of general anesthesia. Because peripheral angiography is viewed as a preparation for vascular surgery, however, only a small fraction of patients with mildly or moderately symptomatic peripheral vascular disease are currently offered the option of peripheral angioplasty.[110]

Dilatation of atherosclerotic or fibromuscular stenoses in the *renal arteries* followed peripheral angioplasty as an application of balloon angioplasty (Fig. 41–18).[6] Renal artery angioplasty continues to be applied with excellent short- and long-term success as an alternative to vascular surgery in patients with renovascular hypertension (p. 835) or renal insufficiency as the result of anatomically suitable stenoses in the main artery or its principal branch.[115,116] Overall, patients with hypertension due to fibromuscular renal arterial disease have an excellent chance of cure (70 per cent), improvement (20 per cent), and lower risk of restenosis (10 to 20 per cent), compared to patients with atherosclerotic renal arterial disease in whom the chances of cure (25 per cent), improvement (40 per cent), and restenosis (40 to 70 per cent) are less favorable. Still, the incidence of major complications from renal angioplasty is low, and these results compare quite favorably with those of renovascular surgery.

In their original paper,[1] Dotter and Judkins predicted that

interventional techniques would ultimately be applied to a variety of other vascular territories, including the *brachiocephalic and cerebral circulation*. Although the underlying disease processes (atherosclerosis and fibromuscular disease) are similar to those treated by balloon angioplasty in other vascular beds, carotid lesions are more likely to exhibit ulceration and adherent thrombus. At the same time, the brain is less tolerant of microembolic debris than any other end organ. Balloon angioplasty, however, continues to be used in inoper-

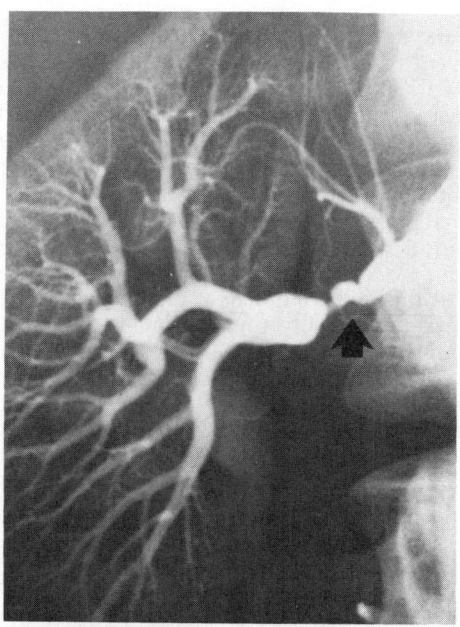

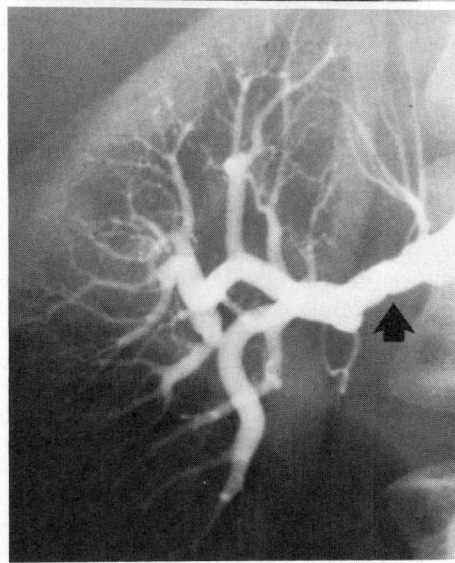

FIGURE 41–18. Renal artery angioplasty. *Top,* Severe stenosis of the right renal artery (arrow) due to fibromuscular disease in a patient with refractory hypertension. *Bottom,* Luminal caliber improved after successful dilatation. (Courtesy of Ducksoo Kim, M.D.)

able lesions of the posterior circulation and in small numbers of patients with stenosis of the extracranial carotid artery.[117,118] Still, use of these applications is likely to increase rapidly over the next decade, since surgical correction of cerebrovascular disease is performed in approximately 100,000 patients per year in the United States and continues to be associated with significant morbidity.

Balloon dilatation of other stenotic vessels has also been used. This includes dilatation of stenoses in pulmonary arteries or veins and vascular shunts.[119-121] A conventional catheter is generally used to cross the target stenosis and place an exchange-length guidewire. The conventional catheter is then removed, and replaced by a balloon dilatation catheter of appropriate diameter. Because of the elasticity of most congenital stenoses, balloon diameters of 10 to 12 mm (slightly larger than the adjacent normal segment) may be required to produce significant dilatation. Balloon dilatation has also

been used to maintain patency of the *ductus arteriosus* in children with cyanotic congenital heart disease and to treat *coarctation of the aorta*. The site of coarctation is crossed with a guidewire, which permits advancement of a diagnostic catheter for performance of baseline angiography and calculation of the aortic diameter adjacent to the area of narrowing. A balloon catheter with a diameter 1 or 2 mm less than that of the normal segment is then advanced over the guidewire, positioned within the stenotic segment, and inflated with dilute contrast material. Successful procedures are marked by at least a 30 per cent increase in the diameter of the treated segment and at least a 50 per cent reduction in the associated pressure gradient. Because primary dilatation of coarctation is associated with a significant incidence of late aneurysm formation,[122] it may be appropriate to reserve balloon dilatation for recurrent stenoses which develop after primary surgical repair (p. 921).[123,124]

Treatment of Valvular Stenosis

PULMONARY BALLOON VALVULOPLASTY

Pulmonary valvular stenosis (p. 931), a relatively common congenital cardiac lesion, was traditionally corrected by surgical "valvuloplasty," i.e., incision of fused commissures under direct vision. Beginning in 1982 pediatric cardiologists began using balloon dilatation catheters with inflated diameters 1 to 2 mm larger than the annulus size (20 to 25 mm) to produce similar commissural splitting by way of a closed transluminal approach.[126] This procedure has been quite successful, with a reduction of the pulmonic valve gradient to approximately one-third of its baseline value. Given the high success rate and low incidence of complication, balloon valvuloplasty has essentially replaced open surgical repair for valvular pulmonic stenosis (p. 933). Application of balloon valvuloplasty for the treatment of *congenital* aortic stenosis has also been reported (p. 1043), with a 70 per cent reduction in valve gradient and no significant increase in aortic regurgitation.[127]

MITRAL BALLOON VALVULOPLASTY

In contrast to *congenital* pulmonic or aortic stenosis, it was believed that adult *acquired* rheumatic and/or calcific stenosis of the mitral or aortic valves would *not* be amenable to balloon valvuloplasty because of (1) the more rigid structure of such lesions, (2) the potential for systemic embolization of valve debris, and (3) the potential for creating severe regurgitation. In 1985, however, balloon valvuloplasty was first applied to young adult patients with acquired (rheumatic) mitral stenosis, using a transseptal approach,[128] and the technique has become widely adapted as an alternative to surgical repair or replacement of stenotic mitral valves.[126]

TECHNIQUE. After puncture of the intraatrial septum with a needle and long sheath (Fig. 7–5, p. 184), a small balloon flotation catheter is advanced from the left atrium to the left ventricle. While it was once common to then advance this catheter across the aortic valve into the descending aorta (Fig. 41–19), a position near the apex of the left ventricle is easier to obtain and adequate for most mitral valvuloplasty procedures. An exchange-length (260 cm) guidewire is then positioned through this catheter to allow removal of the balloon flotation catheter and advancement of a small (8 mm) dilatation catheter for enlargement of the opening made in the intraatrial septum. This step is required to facilitate passage of the larger (23- to 25-mm diameter) valvuloplasty balloon through the intraatrial septum and across the stenotic mitral valve. Inflation of this larger balloon results in separation of the fused commissures analogous to the earlier surgical technique of

closed or open mitral commissurotomy. Subsequent variations of the technique have included the use of two smaller (12 to 18 mm) balloon catheters, which can be advanced individually across the atrial septum and then inflated simultaneously within the mitral orifice[126] or use of a single compliant dumbbell-shaped balloon.[129]

After these encouraging results in young adults with rheumatic mitral stenosis, similar procedures were attempted in adult patients with more rigid calcific lesions (p. 1017). Using this technique, it has been possible to achieve physiologically

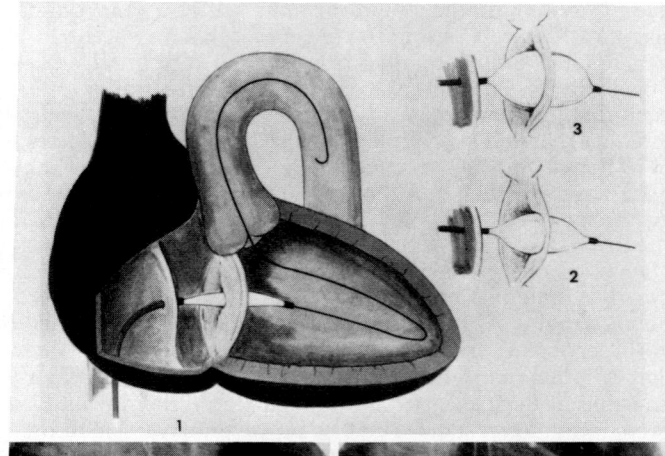

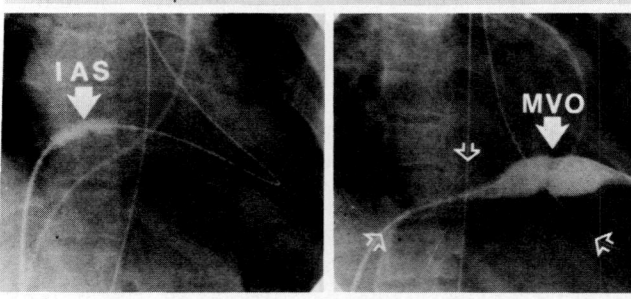

FIGURE 41–19. Mitral balloon valvuloplasty. The *top panel* shows the transseptal approach to mitral valvuloplasty, while the *bottom panel* shows radiographic frames obtained during an actual procedure. After dilatation of the intraatrial septum (IAS) by an 8-mm balloon catheter, a 25-mm dilatation catheter is advanced into the mitral valve orifice (MVO) and inflated. Note the appearance of a "waist" corresponding to the impression of the stenotic mitral orifice on the partially inflated dilatation catheter. This waist resolved with full inflation of the balloon, associated with an increase in mitral valve area from 0.9 to 1.6 cm². The path of the guidewire from right atrium to left atrium, to left ventricle, to descending aorta is shown by the open arrows.

adequate enlargement of the mitral orifice area (from 0.9 to 2.0 cm²). Overall procedural mortality is 1 to 2 per cent, with cardiac perforation by the transseptal needle, guidewire, or dilatation catheter in approximately 1 per cent of patients. A significant increase in the degree of mitral regurgitation is uncommon, as are systemic emboli in patients preselected by transesophageal echocardiography for absence of left atrial thrombus and pretreated with oral warfarin for 2 to 3 months before attenuated valvuloplasty. Approximately 20 per cent of patients show evidence of a small (<2:1) left-to-right shunt at the atrial level, owing to dilatation of the atrial septal puncture during passage of the valvuloplasty balloon. Approximately half of these shunts resolve spontaneously by the time of follow-up catheterization.[130] This minor complication should become even less common as improved technology permits the production of valvuloplasty balloons with smaller collapsed profiles. Similarly, balloon catheters capable of more rapid inflation and deflation will be of value in minimizing the period of systemic arterial hypotension which invariably results from transient occlusion of left ventricular inflow during balloon inflation.

RESULTS. Early (6- to 12-month) follow-up studies have demonstrated preservation of the improved mitral orifice and similar physiological improvements (fall in filling pressures and pulmonary vascular resistance) to those seen after surgical correction of mitral stenosis.[128,131] Both the early and late (1 year) hemodynamic result can be predicted by an "echocardiographic score" in which four unfavorable features (poor leaflet mobility, valvular thickening, subvalvular thickening, and valvular calcification) are each assigned a value of 1 to 4. Patients with a cumulative score below 8 have a greater than 90 per cent chance of a good initial result (valve area > 1.5 cm²) and a low chance (4 per cent) of significant restenosis at 1 year. In contrast, patients with a cumulative score of 8 to 16 have only a 50 per cent chance of a good initial result and a 70 per cent chance of restenosis at 1 year.[126] This pattern may relate to a greater contribution of separation of commissural fusion in patients with pliable leaflets versus a more limited benefit obtained by leaflet cracking and transient stretching of the mitral valve annulus in patients with more rigid valvular and subvalvular structures.

AORTIC BALLOON VALVULOPLASTY
(See also p. 1043)

With evident success of balloon valvuloplasty in the treatment of acquired mitral stenosis and of congenital aortic stenosis in children (p. 925), attention has now been turned to dilatation of calcific aortic stenosis in the adult. This disorder is the principal indication for most of the approximately 20,000 aortic valve replacements performed each year in the United States. Narrowing of the valve orifice is due to a combination of an underlying congenital structural abnormality (e.g., a bicuspid aortic valve), commissural fusion, and stiffening of the leaflets by extensive calcium deposition. Postmortem and intraoperative balloon dilatations have demonstrated separation of fused commissures, increased leaflet pliability due to microfractures and macrofractures through the calcium deposits, and transient stretching of the aortic annulus.[133] These findings suggested that percutaneous aortic valvuloplasty might be possible in advanced aortic stenosis. By 1990 this procedure had been performed in more than 1,000 patients, using principally the retrograde approach (Fig. 41–20).[126]

TECHNIQUE. A conventional catheter is advanced retrogradely across the stenotic valve and into the left ventricle. Through this catheter an exchange-length guidewire is then positioned in the left ventricular apex and used to advance a series of balloon dilatation catheters (12, 15, 18, 20, and, occasionally, 23 mm in diameter) across the stenotic valve. Each balloon is inflated several times using dilute liquid radiographic contrast material. Maintenance of the balloon within

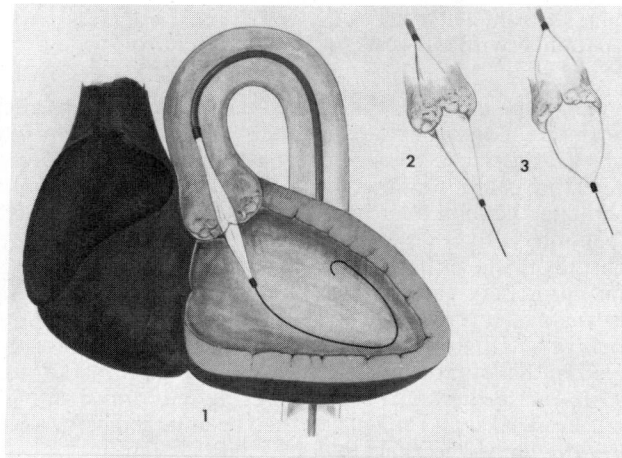

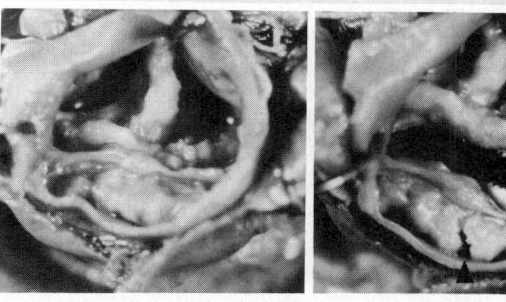

FIGURE 41–20. Aortic balloon valvuloplasty. The *top panel* shows the retrograde approach to aortic valvuloplasty, while the *bottom panels* show the gross appearance of a stenotic aortic valve before (*left*) and after (*right*) postmortem balloon valvuloplasty. Note the fracture through the large calcified nodule (arrow) and the overall improvement in leaflet compliance.

the aortic orifice during inflation is difficult because of a tendency for the balloon to be ejected by the force of left ventricular contraction but is facilitated by the use of catheters with longer (i.e., 6-cm rather than 3-cm) balloon segments. In patients with peripheral vascular disease, aortic balloon valvuloplasty can be performed using an antegrade (transseptal) approach, similar to that used for mitral valvuloplasty.

RESULTS. The magnitude of orifice improvement during aortic valvuloplasty (from 0.6 to 0.9 cm², peak gradient from 60 to 30 mm Hg) appears to be less than that seen with mitral valvuloplasty, but is usually adequate to produce marked improvement in clinical status, filling pressures, and left ventricular performance in patients with severe resting symptoms caused by critical aortic stenosis.[133a,134] Procedural mortality is 5 per cent[134a]; other problems include systemic emboli (1.5 per cent), worsened aortic regurgitation (1 per cent), and vascular injury at the access site (5 to 10 per cent). Balloon inflation seems to cause less hemodynamic compromise than is seen during mitral dilatation because some left ventricular ejection can occur between the inflated balloon and the aortic commissures.

While aortic balloon valvuloplasty is likely to play an increasing role in the treatment of patients whose poor left ventricular function, advanced age, or other medical problems place them at high risk for surgical aortic valve replacement,[135,136,136a] improvement in the orifice area is less than that usually obtained with a valve replacement, and an unacceptably high fraction of patients show evidence of poor long-term (24-month) results[136b] by death (30 to 40 per cent), repeat valvuloplasty (20 per cent), or valve replacement (15 to 20 per cent). Since the predominant effect is by leaflet cracking and annulus stretching, changes in technique (e.g., the use of larger-diameter balloons) have increased the incidence of complications without providing better immediate or long-term results. Valve replacement is thus still preferred in patients with severe aortic stenosis who are candidates for surgery.

OTHER INTERVENTIONAL CATHETERIZATION TECHNIQUES

Some of the earliest applications of interventional cardiology were in patients with congenital heart disease.[121] In 1966 Rashkind described passage of a balloon catheter through a preexisting patent foramen ovale, followed by withdrawal of the inflated balloon to create a functional atrial septal defect in patients with transposition of the great arteries (p. 941), tricuspid atresia, pulmonic atresia, mitral atresia, total anomalous pulmonary venous return, or a single ventricle.[137] Sixteen years later Park and coworkers modified this technique by use of a catheter with a surgical blade, which can be deployed in the left atrium after transseptal puncture and then used to incise the atrial septum during withdrawal.[138] The resulting atrial septal defect can then be enlarged using a balloon catheter as described by Rashkind.

In addition to the creation or enlargement of vascular channels, pediatric cardiologists have also developed devices for closing aberrant vascular channels. Rashkind developed a "double-disc" prosthesis which can be passed across an unwanted atrial septal defect, ventricular septal defect, or patent ductus arteriosus[139–141] (Fig. 41–21). The first disc is deployed on the far side of the defect and then held in place by three spring struts, as the remaining disc and struts are pulled back across the defect and deployed on its near side. The result is sealing of the defect between two layers of prosthetic material.

Methods have also been developed for preoperative closure of unwanted systemic-pulmonary collateral vessels in patients undergoing correction of tetralogy of Fallot, using preformed steel coils or detachable balloons embolized into the unwanted vessel through a catheter delivery system[121,142,143] (Fig. 41–22). These approaches—similar to those used by vascular radiologists to treat arteriovenous malformations or actively bleeding vessels in other beds—lead to occlusion of the target vessel by local thrombosis.

SUMMARY

After the first tentative exploration of mechanical dilatation in the peripheral arterial circulation, the past 15 years have seen the explosive growth of interventional techniques for the treatment of a number of common cardiovascular diseases. Of these techniques, balloon dilatation is the most highly developed. It provides a safe and effective alternative to bypass surgery in up to one-half of patients requiring revascularization of coronary, renal, or peripheral arterial lesions. Extension of this technique to valvular stenosis is of clear value in selected patients and has already made some inroads into current surgical practice. Newer interventional techniques, such as the use of stents, mechanical atherectomy, and thermal or ablative laser devices, have demonstrated early feasibility and will almost certainly enhance one or more existing applications or create entirely new applications for interventional cardiology.

At a time of rising health care costs and an aging population, these interventional techniques frequently offer the chance of equivalent symptomatic improvement with less discomfort, disability, and expense than conventional surgery. As with all new techniques, however, careful validation of their utility in comparison with existing medical and surgical techniques will be necessary to insure their optimal use in patient care.

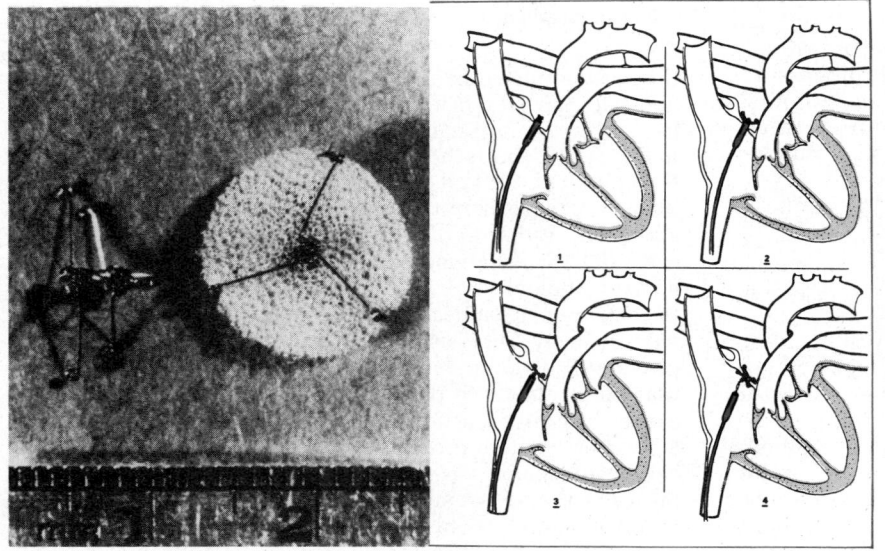

FIGURE 41–21. Closure of an atrial septal defect with the Rashkind double-disc occluder. The Rashkind occluder consists of cloth discs mounted on two pairs of back-to-back spring arms *(left).* The entire device is collapsed for loading into a delivery catheter, which is in turn positioned across the defect. Following extrusion and expansion of the distal arms, the delivery catheter is partially withdrawn so that the proximal arms can be deployed on the near side of the septum.

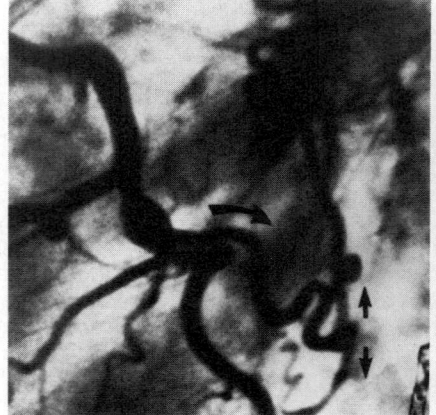 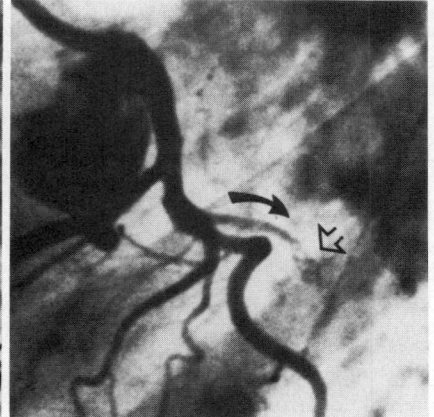

FIGURE 41–22. Coil embolization of a coronary-artery-to-pulmonary-artery fistula. This patient had ischemic chest pain presumed to be due to a persistent fistula from a left atrial branch of the circumflex to the left lower pulmonary artery *(curved arrow, left),* many years following surgical correction of tetralogy. Following placement of a single Gianturco occlusion coil *(open arrow, right)* and selective injection of thrombin, flow through the fistula ceased within 10 minutes.

REFERENCES

TREATMENT OF VASCULAR STENOSIS

1. Dotter, C. T., and Judkins, M. P.: Transluminal treatment of arteriosclerotic objection: Description of a new technique and a preliminary report of its application. Circulation 30:654, 1964.
2. Dotter, C. T., Rosch, J., and Judkins, M. P.: Transluminal dilatation of atherosclerotic stenosis. Surg. Gynecol. Obstet. 127:794, 1968.
3. Dotter, C. T.: Transluminal angioplasty: A long view. Radiology 135:561, 1980.
4. Zeitler, E., Schoop, W., and Zahnow, W.: The treatment of occlusive arterial disease by transluminal catheter angioplasty. Radiology 99:19, 1971.
5. Gruentzig, A., and Kumpe, D. A.: Technique of percutaneous transluminal angioplasty with the Gruentzig balloon catheter. Am. J. Radiol. 132:547, 1979.
6. Gruentzig, A., Kuhlmann, U., Vetter, W., et al.: Treatment of renovascular hypertension with percutaneous transluminal dilatation of a renal-artery stenosis. Lancet 1:801, 1978.

PERCUTANEOUS TRANSLUMINAL CORONARY ANGIOPLASTY

7. Gruentzig, A. R., Senning, A., and Siegenthaler, W. E.: Non-operative dilatation of coronary artery stenosis—percutaneous transluminal coronary angioplasty. N. Engl. J. Med. 301:61, 1979.
8. Kent, K. M., Mullin, S. M., and Passamani, E. R. (eds.): Proceedings of the National Heart, Lung, and Blood Institute workshop on the outcome of percutaneous transluminal angioplasty (June 7–8, 1983). Am. J. Cardiol. 53:1C, 1984.
9. Baim, D. S.: Coronary angioplasty. In Grossman, W., and Baim, D. S. (eds.): Cardiac Catheterization, Angiography, and Intervention, 4th ed. Philadelphia, Lea & Febiger, 1991.
10. Avedissian, M. G., Killeavy, E. S., Garcia, J. M., and Dear, W. E.: Percutaneous transluminal coronary angioplasty: A review of current balloon dilatation systems. Cathet. Cardiovasc. Diagn. 18:263, 1989.
10a. Stammen, F., Piessens, J., Vrolix, M., et al.: Immediate and short-term results of a 1988–1989 coronary angioplasty registry. Am. J. Cardiol. 67:253, 1991.
11. Simpson, J. B., Baim, D. S., Robert, E. W., and Harrison, D. C.: A new catheter system for coronary angioplasty. Am. J. Cardiol. 49:1216, 1982.
12. Detre, K., Holubkov, R., Kelsey, S., et al.: Percutaneous transluminal coronary angioplasty in 1985–1986 and 1977–1981: The NHLBI Registry. N. Engl. J. Med. 318:265, 1988.
13. Holmes, D. R., Holubkov, R., Vlietstra, R. E., et al.: Comparison of complications during percutaneous transluminal coronary angioplasty from 1977 to 1981 and from 1985 to 1986: The NHLBI PTCA Registry. J. Am. Coll. Cardiol. 12:1149, 1988.
14. Detre, K., Holubkov, R., Kelsey, S., et al.: One year follow-up results of the 1985–1986 National Heart, Lung, and Blood Institute's Percutaneous Transluminal Coronary Angioplasty Registry. Circulation 80:421, 1989.
15. Popma, J. J., and Dehmer, G. J.: Care of the patient after coronary angioplasty. Ann. Intern. Med. 110:547, 1989.
16. Ryan, T. J., Faxon, D. P., Gunnar, R. M., et al.: Guidelines for percutaneous transluminal coronary angioplasty—A report of the ACC/AHA Task Force on assessment of diagnostic and therapeutic cardiovascular procedures. J. Am. Coll. Cardiol. 12:529, 1988.
17. Bourassa, M. G., Alderman, E. L., Bertrand, M., et al.: Report of the joint ISFC/WHO task force on coronary angioplasty. Circulation 78:780, 1988.
18. Ellis, S. G., Roubin, G. S., King S. B., et al.: Angiographic and clinical predictors of acute closure after native vessel coronary angioplasty. Circulation 77:372, 1988.
19. Ellis, S. G., Vandormael, M. G., Cowley, M. J., et al.: Coronary morphologic and clinical determinants of procedural outcome with angioplasty for multivessel coronary artery disease. Circulation 82:1193, 1990.
20. Meier, B., Gruentzig, A. R., King, S. B., et al.: Risk of side branch occlusion during coronary angioplasty. Am. J. Cardiol. 53:10, 1984.
21. Meier, B.: Kissing balloon coronary angioplasty. Am. J. Cardiol. 54:918, 1984.
22. Weinstein, J. S., Baim, D. S., Sipperly, M. E., et al.: Salvage of branch vessels during bifurcation lesion angioplasty—acute and long-term follow-up. Cathet. Cardiovasc. Diagn. 22:1, 1991.
23. Dervan, J. P., Baim, D. S., Cherniles, J., and Grossman, W.: Transluminal angioplasty of occluded coronary arteries: Use of a movable guide wire system. Circulation 68:776, 1983.
24. Stone, G. W., Rutherford, B. D., McConahay, D. R., et al.: Procedural outcome of angioplasty for total coronary occlusion: An analysis of 971 lesions in 905 patients. J. Am. Coll. Cardiol. 15:849, 1990.
25. Wohlgelernter, D., Cleman, M., Highman, H. A., and Zaret, B. L.: Percutaneous transluminal coronary angioplasty of the "culprit lesion" for the management of unstable angina pectoris in patients with multivessel coronary artery disease. Am J. Cardiol. 58:460, 1986.
26. Ischinger, T., Gruentzig, A. R., Hollman, J., King, S., et al.: Should coronary arteries with less than 60% diameter stenosis be treated by angioplasty? Circulation 68:148, 1983.
27. de Feyter, P. J.: Coronary angioplasty for unstable angina. Am. Heart J. 118:860, 1989.
28. Leeman, D., McCabe, C. H., Faxon, D. P., et al.: Use of percutaneous transluminal coronary angioplasty and bypass surgery despite improved medical therapy for unstable angina pectoris. Am. J. Cardiol. 61:38G, 1988.
29. Feldman, R. L., Macdonald, R. G., Hill, J. A., et al.: Coronary angioplasty at the time of initial cardiac catheterization. Cathet. Cardiovasc. Diagn. 12:219, 1986.
30. Laskey, M. A., Deutsch, E., Barnathan, E., and Laskey, W. K.: Influence of heparin therapy on percutaneous transluminal coronary angioplasty outcome in unstable angina pectoris. Am. J. Cardiol. 651:425, 1990.
31. Rogers, W. J., Baim, D. S., Gore, J. M., et al.: Comparison of immediate invasive, delayed invasive and conservative strategies following tissue plasminogen activator—results of the Thrombolysis in Myocardial Infarction (TIMI) Phase IIA trial. Circulation 81:1457, 1990.
32. The TIMI Study Group: Comparison of invasive and conservative strategies after treatment with intravenous tissue plasminogen activator: Results of the thrombolysis in myocardial infarction (TIMI) phase II trial. N. Engl. J. Med. 320:618, 1989.
33. O'Keefe, J. H., Rutherford, B. D., McConahay, D. R., et al.: Early results and long-term outcome of direct coronary angioplasty for acute myocardial infarction in 500 consecutive patients. Am. J. Cardiol. 64:1221, 1989.
34. Pinkerton, C. A., Slack, J. D., Orr, C. M., et al.: Percutaneous transluminal angioplasty in patients with prior myocardial revascularization surgery. Am. J. Cardiol. 61:15G, 1988.
35. Cote, G., Myler, R. K., Stertzer, S. H., et al.: Percutaneous transluminal angioplasty of stenotic coronary artery bypass grafts: 5 years' experience. J. Am. Coll. Cardiol. 9:8, 1987.
35a. Plokker, H.W.T., Meester, B. H., and Serruys, P. W.: The Dutch experience in percutaneous transluminal angioplasty of narrowed saphenous veins used for aortocoronary arterial bypass. (In press.)
36. Shimshak, T. M., Giorgi, L. V., Johnson, W. L., et al.: Application of percutaneous transluminal angioplasty to the internal mammary artery graft. J. Am. Coll. Cardiol. 12:1205, 1988.
37. de Feyter, P. J., Serruys, P., van den Brand, M., et al.: Percutaneous transluminal angioplasty of totally occluded venous bypass graft: A challenge that should be resisted. Am. J. Cardiol. 64:88, 1989.
38. Holt, G. W., Sugrue, D. D., Bresnahan, J. F., et al.: Results of percutaneous transluminal coronary angioplasty for unstable angina in patients 70 years of age and older. Am. J. Cardiol. 61:994, 1988.
39. O'Keefe, J. H., Hartzler, G. O., Rutherford, B. D., et al.: Left main coronary angioplasty—early and late results of 127 acute and elective procedures. Am. J. Cardiol. 54:144, 1989.
40. Kahn, J. E., Rutherford, B. D., McConahay, D. R., et al.: Supported "high-risk" coronary angioplasty using intraaortic balloon counterpulsation. J. Am. Coll. Cardiol. 15:1151, 1990.
41. Vogel, R. A., Shawl, F., Tommaso, C., et al.: Initial report of the National Registry of Elective Cardiopulmonary Bypass Supported Coronary Angioplasty. J. Am. Coll. Cardiol. 15:23, 1990.
42. Baim, D. S., and Ignatius, E. J.: Use of percutaneous transluminal coronary angioplasty: Results of a current survey. Am. J. Cardiol. 61:3G, 1988.
43. Weintraub, W. S., Jones, E. L., King, S. B., et al.: Changing use of coronary angioplasty and coronary bypass surgery in the treatment of chronic coronary artery disease. Am. J. Cardiol. 65:183, 1990.
44. Black, A. J. R., Roubin, G. S., Sutor, C., et al.: Comparative costs of percutaneous transluminal coronary angioplasty in multivessel coronary artery disease. Am. J. Cardiol. 62:809, 1988.
45. Ryan, T. J., Klocke, F. J., Reynolds, W. A., et al.: Clinical competence in percutaneous transluminal coronary angioplasty—a statement for physicians from the ACP/ACC/AHA Task Force on Clinical Privileges in Cardiology. Circulation 81:2041, 1990.
46. Hamad, N., Pichard, A. D., Lyle, H. R. P., Lindsay, J.: Results of percutaneous transluminal coronary angioplasty by multiple, relatively low frequency operators: 1986–1987 experience. Am. J. Cardiol. 61:1229, 1988.
47. Wyman, R. M., Safian, R. D., Portway, V., et al.: Current complications of diagnostic and therapeutic cardiac catheterization. J. Am. Coll. Cardiol. 12:1400, 1988.
47a. Plante, S., Laarman, G., de Feyter, P. J., et al.: Acute complications of percutaneous transluminal coronary angioplasty for total occlusion. Am. Heart J. 121:417, 1991.
48. Sanborn, T. A., Faxon, D. P., Waugh, D., et al.: Transluminal angioplasty in experimental atherosclerosis: Analysis for embolization using an in vivo perfusion system. Circulation 66:917, 1982.
49. Sanborn, T. A., Faxon, D. P., Haudenschild, C., et al.: The mechanism of transluminal angioplasty: Evidence for formation of aneurysms in experimental atherosclerosis. Circulation 68:1136, 1983.
50. Castaneda-Zuniga, W. R., Formanek, A., Tadavarthy, M., et al.: The mechanism of balloon angioplasty. Radiology 135:565, 1980.
51. Roubin, G. S., Douglas, J. S., King, S. B., et al.: Influence of balloon size on initial success, acute complications, and restenosis after percutaneous transluminal coronary angioplasty. A prospective randomized study. Circulation 78:557, 1988.
52. Saffitz, J. E., Rose, T. E., Oaks, J. B., and Roberts, W. C.: Coronary artery rupture during coronary angioplasty. Am. J. Cardiol. 51:902, 1983.
53. Kaltenbach, M., Beyer, J., Walter, S., et al.: Prolonged application of pressure in transluminal angioplasty. Cathet. Cardiovasc. Diagn. 10:213, 1984.
54. Wijns, W., Serruys, P. W., Slager, C. J., et al.: Effect of coronary occlusion during percutaneous transluminal angioplasty in humans on left ventricular chamber stiffness and regional diastolic pressure-radius relations. J. Am. Coll. Cardiol. 7:455, 1986.

55. Kent, K. M., Cleman, M. W., Cowley, M. J., et al.: Reduction of myocardial ischemia during percutaneous transluminal coronary angioplasty with oxygenated Fluosol. Am. J. Cardiol. 66:279, 1990.

56. Anderson, H. V., Roubin, G. S., Leimgruber, P. P., et al.: Measurement of transstenotic pressure gradient during percutaneous transluminal coronary angioplasty. Circulation 73:1223, 1986.

57. Black, A. J. R., Namay, D. L., Niederman, A. L., et al.: Tear or dissection after coronary angioplasty—morphologic correlates of an ischemic complication. Circulation 79:1035, 1989.

58. Fischell, T. A., Derby, G., Tse, T. M., and Stadius, M. L.: Coronary artery vasoconstriction after percutaneous transluminal coronary angioplasty: A quantitative arteriographic analysis. Circulation 78:1323, 1988.

59. Sinclair, I. N., McCabe, C. H., Sipperly, M. E., and Baim, D. S.: Predictors, therapeutic options and long-term outcome of abrupt reclosure. Am. J. Cardiol. 61:61G, 1988.

60. Detre, K. M., Holmes, D. R., Holubkov, R., et al.: Incidence and consequences of periprocedural occlusion: The 1985–86 National Heart, Lung, and Blood Institute's Percutaneous Transluminal Coronary Angioplasty Registry. Circulation 82:739, 1990.

61. Talley, J. D., Weintraub, W. S., Roubin, G. S., et al.: Failed elective percutaneous transluminal coronary angioplasty requiring coronary artery bypass surgery: In-hospital and late clinical outcome at 5 years. Circulation 82:1203, 1990.

62. Sundrum, P., Harvey, J. R., Johnson, R. G., et al.: Benefit of the perfusion catheter for emergency coronary artery grafting after failed percutaneous transluminal coronary angioplasty. Am. J. Cardiol. 63:282, 1989.

63. Wilson, R. F., Johnson, M. R., Marcus, M. L., et al.: The effect of coronary angioplasty on coronary flow reserve. Circulation 77:873, 1988.

64. Gruentzig, A. R., King, S. B., III, Schlumpf, M., and Siegenthaler, W.: Long-term follow-up after percutaneous transluminal coronary angioplasty. N. Engl. J. Med. 316:1127, 1987.

65. Bertrand, M. E., LaBlanche, J. M., Thieuleux, F. A., et al.: Comparative results of percutaneous transluminal coronary angioplasty in patients with dynamic versus fixed coronary stenosis. J. Am. Coll. Cardiol. 8:504, 1986.

66. Ellis, S. G., Roubin, G. S., King, S. B., et al.: Importance of stenosis morphology in the estimation of restenosis risk after elective percutaneous transluminal coronary angioplasty. Am. J. Cardiol. 63:30, 1989.

67. Hardoff, R., Shefer, A., Gips, S., et al.: Predicting late restenosis after coronary angioplasty by very early (12–14 h) thallium-201 scintigraphy: Implications with regard to mechanisms of late coronary restenosis. J. Am. Coll. Cardiol. 15:1486, 1990.

68. Liu, M. W., Roubin, G. S., and King, S. B.: Restenosis after coronary angioplasty: Potential biologic determinants and the role of intimal hyperplasia. Circulation 79:1374, 1989.

68a. Veda, M., Becker, A. E., Tsukada, T., et al.: Fibrocellular tissue response after percutaneous transluminal coronary angioplasty. An immuno-cyto-chemical analysis of the cellular composition. Circulation 83:1327, 1991.

68b. Forrester, J. S., Fishbein, M., Helfant, R., and Fagin, J.: A paradigm for restenosis based on cell biology: clues for the development of new preventive therapies. J. Am. Coll. Cardiol. 17:758, 1991.

69. Safian, R. D., Gelbfish, J. S., Erny, R. E., et al.: Coronary atherectomy: Clinical, angiographic and histologic findings and observations regarding mechanism. Circulation 82:69, 1990.

70. Nobuyoshi, M., Kimura, T., Nosaka, H., et al.: Restenosis after successful percutaneous transluminal coronary angioplasty: Serial angiographic follow-up of 220 patients. J. Am. Coll. Cardiol. 12:616, 1988.

71. Beatt, K. J., Serruys, P. W., and Hugenholtz, P. G.: Restenosis after coronary angioplasty: New standards for clinical studies. J. Am. Coll. Cardiol. 15:491, 1990.

72. Schwartz, L., Bourassa, M. G., Lesperance, J., et al.: Aspirin and dipyridamole in the prevention of restenosis after percutaneous transluminal coronary angioplasty. N. Engl. J. Med. 318:1714, 1988.

73. Knudtson, M. L., Flintoft, V. F., Roth, D. L., et al.: Effect of short-term prostacyclin administration on restenosis after percutaneous transluminal coronary angioplasty. J. Am. Coll. Cardiol. 15:691, 1990.

74. Reis, G. J., Boucher, T. M., Sipperley, M. E., et al.: Randomised trial of fish oil for prevention of restenosis after coronary angioplasty. Lancet 2:1777, 1989.

75. Coller, B. S., Folts, J. D., Smith S. R., et al.: Abolition of in vivo platelet thrombus formation in primates with monoclonal antibodies to the platelet GPIIb/IIIa receptor: Correlation with bleeding time, platelet aggregation, and blockage of GPIIb/IIIa receptors. Circulation 80:1766, 1989.

76. Jang, I. K., Gold, H. K., Ziskind, A. A., et al.: Prevention of platelet-rich arterial thrombosis by selective thrombin inhibition (argatroban). Circulation 81:219, 1990.

77. Heras, M., Chesboro, J. H., Webster, M. W. I., et al.: Hirudin, heparin and placebo during deep arterial injury in the pig. Circulation 82:1476, 1990.

78. Kuntz, R. E., Schmidt, D. A., Levine, M. J., et al.: Importance of post-procedure luminal diameter on restenosis following new coronary intervention. Circulation 82: III-314, 1990.

79. Black, A. J. R., Anderson, H. V., Roubin, G. S., et al.: Repeat coronary angioplasty: Correlates of a second restenosis. J. Am. Coll. Cardiol. 11:714, 1988.

80. Teirstein, P. S., Hoover, C. A., Ligon, R. W., et al.: Repeat coronary angioplasty: Efficacy of a third angioplasty for a second restenosis. J. Am. Coll. Cardiol. 13:291, 1989.

81. Waller, B. F.: "Crackers, breakers, stretchers, drillers, scrapers, shavers, burners, welders and melters"—the future treatment of atherosclerotic coronary artery disease. A clinical-morphologic assessment. J. Am. Coll. Cardiol. 13:969, 1989.

81a. Topol, E. J.: Promises and pitfalls of new devices for coronary artery disease. Circulation 83:689, 1991.

82. Baim, D. S., Detre, K., and Kent, K.: Problems in the development of new devices for coronary intervention—Possible role for a multicenter registry. J. Am. Coll. Cardiol. 14:1389, 1989.

83. Dotter, C. T.: Transluminally placed coil-spring endarterial tube grafts: Long-term patency in canine popliteal artery. Invest Radiol. 4:329, 1969.

83a. Goy, J-J., Sigwart, U., Vogt, P., et al.: Long-term follow-up of the first 56 patients treated with intracoronary self-expanding stents (the Lausanne Experience) Am. J. Cardiol. 67:569, 1991.

84. Schatz, R. A.: A view of vascular stents. Circulation 79:445, 1989.

85. Ellis, S. G., and Topol, E. J.: Intracoronary stents: Will they fulfill their promise as an adjunct to angioplasty? J. Am. Coll. Cardiol. 13:1425, 1989.

85a. Schatz, R. A., Baim, D. S., Leon, M., et al: Clinical experience with the Palmaz-Schatz coronary stent—initial results of a multicenter study. Circulation 83: 148, 1991.

85b. Serruys, P. W., Strauss, B. H., Beatt, K. J., et al.: Angiographic follow-up after placement of a self-expanding coronary-artery stent. N. Engl. J. Med. 324: 13, 1991.

86. Levine, M. J., Leonard, B. M., Nash, I. D., et al.: Clinical and angiographic results of balloon-expandable intra-coronary stents in right coronary artery stenoses. J. Am. Coll. Cardiol. 16:332, 1990.

87. Roubin, G. S., King, S. B., Douglas, J. S., et al.: Intracoronary stenting during percutaneous transluminal coronary angioplasty. Circulation 81:IV92, 1990.

88. Sigwart, U., Puel, J., Mirkovitch, V., et al.: Intravascular stents to prevent occlusion and restenosis after transluminal angioplasty. N. Engl. J. Med. 316:701, 1987.

89. Urban, P., Sigwart, U., Gold, S., et al.: Intravascular stenting for stenosis of aortocoronary venous bypass grafts. J. Am. Coll. Cardiol. 13:1085, 1989.

90. Hinohara, T., Selmon, M. R., Robertson, G. C., et al.: Directional atherectomy—new approaches for treatment of obstructive coronary and peripheral vascular disease. Circulation 81:IV79, 1990.

90a. Hinohara, T., Rowe, M., Robertson, G. C., et al.: Effect of lesion characteristics on outcome of directional coronary atherectomy. J. Am. Coll. Cardiol. 17:1112, 1991.

91. von Polnitz, A., Nerlich, A., Berger, H., and Hofling, B.: Percutaneous peripheral atherectomy: Angiographic and clinical follow-up of 60 patients. J. Am. Coll. Cardiol. 15:682, 1990.

92. Rowe, M. H., Hinohara, T., White, N. W., et al.: Comparison of dissection rates and angiographic results following directional coronary atherectomy and coronary angioplasty. Am. J. Cardiol. 66:49, 1990.

93. Stack, R. S., Quigley, P. J., Sketch, M. J., et al.: Extraction atherectomy. In Topol, E. J. (ed.): Textbook of Interventional Cardiology. Philadelphia, W. B. Saunders Company, 1990.

94. Zacca, N. M., Raizner, A. E., Noon, G. P., et al.: Treatment of symptomatic peripheral atherosclerotic disease with a rotational atherectomy device. Am. J. Cardiol. 63:77, 1989.

95. Fourrier, J. L., Bertrand, M. E., Auth, D. C., et al.: Percutaneous coronary rotational atherectomy in humans. Preliminary report. J. Am. Coll. Cardiol. 14:1278, 1989.

95a. Buchbinder, M., Warth, D., O'Neill, W., et al.: Multicenter registry of percutaneous coronary rotational ablation using the rotablator. J. Am. Coll. Cardiol. 17:31A(abstr), 1991.

96. Litvak, F., Grundfest, W. S., Segalowitz, J., et al.: Interventional cardiovascular therapy by laser and thermal angioplasty. Circulation 81:IV109, 1990.

97. Isner, J. M., Donaldson, R. F., Deckelbaum, L. J., et al.: The excimer laser: Gross, light microscopic and ultrastructural analysis of potential advantages for use in laser therapy of cardiovascular disease. J. Am. Coll. Cardiol. 6:1102, 1985.

98. Karsch, K. R., Haase, K. K., Voelker, W., et al.: Percutaneous excimer coronary angioplasty in patients with stable and unstable angina pectoris. Circulation 81:1849, 1990.

99. Litvak, F., Grundfest, W. S., and Goldenberg, T.: Percutaneous excimer laser coronary angioplasty of aortocoronary saphenous vein grafts. J. Am. Coll. Cardiol. 14:803, 1989.

100. Sanborn, T. A., Alexopoulos, D., Marmur, J. D., et al.: Coronary excimer laser angioplasty: Reduced complications and indium-111 platelet accumulation compared with thermal laser angioplasty. J. Am. Coll. Cardiol. 16:502, 1990.

101. Leon, M. B., Almagor, Y., Bartorelli, A. L., et al.: Fluorescence-guided laser-assisted balloon angioplasty in patients with femoropopliteal occlusions. Circulation 81:143, 1990.

102. Tobis, J., Smolin, M., Mallery, J., et al.: Laser-assisted thermal angioplasty in human peripheral artery occlusions: Mechanism of recanalization. J. Am. Coll. Cardiol. 13:1547, 1989.

103. Spears, J. R., Reyes, V. P., Wynne, J., et al.: Percutaneous coronary laser balloon angioplasty: Initial results of a multicenter experience. J. Am. Coll. Cardiol. 16:293, 1990.

104. Lee, B. J., Becker, G. J., Waller, B. F., et al.: Thermal compression and molding of atherosclerotic vascular tissue with use of radiofrequency

energy: Implications for radiofrequency balloon angioplasty. J. Am. Coll. Cardiol. 13:1167, 1989.

105. Meier, B.: Chronic total occlusion angioplasty. Cathet. Cardiovasc. Diagn. 17:212, 1989.

106. Vallbracht, C., Lierman, D., Prignitz, I., et al.: Results of low speed rotational angioplasty for chronic peripheral occlusions. Am. J. Cardiol. 62:935, 1988.

107. Rosenschein, U., Bernstein, J. J., DiSegni, E., et al.: Experimental ultrasonic angioplasty: Disruption of atherosclerotic plaques and thrombi in vitro and arterial recanalization in vivo. J. Am. Coll. Cardiol. 15:711, 1990.

108. Siegel, R. J., Fishbein, M. C., Forester, J., et al.: In vivo ultrasound arterial recanalization of atherosclerotic total occlusions. J. Am. Coll. Cardiol. 15:345, 1990.

109. Palmaz, J. C., Garcia, O. J., Schatz, R. A., et al.: Placement of balloon-expandable intraluminal stents in iliac arteries: First 171 procedures. Radiology 174:969, 1990.

110. Doubilet, P., and Abrams, H. L.: The cost of underutilization—percutaneous transluminal angioplasty for peripheral vascular disease. N. Engl. J. Med. 310:95, 1984.

111. Zairns, C. K.: The vascular wars of 1988: The enemy is met. JAMA 261:416, 1989.

112. Gallins, A., Mahler, F., Probst, P., and Nachbur, B.: Percutaneous transluminal angioplasty of the lower limbs: A 5-year follow-up. Circulation 70:619, 1984.

113. Hewes, R. C., White, R. I., Murray, R. R., et al.: Long-term results of superficial femoral artery angioplasty. A. J. R. 146:1025, 1986.

114. Rooke, T. W., Stanson, A. W., Johnson, C. M., et al.: Percutaneous transluminal angioplasty in the lower extremities: A 5-year experience. Mayo Clin. Proc. 62:85, 1987.

115. Sos, T. A., Pickering, T. G., Saddekni, S., et al.: The current role of renal angioplasty in the treatment of renovascular hypertension. Urol. Clin. North Am. 11:503, 1984.

116. Martin, L. G., Price, R. B., Casarella, W. J., et al.: Percutaneous angioplasty in clinical management of renovascular hypertension: Initial and long-term results. Radiology 155:629, 1985.

117. Motarjeme, A., Keifer, J. W., and Zuska, A. J.: Percutaneous transluminal angioplasty of the vertebral arteries. Radiology 139:715, 1981.

118. Tsai, F. Y., Matovich, V., Hieshima, G., et al.: Percutaneous transluminal angioplasty of the carotid artery. Am. J. Neurol. Radiol. 7:349, 1986.

119. Rothman, A., Perry, S. B., Keane, J. F., and Lock, J. E.: Early results and follow-up of balloon angioplasty for branch pulmonary artery stenoses. J. Am. Coll. Cardiol. 15:1109, 1990.

120. Marx, G. R., Allen, H. D., Ovitt, T. W., and Hanson, W.: Balloon dilation angioplasty of Blalock-Taussig shunts. Am. J. Cardiol. 62:824, 1988.

121. Mullins, C. E.: Pediatric and congenital therapeutic cardiac catheterization. Circulation 79:1153, 1989.

122. Tynan, M., Finley, J.P., Fontes, V., et al.: Balloon angioplasty for the treatment of native coarctation: Results of the valvuloplasty and angioplasty for congenital anomalies registry. Am. J. Cardiol. 65:790, 1990.

123. Cooper, S. G., Sullivan, I. D., and Wren, C.: Treatment of recoarctation: Balloon dilation angioplasty. J. Am. Coll. Cardiol. 14:413, 1989.

124. Rao, P. S.: Which aortic coarctations should we dilate? Am. Heart J. 117:987, 1989.

TREATMENT OF VALVULAR STENOSIS

125. Stanger, P., Cassidy, S. C., Girod, D. A., et al.: Balloon pulmonary valvuloplasty: Results of the valvuloplasty and angioplasty of congenital anomalies registry. Am. J. Cardiol. 65:775, 1990.

126. Block, P. C., and Palacios, I. F.: Aortic and mitral balloon valvuloplasty: The United States experience. In Topol, E. J. (ed.): Textbook of Interventional Cardiology. Philadelphia, W. B. Saunders Company, 1990.

127. Rochini, A. P., Beekman, R. H., Shachar, G. B., et al.: Balloon aortic valvuloplasty: Results of the valvuloplasty and angioplasty congenital anomalies registry. Am. J. Cardiol. 65:784, 1990.

128. Lock, J. E., Khalilullah, M., Shrivastava, S., et al.: Percutaneous catheter commissurotomy in rheumatic mitral stenosis. N. Engl. J. Med. 313:1515, 1985.

128a. Kirklin, J. W.: Percutaneous balloon versus surgical closed commissurotomy for mitral stenosis. (In press.)

128b. Tuzcu, E. M., Block, P. C., and Palacios, I. F.: Comparison of early versus late experience with percutaneous mitral balloon valvuloplasty. J. Am. Coll. Cardiol. 17:1121, 1991.

129. Nobuyoshi, M., Hamasaki, N., Kimura, T., et al.: Indications, complications, and short-term clinical outcome of percutaneous transvenous mitral commissurotomy. Circulation 80:782, 1989.

130. Casale, P., Block, P. C., O'Shea, J. P., and Palacios, I. F.: Atrial septal defect after percutaneous mitral balloon valvuloplasty: Immediate results and follow-up. J. Am. Coll. Cardiol. 15:1300, 1990.

131. Hermann, H. C., Kleaveland, J. P., Hill, J. A., et al.: The M-Heart Percutaneous Balloon Mitral Valvuloplasty Registry: Initial results and early follow-up. J. Am. Coll. Cardiol. 15:1221, 1990.

132. Palacios, I. F., Block, P. C., Wilkins, G. T., and Weyman, A. E.: Follow-up of patients undergoing percutaneous mitral balloon valvotomy: Analysis of factors determining restenosis. Circulation 79:573, 1989.

133. Letac, B., Gerber, L. I., and Koning, R.: Insights on the mechanism of balloon valvuloplasty in aortic stenosis. Am. J. Cardiol. 62:1241, 1988.

133a. McKay, R. G.: The Mansfield Scientific Aortic Valvuloplasty Registry. Overview of acute hemodynamic results and procedural complications. J. Am. Coll. Cardiol. 17:485, 1991.

134. Safian, R. D., Berman, A. D., Diver, D. J., et al.: Balloon aortic valvuloplasty in 170 consecutive patients. N. Engl. J. Med. 319:125, 1988.

134a. Homes, D. R., Jr., Nishimura, R. A., and Reeder, G. S.: In-hospital mortality after balloon aortic valvuloplasty: Frequency and associated factors. J. Am. Coll. Cardiol. 17:189, 1991.

135. Berland, J., Squavin, T., Lefebvre, E., et al.: Percutaneous balloon valvuloplasty in patients with severe aortic stenosis and low ejection fraction. Circulation 79:1189, 1989.

136. Levine, M. J., Berman, A. D., Safian, R. D., et al.: Palliation of valvular aortic stenosis by balloon valvuloplasty as preparation for noncardiac surgery. Am. J. Cardiol. 62:1309, 1988.

136a. Nishimura, R. A., Holmes, D. R., Jr., Michela, M. A., et al.: Follow-up of patients with low output, low gradient hemodynamics after percutaneous balloon aortic valvuloplasty: The Mansfield Scientific Aortic Valvuloplasty Registry. J. Am. Coll. Cardiol. 17:828, 1991.

136b. Bashore, T. M., Davidson, C. J., and the Mansfield Scientific Aortic Valvuloplasty Registry Investigators: Follow-up recatheterization after balloon aortic valvuloplasty. J. Am. Coll. Cardiol. 17:1188, 1991.

137. Rashkind, W. J.: Transcatheter treatment of congenital heart disease. Circulation 67:711, 1983.

138. Park, S. C., Neches, W. H., Mullins, C. E., et al.: Blade atrial septostomy: Collaborative study. Circulation 66:258, 1982.

139. Lock, J. E., Cockerham, J. T., Keane, J. F., et al.: Transcatheter umbrella closure of congenital heart defects. Circulation 75:593, 1987.

140. Lock, J. E., Block, P. C., McKay, R. G., et al.: Transcatheter closure of ventricular septal defects. Circulation 78:361, 1988.

141. Dyck, J. D., Benson, L. N., Smallhorn, J. F., et al.: Catheter occlusion of the persistently patent ductus arteriosus. Am. J. Cardiol. 62:1089, 1988.

142. Gewillig, M., van der Hauwaert, L., and Daenen, W.: Transcatheter occlusion of high-flow Blalock-Taussig shunts with a detachable balloon. Am. J. Cardiol. 65:1518, 1990.

143. Miranda, A. A., Hill, J. A., Mickle, J. P., and Quisling, R. G.: Balloon occlusion of an internal mammary artery to anterior interventricular vein fistula. Am. J. Cardiol. 65:257, 1990.

Rehabilitation of Patients With Coronary Artery Disease

by CHARLES DENNIS, M.D.

Cardiac rehabilitation has traditionally focused on physical reconditioning and risk factor modification for patients recovering from myocardial infarction and coronary artery bypass surgery. Advances in the treatment of coronary artery disease and new data supporting the efficacy of secondary prevention measures have broadened the indications for cardiac rehabilitation services and increased the number of patients who may benefit from these services. Currently only 10 per cent of patients who might benefit from cardiac rehabilitation participate in formal programs.[1] A wider application of these services could potentially reduce the morbidity and mortality of coronary heart disease.

Cardiac rehabilitation has short- and long-term goals. The short-term goals include physical reconditioning sufficient for resumption of customary activities, education of patients and family about the disease process, and psychological support during the early recovery phase of the illness. The long-term goals include identifying and treating risk factors that influence the progression of disease, teaching and reinforcing the health behaviors that improve prognosis, optimizing physical conditioning, and facilitating a return to occupational and avocational activities. Cardiac rehabilitation must be both comprehensive and individualized. The most important factors to be considered in development of a program of rehabilitation are disease severity, medical and surgical therapy, risk factors, physical condition, vocational status, and emotional state.

EXERCISE IN CARDIAC REHABILITATION

PHYSICAL RECONDITIONING

FACTORS INFLUENCING PHYSICAL CAPACITY. Peak exercise capacity is defined as the maximum ability of the cardiovascular system to deliver oxygen to exercising skeletal muscle and of the exercising muscle to extract oxygen from the blood. The most accurate measure of exercise capacity is the maximal oxygen uptake (VO_{2max}), representing the liters of oxygen transported from the lungs per minute and used by skeletal muscle at peak effort. Because measurement of VO_{2max} is cumbersome, multiples of resting oxygen consumption (METS) are used clinically. One MET equals 3.5 ml oxygen uptake per kilogram body weight per minute and represents the approximate metabolic cost to stand quietly.

Exercise tests are calibrated to approximate MET requirements at each stage. The MET capacity on treadmill testing usually overestimates the VO_{2max} for cardiac patients.[2]

The degree of physical incapacity following a cardiac event is related to several factors: physical capacity prior to the event; treatments such as bed rest and medications; intravascular volume depletion; left ventricular dysfunction; residual myocardial ischemia; age; other noncardiac medical problems; and symptoms experienced by the patient during physical activity. Distinguishing the influence of each factor can be difficult, but recognizing their potential effects on physical capacity is paramount to minimizing iatrogenic effects and developing a conditioning program.

IATROGENIC AND PHYSIOLOGICAL FACTORS. While early mobilization is more common than in the past, bed rest remains the initial standard of care for most cardiac patients. Bed rest causes decrements in VO_{2max} of 9 to 30 per cent for several reasons.[3-5] Bed rest causes intravascular volume depletion. Absence of orthostatic stress of upright posture decreases venous capacitance vessel tone and blunts the normal postural vasomotor reflexes. These changes lead to diminished venous return, postural hypotension, and tachycardia.[6] Skeletal muscle mass decreases 10 to 15 per cent with a week of bed rest.[7] Pulmonary abnormalities resulting from bed rest include diminished lung volume and vital capacity and an increased respiratory exchange ratio.[8] Anaerobic metabolism occurs at lower levels of work in individuals placed at bed rest for a week or more. Vigorous exercise training in the supine position during bed rest fails to prevent the deterioration in upright exercise capacity. However, as little as 3 hours of daily upright posture significantly diminishes the deconditioning effects of bed rest.[4,5]

Chronotropic incompetence, the inability to achieve the age-predicted heart rate response to exercise, is common in patients with coronary artery disease.[9] The etiology is not clearly defined but appears to be related to loss of normal vagal reflexes during exercise.[10] Peak heart rate can decrease as much as 25 per cent in the first few weeks after myocardial infarction. Because the heart rate response to exercise is quantitatively the most important mechanism for increasing cardiac output, chronotropic incompetence significantly lowers VO_{2max}. Chronotropic incompetence improves spontaneously over the first 3 to 8 weeks following myocardial infarction, leading to increases in VO_{2max} even in the absence of formal exercise training.[11]

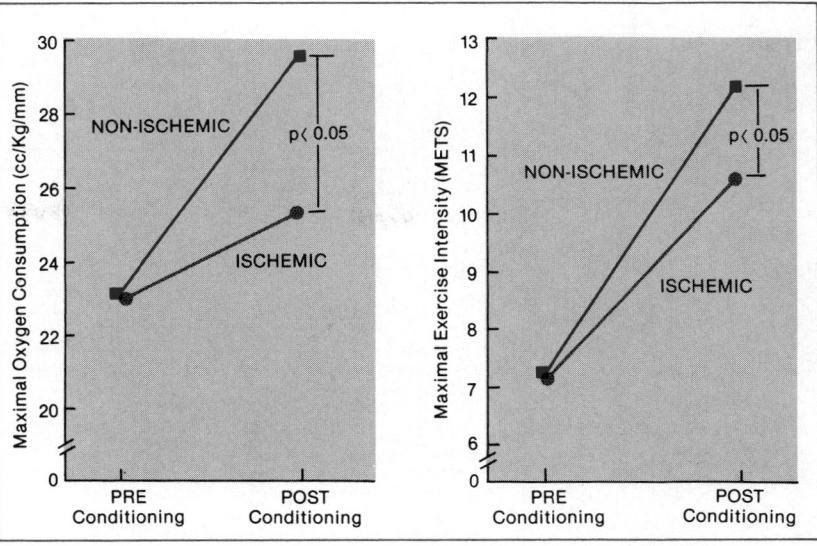

FIGURE 42-1. Maximal oxygen consumption and maximal exercise capacity (in METS) before and after conditioning in patients with and without baseline (before conditioning) exercise-induced ischemia. (From Ades, P. D., Grunvald, M. H., Weiss, R. M., and Hanson, J. S.: Usefulness of myocardial ischemia as predictor of training effect in cardiac rehabilitation after acute myocardial infarction or coronary artery bypass grafting. Am. J. Cardiol. 63:1032, 1989.)

LEFT VENTRICULAR DYSFUNCTION. Left ventricular dysfunction would be expected to impair physical capacity. However, most measures of ventricular performance at rest and during exercise, including left ventricular end-diastolic dimension, velocity of circumferential fiber shortening, systolic time intervals, and ejection fraction,[12] correlate poorly with exercise performance. In patients with left ventricular dysfunction, the two factors most predictive of low exercise capacity are chronotropic incompetence and early onset of anaerobic metabolism during exercise.[13] Central and peripheral mechanisms may preserve exercise capacity even when left ventricular dysfunction is severe. These include a preserved chronotropic response to exercise, increasing stroke volume, ventricular dilation, decreasing peripheral vascular resistance, increased levels of circulating catecholamines, and the ability to tolerate markedly elevated pulmonary artery wedge pressures.[14] Some of these mechanisms may be stimulated by exercise training, whereas others remain unchanged. Because the common clinical measures of resting left ventricular function do not predict exercise capacity, exercise testing is necessary to assess the functional limitation.

MYOCARDIAL ISCHEMIA. If large areas of myocardium become ischemic with exercise, patients may be limited by angina, dyspnea, and/or fatigue. Dyspnea and fatigue in the absence of angina may reflect left ventricular dysfunction at rest or exercise-induced ischemic left ventricular dysfunction, leading to elevated pulmonary vascular pressures and/or inadequate cardiac output.[15] Angina may also limit exercise performance in the absence of exercise-induced left ventricular dysfunction. Because the severity of anginal discomfort and the perception of the discomfort vary among patients, the same severity of myocardial ischemia may limit some patients and be tolerated by others. Amelioration of symptomatic and asymptomatic ischemia by medication may improve exercise capacity even in the absence of formal exercise training[16] (Fig. 42-1).

OTHER FACTORS. Concomitant illnesses, such as chronic obstructive pulmonary disease and peripheral vascular disease, can limit the exercise capacity before the effects of ischemia or left ventricular dysfunction are manifested. The common cardiovascular drugs, including nitrates, beta blockers, and calcium antagonists, increase the exercise capacity by increasing coronary blood flow, decreasing myocardial oxygen demand, or improving hemodynamics during exercise.[17,18]

EFFECTS OF EXERCISE TRAINING

SKELETAL MUSCLE. The primary physiological effects of exercise training are on skeletal muscle performance. Improved skeletal muscle performance is directly related to increases in capillary density, oxidative enzyme content, and increased numbers of mitochondria. These changes increase skeletal muscle perfusion and the efficiency of oxygen extraction.[19]

MYOCARDIAL PERFORMANCE. There is no convincing evidence that low- or moderate-intensity exercise training substantially improves myocardial performance. However, exercise training does cause modest improvements in thallium perfusion.[20,21] Diminished exercise-induced ST-segment abnormalities,[22] increased ejection fraction and stroke volume, and increased ischemic threshold have also been demonstrated with exercise training.[23] Whether these improvements reflect primary effects on myocardial performance or secondary effects due to changes in hemodynamics or skeletal muscle efficiency is debatable. Postulated mechanisms of primary cardiac effects include improved coronary blood flow, development of collateral circulation, and improved oxygen extraction and utilization by myocardium[20-23] (Fig. 42-2).

OTHER EFFECTS. Exercise training lowers heart rate and blood pressure at rest and at submaximal exercise, increases

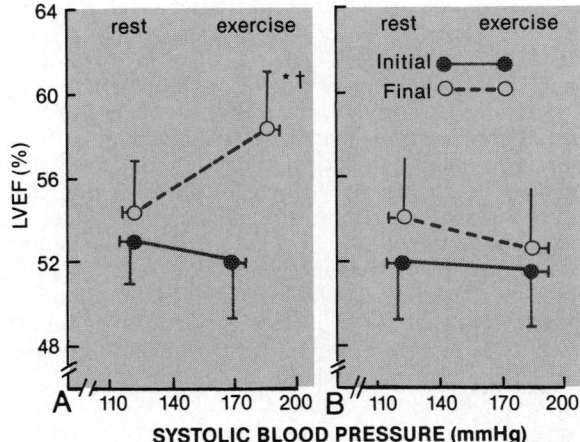

FIGURE 42-2. Effect of training on left ventricular ejection fraction (LVEF). *A,* In the training group, LVEF at rest was not significantly changed after training. During maximal exercise, LVEF increased significantly (*p < .01) above the resting level after (○) but not before (●) training. During maximal exercise, LVEF was significantly higher (†p < .001) after training despite the attainment of higher systolic blood pressure (p < .001). *B,* In the nonexercising patients, LVEF did not change with exercise initially (●) or 12 months later (○). Systolic blood pressure values were also similar. Data are mean ± SE for 25 trained (*A*) and 14 untrained patients (*B*). (From Ehsani, A. A., Biello, D. R., Schultz, J., et al.: Improvement of left ventricular contractile function by exercise training in patients with coronary artery disease. Circulation 74:350, 1986, by permission of the American Heart Association, Inc.)

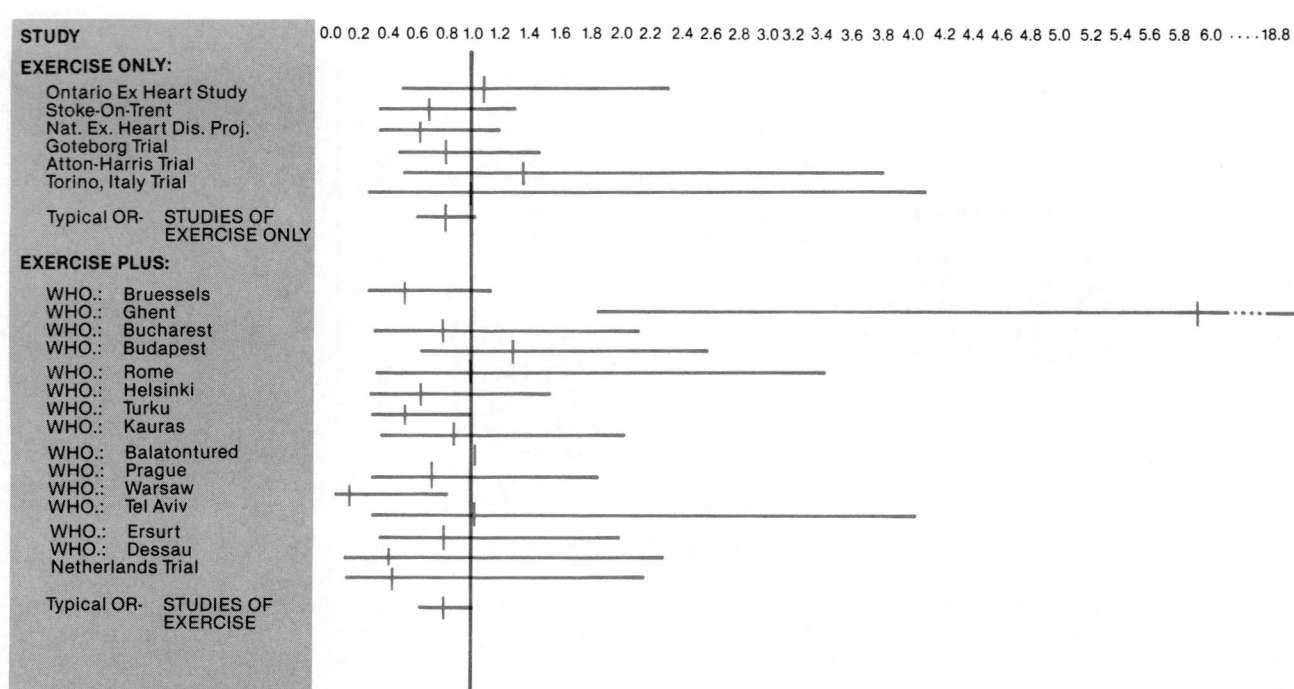

FIGURE 42–3. Chart of effects of pooling from randomized trials of cardiac rehabilitation on the estimate of mortality 3 years after randomization. Short vertical lines indicate the point estimates; horizontal lines depict the 95 per cent confidence intervals. (From O'Connor, G. T., Buring, J. E., Yusuf, S., et al.: An overview of randomized trials of rehabilitation with exercise after myocardial infarction. Circulation 80:234, 1989, by permission of the American Heart Association, Inc.)

peak MET capacity, and increases both endurance and strength. The lower the initial MET capacity, the greater the benefit in most patients.[19,24,25] Patients with a combination of myocardial ischemia and resting left ventricular dysfunction are less likely to benefit from short-term exercise training.[26] Treatment with beta blockers does not prevent a training effect in patients with coronary heart disease,[27] although some studies indicate that the training effect may be blunted.[28] Other benefits of exercise include weight reduction, improved glucose tolerance in diabetic patients, improved HDL cholesterol levels, and psychological benefits, including a greater confidence to resume customary activities more quickly.[29]

MORBIDITY AND MORTALITY. Exercise training has not been shown definitively to reduce morbidity or mortality in patients with coronary heart disease. Only 1 of 22 individual randomized trials of cardiac rehabilitation with exercise training demonstrated a statistically significant reduction in cardiovascular mortality.[30] However, all other studies were limited by inadequate sample size, short follow-up, or crossovers after randomization. Two recent analyses using data pooled from several studies showed that overall mortality and cardiovascular mortality, defined as fatal reinfarction or sudden death, were reduced by 20 to 25 per cent in patients randomized to exercise training (Fig. 42–3). Nonfatal reinfarction rates were similar in exercise and control groups.[31,32] The magnitude of benefit is similar to that seen in the randomized trials of prophylactic beta blockade after myocardial infarction,[33] suggesting that exercise training may be equally beneficial.

SELECTION OF PATIENTS FOR EXERCISE TESTING AND TRAINING

(See also Chap. 6)

PATIENTS ELIGIBLE FOR EXERCISE TRAINING. Exercise training is usually recommended for patients recovering from myocardial infarction or coronary artery bypass graft surgery. Other patients may also benefit, including those with chronic stable angina or compensated congestive heart failure and those recovering from coronary angioplasty, valve surgery, or cardiac transplantation.[19,25,34] Exercise prescription should be based on the results of electrocardiographically monitored exercise tests. Therefore, patients ineligible for exercise testing because of severe angina, uncompensated congestive heart failure, or uncontrolled arrhythmias are not candidates for exercise training. Other limiting noncardiac illnesses such as chronic obstructive pulmonary disease, peripheral vascular disease, stroke, and orthopedic disease do not necessarily obviate exercise testing and training, because specialized techniques such as arm crank ergometry can be used.[35,36]

EXERCISE TESTING. Exercise testing to a symptom or sign limit should be performed as soon after a cardiac event as the patient's condition permits. In uncomplicated cases, testing can be performed 14 to 21 days after myocardial infarction, 14 to 28 days after cardiac surgery, and 3 to 10 days after coronary angioplasty.[37] The advisability of early testing and training after myocardial infarction has been questioned because of experimental and clinical evidence showing abnormal myocardial scar formation, especially in large anterior myocardial infarctions.[38] The clinical relevance of these findings is uncertain and should probably not preclude the current clinical approach.[39] Exercise testing is performed somewhat later after cardiac surgery to minimize the detrimental effects of wound healing and pulmonary dysfunction on exercise performance.

Submaximal exercise testing is commonly used prior to or soon after hospital discharge because of the perceived safety of such testing compared to maximal testing. Maximal testing is then performed at 6 to 8 weeks following hospital discharge. However, there is no evidence that submaximal testing is safer than symptom-limited testing in properly selected patients,[40] and there are disadvantages to submaximal testing. Patients may be inappropriately limited in their customary activities and in exercise training if submaximal testing is used to evaluate physical capacity.[41–43] Return to work may be significantly delayed.[43]

Because exercise capacity is reduced in patients recovering from a cardiac event, a modified treadmill protocol should be used. The Bruce protocol increases by 2 or 3 METS at each stage and quickly surpasses the average capacity of patients recovering from a cardiac event. The modified Naughton protocol starts at a lower MET workload and increases at increments of 1 MET. This gradual progression is better tolerated and provides a more accurate assessment of MET capacity. The usual symptomatic endpoints are dyspnea and fatigue, whereas moderate angina, dizziness, and claudication occur less commonly. Signs that are important endpoints include high-grade ventricular arrhythmias, such as triplets; a fall in systolic blood pressure of 20 mm Hg compared to the previous stage; marked ischemia; and blank facies, suggesting decreased cerebral perfusion.

While the exercise test is the basis of the exercise prescription, certain test results contraindicate exercise training. Severe exercise-induced ischemia, arrhythmias, or left ventricular dysfunction must be corrected before patients are allowed to exercise. Exercise testing should be repeated after treatment to confirm that the abnormalities have resolved. Less severe abnormalities that occur at high heart rates and workloads are not necessarily contraindications to exercise therapy, especially if patients are receiving maximal medical therapy and no other treatment options are available. In those instances, the exercise prescription is modified as discussed below, and more intensive surveillance is used during exercise training.

EXERCISE PRESCRIPTION

INDIVIDUALIZED PRESCRIPTION. The exercise prescription is individualized, based upon the results of the symptom-limited exercise test. The components of the prescription are summarized by the acronym FIT—frequency, intensity, and time. The minimum frequency needed to improve cardiovascular fitness is three times weekly. The intensity is most easily prescribed as a target heart rate. The time or duration of exercise is usually 30 to 60 minutes for each session, but is individually determined.[29,44]

The intensity is based on the peak heart rate achieved during exercise testing. The conditioning effect is a balance between the intensity and duration of exercise. A low intensity is prescribed initially to allow the patient to complete 1 hour sessions without excessive fatigue. A target heart rate of 65 per cent of the peak predicted heart rate is a common starting point. In some instances, especially after cardiac surgery, the resting pulse is high and 65 per cent of the peak heart rate places the target rate near the resting pulse. In those cases, a slightly higher initial target of 75 per cent may be used. Alternatively, 40 to 50 per cent of the difference between the peak and the resting heart rate may be calculated and added to the resting pulse to determine the target. For convenience, the target is given as a 10-sec count. Patients should be taught to measure their pulse during exercise.

COMPONENTS OF EXERCISE SESSIONS. Exercise sessions, whether performed individually or in a group, should last 1 hour. Each session includes a warm-up period, a period of aerobic and muscular conditioning, and a cool-down period. A 10-minute warm-up includes stretching and light calisthenics to prevent musculoskeletal injury and gradually increase the heart rate. A 40-minute conditioning period is best spent in aerobic exercise such as walking, jogging, and bicycling during the first several weeks of the training program. Swimming is excellent aerobic exercise but creates problems with surveillance, pulse monitoring, and response in the event of a cardiovascular emergency. The exercise session is concluded with a 10-minute cool-down using stretching exercises similar to those in the warm-up period. This is especially important in coronary patients, in whom ventricular arrhythmias are commonly precipitated by abrupt cessation of moderate- or high-intensity exercise.[45]

Aerobic conditioning rather than strength training is emphasized in the first several weeks of exercise training. Arm training, especially isometric exercise, is usually proscribed in the early training period because it causes a disproportionate increase in blood pressure compared to heart rate[46] and may compromise sternal wound healing in the first 4 to 6 weeks after cardiac surgery. Standard exercise programs emphasizing dynamic leg training by walking, jogging, and bicycling also increase arm strength and endurance even without specific arm training.[47] If arm and shoulder strength training is important, patients can begin using light hand weights during walk-jog exercises early in the exercise program.

Circuit training, which refers to a series of weight-lifting exercises using moderate weight loads and frequent repetition, emphasizes muscular conditioning in both upper and lower extremities and may be advantageous to some patients later in their training program.[48] This is especially true of those patients who perform a significant amount of upper extremity work in their occupation. The major disadvantage of circuit training is the need for more elaborate equipment.

ADVANCING THE PRESCRIPTION. The Borg scale of Rate of Perceived Exertion (RPE)[49] is a useful tool for advancing the exercise prescription during training. As shown in Table 42–1, the RPE scale gives a numerical value to a perceived level of exertion. Patients should exercise at an RPE of 13 to 15. As patients become more fit, the RPE will fall and the intensity of exercise may then be increased. The target is usually increased by 5 to 10 per cent of the peak heart rate. Ultimately, patients should be able to exercise at 85 per cent of their peak heart rate for the entire session; most patients reach this intensity within 8 to 12 sessions.

Follow-up treadmill testing should be performed 4 to 8 weeks after the beginning of exercise training. Many patients will achieve significantly higher heart rates on subsequent testing. Higher achieved heart rates are related to improvements in chronotropic incompetence in some patients and the ability to achieve a maximal cardiovascular effort in others previously limited by severe skeletal muscle deconditioning.[11] The follow-up treadmill test can be used to advance the exercise prescription for most patients and to allow some to graduate to lower levels of surveillance during exercise.

PATIENTS WITH MYOCARDIAL ISCHEMIA. Patients with exercise-induced myocardial ischemia should receive optimal therapy to eliminate or ameliorate the problem. Some patients will still show evidence of ischemia. Assuming that ischemia does not occur at extremely low workloads, these patients may still exercise safely as long as their target heart rate remains well below that at which ischemia occurs.[50] Limiting the maximal target heart rate to 10 beats per minute below that at which ischemic abnormalities occur is useful clinically. Increased surveillance during exercise, as with continuous ECG monitoring, is also recommended in the initial stages of exercise training.

TABLE 42–1 BORG SCALE OF RATE OF PERCEIVED EXERTION (RPE)[49]

LEVEL OF EXERTION	VALUE
Very, very light	6
	7
	8
Very light	9
	10
Light	11
	12
Somewhat hard	13
	14
Hard	15
	16
Very hard	17
	18
Very, very hard	19
	20

Data from Borg, G., and Linderholm, H.: Exercise performance and perceived exertion in patients with coronary insufficiency, arterial hypertension and vasoregulatory asthenia. Acta Med. Scand. 187:17, 1970.

PATIENTS WITH HEART FAILURE. Patients with heart failure are at higher risk for complications related to exercise but also tend to have the most significant improvements from exercise training. Supervised exercise training has been shown to be safe in patients with heart failure.[25,26,50] The exercise prescription must often be modified for heart failure patients because of limited endurance. Shorter periods of aerobic training, lower target heart rates, and intermittent rest periods can all be used to limit the degree of fatigue felt by these patients. The ultimate target heart rate should also be kept 10 beats per minute below that at which significant symptoms of dyspnea and fatigue occur on exercise testing.

PATIENTS WITH ARRHYTHMIAS. Patients with arrhythmias present a significant challenge to the clinician because of controversies regarding therapy and the uncertainty of the safety of exercise. No definitive data are available regarding the safety of exercise in patients with arrhythmias. The usual clinical approach to cardiac rehabilitation in patients with severe exercise-induced arrhythmias is to exclude them from exercise training until suppression of the arrhythmia is achieved. Higher levels of surveillance are recommended during exercise, using continuous ECG monitoring. Longitudinal studies have shown that arrhythmia frequency and grade are unchanged by exercise training.[51] Stable patterns of arrhythmia during ECG-monitored exercise training are often used as evidence to allow patients to begin supervised, unmonitored exercise. However, the safety of this approach has not been documented.

RISKS OF EXERCISE TRAINING

Exercise training is not without risks. The greatest risk of exercise lies in patients with untreated or unrecognized left ventricular dysfunction, myocardial ischemia, or ventricular arrhythmias. In patients with these abnormalities who have received optimal therapy, the greatest risk lies in exercising at or above the level at which the abnormalities can be elicited by exercise testing.[52] For this reason, the maximum target heart rate used in exercise training must be lower than the heart rate at which abnormalities become evident on testing.

PATIENT SELECTION AND SURVEILLANCE. Safe exercise training is best assured by proper selection of patients and adequate surveillance during exercise. Patients at high risk for cardiovascular complications during exercise have one or more of the characteristics listed in Table 42–2.[34,52,53] In such patients the abnormality should be ameliorated or corrected before starting the exercise program. If the abnormality cannot be corrected, the risks and benefits of exercise training should be carefully considered. If an exercise program is rec-

ommended, the highest level of surveillance during exercise is required. There are some patients in whom the risks of exercise outweigh the benefits despite optimal medical therapy. Such patients should be informed of the risks and counseled not to exercise.

The highest level of surveillance is supervised group exercise with continuous electrocardiographic monitoring. Approximately 15 to 25 per cent of patients eligible for exercise training have one or more of the characteristics in Table 42–2 and require continuous electrocardiographic monitoring.[34,53] The next level of surveillance is unmonitored group exercise training supervised by health professionals with Advanced Cardiac Life Support certification. Patients without high-risk characteristics and those who improve during electrocardiographic monitored training can participate in supervised, unmonitored group training.[53] Very low-risk patients can safely exercise independently after learning the principles of pulse monitoring and symptom recognition. In general, low-risk patients have an exercise capacity of 8 METS or more without symptoms or signs of left ventricular dysfunction, myocardial ischemia, or ventricular arrhythmias. These criteria may be used to graduate patients from supervised programs.[54]

All patients should be taught to monitor their pulse and recognize symptoms during exercise. The concepts of the target heart rate and RPE are conveyed and reinforced during group exercise sessions. These principles and concepts will guide patients in independent, safe, and effective exercise after completion of a formal exercise program. Patients who are unable or unwilling to follow the exercise prescription should receive higher levels of surveillance.

SAFETY OF SUPERVISED PROGRAMS. Despite the potential for cardiovascular complications during exercise training, supervised exercise programs have an extremely good safety record. In a survey of 167 programs, the incidence of fatal events per million patient hours of exercise was 1.3, of myocardial infarction 3.4, and of resuscitated cardiac arrests 8.9. There were no significant differences in these rates for small compared to large programs or continuously electrocardiographically monitored compared to intermittently monitored programs.[55] The event rates in this study were significantly lower than in a survey performed a decade earlier.[56] The reasons for improvement are speculative. Improved risk stratification, improved revascularization and medical therapy, more rigorous standards for cardiac rehabilitation programs, and increased awareness of the necessity for monitoring high-risk patients may all have contributed to the improved safety record.

SECONDARY PREVENTION
(See also Chap. 37)

Increasing evidence supports the widespread application of specific measures to prevent recurrence of cardiac disease after a first cardiac event. In the short term, abstinence from cigarette smoking is extremely effective in reducing morbidity and mortality. In the long term, reduction in serum lipid abnormalities appears to slow the progression of coronary atherosclerosis and may improve the outcome. While controversial, treatment of certain behavioral manifestations, such as Type A behavior, may exert a positive influence on prognosis. There is no definitive evidence that the treatment of hypertension and diabetes positively influences prognosis *after* a cardiac event, although the standard of care is to treat these conditions vigorously.

CIGARETTE SMOKING
(See also p. 1302)

RISKS. Cigarette smoking is an established risk factor for the development of angina and myocardial infarction[57] and increases the risk for recurrence of infarction and death.[58] In survivors of myocardial infarction who continue to smoke, the rate of recurrence of infarction and cardiac death is twice that in patients who quit smoking. The risk of a second

TABLE 42–2   INDICATIONS FOR CONTINUOUS ECG MONITORING DURING EXERCISE TRAINING

CLINICAL INDICATION	OBJECTIVE SIGNS
Severe left ventricular dysfunction	Ejection fraction <30%
Complex ventricular arrhythmia (at rest or exercise induced)	Lown grade 4 or 5
Hypotensive response to exercise	Systolic drop of 20 mm Hg or more at increasing load
Complicated myocardial infarction	Cardiogenic shock Congestive heart failure
Severe exercise-induced ischemia	ST-segment depression ≥ 2 mV Angina at a workload ≤ 5 METS
Low functional capacity	Peak workload ≤ 5 METS
Prior cardiac arrest	
Inability to self-monitor heart rate	

cardiac event declines rapidly after cessation of smoking. Within 3 years of ceasing smoking, the risk of reinfarction is approximately the same in ex-smokers and in survivors who never smoked.[57-59]

PATHOPHYSIOLOGY. The pathophysiology underlying the increased risk for death and reinfarction is uncertain. Platelet aggregation, thrombosis, coronary spasm, and diminished coronary and collateral flow reserve have all been implicated. Coronary flow reserve is significantly lower in smokers than nonsmokers, with heavier smokers having greater reductions than lighter smokers.[60] Fibrinogen levels are significantly higher in smokers than in nonsmokers and increase the primary risk of myocardial infarction.[61] Although the degree of coronary atherosclerosis is not strongly correlated with smoking habits, the risk for myocardial infarction in smokers is strongly correlated with the extent of coronary artery disease and plasma cholesterol levels.[59]

ETIOLOGY OF TOBACCO DEPENDENCE. Smoking is a complex behavior with physiological, psychological, and sociological roots. There are several theories regarding the etiology of tobacco dependence, although no single theory is adequate to explain all aspects of smoking behavior. Physiological dependence on nicotine causes acute craving for cigarettes with abrupt cessation of smoking. Smoking is a habit that minimizes negative emotions such as distress, anger, and fear. It may also be used as a coping mechanism to transfer such negative emotions into socially acceptable behavior. Finally, a smoking habit may have deep sociological origins, such as modeling behavior after parents and peers.[62]

SMOKING CESSATION PROGRAMS. Demographic and psychological factors identify patients more likely to continue smoking after a cardiac event. Lower occupational and educational levels, smoking a greater number of cigarettes, increasing age, and higher rates of alcohol consumption are demographic factors associated with continued smoking. Psychological factors such as a less negative attitude regarding smoking, higher anxiety levels, and a low sense of personal control over life events predict smokers who are less likely to quit smoking after a cardiac event.[62,63]

Smoking cessation is facilitated by treating both the physiological and psychological aspects of the habit. The association between cardiac disease and smoking is well known to the lay public. Myocardial infarction or coronary surgery is a sufficient impetus for 20 to 60 per cent of patients to stop smoking. Patients who receive strong advice from health professionals to stop smoking are more likely to quit and remain abstinent than those who do not receive advice.[64] This is particularly true of individuals who believe that they are at personal risk if they continue smoking. Unfortunately, the high acute cessation rates are also associated with high recidivism rates in the absence of interventions to maintain abstinence.

Hospital confinement for myocardial infarction or coronary surgery usually provides sufficient time for the psychological manifestations of nicotine withdrawal such as irritability, emotionality, inability to concentrate, nausea, and headache to resolve. In patients who continue to crave cigarettes, nicotine dependence is strong, and more gradual nicotine withdrawal may be necessary.[59]

Nicotine withdrawal can be managed by tapering cigarette smoking, gradually changing to lower-nicotine cigarettes, and substituting chewing of nicotine gum. A 2-mg dose of nicotine gum gives average serum nicotine levels of 12 ng/ml compared to 35 to 54 ng/ml from cigarette smoke. This level is usually sufficient to blunt the craving for nicotine, although in heavier smokers higher doses of oral nicotine appear to be more effective.[65] Nicotine gum is prescribed as needed, up to 30 doses per day. The average patient uses 10 doses daily, and the frequency of dosing declines over a 1- to 3-month period. If the patient is still dependent on the gum after 6 months, it is likely being used as a cigarette substitute rather than an aid to abstinence. Aversive techniques, such as smoke holding or rapid puffing, may also be effective in nicotine-dependent patients.

The most effective programs for smoking abstinence address both the physiological and psychological dependence on cigarettes. The prescription of nicotine gum alone does not significantly increase the long-term abstinence rate.[66] Smoking is usually linked to other behaviors, such as eating or talking on the telephone. It is also more common in particular situations, such as stressful activities or social situations.

Teaching patients to recognize the high-risk behaviors or situations in which the desire to smoke is likely is the first step in maintaining abstinence. Using techniques of self-control or substitution of healthful behaviors for smoking assists the patients in abstaining from smoking.[67] Enlisting the social support of family, friends, and coworkers reinforces the nonsmoking behavior. Long-term abstinence rates of up to 70 per cent have been achieved with formal programs.[67,68]

Serum Lipids
(See also p. 1116)

PRIMARY AND SECONDARY PREVENTION. Data from laboratory, epidemiological, and clinical studies have established the role of serum lipids in the genesis of coronary atherosclerosis. There is compelling evidence that reducing serum cholesterol reduces the risk of a primary cardiac event. The Coronary Primary Prevention Trial demonstrated that lowering serum cholesterol with cholestyramine decreased the risk of cardiovascular death and nonfatal myocardial infarction in men with serum cholesterol in the 90th percentile who had no evidence of coronary disease.[69,70] Similar results were obtained in patients treated with gemfibrozil.[71]

The data are less clear regarding the effects of cholesterol reduction on the risk for second cardiac events. Nicotinic acid treatment after myocardial infarction was associated with lower cardiovascular mortality and nonfatal reinfarction rates in the Coronary Drug Project.[72] No other data are yet available definitively linking treatment of increased serum cholesterol with reduction in cardiovascular risk.

PROGRESSION OF ATHEROSCLEROSIS. Progression of atherosclerosis has been linked with higher rates of cardiovascular complications after a first cardiac event.[73] Slowing the progression or causing regression of atherosclerosis would potentially result in a reduction in cardiovascular complications.

Several trials have used quantitative coronary angiography to evaluate the effects of diet and drug therapy on coronary atherosclerosis. The Leiden Intervention Trial evaluated the effect of a vegetarian diet and found that 46 per cent of participants showed no progression of coronary atherosclerosis.[74] The Cholesterol Lowering Atherosclerosis Study was a randomized, placebo-controlled study of the effect of diet plus niacin and colestipol versus diet plus placebo on coronary atherosclerosis in patients who had previously undergone coronary artery bypass surgery. Progression of disease was significantly reduced in native vessels and bypass grafts in the treatment compared to the placebo group. Regression of atherosclerosis was observed in 16.2 per cent of the treatment group as compared to 3.6 per cent of the placebo group. Clinical outcomes were better in the drug group, although the sample size was insufficient to demonstrate an improvement in mortality.[75]

Similar though less conclusive findings were seen in a randomized trial of diet plus cholestyramine versus diet plus placebo in patients with Type II hyperlipidemia and overt coronary disease.[76] These trials suggest that diet and drug therapy can slow the progression of coronary atherosclerosis but do not necessarily reduce morbidity and mortality.

NATIONAL CHOLESTEROL EDUCATION PROGRAM. An expert panel developed recommendations for the evaluation and treatment of hypercholesterolemia that have been publicized as the National Cholesterol Education Program. Low-, moderate-, and high-risk categories of serum cholesterol were established, and treatment within each category was recommended.[77] High-risk patients were those with elevated LDL-cholesterol levels and two or more cardiac risk factors or clinically manifested coronary artery disease. Most patients eligible for cardiac rehabilitation who also have elevated cholesterol levels would be in the high-risk group.

In patients with coronary artery disease, the panel recommends that total cholesterol greater than 200 mg/dl be evaluated with a lipoprotein analysis. Patients with LDL-cholesterol levels greater than 130 mg/dl are recommended for dietary treatment. Patients with LDL-cholesterol greater than 160 mg/dl are recommended for drug therapy in addition to dietary treatment. In both instances, the goal is to reduce LDL-cholesterol below 130 mg/dl. The first-choice drugs are those known to lower LDL-cholesterol that have also lowered the risk of a primary cardiac event.[77] Cholestyramine, colestipol, nicotinic acid, and gemfibrozil all meet these criteria.

The recommendations of the panel have been criticized in some areas. Specific therapy for low HDL-cholesterol levels was not recommended, despite the known increased coronary risk associated with this finding. Data from one primary prevention trial found that increasing the HDL level with gemfibrozil lowered coronary risk independent of any lowering of LDL levels.[71]

No specific recommendations were made regarding modifications of the recommendations in older patients. The benefits of cholesterol treatment in the elderly have been questioned.[78] While drug treatment is recommended at lower LDL-cholesterol levels in patients who manifest coronary disease, some have suggested that the recommendations are too conservative in this subgroup.[79] The panel clearly advises that the guidelines be applied according to the clinical judgments of practicing physicians.[77]

DIETARY TREATMENT. The approach to the dietary treatment of hypercholesterolemia is to lower the intake of total fat, saturated fat, and cholesterol and to achieve ideal weight. A two-step dietary approach is recommended, with the first step restricting total fat to 30 per cent and saturated fat to 10 per cent of caloric intake and cholesterol to 300 mg daily. If the first step is not sufficient to reach desired goals, the second step restricts saturated fat to 7 per cent and cholesterol to 200 mg. A 4- to 12-week period of dietary modification is recommended with at least one reevaluation of serum lipids.[77] The dietary evaluation and treatment plan is best developed by a dietitian with the patient and spouse. Food purchasing and preparation should be emphasized in addition to selection of low-fat and low-cholesterol foods. Information should be provided on selection of foods in restaurants. The cardiac rehabilitation team reinforces the cholesterol management guidelines during rehabilitation sessions.

DRUG TREATMENT. If dietary intervention and exercise are insufficient to meet the goals of treatment of hypercholesterolemia, specific drug therapy should be initiated. The effect of other cardiovascular drugs that may increase serum lipids, such as beta blockers and thiazide diuretics, should be considered. Selection of specific lipid-lowering agents is discussed on page 1142.

EFFECTS OF CARDIAC REHABILITATION. The effect of exercise on serum cholesterol is not clear. Conflicting reports are probably related to the failure of studies to control for effects of changes in body weight, diet, and intensity of exercise.[80] In general, low- to moderate-intensity exercise has little influence on total cholesterol. However, most reports are consistent in demonstrating that all intensities and durations of exercise increase HDL-cholesterol levels.[81] Weight loss resulting from calorie and fat restriction in conjunction with exercise usually results in decreased LDL levels.[80,81]

Other influences are less clear. While moderate alcohol consumption has been associated with a decreased prevalence of coronary heart disease,[83] the reason is unclear. The effects of fish oils are similarly unclear. High concentrations of omega-3 fatty acids either reduce hepatic synthesis of VLDL or increase catabolism. Through this effect, LDL levels may be reduced, especially in hypercholesterolemic states in which VLDL levels are elevated.[84]

PSYCHOLOGICAL FACTORS

COMMON PSYCHIATRIC PROBLEMS. Most professionals providing cardiac rehabilitation believe that exercise training and related services produce significant psychological benefits. In particular, anxiety and depression are improved, and patients have a greater sense of well-being. However, there are few well-performed studies demonstrating psychological benefits of cardiac rehabilitation in the absence of specific interventions, such as stress management or group therapy.[85] In patients with disabling psychiatric symptoms, specific treatment with medications or psychotherapy is indicated. The most common of these symptoms are delirium in the acute setting[86] and anxiety or depression during early recovery.[87] Two areas in which specific interventions might be helpful as an adjunct to cardiac rehabilitation are self-efficacy and Type A behavior.

SELF-EFFICACY. Acute cardiac illnesses have many psychosocial sequelae, including medical restrictions on even the most routine of activities such as driving, climbing stairs, and lifting. These restrictions are reinforced by family, friends, and coworkers, who perceive a poor prognosis and are concerned that physical and emotional stress can further damage the heart. If the patient has a poor understanding of his illness, fear of recurrent cardiac problems leads to a sense of loss of control and a lack of confidence to resume customary activities. This lack of confidence can be a significant impediment to the resumption of a full and active life style.

"Self-efficacy" is a psychological term used to describe how an individual's judgment regarding his capacity for performance of a task or action is an important determinant of whether he will attempt the task or action.[88] Self-efficacy reflects confidence and is highly predictive of action. Self-efficacy for specific tasks can be rated on confidence scales of 0 to 100 per cent. For example, self-efficacy scales that predict whether a coronary patient will be successful with a regular exercise program have been validated for physical activity.[89] The most common areas of low self-efficacy for coronary patients are physical exertion, emotional stress, and sexual activity.[88]

Self-efficacy can be increased in coronary patients by four methods: persuasion, information, vicarious experience, and enactive techniques. Using exercise as an example, physicians can persuade patients that they are capable of exercising. Patients can be informed about what sensations to expect with exercise, so they do not misread normal physiological responses such as tachycardia as grave symptoms. Vicarious experiences can be shared by other patients who have successfully undertaken an exercise program. The most powerful method for increasing exercise self-efficacy is the performance of a supervised exercise test.[88,89]

Self-efficacy is a useful measure for predicting potential success for other important behavioral changes, such as smoking cessation,[67] dietary modification, and exercise training.[89,90] In circumstances of low self-efficacy, informative, persuasive, vicarious, and enactive techniques to raise self-efficacy are helpful for increasing the success rate for behavioral change. Spousal perceptions are equally important. Self-efficacy scales that rate a spouse's perception of the patient's potential for success with a particular task are also highly predictive of success or failure. Support and encouragement by the spouse in behavior change are extremely important for success. Spousal self-efficacy can be raised by means of techniques similar to those used for patients.[88,91]

TYPE A BEHAVIOR. While Type A behavior, i.e., behavior characterized by excesses of competitiveness, pace, and aggressiveness, has been recognized as a risk factor for the development of coronary artery disease,[92] its effect on the prognosis of coronary disease is unknown. Conflicting results are reported in several studies, although there are limitations in each. The major limitations are the populations studied, the instruments used to classify behavior, the duration of follow-up, and the endpoints studied.[93,94] One of the most important concepts that has emerged from the Type A controversy is recognition that the construct probably reflects a collection of behaviors, not all of which are related to either the development or the prognosis of coronary disease. Of the three primary characteristics of Type A behavior—competitive achievement striving, time urgency, and hostility—only the last appears to be independently related to coronary disease outcomes.[95]

Despite the controversy regarding the effect of Type A behavior on prognosis, there is evidence from one intervention trial that modifying Type A behavior reduces risk of recurrent cardiac events in patients recovering from myocardial infarction. The Recurrent Coronary Prevention Project randomized a group of 862 men who had experienced a myocardial infarction to either a control group receiving cardiological counseling or an intervention group receiving cardiological counseling and Type A behavioral counseling. Type A behavior patterns were significantly reduced in the intervention group as compared to the control group. The rate of recurrent cardiac events over 3 years was 13 per cent in control patients and 7.2 per cent in intervention patients. This significant reduction in event rate was primarily related to a reduction in nonfatal myocardial infarctions in the intervention group.[96] The risk reduction is on the same order of magnitude as the benefit of prophylactic beta blockade after myocardial infarction.[33] The results from this single study are encouraging and warrant further investigation of treatment of Type A behavior.

VOCATIONAL REHABILITATION

The cost of cardiovascular disability is high. The direct cost of care for patients with heart disease is estimated at $85 billion annually in the United States.[97,98] Indirect costs, due to goods and services not provided because of cardiovascular illness, are several times greater. Indirect costs can be significantly reduced by increasing the numbers of patients who return to work and shortening the interval between a cardiac event and return to work.

FACTORS RELATED TO EMPLOYMENT. Employment after a cardiac event is related to demographic, medical, and psychosocial factors. Patients unemployed at the time of a cardiac event, those over 60 years of age, and those with blue-collar jobs are significantly less likely to work after the event. Unemployment for 3 months or more before a cardiac event is common in patients with more severe cardiac disease but also may be related to psychological or social causes for unemployment. Retirement and disability benefits are more easily obtained after age 60, encouraging patients to leave the work force. Blue collar workers, especially those who are unskilled, are easily replaced in the work force and consequently lose their jobs more commonly after a cardiac event.[99] After a cardiac event, the medical condition of the patient and the advice provided by the physician regarding return to work are the most important factors influencing the rate of reemployment in previously employed patients.

In the absence of demographic and psychosocial impediments, physicians play a pivotal role in the return-to-work decision.[100] The physician must first ensure that the risk of a cardiovascular complication is low and will not be increased by returning to work and then must determine if the patient has the physical capacity to perform his occupational work. Finally the physician must provide explicit advice regarding the timing of return to work and any work restrictions that the patient and employer must follow.

FACILITATING REEMPLOYMENT. In the majority of patients recovering from cardiac surgery or myocardial infarction, a careful clinical evaluation and a symptom-limited treadmill test are sufficient to guide the physician in the return-to-work decision. Accurate methods to stratify the risk of recurrent coronary events rely on clinical information obtained during hospitalization and specialized testing performed during or shortly after hospitalization. More than half of patients surviving myocardial infarction have no symptoms or signs of congestive heart failure or myocardial ischemia. Their risk of cardiac death, myocardial infarction, or unstable angina in the year following the primary event is less than 10 per cent. A symptom-limited exercise capacity on treadmill

testing of 7 METS or more without ischemia lowers the risk to less than 3 per cent.[101]

The treadmill test also establishes peak physical capacity, which can be related to the patient's occupational work. Individuals can sustain 6 to 8 hours of continuous effort at 40 per cent of their peak MET capacity. Continuous work tolerance declines at higher levels, averaging 4 hours at 60 per cent of peak capacity and 2 hours above 60 per cent of peak capacity.[102] Table 42–3 lists the MET requirements for selected occupational and recreational activities.[103] The average job has an energy requirement well under 5 METS, meaning that a peak capacity of 7 to 10 METS is sufficient for most individuals to perform their occupational work.[102] Only 16 per cent of Americans perform jobs requiring manual labor, and that percentage declines rapidly with age.[104] Most manual labor jobs require only intermittent high-energy expenditure, which significantly prolongs work tolerance.

Intensive physical reconditioning is not necessary for the average patient to return to work. In patients with very low functional capacity and those with higher physical requirements of their job, an exercise training program can hasten their return to work. Unless the patient's job requires lifting and carrying of moderate to heavy loads, the standard aerobic training described previously is sufficient to expedite return to work. In specialized circumstances, exercise programs that include upper extremity isometric training can be provided. Work simulation and specialized training programs may be helpful in unusual circumstances. In the particular circumstance of jobs affecting public safety, such as pilots, police, and fire fighters, more stringent requirements regarding return to work are legislated.[105]

The average interval between uncomplicated myocardial infarction and return to work is 70 to 90 days; it averages 80 to

TABLE 42–3   ESTIMATES OF ENERGY REQUIREMENTS OF AVOCATIONAL AND OCCUPATIONAL TASKS[103]

CATEGORY	SELF-CARE OR HOME	OCCUPATIONAL	RECREATIONAL	PHYSICAL CONDITIONING
Very light < 3 METS < 10 ml/kg/min < 4 kcal	Washing, shaving, dressing, desk work, writing; washing dishes; driving auto	Sitting (clerical, assembly), standing (store clerk, bartender); driving truck, operating crane	Shuffleboard, horseshoes, bait casting, billiards, archery, golf (cart)	Walking (2 mph), stationary bicycle (very low resistance), very light calisthenics
Light 3–5 METS 11–18 ml/kg/min 4–6 kcal	Cleaning windows, raking leaves, weeding, power lawn mowing, waxing floors (slowly), painting, carrying objects (15–30 lb)	Stocking shelves (light objects), light welding, light carpentry, machine assembly, auto repair, paper hanging	Dancing (social and square), golf (walking), sailing, horseback riding, volleyball (6 man), tennis (doubles)	Walking (3–4 mph), level bicycling (6–8 mph), light calisthenics
Moderate 5–7 METS 18–25 ml/kg/min 6–8 kcal	Easy digging in garden, level lawn mowing, climbing stairs (slowly), carrying objects (30–60 lb)	Carpentry (exterior home building), shoveling dirt, using pneumatic tools	Badminton (competitive), tennis (singles), snow skiing (downhill), light backpacking, basketball, skating (ice and roller), horseback riding (gallop)	Walking (4.5–5 mph), bicycling (9–10 mph), swimming (breast stroke)
Heavy 7–9 METS 25–32 ml/kg/min 8–10 kcal	Sawing wood, heavy shoveling, climbing stairs (moderate speed), carrying objects (60–90 lb)	Tending furnace, digging ditches, pick and shovel	Canoeing, mountain climbing, fencing, paddleball, touch football	Jog (5 mph), swim (crawl stroke), rowing machine, heavy calisthenics, bicycling (12 mph)
Very heavy > 9 METS > 32 ml/kg/min > 10 kcal	Carrying loads upstairs, carrying objects (> 90 lb), climbing stairs (quickly), shoveling heavy snow, shoveling 10 min (16 lb)	Lumberjack, heavy laborer	Handball, squash, ski touring over hills, vigorous basketball	Running (≥ 6 mph), bicycle (≥ 13 mph or up steep hills), rope jumping

From Haskell, W. L.: Design and implementation of cardiac conditioning programs. *In* Wenger, N. K., and Hellerstein, H. F. (eds.): Rehabilitation of the Coronary Patient. New York, John Wiley & Sons, pp. 214–215.

100 days after uncomplicated coronary surgery.[100,102,106] These intervals can be substantially shortened with a coordinated approach using risk stratification, treadmill testing, and explicit physician advice regarding the timing of return to work. In employed patients without high-risk clinical characteristics or severe treadmill ischemia, the time from myocardial infarction was shortened from 75 to 51 days in a randomized trial of an early-return-to-work intervention. Recurrent cardiac events averaged 3.5 per cent in the 6 months after infarction and were no higher in patients returning to work earlier than in those returning to work later. Although this study did not include a special intervention for patients performing manual labor, the intervention was as successful in the 11 per cent of the population performing manual labor as it was in the sedentary workers. Higher-risk patients with evidence of congestive heart failure or myocardial ischemia accounted for 23 per cent of all employed patients under the age of 60 and were specifically excluded from the study. Return-to-work decisions in such patients must be individualized.

BENEFITS OF REEMPLOYMENT. The benefits of early return to work are primarily financial; however, the psychological benefits, while more difficult to identify, must not be overlooked. In the trial discussed previously, patients randomized to the return-to-work intervention earned $2100 more than patients randomized to usual care in the 6 months following myocardial infarction. While not specifically examined, financial benefits to employers probably accrued, including increased productivity and reduced costs of temporary employees and disability insurance payments.[107] Interventions that increase the numbers of patients returning to work and shorten the interval between the illness and reemployment will have the greatest impact on reducing the economic burden of cardiovascular disability.

ORGANIZATION OF CARDIAC REHABILITATION SERVICES

For most patients, cardiac rehabilitation begins in the hospital following a cardiac event and continues for several months thereafter. Cardiac rehabilitation has traditionally been provided in phases with activity guidelines based upon the time since the cardiac event. While phased rehabilitation provides a framework, individual patients will progress more slowly or quickly depending upon their age, condition prior to their cardiac event, the severity of illness, and motivation. The rehabilitation program should be individualized to facilitate a rate of recovery commensurate with the patient's status.[108]

INPATIENT REHABILITATION

Hospitalization has been significantly shortened for patients recovering from myocardial infarction and cardiac surgery. Inpatient rehabilitation must make patients self-sufficient in the activities of daily living in a short period of time. Patients must be able to recognize important cardiac symptoms, obtain medical care appropriately, and take prescribed medications. The behavioral changes required for secondary prevention may be introduced in the hospital but are mainly deferred until patients are at home.

EARLY MOBILIZATION. Early mobilization reduces the detrimental effects of bed rest, as discussed previously,[3-7] and maximizes the rate at which customary activities can be resumed. In the coronary care unit, assisted range-of-motion exercises can be initiated in the first 24 to 48 hours for most patients. Patients whose condition is stable should be encouraged to sit in a chair for increasing periods each day to minimize intravascular volume depletion, skeletal muscle deconditioning, and orthopedic impairment. Self-care activities such as shaving, oral hygiene, and sponge bathing can be undertaken in the intensive care unit. These activities have a

low MET requirement (Table 42–3) and encourage patients to resume more activities quickly.[103] There is no specific time frame in which these activities should take place, other than as soon as tolerated by patients within the context of their medical and surgical care.

GRADUATED PHYSICAL ACTIVITY. A graduated program of physical and self-care activities can begin upon transfer from the intensive care unit. Upright posture should be encouraged as much as tolerated. Patients should walk with assistance at least twice daily. While some inpatient programs suggest walking specific distances each day,[108] ambulation can be based upon the patient's tolerance. In that way, patients are neither pushed beyond their tolerance nor held back in their recovery. The target heart rate and RPE scale can be used to individualize the intensity and time of activity. For each session, standing heart rate and blood pressure are obtained, followed by 5 minutes of range-of-motion and flexibility exercises. Patients are then assisted with walking at a rate that keeps the pulse within the range of resting pulse plus 20 beats/min and the RPE less than 14. Most patients will tolerate a minimum of 5 minutes of walking the first day. As long as the pulse and RPE remain within these limits, walking time can be increased until patients are walking for 30 minutes twice daily. At that point, the walking sessions should include stair climbing to ensure that patients can perform that task at home. Patients able to walk unassisted for 30 minutes and climb stairs have sufficient strength and endurance for most activities of daily living.

EDUCATION AND COUNSELING. During the periods of assisted ambulation, the nurse or physical therapist teaches patients how to count their pulse and recognize important symptoms. Before hospital discharge, patients are taught how to obtain emergency medical care; learn the names, dosages, effects, and side-effects of their medications; and have specific questions answered regarding their cardiac status. Basic information regarding the risk factors for coronary disease should be presented, with emphasis on those that affect the patient.

At the time of hospital discharge, patients should receive very specific advice about resumption of activities at home. To exercise safely at home, the patient should be able to count the pulse accurately and understand the use of the RPE scale. Even common sense knowledge should not be presumed by the health professionals caring for the patient. The spouse should receive the advice with the patient because the retention of information by hospitalized patients is limited, and most disagreements between patient and spouse in the early recovery period are related to perceptions of medical advice given.[109,110] A simple approach to providing guidelines for physical activities is to treat them as forms of exercise. Patients can use the rule of resting pulse plus 20 beats/min for most household activities. The patient will learn quickly the heart rate response to each activity and be confident in undertaking such activities at home. Patients should be told what restrictions are placed on common activities, such as climbing stairs, lifting, driving, socializing with visitors, shopping, and walking outdoors. Individual patients may have more specific questions.

Activities that involve more mental than physical stress, such as driving, socializing, and shopping, concern patients and family at the time of hospital discharge. In studies of patients recovering from myocardial infarction who underwent psychological stress testing using standard techniques, the mean resting heart rate rose less than 10 beats/min and the mean systolic blood pressure rose less than 15 mm/Hg with the most stressful intervention. In every case the hemodynamic response to psychological stress was substantially lower than to treadmill exercise testing. In a subset of patients with exercise-induced ST-segment depression, none developed ischemic responses to psychological stress testing.[111] These data suggest that the psychological stress of usual social activities is unlikely to precipitate significant cardiovascular abnormalities in the early recovery period.

EARLY POSTDISCHARGE REHABILITATION AND EXERCISE TRAINING

ACTIVITIES BEFORE EXERCISE TESTING. The interval between hospital discharge and formal cardiac rehabilitation should be as brief as possible. During this period, patients can continue their walking program as it was prescribed in the hospital. They should walk a minimum of 30 minutes twice daily at a target heart rate within the range of resting pulse plus 20 beats/min at an RPE of less than 14. Patients able to tolerate that duration of walking should be encouraged to add a third session or increase the two sessions to 45 minutes each. Secondary prevention efforts can begin, since patients are motivated and have time to begin to make behavioral changes. Initial visits with a dietitian can be scheduled if weight loss or cholesterol reduction is necessary. A smoking abstinence program can begin during this period. Patients should be provided with resources to teach them about coronary disease and risk factor management.

RECOMMENDATIONS FOLLOWING EXERCISE TESTING. A postdischarge exercise test is a good focal point for the subsequent rehabilitation effort. The formal exercise prescription can then be given. Goals for weight loss, serum cholesterol reduction, smoking cessation, and return to work can be established. In the absence of significant abnormalities on the treadmill test, patients may begin most customary activities such as driving, sexual activity, and light lifting. Although lifting is often proscribed for 6 to 8 weeks after myocardial infarction and cardiac surgery, studies suggest that lifting and carrying of moderate loads are not dangerous after uncomplicated myocardial infarction and cardiac surgery. In patients recovering from myocardial infarction, static lifting of 25 to 50 lb and combined static lifting and dynamic treadmill walking were associated with similar or lower double products compared to dynamic treadmill walking alone. In these studies, there was no evidence of myocardial ischemia induced by static lifting alone.[112,113] In another study, static lifting to a double product that elicited ischemia on dynamic treadmill walking was not associated with myocardial ischemia. The conclusion of that study was that the increased diastolic blood pressure response of static lifting increased coronary blood flow and prevented myocardial ischemia.[114]

SEXUAL ACTIVITY. The most common sexual problems of coronary patients are reduction or absence of libido, avoidance of sexual activity even if libido has recovered, impotence, and premature or delayed ejaculation in men. The causes of sexual dysfunction include preexisting conditions, fear of precipitating a cardiac event, depression, and medications, especially beta blockers and diuretics. In addition, the sexual partner may believe that sexual activity could precipitate a cardiac event and therefore may avoid sexual activity. Because patients are reluctant to discuss sexual dysfunction, the physician should address issues of sexuality and consider the effects of medications on sexual drive.[115]

The hemodynamic response to sexual intercourse has been evaluated in patients recovering from myocardial infarction. The maximal heart rate during sexual intercourse averages 120 beats/min, which approximates maximal heart rates attained in the performance of other customary activities.[116] The hemodynamic response to sexual activity is far greater with an unfamiliar than a familiar partner, in unfamiliar settings, and after excessive eating and alcohol consumption.[115] The exercise test can be used to gauge the potential cardiac stress of sexual activity. Patients without significant treadmill abnormalities can be advised to resume sexual activity gradually. Masturbation and mutual caressing can be initiated first, followed by progression to sexual intercourse. Cardiac work associated with sexual intercourse can be minimized by adopting relaxed positions such as side-to-side rather than top-and-bottom postures, which increase the isometric work.[115-117] Patients should be told to report symptoms such as angina, prolonged dyspnea, excessive fatigue, or tachycardia lasting more than 10 minutes after intercourse. In sedentary

individuals, such symptoms may be the only manifestation of exercise-induced or left ventricular dysfunction.

OUTPATIENT REHABILITATION PROGRAMS

Formal cardiac rehabilitation programs typically have both a medical director and a program director. The medical director is a physician, whereas the program director may be trained in a variety of disciplines. The rehabilitation team is multidisciplinary and includes nurses, physical therapists, exercise physiologists, dietitians, vocational counselors, and psychologists. When smaller programs cannot support the broad range of services, a referral network that includes all of the disciplines is necessary. Adequate facilities for outpatient exercise training are needed. If high-risk patients are included, continuous electrocardiographic monitoring must be available. Equipment and training for cardiopulmonary resuscitation are mandatory.

EXERCISE TRAINING. Exercise training guidelines were presented earlier. The type of exercise program the patient enters depends upon medical condition, physical capacity, risk, and ability to self-monitor exercise. Most patients can benefit from group exercise programs. The standard group training program provides three sessions weekly for 8 to 12 weeks. Some patients require more prolonged training, while others may progress to independent exercise more quickly. In such groups, proper techniques of exercise training can be reinforced, and patients can learn how to perform safe and effective exercise independently. The group setting is also an opportunity for patients to receive reliable information from health professionals regarding coronary disease and risk factor modification. While difficult to quantitate, there is an obvious benefit of the social support provided by interactions with other patients in various stages of recovery from coronary illness.[118] Group exercise sessions are often the focal point for the development of educational programs and support groups.

RISK FACTOR MODIFICATION. A comprehensive program of cardiac rehabilitation should combine exercise training with risk factor modification. Smoking abstinence programs and dietary counseling are the two most important additional services a program should provide. Continued reinforcement of the principles of risk factor modification improves compliance with behavioral programs.[85,110]

Current evidence suggests that cardiac rehabilitation programs offering exercise training and facilitation of smoking abstinence and cholesterol lowering can improve the morbidity and mortality in coronary artery disease. Cardiac rehabilitation programs can also facilitate functional recovery. Early risk stratification, including treadmill testing, can identify patients requiring further treatment and hasten the resumption of customary activities of low-risk patients. Education and counseling can improve psychosocial outcomes. Significant economic benefits can be realized when vocational rehabilitation is included in a cardiac rehabilitation program. As the principles of cardiac rehabilitation become more broadly applied, larger numbers of patients with coronary disease will benefit medically, socially, and psychologically.

REFERENCES

EXERCISE IN CARDIAC REHABILITATION

1. Leon, A. S., Certo, C., Comoss, P., et al.: Scientific evidence of the value of cardiac rehabilitation with emphasis on patients following myocardial infarction: I. Exercise conditioning component. J. Cardiopulm. Rehabil. 10:79, 1990.
2. Roberts, J. M., Sullivan, M., Froelicher, V. F., et al.: Predicting oxygen uptake from treadmill testing in normal subjects and coronary artery disease patients. Am. Heart J. 108:1454, 1984.
3. Saltin, B., Blomquist, G., Mitchell, J. H., et al.: Response to exercise after bedrest and after training. Circulation 38:1, 1968.
4. Convertino, V., Hung, J., Goldwater, D., et al.: Cardiovascular responses to exercise in middle-aged men after 10 days of bedrest. Circulation 65:134, 1982.

5. Convertino, V. A., Goldwater, D. J., and Sandler, H.: Bedrest-induced peak VO₂ reduction associated with age, gender, and aerobic capacity. Aviat. Space Environ. Med. 57:17, 1986.
6. Fareeduddin, K., and Abelmann, W. H.: Impaired orthostatic tolerance after bedrest in patients with acute myocardial infarction. N. Engl. J. Med. 280:345, 1969.
7. Dudley, G. A., Gollnick, P. D., Convertino, V. A., et al.: Changes of muscle function and size with bedrest. Physiologist 32:S65, 1989.
8. Landin, R. J., Linnemeier, T. S., Rothbaum, D. A., et al.: Exercise testing and training in the elderly. In Wenger, N. K., and Brest, A. N. (eds.): Exercise and the Heart. 2nd ed. Philadelphia, F. A. Davis Co., 1985, p. 206.
9. Wiens, R. D., Lafia, P., Marder, C. M., et al.: Chronotropic incompetence in clinical exercise testing. Am. J. Cardiol. 54:74, 1984.
10. Thoren, P. N.: Activation of left ventricular receptors with nonmedullated vagal afferent fibers during occlusion of a coronary artery in the cat. Am. J. Cardiol. 37:146, 1976.
11. Haskell, W. L., and DeBusk, R.: Cardiovascular responses to repeated treadmill exercise testing soon after myocardial infarction. Circulation 60:1247, 1979.
12. Franciosa, J. A.: Lack of correlation between exercise capacity and indexes of resting left ventricular performance in heart failure. Am. J. Cardiol. 47:33, 1981.
13. Higginbotham, M. B., Morris, K. G., and Conn, E. H.: Determinants of variable exercise performance among patients with severe left ventricular dysfunction. Am. J. Cardiol. 51:52, 1983.
14. Litchfield, R. L., Kerber, R. E., Benge, W., et al.: Normal exercise capacity in patients with severe left ventricular dysfunction: Compensatory mechanisms. Circulation 129:134, 1982.
15. Ben-Ari, E., Fisman, E. Z., Pines, A., et al.: Painful versus silent myocardial ischemia during leg and arm exercise testing in stable angina pectoris. Am. J. Cardiol. 64:300, 1989.
16. Ades, P. A., Grunvald, M. H., Weiss, R. M., et al.: Usefulness of myocardial ischemia as predictor of training effect in cardiac rehabilitation after acute myocardial infarction or coronary artery bypass grafting. Am. J. Cardiol. 63:1032, 1989.
17. Wenger, N. K.: Cardiovascular drugs: Effects on exercise testing and exercise training of the coronary patient. Cardiovasc. Clin. 15:133, 1985.
18. Ho, S. W. C., McComish, M. H., and Taylor, R. R.: Effect of beta-adrenergic blockade on the results of exercise testing related to the extent of coronary artery disease. Am. J. Cardiol. 55:258, 1985.
19. Franklin, B. A., Wrisley, D., Johnson, S., et al.: Chronic adaptations to physical conditioning in cardiac patients. Clin. Sports Med. 3:471, 1984.
20. Froelicher, V. F., Jensen, D., Atwood, E., et al.: Cardiac rehabilitation: Evidence for improvement in myocardial perfusion and function. Arch. Phys. Med. Rehabil. 61:517, 1980.
21. Hung, J., Gordon, E. P., Houston, N., et al.: Changes in rest and exercise myocardial perfusion and left ventricular function 3 to 26 weeks after clinically uncomplicated acute myocardial infarction: Effects of exercise training. Am. J. Cardiol. 54:943, 1984.
22. Rogers, M. A., Yamamoto, C., Hagberg, J. M., et al.: The effect of 7 years of intense exercise training on patients with coronary artery disease. J. Am. Coll. Cardiol. 10:321, 1987.
23. Ehsani, A. A., Biello, D. R., Schultz, R., et al.: Improvement in left ventricular contractile function in patients with coronary artery disease. Circulation. 74:350, 1986.
24. Laslett, L., Paumer, L., and Amsterdam, E. A.: Exercise training in coronary artery disease. Cardiol. Clin. 5:211, 1987.
25. Dubach, P., and Froelicher, V. F.: Cardiac rehabilitation for heart failure patients. Cardiology 76:368, 1989.
26. Squires, R. W., Lavie, C. J., Brandt, T. R., et al.: Cardiac rehabilitation in patients with severe ischemic left ventricular dysfunction. Mayo Clin. Proc. 62:997, 1987.
27. Laslett, L., Paumer, L., Scott-Baier, P., et al.: Efficacy of exercise training in patients with coronary artery disease who are taking propranolol. Circulation 68:1029, 1983.
28. Ciske, P. E., Dressendorfer, R. H., Gordon, S., et al.: Attenuation of exercise training effects in patients taking beta blockers during early cardiac rehabilitation. Am. Heart J. 112:1016, 1986.
29. Health and Public Policy Committee, American College of Physicians: Cardiac rehabilitation services. Ann. Intern. Med. 109:671, 1988.
30. Kallio, V., Hamalainen, H., Hakkila, J., et al.: Reduction in sudden deaths by a multifactorial intervention programme after acute myocardial infarction. Lancet 2:1091, 1979.
31. Oldridge, N. B., Guyatt, G. H., Fischer, M. E., et al.: Cardiac rehabilitation after myocardial infarction. Combined experience of randomized clinical trials. JAMA 260:945, 1988.
32. O'Connor, G. T., Buring, J. E., Yusuf, S., et al.: An overview of randomized trials of rehabilitation with exercise after myocardial infarction. Circulation 80:234, 1989.
33. Yusuf, S., Peto, R., Lewis, J., et al.: Beta blockade during and after myocardial infarction: An overview of randomized trials. Prog. Cardiovasc. Dis. 27:335, 1985.
34. Position paper on cardiac rehabilitation. Recommendations of the American College of Cardiology. J. Am. Coll. Cardiol. 7:451, 1986.
35. Acker, J., and Martin, D.: Angina and ST-segment depression during treadmill and arm ergometer testing in patients with coronary artery disease. Phys. Ther. 68:195, 1988.
36. Levandoski, S. G., Sheldahl, L. M., Silke, N. A., et al.: Cardiorespiratory responses of coronary artery disease patients to arm and leg cycle ergometry. J. Cardiopulm. Rehabil. 10:39, 1990.
37. Detrano, R., and Froelicher, V. F.: Exercise testing: Uses and limitations considering recent studies. Prog. Cardiovasc. Dis. 31:173, 1988.
38. Jugdutt, B. S., Michorowski, B. L., and Kappagoda, C. T.: Exercise training after anterior Q wave myocardial infarction: Importance of regional left ventricular function or topography. J. Am. Coll. Cardiol. 12:362, 1988.
39. Iskandrian, A. S.: Exercise training after anterior Q wave myocardial infarction: Harmful or beneficial? J. Am. Coll. Cardiol. 12:373, 1988.
40. Hamm, L. F., Stull, G. A., and Crow, R. S.: Exercise testing early after myocardial infarction: Historic perspective and current uses. Prog. Cardiovasc. Dis. 28:463, 1986.
41. Sullivan, I. D., Davies, D. W., and Sowton, E.: Submaximal exercise testing early after myocardial infarction: Difficulty of predicting coronary anatomy and left ventricular performance. Br. Heart J. 53:180, 1985.
42. Weiner, D. A.: Predischarge exercise testing after myocardial infarction: Prognostic and therapeutic features. Cardiovasc. Clin. 15:95, 1985.
43. DeBusk, R. F., and Dennis, C. A.: "Submaximal" predischarge exercise testing after acute myocardial infarction: Who needs it? Am. J. Cardiol. 55:499, 1985.
44. Coplan, N. L., Gleim, G. W., and Nicholas, J. A.: Principles of exercise prescription for patients with coronary artery disease. Am. Heart J. 112:145, 1986.
45. Fagan, E. T., Wayne, V. S., and McConachy, D. L.: Serious ventricular arrhythmias in a cardiac rehabilitation programme. Med. J. Aust. 141:421, 1984.
46. Hanson, P., and Nagle, F.: Isometric exercise: Cardiovascular responses in normal and cardiac populations. Cardiol. Clin. 5:157, 1987.
47. Ben-Ari, E., Kellermann, J. J., Rothbaum, D. A., et al.: Effects of prolonged intensive versus moderate leg training on the untrained arm exercise response in angina pectoris. Am. J. Cardiol. 59:231, 1987.
48. Kelemen, M. H., Stewart, K. J., Gillilan, R. E., et al.: Circuit weight training in cardiac patients. J. Am. Coll. Cardiol. 7:38, 1986.
49. Borg, G., and Linderholm, H.: Exercise performance and perceived exertion in patients with coronary insufficiency, arterial hypertension and vasoregulatory asthenia. Acta Med. Scand. 187:17, 1970.
50. Arvan, S.: Exercise performance of the high risk acute myocardial infarction patient after cardiac rehabilitation. Am. J. Cardiol. 62:197, 1988.
51. Laslett, L., Baier, P. S., and Paumer, L.: Ventricular ectopy frequency and complexity are not altered by exercise training in coronary disease patients. Cardiology 70:284, 1983.
52. Van Camp, S. P., and Peterson, R. A.: Identification of the high risk cardiac rehabilitation patient. J. Cardiopulm. Rehabil. 9:103, 1989.
53. Greenland, P., and Chu, J. S.: Efficacy of cardiac rehabilitation services. With emphasis on patients after myocardial infarction. Ann. Intern. Med. 109:650, 1988.
54. DeBusk, R. F., Haskell, W. L., Miller, N. H., et al.: Medically directed at-home rehabilitation soon after clinically uncomplicated acute myocardial infarction: A new model for patient care. Am. J. Cardiol. 55:251, 1985.
55. Van Camp, S. P., and Peterson, R. A.: Cardiovascular complications of outpatient cardiac rehabilitation programs. JAMA 256:1160, 1986.
56. Haskell, W. L.: Cardiovascular complications during exercise training of cardiac patients. Circulation 57:920, 1978.

SECONDARY PREVENTION

57. Rosenberg, L., Kaufman, D. W., Helmrich, S. P., et al.: The risk of myocardial infarction after quitting smoking in men under 55 years of age. N. Engl. J. Med. 313:1511, 1985.
58. Ronnevik, P. K., Gundersen, T., and Abrahamsen, A. M.: Effect of smoking habits and timolol treatment on mortality and reinfarction in patients surviving acute myocardial infarction. Br. Heart J. 54:134, 1985.
59. Sachs, D. P. L.: Cigarette smoking: Health effects and cessation strategies. Clin. Geriatr. Med. 2:337, 1986.
60. Klein, L. W., Pichard, A. D., Holt, J., et al.: Effects of tobacco smoking on the coronary circulation. J Am. Coll. Cardiol. 1:421, 1983.
61. Wilhelmsen, L., Svardsudd, K., Korsan-Bengfsen, K., et al.: Fibrinogen as a risk factor for stroke and myocardial infarction. N. Engl. J. Med. 311:501, 1984.
62. Ockene, J. K., Hosmer, D., Rippe, J., et al.: Factors affecting cigarette smoking status in patients with ischemic heart disease. J. Chron. Dis. 38:985, 1985.
63. Wilcox, N. S., Prochaska, J. O., Velicer, W. F., et al.: Subject characteristics as predictors of self-change in smoking. Addict. Behav. 10:407, 1985.
64. Nett, L. M.: The physician's role in smoking cessation: A present and future agenda. Chest 97:28S, 1990.
65. McNabb, M. E., Ebert, R. V., and McCusker, K.: Plasma nicotine levels produced by chewing nicotine gum. JAMA 248:865, 1982.
66. Hjalmarson, A. I.: Effect of nicotine chewing gum in smoking cessation: A randomized, placebo-control double-blind study. JAMA 252:2835, 1984.
67. Taylor, C. B., Houston-Miller, N., Haskell, W. L., et al.: Smoking cessation after acute myocardial infarction: The effects of exercise training. Addict. Behav. 13:331, 1988.
68. Garvey, A. J., Heinold, J. W., and Rosner, B.: Self-help approaches to smoking cessation: A report from the normative aging study. Addict. Behav. 14:23, 1989.
69. Lipid Research Clinics Program: The lipid research clinics coronary primary prevention trial results: I. Reduction in incidence of coronary heart disease. JAMA 251:351, 1984.
70. Lipid Research Clinics Program: The lipid research clinics coronary pri-

mary prevention trial results: II. The relationship of reduction in incidence of coronary heart disease to cholesterol lowering. JAMA 251:365, 1984.

71. Frick, M. H., Elo, O., Haapa, K., et al.: Primary-prevention trial with gemfibrozil in middle-aged men with dyslipidemia. Safety of treatment, changes in risk factors and incidence of coronary heart disease. N. Engl. J. Med. 317:1237, 1987.

72. Canner, P. L., Berge, K. G., Wenger, N. K., et al.: Fifteen year mortality in Coronary Drug Project patients: Long-term benefit with niacin. J. Am. Coll. Cardiol. 8:1245, 1986.

73. Moise, A., Bourassa, M. G., Theroux, P., et al.: Prognostic significance of progression of coronary artery disease. Am. J. Cardiol. 55:941, 1985.

74. Artzenius, A. C., Krombout, D., Barth, J. D., et al.: Diet, lipoproteins and progression of coronary atherosclerosis: The Leiden intervention trial. N. Engl. J. Med. 312:805, 1985.

75. Blankenhorn, D. H., Nessim, S. A., Johnson, R. L., et al.: Beneficial effects of combined colestipol-niacin therapy on coronary atherosclerosis and coronary venous bypass grafts. JAMA 257:3233, 1987.

76. Brensike, J. F., Levy, R. I., Kelsey, S. F., et al.: Effects of therapy with cholestyramine on progression of coronary atherosclerosis: Results of the NHLBI type II coronary intervention study. Circulation 69:313, 1984.

77. The expert panel: Report of the National Cholesterol Education Program expert panel on detection, evaluation and treatment of high blood cholesterol in adults. Arch. Intern. Med. 184:36, 1988.

78. Garber, A. M.: Where to draw the line against cholesterol. Ann. Intern. Med. 111:625, 1989.

79. Roberts, W. C.: Lipid-lowering after an atherosclerotic event. Am. J. Cardiol. 65:16F, 1990.

80. Tran, Z. V., and Weltman, A.: Differential effects of exercise on serum lipid and lipoprotein levels seen with changes in body weight. JAMA 254:919, 1985.

81. Krauss, R. M.: Exercise, lipoproteins, and coronary artery disease. Circulation 79:1143, 1989.

82. Dyer, A. R., Stamler, J., Paul, O., et al.: Alcohol consumption and seventeen year mortality in the Chicago Western Electric Company Study. Prev. Med. 9:78, 1980.

83. Haskell, W. L., Camargo, C., Williams, P. T., et al.: The effect of cessation and resumption of moderate alcohol intake on serum high-density-lipoprotein subfractions: A controlled study. N. Engl. J. Med 310:805, 1984.

84. Phillipson, B. E., Rothrock, D. W., Connor, W. E., et al.: Reduction of plasma lipids, lipoproteins and apoproteins by dietary fish oils in patients with hypertriglyceridemia. N. Engl. J. Med. 312:1210, 1985.

85. Godin, G.: The effectiveness of interventions in modifying behavioral risk factors of individuals with coronary heart disease. J. Cardiopulm. Rehabil. 9:223, 1989.

86. Stern, T. A.: Psychiatric management of acute myocardial infarction in the coronary care unit. Am. J. Cardiol. 60:59J, 1987.

87. Tesar, G. E., and Hackett, T. P.: Psychiatric management of the hospitalized cardiac patient. In Krantz, D. S., and Blumenthal, J. A. (eds.). Behavioral Assessment and Management of Cardiovascular Disorders. Sarasota, Fla., Professional Resource Exchange, Inc., 1987.

88. Bandura, A.: Self-efficacy mechanism in human agency. Am. Psychol. 37:122, 1982.

89. Ewart, G. K., Taylor, B., Reese, L. B., et al.: Effects of early postmyocardial infarction exercise testing on self-perception and subsequent physical activity. Am. J. Cardiol. 51:1076, 1983.

90. Ewart, C. K., Stewart, K. J., Gillilan, R. E., et al.: Self-efficacy mediates strength gains during circuit weight training in men with coronary artery disease. Med. Sci. Sports Exerc. 18:531, 1986.

91. Taylor, C. B., Bandura, A., Ewart, C. K., et al.: Exercise testing to enhance wives' confidence in their husbands' cardiac capability soon after clinically uncomplicated acute myocardial infarction. Am. J. Cardiol. 55:635, 1985.

92. The Review Panel on Coronary-Prone Behavior and Coronary Heart Disease: Coronary-prone behavior and coronary heart disease: A critical review. Circulation 63:1199, 1981.

93. Mathews, K. A., and Haynes, S. G.: Type A behavior pattern and coronary disease risk: Update and critical evaluation. Am. J. Epidemiol. 123:923, 1986.

94. Ragland, D. R., and Brand, R. J.: Type A behavior and mortality from coronary heart disease. N. Engl. J. Med. 318:65, 1988.

95. Williams, R. B.: Refining the Type A hypothesis: Emergence of the hostility complex. Am. J. Cardiol. 60:27J, 1987.

96. Friedman, M., Thoresen, C. E., Gill, J. J., et al.: Alteration of Type A behavior and its effect on cardiac recurrences in postmyocardial infarction patients: Summary results of the recurrent coronary prevention project. Am. Heart J. 112:653, 1986.

97. American Heart Association: 1989 Heart Facts. Dallas, American Heart Association, 1988.

98. Wittels, E. H., Hay, J. W., and Gotto, A. M.: Medical costs of coronary artery disease in the United States. Am. J. Cardiol. 65:432, 1990.

99. Guillette, W., Judge, R. D., Koehn, E., et al.: Committee report on economic, administrative and legal factors influencing the insurability and employability of patients with ischemic heart disease: 20th Bethesda conference. J. Am. Coll. Cardiol. 14:1010, 1989.

100. Dennis, C., Houston-Miller, N., Schwartz, R. G., et al.: Early return to work after uncomplicated myocardial infarction: Results of a randomized trial. JAMA 260:214, 1988.

101. Pryor, D. B., Bruce, R. A., Chaitman, B. R., et al.: Task force I: Determination of prognosis in patients with ischemic heart disease: 20th Bethesda conference. J. Am. Coll. Cardiol. 14:1016, 1989.

102. Haskell, W. L., Brachfeld, N., Bruce, R. A., et al.: Task force II: Determination of occupational working capacity in patients with ischemic heart disease: 20th Bethesda conference. J. Am. Coll. Cardiol. 14:1025, 1989.

103. Haskell, W. L.: Design and implementation of cardiac conditioning programs. In Wenger, N. K., and Hellerstein, H. K. (eds.): Rehabilitation of the Coronary Patient. New York. John Wiley & Sons, 1978, pp. 214–215.

104. Bureau of Labor Statistics. Handbook of Labor Statistics. Washington, D.C. U.S. Department of Labor, 1988.

105. DeBusk, R. F.: Determination of cardiac impairment and disability: 20th Bethesda conference. J. Am. Coll. Cardiol. 14:1043, 1989.

106. Smith, G. R., and O'Rourke, D. F.: Return to work after a first myocardial infarction: A test of multiple hypotheses. JAMA 259:1673, 1988.

107. Picard, M. H., Dennis, C., Schwartz, R. G., et al.: Cost-benefit of early return to work after uncomplicated myocardial infarction. Am. J. Cardiol. 63:1308, 1989.

ORGANIZATION OF REHABILITATION SERVICES

108. Wenger, N. K., and Brest, A. N., (eds). Exercise and the Heart. 2nd ed. Philadelphia, F. A. Davis Co., 1985.

109. Beckie, T.: A supportive-educative telephone program: Impact on knowledge and anxiety after coronary artery bypass graft surgery. Heart Lung 18:46, 1989.

110. Wiggins, N. C.: Education and support for the newly diagnosed cardiac family: A vital link in rehabilitation. J. Adv. Nurs. 14:63, 1989.

111. De Busk, R. F., Taylor, C. B., and Agras, W. C.: Comparison of treadmill exercise testing and psychologic stress testing soon after myocardial infarction. Am. J. Cardiol. 43:907, 1979.

112. DeBusk, R. F., Valdez, R., Houston, N., and Haskell, W.: Cardiovascular responses to dynamic and static effort soon after myocardial infarction: Application to occupational work assessment. Circulation 58:368, 1978.

113. Wilke, N. A., Sheldahl, S. G., Levandoski, S. G., et al.: Weight carrying versus handgrip exercise testing in men with coronary artery disease. Am. J. Cardiol. 64:736, 1989.

114. Bertagnoli, K., Hanson, P., and Ward, A.: Attenuation of exercise-induced ST depression during combined isometric and dynamic exercise in coronary artery disease. Am. J. Cardiol. 65:314, 1990.

115. Cooper, A. J.: Myocardial infarction and advice on sexual activity. Practitioner 229:575, 1985.

116. Tardif, G. S.: Sexual activity after a myocardial infarction. Arch. Phys. Med. Rehabil. 70:763, 1989.

117. Papadopoulos, C., Shelley, S. I., Piccolo, M., et al.: Sexual activity after coronary bypass surgery. Chest 90:681, 1986.

118. Fontana, A. F., Kerns, R. D., Rosenberg, R. L., et al.: Support, stress, and recovery from coronary heart disease: A longitudinal causal model. Health Psychol. 8:175, 1989.

The Cardiomyopathies and Myocarditides: Toxic, Chemical, and Physical Damage to the Heart

by JOSHUA WYNNE, M.D., and EUGENE BRAUNWALD, M.D.

The cardiomyopathies constitute a group of diseases, often of unknown etiology, in which the dominant feature is involvement of the heart muscle itself.[1] They are unique in that they are not the result of ischemic,[2]* hypertensive, congenital, valvular, or pericardial diseases (Table 43–1). While the diagnosis of cardiomyopathy requires the exclusion of these etiological factors, the features of cardiomyopathy are often sufficiently distinctive—both clinically and hemodynamically—to allow a positive diagnosis to be made.[1] With increasing awareness of this condition by clinicians, along with improvements in diagnostic techniques, cardiomyopathy is being recognized as a significant cause of morbidity and mortality.[1,3] Whether the result of improved recognition or of other factors, the incidence of cardiomyopathy appears to be increasing.[3,4]

A variety of schemes have been proposed for classifying the cardiomyopathies.[1,5,6] Perhaps the most widely recognized classification scheme is that promulgated by the World Health Organization.[5] In this scheme, the term *cardiomyopathy* is restricted to diseases solely involving the heart muscle that are of unknown cause; other diseases that affect the myocardium but are of known cause or are part of a generalized systemic disorder are termed *specific heart muscle diseases.*[5,6] While conceptually sound, this classification system may be overly rigid for the clinician, because the *clinical* features of a given cardiomyopathy are often identical to those of one of the specific heart muscle diseases.[1] We prefer to use the term

secondary cardiomyopathy to identify those patients with a specific heart muscle disease that clinically closely simulates an idiopathic or "primary" cardiomyopathy. Three basic categories of functional impairment have been described (Table 43–2 and Fig. 43–1): (1) *dilated* (formerly called congestive), characterized by ventricular dilatation, contractile dysfunction, and often symptoms of congestive heart failure; (2) *hypertrophic*, recognized by inappropriate left ventricular hypertrophy, often with asymmetrical involvement of the septum, usually with preserved or enhanced contractile function; and (3) *restrictive*, marked by impaired diastolic filling, in some cases with endocardial scarring of the ventricle. The distinctions between these three functional categories are not absolute, and there is often overlap; in particular, patients with hypertrophic cardiomyopathy also have increased wall stiffness (as a consequence of the myocardial hypertrophy) and thus present some of the features of a restrictive cardiomyopathy.

ENDOMYOCARDIAL BIOPSY

Evaluation of the pediatric or adult patient suspected of suffering from a cardiomyopathy has been facilitated by the use of endomyocardial biopsy (p. 1489).[7-9] Using a flexible bioptome, the clinician easily and safely may obtain tissue samples from the right (and occasionally left) ventricle via a transvenous (or transarterial) approach (Fig. 43–2). The availability of disposable transfemoral bioptomes has further facilitated endomyocardial biopsy.[7] Two-dimensional echocardiography may help guide the placement of the bioptome and reduce radiation exposure.[10] Endomyocardial biopsy results in a small tissue sample (average size 1–4 mm), and multiple

---

* The term *ischemic cardiomyopathy* refers to the condition in which ischemic heart disease causes diffuse fibrosis or multiple infarctions and leads to heart failure with left ventricular dilatation; it may or may not be associated with angina pectoris (p. 1351).

TABLE 43–1   IMPORTANT CAUSES OF CARDIOMYOPATHY AND MYOCARDITIS

1. **Inflammatory**
   a. Infective
      Viral
      Rickettsial
      Bacterial
      Mycobacterial
      Spirochetal
      Fungal
      Parasitic
   b. Noninfective
      Collagen diseases
      Granulomatous
      Kawasaki

2. **Metabolic**
   a. Nutritional
      Thiamine
      Kwashiorkor
      Pellagra
      Scurvy
      Hypervitaminosis D
      Obesity
      Selenium deficiency
      Carnitine deficiency
   b. Endocrine
      Acromegaly
      Thyrotoxicosis
      Myxedema
      Uremia
      Cushing's disease
      Pheochromocytoma
      Diabetes mellitus
   c. Altered metabolism
      Gout
      Oxalosis
      Porphyria
   d. Electrolyte imbalance

3. **Toxic**
   a. Cobalt
   b. Alcohol
   c. Bleomycin
   d. Adriamycin
   e. Phenothiazines and antidepressants
   f. Antimony compounds
   g. Carbon monoxide
   h. Lead
   i. Emetine and dehydroemetine
   j. Chloroquine
   k. Lithium
   l. Cyclophosphamide
   m. Hydrocarbons
   n. Catecholamines
   o. Phosphorus
   p. Mercury
   q. Insect stings
   r. Snake bites
   s. Paracetamol
   t. Reserpine
   u. Corticosteroids
   v. Cocaine
   w. Methylsergide

4. **Infiltrative**
   a. Amyloidosis
   b. Hemochromatosis
   c. Neoplastic
   d. Glycogen storage disorders
   e. Sarcoidosis
   f. Mucopolysaccharidosis
   g. Fabry disease
   h. Whipple disease
   i. Gaucher disease
   j. Sphingolipidoses

5. **Fibroplastic**
   a. Endomyocardial fibrosis
   b. Endocardial fibroelastosis
   c. Löffler's fibroplastic endocarditis
   d. Carcinoid

6. **Hematological**
   a. Sickle cell anemia
   b. Polycythemia vera
   c. Thrombotic thrombocytopenic purpura
   d. Leukemia

7. **Hypersensitivity**
   a. Methyldopa
   b. Penicillin
   c. Sulfonamides
   d. Tetracycline
   e. Phenindione
   f. Phenylbutazone
   g. Antituberculous drugs
   h. Giant cell myocarditis
   i. Cardiac transplant rejection

8. **Genetic**
   a. Hypertrophic cardiomyopathy
      With gradient
      Without gradient

   b. Neuromuscular
      Duchenne muscular dystrophy
      Facioscapulohumeral muscular dystrophy
      Limb-girdle dystrophy of Erb
      Myotonia dystrophica
      Friedreich's ataxia
      Kearns-Sayre syndrome
      Nemaline cardiomyopathy
      Multicore cardiomyopathy

9. **Miscellaneous acquired**
   a. Postpartum cardiomyopathy
   b. Obesity

10. **Idiopathic**
    a. Idiopathic dilated cardiomyopathy
    b. Idiopathic restrictive cardiomyopathy
    c. Idiopathic hypertrophic cardiomyopathy
    d. Idiopathic right ventricular cardiomyopathy

11. **Physical agents**
    a. Heat stroke
    b. Hypothermia
    c. Radiation
    d. Tachycardia

samples are often required, because pronounced topographic variations may be found within the myocardium.[11] It remains controversial as to which patients should be subjected to biopsy, but there is general agreement that biopsy may be of benefit in certain specific situations (Table 43–3).[7,11] Although on occasion endomyocardial biopsy may identify a specific etiological agent in an individual patient with cardiac disease of uncertain cause (Tables 43–4 and 43–5), the clinical utility of routine biopsy in cardiomyopathy remains uncertain, particularly since no definitive pattern has been found in dilated cardiomyopathy (Table 43–6 and Fig. 43–2).[7,11] Although interpretation of biopsy specimens had been plagued by a high degree of interobserver variability, the recent adoption of a near-universally accepted set of histological definitions, the *Dallas criteria*, appears to have substantially improved agreement.[7,11,12] It is hoped that newer histochemical and molecular biological techniques may expand further the diagnostic utility of endomyocardial biopsy.[7]

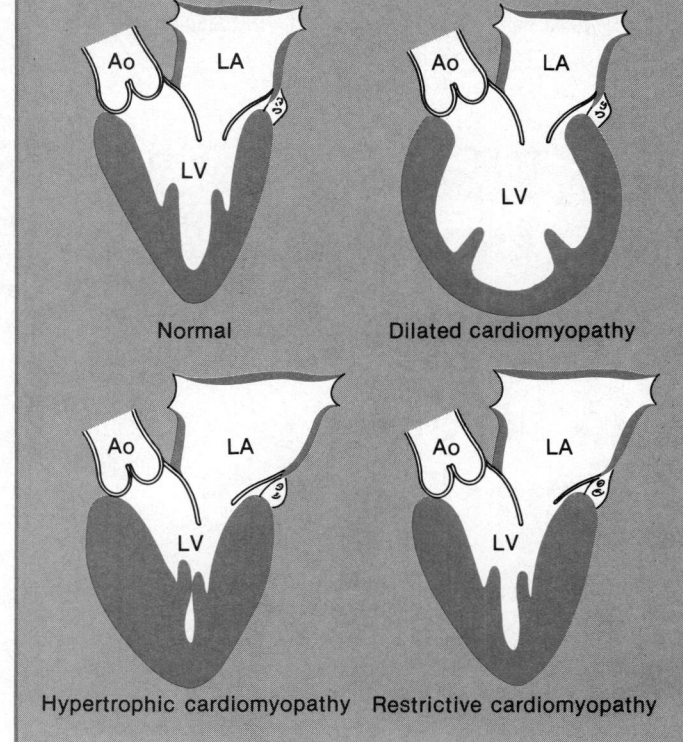

FIGURE 43–1. Diagram comparing three morphologic types of cardiomyopathies of unknown cause. Ao = Aorta, LA = left atrium, LV = left ventricle. (From Waller, B. F.: Pathology of the cardiomyopathies. J. Am. Soc. Echocardiog. *1:*4, 1988.)

TABLE 43-2 FUNCTIONAL CLASSIFICATION OF THE CARDIOMYOPATHIES

	DILATED	RESTRICTIVE	HYPERTROPHIC
Symptoms	Congestive heart failure, particularly left-sided Fatigue and weakness Systemic or pulmonary emboli	Dyspnea, fatigue Right-sided congestive heart failure Signs and symptoms of systemic disease: amyloidosis, iron storage disease, etc.	Dyspnea, angina pectoris Fatigue, syncope, palpitations
Physical Examination	Moderate to severe cardiomegaly; S_3 and S_4 Atrioventricular valve regurgitation, especially mitral	Mild to moderate cardiomegaly: S_3 or S_4 Atrioventricular valve regurgitation; inspiratory increase in venous pressure (Kussmaul's sign)	Mild cardiomegaly Apical systolic thrill and heave; brisk carotid upstroke S_4 common Systolic murmur that increases with Valsalva maneuver
Chest Roentgenogram	Moderate to marked cardiac enlargement, especially left ventricular Pulmonary venous hypertension	Mild cardiac enlargement Pulmonary venous hypertension	Mild to moderate cardiac enlargement Left atrial enlargement
Electrocardiogram	Sinus tachycardia Atrial and ventricular arrhythmias ST-segment and T-wave abnormalities Intraventricular conduction defects	Low voltage Intraventricular conduction defects AV conduction defects	Left ventricular hypertrophy ST-segment and T-wave abnormalities Abnormal Q waves Atrial and ventricular arrhythmias
Echocardiogram	Left ventricular dilatation and dysfunction Abnormal diastolic mitral valve motion secondary to abnormal compliance and filling pressures	Increased left ventricular wall thickness and mass Small or normal-sized left ventricular cavity Normal systolic function Pericardial effusion	Asymmetrical septal hypertrophy (ASH) Narrow left ventricular outflow tract Systolic anterior motion (SAM) of the mitral valve Small or normal-sized left ventricle
Radionuclide Studies	Left ventricular dilatation and dysfunction (RVG)	Infiltration of myocardium (^{201}Tl) Small or normal-sized left ventricle (RVG) Normal systolic function (RVG)	Small or normal-sized left ventricle (RVG) Vigorous systolic function (RVG) Asymmetrical septal hypertrophy (RVG or ^{201}Tl)
Cardiac Catheterization	Left ventricular enlargement and dysfunction Mitral and/or tricuspid regurgitation Elevated left- and often right-sided filling pressures Diminished cardiac output	Diminished left ventricular compliance "Square root sign" in ventricular pressure recordings Preserved systolic function Elevated left- and right-sided filling pressures	Dimished left ventricular compliance Mitral regurgitation Vigorous systolic function Dynamic left ventricular outflow gradient

RVG = Radionuclide ventriculogram; ^{201}Tl = thallium-201

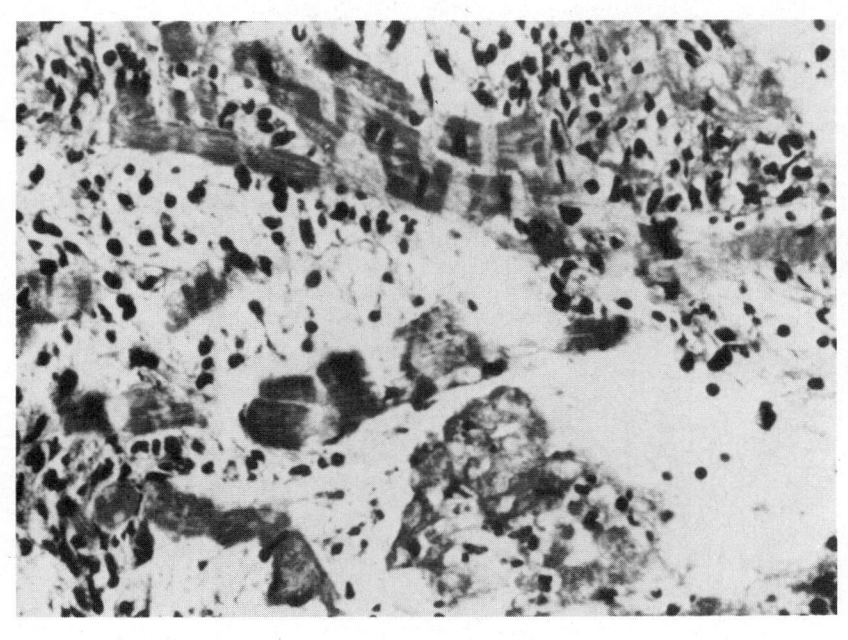

FIGURE 43-2. Endomyocardial biopsy in myocarditis (hematoxylin and eosin, original magnification ×100). Diffuse mononuclear cellular infiltrate with loss and necrosis of myocytes is present. (From Salvi, A., Di Lenarda, A., Dreas, L., et al.: Immunosuppressive treatment in myocarditis. Int. J. Cardiol. 22:329, 1989.)

TABLE 43-3 CLINICAL INDICATIONS FOR ENDOMYOCARDIAL BIOPSY

Definite
Monitoring of cardiac allograft rejection
Monitoring of anthracycline cardiotoxicity
Possible
Detection and monitoring of myocarditis
Diagnosis of secondary cardiomyopathies
Differentiation between restrictive and constrictive heart disease
Uncertain
Unexplained, life-threatening ventricular tachyarrhythmias
AIDS
Formulation of prognosis in idiopathic dilated cardiomyopathy

From Mason, J. W., and O'Connell, J. B.: Clinical merit of endomyocardial biopsy. Circulation 79:971, 1989, reprinted by permission of the American Heart Association, Inc.

TABLE 43-4 SPECIFIC DIAGNOSES THAT CAN BE CONFIRMED BY MYOCARDIAL BIOPSY

Cardiac allograft rejection	Fabry disease of the heart	Henoch-Schönlein purpura
Myocarditis	Carcinoid disease	Rheumatic carditis
Giant cell myocarditis	Irradiation injury	Chagasic cardiomyopathy
Doxorubicin cardiotoxicity	Glycogen storage disease	Chloroquine cardiomyopathy
Cardiac amyloidosis	Cardiac tumors of cardiac origin	Lyme carditis
Cardiac sarcoidosis	Cardiac tumors of noncardiac origin	Carnitine deficiency cardiomyopathy
Cardiac hemochromatosis	Kearns-Sayre syndrome	Right ventricular lipomatosis
Endocardial fibrosis	Cytomegalovirus infection	Hypereosinophilic syndrome
Endocardial fibroelastosis	Toxoplasmosis	

From Mason, J. W., and O'Connell, J. B.: Clinical merit of endomyocardial biopsy. Circulation 79:971, 1989, reprinted by permission of the American Heart Association, Inc.

TABLE 43-5 ENDOMYOCARDIAL BIOPSY DIAGNOSES FOR WHICH THERE IS A PROVEN THERAPY

Cardiac rejection*	Endocardial fibrosis*	Certain malignancies involving the heart
Cardiac sarcoidosis*	Incipient anthracycline cardiotoxicity*	Carnitine deficiency cardiomyopathy
Giant cell myocarditis*	Cardiac hemochromatosis	Lyme carditis
Hypereosinophilic syndrome involving the heart*	Certain infections involving the heart	

*Diagnoses that usually cannot reliably be made without cardiac biopsy.
From Mason, J. W., and O'Connell, J. B.: Clinical merit of endomyocardial biopsy. Circulation 79:971, 1989, reprinted by permission of the American Heart Association, Inc.

TABLE 43-6 ENDOMYOCARDIAL BIOPSY CHARACTERISTICS

DILATED CARDIOMYOPATHY	HYPERTROPHIC CARDIOMYOPATHY
Light microscopy	Light microscopy
Increase in myofiber size	Endocardial thickening and fibrosis
Attenuation of cells	Marked myocardial hypertrophy
Hyperchromatic, irregular shaped nuclei	Large, bizarre nuclei
Interstitial, focal, perivascular fibrosis	Myofiber disorganization
Electron microscopy	Interstitial fibrosis
Hypertrophic changes	Electron microscopy
Increased number of sarcomeres and mitochondria	Myofibrillar disarray
Large, lobulated nuclei	Increased side-to-side junctions
Z-band abnormalities	Increased cell branching
Irregular invaginations of sarcolemma	Increased glycogen
Widened, convoluted, intercalated discs	
Degenerative changes	**MYOCARDITIS**
Myofilament loss	Light and electron microscopy
Aggregation of glycogen and mitochondria	Inflammatory infiltrate, usually lymphocytic
Pleomorphic mitochondria	Necrosis or degeneration of adjacent myocytes
Myelin figures, lipid vacuoles	Uninvolved, normal myocardium
	Absence of severe chronic myocardial changes

From Leatherbury, L., Chandra, R. S., Chapiro, S. R., and Perry, L. W.: Value of endomyocardial biopsy in infants, children, and adolescents with dilated or hypertrophic cardiomyopathy and myocarditis. Reprinted from the American College of Cardiology. J. Am. Coll. Cardiol. 12:1547, 1988.

IDIOPATHIC DILATED CARDIOMYOPATHY

Dilated cardiomyopathy (DCM) is a syndrome characterized by cardiac enlargement and impaired systolic function of one or both ventricles. While formerly it was called congestive cardiomyopathy, the term *dilated cardiomyopathy* is now preferred, since the earliest abnormality usually is ventricular enlargement and systolic contractile dysfunction, with congestive heart failure often (but not invariably) developing later. In an occasional patient, the predominant finding is that of contractile dysfunction with only a mildly dilated left ventricle.[13]

Although the cause is not definable in many cases, more than 75 specific diseases of heart muscle can produce the clinical manifestations of DCM.[1] It is likely that this condition represents a final common pathway that is the end result of myocardial damage produced by a variety of toxic, metabolic, or infectious agents. Alcohol, for example, may lead to severe cardiac dysfunction and may produce clinical, hemodynamic, and pathological findings identical to those present in idiopathic dilated cardiomyopathy (see p. 1402). The course of idiopathic dilated cardiomyopathy is usually one of progressive deterioration, with three-fourths of patients dying within 5 years after the onset of symptoms, although a minority improve, with a reduction in cardiac size and longer survival (Fig. 43–3).[13] A variety of clinical predictors of patients at enhanced risk of death in DCM have been identified (Table 43–7).[1,14-24] However, the predictive reliability of any single feature is not high. Because of considerable variability, it may be difficult to predict with any accuracy the clinical course and outcome in any individual patient.[25] Surprisingly, there is not a good correlation between the extent of impairment of ventricular function and symptoms or mortality,[26] although once advanced biventricular failure has developed, the prognosis is poor.[27] Specific endomyocardial biopsy morphological findings may offer some predictive information regarding prognosis.[25] Children with DCM appear to have a prognosis similar to that of comparable adults; it is controversial whether age at presentation in childhood has any prognostic significance.[28,29]

PATHOLOGY

POSTMORTEM EXAMINATION. This reveals enlargement and dilatation of all four chambers; the ventricles are

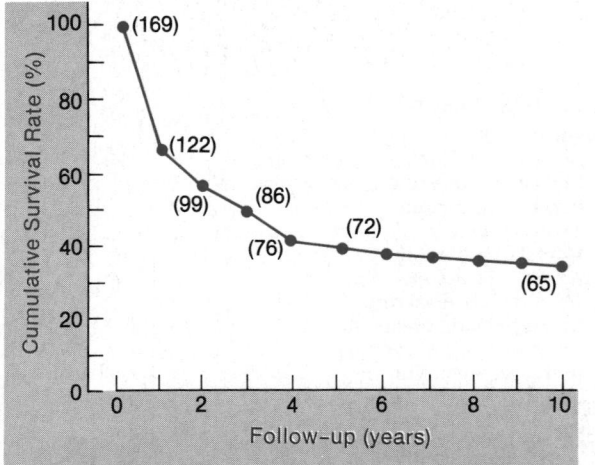

FIGURE 43–3. Ten-year survival curve of 169 patients with dilated cardiomyopathy. Numbers in parentheses are patients alive at the beginning of interval. (From Diaz, R. A., Obasohan, A., and Oakley, C. M.: Prediction of outcome in dilated cardiomyopathy. Br. Heart J. *58*:393, 1987.)

TABLE 43–7   FACTORS ASSOCIATED WITH REDUCED SURVIVAL IN DILATED CARDIOMYOPATHY

S_3
Left ventricular conduction delay
Elevation of filling pressures
Absence of left ventricular thickening
Age > 55 years
Cardiac enlargement
Depressed cardiac output
Depressed ejection fraction
Depressed serum sodium levels
Elevated serum norepinephrine levels
Functional class
Ventricular arrhythmias
Large thallium defects
Myocardial biopsy findings
Ventricular shape (more spherical)

more dilated than the atria[30] (Fig. 43–4). While the thickness of the ventricular wall is increased in some cases, the degree of hypertrophy is often inadequate for the severe dilatation present.[31] The development of left ventricular hypertrophy appears to have a protective or beneficial role in dilated cardiomyopathy, because it may serve to reduce systolic wall stress and protect against further cavity dilatation.[1,32] Scars, usually small, occasionally are found in the left or right ventricle.[30] The cardiac valves are intrinsically normal, and intracavitary thrombi, particularly in the ventricular apex, are common.[31] The coronary arteries are usually normal. The right ventricle is preferentially involved in some cases of dilated cardiomyopathy, sometimes on a familial basis.

HISTOLOGICAL EXAMINATION. Microscopic study reveals extensive areas of interstitial and perivascular fibrosis, particularly involving the left ventricular subendocardium. Small areas of necrosis and cellular infiltrate are seen on occasion, but these typically are not prominent features.[30,31,33] Some myocardial cells are hypertrophied, while others are atrophied (Fig. 43–5).[31] Cardiac biopsy specimens obtained during life by a transvenous or transthoracic approach demonstrate a variety of similar abnormalities, including interstitial fibrosis, cellular infiltrates, cellular hypertrophy, and myocardial cell degeneration.[34,34a,34b] No viruses or other etiological agents have been identified with any regularity in tissue from patients with DCM. Particularly disappointing has been the failure to identify any immunological, histochemical, morphological, ultrastructural, or microbiological markers that might be used to establish the diagnosis of idiopathic dilated cardiomyopathy or to clarify its cause.

ETIOLOGY

It is likely that DCM represents a common expression of myocardial damage that has been produced by a variety of as yet unestablished myocardial insults. While the cause or causes remain unclear,[35] at least four conditions, if not etiologically linked, appear to lower the threshold for the development of cardiomyopathy, and it is possible that in some cases a combination of factors results in severe myocardial damage. Chronic excessive ingestion of alcohol (p. 1402), pregnancy (Chap. 59), systemic hypertension (Chap. 28), and a variety of infections (pp. 1425 to 1434) may each be associated with myocardial dysfunction and congestive failure and are important causes of secondary DCM. Cigarette smoking has also been found to be associated with DCM,[36] independent of its important role as a risk factor in the development of ischemic heart disease.

The precise etiology of contractile dysfunction at the cellular level in patients with DCM remains unclear. While abnormalities in calcium handling by cardiomyopathic tissue is a common finding,[36a] the cause is unestablished.[37] There is a

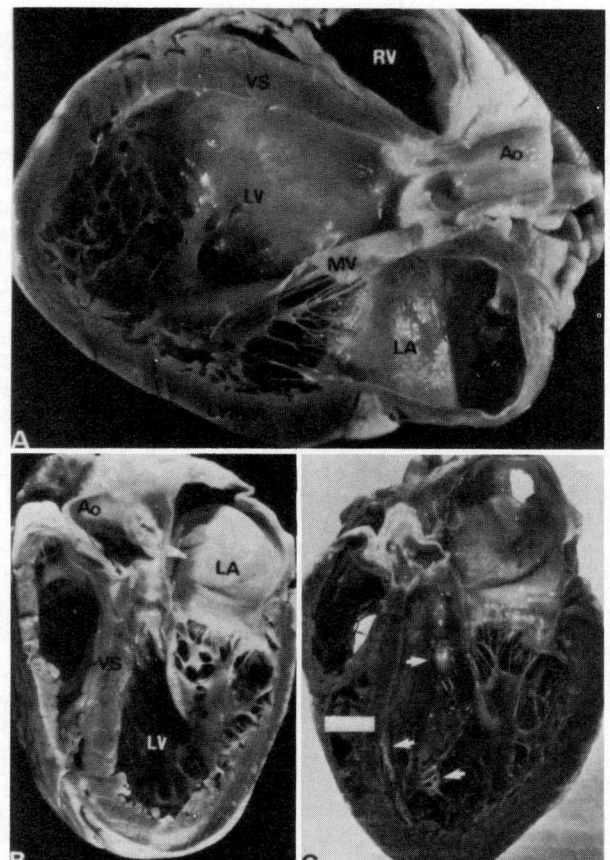

FIGURE 43-4. *A-C,* Three different hearts from patients with dilated cardiomyopathy cut in tomographic planes simulating two-dimensional echocardiographic parasternal long-axis views. In each case, left ventricle (LV) is markedly dilated, but chamber walls vary in thickness. *C,* Whitish endocardial plaques (arrows) ("milk spots") probably represent organized thrombus. Ao = Aorta, LA = left atrium, LVFW = left ventricular free wall, MV = mitral valve, RV = right ventricle, VS = ventricular septum. (From Waller, B. F.: Pathology of the cardiomyopathies. J. Am. Soc. Echocardiog. *1*:4, 1988.)

seems that there is enhanced inhibition of this system in DCM patients, perhaps accounting for their depressed contractile function.[44]

Regardless of possible cellular causes of contractile dysfunction in DCM, there has been wide speculation that an episode of subclinical viral myocarditis initiates an autoimmune reaction that culminates in the development of full-blown DCM.[45-47] While this hypothesis is inviting, it remains largely unsupported; it has been estimated that only 15 per cent of patients with myocarditis progress to DCM.[48] Little evidence exists to suggest prior viral infections in most patients with unequivocal cardiomyopathy.[49] However, there are patients who exhibit the clinical features of DCM in whom endomyocardial biopsy reveals evidence of an inflammatory myocarditis. The reported frequency of finding evidence of an inflammatory infiltrate in DCM varies widely and undoubtedly depends largely on criteria used for diagnosis; using rigorous criteria, only about 5 to 10 per cent of patients with DCM have biopsy evidence of myocarditis.[46,49-51] Other evidence favoring the concept that DCM is a postviral disorder includes the presence of high antibody viral titers,[48] viral-specific RNA sequences,[52] and apparent viral particles[48] in patients with "idiopathic" dilated cardiomyopathy. Dilated cardiomyopathy has been reported as *peripartum cardiomyopathy* when it occurs in this period. This condition is discussed on p. 1798.

Although the findings have not been completely reproducible, abnormalities of both humoral and cellular immunity have been found in patients with DCM, and there is a suggestion of an association with specific HLA antigens.[53] Circulating antimyocardial antibodies[54-57] and abnormalities of various T cells, including cytotoxic T cells, suppressor T lymphocytes, and natural killer cells,[1] have been found in some,[58-62] but not all,[63] studies. It has been suggested that these putative immunological abnormalities may be the consequence of prior viral myocarditis. Viral components may be incorporated into the cardiac sarcolemma, only to serve as an antigenic source that directs the immune response to attack the myocardium.[48]

A variety of other possible causes has been proposed, although none is accepted as *the* cause of DCM (Table 43-8). Thus, endocrine abnormalities as well as the effects of chemicals or toxins, notably doxorubicin, have been suggested as possible etiological factors.[64] It has been suggested that microvascular hyperreactivity (spasm) may lead to myocellular necrosis and scarring, with resultant heart failure, although this remains speculative.[1] From a clinical standpoint, the more important causes of secondary DCM include alcohol, cocaine, human immunodeficiency virus, metabolic abnormalities,

reduction in density of membrane-associated beta-adrenoceptors[38,39] that may be a consequence of the development of anti-beta-adrenoreceptor autoantibodies.[40,41] An alteration in the signal transmission pathway by which the receptors stimulate the contractile apparatus appears likely to occur.[42,43] It

FIGURE 43-5. Diagram showing the various findings commonly observed in sections of left ventricular wall in patients with idiopathic dilated cardiomyopathy. Some myocardial cells are larger than normal, others are smaller than normal and others have been replaced by fibrous tissue, which also is increased in the interstitium between the myocardial cells. (From Roberts, W. C., Siegel, R. J., and McManus, B. M.: Idiopathic dilated cardiomyopathy: Analysis of 152 necropsy patients. Am. J. Cardiol. *60*:1340, 1987.)

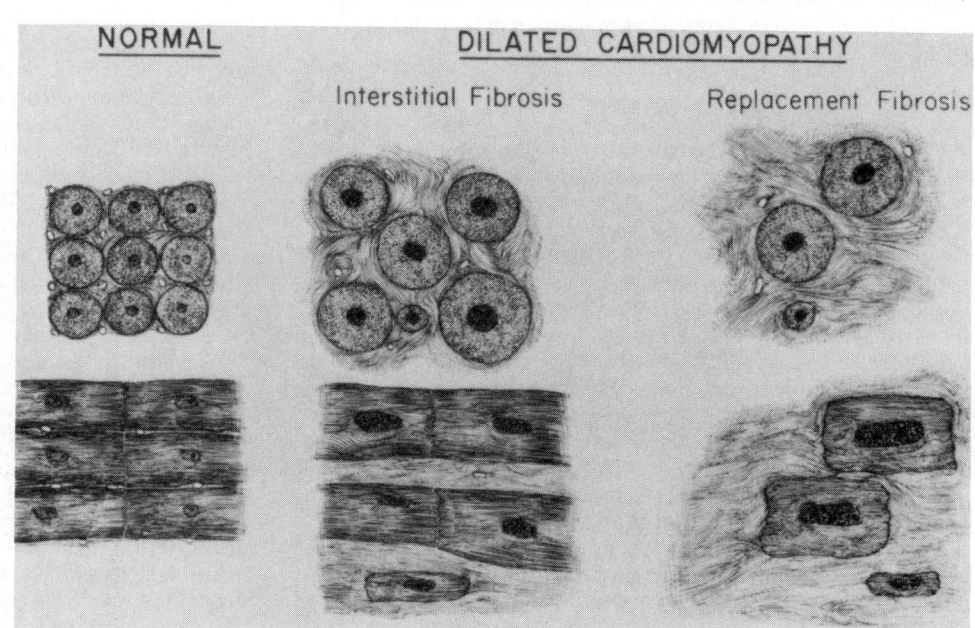

**TABLE 43-8 POSSIBLE CAUSES OR PRECIPITATING FACTORS
IN DILATED CARDIOMYOPATHY**

Hereditary
    X-linked
Nutritional and related deficiencies
    Thiamine deficiency
    Selenium deficiency
    Carnitine deficiency
    Hypophosphatemia
    Hypocalcemia
Toxins and drugs
    Ethanol
    Anthrocyclines
    5-Fluorouracil
Vasoactive agents and microvascular spasm
Decreased coronary flow reserve
Tachyarrhythmia
Calcium overload
Hypocalcemia
Oxygen free radical damage
Pregnancy
Infection
    Viral myocarditis
    HIV virus
    Subacute and chronic myocarditis
Immune/autoimmune mechanisms
Degeneration of cardiac ganglia
Alterations in cardiac cytoskeleton

Adapted from Abelmann, W. H., and Lorell, B. H.: The challenge of cardiomyopathy. Reprinted by permission of the American College of Cardiology.
J. Am. Coll. Cardiol. 13:1219, 1989.

and the cardiotoxicity of a variety of anticancer drugs (especially Adriamycin and 5-fluorouracil).

In contrast to hypertrophic cardiomyopathy, in which it is common, familial transmission is rare in DCM. Occasional instances of autosomal dominant as well as X-linked inheritance in DCM have been reported[65-70]; one intriguing familial metabolic deficiency is that of carnitine, with improvement occurring in the myopathy with carnitine repletion.[71]

An increase of the α subunits of the inhibitory guanine nucleotide-binding protein ($G_{i\alpha}$) has been reported to occur in the membranes of myocytes from failing hearts[72] (Fig. 13-11, p. 360). This abnormality has been shown to be more profound in myocardial membranes from hearts with dilated than in those with ischemic cardiomyopathy.[73] This increase in $G_{i\alpha}$ is associated with a striking reduction of basal adenylate cyclase activity and of the positive inotropic effects of isoproterenol and of the phosphodiesterase inhibitor milrinone (p. 505). These findings suggest that the increase of $G_{i\alpha}$ might contribute to the reduced effects of endogenous catecholamines in DCM.

CLINICAL MANIFESTATIONS

HISTORY. Symptoms usually develop gradually in patients with DCM. Some patients may be asymptomatic yet have left ventricular dilatation for months or even years.[74,75] An unrecognized illness may result in left ventricular dilatation, which is clinically recognized only years later when symptoms develop or when routine chest roentgenography demonstrates cardiomegaly. Other patients, after recovery from what appears to be a systemic viral infection, develop symptoms of heart failure for the first time. In still others, severe heart failure develops acutely during an episode of myocarditis; while some recovery occurs, chronic manifestations of diminished cardiac reserve persist and heart failure reappears months or years later. Although patients of any age may be affected, the disease is most common in middle age and is more frequent in men than in women.

The most striking symptoms are those of left ventricular failure. Fatigue and weakness due to diminished cardiac output are common. Exercise intolerance is common and relates, at least in part, to reduced skeletal muscle perfusion as well as

histological and biochemical alterations in the exercising muscle groups.[76-78] Right heart failure is a late and ominous sign and is associated with a particularly poor prognosis (p. 445). Chest pain occurs in one-fourth to one-half of patients and may suggest concomitant ischemic heart disease.[79] There is a reduction in the vasodilator reserve of the coronary microvasculature in DCM, suggesting that subendocardial ischemia may play a role in the genesis of chest pain despite angiographically normal coronary arteries.[80] Chest pain secondary to pulmonary embolism and abdominal pain secondary to congestive hepatomegaly are frequent in the late stages of the illness.

PHYSICAL EXAMINATION. This usually reveals variable degrees of cardiac enlargement and findings of congestive heart failure. The systolic blood pressure is usually normal or low, and the pulse pressure is narrow, reflecting a diminished stroke volume. Pulsus alternans (p. 24) is common when severe left ventricular failure is present. The jugular veins are frequently distended. Prominent a and v waves are visible— the latter a late manifestation of the presence of tricuspid valvular regurgitation. The liver may be engorged and pulsatile. Peripheral edema and ascites may be present. Wheezing resulting from bronchospasm may be found, apparently as a consequence of bronchial hyperresponsiveness and dilatation of the bronchial vessels.[81]

The precordium usually reveals left and, occasionally, right ventricular impulses, but the heaves are not sustained, as they are in patients with considerable ventricular hypertrophy. The apical impulse is usually displaced laterally, reflecting left ventricular dilatation. A presystolic a wave may be palpable. The second heart sound is usually normally split, although paradoxical splitting (p. 47) may be detected in the presence of left bundle branch block, an electrocardiographic finding that is not unusual in dilated cardiomyopathy. If pulmonary hypertension is present the pulmonary component of the second heart sound may be accentuated, and the splitting may be narrow. Presystolic gallop sounds (S_4) often precede the development of overt congestive heart failure. Ventricular gallops (S_3) are the rule once cardiac decompensation occurs, and a summation gallop is often heard when there is tachycardia. Systolic murmurs are common and are usually due to mitral or, less commonly, tricuspid valvular regurgitation.[74] Mitral regurgitation results from enlargement and abnormal motion of the mitral annulus; ventricular dilatation with resultant distortion of the geometry of the subvalvar apparatus ("papillary muscle dysfunction") plays a lesser role.[82-84] Gallop sounds and regurgitant murmurs can often be elicited or intensified by isometric handgrip exercise with its attendant enhancement of systemic vascular resistance and impedance to left ventricular outflow (p. 62). Systemic emboli resulting from dislodgment of intracardiac thrombi from the left atrium and ventricle and pulmonary emboli that originate in the venous system of the legs are common late complications. Specific abnormalities of blood flow in the left ventricle can be detected by Doppler ultrasonography in patients with echocardiographically demonstrable thrombi.[85]

NONINVASIVE EXAMINATION. To identify potentially reversible secondary causes of dilated cardiomyopathy, several basic screening biochemical tests are often indicated, including determination of serum phosphorus (hypophosphatemia), serum calcium (hypocalcemia), serum creatinine and urea nitrogen (uremia), and serum iron (hemochromatosis).[86] The *chest roentgenogram* usually reveals left ventricular enlargement, although generalized cardiomegaly is often seen. Left ventricular failure may result in signs of pulmonary venous hypertension (i.e., pulmonary vascular redistribution) as well as interstitial and even alveolar edema.[86] Pleural effusions may be present, and the azygos vein and superior vena cava may be dilated when right heart failure supervenes. The *electrocardiogram* often shows sinus tachycardia when heart failure is present. The entire spectrum of atrial and ventricular tachyarrhythmias and atrioventricular conduction disturbances may be seen. Poor R-wave progression and intraventricular conduction abnormalities, especially left bundle branch block, are common.[87] Anterior Q waves may be present when there is extensive left ventricular fibrosis, even without a discrete myocardial scar.[87] ST-segment and T-wave abnormalities are common, as are P-wave changes, especially left atrial abnormality.[87] Ambulatory Holter monitoring often demonstrates ventricular arrhythmias, with about half of monitored patients with DCM exhibiting nonsustained ventricular tachycardia.[88] There is no consensus that complex or frequent ventricular arrhythmias predict sudden (presumably arrhythmic) death, although they do appear to predict total mortality.[89-91] Perhaps ventricular arrhythmias as detected on Holter monitoring are a marker for the extent of myocardial damage in DCM and therefore are *associated* with sudden death without necessarily being its *cause*.[89] In rare cases, particularly in children, recurrent and/or incessant supraventricular or ventricular tachyarrhythmias may actually be the *cause* (rather than the result) of ventricular dysfunction.[92-94] In those cases, restoration of sinus rhythm or slowing of the heart rate may be therapeutic.

Two-dimensional and Doppler *echocardiography* are useful in assessing the degree of impairment of left ventricular function and for excluding concomitant valvular or pericardial disease (Chap. 4).[86] In addition to examining all four cardiac valves for evidence of structural or functional abnormalities, echocardiography allows evaluation of the size of the ventricular cavity and thickness of the ventricular walls and estimation of ventricular function. A pericardial effusion may sometimes be demonstrated. Doppler studies are useful in delineating the severity of mitral (and tricuspid) regurgitation.[74,86,95] *Thallium-201 imaging* at rest may be helpful in distinguishing left ventricular enlargement caused by DCM from that caused by coronary artery disease,[96] although there is not complete agreement on this point.[74,86] However, newer experimental isotopes and positron scanning show great promise for the future[97,98] (Chap. 11). Scanning with gallium or antimyosin antibody may help to identify patients more likely to have myocarditis on biopsy.[99-101]

Radionuclide ventriculography, like echocardiography, reveals increased end-diastolic and end-systolic left ventricular volumes, reduced ejection fractions in both ventricles, and wall-motion abnormalities.[74] In many cases, however, it is not necessary to carry out serial *batteries* of noninvasive tests in order to follow patients with DCM and evaluate their response to treatment.

CARDIAC CATHETERIZATION AND ANGIOCARDIOGRAPHY. The left ventricular end-diastolic, left atrial, and pulmonary artery wedge pressures are usually elevated. Modest degrees of pulmonary arterial hypertension are common.[74] Advanced cases may demonstrate right ventricular dilatation and failure as well, with resultant elevation of the right ventricular end-diastolic, right atrial, and central venous pressures.

Left ventriculography demonstrates enlargement of this chamber, typically with diffuse reduction in wall motion. Segmental wall motion abnormalities during systole and diastole are not uncommon and may simulate the angiographic findings in ischemic heart disease.[102] However, prominent localized wall disorders are more characteristic of ischemic heart disease, while diffuse, global dysfunction is more typical of DCM. The ejection fraction is reduced and the end-systolic volume is increased as a result of the impairment of left ventricular contractility. Sometimes left ventricular thrombi may be visualized within the left ventricle as intracavitary filling defects. Mild mitral regurgitation is often present. On occasion, it may be difficult to distinguish left ventricular dilatation secondary to severe mitral regurgitation from DCM with secondary mitral regurgitation.

Coronary arteriography usually reveals normal vessels, although coronary dilatory capacity may be impaired.[79,80] This examination may be of particular value in patients with abnormal Q waves on the electrocardiogram or regional left ventricular wall motion abnormalities on noninvasive testing.

Coronary arteriography helps to distinguish between myocardial infarction as a result of obstructive coronary artery disease and extensive localized myocardial fibrosis secondary to severe DCM in the absence of coronary artery obstruction.

MANAGEMENT

Since the cause of idiopathic dilated cardiomyopathy is unknown, specific therapy is not possible. Treatment, therefore, is for heart failure, as discussed in Chapter 17. Physical, dietary, and pharmacological interventions may help to control symptoms; only cardiac transplantation (Chap. 18) and specific vasodilator therapy (enalapril and hydralazine plus nitrates) have been shown to prolong life.[1,103-105] Because of the possible link between DCM, microvascular circulatory abnormalities, and abnormal myocardial calcium handling, the use of calcium antagonists is of interest. Diltiazem in particular appears to be safe and preliminary results regarding clinical utility are encouraging, although myocardial depression is an important potential side effect of the calcium antagonists as a group.[1,106] Diuretics may improve symptoms of pulmonary congestion and sometimes can lower ventricular filling pressures without compromising cardiac output.[107]

Certain treatment considerations specific to DCM are worthy of discussion. Because of recent evidence that activation of the sympathetic nervous system may have deleterious cardiac effects (rather than being an important compensatory mechanism as traditionally thought), beta-adrenoceptor blockade (usually with metoprolol) has been suggested as a means to prolong survival.[108] Results to date have been generally favorable, and improvement in symptoms (sometimes dramatic) and survival have been suggested.[108-111] Beta-adrenoceptor blockade has been surprisingly well tolerated, with infrequent aggravation of heart failure (which, on occasion, may be profound). The mechanism of beneficial action of beta blockers may relate to five factors: (1) negative chronotropic effect with reduced myocardial oxygen demand, (2) reduced myocardial damage due to catecholamines, (3) improved diastolic relaxation, (4) inhibition of sympathetically mediated vasoconstriction, and (5) increase in myocardial beta-adrenoceptor density.[112] Assessment of the true clinical efficacy of beta-adrenergic blockage and its impact on mortality in DCM must await the results of an ongoing multicenter trial.[113]

While there is no evidence that antiarrhythmic agents prolong life or prevent sudden death in DCM, it is appropriate to use them in the treatment of symptomatic arrhythmias.[26] Because of the adverse effects of most available agents, many of which depress myocardial contractility and have a proarrhythmic effect (Chap. 23), treatment should be individualized, with both efficacy and toxicity carefully monitored.[114] Unfortunately, electrophysiological testing is of limited utility in DCM, since it is positive in a minority of patients at risk. The lack of inducibility of ventricular tachyarrhythmias does not identify a low-risk group, and pharmacological suppression of provoked arrhythmias does not necessarily predict freedom from recurrences.[115-117] The recording of late potentials by the signal-averaged electrocardiogram has not proved to be especially helpful either.[118] Implantation of the internal defibrillator (p. 750) should be considered in appropriate candidates with symptomatic ventricular tachyarrhythmias. Even in the absence of controlled clinical trials demonstrating their efficacy,[119] anticoagulants are recommended in patients with DCM and heart failure.[120] Anticoagulants should be so used even without direct clinical or echocardiographic evidence of thrombus formation if there are no specific contraindications to these agents.[1,121] In those patients with chronic heart failure secondary to DCM and lymphocytic infiltrate on myocardial biopsy, treatment with corticosteroids and immunosuppressive agents has been advocated. Prednisone therapy does not appear to have a clinically important effect on symptoms, exercise performance, or ejection fraction (in more than just the short term) and is associated with significant complications in half the patients so treated.[122,123] Routine clinical use of immunosuppressive therapy thus cannot be recommended at present, although it is being tested in a prospective randomized clinical trial at the time of this writing.

Surgical repair, mitral annuloplasty, or replacement of regurgitant valves has been attempted in some patients in whom progressive atrioventricular valvular regurgitation (almost always mitral) appeared to result in progressive cardiac enlargement and failure. The results of operation are usually less than satisfactory because of the degree of preexisting cardiac dysfunction and damage. In appropriate patients, cardiac transplantation may be an alternative (Ch. 18), with a 5-year survival rate of about 80 per cent compared with less than 5 per cent in nontransplanted patients.[124]

ALCOHOLIC CARDIOMYOPATHY

Chronic excessive consumption of alcohol may be associated with congestive heart failure, hypertension, arrhythmias, and sudden death; it is the major cause of secondary, nonischemic dilated cardiomyopathy in the Western world.[125,126] It is estimated that two-thirds of the adult population use alcohol to some extent, and more than 10 per cent are heavy users. Therefore, it is not surprising that alcoholic cardiomyopathy is a major problem.[126] Whereas the course in many cases of idiopathic dilated cardiomyopathy relentlessly goes downhill, ceasing consumption of alcohol early in the course of alcoholic cardiomyopathy may halt the progression or even reverse left ventricular contractile dysfunction.[1,127,128]

The consumption of alcohol may result in myocardial damage by three basic mechanisms: (1) a presumed direct toxic effect of alcohol or of its metabolites; (2) nutritional effects, most commonly in association with thiamine deficiency which leads to beriberi heart disease (p. 461); and (3) rarely, toxic effects due to additives in the alcoholic beverage (cobalt)[129,130] (p. 1403). There had been speculation that alcohol caused myocardial damage only through dietary deficiencies, but it is now clear that alcoholic cardiomyopathy occurs in the absence of nutritional deficiencies.[131]

Typical Oriental beriberi may coexist with alcoholic cardiomyopathy, although it is no longer seen with any frequency.[126,130] The distinguishing features of each include peripheral vasodilatation and high output heart failure, often right-sided, in the former and reduced contractility with typically left-sided low output failure in the latter.[1]

Alcohol results in acute as well as chronic depression of myocardial contractility and may produce demonstrable cardiac dysfunction even when ingested by normal individuals in quantities consumed in social drinking[132,133]; compensatory mechanisms such as vasodilatation or sympathetic stimulation are invoked and they may mask the direct myocardial depression produced by alcohol.[130,133,134]

The mechanism of the cardiac depression produced by alcohol remains unclear, and a direct causal relationship between alcohol and the development of cardiomyopathy, while highly likely, has not been proved. In acute studies, alcohol and its metabolite acetaldehyde have been shown to interfere with a number of membrane and cellular functions that involve the transport and binding of calcium, mitochondrial respiration, myocardial lipid metabolism, myocardial protein synthesis, and myofibrillar ATPase.[130,131,135-137] Studies in isolated ferret papillary muscles have shown that ethanol in concentrations similar to those occurring in intoxicated humans depresses myocardial contractility by interfering with excitation-contraction coupling through inhibition of the interaction between calcium and the myofilaments.[138] The accumulation of metabolites of ethanol in the myocardium may interfere with normal myocardial lipid metabolism and may play a role in the pathogenesis of alcohol-induced myocardial damage.[139] The roles that other associated electrolyte imbalances (hypokalemia, hypophosphatemia, hypomagnesemia) may play in alcohol-mediated damage have not been clarified.[131] The major unanswered question is precisely how these metabolic effects result in persistent myocardial injury.

PATHOLOGY. The gross and microscopic pathological findings are nonspecific and similar to those observed in idiopathic dilated cardiomyopathy, although certain ultrastructural details suggest alcoholic cardiomyopathy.[140] Edema of the vascular wall and perivascular fibrosis of the intramyocardial coronary arteries has been observed, and it has been suggested that the myocardial damage in alcoholic cardiomyopathy may be the result of ischemia produced by disease of the small intramural coronary arteries.

Clinical Manifestations

Alcoholic cardiomyopathy most commonly occurs in men 30 to 55 years of age who have been heavy consumers of whiskey, wine, or beer, usually for more than 10 years.[126,140a] While alcoholic cardiomyopathy may be observed in the homeless, malnourished, "skid row" alcoholic man who is a candidate for and often suffers from alcoholic cirrhosis, many patients are well-nourished individuals of middle and even upper socioeconomic status without liver disease or peripheral neuropathy. Therefore, unless a high index of suspicion is maintained, it may be easy to miss a history of alcohol abuse. Persistent questioning of the patient and particularly the relatives of patients with unexplained cardiomegaly or cardiomyopathy is often required to elicit a history of alcoholism.

It is frequently possible to demonstrate mild depression of cardiac function in chronic alcoholics even before cardiac dysfunction becomes clinically manifested.[141] Abnormalities of both systolic function (reduced ejection fraction) and diastolic function (increased myocardial wall stiffness) have been demonstrated in alcoholic patients without cardiac symptoms by a variety of invasive and noninvasive techniques.[141-142a] The typical findings are those of left ventricular dilatation, with reduced ejection fraction.[131] While overt alcoholic liver disease and cardiac involvement often do not occur together, even cirrhotic patients without signs or symptoms of heart disease have inducible evidence of asymptomatic myocardial disease.[141,142]

The development of symptoms may be insidious, although some patients have acute and florid left-sided congestive heart failure. A paroxysm of atrial fibrillation is a relatively frequent initial presenting finding.[130] More advanced cases involve findings of biventricular failure, with left ventricular dysfunction usually dominating. Dyspnea, orthopnea, and paroxysmal nocturnal dyspnea are frequently observed. Palpitations and syncope due to tachyarrhythmias, usually supraventricular, are occasionally present. Angina pectoris does not occur unless there is concomitant coronary artery disease or aortic stenosis.

PHYSICAL EXAMINATION. This usually reveals a narrow pulse pressure, often with an elevated diastolic pressure secondary to excessive peripheral vasoconstriction. There is cardiomegaly, and protodiastolic (S_3) and presystolic (S_4) gallop sounds are common. An apical systolic murmur of mitral regurgitation due to papillary muscle dysfunction is often found. The severity of right heart failure varies, but jugular venous distention and peripheral edema are common. A concomitant skeletal muscle myopathy is a frequent finding.[131,135]

LABORATORY EXAMINATION. The *chest roentgenogram* in the advanced case demonstrates considerable cardiac enlargement (Fig. 43–6), pulmonary congestion, and pulmonary venous hypertension (p. 217). Pleural effusions are often seen. *Electrocardiographic abnormalities* are common and are frequently the only indication of alcoholic heart disease during the preclinical phase. Alcoholic patients without other evidence of heart disease often are seen after developing palpitations, chest discomfort, or syncope typically following a binge of alcohol consumption on a weekend, particularly during the year-end holiday season. This is dubbed the "holiday heart syndrome." The most common arrhythmia observed is atrial fibrillation, followed by atrial flutter and frequent ventricular premature contractions.[143] Alcohol consumption may even predispose to atrial fibrillation or flutter in nonalcoholics.[131,143] Hypokalemia may play a role in the genesis of some of these arrhythmias. Supraventricular arrhythmias are also frequently observed in patients with overt alcoholic cardiomyopathy. Sudden, unexpected death is not uncommon in young adult alcoholics, and it is likely that ventricular fibrillation is responsible.[144]

Atrioventricular conduction disturbances (most commonly first degree heart block), bundle branch block, left ventricular hypertrophy, and repolarization abnormalities are common electrocardiographic findings.[126,130,145] Prolongation of the Q-T

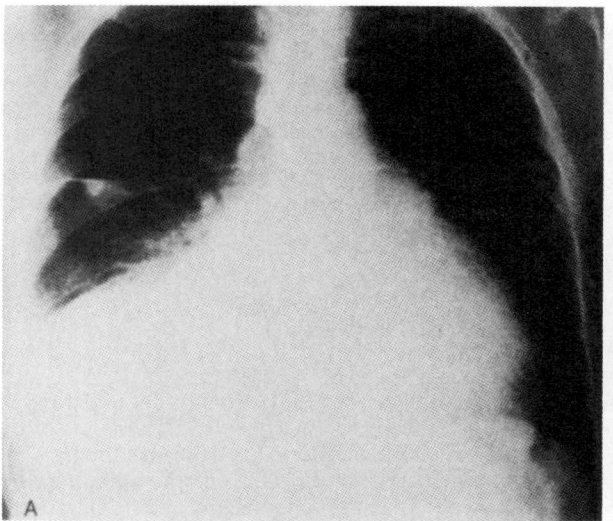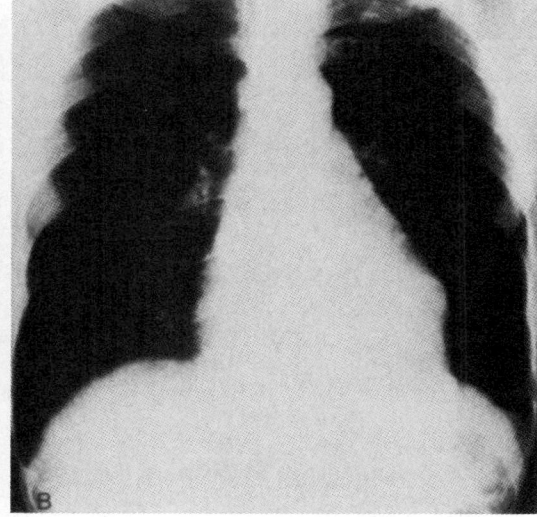

FIGURE 43–6. Chest radiographs of a 36-year-old man with alcoholic cardiomyopathy. *A*, Before abstention, there was marked cardiomegaly and a right pleural effusion. *B*, After 6 weeks of abstention the radiograph was virtually normal. (From Stevenson, L. W., and Perloff, J. K.: The dilated cardiomyopathies: Clinical aspects. Cardiol. Clin. 6:194, 1988.)

interval is noted frequently. ST-segment and T-wave changes are often restored to normal within several days after cessation of alcohol consumption.

The hemodynamic findings observed at cardiac catheterization and the assessment of left ventricular function by noninvasive methods (echocardiography and isotope angiography) resemble those found in idiopathic dilated cardiomyopathy.

The *natural history* of alcoholic cardiomyopathy depends on the drinking habits of the patient. Total abstinence in the early stages of the disease may lead to resolution of the manifestation of congestive heart failure and a return of heart size toward normal,[127,130] although patients with severe heart failure may show no improvement in function or prognosis. Continued alcohol consumption leads to further myocardial damage and fibrosis, with the development of refractory congestive heart failure. Death may also be due to arrhythmia, heart block, and systemic or pulmonary embolism.

MANAGEMENT. The key to the long-term treatment of alcoholic cardiomyopathy is *immediate and total abstinence,* as early in the course of the disease as possible.[146] This may be quite effective (Table 43–6). The prognosis in patients who continue to drink, particularly if they have been symptomatic for a long period, is poor.[130] In the overall population of patients with alcoholic cardiomyopathy, between 40 and 50 per cent succumb within a 3- to 6-year period.[130,145] Prolonged bed rest is also thought to result in functional improvement, although its major benefit may simply be the decreased alcohol consumption.[130]

The management of acute episodes of congestive heart failure is similar to that of idiopathic dilated cardiomyopathy. For patients with severe congestive heart failure, it is prudent to administer thiamine on the chance that beriberi may be contributing to the heart failure. Whether to use chronic anticoagulation (as is usually recommended for idiopathic dilated cardiomyopathy) is controversial[129,143]; we usually do not prescribe coumadin for risk of bleeding due to noncompliance, trauma, and overanticoagulation due to hepatic dysfunction. Animal studies have suggested that ribose and verapamil may improve the myocardial depression found in alcoholic cardiomyopathy,[147,148] but their efficacy in humans is not established.

COBALT CARDIOMYOPATHY

A previously unrecognized syndrome of fulminating congestive heart failure appeared in the mid-1960's, first in Canada, and subsequently in the United States and Europe.[130] The disease was found in people who drank a particular brand of beer to which cobalt sulfate had been added as a foam stabilizer. After cobalt had been removed from the process, no more cases of the disease were reported.

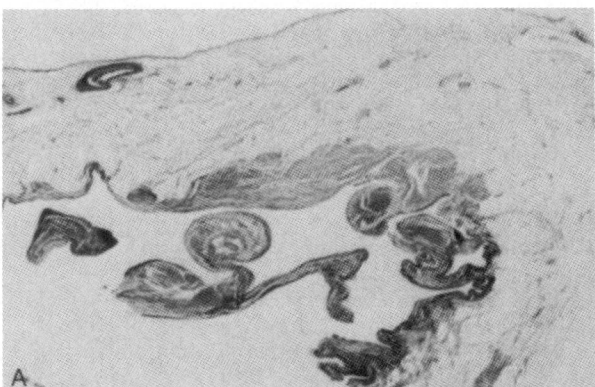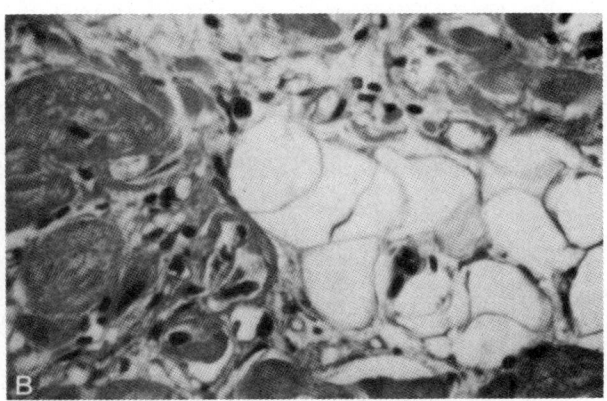

FIGURE 43–7. *A,* Section through the anterior free wall of the right ventricle in a patient with right ventricular cardiomyopathy and sudden death, showing massive lipomatous infiltration (azan, ×5). *B,* Closeup of residual myocardium, showing histological evidence of myocardial degeneration and lipomatous infiltration (hematoxylin-eosin, ×300). (Reproduced by permission from Thiene, G., Nava, A., Corrado, D., et al.: Right ventricular cardiomyopathy and sudden death in young people. N. Engl. J. Med. *318*:129, 1988.)

RIGHT VENTRICULAR CARDIOMYOPATHY (ARRHYTHMOGENIC RIGHT VENTRICULAR DYSPLASIA)

Right ventricular cardiomyopathy is marked by partial or total replacement of right ventricular muscle by adipose or fibrous tissue (Fig. 43–7) and may be associated with ventricular tachyarrhythmias of right ventricular origin (left bundle branch configuration of the QRS)[149–151] (p. 706). The cause of the myocardial changes is unclear — both congenital and acquired factors have been suggested,[150] although probably it is distinct from Uhl's disease, which is marked by extreme thinning of the ventricular wall. Typical clinical features include male predominance, normal physical examination, symptoms of palpitations and syncope, and a risk of sudden death.[149–152] Noninvasive and invasive evaluation demonstrates a dilated, poorly contractile right ventricle, usually with a normal left ventricle.[149–155] Antiarrhythmic therapy appears to control the ventricular arrhythmias, but the influence of therapy on the risk of sudden death is unknown.[149,151,152,156] Electrode catheter ablation (p. 654) has also been successful in patients with drug-resistant ventricular tachycardia.[157]

Hypertrophic Cardiomyopathy

Although first described over one hundred years ago, the unique features of hypertrophic cardiomyopathy (HCM) were not studied systematically until the late 1950's.[158–163] Characteristic findings are inappropriate myocardial hypertrophy, often predominantly involving the interventricular septum of a nondilated left ventricle, with hyperdynamic ventricular function.[161] A distinctive clinical feature was soon recognized in some patients with HCM: a dynamic pressure gradient in the subaortic area that divided the left ventricle into a high-pressure apical region and a lower-pressure subaortic region. Hence the terms *idiopathic hypertrophic subaortic stenosis (IHSS)* and *muscular subaortic stenosis* were suggested, although subsequent findings have indicated that most patients (probably about three-quarters) do not, in fact, ever have obstruction to left ventricular outflow. Since hypertrophy often occurs in the absence of a pressure gradient, the characteristic feature of HCM is myocardial hypertrophy that is out of proportion to the hemodynamic load. Importantly, valvular aortic stenosis or systemic hypertension usually is absent.

The physiological characteristics of HCM differ substantially from those of dilated cardiomyopathy (Table 43–9). The most characteristic pathophysiological abnormality in HCM is *diastolic* dysfunction[158] (see also p. 402 and p. 446). Thus, HCM is characterized by abnormal stiffness of the left ventricle during diastole, with resultant impaired ventricular filling. This abnormality in diastolic relaxation results in elevation of the left ventricular end-diastolic pressure with resulting pulmonary congestion and dyspnea, the most common symptom in HCM, despite typically hyperdynamic left ventricular function. The disease appears to be genetically transmitted in somewhat more than half the patients as a single gene autosomal dominant trait[162] with variable expression

and penetrance.[163,164] In the remainder of patients, the disease appears to occur spontaneously.[165] Evidence of the disease is found in about one-fourth of the first-degree relatives of a patient with HCM; in many of the relatives the disease is milder than in the propositus, the degree of hypertrophy is less and it is more localized, and outflow gradients are usually lacking.[164,166] Symptoms are often absent or minimal, and the disease is detected only by echocardiography. The overall prevalence of HCM is low, and has been estimated to average between 0.02 and 0.2 per cent of the population.[4,167]

PATHOLOGY

MACROSCOPIC EXAMINATION. This typically discloses a marked increase in myocardial mass, and the ventricular cavities are small (Figs. 43–1 and 43–8).[161] The left ventricle is usually more involved with the hypertrophic process than is the right.[168] The atria are dilated and often hypertrophied,[169] reflecting the high resistance to filling of the ventricles caused by diastolic dysfunction and the effects of atrioventricular valve regurgitation. The pattern and extent of left ventricular hypertrophy in HCM vary greatly from patient to patient, and a characteristic feature is heterogenicity in the amount of hypertrophy evident in different regions of the left ventricle.[161] A typical feature found in more than half of the patients with HCM is disproportionate involvement of the interventricular septum and anterolateral wall compared with the posterior segment of the free wall of the left ventricle.[161,170] When hypertrophy is largely localized to the septum, the process has been called asymmetric septal hypertrophy (ASH). Other patterns of hypertrophy are not uncommon, including concentric left ventricular hypertrophy, with symmetrical thickening of the left ventricle, involving the septum and free wall equally. This variant may occasionally be seen in patients with the genetically transmitted as well as the sporadic forms of hypertrophic cardiomyopathy.[161] In some patients with HCM there is substantial hypertrophy in unusual locations, such as the posterior portion of the septum, the posterobasal free wall, and the midventricular level.[170–172] Asymmetric left ventricular hypertrophy is not limited to HCM; 5 to 10 per cent of adult patients with other acquired or congenital defects (especially associated with right ventricular pressure overload) may present with nonuniform, especially septal, hypertrophy.[161]

Apical HCM. A variant with predominant involvement of the apex is common in Japan and is estimated to represent a quarter of Japanese HCM patients.[173] In other parts of the world, apical HCM is uncommon.[174] Typical features include a characteristic spade-like configuration of the left ventricle during angiographic study,[175] giant negative T waves in the precordial electrocardiographic leads, the absence of an intraventricular pressure gradient, mild symptoms, and a generally benign course.[173,176]

Two variants of HCM are seen particularly in elderly women. The first, termed hypertensive hypertrophic cardiomyopathy of the elderly, is characterized by severe concentric left ventricular hypertrophy and small left ventricular cavity size, and is associated with hypertension.[177–180] The second

TABLE 43–9 DIFFERENCES IN SYSTOLIC AND DIASTOLIC FUNCTION IN DILATED (CONGESTIVE) AND HYPERTROPHIC CARDIOMYOPATHY

	DILATED CARDIOMYOPATHY	HYPERTROPHIC CARDIOMYOPATHY
Left ventricular volume		
End-diastolic	Increased	Normal
End-systolic	Markedly increased	Decreased
Left ventricular mass	Increased	Markedly increased
Mass/volume ratio	Decreased	Increased
Systolic function		
Ejection fraction	Decreased	Normal or increased
Myocardial shortening	Decreased	Increased
Wall stress	Increased	Decreased
Diastolic function		
Chamber stiffness	Decreased	Increased
Myocardial stiffness	Increased	Increased

From Chatterjee, K.: Pathophysiology of cardiomyopathy. In Giles, T. D., and Sander, G. E. (eds.): Cardiomyopathy. Middleton, MA, PSG Publishing Co., 1988, p. 65.

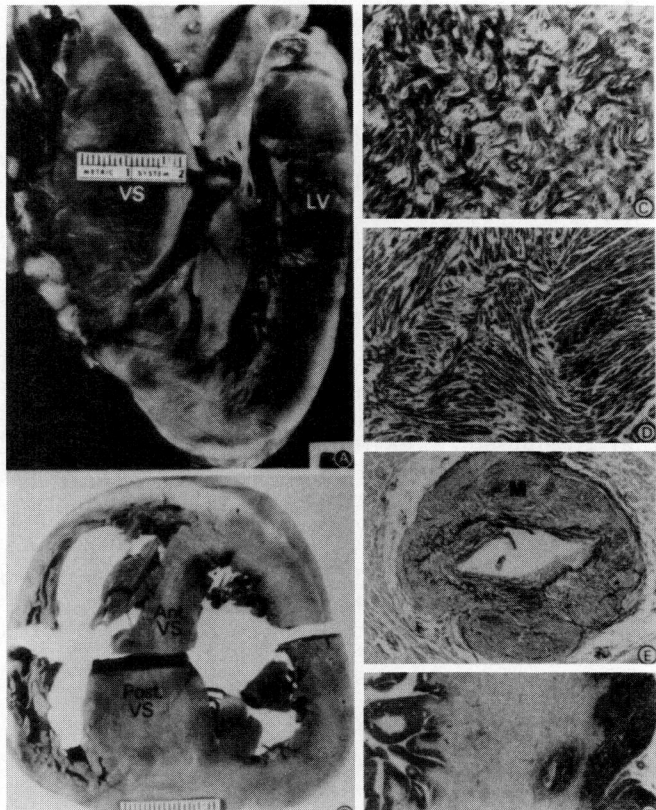

FIGURE 43–8. Morphological components of the underlying disease process in hypertrophic cardiomyopathy. A, Gross heart specimen sectioned in a cross-sectional plane similar to that of the echocardiographic (parasternal) long axis. The pattern of left ventricular hypertrophy is asymmetric, with wall thickening confined primarily to the anterior ventricular septum (VS), which bulges into the left ventricular outflow tract. LV denotes left ventricular free wall. (Reproduced from Maron and Roberts with the permission of the publisher.) B, Heart specimen with a different pattern of hypertrophy; here marked left ventricular wall thickening is localized to the posterior portion of the ventricular septum (Post. VS), whereas the anterior septum (Ant. VS) is only minimally thickened. (Reproduced from Maron with the permission of the publisher.)

C and D, Histology characteristic of the left ventricle in hypertrophic cardiomyopathy. In C, the septal myocardium shows a markedly disordered architecture with adjacent hypertrophied cardiac muscle cells arranged at perpendicular and oblique angles to each other. In D, bundles of hypertrophied cells show a disorganized, interwoven arrangement; E, Intramural coronary artery with an apparently narrowed lumen and thickened wall due primarily to medial (M) hypertrophy; F, Extensive scarring of ventricular septum that is transmural in distribution. (Reproduced by permission from Maron, B. J., Bonow, R. O., Cannon, R. O., et al.: Hypertrophic cardiomyopathy: Interrelations of clinical manifestations, pathophysiology, and therapy. N. Engl. J. Med. 316:780, 1987.)

presentation also is marked by an especially small left ventricular cavity but with relatively mild hypertrophy; other findings include marked anterior displacement of the mitral valve, extensive submitral (annular) calcification, a left ventricular outflow gradient, and the late appearance of severe and progressive symptoms.[181] In contrast to young patients with HCM, the elderly patient is more likely to show a localized septal bulge just below the aortic valve and is less likely to have marked abnormalities in the orientation and curvature of the septum.[182]

A variety of disparate conditions may present similar gross morphological features of HCM, including hyperparathyroidism, infants of diabetic mothers, neurofibromatosis, generalized lipodystrophy, lentiginosis, pheochromocytoma, Friedreich's ataxia, and Noonan syndrome.[161,183–186] Rarely, the findings may be simulated by amyloid or tumor involvement of the septum.[187]

HISTOLOGY. Microscopic findings in HCM are distinc-tive, with myocardial hypertrophy and gross disorganization of the muscle bundles resulting in a characteristic whorled pattern; abnormalities are found in the cell-to-cell arrangement (disarray), and disorganization of the myofibrillar architecture within a given cell[163,188] (Fig. 43–8). Fibrosis is usually prominent[189] and may be extensive enough to produce grossly visible scars.[161] Foci of disorganized cells are often interspersed between areas of hypertrophied but otherwise normal-appearing muscle cells. While abnormally arranged cardiac muscle cells initially were considered specific for HCM, it is now recognized that they may be found in a variety of acquired and congenital heart conditions.[161] What is unique about the disarray in HCM is its ubiquity and frequency. Almost all HCM patients have some degree of disarray and most have involvement of 5 per cent or more of the myocardium; in contrast, disarray in non-HCM patients (when it occurs) usually involves only about 1 per cent of the myocardium (Fig. 43–9).[161]

Abnormal intramural coronary arteries, with a reduction in the size of the lumen and thickening of the vessel wall, are common in HCM,[190] occurring in over 80 per cent of patients (Fig. 43–8).[161,191] This abnormality occurs most frequently in the ventricular septum; it also has been observed in infants who died of this condition and could represent a congenital component of the condition. The prominence of abnormal intramural coronary arteries in areas of extensive myocardial fibrosis is consistent with the hypothesis that these abnormalities may be responsible for the development of myocardial ischemia.[191]

ETIOLOGY

The cause of the myocardial hypertrophy in HCM remains unknown. There are suggestive data linking abnormal myocardial calcium kinetics and specific features of HCM, particularly the abnormalities of diastolic function.[158,192,193] Abnormal calcium fluxes with a resultant increase in intracellular calcium concentration appear to occur as a consequence of an increase in the number of calcium channels.[194] This in turn produces (in an as yet undefined process) hypertrophy and cellular disarray.[192]

Other suggested etiologies of HCM include (1) abnormal sympathetic stimulation because of heightened responsiveness of the heart to or excessive production of circulating

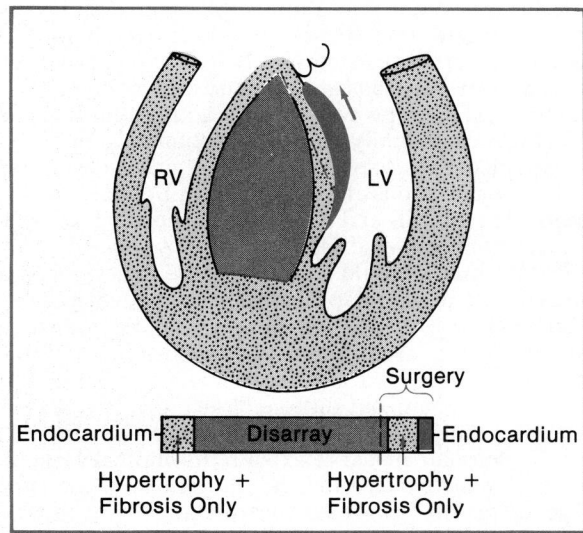

FIGURE 43–9. Diagrammatic representation showing usual location of myocyte disarray in interventricular septum in hypertrophic cardiomyopathy. This explains why disarray is usually deep or absent in septectomy specimen, and why endomyocardial biopsy (3-mm maximum dimension) is also unlikely to sample zone of disarray. RV = right ventricle, LV = left ventricle. (From Tazelaar, H. D., and Billingham, M. E.: The surgical pathology of hypertrophic cardiomyopathy. Arch. Pathol. Lab. Med. 111:257, 1987.)

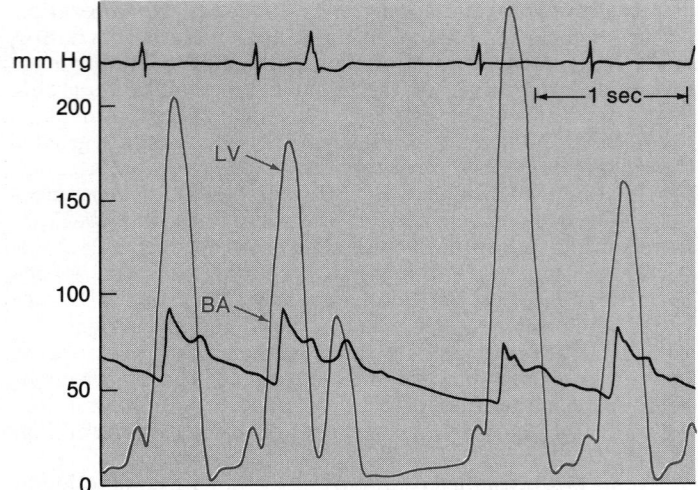

FIGURE 43–10. Simultaneous pressures recorded in the left ventricle (LV) and brachial artery (BA) in a patient with HCM. During the post-premature contraction beat, the pulse pressure in the brachial artery is less than in the control beats. (From Braunwald, E., et al.: Idiopathic hypertrophic subaortic stenosis. Circulation *30*(Suppl. IV):78, 1964, by permission of the American Heart Association, Inc.)

SYSTOLE. Since the initial descriptions of hypertrophic cardiomyopathy, the feature that has attracted the greatest attention is the dynamic pressure gradient (Fig. 43–10). While this pressure gradient was initially thought to be due to a muscular sphincter action in the subaortic region or was an artifact, it appears to be related to further narrowing of an already small outflow tract (narrowed by the prominent septal hypertrophy and possibly abnormal location of the mitral valve) by systolic anterior motion (SAM) of the mitral valve against the septum.[206,207]

There continues to be considerable controversy about the cause and significance of the outflow gradient.[161,208,209] Central to the disagreement is whether there is true obstruction to left ventricular ejection or whether the pressure gradient is simply the consequence of vigorous ventricular emptying.[210,211] Most favor the view that a true mechanical impediment to left ventricular ejection occurs when outflow gradients are present and is the result of distal portions of the mitral valve apparatus moving anteriorly across the outflow tract and contacting the ventricular septum in mid-systole.[161,210,212–217] It is likely that the mitral valve is displaced anteriorly because of Venturi effects or as a result of the increased ejection velocities produced by the abnormal left ventricular outflow tract orientation and geometry (Fig. 43–11).[211,216]

catecholamines[195–197] or reduced neuronal uptake of cardiac norepinephrine[198]; (2) abnormally thickened intramural coronary arteries that do not dilate normally and lead to myocardial ischemia, with resultant fibrosis and abnormal compensatory hypertrophy[197]; (3) subendocardial ischemia, possibly related to abnormalities of the microcirculation, that depletes the energy stores essential for the sequestration of calcium during diastole, resulting in persistent interaction of the contractile elements during diastole and attendant increased diastolic stiffness[199]; and (4) structural abnormalities, including a catenoid configuration of the septum, that lead to myocardial cell hypertrophy and disarray.[197,200]

Mutation of the Myosin Heavy-Chain Gene. Seidman and her collaborators have reported the existence of a gene located on 14 q 1, (i.e., the long arm of the 14th chromosome in the band closest to the centromere) and termed it *FHC-1* (for familial hypertrophic cardiomyopathy); it was believed to be responsible for HCM in two families. Subsequently they found this to be the gene encoding for myosin heavy chain (MHC). Sequencing of this gene in one family with HCM revealed that the abnormality was caused by a gene duplication in which the α and β MHC genes were fused and present in an extra copy. In the second family, there was a point mutation in the β MHC sequence that alters the myosin's arginine to glutamine. Both of these mutations affect the polypeptides crucial to the structure of myofibrils and might be responsible for the myocyte and myofibrillar disarray characteristic of familial HCM.[201–204] Thus, it would appear that the structural organization of the α and β cardiac MHC genes may predispose them to genetic events that produce these two (and perhaps other) mutations, which are ultimately responsible for familial HCM. Seidman et al. have also reported that familial HCM is a genetically heterogeneous disease,[205] i.e., it can be caused by genetic defects in at least two loci. However, the genetic heterogeneity does *not* appear to explain the clinical variability. Further, they have suggested that mutations of the cardiac MHC genes occurring in the myocardial precursor cells of an individual might be responsible for sporadic cases of HCM that would cause a similar phenotype without being responsible for transmission through the germ line (and therefore would not cause familial HCM) (see also pp. 1636 and 1637).

While a genetic test might be developed that could permit early detection of the disease, the demonstrated genetic heterogeneity will require identification of the other gene(s) responsible and ultimately a battery of genetic tests.

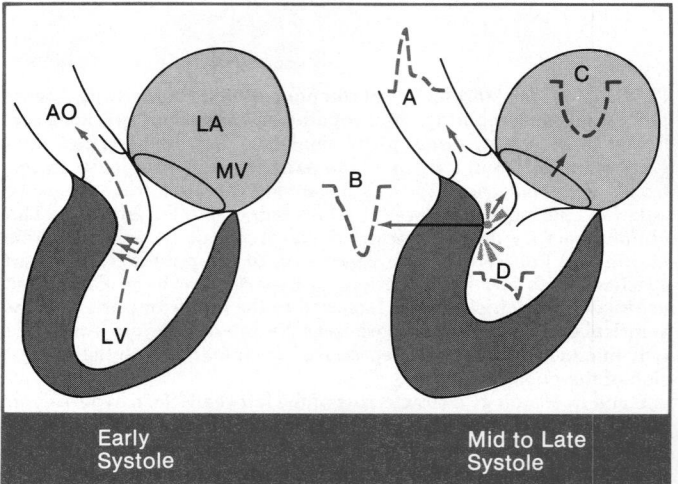

FIGURE 43–11. Left panel illustrates proposed mechanism of mitral leaflet systolic anterior motion (SAM) in early systole in hypertrophic cardiomyopathy (HCM). Ventricular septal hypertrophy causes narrowed outflow tract, as result of which ejection velocity is rapid and path of ejection (dashed line) is closer to mitral leaflets (MV) than is normal. This results in Venturi forces (three short oblique arrows in outflow tract) drawing anterior and/or posterior mitral leaflets toward septum. Subsequent mitral leaflet septal contact results in obstruction to left ventricular (LV) outflow and concomitant mitral regurgitation as seen on right panel. By midsystole, SAM septal contact is well established, causing marked narrowing of LV outflow tract with obstruction to outflow. LA = left atrium.

Proximal to level of SAM-septal contact, converging lines indicate acceleration of jet just proximal to obstruction and narrowing of jet width that occurs. Distal to obstruction, arrow and diverging lines indicate high velocity flow that emanates from site of SAM-septal contact, directed posterolaterally at considerable angle from normal path of aortic outflow. In late systole, although forward flow continues into outflow tract and aorta (AO), the volume of flow is much less than in early nonobstructed systole. Typical Doppler flow velocities that can be recorded are shown.

In right panel, *A*, Integrated Doppler flow signal in ascending aorta; *B*, High outflow tract velocity recorded by continuous wave (CW) Doppler at site of SAM-septal contact; *C*, Presence of mitral regurgitation recorded by CW Doppler; *D*, Late systolic velocity peak that can be recorded in apical region of LV. (From Wigle, E. D.: Hypertrophic cardiomyopathy: A 1987 viewpoint. Circulation *75*:312, 1987, by permission of the American Heart Association, Inc.)

TABLE 43-10 PROPOSED CAUSES OF ISCHEMIA IN HCM DESPITE NORMAL EPICARDIAL CORONARY ARTERIES

Increased muscle mass
Inadequate capillary density
Elevated diastolic filling pressures
Abnormal intramural coronary arteries
Impaired vasodilatory reserve
Systolic compression of arteries
Enhanced myocardial oxygen demand (increased wall stress)

DIASTOLE. Most patients with HCM demonstrate abnormalities of diastolic function whether or not a gradient is present and whether or not they are symptomatic.[210,218] These abnormalities of diastolic filling are largely independent of the extent and distribution of myocardial hypertrophy; patients with mild and apparently localized hypertrophy may demonstrate prominent diastolic dysfunction, suggesting that the myopathic process occurs in ventricular regions that are not macroscopically hypertrophied.[219] Diastolic dysfunction in turn leads to increased filling pressure despite a normal or small left ventricular cavity size and appears to result from abnormalities of left ventricular relaxation and distensibility.[161,210,220] Early diastolic filling is impaired when relaxation is prolonged,[221] perhaps related to abnormal calcium kinetics, subendocardial ischemia, or the abnormal loading conditions found in HCM.[161,222,223] Late diastolic filling is altered when left ventricular distensibility is impaired; as a consequence, filling pressures rise. HCM may cause abnormal distensibility because of fibrosis[191] or cellular disorganization.[161]

MYOCARDIAL ISCHEMIA. Myocardial ischemia is common and multifactorial in HCM (Table 43-10 and Fig. 43-12).[161,210,224-228] Major causes include impaired vasodilator reserve (perhaps related to the thickened and narrowed small intramural coronary arteries found in HCM, see also p. 1405)[190]; increased oxygen demand, especially in patients with outflow gradients; and elevated filling pressures with resultant subendocardial ischemia.[210,224]

CLINICAL MANIFESTATIONS

SYMPTOMS. The majority of patients with HCM are asymptomatic or only mildly symptomatic[229] and often are identified during screening of relatives of a patient with HCM. Unfortunately, the first clinical manifestation of the disease in such individuals may be sudden death. The disease is identified most often in adults in their 30's and 40's; it occurs more often than commonly suspected in elderly patients.[229,229a] The condition has been observed at necropsy in stillborns and both clinically and pathologically in octogenarians. The importance of recognizing this disorder in children at the earliest possible time is highlighted by the higher mortality rate in younger patients; death is often sudden and unexpected.[230] Because syncope and sudden death have been associated with competitive sports and severe exertion in patients with HCM, it is important to diagnose this condition so that these activities may be proscribed. A particularly high index of suspicion of this condition must be maintained to make the clinical diagnosis in the elderly, since their symptoms may easily be confused with those of coronary artery or aortic valve disease. The disease is slightly more common in men,[229] although women may be more likely to be severely disabled and may initially present at a younger age than men.[231]

The clinical picture varies considerably, ranging from the asymptomatic relative of a patient with recognized HCM who has a slightly abnormal echocardiogram but no other manifestation of the illness to the patient with incapacitating symptoms.[230] There is a general relationship between the extent of hypertrophy and the severity of symptoms, but the relationship is not absolute, and some patients have severe symptoms with only mild and apparently localized hypertrophy, and vice versa.[232-234] There is a complex interaction between left ventricular hypertrophy, left ventricular pressure gradient, diastolic dysfunction, and myocardial ischemia that accounts

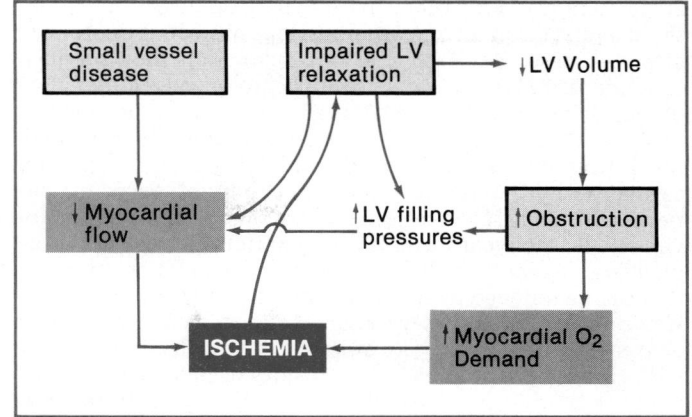

FIGURE 43-12. Determinants of ischemia in hypertrophic cardiomyopathy. (From Maron, B. J., and Epstein, S. E.: Hypertrophic cardiomyopathy: Pathophysiology and therapy. *In* Braunwald, E. (ed.): Heart Disease: A Textbook of Cardiovascular Medicine. 3rd ed. Philadelphia, W. B. Saunders Company, Update No. 7, pp. 157-168, 1989.)

for the great variability in symptoms from patient to patient (Fig. 43-13).

The most common symptom is *dyspnea*, occurring in up to 90 per cent of symptomatic patients, which is largely a consequence of the elevated left ventricular diastolic (and therefore left atrial and pulmonary venous) pressure, which results largely from impaired ventricular filling owing to diastolic dysfunction.[229,230] Angina pectoris (found in about three-fourths of symptomatic patients), fatigue, and presyncope and syncope are also common. Palpitations, paroxysmal nocturnal dyspnea, overt congestive heart failure, and dizziness are found less frequently, although severe congestive heart failure culminating in death may be seen. Exertion tends to exacerbate many of the symptoms.[235] A variety of mechanisms may contribute to the production of angina pectoris. It is at least in part the result of an imbalance between oxygen supply and demand as a consequence of the greatly increased myocardial mass. Transmural infarction may occur in the absence of narrowing in the extramural coronary arteries.[210] Narrowing of the small coronary arteries may contribute to myocardial ischemia,[191,224] particularly during exertion, and perhaps

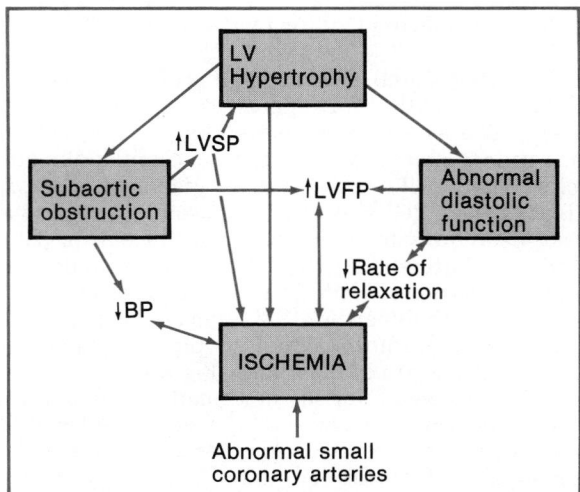

FIGURE 43-13. Pathophysiological and hemodynamic interrelations between left ventricular (LV) hypertrophy, subaortic obstruction, diastolic dysfunction, and myocardial ischemia in hypertrophic cardiomyopathy. The symptoms in any given patient reflect the complex interactions among these pathophysiological mechanisms. LVSP = left ventricular systolic pressure, LVFP = left ventricular filling pressure, BP = blood pressure. (Reproduced by permission from Maron, B. J., Bonow, R. O., Cannon, R. O., et al.: Hypertrophic cardiomyopathy: Interrelations of clinical manifestations, pathophysiology, and therapy. N. Engl. J. Med. 316:780, 1987.)

20 per cent of older patients with hypertrophic cardiomyopathy may have concurrent atheromatous obstructive coronary artery disease. Impaired diastolic relaxation may produce subendocardial ischemia as a result of prolonged maintenance of wall tension with a concomitant slower-than-normal decrease in the impedance to coronary blood flow. Syncope may result from inadequate cardiac output with exertion or from cardiac arrhythmias. It occurs most commonly in young patients with small left ventricular chamber size and evidence of ventricular tachycardia on Holter monitoring.[236] Near-syncopal ("graying out") spells that occur in the erect posture and that can be relieved by immediately lying down are common. However, in contrast to valvular aortic stenosis, syncope or near-syncope may not be an ominous finding in adult patients with HCM; some patients have a history of such episodes dating back many years without deterioration. In children and adolescents, however, presyncope and syncope identify patients at increased risk of sudden death (see Natural History below).

PHYSICAL EXAMINATION. This may be normal in asymptomatic patients without gradients, particularly those with the apical variant of HCM, save for a left ventricular lift and a loud fourth heart sound, but there are usually prominent findings in patients with a left ventricular outflow tract pressure gradient. The apical precordial impulse is often displaced laterally and is usually abnormally forceful and enlarged. Because of decreased left ventricular compliance, a prominent presystolic apical impulse which results from forceful atrial systole is often present.[230] This may result in a double apical impulse as a result of the prominent a wave. A more characteristic but less frequently recognized abnormality is a triple apical beat, the third impulse being a late systolic bulge that occurs when the heart is nearly empty and is performing near-isometric contraction. These findings may be readily recorded by apexcardiography (Fig. 2–17, p. 27).

A systolic thrill may be present (Table 2–1, p. 26), is most frequently palpable at the apex or along the lower left sternal border, and bears only a rough relationship to the severity of the pressure gradient.[231] The jugular venous pulse may demonstrate a prominent a wave, reflecting diminished right ventricular compliance secondary to the massive hypertrophy of the ventricular septum. The carotid pulse typically rises briskly and then declines in midsystole as the gradient develops, followed by a secondary rise. This may be well appreciated on physical examination and can be demonstrated more clearly by means of indirect pulse tracings (Fig. 2–14, p. 24).

The first heart sound is normal and is often preceded by a fourth heart sound that corresponds to the apical presystolic impulse.[231] The second heart sound is usually normally split. In some patients, however, it is narrowly split and in others, particularly those with severe outflow gradients, paradoxical splitting may be noted.[231] A third heart sound is common but does not have the same ominous significance as in patients with valvular aortic stenosis. Systolic ejection sounds relating to rapid acceleration of blood flow may be found on occasion. The auscultatory hallmark of HCM associated with an outflow gradient is a systolic murmur that is typically harsh and crescendo-decrescendo in configuration (Fig. 2–17, p. 27); it usually commences well after the first heart sound and is best heard between the apex and the left sternal border. It often radiates well to the lower sternal border, the axillae, and base of the heart but not into the neck vessels. In patients with large gradients, the murmur usually reflects both outflow tract turbulence and concomitant mitral regurgitation, while in patients without gradients, turbulence in the outflow tract is the only cause. Accordingly, the murmur is often more holosystolic and blowing at the apex and in the axillae (probably due to mitral regurgitation) and midsystolic and harsher along the lower sternal border (due to flow across the outflow tract).[231]

The murmur is labile in intensity and duration, and a variety of maneuvers may be utilized to augment or suppress it (Table 2–8, p. 38, and Fig. 2–27, p. 40).[237] A diastolic rumbling murmur, reflecting increased transmitral flow, may occur in patients with marked mitral regurgitation. The murmur of aortic regurgitation is observed only occasionally in patients with HCM, although mild aortic regurgitation can be demonstrated by Doppler echocardiography in one-third of patients.[238] It may develop after operation to correct the outflow gradient[239] or following infective endocarditis.

It is important to emphasize the features of physical examination that permit differentiation of HCM from fixed orifice obstruction, most commonly due to valvular aortic stenosis (Tables 2–1, p. 26 and 34–11, p. 1039). The character of the carotid pulse and features of the murmur are most useful in this regard. Because there is obstruction to left ventricular emptying from the beginning of systole with fixed valvular stenosis, the carotid upstroke is slowed and of low amplitude (pulsus parvus et tardus). With HCM, initial ejection of blood from the left ventricle is actually enhanced, and therefore the arterial upstroke is brisk. The murmur of HCM, as opposed to that of aortic stenosis, can be reliably identified by its increase with the Valsalva maneuver and during squatting-to-standing action, and its decrease during standing-to-squatting action, passive leg elevation, and handgrip[231] (Table 43–11). Other features that may be helpful but are of considerably less significance are the location of the murmur (it radiates along the carotid arteries in valvular aortic stenosis but not in HCM), and the location of the systolic thrill (most prominent in the second right intercostal space in valvular aortic stenosis and in the fourth interspace along the left sternal border in HCM).

ELECTROCARDIOGRAM. This is usually abnormal in HCM and invariably so in symptomatic patients with left ventricular outflow gradients. Entirely normal electrocardiograms are seen in only about 15 per cent of patients and usually are found in the presence of only localized left ventricular hypertrophy. The most common abnormalities are ST-segment and T-wave abnormalities, followed by evidence of left ventricular hypertrophy, with QRS complexes that are tallest in the midprecordial leads.[240,241] There may be progressive electrocardiographic evidence of hypertrophy over time. Giant negative T-waves in the midprecordial leads of Japanese patients are characteristic of HCM involving the apex,[242] but such a pattern in the West may be found with HCM involving segments other than the apex.[242] Prominent, abnormal Q waves are relatively common, occurring in 20 to 50 per cent of patients. The Q-wave abnormalities often involve the inferior

TABLE 43–11 EFFECTS OF INTERVENTIONS ON OUTFLOW GRADIENT AND SYSTOLIC MURMUR IN HCM

	CONTRACTILITY	PRELOAD	AFTERLOAD
Increase in Gradient and Murmur			
Valsalva maneuver (during strain)	—	↓	↓
Standing	—	↓	—
Postextrasystole	↑	↑	—
Isoproterenol	↑	↓	↓
Digitalis	↑	↓ then ↑	—
Amyl nitrite	— then ↑	↓ then ↑	↓
Nitroglycerin	—	↓	↓
Exercise	↑	↑	↑
Tachycardia	↑	↓	—
Hypovolemia	↑	↓	↓
Decrease in Gradient and Murmur			
Mueller maneuver	—	↑	↑
Valsalva overshoot	—	↑	↑
Squatting	—	↑	↑
Alpha-adrenocepter stimulation (phenylephrine)	—	—	↑
Beta-adrenocepter blockade	↓	↑	—
General anesthesia	↓	—	—
Isometric handgrip	—	—	↑

↑ = increase; ↓ = decrease; — = no major change.

(II, III, aV$_1$) and/or lateral (V$_4$–V$_6$) leads. They appear to be due to depolarization of myopathic cells in the septum that have abnormal electrophysiological properties.[243] A variety of other electrocardiographic abnormalities may occur, including abnormal electrical axis (usually left-axis deviation) and P-wave abnormalities (usually left atrial enlargement). Accessory atrioventricular pathways have been found in HCM, although they are uncommon.[244,245] Clinically significant abnormalities of AV conduction are uncommon but may cause syncope.[246]

Although a hemodynamic mechanism may play a role in the death of patients with HCM (particularly the young), many deaths, particularly those that are known to have been sudden, are probably due to an arrhythmia.[161,247,248] Because of the systolic and diastolic abnormalities in this disorder, rhythm disturbances are less well tolerated.

Ventricular arrhythmias are common in patients with HCM, occurring in over three-fourths of patients undergoing continuous ambulatory electrocardiographic monitoring.[230,249] Ventricular tachycardia is found in about one-fourth of the patients studied, and in some it is a harbinger of subsequent sudden death.[161,229,230] A similar spectrum of arrhythmias may be detected in those asymptomatic relatives of patients with HCM who themselves have the disease (often undiagnosed). Ventricular tachycardia occurs with greater frequency in patients with more pronounced hypertrophy.[250] Treadmill testing may expose arrhythmias that are not present at rest, although continuous ambulatory monitoring is superior in detecting repetitive ventricular tachyarrhythmias. Supraventricular tachycardia may be found in one-fourth to one-half of patients.[249]

Atrial fibrillation occurs in 5 to 15 per cent of patients, and the resultant loss of the atrial contribution to the filling of a hypertrophied, stiff ventricle may result in clinical deterioration. Treatment is often effective in controlling symptoms and restoring sinus rhythm; if this is done, long-term survival usually is not jeopardized.[251–253] The signal-averaged electrocardiogram may prove to be helpful in identifying patients at increased risk of sustained or lethal ventricular arrhythmia, although additional studies are necessary.[254]

Electrophysiological Testing. The role of electrophysiological studies in identifying HCM patients at increased risk of sudden death is evolving.[247,255–258a] These studies identify a variety of abnormalities in HCM patients (Table 43–12), but most important is their ability to induce ventricular tachycardia in two-thirds of patients with syncope or aborted sudden death, compared with 10 per cent in other HCM patients.[256]

CHEST ROENTGENOGRAM. The findings on radiographic examination are variable; heart size, principally the left ventricle, may range from normal to markedly enlarged, but there is little correlation between heart size and the severity of the outflow tract gradient. Left atrial enlargement is frequently observed, especially when significant mitral regurgitation is present. Aortic root enlargement and valvular calcification are not seen unless associated diseases are present, although calcification of the mitral annulus is common in HCM.

ECHOCARDIOGRAPHY. Because echocardiography combines the attributes of high resolution and no known risk, it has been widely utilized in the evaluation of hypertrophic cardiomyopathy (Figs. 4–95, 4–96, and 4–97, p. 100). The two-dimensional study is now standard; M-mode echocardiography may be used as an adjunctive modality.[161] It is useful in the study of patients with suspected HCM and also in the screening of relatives of patients in whom this condition has been documented. The echocardiogram is of value in identifying and quantifying morphological (i.e., distribution of septal hypertrophy) as well as functional features (e.g., hypercontractile left ventricle).

The cardinal echocardiographic feature of HCM is left ventricular hypertrophy. Although the characteristic feature is hypertrophy of the septum and anterolateral free wall, the echocardiogram is useful in identifying involvement of other

TABLE 43–12 ELECTROPHYSIOLOGICAL ABNORMALITIES IN HCM PATIENTS

Abnormal study	81%
Sinoatrial dysfunction	66%
Sustained ventricular tachycardia	43%
His-Purkinje dysfunction	30%
Accessory pathway	5%

Adapted from Fananapazir, L., Tracy, C. M., Leon, M. B., et al.: Electrophysiologic abnormalities in patients with hypertrophic cardiomyopathy: A consecutive analysis in 155 patients. Circulation *80*:1259, 1989, reprinted by permission of the American Heart Association, Inc.

left ventricular locations, including portions of the free wall and the apex.[161] There is considerable variability in the degree and pattern of hypertrophy; in most patients, there is variation in the extent of hypertrophy from left ventricular region to region.[161] Maximal hypertrophy of the septum often occurs midway between the base and apex of the left ventricle. The finding of a thickened septum that is at least 1.3 to 1.5 times the thickness of the posterior wall when measured in diastole just prior to atrial systole has been the time-honored criterion for the diagnosis of asymmetrical septal hypertrophy (ASH). The septum not only is relatively thicker than the posterior wall but is typically at least 15 mm in thickness (normal ≤ 11 mm).

An unusual echocardiographic pattern consisting of a ground-glass appearance has been noted in portions of the hypertrophied myocardium in HCM. Even when abnormalities are not apparent on visual inspection, quantitative texture analysis often identifies them in HCM patients.[259] It has been speculated that this pattern may be related to the abnormal cellular architecture and myocardial fibrosis that has been noted in pathological studies.[259]

A second echocardiographic feature often found in hypertrophic cardiomyopathy in addition to left ventricular hypertrophy is narrowing of the left ventricular outflow tract, which is formed by the interventricular septum anteriorly and the anterior leaflet of the mitral valve posteriorly. The mitral valve apparatus is positioned abnormally close to the septum, possibly the result of the posterior bulging of the septum.[260] When HCM is associated with a pressure gradient, there is abnormal systolic anterior motion (SAM) of the anterior leaflet, and occasionally the posterior leaflet of the mitral valve (Fig. 43–11; also see Fig. 4–95A, p. 100).[260,261] Although the role of SAM in *producing* the gradient is controversial, there is a close relationship between the degree of SAM and the size of the outflow gradient. Prolonged interventricular septal contact of the mitral apparatus is limited to HCM with resting pressure gradients, and there is a close temporal relationship between the onset of the pressure gradient and the onset of septal apposition of the mitral apparatus.

Three explanations have been offered for SAM: (1) the mitral valve is *pulled* against the septum by contraction of the papillary muscles, because of the abnormal location and orientation of these muscles resulting from septal hypertrophy[262]; (2) the mitral valve is *pushed* against the septum (perhaps by the left ventricular posterior wall) because of its abnormal position in the outflow tract; and (3) the mitral valve is drawn toward the septum because of the lower pressure that occurs as blood is ejected at a high velocity through a narrowed outflow tract (Venturi effect).[261] SAM of the mitral valve and dynamic left ventricular gradients is not pathognomonic of HCM but may be found in a variety of other conditions, including hypercontractile states, left ventricular hypertrophy, transposition of the great arteries, and infiltration of the septum. Even mild degrees of left ventricular hypertrophy may be associated with SAM and outflow gradients, particularly under conditions of enhanced sympathetic tone.[263,264] In many cases in conditions other than HCM, SAM is due to buckling of the chordae tendineae rather than to movement of the anterior mitral valve leaflet as occurs in HCM (although the chordae tendineae and papillary muscles may contribute to SAM in HCM).

Several other echocardiographic findings may be present: (1) a small left ventricular cavity; (2) reduced septal motion and thickening during systole, particularly of the upper septum (presumably because of the disarray of the myofibrillar architecture and abnormal contractile function); (3) normal or increased motion of the posterior wall; (4) a reduced rate of closure of the mitral valve in mid-diastole secondary to a decrease in left ventricular compliance or abnormal transmitral flow during diastole; (5) mitral valve prolapse; and (6) partial systolic closure or, more commonly, coarse systolic fluttering of the aortic valve related to turbulent blood flow in the outflow tract. The echocardiographic findings that accompany a left ventricular outflow tract gradient (SAM and aortic valve partial closure) may be quite labile, and provocative measures such as the Valsalva maneuver, pharmacologically induced vasodilatation with amyl nitrite, stimulation of contractility with isoproterenol, or an induced premature ventricular contraction may be required to precipitate the findings.

Abnormalities of diastolic function may be demonstrated by echocardiography in many patients with HCM, independent of the presence or absence of a systolic pressure gradient. The isovolumetric relaxation time, measured from aortic valve closure to mitral valve opening, is frequently prolonged and the peak velocity of left ventricular filling is reduced.[265] Because the septum is typically hypokinetic, the rate of left ventricular filling is determined primarily by the rate of free wall thinning. While there is a general relationship between the extent of hypertrophy and the severity of abnormalities of diastolic function, even nonhypertrophied regions of the HCM ventricle appear to contribute to the impairment of diastolic function seen in HCM.[266]

Doppler ultrasound has confirmed the virtual ubiquity of mitral regurgitation when an outflow gradient is present[267] and has accurately measured the magnitude of the outflow tract gradient.[268] Doppler color flow imaging reveals mitral regurgitation, most prominent in late systole, with the appearance of turbulent flow in the left ventricular outflow tract; in one study, the velocity of the latter was correlated with the degree of SAM, supporting the concept of left ventricular outflow tract obstruction.[269]

RADIONUCLIDE SCANNING. These techniques are gaining popularity in the evaluation of HCM. Thallium-201 myocardial imaging, particularly when tomographic imaging is performed, permits direct determination of the relative thicknesses of the septum and free wall and may be of particular value when technical constraints limit the reliability of echocardiographic evaluation in a given patient with presumed HCM. The utility of rest and exercise thallium-201 scintigraphy in identifying patients with HCM whose angina pectoris is due to obstructive epicardial coronary artery disease is controversial; at least in some patients, thallium-201 defects suggestive of regional myocardial ischemia are found despite angiographically normal coronary arteries.[225,270] Fixed defects, probably indicative of myocardial scarring, occur primarily in patients with impaired systolic function.[161,225] Gated radionuclide ventriculography with blood pool labeling permits the evaluation of not only the size but also the motion of the septum and left ventricle. Disproportionate thickening of the upper septum is a distinctive scintigraphic feature that may be seen in the steep left anterior oblique view. As with the echocardiogram, abnormal diastolic filling of the ventricle has been observed in patients with HCM (both with and without gradients) by computer analysis of the blood pool scan.[271]

HEMODYNAMICS

Cardiac catheterization discloses diminished diastolic left ventricular compliance and in some patients a systolic pressure gradient, when present, within the body of the left ventricle, which is separated from a subaortic chamber by the thickened septum and the anterior leaflet of the mitral valve that abuts the septum[211] (Fig. 43–10). The pressure gradient may be quite labile and may vary between 0 and 175 mm Hg. The pressure tracing may, on occasion, demonstrate a pattern of pulsus alternans.[272] The arterial pressure tracing may demonstrate a "spike and dome" configuration similar to the carotid pulse recording.[211] As a consequence of diminished left ventricular compliance, the mean and particularly the a wave in the left atrial pressure pulse and the left ventricular end-

diastolic pressures are usually elevated. Artifactual outflow gradients may occur if the left ventricular catheter becomes entrapped in the trabeculae of a markedly hypertrophied left ventricle.[207] Proper technique and choice of catheters with side holes should clarify the mechanism of such gradients. Cardiac output may be depressed in patients with longstanding severe gradients. In the majority of patients it is normal; occasionally it is elevated.

Hemodynamic abnormalities in HCM are not limited to the left heart. Approximately one-fourth of patients demonstrate pulmonary hypertension, which is usually mild but in some cases may be moderate to severe. This may be due to elevated mean left atrial pressures. A pressure gradient in the right ventricular outflow tract occurs in approximately 15 per cent of patients who have obstruction to left ventricular outflow[231] and appears to result from muscular contraction of the infundibulum. Right atrial and right ventricular end-diastolic pressures may be slightly elevated.

LABILITY OF GRADIENT. A feature characteristic of HCM is the variability and lability of the left ventricular outflow gradient. A given patient may demonstrate a large outflow gradient on one occasion but have none at another time. In some patients without a resting gradient, it may be temporarily provoked. Three basic mechanisms are involved in the production of dynamic gradients, all of which act by reducing ventricular volume and presumably accentuate the apposition of the anterior mitral leaflet against the septum: (1) increased contractility, (2) decreased preload, and (3) decreased afterload. In a minority of patients with HCM, the gradient is midventricular[273] and may be intensified by increased contractility, which exerts a direct muscular sphincteric action. The stimuli that provoke or intensify left ventricular outflow tract gradients in HCM generally improve myocardial performance in normal subjects and in patients with most other forms of heart disease. Conversely, reductions in contractility or increases in preload or afterload, which increase left ventricular dimensions, reduce or abolish the left ventricular outflow gradient.

Alterations in the magnitude of the gradient are reflected by changes in the findings on physical examination (Table 43–11), noninvasive tests, and left heart catheterization. *It is this dynamic characteristic of HCM that distinguishes it from the discrete forms of obstruction to ventricular outflow.* An increase in the gradient usually results in a louder murmur, a longer ejection period with a more characteristic spike and dome configuration in the carotid pulse, and more flagrant echocardiographic evidence of SAM of the anterior mitral leaflet. In some patients, the intensity of the murmur may *not* track with the gradient, perhaps because in many cases the murmur reflects mitral regurgitation (at least in part).[274]

A number of bedside procedures may be useful in the evaluation of suspected hypertrophic cardiomyopathy.[237] Perhaps the most helpful is sudden standing from a squatting position. Squatting results in an increase in venous return and an increase in aortic pressure, which increases ventricular volume, diminishing the gradient and decreasing the intensity of the murmur. Sudden standing has the opposite effects and results in accentuation of the gradient and the murmur. The Valsalva maneuver is another useful bedside technique for eliciting or exacerbating the gradient. Following a transient increase in arterial pressure that usually lasts for four or five cardiac cycles after the onset of the strain coincident with an increase in heart rate, the arterial systolic and pulse pressures and ventricular volume decline, and the gradient (and murmur) increase. Following release of the strain, there is a compensatory overshoot of arterial pressure and venous return and cardiac slowing, all of which increase ventricular volume and reduce the magnitude of the gradient and the murmur. In occasional patients, there may be paradoxical attenuation of the systolic murmur despite an increase in the pressure gradient, presumably related to a critical reduction in stroke volume. Inhalation of amyl nitrite also intensifies the murmur and the abnormality of the arterial pulse. The murmur of

HCM is attenuated by passive leg elevation, handgrip, and sudden squatting from a standing position.[237]

One of the most potent stimuli for enhancing the gradient is *postextrasystolic potentiation* (p. 380), which may occur following a spontaneous premature contraction or be induced by mechanical stimulation with a catheter. The resultant increase in contractility in the beat following the extrasystole is so marked that it outweighs the otherwise salutary effect of increased ventricular filling caused by the compensatory pause and produces an increase in the gradient and often of the murmur as well. A characteristic change often occurs in the directly recorded arterial pressure tracing, which, in addition to displaying a more marked spike and dome configuration, exhibits a pulse pressure that fails to increase as expected or actually decreases (Fig. 43–10). This is one of the more reliable signs of dynamic obstruction of the left ventricular outflow tract. In some patients, the postextrasystolic murmur is attenuated despite an increase in the outflow gradient, apparently because in this setting the murmur (a hybrid of outflow tract turbulence and mitral regurgitation) is mirroring to a greater degree changes in the degree of mitral regurgitation rather than changes in the outflow tract gradient.[274]

Digitalis glycosides and the beta-adrenoceptor agonist isoproterenol augment the gradient, because they increase myocardial contractility, whereas nitroglycerin and amyl nitrite exaggerate the gradient by decreasing arterial pressure and ventricular volume.[275] Hypovolemia (as a result of hemorrhage or overly aggressive diuresis) may also provoke overt obstruction to left ventricular outflow. The intensity of the murmur and the left ventricular outflow gradient may be decreased by beta-adrenoceptor blockade, although the effect of the latter is often not dramatic and is of most hemodynamic benefit in protecting against the *increase* in the gradient that may be provoked by exercise. In most patients the severity of mitral regurgitation and the intensity of the apical blowing regurgitant murmur vary with the degree of obstruction of left ventricular outflow.

ANGIOCARDIOGRAPHY. Left ventriculography shows a hypertrophied ventricle; when an outflow gradient is present, the anterior leaflet of the mitral valve moves anteriorly during systole and encroaches upon the outflow tract. Associated with this motion of the leaflet is mitral regurgitation, which appears to be a constant finding in patients with gradients. The left ventricular cavity is often small, and systolic ejection is typically vigorous, resulting in virtual obliteration of the cavity at end systole, although the apparent hypercontractile state may relate more to reduced afterload (end-systolic wall stress) than to enhanced inotropy.[276] The papillary muscles are often prominent and may fill the left ventricular cavity in late systole. In patients with apical involvement, the extensive hypertrophy may convey a spade-like configuration to the left ventricular angiogram.[174]

It is often helpful to supplement angiographic evaluation of the left ventricle with simultaneous right ventriculography in a cranially angulated LAO projection in order to obtain optimal visualization of the size, shape, and configuration of the interventricular septum.[277] The left septal surface either is flat or bulges into the left ventricular cavity at its mid or lower portion, in contrast to the normal findings of the septum curving toward the right ventricle.

In patients over 45 years of age, obstructive coronary artery disease is rather common, although the symptoms of ischemic pain are indistinguishable from those of patients with normal coronary angiograms and HCM.[278] The left anterior descending and septal perforator coronary arteries may demonstrate phasic narrowing during systole (myocardial bridging) in the absence of fixed obstructive lesions.[279]

NATURAL HISTORY

The clinical course in HCM is varied; in many patients symptoms are absent or mild, remain stable, and in some instances improve (Fig. 43–14) over a period of 5 to 10 years. The annual attrition is about 3 per cent a year in adults, and 6 per

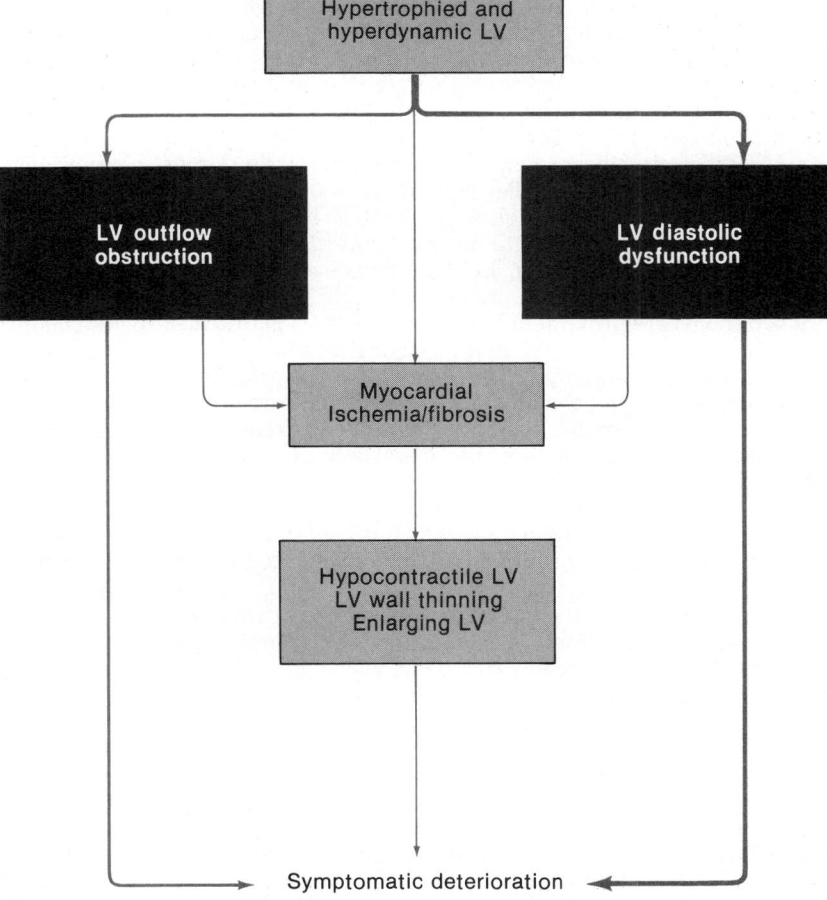

FIGURE 43–14. Possible evolution of disease state in hypertrophic cardiomyopathy. Patients with hypertrophic cardiomyopathy initially have a hypertrophied and hyperdynamic left ventricle. Approximately 20 per cent of patients exhibit left ventricular outflow gradient that can lead to progressive symptomatic deterioration. Patients with gradients, as well as many other patients without them, may have left ventricular diastolic dysfunction that can also lead to progressive symptomatic deterioration. Patients can also proceed through a course characterized by progressive myocardial fibrosis. This may lead to an enlarging and hypocontractile left ventricle and associated symptomatic deterioration. (From Maron, B. J., and Epstein, S. E.: Hypertrophic cardiomyopathy: Pathophysiology and therapy. *In:* Braunwald, E. (ed.): Heart Disease: A Textbook of Cardiovascular Medicine. 3rd ed. Philadelphia, W. B. Saunders Company, Update No. 7, pp. 157–168, 1989.)

cent a year in children[280]; clinical deterioration (aside from sudden death) is usually slow.[161,247,280] Although symptoms are unrelated to the severity or even the presence of a gradient,[210,281] the percentage of severely symptomatic patients does increase with age.[231,280] The onset of atrial fibrillation usually leads to an increase in symptoms, and prompt cardioversion (often pharmacological) is usually indicated.[251] Pregnancy is generally well tolerated, although maternal death has been reported.[282]

Progression of HCM to left ventricular dilatation and dysfunction[283] without a gradient, i.e., dilated cardiomyopathy, occurs in upward of 10 per cent of patients.[210] It appears to result, at least in part, from wall thinning and scar formation as a consequence of myocardial ischemia caused by small vessel coronary artery disease.[284] The extent of left ventricular hypertrophy usually remains stable over time, although a minority of patients may develop increasing degrees of hypertrophy.[285] In some children, the pattern of HCM may develop despite a previous normal echocardiogram; this does not appear to occur in adults.[286] Its occurrence does emphasize that a single normal echocardiogram does *not* exclude HCM in a child or adolescent; cellular disarray and the attendant risk of sudden death may be present even in the absence of left ventricular hypertrophy.[234,287] A marker for the later appearance of clinical HCM may be an initially abnormal electrocardiogram demonstrating increased QRS voltage.[288] Substantial changes in the magnitude of the gradient occur in a small proportion of patients. Both the appearance (or intensification) of a gradient are usually accompanied by an increase in symptoms.[289]

Sudden Death. Death is most often sudden in HCM and may occur in previously asymptomatic patients, in individuals who were unaware they had the disease, or in patients with an otherwise stable course.[231,280] Those features that most reliably identify high-risk patients include young age (<30 years) at diagnosis and family history of HCM with sudden death.[280] The presence or severity of an outflow tract gradient,[290] the degree of functional limitation, and symptoms in general do not correlate with the risk of death.[161] A history of syncope is ominous in children,[247,280,291–293] although not so much in adults. In adults, the single most useful marker of increased risk is nonsustained ventricular tachycardia (NSVT) on 48-hour electrocardiographic monitoring, although most patients (perhaps 75 per cent) with NSVT do *not* die suddenly.[161,210,247,280] In children, the mechanism of death may be different, since preexisting ventricular arrhythmias are much less common.[294] Perhaps in some patients, especially the young, the precipitating event is hemodynamic rather than primarily arrhythmic in origin.[247] Sudden death often occurs during exercise, and strenuous exertion should probably be proscribed in all patients with HCM whether or not symptoms are prominent. Unsuspected HCM is the most common abnormality found at autopsy in young competitive athletes who die suddenly.[295] The development of atrial fibrillation also may be a poor prognostic sign. The degree of left ventricular hypertrophy does not appear to correlate well with prognosis, since patients with massive hypertrophy are often no more than minimally symptomatic and appear to have no more malignant courses than do patients with moderate hypertrophy.[232,247] Sudden death is unlikely, however, in asymptomatic or mildly symptomatic patients with mild hypertrophy.[296]

It is presumed, but not established, that sudden death is due to a ventricular arrhythmia, although atrial arrhythmias may play a role in sensitizing the heart so that ventricular arrhythmias appear subsequently.

MANAGEMENT

Management of patients with HCM is directed toward alleviation of symptoms, prevention of complications, and reduction in the risk of death (Fig. 43–15). Whether asymptomatic patients should be treated is unestablished, because no adequate controlled studies are available.[210] However, reversible

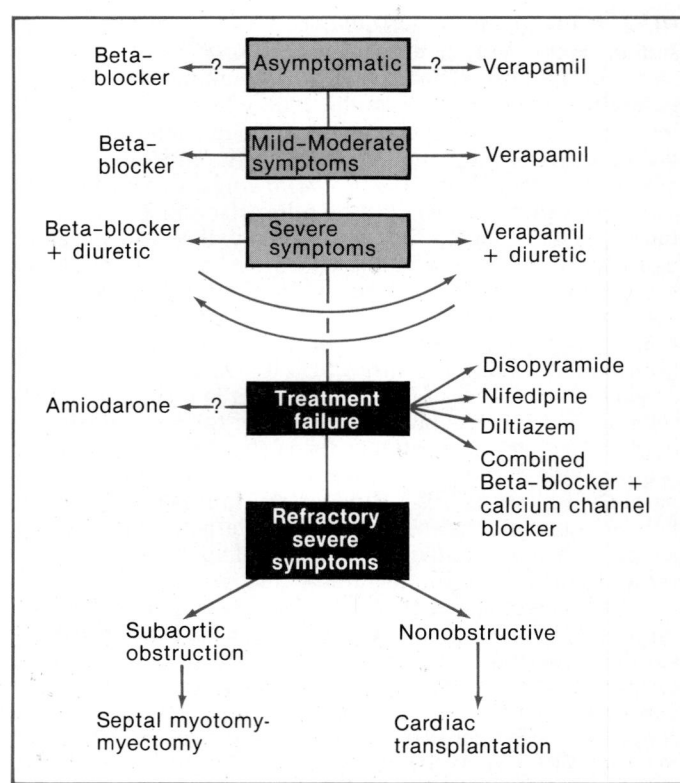

FIGURE 43–15. Therapeutic strategies for patients with hypertrophic cardiomyopathy. Question marks indicate treatment recommendations that are largely unresolved. (From Maron, B. J., and Epstein, S. E.: Hypertrophic cardiomyopathy: Pathophysiology and therapy. *In* **Braunwald, E. (ed.): Heart Disease: A Textbook of Cardiovascular Medicine. 3rd ed. Philadelphia, W. B. Saunders Company, Update No. 7, pp. 157–168, 1989.)**

thallium perfusion defects develop during exercise in half of the asymptomatic patients with HCM,[225] and most of these defects can be improved by the use of verapamil.[297] *Digitalis glycosides* should generally be avoided unless atrial fibrillation or systolic dysfunction develops.[161] *Diuretics* were previously thought to be contraindicated for fear of precipitating or worsening the outflow gradient. More recent experience indicates that cautious use of diuretics often helps reduce symptoms of pulmonary congestion, particularly when combined with beta-adrenergic blockers or calcium antagonists.[161,298] *Beta-adrenergic agonists* may improve diastolic filling but should not be used because they may produce ischemia[299] and usually worsen the outflow gradient.

BETA-ADRENOCEPTOR BLOCKERS. These drugs are the mainstay of medical therapy. With their use, angina, dyspnea, and presyncope may all be improved.[161] Beta blockade may prevent the increase in outflow obstruction that accompanies exercise, although resting gradients are largely unchanged.[298] It decreases the determinants of myocardial oxygen consumption and thus angina pectoris, and perhaps exerts an antiarrhythmic action. Angina pectoris generally responds more favorably to treatment with a beta blocker than does dyspnea.[5] It has also been suggested that beta blockade may prevent sudden death, but its efficacy for this purpose has not been established.[280] Beta blockade also blunts the chronotropic response, thus limiting the demand for increased myocardial oxygen delivery. Beta-adrenoceptor blockade previously was thought to have a beneficial effect on diastolic ventricular filling, but it now appears that any benefit is simply the consequence of a slower heart rate.[161,298] The overall clinical response to beta blockade is variable, however, since only about one-third to two-thirds of patients experience symptomatic improvement[161]; a double-blinded, properly controlled test of this therapy has not been reported. It is reasonable to try large doses of propranolol (greater than 320 mg per day) in patients without contraindications who have not experienced adequate symptomatic improvement with conventional doses. Some patients so treated experience symptomatic improvement and improved exercise capacity.[161]

CALCIUM ANTAGONISTS. These are an increasingly popular alternative to beta-adrenoceptor blockade in the management of HCM[300]; most of the experience has been with verapamil, with more limited use of nifedipine and diltiazem. There is no clear consensus whether therapy should be initiated first with a beta-adrenergic or a calcium antagonist. Exercise performance in particular may be improved when patients are changed from a beta-adrenoceptor blocker to verapamil. Both the hypercontractile systolic function and the abnormalities of diastolic filling may be related to abnormal calcium kinetics, and drugs that block the inward transport of calcium across the myocardial cell membrane may be able to rectify both abnormalities.

Verapamil has been the most widely utilized calcium-channel blocking agent in this condition.[301] Its use was suggested, at least in part, by the observation that it produces a protective and beneficial effect in the hereditary cardiomyopathy of the Syrian hamster, a condition marked by intracellular calcium overload, in which propranolol is ineffective.[197] Although the vasodilator effects of verapamil should not be helpful in HCM, it appears that by depressing myocardial contractility, verapamil can decrease the left ventricular outflow gradient when given intravenously or orally. Perhaps more important from a symptomatic point of view, verapamil improves diastolic filling in HCM,[302,303] at least in part by reducing asynchronous regional diastolic performance.[304] Verapamil appears to improve diastolic filling by improved relaxation rather than by changes in left ventricular diastolic stiffness; at any given diastolic volume, filling pressure is reduced. While variable clinical responses have been reported with verapamil, about two-thirds or more of patients show increased exercise capacity and an improved symptomatic status.[301,305,306] Sustained symptomatic improvement has been noted with the long-term administration of verapamil in ambulatory patients,[303] although important adverse effects, including sudden death, have been observed in a small fraction of patients so treated. Complications with verapamil include suppression of sinus node automaticity and inhibition of atrioventricular conduction, vasodilatation, and negative inotropic effects. These side effects may culminate in hypotension, pulmonary edema, and death; there is a suggestion that antiarrhythmic agents, especially quinidine, may exacerbate the deleterious hemodynamic effects of verapamil. Because of these adverse effects, it has been suggested that verapamil should not be used, or be used only with extreme caution, in patients with high left ventricular filling pressure or symptoms of paroxysmal nocturnal dyspnea or orthopnea. Unfortunately, these are usually the patients who are in greatest need of therapy. In addition, patients with abnormalities of electrical impulse generation or conduction should not receive verapamil unless a pacemaker is in place. We favor initiation of therapy with doses of 240 to 360 mg/day, increasing as needed to higher doses (480 mg/day).

Nifedipine has also been used in HCM, and it may have advantages over verapamil, since it causes less depression of atrioventricular conduction, although it is a more potent vasodilator. Reports of its effect on diastolic function have shown inconsistent results.[161,298,307,308] Nifedipine may also alleviate the chest pain in these patients. Combined administration of nifedipine and propranolol may be of benefit in some patients, particularly those with outflow gradients. However, it should be recognized that the potent vasodilator effects of nifedipine may lead to systemic hypotension and an increase in the outflow gradient,[308] and in high doses it may depress left ventricular function.[309]

Diltiazem has also shown beneficial effects in HCM, producing improved diastolic function.[310] Although the data are not conclusive, there are suggestive findings that calcium-channel blocker therapy may promote regression of left ventricular hypertrophy with a reduction in muscle mass.[311]

OTHER NONSURGICAL MEASURES. *Disopyramide*, an antiarrhythmic drug that alters calcium kinetics, has produced symptomatic improvement and abolition of the pressure gradient in patients with HCM, presumably as a consequence of depression of left ventricular systolic performance.[312-315] Long-term experience with disopyramide is limited, particularly in asymptomatic patients and those without outflow gradients.[161,298]

Beta-adrenoceptor blockers, calcium antagonists, and the conventional antiarrhythmic agents do not appear to suppress serious ventricular arrhythmias or reduce the frequency of supraventricular arrhythmias.[280] However, *amiodarone* is effective in the treatment of both supraventricular and ventricular tachyarrhythmias in HCM without significantly affecting left ventricular function.[316] Although there is some belief that amiodarone improves prognosis in HCM,[317,318] only limited and inconclusive data are available. We do not favor empiric use of amiodarone (or other antiarrhythmic agents for that matter) and share the concern[210] about possible proarrhythmic effects[318a,b] and potential toxicity.[298] In high-risk patients or those surviving a cardiac arrest, insertion of an implantable cardioverter-defibrillator should be considered.[319]

Strenuous exercise should be avoided because of the risk of sudden death; it is the major cause of a fatal outcome in HCM cardiomyopathy. Even though there are many individuals with subclinical HCM who exercise vigorously, the risk of sudden death is sufficiently real that competitive sports are proscribed in patients with marked hypertrophy or other factors believed to be associated with increased risk; e.g., marked left ventricular hypertrophy or a history of sudden death in relatives with HCM, evidence of a marked outflow gradient (>40 mm Hg at rest), and important supraventricular or ventricular arrhythmias.[320] Atrial fibrillation should usually be pharmacologically or electrically converted because of the hemodynamic consequences of loss of the atrial contribution to ventricular filling in this disorder. Infective endocarditis may occur in about 5 per cent of patients, and antibiotic prophylaxis is indicated.[231] The infection usually occurs on the aortic valve or mitral apparatus, on the endocardium, or at the site of the contact lesion on the septum; thus, chronic endocardial trauma may provide a nidus for subsequent infection. Anticoagulants should be given to patients with chronic atrial fibrillation when no contraindication exists.

SURGICAL TREATMENT. A variety of surgical procedures aimed at reducing the outflow gradient have been developed and are most commonly utilized in the markedly symptomatic patient who has not responded well to medical management.[321,321a,321b] The most popular operation for HCM consists of excising a portion of the hypertrophied septum (Figs. 43–16 and 43–17). A transaortic approach with septal myotomy-myectomy is the most widely utilized procedure, although left transventricular as well as combined transaortic and left ventricular approaches have also been employed successfully.[321] Operative management is facilitated by intraoperative echocardiography,[322] and operative mortality is now ≤5 per cent.[321,323] Operation often relieves the obstruction (Fig. 43–18) as well as the mitral regurgitation.[324] The reduction in left ventricular systolic pressure produced by the operation leads to reduced myocardial oxygen demands, especially during stress.[325] Patients over the age of 65 as well as under the age of 10 years have undergone successful operations with benefits and risks comparable to those in the usual patient.[326] Surgery results in long-term improvement in symptoms and exercise capacity in about 70 per cent of patients.[161,327] Furthermore, septal myotomy-myectomy does not produce important impairment of global left ventricular function at rest or during exercise. Myotomy-myectomy may be combined with other necessary operative procedures (particularly coronary artery bypass grafting and mitral valve replacement), although the risk is increased somewhat.[328] Although mitral valve replacement is performed in fewer centers, the long-term results also have been favorable (Fig. 43–18), with symptomatic benefit and an improvement in

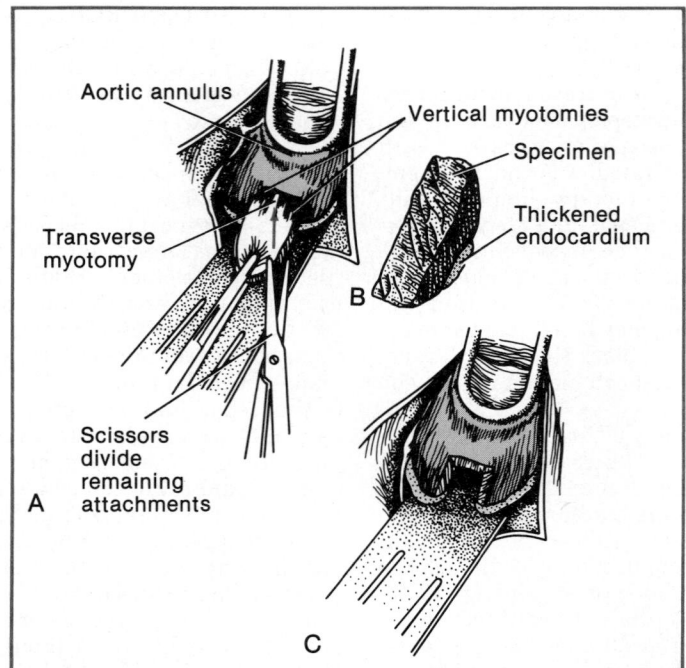

FIGURE 43-16. Illustration of standard ventricular septal myotomy-myectomy operation performed through an aortotomy. *A*, Two vertical and parallel incisions are made in the most basal portion of ventricular septum about 1 cm apart. A third incision is made transversely, connecting the initial two parallel myotomies. Attachments of the muscle bar to the septum are divided. *B*, This segment of muscle is isolated and excised. *C*, At completion of the myotomy-myectomy operation, a rectangular channel is created, about 1 cm wide, 1 cm deep, and 4 cm long, extending from a point 5 to 10 mm below the aortic annulus to a point just distal to the systolic contact between the distal portion of mitral valve leaflets and ventricular septum. In some patients, additional tissue may be resected from the margins of the channel to achieve greater enlargement of the left ventricular outflow tract. (From McIntosh, C. L., and Maron, B. J.: Current operative treatment of obstructive hypertrophic cardiomyopathy. Circulation *78*:487, 1988, reprinted by permission of the American Heart Association, Inc.)

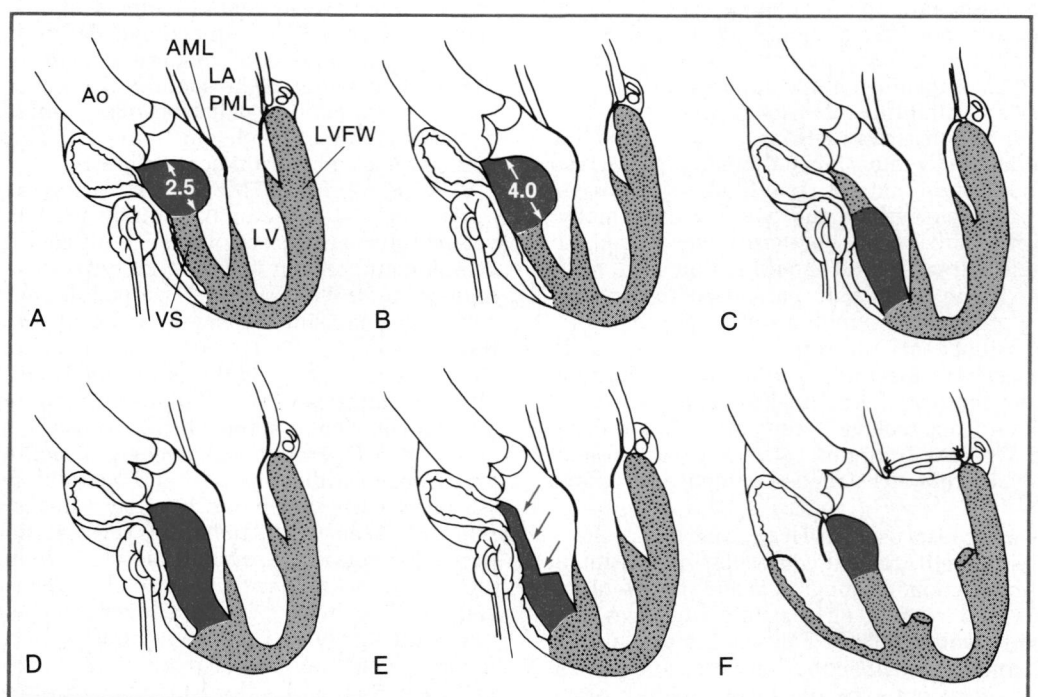

FIGURE 43-17. Illustration of the morphological spectrum of hypertrophic cardiomyopathy and importance of the distribution of ventricular septal (VS) thickening to the myotomy-myectomy operation (shown in diastole). *A–D.* Different distributions of ventricular septal hypertrophy in the longitudinal cross-sectional plane; thickened areas of septum are denoted in red. *A*, Septal hypertrophy is quite localized to the most proximal 2 cm of the anterior basal septum. *B*, Hypertrophy involves the upper and midseptal areas, extending over the proximal 4 cm of anterior septum. *C*, Basal portion of the anterior ventricular septum is relatively thin, whereas substantially increased septal thickness is evident at the point of systolic contact between mitral valve and septum as well as in the more distal portion of the septum. *D*, Hypertrophy is more diffuse and involves the entire septum homogeneously. *E*, Completed myotomy-myectomy channel (arrows) created in the same left ventricle that is depicted in *D*, extending from near the aortic annulus to just beyond the mitral valve tips. *F*, Low-profile disc prosthesis implanted in the mitral position after the native mitral valve has been removed from a patient with relatively thin ventricular septum. AML = anterior mitral leaflet, Ao = aorta, LA = left atrium, LV = left ventricle, LVFW = left ventricular free wall, PML = posterior mitral leaflet. (From McIntosh, C. L., and Maron, B. J.: Current operative treatment of obstructive hypertrophic cardiomyopathy. Circulation *78*:487, 1988, reprinted by permission of the American Heart Association, Inc.)

hemodynamics.[329-332] The rationale for this operation is that it abolishes obstruction by preventing systolic anterior movement (SAM) of the mitral valve (p. 100). It appears to be of particular value in patients with less than severe (18 mm) thickness of the upper septum or other atypical septal morphology, in those with previous myotomy-myectomy with persistent severe symptoms and obstruction, as well as in patients with independent intrinsic mitral valve disease.[331] In appropriate candidates not responding to maximal standard medical and surgical therapy, cardiac transplantation may be an option.[333]

FIGURE 43–18. Plots of hemodynamic alterations associated with ventricular septal myotomy-myectomy (*left*) and mitral valve replacement (*right*) in patients with hypertrophic cardiomyopathy operated on at the National Institutes of Health from 1982 to 1988. Data are from 84 patients (among a total of 156 undergoing operation) who had both preoperative studies and a second cardiac catheterization 6 to 12 months after operation. Data are mean ± SD. LVEDP = left ventricular end-diastolic pressure, LVOT = left ventricular outflow tract, PROV = provocable (with infusion of isoproterenol). PREOP = preoperative patients, POSTOP = postoperative patients, POSTOP ONLY = patients in whom the subaortic gradients recorded under basal conditions preoperatively were 100 mm Hg or more so that measurements of provocable gradients in the catheterization laboratory were not considered to be clinically justified. Therefore, in these patients, provocable gradients were only measured postoperatively at a time when the basal gradient was either absent or small. (From McIntosh, C. L., and Maron, B. J.: Current operative treatment of obstructive hypertrophic cardiomyopathy. Circulation 78:487, 1988, reprinted by permission of the American Heart Association, Inc.)

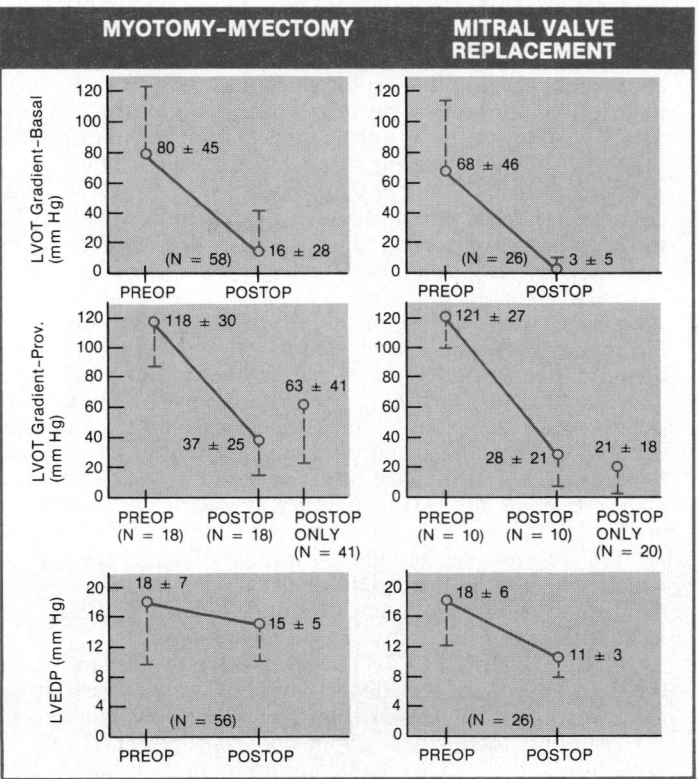

Restrictive and Infiltrative Cardiomyopathies

Of the three major functional categories of the cardiomyopathies (dilated, hypertrophic, and restrictive), the restrictive are the least common in Western countries, although secondary forms of restrictive cardiomyopathy such as endomyocardial disease (see p. 1421) are common in specific geographic regions.[334] The hallmark of the restrictive cardiomyopathies is abnormal diastolic function; the ventricular walls are excessively rigid and impede ventricular filling. Contractile function, on the other hand, is often relatively unimpaired. Thus, restrictive cardiomyopathy bears some functional resemblance to constrictive pericarditis, which is also characterized by normal or near-normal systolic function but abnormal ventricular filling.[334-336] Differentiation of the two conditions is mandatory because of the potential for successful surgical treatment of the latter.[337,338]

A variety of specific pathological processes may result in restrictive cardiomyopathy, although the cause often remains unknown. Myocardial fibrosis, infiltration, or endomyocardial scarring is usually responsible for the abnormal diastolic behavior. Myocardial involvement with amyloid is a common cause of secondary restrictive cardiomyopathy in the Western world, although it can be caused by a variety of other conditions (Table 43–13).[334,339]

Some patients may manifest the features of a restrictive cardiomyopathy and yet exhibit the pathological findings of left ventricular hypertrophy and fibrosis; certainly ventricular hypertrophy, especially hypertrophic cardiomyopathy can cause diminished ventricular compliance but not restrictive cardiomyopathy per se. Findings include biatrial dilatation, often with thrombi in the atrial appendages, and normal left ventricular cavity size.[340] Rare patients may present with findings of restrictive physiology but without fibrosis, infiltration, or other pathological findings demonstrable in the heart. It has been suggested that a defect in myocardial relaxation is present in these patients.[334] Unlike dilated and especially hy-

pertrophic cardiomyopathy, restrictive cardiomyopathy is only rarely familially linked.[341,342]

HEMODYNAMICS. The clinical and hemodynamic features of restrictive heart disease simulate those of chronic constrictive pericarditis; endomyocardial biopsy, CT scanning (Fig. 11–9, p. 317), and especially MR imaging (Fig. 11–31, p. 328) may be particularly useful in differentiating the two diseases by demonstrating myocardial scarring or infiltration (biopsy) or thickening of the pericardium (CT and MR imaging).[334-337,340,343-345] With the use of these modalities,

TABLE 43–13 CLASSIFICATION OF THE RESTRICTIVE CARDIOMYOPATHIES

MYOCARDIAL
A. Noninfiltrative
  Idiopathic
  Scleroderma
B. Infiltrative
  Amyloid
  Sarcoid
  Gaucher disease
  Hurler disease
C. Storage diseases
  Hemochromatosis
  Fabry disease
  Glycogen storage diseases

ENDOMYOCARDIAL
  Endomyocardial fibrosis
  Hypereosinophilic syndrome
  Carcinoid
  Metastatic malignancies
  Radiation
  Anthracycline toxicity

exploratory thoracotomy should be required rarely if at all.[337] The characteristic hemodynamic feature in both conditions is a deep and rapid early decline in ventricular pressure at the onset of diastole, with a rapid rise to a plateau in early diastole.[343] This dip and plateau has been termed the "square root" sign (Fig. 45–14, p. 1483) and is manifested in the atrial pressure tracing as a prominent *y* descent followed by a rapid rise and plateau. The *x* descent may also be rapid, and the combination results in the characteristic M or W waveform in the atrial pressure tracing. The *a* wave is prominent and often is of the same amplitude as the *v* wave.[343] Both systemic and pulmonary venous pressures are elevated, although patients with restrictive heart disease typically have left ventricular filling pressures that exceed right ventricular filling pressure by more than 5 mm Hg, and this difference is accentuated by exercise.[337] In this respect they differ from patients with constrictive pericarditis, in whom diastolic pressures are similar in both ventricles, usually differing by not more than 5 mm Hg. The pulmonary artery systolic pressure is often greater than 45 mm Hg in patients with restrictive cardiomyopathy but is lower in constrictive pericarditis.[334,337] Furthermore, the plateau of the right ventricular diastolic pressure is usually at least one-third of the peak right ventricular systolic pressure in patients with constrictive pericarditis, while it is frequently less in restrictive cardiomyopathy.[334]

CLINICAL MANIFESTATIONS. Exercise intolerance is frequent because of the inability of patients with restrictive cardiomyopathy to increase their cardiac output by tachycardia without further compromising ventricular filling.[337] Weakness and dyspnea are often prominent. Exertional chest pain may be prominent in a small fraction of patients but is usually absent. Particularly in advanced cases, an elevated central venous pressure, with peripheral edema, enlarged liver, ascites, and anasarca may be present.[337] *Physical examination* may reveal jugular venous distention, and an S₃, S₄, or both. An inspiratory increase in venous pressure (Kussmaul sign, p. 1482) may be seen. However, in contrast to constrictive pericarditis, the apex impulse is usually palpable.[334]

Various ancillary laboratory findings in addition to endomyocardial biopsy, CT scanning, and MR imaging may be useful in distinguishing between constrictive and restrictive dis-

ease. While pericardial calcification is neither absolutely sensitive nor specific for constrictive pericarditis (p. 1485), its presence in a patient in whom the differential diagnosis rests between restrictive cardiomyopathy and constrictive pericarditis lends strong support to the latter diagnosis.[337] The echocardiogram may demonstrate thickening of the left ventricular wall and an increase of left ventricular mass in patients with infiltrative disease causing restrictive cardiomyopathy.[334] The pattern of filling of the left ventricle differs in the two conditions, as can be demonstrated by digitized echocardiograms,[346] transthoracic[347,348] and transesophageal Doppler[349] ultrasound, and radionuclide ventriculography (Fig. 43–19).[350,351] In patients with constrictive pericarditis, respiratory variations in left ventricular isovolumic relaxation time and peak mitral valve velocity in early diastole are prominent; however, this finding is not present in patients with restrictive cardiomyopathy (or in normal subjects).[348]

The prognosis in restrictive cardiomyopathy is one of relentless symptomatic progression; only 10 per cent of patients are alive at 10 years.[340] No specific therapy (other than symptomatic) is available,[340] although there is speculation that calcium antagonists may be of some value.[334]

AMYLOIDOSIS

ETIOLOGY AND TYPES. Amyloidosis is a disease complex that results from deposition of unique twisted β-pleated sheet fibrils formed from various proteins by several different pathogenic mechanisms.[334,352] Amyloid may be found in almost any organ, but clinically evident disease does not appear unless there is extensive infiltration. Several classifications systems have been used to characterize the different clinical presentations of amyloidosis. The condition with the traditional designation of *primary amyloidosis* is now known to be caused by the production of an amyloid protein composed of portions of immunoglobulin light chain (designated AL) by a monoclonal population of plasma cells, often as a consequence of multiple myeloma. *Secondary amyloidosis* is due to the production of a nonimmunoglobulin protein, termed AA.[352] Six different forms of *familial amyloidosis* are recognized; they result from the production of a prealbumin protein, and generally present in one of three clinical presentations: progressive neuropathy, cardiomyopathy, or nephropathy.[352] *Senile systemic amyloidosis* also is due to the production of a prealbumin protein and is becoming increasingly common as the average age of the population increases. Scattered deposits of amyloid localized to the aorta or atria

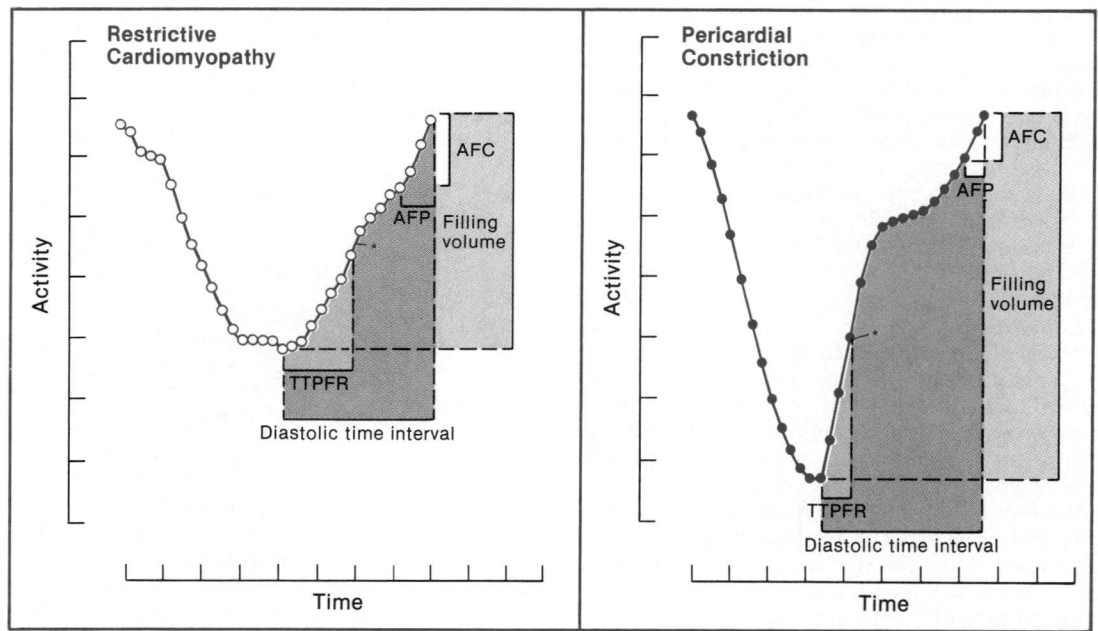

FIGURE 43–19. Time-activity curves showing ventricular emptying and filling for a patient with restrictive cardiomyopathy (*left*), and a patient with pericardial constriction (*right*). Note the slow initial filling in restrictive cardiomyopathy and the rapid initial filling in constriction. * = Peak filling rate, AFC = atrial filling contribution, AFP = atrial filling period, TTPFR = time to peak filling rate. (From Aroney, C. N., Ruddy, T. D., Dighero, H., et al.: Differentiation of restrictive cardiomyopathy from pericardial constriction: Assessment of diastolic function by radionuclide angiography. Reprinted by permission from the American College of Cardiology. J. Am. Coll. Cardiol. **13**:1007, 1989.)

are virtually ubiquitous in individuals over the age of 80; one-fourth have diffuse cardiac involvement.[353] Small deposits of amyloid may often be found in the pulmonary vessels or the vessels of other organs as well.

CARDIAC AMYLOIDOSIS

Involvement of the heart is a common finding and is the most frequent cause of death in amyloidosis associated with an immunocyte dyscrasia.[353] Clinically apparent heart disease is present in one-third to one-half of patients, although the heart is virtually always involved when studied pathologically.[352,353] In secondary amyloidosis, on the other hand, clinically significant cardiac involvement is uncommon (10 per cent or less); the myocardial deposits are typically small and perivascular and usually do not result in significant myocardial dysfunction.[353] Familial amyloidosis is only occasionally associated with overt cardiac involvement and then usually only late in the course of the disease. The clinical course is usually dominated by neurological or renal dysfunction.[353] Cardiac involvement in senile amyloidosis varies from small atrial deposits that do not result in functional impairment to extensive ventricular involvement with resultant cardiac failure.[353]

Cardiac amyloidosis occurs more commonly in men than in women, and it is rare before the age of 30 years.[352,354] Even in the familial form, the onset of clinical cardiac disease usually does not occur before the age of 35 years and generally occurs much later in life.[354]

PATHOLOGY. The pathological findings often include mild atrial enlargement, usually without significant ventricular dilatation (Fig. 43–20). The walls of both ventricles are typically firm, rubbery, noncompliant, and thickened.[334,353,354] Amyloid is present between the myocardial fibers,[353] (Fig. 43–21) with extensive deposition in the papillary muscles occurring commonly. Serial sections of the sinoatrial and atrioventricular nodes and the bundle branches may disclose amyloid deposits, particularly in the familial forms, although fibrosis of these structures is perhaps more common.[354] In addition, endocardial involvement of the atria and ventricles is frequent (Fig. 43–20). Amyloidosis often results in focal thickening of or deposits on the cardiac valves, but these abnormalities do not appear to interfere with valvular function, other than to produce murmurs. The intramural coronary arteries and veins frequently contain amyloid deposits in the media and adventitia, occasionally compromising the lumina of the vessels.[353,354]

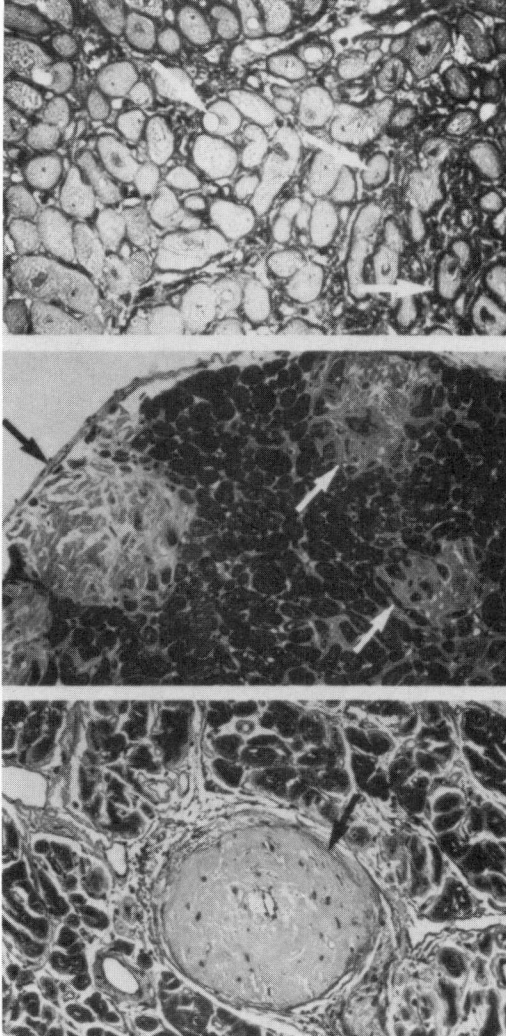

FIGURE 43–21. Patterns of cardiac amyloid deposition. *Top,* pericellular (arrows); *middle,* nodular (arrows); and *bottom,* vascular (arrow). (Top, sulfated alcian blue, ×270; middle and bottom, hematoxylin-eosin, ×135.) (From Pellikka, P. A., Holmes, D. R., Edwards, W. D., et al.: Endomyocardial biopsy in 30 patients with primary amyloidosis and suspected cardiac involvement. Arch. Intern. Med. *148:*662, 1988.)

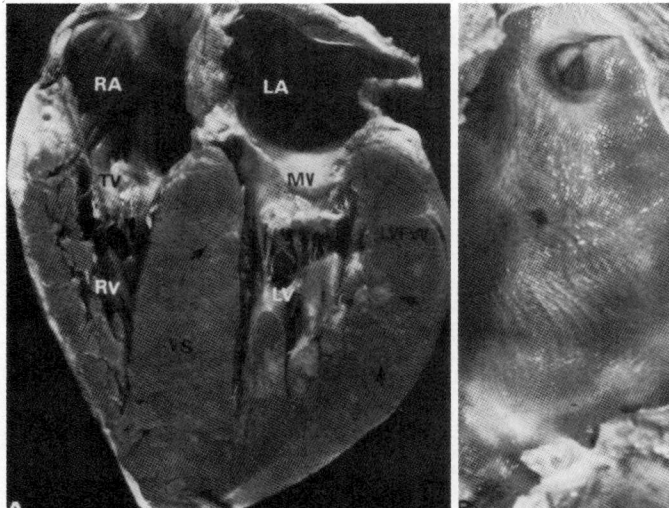

FIGURE 43–20. Amyloid heart disease. *A,* Four-chamber tomographic view of heart showing asymmetrically thickened ventricular septum (VS) compared with left ventricular free wall (LVFW) and grossly visible myocardial and valvular amyloid deposits (arrows). *B,* Close-up of left atrium showing characteristic "gritty" endocardium of cardiac amyloidosis. LA = left atrium, LV = left ventricle, MV = mitral valve, RA = right atrium, RV = right ventricle, TV = tricuspid valve. (From Waller, B. F.: Pathology of the cardiomyopathies. J. Am. Soc. Echocardiog. *1:*4, 1988.)

CLINICAL MANIFESTATIONS. Involvement of the cardiovascular system by amyloidosis occurs in four general forms.

1. The most common presentation of cardiac amyloidosis is that of *restrictive cardiomyopathy.*[353] Right-sided findings dominate the clinical presentation; peripheral edema is a prominent finding while paroxysmal nocturnal dyspnea and orthopnea are absent. Amyloid infiltration of the myocardium results in increased stiffness of the myocardium, producing the characteristic diastolic dip and plateau (square root sign) in the ventricular pressure pulse that may simulate constrictive pericarditis. In contrast to the accelerated early left ventricular diastolic filling found in constrictive pericarditis, cardiac amyloidosis is marked by an impaired rate of early diastolic filling, because of the stiffness of the ventricle.

2. A second common presentation is congestive heart failure due to *systolic dysfunction,* which occurs in many patients. Hemodynamic evidence of restriction of ventricular filling may not be prominent in these patients. The course of this form of the disease is often one of relentless progression, usually poorly responsive to treatment. Angina pectoris occurs on occasion and may be due to amyloid involvement of the coronary arteries or to concomitant atherosclerotic disease.[353,354]

3. *Orthostatic hypotension* is the third mode of presentation, occurring in about 10 per cent of cases. Although most likely

due to amyloid infiltration of the autonomic nervous system or of blood vessels (p. 1647), amyloid deposition in the heart and adrenals may contribute to this manifestation. Hypovolemia as a result of the nephrotic syndrome secondary to renal amyloidosis may aggravate the postural hypotension.[353]

4. An *abnormality of cardiac impulse formation and conduction* is the fourth and least common mode of presentation and may result in arrhythmias and conduction disturbances.[353] Sudden death, presumably arrhythmic in origin, is relatively common.[353,354]

Physical examination often reveals findings of congestive heart failure, especially right-sided; a systolic murmur due to atrioventricular valvular regurgitation may be present.[353] Particularly in patients with the restrictive cardiomyopathic presentation, jugular venous distention, a protodiastolic gallop, hepatomegaly, peripheral edema, and a narrow pulse pressure are found.[334] A fourth heart sound is uncommon, presum-

ably due to amyloid infiltration of the atrium. Patients typically are normotensive or hypotensive; even previously hypertensive individuals usually have a fall in blood pressure as the disease progresses.[353]

The *chest roentgenogram* usually shows cardiomegaly in patients with systolic dysfunction, although heart size may be normal in patients with the restrictive form. Pulmonary congestion may be prominent in patients with congestive heart failure. Pleural effusions are common.[334,353] The *electrocardiogram* is often abnormal; however, the most characteristic feature is diffusely diminished voltage,[353] occurring in approximately half the patients. Myocardial infarction is often simulated because of small or absent R waves in right precordial leads or, less frequently, by Q waves in the inferior leads. Left-axis deviation is seen in more than half the patients.[353] Arrhythmias, particularly atrial fibrillation, are common, although they rarely are the presenting feature of cardiac amyloidosis.[353] Complex ventricular arrhythmias are found frequently in patients with cardiac amyloidosis, and in some may be a harbinger of sudden death.[353,355] Various forms of AV conduction defects are often seen.[353] Abnormalities of AV conduction appear to be particularly common in familial amyloidosis with polyneuropathy.[356] Sinus node involvement is common, and the clinical and electrocardiographic features of the sick sinus syndrome may be present (p. 677).

Echocardiography (Figs. 43–22 and 4–98, p. 101) in advanced cases most commonly reveals increased thickness of the walls of the ventricles, small ventricular chambers, dilated atria, thickening of the interatrial septum, and impaired left ventricular function.[334,353,357,358] Early preclinical unsuspected cardiac involvement may be detectable only by echocardiography or Doppler ultrasound (see below).[334,359] Although the cardiac valves may be thickened, they usually move normally. A pericardial effusion is common but rarely results in tamponade. The appearance of the thickened cardiac walls is often distinctive on two-dimensional echocardiography, demonstrating a granular sparkling texture, presumably due to the amyloid deposit.[353,360] The echocardiographic appearance probably results from the presence of nodules containing amyloid and collagen,[361] and digital image analysis techniques are able to identify a unique tissue signature in cardiac amyloidosis.[259,362] In some cases the pattern of increased wall thickness is nonuniform and may resemble HCM with ASH.[187,353,363] Echocardiographic demonstration of thick left ventricular walls with concomitant low voltage on the electrocardiogram appears to distinguish cardiac amyloidosis from pericardial disease or left ventricular hypertrophy, and this distinctive voltage/mass ratio is characteristic of myocardial infiltration by the amyloid fibrils[334,358,364] (except in the familial forms). Doppler ultrasound[359,365] and radionuclide ventriculography[366] routinely demonstrate abnormalities of diastolic function.[367,367a]

Scintigraphy with technetium-99m-pyrophosphate (p. 315) is often strongly positive with prominent cardiac involvement, although in a minority of cases it is inexplicably falsely negative.[353,368] Positive scans tend to correlate with extensive cardiac involvement; scans are usually negative when the echocardiogram does not demonstrate abnormalities, as well as in the secondary forms of amyloidosis.[353]

Computed tomography may suggest the presence of myocardial amyloid when diffuse ventricular thickening is associated with a radiographic myocardial density lower than that seen when myocardial hypertrophy exists alone; the clinical utility of this modality is uncertain as of this writing.[353]

DIAGNOSIS. Whereas 2 or 3 decades ago the clinical diagnosis of systemic amyloidosis was made correctly antemortem only 25 per cent of the time, with more recent clinical awareness of the disease and the utilization of *biopsy techniques* the diagnosis is now made antemortem in the majority of cases. An abdominal fat aspirate has been the single most useful diagnostic procedure, combining the attributes of ease of performance, sensitivity, and safety.[352,353] Biopsy of rectum, gingiva, bone marrow, liver, kidney, and various other tissues has

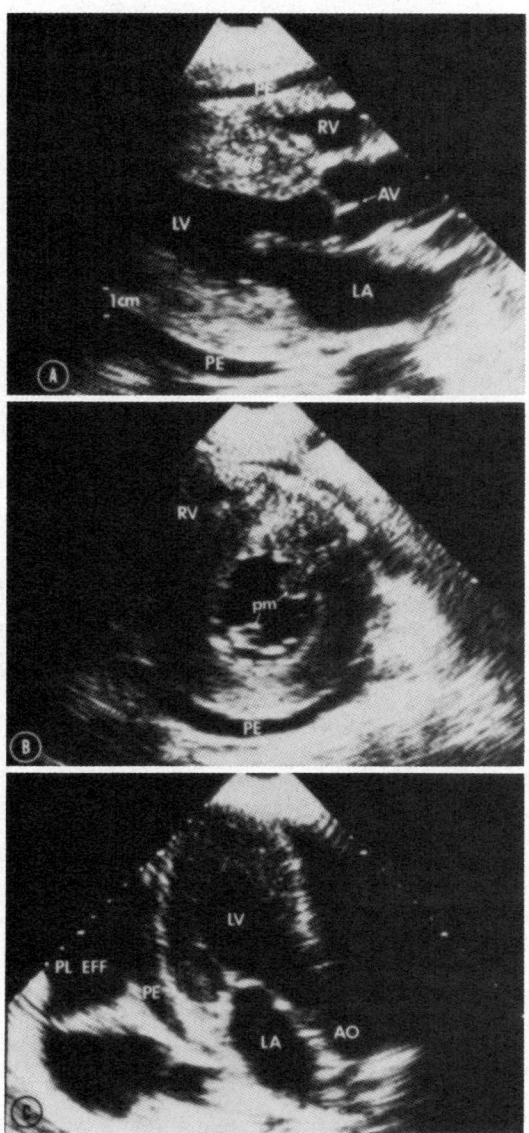

FIGURE 43–22. Parasternal long (A) and short axis (B) and apical long-axis (C) views show typical echocardiographic features of advanced cardiac amyloidosis. Note normal left ventricular cavity size and markedly thickened ventricular walls (ventricular septum = 22 mm, posterior wall = 18 mm, and right ventricular free wall = 15 mm) and the characteristic granular sparkling appearance. Small pericardial effusion (PE) and left pleural effusion (PL EFF) are also present. AO = Aorta, AV = aortic valve, LA = left atrium, LV = left ventricle, pm = papillary muscles, RV = right ventricle, VS = ventricular septum. (From Klein, A. L., Oh, J. K., Miller, F. A., et al.: Two-dimensional and Doppler echocardiographic assessment of infiltrative cardiomyopathy. J. Am. Soc. Echocardiog. *1*:48, 1988.)

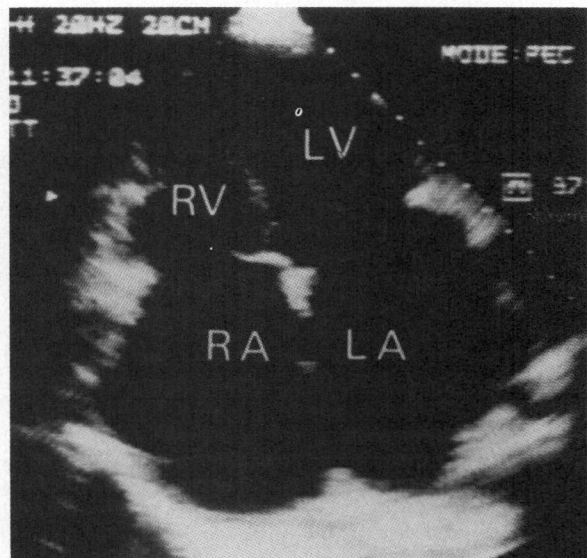

FIGURE 43-23. Two-dimensional echocardiogram (four-chamber apical view) in a 15-year-old boy with idiopathic restrictive cardiomyopathy reveals small right (RV) and left (LV) ventricular cavities with markedly dilated right (RA) and left (LA) atria. (From Child, J. S., and Perloff, J. K.: The restrictive cardiomyopathies. Cardiol. Clin. 6:294, 1988.)

also been employed. Endomyocardial biopsy of the right or left ventricles may be helpful in establishing the diagnosis of cardiac amyloidosis if the abdominal fat aspirate is negative.[334,353]

MANAGEMENT. The treatment of cardiac amyloidosis is generally unsatisfactory and ineffective,[352] although it is speculated that alkylating agents may have some role.[353,355] Digitalis glycosides should be used with caution because patients with cardiac amyloidosis appear to be particularly sensitive to digitalis preparations, and the use of ordinary doses may lead to serious arrhythmias; this may relate to selective binding of digoxin to amyloid fibrils in the myocardium.[353] Similarly, nifedipine binds to amyloid fibrils[369]; its use and that of the other calcium antagonists may lead to exacerbation of congestive heart failure symptoms due to an enhanced negative inotropic effect.[352,370] Insertion of a permanent pacemaker may be beneficial in patients with symptomatic conducting system disease.[353] Careful use of low doses of diuretics and vasodilators may afford some symptomatic benefit,[353] but there is a real risk of hypotension with use of these agents.

INHERITED INFILTRATIVE DISORDERS CAUSING CARDIOMYOPATHY

The intramyocardial accumulation or infiltration of an abnormal metabolic product may result in abnormal systolic contractile performance. However, it may also impair the filling of the ventricles, thereby adding a restrictive component. A variety of infiltrative diseases, often inherited, may result in this hemodynamic picture, including the glycogenoses (p. 1645), the mucopolysaccharidoses (p. 1637), Fabry disease, and Gaucher disease.

FABRY DISEASE

Fabry disease (angiokeratoma corporis diffusum universale) is an X-linked disorder of glycosphingolipid metabolism due to a deficiency of the enzyme ceramide trihexosidase.[371] It is characterized by an intracellular accumulation of a neutral glycolipid, with prominent involvement of the skin and kidneys as well as the myocardium. *Histological examination* often reveals widespread involvement of the myocardium, vascular endothelium, conducting tissues, and valves—particularly the mitral valve.[372] The major clinical manifestations of the disease result from the accumulation of the glycolipid substrate in endothelial cells, with eventual occlusion of small arterioles.[373] The accumulation of the glycolipid occurs in the lysosomes of the cardiac tissues and is responsible for the multiple cardiovascular manifestations of Fabry disease.[374] Symptomatic cardiovascular involvement occurs eventually in most affected males, while female

carriers are usually asymptomatic or only minimally symptomatic, but on occasion may have severe cardiac involvement.[371] Systemic hypertension, renovascular hypertension, mitral valve prolapse, and congestive heart failure are common clinical manifestations. Altered vasomotor activity is found in Fabry disease, resulting in a Reynaud-like picture. Electrocardiographic abnormalities include left ventricular hypertrophy, P-wave abnormalities, conduction defects, and arrhythmias.[374-376] The echocardiogram usually reveals increased left ventricular wall thickness, presumably the result of glycolipid deposition, which may simulate hypertrophic cardiomyopathy and mitral valve prolapse.[374,375] Differentiation from other restrictive or hypertrophic processes (such as cardiac amyloidosis) may not be possible on echocardiographic grounds but may be possible with nuclear magnetic resonance imaging.[374] Endomyocardial biopsy may be of considerable value in making a definitive diagnosis,[374,377] and a low alpha-galactosidase activity in leukocytes is also helpful diagnostically.

Whether renal transplantation prevents progressive cardiac involvement in Fabry disease is not clear.[378]

GAUCHER DISEASE

Gaucher disease is an uncommon, inherited disorder of glycosyl ceramide metabolism. It is secondary to a deficiency of the enzyme beta-glucosidase and results in accumulation of cerebrosides in the spleen, liver, bone marrow, lymph nodes, brain, and myocardium. Diffuse interstitial infiltration of the left ventricle by cells laden with cerebroside occurs in Gaucher disease, associated with reduced left ventricular compliance and cardiac output. Clinical evidence of cardiac involvement is uncommon, but when present it is characterized by left ventricular dysfunction, hemorrhagic pericardial effusion, increase in left ventricular wall mass, and calcification of the left-sided valves.[379-382]

HEMOCHROMATOSIS AND HEMOSIDEROSIS (See also p. 1646.)

Hemochromatosis is characterized by excessive deposition of iron in a variety of parenchymal tissues (heart, liver, gonads, and pancreas). It may occur (1) as a familial or idiopathic disorder, (2) in association with a defect in hemoglobin synthesis resulting in ineffective erythropoiesis, (3) in chronic liver disease, and (4) with excessive oral intake of iron over many years. While patients who have iron deposits in the myocardium almost always have deposits in other organs (e.g., liver, spleen, pancreas, bone marrow), the severity of myocardial involvement varies widely and only roughly parallels that in other organs.[383] Cardiac involvement leads to a mixed dilated/restrictive cardiomyopathic presentation, with both systolic and diastolic dysfunction.[384]

Pathological Findings

(Fig. 57-7 p. 1748.) These consist of a dilated heart with thickened ventricular walls. Myocardial iron deposits are found within the sarcoplasmic reticulum,[385] and are most common in the subepicardial region, followed by the subendocardial region, and are least common in the midmyocardial wall.[386] They are more extensive in ventricular than in atrial myocardium. Involvement of the cardiac conducting system is common.[385] Myocardial degeneration and fibrosis may also occur.

The severity of myocardial dysfunction is proportional to the quantity of iron present in the myocardium.[386] Extensive deposits of cardiac iron (particularly those grossly visible at postmortem examination) are invariably associated with cardiac dysfunction—usually chronic congestive heart failure, which is often the cause of death. Extensive cardiac deposits usually occur in patients who receive more than 100 blood transfusions (unless there is associated iron loss due to bleeding).

Clinical Manifestations

These vary widely, depending on the extent of myocardial involvement. Some patients remain asymptomatic despite echocardiographic evidence of myocardial involvement, which is expressed as normal or increased left ventricular wall thickness, chamber enlargement and contractile dysfunction.[384,386,387] In such cases, a variety of noninvasive techniques, including exercise radionuclide ventriculography, may demonstrate early subclinical myocardial involvement in which treatment is most effective.[384,387,388] Symptomatic cardiac involvement is usually associated with electrocardiographic abnormalities, including ST-segment and T-wave changes, as well as supraventricular arrhythmias; these electrocardiographic changes correlate with the degree of iron deposits in the heart.[384] Atrioventricular conduction disturbances and ventricular arrhythmias are uncommon.

Cardiac involvement usually is evident from the clinical and echocardiographic features; endomyocardial biopsy may be useful to confirm (but not exclude) the diagnosis.[384,386] The diagnosis is aided by finding elevated plasma iron levels (180 to 300 μg/dl; normal = 50 to 150), a normal or low total iron-binding capacity (200 to 300 μg/dl; normal = 250 to 370), and markedly elevated values for saturation of transferrin (80 to 100 per cent; normal = 22 to 46 per cent), serum ferritin (900 to 6000 ng/ml; normal = 3 to 180), urinary iron (9 to 23 mg/24 hr; normal = 0 to 2), and liver iron (600 to 1800 μg/100 mg dry wt; normal = 30 to 140).[389] Repeated phlebotomies or the use of the chelating agent desferrioxamine may be clinically beneficial.[384,390] (For further discussion of the treatment of iron storage disease see p. 1748.).

SARCOIDOSIS

Sarcoidosis is a granulomatous disorder of unknown etiology, characterized by multisystem involvement. Infiltration of the lungs, reticuloendothelial system, and skin usually dominates the clinical picture, but virtually any tissue may be affected. The most important manifestation results from pulmonary involvement. This often leads to diffuse fibrosis that may result in fatal right heart failure. Primary cardiac involvement is not often recognized clinically, although it may be demonstrated at autopsy in 20 to 30 per cent of cases of sarcoid, most of which demonstrate generalized sarcoidosis.[391-394] Clinical manifestations of sarcoid heart disease are present in less than 5 per cent of patients, although myocardial involvement may result in heart block, congestive heart failure, ventricular arrhythmias, and sudden death, particularly in youngsters.[391] Myocardial sarcoidosis may have restrictive as well as congestive features, since cardiac infiltration by sarcoid granulomas results not only in increased stiffness of the ventricular wall but diminished systolic contractile function as well. Myocardial sarcoidosis typically affects young or middle-aged adults of either sex; there is usually evidence of generalized sarcoidosis.[393,395]

Pathology

The typical pathological feature of sarcoidosis is the presence of noncaseating granulomas, which occur in many organs. They infiltrate the myocardium and may eventually become fibrotic scars.[395] The granulomas may involve any region of the heart, although the left ventricular free wall and the interventricular septum are the most common sites, and extensive granulomas and scar tissue in the cephalad portion of the interventricular septum is a constant finding in patients with abnormalities of the conduction system.[395,396] Cardiac effects may range from a few scattered lesions to extensive involvement.[397] Because of the variable cardiac involvement, myocardial biopsy may be positive in only about half of the patients, and therefore a negative biopsy by no means excludes the diagnosis.[398,399] Transmural involvement is common, and large portions of the ventricular wall may be replaced by sarcoid tissue, which may lead to aneurysm formation.[395] While involvement of small coronary artery branches may be found in sarcoidosis, the pathophysiological importance of this observation remains unclear.

CLINICAL MANIFESTATIONS. Sudden death is the most feared and unfortunately one of the more common manifestations of cardiac sarcoidosis.[394-396] Conduction disturbances and congestive heart failure are common manifestations of symptomatic involvement in nonfatal cases, but many patients are apparently asymptomatic despite extensive cardiac involvement.[392-394] Syncope is common and may reflect paroxysmal arrhythmias or conduction disturbances.[334] Atrial and ventricular arrhythmias, especially ventricular tachycardia, are observed frequently.[334] While cor pulmonale as a con-

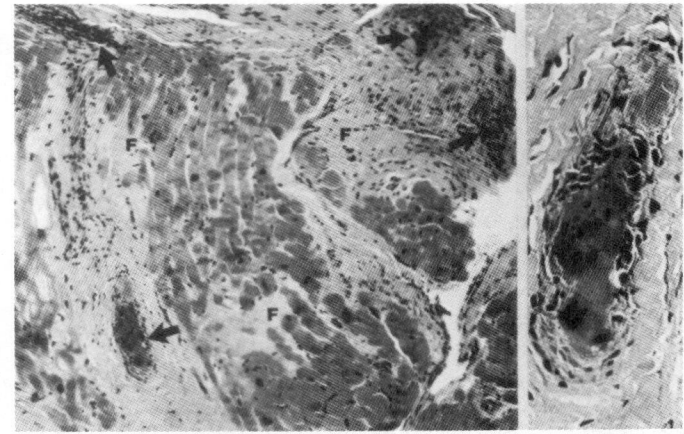

FIGURE 43-24. Under low magnification (left panel) this endomyocardial biopsy sample from a patient with sarcoid shows several foci of intense inflammation (arrows), as well as a marked interstitial infiltrate of mononuclear cells. There is abundant interstitial fibrosis (F). On high power magnification (right panel), a giant cell is clearly discernible in one granuloma. Hematoxylin-phloxine-saffron stain. (Left panel, original magnification ×125; right panel, original magnification ×325.) (From Ratner, S. J., Fenoglio, J. J., and Ursell, P. C.: Utility of endomyocardial biopsy in the diagnosis of cardiac sarcoidosis. Chest **90:**528, 1986.)

sequence of pulmonary sarcoidosis accounts for some of the symptoms of heart failure, many symptoms are caused by direct myocardial involvement by granulomas and scar tissue, and the patients show the clinical features of restrictive or dilated cardiomyopathy.[334] Symptoms of myocardial sarcoid may be present for variable lengths of time; however, the disease may progress rapidly to death, and in some patients the interval from the onset of the cardiac symptoms to death is measured in months.[394] Survival may be considerably longer, however.[393,400]

Cardiac dysfunction is often severe and progressive. Occasionally, patients with extensive involvement develop overt left ventricular aneurysms.[396,400] Pericardial effusions are rare in patients with sarcoidosis.[401,402]

The *physical examination* may reveal findings of extracardiac sarcoid or may be totally normal. A systolic murmur reflecting mitral regurgitation is common. This appears to be more the result of left ventricular dilatation or infiltration than of direct sarcoid involvement of the papillary muscles.

The *electrocardiogram* is frequently abnormal in patients with known sarcoid and most commonly demonstrates T-wave abnormalities.[393] Sarcoidosis appears to have an affinity for involvement of the AV junction and bundle of His, and

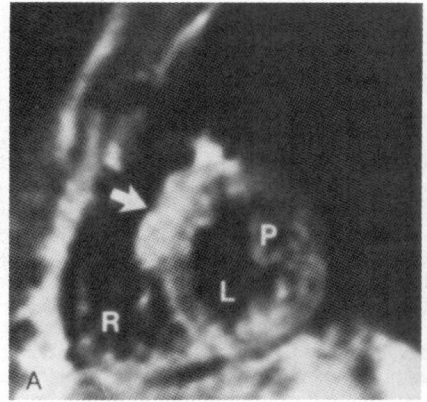
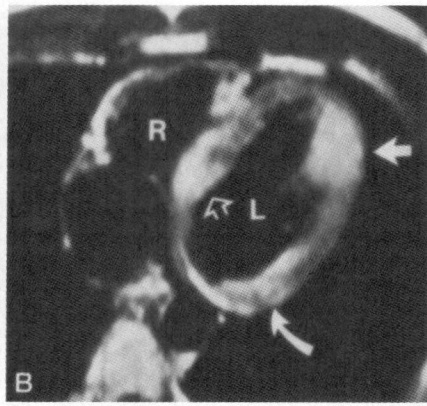
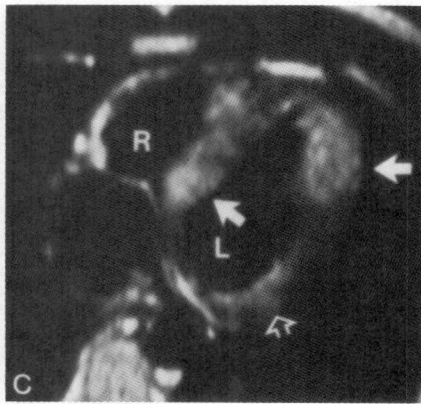

FIGURE 43-25. *A,* Gated cardiac MR image in an oblique sagittal plane from a patient with cardiac sarcoid shows a discrete, high-intensity mass (arrow) arising from basal portion of septum. R = right ventricle, L = left ventricle, P = posterolateral papillary muscle. *B,* Gated cardiac MR image in transverse plane shows discrete high-intensity masses in myocardium of basal portion of septum (open arrow), anterolateral wall (straight closed arrow), and posterolateral wall (curved arrow). *C,* With additional imaging, the normal myocardium has a relative decrease in signal intensity whereas masses (solid arrows) have a higher intensity. Third lesion in posterolateral left ventricle wall (open arrow) is seen better. (From Riedy, K., Fisher, M. R., Belic, N., and Koenigsberg, D. I.: MR imaging of myocardial sarcoidosis. Am. J. Roentgenol. *151:*915, 1988.)

thus varying degrees of intraventricular or AV block are common.[393] With extensive myocardial involvement, pathological Q waves may appear and simulate myocardial infarction.[393] Characteristic features of *echocardiography* include left ventricular dilatation and dysfunction, often with regional wall motion abnormalities suggestive of ischemic heart disease.[393,400]

DIAGNOSIS. In many cases the diagnosis may be suspected in patients with bilateral hilar lymphadenopathy on chest roentgenogram in whom there is clinical or electrocardiographic evidence of myocardial disease. Endomyocardial biopsy may be useful in establishing the diagnosis (Fig. 43–24).[403] Myocardial imaging with thallium-201 may also be helpful in demonstrating segmental perfusion defects that may be due to sarcoid infiltration of the myocardium; there also is speculation that they may reflect a derangement in the microcirculation.[392] Imaging may also indicate the presence of right ventricular hypertrophy in patients with right ventricular overload due to pulmonary fibrosis and pulmonary hypertension. Uptake of technetium pyrophosphate and gallium in myocardial sarcoidosis may aid in the diagnosis, as may nuclear magnetic imaging (Fig. 43–25).[402]

MANAGEMENT. The treatment of myocardial sarcoidosis is difficult. Arrhythmias are often refractory to antiarrhythmic drugs. Permanent pacing may be helpful. While the matter is not settled, it appears that corticosteroids may be of some benefit in treating the conduction disturbances, arrhythmias, and myocardial dysfunction of sarcoidosis.[334,404] Since the risk of sudden death appears to be greatest in patients with extensive myocardial involvement, it may be reasonable to attempt to halt the progression of the disease with steroids before irreversible fibrosis occurs. Formation of a ventricular aneurysm may be a possible side effect of steroid use.[334,396] Insertion of an implantable cardioverter-defibrillator may be considered in appropriate patients at high risk of sudden death.[396]

ENDOMYOCARDIAL DISEASE

Endomyocardial disease (EMD) is a common form of restrictive cardiomyopathy in equatorial Africa and is encountered with less frequency in South America, Asia, and nontropical countries, including the United States.[334,405-408] It is marked by intense endocardial fibrotic thickening of the apex and subvalvular regions of one or both ventricles that results in obstruction to inflow of blood into the respective ventricle, thus producing restrictive physiology. Two variants of the disease have been described, one occurring principally in tropical countries (termed endomyocardial fibrosis, EMF), and the other in temperate countries (Löffler endocarditis parietalis fibroplastica).

Although long considered separate entities, if only because Löffler endocarditis is marked by intense tissue and often peripheral eosinophilia, there is now general agreement that EMF and Löffler endocarditis are different manifestations of the same disease, since the pathological findings in advanced cases are identical.[405-409] Despite the pathological similarities, there are differences in clinical presentation. In addition to the geographic differences, the temperate form of the disease (Löffler endocarditis) acts as a more aggressive and rapidly progressive disorder, affecting principally males, and is associated with hypereosinophilia, thromboembolic phenomena, and generalized arteritis.[410] EMF, conversely, shows no sex predilection, occurs in younger patients, and usually is not associated with an intense eosinophilia.[411]

It has also been postulated that Löffler endocarditis and EMF are different phases in a progressive disease that results from the toxic effect of eosinophils on the heart.[405,412-414] Under this formulation, an initial hypereosinophilia of whatever cause results in damage to the myocardium that produces the first phase of EMD: a necrotic phase, marked by an intense myocarditis, rich in eosinophils, and with an associated arteritis (i.e., Löffler endocarditis). This initial phase

occurs within the first few months of illness. It appears to be followed by a thrombotic stage, occurring about a year after initial presentation, during which the myocarditis has receded, nonspecific thickening of the myocardium is beginning, and there is a variable degree of superimposed thrombus formation. The last stage is one of fibrosis, presenting all of the features of EMF.[405,409] The three stages—necrotic, thrombotic, and fibrotic—have been defined on the basis of postmortem material, and it is not suggested that each patient with advanced disease (manifested by EMF) has necessarily passed through the earlier phases.

The possible role of *eosinophils* in the production of the cardiac abnormalities has intrigued investigators for years.[410,412-414] Eosinophils may damage tissues by direct invasion or the release of toxic substances.[409,415] The presence of degranulated peripheral eosinophils in patients with Löffler endocarditis suggests that the protein constituents of the eosinophil's granule may be cardiotoxic,[412,416] producing first the necrotic phase of EMD, followed by the thrombotic and fibrotic phases after the disappearance of the initial eosinophilia.[405,415]

Since the clinical manifestations of EMD demonstrate geographical and clinical differences, Löffler endocarditis and EMF will be discussed separately, even though they could be part of the same disease continuum.

LÖFFLER ENDOCARDITIS

Hypereosinophilic Syndrome

Marked eosinophilia of any cause may be associated with endomyocardial disease. The typical patient who presents with Löffler endocarditis is a man in his fourth decade who lives in a temperate climate and has the hypereosinophilic syndrome (i.e., persistent eosinophilia with $\geq$ 1500 eosinophils/mm³ for at least 6 months or until death, with evidence of organ involvement).[334,410,412,417] Cardiac involvement in the hypereosinophilic syndrome is the rule, occurring in more than three-fourths of patients.[410,417] Hypereosinophilia and cardiac involvement is also seen in the Churg-Strauss syndrome, which is differentiated by asthma, nasal polyposis, and a necrotizing vasculitis. The cause of the eosinophilia in most patients with Löffler endocarditis is unknown, although in some it may be the result of leukemia, or it may be reactive (that is, secondary to various parasitic, allergic, granulomatous, hypersensitivity, or neoplastic disorders[410,417]). The relationship of the eosinophilia to possible parasitic infestation is unclear.[417]

PATHOLOGY. In the hypereosinophilic syndrome, a variety of organs are usually involved besides the heart, including the lungs, bone marrow, and brain.[334] Cardiac involvement is often biventricular, with mural endocardial thickening of the inflow portions and apex of the ventricles. Histological findings include variable degrees of (1) an acute inflammatory eosinophilic myocarditis involving the myo- and endocardium; (2) thrombosis, fibrinoid change, and inflammatory reaction involving small intramural coronary vessels; (3) mural thrombosis, often containing eosinophils; and (4) fibrotic thickening of up to several millimeters.[412]

CLINICAL MANIFESTATIONS. The principal clinical features include weight loss, fever, cough, skin rash, and congestive heart failure. Although early cardiac involvement may be asymptomatic, overt cardiac dysfunction occurs in more than half the patients and may be right- and/or left-sided.[412] Cardiomegaly, often without overt symptoms of congestive heart failure, may be present, and the murmur of mitral regurgitation is common.[417] Systemic embolism is frequent and may lead to neurological and renal dysfunction. Death is usually due to congestive heart failure, often with associated renal, hepatic, or respiratory dysfunction.

LABORATORY EXAMINATION. The *chest roentgenogram* may reveal cardiomegaly and pulmonary congestion or, less commonly, pulmonary infiltrates. The *electrocardiogram* most commonly shows nonspecific ST-segment and T-wave abnormalities.[417] Arrhythmias, especially atrial fibrillation, and conduction defects, particularly right bundle branch block, may also be present.[412]

The *echocardiogram* commonly demonstrates localized thickening of the posterobasal left ventricular wall, with absent or markedly limited motion of the posterior leaflet of the mitral valve.[334,412] There may be obliteration of the apex by thrombus. Enlargement of the atria may be seen,[418] along with Doppler ultrasound evidence of AV valve regurgitation. The endocardium may be unusually echo-reflective as a consequence of fibrosis.[405]

The *hemodynamic consequences* of the dense endocardial scarring seen in Löffler endocarditis are those of a restrictive cardiomyopathy, as already described (p. 1415), with abnormal diastolic filling due to increased stiffness of the ventricles and a reduction in the size of the ventricular cavity by organized thrombus. Systolic performance usually is largely preserved. Atrioventricular valvular regurgitation may occur because of involvement of the supporting apparatus of the mitral or tricuspid valves.[412] *Cardiac catheterization* reveals markedly elevated ventricular filling pressures, and there may be evidence of tricuspid or mitral regurgitation. A characteristic feature on angiocardiography is largely preserved systolic function with obliteration of the apex of the ventricles. The diagnosis is often confirmed by percutaneous endomyocardial biopsy.[412]

TREATMENT. Medical therapy during the course of early Löffler endocarditis, and surgical therapy during the later phases of fibrosis, may have a positive effect on symptoms and survival. Corticosteroids appear to have a beneficial effect on acute myocarditis,[412] and together with cytotoxic drugs (hydroxyurea in particular), may improve survival substantially.[296,412,417,418] Routine cardiac therapy with digitalis, diuretics, afterload reduction, and anticoagulation as indicated are adjuncts in the management of these patients. Surgical therapy appears to offer significant palliation of symptoms once the fibrotic stage has been reached.[296,417,419]

ENDOMYOCARDIAL FIBROSIS

Endomyocardial fibrosis (EMF) occurs most commonly in tropical and subtropical Africa, particularly Uganda and Nigeria. It is typified by fibrous endocardial lesions of the inflow portion of the right or left ventricle or both and often involves the atrioventricular valves, resulting in regurgitation (Fig. 43–26).[406] It is a relatively frequent cause of heart failure and death in equatorial Africa, accounting for 10 to 20 per cent of deaths due to heart disease.[334,405]

While most prominent in Africa, it is also found in tropical and subtropical regions in the rest of the world, including India, Brazil, Colombia, and Sri Lanka.[406] EMF is most common in specific ethnic groups, notably the Rwanda tribe in Uganda, and in people of low socioeconomic status.[406,420] The disease is equally frequent in both sexes, and, although most common in children and young adults, its reported age range is from 4 to 70 years of age.[334,406,411] It is most common in blacks, but cases have been reported occasionally in whites in temperate climates, rarely in the absence of prior residence in tropical areas.[405]

PATHOLOGY

A pericardial effusion, which may be quite large, may be present.[406] The heart is normal in size or slightly enlarged, but massive cardiomegaly does not occur. The right atrium is often dilated, and in patients with severe right ventricular involvement there may be massive enlargement of this chamber. Indentation of the right border of the heart above the apex as a result of apical scarring may occur.[406]

Combined right and left ventricular disease occurs in about half the cases, with pure left ventricular involvement occurring in 40 per cent and pure right ventricular involvement in the remaining 10 per cent of patients who are examined post mortem.[334] When affected, the right ventricle exhibits extensive, dense, fibrous thickening of the inflow tract and apex, with involvement of the papillary muscles and chordae tendineae. Involvement of the right ventricle may lead to obliteration of the apex, with a mass of thrombus and fibrous tissue filling the cavity.[406] The tricuspid valve is often pulled down and distorted by the fibrous process involving the supporting structures.[421] Right atrial thrombi occur commonly. Left ventricular involvement is similar, with fibrosis extending from the apex up the inflow

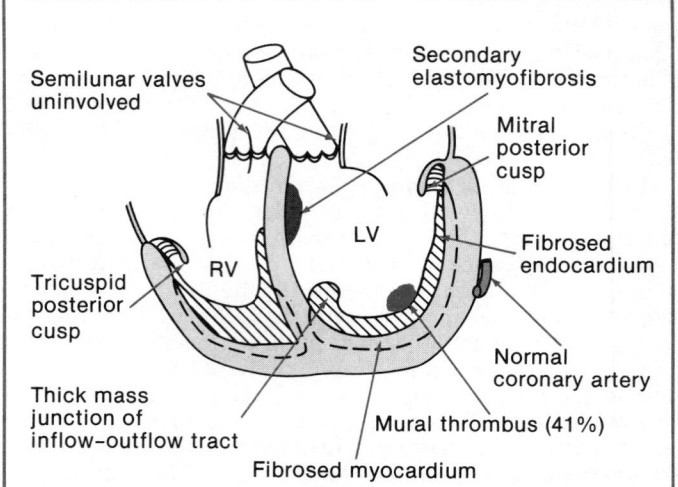

FIGURE 43–26. Cardiac lesions of endomyocardial fibrosis. (From Davies, J. N. P.: Endomyocardial fibrosis. *In* Giles, T. D., and Sander, G. E.: Cardiomyopathy. Littleton, MA, PSG Publishing Co., 1988, p. 188.)

portion of the left ventricle to the posterior mitral valve leaflet. The anterior leaflet of the mitral valve and the outflow portion of the left ventricle are usually spared.[421] Thrombi often overlie the endocardial lesions, and widely distributed endocardial calcific deposits may occur.[422] The coronary arteries are uninvolved, as is the remainder of the body.[334]

Microscopically, the involved endocardium demonstrates a thick layer of collagen tissue on top of a layer of loosely arranged connective tissue.[406] Septa composed of fibrous and granulation tissue extend for variable distances into the myocardium.[334] Interstitial edema is often present, but there is no cellular infiltration. Small patches of fibroelastosis may occur in both ventricular outflow tracts beneath the semilunar valves but are thought to be a secondary phenomenon due to local trauma rather than a result of the basic pathological process.[406]

CLINICAL MANIFESTATIONS

As already noted, EMF may involve both ventricles or either ventricle selectively; left-sided involvement results in symptoms of pulmonary congestion, while predominant right-sided disease may present features of a restrictive cardiomyopathy and therefore simulate constrictive pericarditis. There is often regurgitation of one or both atrioventricular valves. The onset of the disease is usually insidious, but it is sometimes ushered in by an acute febrile illness. Rarely, the disease appears to stabilize, and survival for up to 12 years has been observed, but it is usually relentlessly progressive. Death is due to progressive myocardial failure, often associated with pulmonary congestion, infection, or infarction. The most important immediate cause of death is sudden, unexpected cardiovascular collapse, presumably arrhythmic in origin.[334] Survival appears to be unrelated to site of predominant involvement (right or left ventricle), although those patients presenting in advanced right-sided failure have a worse prognosis than do other patients.[411]

RIGHT VENTRICULAR EMF. Pure or predominant right ventricular involvement is characterized by fibrous obliteration of the right ventricular apex that diminishes the capacity of this chamber. The fibrosis often extends to the supporting apparatus of the tricuspid valve, resulting in tricuspid regurgitation. Therefore, clinical manifestations in patients with right-sided involvement include an elevated jugular venous pressure, a prominent *v* wave, and a rapid *y* descent. A protodiastolic gallop sound may be heard along the lower sternal border,[406] reflecting right ventricular dysfunction. The liver is usually large and pulsatile, and ascites, splenomegaly, and peripheral edema are common. Pulmonary congestion is not present in the absence of left-sided involvement, and the pulmonary artery and pulmonary capillary wedge pressures are normal. A pericardial effusion, which is sometimes quite large, may be present. The right atrium is often enlarged, sometimes massively so.

Laboratory Findings. The *electrocardiogram* is usually abnormal, with diminished QRS voltage (probably resulting from the presence of a pericardial effusion), ST-segment and T-wave abnormalities, and findings of right atrial enlargement, especially a qR pattern in lead V_1.[423] Atrial fibrillation is common.[406] The *chest roentgenogram* demonstrates cardiac enlargement, usually with gross prominence of the right atrium and a pericardial effusion.[406] Calcification in the region of the right ventricular apex may be found.[424] *Echocardiography* may demonstrate right ventricular thickening, obliteration of the apex, dilated atrium, strong echoes emanating from the endocardial surface, and abnormal septal motion in patients with tricuspid regurgitation.[405,406,425] At *angiography* the right ventricular apex is characteristically not visualized because of obliteration by the fibrous endocardium, but tricuspid regurgitation, right atrial enlargement, and filling defects in the right atrium due to intraatrial thrombi are sometimes seen.[334,405] Early angiographic changes that may be present before advanced disease develops include a change in the endocardial appearance, small apical filling defects, and mild tricuspid regurgitation.[406]

LEFT VENTRICULAR EMF. With predominant *left-sided* involvement, the endomyocardial fibrosis invades the apex of the ventricle and usually the chordae tendineae or the posterior mitral valve leaflet as well, leading to mitral regurgitation.[405] The murmur may be confined to late systole, as is characteristic of the papillary muscle dysfunction type of murmur, or it may be pansystolic. Findings of pulmonary hypertension may be prominent. A protodiastolic gallop is commonly heard.[405]

Laboratory Findings. The *electrocardiogram* usually shows T-wave abnormalities and diminished QRS voltage in the presence of a pericardial effusion, although left ventricular hypertrophy may be present.[334] There may be findings of left atrial abnormality.[406] As with right-sided involvement, atrial fibrillation often is present. *Echocardiographic* features include thickening and reduced motion of the posterobasal wall and posterior mitral leaflet, increased echo-reflectivity of the endocardium, preserved systolic wall motion in the presence of apical obliteration, dilated atrium, and Doppler ultrasound evidence of mitral regurgitation (Fig. 43–27).[405,406,425] *Cardiac catheterization* often reveals pulmonary hypertension, with elevated left ventricular filling pressures and a reduced cardiac index.[426] The left ventriculogram usually shows mitral regurgitation, and a filling defect due to an intracavitary thrombus within the ventricle may be seen on occasion[334] (Fig. 43–28). Coronary arteriography does not reveal obstructive disease.

BIVENTRICULAR EMF. This form of endomyocardial fibrosis occurs more frequently than either isolated right- or left-sided disease.[427] If there is more than minimal right ventricular involvement, severe pulmonary hypertension does not occur, and the right-sided findings dominate the clinical presentation. The typical patient with biventricular involvement may have the features of right ventricular endomyocardial fibrosis, as already described, with only a mitral regurgitant murmur to suggest left ventricular involvement. Systemic embolization may occur in up to 15 per cent of patients; infective endocarditis is even less frequent and is found in less than 2 per cent.

DIAGNOSIS

This is based on the presence in an individual of the typical clinical and laboratory features, particularly angiography, from the appropriate geographical area. Eosinophilia is usually not a prominent feature and when present may reflect associated parasitic infestation. *Endomyocardial biopsy* may occasionally be helpful in establishing the diagnosis.[405] However, this risks dislodging a mural thrombus, with resultant embolization, and left-sided biopsy is *not* recommended. In addition, because the disease is often focal, the biopsy may miss the pathological process, particularly if a right ventricular biopsy is performed in a patient with isolated left-sided disease.

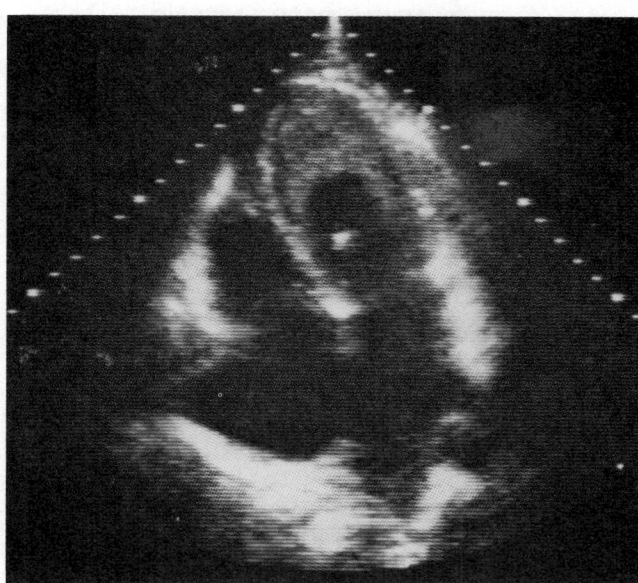

FIGURE 43–27. Apical four-chamber echocardiogram in endomyocardial fibrosis with typical left ventricular apical obliteration. Contrast injection (agitated saline solution) showed right ventricular apical obliteration also. Doppler examination showed moderate mitral regurgitation, severe tricuspid regurgitation, and pulmonary hypertension. (From Acquatella, H., and Schiller, N. B.: Echocardiographic recognition of Chagas' disease and endomyocardial fibrosis. J. Am. Soc. Echocardiog. *1*:60, 1988.)

MANAGEMENT

The medical treatment of EMF is often difficult and not particularly effective. In patients with advanced disease, the outlook is poor, with a 35 to 50 per cent 2-year mortality.[411,427] Substantially better survival may be seen in less symptomatic patients who have milder forms of the disease.[427,428] Digitalis glycosides may be helpful in controlling the ventricular rate in patients with atrial fibrillation, but the response of congestive symptoms is disappointing. Diuretics are not particularly helpful in the treatment of ascites. Once endomyocardial disease has reached the fibrotic stage, surgery offers the possibility of symptomatic improvement and is the treatment of choice.[334] Operative excision of the fibrotic endocardium and replacement of the mitral and/or tricuspid valves have led to substantial symptomatic improvement, especially with predominant left ventricular involvement.[421,423,426,428] Mitral valve repair, rather than replacement, can be accomplished in some patients.[421] Postoperative catheterization has also provided objective evidence of hemodynamic improvement with a reduction in ventricular filling pressures, an increase in cardiac output, and normalization of the angiographic appearance.[421,426] Operative mortality has been high, running between 15 and 25 per cent in the larger series.[421,423,426,428]

FIGURE 43–28. Differences in the apical lesion between endomyocardial fibrosis (EMF), myocardial infarction (MI), and Chagas' heart disease. Both apices can be affected in EMF, but typically LV function is preserved or hypercontractile, and LV obliteration moves inward. In apical MI, dyskinetic apex frequently is combined with septal or anterior wall motion abnormalities, depending on extent of disease of left anterior descending coronary artery. "Neck" of dyskinetic area tends to be large. In chronic Chagas' disease, although apical aneurysm can be as large as in ischemic heart disease, some patients may have typical "small" neck aneurysm. When apical dyskinesis without aneurysm is found, its appearance cannot be used to differentiate between ischemic or Chagas' disease. Chagas' disease with isolated apical aneurysm typically spares all but most apical portion of septum. In Chagas' disease, RV apical dyskinesis or aneurysm may also be present. (From Acquatella, H., and Schiller, N. B.: Echocardiographic recognition of Chagas' disease and endomyocardial fibrosis. J. Am. Soc. Echocardiog. *1*:60, 1988.)

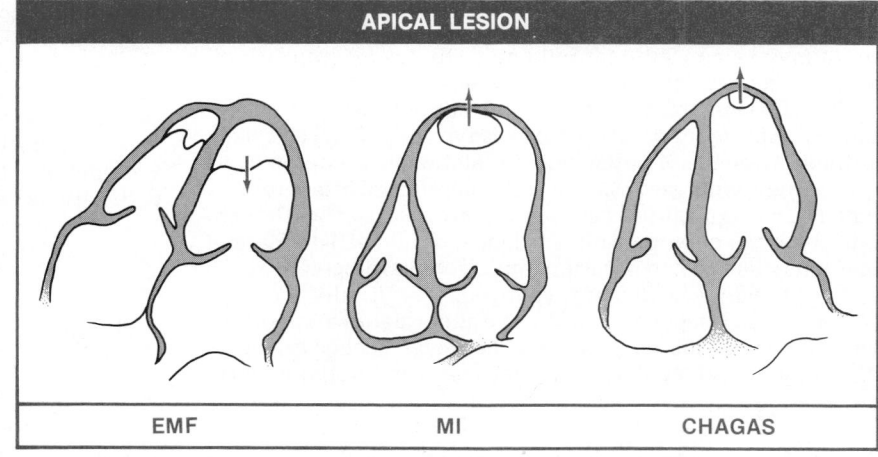

APICAL LESION

EMF   MI   CHAGAS

ENDOCARDIAL FIBROELASTOSIS
(See p. 994)

CARCINOID HEART DISEASE

ETIOLOGY AND PATHOLOGY. The carcinoid syndrome is caused by a metastasizing carcinoid tumor and is characterized by cutaneous flushing, diarrhea, bronchoconstriction, and endocardial plaques composed of a unique type of fibrous tissue. The vasomotor, bronchoconstrictor, and cardiac manifestations are undoubtedly related to circulating humoral substances secreted by the tumor,[429] although the precise substance(s) responsible remains to be elucidated. Virtually all patients develop diarrhea and flushing, while cardiac abnormalities occur in over two-thirds; clinically apparent and severe right-sided disease is seen in a quarter.[430,431]

Sixty to 90 per cent of tumors arise in the appendix, while the rest originate in the ileum, stomach, duodenum, other areas of the gastrointestinal tract, and bronchus.[429] Carcinoid tumors of the ileum are the most likely to metastasize, with involvement of the regional lymph nodes and liver. Also, it is usual that only carcinoid tumors that invade the liver result in carcinoid heart disease.[432] The cardiac lesions may be related to large circulating quantities of serotonin (5-hydroxytryptamine), bradykinin, or other substances secreted by the tumor,[430] which are usually inactivated by the liver, lungs, and brain. Hepatic metastases apparently allow large quantities of tumor products to reach the heart without being inactivated by the liver. Left-sided cardiac involvement occurs in about one-third of patients with fatal cardiac carcinoid; when it occurs, it typically is of little hemodynamic significance, in contrast to right-sided involvement.[429] Many of the left-sided findings are minor; it has been suggested that they are similar to those seen in age-matched normal subjects and do not necessarily indicate carcinoid disease.[430] The preferential right-sided involvement presumably is related to inactivation of the offending humoral substance(s) by the lungs. In rare cases, significant left-sided valvular disease develops, perhaps related to passage of blood directly from the right to the left side of the heart through a patent foramen ovale.[433]

The characteristic *pathological* findings are fibrous plaques that involve the "downstream" aspect of the tricuspid and pulmonic valves, the endocardium of the cardiac chambers, and the intima of the venae cavae, pulmonary artery, and coronary sinus.[429] The fibrous tissue in the plaques results in distortion of the valves, leading to pulmonic stenosis and tricuspid regurgitation, sometimes with some degree of stenosis.[429] Histologically, the plaques consist of deposits of fibrous tissue located superficially on the endocardium with little or no extension into the underlying layers. Ultrastructural and immunohistochemical studies have demonstrated that the plaques are composed of smooth muscle cells embedded in a stroma rich in acid mucopolysacharides and collagen.[434]

CLINICAL MANIFESTATIONS. *Physical examination* usually reveals a systolic murmur along the left sternal border, produced by tricuspid regurgitation; in some cases, there may be concomitant pulmonic stenosis. A murmur of pulmonary regurgitation may be found as well.[429,435]

The *chest roentgenogram* may reveal enlargement of the heart; the pulmonary artery trunk is typically of normal size, without evidence of poststenotic dilatation as occurs in congenital pulmonic stenosis. No specific *electrocardiographic pattern* is diagnostic of carcinoid heart disease,[430] although low voltage is often present. Evidence of right atrial enlargement may be seen on occasion, but electrocardiographic evidence of right ventricular hypertrophy is usually lacking. Nonspecific ST-segment and T-wave abnormalities and intraventricular conduction block may be seen.[430] *Echocardiography* may reveal evidence of tricuspid and/or pulmonary

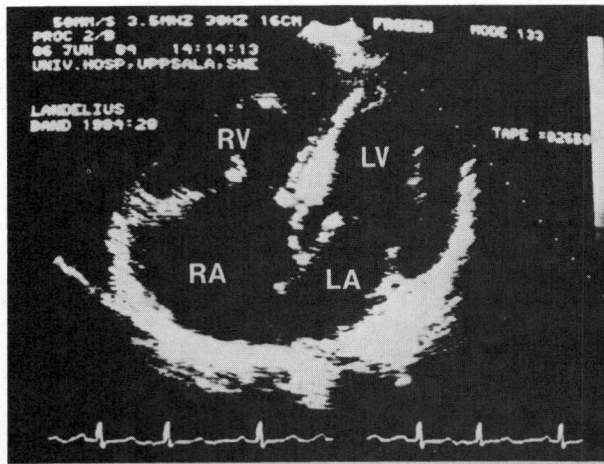

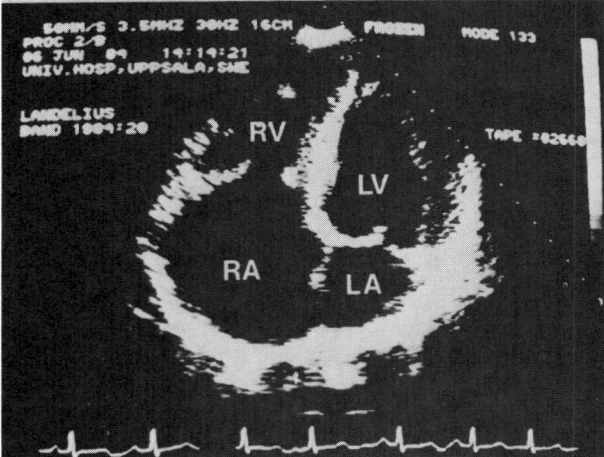

FIGURE 43–29. Echocardiographic apical four-chamber view of a patient with carcinoid heart disease. *Top,* Diastolic frame. *Bottom,* Systolic frame. Note prominent enlargement of right heart cavities and pronounced immobility of tricuspid valve leaflets as compared with the mitral leaflets. LA = left atrium, LV = left ventricle, RA = right atrium, RV = right ventricle. (From Lundin, L., Norheim, I., Landelius, J., et al.: Carcinoid heart disease: Relationship of circulating vasoactive substances to ultrasound detectable cardiac abnormalities. Circulation 77:264, 1988, reprinted by permission of the American Heart Association, Inc.)

valve thickening, along with right atrial and right ventricular dilatation (Fig. 43–29).[430-431]

The *hemodynamic findings* most commonly encountered are those of tricuspid regurgitation (p. 1055) and occasionally pulmonic stenosis. Some patients with the carcinoid syndrome appear to be in a hyperkinetic state, which may lead to high-output heart failure.

MANAGEMENT. In patients with mild congestive heart failure this consists of digitalis and diuretics. Some of the vasomotor symptoms may be controlled with alpha-adrenoceptor blockers and serotonin antagonists. Surgical replacement of the tricuspid valve and pulmonic valvotomy or valvectomy may be beneficial in severely symptomatic patients with serious valvular dysfunction.[436]

OBESITY AND HEART DISEASE
(See p. 1150)

DIABETIC CARDIOMYOPATHY
(See p. 1139)

Myocarditis

When the heart is involved in an inflammatory process, often caused by an infectious agent, myocarditis is said to be present. The inflammation may involve the myocytes, interstitium, vascular elements, and/or pericardium; involvement of the latter structure is discussed in Chapter 45.

Myocarditis has been described during and following a wide variety of viral, rickettsial, bacterial, protozoal, and metazoal diseases; indeed, virtually any infectious agent may produce cardiac inflammation[437,438] (Table 43-14). Infectious agents cause myocardial damage by three basic mechanisms: (1) invasion of the myocardium[439]; (2) production of a myocardial toxin, e.g., diphtheria,[440] and (3) immunologically mediated myocardial damage.[439] The principal mechanism of heart involvement in viral myocarditis is believed to be a cell-mediated immunological reaction to new cell surface changes or a new antigen related to the virus, and not merely resulting from cell damage caused by viral replication.[441,442] Additional evidence for an immune-mediated mechanism is the demonstration of a marked increase in major histocompatibility complex antigen expression in the biopsy specimens from patients with myocarditis.[443] Antibodies against intracellular components may also play a role.[444] Although often mistakenly limited to inflammation due to an infective agent, myocarditis may also be caused by allergic reactions and pharmacological agents, as well as occurring during the course of some systemic diseases such as vasculitis.[440]

Myocarditis may be an acute or a chronic process and may occur during the peripartum period (p. 1798). In North America, viruses are presumed to be the most common agents producing myocarditis, while in South America, Chagas' disease (produced by *Trypanosoma cruzi*) is far more common.[437] The identification of the specific etiological agent responsible for infectious myocarditis usually rests on the associated extracardiac findings, since the cardiovascular signs and symptoms are often nonspecific. The histological findings vary, depending on the stage of the disease, the mechanism of myocardial damage, and the specific etiological agent. Myocardial involvement may be focal or diffuse, but the myocardial lesions are generally randomly distributed in the heart, and thus the clinical consequences depend to a large extent on the size and number of the lesions.[437] However, a single small lesion may have profound consequences if it is located within the cardiac conducting system. The histological findings are usually nonspecific (except for some parasitic and granulomatous forms of myocarditis), and with certain exceptions (Table 43-4), myocardial biopsy seldom elucidates the specific etiological agent.[445]

INFECTIOUS MYOCARDITIS

CLINICAL MANIFESTATIONS. The clinical expression of myocarditis ranges from the asymptomatic state secondary to focal inflammation to fulminant fatal congestive heart failure due to diffuse myocarditis.[437,438] An initial episode of viral myocarditis, perhaps unrecognized and forgotten, may be the initial event that eventually culminates in an "idiopathic" dilated cardiomyopathy.[439] In experimental animals, the structural and functional myocardial alterations that follow viral myocarditis may persist well beyond the stage of viral replication and myocardial inflammatory response,[439] and the late changes resemble those of dilated cardiomyopathy.[440]

The outcome after viral myocarditis is quite variable,[437] perhaps related to differing genetic susceptibility of individual patients.[446] In most patients, the event is entirely self-limited and often unrecognized.[440,447] More overt myocarditis may result in acute congestive heart failure.[439] In others, unrecognized myocarditis may be the cause of arrhythmias in what appears to be a structurally normal heart.[448] Some patients with chest pain and angiographically normal coronary arteries may have had subclinical myocarditis at some point in the past. Most intriguing is the possibility that viral myocarditis may culminate in dilated cardiomyopathy, presumably as a consequence of viral-mediated immunological cardiac damage.[56,296,437,441-444,446]

While transient electrocardiographic abnormalities suggesting myocardial involvement are noted in many patients with infectious diseases, most patients do not have other clinical manifestations of myocarditis.[447] It is postulated that these electrocardiographic changes reflect subclinical myocardial involvement. That unrecognized myocardial involvement occurs with systemic infections is supported by histological evidence of myocarditis during routine postmortem examinations of subjects believed to be free of prior cardiac disease.[448-450] Some degree of myocardial involvement, often subepicardial in location, also frequently occurs in patients with acute pericarditis.[451]

Since myocardial involvement is subclinical in most acute infectious diseases, the majority of patients have no specific complaints referable to the cardiovascular system[447]; the presence of myocarditis is often inferred from the ST-segment and T-wave changes on the electrocardiogram.[439] From a clinical viewpoint, myocardial involvement is associated with nonspecific symptoms, including fatigue, dyspnea, palpitations, and precordial discomfort.[440] Chest pain usually reflects associated pericarditis, but precordial discomfort suggestive of myocardial ischemia is occasionally observed. In some cases, the clinical presentation (with chest pain, electrocardiographic abnormalities, increased muscle enzyme levels, and regional wall motion abnormalities) may simulate an acute myocardial infarction;[452] in others, transient coronary vasospasm has been invoked.[453]

TABLE 43-14 PRINCIPAL INFECTIOUS ETIOLOGICAL AGENTS ASSOCIATED WITH MYOCARDITIS

BACTERIAL INFECTIONS

Streptococcal	Brucellosis
Staphylococcal	Diphtheria
Pneumococcal	Salmonellosis
Meningococcal	Tuberculosis
Hemophilus	Tularemia
Gonococcal	

SPIROCHETAL INFECTIONS

Leptospirosis	Relapsing fever
Lyme disease	Syphilis

FUNGAL INFECTIONS

Aspergillosis	Coccidioidomycosis
Actinomycosis	Cryptococcosis
Blastomycosis	Histoplasmosis
Candidiasis	

PARASITIC INFECTIONS

Cysticercosis	Trichinosis
Schistosomiasis	Trypanosomiasis
Toxoplasmosis	Visceral larva migrans

RICKETTSIAL INFECTIONS

Rocky Mountain spotted fever	Scrub typhus
Q fever	Typhus

VIRAL INFECTIONS

Adenovirus	Mycoplasma pneumoniae
Arbovirus	Poliomyelitis
Coxsackievirus	Psittacosis
Cytomegalovirus	Respiratory syncytial virus
Echovirus	Rabies
Encephalomyocarditis virus	Rubella
Hepatitis	Rubeola
Human immunodeficiency virus	Vaccina
Infectious mononucleosis	Varicella
Influenza	Variola
Mumps	Yellow fever

Adapted from Marboe, C. C., and Fenoglio, J. J.: Pathology and natural history of human myocarditis. Pathol. Immunopathol. Res. 7:226, 1988.

Physical Examination. Tachycardia is usual and may be out of proportion to the temperature elevation.[439] The first heart sound is often muffled, and a protodiastolic gallop may be present. A transient apical systolic murmur may appear,[440] but diastolic murmurs are rare. Clinical evidence of congestive heart failure occurs only in the more severe cases.[439,440] The heart is usually normal in size in the clinically silent cases, but it may be dilated in patients with congestive heart failure. Pulmonary and systemic emboli may occur.

Laboratory Findings. *Electrocardiographic* abnormalities are usually transient and occur far more frequently than does clinical myocardial involvement.[439] The most common changes are abnormalities of the ST segment and T wave, but atrial and in particular ventricular arrhythmias, atrioventricular (AV) and intraventricular conduction defects, and, rarely, Q waves may be seen.[439] Complete AV block is usually transient and resolves without sequelae, but it is occasionally a cause of sudden death in patients with myocarditis.[440] On *radiological examination*, heart size may range from normal to markedly enlarged, and pulmonary congestion may be present in patients with fulminant disease.[440] *Echocardiography* demonstrates some degree of left ventricular dysfunction (surprisingly often regional in nature) in many patients with clinical myocarditis, although wall motion may be normal. Often findings may include increased wall thickness, left ventricular thrombi, and abnormal diastolic filling despite normal systolic function.[454,455] *Radionuclide scanning* after the administration of gallium-67, indium-111 anti-myosin antibody, or technetium-99m pyrophosphate may identify inflammatory and necrotic changes characteristic of myocarditis, as may nuclear magnetic resonance imaging.[101,456-460]

DIAGNOSIS. This is often predicated on the identification of the associated systemic illness and its characteristic features.[447] The diagnosis of viral myocarditis is supported by the identification of the virus in stool, throat washings, blood, myocardium, or pericardial fluid, or by a distinct (usually fourfold) increase in virus neutralizing antibody, complement-fixation, or hemagglutination inhibition titers, but cultures usually are negative and serological tests nondiagnostic.[411] Even in fatal cases, isolation of virus from the myocardium at necropsy is unusual.[437,438] cDNA clones representing various regions of the Coxsackie B virus–specific RNA sequences have been used to detect and quantify virus-specific sequences in tissue.[52] *Endomyocardial biopsy* frequently is used to confirm the diagnosis of myocarditis. A borderline or negative biopsy does not exclude the diagnosis,[461,462] and, if clinically indicated, a repeat biopsy may be appropriate and diagnostic.[463]

PATHOLOGY. Patients with or dying of myocarditis demonstrate a wide spectrum of gross and histological changes, reflecting the range of disease seen clinically. Grossly, the hearts in acute cases are flabby, with focal hemorrhages; in chronic cases, the heart is enlarged and hypertrophied.[440] The histological hallmark of myocarditis is an inflammatory myocardial infiltrate, with associated evidence of myocyte damage.[12,438,440] The inflammatory infiltrate may be composed of a variety of cell types, including polymorphonuclear cells, lymphocytes, macrophages, plasma cells, eosinophils, and/or giant cells.[440] In bacterial myocarditis, polymorphonuclear cells predominate; in viral infections, lymphocytes predominate; and in hypersensitivity myocarditis, eosinophils are seen in abundance.[440] Routine histological examination of the heart rarely provides a specific diagnosis, although in some instances electron microscopic and immunofluorescent techniques may allow elucidation of a specific etiology.

MANAGEMENT. Therapy is often supportive and is usually directed at the more prominent systemic manifestations of the disease. The demonstration of a particular predilection for involvement of the AV conducting system in some forms of myocarditis[439] suggests that patients with suspected myocarditis should be observed closely for any evidence of conduction abnormality. Since exercise intensifies the damage from myocarditis in experimental animals, adequate rest is

important.[464-466] Congestive heart failure responds to routine management, including digitalization and diuresis, although patients with myocarditis appear to be particularly sensitive to digitalis, and toxicity should be watched for. Significant arrhythmias should be treated with antiarrhythmic agents, although beta-adrenoceptor blockers are probably best avoided in view of their negative inotropic action.[467] The use of corticosteroids is controversial.[467a] Although corticosteroids were previously thought to be proscribed in acute viral myocarditis (because increased tissue necrosis and viral replication have been demonstrated following their use in experimental myocarditis), their use in a small number of patients has not been associated with similar dire short-term consequences.[440] Nonsteroidal antiinflammatory agents—indomethacin, salicylates, and ibuprofen,[468,469] along with cyclosporine[470-472a]—are contraindicated during the acute phase of viral myocarditis (the first 2 weeks), because they increase myocardial damage. On the other hand, nonsteroidal antiinflammatory agents appear to be safe in the late phase of myocarditis.[469,473] In experimental models of myocarditis, the converting enzyme inhibitor captopril has beneficial effects in the acute phase of myocarditis; human data are not yet available.[474,474a] Bed rest (or at least restricted activity) is advisable, because exercise in experimental animals with myocarditis is deleterious.[440]

It is hoped that effective antiviral agents,[475,476] immunosuppressive agents, or antilymphocyte monoclonal antibodies for treating viral myocarditis will be available soon for clinical use.[477,478] It may also be possible, in the future, to treat patients with myocarditis with agents that stimulate production of interferon, since this substance affords protection against the effects of viral myocarditis, at least in experimental animals.[479-481] Antibiotics may also be employed with benefit in infections caused by atypical pneumonia and psittacosis.

VIRAL MYOCARDITIS

There are approximately two dozen viruses that may be associated with clinical evidence of myocarditis[440] (Table 43–14). The myocarditis characteristically develops after a lag period of several weeks following the initial systemic infection, suggesting involvement of an immunological mechanism. In animals, a variety of factors appears to enhance susceptibility to myocardial damage, including radiation, malnutrition, steroids, exercise, and previous myocardial injury. Viral myocarditis may be particularly virulent in infants and in pregnant women.[439]

COXSACKIE VIRUS. Both Coxsackie A and B viruses may produce myocarditis, although infection with Coxsackie B is more common, and this agent is the most frequent cause of viral myocarditis.[439] The myocardium appears to be particularly susceptible to the effects of this virus because of the apparent affinity of myocardial membrane receptors for the viral particles.[439] Necropsy often demonstrates a pericardial effusion, pericarditis, cardiac enlargement, and a predominantly mononuclear inflammatory infiltrate, with necrosis of the atrial and ventricular myocardium. In some cases, focal myocardial necrosis simulating myocardial infarction is seen, despite normal coronary arteries.[452]

Although most infections are probably benign, self-limited, and subclinical,[439] Coxsackie myocarditis appears to be particularly virulent in the neonate.[482] In most infections in adults, the other clinical manifestations of viral involvement, such as pleurodynia, myalgia, upper respiratory tract symptoms, and arthralgias, predominate. Severe cases in the adult are characterized by myopericardial involvement with pleuritic or pericarditic chest pain, palpitations, and fever. Many patients with overt myocardial involvement develop congestive heart failure with cardiomegaly and pulmonary edema.

The *electrocardiogram* is virtually always abnormal, with ST-segment and T-wave changes and arrhythmias, often ventricular in origin; AV conduction disturbances are common.[482] Blood levels of myocardial enzymes (serum glutamic oxaloacetic transaminase, creatine kinase) may be normal or elevated, reflecting the absence or presence of variable degrees of myocardial necrosis. *Echocardiography* may reveal diffuse and regional left ventricular wall motion abnormalities[454] that usually improve or disappear over time.

Most patients recover completely within weeks, although the electrocardiogram and ventricular function may require months to return to normal.[483] Rarely, Coxsackie myocarditis is fatal in adults.[484] Some patients become symptomatic following resolution of the infection, and they may present years later with dilated cardiomyopathy.[485,486] Occasionally, patients appear to recover completely only to develop symptoms subsequently.[487]

Treatment is symptomatic, and despite occasional postmortem evidence of intracardiac thrombi, anticoagulation should probably be avoided because of the risk of a hemorrhagic pericardial effusion. Bed rest is indicated during the acute course of myocarditis, but there is no convincing evidence that a period of prolonged rest after apparent resolution of the acute process is useful. Heart failure and cardiac arrhythmias are treated in the usual fashion.

CYTOMEGALOVIRUS. Unrecognized infection with cytomegalovirus (CMV) is extremely common in childhood,[488] and the majority of the adult population have antibodies to CMV. Primary infection after the age of 35 years is uncommon, and generalized infection usually occurs only in immunosuppressed patients with neoplastic disease, after transplantation and with HIV infection.[489,490] The cardiovascular manifestations in adults are generally limited to asymptomatic and transient electrocardiographic changes.[488] Symptomatic cardiac involvement is rare, although a hemorrhagic pericardial effusion or myocarditis with left ventricular dysfunction and attendant congestive heart failure may occur.[488-492] The diagnosis of CMV myocarditis may be suggested by the presence of viral inclusions in myocardial biopsy specimens and confirmed by the detection of viral DNA in the myocardium.[493] While fatalities are unusual, when they do occur histological examination of the heart may reveal focal lymphocytic infiltration and fibrosis.[494]

DENGUE. Although previous dengue epidemics often were associated with symptomatic cardiac involvement, more recent outbreaks have been associated with fewer apparent cardiac complications.[495] Nonspecific electrocardiographic repolarization abnormalities are common but typically benign and transient.[495,496] Transient ventricular arrhythmias may be seen on occasion. Frank myocarditis and clinically significant cardiac involvement appear to be more common in some of the related hemorrhagic fevers, especially those due to arenaviruses.[497]

HEPATITIS. Clinical cardiac involvement in hepatitis is rare; an occasional patient may develop fulminant myocarditis with congestive heart failure, hypotension, and death.[498,499] The characteristic *pathological changes* in the myocardium associated with viral hepatitis are minute foci of necrosis of isolated muscle bundles, often surrounded by lymphocytes, and a diffuse serous inflammation.[498] The ventricles may be dilated, with petechial hemorrhages. Hemorrhage into the myocardium may be a conspicuous finding.[498] Myocardial damage may be produced indirectly through an immune-mediated mechanism or directly by viral invasion of the heart.[498]

Symptomatic myocarditis is generally observed in the first to third week of illness. Patients may have dyspnea, palpitations, and anginal chest pain; fatalities have been reported.[498,500] *Electrocardiographic changes,* including bradycardia, ventricular premature beats, and ST-segment and T-wave changes, may be seen during the course of hepatitis.[498] These abnormalities are usually transient and asymptomatic, although congestive heart failure, cardiomegaly, and sudden death have been reported.[498,499]

Human Immunodeficiency Virus (HIV)

Heart involvement (Table 43–15) in the acquired immunodeficiency syndrome (AIDS) may consist of metastatic involvement from Kaposi's sarcoma (Fig. 43–30), a wide variety of infective and nonspecific forms of myocarditis (Fig. 43–31), pericarditis with or without an effusion, endocarditis, and dilated cardiomyopathy (Fig. 43–32). Cardiac involvement occurs in about one-quarter to one-half of patients (on the basis of echocardiographic, endomyocardial biopsy, and autopsy findings); however, it leads to clinically apparent heart disease in only approximately 10 per cent.[501-513] When there are clinical manifestations, congestive heart failure is the most common finding and is due to left ventricular dilatation and dysfunction, simulating a dilated cardiomyopathy.[505-509] Because of the frequency of opportunistic pulmonary infections, dyspnea may be attributed incorrectly to lung disease rather than congestive heart failure; echocardiography may be useful in identifying left ventricular dysfunction as the cause of the dyspnea.[504,509] Other common clinical and echocardiographic findings that result in symptoms in a minority of patients include pericardial effusion (usually but not invariably without cardiac tamponade), ventricular arrhythmias,

TABLE 43–15 CARDIAC LESIONS IN AIDS 1427

CHAP 43

MYOCARDITIS
  Opportunistic infections
    Pneumocystis carinii
    Mycobacterium tuberculosis
    Mycobacterium avium-intracellulare
    Cryptococcus neoformans
    Aspergillus fumigatus
    Candida albicans
    Histoplasma capsulatum
    Coccidioides immitis
    Toxoplasma gondii
    Herpes simplex
  Viral agents
    Cytomegalovirus
    Human immunodeficiency virus (HIV)
  Lymphocytic myocarditis
  Noninflammatory myocardial necrosis
    Microvascular spasm?

ENDOCARDITIS
  Marantic endocarditis (nonbacterial thrombotic endocarditis)
  Healed bacterial endocarditis
  Aspergillus endocarditis

PERICARDITIS
  Infectious
    Tuberculous
    Herpes simplex
  Noninfectious
  Pericardial effusion

CARDIOMEGALY
  Right ventricular hypertrophy or dilation
  Biventricular dilation (dilated cardiomyopathy)

VASCULAR LESIONS
  Arteriopathy
  Myocardial infarction

MALIGNANCY
  Kaposi's sarcoma
  Malignant lymphoma

TOXIC LESIONS
  Drug-induced
    Drugs used in combating opportunistic infections
    Anti-HIV drugs

From Acierno, L. J.: Cardiac complications in acquired immunodeficiency syndrome (AIDS): A review. Reprinted by permission of the American College of Cardiology. J. Am. Coll. Cardiol. *13*:1144, 1989.

repolarization changes on the electrocardiogram, marantic endocarditis, and right ventricular dilatation and hypertrophy.[502,504,505,507,508,514]

Pathological cardiac findings in AIDS patients are common, with myocarditis the most frequent.[501,507,508,510,511] While opportunistic infections caused by a wide variety of viral, fungal, parasitic, and bacterial pathogens account for some cases of myocarditis, most are unexplained but are suspected to be related to the human immunodeficiency virus (HIV) itself.[508] Isolation of HIV from the myocardium has added further credence to this speculation.[515] It has been speculated that the HIV-related myocarditis may result in the dilated cardiomyopathy found in some patients.[516] Other important postmortem findings include pericardial effusions, right and/or left ventricular dilatation, and nonbacterial thrombotic endocarditis.[507,508,517]

Treatment of AIDS-associated heart disease may afford some degree of symptomatic improvement. Relief of cardiac tamponade, therapy for infective myocarditis, and treatment of congestive heart failure have resulted in at least short-term palliation.[509,518]

INFECTIOUS MONONUCLEOSIS. Evident cardiac involvement in infectious mononucleosis is extremely rare, although nonspecific ST-segment and T-wave abnormalities may be seen.[519] In rare cases, pericarditis and myocarditis (even simulating a myocardial infarction)[520] may be present.[519,521]

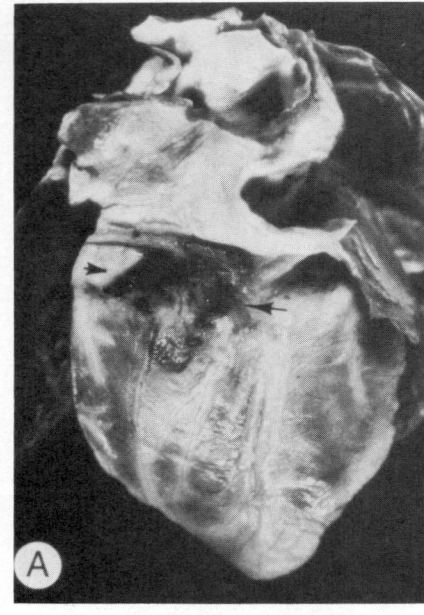

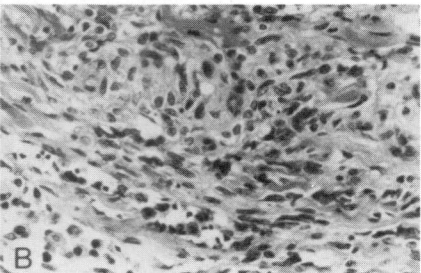

FIGURE 43-30. Kaposi's sarcoma involving the heart in AIDS. *A*, Gross photography of tumor invading the epicardium and superficial myocardium (arrows). *B*, Kaposi's sarcoma of the epicardium. Slit-like vascular clefts (characteristic of Kaposi's sarcoma) were abundant. (Hematoxylin and eosin; original magnification ×250.) (From Lewis, W.: AIDS: Cardiac findings from 115 autopsies. Prog. Cardiovasc. Dis. *32*:207, 1989.)

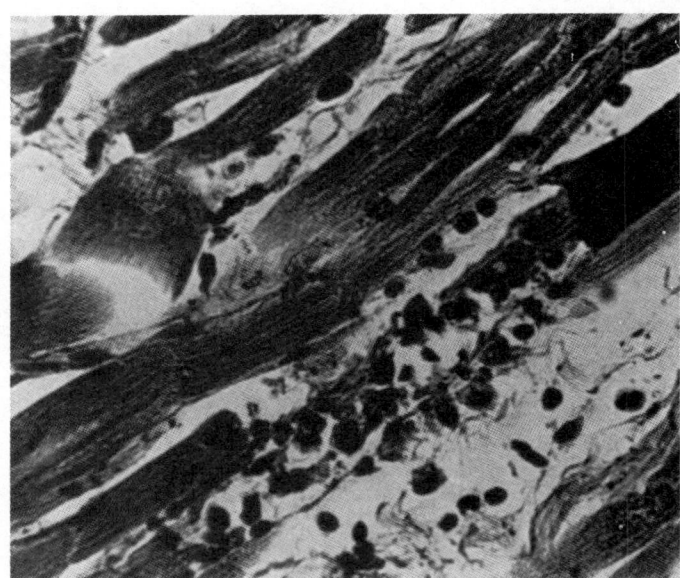

FIGURE 43-31. Example of lymphocytic myocarditis showing myocyte necrosis in AIDS patient (×400, reduced by 5 per cent). (From Baroldi, G., Corallo, S., Moroni, M., et al.: Focal lymphocytic myocarditis in acquired immunodeficiency syndrome (AIDS): A correlative morphologic and clinical study in 26 consecutive fatal cases. Reprinted by permission from the American College of Cardiology. J. Am. Coll. Cardiol. *12*:463, 1988.).

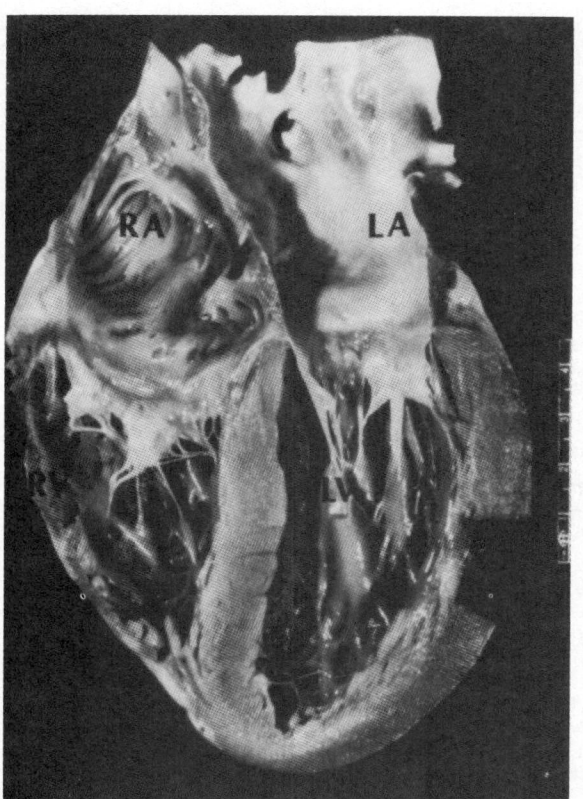

FIGURE 43-32. Marked dilatation of all four chambers of the heart in a patient with AIDS. LA = left atrium, RA = right atrium. (Reproduced by permission from Cohen, I. S., Anderson, D. W., Virmani, R., et al.: Congestive cardiomyopathy in association with the acquired immunodeficiency syndrome. N. Engl. J. Med. *315*:628, 1986.)

INFLUENZA. Although clinically apparent myocarditis is rare in influenza, the presence of preexisting cardiovascular disease greatly increases the risk of morbidity and mortality.[522,523] Postmortem findings in fatal cases include biventricular dilatation,[476] with evidence of a mononuclear infiltrate,[524] especially in perivascular areas.

Cardiac involvement typically occurs within 1 to 2 weeks of the onset of the illness and may be severe, sometimes contributing to mortality.[476] The *clinical manifestations* include dyspnea, palpitations, anginal chest pain, arrhythmia, and heart failure: there may be concomitant involvement of the pericardium.[476,525] Sinus tachycardia or, less commonly, sinus bradycardia may be seen. The *electrocardiogram* may show transient ST-segment and T-wave abnormalities, conduction defects, and even complete AV block[526]; death may be associated with massive hemorrhagic pulmonary edema due to viral or bacterial involvement of the lungs.[527]

LASSA FEVER. Lassa fever, a major cause of death in West Africa that is caused by an arenavirus, often is associated with electrocardiographic abnormalities[528] that may represent subclinical myocardial involvement. More than half the patients demonstrate nonspecific repolarization changes and low voltage.[528] Pericardial involvement may occur.[529] *Pathological findings* include myocardial congestion, edema, and a mononuclear cellular infiltrate.[530] In most cases, however, the putative cardiac involvement does not appear to play a major clinical role.[528]

MUMPS. Myocardial involvement during the course of mumps is rarely recognized.[531,532] The hearts of only a few patients with mumps have come to postmortem examination and they have been found to be both dilated and hypertrophied. Histologically, there is diffuse interstitial fibrosis, with infiltration of mononuclear cells and areas of focal necrosis.[531]

Cardiac involvement is usually unrecognized clinically, and the diagnosis of myocarditis is based on nonspecific electrocardiographic changes.[531] Transient ST-segment and T-wave abnormalities are most common, but extrasystoles and AV conduction block can occur.[531-533] Myocarditis generally occurs in the first week of illness and is transient, in most cases resolving within several weeks. A few patients develop precordial chest pain, dyspnea, palpitations, and fatigue; cardiomegaly and congestive heart failure occur on occasion.[531-534] Tachycardia, a transient apical systolic murmur, and protodiastolic gallop may be present.[531-533]

POLIOMYELITIS. Myocarditis is a frequent finding in fatal cases of poliomyelitis, particularly during epidemics,[537] occurring in half or more of all patients dying with this disease; death may be sudden.[538] While myocardial involvement is usually focal and minimal in extent, some patients with bulbar disease succumb early in the course of the illness, often with cardiovascular collapse.[537,539] These patients all have viral infection of the medulla and severe systemic vasoconstriction that leads to pulmonary edema. Myocarditis appears to contribute to the heart failure.[537] The *electrocardiogram* is frequently abnormal, with ST-segment and T-wave abnormalities, prolongation of the P-R and Q-T intervals,[540] premature contractions, tachycardia, and atrial fibrillation. *Treatment* is symptomatic, with aggressive support of pulmonary function; tracheostomy and prolonged mechanical ventilatory support may be required. Fortunately, this disease has been largely eliminated by immunization.

RESPIRATORY SYNCYTIAL VIRUS. Although respiratory syncytial virus is an important cause of respiratory disease, particularly in children, it rarely results in cardiac involvement.[542] Congestive heart failure and complete heart block have been seen on occasion.[543,544]

RUBELLA AND RUBEOLA. Congenital cardiovascular lesions may develop in the offspring when *rubella* is contracted by the mother during the first trimester of pregnancy, with persistent ductus arteriosus and pulmonary artery maldevelopment as prominent anomalies. Rare cases of myocarditis occur, with attendant conduction defects and heart failure.[545]

In *rubeola,* transient electrocardiographic abnormalities, including prolongation of the P-R interval, ST-segment and T-wave changes, AV conduction abnormalities, and ventricular tachycardia, have been reported.[546,547] Congestive heart failure occurs on rare occasions, and its appearance is a poor prognostic sign, often indicating a fatal outcome.[548] Histological examination of the heart in fatal cases has revealed evidence of myocarditis characterized predominantly by a perivascular lymphocytic infiltrate.[547]

VARICELLA. Clinical myocarditis is a rare finding in varicella, although unsuspected myocarditis is common in fatal varicella.[549] Occasionally a patient may develop overt evidence of myocarditis with congestive heart failure.[549-552] Histological findings include rare but characteristic intranuclear inclusion bodies within the myocardial cells, along with interstitial edema, cellular infiltrates, and myonecrosis. The electrocardiogram may show conduction abnormalities; sudden death occurs rarely.

VARIOLA AND VACCINIA. Cardiac involvement following smallpox is rare, although several cases of myocarditis associated with acute cardiac failure and death have been reported.[553] Myocarditis with pericardial effusion and congestive heart failure has also been observed as a complication of smallpox vaccination[554]; an immunological mechanism has been suggested and dramatic responses to steroids have been reported. The histological changes include a mixed mononuclear infiltrate, with

interstitial edema and occasional degenerating or necrotic muscle bundles.[555]

RICKETTSIAL MYOCARDITIS

The rickettsial diseases frequently are associated with evidence of myocardial involvement, but usually it is subclinical. Transient ST-segment and T-wave alterations in particular are observed commonly. The circulatory collapse that may accompany these diseases is largely a manifestation of abnormalities of the peripheral vascular bed, but a myocardial component may also be present. The basic histopathological process is vasculitis, with a periarterial interstitial infiltrate.

Q FEVER. Endocarditis is the most common cardiac manifestation of infection with *R. burnettii* (Q fever). Myocarditis is not a prominent feature,[556] although dyspnea and chest pain, perhaps reflecting associated pericarditis, occur frequently. The electrocardiogram may demonstrate transient ST-segment and T-wave changes as well as paroxysmal ventricular arrhythmias. Abnormalities of the immune system have been implicated in the pathogenesis of the disease.[557,558]

ROCKY MOUNTAIN SPOTTED FEVER. Clinical evidence of myocarditis is more common than often appreciated in Rocky Mountain spotted fever (caused by *R. rickettsii*), and the heart is often involved in the multisystem damage that occurs as the result of a widespread vasculitis.[559-561] Unsuspected left ventricular dysfunction is common, and echocardiographic evidence of dysfunction may persist in some patients.[559]

SCRUB TYPHUS. Myocarditis is common during the course of scrub typhus (tsutsugamushi disease, caused by *R. tsutsugamushi*).[562] The histological findings are those of a focal panvasculitis involving the small blood vessels. Myocardial necrosis is unusual, but hemorrhage into the heart and subepicardial petechiae may occur. Clinical evidence of myocardial involvement typically is not severe and is usually not associated with residual cardiac damage.[562,563] The electrocardiogram may show nonspecific ST-segment and T-wave abnormalities, as well as first degree AV block. A protodiastolic gallop and apical systolic murmur suggestive of mitral regurgitation are occasionally found.[562]

BACTERIAL MYOCARDITIS

BRUCELLOSIS. Cardiac involvement in the course of brucellosis is uncommon, usually consisting of endocarditis.[564-566] Myocardial involvement, when it occurs, is manifested by T-wave changes and prolongation of AV conduction.[566,567] An occasional patient develops fulminant myocarditis, with a lymphocytic and polymorphonuclear infiltrate.[566,567]

CLOSTRIDIA. Cardiac involvement is common in patients with clostridial infections with multiple organ involvement.[568] The myocardial damage results from the toxin elaborated by the bacteria, but the precise actions of the toxin remain to be elucidated.[569] The *pathological findings* are distinctive, with gas bubbles usually present in the myocardium. Areas of degenerated muscle fibers are apparent, but an inflammatory infiltrate is usually absent.[568] *C. perfringens* may cause myocardial abscess formation with myocardial perforation and resultant purulent pericarditis.[570]

DIPHTHERIA. Myocardial involvement is one of the most serious complications of diphtheria and occurs in up to 20 per cent of cases.[571] Indeed, myocardial involvement is the most common cause of death in this infection, and half of the fatal cases demonstrate cardiac involvement.[571] Cardiac damage is due to the liberation by the diphtheria bacillus of a toxin that inhibits protein synthesis by interfering with the transfer of amino acids from soluble RNA to polypeptide chains under construction.

Pathological findings include a flabby and dilated heart with a myocardium that has a "streaky" appearance. Microscopic examination reveals characteristic fatty infiltration of the myocytes,[571] often with an interstitial inflammatory infiltrate, myocytolysis, and hyaline necrosis of muscle fibers. With time, fibrosis and hypertrophy of the remaining myocardial cells develop. The conduction system is often involved.

Typically, *clinical* signs of cardiac dysfunction appear at the end of the first week of the illness. Cardiomegaly and severe congestive heart failure are often present. A protodiastolic gallop and pulmonary congestion may be prominent features. Elevation of the serum transaminase levels may be seen; a high level is associated with a poor prognosis. Sudden circulatory failure and death may occur. Many patients develop ST-segment and T-wave abnormalities, but atrial and ventricular arrhythmias and conduction defects may also occur.[571] Persistently abnormal electrocardiograms are common following diphtheritic myocarditis, as are cardiomegaly and symptoms of reduced cardiac reserve. Some patients recover fully.

Because of the serious effects of the toxin on the myocardium, antitoxin should be administered as rapidly as possible.[571] Antibiotic therapy is of less urgency. General supportive measures are indicated. Overt congestive heart failure may be resistant to therapy with cardiac glycosides. The development of complete AV block is a serious complication, but it may be amenable to treatment with a transvenous pacemaker. Corticosteroids do not appear to have any place in the treatment of the cardiac abnormalities[572]; treatment with carnitine seems to reduce the incidence of heart failure and the need for pacemaker, and to lower mortality.[573]

INFECTIVE ENDOCARDITIS. Myocardial infection is frequently observed as a consequence of infective endocarditis (Chap. 35).

LEGIONNAIRES' DISEASE. Although pneumonia, rhabdomyolysis, renal failure, and hepatic as well as central nervous system involvement are common with *Legionella pneumophila*, overt cardiac involvement is not. Occasional electrocardiographic changes may be noted, consisting primarily of ST-segment and T-wave abnormalities; ventricular arrhythmias may be seen.[574] Rarely, pericardial effusion or myocarditis with evidence of myocardial necrosis and congestive heart failure may be seen.[575]

MENINGOCOCCUS. Myocardial involvement is common during the course of fatal meningococcal infections but is less commonly recognized in the usual case.[576,577] *Pathological findings* include hemorrhagic myocardial lesions, occasionally associated with intracellular organisms.[577] An interstitial myocarditis composed of lymphocytes, plasma cells, and polymorphonuclear leukocytes is often observed, occasionally with myonecrosis.[577]

Meningococcal myocarditis may result in congestive heart failure, which may be fatal, as well as in pericardial effusion with tamponade.[576,578,579] Death may also occur suddenly and be associated with involvement of the AV node.[577] It is advisable to monitor the heart rhythm of patients with meningococcemia. In milder cases, transient electrocardiographic abnormalities, principally ST-segment and T-wave changes, are often seen and may resolve completely with time.[579]

MYCOPLASMA PNEUMONIAE. Electrocardiographic abnormalities are not uncommon during the course of atypical pneumonia; when carditis occurs, it may be serious, and, rarely, fatal.[535] Nonspecific ST-segment and T-wave abnormalities are the most common manifestation of cardiac involvement. The electrocardiographic findings usually resolve within 1 to 2 weeks. A cell-mediated myocarditis has been postulated as the cause of the changes.[535] Pericarditis may be a prominent finding, and congestive heart failure is occasionally seen.[535,536] A protodiastolic gallop and pericardial friction rub may be noted in occasional cases. No specific treatment for the cardiovascular involvement is usually indicated. Complete recovery is the rule in most patients, although occasional patients may have persistent sequelae, including arrhythmias.[536]

PSITTACOSIS. Myocarditis complicating psittacosis is a relatively common occurrence and is characterized by congestive heart failure and acute pericarditis.[541] *Pathological changes* include fibrinous pericarditis as well as endocarditis and myocarditis. Fever, chest pain, electrocardiographic changes, cardiomegaly, systemic emboli, tachycardia, and hypotension may occur. While most patients recover completely, fatalities have been reported in a small fraction.[541] The systemic infection may be treated effectively with tetracycline, but the effect of the antibiotic on the myocardium is unknown.

SALMONELLA. Symptomatic myocardial involvement during salmonella infections is rare,[580,581] although electrocardiographic abnormalities are often seen, suggesting subclinical myocarditis. *Postmortem findings* in salmonella myocarditis may reveal a shaggy, fibrinous pericarditis and, in some cases, evidence of endocarditis.[582] Myocardial petechiae and hemorrhagic necrosis may occur, with evidence of biventricular dilatation. A polymorphonuclear leukocytic infiltrate with evidence of coronary arteritis may be found. The arteritis may lead to thrombosis, infarction, and death. Other cardiovascular complications include infected mural thrombi, occasionally resulting in pulmonary and systemic emboli, and mycotic aneurysms.[582] Myocardial abscesses often develop and may rupture, producing fatal cardiac tamponade. Myocarditis with congestive heart failure occurs most commonly in children who are severely ill with salmonellosis, and it is associated with a high mortality.[583] When myocarditis occurs, it often develops rapidly, with evidence of biventricular failure, tachycardia, a protodiastolic gallop, an apical systolic murmur of mitral regurgitation, and peripheral edema.

Electrocardiographic abnormalities include ST-segment and T-wave changes, prolonged P-R or Q-T intervals, and low QRS voltage.[580,582,584]

STREPTOCOCCUS. The most commonly detected cardiac finding following beta-hemolytic streptococcal infection is acute rheumatic fever, which is discussed in detail in Chapter 56.

Involvement of the heart by the streptococcus may produce a myocarditis that is distinct from acute rheumatic carditis. It is characterized by an interstitial infiltrate composed of mononuclear cells with occasional polymorphonuclear leukocytes[585]; the infiltrate may be focal or diffuse and may be localized to the subendocardial or perivascular region. There may be small areas of myocardial necrosis.[585] *Electrocardiographic abnormalities,* including prolongation of the P-R and Q-T intervals, occur frequently.[586] While these abnormalities are rarely associated with other clinical manifestations of myocardial involvement, sudden death, conduction disturbances, and arrhythmias may occur.[585,586]

TUBERCULOSIS. Tuberculous involvement of the myocardium (not as a complication of tuberculous pericarditis) is extremely rare, particularly since the introduction of drugs effective against tuberculosis.[587,588] Most cases of myocardial tuberculosis are clinically silent and are diagnosed only at autopsy.[587] Tuberculous involvement of the myocardium may lead to arrhythmias, including atrial fibrillation and ventricular tachycardia, complete AV block, congestive heart failure, left ventricular aneurysms, and sudden death.[587,588]

WHIPPLE DISEASE

Intestinal lipodystrophy, or Whipple disease, may be associated with myocardial involvement, and PAS-positive macrophages may be found in the myocardium, pericardium, and heart valves of patients with this disorder.[589,590] Coronary artery lesions, with smooth muscle necrosis, panarteritis, and medial scarring, are not rare.[591] Unusually, patients may develop pulmonary hypertension.[592] Electron microscopy has demonstrated rod-shaped structures in the myocardium similar to those found in the small intestine, and it has been suggested that they are the causative agent of the myocardial abnormalities. There may be an associated inflammatory infiltrate and foci of fibrosis.[589] The valvular fibrosis may be severe enough to result in aortic regurgitation and mitral stenosis.[591] While asymptomatic, nonspecific electrocardiographic changes are most common; systolic murmurs, pericarditis, and even overt congestive heart failure may occur.[590] Antibiotic therapy appears to be effective in treating the basic disease; however, relapses can occur, often more than 2 years after initial diagnosis.[593,594]

SPIROCHETAL INFECTIONS

LEPTOSPIROSIS (WEIL DISEASE). Cardiac involvement is common in fatal leptospirosis,[595] and almost half of all patients demonstrate transient ST-segment and T-wave abnormalities.[596] The *pathological findings* include petechiae or larger foci of hemorrhage, often located in the epicardium.[597] An interstitial myocardial infiltration, often subendocardial in location, may occur, with involvement of the papillary muscles. Involvement of the AV conduction system, aortitis, and coronary arteritis may be prominent features. The most common manifestations of cardiac involvement are ST-segment and T-wave changes; atrial and ventricular arrhythmias, sinus bradycardia, and conduction defects may occur.[596,598,599] Cardiomegaly, pulmonary congestion, a protodiastolic gallop, pericarditis, and symptoms of congestive heart failure occur rarely.[596]

LYME CARDITIS. Lyme disease is caused by a tickborne spirochete (*Borrelia burgdorferi*).[600] The disease is found principally in areas of tick distribution including most of the United States, Europe, and the Far East.[601] It usually begins during the summer months with a characteristic skin rash (erythema chronicum migrans), followed in weeks to months by neurological, joint, or cardiac involvement; some clinical manifestations may persist for years.[603]

About 10 per cent of patients with Lyme disease develop evidence of transient cardiac involvement, the most common manifestation being variable degrees of AV block.[602,603] The location of the block appears to be at the level of the atrioventricular node.[600] Syncope due to complete heart block is frequent with cardiac involvement, since often there is an asso-

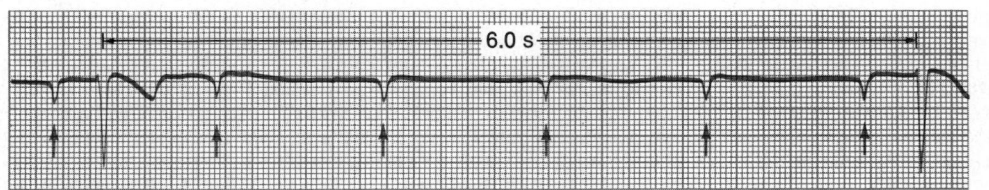

| 6.0 s |

FIGURE 43–33. Complete atrioventricular block with 6-second ventricular asystole in patient with Lyme carditis. P waves, indicated by arrows, are regular at a rate of 50 per minute. (From McAlister, H. F., Klementowicz, P. T., Andrews, C., et al.: Lyme carditis: An important cause of reversible heart block. Ann. Intern. Med. *110*:339, 1989.)

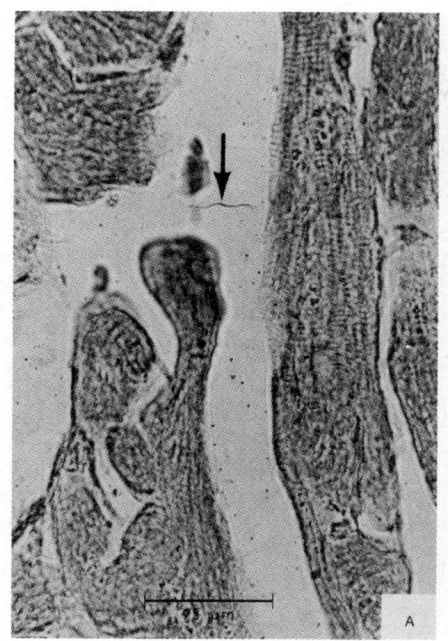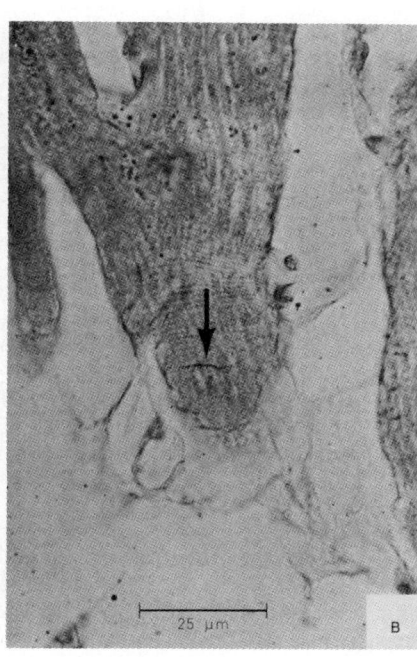

FIGURE 43–34. Human myocardium infected with *B. burgdorferi* (modified Steiner's silver stain). A spirochetal organism is shown in the endomysial space (arrow, Panel A) and apparently within the myocardial cell (arrow, Panel B). (Reprinted with permission from Stanek, G., Klein, J., Bittner, R., and Glogar, D.: Isolation of *Borrelia burgdorferi* from the myocardium of a patient with longstanding cardiomyopathy. N. Engl. J. Med. 322:249, 1990.)

ciated depression of ventricular escape rhythms (Fig. 43–33).[600,604] Ventricular tachycardia occurs uncommonly. Diffuse ST-segment and T-wave abnormalities and transient, usually asymptomatic left ventricular dysfunction may be found in some patients, although cardiomegaly or symptoms of congestive heart failure are rare. A positive[600,601] gallium or indium antimyosin antibody scan may point to suspected cardiac involvement in this disease.[605,606] The demonstration of spirochetes in myocardial biopsies of some patients with Lyme carditis (Fig. 43–34) suggests that the cardiac manifestations are due to a direct toxic effect, although there is speculation that immune-mediated mechanisms may be involved as well.[600,607]

The value of specific therapy in Lyme carditis remains uncertain; however, it is thought that treating the early manifestations of the disease may prevent development of late complications. Patients with second degree or complete heart block should be hospitalized and should undergo continuous electrocardiographic monitoring. Temporary transvenous pacing may be required for up to a week or longer in patients with high-grade block.[600] Although the efficacy of antibiotics in carditis is unestablished, they are utilized routinely (intravenous penicillin G, 20 million units per day, or oral tetracycline, 250 mg four times a day).[600] Whether antiinflammatory agents (salicylates, corticosteroids) can ameliorate heart block is also not clear.[604]

RELAPSING FEVER. Many infections are currently observed in Ethiopia. During pandemics, mortality may be particularly high, reaching 70 per cent, although sporadic cases are often more benign.[608] Cardiac involvement is a common complication and is often implicated as a cause of death. AV conduction defects occur frequently and may be responsible for sudden death, although tachyarrhythmias have also been implicated.[608] Numerous petechiae are observed with a diffuse histiocytic interstitial infiltrate, particularly around small arterioles in the left ventricle.

SYPHILIS. Aortitis is the most common manifestation of luetic involvement of the cardiovascular system. Aortic regurgitation and coronary ostial narrowing are associated findings. Syphilitic involvement of the myocardium itself in the form of gumma formation is rare and is usually unsuspected clinically. Involvement of the interventricular septum may result in damage to the conducting system and AV block.[609] Gummae may also impinge on the heart valves and interfere with their function.[610]

FUNGAL INFECTIONS OF THE HEART

Cardiac fungal infections occur most frequently in patients with malignant disease and/or those receiving chemotherapy, steroids, radiation, or immunosuppressive therapy. Cardiac surgery, intravenous drug abuse, and infection with HIV are also predisposing factors for fungal cardiac involvement.[611]

ACTINOMYCOSIS. Myocarditis is a rare complication of actinomycotic infection, occurring in less than 2 per cent of patients.[612] However, cardiac involvement is quite serious when it does occur. Involvement of the heart most commonly is the result of direct extension of disease within the thorax.[612,613] Initially the pericardium is invaded, with eventual obliteration of the pericardial space. The myocardium may be involved by extension of the pericardial process. Myocardial seeding is less common.[612] The myocardial lesion is a suppurative, necrotizing abscess containing the organism, surrounded by granulation tissue. Both right- and left-sided failure are common manifestations. A pericardial rub may be heard, sometimes associated with clinical evidence of a pericardial effusion or constriction.[612,613]

ASPERGILLOSIS. Myocardial involvement is not uncommon in generalized aspergillosis, and when it occurs it is usually fatal.[614] It is being encountered increasingly in the immunocompromised patient.[615] On pathological examination, myocardial necrosis and infarction caused by thrombosis of vessels that contain fungal mycelia are commonly seen, along with myocardial abscesses and pericardial involvement.[614] The electrocardiogram may be normal in the face of significant myocardial damage but T-wave changes may be present. The *diagnosis* of aspergillus infection is often difficult. Identification of aspergillus through open lung biopsy, aspiration lung biopsy, transtracheal aspiration, or bronchial brush technique may be successful. Treatment with antifungal agents often is unsuccessful.[614]

BLASTOMYCOSIS. Involvement of the heart by the fungus is quite uncommon, even in the immunocompromised heart. When involvement occurs, it is most often by direct extension from the pericardium.

CANDIDIASIS. Disseminated monilial infections are common opportunistic infections, particularly in the compromised host.[616] Endocarditis is the most frequent manifestation of cardiac involvement (p. 1494), occurring most commonly in cardiac surgical patients or drug addicts, although multiple abscesses of the myocardium may occur as associated or independent findings.[617] Complete heart block may be caused by microabscesses of the conduction system.[616]

COCCIDIOIDOMYCOSIS. Involvement of the heart is rare in patients with generalized coccidioidomycosis.[618] The hearts may be grossly normal, although epicardial lesions with resultant pericarditis are common, and progression to constrictive pericarditis may occur (p. 1494). A nonspecific, focal interstitial, and perivascular cellular infiltrate with associated muscle fiber degeneration and interstitial edema is commonly found, although granulomas containing fungi are also seen sometimes.

CRYPTOCOCCOSIS. Cryptococcal infection of the myocardium occurs most commonly in immunocompromised patients with disseminated malignancy or HIV infection.[619] *Pathological examination* may show cardiac dilatation, with epithelial granulomas, giant cells, and an inflammatory infiltrate.[619] When congestive heart failure occurs, pulmonary congestion and muffled heart sounds may be found on physical examination, and cardiomegaly on the chest roentgenogram.[619] The *electrocardiogram* may show first-degree AV block and T-wave inversions; ventricular arrhythmias have been observed.

HISTOPLASMOSIS. Cardiac involvement in histoplasmosis is rare and usually is related to mediastinal fibrosis, the most serious complication of histoplasmosis.[620,621] Pericarditis with effusion may occur[620] (p. 1489) and superior vena caval obstruction has been observed.[621] Myocardial involvement occurs less frequently, although atrial arrhythmias and T-wave abnormalities have been reported.

PROTOZOAL MYOCARDITIS

Trypanosomiasis (Chagas' Disease)

Chagas' disease is caused by the protozoan *Trypanosoma cruzi*. The major cardiovascular manifestation is an extensive myocarditis that typically becomes evident years after the initial infection. The disease is prevalent in Central and South America, particularly in Brazil, Argentina, and Chile, where it is a major public health problem. Perhaps 20 million people in South America may be infected with the parasite.[622] In rare cases, the disease may be found in nonendemic areas as a consequence of transfusion with contaminated blood products.[623]

The natural history of Chagas' disease is characterized by three phases: acute, latent, and chronic. During the *acute phase*, the disease is transmitted to humans (usually below the age of 20 years)[624,625] through the bite of a reduviid bug (subfamily Triatominae), which harbors the parasite in its gastrointestinal tract. This insect acquires the disease from feeding on infected animals, including the armadillo, raccoon, opossum, and skunk as well as domestic dogs and cats. The reduviid bug, popularly known in Argentina as "vinchuca," meaning "to let oneself drop," lives in the walls and roofs of houses and, during nocturnal feedings, drops from the ceiling onto the sleeping person below. The bug then often bites the person around the eyes, and infection of the human host occurs when the trypanosomes in the animal's feces gain entry through abraded skin or through the conjunctivae. Occasionally, this results in unilateral periorbital edema and swelling of the eyelid, termed *Romaña's sign*,[626] while entry through the skin may result in a lesion called a *chagoma*. Transmission may occur through blood transfusions as well as congenitally.

ACUTE TRYPANOSOMIASIS. Following inoculation, the protozoa multiply and then migrate widely throughout the body. In about 1 per cent of cases an acute illness occurs.[625]

Pathological examination during the acute phase often reveals parasites in the cardiac fibers with a marked cellular infiltrate, particularly around cardiac cells that have ruptured and released the parasites.[627] Involvement may extend into the endocardium, resulting in thrombus formation, and into the epicardium, resulting in pericardial effusion. The pathogenesis of the myocardial lesions of acute Chagas' disease appears to relate in large part to immune lysis by antibody and cell-mediated immunity directed against antigens released from *T. cruzi*–infected cells, which become adsorbed onto the surface of infected and noninfected host cells. In experimental acute Chagas' disease there are generalized alterations of the adenylate cyclase complex, but the significance of this observation is not clear.[628]

Clinical Manifestations. These include fever, muscle pains, sweating, hepatosplenomegaly, myocarditis with congestive heart failure, and, occasionally, meningoencephalitis. Most patients recover, and their symptoms resolve over several months. Young children most commonly develop clinical acute disease and generally are more seriously ill than adults.

CHRONIC TRYPANOSOMIASIS. The disease then enters a *latent phase* without clinical symptoms; however, there is evidence of early and progressive subclinical cardiomyopathy. Electrocardiographic changes often appear at this stage and are a marker for the eventual clinical heart disease and increased mortality to become evident later.[624] At an average of 20 years after the initial (and usually unrecognized) infestations, approximately 30 per cent of infected individuals develop findings of *chronic Chagas' disease*, the manifestations of which cover a wide spectrum from asymptomatic but seropositive patients through those with electrocardiographic abnormalities to those with advanced disease characterized by cardiomegaly, congestive heart failure, arrhythmias,

thromboembolic phenomena, atypical chest pain, right bundle branch block, and sudden death.[629–632] In the advanced stage, cardiac dilatation typically involves all the cardiac chambers, although right-sided enlargement may predominate. Even those individuals whose only clinical evidence of the disease is seropositivity often have subclinical cardiac involvement that may be demonstrated by endomyocardial biopsy.[633]

The central paradox in the pathogenesis of this disorder is the negative correlation between the severity of disease and the level of parasitemia. It is not unusual to be unable to detect parasites in patients dying of Chagas' disease.[634] An autoimmune mechanism has been proposed,[634,635] although this has by no means been established.[636] It appears (at least in an animal model) that self-reactive cytotoxic T lymphocytes develop following the initial infection, and these lymphocytes are able to lyse normal host cells, perhaps related to cross-reacting antigens of *T. cruzi* and striated muscle.[1,637,638] A variety of antibodies against myocyte sarcoplasmic reticulum, laminin, and other constituents have also been implicated in the pathogenesis of Chagas' myocarditis. It is thought that the acute phase results in the release from parasite-modified host cells of self components that are immunogenic.[639] Another hypothesis suggests that cardiac parasympathetic denervation leads to eventual chronic Chagas' disease.[640,641]

Pathology. Nerves and autonomic ganglia are frequently abnormal, and megaesophagus and megacolon may occur; less commonly, there is dilatation of the stomach, duodenum, ureter, and bronchi. Different strains of *T. cruzi* may account for the geographic differences in the expression of Chagas' disease; in Brazil, megaesophagus and megacolon are common, but these conditions are unusual in Venezuela.[634] Lesions of the cardiac nerves are routinely found in patients with chronic Chagas' disease, with evidence of cardiac parasympathetic denervation.[642] Pathological cardiac findings include cardiac enlargement with dilatation and hypertrophy of all cardiac chambers. The left ventricular apex is often thin and bulging, resembling an aneurysm[643] (Fig. 43–35). Thrombus formation is frequent and may fill much of the apex; the right atrium also frequently contains thrombus. It has been suggested that this characteristic apical aneurysm may be the result of intravascular platelet aggregation leading to focal myocardial necrosis.[644]

The microscopic findings are principally those of extensive fibrosis, particularly of the left ventricle.[624] A chronic cellular infiltrate composed of lymphocytes, plasma cells, and macrophages is often present. Preferential involvement of the right bundle branch and the anterior fascicle of the left bundle branch by inflammatory and fibrotic changes explains the frequent occurrence of right bundle branch and left anterior fascicular block.[624] The basement membranes of capillaries,

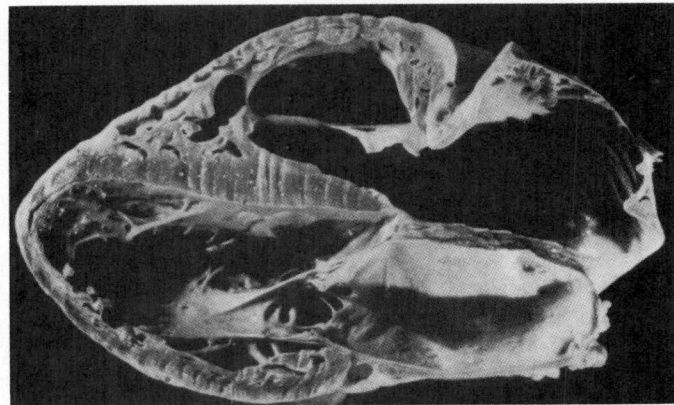

FIGURE 43–35. Long-axis autopsy section of heart from patient who had congestive heart failure caused by chronic Chagas' heart disease. Left ventricular apical and posteroapical thinning and fibrosis with relative septal sparing are evident. Coronary arteries were normal. (From Acquatella, H., Schiller, N. B., Puigbo, J. J., et al.: Circulation 62:790, 1980, reprinted with permission of the American Heart Association, Inc.)

vascular smooth muscle cells, and myocytes are thickened.[645] Parasites may be identified in one-fourth of patients; the frequency with which they are found depends upon the diligence of the search for them.

Clinical Manifestations. Chronic progressive heart failure, often predominantly right-sided, is the rule in advanced cases. Thus, while pulmonary congestion is occasionally noted, the usual findings generally include fatigue due to diminished cardiac output, peripheral edema, ascites, and hepatic congestion. Tricuspid regurgitation is often present, particularly in patients with severe right-sided heart failure, although mitral regurgitation is frequently present as well. The second heart sound is widely split, often with an accentuated pulmonic component, reflecting the combined effects of right bundle branch block and pulmonary hypertension. Autonomic dysfunction is common,[646] with marked abnormalities in the expected reflex changes in heart rate produced by various maneuvers.[647,648]

The *chest roentgenogram* often demonstrates severe cardiomegaly, with or without pulmonary venous hypertension. *Electrocardiographic abnormalities* are the rule[631] particularly in patients who are seroreactive to *T. cruzi* antigen, with right bundle branch block and left anterior hemiblock being the most common changes in patients with chronic Chagas' disease.[43,646,649] ST-segment and T-wave abnormalities are common, while Q waves involving the inferior leads, P-wave abnormalities, and AV block are occasionally seen. Early in the disease, the electrocardiogram may be normal or nearly so. Administration of the antiarrhythmic agent ajmaline may precipitate the appearance of electrocardiographic abnormalities and thus identify patients with as yet clinically silent cardiac involvement. Furthermore, electrophysiological testing of asymptomatic patients, even those with normal electrocardiograms, may demonstrate abnormalities of the conducting system in the majority.

Ventricular arrhythmias are a prominent feature of chronic Chagas' disease.[630] Frequent ventricular premature depolarizations, often with multiple morphologies, are seen frequently, and bouts of ventricular tachycardia may occur.[649] Ventricular arrhythmias are particularly common during and following exercise, occurring in the majority of patients subjected to stress electrocardiographic testing (including some without any clinical evidence of cardiac involvement). Ventricular tachycardia induced by electrophysiological testing is most common in patients with evidence of conduction abnormalities on the electrocardiogram, low ejection fraction and apical left ventricular aneurysm.[639] Syncope and sudden death due to ventricular fibrillation are a constant threat and may develop even before cardiomegaly or heart failure. Sinus bradycardia may also be seen, even in patients with severe heart failure when a tachycardia would be expected, presumably related to cardiac autonomic dysfunction. Atrial arrhythmias, including atrial fibrillation, may also occur. Thromboembolic phenomena are a frequent complication,[643] occurring in more than 50 per cent of the patients.

The *echocardiographic findings* in advanced cases are those of a dilated cardiomyopathy (Fig. 43–28) with dilatation, increased end-diastolic and end-systolic volumes, and reduced ejection fraction, often with enlargement of the left atrium and right ventricle. Diastolic filling of the left ventricle is frequently abnormal, even in those without other clinical or echocardiographic evidence of cardiac involvement.[650,651] In the majority of advanced cases, the echocardiographic appearance is distinctive, with left ventricular posterior wall hypokinesis and relatively preserved interventricular septal motion; an apical aneurysm is often seen on two-dimensional echocardiography. Ten to 15 per cent of asymptomatic patients demonstrate apical dyskinesis.[622]

Radionuclide ventriculography may, like echocardiography, demonstrate right or left ventricular wall motion abnormalities in the absence of an overall depression of global ventricular function.[652]

Left ventricular cineangiography in advanced cases shows a dilated, hypokinetic left ventricle with a large apical aneurysm containing intracavitary thrombus, often with evidence of mitral regurgitation. *Coronary angiography* is usually normal, although abnormalities of the coronary microcirculation have been suggested as the cause of the clinical manifestations of Chagas' disease.[653]

The *complement-fixation* test (Machado-Guerreiro test) is useful in diagnosis; it has high sensitivity and specificity for the identification of chronic Chagas' disease. Also used in diagnosis are the indirect immunofluorescent antibody, the enzyme-linked immunosorbent assay (ELISA), and the hemagglutination tests.[654] Another test that is occasionally useful is the detection of parasites in the blood of patients with chronic Chagas' disease (which occurs in 30 to 40 per cent of cases) by means of *xenodiagnosis*.[625] The patient is bitten by reduviid bugs bred in the laboratory; the subsequent identification of parasites in the intestine of the insect is proof of infection in the human host.

TREATMENT. The management of Chagas' disease remains difficult; although slowly progressive at first, once cardiac decompensation develops there is usually a rapid and inexorable progression to death, which is usually due to arrhythmia, congestive failure, and systemic thromboembolism.[649,655] Major efforts are aimed at interrupting transmission of the parasite to humans; such vector control methods have been generally successful.[622,623,646,656] They may prevent not only the initial infection but also superinfection that may play a role in determining the severity of the resulting cardiomyopathy.[622] Amiodarone appears to be particularly effective in controlling the ubiquitous ventricular arrhythmias seen in Chagas' disease, although whether this translates into improved survival remains unestablished.[625] Anticoagulation may be of some benefit in preventing recurrent thromboembolic episodes. While antiparasitic agents such as nifurtimox and benzimidazole are effective in reducing parasitemia, there is no evidence that they are efficacious in curing the disease.[654] A promising avenue of approach appears to be immunoprophylaxis, although a clinically useful vaccine is not yet available.[626] Insertion of an implantable cardioverter-defibrillator[657] and heart transplantation have been performed in a few patients but are not practical options for the vast majority of patients.

AFRICAN TRYPANOSOMIASIS. African sleeping sickness, due to *Trypanosoma gambiense* or *T. rhodesiense,* may be associated with myocardial abnormalities, although they are of less functional significance than in so-called American trypanosomiasis (Chagas' disease).[658] *T. rhodesiense,* in particular, may lead to cardiac failure,[658] although the central nervous system findings (excessive somnolence) usually dominate the clinical picture.

Pathological examination often reveals pericardial fluid.[658] The heart is not as greatly dilated and hypertrophied as it is in Chagas' disease and may appear grossly to be normal. There is often epicardial thickening with a cellular exudate composed of lymphocytes, plasma cells, and histiocytes. The myocardium typically displays a diffuse interstitial infiltrate, often with zones of patchy fibrosis and interstitial edema.[659]

Nonspecific *electrocardiographic* changes, commonly ST-segment and T-wave abnormalities and prolongation of the Q-T interval, are observed in at least half the patients.[658] Unlike Chagas' disease, arrhythmias and conduction disturbances are usually not prominent features and the arterial pressure is usually normal. Some of the patients have asymptomatic cardiomegaly,[658] although both pulmonary congestion and peripheral edema have been reported.

TOXOPLASMOSIS. *Toxoplasma* infections are caused by an obligate intracellular parasite *(T. gondii);* both congenital and acquired forms may occur.[660] Symptomatic acquired toxoplasmic infections involving the heart are uncommon. They occur most commonly in immunosuppressed patients with malignant diseases, and occasionally in patients with acquired immune deficiency syndrome and following cardiac or bone marrow transplantation.[661,662] An inflammatory infiltrate, often with eosinophils and variable degrees of edema and degeneration of the muscle bundles, and pericardial effusion are often present.[663–665]

Most adult cases are asymptomatic, but *Toxoplasma* infections may produce a severe, fatal disease with multisystem involvement.[661] Toxoplasmic myocarditis, often with pericarditis, may occur as an isolated disease process or as part of a multisystem disseminated disease.[665,666] Manifestations may include arrhythmia (atrial and ventricular), AV block, pericarditis, and heart failure.[660] Large pericardial effusions may be seen on occasion.[663] Diagnosis may be aided by endomyocardial biopsy.[662]

Treatment is with a combination of pyrimethamine and triple sulfonamides, but the response to therapy is variable.[661,662] Corticosteroids may be helpful in treating arrhythmias or conduction defects.

MALARIA. While myocardial changes may be demonstrated during the course of malaria, particularly with *Plasmodium falciparum*, clinical findings to indicate cardiac involvement are rare.[667] The heart generally demonstrates few gross abnormalities. The principal findings are histological. The capillaries are often filled and even distended with an accumulation of parasites, sometimes totally occluding the lumen of the vessels. Thrombosis of the capillaries and ischemic myocardial changes may be seen.[667] Focal myocardial damage may be present, along with an interstitial infiltrate composed of lymphocytes, plasma cells, and macrophages.[667] In rare cases, cardiac failure may contribute to or even cause death.[667] Slight ST-segment and T-wave changes on the electrocardiogram may be the only clinical indications of myocardial involvement.

METAZOAL MYOCARDIAL DISEASE

ECHINOCOCCUS (HYDATID CYST). *Echinococcus* is endemic in many sheep-raising areas of the world, particularly Argentina, Uruguay, New Zealand, Greece, North Africa, and Iceland, but cardiac involvement in hydatid disease is uncommon, occurring in less than 2 per cent of cases.[668,669] The usual host of *Echinococcus granulosus* is the dog, but human beings may serve as intermediate hosts (rather than the sheep, the usual intermediate host) if they accidentally ingest ova from contaminated dog feces.

When cardiac involvement is present, the cysts usually are intramyocardial in the interventricular septum or left ventricular free wall; involvement of the right ventricle or atrium may occur.[668] Involvement of the tricuspid valve may be seen on occasion,[668] and pericardial involvement with compression of the heart is not uncommon.[668] In most cases, a single cardiac cyst is present.[668,669]

A myocardial cyst may degenerate and calcify, develop daughter cysts, or rupture. Rupture of the cyst is the most dreaded complication; rupture into the pericardium may result in acute pericarditis, which may progress to chronic constrictive pericarditis. Rupture into the cardiac chambers may result in systemic or pulmonary emboli.[669] Rapidly progressive pulmonary hypertension may occur with rupture of right-sided cysts, with subsequent embolization of hundreds of scolices into the pulmonary circulation.[668] The liberation of hydatid fluid into the circulation may produce profound, fatal circulatory collapse due to an anaphylactic reaction to the protein constituents of the fluid.[686]

Symptoms depend on the location, size and integrity of the cyst; patients may be asymptomatic or in profound circulatory collapse.[668,669] The *electrocardiogram* may reflect the location of the cyst; T-wave changes and loss of QRS voltage may occur with left ventricular involvement, while AV conduction defects or right bundle branch block may be seen with involvement of the interventricular septum. Chest pain is usually due to rupture of the cyst into the pericardial space with resultant pericarditis. Large cystic masses may sometimes produce right-sided obstruction.[668,669]

Diagnosis. Recognition of an echinococcal cyst of the heart is a relatively simple matter if there is evidence of cysts in other organs, particularly the liver and lung. However, a cardiac cyst may be an isolated, solitary finding. The *chest roentgenogram* frequently shows an abnormal cardiac silhouette or a calcified lobular mass adjacent to the left ventricle. Although computed tomography and nuclear magnetic resonance imaging may aid in the detection and localization of heart cysts, two-dimensional echocardiography is thought to be the best choice.[668,670] *Eosinophilia*, present in some patients, is a useful adjunctive finding. The *Casoni skin test* is not very helpful because both false-positive and false-negative results occur. Serological tests, including hemagglutination and complement-fixation, are more useful.[671]

Management. Until recently, treatment for hydatid disease was limited to surgical excision. Experience suggests that the benzimidazole derivative mebendazole may be somewhat useful in the medical management of this disease.[669] Because of the significant risk of rupture of the cyst and its attendant serious and sometimes fatal consequences, surgical excision is generally recommended, even for asymptomatic patients. The surgical results have been generally favorable.

VISCERAL LARVA MIGRANS. People are occasional accidental hosts of the roundworm infestations of dogs due to *Toxocara canis* but cardiac involvement is rare. Most cases occur in children 1 to 3 years of age.[672] Myocarditis may occur in association with invasion of the myocardium by larvae.[672] The myocardial lesions include granulomas or extensive inflammatory infiltrates (often with eosinophils) with foci of muscle necrosis.[672] Congestive failure and death may occur, although asymptomatic cardiac involvement may be seen as well.[672]

SCHISTOSOMIASIS AND RELATED DISEASES. Direct cardiac involvement in schistosomiasis, heterophyiasis, and cysticercosis is distinctly unusual. The principal cardiovascular manifestation of schistosomiasis is right heart overload as a consequence of embolization of the ova to the pulmonary vasculature, with attendant pulmonary hypertension.

TRICHINOSIS. Infestation with *Trichinella spiralis* is a common human finding. Mild myocarditis is frequent and may be responsible for the majority of fatilities.[673] Less frequently, death is due to pulmonary embolism secondary to venous thrombosis as well as encephalitis.[673]

Although the parasite frequently invades the heart, it does not usually encyst there, and it is rare to find larvae or larval fragments in the myocardium.[673] Nonetheless, *pathological findings* at autopsy may be impressive. The heart may be dilated and flabby and a pericardial effusion may be present. A prominent focal infiltrate composed of lymphocytes and eosinophils, with interstitial edema, hyperemia, and scattered hemorrhages, is commonly found.[673] Areas of muscle degeneration and necrosis are present. The lesions may be due to toxic effects of the products produced in the course of the host reaction.

Clinical Manifestations. Myocarditis usually is mild and goes unnoticed, but in occasional cases it is manifested by congestive heart failure and chest pain, usually appearing around the third week of the disease, when the general constitutional symptoms are abating.[673] Physical examination may be normal, or there may be gross cardiomegaly with severe congestive heart failure. Sudden death may occur, usually in the fourth to eighth week of the illness.

Electrocardiographic abnormalities may be detected in one-fourth of patients with trichinosis and parallel the time course of clinical cardiac involvement, initially appearing in the second or third week and usually resolving by the seventh week of the illness.[674] The most common electrocardiographic abnormalities are repolarization abnormalities and conduction defects.[674] The electrocardiographic changes usually resolve completely.

The definitive *diagnosis* is based on the demonstration of larval forms in tissue biopsy samples, usually of the gastrocnemius muscle.[674] Eosinophilia, when present, is a supportive finding. The skin test is usually but not invariably positive. Treatment is with corticosteroids; dramatic improvement in cardiac function has been reported following their use.[673,674]

TOXIC, CHEMICAL, IMMUNE, AND PHYSICAL DAMAGE TO THE HEART

A wide variety of substances other than infectious agents may act on the heart and damage the myocardium. In some cases, the damage is acute, transient, and associated with evidence of an inflammatory infiltrate with myocyte necrosis (such as with arsenicals and lithium); in other cases, a hypersensitivity reaction occurs, without evidence of necrosis (as with sulfonamides).[675] Other agents that damage the myocardium may lead to chronic changes with resulting histological evidence of fibrosis and a clinical picture of a dilated cardiomyopathy. Furthermore, many offending stimuli may be associated with both acute and chronic phases (e.g., alcohol, Adriamycin). The response often is related to the dose and rate of exposure.

Numerous chemicals and drugs (both industrial and therapeutic) may lead to cardiac damage and dysfunction. Several physical agents (e.g., radiation and excessive heat) may also result in myocardial damage. Furthermore, myocardial involvement may be evident in a variety of systemic diseases, which are described in Part V of this book.

COCAINE (see also p. 1207). The illicit use of this drug is often associated with chest pain, diaphoresis, and palpitations.[676] In a minority of cases, there is evidence of myocardial ischemia or infarction as a consequence of heightened myocardial oxygen demand (increased blood pressure and heart rate), coronary vasoconstriction, accelerated atherosclerosis, or thrombotic occlusion of the coronary artery.[676-679] Associated clinical findings include ventricular arrhythmias, sudden death in some persons, and reversible ventricular myocardial depression (Fig. 43-36).[680-685] Myocarditis, contraction band necrosis, and thickening of the intramural coronary arteries have been found on histological study.[686-689] A variety of mechanisms have been invoked to explain the cardiovascular effects of cocaine, including vasoconstrictor, hypersensitivity, sympathomimetic, and direct actions (Fig. 43-37).[682] Treatment is empirical; beta-adrenergic blockers, combined alpha- and beta-adrenergic blockers, and calcium antagonists have been advocated but without any definite demonstration of their efficacy.[676]

INTERFERON ALPHA. Interferon alpha is a leukocyte-derived protein used therapeutically to treat malignancies and perhaps HIV infections. Cardiotoxicity, usually consisting of hypotension, tachycardia, and transient arrhythmias, occurs in a minority of patients (perhaps up to 10 per cent).[689,690] Several patients have developed congestive heart failure and the clinical picture of a dilated cardiomyopathy during interferon alpha

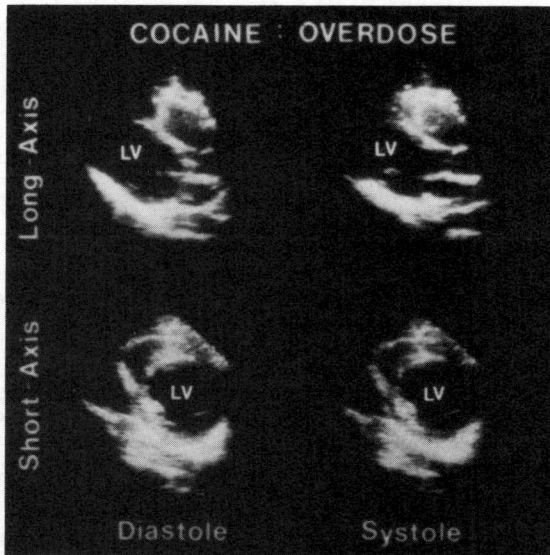

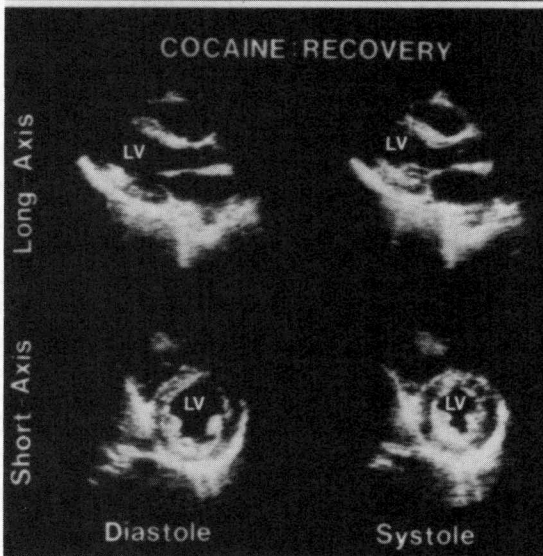

FIGURE 43–36. Two-dimensional echocardiograms recorded in long-axis and short-axis views during systole and diastole in a patient with cocaine cardiotoxicity. *Top,* Echocardiogram recorded shortly after overdose of cocaine shows dilated, globally hypocontractile left ventricle (LV). *Bottom,* Echocardiogram recorded during recovery period shows nondilated left ventricle with markedly improved left ventricular ejection performance. (From Chokshi, S. K., Moore, R., Pandian, N. G., and Isner, J. M.: Reversible cardiomyopathy associated with cocaine intoxication. Ann. Intern. Med. *111:*1039, 1989.)

therapy; in at least some patients, cardiomyopathy resolves rapidly with discontinuation of interferon.[690,691]

TRICYCLIC ANTIDEPRESSANTS. Although sudden death, disturbances in rhythm, and abnormalities of AV conduction may be seen with the tricyclic antidepressants, particularly when taken as an overdose, important depression of left ventricular function is usually not seen, even in patients with preexisting heart disease.[692] It is not clear whether there is a synergistic depression of ventricular function when a tricyclic antidepressant is given with another drug (such as an antiarrhythmic) that also has negative inotropic effects.[693] Postural hypotension may be exacerbated, however, and heart block precipitated in patients with preexisting conduction system disease.[694]

INTERLEUKIN-2 (see also p. 1760). The lymphokine interleukin-2, an antineoplastic agent, has significant cardiovascular toxicity, the most prominent of which is a diffuse capillary leak syndrome with hypotension and oliguria.[695] In about 5 per cent of patients, additional cardiotoxicity is seen,[696] consisting of myocardial ischemia,[695] infarction,[696,697] injury,[698,699] arrhythmias, and eosinophilic myocarditis.[696,700]

PHENOTHIAZINES. The phenothiazines may be associated with a variety of cardiac disturbances, including electrocardiographic changes,

atrial and ventricular arrhythmias, and sudden death.[701] Postural hypotension may also be seen.[693] The cardiac effects are largely dose-dependent. Electrocardiographic abnormalities may be seen with as little as 200 mg of thioridazine per day and consist of lengthening of the Q-T interval and T-wave changes. Prolongation of the Q-T interval may set the stage for the emergence of ventricular arrhythmias, particularly torsades de pointes (p. 707).[701] Higher doses may lead to frank T-wave inversion and increase in the amplitude of the U wave. Changes in the P wave, QRS complex, and ST segment are usually absent. The electrocardiographic abnormalities and arrhythmias resolve with discontinuation of the drug, usually within 48 hours.

Pathological changes in the hearts of patients who have received psychotropic drugs and who have died suddenly include the deposition of acid mucopolysaccharide between muscle bundles in periarteriolar regions as well as the conduction system, with myofibrillar degeneration, and endothelial proliferation in the smaller blood vessels, although a direct causal relationship between drug administration and cardiomyopathic changes is only inferential.[693] A variety of explanations have been invoked for apparent cardiac damage, including direct toxic effects of the phenothiazines on the myocardium, stimulation of higher autonomic centers, and changes in circulating or myocardial levels of catecholamines.

EMETINE. Cardiovascular changes are common with the use of emetine, a drug often employed in the treatment of amebiasis and schistosomiasis, presumably because of its prolonged duration of action and consequent potential for accumulation with resultant toxicity.[693] Myocardial lesions may be observed in some but not all patients at autopsy, and similar cardiac damage is noted in experimental animals given emetine.[702] The myocardial lesions consist of myofibrillar degeneration and necrosis,[702] with an interstitial infiltrate of mononuclear cells and histiocytes.

The *electrocardiogram,* which may be abnormal in 50 per cent of treated patients, most commonly shows reduced T-wave amplitude or inversion. Prolongation of the Q-T interval and ST-segment shifts may also be seen, although abnormalities of the P wave, P-R segment, and QRS complex are infrequent. The electrocardiographic changes usually resolve within weeks or months after cessation of treatment. Sinus tachycardia and hypotension may also be seen, although clinical evidence of myocardial toxicity is usually lacking. Only rare fatalities have been reported. *Dehydroemetine* results in electrocardiographic abnormalities similar to those of emetine, but they are less prominent and of shorter duration.

Emetine and dehydroemetine therapy should be discontinued upon appearance of clinical evidence of cardiac toxicity, but treatment may be continued cautiously if electrocardiographic changes are the only manifestation.

METHYSERGIDE. The widespread fibrotic reactions seen with this drug can also involve the heart. Up to 1 per cent of patients treated long-term may develop typically left-sided valvular lesions resulting in stenosis and regurgitation.[693] Fibrotic endocardial and pericardial lesions are also seen on occasion, producing a hemodynamic picture of restrictive and constrictive disease.[703]

CHLOROQUINE. This drug has been widely used in the prophylaxis and treatment of a variety of parasitic and other diseases and has potent

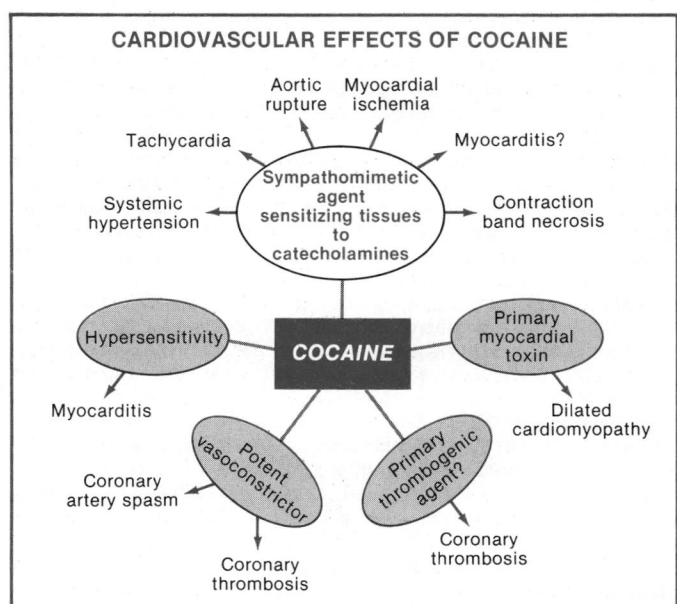

FIGURE 43–37. Diagram showing the effects of cocaine on the heart. (From Waller, B. F.: Cocaine and the heart. Indiana Med. *81:*956, 1988.)

toxic cardiac effects, which appear to be related to its ability to inhibit cellular respiration by blocking the Krebs cycle.[704] It is a myocardial depressant in large doses,[705] although routine doses are not usually associated with clinical evidence of cardiac dysfunction.[704] Electrocardiographic changes may be seen and are similar to those seen with emetine, although they are less pronounced and of shorter duration. In toxic doses, chloroquine may result in depressed cardiac output, bradycardia, arrhythmias, heart block, and death.[704] Characteristic changes are found on endomyocardial biopsy.[704,706]

ANTIMONY COMPOUNDS. Various antimony compounds, such as stibophen and tartar emetic, have been widely used in the treatment of schistosomiasis; less toxic agents are now becoming available. The antimony compounds are associated with electrocardiographic changes in almost all patients.[707] Typical *electrocardiographic changes* include prolongation of the Q-T interval with flattening or inversion of T waves.[707] ST-segment shifts and P-wave changes may be seen, although the QRS complex usually demonstrates no abnormality. The majority of patients do not demonstrate cardiac findings, although chest pain, bradycardia, hypotension, ventricular arrhythmias (including paroxysmal ventricular tachycardia), and sudden death may occur.[707,708]

LITHIUM. Lithium carbonate, used in the treatment of manic-depressive disorders, is associated with T-wave changes in one-fourth or more of patients who receive the drug.[709] Clinical evidence of myocardial involvement is usually lacking, although intoxication with lithium may be associated with ventricular arrhythmias, symptomatic sinus node abnormalities, atrioventricular conduction disturbances, congestive heart failure, and in rare cases, death.[709] In fatal lithium toxicity, the heart is said to be dilated, with evidence of myofibrillar degeneration associated with a lymphocytic interstitial infiltrate and fibrosis, although there is no definite proof that these changes are due to lithium.[709]

HYDROCARBONS. Ingestion of hydrocarbons may result in fragmentation and vacuolization of the muscle fibers with loss of cross-striations.[710] Electrocardiographic changes, arrhythmias, and cardiomegaly may occur. Involvement of the central nervous, renal, hepatic, and pulmonary systems may dominate the clinical presentation and obscure the myocardial damage, which may well contribute to the mortality of hydrocarbon ingestion.[710]

The *fluorinated hydrocarbons*, commonly used as aerosol propellants, appear to be cardiac toxins, contrary to their reputation of being inert. In animal preparations, at least, the aerosol propellants cause ventricular tachyarrhythmias, depress myocardial contractility, and lower systemic vascular resistance and arterial pressure.[711] These cardiovascular effects may be involved in the sudden deaths seen in individuals who abuse aerosols for their psychotropic effect.[711]

CATECHOLAMINES. A severe reversible dilated cardiomyopathy has been observed in conjunction with pheochromocytoma, and the myocardial damage has been attributed to high levels of circulating catecholamines[64,712] (p. 1839). Similar changes have been demonstrated in experimental animals treated with prolonged infusions of L-norepinephrine. Catecholamines also may produce acute myocarditis, with focal myocardial necrosis, inflammation, epicardial hemorrhages, tachycardia, and arrhythmias,[713] as well as indications of a hypertrophic cardiomyopathy.[712] Similar findings have been described with excessive use of beta-adrenergic agonist inhalants and methylxanthines in the treatment of decompensated pulmonary disease.[714]

A variety of mechanisms have been suggested. A direct toxic effect may be involved, or the damage may be secondary to relative tissue hypoxia because of heightened metabolic demands.[715] Alternatively, the damage may result from changes in autonomic tone, enhanced lipid mobility, calcium overload, damaging effects of catecholamine oxidation products, or increased sarcolemmal permeability.[715-718] Aspirin and dipyridamole appear to offer some protection against experimental myocardial necrosis by catecholamines, suggesting that platelet aggregation plays a major role.

LEAD. The prominent features in lead poisoning generally center on the gastrointestinal and central nervous systems. However, myocardial involvement may contribute to or be the principal cause of death in some cases.[719] Electrocardiographic changes, atrioventricular conduction defects, and overt congestive heart failure may occur.[719] The electrocardiographic and myocardial changes appear to be reversible with chelation therapy.[719]

CARBON MONOXIDE. Both acute and chronic carbon monoxide toxicity can occur. While central nervous system findings usually dominate the clinical presentation, significant and occasionally fatal cardiac abnormalities may be present.[720] Because carbon monoxide has a higher affinity for hemoglobin than does oxygen, reduced amounts of oxygen are delivered to the tissues. Thus, the cardiac toxicity may be partially caused by myocardial hypoxia, but a direct toxic effect of the gas on myocardial mitochondria may play an even more important role.[721,722] The *histological features* include focal areas of necrosis, most marked in the subendocardium. Focal perivascular infiltrates and punctate hemorrhages are also seen.[722]

Cardiac involvement may appear promptly after exposure or it may be delayed for up to several days. Palpitations, sinus tachycardia, and various arrhythmias, including ventricular extrasystoles and atrial fibrillation, are common.[723] Bradycardia and AV block may occur in more severe cases.[723] In patients with ischemic heart disease, angina pectoris and myocardial infarction may be precipitated. Electrocardiographic ST-segment and T-wave abnormalities are quite common. Transient right and/or left ventricular wall motion abnormalities may be present.[722] Administration of 100 per cent oxygen, bed rest, and surveillance for serious rhythm or conduction abnormalities will usually permit rapid recovery.

HYPOCALCEMIA (see also pp. 150 and 1841). In rare patients with chronic hypocalcemia (often due to hypoparathyroidism), congestive heart failure may occur and resolve only when the serum calcium level is raised.[724,725] Rapid transfusion of citrated blood can produce hypocalcemia and reversible myocardial depression,[726] as can ambulatory peritoneal dialysis in patients with chronic renal failure.[727]

HYPOPHOSPHATEMIA. A form of reversible left ventricular dysfunction may be seen with severe hypophosphatemia. Restoration of the serum phosphate level to normal results in hemodynamic recovery,[728] although the modest reduction in levels usually seen is associated with normal function.[729]

HYPOMAGNESEMIA. Focal cardiac necrosis is found in experimental magnesium deficiency and may account for the supraventricular and ventricular arrhythmias and electrocardiographic changes that are seen clinically. The ventricular arrhythmias are particularly likely to occur when hypomagnesemia complicates digitalis toxicity.[730,731]

TAURINE DEFICIENCY. A deficiency of taurine, an amino acid found in high concentration in cardiac and retinal tissue, produces a dilated cardiomyopathy in cats that is reversible with oral taurine supplementation.[732] Whether a similar condition exists in humans is unestablished; this has been the subject of speculation.[733]

CARNITINE DEFICIENCY. Carnitine, an essential cofactor for the oxidation of fatty acids, produces a hypertrophic or dilated cardiomyopathy in children when deficient.[71,734-736] Carnitine supplementation can lead to symptomatic and functional improvement[735-738]; determination of carnitine levels therefore is important in children with unexplained cardiomyopathy.[737] Myocardial carnitine levels are reduced in the hearts of patients with dilated cardiomyopathy, but the significance of this observation is unknown at present.[71]

SELENIUM DEFICIENCY. Dietary deficiency of the trace element selenium appears to be one of the principal factors responsible for a form of dilated cardiomyopathy endemic to certain rural areas in China that are deficient in selenium, although others have questioned the etiological role played by selenium.[739] Termed *Keshan disease*, it affects mainly children and young women and apparently is prevented by the prophylactic administration of sodium selenite tablets.[739] A similar cardiomyopathy, occasionally fatal, may be found in Occidentals subjected to prolonged parenteral hyperalimentation.[740]

SCORPION STING. The venom of the scorpion is mainly neurotoxic, but cardiac findings may be prominent and even fatal, particularly in children.[741-744] Hearts are normal on gross examination with prominent microscopic changes usually but not invariably present, particularly in the subendocardial regions and papillary muscles.[745] Degeneration and necrosis of muscle fibers are noted, with interstitial edema and a mononuclear infiltrate. The histological features of scorpion sting suggest high levels of circulating catecholamines and are similar to those seen with experimental catecholamine infusion and in pheochromocytoma.[742] The parasympathetic system appears to be stimulated as well.[742]

The *electrocardiogram* often initially shows tall peaked T waves that progress to inversions and ST-segment shifts. Q waves may appear, and the Q-T interval is usually prolonged.[746] Atrial, junctional, and ventricular arrhythmias may occur. Tachycardia, hypertension, anxiety, diaphoresis, and pulmonary edema—findings resembling those of a massive catecholamine effect—are striking in many patients.[745,746] A smaller number of patients are seen in shock with peripheral vascular collapse. Most deaths are due to pulmonary edema, presumably the result of left ventricular dysfunction.[746a] Occasionally, sudden and unexpected deaths occur in a smaller percentage of patients, presumably as a consequence of arrhythmias. Adrenergic blocking agents and the use of specific antivenom appear to be useful in the management of the cardiovascular manifestation of scorpion stings.[744,747]

WASP AND SPIDER STINGS. Stings by the vespine wasps may lead to hypotension, circulatory collapse, and cyanosis, manifestations of anaphylaxis.[748] Occasional patients may have chest pain and clinical findings compatible with acute myocardial infarction.[748] The mechanism of myocardial damage is unclear; perhaps it merely reflects necrosis from profound hypotension, although a direct toxic effect on the myocardium or an indirect effect on the coronary arteries may be involved.[748]

SNAKE BITE. Cardiac complications are usually not prominent features of snake bites, and the clinical picture is usually dominated by the neurological, hematological, and vascular damage produced by the snakebite toxin.[749,750] Myocardial involvement is seen on occasion and may rarely contribute to morbidity and mortality. T-wave abnormalities are the most common manifestation of myocardial involvement, although ST-segment depression, QRS prolongation, and AV conduction defects may also be seen.[751] The electrocardiographic changes are usually transient, but when persistent they are attributed to direct myocardial damage due to the toxin. Death may occur from circulatory collapse, myocardial depression, or myocardial infarction due to hypotension and coronary artery thrombosis. Coronary artery vasospasm may also be involved.[752-754]

ARSENIC. Arsenicals are currently utilized in pesticides. Myocardial involvement may be seen in both acute and chronic poisoning; the heart may be dilated, with accumulation of pericardial fluid.[755] Multiple local and confluent areas of subepicardial and subendocardial hemorrhage are characteristic findings.[755] The myocardium is usually abnormal, with evidence of a perivascular mononuclear infiltrate.[756]

Clinically unrecognized, toxic, interstitial myocarditis is reflected in T-wave inversions and ST-segment depressions, along with prolongation of the Q-T interval.[755,756] The electrocardiographic changes usually revert to normal within 2 to 4 weeks. The electrocardiographic abnormalities appear to resolve more rapidly when BAL (British antilewisite, dimercaprol) is utilized in therapy.[755,756]

CYCLOPHOSPHAMIDE (see also p. 1759). High doses of cyclophosphamide have been associated with electrocardiographic changes, congestive heart failure, and death from hemorrhagic myocarditis.[757] In the majority of patients treated a reversible decrease of QRS voltage and systolic function is seen, often asymptomatic, although more than 20 per cent may succumb owing to myopericarditis.[758] The myocardial damage appears to result from direct endothelial damage and resultant fibrin microthrombi in the capillaries.

AZIDE. Sodium azide, a chemical preservative that interferes with oxidative phosphorylation, may produce fatal acute cardiotoxicity when accidentally ingested.[759] Pathological findings include marked interstitial edema and myofibrillar degeneration. Clinical features include arrhythmias, myocardial ischemia, left ventricular dysfunction, and hypotension.[759]

PARACETAMOL. Paracetamol, a phenacetin metabolite, may result in massive liver necrosis.[760] On occasion it also results in fatty degeneration and focal necrosis of the myocardium after an overdose.[760]

5-FLUOROURACIL. This antineoplastic agent has been associated with cardiotoxicity manifested by chest pain, electrocardiographic changes, and arrhythmia.[761-764] Swelling of myocardial fibers without an inflammatory infiltrate has been found at necropsy.[763]

DAUNORUBICIN AND ADRIAMYCIN (see p. 1756).

HYPERSENSITIVITY

Hypersensitivity to a variety of agents may result in allergic reactions that involve the myocardium. In addition to anaphylaxis and serum sickness, allergies to a variety of drugs (most commonly the sulfonamides, the penicillins, and methyldopa) or other sensitizers may lead to an allergic myocarditis, characterized by eosinophilia, and a perivascular infiltration of the myocardium by eosinophils, multinucleated giant cells, and leukocytes[765] (Table 43–16). Hypersensitivity myocarditis is rarely recognized clinically and is often first

TABLE 43–16 PRINCIPAL DRUGS CAPABLE OF CAUSING HYPERSENSITIVITY MYOCARDITIS

Antibiotics	**Antiinflammatory**
Amphotericin B	Indomethacin
Ampicillin	Oxyphenbutazone
Chloramphenicol	Phenylbutazone
Penicillin	**Diuretics**
Tetracycline	Acetazolamide
Streptomycin	Chlorthalidone
Sulfonamides	Hydrochlorothiazide
Sulfadiazine	Spironolactone
Sulfisoxazole	**Others**
Anticonvulsants	Amitriptyline
Phenindione	Methyldopa
Phenytoin	Sulfonylureas
Carbamazepine	Tetanus toxoid
Antituberculous	
Isoniazid	
Paraaminosalicylic acid	

From Kounis, N. G., Zavras, G. M., Soufras, G. D., and Kitrou, M. P.: Hypersensitivity myocarditis. Ann. Allergy 62:71, 1989.

TABLE 43–17 CLINICAL FEATURES OF HYPERSENSITIVITY MYOCARDITIS

Cardiac symptoms
Chest discomfort
Dyspnea
Palpitations

Cardiac signs
Irregular pulse
Elevated jugular venous pressure
Gallop rhythm

Electrocardiographic signs
Sinus tachycardia
ST segment elevation
ST segment depression
T-wave inversion
Right bundle branch block
Left bundle branch block
Atrioventricular block
Ventricular tachycardia

Laboratory findings
Increased cardiac enzymes (especially CK-MB)
Cardiomegaly in the chest roentgenogram
Dilated cardiac chambers in echocardiogram
Eosinophils, atypical lymphocytes, and giant cells in biopsy

From Kounis, N. G., Zavras, G. M., Soufras, G. D., and Kitrou, M. P.: Hypersensitivity myocarditis. Ann. Allergy 62:71, 1989.

discovered at postmortem examination, although it is occasionally diagnosed on endomyocardial biopsy.[765] Since some of the clinical courses of patients are marked by sudden death (presumably arrhythmic in origin), it is likely that undiagnosed hypersensitivity myocarditis may have significant clinical effects[766,767] (Table 43–17). Because of the significant deleterious effects, a high index of suspicion for this condition should be maintained; in one unusual case, penicillin residue in pet food led to hypersensitivity myocarditis in a young child.[766] Therapy includes discontinuation of the offending agent, and corticosteroids and/or immunosuppression therapy in severe cases.[765]

METHYLDOPA. Although hepatitis is the most frequently encountered serious adverse reaction to methyldopa, sudden and unexpected death has been reported in a number of patients found at necropsy to have had an unsuspected myocarditis.[765] The *histological findings* have the characteristics of an allergic myocarditis, showing an interstitial inflammatory infiltrate with abundant eosinophils, a vasculitis, and focal myocardial necrosis. Electrocardiographic changes include sinus bradycardia, sinus pauses, and first- and second-degree AV block.[768]

PENICILLIN. Allergic reactions to penicillin are fairly common, but myocardial involvement is rare.[766] *Histological findings* consist of a perivascular and interstitial infiltrate composed of eosinophils and mononuclear cells.[766] Both myocardial infarction and pericarditis may occur and account for some of the electrocardiographic changes.[766,767] Transient electrocardiographic changes may be the only manifestation of cardiac involvement, with sinus tachycardia, ST-segment elevation, and T-wave inversion.[766]

SULFONAMIDES. Sulfonamides may result in myocardial damage owing to a hypersensitivity vasculitis as well as a myocarditis.[767] In fatal cases eosinophilic myocarditis, sometimes with granulomas, usually can be demonstrated. While usually clinically silent, severe and even fatal congestive heart failure may occur.[765] Electrocardiographic changes are usually absent, but nonspecific ST-segment and T-wave abnormalities may be seen.

TETRACYCLINE. Allergic reactions to antibiotics of the tetracycline class include fever, tachycardia, and first degree AV block. Postmortem findings include cardiac dilatation, fibrinoid muscle cell degeneration, and a diffuse interstitial and perivascular infiltrate.[769]

PHENINDIONE. Marked congestive heart failure with cardiomegaly and pulmonary edema has been reported following the use of phenindione. The electrocardiogram may show sinus tachycardia, low QRS voltage, and T-wave inversion.[769]

ANTITUBERCULOUS DRUGS. Most reactions to antituberculous drugs consist of a fever, rash, or both, but serious and fatal cardiac reactions may occur on rare occasions. *Paraaminosalicylic acid* may lead to the development of interstitial edema, acute inflammatory infiltrate, refractory congestive heart failure, hypotension, and ventricular irritability.[770]

Streptomycin has been implicated as an unusual cause of myocarditis. Pathological findings may include cardiac dilatation, myocarditis with necrosis, hemorrhage, and a fibrinous pericardial effusion.[770] Clinically, it may be associated with chest pain, dyspnea, fever, and rash, followed by collapse and death.

GIANT CELL MYOCARDITIS

Giant cell myocarditis is a rare disease of unknown etiology characterized by the presence of multinucleated giant cells in the myocardium. (It is included here because of the possibility that it may be of immune or autoimmune etiology.) Variously called acute isolated myocarditis and granulomatous myocarditis, this condition is typically a rapidly fatal disease, often of young to middle-aged adults.[771,772,772a] *Pathological findings* are usually impressive. The ventricles are dilated, and mural thrombi may be present.[773] A serpiginous area of myocardial necrosis may be seen involving the right as well as the left ventricle.[772] Multinucleated giant cells are found, particularly at the margins of the areas of myocardial necrosis; the giant cells appear to be of macrophage, rather than myocyte origin.[774] An extensive inflammatory infiltrate is present within the necrotic areas, composed of eosinophils, histiocytes, and other cells.[772]

Although giant cell myocarditis appears to be associated with thymoma, systemic lupus erythematosus, and thyrotoxicosis, the cause of the disease remains obscure.[772,774] In many ways the clinical features suggest a viral myocarditis except for the rapid and virulent course. However, despite careful investigation there has been no serological or bacteriological evidence of an infectious etiology.[772] Sarcoid, syphilis, and tuberculosis have all been proposed as possible causes, although these usually present distinctive histological features. It has also been suggested that the cause is an autoimmune reaction,[772] although little evidence aside from the histological findings supports this view.

Both sexes are equally affected; the onset is typically rapid, with dyspnea, chest pain, orthopnea, and hypotension.[772,775] Fever is usually present, with electrocardiographic evidence of widespread myocardial involvement. Sinus tachycardia, left bundle branch block, atrial and ventricular arrhythmias, complete heart block, and findings suggesting acute myocardial necrosis may be seen.[775] Overt congestive heart failure and sudden death may occur.[772] Therapy (other than cardiac transplantation) is invariably unsuccessful, although corticosteroids and immunosuppressive agents have been used.[772a] It has been suggested that cyclosporine might be more effective.[772]

PHYSICAL AGENTS

HEAT STROKE. This condition results from failure of the thermoregulatory center following exposure to high ambient temperature and is manifested principally by hyperpyrexia and central nervous system dysfunction. However, cardiovascular abnormalities (usually electrocardiographic) appear to be common; pulmonary edema and right ventricular dysfunction may occur,[776] along with hypotension and circulatory collapse. *Pathological changes* include dilatation of the right side of the heart, particularly the right atrium. Hemorrhages of the subendocardium and the subepicardium are frequently seen at necropsy and often involve the interventricular septum and posterior wall of the left ventricle.[776] Histological findings include degeneration and necrosis of muscle fibers as well as interstitial edema.[776] Possible factors responsible for myocardial damage include direct thermal injury, myocardial hypoxia secondary to circulatory collapse, decreased coronary blood flow, and metabolic abnormalities resulting from widespread injury to other organs.

Sinus tachycardia is invariably present, while atrial and ventricular arrhythmias are usually absent. Transient prolongation of the Q-T interval may be seen, along with ST-segment and T-wave abnormalities. It may take up to several months for these repolarization abnormalities to resolve. Serum enzyme levels may be elevated and may reflect myocardial damage, at least in part.[776]

HYPOTHERMIA. Low temperature may also result in myocardial damage. Cardiac dilatation may occur with epicardial petechiae and subendo-

cardial hemorrhages. Microinfarcts are present in the ventricular myocardium, and fatty changes are common. The lesions are not due to the low temperature per se but appear to be the result of the circulatory collapse, hemoconcentration, capillary sludging, and depressed cellular metabolism that accompany hypothermia. Clinical manifestations of hypothermia include sinus bradycardia, conduction disturbances, atrial (and occasionally ventricular) fibrillation, and a characteristic deflection of the terminal portion of the QRS pattern (Osborne wave).[777,778]

RADIATION. The employment of ionizing radiation during radiotherapy or, less commonly, after radiation accidents, may result in a variety of acute and chronic cardiac complications including pericarditis with effusion, tamponade, and constriction; coronary artery fibrosis and myocardial infarction; valvular abnormalities; myocardial fibrosis; and conduction disturbances.[779-782] While the heart is thought to be one of the organs most resistant to the effects of radiation, damage to the pericardium (p. 1754), myocardium, and endocardium occurs.[783] Although radiation probably results in some degree of tissue damage in all patients, clinically significant cardiac involvement occurs in the minority of patients. Radiation-induced cardiac damage is related to the dose of radiation, the mass of heart irradiated, and the dose schedule of the radiation.

The late cardiac damage that may follow irradiation appears to result from a long-lasting injury of the capillary endothelial cells, which leads to cell death, capillary rupture, and microthrombi.[780] Because of this damage to the microvasculature, ischemia results and is followed by myocardial fibrosis. In addition to microvascular damage, the major epicardial coronary arteries may become narrowed, especially at the ostia.[780,781,784,785]

Only an occasional patient manifests acute cardiac abnormality clinically with radiation therapy; typically this consists of acute pericarditis.[786] A mild, transient, asymptomatic depression of left ventricular function may be seen early after radiation therapy.[779] The more common clinical expressions of radiation heart disease occur months or years after the exposure.[786] The pericardium is the most common site of clinical involvement, with findings of chronic pericardial effusion or pericardial constriction. Myocardial damage occurs less frequently and is characterized by myocardial fibrosis with or without endocardial fibrosis or fibroelastosis. Left and/or right ventricular dysfunction at rest or with exercise appears to be a common, albeit usually asymptomatic, finding 5 to 20 years after radiation therapy, especially in those in whom the now-outmoded technique of a single anteroposterior port was used.[787]

REFERENCES

1. Abelmann, W. H., and Lorell, B. H.: The challenge of cardiomyopathy. J. Am. Coll. Cardiol. *13*:1219, 1989.
2. Cardiomyopathy. *In* Fowler, N. O.: Diagnosis of Heart Disease. New York, Springer-Verlag, 1991, pp. 239–255.
3. Gillum, R. F.: The epidemiology of cardiomyopathy in the United States. *In* Zipes. D. P., and Rowlands, D. J. (eds.): Progress in Cardiology. Philadelphia, Lea and Febiger, 1989, p. 11.
4. Codd, M. B., Sugrue, D. D., Gersh, B. J., and Melton, L. J., III: Epidemiology of idiopathic dilated and hypertrophic cardiomyopathy. Circulation *80*:564, 1989.
5. WHO Technical Report Series: Cardiomyopathies. Report of a WHO expert committee. Technical Report Series *697*:7, 1984.
6. Goodwin, J. F.: Classification of nonhypertrophic cardiomyopathies. *In* Zipes, D. P., and Rowlands, D. J. (eds.): Progress in Cardiology. Philadelphia, Lea and Febiger, 1989, p. 3.
7. Mason, J. W., and O'Connell, J. B.: Clinical merit of endomyocardial biopsy. Circulation *79*:971, 1989.
8. Yoshizato, T., Edwards, W. D., Alboliras, E. T., et al.: Safety and utility of endomyocardial biopsy in infants, children and adolescents: A review of 66 procedures in 53 patients. J. Am. Coll. Cardiol. *15*:436, 1990.
9. Schmeltz, A. A., Apitz, J., Hort, W., and Maisch, B.: Endomyocardial biopsy in infants and children: Experience in 60 patients. Pediatr. Cardiol. *11*:15, 1990.
10. Miller, L. W., Labovitz, A. J., McBride, L. A., et al.: Echocardiography-guided endomyocardial biopsy: A 5-year experience. Circulation *78*:99, 1988.
11. Lie, J. T.: Myocarditis and endomyocardial biopsy in unexplained heart failure: A diagnosis in search of a disease (editorial). Ann. Intern. Med. *109*:525, 1988.
12. Aretz, H. T., Billingham, M. E., Edwards, W. D., et al.: Myocarditis: A histopathologic definition and classification. Am. J. Cardiovasc. Pathol. *1*:3, 1987.

DILATED CARDIOMYOPATHY

13. Keren, A., Gottlieb, S., Tzivoni, D., et al.: Mildly dilated congestive cardiomyopathy. Use of prospective diagnostic criteria and description of the clinical course without heart transplantation. Circulation *81*:506, 1990.
14. Stevenson, L. W.: Dilated Cardiomyopathy: Principles and Prognosis. *In* Zipes, D. P., and Rowlands, D. J. (eds.): Progress in Cardiology. Philadelphia, Lea and Febiger, 1989, p. 51.
15. Diaz, R. A., Obasohan, A., and Oakley, C. M.: Prediction of outcome in dilated cardiomyopathy. Br. Heart J. *58*:393, 1987.
16. Stevenson, L. W., Fowler, M. B., Schroeder, J. S., et al.: Poor survival of

patients with idiopathic cardiomyopathy considered too well for transplantation. Am. J. Med. 83:871, 1987.

17. Romeo, F., Pelliccia, F., Cianfrocca, C., et al.: Determinants of end-stage idiopathic dilated cardiomyopathy: A multivariate analysis of 104 patients. Clin. Cardiol. 12:387, 1989.

18. Romeo, F., Pelliccia, F., Cianfrocca, C., et al.: Predictors of sudden death in idiopathic dilated cardiomyopathy. Am. J. Cardiol. 63:138, 1989.

19. Juilliere, Y., Danchin, N., Briancon, S., et al.: Dilated cardiomyopathy: Long-term follow-up and predictors of survival. Int. J. Cardiol. 21:269, 1988.

20. Douglas, P. S., Morrow, R., Ioli, A., and Reichek, N.: Left ventricular shape, afterload and survival in idiopathic dilated cardiomyopathy. J. Am. Coll. Cardiol. 13:311, 1989.

21. Tanganelli, P., Di Lenarda, A., Bianciardi, G., et al.: Correlation between histomorphometric findings on endomyocardial biopsy and clinical findings in idiopathic dilated cardiomyopathy. Am. J. Cardiol. 64:504, 1989.

22. Tamai, J., Nagata, S., Nishimura, T., et al.: Hemodynamic and prognostic value of thallium-201 myocardial imaging in patients with dilated cardiomyopathy. Int. J. Cardiol. 24:219, 1989.

23. Keogh, A. M., Baron, D. W., and Hickie, J. B.: Prognostic guides in patients with idiopathic or ischemic dilated cardiomyopathy assessed for cardiac transplantation. Am. J. Cardiol. 65:903, 1990.

24. Chetty, S., and Mitha, A. S.: Arrhythmias in idiopathic dilated cardiomyopathy. A preliminary study. S. Afr. Med. J. 77:190, 1990.

25. Figulla, H. R., Rahlf, G., Nieger, M., et al.: Spontaneous hemodynamic improvement or stabilization and associated biopsy findings in patients with congestive cardiomyopathy. Circulation 71:1095, 1985.

26. Natural history of dilated cardiomyopathy (editorial). Lancet 1:248, 1986.

27. Oakley, C.: Importance of right ventricular function in congestive heart failure. Am. J. Cardiol. 62:14A, 1988.

28. Griffin, M. L., Hernandez, A., Martin, T. C., et al.: Dilated cardiomyopathy in infants and children. J. Am. Coll. Cardiol. 11:139, 1988.

29. Chen, S-C., Nouri, S., Balfour, I., et al.: Clinical profile of congestive cardiomyopathy in children. J. Am. Coll. Cardiol. 15:189, 1990.

30. Roberts, W. C., Siegel, R. J., and McManus, B. M.: Idiopathic dilated cardiomyopathy: Analysis of 152 necropsy patients. Am. J. Cardiol. 60:1340, 1987.

31. Ferrans, V. J.: Pathologic anatomy of the dilated cardiomyopathies. Am. J. Cardiol. 64:9C, 1989.

32. Kuroda, T., Shiina, A., Suzuki, O., et al.: Prediction of prognosis of patients with idiopathic dilated cardiomyopathy: A comparison of echocardiography with cardiac catheterization. Jpn. J. Med. 28:180, 1989.

33. Klein, L. W., and Horowitz, L. N.: Familial right ventricular dilated cardiomyopathy associated with supraventricular arrhythmias. Am. J. Coll. Cardiol. 62:482, 1988.

34. Tazelaar, H. D., and Billingham, M. E.: Leukocytic infiltrates in idiopathic dilated cardiomyopathy. A source of confusion with active myocarditis. Am. J. Surg. Pathol. 10:405, 1986.

34a. Edwards, W. D.: Cardiomyopathies. Hum. Pathol. 18:625, 1987.

34b. Schaper, J., Froede, R., Hein, S., et al.: Impairment of the myocardial ultrastructure and changes of the cytoskeleton in dilated cardiomyopathy. Circulation 83:504, 1991.

35. Bender, J. R.: Idiopathic dilated cardiomyopathy: An immunologic, genetic, or infectious disease, or all of the above? Circulation 83:704, 1991.

36. Hartz, A. J., Anderson, A. J., Brooks, H. L., et al.: The association of smoking with cardiomyopathy. N. Engl. J. Med. 311:1201, 1984.

36a. Wikman-Coffelt, J., Stefenelli, T., Wu, S. T., et al.: [Ca²⁺]ᵢ Transients in the cardiomyopathic hamster heart. Circ. Res. 68:45, 1991.

37. Movsesian, M. A., Bristow, M. R., and Krall, J.: Ca²⁺ uptake by cardiac sarcoplasmic reticulum from patients with idiopathic dilated cardiomyopathy. Circ. Res. 65:1141, 1989.

38. Brodde, O. E., Zerkowski, H. R., Doetsch, N., et al.: Myocardial beta-adrenoceptor changes in heart failure: Concomitant reduction in beta 1- and beta 2-adrenoceptor function related to the degree of heart failure in patients with mitral valve disease. J. Am. Coll. Cardiol. 14:323, 1989.

39. Vago, T., Bevilacqua, M., Norbiato, G., et al.: Identification of alpha 1-adrenergic receptors on sarcolemma from normal subjects and patients with idiopathic dilated cardiomyopathy: Characteristics and linkage to GTP-binding protein. Circ. Res. 64:474, 1989.

40. Limas, C. J., Goldenberg, I. F., and Limas, C.: Autoantibodies against beta-adrenoceptors in human idiopathic dilated cardiomyopathy. Circ. Res. 64:97, 1989.

41. Limas, C. J., Goldenberg, I. F., and Limas, C.: Effect of cardiac transplantation on anti-beta-receptor antibodies in idiopathic dilated cardiomyopathy. Am. J. Cardiol. 63:1134, 1989.

42. Bohm, M., Gierschik, P., Jakobs, K. H., et al.: Localization of a "postreceptor" defect in human dilated cardiomyopathy. Am. J. Cardiol. 64:812, 1989.

43. Limas, C. J., Goldenberg, I. F., and Limas, C.: Influence of anti-beta-receptor antibodies on cardiac adenylate cyclase in patients with idiopathic dilated cardiomyopathy. Am. Heart J. 119:1322, 1990.

44. Maisel, A. S., Michel, M. C., Isel, P. A., et al.: Pertussis toxin treatment of whole blood: A novel approach to assess G protein function in congestive heart failure. Circulation 81:1198, 1990.

45. Muir, P., Nicholson, F., Tilzey, A. J., et al.: Chronic relapsing pericarditis and dilated cardiomyopathy: Serological evidence of persistent enterovirus infection. Lancet 1:804, 1989.

46. O'Connell, J. B., and Mason, J. W.: Immunosuppressive therapy in experimental and clinical myocarditis. Pathol. Immunopathol. Res. 7:292, 1988.

47. Shabetai, R.: Myocarditis and dilated cardiomyopathy: Twins or distant relatives? Cardiology 76:332, 1989.

48. O'Connell, J. B.: Immunosuppression for dilated cardiomyopathy (editorial). N. Engl. J. Med. 321:1119, 1989.

49. Fallon, J. T.: Myocarditis and dilated cardiomyopathy: Different stages of the same disease? Cardiovasc. Clin. 18:155, 1988.

50. Maisch, N., Bauer, E., Hufnagel, G., et al.: The use of endomyocardial biopsy in heart failure. Eur. Heart J. 9:59, 1988.

51. Popma, J. J., Cigarroa, R. G., Buja, L. M., and Hillis, L. D.: Diagnostic and prognostic utility of right-sided catheterization and endomyocardial biopsy in idiopathic dilated cardiomyopathy. Am. J. Cardiol. 63:955, 1989.

52. Bowles, N. E., Rose, M. L., Taylor, P., et al.: End-state dilated cardiomyopathy. Persistence of enterovirus RNA in myocardium at cardiac transplantation and lack of immune response. Circulation 80:1128, 1989.

53. Limas, C. J., and Limas, C.: HLA antigens in idiopathic dilated cardiomyopathy. Br. Heart J. 62:379, 1989.

54. Limas, C. J., Limas, C., Kubo, S. H., and Olivari, M. T.: Anti-beta-receptor antibodies in human dilated cardiomyopathy and correlation with HLA-DR antigens. Am. J. Cardiol. 65:483, 1990.

55. Obrador, D., Ballester, M., Carrio, I., et al.: High prevalence of myocardial monoclonal antimyosin antibody uptake in patients with chronic idiopathic dilated cardiomyopathy. J. Am. Coll. Cardiol. 13:1289, 1989.

56. Schulze, K., Becker, B. F., and Schultheiss, H. P.: Antibodies to the ADP/ATP carrier, an autoantigen in myocarditis and dilated cardiomyopathy, penetrate into myocardial cells and disturb energy metabolism in vivo. Circ. Res. 64:179, 1989.

57. Caforio, A.L.P., Bonifacio, E., Stewart, J. T., et al.: Novel organ-specific circulating cardiac autoantibodies in dilated cardiomyopathy. J. Am. Coll. Cardiol. 15:1527, 1990.

58. Sanderson, J. E., Koech, D., Iha, D., and Ojiambo, H. P.: T-lymphocyte subsets in idiopathic dilated cardiomyopathy. Am. J. Cardiol. 55:755, 1985.

59. Franceschini, R., Messina, V., Petillo, A., et al.: Humoral immunity and lymphocyte subpopulations in patients with dilated cardiomyopathy. Int. J. Cardiol. 8:113, 1985.

60. Anderson, J. L., Carlquist, J. F., and Higashikubo, R.: Quantitation of lymphocyte subsets by immunofluorescence flow cytometry in idiopathic dilated cardiomyopathy. Am. J. Cardiol. 55:1550, 1985.

61. Lowry, P. J., Thompson, R. A., and Littler, W. A.: Cellular immunity in congestive cardiomyopathy. The normal cellular immune response. Br. Heart J. 53:394, 1985.

62. Tatsunori, I., Katsutoshi, Y., Ono, S., et al.: Dilated cardiomyopathy associated with natural killer cell deficiency. Am. Heart J. 115:1326, 1988.

63. Lowry, P. J., Gammage, M. D., Gentle, T. A., et al.: Suppressor T lymphocyte function in patients with idiopathic congestive cardiomyopathy. Br. Heart J. 57:458, 1987.

64. Imperato-McGinley, J., Gautier, T., Ehlers, K., et al.: Reversibility of catecholamine-induced dilated cardiomyopathy in a child with a pheochromocytoma. N. Engl. J. Med. 316:793, 1987.

65. Graber, H. L., Unverferth, D. V., Baker, P. B., et al.: Evolution of a hereditary cardiac conduction and muscle disorder: A study involving a family with six generations affected. Circulation 74:21, 1986.

66. Berko, B. A., and Swift, M.: X-linked dilated cardiomyopathy. N. Engl. J. Med. 316:1186, 1987.

67. Valentine, H. A., Hunt, S. A., Fowler, M. B., et al.: Frequency of familial nature of dilated cardiomyopathy and usefulness of cardiac transplantation in this subset. Am. J. Cardiol. 63:959, 1989.

68. Urie, P. M., and Billingham, M. E.: Ultrastructural features of familial cardiomyopathy. Am. J. Cardiol. 62:325, 1988.

69. Schmidt, M. A., Michels, V. V., Edwards, W. D., and Miller, F. A.: Familial dilated cardiomyopathy. Am. J. Med. Genet. 31:135, 1988.

70. Fragola, P. V., Autore, C., Picelli, A., et al.: Familial idiopathic dilated cardiomyopathy. Am. Heart J. 115:912, 1988.

71. Regitz, V., Shug, A. L., and Fleck, E.: Defective myocardial carnitine metabolism in congestive heart failure secondary to dilated cardiomyopathy and to coronary, hypertensive and valvular heart disease. Am. J. Cardiol. 65:755, 1990.

72. Feldman, A. M., Cates, A. E., Veazey, W. B., et al.: Increase of the 40,000-mol wt pertussis toxin substrate (G Protein) in the failing human heart. J. Clin. Invest. 82:189, 1988.

73. Böhm, M., Gierschik, P., Jakobs, K-H., et al.: Increase in Gᵢₐ in human hearts with dilated but not ischemic cardiomyopathy. Circulation 82:1249, 1990.

74. Rahko, P. S., and Orie, J. E.: The clinical presentation and laboratory evaluation of congestive and ischemic cardiomyopathies. Cardiovasc. Clin. 19:75, 1988.

75. Stewart, R.A.H., McKenna, W. J., and Oakley, C. M.: Good prognosis for dilated cardiomyopathy without severe heart failure or arrhythmia. Q. J. Med. New Series 74:309, 1990.

76. Roubin, G. S., Anderson, S. D., Shen, W. F., et al: Hemodynamic and metabolic basis of impaired exercise tolerance in patients with severe left ventricular dysfunction. J. Am. Coll. Cardiol. 15:986, 1990.

77. Sullivan, M. J., Green, H. J., and Cobb, F. R.: Skeletal muscle biochemistry and histology in ambulatory patients with long-term heart failure. Circulation 81:518, 1990.

78. Caforio, A. L. P., Rossi, B., Risaliti, R., et al.: Type 1 fiber abnormalities in skeletal muscle of patients with hypertrophic and dilated cardiomyopathy: Evidence of subclinical myogenic myopathy. J. Am. Coll. Cardiol. 14:1464, 1989.

79. Cannon, R. O., Cunnion, R. E., Parrillo, J. E., et al.: Dynamic limitation of

coronary vasodilator reserve in patients with dilated cardiomyopathy and chest pain. J. Am. Coll. Cardiol. 10:1190, 1987.

80. Treasure, C. B., Vita, J. A., Cox, D. A., et al.: Endothelium-dependent dilation of the coronary microvasculature is impaired in dilated cardiomyopathy. Circulation 81:722, 1990.

81. Cabanes, L. R., Weber, S. N., Matran, R., et al.: Bronchial hyperresponsiveness to methacholine in patients with impaired left ventricular function. N. Engl. J. Med. 320:1317, 1989.

82. Dickerman, S. A., and Rubler, S.: Mitral and tricuspid valve regurgitation in dilated cardiomyopathy. Am. J. Cardiol. 63:629, 1989.

83. Feldman, M. D., and Beller, G. A.: Is secondary mitral regurgitation in congestive heart failure a marker of clinical importance? J. Am. Coll. Cardiol. 15:181, 1990.

84. Keren, G., Sonnenblick, E. H., and LeJemtel, T. H.:Mitral anulus motion: Relation to pulmonary venous and transmitral flow in normal subjects and in patients with dilated cardiomyopathy. Circulation 78:621, 1988.

85. Maze, S. S., Kotler, M. N., and Parry, W. R.: Flow characteristics in the dilated left ventricle with thrombus: Qualitative and quantitative Doppler analysis. J. Am. Coll. Cardiol. 13:873, 1989.

86. Uretsky, B. F.: Diagnostic considerations in the adult patient with cardiomyopathy or congestive heart failure. Cardiovasc. Clin. 19:35, 1988.

87. Wilensky, R. L., Yudelman, P., Cohen, A. I., et al.: Serial electrocardiographic changes in idiopathic dilated cardiomyopathy confirmed at necropsy. Am. J. Cardiol. 62:276, 1988.

88. Milechman, G., and Scheinman, M. M.: Ventricular dysrhythmias and sudden death in dilated cardiomyopathy. In Zipes, D. P., and Rowlands, D. J. (eds.): Progress in Cardiology. Philadelphia, Lea and Febiger, 1989, p. 85.

89. Anderson, D. P., Freedman, R. A., and Mason, J. W.: Sudden death in idiopathic dilated cardiomyopathy (editorial). Ann. Intern. Med. 107:104, 1987.

90. Liem, L. B., and Swerdlow, C. D.: Value of electropharmacologic testing in idiopathic dilated cardiomyopathy and sustained ventricular tachyarrhythmias. Am. J. Cardiol. 62:611, 1988.

91. Hofmann, T., Meinertz, T., Kasper, W., et al.: Mode of death in idiopathic dilated cardiomyopathy: A multivariate analysis of prognostic determinants. Am. Heart J. 116:1455, 1988.

92. Rakovec, P., Lajovic, J., and Dolenc, M.: Reversible congestive cardiomyopathy due to chronic ventricular tachycardia. PACE 12:542, 1989.

93. Sarembock, I. J., Horak, A. R., and Commerford, P. J.: Tachycardia-induced reversible left ventricular dysfunction: A report of 2 cases. S. Afr. Med. J. 73:484, 1988.

94. Peters, K. G., and Kienzle, M. G.: Severe cardiomyopathy due to chronic rapidly conducted atrial fibrillation: Complete recovery after restoration of sinus rhythm. Am. J. Med. 85:242, 1988.

95. Vanoverschelde, J., Raphael, D. A., Robert, A. R., and Cosyns, J. R.: Left ventricular filling in dilated cardiomyopathy: Relation to functional class and hemodynamics. J. Am. Coll. Cardiol. 15:1288, 1990.

96. Iskandrian, A. S., Hakki, A. H., and Kane, S.: Resting thallium-201 myocardial perfusion patterns in patients with severe left ventricular dysfunction: Differences between patients with primary cardiomyopathy, chronic coronary artery disease, or acute myocardial infarction. Am. Heart J. 11:760, 1986.

97. Eisenberg, J. D., Sobel, B. E., and Geltman, E. M.: Differentiation of ischemic from nonischemic cardiomyopathy with positron emission tomography. Am. J. Cardiol. 59:1410, 1987.

98. Mody, F. V., Brunken, R. C., Stevenson, L. W., et al.: Differentiating cardiomyopathy of coronary artery disease from nonischemic dilated cardiomyopathy utilizing positron emission tomography J. Am. Coll. Cardiol. 17:373, 1991.

99. Bouhour, J. B., Helias, J., de Lajartre, A. Y., et al.: Detection of myocarditis during the first year after discovery of a dilated cardiomyopathy by endomyocardial biopsy and gallium-67 myocardial scintigraphy: Prospective multicentre French study of 91 patients. Eur. Heart J. 9:520, 1988.

100. O'Connell, J. B., and Mason, J. W.: Diagnosing and treating active myocarditis. West. J. Med. 150:431, 1989.

101. Yasuda, T., Palacios, I. F., Dec, G. W., et al.: Indium-111 monoclonal antimyosin imaging in the diagnosis of acute myocarditis. Circulation 76:306, 1987.

102. Sunnerhagen, K. S., Bhargava, V., and Shabetai, R.: Regional left ventricular wall motion abnormalities in idiopathic dilated cardiomyopathy. Am. J. Cardiol. 65:364, 1990.

103. Cohn, J. N., Archibald, D. G., Ziesche, S., et al.: Effect of vasodilator therapy on mortality in chronic congestive heart failure. Results of Veterans Administration Cooperative Study. N. Engl. J. Med. 314:1547, 1986.

104. Massin, E. K.: Current treatment of dilated cardiomyopathy. Texas Heart Inst. J. 18:41, 1991.

105. CONSENSUS Trial Study Group: Effects of enalapril on mortality in severe congestive heart failure. N. Engl. J. Med. 316:1429, 1987.

106. Figulla, H. R., Rechenberg, J. V., Wiegand, V., et al.: Beneficial effects of long-term diltiazem treatment in dilated cardiomyopathy. J. Am. Coll. Cardiol. 13:653, 1989.

107. Stevenson, L. W., and Tillisch, J. H.: Maintenance of cardiac output with normal filling pressures in patients with dilated heart failure. Circulation 74:1303, 1986.

108. Waagstein, F., Caidahl, K., Wallentin, I., et al.: Long-term beta-blockade in dilated cardiomyopathy. Effects of short- and long-term metoprolol treatment followed by withdrawal and readministration of metoprolol. Circulation 80:551, 1989.

109. Heilbrunn, S. M., Shah, P., Bristow, M. R., et al.: Increased beta-receptor density and improved hemodynamic response to catecholamine stimulation during long-term metoprolol therapy in heart failure from dilated cardiomyopathy. Circulation 79:483, 1989.

110. Gilbert, E. M., Anderson, J. L., Deitchman, D., et al.: Long-term beta-blocker vasodilator therapy improves cardiac function in idiopathic dilated cardiomyopathy: A double-blind, randomized study of bucindolol versus placebo. Am. J. Med. 88:223, 1990.

111. Leung, W. H., Lau, C. P., Wong, C. K., et al.: Improvement in exercise performance and hemodynamics by labetalol in patients with idiopathic dilated cardiomyopathy. Am. Heart J. 119:884, 1990.

112. Fowler, M. B., and Bristow, M. R.: Rationale for beta-adrenergic blocking drugs in cardiomyopathy. Am. J. Cardiol. 55:120D, 1985.

113. Lee, H. R., O'Connell, J. B., and Mason, J. W.: Immunosuppression and beta-blockade in heart failure. Cardiol. Clin. 7:171, 1989.

114. Parmley, W. W., and Chatterjee, K.: Congestive heart failure and arrhythmias: An overview. Am. J. Cardiol. 57:34B, 1986.

115. Kulick, D. L., Bhandari, A. K., Hong, R., et al.: Effect of acute hemodynamic decompensation on electrical inducibility of ventricular arrhythmias in patients with dilated cardiomyopathy and complex nonsustained ventricular arrhythmias. Am. Heart J. 119:878, 1990.

116. Milner, P. G., Dimarco, J. P., and Lerman, B. B.: Electrophysiological evaluation of sustained ventricular tachyarrhythmias in idiopathic dilated cardiomyopathy. PACE 11:562, 1988.

117. Constantin, L., Martins, J. B., Kienzle, M. G., et al.: Induced sustained ventricular tachycardia in nonischemic dilated cardiomyopathy: Dependence on clinical presentation and response to antiarrhythmic agents. PACE 12:776, 1989.

118. Fauchier, J. P., Cosnay, P., Moquet, B., et al.: Late ventricular potentials and spontaneous and induced ventricular arrhythmias in dilated or hypertrophic cardiomyopathies. A prospective study about 83 patients. PACE 11:1974, 1988.

119. Falk, R. H.: A plea for a clinical trial of anticoagulation in dilated cardiomyopathy. Am. J. Cardiol. 65:914, 1990.

120. Goodwin, J. F.: Clinical decisions in the management of the cardiomyopathies. Pract. Therapeut. 38:988, 1989.

121. Kyrle, P. A., Korninger, C., Gossinger, H., et al.: Prevention of arterial and pulmonary embolism by oral anticoagulants in patients with dilated cardiomyopathy. Thromb. Haemost. 54:521, 1985.

122. Parrillo, J. E., Cunnion, R. E., Epstein, S. E., et al.: A prospective, randomized, controlled trial of prednisone for dilated cardiomyopathy. N. Engl. J. Med. 321:1061, 1989.

123. Latham, R. D., Mulrow, J. P., Virmani, R., et al.: Recently diagnosed idiopathic dilated cardiomyopathy: Incidence of myocarditis and efficacy of prednisone therapy. Am. Heart J. 117:876, 1989.

124. Heck, C. F., Shumway, S. J., and Kaye, M. P.: The Registry of the International Society for Heart Transplantation: Sixth official report — 1989. J. Heart Transplant. 8:271, 1989.

125. Walsh, T. K., and Vacek, J. L.: Ethanol and heart disease. An underestimated contributing factor. Postgrad. Med. 79:60, 1986.

126. Regan, T. J.: Alcoholic cardiomyopathy. In Zipes, D. P., and Rowlands, D. J. (eds.): Progress in Cardiology. Philadelphia, Lea and Febiger, 1989, p. 129.

127. Pavan, D., Nicolosi, G. L., Lestuzzi, C., et al.: Normalization of variables of left ventricular function in patients with alcoholic cardiomyopathy after cessation of excessive alcohol intake: An echocardiographic study. Eur. Heart J. 8:535, 1987.

128. Auffermann, W., Wu, S., Parmley, W. W., et al.: Reversibility of chronic alcohol cardiac depression: 31P magnetic resonance spectroscopy in hamsters. Magn. Reson. Med. 9:343, 1989.

129. Davidson, M. D.: Cardiovascular effects of alcohol. West. J. Med. 151:430, 1989.

130. McCall, D.: Alcohol and the cardiovascular system. Curr. Probl. Cardiol. 12:351, 1987.

131. Urbano-Marquez, A., Estruch, R., Navarro-Lopez, F., et al.: The effects of alcoholism on skeletal and cardiac muscle. N. Engl. J. Med. 320:409, 1989.

132. Lang, R. M., Borow, K. M., Neumann, A., and Feldman, T.: Adverse cardiac effects of acute alcohol ingestion in young adults. Ann. Intern. Med. 102:742, 1985.

133. Kelbaek, H., Heslet, L., Skagen, K., et al.: Cardiac function after alcohol ingestion in patients with ischemic heart disease and cardiomyopathy: A controlled study. Alcohol Alcohol. 23:17, 1988.

134. Kelbaek, H.: Acute effects of alcohol and food intake on cardiac performance. Prog. Cardiovasc. Dis. 23:347, 1990.

135. Diamond, I.: Alcoholic myopathy and cardiomyopathy (editorial). N. Engl. J. Med. 72:458, 1989.

136. Feldman, A. M., Levine, M. A., Cates, A. E., et al.: Multiple effects of ethanol on cardiac adenylate cyclase. J. Cardiovasc. Pharmacol. 13:774, 1989.

137. Preedy, V. R., and Peters, T. J.: Synthesis of subcellular protein fractions in the rat heart in vivo in response to chronic ethanol feeding. Cardiovasc. Res. 23:730, 1989.

138. Guarnieri, T., and Lakatta, E. G.: Mechanism of myocardial contractile depression by clinical concentrations of ethanol. J. Clin. Invest. 85:1462, 1990.

139. Laposata, E. A., and Lange, L. G.: Presence of nonoxidative ethanol metabolism in human organs commonly damaged by ethanol abuse. Science 231:497, 1986.

140. Tsiplenkova, V. G., Vikhert, A. M., and Cherpachenko, N. M.: Ultrastructural and histochemical observations in human and experimental alcoholic cardiomyopathy. J. Am. Coll. Cardiol. 8:22A, 1986.

140a. Cerqueira, M. D., Harp, G. D., Ritchie, J. L., et al.: Rarity of preclinical alcoholic cardiomyopathy in chronic alcoholics over 40 years of age. Am. J. Cardiol. 67:183, 1991.

141. Dancy, M., Leech, G., Bland, J. M., et al.: Preclinical left ventricular abnormalities in alcoholics are independent of nutritional status, cirrhosis, and cigarette smoking. Lancet I:1122, 1985.

142. Ahmed, S. S., Howard, M., ten Hove, W., et al.: Cardiac function in alcoholics with cirrhosis: Absence of overt cardiomyopathy—myth or fact? J. Am. Coll. Cardiol. 3:696, 1984.

142a. Kupari, M., Koskinen, P., and Suokas, A.: Left ventricular size, mass and function in relation to the duration and quantity of heavy drinking in alcoholics. Am. J. Cardiol. 67:274, 1991.

143. Regan, T. J.: Alcohol and the cardiovascular system (editorial). West. J. Med. 151:454, 1989.

144. Vikert, A. M., Tsiplenkova, V. G., and Cherpachenko, N. M.: Alcoholic cardiomyopathy and sudden cardiac death. J. Am. Coll. Cardiol. 8:3A, 1986.

145. Kinney, E. L., Wright, R. J., and Caldwell, J. W.: Risk factors in alcoholic cardiomyopathy. Angiology 40:270, 1989.

146. Milgaard, H., Kristensen, B. O., and Baandrup, U.: Importance of abstention from alcohol in alcoholic heart disease. Int. J. Cardiol. 26:373, 1990.

147. Clay, M. A., Stewart-Richardson, P., Tassett, D. M., and Williams, J. F.: Chronic alcoholic cardiomyopathy. Protection of the isolated ischaemic working heart by ribose. Biochem. Int. 17:791, 1988.

148. Wu, S., White, R., Wikman-Coiffelt, J., et al.: The preventive effect of verapamil on ethanol-induced cardiac depression: Phosphorus-31 nuclear magnetic resonance and high-pressure liquid chromatographic studies of hamsters. Circulation 75:1058, 1987.

149. Blomstrom-Lundqvist, C., Sabel, K-G., and Olsson, S. B.: A long term follow up of 15 patients with arrhythmogenic right ventricular dysplasia. Br. Heart J. 58:477, 1987.

150. Thiene, G, Nava, A., Corrado, D., et al.: Right ventricular cardiomyopathy and sudden death in young people. N. Engl. J. Med. 318:129, 1988.

151. Mohan, J. C., Chutani, S. K., Sethi, K. K., et al.: Dominant right ventricular dilated cardiomyopathy: Clinical, echocardiographic and haemodynamic profile. Indian Heart J. 41:177, 1989.

152. Brandt, J., Hofvendahl, S., Ljungdahl, L., et al.: Non-invasive recognition of arrhythmogenic right ventricular dysplasia. Acta Med. Scand. 223:281, 1988.

153. Chiddo, A., Locuratolo, N., Gaglione, A., et al.: Right ventricular dysplasia: Angiographic study. Eur. Heart J. 10:42, 1989.

154. Hirooka, Y., Urable, Y., Imaizumi, T., et al.: The usefulness of equilibrium radionuclide ventriculography in the diagnosis of arrhythmogenic right ventricular dysplasia and a report of cases of a familial occurrence. Jpn. Circ. J. 52:511, 1988.

155. Scognamiglio, R., Fasoli, G., Nava, A., et al.: Contribution of cross-sectional echocardiography to the diagnosis of right ventricular dysplasia at the asymptomatic stage. Eur. Heart J. 10:538, 1989.

156. Lemery, R., Brugada, P., Janssen, J., et al.: Nonischemic sustained ventricular tachycardia: Clinical outcome in 12 patients with arrhythmogenic right ventricular dysplasia. J. Am. Coll. Cardiol. 14:96, 1989.

157. Fontaine, G., Frank, R., Rougier, I., et al.: Electrode catheter ablation of resistant ventricular tachycardia in arrhythmogenic right ventricular dysplasia. Heart Vessels 5:172, 1990.

HYPERTROPHIC CARDIOMYOPATHY

158. Braunwald, E.: Hypertrophic cardiomyopathy—continued progress. N. Engl. J. Med. 320:800, 1989.

159. Hypertrophic cardiomyopathy. In Fowler, N. O.: Diagnosis of heart disease. New York, Springer-Verlag, 1991, pp. 256–267.

160. Morrow, A. G., and Braunwald, E.: Functional aortic stenosis: A malformation characterized by resistance to left ventricular outflow without anatomic obstruction. Circulation 20:181, 1959.

161. Maron, B. J., Bonow, R. O., Cannon, R. O., et al.: Hypertrophic cardiomyopathy: Interrelations of clinical manifestations, pathophysiology, and therapy. N. Engl. J. Med. 316:780, and 844, 1987.

162. Jarcho, J. A., McKenna, W., Pare, J.A.P., et al.: Mapping a gene for familial hypertrophic cardiomyopathy to chromosome 14q1. N. Engl. J. Med. 321:1372, 1989.

163. Maron, B. J., and Mulvihill, J. J.: The genetics of hypertrophic cardiomyopathy. Ann. Intern. Med. 105:610, 1986.

164. Greaves, S. C., Roche, A.H.G., Neutze, J. M., et al.: Inheritance of hypertrophic cardiomyopathy: A cross sectional and M mode echocardiographic study of 50 families. Br. Heart J. 58:259, 1987.

165. Autore, C., Fragola, P. V., Picelli, A., et al.: Equivocal and borderline myocardial hypertrophy in relatives of patients with hypertrophic cardiomyopathy: Possible implications in genetics of the disease. Cardiology 75:348, 1988.

166. Maron, B. J., Nichols, P. F., Pickle, L. W., et al.: Patterns of inheritance in hypertrophic cardiomyopathy: Assessment by M-mode and two-dimensional echocardiography. Am. J. Cardiol. 53:1087, 1984.

167. Hada, Y., Sakamoto, T., Amano, K., et al.: Prevalence of hypertrophic cardiomyopathy in a population of adult Japanese workers as detected by echocardiographic screening. Am. J. Cardiol. 59:183, 1987.

168. McKenna, W. J., Kleinebenne, A., Nihoyannopoulos, P., and Foale, R.: Echocardiographic measurement of right ventricular wall thickness in hypertrophic cardiomyopathy: Relation to clinical and prognostic features. J. Am. Coll. Cardiol. 11:351, 1988.

169. Motamed, H. E., and Roberts, W. C.: Frequency and significance of mitral anular calcium in hypertrophic cardiomyopathy: Analysis of 200 necropsy patients. Am. J. Cardiol. 60:877, 1987.

170. Maron, B. J.: Asymmetry in hypertrophic cardiomyopathy: The septal to free wall thickness ratio revisited. Am. J. Cardiol. 55:835, 1985.

171. Wakasugi, S., Shibata, N., Kobayashi, T., et al.: Thallium-201 imaging in a patient with mid-ventricular hypertrophic obstructive cardiomyopathy. J. Nucl. Med. 29:1738, 1988.

172. Zoghbi, W. A., Haichin, R. N., and Quinones, M. A.: Mid-cavity obstruction in apical hypertrophy: Doppler evidence of diastolic intraventricular gradient with higher apical pressure. Am. Heart J. 116:1469, 1988.

173. Maron, B. J.: Apical hypertrophic cardiomyopathy: The continuing saga. J. Am. Coll. Cardiol. 15:91, 1990.

174. Louie, E. K., and Maron, B. J.: Apical hypertrophic cardiomyopathy: Clinical and two-dimensional echocardiographic assessment. Ann. Intern. Med. 106:663, 1987.

175. Gosselin, G., Pasternac, A., Lesperance, J., et al.: Apical hypertrophic cardiomyopathy: Clinical and angiographic characteristics of the first Canadian series. Can. J. Cardiol. 4:258, 1988.

176. Webb, J. G., Sasson, Z., Rakowski, H., et al.: Apical hypertrophic cardiomyopathy: Clinical follow-up and diagnostic correlates. J. Am. Coll. Cardiol. 15:83, 1990.

177. Topol, E. J., Traill, T. A., and Fortuin, N. J.: Hypertensive hypertrophic cardiomyopathy of the elderly. N. Engl. J. Med. 312:277, 1985.

178. Shapiro, L. M.: Hypetrophic cardiomyopathy in the elderly. Br. Heart J. 63:265, 1990.

179. Karam, R., Lever, H., and Healy, B. P.: Hypertensive hypertrophic cardiomyopathy or hypertrophic cardiomyopathy with hypertension? A study of 78 patients. J. Am. Coll. Cardiol. 13:580, 1989.

180. Pearson, A. C., Gudipati, C. V., and Labovitz, A. J.: Systolic and diastolic flow abnormalities in elderly patients with hypertensive hypertrophic cardiomyopathy. J. Am. Coll. Cardiol. 12:989, 1988.

181. Lewis, J. F., and Maron, B. J.: Elderly patients with hypertrophic cardiomyopathy: A subset with distinctive left ventricular morphology and progressive clinical course late in life. J. Am. Coll. Cardiol. 13:36, 1989.

182. Lever, H. M., Karam, R. F., Currie, P. J., and Healy, B. P.: Hypertrophic cardiomyopathy in the elderly: Distinctions from the young based on cardiac shape. Circulation 79:580, 1989.

183. Rheuban, K. S., Blizzard, R. M., Parker, M. A., et al.: Hypertrophic cardiomyopathy in total lipodystrophy. J. Pediatr. 109:301, 1986.

184. Fitzpatrick, A. P., and Emanuel, R. W.: Familial neurofibromatosis and hypertrophic cardiomyopathy. Br. Heart J. 60:247, 1988.

185. Davies, M. J.: Hypertrophic cardiomyopathy: One disease or several? Br. Heart J. 63:263, 1990.

186. Symons, C., Fortune, F., Greenbaum, R. A., and Dandona, P.: Cardiac hypertrophy, hypertrophic cardiomyopathy, and hyperparathyroidism—an association. Br. Heart J. 54:539, 1985.

187. Eriksson, P., Backman, C., Eriksson, A., et al.: Differentiation of cardiac amyloidosis and hypertrophic cardiomyopathy: A comparison of familial amyloidosis with polyneuropathy and hypertrophic cardiomyopathy by electrocardiography and echocardiography. Acta Med. Scand. 221:39, 1987.

188. Davies, M. J.: The current status of myocardial disarray in hypertrophic cardiomyopathy (editorial). Br. Heart J. 51:361, 1984.

189. Factor, S. M., Butany, J., Sole, M. J., et al.: Pathologic fibrosis and matrix connective tissue in the subaortic myocardium of patients with hypertrophic cardiomyopathy. J. Am. Coll. Cardiol. 17:1343, 1991.

190. Tanaka, M., Fujiwara, H., Onodera, T., et al.: Quantitative analysis of narrowings of intramyocardial small arteries in normal hearts, hypertensive hearts, and hearts with hypertrophic cardiomyopathy. Circulation 75:1130, 1987.

191. Maron, B. J., Wolfson, J. K., Epstein, S. E., and Roberts, W. C.: Intramural ("small vessel") coronary artery disease in hypertrophic cardiomyopathy. J. Am. Coll. Cardiol. 8:545, 1986.

192. Pearce, P. C., Hawkey, C., Symons, C., and Olsen, E. G.: Role of calcium in the induction of cardiac hypertrophy and myofibrillar disarray. Experimental studies of a possible cause of hypertrophic cardiomyopathy. Br. Heart J. 54:420, 1985.

193. Gwathmey, J. K., Copelas, L., MacKinnon, R., et al.: Abnormal intracellular calcium handling in myocardium from patients with end-stage heart failure. Circ. Res. 60:70, 1987.

194. Wagner, J. A., Sax, F. L., Weisman, H. F., et al.: Calcium-antagonist receptors in the atrial tissue of patients with hypertrophic cardiomyopathy. N. Engl. J. Med. 320:755, 1989.

195. Koga, Y., Itaya, M., and Toshima, H.: Increased cardiovascular response to epinephrine in hypertrophic cardiomyopathy. Jpn. Heart J. 26:727, 1985.

196. Olsen, E. G.: An endocrine experimental model for myofibrillar disarray as found in hypertrophic cardiomyopathy. J. Mol. Cell. Cardiol. 17:35, 1985.

197. Lawson, J.W.R.: Hypertrophic cardiomyopathy: Current views on etiology, pathophysiology, and management. Am. J. Med. Sci. 294:191, 1987.

198. Brush, J. E., Jr., Eisenhofer, G., Garty, M., et al.: Cardiac norepinephrine kinetics in hypertrophic cardiomyopathy. Circulation 79:836, 1989.

199. Ogata, Y., Hiyamuta, K., Terasawa, M., et al.: Relationship of exercise- or pacing-induced ST segment depression and myocardial lactate metabolism in patients with hypertrophic cardiomyopathy. Jpn. Heart J. 27:145, 1986.

200. Hirzel, H. O., Tuchschmid, C. R., Schneider, J., et al.: Relationship between myosin isoenzyme composition, hemodynamics, and myocardial structure in various forms of human cardiac hypertrophy. Circ. Res. 57:729, 1985.

201. Jarcho, J. A., McKenna, W., Pare, J.A.P., et al.: Mapping a gene for familial hypertrophic cardiomyopathy to chromosome 14q1. N. Engl. J. Med. 321:1372, 1989.

202. Tanigawa, G., Jarcho, J. A., Kass, S., et al.: A molecular basis for familial hypertrophic cardiomyopathy: An α/β cardiac myosin heavy chain hybrid gene. Cell 62:991, 1990.

203. Geisterfer-Lowrance, A.A.T., Kass, S., Tanigawa, G., et al.: A molecular basis for familial hypertrophic cardiomyopathy: A β cardiac myosin heavy chain gene missense mutation. Cell 62:999, 1990.

204. Solomon, S. D., Geisterfer-Lowrance, A.A.T., Vosberg, H-P., et al.: A locus for familial hypertrophic cardiomyopathy is closely linked to the cardiac myosin heavy chain genes, CRI-L436, and CRI-L329 on chromosome 14 at q11-q12. Am. J. Hum. Genet. 47:389, 1990.

205. Solomon, S. D., Jarcho, J. A., McKenna, W., et al.: Familial hypertrophic cardiomyopathy is a genetically heterogeneous disease. J. Clin. Invest. 86:993, 1990.

206. Wigle, E. D.: Hypertrophic cardiomyopathy: A 1987 viewpoint. Circulation 75:311, 1987.

207. Come, P. C., Riley, M. F., Carl, L. V., and Lorell, B.: Doppler evidence that true left ventricular-to-aortic pressure gradients exist in hypertrophic cardiomyopathy. Am. Heart J. 116:1253, 1988.

208. Criley, J. M., and Siegel, R. J.: Has "obstruction" hindered our understanding of hypertrophic cardiomyopathy? Circulation 72:1148, 1985.

209. Pasipoularides, A.: Clinical assessment of ventricular ejection dynamics with and without outflow obstruction. J. Am. Coll. Cardiol. 15:859, 1990.

210. Maron, B. J., and Epstein, S. E.: Hypertrophic cardiomyopathy: Pathophysiology and therapy. In Braunwald, E. (ed.): Heart Disease: A Textbook of Cardiovascular Medicine. 3rd ed. Philadelphia, W. B. Saunders Company. Update No. 7, pp. 157–168, 1989.

211. Murgo, J. P.: The hemodynamic evaluation in hypertrophic cardiomyopathy: Systolic and diastolic dysfunction. Cardiovasc. Clin. 19:193, 1988.

212. Maron, B. J., and Epstein, S. E.: Clinical significance and therapeutic implications of the left ventricular outflow tract pressure gradient in hypertrophic cardiomyopathy. Am. J. Cardiol. 58:1093, 1986.

213. Bonow, R. O.: Left ventricular ejection dynamics and outflow obstruction in hypertrophic cardiomyopathy. J. Am. Coll. Cardiol. 13:1280, 1989.

214. Sasson, Z., Henderson, M., Wilansky, S., et al.: Causal relation between the pressure gradient and left ventricular ejection time in hypertrophic cardiomyopathy. J. Am. Coll. Cardiol. 13:1275, 1989.

215. Bryg, R. J., Pearson, A. C., Williams, G. A., and Labovitz, A. J.: Left ventricular systolic and diastolic flow abnormalities determined by Doppler echocardiography in obstructive hypertrophic cardiomyopathy. Am. J. Cardiol. 59:925, 1987.

216. Hoit, B. D., Penonen, E., Dalton, N., and Sahn, D. J.: Doppler color flow mapping studies of jet formation and spatial orientation in obstructive hypertrophic cardiomyopathy. Am. Heart J. 117:1119, 1989.

217. Stewart, W. J., Schiavone, W. A., Salcedo, E. E., et al.: Intraoperative Doppler echocardiography in hypertrophic cardiomyopathy: Correlation with the obstructive gradient. J. Am. Coll. Cardiol. 10:327, 1987.

218. Maron, B. J., Spirito, P., Green, K. J., et al.: Noninvasive assessment of left ventricular diastolic function by pulsed Doppler echocardiography in patients with hypertrophic cardiomyopathy. J. Am. Coll. Cardiol. 10:733, 1987.

219. Spirito, P., and Maron, B. J.: Relation between extent of left ventricular hypertrophy and diastolic filling abnormalities in hypertrophic cardiomyopathy. J. Am. Coll. Cardiol. 15:808, 1990.

220. Wigle, E. D.: Impaired left ventricular relaxation in hypertrophic cardiomyopathy: Relation to extent of hypertrophy. J. Am. Coll. Cardiol. 15:814, 1990.

221. Alvares, R. F., Shaver, J. A., Gamble, W. H., and Goodwin, J. F.: Isovolumic relaxation period in hypertrophic cardiomyopathy. J. Am. Coll. Cardiol. 3:71, 1984.

222. Betocchi S., Bonow, R. O., Bacharach, S. L., et al.: Isovolumic relaxation period in hypertrophic cardiomyopathy: Assessment by radionuclide angiography. J. Am. Coll. Cardiol. 7:74, 1986.

223. Brutsaert, D. L., Rademakers, F. E., and Sys, S. U.: Triple control of relaxation: Implications in cardiac disease. Circulation 69:190, 1984.

224. Cannon, R. O., Schenke, W. H., Maron, B. J., et al.: Differences in coronary flow and myocardial metabolism at rest and during pacing between patients with obstructive and patients with nonobstructive hypertrophic cardiomyopathy. J. Am. Coll. Cardiol. 10:53, 1987.

225. O'Gara, P. T., Bonow, R. O., Maron, B. J., et al.: Myocardial perfusion abnormalities in patients with hypertrophic cardiomyopathy: Assessment with thallium-201 emission computed tomography. Circulation 76:1214, 1987.

226. Ikeda, H., Shimamatsu, M., Yoshiga, O., et al.: Impaired myocardial perfusion in patients with hypertrophic cardiomyopathy: Assessment with digital subtraction coronary arteriography. Heart Vessels 4:170, 1988.

227. Fine, D. G., Clements, I. P., and Callahan, M. J.: Myocardial stunning in hypertrophic cardiomyopathy: Recovery predicted by single photon emission computed tomographic thallium-201 scintigraphy. J. Am. Coll. Cardiol. 13:1415, 1989.

228. Grover-McKay, M., Schwaiger, M., Krivokapich, J., et al.: Regional myocardial blood flow and metabolism at rest in mildly symptomatic patients with hypertrophic cardiomyopathy. J. Am. Coll. Cardiol. 13:317, 1989.

229. Spirito, P., Chiarella, F., Carratino, L., et al.: Clinical course and prognosis of hypertrophic cardiomyopathy in an outpatient population. N. Engl. J. Med. 320:749, 1989.

229a. Shaver, J. A., Salerni, R., Curtiss, E. I., and Follansbee, W. P.: Clinical

230. Brigden, W.: Hypertrophic cardiomyopathy. Br. Heart J. 58:299, 1987.

231. Frank, S., and Braunwald, E.: Idiopathic hypertrophic subaortic stenosis. Clinical analysis of 126 patients with emphasis on the natural history. Circulation 37:759, 1968.

232. Louie, E. K., and Maron, B. J.: Hypertrophic cardiomyopathy with extreme increase in left ventricular wall thickness: Functional and morphologic features and clinical significance. J. Am. Coll. Cardiol. 8:57, 1986.

233. Spirito, P., Maron, B. J., Bonow, R. O., and Epstein, S. E.: Severe functional limitation in patients with hypertrophic cardiomyopathy and only mild localized left ventricular hypertrophy. J. Am. Coll. Cardiol. 8:537, 1986.

234. McKenna, W. J., Steward, J. T., Nihoyannopoulos, P., et al.: Hypertrophic cardiomyopathy without hypertrophy: Two families with myocardial disarray in the absence of increased myocardial mass. Br. Heart J. 63:281, 1990.

235. Frenneaux, M. P., Porter, A., Caforio, A. L., et al.: Determinants of exercise capacity on hypertrophic cardiomyopathy. J. Am. Coll. Cardiol. 13:1521, 1989.

236. Nienaber, C. A., Hiller, S., Spielmann, R. P., et al.: Syncope in hypertrophic cardiomyopathy: Multivariate analysis of prognostic determinants. J. Am. Coll. Cardiol. 15:948, 1990.

237. Lembo, N. J., Dell-Italia, L. J., Crawford, M. H., and O'Rourke, R. A.: Bedside diagnosis of systolic murmurs. N. Engl. J. Med. 318:1572, 1988.

238. Shiota, T., Sakamoto, T., Takenaka, K., et al.: Aortic regurgitation associated with hypertrophic cardiomyopathy: A colour Doppler echocardiographic study. Br. Heart J. 62:171, 1989.

239. Sasson, Z., Prieur, T., Skrobik, Y., et al.: Aortic regurgitation: A common complication after surgery for hypertrophic obstructive cardiomyopathy. J. Am. Coll. Cardiol. 13:63, 1989.

240. Maron, B. J., Wolfson, J. K., Ciro, E., and Spirito, P.: Relation of electrocardiographic abnormalities and patterns of left ventricular hypertrophy identified by two-dimensional echocardiography in patients with hypertrophic cardiomyopathy. Am. J. Cardiol. 51:189, 1983.

241. Dollar, A. L., and Roberts, W. C.: Usefulness of total 12 lead QRS voltage compared with other criteria for determining left ventricular hypertrophy in hypertrophic cardiomyopathy: Analysis of 57 patients studied at necropsy. Am. J. Med. 87:377, 1989.

242. Alfonso, F., Annopoulos, P. N., Stewart, J., et al.: Clinical significance of giant negative T waves in hypertrophic cardiomyopathy. J. Am. Coll. Cardiol. 15:965, 1990.

243. Cosio, F. G., Moro, C., Alonso, M., et al.: The Q waves of hypertrophic cardiomyopathy: An electrophysiologic study. N. Engl. J. Med. 302:96, 1980.

244. Henderson, M. A., Ruddy, T. D., Makowski, H., and Wigle, E. D.: Left ventricular hypertrophy by ECG in hypertrophic cardiomyopathy. J. Am. Coll. Cardiol. 1:693, 1983.

245. McKenna, W. J., Borggrefe, M., England, D., et al.: The natural history of left ventricular hypertrophy in hypertrophic cardiomyopathy: An electrocardiographic study. Circulation 66:1233, 1982.

246. Khair, G. Z., and Bamrah, V. S.: Syncope in hypertrophic cardiomyopathy. I. Association with atrioventricular block. Am. Heart J. 110:1081, 1985.

247. McKenna, W. J., and Camm, A. J.: Sudden death in hypertrophic cardiomyopathy: Assessment of patients at high risk. Circulation 80:1489, 1989.

248. Nicod, P., Polikar, R., and Peterson, K. L.: Hypertrophic cardiomyopathy and sudden death. N. Engl. J. Med. 318:1255, 1988.

249. Lazzeroni, E., Domenicucci, S., Finardi, A., et al.: Severity of arrhythmias and extent of hypertrophy in hypertrophic cardiomyopathy. Am. Heart J. 118:734, 1989.

250. Spirito, P., Watson, R. M., and Maron, B. J.: Relation between extent of left ventricular hypertrophy and occurrence of ventricular tachycardia in hypertrophic cardiomyopathy. Am. J. Cardiol. 60:1137, 1987.

251. Robinson, K., Frenneaux, M. P., Stockins, B., et al.: Atrial fibrillation in hypertrophic cardiomyopathy: A longitudinal study. J. Am. Coll. Cardiol. 15:1279, 1990.

252. Greenspan, A. M.: Hypertrophic cardiomyopathy and atrial fibrillation: A change of perspective. J. Am. Coll. Cardiol. 15:1286, 1990.

253. Pelliccia, F., Cianfrocca, C., Cristofani, R., et al.: Electrocardiographic findings in patients with hypertrophic cardiomyopathy. J. Electrocardiol. 23:213, 1990.

254. Cripps, T. R., Counihan, P. J., Frenneaux, M. P., et al.: Signal-averaged electrocardiography in hypertrophic cardiomyopathy. J. Am. Coll. Cardiol. 15:956, 1990.

255. Bahl, V. K., Kaul, U., Dev, V., and Bhatia, M. L.: Electrophysiologic evaluation of patients with hypertrophic cardiomyopathy. Int. J. Cardiol. 25:87, 1989.

256. Fananapazir, L., Tracy, C. M., Leon, M. B., et al.: Electrophysiologic abnormalities in patients with hypertrophic cardiomyopathy: A consecutive analysis in 155 patients. Circulation 80:1259, 1989.

257. Kuck, K. H., Kunze, K. P., Schluter, M., et al.: Programmed electrical stimulation in hypertrophic cardiomyopathy. Eur. Heart J. 9:177, 1988.

258. Watson, R. M., Schwartz, J. L., Maron, B. J., et al.: Inducible polymorphic ventricular tachycardia and ventricular fibrillation in a subgroup of patients with hypertrophic cardiomyopathy at high risk for sudden death. J. Am. Coll. Cardiol. 10:761, 1987.

258a. Fananapazir, L., and Epstein, S. E.: Hemodynamic and electrophysiologic evaluation of patients with hypertrophic cardiomyopathy surviving cardiac arrest. Am. J. Cardiol. 67:280, 1991.

259. Lattanzi, F., Spirito, P., Picano, E., et al.: Quantitative assessment of ultra-

sonic myocardial reflectivity in hypertrophic cardiomyopathy. J. Am. Coll. Cardiol. 17:1085, 1991.

260. Madeira, H. C.: The mitral valve in hypertrophic cardiomyopathy—an echocardiographic approach. Postgrad. Med. J. 62:563, 1986.

261. Moro, E., tenCate, F. J., Leonard, J. J., et al.: Genesis of systolic anterior motion of the mitral valve in hypertrophic cardiomyopathy: An anatomical or dynamic event? Eur. Heart J. 8:1312, 1987.

262. Cape, E. G., Simon, D., Jimoh, A., et al.: Chordal geometry determines the shape and extent of systolic anterior mitral motion: In vitro studies. J. Am. Coll. Cardiol. 13:1438, 1989.

263. Miller, W., Walsh, R., and McCall, D.: Eosinophilic heart disease presenting with features suggesting hypertrophic obstructive cardiomopathy. Cathet. Cardiovasc. Diag. 13:185, 1987.

264. Maron, B. J., Epstein, S. E., Bonow, R. O., et al.: Obstructive hypertrophic cardiomyopathy associated with minimal left ventricular hypertrophy. Am. J. Cardiol. 53:377, 1984.

265. Gidding, S. S., Snider, R., Rocchini, A. P., et al.: Left ventricular diastolic filling in children with hypertrophic cardiomyopathy: Assessment with pulsed Doppler echocardiography. J. Am. Coll. Cardiol. 8:310, 1986.

266. Spirito, P., Maron, B. J., Chiarella, F., et al.: Diastolic abnormalities in patients with hypertrophic cardiomyopathy: Relation to magnitude of left ventricular hypertrophy. Circulation 72:310, 1985.

267. Gardin, J. M., Dabestani, A., Glasgow, G. A., et al.: Echocardiographic and Doppler flow observations in obstructed and nonobstructed hypertrophic cardiomyopathy. Am. J. Cardiol. 56:614, 1985.

268. Sasson, Z., Yock, P., Hatle, L. K., et al.: Doppler echocardiographic determination of the pressure gradient in hypertrophic cardiomyopathy. J. Am. Coll. Cardiol. 11:752, 1988.

269. Nishimura, R. A., Tajik, A. J., Reeder, G. S., and Seward, J. B.: Evaluation of hypertrophic cardiomyopathy by Doppler color flow imaging: Initial observations. Mayo Clin. Proc. 61:631, 1986.

270. von Dohlen, T. W., Prisant, L. M., and Frank, M. J.: Significance of positive or negative thallium-201 scintigraphy in hypertrophic cardiomyopathy. Am. J. Cardiol. 64:498, 1989.

271. Chikamori, T., Dickie, S., Poloniecki, J. D., et al.: Prognostic significance of radionuclide-assessed diastolic function in hypertrophic cardiomyopathy. Am. J. Cardiol. 65:478, 1990.

272. Cannon, R. O., Schenke, W. H., Bonow, R. O., et al.: Left ventricular pulsus alternans in patients with hypertrophic cardiomyopathy and severe obstruction to left ventricular outflow. Circulation 73:276, 1986.

273. Blazer, D., Kotler, M. N., Parry, W. R., et al.: Noninvasive evaluation of mid-left ventricular obstruction by two-dimensional and Doppler echocardiography and color flow Doppler echocardiography. Am. Heart J. 114:1162, 1987.

274. Kramer, D. S., French, W. J., and Criley, J. M.: The postextrasystolic murmur response to gradient in hypertrophic cardiomyopathy. Ann. Intern. Med. 104:772, 1986.

275. Sheikh, K. H., Pearce, F. B., and Kisslo, J.: Use of Doppler echocardiography and amyl nitrite inhalation to characterize left ventricular outflow obstruction in hypertrophic cardiomyopathy. Chest 97:389, 1990.

276. Pouleur, H., Rousseau, M. F., van Eyll, C., et al.: Force-velocity-length relations in hypertrophic cardiomyopathy: Evidence of normal or depressed myocardial contractility. Am. J. Cardiol. 52:813, 1983.

277. Kishimoto, C., Kadota, K., Sakurai, T., et al.: Improved evaluation of hypertrophic cardiomyopathy by biventriculography with axial projection. Am. Heart J. 110:77, 1985.

278. Cokkinos, D. V., Krajcer, Z., and Leachman, R. D.: Coronary artery disease in hypertrophic cardiomyopathy. Am. J. Cardiol. 55:1437, 1985.

279. Kimball, B. P., LiPreti, V., Bui, S., and Wigle, E. D.: Comparison of proximal left anterior descending and circumflex coronary artery dimensions in aortic valve stenosis and hypertrophic cardiomyopathy. Am. J. Cardiol. 65:767, 1990.

280. McKenna, W. J.: The natural history of hypertrophic cardiomyopathy. Cardiovasc. Clin. 19:135, 1988.

281. Aron, L. A., Hertzeanu, H. L., Fisman, E. Z., et al.: Prognosis of nonobstructive hypertrophic cardiomyopathy. Am. J. Cardiol. 67:215, 1991.

282. Shah, D. M., and Sunderji, S. G.: Hypertrophic cardiomyopathy and pregnancy: Report of a maternal mortality and review of literature. Obstet. Gynecol. Surv. 40:444, 1985.

283. Fighali, S., Krajcer, Z., Edelman, S., and Leachman, R. D.: Progression of hypertrophic cardiomyopathy into a hypokinetic left ventricle: Higher incidence in patients with midventricular obstruction. J. Am. Coll. Cardiol. 9:288, 1987.

284. Spirito, P., Maron, B. J., Bonow, R. O., and Epstein, S. E.: Occurrence and significance of progressive left ventricular wall thinning and relative cavity dilatation in patients with hypertrophic cardiomyopathy. Am. J. Cardiol. 60:123, 1987.

285. Domenicucci, S., Lazzeroni, E., Roelandt, J., et al.: Progression of hypertrophic cardiomyopathy. A cross sectional echocardiographic study. Br. Heart J. 53:405, 1985.

286. Maron, B. J., Spirito, P., Wesley, Y., and Arce, J.: Development and progression of left ventricular hypertrophy in children with hypertrophic cardiomyopathy. N. Engl. J. Med. 315:610, 1986.

287. Maron, B. J., and Kragel, A. H., and Roberts, W. C.: Sudden death in hypertrophic cardiomyopathy with normal left ventricular mass. Br. Heart J. 63:308, 1990.

288. Panza, J. A., and Maron, B. J.: Relation of electrocardiographic abnormalities to evolving left ventricular hypertrophy in hypertrophic cardiomyopathy during childhood. Am. J. Cardiol. 63:1258, 1989.

289. Ciro, E., Maron, B. J., Bonow, R. O., et al.: Relation between marked changes in left ventricular outflow tract gradient and disease progression in hypertrophic cardiomyopathy. Am. J. Cardiol. 53:1103, 1984.

290. Romeo, F., Pelliccia, F., Cristofani, R., et al.: Hypertrophic cardiomyopathy: Is a left ventricular outflow tract gradient a major prognostic determinant? Eur. Heart J. 11:233, 1990.

291. Romeo, F., Cianfrocca, C., Pelliccia, F., et al.: Long-term prognosis in children with hypertrophic cardiomyopathy: An analysis of 37 patients aged ≤ 14 years at diagnosis. Clin. Cardiol. 13:101, 1990.

292. Nienaber, C. A., Hiller, S., Spielmann, R. P., et al.: Syncope in hypertrophic cardiomyopathy: Multivariate analysis of prognostic determinants. J. Am. Coll. Cardiol. 15:948, 1990.

293. Brandenburg, R. O.: Syncope and sudden death in hypertrophic cardiomyopathy. J. Am. Coll. Cardiol. 15:962, 1990.

294. McKenna, W. J., Franklin, R. C., Nihoyannopoulos, P., et al.: Arrhythmia and prognosis in infants, children and adolescents with hypertrophic cardiomyopathy. J. Am. Coll. Cardiol. 11:147, 1988.

295. Maron, B. J., Epstein, S. E., and Roberts, W. C.: Causes of sudden death in competitive athletes. J. Am. Coll. Cardiol. 7:204, 1986.

296. Spirito, P., and Maron, B. J.: Relation between extent of left ventricular hypertrophy and occurrence of sudden cardiac death in hypertrophic cardiomyopathy. J. Am. Coll. Cardiol. 15:1521, 1990.

297. Udelson, J. E., Bonow, R. O., O'Gara, P. T., et al.: Verapamil prevents silent myocardial perfusion abnormalities during exercise in asymptomatic patients with hypertrophic cardiomyopathy. Circulation 79:1052, 1989.

298. Bonow, R. O., Maron, B. J., Leon, M. B., et al.: Medical and surgical therapy of hypertrophic cardiomyopathy. Cardiovasc. Clin. 19:221, 1988.

299. Udelson, J. E., Cannon, R. O., Bacharach, S. L., et al.: Beta-adrenergic stimulation with isoproterenol enhances left ventricular diastolic performance in hypertrophic cardiomyopathy despite potentiation of myocardial ischemia. Comparison to rapid atrial pacing. Circulation 79:371, 1989.

300. Chatterjee, K.: Calcium antagonist agents in hypertrophic cardiomyopathy. Am. J. Cardiol. 59:146B, 1987.

301. Hopf, R., and Kaltenbach, M.: Ten-year results and survival of patients with hypertrophic cardiomyopathy treated with calcium antagonists. Z. Kardiol. 76:137, 1987.

302. Bonow, R. O., Dilsizian, V., Rosing, D. R., et al.: Verapamil-induced improvement in left ventricular diastolic filling and increased exercise tolerance in patients with hypertrophic cardiomyopathy: Short- and long-term effects. Circulation 72:853, 1985.

303. Shaffer, E. M., Rocchini, A. P., Spicer, R. L., et al.: Effects of verapamil on left ventricular diastolic filling in children with hypertrophic cardiomyopathy. Am. J. Cardiol. 61:413, 1988.

304. Bonow, R. O., Vitale, D. F., Maron, B. J., et al.: Regional left ventricular asynchrony and impaired global left ventricular filling in hypertrophic cardiomyopathy: Effect of verapamil. J. Am. Coll. Cardiol. 9:1108, 1987.

305. Bonow, R. O.: Effects of calcium-channel blocking agents on left ventricular diastolic function in hypertrophic cardiomyopathy and in coronary artery disease. Am. J. Cardiol. 55:172B, 1985.

306. Kaltenbach, M., and Hopf, R.: Treatment of hypertrophic cardiomyopathy: Relation to pathological mechanisms. J. Mol. Cell. Cardiol. 2:59, 1985.

307. Yamakado, T., Okano, H., Higashiyama, S., et al.: Effects of nifedipine on left ventricular diastolic function in patients with asymptomatic or minimally symptomatic hypertrophic cardiomyopathy. Circulation 81:593, 1990.

308. Richardson, P. J.: Calcium antagonists in cardiomyopathy. Br. J. Clin. Pract. 42:4, 1988.

309. Betocchi, S., Bonow, R. O., Cannon, R. O. III, et al.: Relation between serum nifedipine concentration and hemodynamic effects in nonobstructive hypertrophic cardiomyopathy. Am. J. Cardiol. 61:830, 1988.

310. Iwase, M., Sobotata, I., Takagi, S., et al.: Effects of diltiazem on left ventricular diastolic behavior in patients with hypertrophic cardiomyopathy: Evaluation with exercise pulsed Doppler echocardiography. J. Am. Coll. Cardiol. 9:1099, 1987.

311. Rosing, D. R., Idanpaan-Heikkila, U., Maron, B. J., et al.: Use of calcium-channel blocking drugs in hypertrophic cardiomyopathy. Am. J. Cardiol. 55:185B, 1985.

312. Sherrid, M., Delia, E., and Dwyer, E.: Oral disopyramide therapy for obstructive hypertrophic cardiomyopathy. Am. J. Cardiol. 62:1085, 1988.

313. Cokkinos, D. V., Salpeas, D., Ioannou, N. E., and Christoulas, S.: Combination of disopyramide and propranolol in hypertrophic cardiomyopathy. Can. J. Cardiol. 5:33, 1989.

314. Pollick, C., Kimball, B., Henderson, M., and Wigle, E. D.: Disopyramide in hypertrophic cardiomyopathy. I. Hemodynamic assessment after intravenous administration. Am. J. Cardiol. 62:1248, 1988.

315. Duncan, W. J., Tyrrell, M. J., and Bharadwaj, B. B.: Disopyramide as a negative inotrope in obstructive cardiomyopathy in children. Can. J. Cardiol. 7:81, 1991.

316. Sugrue, D. D., Dickie, S., Myers, M. J., et al.: Effects of amiodarone on left ventricular ejection and filling in hypertrophic cardiomyopathy as assessed by radionuclide angiography. Am. J. Cardiol. 54:1054, 1984.

317. McKenna, W. J., Oakley, C. M., Krikler, D. M., and Goodwin J. F.: Improved survival with amiodarone in patients with hypertrophic cardiomyopathy and ventricular tachycardia. Br. Heart J. 53:412, 1985.

318. Counihan, P. J., and McKenna, W. J.: Low-dose amiodarone for the treatment of arrhythmias in hypertrophic cardiomyopathy. J. Clin. Pharmacol. 29:436, 1989.

318a. Fananapazir, L., Leon, M. B., Bonow, R. O., et al.: Sudden death during empiric amiodarone therapy in symptomatic hypertrophic cardiomyopathy. Am. J. Cardiol. 67:169, 1991.

318b. Fananapazir, L., and Epstein, S. E.: Value of electrophysiologic studies in hypertrophic cardiomyopathy treated with amiodarone. Am. J. Cardiol. 67:175, 1991.

319. Cecchi F., Maron, B. J., and Epstein, S. E.: Long-term outcome of patients with hypertrophic cardiomyopathy successfully resuscitated after cardiac arrest. J. Am. Coll. Cardiol. 13:1283, 1989.

320. Maron, B. J., Gaffney, F. A., Jeresaty, R. M., et al.: Task force III: Hypertrophic cardiomyopathy, other myopericardial diseases and mitral valve prolapse. J. Am. Coll. Cardiol. 6:1215, 1985.

321. McIntosh, C. L., and Maron, B. J.: Current operative treatment of obstructive hypertrophic cardiomyopathy. Circulation 78:487, 1988.

321a. Seiler, C., Hess, O. M., Schoenbeck, M., et al.: Long-term follow-up of medical versus surgical therapy for hypertrophic cardiomyopathy: A retrospective study. J. Am. Coll. Cardiol. 17:634, 1991.

321b. Chahine, R. A.: Surgical versus medical therapy of hypertrophic cardiomyopathy: Is the perspective changing? J. Am. Coll. Cardiol. 17:643, 1991.

322. Surgical treatment of hypertrophic obstructive cardiomyopathy. Lancet 1:358, 1989.

323. Mohr, R., Schaff, H. V., Danielson, G. K., et al.: The outcome of surgical treatment of hypertrophic obstructive cardiomyopathy: Experience over 15 years. J. Thorac. Cardiovasc. Surg. 97:666, 1989.

324. Cooper, M. M., Tucker, E., McIntosh, C. L., et al.: Effect of left ventricular septal myectomy on concurrent mitral regurgitation. Ann. Thorac. Surg. 48:251, 1989.

325. Cannon, R. O., McIntosh, C. L., Schenke, W. H., et al.: Effect of surgical reduction of left ventricular outflow obstruction on hemodynamics, coronary flow, and myocardial metabolism in hypertrophic cardiomyopathy. Circulation 79:766, 1989.

326. Mohr, R., Schaff, H. V., Puga, F. J., and Danielson, G. K.: Results of operation for hypertrophic obstructive cardiomyopathy in children and adults less than 40 years of age. Circulation 80:191, 1989.

327. Williams, W. G., Wigle, E. D., Rakowski, H., et al.: Results of surgery for hypertrophic obstructive cardiomyopathy. Circulation 76:V104, 1987.

328. Siegman, I. L., Maron, B. J., Permut, L. C., et al.: Results of operation for coexistent obstructive hypertrophic cardiomyopathy and coronary artery disease. J. Am. Coll. Cardiol. 13:1527, 1989.

329. Leachman, R. D., Krajcer, Z., Azic, T., and Cooley, D. A.: Mitral valve replacement in hypertrophic cardiomyopathy: Ten-year follow-up in 54 patients. Am. J. Cardiol. 60:1416, 1987.

330. Walker, W. S., Reid, K. G., Cameron, E.W.J., et al.: Comparison of ventricular septal surgery and mitral valve replacement for hypertrophic obstructive cardiomyopathy. Ann. Thorac. Surg. 48:528, 1989.

331. Krajcer, Z., Leachman, R. D., Cooley, D. A., et al.: Mitral valve replacement and septal myomectomy in hypertrophic cardiomyopathy: Ten-year follow-up in 80 patients. Circulation 78:35, 1988.

332. McIntosh, C. L., Greenberg, G. J., Maron, B. J., et al.: Clinical and hemodynamic results after mitral valve replacement in patients with obstructive hypertrophic cardiomyopathy. Ann. Thorac. Surg. 47:236, 1989.

333. Warren, S. E., Cohn, L. H., Schoen, F. J., et al.: Advanced diastolic heart failure in familial hypertrophic cardiomyopathy managed with cardiac transplantation. J. Appl. Cardiol. 3:415, 1988.

RESTRICTIVE AND INFILTRATIVE CARDIOMYOPATHY

334. Child, J. S., and Perloff, J. K.: The restrictive cardiomyopathies. Cardiol. Clin. 6:289, 1988.

335. Schoenfeld, M. H., Supple, E. W., Dec, G. W., et al.: Restrictive cardiomyopathy versus constrictive pericarditis: Role of endomyocardial biopsy in avoiding unnecessary thoracotomy. Circulation 75:1012, 1987.

336. Hirota, Y. Shimizu, G., Kita, Y., et al.: Spectrum of restrictive cardiomyopathy: Report of the national survey in Japan. Am. Heart J. 120:188, 1990.

337. Restrictive cardiomyopathy or constrictive pericarditis? (editorial) Lancet 15:372, 1987.

338. Wilmshurst, P. T., and Katritsis, D.: Restrictive cardiomyopathy (editorial). Br. Heart J. 63:323, 1990.

339. Webb-Peploe, M. M.: Obliterative and restrictive cardiomyopathies. Eur. Heart J. 9:159, 1988.

340. Hosenpud, J. D.: Restrictive cardiomyopathy. In Zipes, D. P., and Rowlands, D. J. (eds.): Progress in Cardiology. Philadelphia, Lea and Febiger, 1989, p. 91.

341. Aroney, C., Bett, N., and Radford, D.: Familial restrictive cardiomyopathy. Aust. N.Z. J. Med. 18:877, 1988.

342. Fitzpatrick, A. P., Shapiro, L. M., Rickards, A. F., and Poole-Wilson, P. A.: Familial restrictive cardiomyopathy with atrioventricular block and skeletal myopathy. Br. Heart J. 63:114, 1990.

343. Shabetai, R.: Pathophysiology and differential diagnosis of restrictive cardiomyopathy. Cardiovasc. Clin. 19:123, 1988.

344. Sechtem, U., Tscholakoff, D., and Higgins, C. B.: MRI of the abnormal pericardium. Am. J. Roentgenol. 147:245, 1986.

345. Sechtem, U., Higgins, C. B., Sommerhoff, B. A., et al.: Magnetic resonance imaging of restrictive cardiomyopathy. Am. J. Cardiol. 59:480, 1987.

346. Morgan, J. M., Raposo, L., Clague, J. C., et al.: Restrictive cardiomyopathy and constrictive pericarditis: Non-invasive distinction by digitised M mode echocardiography. Br. Heart J. 61:29, 1989.

347. Appleton, C. P., Hatle, L. K., and Popp, R. L.: Demonstration of restrictive ventricular physiology by Doppler echocardiography. J. Am. Coll. Cardiol. 11:757, 1988.

348. Hatle, L. K., Appleton, C. P., and Popp, R. L.: Differentiation of constrictive pericarditis and restrictive cardiomyopathy by Doppler echocardiography. Circulation 79:357, 1989.

349. Schiavone, W. A., Calafiore, P. A., and Salcedo, E. E.: Transesophageal Doppler echocardiographic demonstration of pulmonary venous flow velocity in restrictive cardiomyopathy and constrictive pericarditis. Am. J. Cardiol. 63:1286, 1989.

350. Gerson, M. C., Colthar, M. S., and Fowler, N. O.: Differentiation of constrictive pericarditis and restrictive cardiomyopathy by radionuclide ventriculography. Am. Heart J. 118:114, 1989.

351. Aroney, C. N., Ruddy, T. D., Dighero, H., et al.: Differentiation of restrictive cardiomyopathy from pericardial constriction: Assessment of diastolic function by radionuclide angiograhy. J. Am. Coll. Cardiol. 13:1007, 1989.

352. Gertz, M. A., and Kyle, R. A.: Primary systemic amyloidosis — a diagnostic primer. Mayo Clin. Proc. 64:1505, 1989.

353. Falk, R. H.: Cardiac amyloidosis. In Zipes, D. P., and Rowlands, D. J. (eds.): Progress in Cardiology. Philadelphia, Lea and Febiger, 1989, p. 143.

354. Smith, T. J., Kyle, R. A., and Lie, J. T.: Clinical significance of histopathologic patterns of cardiac amyloidosis. Mayo Clin. Proc. 59:547, 1984.

355. Olson, L. J., Gertz, M. A., Edwards, W. D., et al.: Senile cardiac amyloidosis with myocardial dysfunction: Diagnosis by endomyocardial biopsy and immunohistochemistry. N. Engl. J. Med. 317:738, 1987.

356. de Freitas, A. F.: The heart in Portuguese amyloidosis. Postgrad. Med. J. 62:601, 1986.

357. Klein, A. L., Oh, J. K., Miller, F. A., et al.: Two-dimensional and Doppler echocardiographic assessment of infiltrative cardiomyopathy. J. Am. Soc. Echocardiogr. 1:48, 1988.

358. Falk, R. H., Plehn, J. F., Deering, T., et al.: Sensitivity and specificity of the echocardiographic features of cardiac amyloidosis. Am. J. Cardiol. 59:418, 1987.

359. Kinoshita, O., Hongo, M., Yamada, H., et al.: Impaired left ventricular diastolic filling in patients with familial amyloid polyneuropathy: A pulsed Doppler echocardiographic study. Br. Heart J. 61:198, 1989.

360. Hongo, M., and Ikeda, S. I.: Echocardiographic assessment of the evolution of amyloid heart disease: A study with familial amyloid polyneuropathy. Circulation 73:249, 1986.

361. Eriksson, P., Eriksson, A., Backman, C., et al.: Highly refractile myocardial echoes in familial amyloidosis with polyneuropathy. Acta Med. Scand. 217:27, 1985.

362. Pinamonti, B., Picano, E., Ferdeghini, E. M., et al.: Quantitative texture analysis in two-dimensional echocardiography: Application to the diagnosis of myocardial amyloidosis. J. Am. Coll. Cardiol. 14:666, 1989.

363. Presti, C. F., Waler, B. F., and Armstrong, W. F.: Cardiac amyloidosis mimicking the echocardiographic appearance of obstructive hypertrophic myopathy. Chest 93:881, 1988.

364. Cueto-Garcia, L., Reeder, G. S., Kyle, R. H., et al.: Echocardiographic findings in systemic amyloidosis: Spectrum of cardiac involvement and relation to survival. J. Am. Coll. Cardiol. 6:737, 1985.

365. Klein, A. L., Hatle, L. K., Burstow, D. J., et al.: Doppler characterization of left ventricular diastolic function in cardiac amyloidosis. J. Am. Coll. Cardiol. 13:1017, 1989.

366. Hongo, M., Fujii, T., Hirayama, J., et al.: Radionuclide angiographic assessment of left ventricular diastolic filling in amyloid heart disease: A study of patients with familial amyloid polyneuropathy. J. Am. Coll. Cardiol. 13:48, 1989.

367. Plehn, J. F., and Friedman, B. J.: Diastolic dysfunction in amyloid heart disease: Restrictive cardiomyopathy or not? J. Am. Coll. Cardiol. 13:54, 1989.

367a. Klein, A. L., Hatle, L. K., Talierco, C. P., et al.: Prognostic significance of Doppler measures of diastolic function in cardiac amyloidosis: A Doppler echocardliography study. Circulation 83:808, 1991.

368. Hongo, M., Hirayama, J., Fujii, T., et al.: Early identification of amyloid heart disease by technetium-99m-pyrophosphate scintigraphy: A study with familial amyloid polyneuropathy. Am. Heart J. 113:654, 1987.

369. Gertz, M. A., Skinner, M., Connors, L. H., et al.: Selective binding of nifedipine to amyloid fibrils. Am. J. Cardiol. 55:1646, 1985.

370. Gertz, M. A., Falk, R. H., Skinner, M., et al.: Worsening of congestive heart failure in amyloid heart disease treated by calcium channel-blocking agents. Am. J. Cardiol. 55:1645, 1985.

371. Hozumi, I., Nishizawa, M., Ariga, T., and Miyatake, T.: Biochemical and clinical analysis of accumulated glycolipids in symptomatic heterozygotes of angiokeratoma corporis diffusum (Fabry's disease) in comparison with hemizygotes. J. Lipid Res. 31:335, 1990.

372. Sakurabab, H., Yanagawa, Y., Igarashi, T., et al.: Cardiovascular manifestations in Fabry's disease. Clin. Genetics 29:276, 1986.

373. Goldman, M. E., Cantor, R., Schwartz, M. F., et al.: Echocardiographic abnormalities and disease severity in Fabry's disease. J. Am. Coll. Cardiol. 7:1157, 1986.

374. Matsui, S., Murakami, E., Takekoshi, N., et al.: Myocardial tissue characterization by magnetic resonance imaging in Fabry's disease. Am. Heart J. 117:472, 1989.

375. Tanaka, H., Adachi, K., Yamashita, Y., et al.: Four cases of Fabry's disease mimicking hypertrophic cardiomyopathy. J. Cardiol. 18:705, 1988.

376. Yokoyama, A., Yamazoe, M., and Shibata, A.: A case of heterozygous Fabry's disease with a short PR interval and giant negative T waves. Br. Heart J. 57:296, 1987.

377. Iwase, M., Yamauchi, K., Maeda, M., et al.: Echocardiographic findings in a case of Fabry's disease with aortic regurgitation and complete AV block, and in his family members. J. Cardiol. 18:589, 1988.

378. Kramer, W., Thormann, J., Mueller, K., and Frenzel, H.: Progressive cardiac involvement by Fabry's disease despite successful renal allotransplantation. Int. J. Cardiol. 7:72, 1985.

379. Casta, A., Hayden, K., and Wolf, W. J.: Calcification of the ascending aorta

and aortic and mitral valves in Gaucher's disease. Am. J. Cardiol. 54:1390, 1984.

380. Platzker, Y., Pisman, E. Z., Pines, A., and Kellermann, J.: Unusual echocardiographic pattern in Gaucher's disease. Cardiology 72:144, 1985.

381. Wilson, E. R., Barton, N. W., and Barranger, J. H.: Vascular involvement in type 3 neuronopathic Gaucher's disease. Arch. Pathol. Lab. Med. 109:82, 1985.

382. Laks, Y., and Passwell, J.: The varied clinical and laboratory manifestations of type II Gaucher's disease. Acta Paediatr. Scand. 76:378, 1987.

383. Barosi, G., Arbustini, E., Gavazzi, A., et al.: Myocardial iron grading by endomyocardial biopsy. A clinico-pathologic study on iron overloaded patients. Eur. J. Haematol. 42:382, 1989.

384. Rahko, P. S., Salerni, R., and Uretsky, B. F.: Successful reversal by chelation therapy of congestive cardiomyopathy due to iron overload. J. Am. Coll. Cardiol. 8:436, 1986.

385. Olson, L. J., Edwards, W. D., McCall, J. T., et al.: Cardiac iron deposition in idiopathic hemochromatosis: Histologic and analytic assessment of 14 hearts from autopsy. J. Am. Coll. Cardiol. 10:1239, 1987.

386. Olson, L. J., Edwards, W. D., Holmes, D. R., Jr., et al.: Endomyocardial biopsy in hemochromatosis: Clinicopathologic correlates in six cases. J. Am. Coll. Cardiol. 13:116, 1989.

387. Dabestani, A., Child, J. S., Henze, E., et al.: Primary hemochromatosis: Anatomic and physiologic characteristics of the cardiac ventricles and their response to phlebotomy. Am. J. Cardiol. 54:153, 1984.

388. Furth, P. A., Futterweit, W., and Gorlin, R.: Refractory biventricular heart failure in secondary hemochromatosis. Am. J. Med. Sci. 290:209, 1985.

389. Powell, L. W., and Isselbacher, K. J.: Hemochromatosis. In Wilson, J. D., et al. (eds.): Harrison's Principles of Internal Medicine. New York, McGraw-Hill, 1990, p. 1825.

390. Strohmeyer, G., Niederau, C., and Stremmel, W.: Survival and causes of death in hemochromatosis. Observations in 163 patients. Ann. N.Y. Acad. Sci. 526:245, 1988

391. Lewin, R. F., Mor, R., Spitzer, S., et al.: Echocardiographic evaluation of patients with systemic sarcoidosis. Am. Heart J. 110:116, 1985.

392. Tellier, P., Paycha, F., Antony, I., et al.: Reversibility by dipyridamole of thallium-201 myocardial scan defects in patients with sarcoidosis. Am. J. Med. 85:189, 1988.

393. Burstow, D. J., Tajik, A. J., Bailey, K. R., et al.: Two-dimensional echocardiographic findings in systemic sarcoidosis. Am. J. Cardiol. 63:478, 1989.

394. Stewart, R. E., Graham, D. M., Godfrey, G. W., et al.: Rapidly progressive heart failure resulting from cardiac sarcoidosis. Am. Heart J. 115:1324, 1988.

395. Temple-Camp, C. R.: Sarcoid myocarditis: A report of three cases. N.Z. Med. J. 102:501, 1989.

396. Bajaj, A. K., Kopelman, H. A., and Echt, D. S.: Cardiac sarcoidosis with sudden death: Treatment with the automatic implantable cardioverter defibrillator. Am. Heart J. 116:557, 1988.

397. Freiman, D. G.: The pathology of sarcoidosis. Semin. Roentgenol. 20:327, 1985.

398. Fleming, H. H.: Sarcoid heart disease (editorial). Br. Med. J. 292:1095, 1986.

399. Lemery, R., McGoon, M. D., and Edwards, W. D.: Cardiac sarcoidosis: A potentially treatable form of myocarditis. Mayo Clin. Proc. 60:549, 1985.

400. Valantine, H., McKenna, W. J., Nihoyannopoulos, P., et al.: Sarcoidosis: A pattern of clinical and morphological presentation. Br. Heart J. 57:256, 1987.

401. Diderholm, E., Eklund, A., Orinius, E., and Widstrom, O.: Exudative pericarditis in sarcoidosis. A case report and echocardiographic study. Sarcoidosis 6:60, 1989.

402. Riedy, K., Fisher, M. R., Belic, N., and Koenigsberg, D. I.: MR imaging of myocardial sarcoidosis. Am. J. Roentgen. 151:915, 1988.

403. Ratner, S. J., Fenoglio, J. J., Jr., and Ursell, P. C.: Utility of endomyocardial biopsy in the diagnosis of cardiac sarcoidosis. Chest 90:528, 1986.

404. Ishikawa, T., Kondoh, H., Nakagawa, S., et al.: Steroid therapy in cardiac sarcoidosis: Increased left ventricular contractility concomitant with electrocardiographic improvement after prednisolone. Chest 85:445, 1984.

405. Moodie, D. S., Baum, J. E., Gill, C. C., and Ratliff, N. B.: Endomyocardial fibrosis: Diagnosis and surgical treatment of two cases occurring in the United States. Cleveland Clin. Q. 53:159, 1986.

406. Valiathan, M. S., Balakrishnan, K. G., and Kartha, C. C.: A profile of endomyocardial fibrosis. Indian J. Pediatr. 54:229, 1987.

407. Valiathan, S. M., and Kartha, C. C.: Endomyocardial fibrosis — the possible connexion with myocardial levels of magnesium and cerium. Int. J. Cardiol. 28:1, 1990.

408. Valiathan, M. S., Kartha, C. C., Eapen, J. T., et al.: A geochemical basis for endomyocardial fibrosis. Cardiovasc. Res. 23:647, 1989.

409. Frustaci, A., Abdulla, A. K., Possati, G., and Manzoli, U.: Persisting hypereosinophilia and myocardial activity in the fibrotic stage of endomyocardial disease. Chest 96:674, 1989.

410. Spry, C. J. F.: The pathogenesis of endomyocardial fibrosis: The role of the eosinophil. Springer Semin. Immunopathol. 11:471, 1989.

411. Gupta, P. N., Valiathan, M. S., Balakrishnan, K. G., et al.: Clinical course of endomyocardial fibrosis. Br. Heart. J. 62:450, 1989.

412. Olsen, E.G.J., and Spry, C.J.F.: Relation between eosinophilia and endomyocardial disease. Prog. Cardiovasc. Dis. 27:241, 1985.

413. Shah, A. M., Brutsaert, D. L., Meulemans, A. L., et al.: Eosinophils from hypereosinophilic patients damage endocardium of isolated feline heart muscle preparations. Circulation 81:1081, 1990.

414. Sasano, H., Virmani, R., Patterson, R. H., et al.: Eosinophilic products lead to myocardial damage. Hum. Pathol. 20:850, 1989.

415. Tai, P. C., Ackerman, S. J., Spry, C. J., et al.: Deposits of eosinophil granule proteins in cardiac tissues of patients with eosinophilic endomyocardial disease. Lancet 21:643, 1987.

416. Spry, C. J., Weetman, A. P., Olsson, I., et al.: The pathogenesis of eosinophilic endomyocardial disease in patients with carcinomas of the lung. Heart Vessels 1:162, 1985.

417. Arnold, M., McGuire, L., and Lee, J. C.: Loeffler's fibroplastic endocarditis. Pathology 20:79, 1988.

418. Hendren, W. G., Jones, E. L., and Smith, M. D.: Aortic and mitral valve replacement in idiopathic hypereosinophilic syndrome. Ann. Thorac. Surg. 46:570, 1988.

419. Blake, D. P., Palmer, I. E., and Olinger, G. N.: Mitral valve replacement in idiopathic hypereosinophilic syndrome. J. Thorac. Cardiovasc. Surg. 89:630, 1985.

420. Olsen, E.G.J.: Pathology of nonhypertrophic cardiomyopathies. In Zipes, D. P., and Rowlands, D. J. (eds.): Progress in Cardiology. Philadelphia, Lea and Febiger, 1989, p. 23.

421. Metras, D., Coulibaly, A. Q., and Quattara, K.: Recent trends in the surgical treatment of endomyocardial fibrosis. J. Cardiovasc. Surg. 28:607, 1987.

422. Lengyel, M., Arvay, A., and Palik, I.: Massive endocardial calcification associated with endomyocardial fibrosis. Am. J. Cardiol. 56:815, 1985.

423. Martinez, E. E., Venturi, M., Buffolo, E., et al.: Operative results in endomyocardial fibrosis. Am. J. Cardiol. 63:627, 1989.

424. Siegel, R. J., and Fishbein, M. C.: Detection of endocardial calcium in endomyocardial fibrosis by computed tomography. Am. J. Cardiol. 60:420, 1987.

425. Pawzy, M. E., Ziady, G., Halim, M., et al.: Endomyocardial fibrosis: Report of eight cases. J. Am. Coll. Cardiol. 5:983, 1985.

426. Valiathan, M. S., Balakrishnan, K. G., Sankarkumar, R., and Kartha, C. C.: Surgical treatment of endomyocardial fibrosis. Ann. Thorac. Surg. 43:68, 1987.

427. Barretto, A. C., da Luz, P. L., de Oliveira, S. A., et al.: Determinants of survival in endomyocardial fibrosis. Circulation 80(Suppl. I): 177, 1989.

428. Mady, C., Pereira Barretto, A. C., de Oliveira, S. A., et al.: Effectiveness of operative and nonoperative therapy in endomyocardial fibrosis. Am. J. Cardiol. 15:1281, 1989.

429. Ross, E. M., and Roberts, W. C.: The carcinoid syndrome: Comparison of 21 necropsy subjects with carcinoid heart disease to 15 necropsy subjects without carcinoid heart disease. Am. J. Med. 79:339, 1985.

430. Lundin, L., Norheim, I., Landelius, J., et al.: Carcinoid heart disease: Relationship of circulating vasoactive substances to ultrasound-detectable cardiac abnormalities. Circulation 77:264, 1988.

431. Lundin, L., Landelius, J., Andren, B., and Oberg, K.: Transesophageal echocardiography improves the value of cardiac ultrasound in patients with carcinoid heart disease. Br. Heart J. 64:190, 1990.

432. Artaza, A., Beiner, J. H., Gonzalez, M., et al.: Carcinoid heart disease: Report of a case secondary to a pure carcinoid tumor of the ovary. Eur. Heart J. 6:800, 1985.

433. Millward, M. J., Blake, M. P., Byrne, M. J., et al.: Left heart involvement with cardiac shunt complicating carcinoid heart disease. Aust. N.Z. J. Med. 19:716, 1989.

434. Lundin, L., Funa, K., Hansson, H. E., et al.: Histochemical and immunohistochemical morphology of carcinoid heart disease. Pathol. Res. Pract. 187:73, 1991.

435. Tornebrandt, K., Eskilsson, J., and Nobin, H.: Heart involvement in metastatic carcinoid disease. Clin. Cardiol. 9:13, 1986.

436. Lundin, L., Hansson, H. E., Landelius, J., and Oberg, K.: Surgical treatment of carcinoid heart disease. J. Thorac. Cardiovasc. Surg, 100:552, 1990.

MYOCARDITIS

437. Weinstein, C., and Fenoglio, J. J.: Myocarditis. Hum. Pathol. 18:613, 1987.

438. Peters, N. S., and Poole-Wilson, P. A.: Myocarditis — continuing clinical and pathologic confusion. Am. Heart J. 121:942, 1991.

439. Reyes, M. P., and Lerner, A. M.: Coxsackievirus myocarditis — with special reference to acute and chronic effects. Prog. Cardiovasc. Dis. 27:373, 1985.

440. Marboe, C. C., and Fenoglio, J. J.: Pathology and natural history of human myocarditis. Pathol. Immunopathol. Res. 7:226, 1988.

441. Gauntt, C. J., Godeny, E. K., and Lutton, C. W.: Host factors regulating viral clearance. Pathol. Immunopathol. Res. 7:251, 1988.

442. Leslie, K. O., Schwarz, J., Simpson, K., and Huber, S. A.: Progressive interstitial collagen deposition in Coxsackievirus B3 – induced murine myocarditis. Am. J. Pathol. 136:683, 1990.

443. Herskowitz, A, Ahmed-Ansari, A., Neuman, D. A., et al.: Induction of major histocompatibility complex antigens within the myocardium of patients with active myocarditis: A nonhistologic marker of myocarditis. J. Am. Coll. Cardiol. 15:624, 1990.

444. Wenger, N. K.: Myocarditis. In Zipes, D. P., and Rowlands, D. J. (eds.): Progress in Cardiology. Philadelphia, Lea and Febiger, 1989, p. 43.

445. Olsen, E. G. J.: Interpretation of endomyocardial biopsies: Infectious agents. Am. J. Cardiovasc. Pathol. 2:329, 1989.

446. Herskowitz, A., Wolfgram, L. J., Rose, N. R., and Beisel, K. W.: Coxsackievirus B₃ murine myocarditis: A pathologic spectrum of myocarditis in genetically defined inbred strains. J. Am. Coll. Cardiol. 9:1311, 1987.

447. Abelmann, W. H.: Myocarditis and dilated cardiomyopathy (editorial). West. J. Med. 150: 458, 1989.

448. Hosenpud, J. D., McAnulty, J. H., and Niles, N. R.: Unexpected myocardial disease in patients with life threatening arrhythmias. Br. Heart J. 56:55, 1986.

449. Claydon, S. M.: Myocarditis as an incidental finding in young men dying from unnatural causes. Med. Sci. Law 29:55, 1989.

450. Phillips, M., Robinowitz, M., Higgins, J. R., et al.: Sudden cardiac death in Air Force recruits. A 20-year review. JAMA 21:2696, 1986.

451. Karjalainen, J., and Heikkila, J.: "Acute pericarditis": Myocardial enzyme release as evidence for myocarditis. Am. Heart J. 111:546, 1986.

452. Miklozek, C. L., Crumpacker, C. S., Royal, H. D., et al.: Myocarditis presenting as acute myocardial infarction. Am. Heart J. 115:768, 1988.

453. Ferguson, D. W., Farwell, A. P., Bradley, W. A., and Rollings, R. C.: Coronary artery vasospasm complicating acute myocarditis: A rare association. West J. Med. 148:664, 1988.

454. Pinamonti, B., Alberti, E., Cigalotto, A., et al.: Echocardiographic findings in myocarditis. Am. J. Cardiol. 62:285, 1988.

455. Arvan, S., and Manalo, E.: Sudden increase in left ventricular mass secondary to acute myocarditis. Am. Heart J. 116:200, 1988.

456. Khaw, B. A., and Haber, E.: Imaging necrotic myocardium: Detection with 99mTc-pyrophosphate and radiolabeled antimyosin. Cardiol. Clin. 7:577, 1989.

457. Rezkalla, S., Kloner, R. A., Khaw, B. A., et al.: Detection of experimental myocarditis by monoclonal antimyosin antibody Fab fragment. Am. Heart J. 117:391, 1989.

458. Matsumori, A., Ohkusa, T., Matoba, Y., et al.: Myocardial uptake of anti-myosin monoclonal antibody in a murine model of viral myocarditis. Circulation 79:400, 1989.

459. Wakafugi, S., Kajiya, S., Hayakawa, M., et al.: Ga-67 myocardial scintigraphy in patients with acute myocarditis. Jpn. Circ. J. 51:1373, 1987.

460. Chandraratna, P. A., Bradley, W. G., Kortman, K. E., and Minagoe, S.: Detection of acute myocarditis using nuclear magnetic resonance imaging. Am. J. Med. 83:1144, 1987.

461. Chow, L. H., Radio, S. J., Sears, T. D., and McManus, B. M.: Insensitivity of right ventricular endomyocardial biopsy in the diagnosis of myocarditis. J. Am. Coll. Cardiol. 14:915, 1989.

462. Hauck, A. J., Kearney, D. L., and Edwards, W. D.: Evaluation of postmortem endomyocardial biopsy specimens from 38 patients with lymphocytic myocarditis: Implications for role of sampling error. Mayo Clin. Proc. 64:1235, 1989.

463. Dec, G. W., Fallon, J. T., Southern, J. F., and Palacios, I.: "Borderline" myocarditis: An indication for repeat endomyocardial biopsy. J. Am. Coll. Cardiol. 15:283, 1990.

464. Ilback, N. G., Fohlman, J., and Friman, G.: Exercise in coxsackie B3 myocarditis: Effects on heart lymphocyte subpopulations and the inflammatory reaction. Am. Heart J. 117:1298, 1989.

465. Lerner, A. M.: A new continuing fatigue syndrome following mild viral illness: A proscription to exercise. Chest 94:901, 1988.

466. Kiel, R. J., Smith, F. E., Chason, J., et al.: Coxsackievirus B3 myocarditis in C3H/HeJ mice: Description of an inbred model and the effect of exercise on virulence. Eur. J. Epidemiol. 5:348, 1989.

467. Rezkalla, S., Kloner, R. A., Khatib, G., et al.: Effect of metoprolol in acute coxsackievirus B3 murine myocarditis. J. Am. Coll. Cardiol. 12:412, 1988.

467a. Chan, K. Y., Iwahara, M., Benson, L. N., et al.: Immunosuppressive therapy in the management of acute myocarditis in children: A clinical trial. J. Am. Coll. Cardiol. 17:458, 1991.

468. Rezkalla, S., Khatib, G., and Khatib, R.: Coxsackievirus B3 murine myocarditis: Deleterious effects of nonsteroidal anti-inflammatory agents. J. Lab. Clin. Med. 107:393, 1986.

469. Rezkalla, S. H., and Kloner, R. A.: Management strategies in viral myocarditis. Am. Heart J. 117:706, 1989.

470. O'Connell, J. B., Reap, E. A., and Robinson, J. A.: The effects of cyclosporine on acute murine Coxsackie B3 myocarditis. Circulation 73:353, 1986.

471. Monrad, E. S., Matsumori, A., Murphy, J. C., et al.: Therapy with cyclosporine in experimental murine myocarditis with encephalomyocarditis virus. Circulation 73:1058, 1986.

472. Kishimoto, C., and Abelmann, W. H.: Absence of effects of cyclosporine on myocardial lymphocyte subsets in Coxsackievirus B3 myocarditis in the aviremic stage. Circ. Res. 65:934, 1989.

472a. Kishimoto, C., Thorp, K. A., and Abelmann, W. H.: Immunosuppression with high doses of cyclophosphamide reduces the severity of myocarditis but increases the mortality in murine coxsackievirus B3 myocarditis. Circulation 82:982, 1990.

473. Rezkalla, S., Khatib, R., Khatib, G., et al.: Effect of indomethacin in the late phase of coxsackievirus myocarditis in a murine model. J. Lab. Clin. Med. 112:118, 1988.

474. Rezkalla, S., Kloner, R. A., Khatib, G., and Khatib, R.: Beneficial effects of captopril in acute coxsackievirus B3 murine myocarditis. Circulation 81:1039, 1990.

474a. Rezkalla, S., Kloner, R. A., Khatib G., and Khatib, R.: Effect of delayed captopril therapy on left ventricular mass and myonecrosis during acute coxsackievirus murine myocarditis. Am. Heart J. 120:1377, 1990.

475. Ray, C. G., Icenogle, T. B., Minnich, L. L., et al.: The use of intravenous ribavirin to treat influenza virus–associated acute myocarditis. J. Infect. Dis. 159:829, 1989.

476. Chan, K. Y., Iwahara, M., Benson, L. N., et al.: Immunosuppressive therapy in the management of acute myocarditis in children: A clinical trial. J. Am. Coll. Cardiol. 17:458, 1991.

477. Gilbert, E. M., O'Connell, J. B., Hammond, M. E., et al.: Treatment of myocarditis with OKT3 monoclonal antibody (letter). Lancet 1:759, 1988.

478. Kishimoto, C., and Abelmann, W. H.: Monoclonal antibody therapy for prevention of acute coxsackievirus B3 myocarditis in mice. Circulation 79:1300, 1989.

479. Kishimoto, C., Crumpacker, C. S., and Abelmann, W. H.: Prevention of murine coxsackie B3 viral myocarditis and associated lymphoid organ atrophy with recombinant human leucocyte interferon alpha A/D. Cardiovasc. Res. 22:732, 1988.

480. Matsumori, A., Tomioka, N., and Kawai, C.: Protective effect of recombinant alpha interferon on coxsackievirus B3 myocarditis in mice. Am. Heart J. 115:1229, 1988.

481. Matsumori, A., Crumpacker, C. S., and Abelmann, W. H.: Prevention of viral myocarditis with recombinant human leukocyte interferon alpha A.D. in a murine model. J. Am. Coll. Cardiol. 9:1320, 1987.

482. Wolfgram, L. J., and Rose, N. R.: Coxsackievirus infection as a trigger of cardiac autoimmunity. Immunol. Res. 8:61, 1989.

483. Rozkovec, A., Cambridge, G., King, M., and Hallidie-Smith, K. A.: Natural history of left ventricular function in neonatal Coxsackie myocarditis. Pediatr. Cardiol. 6:151, 1985.

484. Read, R. B., Ede, R. J., Morgan-Capner, P., et al.: Myocarditis and fulminant hepatic failure from coxsackievirus B infection. Postgrad. Med. J. 61:749, 1985.

485. Remes, J., Helin, M., Vaino, P., and Rautio, P.: Clinical outcome and left ventricular function 23 years after acute coxsackie virus myopericarditis. Eur. Heart J. 11:182, 1990.

486. Levi, G., Scalvini, S., Volterrani, M., et al.: Coxsackie virus heart disease: 15 years after. Eur. Heart J. 9:1303, 1988.

487. O'Connell, J. B., and Robinson J. A.: Coxsackie viral myocarditis. Postgrad. Med. J. 61:1127, 1985.

488. Biton, A., and Herman, J.: Perimyocarditis. Report on an unusual cause. Postgrad. Med. 85:77, 1989.

489. Gonwa, T. A., Capehart, J. E., Pilcher, J. W., and Alivizatos, P. A.: Cytomegalovirus myocarditis as a cause of cardiac dysfunction in heart transplant recipient. Transplantation 47:197, 1989.

490. Shabtai, M., Luft, B., Waltzer, W. C., et al.: Massive cytomegalovirus pneumonia and myocarditis in a renal transplant recipient: Successful treatment with DHPG. Transplant Proc. 20:562, 1988.

491. Markin, R. S., Hollins, S., Wood, R. P., and Shaw, B. W., Jr.: Main autopsy finding in liver transplant patients. Mod. Pathol. 2:339, 1989.

492. Schindler, J. M., and Neftel, K. A.: Simultaneous primary infection with HIV and CMV leading to severe pancytopenia, hepatitis, nephritis, perimyocarditis, myositis, and alopecia totalis. Klin. Wochenschr. 68:237, 1990.

493. Powell, K.F.H., Bellamy, A. R., Catton, M. G., et al.: Cytomegalovirus myocarditis in a heart transplant recipient: Sensitive monitoring of viral DNA by the polymerase chain reaction. J. Heart Transplant 8:465, 1989.

494. Giampalmo, A., Ardoino, S., Borghesi, M. R., et al.: Anatomo-pathologic findings in 25 autopsy cases of AIDS. Pathologica 81:1, 1989.

495. George, R.: Dengue haemorrhagic fever in Malaysia: A review. Southeast Asian J. Trop. Med. Pub. Hlth. 18:278, 1987.

496. Songco, R. S., Hayes, C. G., Leus, C. D., and Manaloto, C.O.R.: Dengue fever/dengue haemorrhagic fever in Filipino children: Clinical experience during the 1983–1984 epidemic. Southeast Asian J. Trop. Med. Pub. Hlth. 18:284, 1987.

497. Milei, J., and Bolomo, N. J.: Myocardial damage in viral hemorrhagic fevers. Am. Heart. J. 104:1385, 1982.

498. Ursell, P. C., Habib, A., Sharma, P., et al.: Hepatitis B virus and myocarditis. Hum. Pathol. 15:481, 1984.

499. Singh, D. S., Gupta, P. R., Gupta, S. S., et al.: Cardiac changes in acute viral hepatitis in Varanasi (India): Case reports. J. Trop. Med. Hyg. 92:243, 1989.

500. Mahapatra, R. K., and Ellis, G. H.: Myocarditis and hepatitis B virus. Angiology 36:116, 1985.

501. Blanchard, D. G., Hagenhoff, C., Chow, L. C., et al.: Reversibility of cardiac abnormalities in human immunodeficiency virus (HIV)-infected individuals: A serial echocardiographic study. J. Am. Coll. Cardiol. 17:1270, 1991.

502. Levy, W. S., Simon, G. L., Rios, J. C., and Ross, A. M.: Prevalence of cardiac abnormalities in human immunodeficiency virus infection. Am. J. Cardiol. 63:86, 1989.

503. Raffanti, S. P., Chiaramida, A. J., Sen, P., et al.: Assessment of cardiac function in patients with the acquired immunodeficiency syndrome. Chest 93:592, 1988.

504. Himelman, R. B., Chung, W. S., Chernoff, D. N., et al.: Cardiac manifestations of human immunodeficiency virus infection: A two-dimensional echocardiographic study. J. Am. Coll. Cardiol. 13:1030, 1989.

505. Corallo, S., Mutinelli, M. R., Moroni, M., et al.: Echocardiography detects myocardial damage in AIDS: Prospective study in 102 patients. Eur. Heart J. 9:887, 1988.

506. Monsuez, J-J., Kinney, E. L., Vittecoq, D., et al.: Comparison among acquired immune deficiency syndrome patients with and without clinical evidence of cardiac disease. Am. J. Cardiol. 62:1311, 1988.

507. Lewis, W.: AIDS: Cardiac findings from 115 autopsies. Prog. Cardiovasc. Dis. 32:207, 1989.

508. Anderson, D. W., Virmani, R., Reilly, J. M., et al.: Prevalent myocarditis in necropsy in the acquired immunodeficiency syndrome. J. Am. Coll. Cardiol. 11:792, 1988.

509. Reilly, J. M., Cunnion, R. E., Anderson, D. W., et al.: Frequency of myocarditis, left ventricular dysfunction and ventricular tachycardia in the acquired immune deficiency syndrome. Am. J. Cardiol. 62:789, 1988.

510. Baroldi, G., Corallo, S., Moroni, M., et al.: Focal lymphocytic myocarditis in acquired immunodeficiency syndrome (AIDS): A correlative morphologic and clinical study in 26 consecutive fatal cases. J. Am. Coll. Cardiol. 12:463, 1988.

511. Acierno, L. J.: Cardiac complications in acquired immunodeficiency syndrome (AIDS): A review. J. Am. Coll. Cardiol. 13:1144, 1989.

512. Grody, W. W., Cheng, L., and Lewis, W.: Infection of the heart by the human immunodeficiency virus. Am. J. Cardiol. 66:203, 1990.

513. Anderson, D. W., and Virmani, R.: Emerging patterns of heart disease in human immunodeficiency virus infection. Hum. Pathol. 21:253, 1990.

514. Stewart, J. M., Kaul, A., Gromisch, D. S., et al.: Symptomatic cardiac dysfunction in children with human immunodeficiency virus infection. Am. Heart. J. 117:140, 1989.

515. Calabrese, L. H., Proffitt, M. R., Yen-Lieberman, B., et al.: Congestive cardiomyopathy and illness related to the acquired immunodeficiency syndrome (AIDS) associated with isolation of retrovirus from myocardium. Ann. Intern. Med. 107:691, 1987.

516. Coplan, N. L., and Bruno, M. S.: Acquired immunodeficiency syndrome and heart disease: The present and the future. Am. Heart J. 117:1175, 1989.

517. Bharati, S., Joshi, V. V., Connor, E. M., et al.: Conduction system in children with acquired immunodeficiency syndrome. Chest 96:406, 1989.

518. Kinney, E. L., Monsuez, J-J., Kitzis, M., and Vittecoq, D.: Treatment of AIDS-associated heart disease. Angiology 40:970, 1989.

519. Frishman, W., Kraus, M. E., Zabkar, J., et al.: Infectious mononucleosis and fatal myocarditis. Chest 72:535, 1977.

520. Tyson, A. A., Jr., Hackshaw, B. T., and Kutcher, M. A.: Acute Epstein-Barr virus myocarditis simulating myocardial infarction with cardiogenic shock. South. Med. J. 82:1184, 1989.

521. Hudgins, J. M.: Infectious mononucleosis complicated by myocarditis and pericarditis. JAMA 235:2626, 1976.

522. Cate, T. R.: Clinical manifestations and consequences of influenza. Am. J. Med. 82:15, 1987.

523. Sprenger, M. J., Van Naelten, M. A., Mulder, P. G., and Masurel, N.: Influenza mortality and excess deaths in the elderly, 1967–1982. Epidemiol. Infect. 103:633, 1989.

524. Engblom, E., Ekfors, T. O., Meurman, O. H., et al.: Fatal influenza A myocarditis with isolation of virus from the myocardium. Acta Med. Scand. 213:75, 1983.

525. Proby, C. M., Hackett, D., Gupta, S., and Cox, T. M.: Acute myopericarditis in influenza A infection. Q. J. Med. 60:887, 1986.

526. Drescher, J., Zink, P., Verhagen, W., et al.: Recent influenza virus A infections in forensic cases of sudden unexplained death. Arch. Virol. 92:63, 1987.

527. Ruben, F. L., and Cate, T. R.: Influenza pneumonia. Semin. Respir. Infect. 2:122, 1987.

528. Cummins, D., Bennett, D., Fisher-Hoch, S. P., et al.: Electrocardiographic abnormalities in patients with Lassa fever. J. Trop. Med. Hyg. 92:350, 1989.

529. McCormick, J. B., King, I. J., Webb, P. A., et al.: Lassa fever: A case-control study of the clinical diagnosis and course. J. Infect. Dis. 155:445, 1987.

530. Walker, D. H., McCormick, J. B., Johnson, K. M., et al.: Pathologic and virologic study of fatal Lassa fever in man. J. Infect. Dis. 107:349, 1982.

531. Ozkutlu, S., Soylemezoglu, O., Calikoglu, A. S., et al.: Fatal mumps myocarditis. Jpn. Heart J. 30:109, 1989.

532. Ward, S. C., Wiselka, M. J., and Nicholson, K. G.: Still's disease and myocarditis associated with recent mumps infection. Postgrad. Med. J. 64:693, 1988.

533. Chaudary, S., and Jaski, B. E.: Fulminant mumps myocarditis. Ann. Intern. Med. 110:569, 1989.

534. Baandrup, U., and Mortensen, S. A.: Fatal mumps myocarditis. Acta Med. Scand. 216:331, 1984.

535. Chen, S. C., Tsai, C. C., and Nouri, S.: Carditis associated with mycoplasma pneumoniae infection. Am. J. Dis. Child. 140:471, 1986.

536. Murray, B. J.: Nonrespiratory complications of M. pneumoniae infection. Am. Fam. Physician 37:127, 1988.

537. Hildes, J. A., Schaberg, A., and Alcock, A.U.W.: Cardiovascular collapse in acute poliomyelitis. Circulation 12:986, 1955.

538. Dunne, J. W., Harper, C. G., and Hilton, J. M.: Sudden infant death syndrome caused by poliomyelitis. Arch. Neurol. 41:775, 1984.

539. Teloth, H. A.: Myocarditis in poliomyelitis. Arch. Pathol. 55:408, 1953.

540. Weinstein, L., and Shelokov, A.: Cardiovascular manifestations of acute poliomyelitis. N. Engl. J. Med. 244:281, 1951.

541. Page, S. R., Stewart, J. T., and Bernstein, J. J.: A progressive pericardial effusion caused by psittacosis. Br. Heart J. 60:87, 1988.

542. Pahl, E., and Gidding, S. S.: Echocardiographic assessment of cardiac function during respiratory syncytial virus infection. Pediatrics 81:830, 1988.

543. Menahem, S., and Uren, E. C.: Respiratory syncytial virus and heart block —cause and effect? Aust. N.Z. J. Med. 15:55, 1985.

544. Martin, J. T., Kugler, J. D., Gumbiner, G. H., et al.: Refractory congestive heart failure after ribavirin in infants with heart disease and respiratory syncytial virus. Nebr. Med. J. 75:23, 1990.

545. Thanopoulos, B. D., Rokas, S., Frimas, C. A., et al.: Cardiac involvement in postnatal rubella. Acta Paediatr. Scand. 78:141, 1989.

546. Goldfield, M., Bayer, N. H., and Weinstein, L.: Electrocardiographic changes during the course of measles. J. Pediatr. 46:30, 1955.

547. Degen, J. A.: Visceral pathology in measles: A clinicopathologic study of 100 cases. Am. J. Med. Sci. 194:104, 1937.

548. Weinstein, L.: Cardiovascular manifestations in some of the common infectious diseases. Mod. Concepts Cardiovasc. Dis. 23:229, 1954.

549. Lorber, A., Zonis, Z., Maisuls, E., et al.: The scale of myocardial involvement in varicella myocarditis. Int. J. Cardiol. 20:257, 1988.

550. Woolf, P. K., Chung, T. S., Stewart, J., et al.: Life-threatening dysrhythmias in varicella myocarditis. Clin. Pediatr. 26:480, 1987.

551. Ettedgui, J. A., Ladusans, E., and Bamford, M.: Complete heart block as a complication of varicella. Int. J. Cardiol. 14:362, 1987.

552. Wagner, D. C., and Murphy, T. V.: Varicella myocarditis. Pediatr. Infect. Dis. J. 9:360, 1990.

553. Anderson, T., Foulis, M. A., Grist, N. R., and Landsman, J. B.: Clinical and laboratory observations in a smallpox outbreak. Lancet 1:1248, 1951.

554. Matthews, A. W., and Griffiths, I. D.: Post-vaccinal pericarditis and myocarditis. Br. Heart J. 36:1043, 1974.

555. Finley-Jones, L. R.: Fatal myocarditis after vaccinations for smallpox. N. Engl. J. Med. 270:41, 1964.

556. Schmeer, N., Krauss, H., Werth, D., and Schiefer, H. G.: Serodiagnosis of Q fever by enzyme-linked immunosorbent assay (ELISA). Zentralbl. Bakteriol. Mikrobiol. Hyg. 267:57, 1987.

557. Maisch, B.: Rickettsial perimyocarditis—a follow-up study. Heart Vessels 2:55, 1986.

558. Koster, F. T., Williams, J. C., and Goodwin, J. S.: Cellular immunity in Q fever: Specific lymphocyte unresponsiveness in Q fever endocarditis. J. Infect. Dis. 152:1283, 1985.

559. Marin-Garcia, J., and Barrett, F. F.: Myocardial function in Rocky Mountain spotted fever: Echocardiographic assessment. Am. J. Cardiol. 51:341, 1983.

560. Marin-Garcia, J., and Mirvis, D. M.: Myocardial disease in Rocky Mountain spotted fever: Clinical, functional, and pathologic findings. Pediatr. Cardiol. 5:149, 1984.

561. Marin-Garcia, J.: Left ventricular dysfunction in Rocky Mountain spotted fever. Clin. Cardiol. 6:501, 1983.

562. Ganjoo, R. K., Sharma, S, N. and Roy, A. K.: Typhus myocarditis (letter). J. Assoc. Physicians India 37:357, 1989.

563. Brown, G. W., Shirai, A., Jegathesan, M., et al.: Febrile illness in Malaysia —an analysis of 1,629 hospitalized patients. Am. J. Trop. Med. Hyg. 33:311, 1984.

564. Valliattu, J., Shuhaiber, H., Kiwan, Y., et al.: Brucella endocarditis. Report of one case and review of the literature. J. Cardiovasc. Surg. 30:782, 1989.

565. Lubani, M., Sharda, D., and Helin, I.: Cardiac manifestations in brucellosis. Arch. Dis. Child. 61:569, 1986.

566. Gur, H., Gefel, D., and Tur-Kaspa, R.: Transient electrocardiographic changes during two episodes of relapsing brucellosis. Postgrad. Med. J. 60:544, 1984.

567. Jubber, A. S., Gunawardana, D. R., and Lulu, A. R.: Acute pulmonary edema in Brucella myocarditis and interstitial pneumonitis. Chest 97:1008, 1990.

568. Roberts, W. C., and Beard, G. W.: Gas gangrene of the heart in clostridial septicemia. Am. Heart J. 74:482, 1967.

569. Stevens, D. L., Troyer, B. E., Merrick, D. T., et al.: Lethal effects and cardiovascular effects of purified alpha- and theta-toxins from Clostridium perfringens. J. Infect. Dis. 157:272, 1988.

570. Guneratre, P.: Gas gangrene (abscess) of heart. N. Y. State J. Med. 75:1766, 1975.

571. Havaldar, P. V., Patil, V. D., Siddibhavi, B. M., et al.: Fulminant diphtheritic myocarditis. Indian Heart J. 41:265, 1989.

572. Thisyakorn, U., Wongvanich, J., and Kumpens, V.: Failure of corticosteroid therapy to prevent diphtheritic myocarditis or neuritis. Pediatr. Infect. Dis. 3:126, 1984.

573. Ramos, H. C., Elias, P. R., Barrucand, L., et al.: The protective effect of carnitine in human diphtheric myocarditis. Pediatr. Res. 18:815, 1984.

574. Castellani Pastoris, M., Nigro, G., and Middulla, M.: Arrhythmia or myocarditis: A novel clinical form of Legionella pneumophila infection in children without pneumonia. Eur. J. Pediatr. 144:157, 1985.

575. Friedland, L., Syndman, D. R., Weingarden, A. S., et al.: Ocular and pericardial involvement in Legionnaires' disease. Am. J. Med. 77:1105, 1984.

576. Brasier, A. R., Macklis, J. D., Vaughan, D., et al.: Myopericarditis as an initial presentation of meningococcemia. Unusual manifestation of infection with serotype W135. Am. J. Med. 82:641, 1987.

577. Sandler, M. A., Pincus, P. S., Weltman, M. D., et al.: Meningococcaemia complicated by myocarditis. A report of 2 cases. S. Afr. Med. J. 75:391, 1989.

578. Ejlertsen T., Vesterlund, T., and Schmidt, E. B.: Myopericarditis with cardiac tamponade caused by Neisseria meningitides serogroup W135. Eur. J. Clin. Microbiol. Infect. Dis. 7:403, 1988.

579. Monsalve, F., Rucabado, L., Salvador, A., et al.: Myocardial depression in septic shock caused by meningococcal infection. Crit. Care Med. 12:1021, 1984.

580. Kovoor, P., Mathew, M., Abraham, T., and Taneja, P. K.: Enteric fever complicated by myocarditis, hepatitis and shock. J. Assoc. Physicians India 36:353, 1988.

581. Delapenha, R. A., Greaves, W. L., Mani, V., and Frederick, W. R.: Typhoid fever with unusual clinical features (letter). South. Med. J. 81:417, 1988.

582. Siwach, S. B., and Nand, N.: Cardiovascular complications of enteric fever. Angiology 34:436, 1983.

583. Le-Van-Diem, A. K.: Typhoid fever with myocarditis. Am. J. Trop. Med. Hyg. 23:218, 1974.

584. Dhar, K. L., Adlakha, A., and Phillips, P. J.: Recurrent seizures and syncope, ventricular arrhythmias with reversible prolonged Q-Tc interval in typhoid myocarditis. J. Indian Med. Assoc. 85:336, 1987.

585. Karjalainen, J.: Streptococcal tonsillitis and acute nonrheumatic myopericarditis. Chest 95:359, 1989.

586. Caraco, J., Arnon, R., and Raz, I.: Atrioventricular block complicating acute streptococcal tonsillitis. Br. Heart J. 59:389, 1988.

587. Rose, A. G.: Cardiac tuberculosis. A study of 19 patients. Arch. Pathol. Lab. Med. 111:422, 1987.

588. Picard, R., Vinceneux, Ph., Lim, D. Q., et al.: Heart failure due to myocardial tuberculosis. Report of three cases. Sem. Hôp. Paris 64:1991, 1988.

589. Southern, J. F., Moscicki, R. A., Magro, C., et al.: Lymphedema, lymphocytic myocarditis, and sarcoid-like granulomatosis. Manifestations of Whipple's disease. JAMA 261:1467, 1989.

590. Sossai, P., DeBoni, M., and Cielo, R.: The heart and Whipple's disease (letter). Int. J. Cardiol. 23:275, 1989.

591. James, T. N., and Bulkley, B. H.: Abnormalities of the coronary arteries in Whipple's disease. Am. Heart J. 105:481, 1983.

592. Morrison, D. A., Gay, R. G., Feldshon, D., and Sampliner, R. E.: Severe pulmonary hypertension in a patient with Whipple's disease. Am. J. Med. 79:263, 1985.

593. Keinath, R. D., Merrell, D. E., Vlietstra, R., and Dobbins, W. O., III: Antibiotic treatment and relapse in Whipple's disease. Long-term follow-up of 88 patients. Gastroenterology 88:1867, 1985.

594. Feldman, M.: Whipple's disease. Am. J. Med. Sci. 291:56, 1986.

595. de Brito, T., Morais, C. F., Yasuda, P. H., et al.: Cardiovascular involvement in human and experimental leptospirosis: Pathologic findings and immunohistochemical detection of leptospiral antigen. Ann. Trop. Med. Parasitol. 81:207, 1987.

596. Lee, M. G., Char, G., Dianzumba, S., and Prussia, P.: Cardiac involvement in severe leptospirosis. West Indian Med. J. 35:295, 1986.

597. De Biase, L., De Curtis, G., Paparoni, S., et al.: Fatal leptospiral myocarditis. G. Ital. Cardiol. 17:992, 1987.

598. Ram, P., and Chandra, M. S.: Unusual electrocardiographic abnormality in leptospirosis: Case reports. Angiology 36:477, 1985.

599. Winearls, C. G., Chan, L., Coghlan, J. D., et al.: Acute renal failure due to leptospirosis: Clinical features and outcome in six cases. Q. J. Med. 53:487, 1984.

600. McAlister, H. F., Klementowicz, P. T., Andrews, C., et al.: Lyme carditis: An important cause of reversible heart block. Ann. Intern. Med. 110:339, 1989.

601. Stanek, G., Klein, J., Bittner, R., and Glogar, D.: Isolation of Borrelia burgdorferi from the myocardium of a patient with longstanding cardiomyopathy. N. Engl. J. Med. 322:249, 1990.

602. van der Linde, M. R., Crijns, H.J.G.M., and Lie, K. I.: Transient complete AV block in Lyme disease: Electrophysiologic observations. Chest 96:219, 1989.

603. van der Linde M. R., Crijns, H.J.G.M., de Koning, J., et al.: Range of atrioventricular conduction disturbances in Lyme borreliosis: A report of four cases and review of other published reports. Br. Heart J. 63:162, 1990.

604. Vlay, S. C., Dervan, J. P., Elias, J., et al.: Ventricular tachycardia associated with Lyme carditis. Am. Heart J. 121:1558, 1991.

605. Rienzo, R. J., Morel, D. E., Prager, D., et al.: Gallium-avid Lyme myocarditis. Clin. Nuc. Med. 12:475, 1987.

606. Kimball, S. A., Janson, P. A., and LaRaia, P. J.: Complete heart block as the sole presentation of Lyme disease. Arch. Intern. Med. 149:1897, 1989.

607. DeKoning, J., Hoogkamp-Korstanje, J.A.A., van der Linde, M. R., and Crijns, H.J.G.M.: Demonstration of spirochetes in cardiac biopsies of patients with Lyme disease. J. Infect. Dis. 160:150, 1989.

608. Wengrower, D., Knobler, H., Gillis, S., Chajek-Shaul, T.: Myocarditis in tick-borne relapsing fever. J. Infect. Dis. 149:1033, 1984.

609. Doscia, J. L., Fisco, J. M., and Brace, W. T.: Complete heart block due to a solitary gumma. Am. J. Cardiol. 13:553, 1964.

610. Spain, D. M., and Johannsen M. W.: Three cases of localized gummatous myocarditis. Am. Heart J. 241:689, 1942.

611. Atkinson, J. B., Robinowitz, M., McAllister, H. H., et al.: Cardiac infections in the immunocompromised host. Cardiol. Clin. 2:671, 1984.

612. Nahass, R. G., Scholz, P., Mackenzie, J. W., and Gocke, D. J.: Chronic constrictive pericarditis. A case report and review of the literature. Arch. Intern. Med. 149:1202, 1989.

613. Slutzker, A. D., and Claypool, W. D.,: Pericardial actinomycosis with cardiac tamponade from a contiguous thoracic lesion. Thorax 44:442, 1989.

614. Schwartz, D. A.: Aspergillus pancarditis following bone marrow transplantation for chronic myelogenous leukemia. Chest 95:1338, 1989.

615. Andersson, B. S., Luna, M. A., and McCredie, K. B.: Systemic aspergillosis as cause of myocardial infarction. Cancer 58:2146, 1986.

616. Hall J. C., and Giltman, L. I.: Candida myocarditis in a patient with chronic active hepatitis and macronodular cirrhosis. J. Tenn. Med. Assoc. 79:473, 1986.

617. Atkinson, J. B., Connor, D. H., Robinowitz, M., et al.: Cardiac fungal infections: Review of autopsy findings in 60 patients. Hum. Pathol. 15:935, 1984.

618. Vartivarian, S. E., Coudron, P. E., and Markowitz, S. M.: Disseminated coccidioidomycosis. Unusual manifestations in a cardiac transplantation patient. Am. J. Med. 83:949, 1987.

619. Lafont, A., Wolff, M., Marche, et al.: Overwhelming myocarditis due to Cryptococcus neoformans in an AIDS patient (letter). Lancet 14:1145, 1987.

620. Loyd, J. E., Tillman, B. F., Atkinson, J. B., and Des Prez, R. M.: Mediastinal fibrosis complicating histoplasmosis. Medicine 67:295, 1988.

621. Garrett, H. E., Jr., and Roper, C. L.: Surgical intervention in histoplasmosis. Ann. Thorac. Surg. 42:711, 1986.

622. Acquatella, H., Catalioti, F., Gomez-Mancebo, J. R., et al.: Long-term control of Chagas disease in Venezuela: Effects on serologic findings, electrocardiographic abnormalities, and clinical outcome. Circulation 76:556, 1987.

623. Grant, I. H., Gold, J.W.M., Wittner, M., et al.: Transfusion-associated acute Chagas' disease acquired in the United States. Ann. Intern. Med. 111:849, 1989.

624. Maguire, J. H., Hoff, R., Sherlock, I., et al.: Cardiac morbidity and mortality due to Chagas' disease: Prospective electrocardiographic study of a Brazilian community. Circulation 75:1140, 1987.

625. Morris, S. A., Tanowitz, H. B., Wittner, M., and Bilezikian, J. P.: Pathophysiological insights into the cardiomyopathy of Chagas' disease. Circulation 82:1900, 1990.

626. Hudson, L., and Britten, V.: Immune response to South American trypanosomiasis and its relationship to Chagas' disease. Br. Med. Bull. 41:175, 1985.

627. Palacios-Pru, E., Carrasco, H., Scorza, C., and Espinoza, R.: Ultrastructural characteristics of different stages of human chagasic myocarditis. Am. J. Trop. Med. Hyg. 41:29, 1989.

628. Morris, S. A., Tanowitz, H., Factor, S. M., et al.: Myocardial adenylate cyclase activity in acute murine Chagas' disease. Circ. Res. 62:800, 1988.

629. Bestetti, R. B., Ramos, C. P., Godoy, R. A., and Oliveira, J. S.: Chronic Chagas' heart disease in the elderly: A clinicopathologic study. Cardiology 74:344, 1987.

630. Carrasco, H. A., Guerrero, L., Prada, H., et al.: Ventricular arrhythmias and left ventricular myocardial function in chronic chagasic patients. Int. J. Cardiol. 28:35, 1990.

631. Casado, J., Davila, D. F., Donis, J. H., et al.: Electrocardiographic abnormalities and left ventricular systolic function in Chagas' heart disease. Int. J. Cardiol. 27:55, 1990.

632. Rossi, M. A.: Microvascular changes as a cause of chronic cardiomyopathy in Chagas' disease. Am. Heart J. 1220:233, 1990.

633. Carrasco, H. A., Palacios-Pru, E., Dagert deScorza, C., et al.: Clinical, histochemical, and ultrastructural correlation in septal endoymocardial biopsies from chronic chagasic patients: Detection of early myocardial damage. Am. Heart J. 113:716, 1987.

634. Oliveira, J. S. M., and Marin-Neto, J. A.: Parasympathetic impairment in Chagas' heart disease: Cause or consequence (editorial)? Int. J. Cardiol. 21:153, 1988.

635. Levin, M. J., Mesri, E., Benarous, R., et al.: Identification of major Trypanosoma cruzi antigenic determinants in chronic Chagas' heart disease. Am. J. Trop. Med. Hyg. 41:530, 1989.

636. Higuchi, M. deL., Lopes, E. A., Saldanha, L. B., et al.: Immunopathologic studies in myocardial biopsies of patients with Chagas' disease and idiopathic cardiomyopathy. Rev. Inst. Med. Trop. Sao Paulo 28:87, 1986.

637. Acosta, A. M., and Santos-Buch, C. A.: Autoimmune myocarditis induced by Trypanosoma cruzi. Circulation 71:1255, 1985.

638. Morato, M. J., Brener, Z., Cancado, J. R., et al.: Cellular immune responses of chagasic patients to antigens derived from different Trypanosoma cruzi strains and clones. Am. J. Trop. Med. Hyg. 35:505, 1986.

639. Sadigursky, M., von Kreuter, B. F., Ling, P. Y., and Santos-Buch, C. A.: Association of elevated anti-sarcolemma, anti-idiotype antibody levels with the clinical and pathologic expression of chronic Chagas myocarditis. Circulation 80:1269, 1989.

640. Fuenmayor, A. J., Rodriguez, L., Torres, A., et al.: Valsalva maneuver: A test of the functional state of cardiac innervation in chagasic myocarditis. Int. J. Cardiol. 18:351, 1988.

641. Davila, D. F., Donis, J. H., Navas, M., et al.: Response of heart rate to atropine and left ventricular function in Chagas' heart disease. Int. J. Cardiol. 21:143, 1988.

642. Oliveira, J.S.M.: A natural human model of intrinsic heart nervous system denervation: Chagas' cardiopathy. Am. Heart J. 110:1092, 1985.

643. Acquatella, H., and Schiller, N. B.: Echocardiographic recognition of Chagas' disease and endomyocardial fibrosis. J. Am. Soc. Echo. 1:60, 1988.

644. Abelmann, W. H.: The dilated cardiomyopathies: Experimental aspects. Cardiol. Clin. 6:219, 1988.

645. Ferrans, V. J., Milei, J., Tomita, Y., and Storino, R. A.: Basement membrane thickening in cardiac myocytes and capillaries in chronic Chagas' disease. Am. J. Cardiol. 61:1137, 1988.

646. Maguire, J. H., Hoff, R., Sleigh, A. C., et al.: An outbreak of Chagas' disease in southwestern Bahia, Brazil. Am. J. Trop. Med. Hyg. 35:931, 1986.

647. Marin-Neto, J. A., Maciel, B. C., Gallo, L., Jr., et al.: Effect of parasympathetic impairment on the haemodynamic response to handgrip in Chagas's heart disease. Br. Heart J. 55:204, 1986.

648. Junqueira, L. F., Jr., Gallo, L., Jr., Manco, J. C., et al.: Subtle cardiac autonomic impairment in Chagas' disease detected by baroreflex sensitivity testing. Braz. J. Med. Biol. Res. 18:171, 1985.

649. de Paola, A.A.V., Horowitz, L. N., Miyamoto, M. H., et al.: Angiographic and electrophysiologic substrates of ventricular tachycardia in chronic chagasic myocarditis. Am. J. Cardiol. 65:360, 1990.

650. Combellas, I., Puigbo, J. J., Acquatella, H., et al.: Echocardiographic features of impaired left ventricular diastolic function in Chagas's heart disease. Br. Heart J. 53:298, 1985.

651. Caeiro, T., Amuchastegui, L. M., Moreyra, E., and Gibson, D. G.: Abnormal left ventricular diastolic function in chronic Chagas' disease: An echocardiographic study. Int. J. Cardiol. 9:417, 1985.

652. Marin-Neto, J. A., Marzullo, P., Sousa, A. C., et al.: Radionuclide angiographic evidence for early predominant right ventricular involvement in patients with Chagas' disease. Can. J. Cardiol. 4:231, 1988.

653. Factor, S. M., Cho, S., Wittner, M., and Tanowitz, H.: Abnormalities of the coronary microcirculation in acute murine Chagas' disease. Am. J. Trop. Med. Hyg. 34:246, 1985.

654. Kirchhoff, L. V.: Is Trypanosoma cruzi a new threat to our blood supply? Ann. Intern. Med. 111:773, 1989.

655. Espinosa, R., Carrasco, H. A., Belandria, F., et al.: Life expectancy analysis in patients with Chagas' disease: Prognosis after one decade (1973–1983). Int. J. Cardiol. 8:45, 1985.

656. Schofield, C. J.: Control of Chagas' disease vectors. Br. Med. Bull. 41:187, 1985.

657. de Paola, A. A., Horowitz, L. N., Miyamoto, M. H., et al.: Automatic im-

plantable defibrillator with VVI pacemaker in a patient with chronic Chagas myocarditis and total atrioventricular block. Am. Heart J. *118*:415, 1989.

658. Tsala Mbala, P., Blackett, K., Mbonifor, C. L., et al.: Functional and immunologic involvement in human African trypanosomiasis caused by *Trypanosoma gambiense*. Bull. Soc. Pathol. Exot. Filiales *81*:490, 1988.

659. Holmes, P. H.: Pathophysiology of parasitic infections. Parasitology *94*:S29, 1987.

660. McCabe, R. E., Brooks, R. G., Dorfman, R. F., and Remington, J. S.: Clinical spectrum in 107 cases of toxoplasmic lymphadenopathy. Rev. Infect. Dis. *9*:754, 1987.

661. Jehn, U., Fink, M., Gundlach, P., et al.: Lethal cardiac and cerebral toxoplasmosis in a patient with acute myeloid leukemia after successful allogenic bone marrow transplantation. Transplantation *38*:430, 1984.

662. Luft, B. J., Billingham, M., and Remington, J. S.: Endomyocardial biopsy in the diagnosis of toxoplasmic myocarditis. Tranplant. Proc. *18*:1871, 1986.

663. Adair, O. V., Randive, N., and Krasnow, N.: Isolated toxoplasma myocarditis in acquired immune deficiency syndrome. Am. Heart J. *118*:856, 1989.

664. Tschirhart, D., and Klatt, E. C.: Disseminated toxoplasmosis in the acquired immunodeficiency syndrome. Arch. Pathol. Lab. Med. *112*:1237, 1988.

665. Tolat, D., and Kim, H. S.: Toxoplasmosis of the brain and heart: Autopsy report of a patient with AIDS. Tex. Med. *85*:40, 1989.

666. Permanyer-Miralda, G., Sagrista-Sauleda, J., and Soler-Soler, J.: Primary acute pericardial disease: A prospective series of 231 consecutive patients. Am. J. Cardiol. *56*:623, 1985.

667. Sharma, S. N., Mohapatra, A. K., and Machave, Y. V.: Chronic falciparum cardiomyopathy (letter). J. Assoc. Physicians India *35*:251, 1987.

668. Oliver, J. M., Sotillo, J. F., Dominguez, F. J., et al.: Two-dimensional echocardiographic features of echinococcosis of the heart and great blood vessels: Clinical and surgical implications. Circulation *78*:327, 1988.

669. Russo, G., Tamburino, C., Cuscuna, S., et al.: Cardiac hydatid cyst with clinical features resembling subaortic stenosis. Am. Heart J. *117*:1385, 1989.

670. Desnos, M., Brochet, E., Cristofini, P., et al.: Polyvisceral echinococcosis with cardiac involvement imaged by two-dimensional echocardiography, computed tomography and nuclear magnetic resonance imaging. Am. J. Cardiol. *59*:383, 1987.

671. Barnard, P. M., MacGregor, L. A., and Weich, H. F. H.: Premere Eichinococcus-sist van die hart 'n Gevalbespreking. S. Afr. Med. J. *76*:275, 1989.

672. Dao, A. H., and Virmani, R.: Visceral larva migrans involving the myocardium: Report of two cases and review of literature. Pediatr. Pathol. *6*:449, 1986.

673. Ursell, P. C., Habib, A., Babchick, O., et al.: Myocarditis caused by *Trichinella spiralis* (letter). Arch. Pathol. Lab. Med. *108*:4, 1984.

674. Lopez-Lozano, J. J., Garcia Merino, J. A., and Liano, H.: Bilateral facial paralysis secondary to trichinosis. Acta Neurol. Scand. *78*:194, 1988.

675. Starling, R. C., and Unverferth, D. V.: Value of endomyocardial biopsy: Indications and applications. *In* Zipes, D. P., and Rowlands, D. J. (eds.): Progress in Cardiology. Philadelphia, Lea and Febiger, 1989, p. 33.

TOXIC, CHEMICAL, IMMUNE AND PHYSICAL DAMAGE

676. Brody, S. L., Slovis, C. M., and Wrenn, K. D.: Cocaine-related medical problems: Consecutive series of 233 patients. Am. J. Med. *88*:325, 1990.

677. Lange, R. A. Cigarroa, R. G., Yancy, C. W., et al.: Cocaine-induced coronary-artery vasoconstriction. N. Engl. J. Med. *321*:1557, 1989.

678. Isner, J. M., and Chokshi, S. K.: Cocaine and vasospasm. N. Engl. J. Med. *321*:1604, 1989.

679. Dressler, F. A., Malekzadeh, S., and Roberts, W. C.: Quantitative analysis of amounts of coronary arterial narrowing in cocaine addicts. Am. J. Cardiol. *65*:303, 1990.

680. Przywara, D. A., and Dambach, G.: Direct actions of cocaine on cardiac cellular electrical activity. Circ. Res. *65*:185, 1989.

681. Chokshi, S. K., Moore, R., Pandian, N. G., and Isner, J. M.: Reversible cardiomyopathy associated with cocaine intoxication. Ann. Intern. Med. *111*:1039, 1989.

682. Waller, B. F.: Cocaine and the heart. Indiana Med. *81*:956, 1988.

683. Fraker, T. D., Jr., Temesy-Armos, P. N., Brewster, P. S., and Wilkerson, R. D.: Mechanism of cocaine-induced myocardial depression in dogs. Circulation *81*:1012, 1990.

684. Abel, F. L., Wilson, S. P., Zhao, R. R., and Fennell, W. H.: Cocaine depresses the canine myocardium. Circ. Shock *28*:309, 1989.

685. Inoue, H., and Zipes, D. P.: Cocaine-induced supersensitivity and arrhythmogenesis. J. Am. Coll. Cardiol. *11*:867, 1988.

686. Majid, P. A., Patel, B., Kim, H-S., et al.: An angiographic and histologic study of cocaine-induced chest pain. Am. J. Cardiol. *65*:812, 1990.

687. Peng, S-K., French, W. J., and Pelikan, P. C. D.: Direct cocaine cardiotoxicity demonstrated by endomyocardial biopsy. Arch. Pathol. Lab. Med. *113*:842, 1989.

688. Isner, J. M., and Chokshi, S. K.: Cardiovascular complications of cocaine. Curr. Prob. Cardiol. *16*:538, 1991.

689. Karch, S. B., and Billingham, M. E.: The pathology and etiology of cocaine-induced heart disease. Arch. Pathol. Lab. Med. *112*:225, 1988.

690. Deyton, L. R., Walker, R. E., Kovacs, J. A., et al.: Reversible cardiac dysfunction associated with interferon alpha therapy in AIDS patients with Kaposi's sarcoma. N. Engl. J. Med. *321*:1246, 1989.

691. Cohen, M. C., Huberman, M. S., and Nesto, R. W.: Recombinant alpha$_2$ interferon-related cardiomyopathy. Am. J. Med. *85*:549, 1988.

692. Levin, R., Burtt, D. M., Levin, W. A., and Ginsberg, M. B.: Ventricular fibrillation in a tetraplegic patient who had a therapeutic level of a tricyclic antidepressant. Paraplegia *23*:354, 1985.

693. Horowitz, J. D.: Drugs that induce heart problems. Which agents? What effects? J. Cardiovasc. Med. *8*:308, 1983.

694. Orme, M. L.: Antidepressants and heart disease (editorial). Br. Med. J. *289*:1, 1984.

695. Margolin, K., Raynor, A., Hawkins, M., et al.: Interleukin-2 and lymphokine-activated killer cell therapy and solid tumors: Analysis and toxicity and management guidelines. J. Clin. Oncol. *7*:486, 1989.

696. Schuchter, L. M., Hendricks, C. B., Holland, K. H., et al.: Eosinophilic myocarditis associated with high-dose interleukin-2 therapy. Am. J. Med. *88*:439, 1990.

697. Nora, R., Abrams, J., and Silverman, H.: Myocardial infarction in patients receiving high-dose recombinant interleukin-2. N. Engl. J. Med. *316*:275, 1987.

698. Osanto, S., Cluitmans, F. H., Franks, H. A., and Cleton, F. J.: Myocardial injury after interleukin-2 therapy. Lancet *2*:48, 1988.

699. Gaynor, E., Vitek, L., Sticklin, L., et al.: The hemodynamic effects of treatment with interleukin-2 and lymphokine-activated killer cells. Ann. Intern. Med. *109*:953, 1988.

700. Samlowski, W. E., Ward, J. H., Craven, C. M., and Freedman, R. A.: Severe myocarditis following high-dose interleukin-2 administration. Arch. Pathol. Lab. Med. *113*:838, 1989.

701. Raehl, C. L., Patel, A. K., and LeRoy, M.: Drug-induced torsade de pointes. Clin. Pharm. *4*:675, 1985.

702. Khan, M. Y., Haider, B., and Thind, I. S.: Emetine-induced cardiomyopathy in rabbits. J. Submicrosc. Cytol. *15*:495, 1983.

703. Harbin, A. D., Gerson, M. C., and O'Connell, J. B.: Simulation of acute myopericarditis by constrictive pericardial disease with endomyocardial fibrosis due to methylsergide therapy. J. Am. Coll. Cardiol. *4*:196, 1984.

704. Ratliff, N. B., Estes, M. L., Myles, J. L., et al.: Diagnosis of chloroquine cardiomyopathy by endomyocardial biopsy. N. Engl. J. Med. *316*:191, 1987.

705. McAllister, H. A., Jr., Ferrans, V. J., Hall, R. J., et al.: Chloroquine-induced cardiomyopathy. Arch. Pathol. Lab. Med. *111*:953, 1987.

706. Estes, M. L., Ewing-Wilson, D., Chou, S. M., et al.: Chloroquine neuromyotoxicity. Clinical and pathologic perspective. Am. J. Med. *82*:477, 1987.

707. Chulay, J. D., Spencer, H. C., and Mugambi, M.: Electrocardiographic changes during treatment of leishmaniasis with pentavalent antimony (sodium stibogluconate). Am. J. Trop. Med. Hyg. *34*:702, 1985.

708. Winship, K. A.: Toxicity of antimony and its compounds. Adverse Drug React. Acute Poisoning Rev. *6*:67, 1987.

709. Brady, H. R., and Horgan, J. H.: Lithium and the heart: Unanswered questions. Chest *93*:166, 1988.

710. James, F. W., Kaplan, S., and Benzig, G., 3rd: Cardiac complications following hydrocarbon ingestion. Am. J. Dis. Child. *121*:431, 1971.

711. Cunningham, S. R., Dalzell, G. W. N., McGirr, P., and Khan, M. M.: Myocardial infarction and primary ventricular fibrillation after glue sniffing. Br. Med. J. *294*:739, 1987.

712. Scott, I., Parkes, R., and Cameron, D. P.: Phaeochromocytoma and cardiomyopathy. Med. J. Austr. *148*:94, 1988.

713. Ferry, D. R., Henry, R. L., and Kern, M. J.: Epinephrine-induced myocardial infarction in a patient with angiographically normal coronary arteries. Am. Heart J. *111*:1193, 1986.

714. Nino, A. F., Berman, M. M., Gluck, E. H., et al.: Drug-induced left ventricular failure in patients with pulmonary disease: Endomyocardial biopsy demonstration of catecholamine myocarditis. Chest *92*:732, 1987.

715. Rona, G.: Catecholamine cardiotoxicity. J. Mol. Cell. Cardiol. *17*:291, 1985.

716. Panagia, V., Pierce, G. N., Dhalla, K. S., et al.: Adaptive changes in subcellular calcium transport during catecholamine-induced cardiomyopathy. J. Mol. Cell. Cardiol. *17*:411, 1985.

717. Downing, S. E., and Lee, J. C.: Contribution of alpha-adrenoceptor activation to the pathogenesis of norepinephrine cardiomyopathy. Circ. Res. *52*:471, 1983.

718. Opie, L. H., Walpoth, B., and Barsacchi, R.: Calcium and catecholamines: Relevance to cardiomyopathies and significance in therapeutic strategies. J. Mol. Cell. Cardiol. *17*:21, 1985.

719. Kopp, S. J., Barron, J. T., and Tow, J. P.: Cardiovascular actions of lead and relationship to hypertension: A review. Environ. Hlth. Perspec. *78*:91, 1988.

720. Kurppa, K., Hietanen, E., Klockars, M., et al.: Chemical exposures at work and cardiovascular morbidity. Atherosclerosis, ischemic heart disease, hypertension, cardiomyopathy and arrhythmias. Scand. J. Work Environ. Hlth. *10*:381, 1984.

721. Penney, D. G.: A review: Hemodynamic response to carbon monoxide. Environ. Hlth. Perspec. *77*:121, 1988.

722. McMeekin, J. D., and Finegan, B. A.: Reversible myocardial dysfunction following carbon monoxide poisoning. Can. J. Cardiol. *3*:118, 1987.

723. Marius-Nunez, A. L.: Myocardial infarction with normal coronary arteries after acute exposure to carbon monoxide. Chest *97*:491, 1990.

724. Levine, S. N., and Rheams, C. N.: Hypocalcemic heart failure. Am. J. Med. *78*:1033, 1985.

725. Rimailho, A., Bouchard, P., Schaison, G., et al.: Improvement of hypocalcemic cardiomyopathy by correction of serum calcium level. Am. Heart J. *109*:611, 1985.

726. Bashour, T. T., Ryan, C., Kabbani, S. S., and Crew, J.: Hypocalcemic acute

myocardial failure secondary to rapid transfusion of citrated blood. Am. Heart J. *108*:1040, 1984.

727. Feldman, A. M., Fivush, B., Zahka, K. G., et al.: Congestive cardiomyopathy in patients on continuous ambulatory peritoneal dialysis. Am. J. Kidney Dis. *11*:76, 1988.

728. Berkelhammer, C., and Bear, R. A.: A clinical approach to common electrolyte problems: 3. Hypophosphatemia. Can. Med. Assoc. J. *130*:17, 1984.

729. Venditti, F. J., Marotta, C., Panezai, F. R., et al.: Hypophosphatemia and cardiac arrhythmias. Mineral Electrolyte Metab. *13*:19, 1987.

730. Berkelhammer, C., and Bear, R. A.: A clinical approach to common electrolyte problems: 4. Hypomagnesemia. Can. Med. Assoc. J. *132*:360, 1985.

731. Seelig, M.: Cardiovascular consequences of magnesium deficiency and loss: Pathogenesis, prevalence and manifestations—magnesium and chloride loss in refractory potassium repletion. Am. J. Cardiol. *63*:4G, 1989.

732. Pion, P. D., Kittleson, M. D., Rogers, Q. R., and Morris, J. G.: Myocardial failure in cats associated with low plasma taurine: A reversible cardiomyopathy. Science *237*:764, 1987.

733. Tenaglia, A., and Cody, R.: Evidence for a taurine-deficiency cardiomyopathy. Am. J. Cardiol. *62*:136, 1988.

734. Carnitine deficiency (unsigned editorial). Lancet *335*:631, 1990.

735. Rodrigues Pereira, R., Scholte, H. R., Luyt-Houwen, I. E. M., and Vaandrager-Verduin, M. H. M.: Cardiomyopathy associated with carnitine loss in kidneys and small intestines. Eur. J. Pediatr. *148*:193, 1988.

736. Bautista, J., Rafel, E., Martinez, A., et al.: Familial hypertrophic cardiomyopathy and muscle carnitine deficiency. Muscle Nerve *13*:192, 1990.

737. Ino, T., Sherwood, W. G., Benson, L. N., et al.: Cardiac manifestations in disorders of fat and carnitine metabolism in infancy. J. Am. Coll. Cardiol. *11*:1301, 1988.

738. Taillard, F., Mundler, O., Tillous-Borde, I., et al.: Value of radionuclide assessment with thallium 201 scintigraphy in carnitine deficiency cardiomyopathy. Eur. Heart J. *9*:811, 1988.

739. Yang, G., Ge, K., Chen, J., and Chen, X.: Selenium-related endemic disease and the daily selenium requirement of humans. Wld. Rev. Nutr. Diet. *55*:98, 1988.

740. Reeves, W. C., Marcuard, S. P., Willis, S. E., and Movahed, A.: Reversible cardiomyopathy due to selenium deficiency. J. Parenter. Enteral Nutr. *13*:663, 1989.

741. Santhanakrishnan, B. R., and Gajalakshmi, B. S.: Pathogenesis of cardiovascular complications in children following scorpion envenoming. Ann. Trop. Paediatr. *6*:117, 1986.

742. Murthy, K.R.K., Zolfagharian, H., Medh, J. D., et al.: Disseminated intravascular coagulation and disturbances in carbohydrate and fat metabolism in acute myocarditis produced by scorpion (*Buthus tamulus*) venom. Indian J. Med. Res. *87*:318, 1988.

743. Brand, A., Keren, A., Kerem, E., et al.: Myocardial damage after a scorpion sting: Long-term echocardiographic follow-up. Pediatr. Cardiol. *9*:59, 1988.

744. Murthy, K.R.K., Vakil, A. E., Yeolekar, M. E., and Vakil, Y. E.: Reversal of metabolic and electrocardiographic changes induced by Indian redscorpion (*Buthus tamulus*) venom by administration of insulin, alpha blocker and sodium bicarbonate. Indian J. Med. Res. *88*:450, 1988.

745. Murthy, K.R.K., Billimoria, F. R., Khopkar, M., and Dave, K. N.: Acute hyperglycaemia and hyperkalaemia in acute myocarditis produced by scorpion (*Buthus tamulus*) venom injection in dogs. Indian Heart J. *38*:71, 1986.

746. Sinha, A. K.: Cardiovascular manifestations of scorpion sting in a case of congenital complete atrioventricular block. J. Indian Med. Assoc. *87*:237, 1989.

746a. Amaral, C.F.S., Lopes, J. A., Magalhaes, R. A., and de Rezende, N. A.: Electrocardiographic, enzymatic and echocardiographic evidence of myocardial damage after *Tityus serrulatus* scorpion poisoning. Am. J. Cardiol. *67*:655, 1991.

747. Amitai, Y., Mines, Y., Aker, M., and Goitein, K.: Scorpion sting in children. A review of 51 cases. Clin. Pediatr. *24*:136, 1985.

748. Jones, E., and Joy, M.: Acute myocardial infarction after a wasp sting. Br. Heart J. *59*:506, 1988.

749. Moore, R. S.: Second-degree heart block associated with envenomation by *Vipera berus*. Arch. Emerg. Med. *5*:116, 1988.

750. Burch, J. M., Agarwal, R., Mattox, K. L., et al.: The treatment of crotalid envenomation without antivenin. J. Trauma *28*:35, 1988.

751. Weiser, E., Wollberg, Z., Kochva, E., and Lee, S. Y.: Cardiotoxic effects of the venom of the burrowing asp, *Atractaspis engaddensis* (*Atractaspididae, Ophidia*). Toxicon *22*:767, 1984.

752. Lee, S. Y., Lee, C. Y., Chen, Y. M., and Kochva, E.: Coronary vasospasm as the primary cause of death due to the venom of the burrowing asp, *Atractaspis engaddensis*. Toxicon *24*:285, 1986.

753. Tibballs, J., Sutherland, S., and Kerr, S.: Studies on Australian snake venoms. Part 1: The haemodynamic effects of brown snake (*Pseudonaja*) species in the dog. Anaesth. Intensive Care *17*:466, 1989.

754. Than-Than, Francis, N., Tin-Nu-Swe, et al.: Contribution of focal haemorrhage and microvascular fibrin deposition to fatal envenoming by Russell's viper (*Vipera russelli siamensis*) in Burma. Acta Trop. *46*:23, 1989.

755. Zaloga, G. P., Deal, J., Spurling, T., et al.: Unusual manifestations of arsenic intoxication. Am. J. Med. Sci. *289*:210, 1985.

756. Hall, J. C., and Harruff, R.: Fatal cardiac arrhythmia in a patient with interstitial myocarditis related to chronic arsenic poisoning. South Med. J. *82*:1557, 1989.

757. Kantrowitz, N. E., and Bristow, M. R.: Cardiotoxicity of antitumor agents. Prog. Cardiovasc. Dis. *27*:195, 1984.

758. Cazin, B., Gorin, N. C., Laporte, J. P., et al.: Cardiac complications after bone marrow transplantation. A report on a series of 63 consecutive transplantations. Cancer *57*:2061, 1986.

759. Judge, K. W., and Ward, N. E.: Fatal azide-induced cardiomyopathy presenting as acute myocardial infarction. Am. J. Cardiol. *64*:830, 1989.

760. Wakeel, R. A., Davies, H. T., and Williams, J. D.: Toxic myocarditis in paracetamol poisoning. Br. Med. J. *295*:1097, 1987.

761. Patel, B., Kloner, R. A., Ensley, J., et al.: 5-Fluorouracil cardiotoxicity: Left ventricular dysfunction and effect of coronary vasodilators. Am. J. Med. Sci. *294*:238, 1987.

762. McKendall, G. R., Shurman, A., Anamur, M., and Most, A. S.: Toxic cardiogenic shock associated with infusion of 5-fluorouracil. Am. Heart J. *118*:184, 1989.

763. Martin, M., Diaz-Rubio, E., Furio, V., et al.: Lethal cardiac toxicity after cisplatin and 5-fluorouracil chemotherapy. Report of a case with necropsy study. Am. J. Clin. Oncol. *12*:229, 1989.

764. Ensley, J. F., Patel, B., Kloner, R., et al.: The clinical syndrome of 5-fluorouracil cardiotoxicity. Invest. New Drugs *7*:101, 1989.

765. Kounis, N. G., Zavras, G. M., Soufras, G. D., and Kitrou, M. P.: Hypersensitivity myocarditis. Ann. Allergy *62*:71, 1989.

766. Markus, C. K., Chow, L. H., Wycoff, D. M., and McManus, B. M.: Pet food-derived penicillin residue as a potential cause of hypersensitivity myocarditis and sudden death. Am. J. Cardiol. *63*:1154, 1989.

767. Taliercio, C. P., Olney, B. A., and Lie, J. T.: Myocarditis related to drug hypersensitivity. Mayo Clin. Proc. *60*:463, 1985.

768. Sadjadi, S. A., Leghari, R. U., and Berger, A. R.: Prolongation of the PR interval induced by methyldopa. Am. J. Cardiol. *54*:675, 1984.

769. Bristow, M. R. (ed.): Drug-Induced Heart Disease. Amsterdam, Elsevier Press, 1980, p. 476.

770. Nariman, S.: Adverse reactions to drugs used in the treatment of tuberculosis. Adv. Drug React. Acute Poison. Rev. *7*:207, 1988.

771. Humbert, P., Faivre, R., Fellman, D., et al.: Giant cell myocarditis: An autoimmune disease? Am. Heart J. *115*:485, 1988.

772. Wilson, M. S., Barth, R. F., Baker, P. B., et al.: Giant cell myocarditis. Am. J. Med. *79*:647, 1985.

772a. Davidoff, R., Palacios, I., Southern, J., et al.: Giant cell versus lymphocytic myocarditis: A comparison of their clinical features and long-term outcomes. Circulation *83*:953, 1991.

773. McKeon, J., Haagsma, B., Bett, J. H. N., and Boyle, C. M.: Fatal giant cell myocarditis after colectomy for ulcerative colitis. Am. Heart J. *111*:1208, 1986.

774. Rabson, A. B., Schoen, F. J., Warhol, M. J., et al.: Giant cell myocarditis after mitral valve replacement: Case report and studies of the nature of giant cells. Hum. Pathol. *15*:585, 1984.

775. McFalls, E. O., Hosenpud, J. D., McAnulty, J. H., et al.: Granulomatous myocarditis. Diagnosis by endomyocardial biopsy and response to corticosteroids in two patients. Chest *89*:509, 1986.

776. Zahger, D., Moses, A., and Weiss, A. T.: Evidence of prolonged myocardial dysfunction in heat stroke. Chest *95*:1089, 1989.

777. Bashour, T. T., Gualberto, A., and Ryan, C.: Atrioventricular block in accidental hypothermia—a case report. Angiology *40*:63, 1989.

778. Solomon, A., Barish, R. A., Browne, B., and Tso, E.: The electrocardiographic features of hypothermia. J. Emerg. Med. *7*:169, 1989.

779. Ikaheimo, M. J., Niemela, K. O., Linnaluoto, M. M., et al.: Early cardiac changes related to radiation therapy. Am. J. Cardiol. *56*:943, 1985.

779a. Carlson, R. G., Mayfield, W. R., Normann, S., and Alexander, J. A.: Radiation-associated valvular disease. Chest *99*:538, 1991.

780. Handle, C. E., Livesey, S., and Lawton, P. A.: Coronary ostial stenosis after radiotherapy: Angioplasty or coronary artery surgery? Br. Heart J. *61*:208, 1989.

781. McEniery, P. T., Dorosti, K., Schiavone, W. A., et al.: Clinical and angiographic features of coronary artery disease after chest irradiation. Am. J. Cardiol. *60*:1020, 1987.

782. Pohjola-Sintonen, S., Totterman, K-J., Salmo, M., and Siltanen, P.: Late cardiac effects of mediastinal radiotherapy in patients with Hodgkin's disease. Cancer *60*:31, 1987.

783. Katayama, T., Irita, A., and Honda, Y.: Pure infundibular pulmonary stenosis induced by radiation therapy—a case report. Angiology *39*:843, 1988.

784. Joensuu, H.: Acute myocardial infarction after heart irradiation in young patients with Hodgkin's disease. Chest *95*:388, 1989.

785. Radwaner, B. A., Geringer, R., Goldmann, A. M. et al.: Left main coronary artery stenosis following mediastinal irradiation. Am. J. Med. *82*:1017, 1987.

786. Joensuu, H., Irjala, K., and Asola, R.: Serum creatine kinase and lactate dehydrogenase during cardiac irradiation. Acta Med. Scand. *222*:247, 1987.

787. Gottdiener, J. S., Katin, M. J., Borer, J. S., et al.: Late cardiac effects of therapeutic mediastinal irradiation. Assessment by echocardiography and radionuclide angiography. N. Engl. J. Med. *308*:569, 1983.

Primary Tumors of the Heart
by WILSON S. COLUCCI, M.D., and EUGENE BRAUNWALD, M.D.

"A diagnosis is easy as long as you think of it."
SOMA WEISS

The incidence of *primary* tumors of the heart* in autopsy series ranges from 0.0017 to 0.28 per cent.[1-5] Thus, these tumors are far less common than metastatic tumors to the heart.[6] The diagnosis is further complicated by the fact that the most common cardiac tumor, myxoma, causes a variety of nonspecific clinical signs and symptoms that often masquerade as many other more common cardiovascular and systemic diseases (Table 44–1). Prior to the advent of modern cardiopulmonary bypass surgical techniques, the correct antemortem diagnosis of an intracardiac tumor was largely academic, since effective therapy was not possible. However, now that many cardiac tumors are curable by operation, it is critically important to establish this diagnosis whenever possible. During the last decade, major advances in noninvasive cardiovascular diagnostic techniques have greatly facilitated this task, and it is now possible safely and readily to screen patients suspected of having a cardiac tumor, in many cases arriving at a definitive diagnosis preoperatively. Nevertheless, a high index of suspicion remains the most important element in diagnosing a cardiac tumor.

HISTORICAL PERSPECTIVE

Although primary tumors of the heart have been recognized since at least as early as the sixteenth century,[7] a correct antemortem diagnosis was not recorded until 1934.[8] The modern era of diagnosis began with the development of angiography, which permitted the visualization of cardiac tumors during life, and, in 1952, Goldberg et al. reported the first angiographic diagnosis of a left atrial myxoma.[9]

Before the development of modern open-heart surgical techniques, there were only rare reports of the successful removal of cardiac tumors, most on the epicardial surface. Prior to the use of cardiopulmonary bypass, most attempts to remove intracardiac tumors were unsuccessful. In 1954, Crafoord performed the first successful excision of an intracardiac tumor, a left atrial myxoma, utilizing total cardiopulmonary bypass under direct vision.[10] The successful surgical excision of a wide variety of cardiac tumors is now possible, and in many instances a complete cure has been achieved.[11,12]

Advances in the field of noninvasive cardiovascular diagnosis have had a major impact on the ability of physicians to recognize cardiac tumors antemortem. A cardiac tumor was first demonstrated by M-mode echocardiography in 1959[13] and, subsequently, echocardiography has become the cornerstone of the noninvasive diagnosis of cardiac tumors. Two-dimensional echocardiography has proved to be even more useful.[14]

---

* Tumors arising elsewhere in the body and metastasizing to the pericardium and heart are discussed in Chap. 45 (Pericardial Disease) and Chap. 57 (Hematologic-Oncologic Disorders and Heart Disease).

Newer diagnostic methods, including radionuclide gated blood pool scanning,[15] digital subtraction angiography, often employing intravenous injection of contrast medium,[16] computed tomography (p. 318),[17] magnetic resonance imaging (p. 328),[18-21] and transesophageal echocardiography[22,23] have been shown to be of value in the diagnosis of cardiac tumors. Magnetic resonance imaging and transesophageal echocardiography may be particularly effective for the precise anatomical characterization of cardiac tumors that are not adequately defined by transthoracic two-dimensional echocardiography. Not surprisingly, the widespread use of echocardiography, as well as some of the newer noninvasive methods, has resulted in a substantial increase in the detection of patients with primary cardiac tumors, many of whom are asymptomatic. Thus, during the past quarter century it has become possible to diagnose and successfully treat the majority of primary cardiac tumors. An appreciation of the clinical features, therefore, is now of far greater importance than heretofore.

CLINICAL PRESENTATION
(Table 44–1)

SYSTEMIC FINDINGS. Cardiac tumors, particularly cardiac myxoma, can produce a broad array of systemic (i.e., noncardiac) findings including fever, cachexia, malaise, arthralgias, Raynaud's phenomenon, rash, clubbing, and episodic bizarre behavior,[24-26] as well as systemic and pulmonary emboli. A variety of laboratory findings has been reported, including hypergammaglobulinemia, an elevated erythrocyte sedimentation rate, thrombocytosis, thrombocytopenia, polycythemia, leukocytosis, and anemia.[24-28] The mechanism by which cardiac tumors cause these systemic manifestations is not known with certainty, but it has been attributed to secretory products of the tumor or to tumor necrosis.

A markedly elevated serum level of interleukin-6 (IL-6), a cytokine implicated in a variety of autoimmune diseases, was observed in a patient with a cardiac myxoma associated with immunologic features. Serum IL-6 levels became undetectable and the immunological features resolved upon removal of the tumor.[29] Increased titers of antibodies to myocardium[30] and neutrophils[31] have also been found in patients with myxoma and were shown to fall after removal of the tumor. A case of multiple myeloma has been attributed to continuous immunological stimulation by a left atrial myxoma.[32] A patient with generalized amyloidosis and cardiac myxoma was found to have an elevated serum level of SAA protein, a serum precursor of AA amyloid.[33] As in the case of autoantibodies associated with myxoma, the level of SAA protein fell markedly after removal of the tumor.[33] Because the cardiac findings are

TABLE 44–1   SYMPTOMS AND SIGNS OF CARDIAC MYXOMA

SYMPTOMS	INCIDENCE %
Dyspnea on exertion	>75
Paroxysmal dyspnea	~25
Fever	~50
Weight loss	~25
Severe dizziness/syncope	~20
Sudden death	~15
Hemoptysis	~15

SIGNS	INCIDENCE %
Mitral diastolic murmur	~75
Mitral systolic murmur	~50
Pulmonary hypertension	~70
Right heart failure	~70
Pulmonary emboli	~25
Anemia	>33
Elevated ESR	>33
Third heart sound (tumor plop)	>33
Atrial fibrillation	~15
Elevated globulins	~10
Clubbing	~5
Raynaud's phenomenon	<5

ESR = Erythrocyte sedimentation rate.
From Fisher, J.: Cardiac myxoma. Cardiovasc. Rev. Rep. 9:1195, 1983.

nonspecific and may be subtle or absent, it is not unusual for these systemic findings to lead to a diagnosis of collagen vascular disease, infection, or noncardiac malignant disease.[34-36] Rarely, myxomas may be superinfected by bacteria or fungi.[37,38]

EMBOLIC PHENOMENA. The embolization of tumor fragments or of thrombi from the surface of a tumor is a frequent and often dramatic clinical occurrence.[39-48] Although myxomas are the source of most tumor emboli because of the combination of their friable consistency and intracavitary location, other types of cardiac tumors occasionally may embolize.

The distribution of tumor emboli depends upon the location of the tumor and the presence or absence of intracardiac shunts. Left-sided tumors embolize to the systemic circulation, resulting in infarction and hemorrhage of viscera, including the heart[46] as well as peripheral limb ischemia and vascular aneurysms.[26,34,40,41,45,47] The diagnosis of an intracardiac tumor may be made after histological examination of systemic embolic material,[39,40,42,49] and therefore it is of critical importance to make every effort to recover and examine embolic material. In some cases, particularly when petechiae are present, biopsy of skin or muscle[26,50] may demonstrate intravascular tumor emboli.

Multiple systemic emboli may mimic systemic vasculitis[26,34,35] or infective endocarditis, especially when associated with other manifestations of a systemic illness such as fever, weight loss, arthralgias, elevated erythrocyte sedimentation rate, and elevated serum gamma globulins. The finding at angiography of multiple vascular aneurysms secondary to tumor emboli in the cerebral, renal, femoral, and coronary arteries is not infrequent,[45,51] and may lead to the mistaken diagnosis of polyarteritis nodosa.[34] The neurological consequences of embolization include transient ischemic attacks, seizures, syncope, and cerebral, cerebellar, brain stem, spinal cord, or retinal infarction.[41,45,47,52] The neurological event may occasionally be the first or only clinical manifestation of a cardiac tumor. An embolic stroke in a young person without evidence of cerebrovascular disease, particularly in the presence of sinus rhythm, should raise the possibility of intracardiac myxoma, as well as infective endocarditis (p. 1078) and prolapse of the mitral valve (p. 1029).

Right-sided cardiac tumors, and left-sided cardiac tumors proximal to left-to-right intracardiac shunts, may result in pulmonary emboli.[43,44,53] Indeed, serious pulmonary hypertension and secondary cor pulmonale due to chronic recurrent pulmonary emboli from a right atrial myxoma have been noted.[44] Clinically, the findings may be indistinguishable from pulmonary emboli secondary to venous thromboembolism (p. 1559). Although the findings on chest roentgenogram are nonspecific, perfusion lung scanning in such patients may be atypical of pulmonary embolism in two respects: (1) The tumor-produced perfusion defects may remain static for long periods, as opposed to typical pulmonary embolic disease in which the defects usually resolve over the course of a few weeks; and (2) there may be complete absence of flow to one lung in the presence of completely normal perfusion of the opposite lung, a pattern unusual with typical pulmonary emboli.

CARDIAC MANIFESTATIONS

The specific signs and symptoms produced by tumors are more closely related to their precise anatomical location than to their histological types.[54] Thus, it is useful to consider the constellation of findings which is typical of each location. The presentation of *pericardial tumors* is considered on page 1506 and will not be discussed here except to point out that primary tumors of the myocardium and endocardium may extend into the pericardial space and produce many of the clinical manifestations of pericardial tumors, including hemorrhagic pericardial effusion and compression of the heart by the effusion or the tumor itself.

MYOCARDIAL TUMORS. When clinically apparent, myocardial tumors most commonly result in disturbances of conduction or rhythm,[55,56] the precise nature of which is determined by the location of the tumor. Thus, tumors in the area of the atrioventricular node, typically angiomas and mesotheliomas, may produce atrioventricular (AV) conduction disturbances, including complete heart block and asystole, and can lead to sudden death.[55,56] A wide variety of arrhythmias may be produced, including atrial fibrillation or flutter, paroxysmal atrial tachycardia with or without block, nodal rhythm, ventricular premature beats, ventricular tachycardia and ventricular fibrillation.[54,57] Intramural tumors may also produce symptoms by virtue of their size and location. Impairment of ventricular performance may simulate congestive, restrictive, or hypertrophic cardiomyopathy (Chap. 43). Tumor infiltration of the myocardial wall occasionally causes myocardial rupture.[58]

LEFT ATRIAL TUMORS. Mobile, pedunculated, left atrial tumors (Fig. 44–1) may prolapse to variable degrees into the mitral valve orifice, resulting in obstruction to atrioventricular blood flow and, frequently, mitral regurgitation. The resultant signs and symptoms often mimic those of mitral valve disease[54,59] (Table 44–2), especially mitral stenosis (Chap. 34)[59a] and include dyspnea, orthopnea, paroxysmal nocturnal dyspnea, acute pulmonary edema, cough, hemoptysis, chest pain, peripheral edema, and fatigue. However, weight loss, pallor, syncope, and sudden death—manifestations uncommon for mitral valve disease—also occur. It is not unusual for the symptoms to be sudden in onset, intermittent, and related to the patient's body position.[54,59] Although the majority of symptoms produced by left atrial tumors are nonspecific, the occurrence of paroxysmal symptoms that arise characteristically in a particular body position and are out of proportion to the clinical findings should raise the possibility of a left atrial tumor. The most common primary cardiac tumor presenting in the left atrium is the benign myxoma, the large majority of which are solitary (p. 1454).

Physical examination may disclose signs of pulmonary congestion, an S_4, a loud S_1 which is often widely split, a holosystolic murmur which is loudest at the apex and resembles mitral regurgitation, and a diastolic murmur resulting from obstruction to flow through the mitral orifice produced by the tumor. The loud S_1 that occurs in patients with left atrial myxoma may be due to the late onset of mitral valve closure resulting from prolapse of the tumor through the mitral valve orifice.[60] Consequently the left ventricular–left atrial pressure crossover occurs at a higher pressure, as in patients with mitral stenosis or a short P-R interval. It has been suggested

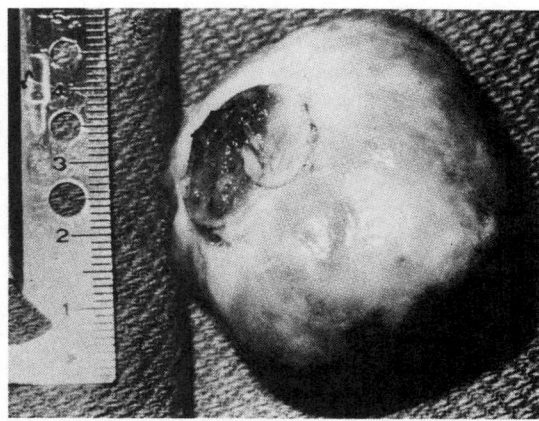

FIGURE 44-1. Gross pathological specimen of a left atrial myxoma removed at operation. The myxoma had a smooth, glistening capsule and measured approximately 5 cm in diameter. By two-dimensional echocardiography, the tumor was seen to prolapse into the left ventricle during diastole. (From Salcedo, E. E., et al.: Echocardiographic findings in 25 patients with left atrial myxoma. Reprinted by permission of the American College of Cardiology. J. Am. Coll. Cardiol. *1*:1162, 1983.)

that the finding of a loud S_1 in the absence of a short P-R interval or a mitral diastolic murmur should raise the suspicion of a left atrial tumor.[60] In many cases an early diastolic sound, termed a tumor plop, can be identified. It is thought to be produced as the tumor strikes the endocardial wall or as its excursion is abruptly halted. Although in most cases the tumor plop occurs later than the opening snap of the mitral valve and earlier than the S_3, it is not surprising that this sound is frequently confused with the opening snap or the S_3.

RIGHT ATRIAL TUMORS. Right atrial tumors frequently produce symptoms of right heart failure, including fatigue, peripheral edema, ascites, hepatomegaly, and prominent a waves in the jugular venous pulse.[53,54] The average time interval from the symptomatic presentation to the correct diagnosis of right atrial tumor may be years. The development of right heart failure may be rapidly progressive and is often associated with new systolic or diastolic murmurs or both. The murmurs are generally the result of tumor obstruction to tricuspid valve flow or of tricuspid regurgitation caused by tumor interference with valve closure or valve destruction caused directly or indirectly by the tumor.[62] It is not surprising that right atrial tumors have been misdiagnosed as Ebstein's anomaly of the tricuspid valve, constrictive pericarditis, tricuspid stenosis, carcinoid syndrome, superior vena caval syndrome, and cardiomyopathy (Table 44-2). Pulmonary embolism and pulmonary hypertension occur and may simulate classic thromboembolic disease.[44,53] Right atrial hypertension may cause right-to-left shunting through a patent foramen ovale, with systemic hypoxia, cyanosis, clubbing, and polycythemia.[63] Whereas myxomas occur much more commonly in the left atrium than the right atrium, sarcomas occur more commonly in the right atrium.[53]

Physical examination may reveal peripheral edema, evidence of superior vena caval obstruction, hepatomegaly, and ascites. An early diastolic rumbling murmur, alone or in combination with a holosystolic murmur secondary to tricuspid regurgitation, may demonstrate respiratory or positional variation. Because of the rarity of *isolated* rheumatic tricuspid valvular disease, the lack of other valvular findings should raise the question of a right atrial tumor. A protodiastolic tumor plop has been described and is thought to be similar in etiology to that produced by the left atrial tumors.[64] The jugular venous pressure may be elevated, and a prominent a wave and steep y descent may be present.

RIGHT VENTRICULAR TUMORS. Right ventricular tumors often present with right heart failure as a result of obstruction to right ventricular filling or outflow. Clinical manifestations include peripheral edema, hepatomegaly, ascites, shortness of breath, syncope, and sudden death.

A systolic ejection murmur at the left sternal border is usually found on physical examination. A presystolic murmur and a diastolic rumble[54] have been noted and are thought to be due to obstruction of the tricuspid valve. An S_3 may be audible, and a low-pitched diastolic sound that coincides with the maximal anterior excursion of the tumor has been ascribed either to tumor or to late closure of the pulmonary valve.[65] P_2 is often delayed, and its intensity may be normal, decreased, or increased. Tumor emboli to the pulmonary arteries may result in pulmonary hypertension, and the presence of tumor in the pulmonic valve orifice may lead to pulmonary regurgitation. The jugular veins are frequently distended with a prominent a wave and may demonstrate Kussmaul's sign (p. 19).

The cardiac findings often lead to a diagnosis of pulmonic stenosis, restrictive cardiomyopathy, or tricuspid regurgitation. Whereas pulmonic stenosis is often asymptomatic and slowly progressive, the symptoms of right ventricular tumors are often rapidly progressive, and there is no poststenotic dilatation or systolic ejection click.

LEFT VENTRICULAR TUMORS. When left ventricular tumors are predominantly intramural in location, they are often asymptomatic, or they may present as conduction disturbances, arrhythmias, or they may interfere with ventricular function. However, when the tumor also has a significant intracavitary component, there may be obstruction to left ventricular outflow, resulting in syncope and findings consistent with left ventricular failure. Atypical chest pain has also been reported and in some cases may reflect obstruction of a coronary artery either directly by tumor involvement or as a result of a tumor embolus to the coronary artery.

On physical examination a systolic murmur may be noted, and both the murmur and the blood pressure may vary with position. Left ventricular tumors may simulate the findings of aortic stenosis, subaortic stenosis, hypertrophic cardiomyopathy endocardial fibroelastosis, and coronary artery disease.

TABLE 44-2 CONDITIONS OFTEN CONFUSED WITH ATRIAL MYXOMA

Left atrium
Rheumatic mitral valve disease (MS, MR)
Pulmonary hypertension (primary, or secondary to mitral valve disease or LV failure)
Intrinsic lung disease
Cerebrovascular disease (CVA, TIA)
Endocarditis
Rheumatic fever
Myocarditis
Vasculitis (polyarteritis, lupus erythematosus)

Right atrium
Rheumatic tricuspid valve disease (TS, TR)
Ebstein's anomaly
Atrial septal defect
Pulmonary hypertension
Pulmonary emboli
Constrictive pericarditis
Pleuropericarditis (rub)
Carcinoid heart disease
Cardiomyopathy

Right ventricle
Pulmonic stenosis
Infundibular stenosis
Pulmonary emboli
Pulmonary hypertension

Left ventricle
Aortic stenosis
Subaortic stenosis
Cerebrovascular disease
Mural thrombus

MS = mitral stenosis; MR = mitral regurgitation; LV = left ventricular; CVA = cerebrovascular accident; TIA = transient ischemic attack; TS = tricuspid stenosis; TR = tricuspid regurgitation.
From Fisher, J.: Cardiac myxoma. Cardiovasc. Rev. Rep. 9:1195, 1983.

TABLE 44-3 RELATIVE INCIDENCE OF TUMORS OF THE HEART

TYPE	NUMBER	PER CENT
Benign		
Myxoma	130	30.5
Lipoma	45	10.5
Papillary fibroelastoma	42	9.9
Rhabdomyoma	36	8.5
Fibroma	17	4.0
Hemangioma	15	3.5
Teratoma	14	3.3
Mesothelioma of the AV node	12	2.8
Granular cell tumor	3	—
Neurofibroma	3	—
Lymphangioma	2	—
Subtotal	319	75.1
Malignant		
Angiosarcoma	39	9.2
Rhabdomyosarcoma	26	6.1
Fibrosarcoma	14	3.3
Malignant lymphoma	7	1.6
Extraskeletal osteosarcoma	5	—
Neurogenic sarcoma	4	—
Malignant teratoma	4	—
Thymoma	4	—
Leiomyosarcoma	1	—
Liposarcoma	1	—
Synovial sarcoma	1	—
Subtotal	106	24.9
TOTAL	425	100.0

Modified from McAllister, H. A., and Fenoglio, J. J.: Tumors of the cardio-vascular system. *In* Atlas of Tumor Pathology. Washington, D.C., Armed Forces Institute of Pathology, 1978. Fasc. 15, 2nd series.

BENIGN VERSUS MALIGNANT TUMORS

The types of benign and malignant mesenchymal tumors that may develop in the heart are typical of those occurring in any mass of striated muscle and connective tissue (Table 44-3). Although the exact incidence of each specific tumor type cannot be stated, about 75 per cent of all cardiac tumors are benign histologically and the remainder are malignant.[3,4] The majority of benign cardiac tumors are myxomas, followed in frequency by a wide variety of other tumors (Table 44-3). Almost all malignant cardiac tumors are sarcomas, and of these the angiosarcoma and rhabdomyosarcoma are the most common forms.

Although it is often difficult or impossible to differentiate histologically benign from malignant tumors prior to operation, certain findings may be helpful. Characteristics suggestive of malignancy include the presence of distant metastases, local mediastinal invasion, evidence of rapid growth in tumor size, hemorrhagic pericardial effusion, precordial pain, location of the tumor on the right side of the heart or on the atrial free wall, evidence of combined intramural and intracavitary location, and extension into the pulmonary veins. Benign tumors are more likely to occur on the left side of the inter-atrial septum and to grow slowly. Although benign tumors do not metastasize, distant tumor emboli may mimic peripheral or pulmonary metastases.[48] The preoperative differentiation between benign and malignant tumors may occasionally be made by examination of peripheral tumor emboli recovered by arteriotomy or by biopsy of skin or muscle.[39,40,42,48,49]

BENIGN CARDIAC TUMORS

Myxomas

As already pointed out, myxomas are the most common type of primary cardiac tumor, comprising 30 to 50 per cent of the total in most pathological series.[3,4,66] Ninety-three per cent of myxomas have been reported to occur sporadically.[67,68] The mean age of patients with sporadic myxoma is 56 years, and 70

per cent are females.[69] However, myxomas have been described in patients ranging in age from 3 to 83 years and are now not infrequently diagnosed in elderly patients in whom the symptoms and signs of cardiac tumor may have been attributed to other causes for a substantial time.[69] Approximately 86 per cent of myxomas occur in the left atrium, and over 90 per cent are solitary.[69] In the left atrium, the usual site of attachment is in the area of the fossa ovalis. Myxomas also may occur in the right atrium, and less often still, in the right or left ventricle. Multiple tumors may occur in the same chamber or in a combination of chambers.[69] Although myxomas may occasionally be found on the posterior left atrial wall, tumors presenting in this location should raise the suspicion of malignancy. Myxomas of the mitral valve have been reported.[70]

The clinical signs and symptoms produced by cardiac myxomas include nonspecific manifestations as just discussed, embolization, and mechanical interference with cardiac function (Table 44-1). Not surprisingly, the symptoms produced by cardiac myxomas may simulate a wide variety of other cardiac and noncardiac conditions (Table 44-2). The clinical presentation of cardiac myxomas in 130 patients reviewed at the Armed Forces Institute of Pathology is summarized in Table 44-4.

FAMILIAL MYXOMAS. These tumors may be familial, and if so, they appear to be transmitted in an autosomal dominant manner.[67,68] In addition, some patients with myxoma may have a syndrome that involves a complex of abnormalities including lentigines or pigmented nevi or both (Fig. 44-2), primary nodular adrenal cortical disease with or without Cushing's syndrome, myxomatous mammary fibroadenomas, testicular tumors, and pituitary adenomas with gigantism or acromegaly[71-77] (Fig. 44-3). Patients may have two or more components of this complex, and generally the first component is diagnosed at a relatively young age (mean age, 18

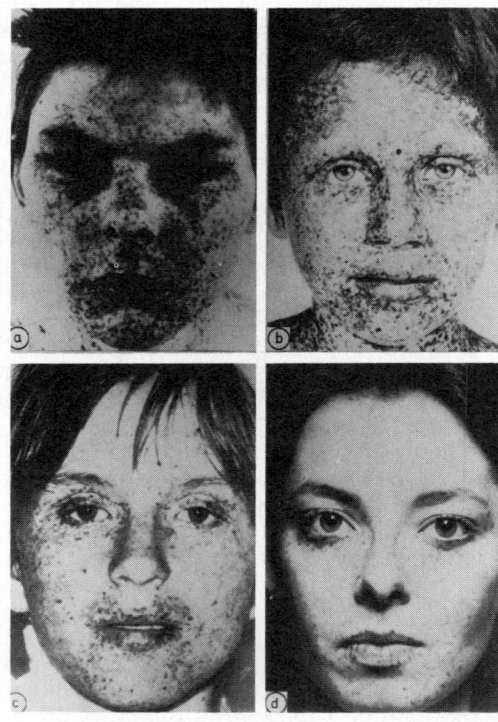

FIGURE 44-2. Four patients with extensive facial freckling, a finding that is associated with "syndrome myxoma." Patients with this syndrome tend to be younger than patients with sporadic myxoma and have a substantially higher incidence of ventricular, multiple, biatrial, recurrent, and familial myxomas of the heart. In addition, these patients, in contrast to patients with sporadic myxoma, may have noncardiac myxomas and endocrine neoplasms. (From Vidaillet, H. J., Jr., Seward, J. B., Fyke, F. E., et al.: "Syndrome myxoma": a subset of patients with cardiac myxoma associated with pigmented skin lesions and peripheral and endocrine neoplasms. Br. Heart J. *57*:247, 1987.)

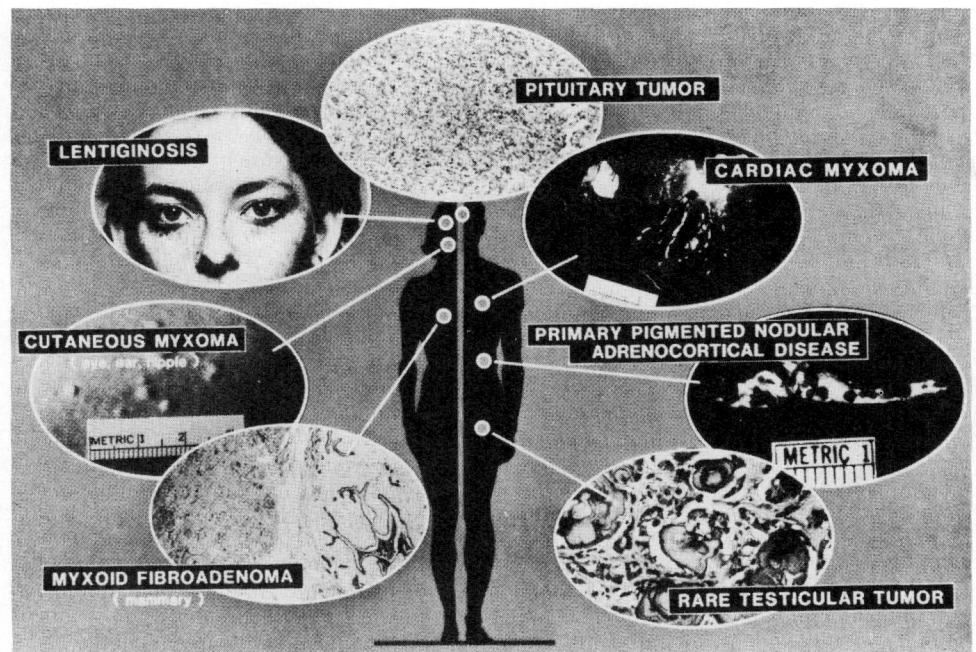

FIGURE 44–3. Clinical elements which may be found in patients with "complex" myxomas. The biological behavior of cardiac myxomas associated with this syndrome differs from that of the more common solitary myxoma. In these patients cardiac myxomas tend to occur at a younger age, are more likely to be familial, and the incidence of multiple and recurrent tumors is higher. (From McCarthy, P. M., et al.: The significance of multiple, recurrent, and "complex" cardiac myxomas. J. Thorac. Cardiovasc. Surg. 91:389, 1986.)

years). Certain aspects of this syndrome have been referred to as the NAME syndrome (nevi, atrial myxoma, myxoid neurofibroma, ephelides)[75] or the LAMB syndrome (lentigines, atrial myxoma and blue nevi).[73] The majority of patients so far described have had cardiac myxomas. Patients with the myxoma syndrome complex, and in particular those with recurrent tumors, have a high incidence of abnormal deoxyribonucleic acid (DNA) ploidy as compared with patients with sporadic tumors.[79]

Taken together, familial myxoma or the complex just described constitutes approximately 7 per cent of all myxomas.[67,78] Compared with patients with sporadic myxoma, these patients are younger (mean age, 20's), are more likely to have multiple myxomas involving chambers other than the left atrium, and are more likely to have recurrence of myxomas postoperatively[67] (Table 44–5). Such "recurrences" most likely represent the multicentric nature of this disease. When multiple myxomas occur simultaneously they are referred to as synchronous, whereas multiple myxomas presenting at different times are referred to as metasynchronous.[67]

Because cardiac myxomas may be familial,[71] routine echocardiographic screening of first degree relatives is appropriate, particularly if the patient is young or has multiple tumors. In patients with a familial history or other components of the syndrome described above, a careful search should be made preoperatively for multiple cardiac myxomas. In addition, these patients should be observed closely postoperatively for

TABLE 44–4 CLINICAL PRESENTATION OF CARDIAC MYXOMA IN 130 PATIENTS*

Signs and symptoms of mitral valve disease	57
Embolic phenomena	36
No cardiac symptoms—incidental finding	16
Signs and symptoms of tricuspid valve disease	6
Sudden unexpected death	5
Pericarditis	4
Myocardial infarction	3
Signs and symptoms of pulmonary valve disease	2
Fever of undetermined origin	2

* One patient with multiple myxomas had signs and symptoms of mitral and tricuspid valve disease.
From McAllister, H. A., and Fenoglio, J. J.: Tumors of the cardiovascular system. In Atlas of Tumor Pathology. Washington, D.C., Armed Forces Institute of Pathology, 1978. Fasc. 15, 2d series.

the development of other tumors (metasynchronous); this occurs in 12 to 22 per cent of such patients.[67]

PATHOLOGY. The pathological features of myxoma are similar to those of an organized thrombus, a finding that has led to the suggestion that myxomas are not true neoplasms but may represent one form of organization of an endocardial thrombus.[80] Although the results of DNA analysis[80a] and most investigators favor the view that myxomas are a true neoplastic process, the cellular origin of the myxoma is not entirely clear. Histological, ultrastructural, and immunohistochemical evidence indicating considerable cellular heterogeneity within the tumor has been interpreted as support for the thesis that myxomas originate by divergent differentiation of mesenchymal cells.[81–86] Some investigators, however, have suggested an origin from endocardial cells.[87] Although histologically benign, myxomas may rarely exhibit malignant biological behavior with invasion of the interatrial septum.[88] Occasional reports suggest that myxomas may have a malignant counterpart[89] as well as the ability to implant and grow at distant foci such as the aorta, brain or bone.[90,91,91a]

Grossly, myxomas may be pedunculated, with a fibrovascular stalk. Most sessile tumors probably represent the base of the pedicle, which remains after the body has embolized.[3] The tumors average 4 to 8 cm in diameter, although tumors of up to 15 cm have been reported. Most myxomas are gelatinous and polypoid, although they may also be smooth and round with a glistening surface; areas of hemorrhage are not unusual (Fig. 44–1).

By *light microscopy,* the cells are uniform, small, and polygonal with round or oval nuclei and a moderate amount of cytoplasm. The cells are surrounded by myxomatous stroma composed predominantly of an eosinophilic matrix which appears to be composed of an acid mucopolysaccharide similar to chondroitin C.[3] The cells and the stroma are frequently positive with PAS stain, whereas only stroma is stained with alcian blue stain. Elastic fibers, reticular fibers, smooth muscle cells, collagen, calcium, and bone may be seen. Other cellular elements include lymphocytes, plasma cells, mast cells, histiocytes, and rarely, fibrocytes. Thin-walled vessels simulating primitive capillaries are present (Fig. 44–4). The surface of the tumor consists of the typical myxoma cells and, in some cases, thrombus.

On *electron microscopic examination,* the myxoma cells demonstrate areas of intracellular junctions (zonulae adherentes), single nuclei with finely dispersed chromatin and nucleoli, rough endoplasmic reticulum, free ribosomes, mito-

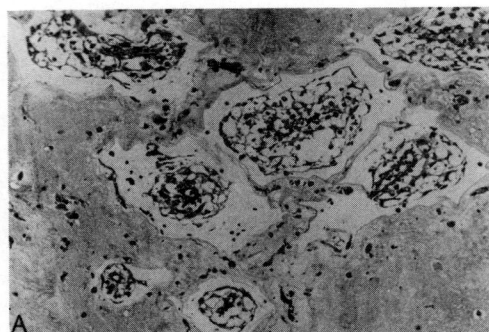
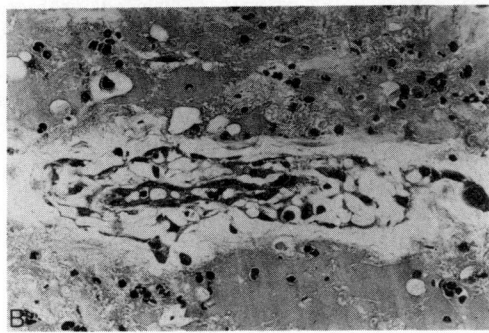

FIGURE 44–4. Light microscopic images of cardiac myxoma cells stained with hematoxylin-eosin, at 20× (Panel A) and 100× (Panel B) powers. Polygonal cells with eosinophilic cytoplasm are embedded in a myxoid matrix composed of an acid mucopolysaccharide-rich stroma. Cells may be arranged singly, often assuming a stellate shape, in small groups in close apposition to capillaries, or in irregular compact clusters, sometimes resembling vascular-like channels. Mitoses are not seen. (From Tanimura Kitazono, M., Nagayama, K., et al.: Cardiac myxoma: Morphologic, histochemical, and tissue culture studies. Hum. Pathol. *19*:316, 1988.)

chondria, Golgi complexes, and cytoplasmic filaments.[3,92–94] On examination with scanning electron microscopy, myxomas are covered by endothelium and possess endothelium-lined crevices and clefts, features not seen in atrial thrombus.[95,96]

PAPILLARY TUMORS OF HEART VALVES. Papillary tumors of the cardiac valves and adjacent endocardium are found, not uncommonly, post mortem and may be identified during life by two-dimensional echocardiography.[3,96] Although the clinical significance of these lesions is debated, there is evidence that they have the potential to cause valvular dysfunction and embolize to vital structures.[3,96,97] These lesions have a characteristic frond-like appearance, may be up to 3 or 4 cm in diameter, are single or multiple, and may occur on any valve; most often the ventricular surface of semilunar valves and the atrial surface of AV valves are affected. Rarely, they may be present on papillary muscle, chordae tendineae, or endocardium.[98] The tricuspid valve is most commonly involved in children and the mitral and aortic valves in adults.[4] Histologically the tumor is covered by endothelium that surrounds a core of loose connective tissue consisting of an acid mucopolysaccharide matrix, smooth muscle cells, and collagen and elastic fibers.[4] The pathogenesis of these lesions is unsettled, but it appears that they may originate from organized mural thrombi.[3,98] Papillary tumors are generally distinguished from Lambl's excrescences, which are ubiquitous acellular deposits covered by a single layer of endothelium and found on heart valves at the site of endothelial damage in over 70 per cent of adults.[3]

RHABDOMYOMAS. These are the most common cardiac tumors of infants and children, the large majority occurring in patients younger than 1 year.[99] Morphological evidence suggests that rhabdomyomas are actually myocardial hamartomas rather than true neoplasms.[100] Consistent with this view is the complete lack of any mitotic activity,[99] the observation at the ultrastructural level that the characteristic glycogen-laden cells are typical of immature myocytes,[100] and the presence of atrial natriuretic peptide.[101] In addition, rhabdomyomas are strongly associated with tuberous sclerosis, a familial syndrome characterized by hamartomas in several organs, epilepsy, mental deficiency, and adenoma sebaceum. Alternatively, it has been suggested that rhabdomyomas may represent a nodular form of a diffuse cardiac glycogen storage disease.[127]

One-third to one-half of patients with cardiac rhabdomyomas are found at autopsy to have tuberous sclerosis; adenoma sebaceum and benign kidney tumors (angiomyolipomas and hamartomas) are seen less fre-

quently.[99] Conversely, approximately 50 per cent or more of patients having tuberous sclerosis but no signs or symptoms of cardiac disease have been shown to have findings on echocardiography that are consistent with rhabdomyoma.[103,104] Rhabdomyomas causing significant intracavitary obstruction may result in death within the first 24 hours of life, whereas patients with less severe involvement may remain asymptomatic, or the tumor may become apparent during infancy or early childhood.[99]

Rhabdomyomas invariably involve the ventricles, affecting the left and right sides equally. Ninety per cent are multiple, and in 30 per cent there is involvement of at least one of the atria. Approximately 50 per cent of rhabdomyomas are large enough to cause significant obstruction of a cardiac chamber or valvular orifice.[99,105] Nonspecific clinical manifestations — including cardiomegaly, right or left ventricular failure or both, an S_3, S_4, and systolic or diastolic murmurs — may mimic mitral stenosis, mitral atresia, aortic stenosis, subaortic stenosis, and infundibular pulmonic stenosis.

Rhabdomyomas are yellow-gray and range from 1 mm to several centimeters in diameter. The microscopic hallmark, termed the spider cell, is a cell containing a central cytoplasmic mass that is suspended by fine fibrillar processing radiating to the periphery, thus giving the appearance of a spider hanging in a net.[3] The cytoplasm is rich in glycogen and stains positively with periodic acid-Schiff reagent.[3] Electron microscopy demonstrates myofibrils, cytoplasmic and mitrochondrial glycogen, and apparent intercellular junctions similar to intercalated discs.[99]

FIBROMAS. Fibromas are benign, connective tissue tumors that occur predominantly in children. The majority occur before the age of 10 years, and about 40 per cent are diagnosed in infants less than 1 year of age.[106] Males and females appear equally affected. Fibromas constitute the second most common type of primary cardiac tumor occurring in infants and children.[106] Whether fibromas represent hamartomas or true neoplasms is debated.[107] The histological criteria for diagnosis are not uniformly agreed upon, and therefore several designations are employed, including fibromyxoma, fibroelastic hamartoma, embryonic mesenchymoma, fibroma, and fibrous rhabdomyoma.

Almost all fibromas occur within the ventricular myocardium — most frequently within the anterior free wall of the left ventricle or the interventricular septum and much less often in the posterior left ventricular wall or right ventricle. Typically, they are gray, firm, circumscribed, not capsulated, and range in size from 3 to 7 cm. Grossly, they resemble fibroids and exhibit a whorled appearance on cut sections. Microscopically, cardiac fibromas consist of elongated fibroblasts admixed with fibrous tissue consisting of collagen and elastin fibers. Their cellularity is variable, and mitotic figures are rarely, if ever, seen. Fibrous tissue is intermingled with adjacent myocardial fibers at the margins of the lesion.[107] Calcification and islands of bone formation may be seen microscopically and occasionally radiographically. The *Gorlin syndrome,* the main features of which are multiple nevoid basal cell carcinomas, cysts of the jaw, and skeletal abnormalities, may be associated in some cases with cardiac tumors, either fibromas or fibrous histiocytomas.[108]

Although fibromas may be incidental findings at postmortem examination, approximately 70 per cent at some time cause mechanical interference with intracardiac flow, ventricular contraction, or conduction disturbances.[3] Clinical manifestations are protean and include murmurs, atypical chest pain, congestive heart failure and signs of subaortic stenosis, valvular or infundibular pulmonic stenosis with right ventricular hypertrophy, tricuspid stenosis, conduction disturbances, ventricular tachycar-

TABLE 44–5 COMPARISON OF THE CLINICAL FEATURES OF SPORADIC MYXOMA AND SYNDROME MYXOMA

FEATURE	SPORADIC	SYNDROME
Age (yr) (range)	56 (39–82)	25 (10–56)
Female/male ratio	2.7:1	1.8:1
Patients (No.)	70	44
Cardiac myxomas (No.)	72	103
Distributions of myxomas (%):		
Atrial/ventricular	100/0	87/13
Single/multiple	99/1	50/50
Biatrial	0	23
Recurrent	0	18
Familial	0	27
Freckling (%)	0	68
Noncardiac tumors (%)	0	57
Endocrine neoplasm (%)	0	30

Vidaillet, H. J., Jr., Seward, J. B., Fyke, F. E. et al.: "Syndrome myxoma": a subset of patients with cardiac myxoma associated with pigmented skin lesions and peripheral and endocrine neoplasms. Br. Heart J. *57*:247, 1987.

dia, and sudden death. As in the case of rhabdomyomas, the increased usage of echocardiography has resulted in the not infrequent detection of cardiac fibromas in patients without cardiac signs or symptoms.[109,110]

LIPOMAS AND LIPOMATOUS HYPERTROPHY OF THE ATRIAL SEPTUM. Lipomas occur at all ages and with equal frequency in both sexes. Most range in diameter from 1 to 15 cm, although some have been reported to weigh more than 2 kg. Most tumors are sessile or polypoid and occur in the subendocardium or subepicardium, although about one-fourth are completely intramuscular.[2] Subendocardial tumors with intracavitary extension produce symptoms that are characteristic of their location, whereas subepicardial tumors may cause compression of the heart and pericardial effusion. The most common chambers affected are the left ventricle, right atrium, and interatrial septum.[4] Intramural tumors may be asymptomatic or result in arrhythmias, AV or intraventricular conduction disturbances, or mechanical interference. Many tumors are clinically silent and are found only at autopsy or become apparent on a routine chest roentgenogram.

Microscopically, the lesions are usually well encapsulated, composed of typical mature fat cells, and occasionally contain fibrous connective tissue (fibrolipoma), muscular tissue (myolipoma), or vacuolated brown fat resembling a hibernoma.

Whereas lipomas are true neoplasms, a condition termed *lipomatous hypertrophy of the interatrial septum* represents the occurrence of an accumulation of mature adipose tissue within the interatrial septum. These lesions range from 1 to 7 cm in dimension, most often protrude into the right atrium, and are more common in obese, elderly, or female patients.[111] A variety of atrial arrhythmias have been attributed to these lesions, but a cause-and-effect relationship has been difficult to establish.[111-113] Since this lesion may occasionally be detected by cineangiography, echocardiography, computed tomography, or other diagnostic techniques, the major clinical dilemma is the differential diagnosis and treatment of an intraatrial filling defect.

ANGIOMAS. Benign vascular tumors, including hemangiomas, lymphangiomas, and angioreticulomas, are extremely rare.[114] Anatomically, they may occur in any part of the heart, but usually are intramural, often in the interventricular septum or AV node, where they may cause complete heart block and sudden death. Cardiac tamponade due to hemopericardium may be the presenting clinical syndrome. More commonly found in the right heart chambers, hemangiomas are generally sessile or polypoid subendocardial nodules ranging from 2 to 4 cm in diameter. Histologically, the tumors consist of endothelium-lined spaces which may contain blood, lymph, or thrombi; they are classified according to the predominant type of proliferating vascular channel.

TERATOMAS. These tumors, which contain elements of all three germ cell layers, occur within the heart less frequently than in the anterior mediastinum. Teratomas are generally observed in children,[130] and when located within the heart, they occur predominantly within the right atrium, right ventricle, or the interatrial or interventricular septum.[115]

BENIGN CYSTIC TUMORS. Benign cystic tumors are small lesions, generally less that 15 mm, that are found in the area of the AV node.[55,56] These lesions are characterized by tubules and cysts lined by flat or cuboidal cells that are devoid of mitotic activity, but may have secretory function. The embryogenic basis and histological classification of these lesions has been controversial,[116,117] as reflected by the variety of terms by which they are called in the literature, including lymphangioendothelioma, mesothelioma, and congenital polycystic tumor.[117]

These lesions present during the first or second decade, exhibit a marked female predominance, and are frequently noted at the time of puberty or pregnancy, thus suggesting a hormonal role in their development and expression. Because of their location in the area of the AV node, they most often present as progressive heart block, syncope, or sudden death, although many are asymptomatic and consistent with a long life. Ventricular tachycardia progressing to ventricular fibrillation has been observed, perhaps explaining the poor results obtained with cardiac pacemakers in this condition.

Epithelium-lined cysts are extremely rare lesions which are usually an incidental postmortem finding.[2-4] They are 4 to 25 mm in diameter and are lined with cuboidal or columnar ciliated epithelium.

ENDOCRINE TUMORS OF THE HEART. Approximately 2 per cent of *paragangliomas* are intrathoracic, and of these most are located in the posterior mediastinum. However, these tumors can also occur in close association with the left atrial or left ventricular epicardium, where they are thought to have arisen from sympathetic fibers to the heart or from ectopic chromaffin cells.[133] More rarely still, paragangliomas may arise within the interatrial septum.[119] Tumors in any of these locations may secrete catecholamines and therefore can be associated with signs and symptoms characteristic of pheochromocytoma (p. 1839).[118,119]

Rarely, benign *thyroid tumors* arise within the heart, presumably from ectopic rests of thyroid tissue.[120] These tumors most often arise from the interventricular septum and present, not infrequently, as obstruction to right ventricular outflow.

About one-fourth of all cardiac tumors exhibit typically malignant histological characteristics and invasive behavior.[2-4] Virtually all of these are sarcomas, thus making these tumors second only to myxomas in overall frequency. Sarcomas may occur at any age, but are most common between the third and fifth decades and show no sex preference. In decreasing order of frequency the sites involved are the right atrium, left atrium, right ventricle, left ventricle, and interventricular septum.

Sarcomas derive from mesenchyme and therefore may display a wide variety of morphological types which may be subtyped as angiosarcoma, rhabdomyosarcoma, fibrosarcoma, and lymphosarcoma.[4]

From a clinical viewpoint, sarcomas characteristically display a rapid downhill course. Death most often occurs from a few weeks to 2 years after the onset of symptoms. These tumors proliferate rapidly and generally cause death through widespread infiltration of the myocardium, obstruction of flow within the heart, or distant metastases. About 75 per cent of all patients with cardiac sarcomas have pathological evidence of distant metastases at the time of death.[121,121a] The most frequent sites are the lungs, thoracic lymph nodes, mediastinum, and vertebral column; less often the liver, kidneys, adrenals, pancreas, bone, spleen, and bowel are involved.

The cardiac findings are determined primarily by the location of the tumor and by the extent of intracavitary obstruction. Typical presentations include progressive, unexplained, congestive heart failure, particularly of the right side; precordial pain; pericardial effusion; tamponade; arrhythmias; conduction disturbances; obstruction of the venae cavae; and sudden death. Tumors limited to the myocardium without intracavitary extension may produce no cardiac symptoms or may cause arrhythmias and conduction disturbances. Because of the rapid growth potential of sarcomas, they commonly extend into the cardiac chambers, the pericardial space, or both. In about 20 per cent of cases, the tumor is sessile or polypoid.[122] When there is extension into the pericardial space, hemorrhagic pericardial effusion is common, and tamponade may occur. Because the right side of the heart is most commonly affected, sarcomas frequently cause signs of right heart failure as a result of obstruction of the right atrium, right ventricle, or tricuspid or pulmonic valves. In addition, obstruction of the superior vena cava may result in swelling of the face and upper extremities, whereas obstruction of the inferior vena cava may result in visceral congestion.

ANGIOSARCOMAS. Included within this category are malignant hemangioendotheliomas, angiosarcomas, Kaposi's sarcomas, angioreticuloendotheliomas, and cavernous angiosarcomas.[4,123,124] All 40 patients in one series were adults.[141] In distinction to most other cardiac sarcomas, in which the sex distribution is equal, there appears to be a 2:1 male-to-female ratio among patients with angiosarcomas. These tumors have a striking predilection for the right atrium, most often arising from the interatrial septum [125] and may be infiltrative or polypoid in nature. Microscopically, angiosarcomas are characterized by ill-defined anastomotic vascular channels lined with atypical, often heaped-up, endothelial cells. By electron microscopy, immature endothelial cells, primitive pericytes, and undifferentiated mesenchymal cells may be identified.[126] Associated cavernous hemangiomas of the liver have been reported.[2]

RHABDOMYOSARCOMAS. These are tumors of striated muscle which often diffusely infiltrate the myocardium but which may also, on occasion, form a polypoid extension into the cardiac chambers and therefore have been clinically mistaken for myxoma.[2] The high incidence of rhabdomyosarcoma in infants and in children, in conjunction with a predilection for the septum in young but not in older patients, has led to the suggestion that in some cases this tumor may arise from embryonic cell rests in the septum.[127] Rhabdomyoblasts are the histological hallmark of this tumor, and 20 to 30 per cent of the tumors have cross-striations.[4] "Strap cells," "tennis racquet cells," and "spider cells" with periodic acid-Schiff-positive cytoplasm may be seen.

FIBROSARCOMAS. Fibrosarcomas of the heart resemble the soft, whitish "fish flesh" characteristic of this tumor type elsewhere in the body. They may contain areas of hemorrhage and necrosis and extensively infiltrate the heart, often involving more than one cardiac chamber. A thrombus may form in an obstructed pulmonary vein or the vena cava or over the mural surface of the tumor.[3]

LYMPHOSARCOMAS. Although cardiac involvement of systemic lymphoma has been reported in 25 to 36 per cent of cases, primary lymphosarcoma involving only the heart or pericardium appears to be much less common.[128] Myocardial infiltration by lymphoma may be nodular or diffuse, and the clinical syndrome of hypertrophic cardiomyopathy has been mimicked.

PULMONARY ARTERY SARCOMAS. Sarcomas of the pulmonary artery trunk, main branches, or pulmonic valve may present as tumor emboli to the lungs or as right ventricular outflow obstruction.[149] These tumors may originate from undifferentiated tissue of the bulbis cordis, usually present after the fourth decade, and show a 2:1 female predominance.[129] Typical symptoms include dyspnea, chest pain, cough, and hemoptysis and may be associated with radiographic findings of a pulmonary hilar mass or cardiomegaly. Right ventricular injection of contrast material helps to delineate the tumor. Although most reported cases were diagnosed post mortem, it is likely that early diagnosis, surgical resection, and possibly chemotherapy may have an impact on survival of patients with this tumor.[129]

DIAGNOSTIC TECHNIQUES

Although certain clinical manifestations may be suggestive of a cardiac tumor, no clinical finding or set of findings is pathognomonic. Furthermore, the majority of cardiac tumors produce signs and symptoms typical of the common forms of heart disease. The development of modern diagnostic methods has had a major impact on the diagnosis and hence the natural history of cardiac tumors. Whereas only 20 years ago the diagnosis of a cardiac tumor was rarely made antemortem, it is now not unusual for cardiac tumors to be diagnosed and cured in patients who are totally asymptomatic or without signs of cardiovascular disease.[130,131] Although cardiac catheterization made possible the definitive preoperative diagnosis of cardiac tumors, it was not until the advent of echocardiography that it was feasible to evaluate all patients suspected of this diagnosis. Both M-mode and two-dimensional echocardiography are effective screening techniques. However, two-dimensional echocardiography, and particularly transesophageal imaging (Fig. 44–5), is more sensitive and provides considerably more information regarding the site of tumor attachment, pattern of tumor movement, and

size. In many centers, the information provided by two-dimensional echocardiography, computed tomography (CT), or magnetic resonance imaging (MRI) (Fig. 44–6) is considered sufficient to proceed directly to surgery without cardiac catheterization and angiography. Catheterization and angiography should not be omitted in the absence of a technically adequate two-dimensional echocardiographic study, CT, or MRI that has visualized all four cardiac chambers.

It is imperative that noninvasive evaluation, preferably by two-dimensional echocardiography (or CT or MRI), be performed whenever cardiac catheterization is planned and the diagnosis of cardiac tumor is considered. Thus, when left atrial myxoma is suspected, it is safest to visualize the left atrium by injecting the contrast agent into the pulmonary artery and film during the levophase. It is particularly important to avoid the transseptal approach, since this risks dislodgment of fragments of tumor that may be attached in the region of the fossa ovalis. Furthermore, since cardiac tumors may be multiple and present in more than one chamber, all four chambers should be visualized noninvasively prior to cardiac catheterization whenever possible.

RADIOLOGICAL EXAMINATION

Cardiac tumors may display several findings on plain chest roentgenograms. These include alterations in cardiac contour, changes in overall cardiac size, specific chamber enlargement, alterations in pulmonary vascularity, and intracardiac calcification.[132,133] The cardiac contour may be normal, may display generalized or specific chamber enlargement that mimics virtually any type of valvular heart disease, or may demonstrate a bizarre appearance. Pericardial effusions are rather common and generally indicate invasion of the pericardial space by a malignant tumor. Mediastinal widening, due to hilar and paramediastinal adenopathy, may indicate spread of a malignant cardiac tumor.[132] A bumpy, irregular, or fuzzy cardiac border may be seen when the pericardium is involved. Cardiac enlargement may reflect rapid tumor growth, particularly in the case of sarcomas, whereas specific chamber enlargement is frequently due to intracavitary obstruction, particularly by pedunculated tumors such as myxomas. Thus, left atrial myxoma may produce the radiological pattern characteristic of mitral stenosis. Occasionally a large tumor mass displaces the heart and may simulate enlargement of a specific chamber.

Calcification visible by roentgenographic methods may occur with several types of cardiac tumor, including rhabdomyomas, fibromas, hamartomas, teratomas, myxomas, and angiomas.[133] Visualization of intracardiac

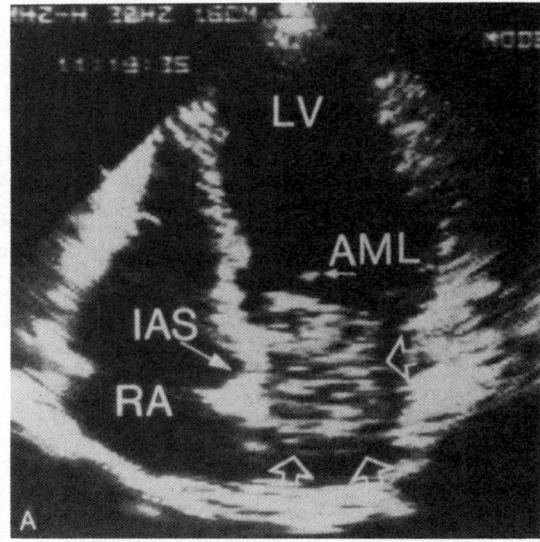
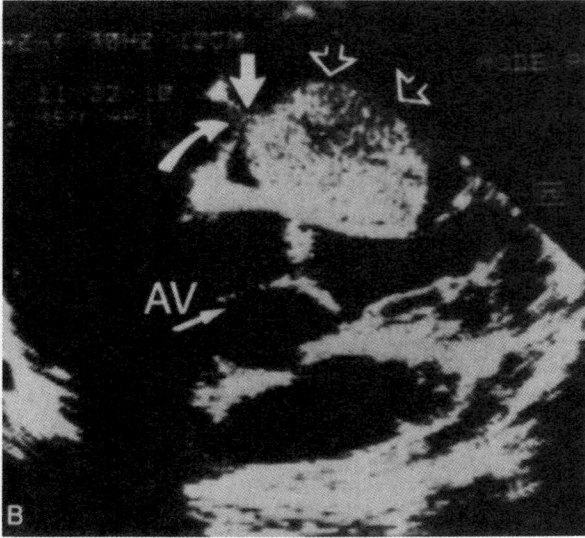

FIGURE 44–5. Transthoracic (Panel A) and transesophageal (Panel B) views of a large left atrial myxoma. Panel A, the transthoracic apical four-chamber view shows a large homogeneous mass in the left atrium (open arrows) in close association with the atrial septum and protruding into the mitral orifice. Panel B, transesophageal examination of the same patient provides substantially better resolution of a large left atrial myxoma (open arrows), and now also delineates a short stalk (thick arrow) and "tenting" of the atrial septum at the fossa ovalis (curved arrow) as the myxoma moves with blood flow during diastole. AML, anterior mitral leaflet; IAS, interatrial septum; LV, left ventricle; RA, right atrium; AV, aortic valve. (From Obeid, A. J., Marvasti, M., Parker, F., and Rosenberg, J.: Comparison of transthoracic and transesophageal echocardiography in diagnosis of left atrial myxoma. Am. J. Cardiol. 63:1006, 1989.)

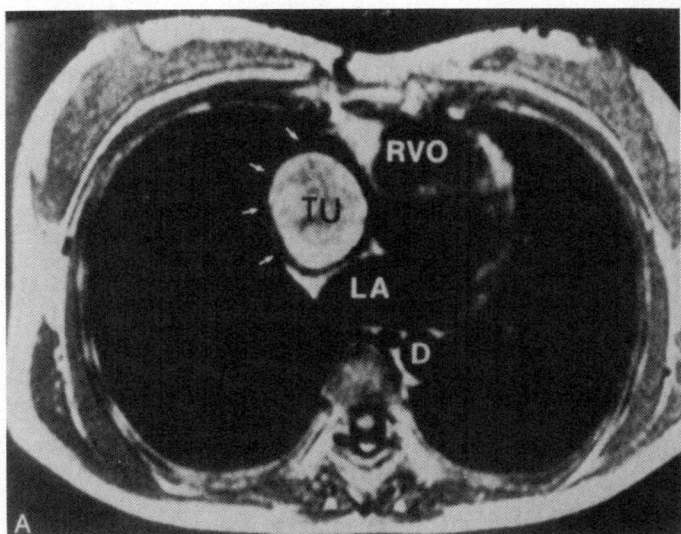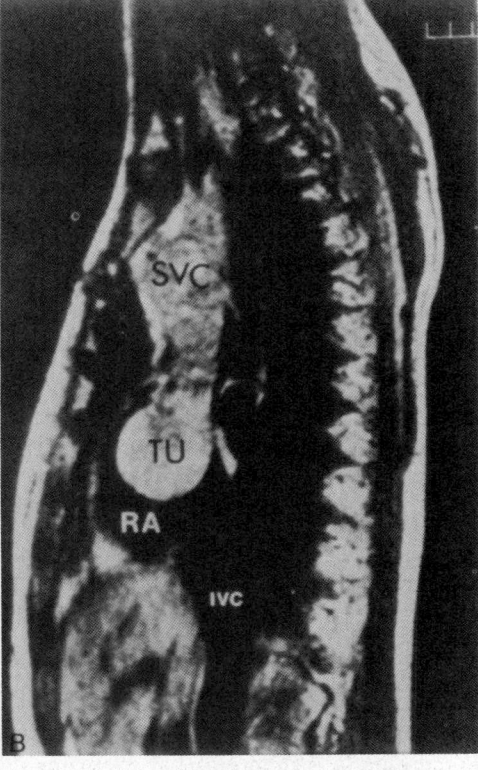

FIGURE 44–6. Magnetic resonance imaging (MRI) tomograms from a patient with a large angiosarcoma involving the right atrium with extension into the superior vena cava, subclavean and innominate veins. *A,* Axial image through the atria showing a large mass within the right atrium (arrows). D, descending aorta; LA, left atrium; RVO, right ventricular outflow tract. *B,* Sagittal image showing the tumor mass within the right atrium, extending into the superior vena cava (SVC). IVC, inferior vena cava. (From Freedberg, R. S., Kronzon, I., Rumancik, W. M., and Liebeskind, D.: The contribution of MRI to evaluations of intracardiac tumors diagnosed by echocardiography. Circulation 77:96, 1988.)

calcium in an infant or a child is unusual and should immediately raise the question of an intracardiac tumor. Cardiac fluoroscopy and laminography may be helpful in differentiating calcification of cardiac tumor from that of other structures, such as cardiac valves, coronary arteries, pericardium, and mural thrombus. Occasionally, calcified atrial polypoid tumors may be seen to prolapse into the ventricle during diastole. Fluoroscopy is also useful in differentiating cardiac tumor from ventricular aneurysm, both of which may result in a localized protrusion on plain chest roentgenograms. However, on fluoroscopic examination, cardiac tumors do not display the paradoxical motion during ventricular contraction that is characteristic of ventricular aneurysm.

NONINVASIVE METHODS

ECHOCARDIOGRAPHY

M-Mode Echocardiography. This technique has been extensively used in the diagnosis and evaluation of cardiac tumors. It is most useful for recognizing pedunculated tumors of the left atrium, primarily left atrial myxomas, and is generally less sensitive for the detection of intramural and sessile tumors.

Left atrial tumors are often pedunculated myxomas that traverse the mitral valve during diastole. Thus, during diastole when the tumor extends into the AV canal, a mass of echoes is visualized behind the anterior leaflet of the mitral valve (Fig. 44–1). During systole, the mitral valve is closed, the tumor is confined to the left atrium, and therefore the mass of echoes is no longer seen in the AV canal. Posterior descent of the anterior mitral leaflet may also be slow as a result of mechanical interference by the tumor. In some cases the tumor is less mobile and therefore may not traverse the mitral orifice; it may be detected only if the left atrium is carefully imaged from several different angles. It has been suggested that to diagnose left atrial tumors reliably the ultrasound beam should be directed in turn (1) through both leaflets of the mitral valve, (2) through the aorta and left atrium, (3) in an intermediate direction through the anterior mitral leaflet and left atrium, and (4) caudally, with a suprasternal transducer position.

Right atrial tumors (p. 1453) generally appear as echoes behind the tricuspid valve, prolapsing into the right ventricle during diastole.[53,62] Be-

cause myxomas frequently occur biatrially, it is vital that when the diagnosis of myxoma is suspected the echocardiographic examination be thorough and include both atria.

Ventricular tumors are less frequently diagnosed by M-mode echocardiography. Left ventricular tumors may be visualized as a mass of echoes interposed between the interventricular septum and the anterior leaflet of the mitral valve, and are present during both systole and diastole. Large left ventricular tumors may cause apparent filling of the left ventricular cavity by an echo-dense mass. *Right ventricular tumors* may be visualized as intracavitary echoes in the right ventricle and, in addition, may result in a paradoxical square wave motion of the interventricular septum.[135] Although reverberations produced by a right ventricular mass may be imaged in a position posterior to the tricuspid valve, the right atrial cavity is free of echoes in such cases.[135]

Two-Dimensional Echocardiography (see Fig. 4–105, p. 105, and 44–5). This technique provides substantial advantages over conventional M-mode echocardiography for the diagnosis and preoperative evaluation of intracardiac tumors.[14,136,137,137a] In the majority of cases of cardiac tumors, the information provided by two-dimensional echocardiography provides adequate information regarding tumor size, attachment, and mobility to allow operative resection without preoperative angiography. This technique is sensitive for detection of small tumors and is especially useful for detection of left ventricular tumors and tumors that do not prolapse through the mitral or tricuspid valve orifices.

According to a recently proposed echocardiographic classification system for left atrial myxomas, Class I tumors are small and prolapse through the mitral valve; Class II tumors are small and nonprolapsing; Class III tumors are large and prolapse; and Class IV tumors are large and nonprolapsing.[138] The increased sensitivity of two-dimensional echocardiography makes possible the diagnosis of cardiac tumors in neonates and in utero.[139] The improved diagnostic power and widespread use of two-dimensional echocardiography have resulted in an increase in the detection of primary cardiac tumors,[131] in many cases prior to the onset of clinical signs or symptoms.

Two-dimensional echocardiography may facilitate the differentiation between left atrial thrombus and myxoma, because the former typically produces a layered appearance and is generally situated in the posterior portion of the atrium, whereas the latter is often mottled in appearance and rarely occurs in the posterior portion of the atrium. In some atrial myxomas, areas of echolucency may be seen within the tumor mass, corresponding to areas of hemorrhage within the tumor. Since these areas of echolucency are not found in thrombotic or infective lesions, this finding may be of value in the differential diagnosis of an intraatrial mass. Continuous-mode Doppler ultrasonography may be useful for evaluating the hemodynamic consequences of valvular obstruction or incompetence caused by cardiac tumors.[140]

Transesophageal Echocardiography. (see Fig. 4–106, p. 105 and 44–5). This approach provides an unimpeded view of both atria[140a] and the atrial septum. Growing experience with the use of this approach to visualize atrial tumors has suggested that it may be superior to transthoracic echocardiography in certain patients.[22,23] Potential advantages of transesophageal echocardiography include improved resolution of the tumor and its attachment (Fig. 44–5), the ability to detect some masses not visualized by transthoracic echocardiography, and improved visualization of right atrial tumors.[22] Although transesophageal echocardiography does not appear warranted on a routine basis, it should be considered when the transthoracic study is suboptimal or confusing.

RADIONUCLIDE IMAGING. Gated blood pool scanning has been used to identify atrial, ventricular, and intramural tumors.[15] Radionuclide ventriculography generally has a lower rate of resolution than does echocardiography or contrast injection angiography and therefore may be less sensitive for the detection of small filling defects. However, radionuclide ventriculography may provide clear visualization of filling defects in some cases when other methods are nondiagnostic, particularly in the case of ventricular or intramural tumors. In some cases, gated blood pool scanning may provide more detailed information regarding myocardial geometry and tumor size and location than that obtained by echocardiography. Mobile left atrial tumors may be seen to prolapse into the left ventricle during diastole. Thus, gated blood pool scanning may, in some cases, provide information complementary to that obtained by echocardiography. In some cases in which the cardiac tumor was not evident by routine static or dynamic radionuclide imaging, it has been possible to delineate the tumor and its movement during a cardiac cycle by use of a computer-generated composite functional image.[15]

COMPUTED TOMOGRAPHY. CT of the heart has been used to demonstrate cardiac tumors[17] (Fig. 11–11, p. 319). Although more experience will be necessary to establish its role, certain advantages are apparent. These include a high degree of tissue discrimination, which may allow definition of the degree of intramural tumor extension; evaluation of the extracardiac structures; and the ability to construct images in any plane. Resolution appears to be improved substantially by gating the computed tomographic acquisition to the cardiac cycle.[17] At present CT appears to be most useful in the evaluation of suspected tumors of the heart to determine the degree of myocardial invasion and the involvement of pericardial and extracardiac structures.

MAGNETIC RESONANCE IMAGING. MRI may be of considerable value in the detection and delineation of cardiac tumors and in some cases may depict the size, shape, and surface characteristics of the tumor more clearly than two-dimensional echocardiography.[18–21] The larger field of view with MRI (Fig. 44–6) provides better definition of tumor prolapse, secondary valve obstruction, and cardiac chamber size than does two-dimensional echocardiography.

OTHER NONINVASIVE METHODS. Cardiac tumors cannot be diagnosed by phonocardiography, apexcardiography, or jugular venous or carotid pulse analysis. However, when valvular or myocardial disease is suspected on clinical grounds, certain atypical findings may raise the question of cardiac tumor. The intensity of the systolic or diastolic murmur caused by a left atrial myxoma is often exquisitely sensitive to positional change, a finding atypical of valvular heart disease. S_1 may be delayed as a consequence of an elevated left atrial pressure, as in mitral stenosis. It is often intense and widely split, and an early systolic sound may occur, representing tumor movement toward the atrium during systole. In addition, a tumor "plop" may be present about 100 msec after S_2, which appears to result from the sudden tension of the tumor stalk as it prolapses into the left ventricle during diastole or from the tumor striking the myocardium. The tumor plop *precedes* the end of the rapid filling wave of the apexcardiogram and can thereby be differentiated from an S_3; as noted, it usually occurs later than an opening snap. Systolic time intervals are usually consistent with a reduced stroke volume. Apexcardiography often shows a deep notch on the upstroke which occurs at the time of extrusion of the tumor through the mitral valve in early systole.

Right atrial tumors may also result in a widely split S_1 and an early systolic sound. The S_2 may be paradoxically split as a result of early pulmonic valve closure. A tumor plop and systolic and diastolic murmurs which are increased by inspiration may also occur with right atrial tumors. The jugular venous pulse tracing may reflect obstruction of the tricuspid orifice, demonstrating an accentuated *a* wave, attenuation of the *x* descent, or an early, broad *v* wave.

ANGIOGRAPHY

Cardiac catheterization and selective angiocardiography are not necessary in all cases of cardiac tumors, since, as already discussed, in many cases adequate preoperative information may be obtained by echocardiography, CT, or MRI. However, several circumstances exist in which the risk and expense of cardiac catheterization are outweighed by the supplemental information it may provide. These situations include cases in which (1) noninvasive evaluation has not been adequate in defining fully tumor location or attachment; (2) all four cardiac chambers have not been adequately visualized noninvasively; (3) a malignant cardiac tumor is considered likely; or (4) other cardiac lesions may coexist with a cardiac tumor and possibly dictate a different surgical approach. For instance, when a malignant cardiac tumor is suspected, cardiac angiography may provide valuable information regarding the degree of myocardial, vascular, and/or pericardial invasion. Likewise, in certain cases, such as the presence of pulmonary hypertension or the coexistence of significant valvular or coronary artery lesions, cardiac catheterization and angiography may provide information that significantly affects the surgical approach.[141]

The major angiographic findings in patients with cardiac tumors include (1) compression or displacement of cardiac chambers or large vessels, (2) deformity of cardiac chambers, (3) intracavitary filling defects, (4) marked variations in myocardial thickness, (5) pericardial effusion, and (6) local alterations in wall motion.[151,152] Displacement of the cardiac chambers or the great vessels without deformation of the internal contour may be observed in both benign and malignant tumors, whereas deformation of a cardiac chamber usually indicates an infiltrating malignant lesion.[152] The most frequent angiographic findings are intracavitary filling defects, which may be either fixed or mobile. Fixed defects may be lobulated or appear as a coarse nodularity of the myocardium often difficult to distinguish from a mural thrombus. Such defects may reflect endocardial tumors with broad attachments or intramural tumors with intracavitary extension. Mobile intracavitary defects are usually pedunculated tumors, typically myxomas, although the stalk may be difficult to visualize. Such tumors may prolapse into the AV valve orifice during diastole or, in the case of ventricular tumors, into the left ventricular outflow tract during systole. An atrial ball thrombus may mimic a pedunculated tumor, but is more likely to be associated with clot in the atrial appendage.

A localized increase in myocardial wall thickness, especially when accompanied by a pericardial effusion, suggests an infiltrating malignant tumor. It is often difficult to differentiate myocardial thickening from pericardial effusion, but this may be aided by observation of the thickness of the right atrial wall. Since the right atrial wall is seldom infiltrated by tumor, the finding of right atrial thickening to greater than 5 mm suggests a pericardial effusion.[133] In myocardial infiltration, localized areas of disordered wall motion may also be noted by cineangiography. Coronary arteriography may in some cases allow visualization of the vascular supply of the tumor, thus demarcating the extent of tumor invasion, the source of its blood supply, and its relation to the coronary arteries.[142,143] However, the vascular pattern of cardiac tumors has not proved to be a useful sign of malignancy.[133]

False-negative angiographic studies generally occur when the diagnosis is not suspected prior to catheterization. False positive studies are most often the result of thrombus, but may also be produced by many entities, such as streaming of non-opaque venous blood, a hematoma in the atrial septum, an aneurysm of the muscular or membranous ventricular septum, Bernheim syndrome, congenital septal dysplasia, and hydatid cysts of the interventricular septum.[133]

The major risk of angiography is peripheral embolization due to dislodgement of a fragment of tumor or of an associated thrombus.[133,144] Therefore, the thorough evaluation of all cardiac chambers by *noninvasive* methods prior to catheterization is recommended in patients suspected of having cardiac tumors so that contrast material can be injected into the chamber proximal (upstream) to the location of the tumor. The transseptal approach to the left atrium (p. 184) is particularly hazardous because of the frequent occurrence of left atrial myxomas in the region of the fossa ovalis.

Growing experience with digital subtraction angiography (p. 1567) indicates that it can provide important diagnostic information in patients with atrial or ventricular tumors having intracavitary projections. The ability to image intracavitary structures during injection of contrast material from a remote site eliminates the risk of catheter-induced tumor embolization and may play an important role in the diagnosis and characterization of a cardiac tumor, particularly in patients in whom the other noninvasive techniques are not technically satisfactory.

TREATMENT AND PROGNOSIS

BENIGN TUMORS

Operative excision is the treatment of choice for most benign cardiac tumors and in many cases results in a complete cure.[11,12,145-147] Although many tumors are histologically benign, all cardiac tumors are potentially lethal as a result of intracavitary or valvular obstruction, peripheral embolization, and disturbances of rhythm or conduction. Unfortunately, it is not unusual for patients to die or experience a major complication while awaiting operation, and therefore it is mandatory to carry out the operation promptly after the diagnosis has been established.[148]

Although some epicardial tumors may be removed without the aid of extracorporeal circulation, most intramural and intracavitary tumors must be excised under direct vision, with use of the heart-lung machine. Closed approaches, although occasionally used in the past, are not now recommended because of increased risk of dislodging tumor fragments. In addition, excision cannot be as complete, and adequate inspection of the other cardiac chambers for additional tumors is not possible.

The dislodgment of tumor fragments constitutes a major risk of operation and may result in peripheral emboli or the dispersion of micrometastases, which may seed peripherally. To reduce this risk, manipulation of the heart prior to cardiopulmonary bypass should be minimized. Some surgeons recommend that venous cannulation for cardiopulmonary bypass be performed via the femoral or azygos vein rather than through the right atrium to avoid dislodging an unsuspected right atrial tumor. In addition, the tumor should be removed

en bloc when possible, and the chamber then irrigated well with saline.

ATRIAL MYXOMAS. Numerous reports document complete cure of left and right atrial myxomas with follow-up periods of 10 to 15 years.[11,12,146-152] In about 1 to 5 per cent of cases a recurrence or second cardiac myxoma has been reported following resection of the initial myxoma.[67,153] Possible causes of the second tumor include incomplete excision of the original tumor with regrowth, growth from a second "pretumorous" focus, i.e., metasynchronous, or intracardiac implantation from the original tumor. Because of the first two possibilities, some surgeons have advocated excision of the entire region of the fossa ovalis and repair of the resultant atrial septal defect to remove presumably high concentrations of "pretumor" cells thought to be located in that region.[150] In one case, the large size of a myxoma, together with its location on the posterior left atrial wall, necessitated complete removal of the heart, followed by autotransplantation, i.e., reimplantation of the patient's excised heart.[153] Laser photocoagulation of a 1 cm area around the stalk attachment site has also been suggested as a way of eradicating pretumorous cells without the necessity of creating an atrial septal defect.[154] Other surgeons have reported equally successful long-term recurrence-free periods with simple excision of the tumor and a small rim at the base.[80] It now appears that in approximately 7 per cent of patients with (1) a familial history of cardiac myxoma, (2) features of the complex of lentigines and other abnormalities described on p. 1454, or (3) synchronous tumor appearance (i.e., multiple tumors at the time of presentation), the incidence of a second tumor occurring at some time in the future is in the range of 12 to 22 per cent, as compared to approximately 1 per cent for patients with sporadic atrial myxoma.[67] It is believed that tumor recurrence in these cases is from a second pretumorous focus of cells. In these high-risk patients, a careful search for multiple tumors preoperatively and more extensive resection of the underlying endocardium, atrial septum, or both is recommended. Careful echocardiographic follow-up for detection of metasynchronous tumors is recommended[67] in all patients following resection of a myxoma. Regardless of the extent of tumor resection performed, such patients should receive periodic long-term follow-up by cross-sectional echocardiography.

OTHER BENIGN TUMORS. Although the majority of operations for cardiac tumors have been performed for atrial myxomas owing to their high frequency, successful excision has also been reported for ventricular myxomas, as well as most other types of benign cardiac tumor, including rhabdomyoma, hamartoma, fibroma, lipoma, hemangioma, and papillary fibroelastoma.[107,155-160] The major surgical considerations in excision of ventricular tumors include preservation of adequate ventricular myocardium, maintenance of proper atrioventricular valve function, and preservation of as much of the conduction system as possible. Often, however, papillary muscles, chordae tendineae, or the AV conduction system must be sacrificed during the resection of a tumor, thereby necessitating replacement of the atrioventricular valve, implantation of a pacemaker, or both. In one case, extensive involvement of the heart by a fibrous histiocytoma that replaced 60 per cent of the left ventricle was treated successfully by cardiac transplantation.[161]

MALIGNANT TUMORS

Operation is not an effective treatment for the great majority of primary malignant tumors of the heart because of the large mass of cardiac tissue involved or the presence of metastases. The major role for surgery in such cases is to establish a diagnosis in order to exclude the possibility of a curable benign tumor. Nevertheless, in some cases palliation of hemodynamics and/or constitutional symptoms and extension of life may be achieved by aggressive therapy. Survivals of from 1 to 3 years have been reported following partial resection, chemotherapy, radiation therapy, or various combinations of these modalities.[126,162-167] In some instances, localized recurrences have been eliminated by multiple operations. Some success in palliation of symptoms has been reported following the combination of chemotherapy and radiation therapy[165] and radiation therapy alone.[168] Lymphosarcoma of the heart frequently responds to chemotherapy, radiation therapy, or both.[169,170] Unfortunately, many other reports indicate a failure to alter the course of cardiac sarcomas despite various combinations of surgery, chemotherapy, and radiation therapy.

REFERENCES

HISTORICAL PERSPECTIVE

1. Straus, R., and Merliss, R.: Primary tumors of the heart. Arch. Pathol. 39:74, 1945.
2. Fine, G.: Neoplasms of the pericardium and heart. In Gould, S. E. (ed): Pathology of the Heart and Blood Vessels. Springfield, Ill., Charles C Thomas, 1968, p. 851.
3. Heath, D.: Pathology of cardiac tumors. Am. J. Cardiol. 21:315, 1968.
4. Lammers, R. J., and Bloor, C. M.: Pathology of cardiac tumors. In Kapoor, A. S. (ed.): Cancer of the Heart. New York, Springer-Verlag, 1986, p. 1.
5. Urba, W. J., and Longo, D. L.: Primary solid tumors of the heart. In Kapoor, A. S. (ed.): Cancer of the Heart. New York, Springer-Verlag, 1986, p. 62.
6. Smith, C.: Tumors of the heart. Arch. Pathol. Lab. Med. 110:1, 1986.
7. Mahaim, I.: Les Tumeurs et les Polypes de Coeur: Étude Anatomo-Clinique. Paris, Masson, 1945.
8. Barnes, A. R., Beaver, D. C., and Snell, A. M.: Primary sarcoma of the heart: Report of a case with E. C. G. and pathological studies. Am. Heart J. 9:480, 1934.
9. Goldberg, H. P., Glenn, F., Dotter, C. T., and Steinberg, I.: Myxoma of the left atrium. Diagnosis made during life with operative and postmortem findings. Circulation 6:762, 1952.
10. Crafoord, C. L.: Case report. In Lam, C. R. (eds.): Proceedings. International Symposium on Cardiovascular Surgery. Philadelphia, W. B. Saunders Company, 1955, p. 202.
11. Reece, I. J., Cooley, D. A., Frazier, O. H., et al.: Cardiac tumors. Clinical spectrum and prognosis of lesions other than classical benign myxoma in 20 patients. J. Thorac. Cardiovasc. Surg. 88:439, 1984.
12. Guiloff, A. K., Flege, J. B., Callard, G. M., et al.: Surgery of left atrial myxomas. Report of eleven cases and review of literature. J. Cardiovasc. Surg. 27:194, 1986.
13. Effert, S., and Domanig, E.: The diagnosis of intra-atrial tumor and thrombi by the ultrasonic echo method. Ger. Med. Mon. 4:1, 1959.
14. Fyke, F. E., Seqard, J. B., Edwards, W. D., et al.: Primary cardiac tumors: Experience with 30 consecutive patients since the introduction of two-dimensional echocardiography. J. Am. Coll. Cardiol. 5:1465, 1985.
15. Bough, E., Bodem, W., Gandsman, E., et al.: Radionuclide diagnosis of left atrial myxoma with computer-generated functional images. Am. J. Cardiol. 52:1365, 1986.
16. Tamari, I., Goldberg, H. L., Moses, J. W., et al.: Left atrial myxoma: Diagnosis by digital substraction intravenous angiography. Cathet. Cardiovasc. Diagn. 12:26, 1986.
17. Jack, C. M., Cleland, J., and Geddes, J. S.: Left atrial rhabdomyosarcoma and the use of digital gated computed tomography in its diagnosis. Br. Heart J. 55:305, 1986.
18. Freedberg, R. S., Kronzon, I., Rumancik, W. M., and Liebeskind, D.: The contribution of magnetic resonance imaging to the evaluation of intracardiac tumors diagnosed by echocardiography. Circulation 77:96, 1988.
19. Brown, J. J., Barakos, J. A., and Higgins, C. B.: Magnetic resonance imaging of cardiac and paracardiac masses. J. Thorac. Imaging 4:58, 1989.
20. Rienmuller, R., Lloret, J. L., Tiling, R., et al.: MR imaging of pediatric cardiac tumors previously diagnosed by echocardiography. J. Comput. Assist. Tomogr. 13:621, 1989.
21. Lund, J. T., Ehman, R. L., Julsrud, P. R., et al.: Cardiac masses: assessment by MR imaging. Am. J. Roentgenol. 152:469, 1989.
22. Obeid, A. I., Marvasti, M., Parker, F., and Rosenberg, J.: Comparison of transthoracic and transesophageal echocardiography in diagnosis of left atrial myxoma. Am. J. Cardiol. 63:1006, 1989.
23. Dittmann, H., Voelker, W., Karsch, K. R., and Seipel, L.: Bilateral atrial myxomas detected by transesophageal two-dimensional echocardiography. Am. Heart J. 118:172, 1989.

CLINICAL PRESENTATION

24. Goodwin, J. F.: Symposium on cardiac tumors. The spectrum of cardiac tumors. Am. J. Cardiol. 21:307, 1968.
25. MacGregor, G. A., and Cullen, R. A.: The syndrome of fever, anaemia and high sedimentation rate with an atrial myxoma. Br. Med. J. 5:158, 1959.
26. Huston, K. A., Combs, J. J., Lie, J. T., and Guiliani, E. R.: Left atrial myxoma simulating peripheral vasculitis. Mayo Clin. Proc. 53:752, 1978.
27. Levinson, J. P., and Kincaid, O. W.: Myxoma of the right atrium associated with polycythemia. N. Engl. J. Med. 264:1187, 1961.
28. Vuopio, P., and Nikkila, E. A.: Hemolytic anemia and thrombocytopenia in a case of left atrial myxoma associated with mitral stenosis. Am. J. Cardiol. 17:585, 1966.

29. Jourdan, M., Bataille, R., Sequin, J., et al.: Constitutive production of interleukin-6 and immunologic features in cardiac myxomas. Arthritis Rheum. 33:398, 1990.
30. Curry H. L. F., Mathews, J. A., and Robinson, J.: Right atrial myxoma mimicking a rheumatic disorder. Br. Med. J. 1:542, 1967.
31. Savige, J. A., Yeung, S. P., Davies, D. J., et al.: Anti-neutrophil cytoplasmic antibodies associated with atrial myxoma. Am. J. Med. 85:755, 1988.
32. Graham, S. L., and Sellers, A. L.: Atrial myxoma with multiple myeloma. Arch. Intern. Med. 139:116, 1979.
33. Wens, R., Goffin, Y., Pepys, M. B., et al.: Left atrial myxoma associated with systemic AA amyloidosis. Arch. Intern. Med. 149:453, 1989.
34. Leonhardt, E. T. G., and Kullenberg, K. P. G.: Bilateral atrial myxomas with multiple arterial aneurysms—A syndrome mimicking polyarteritis nodosa. Am. J. Med. 62:792, 1977.
35. Byrd, W. E., Matthews, O. P., and Hunt, R. E.: Left atrial myxoma presenting as a systemic vasculitis. Arthritis Rheum. 23:240, 1980.
36. Feldman, A. R., and Keeling, J. H.: Cutaneous manifestation of atrial myxoma. J. Am. Acad. Dermatol. 21:1080, 1989.
37. Quinn, T. J., Condini, M. A., and Harris, A. A.: Infected cardiac myxoma. Am. J. Cardiol. 53:381, 1984.
38. Transden, T. M., Prichard, J. G., and Storz, S. O.: Streptococcus viridans bacteremia associated with atrial myxoma. Am. Heart J. 110:180, 1985.
39. Silverman, J., Olwin, J. S., and Graettinger, J. S.: Cardiac myxomas with systemic mobilization. Circulation 26:99, 1962.
40. Koikkalainen, K., Kostiainen, S., and Luosto, R.: Left atrial myxoma revealed by femoral embolectomy. Scand. J. Thorac. Cardiovasc. Surg. 11:33, 1977.
41. Yufe, R., Karpati, G., and Carpenter, S.: Cardiac myxoma: A diagnostic challenge for the neurologist. Neurology 26:1060, 1976.
42. Schweiger, M. J., Hafer, J. G., Jr., Brown, R., and Gianelly, R. E.: Spontaneous cure of infected left atrial myxoma following embolization. Am. Heart J. 99:630, 1980.
43. Gonzalez, A., Altieri, P. I., Marquez, E., et al.: Massive pulmonary embolism associated with right ventricular myxoma. Am. J. Med. 69:795, 1980.
44. Heath, D., and Mackinnon, J.: Pulmonary hypertension due to myxoma of the right atrium. With special reference to the behavior of emboli of myxoma in the lung. Am. Heart J. 68:227, 1964.
45. Semb, B. K., Wexels, J. C., Vatne, K., and Bjornstad, P. G.: Angiographic and echocardiographic observations in surgical patients with atrial myxoma. Cardiovasc. Intervent. Radiol. 8:119, 1985.
46. Rath, S., Har-Zahav, Y., Battler, A., et al.: Coronary arterial embolus from left atrial myxoma. Am. J. Cardiol. 54:1392, 1984.
47. Branch, C. L., Jr., Laster, D. W., and Kelley, D. L., Jr.: Left atrial myxoma with cerebral emboli. Neurosurgery 16:675, 1985.
48. Verkkala, K., Kupari, M., Maamies, T., et al.: Primary cardiac tumors—operative treatment of 20 patients. Thorac. Cardiovasc. Surg. 37:361, 1989.
49. Weerasena, N. A., Groome, D., Pollock, J. G., and Pollock, J. C.: Atrial myxoma as the cause of acute lower limb ischemia in a teenager. Scott. Med. J. 34:440, 1989.
50. Reed, R. J., Utz, M. P., and Terezakis, N.: Embolic and metastatic cardiac myxoma. Am. J. Dermatopathol. 11:157, 1989.
51. Michael, A. S., Mikhael, M. A., and Christ, M.: Myxoma of the heart presenting with recurrent episodes of hemorrhagic cerebral infarction: MR findings. J. Comput. Assist. Tomogr. 13:123, 1989.
52. Knepper, L. E., Biller, J., Adams, H. P., Jr., and Bruno, A.: Neurologic manifestations of atrial myxoma. A 12-year experience and review. Stroke 19:1435, 1988.
53. Panidis, I. P., Kotler, M. N., Mintz, G. S., and Ross, J.: Clinical and echocardiographic features of right atrial masses. Am. Heart J. 107:745, 1984.
54. Harvey, W. P.: Clinical aspects of cardiac tumors. Am. J. Cardiol. 21:328, 1968.
55. James, T. N., and Galakhov, I.: De subitaneis mortibus XXVI. Fatal electrical instability of the heart associated with benign congenital polycystic tumor of the atrioventricular node. Circulation 56:667, 1977.
56. Nishida, K., Kamijima, G., and Nagayama, T.: Mesothelioma of the atrioventricular node. Br. Heart J. 53:468, 1985.
57. Strauss, W. E., Asinger, R. W., and Hodges, M.: Mesothelioma of the AV node: Potential utility of pacing. PACE 11:1296, 1988.
58. Lantz, D. A., Dougherty, T. H., and Lucca, M. J.: Primary angiosarcoma of the heart causing cardiac rupture. Am. Heart J. 118:186, 1989.
59. Greenwood, W. F.: Profile of atrial myxoma. Am. J. Cardiol. 21:367, 1968.
59a. Mitral Stenosis and Left Atrial Myxoma. In Fowler, N. O.: Diagnosis of Heart Disease. New York, Springer-Verlag, 1991, pp. 146–159.
60. Gershlick, A. H., Leech, G., Mills, P. G., and Leatham, A.: The loud first heart sound in left atrial myxoma. Br. Heart J. 52:403, 1984.
61. Bass, N. M., and Sharratt, G. J. P.: Left atrial myxoma diagnosed by echocardiography with observations on tumor movement. Br. Heart J. 35:1332, 1973.
62. Waxler, E. B., Kawai, N., and Kasparian, H.: Right atrial myxoma: Echocardiographic, phonocardiographic and hemodynamic signs. Am. Heart J. 82:251, 1972.
63. Talley, R. C., Baldwin, B. J., Symbas, P. N., and Nutter, D. O.: Right atrial myxoma. Unusual presentation with cyanosis and clubbing. Am. J. Med. 48:256, 1970.
64. Keren, A., Chenzbruna, A., Schuger, L., et al.: The etiology of tumor plop in a patient with huge right atrial myxoma. Chest 95:1147, 1989.
65. Hada, Y., Wolfe, C., Murry, C. F., and Craige, E.: Right ventricular myxoma. Case report and review of phonocardiographic and auscultatory manifestations. Am. Heart J. 100:871, 1980.

66. Bulkley, B. H., and Hutchins, G. M.: Atrial myxomas: A fifty year review. Am. Heart J. 97:639, 1979.

67. McCarthy, P. M., Piehler, J. M., Schaff, H. V., et al.: The significance of multiple, recurrent, and "complex" cardiac myxomas. Thorac. Cardiovasc. Surg. 91:389, 1986.

68. Carney, J. A.: Differences between nonfamilial and familial cardiac myxoma. Am. J. Surg. Pathol. 9:53, 1985.

69. Davison, E. T., Mumford, D., Zaman, Q., and Horowitz, A.: Left atrial myxoma in the elderly. Report of four patients over the age of 70 and review of the literature. J. Am. Geriatr. Soc. 34:229, 1986.

70. Gosse, P., Herpin, D., Roudant, R., et al.: Myxoma of the mitral valve diagnosed by echocardiography. Am. Heart J. 111:803, 1986.

71. Bennett, W. S., Skelton, T. N., and Lehan, P. H.: The complex of myxomas, pigmentation and endocrine overactivity. Am. J. Cardiol. 65:399, 1990.

72. Carney, J. A., Gordon, J., Carpenter, P. C., et al.: The complex of myxomas, spotty pigmentation, and endocrine overactivity. Medicine 64:270, 1985.

73. Rhodes, A. R., Silverman, R. A., Harrist, T. J., and Perez-Atayde, A. R.: Mucocutaneous lentigines, cardiomucocutaneous myxomas, and multiple blue nevi: The "LAMB" syndrome. Am. Acad. Dermatol. 10:72, 1984.

74. Peterson, L. L., and Serrill, W. S.: Lentiginosis associated with a left atrial myxoma. Am. Acad. Dermatol. 10:337, 1984.

75. Vidaillet, H. J., Jr., Seward, J. B., Fyke, E., and Tajik, A. J.: NAME syndrome (nevi, atrial myxoma, myxoid neurofibroma, ephelides): A new and unrecognized subset of patients with cardiac myxoma. Minn. Med. 67:695, 1984.

76. Carney, J. A., Hruska, L. S., Beauchamp, G. D., and Gordon, H.: Dominant inheritance of the complex of myxomas, spotty pigmentation and endocrine overactivity. Mayo Clin. Proc. 61:165, 1986.

77. Michels, V. V.: A new inherited syndrome with cardiac, cutaneous, and endocrine involvement. Mayo Clin. Proc. 61:224, 1986.

78. Vidaillet, H. J., Jr., Seward, J. B., Fyke, F. E. et al.: "Syndrome myoxma": a subset of patients with cardiac myxoma associated with pigmented skin lesions and peripheral and endocrine neoplasms. Br. Heart J. 57:247, 1987.

79. McCarthy, P. M., Schaff, H. V., Winkler, H. Z., et al.: Deoxyribonucleic acid ploidy pattern of cardiac myxomas. Another predictor of biologically unusual myxomas. J. Thorac. Cardiovasc. Surg. 98:1083, 1989.

80. Sayler, W. R., Page, D. L., and Hutchins, G. M.: The development of cardiac myxomas and papillary endocardial lesions from mural thrombus. Am. Heart J. 89:4, 1975.

80a. Seidman, J. D., Berman, J. J., Hitchcock, C. L., et al.: DNA analysis of cardiac myxomas: Flow cytometry and image analysis. Hum. Pathol. 22:494, 1991.

81. Tanimura, A., Tanaka, S., Kitazono, M., and Kosuga, K.: The surface lining of cells of cardiac myxoma. Light, electron microscopic and immunohistochemical observation. Acta Pathol. Jpn. 35:667, 1986.

82. Boxer, M. E.: Cardiac myxoma: An immunoperoxidase study of histogenesis. Histopathology 8:861, 1984.

83. Landon, G., Ordonez, N. G., and Guarda, L. A.: Cardiac myxomas. An immunohistochemical study using endothelial, histiocytic, and smooth-muscle cell markers. Arch. Pathol. Lab. Med. 110:116, 1986.

84. McComb, R. D.: Heterogeneous expression of factor VIII/von Willebrand factor by cardiac myxoma cells. Am. J. Surg. Pathol. 8:539, 1984.

85. Tanimura, A., Kitazono, M., Nagayama, K., et al.: Cardiac myxoma: Morphologic, histochemical, and tissue culture studies. Hum. Pathol. 19:316, 1988.

86. Govoni, E., Severi, B., Cenacchi, G., et al.: Ultrastructural and immunohistochemical contribution to the histogenesis of human cardiac myxoma. Ultrastruct. Pathol. 12:221, 1988.

87. Takagi, M.: Ultrastructural and immunohistochemical characteristics of cardiac myxoma. Acta Pathol. Jpn. 34:1099, 1984.

88. Hannah, H., Eisemann, G., Hiszcyniskyj, R., Wimsky, M., and Cohen, R.: Invasive atrial myxoma. Documentation of malignant potential of cardiac myxoma. Am. Heart J. 104:881, 1982

89. Chen, K. T.: Carcinosarcoma of the heart. Am. Surg. Oncol. 27:48, 1984.

90. Seo, I. S., Warner, T. F. C. S., Colyer, R. A., and Winkler, F. R.: Metastasizing atrial myxoma. Am. J. Surg. Pathol. 4:391, 1980.

91. Budzilovich, G., Aleksic, S., Greco, A., et al.: Malignant cardiac myxoma with cerebral metastases. Surg. Neurol. 11:461, 1979.

91a. Kotani, K., Matsuzawa, Y., Funahashi, T., et al.: Left atrial myxoma metastasizing to the aorta, with intraluminal growth causing renovascular hypertension. Cardiology 78:72, 1991.

92. Ferrans, V. J., and Roberts, W. C.: Structural features of cardiac myxomas. Hum. Pathol. 4:111, 1973.

93. Feldman, P. S., Horvath, E., and Kovacs, K.: An ultrastructural study of seven cardiac myxomas. Cancer 40:2216, 1977.

94. Zhang, P. F., Jones, J. W., and Anderson, W. R.: Cardiac myxomas correlative study by light, transmission, and scanning electron microscopy. Am. J. Cardiovasc. Pathol. 2:295, 1989.

95. Wold, L. E., and Lie, J. T.: Scanning electron microscopy of intracardiac myxoma. Mayo Clin. Proc. 56:198, 1981.

96. Topol, E. J., Bierm, R. O., and Reitz, B. A.: Cardiac papillary fibroelastoma and stroke. Am. J. Med. 80:129, 1986.

97. Pomerance, A.: Papillary "tumours" of the heart valves. J. Pathol. Bacteriol. 81:135, 1961.

98. Lichtenstein, H. L., Lee, J. C. K., and Stewart, S.: Papillary tumor of the heart: Incidental finding at surgery. Hum. Pathol. 10:473, 1979.

99. Fenoglio, J. J., McAllister, H. A., and Ferrans, V. J.: Cardiac rhabdomyoma: A clinicopathologic and electron microscopic study. Am. J. Cardiol. 38:241, 1976.

100. Bruni, C., Prioleau, P. G., Ivey, H. H., and Nolan, S. P.: New fine structural features of cardiac rhabdomyoma: A case report. Cancer 46:2068, 1980.

101. Takatoh, H., Iwamoto, H., Ikezu, M., et al.: Cardiac rhabdomyoma. A case report with reference to atrial natriuretic peptide. Acta Pathol. Jpn. 38:95, 1988.

102. Shrivastava, S., Jacks, J. J., White, R. S., and Edwards, J. E.: Diffuse rhabdomyomatosis of the heart. Arch. Pathol. Lab. Med. 101:78, 1977.

103. Bass, J. L., Breningstall, G. N., and Swaiman, K. F.: Echocardiographic incidence of cardiac rhabdomyoma in tuberous sclerosis. Am. J. Cardiol. 55:137, 1985.

104. Gibbs, J. L.: The heart and tuberous sclerosis. An echocardiographic and electrocardiographic study. Br. Heart J. 54:596, 1985.

105. Howanitz, E. P., Teske, D. W., Qualman, S. J., et al.: Pedunculated left ventricular rhabdomyoma. Ann. Thorac. Surg. 41:443, 1986.

106. Van der Hauwaert, L. G.: Cardiac tumours in infancy and childhood. Br. Heart J. 33:125, 1971.

107. Feldman, P. S., and Meyer, M. W.: Fibroelastic hamartoma (fibroma) of the heart. Cancer 38:314, 1976.

108. Jones, K. L., Wolf, P. L., Jensen, P., et al.: The Gorlin syndrome: A genetically determined disorder associated with cardiac tumor. Am. Heart J. 111:1013, 1986.

109. Takahashi, K., Imamura, Y., Ochi, T., et al.: Echocardiographic demonstration of an asymptomatic patient with left ventricular fibroma. Am. J. Cardiol. 53:981, 1984.

110. deRuiz, M., Potter, J. L., Stavinoha, J., et al.: Real-time ultrasound diagnosis of cardiac fibroma in a neonate. J. Ultrasound Med. 4:367, 1985.

111. Prior, J. T.: Lipomatous hypertrophy of cardiac interatrial septum. Arch. Pathol. 78:11, 1964.

112. Hutter, A. M., Jr., and Page, D. L.: Atrial arrhythmias and lipomatous hypertrophy of the cardiac interatrial septum. Am. Heart J. 82:16, 1971.

113. Simons, M., Cabin, H. S., and Jaffer, C. C.: Lipomatous hypertrophy of the atrial septum: Diagnosis by combined echocardiography and computerized tomography. Am. J. Cardiol. 54:465, 1984.

114. Chao, J. C., Reyes, C. V., and Hwang, M. H.: Cardiac hemangioma. South Med. J. 83:44, 1990.

115. Cox, J. N., Friedli, B., Mechmeche, M., et al.: Teratoma of the heart. Virchows Arch. (A) 402:163, 1983.

116. Duray, P. H., Mark, E. J., Barwick, K. W., et al.: Congenital polycystic tumor of the atrioventricular node. Arch. Pathol. Lab. Med. 109:30, 1985.

117. Linder, J., Shelburne, J. D., Sorge, J. P., et al.: Congenital endodermal heterotopia of the atrioventricular node: Evidence for the endodermal origin of so-called mesotheliomas of the atrioventricular node. Hum. Pathol. 15:1093, 1984.

118. David, T. E., Lenkei, S. C., Marquez-Julio, A., et al.: Pheochromocytoma of the heart. Ann. Thorac. Surg. 41:98, 1986.

119. Hodgson, S. F., Sheps, S. G., Subramanian, R., et al.: Catecholamine-secreting paraganglioma of the interatrial septum. Am. J. Med. 77:157, 1984.

120. Shemin, R. J., Marsh, J. D., and Schoen, F. J.: Benign intracardiac thyroid mass causing right ventricular outflow tract obstruction. Am. J. Cardiol. 56:828, 1985.

121. Whorton, C. M.: Primary malignant tumor of the heart. Cancer 2:245, 1949.

121a. Burke, A. P., and Virmani, R.: Osteosarcomas of the heart. Am. J. Surg. Pathol. 15:289, 1991.

122. Goldberg, H. P., and Steinberg, I.: Primary tumors of the heart. Circulation 11:963, 1955.

123. Glancy, L., Morales, J. B., and Roberts, W. C.: Angiosarcoma of the heart. Am. J. Cardiol. 21:413, 1968.

124. Janigan, D. T., Husain, A., and Robinson, N. A.: Cardiac angiosarcomas. A review and a case report. Cancer 57:852, 1986.

125. Keohane, M. E., Lazzam, C., Halperin, J. L., et al.: Angiosarcoma of the left atrium mimicking myxoma. Case report. Hum. Pathol. 20:599, 1989.

126. Yang, H.-Y., Wasielewski, J. F., Lee, E., and Paik, Y. K.: Angiosarcoma of the heart: Ultrastructural study. Cancer 47:72, 1981.

127. Hui, K. S., Green, L. K., and Schmidt, W. A.: Primary cardiac rhabdomyosarcoma: Definition of a rare entity. Am. J. Cardiovasc. Pathol. 2:19, 1988.

128. Proctor, M. S., Tracy, G. P., and Von Koch, L.: Primary cardiac B-cell lymphoma. Am. Heart J. 118:179, 1989.

129. Bleisch, N., and Kraus, F.: Polypoid sarcoma of the pulmonary trunk. Cancer 46:314, 1980.

DIAGNOSTIC TECHNIQUES

130. Oldershaw, P. J., Sutton, M. St. J., and Gibson, R. V.: Long asymptomatic period of atrial myxomas. Thorax 35:70, 1980.

131. Roberts, W. C.: The echocardiographic diseases. Am. J. Cardiol. 64:1084, 1989.

132. Steiner, R. E.: Radiologic aspects of cardiac tumors. Am. J. Cardiol. 21:344, 1968.

133. Abrams, H. L., Adams, D. F., and Grant, H. A.: The radiology of tumors of the heart. Radiol. Clin. North Am. 9:299, 1971.

134. Sabot, G., Fauvel, J. M., and Bounhoure, J. P.: Echocardiographic diagnosis of mobile left ventricular tumour. Br. Heart J. 42:113, 1979.

135. Nanda, N. C., Barold, S. S., Gramiak, R., et al.: Echocardiographic features of right ventricular outflow tumor prolapsing into the pulmonary artery. Am. J. Cardiol. 40:272, 1977.

136. Green, S. E., Joynt, L. E., Fitzgerald, P. J., et al.: In vivo ultrasonic tissue characterization of human intracardiac masses. Am. J. Cardiol. *51*:231, 1983.

137. Duncan, W. J., Rowe, R. D., Freedom, R. M., et al.: Space-occupying lesions of the myocardium: Role of two-dimensional echocardiography in detection of cardiac tumors in children. Am. Heart J. *104*:780, 1982.

137a. Wrisley, D., Rosenberg, J., Giambartolomei, A., et al.: Left ventricular myxoma discovered incidentally by echocardiography. Am. Heart J. *121*:1554, 1991.

138. Charuzi, Y., Bolger, A., Beeder, C., and Lew, A. S.: A new echocardiographic classification of left atrial myxoma. Am. J. Cardiol. *55*:614, 1985.

139. Dennis, M. A., Appareti, K., Manco-Johnson, M. L., et al.: The echocardiographic diagnosis of multiple fetal cardiac tumors. Ultrasound Med. *4*:327, 1985.

140. Panidis, I. P., Mimtz, G. S., and McAllister, M.: Hemodynamic consequences of the left atrial myxomas as assessed by Doppler ultrasound. Am. Heart J. *111*:927, 1986.

140a. Lyons, S. V., McCord, J., and Smith, S.: Asymptomatic giant right atrial myxoma: Role of transeophageal echocardiography in management. Am. Heart J. *121*:1555, 1991.

141. Fueredi, G. A., Knechtges, T. E., and Czarnecki, D. J.: Coronary angiography in atrial myxoma: Findings in nine cases. Am. J. Roentgenol. *152*:737, 1989.

142. Singh, R. N., Burkholder, J. A., and Magovern, G. J.: Coronary arteriography as an aid in left atrial myxoma diagnosis. Cardiovasc. Intervent. Radiol. *7*:40, 1984.

143. Weyne, A. E., Heyndrickx, G. R., Cuvelier, C. C., et al.: Cardiac imaging techniques in the diagnosis of angiosarcoma of the heart: report of two cases. Postgrad. Med. J. *61*:271, 1985.

144. Pendyck, F., Pierce, E. C., Baron, M. G., and Lukban, S. B.: Embolization of left atrial myxoma after transseptal cardiac catheterization. Am. J. Cardiol. *30*;569, 1972.

TREATMENT AND PROGNOSIS

145. Becker, R. C., Loeffler, J. S., Leopold, K. A., and Underwood, D. A.: Primary tumors of the heart: A review with emphasis on diagnosis and potential treatment modalities. Semin. Surg. Oncol. *1*:161, 1985.

146. Murphy, M. C., Sweeney, M. S., Putnam, J. B., Jr., et al.: Surgical treatment of cardiac tumors: a 25-year experience. Ann. Thorac. Surg. *49*:612, 1990.

147. Dapper, F., Gorlach, G., Hoffmann, C., et al: Primary cardiac tumors—clinical experiences and late results in 48 patients. Thorac. Cardiovasc. Surg. *36*:80, 1988.

148. Semb, B. K.: Surgical considerations in the treatment of cardiac myxoma. J. Thorac. Cardiovasc. Surg. *87*:251, 1984.

149. Marvasti, M. A., Obeid, A. I., Potts, J. L., and Parker, F. B.: Approach in the management of atrial myxoma with long-term follow-up. Ann. Thorac. Surg. *38*:53, 1984.

150. Waller, D. A., Ettles, D. F., Saunders, N. R., and Williams, G.: Recurrent cardiac myxoma: The surgical implications of two distinct groups of patients. Thorac. Cardiovasc Surg. *37*:226, 1989.

151. Bortolotti, U., Maraglino, G., Rubino, M., et al.: Surgical excision of intracardiac myxomas: A 20-year follow-up. Ann. Thorac. Surg. *49*:449, 1990.

152. Larsson, S., Lepore, V., and Kennergren, C.: Atrial myxomas: Results of 25 years' experience and review of the literature. Surgery *105*:695, 1989.

153. Scheld, H. H., Nestle, H. W., Kling, D., et al.: Resection of a heart tumor using autotransplantation. Thorac. Cardiovasc. Surg. *36*:40, 1988.

154. Mesnildrey, P., Bloch, G., Cachera, J. P., and Piwnica, A.: Atrial myxoma: A new surgical approach using neodymium: yttrium-aluminum-garnet laser photocoagulation. J. Thorac. Cardiovasc. Surg. *98*:313, 1989.

155. Parks, F. R., Adams, F., and Longmire, W. P.: Successful excision of a left ventricular hamartoma. Circulation *26*:1316, 1962.

156. Etches, P. C., Gribbin, B., and Gunning, A. J.: Echocardiographic diagnosis and successful removal of cardiac fibroma in 4-year old child. Br. Heart J. *43*:360, 1980.

157. Goldman, S., Lortscher, R., and Pappas, G.: Surgical treatment for rhabdomyoma of the right atrium causing arrhythmias. J. Thorac. Cardiovasc. Surg. *89*:802, 1985.

158. Corno, A., deSimone, G., Catena, G., and Marcelletti, C.: Cardiac rhabdomyoma: Surgical treatment in the neonate. Thorac. Cardiovasc. Surg. *87*:1984.

159. Foster, E. D., Spooner, E. W., Farina, M. A., et al.: Cardiac rhabdomyoma in the neonate: Surgical treatment. Ann. Thorac. Surg. *37*:249, 1984.

160. Orringer, M. B., Sisson, J. C., Glazer, G., et al.: Surgical treatment of cardiac pheochromocytomas. J. Thorac. Cardiovasc. Surg. *89*:753, 1985.

161. Key, T. C., Resnik, R., Dittrich, H. C., and Reisner, L. S.: Successful pregnancy after cardiac transplantation. Am. J. Obstet. Gynecol. *160*:367, 1989.

162. Marvasti, M. A., Bove, E. L., Obeid, A. I., et al.: Primary osteosarcoma of left atrium: Complete surgical excision. Ann. Thorac. Surg. *40*;402, 1985.

163. Sharma, S., Tendolkar, A., and Parulkar, G. B.: Angiosarcoma of the heart. Am. Heart J. *109*:601, 1985.

164. Vergnon, J. M., Vincent, M., Perinetti, M., et al.: Chemotherapy of metastatic primary cardiac sarcomas. Am. Heart J. *110*;682, 1985.

165. Hollingworth, J. H., and Sturgill, B. C.: Treatment of primary angiosarcoma of the heart. Am. Heart J. *78*:254, 1969.

166. Potter, R., Baumgart, P., Greve, H., Schnepper, E.: Primary angiosarcoma of the heart. Thorac. Cardiovasc. Surg. *37*:374, 1989.

167. Dichek, D. A., Holmvang, G., Fallon, J. T., et al.: Angiosarcoma of the heart: Three year survival and follow-up by nuclear magnetic resonance imaging. Am. Heart J. *115*:1323, 1988.

168. Allaire, F. J., Grimm, C. A., Taylor, L. M., and Pfaff, J. P.: Primary hemangioendothelioma of the heart. Rocky Mt. Med. J. *61*:34, 1964.

169. Terry, L. N., and Kilgerman, M. M.: Pericardial and myocardial involvement by lymphomas and leukemias. The role of radiotherapy. Cancer *25*:1003, 1970.

170. Garfein, O. B.: Lymphosarcoma of the right atrium: Angiographic and hemodynamic documentation of response to chemotherapy. Arch. Intern. Med. *135*:325, 1975.

Pericardial Disease
by BEVERLY H. LORELL, M.D., and EUGENE BRAUNWALD, M.D.

ANATOMY

The pericardium forms a strong flask-shaped sac with short tubelike extensions that enclose the origins of the aorta and its junction with the aortic arch, the pulmonary artery where it branches, the proximal pulmonary veins, and venae cavae. Fibrous tissue of the pericardium actually blends with adventitia of the great arteries to form very strong attachments. In addition, the pericardium has firm ligamentous attachments anteriorly to the sternum and xiphoid process, posteriorly to the vertebral column, and inferiorly to the diaphragm.[1,1a]

The human pericardium receives its arterial blood supply from small branches of the aorta and internal mammary and musculophrenic arteries. The pericardium is innervated by the vagus, left recurrent laryngeal nerve, and esophageal plexus and also has rich sympathetic innervation from the stellate and first dorsal ganglia and the cardiac, aortic, and diaphragmatic plexuses. The phrenic nerves course over the pericardium en route to the diaphragm. The afferent nerves responsible for pain perception appear to be transmitted via the phrenic nerve entering the spinal cord at C4–C5.[1] Peripheral sensory fibers that enter the dorsal root ganglia at C8–T2 supply both the brachial plexus and the pericardium, which provides a possible morphological explanation for referred pericardial pain.[2]

THE TWO LAYERS OF THE PERICARDIUM. The pericardium is composed of a fibrous outer layer and an inner serous membrane composed of a single layer of mesothelial cells. The inner serous layer is intimately attached to the surface of the heart and epicardial fat to form the visceral pericardium, and this inner serous membrane reflects back on itself to line the outer fibrous layer to form the parietal pericardium.

The pericardium has two major serosal tunnels: the transverse sinus, which lies posterior to the great arteries and anterior to the atria and superior vena cava, and the oblique sinus, which lies posterior to the left atrium so that the posterior left atrial wall is actually separated from the pericardial space. The serous visceral pericardium is attached to the parietal pericardium by delicate connective tissue with elastin fibers. The parietal pericardium is composed of collagen fibers interlaced with extensive elastic fibers, which are wavy during childhood and become progressively straighter with age, suggesting that young pericardia are more compliant than those of the elderly.

ELECTRON MICROSCOPY. This reveals that exuberant microvilli and long, single cilia project from the serous mesothelium composing the visceral pericardium and the inner lining of the parietal pericardium (Fig. 45–1),[3] which increase markedly the surface area available for fluid transport. Both microvilli and cilia provide a specialized surface to permit movement of the pericardial membranes over each other during each cardiac cycle and to permit the pericardium to accommodate changes in cardiac shape during contraction. In addition, numerous small fenestrations or pores less than 50 μ in diameter provide direct communication between the pericardial and pleural cavities in mammals.[4]

PERICARDIAL FLUID. The human pericardium normally contains up to 50 ml of clear fluid. The visceral pericardium is believed to be the source of normal pericardial fluid and of excessive fluid in disease states. Normal pericardial fluid appears to be an ultrafiltrate of plasma, since electrolytes are present in pericardial fluid in concentrations compatible with such an ultrafiltrate; protein concentrations are about one-third those of the plasma, and albumin is present in a higher ratio in pericardial fluid, reflecting its lower molecular weight. Current data suggest that drainage of the pericardial space occurs both by the thoracic duct via the parietal pericardium and by the right lymphatic duct via the right pleural space.

Pericardial fluid also contains phospholipids that serve as a lubricant to reduce friction between the surfaces of the parietal pericardium and the visceral pericardium.[5] The pericardium appears to produce prostaglandins in response to physiological stimuli that may modulate efferent cardiac sympathetic stimulation and alter cardiac electrophysiological properties.[6] The clinical implications of this potential regulatory effect of the pericardium on electrical conduction of the heart are not yet known.

FUNCTIONS OF THE PERICARDIUM

The pericardium's ligamentous attachments help to fix the heart anatomically and prevent excessive motion with changes in body position. The pericardium also reduces friction between the heart and surrounding organs and provides a barrier against the extension of infection and malignancy from contiguous organs to the heart itself. The role of the pericardium in the regulation of the circulation is controversial, since congenital absence of the pericardium is not associated with overt disturbances of cardiac function. However, observations in both dogs and humans indicate that the pericardium may play a role in (1) the distribution of hydrostatic forces on the heart, (2) the prevention of acute cardiac dilatation, and (3) diastolic coupling of the two ventricles (p. 1468).

The normal pericardium is relatively stiff, and the relationship between pressure within the pericardium and total intrapericardial volume, which is the sum of the volume of the heart itself and the reserve volume of the surrounding pericardial sac, appears as a steep curve when plotted on a graph.[1]

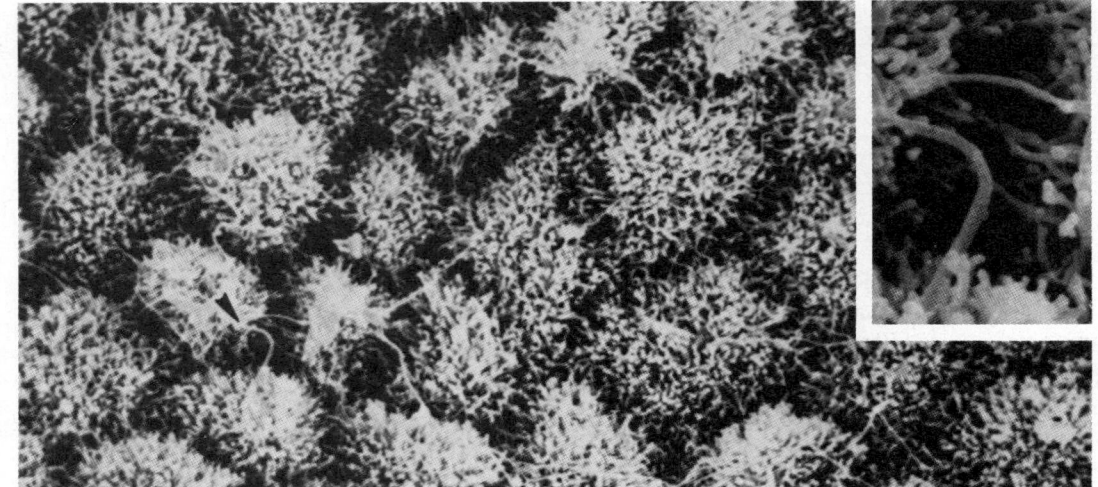

FIGURE 45–1. Scanning electron micrograph of human parietal pericardium. The mesothelial cells are covered with microvilli, and long individual cilia (arrow) are also present. Insert shows cilia at higher magnification. (From Ishihara, T., et al.: Histologic and ultrastructural features of normal human parietal pericardium. Am. J. Cardiol 46:744, 1980.)

Once the pericardium is filled, intrapericardial pressure rises sharply as volume is increased (Fig. 45–2). Thus, the stiffness of the pericardium increases when load is increased, and then it becomes almost inextensible. Although much of our knowledge regarding the physiological role of the pericardium has been derived from experimental studies in dogs, it is important to recognize that the human pericardium is about three times as thick and much less distensible than canine pericardium.[7] Usually, the pericardial sac is filled with a thin film of fluid distributed throughout the pericardial space in such a way that the pericardial reserve volume is not exceeded. This permits respiratory and postural changes in cardiac volume and total intrapericardial volume to occur without significant changes in intrapericardial pressure. When measured with a fluid-filled or micromanometer-tipped catheter, pericardial pressure is nearly equal to intrapleural pressure and varies from −5 to +5 cm H_2O during the respiratory cycle.[8]

INTRAPERICARDIAL PRESSURE. Normal intrapericardial pressure is zero or negative. This has major implications for our understanding of the influence of pericardial pressure on the transmural distending pressure of the cardiac chambers and the operation of the Frank-Starling mechanism in the beat-to-beat regulation of stroke volume.[9] The transmural distending pressure of either ventricle is the difference

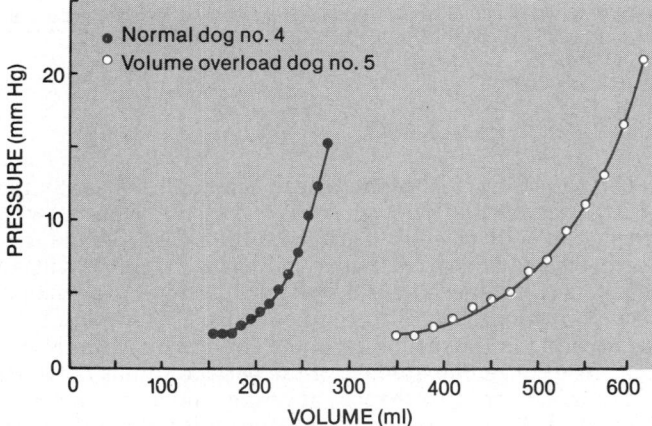

FIGURE 45–2. Pericardial pressure-volume curves from a normal dog (left) and from a dog with chronic volume overload (right). Note that the normal pressure-volume curve (right) is initially flat but becomes extremely steep as total volume within the pericardium increases. In response to chronic cardiac dilatation, the pericardium enlarges in size and mass such that the pericardium can accomodate a large volume at low pressure (right curve). (From Freeman, G. L., and LeWinter, M. M.: Pericardial adaptations during chronic dilation in dogs. Circ. Res. 54:294, 1984.)

between intracardiac and intrapericardial pressures and is independent of gravity. When intrapericardial pressure is assumed to be negative, normally a substantial transmural distending pressure would be expected to exist across both ventricles. For example, when left ventricular end-diastolic pressure is +8 mm Hg and intrapericardial pressure is −2 mm Hg relative to atmosphere, the actual left ventricular distending pressure would be 8 − (−2) = 10 mm Hg, and when right ventricular end-diastolic pressure is 4 mm Hg and intrapericardial pressure is −2 mm Hg relative to atmosphere, the actual right ventricular distending pressure would be 4 − (−2) = 6 mm Hg.

Studies using micromanometer pressure measurements support the view that pericardial pressure is usually very low and thus exerts only a small influence on the average transmural distending pressure of the heart as long as pericardial reserve volume is not exceeded by volume loading.[8] Under normal conditions, it is clear that the pericardium does influence the pattern of venous return and ventricular filling that occurs in every cardiac cycle. Ventricular ejection is accompanied by abrupt descent of the atrioventricular junction (the "base" of the heart) and a reduction in right atrial pressure, manifest by the x descent* in the right atrial pressure pulse as well as by a decline in intrapericardial pressure. These changes result in a surge of venous return during systole, particularly when ventricular and pericardial pressures are increased. This acceleration of venous return during systolic ejection is diminished by opening of the pericardium.

When the volume of the heart or other contents of the pericardial sac increase and exceed the elastic limits of the pericardium during diastole, the heart is shifted to the steep portion of the curve relating intrapericardial pressure and volume, resulting in marked increases in intrapericardial and intracardiac pressures. However, the difference between the two pressures, i.e., the transmural pressure, usually declines. In the extreme case of cardiac tamponade, in which both intrapericardial and intracardiac pressures are markedly increased, the transmural pressure distending the ventricles may fall precipitously toward zero, resulting in decreased ventricular diastolic volumes and preload. These findings, taken together, support the classic view that the pericardium is a distensible "loosely fitting" sac that modestly affects stroke volume by changes in intrapericardial pressure and

---

*It is recognized that the descent in venous pressure after the a wave is usually termed the x descent and, after the c wave, the x' descent. In this chapter, the major systolic venous pressure descent after the a and c waves will be termed the x descent.

transmural pressure and exerts a substantial influence only at higher ventricular and pericardial pressures.

CHALLENGES TO THE "CLASSIC VIEW." This classic view has been seriously challenged by Smiseth and coworkers,[10] who contend that the use of either fluid-filled or micromanometer catheters underestimates pericardial pressure and its influence on transmural distending pressures in normal hearts. They have shown in dogs that the measurement of the *surface contact pressure* of the pericardium against the heart using a flat balloon is more accurate than a fluid-filled catheter in estimating the actual pericardial pressure (the fall in left ventricular pressure observed immediately after opening the pericardium in the absence of any change in chamber volume). Observations from dogs and from humans indicate that when the amount of fluid in the pericardial sac is small, pericardial pressure measured in this way is much higher than intrathoracic pressure or pericardial pressure measured with a fluid-filled or micromanometer catheter, whereas pericardial pressures measured by either a balloon or fluid-filled catheter are similar when a substantial volume of pericardial fluid (40 to 50 ml) is present.[11,12] Thus the controversy regarding the concept of pericardial surface contact pressure does not detract from the accuracy or the clinical utility of measuring intrapericardial pressure with a catheter in patients with large pericardial effusions and cardiac tamponade.

However, these arguments profoundly challenge classic views regarding the normal physiology of the heart and the accurate measurement of the transmural pressure of each ventricle. These studies have emphasized that intrapericardial surface contact pressure is not zero or negative and, to the contrary, is virtually equal to right atrial pressure.[10,11] A further assumption is that differences in pericardial surface contact pressure do not exist over different chambers of the heart. This analysis indicates that left ventricular transmural pressure in normal hearts should be estimated by subtracting right atrial pressure rather than intrathoracic pressure. It also carries the remarkable implication that the transmural distending pressure of the normal right ventricle is extremely small, and negligible or zero at end-diastole.

Experiments by Santamore et al.[13] and Slinker et al.[14] have modified this concept and indicate that closed flat-balloon catheters probably exaggerate the constraining pressure exerted by the normal pericardium on the surface of the heart. Experiments examining right ventricular and left ventricular pressure-volume relationships in arrested canine hearts showed that although right ventricular transmural pressure is always less than left ventricular transmural pressure over the physiological range, measurable right ventricular transmural pressure is always present in the absence of the pericardium even at low volumes, and right heart transmural pressure increases with increments in ventricular volume. In the canine heart the contribution of the pericardium to right ventricular diastolic pressure is substantial (greater than 50 per cent) only at right ventricular filling pressures greater than 10 mm Hg. In addition, experiments indicate that the pressure exerted by the pericardium on the surface of the heart is not uniform over different regions of the heart.[15]

Taken together, these experiments suggest that right atrial pressure cannot be used to estimate precisely the pericardial constraint or to calculate transmural pressures of either ventricle in the normal heart. Furthermore, pericardial catheter measurements tend to underestimate while pericardial balloons tend to overestimate pericardial pressure, which appears to be within the range of 0.2 to 3 mm Hg under normal physiological conditions. Finally, these experiments confirm that the pericardium modifies the filling and intracavitary pressures of both ventricles, particularly when cardiac distention occurs.

LIMITATION OF CARDIAC DISTENTION. The rela-

tively nondistensible pericardium may help to limit acute distention of the heart. This was appreciated as early as 1898 by Bernard, who used a pump to increase pressure in excised hearts with and without the pericardium and noted that hearts unsupported by the pericardium ruptured at lower pressures than did hearts with intact pericardia.[16] Subsequent studies in dogs demonstrated that the pericardium restrains right and left ventricular filling, so that ventricular volume is greater at any given ventricular pressure with the pericardium removed than with the pericardium intact. Thus, acute changes in intracardiac and total intrapericardial volume result in an upward shift of both the left and right ventricular pressure-volume relationships, which is in part mediated by the restraining effect of the pericardium and an increase in intrapericardial pressure.[14,17,18] As ventricular volumes increase, the proportional contribution of the pericardium to end-diastolic pressure of the thin-walled right ventricle increases relative to that of the left ventricle.[14] Thus, as the heart is distended, the pericardium makes a greater contribution to right ventricular end-diastolic pressure than to left ventricular end-diastolic pressure.

The hemodynamic effects of acute volume loading and vasodilators are in part mediated by pericardial constraint. Shirato et al.[19] demonstrated that acute volume loading with dextran in dogs with intact pericardia resulted in an upward shift in the left ventricular pressure–segment length relation, i.e., left ventricular pressure was higher at any given segment length while the reduction of venous return and cardiac volume by means of nitroprusside administration shifted the curves downward toward control levels (Fig. 45–3). This occurred because nitroprusside and other vasodilators that decrease right heart filling reduce the total volume occupied by the heart within the pericardial space and thus reduce the restraining of the left ventricle by the pericardium; in turn, this causes a downward shift of the left ventricular pressure-volume relation so that a given left ventricular volume is associated with lower left ventricular diastolic pressure. After pericardiectomy, volume loading results in a rightward shift in the pressure-segment length relation and, after nitroprusside, a leftward shift along a single curve.[19] When the effect of the pericardium is eliminated by plotting left ventricular transmural pressure versus segment length, the points during all interventions fall along a single curve. Smiseth et al.[20] have extended these findings and have shown that the opposite effects of angiotensin (upward shift) and nitroprusside (downward shift) of the left ventricle pressure-volume relation depend on changes in intrapericardial pressure mediated by shifts in blood volume from the heart to systemic vascular beds.

A restraining effect of the pericardium has been observed early in the course of chronic volume overloading induced by formation of arteriovenous shunts in dogs prior to enlargement of the pericardium by stretch or hypertrophy. However,

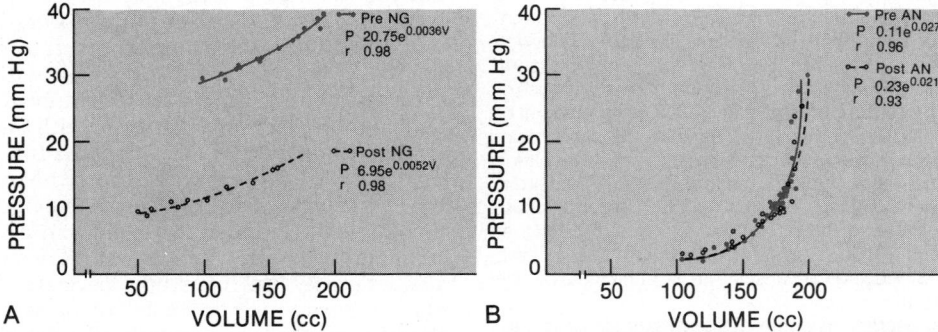

FIGURE 45–3. Left ventricular pressure-volume curves in man (*A*) before and after nitroglycerin (NG) and (*B*) before and after amyl nitrite (AN). Nitroglycerin, which causes venodilation and reduces total intrapericardial volume, shifts the curve downward and leftward. In contrast, the curves before and after amyl nitrite, which causes arterial dilation, can be superimposed. (From Ludbrook, P. A., et al.: Influence of right ventricular hemodynamics on left ventricular diastolic pressure-volume relations in man. Circulation 59:21, 1979, by permission of the American Heart Association, Inc.)

1467
CHAP
45

this restraining effect was not apparent in dogs studied late during the course of chronic volume overload.[21] This occurs because chronic left ventricular enlargement and hypertrophy are accompanied by an increase in the compliance of the pericardial chamber and an increase in total pericardial volume due to the addition of new pericardial tissue.[22] In addition to its effects on ventricular filling, pericardial pressure also appears to influence indices of isovolumic relaxation of the left ventricle. Frais et al.[23] showed that alterations in the asymptote and time constant of left ventricular pressure decay (tau) in dogs subjected to volume loading vary with changes in intrapericardial pressure.

These observations suggest that shifts in the left and right ventricular diastolic pressure-volume relations following volume loading or vasodilator administration are largely due to changes in intrapericardial pressure. However, the pericardium does not affect *intrinsic* myocardial compliance; neither does it account for changes in the left ventricular diastolic pressure-volume relationship observed during ischemia.[24]

VENTRICULAR INTERDEPENDENCE. The pericardium also contributes to diastolic coupling between the two ventricles. The distention of one ventricle alters the distensibility of the other, even in the absence of the pericardium.[25] This effect appears to be mediated in part by shared encircling muscle bands and by the interventricular septum, which tends to bulge into the left ventricle, causing a change in the shape of the left ventricle when the right ventricle is distended.[26] In the absence of the pericardium, large increases in right ventricular volume and pressure are required to cause an appreciable increase in left ventricular filling pressure.[27] In contrast, the presence of an intact pericardium markedly accentuates the coupling between ventricular diastolic pressures.[28] When right ventricular volume and pressure are increased with the normal pericardium intact, right and left ventricular filling pressures are closely correlated, and left ventricular volume is smaller than in the absence of the pericardium. In the absence of the pericardium, cardiac distensibility is primarily related to properties of the myocardium. This effect of the pericardium on the interaction between the two ventricles is accentuated in experimental constrictive pericarditis when the distensibility of the pericardium is decreased.[29] This effect of the pericardium on diastolic ventricular interaction is present at normal filling pressures and becomes of increasing importance at high right ventricular filling pressures. During volume loading in normal conscious dogs, it has been shown that pericardial pressure exerts a disproportionately greater effect on the thin-walled right ventricle, which suggests that the pericardium couples diastolic function of the two ventricles via its influence on right ventricular filling and geometry.[8,14]

Although normal pericardium does not appear to contribute importantly to the interaction of the ventricles during systole at normal filling pressures,[30] it does influence global and regional systolic function during conditions of acute distention of the heart.[31,32] Kanazawa et al.[31] showed that removal of the pericardium in dogs caused insignificant changes in stroke volume, whereas removal of the pericardium during volume loading caused a substantial increase in stroke volume associated with an increase in end-diastolic segment length and systolic excursion. Although pericardial pressure was not measured, it is likely that this increase in stroke volume was due to the Frank-Starling mechanism via an increase of the transmural distending pressure of the ventricle following removal of the pericardium. Furthermore, during volume overload, the pericardium caused an upward shift in the left ventricular end-systolic pressure-volume relationship in the absence of a change in inotropic state. Pericardial constraint also appears to modify regional systolic function during acute right ventricular pressure overload and distention. Goto et al.[32] found that acute right ventricular loading in dogs results in nonuniform decreases in regional left ventricular shortening, an effect that is enhanced by the presence of the pericardium.

The pericardium also appears to limit maximal body oxygen consumption by limiting stroke volume and cardiac output during maximal exercise in conscious dogs.[33] These observations suggest that the normal pericardium exerts a restraining effect and modifies ventricular interaction during systole at high ventricular filling pressures.

In *summary*, there is experimental evidence from canine studies that the pericardium limits acute distention of the heart, mediates changes in the relationship between ventricular pressure and volume, and enhances the effect that distention of one ventricle has on the diastolic pressure-volume relations of the contralateral ventricle.

FUNCTIONS OF THE PERICARDIUM IN HUMANS. There is substantial evidence that the restraining effects of the pericardium are clinically relevant. For example, in humans after pericardiotomy, there is a downward shift of the left ventricular pressure-volume curve that is increasingly prominent as left ventricular volume increases.[34] Similarly, routine pericardial closure after open-heart surgery has been shown to result in an increase in right heart filling pressure associated with a reduction in left ventricular diastolic cavity dimension and cardiac output, whereas opening of the pericardium causes the opposite effects.[35] In addition, angiotensin, nitroprusside, and nitroglycerin infusions, which alter intracardiac volume, cause acute shifts in the left ventricular diastolic pressure-volume relation in humans,[36] an effect that has been shown in animal studies to depend on the presence of the constraint of the pericardium.[20] Ludbrook demonstrated in humans that the downward shift in the left ventricular pressure-volume curve that occurs during nitroglycerin administration is not observed with amyl nitrite, which alters aortic pressure but has little acute effect on intrapericardial volumes (Fig. 45-3).[36,37] After pericardiotomy and loss of the restraining effect of the pericardium, the human left ventricular pressure-volume curve is not altered by nitroprusside administration.[38] These observations indicate that the beneficial effects of interventions such as nitroprusside infusion, in which an augmentation of stroke volume may be observed at a lower ventricular filling pressure, are in part due to an alteration of apparent cardiac distensibility mediated by reducing the restraining effect of the pericardium.[39]

The pericardium may also provide a significant restraining effect on acute cardiac dilatation during acute volume loading in humans.[40] Extrapolating the findings of dog experiments may underestimate the restraining effect of the human pericardium during acute volume loading, since normal human pericardium is thicker and shows much greater viscous responses than canine pericardium.[7] In patients, volume overload due to acute mitral regurgitation is sometimes associated with striking elevation and equilibration of diastolic pressures in all four cardiac chambers similar to that observed in constrictive pericardial disease (p. 1486), but these findings do not appear to be present in patients with chronic volume overload.[41] Similarly, acute right ventricular infarction is sometimes associated with elevation and equilibration of diastolic right and left ventricular pressures[42] that have been shown experimentally to be related to the elevation of intrapericardial pressure.[43]

The role of the pericardium in the pathogenesis of chronic heart failure in patients is controversial and not yet well understood. Although compensatory enlargement and increased capacitance of the pericardium is likely to occur in humans with chronic cardiac enlargement, it is feasible that acute increases in venous return in patients with heart failure could increase the effects of the pericardium on ventricular diastolic and systolic function. Consistent with this hypothesis, Janicki studied the effects of the augmentation of venous return by exercise in 61 patients with chronic heart failure and deduced that pericardial constraint became evident when stroke volume abruptly became invariant and a similar increment in right and left heart filling pressures occurred during progressive exercise.[44] In this study, pericardial constraint became evident during exercise in half of the patients. Thus, it appears that the pericardium can be an important determinant of the limits of systolic pump function and result in the coupling of right and left ventricular diastolic pressures in patients with heart failure.

Acute pericarditis is a syndrome due to inflammation of the pericardium characterized by chest pain, a pericardial friction rub, and serial electrocardiographic abnormalities. The incidence of pericardial inflammation detected in several autopsy series ranges from 2 to 6 per cent, whereas pericarditis is diagnosed clinically in only about 1 of 1000 hospital admissions. This suggests that pericarditis is frequently inapparent clinically, although it may occur in the presence of a vast number of medical and surgical disorders (Table 45–1). The most common causes of the syndrome of acute pericarditis include idiopathic or viral pericarditis, uremia, bacterial infection, acute myocardial infarction, pericardiotomy associated with cardiac surgery, tuberculosis, neoplasm, and trauma. All types of pericarditis are more common in men than in women, and in adults compared with young children. The relative frequency of causes of pericarditis depend on the clinical setting. Presumed viral or idiopathic pericarditis is common in an outpatient setting, while pericarditis related to trauma, neoplasm, and uremia, is seen more frequently in tertiary hospitals.

The *pathological changes* of acute pericarditis are those of acute inflammation, including the presence of polymorphonuclear leukocytes, increased pericardial vascularity, and deposition of fibrin. Inflammation may also involve the superficial myocardium, and fibrinous adhesions may form between the pericardium and epicardium and between the pericardium and adjacent sternum and pleura. The visceral pericardium may also react to acute injury by exudation of fluid. The pathological and clinical features of specific causes of pericarditis are discussed later in this chapter. This section

TABLE 45-1 CAUSES OF PERICARDITIS

1. **IDIOPATHIC (nonspecific)**
2. **VIRAL INFECTIONS:** Coxsackie A virus, Coxsackie B virus, echovirus, adenovirus, mumps virus, infectious mononucleosis, varicella, hepatitis B, AIDS (acquired immunodeficiency syndrome)
3. **TUBERCULOSIS**
4. **ACUTE BACTERIAL INFECTION:** pneumococcus, staphylococcus, streptococcus, gram-negative septicemia, *Neisseria meningitidis, Neisseria gonorrhoeae,* tularemia, *Legionella pneumophila*
5. **FUNGAL INFECTIONS:** histoplasmosis, coccidioidomycosis, *Candida,* blastomycosis
6. **OTHER INFECTIONS:** toxoplasmosis, amebiasis, mycoplasma, *Nocardia,* actinomycosis, echinococcosis, Lyme disease
7. **ACUTE MYOCARDIAL INFARCTION**
8. **UREMIA:** untreated uremia; in association with hemodialysis
9. **NEOPLASTIC DISEASE:** lung cancer, breast cancer, leukemia, Hodgkin's disease, lymphoma
10. **RADIATION**
11. **AUTOIMMUNE DISORDERS:** acute rheumatic fever, systemic lupus erythematosus, rheumatoid arthritis, scleroderma, mixed connective tissue disease, Wegener granulomatosis, polyarteritis nodosa
12. **OTHER INFLAMMATORY DISORDERS:** sarcoidosis, amyloidosis, inflammatory bowel disease, Whipple disease, temporal arteritis, Behçet disease
13. **DRUGS:** hydralazine, procainamide, diphenylhydantoin, isoniazid, phenylbutazone, dantrolene, doxorubicin, methysergide, penicillin (with hypereosinophilia)
14. **TRAUMA:** including chest trauma; hemopericardium following thoracic surgery; pacemaker insertion; cardiac diagnostic procedures; esophageal rupture; pancreatic-pericardial fistula
15. **DELAYED POSTMYOCARDIAL-PERICARDIAL INJURY SYNDROMES:**
    a. **Postmyocardial infarction (Dressler) syndrome**
    b. **Postpericardiotomy syndrome**
16. **DISSECTING AORTIC ANEURYSM**
17. **MYXEDEMA**
18. **CHYLOPERICARDIUM**

TABLE 45-2 PERICARDIAL VERSUS ISCHEMIC PAIN

	ISCHEMIA	PERICARDITIS
Location	Retrosternal; left shoulder, arm	Precordium; left trapezius ridge
Quality	Pressure, burning, buildup	Sharp, pleuritic; or dull, oppressive
Thoracic motion	No effect	Increased by breathing, rotating thorax
Duration	Angina; 1 or 2 to 15 min Unstable angina: ½ hr to hrs	Hours or days
Effort	Stable angina: usually Unstable angina or infarction: usually not	No relation
Posture	No effect; may sit, belch, use Valsalva or knee-chest position for relief	Leaning forward for relief; aggravated by recumbency

From Fowler N. O.: Acute pericarditis. *In* Fowler, N. O. (ed.): The Pericardium in Health and Disease. Mt. Kisco, NY, Futura Publishing Co., 1985, p. 158.

will focus on clinical features common to acute pericarditis of many causes.

HISTORY. *Chest pain* is frequently the chief complaint of patients with acute pericarditis; its quality and location are variable. Pain is often localized to retrosternal and left precordial regions and frequently radiates to the trapezius ridge and neck (Table 45–2). Occasionally it may be localized to the epigastrium, mimicking an "acute abdomen," or have a dull or oppressive quality, with radiation to the left arm similar to the ischemic pain of myocardial infarction. The pain is often aggravated by lying supine, coughing, deep inspiration, and swallowing and is eased by sitting up and leaning forward. Sometimes it is noted with each heartbeat. The pain associated with pericarditis may arise from inflammation of both the pericardium and the adjacent pleura, accounting for the pleuritic nature of the discomfort. Pericardial pain may also be provoked by stretch of the pericardial sac due to the presence of intrapericardial fluid.

Acute pericarditis may also cause *dyspnea.* This symptom is related in part to the need to breathe shallowly to avoid pericardiopleuritic chest pain. Dyspnea may be aggravated by the presence of fever or by the development of a large pericardial effusion that compresses adjacent bronchi and pulmonary parenchyma. Additional symptoms such as cough, sputum production, or weight loss may be due to an underlying systemic disease such as tuberculosis or uremia.

PHYSICAL EXAMINATION. The *pericardial friction rub* (p. 60) is the pathognomonic physical finding of acute pericarditis. It is a scratching, grating, high-pitched sound, described by Laennec's associate Victor Collin as "the squeak of leather of a new saddle under the rider." Although the sound is believed to arise from friction between the roughened pericardial and epicardial surfaces, a loud pericardial rub may also be heard in the presence of scant or large pericardial effusions.[45] The pericardial friction rub is classically described as having three components that are related to cardiac motion during atrial systole (presystole), ventricular systole, and rapid ventricular filling in early diastole. Spodick's prospective analysis of the pericardial friction rub revealed that the presystolic component is present in about 70 per cent of cases, while a ventricular systolic component is the loudest and most easily heard component, present in almost all cases.[46] The rapid diastolic filling component is detected less frequently and may be slurred into that of atrial contraction, resulting in a biphasic "to-and-fro" rub. In this series, a true three-component rub was detected about half the time and at

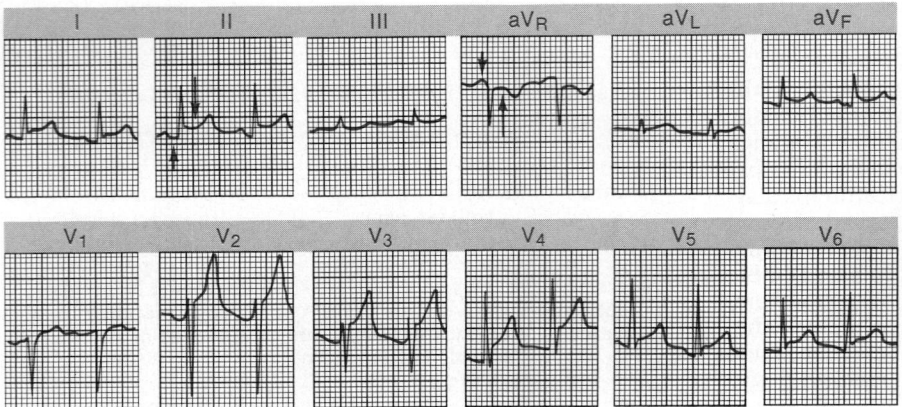

FIGURE 45–4. Stage I electrocardiographic changes from a patient with acute pericarditis. Diffuse ST-segment elevation, which is concave upward, is present in all leads except aV$_R$ and V$_1$. (A short P-R interval unrelated to acute pericarditis is also present.) Depression of the PR segment, an electrocardiographic abnormality that is common in patients with acute pericarditis, is not evident because of the short P-R interval.

the lower left sternal border. The single-component rub is the least common but is likely to be the auscultatory finding in patients with atrial fibrillation.

An important feature of the pericardial friction rub is that it is often evanescent and may change in quality from one examination to the next. Detection of the rub is aided by listening with the stethoscope diaphragm applied firmly to the chest at the lower left sternal border during inspiration and full expiration with the patient sitting up and leaning forward. Occasionally, rubs may be detected with the patient lying supine with arms extended above the head during inspiration or suspended respiration. The single-component pericardial friction rub may be mistaken for a systolic murmur or tricuspid or mitral regurgitation. A pericardial rub may also be confused with the crunch of air in the mediastinum or the artifact of skin scratching against the stethoscope. Pericardial friction rubs may be differentiated from murmurs by (1) the use of exercise to permit detection of a classic three-component rub, (2) the failure of a rub to radiate widely or to vary in timing and duration with inspiration or a change in posture in a manner characteristic of regurgitant murmurs, and (3) by the confirmatory finding of typical electrocardiographic and echocardiographic changes of pericarditis.

ELECTROCARDIOGRAM (see also p. 158). Serial electrocardiograms are extremely helpful in confirming the diagnosis of acute pericarditis. Electrocardiographic changes can occur a few hours or days after the onset of pericardial pain, and the electrocardiographic diagnosis of acute pericarditis is made by detecting the serial appearance of four stages of abnormalities of the ST segments and T waves (Fig. 45–4).[47,48] The etiology of these changes is believed to be related to an actual current of injury caused by superficial myocardial inflammation or epicardial injury. There are four stages in the evolution of acute pericarditis (Table 45–3). Stage I electrocardiographic changes accompany the onset of chest pain and are virtually diagnostic of acute pericarditis. These comprise ST-segment elevation, which, unlike the pattern of ST-seg-

ment elevation in acute myocardial infarction, is concave upward and usually present in all leads except aVr and V1. The T waves are usually upright in the leads with ST-segment elevation. The ST-segment axis in the frontal plane also differs in these two conditions and is reported to range from 30 to 60 degrees in acute pericarditis, unlike acute anterior myocardial infarction in which the ST-segment axis varies from 100 to 120 degrees.[49] Stage II occurs several days later and represents the return of ST segments to baseline, accompanied by T-wave flattening. This change in the ST segments usually occurs prior to the appearance of T-wave inversion. In contrast, T waves in acute myocardial infarction often become inverted before the ST segments return to baseline. Stage III is characterized by inversion of the T waves so that the T-wave vector becomes directed opposite to the ST-segment vector. T-wave inversion is generally present in most leads and is not associated with the loss of R-wave voltage or the appearance of Q waves. These features help to differentiate this stage of nonspecific T-wave inversion from changes associated with the evolution of transmural or subendocardial myocardial infarction. Stage IV represents the reversion of T-wave changes to normal, which may occur up to weeks or months later. T-wave inversion may occasionally persist indefinitely in patients with chronic pericardial inflammation due to tuberculosis, uremia, or neoplastic pericardial disease.

Electrocardiographic abnormalities appear in about 90 per cent of cases of acute pericarditis,[47,50] and the finding of typical Stage I changes or a classic evolution of all four stages can be diagnostic even when other clinical features of pericarditis are misleading. All four stages are detected in about 50 per cent of patients with acute pericarditis. In addition, depression of the PR segment occurs in about 80 per cent of patients with acute pericarditis.[47] Depression of the PR segment occurs during the early stages of ST-segment elevation or T-wave inversion, is usually present in both limb and precordial leads, and may reflect abnormal atrial repolarization due to atrial inflammation.

TABLE 45–3 FOUR-STAGE ("TYPICAL") ECG EVOLUTION OF ACUTE PERICARDITIS

SEQUENCE	LEADS OF "EPICARDIAL" DERIVATION (I, II, aV$_L$, aV$_F$, V$_{3-6}$)			LEADS REFLECTING "ENDOCARDIAL" POTENTIAL aV$_R$, OFTEN V$_1$, SOMETIMES V$_2$		
Stage	J-ST*	T Waves	PR Segment	ST Segment	T Waves	PR Segment
I	Elevated	Upright	Depressed or isoelectric	Depressed	Inverted	Elevated or isoelectric
II early	Isoelectric	Upright	Isoelectric or depressed	Isoelectric	Inverted	Isoelectric or elevated
II late	Isoelectric	Low to flat to inverted	Isoelectric or depressed	Isoelectric	Shallow to flat to upright	Isoelectric or elevated
III	Isoelectric	Inverted	Isoelectric	Isoelectric	Upright	Isoelectric
IV	Isoelectric	Upright	Isoelectric	Isoelectric	Inverted	Isoelectric

* J-ST = junction of S (or T) wave with the end of the QRS complex.
Modified from Spodick, D. H.: Electrocardiographic changes in acute pericarditis. Am. J. Cardiol. *33*:470, 1974.

Variations of the patterns already described are present in slightly less than 50 per cent of patients with pericarditis and include (1) isolated PR-segment depression, (2) the absence of one or more stages of the ST-segment and T-wave changes, (3) evolution of Stage I (ST-segment elevation) directly to Stage IV (reversion of T waves to normal), (4) persistence of T-wave inversion, (5) appearance of ST-segment changes in only a few leads, (6) the appearance of marked T-wave inversion before the ST segments returned to baseline, and (7) the absence of any serial electrocardiographic changes whatsoever.[51] Regional ST-segment deviation may be confused with electrocardiographic changes of regional myocardial ischemia. ST-segment elevation in the right precordial leads has been described in acute pericarditis.[52] The frequency of acute right precordial ST-segment elevation in acute pericarditis has not been systematically studied, and this finding could cause confusion with acute right ventricular infarction.

In addition to the features already described that help to distinguish the ST-segment changes of pericarditis from those of acute myocardial infarction, the changes of Stage I must also be differentiated from the electrocardiographic variant of normal early repolarization (p. 117).[53] This pattern is usually seen in young males, in whom the clinical syndrome of pain and dyspnea suggesting acute pericarditis is absent; PR-segment depression is occasionally present but is uncommon, and most importantly, the electrocardiogram does not evolve through a pattern of the return of ST segments to baseline followed by T-wave inversion. An ST-segment/T wave ratio greater than 0.25 in lead V_6 also appears to discriminate patients with acute pericarditis from those with the normal variant of early repolarization.[54]

Sinus tachycardia is common and may be present in the absence of other contributing factors, such as fever or hemodynamic compromise.[55] Other atrial arrhythmias are infrequent in uncomplicated acute pericarditis and suggest the presence of underlying heart disease.[56] Atrioventricular block, bundle branch block, and ventricular tachycardia are not features of acute pericarditis, and these findings suggest the presence of extensive myocardial inflammation, fibrosis, or acute ischemia.

THE CHEST ROENTGENOGRAM. This is of little diagnostic value in uncomplicated acute pericarditis. If acute pericarditis is complicated by the appearance of a large pericardial effusion, the chest roentgenogram may show both enlargement and changes in configuration of the cardiac silhouette. The chest roentgenogram may provide clues to the underlying etiology of the pericarditis, as in the case of pericarditis secondary to tuberculosis, or malignant disease. Pleural effusions occur in about one-fourth of patients with pericarditis and are usually left-sided in contrast to patients with heart failure in whom right pleural effusions predominate.[50,57] The echocardiogram is at present the most sensitive and accurate tool in the detection and quantification of pericardial fluid and is discussed on pages 102 and 103.

RADIONUCLIDE SCANS. Technetium 99m pyrophosphate scans[58] and gallium radionuclide scans have also been reported to be useful in detecting acute pericarditis,[59] but their sensitivity and specificity have not been clearly established.

BLOOD TESTS. Acute pericarditis is often associated with nonspecific indicators of inflammation, including leukocytosis and elevation of the sedimentation rate. Cardiac isoenzymes are usually normal, but modest elevation of the MB fraction of creatine phosphokinase may occur in the presence of epicardial inflammation accompanying acute pericarditis.[60] For this reason, cardiac isoenzymes cannot always be used to differentiate between acute pericarditis and acute myocardial infarction, particularly non Q-wave infarction.

Based on the history, including recent travel, physical examination, and clinical setting, some patients may require more extensive diagnostic tests to clarify the possibility of an underlying systemic disease. Because of the serious consequences of missing the diagnosis of tuberculous pericarditis, screening for tuberculosis with a tuberculin skin test and a control skin test to exclude anergy is reasonable for patients with acute pericarditis in geographic areas and in patient populations with a low pretest risk of having a positive tuberculin skin test.

Other diagnostic tests that may be indicated in individual patients are based on the clinical presentation: (1) blood cultures to exclude associated possible infective endocarditis and bacteremia; (2) acute and convales-

cent cultures of blood, urine, throat, and feces, if available from the hospital laboratory, to evaluate a suspected viral etiology; (3) HIV test to evaluate the possibility of acquired immunodeficiency syndrome and unusual pathogens in patients with a compatible clinical syndrome; (4) fungal serological tests to evaluate a suspected fungal etiology in patients from endemic areas or in immunocompromised patients; (5) ASO titer in children with suspected rheumatic fever; (6) cold agglutinins to exclude a mycoplasma etiology; (7) heterophile antibody test to exclude mononucleosis; (8) immunofluorescent antibody titers for toxoplasmosis; (9) TSH, T4, and T3 to exclude hypothyroidism; (10) BUN and creatinine to exclude uremic etiology; and (11) antinuclear antibody titer (ANA) and rheumatoid factor, to exclude systemic lupus erythematosus and rheumatoid arthritis.

AORTIC DISSECTION. In middle-aged and elderly patients, close attention should be paid to the history, chest roentgenogram, and echocardiogram for evidence of prior aortic dissection, since subacute inflammatory pericarditis following the slow penetration of blood into the pericardial space can be the initial presentation of aortic dissection.[61]

PERICARDIOCENTESIS AND PERICARDIAL BIOPSY. The issue of the additional diagnostic yields of pericardiocentesis or pericardial biopsy has been addressed by a prospective study of 231 patients with acute pericarditis of inapparent cause.[62] Noninvasive clinical and laboratory studies as described above were done in all patients, while diagnostic pericardiocentesis was done if clinical illnesss and an effusion lasted more than 1 week, and diagnostic biopsy was done if clinical illness lasted more than 3 weeks. This strategy yielded a diagnosis in 14 per cent of patients, which in the majority warranted specific therapy (bacterial pericarditis, tuberculosis, toxoplasmosis, unsuspected malignant disease). The diagnostic yield was substantial when pericardiocentesis or pericardiectomy with biopsy was done to relieve cardiac tamponade (39 and 54 per cent, respectively), and only 5 per cent when these procedures were done only for diagnostic reasons. This experience suggests that there is a higher likelihood of establishing an etiologic diagnosis in patients who develop cardiac tamponade than in those with uncomplicated acute pericarditis, and therapeutic pericardiocentesis or pericardiectomy should always be accompanied by a rigorous examination of fluid or tissue for occult malignant disease or infection. In the immunocompetent patient with uncomplicated acute pericarditis who does not have cardiac tamponade, diagnostic pericardiocentesis or biopsy has a very low yield and is not justified. Pericardiocentesis should be performed for diagnostic reasons in the absence of cardiac tamponade only in patients in whom there is an urgent need to confirm a diagnosis of suspected purulent pericarditis.

MANAGEMENT. The first step in the management of acute pericarditis consists of establishing whether the pericarditis is related to an underlying problem that requires specific therapy. Nonspecific therapy of an initial episode of pericarditis should include bed rest until pain and fever have disappeared, since activity may cause worsening of symptoms. Initial observation in the hospital is warranted for almost all patients with acute pericarditis to exclude an associated myocardial infarction or a pyogenic process and to watch for the development of tamponade, which occurs in about 15 per cent of patients with acute pericarditis.[62]

The pain of pericarditis usually responds to nonsteroidal antiinflammatory agents such as aspirin (650 mg orally every 3 to 4 hours) or indomethacin (25 to 50 mg orally 4 times daily). When pain is severe and does not respond to this therapy within 48 hours, corticosteroids may be employed. If prednisone is used, large doses, such as 60 to 80 mg daily in divided doses, should be given. After 5 to 7 days, if the patient has been free of symptoms for several days, antiinflammatory agents should be tapered. Owing to the adverse consequence of long-term steroid therapy, it is desirable to avoid their use for pain control whenever possible. When long-term steroid administration is needed to control pain and other evidence of inflammation, alternate-day therapy should be attempted. Patients in whom steroids cannot be discontinued may tolerate tapering of steroids and weaning to nonsteroidal antiinflammatory agents.

Antibiotics should be used only to treat documented purulent pericarditis. Oral anticoagulants should not be administered during the acute phase of pericarditis of any cause. If anticoagulants must be continued owing to the presence of a mechanical prosthetic heart valve, we recommend use of intravenous heparin, the action of which can be promptly reversed with protamine, and both physical examination and echocardiography should be performed at regular intervals to watch closely for the development of a pericardial effusion under pressure.

NATURAL HISTORY. Viral pericarditis, idiopathic pericarditis, post-myocardial infarction pericarditis, or the postpericardiotomy syndrome are usually self-limited; clinical and laboratory signs of inflammation abate after 2 to 6 weeks. Sagrista-Sauleda et al.[63] have observed, by physical examination and noninvasive recordings, that about 9 per cent of patients with acute idiopathic pericarditis and pericardial effusion develop signs of mild cardiac constriction within the first 30 days after onset of the illness when signs of acute pericarditis and the effusion have already abated. These findings spontaneously disappear within 3 months and indicate that the development of transient constrictive physiology may occur during the resolution of acute pericardial inflammation.

The most troublesome complication is the development of recurrent episodes of pericardial inflammation at intervals of weeks or months after the initial episode. In two series of patients with acute pericarditis, between 20 and 28 per cent of patients experienced recurrent episodes of pericarditis with severe chest pain.[50,63] The majority of patients can be managed by reinstitution of high-dose nonsteroidal antiinflammatory agents and very gradual tapering over several months to discontinuation or alternate-dose therapy. In rare patients, disabling chest pain associated with fever may recur over a period of years and require steroid administration for pain relief.[64] Pericardiectomy has been proposed for the relief of refractory relapsing pericarditis,[65] but pericardiectomy is not always followed by relief of pain.[64,66]

Pericarditis can also be complicated by the development of disabling or life-threatening hemodynamic complications due to cardiac compression. These include (1) the development of pericardial effusion under pressure, resulting in cardiac tamponade; (2) the development of fibrosis and/or calcification of the pericardium, resulting in chronic constrictive physiology; and (3) a combination of both effusive and constrictive pericardial disease.

Pericardial Effusion

Pericardial effusion may develop as a response to injury of the parietal pericardium with all causes of acute pericarditis. It may be clinically silent, but if the accumulation of fluid causes intrapericardial pressure to increase, resulting in cardiac compression, the symptoms of cardiac tamponade develop. The development of increased intrapericardial pressure secondary to pericardial effusion depends on several factors: (1) the absolute volume of the effusion, (2) the rate of fluid accumulation, and (3) the physical characteristics of the pericardium itself. The pericardial space in humans normally contains between 15 and 50 ml of fluid. If additional fluid accumulates slowly, the pericardium stretches; the pericardial sac can accommodate up to 2 liters without elevation of intrapericardial pressure. However, the normal unstretched pericardial sac can accommodate the rapid addition of only 80 to 200 ml of fluid and still remain on the flat portion of the curve relating intrapericaridial pressure and volume (Fig. 45–2). If additional fluid is rapidly added to a volume exceeding about 150 to 200 ml, a marked rise of intrapericardial pressure occurs. Intrapericardial pressure may also increase markedly after the accumulation of a smaller amount of fluid if the pericardium is excessively stiff because of fibrosis or tumor infiltration.

PERICARDIAL EFFUSION WITHOUT CARDIAC COMPRESSION

HISTORY. Patients who develop pericardial effusion without elevation of intrapericardial pressure may have no symptoms whatsoever. Occasionally these patients complain of a constant oppressive dull ache or pressure in the chest. Large pericardial effusions may cause symptoms by mechanical compression of adjacent structures, including dysphagia from esophageal compression, cough due to bronchial/tracheal compression, dyspnea from lung compression with subsequent atelectasis, hiccups due to phrenic nerve compression, or hoarseness due to recurrent laryngeal nerve compression. Nausea and a sense of abdominal fullness may be present from pressure on adjacent abdominal viscera.

PHYSICAL EXAMINATION. A small pericardial effusion in the absence of an increase in intrapericardial pressure may result in no specific physical findings, whereas a large effusion may produce several characteristic physical findings. First, the heart sounds may be muffled owing to the interposition of fluid between the chest wall and the cardiac chambers. Compression of the base of the left lung by pericardial fluid pro-

duces Ewart's sign, i.e., a patch of dullness on auscultation beneath the angle of the left scapula. Rales may be heard over the lung fields secondary to compression of lung parenchyma. Abnormalities of the arterial pulse, systemic blood pressure, and jugular venous pulse do not occur when a large pericardial effusion is present without significant elevation of the intrapericardial pressure.

CHEST ROENTGENOGRAM. Enlargement of the cardiac silhouette usually does not occur until at least 250 ml of fluid have accumulated in the pericardial space. Therefore, a normal or unchanged chest roentgenogram does not exclude the presence of a hemodynamically important pericardial effusion. This examination may suggest the presence of a pericardial effusion if there is a rapid increase in the size of the cardiac silhouette in the presence of clear lung fields. In some cases the heart may assume a globular or water-bottle shape, blurring the contours along the left cardiac border and obscuring the hilar vessels. Loculated effusions may have a cyst-like appearance (Fig. 45–5).

The parietal pericardial and epicardial fat layers are normally separated by 1 to 2 mm. The presence of effusion may result in more marked separation of the pericardial fat lines,

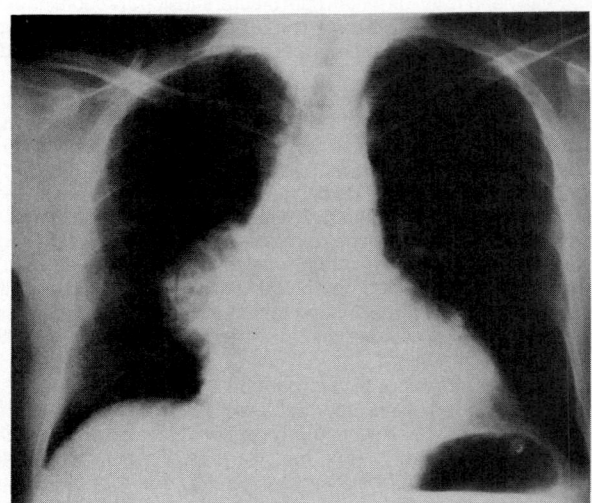

FIGURE 45–5. Posteroanterior chest roentgenogram from a patient with recurrent pericarditis and a loculated pericardial effusion that was subsequently drained surgically. In this patient, the loculated pericardial effusion simulated the roentgenographic appearance of a pericardial cyst.

apparent on high-quality frontal or lateral chest films in about 25 per cent of patients with pericardial effusions.[67] Fluoroscopy may reveal the absence of or weak pulsations and the absence of any changes in the size and shape of the cardiac silhouette during inspiration. These findings are especially useful in the cardiac catheterization laboratory when perforation of the heart is suspected. Computed tomography (p. 317) has also been used to image pericardial effusions, and magnetic resonance imaging (p. 327) can identify effusions, characterize an effusion as hemorrhagic, differentiate fluid from epicardial fat, and delineate other pathology including pericardial thickening and intrapericardial masses[68] (Fig. 11–31, p. 328).

ELECTROCARDIOGRAM. The electrocardiogram may reveal the nonspecific findings of a reduction in QRS voltage and flattening of the T waves as fluid accumulates within the pericardial space.[69] Electrical alternans suggests the presence of massive pericardial effusion and cardiac tamponade.

ECHOCARDIOGRAPHY (see also p. 102). This is the most accurate, rapid, and widely used technique for evaluating pericardial effusion, in following the accumulation or resolution of fluid over time, and in assessing the functional status of the cardiac valves and myocardium. Recognition of pericardial fluid depends on the acoustical differences among the pericardium, cardiac muscle, and pericardial fluid. Accumulation of pericardial fluid results in the appearance of an echo-free space between the posterior left ventricular wall and posterior parietal pericardium and between the anterior wall of the right ventricle and adjacent echoes of the parietal pericardium and chest wall. Posterior and anterior epicardial fat can simulate this echocardiographic appearance of pericardial effusion. M-mode echocardiography appears to be sufficiently sensitive to detect as little as 20 ml of pericardial fluid.[70]

The incidence of small pericardial effusions detected by echocardiography in asymptomatic subjects ranges between 8 and 15 per cent.[71,72] In normal pregnant women, a substantial subset (43 per cent) has been found to have asymptomatic pericardial effusions that resolve within the first weeks after delivery.[72]

Although the quantification of pericardial effusions by echocardiography is not precise, several guidelines of assessment are helpful. Very small effusions are likely to be imaged only posteriorly, with separation of the pericardial and epicardial echoes only in systole. Small-to-moderate-sized effusions are likely to be imaged only posteriorly, with the presence of an echo-free space throughout the cardiac cycle. Pericardial effusions of approximately 300 ml can usually be imaged both anteriorly and posteriorly. Moderate to large effusions may be associated with excessive swinging motion of the heart and the false-positive appearance of mitral valve prolapse and anterior septal motion. Usually, the echo-free space representing a pericardial effusion disappears behind the left atrium owing to the absence of fluid in the oblique pericardial sinus. However, in massive effusions, fluid may also collect in the oblique sinus, resulting in an echo-free space behind the left atrium as well as the left ventricle.

M-mode echocardiography is usually adequate to diagnose pericardial effusion, but occasionally the diagnosis may be confused with a left pleural effusion, giant left atrium, pulmonary infiltrate, or retrograde hiatal hernia. Two-dimensional echocardiography is particularly useful in identifying a loculated pericardial effusion.[73] Blood in the pericardial space can often be differentiated from an effusion of lower acoustical density, and two-dimensional echocardiography is useful in identifying rapidly the presence of hemopericardium with or without thrombus formation secondary to cardiac invasive procedures.[74]

MANAGEMENT. The clinical significance of any pericardial effusion depends on (1) the presence or absence of hemodynamic embarrassment due to increased intrapericardial pressure and (2) the presence and nature of the underlying systemic disease. The use of echocardiography to establish the diagnosis of pericardial effusion is warranted in suspected cases of acute pericarditis, since the presence of effusion is suggestive, although not diagnostic, of pericardial inflammation. Pericardiocentesis (p. 1490) is not indicated unless there is evidence of cardiac compression due to cardiac tamponade or unless analysis of pericardial fluid is necessary to establish a diagnosis such as acute bacterial pericarditis.

CHRONIC PERICARDIAL EFFUSION

Chronic pericardial effusions persisting for more than 6 months may occur in any form of pericardial disease. Often they are surprisingly well tolerated, with no symptoms of cardiac compression, and are discovered when a routine chest roentgenogram discloses an unexpectedly large cardiac silhouette. Chronic pericardial effusions are particularly likely to be found in patients with previous idiopathic or viral pericarditis, uremic pericaditis, and pericarditis secondary to myxedema or neoplasm. Chronic pericardial effusions can also occur in association with ascites and pleural effusions in the setting of chronic salt and water retention of many causes, including chronic heart failure, nephrotic syndrome, and hepatic cirrhosis.[75] Massive idiopathic chronic pericardial effusion is reported to be the initial presentation in about 3 per cent of patients with primary pericardial disease, with predominance in women.[76] The management of chronic pericardial effusion depends in part on the etiology, and occult hypothyroidism should always be excluded. Stable and apparently idiopathic effusions in asymptomatic patients usually require no specific treatment except for avoidance of anticoagulants.

PERICARDIAL EFFUSION WITH CARDIAC COMPRESSION: CARDIAC TAMPONADE

An increase in intrapericardial pressure secondary to fluid accumulation within the pericardial space results in cardiac tamponade, which is characterized by (1) elevation of intracardiac pressures, (2) progressive limitation of ventricular diastolic filling, and (3) reduction of stroke volume and cardiac output.

PATHOPHYSIOLOGY

When intrapericardial pressure is measured using a conventional fluid-filled catheter, usually it is quite close to intrapleural pressure and several millimeters of mercury lower than right and left ventricular diastolic pressures. As already noted (p. 1466), recent studies using special catheters with closed flat balloons indicate that the *constraint* pressure exerted by the normal pericardium is very close to right atrial pressure.[13] However, this controversy regarding the accurate measurement of normal pericardial pressure does not limit the use of fluid-filled catheters in patients with cardiac tamponade, because intrapericardial pressure can be accurately measured by either technique once about 50 ml of free fluid is present in the pericardial space. When the addition of fluid into the pericardial space causes intrapericardial pressure to rise to the level of the right atrial and right ventricular diastolic pressures, the transmural pressure distending these chambers declines to close to zero and cardiac tamponade occurs. The rise of right atrial and intrapericardial pressures is less marked in the presence of hypovolemia, and therefore cardiac tamponade may be masked when hypovolemia is present. Further accumulation of intrapericardial fluid causes both intrapericardial and right ventricular diastolic pressures to rise together to the level of left ventricular diastolic pressure, and all three pressures subsequently rise together in association with a fall in systemic arterial pressure. If left ventricular diastolic pressure is markedly elevated owing to preexisting left ventricular disease, cardiac tamponade occurs when right atrial and right ventricular diastolic and pericardial pressures equalize but at a lower level than the left ventricular diastolic pressure.[77]

CONSEQUENCES OF CARDIAC TAMPONADE. Equalization of intrapericardial and ventricular filling pressures results in markedly diminished transmural distending pressures and diastolic volumes of both ventricles and a fall in stroke volume.[78,79] The reduction in stroke volume is initially compensated for by reflex increases in adrenergic tone; both tachycardia and increases in ejection fraction initially help to maintain forward cardiac output.[78] The importance of the adrenergic support of the heart is reflected in the finding that when beta-adrenergic blockade is carried out in cardiac tamponade, ejection fraction and stroke volume decline.[80] Systemic vascular resistance increases so that, at first, systemic arterial pressure is maintained at the expense of cardiac output. Acute increases in pericardial volume and pressure also reflexly induce a marked decrease in urinary sodium excretion,[81] associated with the inhibition of release of atrial natriuretic factor.[82] With severe cardiac tamponade, as cardiac output declines, compensatory mechanisms are no longer sufficient to maintain systemic arterial pressure, and perfusion of vital organs becomes impaired; reduced coronary perfusion causes selective hypoperfusion of the subendocardium.[83] The superimposition of myocardial ischemia during cardiac tamponade could further compromise left ventricular stroke volume. In extreme cardiac tamponade, transmural diastolic ventricular pressures may actually be less than zero, suggesting that ventricular filling occurs by diastolic suction.[84] Sinus bradycardia, mediated by the cardiac depressor branches of the vagus nerve and by the nonvagal mechanism of sinoatrial node ischemia, may also occur during severe cardiac tamponade.[85] Profound bradycardia often occurs during severe hypotension and precedes the development of electrical-mechanical dissociation and death.

Cardiac tamponade also alters the dynamics of systemic venous return and cardiac filling. Normally, one surge of systemic venous return occurs during ventricular ejection coincident with the systolic x descent of the venous pressure pulse, and a second surge occurs during right atrial emptying with the opening of the tricuspid valve in diastole, corresponding to the y descent. In cardiac tamponade, the heart is compressed throughout the cardiac cycle. During ejection, intracardiac volume decreases, resulting in a transient fall in both intrapericardial and right atrial pressures, manifest as the x descent, which is accompanied by a surge of systemic venous return into the right atrium. However, in early diastole the total volume within the pericardial space remains elevated despite opening of the tricuspid valve; intrapericardial pressure remains elevated and equal to or exceeds early diastolic right atrial pressure so that transmural distending pressure is close to zero or negative. As a result, the usual surge of systemic venous return during early diastole is abolished, right atrial emptying is impeded, and the right atrium is compressed or partially collapsed during diastole. These events are graphically reflected in the right atrial or systemic venous waveform in cardiac tamponade, in that the systolic x descent is prominent while the early diastolic y descent is usually completely absent or attenuated.

REGIONAL TAMPONADE. The individual chambers of the heart resist external compressive force differently, and the magnitude of hemodynamic deterioration during cardiac tamponade critically depends on the specific region of the heart that is compressed during diastole. Fowler and Gable[86] studied regional cardiac tamponade in dogs and showed that isolated tamponade of the right or left ventricle has little hemodynamic effect and that a substantial fall in cardiac output and aortic pressure occurs only when the atria (and intrapericardial veins) are also compressed. A subsequent study of regional tamponade in dogs has shown that right atrial and right ventricular compression causes greater depression of cardiac output and aortic pressure than does left heart compression.[87] In patients with cardiac tamponade, compression of the right heart chambers is likely to be more important than left atrial compression, since pericardial fluid is often not present behind the left atrium during cardiac tamponade, and echocardiographic studies of patients with cardiac tamponade indicate that the presence of left atrial and left ventricular diastolic collapse is variable.[88] For the normal thin-walled right atrium and right ventricle, the critical buckling pressure consists of a negative transmural

pressure of only 0.05 to 0.1 mm Hg.[12] This critical difference between pericardial and right atrial or right ventricular diastolic pressure can occur when pericardial pressure is lower than that of the thick-walled left ventricle, whereas right ventricular collapse may be absent in the presence of severe right ventricular hypertrophy.[89]

RIGHT ATRIAL AND VENTRICULAR COLLAPSE. During the development of tamponade, collapse of the right atrium and right ventricle initially occurs only in early diastole in association with delayed diastolic filling of the right ventricle and a modest fall in cardiac output without hypotension or overt hemodynamic deterioration (Fig. 45-6).[89,90] Pandiastolic right atrial and ventricular buckling occurs when pericardial pressure equals or exceeds right atrial and ventricular pressures throughout diastole so that the ventricles may fill only during atrial systole. This stage is accompanied by a severe reduction in ventricular volumes, a failure of compensatory mechanisms, and hypotension.[89,90] In this setting, pulsus alternans may occur because of beat-to-beat variation in right ventricular output and left ventricular filling.[90] During hypovolemia with low right heart pressures, right ventricular collapse occurs at low intrapericardial pressures while volume expansion delays the development of right ventricular diastolic collapse and hemodynamic deterioration until a higher intrapericardial pressure is achieved.[90,91] Singh et al.[92] have obtained simultaneous hemodynamics and two-dimensional echocardiographic measurements in patients undergoing pericardiocentesis and have shown that hemodynamic improvement first occurs at the point of disappearance of right ventricular diastolic collapse, which is followed by the subsequent disappearance of right atrial collapse and further improvement in cardiac output during continued pericardiocentesis.

PULSUS PARADOXUS. Inspiration and the transmission of negative intrathoracic pressure to the pericardial space further alter the dynamics of right and left ventricular filling and are responsible for pulsus paradoxus, the inspiratory fall of aortic systolic pressure greater than 10 mm Hg (Fig. 45-7). The finding of weakening of the arterial pulse during inspiration was described by Kussmaul in 1873 as the apparent *paradox* of the disappearance of the pulse during inspiration despite persistence of the heartbeat. It should be emphasized that pulsus paradoxus is in fact an exaggeration of the normal inspiratory decline of left ventricular stroke volume by about 7 per cent and of systemic arterial pressure by 3 per cent.[93] Inspiration is normally accompanied by an increase in diastolic dimensions of the right ventricle, a small decrease in left ventricular di-

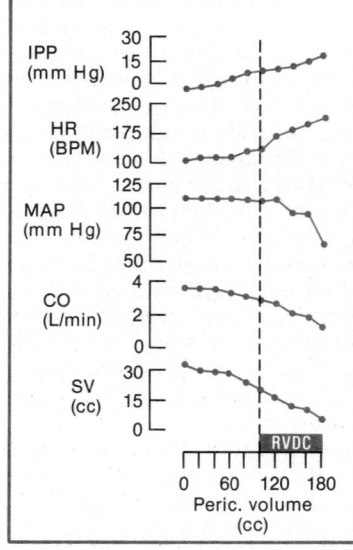

FIGURE 45-6. Hemodynamic measurements from a dog with experimental cardiac tamponade in which two-dimensional echocardiograms showed right ventricular diastolic collapse (RVDC). Mean intrapericardial pressure (IPP) continuously rose as pericardial volume increased, accompanied by a progressive decline of stroke volume (SV). At the time RVDC was first detected, mean arterial pressure (MAP) was well preserved, cardiac output (CO) had only modestly declined, and a compensatory increase in heart rate (HR) was present. Mean arterial pressure fell rapidly late in the course of cardiac tamponade in the decompensated phase. (From Leimgruber, P. P., et al.: The hemodynamic derangement associated with right ventricular diastolic collapse in cardiac tamponade: An experimental echocardiographic study. Circulation **68**:612, 1983, by permission of the American Heart Association, Inc.)

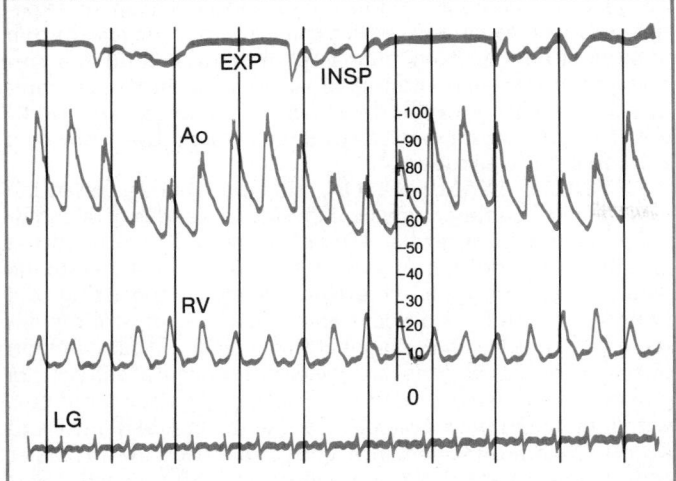

FIGURE 45-7. Recording of aortic (Ao) and right ventricular (RV) pressures in a patient with cardiac tamponade complicated by hypovolemia. Pulsus paradoxus is evident as a marked inspiratory decline in aortic systolic and pulse pressures during inspiration (INSP). RV pressure variation is out of phase with aortic pressure. Note that the RV waveform does not show a dip-and-plateau configuration. (From Shabetai, R., et al.: The hemodynamics of cardiac tamponade and constrictive pericarditis. Am. J. Cardiol. 26:480, 1970.)

pericarditis and restrictive heart disease, and the latter mechanisms may account for its presence in these disorders.

Pulsus paradoxus has also been observed in severe lung disease and massive pulmonary embolism.[101,102] Under these circumstances, pulsus paradoxus is probably related to the transmission of excessively negative intrathoracic pressure during inspiration to the aorta, inspiratory pooling of right ventricular stroke volume in the lungs, and exaggerated right-heart filling with an associated decrease in left-heart filling during inspiration. Pulsus paradoxus may be absent in cardiac tamponade when left ventricular hypertrophy or heart failure causes a marked elevation of left ventricular diastolic pressure so that the two ventricles are unequally compressed. This may occur in atrial septal defect when the increase in systemic venous return during inspiration is shared between the two sides of the heart, and in aortic regurgitation when there is a major component of left ventricular filling that is independent of respiratory variation.[77,103] Pulsus paradoxus may also be absent in the presence of pulmonary hypertension and right ventricular hypertrophy that impedes the inspiratory increase in right ventricular filling; in this unusual clinical situation, the depression of left ventricular diastolic filling and cardiac outcome may depend on regional compression of the left ventricle.[104]

mension, and increased velocity of flow from the venae cavae into the right atrium.[94,95] Pulsus paradoxus in cardiac tamponade appears to result from an exaggeration of these normal findings.

Measurement of intracardiac pressures and flow during experimental tamponade[96] and in humans during cardiac tamponade[93,97] have demonstrated that inspiration causes a decrease in intrapericardial and right atrial pressures. This results in augmentation of flow from the venae cavae into the right atrium and right ventricle and augmentation of pulmonary artery flow and pulmonary artery systolic pressure. The increase in venous return flow during inspiration results in a marked and exaggerated increase in right ventricular dimensions accompanied by a reduction in left ventricular dimensions and flattening and displacement of the septum toward the left ventricle.[98] On the left side of the heart, left atrial and left ventricular diastolic pressures fall, accompanied by a fall in aortic flow and systolic arterial pressure. Thus, *pulsus paradoxus in cardiac tamponade is critically dependent on the inspiratory augmentation of systemic venous return and right ventricular filling.*

Shabetai et al. demonstrated that when experimental cardiac tamponade was induced in dogs, pulsus paradoxus did not develop when either the right heart was bypassed or right ventricular volume was strictly controlled.[96] These experiments also demonstrated that traction on the heart by the diaphragm was not an essential mechanism. These observations indicate that pulsus paradoxus in cardiac tamponade depends on the inspiratory expansion of right-heart filling at the expense of left-heart filling (Fig. 45-8).

The importance of respiratory preload variation is supported by recent observations in patients with cardiac tamponade that showed that left ventricular transmural diastolic pressure falls to or below zero during inspiration.[12] An additional factor that may contribute to the inspiratory fall of left ventricular stroke volume and systolic arterial pressure is a transient reduction in the gradient between the pulmonary venous circulation and the left heart during inspiration causing inspiratory pooling of blood in the lungs (Fig. 45-9).[99] Also the underfilled left ventricle may be operating on the steep ascending limb of the Starling curve so that any inspiratory reduction of left ventricular filling results in marked depression of left ventricular stroke volume and systolic pressure.[100] Pulsus paradoxus is occasionally observed in constrictive

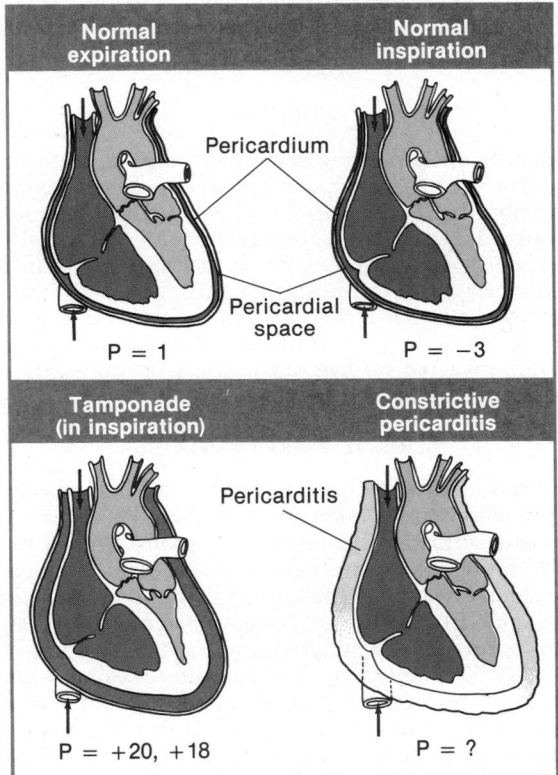

FIGURE 45-8. The hemodynamic effects of respiration. In the normal heart *(upper panel),* inspiration results in a fall in intrathoracic and intrapericardial pressure from +1 to −3 mm Hg, which causes an increase in venous return (heavy black arrows) and a slight increase in right ventricular size at the expense of a slight decrease in left ventricular size due to displacement of the interventricular septum from right to left. During cardiac tamponade *(lower left panel),* inspiration causes a fall in the elevated intrapericardial pressure from +20 to +18 mm Hg. Although both the right and left heart volumes are diminished owing to compression by the pericardial effusion, the inspiratory fall in intrapericardial pressure results in an increase in venous return (heavy black arrow), an increase in right heart volume due to septal bulging, and a further decrease in left heart volume. In constrictive pericarditis *(lower right panel),* the inspiratory fall in intrathoracic pressure is not transmitted to the heart, since the pericardial space is obliterated. For this reason, there is minimal or no increase in venous return (light black arrows) during inspiration. (From Shabetai, R.: The Pericardium. New York, Grune & Stratton, 1981, p. 244.)

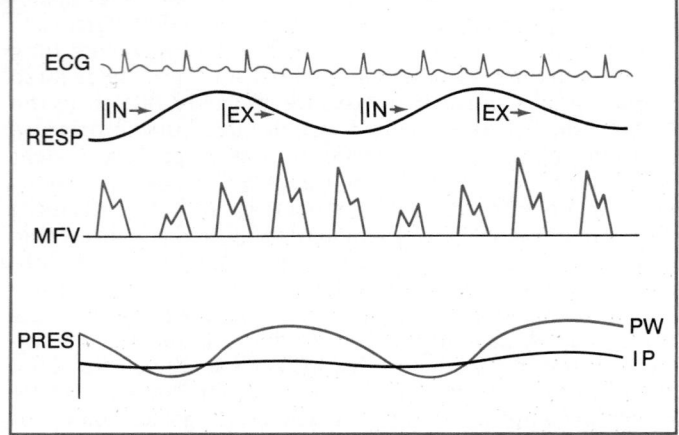

FIGURE 45–9. Relation between mitral flow velocity (MFV) and pericardial and pulmonary wedge pressures. The first beat after the onset of inspiration is associated with a reduced pressure gradient between the pulmonary venous circulation and intrapericardial (and left ventricular diastolic) pressures, which results in an abrupt reduction in mitral flow velocity, as shown, and an increase in tricuspid flow velocity. Opposite changes occur with the onset of expiration. ECG = electrocardiogram, RESP = respiratory phase determined by a nasal thermistor, IN = inspiration, EX = expiration, PRES = pressure, PW = pulmonary capillary wedge, IP = intrapericardial. (From Appleton, C. P., et al.: Cardiac tamponade and pericardial effusion: Respiratory variation in transvalvular flow velocities studied by Doppler echocardiography. J. Am. Coll. Cardiol. *11*:1020, 1988.)

ETIOLOGY

Cardiac tamponade may occur with almost any cause of pericarditis and may exist in either an acute or a chronic form. The distributions of the causes of acute cardiac tamponade in a city hospital between 1963 and 1980[105] and at our institution between 1984 and 1988 are noted in Table 45–4. In these contemporary series the most frequent causes of cardiac tamponade were neoplasm, idiopathic or viral pericarditis, and uremia, followed by pericarditis associated with myocardial infarction, invasive cardiac diagnostic procedures, purulent bacterial infection, and tuberculosis.

CLINICAL MANIFESTATIONS

The triad of (1) a decline in systemic aterial pressure; (2) elevation of systemic venous pressure; and (3) a small, quiet heart was described by the thoracic surgeon Claude S. Beck in 1935.[106] These three features are typical of cardiac tamponade from sudden intrapericardial hemorrhage due to penetrating heart wounds from trauma or invasive diagnostic cardiac procedures, aortic dissection, and intrapericardial rupture of an aortic or cardiac aneurysm. This syndrome develops when the pericardium is not enlarged or stretched, so that the addition of less than 200 ml of fluid or blood causes intrapericardial pressure to rise abruptly to above 20 to 30 mm Hg. In cases that are not immediately fatal, both cardiac output and arterial pressure fall, accompanied by tachycardia and tachypnea. The patient may be stuporous or agitated and restless, and the additional important finding of pulsus paradoxus may be difficult to appreciate when profound hypotension is present. Jugular venous pressure is usually markedly elevated. Precordial heart activity is usually not palpable, and heart sounds are distant or inaudible. Cold, clammy extremities and anuria may be present.

Patients in whom cardiac tamponade develops slowly differ from those with cardiac tamponade due to cardiac penetration or rupture. In the setting of more slowly developing cardiac tamponade, patients usually appear acutely ill but not in extremis, and the major complaint is usually dyspnea.[105] Studies of acute cardiac tamponade in dogs have shown that the elevation of intrapericardial pressure results in the accumulation of interstitial fluid without the development of alveolar

edema or hypoxemia.[107] Thus the sensation of dyspnea experienced by many patients with cardiac tamponade may be due to lung stiffening from increased interstitial fluid that increases the work of breathing. Chest pain may also be present. In patients with chronic development of tamponade, additional systemic symptoms may include weight loss, anorexia, and profound weakness.

PHYSICAL EXAMINATION. Jugular venous distention was the most common physical finding in a series of 56 medical patients whose cardiac tamponade was diagnosed at the bedside.[105] In addition to absolute elevation of the systemic venous pressure, a characteristic waveform consisting of a prominent systolic x descent and absence of diastolic y descent can often be appreciated at the bedside. Other common physical findings include tachypnea (80 per cent), tachycardia (77 per cent), pulsus paradoxus (77 per cent), pulsus paradoxus with total inspiratory disappearance of the brachial pulse and Korotkoff sounds (23 per cent), pericardial friction rub (29 per cent), hepatomegaly (55 per cent), and diminished heart sounds (34 per cent). It is noteworthy that systolic arterial hypotension, consisting of a systolic pressure less than 100 mm Hg, was present in a minority (36 per cent), and the majority of patients were alert, with warm extremities and preservation of urine output.[105]

Pulsus Paradoxus (see p. 24). The finding of pulsus paradoxus is crucial in making the diagnosis of cardiac tamponade, since most patients with slowly developing cardiac tamponade do not have the classic physical findings of a small, quiet heart and severe hypotension. Pulsus paradoxus can be detected on physical examination as an inspiratory decrease in the amplitude of the palpated pulse in the femoral or carotid arteries. Total paradox, i.e., complete disappearance of the palpated pulse during inspiration, occurs during very severe cardiac tamponade or tamponade combined with hypovolemia. The magnitude of the paradoxical pulse can be accurately quantified by means of an intraarterial catheter but may be estimated by cuff sphygmomanometry. The cuff should be inflated 20 mm Hg above systolic pressure and slowly deflated until the Korotkoff sounds are heard only during expiration. The cuff should then be deflated to the point at which Korotkoff sounds are heard equally well in inspiration and expiration. The difference between these pressures is the estimated magnitude of pulsus paradoxus.

Other disorders with systemic venous distention, pulsus paradoxus, and clear lungs that can be confused with cardiac tamponade include obstructive pulmonary disease, constrictive pericarditis, restrictive cardiomyopathy, and massive pulmonary embolism. Pulsus paradoxus is occasionally noted

TABLE 45–4 COMMON CAUSES OF CARDIAC TAMPONADE

DISORDER	%	%
	1980	**1988**
Malignant disease	32	58
Idiopathic pericarditis	14	14
Uremia	9	14
Acute cardiac infarction (receiving heparin)	9	
Diagnostic procedures with cardiac perforation	7.5	
Bacterial	7.5	5
Tuberculosis	5	1
Radiation	4	
Myxedema	4	
Dissecting aortic aneurysm	4	
Postpericardiotomy syndrome	2	
Systemic lupus erythematosus	2	2
Cardiomyopathy (receiving anticoagulants)	2	6

Modified from Guberman, B. A., et al.: Cardiac tamponade in medical patients. Circulation *64*:633, 1981, by permission of the American Heart Association, Inc., and from Levina, M. J., et al.: Implications of echocardiographically-assisted diagnosis of pericardial tamponade in contemporary medical patients. J. Am. Coll. Cardiol. *17*: 59, 1991.

during severe hypovolemia due to hemorrhagic or septic shock, but jugular venous distention is usually absent.[108] Cardiac tamponade may be confused with shock due to right ventricular infarction with jugular venous distention and clear lungs.[42] However, the hemodynamics of right ventricular infarction are more like those of pericardial constriction than of tamponade (p. 1482).

LOW-PRESSURE TAMPONADE. The clinical findings may be further modified in patients with so-called *low-pressure cardiac tamponade* in whom jugular venous distention is absent and the right atrial pressure is low. This syndrome, which occurs in the setting of hypovolemia, represents an early stage in the development of cardiac tamponade in which accumulation of a pericardial effusion causes intrapericardial pressure to rise and equilibrate with low right heart diastolic filling pressures. Pericardiocentesis reduces intrapericardial pressure and causes the separation of right atrial and intrapericardial pressures. Low-pressure cardiac tamponade has been reported in patients with tuberculosis and neoplastic pericarditis complicated by severe dehydration.[109]

TENSION PNEUMOPERICARDIUM. This condition causes hemodynamic changes similar to those of acute hemorrhagic cardiac tamponade.[110] It is being increasingly recognized as a cause of cardiac tamponade with high mortality in infants during mechanical ventilation and in adults as a result of penetrating chest trauma, gastric and esophageal rupture, carcinomatous bronchopericardial fistula, gas production from contiguous infection, and diagnostic procedures such as sternal bone marrow aspiration.[110,111] Characteristic clinical findings include muffled heart sounds, bradycardia, and shifting tympany over the precordium. Unique auscultatory findings can be detected, including a metallic cracking sound, and the bruit de moulin, which was described in the first report of pneumopericardium in 1844 by Bricheteau as "the noise made by floats of a mill wheel as they strike the water,"[112] and which indicates the presence of both air and fluid in the pericardial space.

LABORATORY STUDIES

CHEST ROENTGENOGRAM. There are no roentgenographic features diagnostic of cardiac tamponade. The heart may appear completely normal in size in cardiac tamponade that develops from acute hemopericardium due to cardiac rupture or laceration. On the other hand, if an effusion that accumulates more slowly to more than approximately 250 ml is responsible, the cardiac silhouette may be enlarged with a water bottle configuration (Fig. 8-43, p. 231). This finding suggests the presence of a large pericardial effusion but supplies no information about its hemodynamic significance. In patients with cardiac tamponade due to tension pneumopericardium, the chest roentgenogram usually shows that the heart is surrounded by air delineated by a strip of soft tissue extending up the aorta consisting of the pericardium.

ELECTROCARDIOGRAM. The electrocardiographic abnormalities seen in acute cardiac tamponade include those of acute pericarditis and pericardial effusion *per se* (p. 158). The development of electrical alternans is a more specific indicator of pericardial tamponade and reflects pendular swinging of the heart within the pericardial space.[113] This may not be the only mechanism, since two-dimensional echocardiographic findings suggest that electrical alternans may be related to a beat-to-beat alteration of right and left ventricular filling.[90] Electrical alternans may also occur in constrictive pericarditis, in tension pneumothorax, after myocardial infarction, and with severe cardiac muscle dysfunction. However, the appearance of electrical alternans in a patient with a known pericardial effusion is highly suggestive of cardiac tamponade —a finding that has been confirmed in experimental cardiac tamponade.[114] Electrical alternans of the QRS complex may occur in a 2:1 or 3:1 pattern. Alternans is usually limited to the QRS complex, but alternans of the P wave, QRS complex, and T wave may rarely occur in extreme cardiac tamponade. Both

the abnormal heart motion within the pericardial sac and electrical alternans disappear when pericardial fluid is aspirated.

ECHOCARDIOGRAM (see also p. 102 and Fig. 4-102, p. 103). In patients with jugular venous distention and the possibility of cardiac tamponade, echocardiography is extremely useful and should be performed prior to consideration of pericardiocentesis.[115,116] In a rare patient who is in extremis from the extremely rapid development of cardiac tamponade, the physician may have to rely on the history and physical findings to make a judgment about the need for pericardiocentesis. If echocardiography is readily available and the patient with suspected cardiac tamponade is not moribund, obtaining an echocardiogram will increase the likelihood of diagnosing cardiac tamponade correctly and will prevent inappropriate and potentially lethal attempts at pericardiocentesis or pericardiotomy. First, the echocardiogram helps to document the presence and magnitude of pericardial effusion. The absence of echocardiographic evidence of pericardial effusion virtually excludes the diagnosis of cardiac tamponade (with the important exception of the postoperative cardiac surgery patient in whom loculated fluid or thrombus may cause cardiac compression). Second, the echocardiogram can rapidly differentiate cardiac tamponade from other causes of systemic venous hypertension and hypotension, including constrictive pericarditis, cardiac muscle dysfunction, and right ventricular infarction. The appearance of dense echoes in the pericardial space or extrinsic to the pericardium suggests the presence of compression by material other than free fluid. Echocardiograms can often detect both massive extracardiac hematoma and extrinsic compression of the heart by tumor, which can cause cardiac compression with the physiology of cardiac constriction or cardiac tamponade.

Two-dimensional and Doppler echocardiography can provide additional clues that pericardial effusion is associated with cardiac tamponade. The presence of pulsus paradoxus is associated with sudden leftward motion of the septum during inspiration and an exaggerated increase in right ventricular size with a reciprocal decrease in left ventricular size.[99,116-118] This characteristic respiratory variation in ventricular preload can also be detected by the Doppler ultrasound findings of exaggerated tricuspid and pulmonic flow velocities and reduction of peak mitral flow velocity with the onset of inspiration and the opposite changes after the onset of expiration (Fig. 45-9).[119-121] When the inspiratory reduction in left ventricular filling is extreme, the aortic valve may close prematurely or fail to open[122] and mitral valve opening may be delayed until atrial systole. *Diastolic right atrial and right ventricular compression* or collapse occur early during the development of cardiac tamponade[88-92] (Fig. 45-10). Left atrial diastolic collapse can also occur when pericardial fluid is present behind the left atrium.[88] Right ventricular diastolic collapse appears to be more predictive of cardiac tamponade than pulsus paradoxus, particularly during hypovolemia,[123,124] and these echocardiographic signs may be reversed by volume expansion.[125] Right ventricular diastolic collapse may be absent in the presence of right ventricular hypertrophy. Thus, the echocardiographic findings of pericardial effusion, an inspiratory increase in right ventricular dimensions, and right atrial and ventricular diastolic collapse strongly suggest the diagnosis of cardiac tamponade. However, these changes are not 100 per cent sensitive or specific,[88,90,92,123] and experimental studies indicate that a single echocardiogram cannot always predict the presence or severity of cardiac tamponade.[126] Radionuclide and contrast angiography can also detect right ventricular and right atrial collapse and compression of the superior vena cava as it enters the pericardium,[127] but these findings, while suggestive of cardiac tamponade, also lack complete sensitivity and specificity.

Furthermore, hemodynamic observations at our institution in a consecutive series of 50 patients with suspected cardiac tamponade and echocardiographic evidence of right atrial and ventricular diastolic collapse showed that these echocardio-

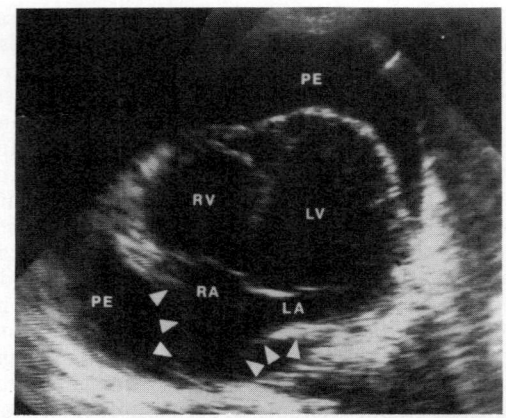

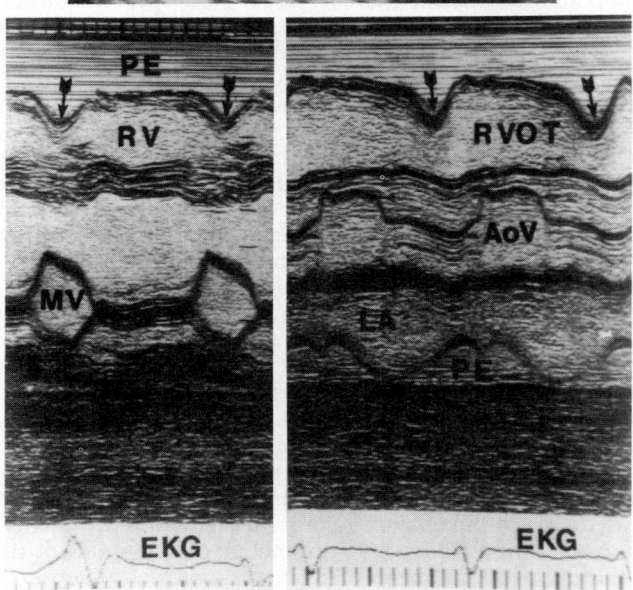

FIGURE 45–10. Two-dimensional *(upper panel)* and M-mode *(lower panels)* echocardiograms from a patient with a malignant pericardial effusion and cardiac tamponade. The two-dimensional image shows a large pericardial effusion (PE) adjacent to the borders of the right ventricle (RV), right atrium (RA), and left ventricle (LV). The effusion is sufficiently large that fluid is also present behind the left atrium (LA). Diastolic compression (white arrows) of both the right and left atria is present. The M-mode images also show striking diastolic compression (dark arrows) of the right ventricle during diastole when the mitral valve (MV) is open and compression of the right ventricular outflow tract (RVOT) in early to mid diastole after aortic valve (AoV) closure.

graphic findings were uniformly associated with elevation of pericardial pressure and the near equilibration of right atrial and right ventricular pressures[128] (Fig. 45–11). However, right heart diastolic collapse was associated with a wide spectrum of hemodynamic derangement, including a subset of patients with minimal elevation of right atrial pressure and the preservation of a normal cardiac output and systemic arterial pressure. Thus, the recognition of patients with cardiac tamponade by echocardiography requires complementary clinical and hemodynamic assessment to distinguish patients with milder degrees of cardiac compression from those with hemodynamic decompensation who require urgent drainage of pericardial fluid. It must be emphasized that cardiac tamponade is a clinical, not an echocardiographic nor a radionuclide, diagnosis that is established definitively by documentation of the elevation and equilibration of intrapericardial and right atrial pressures and the reversal of these findings by evacuation of pericardial fluid.

CARDIAC CATHETERIZATION

Cardiac catheterization is invaluable in establishing the hemodynamic importance of pericardial effusion. Except in ex-

treme emergencies, such as when the patient is moribund, we prefer to catheterize the right heart and pericardial space in conjunction with pericardiocentesis. Cardiac catheterization (1) provides absolute confirmation of the diagnosis of cardiac tamponade; (2) quantitates the hemodynamic compromise; (3) guides pericardiocentesis by documenting that pericardial aspiration is associated with hemodynamic improvement; and (4) permits the detection of coexisting hemodynamic problems, including left ventricular failure, effusive-constrictive pericarditis (p. 1487), and unsuspected pulmonary hypertension in patients with malignant effusions.

Cardiac catheterization typically demonstrates elevation of right atrial pressure with a characteristic preserved systolic x descent and absence of or a diminutive diastolic y descent. When intrapericardial and right atrial pressures are recorded simultaneously, both are elevated and virtually identical (Fig. 45–12); both pressures fall during inspiration, and intrapericardial pressure may fall slightly below right atrial pressure during systolic ejection at the time of the x descent. If intrapericardial pressure is not elevated, and if right atrial and intrapericardial pressures are not virtually identical, the diagnosis of cardiac tamponade must be reconsidered.

Right ventricular mid-diastolic pressure is elevated and equal to right atrial and intrapericardial pressures and lacks the dip-and-plateau configuration characteristic of constrictive percarditis. Since right ventricular and pulmonary artery systolic pressures are equal to the sum of the pressure developed by the right ventricle plus the intrapericardial pressure, right ventricular and pulmonary artery systolic pressures are usually moderately elevated, in the range of 35 to 50 mm Hg. In the case of severe cardiac compression, right ventricular systolic pressure may be reduced and only slightly higher than right ventricular diastolic pressure.

Usually the pulmonary capillary wedge pressure and left ventricular diastolic pressure are elevated and equal to intrapericardial pressure when recorded simultaneously. During expiration, the pulmonary capillary wedge pressure is usually

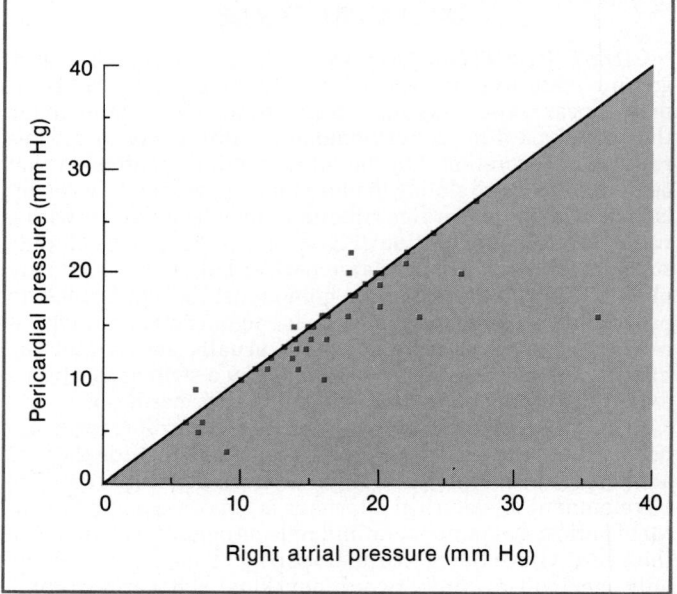

FIGURE 45–11. Relationship between simultaneous measurements of right atrial pressure and intrapericardial pressure in 50 consecutive medical patients with the echocardiographic finding of right atrial diastolic collapse. Although these patients had near-equilibration of right atrial and intrapericardial pressures, the echocardiographic finding of right atrial diastolic collapse was associated with variable degrees of cardiac compression, and 56 per cent of patients had preservation of both a normal cardiac index and systemic arterial pressure. (From Levine, M. J., et al.: Implications of echocardiographically assisted diagnosis of pericardial tamponade in contemporary medical patients: Detection prior to hemodynamic embarrassment. Reprinted by permission of the American College of Cardiology. J. Am. Coll. Cardiol. *17:*59, 1991.)

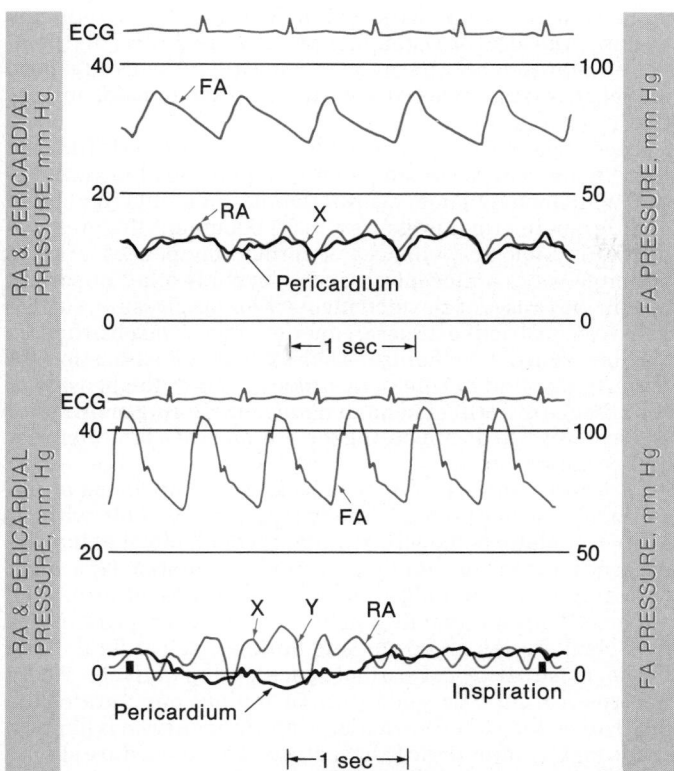

FIGURE 45-12. Simultaneous right atrial (RA) and intrapericardial pressures (scale 0 to 40 mm Hg) and femoral artery pressure (scale 0 to 100 mm Hg) from a patient with decompensated cardiac tamponade. Before pericardiocentesis *(upper panel)*, systemic hypotension is present, and there is elevation and equalization of right atrial and intrapericardial pressures. Note that a systolic *x* descent is present, but the diastolic *y* descent is absent, suggesting that right atrial emptying is impeded by compression of the right ventricle in early diastole. After aspiration of about 300 ml of pericardial fluid *(lower panel)*, cardiac tamponade is relieved as shown by the restoration of intrapericardial pressure to zero, the restoration of right atrial pressure to a normal level, and the improvement in systemic arterial pressure. The right atrial tracing shows the appearance of a diastolic *y* descent, which indicates the relief of cardiac compression and restoration of normal right atrial emptying in early diastole. Although this degree of fluid aspiration relieved tamponade physiology, an additional 1,500 ml of fluid was subsequently aspirated from the pericardial space. (Modified from Lorell, B. H., and Grossman, W.: Profiles in constrictive pericarditis, restrictive cardiomyopathy, and cardiac tamponade. *In* Grossman, W., and Baim, D. S. (eds.): Cardiac Catheterization, Angiography and Intervention. Philadelphia, Lea and Febiger, 1991, p. 644.)

slightly higher than intrapericardial pressure, resulting in a pressure gradient that promotes left-heart filling. During inspiration, the pulmonary capillary wedge pressure may transiently decrease more than intrapericardial pressure such that the pressure gradient between the pulmonary venous circulation and the left heart is reduced or absent. In patients with severe underlying left ventricular dysfunction or hypertrophy and elevation of the left ventricular diastolic pressure, cardiac tamponade can be present when intrapericardial and right atrial pressures are equal but lower than left ventricular diastolic pressure. Depending on the severity of cardiac compression, left ventricular systolic and aortic pressures may be normal or reduced.

Pulsus paradoxus can be easily documented by intraarterial catheterization and pressure measurement. Simultaneous recording of systemic arterial and right ventricular pressures shows that the inspiratory pressure variation is out of phase (Fig. 45-7). Stroke volume is usually markedly depressed. Cardiac output may be normal, owing to the compensatory effect of tachycardia, or it may be markedly reduced when cardiac tamponade is severe; systemic vascular resistance is usually elevated.

Angiographic studies add no additional information if echo-cardiographic findings suggestive of cardiac tamponade were obtained prior to cardiac catheterization. In an otherwise normal heart, right and left ventricular end-diastolic volumes are usually reduced with normal or increased ejection fractions.

Aspiration of pericardial fluid results initially in the lowering of the identical intrapericardial, right atrial, right ventricular, and left ventricular diastolic pressures, followed by a fall of intrapericardial pressure below right atrial pressure and reappearance of the *y* descent in the right atrial waveform (Fig. 45-12). Further aspiration causes intrapericardial pressure to fall to a mean level of zero and to fluctuate with changes in intrathoracic pressure. Since the pressure-volume curve of the pericardium is steep, the initial aspiration of 50 to 100 ml of pericardial fluid usually leads to striking reduction in intrapericardial pressure, marked improvement in systemic arterial pressure and cardiac output, and abolition of pulsus paradoxus. The reduction of intrapericardial pressure is often followed by diuresis, related both to the augmentation of cardiac output and the release of atrial natriuretic factor.[81,82,129]

If intrapericardial pressure falls to zero or becomes negative and right atrial pressure remains elevated, *effusive-constrictive pericarditis* (p. 1489) should be strongly considered, especially in patients with underlying neoplasm or prior radiation. Other causes of continued elevation of right atrial pressure after successful pericardiocentesis include the coexistence of cardiac tamponade and preexisting left ventricular dysfunction causing, in turn, pulmonary hypertension and right atrial hypertension, tricuspid valve disease, and restrictive cardiomyopathy. In patients with suspected malignant disease, pulmonary hypertension due to pulmonary microvascular tumor is an important cause of persistent elevation of right atrial pressure and the failure to relieve dyspnea after complete drainage of the pericardial space.[130]

The distinction between cardiac tamponade and the superior vena cava syndrome must always be made in patients with neoplastic disease in whom these lesions may occur singly or together. In patients with obstruction of the superior vena cava, cardiac tamponade may be suspected from the presence of elevated jugular venous pressure and pulsus paradoxus due to respiratory distress. In this condition (without accompanying cardiac tamponade), pressure in the superior vena cava is markedly elevated, with dampened pulsations, and exceeds right atrial and inferior vena cava pressures. Two-dimensional and Doppler echocardiography may not be successful in distinguishing between these conditions because cardiac tamponade as well as other causes of elevated central venous pressure may modify the appearance and respiratory fluctuation of flow in the venae cavae.[121,131] If elevation of jugular venous pressure persists after relief of cardiac tamponade in patients with neoplastic disease, obstruction of the superior vena cava, as reflected in a pressure gradient between the superior vena cava and right atrium, should be sought. Superior vena caval obstruction may be amenable to radiation therapy.

PERICARDIOCENTESIS

Hemodynamic support during preparation of the patient for pericardiocentesis or pericardiotomy should include administration of intravenous fluid, blood, plasma, or saline. The rationale for volume expansion is that it has been shown to delay the appearance of right ventricular diastolic collapse and hemodynamic deterioration.[91] In experimental cardiac tamponade, administration of norepinephrine and isoproterenol[132] has produced an increase in cardiac output. The vasodilators hydralazine and nitroprusside have also been employed in experimental cardiac tamponade to promote an increase in cardiac output secondary to the reduction of elevated systemic resistance.[133] The administration of vasodilators in conjunction with volume expansion must be done with extreme caution in patients with cardiac tamponade, since it may be hazardous in patients with borderline or frank hypotension. Positive-pressure ventilation should be avoided whenever possible because it has been shown to depress cardiac output further in patients with cardiac tamponade.[134]

Pericardial fluid under pressure causing tamponade can be evacuated by (1) percutaneous pericardiocentesis using a needle or catheter, (2) pericardiotomy via a subxiphoid incision, or (3) partial or extensive surgical pericardiectomy. Considerable controversy exists regarding the exact indications for pericardiocentesis[112] although the procedure has been performed extensively since its initial demonstration in 1840 by the Viennese physician Franz Schuh. The benefits of pericardiocentesis include the rapid relief of cardiac tamponade and the opportunity to obtain accurate hemodynamic measurements before and after pericardial aspiration. The major risk of percutaneous pericardiocentesis is laceration of the heart, coronary arteries, or lung. Prior to the 1970's, pericardiocentesis was usually performed blindly at the bedside using a sharp needle without hemodynamic or echocardiographic monitoring, and the risk of death or life-threatening complications appeared to be as high as 20 per cent.[135]

TECHNIQUE. The modern approach is exemplified by the Stanford experience in 123 patients.[136] In the majority of patients, pericardiocentesis was performed by a cardiologist in the cardiac catheterization laboratory using a subxiphoid approach under fluoroscopic guidance with hemodynamic and electrocardiographic monitoring. In this experience, five deaths occurred in association with pericardiocentesis; nonfatal hemopericardium developed in an additional five patients. Pericardiocentesis in this study was successful in obtaining pericardial fluid in 106 of 123 patients. Importantly, the probability of success in safely obtaining fluid was directly related to the size of the pericardial effusion, since fluid was obtained in 93 per cent of patients with large effusions located both anteriorly and posteriorly on echocardiogram but in only 58 per cent with a small posterior pericardial effusion. In 23 patients a specific etiological diagnosis was possible from analysis of the pericardial fluid. Cardiac tamponade was successfully relieved by pericardiocentesis in 61 per cent, while the remainder required subsequent surgical drainage owing either to failure to relieve tamponade or to recurrence after pericardiocentesis. Surgery was most frequently required in patients with acute traumatic hemopericardium (p. 1503). An unsuspected physiological cause of increased systemic venous pressure other than simple cardiac tamponade was documented in 40 per cent of the patients studied, including effusive-constrictive pericarditis in 17 per cent, congestive heart failure in 16 per cent, and coexisting neoplastic superior vena caval obstruction in 5 per cent. Similar experiences regarding the efficacy and safety of pericardiocentesis have been reported by ourselves[128] and others.[137,138]

Two-dimensional echocardiography is useful in guiding pericardiocentesis. Callahan et al.[139] have reported their experience in 132 consecutive pericardiocenteses guided by two-dimensional echocardiography. Pericardiocentesis was successful in obtaining pericardial fluid in 95 per cent of the procedures. There were no deaths, one pneumothorax, and three minor complications. Partial or complete surgical pericardiectomy was subsequently required in 25 per cent of patients for recurrent effusion, chronic relapsing pericarditis, or effusive-constrictive disease. Two-dimensional echocardiographic guidance is particularly helpful in percutaneous pericardiocentesis in patients with loculated pericardial effusion after cardiac surgery.[140]

RISKS AND COMPLICATIONS. Thus, pericardiocentesis is now safer than it was a decade ago, and when the procedure is performed by an experienced operator, the risk of developing a life-threatening complication is only about 0 to 5 per cent.[128,136-141] The procedure is most likely to be successful and uncomplicated when performed in patients with clear-cut echocardiographic evidence of a large effusion with an anterior clear space of 10 mm or more. Cardiac tamponade associated with malignant pericardial effusion or prior radiation therapy can often be managed with pericardiocentesis alone or with a combination of pericardiocentesis, radiation therapy, and local or systemic chemotherapy.[128,136] This therapeutic approach may be preferable in patients with advanced malignant disease when it is desirable to avoid major surgery that is not definitive.

These recent experiences with pericardiocentesis indicate that the procedure should usually be performed in conjunction with hemodynamic measurements, including right heart and intrapericardial pressures, to (1) document the presence of the physiological changes of cardiac tamponade prior to attempted pericardiocentesis and (2) exclude other important coexisting causes of elevated jugular venous pressure, such as effusive-constrictive disease, superior vena caval obstruction, and left ventricular failure. There is rarely justification for performing blind needle pericardiocentesis at the bedside in the absence of optimal hemodynamic monitoring or of a prior echocardiogram documenting the presence of a large anterior and posterior effusion.

Pericardiocentesis is likely to be either complicated or unsuccessful in improving hemodynamics in patients with (1) acute traumatic hemopericardium in which blood enters the pericardial space as rapidly as it can be aspirated, (2) a small pericardial effusion judged to be less than 200 ml in size, (3) absence of an anterior effusion based on echocardiogram, (4) a loculated effusion, or (5) clot and fibrin as well as fluid filling the mediastinal or pericardial space postoperatively. Acute hemopericardium secondary to laceration, puncture of the heart, or leaking left ventricular or aortic aneurysm is likely to recur rapidly after pericardiocentesis. This procedure should be used only as an emergency temporizing measure prior to surgical pericardial exploration in which repair of the heart or aorta may be necessary.[142] Surgical drainage is also usually preferred in patients with tamponade caused by purulent pericarditis to permit extensive drainage and in patients with suspected or known tuberculous pericarditis to permit bacteriological and histological examination of pericardial biopsy specimens. A very rare complication that may occur after the relief of cardiac tamponade is the development of sudden ventricular dilatation[143] and acute pulmonary edema.[144] The mechanism is probably a sudden increase in pulmonary venous blood flow following the relief of pericardial compression in the presence of underlying ventricular dysfunction.

PROCEDURE OF COMBINED CATHETERIZATION AND PERICARDIOCENTESIS

We prefer the following method of combined catheterization and pericardiocentesis, which allows documentation of increased intrapericardial pressure and assessment of hemodynamic improvement after pericardiocentesis.[145] In contrast to traditional bedside sharp-needle pericardiocentesis, this method utilizes a soft catheter for pericardial aspiration and eliminates the prolonged presence of a sharp needle in the pericardial sac, thereby minimizing the risk of cardiac laceration. If possible, pericardiocentesis should be performed in a cardiac procedure laboratory where radiographic and hemodynamic monitoring facilities are optimal and by cardiologists experienced with hemodynamic measurements and the procedure itself. Before the procedure, the patient's blood should be typed and crossmatched and the cardiac surgery team alerted.

Pericardiocentesis is performed after the recording of baseline hemodynamic variables and cardiac output. Since the equilibration of right and left ventricular diastolic pressures is an important feature of cardiac tamponade, it is often desirable to catheterize both sides of the heart and to record right atrial and right ventricular pressures simultaneously with left ventricular pressure. Care should be taken to use equisensitive transducers and to avoid an underdamped catheter-transducer system. Before pericardiocentesis, the transducer system that will be used to record intrapericardial pressure should be leveled with the other transducers, calibrated, and connected to a short length of fluid-filled tubing and a stopcock.

PATIENT POSITION AND ROUTE. Pericardiocentesis is carried out with the patient's thorax and head tilted up, which enhances the pooling of the effusion anteriorly and inferiorly. Although multiple sites have been advocated for pericardiocentesis, we strongly prefer the subxiphoid route, since it is extrapleural and avoids the coronary, pericardial, and internal mammary arteries. The skin is shaved, cleansed, and prepared in aseptic fashion, and the skin and subcutaneous tissue are anesthetized with 1 per

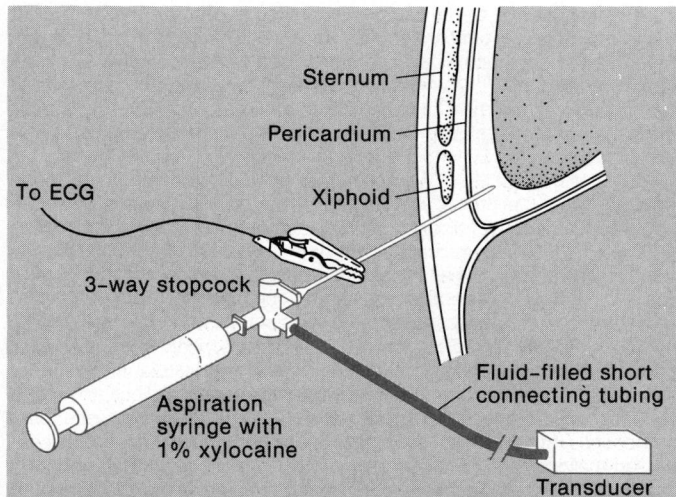

FIGURE 45-13. **Pericardiocentesis using the subxiphoid approach, which avoids the major epicardial vessels. A hollow needle, which is attached via a stopcock to an aspiration syringe and to a short length of connecting tubing to a transducer, is used to enter the pericardial space. When fluid is initially aspirated, the pressure waveform at the needle tip should be briefly examined to confirm that the needle tip is in the pericardial space. A floppy-tipped guidewire is then passed through the hollow needle, the needle is exchanged for a soft flexible catheter with end and side holes to facilitate safe and thorough drainage of the pericardial sac.** (Modified from Lorell, B. H., and Grossman, W.: Profiles in constrictive pericarditis, restrictive cardiomyopathy, and cardiac tamponade. *In* Grossman, W., and Baim, D. S. (eds.): Cardiac Catheterization, Angiography and Intervention. Philadelphia, Lea and Febiger, 1991, p. 643.)

cent lidocaine. The skin is pierced with a No. 11 blade, 0.5 cm below and to the left of the xiphoid process, and the subcutaneous tissues are spread with a small curved clamp.

A long, 8-inch, thin-walled No. 18-gauge pointed needle (pericardiocentesis kit, Mansfield Scientific, Inc., Mansfield, MA) is attached via a stopcock to a hand-held syringe containing 1 per cent lidocaine. One port of the stopcock is connected to the short length of fluid-filled tubing and the transducer that will be used to measure pericardial pressure (Fig. 45-13). The thin-walled needle commonly used for lumbar puncture is not adequate because its long sharp bevel poses some hazard. The metal hub of the needle may be attached by a sterile connector to the V lead of an electrocardiographic machine, and the electrocardiogram should be continuously recorded. *It is essential that the electrocardiogrpahic apparatus have equipotential grounding with no chance of a current wave that could induce ventricular fibrillation.* If this condition cannot be assured, it is safer to omit electrocardiographic monitoring from the needle.

The needle is directed posteriorly until the tip passes posterior to the bony cage. The hub of the needle is then pressed toward the diaphragm, and the needle is advanced with a 15-degree posterior tilt, either directly toward the patient's head or toward the right or left shoulder. As the needle is smoothly and slowly advanced, the operator periodically attempts to aspirate fluid and then injects a small amount of lidocaine to clear the needle and to provide anesthesia of the deep tissues. The needle is advanced until the pericardial membrane is felt to "give" and pericardial fluid is aspirated or until ST-segment elevation and ventricular premature beats appear on the electrocardiogram, indicating that the needle has reached the epicardium. In the latter case, the needle is promptly and smoothly withdrawn while the operator attempts to aspirate pericardial fluid until the needle lies within the fluid-filled pericardial space and the ECG changes disappear. If fluid cannot be freely aspirated, the needle is slowly withdrawn out of the body, avoiding lateral motion; the needle is flushed and the procedure repeated.

If hemorrhagic fluid is freely aspirated and it is not clear whether the needle is in the ventricle, atrium, or pericardial space, a few milliliters of contrast medium may be injected under fluoroscopic observation. If the contrast medium instantly swirls and disappears, the needle is within a cardiac chamber; in contrast, the appearance of sluggish layering of contrast medium inferiorly indicates that the needle is correctly positioned. When fluid can be freely aspirated, the stopcock is turned into its transducer and needle tip, and phasic right atrial pressures are simultaneously displayed. If the needle tip is in the pericardial space, pericardial and right atrial pressures should be equal with identical waveforms. A soft floppy-tip 0.038-inch guidewire is then passed through the hollow needle so that its

tip lies within the pericardial space, as confirmed by fluoroscopy. A soft tapered large-bore lumen No. 6 French or 7 French catheter with multiple sideholes and an end hole is advanced over the guidewire, the guidewire is removed, and a few millimeters of fluid are aspirated. The catheter is then promptly connected to the prepared transducer, and intrapericardial pressure is recorded simultaneously with right atrial and systemic arterial pressure to document the presence of cardiac tamponade.

THE PERICARDIAL FLUID. Fluid samples are then aspirated from the catheter and sent for analysis of protein, amylase, glucose, and cholesterol content; hematocrit and white blood cell count; and bacteriological culture for aerobic and anaerobic bacteria, tuberculosis, and fungi. In most cases, a generous sample of fluid should also be sent in a heparinized container for cytological examination. Right atrial, systemic arterial, and intrapericardial pressures should then be recorded periodically as aliquots of fluid are removed — not only until intrapericardial pressure falls to zero but until no further fluid can be aspirated; intrapericardial pressure may return to normal levels after removal of only 50 to 100 ml of fluid in the presence of an effusion of 1 to 2 liters. In our experience, extremely thorough drainage can be accomplished by connecting the intrapericardial catheter via sterile noncollapsible tubing to a stoppered sterile glass bottle with a vacuum. This should be done only when a soft catheter is in the pericardial space, since vacuum suction would be hazardous with sharp needle drainage. When no further fluid can be aspirated or drained, cardiac output and systemic arterial pressure as well as right atrial, right ventricular, and left ventricular (or pulmonary capillary wedge) pressures should be recorded, the last three simultaneously. The jugular veins should also be examined.

Successful relief of cardiac tamponade is documented by (1) the fall of intrapericardial pressure to levels of −3 and +3 mm Hg, (2) the fall of elevated right atrial pressure and separation between right- and left-heart filling pressures, (3) augmentation of cardiac output, and (4) disappearance of pulsus paradoxus. The presence of continued elevation and equilibration of right and left ventriclar diastolic pressures with the appearance of a prominent y descent in the right atrial pressure tracing strongly suggests the presence of constricting pericardium due to effusive-constrictive pericarditis (p. 1489). Jugular venous distention despite a fall in right atrial pressure should raise the question of coexisting superior vena caval obstruction, particularly in patients with known or suspected malignant disease.

Some cardiologists advocate the routine injection of a small volume of CO_2 or air into the pericardial space to outline the pericardium at the end of the procedure. This procedure has not been shown to be of aid in identifying unsuspected tumor masses,[136] and we do not advocate it. When the pericardial space is nearly obliterated, there is also the risk of injecting gas into a pleural cavity or cardiac chamber or the production of air tamponade.

It is often desirable to leave the intrapericardial catheter in place for several hours to permit repeated aspiration of fluid if cardiac tamponade recurs or to allow instillation of a nonabsorbable corticosteroid or antineoplastic agent in special cases. The catheter may be sutured securely to the skin and attached via a three-way stopcock to a closed drainage system. If the fluid is hemorrhagic or rich in fibrin, the catheter must be cleared frequently with a few millimeters or fluid. Dilute heparin may be instilled into the catheter to prevent clotting. The catheter should usually be removed after 24 to 48 hours because of the risk of introducing infection and producing iatrogenic purulent pericarditis. However, in some patients, continuous catheter drainage for several days has been reported to be necessary and effective in relieving cardiac tamponade.[139,146,147] Percutaneous pericardial drainage in infants and children can be done without complications using a modification of this approach in which a catheter is inserted over a curved guidewire into the pericardial space under fluoroscopic control.[147]

Following pericardiocentesis, the majority of patients should be observed for about 24 hours in an intensive care setting for recurrence of cardiac tamponade. It is frequently helpful to obtain an echocardiogram soon after pericardiocentesis to establish the appearance of the heart and pericardium following aspiration.

PERICARDIECTOMY AND PERICARDIOTOMY

Surgical evacuation of pericardial fluid under pressure can be accomplished for patients who do not require extensive pericardial excision with the subxiphoid limited pericardiotomy. Subxiphoid pericardiotomy can usually be performed under local anesthesia.[142,148] In patients who are not in extremis, the procedure is usually done without initial palliative pericardiocentesis so that the pericardial sac is distended. After a small longitudinal incision is made below the xiphoid process through the linea alba, the diaphragm and pericardium are dissected away from the sternum, and the diaphragm is retracted inferiorly to permit direct exposure of the anterior pericardium. The tense parietal pericardium is visualized, a small incision is made in the pericardium, a small segment of pericardium is resected for drainage, and a tube is inserted into the pericardial space for extrathoracic drainage by gravity into a sterile container.

The use of the term *subxiphoid pericardial window*[142] to describe this operation should probably be avoided, since it creates confusion with a limited pericardiectomy, which is often referred to as a pleuropericardial window or pericardial window. A limited pericardiectomy[149] via a left hemithorax drains the pericardial cavity into the left hemithorax, and all accessible pericardial tissue is not excised. In a complete pericardiectomy the pericardium is resected from the right phrenic nerve to the left pulmonary veins (sparing the left phrenic nerve) and from the great vessels to the mid-diaphragm, while a partial pericardiectomy is limited by the great vessels.[150]

The relative efficacy of these surgical approaches has been reviewed in two recent large series.[149,150] The overall 30-day surgical mortality ranged from 12.5 to 15.5 per cent, and was higher in patients with malignant than benign effusions. The subxiphoid pericardiotomy has some advantages over extensive formal pericardiectomy in that it is simpler and shorter, permits both drainage of pericardial fluid and examination of a small pericardial biopsy specimen, and can usually be performed safely using local anesthesia in critically ill patients.[148] However, in comparison with a significantly higher risk of reoperation for recurrent tamponade or constrictive disease within a few months after surgery.[149] This suggests that the less invasive subxiphoid pericrdiotomy should be chosen as a palliative procedure in patients who are critically ill with limited expected survival. The left thoracotomy partial pericardiectomy appears to offer none of the advantages of the subxiphoid pericardiotomy and is associated with higher operative mortarity.[150] Complete pericardiectomy is usually recomended for the surgical treatment of patients with effusive-constrictive pericardial disease or loculated effusion who are in good general condition and who are expected to survive more than a few months.

PERICARDIOSCOPY. With use of a flexible fiberoptic bronchoscope or endoscope, this procedure has been reported as an adjunct to subxiphoid pericardiotomy following the drainage of the effusion in the operating room.[151,152] Pericardioscopy permits visualization of the parietal pericardium and epicardium on the anterior, posterior, and inferior surfaces of the heart and allows selective biopsies beyond the small region of pericardium that is usually accessible with a subxiphoid incision.

PERICARDIAL BIOPSY. Endrys et al.[153] described a technique for percutaneous pericardial biopsy using an endomyocardial bioptome inserted via a curved sheath after percutaneous pericardiocentesis and distention of the pericardial space with air. These techniques offer new approaches for obtaining diagnostic information in patients with suspected malignant or infectious pericardial disease, but the efficacy and safety of these approaches in comparison with surgical exploration and pericardial biopsy are not yet established.

Constrictive Pericarditis

Constrictive pericarditis is present when a fibrotic, thickened, and adherent pericardium restricts diastolic filling of the heart. It usually begins with an initial episode of acute pericarditis, which may not be detectable clinically, characterized by fibrin deposition, often with a pericardial effusion. This then slowly progresses to a subacute stage of organization and resorption of the effusion, followed by a chronic stage consisting of fibrous scarring and thickening of the pericardium with obliteration of the pericardial space. In the majority of cases, the visceral and parietal layers become completely fused, but in a few cases, the constricting process is produced primarily by the visceral pericardium (epicardium). In the chronic stage of constrictive pericarditis, calcium deposition may contribute to thickening and stiffening of the pericardium. Constrictive pericarditis is usually a symmetrical scarring process that produces uniform restriction of the filling of all heart chambers. Rare cases of strictly localized pericardial thickening have been reported, including constricting bands in the atrioventricular groove surrounding the semilunar valve rings, or in the aortic groove, right ventricular outflow tract, and venae cavae.[154,155]

PATHOPHYSIOLOGY

In classic constrictive pericarditis, the heavily fibrosed or calcified pericardium restricts diastolic filling of all chambers of the heart and determines the diastolic volume of the heart. The symmetrical constricting effect of the pericardium results in elevation and equilibrium of diastolic pressures in all four cardiac chambers (as well as of pulmonary capillary wedge pressures). In early diastole when intracardiac volume is less than that defined by the stiff pericardium, diastolic filling is unimpeded, and early diastolic filling occurs abnormally rapidly because venous pressure is elevated. Rapid early diastolic filling is abruptly halted when the intracardiac volume reaches the limit set by the noncompliant pericardium.

Instantaneous plots of ventricular volume versus time in patients with constrictive pericarditis have shown that virtually all filling of the ventricle occurs very early in diastole. This abnormal pattern of diastolic filling is reflected in the characteristic dip-and-plateau waveforms in both right and left ventricles (Fig. 45–14). The early diastolic dip corresponds to the period of excessively rapid diastolic filling, while the plateau phase corresponds to the period of mid and late diastole when there is little additional ventricular volume expansion. Since the atria are equilibrated with the ventricles in early diastole, the jugular venous waveform and right and left atrial waveforms show a prominent and deep diastolic y descent. The systolic x descent is usually also present, and the venous waveform may therefore exhibit a characteristic M or W configuration.

A bimodal pattern of systemic venous return occurs in constrictive pericarditis with an acceleration of systemic venous blood flow from the venae cavae into the right atrium during both ventricular systolic ejection and early diastole. The greatest acceleration of venous blood flow occurs during early diastole simultaneous with the y descent. This contrasts with the normal filling pattern, in which a bimodal pattern of systemic venous return is also present, but the major surge of venous return occurs during systole. The pattern of systemic venous return in constrictive pericarditis also contrasts with that in cardiac tamponade. Cardiac compression is present throughout diastole in cardiac tamponade, so that the diastolic surge of venous return is blunted, and the venous pressure tracing shows absence of or blunted diastolic y descent and a preserved x descent.

KUSSMAUL'S SIGN. Another striking abnormality of constrictive pericarditis is the failure of intrathoracic pressure changes during respiration to be transmitted to the pericardial space and intracardiac chambers. As a consequence, during inspiration, systemic venous and right arterial pressures do not fall and venous flow into the right atrium does not increase, in contrast to the situation in normal subjects and patients with cardiac tamponade (Fig. 45–8). In some patients, systemic venous pressure may actually increase with inspiration, i.e., *Kussmaul's sign*.[156] This finding may occur in other disorders such as chronic right ventricular failure and restrictive cardiomyopathy, in which right atrial and systemic venous pressures also are markedly elevated. However, Kussmaul's sign does not occur in acute cardiac tamponade, in which the inspiratory fall in intrathoracic pressure is transmitted to the fluid-filled pericardial space.[157] Pulsus paradoxus (p. 1474) is also less common in constrictive pericarditis than in cardiac tamponade, in which the mechanism is thought to be largely the exaggerated increase in right ventricular filling during inspriration at the expense of left ventricular filling. The presence of an inspiratory fall in arterial pressure greater than 10 mm Hg suggests the presence of a tense

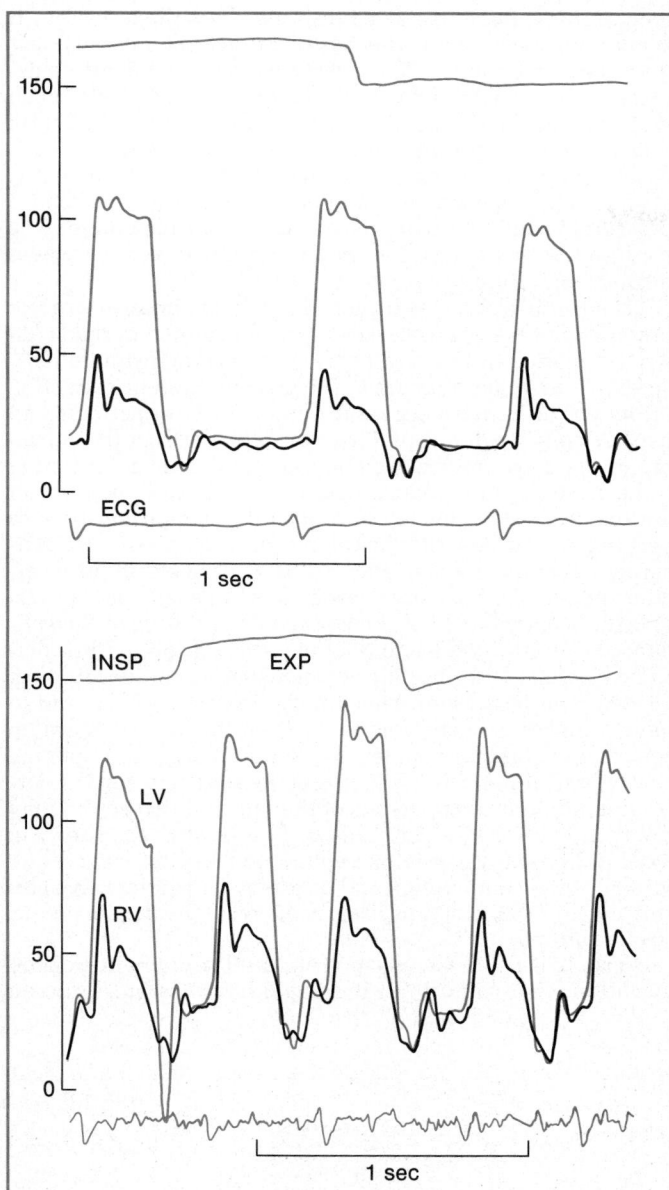

FIGURE 45–14. Left (LV) and right ventricular (RV) pressure recordings from a patient with constrictive pericarditis illustrating that the presence of tachycardia partially obscures evaluation of the diastolic waveforms. The long diastole following a premature beat allows recognition of equilibration of ventricular diastolic pressures before the a wave, as well as detection of a dip-and-plateau configuration of the waveforms. (From Lorell, B. H., and Grossman, W.: Profiles in constrictive pericarditis, restrictive cardiomyopathy, and cardiac tamponade. *In* Grossman, W. (ed.): Cardiac Catheterization and Angiography. Philadelphia, Lea and Febiger, 1986, p. 430.)

pericardial effusion or coexisting pulmonary disease with an exaggerated inspiratory fall in intrathoracic pressure.

Restriction of diastolic filling ultimately results in compensatory renal retention of sodium and water that contributes further to the increase in systemic venous pressure and initially serves to maintain diastolic filling of the ventricles despite pericardial compression. The inhibition of the release of atrial natriuretic factor may contribute to renal fluid retention.[158] In some cases, the pericardial scar is so dense that diastolic ventricular volumes are reduced, which may cause stroke volume and then cardiac output to fall despite compensatory tachycardia. The presence of reduced cardiac output, tachycardia, and elevated right and left heart filling pressures may simulate myocardial failure, and classic ventricular performance curves may show reduced left ventricular stroke volume relative to elevated left ventricular filling pressure. However, systolic contraction of the ventricles and the intrinsic contractile state of the myocardium are usually normal or nearly so.[159] In severe cases of constrictive pericarditis, myocardial systolic function may also be depressed, owing to myocardial atrophy, fibrosis, or compression of superficial coronary arteries in the fibrotic pericardium resulting in myocardial ischemia.[160-162] Although the presence of coexisting cardiomyopathy is usually a factor predictive of a poor outcome after pericardiectomy (p. 1503), a striking improvement of left ventricular ejection fraction may occasionally occur after stripping of a fibrotic and thick pericardium.[163]

SUBACUTE NONCALCIFIC PERICARDITIS. Pathophysiological and hemodynamic findings in patients with subacute noncalcific pericarditis may differ from those in patients with chronic constrictive pericarditis in whom the pericardium resembles a rigid shell. Hancock has suggested that the presence of a thick fluid-fibrin layer in the process of organization leads to relatively elastic compression of the heart, which may be compared to "wrapping the heart tightly with rubber bands."[164] The pathophysiological disturbance caused by this nonrigid fibroelastic form of constrictive pericarditis is similar to that in cardiac tamponade, since fibroelastic constriction compresses the heart continuously throughout the cardiac cycle, and respiratory changes in intrathoracic pressure usually are transmitted to the cardiac chambers.[164] Thus, patterns of ventricular filling and waveforms in the subacute form of fibroelastic compression tend to resemble those of cardiac tamponade rather than of constrictive pericarditis and include a systemic venous waveform with a predominant x descent or equal x and y descents, an inconspicuous early diastolic dip in the ventricular waveform, an inspiratory fall in systemic venous and right atrial pressures, and the presence of pulsus paradoxus (Table 45–5).

ETIOLOGY

Tuberculosis was formerly the leading cause of constrictive pericarditis in Western nations as reported in the classic series

TABLE 45–5   CLINICAL AND HEMODYNAMIC FEATURES OF COMPRESSIVE PERICARDIAL DISEASE

	CARDIAC TAMPONADE	SUBACUTE "ELASTIC" CONSTRICTION	CHRONIC "RIGID" CONSTRICTION
Duration of symptoms	Hours to days	Weeks to months	Months to years
Chest pain, friction rub	Usual	Recent past	Remote
Pulsus paradoxus	Prominent	Usually prominent	Slight or absent
Kussmaul's sign	Absent	Usually absent	Often present
Early diastolic knock	Absent	Usually absent	Often present
Heart size on chest roentgenogram	Usually enlarged	Usually enlarged	Usually normal, sometimes enlarged
Pericardial calcification	Absent	Rare	Often present
Abnormal P waves or atrial fibrillation	Absent	Absent	Often present
Venous (right atrial) waveform	X or Xy	Xy or XY	XY or xY
Pericardial effusion	Always present	Often present	Absent

X and Y = prominent x and y descents, respectively, x and y = inconspicuous x and y descents.
Modified from Hancock, E. W.: On the elastic and rigid forms of constrictive pericarditis. Am. Heart J. *100*:917, 1980.

of Paul[165] and Andrews[166] and their coworkers. In disadvantaged nations, this is still true,[167] whereas with the advent of antituberculosis therapy this disease now accounts for 15 per cent or less of cases in developed nations.[168,169] The largest number of cases of constrictive pericarditis today are of unknown etiology (42 per cent) and attributed to earlier clinically inapparent viral pericarditis.[169] In the past decade, constrictive pericarditis after cardiac surgery has emerged as an important cause (p. 1688). In a series of consecutive patients with constrictive pericarditis seen at Stanford from 1970 to 1985, postsurgical pericarditis accounted for 11 per cent of all cases but constituted 29 per cent of cases between 1980 and 1985.[169] In this series, constrictive pericarditis following mediastinal radiation therapy accounted for 30 per cent of cases, with an average latency period of 11 years after radiotherapy. Other nontubercular causes include chronic renal failure treated with hemodialysis (p. 1868); connective tissue disorders, including rheumatoid arthritis and systemic lupus erythematosus (p. 1501); and neoplastic pericardial infiltration or encasement of the heart due mostly commonly to lung cancer, breast cancer, Hodgkin's disease, and lymphoma. Constrictive pericarditis can develop after incomplete drainage of purulent pericarditis (p. 1494) and as a complication of fungal infections (p. 1494) and parasitic infections (p. 1495). It may occasionally follow pericarditis associated with acute myocardial infarction and the postpericardiotomy syndrome, (p. 1503), and in association with pulmonary asbestosis.[170]

CONSTRICTIVE PERICARDITIS IN CHILDREN (see also p. 1493). Constrictive pericarditis is far less common in children than in adults and may rarely occur following a viral syndrome in a child mistakenly thought to have hepatitis or a protein-losing enteropathy. When constrictive pericarditis occurs in young children, tuberculosis should be strongly considered, since it was a proved or highly likely cause in 56 per cent of 84 children with constrictive pericarditis reported in the literature.[171] Nontraumatic hemopericardium has been reported in children and young adults with congenital bleeding disorders complicated by a second process such as endocarditis or viral syndrome, and constrictive pericarditis has occurred following pericardial bleeding due to congenital afibrinogenemia.[172] The newly described familial syndrome of pericarditis, arthritis, and camptodactyly (flexion contractures) is a rare cause of constrictive pericarditis in children and young adults.[173] A rare congenital cause of constrictive pericarditis is *mulibrey nanism*, an autosomal recessive disorder characterized by dwarfism, constrictive pericarditis, abnormal fundi, and fibrous dysplasia of the long bones.[174,175]

CLINICAL FEATURES

In patients in whom systemic venous and right atrial pressures are modestly elevated (10 to 15 mm Hg), left ventricular filling pressure is also usually only modestly elevated. In this setting, symptoms secondary to systemic venous congestion such as edema, abdominal swelling, and discomfort due to ascites and passive hepatic congestion may predominate. Vague abdominal symptoms such as postprandial fullness, dyspepsia, flatulence, and anorexia may also be present. When both right and left filling pressures are elevated to the level of 15 to 30 mm Hg, symptoms of pulmonary venous congestion, such as exertional dyspnea, cough, and orthopnea, are present. Pleural effusions and elevation of the diaphragm due to ascites may also contribute to dyspnea. Severe fatigue, weight loss, and muscle wasting suggest the presence of fixed or reduced cardiac output.

PHYSICAL EXAMINATION. The single most important finding is elevation of jugular venous pressure. If the neck is examined casually, or if the patient is examined supine so that jugular venous pressure is measured above the angle of the jaw, this important clue to the presence of constrictive pericarditis may be missed. A prominent feature of the elevated jugular venous pressure is the rapidly collapsing negative wave of the diastolic y descent. In patients in sinus rhythm,

both x and y descents can be distinguished; the x descent is synchronous with while the diastolic y descent is out of phase with the carotid pulse. These features may be difficult to detect in patients with tachycardia, tachypnea, or arrhythmia. It may also be difficult to distinguish between right heart failure due to tricuspid regurgitation and chronic constrictive pericarditis by neck vein examination at the bedside. The finding of Kussmaul's sign (an inspiratory increase in systemic venous pressure) is difficult to appreciate at the bedside and may be confused with exaggerated amplitude of the venous waves during inspiration.

The arterial pulse may be normal or show diminished pulse pressure. Severe pulsus paradoxus is uncommon in rigid constrictive pericarditis and rarely exceeds 10 mm Hg unless pericardial fluid under pressure is also present. Systolic retraction of the apical impulse occurs in the majority of patients and usually consists of an unobtrusive diffuse precordial movement. The most impressive abnormality during auscultation is the diastolic pericardial knock, an early diastolic sound that is often heard along the left sternal border in rigid constrictive pericarditis, infrequently heard in subacute constrictive pericarditis of the fibroelastic variety, and not heard in pure cardiac tamponade.[157] The pericardial knock usually occurs 0.09 to 0.12 second after A_2 and corresponds in timing to the sudden cessation of ventricular filling and the premature diastolic plateau of the diastolic ventricular volume curve[176] (Fig. 45–15). The pericardial knock tends to occur earlier and to have a higher acoustic frequency than the typical S_3 gallop sound, and therefore it may be confused with the opening snap of mitral stenosis. Widening of the split between the aortic and pulmonic components of the second heart sound may occur in constrictive pericarditis. This is attributed to (1) a fixed right ventricular stroke volume during inspiration due to pericardial compression and (2) premature aortic valve closure due to a transitory inspiratory decrease in left ventricular stroke volume.

Hepatomegaly is usually present, and prominant hepatic pulsations that conform to the jugular venous pulse can be

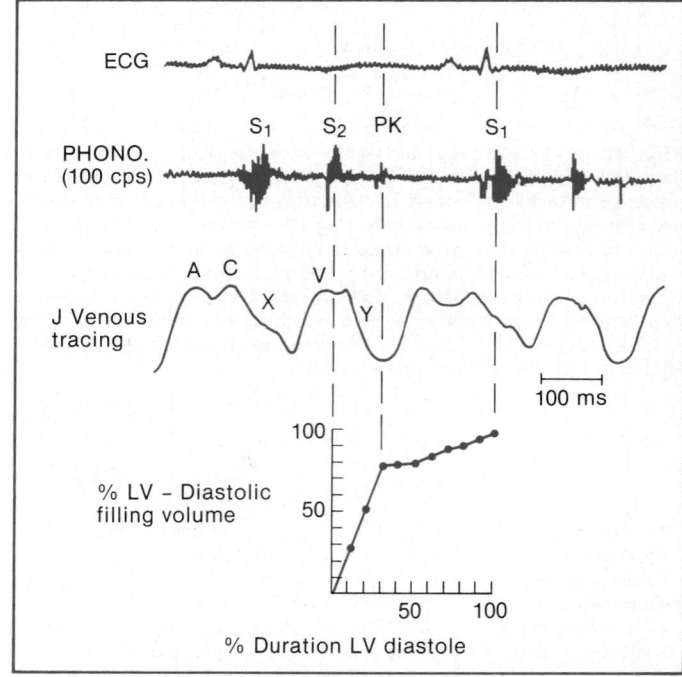

FIGURE 45–15. Electrocardiogram (ECG), phonocardiogram (PHONO), jugular venous pulse tracing, and left ventricular (LV) diastolic filling curve in a patient with constrictive pericarditis and pericardial knock (PN). The pericardial knock (PK) occurs simultaneously with the nadir of the diastolic y descent and sudden plateau of the LV filling curve. (From Tyberg, T. I., et al.: Genesis of pericardial knock in constrictive pericarditis. Am. J. Cardiol. 46:570, 1980.)

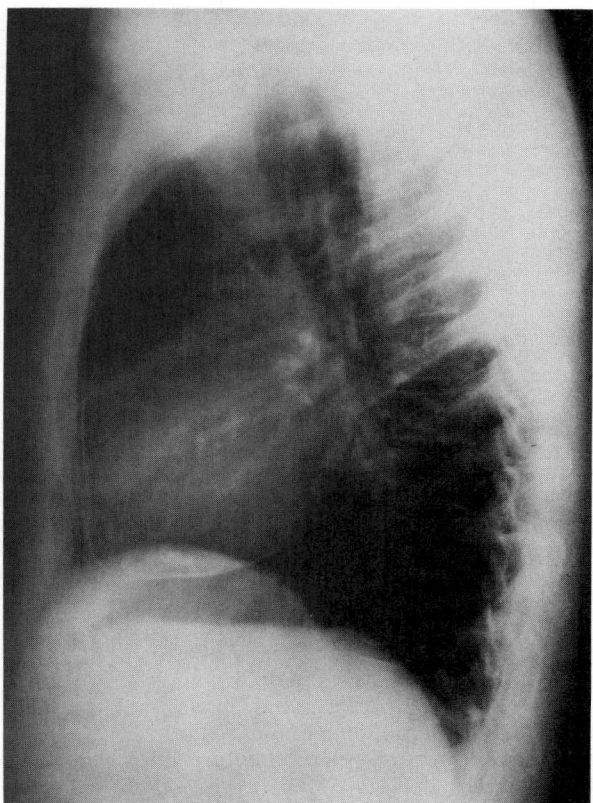

FIGURE 45-16. Lateral chest roentgenogram showing calcification of the pericardium in a patient with chronic constrictive pericarditis of idiopathic (postviral) etiology. The eggshell rim of pericardial calcification is often best appreciated in the lateral projection.

TABLE 45-6 RADIOLOGICAL FEATURES OF CONSTRICTIVE PERICARDITIS

Normal heart size	33%
Enlarged heart	67%
Calcified pericardium	43%
Pleural effusion	83%
Pulmonary venous congestion	86%
Left atrial enlargement	85%

Modified from Pulvaneswary, M., et al.: Constrictive pericarditis. Clinical, hemodynamic, and radiologic correlation. Australas. Radiol. *26*:53, 1982.

about 60 per cent of patients, and unexplained persistent pleural effusion can be the presenting manifestation.[180] Since left atrial pressure is commonly elevated to 15 to 30 mm Hg, there may be evidence of redistribution of blood flow, while Kerley's B lines or infiltrates suggestive of frank pulmonary edema are rare (Table 45-6).

ELECTROCARDIOGRAM. Electrocardiographic findings include low QRS voltage, generalized T-wave inversion or flattening, and left atrial abnormalities suggestive of P mitrale (Fig. 45-17). Atrial fibrillation occurs in less than half the patients with constrictive pericarditis and is thought to be related to longstanding elevation of atrial pressures and atrial enlargement. In a postmortem study of constrictive pericarditis, Levine noted that atrioventricular block, intraventricular conduction defects, and pseudoinfarction patterns with deep wide Q waves seemed to be related to an extension of calcification into the myocardium and around the coronary arteries, compromising coronary blood flow.[161] An unusual pattern that simulates right ventricular hypertrophy with right-axis deviation may be present in about 5 per cent of patients and due to dense pericardial scar overlying the right ventricle in association with compensatory dilation and hyperkinesis of the outflow tract.[181,182]

ECHOCARDIOGRAM. One distinct M-mode echocardiographic pattern of pericardial thickening in constrictive pericarditis consists of two parallel lines representing the visceral and parietal pericardia separated by a clear space of at least 1 mm; another consists of multiple dense echoes.[183] Extreme respiratory variation in the depth of the pulmonic valve a wave[184] and premature pulmonic valve opening secondary to a high right ventricular early diastolic pressure may be present,[185] but these changes are also seen in other disorders with high right ventricular early diastolic pressure, such as tricuspid and pulmonic regurgitation. Other M-mode echocardiographic abnormalities include abrupt posterior motion of the interventricular septum in early diastole, coinciding with the pericardial knock, abrupt posterior motion during atrial systole,[185] and reduced amplitude of left ventricular posterior wall motion.[186] Engle et al.[187] reviewed M-mode echocardiograms from 40 patients with proven constrictive pericarditis and 40 normal subjects. They observed that normal left ventricular size, left atrial enlargement, flattened diastolic ventricular wall motion, and abnormal septal motion were

detected in 70 per cent of patients[177] (Fig. 2-7, p. 19). Other evidence of hepatic dysfunction secondary to passive liver congestion and diminished cardiac output may include ascites, icterus, spider angiomas, and palmar erythema. In young patients with competent venous valves, edema of the extremities may be noticeably absent in the presence of marked abdominal distention. Older patients with longstanding constrictive pericarditis may have enormous ascites and massive edema of the scrotum, thighs, and calves.[177a] In contrast, the upper torso and arms may show evidence of marked muscle wasting and cachexia.

CHEST ROENTGENOGRAM (see also p. 230). The cardiac silhouette may be small, normal, or enlarged. Cardiac enlargement may be apparent because of coexisting pericardial effusion, the contribution of an enormously thickened pericardium, or preexisting cardiac chamber enlargement or hypertrophy. The right superior mediastinum may be prominent as a result of engorgement of the superior vena cava, and left atrial enlargement is common.[178] Extensive calcification of the pericardium is present in approximately half the patients and raises the possibility of a tubercular etiology. The location of calcification is helpful in distinguishing between pericardial and myocardial aneurysm calcium, since pericardial calcification is predominantly located over the right heart chambers and in the atrioventricular grooves, whereas isolated calcification of the left ventricular apex or posterior wall suggests left ventricular aneurysm.[179] However, this finding is not specific for constrictive pericarditis in that *a calcified pericardium is not necessarily a constricted one.* The lateral chest film is particularly useful for the detection of pericardial calcium in the atrioventricular groove or along the anterior and diaphragmatic surfaces of the right ventricle (Fig. 45-16). Fluoroscopy may be helpful in distinguishing pericardial calcification from calcium within the wall of a myocardial aneurysm or thrombus or within the mitral or aortic valves, mitral annulus, or coronary arteries. Pleural effusions are present in

T.D. CONSTRICTIVE PERICARDITIS

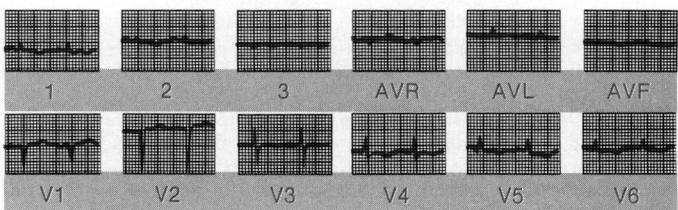

FIGURE 45-17. Electrocardiogram from a patient with surgically proven constrictive pericarditis and normal coronary arteries who had symptoms of chronic fatigue, dyspnea, and chest pain. The electrocardiogram is notable for the presence of a wide, notched P wave and diffuse T-wave inversion. These changes were initially mistakenly thought to be related to coronary insufficiency.

found in most patients, but no single feature was diagnostic of constrictive pericarditis. Computer-assisted digitization of M-mode echocardiograms may be useful in distinguishing the abnormal rapid early diastolic filling of constrictive pericarditis from the more delayed filling pattern of restrictive cardiomyopathy.[188]

Two-dimensional echocardiography in constrictive pericarditis shows an immobile and dense appearance of the pericardium, abrupt displacement of the interventricular septum during early diastolic filling ("septal bounce"), prominent early diastolic filling, and an abnormal contour of the junction of the left ventricle and left atrial posterior wall.[189] Dilatation of the hepatic veins and inferior vena cava,[190] intense and spontaneous contrast in the inferior vena cava,[191] and distention of the inferior vena cava with blunted respiratory fluctuations in diameter ("plethora")[192] have also been described in patients with constrictive pericarditis. Himelman et al.[192] reviewed the diagnostic value of pericardial adhesions, septal bounce, and vena cava plethora and noted that false-positive findings occurred in patients with pacemakers or bundle branch block after pericardiotomy, and with other causes of right heart failure. Studies in an experimental dog model and in patients have confirmed that two-dimensional echocardiography can demonstrate abnormal early diastolic filling but greatly overestimates pericardial thickness.[193]

Doppler echocardiography of the engorged hepatic vein has been reported to show a W-wave pattern that corresponds to the characteristic pattern of right atrial filling and consists of rapid forward flow during early diastole, abrupt deceleration and subsequent reverse flow before the *a* wave, and a second wave of rapid forward flow during early systolic ejection with reverse flow in late systole[194] (Fig. 45–18).

CT AND MR IMAGING (see also Fig. 11–9, p. 317). CT has also emerged as a valuable tool in the evaluation of suspected constrictive pericarditis. The technique is especially useful in identifying pericardial thickening and in identifying other

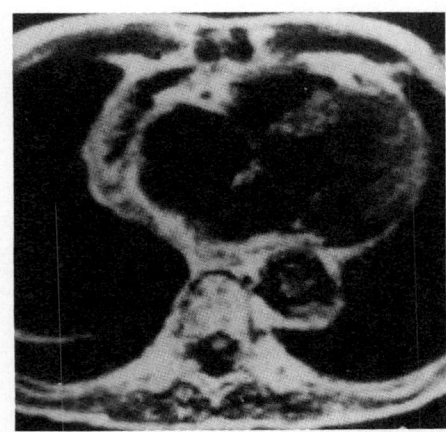

FIGURE 45–19. Magnetic resonance image from a patient with constrictive uremic pericarditis shows irregular thickening of the visceral and parietal pericardial layers, which are separated by low-intensity fluid, overlying the enlarged right atrium. Pericardial fluid is also present behind the left ventricle, which is hypertrophied. (From Soulen, R. L., et al.: Magnetic resonance imaging of constrictive pericardial disease. Am. J. Cardiol. **55**:480, 1985.)

findings compatible with constrictive pericarditis, including dilation of the venae cavae and deformation of the right ventricle.[195,196] Nonvisualization of the left ventricular posterolateral wall by computed tomography suggests coexisting myocardial fibrosis or atrophy and may predict a poor outcome following pericardiectomy.[197]

Experience with MR imaging in patients with constrictive pericarditis suggests that it can detect pericardial thickening, dilation of the venae cavae and hepatic veins, and narrowing of the right ventricle[196,198] (Fig. 45–19). All of these findings are suggestive of constrictive pericarditis.

The use of noninvasive imaging techniques to assist in discrimination between constrictive pericarditis and restrictive cardiomyopathy is discussed later in this chapter (p. 1488).

OTHER LABORATORY FINDINGS. Other abnormal laboratory findings may be present as a result of chronic elevation of right atrial pressure causing passive congestion of the liver, kidneys, and gastrointestinal tract. These include depressed serum albumin, elevated serum globulin, elevated conjugated and unconjugated serum bilirubin, and abnormal hepatocellular function tests. In patients with hepatomegaly and ascites, liver biopsy may show histological features similar to the Budd-Chiari syndrome, including hepatic venule thrombi and ductular proliferation.[199] Chylous ascites may occur because of impedance of lymphatic drainage due to central venous hypertension.[200] Protein-losing enteropathy may be evident from the presence of albumin in the stool and lymphangiectasis on small-bowel biopsy.[201] Elevated systemic venous pressure may also produce variable degrees of albuminuria as well as pronounced protein loss consistent with the nephrotic syndrome.[202] Nonspecific evidence of the presence of chronic disease such as normocytic and normochromic anemia may be found.

DIFFERENTIAL DIAGNOSIS. Constrictive pericarditis should be suspected in patients with jugular venous distention, unexplained pleural effusion, hepatomegaly, systemic edema, or ascites. It must be distinguished from superior vena caval obstruction, nephrotic syndrome, hepatic and intraabdominal disease due to malignancy, and other cardiac causes of right atrial hypertension, including restrictive cardiomyopathy, tricuspid stenosis, tricuspid regurgitation, hypertrophic cardiomyopathy, and right atrial myxoma. It may be extremely difficult to distinguish patients with constrictive pericarditis from those with restrictive physiology due to amyloidosis, sarcoidosis, radiation injury, hemochromatosis, and the hypereosinophilic syndrome, which may involve pericardium as well as the myocardium.[203–205] Both constrictive pericarditis and restrictive cardiomyopathy may show the electrocardiographic changes of atrial fibrillation, left atrial

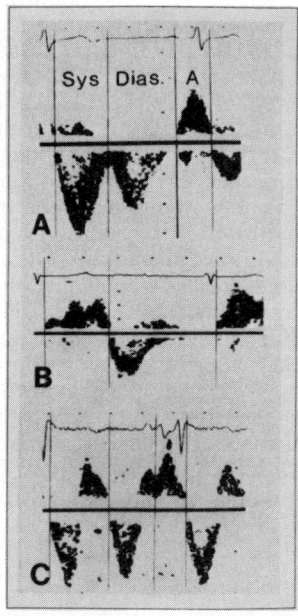

FIGURE 45–18. Pulsed Doppler recordings of central venous flow velocities in the hepatic vein. In *panel A,* a recording of a normal subject shows a normal pattern of biphasic flow with downward deflection of the signal indicative of a normal pattern of biphasic forward flow in systole and diastole with transient reversal of flow during atrial contraction. In *panel B,* a recording of a patient with severe tricuspid regurgitation shows holosystolic reverse flow. In *panel C,* a recording of a patient with constrictive pericarditis shows rapid forward flow in early systole and subsequent reverse flow in late systole, and an abbreviated signal of rapid forward flow in early diastole with abrupt deceleration and subsequent reverse flow that begins in mid-diastole before the *a* wave. (From von Bibra, H., et al.: Diagnosis of constrictive pericarditis by pulsed Doppler echocardiography of the hepatic vein. Am. J. Cardiol. **63**:483, 1989.)

abnormalities, and diffuse low QRS voltage with T-wave flattening. The presence of atrioventricular block and conduction disturbances simulating myocardial infarction favors the diagnosis of restrictive cardiomyopathy. Echocardiography in some patients with restrictive cardiomyopathy may show abnormal thickening of the ventricular myocardium or a peculiar "sparkling" appearance when amyloidosis is present.[206] The simultaneous use of electrocardiography and echocardiography to demonstrate a reduction of the voltage/mass ratio has been described in patients with amyloid restrictive cardiomyopathy in whom diffuse low QRS voltage is associated with increased thickness of the left ventricular wall due to amyloid deposition.[207]

In the presence of findings suggestive of constrictive pericarditis, right- and left-heart catheterization should be performed to document the presence of constrictive physiology and to exclude other causes of right atrial hypertension. Diuresis should be avoided prior to catheterization, since hypovolemia may obscure the characteristic hemodynamic findings. Cardiac catheterization and angiography, often with endomyocardial biopsy, are usually helpful in discriminating between constrictive pericarditis and restrictive cardiomyopathy in many patients, but in a minority exploratory thoracotomy may be required.

CARDIAC CATHETERIZATION AND ANGIOGRAPHY

Cardiac catheterization is useful in the assessment of patients suspected of having constrictive pericarditis to (1) document the presence of elevation and equilibration of diastolic filling pressures, (2) assess the effect of constrictive pericarditis on stroke volume and cardiac output, (3) evaluate myocardial systolic function, (4) assist in the difficult discrimination between constrictive pericarditis and restrictive cardiomyopathy, and (5) exclude compression of the coronary arteries or regional outflow tract compression by the fibrotic pericardium.

Catheterization of both the right and left ventricles should be performed to permit simultaneous recording of right and left heart filling pressures. Typical findings include the elevation and virtual identity (within 5 mm Hg) of right atrial, right ventricular diastolic, left atrial (pulmonary capillary wedge), and left ventricular diastolic pressures before the *a* wave. Right atrial pressure is characterized by a preserved systolic *x* descent, a prominent early diastolic *y* descent, and *a* and *v*

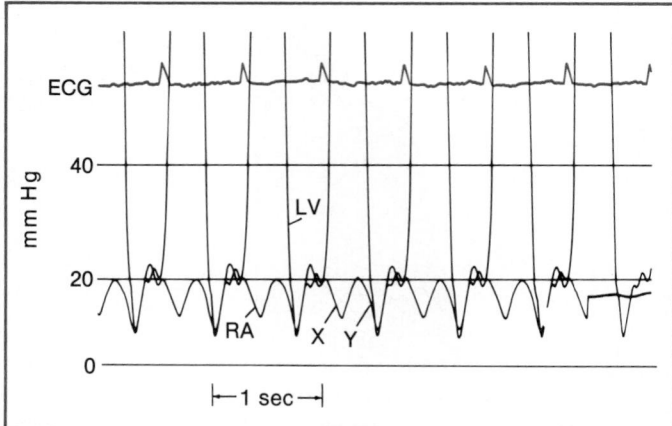

FIGURE 45–20. Simultaneous left ventricular (LV) and right atrial (RA) pressure recordings from a patient with constrictive pericarditis showing that both pressures are elevated and virtually equal throughout diastole. The prominent diastolic *y* descent in the right atrial waveform indicates that right atrial emptying is rapid and unimpeded in early diastole. In contrast, the *y* descent is absent or attenuated in cardiac tamponade because cardiac compression limits right ventricular filling throughout diastole. (From Lorell, B. H., and Grossman, W.: Profiles in constrictive pericarditis, restrictive cardiomyopathy, and cardiac tamponade. *In* Grossman, W., and Baim, D. S. (ed.): Cardiac Catheterization and Angiography. Philadelphia, Lea and Febiger, 1986, p. 440.)

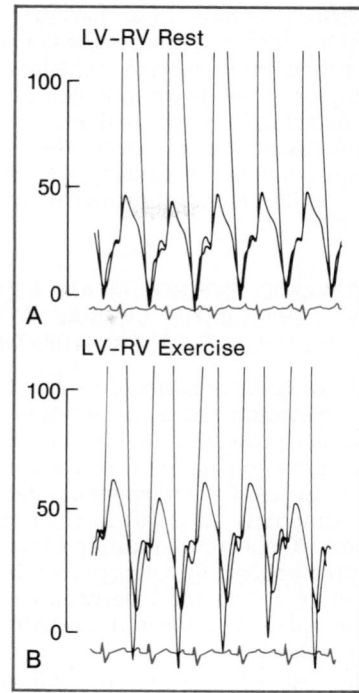

FIGURE 45–21. Representative left (LV) and right ventricular (RV) pressure tracings obtained at rest (*A*) and during exercise (*B*) from a patient with constrictive pericarditis. The diastolic equalization of pressures that is present at rest persists during exercise when the diastolic pressure of both ventricles is substantially higher. (From Robbins, M. A., et al.: Resting and exercise hemodynamics in constrictive pericarditis and a case of cardiac amyloidosis mimicking constriction. Cathet. Cardiovasc. Diagn. 9:463, 1983.)

waves that are small and equal in height and result in the typical M or W configurations (Fig. 45–20). Both the right and left ventricular diastolic pressures show an early diastolic dip followed by a plateau. This sign may be obscured by the presence of tachycardia, although the equilibration of diastolic pressures persists during exercise (Fig. 45–21), and by the damping effect of connecting tubes or bubbles within the catheters and transducers. Right ventricular and pulmonary artery systolic pressures are usually modestly elevated, in the range of 35 to 40 mm Hg, and rarely exceed 60 mm Hg. When hemodynamics in the baseline state are unremarkable, the rapid infusion of about 1000 ml of warmed saline over 6 to 8 minutes may unmask these findings in the rare patient with occult constrictive pericarditis.[208]

Careful recordings during respiration show that mean right atrial pressure fails to decrease normally or actually rises during inspiration. Since inspiration is associated with transient pooling of blood within the pulmonary bed and reduction in right ventricular afterload, inspiration causes a fall in pulmonary artery and right ventricular systolic pressures, pulmonary capillary wedge pressure, and left ventricular diastolic pressure. Because constrictive pericarditis is not associated with marked inspiratory swings in right ventricular filling, pulsus paradoxus is usually absent or less prominent than that observed in cardiac tamponade. Both cardiac output and stroke volume are low-normal or depressed. When they are depressed, compensatory tachycardia and elevation of systemic vascular resistance may be found.

The left ventricular angiogram usually demonstrates that left ventricular end-systolic and end-diastolic volumes are normal or decreased. In the absence of myocardial fibrosis or inflammation, both isovolumic and ejection phase indices of systolic function are normal.[159,209] Venous angiography may demonstrate dilatation of the superior vena cava and straightening of the right heart border; pericardial thickening may be detectable. These findings contrast with those of cardiac tamponade in which diastolic compression of the superior vena cava and right atrium is present. Coronary angiography may demonstrate that the coronary arteries are within the cardiac silhouette rather than on the surface of the heart, and rarely, diastolic pinching or external compression of the coronary arteries may be detected.[210] In rare patients, careful hemodynamic measurements may demonstrate the presence of regional pericardial constriction causing pulmonary outflow tract obstruction, which can be confirmed by right ventricular angiography.[154,155,211]

HEMODYNAMIC DIFFERENTIATION AMONG CONSTRICTIVE PERICARDITIS, CARDIAC TAMPONADE, AND RESTRICTIVE CARDIOMYOPATHY

Although both constrictive pericarditis and tamponade are characterized by elevation and equilibrium of right and left ventricular diastolic pressures, several hemodynamic features differ. In contrast to patients with constrictive pericarditis, patients with cardiac tamponade demonstrate (1) marked pulsus paradoxus, (2) a fall in right atrial pressure during inspiration, (3) elevation of intrapericardial pressure, (4) a right atrial pressure tracing with a predominant x descent and absence of or an attenuated y descent, and (5) lack of a prominent dip-and-plateau pattern in the right and left ventricular pressure pulses.

The findings of cardiac catheterization help to differentiate some but not all patients with constrictive pericarditis from those with restrictive cardiomyopathy (Table 45–7) due to amyloidosis, radiation injury, hemochromatosis, or other causes. In both conditions, right and left ventricular diastolic pressures are elevated, stroke volume and cardiac output are depressed, left ventricular end-diastolic volume is normal or decreased, and diastolic filling is impaired. A diagnosis of restrictive cardiomyopathy is more likely when marked right ventricular systolic hypertension is present (pressure > 60 mm Hg), and left ventricular diastolic pressure exceeds right ventricular diastolic pressure at rest or during exercise by more than 5 mm Hg.[212] However, in some patients with restrictive cardiomyopathy, hemodynamics at rest and during exercise may be indistinguishable from constrictive pericarditis, with equilibration of right and left ventricular diastolic

TABLE 45–7 CONSTRICTIVE PERICARDITIS VERSUS RESTRICTIVE CARDIOMYOPATHY

	CONSTRICTIVE PERICARDITIS	RESTRICTIVE CARDIOMYOPATHY
S₃ gallop	Absent	May be present
Pericardial knock	May be present	Absent
Palpable systolic apical impulse	Absent	May be present
Pericardial calcification	Present 50%	Absent
Pulsus paradoxus	May be present	May be present
Equal RV and LV diastolic pressures	Usually present	LV > RV
Rate of LV filling	80% in first half of diastole	40% in first half of diastole
PEP/LVET	Av. 0.31	Av. 0.48 (congestive failure)
CAT scan, echo, MRI	Thickened pericardium	Normal pericardium

Modified from Fowler, N. O.: Constrictive pericarditis. *In* Fowler, N. O. (ed.): The Pericardium in Health and Disease. Mt. Kisco, NY, Futura Publishing Co., 1985, p. 319.

pressures and a predominant dip-and-plateau pattern in the ventricular waveforms.[145,213–215]

Angiographically, straightening of the right heart border may be present in both conditions, and thickening of the heart border may be detected as a result of either pericardial or myocardial thickening.[216] The finding of a depressed left ventricular ejection fraction in the presence of a small heart has been suggested as a discriminating feature of restrictive cardiomyopathy.[216] However, the left ventricular ejection fraction may be normal in some patients with restrictive cardiomyopathy and, conversely, is occasionally reduced in patients with constrictive pericarditis.[213,214]

Frame-by-frame analysis of left ventricular filling using left ventricular angiograms has been suggested as a method for distinguishing between constrictive pericarditis and restrictive cardiomyopathy.[217] In constrictive pericarditis, early dia-

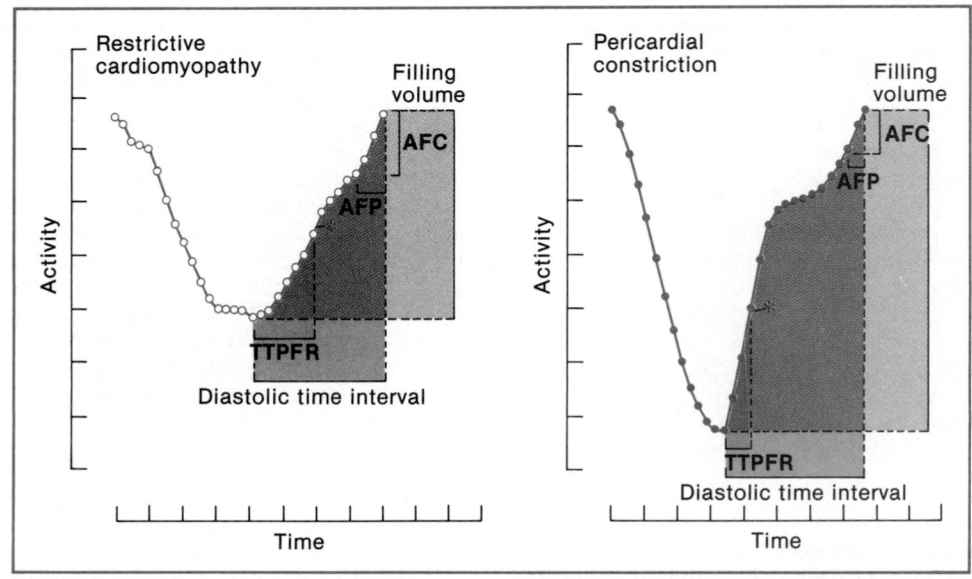

FIGURE 45–22. Time-activity curves obtained using first-pass radionuclide angiography in a patient with restrictive cardiomyopathy *(left panel)* and a patient with constrictive pericarditis *(right panel).* The curve for the patient with constrictive pericarditis is characterized by an increased peak filling rate and an increased extent of ventricular filling, which occurs in early diastole, in contrast with the curve for the patient with restrictive cardiomyopathy that shows a "sluggish" pattern of diastolic filling with slower peak filling rate, a longer time to peak filling rate, and an enhanced atrial contribution to total left ventricular filling volume. * = peak filling rate; AFC = atrial filling contribution; TTPFR = time to peak filling rate. (From Aroney, C. N., et al.: Differentiation of restrictive cardiomyopathy from pericardial constriction: Assessment of diastolic function by radionuclide angiography. J. Am. Coll. Cardiol. *13*:1007, 1989.)

stolic filling tends to be excessively rapid in contrast to restrictive cardiomyopathy, in which early diastolic filling is slower than normal with greater dependence on the atrial contribution to filling. The discrimination between these patterns of left ventricular filling in constrictive pericarditis versus restrictive cardiomyopathy has also been accomplished using noninvasive methods, including the assessment of diastolic filling by radionuclide angiography[218] (Fig. 45–22), digitized M-mode echocardiography,[219] and Doppler echocardiography.[220,221] The use of transthoracic Doppler echocardiography for the analysis of respiratory changes in transvalvular flow velocities[221] and the use of transesophageal Doppler echocardiography to analyze patterns of pulmonary venous flow velocity during respiration[222] have been proposed to distinguish between these conditions. However, the predictive value of these approaches has not yet been established prospectively. Nor has the value of the assessment of filling patterns been clarified in the troublesome patient with suspected restrictive cardiomyopathy who has a dip-and-plateau ventricular waveform that simulates constrictive physiology and itself suggests a pattern of rapid and abruptly attenuated diastolic filling.

ENDOMYOCARDIAL BIOPSY. This technique is very useful in documenting the presence of specific causes of restrictive physiology such as amyloidosis or myocarditis in patients in whom constrictive pericarditis and restrictive cardiomyopathy cannot be differentiated at cardiac catheterization.[213,223] However, normal biopsy findings do not exclude the presence of restrictive cardiomyopathy.[214] Furthermore, pericardial involvement may coexist with several causes of restrictive physiology, including amyloid heart disease, radiation-induced myopathy, and hypereosinophilic syndrome.[169,203–205,224,225] In a minority of patients, exploratory thoracotomy with careful examination of both pericardial and myocardial biopsy specimens is warranted. These examinations will differentiate constrictive pericarditis, a condition that is usually treatable surgically, from restrictive cardiomyopathy, in which treatment is usually expectant.

MANAGEMENT OF CONSTRICTIVE PERICARDITIS

Chronic constrictive pericarditis is a progressive disease without spontaneous reversal of either pericardial thickening or abnormal symptoms and hemodynamics. A minority of patients may survive for many years with modest jugular venous distention and peripheral edema that is controlled by the judicious use of diet and diuretics. The majority of patients who are symptomatic and come to medical attention, however, become progressively more disabled by weakness, ascites, and peripheral edema and subsequently suffer the complications of severe cardiac cachexia. Treatment for constrictive pericarditis is complete resection of the pericardium (p. 1482), which achieves excision of the pericardium from the anterior and inferior surfaces of the right ventricle and the diaphragmatic and anterolateral surfaces of the left ventricle extending to the great vessels and to or across the atrioventricular grooves. Attention must also be paid to the presence of right atrial thrombosis in association with constrictive pericarditis, which should be managed with thrombectomy at the time of pericardiectomy.[226] Changes in technique have included the use of median sternotomy rather than left thoracotomy, cardiopulmonary bypass to permit greater mobilization of the heart,[227] and performance of pericardiectomy earlier in the course of the disease prior to the appearance of cardiac cachexia and dense pericardial calcification. Ultrasonic debridement using an ultrasonic surgical aspiration device has been reported to be a useful adjunct to the complete surgical removal of densely calcified and adherent pericardium.[228]

RESULTS OF PERICARDIECTOMY. In 1980, Culliford et al. reported an operative mortality of 15 per cent with a range of 6 to 25 per cent in over 300 reported cases of pericardiectomy.[229] In over 700 cases reported in 11 series since 1981, the average operative mortality was 11 per cent and ranged from 7 to 19 per cent.[149,230–235] A low-output syndrome occurs in 14 to

28 per cent of patients in the immediate postoperative period, and risk factors predictive of in-hospital mortality and low-output syndrome include the degree of preoperative disability (functional Class III or IV) and severity of constriction as indicated by marked elevation of right ventricular end-diastolic pressure.[230,233] Among patients who survive the operation, symptomatic improvement can be expected in about 90 per cent and complete relief of symptoms in about 50 per cent of patients.[230,231,233–236] Careful actuarial analysis of long-term survival has been available in large series from the Mayo Clinic[230] and Stanford,[233] which have reported a 5-year survival of 84 and 74 per cent, respectively. Long-term survival and symptomatic relief do not appear to be influenced by age, choice of median sternotomy or left thoracotomy, or transient low-output syndrome postoperatively. However, overall outcome is unfavorably influenced by the presence of severe preoperative functional disability (NYHA Class III or IV, diuretic use), renal insufficiency in the preoperative state, the presence of extensive nonresectable calcifications, incomplete pericardial resection, and the presence of radiation pericarditis, which is commonly complicated by myocardial fibrosis and restrictive myocardial disease. These considerations indicate that pericardiectomy should be performed early in the course of constrictive pericarditis in symptomatic patients, since the development of severe clinical disability is associated with a poor surgical outcome.

Pericardiectomy should probably not be routinely attempted in very elderly patients with severe liver dysfunction, cachexia, densely calcified pericardium, and massive cardiac enlargement indicative of underlying myocardial damage or in patients with limited life expectancy. Patients with known or suspected tubercular pericarditis should be treated with multidrug antituberculosis therapy for 2 to 4 weeks before operation; if the diagnosis is confirmed, these drugs should be continued for 6 to 12 months after pericardiectomy.

Striking hemodynamic and symptomatic improvement is apparent in some patients immediately after operation. In others, symptomatic improvement and resolution of elevated jugular venous pressure and abnormal filling patterns may be delayed for weeks to months.[237] This delayed or inadequate response to pericardiectomy has been attributed to incomplete pericardial resection, myocardial damage by the inflammatory process,[230,233] and the development of recurrent cardiac compression by mediastinal inflammation and fibrosis.[238,239] The role of unrecognized constriction by an epicardial peel (visceral pericardium) as a cause for a poor response to pericardiectomy was described by Harrington in 1944[240] and subsequently confirmed.[241] The importance of visceral constriction has also been underscored by the Stanford experience in which 59 per cent of cases had involvement of the visceral pericardium (epicardium) and required visceral decortication.[233] When there is little change in size of the heart or fall in intracardiac pressures after removal of the parietal pericardial layer, consideration should be given to epicardial dissection.

EFFUSIVE-CONSTRICTIVE PERICARDITIS

Effusive-constrictive pericarditis is the condition of a tense pericardial effusion in the presence of visceral pricardial constriction.[242,243] *The hallmark of this condition is continued elevation of right atrial pressure after the aspiration of pericardial fluid and restoration of intrapericardial pressure to zero.* This entity may represent a stage in the development of classic constrictive pericarditis. The most common causes of effusive-constrictive pericarditis are the same as for chronic constrictive pericarditis (p. 1483) and include idiopathic or presumed viral pericarditis, tuberculosis, neoplastic infiltration of the pericardium, and mediastinal irradiation.[243] Symptoms are nonspecific and include atypical chest pain and a heavy sensation over the precordium; in advanced cases, exertional dyspnea may be present.

The physical findings usually resemble those of cardiac tamponade, including pulsus paradoxus, normal or diminished pulse pressure, and jugular venous distention with a predominant x descent and absence of y descent. The chest roentgenogram usually shows cardiac enlargement consistent with the presence of pericardial effusion, and the electrocardiogram may show nonspecific ST- and T-wave abnormalities or diffuse low QRS voltage. Both M-mode and two-dimensional echocardiograms may show a pericardial effusion sandwiched between thickened pericardial membranes with fibrinous pericardial bands.[244]

Although effusive-constrictive pericarditis can be suspected on clinical grounds, the diagnosis is made by recording right heart and intrapericardial pressures both before and after pericardiocentesis.[243] Before pericardiocentesis, the physiology of cardiac tamponade may be present (p. 1473) with elevation and equilibration of intrapericardial, right atrial, right ventricular, and left ventricular diastolic pressures. The right atrial pressure tracing usually shows a prominent x descent and an inspiratory fall in right heart filling pressure. Pericardiocentesis with restoration of intrapericardial pressure to zero may reduce pulsus paradoxus and improve cardiac output, but it does not restore the hemodynamics entirely to normal. After pericardiocentesis, there is persistent elevation and equilibration of right atrial and right and left ventricular diastolic pressures. The waveforms convert to a pattern like that in constrictive pericarditis, with a prominent y descent in the right atrial pressure tracing, a dip-and-plateau pattern in the right ventricular pressure, and the absence of respiratory variation in right heart filling pressures.

Pericardiocentesis may be useful in transiently improving systemic arterial pressure and cardiac output. However, persistent constriction after successful pericardiocentesis indicates the presence of a thickened, constrictive visceral pericardium and the need for further intervention. Treatment consists of total parietal and visceral pericardiectomy.[233,241,243]

Specific Forms of Pericarditis

VIRAL PERICARDITIS

ETIOLOGY AND PATHOGENESIS. The viruses that most commonly cause acute pericarditis are coxsackievirus group B and echovirus type 8.[245,246] There are no clinical features that distinguish acute viral pericarditis from idiopathic pericarditis, and it is likely that the majority of cases of community-acquired idiopathic pericarditis are due to unrecognized viral infections. The seasonal peak incidence of idiopathic pericarditis is in the spring and fall, which coincides with the increased incidence of enterovirus epidemics. Other viruses responsible for acute pericarditis include those that cause mumps, influenza, infectious mononucleosis, poliomyelitis, varicella, rubella, and hepatitis B.[247-251] Infectious mononucleosis may cause acute myopericarditis with the complications of cardiac tamponade, constrictive pericarditis, and severe chest pain, and this etiology can be confirmed by a positive heterophile test.[248] Varicella (chickenpox) may be associated with the complications of severe viral pneumonia, arthritis, and/or acute pericarditis.[249] *Coxiella burnetii*, the rickettsial agent that causes tick-borne Q fever (fever, headache, pneumonitis), is also a cause of pericarditis in endemic areas.[252,253] Rarely, *Mycoplasma pneumoniae*, an important cause of adult nonbacterial pneumonia, causes myopericarditis.[254,255]

Acute pericarditis is now being recognized with increasing frequency in the early stage of acquired immunodeficiency syndrome (AIDS) and may be idiopathic or related to specific viral pathogens.[255-258] Cytomegalovirus may cause pericarditis in otherwise healthy adults with cytomegalovirus mononucleosis[259,260] and in immunocompromised patients,[261] as has been reported in association with AIDS.[262-264] Cytomegalovirus pericarditis has been documented by serial antibody titers and by the demonstration of typical CMV inclusions and dot-blot hybridization with CMV-specific DNA fragments in pericardial biopsy specimens.[260,261] Herpes simplex pericarditis has also been reported in patients with AIDS.[265]

PATHOLOGY. Viral pericarditis causes inflammation of the visceral and parietal pericardial membranes, with infiltration first of polymorphonuclear leukocytes and then of lymphocytes around small vessels. Fibrin is deposited in the pericardial space, giving the pericadium a shaggy, reddened appearance. In some cases the inflammation may result in a serous, serofibrinous, suppurative, or hemorrhagic effusion with a predominance of lymphocytes. Both echoviruses and coxsackieviruses may produce suppurative effusions that resolve by organization, formation of thick adhesions, calcification, and thickening of the pericardium, resulting in constrictive pericarditis.[266]

CLINICAL FINDINGS. A prodromal syndrome of an upper respiratory tract infection that may be described as a "cold" or "the flu" within the preceding weeks is frequently reported by patients with viral pericarditis. The clinical features of viral pericarditis are similar to those of acute pericarditis of many causes, which were described earlier (p. 1469). Viral or idiopathic pericarditis should be suspected in young or otherwise healthy adults with a characteristic prodromal illness and a syndrome of acute pericardial pain. It must be differentiated from pericarditis due to trauma, purulent pericardial infection, myocarditis, and systemic lupus erythematosus. In older patients, the possibility that pericarditis may be due to rheumatoid disorders, myocardial infarction, tuberculosis, or neoplasm should be investigated before one presumes a viral etiology.

The diagnosis of viral infection is strongly supported by the finding of a greater than fourfold rise in serial neutralizing viral antibody titers during the initial 3 weeks of illness. It is rarely productive to attempt to isolate virus from blood, pericardial fluid, pleural fluid, or stool. The development of reverse immunoassays (RIA) of antibodies to enteroviruses holds promise for studies of the role of these viruses in acute pericarditis. Frisk et al. evaluated the incidence of positive coxsackie B-specific IgM RIA titers that were detected in 97 per cent of 30 patients with proven enterovirus infections and in 49 per cent of 37 patients with idopathic myopericarditis, while positive responses were rare in control specimens from normal subjects.[267] A similar incidence (44 per cent) of acute group B coxsackie viral infection has been reported in a cohort of 95 patients with acute myopericarditis.[268] It is of interest that enterovirus-specific IgM and IgA titers indicative of persistent enterovirus infection have been shown in a series of patients with chronic relapsing pericarditis in whom the persistence of chronically high levels of antibody differed from a cohort of patients with a single episode of acute pericarditis.[269]

The diagnosis of acute pericarditis of probable viral etiology is confirmed clinically by the finding of a characteristic pericardial friction rub. Serial electrocardiographic changes of acute pericarditis (p. 1470) are not specific for the etiology of either viral or idiopathic pericarditis; however, the appearance of characteristic electrocardiographic changes may lead to the recognition of pericardial involvement in patients with a viral upper respiratory tract infection. Echocardiographic documentation of substantial pericardial effusion is also supportive evidence of pericardial inflammation in a patient with a viral upper respiratory tract infection and chest pain. Other laboratory findings suggestive of inflammation but not diagnostic of pericarditis include elevation of the sedimentation rate and leukocytosis. Cardiac isoenzymes are frequently abnormally elevated and suggest the presence of extensive associated epicarditis or myocarditis.[60]

NATURAL HISTORY. Acute viral or idiopathic pericarditis is usually a short, dramatic, self-limited illness lasting 1 to 3 weeks. Important complications of acute viral or idiopathic pericarditis include (1) associated myocarditis, (2) recurrent pericarditis, (3) pericardial effusion with cardiac tamponade, and (4) the late development of constrictive pericarditis (p. 1482). Acute myocarditis, which may develop in association with pericarditis due to coxsackieviruses and echoviruses, may result in acute congestive heart failure, arrhythmias, or conduction disturbances, and cardiac enlargement that usually resolves completely or rarely leads to the development of a chronic congestive cardiomyopathy. Pericarditis may recur several weeks later in about 20 to 30 per cent of patients, and a small number of patients develop disabling recurrences over months to years that are extremely difficult to manage. It is unclear whether recurrences of pericardial pain in patients with enterovirus pericarditis are due to an immunological response to the initial viral injury,[267,268] recurrent viral infections of the pericardium,[270] or relapsing chronic viral infection.[269]

MANAGEMENT. Treatment is directed against symptoms, with close observation for the development of cardiac tamponade or myocarditis early in the course of the disease. The management of patients with acute viral pericarditis was already discussed in detail (p. 1471).

TUBERCULOUS PERICARDITIS

ETIOLOGY AND PATHOGENESIS. In industrialized nations, the incidence of tuberculous pericarditis has decreased within the past three decades as a result of effective chemotherapy and public health surveillance. In this setting, it is now a very uncommon cause of acute pericarditis except in patients with AIDS. In a series of 231 consecutive patients whose disease was evaluated prospectively using a rigorous protocol that included pericardiocentesis and biopsy, tuberculosis was diagnosed in only 4 per cent of patients and in 7 per cent of the subset of patients who developed cardiac tamponade.[62] Similarly, tuberculous pericarditis was reported in none of 145 patients who required pericardial drainage[150] and in only 6 per cent of 231 patients who underwent pericardiectomy for chronic constriction[230] at the Mayo Clinic. The incidence of tuberculous pericarditis among patients with pulmonary tuberculosis ranges from about 1 to 8 per cent.[271] The disease continues to be important in immunosuppressed patients[272] and in patients with AIDS.[273-275] Pericarditis can also be caused by atypical mycobacteria in association with AIDS.[264] It is also a major cause of pericarditis among the underprivileged, including South and West African blacks, the black poor of the United States, and Asian and African immigrants.[276-278] For example, in Transkei, South Africa, tuberculous pericarditis with secondary constriction is the second most common cause of "heart failure" after rheumatic heart disease.[277]

Tuberculous pericarditis usually develops by retrograde spread from peribronchial, peritracheal, or mediastinal lymph nodes or by early hematogenous spread from the primary tuberculous infection. Less commonly, the pericardium is involved by the breakdown and contiguous spread of a necrotic tuberculous lesion in the lung, pleura, or spine or by hematogenous spread from distant secondary genitourinary or skeletal infections.[279,280]

PATHOLOGY. Tuberculous pericarditis usually begins with diffuse fibrin deposits, granuloma formation, and the presence of viable acid-fast bacilli.[279] A pericardial effusion then develops, which may be serious but more often contains some blood with a protein content exceeding 2.5 gm/dl. Although polymorphonuclear leukocytes are present early in the development of the effusion, they are later replaced by lymphocytes, monocytes, and plasma cells. Both complement-fixing antimyolemmal and antimyosin types of antibodies have been demonstrated in about 75 per cent of patients with acute tuberculous pericarditis, in contrast to the much lower incidence in patients with viral pericarditis or constrictive pericarditis due to tuberculosis, which suggests that cytolysis mediated by antimyolemmal antibodies may contribute to the development of exudative tuberculous pericarditis.[281] When a tuberculous pericardial effusion accumulates rapidly, even a small effusion may produce cardiac tamponade. As the effusion is absorbed, the pericardium thickens, granulomas proliferate, and a thick coat of fibrin is deposited on the parietal pericardium. At this stage, viable acid-fast bacilli may no longer be present, but caseation may develop and penetrate the myocardium. Finally, fibrous pericarditis develops as the granulomatous reaction is replaced by fibrous tissue and collagen. These changes are followed by the accumulation of cholesterol crystals and the development of pericardial calcification. Constrictive pericarditis develops ultimately in almost all patients with untreated tuberculous pericarditis and in about half or less of the patients who receive antituberculosis chemotherapy.[282-284]

CLINICAL MANIFESTATIONS. Tuberculous pericarditis is usually detected clinically either in the effusive stage or late, i.e., after the development of constrictive pericarditis. It usually develops slowly, with nonspecific systemic symptoms such as fever, night sweats, fatigue, and dyspnea.[277,282,283] In South Africa, right upper abdominal aching due to liver congestion is common in patients with effusive tuberculous pericarditis.[277,282] A torpid course is not invariably present, and an acute illness of less than 2 weeks' duration was described in four to nine patients in whom tuberculous pericarditis was diagnosed during a prospective evaluation of acute pericarditis.[62] Severe pericardial pain of acute onset characteristic of viral and idiopathic pericarditis is uncommon in tuberculous pericarditis.[277,283-286] Heavy sputum production, cough, and hemoptysis—clues to the presence of cavitary pulmonary tuberculosis—are usually absent.

Abnormalities of *physical examination* usually include fever, sinus tachycardia, and pericardial friction rub. In South African patients with tuberculous pericardial effusion, evidence of chronic cardiac compression that mimics heart failure is by far the most common presentation. In one series of 88 patients with effusive tuberculous pericarditis, jugular venous distention was present in 88 per cent, hepatomegaly in 95 per cent, and ascites in 73 per cent, while a pericardial friction rub was heard in only 18 per cent.[277] If the complications of cardiac tamponade or effusive-constrictive pericarditis are present, the physical examination may reveal edema, jugular venous distention, pulsus paradoxus, distant heart sounds, hepatomegaly, and ascites. The chest roentgenogram usually shows an enlarged cardiac silhouette, and pleural effusions may be detected in about half the patients. However, the apices and hila of the lung are usually normal, and pulmonary infiltrates or calcification is present in a minority of the patients.

The clinical presentation of patients with tuberculous pericarditis who develop chronic constrictive pericarditis differs from those with acute or subacute effusive tuberculous pericarditis. Dramatic symptoms such as high fever, night sweats, and precordial pain are uncommon. Findings compatible with severe chronic systemic venous congestion with low output predominate, including jugular venous distention, hypotension with a low pulse pressure, abdominal distention, edema, and muscle wasting. Dyspnea related to large pleural effusions is common.[277,282,287]

During the transition from effusion to constrictive pericarditis, dense, frond-like echoes or transient masses may be appreciated in the pericardial space.[288] Gallium-67 uptake in the pericardium is a nonspecific indicator of pericardial inflammation and can occur in tuberculous, purulent, and acute nonspecific pericarditis.[289]

DIAGNOSIS. Tuberculous pericarditis should be suspected in patients with fever and unexplained cardiomegaly, particularly those who are susceptible to tuberculosis, i.e., the underprivileged or immunosuppressed. It is noteworthy that tuberculous pericarditis may develop during chemotherapy for pulmonary tuberculosis.[290] In a minority of patients with pericarditis, a definitive diagnosis of a tuberculous origin may be made by culture or histological demonstration of tuberculosis outside the pericardium (sputum, gastric wash, pleural fluid, liver or bone marrow biopsy). A definitive diagnosis can be made by isolation of the bacillus from the pericardial fluid or pericardial biopsy. It is difficult to establish a definitive bacteriological diagnosis because of the low yield of the bacillus when pericardial fluid is examined by acid-fast stain on microscopy; the failure of the bacillus to grow on appropriate media or in guinea pigs, even in patients with known tuberculous pericardial effusion; and the need to observe bacterial cultures for at least 8 weeks. The probability of obtaining a definitive diagnosis is greatest if both pericardial fluid and a pericardial biopsy specimen are examined early in the effusive stage.[286,291] However, it must be emphasized that a normal pericardial biopsy result does not exclude tuberculous pericarditis, since in some patients examination of the entire pericardium removed at pericardiectomy or autopsy is required to demonstrate clear-cut evidence of tuberculosis.[286,292] Furthermore, the finding of granulomas and caseous material without viable bacilli is also not diagnostic of tuberculous pericarditis, since these findings can be present in chronic pericardial disease due to rheumatoid arthritis and sarcoidosis. The measurement of a high level of adenosine deaminase activity (>45 units/liter) in pleural or pericardial fluid, although not diagnostic, is supportive of a diagnosis of tuberculous pericarditis.[286,293,294]

It may be necessary to make a presumptive clinical diagnosis of tuberculous pericarditis in severely ill patients with a large hemorrhagic pericardial effusion, a positive tuberculin skin test, and systemic symptoms such as weight loss and anorexia, even when examinations of the pericardial fluid and biopsy do not reveal tuberculosis. In such patients, clinical improvement may occur after initiation of antituberculosis chemotherapy. It should be emphasized that the tuberculin skin test alone is not a reliable indicator of tuberculous pericarditis, since it may be negative in as many as 30 per cent of patients with documented tuberculosis due to anergy, and is positive in about 30 to 40 per cent of patients with acute idiopathic pericarditis and benign natural history.[62,168] Making a presumptive clinical diagnosis of tuberculous pericarditis requires careful judgment, since, on the one hand, treatment should not be withheld from seriously ill patients, while, on the other, it is not prudent to commit patients with nontuberculous effusions to a prolonged course of multiple-drug antituberculosis therapy. The systematic approach suggested by Permanyer-Miralda et al. (p. 1471) appears to have a high likelihood of identifying patients with tuberculous pericarditis with a very low risk of either missing active tuberculosis or inappropriately applying blind antituberculous therapy.[62] This strategy remains to be validated in other populations.

MANAGEMENT. In the era before antituberculosis chemotherapy, tuberculous pericarditis was rapidly fatal, with an early mortality rate greater than 80 per cent; the remaining patients had a protracted course of months to years with frequently fatal outcome due to miliary tuberculosis or constrictive pericarditis. Since the introduction of early chemotherapy, mortality from acute tuberculous pericarditis has fallen to less than 50 per cent, but the effectiveness of antituberculosis chemotherapy in preventing the development of constrictive pericarditis is controversial.[276,282-285] In a recent series of 294 consecutive patients with acute pericarditis, 13 patients were shown to have tuberculous pericarditis and 7 (54 per cent) developed constrictive pericarditis requiring pericardiectomy.[286]

Treatment of tuberculous pericarditis includes hospitalization with bedrest and particular attention to findings of physical examination, electrocardiography, and echocardiography that suggest the development of an enlarging pericardial effusion and tamponade or constrictive pericarditis. Initial

chemotherapy should usually consist of a three-drug regimen, such as oral isoniazid, oral ethambutol, and intramuscular streptomycin. The use of corticosteroids has been advocated to reduce pericardial inflammation and enhance resorption of pericardial effusion.

In a controlled trial in South Africa, 143 patients with tuberculous pericarditis and clinical signs of constrictive physiology were randomized to receive antitubercular drug therapy with prednisolone or placebo added during the first 11 weeks of treatment.[295] In this trial, clinical improvement occurred more rapidly, and there was a lower mortality at 24 months (4 versus 11 per cent) and a lower requirement for pericardiectomy (21 versus 30 per cent) in the prednisolone versus placebo-treated cohort. The use of steroids earlier in the course of tuberculous pericarditis before the development of constrictive physiology has not been studied in a clinical trial. We believe that corticosteroids should be reserved for critically ill patients with recurrent large effusion who do not respond to antituberculosis drugs alone.

In patients with documented cardiac tamponade or with a large pericardial effusion seen on the echocardiogram, the effusion should be drained initially by percutaneous pericardiocentesis with continued catheter drainage. Pericardiectomy should be performed after 4 to 6 weeks of antituberculosis drug therapy if patients develop large recurrent effusions or cardiac compression due to effusive-constrictive disease or early constrictive pericarditis.[271,276,277,283,295] Pericardiectomy should be performed early in the course in patients with clinical and hemodynamic evidence of chronic cardiac compression with anticipation of a good outcome. In a South African study of 113 patients with severe constrictive tuberculous pericarditis, 97 per cent were discharged from the hospital; in the majority, hepatomegaly and edema promptly resolved, whereas resolution of venous congestion required 2 to 3 months in some patients.[287] Mortality is higher among patients who undergo pericardiectomy at the late stage of calcific pericardial constriction.[276,287]

BACTERIAL (PURULENT) PERICARDITIS

Although the clinical spectrum of bacterial purulent pericarditis has changed over the past four decades, mortality remains high. Since the introduction of antibiotics in the 1940's, the incidence of bacterial pericarditis detected at autopsy has decreased.[295,296] Before 1943, purulent pericarditis occurred primarily as a complication of pneumococcal pneumonia or empyema and uncontrolled pleuropulmonary disease due to staphylococci or streptococci. During the antibiotic era, there has been a decline in the incidence of pneumococcal and streptococcal pericarditis, although these organisms continue to cause purulent pericarditis.[297] Acute self-limited pericarditis has also been observed in young adults with acute streptococcal tonsillitis in the absence of rheumatic fever.[298] The incidence of hospital-acquired penicillin-resistant staphylococcal pericarditis in post-thoracotomy patients has increased, and there is a widened spectrum of organisms responsible for bacterial pericarditis, including non-group A streptococcus[299] the gram-negative bacilli (*Proteus, Escherichia coli, Pseudomonas, Klebsiella*),[296] *Brucella melitensis,*[300] *Salmonella* species,[301,302] *Neisseria gonorrhoeae,*[303] *Hemophilus influenzae,*[304] *Francisella tularensis,*[305] anaerobic organisms,[306,307] and other unusual pathogens.[308-310] It is now established that *Neisseria meningitidis*, particularly from serogroup C and W, can cause either a primary infection of the pericardium in the absence of meningitis, or secondary pericarditis complicating meningitis and sepsis.[311-313] *Legionella pneumophila*, the causative organism in legionnaire's disease, has been reported as a cause of purulent pericarditis associated with pneumonia and as a primary infection.[314,315] Important predisposing factors for the development of purulent pericarditis include a preexisting pericardial effusion as in uremic pericarditis, as well as immunosuppression due to burns, immunotherapy, lymphoma, leukemia, or AIDS.

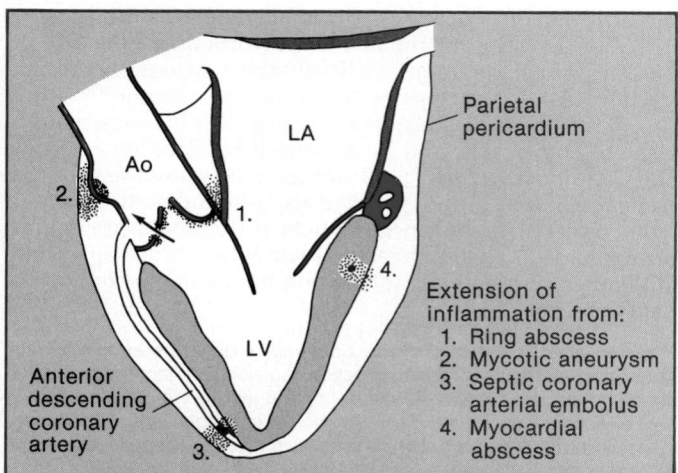

FIGURE 45–23. The pathogenesis of pericarditis in infective endocarditis. Ao = aorta; LV = left ventricle; LA = left atrium. (From Roberts, W. C., and Spray, T. L.: Pericardial heart disease: A study of its causes, consequences, and morphologic features. *In* Spodick, D. H. (ed.): Pericardial Diseases. Philadelphia, F. A. Davis Co., 1976, p. 31.)

The routes of pericardial infection have also changed. Direct pulmonary extension of bacterial pneumonia or empyema now accounts for only about 20 per cent of cases of purulent pericarditis.[307] Today, purulent pericarditis tends to occur in adults via (1) contiguous spread from an early postoperative infection after thoracic surgery or trauma, (2) infection related to infective endocarditis, (3) extension from a subdiaphragmatic suppurative source, and (4) hematogenous spread during bacteremia. In patients with endocarditis, bacterial pericarditis is a life-threatening complication that is detected ante mortem in about 1 of 25 patients with endocarditis,[316] in about 1 of 8 patients with endocarditis studied at autopsy, and in a higher percentage of those with staphylococcal endocarditis.[296] In such patients, bacterial pericarditis may develop (1) by extension from a valve ring abscess, (2) by rupture of an aneurysm, (3) by extension from a myocardial abscess, or (4) from a septic coronary embolus[317,318] (Fig. 45–23). An infected myocardial infarction or aortic aneurysm may also be a source for the development of purulent bacterial pericarditis.[319] Extension of a subdiaphragmatic abscess into the pericardial space is a rare source of purulent pericarditis.[320]

BACTERIAL PERICARDITIS IN CHILDREN. In children, the most common organisms include *Staphylococcus aureus* followed by *Hemophilus influenzae* and *Neisseria meningitis*.[321,322] *Hemophilus influenzae* pericarditis has been increasingly recognized in young children and is usually characterized by a mild prodromal illness followed by the rapid development of cardiac compression and death due to pericardial effusion.[323] Pediatric illnesses associated with the development of bacterial pericarditis include pharyngitis, pneumonia, meningitis, otitis media, impetigo, endocarditis, and bacterial arthritis.[321] The development of bacterial pericarditis in infants and children carries a high mortality—approaching 70 per cent, depending on the organism, and the risk of extremely rapid early development of constrictive pericarditis.[321,324] The high mortality in children appears to be reduced by early diagnosis and combined treatment with parenteral antibiotics and open surgical pericardial drainage, if effusion recurs after initial pericardiocentesis.[321,324] Following this contemporary approach of parenteral antibiotics and early drainage of purulent fluid, a series of purulent pericarditis in children reported a mortality of 18 per cent.[322]

PATHOLOGY. Bacterial pericarditis is usually frankly suppurative by the time it is detected clinically. The inflammation may result in organization and dense adhesions with a loculated pericardial effusion followed by obliteration of the pericardial space, thickening, and eventual calcification of the pericardium. In some patients, the inflammation may involve the adjacent sternum, pleura, and diaphragm with formation of dense adhesions between the parietal pericardium and contiguous structures. The evolution of this inflammatory process has been studied in an animal model of pericarditis caused by the injection of heat-killed staphylococci into the pericardial space.[325]

CLINICAL FEATURES. Bacterial pericarditis is usually an acute fulminant illness of only a few days' duration. In one series,[307] the mean duration of symptoms prior to hospitalization was only 3 days. High fevers, shaking chills, night sweats, and dyspnea are common. In most patients the symptom of typical pericardial chest pain is absent. Tachycardia is present in nearly all patients, but a pericardial friction rub is present in less than half. In many cases the pericarditis remains unsuspected because of the dominant presence of symptoms and signs related to an underlying known infection, such as pneumonia or mediastinitis following complicated thoracic surgery or trauma. The appearance of new jugular venous distention and pulsus paradoxus may be the first evidence of pericardial involvement, and these ominous signs reflect the development of cardiac tamponade due to the acute accumulation of suppurative fluid under pressure. In one series, cardiac tamponade developed acutely in 38 per cent of patients with previously unsuspected purulent pericarditis and contributed to death in the majority.[307]

Laboratory Findings. These usually include a leukocytosis with a marked leftward shift. The chest roentgenogram usually shows enlargement of the cardiac shadow and, less commonly, widening of the mediastinum. In the majority of cases the roentgenogram shows evidence of underlying pneumonia, empyema, or mediastinitis. Electrocardiographic changes typically include ST-segment and T-wave changes characteristic of pericarditis in the majority of patients.[307] The appearance of electrical alternans suggests the possibility of cardiac tamponade. In patients with suspected infective endocarditis, the appearance of a prolonged P-R interval, atrioventricular dissociation, or bundle branch block is strong evidence of extension of infection from the valve ring into the adjacent myocardium. The latter is an important predisposing factor for the development of pericarditis, especially in patients with staphylococcal endocarditis.[307]

Pericardial Fluid. This usually shows polymorphonuclear leukocytosis and sometimes frank pus. Pericardial glucose levels are usually depressed, and the protein content is increased; lactate dehydrogenase values may also be markedly elevated.

Purulent bacterial pericarditis should be suspected in a debilitated patient with unexplained high spiking fevers, dyspnea, markedly elevated white blood cell count, and an increase in the size of the cardiac silhouette on chest roentgenogram. The key to the diagnosis, which unfortunately is frequently not made before death, is a high index of suspicion. An echocardiogram should be promptly obtained to look for evidence of a new pericardial effusion and/or loculation of fluid with adhesions.

Natural History. Despite the lower incidence of purulent bacterial pericarditis in the antibiotic era, overall survival continues to be extremely poor, averaging about 30 per cent in modern series.[307,326] The poor prognosis stems in large part from failure of clinical diagnosis before death. In patients treated only with antibiotics without pericardial drainage, the rapid unsuspected development of a large pericardial effusion may result in sudden cardiovascular collapse and death due to cardiac tamponade. The high mortality from purulent pericarditis can be reduced substantially through the institution of both appropriate parenteral antibiotic therapy and early complete surgical drainage.[307,322,326] Early surgical drainage of the pericardium may help to prevent the complication of constrictive pericarditis. Successful treatment of bacterial endocarditis with long-term simple catheter drainage of the pericardial space has been reported, but experience with this approach is limited.[327]

Meningococcal Pericarditis. The pericardium may become infected early during meningococcal sepsis (in the presence or absence of meningitis), causing purulent pericarditis with cardiac tamponade, as described earlier. In these cases the pericardial fluid is frankly purulent, and viable organisms can usually be isolated. In addition, sterile pericarditis may occur late in the convalescent period in association with arthritis, pleuritis, and ophthalmitis. This syndrome appears to have an immunological etiology, does not require further antibiotic therapy if the primary infection has been adequately treated, and responds to antiinflammatory agents. Febrile, self-limited polyserositis with pericarditis has also been reported after effective treatment of sepsis due to *Staphylococcus aureus*,[328] and in young adults with acute streptococcal tonsillitis in the absense of rheumatic fever.[298]

MANAGEMENT. Suspicion of the presence of purulent pericardial fluid is an indication to explore the pericardial space. This may be done by percutaneous pericardiocentesis only if there is echocardiographic evidence of a large anterior and posterior pericardial effusion that may be safely tapped or, preferably, by a generous subxiphoid pericardiotomy with thorough pericardial drainage. Both pericardial fluid and pericardial tissue should be immediately studied by means of Gram-stained, acid-fast, and fungal smears by an experienced examiner. The fluid should then be cultured for aerobic and anaerobic bacteria with appropriate antibiotic sensitivity testing and for fungi and tuberculosis. Pericardial fluid should also be examined; the number of white blood cells, the differential count, hematocrit, and glucose and protein content should be determined. Cultures of blood, sputum, and recent surgical wounds should also be obtained.

Results of Gram-staining of the pericardial fluid should be used in the selection of antibiotic therapy. If the effusion is purulent but no organisms can be easily identified and tuberculosis is not considered likely, therapy should be initiated with both a semisynthetic antistaphylococcal antibiotic and an aminoglycoside. Depending on the results of the cultures of the pericardial fluid and blood, antibiotic therapy may then be modifed. High concentrations of antibiotics can be achieved in pericardial fluid, so that instillation of antibiotics into the pericardial space is not warranted.[329] However, systemic antibiotics alone are inadequate treatment, and prompt and thorough surgical drainage of the pericardium is essential in almost all patients with bacterial pericarditis.[307,323] Percutaneous aspiration of a large effusion may be extremely helpful in making an initial bacteriological diagnosis and initiating therapy, and percutaneous aspiration followed by catheter drainage is sometimes effective in preventing recurrent effusion.[327,330] However, purulent pericardial effusions are likely to recur, and more extensive surgical drainage may be needed in some patients after antibiotic therapy has been initiated. Open drainage, through creation of a subxiphoid pericardiotomy, is usually adequate when the diagnosis is made early and when the pericardial fluid is thin and the pericardium minimally thickened. This procedure is also the preferred route of drainage in severely disabled patients, since it can be performed under local anesthesia and avoids the pleural cavities. In a patient with a thick purulent effusion and dense adhesions with loculation, extensive pericardiectomy is needed to achieve adequate drainage and to prevent development of constrictive pericarditis,[296,307,324,331] which can occur very early after presentation.[332]

FUNGAL PERICARDITIS

ETIOLOGY AND PATHOPHYSIOLOGY. Histoplasmosis is the most common cause of fungal pericarditis. This diagnosis should be considered in young and otherwise healthy patients suspected of having acute viral or tuberculous pericarditis who live in the Ohio or Mississippi River Valley or the Western Appalachians, where the fungus is endemic.[333] In these areas, histoplasmosis is acquired by inhalation of spores during small rural outbreaks from bird or bat droppings and during major urban outbreaks related to excavation and building demolition. Coccidioidomycosis pericarditis occurs in patients who have inhaled chlamydospores from soil or dust in areas of the American Southwest, particularly the San Joaquin Valley, and Argentina, where it is endemic.[334] Other fungal infections responsible for pericarditis incude aspergillosis, blastomycosis, and those caused by *Candida albicans* and *Candida tropicalis*.[335-338] Groups at increased risk for the development of fungal pericarditis consequent to disseminated infection include drug addicts, patients who are immunosuppressed or who have received potent broad-spectrum antibiotics, and patients recovering from complicated open-heart surgery.

Histoplasmosis pericarditis most commonly develops as a noninfectious inflammatory response to infection confined to adjacent mediastinal lymph nodes and rarely by direct or hematogenous infection in patients with disseminated infection.[333,339] The isolation of organisms from pericardial fluid is unusual, and its predilection for young immunocompetent males suggests that self-limited histoplasmois pericarditis usually represents a sterile immune reaction. Pericarditis due to fungi other than histoplasmosis may occur as a complication of open-heart surgery in adults and children as a result of spread from contiguous infected lymph nodes or pulmonary lesions or hematogenous dissemination in immunosuppressed patients with fungal sepsis.

PATHOLOGY. Pericardial fluid may accumulate extremely rapidly and to massive quantities in patients with histoplasmosis. The fluid can be serous or hemorrhagic with increased protein content and polymorphonuclear leukocytosis. In cases of fungal pericarditis due to agents other than *Histoplasma*, exudative pericardial effusions may accumulate more slowly, so that an effusion may be present for months. Histoplasmosis and other fungal pericardial effusions occasionally become organized, with pericardial thickening, the appearance of granulomas and multinucleated giant cells, and the development of a constricting, calcified pericardium.[333,339]

Histoplasmosis in patients with disseminated infection may rarely cause infection of the myocardium and endocardium as well as of the pericardium.[339] Similarly, aspergillosis, candidiasis, and coccidioidomycosis may cause pericarditis in the context of pulmonary infection, endocarditis, and myocardial abscess.[336,337] Therefore, cardiac decompensation in patients with fungal pericarditis may be due either to the presence of cardiac compression from a pericardial effusion or a constricting pericardium or to an underlying myocardial infection.

CLINICAL FEATURES. The clinical course of histoplasmosis pericarditis is now better understood from two large urban outbreaks in which 6.3 per cent of 712 patients with clinically recognized histoplasmosis had acute pericarditis.[333] Almost all of the patients had a preceding respiratory illness, and pericardial pain and typical electrocardiographic changes at presentation. The chest roentgenogram was always abnormal, an enlarged cardiac silhouette was present in 95 per cent, and pleural effusions and intrathoracic adenopathy were present in two-thirds of the patients. Notably, the "classic" manifestations of histoplasmosis—acute self-limited disseminated infection or severe cavity pulmonary infection—were absent. However, more than 40 per cent of patients had hemodynamic compromise or frank cardiac tamponade consistent with other reports.[333,339] Histoplasmosis pericarditis can rarely occur in the less common setting of severe prolonged disseminated infection evident by fever, anemia, leukopenia, and the syndrome of pneumonitis progressing to pulmonary cavitation, massive hepatomegaly, meningitis, myocarditis, or endocarditis. Severe disseminated infections are especially likely to occur in young infants, elderly males, and immunosuppressed patients.

Coccidioidomycosis Pericarditis. This condition does not occur in the brief self-limited influenza-like form of the infection but is instead a complication of the progressive disseminated form of coccidiodomycosis.[334] Blacks, Filipinos, and Chicanos appear to be especially vulnerable to the development of disseminated coccidioidomycosis. These patients are usually chronically ill and debilitated, with fever, weight loss, and the complications of pulmonary cavitations with lymphadenopathy, osteomyelitis, and meningitis. In immunocompromised patients, the insidious appearance of symptoms of fungal pericarditis and underlying myocardial infection may initially be overlooked because attention is focused on symptoms related to underlying lymphoma, leukemia, or known valvular endocarditis. Physical findings suggestive of cardiac compression (jugular venous distention, hypotension, pulsus paradoxus) may be the first clues to the diagnosis of fungal pericarditis.

DIAGNOSIS.

Histoplasmosis Pericarditis. In young and otherwise healthy adults with evidence of pericarditis, a presumptive clinical diagnosis of histoplasmosis pericarditis can be made on the basis of (1) residence or travel in an endemic area, (2) an elevated complement fixation titer of at least 1:32, and (3) a positive immunodiffusion test.[333] Most patients do not show a progressive rise in titer, since pericarditis usually occurs after initial mild or asymptomatic pneumonitis such that titers are high when first measured. Histoplasmin skin tests are not helpful, and their use may falsely elevate antibody titers.[333] *Histoplasma* may be isolated from specimens from invasive biopsies of mediastinal nodes, but cultures or methenamine silver stains rarely identify the organism in extrapulmonary sites such as the liver, bone marrow, and pericardium in patients with benign, self-limited form of pericarditis. Histoplasmosis pericarditis that occurs in the setting of severe disseminated infection must be differentiated from sarcoidosis, tuberculosis, Hodgkin's disease, and brucellosis. Histological tissue examination and culture are important in disseminated progressive histoplasmosis, and in this setting the organism may be isolated from extrapericardial sites such as the bone marrow, exudate from ulcers, or sputum by inoculation on Sabouraud's medium or by guinea pig inoculation with subsequent subculture of the spleen.

Coccidioidomycosis Pericarditis. A presumptive diagnosis of coccidioidomycosis pericarditis is made in a patient with pericarditis who has (1) a history of dust exposure in an endemic area in the American Southwest, California Central Valley, or South America, (2) a characteristic clinical picture of disseminated coccidioidomycosis involving the lungs and other organs, (3) the appearance of a positive serum precipitin test early in the infection followed by a rising positive complement-fixation antibody titer, and (4) microscopic evidence of the characteristic spherule in biopsy material. A definitive diagnosis is made by culture identification of the organism on Sabouraud's medium. Coccidioidin skin tests are often negative in the presence of progressive disseminated disease.

Other Fungal Pericarditis. If pericarditis due to other fungal organisms is suspected, appropriate complement-fixing antibody titers should be measured. Serology and precipitin tests for *candida* are not sensitive or specific, and the diagnosis of candida pericarditis depends on growth of the fungus from several sites other than superficially contaminated catheters in association with immunosuppression or complicated cardiac surgery.[337] Depending on the clinical setting, it may be important to obtain pericardial fluid and a pericardial biopsy specimen. It must be emphasized that the microscopic finding of granulomas alone is nonspecific and may occur in tuberculosis, fungal and parasitic infections, and sarcoid involvement of the pericardium. Therefore, histological documentation of the characteristic appearance of the fungus and subsequent culture identification are important.

MANAGEMENT. *Histoplasmosis pericarditis* is generally a benign illness that resolves within 2 weeks and does not require treatment with amphotericin.[333] Nonsteroidal antiinflammatory drugs or steroids appear to shorten the duration of chest pain, fever, pericardial friction rub, and effusion.[333] Patients should always be hospitalized, since histoplasmosis may cause the rapid development of massive effusions with acute cardiac tamponade that require emergency pericardiocentesis or pericardiectomy.[333,339] Although pericardial calcification and pericardial constriction have been reported in histoplasmosis pericarditis, these complications are uncommon. Intravenous amphotericin B is required only for patients with histoplasmosis pericarditis and severe systemic disease.

In *nonhistoplasmosis fungal pericarditis* the diagnosis is rarely made before death. Spontaneous remissions do not occur; infection progresses until the patient dies either of the underlying disease or of fungal pericardial and myocardial involvement. Survival from nonhistoplasmosis fungal pericarditis has been reported in occasional patients treated with parenteral antifungal therapy and surgical drainage by pericardiectomy.[337,340] Drug therapy for pericarditis associated with disseminated coccidioidomycosis, aspergillosis, and blastomycosis consists of prolonged intravenous therapy with amphotericin B. The South American form of blastomycosis may require the addition of a sulfonamide. Candida pericarditis associated with fungal sepsis and disseminated infection is treated with amphotericin B, in addition to pericardiectomy.[337] In many cases of nonhistoplasmosis fungal pericarditis, chronic pericardial fungal infection progresses to severe pericardial constriction or, less commonly, cardiac tamponade. Therefore, depending on the patient's underlying medical condition, pericardiectomy is usually indicated. Intrapericardial instillation of antifungal agents has not proved helpful in these diseases. The serious toxicity associated with prolonged amphotericin B administration underscores the importance of making a definitive diagnosis after histological examination or culture.

Pericarditis complicated by the development of cardiac tamponade and chronic constrictive pericarditis may also be caused by *Actinomyces israelii* and *Nocardia asteroides*, which are intermediate forms between fungi and bacteria.[341–343] These organisms may cause indolent infections and invasion of the pericardium from thoracic, abdominal, or cervicofacial abscesses.

OTHER INFECTIOUS PERICARDITIS

The parasite *Toxoplasma gondii*, which is usually acquired by accidental cyst ingestion in endemic areas, is a cause of myocarditis, acute pericarditis, and chronic pericardial effusion.[344] The prevalence of *Toxoplasma* as a cause of acute pericarditis of unknown origin may be underestimated.[62]

Other parasitic causes include amebiasis,[345–347] schistosomiasis,[348] and echinococcosis.[349–351] The diagnosis of amebic pericarditis is facilitated by the demonstration of multiple cystic lesions in the region of the pericardium by chest roentgenography and two-dimensional echocardiography.[346,347] Uncommon causes of parasitic pericarditis include dracunculosis,[352] cysticercosis, and filariasis.[353] These unusual infections rarely cause acute cardiac tamponade but may cause chronic constrictive pericarditis. The spirochetes *Borrelia burgdorferi* and *Babesia microti* are newly recognized as a cause of fatal myopericarditis in association with Lyme disease.[354–356] The psittacosis agent, *Chlamydia psittaci*, an obligate intracellular parasite-like bacterium that causes a febrile pneumonitis via bird-to-human transmission, is also a rare cause of effusive pericarditis.[357]

PERICARDITIS FOLLOWING ACUTE MYOCARDIAL INFARCTION

(See also p. 1263)

Pericarditis is a common occurrence during the first few days after acute myocardial infarction. The incidence of early postmyocardial infarction pericarditis varies from 6 to 25 per cent, although a much higher incidence is detected at autopsy.[358–360] In a prospective study of 703 patients with acute myocardial infarction, pericarditis, defined by the detection of a pericardial friction rub, occurred in 25 per cent of patients with transmural infarction and in 9 per cent of patients with subendocardial (non-Q wave) infarction.[361] Almost all patients with acute transmural myocardial infarction are found to have evidence of a localized fibrinous pericarditis overlying the infarction at autopsy, whereas fibrinous pericarditis is detected in about 10 per cent of patients with subendocardial infarction (non-Q wave infarction) at autopsy.[362] Pericarditis is more prevalent in anterior than in inferior infarction[361] and also occurs following lateral and predominant right ventricular infarction. Other forms of pericardial involvement after myocardial infarction include acute pericardial hemorrhage secondary to cardiac rupture and the late occurrence of Dressler syndrome (p. 1263).

CLINICAL FEATURES. Pericarditis is recognized clinically by the appearance of a pericardial friction rub within 12 hours to 10 days after acute myocardial infarction. In most patients with postinfarction pericarditis, a pericardial friction rub appears on the first, second, or third day after infarction.[359–361] In about 70 per cent of patients, the presence of a pericardial rub is accompanied by pleuritic or positional chest pain.[361] There is usually a slight temperature elevation, but pneumonitis is uncommon. Appearance of a new friction rub more than 10 days after acute infarction probably represents the onset of Dressler syndrome[359] or pericarditis complicating a second infarction. Since pericardial friction rubs are notoriously evanescent, serial auscultatory evaluation of patients in various positions in a quiet room is important for detection. Pericardial rubs with a single systolic component heard near the apex may be confused with a new murmur of mitral regurgitation due to papillary muscle dysfunction or rupture. Postinfarction pericarditis does not directly cause hemodynamic deterioration unless pericardial effusion under pressure develops, causing cardiac tamponade.

In a series of patients with early postinfarction pericarditis,[359] and in a series of patients with acute infarction and pericardial effusion,[363] the use of heparin did not appear to be associated with increased risk. However, hemorrhagic cardiac tamponade related to the use of anticoagulants has been reported as a rare complication in patients with postinfarction pericarditis.[364,365] Constrictive pericarditis has been reported as a sequel of hemopericardium after infarction.[366,367] Acute thrombolytic therapy of acute infarction with streptokinase or tissue plasminogen activator followed by intravenous heparin has not yet been reported to promote the development of hemopericardium after infarction.

The typical diagnostic electrocardiographic changes of acute pericarditis are extremely rare in early postinfarction pericarditis,[360] and the electrocardiogram cannot be used to confirm the diagnosis in this setting. The finding of a small pericardial effusion in a post-myocardial infarction patient in the absence of hemodynamic compromise is also not pathognomonic of acute postinfarction pericarditis. Galve et al. found that a small pericardial effusion could be detected in 28 per cent of patients early after acute infarction in comparison with 8 per cent of asymptomatic patients with unstable angina and 5 per cent of normal subjects.[363] The presence of pericardial effusion correlates highly with the presence of extensive infarction and congestive failure, but not with clinical pericarditis reflected in the appearance of a pericardial rub or pain. Patients who develop pericarditis after infarction experience a more complicated hospital course and more extensive myocardial damage compared to patients without pericarditis, as evidenced by higher myocardial MB-CK enzyme levels and lower ejection fraction.[361] The development of congestive heart failure and a high Killip class are more common in patients with postinfarction pericarditis.[358,359,361] The development of atrial tachyarrhythmias is also more common in patients with pericarditis following infarction.[361,368,369] The appearance of acute postinfarction pericarditis per se does not appear to affect adversely the in-hospital mortality after acute infarction.[358-361] However, pericarditis does appear to be associated with an increase in 12-month mortality, which is probably accounted for by its association with larger infarct size and lower ejection fraction.[361]

Postinfarction pericarditis without cardiac compression must be differentiated from acute stress ulcer, acute pulmonary embolism, and, most importantly, from recurrent myocardial ischemia. Myocardial ischemic pain can usually be differentiated from the pain of postinfarction pericarditis by (1) obvious amelioration of the pain by nitroglycerin and (2) the appearance of new regional ST-segment and T-wave changes with reciprocal changes.

Cardiac Tamponade. The development of cardiac tamponade in patients with myocardial infarction may be related to pericardial hemorrhage secondary to pericarditis or to myocardial rupture within the first 3 days after infarction. Both situations may be associated with cardiovascular collapse, the appearance of dense echoes in the pericardial space or two-dimensional echocardiogram, and an abrupt increase in heart size on the chest roentgenogram. Pericardiocentesis may successfully relieve postinfarction hemorrhagic cardiac tamponade in occasional patients.[370] Massive cardiac hemorrhage secondary to cardiac rupture is usually followed by the rapid development of electromechanical dissociation and death, although survivors have been reported after subacute rupture managed with pericardiocentesis and surgical repair.[371,372] The development of a chronic myocardial rupture (pseudoaneurysm) with effusive-constrictive pericarditis is a rare complication of extensive silent infarction with postinfarction pericarditis.[373]

Acute cardiac tamponade secondary to postinfarction pericarditis must also be differentiated from cardiogenic shock without intrapericardial hemorrhage due to an acute ventricular septal defect or mitral regurgitation. In the setting of an inferior myocardial infarction, the appearance of hypotension, pulsus paradoxus, and jugular venous distention may be related to massive right ventricular infarction rather than to cardiac tamponade. Echocardiographic findings of right ventricular enlargement without a significant pericardial effusion and catheterization findings suggestive of constrictive physiology (right atrial waveform with steep y descent) rather than cardiac tamponade (right atrial waveform with attenuated y descent) help to differentiate these entities and prevent possibly disastrous attempts at pericardiocentesis.

MANAGEMENT. Postinfarction pericarditis may produce mild symptoms that require no specific therapy or severe chest pain that persists for several days. If the pain is severe, high-dose aspirin will relieve pain within 48 hours in most patients. A short course of prednisone may be required in patients whose pain does not improve after a 48-hour trial of nonsteroidal antiinflammatory agents.[374]

There is experimental evidence that indomethacin, ibuprofen, and multiple large doses of corticosteroids interfere with the conversion of the myocardial infarct into a scar, so that thinning of the myocardial wall occurs.[375] Myocardial rupture has been observed in a patient during ibuprofen use for postinfarction percarditis,[376] and there is evidence of a higher incidence of pericardial rupture in postmyocardial infarction patients who receive nonsteroidal antiinflammatory drugs. Therefore, these drugs should be employed with great caution in patients with acute myocardial infarction. Fortunately, aspirin does not appear to cause any of these adverse effects, and postinfarction pericarditis usually responds well to aspirin. Accordingly, we favor use of this drug.

UREMIC PERICARDITIS
(See also p. 1868)

ETIOLOGY. Pericarditis is a frequent and serious complication of chronic renal failure. Before the advent of dialysis, uremic pericarditis was detected in about half of the patients with untreated chronic renal failure and was usually a harbinger of death. Uremic pericarditis is now detected clinically in up to 20 per cent of uremic patients who require chronic dialysis.[377,378] Uremic pericarditis tends to be a complication that occurs either prior to initiation of dialysis or during the first few months of therapy.

The etiology of uremic pericarditis is unknown. Viral causes have been proposed,[379] but there is no consistent evidence to suggest a viral etiology in the majority of cases of uremic pericarditis. The occasional observation of a seasonal clustering of episodes of pericarditis in uremic patients is consistent with a viral etiology. Specific etiological factors, including purulent bacterial infections, are common in patients with uremic pericarditis, and it is unwise to assume that pericarditis in a patient with several renal disease is simply related to uremia. Toxic catabolic nitrogen metabolites and secondary hyperparathyroidism have been suggested mechanisms responsible for uremic pericarditis. This suggestion is supported by the observations that uremic pericarditis is rare in patients with acute mild renal failure and that uremic pericarditis often improves with initiation of dialysis in previously untreated patients. However, there is no clear correlation between the development of pericarditis and the levels of catabolic metabolites in uremic patients. It has also been proposed that pericarditis in dialysis patients may reflect an immunological response. Some support for this hypothesis comes from Maisch and Kochsiek's observations that 64 per cent of 25 patients with chronic uremia and pericarditis had complement-fixing antimyolemmal antibodies with cytolytic properties for cardiac tissue, whereas antimyocardial antibodies were rarely detected in patients with acute renal failure due to surgery or trauma.[380] It is possible that etiological factors in nondialyzed patients differ from those in patients undergoing regular dialysis. In the latter group, systemic and regional heparinization during dialysis itself may exacerbate uremic pericarditis by promoting the tendency of vascular pericardial granulation tissue to bleed into the pericardial space.

Acute uremic pericarditis is characterized by the appearance of shaggy, hemorrhagic, fibrinous exudate on both parietal and visceral pericardial surfaces with little acute inflammatory cellular reaction. In some patients, the friable pericardial surface may bleed, giving rise to hemorrhagic pericardial effusion. Subacute or chronic constrictive pericarditis may develop, coincident with organization of the effusion and formation of thick adhesions within the pericardial space.[381]

CLINICAL FEATURES. The development of pericarditis in patients undergoing dialysis is of clinical importance, since it may (1) cause disability or life-threatening cardiac tamponade in patients who are otherwise well compensated when undergoing dialysis, (2) compromise the status of patients who are candidates for renal transplantation, and (3) cause hemodynamic complications during routine dialysis. Patients with uremic pericarditis usually come to attention because of the development of chest pain. A pericardial friction rub is present on initial presentation in nearly 90 per cent of patients. Fever, leukocytosis, and tachycardia are frequent but nonspecific findings. Dyspnea and cardiac enlargement on the chest roentgenogram are common, but these findings can be related to underlying myocardial dysfunction and volume overload. Uremic pericarditis with a large pericardial effusion may first come to clinical attention when an otherwise asymptomatic patient becomes hypotensive and confused upon fluid removal during ultrafiltration. This occurs because volume depletion may cause an abrupt fall in systemic blood pressure when ventricular filling is already compromised by the presence of a large, tense pericardial effusion. Uremic pericarditis can also present as acute or subacute tamponade with the findings of jugular venous distention, hypotension, and pulsus paradoxus. In a study of 1058 patients undergoing dialysis over a 14-year period, acute cardiac tamponade developed in 17 per cent of 161 episodes of uremic pericarditis.[378]

Echocardiography. The presence of a small pericardial effusion is common in uremic patients, and in the absence of typical pericardial pain and friction rubs it is not diagnostic of pericarditis. Asymptomatic pericardial effusions of small to moderate size occur in 36 to 62 per cent of uremic patients who require dialysis and appear to be related to volume overload and clinical congestive heart failure.[382,383] On the other hand, the presence of a large anterior and posterior pericardial effusion in patients with uremic pericarditis that persists after about 10 days of intensive dialysis is associated with a high likelihood of requiring intervention to relieve tamponade.[377,378,382,384] The presence of a large pericardial effusion in association with echocardiographic findings of right atrial and right ventricular collapse is highly suggestive of cardiac tamponade in a patient with uremic pericarditis. Prior to consideration of pericardiostomy or pericardiectomy, it is important to document that these clinical findings are indeed related to the hemodynamics of cardiac tamponade (elevation and equilibration of pericardial, right and left heart filling pressures) rather than to underlying congestive cardiomyopathy, ischemic heart disease, or excessively vigorous ultrafiltration. It must be remembered that pulsus paradoxus may be absent in uremic patients with cardiac tamponade and coexisting left ventricular failure and elevated left ventricular filling pressures.

MANAGEMENT. Uremic patients who develop symptomatic pericarditis prior to the initiation of dialysis almost always respond to the initiation of vigorous dialysis.[377,382] In patients with acute uremic pericarditis with a large pericardial effusion, a period of 10 days to 3 weeks is usually required for resolution of the effusion after initiation of intensive dialysis.[377,385] In contrast, less than half of patients with asymptomatic pericardial effusions show resolution of effusion after initiation of dialysis.[382] No treatment is required for small, asymptomatic pericardial effusions that can be followed simply by serial echocardiography.[383]

Treatment of symptomatic uremic pericarditis that develops in patients more than 3 months after the initiation of chronic dialysis is controversial, and mutliple approaches have been advocated. About two-thirds of the patients who develop effusive uremic pericarditis following the initiation of dialysis will respond to a program of intensification of dialysis and regional heparinization. The remainder are likely to require operative drainage of the pericardium.[377,386,387] Factors that predict that the strategy of intensive dialysis is likely to fail include the presence of large anterior and posterior effusions, high fever, leukocytosis with left shift, and clinical evidence of the development of cardiac tamponade, such as hypotension and jugular venous distention.[378,385,388] Nonsteroidal antiinflammatory drugs have been widely advocated as therapy for patients with uremic pericarditis. A randomized, double-blind comparison of indomethacin versus placebo in symptomatic patients with uremic pericarditis showed that indomethacin reduced the duration of fever, but it had no significant effect on the duration of chest pain, pericardial rub, pericardial effusion, or need for relief of tamponade, which occurred in 20 per cent of patients.[389] The complications of long-term steroid administration limit its usefulness in the treatment of recurrent uremic pericarditis.

Pericardiocentesis with an indwelling catheter followed by instillation of a nonresorbable steroid into the epicardial space has also been advocated,[390] but this procedure has been complicated by the development of purulent pericarditis.[391] A single pericardiocentesis followed by a one-time instillation of triamcinolone appears to be effective and may eliminate the need for prolonged catheter drainage.[392] There are reports of repetitive pericardiocenteses with low morbidity and mortality in uremic patients,[393]

but other series have reported substantial mortality as a consequence of pericardiocentesis.[377] The presence of a friable visceral pericardium may increase the risk of traumatic intrapericardial hemorrhage in uremic pericarditis, and the status of many patients is also compromised by the presence of left ventricular dysfunction. These considerations warrant special caution during the performance of pericardiocentesis in uremic patients, and this procedure probably should be carried out only by experienced personnel in an optimal environment.

Surgical Treatment. The surgical treatment of uremic patients with pericardial effusions with a subxiphoid pericardiostomy or limited pericardiectomy (window) performed through a left thoracotomy is effective in relieving cardiac tamponade. These approaches do not appear to be associated with an appreciable risk of developing recurrent effusions or constriction.[394,395] The intrapericardial instillation of steroids during surgical drainage has also been advocated,[385] although there is no evidence that this offers any advantage over thorough drainage alone.

Early surgical intervention in uremic patients with a large pericardial effusion has been advocated as a prophylactic measure to prevent the development of cardiac tamponade and to allow the procedures to be carried out at a time when the patient's condition is clinically stable. We feel that this approach is excessively aggressive, since many symptomatic uremic patients with pericardial effusions respond well to intensification of dialysis.

We advocate that patients with hemodynamic instability and with hemodynamic evidence of cardiac tamponade and echocardiographic evidence of a large anterior and posterior effusion may be treated by percutaneous catheter pericardiocentesis with continued catheter drainage of the pericardial sac for 24 to 48 hours. Subxiphoid pericardiotomy or limited pericardiectomy is reserved for patients with hemodynamic instability associated with recurrent pericardial effusions following pericardiocentesis or with loculated pericardial effusions.

NEOPLASTIC PERICARDITIS

(See also p. 1760)

PATHOLOGY. At autopsy, the pericardium is involved in 5 to 15 per cent of patients with malignant neoplasm.[396,397] Lung cancer, breast cancer, leukemia, Hodgkin's disease, and non-Hodgkin's lymphoma account for about 80 per cent of reported cases of malignant pericarditis.[396-402] Other malignant diseases reported to lead to pericardial involvement include gastrointestinal cancer, ovarian cancer, cervical cancer, sarcoma, thymoma, and melanoma[403-406] (Table 45-8). In children the most common etiologic factors are non-Hodgkin's lymphoma, neuroblastoma, sarcomas, and Wilms' tumor,[402] whereas pericardial teratomas are a rare cause of hydrops fetalis in utero and in neonates.[407-409] Primary malignant neoplasms of the pericardium are rare and are predominantly due to mesothelioma, including that arising after asbestos and fiberglass exposure,[410-412] and, less frequently, to benign localized fibrous mesothelioma, malignant fibrosarcoma, angiosarcoma, and benign and malignant teratomas.[413-416] Rare primary neoplasms of the pericardium occasionally have been reported in association with congenital developmental disorders such as tuberous sclerosis.[417] Catecholamine-secreting pheochromocytoma is a rare primary neoplasm of the pericardium.[418]

TABLE 45-8 CAUSES OF TUMORS METASTATIC TO THE PERICARDIUM

PRIMARY MALIGNANT NEOPLASM	FREQUENCY (%)
Lung carcinoma	40
Breast carcinoma	22
Gastrointestinal carcinoma	3
Other carcinomas	6
Leukemia and lymphoma	15
Melanoma	3
Sarcoma	4
Other (including malignant mesothelioma, germ cell tumors)	7

Relative frequency of neoplasms metastatic to the pericardium in 1315 patients.

Data from Goodie, R. B.: Secondary tumors of the heart and pericardium. Br. Heart J. 17:183, 1955; and Scott, R. W., and Garvin, C. F.: Tumors of the heart and pericardium. Am. Heart J. 17:431, 1939.

Pericardial metastases may involve the heart in several ways: (1) extension and attachment to the pericardium of a malignant mediastinal mass, (2) nodular tumor deposits from hematogenous or lymphatic spread, (3) diffuse pericardial thickening and infiltration with tumor, and (4) local infiltration of the pericardium.[398] In the majority of cases, the epicardium and myocardium are *not* involved.

Neoplastic pericarditis may cause several syndromes of cardiac compression. Neoplastic involvement of the pericardium may result in serosanguineous or hemorrhagic effusions, which may develop extremely rapidly, causing acute or subacute cardiac tamponade. Pericardial involvement by tumors such as sarcomas, mesotheliomas, and melanomas can also erode the cardiac chamber or intrapericardial blood vessels, causing acute pericardial distention and abrupt fatal cardiac tamponade. A rare cause of hemorrhagic effusion and cardiac tamponade is intrapericardial extramedullary hematopoiesis associated with preleukemic conditions and with Philadelphia chromosome–positive chronic myeloid leukemia.[419,420] Cardiac compression may also occur as a consequence of the development of both thickened pericardium and pericardial effusion under pressure (effusive-constrictive pericarditis), or it may be caused by thickening of the pericardium produced by tumor encasement of the heart, causing the physiology of constrictive pericarditis.

Not all pericardial effusions associated with mediastinal cancer are malignant. Asymptomatic pericardial effusions are common in patients with mediastinal lymphoma and Hodgkin's disease.[421] These evanescent effusions are frequently detected during staging procedures and presumably develop as a result of impaired lymphatic drainage. Fracp et al. have observed that small, clinically unsuspected pericardial effusions detectable by echocardiography are common in women with metastatic breast cancer.[422] In a prospective study of 38 women with metastatic breast cancer in whom echocardiography was done on a routine basis, 53 per cent were found to have small pericardial effusions that did not progress to cause hemodynamic embarrassment in any patient. It is uncertain whether small pericardial effusions in asymptomatic women with metastatic breast cancer are due to indolent malignant pericardial involvement or impaired lymphatic drainage.

CLINICAL FEATURES. Neoplastic pericarditis is often totally asymptomatic and detected only as an incidental finding at autopsy. However, it is the most common specific cause of acute pericarditis in developed countries. In a prospective series of patients with acute pericarditis of unknown cause, a diagnostic protocol revealed an unsuspected malignant etiology in 5 per cent of patients.[61] In patients with undiagnosed cancer, leukemia, or primary pericardial tumors, cardiac tamponade can be the initial manifestation.[398,412,423] In patients with known malignancy, symptoms resulting from pericardial involvement may be incorrectly attributed to the underlying neoplasm, so that malignant pericarditis is not suspected until symptoms and signs of severe cardiac compression appear.

In patients with malignant pericarditis, dyspnea is by far the most common symptom.[398,401,424] Other frequent symptoms and physical findings include chest pain, cough, orthopnea, and hepatomegaly. Distant heart sounds and a pericardial friction rub are rarely detected, which is in part probably due to a low index of suspicion.[398,424] In the majority of patients the diagnosis is made only when there is evidence of cardiac compression of frank cardiac tamponade, manifest as jugular venous distention, pulsus paradoxus, and hypotension. These findings occur more frequently with neoplastic pericarditis than in patients with an underlying neoplasm and idiopathic or radiation-induced pericarditis.[398]

The chest roentgenogram is abnormal in more than 90 per cent of patients with malignant pericarditis and may show pleural effusion, cardiac enlargement, mediastinal widening, a hilar mass, or, less commonly, an irregular nodular contour of the cardiac silhouette.[398,401] The electrocardiogram is usually abnormal but nonspecific, showing tachycardia, ST- and T-wave changes, low QRS voltage, and occasionally atrial fibrillation. In occasional patients, persistent tachycardia or electrocardiographic changes are the initial findings that lead to the diagnosis.[424] Electrocardiographic findings that are rarely seen in pericarditis, such as atrioventricular conduction disturbances, suggest malignant invasion of the myocardium and conduction system.

DIAGNOSIS. Patients with cancer and pericarditis benefit from a systematic evaluation, and these patients should not be summarily assumed to have a preterminal condition. The diagnosis of malignant pericarditis depends on both documentation of pericardial inflammation and substantiation that pericarditis is due to neoplasm. It is often not appreciated that in approximately half the patients with symptomatic pericarditis and neoplastic disease there is a nonmalignant cause; most commonly the condition is due to prior radiation or to idiopathic causes.[136,398] Many patients with advanced neoplastic disease are immunosuppressed as a consequence of their malignant disease and/or therapy and are therefore also at risk for tuberculous and fungal pericarditis. In a series of 140 patients with acute leukemia, pericarditis was diagnosed clinically or at autopsy in eight patients; it was caused by malignant disease in only one patient and by bacterial, fungal, or tuberculous pericarditis in the other patients.[425] Acute pericarditis has also been rarely reported as a complication of intravenous administration of the chemotherapeutic agents Adriamycin and daunorubicin.

In patients with the acquired immunodeficiency syndrome, the differential diagnosis is complex and includes involvement of the pericardium with Kaposi's sarcoma[426] as well as opportunistic infections with fungus or atypical acid-fast bacilli. Neoplastic pericarditis with cardiac compression must be differentiated from other causes of jugular venous distention, hepatomegaly, and peripheral edema in cancer patients. The most important of these are (1) underlying left ventricular dysfunction secondary to prior cardiac disease or adriamycin cardiac toxicity, (2) superior vena caval obstruction, (3) malignant hepatic involvement with portal hypertension, and (4) microvascular tumor spread in the lungs with secondary pulmonary hypertension.

Echocardiography often provides critical information about the presence and size of a pericardial effusion and the thickness and motion of the pericardium and may suggest the presence of abnormal diastolic filling of the heart due to cardiac compression. Two-dimensional echocardiography may be helpful in the detection of irregular undulating masses that protrude into the pericardial space and define the presence of pericardial space-occupying lesions.[427] Computed tomography and magnetic resonance imaging can also detect the presence of pericardial effusions and, in some instances, may give added information regarding the presence and location of space-occupying masses within the pericardium and adjacent mediastinum and lungs.[410,414,428,429]

We recommend that pericardiocentesis using the catheter drainage technique (p. 1480) should be performed in conjunction with cardiac catheterization in cancer patients with suspected cardiac tamponade in whom a large pericardial effusion is documented by echocardiography. Two additional diagnoses should always be systematically evaluated during cardiac catheterization in these patients. (1) Superior vena caval obstruction may coexist with malignant cardiac tamponade and contribute to the development of facial edema and jugular venous distention and should be systematically excluded at cardiac catheterization in cancer patients. (2) Cyanosis, hypoxemia, and elevation of the pulmonary vascular resistance are not features of cardiac tamponade, and pulmonary microvascular tumor (lymphangitic tumor) should be strongly suspected in a patient with these findings, hypoxemia, or persistent dyspnea following pericardiocentesis. Support for this diagnosis can be obtained at the same setting as pericardiocentesis and right-heart catheterization by obtaining a sample of blood from the pulmonary capillary wedge position for cytological analysis using the right-heart catheter.[430]

The appearance of the pericardial fluid does not differentiate among neoplastic, radiation, or idiopathic causes. Since treatment strategies differ, it is necessary to carry out a meticulous cytological examination of pericardial fluid in an attempt to differentiate malignant pericarditis from radiation-induced or idiopathic pericarditis. Cytological examination of pericardial fluid is diagnostic of a malignant neoplasm in about 85 per cent of the cases of malignant pericarditis.[136,398,431,432] False-negative cytological diagnoses are uncommon in carcinomatous pericarditis but occur more commonly with involvement by lymphoma or mesothelioma.[431,432] The measurement of carcinoembryonic antigen (CEA) may add to the diagnostic yield of the examination of pericardial fluid in patients with suspected neoplastic pericarditis; open pericardial biopsy may be required if the results of cytological examination of pericardial fluid are normal. If a sufficiently large biopsy specimen is obtained, open pericardial biopsy should provide a histological diagnosis in up to 90 per cent of cases. However, false-negative diagnoses may occur if only a small tissue sample is obtained, and in critically ill patients open pericardial biopsy is not without risk.

In patients with echocardiographic evidence of a thickened pericardium and the physical findings of cardiac compression (jugular venous distention, edema, ascites, and hepatomegaly), cardiac catheterization is useful for documenting the presence of constrictive physiology before a decision is made to proceed with aggressive surgical intervention, i.e., extensive pericardiectomy.

NATURAL HISTORY. If cardiac tamponade can be avoided or successfully treated, the mere presence of neoplastic pericarditis does not imply that death is imminent. Since lung cancer and breast cancer are by far the most common causes of malignant pericarditis with cardiac tamponade, both the management strategy and subsequent natural history usually depend on the type of underlying malignant disease. The natural history of neoplastic pericarditis in patients treated for cardiac tamponade was studied using a Kaplan-Meier analysis in two series.[150,398] In both series, the mean survival was 4 months with 25 per cent surviving 1 year. We studied the outcome of a consecutive series of 29 patients with malignant pericardial effusion and tamponade managed with pericardiocentesis in whom the 1-year survival rate was 17 per cent compared with 91 per cent for 21 patients with nonmalignant effusion.[128] These series indicate that a subset of about 25 per cent of patients with cardiac tamponade due to malignant pericarditis who are managed surgically or with pericardiocentesis will enjoy 1 year survival or better. Furthermore, the outcome in patients with malignant pericarditis due to breast cancer is strikingly better than that in patients with lung cancer or other metastatic carcinomas. Following surgical treatment of cardiac tamponade in lung cancer patients, Piehler et al. reported that the mean survival was only 3.5 months in contrast with breast cancer patients in whom mean survival was 9 months with survivorship extending to more than 5 years.[150] In one series of breast cancer patients with malignant pericarditis managed with pericardiectomy or pericardiotomy, the overall median survival was 17 months.[422] A similar prolonged survival in patients with malignant effusion due to breast cancer has been reported by others.[398,432,434–436]

MANAGEMENT. Decisions about the management of neoplastic pericardial effusion depend on the underlying condition of the patient, the presence or absence of clinical manifestations related to cardiac compression, and the prognosis and treatment options available for the specific histology and stage of the underlying malignant disease. At one end of the spectrum are debilitated patients with end-stage malignant disease for whom there is no promising treatment option for the underlying malignant disease and for whom the prognosis is bleak. In this setting, diagnostic procedures should be as brief and painless as possible, and intervention should be directed toward alleviation of symptoms with a goal of improving the quality of the remaining days or weeks of life. In these patients, pericardiocentesis with catheter drainage is indicated for immediate relief of severe dyspnea, chest pain, or orthopnea. At centers experienced in catheter pericardiocentesis, neoplastic cardiac tamponade can be safely relieved with pericardiocentesis in 90 to 100 per cent of cases with a low (< 2 per cent) risk of major complications.[105,128,397,436,437] At centers with a high complication rate with pericardiocentesis or if cardiac tamponade recurs, palliation can be achieved with an equally high success rate and low morbidity by a subxiphoid pericardiotomy under local anesthesia.[150,397] The more invasive and debilitating partial pericardiectomy (window) done via a left thoracotomy has also been advocated, but this procedure appears to have no advantage as a palliative procedure over a subxiphoid pericardiotomy and should rarely be done in patients with end-stage malignancy.[150]

When the general prognosis of the patient is better, several more aggressive treatment options are available, the goals of which are (1) relief of cardiac tamponade, (2) prevention of recurrence of the malignant effusion, and (3) treatment or prevention of constrictive pericardial disease.

In patients with asymptomatic pericardial effusion who have a treatment option of effective chemotherapy or hormonal therapy directed against the underlying malignant disease, treatment with systemic agents alone can be attempted while progression of the effusion is observed by means of echocardiography. In patients with cardiac tamponade and large effusions secondary to neoplastic pericarditis, pericardiocentesis with thorough catheter drainage in combination with systemic chemotherapy can be attempted. Based on small series of patients, the instillation of multiple chemotherapeutic agents, radioisotopes, and lymphokine-activated killer cells into the pericardial space following pericardiocentesis or surgical drainage has been advocated, with the aim being sclerosis of the pericardial membranes and obliteration of the pericardial space.[424,437–441] However, in comparison with complete catheter or surgical pericardial drainage, there is no convincing evidence to date from either a large collective experience or prospective trial to indicate that instillation of drugs into the pericardial space alters the outcome. Side effects of instillation of intrapericardial agents include chest pain, nausea, high fever, and atrial arrhythmias.

External-beam radiation therapy is an important option for patients with radiosensitive tumors who have not yet received extensive mediastinal or cardiac radiation as a treatment modality. Approximately half the patients with malignant pericarditis due to a variety of primary tumors respond to this form of treatment.[436,442] In one series, malignant pericardial effusion improved significantly in 11 of 16 patients with breast cancer, while 6 of 7 patients with malignant pericarditis secondary to leukemia or lymphoma improved with cardiac radiation.

In cancer patients whose overall condition is good and who develop recurrent symptomatic effusions after pericardiocentesis, a limited subxiphoid pericardiotomy should probably not be chosen when the goal is definitive therapy. The procedure has a much higher likelihood of being followed by recurrent tamponade, constriction, or reoperation than does extensive pericardiectomy, and tamponade almost always recurs in less than a year after operation.[150] Since one of four patients with malignant effusive pericarditis is likely to survive at least 1 year, extensive surgical pericardiectomy should be strongly considered in cancer patients with recurrent effusions or pericardial constriction who have (1) potential response to systemic cancer therapy or (2) one or more years of expected survival.

RADIATION PERICARDITIS

ETIOLOGY. Radiation injury to the heart and pericardium is an important complication of radiation therapy used in breast carcinoma, Hodgkin's disease, and non-Hodgkin's lymphoma. Factors that influence the development of radiation-induced heart disease include (1) the radiation dose;

(2) the duration and fractionation of therapy; (3) the volume of the heart included in the radiation field; (4) the use of a ^{60}Co source, with inhomogeneous dose distribution, in comparison with a linear accelerator source; and (5) anterior weighting of the radiation dose.[443,444] When at least 60 per cent of the cardiac silhouette is included within the treatment beam, as occurs in mantle field therapy of patients with Hodgkin's disease, the risk of radiation-induced pericarditis is about 5 to 7 per cent when a dose less than 4000 rads is delivered over 4 weeks and rises sharply in incidence above this dose.[443-446] When the whole pericardium is included in the field, the incidence of pericarditis is about 20 per cent, while the use of a subcarinal block that shields the heart decreases the risk to about 2.5 per cent.[447] This observation has been confirmed in a contemporary series of 590 patients who received mantle irradiation as initial treatment for Hodgkin's disease at the Joint Center for Radiation Therapy; 2.2 per cent of patients developed postirradiation pericarditis.[445]

In patients with Hodgkin's disease who receive radiation therapy using a ^{60}Co source or anterior weighting of the beam, which results in a higher dose to the pericardium, the incidence of pericarditis rises to about 20 per cent.[448] It approaches 50 per cent when a fluid challenge is used to unmask occult constrictive pericarditis.[449] In breast cancer radiation therapy in which the volume of the heart included in the field is usually less than 30 per cent, the incidence of radiation-induced pericarditis is less than 5 per cent, with a tolerance for up to 6000 rads given over 6 weeks.[443]

Pericardial injury may occur during the course of treatment or, more commonly, months later. In one series, 92 per cent of cases in patients presenting with pericardial effusions occurred within 12 months after completion of the course of radiation therapy.[450] However, it is now recognized that radiation pericarditis manifesting as chronic pericardial effusion or constrictive pericarditis may become apparent many years after radiation therapy.[443,446,448-451] In a series of patients with postirradiation constrictive pericarditis referred for pericardiectomy at Stanford, recent cases appeared to have a longer latent period between radiotherapy and presentation with constrictive pericarditis (4.7 years for cases during 1970 to 1980, versus 11 years for cases in 1980 to 1985).[169] The risk and latency period for the later development of constrictive pericarditis in children undergoing mediastinal irradiation is not known. In a study of 17 children observed for 72 months after radiation therapy for Hodgkin's disease, 47 per cent had prominent pericardial thickening on echocardiograms without overt evidence of cardiac constriction.[452]

PATHOLOGY. Radiation pericarditis is associated with fibrin deposition and pericardial fibrosis (Fig. 45–24). The acute inflammatory stage may be accompanied by a pericardial effusion that can be serous, serosanguineous, or hemorrhagic with a high protein and lymphocyte content.[443] The inflammation and initial effusion may resolve spontaneously. Alternatively, the effusion may organize and progress to a stage of dense fibrinous adhesions with gradual obliteration of the pericardial space, thickening of the pericardium, and proliferation of small blood vessels within the pericardium associated with a chronic pericardial effusion or a constricting pericardium. The visceral pericardium may also become fibrotic and thickened, and radiation pericarditis is a common cause of effusive-constrictive pericardial disease. Radiation injury represents an important cause of constrictive pericarditis in children, in whom progression from pericarditis to constriction is otherwise rare.[453]

It is important to recognize that radiation may occasionally injure the heart itself, causing interstitial myocardial fibrosis, valvular thickening, endothelial proliferation, and fibrotic thickening of small intramyocardial arteries. Radiation may also cause premature atherosclerosis of the epicardial coronary arteries.[443,454]

The most important consequence of radiation-induced myocardial fibrosis is the development of restrictive cardiomyopathy, which may coexist with constrictive pericarditis

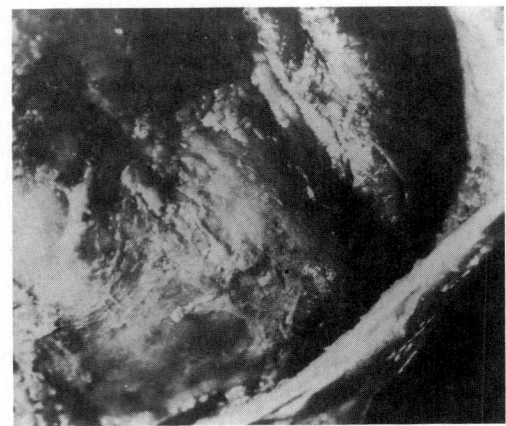

FIGURE 45–24. Anterior surface of the heart from a patient treated with radiation to the mediastinum 29 years before for a malignant thymoma. There is marked thickening of the parietal pericardium which is reflected away from the heart (right), and a thick fibrinous exudate is present on the epicardial surface of the heart. (From Stewart, J. R., and Fajardo, L. F.: Radiation-induced heart disease. Prog. Cardiovasc. Dis. 27:173, 1984.)

and contribute to inadequate relief of symptoms of pulmonary and venous congestion and poor survival after pericardiectomy.

CLINICAL FEATURES. The *acute* form of pericarditis is seldom evident clinically. It usually occurs in the context of irradiation of bulky mediastinal tumor adjacent to the pericardium, which suggests that acute pericarditis is largely related to inflammatory necrosis of the adjacent tumor. Patients may have a syndrome of acute pericarditis consisting of fever, pericardial pain, anorexia, malaise, a pericardial friction rub, and electrocardiographic abnormalities. Acute pericarditis that occurs during radiation therapy usually abates rapidly, does not preclude completion of planned treatment, and correlates poorly with the risk of late pericardial damage.

In the *delayed* form of pericardial injury, the onset of symptoms is usually within 12 months but varies from 4 months to more than 20 years. It may present as the syndrome of acute idiopathic pericarditis or as an asymptomatic pericardial effusion with a coexisting pleural effusion on the chest roentgenogram. In about half of the patients, there is some degree of cardiac compression associated with dyspnea, jugular venous distention, and pulsus paradoxus due to delayed chronic pericardial effusion. The importance of this mode of presentation is underscored by the fact that radiation-induced pericardial effusion now accounts for 10 per cent of patients who undergo surgical drainage of the pericardium.[149,150] In the Stanford experience,[443] about 20 per cent of patients with delayed pericardial injury progress to development of chronic pericarditis that requires pericardiectomy. These patients may present years after radiation therapy with the insidious onset of fatigue, dyspnea, systemic edema, and jugular venous distention due to the development of constrictive pericarditis.[453,454] The clinical recognition and consequences of this delayed form of pericardial injury have become increasingly important as patients with breast cancer and Hodgkin's disease have prolonged survival and cures.

DIAGNOSIS. Radiation-induced pericarditis with pericardial effusion is most often confused with pericarditis due to the underlying malignant disease. However, patients with malignant pericardial effusion are more likely to have massive effusions and cardiac tamponade, and cytological examination of pericardial fluid can identify a malignant origin in about 85 per cent of cases.[398] When symptoms referable to the pericardium occur years after apparently successful treatment of Hodgkin's disease or lymphoma, the pericarditis is much more likely to be related to radiation injury than to recurrent mediastinal malignant disease. Similarly, the development of pericarditis with effusion in women with treated breast cancer with no evidence of metastatic disease is likely to be related to prior radiation, radiation-induced hypothyroidism, or idiopathic (viral) inflammation.[422] Occasionally, histological examination of the pericardium or pericardial fluid may be required to differentiate between radiation-induced pericarditis and recurrent metastatic disease in the pericardium.

MANAGEMENT. Patients in whom an asymptomatic pericardial effusion develops after radiation therapy may be followed up by physical examination and serial echocardiography without the institution of specific therapy. Percutaneous pericardiocentesis by skilled operators should be limited to the treatment of cardiac tamponade or to drainage of a large pericardial effusion when cytological examination is required for management. Radiation-induced thyroid dysfunction occurs in about 25 per cent of patients who undergo mantle irradiation,[445] and hypothyroidism should always be excluded as a cause of effusive pericarditis following radiation therapy. Systemic corticosteroids should be reserved for patients with severe intractable pain or life-threatening effusive disease because of the well-documented risk of unmasking latent radiation-induced lung or heart injury when steroids are withdrawn.[455]

Surgical Treatment. Pericardiectomy is required for that small number of symptomatic patients with large recurrent pericardial effusion or severe effusive-constrictive or constrictive pericarditis. The surgical experience at the Mayo Clinic has shown that late constriction developed in 75 per cent of patients with radiation-induced pericarditis who underwent drainage with a limited left thoracic partial pericardiectomy (window).[150] These data are supported by others[149,233] and suggest that extensive pericardiectomy should be performed in patients with severe effusive or effusive-constrictive radiation-induced pericarditis whose prognosis is otherwise favorable. Operative mortality for pericardiectomy in patients after radiation therapy is 21 per cent, compared with a rate of about 8 per cent in patients with idiopathic constrictive pericarditis.[169] Actuarial analysis has shown that the 5-year survival rate of patients after pericardiectomy for postirradiation pericarditis is 51 per cent, which is inferior to the 83 per cent 5-year survival rate of other patients who underwent pericardiectomy.[233] Factors that contribute to a poor outcome include failure to resect constricting visceral pericardium (epicardium), and underlying myocardial injury and fibrosis causing advanced restrictive cardiomyopathy.[233,456,457] Prospective studies are needed to elucidate the potential role of endomyocardial biopsy for the assessment of myocardial injury and fibrosis to aid in discriminating patients with radiation-induced constrictive pericarditis with a high probability of experiencing a good outcome following pericardiectomy from those with a low probability.

PERICARDITIS RELATED TO HYPERSENSITIVITY OR AUTOIMMUNITY

ACUTE RHEUMATIC FEVER (see also p. 1721)

During the 19th century, acute rheumatic fever was believed to be the most common cause of pericarditis, and it was recognized that rheumatic pericarditis could occur independently of overt rheumatic endocarditis.[458] The condition is now uncommon, but occasionally the development of a pericardial friction rub or effusion is the initial clue to the presence of rheumatic carditis.

PATHOPHYSIOLOGY. Rheumatic pericarditis is characterized by fibrin deposition that can be accompanied by a fibrinous, serofibrinous, or purulent exudate.[458,459] The pericardial reaction usually resolves spontaneously. The deposition of IgG, IgM, and complement on the pericardial surface during active pericarditis has been reported,[459] but it is still unclear whether pericarditis occurs as an immune-mediated mechanism or simply as nonspecific inflammation associated with underlying myocarditis. The development of chronic calcification and constrictive pericarditis, although reported, is very rare.[460]

CLINICAL FEATURES. Rheumatic pericarditis usually occurs at the onset of the initial episode of acute rheumatic fever and may be asymptomatic or associated with typical pericardial pain and other symptoms of acute rheumatic fever, including fever, malaise, and arthralgias (p. 1727). When present, pericarditis usually indicates extensive pancarditis. The diagnosis of rheumatic pericarditis is based on the presence of pericardial chest pain, a pericardial friction rub, or echocardiographic evidence of pericardial effusion in association with the usual serological and clinical criteria for acute rheumatic fever (p. 1728). In children, the onset of pericarditis, which is otherwise rare in this age group, should prompt a rigorous search for evidence of acute rheumatic fever.[460,461] The combination of pericarditis, fever, arthralgias, and rash in a child or young adult may be mistaken for a viral exanthem, Lyme disease, infectious endocarditis, juvenile rheumatoid arthritis, systemic lupus erythematosus, Henoch-Schönlein purpura, Crohn's disease, or sickle cell crisis.

MANAGEMENT. The treatment of rheumatic pericarditis is that of acute rheumatic fever and includes bed rest and penicillin as well as digoxin, if myocardial failure is present. Chest pain associated with rheumatic pericarditis should be treated with aspirin, as described on page 1471. Rarely, corticosteroids are required. Small or moderate-sized pericardial effusions usually resolve spontaneously, and pericardiocentesis should not be performed solely for diagnostic reasons in a patient with documented acute rheumatic fever.

PERICARDITIS ASSOCIATED WITH SYSTEMIC LUPUS ERYTHEMATOSUS (see also p. 1734)

Pericarditis usually occurs during flare-ups of disease activity in patients with systemic lupus erythematosus (SLE) and is the most common cardiovascular manifestation of the disease.[462] Pericarditis is detected clinically in about 20 to 40 per cent of these patients during the course of their disease.[462] Echocardiographic abnormalities can be detected in a higher percentage of these patients, but the clinical significance of this is unclear.[463] The incidence of pericarditis in autopsied patients averages about 62 per cent and ranges from 43 to 100 per cent, whereas the incidence of myocarditis in autopsy series is about 40 per cent.[464,465] The inflammatory process may cause fibrinous or effusive pericarditis with the rare occurrence of pathognomonic hematoxylin bodies in the visceral pericardium. Pericardial fluid may be serous or grossly hemorrhagic with a high protein content, low glucose content, and white cell count below 10,000/mm³ (composed primarily of polymorphonuclear leukocytes). Low pericardial fluid complement levels relative to normal serum values have been reported, but caution must be used in interpreting this finding, since total hemolytic complement levels appear to be normally low in pericardial fluid.[462,466] Cardiospecific antimyosin, antisarcolemmal, and antipericardial antibodies associated with elevated creatine phosphokinase levels have been detected in the serum of a patient with SLE and severe chronic pericarditis prior to steroid treatment and pericardiectomy.[467]

CARDIAC TAMPONADE. This occurs in less than 10 per cent of patients with SLE and clinically recognized pericarditis, while the development of constrictive pericarditis has been reported but is rare.[462,468,469,470] Occasionally, cardiac tamponade is the presenting manifestation of SLE.[470,471] Pericarditis due to SLE may be accompanied by other cardiac lesions, including verrucous endocarditis, inflammation and necrosis involving the conduction system, and coronary artery vasculitis.[462,464]

CLINICAL FEATURES. Pericarditis should be suspected when patients with SLE develop pleuritic chest pain, a pericardial rub, or an enlarging cardiac silhouette on the chest roentgenogram. *Electrocardiographic abnormalities* are those characteristic of acute pericarditis. Since pericarditis usually occurs during periods of active disease, there is typically evidence of increased disease activity on blood tests for complement fixation levels, antinuclear antibodies, lupus erythematosus cell preparations, and sedimentation rate. The *chest roentgenogram* may show enlargement of the cardiac silhouette, pleural effusions, and parenchymal infiltrates. The *echocardiogram* may show evidence of a new pericardial effusion, suggesting the presence of pericardial inflammation. Since many patients with SLE are treated with immunosuppressive drugs, corticosteroids, and cytotoxic agents, a careful physical examination, blood cultures, and tuberculin skin test should be obtained to search for evidence of purulent, fungal, or tuberculous pericarditis. Except when purulent pericarditis is strongly suspected, it is not necessary to confirm the clinical diagnosis of SLE pericarditis by performing pericardiocentesis.

MANAGEMENT. In the majority of patients, pericarditis subsides when the systemic disease becomes inactive following treatment with corticosteroids or immunotherapy. The unusual complication of cardiac tamponade can ordinarily be treated with pericardiocentesis and usually does not require surgical intervention (i.e., pericardiotomy or pericardiectomy). However, since the development of acute cardiac tamponade is unpredictable, symptomatic patients with SLE pericarditis should be hospitalized and under close observation.

RHEUMATOID ARTHRITIS (see also p. 1732)

Although pericarditis is detected at autopsy in up to 50 per cent of patients with rheumatoid arthritis, the clinical incidence of symptomatic pericarditis is less than 10 per cent.[472,473] Based on echocardiographic criteria for the presence of a pericardial effusion, possible effusive pericarditis has been detected in 50 per cent of patients with chronic nodular rheumatoid arthritis, in 15 per cent of patients with typical non-nodular rheumatoid arthritis, and in no patients with typical non-nodular rheumatoid arthritis, and in no patients of comparable age with osteoarthritis.[474] Pericarditis tends to appear in patients with other evidence of severe rheumatoid arthritis, including extensive joint deformity, subcutaneous rheumatoid nodules, pneumonitis, and positive serum rheumatoid factor. On rare occasions, rheumatoid pancarditis with pericarditis can occur in patients with otherwise quiescent well-controlled rheumatoid arthritis.[475] Rheumatoid pericarditis in adults can cause cardiac tamponade and has been recognized as a cause of effusive-constrictive pericarditis and constrictive pericarditis.[243,472,473,476,477] Pericarditis, and the complication of cardiac tamponade, may occur with or without evidence of active joint involvement in children with juvenile rheumatoid arthritis[478-480] and in adults with juvenile rheumatoid arthritis (adult Still's disease).[481-483]

PATHOLOGY. Typical pathological changes in the pericardium are those of nonspecific fibrous thickening of the visceral and parietal pericardium with adhesions. Rarely, small, necrotic granulomatous nodules are detected on the epicardial surface that are histologically identical to the subcutaneous, rheumatoid nodule. Pericardial effusions, whose characteristics are similar to those of pleural effusions associated with rheumatoid arthritis pericarditis, are usually serous or hemorrhagic, with greater than 5 gm/dl of protein, glucose levels less than 45 mg/dl, high cholesterol levels, and white blood cell counts ranging from 20,000 to 90,000/mm³.[472,473] Soluble immune complexes, positive latex fixation titers, and low complement levels in the pericardial fluid as well as immune complex and complement deposits in pericardial vessels with plasma cell infiltration have also been described.[484] Acute pericarditis may progress to cause diffusely constricting fibrotic pericarditis and can coexist with other cardiac lesions, including granulomatous aortic and mitral valve deformity causing chronic aortic or mitral insufficiency.

CLINICAL FEATURES. Rheumatoid arthritis is often associated with fever, precordial chest pain, and dyspnea in association with a pericardial friction rub. Pericarditis commonly coexists with exacerbation of joint inflammation and pleuritis, manifest on the chest roentgenogram as a unilateral or bilateral pleural effusion in about 65 per cent of cases. Children with juvenile rheumatoid arthritis and pericarditis commonly show transient pulmonary infiltrates.[478,479] The *ECG* usually shows nonspecific ST-segment and T-wave changes. The presence of atrioventricular block in patients with rheumatoid pericarditis probably reflects rheumatoid myocardial involvement. On *echocardiography* a pericardial effusion is present in approximately half of patients with nodular rheumatoid arthritis,[472,474,485] but its presence does not always correlate with the presence of symptomatic pericarditis. In some patients, two-dimensional echocardiography can demonstrate the presence of dense fibrinous strands in the pericardial space.[486]

CARDIAC TAMPONADE AND CONSTRICTION. Although rheumatoid pericarditis is usually self-limited and benign, cardiac tamponade may develop abruptly in 3 to 25 per cent of patients[472]; it has been reported as a complication of sudden steroid withdrawal[487] and in association with intravenous anticoagulant therapy.[488] An uncommon but major complication is the rapid onset of subacute effusive-constrictive pericarditis.[472,484] The development of chronic constrictive pericarditis is a well-recognized complication that is more prevalent in men than in women.[243,472,477,489,490]

MANAGEMENT. Patients with symptomatic pericarditis may be treated with aspirin or other nonsteroidal antiinflammatory agents, as described on page 1471.

Pericardiocentesis is indicated for relief of a large anterior-posterior effusion causing cardiac tamponade. Although intrapericardial steroid instillation has been advocated,[491] there is no clear evidence that steroids alter the natural history of effusions or prevent the development of the constrictive pericarditis. There is now an extensive experience in the *surgical management* of rheumatoid pericarditis, and patients with connective tissue disorders (predominantly rheumatoid arthritis) now constitute between 4 and 20 per cent of patients undergoing pericardiectomy.[169,231,232] In patients with documented effusive-constrictive or constrictive pericarditis, pericardiectomy can provide gratifying hemodynamic and symptomatic improvement.[169,232,472,489,490]

PROGRESSIVE SYSTEMIC SCLEROSIS
(see also p. 1736)

Pericardial involvement is found at autopsy in about 50 percent of patients with progressive systemic sclerosis (scleroderma), while pericarditis is detected clinically in about 10 per cent.[492-494] While the pathogenesis of scleroderma pericarditis is unknown, it has been suggested that increased collagen formation by fibroblasts, in combination with tissue hypoxia, may result in aberrant collagen metabolism. Histological changes include nonspecific fibrotic pericardial thickening with adhesions and perivascular inflammatory cells. Pericardial effusions can be detected by means of

echocardiography in about 40 per cent of patients with scleroderma, but in the majority of patients a small pericardial effusion is not associated with symptoms.

When present, the pericardial effusion is straw colored and characterized by a protein content greater than 5 gm/dl, low cell count, and—in contrast with the characteristics of pericardial effusions in SLE and rheumatoid arthritis—the absence of autoantibodies, low complement levels, and immune complexes. Pericardial involvement is often associated with sclerodermatous infiltration of the heart, causing restrictive cardiomyopathy, arrhythmias, and conduction abnormalities.[493]

Scleroderma pericardial disease may present as an acute syndrome resembling viral myocarditis, with fever, chest pain, and pericardial friction rub, and nonspecific electrocardiographic ST- and T-wave changes. In other cases, patients develop a chronic pericardial effusion or pericardial constriction with symptoms of right and left atrial hypertension, cardiomegaly, and pleural effusions on the chest roentgenogram, and low QRS voltage on the electrocardiogram.

MANAGEMENT. There is no definitive treatment for scleroderma pericarditis. Patients with the syndrome of acute pericarditis may be treated with aspirin, as described on pages 1471 and 1496. Rarely, pericardial effusions with cardiac tamponade may develop, necessitating pericardiocentesis.[495] Patients with constrictive pericarditis may require pericardiectomy. Severe recurrent constrictive pericarditis has also been reported as a complication of idiopathic retroperitoneal and mediastinal fibrosis, which are regional expressions of a systemic sclerosing disease.[496] It is especially important to perform cardiac catheterization in patients with scleroderma and suspected cardiac tamponade or constrictive pericarditis, since dyspnea and systemic venous hypertension may be related to sclerodermatous cardiac involvement or to pulmonary hypertension secondary to pulmonary fibrosis. The development of symptomatic pericarditis in patients with scleroderma is ominous, since the 5-year survival rate is about 25 per cent when isolated pericardial or other cardiac involvement is present and about 75 per cent in patients without heart, lung, or kidney involvement.[497]

PERICARDITIS IN OTHER CONNECTIVE TISSUE DISORDERS

Acute pericarditis with pericardial effusions occurs in about 30 per cent of patients with mixed connective tissue and may coexist with other cardiac abnormalities, including myocarditis, conduction systemic degeneration, and intimal hyperplasia of the coronary arteries.[498,499] Cardiac involvement, including pericarditis, is less common in these patients than in patients with systemic sclerosis (scleroderma) or rheumatoid arthritis.

Pericarditis may rarely develop in other connective tissue disorders, including Sjögren's syndrome, dermatomyositis,[500] ankylosing spondylitis,[501] Wegener's granulomatosis,[502] Reiter's syndrome,[503] severe serum sickness,[504] and Felty's syndrome.[505] Pericarditis associated with polyarteritis nodosa may occur in patients who are hepatitis B antigen-positive. It also occurs in disorders of possible autoimmune etiology, including temporal arteritis,[506,507] inflammatory bowel disease,[508,509] Kawasaki's disease,[510] familial Mediterranean fever,[511] Whipple's disease,[512] celiac disease,[513] eosinophilic fasciitis,[514] Behçet's disease, and myasthenia gravis.[515] Amyloidosis is well known as a cause of infiltrative restrictive myopathy, the hemodynamics of which may mimic constrictive pericarditis (p. 1416), but it may also involve the pericardium.[224,225]

Cardiac involvement is present at autopsy in about 25 per cent of patients with sarcoidosis and can involve the pericardium in the absence of significant myocardial infiltration.[516] Sarcoidosis can be a rare cause of cardiac tamponade and constrictive pericarditis;[517,518] in the latter case, the findings of pericardial thickening with noncaseating granulomas may cause confusion with tuberculous or fungal pericarditis (Fig. 45–25).

DRUG- AND TOXIN-RELATED PERICARDITIS

Pericarditis occurs in about 25 per cent of patients with procainamide-related and 2 per cent of those with hydralazine-related development of the SLE syndrome.[519] In these patients, pericarditis may occasionally be complicated by the development of cardiac tamponade or the rapid development of pericardial constriction.[520] Other drugs that may produce pericarditis in association with the drug-induced syndrome of SLE include reserpine, methyldopa, isoniazid, and diphenylhydantoin.[519,521]

Other drugs appear to produce pericarditis through separate mechanisms. Pericarditis has been reported as a complication of a hypersensitivity reaction with peripheral eosinophilia after administration of penicillin[522] and cromolyn sodium.[523] The mechanisms of drug-induced pericarditis following administration of 6-amino-9-D-psicofuranosylpurine,[524] minoxidil,[525] dantrolene sodium,[526] and practolol[527] are not understood. Pericarditis has also been observed in association with polymer fume fever, a syndrome of pleuritis and noncardiogenic pulmonary edema that occurs following inhalation of fumes from the burning of polytetrafluoroethylene (Teflon).[528] Methysergide is well recognized as a cause of constrictive pericarditis as part of a generalized process of mediastinal fibrosis.[529] The

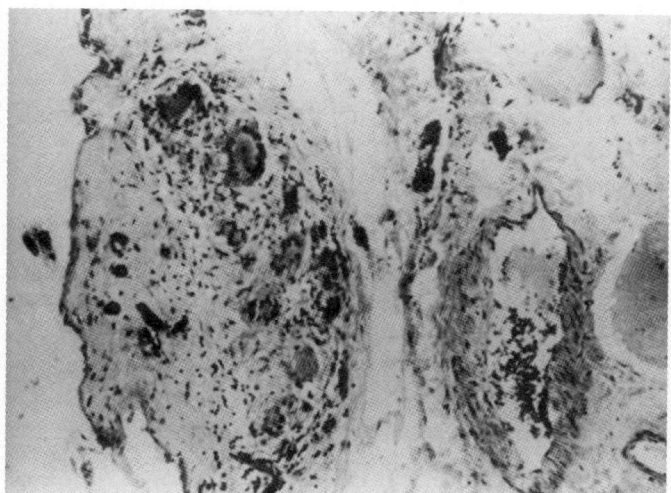

FIGURE 45–25. Photomicrograph of a pericardial biopsy specimen from a patient with cardiac tamponade secondary to cardiac sarcoidosis showing a noncaseating granuloma with several giant cells (250×). (From Verkleeren, J. L., et al.: Cardiac tamponade secondary to sarcoidosis. Am. Heart J. *106*:601, 1983.)

anthracycline neoplastic agents doxorubicin and daunorubicin may cause acute pericarditis as well as myocardial inflammation,[530] and pericarditis has also been reported in association with the use of cytosine arabinoside.[531] Pericarditis has similarly been noted as a foreign body reaction to the presence of silicone[532] and talc[533] within the pericardial space, in association with cardiac iron deposition and pericardial fibrosis in thalassemia,[534] and as a toxic response to scorpionfish sting.[535]

Acute drug-related pericarditis usually resolves when the offending drug is discontinued, and improvement may be accelerated by administration of corticosteroids. The rare development of chronic constrictive pericarditis may be treated by pericardiectomy.

Postmyocardial Infarction (Dressler) Syndrome

(See also p. 1495)

Dressler syndrome is an acute illness with fever, pericarditis, and pleuritis, possibly of autoimmune origin, that occurs weeks to months after an acute myocardial infarction.[536] A similar syndrome of fever and pericarditis has been reported in six patients following pulmonary embolism with infarction.[537] Today, a distinction is usually made between acute postinfarction pericarditis, which occurs during the first week after infarction (p. 1263), and Dressler syndrome, which usually appears 2 to 3 weeks after infarction, with a range of 1 week to several months. Dressler estimated that this syndrome occurred in up to 4 per cent of patients after acute myocardial infarction[538]; however, a more recent series from the same hospital indicates that the incidence of the Dressler syndrome has markedly decreased.[539]

The etiology of Dressler syndrome is unknown. The association of symptoms and the appearance of antimyocardial antibodies has led to the hypothesis that an autoimmune mechanism, with or without a latent viral infection, is the etiologic factor,[539] while some workers have concluded that the development of antimyocardial antibodies is not specific for the presence of Dressler syndrome.[539,540] Leakage of blood into the pericardial space is another proposed mechanism, and the current lower incidence of the syndrome may reflect less use of oral anticoagulants in the postinfarction period.[539] It is likely that there are common factors in the pathogenesis of Dressler syndrome and the postpericardiotomy syndrome, both of which have the following features: (1) an initial insult of endothelial cell injury and entry of blood into the pericardial space; (2) a delayed response after the initial insult, consisting of fever and inflammation of the pericardial surfaces; (3) development of antiheart antibodies; (4) a dramatic re-

sponse to antiinflammatory agents; and (5) a tendency for recurrence.

PATHOLOGY. The histology of the pericardium usually reveals a nonspecific inflammation with fibrin deposition. In contrast to the acute pericarditis following myocardial infarction in which pericardial inflammation is often patchy, overlying the regions of infarction, the pericarditis in Dressler syndrome is usually diffuse.

CLINICAL FEATURES. Patients characteristically have severe malaise, fever, chest pain, and pleurisy.[538,541] The chest pain may be severe enough initially to cause both patient and physician to consider that it is caused by a second myocardial infarction or postinfarction angina.[542] Dressler syndrome is occasionally the initial presentation of a previously undiagnosed infarction.[543] *Physical examination* often discloses a pericardial friction rub and sometimes a pleural friction rub as well. The chest roentgenogram commonly reveals an enlarged cardiac silhouette secondary to pericardial effusion associated with pleural effusions[538] and, occasionally, transient pulmonary infiltrates. The *echocardiographic* evidence of pericardial effusion in the absence of other symptoms is not diagnostic of Dressler syndrome, since asymptomatic small pericardial effusions occur in about one of four patients after myocardial infarction.[363] *Electrocardiographic* abnormalities usually consist of serial ST-segment and T-wave changes strongly suggestive of acute pericarditis, but the electrocardiogram may not be helpful in patients with persistent repolarization abnormalities following infarction. Blood tests usually reveal the nonspecific findings of an increased erythrocyte sedimentation rate and peripheral leukocytosis. Tests for antimyocardial antibodies are not widely available or established as a means of confirming the diagnosis. Gallium scanning has been reported to be ineffective in identifying patients with pericarditis due to Dressler syndrome.[544]

Dressler syndrome can usually be discriminated from recurrent myocardial infarction by (1) the characteristics of the chest pain and its failure to improve with nitroglycerin; (2) the absence of new Q waves on the ECG; and (3) the absence of a marked rise in the CK-MB band. Small increases in cardiac enzyme levels may occur in pericarditis when the underlying epicardium is involved. Dressler syndrome must also be distinguished from hemorrhagic pericarditis secondary to chronic systemic anticoagulation.

MANAGEMENT. A single episode of Dressler syndrome is usually self-limited, but the syndrome does tend to recur. The onset of severe pericarditis usually warrants hospital admission and observation for the development of cardiac tamponade.[545] Oral anticoagulants should be discontinued because of the risk of pericardial hemorrhage. As in other patients with acute pericarditis, patients with severe symptoms with fever and chest pain usually benefit from bed rest and treatment with aspirin or a nonsteroidal antiinflammatory agent. Recurrent episodes of Dressler syndrome may respond only to corticosteroids and occasionally require complete pericardiectomy for relief of intractable pericardial pain or prevention of recurrence. Cardiac tamponade in the absence of anticoagulant therapy can usually be managed with pericardiocentesis.[545] Constrictive pericarditis is a well-recognized complication of Dressler syndrome that may be relieved by pericardiectomy.[546,547]

Postpericardiotomy Syndrome

ETIOLOGY. The postpericardiotomy syndrome is identified by the appearance of fever, pericarditis, and pleuritis more than 1 week after a cardiac operation in which the pericardium has been opened and manipulated. This syndrome was first recognized in patients after mitral commissurotomy for rheumatic heart disease, and it was initially believed to represent reactivation of rheumatic fever.[548] Subsequently, it was realized that the syndrome could occur following cardiac operations in patients without rheumatic heart disease and that the common denominator appeared to be wide incision and manipulation of the pericardium.[549] An identical clinical syndrome has been reported following cardiac perforation by a catheter or transvenous pacemaker, blunt chest trauma, percutaneous diagnostic left ventricular puncture, and epicardial pacemaker implantation.[550] The incidence of postpericardiotomy syndrome following cardiac surgery ranges from 10 to 40 per cent in various series and is higher in children than in adults.[551-553] The observation of a 31 per cent incidence of postpericardiotomy syndrome in patients undergoing cardiac surgery for the Wolff-Parkinson-White syndrome clearly indicates that pericardial damage prior to surgery is not a contributing factor.[553] Furthermore, pericardial drainage techniques do not appear to affect the frequency of development of the syndrome after cardiac surgery.[554]

Analogous to the Dressler syndrome, the etiology of postpericardiotomy syndrome is hypothesized to be an autoimmune reaction directed against the epicardium, possibly in concert with a new or reactivated viral infection. Studies by Engle and colleagues have demonstrated that antiheart antibodies appear in the serum of some patients who undergo pericardiotomy and that there is a positive correlation between the level of the titers and the incidence of the syndrome.[552] Approximately 70 per cent of patients with the postpericardiotomy syndrome and high antiheart antibody titers also develop a fourfold or higher rise in titer against one or more viral antigens, while in patients without the postpericardiotomy syndrome, a rise in viral titers occurs in only 8 per cent of those with normal antiheart antibody titers and in only 19 per cent of those with low levels of antiheart antibody titers; these findings suggest that viral infection may be a triggering or permissive factor. The postpericardiotomy syndrome is rare in children under 2 years of age who undergo cardiac surgery, a finding that may be related to the short exposure time to viruses or to protective maternal antibodies transmitted via the placenta. The development of pleuritis and pleural effusions is believed to reflect involvement of the pleura adjacent to the inflamed pericardium; involvement of serous membranes distant from the heart is uncommon.

PATHOLOGY. There are no pathognomonic histological features of postpericardiotomy syndrome. The presence of blood in the pericardial space adjacent to an injured epicardium may result in later development of pericardial adhesions, thickening of the pericardial membranes, and occasionally fibrinous obliteration of the pericardial space, causing pericardial constriction. Pericardial effusions in patients with postpericardiotomy syndrome may be straw colored, serosanguineous, or frankly hemorrhagic, with a protein content greater than 4.5 gm/dl and a white blood cell count between 3,000 and 8,000/mm³ (composed of both lymphocytes and granulocytes).[555]

CLINICAL FEATURES. Patients typically develop an acute illness characterized by fever, malaise, and chest pain that usually begins during the second or third postoperative week (Fig. 45–26). In some cases, the fever may reflect a continuation of the more common problem of fever in the first week after operation. The chest pain is typical of acute pericarditis (p. 1469) and usually has a pleuritic quality. Nonspecific signs of inflammation, including an elevated sedimentation rate and polymorphonuclear leukocytosis, may also be present. Noncardiac pulmonary edema may also occur.[555a]

Physical examination often reveals a pericardial friction rub. It should be noted that the friction rub present in almost all patients during the first few days after cardiac surgery disappears in most patients who do not develop postpericardiotomy syndrome by the end of the first postoperative week. The *chest roentgenogram* demonstrates left-sided or bilateral pleural effusions in about two-thirds of patients, pulmonary infiltrates in about one-tenth, and transient enlargement of the cardiac silhouette in half.[553] The *ECG* shows nonspecific ST-segment and T-wave changes and episodic atrial tachyarrhythmias. *Echocardiography* is useful in monitoring the appearance and size of a pericardial effusion and in detecting evidence of cardiac compression such as right atrial collapse.

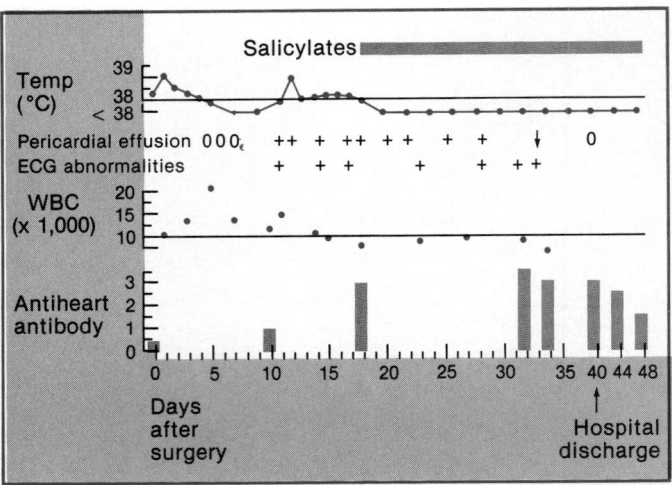

FIGURE 45–26. Representative clinical course of a child with the postpericardiotomy syndrome after cardiac surgery. Note that a febrile illness associated with effusive pericarditis, electrocardiographic changes, and leukocytosis began about 10 days after surgery. The administration of salicylates was followed by prompt relief of fever and pericarditis. The antiheart antibody titer, which was initially high, subsequently declined. (From Engle, M. A., et al.: The postpericardiotomy syndrome. 25 years' experience. J. Cardiovasc. Med. 4:321, 1984.)

However, it should be noted that pericardial effusions are extremely common after cardiac surgery, occurring in 56 to 84 per cent of patients within the first 10 days.[556] Thus, the diagnosis of postpericardiotomy syndrome is made on clinical grounds based on recognition of the distinctive features of the syndrome in the postoperative patient. Other causes of postoperative fever, including infection, as well as the viral-induced postperfusion syndrome of atypical lymphocytosis, fever, and hepatosplenomegaly, must be excluded.[557]

MANAGEMENT. The postpericardiotomy syndrome is a self-limited but often prolonged and disabling illness. Fever and severe chest pain are usually relieved by aspirin or nonsteroidal antiinflammatory drugs. Corticosteroids should be reserved for patients in whom fever and chest pain are not relieved within 48 hours by other antiinflammatory agents. Recurrences tend to appear during the first 6 months after surgery.

Cardiac tamponade is an important and well-recognized complication of the postpericardiotomy syndrome.[555,558,559] In one large series of adult patients who survived cardiac surgery, almost 1 per cent developed cardiac tamponade an average of 49 days after surgery, in association with fever, a pericardial friction rub, and pericardial chest pain typical of the postpericardiotomy syndrome.[555] In contrast to the important role of anticoagulation in early postoperative bleeding after cardiac surgery, the use of anticoagulants did not appear to be a prerequisite for the development of cardiac tamponade in association with the postpericardiotomy syndrome. Cardiac tamponade can be managed conservatively by pericardiocentesis followed by the administration of antiinflammatory agents.[555] Patients with recurrent tamponade require surgical drainage and pericardiectomy. Percutaneous pericardiocentesis should not be attempted in patients with echocardiographic evidence of only a small posterior effusion, a loculated effusion, or an effusion with dense echoes suggesting the presence of both thrombus and free fluid. Constrictive pericarditis is a rare complication that may occur months to years after the postpericardiotomy syndrome.

POSTOPERATIVE HEMOPERICARDIUM. Acute cardiac tamponade and pericardial constriction in the absence of typical features of the postpericardiotomy syndrome also occur secondary to hemopericardium following cardiac surgery and perforation of the heart during cardiac catheterization, pacemaker insertion, pericardiocentesis, and coronary artery angioplasty.[560-563] Acute pericarditis without frank cardiac perforation has been reported in 0.5 per cent of 981 patients who underwent angioplasty, and this complication may be secondary to occult epicardial-pericardial hematoma formation.[564] Other invasive procedures that have been reported to cause hemopericardium and cardiac tamponade include percutaneous aortic and mitral valvuloplasty,[565] sternal bone marrow aspiration,[566] esophagoscopy,[567] and mediastinoscopy.[568] Endoscopic sclerotherapy for esophageal varices is a new cause of both acute hemopericardium and the later development of pericarditis associated with chest pain and the development of cardiac tamponade.[569,570]

In some patients, cardiac tamponade following invasive cardiac procedures and cardiac surgery has been successfully managed with pericardiocentesis alone.[555,571] However, the development of early and late postoperative tamponade is commonly due to the combination of free fluid and organizing thrombus, which usually requires open surgical drainage of the pericardial space. Postoperative cardiac tamponade and thrombus formation can cause localized compression of the heart and have been reported to cause right ventricular outflow obstruction.[572,573]

CONSTRICTIVE PERICARDITIS. This condition is being increasingly recognized as a complication of cardiac surgery and may occur in patients in whom the pericardium is left open but in situ.[574–577] The time from cardiac surgery to definitive diagnosis usually is about 1 year but ranges from less than 1 month to more than 15 years.[575–577] In one review of 5207 adults who underwent cardiac surgery, 0.2 per cent (11 patients) developed constrictive pericarditis, documented by cardiac catheterization, an average of 82 days after operation.[574] An incidence of 0.2 to 0.3 per cent has also been observed in other series.[575]

Etiology. Povidone-iodine irrigation of the heart is postulated to be a triggering factor in some patients. This factor has been absent in most reports, and it is likely that intrapericardial hemorrhage and serosal injury are major contributing factors.[574] In the series of 45 patients reported by Killian et al., transient postpericardiotomy syndrome may have been a contributing factor in about 60 per cent of the patients.[576] There is now strong evidence that postoperative constrictive pericarditis can involve bypass grafts and can contribute to premature graft closure as well as damage to grafts during pericardiectomy.[577–579] The development of constrictive pericarditis, possibly related to both occult hemopericardium and the development of a foreign body reaction to the epicardial patch electrodes, has been observed several months after the placement of automatic implantable cardioverter-defibrillators (AICD).[580] Acute pericarditis as manifested as localized, progressive fibrosis adjacent to the patch electrodes has been found in virtually all patients who have undergone autopsy after AICD placement.[581]

Important clinical features in patients with postsurgical constrictive pericarditis include dyspnea, chest pain, jugular venous distention, pedal edema, and increased roentgenographic heart size, while echocardiographic evidence of pericardial thickening with a posterior pericardial effusion is present in the majority. Magnetic resonance imaging and computed tomography are useful in showing pericardial thickening in some patients.

MANAGEMENT. In patients in whom this syndrome is suspected, the diagnosis of constrictive pericarditis should be confirmed at cardiac catheterization before the pericardium is explored (p. 1478). The majority of these patients (about 85 per cent) improve after undergoing extensive pericardiectomy and are found to have hemorrhage-induced fibrosis of the pericardium, usually associated with a posterior organized hematoma.[575,576] The operative mortality for pericardiectomy in these patients is high, ranging from 5 to 14 per cent.[575]

OTHER FORMS OF PERICARDIAL DISEASE

Myxedema Pericardial Disease

(See also page 1834)

Myxedema is frequently associated with myopathy; pericardial effusion also occurs in up to one-third of patients.[582,583] Since myxedematous patients frequently have ascites, pleural effusions, and uveal edema, it has been suggested that pericardial effusion may be related to a combination of sodium and water retention, slow lymphatic drainage, and increased capillary permeability with protein extravasation.[584] The pericardial fluid is usually clear or straw-colored, with elevated protein and cholesterol concentrations and few leukocytes or red blood cells. Pericardial fluid usually accumulates very slowly and may achieve enormous volumes — as much as 5 to 6 liters. Occasionally, the pericardial effusion may resemble a viscous jelly rather than a clear fluid. Myxedematous pericardial effusions usually do not cause symptoms. Often attention is called to the heart by the finding of unsuspected marked cardiomegaly on a chest roentgenogram, and a large pericardial effusion is occasionally the presenting feature of hypothyroidism.[585]

Since infants and elderly patients with hypothyroidism may be asymptomatic, this etiologic factor should always be excluded in these patients with pericardial effusion of unknown cause. Hypothyroidism should also be considered as the cause of pericardial effusion in patients following mediastinal radiation therapy, in whom 25 per cent develop radiation-induced thyroid dysfunction.[445] The *ECG* often shows nonspecific abnor-

malities, including low QRS voltage and flattened or inverted T waves, due to either myxedematous heart disease or pericardial effusion. In myxedematous patients with cardiac compression from a pericardial effusion, the expected compensatory tachycardia may be absent.

Myxedematous pericardial effusions tend to regress slowly and ultimately disappear over a period of months after patients have been treated with thyroid replacement and have returned to the euthyroid state.[582,585] Cardiac tamponade has been reported, but it is a rare complication.[585–587]

Cholesterol Pericarditis

Cholesterol pericarditis results from pericardial injury associated with deposition of cholesterol crystals and a mononuclear cell inflammatory reaction consisting of foam cells, macrophages, and giant cells. The presence of cholesterol crystals in the pericardial space is believed to provoke a chronic inflammatory response that results in effusion and may ultimately lead to the development of constrictive pericarditis. A pericardial effusion that contains microscopic cholesterol crystals typically has a glittering "gold" appearance. The similarities in the lipid and cholesterol contents of pericardial fluid and serum in some patients with cholesterol pericarditis suggest that simple transudation may explain the high cholesterol content in the pericardial space.

MANAGEMENT. The management of patients with cholesterol pericarditis includes detection and treatment of any underlying predisposing condition associated with the development of cholesterol pericarditis, such as tuberculous, rheumatoid, or myxedematous pericarditis or hypercholesterolemia. However, in the majority of cases, cholesterol pericarditis occurs in the absence of a clear underlying disease.[588] Cholesterol pericardial effusions are usually large, but since they develop slowly, cardiac tamponade is an unusual complication.[589] Pericardiectomy is indicated in the unlikely event of cardiac tamponade as well as in the treatment of massive cholesterol pericardial effusion, which may cause dyspnea and chest pain.[590] The development of constrictive pericarditis requiring pericardiectomy has been reported but is extremely rare.[591]

Chylopericardium

Idiopathic chylopericardium is rare, and chylopericardium is usually associated with mechanical vein obstruction of the thoracic duct or its drainage into the left subclavian vein resulting from (1) surgical or traumatic rupture of the thoracic duct or (2) lymphatic blockage by neoplasms, tuberculosis, or congenital lymphangiomatosis.[592,593] Thoracic duct obstruction with failure of adequate collateral drainage then results in reflux of chyle through lymphatics draining the pericardium. Most patients with chylopericardium are asymptomatic and come to clinical attention when a large, slowly accumulating pericardial effusion is detected on chest roentgenogram or echocardiogram. The presence of a connection between a damaged thoracic duct and the pericardial space can be established by lymphangiography and radionuclide lymphangiography with technetium-99m antimony sulfur colloid, as well as by the recovery of ingested Sudan III, a lipophilic dye, from pericardial aspirate.[592,593] Computed tomography may demonstrate density compatible with fat in the pericardial space.[594] The pericardial fluid is usually milky white with a high cholesterol and triglyceride content, protein content greater than 3.5 gm/dl, and microscopic fat droplets demonstrated with a Sudan III stain.[593] Lymphopericardium, which is due to pericardial angiomas as part of generalized lymphangiectasis, is characterized by clear pericardial fluid.

Cardiac tamponade and constrictive pericarditis are rare complications.[593,594] Chylopericardium has been reported as a rare cause of cardiac tamponade after cardiac surgery.[595,596] The management of symptomatic chylopericardium consists of efforts to reduce the likelihood of recurrence. These include ingestion of a diet rich in medium-chain triglycerides or, if this is unsuccessful, in ligation of the thoracic duct and parietal pericardiectomy to evacuate chylous fluid and prevent reaccumulation.[593,596]

Traumatic Pericarditis

(See also p. 1518)

In addition to penetrating or nonpenetrating cardiac trauma (Chap. 46), other important causes of traumatic pericarditis include rupture of the esophagus into the pericardial space, which may occur from esophageal erosion secondary to esophageal carcinoma or sudden rupture of the esophageal contents into the pericardial space in Boerhaave's syndrome, or as a complication of esophagogastrectomy. Traumatic pericarditis due to esophageal rupture is usually followed by intense erosive pericardial inflammation and infection. Esophageal rupture or perforation may also be followed by the development of an esophagopericardial fistula.[597] These disorders usually require immediate surgical intervention and are associated with a high mortality, although medical management with spontaneous fistula closure has been reported.[597] Pericarditis may also occur secondary to pancreatitis associated with a pericardial effusion with high amylase content and, rarely, the development of cardiac tamponade or a pancreatic-pericardial fistula.[598,599] The incidence of occult pericardial effusion in patients with acute alcoholic pancreatitis is significantly higher (47 per cent) than in control subjects (11 per cent).[598] The development of fistulas to the pericardium in response to ulcer formation, malignant disease, or surgery may occur from other sites, including the stomach,[600] biliary tract,[601] colon,[602] and bronchi.[603]

Pericardial trauma may also give rise to unusual traumatic syndromes, including cardiovascular collapse following herniation of the heart through a rent in the pericardium caused by trauma, or prior pericardiotomy mimicking congenital partial absence of the pericardium with cardiac subluxation,[604,605] and intrapericardial diaphragmatic hernia.[606] Diagnosis of cardiac herniation can be made by computed tomography and magnetic resonance imaging.[605,607] Life-threatening cardiac herniation may also occur following radical left pneumonectomy with partial pericardial resection.[608]

Pericardial Cysts

Pericardial cysts are rare developmental anomalies and are typically located at the right costophrenic angle.[609] Unusual locations include the left costophrenic angle, hilum, and superior mediastinum at the level of the aortic arch. They are usually unilocular and filled with clear liquid, giving rise to the term *springwater cysts*.

Pericardial cysts usually do not cause symptoms or unusual physical findings. Rarely, chest pain may occur owing to torsion of the cyst. These lesions typically come to medical attention as an unsuspected finding of a round, sharply defined mass along the right cardiac border on a chest roentgenogram. The size of the cyst in asymptomatic patients may vary over time.[610,611] In most cases, a cyst can be differentiated from solid tumor or aneurysm by two-dimensional echocardiography or CT (Fig. 45–27).[611] When a suspected pericardial cyst is in an unusual location, angiography may occasionally be needed to discriminate a cyst from an aneurysm or pseudoaneurysm. Pericardial cysts located at the right costophrenic angle can be accurately diagnosed and treated by percutaneous aspiration under fluoroscopic guidance.[612] Because long-term follow-up studies have shown that most asymptomatic patients do not develop symptoms, most patients should be managed conservatively, without surgical exploration.[613]

Other benign developmental abnormalities of the pericardium include benign intrapericardial teratomas and intrapericardial bronchial cysts, which can be identified by computed tomography.[614]

Congenital Absence and Defects of the Pericardium

Congenital absence of the pericardium was first described anatomically by Realdus Columbus in 1559, but its antemortem detection did not occur until 1959.[615] In patients with pericardial agenesis, the anomaly usually involves a partial defect of the left-sided pericardium, which is potentially lethal, in 70 per cent; total absence in 9 per cent; partial absence of the right-sided pericardium, and absence of the inferior pericardium, in 17 per cent.[616] There is a 3:1 male/female predominance among patients with pericardial defects, and about 30 per cent have other congenital anomalies, including atrial septal defect, bicuspid aortic valve, bronchogenic cysts, or pulmonic sequestration. A familial occurrence of congenital absence of the pericardium has been reported.[617]

Total absence of the pericardium is not usually associated with symptoms. Occasionally the patient may complain of chest discomfort and palpitations. The etiology of these symptoms is unknown, but they may be related to torsion of the great vessels due to excess mobility of the heart. Most asymptomatic patients come to attention because of an unexplained heart murmur or abnormal chest roentgenogram. The extremely rare complication of acute chest pain due to strangulation of the heart between the diaphragm and the pulmonary ligament has been reported.[618]

TOTAL ABSENCE. Patients with total absence of the left pericardium often have widened splitting of the second heart sound, a hyperdynamic precordial impulse, leftward displacement of the apical impulse, and a systolic murmur at the upper left sternal border that may be related to turbulent blood flow in an unusually mobile heart. ECG abnormalities include right-axis deviation due to levoposition of the heart, incomplete right bundle branch block, clockwise displacement of the QRS transition zone of the precordial leads, and tall and peaked P waves in the right precordial leads.[619]

The standard posteroanterior view of the chest roentgenogram reveals marked leftward displacement of the cardiac silhouette, prominence of the main pulmonary artery, and interposition of radiolucent lung tissue between the aorta and main pulmonary artery or between the left hemidiaphragm and inferior cardiac border. This anomaly must be differentiated from other conditions that cause prominence of the left hilum or pulmonary artery on the standard chest film, including pulmonic valve stenosis, atrial septal defect, idiopathic dilatation of the pulmonary artery, and hilar adenopathy.

M-mode *echocardiographic findings* simulate those seen in right ventricular volume overload, including dilatation of the right ventricle and paradoxical anterior motion of the septum in systole, which is an artifact related to exaggerated cardiac rotation. Two-dimensional echocardiography can demonstrate localized bulging of the left ventricular contour and the drop-off of pericardial echoes.[620] Radionuclide perfusion imaging can be used to confirm the diagnosis by demonstration of a wedge of lung tissue between the heart and left hemidiaphragm;[621] computed tomography and magnetic resonance imaging can also be used to detect absence of the left pericardium by demonstrating visibility of the right pericardium and absence of the left pericardium, absence of the preaortic recess, and the abnormal presence of a wedge of lung between the aorta and pulmonary artery.[622,623]

Findings at cardiac catheterization are usually normal. Diagnostic left pneumothorax has been used in the past to outline the pericardium, but this procedure is hazardous and is now rarely needed to make the diagnosis of complete absence of the left pericardium if radiological and noninvasive imaging findings are compatible with the diagnosis. Cardiac catheterization with angiography is indicated only if there is a strong suspicion of associated congenital anomalies requiring surgical correction. Usually no specific therapy is required for management of complete absence of the left-sided pericardium.

PARTIAL ABSENCE. Partial left-sided pericardial defects may be complicated by herniation of the left atrial appendage, atrium, or left ventricle through the defect, associated with chest pain, syncope, and sudden death from cardiac strangulation.[624-627] The chest roentgenogram usually shows the nonspecific finding of prominence of the second arch of the left heart border, which must be distinguished from pulmonary artery dilation or aneurysm of the left atrial appendage.[628] Two-dimensional echocardi-

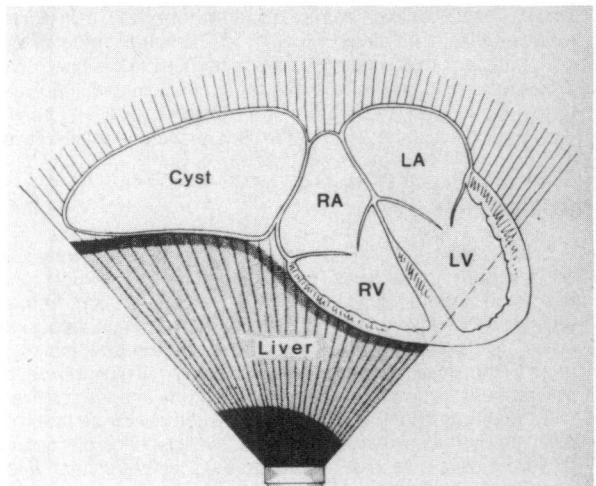
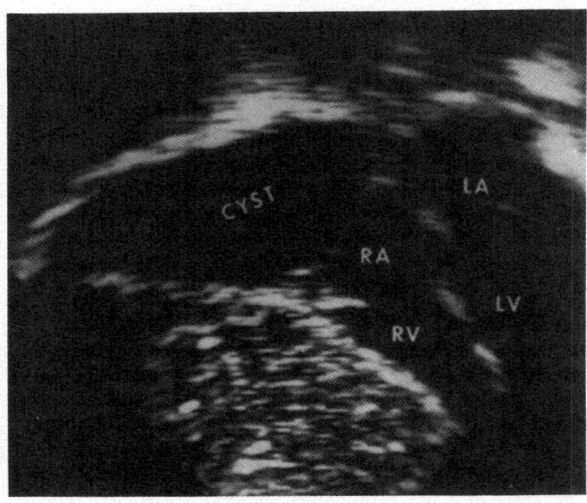

FIGURE 45–27. Two-dimensional subcostal echocardiographic appearance of a well-demarcated benign pericardial cyst adjacent to the right atrial (RA) wall. (From Hynes, J. K., et al.: Two-dimensional echocardiographic diagnosis of pericardial cyst. Mayo Clin. Proc. *58*:60, 1983.)

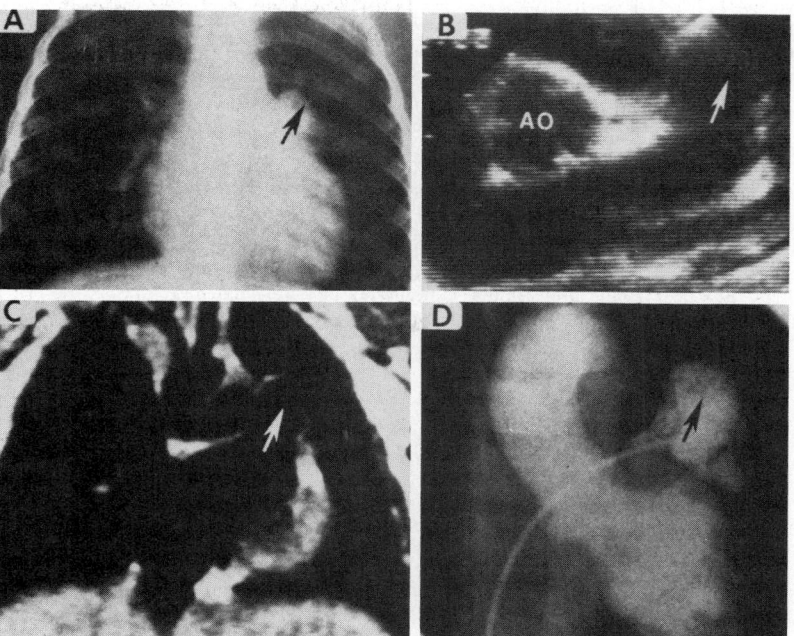

FIGURE 45–28. Noninvasive diagnostic features of partial absence of the left pericardium. The chest roentgenogram (*A*) shows knoblike prominence of the left atrial appendage (arrow). The short-axis cross-sectional 2-D echocardiogram (*B*) shows an enlarged left atrial appendage (arrow) extending beyond the pulmonary artery. The frontal plane magnetic resonance image (*C*) shows enlargement and lateral protuberance of the left atrial appendage (arrow). A contrast cineangiogram (*D*) with the catheter positioned across a patent foramen ovale in the left atrial appendage shows a characteristic wedge of lung between the aorta and pulmonary artery and confirms the herniation of the left atrial appendage (arrow). (From Altman, C. A., et al.: Noninvasive diagnostic features of partial absence of the pericardiaum. Am. J. Cardiol. 63:1536, 1989.)

ography and magnetic resonance imaging are helpful in demonstrating dilation of the left atrial appendage that extends beyond the pulmonary artery (Fig. 45–28).[628,629] Pulmonary artery angiography with follow-through of contrast opacification to the left heart is the standard method of definitively demonstrating herniation of the left atrium or left atrial appendage beyond the left heart border.[628,629] Partial herniation of the heart and diastolic collapse and compression of the coronary arteries through the defect is a complication of this anomaly that uncommonly may contribute to the development of chest pain and coronary artery strictures.[630,631]

The even rarer anomaly of partial right-sided pericardial defect may be associated with inspiratory right-sided chest pain secondary to herniation of the right atrium and right ventricle through the defect or herniation of lung into the pericardial cavity. The chest roentgenogram may show an unusual protuberance of the right heart border, and technetium-99m cardiac blood pool imaging may demonstrate that the abnormal contour of the right heart border fills simultaneously with the right atrium.[632] Right atrial angiography in the left anterior oblique projection is helpful in documenting herniation of the right atrium and right ventricle through the pericardial defect. Surgical treatment of partial left- or right-sided pericardial defects is usually indicated to relieve symptoms and prevent cardiac strangulation. The defect may be approached by excision of the atrial appendage, pericardioplasty, or pericardiectomy.[633]

REFERENCES

ANATOMY AND FUNCTIONS

1. Pericardial Diseases. *In* Fowler, N. O.: Diagnosis of Heart Disease. New York, Springer-Verlag, 1991, pp. 292–313.
1a. Holt, J. P.: The normal pericardium. Am. J. Cardiol. 26;455, 1970.
2. Alles, A., and Dom, R. M.: Peripheral sensory nerve fibers that dichotomize to supply the brachium and the pericardium in the rat. Brain Res. 342:382, 1985.
3. Ishihara, T., Ferrans, V. J., Jones, M., et al.: Histologic and ultrastructural features of normal human parietal pericardium. Am. J. Cardiol. 46:744, 1980.
4. Fukuo, Y., Nakatani, T., Shinohara, H., and Matsuda, T.: Pericardium of rodents: Pores connect the pericardial and pleural cavities. Anat. Res. 220:132, 1988.
5. Hills, B. A., and Butler, B. D.: Phospholipids identified on the pericardium and their ability to impart boundary lubrication. Ann. Biomed. Eng. 13:573, 1985.
6. Miyazaki, T., Pride, H. P., and Zipes, D. P.: Prostaglandins in the pericardial fluid modulate neural regulation of cardiac electrophysiological properties. Circ. Res. 66:163, 1990.
7. Lee, M. D., Fung, Y. C., Shabetai, R., and LeWinter, M. M.: Biaxial mechanical properties of human pericardium and canine comparisons. Am. J. Physiol. 253:H75, 1987.
8. Tyson, G. S., Jr., Maier, G. W., Olsen, C. O., et al.: Pericardial influences on ventricular filling in the conscious dog. Circ. Res. 54:173, 1984.
9. Shabetai, R.: Pericardial and cardiac pressure. Circulation 77:1, 1988.
10. Smiseth, O. A., Frais, M. A., Kingma, I., et al.: Assessment of pericardial constraint in dogs. Circulation 71:158, 1985.
11. Smiseth, O. A., Frais, M. A., Kingma, I., et al.: Assessment of pericardial constraint: The relation between right ventricular filling pressure and pericardial pressure measured after pericardiocentesis. J. Am. Coll. Cardiol. 7:307, 1986.
12. Boltwood, C. M., Jr.: Ventricular performance related to transmural filling pressure in clinical tamponade. Circulation 73:428, 1987.
13. Santamore, W. P., Constantinesco, M., and Little, W. C.: Direct assessment of right ventricular transmural pressure. Circulation 75:744, 1987.
14. Slinker, B. K., Ditchey, R. V., Bell, S. P., and LeWinter, M. M.: Right heart pressure does not equal pericardial pressure in the potassium chloride arrested canine heart in situ. Circulation 7G:357, 1987.
15. Hoit, B. D., Lew, W. Y., and LeWinter, M.: Regional variation in pericardial contact pressure in the canine ventricle. Am. J. Physiol. 255:H1370, 1988.
16. Bernard, H. L.: The functions of the pericardium. J. Physiol. 22:43, 1898.
17. Junemann, M., Smiseth, O. A., Refsum, H., et al.: Quantification of effect of pericardium on LV diastolic PV relation in dogs. Am. J. Physiol. 252:H963, 1987.
18. Gilbert, J. C., and Glantz, S. A.: Determinants of ventricular filling and of the diastolic pressure-volume relation. Circ. Res. 64:827, 1989.
19. Shirato, K., Shabetai, R., Bhargave, V., et al.: Alteration of the left ventricular diastolic pressure-segment length relation produced by the pericardium. Circulation 57:1191, 1978.
20. Smiseth, O. A., Manyari, D. E., Lima, J. A., et al.: Modulation of vascular capacitance by angiotensin and nitroprusside: A mechanism of changes in pericardial pressure. Circulation 76:875, 1987.
21. LeWinter, M. M., and Pavelec, R.: Influence of the pericardium on left ventricular end-diastolic pressure-segment relations during early and later stages of experimental chronic volume overload in dogs. Circ. Res. 50:501, 1982.
22. Freeman, G. L., and LeWinter, M. M.: Pericardial adaptations during chronic cardiac dilation in dogs. Circ. Res. 54:294, 1984.
23. Frais, M. A., Bergman, D. W., Kingma, I., et al.: The dependence of the time constant of left ventricular isovolumic relaxation (tau) on pericardial pressure. Circulation 81:1071, 1990.
24. Serizawa, T., Carabello, B. A., and Grossman, W.: Effect of pacing induced ischemia on left ventricular diastolic pressure-volume relations in dog with coronary stenosis. Circ. Res. 46:430, 1980.
25. Taylor, R. R., Covell, J. W., Sonnenblick, E. H., and Ross, J., Jr.: Dependence of ventricular distensibility on filling of the opposite ventricle. Am. J. Physiol. 213:711, 1967.
26. Brinker, J. A., Weiss, J. L., Lappe, D. L., et al.: Leftward septal displacement during right ventricular loading in man. Circulation 61:626, 1980.
27. Lorell, B. H., Palacios, I., Daggett, W. M., et al.: Right ventricular distention and left ventricular compliance. Am. J. Physiol. 240:H87, 1981.
28. Hoit, B. D., Dalton, N., Bhargava, V., and Shabetai, R.: Pericardial influences on right and left ventricular filling dynamics. Circulation Res. 68:197, 1991.
29. Santamore, W. P., Bartlett, R., Van Buren, S. J., et al.: Ventricular coupling in constrictive pericarditis. Circulation 74:597, 1986.
30. Mangano, D. T.: The effect of the pericardium on ventricular systolic function in man. Circulation 61:352, 1980.
31. Kanazawa, M., Shirato, K., Ishikawa, K., et al.: The effect of pericardium on the end-systolic pressure-segment length relationship in canine left ventricle in acute volume overload. Circulation 68:1290, 1983.
32. Goto, Y., Slinker, B. K., and LeWinter, M. M.: Nonhomogeneous left ventricular regional shortening during acute right ventricular pressure overload. Circ. Res. 65:43, 1989.
33. Stray-Gendersen, J., Musch, T. I., Haidet, G. C., et al.: The effect of pericardiectomy on maximal oxygen consumption and maximal cardiac output in untrained dogs. Circ. Res. 58:523, 1986.
34. Ringertz, H. G., Misbach, G. A., and Tyberg, J. V.: Effect of the normal pericardium on the left ventricular diastolic pressure-volume relationship. Acta Radiol. 22:529, 1981.

35. Jarvinen, A., Peltola, K., Rasanen, J., and Heikkila, J.: Immediate hemodynamic effects of pericardial closure after open-heart surgery. Scand. J. Thorac. Cardiovasc. Surg. 21:131, 1987.

36. Ludbrook, P. A., Byrne, J. D., Kurnik, P. B., and McKnight, R. C.: Influence of reduction of preload and afterload by nitroglycerin on left ventricular diastolic pressure-volume relations and relaxation in man. Circulation 56:937, 1977.

37. Ludbrook, P. A., Byrne, J. D., and McKnight, R. C.: Influence of right ventricular hemodynamics on left ventricular diastolic pressure-volume relations in man. Circulation 59:21, 1979.

38. Wong, C. Y., and Spotnitz, H. M.: Effect of nitroprusside on end-diastolic pressure-diameter relations of the human left ventricle after pericardiotomy. J. Thorac. Cardiovasc. Surg. 82:350, 1981.

39. Ross, J., Jr.: Acute displacement of the diastolic pressure-volume curve of the left ventricle: Role of the pericardium and the right ventricle. Circulation 59:32, 1979.

40. Lee, M. J., and Boughner, D. R.: Mechanical properties of human pericardium. Circ. Res. 57:475, 1985.

41. Bartle, S. H., and Hermann, H. J.: Acute mitral regurgitation in man. Hemodynamic evidence and observations indicating an early role for the pericardium. Circulation 36:839, 1967.

42. Lorell, B. H., Leinbach, R. C., Pohost, G. M., et al.: Right ventricular infarction. Am. J. Cardiol 43:465, 1979.

43. Goldstein, J. A., Vlahakes, G. H., Verrier, E. D., et al.: The role of right ventricular systolic dysfunction and elevated intrapericardial pressure in the genesis of low output in experimental right ventricular infarction. Circulation 65:513, 1982.

44. Janicki, J. S.: Influence of the pericardium and ventricular interdependence on left ventricular diastolic and systolic function in patients with heart failure. Circulation 81(Suppl. II):15, 1990.

ACUTE PERICARDITIS

45. Markiewicz, W., Brik, A., Brook, G., et al.: Pericardial rub in pericardial effusion: Lack of correlation with amount of fluid. Chest 77:643, 1980.

46. Spodick, D. H.: Pericardial rub: Prospective, multiple observer investigation of pericardial friction rub in 100 patients. Am. J. Cardiol. 35:357, 1975.

47. Spodick, D. H.: Diagnostic electrocardiographic sequences in acute pericarditis: Significance of PR segment and PR vector changes. Circulation 48:575, 1973.

48. Surawicz, B., and Lasseter, K. C.: Electrocardiogram in pericarditis. Am. J. Cardiol. 26:471, 1970.

49. Kouvaras, G., Soufras, G., Chronopoulos, G., et al.: The ST segment as a differential diagnostic feature between acute pericarditis and acute inferior myocardial infarction. Angiology 41:207, 1990.

50. Toriya Martinez, R. N., and Gonzalez Hermosillo, J. A.: Acute nonspecific pericarditis. Arch. Inst. Cardiol. Mex. 57:307, 1987.

51. Bruce, M. A., and Spodick, D. H.: Atypical electrocardiogram in acute pericarditis: Characteristics and prevalence. J. Electrocardiol. 13:61, 1980.

52. Carson, W.: Maximal spatial ST vector of ST segment elevation in the right praecordial leads on electrocardiogram due to acute pericarditis. Eur. Heart J. 9:665, 1988.

53. Wanner, W. R., Schaal, S. F., Bashore, T. M., et al.: Repolarization variant vs. acute pericarditis. A prospective electrocardiographic and echocardiographic evaluation. Chest 83:180, 1983.

54. Ginzton, L. E., and Laks, M. M.: The differential diagnosis of acute pericarditis. Circulation 65:1004, 1982.

55. Dressler, N.: Sinus tachycardia complicating and outlasting pericarditis. Am. Heart J. 72:422, 1966.

56. Spodick, D. H.: Frequency of arrhythmias in acute pericarditis determined by Holter monitoring. Am. J. Cardiol. 53:842, 1984.

57. Weiss, J. M., and Spodick, D. H.: Association of left pleural effusion with pericardial disease. N. Engl. J. Med. 308:696, 1983.

58. Olson, H. G., Lyons, K. P., Aronow, W. S., et al.: Technetium-99m stannous pyrophosphate myocardial scintigrams in pericardial disease. Am. Heart. J. 99:459, 1980.

59. Martin, P., Devriendt, J., Goffin, Y., and Verhas, M.: Gallium 67 scintigraphy in fibrinous pericarditis associated with bacterial endocarditis. Eur. J. Nucl. Med. 7:192, 1982.

60. Karjalainen, J., and Heikkila, J.: Acute pericarditis: Myocardial enzyme release as evidence for myocarditis. Am. Heart J. 111:546, 1986.

61. Saner, H. E., Gobel, F. L., Nicoloff, D. M., and Edwairds, J. E: Aortic dissection presenting as pericarditis. Chest. 91:71, 1987.

62. Permanyer-Miralda, G., Sagrista-Sauleda, J., and Soler-Soler, J.: Primary acute pericardial disease: A prospective series of 231 consecutive patients. Am. J. Cardiol. 56:623, 1985.

63. Sagrista-Sauleda, J., Permanyer-Miralda, G., Candell-Riera, J., et al.: Transient cardiac constriction: An unrecognized pattern of evolution in effusive acute idiopathic pericarditis. Am. J. Cardiol. 59:961, 1987.

64. Fowler, N. O., and Harbin, A. D.: Recurrent pericarditis: Follow-up of 31 patients. J. Am. Coll. Cardiol. 7:300, 1986.

65. Hatcher, C. R., Logue, R. B., Logan, W. D., et al.: Pericardiectomy for recurrent pericarditis. J. Thorac, Cardiovasc. Surg. 62:371, 1971.

66. Permanyer-Miralda, G., Sagrista-Sauleda, J., Shabetai, R., et al.: Acute pericardial disease: An approach to etiologic diagnosis and treatment. In Soler-Soler, J., Permanyer-Miralda, G., and Sagrista-Sauleda, J. (eds.): Pericardial Disease: New Insights and Old Dilemmas. Dordrecht, The Netherlands, Kluwer Academic Publishers, 1990, pp. 193–214.

PERICARDIAL EFFUSION

67. Carsky, E. W., Mauceri, R. A., and Azimi, F.: The epicardial fat pad sign: Analysis of frontal and lateral chest radiographs in patients with pericardial effusion. Radiology 137:303, 1980.

68. Miller, S. W.: Imaging pericardial disease. Radiol. Clin. North. Am. 27:1113, 1989.

69. Unverferth, D. V., Williams, T. E., and Fulkerson, P.K.: Electrocardiographic voltage in pericardial effusion. Chest 75:157, 1979.

70. Horowitz, M. S., Schultz, C. S., and Stinson, E. B.: Sensitivity and specificity of echocardiographic diagnosis of pericardial effusion. Circulation 50:239, 1974.

71. Berger, M., Bobak, K., Jelveh, M., and Goldberg, E.: Pericardial effusion diagnosed by echocardiography. Clinical and electrocardiographic findings. Chest 74:174, 1978.

72. Enein, M., Zina, A. A., Kassem, M., and el-Tabbakh, G.: Echocardiography of the pericardium in pregnancy. Obstet. Gynecol. 69:851, 1987.

73. Friedman, M. J., Sahn, D. J., and Haber, K.: Two-dimensional echocardiography and B-mode ultrasonography for the diagnosis of loculated pericardial effusion. Circulation 60:1644, 1979.

74. Iliceto, S., Amtonelli, G., Sorino, M., et al.: Two-dimensional echocardiographic recognition of complications of cardiac invasive procedures. Am. J. Cardiol. 53:846, 1984.

75. Shah, A., and Variyam, E.: Pericardial effusion and left ventricular dysfunction associated with ascites secondary to hepatic cirrhosis. Arch. Intern. Med. 148:585, 1988.

76. Soler-Soler, J.: Massive chronic idiopathic pericardial effusion. In Soler-Soler, J., Permanyer-Miralda, G., and Sagrista-Sauleda, J. (eds.): Pericardial Disease: New Insights and Old Dilemmas. Dordrecht, The Netherlands, Kluwer Academic Publishers, 1990, pp. 153–165.

77. Reddy, P. S., Curtiss, E. I., O'Toole, J. D., and Shaver, J. A.: Cardiac tamponade: Hemodynamic observations in man. Circulation 58:265, 1978.

78. Spodick, D. H.: The normal and diseased pericardium: Current concepts of pericardial physiology, diagnosis, and treatment. J. Am. Coll. Cardiol. 1:240, 1983.

79. Manyari, D. E., Kostuk, W. J., and Purves, P.: Effect of pericardiocentesis on right and left ventricular function and volumes in pericardial effusion. Am. J. Cardiol. 52:159, 1983.

80. Pegram, B. L., Kardon, M. B., and Bishop, V. S.: Changes in left ventricular internal diameter with increasing pericardial pressure. Cardiovasc. Res. 9:707, 1975.

81. Osborn, J. L., and Lawton, M. T.: Neurogenic antinatriuresis during development of acute cardiac tamponade. Am. J. Physiol. 250:H195, 1986.

82. Mancini, G. B. J., McGillem, M. J., Bates, E. R., et al.: Hormonal responses to cardiac tamponade: Inhibition of release of atrial natriuretic factor despite elevation of atrial pressures. Circulation 76:884, 1987.

83. Wechsler, A. S., Auerbach, B. J., Graham, T. C., and Sabiston, D. C.: Distribution of intramyocardial blood flow during pericardial tamponade: Correlation with microscopic anatomy and intrinsic myocardial contractility. J. Thorac. Cardiovasc. Surg. 68:847, 1974.

84. Brecher, G. A.: Critical review of recent work on ventricular diastolic suction. Circ. Res. 6:554, 1958.

85. Kostreva, D. R., Castaner, A., Pedersen, D. H., and Kampine, J. P.: Nonvagally mediated bradycardia during cardiac tamponade or severe hemorrhage. Cardiology 68:65, 1981.

86. Fowler, N. O., and Gabel, M.: The hemodynamic effects of cardiac tamponade: Mainly the result of atrial, not ventricular, compression. Circulation 71:154, 1985.

87. Fowler, N. O., Gabel, M., and Buncher, C. R.: Cardiac tamponade: A comparison of right versus left heart compression. J. Am. Coll. Cardiol. 12:187, 1988.

88. Kronton, I., Cohen, M. L., and Winer, H. E.: Diastolic atrial compression: A sensitive echocardiographic sign of cardiac tamponade. J. Am. Coll. Cardiol. 2:770, 1983.

89. Leimgruber, P. P., Klopfenstein, H. S., Wann, L. S., and Brooks, H. L.: The hemodynamic derangement associated with right ventricular diastolic collapse in cardiac tamponade: An experimental echocardiographic study. Circulation 68:612, 1983.

90. Gaffney, F. A., Keller, A. M., Peshock, R. M., et al.: Pathophysiologic mechanisms of cardiac tamponade and pulsus alternans shown by echocardiography. Am. J. Cardiol 53:1162, 1984.

91. Klopfenstein, H. S., Cogswell, T. L., Bernath, G. A., et al.: Alternations in intravascular volume affect the relation between right ventricular diastolic collapse and the hemodynamic severity of cardiac tamponade. J. Am Coll. Cardiol. 6:1057, 1985.

92. Singh, S., Wann, L. S., Schuchard, G. H., et al.: Right ventricular and right atrial collapse in patients with cardiac tamponade—a combined echocardiographic and hemodynamic study. Circulation 70:966, 1984.

93. Ruskin, J., Bache, R. J., Rembert, J. C., and Greenfield, J. C., Jr.: Pressure-flow studies in man: Effect of respiration on left ventricular stroke volume. Circulation 48:79, 1973.

94. Goldblatt, A., Harrison, D. C., Glick, G., and Braunwald, E.: Studies on cardiac dimensions in intact, unanesthetized man. II. Effects of respiration. Circ. Res. 13:448, 1963.

95. Wexler, L., Bergel, D. H., Gabe, I. T., et al.: Velocity of blood flow in normal human venae cavae. Circ. Res. 23:349, 1968.

96. Shabetai, R., Fowler, N. O., Fenton, J. C., and Masangkay, M.: Pulsus paradoxus. J. Clin. Invest. 44:1882, 1965.

97. Shabetai, R., Fowler, N. O., and Gueron, M.: The effects of respiration on aortic pressure and flow. Am. Heart J. 65:525, 1963.

98. Settle, H. P., Adolph, R. J., Fowler, N. O., et al.: Echocardiographic study of cardiac tamponade. Circulation 56:951, 1977.

99. Gonzales, M. S., Basnight, M. A., Appleton, C. P., et al.: Experimental pericardial effusion: relation of abnormal respiratory variation in mitral flow velocity to hemodynamics and diastolic right heart collapse. J. Am. Coll. Cardiol. 17:239, 1991.

100. Friedman, H. S., Sakurai, H., and Lajam, F.: Pulsus paradosus: A manifestation of marked reduction of left ventricular end-diastolic volume in cardiac tamponade. J. Thorac. Cardiovasc. Surg. 79:74, 1980.

101. Cohen, S. I., Kupersmith, J., Aroesty, J., and Rowe, J. W.: Pulsus paradoxus and Kussmaul's sign in acute pulmonary embolism. Am. J. Cardiol. 32:271, 1973.

102. Settle, H. P., Jr., Engel, P. J., Fowler, N. O., et al.: Echocardiographic study of the paradoxical arterial pulse in chronic obstructive lung disease. Circulation 62:1297, 1980.

103. Winer, H. E., and Kronzon, I.: Absence of paradoxical pulse in patients with cardiac tamponade and atrial septal defects. Am. J. Cardiol. 44:378, 1979.

104. Frey, M. J., Berko, B., Palevsky, H., et al.: Recognition of cardiac tamponade in the presence of severe pulmonary hypertension. Ann. Intern. Med. 111:615, 1989.

105. Guberman, B. A., Fowler, N. O., Engel, P. J., et al.: Cardiac tamponade in medical patients. Circulation 64:633, 1981.

106. Beck, C. S.: Two cardiac compression triads. J.A.M.A. 104:714, 1935.

107. Sznajder, J. I., Evander, E., Pollak, E. R., et al.: Pericardial effusion causes interstitial pulmonary edema in dogs. Circulation 76:843, 1987.

108. Cohn, J. N., Pinkerson, A. L., and Tristani, F. E.: Mechanism of pulsus paradoxus in clinical shock. J. Clin Invest. 46:1774, 1967.

109. Labib, S. B., Udelson, J. E., and Pandian, N. G.: Echocardiography in low pressure cardiac tamponade. Am. J. Cardiol. 63:1156, 1989.

110. Johnston, S. L., and Oliver, R. M.: Cardiac tamponade due to pneumopericardium. Thorax 43:482, 1988.

111. Katzir, D., Klinovsky, E., Kent, V., et al.: Spontaneous pneumopericardium: Case report and review of the literature. Cardiology 76:305, 1989.

112. Bricheteau: Observat d'hydropneumopercarde accompane d'un fluctuation perceptible a l'orielle. Arch. Gen. Med. 4:334, 1844.

113. Usher, B. W., and Popp, R. L.: Electrical alternans: Mechanism in pericardial effusion. Am. Heart. J. 83:459, 1972.

114. Friedman, H. S., Lajam, F., Calderon, J., et al.: Electrocardiographic features of experimental cardiac tamponade in closed-chest dogs. Eur. J.Cardiol. 6:311, 1977.

115. Mazurek, B., Jehle, D., and Martin, M.: Emergency department echocardiography in the diagnosis and therapy of cardiac tamponade. J. Emerg. Med. 9:27, 1991.

116. Chuttani, K., Pandian, N. G., Mohanty, P. K. et al.: Left ventricular diastolic collapse: An echocardiographic sign of regional cardiac tamponade. Circulation 83:1999, 1991.

117. Kronzon, I., Cohen, M. J., and Winer, H. E.: Contribution of echocardiography to the understanding of the pathophysiology of cardiac tamponade. J. Am. Coll. Cardiol. 1:1180, 1983.

118. D'Cruz, I. A., Cohen, H. C., Prabhus, R., and Glick, G.: Diagnosis of cardiac tamponade by echocardiography (changes in mitral valve motion and ventricular dimensions with special reference to paradoxical pulse). Circulation 52:460, 1975.

119. Appleton, C. P., Hatle, L. K., and Popp, R. L.: Cardiac tamponade and pericardial effusion: Respiratory variation in transvalvular flow velocities studied by Doppler echocardiography. J. Am. Coll. Cardiol. 11:1020, 1988.

120. Leeman, D. E., Levine, M. J., and Come, P. C.: Doppler echocardiography in cardiac tamponade: Exaggerated respiratory variation in transvalvular blood flow velocity integrals. J. Am. Coll. Cardiol. 11:572, 1988.

121. Burstow, D. J., Jae, K. O., Baileys, K. R., et al.: Cardiac tamponade: Characteristic Doppler observations. Mayo Clin. Proc. 64:312, 1989.

122. Shindler, D. M., Reddy, K., Shindler, O. I., and Kostis, J. B.: Failure of the aortic valve to open during inspiration in cardiac tamponade. Chest 82:797, 1982.

123. Singh, S., Wann, L. S., Klopfenstein, H. S., et al.: Usefulness of right ventricular diastolic collapse in diagnosing cardiac tamponade and comparison to pulsus paradoxus. Am. J. Cardiol. 57:652, 1986.

124. Cogswell, T. L., Bernath, G. A., Wann, L. S., et al.: Effects of intravascular volume on the value of pulsus paradoxus and right ventricular diastolic collapse in predicting cardiac tamponade. Circulation 72:1076, 1985.

125. Tunick, P. A., Nachamie, M., and Kronzon, I.: Reversal of echocardiographic signs of pericardial tamponade by transfusion. Am. Heart J. 119:199, 1990.

126. Martins, J. B., and Kerber, R. E.: Can cardiac tamponade be diagnosed by echocardiography? Circulation 60:737, 1979.

127. Miller, S. W., Feldman, L., Palacios, I., et al.: Compression of the superior vena cava and right atrium in cardiac tamponade. Am. J. Cardiol. 50:1287, 1982.

128. Levine, M. J., Lorell, B. H., Diver, D. J., and Come, P. C.: Implications of echocardiographically assisted diagnosis of pericardial tamponade in contemporary medical patients: Detection prior to hemodynamic embarrassment. J. Am. Coll. Cardiol. 17:59, 1991.

129. Northridge, D. B., McMurray, J., Ray, S., et al.: Release of atrial natriuretic factor after pericardiocentesis for malignant pericardial effusion. Br. Med. J. 299:603, 1989.

130. Safian, R. D., Come, S. E., Kadin, M., and Lorell, B. H.: Antemortem diagnosis of pulmonary microvascular tumor. Cathet. Cardiovasc. Diagn. 17:112, 1989.

131. Himelman, R. B., Kircher, B., Rockey, D. C., and Schiller, N. B.: Inferior vena cava plethora with blunted respiratory response: A sensitive echocardiographic sign of cardiac tamponade. J. Am. Coll. Cardiol. 12:1470, 1988.

132. Fowler, N. O., and Holmes, J. C.: Hemodynamic effect of isoproterenol and norepinephrine in acute cardiac tamponade. J. Clin. Invest. 48:502, 1969.

133. Kerber, R. E., Jascho, J. A., Litchfield, R., et al.: Hemodynamic effects of volume expansion and nitroprusside compared with the pericardiocentesis in patients with cardiac tamponade. N. Engl. J. Med. 306:929, 1982.

134. Moller, C. T., Schoonbee, C. G., and Rosendorff, C.: Hemodynamics of cardiac tamponade during various modes of ventilation. Br. J. Anaesth. 51:409, 1979.

135. Kilpatrick, Z. M., and Chapman, C. B.: On pericardiocentesis. Am. J. Cardiol. 16:722, 1965.

136. Krikorian, J. G., and Hancock, E. W.: Pericardiocentesis. Am. J. Med. 65:808, 1978.

137. Kaiser, E., and Loewenneck, H.: Pericardial puncture. The most favorable anatomical approach. Munch. Med. Wochenschr. 123:1697, 1981.

138. Heilerh, B., Anderes, U., and Follath, F.: Diagnosis and therapy of cardiac tamponade. An analysis of 50 patients. Schweiz. Med. Wochenschr. 111:735, 1981.

139. Callahan, J. A., Seward, J. B., Nishimura, R. A., et al.: Two-dimensional echocardiographically guided pericardiocentesis: Experience in 117 consecutive patients. Am. J. Cardiol. 55:476, 1985.

140. Pandian, N. G., Brockway, B., Simonetti, J. et al.: Pericardiocentesis under two-dimensional echocardiographic guidance in loculated pericardial effusion. Ann. Thorac. Surg. 45:99, 1988.

141. Morgan, C. D., Marshall, S. A., and Ross, J. R.: Catheter drainage of the pericardium: Its safety and efficacy. Can. J. Surg. 32:331, 1989.

142. Aron, D. C., Richardson, J. D., Webb, G., et al.: Subxiphoid pericardial window in patients with suspected traumatic pericardial tamponade. Ann. Thorac. Surg. 23:545, 1977.

143. Armstrong, N. F., Feigenbaum, H., and Dillon, J. C.: Acute right ventricular dilation and echocardiographic volume overload following pericardiocentesis for relief of cardiac tamponade. Am. Heart J. 107:1266, 1984.

144. Glasser, F., Fein, A. M., Feinsilver, S. H., et al.: Non-cardiogenic pulmonary edema after pericardial drainage for cardiac tamponade. Chest 94:869, 1988.

145. Lorell, B. H., and Grossman, W: Profiles in constrictive pericarditis, restrictive cardiomyopathy, and cardiac tamponade. In Grossman, W., and Baim, D. S. (eds.): Cardiac Catheterization, Angiography, and Intervention. 4th ed. Philadelphia, Lea and Febiger, 1991, pp. 633–653.

146. Erdman, S., Levinsky, L., Derivi, E., and Levy, M. J.: Closed pericardial drainage for relief of cardiac tamponade. Thorac. Cardiovasc. Surg. 34:66, 1986.

147. Lock, J. E., Bass, J. L., Kulif, F. J., and Fuhrman, B. P.: Chronic percutaneous pericardial drainage with modified pigtail catheters in children. Am. J. Cardiol. 53:1179, 1984.

148. Sinzobahamvya, N.: Results of subxiphoid pericardiostomy in pericardial effusion. Acta Chir. Belg. 88:175, 1988.

149. Palatianos, G. M., Thurer, R. J., and Kaiser, G. A.: Comparison of effectiveness and safety of operations on the pericardium. Chest 88:30, 1985.

150. Piehler, J. M., Pluth, J. R., Schaff, H. V., et al: Surgical management of effusive pericardial disease. J. Thorac. Cardiovasc. Surg. 90:506, 1986.

151. Little, A. G., and Ferguson, M. K.: Pericardioscopy as adjunct to pericardial window. Chest 89:53, 1986.

152. Millaire, A., Wurtz, A., Brullard, B., et al.: Value of pericardioscopy in pericardial effusion. Arch. Mal. Coeur 81:1071, 1988.

153. Endrys, J., Simo, M., Shafie, M. Z., et al: New nonsurgical technique for multiple pericardial biopsies. Cathet. Cardiovasc. Diagn. 15:92, 1988.

CONSTRICTIVE PERICARDITIS

154. Nishimura, R. A., Kazmier, F. J., Smith, H. C., and Danielson, G. K.: Right ventricular outflow obstruction caused by constrictive pericardial disease. Am. J. Cardiol. 55:1447, 1985.

155. Nigri, A., Mangieri, E., Martuscelli, E., et al.: Pulmonary trunk stenosis due to constriction by a pulmonary band. Am. Heart J. 114:448, 1987.

156. Meyer, T. E., Sareli, P., Marcus, R. H., et al.: Mechanism underlying Kussmaul's sign in chronic constrictive pericarditis. Am. J. Cardiol. 64:1069, 1989.

157. Hancock, E. W.: Constrictive pericarditis: Modern view of diagnosis and management. J. Cardiovasc. Med. 41:367, 1980.

158. Wolozin, M. W., Ortola, F. V., Spodick, D. H., and Seifter, J. L.: Release of atrial natriuretic factor after pericardiectomy for chronic constrictive pericarditis. Am. J. Cardiol. 61:1323, 1988.

159. Gaasch, W. H., Peterson, K. L., and Shabetai, R.: Left ventricular function in chronic constrictive pericarditis. Am. J. Cardiol. 34:107, 1974.

160. Dines, D. E., Edwards, J. E., and Burchell, H. B.: Myocardial atrophy in constrictive pancarditis. Proc. Staff Meet. Mayo Clin. 33:93, 1958.

161. Levine, H. D.: Myocardial fibrosis in constrictive pericarditis. Electrocardiographic and pathologic observations. Circulation 48:1268, 1973.

162. Gregory, M. A., Whitton, I. D., and Cameron, E. W.: Myocardial ischemia in constrictive pericarditis: A morphometric and electron microscopic study. Br. J. Exp. Pathol. 65:365, 1984.

163. Nichols, D. A., and Peter, R. H.: Constrictive pericarditis as a late complication of meningococcal pericarditis. Am. J. Cardiol. 55:1442, 1985.

164. Hancock, E. W.: On the elastic and rigid forms of constrictive pericarditis. Am. Heart J. *100*:917, 1980.

165. Paul, O., Castleman, B., and White, P. D.: Chronic constrictive pericarditis: A study of 53 cases. Am. J. Med. Sci. *216*:361, 1948.

166. Andrews, G.W.S., Pickering, G. W., and Sellors, T. H.: The aetiology of constrictive pericarditis with special reference to tuberculous pericarditis, together with a note on polyserositis. Q. J. Med. *17*:291, 1948.

167. Bashi, V. V., Ravikumar, J. S., Jairaj, P. S., et al.: Early and late results of pericardiectomy in 118 cases of constrictive pericarditis. Thorax *43*:637, 1988.

168. Blake, S., Bonar, S., O'Neill, H., et al: Aetiology of chronic constrictive pericarditis. Br. Heart J. *50*:273, 1983.

169. Cameron, J., Oesterle, S. N., Baldwin, J. C., and Hancock, E. W.: The etiologic spectrum of constrictive pericarditis. Am. Heart J. *113*:354, 1987.

170. Fischbein, L., Namade, M., Sachs, R. N., et al: Chronic constrictive pericarditis associated with asbestosis. Chest *94*:646, 1988.

171. Van der Horst, R. L.: Pericardial calcification in childhood. Cardiovasc. Radiol. *1*:265, 1978.

172. Bonische, C. H., and Jaffe, J. P.: Spontaneous severe constrictive pericarditis in congenital afibrinogenemia: Mechanism, evaluation and successful surgical management. Am. Heart J. *101*:503, 1981.

173. Laxer, R. M., Cameron, B. J., Chaisson, D., et al.: The camptodactyly-arthropathy-pericarditis syndrome: Case report and literature review. Arthritis Rheum. *29*:439, 1986.

174. Voorhees, M. L., Husson, G. S., and Blackman, M. S.: Growth failure with pericardial constriction. The syndrome of mulibrey nanism. Am. J. Dis. Child. *130*:1146, 1976.

175. Cotton, J. B., Rebelle, C., Bosnio, A., et al.: Familial intrauterine nanism with constrictive pericarditis: The Mulibrey syndrome. Pediatric *43*:197, 1988.

176. Tyberg, T. I., Goodyer, A. V. N., and Langou, R. A.: Genesis of pericardial knock in constrictive pericarditis. Am. J. Cardiol. *46*:570, 1980.

177. Manga, P., Vythilingum, S., and Mitha, A. S.: Pulsatile hepatomegaly in constrictive pericarditis. Br. Heart J. *52*:465, 1984.

177a. Anand, I. S., Ferrari, R., Kalra, G. S., et al.: Pathogenesis of edema in constrictive pericarditis. Circulation *83*:1880, 1991.

178. Plus, G. E., Brower, A. J., and Clagett, O. T.: Chronic constrictive pericarditis: Roentgenologic findings in 35 surgically proved cases. Proc. Staff Meet. Mayo Clinic. *32*:555, 1957.

179. MacGregor, J. H., Chen, J. T., Chiles, C. et al: The radiographic distinction between pericardial and myocardial calcifications. Am. J. Roentgenol. *148*:675, 1987.

180. Tomaselli, G., Gamsu, G., and Stolberg, M. S.: Constrictive pericarditis presenting as pleural effusion of unknown origin. Arch. Intern. Med. *149*:201, 1989.

181. Chesler, E., Mitha, A. S., and Matisonn, R. E.: The ECG of constrictive pericarditis—Pattern resembling right ventricular hypertrophy. Am. Heart J. *91*:420, 1979.

182. Fukuda, K., Nakamura, Y., Ogawa, S., et al.: Constrictive pericarditis with electrocardiographic evidence of right ventricular hypertrophy. Chest *96*:691, 1989.

183. Schnittger, I, Bowden, R. E., Abrams, J., and Popp, R. L.: Echocardiography: Pericardial thickening and constrictive pericarditis. Am. J. Cardiol. *42*:388, 1978.

184. Doi, Y. L., Sugiura, T., and Spodick, D. H.: Motion of pulmonic valve and constrictive pericarditis. Chest *80*:513, 1981.

185. Tei, C., Child, J. S., Tanaka, H., and Shah, P. M.: Atrial systolic notch on the interventricular septal echogram: An echocardiographic sign of constrictive pericarditis. J. Am. Coll. Cardiol. *1*:907, 1983.

186. Trappe, H. J., Herrmann, G., Daniel, W. G., et al.: Reduced diastolic left ventricular posterior wall motion in patients with constrictive pericarditis: Incidence, hemodynamic and clinical correlations. Int. J. Cardiol. *20*:53, 1988.

187. Engle, P. J., Fowler, N. O., Tei, C. W., et al.: M-mode echocardiography in constrictive pericarditis. J. Am. Coll. Cardiol. *6*:471, 1985.

188. Janos, G. G., Arjunan, K., Meyer, R. A., et al.: Differentiation of constrictive pericarditis and restrictive cardiomyopathy using digitized echocardiography. J. Am. Coll. Cardiol. *1*:541, 1983.

189. D'Cruz, I. A., Dick, A., Gross, C. M., et al.: Abnormal left ventricular–left atrial posterior wall contour: A new two-dimensional echocardiographic sign in constrictive pericarditis. Am. Heart J. *118*:128, 1989.

190. Lewis, B. S.: Real time two-dimensional echocardiography in constrictive pericarditis. Am. J. Cardiol. *49*:1789, 1982.

191. Hjemdahl-Monson, C. E., Daniels, J., Kaufman, D., et al.: Spontaneous contrast in the inferior vena cava in a patient with constrictive pericarditis. J. Am. Coll. Cardiol. *4*:165, 1984.

192. Himelman, R. B., Lee, E., and Schiller, N. B.: Septal bounce, vena cava plethora, and pericardial adhesion: Informative two-dimensional echocardiographic signs in the diagnosis of pericardial constriction. J. Am. Soc. Echocadiogr. *1*:333, 1988.

193. Pandian, N. G., Skorton, D. J., Kieso, R. A., and Kerber, R. E.: Diagnosis of constrictive pericarditis by two-dimensional echocardiography: Studies in a new experimental model and in patients. J. Am. Coll. Cardiol. *4*:1164, 1984.

194. Von Bibra, H., Schober, K., Jenni, R., et al.: Diagnosis of constrictive pericarditis by pulsed Doppler echocardiography of the hepatic vein. Am. J. Cardiol. *63*:483, 1989.

195. Sutton, F. J., Whitney, N. O., and Applefeld, M.M.: The role of echocardiography and computed tomography in the evaluation of constrictive pericarditis. Am. Heart J. *109*:350, 1985.

196. Nishimura, R. A., Connolly, D. C., Parkin, T. W., and Stanson, A. W.: Constrictive pericarditis: Assessment of current diagnostic procedures. Mayo Clin. Proc. *60*:397, 1985.

197. Reinmuller, R., Doppman, J. L., Lossner, J. et al.: Constrictive pericardial disease: Prognostic significance of a nonvisualized left ventricular wall. Radiology *156*:753, 1985.

198. Soulen, R. L., Stark, D. D., and Higgins, C. B.: Magnetic resonance imaging of constrictive pericardial disease. Am. J. Cardiol. *55*:480, 1985.

199. Solano, F. X., Young, E., Talamo, T. S., and Dekker, A: Constrictive pericarditis mimicking Budd-Chiari syndrome. Am. J. Med. *80*:113, 1986.

200. Savage, M. P., Munoz, S. J., Herman, W. M., and Kusiak, V. M.: Chylous ascites caused by constrictive pericarditis. Am. J. Gastroenterol. *82*:1088, 1987.

201. Wilkinson, P., Pinto, B., and Senior, J. R.: Reversible protein-losing enteropathy with intestinal lymphangiectasia, secondary to chronic constrictive pericarditis. N. Engl. J. Med. *273*:1178, 1965.

202. Pastor, B. H., and Cahn, M.: Reversible nephrotic syndrome resulting from constrictive pericarditis. N. Engl. J. Med. *262*:872, 1960.

203. Wasserman, A. J., Richardson, D. W., Baird, C. L., and Wyso, E. M.: Cardiac hemochromatosis simulating constrictive pericarditis. Am. J. Med. *32*:316, 1962.

204. Arrillo, J. E., Borer, J. S., Henry, W. L., et al.: The cardiovascular manifestations of the hypereosinophilic syndrome. Am. J. Med. *67*:572, 1979.

205. Lui, C. Y., and Makoui, C.: Severe constrictive pericarditis as an unsuspected cause of death in a patient with idiopathic hypereosinophilic syndrome and restrictive cardiomyopathy. Clin. Cardiol. *11*:502, 1988.

206. Siguera-Filho, A. G., Cunha, C. L. P., Tajik, A. J., et al.: M-mode and two-dimensional echocardiographic features in cardiac amyloidosis. Circulation *63*:188, 1981.

207. Carroll, J. D., Gaasch, W. H., and McAdam, K.P.W.J.: Amyloid cardiomyopathy: Characterization by a distinctive voltage/mass ratio. Am. J. Cardiol. *49*:9, 1982.

208. Bush, C. A., Stang, J. M., Wooley, C. G., and Kilman, J.: Occult constrictive pericardial disease. Diagnosis by rapid volume expansion and correction by pericardiectomy. Circulation *56*:924, 1977.

209. Lewis, B. S., and Gotsman, M. S.: Left ventricular function in systole and diastole in constrictive pericarditis. Am. Heart J. *86*:23, 1973.

210. Goldberg, E., Stein, J., Berger, M., and Berdoff, R. L.: Diastolic segmental coronary artery obliteration in constrictive pericarditis. Cathet. Cardiovasc. Diagn. *7*:197, 1981.

211. Vallance, P.J.T., Gray, H. H., and Oldershaw, P. J.: Diagnostic features of localised pericardial constriction. Int. J. Cardiol. *20*:416, 1988.

212. Meaney, E., Shabetai, R., and Bhargava, V.: Cardiac amyloidosis, constrictive pericarditis and restrictive cardiomyopathy. Am. J. Cardiol. *38*:547, 1976.

213. Swanton, R. H., Brooksby, I.A.B., Davies, M. J., et al.: Systolic and diastolic ventricular function in cardiac amyloidosis. Studies in six cases diagnosed with endomyocardial biopsy. Am. J. Cardiol. *39*:658, 1977.

214. Benotti, J. R., Grossman, W., and Cohn, P. F.: Clinical profile of restrictive cardiomyopathy. Circulation *61*:1206, 1980.

215. Robbins, M. A., Pizzarello, R. A., Stechel, R. P., et al.: Resting and exercise hemodynamics in constrictive pericarditis and a case of cardiac amyloidosis mimicking constriction. Cathet. Cardiovasc. Diagn. *9*:463, 1983.

216. Chew, C., Ziady, G., Raphael, M. J., and Oakley, C. M.: The functional defect in amyloid heart disease. Am. J. Cardiol. *36*:438, 1975.

217. Tyberg, T. I., Goodyer, A.V.N., Hurst, V. W., et al.: Left ventricular filling in differentiating restrictive amyloid cardiomyopathy and constrictive pericarditis. Am. J. Cardiol. *47*:791, 1981.

218. Aroney, C. M., Ruddy, T. D., Dighero, H., et al.: Differentiation of restrictive cardiomyopathy from pericardial constriction. J. Am. Coll. Cardiol. *13*:1007, 1989.

219. Morgan, J. M., Raposo, L., Chow, W. H., and Oldershaw, P. J.: Restrictive cardiomyopathy and constrictive pericarditis: Non-invasive distinction by digitised M mode echocardiography. Br. Heart J. *61*:29, 1989.

220. Klein, A. L., Oh, J. K., Miller, F. A., et al.: Two-dimensional and Doppler echocardiographic assessment of infiltrative cardiomyopathy. J. Am. Soc. Echocardiogr. *1*:48, 1988.

221. Hatle, L. K., Appleton, C. P., and Popp, R. L.: Differentiation of constrictive pericarditis and restrictive cardiomyopathy by Doppler echocardiography. Circulation *79*:357, 1989.

222. Schiavone, W. A., Calafiore, P. A., and Salcedo, E. E.: Transesophageal Doppler echocardiographic demonstration of pulmonary venous flow velocity in restrictive cardiomyopathy and constrictive pericarditis. Am. J. Cardiol. *63*:1286, 1989.

223. Schoenfeld, M. H., Supple, E. W., Dec, G. W., et al.: Restrictive cardiomyopathy versus constrictive pericarditis: Role of endomyocardial biopsy in avoiding unnecessary thoracotomy. Circulation *75*:1012, 1987.

224. Broadarick, S., Paine, R., Higa, E., and Carmichael, K. A.: Pericardial tamponade—A new complication of amyloid heart disease. Am. J. Med. *73*:133, 1982.

225. Kern, M. J., Lorell, B. H., and Grossman, W.: Cardiac amyloidosis masquerading as constrictive pericarditis. Cathet. Cardiovasc. Diagn. *8*:629, 1982.

226. Katagiri, M., Tanabe, Y., Takahashi, M., and Kasuya, S.: Right atrial thrombosis: Association with constrictive pericarditis. Ann. Thorac. Surg. *49*:145, 1990.

227. Copeland, J. G., Stinson, E. B., Griepp, R. B., and Shumway, N. E.: Surgical treatment of chronic constrictive pericarditis using cardiopulmonary bypass. J. Thorac. Cardiovasc. Surg. *69*:236, 1975.

228. Johnson, R. G., Thurer, R. L., Lorell, B. H., and Weintraub R. M.: Ultrasonic

debridement of calcified pericardium in constrictive pericarditis. Ann. Thorac. Surg. 48:855, 1989.

229. Culliford, A. T., Lipton, M., and Spencer, F. C.: Operation for chronic constrictive pericarditis: Do the surgical approach and degree of pericardial resection influence the outcome significantly? Ann. Thorac. Surg. 29:146, 1980.

230. McCaughlin, B. C., Schaff, H. V., Piehler, J. M., et al.: Early and late results of pericardiectomy for constrictive pericarditis. J. Thorac. Cardiovasc. Surg. 89:340, 1985.

231. Robertson, J. M., and Mulder, D. G.: Pericardiectomy: A changing scene. Am. J. Surg. 148:86, 1984.

232. Aagaard, M. T., and Haraldsted, V. Y.: Chronic constrictive pericarditis treated with total pericardiectomy. Thorac. Cardiovasc. Surg. 32:311, 1984.

233. Siefert, F. C., Miller, C. D., Oesterle, S. N., et al.: Surgical treatment of constrictive pericarditis: Analysis of outcome and diagnostic error. Circulation 72 (Suppl. 2):264, 1985.

234. Astrudillo, R., and Ivert, T.; Late results after pericardiectomy for constrictive pericarditis via left thoracotomy. Scand. J. Thorac. Cardiovasc. Surg. 23:115, 1989.

235. Bashi, I., Ravikumar, J. S., Jairaj, P. S., et al.: Early and late results of pericardiectomy in 118 cases of constrictive pericarditis. Thorax 43:637, 1988.

236. Potwar, S. A., Arsiwala, S S., Bhosle, K. N., and Mehta, V. I.: Surgical treatment of chronic constrictive pericarditis. Indian Heart J. 41:30, 1989.

237. Viola, A R.: The influence of pericardiectomy on the hemodynamics of chronic constrictive pericarditis. Circulation 48:1038, 1973.

238. Pick, R. A., Joswig, B. C., and Bloor, C. M.: Recurrent cardiac constriction after pericardiectomy. Arch. Intern. Med. 144:2061, 1984.

239. Kashani, I. A., Higgins, C. B., and Utley, J. R.: Inflammatory constriction following complete pericardiectomy in tuberculous constrictive pericarditis. Clin. Pediatr. 22:219, 1983.

240. Harrington, S. W.: Chronic constrictive pericarditis. Partial pericardiectomy and epicardiolysis in 24 cases. Ann. Surg. 120:468, 1944.

241. Walsh, T. J., Baughman, K. L., Gardner, T. J., and Bulkley, B. H.: Constrictive epicarditis as a cause of delayed or absent response to pericardiectomy. J. Thorac. Cardiovasc. Surg. 83:126, 1982.

242. Spodick, D. H., and Kumar, S.: Subacute constrictive pericarditis with cardiac tamponade. Dis. Chest 54:62. 1968.

243. Hancock, E. W.: Subacute effusive constrictive pericarditis. Circulation 43:183, 1971.

244. Martin, R. P., Bowden, R., Filly, K., and Popp, R. L.: Intrapericardial abnormalities in patients with pericardial effusion. Circulation 61:568, 1980.

SPECIFIC FORMS OF PERICARDITIS

Viral Pericarditis

245. Brodie, H. R., and Marchessault, V.: Acute benign pericarditis caused by Coxsackie virus group B. N. Engl. J. Med. 262:1278, 1960.

246. Celers, J., Celers, P., and Bertocchi, A.: Non-polio enterovirus in France from 1974 to 1985. Pathol. Biol. 36:1221, 1988.

247. Kleinfeld, M., Milles, S., and Lidsky, M.: Mumps pericarditis: Review of the literature and report of a case. Am. Heart J. 55:153, 1958.

248. Cheng, T. C.: Severe chest pain due to infectious mononucleosis. Postgrad. Med. 73:149, 1983.

249. Williams, A. J., Freemont, A. J., and Barnett, D. B.: Pericarditis and arthritis complicating chicken pox. Br. J. Clin. Pract. 37:226, 1983.

250. Adler, R., Takahashi, M., and Wright, H. T., Jr.: Acute pericarditis associated with hepatitis B infection. Pediatrics 61:716, 1978.

251. Fink, C., Schaad, V. B., and Socker, F. P.: Pericarditis as a complication of rubella. Schweiz. Med. Wochenschr. 117:28, 1987.

252. Beaman, M. H., and Hung, J.: Pericarditis associated with tick-borne Q fever. Aust. N. Z. J. Med. 19:254, 1989.

253. Tellez, A, Romero, J. M., and Leon, P.: Pericarditis caused by Q fever. Rev. Clin. Esp. 181:340, 1987.

254. Linz, D. H., Tolle, S. W., and Elliot, D. L.: Mycoplasma pneumoniae. Experience at a referral center. West. J. Med. 140:895, 1984.

255. Balaguer, A, Boronat, M., and Carrascosa, A.: Successful treatment of pericarditis associated with *Mycoplasma pneumoniae* infection. Pediatr. Infect. Dis. J. 9:141, 1990.

256. Malu, K., Longo-Mbenza, B., Lurhuma, Z., and Odio, W.:Pericarditis and the acquired immune deficiency syndrome. Arch. Mal. Coeur. 81:207, 1988.

257. Acierno, L. J.: Cardiac complications in acquired immune deficiency syndrome (AIDS): A review. J. Am. Coll. Cardiol. 13:1144, 1990.

258. Fink, L., Reichek, N., and St. John Sutton, M. G.: Cardiac abnormalities in acquired immune deficiency syndrome. Am. J. Cardiol. 54:1161, 1984.

259. Biton, A., and Herman, J.: Perimyocarditis. Report on an unusual cause. Postgrad. Med. 85:77, 1989.

260. Kassab, A., Demoulin, J. C., Vanlancker, M. A., et al.: Cytomegalovirus hemopericarditis. Acta Cardiol. 42:69, 1987.

261. Einsele, H., Ehninger, G., Vallbracht, A., et al.: Isolated pericardial relapse following allogeneic bone marrow transplantation for acute myelogenous leukemia. Bone Marrow Transplant.4:323, 1989.

262. Cammarosano, C., and Lewis, W.: Cardiac lesions in acquired immune deficiency syndrome (AIDS). J. Am. Coll. Cardiol. 5:703, 1985.

263. Scott, P. J., Conway, S. P., and DaCosta, P.: Cardiac tamponade complicating cytomegalovirus pericarditis in a patient with AIDS. J. Infect. 20:92, 1990.

264. Cohen, I. S., Anderson, D. W., Virmani, R. et al.: Congestive cardiomyopathy in association with the acquired immunodeficiency syndrome. N. Engl. J. Med. 315:628, 1986.

265. Toma, E., Poisson, M., Claessens, M. R., et al.: Herpes simplex type 2 pericarditis and bilateral facial palsy in a patient with AIDS. J. Infect. Dis. 160:553, 1989.

266. Cooper, D.K.C., and Sturridge, M. F.: Constrictive pericarditis following Coxsackie virus infection. Thorax 31:472, 1976.

267. Frisk, G., Torfason, E. G., and Diderholm, H.: Reverse immunoassays of IgM and IgG antibodies to Coxsackie B viruses in patients with acute myopericarditis. J. Med. Virol. 14:191, 1984.

268. Riecansky, I., Schreinerova, Z., Egnerova, A., et al: Incidence of coxsackie virus infection in patients with dilated cardiomyopathy. Cor. Vasa 31:325, 1989.

269. Muir, P., Nicholson, F., Tilzey, A. J., et al.: Chronic relapsing pericarditis and dilated cardiomyopathy: Serologic evidence of persistent enterovirus infection. Lancet 15:804, 1989.

270. Yoneda, S., Ohte, N., Samoto, T., et al.: Two cases of viral myocarditis and one case of viral pericarditis. Jpn. Circ. J. 46:1222, 1982.

Tuberculous Pericarditis

271. Larneu, A. J., Tyers, G. F., Williams, E. H., and Derrick, J. R.: Recent experience with tuberculous pericarditis. Ann. Thorac. Surg. 29:464, 1980.

272. Pogliani, E. M., Cortellaro, M., Foa, P., et al.: Cyclosporin A in the treatment of severe aplastic anemia: Description of a case complicated by the development of tuberculous pericarditis during treatment. Am. J. Hematol. 30:257, 1989.

273. Dalli, E., Quesada, A., Juan, G., et al: Tuberculous pericarditis as the first manifestation of acquired immune deficiency syndrome. Am. Heart J. 114:905, 1987.

274. Kinney, E. L., Monsuez, J. J., Kitzis, M. and Vittecog, D.: Treatment of AIDS-related heart disease. Angiology 40:970, 1989.

275. D'Cruz, I. A., Sengupta, E. E., Abrahams, C., et al.: Cardiac involvement, including tuberculous pericardial effusion, complicating acquired immune deficiency syndrome, Am. Heart J. 5:1100, 1986.

276. Desai, H. N.: Tuberculous pericarditis: A review of 100 cases. S. Afr. Med. J. 55:877, 1979.

277. Strang, J.I.G: Tuberculous pericarditis in Transkei. Clin. Cardiol. 5:667, 1984.

278. Gooi, H. C. and Smith, J. M.: Tuberculous pericarditis in Birmingham. Thorax 33:94, 1978.

279. Peel, A.A.F.: Tuberculous pericarditis. Br. Heart J. 10:195, 1948.

280. Auerbach, O.: Pleural, peritoneal, and pericardial tuberculosis. Am. Rev. Tuberc. 61:845, 1950.

281. Maisch, B., Maisch, S., and Kocksiek, K.: Immune reactions in tuberculous and chronic constrictive pericarditis. Am. J. Cardiol. 50:1007, 1982.

282. Schrire, V.: Experience with pericarditis of Groote Schuur Hospital, Cape Town; An analysis of one hundred and sixty cases over a six-year period. S. Afr. Med. J. 33:810, 1959.

283. Hageman, J. H., D'Esopo, N. D., and Glenn, W.W.L.: Tuberculosis of the pericardium: A long-term analysis of forty-four cases. N. Engl. J. Med. 270:327, 1964.

284. Long, E., Younes, M., Patton, N., and Hershfield, E.: Tuberculous pericarditis: Long-term outcome in patients who received medical therapy alone. Am. Heart J. 117:1133, 1989.

285. Quale, J. M., Lipschik, G. Y., and Heurich, A. E.: Management of tuberculous pericarditis. Ann. Thorac. Surg. 43:653, 1987.

286. Sagrista-Sauleda, J., Permanyer-Miralda, G., and Soler-Soler, J.: Tuberculous pericarditis: Ten year experience with a prospective protocol for diagnosis and treatment. J. Am. Coll. Cardiol. 11:724, 1988.

287. Fennell, W.M.P.: Surgical treatment of constrictive tuberculous pericarditis. S. Afr. Med. J. 62:353, 1982.

288. Agrawal, S., Radhakrishnan, S., and Sinha, N.: Echocardiographic demonstration of resolving intrapericardial mass in tuberculous pericardial effusion. Int. J. Cardiol. 26:240, 1990.

289. Lin, D. S., and Tipton, R. E.: Ga-67 cardiac uptake. Clin. Nucl. Med. 8:603, 1983.

290. Hirasing, R. A., and Van Bel, F.: Tuberculous pericarditis developing during chemotherapy. Eur. J. Resp. Dis. 63:73, 1982.

291. Barr, J. F.: The use of pericardial biopsy in establishing etiologic diagnosis in acute pericarditis. Arch. Intern. Med. 96:693, 1955.

292. Cheitlin, M. D., Serfos, L. J., Sbar, S. S., and Glosser, S. P.: Tuberculous pericarditis: Is limited pericardial biopsy sufficient for diagnosis? Am. Rev. Resp. Dis. 98:287, 1968.

293. Ocana, I., Martinez Vasquez, J. M., Sugura, R. M., et al.: Adenosine deaminase in pleural fluids: A test for the diagnosis of tuberculous pleural effusion. Chest 84:51, 1983.

294. Martinez Vasquez, J. M., Ribera, E., Ocana, I., et al.: Adenosine deaminase activity in tuberculous pericarditis. Thorax 41:888, 1986.

Bacterial (Purulent) Pericarditis

295. Strang, J. I., Kakaza, H. H., Gibson, D. G., et al.: Controlled trial of prednisolone as adjuvant in the treatment of tuberculous constrictive pericarditis in Transkei. Lancet 2:1418, 1987.

296. Klacsmann, P. B., Bulkley, B. H., and Hutchins, G. M: The changed spectrum of purulent pericarditis. An 86 year autopsy experience in 200 patients. Am. J. Med. 63:666, 1977.

297. Berk, S. L., Rice, P. A., Reynolds, C. A., and Finland, M.: Pneumococcal pericarditis: A persisting problem in contemporary diagnosis. Am. J. Med. 70:247, 1981.

298. Karjalainen, J.: Streptococcal tonsillitis and acute nonrheumatic myopericarditis. Chest 95:359, 1989.

299. Marsa, R. J., Blomquist, I. K., Bansal, R. C., et al.: Acute pericarditis due to group C Streptococcus: Report of a medically treated case. Am. J. Med. 86:474, 1989.

300. Rivera, J. M., Garcia-Bragado, F., Gomez, F. A., et al.: Brucellar pericarditis. Infection 16:254, 1988.

301. Haggman, D. L., Rehm, S. J., Moodie, D. S., and MacKenzie, A. H.: Nontyphoidal Salmonella pericarditis: A case report and review of the literature. Pediatr. Infect. Dis. 5:259, 1986.

302. Sanchez-Guerrero, J., and Alarcon-Segovia, D.: Salmonella pericarditis with tamponade in systemic lupus erythematosus. Br. J. Rheumatol. 29:69, 1990.

303. Vietzke, W. M.: Gonococcal arthritis with pericarditis. Arch. Intern. Med. 117:270, 1966.

304. Iggo, R., and Higgins, R.: Bilateral empyema and purulent pericarditis due to Haemophilus influenzae capsular type b. Thorax 43:582, 1988.

305. Evans, M. E., Gregory, D. W., Schaffner, W., and McGee, Z. A.: Tularemia: A 30-year experience with 88 cases. Medicine 64:251, 1985.

306. Finley, R. W., and Marr, J. J.: Anaerobic bacterial abscess following myocardial infarction. Am. J. Med. 78:513, 1985.

307. Rubin, R. H., and Moellering, R. C., Jr.: Clinical, microbiologic, and therapeutic aspects of purulent pericarditis. Am. J. Med. 59:68, 1975.

308. Holoshitz, J., Schneider, M., Yaretsky, A., et al.: Listeria monocytogenes pericarditis in a chronically hemodialyzed patient. Am. J. Med. Sci. 288:34, 1984.

309. Kahn, M. Y.: Subacute constrictive pericarditis from Serratia marcescens. Hum. Pathol. 14:1089, 1983.

310. Lieber, I. H., Rensimer, E. R., and Ericsson, C. D.: Campylobacter pericarditis in hypothyroidism. Am. Heart J. 102:462, 1981.

311. Blaser, M. J., Reingold, A. L., Alsever, R. N., and Hightower, A.: Primary meningococcal pericarditis: A disease of adults associated with serogroup C Neisseria meningitidis. Rev. Infect. Dis. 6:625, 1984.

312. Ejlertsen, T., Vesterlund, T., and Schmidt, E. B.: Myopericarditis with cardiac tamponade caused by Neisseria meningitidis serogroup W135. Eur. J. Clin. Microbiol. Infect. Dis. 7:403, 1988.

313. Brasier, A. R., Macklis, J. D., Vaughan, D., et al.: Myopericarditis as an initial presentation of meningococcemia. Unusual manifestation of infection with serotype W135. Am. J. Med. 82:641, 1987.

314. Luck, P. C., Helbig, J. H., Wunderlich, E., et al.: Isolation of Legionella Pneumophila serogroup 3 from pericardial fluid in a case of pericarditis. Infection 17:388, 1989.

315. Svendsen, J. H., Jonsson, V., and Niebuhr, V.: Combined pericarditis and pneumonia caused by Legionella infection. Br. Heart J. 58:663, 1987.

316. Pititalot, J. P., Allal, J., Thomas, P., et al.: Cardiac complications of infectious endocarditis. Ann. Med. Interne 136:539, 1985.

317. Weinstein, L.: Life-threatening complications of infective endocarditis and their management. Arch. Intern. Med. 146:953, 1986.

318. Suzuki, S., Tajimi, T., Takeshita, A., et al.: Isolated right heart purulent pericarditis forming a large mediastinal mass. Chest 93:667, 1988.

319. Olson, C. J., Edwards, W. D., Olney, B. A., et al.: Hemorrhagic cardiac tamponade: A clinicopathologic correlation. Mayo Clin. Proc. 59:785, 1984.

320. Horton, J. M., and Tucker, W. S., Jr.: Pericarditis with effusion and tamponade complicating left subdiaphragmatic abscess. West. J. Med. 149:213, 1988.

321. Hier-Madsen, K., Suanamaki, K. I., Wulff, J., et al.: Purulent pericarditis in children. Review and case report. Scand. J. Thorac. Cardiovasc. Surg. 19:185, 1985.

322. Sinzobahamvya, N., and Ikeogu, M. O.: Purulent pericarditis. Arch. Dis. Child. 62:696, 1987.

323. Fyfe, D. A., Hagler, D. J., Puga, F. J., and Driscoll, D. J.: Clinical and therapeutic aspects of Hemophilus influenzae pericarditis in pediatric patients. Mayo Clin. Proc. 59:415, 1984.

324. Chun, P. K., and Rocchini, A. P.: Occult constrictive pericarditis in infancy. Chest 78:648, 1980.

325. Leak, L. V., Ferrans, V. J., Cohen, S. R., et al.: Animal model of acute pericarditis and its progression to pericardial fibrosis and adhesions: Ultrastructural studies. Am. J. Anat. 180:373, 1987.

326. Gould, K., Barnett, J. A., and Sanford, J. P.: Purulent pericarditis in the antibiotic era. Arch. Intern. Med. 134:923, 1974.

327. Bouwels, L., Jansen, E., Janssen, J., et al.: Successful long-term catheter drainage in an immunocompromised patient with purulent pericarditis. Am. J. Med. 83:581, 1987.

328. Miller, G. C., and Witham, A. C.: Delayed febrile pleuropericarditis after sepsis. Ann. Intern. Med. 79:194, 1973.

329. Tan, J. S., Holmes, J. C., Fowler, N. O., et al.: Antibiotic levels in pericardial fluid. J. Clin. Invest. 53:7, 1974.

330. Biancaniello, T. M., Anagnostipoulos, C. E., Bernstein, H. E., and Proctor, C.: Purulent meningococcal pericarditis: Chronic percutaneous drainage with a modified catheter aided by echocardiography. Clin. Cardiol. 8:542, 1985.

331. Morgan, R. J., Stephenson, L. W., Woolf, P. K., et al.: Surgical treatment of purulent pericarditis in children. J. Thorac. Cardiovasc. Surg. 85:527, 1983.

332. Laaban, J. P., d'Orbcastel, O. R., Prudent, J., et al.: Primary pneumococcal pericarditis complicated by acute constriction. Intensive Care Med. 10:155, 1984.

Fungal Pericarditis

333. Wheat, L. J., Stein, L., Corya, B. C., et al.: Pericarditis as a manifestation of histoplasmosis during two large urban outbreaks. Medicine 62:110, 1983.

334. Chapman, M. G., and Kaplan, L.: Cardiac involvement in coccidioidomycosis. Am. J. Med. 23:87, 1957.

335. Ross, E. M., Macher, A. M., and Roberts, W. C.: Aspergillus fumigatus thrombi causing total occlusion of both coronary arterial ostia, all four major coronary arteries and coronary sinus and associated with purulent pericarditis. Am. J. Cardiol. 56:499, 1985.

336. Schwartz, D. A.: Aspergillus pancarditis following bone marrow transplantation for chronic myelogenous leukemia. Chest 95:1338, 1989.

337. Kraus, W. E., Valenstein, P. N., and Corey, G. R.: Purulent pericarditis caused by Candida: Report of three cases and identification of high-risk populations as an aid to early diagnosis. Rev. Infect. Dis. 10:34, 1988.

338. Glower, D. D., Douglas, J. M., Jr., Gaynor, J. W., et al.: Candida mediastinitis after a cardiac operation. Ann. Thor. Surg. 49:157, 1990.

339. Prager, R. L., Burney, D. P., Waterhouse, G., and Bender, H. W., Jr.: Pulmonary, mediastinal, and cardiac presentations of histoplasmosis. Ann. Thorac. Surg. 30:385, 1980.

340. Kaufman, L. D., Seifert, F. C., Eilbott, D. J. et al.: Candida pericarditis and tamponade in a patient with systemic lupus erythematosus. Arch. Intern. Med. 148:715, 1988.

341. Holtz, H. A., Lavery, D. P., and Kapila, R.: Actinomycetales infection in the acquired immunodeficiency syndrome. Ann. Intern. Med. 102:203, 1985.

342. Ramsdale, D. R., Gautam, P. C., Perera, B., and Charles, R. G.: Cardiac tamponade due to actinomycosis. Thorax 39:473, 1984.

343. Nahass, R. G., Scholz, P., MacKenzie, J. W., and Gocke, D. J.: Chronic constrictive pericarditis. A case report and review of the literature. Arch. Intern. Med. 149:1202, 1989.

344. Sagrista-Sauleda, J., Permanyer-Miralda, G., Juste-Sanchez, C., et al.: Huge chronic pericardial effusion caused by Toxoplasma gondii. Circulation 66:895, 1982.

345. Baid, C. S., Varma, A. R., and Lakhotia, M.: A case of subacute effusive constrictive pericarditis with a probable amoebic etiology. Br. Heart J. 58:296, 1987.

346. Blackett, K.: Amoebic pericarditis. Int. J. Cardiol. 21:183, 1988.

347. Strang, J. I.: Two-dimensional echocardiography in the diagnosis of amoebic pericarditis. S. Afr. Med. J. 71:328, 1987.

348. van der Horst, R.: Schistosomiasis of the pericardium. J. R. Soc. Trop. Med. Hyg. 73:243, 1979.

349. Chens, W.: Hydatid cysts in the pericardium—a new case and review of the literature. J. Thorac. Cardiovasc. Surg. 30:56, 1982.

350. Hafid, F., Maiza, E., Hammoudi, D., et al: Hydatid cyst of the pericardium and diaphragm. Pediatrie 44:331, 1989.

351. De Martini, M., Nador, F., Binda, A., et al.: Myocardial hydatid cyst ruptured into the pericardium: Cross-sectional echocardiographic study and surgical treatment. Eur. Heart J. 9:819, 1988.

352. Kinare, S. G., Parulkar, G. B., and Sen, P. K.: Constrictive pericarditis resulting from dracunculosis. Br. Med. J. 1:845, 1962.

353. Charon, A., and Sinha, K.: Constrictive pericarditis following filiariasis. Indian Heart J. 25:213, 1973.

354. Marcus, L. C., Steere, A. C., Duray, P. H., et al.: Fatal pancarditis in a patient with coexistent Lyme disease and babesiosis. Intern. Med. 103:374, 1985.

355. Lorcerie, B., Boutron, M. C., Portier, H., et al.: Pericardial manifestations of Lyme disease. Ann. Med. Interne 138:601, 1987.

356. Veyssier, P., Davous, N., Kaloustian, E, et al.: Cardiac involvement in Lyme disease. Rev. Med. Interne 8:357, 1987.

357. Page, S. R., Stewart, J. T., and Bernstein, J. J.: A progressive pericardial effusion caused by psittacosis. Br. Heart J. 60:87, 1988.

Pericarditis Following Acute Myocardial Infarction

358. Dubois, C., Smeets, J. P., Demoulin, J. C., et al.: Frequency and clinical significance of pericardial friction rubs in the acute phase of myocardial infarction. Eur. Heart J. 6:766, 1985.

359. Lichstein, E., Arsura, E., Hollander, G., et al.: Current incidence of postmyocardial infarction (Dressler's) syndrome. Am. J. Cardiol. 50:1269, 1982.

360. Krainin, F. M., Flessas, A. P., and Spodick, D. H.: Infarction-associated pericarditis. N. Engl. J. Med. 311:1211, 1984.

361. Tofler, G. H., Muller, J. A., Stone, P. H., et al.: Pericarditis in acute myocardial infarction: Characterization and clinical significance. Am. Heart J. 117:86, 1989.

362. Levine, H. D.: Subendocardial infarction in retrospect: Pathologic, cardiographic, and ancillary features. Circulation 72:790, 1985.

363. Galve, E., Garcia-del-Castillo, H., Evangelista, A., et al.: Pericardial effusion in the course of myocardial infarction: Incidence, natural history, and clinical relevance. Circulation 73:294, 1986.

364. Aarseth, S, and Lange, H. F.: The influence of anticoagulant therapy on the occurrence of cardiac rupture and hemopericardium following heart infarction: I. A study of 89 cases of hemopericardium. Am. Heart J. 56:250, 1958.

365. Lange, H. F., and Aarseth, S: The influence of anticoagulant therapy on the occurrence of cardiac rupture and hemopericardium following heart infarction. II. A controlled study of a selected treated group based on 1,044 autopsies. Am. Heart J. 56:257, 1958.

366. Karim, A. M., and Solomon, J.: Constrictive pericarditis after myocardial infarction. Am. J. Med. 79:389, 1985.

367. Low, R. I., Arthur, A., Kelly, P. B., and Takeda, P. A: Clotted hemopericardium post myocardial infarction presenting as effusive constrictive pericarditis. Am. Heart J. 109:905, 1985.

368. Liberthson, R. R., Salisbury, K. W., and Hutter, A. M., Jr.: Atrial tachyarrhythmias in acute myocardial infarction. Am. J. Med. 60:956, 1976.

369. Liem, K. L., Durrer, D, and Lie, K. L.: Pericarditis in acute myocardial infarction. Lancet 2:1004, 1975.

370. Limaye, S. B., and Stubberfield, J.: Cardiac tamponade following infarction: Management with pericardiocentesis and surgery. Aust. N. Z. J. Med. 15:446, 1985.

371. Coma-Canella, I., Lopez-Sendon, J., Gonzalez-Garcia, A, and Jadraque, L. M.: Hemodynamic effect of dextran, dobutamine, and pericardiocentesis in cardiac tamponade secondary to subacute heart rupture. Am. Heart J. 114:78, 1987.

372. Stryjer, D., Friedensohn, A., and Hendler, A.: Myocardial rupture in acute myocardial infarction: Urgent management. Br. Heart J. 59:73, 1988.

373. Sehgal, E., Sherman, W., Isom, O.W., et al.: Left ventricular pseudoaneurysm causing superior vena caval obstruction and effusive-constrictive pericarditis. J. Nucl. Med. 28:918, 1987.

374. Berman, J., Haffajee, C. I., and Alpert, J. S.: Therapy of symptomatic pericarditis after myocardial infarction: Retrospective and prospective studies of aspirin, indomethacin, prednisone, and spontaneous resolution. Am. Heart J. 101:750, 1981.

375. Hammerman, H., Kloner, R. A., Schoen, F. J., et al.: Indomethacin-induced scar thinning following experimental myocardial infarction. Circulation 67:1290, 1983.

376. Boden, W. E., and Sadaniantz, A.: Ventricular septal rupture during ibuprofen therapy for pericarditis after acute myocardial infarction. Am. J. Cardiol. 55:1631, 1985.

Uremic Pericarditis

377. Suki, W. N.: Pericarditis. Kidney Int. (Suppl.) 24:510, 1988.

378. Rutsky, E. A., and Rostand, S. G.: Treatment of uremic pericarditis and pericardial effusion. Am. J. Kidney Dis. 10:2, 1987.

379. Joffe, P., and Johannesen, A. C.: Uraemic pericarditis, an epidemic disease? Dan. Med. Bull. 34:117, 1987.

380. Maisch, B., and Kochsiek, K.: Humoral immune reactions in uremic pericarditis. Am. J. Nephrol. 3:264, 1983.

381. Lindsay, J., Jr., Crawley, I. S., and Callaway, G. M.: Chronic constrictive pericarditis following uremic hemopericardium. Am. Heart J. 79:390, 1970.

382. Frommer, J. P., Young, J. B., and Ayus, J. C.: Asymptomatic pericardial effusion in uremic patients: Effect of long-term dialysis. Nephron 39:296, 1985.

383. Yoshida, K., Shiina, A., Asano, Y. and Hosoda, S.: Uremic pericardial effusion: Detection and evaluation of uremic pericardial effusion by echocardiography. Clin. Nephrol. 13:260, 1980.

384. Leehey, D. J., Daugirdas, J. T., Popli, S., et al.: Predicting need for surgical drainage of pericardial effusion in patients with end-stage renal disease. Int. J. Artif. Organs 12:618, 1989.

385. Morlans, M.: Pericardial involvement in end stage renal disease. In Soler-Soler, J., Permanyer-Miralda, G., and Sagrista-Sauleda, J.: Pericardial Disease: New Insights and Old Dilemmas. Dordrecht, The Netherlands, Kluwer Academic Publishers, 1990, p. 123–139.

386. Masson, J. F., Maes, M. L., and Zilberman, C.: Pericarditis in chronic renal insufficiency treated by periodic hemodialysis. Rev. Med. Intern. 2:447, 1981.

387. Kwasnik, E. M., Koster, J. K., Lazarus, J.M., et al.: Conservative management of uremic pericardial effusions. J. Thorac. Cardiovasc. Surg. 76:629, 1978.

388. Rotler, M. N., and Swartz, C.: Predicting success of intensive dialysis in the treatment of uremic pericarditis. Am. J. Med. 76:38, 1984.

389. Spector, D, Alfred, H., Seidlecki, M., and Briefel, G.: A controlled study of the effect of indomethacin in uremic pericarditis. Kidney Int. 24:663, 1983.

390. Buselmeir, T. J., Davin, T. D., and Simmons, R. L.: Treatment of intractable uremic pericardial effusion: Avoidance of pericardiectomy with local steroid instillation. JAMA 240:1358, 1978.

391. Feinroth, M. V., Goldstein, E J., Josephson, A., and Friedman, E. A.: Infection complicating intrapericardial steroid instillation in uremic pericarditis. Clin. Nephrol. 15:331, 1981.

392. Quigg, R. J., Idelson, B. A., Yoburn, D. C., et al.: Local steroids in dialysis-associated pericardial effusion. Arch. Intern. Med. 145:2249, 1985.

393. Beaudry, C., Nakamoto, S., and Koloff, W. J.: Uremic pericarditis and cardiac tamponade in chronic renal failure. Ann. Intern. Med. 64:990, 1966.

394. Frame, J. R., Lucas, S. K., Pederson, J. A., and Elkins, R. C.: Surgical treatment of pericarditis in the dialysis patient. Am. J. Surg. 146:300, 1983.

395. Prager, R. L., Wilson, C. H., and Bender, H. W., Jr.: The subxiphoid approach to pericardial disease. Ann. Thorac. Surg. 34:6, 1982.

Neoplastic Pericarditis

396. Mukai, K., Shinkai, T., Tominaga, K., and Shimosato, Y.: The incidence of secondary tumors of the heart and pericardium: A ten-year study. Jpn. J. Clin. Oncol. 18:195, 1988.

397. Press, O. W., and Livingston, R.: Management of malignant pericardial effusion and tamponade. JAMA. 257:1088, 1987.

398. Posner, M. R., Cohen, G. I., and Skarin, A. T.: Pericardial disease in patients with cancer. Am. J. Med. 71:407, 1981.

399. Roberts, W. C., Bodey, G. P., and Wertlake, P. T.: The heart in acute leukemia: A study of 420 autopsy cases. Am. J. Cardiol. 21:388, 1968.

400. Roberts, W. C., Glancy, D. L., and DeVita, V. T.:Heart in malignant lymphoma (Hodgkin's disease, lymphosarcoma, reticulum cell sarcoma and mycosis fungoides): A study of 196 autopsy cases. Am. J. Cardiol. 22:85, 1968.

401. Thurber, D. L., Edwards, J. E., and Achor, R. W.: Secondary malignant tumors of the pericardium. Circulation 26:228, 1962.

402. Chan, H. S., Sonley, M. J., Moes, C. A., et al.: Primary and secondary tumors of childhood involving the heart, pericardium, and great vessels. Cancer 56:825, 1985.

403. Wilding, G., Green, H. L., Longo, D. L., and Urba, W. J.: Tumors of the heart and pericardium. Cancer Treat. Rev. 15:165, 1988.

404. Rudoff, J., Percy, R., Benrubi, G., and Ostrowski, M. L.: Recurrent squamous cell carcinoma of the cervix presenting as cardiac tamponade: Case report and subject review. Gynecol. Oncol. 34:226, 1989.

405. Malviya, V. K., Casselberry, J. M., Parekh, N., and Deppe, G.: Pericardial metastases in squamous cell cancer of the cervix. J. Reprod. Med. 35:49, 1990.

406. Venegas, R. J., and Sun, N. C.: Cardiac tamponade as a presentation of malignant thymoma. Acta Cytol. 32:257, 1988.

407. Skyggebjerg, K. D.: Hydrops fetalis caused by intrapericardial teratoma. Acta Obstet. Gynecol. Scand. 67:653, 1988.

408. Webber, H. S., Kleinman, C. S., Hellenbrand, W. E., et al.: Development of a benign intrapericardial tumor between 20 and 40 weeks of gestation. Pediatr. Cardiol. 9:153, 1988.

409. Brabham, K. R., and Roberts, W. C.: Cardiac-compressing intrapericardial teratoma at birth. Am. J. Cardiol. 63:386, 1989.

410. Gossinger, H. D., Siostrzonek, P., Zangeneh, M., et al.: Magnetic resonance imaging finding in a patient with pericardial mesothelioma. Am. Heart J. 115:1321, 1988.

411. Lund, O., Hansen, O. K., Ardest, S., and Baandrup, V.: Primary malignant pericardial mesothelioma mimicking left atrial myxoma. Scand. J. Thorac. Cardiovasc. Surg. 21:273, 1987.

412. Pasqual, M. A., Povar, J., Munoz, J. R., et al.: Pericardial mesothelioma. Rev. Esp. Cardiol. 42:559, 1989.

413. el-Naggar, A. K., Ro, J. Y., Ayala, A. G., et al.: Localized fibrous tumor of the serosal cavities. Immunohistochemical, electron microscopic, and flow-cytometric DNA study. Am. J. Clin. Pathol. 92:561, 1989.

414. Kim, E. E., Wallace, S., Abello, R., et al.: Malignant cardiac fibrous histiosarcomas and angiosarcomas: MR features. J. Comput. Assist. Tomogr. 13:627, 1989.

415. Montalescot, G., Chapelon, C., Drobinski, G., et al.: Diagnosis of primary cardiac sarcoma. Report of 4 cases and review of the literature. Int. J. Cardiol. 20:209, 1988.

416. Meissner, A., Kirch, W., Regensburger, D., et al.: Intrapericardial teratoma in an adult. Am. J. Med. 84:1089, 1988.

417. Naramoto, A, Itoh, N., Nakano, M., and Shigematsu, H.: An autopsy case of tuberous sclerosis associated wth primary pericardial mesothelioma. Acta Pathol. Jpn. 39:400, 1989.

418. Shimoyama, Y., Kawada, K., and Imamura, H.: A functioning intrapericardial paraganglioma (pheochromocytoma). Br. Heart J. 57:380, 1987.

419. Haedersdal, C., Hasselbalch, H., Devantier, A., and Saunamaki, K.: Pericardial haematopoiesis with tamponade in myelofibrosis. Scand. J. Haematol. 34:270, 1985.

420. Shih, L. Y., Lin, F. C., and Kuo, T. T.: Cutaneous and pericardial extramedullary hematopoiesis with cardiac tamponade in chronic myeloid leukemia. Am. J. Clin. Pathol. 89:693, 1988.

421. Markiewicz, W., Gladstein, E., London, E. J., and Popp, R. L.: Echocardiographic detection of pericardial effusion and pericardial thickening in malignant lymphoma. Radiology 123:161, 1977.

422. Fracp, M. B., Ingle, J. N., Giuliani, E. R., et al.: Pericardial effusion in women with breast cancer. Cancer 60:263, 1987.

423. Lopez, J. M., Delgado, J. L., Tovar, E., and Gonzalez, A. G.: Massive pericardial effusion produced by extracardiac malignant neoplasms. Arch. Intern. Med. 143:1815, 1983.

424. Theologides, A.: Neoplastic cardiac tamponade. Semin. Oncol. 5:181, 1978.

425. Nowicka, J., Haus, O., Dzik, T., et al.: Pericarditis in the course of acute leukemia. Folia Haematol. 114:220, 1987.

426. Steigman, C. K., Anderson, D. W., Macher, A. M., et al.: Fatal cardiac tamponade in acquired immunodeficiency syndrome with epicardial Kaposi's sarcoma. Am. Heart. J. 116:1105, 1988.

427. Engberding, R., Schulze-Waltrup, N., Grosse-Heitmeyer, W., and Stoll, V.: Transthoracic and transesophageal 2-D echocardiography in the diagnosis of peri- and paracardiac tumors. Dtsch. Med. Wochenschr. 112:49, 1987.

428. Pizzarello, R. A., Goldberg, S. M., Goldman, M. A., et al.: Tumor of the heart diagnosed by magnetic resonance imaging. J. Am. Coll. Cardiol. 5:989, 1985.

429. Brown, J. J., Barakos, J. A., and Higgins, C. B.: Magnetic resonance imaging of cardiac and paracardiac masses. J. Thorac. Imaging 4:58, 1989.

430. Safian, R. D., Come, S. E., Kadin, M., and Lorell, B. H.: Use of pulmonary capillary wedge aspirates for the antemortem diagnosis of pulmonary microvascular tumor. Cathet. Cardiovasc. Diagn. 17:112, 1989.

431. King, D. T., and Nieberg, R. K.: The use of cytology to evaluate pericardial effusions. Ann. Clin. Lab. Sci. 9:18, 1979.

432. Yazdi, H. M., Hajdu, S. I., and Melamed, M. R.: Cytopathology of pericardial effusions. Acta Cytol. J. 24:401, 1980.

433. Tatsuda, M., Yamamura, H., Yamamoto, R., et al.: Carcinoembryonic antigens in the pericardial fluid of patients with malignant pericarditis. Oncology 41:328, 1984.

434. Yancik, R., Reis, L. G., and Yates, J. W.: Breast cancer in aging women. A population-based study of contrasts in stage, surgery, and survival. Cancer 63:976, 1989.

435. Carter, C. L., Allen, C., and Henson, D. E.: Relation of tumor size, lymph node status, and survival in 24,740 breast cancer cases. Cancer 63:181, 1989.

436. Sundareswaren, R., Marshall, A. J., Pickard, J. G., and Tyrrell, C. J.: Pericardiocentesis and systemic cytotoxic therapy in the management of cardiac tamponade secondary to disseminated breast carcinoma. Br. Heart J. 60:162, 1988.

437. Shepherd, F. A., Morgan, C., Evans, W. K., et al.: Medical management of malignant pericardial effusion by tetracycline sclerosis. Am. J. Cardiol. 60:1161, 1987.

438. Hawkins, J. W., and Vacek, J. L.: What constitutes definitive therapy of malignant pericardial effusion? "Medical" versus surgical treatment. Am. Heart. J. 118:428, 1989.

439. Florentino, M. V., Daniele, O., Morandi, P., et al.: Intrapericardial instillation of platin in malignant pericardial effusion. Cancer 62:1904, 1988.

440. Figoli, F., Zanette, M. L., Tirelli, V., et al.: Pharmacokinetics of VM26 given intraperitoneally or intravenously in patients with malignant pericardial effusion. Cancer Chemother. Pharmacol. 20:239, 1987.

441. Ueno, Y., Kohgo, Y., Sasagawa, Y., et al.: A case of pericarditis carcinomatosa showing good response following local transfer of lymphokine-activated killer cells. Gan To Kagaku Ryoho 14:2579, 1987.

442. Cham, W. C., Freiman, A. H., and Carstens, P. H. B.: Radiation therapy of cardiac and pericardial metastases. Ther. Radiol. 114:701, 1975.

443. Stewart, J. R., and Fajardo, L. F.: Radiation-induced heart disease: An update. Prog. Cardiovasc. Dis. 27:173, 1984.

Radiation Pericarditis

444. Cosset, J. M., Henry-Amar, M., Girinski, T., et al.: Late toxicity of radiotherapy in Hodgkin's disease. The role of fraction size. Acta Oncol 27:123, 1988.

445. Tarbell, N. J., Thompson, L., and Mauch, P.: Thoracic irradiation in Hodgkin's disease: Disease control and long-term complications. Int. J. Radiat. Oncol. Biol. Phys. 18:275, 1990.

446. Mill, S. B., Baglan, R. J., Kurichety, P., et al.: Symptomatic radiation-induced pericarditis in Hodgkin's disease. Int. J. Radiat. Oncol. Biol. Phys. 10:2061, 1984.

447. Carmel, R. J., and Kaplan, H. S.: Mantle irradiation in Hodgkin's disease. Cancer 37:2813, 1976.

448. Coltart, R. S., Roberts, J. T., Thom, C. H., and Petch, M. C.: Severe constrictive pericarditis after single 16 MeV anterior mantle irradiation for Hodgkin's disease. Lancet 1:488, 1985.

449. Applefeld, M. M., Slawson, R. G., Spicer, K. M., and Singleton, R. T.: Long-term cardiovascular evaluation of patients with Hodgkin's disease treated by thoracic mantle radiation therapy. Cancer Treat. Rep. 66:1003, 1982.

450. Martin, R. G., Ruckdeschel, J. C., Chang, P., et al.: Radiation-related pericarditis. Am. J. Cardiol 35:216, 1975.

451. Applefeld, M. M., Slawson, R. G., Hall-Craigs, M., et al.: Delayed pericardial disease after radiotherapy. Am. J. Cardiol. 47:210, 1981.

452. Green, D. M., Gingell, R. L., Pearce, J., et al.: The effect of mediastinal irradiation on cardiac function of patients treated during childhood and adolescence for Hodgkin's disease. J. Clin. Oncol. 5:239, 1987.

453. Greenwood, R. D., Rosenthal, A., Cassedy, R., et al.: Constrictive pericarditis in childhood due to mediastinal irradiation. Circulation 50:1033, 1974.

454. Brosius, F. C., Waller, B. F., and Roberts, W. C.: Radiation heart disease. Am. J. Med. 70:519, 1981.

455. Castellino, R. A., Gladstein, E., and Turbow, M. M.: Latent radiation injury of lungs or heart activated by steroid withdrawal. Ann. Intern. Med. 80:593, 1974.

456. Morton, D. L., Kagan, A. R., Roberts, W. C., et al.: Pericardiectomy for radiation-induced pericarditis with effusion. Ann. Thorac. Surg. 8:195, 1969.

457. Ni, Y., von Segesser, L. K., and Turina, M.: Futility of pericardiectomy for postirradiation constrictive pericarditis? Ann. Thorac. Surg. 49:445, 1990.

PERICARDITIS RELATED TO HYPERSENSITIVITY OR AUTOIMMUNITY

458. Osler, W.: The Principles and Practice of Medicine. New York, D. Appleton and Company, 1892, p. 273.

459. Persellin, S. T., Ramirez, G., and Moatamed, F.: Immunopathology of rheumatic pericarditis. Arthritis Rheum. 25:1054, 1982.

460. Przybojewski, J. Z.: Rheumatic constrictive pericarditis. A case report and review of the literature. S. Afr. Med. J. 59:682, 1981.

461. Rathore, M. H., and Barton, L. L.: Acute rheumatic pericarditis. Pediatr. Infect. Dis. J. 8:183, 1989.

462. Ansari, A., Larson, P. H., and Bates, H. D.: Cardiovascular manifestations of systemic lupus erythematosus: Current perspective. Prog. Cardiovasc. Dis. 27:421, 1985.

463. Chang, R. W.: Cardiac manifestation of systemic lupus erythematosus. Clin. Rheum. Dis. 8:197, 1982.

464. Doherty, N. E., and Siegel, R. J.: Cardiovascular manifestations of systemic lupus erythematosus. Am. Heart. J. 110:1257, 1985.

465. Bulkley, B. H., and Roberts, W. C.: The heart in systemic lupus erythematosus and the changes induced in it by corticosteroid therapy. Am. J. Med. 58:243, 1975.

466. Kinney, E., Wynn, J., Hinton, D. M., et al.: Pericardial-fluid complement. Normal values. Am. J. Clin. Pathol. 72:972, 1979.

467. Wolf, R. E., King, J. W., and Brown, T. A.: Antimyosin antibodies and constrictive pericarditis in lupus erythematosus. J. Rheumatol. 15:1284, 1988.

468. Jacobsen, E. J., and Reza, M. J.: Constrictive pericarditis in systemic lupus erythematosus. Demonstration of immunoglobulins in the pericardium. Arthritis Rheum. 21:972, 1978.

469. Starkey, R. H., and Hahn, B. H.: Rapid development of constrictive pericarditis in a patient with systemic lupus erythematosus. Chest 63:448, 1973.

470. Ehrenfeld, M., Asman, A., Shpilberg, O., and Samra, Y.: Cardiac tamponade as the presenting manifestation of systemic lupus erythematosus. Am. J. Med. 86:626, 1989.

471. Porcel, J. M., Selva, A., Tornos, M. P., et al.: Resolution of cardiac tamponade in systemic lupus erythematosus with indomethacin. Chest 96:1193, 1989.

472. Thadani, U., Iveson, J. M., and Wright, V.: Cardiac tamponade, constrictive pericarditis and pericardial resection in rheumatoid arthritis. Medicine 54:261, 1975.

473. Escalante, A., Kaufman, R. L., Quismorio, F. P., Jr., et al.: Cardiac compression in rheumatoid arthritis. Semin. Arthritis Rheum. 20:148, 1990.

474. Kirk, J., and Cosh, J.: The pericarditis of rheumatoid arthritis. Q. J. Med. 38:397, 1969.

475. Sigel, L. H., and Friedman, H. D.: Rheumatoid pancarditis in a patient with well controlled rheumatoid arthritis. J. Rheumatol. 16:368, 1989.

476. Stables, R. H., Campbell, S., and Ormerod, O.J.M.: Haemopericardium in rheumatoid arthritis. Int. J. Cardiol. 23:268, 1989.

477. Breut, C., Drouelle, S., Lognone, S., et al.: Complications of rheumatoid pericarditis: Constriction and tamponade. Presse Med. 18:1151, 1989.

478. Alukal, M. K., Costello, P. B., and Green, F. A.: Cardiac tamponade in systemic juvenile rheumatoid arthritis requiring emergency pericardiectomy. J. Rheumatol. 11:222, 1984.

479. Newman, B., Park, S. C., and Oh, K. S.: Coexistent transient pulmonary edema and pericardial effusion. Pediatr. Radiol. 18:455, 1988.

480. Bagga, A., Kabra, S. K., Shankar, V., and Kalra, V.: Cardiac tamponade in juvenile rheumatoid arthritis. Indian Pediatr. 25:875, 1988.

481. Esdaile, J. M., Tannenbaum, H., and Hawkins, D.: Adult Still's disease. Am. J. Med. 68:825, 1980.

482. Jamieson, T. W.: Adult Still's disease complicated by cardiac tamponade. JAMA 249:2065, 1983.

483. Shimomoto, H., Imaizumi, K., Mizoguchi, K., and Ikeda, T.: A case of adult Still's disease with severe pulmonary complications. Nippon Kyobu Shikkan Gakkai Zasshi 27:1092, 1989.

484. Butman, S., Espinoza, L. R., Carpio, J. D., and Osterland, C. K.: Rheumatoid pericarditis. Rapid deterioration with evidence of local vasculitis. JAMA 238:2394, 1977.

485. Parkash, R., Atassi, A., Poske, R., and Rosen, K. M.: Prevalence of pericardial effusion and mitral valve involvement in patients with rheumatoid arthritis without cardiac symptoms. N. Engl. J. Med. 289:597, 1973.

486. Lam, D., and Rapaport, E.: Two-dimensional echocardiographic demonstration of intrapericardial fibrinous strands in rheumatoid pericarditis. Am. Heart J. 114:442, 1987.

487. Mathew, P. K.: Pericardial tamponade secondary to sudden steroid withdrawal in chronic rheumatoid arthritis. Chest 75:532, 1977.

488. Cotton, D. W., Cooper, C., Searle, M., et al.: Fatal cardiac tamponade complicating anticoagulant therapy in rheumatoid arthritis. Clin. Exp. Rheumatol. 5:367, 1987.

489. Thould, A. K.: Constrictive pericarditis in rheumatoid arthritis. Ann. Rheum. Dis. 45:89, 1986.

490. Keith, T. A.: Chronic constrictive pericarditis in association with rheumatoid disease. Circulation 25:477, 1962.

491. Nakano, T., Konishi, T., Yamamuro, M., et al.: Cardiac tamponade in rheumatoid arthritis. Successful treatment with intrapericardial steroid administration. Jpn. Heart J. 28:287, 1987.

492. Nassar, W. K., Miskin, M. E., and Rosenbaum, D.: Pericardial and myocardial disease in progressive systemic sclerosis. Am. J. Cardiol. 22:538, 1968.

493. Janosik, D. L., Osborn, T. G., Moore, T. L., et al.: Heart disease in systemic sclerosis. Semin. Arthritis Rheum. 19:191, 1989.

494. Smith, J. W., Clements, P. J., Levisman, J., et al.: Echocardiographic features of progressive systemic sclerosis. Am. J. Med. 66:28, 1979.

495. Uhl, G. S., and Kippes, G. M.: Pericardial tamponade in systemic sclerosis (scleroderma). Br. Heart J. 42:345, 1979.

496. Hanley, P. C.: Constrictive pericarditis associated with combined retroperitoneal and mediastinal fibrosis. Mayo Clin. Proc. 59:300, 1984.

497. Medsger, T. A., Jr., Masi, A. T., and Rodnan, G. P.: Survival with systemic sclerosis (scleroderma). A life-table analysis of clinical and demographic factors in 309 patients. Ann. Intern. Med. 75:369, 1971.

498. Alpert, M. A., Goldberg, S. H., Singsen, B. H., et al.: Cardiovascular complications of mixed connective tissue disease in adults. Circulation 69:1182, 1983.

499. Purice, S., Luca, R., Vintila, M., et al.: Cardiac involvement in progressive

systemic sclerosis and polymyositis: A comparative study in 116 patients. Med. Interne 27:209, 1989.

500. Tamir, R., Pick, A. J., and Theodor, E.: Constrictive pericarditis complicating dermatomyositis. Ann. Rheum. Dis. 47:961, 1988.

501. Shah, A., and Askari, A. D.: Pericardial changes and left ventricular function in ankylosing spondylitis. Am. Heart J. 113:1529, 1987.

502. Maryhew, N. L., Bache, R. J., and Messner, R. P.: Wegener's granulomatosis with acute pericardial tamponade. Arthritis Rheum. 31:300, 1988.

503. Csonka, G. W., and Oates, J. K.: Pericarditis and electrocardiographic changes in Reiter's syndrome. Br. Med. J. 1:866, 1957.

504. Goldman, M. J., and Lau, F. Y. K.: Acute pericarditis associated with serum sickness. N. Engl. J. Med. 250:278, 1954.

505. Shapiro, L., and Buckingham, R. B.: Septic rheumatoid pericarditis complicating Felty's syndrome. Arthritis Rheum. 24:1435, 1981.

506. Clementz, G. L., Gold, F., Khaiser, N., et al.: Giant cell arteritis associated with pericarditis and pancreatic insufficiency in a patient with psoriatic arthritis. J. Rheumatol. 16:128, 1989.

507. Sonnenblick, M., Nesher, G., and Rosin, A.: Nonclassical organ involvement in temporal arteritis. Semin. Arthritis Rheum. 19:183, 1989.

508. Granot, E., Rottem, M., and Rein, A. J.: Carditis complicating inflammatory bowel disease in children. Case report and review of the literature. Eur. J. Pediatr. 148:203, 1988.

509. Birnbaum, Y., and Shpirer, Z.: Cardiac involvement in inflammatory bowel disease. Harefuah 1:235, 1989.

510. Cullen, S., Duff, D. F., Denham, B., and Ward, O. C.: Cardiovascular manifestations in Kawasaki disease. Ir. J. Med. Sci. 158:253, 1989.

511. Erol, C., Sonel, A., Candan, I., et al.: Pericardial involvement in familial Mediterranean fever. Postgrad. Med. J. 64:453, 1988.

512. Crake, T., Sandie, G. I., Crisp, A. J., and Record, C. O.: Constrictive pericarditis and intestinal hemorrhage due to Whipple's disease. Postgrad. Med. J. 59:194, 1983.

513. Dawes, P. T., and Atherton, S. T.: Coeliac disease presenting as recurrent pericarditis. Lancet 1:1021, 1981.

514. Naschitz, J. E., Yeshurun, D., Miselevich, I., and Boss, J. H.: Colitis and pericarditis in a patient with eosinophilic fasciitis. A contribution to the multisystem nature of eosinophilic fasciitis. J. Rheumatol. 16:688, 1989.

515. Wanner, W. R., Williams, T. E., Fulkerson, P. K., et al.: Postoperative pericarditis following thymectomy for myasthenia gravis. A prospective study. Chest 83:647, 1983.

516. Silverman, K. J., Hutchins, G. M., and Bulkley, B. H.: Cardiac sarcoid: A clinicopathologic study of 84 unselected patients with systemic sarcoidosis. Circulation 58:1204, 1978.

517. Garrett, J., O'Neill, H., and Blake, S.: Constrictive pericarditis associated with sarcoidosis. Am. Heart J. 107:394, 1984.

518. Diderholm, E., Eklund, A., Orinius, E., and Widstrom, O.: Exudative pericarditis in sarcoidosis. Sarcoidosis 6:60, 1989.

519. Alarcon-Segovia, D.: Drug-induced lupus syndromes. Mayo Clin. Proc. 44:664, 1969.

520. Browning, C. A., Bishop, R. L., Heilpern, R. J., et al.: Accelerated constrictive pericarditis in procainamide-induced systemic lupus erythematosus. Am. J. Cardiol. 53:376, 1984.

521. Harrington, T. M., and Davis, D. E.: Systemic lupus-like syndrome induced by methyldopa therapy. Chest 79:696, 1981.

522. Schoenwetter, A. H, and Silber, E. N.: Penicillin hypersensitivity, acute pericarditis and eosinophilia. J.A.M.A. 191:136, 1965.

523. Slater, E. E.: Cardiac tamponade and peripheral eosinophilia in a patient receiving cromolyn sodium. Chest 73:878, 1978.

524. Yates, R. C., and Olson, K. B.: Drug-induced pericarditis. Report of three cases due to 6-amino-9-D-psicofuranosylpurine. N. Engl. J. Med. 265:274, 1961.

525. Krehlik, J. M., Hindson, D. A., Crowley, J. J., Jr., and Knight, L. L.: Minoxidil-associated pericarditis and fatal cardiac tamponade. West. J. Med. 143:527, 1985.

526. Miller, D. H., and Haas, L. F.: Pneumonitis, pleural effusion and pericarditis following treatment with dantrolene. J. Neurol. Neurosurg. Psychiatry 47:553, 1984.

527. Lipworth, B. J., and Oakley, D. G.: Surgical treatment of constrictive pericarditis due to practolol. A case report. J. Cardiovasc. Surg. 29:408, 1988.

528. Haugtomt, H., and Haerem, J.: Pulmonary edema and pericarditis after inhalation of teflon fumes. Tidsskr. Nor. Laegeforen 109:584, 1989.

529. Harbin, A. D., Gerson, M. C., and O'Connell, J. B.: Simulation of acute myopericarditis by constrictive pericardial disease with endomyocardial fibrosis to methysergide therapy. J. Am. Coll. Cardiol. 4:196, 1984.

530. Bristow, M. R., Thompson, P. D., Martin, R. P., et al.: Early anthracycline toxicity. Am. J. Med. 65:823, 1978.

531. Cazin, B., Gorin, N. C., Laporte, J. P., et al.: Cardiac complications after bone marrow transplantation. Cancer 57:2061, 1986.

532. Ratliff, N. B., McMahon, J. T., Shirey, E. K., and Groves, L. K.: Silicone pericarditis. Cleve. Clin. Q. 51:185, 1984.

533. Fraker, T. D., Jr., Walsh, T. E., Morgan, R. J., and Kim, K.: Constrictive pericarditis after the Beck operation. Am. J. Cardiol. 54:931, 1984.

534. Sonakul, D., Thakerngpol, K., and Pocaree, P.: Cardiac pathology in 76 thalassemic patients. Birth Defects 23:177, 1988.

535. Abdun Nur, D., Marcus, C. S., and Russell, F. E.: Pericarditis associated with scorpionfish (Scorpaena buttata) sting. Toxicon 19:579, 1981.

536. Dressler, W.: A postmyocardial infarction syndrome. Preliminary report of a complication resembling idiopathic recurrent benign pericarditis. JAMA 160:1379, 1956.

537. Jerjes-Sanchez, C., Ibarra-Perez, C., Ramirez-Rivera, A., et al.: Dressler-like syndrome after pulmonary embolism and infarction. Chest 92:115, 1987.

538. Dressler, W.: The post-myocardial infarction syndrome. A report of forty-four cases. Arch. Intern. Med. 103:28, 1959.

539. Van der Geld, H.: Anti-heart antibodies in the post-pericardiotomy and the post-myocardial infarction syndrome. Lancet 2:617, 1964.

540. Liem, K. L., ten Veen, J. H., Lie, K. I., et al.: Incidence and significance of heart muscle antibodies in patients with acute myocardial infarction and unstable angina. Acta Med. Scand. 206:473, 1971.

541. Weiser, N. J., Kantor, M., and Russell, H. K.: Post-myocardial infarction syndrome. Circulation 20:371, 1959.

542. Holloway, J. D.: Post-infarction pericarditis. Chronic symptoms in a middle-aged man. Postgrad. Med. 15:57, 1989.

543. Streifer, J., Pitlik, S., Dux, S., et al.: Dressler's syndrome after right ventricular infarction. Postgrad. Med. J. 60:298, 1984.

544. Hutchison, S. J., McKillop, J. H., and Hutton, I.: Failure of gallium-67 citrate imaging to diagnose post-myocardial infarction (Dressler's) syndrome. Eur. J. Nucl. Med. 13:52, 1987.

545. Hertzeanu, H., Almog, C., and Algom, M.: Cardiac tamponade in Dressler's syndrome. Cardiology 70:31, 1983.

546. Goldhaber, S. Z., Lorell, B. H., and Green, L. H.: Constrictive pericarditis. A case requiring pericardiectomy following Dressler's postmyocardial infarction syndrome. J. Thorac. Cardiovasc. Surg. 81:793, 1981.

547. Kanawaty, D. S., Burggraf, G. W., and Abdollah, H.: Constrictive pericarditis and anemia post myocardial infarction. Can. J. Cardiol. 5:147, 1989.

548. Soloff, L. A., Zatuchni, J., Janton, D. H., et al.: Reactivation of rheumatic fever following mitral commissurotomy. Circulation 8:481, 1953.

549. Engle, M. A., and Ito, T.: The postpericardiotomy syndrome. Am. J. Cardiol. 7:73, 1961.

550. Peters, R. W., Scheinman, M. M., Raskin, S., and Thomas, A. N.: Unusual complications of epicardial pacemakers. Am. J. Cardiol. 45:1088, 1980.

551. Livelli, F. D., Jr., Johnson, R. A., McEnany, M. T., et al.: Unexplained in-hospital fever following cardiac surgery: Natural history, relationship to postpericardiotomy syndrome and a prospective study of therapy with indomethacin versus placebo. Circulation 57:968, 1978.

552. Engle, M. A., Gay, W. A., Jr., Zabriskie, J. B., and Senterfit, L. B.: The postpericardiotomy syndrome: 25 years' experience. J. Cardiovasc. Med. 4:321, 1984.

553. Kaminsky, M. E., Rodan, B. A., Osborne, D. R., et al.: Postpericardiotomy syndrome. Am. J. Radiol. 138:503, 1982.

554. DeSaulniers, D., Gervais, N., and Rouleau, J.: Does pericardial drainage decrease the frequency of the postpericardiotomy syndrome? Can. J. Surg. 24:265, 1981.

555. Ofori-Krakye, S. K., Tyberg, T. I., Geha, A. S., et al.: Late cardiac tamponade after open heart surgery: Incidence, role of anticoagulants in its pathogenesis and its relationship to the postpericardiotomy syndrome. Circulation 63:1323, 1981.

555a. Kassanoff, A. H., and Martirossian, M. G.: Postpericardiotomy and post-myocardial infarction syndrome presenting as noncardiac pulmonary edema. Chest 99:1410, 1991.

556. Weitzman, L. B., Tinkler, W. P., Kronzon, I., et al.: The incidence and natural history of pericardial effusion after cardiac surgery—an echocardiographic study. Circulation 69:506, 1984.

557. Wheeler, E. O., Turner, J. D., and Scannell, J. G.: Fever, splenomegaly, and atypical lymphocytes. A syndrome observed after cardiac surgery utilizing a pump oxygenator. N. Engl. J. Med. 266:454, 1962.

558. Berger, R. L., Loveless, G., and Warner, O.: Delayed and latent postcardiotomy tamponade: Recognition and nonoperative treatment. Ann. Thorac. Surg. 12:22, 1971.

559. King, T. E., Jr., Stelzner, T. J., and Sahn, S. A.: Cardiac tamponade complicating the postpericardiotomy syndrome. Chest 83:500, 1983.

560. Gehl, L., Iskandrian, A. S., Goel, I., et al.: Cardiac perforation with tamponade during cardiac catheterization. Cathet. Cardiovasc. Diagn. 8:293, 1982.

561. B-Lundqvist, C., Olsson, S. B., and Varnauskas, E.: Transseptal left heart catheterization: A review of 278 studies. Clin. Cardiol. 9:21, 1986.

562. Foster, C. J.: Constrictive pericarditis complicating an endocardial pacemaker. Br. Heart J. 47:497, 1982.

563. Goldbaum, T. S., Jacob, A. S., Smith, D. F., et al.: Cardiac tamponade following percutaneous transluminal coronary angioplasty. Cathet. Cardiovasc. Diagn. 11:413, 1985.

564. Slack, J. D., Pinkerton, C. A., and Nassar, W. K.: Acute pericarditis after percutaneous transluminal coronary angioplasty. Am. J. Cardiol. 55:843, 1985.

565. Koller, H.: Pericardial tamponade as a lethal complication following dilation of aortic valve stenosis. Wien Med. Wochenschr. 137:255, 1987.

566. Bichel, J.: Serious complications of sternal puncture. Ugeskr. Laeger 151:442, 1989.

567. Mellon, J. K., Galvin, J. F., Bowe, P. C., et al.: Oesophago-pericardial fistula and cardiac tamponade after oesophagoscopy. Eur. J. Cardiothorac. Surg. 2:282, 1988.

568. Puhakka, H. J.: Complications of mediastinoscopy. J. Laryngol. Otol. 103:312, 1989.

569. Knauer, C. M., and Fogel, M. R.: Pericarditis: Complication of esophageal sclerotherapy. A report of three cases. Gastroenterology 93:287, 1987.

570. Brown, D. L., and Luchi, R. J.: Cardiac tamponade and constrictive pericarditis complicating endoscopic sclerotherapy. Arch. Intern. Med. 147:2169, 1987.

571. Lindenau, K. F., Warnke, H., and Bergmann, U.: Cardiac tamponade following open heart surgery. Zentralbl. Chir. 104:1345, 1979.

572. Marx, P., Jaffe, C., Laks, H., and Wolfson, S.: Delayed post-cardiac-surgery

tamponade producing localized right atrial compression. Cathet Cardiovasc. Diagn. 7:275, 1981.

573. Huwer, H., Vokmer, I., and Dyckmans, J.: Late pericardial tamponade after aortic and mitral valve replacement. Thorac. Cardiovasc. Surg. 36:54, 1988.

574. Ng, A. S. H., Dorosti, K., and Sheldon, W. C.: Constrictive pericarditis following cardiac surgery—Cleveland Clinic experience: Report of 12 cases and review. Cleve. Clin. Q. 50:39, 1984.

575. Cimino, J. J., and Kogan, A. D.: Constrictive pericarditis after cardiac surgery: Report of three cases and review of the literature. Am. Heart J. 118:1292, 1989.

576. Killian, D. M., Furiasse, J. G., Scanlon, P. J., et al.: Constrictive pericarditis after cardiac surgery. Am. Heart J. 118:563, 1989.

577. Ribiero, P., Sapsford, R., Evans, T., et al.: Constrictive pericarditis as a complication of coronary artery bypass surgery. Br. Heart J. 51:205, 1984.

578. Kabbani, S. S., Bashour, T., Ellertson, D. G., et al.: Constrictive pericarditis following myocardial revascularization: A possible cause of graft occlusion. Am. Heart J. 110:493, 1985.

579. Bewtra, C., and Schultz, R. D.: Constrictive calcific pericarditis following coronary arterial bypass surgery. Hum. Pathol. 16:522, 1985.

580. Almassi, G. H., Chapman, R. D., Troup, P. J., et al.: Constrictive pericarditis associated with patch electrodes of the automatic implantable cardioverter-defibrillator. Chest 92:369, 1987.

581. Singer, I., Hutchins, G. M., Mirowski, M., et al.: Pathologic findings related to the lead system and repeated defibrillations in patients with the automatic implantable cardioverter-defibrillator. J. Am. Coll. Cardiol. 10:382, 1987.

582. Kerber, R. E., and Sherman, B.: Echocardiographic evaluation of pericardial effusion in myxedema. Incidence and biochemical and clinical correlations. Circulation 52:823, 1975.

583. Hardisty, C. A., Naik, D. R., and Munro, D. S.: Pericardial effusion in hypothyroidism. Clin. Endocrinol. 13:349, 1980.

584. Parving, H., Hansen, J. M., Nielsen, S. V., et al.: Mechanisms of edema formation in myxedema-increased protein extravasation and relatively slow lymphatic drainage. N. Engl. J. Med. 301:460, 1981.

585. Zimmerman, J., Yahalom, J., and Bar-On, H.: Clinical spectrum of pericardial effusion as the presenting feature of hypothyroidism. Am. Heart J. 106:770, 1983.

586. Das, S., Lieberman, A. N., and Schussler, G. C.: Prolonged persistence of a large pericardial effusion and hemodynamic evidence of cardiac tamponade during treatment of myxedema. Clin. Cardiol. 5:459, 1982.

587. Manolis, A. S., Varriale, P., and Ostrowski, R. M.: Hypothyroid cardiac tamponade. Arch. Intern. Med. 147:1167, 1987.

588. Rosenbau, D. L., and Yu, P. N.: Idiopathic cholesterol pericarditis with effusion. Am. Heart J. 70:515, 1965.

589. Van Buren, P. C., and Roberts, W. C.: Cholesterol pericarditis and cardiac tamponade with congenital hypothyroidism in adulthood. Am. Heart J. 119:697, 1990.

590. Ridenhouse, C. E., and Kiphart, R. J.: Idiopathic cholesterol pericarditis treatment with pericardiectomy. Ann. Thorac. Surg. 4:360, 1967.

591. Stanley, R. J., Subramanian, R., and Lie, J. T.: Cholesterol pericarditis terminating as constrictive calcific pericarditis. Follow-up study of patient with 40-year history of disease. Am. J. Cardiol. 46:511, 1980.

592. Bhatti, M. A., Ferrante, J. W., Gielchinsky, I., and Norman, J. C.: Pleuropulmonary and skeletal lymphagiomatosis with chylothorax and chylopericardium. Ann. Thorac. Surg. 40:398, 1985.

593. Rose, D. M., Colvin, S. B., Danilowicz, D., and Isom, O. W.: Cardiac tamponade secondary to chylopericardium following cardiac surgery: Case report and review of the literature. Ann. Thorac. Surg. 34:333, 1982.

594. Morishita, Y., Taira, A., Furoi, A., et al.: Constrictive pericarditis secondary to primary chylopericardium. Am. Heart J. 109:373, 1985.

595. Pereira, W. M., Kalil, R. A., Prates, P. R., and Nesralla, I. A.: Cardiac tamponade due to chylopericardium after cardiac surgery. Ann. Thorac. Surg. 46:572, 1988.

596. Bar-El, Y., Smolinksy, A., and Yellin, A.: Chylopericardium as a complication of mitral valve replacement. Thorax 44:74, 1989.

597. Naggar, C. Z., Daly, P. A., Burke, M. J., and Swartz, M. R.: Successful medical management of esophagopericardial fistula. Heart Lung 16:47, 1987.

598. Variyam, E. P., and Shah, A.: Pericardial effusion and left ventricular function in patients with acute alcoholic pancreatitis. Arch. Intern. Med. 147:923, 1987.

599. Jones, B., Haponik, E. F., and Katz, R.: Fibrinous pericarditis: An uncommon complication of acute pancreatitis. South. Med. J. 80:377, 1987.

600. Letoquart, J. P., Fasquel, J. L., L'Huillier, J. P., et al.: Gastropericardial fistula. Review of the literature apropos of an original case. J. Chir. 127:6, 1990.

601. Song, Z. L.: Cholangiothoracic fistulae. Chung Hua Wai Ko Tsa Chih 27:269, 1989.

602. Isolauri, J., and Markkula, H.: Recurrent ulceration and colopericardial fistula as late complications of colon interposition. Ann. Thorac. Surg. 44:84, 1987.

603. Ali, I., and Beg, M. H.: Traumatic bronchopericardial fistula presenting as cardiac tamponade. J. Thorac. Cardiovasc. Surg. 95:740, 1988.

604. Aho, A. J., Vanttinen, E. A., and Nelimarkka, O. I.: Rupture of the pericardium with luxation of the heart after blunt trauma. J. Trauma 27:560, 1987.

605. Rothschild, P. A., Tarver, R. D., Boyko, O. B., and Conces, D. J., Jr.: MR diagnosis of herniation of the left ventricle through a pericardial window. Comput. Radiol. 11:15, 1987.

606. Callejas, M. A., Mestres, C. A., Catalan, M., and Sanchez-Lloret, J.: Traumatic intrapericardial diaphragmatic rupture. Thorac. Cardiovasc. Surg. 32:376, 1984.

607. Kirsch, J. D., and Escarous, A.: CT diagnosis of traumatic pericardium rupture. J. Comput. Assist. Tomogr. 13:523, 1989.

608. Cassorla, L., and Katz, J. A.: Management of cardiac herniation after intrapericardial pneumonectomy. Anesthesiology 60:362, 1984.

609. Feigin, D. S., Fenoglio, J. J., McAllister, H. A., and Madewell, J. E.: Pericardial cysts: A radiologic-pathologic correlation and review. Radiology 125:15, 1977.

610. Kruger, S. R., Michaud, J., and Cannom, D. S.: Spontaneous resolution of a pericardial cyst. Am. Heart J. 109:1390, 1985.

611. Hynes, J. K., Tajik, A. J., Osborn, M. J., et al.: Two-dimensional echocardiographic diagnosis of pericardial cyst. Mayo Clin. Proc. 58:60, 1983.

612. Klatte, E. C., and Yune, H. Y.: Diagnosis and treatment of pericardial cysts. Radiology 104:541, 1972.

613. Unverferth, D. V., and Wooley, C. F.: The differential diagnosis of paracardiac lesions: Pericardial cysts. Cathet. Cardiovasc. Diagn. 5:31, 1979.

614. Moncada, R., Baglia, K., Moguillansky, S. J., et al.: CT diagnosis of congenital intrapericardial masses. J. Comput. Assist. Tomogr. 9:56, 1985.

615. Ellis, K., Leeds, N. E., and Himmelstein, A.: Congenital deficiencies in partial pericardium: Review of two new cases including successful diagnosis by plain roentgenography. Am. J. Roentgenol. 82:125, 1959.

616. Letanche, G., Gayet, C., Souguet, P. J., et al.: Agenesis of the pericardium: Clinical, echocardiographic and MRI aspects. Rev. Pneumol. Clin. 44:105, 1988.

617. Taysi, K., Hartmann, A. F., Shackelford, G. D., and Sundarum, V.: Congenital absence of the pericardium in a family. Am. J. Med. Genet. 21:77, 1985.

618. Gehlmann, H. R., and van Ingen, G. J.: Symptomatic congenital complete absence of the left pericardium. Case report and review of the literature. Eur. Heart J. 10:670, 1989.

619. Inoue, H., Fujii, J., Mashima, S., and Marao, S.: Pseudo right atrial overloading pattern in complete defect of the left pericardium. J. Electrocardiol. 14:413, 1981.

620. Candan, I., Erol, C., and Sonel, A.: Cross sectional echocardiographic appearance in presumed congenital absence of the left pericardium. Br. Heart J. 55:405, 1986.

621. D'Altoria, R. A., and Caro, J. Y.: Congenital absence of the left pericardium detected by imaging of the lung: Case report. J. Nucl. Med. 18:267, 1977.

622. Gutierrez, F. R., Shackelford, G. D., McKnight, R. C., et al.: Diagnosis of congenital absence of left pericardium by MR imaging. J. Comput. Assist. Tomogr. 9:551, 1985.

623. Millaire, A., Goullard, L., Tison, E., et al.: Unilateral agenesis of the pericardium. Arch. Mal. Coeur. 83:275, 1990.

624. Saito, R., and Hotta, F.: Congenital pericardial defect associated with cardiac incarceration: Case report. Am. Heart J. 100:866, 1980.

625. Chapman, J. E., Rubin, J. W., Gross, C. M., and Janssen, M. E.: Congenital absence of pericardium: An unusual cause of atypical angina. Ann. Thorac. Surg. 45:191, 1988.

626. Jones, J. W., and McManus, B. M.: Fatal cardiac strangulation by congenital partial pericardial defect. Am. Heart. J. 107:183, 1984.

627. Auch-Schweik, W., Bonzel, T., Krause, T., et al.: Differential diagnosis of chest pain and diagnostic findings in pericardial defects combined with coronary artery disease. Clin. Cardiol. 11:650, 1988.

628. Altman, C. A., Ettedgui, J. A., Wozney, P., and Beerman, L. B.: Noninvasive diagnostic features of partial absence of the pericardium. Am. J. Cardiol. 63:1536, 1989.

629. Ruys, F., Paulus, W., Stevens, C., and Brutsaert, D.: Expansion of the left atrial appendage is a distinctive cross-sectional echocardiographic feature of congenital defect of the pericardium. Eur. Heart J. 4:738, 1983.

630. Wolff, F., Fritz, A., Dumeny, P., and Eisenmann, B.: Diastolic coronary prolapse in partial left pericardial agenesis. Arch. Mal. Coeur. 80:206, 1987.

631. Amiri, A., Weber, C., Schlosser, V., and Meinertz, T. H.: Coronary artery disease in a patient with a congenital pericardial defect. Thorac. Cardiovasc. Surg. 37:379, 1989.

632. Minocha, G. K., Falicov, R. E., and Nijensohn, E.: Partial right-sided congenital pericardial defect with herniation of the right atrium and right ventricle. Chest 76:484, 1979.

633. Bernal, J. M., Lepiedra, J. O., Gonzalez, I., et al.: Angiocardiographic demonstration of a partial defect of the pericardium with herniation of the left atrium and ventricle. J. Cardiovasc. Surg. 27:344, 1986.

Traumatic Heart Disease

by PETER F. COHN, M.D., and EUGENE BRAUNWALD, M.D.

Unfortunately, traumatic heart disease is still regarded as an uncommon and even esoteric form of heart disease of interest primarily to emergency physicians or those in the military service. That this is not the case is attested to by the statistics —violent injury accounts for the majority of deaths in persons under 40 years of age,[1] and among these victims cardiac trauma is one of the leading causes of death.[2,3] For example, chest injuries are directly responsible for more than 25 per cent of the 50,000 to 60,000 deaths that result annually from automobile accidents and contribute significantly to another 25 per cent of these deaths.[4] The increasing frequency of physical violence has also resulted in a corresponding increase in the incidence of traumatic heart disease, especially in *young adult males*. These are the most frequent victims, since they are more likely to have automobile and motorcycle accidents, to incur injuries while performing heavy labor, and to be involved in or victims of acts of physical violence.

There is, regrettably, no evidence that the frequency of these mishaps is declining. At Boston City Hospital, for example, the annual incidence of penetrating wounds of the heart rose from 2.8 cases during the period from 1956 through 1964 to 8.0 cases from 1965 through 1976.[5] In Houston,[6] a 30-year analysis of 4459 patients with cardiovascular injuries (86 per cent of whom were males) showed a steady rise between 1958 (averaging 27 patients/yr) and 1988 (213 patients/yr) (Table 46–1). In addition, the incidence of medically related cardiac trauma is also rising, such as increased use of intravascular and intracardiac catheters leading to penetrating injuries of the heart and great vessels, and resuscitative cardiac massage causing a variety of nonpenetrating injuries of these organs.

The two principal, immediate consequences of cardiac injury are *exsanguinating hemorrhage* and *cardiac tamponade*. Effective treatment has resulted in an increasing number of immediate survivors, and later sequelae—including myocardial infarction, ventricular aneurysm and pseudoaneurysm, ventricular septal defect, valvular damage, recurrent pericarditis, and constrictive pericarditis—are becoming far more common. Serious cardiac trauma is frequently overlooked in patients with nonpenetrating injury, particularly when other structures such as the thoracic cage and lungs are obviously damaged. Such oversight can be tragic, because the lethal consequences of cardiac injury may suddenly emerge after the superficial injuries have been attended to. Clearly, a much higher index of suspicion of this possibility is necessary if the increasing magnitude of this problem is to be halted and reversed.

NONPENETRATING CARDIAC INJURY

Nonpenetrating injuries result from the effects of external physical forces, but it is important to recognize that these forces need not necessarily be applied directly to the chest, since injuries to the heart and great vessels may also occur with trauma to other parts of the body. Parmley et al. have summarized the mechanisms of nonpenetrating injuries to the heart as follows: (1) direct force against the chest; (2) bidirectional force against the thorax; (3) indirect forces resulting in a marked increase in intravascular pressure, as from sudden compression in the abdomen and lower extremities; (4) decelerative forces; (5) blast forces; (6) concussive forces; and (7) combinations of these.[6]

The most common cause of nonpenetrating injury in civilian life is probably that directly related to *vehicular impact,*[7] either by direct compression, usually with the steering wheel squeezing the heart between the sternum and the spine, or by indirect compression. Causes of nonpenetrating injuries other than automobile and motorcycle accidents include direct blows to the chest by any kind of blunt object or missile, such as a clenched fist and various kinds of sporting equipment, as well as by the kicks of animals, falls, and cardiac resuscitative procedures. Fractures of the bony structures of the chest wall are *not* necessary accompaniments of cardiac injury in any of these situations. This point is of critical importance, since *the absence of such obvious injuries following trauma should by no*

TABLE 46–1 ETIOLOGY OF CARDIOVASCULAR INJURIES PER 5-YEAR TIME INTERVAL

Etiology	1958–63	1964–69	1970–73	1974–78	1979–83	1984–88	Total
Gunshot wound	42	236	436	501	625	456	2296
Stab/laceration	64	110	161	229	362	463	1389
Blunt trauma	1	17	58	90	62	76	304
Shotgun wound	1	15	45	55	61	37	214
Iatrogenic	1	1	0	0	4	25	31
Other/unknown	54	20	111	25	3	12	225
Total	163	399	811	900	1117	1069	4459

From Mattox, K. L., et al.: Five thousand seven hundred sixty cardiovascular injuries in 4459 patients: Epidemiologic evolution 1958 to 1987. Ann. Surg. *209:*698, 1989.

TABLE 46–2 TYPES OF CARDIAC INJURY FROM BLUNT TRAUMA

A. MYOCARDIUM
1. Contusion
2. Laceration
3. Rupture
4. Septal perforation
5. Aneurysm, pseudoaneurysm
6. Hemopericardium, tamponade
7. Thrombosis, systemic embolism

B. PERICARDIUM
1. Pericarditis
2. Postpericardiotomy syndrome
3. Constrictive pericarditis
4. Pericardial laceration
5. Hemorrhage
6. Cardiac herniation

C. ENDOCARDIAL STRUCTURES
1. Rupture of papillary muscle
2. Rupture of chordae tendineae
3. Rupture of atrioventricular and semilunar valves

D. CORONARY ARTERY
1. Thrombosis
2. Laceration
3. Fistula

From Jackson, D. H., and Murphy, G. W.: Nonpenetrating cardiac trauma. Mod. Conc. Cardiovasc. Dis. 45:123, 1976, by permission of the American Heart Association, Inc.

means exclude the possibility of nonpenetrating injury to the heart. The clinical manifestations may not be apparent for days or even weeks after the accident.

Pathological findings following nonpenetrating cardiac injury usually include some degree of pericarditis, which may be associated with the late development of pericardial constriction. Changes in the heart itself range from minute ecchymotic areas in the subepicardium or subendocardium to transmural contusions with edematous, fragmented, or necrotic muscle fibers, surrounded at first by red blood cells and invaded soon thereafter by polymorphonuclear leukocytes. The external appearance of the heart may be misleading in the case of nonpenetrating injury, since large areas of intramural contusion, including involvement of the interventricular septum, may not be apparent.[4,8] In patients who survive the injury, healing is by scar formation resembling that following acute myocardial infarction, and post-traumatic aneurysms resembling postinfarction aneurysms may develop.[9] The types of cardiac injury resulting from blunt (nonpenetrating) trauma are listed in Table 46-2, the most severe forms being rupture of the aortic or mitral valve and rupture of the interventricular septum or even of the free wall of a cardiac chamber. While these injuries are frequently fatal, fortunately they constitute only a small fraction of all nonpenetrating injuries (Table 46-3).

PERICARDIUM

Injury to the pericardium in blunt trauma may range from contusion to laceration or rupture. Whether the pericardium tears or not, some degree of traumatic pericarditis is found at autopsy or operation in most patients sustaining severe blunt trauma of the chest, especially of the precordial area. Parmley et al. reported pericardial laceration or rupture in 249 of 546 autopsy cases of nonpenetrating trauma to the heart,[6] but it should be noted that this rarely occurs as an isolated lesion (Table 46-3) and is usually associated with cardiac contusion and even more serious cardiac injury. On the basis of a series of experiments in a canine model, in which 14 of 18 dogs receiving sublethal blunt chest trauma developed pericardial rents, DeMuth et al. suggested that a higher frequency of pericardial tears than is generally appreciated occurs in survivors of chest trauma.[10] Herniation of the heart or a portion of it through the defect may result from such injuries.[11] Clinically, a rent in the pericardium can occur as a consequence of blunt trauma, and delayed herniation of the heart through the rent may then compromise circulatory function acutely.

CLINICAL FEATURES AND DIAGNOSIS. Clinically, traumatic pericarditis is manifested by the development of a typical pericardial friction rub and ST-T–wave changes on the electrocardiogram characteristic of pericarditis (p. 1470). During and immediately following the acute episode, the major problem is not the pericarditis itself but its most common complications, i.e., hemopericardium and resultant tamponade, discussed on p. 1473. Commonly, the patient is restless, with hypotension, oliguria or anuria, distant heart sounds, and pulsus paradoxus. There is usually diffuse low voltage on the electrocardiogram. Pericardial fluid on the echocardiogram (p. 1473) is a key finding.[12]

TREATMENT AND PROGNOSIS. As a rule, uncomplicated pericarditis secondary to cardiac trauma simply resolves. Tamponade, however, requires emergency operative treatment, as discussed below. Recurrent pericardial effusions sometimes associated with chest pain and fever, i.e., the so-called postcardiotomy syndrome, occur in a small number of patients. The cause of this syndrome is not clear (p. 1473). Although patients with recurrent effusion usually respond to aspirin or nonsteroidal antiinflammatory agents, occasionally glucocorticosteroids are necessary. Constrictive pericarditis (p. 1482) occurs as a rare complication of traumatic pericarditis, with or without recurrent effusions.

MYOCARDIUM

CONTUSION. Myocardial contusion usually produces no significant symptoms and often goes unrecognized. At times, manifestations of the injury are masked by injury to the chest wall or other organs.[13-16] This is important because as many as 75 per cent of patients with myocardial contusion can have

TABLE 46–3 NONPENETRATING CARDIAC TRAUMA

TYPE AND/OR SITE OF INJURY	NUMBER OF CASES	CASES COMBINED WITH AORTIC RUPTURE	TOTAL
Rupture	**273**	**80**	**353**
Right ventricle	56	10	66
Left ventricle	46	13	59
Right atrium	35	6	51
Left atrium	24	2	26
IV septum	25(20*)	7(4*)	30(24*)
IA septum	18(10*)	5(3*)	25(13*)
Multiple chamber ruptures	69	37	106
			128
Contusion/laceration	**105**	**24**	
Pericardial laceration	**18**	**18**	**36**
Hemopericardium	**13**	**12**	**25**
Valvular laceration/rupture	**1(2†)**	**0(4†)**	**1(6†)**
Aortic valve	1(1†)	0(2†)	1(3†)
Pulmonic valve	0(4†)	0	0(4†)
Tricuspid valve	0(8†)	0	0(8†)
Mitral valve	0(8†)	0(1†)	0(9†)
Mitral and tricuspid valves	0(1†)	0(1†)	0(2†)
Coronary artery laceration/ rupture	**0(7†)**	**1(2†)**	**1(9†)**
Papillary muscle laceration/ rupture	**1(23†)**	**0**	**1(23†)**
TOTAL	**411**	**135**	**546**

Numbers in parentheses indicate more significant associated cardiac injuries (tabulated in another column).
* Associated with other sites of cardiac rupture.
† Combined with cardiac rupture or other cardiac injury.
From Parmley, L. F., et al.: Nonpenetrating traumatic injury of the heart. Circulation 18:371, 1958, by permission of the American Heart Association, Inc.

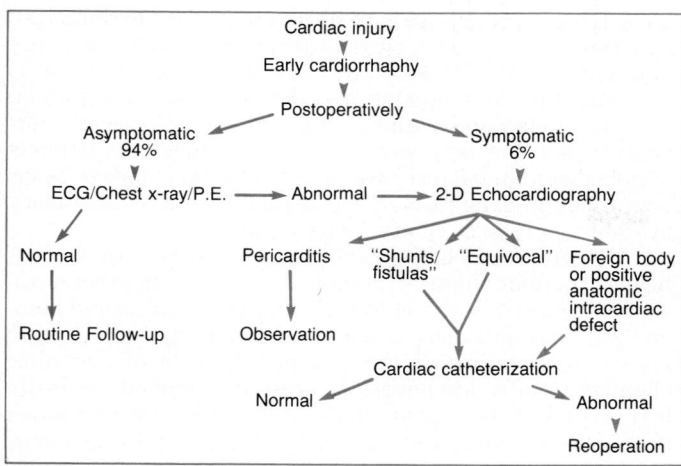

FIGURE 46–1. A recommended decision schema for post-traumatic cardiac evaluation. Following cardiac injury repair is generally carried out by simple cardiorrhaphy. This algorithm shows a suggested approach to detect residual damage following emergency cardiorrhaphy. (From Mattox, K. L., et al.: Cardiac evaluation following heart injury. J. Trauma 25:758, © by Williams and Wilkins, 1985.)

signs of external chest injury.[17] Thus there is a higher frequency of diagnosis of cardiac contusion associated with increasing awareness of the lesion.

Clinical Features and Diagnosis. The most common symptom of myocardial contusion is precordial pain resembling that of myocardial infarction, but the pain from other sites of chest trauma can confuse the clinical picture.[15,17] As with myocardial infarction, nitroglycerin and related drugs have little effect in relieving the pain. The *electrocardiogram* probably represents one of the most helpful tools for recognizing contusion of the left ventricle. Either nonspecific ST-T abnormalities or the classic findings of pericarditis are the most common changes noted. Initially, electrocardiographic signs of deeper injury to the myocardium, i.e., pathological Q waves, may be dwarfed by pericardial inflammation; only as the latter subsides does injury to the myocardium become more evident. However, because the possibility of cardiac trauma is often not considered in trauma victims, an electrocardiogram is often not recorded immediately on patients with chest injuries and the diagnosis may be missed. Just as in acute myocardial infarction, serial findings, i.e., the evolution of Q waves and the subsidence of the ST-segment and T-wave abnormalities, are of critical importance. The sensitivity and specificity of electrocardiographic findings are less than 100 per cent, however; hence the need for additional tests.

A recommended decision schema for evaluating cardiac injury immediately after early cardiorrhaphy is depicted in Figure 46–1.

SERUM ENZYMES. *Since enzyme levels* may be elevated by trauma to noncardiac as well as to cardiac tissue, they too are of limited diagnostic value. With the widespread availability of reliable measurements of the MB band of creatine kinase (CK), the presence or absence of cardiac necrosis can be better documented in patients with blunt trauma.[18] Indeed, with the electrocardiogram and CK-MB as screening tests, the detection of myocardial contusion has increased from 7 to 17 per cent in patients with blunt chest trauma entering the Henry Ford Hospital.[19] Similarly, at the Mayo Clinic 58 of 291 such patients (20 per cent) had elevations of CK-MB.[20] However, false-positive elevations of the CK-MB isoenzyme can also be seen if the total CK is greater than 20,000 units; this can occur after massive injury to skeletal muscle.

RADIONUCLIDE IMAGING (see Chap. 10). Myocardial perfusion is reduced in areas of myocardial contusion.[18] Chiu et al. have used technetium-labeled pyrophosphate to demonstrate images of positive uptake that were then correlated with postmortem angiograms showing extravasation of contrast material.[21] Images usually became negative 1 week after the trauma. Contused myocardium concentrates ^{99m}Tc-pyrophosphate in amounts comparable to those observed in ischemic injury. Scanning following injection of radioactive thallium to detect areas of reduced perfusion and of labeled pyrophosphate to locate areas of recent necrosis may be expected to identify patients with myocardial damage following blunt injury, to localize this damage, and to indicate the extent of the damage. Radionuclide ventriculography often shows a reduced ventricular ejection fraction in such patients.[22] These tests show changes similar to those observed in patients with acute myocardial infarction (Chap. 39). Sutherland et al.[22] used radionuclide ventriculography to define focal defects in ventricular wall motion. They subgrouped the 43 patients whom they studied into those with right ventricular abnormalities (18), left ventricular abnormalities (4), biventricular abnormalities (6), and neither kind (15). They described the state of right ventricular pump function using modified ventricular function curves and found it to be surprisingly well preserved (Fig. 46–2). Schamp et al. also found a high (83 per cent) frequency of right ventricular abnormalities in the 40 patients they studied.[23]

ECHOCARDIOGRAPHY. In addition to identifying pericardial effusion, *two-dimensional echocardiography* is also useful in evaluating cardiac injuries, including myocardial contusion. Such findings as abnormal wall motion and chamber enlargement can be detected with this technique.[24] Echocardiography is useful when the patient with suspected cardiac injury first undergoes testing, as well as after emergency thoracotomy and cardiac repair in an effort to detect residual cardiac damage. When confirmed with pulsed-Doppler echocardiography, intracardiac shunts and regurgitant lesions can be demonstrated.

ARRHYTHMIAS. A wide variety of arrhythmias is common with areas of extensive contusion,[25] and ventricular tachycardia that degenerates into ventricular fibrillation represents a frequent cause of death in these patients. The precise mechanism responsible for these arrhythmias has not been defined, but in the dog, increasing frequencies of ventricular premature beats were observed with increasing grades of trauma.[13] In addition, both atrioventricular and intraventricular conduction defects, as well as sinus node dysfunction, are seen.[26,27] In contrast to acute myocardial infarction, cardiac contusion rarely leads to severe *heart failure* unless massive damage to a valve or rupture of the interventricular septum has

FIGURE 46–2. Left and right ventricular (LV and RV) myocardial function curves in 43 patients who sustained acute myocardial contusion complicating blunt chest injury. Patients with RV contusion (●) maintained an RV stroke work index (RVSWI) similar to that of patients without RV contusion (○) by virtue of a larger RV end-diastolic volume index (RVEDVI) (preload). Hence, RV performance was well-maintained albeit at a greater preload and the two groups of patients appeared to have identical LV function. NS = not significant; SD = standard deviation. (From Sutherland, G. R., et al.: Hemodynamic adaptation to acute myocardial contusion complicating blunt chest injury. Am. J. Cardiol. 57:291, 1986.)

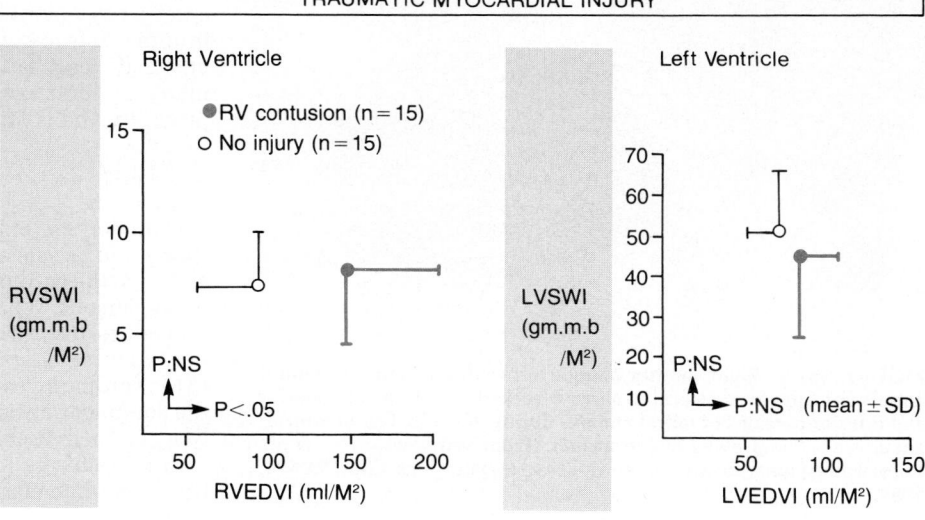

occurred.[28] However, some impairment of right and/or left ventricular function, as reflected in depressed ejection fractions and ventricular function (myocardial performance) curves, may be found.[22,29] In the animal model, alcohol ingestion potentiates the effect of blunt trauma on the myocardium.[30] This gives added strength to the warning not to mix drinking and driving.

Treatment and Prognosis. In this era of progressively earlier ambulation of patients with acute myocardial infarction, a similar approach appears to be reasonable after several days of close observation for myocardial contusion. Several groups have concluded that in trauma patients in stable condition, contusion neither increases the complication rate nor necessitates intensive care unit monitoring.[31,32] Hossack et al. have even questioned the need for routine imaging studies.[33] From the point of view of physical activity, we recommend treating these patients in a manner similar to that for those with acute myocardial infarction with comparable extent of myocardial damage (Chap. 39). However, *treatment with anticoagulants and obviously with thrombolytics is contraindicated*, since intramyocardial or intrapericardial hemorrhage may be precipitated or exacerbated. Atrial fibrillation, when present, usually reverts to sinus rhythm spontaneously. If it does not, digitalis glycosides may be used to slow the ventricular rate and may also cause reversion to sinus rhythm. Chest pain is best treated with analgesics; nonsteroidal anti-inflammatory agents are not advised because they might interfere with myocardial healing (p. 1215).

As already noted, the prognosis from complete or partial recovery is generally excellent, but these patients require careful follow-up, since late complications, ranging from ventricular arrhythmias to cardiac rupture, may occur. Coronary occlusion[34-36] aorto-right atrial fistula,[37] and ventricular aneurysms (Fig. 46-3)[9] are occasional sequelae, and there is no agreement about whether or not surgical resection of the last-named is required. It is our policy to use the presence of heart failure as an indication for operation of aneurysms analogous to that in patients with postinfarct aneurysms (p. 1260). Pseudoaneurysms, however, require immediate repair (p. 227).

Although many analogies can be drawn between the cardiac necrosis caused by trauma and that caused by ischemic heart disease, a number of critically important differences must be emphasized. Patients with acute myocardial infarction secondary to coronary artery disease generally have diffuse, obstructive, gradually progressive coronary atherosclerosis, are frequently middle-aged or elderly, and may have underlying heart disease such as that secondary to prolonged hypertension or diabetes mellitus; patients with traumatic myocardial contusion generally have normal coronary vessels and only a discrete area of myocardial damage; most often, they are young and without underlying cardiovascular illness. Hence, the long-term prognosis in surviving patients with myocardial necrosis secondary to trauma tends to be far better than in patients with myocardial infarction secondary to atherosclerotic coronary artery disease.

CARDIAC RUPTURE. There appear to be two mechanisms of cardiac rupture: (1) acute laceration due to compression of the heart by direct force,[38] and (2) contusion and hemorrhage that proceed to necrosis, softening, and rupture several days following the trauma. Rupture of a cardiac chamber usually, but not always, results in immediate death. It is this minority of patients that survive the initial trauma that must be assessed and treated immediately in the emergency room setting.

Clinical Features and Diagnosis. In the patient who survives the first few minutes of cardiac rupture, the clinical picture of cardiac tamponade described above is common. Although ventricular rupture is far more common than is atrial rupture,[3] the latter occurs particularly following automobile accidents. Rupture of the interventricular septum should be suspected in patients who develop severe congestive heart failure immediately or within several days of the trauma, together with a new holosystolic murmur along the left sternal border; however, trauma to the mitral valve apparatus, which may be manifested with a similar picture clinically, must be excluded. On the basis of a series of 546 autopsy cases of nonpenetrating injury to the heart, the incidence of rupture of the ventricular septum has been estimated by Parmley et al. to be almost 10 per cent, with a similar number of patients experiencing rupture of the atrial septum (Table 46-3).[6] These lesions may occur without other serious cardiac injuries, but occasionally other abnormalities are present, including valve cusp perforations and a variety of intracardiac shunts.[39] Although the predilection for perforation of the ventricular septum is highest at the apex, any portion of the muscular septum may be involved, and multiple perforations are not uncommon. The diagnosis of ventricular septal defect and of damage to the mitral valve apparatus can be confirmed by means of catheterization, demonstration of an oxygen step-up in the right ventricle, left ventricular angiography,[40] as well as by color-flow Doppler echocardiography[24] (p. 1523).

Treatment and Prognosis. Patients with external rupture of the heart obviously require emergency surgery if they are to have any chance of survival. Although operation should not be postponed, pericardiocentesis and expansion of the intravascular volume can be carried out while the most rapid preparations possible for operation are undertaken. Successful surgical treatment of external cardiac rupture has been reported in a small number of cases.[41] In contrast, patients with rupture of the interventricular septum do not always require emergency operation. Indeed, many defects are small, with minimal left-to-right shunts, and may even heal spontaneously. If heart failure develops subsequently, as occurs in many patients, surgical correction should be carried out promptly and is often successful.

COMPLICATIONS OF CARDIAC RESUSCITATION

Closed-chest (external) cardiac massage (p. 776) is generally thought to be safe and simple—so much so that it is included as part of the cardiopulmonary resuscitation technique taught to lay persons. What is not sufficiently appreciated is that the procedure itself can result in serious complications, which may go unrecognized because many of the patients succumb to the cardiac arrest itself.[42] Even at postmortem examination, the complications may be improperly attributed to the underlying cardiac disease.

Rupture of the left ventricle is a more common complication of cardiac massage than is rupture of the right ventricle.

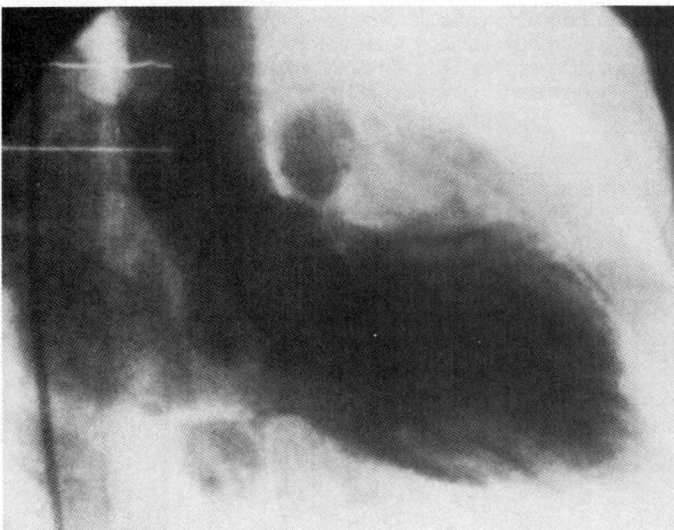

FIGURE 46-3. Right anterior oblique left ventriculogram. Submitral aneurysms appear as saccular narrow-necked structures at superior and inferior portions of mitral annulus during diastole. Top of inferior aneurysm is compressed by left atrium. (From Matthews, R. V., et al.: Chest trauma and subvalvular left ventricular aneurysms. Chest 95:474, 1989.)

However, rupture of either chamber may occur and may be life-threatening if the patient survives the arrhythmia that necessitated massage in the first place. Since in most instances external resuscitation is performed for patients with myocardial infarction, it may not always be clear whether the left ventricular rupture preceded the massage or occurred as a consequence of it.

Rupture of right ventricular papillary muscles with acute tricuspid regurgitation has also been reported as a complication of closed-chest cardiac massage,[43] as has rupture of the atria and aorta and dissecting hematoma of a coronary artery.[44] A variety of noncardiovascular traumatic lesions, such as fracture of the sternum, hemothorax, pneumothorax, and laceration of abdominal organs may occur. Because of the efficacy of cardiopulmonary resuscitation and its increasing use by paramedical personnel and laymen, an increasing number of such complications may be anticipated in the future. This increased incidence will be stemmed only by educational programs for all individuals likely to employ this technique.

PENETRATING CARDIAC INJURY

Penetrating cardiac injuries occurring in civilian life are due to a variety of objects, such as bullets, knives, ice picks, and the like. The demographics of penetrating cardiac trauma in Jefferson County, Alabama were reviewed by Naughton, et al.[45] As with blunt trauma, male victims predominated and gunshot wounds were the major mechanism of injury. Penetrating injuries may also be due to the inward displacement of ribs or sternal fragments accompanying chest injuries. The chamber most commonly involved in this type of injury is the right ventricle because of its anterior position, followed, in descending order of frequency, by the left ventricle, the right atrium, and the left atrium.[46] However, penetrating wounds of the precordium are not the only types of wounds that may result in cardiac injury. Occasionally, wounds of other areas of the chest, as well as of the neck and upper abdomen, are associated with penetration of the heart. In addition, intravenous or intracardiac catheters may fracture and become impaled within the walls of a great vessel or cardiac chamber (Chap. 7). Migration of an indwelling venous catheter into the pulmonary artery, which may ultimately lead to perforation of this vessel, is another complication that has increased in frequency with its widespread use in intensive care units. Formerly, thoracotomy was necessary to remove these catheter fragments, but catheters with snares and other devices are now available for this purpose.[47,48]

Perforation of the right ventricle with a transvenous pacing electrode is not uncommon, but tamponade is rare. During cardiac catheterization, perforation of the thin-walled right atrium or outflow tract of the right ventricle has been reported. Such patients usually require only careful observation, but when tamponade occurs, immediate drainage is mandatory.[49] Coronary angioplasty[50] and endomyocardial biopsy[51,52] can also result in tamponade. Dissection of the aorta or arch vessels has been reported as a complication of retrograde arterial catheterization and occasionally is also severe enough to require operative intervention.

Penetrating wounds of the heart often result in laceration of the pericardium, sometimes occurring alone but usually associated with laceration of the myocardium itself. One or more chambers but also the cardiac valves and their accessory structures, as well as the interventricular and interatrial septa, may be perforated. Cardiac tamponade resulting from pneumopericardium has been reported.[53] When laceration of the pericardium occurs as an isolated lesion, acute compromise of cardiac function resulting from herniation of the heart may be the presenting manifestation. Occasionally, low-velocity missiles may penetrate the cardiac chambers but may be retained within the myocardium.

The most common penetrating injuries resulting from physical violence are stab and gunshot wounds.[45,54] The former do not necessarily cause extensive cellular destruction adjacent to the wound; they resemble surgical incisions, and transmural wounds in the thick-walled left ventricle may actually seal quickly without disastrous consequences. In contrast, bullet wounds are associated with bleeding that is not usually self-limited and extensive cellular destruction in and adjacent to the path of the bullet. When a coronary artery is lacerated or perforated, myocardial infarction may ensue.

CLINICAL FEATURES AND DIAGNOSIS. The clinical picture of a penetrating wound of the heart depends on several factors, including the object responsible for the injury (e.g., bullet, knife, ice pick), the size of the wound, and the precise location of the structures injured. Pericardial laceration occurring by itself is uncommon and of relatively little significance unless infection supervenes. Rather, the injuries to underlying cardiac structures usually determine the clinical presentation, course, and choice of treatment. However, the nature of the pericardial wound is important, i.e., whether or not the wound is open and allows free drainage of intrapericardial blood. If the pericardium remains open and extravasated blood can pass freely into the pleural cavities or mediastinum, cardiac tamponade will not develop, at least initially, and the presenting signs and symptoms will be those of hemorrhage and hemothorax. On the other hand, if the pericardium does *not* permit free drainage because its opening has been obliterated by a blood clot, adjacent lung tissue, or other structures, or because a flap develops in the pericardial rent, immediate exsanguination may be averted, but tamponade may occur minutes or hours later. In some instances, blood accumulates both intra- and extrapericardially.

Whether the hemorrhage is intra- or extrapericardial, its severity can often be surmised from the clinical picture. Traumatic penetrating lesions of the heart are usually associated with injuries to the lungs and other organs, which may predominate at first; a high index of suspicion of cardiac penetration is necessary when patients are evaluated following thoracic or upper abdominal trauma. Although extensive injuries to the pericardium and underlying heart are usually immediately fatal or result in shock, delayed clinical manifestations of cardiac injury as a result of hemorrhage, infection, retained foreign bodies, or arrhythmias may become apparent after the other bodily injuries have been attended to. Failure to give serious consideration to the possibility that *cardiac* damage has occurred in a patient with obvious noncardiac trauma may lead to an unanticipated catastrophe.

Although echocardiography is extremely valuable in the recognition of pericardial effusion[12,24,27,55] (p. 102), foreign bodies in the heart,[56] and intracardiac shunts,[12,24,57,58] it is not always readily available in an emergency setting. When agitation, cool and clammy skin, neck vein distention, pulsus paradoxus, and other classic findings of tamponade (considered earlier) are present, the diagnosis can be relatively simple; in patients without such typical findings, the clinical picture may be attributed to blood loss, especially since volume expansion can improve the hemodynamic state, at least temporarily. Whether or not pericardiocentesis should be performed as a diagnostic test is controversial. If nonclotting blood is obtained, the diagnosis of hemopericardium is confirmed, and the accompanying decompression may constitute effective, albeit temporary, initial treatment. If the pericardiocentesis is negative, however, cardiac tamponade cannot be ruled out. Since, as discussed below, the primary management in any event is thoracotomy, it seems pointless to waste valuable time with pericardial aspiration unless there is doubt regarding the diagnosis.

TREATMENT. The definitive treatment of cardiac wounds *accompanied by severe hemorrhage* is immediate thoracotomy and cardiorrhaphy.[59] Although multiple pericardiocenteses are no longer considered a substitute for thoracotomy in the treatment of cardiac wounds associated with cardiac tamponade, there may still be a role for pericardial aspiration *while the patient is being prepared for operation.* Algorithms for management of patients with penetrating

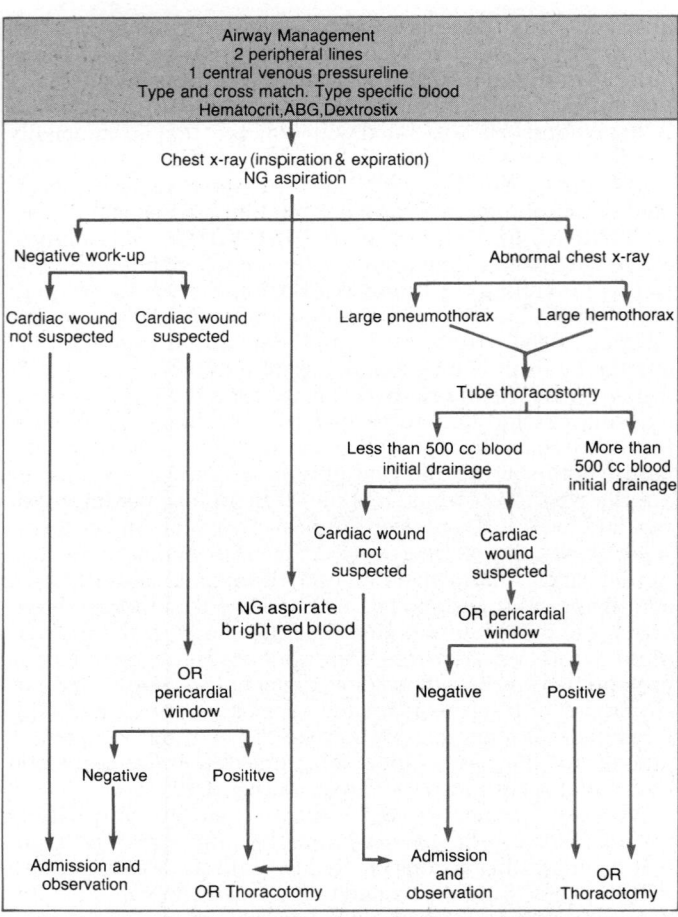

FIGURE 46–4. Algorithm for management of penetrating chest wound with stable vital signs on admission. ABG = arterial blood gases; NG = nasogastric. (From Karrel, R., et al.: Emergency diagnosis, resuscitation, and treatment of acute penetrating cardiac trauma. Ann. Emerg. Med. *11*:504, 1982.)

chest wounds—with either stable or unstable vital signs—have been proposed (Figs. 46–4 and 46–5). The availability in many hospitals of surgical teams and equipment for cardiopulmonary bypass has permitted the safe and effective repair of many penetrating injuries of the heart. Marshall and associates[54] described a 10½-year experience with 47 patients admitted after penetrating cardiac trauma (stab wounds and gunshot wounds); 46 underwent immediate surgery and 10 died. The one patient who refused surgery also died, resulting in a total mortality of 11/47, or 23 per cent. Mortality was 26 per cent in patients with shunts and 15 per cent in those with tamponade.

Occasionally, thoracotomy may be performed in moribund patients for whom general anesthesia is unnecessary. However, adequate ventilation must be maintained. Administration of antibiotics and tetanus prophylaxis should also be instituted as routine measures. Operative treatment includes repair of the pericardium, myocardium, aorta, and valves as well as of any lacerations of the coronary arteries. At operation, the heart and great vessels should be thoroughly examined for the presence of multiple wounds. When the bullet has penetrated the anterior wall of the heart, the posterior wall should always be inspected for an exit wound before the chest is closed. Many victims of penetrating cardiac injury, young and otherwise in good health, can withstand relatively long periods of hypoperfusion without irreversible brain, renal, or cardiac damage. Therefore, one should err on the side of aggressive attempts at resuscitation in patients who arrive moribund in the operating room. Retained foreign bodies in the heart are less of a problem in civilian than in military injuries, because shootings in civilian life usually occur at short range and thus result in through-and-through wounds.

There is disagreement concerning whether or not retained foreign bodies should be removed. Certainly, if the projectile is accessible, it should be removed; echocardiography (Fig. 46–6) can be helpful in locating foreign bodies.[56,60] If deemed not dangerous, they can probably be left in place, although there is some risk of later infection, pain, aneurysm formation, or migration of the foreign body.[60,61] In addition, dealing with a patient who is preoccupied with the knowledge that he has a foreign body retained in or close to the heart may present some difficulty; indeed, anxiety can become excessive, impairing the patient's function more than the physical damage and, occasionally, becoming an indication for reoperation and extraction of the object. The serious consequences of a foreign body embolus from the left ventricle also encourage a more aggressive surgical policy toward foreign bodies lodged in that chamber than in the right ventricle. Foreign bodies embedded at strategic points in great vessels may erode the vessel and cause potentially severe hemorrhage or may embolize[60] and should, if possible, be removed.

Late complications of penetrating wounds of the heart are quite common and include post-traumatic pericarditis and infection as well as arrhythmias, ventricular septal defect, and ventricular aneurysm.

PROGNOSIS. The outlook following a penetrating wound depends, first and foremost, on the extent of the injury. Gunshot wounds of the heart are more usually fatal than are stab wounds, while among the latter, knife wounds are more serious than are ice pick wounds. Salvage rates are lower in patients with extrapericardial hemorrhage compared with tamponade and also with penetrating wounds involving thin-walled structures such as the atria or the pulmonary artery, since they rarely seal off spontaneously, whereas injury

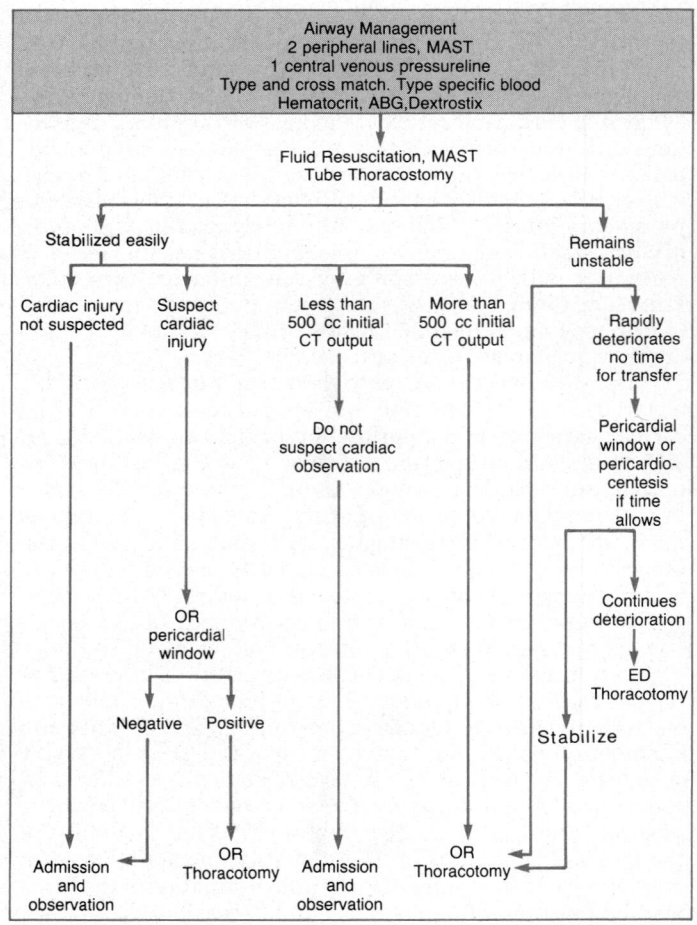

FIGURE 46–5. Algorithm for penetrating chest wound with unstable vital signs on admission. MAST = military anti-shock trousers. (From Karrel, R., et al.: Emergency diagnosis, resuscitation, and treatment of acute penetrating cardiac trauma. Ann. Emerg. Med. *11*:504, 1982.)

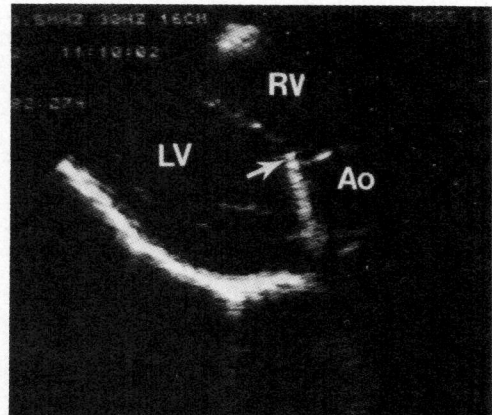

FIGURE 46-6. Two-dimensional echocardiographic image in the left parasternal long-axis view. A bullet fragment (arrow) is located high in the interventricular septum and has the typical appearance of such missiles with dense trailing reverberations. Ao = aortic root; LV = left ventricle; RV = right ventricle. (From Hassett, A., et al.: Utility of echocardiography in the management of patients with penetrating missile wounds of the heart. Reprinted with permission of the American College of Cardiology. J. Am. Coll. Cardiol. 7:1151, 1986.)

to the ventricles is associated with distinctly higher survival. The state of consciousness and the extent of damage, if any, to the central nervous system at the time the patient is brought to the hospital also affect prognosis. It is clear that delay in performing the initial thoracotomy also adversely influences the chances for survival.

Rupture of the interventricular septum (Fig. 46-7) is often a late complication of penetrating injury as it is with blunt injury. Asfaw et al. described 12 patients with stab wounds who presented with cardiac tamponade and who had epicardial and pericardial wounds that were repaired at thoracotomy.[62] Days to years later, septal defects were diagnosed, but only four patients were symptomatic enough to warrant subsequent reoperation for closure of the defect. Residual injuries requiring reoperation can often be detected with color-flow Doppler echocardiography.[24]

Patients with preexisting valvular heart disease may be at higher risk than those with normal valves for the development of valvular injury following blunt trauma. Parmley et al. cited a 9 per cent incidence of valvular injury in their report of 546 cases of nonpenetrating chest trauma (Table 46-3).[6] Damage to the aortic valve is by far the most common of these lesions (Fig. 46-8). (Parmley's series appears to be an exception in this regard.) This is followed, in order, by damage to the mitral and tricuspid valves, presumably owing to the higher pressures generated by blunt trauma to the aorta. Indeed, sustained damage of the aortic valve should be suspected in any patient without a history of heart disease who presents with a heart murmur after severe blunt trauma to the chest. Damage to cardiac valves may also occur as a consequence of penetrating wounds of the heart, but, in contrast to the damage caused by nonpenetrating injury, these are rarely solitary lesions.[63,64] Blunt chest trauma has also been reported to cause bioprosthetic valve dysfunction.[65,66]

CLINICAL FEATURES AND DIAGNOSIS. New, loud, musical murmurs are characteristic of injury to the valves and their supporting structures. The combination of a high-pitched diastolic blowing murmur with a widened pulse pressure following blunt trauma to the chest suggests rupture of the *aortic valve*. The murmur and the hemodynamic consequences of the rupture may not appear for several days following the trauma. Aortic regurgitation may also occur transiently owing to perivalvular edema or hemorrhage.

Rupture of the *mitral valve* or of a papillary muscle appears to occur as a consequence of sudden obstruction of left ventricular outflow due to blunt injury in early diastole. It is usually associated with the development of precordial pain and a loud, harsh holosystolic murmur that radiates to the apex. Fulminant pulmonary edema quickly develops; compensation in those patients with lesser degrees of regurgitation due to torn leaflets or chordae tendineae may remain for longer periods of time, although they may eventually show signs of decompensation.

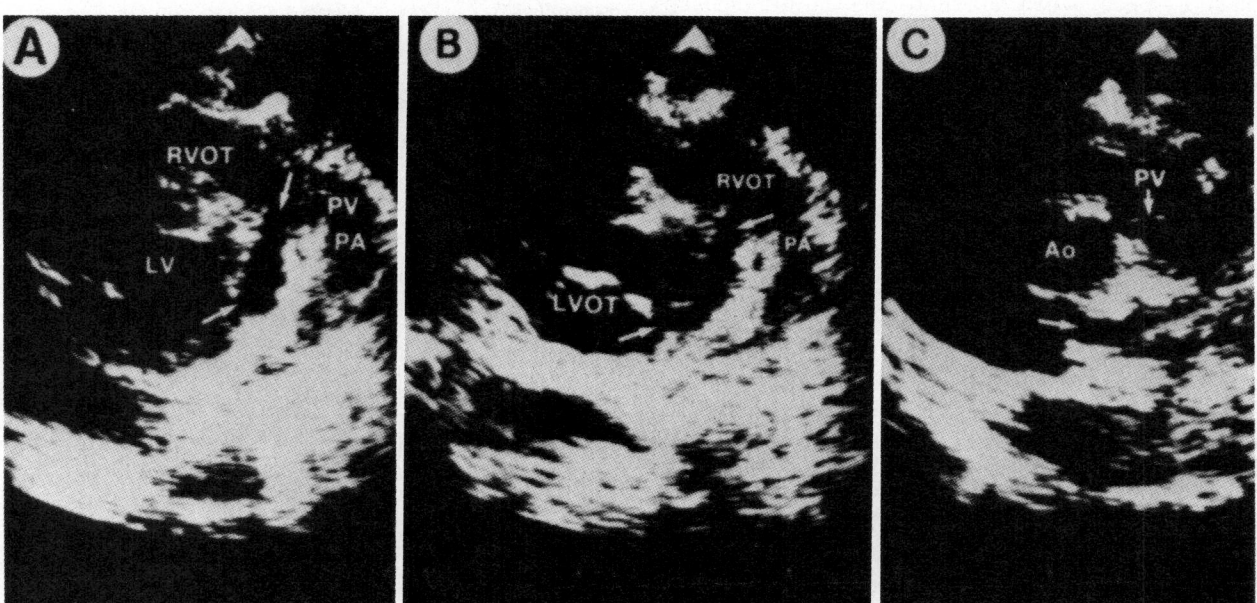

FIGURE 46-7. Two-dimensional echocardiogram from the parasternal short-axis position in a patient with a ventricular septal defect caused by knife stabbing. *A,* A defect is seen in the interventricular septum (arrows) between the left ventricle (LV) and the right ventricular outflow tract (RVOT) just proximal to the pulmonary valve (PV). *B,* At a slightly higher level the defect originates in the left ventricular outflow tract (LVOT) and exits in the distal right ventricular outflow tract. *C,* At an even higher level, but just below the aorta (Ao) and left atrium, a portion of the defect is seen (arrow). PA = pulmonary artery. (From Goldfarb, M. S., et al.: Two-dimensional Doppler echocardiographic diagnosis of a traumatic intracardiac shunt. Am. J. Cardiol. 57:494, 1986.)

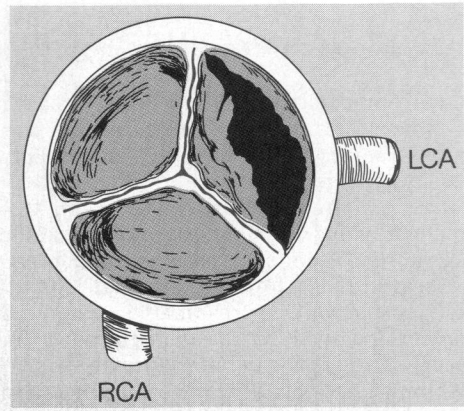

FIGURE 46–8. Diagram showing avulsion of the left coronary cusp of the aortic valve due to blunt chest trauma. (From Devineni, R., and McKenzie, F. N.: Avulsion of a normal aortic valve cusp due to blunt chest injury. J. Trauma *24*:910, © by Williams and Wilkins, 1984.)

Rupture of the *tricuspid valve* is not as rare as previously thought[67,68] and is more benign than mitral valve rupture, with symptoms ranging from fatigue to ascites and edema. Physical findings can be striking, with prominent systolic venous pulsations, hepatic pulsations, and a typical holosystolic murmur with inspiratory accentuation.

TREATMENT AND PROGNOSIS. The prognosis depends largely on the severity of the regurgitation. Since the lesion usually develops suddenly, the ventricle does not have the opportunity to adapt to this burden, as it does in most forms of chronic valvular regurgitation. Obviously, the baseline condition of the ventricle prior to the trauma, the presence of other injuries occurring simultaneously, and the severity of the regurgitation affect the heart's ability to tolerate the insult. When effective surgical treatment is not possible, survival without the need for operation is not uncommon in patients with mild or moderate regurgitation. With severe left ventricular failure due to a ruptured mitral valve or papillary muscle, however, early surgery is mandatory.

The diagnosis of acute left ventricular failure may be difficult immediately after serious trauma, because fractured ribs and pulmonary contusions may be blamed for the shortness of breath and dyspnea. When left ventricular failure develops slowly or the lesion is not hemodynamically significant, as with lesser degrees of injury, medical therapy may suffice. Hemorrhage into a papillary muscle may cause late necrosis and delayed rupture, and these patients must be observed carefully.

Post-traumatic *tricuspid* regurgitation appears to have a more benign course, and many patients survive for long periods with supportive treatment. However, when failure does occur, valve replacement is the procedure of choice.

INJURIES TO THE CORONARY ARTERIES AND GREAT VESSELS

CORONARY ARTERIES

Transmural myocardial infarctions have been reported following blunt trauma, (including trauma to the head)[69] but angiographic confirmation of coronary obstruction is uncommon, and, when found, its relationship to preexisting coronary atherosclerosis may be difficult to determine. When infarction occurs, it may not be clear whether it results directly from myocardial contusion, from trauma to a coronary artery, or from some combination of these two processes. In many cases of myocardial infarction, preexisting coronary artery disease has been present, and it is reasonable to postulate that the injury dislodges a plaque, which then obstructs the vessel completely. However, it is also possible that a normal coronary artery becomes occluded, by either a traumatically induced intimal tear or hemorrhage.[70] Indeed, coronary arteriography has provided strong evidence that myocardial infarction follows blunt chest trauma in previously asymptomatic persons with normal vessels except for complete obstruction of the vessel supplying the infarcted area (Fig. 46–9).[36] The complications of myocardial infarction — arrhythmias, pump failure, and late devel-

opment of aneurysms — are similar when the lesion has an atherosclerotic basis, and treatment is similar as well. However, it may be anticipated that *following survival from the initial episode, the long-term prognosis will be more favorable in patients with traumatic damage of a coronary artery,* because the remaining vessels are usually normal. There are exceptions, however.[71]

ANEURYSM. Left ventricular *aneurysm and pseudoaneurysm* following injury to the coronary arteries can lead to ventricular rupture, cardiac failure, embolism, or arrhythmia. Operative intervention is indicated in the presence of a pseudoaneurysm, in which the myocardium has actually ruptured but in which a thrombus, fibrous tissue, and/or pericardium prevent exsanguination, since external rupture — an event that is usually fatal — is likely to occur ultimately if the condition is left untreated. Pseudoaneurysm can often be differentiated from true aneurysm by contrast or radionuclide angiography (p. 1349).

FISTULA. Formation of an *arteriovenous fistula* is an unusual complication of traumatic damage of a coronary artery.[72] Injury to the right coronary artery is more commonly followed by an arteriovenous fistula than is injury to the left. The venous side of the fistula may be the coronary sinus, the great cardiac vein (Fig. 46–10), the right atrium, or the right ventricle; in the last instance, the fistula should be termed an "arteriocameral fistula." The murmur in traumatic coronary arteriovenous or arteriocameral fistula is usually loud, widely radiating, and continuous; the electrocardiogram frequently shows transmural myocardial infarction, and the roentgenogram exhibits cardiomegaly with increased pulmonary vascularity. In patients who do not undergo surgical repair, symptoms of congestive heart failure and chest pain are frequent unless the shunt is minimal.

Espada et al. reported nine patients with *coronary artery lacerations* among a series of 76 penetrating wounds of the heart, including seven patients with stab wounds and two with gunshot wounds.[73] The left anterior descending coronary artery is the vessel most commonly involved, and at operation, the treatment of choice is suture-ligation of the cut vessel with coronary artery bypass grafting if the lacerated vessel is large and the lesion is a proximal one. Angiography is not advised in the emergency setting, as it is with nonpenetrating trauma. However, postoperative angiography is useful in localizing the presence of possible residual injuries such as a coronary arteriocameral fistula.

INJURIES TO THE GREAT VESSELS (See also p. 1551)

Rupture of the aorta is one of the most common traumatic lesions involving the heart or great vessels. In one of every six automobile accident victims dying from blunt chest trauma the aorta is ruptured.[74] To a lesser extent, aortic rupture also occurs with falls from heights and other types of crushing injuries.[75] Rupture occurs in the isthmus in 90 per cent of

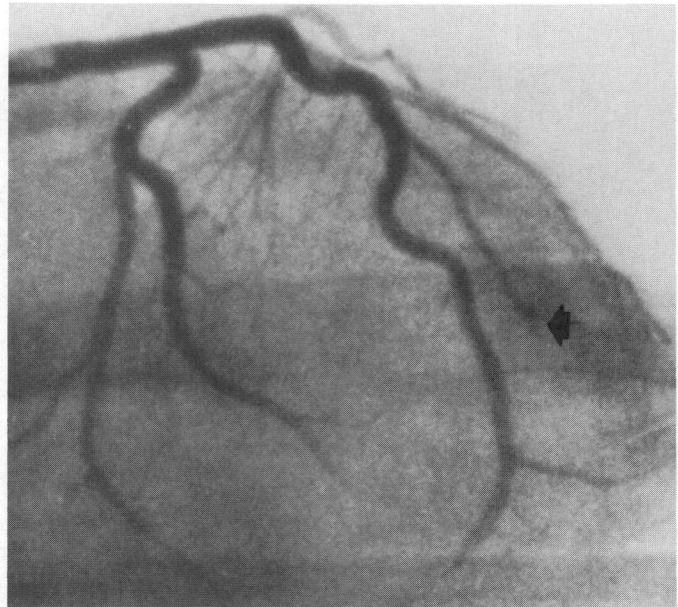

FIGURE 46–9. Coronary angiography of the left coronary artery (RAO projection) 3 days after an auto accident shows a nonocclusive thrombus in the left main artery and distal occlusion of the left anterior descending coronary artery (arrow) and of a diagonal branch. (From Unterberg, C., et al.: Traumatic thrombosis of the left main coronary artery and myocardial infarction caused by blunt chest trauma. Clin. Cardiol. *12*:672, 1989. Copyrighted and reprinted with permission of Clinical Cardiology Publishing Co., Inc., and/or the Foundation for Advances in Medicine and Science.)

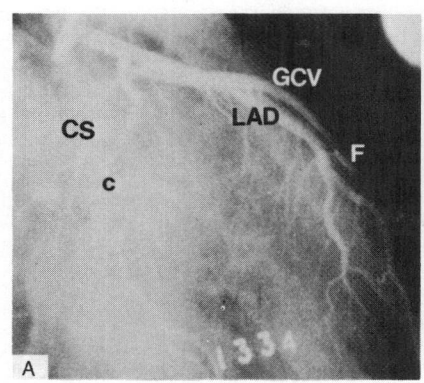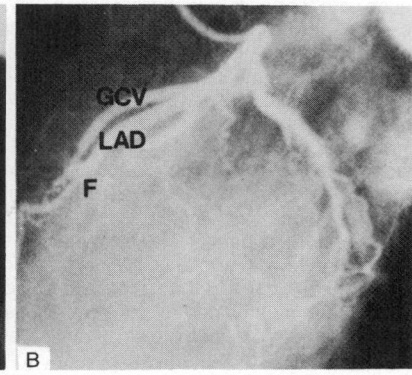

FIGURE 46-10. Left coronary arteriograms *(A)* in the right anterior oblique projection and *(B)* in the left anterior oblique projection in a patient six weeks after a penetrating chest injury. The fistula (F) can be seen arising from the second diagonal branch of the left anterior descending coronary artery (LAD) with early opacification of the great cardiac vein (GCV) and coronary sinus (CS). C = circumflex branch. (From Martin, R., et al.: Late pericardial tamponade and coronary arteriovenous fistula after trauma. Br. Heart J. *55*:216, 1986.)

cases. Multiple tears may be present in some patients, and in others the edges of the torn aorta may be separated by several centimeters, producing a mediastinal hematoma or pseudoaneurysm.

It has been estimated that 10 to 20 per cent of patients with ruptured aortas live long enough to be treated successfully under ideal circumstances, which include a high level of awareness of the possibility of aortic rupture in victims of automobile accidents as well as a well-coordinated team approach.[76] As with cardiac injury, rupture of the aorta may be overshadowed by injuries to other organs, and the diagnosis may be overlooked.[77] Common clinical and radiological findings are listed in Table 46-4. Patients with aortic rupture often complain of pain in the back in addition to the chest, as do patients with aortic dissection (p. 1535). If the expanding mediastinal hematoma or false aneurysm narrows the aortic lumen, or if the torn intima and media cause partial aortic obstruction, ischemia of the spinal cord and kidneys may ensue. A systolic murmur may be heard in the midscapular region, and widening of the superior mediastinum is visible on the chest roentgenogram (Fig. 47-23, p. 1550) along with other findings.[78,79]

A diagnostic triad that occurs in well over half the cases of ruptured aorta consists of (1) increased arterial pressure and pulse amplitude in the upper extremities, (2) decreased pressure and pulse amplitude in the lower extremities, and (3) radiological evidence of widening of the superior mediastinum.[80] Chronic rupture of the aorta may be manifested by hoarseness, dysphagia, and cough. The diagnosis can be confirmed by aortography, which should be performed as soon as the nature of the injury is suspected. CT scanning is *not* a useful screening procedure;[80] aortography is very useful for diagnosing and localizing the injury. The entire thoracic aorta and its branches should be visualized so as not to overlook a rupture occurring at an unusual site or multiple sites of rupture (Fig. 46-11).[82]

PENETRATING TRAUMA TO THE GREAT VESSELS. This is usually the result of bullet or stab wounds and occurs most commonly in conjunction with cardiac wounds. Cardiac tamponade is a frequent complication of injury to the intrapericardial segment of one of the great vessels, but when it is extrapericardial, massive hemothorax is usually the presenting finding. The superior vena cava, trachea, or esophagus or some combination of these structures may be compressed if a large mediastinal hematoma forms as a result of bleeding. Injury to the innominate or carotid arteries may compress these vessels, with resultant neurological signs. An arteriovenous fistula may develop with symptoms of congestive heart failure accompanied by a systolic or, more commonly, a continuous murmur.[83] These fistulous connections may also involve the systemic and pulmonary vessel.[84] Blunt trauma has also been reported to cause transection of the inferior vena cava.[85]

Penetrating injury to the great vessels should be suspected in any patient in whom a projectile traverses the mediastinum and is suggested by radiological evidence of a widened mediastinum. Aortography should be performed immediately, provided that emergency thoracotomy for shock or tamponade can be deferred briefly. Immediate operation, sometimes using a heparinized shunt between the ascending and descending aorta, should be carried out as soon as the diagnosis of thoracic aortic disruption has been established.[86] Pickard et al. described their experi-

TABLE 46-4 CLINICAL AND RADIOLOGICAL FINDINGS IN PATIENTS WITH AORTIC INJURY

A. CLINICAL FINDINGS	PERCENTAGE OF PATIENTS
Bone fractures (other than ribs)	75
External evidence of thoracic injury	66
Upper extremity hypertension	30-45
Systolic murmur	20-45
Dyspnea	10
Paralysis	10
Back pain	7
Dysphagia	4

B. RADIOLOGICAL FINDINGS	PERCENTAGE OF PATIENTS
Abnormal aortic outline	100
Mediastinal widening	50-100
NG tube displaced to right	100
Displaced SVC	85
Left apical cap	65-93
Opacification of AP clear space	60
First or second rib fractures	50
Depressed left bronchus	35-80
Pneumothorax/pneumomediastinum	35-50
Hemothorax	20-65
Displaced right paraspinous line	15-55
Pulmonary contusion	15-50
Displaced left paraspinous line	15-25
Deviation of trachea to right	10-55

SVC = superior vena cava; NG = nasogastric; AP = anteroposterior.
Adapted from Barcia, T. C., and Livoni, J. P.: Indications for angiography in blunt thoracic trauma. Radiology *147*:15, 1983.

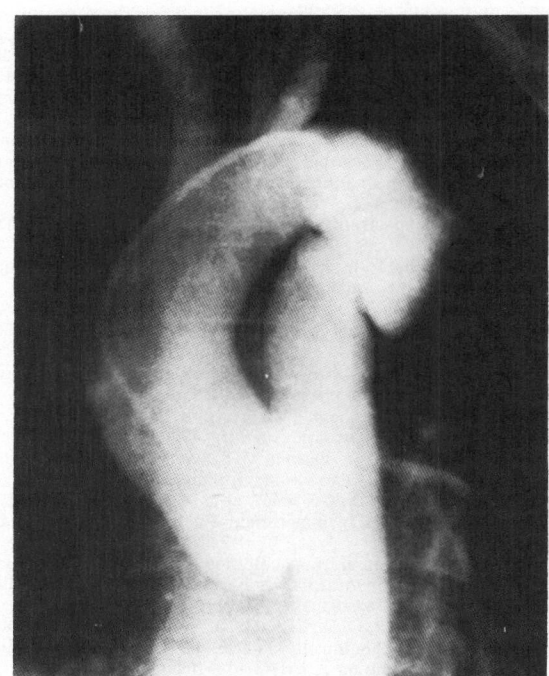

FIGURE 46-11. In a 27-year-old male, acute false and irregular aneurysm of the thoracic aorta just distal to the left subclavian artery. (Reproduced with permission from Andresen, J., and Axelsen, F.: Traumatic rupture of the thoracic aorta. Scand. J. Thorac. Cardiovasc. Surg. *14*:281, 1980.)

ence with 22 patients with transection of the descending thoracic aorta secondary to blunt trauma who reached the hospital alive; five patients died shortly after admission, three died in the operating room, three died within 30 days of operation, and one died more than 1 year after the injury.[87] Ten patients were long-term survivors. A Dacron tube graft was utilized to bridge the defect in the majority of patients.

In order to avoid the problem inherent in heparinization, i.e., bleeding from what are often multiple sites of trauma, tears of the descending thoracic aorta may often be repaired without cardiopulmonary bypass by simple aortic cross-clamping, as long as the cross-clamp time is restricted to less than 30 minutes.[88,89] An experienced surgeon can interpose a graft into the aorta with a total occlusion time ranging from 13 to 21 minutes, and ischemic injury to the spinal cord or kidneys should not occur. This technique may be aided by the intravenous administration of nitroprusside, which can maintain proximal aortic systolic pressure below 140 mm Hg.

Antiadrenergic agents such as guanethidine, reserpine, and propranolol, which have been utilized in the treatment of spontaneous dissection of the aorta (p. 1540), may also have a role in treatment of patients with aortic rupture if, for logistical reasons, operation must be deferred.

REFERENCES

1. Committee on Trauma and Committee on Shock: Accidental death and disability: The neglected diseases of modern society. Washington, D.C., National Academy of Sciences, 1965, p. 5.
2. Cheitlin, M. D.: Cardiovascular trauma. Circulation 65:1529, 1982, and Circulation 66:244, 1982.
3. Mayfield, W., and Hurley, E. J.: Blunt cardiac trauma. Am. J. Surg. 148:162, 1984.
4. Sherman, M. M., Saini, V. K., Yarnoz, M. D., Ramp, J., Williams, L. F., and Berger, R. L.: Management of penetrating heart wounds. Am. J. Surg. 135:553, 1978.
5. Mattox, K. L., Feliciano, D. V., Burch, J., et al.: Five thousand seven hundred sixty cardiovascular injuries in 4459 patients: Epidemiologic evolution 1958 to 1987. Ann. Surg. 209:698, 1989.

NONPENETRATING CARDIAC INJURY

6. Parmley, L. F., Manion, W. C., and Mattingly, T. W.: Nonpenetrating traumatic injury of the heart. Circulation 18:371, 1958.
7. Glock, Y., Massabuau, P., and Puel, P.: Cardiac damage in non-penetrating chest injuries. J. Cardiovasc. Surg. 30:27, 1989.
8. Rothstein, R. J.: Myocardial contusion. J.A.M.A. 250:2189, 1983.
9. Matthews, R. V., French, W. J., and Criley, J. M.: Chest trauma and subvalvular left ventricular aneurysms. Chest 95:474, 1989.
10. DeMuth, W. E., Lerner, E. H., and Liedtke, A. J.: Nonpenetrating injury of the heart: An experimental model. J. Trauma 13:639, 1973.
11. Clifford, R. P., and Gill, K. S.: Traumatic rupture of the pericardium with dislocation of the heart. Injury 16:123, 1984.
12. Miller, F. A., Jr., Seward, J. B., Gersh, B. J., et al.: Two-dimensional echocardiographic findings in cardiac trauma. Am. J. Cardiol. 50:1022, 1982.
13. Lau, V.-K., Viano, D. C., and Doty, D. B.: Experimental cardiac trauma — Ballistics of a captive bolt pistol. J. Trauma 21:39, 1982.
14. Pandian, N. G., Skorton, D. J., Doty, D. B., and Kerber, R. E.: Immediate diagnosis of acute myocardial contusion by two-dimensional echocardiography: Studies in a canine model of blunt chest trauma. J. Am. Coll. Cardiol. 2:488, 1983.
15. Tenzer, M. L.: The spectrum of myocardial contusion: A review. J. Trauma 25:620, 1985.
16. Frazee, R. C., Mucha, P., Jr., Farnell, M. B., and Miller, F. A., Jr.: Objective evaluation of blunt cardiac trauma. J. Trauma 26:510, 1986.
17. Snow, N., Richardson, J. D., and Flint, L. M., Jr.: Myocardial contusion: Implications for patients with multiple traumatic injuries. Surgery 92:744, 1982.
18. Kumar, S. A., Puri, V. K., Mittal, V. K., and Cortez, J.: Myocardial contusion following nonfatal blunt chest trauma. J. Trauma 23:327, 1983.
19. Torres-Mirabal, P., Gruenberg, J. C., Brown, R. S., and Obeid, F. N.: Spectrum of myocardial contusion. Am Surg. 48:383, 1982.
20. Frazee, R. C., Mucha, P., Jr., Farnell, M. B., and Miller, F. A., Jr.: Objective evaluation of blunt cardiac trauma. J. Trauma 26:510, 1986.
21. Chiu, C. L., Roelofs, J. D., Go, R. T., et al.: Coronary angiographic and scintigraphic findings in experimental cardiac contusion. Radiology 116:679, 1975.
22. Sutherland, G. R., Cheung, H. W., Holliday, R. L., et al.: Hemodynamic adaptation to acute myocardial contusion complicating blunt chest injury. Am. J. Cardiol. 57:291, 1986.
23. Schamp, D. J., Plotnick, G. D., Croteau, D., et al.: Clinical significance of radionuclide angiographically-determined abnormalities following acute blunt chest trauma. Am. Heart J. 116:500, 1988.
24. Mattox, K. L., Limacher, M. C., Feliciano, D. V., et al.: Cardiac evaluation following heart injury. J. Trauma 25:758, 1985.
25. Fox, K. M., Rowland, E., Krikler, D. M., et al.: Electrophysiological manifestations on nonpenetrating cardiac trauma. Br. Heart J. 43:458, 1980.
26. Cooperman, Y., Low, S., and Laniado, S.: Traumatic heart block. PACE 12:25, 1989.
27. Bognolo, D. A., Rabow, F. I., Vijayanagar, R. R., and Eckstein, P. F.: Traumatic sinus node dysfunction. Ann. Emerg. Med. 11:319, 1982.
28. Évora, P. R. B., Ribeiro, P. J. F., Brasil, J. C. F., et al.: Late surgical repair of ventricular septal defect due to nonpenetrating chest trauma: Review and report of two contrasting cases. J. Trauma 25:1007, 1985.
29. Torres-Mirabal, P., Gruenberg, J. C., Talbert, J. G., and Brown, R. S.: Ventricular function in myocardial contusion: A preliminary study. Crit. Care Med. 10:19, 1982.
30. Desiderio, M. A.: The potentiation of the response to blunt cardiac trauma by ethanol in dogs. J. Trauma 26:467, 1986.
31. Dubrow, T. J., Mihalka, J., Eisenhauer, D. M., et al.: Myocardial contusion in the stable patient: What level of care is appropriate? Surgery 106:267, 1989.
32. Soliman, M. H., and Waxman, K.: Value of a conventional approach to the diagnosis of traumatic cardiac contusion after chest injury. Crit. Care Med. 15:218, 1987.
33. Hossack, K. F., Moreno, C. A., Vanway, C. W., and Burdick, D. C.: Frequency of cardiac contusion in nonpenetrating chest injury. Am. J. Cardiol. 61:391, 1988.
34. Watt, A. H., and Stephens, M. R.: Myocardial infarction after blunt chest trauma incurred during rugby football that later required cardiac transplantation. Br. Heart J. 55:408, 1986.
35. Espinosa, R., Badui, E., Castaño, R., and Madrid, R.: Acute posterior wall myocardial infarction secondary to football chest trauma. Chest 88:928, 1985.
36. Unterberg, C. Buchwald, A., and Viegand, V.: Traumatic thrombosis of the left main coronary artery and myocardial infarction caused by blunt chest trauma. Clin. Cardiol. 12:672, 1989.
37. Chang, H., Chu, S-H., and Lee, Y-T.: Traumatic aorto-right atrial fistula after blunt chest injury. Ann. Thorac. Surg. 45:778, 1989.
38. Getz, B. S., Davies, E., Steinberg, S. M., et al.: Blunt cardiac trauma resulting in right atrial rupture. J.A.M.A. 255:761, 1986.
39. Hines, G. L., Doyle, E., and Acinapura, A. J.: Post-traumatic ventricular septal defect, mitral insufficiency, and multiple coronary cameral fistulas. J. Trauma 17:234, 1977.
40. Pickard, L. R., Mattox, K. L., and Beall, A. C., Jr.: Ventricular septal defect from blunt chest injury. J. Trauma 20:329, 1980.
41. Leavitt, B. J., Meyer, J. A., Morton, J. R., et al.: Survival following nonpenetrating traumatic rupture of cardiac chambers. Ann. Thorac. Surg. 44:532, 1987.
42. Eisenberg, M. S., Horwood, B. T., Cummins, R. O., et al.: Cardiac arrest and resuscitation: A tale of 29 cities. Ann. Emerg. Med. 19:179, 1990.
43. Gerry, J. L., Bulkley, B. H., and Hutchins, G. M.: Rupture of the papillary muscle of the tricuspid valve. A complication of cardiopulmonary resuscitation and a rare cause of tricuspid insufficiency. Am. J. Cardiol. 40:825, 1977.
44. Baker, P. B., Keyhani-Rofagha, S., Graham, R. L., and Sharma, H. M.: Dissecting hematoma (aneurysm) of coronary arteries. Am. J. Med. 80:317, 1986.

PENETRATING CARDIAC INJURY

45. Naughton, M. J., Brissie, R. M., Bessey, P. Q., et al.: Demography of penetrating cardiac trauma. Ann Surg. 209:676, 1989.
46. Fallahnejad, M., Kutty, A. C. K., and Wallace, H. W.: Secondary lesions of penetrating cardiac injuries. Ann. Surg. 191:228, 1980.
47. Auge, J. M., Oriol, A., Serra, C., and Crexells, C.: The use of pigtail catheters for retrieval of foreign bodies from the cardiovascular system. Cathet. Cardiovasc. Diagn. 10:625, 1984.
48. McIvor, M. E., Kaufman, S. L., Satre, R., et al.: Search and retrieval of a radiolucent foreign object. Cath. Cardiovasc. Diagn. 16:19, 1989.
49. Gehl, L., Iskandrlann, A. N., Goel, I., et al.: Cardiac perforation with tamponade during cardiac catheterization. Cathet. Cardiovasc. Diagn. 8:293, 1982.
50. Goldbaum, T. S., Jacob, A. S., Smith, D. F., et al.: Cardiac tamponade following percutaneous transluminal coronary angioplasty: Four case reports. Cathet. Cardiovasc. Diagn. 11:413, 1985.
51. Przybojewski, J. Z.: Endomyocardial biopsy: a review of the literature. Cathet. Cardiovasc. Diagn. 11:287, 1985.
52. Anastasious-Nana, M. I., O'Connell, J. B., Nanas, J. N., et al.: Relative efficiency and risk of endomyocardial biopsy: Comparisons in heart transplant and nontransplant patients. Cath. Cardiovasc. Diagn. 16:7, 1989.
53. Cummings, R. G., Wesly, R. L. R., Adams, D. H., and Lowe, J. E.: Pneumopericardium resulting in cardiac tamponade. Ann. Thoracic Surg. 37:511, 1984.
54. Marshall, W. G., Jr., Bell, J. L., and Kouchoukos, N. T.: Penetrating cardiac trauma. J. Trauma 24:147, 1984.
55. Whye, D., Barish, R., Almquist, T., et al.: Echocardiographic diagnosis of acute pericardial effusion in penetrating chest trauma. Am. J. Emerg. Med. 6:21, 1988.
56. Hassett, A. Moran, J., Sabiston, D. C., and Kisslo, J.: Utility of echocardiography in the management of patients with penetrating missile wounds of the heart. J. Am. Coll. Cardiol. 7:1151, 1986.
57. Miller, J. T., Richards, K. L., Miller, J. F., and Crawford, M. H.: Doppler echocardiographic determination of the cause of a systolic murmur following penetrating chest trauma. Am. Heart J. 111:988, 1986.
58. Goldfarb, M. S., Walpole, H. T., Jr., Landolt, C. C., et al.: Two-dimensional Doppler echocardiographic diagnosis of a traumatic intracardiac shunt. Am. J. Cardiol. 57:494, 1986.

59. Martin, L. F., Mavroudis, C., Dyess, D. L., et al.: The first 70 years' experience managing cardiac disruption due to penetrating and blunt injuries at the University of Louisville. Am. Surg. 52:14, 1986.

60. Bergin, P. J.: Aortic thrombosis and peripheral embolization after thoracic gunshot wound diagnosed by transesophageal echocardiography. Am. Heart J. 119:688, 1990.

61. Alsofrom, D. J., Marcus, N. H., Seigel, R. S., et al.: Shotgun pellet embolization from the chest to the middle cerebral arteries. J. Trauma 22:155, 1982.

62. Asfaw, I., Thoms, N. W., and Arfulu, A.: Interventricular septal defects from penetrating injuries of the heart. A report of 12 cases and review of the literature. J. Thorac. Cardiovasc. Surg. 69:450, 1975.

63. Rustad, D. G., Hopeman, A. R., Murr, P. C., and VanWay, C. W., III: Aorta-cardiac fistula with aortic valve injury from penetrating trauma. J. Trauma 26:266, 1986.

64. Werne, C., Sagraves, S. G., and Costa, C.: Mitral and tricuspid valve rupture from blunt trauma sustained during a motor vehicle collision. J. Trauma 29:15, 1989.

65. Reinfeld, H. B., Agatston, A. S., Robinson, M. J., and Hildner, F. J.: Bioprosthetic mitral valve dysfunction following blunt chest trauma. Am. Heart J. 111:800, 1986.

66. Rumisek, J. D., Robonowitz, M., Virmani, R., et al.: Bioprosthetic heart valve rupture associated with trauma. J. Trauma 26:276, 1986.

67. Eskilsson, J.: Tricuspid insufficiency caused by nonpenetrating chest trauma: Report of two cases diagnosed by Doppler cardiography. Acta Med. Scand. 218:347, 1985.

68. Gayet, C., Pierre, B., Delahaye, J-P., et al.: Traumatic tricuspid insufficiency: An underdiagnosed disease. Chest 92:429, 1987.

69. Bashour, T. T., Morelli, R. L., Cunningham, T., and Budge, W. R.: Acute coronary thrombosis following head trauma in a young man. Am. Heart J. 119:676, 1990.

70. Sabbah, H. N., Mohyi, J., and Stein, P. D.: Coronary arteriography in dogs following blunt cardiac trauma: A longitudinal assessment. Cath. Cardiovasc. Diagn. 15:155, 1988.

71. Watt, A. H., and Stephens, M. R.: Myocardial infarction after blunt chest trauma incurred during rugby football that later required cardiac transplantation. Br. Heart J. 55:408, 1986.

72. Martin, R., Mitchell, A., and Dhalla, N.: Late pericardial tamponade and coronary arteriovenous fistula after trauma. Br. Heart J. 55:216, 1986

73. Espada, R., Whisennard, H. H., Mattox, K. L., and Beall, A. C., Jr.: Surgical management of penetrating injuries to the coronary arteries. Surgery 78:755, 1975.

74. Greendyke, R. M.: Traumatic rupture of the aorta. Special reference to automobile accidents. J.A.M.A. 195:527, 1966.

75. Shaikh, K. A., Schwab, C. W., and Camishion, R. C.: Aortic rupture in blunt trauma. Am. Surg. 52:47, 1986.

76. Ayella, R. J., Hankins, J. R., Turney, S. Z., and Cowley, R. A.: Ruptured thoracic aorta due to blunt trauma. J. Trauma 17:199, 1977.

77. Barcia, T. C., and Livoni, J. P.: Indications for angiography in blunt thoracic trauma. Radiology 147:15, 1983.

78. Gundry, S. R., Burney, R. E., Mackenzie, J. R., et al.: Assessment of mediastinal widening associated with traumatic rupture of the aorta. J. Trauma 23:293, 1983.

79. Heystraten, F. M., Rosenbusch, G., Kingma, L. M., et al.: Chest radiography in acute traumatic rupture of the thoracic aorta. Acta Radiolog. 29:411, 1988.

80. Symbas, P. N., Tyras, D. H., Ware, R. E., and Hatcher, C. R., Jr.: Rupture of the aorta. A diagnostic triad. Ann. Thorac. Surg. 15:405, 1973.

81. Miller, F. B., Richardson, J. D., Thomas, H. A., et al.: Role of CT in diagnosis of major arterial injury after blunt thoracic trauma. Surgery 106:596, 1989.

82. Kirsh, M. M., Orringer, M. B., Behrendt, D. M., et al.: Management of unusual traumatic ruptures of the aorta. Surg. Gynecol. Obstet. 146:365, 1978.

83. Machiedo, G. W., Jain, K. M., Swan, K. G., et al.: Traumatic aorto-caval fistula. J. Trauma 23:243, 1983.

84. Arom, K. V., and Lyons, G. W.: Traumatic pulmonary arteriovenous fistula. J. Thorac. Cardiovasc. Surg. 70:918, 1975.

85. Peitzman, A. B., Udekwu, A. O., Pevec, W., and Albrink, M.: Tansection of the inferior vena cava from blunt thoracic trauma: Case reports. J. Trauma 29:534, 1989.

86. Akins, C. W., Buckley, M. J., Daggett, W., et al.: Acute traumatic disruption of the thoracic aorta: A ten-year experience. Ann. Thorac. Surg. 31:305, 1981.

87. Pickard, L. R., Mattox, K. L., Espada, R., et al.: Transection of the descending thoracic aorta secondary to blunt trauma. J. Trauma 17:749, 1977.

88. Vasko, J. S., Raess, D. H., Williams, T. E., Jr., et al.: Nonpenetrating trauma to the thoracic aorta. Surgery 82:400, 1977.

89. Turney, S. Z., Attar, S., Ayella, R., et al.: Traumatic rupture of the aorta. A five-year experience. J. Thorac. Cardiovasc. Surg. 72:727, 1976.

Diseases of the Aorta

by KIM A. EAGLE, M.D., and ROMAN W. DE SANCTIS, M.D.

THE NORMAL AORTA

FUNCTION. Appropriately called "the greatest artery" by the ancients, the aorta is admirably suited for its task. This thin but large and remarkably tough vessel must absorb the impact of 2.5 to 3 billion heartbeats in an average lifetime while carrying roughly 200,000,000 liters of blood to the body.

Arteries can be categorized as either "conductance" or "resistance" vessels. Conductance vessels are the conduits for blood, and the aorta is the ultimate conductance vessel. It is composed of three layers: a thin, inner tunica intima; a thick middle layer, the tunica media; and a rather thin outer layer, the tunica adventitia. The strength of the aorta lies in the tunica media, which is composed of laminated but intertwining sheets of elastic tissue arranged in a spiral manner that affords maximum tensile strength. As thin as it is, the wall of the aorta can withstand the experimental pressure of thousands of millimeters of mercury without bursting. In contrast to peripheral arteries, the aortic media contains very little smooth muscle, although there is a network of some smooth muscle and collagen between the elastic layers. This tremendous accretion of elastic tissue in the aorta gives it not only great tensile strength but also elasticity, which serves a vital circulatory role. The aortic intima is a thin, delicate layer lined by endothelium and easily traumatized. The adventitia contains mainly collagen but also houses the important vasa vasorum and lymphatics, which nourish the aortic wall.

As systole develops, part of the force generated by the contracting ventricle is converted into potential energy stored in the wall of the aorta as it is distended by the blood ejected into it. In diastole, this potential energy in the stretched aortic wall is transformed into kinetic energy as the resilient aorta decompresses, and the force that is created acts against the column of blood contained within the lumen. With a competent aortic valve proximally, the blood is propelled distally into the arterial bed. Thus, the aorta plays a major role in circulating the blood after it is delivered into the aorta by the heart. The pulse wave itself with its milking effect is transmitted along the aorta to the periphery at a speed of about 5 meters per second. This is much faster than the velocity of the intraluminal blood, which travels only 40 to 50 cm per second.

The systolic pressure developed within the aorta is a function of the volume of blood ejected into the aorta, the compliance or distensibility of the aorta, and the resistance to blood flow. Resistance is determined primarily by the tone in the peripheral muscular arteries and arterioles and to a slight extent by the inertia of the column of blood in the aorta when systole commences. The aorta and its branches tend to stiffen with age, accounting for the increase in systolic blood pressure with advancing age.

In addition to its conductance and pumping functions, the aorta plays a role in the control of systemic vascular resistance and heart rate. Pressure-responsive receptors analogous to those in the carotid sinus lie in the ascending aorta and the aortic arch and send afferent signals to the vasomotor center in the brain stem by way of the vagus nerves. Raising the aortic pressure causes reflex bradycardia and reduction of systemic vascular resistance, whereas lowering the pressure increases the heart rate and systemic resistance.

ANATOMICAL CONSIDERATIONS. The *ascending aorta* in a normal adult is about 3 cm wide at its origin from the base of the heart and extends 5 to 6 cm cephalad to join the aortic arch. Normally, the ascending aorta lies just to the right of the midline. Its proximal portion is within the pericardial cavity. Nearby structures include the pulmonary trunk in front and the left atrium, right pulmonary artery, and right main stem bronchus behind.

The *arch of the aorta* gives rise to all the brachiocephalic vessels. It courses slightly leftward in front of the trachea and then proceeds dorsally and inferiorly above the left main stern bronchus to the left of the trachea and esophagus. The arch assumes almost a directly anteroposterior orientation in the superior mediastinum. Other closely related structures are the left phrenic and vagus nerves to the left of the arch; inferiorly lie the bifurcation of the pulmonary trunk and most of the left lung. The left recurrent laryngeal nerve also loops underneath it distally.

The *descending thoracic aorta* is the continuation of the aorta beyond the arch. It lies in the posterior mediastinum to the left of the vertebral column, gradually courses in front of the vertebral column as it descends, occupying a position behind the esophagus, and passes through the diaphragm, usually at the level of the 12th thoracic vertebra.

A small but important segment called the *aortic isthmus* is the point at which the arch and descending thoracic aorta join. This is where coarctations of the aorta are usually located, and it is also the point at which the mobile portion of the aorta—the ascending aorta and arch—becomes relatively fixed to the thorax by the pleural reflections, intercostal arteries, and left subclavian artery. The aorta is especially vulnerable to trauma at this point.

The *abdominal aorta* forms the continuation of the thoracic aorta, giving off the important splanchnic vessels and ending in the aortic bifurcation at the level of the 4th lumbar vertebra.

EXAMINATION OF THE AORTA

Unless the aorta is abnormally enlarged, the only location at which it can be palpated is in the abdomen. The ease with which it can be felt depends largely on the body habitus and on the pulse pressure; it is readily felt in thin individuals. It is quite sensitive to pressure. Auscultation usually is unrevealing in aortic diseases, except for occasional bruits at sites of narrowing of the aorta or its tributary branches. Diseases of the proximal ascending aorta sometimes involve the aortic valve, with resultant aortic insufficiency.

Chest roentgenography and fluoroscopy are valuable and simple procedures for assessing the aorta. Normally, the ascending aorta is not visible on the direct anteroposterior chest roentgenogram. The aortic arch is seen as the aortic "knob" or "knuckle" in the superior mediastinum just to the left of the vertebral column (Fig. 8–6, p. 205). The edge of the descending thoracic aorta can often be recognized to the left of the spine.

On the lateral chest roentgenogram, the proximal ascending aorta can be seen as an indistinct shadow in the middle mediastinum arising from the base of the heart. The ascending

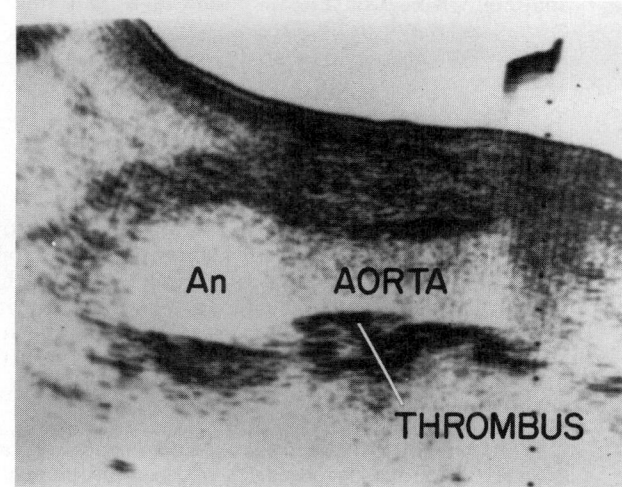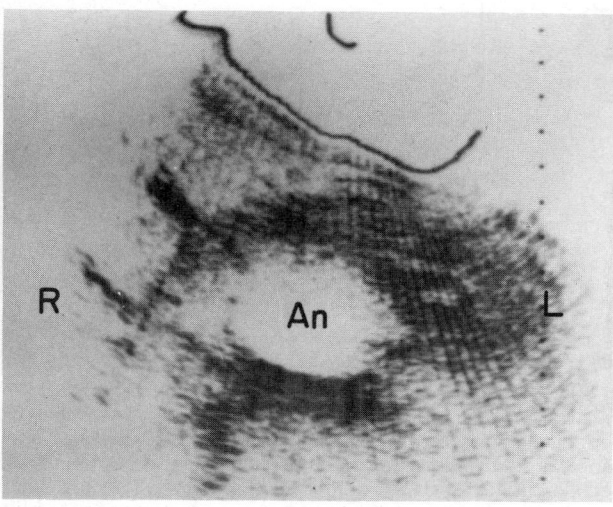

POSTERIOR

FIGURE 47–1. Cross-sectional echocardiograms of an abdominal aortic aneurysm in a 62-year-old man. *Left,* Lateral view showing a 5-cm aneurysm (An), with dilatation of the aorta distal to the aneurysm. The widened aorta is visualized down to the aortic bifurcation. Note the thrombus in the wall of the aneurysm. The dense echoes between the aneurysm and skin are made up of subcutaneous fat, muscle, and mesenteric contents. *Right,* Echocardiogram with the ultrasound beam oriented in the anteroposterior direction showing the aneurysm clearly. R and L indicate the patient's right and left sides. The distance between each of the dots aligned vertically on the right in both scans represents 1 cm. (Courtesy of Rob Kirkpatrick, M.D., Department of Radiology, Massachusetts General Hospital, Boston.)

aorta and arch are best demonstrated in a left anterior oblique projection — a view that should always be included when disease of the thoracic aorta is suspected (Fig. 8–15, p. 214).

Calcification in the aortic knob is often present, particularly in older people and patients with hypertension. It has little significance. Arteriosclerosis often results in extensive aortic calcification. The location of aortic calcification is useful in the differential diagnosis of aortic disease. Syphilis causes calcification predominantly of the ascending aorta, whereas arteriosclerotic calcification is ordinarily densest in the arch and the descending thoracic and abdominal aorta. Aneurysms of the abdominal aorta can often be seen radiographically if they are calcified. A lateral film of the abdomen is the most useful view for demonstrating them.

Normally, the aorta tends to elongate and widen slightly with age, a process which is accelerated by hypertension. Aneurysms, of course, appear as localized dilatations of the aorta. It is sometimes difficult to distinguish aneurysms from other mediastinal masses. In such cases fluoroscopy or real-time ultrasound may be very helpful by showing the presence or absence of pulsations in the mass.

Angiographic study of the aorta is of critical importance in the evaluation of aortic diseases. Aneurysms, aortic dissections, and occlusive disease of the aorta and its arterial branches can usually be readily demonstrated by a contrast study. With technical improvements in digital subtraction angiography, performed by venous injection of contrast material, adequate aortic definition should be possible while obviating catheterization of the aorta. However, this technique is limited by poor spatial resolution, artifacts caused by patient movement, and difficulty in defining anatomical detail because of overlapping blood vessels.[1]

Ultrasonography is a very important tool in the diagnosis of aortic disease (p. 106). The presence or absence of an abdominal aortic aneurysm can be definitively established by this simple noninvasive technique. In particular, two-dimensional echocardiography is extremely accurate in both diagnosing and sizing abdominal aortic aneurysms (Fig. 47–1) and can also provide valuable information about the location and size of aortic root aneurysms. Transesophageal echocardiography, particularly when combined with Doppler color flow imaging, now allows the highly accurate ultrasound assessment of both proximal and distal aortic dissection.[2,3]

Computed tomographic scanning of the body (CT scan), enhanced by intravenous injection of contrast material, is an excellent technique for noninvasive visualization of the aorta (Fig. 47–2, and Fig. 11–16, p. 320). CT scans are particularly useful for the diagnosis and sizing of thoracic and abdominal aortic aneurysms and for the diagnosis of aortic dissection and traumatic aneurysms of the aorta.[4-7] The CT scan is even more accurate than ultrasonography in determining the size of abdominal aortic aneurysms.[8] Magnetic resonance imaging (MRI) is another excellent noninvasive technique for evaluating aortic disease (Fig. 11–46, p. 336). It has advantages over CT scanning in that imaging can be performed in multiple planes (i.e., coronal and sagittal planes) and contrast agents are

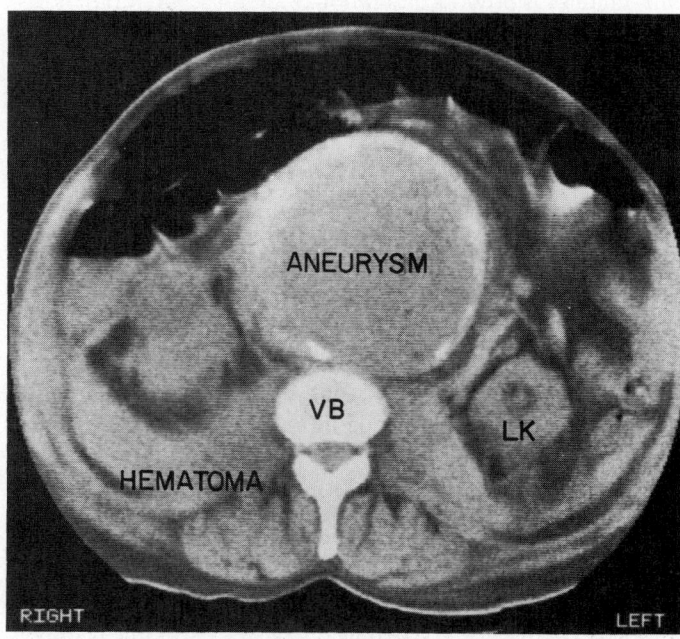

FIGURE 47–2. Abdominal CT scan showing a large, leaking abdominal aortic aneurysm. The aneurysm measures approximately 11 cm in diameter and abuts the vertebral body (VB) posteriorly. The light areas in the periphery of the aneurysm are calcific deposits in the aortic wall. The lower pole of the left kidney is identified (LK); behind the right kidney is a retroperitoneal hematoma. (Courtesy of Jack Wittenberg, M.D., Department of Radiology, Massachusetts General Hospital, Boston.)

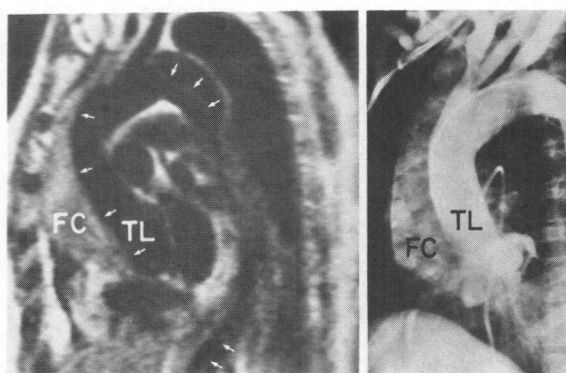

FIGURE 47–3. Nuclear magnetic resonance image in long axis (left), with corresponding aortogram (right) in a 55-year-old woman with a Type A dissection. The arrows indicate the partition between the false channel (FC) of the dissection and the true lumen (TL) of the aorta. The dissection extends into the descending thoracic aorta. The false channel shows up densely in the NMR scan because of stagnant blood blow within it. (Courtesy of Robert E. Dinsmore, M.D., Massachusetts General Hospital, Boston. NMR scan from Dinsmore, R. E., et al.: A. J. R. *146*:1286, 1986.)

unnecessary. Many studies confirm its accuracy in locating and sizing aortic aneurysms and dissections (Fig. 47–3).[9-16]

PATHOGENESIS OF DISEASES OF THE AORTA

Diseases of the aorta are either congenital or acquired.[16a] Congenital defects in turn are either gross anatomical abnormalities, such as coarctation, right aortic arch, anomalous arterial branches, double aortic arches, and so on, or histological disorders, such as degenerative abnormalities in the aortic wall that predispose to later problems (e.g., cystic medial degeneration in the Marfan syndrome and other inherited connective tissue disorders).

The only congenital gross anatomical disease considered in this chapter is pseudocoarctation (p. 1549). *Coarctation* is discussed on pages 920, 967, and 1550. All other conditions discussed either are acquired or result from congenital histological changes in the aortic wall.

Acquired diseases of the aorta are primarily the result of degenerative changes in the aortic wall. Prominent among the factors that lead to this degeneration are aging, arteriosclerosis, hypertension, and specific infectious, inflammatory, or autoimmune diseases that involve the aorta focally or diffusely. Some of these processes may affect the aortic root, with resultant aortic insufficiency, or the major arterial branches arising from the aorta. The importance of the velocity at which blood is ejected from the left ventricle (dV/dt) as a major shearing stress on the aortic wall has also been emphasized as promoting aortic dissection.

Some patients with aortic aneurysms have been shown to have decreased ratios of type III collagen as compared with type I collagen.[16b] In these instances it is not unusual to find a family history of aneurysm, particularly in women, with up to 18 per cent of first-degree relatives affected.[16c,16d] Several investigators have proposed that polymorphic variants in collagen type III genes are responsible for these observations, much as has been seen in Ehlers-Danlos Type IV syndrome.[16e]

Arteriosclerosis is especially important in the pathogenesis of aortic aneurysms. Hypertension may be particularly important in causing diseases of the aorta. Experimental work suggests that hypertension leads to structural aortic changes that may accelerate medial degeneration in certain patients; may decrease the blood flow in the vasa vasorum, with resultant ischemia of the aortic wall; and may initiate a response that stiffens the aorta and serves to perpetuate the hypertensive state. Although some degree of aortic medial degeneration is common with aging, the extent and severity of these changes are much greater in hypertensive individuals.[17-19]

ARTERIOSCLEROTIC AORTIC ANEURYSMS

ABDOMINAL AORTIC ANEURYSMS

Approximately three-fourths of all arteriosclerotic aortic aneurysms are confined to the abdominal aorta. Normally, in the adult, the aorta measures 2 cm in diameter at the level of the celiac axis and 1.8 cm just below the renal arteries; it then tapers slightly to the iliac vessels. Most abdominal aneurysms arise in the area between the renal arteries and the aortic bifurcation. Clinically significant aneurysms measure 4 cm or more in diameter.

ETIOLOGY AND PATHOGENESIS. Abdominal aortic aneurysms arise in areas of dense atherosclerosis. The atherosclerotic process erodes the aortic wall, destroying the medial elastic elements.[20] This causes weakening of the aortic wall and eventually leads to fusiform or, rarely, saccular dilation of the abdominal aorta. As the aorta widens, tension in the wall of the aorta rises in accordance with Laplace's law, which states that tension is proportional to the product of pressure and radius. Further widening results in greater tension, which in turn leads to acceleration in the rate of enlargement of the aneurysm. A vicious circle is thus established and produces dilatation that is often rapidly progressive. Hypertension may also contribute to the pathogenesis of these aneurysms. Epidemiological studies suggest that there is a familial occurrence of abdominal aortic aneurysms.[21]

Most abdominal aortic aneurysms arise just below the renal arteries and extend to, and often involve, the aortic bifurcation. Only 2 to 5 per cent of abdominal aortic aneurysms are suprarenal, and these usually result from the distal extension of a thoracic aneurysm into the abdomen. As aneurysms expand they may compress contiguous structures. Laminated thrombi frequently form in areas of stagnant flow within the aneurysm. Thrombotic and arteriosclerotic debris may embolize distally (p. 1551) and compromise the circulation of tributary arteries. Finally, the aneurysm may rupture. Of those aneurysms which do rupture, 80 per cent rupture retroperitoneally, and most of the remainder rupture into the peritoneal cavity, causing rapid circulatory collapse.[22] Rarely, an aneurysm may rupture into the inferior vena cava, iliac vein, or renal vein.[23,24]

CLINICAL MANIFESTATIONS. The majority of abdominal aneurysms are asymptomatic and are discovered on routine physical examination or on a routine abdominal roentgenogram.[25] Aneurysms may cause a sense of fullness in the epigastrium. If pain is present, it is usually located in the hypogastrium and lower back. The pain is usually steady, with a gnawing quality, and may last for hours or days at a time. In contrast to musculoskeletal back pain, it is not affected by movement, although patients may be more comfortable in certain positions, such as with the legs drawn up. Some astute patients may suspect an aneurysm by recognizing an abnormal pulsation of the aorta, as when lying down reading a book perched on the abdomen. Expansion and impending rupture are heralded by the development of pain, often of sudden onset, which is characteristically constant, severe, and located in the back or lower abdomen, sometimes with radiation into the groin, buttocks, or legs. Actual rupture is associated with the abrupt onset of back pain with abdominal pain and tenderness. Most patients have a palpable, pulsatile abdominal mass and many are hypotensive.[26]

Many aneurysms can be detected on physical examination, although even large aneurysms may be difficult or impossible to detect in obese individuals. When palpable, a pulsatile mass extending variably from between the xiphoid process to the umbilicus may be appreciated. Owing to difficulty in distinguishing the abdominal aorta from surrounding structures by palpation, the size of an aneurysm tends to be overestimated on physical examination. Moreover, it may sometimes be difficult to differentiate a tortuous, ectatic aorta from true aneurysmal dilatation. Aneurysms are often sensitive to palpation and may be quite tender if they are rapidly expanding or about to rupture. Aneurysms should always be palpated cautiously, particularly if they are tender.

Associated occlusive arterial disease is sometimes present in the femoral pulses and distal pulses in the legs or feet. Bruits arising from associated narrowed arteries may be heard over the aneurysm. Rarely, an aneurysm may expand in such a way as to occlude the inferior vena cava or one of the iliac veins, resulting in venous congestion and edema in one or both legs. Occasionally an arteriovenous fistula may be formed by spontaneous rupture into the inferior vena cava, iliac vein, or renal vein and a syndrome of hemodynamic collapse and acute high-output cardiac failure results.[24,27]

Patients who suffer rupture of an abdominal aortic aneurysm are critically ill.[28] Hemorrhagic shock may ensue rapidly and is manifested by hypotension, vasoconstriction, mottled skin, diaphoresis, mental obtundation, oliguria, and terminally by arrhythmias and cardiac arrest.[26] Retroperitoneal hemorrhage may be signaled by hematomas in the flanks and groin. Rupture into the abdominal cavity may result in abdominal distention, whereas rupture into the duodenum presents as massive gastrointestinal hemorrhage.

DIAGNOSIS AND SIZING OF ANEURYSMS. Currently, aneurysms may be detected and their size estimated by seven methods: (1) physical examination, (2) routine roentgenography, (3) abdominal ultrasound, (4) abdominal aortic angiography, (5) digital subtraction angiography, (6) CT scan, and (7) MRI.

Brewster and colleagues have carefully compared results on physical examination, routine roentgenography, two-dimensional echocardiography, and aortic angiography for sizing abdominal aortic aneurysms.[29] *Physical examination* is clearly the least accurate. *Lateral x-ray examination* of the lumbar spine is inexpensive and reliably detects the outline of the aneurysm if its wall is calcified (Fig. 47–4). However, this is not the case in at least one-fourth of all patients with aneurysms, so that these cannot be visualized radiographically.[30] *Cross-sectional ultrasound* is very accurate and is easily and atraumatically performed (Fig. 47–1). Refinements in ultrasonic techniques have permitted precise definition of the aortic adventitial border. Thus, abdominal ultrasound is currently the simplest and best way to detect and size an abdominal aortic aneurysm.

Abdominal aortic angiography is less accurate in predicting size because the full width of an aneurysm may be masked by the presence of nonopacified mural thrombus. Moreover, angiography carries with it a small but definite risk of complications, including hematoma, localized dissection, infection, embolization, and renal failure. Nevertheless, when angiography is performed by experienced hands, morbidity from the procedure is minimal, and valuable information is often gleaned from it. Thus, in a survey of 190 patients, angiography of the aorta and distal circulation resulted in only minor complications in 2 per cent; averted an incorrect diagnosis in 11 per cent; revealed extension of the aneurysm above the renal arteries in 5 per cent; showed renal artery stenosis in 22 per cent and atypical renal arterial anatomy in 17 per cent; delineated significant occlusive vascular disease in 48 per cent; and demonstrated associated aneurysms of the iliac, hypogastric, femoral, and popliteal vessels in 50 per cent.[31] Thus, aortography — if performed by experienced angiographers — is currently recommended for patients in whom there is any question of a correct diagnosis, for hypertensive patients with possible renal arterial disease, when the extent of the aneurysm is unclear, and for patients with suspected associated occlusive or aneurysmal diseases. In fact, at our institution, it is done routinely in most patients under consideration for surgery in order to facilitate perioperative management.

Experience with *digital subtraction angiography* (p. 1567) is still being accumulated, and it is hoped that this technique will eventually yield information as detailed as that provided by aortography, while eliminating the need for intraarterial injection. *CT scanning* has proved to be as useful and accurate as ultrasound in the diagnosis and measurement of abdominal aortic aneurysms (Fig. 47–2). Additional advantages over ultrasound are that it provides better definition of the intraluminal characteristics of the aneurysm and relationships to surrounding structures such as renal arteries, retroperitoneum, and spine.[4] It also provides potentially useful information about other abdominal organs.[4] However, it does involve the use of radiation and is more costly and time-consuming than ultrasound. Studies of MRI (p. 332) (Fig. 47–3) demonstrate close correlation between this technique and both CT scanning and ultrasound with regard to estimating the size of aneurysms and their relationship to the renal and iliac arteries. Its major limitations have included prolonged imaging time and a greater cost. However, the newer generation magnets may require much less imaging time than older models. For these reasons, ultrasound remains the procedure of choice for the screening of patients with suspected aneurysms.

NATURAL HISTORY. There is a crucial relationship between the size of aneurysms and their natural history, which is why it is so important to determine their width. Half of all aneurysms greater than 6 cm in diameter rupture within 1 year, compared with 15 to 20 per cent of aneurysms less than 6

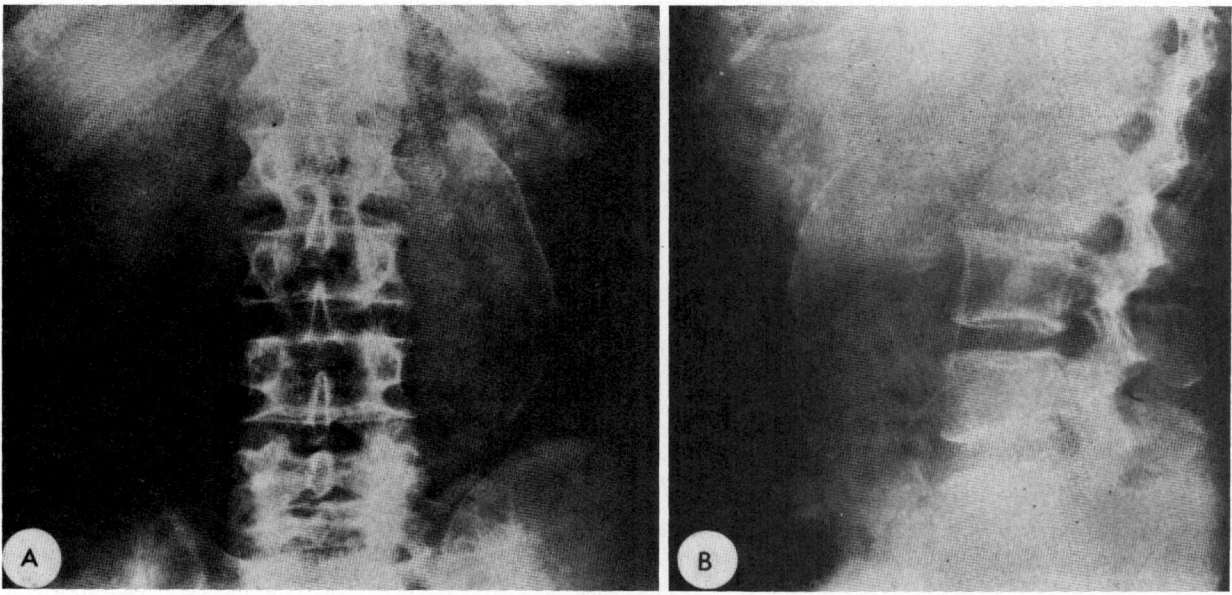

FIGURE 47–4. Anteroposterior (*A*) and lateral (*B*) views of the lumbar spinal column and the abdomen, disclosing a soft tissue mass with curvilinear calcification. (From Estes, J. E., Jr.: Abdominal aortic aneurysm: A study of one hundred and two cases. Circulation 2:261, 1950, by permission of the American Heart Association, Inc.)

cm.[32] In a review of 24,000 consecutive autopsies, Darling et al. found that in aneurysms 10 cm or larger the incidence of rupture was 60 per cent; for those 7 to 10 cm the incidence was 45 per cent; and for those measuring 4 to 7 cm the rate was 25 per cent.[33] Two recent reports suggest an "average" aneurysm expansion rate of 0.4 to 0.5 cm in diameter per year,[34,35] while another population-based study suggested an average expansion rate of 0.21 cm in diameter per year.[36] Despite this seeming discrepancy, all three studies confirm that the rate of aneurysm expansion increases as aneurysms become larger and the risk of rupture becomes prohibitive (more than 25 per cent) when aneurysm diameter exceeds 4 to 5 cm.

SURGICAL MANAGEMENT. At present, elective surgery is advised for all abdominal aortic aneurysms 6 cm in diameter or wider, assuming that surgical risks are not prohibitive because of other medical problems. The management of asymptomatic aneurysms less than 6 cm in diameter remains controversial. Pasch and coworkers have argued that elective resection of such lesions would result in the saving of lives and is economically viable because it obviates the tremendously costly care associated with aneurysm rupture.[37] Cooley has argued that improvements in surgical management of acute rupture now allow salvage of nearly 80 per cent of patients,[38] but the experience of others would appear to favor elective resection of aneurysms larger than 4 cm in otherwise good surgical candidates.[32,33] In poor-risk patients with aneurysms of 4 to 6 cm, close follow-up is advised, with immediate surgery if the aneurysm expands or shows signs of impending rupture, such as the sudden onset of pain.

Surgery consists of resection of the aneurysm and insertion of a synthetic prosthesis, usually of Dacron. Sometimes a simple tube graft is all that is necessary, although frequently the operation must be carried distally into one or both iliac arteries in order to excise the aneurysm completely. With large aneurysms, much of the wall of the aneurysm may be left in situ ("intrasaccular approach of Creech"). This reduces the need for extensive dissection, thereby decreasing aortic cross-clamping time, and has significantly ameliorated the problem of postoperative sexual dysfunction.

Expanding or ruptured abdominal aortic aneurysms are true surgical emergencies. In the case of rupture, patients can sometimes be stabilized by using a compression G-suit, a garment that may diminish the rate of bleeding by exerting counterforce externally against the abdomen. However, operation must be undertaken as soon as possible.

Perioperative Management. Advances in perioperative management have improved survival rates in patients undergoing surgical resection of abdominal aortic aneurysms. Many of these patients have significant heart disease, and monitoring of arterial blood pressure, cardiac output, cardiac filling pressures, and urine output may help enormously in their operative management. These measurements provide a valuable guide to volume replacement. So-called "declamping shock" has been virtually eliminated by volume replacement guided by monitored pressures. This term is applied to a syndrome characterized by marked hypotension upon release of the aortic cross clamp at the completion of surgery; the cause is believed to be pooling of blood in the dilated distal vascular bed and release of vasodepressor substances that have accumulated during surgery distal to the aortic clamp. The use of vasodilators such as nitroprusside or intravenous nitroglycerin may also improve and protect cardiac function by attenuating the changes in left ventricular afterload caused by clamping and unclamping the aorta.[39] Administration of mannitol and potent loop diuretics such as intravenous furosemide has reduced the frequency of postoperative renal failure.[40] The occurrence of renal failure postoperatively in patients with ruptured abdominal aortic aneurysms has correlated with very poor survival rates. Autotransfusion has led to less frequent occurrence of hepatitis and fewer transfusion reactions,[41] and antibiotic coverage has reduced the frequency of infections. Hypothermia has been better controlled,

and better understanding of the clotting system has improved management of hemostasis.

Many patients with abdominal aortic aneurysms are heavy smokers and have serious chronic obstructive lung disease. Such patients have benefited greatly from improvements in postoperative respiratory care. Preoperative preparation of pulmonary patients is also important, and smokers should abstain from tobacco use for at least 1 month before surgery.

If there is evidence of carotid artery disease in patients facing elective aneurysm resection, preoperative evaluation and surgery for critical carotid stenoses, if indicated, have resulted in fewer strokes. In patients with severe coronary artery disease, it may be important to evaluate the extent of coronary narrowing before aneurysm resection. Since half the perioperative deaths in this setting are due to myocardial infarction,[42] Hertzer and others have recommended routine coronary angiography and selective coronary bypass surgery before aneurysm resection in patients with severe correctable coronary disease.[43] Studies by Boucher et al.[44] and Eagle et al.[45] have suggested that dipyridamole-thallium cardiac scanning (p. 1712) is an effective noninvasive means of identifying patients at highest risk for perioperative ischemic events. In recent reports, these investigators have shown that further preoperative testing is unnecessary in patients without overt clinical evidence of left ventricular dysfunction, coronary artery disease, or diabetes.[46] However, in patients with one or more of these clinical markers, dipyridamole-thallium testing is quite useful in separating patients into low- and high-risk categories.[46] In particular, patients with thallium redistribution in multiple segments of myocardium are at highest risk.[47] It is in this subgroup that coronary angiography and selective bypass surgery or coronary artery angioplasty, is likely to be most helpful.[48] Others have evaluated exercise stress testing[49] (Chap. 6), gated blood pool scanning,[50] and Holter monitoring for silent ischemia[51] to identify patients at high risk. Further experience with these methods and their comparison with each other is necessary before the best and most cost-effective ways of assessing cardiac risk can be determined.

In cases of associated severe renal artery stenosis causing renin-dependent hypertension or jeopardizing renal function, simultaneous renal artery reconstruction is often performed.[52]

OPERATIVE RISK. The risk of operation obviously depends on the general status of the patient and on whether the aneurysm has ruptured. Prompt recognition and immediate operation for patients with rupture have markedly improved survival. In low-risk patients, the mortality from the elective resection of abdominal aortic aneurysms should be 2 to 5 per cent. With expanding aneurysms, mortality is 5 to 15 per cent, and with rupture, mortality has reached a plateau at approximately 50 per cent, the major determinant of survival being the speed with which surgery is accomplished.[40,52-54]

Age and preexisting cardiac, pulmonary, cerebrovascular, and/or renal diseases all add to the surgical risk. Congestive heart failure, diabetes, and evidence of coronary artery disease are particularly important, whereas advanced age per se should not be a deterrent to surgery in an otherwise healthy patient.[45,55]

An alternative to aneurysmectomy for patients at very high risk has been reported by Karmody et al.[56] This group has combined thrombosis of the aortic aneurysm with right axillary to bilateral femoral artery bypass conduits. Thrombosis of the aneurysm usually followed the interruption of flow below the aortic bifurcation achieved by ligation of the iliac outflow vessels. If the aneurysm did not thrombose within 72 hours, the iliac outflow vessels responsible for continued patency were identified by angiography and were occluded by intraarterial injection of bucrylate. Although the perioperative and late mortality in these patients was high (17 deaths among 42 patients), the deaths were related mostly to associated diseases and not to the operative procedure itself.

The statistics showing better survival with elective resection of aneurysms are impressive. From several reports, the 5-year survival rate is only 5 to 10 per cent in patients with unexcised aneurysms larger than 6 cm compared with over 50 per cent for those who undergo resection and 80 per cent for the age-matched "normal" population. *Late* survival is unaffected by whether the aneurysm was electively resected, acute, or ruptured.[54] With aneurysms smaller than 6 cm, the 5-year unoperated survival rate is about 50 per cent, as opposed to 60 to 70 per cent for those who undergo resection.[57]

COMPLICATIONS. The rate of late complications of aneurysmectomy is approximately 10 per cent.[58,59] These complications include stenosis or occlusion of the prosthetic graft, false aneurysm formation, enteric fistula formation, infection, and rupture. Patients with graft occlusion usually have evidence of prior distal vascular disease that impedes aortic runoff. *Occlusions* occur mainly at the sites of anastomosis, and patients usually develop ischemic symptoms distal to the graft site. These stenoses may be amenable to correction by balloon catheter angioplasty.[60] *False aneurysms* may be caused by infection but others arise spontaneously and present as expanding masses in the groin, abdomen, or lower back. *Enteric fistulas* are caused by rupture of the graft into the duodenum, resulting in gastrointestinal hemorrhage, and are associated with a high mortality. This complication can occur anywhere from 1 day to several years after operation, and the diagnosis must be suspected in any patient who has undergone abdominal aneurysmectomy and who presents with melena, hematemesis, hematochezia, or abdominal pain.[24,61,62] Recognition is obtained by gastrointestinal series, endoscopy, colonoscopy, or angiography. *Infections* most commonly are seen as a painful or tender groin mass, with or without a draining sinus. Recommended therapy involves administration of antibiotics, removal of the infected prosthetic material, and reestablishment of the circulation by an alternate route, usually axillofemoral bypass.

Attention has been called to the occasional occurrence of *colonic ischemia* following aneurysm surgery, caused by the intraoperative sacrifice of the inferior mesenteric artery in patients with concomitantly diseased superior or mesenteric and hypogastric arteries, resulting in inadequate perfusion of the colon.[63] This complication is best avoided by paying careful attention to collateral blood flow to the colon, maintaining adequate blood pressure during surgery, and handling the distal colon carefully at the time of operation. If necessary, reimplantation of the inferior mesenteric artery can be performed if collateral circulation is inadequate. Doppler ultrasound measurement of inferior mesenteric arterial flow or direct measurement of the inferior mesenteric arterial stump pressure may be useful in identifying patients likely to benefit from such reimplantation.[63]

THORACIC AORTIC ANEURYSMS

About one-fourth of all arteriosclerotic aneurysms involve the thoracic aorta. Dilatation may occur anywhere along the thoracic aorta—that is, the ascending segment, the arch, or the descending portion; the latter two sites are the more common ones. This contrasts with luetic aneurysms, which are located predominantly in the ascending aorta. Sometimes the entire aorta is ectatic, with localized aneurysms at many sites in both the thoracic and the abdominal aorta. Aneurysms of the descending thoracic aorta not infrequently extend into the abdominal aorta, creating a thoracoabdominal aneurysm.

PATHOGENESIS. The pathogenesis of arteriosclerotic aneurysms is identical to that of aneurysms in the abdominal aorta. The arteriosclerotic process leads to weakening of the aortic wall, medial degeneration, and localized dilatation. Hypertension often coexists and contributes to both undermining the strength of the aortic wall and expansion of the aneurysm. In the thorax, localized saccular aneurysms are somewhat more common than circumferential or fusiform aneurysms. The natural history of thoracic aneurysms differs

somewhat from that of abdominal aortic aneurysms in that spontaneous rupture without warning is less common, because evidence of a growing thoracic aneurysm is usually afforded by symptoms caused by compression of the surrounding structures.[64]

CLINICAL MANIFESTATIONS. Thoracic aneurysms are frequently associated with widespread atherosclerosis, particularly of the renal, cerebral, and coronary arteries. In fact, the consequences of arterial obliterative disease in these other areas may dominate the clinical picture.

Symptoms and signs of thoracic aneurysms are related to their size and location and are caused primarily by their impingement upon adjacent structures. Thus, tracheal deviation, wheezing, cough, dyspnea, stridor, hemoptysis, recurrent pneumonitis, and intrapulmonary hemorrhage are the direct result of compression of the tracheobronchial tree and contiguous lung, especially the left main stem bronchus, by aneurysms of the descending thoracic aorta. Occasionally, an asymptomatic arch aneurysm will be visible or palpable rising above the suprasternal notch. Hoarseness may follow compression of the recurrent laryngeal nerve. Arch aneurysms sometimes produce a tracheal tug. Dysphagia arises from pressure against the nearby esophagus. The superior vena caval syndrome can develop as a consequence of obstruction of venous return from the superior vena cava or innominate veins.

Pain is due to compression and erosion of adjacent musculoskeletal structures. It is usually steady and boring—occasionally pulsating—and may be extremely severe. Erosion of the sternum and right thoracic cage may result from large aneurysms of the ascending aorta, while erosion of the vertebral column and posterior left ribs may result from descending thoracic aortic aneurysms. Visible and pulsatile masses are evident when aneurysms reach and begin to erode through the chest wall. Rupture of an aneurysm is heralded by the dramatic onset of excruciating pain, usually in the area where some pain had existed previously.

DIAGNOSIS. Most thoracic aortic aneurysms are readily visible on chest roentgenograms, with fluoroscopy helping to differentiate an aneurysm from other types of mediastinal masses, such as neoplasms. However, some aneurysms are small, especially saccular aneurysms, and may rupture without having been visible on chest roentgenogram (Fig. 47–5). Aortic angiography is clearly the definitive procedure for outlining an aneurysm to make a diagnosis and to reveal the anatomical features of the aneurysm (Fig. 47–6). It should be performed in all patients under consideration for surgical repair. Although digital subtraction angiography continues to undergo evaluation as an alternative to conventional angiography, its inability to define the anatomy of small arteries (such as coronary arteries) and susceptibility to motion artifact limit its general application at this time.[1] CT scanning (Fig. 11–15, p. 320) enhanced by the use of a contrast medium can be used to identify and size aneurysms of both the ascending and the descending thoracic aorta.[4] Alternatively, significant aneurysms of either the ascending or the descending thoracic aorta can be defined by cross-sectional ultrasonography, but in the thoracic aorta, unlike the abdominal aorta, this technique is not as accurate as the CT scan, especially in the descending thoracic aorta. Transesophageal echocardiography has emerged as a better ultrasonographic method for imaging the thoracic aorta. Studies suggest that it is comparable to CT scanning in defining thoracic aneurysms (Fig. 4–13, p. 69). MRI is also an excellent technique that does not require administration of contrast agents. It is very reliable in defining the infarct and size of thoracic aneurysms.[9,11]

NATURAL HISTORY. Data for natural history of arteriosclerotic thoracic aortic aneurysms are somewhat scanty, but, as with abdominal aneurysms, ultimate survival is related to the size of the aneurysm. Thoracic aneurysms greater than 7 cm in diameter are more prone to rupture than are smaller ones.[64] Aneurysms that indicate expansion by producing

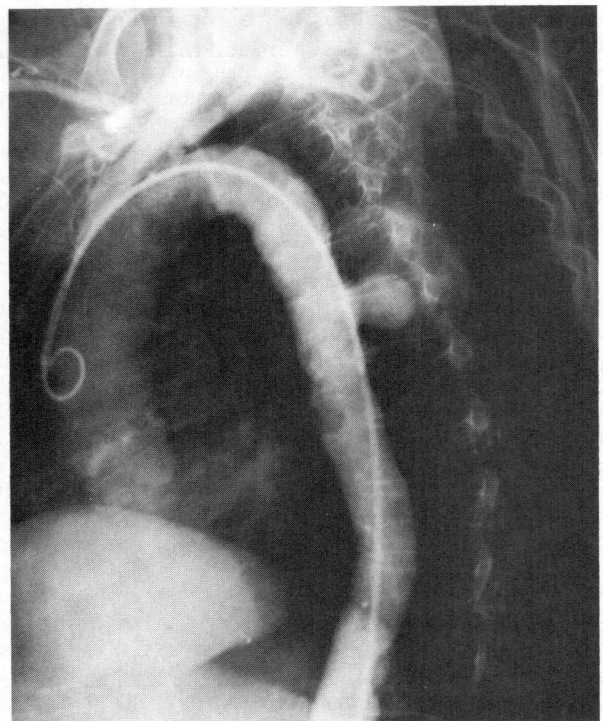

FIGURE 47–5. A localized saccular aneurysm in the descending thoracic aorta is clearly shown in the aortic angiogram of this 62-year-old man. The aneurysm had leaked, and a faint halo caused by the hematoma can be seen surrounding the aneurysm. The routine chest film appeared normal in this patient. (Courtesy of Christos Athanasoulis, M.D., and Arthur Waltman, M.D., Section of Vascular Radiology, Massachusetts General Hospital, Boston.)

symptoms of compression of surrounding structures are obviously diagnosed and treated earlier than aneurysms at "silent" sites. As noted, thoracic aneurysms are frequently associated with severe generalized arteriosclerosis, and many patients die of complications of arteriosclerosis before an aneurysm can rupture. When aneurysms do pursue a natural course, it has been found that symptomatic aneurysms are more prone to rupture than are asymptomatic ones. In the classic natural history study by Joyce et al., patients with symptomatic thoracic aneurysms had a 27 per cent 5-year survival compared with 58 per cent in asymptomatic patients. One-third of the deaths were attributed to rupture, while more than half were caused by complications of arteriosclerosis unrelated to the aneurysm.[65]

MANAGEMENT. Historically, surgical therapy once consisted of the introduction of long lengths of thrombogenic wire into an aneurysm, with the resultant thrombus buttressing the wall of the aneurysm. Direct wrapping of the aneurysm has also been tried. Currently, surgical excision is the procedure of choice whenever possible and is advised for aneurysms measuring 7 cm or more in diameter in the ascending and descending thoracic aorta. Clearly, even smaller aneurysms should be resected if they are producing symptoms. The aggressiveness with which surgical repair is undertaken depends greatly upon the general condition of the patient. The surgical procedure must be tailored to the specific aneurysm. Saccular aneurysms can sometimes be excised directly without resection of the aorta. Fusiform aneurysms in the ascending and descending thoracic aorta are best resected and replaced with a prosthetic tubular sleeve of appropriate size. Total cardiopulmonary bypass is necessary for the removal of ascending aortic aneurysms, and partial bypass to support the circulation distal to the aneurysm is often advisable in resection of descending thoracic aortic aneurysms. A temporary shunt (Gott shunt) may be used from the proximal aorta to the aorta beyond the aneurysm to divert blood around the site of the aneurysm while it is being repaired,[66] although the use of such adjuncts is less important than are the nature and extent of the aneurysm in determining the incidence of postoperative complications.[67]

The use of a composite graft consisting of a Dacron tube with a prosthetic aortic valve sewn into one end represents a major advance in therapy of proximal aortic aneurysms extending to the aortic annulus and associated with aortic regurgitation. The valve and graft are sewn into the annulus, and the coronary arteries are reimplanted into the Dacron aortic graft or onto separate Dacron tubes.[68,69] (Fig. 47–16).

Fusiform aneurysms of the arch have been successfully excised surgically; however, the risks of operation in this area are high. Arch aneurysmectomy requires excision of the aneurysm and in some instances reimplantation of all the brachiocephalic vessels. Each of these important arteries is selectively perfused by local cannulation while they are being reimplanted. Alternatively, resection of the aneurysm using profound hypothermia and circulatory arrest, a technique that is now favored by many surgical groups, has been used successfully.[70,71] In some centers both selective cerebral perfusion and hypothermic cardiopulmonary bypass are utilized.[72]

Surgical results have improved considerably in recent years, with a nearly 90 per cent survival rate for the elective resection of ascending and descending thoracic aortic aneurysms being reported in most major centers.[68,69,73,74] Moreno-Cabral reported a 94 per cent early and an 80 per cent late survival rate[75] in 214 patients with arteriosclerotic aneurysms of the ascending aorta. In a report on 82 patients with thoraco-

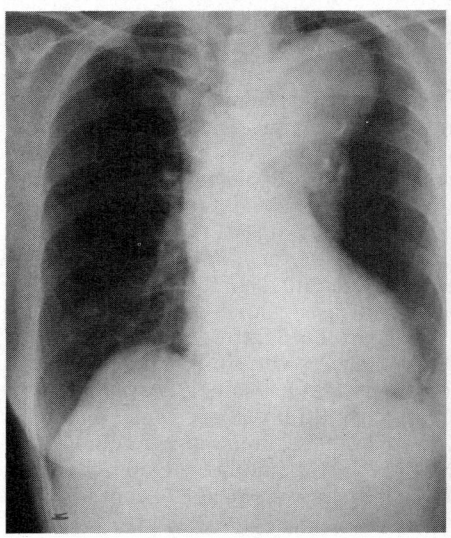
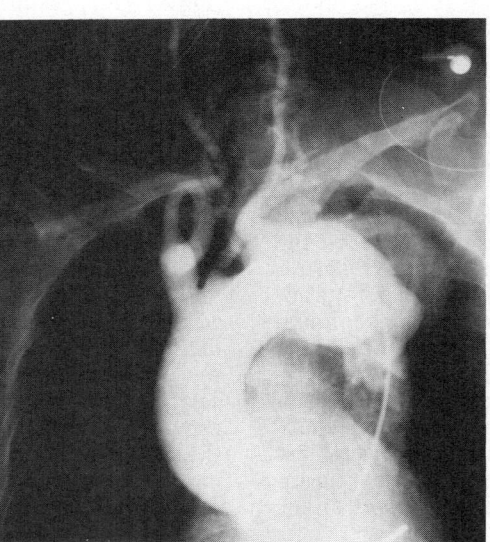

FIGURE 47–6. *Left,* **Posteroanterior chest roentgenogram in a 66-year-old woman with an arteriosclerotic aneurysm of the descending thoracic aorta.** *Right,* **Aortographic appearance in the left oblique anterior projection. The aneurysm arises just at the site of origin of the left subclavian artery. Thrombus is evident in the outer wall of the aneurysm on the angiogram. (Courtesy of Christos Athanasoulis, M.D., and Arthur Waltman, M.D., Section of Vascular Radiology, Massachusetts General Hospital, Boston.)**

abdominal aneurysms, the survival rate was 94 per cent.[76] More recently, in a large series of patients with aneurysm and/or dissection involving the ascending aorta or arch, Crawford reported a 91 per cent 30-day and 66 per cent 5-year survival.[74]

Major complications of the operation are technical, especially hemorrhage from tearing of the diseased aorta. A catastrophic complication of resection of descending thoracic aortic aneurysms is paraplegia from inadvertent interruption of the arterial blood supply to the spinal cord. This problem has been reduced by maintaining distal aortic perfusion during surgery[77]; by reducing the period of aortic cross clamping; by removal of minimal segments of aorta with the attendant intercostal arteries, especially in the areas of T7 through T9; by prompt treatment of hypertension in the proximal aorta, which elevates cerebrospinal fluid pressure, thus reducing collateral blood flow to the spinal cord; and possibly by perfusion cooling of the spinal cord during surgery. Recent studies report that the spinal cord is injured in at least 5 per cent of patients despite these and other precautions.[68,73,78,79]

Complications of associated arteriosclerosis, such as myocardial infarction, cerebrovascular infarcts, and renal failure, often manifest themselves under the massive physiological stress of surgery. The most frequent causes of early postoperative deaths are myocardial infarction, congestive heart failure, stroke, renal failure, hemorrhage, respiratory failure, and sepsis. Advanced age, emergency operation, prolonged aortic cross-clamp time, extent of aneurysm, diabetes, previous aortic operation, aneurysm symptoms, and intraoperative hypotension are the most important factors determining early perioperative morbidity and mortality.[75] Late postoperative deaths are usually associated with cardiac complications, aneurysm rupture respiratory failure, or stroke.[74,75] Aneurysm rupture may be due to aneurysm formation at the graft margins or formation of aneurysms at other aortic sites.[73]

Many patients with arteriosclerotic aneurysms are heavy smokers, and pulmonary complications are frequent. The left lung may be severely traumatized by compression during resection of large aneurysms of the descending thoracic aorta, a complication that may seriously jeopardize the patient's survival, particularly if there is underlying pulmonary disease.

Widespread aneurysmal dilatation of the aorta often precludes operation, although there are reports of successful surgical replacement of essentially the entire diseased thoracic and abdominal aorta. Associated diseases—especially pulmonary—preclude any operation in still others. Although it seems logical to reduce blood pressure vigorously in patients

with aneurysms and to reduce the velocity of ventricular ejection, the long-term impact of such therapy on retarding the expansion of aneurysms and improving survival is unknown.

AORTIC DISSECTION

Acute aortic dissection is a relatively common catastrophic illness and occurs at the rate of at least 2000 new cases per year in the United States.[80-82] Over the past two decades, great strides have been made in the diagnosis and the medical and surgical treatment of this highly lethal disease.[74,83,83a] It has been cogently pointed out that the term *dissecting hematoma* describes this entity more accurately than does the commonly used term dissecting aneurysm. More recently, the simpler term *aortic dissection* has gained favor.

Aortic dissection is caused by the sudden development of a tear in the aortic intima, opening the way for a column of blood driven by the force of the arterial pressure to enter the aortic wall, destroying the media and stripping the intima from the adventitia for variable distances along the length of the aorta.[84] It is uncertain whether the primary event in aortic dissection is rupture of the intima, with secondary dissection into the media, or hemorrhage within a diseased media followed by disruption of the subjacent intima and subsequent propagation of the dissection through the intimal tear (Fig. 47–7). However, occasional cases of extensive aortic dissection can occur without any identifiable intimal tear.[85]

The manifestations of aortic dissection in any given patient are determined by its path as it progresses through the aorta. Thus, the circulation of any major artery arising from the aorta may be compromised; disruption of the support of the aortic valve by extension into the aortic root may cause aortic incompetence; and finally the dissecting column may rupture through the adventitia anywhere along the aorta, although the two most common sites of rupture are the pericardial space and the left pleural cavity.

CLASSIFICATION. Most classification schemes for aortic dissection are based upon the fact that over 95 per cent of all dissections arise in one of two locations: (1) the ascending aorta within several centimeters of the aortic valve and (2) the descending thoracic aorta, usually just beyond the origin of the left subclavian artery at the site of the ligamentum arteriosum.[81] The widely used classification of DeBakey et al. recognizes three groups (Fig. 47–8). Types I and II both begin in the ascending aorta: Type I extends beyond the ascending aorta and arch, whereas Type II is confined to the ascending aorta.

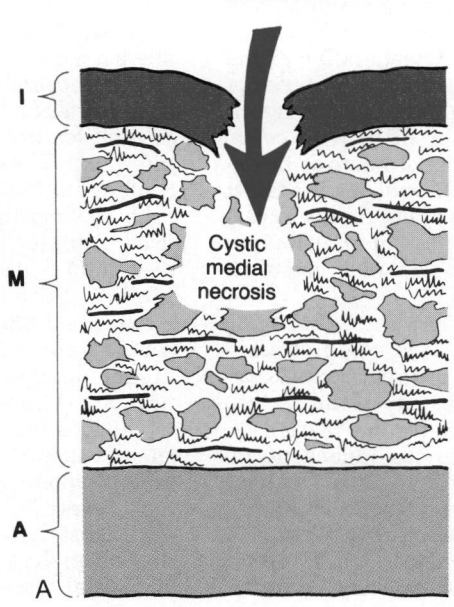
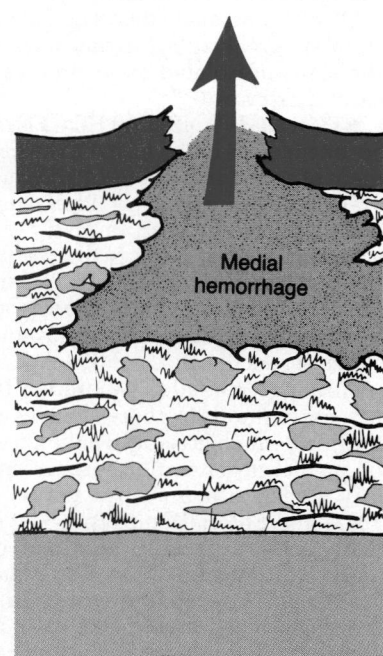

FIGURE 47–7. Proposed mechanisms of initiation of aortic dissection. In both cases, cystic medial necrosis is present. In *A*, an intimal tear is the initial event, allowing aortic blood to enter the media. In *B*, the primary event is hemorrhage into the media, with secondary rupture of the overlying intima. I = intima; M = media; A = adventitia.

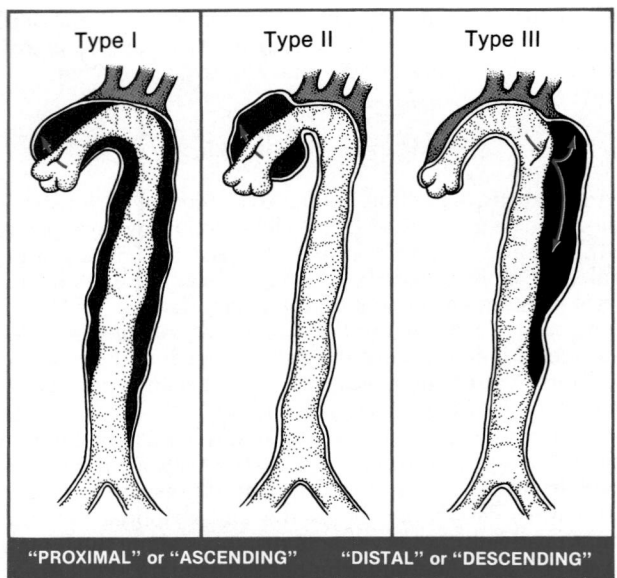

Type I	Type II	Type III

"PROXIMAL" or "ASCENDING" "DISTAL" or "DESCENDING"

FIGURE 47–8. The DeBakey classification of aortic dissections.

Type III originates in the descending thoracic aorta and usually propagates distally for a variable distance. It uncommonly extends retrograde into the arch and ascending aorta. In Type IIIa dissection, the process is limited to the thoracic aorta, while a IIIb designation connotes extension of the dissection below the diaphragm.[86]

Another classification, based upon approach to therapy and proposed by Daily et al., delineates two types, A and B.[87] Type A includes all proximal dissections and those distal dissections that extend retrograde to involve the arch and ascending aorta; Type B refers to all other distal dissections without proximal extension.

Since the behavior and managment of Types I and II dissections are similar, many investigators, including ourselves, have adopted a simple two-category classification into "proximal" (DeBakey Types I and II) and "distal" (DeBakey Type III) dissections.[88] "Ascending" and "descending" have also been used synonymously with "proximal" and "distal." Proximal dissections occur more frequently than distal dissections in a ratio of almost two to one in autopsy series.[89] However, because proximal dissections are more rapidly lethal, many clinical series report larger numbers of patients with distal than proximal dissection.[88,90]

Other occasional sites of origin include the aortic arch and the abdominal aorta. Furthermore, individual arteries may be the locus of isolated dissection, especially the coronary and carotid arteries.[91-93]

ETIOLOGY AND PATHOGENESIS. Degeneration of the aortic media is believed to be the prerequisite for the development of aortic dissection.[81-84,94] Usually, this consists of deterioration of the collagen and elastic tissue, often with cystic changes. This process, termed cystic medial necrosis or degeneration, most often is the result of chronic stress against the aortic wall, such as might occur with longstanding hypertension. Indeed, hypertension is an important contributing factor to aortic dissection and is found in well over half of all cases, especially those of distal dissection.

Although medial degeneration is part of the normal aging process in the aorta, these changes are qualitatively and quantitatively much greater in patients with aortic dissection. Cystic medial degeneration is an intrinsic feature of the hereditary defects of connective tissue, especially the Marfan (p. 1641) and Ehlers-Danlos (p. 1643) syndromes. Indeed, aortic dissection—especially proximal dissection—is a frequent and serious complication of the Marfan syndrome. However, cystic medial degeneration and aortic dissection may occur in the absence of an associated phenotypic syndrome.[95] Certain congenital cardiovascular abnormalities, especially coarcta-

tion of the aorta and bicuspid aortic valves, predispose to aortic dissection. A combination of bicuspid aortic valve, cystic medial degeneration, and aortic root dissection in the absence of the Marfan syndrome has been described.[96] Recent reports of aortic dissection in patients with Noonan syndrome and Turner syndrome have also appeared.[97,98] Also, a family in which nine members developed aortic dilatation or dissection over two generations has recently been described.[99] Cystic medial degeneration appears to be a common theme in all these patients.

An unexplained relationship exists between pregnancy and aortic dissection (p. 1801). About half of all aortic dissections in women under the age of 40 occur during pregnancy, usually in the last trimester.[100,101] Isolated coronary artery dissection also usually occurs during pregnancy.

In older patients, dissections occasionally originate by way of perforation through an intimal atheromatous plaque. Trauma almost never causes a classic aortic dissection, although a localized tear in the region of the aortic isthmus is not uncommon following massive chest trauma. Rarely, dissection of the aorta is a complication of other forms of vasculitis, including granulmatous arteritis (p. 1547).

Although strenuous physical exertion and emotional stress have been linked to aortic dissection, such a relationship is not usual. In a series of 124 cases of aortic dissection that we reviewed, we found such a history in only 14 per cent.[88]

The role played by chemicals toxic to connective tissue in the etiology of dissecting aneurysm in human beings is unknown. It is well known that the seeds of *Lathyrus odoratus* (sweet pea), which contain aminopropionitrile, cause cystic medial degeneration and aortic dissection in rats.[102] We have encountered a proximal dissection in a young man with no obvious predisposing factors other than prolonged industrial exposure to dimethyl hydrazine, a connective tissue toxin.[88]

CLINICAL MANIFESTATIONS

Aortic dissection afflicts men more frequently than women in a ratio of approximately two to one and has a peak incidence in the sixth and seventh decades, with a range from childhood well into the 90's.[103] Patients with proximal dissection are on the average somewhat younger. By far the most common presenting symptom of aortic dissection is *severe pain*, which is found in over 90 per cent of cases.[104] In fact, those patients without pain usually have suffered some disturbance of consciousness as a result of the dissection that renders them unable to perceive pain. Nonetheless, painless dissection can and does occur rarely.[105]

Cataclysmic in onset, the pain of aortic dissection is often as severe at its inception as it ever becomes. This feature contrasts with that of myocardial infarction, where the pain usually has a crescendo-like onset. The pain of dissection may be all but unbearable, forcing the patient to writhe in agony or to pace restlessly in an attempt to gain some measure of relief. Several features of the pain may arouse suspicion of aortic dissection. The quality of the pain as described by the patient is often morbidly appropriate to the actual event. Adjectives such as "tearing," "ripping," and "stabbing" are frequently used. Another important characteristic of the pain of aortic dissection is its tendency to migrate from its point of origin to other sites, following the path of the dissecting hematoma as it extends through the aorta. This feature was noted in 70 per cent of our cases.[88] Vasovagal manifestations, such as a drenching sweat, apprehension, nausea, vomiting, and faintness, are common at the outset.

The location of pain may be of some help in suggesting the site of origin.[88] Pain felt maximally in the anterior thorax is more frequent with proximal dissection, whereas pain that is most severe in the interscapular area is much more common with a distal site of origin. Although pain may be felt simultaneously in the anterior and posterior chest with both proximal and distal dissection, the *absence* of posterior interscapular pain strongly militates against a distal dissection, since over 90 per cent of patients with distal dissection report some back pain. Pain in the neck, throat, jaw, or teeth often occurs in dissections involving the ascending aorta or arch.

Less common modes of presentation include congestive heart failure with or without associated chest pain, cerebrovascular accidents, syncope, paraplegia, and pulse loss with or without ischemic pain. Heart failure usually results from severe aortic regurgitation secondary to the dissection. The occurrence of syncope in aortic dissection may bear special significance. Syncope without focal neurological signs occurred in 6 of 124 patients in our series. In each case, there was evidence for rupture of the dissection into the pericardial cavity with cardiac tamponade.[88]

Diagnosis

PHYSICAL FINDINGS. The diagnosis of aortic dissection can often be made with reasonable assurance from the *physical examination* alone. Patients with aortic dissection may appear to be in shock; however, the blood pressure when measured is frequently elevated. More than half the patients with distal dissection are hypertensive on initial presentation. Hypotension usually results from cardiac tamponade, intrapleural or intraperitoneal rupture, or dissection of the brachiocephalic vessels resulting in "pseudohypotension," i.e., the inability to measure the blood pressure accurately because of occlusion of the brachial arteries.

Those physical findings most typically associated with aortic dissection, namely, pulse deficits, aortic insufficiency, and neurological manifestations, are more characteristic of proximal than distal dissection. Pulse abnormalities, which include the absence, diminution, or reduplication of pulses, occur in approximately one-half of patients with proximal dissection and most commonly involve the brachiocephalic vessels. Pulse deficits are much less common in patients with distal dissection and tend to involve the left subclavian and femoral arteries, although the femoral vessels are equally affected by the distal propagation of a proximal dissection. Pulses may be lost either by direct compression of the lumen of an artery through extension of the dissection into it or by blockade due to a flap of intima overlying the vessel orifice. Rarely, intimointimal intussusception may occur.[106] Whatever the cause, pulse deficits in aortic dissection may be transitory, owing to decompression of the hematoma by distal reentry into the true lumen or by movement of the intimal flap away from the occluded orifice.

Aortic regurgitation is an important feature of proximal dissection and occurs in over 50 per cent in most series.[107] It was present in two-thirds of our patients with proximal dissection.[88] When aortic regurgitation is present in patients with distal dissection, it most commonly antedates the dissection and results from preexisting dilatation of the aortic root due to severe hypertension or annuloaortic ectasia. The murmur of aortic regurgitation in aortic dissection often has a musical quality and may be heard better along the right than the left sternal border. It may wax and wane, the intensity varying directly with the height of the arterial blood pressure. Depending upon the severity of the regurgitation, other peripheral signs of aortic incompetence may be present, such as collapsing pulses and a wide pulse pressure. There are three mechanisms of aortic regurgitation in proximal dissection (Fig. 47–9). First, the dissection may dilate the aortic root, widening the annulus so that aortic leaflets are unable to coapt in diastole; second, in an asymmetrical dissection, pressure from the dissecting hematoma may depress one leaflet below the line of closure of the others; and third, the annular support of the leaflets or the leaflets themselves may be torn so as to render the valve incompetent.

As noted, patients with proximal dissection sometimes have heart failure, which is almost always due to the sudden onset of severe aortic insufficiency. In rare cases, the conges-

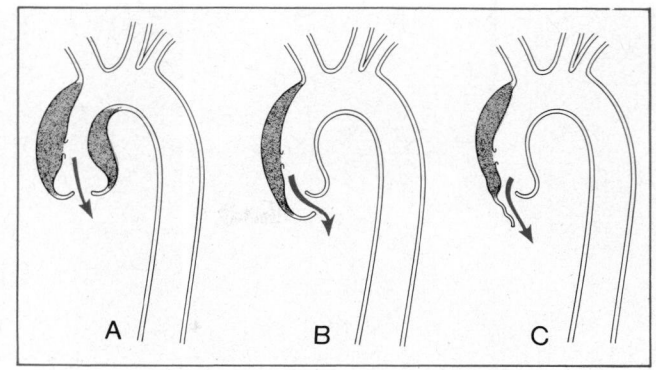

FIGURE 47–9. Mechanisms of aortic regurgitation in proximal dissecting aortic aneurysm. *A,* A circumferential tear pulls the annulus apart, preventing the leaflets from coapting. *B,* With asymmetrical dissection, pressure from the hematoma depresses one leaflet below the line of closure of the other. *C,* The annular support is disrupted, resulting in a flail aortic leaflet and aortic regurgitation.

tive failure may be so severe as to mask the murmur and other usual signs of aortic regurgitation. In a few such patients whom we have encountered, the presence of disproportionately bounding pulses in the face of severe heart failure, coupled with a history highly suggestive of aortic dissection, served as a clue to the correct diagnosis.

Neurological deficits associated with aortic dissection include cerebrovascular accidents, ischemic peripheral neuropathy, ischemic paraparesis, and disturbances of consciousness. Each of these is more common with proximal dissection, but deficits in the lower extremities are equally frequent in proximal and distal dissection.

Other occasionally encountered clinical manifestations of aortic dissection include pulsation of one of the sternoclavicular joints, Horner syndrome due to compression of the superior cervical sympathetic ganglion, vocal cord paralysis and hoarseness from pressure against the left recurrent laryngeal nerve, superior mediastinal syndrome from superior vena caval compression,[108] pulsating neck masses, tracheal or bronchial compression with bronchospasm,[81] hemorrhage into the tracheobronchial tree with hemoptysis,[109] hematemesis due to perforation into the esophagus,[110] heart block from retrograde burrowing of a dissection into the interatrial septum and thence down to the AV node,[111] and a continuous murmur due to rupture into the right atrium or ventricle.[112] Pleural effusions result from rupture of the dissection into one of the pleural spaces—usually the left—or simply from an exudative inflammatory reaction around the involved aorta. Additional complications may result from occlusion of important arteries by the dissection. Mesenteric infarction, renal infarction with severe renovascular hypertension, and myocardial infarction (seen in 1 to 2 per cent of patients with proximal dissection) are among the more serious occlusive events. Occasionally, high fever results, presumably from the release of pyrogenic substances from the hematoma or from associated effusions.

A variety of conditions may mimic aortic dissection. These include myocardial infarction, acute aortic regurgitation without dissection, thoracic nondissecting aneurysm, musculoskeletal pain, mediastinal tumors, pericarditis, and coronary insufficiency.[113] Confusion usually arises in these conditions when chest pain suggesting aortic dissection is coincidentally associated with other clinical manifestations of that entity, such as aortic regurgitation, deficient pulses, neurological abnormalities, or an abnormally widened aortic contour.[113]

Routine laboratory studies are not very helpful in making the diagnosis of aortic dissection. Anemia may develop from significant hemorrhage or sequestration of blood in the false channel. A mild to moderate polymorphonuclear leukocytosis (10,000 to 14,000/mm³) is common. Lactic acid dehydro-

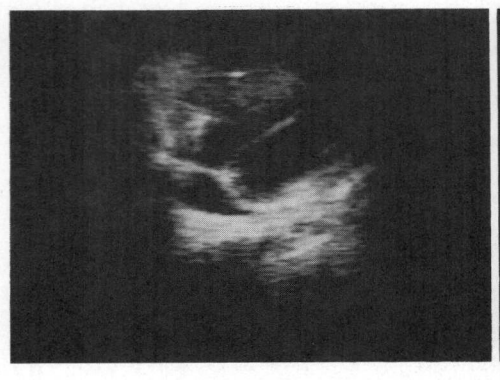
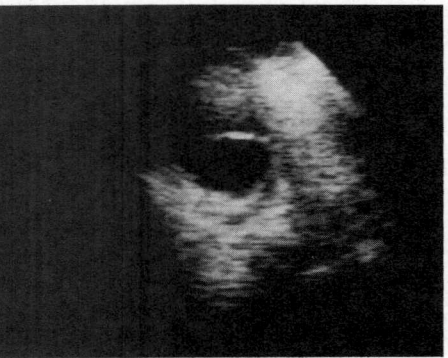

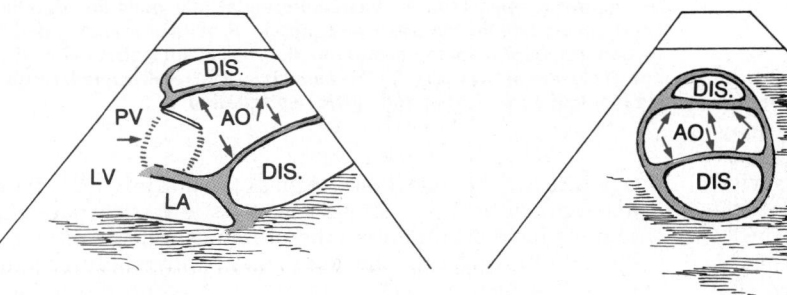

FIGURE 47–10. Cross-sectional echogram of the proximal aorta in a 63-year-old woman with dissection of the proximal aorta occurring 12 years after implantation of a Starr-Edwards aortic valve prosthesis. A, Parasternal long-axis recording. B, Short-axis recording. The actual recordings are shown above, and diagrammatic representations of the findings are pictured below. The echodense prosthetic valve (PV) is easily seen on the long-axis recording. Surrounding the aorta (AO) is the false channel of the dissection (DIS). (From Weyman, A. E.: Cross-sectional Echocardiography. Philadelphia, Lea and Febiger, 1982.)

genase (LDH) and bilirubin levels are sometimes elevated because of hemolysis of blood trapped within the false lumen. Serum glutamic oxaloacetic transaminase (SGOT) and creatine phosphokinase (CK or CK-MB) values are usually normal. Disseminated intravascular coagulation has been reported rarely.[114] The electrocardiogram frequently shows left ventricular hypertrophy from preexistent hypertension and usually the absence of acute ischemic changes. The absence of electrocardiographic changes of myocardial ischemia or infarction in a patient with severe chest pain is a helpful point in the differential diagnosis from myocardial infarction.

IMAGING TECHNIQUES: ULTRASOUND, CT, AND MRI. Diagnostic ultrasound (M-mode), in combination with cross-sectional (2-D) echocardiography, is helpful in the detection of a proximal dissection by revealing a widened aortic root, with delineation of the dissecting hematoma[115-117] (Figs. 4–109 and 47–10). The delineation of descending aortic dissection is now possible using transesophageal ultrasound (Fig. 47–11). One large multicenter study reported a sensitivity and specificity of 99 and 98 per cent respectively with transesophageal echocardiography in the diagnosis of aortic dissection.[118,118a] The addition of Doppler color flow imaging can identify sites of communication between true and false lumen and define flow characteristics in both lumina. CT scanning with contrast injection (Fig. 11–15, p. 320) is quite accurate in defining both ascending and descending dissections, provided that there is identification of a false lumen to distinguish the dissection from a fusiform aneurysm.[116,119] MRI is another noninvasive technique that may be useful in defining aortic dissection. Identification of an intimal flap is possible in most cases, as is characterization of the extent of the dissection and involvement of major branch vessels.[9-12,122] Unlike CT scanning, it does not require administration of potentially toxic contrast material. Its major limitations are necessity for prolonged imaging time, cost, and inability to use metallic objects such as medication pumps, pacemakers, and others in and around the magnet. Although ultrasounds, CT, and MRI

clearly offer the advantage of noninvasive diagnosis,[120,121] angiography is generally required to define the full extent of the dissection, to outline the relationship of the dissection to the major aortic branches, to evaluate aortic valve competency, and to identify the site of the intimal tear. However, these noninvasive techniques—especially the CT scan or MRI—are quite useful in the long-term follow-up of treated patients with aortic dissection to detect evidence of localized aneurysm formation. Chest roentgenography or two-dimensional echocardiography and aortic angiography provide the most substantive laboratory tests for initial suspicion and definitive diagnosis, respectively. Chest roentgenography almost always

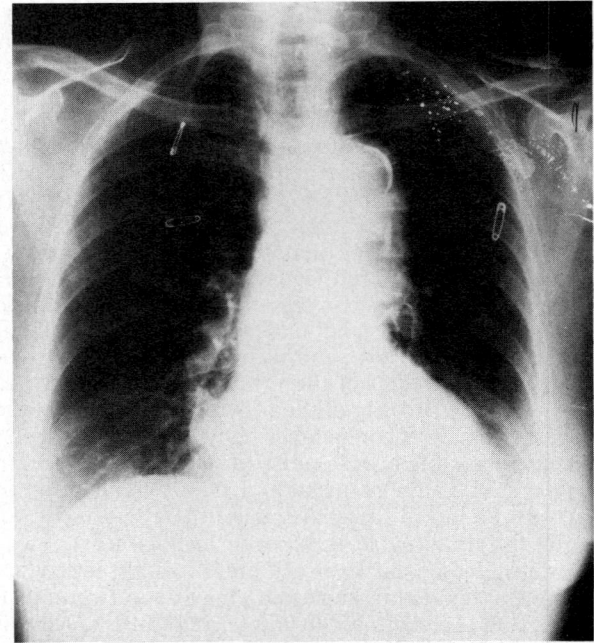

FIGURE 47–12. "Calcium sign" in distal dissection in an 80-year-old woman with longstanding hypertension. Note the marked separation of the calcification in the aortic knob and descending thoracic aorta from the outer wall of the aorta. This distance is normally no greater than 0.5 cm.

Figure 47–11. See color plate 10

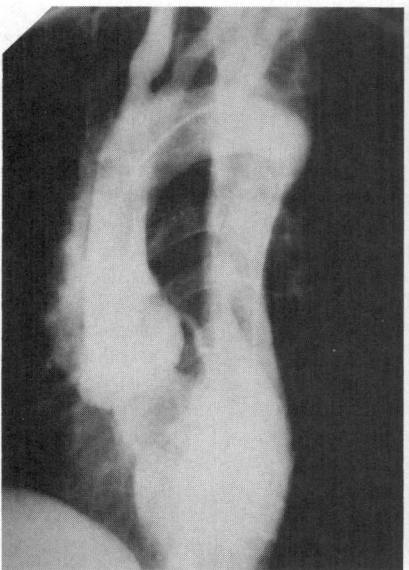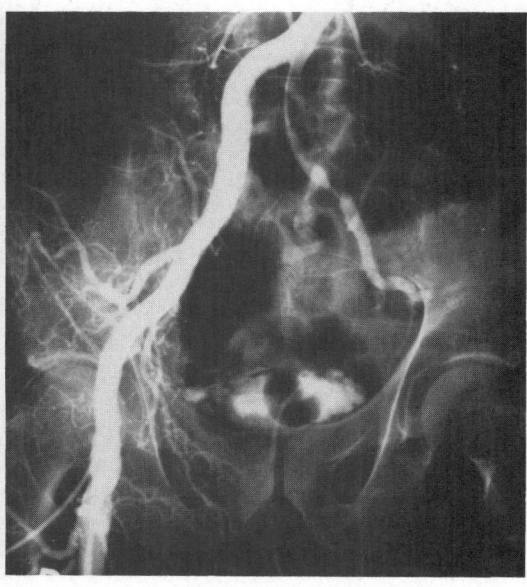

FIGURE 47-13. *Left,* Thoracic aortogram in the left anterior oblique projection showing a dissection beginning in the ascending aorta and spiraling through the aortic arch into the descending aorta. The false lumen can be faintly visualized. *Right,* Angiogram of the distal aorta showing virtual obstruction of the left iliac artery by the dissection. (Courtesy of Christos Athanasoulis, M.D., and Arthur Waltman, M.D., Section of Vascular Radiology. Massachusetts General Hospital, Boston.)

reveals an abnormally widened aortic contour. A localized bulge may overlay the site of origin, and the aortic silhouette may be widened wherever the dissection extends. If the aortic knob is calcified, separation of the intimal calcification from the adventitial border exceeding 1 cm (the "calcium sign") is virtually pathognomonic of aortic dissection (Fig. 47-12). Tracheal deviation or a left pleural effusion may be seen. Comparison with previous films is most helpful. On the other hand, it is possible for extensive aortic dissection to occur without radiographic abnormalities. For suspected proximal dissection, two-dimensional echocardiography can be rapidly performed and frequently will show the dissection.

AORTIC ANGIOGRAPHY. The single most important study in the diagnosis of aortic dissection is *aortic angiography.* Although originally performed by injection of contrast material into the pulmonary artery, with aortic opacification following the pulmonary venous phase, retrograde angiography is now the method of choice. The hazards of this approach have proved minimal, provided the catheter is carefully inserted and contrast material is not injected into the false channel. Aortic angiography has three objectives: (1) to establish a definite diagnosis, (2) to identify the site of origin of the dissection, and (3) to delineate the extent of the dissection and the distal circulation to vital organs (Figs. 47-13 and 47-14).

One additional feature to be assessed by angiography is the degree to which the false channel is opacified. There is evidence that the prognosis in medically treated patients is better in those with a nonopacified false channel, presumably an indication of thrombus formation in the channel that may serve to buttress the wall of the dissected aorta.[123] Although highly accurate, angiography is not without occasional pitfalls in the detection of aortic dissection.[113] Angiography may fail to show a dissection if there is faint opacification of the false lumen, unusual tearing of the intima, a small and localized dissection, or equal simultaneous opacification of both channels.[124] Nevertheless, when properly obtained and interpreted, angiograms provide a definite diagnosis in almost every case, and the procedure is well tolerated by even critically ill patients.

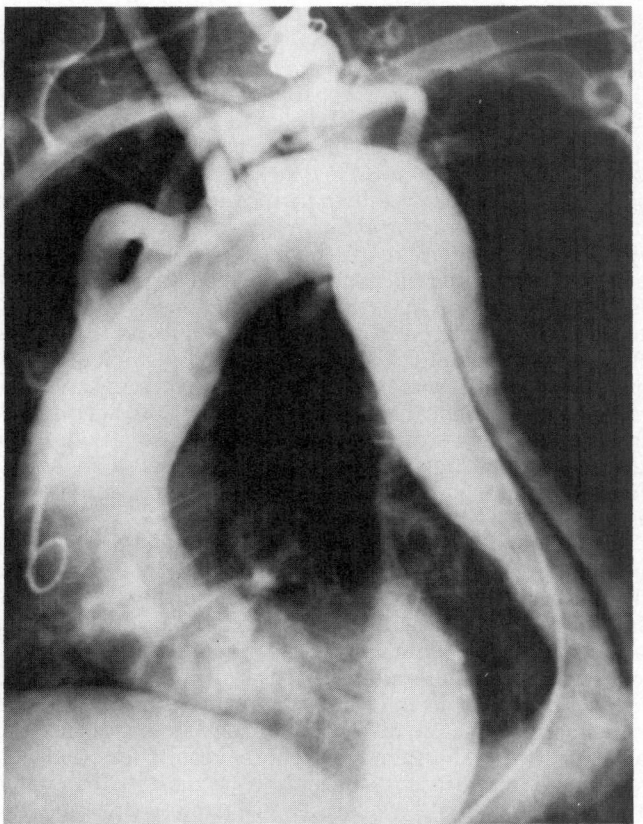

FIGURE 47-14. Left oblique anterior view of the aorta outlined angiographically showing a distal aortic dissection in a 63-year-old man. The true and false channels are clearly seen. The false channel is heavily opacified.

MANAGEMENT

Therapy for aortic dissection is directed at halting the progression of the dissecting hematoma, since fatal complications arise not from the intimal tear itself but rather from the subsequent course taken by the dissection.[125] Without treatment, aortic dissection is highly fatal. In a collective review of long-term survival in untreated aortic dissection, more than one-fourth of all patients were dead within 24 hours, more than one-half died within the first week, more than three-fourths died within 1 month, and more than 90 per cent died within 1 year.[126]

The first surgical approach to aortic dissection was the so-called fenestration procedure in which the dissected aorta was incised and a distal communication was created between the true and false channels, thereby decompressing the false lumen.[127,128] Definitive surgical therapy was pioneered by De-Bakey and colleagues in the early 1950's.[129] Its principles are to excise the intimal tear, obliterate the false channel by oversewing aortic edges, reconstitute the aorta with or without interposition of a synthetic graft, and, in the case of proximal dissection, restore aortic valve competence by resuspension of the displaced aortic leaflets or by prosthetic aortic valve replacement.

Aggressive medical treatment of aortic dissection was first advocated by Wheat, Palmer, and collaborators.[130] They established two goals for pharmacological therapy: (1) reduction of the systolic blood pressure, and (2) diminution of the velocity of left venticular ejection (dV/dt), which is thought to be a major stress acting upon the aortic wall that contributes to the genesis and propagation of aortic dissection. Originally introduced for patients too ill to withstand surgery, medical therapy now forms the basis for the initial treatment of virtually all patients with aortic dissection before definitive diagnosis by angiography and serves as primary long-term therapy in additional subsets of patients.

EARLY EMERGENCY TREATMENT. All patients in whom there is a strong suspicion of aortic dissection should be admitted immediately to an intensive care unit, where blood pressure, cardiac rhythm, central venous pressure, urine output, and, when necessary, pulmonary wedge pressure and cardiac output can be monitored. Initial therapeutic goals are the elimination of pain and the reduction of systolic blood pressure to 100 to 120 mm Hg (mean of 60 to 75 mm Hg) or to the lowest level commensurate with adequate vital organ (cardiac, renal, and cerebral) perfusion. Simultaneously, arterial dV/dt, which reflects the velocity of left ventricular ejection, should be reduced by beta-adrenergic blockade regardless of whether systolic hypertension or pain is present.

For acute reduction of arterial pressure, the potent vasodilator sodium nitroprusside is very effective, mixed as 50 to 100 mg in 500 ml of 5 per cent dextrose in water and infused initially at 25 to 50 μg/min, with dosages varying according to blood pressure response. Side effects include nausea, restlessness, somnolence, hypotension, and cyanide or thiocyanate toxicity, which can develop after more than 48 hours of continuous use. Sodium nitroprusside alone can cause an increase in dV/dt, which can potentially contribute to propagation of the dissection.[131] Thus, adequate simultaneous beta-adrenergic blockade is essential when this drug is used.[132]

If sodium nitroprusside is ineffective or poorly tolerated, the ganglionic blocking agent trimethaphan (Arfonad), mixed as 500 mg to 2.0 gm in 500 ml of 5 per cent glucose and water, can be used. The initial infusion rate is 1 mg/min, with the dose titrated against the blood pressure response, which is enhanced by the orthostatic maneuver of elevating the head of the bed. Limitations in the use of this powerful agent include severe hypotension, tachyphylaxis, somnolence, and sympathoplegia with urinary retention, constipation, ileus, and pupillary dilation. In contrast to sodium nitroprusside, trimethaphan depresses dV/dt, which should provide a relative advantage in the treatment of aortic dissection. However, its unpleasant side effects and rapid tachyphylaxis have relegated this drug to a position of second choice in acute therapy in most centers.

To reduce dV/dt acutely, propranolol or a comparable intravenous beta blocker should be used in incremental doses of 1 mg intravenously every 5 minutes until there is evidence of satisfactory beta blockade, usually indicated by a pulse rate of 60 to 80 beats/min in the acute setting. A test dose of 0.5 mg intravenously is advised. The maximum initial total dose should not exceed 0.15 mg/kg. Additional propranolol should be given intravenously every 4 to 6 hours in order to maintain adequate beta blockade, as reflected in heart rate, usually in dosages somewhat lower than the initial amount, i.e., 2 to 6 mg. In chronic stable dissection, propranolol (or an alternative beta blocker) can be started orally, using 20 to 40 mg every 6 hours. Propranolol is contraindicated in the presence of bradycardia, asthma, or heart failure. Since propranolol was the first generally available beta-adrenoceptor blocking drug, it is the one that has been used most widely in aortic dissection. However, there is good reason to believe that other beta blockers are equally effective if used in equivalent doses. In particular, those which are cardioselective, such as atenolol and metoprolol, may be preferable in patients with chronic obstructive lung disease or a history of bronchial asthma. Labetolol, a recently released alpha- and beta-adrenergic receptor blocker (p. 1308), has great promise for the treatment of aortic dissection.[133] It combines selective alpha blockade and nonselective beta blockade, which lowers both blood pressure and dV/dt.

Labetalol is given intravenously in a first dose of 5 to 20 mg; further doses of 20 to 40 mg can be administered every 10 to 15 minutes until blood pressure returns to usual levels or a total dose of 300 mg has been given.

Refractory hypertension can follow occlusion of one or both renal arteries, with resultant release of large amounts of renin. In this situation, the intravenous ACE inhibitor, enalapril, may be quite effective in doses of 1 to 2 mg every 4 to 6 hours.

The initial experience with calcium-channel antagonists in the treatment of aortic dissection is encouraging. Use of these agents in managing hypertensive crisis has been favorable (p. 870).[134] Sublingual nifedipine has been used successfully to treat refractory hypertension associated with aortic dissection.[135] The combined vasodilator and negative inotropic effects of these drugs are ideally suited for this disease. Once the patient's condition is stabilized, angiography should be performed for a definitive diagnosis. Angiography should be performed as soon as possible after admission, unless a life-threatening complication such as aortic rupture, free aortic regurgitation, cardiac tamponade, or compromise of a vital organ has supervened. If any of these potentially lethal problems arises, surgery must be undertaken immediately, with angiography performed if possible while the operating room is being readied.

DEFINITIVE SUBSEQUENT THERAPY. Despite minor variations from center to center, a reasonable consensus as to the definitive therapy of aortic dissection has evolved over the past two decades. Although either medical or surgical therapy can be associated with an extremely successful outcome, it can be generally stated that *surgical results are superior to medical results in acute proximal dissection*, and, conversely, *medical therapy offers a relative advantage over surgery in most cases of uncomplicated acute distal dissection.*[136-138] These differences are based largely upon the disparate natural history of proximal and distal disease. Even minute progression of a proximal dissection poses potentially devastating consequences such as pulse loss, aortic regurgitation, neurological compromise, or cardiac tamponade. Thus, immediate surgical repair promises a better outcome. In contrast, patients with distal dissection are for the most part older and have a relatively increased incidence of advanced atherosclerotic or cardiopulmonary disease, thus rendering their surgical risks considerably higher. Medical therapy has proved to be quite effective in this group. Agreement on these principles is not unanimous, with some investigators advocating surgical treatment of all acute dissections, both proximal and distal.[138] However, a recent study involving patients from both Duke and Stanford has shown that medical therapy provides equivalent outcome to surgical treatment of uncomplicated distal dissection.[139]

A hospital survival of approximately 80 to 90 per cent has been reported for patients with acute proximal dissection treated surgically and 80 per cent for those with acute distal dissection treated medically.[139,140] Hospital survival for patients with chronic dissection (defined as presentation 2 weeks or more after the onset of dissection) treated either surgically—usually because of aortic insufficiency or an enlarging aneurysm—or medically exceeds 90 per cent.[136-138,140,141] The somewhat poorer results for surgically treated patients with acute dissection are mostly attributable to complications that have already occurred as a result of the dissection before definitive therapy,[137] although the fragility of the aortic wall in acute dissection often presents a serious problem to surgeons, adding to the risks of operation. The

TABLE 47–1 INDICATIONS FOR DEFINITIVE SURGICAL AND MEDICAL THERAPY IN AORTIC DISSECTION

Surgical
1. Treatment of choice for acute proximal dissection
2. Treatment for acute distal dissection complicated by the following:
   a. Progression with vital organ compromise
   b. Rupture or impending rupture (e.g., saccular aneurysm formation)
   c. Aortic regurgitation (rare)
   d. Retrograde extension into the ascending aorta
   e. Dissection in Marfan syndrome

Medical
1. Treatment of choice for uncomplicated distal dissection
2. Treatment for stable, isolated arch dissection
3. Treatment of choice for stable chronic dissection (uncomplicated dissection presenting 2 weeks or later after onset)

better survival in patients with chronic dissection derives from this same principle, i.e., they have already selected themselves out as a group destined to do well because they have survived the initial high mortality that occurs within the first 2 weeks of onset of the dissection.[136,137] The results of long-term follow-up will be discussed below.

The generally advocated *indications for definitive surgical therapy* are summarized in Table 47–1. Note that occasional patients with proximal dissection who refuse surgery or for whom surgery is contraindicated by age or prior debilitating illness can be treated successfully by medical therapy. Moreover, both early and late medical therapy are usually required in *all* patients, inlcuding those treated surgically, to provide stabilization initially and to protect against later redissection.

SURGICAL THERAPY. Although the precise timing of surgery in patients without life-threatening complications is somewhat controversial, prompt repair is generally recommended to prevent even minimal progression of the dissection that might lead to further complications.[137a] Surgical risk for all patients is obviously increased by age; associated diseases, especially pulmonary emphysema; aneurysm leakage; cardiac tamponade; shock; or vital organ compromise as a result

of such conditions as myocardial infarction, cerebrovascular accident, and particularly renal failure.[138]

As noted, the usual objectives of definitive surgical therapy are excision of the intimal tear and obliteration of entry into the false lumen by suturing together the edges of the dissected aorta proximally and distally. Aortic continuity is then reestablished either by joining the edges of the aorta directly or by interposing a prosthetic sleeve graft between the two ends of the aorta (Fig. 47–15). Determining the routes of perfusion of vital organs distal to the surgical site by preoperative angiography may be of importance. For example, one or both renal arteries occasionally are found to be fed from the false lumen, in which case the false channel at the distal end of the surgically transected aorta might be left unclosed.

There is growing consensus favoring more aggressive surgical repair of dissections involving the proximal aorta, regardless of the site of intimal tear, to prevent extension and rupture into the pericardial cavity. This applies even if the dissection originates in the distal aorta and extends proximally.[138,140]

When aortic regurgitation complicates aortic dissection, simple decompression of the false channel may be all that is necessary to resuspend the leaflets and restore valvular competence. However, most surgeons have become increasingly aggressive about replacing the aortic valve if it appears that even moderate aortic regurgitation will be present after the leaflets are decompressed. This avoids the high risk of having to replace the aortic valve in a second operation through a diseased aorta at some later date.

For repair of a proximal dissection, total cardiopulmonary bypass is necessary. On occasion, because of extensive dissection of the aorta, it may be difficult to find a safe site for placement of a perfusion cannula. In rare cases, we have had to abandon plans for surgical repair of a proximal dissection for this reason. In the repair of dissections of the descending thoracic aorta, support of the distal circulation may be necessary and can be achieved either by partial left heart bypass or by using a conduit that carries blood from the proximal to the distal aorta, circumventing the site of the dissection.

The actual operative procedure itself, in aortic dissection, is technically demanding. The wall of the diseased aorta is often

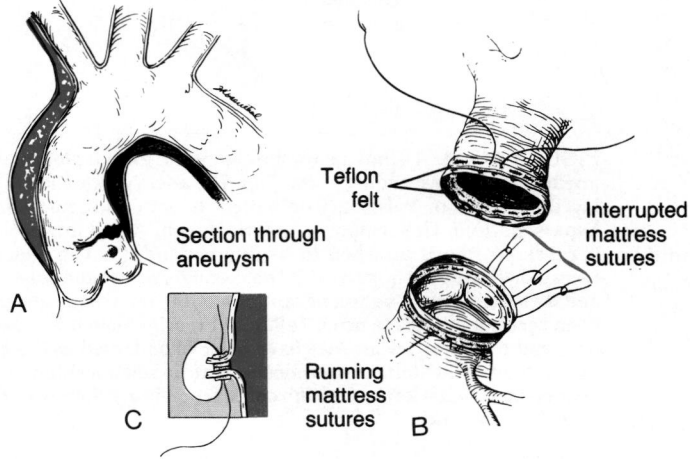

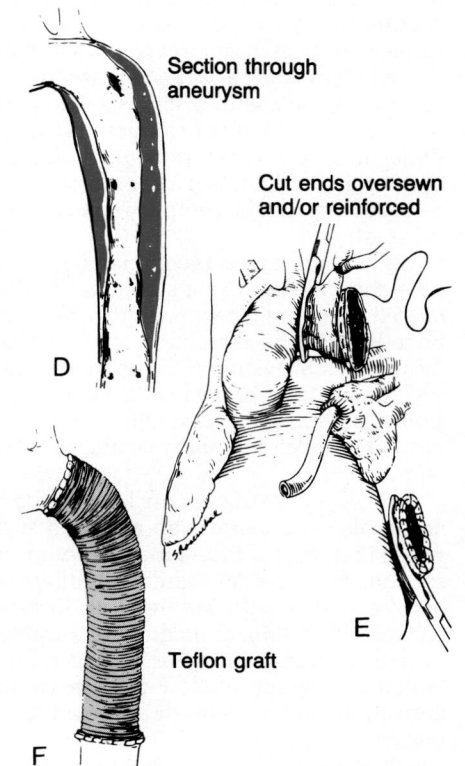

FIGURE 47–15. Several steps in the surgical repair of a proximal (*A, B,* and *C*) and a distal (*D, E,* and *F*) aortic dissection. *A* and *D* show the dissections and the intimal tears. *B,* The aorta has been transected, and the ends of the aorta have been oversewn to obliterate the false lumen and have been buttressed with Teflon felt to prevent the sutures from tearing through the fragile tissue. *C,* The aortic ends are brought together in such a way that the Teflon is again used to reinforce the suture line between the two ends of the aorta or between the aorta and a sleeve graft, if such a graft is necessary for reconstitution of the aorta. *E* shows resection of a distal dissection, with a Teflon graft interposed in *F.* (*D, E,* and *F* reprinted by permission from Austen, W. G., and DeSanctis, R.: Surgical treatment of dissecting aneurysm of the thoracic aorta. N. Engl. J. Med. 272:1314, 1965.)

friable, and the repair must be performed with meticulous care. The use of Teflon felt to buttress the wall and prevent sutures from tearing through the fragile aorta has represented a significant technical advance (Fig. 47–15B). An alternate surgical approach consists of the wrapping of an unstable arch dissection with Dacron.[142] Bleeding, infection, and pulmonary or renal insufficiency consititute the most common early complications of surgical therapy. Spinal cord ischemia with resultant paraplegia due to inadvertent interruption of blood supply from the anterior spinal or intercostal arteries is a rare but dreaded consequence. Late complications include progressive aortic regurgitation if the aortic valve has not been replaced, localized aneurysm formation, and redissection at the original site of repair or at an independent secondary site.[143]

Several innovative techniques for the surgical treatment of aortic dissection have been reported. One utilizes an intraluminal sutureless prosthesis.[144,145] Another, applied especially to distal but also to proximal dissection, consists of bypassing the dissected aorta with a Dacron sleeve, ligating the aorta at the site of proximal extension of the dissection, and creating reversal of flow in the distal aorta to perfuse the major arterial branches arising from the dissected segment.[146] Tanabe and coworkers have inserted strips of Ivalon sponge in the false channel, with the intention of stimulating the organization of blood and the formation of thrombus, thus strengthening the wall of the dissected aorta.[147] Finally, Carpentier and colleagues have reported the use of a gelatin-resorcin-formaldehyde glue to stick the dissected layers of proximal aortic dissections together, thus avoiding the necessity of prosthetic graft replacement.[148] These techniques have been used in only small numbers of patients, and long-term follow-up is lacking.

In proximal dissection, when the aorta is fragile and badly torn, replacement of the aorta and the aortic valve using a composite graft into which the coronary arteries are reimplanted has been a valuable technique (Fig. 47–16).[66]

MEDICAL THERAPY. Indications for *definitive* medical therapy are summarized in Table 47–1. Clearly, operation must be performed if there is medical failure, such as rupture or impending rupture, progression of the dissection with vital organ compromise, aortic regurgitation, or inability to control pain or blood pressure with drugs. Although we prefer medical therapy for low-risk patients with stable distal dissection, some centers advise surgery in this group as well.[136,143] Controlled studies of medical versus surgical treatment of comparable patients with distal dissection are lacking. Because of the extreme difficulty of surgery involving aortic arch dissections, medical therapy is usually advocated in those rare dissections that originate in the arch, with operative intervention reserved for serious complications that might occur on medical treatment.

Medical therapy is recommended for patients with chronic dissection, defined as a stable aortic dissection that has occurred 2 or more weeks prior to presentation, unless late complications of the dissection, such as aortic insufficiency or localized aneurysm formation, necessitate surgery.

Complications of medical therapy include severe hypotension related to the drugs, with possible precipitation of acute tubular necrosis, cerebrovascular accident, or myocardial infarction.[137]

Late follow-up of patients leaving the hospital with treated aortic dissection shows an actuarial survival rate not much worse than that of individuals of comparable age without dissection; there are no significant differences in these patients between those with proximal vs. distal dissection, acute vs. chronic dissection, or medical vs. surgical treatment.[137] Thus, initially successful surgical or medical therapy is usually sustained on long-term follow-up. Late complications include redissection, aortic regurgitation, and localized aneurysm formation.

Long-term medical therapy to control hypertension and reduce dV/dt is indicated for all patients who have sustained an

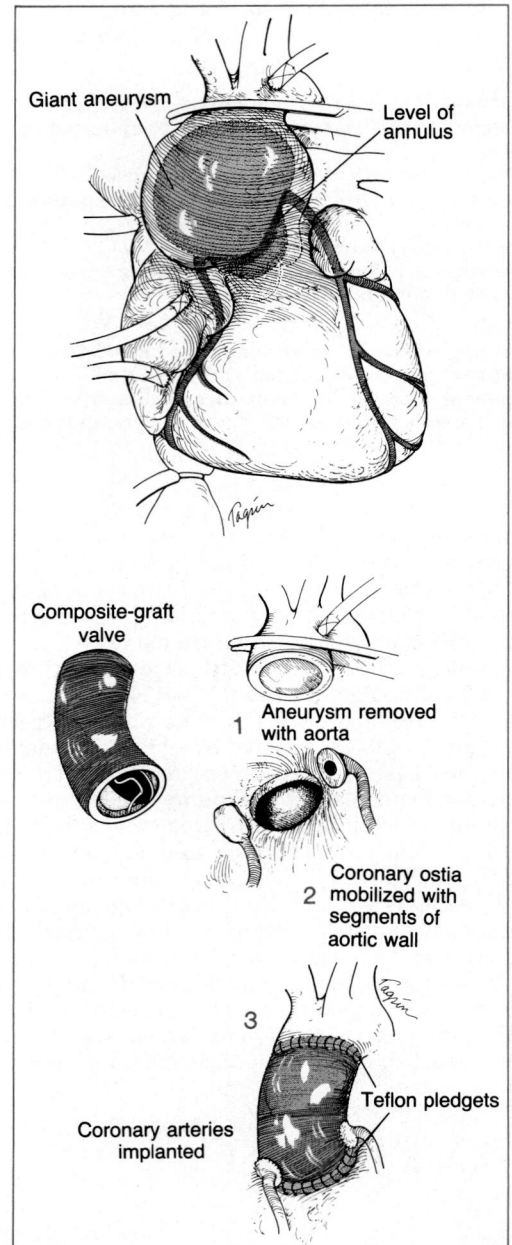

FIGURE 47–16. Technique for the composite graft replacement of an aneurysm of the ascending aorta. *Top,* The aneurysm is shown, involving the sinuses of Valsalva. The patient is on total cardiopulmonary bypass. *Bottom,* The composite graft is shown, with a low profile, tilting-disc prosthesis attached to its inferior end. (1) The aneurysm is resected with the aortic valve; (2) The coronary ostia have been excised, and mobilized with a button or aortic wall; (3) The composite graft has been secured into place using Teflon felt reinforcement for the suture line, and the coronary arteries have been reimplanted as the graft. In the method of Bentall, the composite graft is sewn inside the incised aneurysm, which is left in situ. The coronary ostia are then anastomosed directly to the graft.

aortic dissection, regardless of whether they have received definitive surgical or medical therapy. Systolic blood pressure should be controlled at or below a level of 130 to 140 mm Hg, or even lower if tolerated. Preferred agents are those with a negative inotropic as well as hypotensive effect, such as beta blockers and calcium-channel antagonists, together with a diuretic if necessary to control blood pressure. Hydralazine and minoxidil increase cardiac output and arterial dV/dt and should be used only in the presence of adequate beta blockade. Angiotensin-converting enzyme inhibitors and other drugs such as clonidine and guanabenz are powerful antihypertensive agents and should be useful, especially in combination with beta blockers.

Follow-up of patients who have sustained an aortic dissection should include careful and repeated physical examinations, periodic chest roentgenograms, and CT or MRI scans if localized aneurysm formation is suspected.

ANNULOAORTIC ECTASIA

In a number of patients with pure aortic regurgitation the cause is idiopathic dilatation of the proximal aorta and the aortic annulus. The term *annuloaortic ectasia* was first used by Ellis et al. in 1961 to describe this clinicopathological condition.[149] The entity has been subsequently recognized with increasing frequency and makes up about 5 to 10 per cent of the population of patients who currently undergo aortic valve replacement for pure aortic regurgitation.

ETIOLOGY AND PATHOGENESIS. The common pathological feature shared by patients with annuloaortic ectasia is that of severe degenerative changes (usually cystic medial necrosis) in the wall of the afflicted aorta. Some degree of cystic medial necrosis with annuloaortic ectasia is found in virtually all cases of Marfan syndrome.[150] In fact, it can be severe and is a frequent cause of death from fatal aortic rupture or dissection in this syndrome (p. 1641). There is some evidence to suggest that abnormalities in collagen cross linkage may play a role in this phenomenon,[151] while others have identified abnormalities in elastin.[152] In most reported series of patients with annuloaortic ectasia, however, patients with classic Marfan syndrome have been excluded. Careful examination of patients with annuloaortic ectasia usually reveals that about one-fourth to one-half have other stigmata of Marfan syndrome, indicating that many patients represent a forme fruste of that connective tissue disorder. In a clinicogenetic study of 18 patients with severe aortic regurgitation and dilatation of the ascending aorta but without other evidence of the Marfan syndrome except on pathological examination of the aorta, Emanuel et al. reported that 37.3 per cent of 126 first-degree relatives had one or more stigmata of Marfan syndrome.[153] Thus, it appears that many of these patients have primarily the aortic abnormalities of Marfan syndrome without the other manifestations of the disease. In summary, then, patients with annuloaortic ectasia appear to fall into three groups: (1) those with classic Marfan syndrome, (2) those with a forme fruste of Marfan syndrome, and (3) those with cystic medial necrosis and no obvious underlying cause.

As the media degenerates, the aorta widens. The aortic root is involved, and the annulus dilates, drawing the aortic leaflets apart and leading to aortic regurgitation. The weakened aorta may dissect and this may aggravate the aortic regurgitation.

CLINICAL MANIFESTATIONS. Men predominate over women in virtually all series by a ratio of anywhere between 2 and 8 to 1. Patients without obvious Marfan syndrome usually are encountered in the fourth, fifth, and sixth decades with progressively more severe aortic regurgitation. Patients with the classic Marfan syndrome or its forme fruste are generally younger. Some patients with annuloaortic ectasia experience sudden onset and rapid progression of symptoms, which sometimes but not always are due to severe aortic regurgitation secondary to aortic dissection. In the study of Lemon and White, recent aortic root dissection was found in 11 of 25 patients with annuloaortic ectasia who came to surgery.[154] All 11 of these patients had experienced chest pain before operation, although chest pain was also present in several patients without aortic dissection.

The physical examination may reveal abnormal pulsation of the dilated aorta over the 2nd and 3rd right intercostal spaces, especially if the examination is done with the patient sitting and in full expiration. We have seen three patients with annuloaortic ectasia who had pulsation of the right sternoclavicular joint.

There is nothing unique about the signs of aortic regurgitation in patients with annuloaortic ectasia as opposed to those with regurgitation from other causes, except for the greater intensity of the diastolic murmur to the right of the sternum in the former group and to the left in patients with a primary valvular abnormality. Lemon and White did find that the two features—acute or subacute development of symptoms and the presence of chest pain—were more frequent in the group of patients with annuloaortic ectasia than in those with pure valvular aortic regurgitation, presumably on a rheumatic

basis.[154] Features of Marfan syndrome should be sought and may be obvious, subtle, or absent.

The chest film usually shows a grossly dilated aortic root and ascending aorta with left ventricular enlargement proportionate to the severity of aortic regurgitation. Calcification in the aortic valve and dilated aorta is usually absent. Echocardiography, CT scan, or MRI demonstrate an abnormally widened aortic root. The huge aorta and aortic regurgitation are easily demonstrated angiographically. Lemon and White identified three types of angiographic aortic enlargement: (1) "pear-shaped" enlargement (56 per cent) (Fig. 47–17), (2) diffuse symmetrical dilatation (27 per cent), and (3) dilatation limited to the sinuses of Valsalva (6 per cent). In our own unpublished experience, aneurysmal dilatation of the sinuses of Valsalva is typically seen in those with Marfan syndrome. The mean maximal aortic diameter in Lemon and White's patients was 7.6 ± 2.7 cm and ranged from 4.8 to 15 cm. This is two to five times the normal aortic diameter. Because dissections are characteristically small, circumscribed, and confined to the ascending aorta, they may not be easy to identify angiographically.

MANAGEMENT. Surgical correction using total cardiopulmonary bypass is usually undertaken for relief of aortic regurgitation when it is severe and responsible for symptoms of left ventricular failure or when the left ventricle or ascending aorta is increasing in size. However, in addition to replacement of the aortic valve, resection of the aneurysmal aorta with insertion of a prosthetic graft is generally required. Some surgeons advise sewing an artificial aortic valve to one end of a long prosthetic sleeve and suturing this in place from the aortic annulus at one end to the ascending aorta where it narrows beyond the aneurysm at the other. This reconstruction necessitates reimplantation of the coronary arteries (Fig. 47–16). In fact, with aneurysmal sinuses of Valsalva, the coronary ostia may be carried cephalad by the enlarging sinuses, again necessitating ligation and reimplantation of the coronary arteries or the construction of saphenous vein bypass conduits from the aorta to the ligated coronary arteries. Because of the magnitude of the operation and the frequently friable tissues

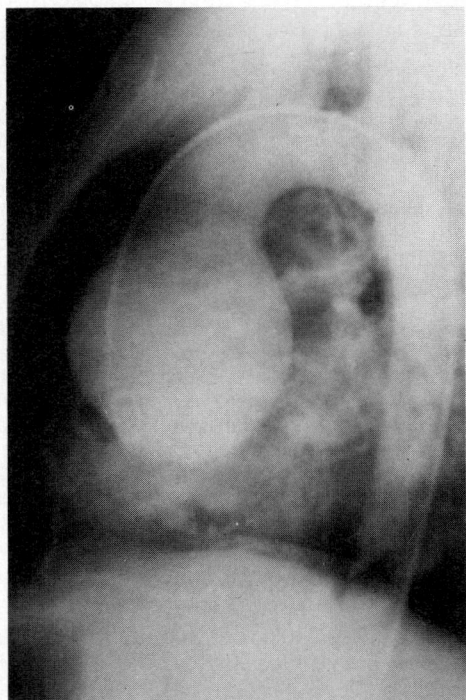

FIGURE 47–17. Lateral aortogram in a man with annuloaortic ectasia. The bulbous, pear-shaped aortic root can be easily seen. The left ventricle is opacified consequent to aortic regurgitation. (Courtesy of Christos Athanasoulis, M.D., and Arthur Waltman, M.D., Section of Vascular Radiology, Massachusetts General Hospital, Boston.)

that make operation difficult, the risks of failure of aortic valve replacement and aneurysm resection are between 10 and 15 per cent in most centers; 5- and 10-year survival rates have been reported at approximately 75 per cent and 55 per cent, respectively.[155,156] Gott et al. reported a 90 per cent 8-year survival in 49 patients operated on for ascending aortic aneurysms associated with Marfan syndrome[157]; they recommend elective repair of the aorta in patients with Marfan syndrome and aortic root diameter greater than 6.0 cm.[157] However, this policy remains controversial.[158] The relative risk of dissection, based on aortic site, appears to be variable. In an echocardiographic study, 3 of 11 patients with annuloaortic ectasia developed dissection during a mean follow-up of 18 months. All three had aortic root diameters exceeding 5.0 cm; however, four other patients with aortic diameters greater than 5.0 cm did not develop dissections.

Although postoperative results in survivors may be excellent, there is a disturbing occurrence of late sudden deaths, mostly from aortic dissection.[159] Late reoperation for adjacent aneurysm formation or dissection is necessary in more than 20 per cent of patients.[156] Death from progressive heart failure and sudden cardiac deaths also occur.

AORTIC ARTERITIS SYNDROMES

Takayasu's Arteritis

This peculiar arteritis was first noted in 1908 by the Japanese ophthalmologist Takayasu, who described a young woman with cataracts and unusual wreathlike arteriovenous anastomoses surrounding the optic papillae. In discussing this case, Takayasu's colleagues called attention to two patients with similar ocular findings who also had absent radial pulses. Subsequently, this disease entity has been described by a variety of terms that reflect some of its many features, such as "aortic arch syndrome," "pulseless disease," "reversed coarctation," "occlusive thromboaortopathy," "young female arteritis," as well as Takayasu's arteritis.[160]

PATHOPHYSIOLOGY AND ETIOLOGY. This disease occurs worldwide, although the majority of cases have been reported from Asia and Africa and most large series consist of Asians, with a heavy predilection for women.[161]

The basic pathological process is that of marked intimal proliferation and fibrosis and fibrous scarring and degeneration of the elastic fibers of the media, with round cell infiltration of variable intensity. However, fibrosis predominates over cellular reaction. The adventitia and intima become markedly thickened and vasa vasorum are destroyed. In its advanced cicatricial stage, the gross appearance of the aorta strikingly resembles the tree-bark–like appearance of luetic aortitis. The proliferative process leads to obliterative luminal changes in the aorta and involved arteries. Localized aneurysm formation, poststenotic dilatation, and calcification in the aortic and arterial walls are late complications. The process most often involves the arch of the aorta and its major branches, usually with changes that are most marked at the points of origin of the arteries from the aorta. It may present as multisegmental aortic disease with areas of normal wall between affected sites, diffuse involvement of the aorta, or disease of individual arteries arising from the aorta. The pulmonary arterial tree may also be affected. In a report from the United States, the most frequently affected arteries were the subclavian (90 per cent), carotid (45 per cent), vertebral (25 per cent), and renal (20 per cent).[162] In another series from the United States, the subclavian arteries, mesenteric arteries, and abdominal aorta were most commonly involved, each in nearly 80 per cent of cases.[163]

Ueno et al. have subdivided the disease into three types, depending upon the sites of involvement[164] (Fig. 47–18). Type I involves primarily the aortic arch and its branches; Type II spares the aortic arch, involving the thoracoabdominal aorta and its branches; Type III combines features of both. Lupi-Herrera and colleagues have suggested a fourth category, Type IV, in which there is pulmonary arterial involvement.[161] In their series of 107 cases, the incidences of the various types were 8, 11, 65, and 45 per cent for Types I, II, III, and IV, respectively.

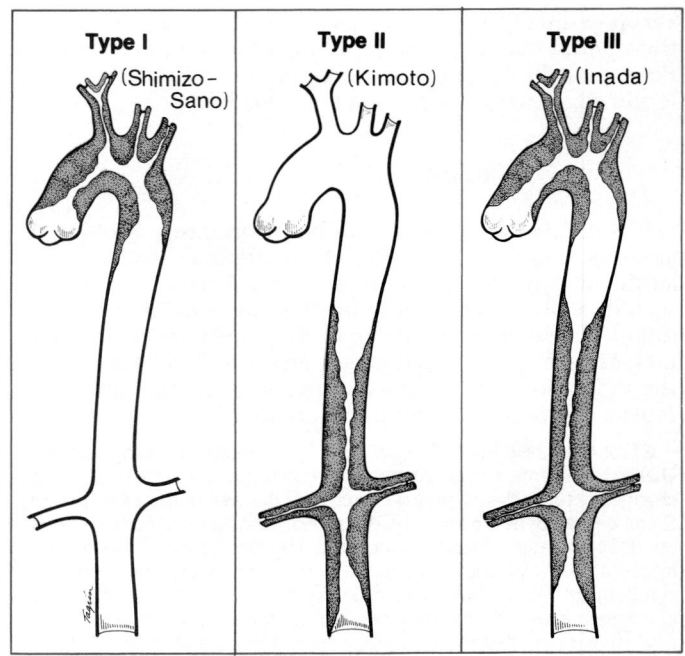

FIGURE 47–18. Types of Takayasu's arteritis. Type I involves primarily the aortic arch and brachiocephalic vessels. Type II affects the thoracoabdominal aorta and particularly the renal arteries. Type III combines features of both Types I and II. Types I and III may be complicated by aortic regurgitation. The eponyms for each type are noted.

A specific etiology for Takayasu's arteritis has not been found.[162] It has been linked to rheumatic fever, streptococcal infections, rheumatoid arthritis, and other collagen vascular diseases. Although giant cells are occasionally found in pathological specimens of vessels involved by the disease, the entity seems clearly distinct from giant cell arteritis, which affects predominantly patients over the age of 50 and involves mainly medium-sized muscular arteries. Although the aortic scarring of advanced Takayasu's arteritis resembles that of syphilis, nothing else suggests a causal relationship. Some investigators have reported a strikingly higher incidence of tuberculin skin reactivity to both *Mycobacterium tuberculosis* and atypical mycobacteria in patients with Takayasu's arteritis compared with the general population, raising the possibility of a relationship to tuberculosis,[165] but this observation has not been confirmed.[163] Although antiaortic antibodies have been detected in patients with this disease, their etiological role is uncertain. Overall, the bulk of evidence favors an autoimmune etiology. It is likely that the arteritis represents the final common pathological expression of a number of different antigenic stimuli in susceptible patients. An association between Takayasu's arteritis and certain HLA subtypes has been reported,[166,167] although the importance of the association remains unclear.[162,163]

CLINICAL MANIFESTATIONS. The disease affects women more frequently than men, in a ratio of 8 to 1. In as many as three-fourths of cases, onset is in the teenage years, although cases beginning in infancy or late middle age have been reported.[161,168,169] More than half the patients with this disease develop an initial systemic illness characterized by symptoms such as fever, anorexia, malaise, weight loss, night sweats, arthralgias, pleuritic pain, and fatigue. Localized pain and tenderness may be noted over affected arteries. This phase subsides, and these patients—as well as those who do not go through this so-called initial "systemic phase"—after a latent period of variable duration show symptoms and signs referable to the obliterative and inflammatory changes in the vessels. These late manifestations include diminished or absent pulses in 96 per cent, bruits in 94 per cent, hypertension in 74 per cent, and heart failure in 28 per cent.[161] The retinopathy originally described by Takayasu is seen in only about 25 per cent and is usually associated with carotid arterial involvement. The ocular process may lead to retinal detachment and loss of vision.

Patients with Types I and III exhibit those findings which are considered to be most typical of this disease, namely "reversed" coarctation of the aorta with absent or diminished upper body pulses and barely detectable blood pressure in the arms, higher pressures in the lower extremities, bruits overlying diseased arteries, manifestations of ischemia at various affected sites, and syncope. Patients with Type II arteritis may have abdominal angina and claudication of the limbs but also tend to develop hypertension because of renal arterial involvement. In fact, hypertension is an extremely important complication of this disease, and it may be difficult to recognize because of the diminished pulsations in the arms. Hypertension appears to arise through several mechanisms, the two most important of which are hemodynamically significant acquired coarctation of the aorta and renal artery stenosis. Decreased aortic capacitance and reduced baroreceptor reactivity may be contributory.[170,171]

Heart failure, when present, is usually seen in very young patients and appears to be a consequence of systemic hypertension. Rarely, aortic regurgitation can also contribute to congestive failure and is due to severe hypertension or to inflammation with scarring of the aortic valve by the inflammatory process.[172] Myocarditis has recently been described in several patients with congestive heart failure without hypertension or aortic regurgitation.[173] Whether this is a frequent cause of heart failure is unknown. The ostia and proximal segments of the coronary arteries can be affected, resulting in angina or myocardial infarction.[174,174a] Rarely, aneurysms are palpable or arteriovenous fistulas occur.[168] Takayasu's arteritis may be a common cause of atypical coarctation syndromes in adults.[175] The frequent absence of antecedent systemic symptoms and the more equal sex distribution of this form of the disease have been stressed. It is also believed that Takayasu's arteritis may be responsible for some cases of what appear to be primary pulmonary hypertension,[176] and occasionally fever of unknown origin.[177]

Laboratory abnormalities during the systemic phase are frequent.[163,165] The sedimentation rate is elevated, and a low-grade leukocytosis and mild anemia of chronic disease are common. These return toward normal when the systemic phase resolves. IgG or IgM values are elevated in more than half the patients. Immune complexes are infrequently present.[162] Other serological abnormalities are common but not specific. These include elevated levels of C-reactive protein, increased antistreptolysin-O titers, the occasional presence of rheumatoid factor and antinuclear antibodies, and elevated fibrinogen levels.[178]

Chest roentgenograms are usually unrevealing, although a rim of calcification is sometimes seen in the walls of the affected arteries. Arteriography reveals typical findings of an irregular intimal surface, with stenosis of the aorta or its tributary arteries, poststenotic dilatations, saccular aneurysms, and even complete occlusion of vessels (Fig. 47–19). Lande and Rossi have described the affected thoracic aorta as having a typical, narrowed, "rat-tail" angiographic appearance (Fig. 47–20).[179]

DIAGNOSIS. Proposed criteria for the clinical diagnosis of Takayasu's arteritis are shown in Table 47–2.[180] An obligatory criterion is age ≤ 40 years at diagnosis. The two major criteria reflect involvement of either subclavian artery. There are nine minor criteria. A high probability of the disease exists if, in addition to age ≤ 40 years, the patient meets two major criteria; one major and two or more minor criteria; or four or more minor criteria.[180]

TREATMENT AND PROGNOSIS. Adrenal corticosteroids are often effective in relieving constitutional symptoms and halting progression in patients with the systemic phase of the disease.[162,163] Fever, malaise, and fatigue are often dramatically relieved by steroids, and the sedimentation rate, which is a sensitive indicator of the activity of the disease, falls toward normal. In patients with continued systemic symptoms and/or documented disease progression, cyclophosphamide can be added. This usually results in clinical improvement and the ability to reduce corticosteroids to every other day dosing.[164] The recommended dose of cyclophosphamide is

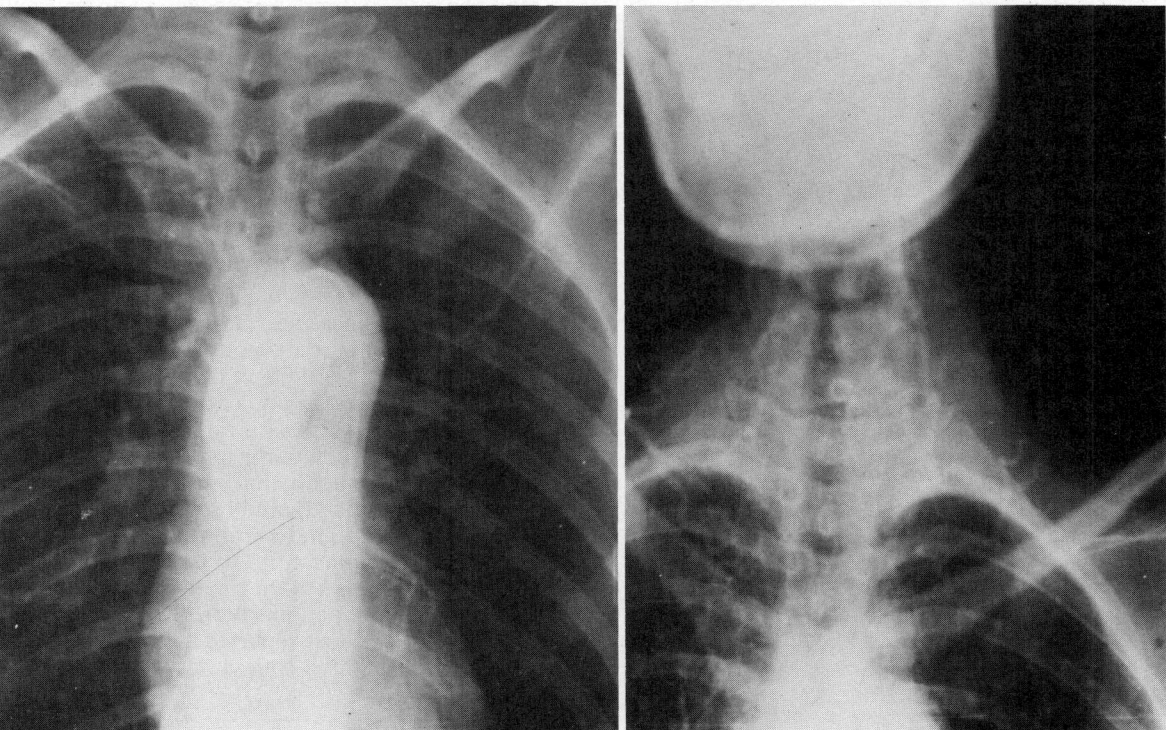

FIGURE 47–19. Thoracic aortogram *(left)* and late films of the head, neck, and upper thorax *(right)* in a 34-year-old Chinese woman with Takayasu's arteritis and no palpable pulses in the upper half of her body. The aortogram shows no direct filling of any of the major arteries arising from the aorta except the coronary arteries. In the delayed film *(right)* collateral channels faintly fill the carotid and vertebral systems.

TABLE 47–2 PROPOSED CRITERIA FOR THE CLINICAL DIAGNOSIS OF TAKAYASU'S DISEASE*

CRITERION	DEFINITION
Obligatory criterion	
Age ≤ 40 yr	Age ≤ 40 yr at diagnosis or at onset of "characteristic signs and symptoms"† of 1 month duration in patient history.
Two major criteria	
1. Left mid subclavian artery lesion	The most severe stenosis or occlusion present in the mid portion from the point 1 cm proximal to the left vertebral artery orifice to that 3 cm distal to the orifice determined by angiography.
2. Right mid subclavian artery lesion	The most severe stenosis or occlusion present in the mid portion from the right vertebral artery orifice to the point 3 cm distal to the orifice determined by angiography.
Nine minor criteria	
1. High ESR	Unexplained persistent high ESR ≥ 20 mm/h (Westergren) at diagnosis or presence of the evidence in patient history.
2. Carotid artery tenderness	Unilateral or bilateral tenderness of common carotid arteries by physician palpation: neck muscle tenderness is unacceptable.
3. Hypertension	Persistent blood pressure ≥ 140/90 mm Hg brachial or ≥ 160/90 mm Hg popliteal at age ≤ 40 yr or presence of the history at age ≤ 40 yr.
4. Aortic regurgitation	By auscultation or Doppler echocardiography or angiography.
or Annuloaortic ectasia	By angiography or two-dimensional echocardiography.
5. Pulmonary artery lesion	Lobar or segmental arterial occlusion or equivalent determined by angiography or perfusion scintigraphy; or presence of stenosis, aneurysm, luminal irregularity or any combination in pulmonary trunk or in unilateral or bilateral pulmonary arteries determined by angiography.
6. Left mid common carotid lesion	Presence of the most severe stenosis or occlusion in the mid portion of 5 cm in length from the point 2 cm distal to its orifice determined by angiography.
7. Distal brachiocephalic trunk lesion	Presence of the most severe stenosis or occlusion in the distal third determined by angiography.
8. Descending thoracic aorta lesion	Narrowing, dilation or aneurysm, luminal irregularity, or any combination determined by angiography: tortuosity alone is unacceptable.
9. Abdominal aorta lesion	Narrowing, dilation or aneurysm, luminal irregularity, or any combination and absence of lesion in aortoiliac region consisting of 2 cm of terminal aorta and bilateral common iliac arteries determined by angiography; tortuosity alone is unacceptable.

* The proposed criteria consist of one obligatory criterion, two major criteria, and nine minor criteria. In addition to the obligatory criterion, the presence of two major criteria, or one major and two or more minor criteria, or four or more minor criteria suggests a high probability of the presence of Takayasu's disease.

† "Characteristic signs and symptoms" are explained in the text (Methods). ESR = erythrocyte sedimentation rate.

From Ishikawa, K.: Diagnostic approach and proposed criteria for the clinical diagnosis of Takayasu's arteriopathy J. Am. Coll. Cardiol. *12*:964, 1988.

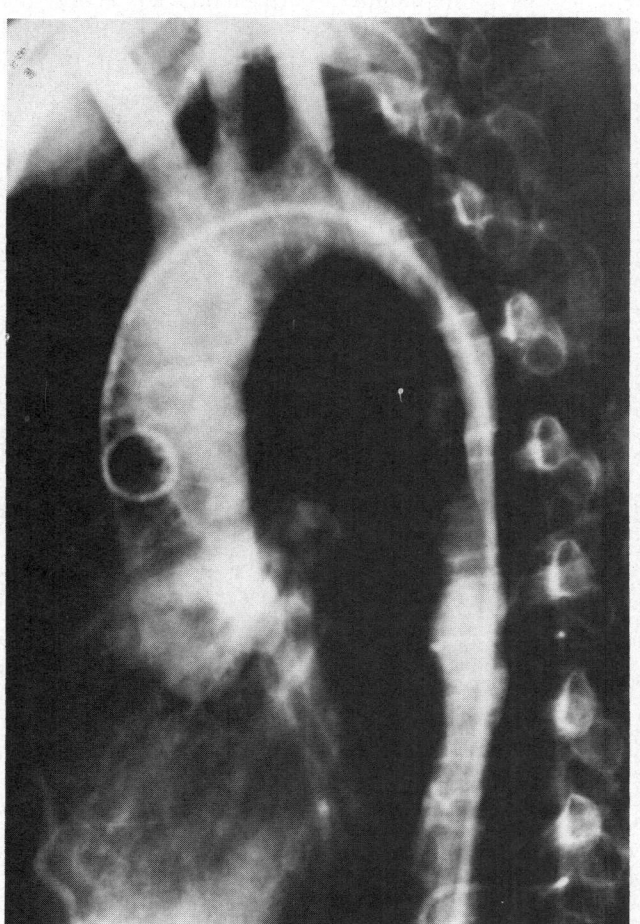

2 mg/kg/day, adjusted to maintain the peripheral leukocyte count above 3000/mm³. Anticoagulant drugs, including those of the warfarin family, and drugs that inhibit platelet function, such as aspirin and dipyridamole, are recommended both to treat transient ischemic symptoms and to prevent progression of the disease. Their efficacy is not established. Aggressive treatment of hypertension, when present, is important. In cases related to renovascular disease, the angiotensin-converting enzyme inhibitors may be particularly effective.[181,182] A variety of *surgical treatments* may be needed to deal with late complications of Takayasu's arteritis,[162,163,183,184] including endarterectomy, bypass of obstructed arteries (especially the renal arteries), resection of localized coarctations, excision of saccular aneurysms, and, rarely, aortic valve replacement. Successful use of percutaneous transluminal angioplasty for dilation of stenotic lesions in carotid, subclavian, renal, and mesenteric arteries has also been reported.[163,185]

The course of the disease is unpredictable, but slow progression over a period of months to years is usual. Morbidity and mortality depend upon the presence or absence of severe complications, which include retinopathy, secondary hypertension, aortic regurgitation, and aortic or arterial aneurysms. In several series, uneventful survival over 5 to 7 years was 97 per cent in patients without major complications compared with 59 per cent in patients with complications.[186,187] In a follow-up study, Ishikawa reported 9-year survival of 94 per cent in patients with stable symptoms but 60 to 70 per cent in

FIGURE 47–20. Aortogram in a 28-year-old Korean man with the clinical features of coarctation of the aorta that proved to be the result of Takayasu's arteritis. Note the typical "rat-tail" angiographic appearance of the descending thoracic aorta.

patients with crescendo symptom patterns.[188] Heart failure and cerebrovascular accidents are common causes of death. However, the combination of corticosteroid therapy, cytotoxic agents, and surgery when needed have led to 5-year survival rates that now may approximate 100 per cent.[162,163]

GIANT CELL ARTERITIS

This disease of unknown cause is predominantly found in elderly people and characteristically involves medium-sized arteries. However, the aorta and its major branches are affected in about 15 per cent of cases.[189] The disease is also referred to as "granulomatous arteritis," "cranial" or "temporal" arteritis, and "arteritis of the aged." It is closely allied to a syndrome characterized by diffuse muscular aching and stiffness called polymyalgia rheumatica.

PATHOPHYSIOLOGY AND ETIOLOGY. The many names given this disease describe its important features. The characteristic pathological lesion that distinguishes it from other arteritis syndromes is granulomatous inflammation of the media of small- to medium-caliber arteries, about the size of the temporal artery, with special predilection for vessels of the head and neck.[190] In addition to granulomas, an inflammatory infiltrate is usually found, composed largely of eosinophils, plasma cells, and other mononuclear cells. Endarteritis is not an important feature, but the mural involvement can lead to obstruction of involved arteries. Rarely, the aortic wall may be weakened by the inflammatory process, leading to localized aneurysm formation, aortic annular dilatation, and aortic regurgitation.[191]

Involvement of the aorta[192] and its major tributaries, when it occurs, usually coexists with the more classic and prevalent syndromes of temporal arteritis and polymyalgia rheumatica, although the aorta may rarely serve as the primary target of this disease.

The etiology of giant cell arteritis is unknown, although the generalized systemic manifestations of the disease and its occasional apparent temporal relationship to prior immunization or a viral illness suggest a possible infectious or autoimmune origin.[193] Klein et al. point out that involvement of the aorta and larger arteries may often arise as corticosteroid therapy for the more classic forms of this disease is being tapered.[189]

CLINICAL MANIFESTATIONS. Giant cell arteritis typically affects patients over the age of 50 and occurs predominantly in women. The disorder is more common in black women and appears to be distinctly uncommon in Hispanics.[194] The classic presentation is a triad of severe headache, marked malaise, and fever. Other common constitutional symptoms include anorexia, weight loss, lassitude, myalgias, and night sweats. Headaches are often intense and almost unbearable. Headache typically occurs over involved arteries, usually the temporal arteries but occasionally the occipital region. The area around the arteries is exquisitely sensitive to pressure, and complaints such as being unable to rest the head comfortably against a pillow, wear a hat, or comb one's hair are common. Claudication in the jaw muscles while chewing occurs in up to two-thirds of patients and is most suggestive of the diagnosis. A serious complication that may occur anywhere in the course of the disease is the onset of blindness from involvement of the ophthalmic artery— blindness that is often irreversible. Visual symptoms ranging from blurring to diplopia and visual loss occur in 25 to 50 per cent of patients. In its milder forms, patients may complain only of generalized muscular aches and pains and unusual fatigue, the syndrome of polymyalgia rheumatica. Blindness in these cases is uncommon. Polymyalgia rheumatica is seen in nearly 40 per cent of patients with giant cell arteritis.[195]

On rare occasions, consequences of involvement of the aorta or its major tributaries may be the first manifestations of the disease, although more typically, when such involvement occurs, it is part of the more generalized syndrome. However, when aortic or major branch disease is present, the symptoms are similar to those of Takayasu's arteritis and are the result of ischemia in the structures supplied by the involved arteries. Specifically, symptoms may include claudication of either upper or lower extremities, paresthesias, Raynaud's phenomenon, abdominal angina, coronary ischemia, transient cerebral ischemic attacks, and aortic arch and great vessel "steal"

syndromes. More rarely, aortic aneurysms, aortic regurgitation, and aortic dissection may occur.[196] Interestingly, renal artery involvement is almost never seen, in contrast with Takayasu's arteritis.[189] Rarely, death can occur from aortic rupture or dissection.

On *physical examination*, fever is almost universal and patients appear ill. Involved vessels are thickened and very tender. Indeed, an experienced examiner can make the diagnosis of temporal arteritis with virtual certainty at the bedside simply by palpating an indurated, beaded, tender, temporal artery. Pulses may be lost, and bruits may occur over sites of arterial occlusion. Signs of aortic regurgitation are rarely present.

Laboratory tests may be helpful in making the diagnosis. A very high sedimentation rate is virtually a sine qua non for this disease and is a valuable guide to the activity of the process. A moderate normochromic, normocytic anemia is the rule. Acute phase reactants such as alpha$_2$ globulin are increased, and IgG and C3, and C4 (complement) levels are often elevated.[197]

The *diagnosis* is confirmed by biopsy of an involved artery, usually the temporal artery. In cases of larger vessel and aortic involvement, angiography may serve to differentiate arteritis from arteriosclerosis by the following features, as described by Klein et al.: (1) long, smooth, tapering stenosis alternating with segments of normal or even slightly increased diameter; (2) the absence of irregular ulcerated atheromatous plaques seen in profile; and (3) the more typical anatomical distribution of arteritis to include the subclavian, axillary, and brachial arteries.[189]

MANAGEMENT. High-dose steroid therapy, e.g., 60 to 80 mg of prednisone per day, is recommended in all patients with granulomatous arteritis. The intent of therapy is not only to reverse the disease but also to prevent progression, especially in the ophthalmic arteries, in order to prevent blindness. With constitutional symptoms and the sedimentation rate used as a guide, steroids can usually be reduced gradually to a maintenance dose of 5 to 15 mg/day (or every other day) for 1 to 2 years. The overall course is one of progressive improvement and eventual complete resolution. However, in many patients, the course of the disease may be protracted for months or years. Methotrexate in doses of 7.5 to 12.5 mg per week may be beneficial in patients with steroid-resistant symptoms or can be steroid-sparing in patients needing protracted treatment.[198] Very rarely, surgical resection of an expanding aneurysm or replacement of a regurgitant aortic valve is necessary.[191,196]

OTHER ARTERITIS SYNDROMES

In addition to the aortic inflammation of Takayasu's and giant cell arteritis, isolated aortic regurgitation due to dilatation of the aortic valve ring with associated aortic root involvement may occur during the course of ankylosing spondylitis, psoriatic arthritis, arthritis associated with ulcerative colitis, relapsing polychondritis, and Reiter's syndrome (Chap. 56).[199-201] In addition, aneurysms of the aorta, pulmonary artery, and other major vessels can complicate Behçet's syndrome.[202]

Reported instances of aortitis complicating each of these diseases are rare. For example, it is seen in 1 to 4 per cent of patients with ankylosing spondylitis (p. 1731), and only a small number of well-described cases of Reiter's syndrome with aortic regurgitation have been documented (p. 1732). Nevertheless, the symptoms of aortic regurgitation and resultant heart failure may eventually dominate the clinical picture. In each case of arthritis-associated aortitis, the underlying arthritic disease is particularly fulminant and prolonged, and multiple extraarticular features are usually manifest.

PATHOLOGICAL FEATURES. These appear to be similar in each of the aforementioned diseases. In the early stages of inflammation there is marked dilatation of the aortic valve ring with patchy elastic tissue disruption, an active inflammatory cell infiltrate, and subendothelial fibrosis.[199] These changes are most marked in the aortic root. Later, the proximal ascending aorta appears similar to that in luetic aortitis, with intimal thickening, coarse granular plaque formation, and characteristic obliterative endarteritis of the vasa vasorum. The aortic root dilates but usually without frank aneurysm formation. Early, the aortic valve cusps remain essentially normal and later become thickened and retracted, presumably as a result of the incompetence that arises from root dilatation. Echocardiographic data suggest that patients with subclinical aortitis may be identified by the presence of subaortic fibrous ridging or marked leaflet thickening, even when aortic root dimensions are normal.[203]

The clinical features are those of aortic regurgitation and resemble those of annuloaortic ectasia. However, it is worth noting that the course of this disease is variable. Some patients exhibit a rapid progressive course of cardiac decompensation, whereas others have a more indolent and stable natural history. Thus, the development of aortic regurgitation does not necessarily signify an irreversible downhill course. There is some evidence that the inflammation of the aortic root may be episodic; worsening of aortic regurgitation may also pursue an intermittent course.

Treatment consists of that required for the underlying arthritis or other disease. Aortic valve replacement should be performed when indicated, although special problems may be encountered in these patients. For example, pulmonary function is often impaired in ankylosing spondylitis as a result of rigidity of the thoracic spine and chest wall. In the rare patient with ulcerative colitis who requires aortic valve replacement, a porcine valve is recommended so that anticoagulation will be unnecessary. In contrast to annuloaortic ectasia, replacement of the ascending aorta itself is almost never necessary.

CARDIOVASCULAR SYPHILIS

Once accounting for 5 to 10 per cent of all cardiovascular deaths, syphilitic disease of the heart and aorta has become a rarity in most major medical centers today as a result of aggressive antibiotic treatment of lues in its early stages. Cardiovascular complications occur in approximately 10 per cent of cases of untreated lues. The latent period may extend from 5 to 40 years after the initial spirochetal infection, with a usual time of 10 to 25 years.

PATHOLOGY. The consequences of lues are the direct results of spirochetal infection of the aortic media, thought to occur usually during the secondary phase of the disease, with subsequent inflammation and scarring of the aortic wall. Although the aorta may be invaded anywhere along its course, the most common location is the ascending aorta. It is postulated that this area has a proclivity for syphilitic involvement because it is richer in lymphatics than any other portion of the aorta. The muscular and elastic tissues of the media are destroyed by the spirochetes and the resultant inflammatory process and are replaced by vascular fibrous tissue.

The aortic wall becomes progressively weakened by the inflammatory process, and it may become calcified. Such weakening leads to aneurysmal dilatation. The overlying intima becomes furrowed and wrinkled and is covered with large plaques of a glistening, pearly material. This accounts for the "tree-bark" appearance of the involved aorta characteristic of luetic aortitis.

The infection may extend into the aortic root, resulting in aortic regurgitation due to dilatation of the aortic annulus and separation of the aortic valve commissures. Luetic aortic regurgitation is usually associated with an aortic aneurysm. An obliterative endarteritis may also obstruct the ostia of the coronary arteries. The scarring and injury from lues may progress long after the spirochetal organisms have been eradicated.

There are four categories of syphilitic heart disease[204]: (1) uncomplicated syphilitic aortitis, (2) syphilitic aortic aneurysm, (3) syphilitic aortic valvulitis with aortic regurgitation, and (4) syphilitic coronary ostial stenosis. Based on autopsy studies, about one-third of patients with pathological incidence of cardiovascular lues are asymptomatic; half have a significant aortic aneurysm, and, of these, one-half to one-third have associated aortic regurgitation. Five to 10 per cent will have essentially pure aortic regurgitation, and 26 per cent will have significant luetic coronary ostial stenosis, often in association with aortic regurgitation or an aortic aneurysm.

CLINICAL MANIFESTATIONS. Luetic aneurysms can arise anywhere along the aorta (including the abdomen), but the classical location is in the ascending aorta. They are usually saccular but may be fusiform. In the absence of aortic regurgitation, aneurysms may undergo significant enlargement without producing symptoms. Eventually, aneurysms may expand enough to reach, compress, and even erode contiguous structures, particularly the sternum and anterior right thoracic cage in the case of aneurysms of the ascending aorta. A thrusting, pulsating mass may be seen and palpated. Erosion of the bony structures of the chest wall causes pain at the point of involvement. Ascending aortic aneurysms and those involving the arch may produce a tracheal tug, stridor, and dysphagia. Aneurysms elsewhere may cause symptoms from compression of adjacent structures similar to those of any type of aneurysm located in the same area.

Luetic aortic regurgitation tends to occur in older patients with luetic cardiovascular disease, presumably because the disease has been present longer in these individuals. The earliest auscultatory sign of luetic aortic valve involvement is a tambour-like aortic valve closure sound. Because of the dilated aortic root, the murmur of luetic aortic regurgitation may be more prominent along the right sternal border rather than the left. It is often musical in quality and in rare instances of aortic cusp eversion may be particularly loud, with an associated thrill.

Because there is often considerable calcification in the aortic annulus, stiffness of the base of the aortic leaflets, and usually a dilated proximal aorta, a loud systolic ejection murmur, sometimes with a thrill, is often present in luetic aortic valve disease in the absence of any significant aortic stenosis. Also, a loud, slapping ejection sound is sometimes caused by sudden distention of the dilated aorta in early systole.

Luetic aortic regurgitation is associated with an aneurysm of the ascending aorta. Because of concomitant coronary ostial stenosis, angina pectoris may be particularly troublesome. Atrial fibrillation is seen more commonly than in other types of pure aortic regurgitation. Otherwise, the signs and symptoms are typical for those of aortic regurgitation.

DIAGNOSIS. Usually, there is a history of syphilis, and other manifestations of tertiary lues are found in 10 to 30 per cent of patients with cardiovascular syphilis. Fifteen to 30 per cent of patients have negative routine serological tests for syphilis (Wasserman, Hinton, Kahn, Venereal Disease Research Laboratories [VDRL], and Kolmer). On the other hand, serological tests directed against a specific treponema antigen, such as the *Treponema pallidum* immobilization (TPI) test or the fluorescent treponemal antibody absorption (FTA-ABS) test, are almost invariably positive. The chest roentgenogram may afford extremely valuable clues to the diagnosis of luetic aortitis. In sharp contrast to arteriosclerosis, calcification in the ascending aorta proximal to the brachiocephalic vessels is almost always much more extensive than that elsewhere.

Angiography may delineate the aneurysm (Fig. 47–21) and help to quantify the severity of aortic regurgitation. In patients suspected of having coronary ostial stenosis and in any patient with cardiovascular syphilis in whom surgical correction is contemplated, the coronary artery anatomy — and particularly the ostia — should be visualized by angiography if possible.

TREATMENT. All patients with syphilis, including cardiovascular syphilis, who are seen 1 year or more after the initial contact should be given a course of antibiotic therapy aimed at curing the spirochetal infection. Penicillin is still the most effective antibiotic and is given as benzathine penicillin G (Bicillin), 2.4 million units intramuscularly weekly for 3 weeks (total of 7.2 million units). For patients allergic to penicillin, the recommended therapy is doxycycline, 200 mg orally two times daily for 21 days. In penicillin-allergic patients who cannot tolerate doxycycline, the penicillin allergy should be confirmed. In such patients, the alternative regimen is erythromycin, 500 mg orally four times daily for 30 days. Compliance and serological follow-up must be confirmed, especially with the latter regimen.[205] The effectiveness of treatment can be monitored by a decrease in VDRL titer, with the desired result being a fourfold reduction in titer in 12 to 24 months.

Although a course of antibiotics is recommended in any previously untreated patient with cardiovascular syphilis, even those with a negative serology, there is no good evidence that such treatment reverses, or even halts, the progression of aortitis or aortic regurgitation. In cases of cardiovascular syphilis, cerebrospinal fluid examination should also be performed, and, if positive, this too should be followed to assure the adequacy of therapy. Since the efficacy of antibiotics other than penicillin against syphilis is not well studied beyond 1 year, close follow-up of patients treated with these alternative modes is necessary.

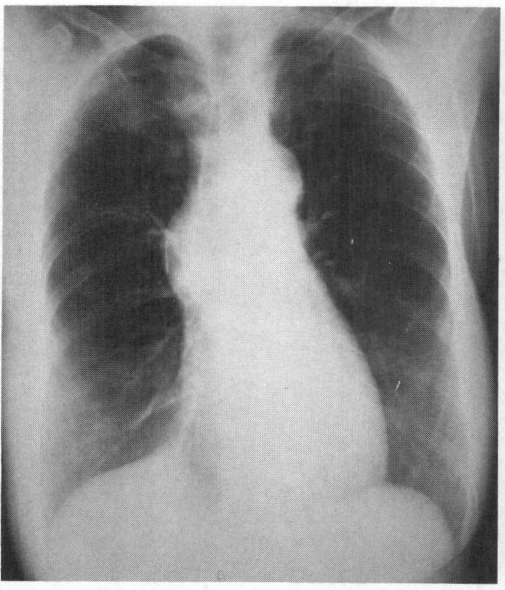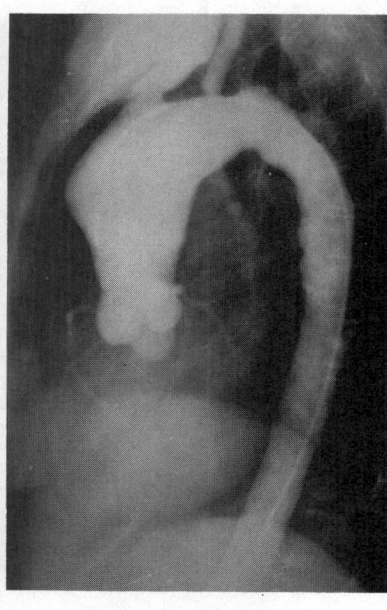

FIGURE 47–21. Films obtained from a 58-year-old woman with luetic aortitis. *Left,* Posteroanterior chest film showing an aneurysm of the ascending aorta with a faint rim of calcification. *Right,* Angiographic appearance of the aneurysm in the lateral view. (Courtesy of Christos Athanasoulis, M.D., and Arthur Waltman, M.D., Section of Vascular Radiology, Massachusetts General Hospital, Boston.)

Indications for excision of the luetic aneurysms are similar to those for other thoracic aortic aneurysms (p. 1533): a diameter of 7 cm or larger or an aneurysm of any size that produces symptoms or is expanding rapidly. Since many luetic aneurysms are saccular, aneurysmorrhaphy is occasionally adequate. However, since ongoing aortitis and scarring are possible, it is probably wiser to replace as much as possible of the diseased aorta with a prosthetic graft. Replacement of the aortic valve is indicated for significant aortic regurgitation, and the results are as good as in aortic regurgitation of other causes. Since the coronary artery disease of syphilis is usually ostial, a localized endarterectomy at the orifices of the coronary arteries may be possible. If an adequate lumen cannot be obtained by endarterectomy, bypass may be necessary.

PSEUDOCOARCTATION

Pseudocoarctation of the aorta is a rare condition resulting from elongation of the aortic arch, with redundancy and kinking of the aorta just distal to the origin of the left subclavian artery at the level of the ligamentum arteriosum.[206,207] Other terms used to describe this entity have included "mild coarctation," "atypical coarctation," or "subclinical coarctation." The etiology is believed to be congenital, with a lack of compression and fusion of certain of the segments of the dorsal aortic root and fourth arch. It is of interest that the incidence and distribution of associated cardiac anomalies parallel those seen in true coarctation. These anomalies include bicuspid aortic valve, sinus of Valsalva aneurysms, ventricular septal defect, corrected transposition, and Turner syndrome.[208,209]

CLINICAL MANIFESTATIONS. The pressure gradient across the deformed area is usually trivial or absent. Thus, the clinical features of true coarctation—upper extremity hypertension, lower extremity hypotension, and the development of collateral arterial circulation—are absent. Physical findings are often those of the associated lesions, although a murmur is sometimes heard over the aortic kink in the interscapular area. With mild degrees of obstruction, blood pressure in the lower extremities may be slightly reduced, and there may be a subtle pulse lag between the radial and femoral arteries.

The entity can usually be recognized on chest roentgenography. The typical appearance is that of a double, rounded density in the left superior mediastinum. Pitfalls in interpreting the x-ray films are common. The upper density, though relatively translucent, represents the uppermost extension of redundant aorta and is often mistaken for tumor or aneurysm. The lower density is the area of the aorta involved by poststenotic dilatation, and it is often misinterpreted as the aortic knob. Calcification may occur in the area of narrowing. Angiography confirms the diagnosis.

SIGNIFICANCE. Problems may arise in pseudocoarctation from the formation of aneurysms either proximal or distal to the kink (Fig. 47–22). Associated aneurysms of the left subclavian artery have been reported.[210] Rarely, thrombus forms at the site of atheromatous degeneration and calcification in the kinked segment.[211] Complete thrombosis can produce a picture mimicking true coarctation, although collateral arterial circulation is notably absent. Thrombus can also propagate directly into tributary vessels or embolize distally. The left subclavian artery is particularly vulnerable because of its proximity to the pseudocoarctation. Infection at the site of aortic narrowing is a rare problem.

TREATMENT. Therapy is necessary only for complications of pseudocoarctation. In the absence of complications, surgical resection is not indicated. If a bruit or pressure gradient is present over an area of pseudocoarctation, antibiotic prophylaxis for endocarditis should be given before dental or surgical procedures.

AORTIC TRAUMA

(See also p. 1524)

Blunt Trauma

Aortic injuries are associated with severe blunt trauma,[212] and they are far from rare. In one autopsy series of fatal automobile accidents, rupture of the aorta was found in one-sixth of all victims.[213]

ETIOLOGY AND PATHOGENESIS. Aortic trauma most commonly results from injuries associated with sudden high-speed deceleration upon impact, such as that resulting from motor vehicle accidents, blast injuries, cave-ins, crush injuries, or severe falls.[213–216] The abrupt deceleration of the body as it crashes to a sudden stop creates enormous shearing forces that act maximally at those points where a highly mobile portion of the aorta joins a fixed segment. Less frequently, pressure or blast injuries may produce rupture of the aorta, believed to be caused by an acute increase in intraaortic pressure generated by the compression of blood contained within the aorta and further increased by the force imparted by cardiac systole.

Although the aorta may be torn anywhere along its length, the most frequent point of rupture (the site in 90 per cent of cases) is in the aortic isthmus at the site of insertion of the ligamentum arteriosum, just distal to the origin of the left subclavian artery. Here, the relatively mobile descending thoracic aorta sweeps dorsally to become fixed to the thoracic cage by the ligamentum arteriosum, the intercostal arteries, and the left subclavian artery. The injury may vary from a minuscule rent in the aortic wall to a complete circumferential transection of all three layers of the aorta. In a series of 296 cases of aortic trauma studied by Parmley et al., a circumferential tear was evident in 80 per cent.[214] If the aorta is partially transected and the patient survives, a localized saccular aneurysm or pseudoaneurysm may subsequently develop at the site of the tear. Pseudoaneurysms may also form between the two ends of a totally transected aorta.

In addition to the aortic isthmus, other areas of injury include the supravalvular portion of the ascending aorta; the innominate artery, which may be avulsed from the aorta; the aortic arch; other portions of the descending thoracic aorta; the abdominal aorta; and combinations of these.[217]

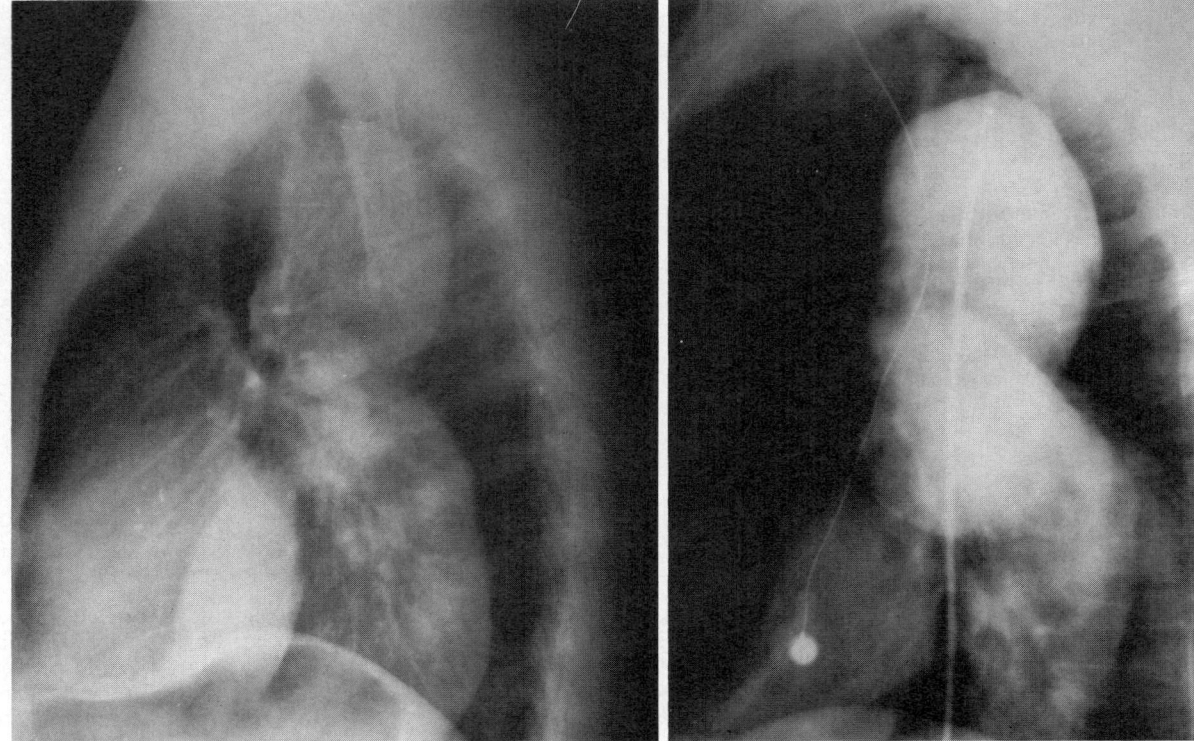

FIGURE 47–22. Pseudocoarctation of the aorta, with aneurysmal dilatation of the aorta proximal and distal to the point of narrowing. *Left,* Lateral chest roentgenogram. *Right,* The aorta is outlined with contrast material.

CLINICAL MANIFESTATIONS. The diagnosis of aortic trauma is often obscured by the presence of other serious injuries, such as central nervous system damage, visceral injury, and multiple skeletal fractures.[218] About two-thirds of patients with aortic rupture have clear-cut evidence of other thoracic trauma, such as chest or cardiac contusions, rib or vertebral fractures, pulmonary contusions, and hemorrhagic pleural effusions. The remaining one-third are surprisingly free of overt evidence of chest wall injury.

Few symptoms are directly attributable to the aortic trauma per se. Pressure from a localized hematoma can cause dyspnea and stridor from tracheal or bronchial compression, dysphagia from esophageal compression, or superior vena caval syndrome from caval compression. Although it is uncommon, the syndrome of so-called "acute coarctation" with upper extremity hypertension, reduced blood pressure in the lower extremities, a systolic murmur over the precordium or in the interscapular area, and a palpable radial-femoral pulse lag is virtually classic for the diagnosis. An interscapular systolic bruit may be heard. Otherwise, the physical examination is relatively unrevealing. Localized aneurysms developing in the aortic isthmus late after trauma may cause hoarseness, cough, and dysphagia from compression of the adjacent recurrent laryngeal nerve, bronchus, and esophagus.

DIAGNOSIS. Because the diagnosis is so frequently overshadowed by the presence of other severe injuries, rupture of the aorta is often overlooked. *A high index of suspicion is crucial, and evidence of aortic trauma should be sought in any patient with severe bodily injuries.* In the absence of classic physical findings—a common situation—the diagnosis is best suspected from the chest roentgenogram, which, if properly obtained and interpreted, is abnormal in over 90 per cent of patients with traumatic aortic rupture. Marsh and Sturm have delineated criteria for rupture of the aorta based upon a 40-degree anteroposterior supine chest film. The numbers on Figure 47–23 correspond to these criteria: (1) mediastinum measuring greater than 8 cm at the level of the aortic knob, (2) shift of the trachea toward the right, (3) blurring of the normally sharp outline of the aorta, (4) obliteration of the medial aspect of the apex of the upper lobe of the left lung, (5) opacifi-

cation of the clear space between the aorta and pulmonary artery, and (6) depression of the left main stem bronchus below 40 degrees.[219] In a follow-up report, these authors identified indistinct aortic contour, opacification of the clear space between aorta and pulmonary artery, and mediastinal widening (mean diameter = 9.4 cm) as the most sensitive markers for aortic injury.[220] Others have shown that deviation of the trachea (or a nasogastric tube) to the right, depression of the main left bronchus, and widening of the left paraspinal line are also important.[221-223] The concept of increased mediastinal width compared to chest width (m/c ratio) has also been advocated

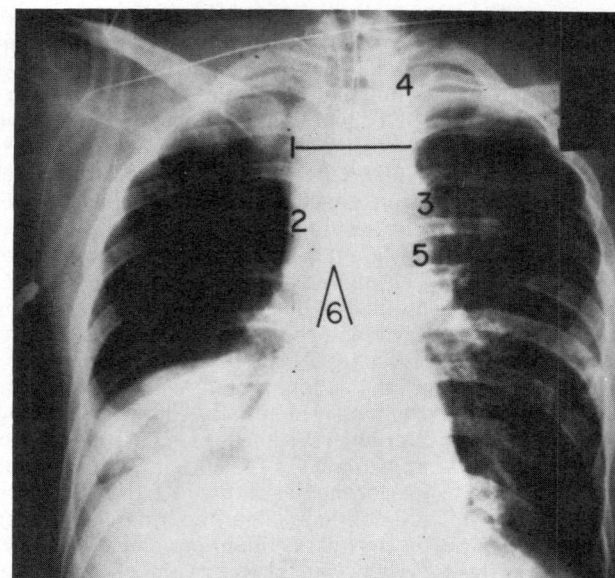

FIGURE 47–23. Aortic trauma. Roentgenographic characteristics of rupture of the proximal descending thoracic aorta in the supine anteroposterior projection (film-to-tube distance = 40 inches). The M/C ratio is 0.32. See text for key to numbers. (From Marsh, D. G., and Sturm, J. T.: Traumatic aortic rupture: Roentgenographic indications for angiography. Ann. Thorac. Surg. *21:*337, 1976.)

as a helpful sign for quantifying the magnitude of mediastinal widening and likelihood of aortic injury.[224] While any m/c ratio greater than 0.20 is considered abnormal, the specificity of the test for identifying patients with aortic injury increases from less than 25 per cent to nearly 90 per cent when the ratio is greater than 0.28. In cases of thoracic trauma, as the ratio increases from 0.25 to 0.28, the threshold for performing angiography should be lower; whenever the m/c ratio exceeds 0.28, additional studies should be carefully considered. It is also important to remember that occasional patients with aortic injury will have no specific signs of mediastinal hemorrhage.[225] CT scanning with contrast injection may confirm the diagnosis and should be performed as expeditiously as possible in a stable patient who has sustained severe chest trauma.[226] Should the diagnosis remain in question or if the patient's condition is unstable, the threshold for performing angiography in suspected cases should be low (Fig. 47–24 and Fig. 46–11, p. 1525). As with chest radiography, CT scanning can occasionally miss severe injuries, including aortic transection.[227]

COURSE AND PROGNOSIS. Approximately 80 per cent of patients with aortic rupture die instantly, although usually from other injuries, such as massive hemorrhage from other sites, trauma to other vital organs, or brain damage. Of those who survive the initial event, death often occurs within the first week from progressive hemorrhage at the site of the aortic tear. However, even with complete transection of the aorta, patients may be remarkably stable. About 2 to 5 per cent of patients with partial tears of the aorta go on to develop a localized aneurysm or pseudoaneurysm over a period of months or years, usually anterior to the aortic isthmus. This may either remain stable or ultimately expand. Such traumatic aneurysms frequently calcify or may become infected.

TREATMENT. The treatment of aortic trauma is operative repair, which should be undertaken as soon as possible once the condition is recognized. Occasionally, other serious injuries make it necessary to delay operation in order to stabilize the patient's condition, but even in the face of other severe trauma, surgery should be performed if there is evidence of progressive hemorrhage from the aorta. Some centers have advocated use of thoracic aortic occlusion with an intraaortic balloon pump to stabilize critically ill patients before definitive surgery.[228] Rupture of the aorta is usually treated by resecting the torn segment of the aorta and interposing a prosthetic graft between the two ends of the aorta. It may be necessary to support the distal circulation with a pump oxygenator or conduit bypass from the left ventricle or proximal aorta to the distal aorta around the rupture in order to reduce ischemic damage to the spinal cord, abdominal viscera, and kidneys.[229,230] Prompt recognition and operation for a ruptured aorta has resulted in survival of nearly 70 per cent of patients with this injury who reach the hospital alive.[218,229,231]

In cases of localized saccular aneurysms developing late after trauma, surgical excision is advised if the patient is an otherwise reasonable operative candidate. Long-term follow-up of patients with such lesions indicates that about half the aneurysms slowly expand and may even rupture. Surgery is curative and can be undertaken at a small risk (1 to 3 per cent).

Penetrating Trauma

Penetrating trauma of the aorta or any of its major arterial trunks is caused by puncture or laceration by missiles or knives, particularly bullet and stab wounds. Massive hemorrhage, often leading to rapidly fatal exsanguination, ensues. The consequences of the trauma depend upon the site and severity of perforation. Thus, perforation of the aorta within the pericardial sac may lead to cardiac tamponade. Perforation of the aorta elsewhere may cause massive hemorrhage, with compression of surrounding structures by the hematoma, such as the vena cava, tracheobronchial tree, and esophagus. Occlusion of a lacerated artery itself or of adjacent vessels may occur, producing focal signs and symptoms such

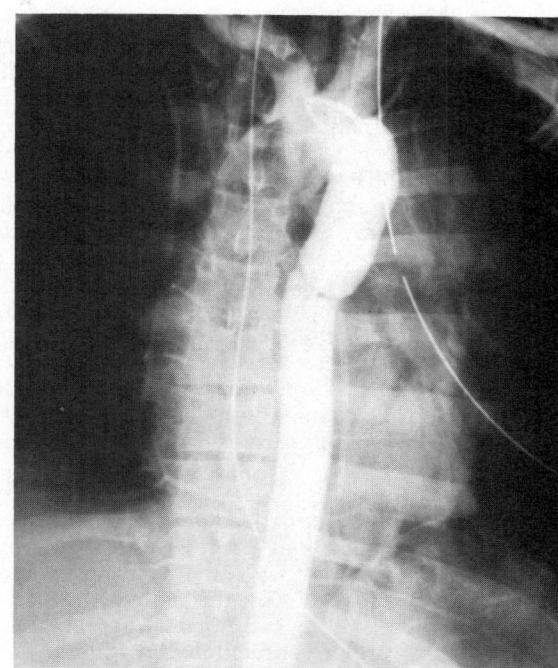

FIGURE 47–24. Thoracic aortogram in a 26-year-old man injured in a motor vehicle accident, showing traumatic transection of the aorta. The site of the tear can be clearly seen. (Courtesy of Robert Dinsmore, M.D., Massachusetts General Hospital, Boston.)

as loss of the right carotid and brachial pulses, with right hemispheric neurological signs in the case of occlusion of the innominate artery. Occasionally, simultaneous penetration of an adjacent artery and vein may cause an arteriovenous fistula, with a resultant continuous murmur, wide pulse pressure, and increased cardiac output.[232,233]

MANAGEMENT. Immediate surgical repair should be undertaken in any patient suspected of having a penetrating wound of the aorta, i.e., one with a missile or stab wound of the chest associated with a wide mediastinum on roentgenogram. If the patient's condition allows it, emergency angiography can usually pinpoint the site of perforation. However, in most patients who survive to reach the hospital, immediate operation for closure of the wound and evacuation of the hematoma is necessary. Similarly, laceration or penetrating wounds of arteries require urgent surgical correction.

AORTIC THROMBOEMBOLIC DISEASE

Aortic Embolism

Between 10 and 25 per cent of peripheral arterial emboli affect the aortic bifurcation, resulting in what are termed "saddle emboli." At least 90 per cent of these emboli originate within the chambers of the left side of the heart; 5 per cent come from the aorta itself, usually from thrombus overlying an arteriosclerotic plaque; and the remainder come from undetermined sites.[234] Rarely, paradoxical systemic embolism from the venous circulation occurs through a patent foramen ovale or atrial septal defect. Conditions that predispose to peripheral embolism are myocardial infarction with mural thrombus, ventricular aneurysm, prosthetic valves, congestive cardiomyopathy, and atrial fibrillation, especially in patients with rheumatic mitral stenosis. So-called "marantic endocarditis" is occasionally encountered in chronically ill patients, especially those with malignant disease, and consists of sterile intracardiac thrombi that may dislodge and travel to distal sites. Other less common conditions that serve to cause arterial emboli are left atrial myxomas and acute and subacute bacterial endocarditis. Emboli in endocarditis are usually small, although large emboli are seen in acute bacterial endocarditis and fungal (*Candida*) endocarditis. This can rarely be seen in disseminated *Aspergillus* infection.[235] An increased tendency to thromboembolism is encountered in women taking contraceptive pills and estrogens; in patients with malignant diseases, particularly carcinoma of the pancreas; and, rarely, in patients with antithrombin III deficiency.[236]

CLINICAL MANIFESTATIONS. Aortic bifurcation embolism is heralded by the sudden onset of excruciating pain in both legs. The pain usually extends distally from the midthigh area but can also involve the buttocks, lumbosacral area, and perineum. Associated with the intense pain are numbness, symmetrical weakness, and paresthesias. Schatz and Stanley have summarized in alliteration this classic presentation as "Pain, Paralysis, Paresthesias, Pulselessness, and Pallor."[237] Additional nonclassic presentations may include sudden onset of bilateral lower extremity weakness, severe hypertension, and acute abdominal pain simulating a perforated viscus.[238]

Examination reveals cold, pale extremities that are cyanotic and often exhibit a mottled, reticulated, reddish-blue appearance. These changes may progress to the blue-black color of gangrene, beginning first in the toes and extending proximally. Pulses are absent below the abdominal aorta. Initially sluggish, capillary filling is ultimately absent. Signs of ischemic neuropathy are present and include diminished or absent deep tendon reflexes, symmetrical weakness, and loss of all modalities of sensation, usually with demarcation at the level of the midthigh. If ischemia persists long enough, there may be myonecrosis with the release of products of muscle breakdown into the bloodstream, causing shock, hypotension, hyperkalemia, myoglobinuria, and acute tubular necrosis. Sepsis may add a serious further dimension to an already desperate problem. If perfusion is not reestablished within hours, death is almost inevitable.

The *differential diagnosis* includes acute aortic thrombosis from arteriosclerotic disease and aortic dissection. With thrombosis, there is usually a history of prior claudication, and an embolic source is lacking. With aortic dissection, a history of severe chest or back pain and an abnormal aortic contour on chest x-ray film usually provide distinguishing features.

The diagnosis is confirmed by angiography. However, most investigators advise prompt surgical intervention without angiography if the diagnosis is strongly suspected, since a delay could lead to irreversible ischemic damage to the limbs.

THERAPY. Most emboli can be removed by using Fogarty balloon-tipped catheters inserted through a transfemoral arterial approach under local anesthesia. In addition to retrieving the embolic material, passage of the Fogarty catheters into the distal arterial bed may result in the removal of any thrombus that may have formed as a result of the stagnant flow beyond the embolus. If the embolus cannot be retrieved with Fogarty catheters, removal by direct transabdominal aortotomy is necessary. Operative mortality ranges from 15 to 30 per cent, with death due to the underlying cardiac disease[238]; limb salvage is estimated at 80 to 90 per cent in most series.[238] Anticoagulation with constant intravenous heparin is instituted upon completion of the operation and is continued until therapeutic levels are achieved with one of the warfarin sodium family of drugs. Depending upon the clinical situation, long-term anticoagulant therapy using warfarin or antiplatelet agents may be required. Reembolization may occur in up to 25 per cent of patients, and some series suggest a reduced incidence if long-term anticoagulants are used. Using the transfemoral approach, surgery can be carried out with a low mortality even in patients whose other disease makes them poor operative risks. Limbs are almost uniformly salvaged if operation is undertaken promptly. All embolic debris should be cultured and examined microscopically. Left atrial myxomas are sometimes first recognized by the pathological examination of embolic specimens.

Aortic Thrombosis

Rarely, primary thrombosis of the distal abdominal aorta may be seen as a result of atheromatous disease or in rare patients with antithrombin III deficiency. In such patients, treatment is generally surgical, although an occasional case of successful balloon catheter dilatation has been reported.[236,239,240] Studies in experimental animals using tissue plasminogen activator (t-PA) for the treatment of aortic thrombotic occlusion suggest that this drug may have a potential role in treating patients with both peripheral emboli and aortic thrombosis.[241]

Atheromatous Emboli

Embolism of atheromatous debris from the disruption of arteriosclerotic plaques in the aorta or its major arterial trunks has been noted with increasing frequency. Usually, such embolism takes the form of showers of microemboli, each between 150 and 600 μm in size, into small arterial branches — an entity that is also termed "cholesterol embolism." However, obstruction of large arteries by embolic arteriosclerotic material may also occur.[242] By far the most common cause of cholesterol embolism is surgery or angiography that involves an atherosclerotic aorta.[243] Atheromatous embolism into the renal and splanchnic vascular beds is common after major abdominal vascular procedures, particularly resection of abdominal aortic aneurysms. Embolism of atheromatous material also occurs as an occasional complication of intraarterial cannulation, cardiac catheterization,[244] and cardiopulmonary bypass. In addition to these iatrogenic causes, however, spontaneously occurring cholesterol embolism is encountered, particularly from the aorta into the femoral-popliteal system. Studies have suggested a causal relationship between cholesterol embolism and anticoagulant therapy, especially long-term anticoagulation with warfarin sodium–type drugs.[245] Presumably, anticoagulation promotes hemorrhage into plaques, leading to their disruption, or prevents the formation of protective thrombus over ulcerated plaques. Finally, atheromatous embolism has followed blunt trauma to the aorta.

CLINICAL MANIFESTATIONS. The consequences of cholesterol embolism depend upon the vascular bed involved as well as the extent to which the small arterial vessels are occluded. Two important complications of cholesterol embolism following abdominal aortic surgery are pancreatitis and renal failure from diffuse microinfarction of the pancreas and kidneys, respectively. Renal failure may be severe and irreversible (p. 1835). Occasionally, cholesterol embolism has been implicated as a cause of severe renovascular hypertension. Gastrointestinal hemorrhage from microinfarction of abdominal viscera is also encountered. Showers of atheromatous emboli may affect the cerebral circulation, producing either focal neurological defects or a diffuse encephalopathic picture. In such cases, shiny cholesterol particles are sometimes visible in the retinal arteries.[246]

Spontaneously occurring cholesterol embolism in the lower extremities is manifested by bilateral pain, livedo reticularis, and purpuric and ecchymotic lesions in the lower legs, feet, and toes. These manifestations may be paroxysmal as emboli intermittently dislodge from their sites of origin. Skin necrosis and ischemic gangrene are common, especially in the toes ("blue toe syndrome").[245,247] With this clinical evidence of severe ischemia, arterial pulses are characteristically well preserved unless there is coincidental peripheral vascular disease.

The clinical picture may mimic that of a vasculitis or septic embolism from neisserial organisms — especially meningococcemia — or bacterial endocarditis. The absence of fever and other signs of systemic illness and the localized distribution of the lesions serve to distinguish cholesterol embolism from these other entities. The diagnosis has been made by muscle biopsy, which may show cholesterol particles in the arterioles.

THERAPY. For the most part, there is no specific treatment for cholesterol microembolism. Careful attention to the prevention of necrosis and infection in the involved extremities is important. Although the amputation of gangrenous digits is occasionally necessary, the ultimate prognosis for recovery is quite good, unless embolism is frequent and recurrent. Pancreatitis often subsides, even though it may be severe. Renal failure may be irreversible.

The use of anticoagulants in the prevention of further embolism is controversial, with some investigators advocating that they be given and others contending that they promote further atheromatous emboli. Overall, it appears that they are not of much value. In instances of recurrent atheromatous embolism, it may be possible to pinpoint the source of the cholesterol particles by angiography and to perform an endarterectomy or to excise the involved segment and replace it with a prosthetic graft. It has been suggested that use of a blood filtering device during aortoiliac reconstruction might reduce or prevent cholesterol embolism in that setting.[248]

AORTIC BACTERIAL INFECTIONS

The term "infected aneurysm" has gradually replaced the original designation of "mycotic aneurysm" used by Osler to define any localized dilation caused by sepsis in the wall of the aorta or any artery and thus to avoid confusion with infections of truly fungal origin. Infection can cause virtually any kind of aneurysmal dilatation, including fusiform, saccular, and false aneurysms. Rupture into the venous system may cause arteriovenous fistulas. Alternatively, infection may arise within preexisting arteriosclerotic aneurysms. Infected aortic aneurysms are rare, with only 1 or 2 cases per year recently being reported from a large general hospital.[249]

PATHOGENESIS. Vascular infection may arise by any of three different mechanisms. First, septic emboli from bacterial endocarditis or diffuse bacteremia may infect normal or diseased tissue. This mechanism of infection has become less frequent owing to the widespread use of effective antibiotics for the control of septicemia. Second, there may be contiguous spread from adjacent abscesses, infected lymph nodes, empyema, and so on. This is the usual cause for rare cases of tuberculous vascular involvement. Third, sepsis may be introduced directly from an external source, such as trauma, intravenous injections, or surgery. The incidence of this type of infection is increasing because of more frequent motor vehicle accidents, the widespread use of intravenous narcotics by drug addicts, and the performance of more intravascular procedures that may produce a portal for infection, such as intraarterial catheterization and intraaortic balloon counterpulsation. With this type of sepsis, the peripheral arteries are obviously more frequently involved than the aorta per se.

Although virtually any organism may infect the arterial tree, certain bacteria seem to have a proclivity for this type of infection. In particular, this is true of the Salmonella group, which tends to infect arteriosclerotic aneurysms. Staphylococcus aureus was the most common organism identified in a recent series, followed by Salmonella.[250]

CLINICAL MANIFESTATIONS. Most patients with infected aortic aneurysms are febrile; the height of the fever depends upon the severity of infection, the organism, and the site of the infection. Extremely high fever and rigors are common. Symptoms may arise from localized expansion of an infected aneurysm, such as dysphagia from esophageal compression and pain in areas contiguous to the infected sac. If palpable, infected aneurysms are almost always tender. A tender and pulsatile mass in a febrile patient should be considered an infected aneurysm until proved otherwise. Jarrett et al. have suggested that infected aortic aneurysms can be differentiated from sterile ones by the presence of fever, relative preponderance in women, tenderness, lack of calcification, and a tendency for early vertebral erosion.[249] With tuberculous involvement, evidence is almost always seen on the chest x-ray. This, coupled with a pulsating mass lesion, should elicit the correct diagnosis.

Sepsis in more peripheral arteries presents most commonly as fever with a palpable, painful, pulsating mass. Symptoms of compression of contiguous structures may also be present, such as arterial regurgitation or a neuropathy. Small abscesses in the distribution of the artery are often seen in staphylococ-

cal infections. The most common sites for infected aneurysms are the following arteries: femoral, abdominal aorta, superior mesenteric, brachial, iliac, and carotid arteries. Together, the femoral arteries and abdominal aorta account for nearly 70 per cent of all mycotic aneurysms.[250]

Leukocytosis, an elevated sedimentation rate, and positive blood cultures are present in most cases. Commonly reported organisms other than Staphylococcus aureus and Salmonella species are other gram-positive and gram-negative organisms, such as pneumococcus,[251] Pseudomonas, and anaerobes. Rarely, fungal infections with Candida or Aspergillus may occur.[235] Localization of suspected infected aneurysms in a patient with sepsis can be aided by angiography. Valuable information can sometimes be obtained from ultrasound, gallium, and CT scans.[252]

The natural history of infected aneurysms is that of progressive expansion, thinning of the aneurysm wall, and eventual rupture. Jarrett et al. found a more rapid progression in patients with gram-negative infections.[249]

THERAPY. Treatment is always surgical excision combined with appropriate antibiotic or antituberculous chemotherapy. Wide excision of infected tissue is advised.[249,250] Usually a prosthetic tube graft must be inserted if the aorta or a major artery is involved. Early recognition and therapy clearly alter the outcome favorably.

AORTIC TUMORS

One review cites 27 cases of primary aortic tumors recorded in the world's literature.[253] Clearly, secondary tumors can arise from direct extension and invasion from adjacent lung or abdominal neoplasms or from embolic spread. Histological types include fibrosarcoma (most commonly), fibromyxosarcoma, myxosarcoma, fibromyxoma, angiosarcoma, malignant fibrous histiocytoma, leiomyosarcoma, myxoma and endothelioma.[253,254] In the 27 cases of primary aortic tumors, the age of the patients ranged from infancy to 75 years, with a mean of 54 years; male sex predominated by 2:1. Presentation in over half the cases consisted of abdominal or leg pain, proximal hypertension due to the acquired coarctation, decreased femoral pulses, fever, claudication, and occasionally bruits are also seen. Diagnosis is made by the usual noninvasive or angiographic techniques, with key features being the irregular appearance of the lumen and lack of enlargement of the outer diameter of the aorta.

REFERENCES

EXAMINATION OF THE AORTA

1. Grossman, L. B., Buonocore, E. Modic, M. T., and Meaney, T. F.: Digital subtraction angiography of the thoracic aorta. Radiology 150:323, 1984.
2. Seward, J. B., Khandheria, B. K., Oh, J. K. et al.: Transesophageal echocardiography: Technique, anatomic correlations, implementation, and clinical applications. Mayo Clin. Proc. 63:649, 1988.
3. Taams, M. A., Gussenhoven, W. J., Schippers, L. A. et al.: The value of transesophageal echocardiography for diagnosis of thoracic aorta pathology. Eur. Heart J. 9:1308, 1988.
4. Brundage, B. H., Rich, S., and Spigos, D.: Computed tomography of the heart and great vessels: Present and future. Ann. Intern. Med. 101:801, 1984.
5. Singh, H., Fitzgerald, E., and Ruttley, M. S.: Computed tomography: The investigation of choice for aortic dissection? Br. Heart J. 56:171, 1986.
6. White, R. D., Lipton M. J., Higgins, C. B. et al.: Noninvasive evaluation of suspected thoracic aortic disease by contrast-enhanced computed tomography. Am. J. Cardiol. 57:282, 1986.
7. Demos, T. C., Posniak, H. V., and Marsan, R. E.: CT of aortic dissection. Semin. Roentgenol. 24:22, 1989.
8. Gomes, M. N., and Choyke, P. L.: Pre-operative evaluation of abdominal aortic aneurysms: Unltrasound or computed tomography? J. Cardiovasc. Surg. 28:159, 1987.
9. Dinsmore, R. E., Liberthson, R. R., Wismer, G. L. et al.: Magnetic resonance imaging of thoracic aortic aneurysms: Comparison with other diagnostic techniques. A. J. R. 146:309, 1986.
10. Valk, P. E., Hale, J. D., Kaufman, L. et al.: MR imaging of the aorta with three dimensional vessel reconstruction: Validation by angiography. Radiology 157:721, 1985.
11. Glazer, H. S., Gutierrez, F. R., Levitt, R. E. et al.: The thoracic aorta studied by MR imaging. Radiology 157:149, 1985.
12. Goldman, A. P., Kotler, M. N., Scanlon, M. H. et al.: The complementary role of magnetic resonance imaging, Doppler echocardiography, and computed tomography in the diagnosis of dissecting thoracic aneurysms. Am. Heart J. 111:970, 1986.
13. Mossard, J. M., Baruthio, J., Germain, P. et al.: Nuclear magnetic reso-

nance in the diagnosis of aortic diseases. Arch. Mal. Coeur. 79:456, 1986.

14. Goldman, A. P., Kotler, M. N., Scanlon, M. H. et al.: Magnetic resonance imaging and two-dimensional echocardiography. Alternative approach to aortography in diagnosis of aortic dissecting aneurysm. Am. J. Med. 80:1225, 1986.

15. Lois, J. F., Gomes, A. S., Brown, K. et al.: Magnetic resonance imaging of the thoracic aorta. Am. J. Cardiol. 60:358, 1987.

16. Gefter, W. B.: Chest applications of magnetic resonance imaging: An update. Radiol. Clin. North Am. 26:573, 1988.

16a. Aortic diseases. In Fowler, N. O.: Diagnosis of Heart Disease. New York, Springer-Verlag, 1991, pp. 375–388.

16b. Powell, J. T., and Greenhalgh, R. M.: Cellular, enzymatic, and genetic factors in the pathogenesis of abdominal aortic aneurysms. J. Vasc. Surg. 1989; 9:297, 1989.

16c. Powell, J. T., and Greenhalgh, R. M.: Multifactorial inheritance of abdominal aortic aneurysm. Eur. J. Vasc. Surg. 1:29, 1987.

16d. Johnston, K. W., and Scobie, T. K.: Multicenter prospective study of nonruptured abdominal aortic aneurysms. I. Population and operative management. J. Vasc. Surg. 7:69, 1988.

16e. Tsipouras, P., Byers, P. H., Schwartz, R. C. et al.: Ehlers-Danlos syndrome Type IV: Cosegregation of the phenotype to a COL3AI allele of Type III collagen. Hum. Genet. 74:41, 1986.

PATHOGENESIS OF DISEASES OF THE AORTA

17. Iwatsuki, K., Cardinale, G. J., Spector, S., and Udenfriend, S.: Reduction of blood pressure and vascular collagen in hypertensive rats by β-aminopropionitrile. Proc. Natl. Acad. Sci. USA 74:360, 1977.

18. Schlatmann, T.J.M., and Becker, A. E.: Pathogenesis of dissecting aneurysm of the aorta. Am. J. Cardiol. 39:21, 1977.

19. Heistad, D. D., Marcus, M. L., Law, E. G., Armstrong, M. L., Ehrhardt, J. C., and Abboud, F. M.: Regulation of blood flow to the aortic media in dogs. J. Clin. Invest. 62:133, 1978.

20. Thurmond, A. S., and Semler, H. J.: Abdominal aortic aneurysm: Incidence in a population at risk. J. Cardiovasc. Surg. (Torino) 27:457, 1986.

21. Darling, R. C. III, Brewster, D. C., Darling, R. C. et al.: Are familial abdominal aortic aneurysms different? J. Vasc. Surg. 10:39, 1989.

ARTERIOSCLEROTIC AORTIC ANEURYSMS

22. Darling, R. C.: Ruptured arteriosclerotic abdominal aortic aneurysms. Am. J. Surg. 119:397, 1970.

23. Rantakokko, V., Havia, T., Inberg, M. V., and Vänttinen, E.: Abdominal aortic aneurysms: A clinical and autopsy study of 408 patients. Acta Chir. Scand. 149:151, 1983.

24. Astarita, D., Filippone, D. R., and Cohn, J. D.: Spontaneous major intra-abdominal arteriovenous fistulas: A report of several cases. Angiology 36:656, 1985.

25. Bickerstaff, L. K., Hollier, L. H., Van Peenen, H. J. et al.: Abdominal aortic aneurysms: The changing natural history. J. Vasc. Surg. 1:6, 1984.

26. Crew, J. R., Bashour, T. T., Ellertson, D. et al.: Ruptured abdominal aortic aneurysms: Experience with 70 cases. Clin. Cardiol. 8:433, 1985.

27. Jenkins, A. M., Ruckley, C. V., and Nolan, B.: Ruptured abdominal aortic aneurysm. Br. J. Surg. 73:395, 1986.

28. Martinussen, H. J., Lolk, A., Rohr, N. et al.: Ruptured abdominal aortic aneurysm with fistula into the inferior vena cava. J. Cardiovasc. Surg. (Torino) 27:298, 1986.

29. Brewster, D. C., Darling, R. C., Raines, J. K. et al.: Assessment of abdominal aortic aneurysm size. Circulation 56:164, 1977.

30. Retief, P. J., and Loubser, J. S.: Diagnosis and treatment of abdominal aortic aneurysm. A report of 82 cases. S. Afr. Med. J. 56:67, 1979.

31. Brewster, D. C., Retana, A., Waltman, A. C., and Darling, R. C.: Angiography in the management of aneurysms of the abdominal aorta. Its value and safety. N. Engl. J. Med. 292:822, 1975.

32. Gliedman, M. L., Ayers, W. B., and Vestal, B. L.: Aneurysms of the abdominal aorta and its branches: A study of untreated patients. Ann. Surg. 217:1537, 1982.

33. Darling, R. C., Messina, C. R., Brewster, D. C., and Ottinger, L. W.: Autopsy study of unoperated abdominal aortic aneurysms. The case for early resection. Circulation 56(Suppl. II):161, 1977.

34. Delin, A., Ohlsén, H., and Swedenborg, J.: Growth rate of abdominal aortic aneurysms as measured by computed tomography. Br. J. Surg. 72:530, 1985.

35. Bernstein, E. F., and Chan, E. L.: Abdominal aortic aneurysm in high risk patients. Ann. Surg. 200:255, 1985.

36. Nevitt, M. P., Ballard, D. J., and Hallett, J. W., Jr.: Prognosis of abdominal aortic aneurysms: A population-based study. N. Engl. J. Med. 321:1009, 1989.

37. Pasch, A. R., Ricotta, J. J., May, A. G. et al.: Abdominal aortic aneurysm: The case for elective resection. Circulation 70(Suppl. I):1, 1984.

38. Cooley, D. A., and Carmichael, M. J.: Abdominal aortic aneurysm. Circulation 70(Suppl. I):5, 1984.

39. Shenaq, S. A., Chelly, J. E., Karlberg, et al.: Use of nitroprusside during surgery for thoracoabdominal aortic aneurysm. Circulation 70(Suppl. I):7, 1984.

40. Thompson, J. E., Hollier, L. H., Patman, R. D., and Persson, A. V.: Surgical management of abdominal aortic aneurysms: Factors influencing mortality and morbidity—A 20-year experience. Ann. Surg. 181:654, 1975.

41. Brener, B. J., Raines, J. K., and Darling, R. C.: Intraoperative autotransfusion in abdominal aortic resections. Arch. Surg. 107:78, 1973.

42. Hertzer, N. R.: Fatal myocardial infarction following abdominal aortic aneurysm resection. Three hundred forty-three patients followed 6–11 years postoperatively. Ann. Surg. 192:671, 1980.

43. Hertzer, N. R., Bevin, E. G., Young, J. R. et al.: Coronary artery disease in peripheral vascular patients. Ann. Surg. 199:223, 1984.

44. Boucher, C. A., Brewster, D. C., Darling, R. C. et al.: Determination of cardiac risk by dipyridamole-thallium imaging before peripheral vascular surgery. N. Engl. J. Med. 312:389, 1985.

45. Eagle, K. A., Singer, D. E., Brewster, D. C. et al.: Dipyridamole thallium scans in the preoperative evaluation of patients undergoing vascular surgery. JAMA 257:2185, 1987.

46. Eagle, K. A., Coley, C. M., Newell, J. B. et al.: Combining clinical and thallium data optimizes preoperative assessment of cardiac risk before major vascular surgery. Ann. Intern. Med. 110:859, 1989.

47. Levinson, J. R., Boucher, C. A., Coley, C. M. et al.: Semiquantitative analysis of dipyridamole-201thallium redistribution improves risk stratification before vascular surgery. Am. J. Cardiol. 66:406, 1990.

48. Eagle, K. A., and Boucher, C. A.: Cardiac risk of noncardiac surgery. N. Engl. J. Med. 321:1330, 1989.

49. Leppo, J., Plaja, J., Gionet, M. et al.: The noninvasive evaluation of cardiac risk prior to vascular surgery. Circulation 72(Suppl. III):147A, 1985.

50. Pasternack, P. F., Imparato, A. M., Riles, T. S. et al.: The value of radionuclide angiogram in the prediction of perioperative myocardial infarction in patients undergoing lower extremity revascularization procedures. Circulation 72(Suppl. II):13, 1985.

51. Raby, K. E., Goldman, L., Creager, M. A. et al.: Correlation between preoperative ischemia and major cardiac events after peripheral vascular surgery. N. Engl. J. Med. 321:1296, 1989.

52. Brewster, D. C., Bluth, J., Darling, R. C., and Austen, W. G.: Combined aortic and renal artery reconstruction. Am. J. Surg. 131:457, 1976.

53. Crawford, E. S., Saleh, S. A., Babb, J. W., III et al.: Infrarenal abdominal aortic aneurysm: Factors influencing survival after operation performed over a 25-year period. Ann. Surg. 193:699, 1981.

54. Fielding, J.W.L., Black, J., Ashton, F. et al.: Diagnosis and management of 528 abdominal aortic aneurysms. Br. Med. J. 283:355, 1981.

55. O'Donnell, T. F., Darling, R. C., and Linton, R. R.: Is 80 years too old for aneurysmectomy? Arch. Surg. 111:1250, 1976.

56. Karmody, A. M., Leather, R. P., Goldman, M. et al.: The current position of nonresective treatment for abdominal aortic aneurysm. Surgery 94:591, 1983.

57. Soreide, O., Lillestol, J., Christensen, O. et al.: Abdominal aortic aneurysms: Survival analysis of four hundred thirty-four patients. Surgery 91:188, 1982.

58. Plate, G., Hollier, L. A., O'Brien, P. et al.: Recurrent aneurysms and late vascular complications following repair of abdominal aortic aneurysms. Ann. Surg. 120:590, 1985.

59. Hollier, L. A., Plate, G., O'Brien, P. et al.: Late survival after abdominal aortic aneurysm repair: Influence of coronary artery disease. J. Vasc. Surg. 1:290, 1984.

60. Mitchell, E., Kadir, S., Kaufman, S. L. et al.: Percutaneous transluminal angioplasty of aortic graft stenoses. Radiology 149:439, 1983.

61. O'Donnell, T. F., Scott, G., Shepard, A. et al.: Improvements in the diagnosis and management of aortoenteric fistula. Am. J. Surg. 149:481, 1985.

62. Kierman, P. D., Pairolero, P. C., Hubert, J. P., Jr. et al.: Aortic graft-enteric fistula. Mayo Clin. Proc. 55:731, 1980

63. Ernst, C. B.: Prevention of intestinal ischemia following abdominal aortic reconstruction. Surgery 93:102, 1983.

64. Collins, J. J., Koster, J. K., Cohn, L. H., and Van Devanter, S. H.: Common aortic aneurysms: when to intervene. J. Cardiovasc. Med. 8:245, 1983.

65. Joyce, J. W., Fairbairn, J. F., Kincaid, O. W., and Juergens, J. L.: Aneurysms of the thoracic aorta—A clinical study with special reference to prognosis. Circulation 29:176, 1964.

66. Culliford, A. T., Ayvaliotis, B., Shemin, R. et al.: Aneurysms of the descending aorta. J. Thorac. Cardiovasc. Surg. 85:98, 1983.

67. Livesay, J. J., Cooley, D. A., Ventimiglia, R. A. et al.: Surgical experience in descending thoracic aneurysmectomy with and without adjuncts to avoid ischemia. Ann. Thorac. Surg. 39:37, 1985.

68. Cabrol, C., Pavie, A., Mesnildrey, P. et al.: Long-term results with total replacement of the ascending aorta and reimplantation of the coronary arteries. J. Thorac. Cardiovasc. Surg. 91:17, 1986.

69. Coselli J. S., and Crawford, E. F.: Composite valve-graft replacement of aortic root using separate Dacron tube for coronary artery reattachment. Ann. Thorac. Surg. 47:558, 1989.

70. Antunes, M. J., Colson, P. R., and Kinsley, R. H.: Hypothermia and circulatory arrest for surgical resection of aortic arch aneurysms. J. Thorac. Cardiovasc. Surg. 86:576, 1983.

71. Crawford, E. S., and Snyder, D. M.: Treatment of aneurysms of the aortic arch. J. Thorac. Cardiovasc. Surg. 85:237, 1983.

72. Matsuda, H., Nakano, S., Shirakura, R. et al.: Surgery for aortic arch aneurysm with selective cerebral perfusion and hypothermic cardiopulmonary bypass. Circulation 80(Suppl. I):243, 1989.

73. Pressler, V., and McNamara, J. J.: Aneurysms of the thoracic aorta. J. Thorac. Cardiovasc. Surg. 89:50, 1985.

74. Crawford, E. F., Svensson, L. G., Coselli, J. S. et al.: Surgical treatment of aneurysm and/or dissection of the ascending aorta, transverse aortic arch, and ascending aorta and transverse aortic arch: Factors influencing survival in 717 patients. J. Thorac. Cardiovasc. Surg. 98:659, 1989.

75. Moreno-Cabral, C. E., Miller, C., Mitchell, S. et al.: Degenerative and atherosclerotic aneurysms of the thoracic aorta. J. Thorac. Cardiovasc. Surg. 88:1020, 1984.

76. Crawford, E. S., Snyder, D. M., Cho, G. C., and Roehm, J.O.F., Jr.: Progress in treatment of thoracoabdominal and abdominal aortic aneurysms involving celiac, superior mesenteric, and renal arteries. Ann. Surg. 188:404, 1978.

77. Verdant, A., Page, A., Cossette, R. et al.: Surgery of the descending thoracic aorta: Spinal cord protection with the Gott shunt. Ann. Thorac. Surg. 46:147, 1988.

78. Laschinger, J. C., Cunningham, J. N., Nathan, I. N. et al.: Experimental and clinical assessment of the adequacy of partial bypass in maintenance of spinal cord blood flow during operations on the thoracic aorta. Ann. Thorac. Surg. 36:416, 1983.

79. Crawford, E. S., Mizrahi, E. M., Hess, K. R. et al.: The impact of distal aortic perfusion and somatosensory evoked potential monitoring on prevention of paraplegia after aortic aneurysm operation. J. Thorac. Cardiovasc. Surg. 95:357, 1988.

AORTIC DISSECTION

80. Wheat, M. W., Jr.: Acute dissecting aneurysms of the aorta: Diagnosis and treatment—1979. Am. Heart J. 99:373, 1980.

81. Roberts, W. C.: Aortic dissection: Anatomy, consequences, and causes. Am. Heart J. 101:195, 1981.

82. Doroghazi, R. M., and Slater, E. E. (eds.): Aortic Dissection. New York, McGraw-Hill Book Company, 1983.

83. Cooke, J. P., and Safford, R. E.: Progress in the diagnosis and management of aortic dissection. Mayo Clin. Proc. 61:147, 1986.

84. Wheat, M. W., Jr.: Pathogenesis of aortic dissection. In Doroghazi, R. M., and Slater, E. E. (eds.): Aortic Dissection. New York, McGraw-Hill Book Company, 1983, p. 55.

85. Yamada, T., Tada, S., and Harada, J.: Aortic dissection without intimal rupture: Diagnosis with MR imaging and CT. Radiology 168:347, 1988.

86. DeBakey, M. E., McCollum, C. H., Crawford, E. S. et al.: Dissection and dissecting aneurysms of the aorta: 20-year follow-up of 527 patients treated surgically. Surgery 92:1118, 1982.

87. Daily, P. O., Trueblood, H. W., Stinson, E. B. et al.: Management of acute aortic dissection. Ann. Thorac. Surg. 10:237, 1970.

88. Slater, E. E., and DeSanctis, R. W.: The clinical recognition of dissecting aortic aneurysm. Am. J. Med. 60:625, 1976.

89. Larson, E. W., and Edwards, W. D.: Risk factors for aortic dissection: A necropsy study of 161 cases. Am. J. Cardiol. 53:849, 1984.

90. Leonards, J. C., and Hasleton, P. S.: Dissecting aortic aneurysms: A clinicopathological study. Q. J. Med. 48:55, 1979.

91. Bulkley, B. H., and Roberts, W. C.: Dissecting aneurysm (hematoma) limited to coronary artery. Am. J. Med. 55:747, 1973.

92. Hochberg, F. H., Bean, C., Fisher, C. M., and Roberson, G. H.: Stroke in a 15-year-old girl secondary to terminal carotid dissection. Neurology 25:725, 1980.

93. Demaio, S. J., Jr., Kinsella, S. H., and Silverman, M. E.: Clinical course and long-term prognosis of spontaneous coronary artery dissection. Am. J. Cardiol. 64:471, 1989.

94. Dalen, J. R., Pape, L. A., Cohn, L. H. et al.: Dissection of the aorta: Pathogenesis, diagnosis, and treatment. Prog. Cardiovasc. Dis. 23:237, 1980.

95. Loeppky, C. B., Alpert, M. A., Hamel, P. C. et al.: Extensive aortic dissection from combined-type cystic medial necrosis in a young man without predisposing factors. Chest 79:116, 1981.

96. McKusick, V. A., Logue, R. B., and Bahnson, H. T.: Association of aortic valvular disease and cystic medial necrosis of the ascending aorta; report of four instances. Circulation 16:188, 1957.

97. Shachter, N., Perloff, J. K., and Mulder, D. G.: Aortic dissection in Noonan's syndrome. Am. J. Cardiol. 54:464, 1984.

98. Price, W. H., and Wilson J.: Dissection of the aorta in Turner's syndrome. J. Med. Genetics 20:61, 1983.

99. Nicod, P., Bloor, C., Godfrey, M. et al.: Familial aortic dissecting aneurysm. J. Am. Coll. Cardiol. 13:811, 1989.

100. Pumphrey, C. W., Fay, T., and Weir, I.: Aortic dissection during pregnancy. Br. Heart J. 55:106, 1986.

101. Williams, G. M., Gott, V. L., Brawley, R. K. et al.: Aortic disease associated with pregnancy. J. Vasc. Surg. 8:470, 1988.

102. Ponseti, I. V., and Baird, W. A.: Scoliosis and dissecting aneurysm of the aorta in rats fed with Lathyrus odoratus seeds. Am. J. Pathol. 28:1059, 1952.

103. Fikar, C. R., Amrhein, J. A., Harris, J. P., and Lewis, E. R.: Dissecting aortic aneurysm in childhood and adolescence. Clin. Pediatr. 20:578, 1981.

104. Slater, E. E.: Aortic dissection: Presentation and diagnosis. In Doroghazi, R. M., and Slater, E. E. (eds.): Aortic Dissection. New York, McGraw-Hill Book Company, 1983, p. 61.

105. Cohen, S., and Littman, D.: Painless dissecting aneurysm of the aorta. N. Engl. J. Med. 271:143, 1964.

106. Symbas, P. N., Kelly, T. F., Vlasis, S. E. et al.: Intimo-intimal intussusception and other usual manifestations of aortic dissection. J. Thorac. Cardiovasc. Surg. 79:926, 1980.

107. Hirst, A. E., and Gore, I.: The etiology and pathology of aortic regurgitation. In Doroghazi, R. M., and Slater, E. E. (eds.): Aortic Dissection. New York, McGraw-Hill Book Company, 1983, p. 13.

108. Riley, D. J., Liv, R. T., and Saxanoff, S.: Aortic dissection: A rare cause of the superior vena cava syndrome. J. Med. Soc. N. J. 78:187, 1981.

109. McCarthy, C., Dickson, G. H., Besterman, E. M. M. et al.: Aortic dissection with rupture through ductus arteriosus into pulmonary artery. Br. Heart J. 34:284, 1972.

110. Roth, J. A., and Parekh, M. A.: Dissecting aneurysms perforating the esophagus. N. Engl. J. Med. 299:776, 1978.

111. Thiene, G., Rossi, L., and Becker, A. E.: The atrioventricular conduction system in dissecting aneurysm of the aorta. Am. Heart J. 98:447, 1979.

112. Morris, A. L., and Barwinsky, J.: Unusual vascular complications of dissecting thoracic aortic aneurysm. Cardiovasc. Radiol. 1:95, 1978.

113. Eagle, K. A., Quertermous, T., Kritzer, G. A. et al.: Spectrum of conditions initially suggesting acute aortic dissection but with negative aortograms. Am. J. Cardiol. 57:322, 1986.

114. ten Cate, J. W., Timmers, H., and Becker, A. E.: Coagulopathy in ruptured or dissecting aortic aneurysms. Am. J. Med. 59:171, 1975.

115. Granato, J. E., Dee, P., and Gibson, R. S.: Utility of two-dimensional echocardiography in suspected ascending aortic dissection. Am. J. Cardiol. 56:123, 1985.

116. Perez, J. E.: Noninvasive diagnosis: Computed tomography and ultrasound. In Doroghazi, R. M., and Slater, E. E. (eds.): Aortic Dissection. New York, McGraw-Hill Book Company, 1983, p. 133.

117. Iliceto, S., Nanda, N. C., Rizzon, P. et al.: Color Doppler evaluation of aortic dissection. Circulation 75:748, 1987.

118. Erbel, R., Engberding, R., Daniel, W. et al.: Echocardiography in diagnosis of aortic dissection. Lancet I:457, 1989.

118a. Adachi, H., Kyo, S., Takamoto, S., et al.: Early diagnosis and surgical intervention of acute aortic dissection by transesophageal color flow mapping. Circulation 82(Suppl. IV):IV19, 1990.

119. Thorsen, M. K., San Dretto, M. A., Lawson, T. L. et al.: Dissecting aortic aneurysms: Accuracy of computed tomographic diagnosis. Radiology 148:773, 1983.

120. Smith, D. C., and Jang, G. C.: Radiological diagnosis and aortic dissection. In Doroghazi, R. M., and Slater, E. E. (eds.): Aortic Dissection. New York, McGraw-Hill Book Company, 1983, p. 71.

121. Vasile, N., Mathieu, D., Keita, K. et al.: Computed tomography of thoracic aortic dissection: Accuracy and pitfalls. J. Comput. Assist. Tomogr. 10:211, 1986.

122. Amparo, E. G., Higgins, C. B., Hricak, L, and Sollitto, R.: Aortic dissection: Magnetic resonance imaging. Radiology 155:399, 1985.

123. Dinsmore, R. E., Willerson, J. T., and Buckley, M. J.: Dissecting aneurysm of the aorta. Aortographic features affecting prognosis. Diagn. Radiol. 105:567, 1972.

124. Shuford, W. H., Sybers, R. G., and Weens, H. S.: Problems of the aortographic diagnosis of dissecting aneurysms of the aorta. N. Engl. J. Med. 280:225, 1969.

125. Collins, J. J., Jr., Koster, J. K., Jr., Cohn, L. H., and VanDevanter S. H.: Common arotic aneurysms: When to intervene. J. Cardiovasc. Med. 8:245, 1983.

126. Anagnostopoulos, C. E., Prabhakar, M. J. S., and Kittle, C. F.: Aortic dissections and dissecting aneurysms. Am. J. Cardiol. 30:263, 1972.

127. Gurin, D., Bulmer, J. W., and Derby, R.: Dissecting aneurysm of the aorta. Diagnosis and operative relief of acute arterial obstructions due to this course. N. Y. State J. Med. 35:1200, 1935.

128. Shaw, R. W.: Acute dissecting aortic aneurysms: Treatment by fenestration of the internal wall of the aneurysm. N. Engl. J. Med. 253:331, 1955.

129. DeBakey, M. E., Cooley, D. A., and Creech, O., Jr.: Surgical considerations of dissecting aneurysms of the aorta. Ann. Surg. 142:586, 1955.

130. Wheat, M. W., Jr., Palmer, R. F., Barley, T. D., and Seelman, R. C.: Treatment of dissecting aneurysms of the aorta without surgery. J. Thorac. Cardiovasc. Surg. 50:364, 1965.

131. Palmer, R. F., and Lasseter, K. C.: Nitroprusside and aortic dissecting aneurysm (letter). N. Engl. J. Med. 294:1403, 1976.

132. Wheat, M. W.: Intensive drug therapy. In Doroghazi, R. M., and Slater, E. E. (eds.): Aortic Dissection. New York, McGraw-Hill Book Company, 1983, p. 165.

133. Grubb, B. P., Sirio, C., and Zelis, R.: Intravenous labetalol in acute aortic dissection. JAMA 258:78, 1987.

134. Frishman, W. B., Weinberg, P., Peled, H. B. et al.: Calcium entry blockers for the treatment of severe hypertension and hypertensive crisis. Am. J. Med. 77(Suppl. 2B):35, 1984.

135. White, S. R., and Hall, J. B.: Control of hypertension with nifedipine in the setting of aortic dissection. Chest 88:781, 1985.

136. Miller, D. C., Stinson, E. B., Oyer, P. E. et al.: The operative treatment of aortic dissections: Experience with 125 patients over a sixteen year period. J. Thorac. Cardiovasc. Surg. 78:365, 1979.

137. Doroghazi, R. M., Slater, E. E., DeSanctis, R. W. et al.: Long-term survival patients treated with aortic dissection. J. Am. Coll. Cardiol. 3:1026, 1984.

137a. Svensson, L. G., Crawford, E. S., Hess, K. R., et al.: Dissection of the aorta and dissecting aortic aneurysms: Improving early and long-term surgical results. Circulation 82(Suppl. IV):IV24, 1990.

138. Miller, D. C., Mitchell, R. C., Oyer, P. E. et al.: Independent determinants of operative mortality for patients with aortic dissections. Circulation 70(Suppl. I):153, 1984.

139. Glower, D. D., Fann, J. I., Speier, R. H. et al.: Comparison of medical and surgical therapy for uncomplicated descending aortic dissection. Circulation 80(Suppl. II):24, 1989.

140. Crawford, E. S., Svensson, L. G., Coselli, J. S. et al.: Aortic dissection and dissecting aortic aneurysms. Ann. Surg. 208:254, 1988.

141. Cachera, J. P., Vouhe, P. R., Loisance, D. Y. et al.: Surgical management of acute dissections involving the ascending aorta. J. Thorac. Cardiovasc. Surg. 82:576, 1981.

142. Kolff, J., Bates, R. J., Balderman, S. C. et al.: Acute aortic arch dissection: Reevaluation of the indication for medical and surgical therapy. Am. J. Cardiol. 39:727, 1977.

143. Haverich, A., Miller, D. C., Scott, W. C. et al.: Acute and chronic aortic

dissections—determinants of long-term outcome for operative survivors. Circulation 72(Suppl. II):22, 1985.

144. Lemole, G. M., Strong, M. D., Spagna, P. M., and Karmilowicz, N. P.: Improved results for dissecting aneurysms: Intraluminal sutureless prosthesis. J. Thorac. Cardiovasc. Surg. 83:249, 1982.

145. Diehl, J. T., Moon, B., LeClerc, Y. et al.: Acute type A dissection of the aorta: surgical management with the sutureless intraluminal prosthesis. Ann. Thorac. Surg. 43:502, 1987.

146. Carpentier, A., Deloche, A., Fabiani, J. N. et al.: New surgical approach to aortic dissection: Flow reversal and thromboexclusion. J. Thorac. Cardiovasc. Surg. 81:659, 1981.

147. Tanabe, T., Hashimoto, M., Sakai, K. et al.: Surgical treatment of aortic dissection: Application of Ivalon sponge to the dissected lumen. Ann. Thorac. Surg. 41:169, 1986.

148. Fabiani, J. -N., Jebara, V. A., Deloche, A. et al.: Use of surgical glue without replacement in the treatment of type A aortic dissection. Circulation 80(Suppl. I):264, 1989.

ANNULOAORTIC ECTASIA

149. Ellis, P. R., Cooley, D. A., and DeBakey, M. E.: Clinical consideration and surgical treatment of annulo-aortic ectasia. J. Thorac. Cardiovasc. Surg. 42:363, 1961.

150. Pyeritz, R. E., and McKusick, V. A.: The Marfan syndrome: Diagnosis and management. N. Engl. J. Med. 300:772, 1979.

151. Boucek, R. J., Noble, N. L., Gunja-Smith, Z., and Butler, W. T.: The Marfan syndrome: A deficiency of chemically stable collagen cross links. N. Engl. J. Med. 305:988, 1981.

152. Abraham, P. A., Perejda, A. J., Carnes, W. H., and Uitto, J.: Marfan syndrome: Demonstration of abnormal elastin in the aorta. J. Clin. Invest. 70:1245, 1982.

153. Emanuel, R., Ng, R.A.L., Marcomichelakis, J. et al.: Formes frustes of Marfan's syndrome presenting with severe aortic regurgitation. Clinicogenetic study of 18 families. Br. Heart J. 39:190, 1977.

154. Lemon, D. K., and White, C. W.: Annulaortic ectasia: Angiographic, hemodynamic and clinical comparison with aortic valve insufficiency. Am. J. Cardiol. 41:482, 1978.

155. Miller, D. C., Stinson, E. B., Oyer, P. E. et al.: Concomitant resection of ascending aortic aneurysm and replacement of the aortic valve. J. Thorac. Cardiovasc. Surg. 79:388, 1980.

156. Svensson, L. G., Crawford, S., Coselli, J. S. et al.: Impact of cardiovascular operation on survival in the Marfan patient. Circulation 80(Suppl. I):233, 1989.

157. Gott, V. L., Pyeritz, R. E., Magovern, G. J., Jr. et al.: Surgical treatment of aneurysms of the ascending aorta in the Marfan syndrome. Results of composite-graft repair in 50 patients. N. Engl. J. Med. 314:1070, 1986.

158. Pyeritz, R. E., Gott, V. L., McDonald, G. R. et al.: Surgical repair of the Marfan aorta: Technique, indications, and complications. Johns Hopkins Med. J. 151:71, 1982.

159. Crawford, E. S.: Marfan's syndrome: Broad spectral surgical treatment of cardiovascular manifestations. Ann. Surg. 198:487, 1983.

AORTIC ARTERITIS SYNDROMES

160. Takayasu, M.: Case with unusual changes of the central vessels in the retina. Acta Soc. Ophthalmol. Jpn. 12:554, 1908.

161. Lupi-Herrera, E., Sanchez-Torres, G., Marcushamer, J. et al.: Takayasu's arteritis. Clinical study of 107 cases. Am. Heart J. 93:94, 1977.

162. Shelhamer, J. H., Volkman, D. J., Parillo, J. E. et al.: Takayasu's arteritis and its therapy. Ann. Intern. Med. 103:121, 1985.

163. Hall, S., Barr, W., Lie, J. T. et al.: Takayasu arteritis. Medicine 64:89, 1985.

164. Ueno, A., Awane, G., and Wakahayachi, A.: Successfully operated obliterative brachiocephalic arteritis (Takayasu) associated with the elongated coarctation. Jpn. Heart J. 8:538, 1967.

165. Kakao, K., Ikeda, M., Kimata, S. et al.: Takayasu's arteritis—Clinical report of 84 cases and immunological studies of 7 cases. Circulation 35:1141, 1967.

166. Volkman, D. J., Mann, D. L., and Fauci, A. S.: Association between Takayasu's arteritis and a B-cell alloantigen in North Americans. N. Engl. J. Med. 306:464, 1982.

167. Numano, F., Isohisa, I., Egami, M. et al.: HLA-DR MT and MB antigens in Takayasu disease. Tissue Antigens 21:208, 1983.

168. Gronemeyer, P. S., and deMello, D. E.: Takayasu's disease with aneurysm of right common iliac artery and iliocaval fistula in a young infant: Case report and review of the literature. Pediatrics 69:626, 1982.

169. Morooka, S., Saito, Y., Nonaka, Y. et al.: Clinical features of aortitis syndrome in Japanese women older than 40 years. Am. J. Cardiol. 53:859, 1984.

170. Swinton, N. W., and Cook, G. A.: Systolic hypertension and cardiac mortality of Takayasu's aortoarteritis. Angiology 27:568, 1976.

171. Takishita, A., Tanaka, S., Orita, G. et al.: Baroflex sensitivity in patients with Takayasu's aortitis. Circulation 55:803, 1977.

172. Akikusa, B., Kondo, Y., and Muraki, N.: Aortic insufficiency caused by Takayasu's arteritis without usual clinical features. Arch. Pathol. Lab. Med. 105:650, 1981.

173. Talwar, K. K., Chopra, P., Narula, J. et al.: Myocardial involvement and its response to immunosuppressive therapy in nonspecific aortoarteritis (Takayasu's disease)—a study by endomyocardial biopsy. Int. J. Cardiol. 23:323, 1988.

174. Cipriano, P. R., Silverman, J. F., Perlroth, M. G. et al.: Coronary arterial narrowing in Takayasu's aortitis. Am. J. Cardiol. 39:744, 1977.

174a. Hashimoto, Y., Numano, F., Maruyama, Y., et al.: Thallium-201 stress scintigraphy in Takayasu Arteritis. Am. J. Cardiol. 67:879, 1991.

175. Slater, E. E., and Fallon, J. T.: Upper extremity hypertension in a 28-year-old Korean man. Case Records of the Massachusetts General Hospital. N. Engl. J. Med. 299:1002, 1978.

176. Lupi, H. E., Sanchez, T. G., Horwitz, S., and Gutierrez, F. E.: Pulmonary artery involvement in Takayasu's arteritis. Chest 67:69, 1975.

177. Wu, Y.-J.J., Martin, B., Ong, K. et al.: Takayasu's arteritis as a cause of fever of unknown origin. Am. J. Med. 87:476, 1989.

178. Kanaide H., Takeshita, A., and Nakamura, M.: Etiologic aspects of coagulopathy in Takayasu's aortitis. Am. Heart J. 104:1039, 1982.

179. Lande, A., and Rossi, P.: The value of total aortography in the diagnosis of Takayasu's arteritis. Radiology 114:287, 1975.

180. Ishikawa, K.: Diagnostic approach and proposed criteria for the clinical diagnosis of Takayasu's arteriopathy. J. Am. Coll. Cardiol. 12:964, 1988.

181. Grossman, E., Morag, B., Nussinovitch, N. et al.: Clinical use of captopril in Takayasu's disease. Arch. Intern. Med. 144:95, 1984.

182. Huddle, K. R., Doodha, M. I., and Mackenzie, M.: Captopril in the treatment of renovascular hypertension secondary to Takayasu's arteritis. S. Afr. Med. J. 69:58, 1986.

183. Duncan, J. M., and Cooley, D. A.: Surgical consideration in aortitis with special emphasis on Takayasu's arteritis. Texas Heart Inst. J. 10:233, 1983.

184. Pajari, R., Hekeli, P., and Harjola, P. T.: Treatment of Takayasu's arteritis: An analysis of 29 operated patients. Thorac. Cardiovasc. Surg. 34:176, 1986.

185. Hodgins, G. W., and Dutton, J. W.: Transluminal dilatation of Takayasu's arteritis. Can. J. Surg. 27:355, 1984.

186. Ishikawa, K.: Survival and morbidity after diagnosis of occlusive thromboaortopathy (Takayasu's disease). Am. J. Cardiol. 47:1026, 1981.

187. Subramanyan, R., Joy, J., and Balakrishnan, K. G. Natural history of aortoarteritis (Takayasu's disease). Circulation 80:429, 1989.

188. Ishikawa, K.: Patterns of symptoms and prognosis in occlusive thromboaortopathy (Takayasu's disease). J. Am. Coll. Cardiol. 8:1041, 1986.

189. Klein, R. G., Hunder, G. G., Stanson, A. W., and Sheps, S. G.: Larger artery involvement in giant cell (temporal) arteritis. Ann. Intern. Med. 83:806, 1975.

190. Vincent, F. M., and Vincent, T.: Bilateral carotid siphon involvement in giant cell arteritis. Neurosurgery 18:773, 1986.

191. Austen, W. G., and Blennerhassett, M. B.: Giant cell aortitis causing an aneurysm of the ascending aorta and aortic regurgitation. N. Engl. J. Med. 272:80, 1965.

192. Perruquet, J. L., Davis, D. E., and Harrington, T. M.: Aortic arch arteritis in the elderly. An important manifestation of giant cell arteritis. Arch. Intern. Med. 146:289, 1986.

193. Ghose, M. K., Shensa, S., and Lerner, P. I.: Arteritis of the aged (giant cell arteritis) and fever of unexplained origin. Am. J. Med. 60:429, 1976.

194. Gonzalez, E. B., Varner, W. T., Lisse, J. R. et al.: Giant-cell arteritis in the southern United States: An 11-year retrospective study from the Texas Gulf Coast. Arch. Intern. Med. 149:1561, 1989.

195. Chuang, T., Hunder, G. G., Ilstrup, D. M., and Kurland, L. T.: Polymyalgia rheumatica. Ann. Intern. Med. 97:672, 1982.

196. Salisbury, R. S., and Hazleman, B. L.: Successful treatment of dissecting aortic aneurysm due to giant cell arteritis. Ann Rheum. Dis. 40:507, 1981.

197. Malmvall, B. E., and Bengtsson, B. A.: Serum levels of immunoglobin and complement in giant cell arteritis. JAMA 236:1876, 1976.

198. Krall, P. L., Mazanec, D. J., and Wilke, W. S.: Methotrexate for corticosteroid-resistant polymyalgia rheumatica and giant cell arteritis. Cleveland Clin. J. Med. 56:253, 1989.

199. Paulus, H. E., Pearson, C. M., and Pitts, W.: Aortic insufficiency in five patients with Reiter's syndrome. A detailed clinical and pathologic study. Am. J. Med. 53:464, 1972.

200. Muna, W. F., Roller, D. H., Craft, J. et al.: Psoriatic arthritis and aortic regurgitation. JAMA 244:363, 1980.

201. Morgan, S. H., Asherson, R. A., and Hughes, G. V.: Distal aortitis complicating Reiter's syndrome. Br. Heart J. 52:115, 1984.

202. Park, J. H., Han, M. C., and Bettman, M. A.: Arterial manifestations of Behçet disease. A. J. R. 143:821, 1984.

203. LaBresh, K. A., Lally, E. V., Sharma, S. C., and Ho, G.: Two-dimensional echocardiographic detection of preclinical aortic root abnormalities in rheumatoid variant diseases. Am. J. Med. 78:908, 1985.

CARDIOVASCULAR SYPHILIS

204. Heggtveit, H. A.: Syphilitic aortitis. A clinicopathologic autopsy study of 100 cases, 1950 to 1960. Circulation 29:346, 1964.

205. Center for Disease Control Recommended Treatment Schedules, 1985. The Sexually Transmitted Diseases Advisory Committee. Morbid. Mortal. Weekly Rep. 34:94s, 1985(Suppl. 4S).

206. Steinberg, I.: Anomalies (pseudocoarctation) of the arch of the aorta—Report of 8 new and review of 8 previously published cases. A. J. R. 88:73, 1962.

207. Brinsfield, D. E., Shuford, W. M., Plauth, W. H., Jr., and Sybers, R. G.: Congenital anomalies of the aorta. In Lindsay, J., Jr., and Hurst, J. W. (eds.): The Aorta. New York, Grune and Stratton, 1979, p. 271.

208. Lajos, T. Z., Meckstroth, C. V., Klassen, K. P., and Sherman, N. J.: Pseudocoarctation of the aorta. A variant or an entity? Chest 58:571, 1970.

209. Wolf, W. J.: Pseudocoarctation of the aortic arch in a patient with Turner's syndrome. Clin. Cardiol. 9:A5, 1986.
210. Bahabozorgui, S., Bernstein, R. G., and Frater, R.W.M.: Pseudocoarctation of the aorta associated with aneurysm formation. Chest 60:616, 1971.
211. Bland, E. F., and Castleman, B.: Vascular collapse in a woman with an unusual calcified ring in the aortic arch. N. Engl. J. Med. 280:1466, 1969.

AORTIC TRAUMA

212. Shaikh, K. A., Schwab, C. W., Camishion, R. C.: Aortic rupture in blunt trauma. Am. Surg. 52:47, 1986.
213. Greendyke, R. M.: Traumatic rupture of aorta: Special reference to automobile accidents. JAMA 195:527, 1966.
214. Parmley, L. F., Mattingly, T. W., Manion, W. C., and Jahnke, E. J.: Nonpenetrating traumatic injury of the aorta. Circulation 17:1086, 1958.
215. Fleming, A. W., and Green, D. C.: Traumatic aneurysms of the thoracic aorta: Report of 43 patients. Ann. Thorac. Surg. 18:91, 1974.
216. Shorr, R. M., Crittenden, M., Indeck, M. et al.: Blunt thoracic trauma: Analysis of 515 patients. Ann. Surg. 206:200, 1987.
217. Faro, R. S., Monson, D. O., Weinberg, M., and Javid, H.: Disruption of aortic arch branches due to nonpenetrating chest trauma. Arch. Surg. 118:1333, 1983.
218. Sturm, J. T., Billiar, T. R., Dorsey, J. S. et al.: Risk factors for survival following surgical treatment of traumatic aortic rupture. Ann. Thorac. Surg. 39:418, 1985.
219. March, D. G., and Sturm, J. T.: Traumatic aortic rupture: Roentgenographic indications for angiography. Ann. Thorac. Surg. 21:337, 1976.
220. Sturm, J. T., Olson, F. R., and Cicero, J. J.: Chest roentgenographic findings in 26 patients with traumatic rupture of the thoracic aorta. Ann. Emerg. Med. 12:598, 1983.
221. Woodring, J. H., and Dillon, M. L.: Radiographic manifestations of mediastinal hemorrhage from blunt chest trauma. Ann. Thorac. Surg. 37:171, 1984.
222. Heystraten, F. M., Rosenbusch, G., Kingma, L. M. et al.: Chest radiography in acute traumatic rupture of the thoracic aorta. Acta Radiologica 29:411, 1988.
223. Mirvis, S. E., Bidwell, J. K., Buddemeyer, E. U. et al.: Value of chest radiography in excluding traumatic aortic rupture. Radiology 163:487, 1987.
224. Stark, P.: Traumatic rupture of the thoracic aorta: A review. Crit. Rev. Diagn. Imaging 21:229, 1983.
225. Woodring, J. H., and King, J. G.: The potential effects of radiographic criteria to exclude aortography in patients with blunt chest trauma. J. Thorac. Cardiovasc. Surg. 97:456, 1989.
226. Brooks, A. P., Olson, L. K., and Shackford, S. R.: Computed tomography in the diagnosis of traumatic rupture of the thoracic aorta. Clin. Radiol. 40:133, 1989.
227. Miller, F. B., Richardson, J. D., Thomas, H. A. et al.: Role of CT in diagnosis of major arterial injury after blunt thoracic trauma. Surgery 106:596, 1989.
228. Gupta, B. K., Khaneja, S. C., Flores, L. et al.: The role of intra-aortic balloon occlusion in penetrating abdominal trauma. J. Trauma 29:861, 1989.
229. Atkins, C. W., Buckley, M. J., Daggett, W. et al.: Acute traumatic disruption of the thoracic aorta: A ten-year experience. Ann. Thorac. Surg. 31:305, 1981.
230. Marvasti, M. A., Meyer, J. A., Ford, B. E., and Parker, F. B., Jr.: Spinal cord ischemia following operation for traumatic aortic transection. Ann. Thorac. Surg. 42:425, 1986.
231. Stiles, Q. R., Cohlmia, G. S., Smith, J. H. et al.: Management of injuries of the thoracic and abdominal aorta. Am. J. Surg. 150:132, 1985.
232. Haskell, R. J., French, W. J., and Harley, D. P.: Traumatic aorto-right ventricular fistula presenting with a diastolic murmur. Am. Heart J. 109:1110, 1985.
233. Snow, N., and Johnson, P.: Traumatic fistula between the descending thoracic aorta and left main pulmonary artery. J. Trauma 25:263, 1985.

AORTIC THROMBOEMBOLIC DISEASE

234. Heiskell, C. A., and Conn, J., Jr.: Aortoarterial emboli. Am. J. Surg. 132:4, 1976.
235. Byard, R. W., Jimenez, C. L., Carpenter, B. F., and Hsu, E.: Aspergillus-related aortic thrombosis. Can. Med. Assoc. J. 136:155, 1987.
236. Shapiro, M. E., Rodvien, R., Bauer, K. A., and Salzman, E. W.: Acute aortic thrombosis in antithrombin III deficiency. JAMA 245:1759, 1981.
237. Schatz, I. J., and Stanley, J. C.: Saddle embolus of the aorta. JAMA 235:1262, 1976.
238. Babu, S. C., Shah, P. M., Sharma, P. et al.: Adequacy of central hemodynamics versus restoration of circulation in the survival of patients with acute aortic thrombosis. Am. J. Surg. 154:206, 1987.
239. Tegtmeyer, C. J., Wellons, H. A., and Thompson, R. N.: Balloon dilation of the abdominal aorta. JAMA 244:2636, 1980.
240. Deriu, G. P., and Ballotta, E.: Natural history of ascending thrombosis of the aorta. Am. J. Surg. 145:652, 1983.
241. Topol, E. J., Ciuffo, A. A., Pearson, T. A. et al.: Thrombolysis with recombinant tissue plasminogen activator in atherosclerotic thrombotic occlusion. J. Am. Coll. Cardiol. 5:85, 1985.
242. Machleder, H. I., Takiff, H., Lois, J. F., and Holburt, E.: Aortic mural thrombus: An occult source of arterial thromboembolism. J. Vasc. Surg. 4:473, 1986.
243. Dahlberg, P. J., Frecentese, D. F, and Cogbill, T. H.: Cholesterol embolism: Experience with 22 histologically proven cases. Surgery 105:737, 1989.
244. Colt, H. G., Begg, R. J., Saporito, J. J. et al.: Cholesterol emboli after cardiac catheterization. Medicine 67:389, 1988.
245. Hyman, B. T., Landas, S. K., Ashman, R. F. et al.: Warfarin-related purple toes syndrome and cholesterol microembolization. Am. J. Med. 82:1233, 1987.

ATHEROMATOUS EMBOLI

246. Coppetto, J. R., Lessell, S., Greco, T. P., and Eisenberg, M. S.: Diffuse disseminated atheroembolism. Arch. Ophthalmol. 102:255, 1984.
247. Fisher, D. F., Clagett, G. P., Brigham, R. A. et al.: Dilemmas in dealing with the blue toe syndrome: Aortic vs. peripheral source. Am. J. Surg. 148:836, 1984.
248. Robicsek, F.: Prevention of cholesterol embolism (trash foot) during aorto-iliac reconstruction using a blood filtering device. J. Cardiovasc. Surg. (Torino) 27:63, 1986.

AORTIC BACTERIAL INFECTIONS

249. Jarrett, F., Darling, R. C., Mundth, E. D., and Austen, W. G.: Experience with infected aneurysms of the abdominal aorta. Arch. Surg. 110:1281, 1975.
250. Brown, S. L., Busuttil, R. W., Baker, J. D. et al.: Bacteriologic and surgical determinants of survival in patients with mycotic aneurysms. J. Vasc. Surg. 1:541, 1984.
251. Worrell, J. T., Buja, L. M., and Reynolds, R. C.: Pneumococcal aortitis with rupture of the aorta: Report of a case and review of the literature. Am. J. Clin. Pathol. 89:565, 1988.
252. Vogelzang, R. L., and Sohaey, R.: Infected aortic aneurysms: CT appearance. J. Comput. Assist. Tomog. 12:109, 1988.
253. Schipper, J., van Oostayen, J. A., den Hollander, J. C., and van Seyen, A. J.: Aortic tumours: Report of a case and review of the literature. Br. J. Radiol. 62:35, 1989.

AORTIC TUMORS

254. Schmid, E., Port, J. S., Carroll, R. M., and Friedman, N. B.: Primary metastasizing aortic endothelioma. Cancer 54:1407, 1984.

Pulmonary Embolism

by SAMUEL Z. GOLDHABER, M.D., and EUGENE BRAUNWALD, M.D.

Pulmonary embolism (PE) is the third most common cardiovascular disease, after acute ischemic syndromes and stroke. However, venous thromboembolism (VTE) receives less attention than is warranted because PE and deep venous thrombosis (DVT) are managed by physicians in many different specialties (e.g., cardiologists, pulmonologists, hematologists, vascular medicine specialists, vascular surgeons, general internists, and family practitioners). Nevertheless, during the past few years, major advances have been made in optimizing strategies for diagnosis and prevention of this illness, which accounts for approximately 300,000 hospitalizations annually in the United States.[1,2] Unfortunately, PE causes as many as 50,000 deaths per year and, during the past 15 years, the mor-

tality rate has not declined.[3] PE affects men more commonly than women and occurs with increasing frequency in older age groups. However, the death rate is relatively high even among younger patients (Fig. 48–1). Furthermore, recognized cases of VTE constitute only a minority of actual episodes because the diagnosis is elusive and, despite advances in diagnostic imaging, the condition commonly goes undetected until postmortem examination.[4] Therefore, prompt and accurate diagnosis remains the most important step toward managing this illness.[4a] Major controversy and uncertainty persist concerning the proper role of thrombolytic therapy in the overall treatment strategy for PE. Clinical trials are being undertaken to address this important but troublesome issue.

Pathophysiology of Pulmonary Embolism

In 1856, Rudolf Virchow postulated that a triad of factors led to intravascular coagulation: (1) local trauma to the vessel wall, (2) hypercoagulability, and (3) stasis.[5] One useful approach to classifying hypercoagulable states is to consider

them as either primary or secondary.[6] Primary hypercoagulable states are usually inherited abnormalities, whereas secondary states are usually acquired clinical conditions associated with an increased risk for PE (Table 48–1).

HYPERCOAGULABLE STATES
(See also Chap. 57)

PRIMARY HYPERCOAGULABLE STATES. Antithrombin III (AT-III) is the major inhibitor of thrombin (which converts circulating fibrinogen to fibrin clot) and other activated clotting factors (Fig. 48–2). The most frequent manifestations of AT-III deficiency are recurrent PE and DVT.[6] Inheritance is autosomal dominant, with partial gene penetration. Congenital deficiencies of protein C (which consumes factors Va and VIIIa and also stimulates fibrinolysis)[7] and protein S (a cofactor for activated protein C) also predispose to recurrent venous thromboembolism at a young age. Defective fibrinolysis, whether due to defective release of tissue plasminogen activator (t-PA)[8] or an excess of t-PA inhibitor,[9] is also associated with venous thrombosis. "Lupus anticoagulant," often encountered in patients without lupus, is usually associated with a prolonged partial thromboplastin time (PTT) but paradoxically increases the risk of venous thromboembolism.[10,11] Lupus anticoagulants are antibodies that interfere with phospholipid-dependent coagulation reactions. Sensitive assays that employ the negatively charged phospholipid cardiolipin as the antigen have identified patients with elevated levels of

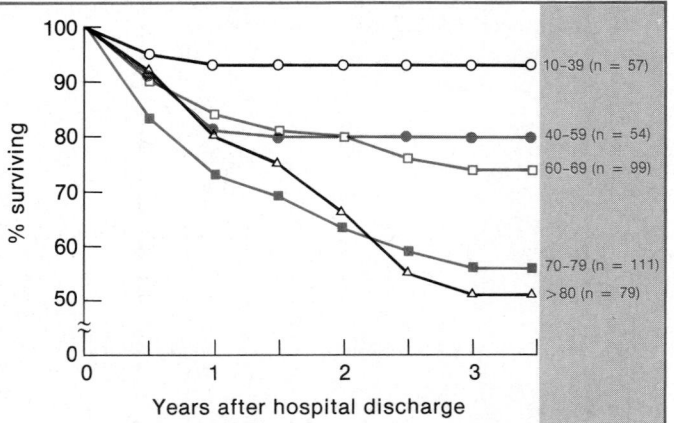

FIGURE 48–1. Age-specific survival rates in 400 patients discharged with the first episode of clinically recognized DVT and/or PE. (From Anderson, F. A., Jr., Wheeler, H. B., Goldberg, R. J., et al.: A population-based perspective of the incidence and case fatality rates of deep vein thrombosis and pulmonary embolism: the Worcester DVT Study. Arch. Intern. Med. *157*:933, 1991.

TABLE 48-1 HYPERCOAGULABLE STATES

PRIMARY
Antithrombin III deficiency
Protein C deficiency
Protein S deficiency
Lupus anticoagulant
Anticardiolipin antibodies

SECONDARY
Abnormalities of coagulation
Cancer
Pregnancy
Oral contraceptives
Nephrotic syndrome
Abnormalities of platelets
Heparin associated thrombocytopenia
Myeloproliferative disorders
Paroxysmal nocturnal hemoglobinuria
Abnormalities of blood vessels and rheology
Conditions promoting venous stasis (immobilization, postoperative state, obesity, advanced age)
Central venous and long-term in-dwelling catheters
Hyperviscosity (polycythemia, leukemia, sickle cell disease, leukoagglutination)

anticardiolipin antibodies (ACA)—especially IgG and IgM ACA—that are associated with increased frequency of clinical thrombosis and fetal loss.[12,13] Some but not all patients with elevated ACA have demonstrable lupus anticoagulants. The titer of the ACA appears to correlate with the degree of PTT prolongation and with the risk of thrombosis. Investigation of potential primary hypercoagulable states (Table 48-1) has the highest yield in patients younger than 45 years old who have "idiopathic" PE or DVT. Among such patients, approximately 15 per cent may have an identifiable disorder related to defective fibrinolysis or deficiencies in protein C, protein S, or AT-III.[14]

SECONDARY HYPERCOAGULABLE STATES. Some of the most readily recognized risk factors for PE occur in secondary hypercoagulable states (Table 48-1), in which the molecular mechanisms causing thrombosis are not known, as they are in the primary conditions. When investigating the possibility of PE, clinicians may find these clinical settings to be more useful than are symptoms and signs of PE, which are often nonspecific. Among hospitalized patients, the most common setting for PE is after a recent surgical procedure in which vessel trauma is combined with immobilization. Obesity, with its associated venous stasis, may be a long-term risk factor for PE[15] and may also increase the risk of PE among hospitalized patients undergoing surgery.

Neoplastic disease is another well-established risk factor for PE. Patients with known malignancy in whom PE is suspected may have either thrombotic or tumor emboli. Furthermore, PE[16] or DVT[17] (especially bilateral limb DVT) in patients without overt cancer may herald the presence of occult malignancy that will become manifested clinically within the next several years. This suggests that patients with VTE should be screened and followed carefully for cancer when no cause for the PE or DVT is clinically apparent.[18]

PE is also associated with oral contraceptive use and pregnancy,[19] particularly among women confined to bed because of preeclampsia or eclampsia or those who have had a cesarean section.[19] The risk of VTE is actually much greater during the first 6 weeks after delivery than during the pregnancy itself. With respect to maternal mortality, PE is the leading cause (after trauma) and is four times more common than death from hemorrhage or an anesthetic accident and twice as common as death from an ectopic pregnancy or infection.[20]

Indwelling central venous lines can be a nidus for right atrial thrombus that serves as a souce of PE. These catheters are being used with increasing frequency to provide alimentation for chronically ill patients and as venous access for long-term cancer chemotherapy protocols[21,22] (Fig. 48-3). An increasing number of reports have also noted large right atrial thrombi due to acute myocardial infarction, congestive heart failure, atrial fibrillation, or a combination of predisposing factors.[23] In fact, the detection of right atrial thrombus (usually with two-dimensional echocardiography) in most cases should prompt a search for concomitant PE.

DEEP VENOUS THROMBOSIS

RELATIONSHIP OF DVT TO PE. Although the risk of PE among patients with DVT proximal to the calf is high (approxi-

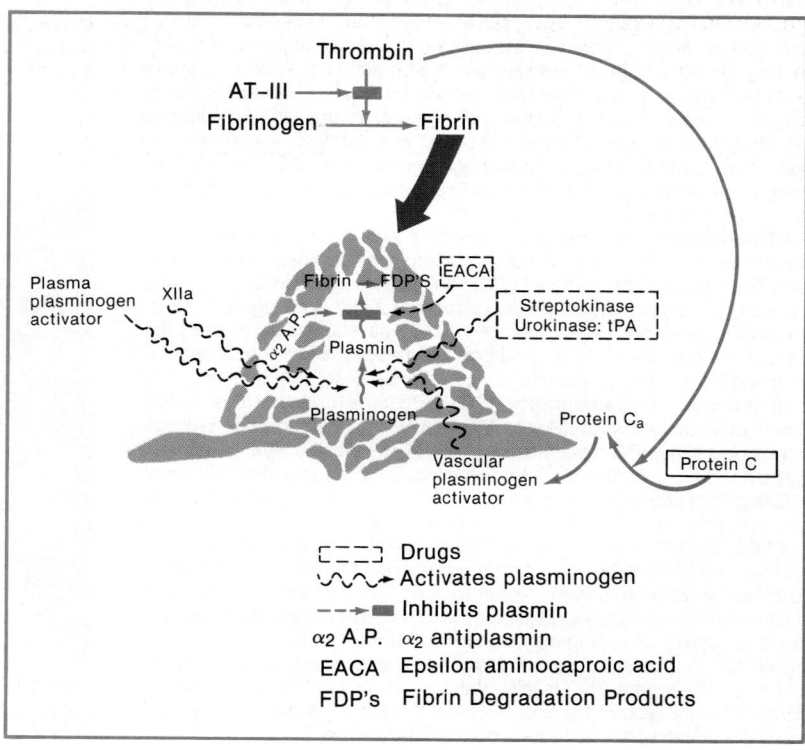

FIGURE 48-2. Schematic view of the fibrinolytic system. Vascular and plasma plasminogen activators as well as pharmacological agents can activate plasmin trapped within the clot. Plasmin dissolves the fibrin clot. Inhibitors of plasmin include alpha²-antiplasmin, also trapped within the clot, and pharmacological agents. (From Stead, R. B.: Regulation of hemostasis. In Goldhaber, S. Z. [ed]: Pulmonary Embolism and Deep Venous Thrombosis. Philadelphia, W. B. Saunders Co., 1985, p. 38).

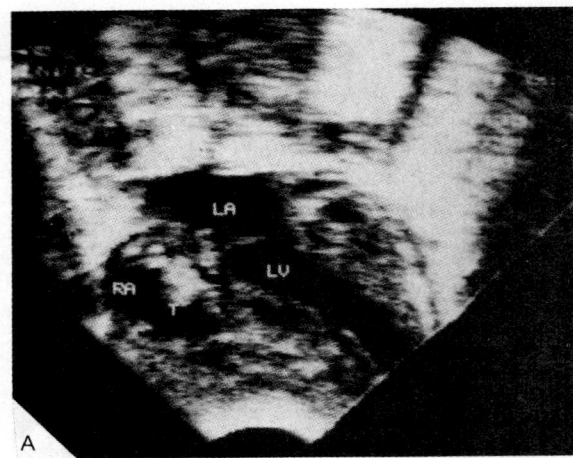
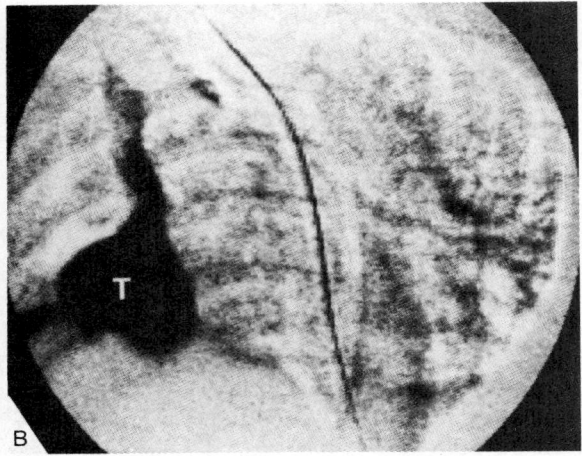

FIGURE 48–3. *A,* Two-dimensional echocardiogram from the subxiphoid position in a 9-month-old boy with *Staphylococcus epidermidis* septicemia and a central hyperalimentation line. A large thrombus (T) can be seen low in the right atrium (RA), just above the tricuspid valve. The mass, acting as a partial ball-valve thrombus, obstructed right ventricular outflow. LA = left atrium; LV = left ventricle. *B,* Digital subtraction angiogram, with contrast material injected through the hyperalimentation catheter. With the catheter tip in the superior aspect of the RA, contrast enters a large cavitary RA thrombus (T), which acts as a cul-de-sac. Thus, contrast cannot be seen in the RA or right ventricle. This thrombus is an ominous nidus for potential pulmonary embolization. (From Fulton, D. R.: Venous thromboembolism in children. *In* Goldhaber, S. Z. [ed.]: Pulmonary Embolism and Deep Venous Thrombosis. Philadelphia, W. B. Saunders Company, 1985, p. 249.)

mately 50 per cent),[24] this risk is lower (approximately one in three) when DVT remains confined to calf veins.[25] In contrast to leg DVT, superficial thrombophlebitis and upper extremity thrombosis are less often associated with PE.

DIAGNOSIS. DVT often occurs without any symptoms or signs. When present, however, the major symptoms are leg pain, tenderness, and swelling, while the major signs are leg edema, discomfort in the calf upon forced dorsiflexion of the foot (Homans' sign), venous distention of subcutaneous vessels, discoloration, and a palpable cord (i.e., thrombus). Unfortunately, these symptoms and signs are not specific for DVT, so that diagnoses based on clinical findings are often incorrect. Therefore, clinical suspicion of DVT should prompt definitive radiological evaluation.

B-mode Ultrasonography. The introduction of B-mode ultrasonography has revolutionized the diagnosis of DVT. When the ultrasound transducer is placed over the common femoral and popliteal veins, the inability to compress these veins is a highly accurate indication of DVT proximal to the calf.[26] The entire ultrasonographic procedure can be completed on both legs within 15 minutes. At times, thrombus can be demonstrated within the lumen (Fig. 48–4). With more expensive and sophisticated machines, color Doppler imaging can be added to the ultrasound examination, and resolution of calf vein thrombi 1 mm^2 can be achieved.[27] Nevertheless, use of a relatively inexpensive high-resolution real-time scanner equipped with a 5-MHz electronically focused linear-array transducer is adequate for reliable diagnosis of DVT proximal to the calf. Experienced ultrasonographers can often use this machine to image adequately the calf veins as well. B-mode ultrasonography is so reliable, inexpensive, safe, and nontraumatic that it is rapidly supplanting leg phlebography as the "gold standard."

Phlebography. Venography is costly, invasive, and occasionally results in complications such as contrast allergy and contrast-induced phlebitis. Patients with massive leg DVT often have nondiagnostic venograms because the contrast agent simply cannot reach the deep leg veins. Consequently, we reserve phlebography for those situations in which the ultrasound examination is equivocal or, alternatively, when the ultrasound examination is normal despite a high clinical suspicion for DVT.

Impedance Plethysmography (IPG). IPG, which was the most widely used noninvasive test to detect DVT, has been superseded by B-mode ultrasonography. IPG measures changes in electrical resistance caused by obstruction to venous outflow. Two studies have suggested that serial IPG testing repeated three to six times over 10 to 14 days will accurately detect calf vein DVT that extends proximally.[28,29]

TREATMENT. For all cases of DVT proximal to the calf and for symptomatic calf DVT,[30] the usual treatment is initial heparin anticoagulation followed by warfarin therapy. Asymptomatic DVT limited to the calf need not be treated with anticoagulation as long as serial noninvasive monitoring for 2 weeks after diagnosis confirms that the clot has not extended proximally. Anticoagulation reduces the risk of proximal propagation of clot and subsequent PE. Usually, therapy is initiated with a continuous intravenous infusion of heparin, because this appears to be more efficacious than intermittent subcutaneous administration.[31]

The proper role of thrombolytic therapy in the treatment of DVT remains uncertain. Two potential advantages of thrombolysis are the prevention of PE by dissolution in situ of the source of embolization in the pelvic or upper extremity veins or the deep veins of the leg, and the prevention of chronic venous insufficiency. The potential benefits of these preventive measures, neither of which has been proved, must be weighed against the risks of hemorrhage. More than 80 per cent of our DVT patients have a contraindication to thrombolysis. These patients are treated with heparin and warfarin or with an inferior vena caval filter. Among those without contraindications to thrombolysis, we consider the use of thrombolytic therapy followed by a full course of heparin anticoagulation and warfarin. As an adjunctive measure, we prescribe thigh-high compression (30 to 40 mm Hg) stockings to our DVT patients when they ambulate. The stockings help prevent distention of the vein wall and may moderate the syndrome of chronic venous insufficiency that two-thirds of DVT patients treated with standard anticoagulation therapy inevitably experience.[32]

Although chronic anticoagulation (usually for 3 months) is prescribed to avert recurrent VTE, the optimal length of such treatment is unknown. One-fifth of patients with DVT may experience a recurrence despite 3 months of anticoagulation.[33] Therefore, in our practice, we anticoagulate those patients who have no long-term risk factors for 6 months, with (rabbit brain thromboplastin) PT maintained at 15 to 16 sec. For those patients with risk factors such as massive obesity, cancer, and previous DVT, anticoagulants are given for an indefinite period of time.

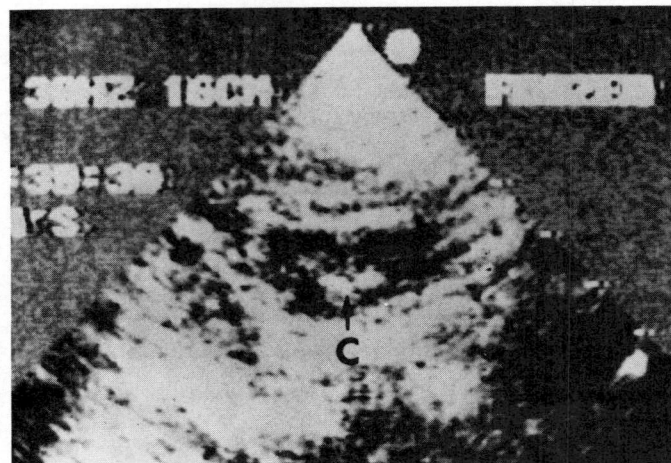

FIGURE 48–4. Left common femoral vein thrombus visualized with high resolution B-mode ultrasonography in a 30-year-old woman. This vein also lacked compressibility. c = clot.

PATHOPHYSIOLOGY

When venous thrombi become dislodged from their site of formation, they flow through the venous system to the pulmonary arterial circulation. If an embolus is extremely large, it may lodge at the bifurcation of the pulmonary artery, forming a "saddle embolus" (Fig. 48–5 *Top*). More commonly, a major pulmonary vessel is occluded (Fig. 48–5 *Bottom*).

The pathophysiological response to acute PE depends on the extent to which pulmonary artery blood flow is obstructed, on preexisting cardiopulmonary disease, and on the release of vasoactive humoral factors from activated platelets that accumulate at the site of new clot (p. 1767). In patients without previous cardiopulmonary disease, right ventricular afterload increases when pulmonary artery obstruction reduces the pulmonary vascular bed by 25 per cent or more. To compensate for this impairment, right ventricular and pulmonary ar-

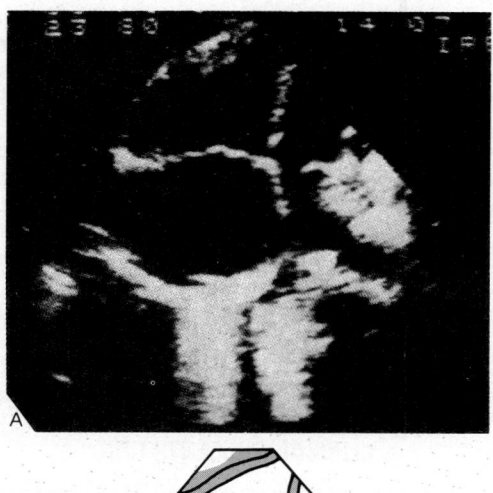
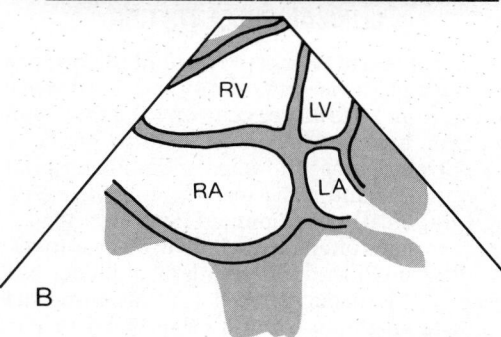

FIGURE 48–6. Apical four-chamber two-dimensional echocardiogram (*A*) and schematic drawing (*B*) from a patient with massive pulmonary embolism. There is marked dilatation of the right atrium (RA) and right ventricle (RV). (The apparent mass in the region of the left atrium (LA) is an imaging defect.) (From Hoagland, P. M.: Massive pulmonary embolism. *In* Goldhaber, S. Z. [ed.]: Pulmonary Embolism and Deep Venous Thrombosis. Philadelphia, W. B. Saunders Company, 1985, p. 187.)

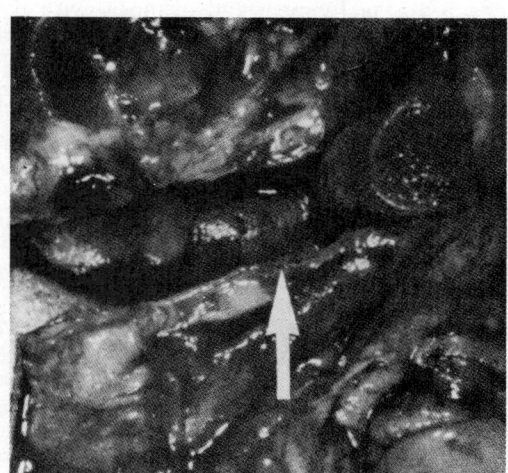
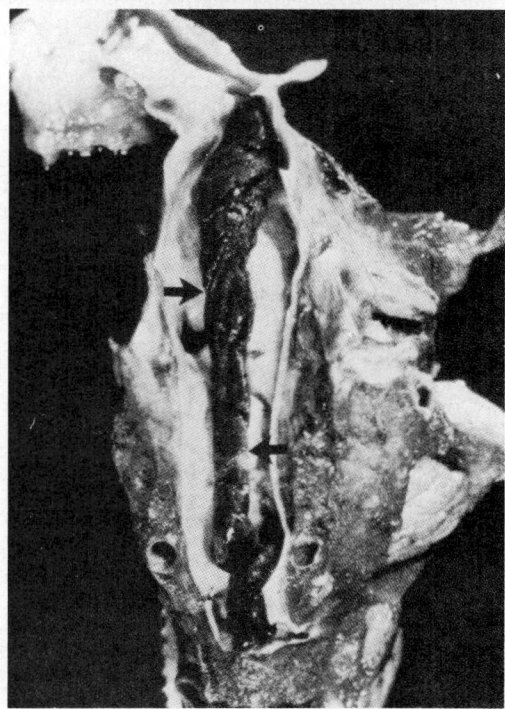

FIGURE 48–5. *Top*, Saddle embolus at the bifurcation of the pulmonary artery. *Bottom*, Pulmonary embolus in left lower lobe pulmonary artery, with minimal attachment to the wall of the vessel. The embolus was dark red, typical of venous thrombi, and had indentations believed to represent impressions of the venous valves (arrows). (From Godleski, J. J.: Pathology of deep venous thrombosis and pulmonary embolism. *In* Goldhaber, S. Z. [ed.]: Pulmonary Embolism and Deep Venous Thrombosis. Philadelphia, W. B. Saunders Company, 1985, p. 17.)

tery pressures rise. As right ventricular afterload increases acutely, this chamber dilates (leading in turn to tricuspid regurgitation) and becomes hypokinetic. These findings can be observed on two-dimensional (Fig. 48–6) and Doppler echocardiography, which can be used to estimate pulmonary artery pressure. As the right ventricle fails, right atrial pressure rises and cardiogenic shock ensues. When cardiac function has been compromised by previous cardiopulmonary illness, relatively smaller emboli obstructing only one or two pulmonary segments can exert a similar hemodynamic effect.

Although preload, afterload, heart rate, and contractility have traditionally been considered the determinants of left ventricular systolic performance (Chap. 13), acute increases in right ventricular pressure can also affect left ventricular function. In a canine model, acutely induced moderate right ventricular hypertension displaces the interventricular septum toward the left ventricle. Therefore, during pressure overload of the right ventricle, the anatomical juxtaposition of the two ventricles (i.e., ventricular interdependency) results in decreased left ventricular diastolic filling and end-diastolic volume.[34] Increased pericardial restraint during PE may also impair left ventricular function by reducing preload.[35]

Among 14 patients with acute massive PE, echocardiography revealed increased right ventricular end-systolic and end-diastolic areas, reduced right ventricular fractional area contraction, interventricular septal flattening at both end-systole and end-diastole, and markedly decreased left ventricular end-diastolic dimensions. Left ventricular fractional area contraction remained normal. During treatment, the interventricular septum progressively returned to a more normal configuration at both end-systole and end-diastole, and left ventricular diastolic dimension steadily increased. Thus, it appeared that circulatory failure due to massive PE is mediated through a profound decrease in left ventricular preload. Acute dilation of the right ventricle with the concomitant restraining action of the pericardium accounted for the leftward shift of the interventricular septum and reduced left ventricular compliance.[36]

After pulmonary embolization, the release of neurohumoral factors causes pulmonary vasoconstriction and bronchospasm that can affect outcome adversely. Experimental studies suggest that during acute PE the two most important vasoactive humoral factors are serotonin and thromboxane A_2 (TxA_2).[37] Serotonin, a potent neural and smooth muscle agonist, is stored primarily in the dense bodies of platelets and mediates bronchospasm in the small airways, either by direct bronchial smooth muscle constriction or by stimulation of a reflex that induces bronchospasm. Activated platelets also release TxA_2, a potent vasoconstrictor and bronchoconstrictor. Increased dead space and reflex airway constriction from PE result in wasted ventilation. The surfactant concentration can decrease, with attendant alveolar collapse and atelectasis, especially during the first few days after embolization.

Diagnosis of Pulmonary Embolism

CLINICAL PRESENTATION

Clinical suspicion of PE is of paramount importance to guide diagnostic testing. In various autopsy series, rates of overdiagnosis ranged from 32 to 62 per cent, and the rate of underdiagnosis has been reported to be as high as 84 per cent.[38] In the Urokinase-Streptokinase Pulmonary Embolism Trial (UPET), clinical symptoms and signs were tabulated in 327 patients with angiographically documented PE (Table 48–2). Because symptoms and signs often do not help to discriminate between patients with true PE and those with no evidence of PE on the arteriogram,[39] the diagnosis with ventilation-perfusion lung scanning or angiography should be pursued in virtually all cases in which PE is suspected (Fig. 48–7).

DIFFERENTIAL DIAGNOSIS. The wide differential diagnosis justifies the reputation of PE as "The Great Masquerader" (Table 48–3). When established pneumonia (with an infiltrate on chest x-ray), congestive heart failure, or myocardial infarction does not respond to appropriate therapy, it may be prudent to rule out coexisting PE. Recurrent PE can increase pulmonary artery pressure[40] and may be mistaken for primary pulmonary hypertension (p. 806)[41,42] (Table 48–4). Although these two conditions share many similarities, certain other features can be used to differentiate them (Table 48–4).

CLINICAL SYNDROMES OF PE

MASSIVE PE. This can be defined as sufficient obstruction of pulmonary arterial blood flow to cause a substantial increase in right ventricular afterload and consequent elevation of pulmonary arterial systolic pressure. Such patients are at highest risk for sudden death from PE or, over the long term, for chronic pulmonary hypertension due to pulmonary arterial clot that has failed to lyse. The most common features that suggest this diagnosis are syncope, profound dyspnea, cor pulmonale, cardiogenic shock, and cardiac arrest (particularly with electromechanical dissociation). Severe pleuritic chest pain usually indicates that the patient does not have massive PE. When syncope occurs, it may at times be caused by associated vagal bradyarrhythmias.[43] Patients also frequently display tachycardia, tachypnea, and cyanosis with distended neck veins; cardiogenic shock (Chap. 21) may be present or incipient. Less common presentations include fever, wheezing, disseminated intravascular coagulation, and paradoxical arterial embolism.[44,45] The differential diagnosis may include septic shock, superior vena caval syndrome, pericardial tamponade (p. 1473), constrictive pericarditis (p. 1486), and right ventricular infarction.

SUBMASSIVE PE. This can be defined as embolism to one or more pulmonary segments not accompanied by substantial elevations in right ventricular and pulmonary artery systolic pressures. Although these patients are not likely to succumb to an acute episode, unlysed thrombi in the pulmonary arteries can eventually lead to chronic pulmonary hypertension. The most frequent symptom is pleuritic chest pain.

PULMONARY INFARCTION. With occlusion of small peripheral pulmonary arteries, bronchoconstriction frequently occurs, and collateral blood flow via the bronchial arteries may not be preserved, leading to pulmonary infarction. The clinical diagnosis of pulmonary infarction due to PE cannot be established unless an infiltrate is present on chest X-ray and the usual criteria for PE on lung scan or pulmonary angiography are met. The primary alternative diagnosis based on clinical presentation is pneumonia. Some PE patients with pulmonary infarction present with hemoptysis; virtually all experience intense pleuritic pain but tend to have a unilateral, distal embolism that is less extensive on angiography than in PE patients without pulmonary infarction.[46] Typically, symptoms and signs develop 3 to 7 days after the onset of embolism.

CHRONIC PULMONARY HYPERTENSION. Recurrent PE may cause chronic pulmonary hypertension associated

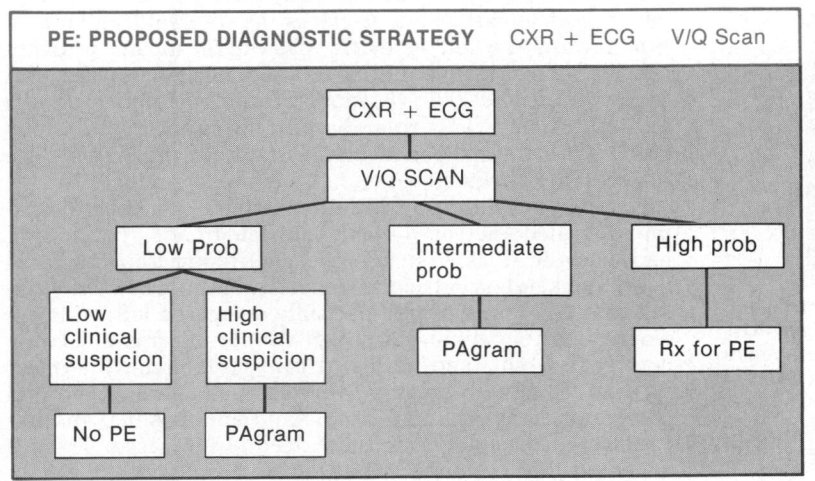

FIGURE 48–7. Diagnostic strategy in suspected pulmonary embolism. CXR = chest x-ray; V/Q = ventilation/perfusion; prob = prob; PAgram = pulmonary arteriogram.

TABLE 48–2 SYMPTOMS AND SIGNS IN 327 PATIENTS WITH PULMONARY EMBOLISM

	PERCENTAGE AFFECTED
SYMPTOMS	
Chest pain	88
Pleuritic chest pain	74
Dyspnea	84
Apprehension	59
Cough	53
Hemoptysis	30
Diaphoresis	36
Syncope	13
SIGNS	
Tachypnea (RR > 16/min)	92
Rales	48
Accentuated 2nd heart sound	53
Tachycardia (HR > 100/min)	44
Fever (Temp > 37.8°C)	43
Phlebitis	32
Cyanosis	19

From Bell, W. R., Simon, T. L., and DeMets, D. L.: The clinical features of submassive and massive pulmonary emboli. Am. J. Med. 52:355, 1977. (Data based on the Urokinase-Streptokinase Pulmonary Embolism Trial.)

TABLE 48–3 DIFFERENTIAL DIAGNOSIS OF PULMONARY EMBOLISM

Myocardial infarction
Pneumonia
Congestive heart failure
Asthma
Chronic obstructive pulmonary disease
Intrathoracic cancer
Rib fracture
Pneumothorax
"Musculoskeletal pain"

with a clinical syndrome of progressive right heart failure and cor pulmonale. This condition tends to develop insidiously when PE either is not diagnosed or is treated inadequately. It is hypothesized that the use of thrombolytic agents to treat PE may reduce the incidence of this complication. On examination, the lung fields may be clear despite the presence of dyspnea, cyanosis, jugular venous distention, v waves due to tricuspid regurgitation, hepatic enlargement, ascites, and lower extremity edema. Chronic pulmonary hypertension due to recurrent PE is a feared complication of venous thromboembolism and has a poor prognosis. Nevertheless, it is important to recognize this clinical syndrome so that these patients can be evaluated for potential pulmonary thromboendarterectomy (p. 1574).

NONTHROMBOTIC PE. Sources of nonthrombotic PE[47] include tumor,[48] fat, amniotic fluid,[49] air, and particulate matter such as cotton and catheters.

NONIMAGING MODALITIES

ARTERIAL BLOOD GASES. Hypoxemia, determined by means of arterial blood gas measurement, has traditionally been considered an important screening test for PE. Yet patients suspected of PE who are then found to have normal lung scans or pulmonary angiograms may be as or more hypoxemic than those with documented PE. Conversely, a high arterial PO_2 can cause the physician mistakenly to refrain from pursuing the diagnosis of PE. More recently, it has been suggested that the inaccuracy of hypoxemia can be overcome by analyzing arterial blood gases for the presence of an increased alveolar-arterial oxygen gradient because, in PE, both a ventilation-perfusion mismatch and an increase in true intrapulmonary shunt should increase this gradient.[50] However, others have found that a normal A-a oxygen gradient does not exclude the diagnosis of PE.[51] Therefore, we believe that arterial blood gases, while of value for many aspects of patient care, are so misleading in the investigation of suspected PE that they should not be part of the diagnostic strategy.

ANALYSIS OF PLEURAL FLUID. The results of pleural fluid analysis are so variable[52] that thoracentesis need not be undertaken in patients with suspected PE unless a concomitant infectious process is considered likely. (If thoracentesis has been performed, thrombolytic agents usually should not be administered for 10 days.)

TABLE 48–4 PRIMARY PULMONARY HYPERTENSION (PPH) VS. RECURRENT PE

SIMILARITIES		
Symptoms	Fatigue, dyspnea on exertion—most common Chest pain, syncope, hemoptysis, cyanosis—also common	
Clinical course	Progressive dyspnea, right heart failure	
Hemodynamics	Elevated right heart pressures, normal pulmonary capillary wedge pressure	
DIFFERENCES	**PPH**	**Recurrent PE**
Age	20 to 40 years	>50 years
Female:male ratio	4:1	1:1
Clinical course	Continued downhill	Downhill, with stabilization between episodes
Lung scan	No segmental perfusion defects	Segmental or larger perfusion defects
Pulmonary artery systolic pressure	>60 mm Hg	<60 mm Hg
Pulmonary arteriogram	"Pruning"	Intraluminal filling defects
Confounding problems with arteriogram	Thrombi may occur on or distal to PPH lesions	"Pruning," a common angiographic finding in PPH, can also indicate PE. Arteriogram may not show emboli late in the clinical course
Diagnostic alternatives	Open lung biopsy	Pulmonary angioscopy
Therapy	Isoproterenol Hydralazine Nifedipine Anticoagulation	Anticoagulation IVC interruption Thromboendarterectomy

From Goldhaber, S. Z.: Strategies for diagnosis. In Goldhaber, S. Z. (ed.): Pulmonary Embolism and Deep Vein Thrombosis. Philadelphia, W. B. Saunders Company, 1985, p. 89.

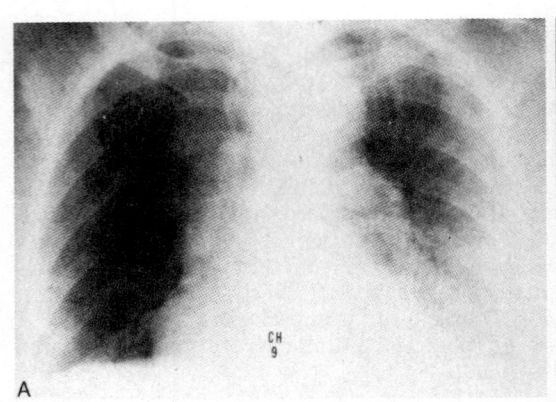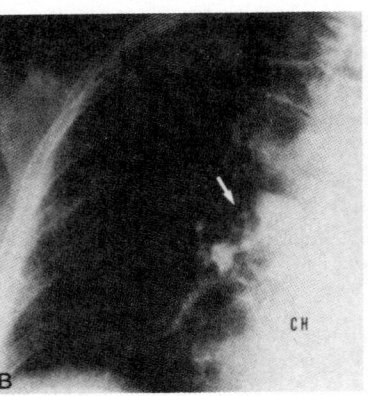

FIGURE 48-8. *A*, Chest x-ray of patient with clinical signs of pulmonary embolism showing marked oligemia (Westermark's sign) in the entire right lobe. *B*, arteriogram from same patient showing massive saddle embolus in the right main pulmonary artery (arrow). (Courtesy of Jack L. Westcott, M.D., The New York Hospital and Cornell University Medical College.)

ELECTROCARDIOGRAM. The electrocardiogram tends to show characteristic abnormalities only in patients with massive PE. Traditional manifestations of acute cor pulmonale such as $S_1Q_3T_3$ (Fig. 5-13, p. 127), right bundle branch block, P pulmonale, or right-axis deviation occurred in 26 per cent of the patients evaluated in the Urokinase Pulmonary Embolism Trial (UPET).[53] Usually, when the electrocardiogram suggests PE, the diagnosis tends to be apparent for other reasons.

BLOOD TESTS. To date, no rapid, inexpensive, and accurate blood test to screen for PE or DVT (analogous to the CK-MB enzyme assays used to diagnose acute myocardial infarction) has been found. The most promising blood test appears to be the D-dimer, which needs further refinement before it becomes a reliable clinical tool. In thrombotic conditions such as PE, endogenous plasmin-mediated proteolysis of cross-linked human fibrin tends to occur, with release of unique products that can be quantified, including D-D and Y-D dimeric fragments. With the use of monoclonal antibodies, immunoassays for human D-dimer have been developed. In a study of 19 patients with angiographically proven PE and 50 patients with completely normal lung scans who were suspected of having PE, elevated levels of D-dimer were present in 89 per cent of patients with PE. However, D-dimer elevation was also present in 56 per cent of patients who did not have PE.[54]

PULMONARY FUNCTION TESTS. PE causes an increase in both the physiological deadspace (V_D) and in the ratio of V_D to tidal volume (V_T). In a study of 16 patients with angiographically diagnosed PE and 29 patients in whom PE was excluded, a $V_D/V_T > 40$ per cent in the presence of a normal spirogram was highly suggestive of PE, whereas a $V_D/V_T < 40$ per cent made the diagnosis of PE very unlikely.[55]

CONVENTIONAL IMAGING MODALITIES

Chest Roentgenography

Occlusion of a lobar or segmental artery will cause a relative local hyperlucency on plain film, with diminished vascular markings (Fig. 48-8). An engorged major hilar artery on a plain film is another important clue to massive PE, especially when serial studies are available. The sudden appearance of a "plump" vessel, particularly the right descending pulmonary artery, may suggest embolic disease. In most cases, hilar signs are right-sided because cardiac and main pulmonary artery shadows make it difficult to visualize left-sided hilar signs. Abrupt tapering or termination of a vessel, termed the "knuckle sign," although rarely noted, can be diagnostic of PE. Nonspecific signs include diminished volume of a lower lobe with displacement of a major fissure or elevation of a hemidiaphragm. Obviously, these findings on chest roentgenography are not diagnostic, but in the proper clinical setting they may increase or even arouse suspicion.[56]

In *pulmonary infarction*, parenchymal consolidation is observed as an increased radiographic density. This finding may be due to actual tissue necrosis or to so-called reversible infarction (i.e., hemorrhage and edema) that clears within 3 to 7 days. However, if infarction leads to necrosis, the average time of resolution is about 3 weeks, usually with permanent residual fibrotic changes. The classic configuration is a homogeneous wedge-shaped density in the peripheral region of the lung with a rounded, convex apex pointing toward the hilum —commonly referred to as "Hampton's hump" (Fig. 48-9).[57] *Absence of an air bronchogram* in a parenchymal consolidation is suggestive of infarction as opposed to a pneumonic process; on the other hand, the *presence* of an air bronchogram is inconclusive because it is sometimes observed in patients with PE.

The chest roentgenogram may also provide an important clue that pulmonary artery hypertension is due to chronic PE when there is right-sided cardiomegaly, mosaic oligemia, or right descending pulmonary artery enlargement.[58] Overall, however, chest roentgenography is an insensitive screening test for PE. Its major diagnostic utility lies in its capacity to suggest diagnoses *other* than PE, such as pneumonia, heart failure, or pneumothorax.

Lung Scanning

Ventilation-perfusion lung scanning is the key diagnostic test in screening for PE.[58a] A normal perfusion scan essentially rules out all but trivial-sized PE and helps direct clinical attention to other diagnostic possibilities. It is usually safe to withhold anticoagulant therapy in patients with suspected PE and normal perfusion scans, regardless of the clinical manifestations; ordinarily, such patients do not need to undergo pulmonary angiography.[59]

For patients with perfusion defects that are segmental or greater in size, normal ventilation on scintigraphy in the same areas as the perfusion defects increases the likelihood of PE. Abnormal scans are usually categorized as having a low, moderate, high, or indeterminate probability for PE. At the Brigham and Women's Hospital, low probability scans are defined as showing multiple subsegmental perfusion defects without a ventilation study, or subsegmental or larger perfusion defects with abnormal ventilation correlating with the perfusion defects (a ventilation-perfusion [V̇/Q̇] "match"). Moderate probability scans show multiple subsegmental perfusion defects with normal ventilation, or segmental or larger

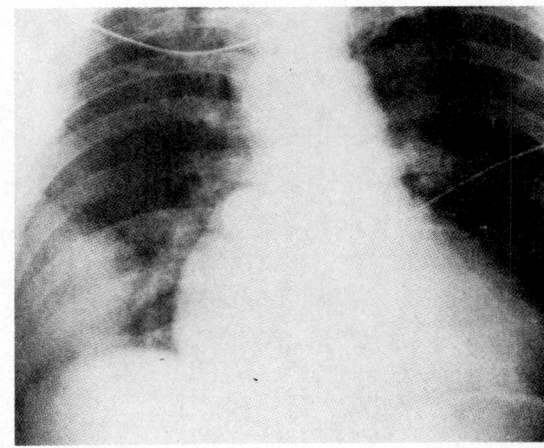

FIGURE 48-9. Posteroanterior chest x-ray of patients with pulmonary embolism showing "Hampton's hump" in right lower lung field, a homogeneous, wedge-shaped density in the peripheral field, convex to the hilum. (Courtesy of Jack L. Westcott, M.D., The New York Hospital and Cornell University Medical College.)

| | PULMONARY EMBOLISM | | | NO | TOTAL |
	Present	Absent	Uncertain	ANGIOGRAM	N
Scan Category					
High	102	14	1	7	124
Intermediate	105	217	9	33	364
Low	39	199	12	62	312
Near-normal/normal	5	50	2	74	131
Total	251	480	24	176	931

From the PIOPED Investigators: Value of the ventilation/perfusion scan in acute pulmonary embolism. JAMA 263:2756, 1990.

perfusion defects without a ventilation study. High probability scans show segmental or larger perfusion defects with normal ventilation (V̇/Q̇ "mismatch"). Alternatively, a scan can be high probability with two or more large perfusion defects that are substantially larger than either ventilation or chest x-ray abnormalities. Scans are of indeterminate probability when the chest x-ray either demonstrates COPD or is abnormal in the region(s) of the perfusion defect.

Hull and colleagues at McMaster University in Hamilton, Ontario compared abnormal ventilation-perfusion lung scans with results of pulmonary angiography among patients suspected of having PE.[60] Their findings support the traditional definition of a high-probability lung scan (e.g., 86 per cent accuracy) but they found that 37 of 116 (32 per cent) of their patients with non–high-probability scans also had PE at angiography. More recently, under the auspices of the National Heart, Lung, and Blood Institute, a multicenter study was undertaken to determine the diagnostic usefulness of the ventilation-perfusion lung scan in acute PE.[61,61a] The Prospective Investigation of Pulmonary Embolism Diagnosis (PIOPED) recruited 931 patients, of whom 81 per cent completed mandatory angiography within a day of obtaining an abnormal lung scan. Among the 755 patients who completed angiography, 33 per cent had PE. The most important finding in PIOPED is that of the 251 patients with positive angiograms, only 102 (41 per cent) had high-probability lung scans. Therefore, the sensitivity of high-probability lung scans for PE at angiography is only 41 per cent. Accordingly, if high-probability lung scans are relied upon to establish the diagnosis, PE will not be recognized in more than half (59 per cent) of patients who present with it.

In PIOPED, the positive predictive value of lung scanning for PE at angiography was as follows: 87 per cent for high, 32 per cent for intermediate, 16 per cent for low, and 9 per cent for near-normal scans (Table 48–5). When the "clinical probability" was factored into the interpretation of the lung scan, it was evident that some patients suspected of having PE would not require further work-up before a disposition was made. For example, among patients who had both high-probability lung scans and a clinical suspicion for PE of more than 80 per cent, the likelihood of PE at angiography was 96 per cent. Conversely, among patients who had both a low probability lung scan and a clinical suspicion for PE of less than 20 per cent, the likelihood of PE at angiography was only 4 per cent (Table 48–6). The majority of patients will not fit neatly into

either of these categories and, in most circumstances, such as an intermediate- or low-probability scan with high clinical suspicion, the diagnosis of PE should be pursued with angiography (Fig. 48–7). Lung imaging for suspected PE is usually a low-yield strategy, unless the patient has symptoms or signs of DVT or cancer.

Given the limitations of lung scanning, clinicians normally should not defer pulmonary angiography after obtaining a nondiagnostic scan, particularly when the results of the scan differ sharply from the clinical impression obtained by integrating history, symptoms, signs, and findings on the chest roentgenogram and electrocardiogram. Therefore, in estimating the probability of PE, the physician should interpret the lung scan on the basis of clinical assessment of the likelihood of disease.

Pulmonary Angiography

INDICATIONS. When a ventilation-perfusion lung scan is entirely normal, the diagnosis of PE can be excluded reliably. Conversely, when ventilation-perfusion lung scanning indicates a high probability of PE and clinical suspicion is high before scanning, it is not necessary to proceed with pulmonary angiography unless there is some mitigating factor that obscures the diagnosis, such as asthma, intrathoracic cancer, or previous PE. Usually, multiple segmental or lobar perfusion defects in areas of normal ventilation will correspond with angiographically documented PE. (However, if thrombolytic therapy or inferior vena caval interruption is being considered, one may wish to eliminate even the slightest diagnostic uncertainty by obtaining a pulmonary angiogram.) It is also worth emphasizing that perfusion scan findings understate the severity of angiographic and hemodynamic compromise among patients with chronic thromboembolic pulmonary hypertension.[62] For patients with low probability scans, we do not obtain pulmonary angiograms unless clinical suspicion of PE is high.

In general, pulmonary angiography is reserved for patients with nondiagnostic moderate probability or indeterminate lung scans, except when clinical suspicion for PE is high despite low probability scan results. The use of pulmonary angiography is increasing because the limitations of lung scanning and clinical diagnosis are becoming more widely appreciated, especially since results of the McMaster and PIOPED studies were disseminated. However, unless the patient's condition is

TABLE 48-6 PIOPED: PULMONARY EMBOLISM STATUS

| | CLINICAL PROBABILITY (%) | | | |
	80–100 No. PE/PTS (%)	20–79 No. PE/PTS (%)	0–19 No. PE/PTS (%)	All Probabilities No. PE/PTS (%)
Scan category				
High	28/29 (96)	70/ 80 (88)	5/ 9 (56)	103/118 (87)
Intermediate	27/41 (66)	66/236 (28)	11/ 68 (16)	104/345 (30)
Low	6/15 (40)	30/191 (16)	4/ 90 (4)	40/296 (14)
Near-normal/normal	0/ 5 (0)	4/ 62 (6)	1/ 61 (2)	5/128 (4)
Total	61/90 (68)	170/569 (30)	21/228 (9)	252/887 (28)

From the PIOPED Investigators: Value of the ventilation/perfusion scan in acute pulmonary embolism. JAMA 263:2757, 1990.

hemodynamically unstable or unless empirical heparinization is absolutely contraindicated (e.g., active gastrointestinal bleeding), these studies need not be done on an emergency basis.

We do not substitute leg ultrasonography, impedance plethysmography (IPG), or venography for pulmonary angiography unless the patient is pregnant or has an important relative contraindication to angiography such as right atrial thrombus or previous anaphylaxis to contrast agent. In the prospective study by Hull et al.,[60] only 71 per cent of patients with positive pulmonary angiograms had positive venograms; conversely, 33 per cent of patients with normal pulmonary angiograms had positive venograms. Another strategy that we avoid is empirical anticoagulation followed by serial lung scanning to determine whether pulmonary perfusion has improved over time. Such improvement, if observed, could be due to resolving asthma or viral pneumonia as well as PE.

To summarize, except for extenuating circumstances (such as terminal illness, a history of life-threatening anaphylaxis to contrast medium, or pregnancy), we usually recommend pulmonary angiography when lung scans are inconclusive (i.e., moderate or indeterminate probability for PE). We also pursue angiography when our clinical suspicion for the condition is discordant with the result of the lung scan.

PERFORMANCE OF PULMONARY ANGIOGRAPHY

The pulmonary angiogram is the most specific examination available for establishing the clinical diagnosis of PE and serves as a template against which other techniques and approaches are measured.[63] The procedure is generally safe, except in patients who have a contrast allergy, right ventricular end-diastolic pressure more than 20 mm Hg,[64] or amiodarone-induced pulmonary toxicity (p. 646).[65] Newer contrast agents of lower osmolality are less toxic than conventional angiographic dye in patients with pulmonary hypertension.[66] We always employ low osmolar contrast rather than conventional angiographic dye, despite the higher cost of these newer agents. In addition to enhancing patient safety, low osmolar contrast agents virtually abolish the heat sensation and urge to cough. Low osmolar contrast agents may be cost-effective in pulmonary angiography because, unlike conventional contrast agents, the angiographic views almost never have to be repeated because of patient coughing and consequent blurring of the films.

As with any procedure, there is a learning curve for proper and safe performance of pulmonary angiography. Of the 755 patients in PIOPED who completed angiography, the procedure was a contributing cause of death in two (0.3 per cent), both of whom were seriously ill before angiography.[61] At the University of California in San Diego, which has a team of physicians and nurses experienced in managing PE patients with severe chronic pulmonary hypertension, 67 consecutive patients with moderate or severe pulmonary hypertension underwent pulmonary angiography. No major rhythm disturbances or systemic hypotension requiring therapy occurred, and there were no deaths. Thus, pulmonary angiography can be carried out safely despite the presence of severe pulmonary hypertension and right ventricular failure, as long as the procedure is performed by an experienced medical team.[67]

PREPARATION OF THE PATIENT. The rationale for performing this test should be explained to the patient and family. Those with high-proba-

bility lung scans should understand that, while there is a 5 to 15 per cent chance that they do not have PE, this determination can be made only with pulmonary angiography. The patient should be told that the procedure may cause discomfort. The injection of conventional contrast medium causes a transient hot, flushed feeling coupled with an almost irresistible urge to cough. Patients should also be informed that pulmonary angiography usually requires between one and four sets of injections in different views (Fig. 48–10).

A history of allergy to contrast medium should be sought. Patients should avoid heavy meals for at least 4 hours before angiography. Heparin can be discontinued for several hours before the procedure. Premedication may include 25 to 50 mg of oral diphenhydramine or 5 to 10 mg of diazepam 30 to 60 minutes before the procedure; when there is a history of adverse reactions to contrast medium, high-dose steroids may be added. If true anaphylaxis to dye has occurred in the past, the decision to proceed with the study must be questioned.

THE ANGIOGRAPHIC PROCEDURE. Our preferred approach is via the right femoral vein. Percutaneous cannulation of the femoral vein permits rapid access to a large vessel and avoids the problems of using small brachial veins, which may be difficult to cannulate with a No. 7 French catheter and which are prone to venospasm. To avoid inadvertent perforation of the right ventricle, a catheter with a pigtail configuration can be used rather than one with a straight end.[68] A pigtail catheter can be manipulated easily into the pulmonary artery in a number of ways: (1) a deflector wire (Cook, Inc., Bloomington, IN) or a curve applied to the stiff end of a 0.038-inch guidewire can be used to bend the catheter in the heart to facilitate its placement into the pulmonary artery (Fig. 48–11); (2) a precurved pigtail catheter such as a Grollman catheter can be used; or (3) a No. 7 French double-lumen Swan-Ganz catheter can be positioned first in the pulmonary artery and can then be replaced by a pigtail catheter over a 0.035 inch-diameter exchange guidewire.

Ordinarily, right atrial, right ventricular, and pulmonary artery pressures are recorded through a pigtail catheter before pulmonary arteriography. Perfusion defects on the lung scan are used to determine which lung to study initially.

Selective angiography should be used rather than main pulmonary artery injection. Once the catheter has been positioned and the patient has been placed in the desired projection, a test dose of 5 to 10 ml is administered. A plain scout film is then obtained to ensure satisfactory exposure and field of view. Before the injection, the patient should be instructed carefully about proper breathing technique and should be reminded to try to suppress the urge to cough. Filming is carried out during maximal inspiration.

Twenty to 25 ml of contrast medium per second is injected for 2 seconds. The exposure rates for this phase are 3 per second for 3 seconds and then 1 per second for the pulmonary venous phase, which occurs 5 to 7 seconds after injection. After the selective pulmonary artery injection, pulmonary artery pressures are rechecked to monitor a possible pulmonary hypertensive response, and systemic arterial pressure should be rechecked to detect potential hypotension. The "large film" method that we use offers high-resolution clarity of vascular detail and versatility in field size. An alternative approach utilizes cineangiography.

INTERPRETING THE ANGIOGRAM. PE cannot be excluded unless the vasculature appears normal on two different oblique views (Fig. 48–10). A definitive diagnosis of PE depends on visualization of a clot. Primary arteriographic signs of emboli are persistent lucent defects without obstruction to flow or a trailing edge of an intraluminal lucency if there is complete obstruction to flow distally. Secondary signs—not diagnostic in themselves but simply indicators of decreased pulmonary perfusion—

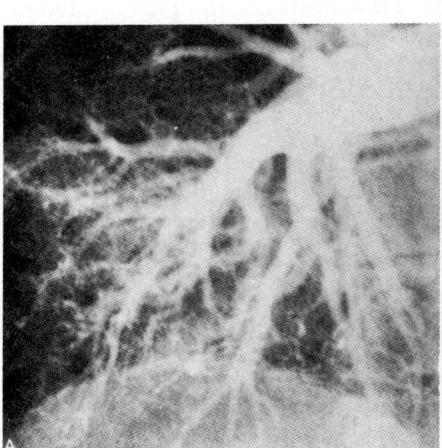
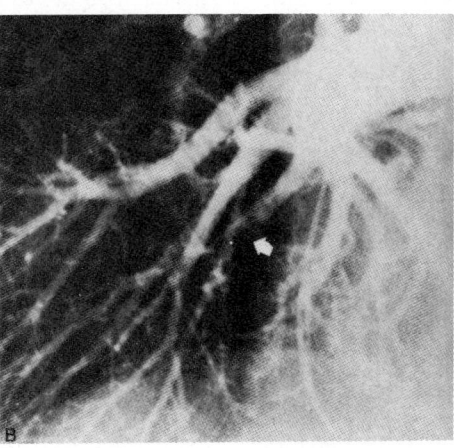

FIGURE 48–10. Selective right pulmonary arteriogram. *A,* Left posterior oblique projection of right lower lobe with normal-appearing pulmonary arteriogram due to overlap of vasculature. *B,* Right posterior oblique projection of the same area exhibiting an intravascular filling defect (arrow) in the artery to the lateral basal segment of the right lower lobe. (Courtesy of Thomas A. Sos, M.D., The New York Hospital and Cornell University Medical Center.)

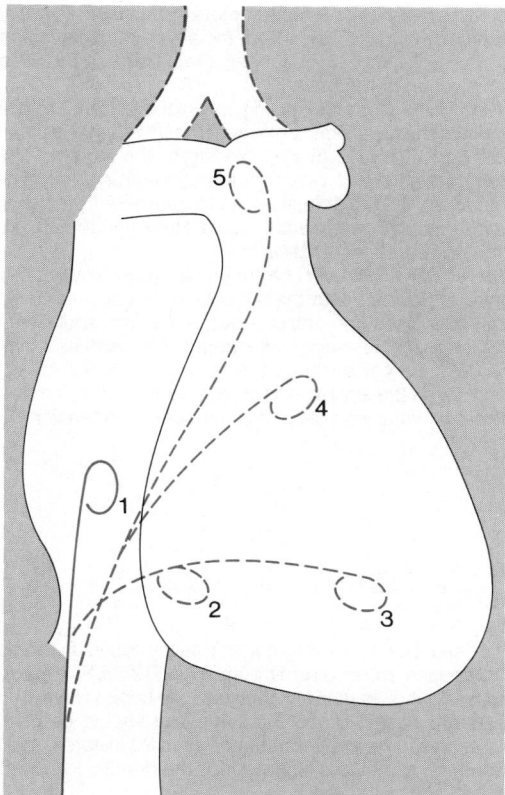

FIGURE 48–11. Technique for pulmonary artery catheterization. The pigtail catheter is advanced into the right atrium (1). A deflector guidewire is inserted into the catheter, the tip of the wire lying immediately proximal to the pigtail loop. The guidewire is deflected using the external handle, so that the catheter is curved toward the tricuspid valve (2). With the deflected guidewire fixed, the catheter is stripped off the wire and into the right ventricle (3). After deflection is released, the catheter will assume a straighter course, pointing toward the right ventricular outflow tract (4). As counterclockwise torque is applied, the catheter is advanced into the main pulmonary artery (5). With further advancement, the catheter will usually enter the left pulmonary artery. To select the right pulmonary artery, the deflector wire can be used to deflect the catheter toward the right, just below the level of the tracheal bifurcation. Pressure measurements are obtained in each right-sided cardiac chamber between each of the maneuvers described here. (From Meyerovitz, M.: How to maximize the safety of coronary and pulmonary angiography in patients receiving thrombolytic therapy. Chest 97:134S, 1990.)

include areas of avascularity or oligemia, a prolonged arterial phase, tortuosity of peripheral vessels, and delayed visualization of the pulmonary venous circulation. These signs are often associated with PE but can occur in other conditions (e.g., bronchial asthma, severe mitral stenosis with associated pulmonary hypertension, or left ventricular failure) and thus are not specific. A primary sign of embolus is mandatory to prevent false-positive diagnoses. Not all pulmonary artery filling defects or occlusions are due to PE. Other causes include pulmonary Takayasu's arteritis (p. 1544), angiosarcoma, and sarcoidosis.[69]

Angiographic methods for quantitation of the severity of PE have been problematic. The Walsh scoring system,[70] which is most commonly used in the United States, does not take into account impairment of peripheral perfusion. The Miller index,[71] which is commonly used in Europe, can overestimate the extent of pulmonary vascular obstruction among patients with massive PE.

Both methods fail to differentiate adequately between clot size and the degree of vascular occlusion. This limitation can be problematic when a small thrombus causes only a partial filling defect with little effect on blood flow. A newer method for quantitating pulmonary angiograms has been proposed and may be more precise than either the Walsh or Miller indices.[72] However, this newer method appears to be more complex and has not been utilized in any therapeutic trials of PE.

In summary, pulmonary angiography is an underutilized procedure that provides maximal diagnostic accuracy. Because the use of stiff catheters that occasionally cause perforation of the right heart and cardiac tamponade has been abandoned, morbidity at present is predominantly related to

toxicity of the contrast agent rather than the catheterization. With proper technique and judicious use of nonionic contrast agents, the mortality rate should not exceed 0.2 to 0.3 per cent.[61,63]

OTHER IMAGING MODALITIES

ECHOCARDIOGRAPHY. The diagnosis of massive PE can sometimes be established by means of two-dimensional echocardiography (Fig. 48–12).[73] The technique of transesophageal two-dimensional echocardiography is particularly well suited for the detection of massive central PE.[74]

Echocardiographic features that suggest acute PE include a dilated, hypokinetic right ventricle, absence of right ventricular hypertrophy, the presence of tricuspid regurgitation with increased flow velocity compatible with mild to moderate elevation of pulmonary arterial systolic pressure, and the absence of important left heart pathological conditions. Features suggestive of chronic pulmonary hypertension that could be caused by chronic PE include a dilated right ventricle that may be hypokinetic, right ventricular hypertrophy, and tricuspid regurgitation with increased flow velocity compatible with moderate to severe elevation of pulmonary arterial systolic pressure.[75]

For patients with dyspnea of unknown cause, it is useful to obtain an echocardiogram. Two-dimensional and Doppler echocardiography can either confirm the presence of left-sided cardiac dysfunction or suggest PE due to the findings of acute pulmonary hypertension.[76]

DIGITAL SUBTRACTION PULMONARY ANGIOGRAPHY (DSA). Although DSA is a useful technique for diagnosing PE in patients suspected of having massive central embolism, it cannot exclude clinically important peripheral PE. Whether DSA remains a research procedure for detecting PE will depend mostly on whether further technological modifications can reduce motion artifacts and improve the images of segmental and subsegmental pulmonary arteries.[77] At present, the only possible niche for DSA performed via a peripheral vein would be in screening patients who present with suspected life-threatening PE.[78]

COMPUTED TOMOGRAPHY (CT). This technique has been used to demonstrate PE[79] and pulmonary infarction.[80] CT scanning should be considered an inadequately validated diagnostic modality that may be appropriate for patients with pulmonary hypertension when the risks associated with conventional angiography are considered prohibitively high. CT scanning is more properly utilized for serial noninvasive evaluation after thrombolysis or surgical embolectomy among patients who have undergone baseline pulmonary angiography.

MAGNETIC RESONANCE IMAGING (MRI). This technique does not image rapidly flowing blood and may therefore be uniquely suited for

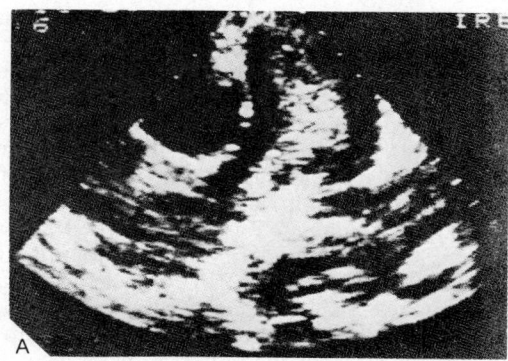

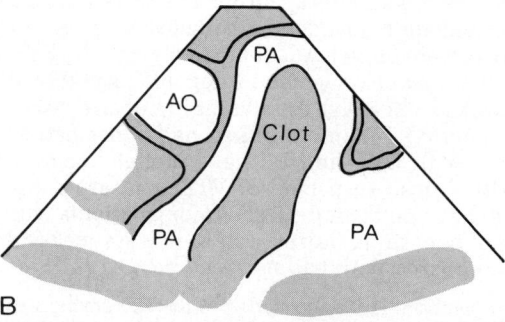

FIGURE 48–12. Two-dimensional echocardiogram in the short-axis parasternal view (*A*) and schematic drawing (*B*) showing a thrombus in the pulmonary artery in a patient with massive pulmonary embolism (seen in Figure 47–4). (From Hoagland, P. M.: Massive pulmonary embolism. *In* Goldhaber, S. Z. [ed.]: Pulmonary Embolism and Deep Venous Thrombosis. Philadelphia, W. B. Saunders Company, 1985, p. 187.)

detecting PE. Initial case reports have been encouraging.[81] The diagnostic niche for MRI may be in differentiating acute from chronic PE.[82]

RADIOISOTOPE IMAGING. The physical half-life of indium-111 (2.8 days) and the biological life of the injected platelet (8 to 10 days) permit imaging of PE and DVT[83] for at least 5 days after injection of the platelet suspension. Therefore, the technique may be useful for surveillance of high-risk patients[84] and for monitoring the therapeutic response once PE and DVT have been detected and treated.[85] However, a prospective study of 65 patients with suspected DVT who underwent indium-111 platelet scintigraphy 2 hours after injection demonstrated a disappointingly low sensitivity of approximately 40 per cent, although the specificity was excellent (greater than 90 per cent) when compared with contrast venography. In this study, the early images were problematic because of slow incorporation of platelets into the thrombi. In addition, limbs with varicose veins and postphlebitic changes presented difficulties in distinguishing platelet uptake into active thrombus.[86]

A promising imaging technique is indium-111–labeled monoclonal anti-fibrin antibodies for the detection of DVT. A study of 52 patients suspected of having DVT indicated greater than 90 per cent sensitivity in the calf but progressively less accuracy more proximally. The monoclonal antifibrin antibody binds specifically to the amino terminal region of fibrin but does not cross-react with fibrinogen. Diagnosis can be made within 2 hours after injection of the tracer.[87]

Another intriguing isotopic imaging technique utilizes an iodine-125–labeled mutant of tissue plasminogen activator (t-PA) that is fibrinolytically inactive to bind to thrombi. In vitro binding of the mutant t-PA to clots formed from human blood was concentration-dependent, time-dependent, and specific. The rapid clearance of mutant t-PA from the circulation may make it a useful clinical imaging agent. However, to date, in vivo use of this agent has not been reported.[88]

FIBEROPTIC ANGIOSCOPY. After jugular venotomy and insertion of the fiberoptic angioscope into the superior vena cava, the balloon is inflated to displace blood and obtain a clear view. The angioscope is then guided with fluoroscopic assistance into the right heart and main pulmonary artery. Pulmonary artery branches as distal as segmental arteries can be examined. While the technique is complicated to learn, it may be particularly useful in patients with chronic pulmonary hypertension.[89]

Treatment of Pulmonary Embolism

ANTICOAGULATION

Heparin
(See also p. 1761)

Heparin accelerates the action of antithrombin III 1000-fold to prevent further fibrin deposition (Fig. 48–2) and to allow for the body's natural fibrinolytic mechanisms to lyse clot that has already formed. Heparin does *not* dissolve thrombus that already exists. One placebo-controlled randomized trial has been carried out in PE patients.[90] The mortality rate was significantly lower among the treated patients, and the randomized trial was discontinued for ethical reasons. No randomized placebo-controlled trial with heparin has ever been undertaken in DVT.[27]

To achieve an effective antithrombotic state, a certain minimal level of heparin anticoagulation appears necessary. In practice, an effective level of heparin anticoagulation can be inferred from an activated partial thromboplastin time (PTT) that is at least 1½ times greater than the control value.[91]

Unfortunately, physicians tend to administer inadequate doses of heparin to patients with DVT and PE. In a review of physician practices at Vanderbilt University School of Medicine, 60 per cent of patients with venous thromboembolism (VTE) did not have a single PTT greater than 1.5 times control within the first 24 hours of heparin therapy. Not until day 8 of treatment were 90 per cent of the PTTs within the therapeutic range.[92] It is apparent that the usual practice of administering an initial 5000 unit bolus of heparin followed by an initial infusion of 1000 U/hr is inadequate therapy for most patients with VTE. When subtherapeutic PTTs were obtained in this study, physicians responded with modest increases in heparin dosing that were often inadequate to elevate the PTT into the therapeutic range. Conversely, when unacceptably high PTTs were obtained, excessive reductions in heparin dosage caused subtherapeutic PTTs in more than half of the patients.

Patients with DVT and PE have higher heparin requirements than those suspected of VTE who are subsequently proved to have no thrombosis.[93] Among patients with PE, the half-life of heparin is shorter and the clearance of heparin is greater compared with patients who have DVT.[94]

A unique problem is the monitoring of therapy among patients with elevated PTTs at baseline due to the presence of the lupus anticoagulant or anticardiolipin antibodies. Obviously, the usual criterion of a PTT greater than 1½ times control cannot be utilized in this population. To obviate this problem, we measure quantitatively the heparin level by having our chemistry laboratory use an HEPRN pack (Dupont Co., Wilmington, DE) in the automated clinical analyzer used for other chemistry tests.

The plasma heparin level is a chromogenic assay based on the inhibition of factor X_a by heparin-activated antithrombin III. The HEPRN pack contains excess factor X_a and, essentially, analyzes the heparin level by means of an anti-factor X_a assay. Blood for this assay should be drawn into a citrated tube, placed on ice, centrifuged within 30 minutes, and analyzed within 4 hours. The therapeutic range for the heparin level is 0.2 to 0.5 U/ml.

For pregnant women with DVT and PE, we treat initially with continuous intravenous heparin and then teach the patient to self-administer full-dose subcutaneous heparin for the remainder of the pregnancy. With subcutaneous injections, peak heparin levels are usually obtained at approximately 3 hours, and the effect may last for 12 hours if the heparin dose is adequate. To monitor the heparin, our target is either a mid-interval PTT of approximately 1.5 times control or a "trough" PTT that is at least several seconds elevated above the upper limit of normal. We have found this approach safe for both the mother and fetus.[95] Although there has been some enthusiasm for administering continuous intravenous heparin to pregnant women by utilizing a portable infusion pump,[96] we have abandoned this approach at Brigham and Women's Hospital because of bleeding complications that occurred despite therapeutic PTT levels.[97]

A correlation between hemorrhagic risk and excessively prolonged PTT (e.g., more than 3 times control) seems logical but is not well documented in prospective trials. However, a retrospective analysis of anticoagulated patients at Brigham and Women's Hospital found that bleeding does correlate with the intensity of therapy.[98] Compared with patients whose maximal PTT (or prothrombin time) was less than twice the control value, major bleeding was 3 times as frequent in patients with a maximal PTT (or prothrombin time) that was 2.0 to 2.9 times control and 7.9 times as frequent among patients with a PTT (or prothrombin time) prolonged to 3.0 or more times control. Other independent risk factors for major in-hospital bleeding among anticoagulated patients included the presence of comorbid conditions, age exceeding 60 years, and liver dysfunction that worsened during treatment.

In the majority of studies in which continuous and intermittent infusion of heparin have been compared, the frequency of major hemorrhage was lower with continuous intravenous infusion.[33] However, the patients who were given continuous intravenous heparin infusions tended to receive lower total doses of heparin than those allocated to subcutaneous injections. Theoretically, intermittent intravenous or subcutaneous heparin administration is disadvantageous because it temporarily causes excessive anticoagulation, as reflected by highly elevated peak PTT levels. Therefore, whenever feasible, for patients with suspected acute PE our practice is to administer heparin therapy by continuous intravenous infusion after an initial bolus of heparin.

INITIATION OF HEPARIN THERAPY. Heparin is the cornerstone of treatment for acute PE. Before heparin therapy is begun, the most important first step is to obtain a careful history. In particular, one should consider risk factors such as history of coagulopathy, thrombocytopenia, vitamin K deficiency, older age, underlying diseases, and concomitant drug therapy. The most frequently overlooked portion of the physical examination is a rectal examination for occult blood. The results of the examination should be recorded in the patient's chart. When a stool guaiac examination is equivocal (i.e., "trace"), we proceed with heparin anticoagulation but maintain an even higher state of vigilance than usual for potential bleeding complications.

If results of the history and physical examination are benign, heparin can be started before lung scanning or pulmonary angiography in situations when clinical suspicion of PE is high. However, if a severe bleeding problem is detected, such as active gastrointestinal bleeding, heparin therapy should be withheld and if the diagnosis of PE is confirmed, nonpharmacological treatment with insertion of an inferior vena cava (IVC) filter should be considered. Interestingly, we have modified our practice and no longer automatically place an inferior vena cava filter in patients with nonhemorrhagic brain tumors. Many of these patients can be anticoagulated safely.[99] For patients at high risk of bleeding from heparin, the angiographer should be alerted to the possible need to insert an IVC filter on short notice.

The dosage regimen for achieving optimal heparinization is empirical. For an average-sized adult in whom there is only a modest suspicion of PE, the usual initial dose would be a 5000-unit intravenous bolus followed by a continuous intravenous infusion of 1000 units per hour. In a patient suspected of having massive PE, a more appropriate initial dose is a 10,000-unit bolus followed by an infusion of 1500 units per hour. For maintenance heparin anticoagulation, the PTT should remain 1.5 to 2.5 times the control level and should be checked every 4 hours until the target PTT level is obtained. When the PTT is less than 1.5 times control, the continuous infusion dose should be increased rapidly, by an increment of at least 25 per cent. Conversely, if a PTT level exceeds 3 times the control value, a reduction in the infusion rate of no more than 25 per cent of the dose should be made. Otherwise, if too much of an adjustment is made, a rebound effect to a subtherapeutic level of anticoagulation can be anticipated. In general, heparin infusion rates of 1500 to 2000 units per hour are quite common for achieving adequate anticoagulation, particularly during the first few days of treatment.

COMPLICATIONS. The most important adverse effect of heparin is hemorrhage. Major bleeding during anticoagulation may unmask a previously silent lesion such as bladder or colon cancer. For most cases of moderate bleeding, cessation of heparin therapy will suffice, and the PTT level will usually return to normal within 2 to 3 hours because the half-life of heparin is only 60 to 90 minutes. Resumption of heparin at a lower dose or alternative means of therapy depends on the severity of the bleeding, the risk of recurrent thromboembolism, and the extent to which bleeding may have resulted from excessive anticoagulation (i.e., a PTT greater than 3 times the baseline value). In the event of life-threatening or intracranial hemorrhage, protamine sulfate can be administered when heparin is discontinued. Protamine, a strongly basic protein, will immediately reverse anticoagulant activity by forming a stable complex with the acidic heparin. For life-threatening hemorrhage, the usual dose is approximately 1 mg per 100 units of heparin, administered slowly (e.g., 50 mg over 10 to 30 minutes). Protamine sulfate can cause allergic reactions that vary from mild to life-threatening.[100]

Mild thrombocytopenia that may develop with heparin therapy probably represents a direct, nonimmune-mediated effect of heparin and is not associated with serious clinical consequence. Heparin-associated thrombocytopenia[101] (p. 1782) occurs more frequently with beef lung than with pork gut heparin.[102] The frequency of heparin-associated thrombocytopenia can vary according to the specific lot of heparin that is obtained from the manufacturing plant.[103] When the thrombocytopenia is associated with thrombosis, the condition is immune-mediated and may be life-threatening. Heparin-induced thrombosis can occur even with small doses of prophylactic heparin (e.g., 5000 U subcutaneously every 8 hours).[104]

The thrombotic events are often distinctly unusual and may involve the skin[105] or major arteries,[106] such as the femoral or radial arteries.

Patients undergoing prolonged heparin therapy at relatively high doses may develop osteopenia, osteoporosis, and pathological bone fractures.[107,108] In addition, continuous heparin infusion causes aldosterone depression by an unknown mechanism within 4 to 8 days after initiation of therapy.[109] In patients with a normally functioning renin-angiotensin-aldosterone axis, this is probably of no clinical significance, although serum sodium levels may drop slightly. However, it may cause clinically important hyperkalemia in certain patients, such as those with diabetes[110] or renal failure.[111]

Heparin-associated elevations in transaminase levels are being recognized with increasing frequency. The increases occur more often in men, have no relation to whether the heparin is of bovine or porcine origin, and usually do not appear to be associated with clinical toxicity.[112] In our multicentered trial of DVT therapy, it was found that, one week after therapy with heparin alone, patients experienced a mean doubling of serum glutamic oxaloacetic transaminase levels. No similar trend in other measures of liver function (e.g., bilirubin, akaline phosphatase, lactic dehydrogenase) was observed.[101]

Warfarin Sodium
(see p. 1782)

OVERLAP WITH HEPARIN. In the early stage of warfarin administration, the level of protein C falls and this creates a thrombogenic potential. By the overlapping of heparin and warfarin for 4 to 5 days, this theoretically procoagulant effect of warfarin can be counteracted. It is our practice to overlap heparin and warfarin administration for at least 5 days. An Australian study of VTE patients treated everyone initially with heparin and randomly allocated patients to an "early warfarin" or "late warfarin" treatment group. The "early" group initiated warfarin on average after one day of hospitalization. The "late" group began warfarin after 7 days of continuous intravenous heparin. The efficacy and safety of heparin was similar in both groups, and early warfarin treatment shortened overall hospital stay by an average of 4 days.[113] These findings are consistent with the results of a more recent randomized trial at McMaster University. Patients with DVT were treated with either 5 days of heparin (with warfarin begun on the first day) or 10 days of heparin (with warfarin begun on the fifth day). The rate of recurrent DVT and bleeding was the same in both groups.[114] It is our practice to treat with 5 to 7 days of heparin and to initiate warfarin on the first or second hospital day.

DURATION AND INTENSITY OF THERAPY. Chronic anticoagulation is prescribed in PE to avert recurrent venous thromboembolism. In Phase I of UPET, one-fifth of the patients enrolled in the trial suffered recurrent PE during the first 2 weeks of therapy.[115] Recurrence appeared to correlate with lack of adequate intensity of anticoagulation. Although PE patients often receive chronic oral warfarin therapy for 6 months, its optimal duration and intensity are unknown. In patients with a transiently incurred risk for the development of PE, such as an operation, the utility of continuing anticoagulation indefinitely is probably low. However, for patients with a risk factor that is irreversible (i.e., metastatic cancer) or not easily modified (e.g., massive obesity), a stronger case can be made for continuing anticoagulants indefinitely.

The American College of Chest Physicians (ACCP) in conjunction with the National Heart, Lung, and Blood Institute (NHLBI) appointed a special panel to evaluate the indications for anticoagulation in a variety of cardiovascular illnesses. For venous thromboembolism (including DVT and PE) a therapeutic range for oral anticoagulation was determined in which the PT was prolonged 1.3 to 1.5 times the baseline value (using the Simplastin assay).[33] However, this recommendation, which we follow for DVT patients, is based on trials of DVT therapy[116] rather than PE (for which adequate trials are lacking). With regard to duration of therapy, the ACCP-NHLBI group recommended that patients with slowly resolving risk factors (e.g., prolonged immobilization) should be treated for at least 3 months, whereas patients with tumors, AT-III or protein C deficiency, or recurrent venous thromboembolism should be treated indefinitely. The panel implied that no more than 3 months of treatment was necessary for patients with risk factors that are readily reversible, such as estrogen use or transient immobilization.

We usually initiate warfarin therapy with 10 mg daily for 3 days and tend to treat patients with PE more aggressively than those with DVT, in terms of both intensity and duration of anticoagulation, maintaining the PT within the range of 16 to 20 seconds. If risk factors are transient, we treat with warfarin for one year. Otherwise, we advise indefinite anticoagulation.

COMPLICATIONS. The major toxic effect of warfarin is bleeding that tends to be proportional to the intensity of anticoagulation and may be increased by the presence of risk factors such as severe hepatic or renal disease, alcoholism, drug interactions, trauma, malignancy, and known previous bleeding sites in the gastrointestinal tract. A study at Brigham and Women's Hospital demonstrated that the risk of bleeding increases as the PT increases. Of 130 cases of bleeding, 38 per cent were due to remediable lesions, half of which were occult before warfarin administration.[117]

Major life-threatening bleeding requires immediate treatment with enough cryoprecipitate or fresh frozen plasma (FFP, usually 2 units) to normalize the PT and achieve immediate hemostasis.[100] To treat less serious bleeding, vitamin K may be administered parenterally; a dose of 10 mg subcutaneously or intramuscularly will usually reverse the effects of warfarin in 6 to 12 hours. However, this approach will make the patient's condition relatively refractory to warfarin for up to 2 weeks, so that reinstitution of warfarin becomes more difficult.

Minor bleeding with a prolonged PT may merely require interruption of warfarin therapy, without administration of FFP, until the PT has returned to the therapeutic range. If bleeding occurs when the PT is within the therapeutic range, occult malignancy should be suspected and ruled out. Evaluation of patients with minor bleeding and a PT above the therapeutic range is less productive. A study at Boston City Hospital showed that changing from Coumadin to generic warfarin was associated with increased morbidity and increased expense owing to widely fluctuating PT levels.[118] Our practice is to prescribe Coumadin.

Warfarin-induced skin necrosis[119] is a rare but important complication that may be related to a warfarin-induced reduction of protein C. In patients suspected of protein C deficiency, warfarin should be initiated with a lower dose than usual (e.g., 5 mg daily), with full heparin anticoagulation maintained until warfarin's therapeutic effect is achieved.

The "purple toes syndrome" is another rare complication of warfarin that appears to be caused by cholesterol microembolization.[120] In this syndrome, crystals are released from ulcerated atherosclerotic plaques. It appears that warfarin may worsen cholesterol microembolic disease by interfering with the healing of ulcerated atherosclerotic plaques. Therefore, warfarin should be discontinued in patients in whom the purple toes syndrome or other evidence of cholesterol microembolization develops.

During pregnancy, heparin should be used instead of warfarin because warfarin is associated with a 10-fold higher rate of congenital anomalies.[121] The fetus is particularly susceptible to warfarin embryopathy during the sixth through twelfth week of gestation.[122] The main features are saddle nose, nasal hypoplasia, frontal bossing, short stature, stippled epiphyses, optic atrophy, cataracts, mental retardation, and flexion contractures. Intracranial bleeding may also lead to secondary central nervous system deformities. We never prescribe warfarin during any portion of a pregnancy. If pregnancy is diagnosed after the sixth week of gestation, we counsel the parents about the risks of warfarin embryopathy, which occurs in 25 to 30 per cent of fetuses exposed during this vulnerable period of gestation.[122]

Although it was thought that women taking warfarin postpartum could not breast feed, it is now evident that breast feeding can be undertaken safely. The level of warfarin in breast milk is so low (25 ng/ml)[123] that it cannot be detected in the baby's plasma.[123,124]

PROTHROMBIN TIME CONTROL. Most warfarin is administered in the outpatient setting. Until recently, we adjusted the dosage of warfarin on the basis of the plasma PT. When the laboratory telephoned us with PT results, we had to contact patients to either reassure them that their dosing regimen was appropriate or make dosage adjustments. We found that it was quite difficult to explain changes in anticoagulation dosing by telephone. We can now make in-office assessments of warfarin dosing

with the Coumatrak (Dupont Co, Wilmington, DE), which provides the PT result in 2 minutes by use of a drop of whole blood obtained from a fingertip puncture.[125] Substantial saving of time has resulted, and patients have left the office with greater peace of mind and with a more accurate understanding of their warfarin dosing regimen. The Coumatrak has also been used at home by anticoagulated patients,[126] much like fingerstick glucose monitors in the management of diabetes mellitus.

THROMBOLYTIC THERAPY
(See also p. 1230 and 1785)

Streptokinase and Urokinase (First-Generation Agents)

Streptokinase (SK) and urokinase (UK) are proteins that indirectly (SK) or directly (UK) activate endogenous plasminogen to form plasmin, which actually lyses clot that has recently formed (Fig. 48–2). In almost all patients, a lytic state will rapidly develop with SK or UK. For SK, the standard regimen to treat PE is 250,000 IU over 30 minutes followed by 100,000 IU per hour for 24 hours. For UK, the standard dose is 4400 IU/kg (i.e., 2000 IU/lb/hr) over 10 minutes followed by 4400 IU/kg/hr (i.e., 2000 IU/lb/hr) for 12 to 24 hours. Although single-bolus therapy with UK has been proposed and appears promising,[127] experience with regimens such as 15,000 IU/kg over 10 minutes has been limited.[128]

Laboratory monitoring is directed toward verifying that the lytic state has been achieved, which is required for drug efficacy. In the presence of a lytic state, there is no need to titrate the dose. The lytic state can be verified by measuring increases in fibrin degradation products, thrombin time, whole blood euglobulin lysis time, PT, or PTT. Among patients with DVT who are treated with SK, an increase in the bleeding time may correlate with thrombolytic efficacy.[129] The most sensitive, widely available test is the thrombin time. Any one of these tests will suffice if the pretreatment value is normal and if a value obtained 4 or more hours after the initiation of fibrinolytic therapy is abnormal. In general, the dosage of the lytic agent can be doubled if a lytic state cannot be documented using standard regimens. Interestingly, the risk of bleeding from SK and UK has not been shown to correlate closely with any specific laboratory abnormality or with the dosage of the lytic agent.[130]

INDICATIONS AND CONTRAINDICATIONS. Whereas heparin acts primarily to prevent thrombus extension, thrombolytic agents promote dissolution of recently formed clots. Only three randomized trials comprising a total of 210 patients have compared SK or UK with heparin for PE treatment.[115,131,132]

In these trials, no reduction in mortality from PE was apparent with SK or UK, even though clots lysed more quickly when these agents were used. In two of the three studies, bleeding complications occurred more often after thrombolysis.[115,132] Increases in pulmonary capillary diffusing capacity and pulmonary capillary blood volume were demonstrated on 2-week and 1-year follow-up in patients treated with SK or UK as compared with heparin-treated patients.[133]

Many patients suspected of having PE receive heparin by continuous infusion while undergoing diagnostic evaluation. After a definitive diagnosis is established, the physician must decide whether to continue heparin anticoagulation or to interrupt heparin treatment for a course of thrombolytic therapy. For patients with venous thromboembolism, the benefit-to-risk ratio of thrombolytic agents is highest in those with massive PE; however, patients with moderate-sized or large emboli may also benefit from this treatment. Heparin should be discontinued several hours before thrombolytic therapy is initiated. Physical handling of the patient and arterial and venous punctures should be minimized because no thrombolytic agent can discriminate between "bad" clot due to PE and "good" clot required for normal hemostasis. Upon discontinuation of SK or UK, heparin should be given by continuous infusion without a loading dose when the thrombin time or

PTT decreases to approximately twice the control value. Contraindications to the use of SK or UK include intracranial or intraspinal disease, recent surgery, or trauma. However, we do not adhere to any upper age limit, and we do not consider the presence of cancer an exclusion criterion.

COMPLICATIONS. Trivial superficial oozing at venipuncture or arterial catheter insertion sites may be considered an index of drug efficacy rather than a complication of thrombolytic therapy. Such bleeding can be controlled with manual compression followed by a pressure dressing. In the UPET, severe bleeding, defined as the need for transfusion of more than 2 units of blood or a decrease in hematocrit of more than 10 points, occurred in 22 of the 82 (27 per cent) UK-treated patients in Phase I. The large amount of blood drawn during the first 24 hours of Phase I (about 200 ml) contributed to the fall in hematocrit; during Phase II,[134] fewer patients (12 per cent) had severe bleeding. In many instances, bleeding occurred at the vascular puncture sites for pulmonary angiography.

Of greatest concern is the risk of intracranial bleeding, which occurs in two to six of every 1000 patients treated with thrombolytic therapy. Retroperitoneal hemorrhage can also be life-threatening because the bleeding is often sustained and brisk, and the source often is difficult to locate. This complication can occur during the femoral catheterization if an artery is inadvertently punctured above the inguinal ligament. Genitourinary and other internal bleeding generally can be well managed; however, if internal bleeding is excessive, therapy should be discontinued. If bleeding is brisk or potentially life-threatening, 10 units of cryoprecipitate should be ordered from the blood bank. Each unit contains 200 to 500 mg of fibrinogen and 80 units of Factor VIII in a volume of 10 to 15 ml. A dose of 10 units will increase the fibrinogen level by about 70 mg/dl and the Factor VIII level by about 30 per cent of normally circulating levels. Cryoprecipitate can be thawed rapidly and should be available within 10 minutes of a request.

In addition, two units of fresh frozen plasma (FFP) should be ordered. FFP, which may take 45 minutes to thaw, is a source of Factors V and VIII as well as alpha $_2$-antiplasmin, fibrinogen, and other active coagulation factors.[100] Minor allergic reactions due to SK or (less often) UK occur occasionally and are manifested by fever and chills. To suppress this reaction, steroids, diphenhydramine (Benadryl), and acetaminophen can be administered prophylactically. If chills occur despite premedication, we have found 50 to 100 mg of intravenous meperidine to be quite effective in suppressing them.

Tissue Plasminogen Activator (t-PA)

(See also p. 1231)

In experimental canine and rabbit models of venous thrombosis, t-PA caused more fibrin-specific thrombolysis and less hemorrhage than did either UK or SK.[135] These experiments have served as the basis for clinical use of t-PA in patients with venous thromboembolism. Its use in acute PE was first reported in a 63-year-old man with massive PE (documented angiographically) who had undergone renal transplantation 5 weeks before t-PA treatment[136]; 30 mg (0.5 mg/kg) of t-PA was infused over 90 minutes through a catheter inserted into the right ventricle. The patient, who had been moribund, recovered dramatically.

In the authors' initial investigation, the short-term efficacy and safety of acutely administered t-PA in acute PE[137,138] were studied. Of 47 patients with angiographically documented PE, 44 had significant clot lysis after 2 to 6 hours of t-PA administered through a peripheral vein. Average pulmonary artery pressures decreased significantly after t-PA therapy, and lung scanning indicated marked improvement in pulmonary perfusion after treatment.[139] In some patients, right ventricular dysfunction and tricuspid regurgitation were documented by Doppler echocardiography before treatment but resolved rapidly after t-PA therapy.[140] In the authors' second PE Trial, the infusion time for t-PA was compressed from 6 to 2 hours. Patients were randomized to a fixed dose of t-PA (100 mg/2 h) or an FDA-approved 24-hour dose of weight-adjusted urokinase. t-PA achieved clot lysis more rapidly (Fig. 48–13A and Fig. 48–13B) and was safer.[141]

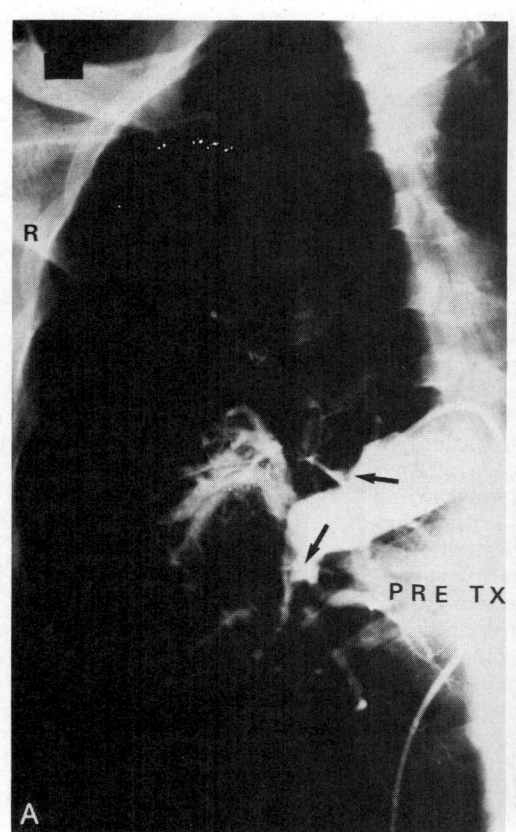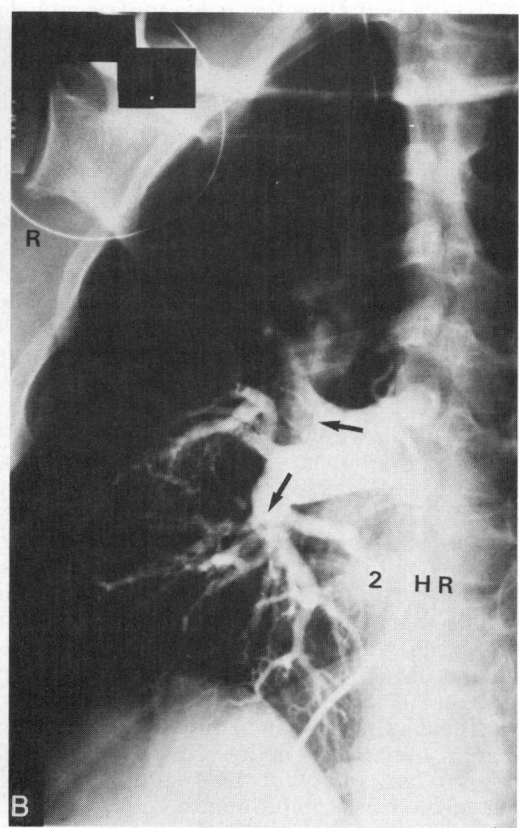

FIGURE 48–13. *A,* Baseline right lung pulmonary angiogram in a 58-year-old man with a 5-day history of dyspnea. Intraluminal clot is visualized in the right upper and lower lobe arteries (arrows) before treatment. The pulmonary artery pressure was 118/40 mm Hg with a mean PA pressure of 65 mm Hg. *B,* Follow-up pulmonary angiogram demonstrates moderate clot lysis immediately after a 2-hour course of peripheral intravenous t-PA administered in a dose of 100 mg as a continuous infusion. The pulmonary artery pressure is now 53/19 with a mean PA pressure of 34 mm Hg. There has been no change in the systemic arterial pressure. (From Goldhaber, S. Z., Kessler, C. M., Heit, J., et al.: A randomized controlled trial of recombinant tissue plasminogen activator versus urokinase in the treatment of acute pulmonary embolism. Lancet 2:293, 1988.)

Recently, Levine et al. published the results of a clinical trial[142] suggesting that weight-adjusted bolus t-PA (0.6 mg/kg ideal body weight with a maximum dose of 50 mg), administered over 2 minutes, can achieve comparable efficacy (assessed by pulmonary reperfusion on pre- and post-treatment perfusion lung scans) to the efficacy we achieved in our prior t-PA vs. urokinase trial[137] and to the pulmonary reperfusion observed in UPET.[115] No major bleeding episodes occurred with bolus t-PA, and there was an approximate one-third decrease from the baseline fibrinogen level at 30 minutes. The theory supporting bolus t-PA as safer than a prolonged infusion is that the bolus is cleared rapidly, thus preventing large amounts of circulating t-PA from interacting with the fibrinogen degradation products (FDPs) of the PE being lysed and therefore limiting the potential of the FDPs to promote fibrinogenolysis.[143-145] Other investigators have studied bolus t-PA in a rabbit jugular vein thrombosis model[146] and in a canine model of PE.[147-149]

Clozel et al.[146] found that the extent of thrombolysis was similar regardless of whether the same dose of t-PA was administered as a bolus or as a continuous 4-hour infusion. Prewitt's group found that the rate of thrombolysis is markedly increased with a 15-minute t-PA infusion compared with a 90-minute infusion, although the total clot lysis was similar in both sets of dogs.[147] However, they found in a subsequent study that a 15-minute t-PA infusion caused more thrombolysis than a 5-minute infusion.[148] This latter study suggests an upper limit to the dose-thrombolytic rate relation with t-PA. In an even more recent study,[149] Prewitt et al. found that a 15-minute infusion of 2 mg/kg of t-PA did not cause significantly more clot lysis than a 15-minute infusion of 1 mg/kg of t-PA. Thus, a bolus of t-PA appears to be a very promising treatment strategy for patients with PE. However, its safety and efficacy have not been tested in a randomized trial against the FDA-approved 100 mg/2 hr regimen of t-PA.

ANTICOAGULATION VS. THROMBOLYTIC THERAPY

Standard therapy for PE has employed heparin anticoagulation followed by warfarin, without thrombolytic therapy. The rationale for anticoagulation therapy is to provide prophylaxis against additional thromboembolic events while natural fibrinolytic mechanisms gradually lyse the previously formed pulmonary artery clot(s). In contrast, the rationale for thrombolytic therapy (followed by anticoagulation) is that thrombolysis actively dissolves clot that has already formed, thereby restoring cardiopulmonary function to normal as quickly as possible.[149a] Thrombolysis relieves the obstruction to pulmonary artery blood flow and thus improves right ventricular function and pulmonary perfusion and reduces pulmonary artery pressures. Lytic therapy may also improve pulmonary function over the long term,[133] may help prevent the development of chronic pulmonary hypertension, and may reduce the source of embolus in the peripheral venous system as well as in the pulmonary artery, thereby preventing recurrent PE.

For patients with major PE who are treated with anticoagulants alone, pulmonary artery clot may fail to resolve in 75 per cent after 1 to 4 weeks[150] and in 50 per cent after 4 months[151] of follow-up. In the UPET, the UK-treated patients initially exhibited significantly greater hemodynamic and anatomical improvement than the heparin-treated patients. However, 7 days after treatment, no difference between the two groups could be demonstrated on lung scans.[115] Unfortunately, no large-scale trial has yet been undertaken to determine whether thrombolytic therapy can reduce the mortality and recurrent PE rate compared with standard heparin treatment.

Although the Food and Drug Administration approved 24-hour SK and 12- to 24-hour UK in 1977 to treat PE, these agents are used only rarely for this condition, probably because of fear of bleeding complications. t-PA (100 mg/2 h) was approved by the FDA in 1990 for use in PE. In 1980, an NIH Consensus Development Conference[152] concluded that thrombolytic therapy was not being utilized often enough for patients with PE who (1) had obstruction of blood flow to a lobe or multiple pulmonary segments or (2) were hemodynamically compromised, regardless of the anatomical size of the PE.[152a] Nevertheless, use of thrombolytic therapy for PE has continued to languish. As of this writing, outside of a research setting, we advocate utilization of thrombolytic therapy according to these NIH guidelines.

ADJUNCTIVE MEDICAL THERAPY

Although the cornerstone of PE treatment involves anticoagulation or thrombolysis, adjunctive measures are also useful. Hypoxia should be treated with supplemental oxygen. In most cases, two to four liters of oxygen via nasal prongs will suffice, but the threshold for intubation and ventilatory support should be low. Right heart failure due to PE should be treated with alpha-range dopamine to alleviate hypotension, dobutamine to increase the cardiac index and stroke index,[153] and possibly amrinone[154] because of its vasodilatory and inotropic properties.

Discomfort due to PE can be intense and can cause chest wall splinting, making the patient susceptible to pneumonia and increased hypoxia owing to poor ventilation. Therefore, pain should be controlled aggressively, with either narcotic analgesia or nonsteroidal antiinflammatory agents. Despite the theoretical concern that nonsteroidal antiinflammatory agents might affect platelet function adversely and predispose to bleeding during anticoagulant or thrombolytic therapy, we use these antiinflammatory drugs liberally and find that they are often more effective than narcotics, presumably because the pleuritic pain of PE is due to inflammation. Fever often accompanies PE and not only should be suppressed with acetaminophen but also should lead to a search for accompanying infection, particularly pneumonia.

INFERIOR VENA CAVAL (IVC) INTERRUPTION

INDICATIONS. Most IVC interruption is undertaken with IVC filters, which normally can be inserted percutaneously by an interventional angiographer (Table 48-7). IVC ligation or external clips placed at laparotomy are rarely utilized. However, no randomized clinical trial has compared medical therapy with IVC interruption nor has any study been done to compare the different modes of IVC interruption (i.e., ligation, external clips, filters).[155,156] Certain disadvantages of IVC in-

TABLE 48-7 PERCUTANEOUS INSERTION OF INFERIOR VENAL CAVAL FILTERS

INDICATIONS

1. Anticoagulation contraindicated in patients with known pulmonary emboli:
   a. Bleeding, or known risk of bleeding (e.g., gastrointestinal)
   b. Patients with complications of anticoagulation (e.g., hemorrhage, heparin-induced thrombocytopenia)
2. Anticoagulation failure despite adequate therapy (e.g., recurrent pulmonary embolism)
3. Prophylactic for high-risk patients:
   a. Extensive or progressive deep vein thrombophlebitis
   b. Following surgical pulmonary embolectomy
   c. Severe pulmonary hypertension; cor pulmonale

CONTRAINDICATIONS (i.e., SURGICAL VENOTOMY PREFERRED)

1. Severe coagulopathy, predisposing to bleeding from the puncture site
2. Anticipated patient noncompliance with post-procedure rest orders (especially with a 24-French filter system)
3. Obstructing thrombus along the available route(s) of insertion

From Goldhaber, S. Z., and Grassi, C. J.: Management of pulmonary embolism. In Sabiston, D. C., Jr.: Textbook of Surgery. 14th ed. Philadelphia, W. B. Saunders Company. Update No. 8, pp. 115-127, 1990.

terruption devices should be recognized. First, anticoagulation should be continued whenever possible as adjunctive therapy to help prevent thrombosis at the site of the device and to help prevent limb DVT. Second, if the device becomes occluded with thrombus, large paravertebral venous collateral channels may develop and permit recurrent embolization. Third, it is unknown whether the currently employed interruption devices will cause long-term complications (i.e., perforation or migration). All other implanted devices, whether they be heart valves, pacemakers, or artificial hips, have a lifespan beyond which they require replacement or revision. Therefore, indications for IVC interruption in relatively young patients should be particularly stringent.

LIGATION. There are two possible indications for complete ligation of the inferior vena cava. One is septic embolization, since these emboli are usually small and would pass through all contemporary devices that maintain partial caval patency. In the presence of intravascular sepsis, no foreign material should be placed in the inferior vena cava. However, small emboli should theoretically have little difficulty traversing the collateral circulation around the ligated vessel, and patients with septic pelvic thrombophlebitis can almost always be treated successfully with heparin anticoagulation and antibiotics alone.[157] The second possible use of ligation is the rare case of documented or potential paradoxical emboli-

From Goldhaber, S. Z., and Grassi, C. J.: Management of pulmonary embolism. In Sabiston, D. C., Jr.: Textbook of Surgery. 14th ed. Philadelphia, W. B. Saunders Company. Update No. 8, pp. 115–127, 1990.

TABLE 48–8 THE "IDEAL" VENA CAVAL FILTER

1. Biocompatible, nonthrombogenic construction
2. High filtering efficiency (large and small emboli)
3. Does not impede flow (e.g., paraxial flow)
4. Rapid percutaneous insertion
   (a) Small caliber
   (b) Release mechanism sample and controlled
   (c) Amenable to repositioning
5. Secure fixation within the vena cava
6. Retrievability

zation[44] because of the devastating neurological effects of even a small paradoxical embolus.

EXTERNAL CLIPS. If a laparotomy is performed, the external clip, such as the Adams-DeWeese device, is preferred to ligation because of its fewer hemodynamic and venous complications and the low frequency of recurrent pulmonary embolization.[158]

TRANSVENOUS DEVICES (Fig. 48–14). Currently, no single type of filter device is ideal (Table 48–8). The Mobin-Uddin filter was used commonly from 1969 to 1977 but is no longer available in the United States. Although the recurrent

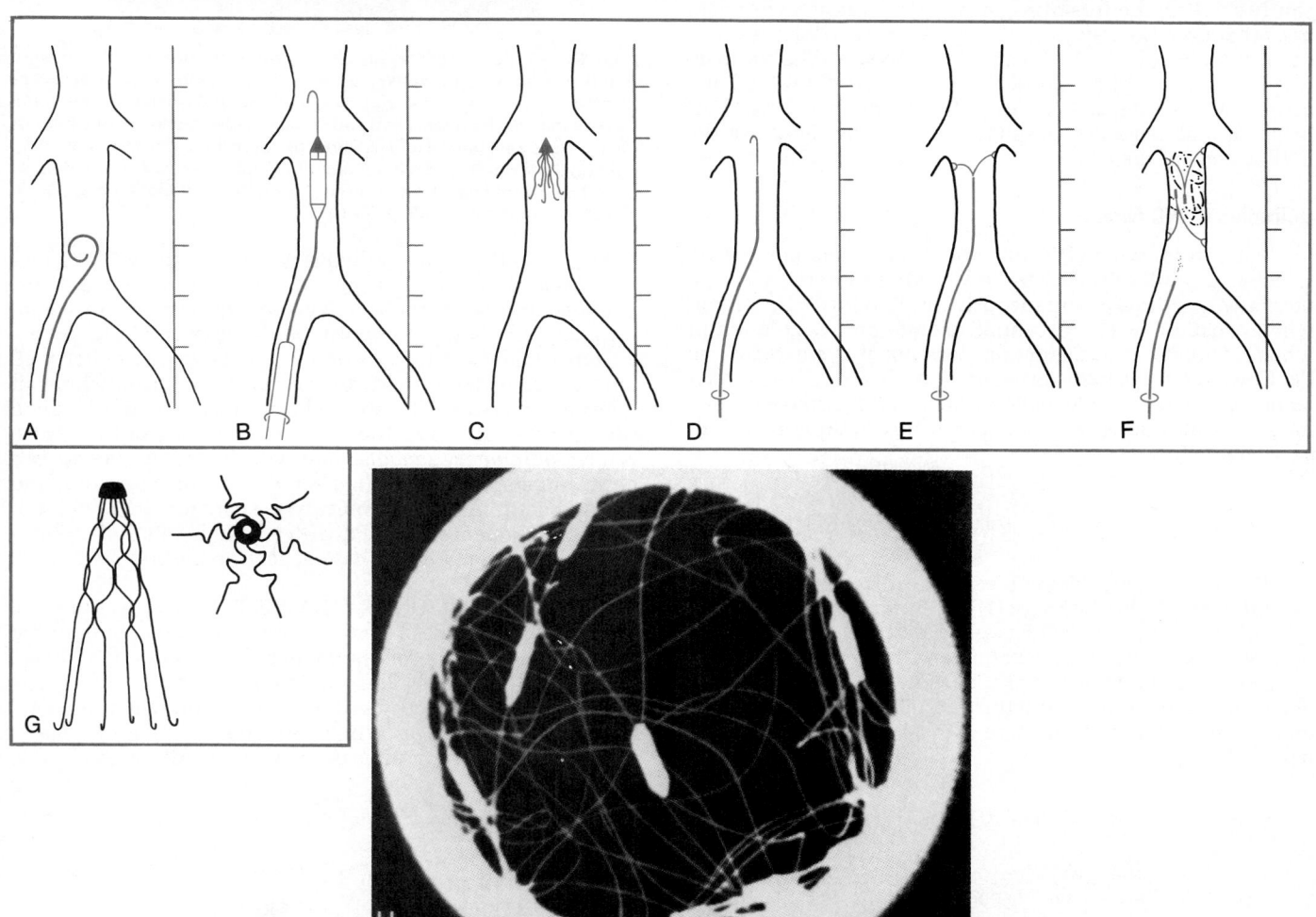

FIGURE 48–14. Technique for insertion of inferior vena caval filters. *A,* After the vena cavagram is completed with the pigtail catheter, *B,* the filter-introducer system is positioned. *C,* The stainless steel Greenfield filter is released just inferior to the renal veins; alternatively, the following procedure is undertaken if a Bird's Nest filter is preferred to a Greenfield filter. *D,* Following the cavagram, the free-form filter system is inserted over a guidewire, *E,* the Bird's Nest filter is positioned and fixation is started, and, *F,* the mesh is reformed below the renal veins, detached, and the introducer is withdrawn. *G,* Greenfield filter lateral (left hand panel) and axial (right hand panel) views. This device consists of six 0.15 inch stainless steel wires in a conical shape extending from a central hub. These wires form a cone with a maximal apical angle of 35 degrees, and the tips form a circular base with a maximum diameter of 30 mm. At the inferior ends, hooks engage the vena caval wall and prevent filter migration, with the filter apex directed cephalad. *H,* Bird's Nest filter in the axial view demonstrating the mesh-like shape. The filter wire mesh consists of a set of four 25 cm long 0.018 inch stainless steel wires which have preshaped random bends. These are fixed to proximal and distal V-struts, which affix the mesh to the vena caval wall. (From Goldhaber, S. Z., and Grassi, C. J.: Management of pulmonary embolism. *In* Sabiston, D. C., Jr.: Textbook of Surgery. 14th ed. Philadelphia, W.B. Saunders Company. Update No. 8, pp. 115–127, 1990.)

PE rate was low (0.5 per cent),[159,160] the frequency of IVC occlusion was high, up to 60 per cent. The Adams-DeWeese Teflon vena caval clip is available and is designed to narrow the IVC to four serrated transverse slits, 3 to 5 mm in diameter. However, it is rarely used at this time.

The Greenfield filter (GF) (Medi-Tech, Watertown, MA) (Fig. 48–14G), constructed of stainless steel, permits filling of 70 per cent of the filter cone by thrombus with a reduction in its effective cross-sectional area of only 50 per cent.[161,162] With the increased popularity of transfemoral radiological placement and a reported 10 to 24 per cent incidence of clinically symptomatic femoral vein thrombosis,[163,164] the main disadvantage of the GF has been its large 24 French introducer-sheath. Other complications include penetration of the vena caval wall by the filter foot prongs, filter tilting within the vena cava, retroperitoneal hemorrhage, and IVC occlusion in 3 to 5 per cent of cases.[162,164] The frequency of clinically evident recurrent PE averages 2 to 3 per cent.[162,165]

The Gianturco-Roehm Bird's Nest filter (BNF), in clinical trials since 1982 (Cook, Inc., Bloomington, IN), has a small sheath size, 12 French, with an 11 French preloaded filter catheter, thus avoiding the necessity of handling the filter.[166] After the formation of the filter, the wires resemble the shape of a bird's nest (Fig. 48–14H). The BNF design has several advantages over the GF. The introducer-sheath is significantly smaller; the freeform mesh of the filtration wire does not suffer from the requirements of centering within the vena caval lumen; and the BNF can accommodate IVCs up to 40 mm in diameter. The reported rate of recurrent PE is 2.7 per cent and the rate of IVC occlusion is 2.9 per cent.[166] At Brigham and Women's Hospital, we now routinely use the BNF instead of the GF.

Utilization of IVC Filters

Patients for whom IVC interruption is recommended are selected carefully (Table 48–7). We advise interruption (almost always with a percutaneously inserted Bird's Nest filter) when a patient with PE cannot tolerate anticoagulation or when adequate anticoagulation does not prevent recurrent PE. However, we usually do not employ these devices prophylactically in patients who have sustained a single large pulmonary embolus that is responding clinically to thrombolysis or anticoagulation.

PULMONARY EMBOLECTOMY

Pulmonary embolectomy can be utilized to treat PE in two different clinical settings: (1) during acute PE in the critically ill patient (i.e., when PE is associated with shock), and (2) to treat disabling dyspnea in patients with chronic pulmonary hypertension due to occult or recurrent PE. In patients with persistent right ventricular failure despite embolectomy, pulmonary artery counterpulsation with a balloon pump may be useful.[167]

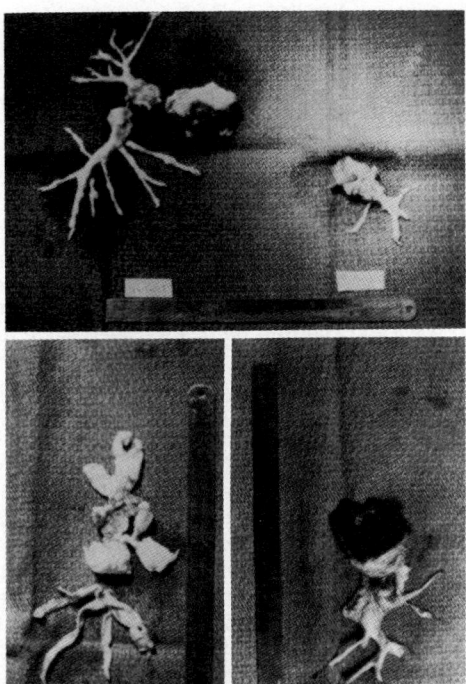

FIGURE 48–15. Large segments of chronic organized clot that were removed from the pulmonary arteries of two patients with excellent results (i.e., they improved from New York Heart Association functional class IV to I). Both patients had had complete obstruction of one pulmonary artery and partial obstruction of the other. (From Utley, J. R.: Pulmonary thromboendarterectomy. *In* Goldhaber, S. Z. (ed.): Pulmonary Embolism and Deep Venous Thrombosis. Philadelphia, W. B. Saunders Company, 1985, p. 278.)

ACUTE PE. Open pulmonary embolectomy[168] is associated with a mortality of approximately 30 per cent and normally should be reserved for patients in extremis in whom thrombolytic therapy is contraindicated or is failing. Embolectomy should also be considered in patients with massive PE due to right atrial or right ventricular thrombus in whom an inferior vena caval filter would be useless, particularly when thrombolytic agents fail to lyse these sources of PE. *Transvenous pulmonary embolectomy* with catheter suction is a promising approach[169,170] that requires further research and development. Another innovative approach involves mechanical fragmentation of PE with a flexible rotating tip catheter.[171] This latter strategy has not been applied clinically as of this writing.

CHRONIC PULMONARY HYPERTENSION (see also p. 790). Recurrent PE can lead to chronic, persistent pulmonary artery clot with attendant pulmonary hypertension, dyspnea, and cor pulmonale.[172] This major complication occurs most often when endogenous fibrinolysis fails and when the diagnosis of recurrent PE is initially overlooked and anticoagulation is withheld for months or even years. Although chronic

TABLE 48–9 AVERAGE HEMODYNAMIC VALUES IN 34 PATIENTS BEFORE AND IMMEDIATELY AFTER THROMBOENDARTERECTOMY AND AT FOLLOW-UP

	PREOPERATIVE	IMMEDIATELY POSTOPERATIVE	FOLLOW-UP*
Mean pulmonary artery pressure (mm Hg)	49	27	24
Mean pulmonary artery systolic press (mm Hg)	80	43	38
Cardiac output (L/min)	3.8	5.9	4.9
Pulmonary vascular resistance (dynes-sec-cm⁻⁵)	997	230	272

* Follow-up 3 months to 16 years after thromboendarterectomy.
Modified from Moser, K. M., Auger, W. R., and Fedullo, P. F.: Chronic major-vessel thromboembolic pulmonary hypertension. Circulation 81:1735, 1990, by permission of the American Heart Association.

obstruction of the pulmonary arteries can occur despite prompt anticoagulation, it is probably less frequent when thrombolysis is employed. Chronic pulmonary hypertension due to PE is usually refractory to anticoagulants and thrombolytic agents but can sometimes be managed with pulmonary thromboendarterectomy.[173,174] Surgical success leads to a dramatic reduction in symptoms, with associated improvements noted on lung scanning and pulmonary angiography. Pulmonary thromboendarterectomy produces an early marked reduction of pulmonary hypertension, which is often sustained (Table 48-9). There is an early reduction in the size of the pulmonary artery, right ventricle, right atrium, and inferior vena cava with a normalization of the interventricular septal position. This suggests that some changes in cardiac geometry may be afterload dependent and reversible soon after marked afterload reduction.[175,176] The results of embolectomy tend to

be most successful when an embolized thrombus can be removed in large segments that form a cast of the pulmonary vascular tree (Fig. 48-15). In the future, balloon angioplasty may be useful in treating some of these patients.[177]

INDICATIONS FOR PULMONARY EMBOLECTOMY. Despite progress in the technique of pulmonary embolectomy for PE, we regard this operation as a treatment of last resort. For acute massive PE, thrombolytic therapy should be attempted first unless there is an absolute contraindication to its use. For chronic PE, we would not recommend embolectomy unless progressive incapacity due to chronic pulmonary hypertension is well documented. The potential for postoperative rehabilitation must be good, and candidates must be willing to accept the risk of death or of failure to improve that accompanies this "high-stakes" operation.

Prevention of Pulmonary Embolism

RATIONALE

PE is difficult to diagnose, expensive to treat, and occasionally lethal despite therapy. Fortunately, a wide array of effective preventive techniques are available, including pharmacological, mechanical, and combined pharmacological and mechanical measures.[178] Until recently, these measures were widely underutilized. However, with the publication of the 1986 NIH Consensus Development Conference recommendations, the implementation of VTE prophylaxis has become mandatory, from a medicolegal viewpoint, among moderate- and high-risk hospitalized patients.[179] It appears that among postoperative patients, the risk of developing DVT persists after hospital discharge as well.[180] This problem is being addressed by use of prophylactic strategies, such as graduated compression stockings and low-dose warfarin, that are prescribed during the first month after hospital discharge.

PHARMACOLOGICAL AGENTS

LOW-DOSE HEPARIN. The most comprehensive randomized controlled trial of low-dose heparin (5000 units of subcutaneous heparin 2 hours preoperatively and every 8 hours thereafter for 7 days) as postoperative prophylaxis against fatal PE was organized by Kakkar in the International Multicentre Trial (IMT) involving 4121 patients.[181] Eligible patients were over age 40 and were scheduled to undergo elective major surgery. Of the autopsied subjects, 16 controls died of PE versus only two patients in the heparin group. Although more wound hematomas occurred among heparin-treated patients, the number of deaths due to hemorrhage was not increased among those who received heparin. Collins and colleagues have reviewed data from 78 randomized controlled trials with 15,598 patients that have confirmed the IMT result.[182] There was a 40 per cent reduction in nonfatal PE and 64 per cent reduction in fatal PE among heparin-treated patients. The heparin-treated patients also had about one-third as many instances of DVT as control patients, regardless of whether they had undergone general, urological, elective orthopedic, or traumatic orthopedic surgery. There was no significant difference in fatal hemorrhage between the heparin and control groups. Although excessive bleeding was more likely to occur among patients assigned to heparin therapy—especially those who underwent urological procedures—the absolute excess in bleeding was only about 2 per cent.

WARFARIN. In patients at high risk for DVT or PE, low- or moderate-dose warfarin may be appropriate. In a randomized trial at McMaster University, moderate-dose warfarin therapy (target PT of 16 to 18 seconds) reduced the frequency of DVT in patients who had undergone surgery for hip fractures.[185] We use warfarin routinely (in combination with intermittent pneumatic compression) for VTE prophylaxis among patients who undergo total hip replacement, total knee replacement, or osteotomy. Warfarin is initiated the evening before operating in a dose of 5 to 10 mg; 5 mg is given on the night of operation; the dose is then adjusted to achieve a target PT of 15 to 17 seconds. Warfarin is continued after discharge for approximately 1 month.

DEXTRAN. This glucose polymer impairs platelet function by causing decreased platelet aggregability. Dextran 40, with a mean molecular weight of 40,000 (known also as low molecular weight dextran), is approved for prophylaxis against venous thromboembolism. Potential adverse effects include anaphylaxis, volume overload, nephrotoxicity, and (ironically) bleeding. Dextran's efficacy appears comparable to that of

low-dose heparin.[183-184] Its particular niche appears to be among patients who require pharmacological VTE prophylaxis but who are unable to receive heparin because of a bleeding problem or previous adverse reaction to heparin, such as heparin-associated thrombocytopenia.

LOW MOLECULAR WEIGHT HEPARIN (LMWH). LMWH, not yet commercially available, has three major potential advantages over unfractionated heparin: (1) a lower frequency of heparin-associated thrombocytopenia, (2) effective prophylaxis with administration only once daily, and (3) a greater efficacy than unfractionated heparin. In a double-blind British study comparing LMWH with unfractionated heparin among 295 patients undergoing elective major abdominal surgery, the rate of DVT as detected on leg scanning with ^{125}I-labeled fibrinogen was 2.5 per cent among those who received LMWH compared with 7.5 per cent among those who received unfractionated heparin (p < 0.05).[187] LMWH is also very effective in preventing DVT among patients undergoing elective hip surgery.[188]

ASPIRIN. An overview of antiplatelet trials in the prevention of VTE indicates that antiplatelet therapy is effective in reducing the frequency of DVT by about one-third and in reducing the frequency of PE by about two thirds.[186] However, this finding has not been established in randomized controlled trials of aspirin that focus specifically upon PE as a primary endpoint. Therefore, further data are needed before long-term aspirin prophylaxis can be considered standard therapy for prevention of PE.

MECHANICAL MEASURES

GRADED ELASTIC COMPRESSION STOCKINGS. The most popular type of graded elastic compression is called a TED (thromboembolism-deterrent) stocking. Pressure exerted by the TED stocking is graded: 18 mm Hg at the ankle, 14 mm Hg at midcalf, 8 mm Hg in the popliteal region, 10 mm Hg at the lower thigh, and 8 mm Hg at the upper thigh. Thigh-high TED stockings reduce the frequency of DVT in general surgery patients[189] and appear to be cost-effective as well.[190]

INTERMITTENT PNEUMATIC COMPRESSION (IPC). Intermittent pneumatic compression of the legs (Fig. 48-16) has become an increasingly popular nonpharmacological method for preventing postoperative DVT. IPC devices expel blood from the legs, and the mechanical force may enhance fibrinolytic activity. To test this latter hypothesis, patients undergoing general surgery were randomized either to specially designed intermittent compression devices applied to the *arms* or no prophylaxis. Postoperatively, the frequency of *leg* DVT was assessed with fibrinogen leg scanning. Leg DVT developed in 32 per cent of the control group compared with 14 per cent of the group treated with intermittent arm compression. The reduction of distant thrombosis suggests that an increase in fibrinolytic activity is caused by IPC.[191]

IPC may be even more effective in preventing DVT when graduated compression stockings are used simultaneously.[192] Among patients who have undergone total hip replacement, thigh-high IPC using a sequential compression device has proved efficacy in halving the rate of proximal DVT, from 27 per cent to 14 per cent.[193] IPC has also been proved to be cost-effective in preventing DVT among patients undergoing major orthopedic surgery.[194]

INFERIOR VENA CAVAL (IVC) INTERRUPTION. Interruption of the IVC should be used prophylactically as a preoperative measure only under exceptional circumstances. Patients must be at high risk for PE (e.g., recent prior PE) and must have a contraindication to pharmacological prophylaxis (e.g., active gastrointestinal bleeding, chemotherapy-induced

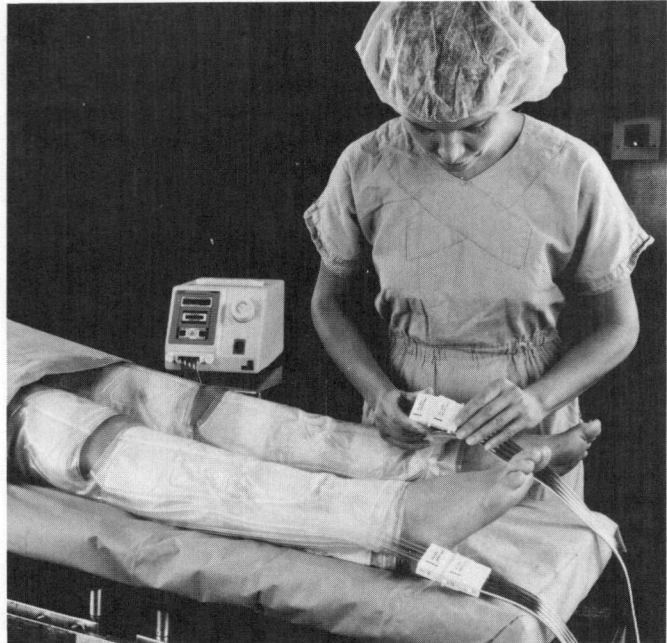

FIGURE 48–16. The Kendall Sequential Compression Device (SCD) expels blood from the legs, and its mechanical force may enhance fibrinolytic activity. The three compartments produce graded sequential compression of the ankles, calves, and thighs, with pressures of 35, 30, and 20 mm Hg, respectively, causing a 240 per cent increase in peak blood flow velocity.

thrombocytopenia, or neurosurgery) and to mechanical prophylaxis (e.g., recent DVT).

COMBINED MODALITIES. No prophylaxis strategy can abolish the risk of DVT. Therefore, combined modalities — especially combined pharmacological and mechanical measures — are useful in VTE prophylaxis, especially among high-risk patients. Among general surgical patients, the combination of heparin plus graduated compression stockings appears particularly effective both in individual trials[195] and in pooled overviews.[196] Among orthopedic surgical patients, the most frequently employed prophylaxis combination is IPC plus low- to moderate-dose warfarin.

RECOMMENDED APPROACH TO PROPHYLAXIS OF PULMONARY EMBOLISM

The NIH Consensus Development Conference on Prevention of Venous Thrombosis and PE has issued recommendations for many specific conditions.[179] Table 48–10 sets forth a general strategy for prevention of PE. However, the intensity of prophylaxis must be assessed separately for each patient on the basis of the patient's level of risk. Therefore, the particular recommendations in Table 48–10 are less important than the idea of providing VTE prophylaxis for every hospitalized patient at high or moderate risk.

SURGICAL PATIENTS

GENERAL SURGERY. Among patients over 40, the average frequency of DVT is 25 per cent based on fibrinogen leg scanning and 19 per cent based on venography in control patients who do not receive prophylaxis. Clinically significant PE occurs in approximately 1.6 per cent of the general surgical population.[179] The NIH Consensus statement recommends prophylaxis in all general surgical patients when any one of the following criteria apply:

- the patient is 40 years of age or older, *or*
- the patient will undergo a surgical procedure of more than 1 hour's duration, *or*
- the patient has cancer, *or*
- the patient has suffered prior PE or DVT

The recommended modality is heparin, 5000 units subcutaneously every 8 to 12 hours, beginning before operation and continuing at least until the patient is ambulatory. Alternative prophylactic modalities include dextran, IPC, and graded compression stockings. Our approach to prophylaxis consists of either graded compression stockings plus low-dose heparin or IPC (Table 48–10).

ORTHOPEDIC SURGERY. In hip surgery and knee reconstruction, DVT rates range from 45 to 70 per cent without prophylaxis. Among patients undergoing hip surgery or total knee replacement, the frequency of fatal PE is 1 to 3 per cent.[179,197] Our approach for lower extremity orthopedic surgery is to use both IPC and warfarin.

UROLOGICAL SURGERY. The overall risk of venous thromboembolism in urological surgery is 25 per cent, similar to that in general surgery. Open prostatectomy is associated with a rate of DVT of 40 per cent, whereas for transurethral prostatectomy the rate is 10 per cent.[179] For urological patients, we normally recommend IPC.

GYNECOLOGICAL SURGERY. The guidelines for prophylaxis in benign gynecological surgery are the same as for general surgery. However, patients with gynecological cancer should be considered at high risk for venous thromboembolism and may benefit from the combination of IPC plus warfarin.

NEUROSURGERY. The risk of PE and DVT in neurosurgical patients is similar to that in other surgical high-risk groups. For patients with intracranial or spinal cord lesions, even minor bleeding could have disastrous consequences. Therefore, IPC is recommended.

PREGNANCY. For pregnant women with prior VTE, we assess the level of risk and often attempt to avoid low-dose heparin because of its potential effect of bone demineralization. We recommend that pregnant women at high risk engage in 60 minutes per day of walking, biking, or swimming if feasi-

TABLE 48–10   STRATEGY FOR PE PROPHYLAXIS

CONDITION	STRATEGY
Orthopedic or gynecological cancer surgery	IPC plus low-dose Coumadin
General surgery for patients with prior VTE, cancer, or obesity	IPC *or* graded-compression stockings plus low-dose subcutaneous heparin
General or urological surgery (without prior VTE) or gynecologic surgery for benign condition	Graded-compression stockings plus low-dose subcutaneous heparin *or* IPC
Neurosurgery, eye surgery, or other surgery for patients in whom pharmacological prophylaxis is contraindicated	Graded-compression stockings ± IPC
Pregnancy with prior VTE	Antepartum: graded-compression stockings plus daily exercise program plus serial leg examinations *or* subcutaneous heparin Peripartum: intermittent pneumatic compression plus low-dose subcutaneous heparin Postpartum: Coumadin for 6 weeks
Medical conditions	Graded-compression stockings ± low-dose subcutaneous heparin *or* IPC

IPC = intermittent pneumatic compression; VTE = venous thromboembolism.

ble. We prescribe maternity-style graded compression stockings with high compression levels of 30 to 40 mm Hg. We have these women return for frequent follow-up evaluation during the pregnancy with emphasis on leg examination and ultrasonographic testing. For women who are at very high risk of VTE or who are unable to comply with an exercise program and frequent office visits, we prescribe prophylactic subcutaneous heparin.

MEDICAL PATIENTS

The general medical population has been the least studied group with regard to DVT. These patients are frequently immobilized for prolonged periods; those who have cancer are likely to be hypercoagulable. For patients with nonhemorrhagic stroke, we usually employ IPC; for other medical patients, such as those with chronic congestive heart failure, we usually prescribe graded compression stockings and/or low-dose heparin.

REFERENCES

PATHOPHYSIOLOGY OF PULMONARY EMBOLISM

1. Gillum, R. F.: Pulmonary embolism and thrombophlebitis in the United States, 1970–1985. Am. Heart J. 114:1262, 1987.
2. Anderson, F. A., Jr., Wheeler, H. B., Goldberg, R. J., et al.: A population-based perspective of the incidence and case-fatality rates of venous thrombosis and pulmonary embolism: The Worcester DVT study. Arch. Intern. Med. (in press).
3. Goldhaber, S. Z.: Pulmonary embolism death rates. Am. Heart J. 115:1342, 1988.
4. Goldman, L., Sayson, R., Robbins, S., et al.: The value of the autopsy in three medical eras. N. Engl. J. Med. 308:1000, 1983.
4a. Pulmonary Embolism. In Fowler, N. O.: Diagnosis of Heart Disease. New York, Springer-Verlag, 1991, pp. 283–291.
5. Virchow, R.: Gesammelte Abhandlungen zur Wissenschaftlichen Medizin. Frankfurt, Meidinger Sohn, 1856, p. 219.
6. Schafer, A. L.: The hypercoagulable states. Ann. Intern. Med. 102:814, 1985.
7. Clouse, L. H., and Comp, P. C.: The regulation of hemostasis: The protein C system. N. Engl. J. Med. 314:1298, 1986.
8. Stead, N. W., Bauer, K. A., Kinney, T. R., et al.: Venous thrombosis in a family with defective release of vascular plasminogen activator and elevated plasma factor VIII/von Willebrand's factor. Am. J. Med. 74:33, 1983.
9. Pizzo, S. V., Fuchs, H. E., Doman, K. A., et al.: Release of tissue plasminogen activator and its fast-acting inhibitor in defective fibrinolysis. Arch. Intern. Med. 146:188, 1986.
10. Branch, D. W., Scott, J. R., Kochenour, N. K., and Hershgold, E.: Obstetric complications associated with lupus anticoagulant. N. Engl. J. Med. 313:1322, 1985.
11. Petri, M., Rheinschmidt, M., Whiting-O'Keefe, Q., et al.: The frequency of lupus anticoagulant in systemic lupus erythematosus. A study of 60 consecutive patients by activated partial thromboplastin time, Russell viper venom time, and anticardiolipin antibody level. Ann. Intern. Med. 106:524, 1987.
12. Triplett, D. A., Brandt, J. T., Musgrave, K. A., and Orr, C. A.: The relationship between lupus anticoagulants and antibodies to phospholipid. JAMA 259:550, 1988.
13. Alving, B. M., Barr, C. F., and Tang, D. B.: Correlation between lupus anticoagulants and anticardiolipin antibodies in patients with prolonged activated partial thromboplastin times. Am. J. Med. 88:112, 1990.
14. Gladson, C. L., Scharrer, I., Hach, V., et al.: The frequency of type I heterozygous protein S and protein C deficiency in 141 unrelated young patients with venous thrombosis. Thromb. Haemost. 59:18, 1988.
15. Goldhaber, S. Z., Savage, D. D., Garrison, R. J., et al.: Risk factors for pulmonary embolism: The Framingham Study. Am. J. Med. 74:1023, 1983.
16. Gore, J. M., Appelbaum, J. S., Greene, H. L., et al.: Occult cancer in patients with acute pulmonary embolism. Ann. Intern. Med. 96:556, 1982.
17. Goldberg, R. J., Seneff, M., Gore, J. M., et al.: Occult malignancy in patients with deep venous thrombosis. Arch. Intern. Med. 147:251, 1987.
18. Goldhaber, S. Z., Buring, J. E., and Hennekens, C. H.: Cancer and venous thromboembolism. Arch. Intern. Med. 147:216, 1987.
19. Dixon, J. E.: Pregnancies complicated by previous thromboembolic disease. Br. J. Hosp. Med. 37:449, 1987.
20. Sachs, B. P., Brown, D.A.J., Driscoll, S. G., et al.: Maternal mortality in Massachusetts: Trends and prevention. N. Engl. J. Med. 316:667, 1987.
21. Anderson, A. J., Krasnow, S. H., Boyer, M. W., et al.: Hickman catheter clots: A common occurrence despite daily heparin flushing. Cancer Treat. Rep. 71:651, 1987.
22. Anderson, A. J., Krasnow, S. H., Boyer, M. W., et al.: Thrombosis: The major Hickman catheter complication in patients with solid tumor. Chest 95:71, 1989.

23. Farfel, Z., Shecter, M., Vered, Z., et al.: Review of echocardiographically diagnosed right heart entrapment of pulmonary emboli-in-transit with emphasis on management. Am. Heart J. 113:171, 1987.
24. Huisman, M. V., Buller, H. R., ten Cate, J. W., et al.: Unexpected high prevalence of silent pulmonary embolism in patients with deep venous thrombosis. Chest 95:498, 1989.
25. Doyle, D. J., Turpie, A.G.G., Hirsh, J., et al.: Adjusted subcutaneous heparin or continuous intravenous heparin in patients with acute deep vein thrombosis: A randomized trial. Ann. Intern. Med. 107:441, 1987.
26. Lensing, A.W.A., Prandoni, P., Brandjes, D., et al.: Detection of deep-vein thrombosis by real-time B-mode ultrasonography. N. Engl. J. Med. 320:342, 1989.
27. Polak, J. F., Cutler, S. S., and O'Leary, D. H.: Deep veins of the calf: Assessment with color Doppler flow imaging. Radiology 171:481, 1989.
28. Hull, R. D., Hirsh, J., Carter, C. J., et al.: Diagnostic efficacy of impedance plethysmography for clinically suspected deep-vein thrombosis: A randomized trial. Ann. Intern. Med. 102:21, 1985.
29. Huisman, M. V., Buller, H. R., ten Cate, J. W., and Vreeken, J.: Serial impedance plethysmography for suspected deep venous thrombosis in outpatients. The Amsterdam General Practitioner Study. N. Engl. J. Med. 314:823, 1986.
30. Lagerstedt, C. I., Olsson, C. -G., Fagher, B. O., et al.: Need for long-term anticoagulant treatment in symptomatic calf-vein thrombosis. Lancet 2:515, 1985.
31. Hull, R. D., Raskob, G. E., Hirsh, J., et al.: Continuous intravenous heparin compared with intermittent subcutaneous heparin in the initial treatment of proximal-vein thrombosis. N. Engl. J. Med. 315:1109, 1986.
32. Strandness, D. E., Langlois, Y., Cramer, M., et al.: Long-term sequelae of acute venous thrombosis. JAMA 250:1289, 1983.
33. Hyers, T. M., Hull, R. D., and Weg, J. G.: Antithrombotic therapy for venous thromboembolic disease. Chest 95:37S, 1989.
34. Visner, M. S., Arentzen, C. E., O'Connor, M. D., et al.: Alterations in left ventricular three-dimensional dynamic geometry during acute right ventricular hypertension in the conscious dog. Circulation 67:353, 1983.
35. Belenkie, I., Dani, R., Smith, E. R., and Tyberg, J. V.: Ventricular interaction during experimental acute pulmonary embolism. Circulation 78:761, 1988.
36. Jardin, F., Dubourg, O., Gueret, P., et al.: Quantitative two-dimensional echocardiography in massive pulmonary embolism: Emphasis on ventricular interdependence and leftward septal displacement. J. Am. Coll. Cardiol. 10:1201, 1987.
37. Manny, J., and Hechtman, H. B.: Vasoactive humoral factors. In Goldhaber, S. Z. (ed.): Pulmonary Embolism and Deep Venous Thrombosis. Philadelphia, W.B. Saunders Company, 1985, p. 283.

DIAGNOSIS OF PULMONARY EMBOLISM

38. Goldhaber, S. Z.: Strategies for diagnosis. In Goldhaber, S. Z. (ed.): Pulmonary Embolism and Deep Venous Thrombosis. Philadelphia, W.B. Saunders Company, 1985, p. 79.
39. Stein, P. D., Willis, P. W. III, and DeMets, D. L.: History and physical examination in acute pulmonary embolism in patients without preexisting cardiac or pulmonary disease. Am. J. Cardiol. 47:218, 1981.
40. Rich, S., Levitsky, S., and Brundage, B. H.: Pulmonary hypertension from chronic pulmonary thromboembolism. Ann. Intern. Med. 108:425, 1988.
41. Rich, S., Dantzker, D. R., Ayres, S. M., et al.: Primary pulmonary hypertension: A national prospective study. Ann. Intern. Med. 107:216, 1987.
42. Newman, J. H., and Ross, J. D.: Primary pulmonary hypertension: A look at the future. J. Am. Coll. Cardiol. 14:551, 1989.
43. Simpson, R. J., Jr., Podolak, R. P., Mangano, C. A., Jr., et al.: Vagal syncope during recurrent pulmonary embolism. J.A.M.A. 249:390, 1983.
44. Loscalzo, J.: Paradoxical embolism: Clinical presentation, diagnostic strategies, and therapeutic options. Am. Heart J. 112:141, 1986.
45. Lechat, P., Mas, J. L., Lascault, G., et al.: Prevalence of patent foramen ovale in patients with stroke. N. Engl. J. Med. 318:1148, 1988.
46. Tsao, M. S., Schraufnagel, D., and Wang, N. -S.: Pathogenesis of pulmonary infarction. Am. J. Med. 72:599, 1982.
47. Adler, D. S.: Nonthrombotic pulmonary embolism. In Goldhaber, S. Z. (ed.): Pulmonary Embolism and Deep Venous Thrombosis. Philadelphia, W.B. Saunders Company, 1985, p. 209.
48. Goldhaber, S. Z., Dricker, E., Buring, J. E., et al.: Clinical suspicion of autopsy-proven thrombotic and tumor pulmonary embolism in cancer patients. Am. Heart J. 114:1432, 1987.
49. Sperry, K.: Amniotic fluid embolism: To understand an enigma. JAMA 255:2183, 1986.
50. Cvitanic, O., and Marino, P. L.: Improved use of arterial blood gas analysis in suspected pulmonary embolism. Chest 95:48, 1989.
51. Overton, D. T., and Bocka, J. J.: The alveolar-arterial oxygen gradient in patients with documented pulmonary embolism. Arch. Intern. Med. 148:1617, 1988.
52. Bynum, L. J., and Wilson, J. E. III: Characteristics of pleural effusions associated with pulmonary embolism. Arch. Intern. Med. 136:159, 1976.
53. Stein, P. D., Dalen, J. E., McIntyre, K. M., et al.: The electrocardiogram in acute pulmonary embolism. Prog. Cardiovasc. Dis. 17:247, 1975.
54. Goldhaber, S. Z., Vaughan, D. E., Tumeh, S. S., and Loscalzo, J.: Utility of cross-linked fibrin degradation products in the diagnosis of pulmonary embolism. Am. Heart J. 116:505, 1988.

55. Burki, N. K.: The dead space to tidal volume ratio in the diagnosis of pulmonary embolism. Am. Rev. Respir. Dis. 133:679, 1986.

56. Markisz, J. A.: Radiologic and nuclear medicine diagnosis. In Goldhaber, S. Z. (ed.): Pulmonary Embolism and Deep Venous Thrombosis. Philadelphia, W.B. Saunders Company, 1985, p. 41.

57. Hampton, A. O., and Castleman, B.: Correlation of postmortem chest teleroentgenograms with autopsy findings with special reference to pulmonary embolism and infarction. A.J.R. 43:305, 1940.

58. Woodruff, W. W. III, Hoeck, B. E., Chitwood, W. R., Jr., et al.: Radiographic findings in pulmonary hypertension from unresolved embolism. A.J.R. 144:681, 1985.

58a. Kelley, M. A., Carson, J. L., Palevsky, H. I., and Schwartz, J. S.: Diagnosing pulmonary embolism: New facts and strategies. Ann. Intern. Med. 114:300, 1991.

59. Hull, R. D., Raskob, G. E., Coates, G., and Panju, A. A.: Clinical validity of a normal perfusion lung scan in patients with suspected pulmonary embolism. Chest 97:23, 1990.

60. Hull, R. D., Hirsh, J., Carter, C. J., et al.: Diagnostic value of ventilation-perfusion lung scanning in patients with suspected pulmonary embolism. Chest 88:819, 1985.

61. The PIOPED Investigators: Value of the ventilation/perfusion scan in acute pulmonary embolism: Results of the prospective investigation of pulmonary embolism diagnosis (PIOPED). JAMA 263:2753, 1990.

61a. Stein, P. D., Alavi, A., Gottschalk, A., et al.: Usefulness of noninvasive diagnostic tools for diagnosis of acute pulmonary embolism in patients with a normal chest radiograph. Am. J. Cardiol. 67:1117, 1991.

62. Ryan, K. L., Fedullo, P. F., Davis, G. B., et al.: Perfusion scan findings understate the severity of angiographic and hemodynamic compromise in chronic thromboembolic pulmonary hypertension. Chest 93:1180, 1988.

63. Kramer, F. L., Teitelbaum, G., and Merli, G. J.: Panvenography and pulmonary angiography in the diagnosis of deep venous thrombosis and pulmonary thromboembolism. Radiol. Clin. North Am. 24:397, 1986.

64. Perlmutt, L. M., Braun, S. D., Newman, G. E., et al.: Pulmonary arteriography in the high-risk patient. Radiology 162:187, 1987.

65. Wood, D. L., Osborn, M. J., Rooke, J., and Holmes, D. R.: Amiodarone pulmonary toxicity: Report of two cases associated with rapidly progressive fatal adult respiratory distress syndrome after pulmonary angiography. Mayo Clin. Proc. 60:901, 1985.

66. Low osmolality contrast agents. Med. Lett. 31:85, 1989.

67. Nicod, P., Peterson, K., Levine, M., et al.: Pulmonary angiography in severe chronic pulmonary hypertension. Ann. Intern. Med. 107:565, 1987.

68. Meyerovitz, M.: How to maximize the safety of coronary and pulmonary angiography in patients receiving thrombolytic therapy. Chest 97:132S, 1990.

69. Cassling, R. J., Lois, J. F., and Gomes, A. S.: Unusual pulmonary angiographic findings in suspected pulmonary embolism. A.J.R. 145:995, 1985.

70. Walsh, P. N., Greenspan, R. H., Simon, M., et al.: An angiographic severity index for pulmonary embolism. Circulation 47:II-101, 1973.

71. Miller, G.A.H., Sutton, G. C., Kerr, I.I.H., et al.: Comparison of streptokinase and heparin in treatment of isolated acute massive pulmonary embolism. Br. Med. J. 2:681, 1971.

72. Simon, M., Sharma, G.V.R.K., and Sasahara, A.A.: An angiographic method for quantitating the severity of pulmonary embolism and the effects of therapy. Int. Angiol. 3:389, 1984.

73. Kasper, W., Meinertz, T., Henkel, B., et al.: Echocardiographic findings in patients with proved pulmonary embolism. Am Heart J. 112:1284, 1986.

74. Nixdorff, E., Erbel, R., Drexler, M., and Meyer, J.: Detection of thromboembolus of the right pulmonary artery by transesophageal two-dimensional echocardiography. Am. J. Cardiol. 61:488, 1988.

75. Come, P. C.: Echocardiographic recognition of pulmonary arterial disease and determination of its cause. Am. J. Med. 84:384, 1988.

76. Goldhaber, S. Z.: Optimal strategy for diagnosis and treatment of pulmonary embolism due to right atrial thrombus. Mayo Clin. Proc. 63:1261, 1988.

77. Pond, G. D.: Pulmonary digital subtraction angiography. Radiol. Clin. North Am. 23:243, 1985.

78. Mussett, D., Rosso, J., Petitprez, P., et al.: Acute pulmonary embolism: Diagnostic value of digital subtraction angiography. Radiology 166:455, 1988.

79. Chintapalli, K., Thorsen, M. K., Olson, D. L., et al.: Computed tomography of pulmonary thromboembolism and infarction. J. Comput. Assist. Tomogr. 12:553, 1988.

80. Balakrishnan, J., Meziane, M. A., Siegelman, S. S., and Fishman, E. K.: Pulmonary infarction: CT appearance with pathologic correlation. J. Comput. Assist. Tomogr. 13:941, 1989.

81. Szucs, R. A., Rehr, R. B., and Tatum, J. L.: Pulmonary artery thrombus detection by magnetic resonance imaging. Chest 95:232, 1989.

82. Posteraro, R. H., Sostman, H. D., Spritzer, C. E., and Herfkens, R. J.: Cine-gradient-refocused MR imaging of central pulmonary emboli. A.J.R. 152:465, 1989.

83. Ezekowitz, M. D., Pope, C. F., Sostman, H. D., et al.: Indium-111 platelet scintigraphy for the diagnosis of acute venous thrombosis. Circulation 73:668, 1986.

84. Clarke-Pearson, D. L., Coleman, R. E., Siegel, R., et al.: Indium-111 platelet imaging for the detection of deep venous thrombosis and pulmonary embolism in patients without symptoms after surgery. Surgery 98:98, 1985.

85. Ezekowitz, M. D., Pope, C. F., and Smith, E. O.: Indium-111 platelet imaging. In Goldhaber, S. Z. (ed.): Pulmonary Embolism and Deep Venous Thrombosis. Philadelphia, W. B. Saunders Company, 1985, p. 261.

86. Farlow, D. C., Ezekowitz, M. D., Rao, S. R., et al.: Early image acquisition after administration of indium-111 platelets in clinically suspected deep venous thrombosis. Am. J. Cardiol. 64:363, 1989.

87. Jung, M., Kletter, K., Dudczak, R., et al.: Deep vein thrombosis: Scintigraphic diagnosis with in-111-labeled monoclonal antifibrin antibodies. Radiology 173:469, 1989.

88. Fry, E.T.A., Mack, D. L., Monge, J. C., et al.: Labeling of human clots in vitro with an active-site mutant of t-PA. J. Nucl. Med. 30:187, 1990.

89. Shure, D., Gregoratos, G., and Moser, K. M.: Fiberoptic angioscopy: Role in the diagnosis of chronic pulmonary arterial obstruction. Ann. Intern. Med. 103:844, 1985.

TREATMENT OF PULMONARY EMBOLISM

90. Barritt, D. W., and Jordan, S. C.: Anticoagulant drugs in the treatment of pulmonary embolism. A controlled trial. Lancet 1:1309, 1960.

91. Basu, D., Gallus, A., Hirsh, J., and Cade, J.: A prospective study of the value of monitoring heparin treatment with the activated partial thromboplastin time. N. Engl. J. Med. 287:324, 1972.

92. Wheeler, A. P., Jaquiss, R.D.B., and Newman, J. H.: Physician practices in the treatment of pulmonary embolism and deep venous thrombosis. Arch. Intern. Med. 148:1321, 1988.

93. Beaver, B. L., Young, D., and Satiani, B.: Prediction of heparin requirements in acute thromboplastic venous disease. Arch. Surg. 120:436, 1985.

94. Hirsh, J., van Aken, W. G., Gallus, A. S., et al.: Heparin kinetics in venous thrombosis and pulmonary embolism. Circulation 53:691, 1976.

95. Ginsberg, J. S., Kowalchuk, G., Hirsh, J., et al.: Heparin therapy during pregnancy. Arch. Intern. Med. 149:2233, 1989.

96. Brabeck, M. C.: Ambulatory management of thromboembolic disease during pregnancy with continuous infusion heparin. JAMA 257:1790, 1987.

97. Barss, V. A., Schwartz, P. A., Greene, M. F., et al.: Use of the subcutaneous heparin pump during pregnancy. J. Reprod. Med. 30:899, 1985.

98. Landefeld, C. S., Cook, E. F., Flatley, M., et al.: Identification and preliminary validation of predictors of major bleeding in hospitalized patients starting anticoagulant therapy. Am. J. Med. 82:703, 1987.

99. Olin, J. W., Young, J. R., Graor, R. A., et al.: Treatment of deep vein thrombosis and pulmonary emboli in patients with primary and metastatic brain tumors. Arch. Intern. Med. 147:2177, 1987.

100. Sane, D. C., Califf, R. M., Topol, E. J., et al.: Bleeding during thrombolytic therapy for acute myocardial infarction: Mechanisms and management. Ann. Intern. Med. 111:1010, 1989.

101. Goldhaber, S. Z., Meyerovitz, M. F., Green, D., et al.: Randomized controlled trial of tissue plasminogen activator in proximal deep venous thrombosis. Am. J. Med. 88:235, 1990.

102. Rao, A. K., White, G. C., Sherman, L., et al.: Low incidence of thrombocytopenia with porcine mucosal heparin. Arch. Intern. Med. 149:1285, 1989.

103. Stead, R. B., Schafer, A. I., Rosenberg, R. D., et al.: Heterogeneity of heparin lots associated with thrombocytopenia and thromboembolism. Am. J. Med. 77:185, 1984.

104. Rankin, J. A.: Heparin-induced thrombosis (white clot syndrome) secondary to prophylactic subcutaneous administration of heparin. Can. J. Surg. 31:33, 1988.

105. Kelly, R. A., Gelfand, J. A., and Pincus, S. H.: Cutaneous necrosis caused by systemically administered heparin. JAMA 246:1582, 1981.

106. Cimo, P. L., Moake, J. L., Weinger, R. S., et al.: Heparin-induced thrombocytopenia: Association with a platelet aggregating factor and arterial thromboses. Am. J. Hematol. 6:125, 1976.

107. Squires, J. W., and Pinch, L. W.: Heparin-induced spinal fractures. JAMA 241:2417, 1979.

108. de Swien, M., Ward, P. D., Fidler, J., et al.: Prolonged heparin therapy in pregnancy causes bone demineralization. Br. J. Obstet. Gynaecol. 90:1129, 1983.

109. O'Kelly, R., Magee, F., and McKenna, T. J.: Routine heparin therapy inhibits adrenal aldosterone production. J. Clin. Endocrinol. Metab. 56:108, 1983.

110. Phelps, K. R., Oh, M. S., and Carroll, H. J.: Heparin-induced hyperkalemia: Report of a case. Nephron 25:254, 1980.

111. Leekey, D., Gantt, C., and Lim, V.: Heparin-induced hypoaldosteronism —Report of a case. JAMA 246:2189, 1981.

112. Dukes, G. E., Sanders, S. W., Russo, J., et al.: Transaminase elevations in patients receiving bovine or porcine heparin. Ann. Intern. Med. 100:646, 1984.

113. Gallus, A., Jackaman, J., Tillett, J., et al.: Safety and efficacy of warfarin started early after submassive venous thrombosis or pulmonary embolism. Lancet 2:1293, 1986.

114. Hull, R. D., Raskob, G. E., Rosenbloom, D., et al.: Heparin for 5 days as compared with 10 days in the initial treatment of proximal venous thrombosis. N. Engl. J. Med. 322:1260, 1990.

115. Urokinase Pulmonary Embolism Trial: A National Cooperative Study. Circulation 47 and 48(Suppl. II):1, 1973.

116. Hull, R., Hirsh, J., Jay, R., et al.: Different intensities of oral anticoagulant therapy in the treatment of proximal-vein thrombosis. N. Engl. J. Med. 307:1676, 1982.

117. Landefeld, C. S., Rosenblatt, M. W., and Goldman, L.: Bleeding in outpatients treated with warfarin: Relation to the prothrombin time and important remediable lesions. Am. J. Med. *87*:153, 1989.

118. Richton-Hewett, S., Foster, E., and Apstein, C. S.: Medical and economic consequences of a blinded oral anticoagulant brand change at a municipal hospital. Arch. Intern. Med. *148*:806, 1988.

119. Broekmans, A. W., Bertina, R. M., Leoliger, E. A., et al.: Protein C and the development of skin necrosis during anticoagulant therapy. Thromb. Haemost. *49*:251, 1983.

120. Hyman, B. T., Landas, S. K., Ashman, R. F., et al.: Warfarin-related purple toes syndrome and cholesterol microembolization. Am. J. Med. *82*:1233, 1987.

121. Hall, J. G., Pauli, R. M., and Wilson, K. M.: Maternal and fetal sequelae of anticoagulation during pregnancy. Am. J. Med. *68*:122, 1980.

122. Iturbe-Alessio, I., Fonseca, M.D.C., Mutchinik, O., et al.: Risks of anticoagulant therapy in pregnant women with artificial heart valves. N. Engl. J. Med. *315*:1390, 1986.

123. Orme, M.L'E., Lewis, P. J., de Swiet, M., et al.: May mothers given warfarin breast-feed their infants? Br. Med. J. *1*:1564, 1977.

124. McKenna, R., Cole, E. R., and Vasan, U.: Is warfarin sodium contraindicated in the lactating mother? J. Pediatr. *103*:325, 1983.

125. Lucas, F. V., Duncan, A., Jay, R., et al.: A novel whole blood capillary technic for measuring the prothrombin time. Am. J. Clin. Pathol. *88*:442, 1987.

126. Ansell, J., Holden, A., and Knapic, N.: Patient self-management of oral anticoagulation guided by capillary (fingerstick) whole blood prothrombin times. Arch. Intern. Med. *149*:2509, 1989.

127. Dickie, K. J., de Groot, W. J., Cooley, R. N., et al.: Hemodynamic effects of bolus infusion of urokinase in pulmonary thromboembolism. Am. Rev. Respir. Dis. *109*:48, 1974.

128. Petipretz, P., Simmoneau, G., Cerrina, J., et al.: Effects of a single bolus of urokinase in patients with life-threatening pulmonary embolism: A descriptive trial. Circulation *70*:861, 1984.

129. Hirsch, D. R., and Goldhaber, S. Z.: The bleeding time: Its potential utility among patients receiving thrombolytic therapy. Am. Heart J. *119*:158, 1990.

130. Stead, R. B.: Clinical pharmacology. *In* Goldhaber, S. Z. (ed.): Pulmonary Embolism and Deep Venous Thrombosis. Philadelphia, W. B. Saunders Company, 1985, p. 99.

131. Tibbutt, D. A., Davies, J. A., Anderson J. A., et al.: Comparison by controlled clinical trial of streptokinase and heparin in treatment of life-threatening pulmonary embolism. Br. Med. J. *1*:343, 1974.

132. Ly, B., Arnesen, H., Eie, H., and Hol, R.: A controlled clinical trial of streptokinase and heparin in the treatment of major pulmonary embolism. Acta Med. Scand. *203*:465, 1978.

133. Sharma, G.V.R.K., Burleson, V. A., and Sasahara, A. A.: Effect of thrombolytic therapy on pulmonary-capillary blood volume in patients with pulmonary embolism. N. Engl. J. Med. *303*:842, 1980.

134. Urokinase-Streptokinase Embolism Trial: Phase 2 results. A cooperative study. JAMA *229*:1606, 1974.

135. Agnelli, G., Buchanan, M. R., Fernandez, F., et al.: A comparison of the thrombolytic and hemorrhagic effects of tissue-type plasminogen activator and streptokinase in rabbits. Circulation *72*:178, 1985.

136. Bounameaux, H., Vermylen, J., and Collen, D.: Thrombolytic treatment with recombinant tissue-type plasminogen activator in a patient with massive pulmonary embolism. Ann. Intern. Med. *103*:64, 1985.

137. Goldhaber, S. Z., Vaughan, D. E., Markis, J. E., et al.: Acute pulmonary embolism treated with tissue plasminogen activator. Lancet *2*:886, 1986.

138. Goldhaber, S. Z., Meyerovitz, M. F., Markis, J. E., et al.: Thrombolytic therapy of acute pulmonary embolism: Current status and future potential. J. Am. Coll. Cardiol. *10*:96B, 1987.

139. Parker, J. A., Markis, J. E., Palla, A., et al.: Pulmonary perfusion after rt-PA therapy for acute embolism: Early improvement assessed with segmental perfusion scanning. Radiology *166*:441, 1988.

140. Come, P. C., Kim, C., Parker, J. A., et al: Early reversal of right ventricular dysfunction in patients with acute pulmonary embolism after treatment with intravenous tissue plasminogen activator. J. Am. Coll. Cardiol. *10*:971, 1987.

141. Goldhaber, S. Z., Kessler, C. M., Heit, J., et al.: A randomized controlled trial of recombinant tissue plasminogen activator versus urokinase in the treatment of acute pulmonary embolism. Lancet *2*:293, 1988.

142. Levine, M. N., Hirsh, J., Weitz, J., et al.: A randomized trial of a single bolus dosage regimen of recombinant tissue plasminogen activator in patients with acute pulmonary embolism. Chest *98*:1473, 1990.

143. Agnelli, G.: The rationale for bolus t-PA therapy to improve efficacy and safety. Chest *97*:161S, 1990.

144. Agnelli, G., Buchanan, M. R., Fernandez, F., et al: Sustained thrombolysis with DNA-recombinant tissue type plasminogen activator in rabbits. Blood *66*:399, 1985.

145. Agnelli, G., Buchanan, M. R., Fernandez, F., and Hirsh, J.: The thrombolytic and hemorrhagic effects of tissue type plasminogen activator: Influence of dosage regimens in rabbits. Thromb. Res. *40*:769, 1985.

146. Clozel, J-P., Tschopp, T., Luedin, E., and Holvoet, P.: Time course of thrombolysis induced by intravenous bolus or infusion of tissue plasminogen activator in a rabbit jugular vein thrombosis model. Circulation *79*:125, 1989.

147. Shiffman, F., Ducas, J., Hollett, P., et al.: Treatment of canine embolic pulmonary hypertension with recombinant tissue plasminogen activator: Efficacy of dosing regimes. Circulation *78*:214, 1988.

148. Prewitt, R. M., Shiffman, F., Greenberg, D., et al.: Recombinant tissue-type plasminogen activator in canine embolic pulmonary hypertension. Effects of bolus versus short-term administration on dynamics of thrombolysis and on pulmonary vascular pressure-flow characteristics. Circulation *79*:929, 1989.

149. Prewitt, R. M., Hoy, C., Kong, A., et al.: Thrombolytic therapy in canine pulmonary embolism. Comparative effects of urokinase and recombinant tissue plasminogen activator. Am. Rev. Respir. Dis. *141*:290, 1990.

149a. Goldhaber, S. Z.: Recent advances in the diagnosis and lytic therapy of pulmonary embolism. Chest *99*:1735, 1991.

150. Dalen, J. E., Banas, J. S., Brooks, H. L., et al.: Resolution rate of acute pulmonary embolism in man. N. Engl. J. Med. *280*:1194, 1969.

151. Tow, D. E., and Wagner, N. H., Jr.: Recovery of pulmonary artery flow in patients with pulmonary embolism. N. Engl. J. Med. *276*:1053, 1967.

152. Thrombolytic Therapy in Thrombosis: A National Institutes of Health Consensus Development Conference. Ann. Intern. Med. *93*:141, 1980.

152a. Mitchell, J. P., and Trulock, E. P.: Tissue plasminogen activator for pulmonary embolism resulting in shock: Two case reports and discussion of the literature. Am. J. Med. *90*:255, 1991.

153. Jardin, F., Genevray, B., Brun-Ney, D., and Margairaz, A.: Dobutamine: A hemodynamic evaluation in pulmonary embolism shock. Crit. Care Med. *13*:1009, 1985.

154. Spence, T. H., and Newton, W. D.: Pulmonary embolism: Improvement in hemodynamic function with amrinone therapy. South. Med. J. *82*:1267, 1989.

155. Grassi, C. J., and Goldhaber, S. Z.: Interruption of the inferior vena cava for prevention of pulmonary embolism: Transvenous filter devices. Herz *14*:182, 1989.

156. Goldhaber, S. Z., Buring, J. E., Lipnick, R. J., and Hennekens, C. H.: Interruption of the inferior vena cava by clip or filter. Am. J. Med. *76*:512, 1984.

157. Josey, W. E., and Staggers, S. R.: Heparin therapy in septic pelvic thrombophlebitis. A study of 46 cases. Am. J. Obstet. Gynecol. *120*:228, 1974.

158. Askew, A. R., and Gardner, A.M.N.: Long-term follow-up of partial caval occlusion by clip. Am. J. Surg. *140*:441, 1980.

159. Mobin-Uddin, K., Utley, J. R., and Bryant, L. R.: The inferior vena cava umbrella filter. Prog. Cardiovasc. Dis. *17*:391, 1975.

160. McIntyre, A. B., McCready, R. A., Hyde, G. L., and Mattingly, W.: A ten-year follow-up study of the Mobin-Uddin filter for vena cava interruption. Surg. Gynecol. Obstet. *158*:513, 1984.

161. Greenfield, L. J., and Michna, B. A.: Twelve-year clinical experience with the Greenfield vena caval filter. Surgery *104*:706, 1988.

162. Messmer, J. M., and Greenfield, L. J.: Greenfield caval filters: Long-term radiographic follow-up study. Radiology *156*:613, 1985.

163. Kantor, A., Glanz, S, Gordon, D. H., and Sclafani, S.J.A: Percutaneous insertion of the Kimray-Greenfield filter: Incidence of femoral vein thrombosis. A.J.R. *149*:1065, 1987.

164. Pais, S. O., Mirvis, S. E., and De Orchis, D. F.: Percutaneous insertion of the Kimray-Greenfield filter: Technical considerations and problems. Radiology *165*:377, 1987.

165. Geisinger, M. A., Zelch, M. G., and Risius, B.: Recurrent pulmonary emboli after Greenfield filter placement. Radiology *165*:383, 1987.

166. Roehm, J.O.F., Johnsrude, I. S., Barth, M. H., and Gianturco, C.: The Bird's Nest inferior vena cava filter: Progress report. Radiology *168*:745, 1988.

167. Gold, J. P., Shemin, R. J., DiSesa, V. J., et al.: Balloon pump support of the failing right heart. Clin. Cardiol. *8*:599, 1985.

168. Gray, H. H., Morgan, J. M., Paneth, M., and Miller, G.A.H.: Pulmonary embolectomy for acute massive pulmonary embolism: An analysis of 71 cases. Br. Heart J. *60*:196, 1988.

169. Moore, J. H., Jr., Koolpe, H. A., Carabasi, R. A., et al.: Transvenous catheter pulmonary embolectomy. Arch. Surg. *120*:1372, 1985.

170. Feitelberg, S. P., Kahn, S. E., Kotler, M. N., et al.: Transfemoral embolectomy for massive pulmonary embolus and associated myocardial infarction. Am. Heart J. *113*:819, 1987.

171. Stein, P. D., Sabbah, H. N., Basha, M. A., et al.: Mechanical fragmentation of pulmonary thromboemboli in dogs by means of a flexible rotating tip catheter (Kensey catheter). J. Am. Coll. Cardiol. *15*:189A, 1990.

172. Rich, S., Levitsky, S., and Brundage, B. H.: Pulmonary hypertension from chronic pulmonary thromboembolism. Ann. Intern. Med. *108*:425, 1988.

173. Chitwood, W. R., Jr., Lyerly, H. K., and Sabiston, D. C., Jr.,: Surgical management of chronic pulmonary embolism. Ann. Surg. *201*:11, 1985.

174. Moser, K. M., Daily, P. O., Peterson, K., et al.: Thromboendarterectomy for chronic, major-vessel thromboembolic pulmonary hypertension. Immediate and long-term results in 42 patients. Ann. Intern. Med. *107*:560, 1987.

175. Dittrich, H. C., Nicod, P. H., Chow, L. C., et al.: Early changes of right heart geometry after pulmonary thromboendarterectomy. J. Am. Coll. Cardiol. *11*:937, 1988.

176. Moser, K. M., Auger, W. R., Fedullo, P. F.: Chronic major-vessel thromboembolic pulmonary hypertension. Circulation *81*:1735, 1990.

177. Voorburg, J.A.I., Cats, V. M., Buis, B., and Bruschke, A.V.G.: Balloon angioplasty in treatment of pulmonary hypertension caused by pulmonary embolism. Chest *94*:1249. 1988.

PREVENTION OF PULMONARY EMBOLISM

178. Goldhaber, S. Z.: Venous thromboembolism: How to prevent a tragedy. Hospital Practice *23*:164, 1988.

179. NIH Consensus Development Statement. Prevention of venous thrombosis and pulmonary embolism. JAMA 256:744, 1986.

180. Scurr, J. H., Coleridge-Smith, P. D., and Hasty, J. H.: Deep venous thrombosis: A continuous problem. Br. Med. J. 297:28, 1988.

181. An International Multicentre Trial: Prevention of fatal postoperative pulmonary embolism by low doses of heparin. Lancet 2:45, 1975.

182. Collins, R., Scrimgeour, A., Yusuf, S., and Peto, R.: Reduction in fatal pulmonary embolism and venous thrombosis by perioperative administration of subcutaneous heparin: Overview of results of randomized trials in general, orthopedic, and urologic surgery. N. Engl. J. Med. 318:1162, 1988.

183. Bergqvist, D.: Dextran in the prophylaxis of deep-vein thrombosis. JAMA 258:324, 1987.

184. Ljungstrom, K. G.: The antithrombotic efficacy of dextran. Acta Chir. Scand. 543:26, 1988.

185. Powers, P. J., Gent, M., Jay, R. M., et al.: A randomized trial of less intense postoperative warfarin or aspirin therapy in the prevention of venous thromboembolism after surgery for a fractured hip. Arch. Intern. Med. 149:771, 1989.

186. Anti-platelet Trialists Collaboration: Personal communication.

187. Kakkar, V. V.: Prevention of post-operative venous thromboembolism by a new low molecular weight heparin fraction. Nouv. Rev. Fr. Hematol. 26:277, 1984.

188. Turpie, A.G.G., Levine, M. N., Hirsh, J., et al.: A randomized controlled trial of low-molecular-weight heparin (enoxaparin) to prevent deep-vein thrombosis in patients undergoing elective hip surgery. N. Engl. J. Med. 315:925, 1986.

189. Allan, A., Williams, J. T., Bolton, J. P., and Le Quesne, L. P.: The use of graduated compression stockings in the prevention of postoperative deep vein thrombosis. Br. J. Surg. 70:172, 1983.

190. Oster, G., Tuden, R. L., and Colditz, G. A.: Prevention of venous thromboembolism after general surgery. Cost-effectiveness analysis of alternative approaches to prophylaxis. Am. J. Med. 82:889, 1987.

191. Knight, M.T.N., and Dawson, R.: Effect of intermittent compression of the arms on deep venous thrombosis in the legs. Lancet. 2:1265, 1976.

192. Scurr, J. H., Coleridge-Smith, P. D., and Hasty, J. H.: Regimen for improved effectiveness of intermittent pneumatic compression in deep venous thrombosis prophylaxis. Surgery 102:816, 1987.

193. Hull, R. D., Raskob, G. E., Gent, M., et al.: Effectiveness of intermittent pneumatic leg compression for preventing deep vein thrombosis after total hip replacement. JAMA 263:2313, 1990.

194. Oster, G., Tuden, R. L., and Colditz, G. A.: A cost-effectiveness analysis of prophylaxis against deep-vein thrombosis in major orthopedic surgery. JAMA 257:203, 1987.

195. Wille-Jorgensen, P., Thorup, J., Fischer, J. A., et al.: Heparin with and without graded compression stockings in the prevention of thromboembolic complications of major abdominal surgery: A randomized trial. Br. J. Surg. 72:579, 1985.

PROPHYLAXIS

196. Colditz, G. A., Tuden, R. L., and Oster, G.: Rates of venous thrombosis after general surgery: Combined results of randomized clinical trials. Lancet 2:143, 1986.

197. Foley, F., Maslack, M. M., Rothman, R. H., et al.: Pulmonary embolism after hip or knee replacement: Postoperative changes on pulmonary scintigrams in asymptomatic patients. Radiology 172:481, 1989.

Cor Pulmonale

by E. REGIS McFADDEN, Jr., M.D., and EUGENE BRAUNWALD, M.D.

Chronic cor pulmonale is defined as a combination of hypertrophy and dilatation of the right ventricle (RV) secondary to pulmonary hypertension; the latter is caused by disease of the pulmonary parenchyma and/or pulmonary vascular system between the origins of the main pulmonary artery and the entry of the pulmonary veins into the left atrium.[1] *Acute cor pulmonale* is defined as acute right heart strain or overload resulting from the pulmonary hypertension that usually follows massive pulmonary embolism. Cor pulmonale encompasses many disease states with diverse etiologies, pathophysiological mechanisms, and clinical characteristics that have in common only a disturbance of the pulmonary circulation.[2] This chapter focuses on those conditions that produce pulmonary hypertension by acting primarily on the gas-exchanging, neuromuscular, and ventilatory control functions of the respiratory system. Primary pulmonary hypertension and pulmonary thromboembolism, two important causes of cor pulmonale, are discussed in Chaps. 27 and 49, respectively.

ANATOMICAL AND PATHOPHYSIOLOGICAL CORRELATES

RIGHT VENTRICULAR ANATOMY

For the first 3 months of life in infants born at or near sea level, the RV is larger and heavier and has a greater end-diastolic volume than the left.[3,7] With advancing age, the left ventricle (LV) becomes dominant, and in the adult, the right ventricular wall is relatively thin and has a crescentic configuration on cross section. However, in high-altitude dwellers, the situation is different. The degree of RV preponderance, both at birth and for the first 3 months of life, is greater than that seen in low-altitude residents, and the normal regression in size is so delayed that right ventricular enlargement can persist through the first decade.[6] In native adults living above 12,000 feet, 93 per cent of the hearts in a necropsy series showed some degree of right ventricular enlargement.[8] These morphological findings have a close relationship to the hemodynamic characteristics of persons at high altitudes and can be related to the degree of pulmonary arterial hypertension.[9]

Several methods may be used to ascertain the characteristics, presence, and severity of right ventricular hypertrophy; the two traditional methods involve the measurement of ventricular weight and wall thickness. Many investigators believe that wall thickness determinations are not sufficiently precise. Fulton et al. have provided weight criteria that are used widely.[10] In their technique, the RV is dissected free, and the septum is weighed together with the LV. Right ventricular weight can then be described in absolute terms or as a ratio of the LV plus the septum (S) [i.e., (LV + S)/RV]. Using these criteria, a heart is considered normal only if the total ventricular weight is less than 250 gm, the free wall of the RV weighs less than 65 gm in men and 50 gm in women, and the ratio of (LV + S)/RV is between 2.3 : 1 and 3.3 : 1. If left ventricular hypertrophy also is present,

the ratio may be within normal limits or even raised. Using this method, Mitchell and colleagues found that the upper limits of normal (as defined by the mean plus 2 standard deviations) in men 40 or more years of age at death were 69 gm for the RV and 203 gm for the LV plus septum. These observers also noted that in their study, right ventricular thickness was a relatively poor index of hypertrophy.[11]

Others have determined muscle fiber size morphometrically and found the distribution of myocardial fiber diameters to be uniform, with a distinct bell-shaped distribution noted for the RV, LV, and septum.[12] In cases of pure RV hypertrophy, the distribution always shifted, so that the mean diameter of the muscle fibers from the RV exceeded that of the septum or normal LV. An example of an enlarged RV in cor pulmonale is shown in Figure 49–1.

RIGHT VENTRICULAR FUNCTION

Because RV hypertrophy occurs most commonly in association with longstanding elevations in pulmonary arterial pressures, an analogy often has been made between the LV in systemic hypertension and the RV in pulmonary hypertension. Because there is no fundamental difference in either the configuration or the pumping action of the two ventricles before birth, the differences that exist in the adult have been attributed to the flow resistances in the respective circula-

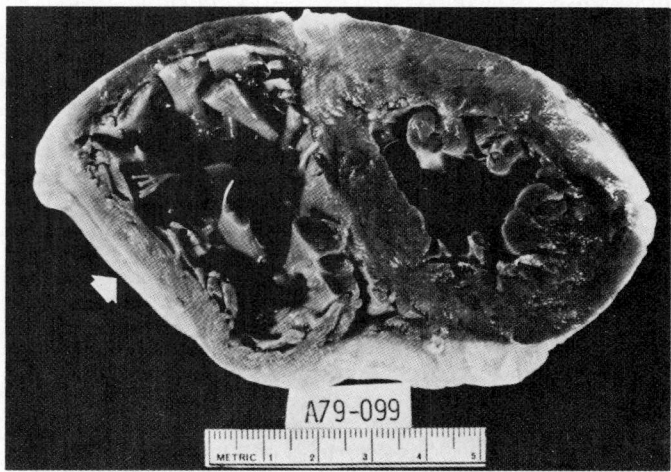

FIGURE 49–1. Cor pulmonale, heart cut in cross section. Notice the rounded contour of the right ventricular cavity (indicated by arrow), which is typical of dilation. The normal right ventricle is a crescent-shaped thin-walled structure. Both hypertrophy and dilatation of the right ventricle are present in this case. (From Taylor, W. E.: Pathology of pulmonary heart disease. In Rubin, L. J. [ed.]: Pulmonary Heart Disease. Boston, Martinus Nijhoff, 1984, p. 65.)

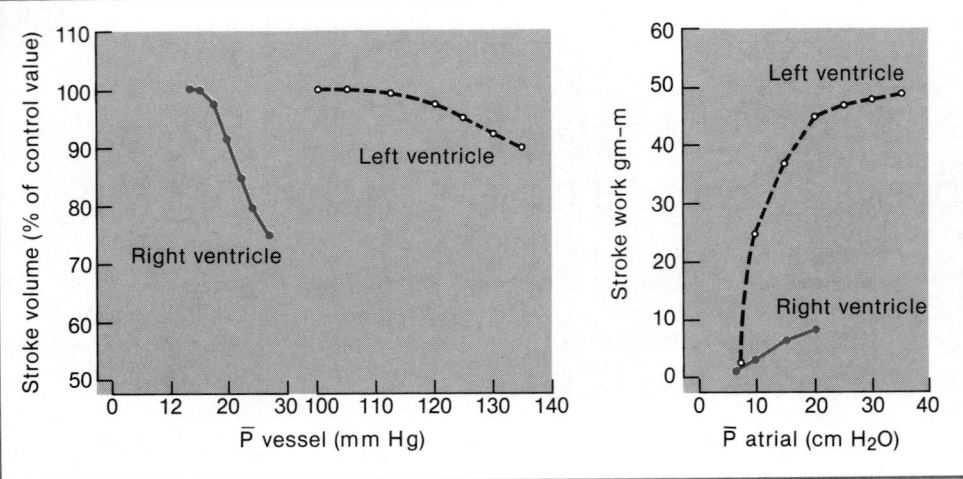

FIGURE 49-2. Effects of increasing preload and afterload on right and left ventricular function. The data in the left panel were obtained by constricting the main pulmonary artery and aorta in dogs. The right panel demonstrates the effect of increasing preloads. RV = right ventricle; LV = left ventricle.

tions.[13] As already noted, the normal adult RV has thin walls and a crescentic shape; its pumping action is akin to that of a bellows working in series with a low-pressure circuit, in contrast to the concentric contraction of the left ventricle.[13-15] Because it is much thinner than the LV, the RV is more compliant,[16] and in comparison with the left, it is better able to handle an increase in volume than in pressure load. The evidence in support of this statement is derived in the main from animal data[17-20] (Fig. 49-2), which contrast the effects of increasing preload and afterload on right and left ventricular function. In the left-hand panel, stroke volume is plotted as a function of various afterloads that were produced by actively constricting the main pulmonary artery and aorta in the dog.[17,18] Small increments in pulmonary artery pressure are associated with sharp decreases in RV stroke volume. In contrast, the LV, which normally works against high initial pressures, continues to maintain stroke volume despite substantial increases in systemic arterial pressure.

The right-hand portion of this figure demonstrates the effects of increasing preload. These ventricular function curves were obtained by volume infusions into the atria of dogs.[20] Note the marked differences in the respective ventricular stroke work that occur as right and left atrial pressures are increased. For a fourfold elevation in filling pressure (i.e., from 5 to 20 cm H_2O), the increase in left ventricular work was about five times that of the right.

In response to chronic pressure loads, significant changes develop in the configuration, mass, and functional characteristics of the RV. The rate at which these occur in humans and the magnitude of the pressures needed to produce them are unknown. Animal studies indicate that alterations in structure and function can be quite rapid after experimental outflow tract obstruction. Spann et al. observed a 71 per cent increase in right ventricular weight in cats 2 days after the pulmonary artery was banded, and within a month, right ventricular weight had risen by 150 per cent of control.[21] Response may not be as rapid in humans but is qualitatively similar.

The lumen of the main pulmonary artery can be reduced acutely by 60 to 80 per cent before aortic pressure declines as a consequence of a fall in cardiac output.[22-24] Because these experiments ignored the effects of neurohumoral compensations that support the systemic circulation, the impression has arisen that the acute right ventricular response is an abrupt, all-or-none event. However, as suggested in Figure 49-2, right ventricular decompensation is really a continuum.[17,20] At right ventricular systolic pressures of 60 to 80 mm Hg, right ventricular dilatation and failure occur with systemic hypotension and hypoperfusion.[25] The rate and/or absolute level of outflow tract obstruction at which these alterations develop can be greatly amplified or attenuated by respectively decreasing or increasing right coronary artery blood flow.[25] The relative roles played by changes in coronary blood flow in acute right heart failure in humans have yet to be determined.

PULMONARY VASCULAR ANATOMY

WALL STRUCTURE. Starting from the pulmonary artery and proceeding distally toward the capillaries, four structural regions can be identified: elastic, muscular, partially muscular, and nonmuscular[29] (Fig. 27-8, p. 800). In keeping with its embryological derivation, the main pulmonary artery and the first five generations are elastic in nature but less so than the aorta and major systemic arteries. These vessels, by definition, have more than five elastic laminae in their media and are more than 2000 μm in diameter in the adult. In the axial pathway, the next three generations are said to be transitional.

Muscular arteries have between 2 and 5 elastic laminae and a continuous muscle coat. These arteries form the majority of vessels in the lung and are found in a diameter range of 150 to 2000 μm in the adult. The medial muscle coat is very thin compared with the arterioles in the systemic circulation. These vessels give way to partially muscular arteries in which the muscle is arranged in a spiral, so that in cross section it appears as a crescent, with the rest of the wall being like a capillary. Nonmuscular arteries are larger than capillaries and range from 30 to 75 μm in diameter in adults. Partially muscular and nonmuscular arteries all lie within the alveolar units in adults. The smallest muscular and partially muscular arteries are thought to represent the resistance arteries.[29]

Although there is great variation in the sizes of arteries that accompany conducting airways such as lobar bronchi, those that follow the respiratory bronchi and alveolar ducts are muscular or partially so.[29] The implications for function of these observations are severalfold. It is known that gas exchange occurs in respiratory bronchi and alveolar ducts through the arteries that accompany these structures.[30] When this information is coupled with the fact that hypoxia acts directly to constrict muscular arteries, it is apparent that this area of the lung has the propensity for active control of pulmonary blood flow. Further, since the spiral of muscle in the partially muscular arteries is directly contiguous with the muscle encircling the larger vessels, retrograde propagation of the hypoxic stimulus can occur in the intracellular pathways of the muscle syncytium,[29] and a wider and more severe response can develop.

INNERVATION. In further contrast to the peripheral circulation, it has proved difficult to demonstrate a nerve supply in the pulmonary circulation. Evidence suggests that although both adrenergic and cholinergic fibers are present, they are sparse in comparison with those innervating systemic vessels of similar size, and their distribution tends to be concentrated in the larger vessels at the hilum.[30,31] Recent data indicate that these nerves contain other neurotransmitters, such as vasoactive intestinal peptide in parasympathetic fibers, substance P, the neurokinins, calcitonin gene-related peptide in sensory fibers, and neuropeptide tyrosine in sympathetic fibers.[32] Some studies in children indicate that the predominant neuropeptide transmitter is tyrosine and that, during growth and development, the relative density of nerve fibers increases only in the arteries of the respiratory unit.[32] In this work, pulmonary hypertension in infants was associated with premature innervation of these arteries.

In *summary*, the structure of the pulmonary circulation is in keeping with its hemodynamics. The thin-walled, sparsely innervated vessels which contain relatively small amounts of smooth muscle (Fig. 27-4, p. 795) do not favor the development of marked vasomotor responses, and, indeed, vasoconstriction alone is not sufficient to overload the RV to the point of producing acute cor pulmonale.[33] Consequently, mechanical obstruction of the pulmonary circulation can be inferred when there is acute cor pulmonale, and structural alterations in the pulmonary vascular bed must be present in the chronic form.

PHYSIOLOGY OF THE PULMONARY CIRCULATION
(See also Chap. 27)

The physiology of the pulmonary circulation is unique from several standpoints. Most of this vascular bed is contained within the parenchyma of the lung, and thus the vessels are subjected to external distending and compressive forces which can act independently of any intrinsic properties of the vessels themselves. In addition, the pulmonary circulation is in series with a pump capable of developing only low pressures, yet it must accommodate the entire cardiac output under all states of physical activity. Consequently, it must adjust to wide variations in blood flow without much change in pressure so as not to overload the RV.

PRESSURE-VOLUME RELATIONS. Historically, it has been thought that the pulmonary circulation is highly distensible and that the vessels dilate to accommodate increases in cardiac output, thus preventing an increase in pulmonary artery pressure in high-flow states.[34,35] Actual measurements of the compliance of the pulmonary vessels have shown that this vascular bed is significantly stiffer than its systemic counterpart,[36,37] and only small increments in blood volume can be accepted by the large pulmonary vessels.[38-41] The major mechanism which accommodates increased blood flow and volume is the recruitment of previously unperfused vessels.[36,42] Morphological evidence suggests that both recruitment and distention occur with an increase in pulmonary blood flow and that the transmural pressures to which the vessel is subjected are what determine which one predominates.[43] In superior portions of the lung where the vessels are collapsed or where alveolar pressure is greater than pulmonary venous pressure, recruitment appears to be the major mechanism. Distention is more important in dependent portions of the lung in which pulmonary venous pressure is greater than alveolar pressure (see below)[30] (Fig. 20–8, p. 555).

PRESSURE-FLOW RELATIONS. Evaluation of the pressure-flow relations of the pulmonary circulation in normal humans at any given lung volume demonstrates a hyperbolic configuration in which large changes in pulmonary blood flow are associated with small elevations in pulmonary artery pressure (Fig. 49–3A). The net result is that as flow increases, pulmonary vascular resistance decreases (Fig. 49–3B).[33] Consequently, irrespective of whether distention or recruitment occurs, both mechanisms maintain a low-pressure circuit during situations of increased blood flow.

A U-shaped curve describes pulmonary vascular resistance as a function of lung volume (Fig. 49–3C).[40] At the extremes of lung volume of full inflation and deflation, vascular resistance is high, and it reaches its nadir at about the resting end-expiratory position (i.e., at functional residual capacity). These findings can be explained by considering the geometry assumed by the alveolar and intrapulmonic but extraalveolar vessels in response to the transmural pressures to which they are exposed.

Because the pulmonary vessels are within the substance of the lung, their dimensions reflect the forces exerted on them by the pulmonary parenchyma. At low lung volumes, the extraalveolar vessels tend to collapse because radial traction no longer supports them. Simultaneously, the alveolar vessels are pulled open by the increased recoil forces generated by the tendency of the alveoli to become smaller. As the lung is inflated to volumes above functional residual capacity, the larger vessels tend to be pulled open, but there is now a progressive increase in the resistance of the small vessels as they are squeezed and lengthened by enlarging alveoli. In addition to this deformation, alterations in alveolar pressure also can influence dynamically the lumina of small vessels. When alveolar pressure is positive, as it is during expiration or with the Valsalva maneuver, vessels are compressed. Alternatively, with negative pressure, as with inspiration or the Mueller maneuver, small vessels are subjected to a proportional distending pressure. It is therefore apparent that alveolar pressure can play a critical role in determining the distribution of pulmonary blood flow and, accordingly, gas exchange.

DETERMINANTS OF PULMONARY GAS EXCHANGE

DISTRIBUTION OF PULMONARY BLOOD FLOW. In the normal human in the upright position, blood flow per unit volume of lung increases progressively from the apex to the base, with flow at the apex being virtually absent[44,45] (Fig. 20–8, p. 555). This distribution is affected by changes of posture and by exercise. When a subject is in the supine position, apical blood flow increases but the basal flow remains virtually unchanged, with the result that the distribution from apex to base becomes almost uniform. In this posture, flow in the posterior or dependent regions exceeds that in the anterior parts. During mild exercise in the upright position, flow to both the upper and the lower zones increases but more so to the upper, so that flow becomes more evenly distributed.

West[44,45] and Permutt and Riley[46] have demonstrated that the pressure-flow relations through the lung can be analogous to those of a "waterfall" or Starling resistor. The basic point of these studies is that the effective pressure drop in the pulmonary vasculature is not always the difference between inflow (pulmonary artery) and outflow (left atrial) pressures but often is between the inflow pressure and the closing pressure of small vessels downstream.

In normal human lungs, pulmonary arterial and venous pressures both increase from superior to dependent regions because of hydrostatic ef-

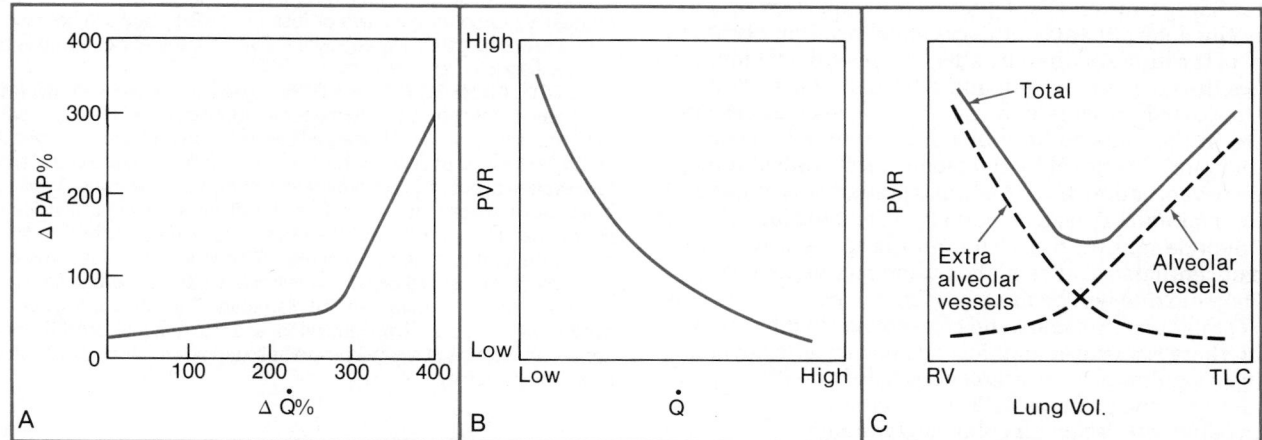

FIGURE 49–3. Some aspects of pulmonary vascular physiology. *A,* Pressure-flow relation. *B,* Resistance-flow relation. *C,* Pulmonary vascular resistance (PVR) as a function of lung volume for the total system and for extraalveolar and alveolar vessels. $\triangle$PAP = percentage of change of mean pulmonary artery pressure from control; $\triangle$Q = percentage of change in cardiac output; 100 = normal cardiac output; RV = residual volume; TLC = total lung capacity.

fects resulting from gravity acting on the blood.[44,45] Alveolar pressures remain essentially constant throughout the lung. Alveolar pressure exceeds venous pressure at a more dependent portion of the lung than does arterial pressure. This results in distribution of blood flow to three major areas.

In the most superior area (zone I), no flow occurs because alveolar pressure exceeds pulmonary arterial pressure. Presumably, this is because thin-walled collapsible vessels are directly exposed to alveolar pressure. In humans, the pulmonary artery pressure is sufficiently high to bring blood to the apex of the lung so that no zone I is present under normal conditions. Flow in the upper segments of the lung may disappear, however, if pulmonary artery pressure falls or if alveolar pressure is elevated, as it is in obstructive airway disease. In the middle zone (zone II), arterial pressure exceeds alveolar pressure, but the latter is greater than venous pressure. Here, flow through the capillaries is proportional to the difference between arterial and alveolar pressure. In the lowest zone, zone III, venous pressure exceeds alveolar pressure, the vessels are held open, and flow is determined in the usual way by the arterial-venous pressure difference. A small zone of reduced flow at the very base of the lung also has been observed and attributed to a possible increase in the interstitial pressure as a consequence of the reduced expansion of the lung parenchyma in the lower zone. This has, therefore, been called zone IV. There is still some uncertainty about the cause of the reduced flow in this area, but the concept of reduction in flow caused by an increased interstitial pressure is almost certainly important in mitral stenosis and may be responsible for the reduction in basilar blood flow observed in that condition.

Distribution of Ventilation

The distribution of ventilation, like that of perfusion, decreases from base to apex in the normal lung, but the rate of change is only about one-third that seen with blood flow.[44] Here, too, gravity plays a role, and changes in posture have an influence. Thus, when normal subjects lie supine, the difference in ventilation between the anatomical upper and lower zones is abolished,[44] and in the inverted lung, the apex ventilates better than the base, so the normal pattern is reversed.

Evaluation of the relative rates of expansion of the upper and lower zones in the upright position reveals different patterns of distribution, depending on the lung volume from which inspiration is initiated.[47] As a consequence of the effect of gravity and the shape of the pressure-volume curve of the lung, when a normal subject takes a breath from functional residual capacity (FRC), ventilation is preferentially distributed to the dependent lung zones. Because blood flow in the resting state also is preferentially distributed to this area, this matching of ventilation to perfusion in different body positions ensures efficient gas exchange under a variety of physiological conditions.

If breathing takes place at lung volumes lower than FRC, the distribution of ventilation is quite different. Because of closure of dependent airways, the most inferior portions of the lung do not ventilate, and all of the inspired gas goes preferentially to the upper zones. The phenomenon of airway closure at low lung volumes has major physiological significance and can produce substantial alterations in ventilation-perfusion relations and arterial hypoxia.[48,49]

Ventilation-Perfusion Ratios

Ventilation-perfusion ($\dot{V}_A/\dot{Q}$) ratios are important because they are the determinants of the gas exchange that occurs in any part of the lung and thereby affect the overall efficiency of the lungs in taking up oxygen and eliminating carbon dioxide.[44] The partial pressure of oxygen in the alveolar gas (and therefore in the end-capillary blood) is set by a balance between the rate of removal by the blood and its rate of replenishment by ventilation. If ventilation is gradually reduced and perfusion maintained to an alveolus, oxygen tension falls and carbon dioxide tension rises. The limit is reached when the unit is not ventilated at all, and the pulmonary venous oxygen and carbon dioxide will be those of mixed venous blood. This is a $\dot{V}_A/\dot{Q}$ relationship of zero and corresponds to the situation in which there is a true anatomical pulmonary arteriovenous shunt (e.g., a pulmonary arteriovenous fistula or a functional one such as produced by atelectasis). By contrast, if perfusion to a normally ventilating alveolus is gradually reduced, the oxygen tension in the venous blood draining this alveolus rises and the partial pressure of carbon dioxide falls. The limit now occurs when the unit is unperfused. This is a $\dot{V}_A/\dot{Q}$ of infinity and is seen in situations in which blood supply is disrupted, such as by pulmonary emboli or other disease in

which occlusion of the pulmonary arterial circulation occurs. Between these two extreme examples, a wide range of $\dot{V}_A/\dot{Q}$ abnormalities is possible.

The alveoli hypoventilated in relation to their perfusion (i.e., low $\dot{V}_A/\dot{Q}$ ratio) cause hypoxemia, and their presence has the same effect as mixing venous and arterial blood. This is termed venous admixture or "wasted blood"; it is evaluated clinically by determining the oxygen tension difference between ideal alveolar gas and arterial blood. Normally, venous admixture or "shunt effect" is only about 2 to 3 per cent of the cardiac output, but in severe disease it may rise to 30 per cent or more. The normal alveolar arterial difference of oxygen (A-aDO$_2$) is 20 mm Hg or less.[50,51]

The alveoli which are hyperventilated in relation to their perfusion (i.e., high V_A/Q ratio) mainly affect CO_2 elimination. They behave as if part of the inspired gas bypassed the alveoli, so this effect has been called "wasted ventilation" or an increase in "physiological dead space." It is evaluated by comparing mixed expired and arterial CO_2, using the Bohr equation. The physiological dead space normally is less than 30 per cent of the tidal volume.[51,52] In severe lung disease, it can rise to 50 per cent or more. Every pathological condition that directly affects the pulmonary parenchyma or its vascular bed results in mismatched ventilation and blood flow. Consequently, this abnormality is by far the most common cause of arterial hypoxemia in disease states. Both venous admixture and physiological dead space are typically increased in chronic obstructive and infiltrative lung diseases. In pulmonary thromboembolism, an increase in dead space predominates.

In many pulmonary parenchymal diseases, blood supply to poorly ventilated areas tends to be reduced, so that the V_A/Q ratios are not as low as they would otherwise be. One reason for this is that the local pathological process tends to disturb both ventilation and perfusion by its mechanical effects. Another is local hypoxic vasoconstriction, which shunts blood away from the involved alveoli.[53-55] In the case of thromboembolic phenomena, the regional decreases in CO_2 concentration that occur cause local increases in the resistance of small airways and thus reduce ventilation to the affected region.

Other Causes of Abnormal Arterial Blood Gases

In addition to $\dot{V}_A/\dot{Q}$ inequalities, there are four other causes of arterial hypoxemia: (1) anatomical right-to-left intracardiac or intrapulmonary shunts usually caused by congenital heart disease (Chaps. 31 and 32); (2) reductions in the inspired concentration of oxygen; (3) defects in the diffusion of oxygen from the alveolus to the blood; and (4) alveolar hypoventilation.

Although it was originally thought that measurements of the *diffusing capacity* of the lung for oxygen could demonstrate a specific impairment in the transfer of molecular oxygen across a thickened membrane (i.e., alveolar-capillary block), it is now appreciated that single breath tests of diffusing capacity that use carbon monoxide are profoundly influenced by three variables: (1) the surface area available for diffusion, (2) the volume of blood within the capillaries, and (3) the rate of combination of CO_2 and hemoglobin.[56] Other factors, such as the molecular path for diffusion and the stratified heterogeneity of gas mixtures, also play a role.[57] In addition to the above, steady-state methods also are influenced by regional V_A/Q relations.[56] Thus these techniques do not measure the thickness of the alveolar-capillary membrane, and in any disease associated with a loss of elastic recoil (loss of surface area through disruption of alveolar walls), marked V_A/Q heterogeneities or loss of capillary bed will be associated with a reduced "diffusing capacity." Even so, the effect that this has on gas exchange is, at most, small.

ALVEOLAR HYPOVENTILATION. This is a condition in which insufficient gas exchange occurs to meet metabolic demands. It can result from many causes: severe $\dot{V}_A/\dot{Q}$ inequalities; reduced drive from the respiratory center so that the patient "will not breathe"; failure of the patient's respiratory system to act on the information sent from the central nervous system because of severe intrinsic pulmonary disease; or abnormalities of the neuromuscular apparatus of the chest wall or diaphragm.[58] In the latter cases, the patient "cannot breathe." Regardless of cause, the cardinal features of the arterial blood are hypoxemia and hypercapnia, and both must be present to establish the diagnosis. The various diseases associated with alveolar hypoventilation and the mechanisms by which it comes about in each are discussed as examples of chronic cor pulmonale later in this chapter.

EFFECTS OF ALVEOLAR GAS TENSIONS ON THE PULMONARY CIRCULATION

HYPOXIA. The most potent stimulus for the development of pulmonary vasoconstriction is alveolar hypoxia[30,53,54,59]

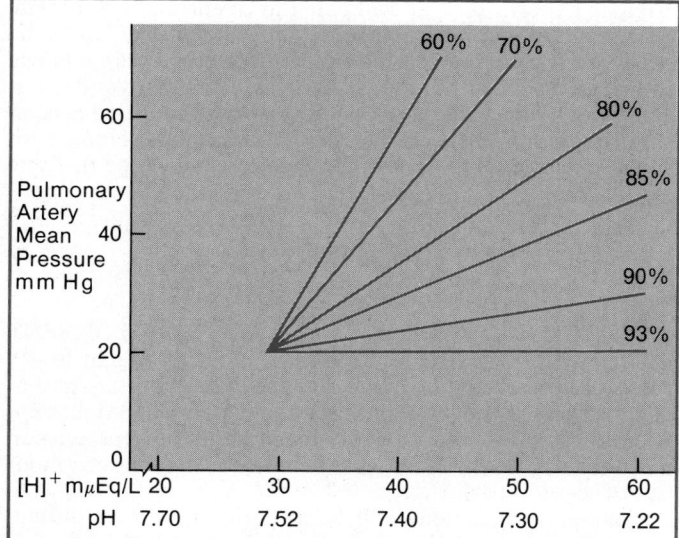

FIGURE 49–4. Relation of arterial oxygen saturation and hydrogen ion concentration to pulmonary artery pressure. (Reproduced from Enson, Y., et al.: The influence of hydrogen ion concentration and hypoxia on the pulmonary circulation. J. Clin. Invest. *43*:1146, 1964, by copyright permission of the American Society for Clinical Investigation.)

(Fig. 27–4, p. 795). Although acute vasoconstriction appears when the alveolar pO_2 is 60 mm Hg or lower, this response is found only in about two-thirds of normal subjects.[60] It is speculated that the subjects who respond to hypoxemia with pulmonary vasoconstriction are those who would be prone to develop chronic cor pulmonale if they developed a disease that interfered with effective alveolar ventilation.[61] The pulmonary constrictor response to hypoxia appears to be locally mediated since it can be elicited both in denervated lungs and isolated perfused lungs.

ACIDOSIS. This also has been shown to produce significant increases in pulmonary vascular resistance as well as to act synergistically with hypoxia.[62] In contrast, an increase in arterial pCO_2 seems to exert no direct effect. Instead, it seems to operate by way of the increase in hydrogen ion concentration that it induces. The interaction of hypoxia and acidemia is clinically important; these two conditions frequently coexist, and their interplay follows a predictable pattern (Fig. 49–4). At minor degrees of oxygen unsaturation, pulmonary artery pressure is relatively insensitive to hydrogen ion concentration, whereas it is extremely sensitive at high levels of unsaturation. On the other hand, when the pH is high, the pressor effect of hypoxia is blunted.

Although the localization of the pulmonary vascular pressor response within the lung is still controversial, most studies indicate that it occurs in partially muscular arteries less than 200 μm in diameter.[29,53,55,63] The mechanism by which hypoxia causes pulmonary arterial smooth muscle to constrict is unclear.

The available information points toward two major alternatives: an indirect effect by which hypoxia might cause endothelial cells to generate various eicosanoids or other cells in the pulmonary parenchyma to release vasoactive substances (e.g., histamine from mast cells), or a direct effect of hypoxia on pulmonary arterial smooth muscle. Other influences may enhance hypoxic pulmonary vasoconstriction. For example, it is possible that extrapulmonic reflexes or the adrenergic neurotransmitter norepinephrine may augment the pressor response.

PULMONARY HYPERTENSION. The precise mechanism by which the resting tone of the pulmonary circulation is controlled is unknown. The smooth muscle and connective tissue elements in the walls of the vessels certainly contribute. The relative roles of other potential controlling factors such as the

neuropeptides of the nonadrenergic noncholinergic nervous system, or locally formed or circulating mediators such as the eicosanoids (prostacyclin, thromboxane, leukotrienes), catecholamines (epinephrine, norepinephrine), and autacoids (histamine, bradykinin), and endothelial-derived relaxing and contrasting factors have yet to be explored.[64]

Pulmonary vasoconstriction produces an acute rise in pressure, and it is now known that continuing constriction with pulmonary hypertension of even a few days' duration is associated with structural changes in the vessels.[29] Luminal narrowing is brought about by an increase in the thickness of the medial coat, endothelial swelling, hypertrophy, and the appearance of muscle at more peripheral levels than normal. With continued insult, a reduction in cross-sectional area of the vascular bed develops in association with an increase in RV weight. Although these structural and functional changes occur with all forms of pulmonary hypertension, different time sequences of development or ultrastructural patterns may be seen with different disease processes.

CHRONIC COR PULMONALE

INCIDENCE

Because of its association with chronic lung disease, chronic cor pulmonale is a common type of heart disease.[1,5,7,65] The U.S. Public Health Service estimates that chronic lung disease affects 47 million people in the United States alone and accounts for more than 80,000 deaths every year.[66] Although precise figures on the prevalence of cor pulmonale are lacking, it is possible to appreciate the potential magnitude of the problem by recognizing that chronic bronchitis and emphysema are its most common causes and that these two diseases result in about 30,000 deaths per year.[67] In one study in England, cor pulmonale was responsible for 30 to 40 per cent of all clinical cases of heart failure and of a total of 487 cases of cardiac disease;[68] in the United States 10 to 30 per cent of hospital admissions for congestive heart failure are due to cor pulmonale.[69] Most patients are 45 years of age or older, and men are affected more frequently than women.

The presence of pulmonary hypertension with chronic respiratory disease contributes significantly to mortality. The available data suggest that the severity of pulmonary hypertension correlates more closely with survival than any other variable studied[70–72] (Fig. 49–5). Patients with severe airway obstruction ($FEV_1 < 1$ liter) without pulmonary hypertension

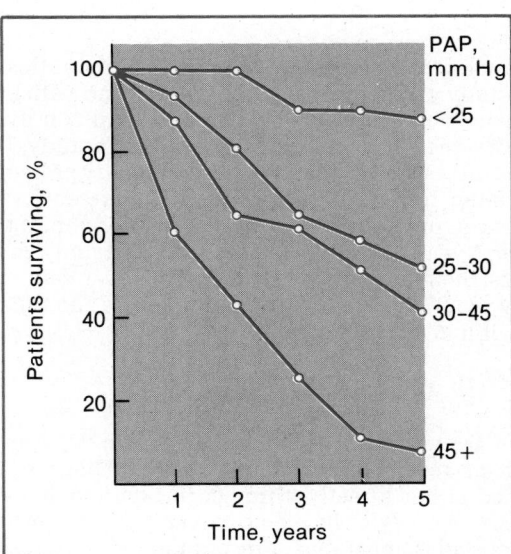

FIGURE 49–5. Correlation between survival (years) and baseline measurement of mean pulmonary arterial pressure (PAP) in patients with chronic bronchitis. (From Bishop, J. M.: Hypoxia and pulmonary hypertension in chronic bronchitis. Prog. Resp. Res. *9*:10, 1975.)

TABLE 49-1 ETIOLOGIES OF PULMONARY HEART DISEASE

1. **Diseases Affecting Air Passages of the Lung and Alveoli**
   a. Chronic obstructive pulmonary diseases
   b. Cystic fibrosis
   c. Congenital developmental defects
   d. Infiltrative or granulomatous diseases
      (1) Idiopathic pulmonary fibrosis
      (2) Sarcoidosis
      (3) Pneumoconiosis
      (4) Scleroderma
      (5) Mixed connective tissue disease
      (6) Systemic lupus erythematosus
      (7) Rheumatoid arthritis
      (8) Polymyositis
      (9) Eosinophilic granuloma
      (10) Malignant infiltration
      (11) Radiation
   e. Upper airways obstruction
   f. Pulmonary resection
   g. High-altitude disease

2. **Diseases Affecting Thoracic Cage Movement**
   a. Kyphoscoliosis
   b. Thoracoplasty
   c. Pleural fibrosis
   d. Neuromuscular weakness
   e. Sleep apnea syndromes
   f. Idiopathic hypoventilation

3. **Diseases Affecting the Pulmonary Vasculature**
   a. Primary diseases of the arterial wall
      (1) Primary pulmonary hypertension
      (2) Granulomatous pulmonary arteritis
      (3) Toxin-induced pulmonary hypertension
         a) Aminorex fumarate
         b) Intravenous drug abuse
      (4) Chronic liver disease
      (5) Peripheral pulmonic stenosis
   b. Thrombotic disorders
      (1) Sickle cell diseases
      (2) Pulmonary microthrombi
   c. Embolic disorders
      (1) Thromboembolism
      (2) Tumor embolism
      (3) Other embolism (amniotic fluid, air)
      (4) Schistosomiasis and other parasites

4. **Pressures on Pulmonary Arteries by Mediastinal Tumors, Aneurysms, Granulomata, or Fibrosis**

From Rubin, L. J.: Introduction. Pulmonary Heart Disease. Boston, Martinus Nijhoff, 1984, p. 1.

tricular hypertrophy, and impair right ventricular function. Fortunately, most disorders affect too small a segment of the lungs or are too circumscribed in their effects on gas exchange to initiate the chain of events that leads to right ventricular hypertrophy and failure. A list of the various disease categories commonly associated with cor pulmonale, along with some specific examples of each process, is presented in Table 49-1.

PATHOPHYSIOLOGY
(Table 49-2)

FACTORS CONTRIBUTING TO THE DEVELOPMENT OF PULMONARY HYPERTENSION. (Figs. 49-6 and 49-7). Most researchers would agree that the most important pathogenetic mechanisms that produce abnormalities in right ventricular structure and function are pulmonary hypertension and abnormal concentrations of blood gases that directly modify myocardial performance.[71,76]

Some paradoxes remain. In some patients with cor pulmonale and hypoxemic obstructive lung disease (see later discussion), the pulmonary artery pressure does not reach levels high enough to lead to reduced ejection fractions of the RV. Nonetheless, such patients develop clinical signs of RV overload.[77,78] Further, pathophysiological studies in selected patients suggest that cor pulmonale, in association with obstructive airway disease, may not be closely related at death to many of the physiological parameters thought to be important in its development (i.e., pulmonary hypertension, right ventricular hypertrophy, and low cardiac output). These features are in fact inconsistent terminal features in this group.[79]

As already noted, the normal pulmonary circulation is a low-resistance system with considerable reserve; therefore, substantial reductions in the size of the effective vascular bed must occur before pulmonary hypertension develops and becomes sustained. The pathogenetic sequence is unknown, and probably a number of mechanisms interact to produce pulmonary hypertension. Any theory regarding the development of cor pulmonale must take into account the effects of the anatomical loss of vessels (i.e., anatomical restriction of the pul-

have much greater longevity than those without this finding. In the study of Burrows and colleagues,[70] no patient with a pulmonary vascular resistance greater than 550 dynes-sec-cm^{-5} survived 3 years. Similarly, in Bishop's study,[71] mortality rates increased progressively as pulmonary pressures rose. In the latter investigation, less than 10 per cent of patients with a mean pulmonary artery pressure of 45 mm Hg or more survived 5 years. Finally, Traver et al.,[72] in a study on patients with obstructive lung disease, found a 50 per cent mortality rate of 7 years in patients with cor pulmonale and 13.5 years in those without cor pulmonale.

ETIOLOGY

There are many causes of cor pulmonale.[73,74] Any disease that affects ventilatory mechanics, gas exchange, or the vascular bed either directly, through intrapulmonic events, or indirectly, by way of its effect on ventilatory control or the neuromuscular apparatus of respiration, may cause cor pulmonale.[75] Because this is true of essentially all primary pulmonary disorders, the development of cor pulmonale simply indicates that the primary pulmonary disease was sufficiently advanced to raise pulmonary artery pressure, cause right ven-

TABLE 49-2 POTENTIAL PATHOGENETIC MECHANISMS LEADING TO PULMONARY ARTERIAL HYPERTENSION AND COR PULMONALE

MECHANISMS	EXAMPLE
Primary	
Anatomical decrease in cross-sectional area (vessel destruction; encroachment on lumen by hypertherapy) of the pulmonary resistance vessels	Interstitial fibrosis and granuloma
Vasoconstriction of pulmonary resistance vessels	Hypoxia and acidosis
Contributory	
Large increments in pulmonary blood flow	Exercise
Increased pressures on the left side of the heart and pulmonary veins	Left ventricular failure or pulmonary veno-occlusive disease
Increased viscosity of the blood	Secondary polycythemia of chronic hypoxia
Unproved	
Compression of pulmonary resistance vessels by raised alveolar pressures in their vicinity	Asthmatic bronchitis
Bronchial arterial-pulmonary arterial anastomoses	Expanded bronchial circulation

From Fishman, A. P.: Pulmonary hypertension and cor pulmonale. *In* Fishman, A. P.: Pulmonary Diseases and Disorders, 2nd ed. New York, McGraw-Hill Book Co., 1988, p. 1001.

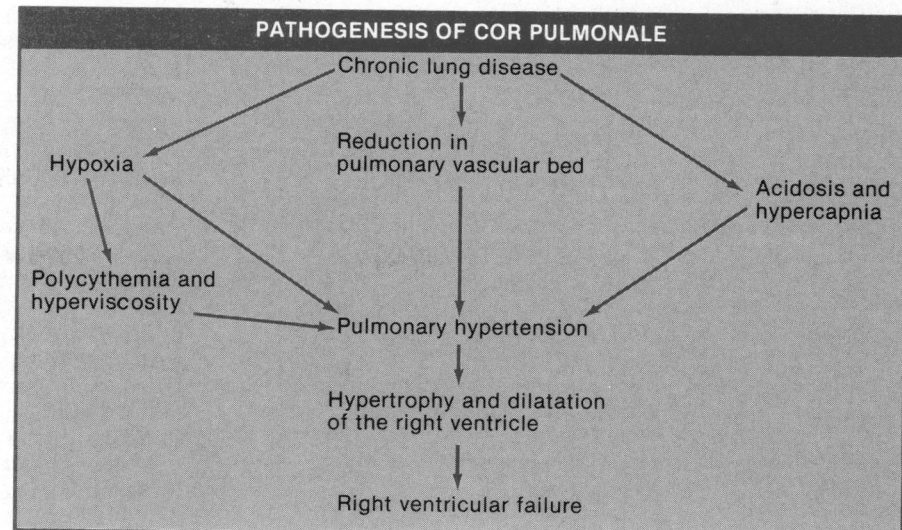

PATHOGENESIS OF COR PULMONALE

Chronic lung disease

Hypoxia

Reduction in
pulmonary vascular bed

Acidosis and
hypercapnia

Polycythemia and
hyperviscosity

Pulmonary hypertension

Hypertrophy and dilatation
of the right ventricle

Right ventricular failure

FIGURE 49–6. Pathogenesis of cor pulmonale. (From Summer, W. R.: Acute cor pulmonale. *In* Rubin, L. J. [ed.]: Pulmonary Heart Disease. Boston, Martinus Nijhoff, 1984, p. 285.)

monary vascular bed), pulmonary arteriolar constriction, increased blood viscosity, and increased blood flow, although the relative roles of these several factors have not been clearly defined and probably vary from patient to patient.[85]

It has long been thought that the essential pathology in chronic cor pulmonale is a *physical loss of vessels*, leading to a restricted vascular bed. Although it is certainly true that this mechanism contributes to the pulmonary hypertension observed in vascular occlusion resulting from multiple pulmonary emboli (Chap. 48), aplasia, or extensive excision of lung tissue,[23,59] other factors also must be considered, since emphysema, a disease in which alveolar vessels are widely destroyed, typically is associated with resting pulmonary hypertension and cor pulmonale only late in its course.[80] Thus, a decrease in the anatomical extent of the pulmonary vascular bed does not play a major role in the development of pulmonary hypertension unless the reduction is extreme. Other processes (i.e., a constricted vascular bed) can *decrease the effective cross-sectional area without a loss of vessels.* The effective area can be reduced by arteriolar constriction se-

condary to alveolar hypoxemia and acidosis[59,61,62,64] and by the various pathological changes responsible for pulmonary hypertension[29,81–83] (Chap. 27).

The potent vasoconstricting influence resulting from alveolar hypoxia is shared by the disease entities responsible for chronic cor pulmonale and listed in Table 49–1. The resulting pulmonary hypertension, when persistent, can make the vessels rigid and reduce their lumina by producing intimal thickening, inflammatory changes, and medial hypertrophy.[29,79]

Intimal thickening of the pulmonary arterioles, regardless of its cause, often has a patchy distribution and is a frequent postmortem finding in patients beyond the age of 40 years who were free of pulmonary hypertension during life.[84] Its extent must be great to account for the perpetuation or worsening of pulmonary hypertension. Intimal thickening can be both a cause and a result of pulmonary hypertension. The reversibility of this process is unknown, but the fibrotic component is presumably permanent. Inflammatory changes vary from cellular infiltrates to fibrinoid necrosis and fibrosis. Most often these types of alterations are found in diffuse inflammatory lung lesions or with systemic illness with vasculitis. They have been noted, however, secondary to pulmonary hypertension of any cause.[82,84] Hypertrophy and hyperplasia of the smooth muscle in the media of the arterioles are regular findings in longstanding pulmonary hypertension (p. 790) and have been found to be partially reversible.[29,81–83]

The *structural* changes induced by hypoxia are believed to account for half of the rise in pulmonary artery pressure that persists when the patient breathes room air. These changes also set the stage for further reactivity. Acute hypoxia superimposed on a vascular bed in which structural remodeling has occurred is known to produce a greater hemodynamic effect than that seen in a normal circulation.[29]

An *increase in the viscosity of blood* has been shown experimentally to raise pulmonary vascular resistance.[85] Viscosity usually is elevated as a result of chronic hypoxemia stimulating red cell production through erythropoietin release. It represents an adaptation that tends to restore arterial oxygen delivery. However, the compensatory mechanism is useful only up to a point because at very high levels of hematocrit, the high viscosity of the blood can impair capillary flow.[86] With high hematocrits the shear rates are low, and as the blood flow slows in the capillaries, viscosity increases even further, requiring a greater driving pressure. In laboratory animals, polycythemia contributes significantly to the rise in pulmonary resistance during both acute hypoxia and recovery.[29] These considerations have served as the rationale for phlebotomy in selected patients with cor pulmonale.

The final traditional factor that has been proposed as contributing to pulmonary hypertension is an increase *in pulmonary blood flow.* Extensive intimal hypertrophy and pathological medial necrosis have been created in the pulmonary circulation of animals by anastomosing a pulmonary artery either to the aorta or to one of its main branches.[87] Although studies demonstrate that collateral channels develop between the bronchial and pulmonary vascular beds in chronic obstructive pulmonary disease,[88,89] except in the case of bronchiectasis, these channels seldom are large enough to contribute importantly to pulmonary hypertension.[89] As discussed below, increased cardiac output can raise pulmonary pressures in patients with both constricted and restricted vascular beds.

One area in which high pulmonary blood flow appears to play an impor-

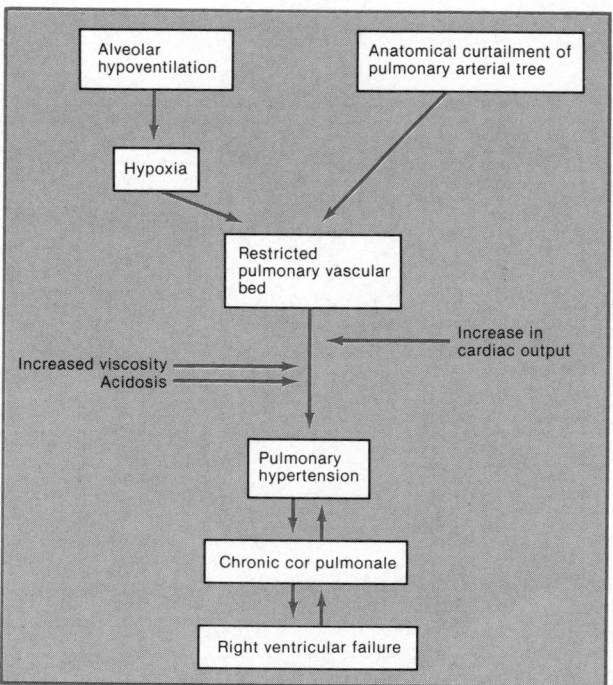

Alveolar
hypoventilation

Anatomical curtailment of
pulmonary arterial tree

Hypoxia

Restricted
pulmonary vascular
bed

Increase in
cardiac output

Increased viscosity
Acidosis

Pulmonary
hypertension

Chronic cor pulmonale

Right ventricular failure

FIGURE 49–7. Pathogenesis of pulmonary hypertension and cor pulmonale in kyphoscoliosis. (From Fishman, A. P.: Pulmonary hypertension and cor pulmonale. *In* Fishman, A. P.: Pulmonary Diseases and Disorders. 2nd ed. New York, McGraw-Hill Book Co., 1988, p. 1033.)

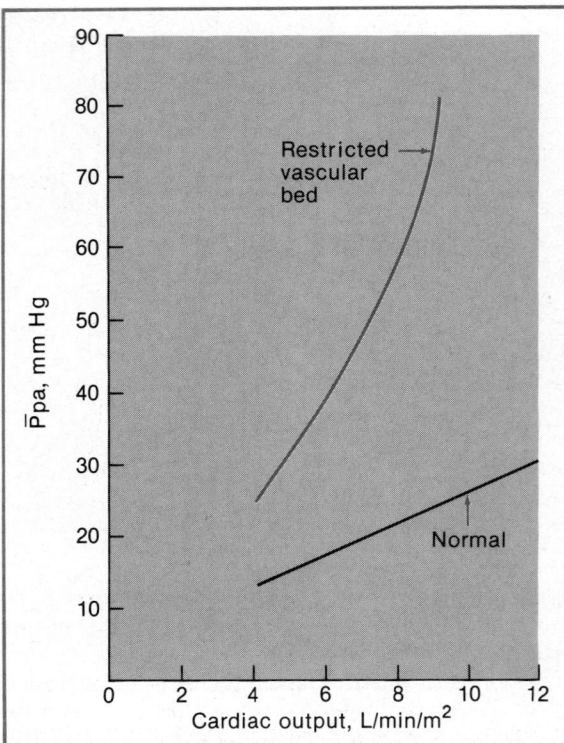

FIGURE 49-8. Pulmonary circulation at sea level, at rest, and during exercise. Restriction of the pulmonary arterial tree causes higher pulmonary arterial pressures at any level of blood flow. (From Fishman, A. P.: Pulmonary hypertension and cor pulmonale. *In* Fishman, A. P.: Pulmonary Diseases and Disorders. 2nd ed. New York, McGraw-Hill Book Co., 1988, p. 999.)

tant role in the development of elevated pulmonary artery pressure and resistance is in congenital heart diseases associated with left-to-right shunts[90] (p. 906): Once established, the anatomical changes in the pulmonary vascular bed may not be completely reversible, even when pulmonary blood flow is restored to normal surgically. Morphological examination of the lungs of patients with congenital cardiac disease and high pulmonary flow shows a gradation of pathological changes that reflects the duration and severity of the condition[90,91] (p. 896).

It is not clear how the above-described pathogenetic mechanisms interrelate in the development of pulmonary hypertension. It is easy to appreciate that the loss of vessels and diffuse constriction of the arterioles with the attendant pathological changes in their walls and lumina can combine to cause a reduction of the pulmonary vascular bed, which in turn causes an increase in pulmonary vascular resistance. These changes need not be manifested at rest as an elevated pulmonary artery pressure. As shown in Figure 49-3, the normal pulmonary vascular bed has the ability to accept large increases in flow without marked increases in pressure, probably through the recruitment of parallel vascular channels. In the case of a restricted vascular bed, this reserve is lost and the patients' physiological response is as though they were starting at the bend of the normal pressure-flow relation (Fig. 49-8). The importance of hypoxia as a determinant of pulmonary artery pressure is demonstrated in Figure 49-9.

Under these circumstances, pressure can rise dramatically with exercise or any other condition that causes pulmonary blood flow to increase. As the secondary changes in the vessels develop with progression of the underlying disease, further raising of pulmonary vascular resistance causes elevation of pulmonary artery pressure, sometimes even at rest. The pressure-flow relation (Fig. 49-3A) is shifted upward and to the left, as in a constricted bed, so that small increments in flow produce large increases in pressure over the entire range of cardiac output. It may be inferred that small increases in output are accompanied by large increases in right ventricular work. Increases in viscosity, collateral blood flow, hypoxemia, and acidemia worsen the situation by further increasing pulmonary artery pressure.[70,92,93]

RIGHT VENTRICULAR DYNAMICS. The hemodynamic findings in cor pulmonale depend, to some extent, on the cause and duration of the underlying pathological process. Most patients with relatively mild obstructive lung disease without severe hypoxemia have normal mean right atrial and

right ventricular end-diastolic pressures, normal cardiac outputs, normal or slightly elevated pulmonary artery pressures, and slightly elevated pulmonary vascular resistances at rest.[29,70,94-96] Right ventricular ejection fraction, as determined by radionuclide angiography, tends to be normal.[97,98] With exercise, pulmonary artery pressure rises further, right ventricular stroke work increases (Fig. 49-9), and right ventricular ejection fraction falls.[97,98] Relating end-diastolic pressure to stroke work suggests that these patients function on an extension of the normal right ventricular function curve.[99] These findings need not be accompanied by clinical or electrocardiographic evidence of right ventricular hypertrophy,[95] although evidence of right ventricular enlargement may be seen on two-dimensional echocardiography. Acute right ventricular failure can develop in these patients if respiratory failure, hypoxia, and further elevation of pulmonary artery pressure are precipitated by a pulmonary infection.

Progression of the airway obstruction tends to accentuate these findings. As the ventilatory impairment worsens, the hemodynamic alterations, including elevations of the right ventricular end-diastolic and end-systolic volumes, follow.[100,101] At the stage when severe chronic hypoxemia develops, usually in association with chronic hypercapnia, there is moderate pulmonary hypertension at rest, which becomes more severe during exercise in association with abnormal right ventricular filling pressures and function in most patients[70-72,97-102] (Fig. 49-10). Cardiac output tends to be normal or even slightly elevated at rest[103] but increases little with exercise when the patient breathes room air. Oxygen admin-

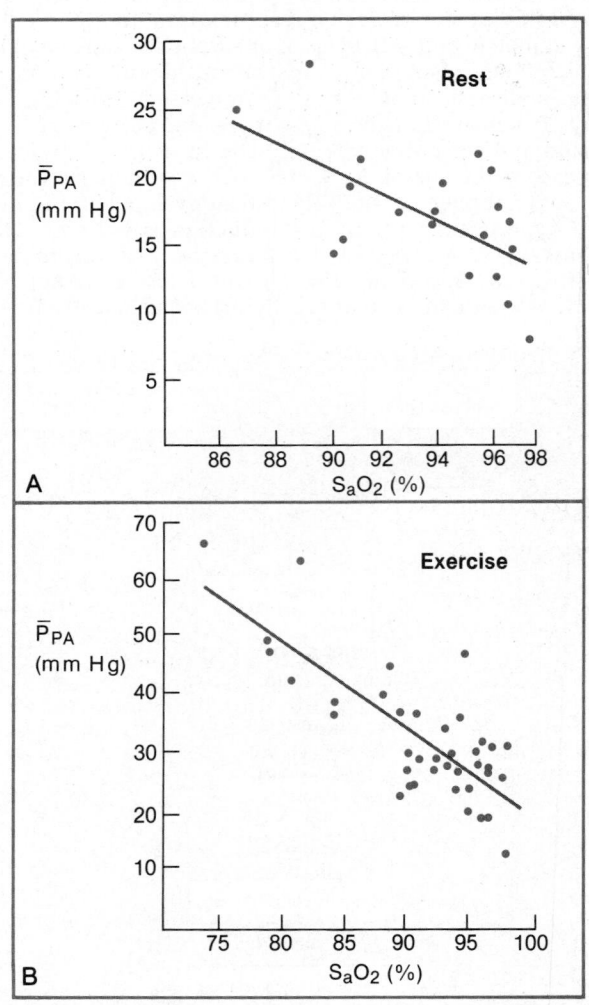

FIGURE 49-9. The correlation between arterial oxygen saturation (SaO$_2$) and mean pulmonary artery pressures (P̄$_{pa}$) at rest and during exercise in patients with chronic obstructive lung disease. (From Stewart, R. I., et al.: Cardiac output during exercise in patients with COPD. Chest 89:199, 1986.)

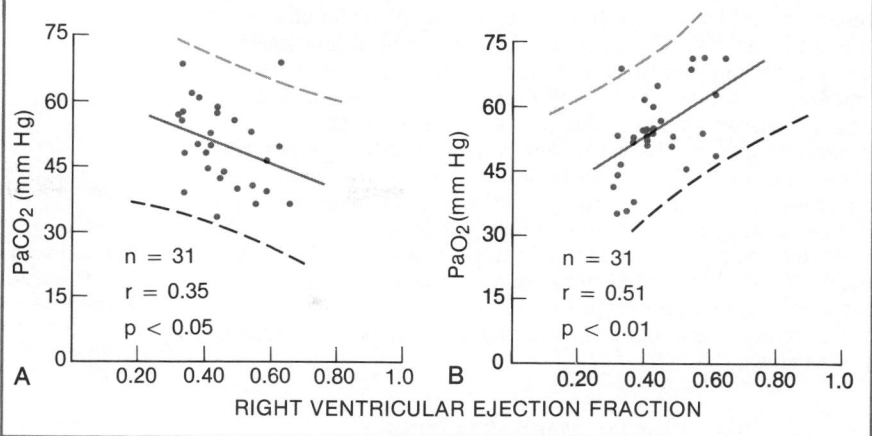

FIGURE 49-10. Relation between arterial carbon dioxide tension (P_{CO_2}) (left panel), arterial oxygen tension (PaO_2) (right panel), and right ventricular ejection fraction in patients with chronic bronchitis and emphysema. These data represent air breathing at rest. (From Flenley, D. C., and Muir, A. L.: Cardiovascular effects of oxygen therapy for pulmonary arterial hypertension. Clin. Chest Med. *4*:297, 1983.)

istration may lower pulmonary artery pressure and raise the right ventricular ejection fraction.[102] Systolic pulmonary artery pressures can reach levels of 80 mm Hg, and these patients are likely to show the clinical and electrocardiographic changes usually ascribed to cor pulmonale. Failure of the RV is associated with an expanded circulating blood volume. In contrast to left ventricular failure, the pulmonary blood volume-total volume ratio remains essentially normal (about 1 to 10) even though red cell mass may be considerably increased.[95] Both circulating plasma volume and lung water increase,[104,105] and each has been shown to decrease as pulmonary artery pressure is lowered with therapy.

LEFT VENTRICULAR DYNAMICS. Abnormally elevated pulmonary venous pressures, with or without overt left ventricular failure, invariably produce alterations in pulmonary mechanics and gas exchange, even in patients with normal lungs. Consequently, left ventricular dysfunction could have deleterious effects in cor pulmonale. Controversy persists about whether the disease affecting the lungs and RV in these patients produces left ventricular disease, or whether the latter results from independent causes.[103] Evidence exists that many patients with cor pulmonale who are over the age of 65 are hypertensive and have reduced left ventricular compliance and/or regional left ventricular wall motion disorders secondary to ischemic heart disease.

The view that disorders of the RV may result in left ventricular disease has gained support from several sources. Animal experiments have shown that (1) right ventricular failure after banding of the pulmonary artery leads to similar morphological and biochemical changes in both cardiac chambers and to reduced contractility of the LV[106-108]; (2) in both isolated hearts and intact animals, alterations in right ventricular compliance or dimensions also change the mechanical properties of the left ventricle, perhaps acting in part through changes in the thickness or position of the interventricular septum (Fig. 49-11)[16,109,110]; and (3) cattle at high altitude with severe pulmonary hypertension have elevated left ventricular end-diastolic pressures.[111] Although these observations are provocative, their relevance to human disease is uncertain.

Autopsy studies have shown that left ventricular hypertrophy frequently occurs in patients with cor pulmonale,[112-114] and left ventricular dysfunction of varying degrees has been observed in vivo.[106,114-116,116a] In all of these investigations, none of the usual causes of left ventricular disease were apparent. Thus, it appears that the structure and function of the left ventricle can become abnormal in association with the pathogenetic mechanisms underlying cor pulmonale. This is probably an uncommon occurrence, and the weight of current evidence indicates that cor pulmonale per se usually does *not* seriously impair left ventricular performance.[70,99,113,117-125]

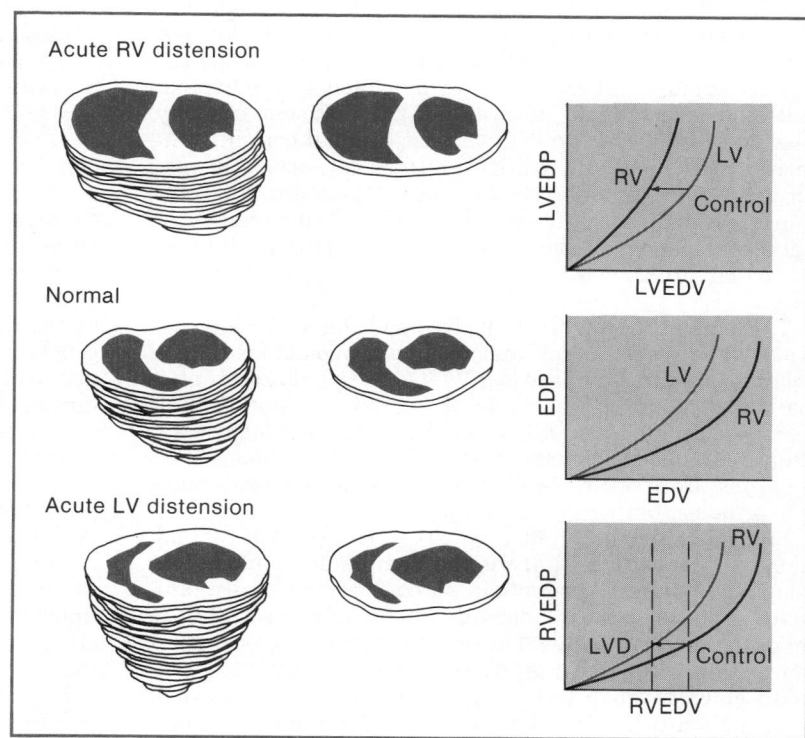

FIGURE 49-11. Alterations in compliance by distention of the contralateral ventricle. Note that acute distention of either ventricle changes not only that ventricle's pressure-volume curve but alters the compliance of the other ventricle as well. The middle graph shows the end-diastolic volume-pressure relations for the right ventricle (RV) and left ventricle (LV). The top graph shows these relations for the LV with a normal RV (right curve) and after the RV has been acutely distended (RVD, left curve). The bottom graph shows the relations for the RV with a normal LV (right curve) and after the LV has been acutely distended (LVD). (From Weber, K. T., et al.: Contractile mechanics and interaction of the right and left ventricles. Am. J. Cardiol. *47*:686, 1981.)

When abnormalities in the latter have been found, they could be explained by a reduction in the apparent distensibility of the left ventricle secondary to right ventricular dilatation (Fig. 49–11),[126,127] by a reduction in right ventricular stroke volume causing diminished left-sided filling, or by independent disease processes such as coronary artery disease aggravated by hypoxemia.[106,125] Given the heterogeneity of the population with cor pulmonale and the variance of its natural history, the controversy will undoubtedly continue. An uncommon syndrome of drug-induced left ventricular failure has been described in patients with chronic lung disease. Some right ventricular endomyocardial biopsies have been compatible with catecholamine myocarditis (p. 1436) in those patients who had been on large doses of adrenergic agonist inhalants and methylxanthines.

CLINICAL MANIFESTATIONS

Chronic Obstructive Pulmonary Disease (COPD)[73,103,123,124]

COPD, by far the most common form of pulmonary parenchymal disease responsible for chronic pulmonary hypertension, consists of chronic bronchitis, emphysema, and in some instances bronchial asthma. Atopic asthma does *not* produce chronic cor pulmonale,[80] and intrinsic, or nonatopic, asthma often is a variant of chronic bronchitis. In this discussion, COPD refers exclusively to chronic bronchitis and/or emphysema.

In most patients with COPD, chronic bronchitis and emphysema coexist, but cor pulmonale is restricted to those with functionally significant airway disease with or without emphysema.[80] This admixture has given rise to a great deal of confusion in terminology in the literature, and until the matter was sorted out by Burrows and colleagues[128] and Mitchell and Filley,[129] the terms bronchitis and emphysema frequently were considered to be synonymous. These workers described fundamental differences in the clinical, physiological, and pathological features of the two conditions and laid the groundwork for a better understanding of these conditions.

CHRONIC BRONCHITIS. It is possible to think of COPD as a continuum, with chronic bronchitis at one extreme and emphysema at the other and the majority of patients having features of both conditions. The distinctions between the two groups are presented in Table 49–3. In the *chronic bronchitis* variety ("blue bloater," "nonfighter"), chronic cough with sputum production, frequently recurring chest infection, secondary erythrocytosis, and repeated bouts of right heart failure are common. Physiologically, the patients have hypoxemia and hypercapnia at rest, normal diffusion capacity, elevated residual volume, functional residual capacity, and airway resistance, with relatively normal values for total lung capacity and pulmonary compliance. Maximum flow rates and forced expiratory volumes are abnormally depressed. The chest roentgenogram shows moderately hyperinflated lungs, increased bronchovascular markings, and sometimes cardiomegaly.

The basic abnormality is widespread but regionally unequal airway obstruction that results in mismatched $\dot{V}_A/\dot{Q}$ relationships. In regions of low $\dot{V}_A/\dot{Q}$ ratios, pulmonary arterial constriction on the basis of hypoxia and/or acidosis occurs. With progression, alveolar hypoventilation develops, the vascular bed becomes constricted, and the pulmonary artery pressure at rest rises. The main pulmonary artery and its two principal branches are enlarged.

EMPHYSEMA. In the emphysematous type ("pink puffer," "fighter"), dyspnea is the dominant symptom, and cough and sputum production are considerably less prominent. Erythrocytosis is uncommon, and right heart failure tends to occur as a terminal event. In keeping with the hyperventilation, the alveolar-arterial gradient for oxygen is abnormally elevated, but arterial oxygen tension usually is normal or only slightly depressed; hypocapnia is common. Standard

TABLE 49-3 COMPARISON OF THE CLINICAL AND PHYSIOLOGICAL FEATURES OF EMPHYSEMA AND CHRONIC BRONCHITIS

	EMPHYSEMA	CHRONIC BRONCHITIS
Synonyms	Pink puffer Fighter	Blue bloater Nonfighter
Signs and Symptoms		
Cough and sputum	Scant	Marked
Dyspnea at rest	Marked	Usually absent
Recurrent chest infections	Unusual	Frequent
Habitus	Often thin, wasted	Often obese
Cyanosis	No	Yes
Edema	No	Yes
Increased AP diameter of thorax	Marked	Mild
Hyperresonance to percussion	Marked	Mild
Breath sounds	Absent to depressed	Rales and rhonchi
Chest x-ray	Hyperinflation; no cardiomegaly	No hyperinflation; cardiomegaly
Electrocardiogram	RVM uncommon	RVM common
Pulmonary Gas Exchange		
Hematocrit	Normal	Elevated
PaO_2	Slight reduction	Marked reduction
$PaCO_2$	Low or normal	Elevated
Diffusing capacity	Markedly decreased	Normal or slightly reduced
Pulmonary Mechanics		
Expiratory flow rates	Reduced	Reduced
Elastic recoil	Markedly reduced	Normal or slightly reduced
Lung volume	Marked hyperinflation	Mild hyperinflation
Pulmonary Circulation		
Pulmonary hypertension at rest with exercise	None or mild	Marked
Right heart failure	Terminal	Repeated

spirometric indices cannot differentiate this group from those with chronic bronchitis, since the degree of obstruction as measured by this technique may be similar. However, the pink puffer has abnormally low diffusing capacity and greatly increased lung volumes and pulmonary compliance. Roentgenograms of the chest reveal marked pulmonary hyperinflation with flattened diaphragms, oligemia of the peripheral lung fields, and a small heart[130] (Fig. 49–12). With the onset of cor pulmonale, the prominence of the vascular markings increases, but RV enlargement may be difficult to observe.

Although there is some airway disease in this condition, the primary pathological defect is widespread destruction of alveolar septa. As a result, the surface area for gas exchange is lost more or less in proportion to alveolar vessels, and arterial gas tensions can be reasonably well maintained for a period of time by increasing ventilation. The destruction of the parenchyma results in loss of lateral traction of small airways, so that they narrow and collapse. Then the regional distribution of inspired air becomes more impaired, with resultant worsening of the abnormalities in $\dot{V}_A/\dot{Q}$ ratios. These patients ini-

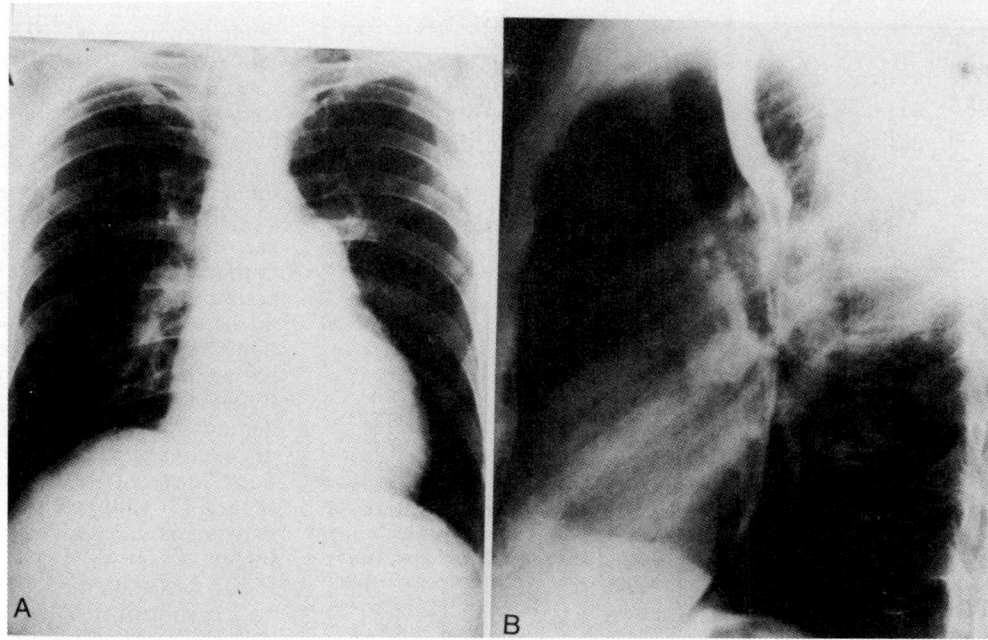

FIGURE 49–12. X-ray changes in cor pulmonale. *A,* Posteroanterior chest x-ray showing cardiomegaly, a definitely enlarged main pulmonary artery, and an enlarged right pulmonary artery. *B,* Lateral chest x-ray shows filling in of the retrosternal space and an enlarged left pulmonary artery. (From Murphy, M. L., Dinh, H., and Nicholson, D.: Chronic cor pulmonale. *In* Bone, R. C. [ed.]: Disease-a-Month, Oct 1989 p. 687.)

tially have a restricted vascular bed, with normal or near-normal pulmonary artery pressures at rest. As their disease process worsens with the development of airway disease and further deterioration of gas exchange, secondary changes in the vasculature occur and resting pulmonary artery hypertension and cor pulmonale develop.

CLINICAL MANIFESTATIONS OF COR PULMONALE WITH HEART FAILURE. These include increasing dyspnea; paroxysmal cough, occasionally with syncope; and fluid retention with edema and sometimes ascites. The distended neck veins exhibit prominent *a* and *v* waves and do not collapse with inspiration. Central cyanosis frequently is present, and hypoxemia, as measured by arterial oxygen saturation, correlates with the pulmonary artery pressure[131] (Fig. 49–8). Pulsus paradoxus (pp. 24 and 1476) may be present. Right ventricular hypertrophy is indicated by a palpable parasternal or subxiphoid heave. On auscultation, a (right-sided) S_3 gallop (heard along the left sternal edge or in the epigastrium and accentuated by inspiration) and a loud pulmonic second sound frequently are present. A holosystolic murmur along the lower left parasternal edge, accentuated by inspiration, usually indicates tricuspid regurgitation; its presence can be confirmed by Doppler echocardiography.[132] These cardiac findings can be evanescent and can develop quickly when acute respiratory failure is superimposed on COPD. Radionuclide techniques have shown that RV ejection fractions are correlated positively with arterial oxygen tension and inversely with arterial pCO_2[133] (Fig. 49–10). Examination of the lungs reveals diffuse inspiratory and expiratory rhonchi and wheezes, and the liver is enlarged and frequently pulsatile. If acute respiratory failure is present in addition, papilledema, confusion, a hyperkinetic circulation, and asterixis also may be present.

It is important to recognize that the hypoxemia of patients with COPD may be profoundly worsened during sleep.[134] This phenomenon may cause a further rise in pulmonary artery pressure and nocturnal cardiac arrhythmias.[135,136] The possible pathogenetic role of these phenomena in the development of cor pulmonale is discussed below.

Treatment

REDUCTION OF AIRWAY OBSTRUCTION. The management of cor pulmonale in COPD is to relieve pulmonary hypertension by improving gas exchange.[136–138] This is accomplished by reducing bronchial smooth muscle constriction, promoting drainage of retained secretions, promptly and

vigorously treating respiratory tract infections, and providing supplemental oxygen. The first two goals can be achieved simultaneously with the use of bronchodilators. In addition to relieving smooth muscle spasm, the sympathomimetics also increase mucociliary transport.[139] The net effect of these measures is to reduce airway obstruction and improve the regional distribution of inspired air and, in that manner, $\dot{V}_A/\dot{Q}$ relationships. Methylxanthines may provide benefits above and beyond the usual bronchodilatation, for this class of compounds has been reported to produce favorable hemodynamic effects as well. In one study, the intravenous administration of aminophylline in patients with cor pulmonale was shown to reduce mean pulmonary artery and right and left ventricular end-diastolic pressures significantly without inducing a change in the cardiac index,[140] and in another, right and left ventricular ejection fractions were increased.[141] The use of methylxanthines to improve diaphragmatic function has been in vogue for a number of years. Although this effect does occur, it is quite limited and of questionable clinical significance. Moreover, the effect is nonspecific and also has been observed with beta-adrenergic agonists.

OXYGEN ADMINISTRATION. The administration of supplemental oxygen in a controlled manner represents a major advance in the treatment of cor pulmonale. In acute respiratory failure, supplemental oxygen results in prompt and often dramatic improvement in pulmonary hemodynamics.[70] In fact, long-term oxygen therapy is the only treatment thus far shown to decrease mortality in COPD and to stop the progression of pulmonary hypertension.[142–144] In patients with progressive RV hypertrophy or recurrent heart failure from cor pulmonale associated with severe hypoxemia ($PaO_2 < 50$ mm Hg) and severe pulmonary hypertension, marked improvement has been found when oxygen was administered for 12 to 15 hours per day.[145,146]

Two major controlled studies of different aspects of long-term oxygen therapy in patients with COPD have been carried out. The U.S. (NIH-sponsored) Nocturnal Oxygen Therapy Trial[142] sought to determine if oxygen given for 19 hours a day improved survival over that observed with predominant nocturnal therapy (12 hr/day). The English (MRC) trial, on the other hand, sought to discover whether oxygen administration for 15 to 24 hours of the day had a positive effect on survival as compared with no oxygen.[143] The composite data are contained in Figure 49–13. Survival was poorest in those who did not receive supplemental oxygen and best in those who received it for the longest portion of the day.

According to recent data, survival tends to be greatest in

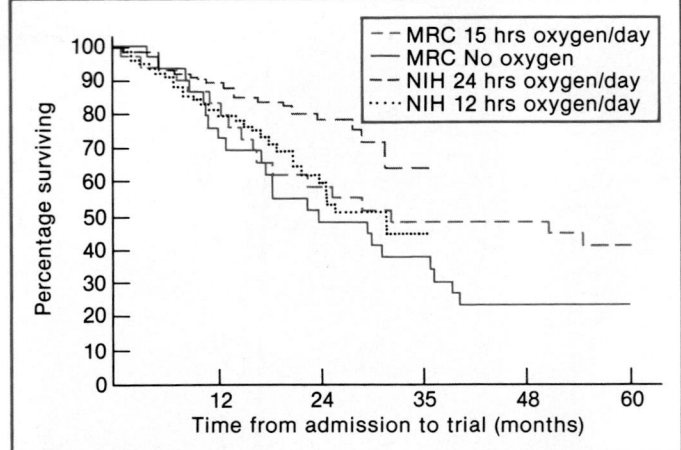

FIGURE 49-13. Survival curves in the MRC (British) and NIH (U.S.) long-term oxygen therapy trials in patients with severe hypoxemia and cor pulmonale. (From Flenley, D. C., and Muir, A. L.: Cardiovascular effects of oxygen therapy for pulmonary arterial hypertension. Clin. Chest Med. 4:297, 1983.)

younger patients (<60 years of age) with only moderate pulmonary artery hypertension at the time of therapy (mean pulmonary artery pressure <30 mm Hg).[144]

The criterion most commonly used to initiate chronic oxygen therapy is an arterial oxygen tension of 55 mm Hg or less. The inspired oxygen concentration is adjusted to produce a pO_2 of 60 mm Hg or greater. If chronic oxygen therapy is contemplated, it is *mandatory* to demonstrate that the supplemental oxygen will not result in worsening of alveolar hypoventilation with progressive hypercapnia and deterioration of the patient's mental status.

With the widespread availability of pulse oximetry, the place of this technique in the assessment of patients on long-term oxygen therapy is questioned. Although these devices are reasonably accurate under steady-state conditions, they can give false readings during exercise and in the presence of hemodynamic instability, dark skin pigmentation, jaundice, carboxyhemoglobin, and systemic alkalosis.[147] Equally important, pulse oximetry cannot detect acidosis or hypercapnia. Hence arterial blood gases, and not pulse oximetry, should be the means of selecting patients for long-term oxygen therapy. Once the patient's gas exchange is stable on oxygen, oximetry can then be used for monitoring.

VASODILATORS. Another proposed means of reducing pulmonary artery pressure is afterload reduction with vasodilators. This approach assumes that the RV failure seen with COPD results from increased afterload and that a significant feature of the latter is related to active vasoconstriction.[148] A number of drugs have been tried with varying degrees of effectiveness: isoproterenol,[149] phentolamine,[150] diazoxide,[151] prazosin,[152] hydralazine,[153,154] pirbuterol,[155] methyldopa,[156] and the calcium antagonists diltiazem, nifedipine, and nitrendipine.[157-159] During acute testing these have all been reported to improve pulmonary vascular hemodynamics.[160] Hydralazine (Fig. 49-14) and nifedipine appear to be particularly beneficial, and have been found to reduce pulmonary vascular resistance and increase cardiac output in patients with pulmonary hypertension from various causes[153-160] (p. 811). Nifedipine also has been shown to inhibit hypoxic vasoconstriction in patients with acute respiratory failure.[160]

Although there is no question that the aforementioned agents can increase RV stroke volume and reduce pulmonary vascular resistance acutely in patients with severe pulmonary hypertension, unfortunately this hemodynamic benefit does not carry over to the long run. To date, none of these drugs have lead to long-term clinical improvement or to improved survival.[155,157,161,162] In addition, vasodilator therapy can have significant side effects, such as worsening hypoxemia and sys-

temic hypotension.[163] This form of treatment, although theoretically attractive, has not yet lived up to its promise.

OTHER MEASURES. The indications for the use of other therapeutic measures, such as phlebotomy, diuretics, and cardiac glycosides, are considerably less clear. In the case of *phlebotomy*, most older studies have demonstrated an improvement in the subjective complaints related to vascular engorgement, but no evidence of improvement in pulmonary gas exchange, mechanics, or hemodynamics has been found.[164,165] Newer evidence suggests that erythropheresis in patients with secondary polycythemia and cor pulmonale reduces blood viscosity and improves right ventricular function.[166,167] *Diuretics* are commonly used for cor pulmonale with failure, and although there is little question of their effectiveness in reducing fluid retention, there are scant data to demonstrate that they improve pulmonary hemodynamics or gas exchange in the absence of left ventricular decompensation. Excessive use of potent diuretics can aggravate the loss of H^+ and Cl^- induced by chronic hypercapnia and cause a severe metabolic alkalosis. Hence, they should be used sparingly.

The use of *cardiac glycosides* in patients with cor pulmonale is controversial (p. 489). Digitalis apparently is effective in raising cardiac output in patients with cor pulmonale at rest but only at the expense of concomitant increases in pulmonary artery pressures. The consensus is that there is no clearcut evidence that cardiac glycosides are of substantial benefit *unless left ventricular failure coexists*.[168] Sympathomimetics such as terbutaline may, in addition to their beneficial effects on the tracheobronchial tree, exert a positive inotropic effect.[169]

PROGNOSIS. The outlook for patients with cor pulmonale secondary to COPD is difficult to state with certainty, for it is inextricably linked to the underlying disorder. When cor pulmonale develops in patients with emphysema, life expectancy is quite short, yet patients with bronchitis usually tolerate three to five episodes of failure before ultimately succumbing to the disease. Although long-term survival has been reported after the onset of cor pulmonale with heart failure, the 2- to 3-year survival rates range from 33 to 50 per cent[170-173] but may be improved with continuous oxygen therapy.

In both the NIH and MRC trials cited above, pulmonary vascular resistance and pulmonary artery pressure either declined or remained constant in those patients treated with

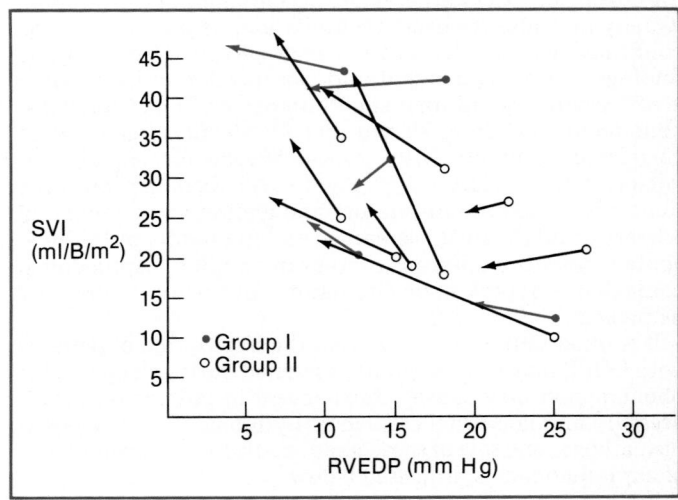

FIGURE 49-14. The relationship between right ventricular end-diastolic pressure (RVEDP) and stroke volume index (SVI) in 14 patients with right ventricular failure treated with oral hydralazine. Circles represent control and arrows represent post-hydralazine measurements. Patients in group I had significant reductions in mean pulmonary arterial pressure, while those in group II did not. (From Rubin, L. J.: Cardiovascular effects of vasodilator therapy for pulmonary arterial hypertension. Clin. Chest Med. 4:309, 1983.)

TABLE 49-4 CAUSES OF CHRONIC HYPOVENTILATION SYNDROME

(1) Impaired Ventilatory Control
- a. **Functional**
  - **Obesity-hypoventilation syndrome**
  - **Myxedema**
  - **Drugs (narcotics, sedatives)**
  - **Metabolic abnormalities (hypokalemia, hypophosphatemia, hypomagnesemia, metabolic alkalosis)**
- b. **Structural**
  - **Brain stem infarction or neoplasm**
- c. **Idiopathic**
  - **Primary alveolar hypoventilation**

(2) Neuromuscular disorders
- a. **Myopathies**
  - **Muscular dystrophy**
- b. **Neuropathies**
  - **Bilateral diaphragm paralysis**
  - **Poliomyelitis**
  - **Amyotrophic lateral sclerosis**
  - **Cervical spinal cord injury**
  - **Guillain-Barré syndrome**
- c. **Disorders of neuromuscular junction**
  - **Myasthenia gravis**

(3) Chest-wall Abnormalities
- a. **Kyphoscoliosis**
- b. **Thoracoplasty**

(4) Airway Obstruction
- a. **Upper airway**
  - **Tracheal stenosis**
  - **Obstructive sleep apnea**
  - **Laryngeal or nasal polyps**
  - **Tonsillar hypertrophy**
- b. **Lower airway**
  - **Chronic obstructive pulmonary disease**

(5) Parenchymal Lung Disease
- a. **Interstitial lung disease**
- b. **Surgical resection**

From Strumpf, D. A., Millman, R. P., and Hill, N. S.: The management of chronic hypoventilation. Chest *98*:474, 1990.

oxygen, suggesting a stabilization of the disease process. In those not so treated, mean pulmonary pressure and total pulmonary vascular resistance rose, on the average, 3 mm Hg and 100 dynes-sec-cm^{-5} per year, respectively.

Inadequate Ventilatory Drive

(Table 49-4)

The common denominator in this category of disorders causing cor pulmonale is a depressed output from the respiratory center, with resultant generalized alveolar hypoventilation. Cor pulmonale is then the result of pulmonary hypertension caused by chronic hypoxemia and acidemia.

OBESITY-HYPOVENTILATION SYNDROME. The association of extreme obesity with alveolar hypoventilation was originally made by Sir William Osler; Burwell et al. subsequently coined the term "pickwickian syndrome" to describe the combination of obesity, somnolence, plethora, and edema.[174] Despite many investigations, the pathogenesis of the hypoventilation in this syndrome remains obscure.[175] Excessive reduction of chest-wall compliance and muscle weakness secondary to obesity may account in part for this syndrome, but many extremely obese people with these defects do not hypoventilate. These patients may have abnormally low ventilatory responses to hypercapneic and anoxic stimulation, which improve with treatment.[176] Consequently hyposensitivity of the respiratory center with depressed ventilatory drive, whether acquired or preexistent, is probably a background factor.

The primary *treatment* of this disorder consists of weight reduction. The respiratory stimulant progesterone and its congeners have been shown to increase alveolar ventilation so that hypoxemia, hypercapnia, and cor pulmonale all improve substantially.[177,178] This may prove to be a useful adjunct until weight is reduced. If respiratory and cardiac failure are life-threatening, ventilatory assistance may be required.

SLEEP APNEA SYNDROME. After the description of the pickwickian syndrome, variant manifestations such as periodic respirations and hypersomnia were recognized, and it soon became apparent that patients with disturbed respirations during sleep could develop pulmonary hypertension and cor pulmonale.[179,179a] This has been designated the sleep apnea syndrome. Three types of patterns have been recorded (Fig. 49-15): (1) *central apnea*, in which airflow stops in conjunction with cessation of all respiratory muscle effort; (2) *obstructive apnea*, in which upper airway obstruction causes airflow to cease despite continuing or increasing efforts of the inspiratory muscles. The obstruction is believed to result from relaxation or discoordination of the buccal and pharyngeal muscles, from collapse of the walls of the pharynx due to failure of the genioglossus muscle, from greatly enlarged tonsils or adenoids, from backward movement of the tongue during sleep, and from narrowing of the upper airway secondary to marked obesity;[180] and (3) *mixed apnea*, in which airflow and respiratory effort stop early in the episode, followed by a resumption of unsuccessful respiratory effort.[179,180,180a]

The apneic periods, which can occur 40 to 60 times per hour,[180] are associated with phasic hypoxemia and hypercapnia. Alterations in gas exchange may be quite striking, and the pO$_2$ can fall to 20 to 25 mm Hg with saturations below 50 per cent. Pulmonary and systemic arterial pressures rise with each apneic period, and stroke volume, heart rate, and cardiac output fall.[176] With repetitive episodes, the pulmonary artery pressures progressively increase throughout the night[176] (Fig. 49-16). Hence, pulmonary hypertension is most severe in the morning. During the day, the pressures fall only to rise again with sleep the next night. Eventually hypoxemia, hypercapnia, and pulmonary hypertension become permanent and gradually worsen while the patient is awake.

In association with the fluctuation in gas exchange, patients often have severe bradyarrhythmias and tachyarrhythmias.[181] The former usually occur during periods of apnea, whereas the latter begin with the onset of breathing. The type of arrhythmias found consist of sinus bradycardia, sinus arrest, long asystolic periods (ranging from 2 to 13 seconds), sinoatrial block, premature atrial contractions, atrial fibrillation, ventricular premature beats with bigeminy and trigeminy, multifocal premature beats, and ventricular tachycardia.[181-183] Pulmonary capillary wedge pressures also may increase during periods of apnea.[184] The clinical symptomatology differs, depending on the type, frequency, and intensity of the abnormal, sleep-related respiratory pattern.

The patient rarely reaches the deep stages of sleep because of hypoxic arousal and therefore is chronically sleep-deprived. The other common clinical manifestations are loud

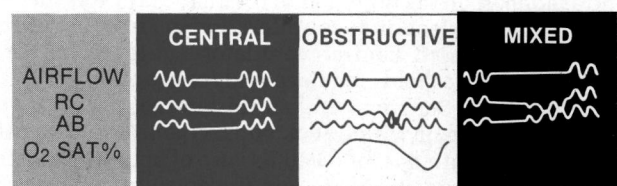

FIGURE 49-15. Schematic representation of the three patterns of apnea that develop during sleep in humans. RC and AB represent ribcage and abdominal displacement, respectively. O$_2$ sat = oxygen saturation. In each type, airflow at the nose and mouth is absent, indicating apnea. In central apneas, respiratory efforts as measured by the movement of the ribcage and abdomen are absent. During obstructive apneas, the efforts by the chest-wall muscles are present throughout the entire episode. In mixed apneas, both central and obstructive patterns are present. (From Strohl, K. P., et al.: Physiologic basis of therapy for sleep apnea. Am. Rev. Resp. Dis. *134*:791, 1986.)

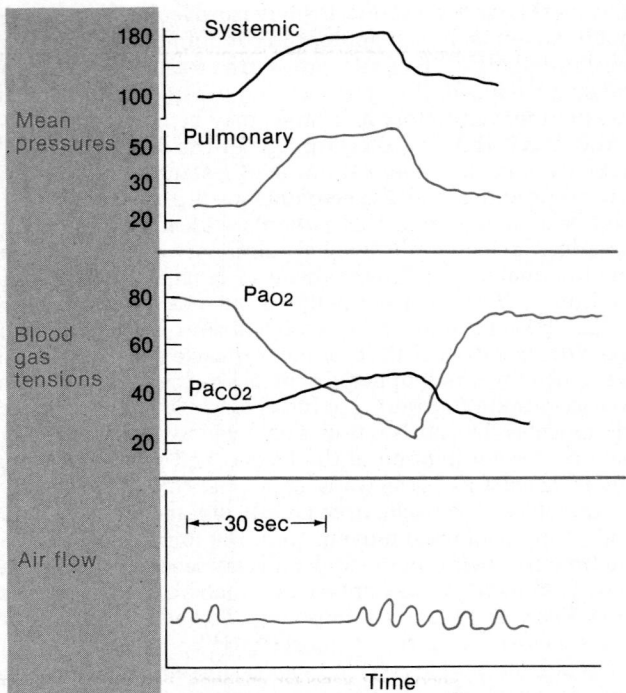

FIGURE 49–16. Schematic representation of hemodynamic and blood gas events during an apneic period. Respiratory pauses are associated with a fall in PaO_2 that usually exceeds the rise in $PaCO_2$. The combined hypoxia and hypercapnia are probably responsible for the rise in pulmonary arterial pressure which occurs with each apnea. Note that baseline pulmonary arterial pressure is slightly higher after the apneic episode. (From Weil, J. V.: Pulmonary hypertension and cor pulmonale in hypoventilating patients. *In* Weir, E. K., and Reeves, J. T. [eds.]: Pulmonary Hypertension. Mount Kisco, N.Y., Futura Publishing Co., 1984, p. 321.)

snoring, abnormal behavior during sleep (somnambulism, tremors, or myoclonus), altered states of consciousness, nocturnal enuresis, morning headache, daytime hypersomnolence, hypnagogic hallucinations, and systemic hypertension (Fig. 49–17). Most patients with sleep apnea are *not obese* and ventilate normally when awake. Patients with obstructive apnea tend to have less severe hypoventilation and fewer hemodynamic abnormalities than do patients with the other varieties. The diagnosis is readily established by performing polysomnography during sleep.

Several well-controlled studies indicate that about 20 per cent of patients with sleep apnea syndrome will have coexistent COPD and that most of these patients will develop pulmonary hypertension.[185,186] Diagnosis of the combined problem can be difficult unless specifically sought, and treatment of both problems is required to control the patient's symptoms.

The cause of sleep apnea is unknown. The weight of current evidence indicates that obstructive apneas occur because of occlusion of the upper airway in the region of the pharynx.[180] Central apneas, on the other hand, may have multiple mechanisms, including sleep-induced alteration in respiratory muscle drive, depressed central ventilatory output, and/or a change in the thresholds for sleep and/or arousal.[180]

Management. Sedatives and antihistamines should be assiduously avoided or withdrawn, and oxygen should be used with caution. Death has followed the use of both narcoleptics and oxygen administered in an uncontrolled manner.[180] Treatment of central apnea consists of respiratory stimulants or nocturnal ventilatory support with respirators.[180] Phrenic nerve or diaphragmatic pacing also has been recommended.[189] In obstructive apnea, tracheostomy and nasal CPAP (continuous positive airway pressure applied to the nose during sleep) are the most commonly used therapeutic modalities.[180] The former bypasses the area of obstruction, whereas the latter is believed to act as a pneumatic splint that prevents upper airway collapse. In an obese patient with obstructive apnea,

weight reduction may obviate the need for a permanent tracheal cannula. Removal of enlarged tonsils and/or adenoids or surgical enlargement of the entrance to the airway may be enormously helpful. Nocturnal oxygen therapy may be helpful in some patients by reducing the duration of the apneic periods and decreasing the related arrhythmias but, as already indicated, should be used with care.[187]

PRIMARY ALVEOLAR HYPOVENTILATION. Generalized alveolar hypoventilation in the absence of obesity or intrinsic disease of the lungs, chest wall, or neuromuscular apparatus has been ascribed to a failure of the autonomic control of ventilation. Most cases are acquired and are seen after encephalitis, brain stem surgery, meningitis, and the like, but congenital occurrence has been reported.[188] In this rare condition, the respiratory center does not respond normally to its chemical stimuli, and the patient has a flat or markedly depressed ventilatory–carbon dioxide response curve. An affected patient can improve alveolar ventilation and restore the arterial oxygen and carbon dioxide to normal by voluntary hyperventilation. This syndrome has been called *Ondine's curse.* The pathogenesis and treatment are similar to that outlined for other forms of generalized alveolar hypoventilation. An interesting therapeutic development is long-term pacing of the diaphragm by means of electrical stimulation of the phrenic nerves.[189]

CHRONIC MOUNTAIN SICKNESS. Some acclimatized residents of high altitudes suffer a transient loss of their adaptation after short stays at sea level and, on return to altitude, develop acute pulmonary edema with circulatory and electrocardiographic changes similar to those seen in acute cor pulmonale.[190] Some people who remain at high altitude lose their acclimatization and develop signs and symptoms of generalized alveolar hypoventilation with chronic cor pulmonale. This syndrome is variously called *chronic mountain sickness, soroche,* or *Monge disease.*[191] The mechanism for the hypoventilation is unknown, but it has been postulated that it is due to an adaptation or desensitization of the hypoxic chemoreceptors in the carotid body to chronic hypoxia.[192] The only treatment is removal of the patient to sea level, where pulmonary artery pressure usually falls acutely. With prolonged residence at sea level, polycythemia disappears, and

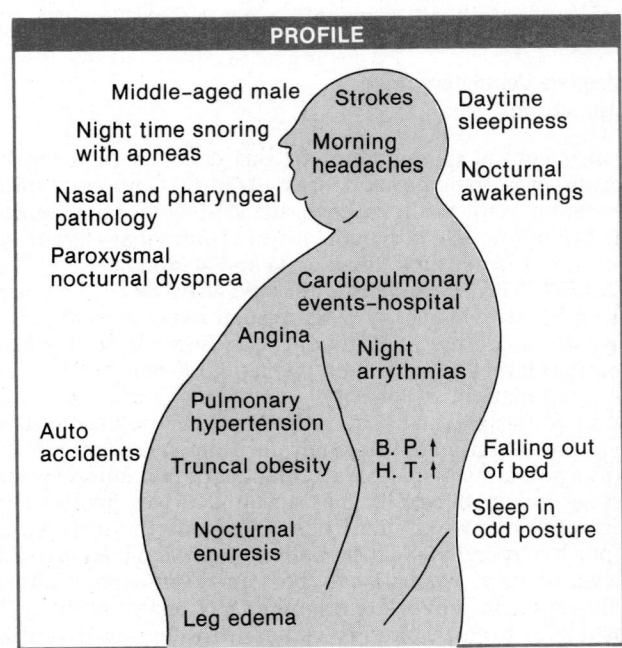

FIGURE 49–17. Clinical profile in patients with hypersomnia-sleep apnea syndromes. BP = blood pressure; HT = hematocrit. (From Burack, B.: The hypersomnia–sleep apnea syndrome: Its recognition in clinical cardiology. Am. Heart J. *107*:543, 1984.)

there is believed to be some involution of the structural changes of the pulmonary vessels.

UPPER AIRWAY OBSTRUCTION. Obstruction of the upper airways may be responsible for an inadequate ventilatory drive, global alveolar hypoventilation, and cor pulmonale. For the most part, this occurs in children,[193] especially black children, who have enlarged tonsils and adenoids; however, cor pulmonale has been reported to follow acute tonsillitis in adults.[194] Other causes include vascular ring (p. 954), macroglossia, micrognathia, laryngotracheomalacia, laryngeal web, Crouzon disease, Hurler syndrome, and severe Pierre Robin syndrome,[195,196] but it also can develop with obstruction of the upper airway during sleep in both children and adults.[197] The mechanism for the hypoventilation is not clear. It has been suggested that an abnormally reactive pulmonary vascular bed, a defect in the central control of respiration, and an interference with normal sleep physiology, as in the sleep apnea syndrome, may play a part, singly or in combination. There is little direct evidence for the first mechanism. However, it is known that ventilatory responsiveness to carbon dioxide is blunted in these patients and that it does not return to normal after therapy.[198]

The clinical features may mimic asthma, but more often the patients display somnolence, respiratory stridor, and recurrent respiratory tract infections. Treatment consists of surgical removal of the obstruction.

PULMONARY VASCULAR DISORDERS (see also Chap. 27). This category consists of diseases such as primary pulmonary hypertension that primarily affect the pulmonary vasculature, with minimal or no parenchymal involvement. These diseases represent the most straightforward pathogenetic sequence in which pulmonary hypertension and RV overloading are consequences of a progressive increase in pulmonary vascular resistance resulting from gradual obliteration of the pulmonary vascular bed. In addition to their pathophysiology, these diseases share in common the symptom of dyspnea and strikingly high pulmonary artery pressures, despite the fact that both vital capacity and pulmonary gas exchange may be only minimally impaired.[199] The latter finding frequently is of considerable diagnostic importance.

Chronic Suppurative Pulmonary Disease Associated with Cor Pulmonale

The two prime examples of chronic suppurative disease associated with chronic cor pulmonale are bronchiectasis and cystic fibrosis.

BRONCHIECTASIS. This chronic inflammatory disease is characterized clinically by cough and the production of copious amounts of purulent sputum and pathologically by cylindrical and saccular dilatation of airways.[200,201] In most patients one can elicit a history of pneumonia developing as a complication of measles, pertussis, or some other contagious disease of childhood. It is thought that bacterial pneumonia and associated atelectasis are responsible for the destruction and dilatation of the bronchial walls. A small percentage of cases are associated with congenital defects such as Kartagener triad and either congenital or acquired defects in immune mechanisms. Cor pulmonale develops in far-advanced cases in which destruction of lung tissue and fibrosis is extensive. The mechanisms for pulmonary hypertension are believed to be capillary loss, hypoxia, and increased bronchial-pulmonary collateral blood flow. Formerly this was a relatively common affliction, but bronchiectasis has decreased considerably in incidence during the past three decades, presumably because of the increasing use of antibiotics.

CYSTIC FIBROSIS. This genetic (autosomal recessive) defect is characterized by the secretion from exocrine glands of thick, tenacious mucus in which the mucopolysaccharide content is relatively insoluble and easily denatured. The lungs are involved to some extent in virtually all patients with the disease, and the thick mucus throughout the tracheobronchial tree partially or completely obstructs air passages, giving rise to focal atelectasis, pneumonia, bronchiectasis, and abscess formation.[202] Cor pulmonale is an important feature in the natural history, and it contributes to 70 per cent of the deaths.[203] Clinical recognition of the cardiac involvement in cystic fibrosis can be difficult in the early stage of the disease. Many investigators use noninvasive radionuclide scanning and/or echocardiography to improve detection.[204] One group has developed an echo-

cardiographic scoring system that provides a method for assessing the progression of the cardiac involvement and for evaluating prognosis.[205] Physiological studies have suggested that hypoxia is the principal stimulus to the production of pulmonary hypertension, and pathological data have supported this.[206-208] In the past, the development of cardiac failure usually presaged death within a few months. In recent years, however, the prognosis has been improving, and a number of patients have survived for considerable periods into their twenties. These patients have been maintained on a vigorous, comprehensive pulmonary care program with postural drainage, antibiotics, and bronchodilators.

Restrictive Lung Diseases

This category encompasses a multitude of diseases which have in common a destruction of functioning pulmonary parenchyma with restriction of the pulmonary vascular bed. The latter results from a physical loss of vessels as well as from intrinsic abnormalities in the lumina and walls of those remaining. Essentially, five types of processes alone or in combination can produce this effect: (1) diffuse interstitial, (2) diffuse alveolar, (3) mixed alveolar-interstitial, (4) chest wall and pleural, and (5) extensive resection of lung tissue with disease in the residual parenchyma. Specific examples of the first three categories are sarcoidosis, radiation fibrosis, connective tissue disorders with primary or secondary lung involvement, fibrosing alveolitis, alveolar proteinosis, pneumoconiosis, and progressive massive fibrosis. The prototypes for the fourth and fifth categories are thoracoplasty for chronic tuberculosis and surgical resections for granulomatous disease or bronchiectasis.

Pulmonary parenchymal disease, especially when complicated by fibrosis of tissue and secondary vascular changes, can lead to severe pulmonary hypertension. As with the other conditions with a restricted vascular bed, the pulmonary hypertension is initially confined to circumstances in which the cardiac output is elevated. As the vascular bed becomes further restricted and the vessels stiffen, pulmonary hypertension persists at rest and intensifies with increased blood flow. As long as hypoxemia remains mild, pulmonary hypertension is modest, but cor pulmonale develops with respiratory failure. Fortunately, the sequence is not inevitable in most patients with these problems. If the pathological process stabilizes, as is often the case, the patient is left with modest pulmonary hypertension at rest, which is usually well tolerated.[59]

PATHOPHYSIOLOGY. In these diseases, the lungs are stiff, with reduced volumes, and minute ventilation is high, with or without an elevated alveolar ventilation. Arterial oxygen tension usually is moderately reduced at rest, but severe hypoxemia may develop with exercise. The diffusing capacity is low and fails to increase normally as cardiac output rises. In contrast to the chronic obstructive syndromes, the correlation between arterial blood gases and pulmonary artery pressure is poor,[209] and there seems to be a parallel deterioration in pulmonary mechanics and hemodynamics.[210] As a general rule, when the vital capacity exceeds 80 per cent of normal, hemodynamics are normal. When vital capacity is between 50 and 80 per cent, vascular resistance is increased and pulmonary artery pressure in the resting state is at the upper limits of normal. When vital capacity is below 50 per cent, pulmonary hypertension usually is present at rest. The role of hypoxic vasoconstriction in these patients has been difficult to clarify. Experimental evidence indicates that the ability of the pulmonary vasculature to respond to alveolar hypoxia is abnormal in diseased regions, so that when hypoxia does occur, blood is shifted toward the affected areas, thus worsening net gas exchange.[18] In any event, the development of severe hypoxemia and carbon dioxide retention heralds the onset of right ventricular failure, which usually is seen late in the course.

CLINICAL FEATURES. In keeping with the pathophysiology, the prominent symptoms of restrictive lung disease are tachypnea at rest and severe dyspnea on exertion. Fine inspiratory rales are found, along with the previously mentioned signs of pulmonary hypertension and right ventricular hypertrophy and/or failure. Early in the course of patients with pulmonary fibrosis, glucocorticoids or immunosuppressive drugs may be helpful if noninfectious inflammatory processes are believed to be present. In the late stages with extensive pulmonary fibrosis, these modalities are unsuccessful; all that can be offered is continuous oxygen therapy, diuretics, and cardiac glycosides. Vasodilator therapy is still experimental but may offer some hope in selected patients.[148] Although many of the diseases in this category progress slowly, once cor pulmonale develops, the prognosis is poor and lung transplantation may be the only hope.

Disorders of the Neuromuscular Apparatus and Chest Wall

These disorders have in common the mechanical failure of the bellows apparatus, through weakness or paralysis of the respiratory muscles or through distortion of the geometry of the thorax. Several factors contribute to the development of cor pulmonale.

FAILURE OF THE NEUROMUSCULAR APPARATUS. Respiratory muscle weakness can result from generalized diseases of muscles such as myopathic infiltrating diseases or muscular dystrophy, but it more commonly follows a neurological disorder, such as a cord lesion at or below the third cervical vertebra, amyotrophic lateral sclerosis, myasthenia gravis, poliomyelitis, or Guillain-Barré syndrome.[199] In all of these diseases, the primary derangement is *generalized alveolar hypoventilation* from mechanical impedance to the movement of the rib cage, diaphragm, or both. The lungs and airways usually are not diseased, although they can become so with retained secretions and multiple aspirations. Although acute respiratory failure is common in these diseases, for cor pulmonale to develop in response to the hypoxic and hypercapneic stimuli the disorder must be chronic; consequently, this complication tends to be seen more often with cord lesions than with the other conditions just noted. Mechanical ventilatory support is the only treatment for the hypoventilation; a cuirass type of respirator is effective in these patients. Along with this, vigorous bronchial toilet facilitates the impaired handling of secretions that frequently coexists.

DIAPHRAGMATIC PARALYSIS. Bilateral diaphragmatic paralysis is an uncommon but insidious and frequently unrecognized cause of cor pulmonale.[211] In the upright position ventilation may be normal or almost so, but with assumption of the supine position gas exchange deteriorates. The diagnosis may be suspected in the patient with supine breathlessness, a disturbed sleep pattern, paradoxical (i.e., inward) motion of the abdomen on inspiration, and a low vital capacity in the erect position. Treatment consists of assisting ventilation when the patient is supine or during sleep. This can easily be accomplished under most circumstances with a rocking bed. When this is inadequate, electrical pacing of the diaphragm may be used.[189] Occasionally, diaphragmatic fatigue can contribute to the respiratory failure of COPD.[212] Bilateral diaphragmatic paralysis can occur after cardiac surgery.[213] The use of ice cardioplegia can damage the phrenic nerves and result in respiratory failure that becomes manifest as soon as the patient is removed from the ventilator postoperatively. This complication usually is transitory, and diaphragmatic function returns.

CHEST-WALL DISORDERS. The common congenital or acquired abnormalities that distort the geometry of the thoracic cage include kyphoscoliosis, pectus excavatum, pectus carinatum, and ankylosing spondylitis; of these, only kyphoscoliosis is associated with cor pulmonale.[214] *Kyphosis* refers to any posterior angulation of the spine, and *scoliosis* consists of a lateral displacement with at least one compensatory curve in the opposite direction. A kyphotic angle exceeding 100 degrees or an angle of scoliosis in excess of 120 degrees may be associated with cor pulmonale.[215] Such marked structural abnormalities of the thorax lead to abnormal positioning and functioning of the respiratory muscles, compression of the lung and pulmonary vasculature, and abnormal gas exchange.[215,216] In addition, it has been suggested that scoliosis interferes with the growth and development of alveoli and pulmonary arteries[217]; dyspnea is the major symptom of these disorders.

Therapy is directed toward avoiding complicating infections; episodes of acute respiratory failure are treated with mechanical ventilation. Surgical improvement of the thoracic deformity often is not associated with a commensurate change in cardiorespiratory function.[218]

NONINVASIVE ASSESSMENT OF COR PULMONALE

Echocardiography

M-mode echocardiography in adults with obstructive airway disease has been disappointing because the pulmonary hyperinflation associated with these conditions frequently precludes adequate visualization of the cardiac valves and chambers. Two-dimensional techniques can overcome this deficiency and permit visualization of right atrial and ventricular cavity dimensions and wall thickness (Fig. 49–18). These parameters are markedly influenced by the state of ventricular function and correlate well with radionuclide parameters of size and function.[219] The right atrium, right ventricle, and pulmonary artery are dilated. The two-dimensional echocardiogram also is useful in excluding left-sided heart disease as a cause of pulmonary hypertension and RV enlargement.

Various echocardiographic techniques available for the noninvasive assessment of pulmonary artery pressure are discussed on p. 80. The most useful of these is the Doppler echocardiographic assessment of the velocity of tricuspid regurgitant blood flow, which, when used in the Bernoulli equation, can be used to determine the right ventricular–right atrial pressure gradient. When this is added to the right atrial pressure, which is assessed clinically, the pulmonary artery systolic pressure can be estimated. This technique is quite useful in the identification of patients with chronic lung disease who have cor pulmonale.[220–224,224a]

Electrocardiographic Findings

(Table 49–5)

In the past, the use of the electrocardiogram to make the diagnosis of cor pulmonale has centered on the electrocardiographic demonstration of right ventricular hypertrophy (p. 126). The classic criteria of a shift of the mean QRS axis to the right (right axis deviation greater than +110 degrees), an R:S ratio in V$_1$ greater than 1, and an R:S ratio in V$_6$ of less than 1 were derived from patients with congenital heart disease[225,226] and have proved to be relatively poor criteria of cor pulmonale in patients with chronic obstructive lung disease.[227,228] The reason is that moderate RV hypertrophy is a late manifestation of cor pulmonale and occurs only after prolonged dilatation of the ventricle.[229]

Kilcoyne and associates studied 200 patients with chronic obstructive lung disease and demonstrated that when the arterial oxygen saturation fell below 85 per cent and mean pulmonary pressure rose to 25 mm Hg or greater, one or more of the following changes would develop in the electrocardiogram: (1) a rightward shift of the mean QRS axis of 30 degrees or more from its previous position; (2) inverted, biphasic, or flattened T waves in the right precordial leads; (3) depressed ST segments in leads II, III, and aV$_f$; and (4) incomplete or complete right bundle branch block.[228]

PRE

POST

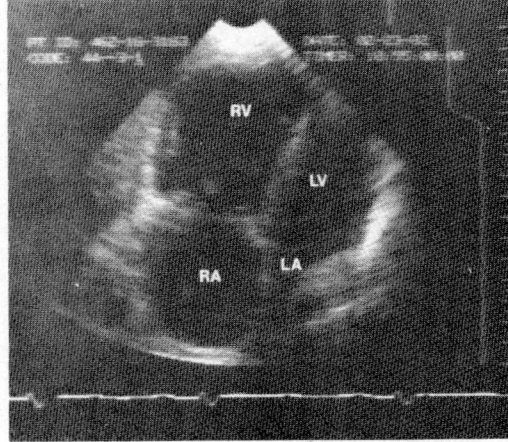
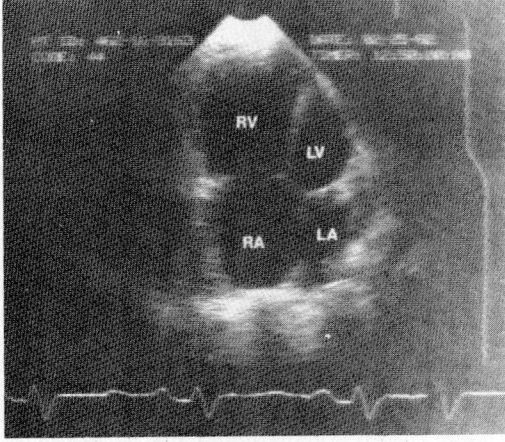

FIGURE 49–18. Echocardiogram from a 47-year-old man with pulmonary hypertension before *(left)* and 48 hours after *(right)* beginning therapy with nifedipine. The right atrium and right ventricle are greatly increased in size before treatment and are reduced in size by therapy. (From Rubin, L. J.: Cardiovascular effects of vasodilator therapy for pulmonary arterial hypertension. Clin. Chest Med. *4*:309, 1983.)

TABLE 49-5 ELECTROCARDIOGRAPHIC CHANGES IN COR PULMONALE

ECG CRITERIA FOR COR PULMONALE WITHOUT OBSTRUCTIVE DISEASE OF THE AIRWAYS*

1. Right-axis deviation with a mean QRS axis to the right of $+110°$
2. R/S amplitude ratio in $V_1 > 1$
3. R/S amplitude ratio in $V_6 < 1$
4. Clockwise rotation of the electrical axis
5. P-pulmonale pattern
6. S_1Q_3 or $S_1S_2S_3$ pattern
7. Normal voltage QRS

ECG CHANGES IN CHRONIC COR PULMONALE WITH OBSTRUCTIVE DISEASE OF THE AIRWAYS†

1. Isoelectric P waves in lead I or right-axis deviation of the P vector
2. P-pulmonale pattern (an increase in P-wave amplitude in II, III, AV_f)
3. Tendency for right-axis deviation of the QRS
4. R/S amplitude ratio in $V_6 < 1$
5. Low-voltage QRS
6. S_1Q_3 or $S_1S_2S_3$ pattern
7. Incomplete (and rarely complete) right bundle branch block
8. R/S amplitude ratio in $V_1 > 1$
9. Marked clockwise rotation of the electrical axis
10. Occasional large Q wave or QS in the inferior or midprecordial leads, suggesting healed myocardial infarction

*Any one of the first three criteria suffices to raise suspicion of right ventricular hypertrophy. The diagnosis becomes more certain if two or more of these findings are present (2 and 7). The last four criteria commonly occur in cor pulmonale secondary to primary alveolar hypoventilation, interstitial disease of the lung, or pulmonary vascular disease.

†The first seven criteria are suggestive but nonspecific; the last three are more characteristic of cor pulmonale in obstructive disease of the airways.

Reproduced with permission from Holford, F. D.: The electrocardiogram in lung disease. *In* Fishman, A. P. (ed.): Pulmonary Diseases and Disorders. New York, McGraw-Hill Book Co., 1980, p. 140.

With an increase in arterial saturation, these alterations disappeared. The T-wave changes in the right precordial leads and the axis shifts to the right occurred with only modest elevations of pulmonary artery pressure, but if these elevations became more severe, and if recurrences were frequent, then the rightward rotation of the QRS axis and the T-wave changes in the right precordial leads tended to become persistent. If pulmonary function were not improved, true right-axis deviation (a frontal plane axis greater

than $+90$ degrees) and increased R-wave voltage in the right precordial leads developed (Fig. 49–19). Once the latter occurred, the electrocardiogram was less likely to mirror any physiological variability, as reversion of the increased voltage to normal rarely occurred after improvement in arterial blood gases.

Other studies have suggested that clockwise rotation, right-axis deviation, a qR pattern in aV_r, and electrocardiographic evidence of right atrial enlargement (P pulmonale), in that order, also would point to right ventricular hypertrophy in patients with chronic cor pulmonale. Occasionally in chronic obstructive lung disease, the mean QRS axis may be directed posteriorly, superiorly, and to the right, so that there is apparent left-axis deviation in the standard limb leads. This pattern, along with low voltage, most often is associated with emphysema.

The electrocardiogram is far more accurate in detecting RV hypertrophy in patients with primary pulmonary hypertension than it is in detecting such hypertrophy in patients with chronic lung disease. The latter causes flattening of the diaphragms and hyperinflation of the lung, which produces changes in the electrocardiogram resembling right ventricular hypertrophy.[103]

Electrocardiographic features of prognostic importance in severe chronic bronchial obstruction have been outlined by Kok-Jensen.[230] In a study of 288 patients, survival was found to be very poor in patients with a QRS axis of $+90$ to $+180$ degrees and an amplitude of the P wave in lead II of 0.20 mV or more; only 37 and 42 per cent, respectively, of the patients with these changes were alive after 4 years.

Arrhythmias. Ambulatory electrocardiograms obtained in 69 stable patients enrolled in the nocturnal oxygen therapy trial described earlier (p. 1591) showed multiple patterns.[231] Ventricular premature beats were found in 83 per cent, ventricular bigeminy in 68 per cent, paired ventricular premature beats in 61 per cent, and nonsustained ventricular tachycardia in 22 per cent of the patients. Sixty-nine per cent had supraventricular tachycardia. Repetitive ventricular arrhythmia occurred in 64 per cent of the patients and tended to be found in those with hypercapnia and edema.

Vectorcardiograms. The vectorcardiogram has been correlated with hemodynamics in patients with COPD, and a linear correlation has been found between terminal rightward QRS forces and mean pulmonary artery pressure during exercise. Because in one such correlation[232] no patient met the electrocardiographic criteria for RV hypertrophy, it was suggested that the vectorcardiogram may be more selective in identifying early hemodynamic abnormalities in the pulmonary circulation.

Radioisotope Imaging

A frequently used radionuclide for RV imaging is thallium-201. The distribution of this isotope is a function of regional myocardial blood flow and myocardial mass, and so only the left ventricle tends to be visualized at rest. Imaging of the right ventricle at rest usually signifies that hypertrophy and dysfunction of the RV are present.[233]

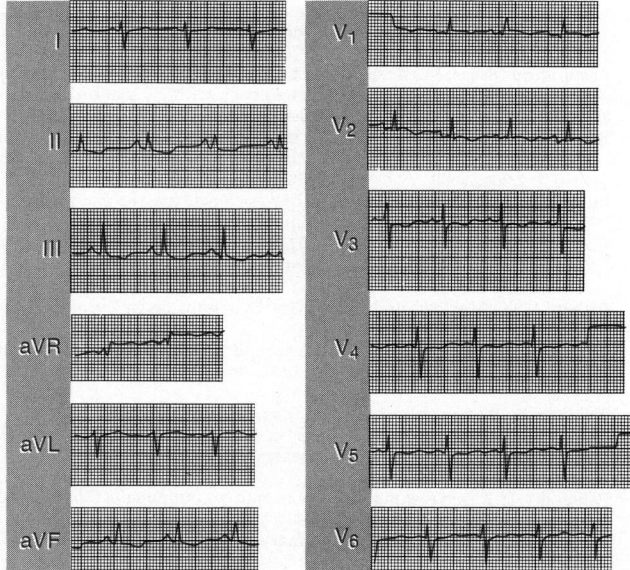

FIGURE 49–19. Electrocardiogram in a patient with emphysema and diffuse lung disease; there is right axis deviation, "P pulmonale," a QR pattern in V_1 and an rS pattern in V_6. (From McGowan, F. X., and Wagner, G. S.: The electrocardiogram in chronic lung disease. *In* Rubin, L. J. [ed.]: Pulmonary Heart Disease. Boston, Martinus Nijhoff, 1984, p. 117.)

REFERENCES

ANATOMICAL AND PATHOPHYSIOLOGICAL CORRELATES

1. Chronic cor pulmonale: Report of an expert committee. Wld. Hlth. Org. Tech. Rep. Ser. *213*:1, 1961.
2. Chronic Cor Pulmonale. *In* Fowler, N. O.: Diagnosis of Heart Disease. New York, Springer-Verlag, 1991, pp. 268–282.
3. Lewis, T.: Observations upon ventricular hypertrophy with especial reference to preponderance of one or other chamber. Heart *5*:367, 1914.
4. Emery, J. L., and Mithal, A.: Weight of cardiac ventricles at and after birth. Br. Heart J. *23*:313, 1961.
5. Keen, E. N.: The post-natal development of the human cardiac ventricles. J. Anat. *89*:484, 1955.
6. Arias-Stella, J., and Recavarren, S.: Right ventricular hypertrophy in native children living at high altitude. Am. J. Pathol. *41*:55, 1962.
7. Mathew, R., Thilenius, O. G., and Arcilla, R. A.: Comparative response of right and left ventricles to volume overload. Am. J. Cardiol. *38*:239, 1976.
8. Recavarren, S., and Arias-Stella, J.: Right ventricular hypertrophy in people born and living at high altitudes. Br. Heart J. *26*:806, 1964.
9. Penaloza, D., Sime, F., Banchero, N., et al.: Pulmonary hypertension in healthy men born and living at high altitudes. Am. J. Cardiol. *11*:150, 1963.
10. Fulton, R. M., Hutchinson, E. C., and Jones, A. M.: Ventricular weight in cardiac hypertrophy. Br. Heart J. *14*:413, 1952.
11. Mitchell, R. S., Stanford, R. E., Silvers, G. W., and Dart, G.: The right ventricle in chronic airway obstruction: A clinicopathologic study. Am. Rev. Respir. Dis. *114*:147, 1976.
12. Ishikawa, S., Fattal, G. A., Popiewicz, J., and Wyatt, J. P.: Functional morphometry of myocardial fibers in cor pulmonale. Am. Rev. Respir. Dis. *105*:358, 1972.
13. Brecher, G. A., and Galletti, P. M.: Functional anatomy of cardiac pumping. *In* Hamilton, A. F., and Dow, P. (eds.): Handbook of Physiology; Circulation. Vol. II. Washington, D.C., American Physiological Society, 1963, p. 759.

14. Visner, M. S., Arentzen, C. E., O'Connor, M. J., et al.: Alterations in left ventricular three-dimensional dynamic geometry and systolic function during acute right ventricular hypertension in the conscious dog. Circulation 67:353, 1983.

15. Barnard, D., and Alpert, J. S.: Right ventricular function in health and disease. Current Problems in Cardiology 12:417, 1987.

16. Laks, M. M., Garner, D., and Swan, H. J. C.: Volumes and compliances measured simultaneously in the right and left ventricles of the dog. Circ. Res. 20:565, 1967.

17. Abel, F. L., and Waldhausen, J. A.: Effects of alterations in pulmonary vascular resistance on right ventricular function. J. Thorac. Cardiovasc. Surg. 54:886, 1967.

18. Abel, F. L.: Effects of alterations in peripheral resistance on left ventricular function. Proc. Soc. Exp. Biol. Med. 120:52, 1965.

19. Morrison, D., Goldman, S., Wright, A. L., et al.: The effect of pulmonary hypertension on systolic function of the right ventricle. Chest 84:250, 1983.

20. Sarnoff, S. J., and Berglund, E.: Ventricular function. I. Starling's law of the heart studied by means of simultaneous right and left ventricular function curves in the dog. Circulation 9:706, 1954.

21. Spann, J. R., Buccino, R. A., Sonnenblick, E. H., and Braunwald, E. B.: Contractile state of cardiac muscle obtained from cats with experimentally produced ventricular hypertrophy and heart failure. Circ. Res. 21:341, 1967.

22. Haggart, G. E., and Walker, A. M.: The physiology of pulmonary embolism as disclosed by quantitative occlusion of the pulmonary artery. Arch. Surg. 6:764, 1923.

23. Gibbons, J. H., Hopkinson, M., and Churchill, E. D.: Changes in the circulation produced by gradual occlusion of the pulmonary artery. J. Clin. Invest. 11:543, 1932.

24. Fineberg, M. H., and Wiggens, C. J.: Compensation and failure of the right ventricle. Am. Heart J. 11:255, 1936.

25. Brooks, H., Kirk, E. S., Vokonas, P. S., et al.: Performance of the right ventricle under stress: Relation to right coronary flow. J. Clin. Invest. 50:2176, 1971.

26. Krahl, V. E.: Anatomy of the mammalian lung. In Fenn, O. W., and Rahn, H. (eds.): Handbook of Physiology; Respiration. Vol. I. Washington, D.C., American Physiological Society, 1964, p. 224.

27. Hislop, A., and Reid, L.: Intrapulmonary arterial development during fetal life–branching pattern and structure. J. Anat. 113:35, 1972.

28. Boyden, E. A., and Tompsett, D. H.: The changing patterns in the developing lungs of infants. Acta Anat. 61:164, 1965.

29. Meyrick, B., and Reid, L.: Pulmonary hypertension: Anatomic and physiologic correlations. Clin. Chem. Med. 4:199, 1983.

30. Fishman, A. P.: The normal pulmonary circulation. In Fishman, A. P. (ed.): Pulmonary Diseases and Disorders, 2nd ed. New York, McGraw-Hill Book Co., 1991, pp. 975–998.

31. Hebb, C.: Motor innervation of the pulmonary blood vessels of mammals. In Fishman, A. P., and Hecht, H. H. (eds.): The Pulmonary Circulation and the Interstitial Space. Chicago, University of Chicago Press, 1969, p. 195.

32. Allen, K. M., Wharton, J., Polak, J. M., and Ghaworth, S. G.: A study of nerves containing peptides in the pulmonary vasculature of healthy infants and children and those with pulmonary hypertension. Br. Heart J. 62:353, 1989.

33. Fishman, A. P.: Dynamics of the pulmonary circulation. In Hamilton, W. F., and Dow, P. (eds.): Handbook of Physiology; Circulation. Vol. II. Washington, D.C., American Physiological Society, 1963, p. 1667.

34. Bard, P.: The pulmonary circulation and respiratory variations in the systemic circulation. In Bard, P. (ed.): Medical Physiology. St. Louis, C. V. Mosby, 1961, p. 231.

35. Brofman, B. L., Charms, B. L., Kohn, P. M., et al.: Unilateral pulmonary artery occlusion in man. Control studies. J. Thorac. Surg. 34:206, 1957.

36. Guyton, A. C.: Circulatory Physiology: Cardiac Output and Its Regulation. Philadelphia, W. B. Saunders Company, 1963.

37. Maseri, A., Caldini, P., Howard, P., et al.: Determinants of pulmonary vascular volume–recruitment versus distensibility. Circ. Res. 31:218, 1972.

38. Lanari, A., and Agrest, A.: Pressure-volume relationship in the pulmonary vascular bed. Acta Physiol. Lat. Am. 4:116, 1954.

39. Caro, C. G.: Extensibility of blood vessels in isolated rabbit lung. J. Physiol. (Lond.) 178:193, 1865.

40. Howell, J. B. L., Permutt, S., Proctor, D. F., and Riley, R. L.: Effect of inflation of the lung on different parts of the pulmonary vascular bed. J. Appl. Physiol. 16:71, 1961.

41. Engelberg, J., and DuBois, A. B.: Mechanics of pulmonary circulation in isolated rabbit lungs. Am. J. Physiol. 186:401, 1959.

42. Maseri, A., Caldini, P., Permutt, S., and Zierler, K. L.: Pressure volume relationship in the pulmonary circulation. In Widimsky, J., Daum, S., and Herzog, H. (eds.): Progress in Respiration Research. Vol. 5. Basel, S. Karger, 1970, p. 53.

43. Glazier, J. B., Hughes, J. M. B., Maloney, J. E., and West, J. B.: Measurements of capillary dimensions and blood volume in rapidly frozen lungs. J. Appl. Physiol. 26:65, 1969.

44. West, J. B.: Ventilation/Blood Flow and Gas Exchange. 2nd ed. Philadelphia, F. A. Davis Co., 1970.

45. Zapol, W. M.: Acute respiratory failure in the surgical patient. In Fishman, A. P. (ed.): Pulmonary Diseases and Disorders. 2nd ed. New York, McGraw-Hill Book Co., 1991, pp. 2433–2442.

46. Permutt, S., and Riley, R. L.: Hemodynamics of collapsible vessels with tone: The vascular waterfall. J. Appl. Physiol. 18:924, 1963.

47. Klocke, R. A.: Ventilation, pulmonary blood flow, and gas exchange. In Fishman, A. P. (ed.): Pulmonary Diseases and Disorders. 2nd ed. New York, McGraw-Hill Book Co., 1991, pp. 185–198.

48. LeBlanc, P., Ruff, F., and Milic-Emili, J.: Effect of age and body position on airway closure in man. J. Appl. Physiol. 28:448, 1970.

49. Craig, D. B., Wahba, W. M., Don, H. F., et al.: Closing volume and its relationship to gas exchange in seated and supine position. J. Appl. Physiol. 31:717, 1971.

50. Lenfant, C.: Measurements of ventilation-perfusion distribution with alveolar-arterial differences. J. Appl. Physiol. 18:1090, 1963.

51. Raine, J. M., and Bishop, J. M.: A-a difference in O_2 tension and physiologic dead space in normal man. J. Appl. Physiol. 18:284, 1963.

52. Severinghaus, J. W., and Stupfel, M.: Alveolar dead space as an index of distribution of blood flow in pulmonary capillaries. J. Appl. Physiol. 10:335, 1957.

53. Grover, R. F.: Chronic hypoxic pulmonary hypertension. In Fishman, A. P. (ed.): The Pulmonary Circulation: Normal and Abnormal. Philadelphia, University of Pennsylvania Press, 1990, pp. 283–299.

54. Fishman, A. P.: Hypoxia and its effects on the pulmonary circulation. Circ. Res. 38:221, 1976.

55. Bergofsky, E. H.: Mechanisms underlying vasomotor regulation of regional pulmonary blood flow in normal and disease states. Am. J. Med. 57:378, 1974.

56. Bates, D. V., Macklem, P. T., and Christie, R. V.: Respiratory Function in Disease. 2nd ed. Philadelphia, W. B. Saunders Company, 1971, p. 75.

57. Engel, L. A., and Macklem, P. T.: Gas mixing and distribution in the lung. In Widdicombe, J. G. (ed.): Respiratory Physiology II. International Review of Physiology. Vol. 14. Baltimore, University Park Press, 1977, p. 37.

58. Sykes, M. K., McNicol, M. W., and Campbell, E. J. M.: Respiratory Failure. Oxford, Blackwell Scientific Publications, 1971, p. 56ff.

59. Habb, P. E., and Durand-Arczynska, W. Y.: Carbon monoxide effects on oxygen transport. In Crystal, R. G., et al. (eds.): The Lung: Scientific Foundations. New York, Raven Press, 1991, pp. 1267–1276.

60. Fowler, K. T., and Read, J.: Effect of alveolar hypoxia on zonal distribution of pulmonary blood flow. J. Appl. Physiol. 18:244, 1963.

61. Lindsay, D. A., and Reed, J.: Pulmonary vascular responsiveness in the prognosis of chronic obstructive lung disease. Am. Rev. Respir. Dis. 105:242, 1972.

62. Enson, Y., Guintini, C., Lewis, M. L., et al.: The influence of hydrogen ion concentration and hypoxia on the pulmonary circulation. J. Clin. Invest. 43:1146, 1964.

63. Bergofsky, E. H., Haas, F., and Procelli, R. J.: Determination of the sensitive vascular sites from which hypoxia and hypercapnia elicit rises in pulmonary arterial pressure. Fed. Proc. 27:1420, 1968.

64. Bergofsky, E. H.: Humoral control of the pulmonary circulation. Ann. Rev. Physiol. 42:221, 1980.

CHRONIC COR PULMONALE

65. Fishman, A. P.: Pulmonary hypertension and cor pulmonale. In Fishman, A. P. (ed.): Pulmonary Diseases and Disorders. 2nd ed. New York, McGraw-Hill Book Co., 1988, pp. 999–1048.

66. U. S. Department of Health and Human Services, National Heart, Lung and Blood Institute, Division of Lung Diseases: Progress report, 1980, p. 121.

67. Respiratory Disease. Task force report on prevention, control and education. Washington, D.C., U.S. Department of Health, Education and Welfare, Public Health Service, National Institute of Health, 1977, p. 83.

68. Stuart-Harris, C. H., Twidle, R. H. S., and Clifton, M. A.: Hospital study of congestive heart failure with special reference to cor pulmonale. Br. Med. J. 2:201, 1959.

69. Inter-Society Commission for Heart Disease Resources: Primary prevention of pulmonary heart disease. Circulation 41:A-17, 1970.

70. Burrows, B., Kettel, L. J., Niden, A. H., et al.: Patterns of cardiovascular dysfunction in chronic obstructive lung disease. N. Engl. J. Med. 286:912, 1972.

71. Bishop, J. M.: Hypoxia and pulmonary hypertension in chronic bronchitis. Prog. Resp. Dis. 9:10, 1975.

72. Traver, G. A., Cline, M. G., and Burrows, B.: Predictors of mortality in chronic obstructive pulmonary disease. Am. Rev. Respir. Dis. 119:895, 1979.

73. Fishman, A. P.: Cor pulmonale. Am. Rev. Respir. Dis. 114:775, 1976.

74. Enson, Y.: Pulmonary heart disease. In Baum, G. L. and Wolinsky, E. (eds.): Textbook of Pulmonary Diseases. 4th ed. Boston, Little, Brown, 1989, pp. 1181–1197.

75. Palevesky, H. I., and Fishman, A. P.: Chronic cor pulmonale: Etiology and management. JAMA 263:2347, 1990.

76. Berbel, L. N., and Miro, R. E.: Pulmonary hypertension in the pathogenesis of cor pulmonale. Cardiovasc. Rev. 4:359, 1983.

77. Weitzenblum, E., Hirth, C., Duculone, A., et al.: Prognostic value of pulmonary artery pressure in chronic obstructive pulmonary disease. Thorax 36:752, 1981.

78. Finlay, M., Middleton, H. C., Peake, M. D., and Howard, P.: Cardiac output, pulmonary hypertension, hypoxemia and survival in patients with chronic obstructive airways disease. Eur. J. Respir. Dis. 64:252, 1983.

79. Wilkinson, M., Langhorne, C. A., Heath, D., et al.: A pathophysiological

study of 10 cases of hypoxia cor pulmonale. Q. J. Med. (New Series) 66:65, 1988.

80. Thurlbeck, W. M., Henderson, J. A., Fraser, R. G., and Bates, D. V.: Chronic obstructive lung disease. A comparison between clinical, roentgenologic, functional and morphologic criteria in chronic bronchitis, emphysema, asthma and bronchiectasis. Medicine 48:81, 1970.

81. Edwards, J. E.: Pathology of chronic pulmonary hypertension. Pathol. Annu. 9:1, 1974.

82. Wagenvoort, C. A., and Wagenvoort, N.: Hypoxic pulmonary vascular lesions in man at high altitude and in patients with chronic respiratory disease. Pathol. Microbiol. 39:276, 1973.

83. Semmens, M., and Reid, L.: Pulmonary arterial muscularity and right ventricular hypertrophy in chronic bronchitis and emphysema. Br. J. Dis. Chest. 68:253, 1974.

84. Wagenvoort, C. A., Heath, D., and Edwards, J. E.: The Pathology of the Pulmonary Vasculature. Springfield, Ill., Charles C Thomas, 1964.

85. Roos, A.: Poiseuille's law and its limitation in vascular systems. In Grover, R. F. (ed.): Progress in Research in Emphysema and Chronic Bronchitis. Basel, Karger, 1963, p. 32.

86. Wells, R. E., and Merrill, E. W.: Influence of flow properties of blood upon viscosity hematocrit relationships. J. Clin. Invest. 41:1591, 1962.

87. Rendas, A., Lennar, S., and Reid, L.: Aorto-pulmonary shunts in growing pigs: Functional and structural assessment of the changes in the pulmonary circulation. J. Thorac. Cardiovasc. Surg. 77:109, 1979.

88. Balchum, O. J., Jung, R. C., Turner, A. F., and Jacobson, G.: Pulmonary artery to vein shunts in obstructive pulmonary disease. Am. J. Med. 43:178, 1967.

89. Boushy, S. F., North, L. B., and Trice, J. A.: The bronchial arteries in chronic obstructive pulmonary disease. Am. J. Med. 46:506, 1969.

90. Meyrick, B., and Reid, L.: Ultrastructural findings in lung biopsy material from children with congenital heart defects. Am. J. Pathol. 101:527, 1980.

91. Rabinovitz, M., Haworth, S., Vanck, Z., et al.: Early pulmonary vascular changes in congenital heart disease studied in biopsy tissue. Hum. Pathol. 11:499, 1980.

92. Marcus, J. H., McLean, R. L., Duffell, G. M., and Ingram, R. H.: Exercise performance in relation to the pathophysiologic type of chronic obstructive pulmonary disease. Am. J. Med. 49:14, 1970.

93. Harris, P., Segal, N., and Bishop, J. M.: The relation between pressure and flow in the pulmonary circulation in normal subjects and in patients with chronic bronchitis and mitral stenosis. Cardiovasc. Res. 2:73, 1968.

94. Seibold, H., Henze, E., Kohler, J., et al.: Right ventricular function in patients with chronic obstructive pulmonary disease. Klin. Wochenschr. 63:1041, 1985.

95. Kawakami, Y., Kishi, F., Yamamoto, H., and Miyamoto, K.: Relation of oxygen delivery, mixed venous oxygenation and pulmonary hemodynamics to prognosis in chronic obstructive pulmonary disease. N. Engl. J. Med. 308:1045, 1983.

96. Bergofsky, E. H.: Tissue oxygen delivery and cor pulmonale in chronic obstructive pulmonary disease. N. Engl. J. Med. 308:1092, 1983.

97. Klinger, J. R., and Hill, N. S.: Right ventricular dysfunction in chronic obstructive pulmonary disease: Evaluation and management. Chest 99:715, 1991.

98. Olvey, S. K., Redufo, L. A., Stevens, P. M., et al.: First pass radionuclide assessment of right and left ventricular ejection fraction in chronic pulmonary disease. Effect of oxygen upon exercise response. Chest 78:4, 1980.

99. Khaja, F., and Parker, J. D.: Right and left ventricular performance in chronic obstructive lung disease. Am. Heart J. 82:319, 1971.

100. Brunet, F., Dhainaut, J. F., Devaux, J. Y., et al.: Right ventricular performance in patients with acute respiratory failure. Intensive Care Med. 14:474, 1988.

101. Biernacki, W., Flenley, D. C., Muir, A. L., and MacNee, W.: Pulmonary hypertension and right ventricular function in patients with COPD. Chest 94:1169, 1988.

102. Stewart, R. I., and Lewis, C. M.: Cardiac output during exercise in patients with COPD. Chest 89:199, 1986.

103. Murphy, M. L., Dinh, H., and Nicholson, D.: Chronic cor pulmonale. Disease-a-Month 35:653, 1989.

104. Samet, P., Fritts, H. W., Jr., Fishman, A. P., and Cournand, A.: The blood volume in heart disease. Medicine 36:211, 1957.

105. Turino, G. M., Edelman, N. H., Richards, E. C., and Fishman, A. P.: Extravascular lung water in cor pulmonale. Bull. Physiol. Pathol. Respir. 4:47, 1968.

106. Meerson, F. Z.: The myocardium in hyperfunction, hypertrophy, and heart failure. Circ. Res. 25(Suppl. 2):1, 1969.

107. Chidsey, C. A., Kaiser, G. A., Sonnenblick, E. H., et al.: Cardiac norepinephrine stores in experimental heart failure in the dog. J. Clin. Invest. 43:2386, 1964.

108. Chandler, B. M., Sonnenblick, E. H., Spann, J. F., Jr., and Pool, P. E.: Association of depressed myofibrillar adenosine triphosphatase and reduced contractility in experimental heart failure. Circ. Res. 21:717, 1967.

109. Kelly, D. T., Spotnitz, H. M., Beiser, G. D., et al.: Effects of chronic right ventricular volume and pressure loading on left ventricular performance. Circulation 44:403, 1971.

110. Feneley, M. P., Olsen, C. D., Glower, D. D., and Rankin, J. S.: Effect of acutely increased right ventricular afterload on work output from the left ventricle in conscious dogs. Circ. Res. 65:135, 1989.

111. Hecht, H. H., Kuida, H., and Tsagaris, T. J.: Brisket disease. IV. Impairment of left ventricular function in a form of cor pulmonale. Trans. Assoc. Am. Physicians 75:263, 1962.

112. Fluck, D. C., Chandrasekar, R. G., and Gardner, F. U.: Left ventricular hypertrophy in chronic bronchitis. Br. Heart J. 28:92, 1966.

113. Murphy, M. L., Adamson, J., and Hutcheson, F.: Left ventricular hypertrophy in patients with chronic bronchitis and emphysema. Ann. Intern. Med. 81:307, 1974.

114. Rao, S. B., Cohn, K. E., Eldridge, F. L., and Hancock, E. W.: Left ventricular failure secondary to chronic pulmonary disease. Am. J. Med. 45:229, 1968.

115. Jezek, V., and Schrijen, F.: Left ventricular function in chronic obstructive pulmonary disease with and without cardiac failure. Clin. Sci. Mol. Med. 45:267, 1973.

116. Seibold, H., Roth, U., Lippert, R., et al.: Left heart function in chronic obstructive lung disease. Klin. Wochenschr. 64:433, 1986.

116a. Johnson, G. L., Kanga, J. F., Moffett, C. B., and Noonan, J. A.: Changes in left ventricular diastolic filling patterns by Doppler echocardiography in cystic fibrosis. Chest 99:646, 1991.

117. Frank, M. J., Weisser, A. B., Moschos, C. B., and Levinson, G. E.: Left ventricular function, metabolism, and blood flow in chronic cor pulmonale. Circulation 48:798, 1973.

118. Williams, J. F., Childress, R. H., Boyd, D. L., et al.: Left ventricular function in patients with chronic obstructive pulmonary disease. J. Clin. Invest. 47:1143, 1968.

119. Unger, K., Shaw, D., Karliner, J. S., et al.: Evaluation of left ventricular performance in acutely ill patients with chronic obstructive lung disease. Chest 68:135, 1975.

120. Steele, P., Ellis, J. H., Jr., Van Dyke, D., et al.: Left ventricular ejection fraction in severe chronic obstructive airways disease. Am. J. Med. 59:21, 1975.

121. Christianson, L. C., Shah, A., and Fisher, V. J.: Quantitative left ventricular cineangiography in patients with chronic obstructive pulmonary disease. Am. J. Med. 66:399, 1979.

122. Gabinski, C., Courty, G., Besse, P., and Castaing, R.: Left ventricular function in chronic obstructive lung disease. Bull. Eur. Physiopathol. Resp. 15:755, 1979.

123. Rubin, L. J.: Clinical evaluation. In Rubin, L. J. (ed.): Pulmonary Heart Disease. Boston, Martinus Nijhoff, 1984, p. 107.

124. Murphy, M. L., and Bone, R. C.: Cor Pulmonale in Chronic Bronchitis and Emphysema. Mount Kisco, N.Y., Futura Publishing Co., 1984, 276 pp.

125. Slutsky, A., Hooper, W., Ackerman, W., et al.: Evaluation of left ventricular function in chronic pulmonary disease by exercise gated equilibrium radionuclide angiography. Am. Heart J. 101:414, 1981.

126. Nino, A. F., Berman, M. M., Gluck, E. H., et al.: Drug-induced left ventricular failure in patients with pulmonary disease: Endomyocardial biopsy demonstration of catecholamine myocarditis: Chest 92:732, 1987.

127. Lavine, S. J., Tami, L., and Jawad, I.: Pattern of left ventricular diastolic filling associated with right ventricular enlargement. Am. J. Cardiol. 62:444, 1988.

128. Burrows, B., Fletcher, C. M., Heart, B. E., et al.: Emphysematous and bronchial types of chronic airways obstruction: Clinico-pathological study of patients in London and Chicago. Lancet 1:830, 1966.

129. Mitchell, R. S., and Filley, G. F.: Chronic obstructive bronchopulmonary disease. I. Clinical features. Am. Rev. Respir. Dis. 89:360, 1964.

130. Stanford, W., and Galvin, J. R.: The radiology of right heart dysfunction: Chest roentgenogram and computed tomography. J. Thorac. Imag. 4:7, 1989.

131. Bishop, J. M., and Grass, K. W.: Use of other physiologic variables to predict pulmonary artery pressure in patients with chronic respiratory distress. Multicenter study. Eur. Heart J. 2:509, 1981.

132. Venditho, M. A., Pisano, D., Simelans, J. P., and Dickerson, C. N.: The incidence of tricuspid valvular regurgitation in patients with severe chronic obstructive pulmonary disease as determined by two-dimensional echocardiography. JAMA 84:264, 1984.

133. Flenley, D. C., and Muir, A. L.: Cardiovascular effects of oxygen therapy for pulmonary arterial hypertension. Clin. Chem. Med. 4:297, 1983.

134. Douglas, N. J., Calvertey, P. M. A., Leggett, R. J. E., et al.: Transient hypoxemia during sleep in chronic bronchitis and emphysema. Lancet 1:1, 1979.

135. Tinlapun, V. G., and Mir, M. A.: Nocturnal hypoxemia and associated electrocardiographic changes in patients with chronic obstructive airway disease. N. Engl. J. Med. 306:125, 1982.

136. Ingram, R.: Chronic bronchitis, emphysema, and chronic airways obstruction. In Wilson, J. E., et al. (eds.): Harrison's Principles of Internal Medicine. 12th ed. New York, McGraw-Hill Book Co., 1991, p. 1074.

137. Rubin, L. J., and Peter, R. H.: Therapy of pulmonary heart disease. In Rubin, L. J. (ed.) Pulmonary Heart Disease. Boston, Martinus Nijhoff, 1984, p. 325.

138. Myers, K. E., and Bogden, P. E.: Bronchodilators for patients with chronic heart disease. Postgrad. Med. 86:324, 1989.

139. McFadden, E. R., Jr.: Inhaled Aerosol Bronchodilators. Baltimore, Williams and Wilkins, 1986, p. 99.

140. Parker, J. O., Kelkar, K., and West, R. S.: Hemodynamic effects of aminophylline in cor pulmonale. Circulation 33:17, 1966.

141. Matthay, R. A., Berger, H. J., Locke, J., et al.: Effect of aminophylline upon right and left ventricular performance in chronic obstructive pulmonary disease. Noninvasive assessment by radionuclide angiocardiography. Am. J. Med. 65:903, 1978.

142. Nocturnal Oxygen Therapy Trial Group. Continuous or nocturnal oxygen therapy in hypoxemic chronic obstructive lung disease. A clinical trial. Ann. Intern. Med. 93:391, 1980.

143. MRC Working Party: Long-term ancillary oxygen therapy in chronic hy-

poxic cor pulmonale complicating chronic bronchitis and emphysema. A clinical trial. Lancet 1:681, 1981.

144. Weitzenblum, E., Sautegeau, A., Ehrhart, M., et al.: Long term oxygen therapy can reverse the progression of pulmonary hypertension in patients with chronic obstructive pulmonary disease. Am. Rev. Respir. Dis. 131:493, 1985.

145. Hall, J., and Wood, L. D. H.: Oxygen therapy. In Crystal, R.G., et al. (eds.): The Lung: Scientific Foundations. New York, Raven Press, 1991, pp. 2143–2154.

146. Morrison, D., Caldwell, J., Lakshminaryan, S., et al.: The acute effects of low flow oxygen and isosorbide dinitrate on left and right ventricular ejection fractions in chronic obstructive pulmonary disease. J. Am. Coll. Cardiol. 2:652, 1983.

147. Wuertemberger, G., Zielinsky, J., Sliwinsky, P., et al.: Survival in chronic obstructive pulmonary disease after diagnosis of pulmonary hypertension related to long term oxygen therapy. Lung 168(Suppl.):762, 1990.

148. Rubin, L. J.: Vasodilator therapy (general aspects). In Fishman, A. P. (ed.): The Pulmonary Circulation: Normal and Abnormal. Philadelphia, University of Pennsylvania Press, 1990, pp. 479–483.

149. Lupi-Herrera, E., Bialostozky, D., and Sobrino, A.: The role of isoproterenol in pulmonary artery hypertension of unknown etiology. Chest 79:292, 1981.

150. Ruskin, J., and Hutter, A. M.: Primary pulmonary hypertension treated with oral phentolamine. Ann. Intern. Med. 90:772, 1979.

151. Klinke, W. P., and Gilbert, J. A. L.: Diazoxide in primary pulmonary hypertension. N. Engl. J. Med. 302:91, 1980.

152. Vik-Mo, H., Walde, N., Jentoft, H., and Halvorsen, F. J.: Improved haemodynamics but reduced arterial blood oxygenation at rest and during exercise after long-term oral prazosin therapy in chronic cor pulmonale. Eur. Heart J. 6:1047, 1985.

153. Rubin, L. J., Handel, F., and Peter, R. H.: The effects of oral hydralazine on right ventricular and diastolic pressure in patients with right ventricular failure. Circulation 65:1369, 1982.

154. Brent, B. N., Berger, J., Matthay, R. A., et al.: Contrasting acute effects of vasodilators (nitroglycerin, nitroprusside and hydralazine) on right ventricular performance in patients with chronic obstructive pulmonary disease and pulmonary hypertension: A combined radionuclide-hemodynamic study. Am. J. Cardiol. 51:1682, 1983.

155. Biernacki, W., Prince, K., Whyte, K., et al.: The effects of six months of daily treatment with the beta-2 agonist oral pirbuterol on pulmonary hemodynamics in patients with chronic hypoxic cor pulmonale receiving long term oxygen therapy. Am. Rev. Respir. Dis. 139:492, 1989.

156. Evans, T. W., Waterhouse, J., Finlay, M., et al.: The effects of long-term methyldopa in patients with hypoxic cor pulmonale. Br. J. Dis. Chest 82:405, 1988.

157. Rubin, L. J., and Moser, K.: Long-term effects of nitrendipine on hemodynamics and oxygen transport in patients with cor pulmonale. Chest 89:141, 1986.

158. Singh, H., Ebejer, M. J., Higgins, D. A., et al.: Acute haemodynamic effects of nifedipine at rest and during maximum exercise in patients with chronic cor pulmonale. Thorax 40:910, 1985.

159. Crevey, B. J., Dantzker, D. R., Bower, J. S., et al.: Hemodynamic and gas exchange effects of intravenous diltiazem in patients with pulmonary hypertension. Am. J. Cardiol. 49:578, 1982.

160. Weir, E. K.: Acute vasodilator testing and pharmacological treatment of primary pulmonary hypertension. In Fishman, A. P. (ed.): The Pulmonary Circulation: Normal and Abnormal. Philadelphia, University of Pennsylvania Press, 1990, pp. 485–499.

161. Morley, T. F., Zappasodi, S. J., Belli, A., and Giudice, J. C.: Pulmonary vasodilator therapy for chronic obstructive pulmonary disease and cor pulmonale. Chest 92:71, 1987.

162. Vestri, R., Philip-Joet, F., Surpas, P., et al.: One year clinical study on niphedipine in the treatment of pulmonary hypertension in chronic obstructive lung disease. Respiration 54:139, 1988.

163. Packer, M., Greenberg, B., Massiz, B., and Dash, H.: Deleterious effects of hydralazine in patients with pulmonary hypertension. N. Engl. J. Med. 306:1326, 1982.

164. Dayton, L. M., McCullough, R. E., Scheinhorn, D. J., and Weil, J. V.: Symptomatic and pulmonary response to acute phlebotomy in secondary polycythemia. Chest 68:785, 1975.

165. Rakita, L., Gillespie, D. G., and Sancetta, S. M.: The acute and chronic effects of phlebotomy on general hemodynamics and pulmonary function of patients with secondary polycythemia associated with pulmonary emphysema. Am. Heart J. 70:466, 1965.

166. Wallis, P. J. W., Skehan, J. D., Newland, A. C., et al.: Effect of erythropheresis on pulmonary hemodynamics and O_2 transport in patients with secondary polycythemia and cor pulmonale. Clin. Sci. 70:91, 1986.

167. Erickson, A. D., Golden, W. R., Claunch, B. C., et al.: Acute effects of phlebotomy on right ventricular size and performance in polycythemic patients with chronic obstructive pulmonary disease. Am. J. Cardiol. 52:163, 1983.

168. Mathur, P. N., Powles, A. C. P., Pugsley, S. O., et al.: Effect of digoxin on right ventricular function in severe chronic airway obstruction. Ann. Intern. Med. 95:283, 1981.

169. Sunderrajan, E. V., Byron, W. A., McKenzie, W. N., et al.: The effect of terbutaline on cardiac function in patients with stable chronic obstructive lung disease. JAMA 250:2151, 1983.

170. Gottlieb, L. S., and Balchum, O. J.: Course of chronic obstructive pulmonary disease following first onset of respiratory failure. Chest 63:5, 1973.

171. Stevens, P. M., Terplan, M., and Knowles, J. H.: Prognosis of cor pulmonale. N. Engl. J. Med. 269:1289, 1963.

172. Burrows, B., and Earle, R. H.: Course and prognosis of chronic obstructive lung disease. A prospective study of 200 patients. N. Engl. J. Med. 280:397, 1969.

173. Mitchell, R. S., Webb, N. C., and Filley, G. F.: Chronic obstructive lung disease. III. Factors influencing prognosis. Am. Rev. Respir. Dis. 89:878, 1964.

174. Burwell, C. S., Robin, E. D., Whaley, R. D., and Bickelman, A. G.: Extreme obesity associated with alveolar hypoventilation—a pickwickian syndrome. Am. J. Med. 21:811, 1956.

175. Rochester, D. F., and Enson, Y.: Current concepts in the pathogenesis of the obesity-hypoventilation syndrome. Am. J. Med. 57:402, 1974.

176. Weil, J. V.: Pulmonary hypertension and cor pulmonale in hypoventilating patients. In Weir, E. K., and Reeves, J. T. (eds.): Pulmonary Hypertension. Mount Kisco, N.Y., Futura Publishing Co., 1984, p. 321.

177. Lyons, H. A., and Huang, C. T.: Therapeutic use of progesterone in alveolar hypoventilation associated with obesity. Am. J. Med. 44:881, 1968.

178. Sutton, F. D., Zwillich, C. W., Creagh, C. E., et al.: Progesterone for outpatient treatment of pickwickian syndrome. Ann. Intern. Med. 83:476, 1975.

179. Cherniack, N. S.: Respiratory dysrhythmias during sleep. N. Engl. J. Med. 305:325, 1981.

179a. Millman, R. P., and Fishman, A. P.: Sleep apnea syndromes. In Fishman, A. P. (ed.): Pulmonary Diseases and Disorders. 2nd ed. New York, McGraw-Hill Book Co., 1991, pp. 1347–1362.

180. Strohl, K. P., Cherniack, N. S., and Gather, B.: Physiologic basis of therapy in sleep apnea. Ann. Rev. Respir. Dis. 134:791, 1986.

180a. Khoo, M. C. K.: Periodic breathing. In Crystal, R. G., et al. (eds.): The Lung: Scientific Foundations. New York, Raven Press, 1991, pp. 1419–1432.

181. Burrek, B.: The hypersomnia-sleep apnea syndrome: Its recognition in clinical cardiology. Am. Heart J. 107:543, 1984.

182. Guilleminault, C., Cannally, S. J., and Winkler, R. A.: Cardiac arrhythmia and conduction disturbances during sleep in 400 patients with sleep apnea syndrome. Am. J. Cardiol. 52:490, 1983.

183. Peiser, J., Ovnat, A., Uwyyed, K., et al.: Cardiac arrhythmias during sleep in morbidly obese sleep-apneic patients before and after gastric bypass surgery. Clin. Cardiol. 8:519, 1985.

184. Buda, A. J., Schroeder, J. S., and Guilleminault, C.: Abnormalities of pulmonary wedge pressures in sleep-induced apnea. Int. J. Cardiol. 1:67, 1981.

185. Fletcher, E. C., Schaaf, J. W., Miller, J., and Fletcher, J. G.: Long term cardiopulmonary sequelae in patients with sleep apnea and chronic lung disease. Am. Rev. Respir. Dis. 135:525, 1987.

186. Weitzenblum, E., Krieger, J., Apprill, M., et al.: Daytime pulmonary hypertension in patients with obstructive sleep apnea syndrome. Am. Rev. Respir. Dis. 138:345, 1988.

187. Martin, R. J., Sanders, M. H., Gray, B. A., and Pennock, B. E.: Acute and long-term ventilatory effects of hyperoxia in the adult sleep apnea syndrome. Am. Rev. Respir. Dis. 125:175, 1982.

188. Mellins, R. B., Balfour, H. H., Jr., Turino, G. M., and Winters, R. W.: Failure of automatic control of ventilation (Ondine's curse). Medicine 49:487, 1970.

189. Glenn, W. W. L., Holcomb, W. C., Hogan, J., et al.: Diaphragm pacing by radiofrequency transmission in the treatment of chronic ventilatory insufficiency: Present status. J. Thorac. Cardiovasc. Surg. 66:505, 1973.

190. Penaloza, D., and Sime, F.: Circulatory dynamics during high altitude pulmonary edema. Am. J. Cardiol. 23:369, 1969.

191. Penaloza, D., and Sime, F.: Chronic cor pulmonale due to loss of altitude acclimatization (chronic mountain sickness). Am. J. Med. 50:728, 1971.

192. Severinghaus, J. W., Bainton, C. R., and Carcelen, A.: Respiratory insensitivity to hypoxia in chronically hypoxic man. Respir. Physiol. 1:308, 1966.

193. Bland, J. W., Edwards, F. K., and Brainsfield, D.: Pulmonary hypertension and congestive heart failure in children with chronic upper airway obstruction. New concepts and etiologic factors. Am. J. Cardiol. 23:830, 1969.

194. Randall, C. S., Braman, S. S., and Millman, R. P.: Rapid development of cor pulmonale following acute tonsillitis in adults. Chest 95:462, 1989.

195. Noonan, J. A.: Pulmonary heart disease. Pediatr. Clin. North Am. 18:1255, 1971.

196. Johnson, G. M., and Todd, D. W.: Cor pulmonale in severe Pierre Robin syndrome. Pediatrics 65:152, 1980.

197. Glenn, W. W. L., Gee, J. B. L., Cole, D. R., et al.: Combined central alveolar hypoventilation and upper airway obstruction. Treatment by tracheostomy and diaphragm pacing. Am. J. Med. 64:50, 1978.

198. Ingram, R. H., Jr., and Bishop, J. B.: Ventilatory response to carbon dioxide after removal of chronic upper airway obstruction. Am. Rev. Respir. Dis. 102:645, 1970.

199. Williams, M. H., Jr., Adler, J. J., and Colp, C.: Pulmonary function studies as an aid in the differential diagnosis of pulmonary hypertension. Am. J. Med. 47:378, 1969.

200. Glauser, E. M., Cook, C. D., and Harris, C. B. C.: Bronchiectasis. A review of 187 cases in children with follow-up pulmonary function studies in 58. Acta Paediatr. Scand. (Suppl.) 165:1, 1966.

201. Reid, L.: Reduction in bronchial subdivisions in bronchiectasis. Thorax 5:233, 1950.

202. Colten, H. R.: Cystic fibrosis. In Wilson, J. E., et al. (eds.): Harrison's Principles of Internal Medicine, 12th ed. New York, McGraw-Hill Book Co., 1991, p. 1072.

203. Moss, A. J.: The cardiovascular system in cystic fibrosis. Pediatrics 70:728, 1982.

204. Moskowitz, W. B., Gewitz, M. H., Heyman, S., et al.: Cardiac involvement in cystic fibrosis: Early noninvasive detection and vasodilator therapy. Ped. Pharmacol. 5:139, 1985.

205. Lester, L. A., Egge, A. C., Hubbard, V. S., Camerini-Otero, C. S., and Fink, R. J.: Echocardiography in cystic fibrosis: A proposed scoring system. J. Pediatr. 97:742, 1980.

206. Ryland, D., and Reed, L.: The pulmonary circulation in cystic fibrosis. Thorax 30:285, 1975.

207. Benesova, D., Voriskova, M., Hrobonova, V., and Vavrova, V.: Cardiovascular complications of cystic fibrosis. Cesk. Pediatr. 38:458, 1983.

208. Sahilahti, E., and Rapola, J.: Frequent myocardial lesions in Schwachman's syndrome. Eight fatal cases among 16 Finnish patients. Acta Pediatr. Scand. 73:642, 1984.

209. Emirgil, C., Sobol, B. J., Herbert, W. H., and Trout, K.: The lesser circulation in pulmonary fibrosis secondary to sarcoidosis and its relationship to respiratory function. Chest 60:371, 1971.

210. Enson, Y., Thomas, H. M., III, Bosken, C. H., et al.: Pulmonary hypertension in interstitial lung disease: Relationship of vascular resistance to abnormal lung structure. Trans. Assoc. Am. Physicians 88:248, 1975.

211. Newsom Davis, J., Goldman, M., Loh, L., and Casson, M.: Diaphragm function and alveolar hypoventilation. Q. J. Med. 45:87, 1976.

212. Aubier, M., DeTroyer, A., Sampson, M., et al.: Aminophylline improves diaphragmatic contractility. N. Engl. J. Med. 305:249, 1981.

213. Chandler, K. W., Rozas, C. J., Kory, R. C., and Goldman, A. L.: Bilateral diaphragmatic paralysis complicating local cardiac hypothermia during open heart surgery. Am. J. Med. 77:243, 1984.

214. Bergofsky, E. H.: Respiratory failure in disorders of the thoracic cage. Am. Rev. Respir. Dis. 119:643, 1979.

215. Bergofsky, E. H., Turino, G. M., and Fishman, A. P.: Cardiorespiratory failure in kyphoscoliosis. Medicine 38:263, 1959.

216. Bijure, J., Grimby, G., Kasalicky, J., Lindh, M., and Nachemson, A.: Respiratory impairment and airway closure in patients with untreated idiopathic scoliosis. Thorax 25:451, 1970.

217. Davies, G., and Reid, L.: Effect of scoliosis on growth of alveoli and pulmonary arteries and on the right ventricle. Arch. Dis. Child. 46:623, 1971.

218. Westgate, H. D., and Moe, J. H.: Pulmonary function in kyphoscoliosis before and after correction by the Harrington instrumentation method. J. Bone Joint Surg. 51:935, 1969.

219. Starling, M. R., Crawford, M. H., Sorensen, S. G., and O'Rourke, R. A.: A new two-dimensional echocardiographic technique for evaluating right ventricular size and performance in patients with obstructive lung disease. Circulation 66:612, 1982.

220. Ferrazza, A., Marino, B., Giusti, V., et al.: Usefulness of left and right oblique subcostal view of the echo-Doppler investigation of pulmonary arterial blood flow in patients with chronic obstructive pulmonary disease. Chest 98:286, 1990.

221. Migueres, M., Escamilla, R., Coca, F., et al.: Pulsed Doppler echocardiography in the diagnosis of pulmonary hypertension in COPD. Chest 98:280, 1990.

222. Himelman, R. B., Abbott, J. A., Lee, E., et al.: Doppler echocardiography and ultrafast cine-computed tomography during dynamic exercise in chronic parenchymal pulmonary disease. Am. J. Cardiol. 64:528, 1989.

223. Danchin, N., Cornette, A., Henriquez, A., et al.: Two-dimensional echocardiographic assessment of the right ventricle in patients with chronic obstructive lung disease. Chest 92:229, 1987.

224. Bertoli, L., Mantero, A., Alpago, R., et al.: Value of two-dimensional echocardiography in the identification of pulmonary hypertension in chronic obstructive lung disease. Respiration 55:193, 1989.

224a. Tramarin, R., Torbicki, A., Marchandise, B., et al.: Doppler echocardiographic evaluation of pulmonary artery pressure in chronic obstructive pulmonary disease. A European multicentre study. Eur. Heart J. 12:103, 1991.

225. McGowan, F. X., and Wagner, G. S.: The electrocardiogram in chronic lung disease. In Rubin, L. J. (ed.): Pulmonary Heart Disease. Boston, Martinus Nijhoff, 1984, p. 117.

226. Goodwin, J. F., and Abdin, Z. N.: The cardiogram of congenital and acquired right ventricular hypertrophy. Br. Heart J. 21:523, 1959.

227. Phillips, R. W.: The electrocardiogram in cor pulmonale secondary to pulmonary emphysema: A study of 18 cases proved by autopsy. Am. Heart J. 56:352, 1958.

228. Kilcoyne, M. M., Davis, A. L., and Ferrer, M. I.: A dynamic electrocardiographic concept useful in the diagnosis of cor pulmonale. Circulation 42:903, 1970.

229. Holford, F. D.: The electrocardiogram in pulmonary disease. In Fishman, A. P. (ed.): Pulmonary Diseases and Disorders. 2nd ed. New York, McGraw-Hill Book Company, 1991, pp. 471–478.

230. Kok-Jensen, A.: Simple electrocardiographic features of importance for prognosis in severe chronic bronchial obstruction. Scand. J. Respir. Dis. 56:273, 1975.

231. Shih, H. T., Webb, C. R., Conway, W. A., et al.: Frequency and significance of cardiac arrhythmias in chronic obstructive lung disease. Chest 94:44, 1988.

232. Wilson, J. R., Mason, U. G., Bahler, R. C., et al.: Vectorcardiographic detection of early hemodynamic abnormalities in chronic obstructive pulmonary disease. Chest 76:160, 1979.

233. Shuk, J. W., Walder, J., Oetgen, W., and Thomas, H. M.: Right ventricular visualization by thallium 201 myocardial scintigraphy in chronic obstructive pulmonary disease. South. Med. J. 78:1435, 1985.

PART IV

BROADER PERSPECTIVES ON HEART DISEASE AND CARDIOLOGIC PRACTICE

50

General Principles of Cardiovascular Cellular and Molecular Biology

by BERNARDO NADAL-GINARD, M.D., Ph.D, and VIJAK MAHDAVI, Ph.D.

As is the case for other organ systems, the development, structure, and function of the cardiovascular system depend on the proper functioning of its constituent cellular elements. Derangement of these cellular functions is at the basis of all cardiovascular disease. Every normal and disordered physiological process at the levels of cell, tissue, and organ is the result of complex biochemical reactions. These biochemical reactions involve proteins that, in turn, are the products of specific genes. Therefore, at some point in the future it should

be possible to describe cardiovascular physiological and pathological processes at the cellular, molecular, and genetic levels; this remains an elusive goal for most cardiovascular processes. As a consequence, many diagnostic and therapeutic approaches to cardiovascular disease are still based on empirical observations rather than on an understanding of the precise molecular dysfunction that is at the basis of the disease and the manner in which it is affected by therapeutic agents.

Molecular Biology and the Cardiovascular System

Until recently, the view prevailed that the heart is a relatively static organ biochemically and it therefore did not seem to be either particularly interesting or suitable as a subject for major questions of cellular and molecular biology. As a consequence, the impact of newly developed techniques of recombinant DNA and genetic manipulation on the understanding of the cellular and molecular biology of the heart has lagged behind that of other organs. However, the power of these new techniques and approaches is just beginning to be felt in the field of cardiovascular biology.

MOLECULAR BASIS OF GENE EXPRESSION

All of the genetic information required to produce a human is stored in the nucleus of each cell in the form of deoxyribonucleic acid (DNA). In humans, DNA is packaged in 23 pairs of chromosomes as a double-stranded linear molecule composed of purine (adenosine, A, and guanosine, G) and pyrimidine (thymidine, T, and cytosine, C) bases. These bases pair with each other according to Watson and Crick's rules so that an A

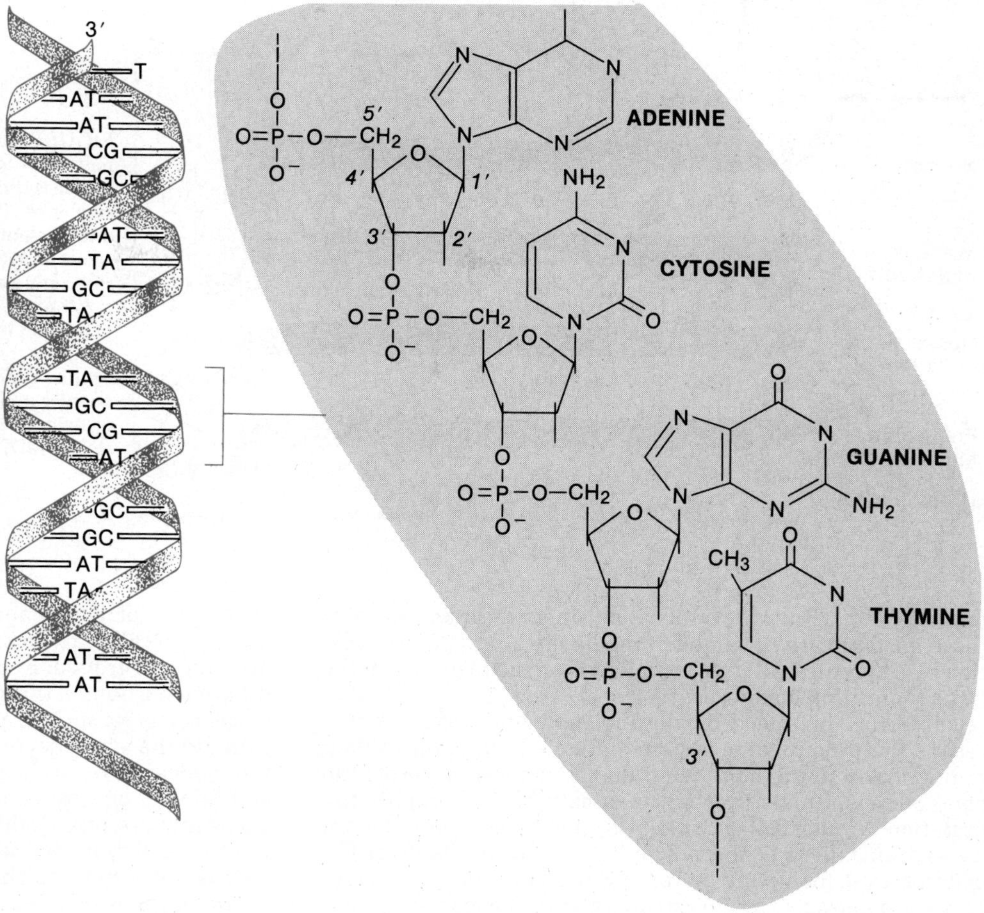

FIGURE 50–1. The structure of DNA. *Left,* a schematic drawing of the DNA double helix, showing the sugar-phosphate backbone as a ribbon, with the bases arranged toward the middle. Note that A always pairs with T and C always pairs with G. *Right,* an expanded view of four nucleotides along one strand, showing the complete chemical structure of the sequence 5'-ACGT-3'. (A nucleotide consists of a sugar, a phosphate group, and an attached base.) Note that the 5' and 3' designations, used to indicate the polarity of a DNA strand, refer to the numbering of carbons on the deoxyribose ring. The four nucleotide bases comprising DNA are adenine, cytosine, guanine, and thymine. Adjacent bases in a DNA single-stranded molecule are joined by phosphate group linkages between the 5' and 3' carbons of their respective deoxyribose sugar moieties. In DNA, adenine will pair with its complementary nucleotide thymine, and guanine with cytosine, by hydrogen bond formation between their respective purine and pyridamine rings. In this manner, complementary DNA strands pair to form a double helix (*left*). The 5' to 3' order of the phosphate linages in the DNA strands of the double helix are reciprocal; i.e., the DNA strands are antiparallel. (From Gelehrter, T. D., and Collins, F. S.: *Principles of Medical Genetics.* Baltimore, Williams and Wilkins, 1990, p. 10.)

is always paired with a *T* and a *G* with a *C* (Fig. 50–1). As a consequence of this complementary characteristic, knowing the sequence of one strand of DNA allows prediction of the other. In this simple manner, each strand carries the information needed for its faithful duplication and provides the basis for heredity. The rules of base pairing assure that individual cells and whole organisms transmit an identical copy of the DNA sequence stored in the nucleus to their descendants.

The capacity of DNA to store information in a continuous string of *A*s, *T*s, *C*s, and *G*s (the letters of the genetic alphabet) is enormous because the string of DNA is decoded into three letter words called *codons* (Fig. 50–2). Each codon, in turn, specifies either one of the 20 different amino acids that constitute the building blocks of proteins or is used as a punctuation

signal to indicate the end of coding information. A *gene* is constituted by the string of bases in the DNA that codes for the amino acid sequence of a protein molecule together with the DNA sequences needed for the regulation of the gene. These regulatory sequences, in general, flank the coding sequences. The gene is the basic functional unit of heredity that is transmitted from one generation to the next.

The simplicity of the system evolved by DNA to store and transmit information is what ensures its accuracy and fidelity. Each second, many millions of cells in the body divide. One of the marvels of DNA is that each time a cell divides, two strands of DNA, each containing approximately one and a half billion bases that have the capacity to code for approximately 100,000 different proteins, are copied faithfully, in a matter of

FIGURE 50–2. The genetic code. The table shows the correspondence (the genetic code) between three-base codons in mRNA and the amino acid inserted into the polypeptide. Amino acids are represented by two types of abbreviations: a three-letter and a single-letter abbreviation. The triplet code of RNA bases that specifies the utilization of amino acids in protein is shown. The triplets are called codons and are "degenerate"; i.e., some amino acids are designated by more than one triplet sequence. All proteins start with a methionine; therefore, its coding sequence, AUG, is also the "start" codon (marked *). Three codons, UAA, UAG and UGA, are "stop" codons and serve to terminate protein translation. The one-letter shorthand notations for the designation of amino acids in primary protein sequences are also shown. Amino acid abbreviations: Ala, alanine; Arg., arginine; Asp, aspartic acid; Cys, cysteine; Gln, glutamine; Glu, glutamic acid; Gly, glysine; His, histidine; Ile, isoleucine; Leu, leucine; Met, methionine; Phe, phenylalanine; Pro, proline; Ser, serine; Thr, threonine; Trp, tryptophan; Tyr, tyrosine; Val, valine. (From Hartl, D. L.: *Human Genetics.* Hagerstown, MD, Harper and Row, 1983, p. 278.)

THE GENETIC CODE

First nucleotide in codon (5' end)	Second nucleotide in codon							
	U		**C**		**A**		**G**	
U	UUU phe / UUC phe — F		UCU ser / UCC ser / UCA ser / UCG ser — S		UAU tyr / UAC tyr — Y		UGU cys / UGC cys — C	
	UUA leu / UUG leu — L				UAA (stop) / UAG (stop)		UGA (stop) / UGG trp W	
C	CUU leu / CUC leu / CUA leu / CUG leu — L		CCU pro / CCC pro / CCA pro / CCG pro — P		CAU his / CAC his — H		CGU arg / CGC arg / CGA arg / CGG arg — R	
					CAA gln / CAG gln — Q			
A	AUU ile / AUC ile / AUA ile — I		ACU thr / ACC thr / ACA thr / ACG thr — T		AAU asn / AAC asn — N		AGU ser / AGC ser — S	
	AUG* met M				AAA lys / AAG lys — K		AGA arg / AGG arg — R	
G	GUU val / GUC val / GUA val / GUG val — V		GCU ala / GCC ala / GCA ala / GCG ala — A		GAU asp / GAC asp — D		GGU gly / GGC gly / GGA gly / GGG gly — G	
					GAA glu / GAG glu — E			

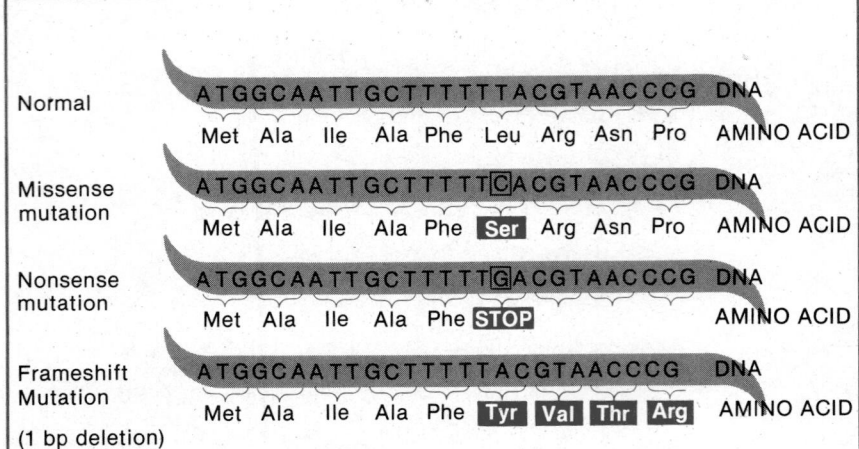

FIGURE 50–3. Examples of mutation; bd = base pair. The "sense" strand DNA sequence of a coding region is shown, together with the encoded amino acid sequence. Three different mutations affecting the second nucleotide of a leucine codon are shown. A missense mutation results in the substitution of an incorrect amino acid, while a nonsense mutation generates a "stop" codon and results in premature termination of protein translation. Addition or deletion of nucleotides can result in a change in the reading frame of the triplet codons (frameshift mutation), and consequently a change in the amino acid sequence of the protein. (From Hartl, D. L.: Human Genetics. Hagerstown, MD, Harper and Row, 1983, p. 22.)

minutes and with (on average) one single mistake. Many of these mistakes are corrected immediately after DNA replication by a "proofreading" system that is an intrinsic part of the DNA replication apparatus.

The errors produced during the replication of DNA that escape the proofreading system are called *mutations*. When mutations occur in somatic cells in most cases they are of little consequence, unless they occur in cells able to amplify the mutation through cell division. Although these mutations are never transmitted to the progeny, they are heritable at the cellular level. (In fact, an increasing number of neoplastic processes are known to originate through this mechanism.) Only when the change in the DNA is present in the reproductive cells does the mutation become transmitted to the progeny. In a genetic sense, therefore, a mutation is a stable and heritable change in the DNA sequence.

Mutations can involve gross rearrangements in the DNA sequence produced by deletions, duplications, and translocations or may involve a single base change in which one base is substituted for another (Fig. 50–3). Many of these point mutations have no detectable physiological and biochemical effects because they do not change the meaning of the codon they affect. This is because of the "degeneracy of the genetic code" in which a given amino acid can be encoded by more than one specific codon; for example, leucine and proline are each encoded by six different codons. Changes in the DNA sequence that do not change the coding content of the gene are called *silent mutations*. When they change the meaning of the codon, they either change the amino acid that is specified (missense mutation) or introduce a stop signal that truncates the coding sequence (nonsense mutation). Many of the human mutations identified so far represent missense mutations that produce an amino acid change in the protein specified by the mutant gene. In some cases, these substitutions have little or no effect on the function of the protein. In other cases, however, the function of the protein is impaired or totally abolished. This latter class of mutations may be responsible for the inherited diseases.

DECODING THE INFORMATION STORED IN DNA

With the exception of the cells of the immune system, all somatic cells contain the same genetic information in their nuclear DNA. In fact, the nucleus of a single somatic cell contains the information necessary to produce a complete organism. However, despite the fact that all cells have the same genotype, multicellular organisms are composed of many different cell types that differ dramatically from one another. These different phenotypes are the result of each cell type making selective use of the common genetic information stored in its nucleus. This selective use of the genome by different cell types at particular stages of development or in dif-

ferent physiological states is the basis of development in general and of cell differentiation in particular. Specific cell types are different from one another because they use specifically different portions of the genome. Genes that are expressed in a single cell type, such as albumin in the hepatocyte, the globin genes in the erythrocyte, and cardiac myosin heavy chain in the myocardium, are cell *type–specific* genes (Fig. 50–4). In addition, all or most cell types share the expression of many genes that are responsible for carrying out the cellular functions necessary for cell survival and proliferation, such as glycolysis, oxidative metabolism, and cell division. This set of common genes is called *housekeeping genes*.

The genetic information that encodes the linear sequence of amino acids in a protein is co-linear with the final protein product; that is, the codons that specify each of the amino acids from the amino to the carboxyl terminus are found in the gene in the same order found in the protein. Surprisingly, with very few exceptions this linear sequence of codons is interrupted by noncoding sequences that disrupt the reading frame of the gene. Consequently, the message specifying a protein encoded by the gene is encrypted in a manner so that it can be read only after the noncoding sequences interspersed between the coding ones have been removed. The sequences containing coding information are called *exons*, because these sequences normally exit the nucleus and accumulate in the cytoplasm. The portions of the gene between the exons are called *introns*, because normally they cannot be transported and remain inside the nucleus (Fig. 50–5). Therefore, in order to decode a gene successfully, the introns need to be removed and the exons joined together to provide an uninterrupted co-linear protein sequence.

TRANSCRIPTION

The selective use by different cells of the genetic information stored in the DNA is made possible because this information is not used directly but is transcribed into a molecule that can be read by the protein synthetic machinery of the cell. By a complex enzymatic process called *transcription*, the double-stranded DNA of each gene expressed in a given cell is copied into a single-stranded ribonucleic acid (RNA) (Fig. 50–6). This molecule of RNA uses the same genetic code as the DNA, but its bases contain the sugar ribose instead of deoxyribose that forms part of DNA. This molecule, which is the intermediate between the gene and the protein, is called *pre-messenger RNA* (pre-mRNA). The pre-mRNA is synthesized in the nucleus of the cell as a faithful copy of the gene and therefore contains both the exons and the introns. After transcription, the introns are removed from each of the transcripts by a process called *pre-mRNA splicing*. After the introns are completely spliced out and further processed in the nucleus, the pre-mRNA has been converted into a mature mRNA that con-

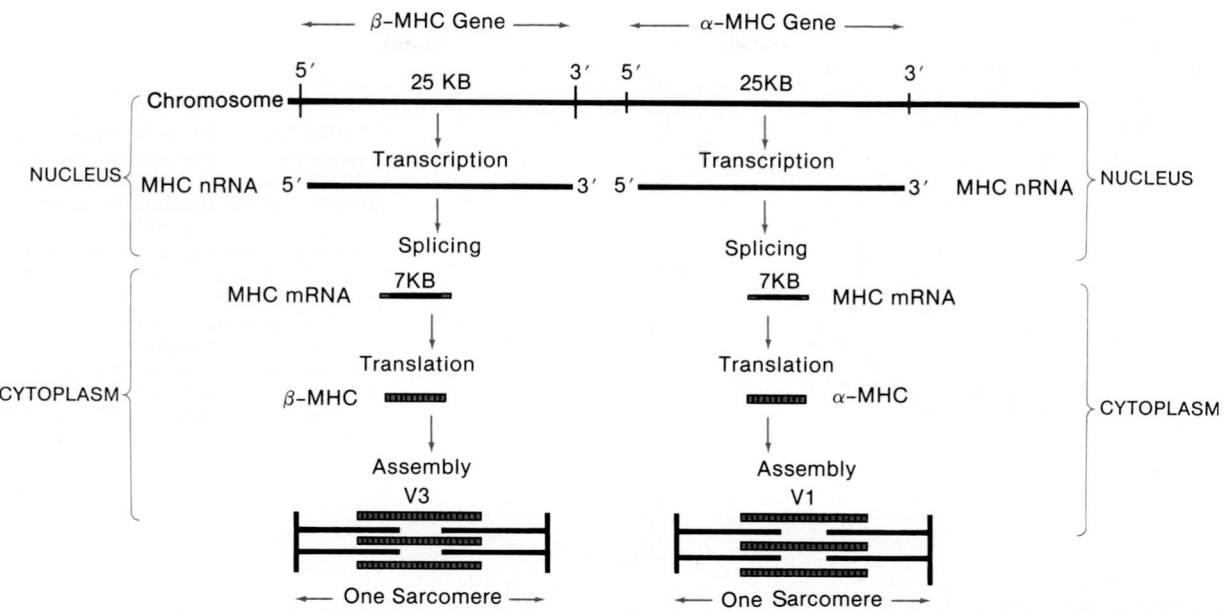

FIGURE 50-4. Decoding the information stored in the DNA. The steps involved in the regulation of gene expression are illustrated for the cardiac myosin heavy chain (MHC) genes. These genes are organized in tandem on the chromosome, and their expression, at the transcriptional level, is regulated by tissue, developmental, hormonal, physiological, and pathological stimuli. The DNA sequences coding for the α- and β-myosin heavy chains (MHC) are each contained in a 25 kilobase (KB) region of human chromosome 14. A primary RNA transcript (nRNA) is transcribed in the nucleus of cardiocytes. Noncoding sequences are spliced out and the 7 KB mature messenger RNA (mRNA) transported to the cytoplasm. The protein subunit chains are translated from the mRNA on ribosomes and the multimeric myosin proteins are assembled and organized in the sarcomeres. The similarity in DNA sequence of the adjacent MHC genes can lead to mispairing of chromosomes during DNA replication and the generation of deletion mutations. nRNA, nuclear ribonucleic acid or pre-messenger RNA (mRNA); KB, kilobases.

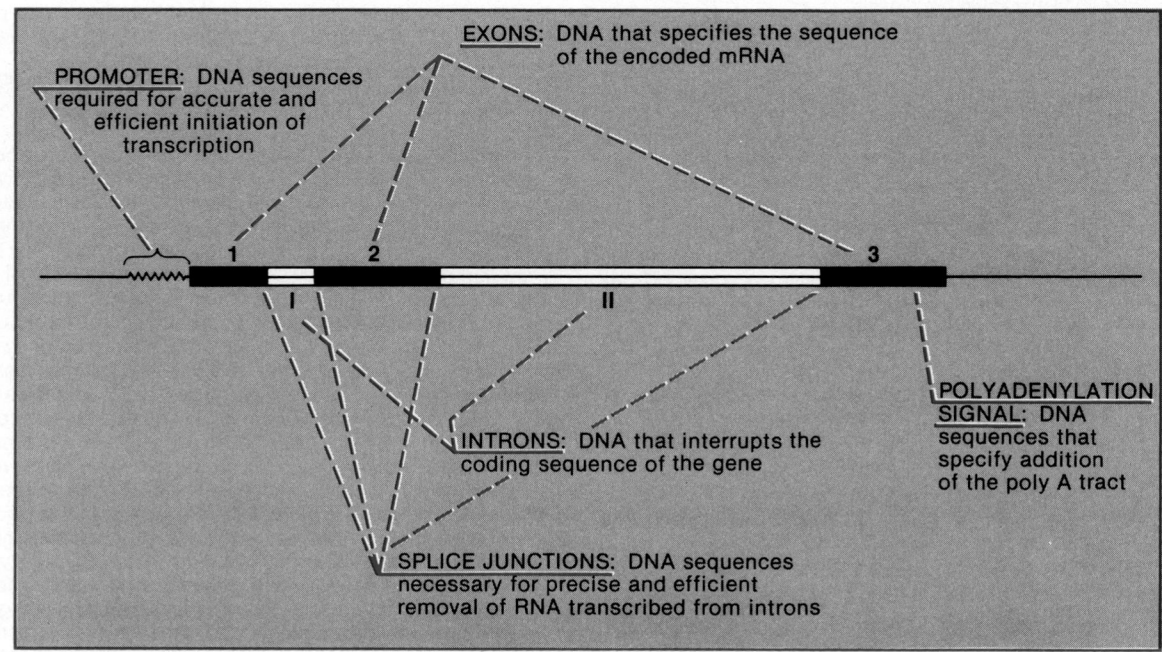

FIGURE 50-5. Functional elements of the β-globin gene. Expression of β-globin in specific cell lineages is regulated by tissue-specific enhancer sequences, which can be located at a distance from the coding sequences and are not shown. The promoter sequences facilitate binding of RNA polymerase and the initiation of RNA transcription at the mRNA start site. Non-coding intron sequences are present in the primary RNA transcript, but are spliced out of the mature mRNA, which contains only exons. The polyadenylation signal sequence directs the addition of a poly-adenine "tail" to the 3' end of the mRNA. Mutations that affect β-globin expression have been found in its enhancer, promoter, exon, splice-junction and polyadenylation signal sequences. (From Stamatoyannopoulos, G., Nienhuis, A. W., Leder, P., and Majerus, P. W. (eds): The Molecular Basis of Blood Diseases. Philadelphia, W.B. Saunders Company, 1987, p. 29)

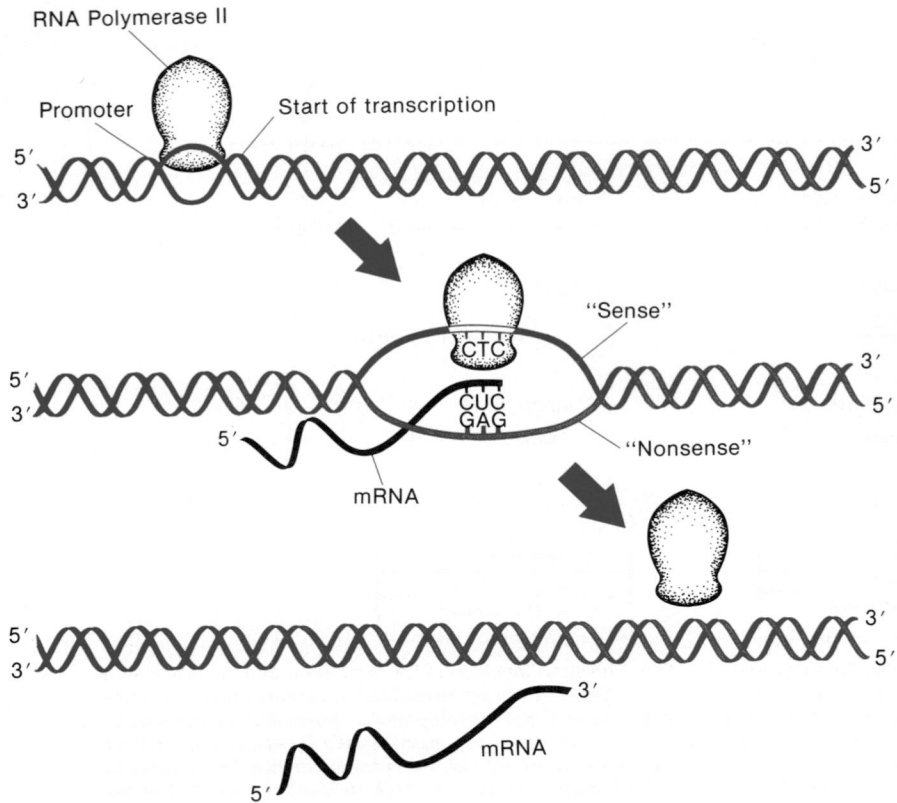

FIGURE 50-6. Schematic drawing of the transcription process. RNA polymerase II recognizes a specific sequence at the 5′ end of a gene (the promoter) and begins to transcribe it into the messenger RNA (mRNA). The mRNA is synthesized in the 5′ to 3′ direction and has the same sequence as the 5′ to 3′ DNA strand, also known as the "sense" strand. The mechanism of RNA formation presumably depends on base pairing of the newly formed RNA with the "nonsense" strand of the DNA, which acts as a template for copying. (From Gelehrter, T. D., and Collins, F. S.: Principles of Medical Genetics. Baltimore, Williams and Wilkins, 1990, p. 14.)

tains a methylated guanosine at its 5′ end (the cap site) and a string of adenosines at the 3′ end, known as the poly(A) tail. This mRNA is then transported to the cytoplasm, where it can be read by the translation machinery and may serve as a template for multiple rounds of translation to generate multiple copies of the protein.

It is now evident that splicing serves an important regulatory function because through this mechanism a single gene can produce several protein isoforms that might have different function or subcellular location. This is so because in some cases exons encoding a particular domain of the protein are present in the gene in several copies, each encoding a different variant of the sequence. These exons can be incorporated into the mature mRNA in different combinations and each will give rise to a different variant of the corresponding protein. The mechanism by which the cell makes selective use of particular exons is called *alternative splicing*. This mode of posttranscriptional gene regulation is particularly prevalent in skeletal and cardiac muscle and plays an important role in the generation of sarcomeric diversity.

The flow of genetic information from the nucleus to the cytoplasm of the cell is ideally suited for two main purposes: selective use and amplification of the genetic information encoded by the DNA. Due to transcription that is specific for the cell, the developmental stage, and the physiological state, the genome common to all cells is used to produce cells with widely different functions. Although most genes are present in the genome in a single copy, their informational content can be amplified several thousandfold by making multiple mRNA copies. Each of these mRNAs is, in turn, further amplified when it undergoes multiple rounds of translation to generate multiple copies of the protein. This amplification mechanism makes it possible for genes such as β-globin and myosin heavy chain to represent a large percentage of the protein content of erythrocytes or cardiac myocytes, respectively, despite the fact that each isoform of these proteins is encoded by a gene present in a single copy per haploid genome. (For further details on these general topics, see references 2 to 4.)

RECOMBINANT DNA TECHNOLOGY AS A TOOL OF CARDIOVASCULAR BIOLOGY

Although by the early 1970's most of the basic facts about the structure and function of DNA and RNA were known, progress in elucidating the regulatory mechanisms of gene expression was hampered by the inability, with the technology then available, to isolate and purify the DNA and mRNA sequences corresponding to a single gene. It soon became apparent that cloning of particular DNA sequences in bacterial cells would be necessary to produce sufficiently large and homogeneous quantities of DNA to be suitable for the characterization required to understand the regulatory processes. The discovery of restriction endonucleases was crucial in making possible the development of cloning technology. Smith and Wilcox[5] were the first to report a bacterial enzyme able to cut DNA at a specific nucleotide sequence (restriction site). The existence of a large family of these molecules soon became apparent; each molecule recognizes a specific DNA sequence with an extremely high level of specificity and efficiency. Danna and Nathans[6] realized that these specific cuts could be exploited to characterize a DNA molecule by digestion into several fragments with specific restriction enzymes, followed by separation of these fragments according to their electrophoretic mobility. Because individual DNA molecules contain unique sequences, the pattern of digestion provided a set of fragments that was unique for a specific gene. Using this strategy, Danna and Nathans[6] generated the first restriction map of the DNA tumor virus *SV-40* (Fig. 50-7). This accomplishment, together with the discovery of an enzyme that can join separate ends of DNA (*DNA ligase*), opened the way for the cloning of DNA molecules.

GENE CLONING. In 1972 Berg, Boyer, Cohen, and their collaborators[7,8] inserted a fragment of DNA that had been cut with the *E. coli* restriction enzyme Eco RI into a *plasmid vector* that had also been cut with Eco RI. Plasmid vectors are circular DNA molecules that can replicate autonomously in bacterial cells. After ligation of the cohesive ends of the two molecules generated by Eco RI with DNA ligase, a new plasmid

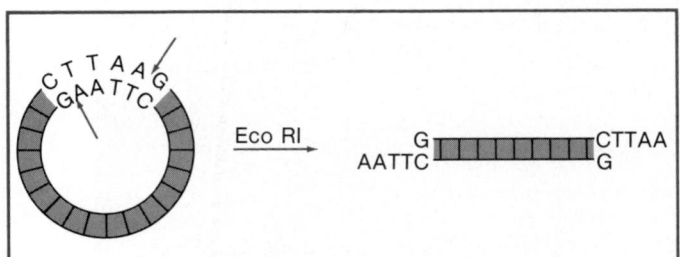

FIGURE 50-7. DNA cloning. The restriction endonuclease EcoR1 will recognize and cut a circular or linear DNA molecule at the palindromic nucleotide sequence 5′-CTTAAg-3′. Since the digestion is asymmetric, the resulting fragments will have overhanging unpaired nucleotides, called "sticky ends," which can pair with a complementary strand and be ligated to form a recombinant DNA molecle. (From Suzuki, D. T., Griffiths, A. J. F., Miller, J. H., and Lewontin, R. C.: An Introduction to Genetic Analysis. 4th ed, New York, W.H. Freeman and Co., 1989, p. 396.)

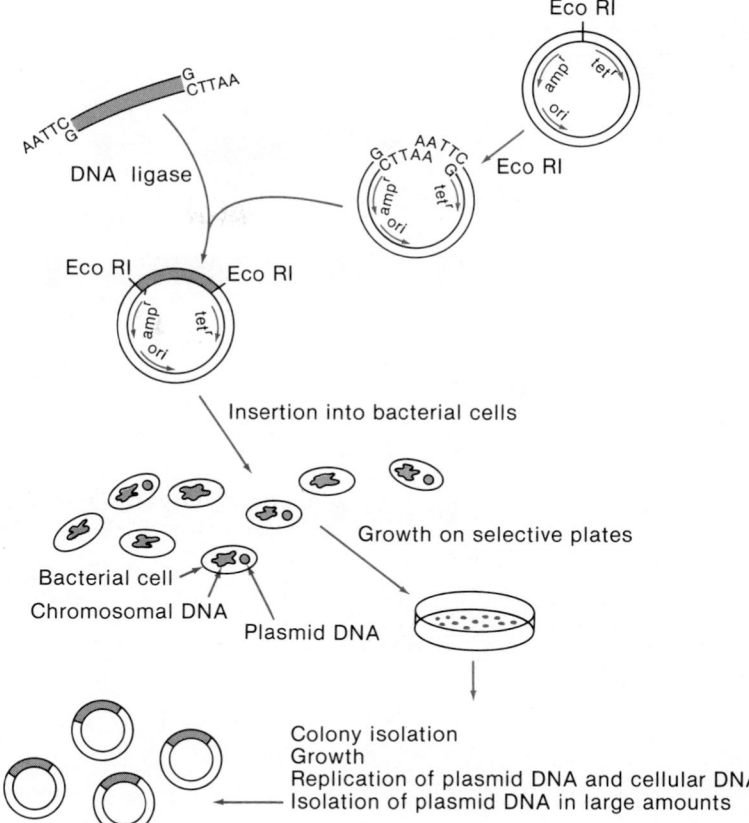

FIGURE 50–8. The process of cloning a DNA fragment into a plasmid cloning vector. A fragment of interest is cut with a restriction endonuclease and ligated into a plasmid vector. The vector contains an origin of replication ("ori") so that it can be grown in bacteria, and an antibiotic resistance gene, so that cells containing the plasmid can be selectively amplified. The recombinant plasmid is mixed with antibiotic-sensitive bacteria that have been treated to permeabilize their cell membranes to facilitate plasmid DNA uptake, a process called bacterial transformation. Bacterial clones carrying the plasmid are antibiotic resistant and grow on selective plates. Individual clones can be grown to abundance in liquid culture, and the recombinant plasmid DNA isolated and purified in quantity. (From Fritsch, E. F., and Maniatis, J.: Methods of Molecular Genetics. *In* Stamatoyannopoulos, G., Nienhuis, A. W., Leder, P., and Majerus, P. W. (eds.): The Molecular Basis of Blood Diseases. Philadelphia, W.B. Saunders Company, 1987, p. 5.)

molecule was produced that contained a piece of foreign DNA. After this recombinant plasmid DNA was reintroduced into bacterial cells (a process called *transformation*), it could be grown and purified in large and homogeneous quantities, taking advantage of the different physical characteristics of plasmid and genomic DNA that allow for their easy separation by physical means. This seemingly simple cloning process, in essence the same that is used today, ushered in the era of recombinant DNA (Fig. 50–8).

USE OF REVERSE TRANSCRIPTASE

A modification of the cloning procedure already outlined was rapidly developed to allow for the cloning of mRNA sequences (Fig. 50–9A). This procedure takes advantage of *reverse transcriptase,* the enzyme discovered by Baltimore[9] and Temin[10] and used by RNA viruses to convert the RNA into DNA. By means of this enzyme, the usual flow of genetic information from DNA to RNA that occurs in the cell nucleus can be reversed in the test tube. The single-stranded mRNA molecule that normally is not replicated can be converted into a double-stranded DNA molecule that may be replicated indefinitely. This DNA molecule is a faithful copy of the mRNA and is called *copy DNA (cDNA).* The cDNA produced in this manner, however, cannot be cloned into the plasmid vector, because it is not flanked by restriction enzyme sites. Therefore, compatible cohesive termini on the cDNA and plasmid DNA need to be created in order to ligate the two molecules together. This is accomplished by the thymic enzyme terminal transferase, which is able to incorporate a string of nucleotides at the free end of a DNA molecule. When a string of Gs is added to the ends of the plasmid molecule and a string of Cs is added to the end of the cDNA, because of the base-pairing rules, the two molecules can be annealed together and ligated to form a new recombinant plasmid ready to be amplified when introduced into bacteria (Fig. 50–9A).

One of the shortcomings of plasmids as cloning vectors is their low capacity for foreign DNA that allows for the cloning of relatively short sequences. This too has been addressed by the development of new cloning vectors that accommodate quite long DNA sequences. These vectors use bacterial phages or yeast chromosomal sequences as recipients of the foreign DNA sequences. In some cases, vectors are engineered so that the bacteria will produce a protein, or a portion thereof, from the fragment of inserted DNA. To accomplish this, the cDNA sequence is inserted and fused downstream from a bacterial gene that is readily induced by a drug or metabolite (Fig. 50–9B). When induced, this gene produces large quantities of the corresponding fusion protein. These *bacterial expression vectors* have the advantage that the gene of interest can be screened using antibodies against the cognate protein or, in some cases, using radiolabeled ligands specific for the protein being cloned. In addition, these vectors are used to produce the corresponding fusion protein in large quantities that can be easily isolated and purified.

GENE ISOLATION

With use of the aforementioned methods, it has become routine practice to isolate genes coding for a large variety of proteins. Once a partial sequence of a protein is known or a specific antibody against it is available, it is possible to produce a synthetic oligonucleotide that contains the codons required to produce the corresponding amino acid sequence (Fig. 50–9B). In addition, if the protein is available in small quantities, a synthetic peptide can be produced and used to raise antibodies against this portion of the protein sequence. With these two reagents at hand it is a straightforward task to screen a cDNA or genomic library for the clones that contain the cDNA for this protein using a DNA sequence corresponding to the known amino acid sequence, an antibody against the protein, or a ligand recognized by the protein. This protocol for gene isolation and characterization requires some knowledge of the protein investigated. For this reason, it is called a *direct* method of gene isolation, as compared with the *reverse genetics* method described below that requires no knowledge of the protein sequence or function.

GENE MAPPING

The ready availability of DNA fragments homogeneous in length and sequence allowed the development of efficient techniques of *DNA sequencing.* In 1975 Sanger[11] developed an effective approach to sequencing of single-stranded DNA by elongating nascent DNA chains with DNA polymerase and terminating them at a specific base through incorporating a modified nucleotide that cannot be elongated (a chain terminator). The first complete nucleotide sequence of a natural gene was obtained using this approach. Two years later Maxam and Gilbert[12] developed a different approach to sequencing of double-stranded DNA by specific chemical modification of bases to induce specific cleavages at a particular base. With these two techniques, the sequencing of long genomic and cDNA molecules rapidly became routine. The number of genes sequenced in the following decade runs into the thousands. Further developments and improvements of the Sanger technique[13] have led to the automation of many of the procedures involved in DNA sequencing to the point that sequencing the complete human genome has become a practical goal for the end of the century. However, before this task is accomplished, it will be necessary to produce an accurate and detailed physical map of the human genome.

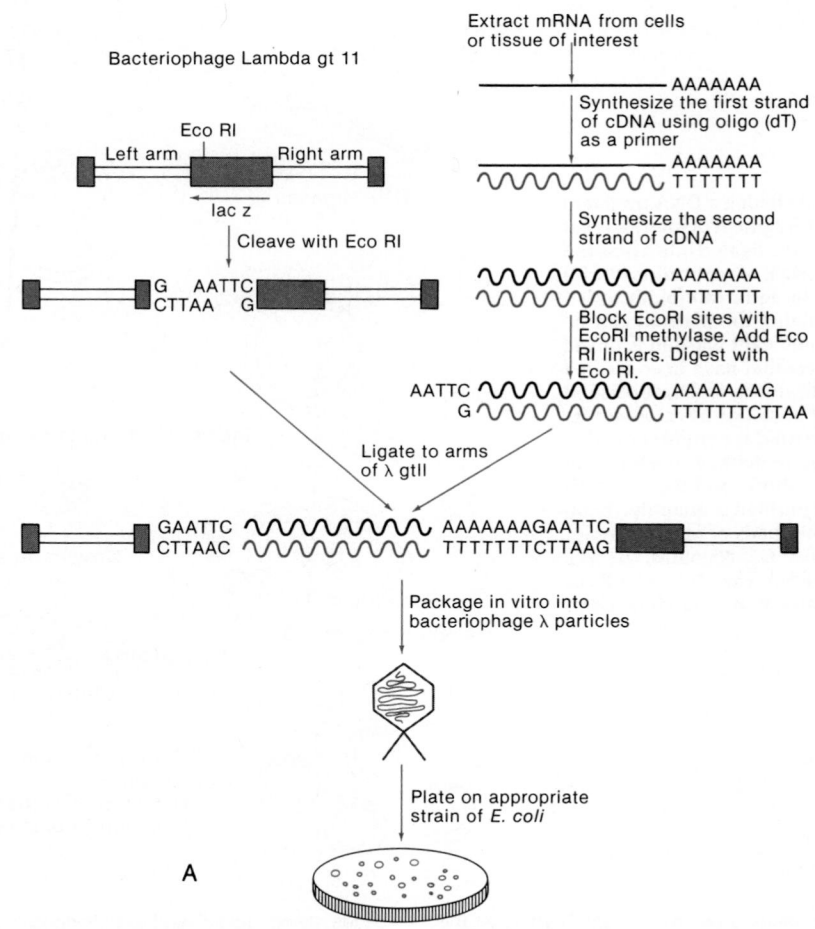

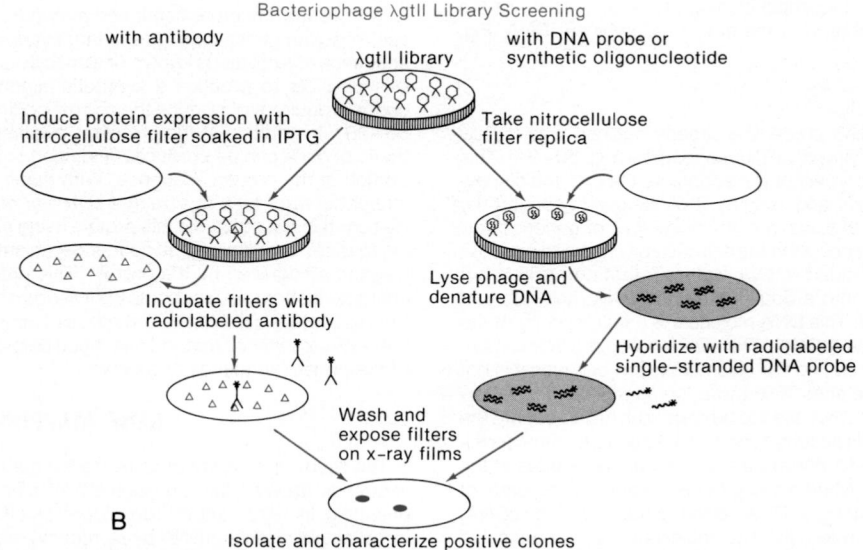

FIGURE 50-9. Cloning in an expression bacteriophage vector. *A.*, The bacteriophage gt11 expression vector contains an Eco R1 cloning site within an inducible gene (lac z or β-galactosidase). A functional coding sequence can be cloned into this site by preparing complementary DNA (cDNA) from messenger RNA using reverse transcriptase. A double-stranded fragment of cDNA can be modified to facilitate cloning by the addition of "linkers" which contain sequences that can be ligated to the "sticky ends" of the vector. Recombinant bacteriophage containing cDNA is mixed in vitro with bacteriophage coat protein, reconstituting infectious virus. *B.*, Recombinant bacteriophage carrying a particular cDNA can be identified by either expression or hybridization screening. Bacteria containing the bacteriophage can be stimulated to make the cDNA-encoded protein by adding an inducer (IPTG) of lac z into which the cDNA has been cloned. The presence of the synthesized protein on nitrocellulose filter replicas of the bacterial plate can be detected by binding of radiolabelled antibodies. Alternatively, recombinant bacteriophage carrying the cDNA sequence can be identified by hybridization to the filter of oligonucleotides or cloned DNA sequences. When a positive signal is detected on the replica filter, the corresponding bacteriophage plaque can be picked from the bacterial plate. The bacteriophage can then be amplified and its DNA characterized by restriction enzyme or DNA sequencing analysis.

RESTRICTION FRAGMENT LENGTH POLYMORPHISMS. The map of the human genome, which is now being constructed, consists of identification of landmarks in human DNA; this process allows the allocation of a given DNA fragment to a specific chromosome and to a particular location within the chromosome. This is accomplished by pinpointing of particular DNA polymorphisms that can differentiate between the two alleles of a given gene. These polymorphisms, called *restriction fragment length polymorphisms* (RFLPs),[14] are a result of the normal variability in the DNA among different individuals that can be recognized by specific restriction endonucleases. On the average, one in every 500 nucleotides has differences between two randomly selected alleles,[15] and approximately 5 per cent of these differences can be detected by restriction enzymes.

A restriction enzyme will cut the DNA at a particular site in one chromosome but not at the same place in the homologous chromosome because of differences in the DNA sequence in the chromosome inherited from each parent. This difference in the restriction enzyme sites is reflected in the size of the DNA fragments generated by the enzyme and visualized on Southern blot testing when hybridized to a DNA probe. The ability of this procedure to distinguish between the paternal and the maternal chromosomes is of great clinical significance. Moreover, it permits the identification of RFLPs that segregate with a particular trait in heterozygous individuals. Therefore, with this technique it is possible to determine whether the pattern of inheritance of a given disorder segregates with a particular chromosome. If this is the case, this particular trait has been mapped to the chromosome. Many different RFLPs for each human chromosome have now been identified; this may facilitate the assignment of any trait that segregates in a large family to a specific chromosome. Because of the abundance of the DNA polymorphisms, when a gene responsible for a disease is cloned, RFLPs may be found within or around the gene that allow distinction between the normal and defective genes in heterozygous individuals.

This process of mapping individual genes in the genome has led to the development of powerful techniques to search for genes whose biochemical function is not known but whose mutation produces a well-defined phenotype. By taking advantage of RFLPs, it is possible, in many cases, to determine which member of a chromosome pair is inherited from the mother and which one has been inherited from the father. Therefore, if a trait is inherited in a mendelian manner in a given family (Chap. 51), when the pattern of inheritance of the disease or trait as well as the origin (paternal or maternal) of each of the chromosomes in the affected and nonaffected members of the family is known, it is possible to map the gene responsible for the trait to a specific chromosome. This may be accomplished even when the function and nature of the gene are unknown. This process is called *gene* or *chromosome mapping.*

Once the chromosome is identified, it is possible to pinpoint the gene in question and isolate its sequence by a process called *chromosome walking.* This approach is known as *reverse genetics* because, in contrast to the direct approach in which the function of the gene and its protein product are already known and used to identify the gene sequences. In this case neither the biochemical function of the gene nor its protein product is known. The normal or abnormal phenotype produced by the gene is the only available clue. The gene is isolated first in order to determine its function. Although this approach is still in its infancy, it holds tremendous promise for the identification of genes responsible for many pathological processes that have obscure and/or complex biochemical nature. Gene mapping has been used to localize the gene responsible for Huntington's chorea,[16] and reverse genetics has been utilized to identify and clone the genes for Duchenne muscular dystrophy[17] and cystic fibrosis.[18]

In the cardiovascular system, reverse genetics using RFLPs has been successfully applied to identify the myosin heavy-chain gene as the locus responsible for certain forms of familial hypertrophic cardiomyopathy in humans[19] (p. 1406), and genetic mapping has been used to identify the locus associated with situs inversus in the iv/iv mouse.[20]

GENE MAPPING BY HYBRIDIZATION

In addition to the RFLP mapping method, a gene can be readily mapped to a chromosome once cDNA and/or genomic sequences of the gene have been cloned, using hybrid chromosome panels or in situ hybridization of the metaphase chromosomes. Hybrid chromosome panels consist of a collection of hybrid cell clones (usually mouse X human hybrid cells). In these combinations, human chromosomes are preferentially and randomly lost from the hybrid cells, and clones that contain only a subset of human chromosomes can be isolated. Panels of these clones are constituted so that it is possible to include and exclude every possible chromosome. DNA from these cells is isolated, digested with a battery of restriction enzymes, separated by gel electrophoresis, and transferred to a membrane support. This is a blotting procedure that can be used for DNA, RNA, or protein. This process, which was first described for analysis of DNA by Southern,[21] is called *Southern blot* when the filter immobilized molecule is DNA, *Northern blot* when it is RNA, and *Western* or *South-*

western blot when proteins are blotted. The electrophoretically size-separated DNA is then *hybridized* to the radiolabeled cDNA or genomic DNA from the gene to be mapped.

Under the appropriate conditions, the labeled DNA will only hybridize to its cognate sequences blotted to the membrane, despite the fact that it contains DNA from the entire genome. The radiolabeled probe will produce a characteristic pattern of bands that can be visualized when the membrane is exposed to a radiographic film (autoradiograph). In somatic cell hybrid panels, it is possible to distinguish the band produced by hybridization to the mouse genes from the bands produced by the human genes. When the hybridization pattern produced by the human genes is compared with the known chromosome composition of each clone, it is possible to assign the gene sequence to a particular chromosome. An alternative process is to hybridize the radiolabeled cDNA or genomic probe to a mitotic metaphase chromosome spread. The site of hybridization of the probe to the cognate chromosome is visualized by photographic emulsion autoradiography, in which the density of the silver grains indicates not only the chromosomal location of the gene, but also its subchromosomal location.

USE OF CLONED DNA FOR DIAGNOSIS AND TREATMENT OF GENETIC DISORDERS

Substantial progress has been made in identifying genetic loci in humans (Fig. 51–1, p. 1624). In the last edition of McKusick's "Mendelian Inheritance in Man," more than 1500 genes had been mapped to a specific human chromosome.[22] The rate of gene mapping is accelerating rapidly and has now reached more than one gene a day. The valuable contribution of gene mapping to clinical medicine is obvious, although as of this writing it is at the earliest stages of development. However, in the past few years, more than a dozen clinically important genes causative of mendelian-inherited diseases have been mapped, including Huntington's chorea on chromosome 4, adenomatous polyposis of the colon on chromosome 5, cystic fibrosis on chromosome 7, certain forms of familial hypertrophic cardiomyopathy on chromosome 14, retinoblastoma on chromosome 13, neurofibromatosis on chromosome 17, one form of Alzheimer's disease on chromosome 21, and Duchenne muscular dystrophy to the short arm of the X chromosome.

At the time of mapping, there was little information as to the nature of the biochemical defect in some cases. For this reason, there were no reliable diagnostic tests for many of these diseases; moreover, patient testing could not be done during fetal or postnatal life before the appearance of clinical manifestations of the disease. This lack of basic information also made it difficult to design therapeutic approaches to attack the biochemical processes involved or their consequences. However, once the gene had been mapped, it rapidly became possible to use this information for prenatal diagnosis, premorbid diagnosis, and carrier detection for conditions such as cystic fibrosis, muscular dystrophy, and Huntington's chorea, among others.

Despite this progress and the expectations raised by these methods, most of the progress thus far has related to disorders caused by defects in a single gene in which there is a clear mendelian inheritance of the characteristic phenotype.[22] Since many of the significant diseases affecting the cardiovascular system (such as hypertension and atherosclerosis) are *multigenic* and multifactorial, it is not surprising that the impact of the genetic approach in diagnosis and patient management is lagging compared with other areas of medicine, such as immunology, oncology, and metabolism.

MUTATIONS. Two main types of genetic lesions (mutations) are responsible for inherited diseases: gross abnormalities of genes or chromosomes (deletions, insertions, and rearrangements), and a single- or few-base substitution or deletion in critical regions of the gene (point mutations) (Fig. 50–3). The gross abnormalities of genes are the easiest to detect using Southern blot analysis and are simple to explain pathogenetically. The gene does not function because it has been partially or completely deleted or it has been inactivated because an extraneous piece of DNA has been inserted in a crucial area (coding or regulatory). Gross rearrangements can occur in genes that are duplicated in tandem; that is, when there are two quite similar copies of a gene on neighboring regions of the same chromosome. One example of this type of genetic defect involves the α-globin gene cluster, in which rearrangements between the several copies of the α-globin genes can occur by unequal crossover during meiosis, which then gives rise to a mutation that causes α-thalassemia. In the cardiovascular system, affected members of a family with familial hypertrophic cardiomyopathy carry a hybrid myosin heavy-chain (MHC) gene produced by a crossover between the α- and β-MHC genes,[23] which are normally located next to each other on the same chromosome.[24,25]

Point Mutations. Caused by substitution, deletion, or insertion of a single or few nucleotides, point mutations are the most common cause of genetic defect identified so far. Even when they affect only a single nucleotide, these point mutations can have important consequences for the expression of the gene involved. They might completely or partially eliminate the gene product. This can occur because the mutation affects transcription, splicing, or translation of the mRNA. In many cases, however, the effect of the mutation is limited to the substitution of one amino acid for another. The phenotypic consequences of this can be as serious as those of the gross gene rearrangements, or they can be less drastic, depending on the nature of the substitution.

OLIGONUCLEOTIDE PROBES. Point mutations can be identified by restriction enzyme analysis, when the change in nucleotide sequence they produce either creates or abolishes a restriction endonuclease recognition site. At most, 5 to 10 per cent of all point mutations can be detected directly by restriction analysis.[26] For this reason, an alternative method of detection has been devised with synthetic oligonucleotides used as probes to recognize directly the mutated sequence and to distinguish between mutant and normal alleles. These oligonucleotides, specifically tailored for each mutation, will, under optimal conditions, recognize only their identical homologous sequence but will not recognize a sequence that varies at one or more nucleotides. In this manner, the normal gene will be identified only by the normal sequence, while the mutant gene will be recognized only by its mutant counterpart.[27] Although this technique is quite powerful, it has the obvious limitation that it can be used only when the molecular basis of the genetic lesion has already been identified and the proper sequence is known.

In theory, this type of oligonucleotide analysis should allow for the diagnosis of all the known point mutations in a particular gene. In practice, however, its applicability is more limited for several reasons: in many cases of single gene disorders, such as cystic fibrosis[28] and osteogenesis imperfecta,[29] there are many different mutations causing the disease and each family has a different mutation. In other cases, the probes are specific for a single family and cannot be used for anyone else. This is the case for a type of familial hypertrophic cardiomyopathy caused by a single-base substitution in the β-MHC gene.[30]

PRENATAL DIAGNOSIS. Genetic defects, caused by either gross rearrangements or point mutations, can be diagnosed by Southern blot analysis using the methods already described and cloned genes or synthetic oligonucleotides as probes. For this test a significant amount of genomic DNA is needed, which necessitates a long waiting time to grow cells obtained by amniocentesis or chorion villus sampling. These limitations have been eliminated by recently developed methodology. The *polymerase chain reaction* (PCR)[31] allows for the rapid amplification of very small samples of DNA (even a single molecule) by repeated cycles of DNA synthesis using a temperature-resistant DNA polymerase.[32] In this manner, it is possible to amplify a region of a gene starting with the DNA from a single cell or very few cells, followed by hybridization of a diagnostic DNA probe to the amplified DNA. This procedure, which can be completed in a day, has rapidly become the method of choice for the diagnosis of single-gene dis-

orders. The sensitivity and efficiency of the procedure have allowed its application to embryos grown in vitro before implantation in order to identify carriers of known disorders affecting one of the parents. In those cases, a single cell removed from the embryo before transfer to the uterus is sufficient for the procedure. For prenatal diagnosis it is not necessary to know the precise molecular defect that has caused the disease in a given family or individual. It is sufficient to identify the abnormal gene and to be able to follow its pattern of inheritance. As already indicated, in the absence of a cloned gene, the availability of RFLPs located close to the responsible gene is sufficient for this type of analysis.

USE OF CLONED GENES FOR RESEARCH AND THERAPY

Once cDNA clones containing the complete coding sequence for a particular protein have been isolated, they can be used to express the protein product in a variety of cell types. This approach is particularly useful for several purposes: to determine the physiological role of the particular protein, to analyze its structure-function relationships in detail, and to produce large quantities of a natural gene product or its mutants. This is especially useful when these products are synthesized in small amounts by the original source, as is the case for insulin, growth hormone, tissue-type plasminogen activator (t-PA), and erythropoietin, all of which have been produced from cloned DNA and are currently in clinical use.

The advantages of this approach are exemplified by the development of t-PA as a research and therapeutic tool (p. 1231). Although the effect of t-PA as a fibrinolytic agent had been known for several years, its effect on thrombi was tested using t-PA secreted by a tumor cell line in culture.[33] Given the promising results, it became clear that an alternative and more efficient mode of production was required if the role of this substance in acute myocardial infarction was to be assessed. For this reason, the protein secreted by melanoma cell lines was first purified. With use of limited proteolysis followed by peptide sequencing, the sequence of a small portion of the protein was obtained. This sequence was used to synthesize a DNA oligonucleotide containing all possible codon combinations able to code for the t-PA peptide sequence available. This synthetic DNA was used to screen a cDNA library from melanoma cells that contained several hundred thousand different cDNA sequences. Based on the specific hybridization of the synthetic cDNA probes, clones containing the complete sequence coding for t-PA were isolated and remain a source for t-PA production.

Once the cDNA clones have been isolated, it is necessary to produce the corresponding protein. It is possible to carry out the whole process in vitro using cell-free systems that carry out the transcription and translation required to make the protein product. However, this process is quite inefficient and only limited quantities of protein for analytical analyses can be obtained in this manner. To produce large quantities, it is essential to use a host cell capable of using a foreign gene as one of its own. The two most effective expression cell systems use either bacteria or animal cells as the hosts for the cloned gene. In both cases it is important to use strategies that will "trick" the cell into making this foreign gene product in large quantities. In the case of bacteria, the most common strategy is to fuse the cDNA coding for the protein of interest to the coding portion of a gene whose expression can be induced at will to a very high level in response to a drug or metabolite in the medium. In this manner, a fusion protein is obtained that has the amino terminus of the bacterial protein and the carboxyl terminus of the cloned gene; when the host gene is induced, the cloned protein is made in large amounts as a byproduct.

Although recombinant proteins formed by bacteria often have many of the biological functions of the native protein, this is not always the case. Usually, this is because bacterial cells do not produce the postsynthetic modification such as glycosylation or acetylation that is characteristic of the product from animal cells. For this reason, ingredients intended for pharmacological use are commonly produced by expressing the cloned gene in animal cells. To accomplish this, the cloned cDNA to be expressed is ligated to a plasmid vector containing the regulatory sequences (promoter) of an animal gene that is normally expressed at high levels. This DNA is then introduced into the animal cell by a process called *transfection*. In the case of t-PA, it soon became obvious that not enough t-PA could be produced by the transfected cells for clinical trials. To address this problem, Kaufman et al.[35] devised means to produce more t-PA in animal cells by means of the ability of most cells to make multiple copies of the gene coding to dehydrofolate reductase (DHFR) when grown in the presence of the antitumor drug methotrexate.[36] This gene amplification in response to the drug results in the presence of several hundred copies of the DHFR gene in each cell. Kaufman ligated the t-PA cDNA to a cloned DHFR gene in an expression vector. After the gene had been transfected into the host cells, it was amplified by exposing the cells to increasing levels of methotrexate. The augmented DHFR gene sequences produced amplification of the neighboring t-PA cDNA sequences, resulting in a ~100 fold increase in the amount of t-PA secreted into the medium.

The availability of t-PA cDNA sequences has also served to elucidate structure-function relationships in the molecule. By mutation or deletion or both of particular residues or whole domains of the protein, a large number of variant t-PA molecules have been produced. These molecules have different primary structures and/or posttranslational modifications, such as glycosylation, that in many cases change the enzymatic properties or the half-life of the enzyme.

The use of cloned genes for the study of structure-function relationships is a particularly powerful tool for dissection of molecules relevant to the structure and function of the cardiovascular system. Williams et al. used this approach to perform a detailed analysis of the signaling mechanisms involved in the pathway of growth factor signaling using the platelet-derived growth factor (PDGF) receptor as the model system.[37] By this mechanism they elucidated elements in the cellular machinery responsive to receptor stimulation, as well as the structurally and functionally important features of the receptor involved in ligand binding, activation, and interaction with other cellular components.[38] A similar approach has been used by Lefkowitz and colleagues to study the relevant functional elements of the beta-adrenoceptors[39] and Numa et al. for the acetylcholine receptor as well as the sodium and calcium channels,[40] among others.

EXPRESSION OF CLONED GENES IN INTACT ANIMALS. The ability to introduce and target the expression of individual genes to individual cell types and tissues of the living animal or human is one of the most promising developments of molecular biology. Although the value of this technique in analysis of basic mechanisms of gene expression is high, this is overshadowed by its possible practical applications for gene therapy. Brinster and colleagues were the first to demonstrate that it is possible to inject cloned genes into the nucleus of a fertilized egg to produce animals that express the transfected gene (*transgene*) during development and are able to transmit it to their progeny in an inheritable mendelian manner,[41] i.e., the creation of transgenic animals. In most cases the information required to direct the expression of a cloned gene to the proper tissue in which the endogenous gene is expressed is located in the 5′ flanking region of the gene. In this manner, it has been shown that, if a gene containing the 5′ flanking sequences of the atrial natriuretic factor is injected into mouse oocytes, it is exclusively expressed in the cardiac tissues of the resulting mice in a pattern similar to that of the endogenous gene.[42] In these experiments, the transgene responds to physiological stimuli, such as work-overload hypertrophy, in a manner indistinguishable from the natural gene, by reintroduction of its expression in the ventricles of adult animals.[43] A similar result has been obtained with constructs containing the 5′ flanking region of the α-MHC gene. Therefore, with this approach, it is possible to analyze the role of

different regulatory sequences in the gene in a natural context, during development and under conditions that are physiologically relevant.

From these experiments it became clear that only selected portions of the gene were required to direct the expression of a foreign gene to the proper cell type. In most, but not all, cases the sequences required and sufficient to direct the proper expression of a gene are located outside the coding regions in the so-called 5′ flanking sequences. These sequences, which contain all of the elements required to direct the proper transcription of the gene, include the promoter sequence and the transcription start site. In some genes many of the important sequences needed for transcription are clustered together in a region of the chromosome and constitute a *tissue-specific enhancer*. These tissue-specific enhancers are the binding sites for transcription factors that are specific for a given cell type or a particular stage of development or both. In some cases these enhancers are not located in the 5′ flanking sequences but rather within the coding region of the gene or at the 3′ flanking region.[44]

These enhancer sequences are able to stimulate (enhance) the expression of any gene even when located at a great distance from the gene. With this type of sequence it has been possible to create hybrid genes and direct their expression to cardiac cells. In this manner the expression of gene products not normally found in the myocardium can be induced. One of the most spectacular outcomes of this approach has resulted from directing the expression of different oncogenes to the myocardium. Unregulated expression of c-myc during development produces cardiac hyperplasia, generating hearts that have an abnormally large number of cells.[45] Even more striking, when the expression of the T antigen oncogene from the simian virus (SV) 40 is directed in mice toward the atria by the atrial natriuretic factor gene promoter and flanking sequences, the resulting mice develop atrial tumors.[46] If the same oncogene is directed toward the atria and ventricle by the α-MHC promoter and flanking sequences, the mice develop atrial and ventricular tumors.[47] The myocardial cells from these hearts are constituted to express the T antigen and have many properties of a tumor cell. However, these properties have been exploited to generate atrial and ventricular myocyte cell lines that cause growth for many passages in tissue culture dishes while retaining many of the differentiated properties of normal cardiac myocytes. The production of these cell strains has been a longstanding goal in the field of cellular and molecular cardiology and should provide a valuable tool to study the biology of these cells.

Gene Therapy

INSERTION OF GENES INTO THE GERM LINE. In addition to its use for the study of gene expression, the potential application of gene transfer technology to correct genetic defects has been obvious for many years and has proved to be successful in experimental animals, when the normal gene was injected into oocytes of mutant animals. In these cases, the gene is present in all cells of the transgenic organism, including the germ cells, and is transmitted to its progeny in a mendelian manner. Obviously, this approach is not feasible in humans because of ethical and practical considerations: the rate of success of this approach is too low, the long-term consequences of harboring the transgene in all cells of the body remain unknown, and tampering with human germ plasm is unacceptable ethically. Therefore, gene therapy in humans is likely to be limited to somatic cells.

INSERTION OF GENES INTO SOMATIC CELLS. Theoretically, a large number of inherited human diseases should be correctable by the introduction of new genes in appropriate cell types. However, since most current models of gene transfer result in the random insertion of the incoming sequence into the genome without correction of the endogenous mutant gene, the ideal candidate diseases are single-gene recessive disorders. A principal requirement for performing somatic gene therapy is the availability of a safe and efficient method of inserting the gene into the appropriate cells. In addition, in the best circumstances the recipient cells should be long lived, so that they produce the permanent correction of the disorder. Therefore, it is not surprising that most of the effort in human gene therapy has been directed toward the introduction of corrective genes into somatic cells. This approach is particularly promising for the correction of hematological disorders because of the relative ease of obtaining stem cells that might be genetically engineered and reintroduced into the body, where they would repopulate the bone marrow and differentiate into different cell types. Combined immunodeficiency caused by adenosine deaminase (ADA) deficiency, beta-thalassemia, and lipid storage diseases such as Gaucher's disease are particularly suitable for this type of therapy. This approach, however, has been hindered by two main problems. First, since the number of target stem cells is quite low, an efficient delivery system is required for this strategy. Second, the transgene needs to be regulated properly during development and in response to different physiological stimuli.

GENE INSERTION USING RETROVIRUSES. In the past few years significant progress has been made in the delivery of genes using a variety of viral vectors. Replication-defective retroviral vectors and cell lines that package the vectors into viral particles have been developed and have proved highly efficient.[48–50] Although thus far the attempts to perform retroviral gene transfer in nonhuman primates have been disappointing, there is evidence that most of the problems hampering progress can be solved.[51] In the meantime, gene transfer has been used to mark autologous tumor-infiltrating lymphocytes (TIL) by means of retrovirus-mediated gene transfer in a series of patients with melanoma. This represents the first report of approved gene transfer in humans and clearly indicates the potential value and relative safety of using retroviral gene markers to study the biology of human cells. As indicated by Rosenberg et al., it should be possible to transduce these TIL cells or other populations of lymphocytes with vectors expressing cytokines or other molecules whose increased concentration would be beneficial.[52]

GENE INSERTION INTO ENDOTHELIAL CELLS. In the cardiovascular system, the endothelial cells appear to be the most promising target for retroviral gene therapy because of their long life and easy accessibility. Nabel et al. demonstrated that endothelial cells genetically modified to express an indicator gene could be used to seed denuded iliofemoral arteries in the in vivo swine model and that they continued to express the indicator gene for at least 4 weeks after implantation.[53] In a similar experiment, Wilson et al. seeded Dacron grafts with endothelial cells genetically engineered to express an indicator gene.[54] The indicator gene was expressed in these carotid artery grafts for at least 5 weeks after implantation. More recently, Dichek et al. seeded endothelial cells that had been modified to produce t-PA onto vascular stents in vitro.[55] The genetically modified endothelial cells continued to express t-PA at significantly higher levels than normal endothelial cells while attached to the stent, and they remained in place when the stent was expanded by balloon dilatation. The number of cells implanted with the stent would not be expected to produce a systemic anticoagulant effect; however, the increased local concentration of t-PA might be sufficient to produce a local thrombolytic effect at the surface of the stents and might make them less subject to thrombosis when implanted in vivo. Although significantly much more data are required to determine the clinical efficacy of this form of gene therapy, it is clear that this approach is potentially useful. Interestingly, catheter-directed delivery of retroviruses to endothelial cells in situ has recently been reported with encouraging results.[56] If this method of delivery proves to be of general applicability, it would simplify greatly this approach to gene therapy and broaden its application.

Recent reports from several laboratories have demonstrated that functional genes can be administered by direct injection into living animals without the use of retroviruses. In some of these cases long-term expression has been obtained in vivo without the need to integrate the foreign gene into the genome of the host cell. The level and duration of expression obtained suggest that these approaches will have scientific and therapeutic applications. Wolff and colleagues demonstrated expression of marker genes following direct injection into skeletal muscle in vivo.[57] Although there was no evidence of integration into the host genome, expression persisted for more than 6 months. Similar results in cardiac muscles using viral promoters to direct the expression of the marker gene were subsequently reported.[58] High levels of expression can be obtained when the marker gene is linked to a myocardial-specific promoter gene sequence as has been demonstrated by several groups, including the authors' own.

HOPES FOR HUMAN GENE THERAPY. Although the studies just mentioned are still in the experimental phase, they provide a glimpse of what is likely to become possible in the near future. It is now clear that many genes coding for physiologically and therapeutically important proteins can be introduced into the cardiovascular system either through the endothelial cells or through direct injection into the myocardium to provide for their local or systemic release in vivo. Proteins that induce angiogenesis, inhibit smooth muscle proliferation, lower plasma levels of cholesterol, affect the thrombogenic properties of the endothelial wall, or produce vasodilation are only a few of the gene products that are candidates for use in gene therapy. Patients with certain forms of cardiomyopathy, such as in muscular dystrophy (p. 1813), may be candidates for direct gene therapy into the myocardium. More tantalizing is the prospect of manipulating the genes responsible for the cell cycle to induce cell division of the differentiated cardiac myocytes at the borders of a ischemic injury to regenerate cardiac muscle. Therefore, "in vivo" gene delivery could allow for creation of customized, discretely localized "cellular factories" in individual patients for the endogenous production of therapeutically efficacious drugs targeted at specific disease processes. Although formidable obstacles such as the regulation of production of gene products obscure the path to routine use of gene therapy in human disease, the first steps down that path recently have been taken successfully.[59]

Molecular Biology of the Cardiac Contractile System

Despite the contributions of molecular biology to the understanding of many processes affecting the cardiovascular system, the cellular and molecular bases of cardiac performance remain poorly understood for the most part. As indicated at the beginning of this chapter, this situation is due, at least in part, to the fact that the myocardium is a less-than-ideal tissue for the application of genetic and molecular approaches.

Given the essential role of the myocardium in the survival of the organism, most of the genetic mutations that significantly affect its development or function or both are likely to be lethal. This feature explains the relatively small number of mutations that affect the myocardium either in humans or animal models described thus far. This contrasts with the large number of mutations affecting blood cells, the endocrine system, and metabolic pathways, among others. The existence of these mutations has provided the means of entry for the molecular dissection of these systems. In addition to the relative unavailability of mutations in the cardiovascular system, the difficulty in obtaining repeated samples of the myocardium from the same animal that are suitable for biochemical and molecular analysis has also slowed progress.

Furthermore, the existence of well-characterized cell lines that can be grown in homogeneous populations and mutated at will are an almost essential requirement for the exploitation of recombinant DNA technology to elucidate regulatory pathways. Given that the cardiac myocyte is a terminally differentiated cell that has lost its ability to replicate in vivo or in vitro shortly after birth,[1] no cell lines with well-defined characteristics of cardiac myocytes have been available until now. The aforementioned combination of characteristics has played an important role in delaying the dissection of the cellular and molecular basis of cardiac performance in physiological and pathological states. Yet it is clear that the application of modern techniques of cellular and molecular biology holds great promise for solving some of the major problems in clinical cardiovascular medicine. In addition, it is becoming increasingly clear that the cardiovascular system in general, and the myocardium in particular, is an excellent model with which to address some broad biological questions that have general significance.

Some recent advances in the understanding of the molecular biology of the cardiac contractile system and its response to physiological and pathological stimuli are presented below. Particular emphasis is placed on the contractile apparatus and on those areas that highlight the extraordinary plasticity of this tissue at the biochemical level and that highlight the insight obtained through new molecular approaches.

THE CARDIAC CONTRACTILE APPARATUS

The sarcomere (Figs. 13–1, p. 353, and 13–4, p. 355) is the basic contractile unit of both the myocardium and skeletal

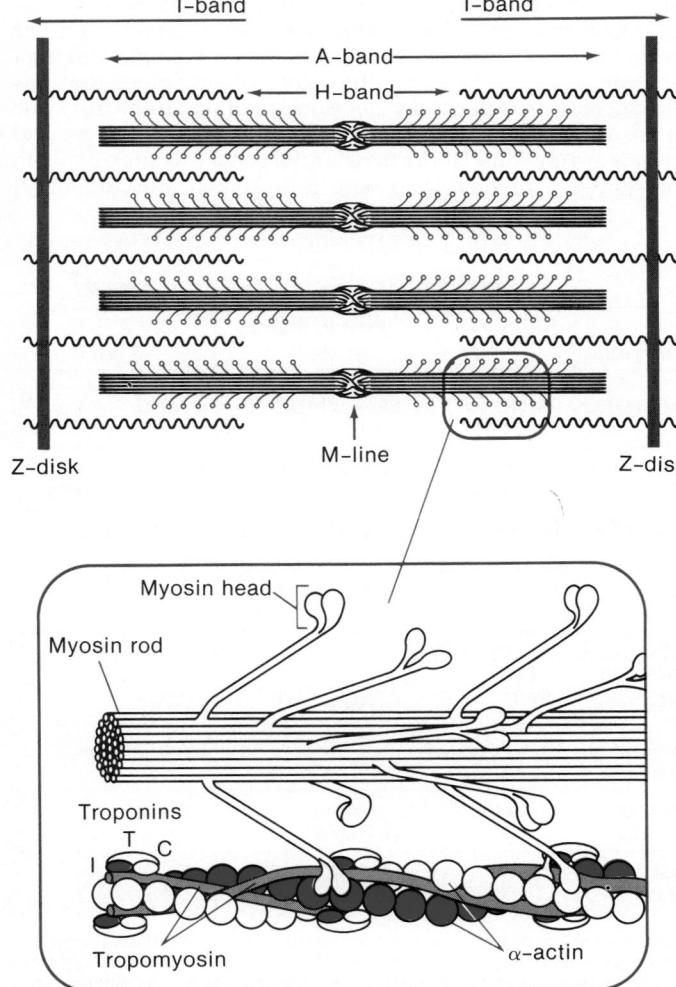

FIGURE 50–10. **Structural organization of a sarcomere. Each sarcomere (top panel) is constituted by sets of parallel thick and thin filaments (bottom panel) which partially overlap and are connected to one another.**

muscle.[60] The contractile properties of the myocardium—in terms of force generated and velocity of contraction—are dependent on the number as well as the biochemical composition of its sarcomeres. The sarcomere, in turn, is made up of seven major proteins and several minor ones organized into thick and thin filaments. The thin filaments, anchored at the Z lines (Fig. 50–10), are formed by a double helix of polymerized sarcomeric actin molecules. In the major groove of this double helix is located a continuous coil of tropomyosin (TM) dimers. Every tropomyosin dimer interacts with seven actins and it is associated with a troponin (Tn) complex (Fig. 13–4, p. 355). Each complex in turn is composed of one molecule of each of the three troponins—T, C, and I. This tropomyosin-troponin complex is responsible for the calcium sensitivity of the contractile apparatus. It regulates the interaction between the heads of the myosin molecule, located in the thick filament, and actin, the main constituent of the thin filament. Although much is known about this interaction, the precise molecular mechanisms responsible for the biochemical-mechanical transduction have not yet been fully elucidated.

The thick filament contains the molecular motor of contraction, the myosin heavy chain (MHC). This is a bifunctional molecule that exists in a dimeric form (Fig. 13–5, p. 355). The two functional domains are constituted of the rod portion and the head; the rod is composed of the carboxyl-terminal half of the molecule and is a regular coiled helix responsible for the assembly of myosin into an organized antiparallel thick filament with heads regularly spaced every 14.3 Å at both ends with a bare zone in the middle. The rod carries the load during contraction; its antiparallel organization makes possible the shortening of the sarcomere by pulling together two thin filaments pointing in opposite direction and attached to two neighboring Z lines. During the contraction cycle, the head of MHC—composed of the amino-terminal half of the molecule—interacts directly with the actin molecules in the thin filament and carries the ATPase activity required to produce the physical translocation needed for fiber shortening. The ATPase activity of MHC is modulated by two smaller protein subunits bound to each MHC head—the alkali and essential myosin light chains (MLC). As originally pointed out by Barany, there is a direct correlation between the unloaded maximum velocity of shortening of a muscle fiber (V_{max}) and the actin-activated ATPase activity of its MHC.[61] Although there are some apparent exceptions to this rule, fibers with an MHC with high ATPase activity contract faster than those with a lower enzymatic activity.[62,63] As might be anticipated, there is an inverse correlation between ATPase activity of the MHC in a fiber and the energetic cost to perform a given workload.[62-64] The more rapidly the fiber contracts, the higher the energetic cost of producing the same amount of work. It is clear, therefore, that the *type* of MHC and its ATPase activity present in the sarcomeres are physiologically significant and have a profound effect on the contractile properties of the myocardium.

In addition to the seven major proteins mentioned earlier, the sarcomere contains a number of other proteins, such as α-actinin, C protein, titin, and nebulin,[65,66] that are present in smaller concentrations and are thought to play important roles either in sarcomeric organization or modulation of function. However, with the exception of α-actinin, which is the main constituent of the Z line and serves to anchor the actin filament,[65] the precise function of these minor components of the sarcomere remains to be defined.

The intrinsic properties of the sarcomere are the main determinants of the contractile state. However, a number of other molecules, such as adrenoceptors[67] (p. 363), ion channels[68] (p. 358), Na+, K+-ATPase (p. 359), sarcolemmal and sarcoplasmic calcium pumps (p. 361), and sarcoplasmic calcium–release channels,[69-71] are also involved in its modulation. Most of these molecules exert their effect on contractility by directly or indirectly modulating either the availability or the response to calcium by the contractile proteins. Each of the cardiac contractile proteins is a member of a family of *isoforms* that is specific to the cell type and stage of development.

EXPRESSION OF MULTIPLE ISOFORMS

The regulated expression of cell type–specific protein isoforms that are structurally distinct and developmentally regulated is a fundamental characteristic of higher organisms. The molecular mechanisms responsible for the generation of this protein diversity can be broadly categorized into two main systems: those that select a particular gene among the members of a multigene family for expression in a particular cell and those that generate several different isoforms from a single gene. This latter mechanism includes DNA rearrangement and alternative pre-mRNA splicing. Both mechanisms involve the differential use of intragenic sequences that lead to the production of multiple protein isoforms from a single gene. DNA rearrangement appears to be restricted to a quite limited set of genes coding for immunoglobulins and T-cell receptors.[72,73] In contrast, increasing numbers of genes in organisms ranging from insects to humans, including their DNA and RNA viruses, are known to be alternatively spliced.

Alternative pre-mRNA splicing is particularly prevalent in striated muscle, including the myocardium. Among the contractile protein genes, this mode of gene regulation has been documented for alpha- and beta-tropomyosin, troponin T, and the myosin light chains, in addition to a number of other genes.[74,75] Furthermore, the major constituents of the thick (MHCs and MLCs) and thin (actin, tropomyosins, and troponins [C, T, and I]) filaments of mammalian sarcomeres are each encoded by a multigene family of moderate size, ranging from four to eight members.[60,66,76] The expression of each member of these multigene families is regulated at the transcriptional level in a tissue-specific and developmentally regulated manner. The different isoforms of sarcomeric contractile proteins, generated either through the transcription of different genes or from the same gene by alternative pre-mRNA splicing, are able to substitute for one another and

when present to combine in the same cell. The restricted combined use of the different members of these multigene families allows for the generation of a moderate number of qualitatively different sarcomere types that exhibit significantly different physiological characteristics, at least in some cases.[66,67,76,77] This potential for the production of different sarcomeres is greatly increased by the generation of multiple protein isoforms by individual MLC and TNT genes. Therefore, in order to understand the mechanisms involved in generating myocardial protein diversity, it is necessary to know the elements responsible for the selective transcription of a given gene in a particular cell type at a particular time in development or physiological state as well as the factors that regulate alternative pre-mRNA splicing in the same cell.

Most of the genes coding for contractile proteins have now been identified; cDNA and genomic sequences have been obtained, mapped to the human genome, and characterized for their potential to generate multiple protein isoforms by alternative splicing. Although some of these genes are closely clustered on the same chromosome, as is the case for the cardiac and skeletal MHCs,[78–80] most other contractile protein gene families are not linked but are scattered on several chromosomes.[81,82] Therefore, although the contractile proteins are assembled in the sarcomere in quite precise stoichiometric quantities, their regulation is of necessity complex, because it involves multiple genes that are located in different regions of the genome that, with few exceptions, do not seem to have common regulatory sequences.

Some of the contractile protein isoforms expressed in the myocardium are shared with skeletal muscle, while others are expressed exclusively in the heart[60,66,67] (Table 50–1). Moreover, for several of these proteins, the atrial and ventricular isoforms are different from one another and both differ from the ones expressed in the conduction system. Although the physiological basis for the selective advantage that has produced this isoform distribution is not apparent from our present understanding of contractility, two main general trends are obvious: (1) the myocardial genes are more likely to be shared with slow than with fast skeletal muscle and (2)

TABLE 50–1 EXPRESSION OF CONTRACTILE PROTEIN GENES IN STRIATED SKELETAL AND CARDIAC MUSCLES OF SMALL MAMMALS

	SKELETAL MUSCLES			VENTRICLE			ATRIUM
	Embryonic/ Neonatal	Adult Fast	Adult Slow	Embryonic	Adult	Pressure Overload Adult	Adult
Myosin heavy chain (MHC)	Embryonic MHC Neonatal MHC	Fast II A MHC Fast II B MHC	Slow I = βMHC	Slow/βMHC	αMHC + ~βMHC	Slow/βMHC + αMHC	α MHC
Myosin light chain (LC)	LC1e LC1f	LC1f LC3f	LC1slow/ cardiac	LC1e	LC1slow/ cardiac	LC1slow/cardiac + LCe	LC1e LC1slow/cardiac
Myosin light chain 2	LC2sk	LC2sk	LC2sk	LC2 cardiac	LC2 cardiac	LC2 cardiac	LC2 cardiac
Tropomyosin	ββ	α/β α/α	α/β	β/α	α/α	α/β	α/α
Troponins T	Fast TnT Slow TnT	Fast TNT	Slow TNT	(Emb)cardiac TNT	(Adult)cardiac TNT		Cardiac TNT
C	c TNC (slow/ cardiac)	skTNC (skeletal)	cTNC	cTNC	cTNC	cTNC	cTNC
I	Fast TNI	Fast TNI	Slow/cardiac TNI	Slow/cardiac TNI	Slow/cardiac TNI		Slow/cardiac
Actin	c α-actin sk α-actin	sk α-actin	sk α-actin	sk α-actin c α-actin	c α-actin	c α-actin sk α-actin	c α-actin
Creatine kinase	BB ck BM ck	MM ck	MM ck	BB ck MM ck	MM ck	MM ck BB ck	

MHC = Myosin heavy chain; each member of this gene family is indicated by a prefix indicating the most common nomenclature used to duplicate the gene. MLC = myosin light chain gene products: LC1e = light chain 1 embryonic, LC1 slow/cardiac = light chain specific for slow and cardiac tissues. LC1f and LC3f are the two products for the myosin light chain 1/3 that is predominantly expressed in fast muscle. LC2sk and LC2 cardiac denote the light chain 2 characteristic of skeletal (sk) and cardiac muscle, respectively. Tropomyosin α and β designate these products of these two genes. α-TM is characteristic of differentiated striated muscle while β is characteristic of the undifferentiated cells. TNC, TNT, TNI indicate troponin C, T, and I, respectively. The prefixes cardiac, skeletal, slow, and embryonic indicate the tissue and or developmental stage in which this gene product is predominantly expressed. cα-Actin and skα-actin indicate the isoform characteristic of adult normal cardiac and skeletal muscle, respectively. Creatine kinase B and M isoform indicate the muscle-specific (M) and nonmuscle (B) isoforms.

embryonic and fetal cardiac isoforms are shared more often with striated muscle than are their adult cardiac counterparts.

1615

CHAP 50

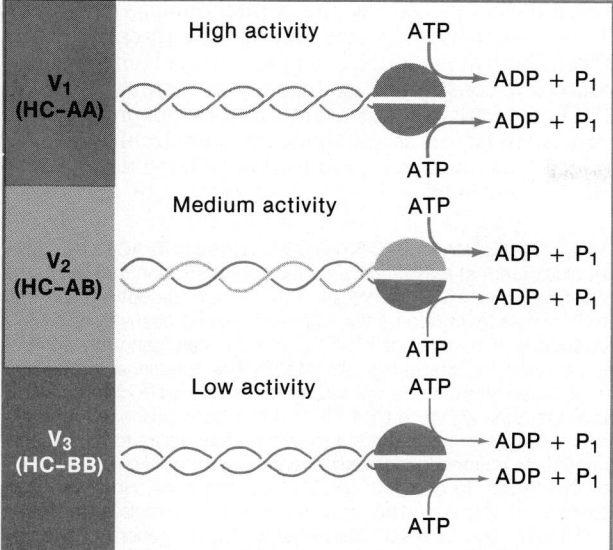

FIGURE 50–11. The three ventricular myosin isoenzymes, designated V1, V2, and V3, originate from combinations of two heavy-chain subunits (HC-A and HC-B), which differ in amino acid sequence. Functionally, these differences are expressed in the level of myosin ATPase activity and contractile performance. Thus, hydrolysis of ATP and release of reaction products are most rapid for V1 and slowest for V3; V2 is intermediate. (From Morkin, E.: Contractile proteins of the heart. Hosp. Pract. *18*:107, 1983.)

ISOFORM SWITCHES IN RESPONSE TO PHYSIOLOGICAL AND PATHOLOGICAL STIMULI

In the ventricles of most mammalian species, including the human, three myosin isoforms have been identified on the basis of their electrophoretic mobility—V1, V2, and V3.[82,83] However, these three myosins are composed of only two distinct types of MHCs, referred to as α and β. V1 and V3 are composed of $\alpha\alpha$ and $\beta\beta$ homodimers, respectively, while V2 is an $\alpha\beta$ heterodimer (Fig. 50–11). These two myosins are produced by two different genes that are closely linked[78,79] and are located on chromosomes 3 and 14 in human and mouse, respectively.[79]

As for all muscle types, the myosin composition of the myocardium is of physiological importance, because the relative distribution of α- and β-MHC is directly correlated with the contractile properties of the heart. The α-MHC, which has high Ca^{++}- and actin-activated ATPase activity,[83,84] is associated with an increased shortening velocity of the cardiac fibers.[84,85] In contrast, the β-MHC, which has lower ATPase activity,[83,84] is associated with slower shortening velocity[84,85] (Fig. 50–12, top). It is therefore interesting that the ratio of these two different cardiac isoforms is developmentally regulated. In the ventricles of all mammalian species studied so far,

FIGURE 50–12. Correlation of the ventricular myosin heavy chain phenotype and contractile performance of the myocardium in response to physiological, pathological, and developmental stimuli.

CARDIAC MYOSIN HEAVY-CHAIN ISOFORMS			
	ATPase activity	Shortening velocity	Efficiency of force production
α-MHC (V$_1$)	High	Fast	Low
β-MHC (V$_3$)	Low	Slow	High
ISOFORM SWITCHES			
	Thyroid hormone	Exercise	Work overload	Aging
α-MHC (V$_1$)	↑	↑	↓	↓
β-MHC (V$_3$)	↓	↓	↑	↑

FIGURE 50–13. Effect of thyroid hormone on cardiac myosin expression.

		Ventricles			Atria			Isoform
		Hyper	Normal	Hypo	Hyper	Normal	Hypo	
Human large mammals								V$_3$ $\beta\beta$
								V$_2$ $\alpha\beta$
								V$_1$ $\alpha\alpha$
Rat small mammals								V$_3$ $\beta\beta$
								V$_2$ $\alpha\beta$
								V$_1$ $\alpha\alpha$

β-MHC is the most abundant isoform in utero until late fetal life.[86] In small mammals such as the rat and mouse, α-MHC increases immediately before birth and becomes the predominant form throughout perinatal and adult life.[86,87] In contrast, in large mammals such as humans, α-MHC is predominant only transiently shortly after birth, with β-MHC then becoming and remaining the most abundant isoform.[86,88] The situation is different in the atria, in which α-MHC is the predominant isoform throughout life in both small and large species[60,87,88] (Fig. 50–13). In all species studied, including humans, the distribution of the cardiac MHC isoforms changes in response to certain pathological and experimental conditions such as work overload,[85,89–92] diabetes,[93] gonadectomy,[94] and, more importantly, changes in thyroid hormone levels (Figs. 50–12 and 50–13).[82,84,87,95,97] These changes are regulated at the level of transcription of the respective genes, because there is a direct correlation between the levels of α- and β-MHC and the corresponding mRNAs[87,97] and between these and the rate of transcription.[98]

REGULATION OF CARDIAC MHC GENES BY THYROID HORMONE
(See also p. 1830)

Thyroid hormone plays a fundamental role in the regulation of the MHC phenotype, both in the myocardium and in skeletal muscle.[97] In mammals at least, all the genes of the striated MHC multigene family are, without exception, responsive to thyroid hormone. Surprisingly, however, whether the hormone induces or represses the expression of a given MHC depends on the gene itself and the muscle in which it is expressed. The same gene can be induced by the hormone in one muscle and repressed in another,[97] indicating that the regulation of this gene family by thyroid hormone is likely to be more complex than described so far for a variety of steroid hormones.[98] In the heart, there is a precise correlation between the levels of circulating thyroid hormone and the relative levels of α- and β-MHC in the ventricles.[87] The expression of α-MHC is dependent on the presence of thyroid hormone (Fig. 50–12, *bottom*). In its absence the α-MHC gene is not transcribed. The converse is true for β-MHC; the expression of this gene is repressed by thyroid hormone and it is induced in hypothyroid states.[87,97] The induction of α-MHC at the time of birth is directly correlated with the surge in the circulating thyroid hormone that occurs at this time.[87] This effect of thyroid hormone on cardiac MHC expression can be directly demonstrated in experimental animals by manipulation of their thyroid state. After surgical or chemical (5-thiouracil) thyroidectomy, the expression of α-MHC is completely suppressed and only β-MHC is expressed in the myocardium.

Replacement therapy restores the normal phenotype. On the other hand, hyperthyroid states repress the expression of the β-MHC gene both at the mRNA and protein levels and produce a myocardium constituted exclusively by α-MHC[87,97] (Fig. 50–13). These results are not indirect and are not produced by changes in such factors as metabolic state, or circulating catecholamines. They can be reproduced in isolated tissue slices and cells in culture.[100]

MOLECULAR MECHANISM OF THYROID HORMONE ACTION. This has been elucidated, at least in part, by the demonstration that the c-erb proto-oncogenes (p. 1618) serve as the nuclear receptors for this hormone.[101–104] At least two genes with well-defined tissue-specific expression encode this receptor,[101–103] and each can generate several different isoforms by alternative splicing.[103] The functional properties of some of these alternatively spliced isoforms are quite different, and some have lost their ability to bind T3.[104] It has been proposed recently that some of the isoforms that are impaired in their ability to bind ligand might function as antioncogenes and/or antireceptor molecules[105,106] because of their ability to compete for DNA binding sites. However, due to the absence of ligand binding, they are unable to stimulate transcription.[104–106] It remains to be determined whether this is a general phenomenon. The functional T3 receptors are hormone-dependent transcriptional factors that exercise their effect through binding to a thyroid hormone responsive element (TRE) in the responsive gene.[104,106,107] The TRE for the human and rat β-MHC genes has been determined by a combination of deletion mapping, site-directed mutagenesis, and in vitro and in vivo hormone receptor binding assays.[100,104,108] The two genes have a TRE with identical sequence, and both are able to confer thyroid hormone sensitivity to heterologous genes.[42,46,50] Therefore, the sequence containing the TRE is both required and sufficient to confer T3 responsiveness on a gene.

T3 REPRESSION OF MHC GENES. The mechanism of T3 repression of MHC gene expression is less well understood. Both the human and rat β-MHC genes have sequences with a high degree of homology to the TRE of the α-MHC genes.[100,108] These sequences do not have an effect on the heterologous gene promoters so far tested, and it is not clear whether or not they are specifically recognized by the thyroid hormone receptor. Since these putative TRE sequences in the β-MHC genes are overlapping with the CAAT box sequences,[100] an essential promoter element in these genes, the possibility that T3 exerts its negative regulatory role by sterically hindering the binding of an essential transcription factor is presently being investigated.

The results summarized above demonstrate that thyroid hormone plays an important role in regulating cardiac MHC expression and raise the question of whether this hormone is solely responsible for the regulation of these genes (Fig. 50–14). Several lines of evidence indicate that this is *not* the case. First, it is clear that the α- and β-MHC genes respond to thyroid hormone in a tissue-dependent manner. For example, in the ventricle, the α-MHC gene is exquisitely sensitive to T3 and it is not expressed at all in the hypothyroid state. However, in the atria of the same heart, this gene is practically unresponsive to the hormone. The different behavior in the

GENE SWITCHES IN CARDIAC VENTRICLES

	Fetus & neonates	Normal adult	Work overload	Hypo-thyroid	Hyper-thyroid
Myosin heavy chain	β, α	α	$\beta\alpha$	β	α
α–Actin	Skeletal cardiac	Cardiac	Cardiac skeletal		
Tropomyosin	α,β	α	α, β	Same as normal adult	
Na$^+$, K$^+$-ATPase	α_1, α_2	α_1	α_1, α_2		
ANF	+	−	+ +		

FIGURE 50–14. Gene switches in cardiac ventricles.

two tissues is not due to the lack of functional thyroid hormone receptors in the atria, since other genes in this structure are readily responsive to the hormone. A similar phenomenon is apparent for the β-MHC gene. As already indicated, in the ventricle the expression of this gene is repressed by thyroid hormone. Yet in the same animals, its expression continues at almost normal level in the slow fibers of skeletal muscle. Moreover, the TRE of these genes does not explain their tissue specificity because they act as positive regulators of transcription in the presence of receptor and T3, irrespective of the cell type in which they are expressed. In fact, the tissue specificity of these genes is conferred by a combination of positive and negative transcriptional regulatory elements.[108] These other regulatory elements are likely to be responsible for the species-specific differences in the expression of these genes.

WORK-OVERLOAD HYPERTROPHY INDUCES MHC GENE ISOFORM SWITCHES IN THE MYOCARDIUM

The involvement of different regulatory pathways in the expression of the cardiac MHC genes becomes evident when the changes produced by work-overload hypertrophy are analyzed. In small mammals, particularly in rats, in response to a moderate increase in mean aortic pressure (~30 mm Hg) produced by aortic coarctation[109] there is a rapid induction of β-MHC mRNA. This is followed by the appearance of comparable levels of β-MHC protein, in parallel with an increase in left ventricular weight. A similar change is not detectable in larger mammals, including the human, because β-MHC is the predominant isoform expressed in the normal ventricle of such mammals. However, in human atria, which normally express α-MHC, a switch to β-MHC is readily apparent in response to increased pressure.[110] Therefore, the hypertrophied myocardium induces the expression of β-MHC and represses the expression of the α-gene. With respect to the MHC phenotype, it resembles the fetal and hypothyroid states. Yet in these animals the circulating level of thyroid hormone remains normal, and their metabolic state argues against hypothyroidism. Other features argue persuasively that this isoform switch produced in response to work-overload hypertrophy is not regulated through the thyroid hormone pathway.[109]

WORK-OVERLOAD HYPERTROPHY INDUCES MANY FETAL ISOFORMS. The isoform switches produced in response to increased afterload are not limited to MHC. In fact, a general myocardial response to work overload occurs rapidly and affects a number of cellular compartments.[111] This response is characterized by the reexpression of the protein isoforms that are normally expressed in fetal life and normally suppressed in adulthood. This phenomenon has been demonstrated for all the gene phenotypes analyzed so far, including other contractile proteins such as skeletal α-actin,[111,112] myosin light chain 1,[113] and tropomyosin[111]; membrane proteins such as Na+, K+-ATPase (the cardiac glycoside receptor)[114]; secreted molecules such as atrial natriuretic peptide (ANP)[111]; and those involved in ATP regeneration, such as creatine kinase.[116] With the exception of ANF, all of these examples represent the reexpression of an isoform normally expressed only during fetal and early postnatal life that is later replaced by the corresponding adult isoform. ANF expression in the ventricles is normally suppressed after birth and is not replaced by another isoform. Its expression, however, is rapidly reinduced in response to the hypertrophic stimulus.

From these observations it is clear that myocardial hypertrophy is not only a quantitative phenomenon involving an increase in cardiac mass but, more importantly, it also results in a significant qualitative change in important constituents of the myocardium. In general, these changes produce a muscle that has many of the biochemical characteristics of fetal myocardium.

What is the stimulus for this dramatic and concerted change

in myocardial gene expression in response to work overload? One possibility is thyroid hormone itself. However, as already indicated, no changes in thyroid hormone levels are detected in these animals. Furthermore, if thyroid hormone were responsible, the normal phenotype could be reestablished in response to thyroid hormone therapy. This is not the case. Thyroid hormone can overcome the effect of pressure overload on MHC gene expression but cannot influence the other phenotypic changes.[109,111] Administration of high doses of T3 in hypertrophic animals produces a rapid de-induction of the β-MHC gene with the concomitant induction of the α-MHC, despite the fact that these animals have a higher degree of hypertrophy than do those with simple hemodynamic overload.[109,111] None of the changes in the expression of other genes are affected by the hormone. These results give further support to the contention that the changes induced by hemodynamic overload are not secondary to thyroid hormone changes. However, in the case of the MHC genes, T3 has a dominant effect and can overcome the regulatory mechanisms induced by the hypertrophic stimulus. This behavior highlights the complex interplay that exists between hemodynamic and hormonal stimuli in the expression of myocardial genes.

It is noteworthy that in animals with aortic banding (experimental coarctation), the most commonly used model system, increased afterload, is not the only consequence of the manipulation. Aortic binding might produce an elevation in circulating catecholamine levels and/or activation of the renin-angiotensin system secondary to decreased renal blood flow. Norepinephrine[116,117] and possibly angiotensin II might directly stimulate myocardial cell hypertrophy independently of the hemodynamic effects. The effect of norepinephrine on cardiac cell growth in culture has been shown to be mediated by stimulation of the α1-adrenoceptor,[116] which couples the hydrolysis of membrane phosphatidylinositol followed by the release of IP3 [118] and activation of protein kinase C (Fig. 13–12, p. 360).[119] Furthermore, phorbol esters, which are direct activators of protein kinase C, can produce hypertrophy and isoform switches when administered to cultured neonatal cardiac cells.[120] However, the fact that the atria and right ventricles of the animals with aortic banding do not exhibit the isoform transitions already described strongly suggests that these humoral mechanisms do not play an important role, if they are involved at all, in the processes described here.

MOLECULAR BASIS FOR CERTAIN FORMS OF HYPERTROPHIC CARDIOMYOPATHY

(See p. 1636)

Until recently, not a single mutation for any of the genes coding for contractile proteins had been identified in vertebrates. This contrasts with the large number of mutations with impaired function detected in lower organisms. The lack of phenotypic mutants in vertebrates could be explained by assuming that either most mutations are lethal or that they lack a distinctive phenotype because the mutant isoform is replaced by another from the same multigene family. The latter hypothesis was given credence by the finding of a mouse strain that lacks a functional cardiac α-actin gene. These animals have a normal life span and apparent cardiac performance and express the skeletal α-actin gene in the myocardium at all stages of development and physiological states. This phenotype, together with the changes induced by thyroid hormone and work overload hypertrophy, strongly supports the concept that different isoforms are interchangeable, although they might result in subtle changes in cardiac performance.

For this reason it is surprising that the mutation responsible for certain forms of familial hypertrophic cardiomyopathy maps to the cardiac myosin genes. This disease is a dominant disorder characterized by cardiac hypertrophy, a wide spectrum of clinical symptoms, and a high rate of sudden death (p. 1411). Pathological findings include increased myocardial mass with myocyte and myofibrillar disarray. It has recently been demonstrated that at least two different mutations can produce the disease. In one case there is a novel α/β cardiac MHC hybrid,[23] while in the other a single base pair mutation produces a missense mutation in the β-MHC.[30] From the sequence it appears that both mutant MHCs should be functional, although the mutation maps to an amino acid residue that is conserved in all the MHC sequenced thus far, ranging from unicellular organisms to humans. Although the molecular mechanisms responsible for the production of the anatomical changes in familial hypertrophic cardiomyopathy remain to be elucidated, the dominant character of the phenotype suggests that the assembly of the thick filament is affected by the mutation. Because not all cases of this disease map to the MHC locus, it is likely that mutations in other genes encoding contractile proteins can also produce the same clinical syndrome.

EXPRESSION OF PROTO-ONCOGENES BY WORK OVERLOAD

(See p. 1617)

The cardiac response to normal growth requirements, as well as to work overload, depends on the developmental state of the organ. During fetal and early postnatal life, the demand for an increased cardiac mass is filled mainly by an increase in the number of myocytes (hyperplasia). However, soon after birth, cardiac myocytes lose their ability to divide.[1] Later in life, demand for an increased myocardial mass is met exclusively by an increase in the size of a fixed number of preexisting myocytes. The molecular mechanisms responsible for the loss of replicative ability (terminal differentiation) remain unknown. Genes involved in determining the myogenic lineage and terminal differentiation in skeletal muscle, such as $MyoD$,[121] myogenin,[122] and Mif[123] that function as tissue-specific transcriptional factors, are not involved in the determination and differentiation of the cardiac myocytes, because they are not expressed in these cells. It is likely that a family of genes with functional similarities but with significant sequence divergence from the ones identified in skeletal muscle is responsible for the cardiac phenotype.

What is the mechanism involved in inducing cell growth and isoform switches in response to work overload? The observed reexpression of fetal isoforms in cardiac hypertrophy is reminiscent of the mitogenic response of many differentiated cell types, such as hepatocytes, which often involves the suppression of the adult phenotype and reexpression of the fetal pattern, as is the case in the inhibition of albumin and induction of α-protein expression during liver regeneration.[124] In a general biological context, cardiac hypertrophy could be considered the equivalent of the growth response exhibited by most cell types in response to mitogens. In this particular case the growth response is carried out by terminally differentiated cells (myocytes) that are unable to undergo cell division and have only the hypertrophic response open to them. If this hypothesis were correct, it would be expected that the initial response to the hypertrophic stimuli would mimic early events of cell division induced by growth factors in a large variety of cell types.

One of the early responses of stationary cells to growth stimuli is the induction of a series of proto-oncogenes, such as c-fos and c-myc, among others, that directly or indirectly turn on the cascade of events that leads to cell division. These molecules owe their name to the fact that they are the cellular counterpart of viral oncogenes and their regulation is usually altered in neoplastic cells. Recently, however, it has been demonstrated that these proto-oncogenes are bona fide transcriptional factors that in most cases form part of the normal growth induction machinery of the cell in response to growth stimuli.[125] Furthermore, c-myc is able to induce a family of heat shock or stress proteins that are involved in protecting the viability of cells under adverse conditions. This occurs by mechanisms that are not fully elucidated but might affect proper protein folding[126] and/or modulation of gene transcription.[127]

ROLE OF PROTO-ONCOGENES. Not surprisingly, c-fos and c-myc mRNAs begin to accumulate within 1 hour after the increase in afterload, reach high levels within 3 hours, and return to basal levels in less than 24 hours. Similarly, the mRNA for one of the major stress proteins, HSP 70, is also increased within 30 minutes of increasing aortic pressure.[111] Thus, similar to the mitogenic response of a variety of cell types, induction of the cellular proto-oncogenes and major stress protein genes reflects early changes occurring in the nuclei of myocardial cells in response to acute pressure overload and appears to play an important role in mediating the hypertrophic response. That this factor has a causative role in the hypertrophic response is suggested by the fact that the overexpression of c-myc in the myocardium of transgenic animals induces cardiac enlargement and cellular hyperplasia.[128] Several growth factors, including transforming growth factor β (TGFβ) and basic fibroblast growth factor (bFGF), applied to cardiocytes in culture induce a pattern of contractile protein and proto-oncogene expression that is quite similar to that produced by work overload in the intact heart.[127] These results demonstrate that the lack of mitogenic response by cardiac myocytes is not due to a loss of receptors for growth factors. They also give further support to the hypothesis that work overload affects gene expression through mechanisms similar to or shared by the growth factor receptors.

The inability of the cardiocytes to mount a full mitogenic response when challenged by work overload or growth factors remains to be explained, as it does in all other terminally differentiated cells, such as neurons and certain epithelial cells. On the one hand, these cells could have irreversibly lost the expression of some of the genes required to traverse the cell cycle. In that case it should be impossible for them to reenter the cell cycle in response to any stimulus. On the other hand, the terminally differentiated program could induce an inhibitor of the cell cycle. In that case, repression or neutralization of the inhibitor should enable the cells to cycle again. Recently, recessive cellular oncogenes with many of the properties required for this role have been described. One of them, the product of the retinoblastoma (Rb) gene, has been shown to belong to this class. The activity of this gene product is neutralized by certain viral oncogenes: SV40 T antigen[129] and adenovirus EiA.[130] Based on the finding that SV40 T antigen is able to reinduce the ability to cycle to differentiated myotubes,[131] it has been possible to reinduce the cell cycle in terminally differentiated cardiocytes and to create cell lines that express many of the differentiated characteristics. These results suggest the presence of inhibitors in differentiated cardiocytes. Identification of the molecule(s) involved could provide the tool required to induce cardiac muscle regeneration.

WALL STRESS AS A DETERMINANT OF HYPERTROPHY. In various models of cardiac hypertrophy, systolic and diastolic wall stress have been implicated as major determinants of the degree and pattern of hypertrophy during pressure and volume overload.[132] In addition, studies using isolated heart preparations have demonstrated that increased wall tension alone can stimulate protein synthesis[60] directly. Although the precise molecular mechanisms by which wall stress is communicated to the myocyte nucleus remain to be elucidated, the recently discovered stretch-sensitive ion channels[133] provide a likely candidate for the sensor mechanism. These channels could provide a very sensitive measure of wall stress. The ionic changes produced by their opening or closing could trigger a second messenger cascade (perhaps involving IP3) that results in the changes in gene expression already described. The recent demonstration that stretching of isolated cardiocytes in culture induces the changes of contractile gene and proto-oncogene expression[134] described for work overload and growth factors supports this hypothesis.

In physiological terms, the reexpression of the fetal isogenes might be a beneficial adaptation to hemodynamic overload. As a consequence of the changes induced in the thin and thick filaments during cardiac hypertrophy, sarcomeres with significantly different functional properties are produced. For the myocardium, the fetal isoform of MHC has been shown to be energetically more efficient than that of the adult. Moreover, because ANP has potent natriuretic, diuretic, and vasodilatory effects, the marked induction of this molecule in the ventricle in response to increased wall tension might be interpreted as an adaptational response to reduce hemodynamic load imposed on the ventricle.

CONCLUSIONS

It has become apparent that the myocardium is now amenable to cellular and molecular "dissection." It can serve as a good experimental model to address questions that are relevant not only to the cardiovascular system but are also of general biological significance. In addition, it is clear that cardiac hypertrophy is not a simple quantitative increase in ventricular mass but a qualitatively different and heterogeneous process that is influenced strongly by the nature of the hypertrophic stimulus and the developmental stage of the myocardium. Induction of cellular proto-oncogenes that play a role in cell growth in the very early stages of work overload hypertrophy mimics the mitogenic response to growth factors by a variety of cells. The quantitative and qualitative changes in the expression of contractile and regulatory genes that occur later probably represent only a small sample of the changes produced in the myocardium in response to the hypertrophic stimuli. The finding that each fetal gene examined so far is reexpressed in response to pressure overload hypertrophy suggests that reinduction of the fetal program might be a general adaptive process to hemodynamic stress.

Further work is needed, however, to elucidate the precise mechanisms by which the hemodynamic and/or mechanical stimuli are converted into biochemical signals that lead to quantitative as well as qualitative changes in gene expression. A better understanding is also required of the genes involved in converting precursor mesenchymal cells into the cardiogenic pathway, and of the cell-specific transcriptional factors responsible for the expression of cardiac specific genes, as well as of the genes involved in blocking these cells in the terminally differentiated myocytes. This information is essential in order to be able to manipulate the process of cardiac hypertrophy and changes of contractile state to physiological advantage.

REFERENCES

MOLECULAR BIOLOGY AND THE CARDIOVASCULAR SYSTEM

1. Zak, R.: Development and proliferative capacity of cardiac muscle cells. Circ. Res. 35 (Suppl. II):17, 1974.
2. Watson, Hopkins, Roberts, et al.: Molecular Biology of the Gene. 4th Ed. The Benjamin/Cummings Publishing Co., Inc., 1987.
3. Darnell, J., Lodish, H., and Baltimore, D. (eds.): Molecular Cell Biology. New York, Scientific American Books, Inc., 1986.
4. Chien, K. R., and Knowlton, K. V.: Cardiovascular molecular biology. Introduction to the Series. Circulation 80:219, 1989.
5. Smith, H. O., and Wilcox, K. W.: A restriction enzyme from Hemophilus influenzae. Purification and general properties. J. Mol. Biol. 51:379, 1970.
6. Danna, K., and Nathans, D.: Specific cleavage of simian virus 40 DNA by restriction endonuclease of Hemophilus influenzae. Proc. Natl. Acad. Sci. USA 68:2913, 1971.
7. Cohen, S. N., Chang, A. C., Boyer, M. W., and Melling, R. B.: Construction of biologically functional bacterial plasmids in vitro. Proc. Natl. Acad. Sci. 70:3240, 1973.
8. Jackson, D. A., Symons, R. H., and Berg, P.: Biochemical method for inserting new genetic information into DNA of simian virus 40: Circular SV40 molecules containing lambda phage genes and the galactose operon of Escherichia coli. Proc. Natl. Acad. Sci. USA 69:2904, 1973.
9. Baltimore, D.: Viral RNA-dependent DNA polymerase. Nature 226:1209, 1970.
10. Temin, H. M., and Mizutani, S.: RNA-dependent DNA polymerase in virions of Rous sarcoma virus. Nature 226:1211, 1975.
11. Sanger, F., and Coulson, A. R.: A rapid method for determining the sequences in DNA by primed synthesis with DNA polymerase. J. Mol. Biol. 94:441, 1975.
12. Maxam, A. M., and Gilbert, W.: A new method for sequencing DNA. Proc. Natl. Acad. Sci. USA. 74:560, 1977.
13. Sanger, F., Nicklen, S., and Coulson, A. R.: DNA sequencing with chain-termination inhibitors. Proc. Natl. Acad. Sci. USA. 74:5463, 1977.
14. Botstein, D., White, R. L., Skolnick, M., and Davis, R. W.: Construction of a genetic linkage map in man using restriction fragment length polymorphisms. Am J. Hum. Genet. 32:314, 1980.
15. Mckusick, V. A.: Mapping and sequencing the human genome. N. Engl. J. Med. 320:910, 1989.
16. Gusella, J. F.: DNA polymorphism and human disease. Annu. Rev. Biochem. 55:831, 1986.
17. Hoffman, E. P., Brown, R. H., Jr., and Kunkel, L. M.: Dystrophin, the protein product of the Duchenne muscular dystrophy locus. Cell 51:919–928, 1988.
18. Rommens, J. M., Iannuzzi, M. C., Kerem, Bat-Sheva, et al.: Identification of the cystic fibrosis gene: Chromosome walking and jumping. Science 245:1059, 1989.
19. Watkins, M. C., Jardro, J. A., Solomon, S. D., et al.: Mapping of the gene for familial hypertrophic cardiomyopathy and analysis of genetic heterogeneity. Eur. Heart J. 11 (Abst. suppl.) 1990.
20. Brueckner, M., D'Eustachio, P., and Horwich, A. L.: Linkage mapping of a mouse gene, iv, that controls left-right asymmetry of the heart and viscera. Proc. Natl. Acad. Sci. USA 86:5035, 1989.

USE OF CLONED DNA FOR DIAGNOSIS AND TREATMENT OF GENETIC DISORDERS

21. Southern, E.: Detection of specific sequences among DNA fragments separated by gel electrophoresis. J. Mol. Biol. 98:503, 1975.
22. McKusick, V. A.: Mendelian Inheritance in Man: Catalogs of Autosomal Dominant, Autosomal Recessive, and X-Linked Phenotypes. 9th Ed. Baltimore, Johns Hopkins University Press, 1990.
23. Tanigawa, G., Jarcho, J. A., Kass, S., et al.: A molecular basis for familial hypertrophic cardiomyopathy: An α - β cardiac myosin heavy chain gene. Cell 62:991, 1990.
24. Mahdavi, V., Chambers, A., and Nadal-Ginard, B.: The ventricular α- and β-MHC genes are linked in the genome and organized according to their developmental expression. Proc. Natl. Acad. Sci. USA. 81:2626, 1984.
25. Saez, L. J., Gianola, K. M., McNally, E. M., et al.: Human cardiac myosin heavy chain genes and their linkage in the genome. Nucl. Acids Res. 15:5443, 1989.
26. Antonarakis, S. E.: Diagnosis of genetic disorders at the DNA level. N. Engl. J. Med. 320:153, 1989.
27. Studenski, A. B., and Wallace, R. B.: Allele-specific hybridization using oligonucleotide probes of very high specific activity: Discrimination of the human β A- and β S-globin genes. DNA 3:7, 1984.
28. Cutting, G. R., Kasch, L. M., Rosenstein, B. J., et al.: A cluster of cystic fibrosis mutations in the first mucustide-binding fold of the cystic fibrosis conductance regulatory protein. Nature 346:366, 1990.
29. Sykes, B.: Bone disease cytogenetics. Nature 348:18, 1990.
30. Geisterfer-Lowrance, A. A. T., Kass, S., Tanigawa, G., et al.: A molecular basis of familial hypertrophic cardiomyopathy. A β cardiac myosin heavy chain missense mutation. Cell 62:999, 1990.
31. Saiki, R. K., Scharf, S., Faloona, F., et al.: Enzymatic amplification of β-globin genomic sequences and restriction site analysis for diagnosis of sickle cell anemia. Science 230:1350, 1985.
32. Saiki, R. K., Gelfand, D. H., Staffel, S., et al.: Primer-directed enzymatic amplification of DNA with a thermastable DNA polymerase. Science 239:487, 1988.
33. Van der Werf, F., Ludbrook, P. A., Bergmann, S. R., et al.: Coronary thrombolysis with tissue-type plasminogen activator in patients with evolving myocardial infarction. N. Engl. J. Med. 310:609, 1984.
34. Penmica, D., Holmes, W. E., Kohr, W. J., et al.: Cloning and expression of human tissue-type plasminogen activator cDNA in E. coli. Nature 301:214, 1983.
35. Kaufman, R. J., Wasley, L. C., Spilioles, A. J., et al.: Coamplification and coexpression of human-type plasminogen activator and murine dehydrofolate reductase sequences in Chinese hamster ovary cells. Mol. Cell. Biol. 5:1750, 1985.
36. Alt, K. W., Kellems, R. E., Bertino, J. R., and Schimke, R. T.: Selective multiplication of dehydrofolate reductase genestin methotrexate-resistant variants of cultured murine cells. J. Biol. Chem. 253:1351, 1978.
37. Yarden, Y., Escobedo, J. A., Kuang, W. J., et al.: Structure of the receptor for platelet-derived growth factor helps define a family of closely related growth factor receptors. Nature 323:226, 1986.
38. Escobedo, J. A., and Williams, L. T.: A PDGF receptor domain essential for mitogensis but not for many other responses to PDGF. Nature 335:85, 1988.
39. O'Dowd, B. F., Hnatowich, M., Regan, J. W., et al.: Site directed mutagenesis of the cytoplasmic domains of the human β2-adrenergic receptor. J. Biol. Chem. 263:1598, 1988.
40. Noda, M., Ikeda, T., Suzuki, M., et al.: Expression of functional sodium channels from cloned cDNA. Nature 322:826, 1986.
41. Brinster, R. L., Chen, M. Y., Trumbauer, M., et al.: Somatic expression of herpes thymidine kinase in mice following injection of a fusion gene into eggs. Cell 27:223, 1981.
42. LaPointe, M. C., Wu, J. P., Greenberg, B., and Gardner, D. G.: Upstream sequences confer atrial-specific expression on the human atrial natriuretic factor gene. J. Biol. Chem. 263:9075, 1988.
43. Seidman, C. E., Wong, D. W., Jarcho, J. A., et al.: Cis-Acting sequences that mediate atrial natriuretic factor gene expression. Proc. Natl. Acad. Sci. USA 85:4104, 1988.
44. Gluzman, Y., and Shenk, T. (eds.): Enhancers and Eukaryotic Gene Expression. Current Communications in Molecular Biology. Cold Spring Harbor Laboratory, 1983.
45. Jackson, T., Allard, M. F., Sreenan, C. M., et al.: The c-myc proto-oncogene regulates cardiac development in transgenic mice. Mol. Cell. Biol. 10:3709–3716, 1990.
46. Field, L. J.: Atrial natriuretic factor—SV40 T antigen transgenes produce tumors and cardiac arrhythmias in mice. Science 239:1029, 1988.
47. Steinhelper, M. E., Katz, E., Lanson, N., et al.: Myocardial hyperplasia in transgenic mice. J. Cell Biochem. (abstr.) (Supp. 15C):H14, 1991.

48. Mann, R., Mulligan, R. C., and Baltimore, D.: Construction of a retroviral packaging mutant and its use to produce helper-free defective retrovirus. Cell 33:153, 1983.

49. Miller, A. D., Jolly, D. J., Friedman, T., and Verma, I. M.: A transmissible retrovirus expressing human hypoxanthine phosphoribosyltransferase (HPRT): Gene transfer into cells obtained from humans deficient in HPRT. Proc. Natl. Acad. Sci. USA 80:4709, 1983.

50. Dzierzak, E. A., Papayannopoulou, T., and Mulligan, R. C.: Lineage-specific expression of a human β-globin gene in murine marrow transplant recipients reconstituted with retrovirus-transduced stem cells. Nature 331:35, 1988.

51. Cournoyer, D., and Caskey, C. T.: Gene transfer into humans. A first step. N. Engl. J. Med. 323:601, 1990.

52. Rosenberg, S. A., Aebersold, P., Cornetta, K., et al.: Gene transfer into humans — immunotherapy of patients with advanced melanoma using tumor-infiltrating lymphocytes modified by retroviral transduction. N. Engl. J. Med. 323:570, 1990.

53. Nabel, E. G., Plautz, G., Boyce, F. M., et al.: Recombinant gene expression in vivo within endothelial cells of the arterial wall. Science 244:1342, 1989.

54. Wilson, J. M., Birinyi, L. K., Salomon, R. N., et al.: Implantation of vascular grafts lined with genetically modified endothelial cells. Science 244:1344, 1989.

55. Dichek, D. A., Neville, R. F., Zwiebel, J. A., et al.: Seeding of intravascular stents with genetically engineered endothelial cells. Circulation 80:1347, 1989.

56. Nabel, E. G., Plautz, G., and Boice, F. M.: Site-specific gene expression in vivo by direct gene transfer into the arterial wall. Science 249:1285, 1990.

57. Wolff, J. A., Malone, R. W., Williams, P., et al.: Direct gene transfer into mouse muscle in vivo. Science 247:1465, 1990.

58. Lin, M., Parmacek, M. S., Marle, G., et al.: Expression of recombinant genes in myocardium in vivo after direct injection of DNA. Circulation 82:2217, 1990.

59. Swain, J. L.: Gene therapy — A new approach to the treatment of cardiovascular disease. Circulation 80:1495, 1989.

MOLECULAR BIOLOGY OF THE CARDIAC CONTRACTILE SYSTEM

60. Swynghedauw, B.: Developmental and functional adaptation of contractile proteins in cardiac and skeletal muscles. Physiol. Rev. 66:710, 1986.

61. Barany, M.: ATPase activity of myosin correlated with speed of muscle shortening. J. Gen. Physiol. 50(Suppl.):197, 1967.

62. Scheuer, J., and Bhan, A. K.: Cardiac contractile proteins. Adenosine triphosphatase activity and physiological function. Circ. Res. 45:1, 1979.

63. Schwartz, K., Lecarpentier, Y., Martin et al. Myosin isoenzymic distribution correlates with speed of myocardial contraction. J. Mol. Cell Cardiol. 13:1071, 1981.

64. Alpert, N. R., and Mulieri, L. A.: Increased myothermal economy of isometric force generation in compensated cardiac hypertrophy induced by pulmonary artery constriction in the rabbit. A characterization of heat liberation in normal and hypertrophied right ventricular papillary muscles. Circ. Res. 50:491, 1982.

65. Obinata, T., Maruyama, K., Sugita, H., et al.: Dynamic aspects of structural proteins in vertebrate skeletal muscle. Muscle Nerve 4:456, 1981.

66. Emerson, C., Fischman, D. A., Nadal-Ginard, B., and Siddiqui, M. A. Q. (eds.): Molecular Biology of Muscle Development. UCLA Symposia on Molecular and Cellular Biology. New Series, 29. New York, Alan R. Liss, 1986.

67. Stiles, G. L., and Lefkowitz, R. J.: Cardiac adrenergic receptors. Annu. Rev. Med. 35:149, 1984.

68. Catterall, W. A.: Molecular properties of voltage-sensitive sodium channels. Annu. Rev. Biochem. 55:953, 1986.

69. Herrera, V. L., Emanuel, J. R., Ruiz-Opazo, N., et al.: Three differentially expressed Na, K-ATPase α subunit isoforms: Structural and functional implications. J. Cell. Biol. 105:1855, 1987.

70. MacLennan, D. H., Brandl, C. J., Korczak, B., and Green, N. M.: Amino-acid sequence of a $Ca^{2+} + Mg^{2+}$-dependent ATPase from rabbit muscle sarcoplasmic reticulum, deduced from its complementary DNA sequence. Nature 316:696, 1985.

71. Brandl, C. J., Green, N. M., Korczak, B., and MacLennan, D. H.: Two Ca^{2+} ATPase genes: Homologies and mechanistic implications of deduced amino acid sequences. Cell 44:597, 1986.

72. Siu, G., Kronenberg, M., Strauss, E., et al.: The structure, rearrangement, and expression of Dβ gene segments of the murine T-cell antigen receptor. Nature 311:344, 1984.

73. Honjo, T., and Habu, S.: Origin of immune diversity: Genetic variation and selection. Annu. Rev. Biochem. 54:803, 1985.

74. Breitbart, R. E., Andreadis, A., and Nadal-Ginard, B.: Alternative splicing: A ubiquitous mechanism for the generation of multiple protein isoforms from single genes. Annu. Rev. Biochem. 56:467, 1987.

75. Smith, C. W. J., Patton, J. G., and Nadal-Ginard, B.: Alternative splicing in the control of gene expression. Annu. Rev. Genet. 23:527, 1989.

76. Kedes, L. H., and Stockdale, F. E. (eds.): UCLA Symposia on Molecular and Cellular Biology of Muscle Development. New York, Alan R. Liss, 1988.

77. Pette, D., and Vrbova, G.: Neural control of phenotypic expression in mammalian muscle fibers. Muscle Nerve 8:676, 1985.

78. Leinwand, L. A., Fournier, R. E., and Nadal-Ginard, B.: TB multigene family for sarcomeric myosin heavy chain in mouse and human DNA: Localization on a single chromosome. Science 221:766, 1983.

79. Mahdavi, V., Chambers, A. P., and Nadal-Ginard, B.: Cardiac α and β myosin heavy chain genes are organized in tandem. Proc. Natl. Acad. Sci. USA 81:2626, 1984.

80. Saez, L. J., Gianola, K. M., McNally, E. M., et al.: Human cardiac myosin heavy chain genes and their linkage in the genome. Nucleic Acids Res. 15:5443, 1987.

81. Czosnek, H., Nudel, U., Shani, M., et al.: The genes coding for the muscle contractile proteins, myosin heavy chain, myosin light chain 2, and skeletal muscle actin are located on three different mouse chromosomes. EMBO J. 1:1299, 1982.

82. Hoh, J. F., McGrath, P. A., and Hale, P. T.: Electrophoretic analysis of multiple forms of rat cardiac myosin: Effects of hypophysectomy and thyroxine replacement. J. Mol. Cell Cardiol. 10:1053, 1978.

83. Pope, B., Hoh, J. F., and Weeds, A.: The ATPase activities of rat cardiac myosin isoenzymes. FEBS Lett. 118:205, 1980.

84. Schwartz, K., Lecarpentier, Y., Martin, J. L., et al.: Myosin isoenzymic distribution correlates with speed of myocardial contraction. J. Mol. Cell Cardiol. 13:1071, 1981.

85. Lompre, A. M., Schwartz, K., d'Albis, A., et al.: Myosin isoenzyme redistribution in chronic heart overload. Nature 282:105, 1979.

86. Lompre, A. M., Mercadier, J. J., Wisnewsky, C., et al.: Dev. Biol. 84:286, 1981.

87. Lompre, A. M., Mahdavi, V., and Nadal-Ginard, B.: Expression of the cardiac ventricular α and β myosin heavy chain genes is developmentally and hormonally regulated. J. Biol. Chem. 259:6437, 1984.

88. Chizzonite, R. A., and Zak, R.: Regulation of myosin isoenzyme composition in fetal and neonatal rat ventricle by endogenous thyroid hormones. J. Biol. Chem. 259:12628, 1984.

89. Mercadier, J. J., Lompre, A. M., Wisnewsky, C., et al.: Myosin isoenzyme changes in several models of rat cardiac hypertrophy. Circ. Res. 49:525, 1981.

90. Gorza, L., Pauletto, P., Pessina, A. C., et al.: Isomyosin distribution in normal and pressure-overloaded rat ventricular myocardium. An immunohistochemical study. Circ. Res. 49:1003, 1981.

91. Litten, R. Z., 3rd, Martin, B. J., Low, R. B., and Alpert, N. R.: Altered myosin isozyme patterns from pressure-overloaded and thyrotoxic hypertrophied rabbit hearts. Circ. Res. 50:856, 1982.

92. Scheuer, J., Malhotra, A., Hirsch, C., et al.: Physiologic cardiac hypertrophy corrects contractile protein abnormalities associated with pathologic hypertrophy in rats. J. Clin. Invest. 70:1300, 1982.

93. Dillmann, W. H.: Diabetes mellitus induces changes in cardiac myosin of the rat. Diabetes 29:579, 1980.

94. Malhotra, A., Penpargkul, S., Fein, F. S., et al.: The effect of streptozotocin-induced diabetes in rats on cardiac contractile proteins. Circ. Res. 49:1243, 1981.

95. Everett, A. W., Clark, W. A., Chizzonite, R. A., and Zak, R.: Change in synthesis rates of α and β myosin heavy chains in rabbit heart after treatment with thyroid hormone. J. Biol. Chem. 258:2421, 1983.

96. Chizzonite, R. A., Everett, A. W., Clark, W. A., et al.: Isolation and characterization of two molecular variants of myosin heavy chain from rabbit ventricle. Change in their content during normal growth and after treatment with thyroid hormone. J. Biol. Chem. 257:2056, 1982.

97. Izumo, S., Mahdavi, V., and Nadal-Ginard, B.: All members of the MHC multigene family respond to thyroid hormone in a highly tissue-specific manner. Science 231:597, 1986.

98. Umeda, P. K., Levin, J. E., Shinha, A. M., et al.: In Emerson, C., et al. (eds.): Molecular Biology of Muscle Development. New York, Alan R. Liss, 1986, pp. 809–823.

99. Evans, R. M.: The steroid and thyroid hormone receptor superfamily. Science 240:889, 1988.

100. Mahdavi, V., Koren, G., Michaud, S., et al.: In Kedes, L. H., and Stockdale, F. E. (eds.): Cellular and Molecular Biology of Muscle Development. New York, Alan R. Liss, 1989, pp. 369–379.

101. Sap, J., Munoz, A., Damm, K., et al.: The c-erb-A protein is a high-affinity receptor for thyroid hormone. Nature 324:635, 1986.

102. Weinberger, C., Thompson, C. C., Ong, E. S., et al.: The c-erb-A gene encodes a thyroid hormone receptor. Nature 324:641, 1986.

103. Thompson, C. C., Weinberger, C., Lebo, R., and Evans, R. M.: Identification of a novel thyroid hormone receptor expressed in the mammalian central nervous system. Science 237:1610, 1987.

104. Izumo, S., and Mahdavi, V.: Thyroid hormone receptor isoforms generated by alternative splicing differentially activate myosin HC gene transcription. Nature 334:539, 1988.

105. Damm, K., Thompson, C. C., and Evans, R. M.: Protein encoded by c-erbA functions as a thyroid hormone receptor antagonist. Nature 339:593, 1989.

106. Koenig, R. J., Lazar, M. A., Hodin, R. A., et al.: Inhbition of thyroid hormone action by a non-hormone binding c-erbA protein generated by alternative mRNA splicing. Nature 337:659, 1989.

107. Glass, C. K., Franco, R., Weinberger, C., et al.: A c-erb-A binding site in rat growth hormone gene mediates transactivation by thyroid hormone. Nature 329:738, 1987.

108. Thompson, W. R., Koren, G., Izumo, S., et al.: Molecular recognition of myosin heavy chain switches: A model for study of cardiac gene expression. In Clarck, E. B., and Takao, A. (eds.): Developmental Cardiology: Morphogenesis and Function. Mount Kisco, NY, Futura Publishing Co., 1990, pp. 13–25.

109. Izumo, S., Lompre, A. M., Matsuoka, R. et al.: Myosin heavy chain messenger RNA and protein isoform transitions during cardiac hypertrophy. Interaction between hemodynamic and thyroid hormone-induced signals. J. Clin. Invest. 79:970, 1987.

110. Mercadier, J. J., Bouveret, P., Gorza, L., et al.: Myosin isoenzymes in normal and hypertrophied human ventricular myocardium. Circ. Res. *53*:52, 1983.

111. Izumo, S., Mahdavi, V., and Nadal-Ginard, B.: Proto-oncogene induction and reprogramming of cardiac gene expression produced by pressure overload. Proc. Natl. Acad. Sci. USA *85*:339, 1988.

112. Schwartz, K., Lompre, A. M., Bouveret, P., et al.: Accumulation of skeletal actin mRNA in experimental cardiac hypertrophy. J. Mol. Cell. Cardiol. *17* (Suppl. 3) abstract 22, 1985.

113. Hirzel, H. O., Tuckschmid, C. R., Schneider, J., et al.: Relationship between myosin isoenzyme composition, hemodynamics, and myocardial structure in various forms of human cardiac hypertrophy. Circ. Res. *57*:729, 1985.

114. Cantley, L. C.: Structure and Mechanism of the (Na,K)-ATPase. Curr. Top. Bioenergetics. *11*:201, 1981.

115. Ingwall, J. S., Kramer, M. F., Fifer, M. A., et al.: The creatine kinase system in normal and diseased human myocardium. N. Engl. J. Med. *313*:1050, 1985.

116. Simpson, P.: Norepinephrine-stimulated hypertrophy of cultured rat myocardial cells is an α1-adrenergic response. J. Clin. Invest. *72*:732, 1983.

117. Lacks, M. M., and Morady, F.: Norepinephrine — the myocardial hypertrophy hormone. Am. Heart J. *91*:674, 1976.

118. Berridge, M. J., and Irvine, R. F.: Inositol triphosphate, a novel second messenger in cellular signal transduction. Nature *312*:315, 1984.

119. Nishizuka, Y.: The role of protein kinase C in cell surface signal transduction and tumour promotion. Nature *308*:693, 1984.

120. Simpson, P. C., and Karliner, J. S.: Regulation of cardiac myocyte hypertrophy by a tumor-promoting phorbol ester. Clin. Res. *33*:229A (abstr) 1985.

MOLECULAR BASIS FOR CERTAIN FORMS OF HYPERTROPHIC CARDIOMYOPATHY

121. Lassar, A. B., Paterson, B. M., and Weintraub, H.: Transfection of a DNA locus that mediates the conversion of 10T1/2 fibroblasts to myoblasts. Cell *47*:649, 1986.

122. Wright, W. E., Sassoon, D. A., and Lin, V. K.: Myogenin, a factor regulating myogenesis, has a domain homologous to MyoD. Cell *56*:607, 1989.

123. Braun, T., Buschhausen-Denker, G., Bober, E., et al.: A novel human muscle factor related to but distinct from MyoD1 induces myogenic conversion in 10T1/2 fibroblasts. EMBO J. *8*:701, 1989.

124. Ruoslahti, E., Pihko, H., and Seppala, M.: Alpha-fetoprotein: Immunochemical purification and chemical properties. Expression in normal state and in malignant and nonmalignant liver disease. Transplant Rev. *20*:38, 1974.

125. Johnson, P. F., and McKnight, S. L.: Eukaryotic transcriptional regulatory proteins. Annu. Rev. Biochem. *58*:799, 1989.

126. Rothman, J. E.: Signal-peptide recognition. GTP and methionine bristles (news). Nature *340*:433, 1989.

127. Schneider, M. D., Shih, H. T., and Parker, T. G.: Peptide growth factors and activated oncogenes can selectively induce expression of "fetal" contractile protein genes. J. Mol. Cell. Cardiol. *21*: (Suppl. III) abstract 67.

128. Jackson, T., Allard, M. F., Sreenan, C. M., et al.: The c-myc proto-oncogene regulates cardiac development in transgenic mice. Molec. Cell. Biol. *10*:3709, 1990.

129. DeCaprio, J. A., Ludlow, J. W., Figge, J., et al.: SV40 large tumor antigen forms a specific complex with the product of the retinoblastoma susceptibility gene. Cell *54*:275, 1988.

130. Whyte, P., Buchkovich, K. J., Horowitz, J. M., et al.: Association between an oncogene and an anti-oncogene: the adenovirus E1A proteins bind to the retinoblastoma gene product. Nature *334*:124, 1988.

131. Endo, T., and Nadal-Ginard, B.: In Kedes, L. H. and Stockdale, F. E. (eds.): UCLA Symposia on Molecular and Cellular Biology. New Series, vol. 93. New York, Alan R. Liss, 1989, pp. 95–104.

131a. Thompson, R.: Unpublished observation.

132. Grossman, W.: Cardiac hypertrophy: Useful adaptation of pathologic process? Am. J. Med. *69*:576, 1980.

133. Guharay, F., and Sachs, F.: Stretch-activated single ion channel currents in tissue-cultured embryonic chick skeletal muscle. J. Physiol. (Lond.) *352*:685, 1984.

134. Komuro, I., Kurabayashi, M., Takaku, F., and Yazaki, Y.: Expression of cellular oncogenes in the myocardium during the developmental stage and pressure-overloaded hypertrophy of the rat hearts. Circ. Res. *62*:1075, 1988.

Genetics and Cardiovascular Disease
by REED E. PYERITZ, M.D., Ph.D.

GENETIC FACTORS IN DISEASE

Genes contribute to both the cause and the pathogenesis of virtually any abnormality of human physiology and behavior including, of course, disorders of the heart and vascular system. This statement carries two messages in addition to the obvious one. First, the pathology associated with even the most "environmental" of causes, such as trauma, malnutrition, and drug abuse, can be defined only in terms of the human body's response to the insult. How the stress of the initial insult is expressed (the *phenotype*) and how the patient suffers and perhaps recovers are, to varying and as yet often poorly defined degrees, dependent on the patient's *genotype*. This idea seems self-evident and verges on the trite, but it is frequently neglected. Some environmental insults, such as massive trauma or poisoning, will be lethal to all, regardless of genotype. Nonetheless, as fields such as *pharmacogenetics* and *ecogenetics* develop, genetic susceptibilities to human disease will be better and more simply defined, and the physician must become increasingly attuned to the importance of the genotype.

Second, the introductory statement stresses that genetic factors play roles in *both* cause and process and that etiology and pathogenesis, while related, are conceptually distinct. For example, the cause of sickle cell anemia is clearly a single mutant gene, whereas whether a patient homozygous for this mutation expresses all, some, or none of the manifestations of the disease is dependent on many other genetic and nongenetic factors. Conversely, the cause of pneumococcal pneumonia is equally evident, but the severity and resolution of the disease depend on the patient's immune competency (which in turn is dependent on genetic and nongenetic factors) as much as on treatment with an antibiotic.

The genotype, therefore, can be detrimental in at least two distinct ways. First, mutant genes can so upset embryology or physiology that a clinical abnormality occurs. Whereas the phenotype of any particular mutation will depend on a host of factors, including which homeostatic systems are available to modulate the action of the defect, the genotype has the principal role in causing the disease. It is this class of mutations that are usually referred to as genetic diseases. Second, a mutation can facilitate the action of an extrinsic cause in producing disease. Inherited susceptibilities are part of the pathogenesis of disease and are what are sought, and often revealed, in taking the patient's family history. Unfortunately, until recently there has been little that the clinician could do to pursue tantalizing facts, such as multiple relatives under age 50 suffering myocardial infarction. The long-touted prospect of detecting a patient's inherited susceptibilities and intervening before irreversible clinical sequelae occur is slowly becoming reality.

DISORDERS DUE TO MICROSCOPIC ALTERATIONS IN CHROMOSOMES

Estimates of the total number of human genes range between 50,000 and 100,000. Two copies (termed *alleles*) of each gene are arrayed along 23 pairs of *chromosomes*. Twenty-two of the chromosomes are called *autosomes* (numbered 1 through 22), while the 23rd pair are the *sex chromosomes*, X and Y. Females have two X chromosomes and males have an X and a Y chromosome. Both autosomal alleles are potentially active in specifying RNA copies of their DNA sequences; whether a gene is active depends on the cell type, developmental stage of the organism, and the regulatory molecules that interact with promoter and enhancer nucleotide sequences that control transcription of the gene. In cells with two X chromosomes (i.e., in all females, in the Klinefelter syndrome in which two X's and one Y occur, and in other rare conditions), only one X is active after early embryogenesis.

Human chromosomes can be examined by culturing cells capable of mitosis; T-lymphocytes obtained from venous blood are the usual source, but fibroblasts, cells from chorionic villi, amniocytes, and leukocyte precursors present in bone marrow are also used clinically. Chromosomes are distinguished from one another by their size, shape (determined by the position of a constriction called the *centromere*, which functions as the attachment of the mitotic apparatus), and characteristic banding pattern as revealed by any of several staining techniques. The chromosomes are photographed, cut out, and arranged in pairs, from 1 through 22 and the sex chromosomes, in a display called the *karyotype*. This display and its interpretation are the end results of a clinical study of a patient's chromosomes. The chromosome constitution of a cell is designated by first specifying the number of chromosomes present (46 being normal in diploid cells), then specifying the sex chromosomes, and finally describing any abnormalities. For example, a normal male is designated 46,XY, and a female with an extra chromosome 21 is designated 46,XX,+21.

Chromosome aberrations, especially too many or too few chromosomes *(aneuploidy)*, are extremely common in human embryos; more than one-half of all conceptuses are spontaneously aborted in early pregnancy, and at least one-half of them are aneuploid. Among live-born infants, about 0.5 per cent have a chromosome aberration.

ANEUPLOIDY. Gain or loss of chromosomes generally happens by nondisjunction, or the failure of a homologous pair of chromosomes to separate. Absence of one chromosome is termed *monosomy;* all autosomal monosomies are embryonic lethals, as is presence of only a Y sex chromosome. Presence of three chromosomes is *trisomy,* and presence of an entire extra set of chromosomes (for a total of 69) is *triploidy.* The most common autosomal aneuploidy, trisomy 21 associated with the Down syndrome, and aneuploidy for sex chromosomes are all compatible with survival into adulthood.

CHROMOSOME REARRANGEMENTS. A chromosome can break and rejoin within itself, potentially giving rise to an *inversion* of genetic material. Often no apparent phenotypic effect is seen in people with an inversion, but because inversions may disrupt chromosome pairing during meiosis, their offspring may have more profound aberrations.

DELETIONS AND DUPLICATIONS. Just as their names imply, these aberrations are losses or gains of chromosomal material. Many clinical syndromes have been associated with aberrations of specific chromosome regions.[1,2] The smallest deletion detectable by light microscopy is associated with loss of considerable DNA, on the order of one million base pairs, so more than one gene is potentially disrupted or lost.

A number of conditions, each thought to be due to a mutation in a single locus, are associated with small interstitial chromosome deletions (Table 51–1). So rather than pleiotropic manifestations of one mutation, these conditions are likely to be due to the effects of several, and perhaps many, mutations and are therefore called *contiguous gene deletion syndromes.*[3] Such deletions are potentially heritable, and the occurrence of the disorder in a family behaves as a mendelian dominant.

DISORDERS DUE TO CHANGES IN SINGLE NUCLEAR GENES

(See also Chap. 50)

Mutations of genes located on the 22 pairs of autosomes and the two sex chromosomes produce phenotypes inherited according to the two principal tenets of Mendel: alleles segregate and nonalleles assort. The first statement refers to gametes receiving as a result of meiosis only one of the two alleles at a given locus. The second statement describes the results of recombination, the meiotic process of rearranging DNA between the two chromosomes of the pair *(homologous chromosomes);* if two loci are widely spaced along a chromosome, their chances of being separated by recombination are 50–50, and they are said to be *unlinked.*

More than 5000 individual loci have been identified on the basis of the phenotype that mutations in single genes produce. The presumption of single-gene defects is based in most instances on the pattern of inheritance in families; segregation of the phenotype according to mendelian principles is the central piece of evidence. For an increasing number of loci, however, molecular genetic techniques have mapped the phenotype to a single gene, or even revealed the actual alteration in nucleotide sequence.[4,5] The range of known mendelian variation in humans and information about gene mapping and molecular defects are routinely catalogued[6] and available online.[7] Based on current estimates of the size of the human genome, about 5 to 10 per cent of loci have been identified through the effects their mutations have on phenotype.

More than 2000 loci have been mapped to a restricted region of the genome. Many of these loci cause specific mendelian disorders, and the genetic map of these loci represents the "morbid anatomy of the human genome." All of the cardiovascular and hemostatic disorders that have been mapped by early 1991 are shown in Figure 51–1.

Dominance and Recessiveness

These related concepts are characteristics of the phenotype, *not of the gene.* A phenotype is dominant when the patient is *heterozygous* for a mutation, i.e., when one copy of the mutant allele, and one copy of the normal allele, are present; this holds for genes on both autosomes and the X chromosome. A phenotype is recessive when the patient has two mutant alleles at the locus causing the condition. If the mutant alleles are identical, the patient is *homozygous* at that locus, a situation usually present either when the allele is identical by descent through both parents (i.e., the parents had a common ancestor and are *consanguineous)* or when the mutant allele is common in the population (e.g., the most prevalent mutation for cystic fibrosis and the mutation for sickle cell anemia). Biochemical and molecular genetic assessment of mutant alleles has shown that the majority of recessive phenotypes are due to two distinct mutant alleles, a situation termed a *genetic compound,* indicative of the widespread heterogeneity in mutations at each locus. Males have but one X chromosome, and each locus is therefore *hemizygous;* a mutant locus is always expressed in the phenotype of a male. Dominance and recessiveness for X-linked traits refer to expression in heterozygous and homozygous women, respectively.

Whether a disorder is called dominant or recessive depends on how carefully the phenotype is assessed and how it is defined. For example, familial hypercholesterolemia is a relatively common hereditary disorder due to defects in the receptor for low-density lipoprotein (LDL, p. 1128). The vast majority of patients are heterozygous for a mutant allele at the LDLR locus on chromosome 19,[8] and the disease is inherited as a mendelian dominant trait. However, if a man and a woman, each heterozygous for an LDLR mutation, mate, they have a 25 per cent risk of having a child who inherits both of the mutant alleles and will thereby be either homozy-

TABLE 51–1 CONTIGUOUS GENE DELETION SYNDROMES

	LOCUS	CARDIOVASCULAR ABNORMALITIES
Syndromes with Cardiovascular Involvement		
Arteriohepatic dysplasia	20p11.2	Peripheral pulmonic stenosis
DiGeorge sequence	22q11	Truncus arteriosus, right aortic arch, TOF, PDA
Miller-Dieker syndrome	17p13	Patent ductus arteriosus ± complex anomalies
Prader-Willi syndrome	15q11–q13	Cor pulmonale (2° to obesity and central apnea)
WAGR syndrome	11p13	Hypertension (2° to Wilms tumor)
Syndromes Without Frequent Cardiovascular Involvement		
Angelman syndrome	15q11–q13*	
Smith-Magenis syndrome	17p11.2	

TOF = tetralogy of Fallot; PDA = patent ductus arteriosus.
WAGR = Wilms tumor, aniridia, genitourinary, and retardation.
* The deletion is indistinguishable from that of the Prader-Willi syndrome; genetic imprinting is thought to account for the phenotypic differences. In Prader-Willi, the deleted chromosome is always the chromosome 15 inherited from father, while in Angelman syndrome, the deletion affects the maternal chromosome 15.

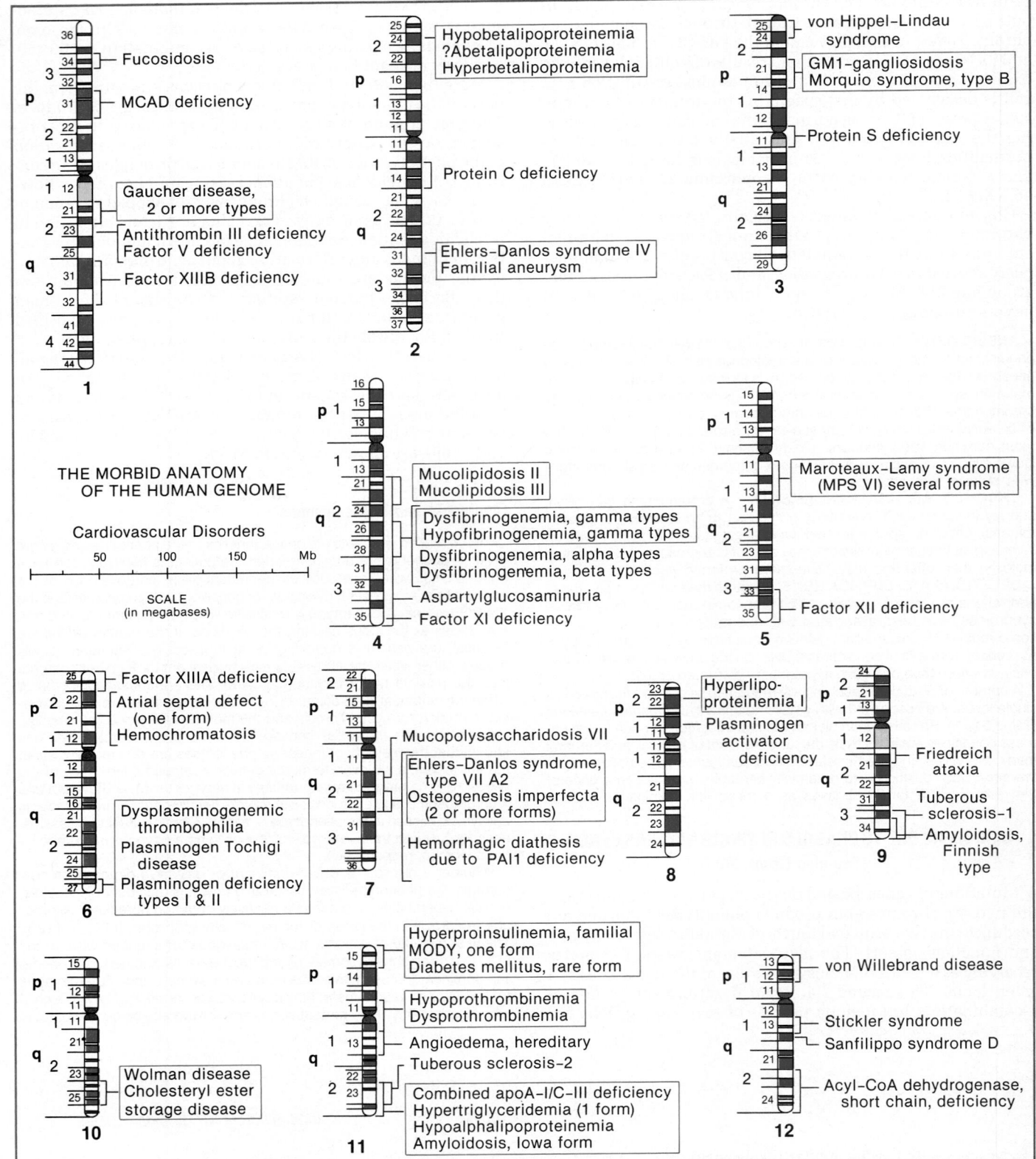

FIGURE 51-1. Chromosomal location of human genes associated with disorders of the cardiovascular system. These 76 genes affect the structure, function, and metabolism of the heart and blood vessels and hemostasis and have been identified by the deleterious effects of mutations. Numerous additional genes that encode structural proteins important to the cardiovascular system have been identified but not yet associated with disease. In the figure, brackets next to the chromosome show the regional localization of the gene causing a particular disorder. Brackets next to two or more disorders indicate that all of the genes causing the disorders map to the same region. Disorders surrounded by boxes are caused by different mutations at the same gene.

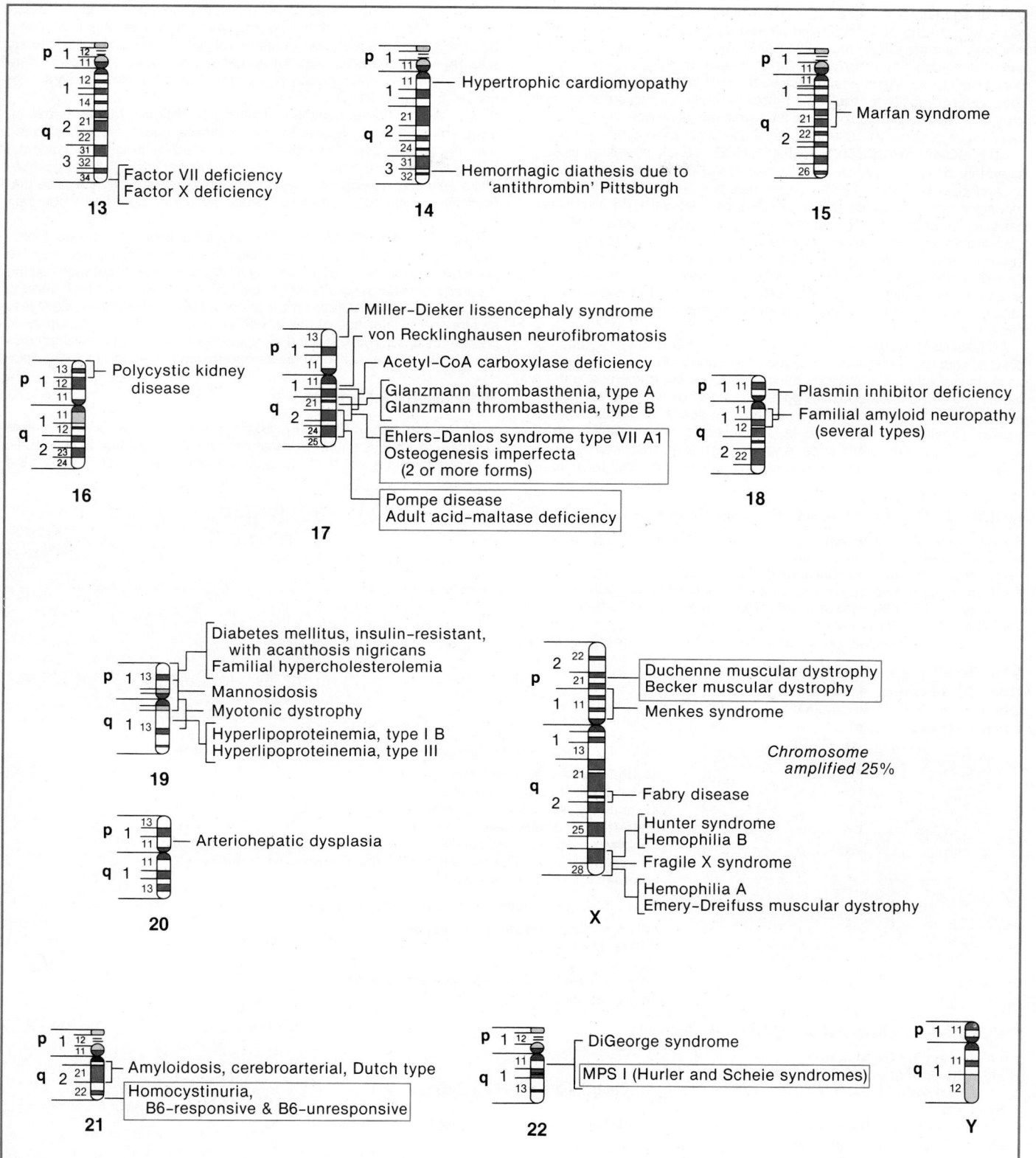

FIGURE 51–1 *Continued*

gous or a genetic compound at the LDLR gene. This child will have a much more severe form of familial hypercholesterolemia (see p. 1145) that is inherited as a mendelian recessive trait. Similarly, homozygosity for the sickle hemoglobin mutation at the β-globin locus on chromosome 11 produces the familiar autosomal recessive disease, sickle cell anemia. However, heterozygosity for the same mutation rarely produces disease but produces sickling of erythrocytes if they are examined under conditions of low oxygen tension; this phenotype is transmitted as a dominant trait.

AUTOSOMAL RECESSIVE INHERITANCE. Nearly all deficiencies of enzymatic activity—the classic inborn errors of metabolism first defined by Archibald Garrod in 1903—cause recessive phenotypes. Most homeostatic systems, which include all metabolic pathways, have sufficient flexibility to function well if one of the enzymatic steps functions at half-normal efficiency, as would occur in heterozygosity for a mutant allele at a structural gene for an enzyme. However, homeostasis cannot cope if two mutant alleles cause a reduction in enzymatic activity to a few percent or less of normal activity. The characteristics of autosomal recessive inheritance, features common to such phenotypes, and a typical pedigree are shown in Figure 51–2.

AUTOSOMAL DOMINANT INHERITANCE. Only a few enzyme deficiencies, but many disorders of development and structure, are inherited as dominant traits. The reasons for this are probably numerous and are certainly poorly understood. One possibility is that developmental homeostasis has a limited repertoire of responses to stress, and when a structural or regulatory macromolecule is reduced to only one-half normal amount, the system cannot cope. Another possibility, illustrated by mutations in procollagen molecules, pertains to gene products that must inter-

act before becoming functional; an aberrant protein combined with a normal one would be a defective multimer, and the effect of being heterozygous for a mutation would be magnified (the concept of *protein suicide*).[9] The characterisitics of autosomal dominant inheritance, features common to many such phenotypes, and a typical pedigree are shown in Figure 51–3.

With the notable exception of Huntington disease, human dominant traits are *incomplete,* in that the heterozygote is less severely affected than the homozygote. Defects of the LDLR are illustrative, in which the heterozygote has classic type IIa hyperlipidemia, while the homozygote has a quantitatively worse form of the same disease.[8] It may well be that homozygosity for most alleles that cause dominant disorders is incompatible with life.

X-LINKED INHERITANCE. The characterisitics of X-linked inheritance, features common to such phenotypes, and a typical pedigree are shown in Figure 51–4. While virtually all diseases due to mutations on the X chromosome are more severe in hemizygous males, women heterozygous for the same mutations often show some manifestations, albeit less severe and of later age of onset. For example, most women carriers of α-galactosidase A deficiency (Fabry's disease) eventually develop cerebrovascular disease or renal failure due to accumulation of sphingolipid.

Mitochondrial Inheritance

Energy generation through oxidative phosphorylation occurs in mitochondria in the cytoplasm of most cell types. Numerous mitochondria, each containing a single chromosome, exist in each cell. Some of the

---

FIGURE 51–2. *Characteristics of autosomal recessive inheritance*

A single generation affected
Sexes affected equally frequently
Each parent heterozygous (a carrier)
Each offspring of two carriers has a 25% chance of being affected, a 50% chance of being a carrier, and a 25% chance of inheriting neither mutant allele
Two-thirds of clinically normal offspring are carriers
The rarer the phenotype, the greater the likelihood of consanguinity

Characteristics of autosomal recessive phenotypes

Often due to enzyme deficiencies
Often more severe than dominant disorders
Often early age of onset

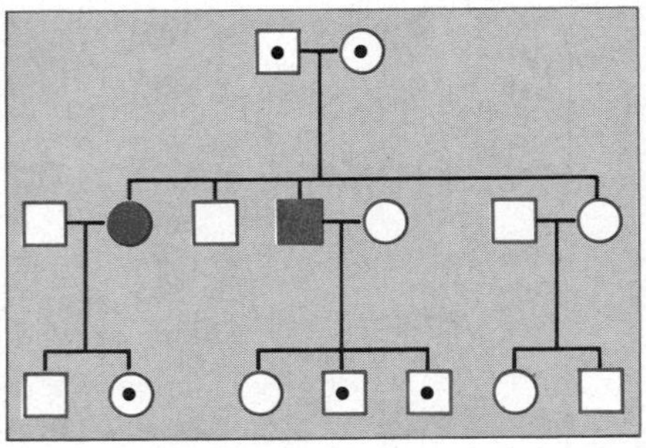

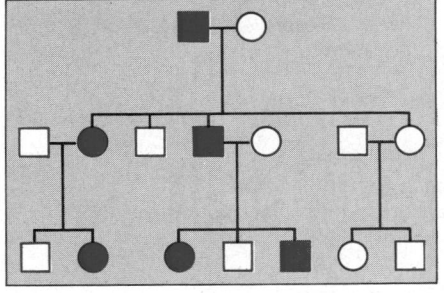

FIGURE 51–3. *Characteristics of autosomal dominant inheritance*

Multiple generations affected
Sexes affected equally frequently
In familial cases, only one parent need be affected
Male-to-male transmission occurs
Offspring of an affected parent have a 50% chance of being affected
Frequency of sporadic cases higher the more severe the condition
Paternal age effect in sporadic cases

Characteristics of autosomal dominant phenotypes

Often associated with malformations
Often pleiotropic
Usually variable
Often less severe than recessive phenotypes
Often age-dependent

FIGURE 51–4. *Characteristics of X-linked inheritance*

No male-to-male transmission
All daughters of affected males are carriers
Sons of a carrier mother have a 50% chance of being affected; daughters have a 50% chance of being carriers
Some mothers of an affected male will not be carriers, but they may have more affected sons if germinal mosaicism is present

Characteristics of X-linked phenotypes

More severe in males
Heterozygous females may be unaffected
Variable, especially in females

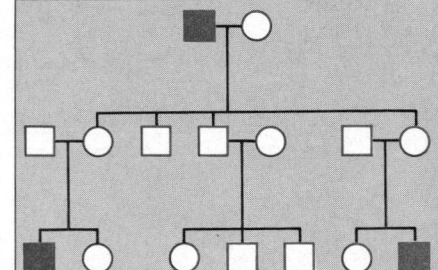

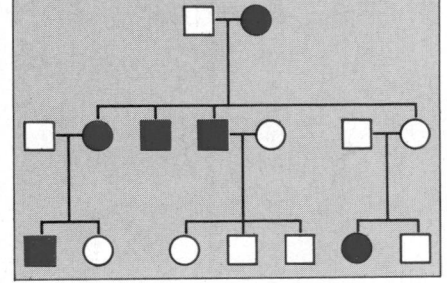

FIGURE 51–5. *Characteristics of disorders due to a mutation of the mitochondrial chromosome*

Sexes equally frequently and severely affected
Transmission only through women; offspring of affected men are unaffected
All offspring of an affected woman may be affected
Variability of expression can be extreme in a family, including apparent nonpenetrance
Phenotypes may be age-dependent

enzymes of oxidative phosphorylation are encoded by genes on the nuclear chromosomes and the proteins transported into the mitochondrion; the rest of the proteins are encoded by genes on the mitochondrial chromosome. Thus, genetic defects of oxidative phosphorylation can be due to mutations of genes on the autosomes or the X chromosome, and the resulting diseases behave as mendelian recessive traits, and to mutations of genes on the mitochondrial chromosome, and the resulting diseases do not behave as mendelian traits.[10,11] The differences are explicable by the events of conception. The spermatocyte contributes virtually no mitochondria to the zygote, and the entire complement of mitochondria that will ever by present in the fetus are derived from the mitochondria already present in the cytoplasm of the oocyte. Thus, phenotypes due to mutations of the mitochondrial chromosome show *maternal inheritance,* the characteristics of which are shown in Figure 51–5.

PRINCIPLES OF CLINICAL GENETICS

PLEIOTROPY. Most mutant alleles have effects on more than one organ system, and a mendelian phenotype frequently displays multiple, often diverse, manifestations.[12] For example, the Marfan syndrome (p. 1641) is defined by abnormalities in the eye, skeleton, skin, heart, and aorta, and until the recent recognition of a defect in extracellular microfibrils,[13] the findings could not be linked either etiologically or pathogenetically.[14]

VARIABILITY. The effect of the same mutant allele on phenotype can be different among people heterozygous (for dominant traits), homozygous (for autosomal recessive traits), or hemizygous (for X-linked traits) for the allele. Variability can be described in terms of the frequency of a particular pleiotropic manifestation among patients with the mutation; the severity of the phenotype; and the age of onset of manifestations. If a person has the mutant allele(s) but shows no phenotypic effect, the trait is called *nonpenetrant.* To an important degree, whether a clinical phenotype is called nonpenetrant or not depends on the sensitivity of the techniques employed for detection. For example, two decades ago, based on bedside examination, cardiovascular abnormalities were thought to affect about half of people with the Marfan syndrome; echocardiography now reveals aortic dilatation in more than 90 per cent. The term *incomplete penetrance* should not be used with reference to individuals but to mean a prevalence of the phenotype in less than 100 per cent of people known to carry the mutation(s). The Holt-Oram syndrome (see p. 1633) is an instructive example. In this autosomal dominant syndrome of reduction anomalies of the upper limb and congenital heart defect, patients in the same family can have only arm anomalies, only a heart defect, or both. Moreover, the severity of the reduction defect varies widely, from a proximally placed thumb to near-total absence of the arm. The cardiac feature is incompletely penetrant because only about 50 per cent of patients have it, but in any individual with the Holt-Oram allele, the heart is either structurally normal or not.

Numerous genetic and environmental factors can affect expression of a gene (Table 51–2), and it is often impossible to determine which of these factors are most important in a specific patient or particular disease. However, the pervasiveness of variable expression emphasizes that phenotypes determined by single genes are to some extent really "multifactorial."

GENETIC HETEROGENEITY. Similar or even identical phenotypes can be due to fundamentally distinct mutations, a phenomenon termed genetic heterogeneity. For example, Marfan syndrome and homocystinuria were long thought to be the same disorder, despite what now appear in retrospect to be obvious differences in inheritance pattern and intelligence.[15] As in the case of these two disorders, the causes may lie in two different genes whose products are functionally distinct. Osteogenesis imperfecta exemplifies a disorder in which mutations in two genes, $\alpha 1(I)$ and $\alpha 2(I)$ procollagen, can each produce the same phenotype because the two proteins interact to form type I collagen.[16] Genetic heterogeneity is pervasive at the intragenic level of analysis; except for sickle

TABLE 51-2 CAUSES OF VARIABILITY OF GENE EXPRESSION

1627

CHAP
51

Genetic background
Age dependency
Sex influence
Sex limitation
Modifying loci: hypostasis and epistasis
Gene alteration
    Somatic mutation
    Somatic amplification
    Transpositions and rearrangements

    Mutations
    Physiological rearrangements
Variation in X-inactivation*
Endogenous complementation*
Maternal factors
    Effects of mitochondrial genome
    Intrauterine environment
Imprinting
Exogenous and ecological factors
    Ecology — temperature, diet
    Teratogens
    Medical intervention
    Chance
    Chaos

* Pertains to female heterozygotes for X-linked disorders.

cell anemia, virtually all single-gene disorders are due to a variety of mutations at a given locus.[17–20]

NONPATHOLOGICAL VARIATION IN THE CARDIOVASCULAR SYSTEM

CARDIAC STRUCTURE AND PHYSIOLOGY. All aspects of the ontogeny of the cardiovascular system are dictated by the genome. If, as seems most credible, few genes have a large effect and many have small contributions, any specific aspect of "normal" cardiovascular phenotype — size, shape, function — will exhibit multifactorial inheritance. In other words, to the extent that any given phenotype can be quantified, it will show a normal distribution within the population, and near-relatives will be more similar to each other than they will to distant relatives and the rest of the population. The twin method should demonstrate a higher concordance of the trait in monozygotic than dizygotic twins. However, surprisingly few phenotypes have been examined.

Preliminary data on left ventricular dimensions measured echocardiographically showed higher correlations between parent and child than between matched controls, suggesting a genetic contribution[21]; however, as in many such studies, the effect of shared environment was not estimated. In an attempt to minimize environmental contributions, left ventricular sizes of twins who were not exercise trained were compared; the mean intrapair differences in echocardiographic dimensions were less in the monozygotic than in the dizygotic twins and nontwin sibs.[22] The caliber and branch geometry of coronary arteries show familial resemblance, and both parameters are much more similar in monozygotic twins than in other relatives.[23]

Measures of cardiac electrophysiology show familial resemblance. Studies of both nuclear families[24] and twins[25,26] suggest a genetic contribution to resting heart rate, conduction times, and repolarization time. Genetic control of normal cardiovascular function has been especially difficult to study because of the multitude of environmental (training, diet), stochastic (age), and clinical (subtle, unrecognized pathology) issues that confound comparisons of relatives and controls. Thus far, no strong genetic contribution to an individual's response to physical conditioning has emerged.[22]

VASCULAR SYSTEM. All members of certain inbred animal strains show little variation in arterial anatomy, especially branch angles, and considerable variation with other strains of the same species. Except for the study of coronary arterial anatomy already noted,[23] similar studies of humans have not been reported.

One intriguing question of clinical importance is whether certain people are predisposed to arterial spasm and if this susceptibility has a genetic basis. An examination of hereditary pathological and polymorphic variation in factors elaborated by endothelial cells, platelets, and leukocytes to maintain patency of blood vessels, such as prostacyclin, endothelium-derived relaxing factor, and endothelin-1, may prove enlightening.[27,28]

CARDIOVASCULAR DISORDERS ASSOCIATED WITH CHROMOSOME ABERRATIONS

Chromosome aberrations cause primarily structural defects of the cardiovascular system that are evident at birth. The frequency of chromosome aberrations among live-born children with congenital heart defects has been found to range from 5 to 13 per cent.[29,30] Upward of 40 per cent of all fetuses with heart defects detected by ultrasonography at 18 to 20 weeks' gestation have chromosome aberrations; most are spontaneously aborted. Most forms of aneuploidy and most duplications and deletions of more than a chromosome band are associated with defects of the cardiovascular system[32] (Tables 51–1 and 51–3). Exceptions are 47,XXX, 47,XYY, and 47,XXY (Klinefelter syndrome), in which the incidence of congenital heart disease is probably not elevated over the population baseline.

ANEUPLOIDY. How the abnormal phenotypes caused by autosomal aneuploidy develop remains controversial. One view holds that disturbance of the dosage of the genes present on the specific aneuploid chromosome segments is the central issue. The other view is that any aneuploid state disturbs developmental homeostasis in a nonspecific manner. The former theory would predict some distinctiveness of phenotype among the trisomy syndromes that occur in live-born children, whereas the latter would predict shared manifestations. At a coarse level, the clinical pictures are similar, with grave problems of the craniofacies, central nervous system, genitalia, distal limbs, and heart usually present. But when a more refined examination of the phenotypes is obtained, considerable distinctiveness emerges. The three most common autosomal trisomies[8,10,13] can be distinguished readily at the bedside. In all three, membranous ventricular and atrial sep-

tal defects are common. However, the detailed accounting of cardiovascular lesions among large numbers of patients with these trisomies reveals important differences that suggest that aneuploidy exerts more than a global effect on development. In this and most other analyses of congenital heart defects, the system of classification based on the presumed pathogenetic mechanisms proves most instructive and is a useful approach to comparing different causative factors (Table 51–4). About one-quarter of the defects in trisomies 13 and 18 are due to cell migration abnormalities, and two-thirds are flow lesions; when combined, these two mechanisms account for considerably more of these classes of defects than in the general population with congenital heart disease. By contrast, in trisomy 21 left-sided flow lesions are much less common, whereas abnormal closure of endocardial cushions is strikingly frequent; indeed, in contrast to endocardial cushion defects without a chromosome 21 anomaly, left-sided flow lesions are rarely seen in Down syndrome patients with endocardial cushion defects.[30,34,35] Furthermore, the high incidence of endocardial cushion defects and low incidence of conotruncal and distal aortic anomalies has suggested a distinct pathogenetic mechanism in trisomy 21, potentially involving cell adhesiveness and the extracellular matrix.[33,36]

TRISOMY 21—DOWN SYNDROME. This most common phenotype due to a human chromosome aberration occurs about once in every 600 births. Most patients have trisomy 21, and the risk of this aberration is exponentially related to maternal age; the risk is lowest for young women and rises steeply after age 35, reaching 4 per cent for women over age 45. A small minority (3 per cent) of Down syndrome results from an extra copy of all or part of the long arm of chromosome 21 translocated to another chromosome. This situation is relatively more common in mothers under age 30. The pheno-

TABLE 51–3 CARDIOVASCULAR MANIFESTATIONS ASSOCIATED WITH CHROMOSOME ABERRATIONS

CHROMOSOME ABERRATION	EPONYM	CARDIOVASCULAR MANIFESTATIONS
Triploidy		
69,XXX (or XXY or XYY)		>50% have CHD: ASD and VSD
Aneuploidy		
+13	Patau	~80% have CHD; 75% of CHD is complex: PDA, VSD, ASD, PS, AS, dextrocardia, CoA
+18	Edwards	~90% have CHD: most CHD is complex: VSD, PDA, ASD, bicuspid PV and AV, CoA
+21	Down	~40% have CHD: ECD, TOF; MVP in ~20%; AR
+8 mosaicism		~25% have CHD, most of little clinical consequence: VSD, PDA, CoA, PS
+9 mosaicism		~70% have CHD, usually complex: VSD, PDA, PLSVC
45,X	Turner	~10% have clinically important CHD: 50% of these have CoA; mild CoA is likely much more common; also AS, ARD, VSD, ASD, dextrocardia
47,XXX		CHD not increased
47,XXY	Klinefelter	CHD possibly slightly increased; ? mild conduction changes; venous thromboembolic disease
47,XYY		CHD not increased; ? mild conduction changes
Deletions		
4p−	Wolf-Hirschhorn	~50% have CHD, usually complex: VSD, ASD, PDA, PS
5p−	Cri du chat	~20% have CHD, usually single: VSD, PDA, ASD, PS
7q−		~20% have CHD, various, often complex
13q−		CHD common, often severe, but depend on region deleted
18p−		CHD uncommon
18q−		~25% have CHD, usually single, of little consequence: VSD, PDA, ASD, PS
ring 18		~20% have CHD: CoA, PA hypoplasia, HLH, PLSVC
Duplications		
4p trisomy		~10% have CHD, usually single: no defect predominates
9 p trisomy		<10% have CHD: VSD, ASD, AS, PS
10p trisomy		~30% have CHD, usually single: no defect predominates
10q24–qter trisomy		~50% have CHD, usually complex: ECD, VSD, TOF
22pter–q11 trisomy or tetrasomy	Cat eye	~50% have CHD, usually complex: TAPVR, VSD, TOF
Other Aberrations		
Marker Xq27.3	Fragile X syndrome	~50% have aortic root dilatation, MVP, or both

CHD = congenital heart defect(s); ASD = atrial septal defect; VSD = ventricular septal defect; PDA = patent ductus arteriosus; PS = valvular pulmonic stenosis; AS = aortic stenosis; CoA = coarctation of aorta; PV = pulmonic valve; AV = aortic valve; ECD = endocardial cushion defect; TOF = tetralogy of Fallot; MVP = mitral valve prolapse; AR = aortic regurgitation; PLSVC = persistence of left superior vena cava; ARD = aortic root dilatation; PA = pulmonary artery; HLH = hypoplastic left heart; TAPVR = totally anomalous pulmonary venous return.

TABLE 51-4 CLASSIFICATION OF CONGENITAL HEART DEFECTS BASED ON PATHOGENETIC MECHANISMS[33]

PATHOGENETIC MECHANISM	EXAMPLES OF DEFECTS
Embryonic blood flow defects	
Left-sided lesions	HLH; bicuspid aortic valve; IAA type A; CoA; PDA
Right-sided lesions	Secundum ASD; PS
Mesenchymal tissue migration defects	TOF; D-TGA
Extracellular matrix defects	ECD
Abnormal cellular death	Ebstein anomaly; muscular VSD
Defects of looping and situs	L-TGA
Abnormalities of targeted growth	TAPVR

HLH = hypoplastic left heart; IAA = interrupted aortic arch; CoA = coarctation of aorta; PDA = patent ductus arteriosus; ASD = atrial septal defect; PS = valvular pulmonic stenosis; TOF = tetralogy of Fallot; TGA = transposition of great arteries; ECD = endocardial cushion defect; VSD = ventricular septal defect; TAPVR = totally anomalous pulmonary venous return.

types of the two forms of Down syndrome do not differ. The phenotype tends to be less severe if the trisomy is mosaic (3 per cent of Down syndrome) as a result of a mitotic nondisjunctional error in the embryo.

The most common causes of morbidity and mortality in Down syndrome patients are congenital heart defects present in 40 to 50 per cent of cases, hematological malignant disease, and duodenal atresia. If the patient either escapes or survives these problems, survival into the fifth decade and beyond is likely, but complicated by progressive dementia of the Alzheimer type. Premature aging may also affect the vasculature, although definitive studies are lacking.

The most characteristic cardiac anomaly in the Down syndrome is a defect of closure of the endocardial cushions. Complicating the clinical problems in such patients and those with simple septal defects is a seeming predisposition to pulmonary hypertension in the face of elevated right-sided flow.[37] About one-third of congenital heart defects are complex, and these patients tend not surprisingly to be the most ill patients. Mitral valve prolapse is found with a frequency exceeding that in age- and sex-matched controls.[38,39] The aortic and pulmonary valve cusps seem predisposed to fenestrations in adulthood.

The medical management of patients with the Down syndrome has undergone evolution to more aggressive measures in recent years. Objections and hesitations on medical, societal, and ethical grounds to operative repair of heart defects in the Down syndrome have been mollified substantially.[40] More follow-up data are becoming available, and early and late postoperative survival in Down syndrome patients appears to be no different from that in other patients with similar defects.[37,40,41]

TRISOMY 18. *Edwards syndrome* is the second most common autosomal trisomy. Most cases are due to meiotic disjunction, and there is a strong relationship to maternal age. Routine prenatal diagnostic testing of women over age 34 could detect at least one-third of all autosomal trisomies, but less than one-half of all women of this advanced age undergo testing. Currently prenatal detection of trisomies followed by termination of pregnancy is having a small but measurable impact on decreasing the incidence of *Down, Edwards, and Patau* syndromes.

Although the severity of the phenotype rarely enables survival beyond a few months, 10 per cent of patients live to 1 year, and a few survive to adulthood, perhaps because of undetected mosaicism for a chromosomally normal cell line. However, central nervous system function is far less than that in the Down syndrome and leads to complex medical management and supportive care for long-term survivors.[42] Cardiovascular defects occur in at least 90 per cent of cases and contribute to death. Complex lesions, usually involving septal defects, dysplastic valves that are rarely hemodynamically important, patent ductus arteriosus, and persistence of the left superior vena cava are common.[43,44] Right ventricular enlargement is common and may indicate not only shunting from left to right, but pulmonary hypertension due to anomalies of the pulmonary vasculature.[43] As in the Down syndrome, transposition of the great ar-

teries is virtually unknown in trisomy 18.[44] Rarely should invasive diagnostic procedures or aggressive supportive measures be undertaken in Edwards syndrome.

TRISOMY 13. *Patau syndrome* occurs in about 0.01 per cent of live births and in progressively higher frequencies in stillbirths and spontaneous abortions. The external phenotype is usually severe, but occasionally not as characteristic as other trisomies; survival beyond a few weeks is rare, and the causes of death involve multiple organ systems, especially the heart. Cardiovascular anomalies are a bit less frequent than in trisomy 18 and have a slightly different spectrum.[32,43] Septal defects are the most common isolated lesions; dextrocardia and bicuspid semilunar valves occur in association with other anomalies.

Patients who survive beyond a month most often are mosaic for a chromosomally normal cell line; thus, prognosis is fraught with uncertainty until detailed analysis is completed. Whether invasive cardiological studies are performed or aggressive management undertaken can be determined by the severity of involvement of other organ systems, especially the brain, pending cytogenetic investigation.

TURNER SYNDROME. About one in every 2500 females lacks an X chromosome and has a 45,X karyotype. The frequency of a nonmosaic 45,X karyotype is much higher in spontaneous abortuses than in liveborns, and probably less than 2 per cent of such conceptuses come to term. The clinical phenotype is variable and often mild; the diagnosis is often not suspected until a child's short stature is evaluated or a woman complains of amenorrhea. Many cases are mosaic for cell lines with 46,XX or 46,XY constitutions. A variety of structural aberrations involving the X chromosome can cause partial or complete Turner syndrome.

Among patients with the 45,X karyotype, reported frequencies of congenital cardiovascular defects vary from 20 to 50 per cent, depending on how patients were ascertained. Fifty to 70 per cent of those with cardiovascular defects have clinically important aortic coarctation, usually of the postductal form.[45] As noninvasive imaging studies of asymptomatic patients become routine, the frequency of coarctation may increase. A variety of other cardiac malformations may occur, either singly or combined with coarctation. However, there is strong support for left-sided flow abnormalities as a major pathogenetic mechanism. Bicuspid aortic valve and dilatation of the ascending aorta (with a risk of dissection and histopathology showing elastic fiber disruption) occur even in the absence of coarctation,[46,47] and hypoplastic left heart has been reported.[48] Partial anomalous pulmonary venous drainage without an atrial septal defect is fairly common and should be suspected when right ventricular overload is detected on echocardiography.[49]

Postmortem examination of midtrimester abortuses with 45,X showed a higher incidence of left-sided flow lesions than found at birth, and the authors speculate on an association between the pathogenesis of the cardiovascular anomalies and the uniform presence of lymphatic obstruction at the base of the heart.[45]

Blood pressure elevation is common, even without coarctation or after its repair; a high frequency of renal anomalies is one likely cause, but not the sole explanation, for the prevalence of hypertension.

Women with mosaic karyotypes are less likely to have cardiovascular defects.

CONGENITAL HEART DISEASE
(See Chaps. 31 and 32)

In the past few decades, the reported incidence of structural heart defects in newborns has increased from 5 to 7 per 1000 live births, probably as the result of increased diagnostic sensitivity (especially cross-sectional and Doppler echocardiography and magnetic resonance imaging).[50-54] Supporting this explanation is the lack of change over the same period in the incidence of critical defects at 3.1 to 3.5 per 1000.[50] This enhanced resolving power of noninvasive methods should prove particularly useful in the study of familial structural defects, because apparently unaffected relatives can be evaluated for subclinical evidence of anomalies. Few investigations to date have capitalized on this approach.[55,56]

As is evident from the previous section, gross aberrations of chromosomes produce an extensive and varied array of structural heart disease, an observation as true for spontaneous abortuses as for liveborn children.[57] Unfortunately, the complexity and inscrutability of the human genome severely limit the insight that cytogenetic aberrations provide into etiology and pathogenesis of congenital malformations. This situation is little improved, however, in considering the other two mechanisms by which genes cause congenital heart defects — multifactorial processes and mutations of single genes. The latter group should prove instructive soon, as the protein products of the mutant loci are identified and their normal function and regulation are defined.

MULTIFACTORIAL PROCESSES. The empirical risks of recurrence of congenital heart defects have increased in recent years,[58,59] in keeping with the overall higher incidence noted above. However, this conclusion has been criticized because the studies focused on the offspring of women probands, in whom the recurrence risk appears higher than in men with congenital heart defects.[60] In addition to this unexplained maternal influence, other factors may be at work. For example, improved detection of subtle lesions, more faithful reporting of patients, and the assiduousness of epidemiologists may have shown a systematic variation. It is true that some patients with cardiovascular problems now survive[61,61a] to bear children because of improved medical and surgical care; their offspring might be at increased risk because of the severity of the parents' problems, but some evidence against this idea exists.[62]

As mentioned earlier, the familial aggregation of congenital heart defects has been employed to validate many of the predictions of the threshold liability model of multifactorial inheritance.[56,63-66] In most studies, whether focused on populations or families, defects were classified by their pathology; for example, all ventricular septal defects were considered as one group. There has been bias in reporting families in which one type of defect aggregates, which has led to many reports of "familial atrial septal defect," "familial cardiomyopathy," and so on, without regard to the fact that not all septal defects or cardiomyopathies have the same structure on careful scrutiny, let alone the same cause.

A major advance has been the movement to examine familial aggregation of defects based on presumed pathogenesis.[67-69] The scheme developed by Clark,[33] and since modified and expanded[70] (Table 51-4), has become widely used. Under this approach, some anatomically distinct lesions will be related by common pathogenesis; if it is the pathogenetic mechanism that is under abnormal genetic control, then the occurrence of the distinct defects in the same family would not be troublesome in a genetic model. Alternatively, defects unrelated by pathogenesis would require a different interpretation. This model also focuses on the examination of apparently unaffected relatives and hence increases the chances of detecting subtle manifestations of defective development of cardiovascular structures.

ERRORS IN MESENCHYMAL TISSUE MIGRATION. Included in this category are a wide range of anomalies of the outflow tract, some due to failure of fusion and others due to failure of septation. Relatives of probands with interruption of the aortic arch type B or truncus arteriosus, both uncommon conotruncal malformations, had 2.5 per cent and 6.6 per cent incidences, respectively, of congenital heart defects.[71] Both recurrence rates were higher than expected. The frequency of congenital malformations was much lower in relatives of patients with other forms of interrupted aortic arch. Moreover, relatives of probands with truncus arteriosus and other defects had a recurrence rate of 13 per cent, the majority in the spectrum of conotruncal lesions. Here is an instance in which refined empirical risk data should improve the accuracy of genetic counseling.

Categorizing anatomical defects by presumed pathogenesis

emphasizes that all ventricular septal defects are not alike. If there is a strong genetic component to the etiology of tetralogy of Fallot, for example, one might find in close relatives an increased risk not only of tetralogy but of truncus arteriosus and supracristal ventricular septal defects, but not of other forms of septal defects.

FLOW DEFECTS. Left-sided flow lesions comprise a spectrum that includes hypoplastic left heart, congenital aortic stenosis, bicuspid aortic valve, interrupted aortic arch type A, and aortic coarctation. Various components of this spectrum can be present in the same patient.[72] Data from the Baltimore-Washington Infant Study,[73,74] a population-based case-control study of congenital cardiovascular malformations, were used to show that in first-degree relatives of probands with isolated hypoplastic left heart, incidence of bicuspid aortic valve was 12 per cent; most of the cases were asymptomatic and unrecognized before they were detected by echocardiography as part of this investigation.[55] In an exceptional family, four instances of aortic coarctation occurred in four generations.[75]

The association of coarctation of the aorta, bicuspid aortic valve, and dilatation of the ascending aorta, which may occur as part of the *Turner syndrome*,[46] is well known in the general population.[76,77] Several intriguing questions need to be addressed regarding the genetics and pathogenesis of this association. To what extent is the ascending aorta intrinsically abnormal, and hence predisposed to dilate, and to what extent is the dilatation simply a result of abnormal turbulence created by a bicuspid aortic valve? The fact that some patients with this association also have subtle evidence of a systemic connective tissue abnormality, reminiscent of Marfan syndrome, supports the former hypothesis. It will be of interest to extend the study of left-sided flow lesions to include probands with coarctation or congenital aortic stenosis and to evaluate close relatives with techniques capable of detecting the entire range of flow defects.

EXTRACELLULAR MATRIX ABNORMALITIES. Enough is known about the biochemistry and cell biology of cardiac embryology to state with some confidence that the extracellular matrix ("connective tissue") plays an important role. The endocardial cushions have received the most attention as an area where defects in the extracellular matrix might produce malformations.[33] The high frequency of endocardial cushion defects and atrioventricular septal defects in Down syndrome has been noted (p. 1629). Of interest is the finding of increased adhesiveness of fibroblasts from trisomy 21 patients, a phenomenon that could reflect interaction with the extracellular matrix.[78] The distinctiveness of endocardial cushion defects in patients with normal chromosomes and in those with trisomy 21 has been suggested because of differences in associated cardiovascular malformations. However, of six families in which the proband had an endocardial cushion defect, three had recurrence of the same type of defect in a relative, including two with trisomy 21.[69]

SITUS AND LOOPING DEFECTS. This is an area fraught with difficulties of nomenclature, diagnosis, and heterogeneity of both etiology and pathogenesis. In analysis of clinical data, the most informative approach, but clearly arduous because of the large amount of data required, would be to categorize probands and their relatives by the type of situs (solitus, inversus, dextroversion, and levoversion, p. 941), and each of those by the presence or absence of other cardiac and visceral defects. This has not been done on epidemiological cohorts, and in family studies relatives have rarely been subjected to evaluations sufficiently detailed to characterize their phenotypes in detail.[79]

Several mendelian phenotypes point to single genes that have a major effect on determining laterality. In the autosomal recessive *Kartegener syndrome*, a randomization of lateralization of the heart (situs solitus and situs inversus are equally likely in homozygotes)[80] coexists with a defect in ciliary motility, which leads to sinusitis, bronchiectasis, and sperm immotility.[81,82] Not all morphological defects of cilia are associated with aberrations of cardiac situs.[6] Situs inversus with splenic and other cardiac defects, particularly of the position of the great vessels, can be inherited as an autosomal recessive,[83-85] as an autosomal dominant,[86] and as an X-linked recessive.[87,88] Some of the families with these apparently single-gene disorders have concordance of phenotype, but many do not, suggesting that in some cases various types of situs defects, polysplenia, and asplenia are different manifestations of the same mutation.

There is a paucity of data on the recurrence risks of defects in the *cell death* and *abnormal targeted growth* categories. Preliminary data from the Baltimore-Washington Infant Study do not show an increased risk of any cardiovascular defect in the relatives of a proband with a defect in either of these categories.[70]

DISORDERS OF UNCLEAR ETIOLOGY. A number of disorders include an important likelihood of malformation of the cardiovascular system but are of unclear cause (Table 51-5). Familial recurrence is so low as to be *incompatible* with multifactorial inheritance. Several of these disorders deserve comment.

Certain congenital cardiac defects and other malformations occur together more frequently than expected by chance; this *association* of de-

TABLE 51–5 DISORDERS OF UNCERTAIN CAUSE AND INHERITANCE THAT ARE ASSOCIATED WITH A HIGH INCIDENCE OF CARDIOVASCULAR ABNORMALITIES

DISORDER AND PHENOTYPE	MIM NO.*	CARDIOVASCULAR ABNORMALITIES†
Aase syndrome (Congenital anemia, triphalangeal thumbs)	205600	VSD
Bilateral left-sidedness sequence (Polysplenia syndrome)	208530	ASD
Bilateral right-sidedness sequence (Asplenia syndrome; Ivemark syndrome)	208530	Situs inversus, ECD, VSD
CHARGE association (Coloboma, heart anomaly, choanal atresia, retardation, genital, and ear anomalies)	214800	TOF, PDA, ECD, VSD
Cornelia de Lange syndrome (Short stature, retardation, synophrys, hypertrichosis, micromelia, genital anomalies)	122470	~20% have CHD: VSD, PDA, ASD, PLSVC, TOF
DiGeorge sequence‡ (Abnormalities of derivatives of 3rd and 4th pharyngeal pouches and 4th branchial arch: hypoplastic thymus with cellular immune deficiency, hyoplastic parathyroids with hypocalcemia)	188400	CHD in ~100%: aortic arch anomalies (especially IAA type B and right-sided aortic arch); PDA, TOF
Goldenhar syndrome (Abnormalities of derivatives of 1st and 2nd branchial arch: hemifacial microsomia, microtia, vertebral anomalies)	141400, 164210, 257700	~50% have CHD: VSD, TOF, PDA, CoA, right-sided aortic arch, PLSVC
Klippel-Feil sequence (Short neck, limited rotation of the head, cervical anomalies)	118100, 148900, 214300	Variable estimates (5–70%) of CHD: VSD, dextrocardia
"Kabuki make-up" syndrome (Dwarfism, peculiar facies, scoliosis, mental retardation)	147920	30% have CHD: ASD, VSD, TOF, CoA, PDA
Pallister-Hall syndrome (Hypothalamic hamartoblastoma, hypopituitarism, imperforate anus, postaxial polydactyly)	146510	ECD
Poland sequence (Unilateral absence of sternocostal pectoralis major, ipsilateral synbrachydactyly)	173800	~10% have dextrocardia or dextroversion
Rubinstein-Taybi syndrome (Short stature, retardation, microcephaly, characteristic facies, broad thumbs)	268600	~20% have CHD: ECD, ASD, TOF, PDA, VSD
VATER association (Vertebral defects, anal atresia, tracheo-esophageal fistula, radial dysplasia, renal anomaly)	192350	VSD

VSD = ventricular septal defect; ASD = atrial septal defect; TOF = tetralogy of Fallot; PDA = patent ductus arteriosus; ECD = endocardial cushion defect; CHD = congenital heart defect(s); PLSVC = persistence of left superior vena cava; IAA = interrupted aortic arch; CoA = coarctation of aorta; VSD = ventricular septal defect.

* None of these disorders is evidently due to a mutation in a single gene; however, most are listed in Mendelian Inheritance in Man (MIM),[6] and the MIM no. is provided as a ready source to the literature.

† Cardiovascular defects listed in approximate order of decreasing frequency.

‡ Some cases associated with del(22)(q11), raising the possibility of a contiguous gene deletion defect.

fects suggests a common cause, pathogenesis, or both, but the following disorders and those in Table 51–6 remain enigmatic on most of these counts. Designation as a *sequence* implies that some evidence exists for a common developmental problem to account for the features.

CHARGE Association (Table 51–5). Patients with this condition by definition have congenital heart defects.[89,90] The spectrum of cardiovascular malformations suggests not so much a common pathogenetic scheme as a common time of abnormal development. During gestational

days 32 to 45, cardiac septation, fusion of the endocardial cushions and membranous ventricular septum, and formation of the outflow tracts and valves occur. An environmental insult or a breakdown in developmental homeostasis during this period could result in the malformation spectrum of this disorder. The defects in other systems could also arise during this embryological window and would be consistent with either environmental or intrinsic factors.

DiGeorge Sequence. This involves developmental anomalies of the

TABLE 51–6 CONGENITAL HEART DEFECTS OCCASIONALLY SHOWING FAMILIAL AGGREGATION CONSISTENT WITH MENDELIAN INHERITANCE

DEFECT	MIM NO.*	DEFECT	MIM NO.
Aneurysm, intracranial berry	105800	Hypoplastic left heart	140500, 241550
Aneurysm, abdominal aortic	100070	Hypoplastic right heart	277200
Angioma	106050, 106070, 206570	Lymphedema, congenital	153000, 153100, 153400, 214900, 247440
ASD, ostium primum	209400		
ASD, ostium secundum	108800, 108900, 178650	Mitral valve prolapse	157700
Bicuspid aortic valve	109730	Patent ductus arteriosus	169100
Cardiomyopathy, dilated	108770, 115200, 115250, 212110	Pulmonary venous return, anomalous	106700
Cardiomyopathy, hypertrophic	192600		
Conotruncal defect	231060	Pulmonic stenosis	126190, 178650, 193520, 265500, 265600, 270460
Dextrocardia	244400, 304750		
Ebstein anomaly	224700	Subaortic stenosis	271950, 271960
Endocardial fibroelastosis	226000, 227280, 305300	Supravalvular aortic stenosis	185500, 194050
Hemangioma	106070, 140800, 140900, 234800	Tetralogy of Fallot	187500
Hemangioma, cavernous	116860, 140850	Ventricle, single	234750

* Data from Mendelian Inheritance in Man.[6]

fourth branchial arch and derivatives of the third and fourth pharyngeal pouches that give rise to the characteristic features. Cardiovascular defects are common, fall into the mesenchymal tissue migration error (conotruncal) spectrum,[33] and frequently cause death in the first month of life. The malformations range from tetralogy of Fallot to ventricular septal defect, truncus arteriosus, patent ductus arteriosus, interrupted aorta, and right aortic arch.[91] Recently several cases have been found to have a small deletion of the proximal long arm of chromosome 22, raising the possibility that this sequence is a contiguous gene deletion syndrome, at least in some instances (Table 51–1).

VATER Association (Table 51–5). This condition has expanded over the years to include *v*ertebral, ventricular septal, *a*nal, *t*racheo-*e*sophageal, *r*adial, and *r*enal defects. Omitted from the mnemonic is the single umbilical artery often present.[92,93] Cardiac defects are present in about one-half of patients with more than two components of this association but usually are not life threatening. Although infants with this condition often fail to thrive initially, the long-term prognosis for health and mental function is good, so aggressive management of the multiple malformations is warranted. It is important to separate as soon as possible those patients who have the features of trisomy 18 or 13q- chromosome aberrations, as prognosis in these cases is distinctly unfavorable.

MENDELIAN DISORDERS

Some congenital cardiovascular defects segregate in occasional families as predicted of a mendelian phenotype. There is strong bias favoring reporting such occurrences and an equally strong temptation to conclude that, at least in some cases, the defect is caused by mutation in a single gene. However, rarely and by chance alone, a multifactorial trait will recur in a family in a pattern mimicking mendelian segrega-

tion. This potential confusion and the resultant uncertainty in counseling patients and families pertains equally well to disturbances of conduction and rhythm, to various cardiomyopathies, to vascular anomalies, and to hypertension, all discussed subsequently. The true cause of the cardiovascular diseases in such families may not become clarified until each is investigated in detail, perhaps as a result of efforts to map and sequence the entire human genome.

The subject of this section can therefore be parsed into three broad classes of conditions: congenital cardiac defects that occasionally seem to be inherited as mendelian traits (Table 51–6), pleiotropic mendelian syndromes that always or frequently affect the structure of the cardiovascular system (Table 51–7), and mendelian syndromes that occasionally affect the cardiovascular system (Table 51–8).

FAMILIAL ATRIAL SEPTAL DEFECT. Two mendelian forms of atrial septal defect exist as autosomal dominant traits. One has no associated problems and has been described in few pedigrees.[94] Preliminary and unsubstantiated evidence places the gene for this form of secundum atrial septal defect on chromosome 6 linked to the HLA complex.[95]

The second, and more common, condition has atrioventricular conduction delay as the only pleiotropic feature.[96,97] The defect is of the secundum type, and relatives do not seem to be at increased risk of other cardiac malformations. The severity of heart block rarely progresses to third degree. The electrocardiographic abnormality in a patient with apparently sporadic atrial septal defect should prompt a detailed family history and evaluation of close relatives. Attention should be

TABLE 51–7 MENDELIAN DISORDERS WITH CONGENITAL DEFECTS OF CARDIOVASCULAR STRUCTURE AS FREQUENT MANIFESTATIONS

DESCRIPTIVE NAME	EPONYM	MIM NO.*	CARDIOVASCULAR ABNORMALITIES
Adult polycystic kidney disease		173900	MVP, dilated aortic root, intracranial berry aneurysm
Arteriohepatic dysplasia	Alagille syndrome	118450	PPS
Cataract and cardiomyopathy		212350	HCM
Chondroectodermal dysplasia	Ellis–van Creveld syndrome	225500	ASD (ostium primum), common atrium
Deafness, mitral regurgitation, and short stature	Forney syndrome	157800	MR
Familial collagenoma syndrome		115250	DCM
Heart-hand syndrome	Holt-Oram syndrome	142900	ASD (ostium secundum), VSD, MVP, HLH
Keratosis palmoplantaris	Mal de Meleda	248300	DCM, dysrhythmia
Malignant hyperthermia and skeletal defects	King syndrome	145600	malignant hyperthermia → cardiac arrest
	Noonan syndrome	163950	PS, HCM
Pulmonic stenosis and deafness		178651	PS
	Smith-Lemli-Opitz syndrome	270400	PDA, ASD, VSD, TOF, ECD, CoA
Velocardiofacial syndrome	Shprintzen syndrome	192430	TOF, tortuous retinal vasculature

MVP = mitral valve prolapse; PPS = peripheral pulmonic stenosis; HCM = hypertrophic cardiomyopathy; ASD = atrial septal defect; MR = mitral regurgitation; DCM = dilated cardiomyopathy; VSD = ventricular septal defect; HLH = hypoplastic left heart; PS = valvular pulmonic stenosis; PDA = patent ductus arteriosus; TOF = tetralogy of Fallot; ECD = endocardial cushion defect; CoA = coarctation of aorta.
* Data from Mendelian Inheritance in Man.[6]

TABLE 51–8 MENDELIAN DISORDERS WITH CARDIOVASCULAR ABNORMALITIES OCCASIONAL MANIFESTATIONS

SYNDROME	EPONYM	MIM NO.*	CARDIOVASCULAR ABNORMALITIES
Acrocephalosyndactyly type I	Apert syndrome	101200	PS, PPS, VSD, EFE
Acrocephalopolysyndactyly type II	Carpenter syndrome	201000	PDA, VSD, PS, TGV
Hereditary angioedema		106100	Coronary arteritis
Imperforate anus with hand, foot, and ear anomalies	Townes-Brocks syndrome	107480	Sporadic cases have CHD: VSD, ASD
Mandibulofacial dysostosis	Treacher Collins syndrome	154500, 248390	10% have CHD: variable
Neuronal ceroid lipofuscinosis	Batten disease	204200	HCM
Orofacial digital syndrome type II	Mohr syndrome	252100	Variable
Short rib–polydactyly syndrome	Saldino-Noonan syndrome	263530	TGV, ECD, hypoplastic right heart
Thrombocytopenia–absent radius syndrome		274000	TOF

PS = valvular pulmonic stenosis; PPS = peripheral pulmonic stenosis; VSD = ventricular septal defect; EFE = endocardial fibroelastosis; PDA = patent ductus arteriosus; TGV = transposition of great arteries; CHD = congenital heart defect(s); ASD = atrial septal defect; HCM = hypertrophic cardiomyopathy; ECD = endocardial cushion defect; TOF = tetralogy of Fallot.
* Data from Mendelian Inheritance in Man.[6]

directed to the upper limbs, particularly the thumbs, to rule out the Holt-Oram syndrome; radiographic examination of the entire limbs of the proband is helpful on this account.

When patients with atrial septal defect due to aneuploidy (a syndrome with extracardiac features), and one of the autosomal dominant forms are excluded, the recurrence risk of atrial septal defect is about 3 per cent, a value that conforms closely to the multifactorial threshold model.[63,66] Several pleiotropic mendelian conditions have defects of the atrial septum as frequent manifestations.

HOLT-ORAM SYNDROME. This autosomal dominant condition, first elaborated in 1960, shows marked variability within a pedigree.[98] The cardinal manifestations are dysplasia of the upper limbs and atrial septal defect. In heterozygotes for the mutation, arm deformity ranges from undetectable through distally placed thumbs and hypoplastic thenar eminences, triphalangeal thumbs, anomalies of the carpus, and radial aplasia, to phocomelia and hypoplasia of the clavicles and shoulders. Upper extremity deformity is usually bilateral but may be asymmetrical in severity, with the left side the worse.[99] Similarly, the atrial involvement ranges from none to a large secundum defect with early, severe hemodynamic compromise. Other cardiac malformations have been reported, with ventricular septal defects the most frequent. The skeletal and cardiac manifestations are not correlated in individuals, and how a parent is affected is not a reliable predictor of effects on an offspring. Prenatal diagnosis by ultrasound was reported in a fetus with severe limb anomalies;[100] presumably a large septal defect could be detected as well. Other manifestations include dermatoglyphic abnormalities,[98,101] pectus excavatum,[98] hypoplastic peripheral arteries,[99] and cardiac conduction disturbance, the last usually involving the AV node and present in patients with septal defects.[98,99,101] Although the Holt-Oram syndrome bears some resemblance to the VATER association, the clear mendelian nature and lack of more extensive organ system involvement of the former indicate that the two conditions do not represent a pathogenetic spectrum.

The diagnosis of Holt-Oram syndrome is most likely to be missed in a patient with an unknown or unremarkable family history, a secundum septal defect, and minimal or no thumb anomaly. In any "sporadic" case of an atrial septal defect, the patient and the parents should be carefully examined for limb malformations and the family history studied in detail. Detection of a subtle limb defect will alter the recurrence risk in offspring of the proband from the empirical risk of an isolated septal defect of 3 per cent to the 50 per cent of an autosomal dominant trait.

ELLIS-VAN CREVELD SYNDROME (Fig. 51-6). This rare, autosomal recessive chondrodysplasia is found among the old order Amish because of a founder effect and consanguinity. Short stature, metaphyseal dysplasia, dysplastic nails and teeth, and postaxial polydactyly are the pleiotropic manifestations in addition to congenital heart disease.[102] The last is present in more than one-half of homozygotes, and most of the defects affect the atrial septum. The majority are defects of endocardial cushion closure, including ostium primum defects of widely varying size up to a single atrium. This disorder has long been thought to be due to an as yet unknown defect in the extracellular matrix, which would fit with the high frequency of endocardial cushion lesions. However, defects thought due to abnormal embryonic flow (coarctation, hypoplastic left heart, and patent ductus arteriosus) occur in about 20 per cent of cases. Ellis-van Creveld syndrome can be diagnosed prenatally by detection of polydactyly by ultrasonography.

VENTRICULAR SEPTAL DEFECT. This malformation does not seem to be inherited as an isolated mendelian malformation, and no syndromes include it as a common, isolated manifestation. One intriguing pedigree showed maternal transmission of a risk for atrial or ventricular septal defects to at least 11 of 13 offspring; the suggestion was made that phenotype was determined by the mitochondrial chromosome.[103] Subsequent study of the mitochondrial chromosome has not uncovered a candidate gene,[11] and the family has not been studied molecularly. Many other isolated defects have been described in families in patterns suggestive of mendelian inheritance, but only for supravalvular aortic stenosis and mitral valve prolapse is there convincing evidence for the action of a single mutant gene.

SUPRAVALVULAR AORTIC STENOSIS (see also p. 94). This congenital lesion, which may be asymptomatic and detected long after birth because of an ejection murmur, occurs in at least three settings. It can be a sporadic anomaly, a component of Williams syndrome (itself of heterogeneous cause), or an autosomal dominant trait associated with peripheral

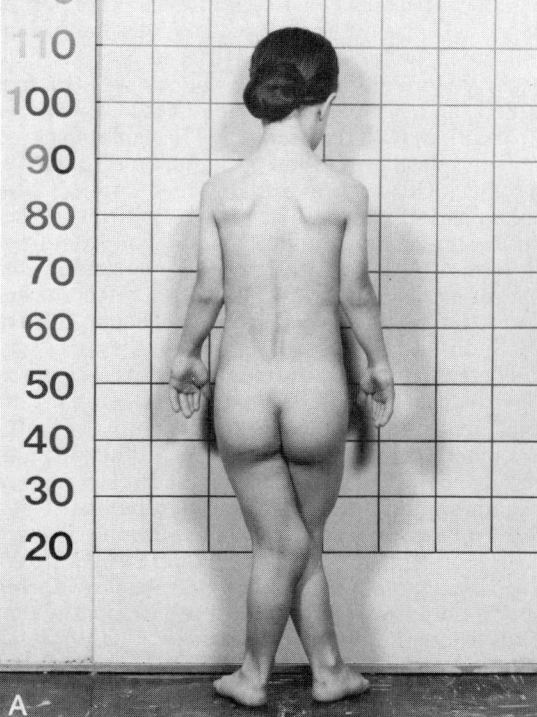

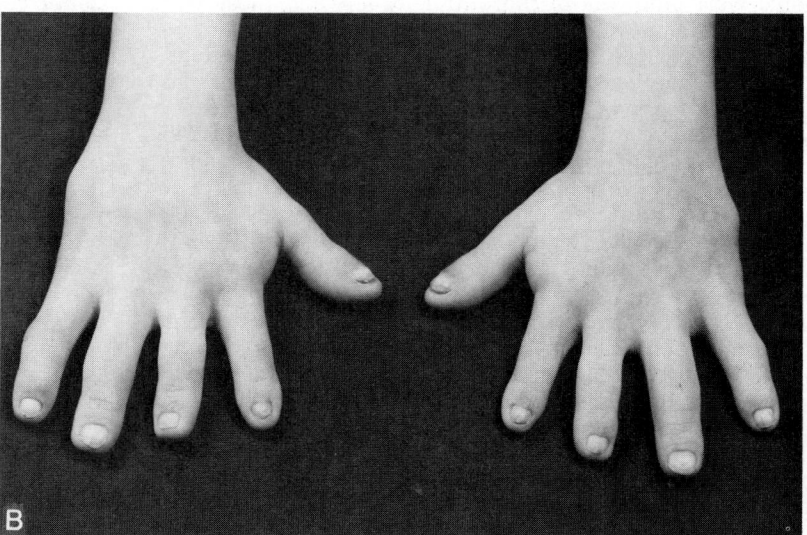

FIGURE 51-6. Ellis-van Creveld syndrome in a young woman. *A,* Note short stature, joint contractures at the elbows, and marked genu valgum. *B,* The fingers are short and the nails dysplastic. Note the protuberances along the ulnar edges of the hands where sixth digits were amputated.

pulmonic stenoses. Cause of the sporadic anomaly is unclear, and counseling about recurrence is difficult. Undetected hypercalcemia during the vulnerable period of gestation or neonatal life has been suggested as one cause.

Williams syndrome is usually sporadic but, in more instances than previously recognized, is a highly variable autosomal dominant condition. The full spectrum includes infantile hypercalcemia, abnormal ("elfin") facies, mental deficiency, short stature, multiple peripheral pulmonic stenoses, and supravalvular aortic stenosis.[104] Occasional cardiovascular manifestations are mitral valve prolapse, bicuspid aortic valve, and hypertension.[105,106] Although patients usually survive the problems of infancy and show catch-up growth, progressive problems of joint contractures, genitourinary and gastrointestinal dysfunction, and psychosocial adjustment define the long-term prognosis.[107] As there are a number of causes of infantile hypercalcemia (including exposure to excessive vitamin D during pregnancy), the clinical entity should be called the Williams phenotype, with the designation "syndrome" reserved for the autosomal dominant variety.

Autosomal dominant supravalvular aortic stenosis is now recognized as an entity distinct from Williams syndrome.[108-110] Mental retardation and abnormal facies should prompt rejection of the diagnosis of this "pure" cardiovascular disorder. Peripheral pulmonary artery stenoses may be present but rarely cause hemodynamic problems. The aortic lesion requires surgery in less than half of patients. Screening of relatives is essential and easily conducted with echocardiography.

MITRAL VALVE PROLAPSE (see also p. 1029). This trait is of heterogeneous cause and pathogenesis; although it has been called the most common abnormality of human heart valves,[111,112] mitral valve prolpase (MVP) is equally clearly not always an "abnormality." Here only the heritable forms of MVP will be discussed. These can be classified into three groups. The first is an autosomal dominant form with minimal extracardiac involvement. The second is an autosomal dominant condition that is clinically variable, and at one end of its spectrum merges with the Marfan syndrome; it could just as well be discussed as a heritable disorder of connective tissue. The third category is composed of the various mendelian syndromes that include mitral valve prolapse as a pleiotropic manifestation.

The first category, which some have called mitral valve prolapse syndrome[113] or familial mitral valve prolapse,[114] includes a condition that is centered on the mitral valve. The development of actual prolapse shows the age- and sex-dependent behavior characteristic of the "idiopathic" form so common in the general population.[114,115] Formal genetic studies confirm *autosomal dominance with variable expression.*[114,115] This category has been partitioned into those patients with billowing of the mitral leaflets and those with excessive systolic mitral annular expansion; because this phenotype breeds relatively true, two distinct autosomal dominant forms may exist.[116] The cause(s) of these entities is unknown.[117] Moreover, when and how the phenotype of this condition can be distinguished from the sporadic cases of MVP and the cases with obvious evidence of a systemic disorder of connective tissue are unclear. The only consistent extracardiac manifestations are excessive arm span in women and relatively low body weight and systolic blood pressure.[118,119]

Many clinical geneticists and cardiologists are referred patients with a suspicion of Marfan syndrome (p. 1641) or Ehlers-Danlos syndrome (p. 1643). Some of these patients do not meet minimal diagnostic criteria for a recognized connective tissue disorder[120] but clearly have extracardiac features consistent with a defect of the extracellular matrix described below. MVP is commonly but not always present; when it is, and evidence of a systemic abnormality of connective tissue is lacking, the patient should be considered as having the condition described in the preceding paragraph, what some call primary mitral valve prolapse.[121] The clinical spectrum of the

patients with syndromic MVP includes abnormal striae atrophicae, excessive arm span and leg length, joint hypermobility, pectus excavatum, scoliosis, reduction in thoracic kyphosis ("straight back"), myopia, and mild aortic root dilatation.[122] Aortic dilatation beyond 3 SD above the mean for body surface area, aortic dissection, ectopia lentis, or a family history of any of these three features *removes a* patient from this category. For the remainder of patients, the acronym MASS phenotype, for mitral valve, aorta, skin, and skeletal, describes what certainly is a heterogeneous grouping of patients and families. Aorta is mentioned specifically because of the appropriate concern that progressive dilatation and dissection will occur; in fact, neither has been the case, although prospective evaluation has been brief. Many of the associations between MVP and deformity of the thoracic cage and spontaneous pneumothorax are explained by the MASS phenotype.[123-125]

Finally, as described below, MVP frequently accompanies the Marfan syndrome, several of the Ehlers-Danlos syndromes, and cutis laxa and occurs more often than expected in osteogenesis imperfecta, Larsen syndrome, pseudoxanthoma elasticum, and other mendelian syndromes (see Table 51-11). In addition, occasional families with otherwise unclassified heritable disorders of connective tissue have prominent involvement of the mitral apparatus, with myxomatous deterioration or calcification, or both.[126]

NOONAN SYNDROME. Among the pleiotropic mendelian syndromes that have frequent cardiovascular involvement, the Noonan syndrome is important because of its relatively high prevalence and clinical variability. This autosomal dominant condition has been called the male Turner syndrome in the past because of the short stature, cubitus valgus, neck webbing, congenital lymphedema, and congenital heart defects that coexist in the 45, X Turner syndrome. However, the Noonan syndrome is distinct, not simply because both men and women are affected. Patients with Noonan syndrome often have an unusual deformity of the sternum, mental dullness, hypertelorism, ptosis, and cryptorchidism.[127] The cardiovascular defects, while widely varied, do not include an increased incidence of coarctation of the aorta.[128] Because of the dysmorphism of the facies and the cardiac involvement, Noonan syndrome is often classified, along with Williams, LEOPARD, King, and Watson syndromes, as a cardiofacial syndrome.

The entire phenotype of the Noonan syndrome is highly variable, and affected people can escape clinical problems (or accurate diagnosis), even if they have obvious manifestations.[129] Similarly, a wide range of cardiovascular involvement can occur.[130] *Valvular pulmonic stenosis* was the first defect identified, and Noonan syndrome should always be considered in a patient with this lesion.[131] The valve cusps are thickened and dysplastic, even in the absence of hemodynamic compromise. Obstruction to right-sided flow can also occur in Noonan patients because of pulmonary artery hypoplasia[132] or infundibular subvalvular changes. The latter finding reflects a generalized predisposition to hypertrophic cardiomyopathy, often asymmetrical, that can affect either ventricle.[133,134] Atrial septal defect occurs in about one-third of patients, usually in association with pulmonic stenosis. Ventricular septal defects and patent ductus arteriosus each occur in about 10 per cent. Congenital anomalies of coronary arteries are occasionally and unexpectedly found during evaluation of more obvious defects.[134a] The electrocardiogram often shows left anterior hemiblock and a deep precordial S wave, a pattern not common in pulmonic stenosis of other causes.

Lymphatic dysplasia, especially of the lower limbs, is common but causes clinical difficulties in less than 20 per cent.[127] While evidence of lymphedema often disappears during childhood, chylothorax and a protein-losing enteropathy represent the severe end of the spectrum.[135]

Noonan syndrome shares features with other cardiofacial syndromes, and in sporadic cases (which account for 50 per cent of Noonan syndrome) diagnosis can be difficult. All are autosomal dominant, so genetic counseling is somewhat easier. Affected males have reduced reproductive capabilities because of testicular abnormalities. Susceptibility to malignant hyperthermia can be detected by family history, elevated skeletal muscle creatine kinase levels, or muscle biopsy. Despite the relatively high frequency of the Noonan syndrome, estimated up to 1 per 1000, neither its cause nor its pathogenesis is clear. The gene has not been mapped, and interlocus genetic heterogeneity is possible. Intriguing issues that may shed light on these uncertainties are the overlap in phenotype with type I neurofibromatosis[136] (the gene for which is on chromosome 17 and has been cloned) and the frequent coexistence of Noonan syndrome and deficiency of coagulation factor XI.[137]

TERATOGENIC EFFECTS

A teratogen is any agent that adversely affects embryonic or fetal development, such as infectious vectors, radiation, drugs, and other chemicals (Table 51–9). Teratogenic effects on the cardiovascular system are considered in this chapter for several reasons: (1) The phenotypes are often reminiscent of those due to chromosomal aberrations and single-gene mutations. (2) Clinical geneticists and dysmorphologists are involved in diagnosing, managing, and investigating both teratogenic and genetic syndromes. (3) How the organism responds to an encounter with a potential teratogen is largely determined by its genome. The entire field of ecogenetics and part of pharmacogenetics are concerned with these issues.

The abilities to resist disruption of normal human embryogenesis and development involve systems quite distinct from physiologic homeostasis and related only in part with developmental homeostasis. Genetic susceptibilities to teratogens can be illustrated by diverse mechanisms: reduced or inaccurate repair of radiation-induced DNA damage; enhanced receptiveness to viral entry or replication; immune deficiencies that prevent inactivation of infectious vectors or maintenance of immunity; slow inactivation of a compound that exerts a direct deleterious effect; or rapid conversion of an inoffensive drug to a teratogenic metabolite. These types of hereditary variation may be determined by single genes, with susceptibility inherited as a mendelian trait, or by many genes, each of small effect. Either situation can account for the well-known fact that only a fraction of pregnancies exposed to a given agent will be affected adversely. Variation in dose and timing of exposure also confound interpretation of epidemiological and family data. It is not surprising, then, that the actual appearance of the abnormal phenotype is not amenable to traditional pedigree analysis. Rather, examination of the biochemical susceptibilities has proved, and will continue to prove, more enlightening.

Some teratogens, such as warfarin, have a clear action that explains how the pleiotropic manifestations emerge. The action of other teratogens, such as alcohol, is obscure. Finally, in some teratogenic syndromes, such as that in offspring of women with diabetes mellitus, the actual offensive agent is unclear, and multiple pathogenetic mechanisms seem to pertain.[138,139] Regardless of cause and pathogenetic mechanism, the phenotypes of many teratogens often share manifestations, especially prenatal growth retardation, abnormalities of the craniofacies, and mental retardation. The following syndromes have prominent consequences on the cardiovascular system.

FETAL ALCOHOL SYNDROME. Ethanol is the most common teratogen to which the human embryo and fetus are exposed. The period of greatest vulnerability is during the first trimester, and the risks are clearly related to the amount of alcohol consumed; the risk of the fetal alcohol syndrome occurring in an offspring of a chronic alcoholic woman is 30 to 50 per cent. The features are highly variable and include growth retardation, mild to moderate mental retardation, hyperactivity, short palpebral fissures, a smooth philtrum with a thin upper lip, and small distal phalanges.[140] Congenital heart defects occur in more than one-half of children with the full spectrum of the phenotype; ventricular septal defects are most common and often insignificant, but atrial septal defects, tetralogy of Fallot, and aortic coarctation can occur.

FETAL HYDANTOIN SYNDROME. Virtually all antiseizure medications can affect the fetus. Hydantoin was the first to be identified as a teratogen. The risk to the fetus depends in part on the genotype of the fetus; defects in arene oxidase predisposes to the full syndrome.[141,142] The features include prenatal and postnatal growth retardation, mild mental retardation, a broad face with a short nose, short distal phalanges with small nails, and hip dislocation. Cardiovascular defects, which are an inconstant part of the syndrome, include septal defects, right- and left-sided flow defects, and a single umbilical artery.

RETINOIC ACID EMBRYOPATHY. Isotretinoin was not recognized as a teratogen until after it was licensed for the treatment of acne. The vulnerable period extends from the first week through the fourth month of gestation. The risks of miscarriage and stillbirth are elevated. The phenotype includes anomalies of the craniofacies and gross neuroanatomical disruption. Cardiovascular defects are common and emphasize a variety of conotruncal malformations.[143] Liveborn infants often succumb to the cardiac and brain anomalies. Although the mechanism of action is not certain, vitamin A derivatives such as retinoic acid function as morphogens during embryogenesis, serving as signals for cell migration. The fact that the cardiovascular defects are primarily those of rotation and folding suggest disruption of a normal developmental homeostatic system.

WARFARIN EMBRYOPATHY. Coumarin-related vitamin K antagonists are usually prescribed for a variety of cardiovascular problems to women of childbearing age (p. 1805) and can cause a variety of cardiovascular and other organ damage to the fetus. Coumarin interferes with embryogenesis directly when administered during gestational weeks 6 through 9. The most pronounced effects are on cartilage because of inhibition of enzymes of extracellular matrix metabolism. Congenital cardiac defects are perhaps increased in frequency but fit no specific pathogenetic mechanism.[144] The second pattern of coumarin effects involves exposure during the second and third trimester and includes spontaneous abortion, stillbirth, and various central nervous system defects. The last are not due simply to intracranial hemorrhage as was once assumed.[144]

What predisposes to the adverse fetal effects of coumarin remains to be discovered. First, more than 75 per cent of women who take coumarin derivatives throughout pregnancy have normal offspring; reassuring most women while identifying those at risk for adverse effects has obvious advantages. Second, placing all pregnant women on a regimen of heparin is not an acceptable solution, because heparin can cause stillbirth or premature fetal loss in about 20 per cent of exposures, is not as effective as coumarin in some indications for anticoagulation, and is more trouble to administer and regulate.

MATERNAL PKU. The inborn error of metabolism phenylketonuria

TABLE 51–9 CARDIOVASCULAR DEFECTS ASSOCIATED WITH PRENATAL EXPOSURE TO TERATOGENS

TERATOGEN	CARDIOVASCULAR ABNORMALITIES*
Ethanol	~50% have CHD: VSD (~50% close spontaneously), TOF, ASD, ECD, absence of a pulmonary artery
Hydantoin	~10% have CHD: VSD, ASD, PS
Lithium	<3% have Ebstein anomaly
Phenylalanine	~20% have CHD: TOF
Retinoic acid	>50% have CHD: TGA, TOF, VSD, IAA
Rubella	>50% have CHD: PDA with or without ASD, VSD, PPS, IAA
Trimethadione	~50% have CHD: complex combinations most frequent (involving VSD, ASD, PDA, AS, PS), VSD, TOF
Valproic acid	>50% have CHD: left- and right-sided flow lesions: CoA, HLH, ASD, VSD, pulmonary atresia
Vitamin D	supravalvular aortic stenosis is the cardinal manifestation; PPS
Warfarin	~10% have CHD: PDA, PS; rarely, intracranial hemorrhage

CHD = congenital heart defect(s); VSD = ventricular septal defect; TOF = tetralogy of Fallot; ASD = atrial septal defect; ECD = endocardial cushion defect; PS = valvular pulmonic stenosis; TGA = transposition of great arteries; IAA = interrupted aortic arch; PPS = peripheral pulmonic stenosis; PDA = patent ductus arteriosus; AS = aortic stenosis; CoA = coarctation of aorta; HLH = hypoplastic left heart.

* Among patients with the full clinical spectrum associated with each teratogen; cardiovascular defects listed in decreasing order of prevalence.

produces severe mental retardation unless the phenylalanine content of the diet is markedly reduced soon after birth.[145] Deficiency of phenylalanine hydroxylase in the fetus produces no harm because fetal blood levels of phenylalanine are regulated by the heterozygous mother's enzyme. Since neonatal screening for this disease is now routine in all states, virtually all patients receive treatment and grow to adulthood with average intelligence. Many patients discontinue the rigorous dietary therapy during adolescence when the elevated phenylalanine levels have far less deleterious effects. The embryopathy occurs when a woman with homozygous deficiency for phenylalanine hydroxylase becomes pregnant and her fetus is exposed to high levels of the amino acid that overwhelm its ability to metabolize. The result is highly predictable if the mother does not restart dietary restriction of phenylalanine for the entire gestation: moderate to severe mental retardation, prenatal and postnatal growth retardation, microcephaly, and a variety of cardiovascular defects in 15 to 20 per cent.[146] This condition can largely be prevented by effective counseling of female patients with phenylketonuria.

FETAL RUBELLA EFFECTS (see p. 888). About 50 per cent of fetuses become infected with the rubella virus when the mother is infected during the first trimester. Not only does the infected fetus suffer varied and severe interference with development and organogenesis, but it acquires a chronic viral illness that can persist for years. The most common features of the embryopathy are mental deficiency, deafness, cataract, and cardiovascular defects. Patent ductus arteriosus is common as are septal defects. Peripheral pulmonary stenosis and fibromuscular proliferation of medium and small arteries often improve postnatally.

CARDIOMYOPATHIES

(See also Chap. 43)

Each of the three clinical categories of primary cardiomyopathy—hypertrophic, dilated, and restrictive—can be caused by mutations in single genes as judged by mendelian inheritance of a consistent phenotype in multiple families. Many other mendelian disorders also cause cardiomyopathies as a secondary consequence of their basic metabolic disturbance.

HYPERTROPHIC CARDIOMYOPATHY

(See also p. 1404)

In the more than 30 years since the recognition of hypertrophic cardiomyopathy as a clinical entity, many aspects of its natural history, pathology, and management have been substantially clarified.[147] The phenotype is most clearly defined anatomically and histologically and consists of myocardial hypertrophy without secondary cause; cellular and myofiber disarray; myocardial fibrosis; and mediointimal proliferation of small coronary arteries. None of these features is pathognomonic; for example, myofiber disorganization is present in the normal human heart during embryogenesis and in congenital heart defects that place strain on the right-sided circulation.[148]

About half of probands with idiopathic hypertrophic cardiomyopathy of any segment of the left ventricle have affected first-degree relatives, and in those families the phenotype is inherited as an autosomal dominant.[149-151] There is wide variability of expression within a family, in part due to age-dependency of the trait.[151a] Later generations of relatives in adolescence and childhood may not have developed echocardiographic evidence of hypertrophy. Hence, pedigree screening for clinical, counseling, or investigative purposes should not be considered complete until the following criteria are satisfied: two-dimensional echocardiography is used to insure that segmental hypertrophy is detected; a person at risk has a normal echocardiographic study and no evidence of electrocardiographic abnormality or important dysrhythmia after about age 20; and a person of any age has left ventricular hypertrophy without any other explanation, such as hypertension or aortic stenosis.[151b]

In about one-half of families with more than one affected person, the oldest patient appears to be the first affected relative, with neither parent involved.[149,150] Some of these patients may have hypertrophic cardiomyopathy on account of a new mutation rendering them heterozygous; they would have

a 50:50 chance of having affected offspring. Others may be phenocopies, that is, have environmental causes of hypertrophy that remain obscure. The possibility of autosomal recessive inheritance has been raised,[147] but convincing pedigrees, in which all parents and offspring of multiple affected sibs have normal echocardiographic findings, have not been found.[149,152]

Given the variability in segmental pattern of hypertrophy within families,[153] the two pedigrees that show *only* apical cardiomyopathy suggest that multiple genetic forms exist.[154] Genetic heterogeneity is also supported by linkage studies that identify potential loci on two different human chromosomes. With cloned DNA probes and restriction fragment site polymorphisms,[5] the phenotype in one large family was linked tightly and with a good statistical power to chromosome band 14q11.[155] Subsequently, the genes for the cardiac α and β myosin heavy chains were linked to the same polymorphism, and are the leading candidates as the site of the basic defect.[155a] However, hypertrophic cardiomyopathy is clearly of heterogeneous genetic cause, as some families show no linkage of the phenotype with 14q11.[155b] In one family, indistinguishable clinically from typical hypertrophic cardiomyopathy, the disease was found only in relatives who had a fragile-site marker on chromosome 16, whereas unaffected relatives lacked the marker.[156] It is possible, but unlikely, that the fragile site itself has something to do with the mutation. More likely the fragile site is close to the gene and therefore serves simply as a pointer, just like the restriction fragment polymorphisms did in the previous example. It is also possible, because the pedigree is relatively small, that the result is fortuitous but incorrect. In appropriate families, availability of tightly linked DNA markers permits prenatal diagnosis and presymptomatic detection superior to echocardiography.

DILATED CARDIOMYOPATHY

(See also p. 1398)

The prevalence of idiopathic dilated cardiomyopathy is about double that of the hypertrophic form.[157] No population-based studies have explored the family history of probands with the dilated, congestive form, and the frequency of hereditary forms is virtually unknown. Although numerous occurrences of familial dilated cardiomyopathy are reported, few investigations have been conducted of an unselected series of probands for clinical and subclinical evidence of cardiac disease.[158] Thus, it is unclear what fraction of patients with idiopathic dilated cardiomyopathy have a mendelian disease, how many have a new mutation for a mendelian disease, and how many have phenocopies of nongenetic causes. Estimates of a positive family history, which could suggest a mendelian condition or a shared environmental cause, range from 7 to 30 per cent.[158-161]

Because of the risk of severe dysrhythmia in dilated cardiomyopathy, early detection of people with the disorder can be life saving. Two-dimensional echocardiography is a sensitive method for detecting affected relatives with subclinical disease. Individuals who have equivocal left ventricular enlargement or dysfunction can have ambulatory electrocardiographic monitoring and, if the diagnosis is still uncertain, can have serial examinations. Certainly every patient with idiopathic dilated cardiomyopathy should have a detailed family history. If any close relative has a history consistent with cardiomyopathy, dysrhythmia, or sudden death at a relatively young age, counseling about the risk of a familial disease and the potential benefits of pedigree screening should be offered.

The majority of instances of familial occurrence fit autosomal dominant inheritance.[161-166] Considerable clinical variability characterizes virtually all pedigrees; variation in severity, clinical phenotype, and age of onset is typical. Several pedigrees suggest autosomal recessive inheritance,[162,167,168] but nonpenetrance and germinal mosaicism are potential explanations for what is really a dominant trait. Recurrence of congestive cardiomyopathy of early onset in an inbred pedigree is more convincing for an autosomal recessive condition.[169] In one pedigree with relatively early onset of symptoms (15 to 21 years of age) in males, much later onset in females, and lack of transmission of cardiomyopathy from father to son (although there was only one opportunity in this family), inheritance is most compatible with X linkage.[170]

The causes of these various hereditary forms of dilated cardiomyopathy are unknown. In some families with autosomal dominant disease, a mild proximal skeletal myopathy of type I fibers coexists with cardiac involvement.[164,171,172] Skeletal muscle changes might serve not only as an early clinical marker of heterozygosity for the mutant gene in some individuals at risk but also indicate that the search for cause should address structural components or metabolites common to both cardiac and skeletal myofibers. Histological examination of myocardium generally shows nonspecific hypertrophy and fibrosis. By electron microscopy, however, mitochondria are distinctly abnormal, a finding not seen in congestive heart failure of other causes.[172,173] Because the inheritance pattern in these cases does not suggest a mutation of the mitochondrial genome, focus could be directed on nuclear genes that encode structural components of the mitochondrion, components of the respiratory chain found in the mitochondrion, or enzymes that regulate and facilitate free fatty acid metabolism in the mitochondrion. As with virtually every common disease, associations with immune response factors have been investigated in dilated cardiomyopathy. Weak associations with HLA-DR loci were found that seemed to predispose to the disease in some cases,[174] but these results remain unconfirmed and unexplained.

In one family, cardiomyopathy developed only in association with pregnancy.[175] Although peripartum cardiomyopathy is a well-recognized, usually sporadic, disorder (see p. 1798), its occurrence in five women in two generations suggests a hereditary predisposition.

RESTRICTIVE CARDIOMYOPATHY
(See also p. 1415)

The pathogenesis of the majority of cases of restrictive cardiomyopathy involves infiltration or replacement of the myocardium or both. The causes are varied and can be nongenetic or genetic; the latter are mostly metabolic diseases with secondary effects on the heart and are summarized in Table 51–10; some are reviewed subsequently. A common form of restrictive cardiomyopathy that has primary genetic forms among many other causes is endocardial fibroelastosis. Other mutations produce restriction through pericardial constriction. Isolated pedigrees of primary myocardial fibrosis without secondary cause and leading to restrictive hemodynamics are not classifiable.[176,177]

ENDOCARDIAL FIBROELASTOSIS (see also p. 944). This abnormality is characterized by thickening of the endocardium, which leads to decreased compliance and impaired diastolic function. Primary forms, discussed here, are unassociated with other cardiac anomalies (Table 51–11). When congenital, endocardial fibroelastosis accounts for somewhat under 10 per cent of childhood deaths from heart disease. In infants there is often an indolent course of failure to thrive, tachypnea, and tachycardia, until a precipitant such as an upper respiratory infection leads to rapid cardiac decompensation. Treatment of children with primary endocardial fibroelastosis is ineffective; cardiac transplantation now offers some hope. Autopsy shows enlargement of the left ventricle and perhaps other chambers, no abnormality of lung vessels, and collapse of the left lower lobe. Histopathological study reveals extensive deposition of extracellular matrix, primarily collagen and elastic fibers, in the endocardium.

X-linked recessive inheritance is the most firmly established of the single-gene causes, and even here there may be heterogeneity. Some pedigrees show mainly small, contracted cardiac chambers, while others have chamber dilatation; both are compatible with the functional pathophysiology described

by the term "restrictive." Males are affected earlier and more severely by both forms, with death in infancy not unusual.[178] In other families, the ventricles are dilated, and the condition is distinguished from X-linked dilated cardiomyopathy by the presence of endocardial fibroelastosis and an immune deficiency due to defective granulocyte function in the former.[179] Morphological abnormalities of mitochondria were present on ultrastructural studies of heart and leukocytes. Insufficient longitudinal experience is recorded to know whether females heterozygous for this mutation develop a dilated restrictive cardiomyopathy later in life.

Several pedigrees suggestive of autosomal recessive inheritance of primary endocardial fibroelastosis were reported before the routine availability of laboratory methods to diagnose metabolic derangements, especially defects in fatty acid catabolism.[180-182] Endocardial fibroelastosis can be a prominent finding at autopsy in patients with autosomal dominant dilated cardiomyopathy[183]; whether the endocardial changes are primary, representing yet another mendelian form of this disorder, or secondary is unclear.

CARDIOMYOPATHIES SECONDARY TO OTHER CAUSES

INBORN ERRORS OF METABOLISM. These can affect the left ventricle by various mechanisms and produce diverse anatomical, histological, and functional disturbances. The most common anatomical result is an apparent hypertrophic cardiomyopathy, which is actually *pseudohypertrophic*, because the thickened walls are not due to myocardial cell hypertrophy, but to cellular or interstitial infiltration by metabolites. Abnormalities of both systolic and diastolic function result, outflow obstruction may occur, and in some cases the hemodynamic characteristics resemble a restrictive cardiomyopathy. The offending metabolite may be an incompletely degraded macromolecule such as glycogen (*glycogen storage disorder II* [Pompe's disease] and *glycogen storage disorder III*), proteoglycan and glycosaminoglycan (*mucopolysaccharidoses I, III, IV, VI, and VII*), sphingolipid (*Fabry's disease, Tay-Sachs disease, Farber's disease, Refsum's disease,* and *Gaucher's disease*), glycoprotein (*fucosidosis* and *mannosidosis*), and amyloid (*familial amyloidoses I and III*) or a small molecule such as iron in *hemochromatosis.* Some of these disorders are discussed later. True myocardial hypertrophy occurs as a part of mendelian syndromes of unclear cause, such as *Noonan syndrome, von Recklinghausen neurofibromatosis,*[184] and *LEOPARD syndrome,*[185,186] and monogenic errors of metabolism, notably those producing *hyperthyroidism* and *pheochromocytoma.* Any of the mendelian disorders that cause hypertension (Table 51–12) may, over time, produce true myocardial hypertrophy.

Dilated cardiomyopathy often results from inborn errors of energy production, especially fatty acid metabolism. Various disorders associated with *carnitine deficiency, mitochondrial* and *peroxisomal dysfunction,* and *muscle dysfunction* can present with symptoms of congestive heart failure or dysrhythmia.

Restrictive cardiomyopathy often occurs with both hemodynamic evidence of impaired diastolic filling and wall thickening; any of the conditions causing pseudohypertrophy of the myocardium can eventually exhibit restrictive pathophysiology. Hemochromatosis and the amyloidoses, both hereditary and acquired forms, are especially likely to present in this manner. Connective tissue replaces myocytes or infiltrates the interstitium in a number of conditions. Fibrosis of the myocardium may cause pseudohypertrophy, but the clinical consequences are more those of restriction. Disorders in this category are those that cause coronary artery disease (*diabetes mellitus,* the *hemoglobinopathies* associated with sickling, *Fabry disease* and the *mucopolysaccharidoses*) and some of the *muscular dystrophies,* in which myocardial fibers are replaced by extracellular matrix. Finally, a number of hereditary conditions are associated with endocardial fibroelastosis (Table 51–11).

CONSTRICTIVE PERICARDITIS (see also Chap. 35). Two rare autosomal recessive disorders include fibrous thickening of the pericardium as a manifestation. In both, signs and symptoms of constrictive pericarditis develop insidiously, and treatment by pericardiotomy is life saving. One condition was first described in Finland and given the name *MULIBREY nanism,* a combination of a mnemonic for *muscle, liver, brain,* and *eye* and an archaic word for dwarfism (nanism).[44] Growth failure from an early age is common, and growth does not improve once pericardial constriction is abated. Subsequently, more than a dozen patients, generally with consanguineous parents, have been reported from around the world.[187]

The *arthropathy-camptodactyly syndrome* previously had been reported because of the skeletal and rheumatological manifestations before pericardial effusion and fibrous thickening of the pericardium were recognized as manifestations.[188-190] Its cause is unknown.

DISORDER	EPONYM OR COMMON NAME	MIM NO.*	PATHOGENESIS	CARDIOVASCULAR INVOLVEMENT	BIOCHEMICAL DEFECT	GENE LOCUS†	ANIMAL MODEL
Aminoacidopathies							
Alkaptonuria	Ochronosis	203500	Deposition of homogentisic acid in connective tissue	AS; atherosclerosis			
Cystinosis, nephropathic type		219800	Lysosomal storage	Hypertension from renal failure, vascular wall thickening	?	?	
Homocystinuria		236200	Unknown	Early CAD; venous thrombosis; pulmonary embolism	Cystathionine-β-synthase	CBS; 21q21-q22.1	
Oxalosis I	Hyperoxaluria	259900	Vascular and tissue accumulation of oxalate	Conduction defect; vascular occlusions; Raynaud phenomenon	Peroxisomal alanine: Glyoxylate aminotransferase	AGT	
Defects in fatty acid metabolism							
Carnitine transport defect	Primary carnitine deficiency	212140	Lipid myopathy; defective energy generation	DCM: ECF	?	?	Syrian hamster
MCAD deficiency		201450	Lipid myopathy; defective energy generation	DCM	Medium-chain acyl-CoA dehydrogenase	ACADM,1p	
LCAD deficiency		201460	Lipid myopathy; defective energy generation	DCM	Long-chain acyl-CoA dehydrogenase	ACADL,7	
Glycogen storage disorders							
GSD I	Pompe	252300	Lysosomal storage	Pseudohypertrophic CM; short P-R interval; ECF	α-1,4-glucosidase	GAA: 17q21-q25	Canine & bovine
GSD II	Adult acid maltase deficiency	232300	Lysosomal storage	Primarily skeletal muscle; respiratory insufficiency; cor pulmonale	α-1,4-glucosidase		
GSD III	Forbes; debrancher deficiency	232400	Intracellular glycogen accumulation fibrosis	Pseudohypertrophic CM	Amylo-1,6-glucosidase		
Phosphorylase kinase deficiency	GSD of the heart		Hypoglycemia	DCM	Phosphorylase kinase		
Glycoproteinoses							
Fucosidosis, severe		230000	Lysosomal storage	Myocardial thickening	α-fucosidase	FUCA1; 1p34	
Fucosidosis, mild		230000	Lysosomal storage	Angiokeratoma	α-fucosidase	FUCA1; 1p34	
Mannosidosis		248500	Lysosomal storage	Myocardial thickening; valvular thickening; conduction disturbance	α-mannosidase	MANB, 19p13.2-12	
Aspartylglycosaminuria		208400	Lysosomal storage	Valvular thickening	Aspartylglycosylamine amino hydrolase	AGA, 4q21-qter	
Mucolipidoses							
ML II	I-cell	252500	Lysosomal storage	Same as MPS IH	Acetylglucosamine-1-phosphotransferase	GNPTA; 4q21-q23	
ML III	Pseudo-Hurler polydystrophy	252500	Lysosomal storage	Valvular thickening and dysfunction, esp. AS, AR	Acetylglucosamine-1-phosphotransferase	GNPTA; 4q21-q23	
Mucopolysaccharidoses							
MPS IH	Hurler	252800	Lysosomal storage	Early CAD; PH and OAD→CP; valvular dysfunction, esp. MR, AR; pseudohypertrophic CM	α-L-iduronidase	IDUA, 22q11-pter	Canine and feline
MPS IS	Scheie	252800	Lysosomal storage	Valvular dysfunction, esp. AS	α-L-iduronidase	IDUA, 22q11-pter	
MPS IH/S	Hurler-Scheie	252800	Lysosomal storage	Same as MPS IH	α-L-iduronidase	IDUA, 22q11-pter	
MPS II	Hunter	209900	Lysosomal storage	Same as MPS IH; less severe in mild MPS II variant	Sulfoiduronate sulfatase	IDS, Xq28	
MPS III A	Sanfilippo A	252900	Lysosomal storage	Valvular thickening and occasional dysfunction	Heparin sulfate sulfatase	?	
MPS III B	Sanfilippo B	252920	Lysosomal storage	Valvular thickening and occasional dysfunction	N-acetyl-α-D-glucosaminidase	?	
MPS III C	Sanfilippo C	252930	Lysosomal storage	Valvular thickening and occasional dysfunction	acetyl-CoA: α-glucosaminidase N-acetyltransferase	?	

DISORDER	EPONYM OR COMMON NAME	MIM NO.*	PATHOGENESIS	CARDIOVASCULAR INVOLVEMENT	BIOCHEMICAL DEFECT	GENE LOCUS†	ANIMAL MODEL
MPS III D	Sanfilippo D		Lysosomal storage	Valvular thickening and occasional dysfunction	N-acetylglucosamine-6-sulfatase	G6S, 12q14	
MPS IV A	Morquio A	253000	Lysosomal storage	Valvular dysfunction, esp. AR	Galactosamine-6-sulfatase		
MPS IV B	Morquio B	253010	Lysosomal storage	Milder than MPS IV A	β-galactosidase		
MPS VI	Maroteaux-Lamy	253200	Lysosomal storage	Same as MPS IH	Arylsulfatase B	5p11-qter	Feline
MPS VII	Sly	253220	Lysosomal storage	Valvular thickening	β-glucuronidase	GUSB;7q	Mouse and canine
Sphingolipidoses α-Galactosidase A deficiency	Fabry	301500	Cellular accumulation of trihexosylceramide, esp. endothelium	Early CAD, valvular thickening and dysfunction; pseudohypertrophic CM; short P-R interval; arteriolar occlusion; angiokeratoma	α-galactosidase A	GLA; Xq22	
Ceramidase deficiency	Farber	228000	Histiocytic infiltration	Nodular thickening of valves	Ceramidase	?	
Glucocerebrosidase deficiency	Gaucher, adult form	230800	Cellular accumulation of glucocerebroside	PH→CP; interstitial infiltration of myocytes by Gaucher cells; constrictive pericarditis	β-glucocerebroside	GBA; 1q21	
Miscellaneous disorders Acid lipase deficiency	Wolman	278000	↑ Cholesterol; foam cell infiltration	Atherosclerosis	Lysosomal acid lipase	LIPA, 10q	
Acid lipase deficiency	Cholesterol ester storage disease	278000	↑ Cholesterol, foam cell infiltration	Atherosclerosis; PH	Lysosomal acid lipase	LIPA, 10q	
Geleophysic dysplasia		231050	Lysosomal storage	Valvular dysfunction	?		
Hereditary angioedema		106100	Complement and kinin activation	Angioedema	C1 esterase inhibitor	CINH, 11p11.2-q13	
Multiple sulfatase deficiency	Juvenile sulfatidosis	272200	Lysosomal storage		?		

CAD = coronary artery disease; DCM = dilated cardiomyopathy; ECF = endocardial fibroelastosis; CM = cardiomyopathy; AS = aortic stenosis; AR = aortic regurgitation; PH = pulmonary hypertension; OAD = obstructive airway disease; CP = cor pulmonale; MR = mitral regurgitation; GSD = glycogen storage disease.
* Data from Mendelian Inheritance in Man.[6]
† Gene symbol followed by chromosomal locus.

TABLE 51-11 DISORDERS ASSOCIATED WITH RESTRICTIVE CARDIOMYOPATHY

	MIM NO.*
Primary endocardial fibroelastosis	
Familial endocardial fibroelastosis	226000, 305300
Faciocardiorenal syndrome	227280
Secondary endocardial fibroelastosis	
as a relatively common manifestation	
Maternal lupus erythematosus	
Pseudoxanthoma elasticum	177850, 264800
Systemic carnitine deficiency	212140
Trisomy 18	
as a relatively infrequent manifestation	
Cornelia de Lange syndrome	122470
Rubinstein-Taybi syndrome	268600
Secondary infiltrative cardiomyopathy	
Familial amyloidoses I and III	176300
Fabry's disease	301500
Gaucher's disease type I	230800
Glycogen storage disorder II	232300
Glycogen storage disorder III	232400
Hemochromatosis	235200
Mucopolysaccharidosis IH	252800
Mucopolysaccharidosis II	309900

* Data from Mendelian Inheritance in Man.[6]

TABLE 51–12 MENDELIAN CONDITIONS AND MOLECULAR DEFECTS PREDISPOSING TO ATHEROSCLEROSIS

PHENOTYPE	GENE	LOCUS	MIM NO.
Cholesterol ester storage disease	Acid lipase	LIPA; 10q24-q25	278000
Hypoapo A-I; ↓ HDL	Apolipoprotein A-I	APOA1; 11q23-qter	107680
Hyperapo B; ↑ LDL	Apolipoprotein B	APOB; 2p24	107730
Hyperlipoproteinemia Ib; ↓ TG	Apolipoprotein C-II	APOC2; 19q13.1	207750
Hypoapo C-III; low HDL	Apolipoprotein C-III	APOC3; 11q23-qter	107720
Hyperlipoproteinemia III	Apolipoprotein E-II	APOE; 19q13.1	107741
Hyperlipoproteinemia Lp(a)	Apolipoprotein Lp(a)	LPA; 16q26-q27	152200
Hyperlipoproteinemia I; ↑ chylomicrons	Lipoprotein lipase	LPL; 8p22	238600
Hyperlipoproteinemia II; ↑ LDL	LDL receptor	LDLR; 19p13.2-p13.1	143890
Analpha-lipoproteinemia (Tangier disease); ↓ HDL	?	?	205400
Hyperlipidemia V; combined hyperlipidemia	?; probably heterogeneous	?	238400
Hyperlipidemia VI; familial hyperchylomicronemia & hyperprebeta-lipoproteinemia	?; probably heterogeneous	?	238500
Werner syndrome	?	?	277700

PRIMARY DISORDERS OF RHYTHM AND CONDUCTION

Virtually every dysrhythmia and conduction abnormality has been reported to occur in relatives. For example, *familial disturbance of conduction* occurs, without evident cause, at the sinus node,[191–196] atrioventricular node,[197–200] and bundle branches.[201–205] However, understanding the genetics of cardiac electrophysiology has been hampered by several characteristics of this extensive literature: Most families have been small, so that mode of inheritance, or even whether the inheritance is mendelian, is uncertain; many of the families show a mixture of different defects, partly because the disease is progressive[206,207]; and some specific conduction defects are associated with hereditary myocardial diseases, such as hypertrophic cardiomyopathy,[208] atrial cardiomyopathy,[209,210] and familial amyloidosis.[211] As noted earlier, there seems to be genetic control of normal electrical conduction, so it would not be surprising to find mutations in single genes that produced clinically important disturbance.

An important cause of complete heart block, though not mendelian, nonetheless involves genetic factors. The association between rheumatic diseases and heart block was clearly established when the offspring of mothers with acquired disorders of connective tissue, especially lupus erythematosus, were found to have complete heart block.[212–214] Many examples of "autosomal recessive" congenital heart block represent this familial, but nonmendelian, etiology. The risk is not related to severity of the maternal disease but is highest in children of women with antibodies to ribonucleoprotein (anti-Ro[SS-A])[215] and at least one allele for HLA-DR3.[216] Thus, it may be the maternal genotype that determines susceptibility to inflammation of the fetal heart at vulnerable periods, such as gestational weeks 3 to 4 when the atrioventricular node is forming. Genetic susceptibility to inflammation of the atrioventricular node of patients themselves is suggested by the relatively high association of HLA-B27 in adults requiring permanent pacemakers[217,218]; not all of these patients have overt evidence of HLA-B27–associated rheumatic diseases.

Familial dysrhythmia is also not uncommon. Nodal rhythm,[219] ventricular irritability,[220] and tachydysrhythmia associated with accessory atrioventricular pathways[221–223] have been reported in families. Hereditary cardiomyopathies are another cause of familial dysrhythmia, and a notable example is arrhythmogenic right ventricular dysplasia, an autosomal dominant condition with variable expression[224–226] (see also p. 763). In addition to these disorders, several syndromes involving prolongation of the Q-T interval deserve comment.

WARD-ROMANO SYNDROME (see also p. 1640). Familial syncope and sudden death have long been associated with ventricular dysrhythmia, but a distinct syndrome was not recognized until Ward[227] and Romano,[228] working independently nearly three decades ago, reported the characteristic prolonged Q-T interval. Subsequent investigations of numerous families have clearly established that the defect in repolarization is inherited as an *autosomal dominant.* Although a long Q-T$_c$ is consistently present, other abnormalities of conduction also occur, although they may not be evident on the resting electrocardiogram.[229] Ward-Romano syndrome is distinguished from the Jervell and Lange-Nielsen syndrome by inheritance pattern and the absence of hearing deficiency. Early suggestions of linkage of Ward-Romano syndrome to HLA[230] have not been substantiated,[231] and neither the gene locus nor the cause is known. Treatment with beta-adrenergic blockade or an automatic implanted defibrillator is effective. Individuals heterozygous for the mutant gene should be identified through a detailed family history and counseled appropriately.

JERVELL AND LANGE-NIELSEN SYNDROME (see also p. 1640). The association of familial syncope, sudden death, and congenital deafness was codified in 1957,[232] although as with most eponymous syndromes, reports of affected individuals occurred previously. As would be expected for a rare, autosomal recessive condition, the parents of affected children are more likely than average to be consanguineous. Although heterozygotes have normal hearing and no overt primary rhythm disturbance, the Q-T$_c$ intervals may be slightly prolonged.[233] The frequency of a long Q-T$_c$ among deaf children is about 1 per 100, so routine electrocardiographic screening of anyone with congenital deafness is warranted.

Neither the cause nor the pathogenesis is known. Fright and rage clearly precipitate syncope and sudden death, leading to the proposal of autonomic dysfunction as the basic defect. However, allotransplantation of the heart, thereby causing complete denervation, failed to correct the underlying problem in one patient.[234]

DISORDERS OF CONNECTIVE TISSUE

The two broad classes of disorders of connective tissue are those due to mutations in single genes that determine or somehow affect components of the extracellular matrix and those due to extrinsic factors affecting the extracellular matrix, such as rheumatoid arthritis and systemic lupus erythematosus. The former category includes many disorders that affect the cardiovascular system. Susceptibility to so-called acquired disorders of connective tissue is, in part, determined by genes, and this specific aspect will be reviewed. Disorders due to intrinsic factors acting on the extracellular matrix are discussed in Chapter 56.

Mendelian Disorders of the Extracellular Matrix

Close to 200 distinct phenotypes now comprise this category, which was first defined less than four decades ago with fewer than 10 disorders.[235] Several reviews and textbooks describe the phenotypes of many of the conditions, including their frequent cardiovascular matrix (Table 51–13).[16,236–242]

TABLE 51–13 CARDIOVASCULAR MANIFESTATIONS OF HERITABLE DISORDERS OF CONNECTIVE TISSUE

DISORDER		MIM NO.*	CARDIOVASCULAR MANIFESTATIONS
Cutis laxa		219100	PS, PPS, CP
		123700	MVP
Ehlers-Danlos	I	130000	MVP
	II	130010	MVP
	III	130020	MVP
	IV	130050	Arterial rupture, MVP
	VI	225400	MVP
	VIII	130080	MVP
	X	225310	MVP, aortic root dilatation
Osteogenesis imperfecta	I	166200	MVP, mild aortic root dilatation
	II	166210	CP, arterial calcification
	III	259420	MVP
	IV	166220	Aortic root dilatation
Marfan syndrome		154700	MVP, aortic root dilatation, aortic dissection
MASS phenotype		157700	MVP, mild aortic root dilatation
Pseudoxanthoma elasticum		177850	Arteriosclerosis

PS = valvular pulmonic stenosis; PPS = peripheral pulmonic stenosis; CP = cor pulmonale; MVP = mitral valve prolapse
* Data from Mendelian Inheritance in Man.[6]

MARFAN SYNDROME

(See also p. 1627)

This *autosomal dominant* disorder is relatively frequent (~1 per 10,000), occurs in all races and ethnic groups, and is often not diagnosed during life.[243-245] In light of the classic phenotype, failure to diagnose the Marfan syndrome may seem surprising; however, marked clinical variability, age dependency of all of the manifestations, and a high (~30 per cent) rate of new mutation all conspire to make detection of mildly affected, young, sporadic patients challenging.[246] The diagnosis remains based solely on clinical criteria, although progress on defining the biochemical basis[13] and the genetic locus[247] raises the hope of more definitive criteria. Current criteria (Table 51–14) depend on the manifestations in the cardinal organ systems—the eye, the skeleton, the heart, and the aorta—and other systems, and the family history[120] (Fig. 51–7). The presence of manifestations more specific for the Marfan syndrome ("hard criteria"), such as aortic dilatation, aortic dissection in a nonhypertensive young person, ectopia lentis, and dural ectasia, clearly are more important diagnostically than features common in other connective tissue disorders and in the general population, such as scoliosis, joint hypermobility, myopia, and MVP.

The most common cardiovascular features are MVP and dilatation of the sinuses of Valsalva.[243-246,248-250] Associated clinical problems of mitral regurgitation, aortic regurgitation, and aortic dissection account for most of the early mortality that results in an average age of death in the fourth and fifth decades.[251] Children tend to be more severely affected by mitral valve disease,[252-256] while aortic problems are progressive and more likely in adolescence and beyond.

MITRAL VALVE INVOLVEMENT. Mitral valve prolapse is age dependent and more common in women with the Marfan syndrome. The incidence reaches 60 to 80 per cent when patients are studied by two-dimensional echocardiography,[121,257] and generally the valve leaflets have an elongated and redundant appearance. Progression of severity, as judged by appearance or worsening of mitral regurgitation by clinical and echocardiographic criteria, occurs in at least one-quarter of patients,[258] a much higher rate than in MVP found in the general population.[259] The mitral annulus dilates and contributes to the regurgitation, as do stretching and occasional rupture of chordae. About 10 per cent of patients with marked prolapse have calcification of the mitral annulus. Standard treatment for chronic mitral regurgitation is indicated, but coexistent aortic root dilatation usually requires that increasing inotropy be avoided. When mitral regurgitation becomes severe enough to warrant surgical intervention, two considerations must be added to the balance: (1) Repair of the mitral apparatus is often successful in the Marfan syndrome,[260-262] although long-term prospective studies are not yet complete.

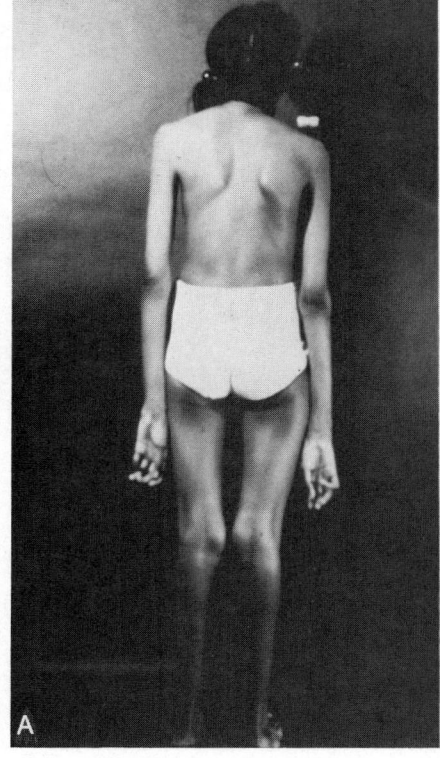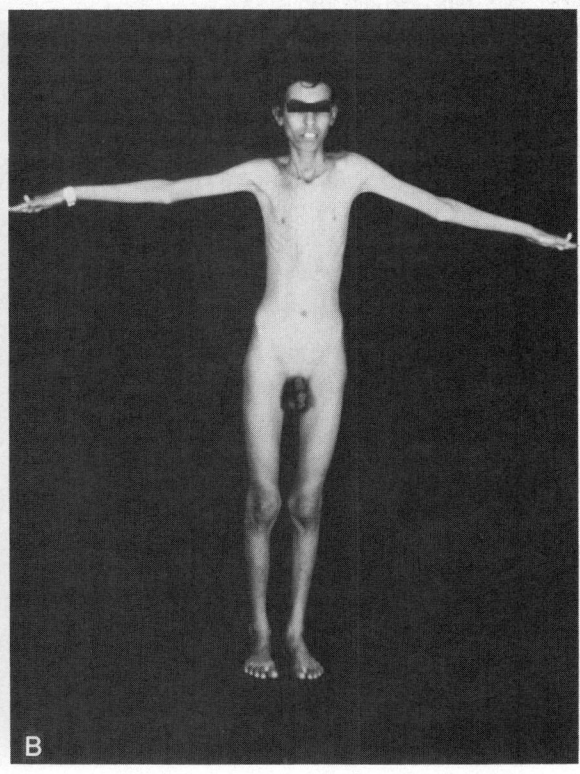

FIGURE 51–7. External phenotype of a boy with Marfan syndrome, showing long extremities and digits, tall stature, and pectus carinatum.

TABLE 51-14 DIAGNOSTIC CRITERIA FOR THE MARFAN SYNDROME:[120] PHENOTYPIC MANIFESTATIONS*

Skeleton
Joint hypermobility, tall stature, pectus excavatum, reduced thoracic kyphosis, scoliosis, arachnodactyly, dolichostenomelia, pectus carinatum, erosion of the lumbosacral vertebrae from dural ectasia†

Eye
Myopia, retinal detachment, elongated globe, ectopia lentis†

Cardiovascular
Mitral valve prolapse, endocarditis, dysrhythmia, dilated mitral annulus, mitral regurgitation, tricuspid valve prolapse, aortic regurgitation, aortic dissection,† dilatation of the aortic root†

Pulmonary
Apical blebs, spontaneous pneumothorax

Skin and integument
Inguinal hernias, incisional hernias, striae atrophicae

Central nervous system
Attention deficit disorder, hyperactivity, verbal-performance discrepancy, dural ectasia†, anterior pelvic meningocele†

If the family history is positive for a close relative clearly affected by the Marfan syndrome, to make the diagnosis in the patient, manifestations should be present in the skeleton and one of the other organ systems.

If the family history is negative or unknown, to make the diagnosis, the patient should have manifestations in the skeleton, the cardiovascular system, and one other system, and at least one of the manifestations indicated by †.

* Manifestations are listed within each organ system in increasing specificity for Marfan syndrome, although none is completely specific; those indicated by † are the most specific.

Repair is less easily accomplished when the cusps are extremely redundant, there is marked chordal damage, or the annulus is heavily calcified. (2) The aorta may be enlarged enough to permit concomitant replacement. We have often delayed mitral valve surgery for a time, carefully following ventricular function, until the sinuses of Valsalva dilated enough to make composite graft repair feasible.[263] On the other hand, when operation is primarily because of aortic dilatation, a mitral annuloplasty can be performed if there is more than trivial mitral regurgitation.[262] In Marfan syndrome, as in virtually all of the heritable disorders of connective tissue, there is an increased susceptibility to dehiscence of prosthetic mitral valves, regardless of the care taken in placing them.

AORTIC ROOT INVOLVEMENT. The sinuses of Valsalva are often dilated at birth, and the rate of progression varies widely among patients in general and also among relatives (Fig. 51-8). Thus, predicting long-term risks of developing aortic regurgitation (which is clearly positively associated with aortic root diameter[264]), suffering aortic dissection (which is less clearly associated with diameter), or requiring aortic surgery is fraught with uncertainty. Regular echocardiography is sufficient for detecting and monitoring changes in diameter, because in the absence of dissection, dilatation is limited to the proximal ascending aorta, and the rate of change is slow, measured in millimeters per year. Rare exceptions have been reported.[265-267] Patients with dilatation less than 1.5 times the mean diameter predicted for their body size[122,268] can be observed annually; as the diameter increases, more frequent evaluation is necessary. Aortic regurgitation often appears in adults at a diameter of 50 mm but may be absent at diameters of more than 60 mm.[264] The risk of dissection increases with the size of the aorta and fortunately occurs infrequently below a diameter of 60 mm. By that diameter, the coronary ostia have usually migrated distally in the sinuses, and the technical nuances of emplacing a composite graft are thereby eased. Many surgeons have adopted the criterion of a 60-mm maximal aortic root dimension for performing elective composite graft repair in Marfan syndrome patients, regardless of the severity of the aortic regurgitation,[263] although some operate even sooner.[269] The perioperative results of both elective and emergency repair of the aortic root have been excellent and a marked improvement from the pre-composite graft era that ended in the mid 1970's. Long-term results of operation are limited by the problems of endocarditis and anticoagulation, common to all prosthetic valves, but in the absence of chronic aortic dissection appear favorable for patients with Marfan syndrome.[265,269,270]

THORACIC ABNORMALITIES. Severe *pectus excavatum* may complicate cardiovascular surgery by making exposure of the heart by median sternotomy difficult. For elective cardiovascular surgery, repair of the sternal deformity some months in advance permits sufficient healing of the costochondral junctions that a stable and functionally and cosmetically improved thoracic cage will facilitate further surgery and postoperative recovery.[271] Simultaneous repair of cardiac and sternal defects, while possible,[271,272] is a long procedure, and intraoperative bleeding from bone can be considerable because of the anticoagulation associated with cardiopulmonary bypass.

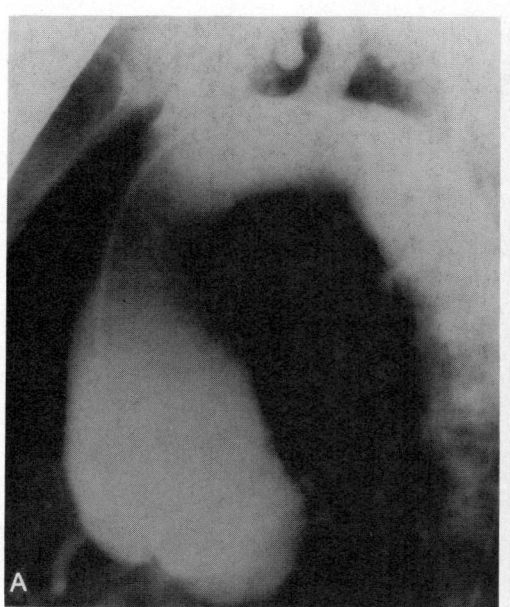

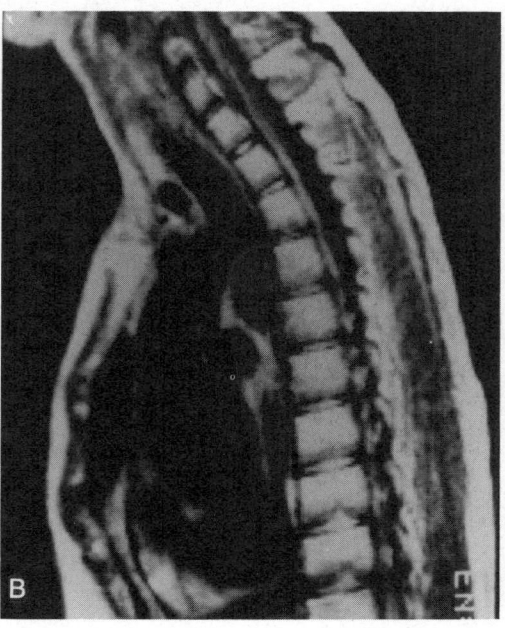

FIGURE 51-8. Dilatation of the aortic root in Marfan syndrome. *A,* Lateral angiogram of the ascending aorta showing dilatation of the sinuses of Valsalva and proximal ascending aorta and relatively normal caliber of the distal ascending aorta. *B,* Lateral magnetic resonance imaging of the same patient.

AORTIC DISSECTION (see also p. 1535). This complication usually begins just above the coronary ostia and extends the entire length of the aorta (type I in the DeBakey scheme) (p. 1535). About 10 per cent of dissections begin distal to the left subclavian (type III), but rarely is dissection limited to the abdominal aorta. Angiography (Fig. 47–13, p. 1539), magnetic resonance imaging (Fig. 11–40, p. 332), and transesophageal echocardiography all have a role in the diagnosis of acute dissection in the Marfan syndrome, with the capabilities and experience of the medical center and the stability of the patient important determinants of the approach. As many acute dissections of the ascending aorta in Marfan syndrome have a stuttering course that culminates in death from rupture or hemopericardium, rapid transfer to a facility prepared to perform immediate repair is essential.

Not all acute dissections in Marfan syndrome involve severe, tearing chest pain that radiates to the back; indeed, some extensive dissections have been occult.[263] This experience reinforces the need for a high index of suspicion by physicians whenever a tall, nearsighted young person with thoracic cage deformity arrives at an emergency department with vague complaints of lightheadedness, chest or abdominal discomfort, or a murmur of aortic regurgitation. Similarly, patients known to have Marfan syndrome and their close relatives need to be educated about the signs and symptoms of aortic dissection. In general, the management of acute and chronic dissection in the Marfan syndrome follows standard practice,[273] with several departures. First, all dissections of the ascending aorta should be repaired promptly, preferably with a composite graft. Second, regular evaluation with magnetic resonance imaging is important, as the diameter of any region of dissected aorta is likely to expand over time.[274,275] Third, reduction of systolic blood pressure and administration of negative-inotropic doses of beta-adrenergic blockers, regardless of blood pressure, should be even more strictly adhered to than in dissections without a connective tissue abnormality. In most instances, any region of the aorta should be repaired when complications of further dissection, branch vessel occlusion, or dilatation beyond about 60 mm occur. A staged approach to total replacement of the Marfan aorta is now both feasible and successful.[276]

DYSRHYTHMIAS. Some patients develop serious ventricular or supraventricular dysrhythmia. The latter often accompanies chronic mitral regurgitation, but the former may be of high grade and difficult to suppress when only mitral valve prolapse is present. Some patients have the syndrome of autonomic dysfunction, atypical chest pain, and palpitations seen in patients with mitral valve prolapse unassociated with a flagrant connective tissue abnormality.

MANAGEMENT. The routine cardiological management of the Marfan syndrome is multifaceted: regular clinical and echocardiographic examinations; routine endocarditis prophylaxis for dental and other procedures; restriction of activity from heavy weightlifting, contact sports and any exertion at maximal capacity; and chronic beta-adrenergic blockade form the basic approach, with individual variation often appropriate. Support for the role of beta-blockade comes from several prospective studies, as yet unpublished in full, that show a reduction in the rate of aortic dilatation and the risk of aortic dissection in patients treated with negatively inotropic doses of propranolol or atenolol.[277,278] However, short-term administration of propranolol to patients with large sinus of Valsalva aneurysms, while reducing heart rate and peak systolic pressure, did not improve the impedance characteristics recorded in the ascending aorta.[279]

A woman with Marfan syndrome has two concerns regarding pregnancy (see also p. 1797). The first is the 50 : 50 risk that any child will inherit the condition; currently prenatal diagnosis is not possible but will become available in the near future for most couples. The second is the risk of dissection that the hemodynamic stresses of pregnancy place on the aorta. Several dozen case reports attest the heightened incidence of dissection during the third trimester, parturition, and the month post partum.[280-286] However, in the majority of instances, serious aortic dilatation was present. The author observed 20 women with classic Marfan syndrome, whose aortic root dimensions were less than 42 mm, through 28 successful pregnancies with no change in the caliber of their aortas (unpublished data). Nonetheless, aortic dissection of the descending aorta has occurred during pregnancy in a woman who had little root dilatation.[281]

ETIOLOGY. The cause of Marfan syndrome seems likely to involve microfibrils, components of the extracellular matrix that are widely dispersed and perform multiple function.[13,287] Microfibrils form the scaffolding upon which elastin is deposited to form elastic fibers. Fragmentation and disorganization of elastic fibers in the aortic media have long been a histological marker (inappropriately called cystic medial necrosis) of Marfan syndrome,[243,288] although similar microscopic pathology occurs in familial aortic aneurysms and aging aortas of the normal population.[289] A defect in a component of microfibrils would explain all of the pleiotropic manifestations of Marfan syndrome.[14] In fibroblast lines from many patients, defects in the synthesis, secretion, or matrix assembly of fibrillin have been described.[289a] In addition, the gene for fibrillin maps close to the 15q15–q21.3 region[289b] previously identified as the site of the Marfan syndrome gene.[247a] Work is under way to define mutations in the fibrillin gene in patients.

MITRAL VALVE PROLAPSE AND THE MASS PHENOTYPE. This heterogeneous group of conditions, described above (p. 1634) likely contains large numbers of patients and families who have a defect of the extracellular matrix underlying the phenotypes. Whether some or many of these defects are related to the cause of Marfan syndrome should become clear in the near future.

EHLERS-DANLOS SYNDROMES

This group of heterogeneous conditions is linked by variable involvement of the skin and the joints, with hyperelasticity and fragility of the former occurring with hypermobility of the latter.[6,120,236] Mitral valve prolapse is clearly increased in frequency in most of the clinical types,[238,290,291] but aortic root dilatation is an uncommon finding. The most serious cardiovascular problems occur in *Ehlers-Danlos type IV* in the form of spontaneous rupture of large- and medium-caliber arteries. Various defects of type III collagen are the cause of the phenotype in virtually all patients studied.[16,292,293] In the classic syndrome, true aneurysms rarely form; rather, a rupture without dissection usually occurs as a catastrophic event. Most prone are the abdominal aorta and its branches, the great vessels of the aortic arch, and the large arteries of the limbs. False aneurysms[292] and fistulas[294] may be one result in those patients who do not die from the initial rupture. Vascular surgery is difficult, as the normal-appearing vessels around the rent fail to hold sutures. As a consequence, elective surgery to repair vascular anomalies, such as false aneurysms, that are causing no immediate problem is contraindicated in most cases. Ehlers-Danlos type IV is often sporadic but, when familial, is usually autosomal dominant. This genetic experience and studies of the type III collagen molecule and its gene all show that nearly all patients are heterozygous for a mutation in the type III collagen locus on human chromosome 2. The reason a defect in one-half of the type III procollagen being produced causes such a severe phenotype is the phenomenon of "protein suicide"; each mature type III collagen molecule is a triple helix of three procollagen chains, and the stoichiometry when half of the chains are defective predicts that only one in eight mature molecules will contain no mutant chain; this prediction has been verified by biochemical analysis.[16] Prenatal diagnosis is possible by examining collagen production in amniocytes. However, pregnancy is particularly hazardous to women with Ehlers-Danlos type IV because of vascular rupture and should be avoided on medical grounds.[295]

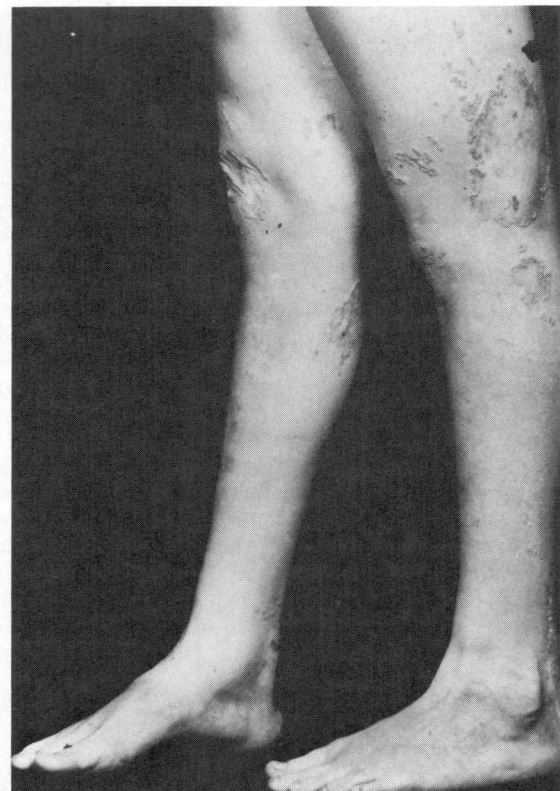

FIGURE 51–9. Legs of a patient with Ehlers-Danlos type IV who died of rupture of the subclavian artery. Note the mild joint hypermobility and the striking dermal abnormalities — elastosis perforans serpiginosa and thin, atrophic scars over areas of recurrent trauma.

PSEUDOXANTHOMA ELASTICUM

This is a clinically variable and genetically heterogeneous disorder of unknown cause. Histopathological examination of affected tissues show fragmentation and calcification of elastic fibers. The skin, the eye, the gastrointestinal system, and the cardiovascular system are the organs most severely affected.[120,236,296] The skin shows highly characteristic raised, yellowish papules (pseudoxanthoma) overlying areas of flexural stress, such as the neck, cubital and popliteal fossae, and

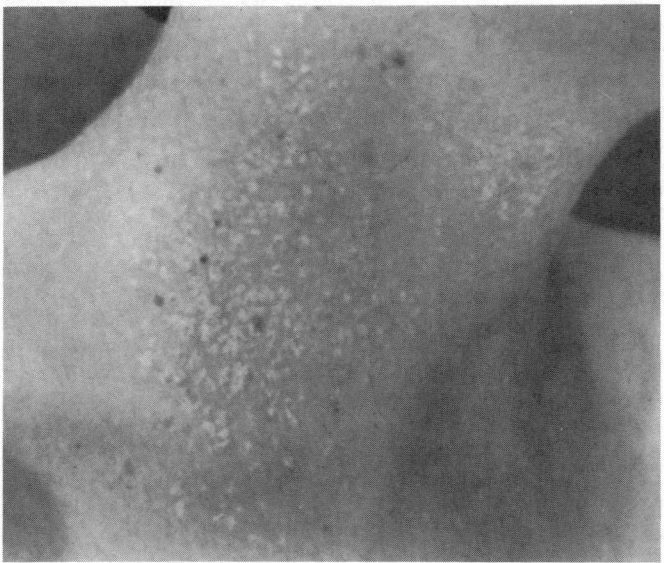

FIGURE 51–10. Skin of a young man with pseudoxanthoma elasticum. The neck is a typical location to notice the raised, yellowish papules from which the name of the condition derives.

groin. Breaks in the elastic lamella, Bruch's membrane of the choroid produce the funduscopic finding of angioid streaks. Gastrointestinal hemorrhage is common and potentially fatal; mucosal arterioles bleed, and because the calcified elastic fibers prevent effective vessel retraction, hemostasis is difficult. Selective arterial embolization was life saving in one instance.[297] The heart is affected in a number of ways. Endocardial fibroelastosis is common, but because primarily the atria are involved, a restrictive cardiomyopathy is uncommon. Mitral valve prolapse may be increased in frequency[298,299] but is rarely a clinical problem. Coronary artery disease with myocardial ischemia and infarction is the major problem and a common cause of early death.[236,300] Elastic and muscular arteries, including the coronaries, develop a type of arteriosclerosis similar to Mönckeberg's; progressive luminal narrowing occurs and can produce complete occlusion. Initially this is most evident at the radial and ulnar arteries, where absence of pulses and a positive Allen test are noted early in the course.[300] Because narrowing progresses slowly, collaterals form, and peripheral ischemia is a late complication. Because the arterial stenoses tend to be diffuse, bypassing them often involves extensive surgery. One patient with marked endocardial fibroelastosis was helped by resection of calcified elastic bands within the left ventricle.[301] Because the basic defect is unknown, no specific treatment is available. Because of a positive association between phenotypic severity and dietary calcium intake, patients can be advised to restrict consumption of dairy products and to avoid calcium supplements.[302] Hypertension and all risk factors for atherosclerosis should be aggressively controlled.

GENETIC SUSCEPTIBILITY TO ACQUIRED DISORDERS OF CONNECTIVE TISSUE

Genetic factors are clearly implicated in the susceptibility to many of the rheumatic disorders and to specific complications of specific conditions. The cardiovascular manifestations of these disorders are particularly interesting in this regard (p. 1723). For example, study of HLA-DR antigen frequencies suggests that immune-response factors are involved in the pathogenesis of chronic rheumatic heart disease in blacks.[303]

INBORN ERRORS OF METABOLISM THAT AFFECT THE CARDIOVASCULAR SYSTEM

The hundreds of biochemical defects that affect human metabolism have direct or secondary impact on the cardiovascular system (Table 51–10). Several examples will be reviewed, selected for their relevance to clinical practice or their instructive lessons about pathophysiology.

AMINOACIDOPATHIES

Inborn errors of amino acid metabolism result in the accumulation of precursors and a deficit of end products, either or both of which can be detrimental. In *alkaptonuria*,[304] an intermediate of tyrosine catabolism polymerizes to homogentisic acid, which readily accumulates in the extracellular matrix. Over many years, connective tissue of cartilage, heart valves, and arteries becomes increasingly abnormal. Aortic stenosis and arteriosclerosis are the cardiological sequelae.

Homocystinuria

This condition is caused by a deficiency of cystathionine β-synthase; the pathogenesis of the pleiotropic manifestations is largely unknown.[305] Perhaps the amino acid sulfhydryl groups bind to collagen and other macromolecules and interfere with cross-linking. The clinical features, once confused with the Marfan syndrome, include tall stature, skeletal deformity, ectopia lentis, mental retardation, psychiatric distur-bances, and a predilection for venous and arterial thromboses. Those patients with mutations that render the enzyme activity able to be increased by pharmacological doses of pyridoxine are less severely affected; early treatment can prevent most aspects of the phenotype.[306] Patients unresponsive to pyridoxine can be helped by a low-protein diet to reduce intake of methionine.

Myocardial infarction, pulmonary embolism, and stroke are the most common causes of death. The pathogenesis of the vascular complications was once thought to involve abnormal platelet function, but platelet survival in untreated patients is normal.[307] Controversy continues about susceptibility of heterozygotes, who have none of the external phenotype of the disease, to vascular disease.[308-310] Some epidemiological evidence suggests an increased risk of stroke, while challenging individuals with a methionine load appears to identify those who accumulate more homocysteine than normal and who have an increased chance of having atherosclerosis.[311]

DISORDERS OF FATTY ACID METABOLISM

While most organs can metabolize fatty acids when faced with hypogly-cemia, only the heart depends on fatty acids as the primary source of energy generation. Thus, it is not surprising that virtually all genetic defects in fatty acid metabolism, including generalized defects in mitochondria and peroxisomes, are associated with myocardial dysfunction. Other substrates—glucose, lactate, and oxaloacetate—also generate energy in myocardial cells by entry into mitochondria and the tricarboxylic acid (Krebs) cycle. Thus, defects in conversion of pyruvate to acetylcoenzyme A and in any point along the tricarboxylic acid cycle and the respiratory chain will have a major impact on myocardial energy generation. Quite likely, some sporadic and familial instances of idiopathic cardiomyopathy may represent undiagnosed or undefined metabolic disorders.

PRIMARY CARNITINE DEFICIENCIES. Carnitine is a required cofactor for entry of long-chain fatty acids into mitochondria and is both synthesized endogenously and available from dietary sources.[312] Deficiency of carnitine effectively blocks metabolism of long-chain fatty acids throughout the body and hepatic metabolism of ketones. Because of their relative dependency on fatty acids, muscle cells, including myocytes, suffer out of proportion to other tissue when carnitine levels are low for any reason. Cytoplasmic inclusions of lipid are characteristic findings in myocytes and hepatocyes.

Several mendelian defects exist leading to actual or relative carnitine deficiency. An autosomal recessive defect in carnitine palmitoyltransferase I leads to a skeletal muscle myopathy with little effect on the heart.[313] So-called systemic carnitine deficiency can be due to a variety of causes: primary deficiency of intake, synthesis, or function, and secondary deficiency, the majority now known to be a result of defects in fatty acid metabolism (especially medium-chain acylcoenzyme A dehydrogenase deficiency).[312,314,315] The latter group of conditions often do not respond to pharmacological doses of carnitine, whereas primary deficiencies often do.[315,316]

Primary carnitine deficiency usually presents in infancy with hypoglyce-mia, coma, and congestive heart failure due to dilated cardiomyopathy. In the few cases reported, problems largely resolve; they can be prevented from recurring by oral supplementation with l-carnitine[315-317] (p. 1436). Some of the infants with systemic carnitine deficiency have been shown to have a defect in carnitine transport, which leads to excessive urinary loss and which affects muscle but not liver.[315] Thus, muscle cells still may be relatively deficient in carnitine, despite supplementation, and long-term prognosis is uncertain at this time.[315,317]

MITOCHONDRIAL MYOPATHIES (see also Chap. 14). All of the enzymes of fatty acid oxidation are encoded by genes located on nuclear chromosomes, but the components of the electron transport chain are encoded by both nuclear and mitochondrial genes. Several syndromes involving various types of myopathies have been shown to be due to mutations in the mitochondrial chromosome.[11] The *Kearns-Sayre* syndrome includes pigmentary degeneration of the retina, ophthalmoplegia, and cardiomyopathy as its most prominent manifestations; all of the affected tissue have nearly exclusive reliance on oxidative phosphorylation for energy generation. Variations in both the actual mutations and the fraction of abnormal mitochondria in the cells of the different organs (heteroplasmy) account for many of the clinical differences in phenotype, severity, and age of onset among patients with this disorder. Inheritance is maternal for patients with mitochondrial mutations; apparent autosomal recessive and dominant inheritance may indicate that mutations of nuclear genes can impair electron transport similarly to mitochondrial mutations.[6]

The disease has been treated with moderate success over the short term with coenzyme Q[318] and with cardiac transplantation in one case.[319]

1645

CHAP
51

GLYCOGENOSES

Three of the glycogen storage disorders affect cardiac muscle.

GLYCOGEN STORAGE DISEASE II (see also p. 995). This *autosomal recessive* condition is due to deficiency of the lysosomal enzyme α-1,4-glucosidase and results in the lysosomal accumulation of glycogen in most tissues. Several allelic variants occur.[320,321] The condition with infantile onset is called *Pompe disease*, and cardiac involvement is profound.[322] The infant with Pompe disease appears well initially but soon fails to thrive and develops hypotonia, tachypnea, and tachycardia; the disease progresses during the first year to irreversible congestive heart failure and death from pneumonia or cardiopulmonary failure. Typically, auscultation reveals no murmurs until late in the course when obstruction develops, and hypoglycemia does not appear because the nonlysosomal pathway of glycogen catabolism is intact. The diagnosis is suggested by massive cardiomegaly on examination and chest radiography and by characteristic echocardiographic abnormalities of a short P-R interval and markedly increased QRS voltage.[239] Echocardiography shows tremendously thickened (pseudohypertrophic) ventricles, and Doppler interrogation or catheterization may reveal subaortic and subpulmonic pressure gradients characteristic of obstructive cardiomyopathy.

Reduced diastolic function of a restrictive cardiomyopathy develops eventually, and endocardial fibroelastosis is common.[323,324] With these findings, the diagnosis of Pompe disease is virtually certain, but it can be confirmed by analysis of α-1,4-glucosidase activity in cultured fibroblasts. Prenatal diagnosis is possible by enzymatic assay of amniocytes. Treatment is supportive, but cardiac transplantation could correct the cardiac problem; unfortunately, involvement of other organs, including the lungs, liver, and skeletal muscle might eventually prove just as serious as the cardiomyopathy. Bone marrow transplantation might be a solution if performed early in the course. An animal model of α-1,4-glucosidase deficiency exists in cattle and develops cardiac pathology typical of human Pompe disease.[325]

Cardiomyopathy may develop in the juvenile-onset form of α-1,4-glucosidase deficiency,[326] but it is not invariable because of allelic heterogeneity. In one sibship without cardiac involvement, three brothers had extensive hepatic, skeletal muscle, and arterial smooth muscle accumulation of glycogen, and each died of rupture of a basilar artery aneurysm.[327] The adult-onset form usually presents with insidious onset of respiratory insufficiency, and clinically important cardiac disease is rare.

GLYCOGEN STORAGE DISEASE III (see p. 1638). This autosomal recessive deficiency of amylo-1,6-glucosidase results in infantile- and juvenile-onset syndromes of muscular weakness, wasting, and hepatomegaly. Clinical cardiac disease is not common, although both cytoplasmic (nonlysosomal) and intermyofibril glycogen is routinely present in the heart and causes pseudohypertrophy. The diagnosis has been established by enzymatic assay of an endomyocardial biopsy specimen.[328]

GLYCOGEN STORAGE DISEASE IV. This is caused by deficiency of α-1,4-glucan:α-1,4-glucan 6-glycosyl transferase. It usually causes a fatal disorder of early childhood characterized by hepatic failure; although extensive deposition of polysaccharide occurs in the heart, death intervenes before cardiac symptoms appear. A child who developed exertional dyspnea and exercise intolerance at 7 years was found to have a dilated cardiomyopathy; this enzyme deficiency was diagnosed by endomyocardial biopsy.[329]

CARDIAC PHOSPHORYLASE KINASE DEFICIENCY. A single case of this enzyme deficiency has been reported; deposition of glycogen was confined to the heart, which was massively thickened and enlarged, and had caused the death of the 5-month-old infant.[330]

Glycoproteinoses

As shown in Table 51–10, this group of disorders results in the lysosomal accumulation of a variety of compounds that cannot be catabolized further because of the specific enzyme deficiency. Some have prominent cardiac pathology, generally of pseudohypertrophy and valvular thickening, which present with congestive failure, valvular dysfunction, conduction defects, or dysrhythmia.

HEMATOLOGICAL DISORDERS
(See Chap. 57)

HEMOCHROMATOSIS (See pp. 1419 and 1747). This is an autosomal recessive disorder of unknown cause that results in iron deposition in many tissues, including the myocardium. The manifestations include diabetes mellitus, skin hyperpigmentation, hypogonadism, hepatic failure with cirrhosis, hepatoma, and congestive heart failure; severity is considerably worse, and age of onset earlier, in men because of the autophlebotomy provided by menstruation.[331,332] The gene is located close to the HLA complex on chromosome 6, and presymptomatic diagnosis can be made in a family, even prenatally, by determining HLA antigen haplotypes and performing linkage analysis. Diagnosis in sporadic cases depends on finding increased serum iron, ferritin, and, especially, transferrin saturation in the absence of any obvious cause of excessive iron intake.[333] Fully 10 per cent of the population is heterozygous for the hemochromatosis mutation, suggesting that at an incidence of 2 to 3 per 1000, this disease is underdiagnosed.

Cardiac involvement often appears first as dysrhythmia or congestive heart failure. Dysrhythmia, conduction abnormalities, and low QRS voltage are typical electrocardiographic findings; cardiomegaly is seen on chest radiography; and a dilated cardiomyopathy with reduced systolic function can be documented on echocardiography.[334] Occasional patients have a restrictive pattern on cardiac catheterization.[335]

Treatment by repeated phlebotomy is most effective if begun before organ damage is irreversible. If a patient with congestive heart failure has not yet developed serious compromise in other organs, cardiac transplantation may be contemplated, as may combined heart-liver replacement.

HEMOGLOBINOPATHIES (see p. 1744). *Sickle cell disease* and other hemoglobinopathies associated with sickling can produce ischemia and infarction in multiple organs by occlusion of small vessels; however, the heart is relatively resistant.[336] Nonetheless, the combination of chronic hypoxemia and anemia produces a chronic high-output state that leads to congestive heart failure in many adults. The cardiovascular system can also be compromised by hypertension from renal infarction, pulmonary embolism and infarction (the chest pain of which often causes concern about myocardial ischemia), stroke, and hemosiderosis from chronic transfusions. In addition to a hyperdynamic congestive failure, iron overload is the principal risk to the myocardium in other causes of decreased erythrocyte production (*thalassemias*) and increased erythrocyte consumption (*hemolytic anemias*) requiring repeated transfusions.

MUCOPOLYSACCHARIDOSES AND DISORDERS OF TARGETING LYSOSOMAL ENZYMES

Many of the specific disorders in these two groups share phenotypic manifestations and are caused by various defects in the ability of lysosomes to catabolize proteoglycan and glycosaminoglycan. Short stature, progressive coarsening of facial features, a skeletal dysplasia termed dysostosis multiplex, corneal clouding, and protean effects on the cardiovascular system are common[236,238,337–340,340a] (Fig. 51–11). Only MPS IS

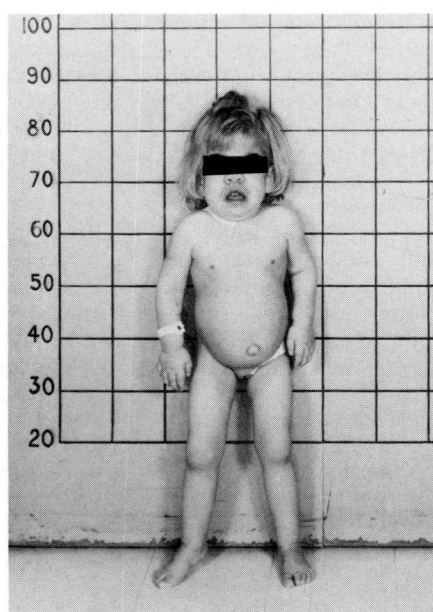

FIGURE 51–11. The Hurler syndrome in a 4-year-old girl. Note short stature and coarse facial features.

(Scheie syndrome), the mild form of MPS II (mild Hunter syndrome), MPS IV (Morquio syndrome), and MPS VI (Maroteaux-Lamy syndrome) have minimal or no mental impairment.

The cardiovascular complications (Table 51–10), which are all progressive and usually insidious, arise from engorgement of cells and tissues with macromolecular storage material.[238,341] First, the ventricular walls become pseudohypertrophic, and systolic function gradually deteriorates. The electrocardiogram shows reduced QRS voltages; rarely is any conduction disturbance present. Second, coronary arteries narrow because of intimal and medial thickening.[342] Myocardial infarction is common in MPS IH and the severe form of MPS II, although the patients are usually too retarded to complain of classic symptoms, and the diagnosis is made post mortem.[343] Third, valve leaflets thicken and cause progressive dysfunction that is oddly specific for individual disorders. For example, aortic stenosis is common in MPS IS, and mitral regurgitation is found frequently in MPS IH and MPS IV. Finally, narrowing of the upper and middle airways causes obstructive apnea, chronic hypoxemia and hypercarbia, pulmonary hypertension, and eventually cor pulmonale.[344,345,345a]

Until recently, treatment of children with those conditions that caused mental retardation has been supportive. Increasing experience with bone marrow transplantation in many of the conditions shows that, in the relatively few survivors of the transplant, somatic accumulation of mucopolysaccharide can be reduced, with clinical improvement in cardiopulmonary function.[337] However, improvement of central nervous system function has been marginal or absent. Nonetheless, bone marrow transplantation may have a role, especially in MPS IV and MPS VI, in which cardiopulmonary compromise can greatly shorten otherwise productive lives. Attempts at cardiovascular surgery, indeed of any procedure requiring general anesthesia, are fraught with risks of difficult intubation, hyperextension of the neck with cervical cord damage (the odontoid process is often hypoplastic), and prolonged efforts to wean from mechanical ventilation.[344]

SPHINGOLIPIDOSES

Fabry Disease
(See also p. 1626)

This X-linked condition deserves comment because the diagnosis is often not made until adulthood when serious end-organ damage has occurred.[346,347] As a result of deficiency of α-galactosidase A, ceramide trihexoside and other glycosphingolipids accumulate in lysosomes of many cells and organs, especially endothelial cells, glomerular and tubular cells of the kidney, and the heart. Microangiopathy causes the characteristic skin lesion, angiokeratoma, and may contribute, along with primary nerve involvement, to acroparesthesias and painful crises. Proteinuria and hypertension precede renal failure, which often has led to death in males and often leads by the fourth decade to the necessity for long-term dialysis or renal transplantation. A successful kidney allograft does not correct the systemic metabolic defect,[348] and the disease usually progresses in other organs.[349]

Structural and functional cardiac involvement is similar qualitatively to that in the mucopolysaccharidoses. Thickening of the myocardium is pseudohypertrophy from deposition of glycosphingolipid in lysosomes; the diagnosis has been made by endocardial biopsy during the evaluation of unexplained ventricular hypertrophy or frank obstructive cardiomyopathy.[350,350a] Chronic hypertension can exaggerate left ventricular dysfunction, as can ischemia and infarction from diffuse luminal narrowing of the coronary arteries. Two-dimensional echocardiography is useful for serial documentation of myocardial function.[351] Although valvular thickening and MVP are common, hemodynamically important mitral regurgitation is not.[351,352] The pulmonary vasculature becomes narrowed and right-sided pressures rise, but cor pulmonale is rarely a problem. The electrocardiogram often shows a shortened P-R interval, increased left ventricular voltages, and dysrhythmia. Medium-sized arteries throughout the body develop luminal narrowing, with cerebrovascular disease the most common cause of death after renal failure.

Heterozygous females generally show some clinical manifestations, especially in the eye, and at much later ages than hemizygous males develop renal, cerebrovascular, and cardiac disease.[346,351-353] Prenatal diagnosis is possible, and a detailed family history and genetic counseling are essential whenever the disease is found. The gene for α-galactosidase A has been cloned, and a variety of mutations identified, illustrating allelic genetic heterogeneity.[350a,354]

Familial Amyloidoses

(See also p. 1451)

A variety of disorders, defined initially by clinical phenotype and due to progressive accumulation of amyloid in organs and tissues, are beginning to be categorized by the underlying biochemical and genetic defects.[6,355] The several conditions termed familial amyloidosis with polyneuropathy, and originally classified as separate autosomal dominant disorders, are now known to be due to different mutations in the same gene encoding transthyretin, a thyroxine- and retinol-binding protein also called prealbumin. Although polyneuropathy dominates the early course during young adulthood, renal failure and restrictive cardiomyopathy supervene later and cause death in most cases. The age of onset, severity, and predilection for kidney and cardiac involvement are determined by the type of mutation, with males affected earlier and more severely.[356-358]

NEUROMUSCULAR DISORDERS

(See Chap. 60)

CARDIAC TUMORS

(See Chap. 44)

The three most common tumors that originate in the heart are myxomas, fibromas, and rhabdomyomas. All occur as part of hereditary syndromes and as sporadic events. The new occurrence of any of these tumors, especially in a child, may represent the first manifestation of a systemic condition, so a

detailed general examination and family history are always indicated.[359] For example, 51 to 86 per cent of cardiac rhabdomyomas occur because of tuberous sclerosis.[359a] Tumors due to hereditary disorders tend to be multiple and to recur after resection.

INHERITED DISORDERS OF THE CIRCULATION

Hereditary Hemorrhagic Telangiectasia

This autosomal dominant condition, often called Osler-Rendu-Weber disease, is more common than appreciated. Because of marked intrafamilial- and interfamilial variability, the condition may go undiagnosed in affected patients for years despite mild manifestations.[360] Mucocutaneous telangiectases occur on the tongue, lips, and fingertips most commonly (Fig. 2–4, p. 17). Small and moderate-sized arteriovenous fistulas occur in the nose, leading to recurrent epistaxis, in the gastrointestinal system, where they cause recurrent bleeding and occult anemia, and in the lung, resulting in hypoxemia, hemoptysis, polycythemia, clubbing, paradoxical embolization through the right-to-left shunt, and a hyperdynamic circulation. Less common sites of vascular malformations are the liver[361] and the kidney.[362] Diffuse ectasia of the coronary arteries was noted in one patient.[363]

Patients with this condition, and their close relatives, should be screened for pulmonary arteriovenous malformations through auscultation and a chest x-ray. A low arterial PO$_2$ should prompt consideration of angiography and therapeutic balloon occlusion of the feeding arteries of any sizable malformation to prevent systemic embolization, especially to the brain.[364] Danazol helps to reduce epistaxis.[365] Neither the biochemical defect nor the gene for hereditary hemorrhagic telangiectasia has been identified, and prenatal diagnosis is not yet possible.

Von Hippel-Lindau Syndrome

The features of this *autosomal dominant* condition involve malformations and abnormal growth of small blood vessels. Retinal angioma, hemangioblastoma of the cerebellum, and hemangioma of the spinal cord occur in association with renal cell carcinoma, pancreatic and epididymal cystadenomas, and pheochromocytoma.[366-369] Secondary hypertension due to renal disease and pheochromocytoma, which is often bilateral, occurs. The basic cause is unclear, but the gene has been mapped to the short arm of chromosome 3, so that prenatal diagnosis by means of linkage analysis is possible.

DISORDERS AFFECTING PRIMARILY ARTERIES

Mendelian disorders are associated with a diverse array of arterial pathology, and some have been described or catalogued earlier in this chapter. This section deals with two categories of disorders caused by a single mutant gene: pleiotropic syndromes better known for affecting organ systems other than the vasculature, and primary abnormalities of arteries.

ADULT POLYCYSTIC KIDNEY DISEASE. In the United States, this relatively common autosomal dominant disease affects a half million people and accounts for about 3 per cent of all long-term hemodialysis. Development of renal cysts is age dependent, and presymptomatic detection of heterozygotes, even by ultrasonography, can be uncertain into adulthood.[369a] About one-half of patients are hypertensive, one-half have hepatic cysts, one-half eventually develop severe renal failure, and an unknown (but probably high) fraction have colonic diverticula. Elevated plasma renin levels contribute to hypertension long before renal failure occurs.[369b] The cardiovascular manifestations include MVP in one-quarter, mild dilatation of the aortic root, occasional thoracic and abdominal aneurysms, and a predisposition to regurgitation of the aortic, mitral, and tricuspid valves.[370-372] The association of diverticula, organ cysts, and cardiovascular lesions reminiscent of, but milder than, the Marfan syndrome suggests an underlying connective tissue disorder.

The most serious vascular problem is typical "berry" aneurysms of the cerebral circulation, which occur in about 10 per cent of heterozygotes but which may remain asymptomatic throughout life. Hypertension predisposes to subarachnoid hemorrhage. How to screen for and treat intracranial aneurysms in patients without neurological symptoms remains controversial, with some advocating angiography and prophylactic surgery,[373] and others concluding that such aggressive management carries more risk than doing nothing.[374] The advent of high-resolution noninvasive screening techniques, such as magnetic resonance imaging, may well have altered the balance, and the analysis is worth repeating.

The gene for most cases of adult polycystic kidney disease has been mapped to a locus, PkD1, on human chromosome 16, but neither the biochemical nor the gene defect is known. In these families, presymptomatic and prenatal diagnoses are possible using DNA probes around the region where the gene is located.[375] In rare families, renal disease is unlinked to chromosome 16 markers,[376] and tends to occur later than in cases due to a mutation of PkD1.[369a]

ARTERIOHEPATIC DYSPLASIA. An autosomal dominant disorder of marked variability, *Alagille syndrome* causes neonatal jaundice and congestive heart failure in the most severely affected infants but may be asymptomatic in heterozygous relatives.[377,378] The cardiovascular findings include peripheral pulmonary artery stenosis in the majority, occasionally associated with septal defects or patent ductus arteriosus. Renal disease may produce hypertension. In some cases, a small deletion of the short arm of chromosome 20 (del[20][p11.2]) has been detected, suggesting the possibility that this complex phenotype is a contiguous gene deletion syndrome.[3]

ARTERIAL ECTASIA AND DISSECTION. Pedigrees abound in which dilatation of the aortic root, aneurysm of the abdominal aorta, aortic dissection without dilatation, or a combination of these problems occurs in an autosomal dominant pattern without evidence of a recognized heritable disorder of connective tissue.[379-381] Because of the variable presentation and natural history of the aortic disease, presymptomatic detection of presumed heterozygotes is uncertain, as is reassurance of relatives at risk who are of childbearing age and would prefer not to pass this condition to offspring. Until recently, no basic defect had been identified. In two families with autosomal dominant transmission of arterial aneurysms and mild increased skin fragility and bruisability, different mutations in the gene encoding type III procollagen have been found.[382,383] Thus, depending on the mutation, deficiency of type III collagen can cause the classic syndrome of Ehlers-Danlos type IV (p. 1643) or a form of the much subtler but just as deadly syndrome, familial arterial rupture. For these families in which the mutations have been defined, reliable presymptomatic and prenatal diagnoses are at hand.

Formal genetic analysis of 91 families ascertained through a proband with abdominal aortic aneurysm suggests an autosomal recessive predisposition exists for late-onset aneurysms.[383a] This study provides a rationale for offering ultrasound screening to sibs of patients with abdominal aortic dilatation.

FAMILIAL ARTERIAL TORTUOSITY. This is a rare, possibly autosomal recessive, condition of unknown cause. Diffuse ectasia of all systemic arteries occurs with, paradoxically, peripheral pulmonic stenoses.[384]

FAMILIAL INTRACRANIAL HEMORRHAGE. In addition to adult polycystic kidney disease, three syndromes predispose to subarachnoid or cerebral hemorrhage. *Berry aneurysms* without pleiotropic manifestations in other organs are a rare, but well documented, autosomal dominant trait.[385,386] A defect in type III collagen has been suggested by linkage analysis, but not by biochemical investigation, in several families.[387]

The *cerebral arterial type of familial amyloidosis* (type VI) is an autosomal dominant condition due to a defect in the proteinase inhibitor cystatin C.[388] This disease is rare outside of Iceland and Holland. The walls of cerebral arteries are thickened by a material resembling amyloid, and the vessels become tortuous and fragile. Recurrent cerebral hemorrhage is common in the fifth and sixth decades.[389]

TABLE 51-15   MENDELIAN DISORDERS ASSOCIATED WITH ABNORMAL BLOOD PRESSURE

DISORDER	MIM NO.*	PATHOGENESIS
Primarily elevated blood pressure		
Adrenal hyperplasia IV	202010	11-β-hydroxylase deficiency → ↑ 11-deoxycorticosterone
Adrenal hyperplasia V	202110	17-α-hydroxylase deficiency → ↑ 11-deoxycorticosterone
Aldosteronism	103900	↑ Aldosterone
Alport syndrome	104200	Renal failure
	301050	
Amyloidosis, familial visceral (amyloidosis VIII)	105200	Nephropathy
Arterial calcification of infancy	208000	Arteriosclerosis
Arterial fibromuscular dysplasia	135580	Renal artery stenosis → ↑ renin
Arteriohepatic dysplasia	118450	Renal dysplasia; renal arterial stenosis
Bartter syndrome	241200	2° to hyperaldosteronism
Fabry disease	301500	Renal failure; renal arterial stenosis; arteriolar stenosis → ↑ peripheral resistance
Multiple endocrine neoplasia I	131100	Adrenocortical adenoma → ↑ Cushing syndrome
Multiple endocrine neoplasia II	171400	Pheochromocytoma → ↑ catecholamines
Nail-patella syndrome	161200	Nephropathy
Neurofibromatosis type I	162200	Pheochromocytoma → ↑ catecholamines; and renal arterial fibromuscular dysplasia
Paraganglioma	168000	↑ Catecholamines
		Pheochromocytoma → ↑ catecholamines
Pheochromocytoma, familial	171300	↑ Catecholamines
Polycystic kidney disease, adult	173900	↑ Renin; renal failure
	173910	
Porphyria, acute intermittent	176000	?, but only during acute attacks
Pseudohypoaldosteronism, type I	264350	Aldosterone receptor deficiency
Pseudohypoaldosteronism, type II	145260	Defective renal secretion of potassium
Pseudoxanthoma elasticum	177850	Arteriosclerosis
	264800	
Riley-Day syndrome	223900	Dysautonomia
von Hippel-Lindau syndrome	193300	Pheochromocytoma → ↑ catecholamines
Wilms' tumor	194070	?
	194071	
	194090	
Primarily low blood pressure†		
Dopamine β-hydroxylase deficiency	223360	↑ Synthesis of epinephrine
Fabry disease	301500	↓ Peripheral vascular tone
Hyperbradykininism	143850	↑ Bradykinin
Pelizaeus-Merzbacher, late-onset	169500	?
Peripheral motor neuropathy and dysautonomia	252320	?
Pheochromocytoma, familial	171300	↑ Catecholamines (epinephrine)
Shy-Drager syndrome	146500	1° Autonomic insufficiency

* Data from Mendelian Inheritance in Man.[6]

† Does not include hypovolemia, obstruction of blood flow, and cardiogeneic causes of hypotension, each of which subsumes numerous hereditary disorders as primary causes.

Familial hemangiomas have been reported infrequently to occur as an autosomal dominant condition.[390] The brain and retina are the principal sites of vascular malformation, although in some pedigrees, cutaneous lesions occur. The intracranial hemangioma can be large and present with varied neurological symptoms, including hemorrhage.

FAMILIAL ARTERIAL OCCLUSIVE DISEASES. *Fibromuscular dysplasia* of the renal and other arteries occurs in *von Recklinghausen neurofibromatosis,* and along with pheochromocytoma can be a cause of hypertension.[391,392] The arterial lesion can occur by itself in families and produce stroke, myocardial infarction, intermittent claudication, and hypertension at young ages ranging down to childhood.[393] Inheritance is most consistent with autosomal dominance.[394,395]

Familial hypoplasia of the carotid arteries,[396] *familial arteriopathy* caused by concentric thickening of systemic and pulmonic arteries,[397] and generalized *arterial calcification of infancy*[398] are all rare, possibly mendelian, syndromes of unknown cause.

FAMILIAL PULMONARY HYPERTENSION (see also p. 804). Primary pulmonary hypertension is occasionally familial.[399–401] Inheritance is most consistent with an autosomal dominant predisposition with sex influence favoring expression in females.[6] The cause is unknown, but molecular defects favoring recurrent microemboli to the pulmonary circulation afford one area to explore.

Pulmonary hypertension can occur in *neurofibromatosis* due to pulmo-

DISORDERS AFFECTING PRIMARILY VEINS

VARICOSE VEINS. Although a familial susceptibility to varicosities of the lower extremity clearly exists, and favors women in a ratio of 2:1, mendelian inheritance has not been confirmed. *Marfan syndrome,* various *Ehlers-Danlos syndromes,* and an autosomal recessive condition featuring distichiasis (a double row of eyelashes)[403] predispose to varicose veins.

ATRETIC VEINS. Some patients with the *Klippel-Trenaunay-Weber syndrome* of cutaneous hemangioma and hemihypertrophy have atresia of the deep venous system.[404] The concomitant superficial varicosities should not be stripped, lest the remaining venous drainage of the lower extremity be removed. This is a confusing syndrome that overlaps with several others; mendelian inheritance is uncertain. Renal arterial aneurysm and hemangioma occurred in one patient.[405]

DISORDERS AFFECTING PRIMARILY LYMPHATICS

Several forms of *hereditary lymphedema* exist, with the best studied inherited as autosomal dominants.[6] An early-onset form bears the eponym *Nonne-Milroy lymphedema* and can cause a protein-losing enteropathy and pleural effusion. *Meige lymphedema* does not appear until about the time of puberty and is most severe in the legs, although one family with late-onset edema had involvement of the arms and face.[406]

GENETIC FACTORS PREDISPOSING TO ATHEROSCLEROSIS

A variety of genetic factors, in addition to the well-studied errors of lipid metabolism clearly predispose to atherosclerosis (Table 51–12; see also Chap. 37). Few genes outside of those involved in lipid metabolism have such an overwhelming impact as to be identifiable from family studies. However, genes that predispose to hypertension and diabetes mellitus, control arterial diameter, reactivity, and branching angles, affect platelet adhesiveness, and regulate endothelial and smooth muscle function can all be considered candidate genes for study in families predisposed to atherosclerosis.

ESSENTIAL HYPERTENSION

The role of genetic factors in essential hypertension is discussed on page 826. Blood pressure is a quantifiable trait that shows continuous variation within the population. Although many genes and environmental factors undoubtedly affect a person's blood pressure, familial transmission of some arbitrarily defined disease "hypertension" follows neither mendelian nor multifactorial inheritance.[407] A variety of cybernetic systems operate to maintain the blood pressure within tolerable limits. When this physiological homeostasis goes awry, or its limits are too lax, pathological and clinical consequences occur.[408]

A number of mendelian conditions, most of which are rare, cause major deviations of blood pressure from an appropriate physiological range (Table 51–15). These disorders are likely to be underdiagnosed.

Acknowledgment

Preparation of this chapter was supported by grant HL35877 from the National Institutes of Health.

REFERENCES

GENETIC FACTORS IN DISEASE

1. deGrouchy, J., and Turleau, C.: Clinical Atlas of Human Chromosomes. 2nd ed. New York, John Wiley & Sons, 1984.
2. Gardner, R. J., and Sutherland, G. R.: Chromosome Abnormalities and Genetic Counseling. New York, Oxford University Press, 1989.
3. Emanuel, B. S.: Molecular cytogenetics: Toward dissection of the contiguous gene syndromes. Am. J. Hum. Genet. 43:575, 1988.
4. Orkin, S. H.: Molecular genetics and inherited human disease. In Scriver, C.R., Beaudet, A. L., Sly, W. S., and Valle, D. (eds.): The Metabolic Basis of Inherited Disease. 6th ed. New York, McGraw-Hill Book Co., 1989, p. 165.
5. White, R. and Lalouel, J. M.: Genetic markers in medicine: DNA sequence variants in the human population reveal genetic basis for metabolic variation. In Scriver, C. R., Beaudet, A. L., Sly, W. S., and Valle, D. (eds.): The Metabolic Basis of Inherited Disease. 6th ed. New York, McGraw-Hill Book Co., 1989, p. 277.
6. McKusick, V. A.: Mendelian Inheritance in Man. 9th ed. Baltimore, Johns Hopkins University Press, 1990.
7. McKusick, V. A.: Online Mendelian Inheritance in Man [OMIM™]; contact OMIM User Support, Welch Medical Library, 1830 East Monument Street, Third Floor, Baltimore, MD 21205, Tel: 301-955-7058.
8. Goldstein, J. L., and Brown, M. S.: Familial hypercholesterolemia. In Scriver, C. R., Beaudet, A. L., Sly, W. S., and Valle, D. (eds.): The Metabolic Basis of Inherited Disease. 6th ed. New York, McGraw-Hill Book Co., 1989, p. 1215.
9. Prockop, D. J.: Mutations in collagen genes: Consequences for rare and common diseases. J. Clin. Invest. 75:783, 1985.
10. Clarke, A.: Mitochondrial genome: Defects, disease, and evolution. J. Med. Genet, 27:451, 1990.
11. Wallace, D. C.: Mitochondrial DNA mutations and neuromuscular disease. Trends Genet. 5:9, 1989.
12. Costa, T., Scriver, C. R., and Childs, B.: The effect of mendelian disease on human health: A measurement. Am. J. Med. Genet. 21:231, 1985.
13. Hollister, D. W., Godfrey, M., Sakai, L. Y., et al.: Marfan syndrome: Immunohistologic abnormalities of the elastin-associated microfibrillar fiber system. N. Engl. J. Med. 323:152, 1990.
14. Pyeritz, R. E.: Pleiotropy revisited: Molecular explanations of a classic concept. Am. J. Med. Genet. 34:124, 1989.
15. Schimke, R. N., McKusick, V. A., Huang, T., et al.: Homocystinuria. JAMA 193:87, 1965.
16. Byers, P. H.: Disorders of collagen biosynthesis and structure. In Scriver, C. R., Beaudet, A. L., Sly, W. S., and Valle, D. (eds.): The Metabolic Basis of Inherited Disease. 6th ed. New York, McGraw-Hill Book Co., 1989, p. 2805.
17. Antonarakis, S. E., and Kazazian, H. H., Jr.: The molecular basis of hemophilia A in man. Trends Genet. 4:233, 1988.
18. Kazazian, H. H., Jr., and Boehm, C. D.: Molecular basis and prenatal diagnosis of β-thalassemia. Blood 72:1107, 1988.
19. Südhof, T. C., Goldstein, J. L., Brown, M. S., et al.: The LDL receptor gene: A mosaic of exons shared with different proteins. Science 228:815, 1985.
20. Antonarakis, S. E., Waber, P. G., Kittur, A. S., et al.: Hemophilia A: Detection of molecular defects and of carriers by DNA analysis. N. Engl. J. Med. 131:842, 1985.
21. Diano, R., Bouchard, C., Dumesnil, J., et al.: Parent-child resemblance in left ventricular echocardiographic measurements. Can. J. Appl. Sport. Sci. 5:4, 1980.
22. Adams, T. D., Yanowitz, F. G., Fisher, A. G., et al.: Heritability of cardiac size: An echocardiographic and electrocardiographic study of monozygotic and dizygotic twins. Circulation 71:39, 1985.
23. Herrington, D. M., and Pearson, T. A.: Clinical and angiographic similarities in twins with coronary artery disease. Am. J. Cardiol. 59:366, 1987.
24. Moller, P., and Heiberg, A.: Atrioventricular conduction time—a heritable trait? I. Family studies. Clin. Genet. 18:454, 1980.
25. Moller, P., Heiberg, A., and Berg, K.: The atrioventricular conduction time—a heritable trait? III. Twin studies. Clin. Genet. 21:181, 1982.
26. Hawlik, R. J., Garrison, R. J., Fabsitz, R., et al.: Variability of heart rate, P-R, QRS and QT durations in twins. J. Electrocardiol. 13:45, 1980.
27. Dinerman, J. L., and Mehta, J. L.: Endothelial, platelet and leukocyte interactions in ischemic heart disease: Insights into potential mechanisms and their clinical relevance. J. Am. Coll. Cardiol. 16:207, 1990.
28. Yang, Z., Richard, V., von Segesser, L., et al.: Threshold concentrations of endothelin-1 potentiate contractions to norepinephrine and serotonin in human arteries: A new mechanism of vasospasm? Circulation 82:188, 1990.

29. Eriksen, N. L., Buttino, L., and Juberg, R. C.: Congenital pulmonary atresia with intact ventricular septum, tricuspid insufficiency, and patent ductus arteriosus in two sibs. Am. J. Med. Genet. 32:187, 1989.

30. Ferencz, C., Neill, C. A., Boughman, J. A., et al.: Congenital cardiovascular malformations associated with chromosome abnormalities: An epidemiologic study. J. Pediatr. 114:79, 1989.

31. Berg, K. A., Clark, E. B., Astemborski, J. A., et al.: Prenatal detection of cardiovascular malformations by echocardiography: An indication for cytogenetic evaluation. Am. J. Obstet. Gynecol. 159:477, 1988.

32. Schinzel, A. A.: Cardiovascular defects associated with chromosomal aberrations and malformation syndromes. Prog. Med. Genet. 5:301, 1983.

33. Clark, E. B.: Mechanisms in the pathogenesis of congenital cardiac malformations. In Pierpont, M. E. M., and Moller, J. H. (eds): Genetics of Cardiovascular Disease. Boston, Martinus Nijhoff Publishing, 1986, p. 3.

34. Hersh, J. H., Rees, A. H., Bloom, A. S., et al.: Cardiac malformations in trisomy 18 and 13: Specificity or nonspecificity? (abstr.) Proc. Greenwood Genet. Cen. 9:66, 1990.

35. De Biase, L., Di Ciommo, V., Ballerini, L., et al.: Prevalence of left-sided obstructive lesions in patients with atrioventricular canal without Down syndrome. J. Thorac. Cardiovasc. Surg. 91:467, 1986.

36. Kurnit, D. M., Aldridge, J. F., Matsuoka, R., et al.: Increased adhesiveness of trisomy 21 cells and atrioventricular canal malformations in Down syndrome: A stochastic model. Am. J. Med. Genet. 20:385, 1985.

37. Clapp, S., Perry, B. L., Farooki, Z. Q., et al.: Down's syndrome, complete atrioventricular canal, and pulmonary vascular obstructive disease. J. Thorac. Cardiovasc. Surg. 100:115, 1990.

38. Goldhaber, S. Z., Rubin, I. L., Brown, W., et al.: Valvular heart disease (aortic regurgitation and mitral valve prolapse) among institutionalized adults with Down's syndrome. Am. J. Cardiol. 57:278, 1986.

39. O'Brien, J. S., Geggel, R., and Feingold, M.: Mitral valve prolapse in Down syndrome (abstr.). Proc. Greenwood Genet. Cen. 9:96, 1990.

40. Schneider, D. S., Zahka, K. G., Clark, E. B., et al.: Patterns of cardiac care in infants with Down syndrome. Am. J. Dis. Child. 143:363, 1989.

41. Greenwood, R. D., and Nadas, A. S.: The clinical course of cardiac disease in Down's syndrome. Pediatrics 58:893, 1976.

42. Van Dyck, D. C., and Allen, M.: Clinical management considerations in long-term survivors with trisomy 18. Pediatrics 58:893, 1976.

43. Musewe, N. N., Alexander, D. J., Teshima, I., et al.: Echocardiographic evaluation of the spectrum of cardiac anomalies associated with trisomy 13 and trisomy 18. J. Am. Coll. Cardiol. 15:673, 1990.

44. Van Praagh, S., Truman, T., Firpo, A., et al.: Cardiac malformations in trisomy-18: A study of 41 postmortem cases. J. Am. Coll. Cardiol. 13:1586, 1989.

45. Lacro, R. V., Lyons Jones, K., and Benirschke, K.: Coarctation of the aorta in Turner syndrome: A pathologic study of fetuses with nuchal cystic hygromas, hydrops fetalis and female genitalia. Pediatrics 81:445, 1988.

46. Lin, A. E., and Garver, K. L.: Genetic counseling for congenital heart defects. J. Pediatr. 113:1105, 1988.

47. Allen, D. B., Hendricks, S. A., and Levy, J. M.: Aortic dilation in Turner syndrome. J. Pediatr. 109:302, 1986.

48. Natowicz, M., and Kelley, R. I.: Association of Turner syndrome with hypoplastic left-heart syndrome. Am. J. Dis. Child. 141:218, 1987.

49. Moore, J. W., Kirby, W. C., Rogers, W. M., et al.: Partial anomalous pulmonary venous drainage associated with 45,X Turner's syndrome. Pediatrics 86:273, 1990.

CONGENITAL HEART DISEASE

50. Fixler, D. E., Pastor, P., Chamberlin, M., et al.: Trends in congenital heart disease in Dallas County births: 1971–1984. Circulation 81:137, 1990.

51. Hagler, D. J., Edwards, W. D., Seward, J. B., et al.: Standardized nomenclature of the ventricular septum and ventricular septal defects, with applications for two-dimensional echocardiography. Mayo Clin. Proc. 60:741, 1985.

52. Helmcke, F., de Souza, A., Nanda, N. C., et al.: Two-dimensional and color Doppler assessment of ventricular septal defect of congenital origin. Am. J. Cardiol. 63:1112, 1989.

53. Lowell, D. G., Turner, D. A., Smith, S. M., et al.: The detection of atrial and ventricular septal defects with electrocardiographically synchronized magnetic resonance imaging. Circulation 73:89, 1986.

54. Simpson, I. A., Sahn, D. J., Valdes-Cruz, L. M., et al.: Color Doppler flow mapping in patients with coarctation of the aorta: New observations and improved evaluation with color flow diameter and proximal acceleration as predictors of severity. Circulation 77:736, 1988.

55. Brenner, J. I., Berg, K. A., Schneider, D. S., et al.: Cardiac malformations in relatives of infants with hypoplastic left-heart syndrome. Am. J. Dis. Child. 143:1492, 1989.

56. Pyeritz, R. E., and Murphy, E. A.: The genetics of congenital heart disease: Perspectives and prospects. J. Am. Coll. Cardiol. 13:1458, 1989.

57. Ursell, P. C., Byrne, J. M., and Strombino, B. A.: Significance of cardiac defects in the developing fetus: A study of spontaneous abortuses. Circulation 72:1232, 1985.

58. Whittemore, R. Hobbins, J. C., and Engle, M. A.: Pregnancy and its outcome in women with and without surgical treatment of congenital heart disease. In Engle, M. A., and Perloff, J. K. (eds.): Congenital Heart Disease After Surgery. New York, Yorke Medical Books, 1983, p. 362.

59. Rose, V. R., Gold, J. M., Lindsay, G., et al.: A possible increase in the incidence of congenital heart defects among the offspring of affected parents. J. Am. Coll. Cardiol. 6:376, 1985.

60. Nora, J. J., and Nora, A. H.: Update on counseling the family with a first-degree relative with a congenital heart defect. Am. J. Med. Genet. 29:137, 1988.

61. Boughman, J. A.: Familial risks of congenital heart defects (letter). Am. J. Med. Genet. 29:233, 1988.

61a. Murphy, J. G., Gersh, B. J., McGoon, M.D., et al.: Long-term outcome after surgical repair of isolated atrial septal defect: Follow-up at 27 to 32 years. N. Engl. J. Med. 323:1645, 1990.

62. Gold, R.J.M., Rose, V., and Yau, Y.: Severity and recurrence risk of congenital heart defects exemplified by atrial septal defect secundum. Clin. Genet. 32:148, 1987.

63. Nora, J. J., and Nora, A. H.: Recurrence risks in children having one parent with a congenital heart disease. Circulation 53:701, 1976.

64. Nora, J. J., and Nora, A. H.: The evolution of specific genetic and environmental counseling in congenital heart disease. Circulation 57:205, 1978.

65. Nora, J. J., and Nora, A. H.: Genetic epidemiology of congenital heart disease. Prog. Med. Genet. 5:91, 1983.

66. Sanchez-Cascos, A.: The recurrence risk in congenital heart disease. Eur. J. Cardiol. 7:197, 1978.

67. Corone, P., Bonaiti, C., Feingold, J., et al.: Familial congenital heart disease: How are the various types related? Am. J. Cardiol. 51:942, 1983.

68. Boughman, J. A., Berg, K. A., Astemborski, J. A., et al.: Familial risks of congenital heart defect assessed in a population-based epidemiologic study. Am. J. Med. Genet. 26:839, 1987.

69. Ferencz, C., Boughman, J. A., Neill, C. A., et al.: Congenital cardiovascular malformations: Questions on inheritance. J. Am. Coll. Cardiol. 14:756, 1989.

70. Maestri, N. E., Beaty, T. H., Liang, K.-Y., et al.: Assessing familial aggregation of congenital cardiovascular malformations in case-control studies. Genet. Epidemiol. 5:343, 1988.

71. Pierpont, M.E.M., Gobel, J. W., Moller, J. H., et al.: Cardiac malformations in relatives of children with truncus arteriosus or interruption of the aortic arch. Am. J. Cardiol. 61:423, 1988.

72. Natowicz, M., Chatten, J., Clancy, R., et al.: Genetic disorders and major extracardiac anomalies associated with the hypoplastic left heart syndrome. Pediatrics 82:698, 1988.

73. Rubin, J. D., Ferencz, C., McCarter, R. J., et al.: Congenital cardiovascular malformations in the Baltimore-Washington area. Md. State Med. J. 34:1079, 1985.

74. Ferencz, C., Rubin, J. D., McCarter, R. J., et al.: Congenital heart disease: Prevalence at livebirth (The Baltimore-Washington Infant Study). Am. J. Epidemiol. 122:31, 1985.

75. Beekman, R. H., and Robinow, M.: Coarctation of the aorta inherited as an autosomal dominant trait. Am. J. Cardiol.56:818, 1985.

76. McKusick, V. A., Logue, R. B., and Bahnson, H. T.: Association of aortic valvular disease and cystic medial necrosis of the ascending aorta: Report of four instances. Circulation 16:188, 1957.

77. Lindsay, J., Jr.: Coarctation of the aorta, bicuspid aortic valve and abnormal ascending aortic wall. Am. J. Cardiol. 61:182, 1988.

78. Wright, T. C., Orkin, R. W., Destrempes, M., et al.: Increased adhesiveness of Down syndrome fetal fibroblasts in vitro. Proc. Natl. Acad. Sci. USA 81:2426, 1984.

79. Weigel, W. J., Driscoll, D. J., and Michels, V. V.: Occurrence of congenital heart defects in siblings of patients with univentricular heart and tricuspid atresia. Am. J. Cardiol. 64:768, 1989.

80. Moreno, A., and Murphy, E. A.: Inheritance of Kartagener syndrome. Am. J. Med. Genet. 8:305, 1981.

81. Afzelius, B. A.: A human syndrome caused by immotile cilia. Science 193:317, 1976.

82. Afzelius, B. A., and Mossberg, B.: Immotile-cilia syndrome (primary ciliary dyskinesia), including Kartagener syndrome. In Scriver, C. R., Beaudet, A. L., Sly, W. S., and Valle D. (eds.): The Metabolic Basis of Inherited Disease. 6th ed. New York, McGraw-Hill Book Co., 1989, p. 2739.

83. Arnold, G. L., Bixler, D., and Girod, D.: Probable autosomal recessive inheritance of polysplenia, situs inversus and cardiac defects in an Amish family. Am. J. Med. Genet. 16:35, 1983.

84. Czeizel, A.: Familial situs inversus and congenital heart defects. Am. J. Med. Genet. 28:227, 1981.

85. Zlotogora, J., and Elian, E.: Asplenia and polysplenia syndromes with abnormalities of lateralization in a sibship. J. Med. Genet. 18:301, 1981.

86. Niikawa, N., Kohsaka, S., Mizumoto, M., et al.: Familial clustering of situs inversus totalis, and asplenia and polysplenia syndrome. Am. J. Med. Genet. 16:43, 1983.

87. Soltan, H. C., and Li, M. D.: Hereditary dextrocardia associated with congenital heart defects: Report of a pedigree. Clin. Genet. 5:51, 1974.

88. Mathias, R. S., Lacro, R. V., and Jones, K. L.: X-linked laterality sequence: Situs inversus, complex cardiac defects, splenic defects. Am. J. Med. Genet. 28:111, 1987.

89. Cyran S. E., Martinez, R., Daniels, S., et al.: Spectrum of congenital heart disease in CHARGE association. J. Pediatr. 110:576, 1987.

90. Oley, C. A., Baraitser, M., and Grant, D. B.: A reappraisal of the CHARGE associaton. J. Med. Genet. 25:147, 1988.

91. Freedom, R. M., Rosen, F. S., and Nadas, A. S.: Congenital cardiovascular

disease and anomalies of the third and fourth pharyngeal pouch. Circulation 46:165, 1972.

92. Temtamy, S. A., and Miller, J. D.: Extending the scope of the VATER associaton: Definition of a VATER syndrome. J. Pediatr. 85:345, 1974.

93. Weaver, D. D., Mapstone, C. L., Yu, P.: The VATER association: Analysis of 46 patients. Am. J. Dis. Child. 140:225, 1986.

94. Lynch, H. T., Bachenberg, K., Harris, R. E., et al.: Hereditary atrial septal defect: Update of a large kindred. Am. J. Dis. Child. 132:600, 1978.

95. Mohl, W., and Mayr, W. R.: Atrial septal defect of the secundum type and HLA. Tissue Antigens 10:121, 1977.

96. Kahler, R. L., Braunwald, E., Plauth, W. H., Jr., et al.: Familial congenital heart disease. Am. J. Med. 40:384, 1966.

97. Pease, W. E., Nordenberg, A., and Ladda, R. L.: Genetic counseling in familial atrial septal defect with prolonged atrioventricular conduction. Circulation 53:759, 1976.

98. Gall, J. C., Stern, A. M., Cohen, M. M., et al.: Holt-Oram syndrome: Clinical and genetic study of a large family. Am. J. Hum. Genet. 18:187, 1966.

99. Smith, R.R.L., Hutchins, G. M., Sack, G. H., Jr., et al.: Unusual cardiac, renal and pulmonary involvement in Gaucher's disease: Interstitial glucocerebroside accumulation, pulmonary hypertension and fatal bone marrow embolization. Am. J. Med. 65:352, 1978.

100. Muller, L. M., De Jong, G., and Van Heerden, K.M.M.: The antenatal ultrasonographic detection of the Holt-Oram syndrome. S. Afr. Med. J. 68:313, 1985.

101. Zhang, K-Z., Sun, Q-B, and Cheng, T. O.: Holt-Oram syndrome in China: A collective review of 18 cases. Am. Heart J. 111:572, 1986.

102. McKusick, V. A., Egeland, J. A., Eldridge, R., et al.: Dwarfism in the Amish: I. The Ellis-van Creveld syndrome. Bull. Johns Hopkins Hosp. 115:306, 1964.

103. Sherman, J., Angulo, M., Boxer, R. A., et al.: Possible mitochondrial inheritance of congenital cardiac septal defect (letter). N. Engl. J. Med. 313:186, 1985.

104. Preus, M.: The Williams syndrome: Objective definition and diagnosis. Clin. Genet. 25:422, 1984.

105. Maisuls, H., Alday, L. E., and Thuer, O.: Cardiovascular findings in the Williams-Beuren syndrome. Am. Heart J. 114:897, 1987.

106. Hallidie-Smith, K. A., and Karas, S.: Cardiac anomalies in Williams-Beuren syndrome. Arch. Dis. Child. 63:809, 1988.

107. Morris, C. A., Demsey, S. A., Leonard, C. O., et al.: Natural history of Williams syndrome: Physical characteristics. J. Pediatr. 113:318, 1988.

108. Chiarella, F., Bricarelli, F. D., Lupi, G.: Familial supravalvular aortic stenosis: A genetic study. J. Med. Genet. 26:86, 1989.

109. Ensing, G. J., Schmidt, M. A., Hagler, D. J., et al.: Spectrum of findings in a family with nonsyndromic autosomal dominant supravalvular aortic stenosis: A Doppler echocardiographic study. J. Am. Coll. Cardiol. 13:413, 1989.

110. Schmidt, M. A., Ensing, G. J., Michels, V. V., et al.: Autosomal dominant supravalvular aortic stenosis: Large three-generation family. Am. J. Med. Genet. 32:384, 1989.

111. Procacci, P. M., Savran, S. V., Schreiter, S. L., et al.: Prevalence of clinical mitral-valve prolapse in 1169 young women. N. Engl. J. Med. 294:1086, 1976.

112. Devereux, R. B., Kramer-Fox, R., Shear, M. K., et al.: Diagnosis and classification of severity of mitral valve prolapse: Methodologic, biologic, and prognostic considerations. Am. Heart J. 113:1265, 1987.

113. Wooley, C. F., and Boudoulas, H.: Mitral valve prolapse: A classification. In Boudoulas, H., and Wooley, C. F. (eds.): Mitral Valve Prolapse and the Mitral Valve Prolapse Syndrome. Mt. Kisco, N.Y., Futura Publishing Co., 1988, p. 3.

114. Devereux, R. B., and Kramer-Fox, R.: Inheritance and phenotypic features of mitral valve prolapse. In Boudoulas, H., and Wooley, C. F. (eds.): Mitral Valve Prolapse and the Mitral Valve Prolapse Syndrome. Mt. Kisco, N.Y., Futura Publishing Co., 1988, p. 109.

115. Strahan, N. V., Murphy, E. A., Fortuin, N. J., et al.: Inheritance of the mitral valve prolapse syndrome. Discussion of a three-dimensional penetrance model. Am. J. Med. 74:967, 1983.

116. Pini, R., Greppi, B., Kramer-Fox, R., et al.: Mitral valve dimensions and motion and familial transmission of mitral valve prolapse with and without mitral leaflet billowing. J. Am. Coll. Cardiol. 12:1423, 1988.

117. Henney, A. M., Schwartz, R. C., Child, A. H., et al.: Genetic evidence that mutations in the COL1A2, COL3A1 or COL5A2 collagen genes are not responsible for mitral valve prolapse. Br. Heart J. 61:292, 1989.

118. Hickey, A. J., Narunsky, L., and Wilcken, D.E.L.: Bodily habitus and mitral valve prolapse. Aust. N. Z. J. Med. 15:326, 1985.

119. Devereux, R. B., Brown, W. T., Lutas, E. M., et al.: Association of mitral valve prolapse with low body weight and low blood pressure. Lancet 2:792, 1982.

120. Beighton, P., de Paepe, A., Danks, D., et al.: International nosology of heritable disorders of connective tissue, Berlin, 1986. Am. J. Med. Genet. 29:581, 1988.

121. Roman, M. J., Devereux, R. B., Kramer-Fox, R., et al.: Comparison of cardiovascular and skeletal features of primary mitral valve prolapse and the Marfan syndrome. Am. J. Cardiol. 3:317, 1989.

122. Glesby, M. J., and Pyeritz, R. E.: Association of mitral valve prolapse and systemic abnormalities of connective tissue: A phenotypic continuum. J.A.M.A. 262:523, 1989.

123. Hirschfeld, S. S., Rudner, C., Nash, C. L. Jr., et al.: Incidence of mitral valve prolapse in adolescent scoliosis and thoracic kyphoscoliosis. Pediatrics 70:451, 1982.

124. Chen, W.W.C., Chan, F. L., Wong, P.H.C., et al.: Familial occurrence of

125. Shamberger, R. C., Welch, K. J., and Sanders, S. P.: Mitral valve prolapse associated with pectus excavatum. J. Pediatr. 111:404, 1987.

126. Rogan, K., Sears-Rogan, P., Vermani, R., et al.: Familial myxomatous valvular disease. Am. J. Cardiol. 63:1149, 1989.

127. Mendez, H.M.M., and Opitz, J. M.: Noonan syndrome: A review. Am. J. Med. Genet. 21:493, 1985.

128. Caralis, D. G., Char, F., Graber, J. D., et al.: Delineation of multiple cardiac anomalies associated with the Noonan syndrome in an adult and review of the literature. Johns Hopkins Med. J. 134:346, 1974.

129. Allanson, J. E., Hall, J. G., Hughes, H. E., et al.: Noonan syndrome: The changing phenotype. Am. J. Med. Genet. 21:507, 1985.

130. Van Der Hauwaert, L. G., Fryns, J. P., Dumoulin, M., et al.: Cardiovascular malformations in Turner's and Noonan's syndrome. Br. Heart J. 40:500, 1978.

131. Noonan, J. A., and Ehmke, D. A.: Associated noncardiac malformations in children with congenital heart disease. J. Pediatr. 63:468, 1963.

132. Pearl, W.: Cardiovascular anomalies in Noonan's syndrome. Chest 71:677, 1977.

133. Phornphutkul, C., Rosenthal, A., and Nadas, A. S.: Cardiomyopathy in Noonan's syndrome. Br. Heart J. 35:99, 1973.

134. Battiste, C. E., Feldt, R. H., and Lie, J. T.: Congestive cardiomyopathy in Noonan's syndrome. Mayo Clin. Proc. 52:661, 1977.

134a. Wong, C.-K., Cheng, C.-H., Lau, C.-P., et al.: Congenital coronary artery anomalies in Noonan's syndrome. Am. Heart J. 119:396, 1990.

135. Miller, M., and Motulsky, A. G.: Noonan syndrome in an adult family presenting with chronic lymphedema. Am. J. Med. 65:379, 1978.

136. Quattrin, T., McPherson, E., and Putnam, T.: Vertical transmission of the neurofibromatosis/Noonan syndrome. Am. J. Med. Genet. 26:645, 1987.

137. Kitchens, C. S., and Alexander, J. A.: Partial deficiency of coagulation factor XI as a newly recognized feature of Noonan syndrome. J. Pediatr. 102:224, 1983.

138. Khoury, M. J., Becerra, J. E., Cordero, J. F., et al.: Clinical-epidemiologic assessment of patterns of birth defects associated with human teratogens: Application to diabetic embryopathy. Pediatrics 83:658, 1989.

139. Beckman, D. A., and Brent, R. L.: Mechanisms of teratogenesis. Annu. Rev. Pharmacol. Toxicol. 24:483, 1984.

140. Jones, K. L.: Fetal alcohol syndrome. Pediatr. Rev. 8:122, 1986.

141. Finnell, R. H., and Chernoff, G. F.: Genetic background. The elusive component in the fetal hydantoin syndrome. Am. J. Med. Genet. 19:459, 1984.

142. Strickler, S. M., Dansky, L. V., Miller, M. A., et al.: Genetic predisposition to phenytoin-induced birth defects. Lancet 2:746, 1985.

143. Lammer, E. J.: Retinoic acid embryopathy. N. Engl. J. Med. 313:837, 1985.

144. Hall, J. G., Pauli, R. M., and Wilson, K. M.: Maternal and fetal sequelae of anticoagulation during pregnancy. Am. J. Med. 68:122, 1980.

145. Scriver, C. R., Kaufman, S., and Woo, S.L.C.: The hyperphenylalaninemias. In Scriver, C. R., Beaudet, A. L., Sly, W. S., and Valle, D. (eds.): The Metabolic Basis of Inherited Disease, 6th ed. New York, McGraw-Hill Book Co., 1989, p. 495.

146. Lenke, R. R., and Levy, H. L.: Maternal phenylketonuria and hyperphenylalaninemia. N. Engl. J. Med. 303:1202, 1980.

CARDIOMYOPATHIES

147. Maron, B. J., Bonow, R. O., Cannon, R. O., III, et al.: Hypertrophic cardiomyopathy: Interrelations of clinical manifestations, pathophysiology, and therapy. N. Engl. J. Med. 316:780;844, 1987.

148. Bulkley, B. H., Weisfeldt, M. L., and Hutchins, G. M.: Asymmetric septal hypertrophy and myocardial fiber disarray: Features of normal, developing, and malformed hearts. Circulation 56:292, 1977.

149. Maron, B. J., Nichols, P. F., III, Pickle, L. W., et al.: Patterns of inheritance in hypertrophic cardiomyopathy: Assessment by M-mode and two-dimensional echocardiography. Am. J. Cardiol. 53:1087, 1984.

150. Maron, B. J., and Mulvihill, J. J.: The genetics of hypertrophic cardiomyopathy. Ann. Intern. Med. 105:610, 1986.

151. ten Cate, F. J., Hugenholtz, P. G., van Dorp, W. G., et al.: Prevalence of diagnostic abnormalities in patients with genetically transmitted asymmetric septal hypertrophy. Am. J. Cardiol. 43:731, 1979.

151a. Ferraro, M., Scarton, G., and Ambrosini, M.: Cosegregation of hypertrophic cardiomyopathy and a fragile site on chromosome 16 in a large Italian family. J. Med. Genet. 27:363, 1990.

151b. Epstein, N. D., Lin, H. J., and Fananapazir, L.: Genetic evidence of dissociation (generational skips) of electrical from morphologic forms of hypertrophic cardiomyopathy. Am. J. Cardiol. 66:627, 1990.

152. Greaves, S. C., Roche, A.H.G., Neutze, J. M., et al.: Inheritance of hypertrophic cardiomyopathy: A cross sectional and M mode echocardiographic study of 50 families. Br. Heart J. 58:259, 1987.

153. Cirò, E., Nichols, P. F., and Maron, B. J.: Heterogeneous morphologic expression of genetically transmitted hypertrophic cardiomyopathy: Two-dimensional echocardiographic analysis. Circulation 67:1227, 1983.

154. Penas, M., Fuster, M., Fabregas, R., et al.: Familial apical hypertrophic cardiomyopathy. Am. J. Cardiol. 62:821, 1988.

155. Jarcho, J. A., McKenna, W., Pare, J.A.P., et al.: Mapping a gene for familial hypertrophic cardiomyopathy to chromosome 14q1. N. Engl. J. Med. 321:1372, 1989.

155a. Solomon, S. D., Geisterfer-Lowrance, A.A.T., Vosberg, H.-P., et al.: A locus for familial hypertrophic cardiomyopathy is closely linked to the cardiac myosin heavy chain genes, CRI-L436, and CRI-L329 on chromosome 14 at q11-q12. Am. J. Hum. Genet. 47:389, 1990.

155b. Solomon, S.D., Jarcho, J. A., McKenna, W., et al.: Familial hypertrophic cardiomyopathy is a genetically heterogeneous disease. J. Clin. Invest. 86:993, 1990.

156. Ferraro, M., Scarton, G., and Ambrosini, M.: Cosegregation of hypertrophic cardiomyopathy and a fragile site on chromosome 16 in a large Italian family. J. Med. Genet. 27:363, 1990.

157. Codd, M. B., Sugrue, D. D., Gersh, B. J., et al.: Epidemiology of idiopathic dilated and hypertrophic cardiomyopathy: A population-based study in Olmsted County, Minnesota, 1975–1984. Circulation 80:564, 1989.

158. Michels, V. V., Moll, P. P., Miller, F. A., et al.: Frequency of familial dilated cardiomyopathy in an unselected series of patients with idiopathic dilated cardiomyopathy (abstr.). Am. J. Hum. Genet. 45:A55, 1989.

159. Fragola, P. V., Autore, C., Picelli, A., et al.: Familial idiopathic dilated cardiomyopathy. Am. Heart J. 115:912, 1988.

160. Valantine, H. A., Hunt, S. A., Fowler, M. B., et al.: Frequency of familial nature of dilated cardiomyopathy and usefulness of cardiac transplantation in this subset. Am. J. Cardiol. 63:959, 1989.

161. Michels, V. V., Driscoll, D. J., and Miller, F. A., Jr.: Familial aggregation of idiopathic dilated cardiomyopathy. Am. J. Cardiol. 55:1232, 1985.

162. Emanuel, R., Withers, R., and O'Brien, K.: Dominant and recessive modes of inheritance in idiopathic cardiomyopathy. Lancet 2:1065, 1971.

163. Graber, H. L., Unverferth, D. V., Baker, P. B., et al.: Evolution of a hereditary cardiac conduction and muscle disorder: A study involving a family with six generations affected. Circulation 74:21, 1986.

164. Gardner, R.J.M., Hanson, J. W., Ionasescu, V. V., et al.: Dominantly inherited dilated cardiomyopathy. Am. J. Med. Genet. 27:61, 1987.

165. Maclennan, B. A., Tsoi, E. Y., Maguire, C., et al.: Familial idiopathic congestive cardiomyopathy in three generations: A family study with eight affected members. Q. J. Med. 63:335, 1987.

166. Schmidt, M. A., Michels, V. V., Edwards, W. D., et al.: Familial dilated cardiomyopathy. Am. J. Med. Genet. 31:135, 1988.

167. Koike, S., Kawa, S., Yabu, K., et al.: Familial dilated cardiomyopathy and human leucocyte antigen: A report of two family cases. Jpn. Heart J. 28:941, 1987.

168. Przybojewski, J. Z., Vanderwalt, J. J., Vaneeden, P. J., et al.: Familial dilated (congestive) cardiomyopathy. Occurrence in two brothers and an overview of the literature. S. Afr. Med. J. 66:26, 1984.

169. Goldblatt, J., Melmed, J., and Rose, A. G.: Autosomal recessive inheritance of idiopathic dilated cardiomyopathy in a Madeira Portuguese kindred. Clin. Genet. 31:249, 1987.

170. Berko, B. A., and Swift, M.: X-linked dilated cardiomyopathy. N. Engl. J. Med. 316:1186, 1987.

171. Caforio, A.L.P., Rossi, B., and Risaliti, R.: Type 1 fiber abnormalities in skeletal muscle of patients with hypertrophic and dilated cardiomyopathy: Evidence of subclinical myogenic myopathy. J. Am. Coll. Cardiol. 14:1464, 1989.

172. Hubner, G., and Grantzow, R.: Mitochondrial cardiomyopathy with involvement of skeletal muscles. Virchows Arch 399:115, 1983.

173. Urie, P. M., and Billingham, M. E.: Ultrastructural features of familial cardiomyopathy. Am. J. Cardiol. 62:325, 1988.

174. Anderson, J. L., Carlquist, J. F., Lutz, J. R., et al.: HLA A, B and DR typing in idiopathic dilated cardiomyopathy: A search for immune response factors. Am. J. Cardiol. 53:1326, 1984.

175. Voss, E. G., Reddy, C.V.R., Detrano, R., et al.: Familial dilated cardiomyopathy. Am. J. Cardiol. 54:456, 1984.

176. Aroney, C., Bett, N., and Radford, D.: Familial restrictive cardiomyopathy. Aust. N. Z. J. Med. 18:877, 1988.

177. Fitzpatrick, A. P., Shapiro, L. M., Rickards, A. F., et al.: Familial restrictive cardiomyopathy with atrioventricular block and skeletal myopathy. Br. Heart J. 63:114, 1990.

178. Hodgson, S., Child, A., and Dyson, M.: Endocardial fibroelastosis: Possible X-linked inheritance. J. Med. Genet. 24:210, 1987.

179. Barth, P. G., Scholte, J. A., Berden, J. A., et al.: An X-linked mitochondrial disease affecting cardiac muscle, skeletal muscle and neutrophil leukocytes. J. Neurol. Sci. 62:327, 1983.

180. Chen, S.-H, Thompson, M. W., and Rose, V.: Endocardial fibroelastosis: Family studies with special reference to counseling. J. Pediatr. 79:385, 1971.

181. Hallidie-Smith, K. A., and Olsen, E.G.J.: Endocardial fibro-elastosis, mitral incompetence, and coarctation of abdominal aorta: A report of 3 sibs. Br. Heart J. 30:850, 1968.

182. Opitz, J. M.: Genetic aspects of endocardial fibroelastosis. Am. J. Med. Genet. 11:92, 1982.

183. Ross, R. S., Bulkley, B. H., Hutchins, G. M., et al.: Idiopathic familial myocardiopathy in three generations: A clinical and pathologic study. Am. Heart J. 96:170, 1978.

184. Fitzpatrick, A. P., and Emanuel, R. W.: Familial neurofibromatosis and hypertrophic cardiomyopathy. Br. Heart J. 60:247, 1988.

185. Sommer, A., Contras, S. B., Craenen, J. M., et al.: A family study of the leopard syndrome. Am. J. Dis. Child. 121:520, 1971.

186. St. John Sutton, M. G., Tajik, A. J., Giuliani, E. R., et al.: Hypertrophic obstructive cardiomyopathy and lentiginosis: A little known neural ectodermal syndrome. Am. J. Cardiol. 47:214, 1981.

187. Voorhees, M. L., Hussan, G. S., and Blackman, M. S.: Growth failure with pericardial constriction: The syndrome of mulibrey nanism. Am. J. Dis. Child. 130:1146, 1976.

188. Martinez-Lavin, M., Buendia, A., Delgado, E., et al.: A familial syndrome of pericarditis, arthritis and camptodactyly. N. Engl. J. Med. 309:224, 1983.

189. Laxer, R. M., Cameron, B. J., Chaisson, D., et al.: The camptodactyly-arthropathy-pericarditis syndrome: Case report and literature review. Arthritis Rheum. 29:439, 1986.

190. Bulutlar, G., Yazici, H., Ozdogan, H., et al.: A familial syndrome of pericarditis, arthritis, camptodactyly, and coxa vara. Arthritis Rheum. 29:436, 1986.

DISORDERS OF RHYTHM AND CONDUCTION

191. Gambetta, M., Weese, J., Ginsburg, M., et al.: Sick sinus syndrome in a patient with familial PR prolongation. Chest 64:520, 1973.

192. Livesley, B., Catley, P. F., and Oram, S.: Familial sinuatrial disorder. Br. Heart J. 34:668, 1972.

193. Mackintosh, A. F.: Sinuatrial disease in young people. Br. Heart J. 45:62, 1981.

194. Nordenberg, A., Varghese, P. J., and Nugent, E. W.: Spectrum of sinus node dysfunction in two siblings. Am. Heart J. 91:507, 1976.

195. Spellberg, R. D.: Familial sinus node disease. Chest 60:246, 1971.

196. Caralis, D. G., and Varghese, P. J.: Familial sinoatrial node dysfunction: Increased vagal tone a possible aetiology. Br. Heart J. 38:951, 1976.

197. Balderston, S. M., Shaffer, E. M., Sondheimer, H. M., et al.: Hereditary atrioventricular conduction defect in a child. Pediatr. Cardiol. 10:37, 1989.

198. Khorsandian, R. S., Moghadam, A.-N., and Müller, O. F.: Familial congenital A-V dissociation. Am. J. Cardiol. 14:118, 1964.

199. Wagner, C. W., and Hall, R. J.: Congenital familial atrioventricular dissociation: Report of three siblings. Am. J. Cardiol. 19:593, 1967.

200. Wolkowicz, J., and Burgess, J. H.: Complete heart block in an Inuit family. Can. J. Cardiol. 4:352, 1988.

201. Stephan, E.: Hereditary bundle branch system defect: Survey of a family with four affected generations. Am. Heart J. 95:89, 1978.

202. Steenkamp, W.F.J.: Familial trifascicular block. Am. Heart J. 84:758, 1972.

203. Mézáros, M., and Czeizel, A.: ECG conduction disturbance in the first-degree relatives of children with ventricular septal defect. Clin. Genet. 19:298, 1981.

204. Kennel, A. J., Callahan, J. A., Maloney, J. D., et al.: Adult-onset familial infra-Hisian block. Am. Heart J. 102:447, 1981.

205. Lorber, A., Maisuls, E., and Naschitz, J.: Hereditary right axis deviation: Electrocardiographic pattern of pseudo left posterior hemiblock and incomplete right bundle branch block. Int. J. Cardiol. 20:399, 1988.

206. Van Der Merwe, P.-L., Weymar, H. W., Torrington, M., et al.: Progressive familial heart block (type I): A follow up study after 10 years. S. Afr. Med. J. 73:275, 1988.

207. Torrington, M., Weymar, H. W., van der Merwe, P.-L., et al.: Progressive familial heart block: Pt I. Extent of the disease. S. Afr. Med. J. 70:354, 1986.

208. Kothari, S. S., Agrawal, S. M., and Krishnaswami, S.: Familial complete heart block in hypertrophic cardiomyopathy. Int. J. Cardiol. 20:294, 1988.

209. Stables, R. H., Bailey, C., and Ormerod, O.J.M.: Idiopathic familial atrial cardiomyopathy with diffuse conduction block. Q. J. Med. 264:325, 1989.

210. Williams, D. O., Jones, E. L., Nagle, R. E., et al.: Familial atrial cardiomyopathy with heart block. Q. J. Med. 41:491, 1972.

211. Olofsson, B.-V., Eriksson, P., and Eriksson, A.: The sick sinus syndrome in familial amyloidosis with polyneuropathy. Int. J. Cardiol. 4:71, 1983.

212. Winkler, R. B., Nora, A. H., and Nora, J. J.: Familial congenital complete heart block and maternal systemic lupus erythematosus. Circulation 56:1103, 1977.

213. McCue, C. M., Mantakas, M. E., Tingelstad, J. B., et al.: Congenital heart block in newborns of mothers with connective tissue disease. Circulation 56:82, 1977.

214. Chameides, L., Truex, R. C., Vetter, V., et al.: Association of maternal systemic lupus erythematosus with congenital complete heart block. N. Engl. J. Med. 297:1204, 1977.

215. Scott, J. S., Maddison, P. J., Taylor, P. V., et al.: Connective-tissue disease, antibodies to ribonucleoprotein, and congenital heart block. N. Engl. J. Med. 309:209, 1983.

216. Lockshin, M. D., Gibofsky, A., Peebles, C. L., et al.: Neonatal lupus erythematosus with heart block: Family study of a patient with anti-SS-A and SS-B antibodies. Arthritis Rheum. 26:210, 1983.

217. Bergfeldt, L., and Möller, E.: Complete heart block—another HLA B27 associated disease manifestation. Tissue Antigens 21:385, 1983.

218. Bergfeldt, L., Vallin, H., and Edhag, O.: Complete heart block in HLA B27 associated disease. Electrophysiological and clinical characteristics. Br. Heart J. 51:184, 1984.

219. Bacos, J. M., Eagan, J. T., and Orgain, E. S.: Congenital familial nodal rhythm. Circulation 22:887, 1960.

220. Gault, J. H., Cantwell, J., Lev, M., et al: Fatal familial cardiac arrhythmias. Am. J. Cardiol. 29:548, 1972.

221. Gulotta, S. J., das Gupta, R., Padmanabhan, V. T., et al.: Familial occurrence of sinus bradycardia, short PR interval, intraventricular conduction defects, recurrent supraventricular tachycardia, and cardiomegaly. Am. Heart J. 93:19, 1977.

222. Chia, B. L., Yew, F. C., Chay, S. O., et al.: Familial Wolff-Parkinson-White syndrome. J. Electrocardiol. 15:195, 1982.

223. Vidaillet, H. J., Pressley, J. C., Henke, E., et al.: Familial occurrence of accessory atrioventricular pathways: Preexcitation syndrome. N. Engl. J. Med. 317:65, 1987.

224. Ibsen, H.H.W., Baandrup, U., and Simonsen, E. E.: Familial right ventricular dilated cardiomyopathy. Br. Heart J. 54:156, 1985.

225. Laurent, M., Descases, C., Biron, Y., et al.: Familial form of arrhythmogenic right ventricular dysplasia. Am. Heart J. *113*:827, 1987.

226. Ruder, M. A., Winston, S. A., Davis, J. C., et al.: Arrhythmogenic right ventricular dysplasia in a family. Am. J. Cardiol. *56*:799, 1985.

227. Ward, O. C.: A new familial cardiac syndrome in children. J. Ir. Med. Assoc. *54*:103, 1964.

228. Romano, C.: Congenital cardiac arrhythmia. Lancet *1*:658, 1965.

229. Greenspon, A. J., Kidwell, G. A., Barrasse, L. D., et al.: Hereditary long QT syndrome associated with cardiac conduction system disease. PACE *12*:479, 1989.

230. Itoh, S., Munemura, S., and Satoh, H.: A study of the inheritance pattern of Romano-Ward syndrome. Clin. Pediatr. *21*:20, 1982.

231. Weitkamp, L. R., Moss, A. J., Schwartz, P. J., et al.: Analysis of HLA haplotypes in long QT syndrome: withdrawal of the preliminary assignment of LQT to the HLA linkage group (abstr.). Cytogenet. Cell Genet. *51*:1106, 1989.

232. Jervell, A., and Lange-Nielsen, F.: Congenital deaf-mutism, functional heart disease with prolongation of Q-T interval and sudden death. Am. Heart J. *54*:59, 1957.

233. Fraser, G. R., Froggatt, P., and Murphy, T.: Genetical aspects of the cardioauditory syndrome of Jervell and Lange-Nielsen (congenital deafness and electrocardiographic abnormalities). Ann. Hum. Genet. *28*:133, 1964.

234. Till, J. A., Shinebourne, E. A., Pepper, J., et al.: Complete denervation of the heart in a child with congenital long QT and deafness. Am. J. Cardiol. *62*:1319, 1988.

DISORDERS OF CONNECTIVE TISSUE

235. McKusick, V. A.: Heritable Disorders of Connective Tissue. St. Louis, C. V. Mosby Co., 1956.

236. McKusick, V. A.: Heritable Disorders of Connective Tissue, 4th ed. St. Louis, C. V. Mosby Co., 1972

237. Bowen, J., Boudoulas, H., and Wooley, C. F.: Cardiovascular disease of connective tissue origin. Am. J. Med. *82*:481, 1987.

238. Pyeritz, R. E.: Cardiovascular manifestation of heritable disorders of connective tissue. Prog. Med. Genet. *5*:191, 1983.

239. Pyeritz, R. E.: Storage disorders. In Pierpont, M. E., and Moller, J. H. (eds.): The Genetics of Cardiovascular Disease. Boston, Martinus Nijhoff Publishing, 1987, p. 215.

240. Pyeritz, R. E.: Heritable disorders of connective tissue. In Pierpont, M. E., Moller, J. H. (eds.): The Genetics of Cardiovascular Disease. Boston, Martinus Nijhoff Publishing, 1987, p. 265.

241. Royce, P. M., and Steinmann, B.: Extracellular Matrix and Inheritable Disorders of Connective Tissue. New York, Wiley-Liss (in press).

242. Beighton, P. (ed.): Heritable Disorders of Connective Tissue. 5th ed. St. Louis, C. V. Mosby (in press).

243. McKusick, V. A.: The cardiovascular aspects of Marfan's syndrome: A heritable disorder of connective tissue. Circulation *11*:321, 1955.

244. Pyeritz, R. E., and McKusick, V. A.: The Marfan syndrome—diagnosis and management. N. Engl. J. Med. *300*:772, 1979.

245. Roberts, W. C., and Honig, H. S.: The spectrum of cardiovascular disease in the Marfan syndrome: A clinicomorphologic study of 18 necropsy patients and comparison to 151 previously reported necropsy patients. Am. Heart J. *104*:115, 1982.

246. Pyeritz, R. E.: The Marfan syndrome. In Royce, P. M., and Steinmann, B. (eds.) Extracellular Matrix and Inheritable Disorders of Connective Tissue. New York, A. R. Liss (in press).

247. Kainulainen K., Pulkkinen, L., Savolainen, A., et al.: The gene defect causing Marfan syndrome is located in chromosome 15. N. Engl. J. Med. *323*:935, 1990.

247a. Dietz, H. C., Pyeritz, R. E., Hall, B. D., et al.: The Marfan syndrome locus: Confirmation of assignment to chromosome 15 and identification of tightly linked markers at 15q15-q21.3. Genomics *9*:355, 1991.

248. Pyeritz, R. E.: Conference report: First international symposium on the Marfan syndrome. Am. J. Med. Genet. *32*:233, 1989.

249. Marsalese, D. L., Moodie, D. S., Vacante, M., et al.: Marfan's syndrome: Natural history and long-term follow-up of cardiovascular involvement. J. Am. Coll. Cardiol. *14*:422, 1989.

250. Child, J. S., Perloff, J. K., and Kaplan, S.: The heart of the matter: Cardiovascular involvement in Marfan's syndrome. J. Am. Coll. Cardiol. *14*:429, 1989.

251. Murdoch, J. L., Walker, B. A., Halpern, B. L., et al.: Life expectancy and causes of death in the Marfan syndrome. N. Engl. J. Med. *286*:804, 1972.

252. Phornphutkul, C., Rosenthal, A., and Nadas, A. S.: Cardiac manifestations of Marfan syndrome in infancy and childhood. Circulation *47*:581, 1973.

253. Sisk, H. E., Zahka, K. G., and Pyeritz, R. E.: The Marfan syndrome in early childhood: Analysis of 15 patients diagnosed less than 4 years of age. Am. J. Cardiol. *52*:353, 1983.

254. Gross, D. M., Robinson, L. K., Smith, L. T., et al.: Severe perinatal Marfan syndrome. Pediatrics *84*:83, 1989.

255. Geva, T., Hegesh, J., and Frand, M.: The clinical course and echocardiographic features of Marfan's syndrome in childhood. Am. J. Dis. Child. *141*:1179, 1987.

256. Morse, R. P., Rockenmacher, S., Pyeritz, R. E., et al.: Diagnosis and management of Marfan syndrome in infants. Pediatrics *86*:888, 1990.

257. Pyeritz, R. E.: Heritable disorders of connective tissue. In Boudoulas, H., and Wooley, C. F. (eds.): Mitral Valve Prolapse and the Mitral Valve Prolapse Syndrome. Mt. Kisco, N. Y., Futura Publishing Co., 1988, p. 129.

258. Pyeritz, R. E., and Wappel, M. A.: Mitral valve dysfunction in the Marfan syndrome. Am. J. Med. *74*:797, 1983.

259. Kolibash, A. J., Jr.: Natural history of mitral valve prolapse. In Boudoulas, H., and Wooley, C. F. (eds.): Mitral Valve Prolapse and the Mitral Valve Prolapse Syndrome. Mt. Kisco, N. Y., Futura Publishing Co., 1988, p. 257.

260. Crawford, E. S., and Coselli, J. S.: Marfan's syndrome: Combined composite valve graft replacement of the aortic root and transaortic mitral valve replacement. Ann. Thorac. Surg. *45*:296, 1988.

261. Cohn, L. H. DiSesa, V. J., Couper, G. S., et al.: Mitral valve repair for myxomatous degeneration and prolapse of the mitral valve. J. Thorac. Cardiovasc. Surg. *98*:987, 1989.

262. Gott, V. L., Pyeritz, R. E., Cameron, D., et al.: Ascending aortic aneurysm in the Marfan syndrome: Results of composite graft repair in 100 patients. Ann. Thorac. Surg. (in press).

263. Gott, V. L., Pyeritz, R. E., Magovern, G. J., Jr., et al.: Surgical treatment of aneurysms of the ascending aorta in the Marfan syndrome. Results of composite-graft repair in 50 patients. N. Engl. J. Med. *314*:1070, 1986.

264. Lima, S. D., Lima, J.A.C., Pyeritz, R. E., et al.: Relationship of mitral valve prolapse to left ventricular size in Marfan's syndrome. Am. J. Cardiol. *55*:739, 1985.

265. Lafferty, K., McLean, L., Salisbury, J., et al.: Ruptured abdominal aortic aneurysm in Marfan's syndrome. Postgrad. Med. J. *63*:685, 1987.

266. Pruzinsky, M. S., Katz, N. M., and Green, C. E., et al.: Isolated descending thoracic aortic aneurysm in Marfan's syndrome. Am. J. Cardiol. *51*:1159, 1988.

267. van Ooijen, B.: Marfan's syndrome and isolated aneurysm of the abdominal aorta. Br. Heart J. *59*:81, 1988.

268. Henry, W. L., Gardin, J. M., and Ware, J. H.: Echocardiographic measurements in normal subjects from infancy to old age. Circulation *62*:1054, 1980.

269. Crawford, E. S.: Marfan's syndrome: Broad spectral surgical treatment cardiovascular manifestations. Ann. Surg. *198*:487, 1983.

270. Svensson, L. G., Crawford, E. S., Coselli, J. S., et al.: Impact of cardiovascular operation on survival in the Marfan patient. Circulation *80*:233, 1988.

271. Arn, P. H., Scherer, L. R., Haller, J. A., Jr., et al.: Outcome of pectus excavatum in patients with Marfan syndrome and in the general population. J. Pediatr. *115*:954, 1989.

272. Pyeritz, R. E., Gott, V. L., McDonald, G. R., et al.: Surgical repair of the Marfan aorta: Technique, indications, and complications. Johns Hopkins Med. J. *151*:71, 1982.

273. deSanctis, R., Doroghazi, R. M., Austen, W. G., et al.: Aortic dissection. N. Engl. J. Med. *317*:1060, 1987.

274. Schaefer, S., Peshock, R. M., Malloy, C. R., et al.: Nuclear magnetic resonance imaging in Marfan's syndrome. J. Am. Coll. Cardiol. *9*:70, 1987.

275. Soulen, R. L., Fishman, E., Pyeritz, R. E., et al.: Evaluation of the Marfan syndrome: MR imaging versus CT. Radiology *165*:697, 1987.

276. Crawford, E. S., Crawford, J. L., Stowe, C. L., et al.: Total aortic replacement for chronic aortic dissection occurring in patients with and without Marfan's syndrome. Ann. Surg. *199*:358, 1984.

277. Pyeritz, R. E.: Effectiveness of beta-adrenergic blockade in the Marfan syndrome: Experience over 10 years (abstr.). Am. J. Med. Genet. *32*:245, 1989.

278. Zahka, K. G., Hensley, C., and Glesby, M., et al.: The impact of medical therapy on the cardiovascular prognosis of the Marfan syndrome in early childhood (abstr). J. Am. Coll. Cardiol. *13*:119, 1989.

279. Yin, F.C.P., Brin K. P., Ting, C.-T, et al.: Arterial hemodynamics in the Marfan syndrome. Circulation *79*:854, 1989.

280. Pyeritz, R. E.: Maternal and fetal complications of pregnancy in the Marfan syndrome. Am. J. Med. *71*:784, 1981.

281. Rosenblum, N., Grossman, A., and Gabbe, S.: Failure of serial echocardiographic studies to predict dissection in a pregnant woman with Marfan's syndrome. Am. J. Obstet. Gynecol. *146*:490, 1983.

282. Smith, V. C., Eckenbrecht, P.D., Hankins, G.D.V., et al.: Marfan's syndrome, pregnancy, and the cardiac surgeon. Milit. Med. *154*:404, 1989.

283. Mor-Yosef, S., Younis, J., Granat, J., et al.: Marfan's syndrome in pregnancy. Obstet. Gynecol. Surv. *43*:382, 1988.

284. Ferguson, J. E., II, Ueland, K., Stinson, E. G., et al.: Marfan's syndrome: Acute aortic dissection during labor, resulting in fetal distress and cesarean section, followed by successful surgical repair. Am. J. Obstet. Gynecol. *147*:759, 1983.

285. Cola, L. M., and Lavin, J. P., Jr.: Pregnancy complicated by the Marfan syndrome with aortic arch dissection, subsequent arch replacement and triple coronary artery bypass grafts. J. Reprod. Med. *30*:685, 1985.

286. Bailey, M. K., Hwu-Yun, R., Baker, J. D., III, et al.: Marfan syndrome in the parturient. J. S.C. Med. Assoc. *8*:327, 1989.

287. Sakai, L. Y., Keene, D. R., Engvall, E.: Fibrillin, a new 350-kD glycoprotein, is a component of extracellular microfibrils. J. Cell. Biol. *103*:2499, 1986.

288. Perejda. A. J., Abraham, P. A., Carnes, W. H., et al.: Marfan's syndrome: Structural, biochemical and mechanical studies of the aortic media. J. Lab. Clin. Med. *106*:376, 1985.

289. Becker, A. E.: Medionecrosis aortae. Pathol. Microbiol. *43*:124, 1975.

289a. McGookey, D. J., Pyeritz, R. E., and Byers, P. H.: Marfan syndrome: altered synthesis, secretion or extracellular incorporation of fibrillin. Am. J. Hum. Genet. *47*:A67, 1991.

289b. Magenis, E., and Sakai, L. Y.: The gene for fibrillin maps by in situ hybridization to 15q. Genomics (in press).

290. Leier, C. V., Call, T. D., Fulkerson, P. K., et al.: The spectrum of cardiac defects in the Ehlers-Danlos syndrome, types I and III. Ann. Intern. Med. *92*:171, 1980.

291. Jaffe, A. S., Geltman, E. M., Rodey, G. E., et al.: Mitral valve prolapse: A consistent manifestation of type IV Ehlers-Danlos syndrome. Circulation 64:121, 1981.

292. Pyeritz, R. E., Stolle, C. A., Parfrey, N. A., et al.: Ehlers-Danlos syndrome IV due to a novel defect in type III procollagen. Am. J. Med. Genet. 19:607, 1984.

293. Nicholls, A. C., De Paepe, A., Narcisi, P., et al.: Linkage of a polymorphic marker for the type III collagen gene (COL3A1) to atypical autosomal dominant Ehlers-Danlos syndrome type IV in a large Belgian pedigree. Hum. Genet. 78:276, 1988.

294. Fox, R., Pope, F. M., Narcisi, P., et al.: Spontaneous carotid cavernous fistula in Ehlers-Danlos syndrome. J. Neurol. Neurosurg. Psychiat. 51:984, 1988.

295. Rudd, N. L., Nimrod, C., Holbrook, K. A., et al.: Pregnancy complications in type IV Ehlers-Danlos syndrome. Lancet 1:50, 1983.

296. Viljoen, D. L., Pope, F. M., and Beighton, P.: Heterogeneity of pseudoxanthoma elasticum: Delineation of a new form? Clin. Genet. 32:100, 1987.

297. Cunningham, J. R., Lippman, S. M., Renie, W. A., et al.: Pseudoxanthoma elasticum: Treatment of gastrointestinal hemorrhage by arterial embolization and observations of autosomal dominant inheritance. Johns Hopkins Med. J. 147:168, 1980.

298. Lebwohl, M. G., Distefano, D., Prioleau, P. G., et al.: Pseudoxanthoma elasticum and mitral valve prolapse. N. Engl. J. Med. 307:228, 1982.

299. Pyeritz, R. E., Weiss, J. L., Renie, W. A., et al.: Pseudoxanthoma elasticum and mitral-valve prolapse. N. Engl. J. Med. 307:1451, 1982.

300. Goodman, R. M., Smith, E. W., Paton, D., et al.: Pseudoxanthoma elasticum: A clinical and histopathological study. Medicine 42:297, 1963.

301. Challenor, V. F., Conway, N., and Monro, J. L.: The surgical treatment of restrictive cardiomyopathy in pseudoxanthoma elasticum. Br. Heart J. 59:266, 1988.

302. Renie, W. A., Pyeritz, R. E., Combs, J., et al.: Pseudoxanthoma elasticum: High calcium intake in early life correlates with severity. Am. J. Med. Genet. 19:235, 1984.

303. Maharaj, B., Hammond, M. G., Appadoo, B., et al.: HLA-A, B, DR, and DQ antigens in black patients with severe chronic rheumatic heart disease. Circulation 76:259, 1987.

INBORN ERRORS OF METABOLISM THAT AFFECT THE CARDIOVASCULAR SYSTEM

304. La Du, B. N.: Alcaptonuria. In Scriver, C. R., Beaudet, A. L., Sly, W. S., and Valle, D. (eds.): The Metabolic Basis of Inherited Disease. 6th ed. New York, McGraw-Hill Book Co., 1989, p. 775.

305. Mudd, S. H., Levy, H. L., and Skovby, F.: Disorders of transsulfuration. In Scriver, C. R., Beaudet, A. L., Sly, W. S., and Valle, D. (eds.): The Metabolic Basis of Inherited Disease. 6th ed. New York, McGraw-Hill Book Co., 1989, p. 693.

306. Mudd, S. H., Skovby, F., Levy, H. L., et al.: The natural history of homocystinuria due to cystathionine beta-synthase deficiency. Am. J. Hum. Genet. 37:1, 1985.

307. Hill-Zobel, R. L., Pyeritz, R. E., Scheffel, U., et al.: Kinetics and biodistribution of ^{111}In-labeled platelets in homocystinuria. N. Engl. J. Med. 307:781, 1982.

308. Mudd, S. H.: Vascular disease and homocysteine metabolism (editorial). N. Engl. J. Med. 313:751, 1985.

309. Murphy-Chutorian, D. R., Wexman, M. P., Grieco, A. J., et al.: Methionine intolerance: A possible risk factor for coronary artery disease. J. Am. Coll. Cardiol. 6:725, 1985.

310. Kang, S. S., Wong, P.W.K., Cook, H. Y., et al.: Protein-bound homocyst(e)ine: A possible risk factor for coronary artery disease. J. Clin. Invest. 77:1482, 1986.

311. Wilcken, D. E., and Wilcken, B.: The pathogenesis of coronary artery disease: A possible role for methionine metabolism. J. Clin. Invest. 57:1079, 1976.

312. Roe, C. R., and Coates, P. M.: Acyl-CoA dehydrogenase deficiencies. In Scriver, C. R., Beaudet, A. L., Sly, W. S., and Valle, D. (eds.): The Metabolic Basis of Inherited Disease. 6th ed. New York, McGraw-Hill Book Co., 1989, p. 889.

313. Harper, P. S.: The muscular dystrophies. In Scriver, C. R., Beaudet, A. L., Sly, W. S., and Valle, D. (eds.): The Metabolic Basis of Inherited Disease. 6th ed. New York, McGraw-Hill Book Co., 1989, p. 2869.

314. Rebouche, C. J., and Engel, A. G.: Carnitine metabolism and deficiency syndromes. Mayo Clin. Proc. 58:533, 1983.

315. Treem, W. R., Stanley, C. A., Finegold, D. N., et al.: Primary carnitine deficiency due to a failure of carnitine transport in kidney, muscle, and fibroblasts. N. Engl. J. Med. 319:1331, 1988.

316. Waber, L. J., Valle, D., Neill, C., et al.: Carnitine deficiency presenting as familial cardiomyopathy: A treatable defect in carnitine transport. J. Pediatr. 101:700, 1982.

317. Tripp, M. E., Katcher, M. L., Peters, H. A., et al.: Systemic carnitine deficiency presenting as familial endocardial fibroelastosis. N. Engl. J. Med. 305:385, 1981.

318. Ogasahara, S., Engel, A. G., Frens, D., et al.: Muscle coenzyme Q deficiency in familial mitochondrial encephalomyopathy. Proc. Natl. Acad. Sci. USA 86:2379, 1989.

319. Channer, K. S., Channer, J. L., Campbell, M. J., et al.: Cardiomyopathy in the Kearns-Sayre syndrome. Br. Heart J. 59:486, 1988.

320. Hers, H.-G., Van Hoof, F., and de Barsy, T.: Glycogen storage diseases. In Scriver, C. R., Beaudet, A. L., Sly, W. S., and Valle, D. (eds.): The Meta-

bolic Basis of Inherited Disease. 6th ed. New York, McGraw-Hill Book Co., 1989, p. 425.

321. Bashan, N., Potashnik, R., Barash, V., et al.: Glycogen storage disease type II in Israel. Isr. J. Med. Sci. 24:224, 1988.

322. Ehlers, K. H., Hagstrom, J.W.C., Lukas, D. S., et al.: Glycogen-storage disease of the myocardium with obstruction to left ventricular outflow. Circulation 25:96, 1962.

323. Bharati, S., Serratto, M., Du Brow, I., et al.: The conduction system in Pompe's disease. Pediatr. Cardiol. 2:25, 1982.

324. Bonnici, F., Shapiro, R., Joffe, H. S., et al.: Angiocardiographic and enzyme studies in a patient with type II glycogenosis. S. Afr. Med. J. 58:860, 1980.

325. Robinson, W. F., Howell, J. M., and Dorling, P. R.: Cardiomyopathy in generalised glycogenosis type II in cattle. Cardiovasc. Res. 17:238, 1982.

326. Suzuki, Y., Tsuji, A., Omura, K., et al.: Km mutant of acid alpha-glucosidase in a case of cardiomyopathy without signs of skeletal muscle involvement. Clin. Genet. 33:376, 1988.

327. Makos, M. M., McComb, R. D., Hart, M. N., et al.: Alpha-glucosidase deficiency and basilar artery aneurysm: Report of a sibship. Ann. Neurol. 22:629, 1987.

328. Olson, L. J., Reeder, G. S., Noller, K. L., et al.: Cardiac involvement in glycogen storage disease III. Morphologic and biochemical characterization with endomyocardial biopsy. Am. J. Cardiol. 53:980, 1984.

329. Servidei, S., Metlay, L. A., Chodosh, J., et al.: Fatal infantile cardiopathy caused by phosphorylase b kinase deficiency. J. Pediatr. 113:82, 1988.

330. Eishi, Y., Takemura, T., Sone, R., et al.: Glycogen storage disease confined to the heart with deficient activity of cardiac phosphorylase kinase: a new type of glycogen storage disease. Hum. Pathol. 16:193, 1987.

331. Bothwell, T. H., Charlton, R. W., and Motulsky, A. G.: Hemochromatosis. In Scriver, C. R., Beaudet, A. L., Sly, W. S., and Valle, D. (eds.): The Metabolic Basis of Inherited Disease. 6th ed. New York, McGraw-Hill Book Co., 1989, p. 1433.

332. Valberg, L. S., and Ghent, C. N.: Diagnosis and managment of hereditary hemochromatosis. Annu. Rev. Med. 36:27, 1985.

333. Edwards, C. Q.: Early detection of hereditary hemochromatosis. Ann. Intern. Med. 101:707, 1984.

334. Olson, L. J., Baldus, W. P., and Tajik, A. J.: Echocardiographic features of idiopathic hemochromatosis. Am. J. Cardiol. 60:885, 1987.

335. Cutler, D. J., Isner, J. M., Bracey, A. W., et al.: Hemochromatosis heart disease: An unemphasized cause of potentially reversible restrictive cardiomyopathy. Am. J. Med. 69:923, 1980.

336. Weatherall, D. J., Clegg, F. B., Higgs, D. R., et al.: The hemoglobinopathies. In Scriver, C. R., Beaudet, A. L., Sly, W. S., and Valle, D. (eds.): The Metabolic Basis of Inherited Disease. 6th ed. New York, McGraw-Hill Book Co., 1989, p. 2281.

337. Neufeld, E. F., and Muenzer, J.: The mucopolysaccharidoses. In Scriver, C. R., Beaudet, A. L., Sly, W. S., and Valle, D. (eds.). The Metabolic Basis of Inherited Disease. 6th ed. New York, McGraw-Hill Book Co., 1989, p. 1565.

338. Nolan, C. M., and Sly, W. S.: I-cell disease and pseudo-Hurler polydystrophy: Disorders of lysosomal enzyme phosphorylation and localization. In Scriver, C. R., Beaudet, A. L., Sly, W. S., and Valle, D. (eds.): The Metabolic Basis of Inherited Disease. 6th ed. New York, McGraw-Hill Book Co., 1989, p. 1589.

339. Johnson, G. L., Vine, D. L. Cottrill, C. M., et al.: Echocardiographic mitral valve deformity in the mucopolysaccharidoses. Pediatrics 67:401, 1981.

340. Gross, D. M., Williams, J. C., Caprioli, J., et al.: Echocardiographic abnormalities in the mucopolysaccharide storage diseases. Am. J. Cardiol. 61:170, 1988.

340a. John, R. M., Hunter, D., and Swanton, R. H.: Echocardiographic abnormalities in type IV mucopolysaccharidosis. Arch. Dis. Childhood 65:746, 1990.

341. Nelson, J., Shields, M. D., and Mulholland, H. C.: Cardiovascular studies in the mucopolysaccharidoses. J. Med. Genet. 27:94, 1990.

342. Brosius, F. C., III, and Roberts, W. C.: Coronary artery disease in the Hurler syndrome: Qualitative and quantitative analysis of the extent of coronary narrowing at necropsy in six children. Am. J. Cardiol. 47:649, 1981.

343. Renteria, V. G., Ferrans, V. J., and Roberts, W. C.: The heart in the Hurler syndrome: Gross, histologic and ultrastructural observations in five necropsy cases. Am. J. Cardiol. 38:487, 1976.

344. Semenza, G. L., and Pyeritz, R. E.: Respiratory complications of the mucopolysaccharide storage disorders. Medicine 67:209, 1988.

345. Young, I. D., and Harper, P.S.: Long-term complications in Hunter's syndrome. Clin. Genet. 16:125, 1979.

345a. Lenarsky, C., Kohn, D. B., Weinberg, K. I., et al.: Bone marrow transplantation for genetic diseases. Hematol./Oncol. Clin. North Am. 4:589, 1990.

346. Desnick, R. J., and Bishop, D. F.: Fabry disease: α-Galactosidase deficiency; Schindler disease: α-N-acetylgalactosaminidase deficiency. In Scriver, C. R., Beaudet, A. L., Sly, W. S., and Valle, D. (eds.): The Metabolic Basis of Inherited Disease. 6th ed. New York, McGraw-Hill Book Co., 1989, p. 1797.

347. Morgan, S. H., and Crawford, M. d'A.: Anderson-Fabry disease. A commonly missed diagnosis. Br. Med. J. 297:872, 1988.

348. Spence, M. W., MacKinnon, K. E., Burgess, J. K., et al.: Failure to correct the metabolic defect by renal allotransplantation in Fabry's disease. Ann. Intern. Med. 84:13, 1976.

349. Kramer, W., Thormann, J., Mueller, K., et al.: Progressive cardiac involvement by Fabry's disease despite successful renal allotransplantation. Int. J. Cardiol. 7:72, 1985.

350. Colucci, W. S., Lorell, B. H., Schoen, F. J., et al.: Hypertrophic obstructive cardiomyopathy due to Fabry's disease. N. Engl. J. Med. 307:926, 1982.

350a. von Scheidt, W., Eng., C. M., Fitzmaurice, T. F., et al.: An atypical variant of Fabry's disease with manifestations confined to the myocardium. N. Engl. J. Med. *324*:395, 1991.

351. Goldman, M. E., Cantor, R., Schwartz, M. F., et al.: Echocardiographic abnormalities and disease severity in Fabry's disease. J. Am. Coll. Cardiol. *7*:1157, 1986.

352. Sakuraba, H., Yanagawa, Y., Igarashi, T., et al.: Cardiovascular manifestations in Fabry's disease: A high incidence of mitral valve prolapse in hemizygotes and heterozygotes. Clin. Genet. *29*:276, 1986.

353. Mutoh, T., Senda, Y., Sugimura, K., et al.: Severe orthostatic hypotension in a female carrier of Fabry's disease. Arch. Neurol. *34*:468, 1988.

354. Bernstein, H. S., Bishop, D. F., Astrin, K. H., et al.: Fabry disease: Six gene rearrangements and an exonic point mutation in the alpha-galactosidase gene. J. Clin. Invest. *83*:1390, 1989.

355. Benson, M. D., and Wallace, M. R.: Amyloidosis. *In* Scriver, C. R., Beaudet, A. L., Sly, W. S., and Valle, D. (eds.): The Metabolic Basis of Inherited Disease. 6th ed. New York, McGraw-Hill Book Co., 1989, p. 2439.

356. Benson, M. D., Wallace, M. R., Tejada, E., et al.: Hereditary amyloidosis: Description of a new American kindred with late onset cardiomyopathy: Appalachian amyloid. Arthritis Rheum. *30*:195, 1987.

357. Backman, C., and Olofsson, B. O.: Echocardiographic features in familial amyloidosis with polyneuropathy. Acta Med. Scand. *214*:273, 1983.

358. Eriksson, A., Eriksson, P., Olofsson, B.-O., et al.: The cardiac atrioventricular conduction system in familial amyloidosis with polyneuropathy: A clinico-pathologic study of six cases from Northern Sweden. Acta Pathol. Microbiol. Immunol. Scand. *91*:343, 1983.

359. Vidaillet, H. J., Jr.: Cardiac tumors associated with hereditary syndromes. Am. J. Cardiol. *61*:1355, 1988.

359a. Harding, C. O., and Pagon, R. A.: Incidence of tuberous sclerosis in patients with cardiac rhabdomyoma. Am. J. Med. Genet. *37*:443, 1990.

INHERITED DISORDERS OF THE CIRCULATION

360. Peery, W. H.: Clinical spectrum of hereditary hemorrhagic telangiectasia (Osler-Weber-Rendu disease). Am. J. Med. *82*:989, 1987.

361. Nikolopoulos, N., Xynos, E., and Vassilakis, J. S.: Familial occurrence of hyperdynamic circulation status due to intrahepatic fistulae in hereditary hemorrhagic telangiectasia. Hepatogastroenterology *35*:167, 1988.

362. Cooke, D.A.P.: Renal arteriovenous malformation demonstrated angiographically in hereditary haemorrhagic telangiectasia (Rendu-Osler-Weber disease). J. R. Soc. Med. *79*:744, 1986.

363. Kurnik, P. B., and Heymann, W. R.: Coronary artery ectasia associated with hereditary hemorrhagic telangiectasia. Arch. Intern. Med. *149*:2357, 1989.

364. Terry, P. B., White, J. I., Jr., Barth, K. H., et al.: Pulmonary arteriovenous malformations: Physiologic observations and results of therapeutic balloon embolization. N. Engl. J. Med. *308*:1197, 1983.

365. Haq, A. U., Glass, J., Netchvolodoff, C. V., et al.: Hereditary hemorrhagic telangiectasia and danazol. Ann. Intern. Med. *109*:171, 1988.

366. Green, J. S., Bowmer, M. I., and Johnson, G. J.: Von Hippel-Lindau disease in a Newfoundland kindred. Can. Med. Assoc. J. *134*:133, 1986.

367. Griffiths, D.F.R., Williams, G. T., and Williams, E. D.: Duodenal carcinoid tumours, phaeochromocytoma and neurofibromatosis: Islet cell tumour, phaeochromocytoma and the von Hippel-Lindau complex: Two distinctive neuroendocrine syndromes. Q. J. Med. *245*:769, 1987.

368. Jennings, A. M., Smith, C., Cole, D. R., et al.: Von Hippel-Lindau disease in a large British family: Clinicopathological features and recommendations for screening and follow-up. Q. J. Med. *66*:233, 1988.

369. Lamiell, J. M., Salazar, F. G., and Hsia, Y. E.: Von Hippel-Lindau disease affecting 43 members of a single kindred. Medicine *68*:1, 1989.

369a. Parfrey, P. S., Bear, J. C., Morgan, J., et al.: The diagnosis and prognosis of autosomal dominant polycystic kidney disease. N. Engl. J. Med. *323*:1085, 1990.

369b. Chapman, A. B., Johnson, A., Gabow, P. A., et al.: The renin-angiotensin-aldosterone system and autosomal dominant polycystic kidney disease. N. Engl. J. Med. *323*:1091, 1990.

370. Leier, C. V., Baker, P. B., Kilman, J. W., et al: Cardiovascular abnormalities associated with adult polycystic kidney disease. Ann. Intern. Med. *100*:683, 1984.

371. Hossack, K. F., Leddy, C. L., Johnson, A. M., et al: Echocardiographic findings in autosomal dominant polycystic kidney disease. N. Engl. J. Med. *319*:907, 1988.

372. Chapman, J. R., and Hilson, A.J.W.: Polycystic kidneys and abdominal aortic aneurysms. Lancet *1*:646, 1980.

373. Wakabayashi, T., Fujita, S., Ohbora, Y., et al.: Polycystic kidney disease and intracranial aneurysms: Early angiographic diagnosis and early operation for the unruptured aneurysm. J. Neurosurg. *58*:488, 1983.

374. Levey, A. S., Pauker, S. G., and Kassirer, J. P.: Occult intracranial aneurysms in polycystic kidney disease: When is cerebral arteriography indicated? N. Engl. J. Med. *308*:986, 1983.

375. Germino, G. G., Barton, N. J., Lamb, J., et al.: Identification of a locus which shows no genetic recombination with the autosomal dominant polycystic kidney disease gene on chromosome 16. Am. J. Hum. Genet. *46*:925, 1990.

376. Elles, R. G., Read, A. P., Hodgkinson, K. A., et al.: Recombination or heterogeneity: Is there a second locus for adult polycystic kidney disease? J. Med. Genet. *27*:413, 1990.

377. Shulman, S. A., Hyams, J. S., Gunta, R., et al.: Arteriohepatic dysplasia (Alagille syndrome): Extreme variability among affected family members. Am. J. Med. Genet. *19*:325, 1984.

378. Mueller, R. F.: The Alagille syndrome (arteriohepatic dysplasia). J. Med. Genet. *24*:621, 1987.

379. Nicod, P., Bloor, C., Godfrey, M., et al.: Familial aortic dissecting aneurysms. J. Am. Coll. Cardiol. *13*:811, 1989.

380. Toyama, M., Amano, A., and Kameda, T.: Familial aortic dissection: A report of rare family cluster. Br. Heart J. *61*:204, 1989.

381. Bixler, D., and Antley, R. M.: Familial aortic dissection with iris anomalies — a new connective tissue disease syndrome? Birth Defects *12*(5):229, 1976.

382. Kontusaari, S. Tromp, G., Kuivaniemi, H., et al.: Inheritance of RNA splicing mutation (G^{+1} ^{IVS20}) in the type III procollagen gene (COL3AI) in a family having aortic aneurysms and easy bruisability: Phenotypic overlap between familial arterial aneurysms and Ehlers-Danlos syndrome type IV. Am. J. Hum. Genet. *47*:112, 1990.

383. Kontusaari, S., Tromp, G., Kuivaniemi, H., et al.: A mutation in the gene for type III procollagen (COL3AI) in a family with aortic aneurysms. J. Clin. Invest. *86*:1465, 1990.

383a. Majumder, P. P., St. Jean, P. L., Ferrell, R. E., et al.: On the inheritance of abdominal aortic aneurysm. Am. J. Hum. Genet. *48*:164, 1991.

384. Welch, J. P., Aterman, K., and Day, E.: Familial aggregation of a 'new' connective disorder, a nosologic problem. Birth Defects *7*(8):204, 1971.

385. Fox, J. L., and Ko, J. P.: Familial intracranial aneurysms: Six cases among 13 siblings. J. Neurosurg. *52*:501, 1980.

386. Halal, F., Mohr, G., Toussi, T., et al.: Intracranial aneurysms: A report of a large pedigree. Am. J. Med. Genet. *15*:89, 1983.

387. De Paepa, A., Van Landeghem, W., De Keyser, F., et al.: Collagen type III deficiency associated with multiple intracranial aneurysms (abstr.) Clin. Genet. *33*:462, 1988.

388. Abrahamson, M.: Human cysteine proteinase inhibitors: Isolation, physiological importance, inhibitory mechanism, gene structure and relation to hereditary cerebral hemorrhage. Scand. J. Clin. Lab. Invest. *48*:21, 1988.

389. Wattendorff, A. R., Bots, G.T.A.M., Went, L. N., et al.: Familial cerebral amyloid angiopathy presenting as recurrent cerebral haemorrhage. J. Neurol. Sci. *55*:121, 1982.

390. Pasyk, K. A., Argenta, L. C., and Erickson, R. P.: Familial vascular malformations: Report of 25 members of one family. Clin. Genet. *26*:221, 1984.

391. Stanley, J. C.: Arterial fibrodysplasia. Arch. Surg. *110*:561, 1975.

392. Kousseff, B. G., and Gilbert-Barness, E. F.: Vascular neurofibromatosis and infantile gangrene. Am. J. Med. Genet. *34*:221, 1989.

393. Petit, H., Bouchez, B., Destee, A., et al.: Familial form of fibromuscular dysplasia of the internal carotid artery. J. Neuroradiol. *10*:15, 1983.

394. Gladstein, K., Rushton, A. R., and Kidd, K. K.: Penetrance estimates and recurrence risks for fibromuscular dysplasia. Clin. Genet. *17*:115, 1980.

395. Rushton, A. R.: The genetics of fibromuscular dysplasia. Arch. Intern. Med. *140*:233, 1980.

396. Austin, J. G., and Stears, J. C.: Familial hypoplasia of both internal carotid arteries. Arch. Neurol. *24*:1, 1971.

397. McDonald, A. H., Gerlis, L. M., and Somerville, J.: Familial arteriopathy with associated pulmonary and systemic arterial stenoses. Br. Heart J. *31*:375, 1969.

398. Van Dyck, M., Proesmans, W., VanHollebeke, E., et al.: Idiopathic infantile arterial calcification with cardiac, renal and central nervous system involvement. Eur. J. Pediatr. *148*:374, 1989.

399. Melmon, K. L., and Braunwald, E.: Familial pulmonary hypertension. N. Engl. J. Med. *269*:770, 1963.

400. Kingdon, H. S., Cohen, L. S., Roberts, W. C., et al.: Familial occurrence of primary pulmonary hypertension. Arch. Intern. Med. *118*:422, 1966.

401. Loyd, J. E., Primm, R. K., and Newman, J. H.: Familial primary pulmonary hypertension: Clinical patterns. Am. Rev. Respir. Dis. *129*:194, 1984.

402. Porterfield, J. K., Pyeritz, R. E., and Traill, T. A.: Pulmonary hypertension and interstitial fibrosis in von Recklinghausen neurofibromatosis. Am. J. Med. Genet. *25*:531, 1986.

403. Goldstein, S., Qazi, Q. H., Fitzgerald, J., et al.: Distichiasis, congenital heart defects and mixed peripheral vascular anomalies. Am. J. Med. Genet. *20*:283, 1985.

404. Lindenauer, S. M.: The Klippel-Trenaunay-Weber syndrome: Varicosity, hypertrophy and hemangioma with no arteriovenous fistula. Ann. Surg. *162*:303, 1965.

405. Campistol, J. M., Agusti, C., Torras, A., et al.: Renal hemangioma and renal artery aneurysm in the Klippel-Trenaunay syndrome. J. Urol. *140*:134, 1988.

406. Herbert, F. A., and Bowen, P. A.: Hereditary late-onset lymphedema with pleural effusion and laryngeal edema. Arch. Intern. Med. *143*:913, 1983.

407. Childs, B.: Causes of essential hypertension. Prog. Med. Genet. *5*:1, 1983.

408. Murphy, E. A., and Pyeritz, R. D.: Homeostasis: VII. A conspectus. Am. J. Med. Genet. *24*:735, 1986.

Aging and the Heart

by MYRON L. WEISFELDT, M.D., EDWARD G. LAKATTA, M.D.,
and GARY GERSTENBLITH, M.D.

CONCEPTS AND THEORIES OF CHANGES WITH AGE

Students of cardiovascular medicine often are presented with two distinct issues concerning the burden imposed on the cardiovascular system by advanced age. The first is that represented by the aged, infirm patient with severe heart failure. At times no clear cause can be defined, and even when one is, the diagnostic and therapeutic management often is more challenging than is the case with the younger patient with the same disease. The issue presented by these patients, therefore, is that the cardiovascular limitations associated with aging itself are significant and often severe. There also is the observation represented by the elderly marathon runner, swimmer, or master athlete whose physical abilities are equal or superior to those of people 30 years younger. The findings in such people suggest that if there is any limitation of cardiovascular reserve imposed by the aging process per se, it is minor. There is some evidence that age-associated musculoskeletal, pulmonary, or psychological factors are more important than cardiovascular consideration in these patients.

AGING, DISEASE, AND LIFE STYLE. Attempts to solve the dilemma posed by the seemingly varied effects of age in the two subject subsets noted above are handicapped by the additional effects of both an increasing prevalence of disease and the altered life style associated with aging. The most prevalent disease, coronary atherosclerosis, is present in up to 60 per cent of elderly people in Western society,[1,2] has a profound effect on measurements of cardiovascular function during stress, but is difficult to diagnose in the absence of overt symptoms or electrocardiographic abnormalities. The most important life style variable is physical activity status. Exercise conditioning and deconditioning studies have indicated that even short periods of changes in physical activity can have a profound influence on cardiovascular function.[3] Toxins from food and chemical exposure (including cumulative effects of cigarette smoking and radiation, as well as malnutrition) are other life style variables whose effects may merge into those of disease. There is considerable evidence, therefore, that changes in the prevalence of disease and altered life style accompanying aging may have accounted for some of the previously described alterations attributed to aging alone.

In summary, changes in cardiovascular function accompanying aging in an unselected population may be due to changes in disease patterns and life style variables as well as those resulting simply from aging. Of the three, aging appears to be the least potent and, therefore, the most difficult to define. Although age-induced changes in cardiac structure, function, and neurohumoral responses do modify cardiovascular function, they are most important clinically when they are superimposed on significant disease or other cardiovascular stresses. The effects of aging alone on cardiovascular function should be examined in the subjects who are free of cardiovascular disease and who have a relatively homogeneous level of physical conditioning. It is relatively easy to exclude people who have symptomatic disease, but identification of atherosclerosis is more difficult in many people because of its high prevalence and because it often is asymptomatic.

INTERPRETATION OF STUDIES OF AGING. The best information concerning aging comes from longitudinal, or repeated, studies of healthy people who have active life styles. Because longitudinal studies require a prolonged time to perform, most aging studies in humans have used cross-sectional methodology. In any aging study it is important to note that data expressed as a ratio (e.g., cardiac index or myosin adenosine triphosphatase activity per milligram protein) may change with age because of changes in the denominator (for the examples given, body mass and total protein content) rather than because of a change in the parameter itself. The interpretation of cross-sectional studies also is limited by the possibility that the older volunteers may represent a subset of the general population selected for longevity and/or high motivational factors.

CARDIOVASCULAR CHANGES IN AGING

After neonatal development, the number of myocardial cells in the heart does not increase.[4] Detailed studies of biochemical and anatomical changes accompanying aging have been performed. It is important, though, to assess the physiological importance of these findings. Although one step in a complex biochemical pathway may be altered with age, the alteration may have no physiological significance if that step does not limit the rate of the overall reaction. Clearly, important general conclusions about cardiovascular aging are as follows:

1. There is moderate hypertrophy of left ventricular myocardium, probably in response to increased arterial vascular stiffness and dropout of myocytes.[5-7]
2. When myocardial hypertrophy occurs, it is out of proportion to capillary and vascular growth.[8]
3. The ability of myocardium to generate tension is well maintained as a result of prolonged duration of contraction and greater stiffness, despite a modest decrease in the velocity of shortening of cardiac muscle.

4. There is a selective decrease in beta-adrenoceptor–mediated inotropic, chronotropic, and vasodilating cardiovascular responses with aging.[9,10]

5. Increased pericardial and myocardial stiffness and delayed relaxation during aging may limit left early ventricular filling during stress,[10a] although end-diastolic volume is not compromised in healthy individuals.

GENERAL THEORIES OF AGING: CARDIOVASCULAR APPLICATION

As organized and discussed by Hayflick,[11] current broadly accepted theories of aging can be grouped by level of integration into genome, physiological, and organ theories. Most work to date on the cardiovascular system has been at the latter two levels.

GENOME THEORIES. The most popular current genome theory proposes that genes are programmed for aging and/or death of the organism.[12-14] Each species as well as cells in culture has what appears to be unmodifiable general boundaries for the duration of survival. Because cardiac function with age does not limit survival in the absence of disease or toxin exposure, little testing of this hypothesis is feasible in the cardiovascular system. Programmed dysfunction or cell destruction may account for neurohormonal regulatory dysfunction, but these notions are remote from the fundamental tenets of the hypothesis. Two other related genomic theories of aging are somatic mutation (related or not to environmental irradiation) and the error theories. Owing to either programmed DNA variability or toxic agents, there is an accumulation of cell components with errors in protein structure and/or sequence. The error theories may not be relevant, however, since searches for such errors have not been successful. In the heart certain aspects of function are so well maintained that it is difficult to use such a general theory to explain the relatively selective cardiovascular age changes.

PHYSIOLOGICAL THEORIES. Physiological theories of aging clearly appear more attractive as explanations for cardiovascular changes.[15-17] One, the cross-linkage theory of aging, points to the importance of time-related changes in the extracellular protein matrix, particularly of collagen and ground substance. Such changes are certainly at the basis of age-associated increases in stiffness of pericardial, valvular, and perhaps myocardial and vascular tissues. Secondary responses probably include myocardial hypertrophy and vascular smooth muscle changes. Neurohormonal changes would be more difficult to explain. Alternatively, physiological theories related to injury by free radicals and/or accumulation of waste product could explain the selectivity of aging changes in terms of selective sensitivity of specific enzymes to free radical injury or specific detrimental effects of waste product buildup, tissue by tissue.

ORGAN THEORIES. Organ theories are attractive in their simplicity and ease of understanding and demonstration. There are two major theories: immunological and neuroendocrine.[17,18] The immunological theory offers an explanation for survival duration characteristics of species in terms of programmed immunological dysfunction leading to autoimmune cellular injury but offers little to explain specific selective changes in the cardiovascular system. The neuroendocrine theory, perhaps in combination with the cross-linkage theory, would provide explanations for many of the observed changes in the characteristics of cardiac function with aging. In the neuroendocrine theory, changes in hypothalamic function, possibly genetically-induced, lead to changes in nerves and mediators. Major alterations in physiological function and the response to stress reflect the long-term and progressive summation effects of changes in individual neurohormonal mediators.

CARDIAC MUSCLE FUNCTION IN AGING

EXCITATION-CONTRACTION COUPLING

Our current understanding of how aging affects the myocardial contraction at the tissue-cellular levels is derived from studies in animal models. In cardiac muscles of senescent animals, contraction and relaxation times are prolonged. Figure 52–1B shows twitch recordings from adult rats (7 months) and aged rats (24 months).[18-28] Prolonged duration of contraction and relaxation can be attributed to alterations in mechanisms that govern excitation-contraction coupling in the heart (p. 357). Excitation of cardiac muscle results in a transient rise in cytosolic [Ca++]. This activates myofilaments which stiffen, shorten, and produce force. The rate of decline in force or muscle lengthening reflects, in part, the rate and time course of decline in [Ca++].

CALCIUM TRANSIENT. The time course of the Ca++–myofilament interaction is a major determinant of duration of

contraction and the time course of relaxation. This is determined in part by the extent and rate of myofilament shortening during the contraction, which is itself, in part, determined by the amount of Ca++ bound to troponin before the onset of contraction. The extent and rate of myofilament shortening are determined in part by the rate of myofilament hydrolysis of adenosine triphosphate (ATP) and crossbridge cycling rate and in part by the time course of the myoplasmic [Ca++] transient, the duration of which is determined by sarcolemmal depolarization and by the rates of sarcoplasmic reticulum Ca++ release and pumping. The myoplasmic [Ca++] transient that follows sarcolemmal depolarization in cardiac muscle has been monitored by injecting the chemiluminescent protein aequorin into multiple cells of that tissue and measuring the light transient that precedes contraction.[28] The duration of the myoplasmic [Ca++] transient, measured as the time course of aequorin luminescence, is prolonged in isometric muscle isolated from aged versus younger adult rats (Fig. 52–1C). The myoplasmic free [Ca++] transient results primarily from the sarcoplasmic reticulum Ca++ release and is the net result of the amount of Ca++ released and the extent of Ca++ binding to cell proteins. The rate at which the sarcoplasmic reticulum pumps Ca++ is diminished in hearts of senescent versus younger animals (Fig. 52–1D),[21,29] and this appears to be a major contributor to the prolonged transient and the prolonged time course of cardiac muscle relaxation. The reduction in sarcoplasmic reticulum Ca++ transport rate may be related to a decrease in the density of pump sites, as mRNA coding for the sarcoplasmic reticulum pump protein (Ca++ ATPase) is reduced by about 50 per cent in senescent versus younger adult hearts.[30]

The transmembrane action potential of working cardiac muscle from both right and left ventricles of senescent rats is markedly prolonged compared with young controls (Fig. 52–1A).[20,24] The magnitude of action potential prolongation in right ventricular isometric muscle from senescent rats is as great as that in left ventricular muscle and as great as that in muscle from experimentally hypertrophied rat hearts.[31] The overshoot and level of depolarization at all relative repolarization times are also greater in older than in younger Wistar rat cardiac muscles.[20] The mechanism for the prolonged action potential appears to be caused by a reduction in outward currents, as the magnitude of the Ca++ current (under conditions in which Na+ current is blocked) is not markedly changed with age.[32] The larger action potential in intact senescent muscle may serve to reduce Ca++ efflux by means of Na/Ca exchange, which is voltage-sensitive and occurs during the action potential of each heartbeat.[33] This would "conserve" cytosolic calcium content and would allow more Ca++ to be pumped by the sarcoplasmic reticulum. Alternatively, the changes in the action potential could be the result of age-related differences in the cytosolic [Ca++] transient (i.e., the prolonged [Ca++] transient may cause a prolonged action potential).[34]

DURATION OF CONTRACTION, RELAXATION, AND MUSCLE STIFFNESS. The prolonged time course of the myoplasmic free Ca++ transient also may affect other aspects of the cardiac contraction that depend on Ca++–myofilament interactions (i.e., the time to peak force [Fig. 52–1B] and the ability of myofilaments to shorten and stiffen at differing times after excitation). The time to peak stiffness and half-relaxation time of peak stiffness are prolonged in senescent versus younger adult cardiac muscle,[23,25,26,35] probably reflecting the prolonged [Ca++] transient and slowed Ca++ uptake by the sarcoplasmic reticulum. Muscle stiffness is measured as the ratio of the change in force in response to a length change. Stiffness measured in response to small sinusoidal changes in muscle length made during the contraction has been referred to as "active dynamic" stiffness. The active dynamic stiffness is a linear function of the force and increases as force increases with time during a contraction. The slope coefficient (a) of the active stiffness–force relation, but not its intercept, increases in senescence. Enhanced dynamic stiffness in senescent muscle is present only during contractile activation by Ca++.[23,25] A

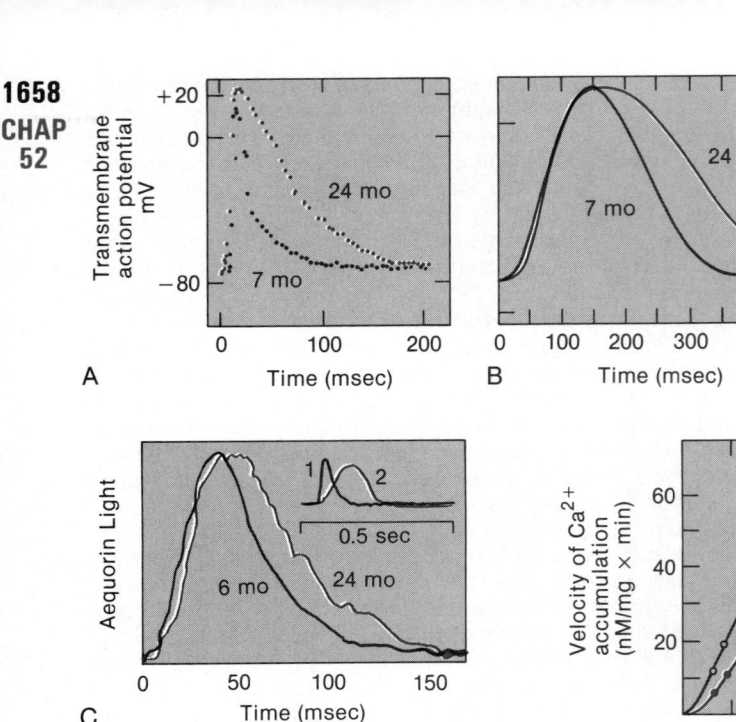

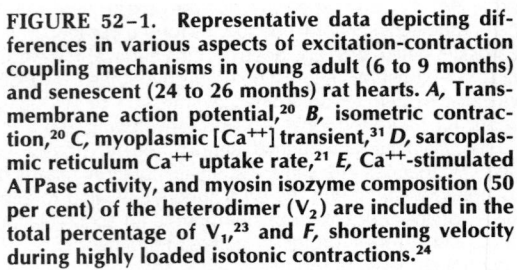

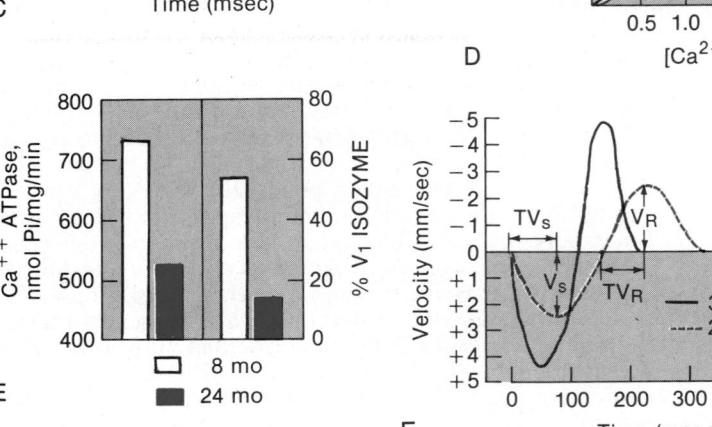

FIGURE 52-1. Representative data depicting differences in various aspects of excitation-contraction coupling mechanisms in young adult (6 to 9 months) and senescent (24 to 26 months) rat hearts. *A*, Transmembrane action potential,[20] *B*, isometric contraction,[20] *C*, myoplasmic [Ca++] transient,[31] *D*, sarcoplasmic reticulum Ca++ uptake rate,[21] *E*, Ca++-stimulated ATPase activity, and myosin isozyme composition (50 per cent) of the heterodimer (V₂) are included in the total percentage of V₁,[23] and *F*, shortening velocity during highly loaded isotonic contractions.[24]

possible explanation for the increase in the slope stiffness during contraction is as follows: at times during contraction when force is still increasing and myoplasmic [Ca++] is decreasing, myoplasmic [Ca++] remains higher in senescent than in younger muscles. This may result in a relative increase in Ca++–myofilament interaction in senescent versus younger muscles during this phase of contraction, but not at earlier times. The steady-state myofilament response to Ca++ is not altered with age, and neither the maximum force nor the shape of the force-pCa relation differs with age.[19]

FORCE GENERATION. The amplitude of the twitch (Fig. 52–1B) and aequorin luminescence (Fig. 52–1C) do not decline in senescent muscles as long as the [Ca++] in the superfusate is in the physiological range and the rate of stimulation is low. In addition, peak twitch force at relatively low rates of stimulation (6 to 48 min/liter) does not differ with age across a broad range of resting lengths.[18,20,21,24,26–28,31,36–38] Postextrasystolic twitch potentiation during continual paired stimulation also is preserved in senescent muscles.[39] The relatively low rates of stimulation required for studies in papillary muscles do not permit assessment of the extent of Ca++ release at rates approaching those in the rat in vivo (e.g., 300 per minute). In addition, the stability of isolated bulk muscle preparations requires that the temperature be maintained typically at 30°C or less. The maintenance of peak twitch force at low stimulation frequencies and temperature in senescent muscle may, in part, result from the prolonged myoplasmic [Ca++] transient (Fig. 52–1C). In rat muscles bathed in physiological [Ca++], in the absence of drugs the amplitude of Ca++ release and twitch force declines as the stimulation frequency is in-

creased. The magnitude of this decline is not different in senescent and young adult muscles.[28] However, in bathing medium containing higher [Ca++], whereas muscles from younger adult rats are able to produce the same Ca++ release and twitch force at low and higher rates of stimulation, at the higher stimulation rate, senescent muscles cannot.[28] In addition, in physiologic bathing Ca++ solution, when the coupling interval of paired stimulation is decreased below 200 msec, senescent, but not adult, muscles fail to generate a twitch response to the second stimulus.[26] These deficits of the senescent muscle may be related, in part, to the diminished Ca++ pumping rate by sarcoplasmic reticulum in senescent muscle (Fig. 52–1D).

CONTRACTILE PROTEINS
(See also p. 406)

A decrease in the rate of ATP hydrolysis has been observed in various contractile protein preparations isolated from the myocardium of aged as compared with younger animals.[19,22,36,40–43] The rate and extent of this decline vary with the particular preparation studied. The Ca++-activated myosin ATPase activity has been found to decline progressively with age from maturation through senescence.[22,36,43a,43b] Myosin ATPase activity is modulated by the myosin heavy chain isoform type.[44] The percentage of the alpha heavy chain myosin (i.e., that which has the most rapid ATP hydrolytic rate [i.e., V₁ isomyosin]) declines progressively with age in rats from maturation through senescence, whereas the proportion of the beta myosin heavy chain with a slower ATP hydrolytic rate (V_3 isoform) progressively increases with age.[22,36] By 24 months of age V_1 constitutes less than 20 per cent of the total myosin content (Fig. 52–1E). This shift in myosin isoform (V_1 to V_3) is regulated at the transcriptional level, in part at least, as mRNA levels coding for the alpha and beta heavy chains markedly decrease and increase, respectively, with adult aging.[43a,43b,45]

The myosin isozyme shift to a greater percentage of V_3 with aging is accompanied by a reduction in the velocity of isotonic shortening (Fig. 52–1F).[24,40,46] In the isometric contraction, the time to peak tension and duration of the contraction are directly related to the percentage of V_3 or inversely related to the percentage of V_1.[22] The increase in the stiffness during the twitch in senescent versus younger adult rat cardiac muscle[23,25,35] might be related to differences in isozymes.

MORPHOLOGICAL PROPERTIES

The senescent Wistar rat heart exhibits moderate cardiac hypertrophy compared with hearts from young and middle-age animals.[6,35] This occurs in the absence of systemic hypertension.[47] In hearts of male Fischer 344 rats, collagen accumulates in relation to ventricular protein after 3 months of age and continues in that mode with increased age of the animal, leveling off at about 12 per cent at 22 to 26 months, a twofold increase over that at 1 month.[48] With advancing age papillary muscles of the left heart become fibrosed to a greater extent than in the right heart of Fischer rats.[48] In Wistar rats the average left ventricular collagen content doubles between adulthood and senescence.[37] Still, the volume fraction of collagen is less than 5 to 10 per cent of the cardiac mass. Collagen accumulates in intrinsic collagenous structures, including perimysial weaves, coiled perimysial fibers, and struts, where the preexisting fibers are thicker and more extensive. Regions of fibrosis also are increased in size and volume in older animals.[48] In the Sprague-Dawley strain an age-associated increase in the extent of myocardial fibrosis, involving 60 per cent of the rats at the time of spontaneous death, has been observed.[49] This fibrosis appears rather diffuse, with hypertrophied bundles intermingled among the fibrous tissue. The fibrosis is dispersed rather widely within the myocardium, but some concentration is noted in the subendocardial and subepicardial regions.

The majority of the increase in cardiac mass with aging in the Wistar rat can be explained by myocardial cell enlargement. In individual myocytes isolated from Wistar rats of 2, 6 to 9, and 24 to 25 months of age, the average myocyte length measured under high-power light microscopy increased from 133 μm at 2 months to 146 μm at 6 to 9 months to 162 μm at 24 to 25 months of age. The average slack sarcomere length does not vary with age. The average cell volume, measured by means of Coulter counter techniques, approximately doubles between 2 and 24 months.[50] In male Sprague-Dawley rats in the interval between 3 and 10 to 12 months the mean myocyte cell volume per nucleus increases 53 and 26 per cent in the left and the right ventricle, respectively. The total number of myocyte nuclei remains constant in either ventricle. By 19 to 20 months a further (39 per cent) cellular hypertrophy of the left ventricle of the heart occurs found in association with an 18 per cent loss in cell number. Cell loss was accompanied by discrete areas of interstitial and replacement fibrosis in the subendocardium.[7] In contrast to the left ventricle, in the right ventricle no focal myocardial damage was observed, and the measured 35 per cent additional enlargement of myocytes occurred without a change in cell number. These cellular changes in this strain over the age range occurred without an increase in the ratio of heart weight to body weight. Thus the aging left ventricle is composed of a smaller number of hypertrophied cells. As this strain, like the Wistar strain discussed above, is not hypertensive, the stimulus for cell loss and hypertrophy of remaining cells with aging is not known.

PASSIVE MUSCLE PROPERTIES

Classic studies of muscle mechanics denote as "passive"[51] those tissue properties that do not directly depend on excitation. These properties are important because they influence the rate, time course, and extent of shortening and force development. The manner in which the myofilaments are coupled to passive components of the tissue also is a determinant of the viscoelastic properties of muscle.[52,53] Even with detailed information on the amount of collagen, its physical characteristics, and the characteristics of the network weave, direct cause-effect relations between structural and functional alterations are difficult to substantiate.[18]

Estimation of the elastic or viscoelastic modulus is a more meaningful method of assessing passive muscle properties than measurement of resting force at L_{max} or examination of the passive length-tension curve.[54,55] No alteration in passive viscoelastic stiffness parameters can be demonstrated.[23,25,35] In intact ventricles of various species the effect of advanced age on the modulates of viscoelastic stiffness is inconclusive,

with no change,[56] an increase,[57,58] and a decrease[59] having been observed.

SIMILARITIES BETWEEN AGING AND EXPERIMENTAL CARDIAC OVERLOAD IN YOUNGER ANIMALS

Many of the changes that occur with senescence in the normotensive rat also occur in the myocardium of younger animals in which experimental hypertension has caused cardiac hypertrophy (cf. ref. 60 for review). The strikingly similar pattern of alteration in excitation-contraction coupling mechanisms in the young hypertensive heart and those occurring in senescence are summarized in Table 52–1. The myocardial hypertrophy in pressure overload is a manifestation of an enhanced net protein synthesis owing to enlargement of a relatively constant number of cardiac myocytes, and reflects global activation of cardiac genes at the translational and posttranslational levels.[61] Because similar changes in cellular ribonucleic acid (RNA) concentration and the rate of protein synthesis have been observed with aging and chronic myocardial overload, it has been suggested that the latter (which usually is accompanied by myocardial hypertrophy) represents "accelerated aging."[62]

There is evidence that the signal that transduces the stress of an enhanced pressure load is mechanical (i.e., stretch or tension).[63-69] In this regard, stimulation of protein synthesis for both systolic and diastolic tension is described by a single linear function.[69] The tension effect may be mediated in part by enhanced coronary flow[70] or hormonal stimulation.[65,66,68,71] There is evidence for an interaction of stretch- and hormone receptor–mediated intracellular signal transduction (e.g., cyclic adenosine monophosphate [cAMP] or phosphatidylinositol turnover[66,72]) or ion flux (e.g., Na^+[63]), possibly related to stretch-induced activation of ionic channels.[73] Reorganization of intracellular matrix proteins, desmin and tubulin, also may mediate the stretch response.[74] Additionally, stretch of extracellular matrix and ventricular and cardiac endothelium may lead to the production of growth factors which can initiate protein synthesis.

It is tempting to speculate that because the *pattern* of changes in cell mechanisms occurs in both experimental pressure overload and aging, it may reflect a "logic" within the genome that regulates the expression of multiple genes for cellular adaptation to occur. This particular adaptive constellation allows for an energy-efficient and prolonged contraction. In the hypertensive heart it can be inferred that these adaptations occur in response to an increased afterload; however, with aging, whether the pattern that occurs is adaptive or degenerative is uncertain because the stimuli for these changes remain to be identified. If these changes were to occur in human myocardium with aging, they could easily be attributed to the stiffer arterial system and increases in arterial pressure and impedance. There is no data, however, to indicate that arterial stiffening or vascular impedance occurs with aging in rats, and the changes depicted in Table 52–1 have been described in two strains of rats that do not become hypertensive with aging.[7,47] Although peripheral resistance increases with age in rats, it appears to plateau at 10 to 12 months (cf. ref. 18 for review) and cannot be directly related to the changes in Figure 52–1, which are progressive with advancing age.

The increased left ventricular mass that occurs in the Wistar strain with

TABLE 52–1 ALTERATIONS OF CARDIAC MUSCLE FUNCTION IN AGING AND HYPERTENSION

FUNCTIONAL MEASURE	EXPERIMENTAL LV PRESSURE LOADING	NORMO-TENSIVE
Contraction duration	↑	↑
Contraction velocity	↓	↓
Myosin isozyme composition	↓ V_1, ↑ V_3	↓ V_1, ↑ V_3
Sarcoplasmic reticulum Ca^{++} pumping rate	↓	↓
Cytosolic Ca^{++} transient duration	↑ (Ferret)	↑
Myofilament Ca^{++} sensitivity	↔	↔
Action potential repolarization time	↑	↑
β-Adrenergic inotropic response	↓	↓
Cardiac glycoside response	↓	↓

The phenotypic pattern of adult aging bears a striking resemblance to that of experimental pressure loading in young animals and suggests that the molecular mechanisms may be similar in both cases.[60]

aging is largely due to an increase in left ventricular cavity size with the wall thickness appearing to remain normal.[5] Still, as is the case in the young hypertensive rodent, cardiac myocytes become enlarged in the senescent heart, and it may be argued that mechanical hormonal stimulation for cardiac hypertrophic response is present within the aging heart. It may be hypothesized that the dropout of myocardial cells with aging leads to augmented stretch on the remaining cells, and that this is the stimulus for cellular hypertrophy and the adaptive mechanisms that accompany this hypertrophy, as identified for the hypertensive heart, lead to a prolonged efficient contraction. On the other hand, prolonged contraction with aging persists in transplanted, mechanically unloaded atrophied hearts and also in right ventricular muscle in which no cell dropout has been observed.[7]

CHANGES IN THE THYROID STATE. Alterations of thyroid status can produce alterations in the variables depicted in Figure 52–2 (see also Chap. 61). In this regard the changes observed in the aging heart mimic to some extent those observed in the hypothyroid state.[44,75–77] Whether a relative hypothyroid state accompanies aging is uncertain. An age-associated decline in plasma thyroxine levels occurs in at least two rat strains,[22,78] but the magnitude of the decline is small. Still, it has been reported that administration of sufficient thyroxine to restore plasma levels in older rats to those levels that occur in younger rats can abolish the

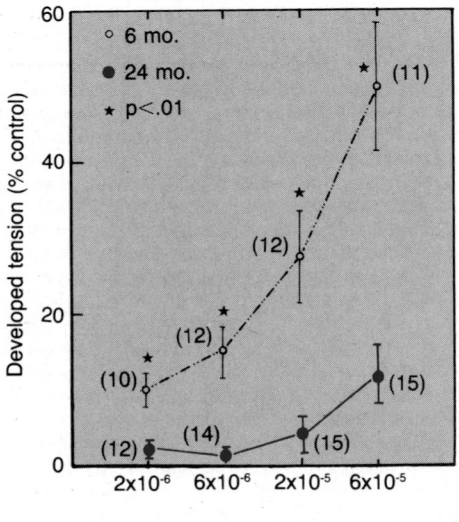

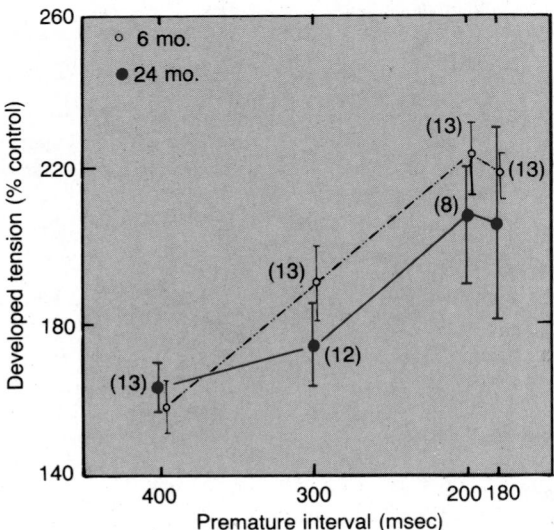

FIGURE 52–2. *Top,* The effect of age of the relative increase on twitch tension in response to incremental concentrations of ouabain in isolated left ventricular trabeculae from 6- to 24-month-old rats. Before drug, twitch tension did not vary with age. *Bottom,* Same muscles show no decrease in inotropic response to post extrasystolic potentiation. (From Gerstenblith, G., et al.: Diminished inotropic responsiveness to ouabain in aged rat myocardium. Circ. Res. *44*:577, 1979, by permission of the American Heart Association, Inc.)

age-associated decline in myosin ATPase activity[78]; however, reversal of the isozyme pattern did not occur with small doses of thyroxine.[78] High doses of thyroxine for a short period of time can increase the myosin V_1 content of senescent hearts but cannot fully restore this to the level observed in the younger heart.[22] Thus failure of cells to respond to thyroxine (e.g., deficits in nuclear receptors or DNA binding sites) may occur with aging and, in part, underlie the pattern of change depicted in Table 52–1.

GLUCOSE INTOLERANCE. This has been observed to occur in aged rats[79] and could possibly relate to some of the alterations noted in Table 52–1 because, in rats made diabetic, marked shifts occur in the myosin isoform pattern (increases in V_3 isoform) and in actomyosin and ATPase activity.[80–82] Additionally, the sarcoplasmic reticulum Ca^{++} ATPase activity and Ca^{++} uptake of isolated sarcoplasmic reticulum are depressed in diabetic hearts,[83–85] and the contraction time is prolonged.[86]

PHYSICAL CONDITIONING EFFECTS ON SENESCENT CARDIAC MUSCLE

A reduction of physical activity occurs with age even in rats in captivity.[87,88] Many of the cardiac mechanisms depicted in Figure 52–1 can be modulated by physical conditioning, and physical conditioning of older animals has been shown to modify some of the changes in Table 52–1 but not others.[89]

Chronic exercise in senescent rats abolishes prolonged contraction and reduces the active dynamic stiffness without altering myocardial mass.[24] This chronic (5 months' duration) mild wheel exercise protocol, which was insufficient to alter the body or heart weight in adult (6 to 9 months) and senescent (24 to 26 months) rats at sacrifice, did not alter twitch amplitude in isolated left ventricular trabecular measured across a range of $[Ca^{++}]$ at either age. In the younger animals, this exercise protocol was ineffective in altering the duration of contraction or dynamic stiffness measured during contraction in muscles. In senescent muscles, however, it eliminated the age-associated increase in these parameters to the levels observed in the younger adult muscle. The reduction in both the slope stiffness coefficient and duration of contraction is consistent with an effect of exercise to reduce the duration of the myoplasmic Ca^{++} transient. Indeed, recent studies suggest that the duration of the Ca^{++} transient in senescent cardiac muscle is reduced after chronic exercise.[90] The reduced rate of sarcoplasmic reticulum Ca^{++} sequestration in the senescent heart also can be reversed by chronic physical conditioning.[91]

BIOCHEMICAL CHANGES. A greater relative effect of chronic exercise on some other aspects of cardiac biochemistry in senescent as compared with young adult rat myocardium also has been observed. Although chronic exercise usually does not augment cytochrome *c* oxidase activity in cardiac muscle of younger animals as it does in skeletal muscle,[92] a modest augmentation of cytochrome *c* oxidase has been observed in hearts of senescent animals.[92] This was accompanied by exercise-induced increases in the rates of glutamate-malate, palmitoylcarnitine, and succinate oxidation.[92] Thus, exercise can partially reverse the decline in the oxidation.[92]

Marked age-related declines in cardiac aldolase and superoxide dismutase activities in mice between 9 and 27 months are prevented by chronic exercise begun at 6 months of age and continued into old age.[94] The progressive decline in myocardial Ca^{++}-activated actomyosin ATPase activity that begins during maturation (after 1 month in the rat) and progresses with advancing adult age can be retarded by a chronic (3 months) period of exercise. This relatively small, beneficial effect of exercise, however, was observed only through 12 to 15 months.[94] In older animals that began exercise at 17 to 22 months and were sacrificed at 20 to 25 months, a decline in this ATPase occurred.[95] The altered myosin isoform profile in the senescent heart is not affected by chronic physical conditioning.[96] The insulin resistance of the aging rat also is ameliorated by chronic exercise,[79] as is the response of senescent cardiac muscle to reoxygenation after hypoxia.[97]

RESPONSE OF THE OLDER HEART TO CHRONIC HEMODYNAMIC OVERLOAD

Whereas the relative adaptive response of the senescent versus younger heart to moderate exercise is enhanced, the response to mechanical stresses that evoke substantial myocardial hypertrophy (e.g., pressure or volume overload) appears, in some instances, to be reduced. The extent of hypertrophy after aortic banding,[98] volume overload,[99] or the creation of renal hypertension[36] in senescent rats appears to be reduced. (In the latter study the significance is unclear, because of four groups tested, one younger age group also showed a reduction in the extent of hypertrophy. Additionally, a subsequent study in the same pressure-loading model of the same rat strain observed that the hypertrophic response of senescent heart was not decreased.[100]) The extent to which myosin isoform ATPase activity, action potential, and contraction duration become altered appears to be correlated with the extent of hypertrophy, regardless of age.[36] The hypertrophic response to chronic AV block, causing a 50 per cent reduction in heart rate and 50 per cent hypertrophy, decreases with age and is accompanied by a reduced contractile adaptation.[101] Furthermore, the contractile response to stressful conditions (high pacing rate and high bathing calcium concentration) is reduced in senescent hearts that had responded to mild aortic banding[102] with an appropriate degree of hypertrophy.

Thus it appears that the adaptive reserve capacity with respect to an increase in cardiac mass may become diminished with advancing age. This may indicate that some cardiac adaptations (e.g., an increase in myocyte size or heart size) become utilized with aging such that the reserve capacity of the aged heart to respond to these stressful situations is diminished. This could be in part related to cell death and fibrosis when cell size becomes limiting, owing to ischemia or inadequacy of cell ionic or energy homeostasis for other reasons. A relative reduction in the extent of cardiac hypertrophy in response to a given increment of arterial pressure also could indicate age-associated reduction in the efficiency of global activation of protein synthesis.

DIMINISHED MYOCARDIAL RESPONSE TO BETA-ADRENOCEPTOR STIMULATION

Although the effect of beta-adrenergic agonists to abbreviate the duration of contraction duration is not age-related in isolated cardiac cells, muscle, or perfused rat myocardium, their effect to enhance contractile force is diminished.[27,38,103] Age-related changes that are, in part, distal to the receptor-cyclase system are required to explain the diminished myocardial contractile response to isoproterenol. Neither the number of myocardial beta receptors nor their affinity for antagonists or for isoproterenol appears to be altered with age, and neither basal levels of cAMP nor the increased level achieved during the peak contractile response were age-related. Furthermore, the age-related deficit in enhancement of contractility observed with isoproterenol persisted when dibutyryl cAMP was used as the agonist. Dibutyryl cAMP bypasses the receptor-cyclase system. Neither basal nor stimulated levels of protein kinase activity in the same myocardial preparations in which the contractile responses were studied varied with age. Thus, an explanation for the depressed inotropic response is that one or more steps distal to protein kinase activation differ with age. The possibilities include differences in the extent of phosphorylation of various proteins or differences in ion flux or binding that results from a given level of phosphorylation, or age differences in phosphoprotein phosphatase activity, an enzyme that dephosphorylates proteins and organelles. An age-associated deficit in the ability of norepinephrine to augment troponin I phosphorylation has recently been observed.[104] This was attributed, however, to an apparent net decrease in cAMP production. A 20 per cent increase in phosphoprotein phosphatase activity in the senescent heart has been measured.[38] Enhanced adenosine in coronary effluent isolated from older versus younger rats has been observed and has been related to a reduction in the response to beta-adrenergic stimulation in these hearts.[105] An alternative explanation (i.e., that the Ca^{++}-myofilament interaction that leads to force production is altered with age) can be excluded, since in both intact and skinned preparations[19] the effect of Ca^{++} on force production, from threshold to maximum, is not altered with age.

DIMINISHED RESPONSE TO DIGITALIS GLYCOSIDES

The contractile response to ouabain is diminished in the senescent as compared with the adult myocardium (Fig. 52–2, top).[41] The response to paired stimulation (which causes a much greater increase in contractility than ouabain) in the

same muscles is not age-related (Fig. 52–2, bottom). Thus, the depressed response to ouabain of senescent muscle cannot readily be attributed to a nonspecific failure of the excitation-contraction process, to an inability of the myofilaments to generate additional force, or to a failure in energy necessary for a sustained inotropic response. The mechanism for the effect of age may be at the Na^+, K^+-ATPase receptor (p. 480, i.e., an age-related difference in receptor density, ouabain binding, resultant enzyme inhibition) or in the extent of enhanced Ca^{++} loading caused by this inhibition. The relative ouabain inhibition of Na^+, K^+-ATPase in crude membrane preparations is not dependent on age over the adult range.[41] In the intact senescent (11 to 13 years) beagle, as compared with the adult (1 to 3 years) dog, a decrement in the contractile response to acetylstrophanthidin with no difference in glycoside Na^+, K^+-ATPase inhibition also has been demonstrated.[106]

SUMMARY OF ANIMAL STUDIES

Most information regarding age of the myocardium comes from studies in the rat model. Isometric force production, at least at low frequencies of stimulation, is preserved. There is no clear-cut indication that passive stiffness is increased. Whereas the affinity of the myofibrils for Ca^{++} is preserved in senescent muscle, the inotropic responses to cardiac glycosides and beta-adrenergic stimulation are reduced. The latter may underlie, in part, the alterations in cardiodynamics (i.e., greater utilization of the Frank-Starling mechanism) during vigorous exercise in older men. In senescence, contraction is prolonged in part because the Ca^{++} released into the myoplasm during systole is removed more slowly than in the younger heart. A major cause of this appears to be a reduced rate of Ca^{++} sequestration by the sarcoplasmic reticulum. Although the duration of action potential also is longer in senescent than in younger cardiac muscle, its role in the prolonged contraction is less clear. The action potential changes could reflect age-related changes in the sarcolemmal ionic conductances or be the result of the prolonged myoplasmic Ca^{++} transient. In the older rat heart, myosin isozymes shift to slower forms and ATPase activity declines. These changes appear to underlie the observed decline in shortening velocity in senescent muscle contracting in the isotonic mode. The interrelated alterations in excitation-contraction mechanisms and myofibrillar biochemistry that occur in senescence are adaptive. The same constellation of changes is observed in the myocardium of young rats in which myocardial hypertrophy is induced by chronic hypertension or aortic banding. Some of these changes (e.g., the prolonged contraction duration and decline in sarcoplasmic reticulum pumping ability) can be reversed by chronic exercise in senescent animals.

CARDIAC FUNCTION IN NORMAL AGING HUMANS

The effect of age on cardiac function in humans can be addressed only in the context of the population studied and the variable used to define and measure cardiac function. One of the most consistent findings in studies of the influence of aging is the large variation in the older population for nearly every cardiovascular variable. There are many older people whose measured performance is equal to, or in some instances superior to, their middle-aged counterparts as well as some who are considerably below the mean for their age group. This variation must be related to differences in factors other than age which influence cardiovascular performance. The most important of these are the presence of cardiovascular disease, primarily hypertension and coronary atherosclerosis, and physical conditioning status. Therefore, the results of studies in humans must be related to the certainty of freedom from the effects of superimposed disease and the physical conditioning status of the subjects. This is particularly true when quantitating the "effect of age" on measured left ventricular performance.

ASSESSMENT OF PERFORMANCE

Another equally important consideration is the measured variable. Although maximum oxygen consumption is considered to be the best index of cardiovascular performance, there are several potential difficulties in determining the age effect on this important parameter. The first is that to be certain that any person's oxygen consumption during exercise is the maximum, it is necessary to demonstrate no significant increase in oxygen consumption despite an increase in workload. This often is not found in studies of older age groups, and suggests that musculoskeletal or some other noncardiovascular parameters are limiting exercise before the true maximum oxygen consumption can be achieved. Even if a plateau is reached, it is possible that age differences in muscle mass or in the ability of the muscles to extract and use oxygen may be the limiting factor rather than cardiovascular function per se. This is suggested by recent evidence that age differences in maximum oxygen consumption are minimized or abolished when the values are adjusted for lean body mass.[107]

Studies of "normal" aging have been handicapped until recently by a natural reluctance to use invasive methodology in people who are thought to be free of cardiovascular disease. This resulted in two major limitations in some earlier work. The first is that it was difficult to exclude patients with occult coronary disease. This is an important consideration because the prevalence of autopsy-documented disease is much higher than the prevalence of clinically obvious disease.[2,108,109] Many people thought to be free of coronary disease on screening using routine history, physical examination, and resting electrocardiogram undoubtedly were not. Because there is an age-related increase in the incidence of inapparent disease, many older study participants with latent coronary disease were included in study protocols. A second limitation resulting from the hesitancy to use invasive methodology was an inability to measure central circulatory function (i.e., stroke volume or its determinants, end-diastolic and end-systolic volumes) in relatively large numbers of volunteers. The recent introduction of nuclear cardiology techniques, specifically the use of thallium scintigraphy to diagnose the presence of coronary disease, and gated blood pool scans to measure cardiac volumes during exercise, provided significant additional information concerning the effect of normal aging on cardiac function during rest and exercise stress.

HEMODYNAMICS AT REST: NO CHANGE IN STROKE VOLUME OR EJECTION FRACTION. Although invasive studies have indicated that aging is associated with a decline in cardiac output at rest,[110-112] these results may have been due to the selection of subjects not free of disease or to the methodology used. Cardiac output may increase more in younger people because of an age difference in the stress response to the invasive procedure itself. Several studies using noninvasive techniques have shown no age-related decrement in cardiac output, heart rate, stroke volume, or ejection fraction at rest.[113-116]

One of the more significant age-associated changes in resting cardiovascular parameters is an increase in systolic arterial pressure (Fig. 28-3, p. 820). This is probably secondary to age-associated changes in arterial stiffening, since the rise in blood pressure varies directly with vascular stiffness in different populations.[117] The increased systolic pressure is probably responsible, in part, for the mild left ventricular hypertrophy associated with aging (Fig. 52-3)[116,118]; it also is seen in laboratory animals, as discussed earlier. This hypertrophy tends to normalize wall stress and may preserve indices of left ventricular function, including resting ejection fraction and the velocity of circumferential fiber shortening.[116] Apart from the increase in systolic pressure, the most striking and consistent change in resting indices is a slowed, delayed, and more heterogeneous pattern of early diastolic filling.[119-121] This is probably due to prolonged cardiac muscle relaxation, and is a consistent characteristic of aging which has been found in many species and experimental preparations, as discussed above. Increased mitral valve stiffness also may play a role. The functional importance of this alteration under normal conditions is not great, since end-diastolic volume is either not age-related or slightly increased with age at rest[113,116,122] and during exercise.[113] However, it probably renders older persons more susceptible to hemodynamic compromise in the presence of a tachycardiac arrhythmic stress[123] or in the presence of superimposed ischemic or hypertensive disease, both of which independently impair diastolic filling.

HEMODYNAMICS DURING EXERCISE: LOWER HEART RATE AND GREATER END-SYSTOLIC AND END-DIASTOLIC VOLUMES. In contrast to the subtle age effect on resting hemodynamic indices, there are more dramatic changes during exercise stress. Most investigators have reported a decline in maximum oxygen uptake and heart rate with aging,[124] even in athletes.[125] Several have reported a decline in exercise cardiac output with increasing age because of a decrease in both heart rate and stroke volume.[111,112] In one study in persons carefully screened to eliminate ischemic heart disease, no age effect was found on cardiac output at comparable and peak workloads because an increase in stroke volume compensated for the decline in heart rate in the older people.[113] In this study end-systolic and end-diastolic volumes also were measured, and the increase in stroke volume was achieved by greater use of the Frank-Starling mechanism (i.e., an increase in end-diastolic volume). Additionally, in younger people there was greater systolic emptying with a decrease in end-systolic volume, as compared with the resting values (Fig. 52-4). Ejection fraction increased more from rest to exercise in younger than in older people. In most older people who were free of disease ejection fraction did increase with exercise, but by only a small amount.

These age-associated changes in the mechanisms used to augment cardiac output with exercise can be interpreted in the light of data showing an age-associated decrease in the inotropic,[27,38] chronotropic,[126] and arterial vasodilating effects of catecholamine stimulation.[127,128] During exercise, heart rate increases less in older people, probably, in part, because of a decreased cardiovascular response to catecholamines (Fig. 52-4). End-systolic volume (Fig. 52-4) also decreases less, owing to a diminished inotropic and vasodilating re-

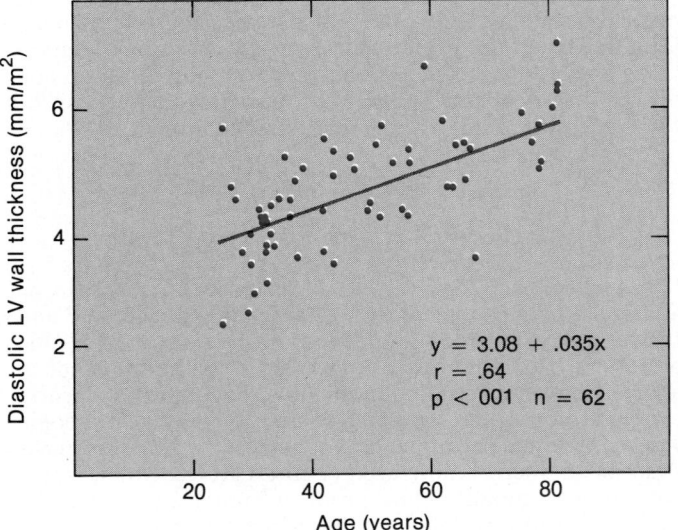

FIGURE 52-3. Linear regression plot of the relationship between age and diastolic left ventricular wall thickness (mm/M²) in male participants of the Baltimore Longitudinal Aging Population. Increased age is associated with mild left ventricular hypertrophy.[116] (From Gerstenblith, G., Frederiksen, J., Yin, V.C.P., et al.: Echocardiographic assessment of a normal adult aging population. Circulation 56:273, 1977, reprinted by permission of the American Heart Association, Inc.)

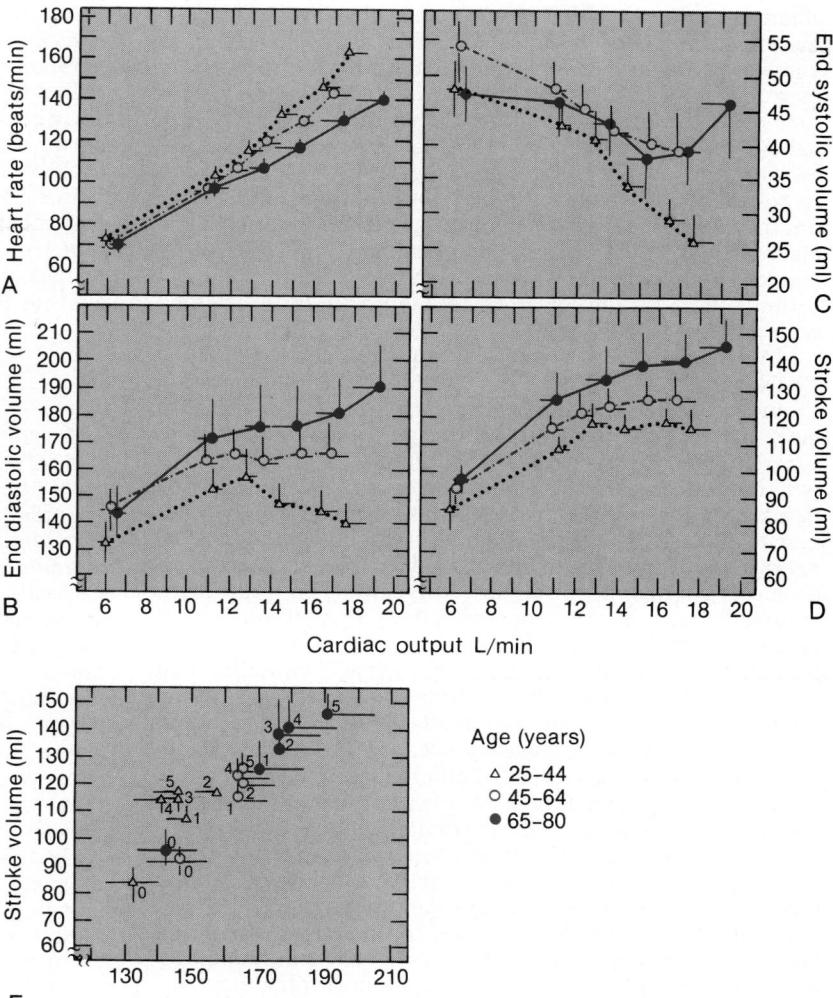

FIGURE 52–4. The relationship between cardiac output (plotted in L/min along the abscissa in Panels A to D) and heart rate (Panel A), end-diastolic volume (Panel B), end-systolic volume (Panel C), and stroke volume (Panel D) and the stroke volume–end-diastolic volume relationship (Panel E) at rest and during graded upright bicycle exercise measured by means of gated blood pool scans. The subjects are divided into three age groups, 25 to 44 years old (n = 22), 45 to 64 years old (n = 23), and 65 to 79 years old (n = 16). The number of subjects able to complete the exercise periods decreased with increasing workload; at a workload of 125 watts, n = 16 in group 1, n = 15 in group 2, and n = 11 in group 3. When the data were analyzed including only those who were able to achieve the 125 watt workload, a similar pattern was observed in all parameters and the significance of the age effect was unchanged. (From Rodeheffer, R. J., Gerstenblith, G., Becker, L. C., et al.: Exercise cardiac output is maintained with advancing age in healthy human subjects: Cardiac dilatation and increased stroke volume compensate for a diminished heart rate. Circulation 69:203, 1984, reprinted by permission of the American Heart Association, Inc.)

sponse to catecholamines.[113] Finally, the benefit of the Frank-Starling mechanism is unaltered with age and used effectively during exercise to maintain output through a higher stroke volume at a greater end-diastolic volume (Fig. 52–4B and D).[113] The decrease in catecholamine-mediated effects during exercise is probably not caused by decreased elaboration of catecholamines, since plasma levels are higher, not lower, in humans during exercise.[129]

AGING, DISEASE, AND CARDIAC FUNCTION

ISCHEMIC HEART DISEASE

DIAGNOSIS. The prevalence and severity of coronary atherosclerosis increase so dramatically with age that more than one-half of all deaths in people aged 65 years or older are due to coronary disease and about three-fourths of all deaths from ischemic heart disease occur in the elderly.[130] The diagnosis of ischemic heart disease may be more difficult in the older person, since the prevalence of diagnosed disease[109] is only one-third to one-half the prevalence of autopsy-documented significant atherosclerosis.[108] The lack of classic symptomatology may be related to an age-associated decline in physical activity to the point at which ischemic symptoms are not present. In addition, dyspnea, rather than pain, may be the most prominent feature of the clinical picture in angina as well as infarction (p. 1293),[131] possibly because of the age-related changes in myocardial and pericardial compliance and diastolic relaxation discussed above. The physical examination is of limited usefulness in the diagnosis of ischemic heart disease. It should be remembered, however, that the transient features associated with acute ischemia (i.e., an S₄ gallop, reversed splitting

of the second sound, and a systolic murmur owing to mitral regurgitation) often are present in older people, even in the absence of ischemia.[132–134]

Stress testing (Chap. 6) also is useful in the diagnosis of an older patient with suspected coronary disease but with certain caveats. The presence of resting ST-segment abnormalities or the use of digitalis, both of which are more common in the elderly, may invalidate the interpretation of the stress electrocardiogram, and in this setting stress testing using thallium scintigraphy is helpful. Thallium imaging also is helpful when the stress test is unexpectedly negative in an older person whose history suggests the presence of ischemia, since the predictive accuracy of a negative test is low in a population with a high prevalence of disease. Finally, many elderly patients may not be capable of exercising to 85 to 90 per cent of their predicted maximal heart rate. In this setting a thallium scan after dipyridamole administration may provide similar diagnostic information.[135]

MANAGEMENT OF CHRONIC ISCHEMIC HEART DISEASE (see also Chap. 40). The approaches to treatment of angina in older and younger patients are similar. After diagnosis, reversible factors should be identified and treated. Of these, anemia, hyperthyroidism, hypertension, congestive heart failure, and supraventricular arrhythmias may all be more common in the elderly. It also should be remembered that atherosclerosis is a progressive disease, and that although it has been stated that risk factor reduction is less important in the older patient, more recent evidence suggests that both successful treatment of hypertension[136,137] and smoking cessation[138] decrease cardiovascular mortality in the elderly. The use of specific anti-ischemic agents is discussed below. If medical therapy fails to adequately control symptoms, percutaneous transluminal coronary angioplasty (PTCA) should be considered. Although some reports indicate that in-hospital mortality associated with PTCA is higher in older than in younger patients,[139] low mortality (0.8 per cent) also has been reported, which does not differ from that in younger patients.[140] If the coronary anatomy is not suitable for PTCA in patients in whom medical therapy has failed, surgery should be performed. Although coronary bypass is associated with increased perioperative mortality[141] and morbidity and longer duration of hospitalization, as well as increased costs in the older patient,[142] the risks of complications are decreasing[143] and long-term pain relief and survival are good.[143,144] In most patients these results compare favorably with those attained with medical therapy (Fig. 52–5).[145]

MANAGEMENT OF ACUTE MYOCARDIAL INFARCTION (see also Chap. 39). The treatment of acute infarction should be undertaken with the realization that the risk of mortality, congestive heart failure, pulmonary edema, and ventricular rupture is higher in the elderly.[146-148] It is unclear whether the increased incidence of these complications is due to intrinsic age-related changes in the response to the ischemic insult itself, poorer reserve in the remaining noninfarcted regions, perhaps owing to diminished catecholamine responsiveness, the higher prevalence of hypertension, prior myocardial damage, and/or large infarctions. In addition, important topographical changes develop hours to days after an infarction which importantly affect overall mortality and morbidity. Animal and clinical studies have defined regional dilatation and wall thinning at the site of the infarction,[149] and compensatory hypertrophy may occur in the region remote from the infarction. Age-related differences in these architectural changes accompanying an infarction could result from preexisting changes in left ventricular wall thickness,[116,118] peripheral impedance,[127] collagen content,[37] capability of undergoing compensatory hypertrophy, and/or the inflammatory and healing response to the infarct itself.

The demonstration that coronary thrombus is present in a large proportion of patients with early transmural infarction[150] has prompted a number of placebo-controlled randomized studies evaluating the ability of thrombolytic therapy to improve survival.[151-155] These studies also show a several fold, age-related increase in mortality in patients assigned to placebo therapy. Although the magnitude of the benefit confirmed by thrombolytic therapy has been reported to be low in patients over 75 years of age,[151] other studies indicate large survival differences for those over age 65.[152-154] The prevalence of contraindications to thrombolytic treatment increases with age, particularly hypertension, history of stroke, and gastrointestinal bleeding.

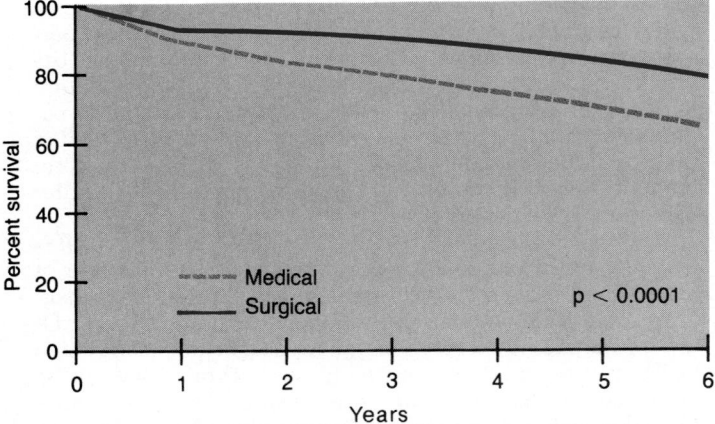

FIGURE 52–5. Cumulative 6-year survival in surgical and medical groups in 1491 patients 65 years or older from the CASS registry. Survival is adjusted for left ventricular wall motion, congestive heart failure, number of diseased vessels, number of associated medical diseases, and age at angiography. (Reprinted with permission from Gersh, B. J., Kronmal, R. A., Schaff, H. V., et al.: Comparison of coronary artery bypass surgery and medical therapy in patients 65 years of age or older. N. Engl. J. Med. *313:*217, 1985.)

Additional considerations regarding treatment of acute myocardial infarction include the higher likelihood of central nervous system side effects from lidocaine[156] and an increased risk of heparin-induced bleeding in older women.[157] The elderly benefit as much as younger patients do from the secondary prevention effects of beta blockade.[158] In a Netherlands multicenter double-blind randomized trial involving more than 800 patients over the age of 60 years, oral anticoagulation was associated with a significantly lower incidence of recurrent myocardial infarction and death.[159] Successful aggressive management of complications, including septal rupture,[160] also has been reported.

ARRHYTHMIAS

(See also Chap. 24)

In part because of the increasing prevalence of hypertension and coronary disease, arrhythmias occur more frequently and more often are associated with hemodynamic compromise in the older age groups. In one study the incidences of supraventricular and ventricular ectopic activity (> 100 beats/24 hours of ambulatory monitoring) were 26 per cent and 17 per cent, respectively, in 98 healthy subjects 60 to 85 years of age.[161] Ventricular couplets occurred in 11 per cent but ventricular tachycardia in only 4 per cent of the population. The incidence of asymptomatic ventricular tachycardia on routine treadmill testing in elderly people without other evidence of organic heart disease has been reported to be 4 per cent.[162] These arrhythmias were not associated with symptoms or subsequent sudden death. It should be recognized, however, that arrhythmias may be more ominous in the presence of disease. Even in the absence of disease, slowed and delayed early diastolic relaxation and filling owing to age alone[119,120] may result in greater compromised cardiac output in the older person with a tachyarrhythmia. Any compromise of cardiac output and blood pressure may, in turn, be associated with more critical decreases in cerebral flow in the older patient because of impaired cardiovascular reflex responses to hypotension,[122] an increased likelihood of preexisting cerebrovascular disease, and increased vascular stiffness.

The diagnosis of an arrhythmia in an older patient differs only in that the index of suspicion should perhaps be higher for any complaints relating to transient cerebral ischemia, angina, heart failure, or mental status changes. Long-term ambulatory monitoring often is useful. The urgency of therapy depends on the associated hemodynamic changes, and emergency treatment is the same in all age groups. The routine work-up should include a search for reversible precipitating factors. Some of these, including electrolyte imbalance, digitalis excess, hyperthyroidism, anemia, pulmonary embolism, and congestive heart failure, are more common in the older population. Specific therapy for the arrhythmia is guided by the severity of associated symptoms, the presence and type of underlying heart disease, and the recognition of the age-associated changes in the pharmacokinetics of the antiarrhythmic drugs, as discussed below.

BRADYARRHYTHMIAS. Sinus bradycardia often is present in older people in both the presence and absence of cardiac disease. It may be related to age-associated histological changes in the sinus node, a hypersensitive carotid sinus reflex, or medications, including digitalis, calcium- or beta-blocking drugs, and some other antihypertensives. Evaluation should be undertaken if the patient is symptomatic, and in this instance it is important to determine whether the transient symptoms are in fact caused by the bradyarrhythmia, since other causes for neurological symptoms often are present in this age group. Long-term ambulatory monitoring is most useful in this regard. If the patient is symptomatic, immediate therapy depends on the degree of hemodynamic compromise. Emergency temporary measures, including the administration of atropine and isoproterenol and the insertion of a temporary pacemaker, can be used. If no reversible factors are present, the only effective long-term therapy is permanent pacing. Pacemakers which allow for proper sequencing of atrial and ventricular events may be particularly useful in the elderly because of an increased reliance on late diastolic filling and hence atrial systole.

VALVULAR HEART DISEASE
(See also Chap. 34)

The diagnosis of valvular heart disease in the elderly often is obscured by age-related but benign systolic murmurs,[134] changes in S_2, and increased stiffness of the central arteries. This stiffness may prevent the appearance of the slow anacrotic shoulder and small pulse pressure which would otherwise be seen in significant *aortic stenosis*. The other findings, however, particularly in the presence of a late-peaking systolic murmur, electrocardiographic evidence of left ventricular hypertrophy, and echocardiographic demonstration of valve narrowing and calcification, all retain their significance. Doppler examination may be particularly useful in assessing the severity of obstruction.[163] The usual causes are calcification of a congenitally bicuspid valve and, in those over 75 years of age, degenerative calcification.[164] Aortic valve replacement should be recommended for the usual indications (i.e., syncope, angina, and failure) and is associated with low mortality and excellent results in terms of quality of life.[165,166] Balloon aortic valvuloplasty (p. 1376) provides only palliative relief in patients with aortic stenosis,[167] and should be considered only in those with definite contraindications to surgery.

The diagnosis of *aortic regurgitation* is not more difficult in the older age groups, but the timing of aortic valve replacement may be because of the often benign course of the disease. Surgery usually is recommended only for those patients who continue to be symptomatic on medical therapy.

Mitral stenosis usually is due to rheumatic disease, whereas regurgitation can be due to rheumatic disease as well as calcification of the mitral annulus, mitral valve prolapse (at times with superimposed endocarditis), and ischemic papillary muscle dysfunction. Survival is considerably shortened in the presence of atrial fibrillation and failure,[168] and the results of mitral valve surgery are satisfactory.[169,170] Balloon mitral valvuloplasty in elderly patients with heavily calcified valves is associated with slightly higher morbidity and mortality than in younger patients with pliable valves and no subvalvular stenosis.

HYPERTENSION
(See also Chap. 28)

The importance of the diagnosis and effective treatment of hypertension in the elderly cannot be overemphasized. It is the major remediable risk factor for cardiovascular morbidity and mortality, and successful therapy decreases the incidence of death and cerebrovascular events.[137,171-176,176a,176b] The prevalence of hypertension, defined by a blood pressure of 160/95 or greater, is 30 per cent in elderly men, and an additional 10 to 15 per cent of the total elderly population have isolated systolic hypertension, defined by a systolic pressure exceeding 160 mm Hg and a diastolic of less than 90 mm Hg. Convincing evidence of the effectiveness of therapy for even mild diastolic hypertension in the elderly is provided by the results of the Hypertension Detection and Follow-up Program Trial[136] (a 17.2 per cent reduction in mortality and 45 per cent reduction in cerebrovascular events), the Australian National Blood Pressure Study[172] (a 30 per cent reduction in trial end points), and the European Working Party on High Blood Pressure in the Elderly Trial.[137] In the latter study there were a 38 per cent reduction in cardiac mortality and a 27 per cent reduction in total cardiovascular mortality using an intention-to-treat analysis.

There are no data concerning the effectiveness of therapy for isolated systolic hypertension. However, in view of the fact that systolic blood pressure is the best discriminator of risk in people over age 45[176] and that systolic blood pressure can be controlled effectively with minimal side effects,[177] the Joint National Committee on Detection, Evaluation, and Treatment of High Blood Pressure has recommended that therapy be instituted in the elderly with isolated systolic hypertension.[178]

Thiazides have been used as the step one antihypertensive agent in all of the major trials that have documented a decline in cardiovascular morbidity and mortality. There are several concerns, however, regarding an increase in other cardiovascular risk factors and possibly mortality in patients with baseline electrocardiographic abnormalities.[179] Although beta blockers are effective antihypertensive agents in some populations, elderly patients respond less often than do young hypertensives.[180] Calcium channel antagonists[181] and angiotensin-converting enzyme inhibitors[182] may be especially well suited for use in the older population. They have the potential for effectively controlling blood pressure as either single agents or in combination and also to reduce left ventricular hypertrophy.

The importance of left ventricular hypertrophy as a risk factor for the development of coronary artery disease was reported by Levy et al.[183] in data from the Framingham study. These investigators reported a severalfold increase in the development of coronary disease in elderly hypertensives conferred by the presence of advanced left ventricular hypertrophy. The increase was independent of the risk afforded by pressure elevation alone. A study reported by Schulman et al.[184] compared the ability of the calcium channel blocker verapamil and the beta blocker atenolol to induce regression of left ventricular mass in older hypertensives and the effect of regression on left ventricular function and diastolic filling parameters. This study showed that the calcium antagonist was better able to induce regression than the beta blocker. In addition, regression was associated with an increase in peak diastolic filling rate and did not handicap either cardiac output or ejection fraction at rest or during mild upright bicycle exercise.

An interesting small group of elderly patients with hypertensive hypertrophic cardiomyopathy also has been described.[185] Females made up more than three-fourths of the reported group, and symptoms consisted primarily of dyspnea and chest pain. The diagnosis is made by echocardiography, which shows exaggerated contractile function, small systolic and diastolic cavity dimensions, and prolonged and reduced early diastolic filling. The importance of the recognition of this patient subset is that therapy with vasodilators was associated with clinical deterioration, whereas patients treated with beta blockers or calcium antagonists were markedly improved.

USE OF CARDIOVASCULAR DRUGS IN THE ELDERLY

As a consequence of the increased prevalence of cardiovascular (and other) diseases in the elderly, the percentage of total expenditures for drugs in this age group is severalfold higher than in the total population.[186] In considering the effects of age on the pharmacokinetics and pharmacodynamics of cardiovascular agents,[187-189] it is important to note the heterogeneity of response in the older population. There are no strict age-related rules, therefore, which apply to the entire geriatric population, and it is clear that the commitment of the physician to assess carefully the therapeutic results and side effects of medical therapy must be greater in older than in younger age groups.

Although age-related changes in gastric pH and absorptive surface have been described, these have relatively unimportant effects for most cardiovascular drugs. The distribution of cardiovascular agents, however, is affected by age-associated decreases in serum albumin[189] and lean body mass[190] and increases in alpha$_1$-acid glycoproteins[191] and body fat.[190] A decrease in albumin results in increased free drug for those agents which are highly protein-bound, which will, in turn, increase plasma concentrations for those agents whose metabolism is independent of the available free drug (e.g., lidocaine and propranolol). An increase in alpha$_1$-acid glycoprotein results in a decrease in the free fractions of acidic drugs such as phenytoin.[191] A change in body mass results in an increased distribution volume for fat-soluble drugs and a decreased distribution volume for water-soluble agents.

The effect of age on metabolism and excretion relates to its effect on renal and hepatic function. The influence of age on renal function has been extensively studied, and includes a diminished glomerular filtration rate of 30 to 40 per cent over a broad age range[192] as well as decreased renal tubular secretion and concentration ability. Because lean body mass decreases with age, renal function cannot be indexed using serum creatinine alone in older patients. These changes result in decreased clearance of quinidine, procainamide, digoxin, and the water-soluble beta blockers including atenolol. Diminished renal excretion of furosemide[193] results in a diminished diuretic response to this drug and presumably other agents which act on the luminal side of the kidney tubule. The effect of age on hepatic metabolism has been evaluated less extensively but is undoubtedly influenced by the decrease in hepatic mass, blood flow, and activity of the microsomal fixed-function oxidizing system. These changes result in increased half-lives of lidocaine and the lipid-soluble beta blockers, including propranolol.[194]

In addition to its effects on pharmacokinetics, age may influence the cardiac response to any given level of drug. Thus, a diminished response to beta agonists,[10,27,38] beta blockers,[194] and digitalis preparations[39,106] has been observed in human and/or animal models. The increased prevalence of other disease associated with aging may render the older person more sensitive to the side effect profile of cardiovascular agents as well. Preexisting decreased plasma volume and decreased baroreflex activity may render older patients more susceptible to the hypotensive effects of nitrates and diuretics. Preexisting conduction system disease or left ventricular dysfunction also may increase the likelihood of side effects with some beta blockers and calcium antagonists.

SUMMARY

The characterization of those cardiovascular changes in humans that are due to aging alone is difficult because of the age-related increasing prevalence of overt and latent cardiovascular disease and sedentary life style. It appears, however, that age does not significantly alter left ventricular performance except in the presence of a superimposed stress which can take the form of severe exercise or disease, particularly ischemia, a tachycardic arrhythmia, or hypertension. In these instances, impaired diastolic relaxation and systolic emptying, the latter probably related to a diminished responsiveness to beta-adrenoceptor stimulation, may occur.

The diagnostic and therapeutic principles used in the management of cardiac disease do not differ in older and younger patients. The presence of other associated diseases, changed life style habits, and altered pharmacokinetics and pharmacodynamics, however, require a more careful, skilled, conscientious, and often time-consuming application of these principles in the treatment of older patients. This is especially true in the management of hypertension, the successful treatment of which has the potential to cause an enormous reduction in the prevalence of cardiovascular disease and its complications. The treatment of ischemic disease should be adjusted to the life style of the individual patient. Nevertheless, those older patients whose life style is significantly impaired by ischemic symptoms or the side effects of medical therapy should not be denied the benefits of PTCA and bypass surgery simply because of their age.

REFERENCES

CONCEPTS AND THEORIES OF CHANGES WITH AGE

1. Elveback, L., and Lie, J. T.: Continued high incidence of coronary artery disease at autopsy in Olmstead County, Minnesota, 1950–1979. Circulation 70:345, 1984.
2. White, N. K., Edwards, J. E. and Dry, T. J.: The relationship of the degree of coronary atherosclerosis with age in men. Circulation 1:645, 1950.
3. Saltin, B., Blomquist, G., Mitchell, J. H., et al.: Response to exercise after bed rest and after training. A longitudinal study of adaptive changes in oxygen transport and body composition. Circulation 38(Suppl. 7):vii, 1968.
4. Moore, G. W., Hutchins, G. M., and Prito, J. C.: Cardiac hypertrophy occurs by myocyte enlargement, no repletion [abstr.]. Fed. Proc. 39:1111, 1980.
5. Weisfeldt, M. L., Wright, J. R., Shreiner, D. P., et al.: Coronary flow and oxygen extraction in perfused hearts of senescent male rats. J. Appl. Physiol. 30:44, 1971.
6. Yin, F.C.P., Spurgeon, H. A., Rakusan, K., et al.: Use of tibial length to quantify cardiac hypertrophy: Application in the aging rat. Am. J. Physiol. 243:H941, 1982.

7. Aversa, P., Hiler, B., Ricci, R., et al.: Myocyte cell loss and myocyte hypertrophy in the aging rat heart. J. Am. Coll. Cardiol. 8:1441, 1986.
8. Tomanek, R. J.: Effect of age and exercise on the extent of the myocardial capillary bed. Anat. Rec. 167:55, 1970.
9. Gerstenblith, G., Lakatta, E. G., and Weisfeldt, M. L.: Age changes in myocardial function and exercise response. Prog. Cardiovasc. Dis. 19:1, 1976.
10. Lakatta, E. G.: Catecholamines and cardiovascular function in aging. In Sacktor (ed.): Endocrinology and Metabolism Clinics. Vol. 16, Endocrinology and Aging. Philadelphia, W. B. Saunders, 1987, pp. 877–891.
10a. Pearson, A. C., Gudipati, C. V., and Labovitz, A. J.: Effects of aging on left ventricular structure and function. Am. Heart J. 121:871, 1991.
11. Hayflick, L.: Theories of biological aging. In Andres, R., Bierman, E. L., and Hazzard, W. R. (eds.): Principles of Geriatric Medicine. New York, McGraw-Hill Book Co., 1985, p. 9.
12. Roth, G. S.: Age-associated changes in hormone action: The role of receptors. In Schimke, R. T. (ed.): Biological Mechanisms in Aging. Washington, D.C., Department of Health and Human Services, 1980, p. 678.
13. Medvedev, Z. A.: Repetition of molecular-genetic information as a possible factor in evolutionary changes of life-span. Exp. Gerontol. 7:227, 1972.
14. Hayflick, L.: The limited in vitro life-time of human diploid cell strains. Exp. Cell. Res. 25:585, 1961.
15. Harman, D.: The aging process. Proc. Natl. Acad. Sci. USA 78(11):7124, 1981.
16. Bjorksten, J.: The crosslinkage theory of aging. Finska Kemists Medd. 80(2):23, 1971.
17. Schimke, R. T. (ed.): Biological Mechanisms in Aging. Washington, D.C., U.S. Department of Health and Human Services, 1980.
18. Lakatta, E. G., and Yin, F.C.P.: Myocardial aging: Functional alterations and related cellular mechanisms. Am. J. Physiol. 242:H927, 1982.

CARDIAC MUSCLE FUNCTION IN AGING

19. Bhatnagar, G. M., Walford, G. D., Beard, E. S., et al.: ATPase activity and force production in myofibrils and twitch characteristics in intact muscle from neonatal, adult, and senescent rat myocardium. J. Mol. Cell. Cardiol. 16:203, 1984.
20. Wei, J. Y., Spurgeon, H. A. and Lakatta, E. G.: Excitation-contraction in rat myocardium: Alterations with adult aging. Am. J. Physiol. 246:H784, 1984.
21. Froehlich, J. P., Lakatta, E. G., Beard, E., et al.: Studies of sarcoplasmic reticulum function and contraction duration in young adult and aged rat myocardium. J. Mol. Cell. Cardiol. 10:427, 1978.
22. Effron, M. B., Bhatnagar, G. M., Spurgeon, H. A., et al.: Changes in myosin isoenzymes, ATPase activity, and contraction duration in rat cardiac muscle with aging can be modulated by thyroxine. Circ. Res. 60:238, 1987.
23. Spurgeon, H. A., Steinbach, M. F., and Lakatta, E. G.: Chronic exercise prevents characteristic age-related changes in rat cardiac contraction. Am. J. Physiol. 244:H513, 1983.
24. Capasso, J. M., Malhotra, A., Remily, R. M., et al.: Effects of age on mechanical and electrical performance of rat myocardium. Am. J. Physiol. 245:H72, 1983.
25. Spurgeon, H. A., Thorne, P. R., Yin, F.C.P., et al.: Increased dynamic stiffness of trabeculae carneae from senescent rats. Am. J. Physiol. 232:H373, 1977.
26. Lakatta, E. G., Gerstenblith, G., Angell, C. S., et al.: Prolonged contraction duration in aged myocardium. J. Clin. Invest. 55:61, 1975.
27. Lakatta, E. G., Gerstenblith G., Angell, C. S., et al.: Diminished inotropic response of aged myocardium to catecholamines. Circ. Res. 36:262, 1975.
28. Orchard, C. H., and Lakatta, E. G.: Intracellular calcium transients and developed tensions in rat heart muscle. A mechanism for the negative interval-strength relationship. J. Gen. Physiol. 86:637, 1985.
29. Narayanan, N.: Differential alterations in ATP-supported calcium transport activities of sarcoplasmic reticulum and sarcolemma of aging myocardium. Biochem. Biophys. Acta 678:442, 1981.
30. Maciel, I.M.Z., Polikar, R., Rohrer, D., et al.: Age-induced decreases in the messenger RNA coding for the sarcoplasmic reticulum Ca²⁺-ATPase of the rat heart. Circ. Res. 67:230, 1990.
31. Lakatta, E. G.: Do hypertension and aging similarly affect the myocardium? Circulation 75(Suppl. I):69, 1987.
32. Walker, K. E., Lakatta, E. G., and Houser, S. R.: Calcium currents in senescent rat ventricular myocytes. Circulation 80(Suppl. II):142, 1989.
33. Noble, D.: The surprising heart: A review of recent progress in electrophysiology. J. Physiol. 353:1, 1984.
34. Boyett, M. R., Capogrossi, M. C., duBell, W. H., et al.: Cytosolic Ca²⁺ modulation of the action potential in rat ventricular myocytes. J. Physiol. (Lond) 415:109P, 1989.
35. Yin, R.C.P., Spurgeon, H. A., Weisfeldt, M. L., and Lakatta, E. G.: Mechanical properties of myocardium from hypertrophied rat hearts. A comparison between hypertrophy induced by senescence and by aortic banding. Circ. Res. 46:292, 1980.
36. Capasso, J. M., Malhotra, A., Scheuer, J., and Sonnenblick, E. H.: Myocardial biochemical, contractile and electrical performance following imposition of hypertension in young and old rats. Circ. Res. 58:445, 1986.
37. Weisfeldt, M. L., Loeven, W. A., and Shock, N. W.: Resting and active mechanical properties of trabeculae carneae from aged male rats. Am. J. Physiol. 220:H1921, 1971.
38. Guarnieri, T., Filburn, C. R., Zitnik, G., et al.: Contractile and biochemical

correlates of beta-adrenergic stimulation of the aged heart. Am. J. Physiol. *239*:H501, 1980.

39. Gerstenblith, G., Spurgeon, H. A., Froehlick, J. P., et al.: Diminished inotropic responsiveness to ouabain in aged rat myocardium. Circ. Res. *44*:517, 1979.

40. Alpert, N. R., Gale, H. H., and Taylor, N.: The effect of age on contractile protein ATPase activity and the velocity of shortening. *In* Tanz, R. D., Kavaler, F., and Roberts, J. (eds.): Factors Influencing Myocardial Contractility. New York, Academic Press, 1967, pp. 127–133.

41. Jacob, R., Kissling, G., Ebrecht, G., et al.: Adaptive and pathological alterations in experimental cardiac hypertrophy. *In* Chazov, E., Saks, V., and Rona, G.(eds.): Advances in Myocardiology. Vol. 5. New York, Plenum Medical, 1983, p. 55.

42. Mercadier, J-J., Lompre, A-M., Wisnewsky, C., et al.: Myosin isoenzyme changes in several models of rat cardiac hypertrophy. Circ. Res. *49*:525, 1981.

43. Rockstein, M., Chesky, J. A., and Lopez, T.: Effects of exercise on the biochemical aging of mammalian myocardium. I. Actomyosin ATPase. J. Gerontol. *36*:294, 1981.

43a. Buttrick, P., Malhotra, A., Factor, S., et al.: Effect of aging and hypertension on myosin biochemistry and gene expression in the rat heart. Circ. Res. *68*:645, 1991.

43b. O'Neill, L., Holbrook, N. J., Fargnoli, J., and Lakatta, E. G.: Progressive changes from young adult age to senescence in mRNA for rat cardiac myosin heavy chain genes. Cardioscience *2*:1, 1991.

44. Hoh, J.F.Y., and Rossmanith, G. H.: Ventricular isomyosins and the tonic regulation of cardiac contractility. *In* Stone, H. L., and Weglicki, W. B. (eds.): Pathobiology of Cardiovascular Injury. Boston, Martinus Nijhoff, 1985, p. 476.

45. O'Neill, L., Holbrook, N. J., and Lakatta, E.G.: Progressive changes in steady state mRNA levels of rat cardiac myosin chain genes from young adult to senescence. J. Mol. Cell. Cardiol. *22*(Suppl. 1):S34, 1990.

46. Ebrecht, G., Rupp, H., and Jacob, R.: Alterations of mechanical parameters in chemically skinned preparations of rat myocardium as a function of isoenzyme pattern of myosin. Basic Res. Cardiol. *77*:220, 1982.

47. Rothbaum D. A., Shaw, D. J., Angell, C. S., and Shock, N. W.: Cardiac performance in unanesthetized senescent male rat. J. Gerontol. *28*:287, 1973.

48. Eghbali, M., Robinson, T. F., Seifer, S., and Blumenfeld, O. O.: Collagen accumulation in heart ventricles as a function of growth and aging. Cardiovasc. Res. *23*:723, 1989.

49. Wilens, S. L., and Sproul, E. E.: Spontaneous cardiovascular disease in the rat. Am. J. Pathol. *14*:177, 1938.

50. Fraticelli, A., Josephson, R., Danziger, R., et al.: Morphological and contractile characteristics of rat cardiac myocytes from maturation to senescence. Am. J. Physiol. *257*:H259, 1989.

51. Simmons, R. M., and Jewell, B. R.: Mechanics and models of muscular contraction. *In* Linden, R. J. (ed.): Recent Advances in Physiology. New York, Longman, 1973, p. 87.

52. Borg, T. K., and Caulfield, J. B.: The collagen matrix of the heart. Fed. Proc. *40*:2037, 1981.

53. Borg, T. K., Ranson, W. F., Moslehy, F. A., and Caulfield, J. B.: Structural basis of ventricular stiffness. Lab. Invest. *44*:49, 1981.

54. Pinto, J. G., and Fung, Y. C.: Mechanical properties of the heart muscle in the passive state. J. Biomech. *6*:597, 1973.

55. Mirsky, I., and Laks, M. M.: Time course of changes in the mechanical properties of the canine right and left ventricles during hypertrophy caused by pressure overload. Circ. Res. *46*:530, 1980.

56. Kane, R. L., McMahon, T. A., Wagner, R. L., and Abelmann, W. H.: Ventricular elastic modulus as a function of age in the Syrian golden hamster. Circ. Res. *38*:74, 1976.

57. Templeton, G. H., Platt, M. R., Willerson, J. T., and Weisfeldt, M. L.: Influence of aging on left ventricular hemodynamics and stiffness in beagles. Circ. Res. *44*:189, 1979.

58. Bryg, R. J., Williams, G. A., and Labovitz, A. J.: Effect of aging on left ventricular diastolic filling in normal subjects. Am. J. Cardiol. *59*:971, 1987.

59. Janz, R. F., Kubert, R. B., Mirsky, I., et al.: Effect of age on passive elastic stiffness of rat heart muscle. Biophys. J. *16*:281, 1976.

60. Lakatta, E. G.: Regulation of cardiac excitation-contraction relaxation mechanisms in the hypertensive heart. *In* Cox, R. H. (ed.): Cellular and Molecular Mechanisms of Hypertension. New York, Plenum, *(in press).*

61. Schwartz, K. Lompre, A. M., de la Bastie, D., and Mercadier, J. J.: Mechano-genic transduction in the hypertrophied heart. J. Mol. Cell. Cardiol. *21*(Suppl. III):S24, 1989.

62. Meerson, F. Z., Javich, M. P., and Lerman, M. I.: Decrease in the rate of RNA and protein synthesis and degradation in the myocardium under long-term compensatory hyperfunction and aging. J. Mol. Cell. Cardiol. *10*:145, 1978.

63. Kent, R. L., Hoober, J. K., and Cooper, G.: Load responsiveness of protein synthesis in adult mammalian myocardium: Role of cardiac deformation linked to sodium influx. Circ. Res. *64*:74, 1989.

64. Mann, D. L., Kent, R. L., and Cooper, G., IV: Load regulation of the properties of adult feline cardiocytes: Growth induction by cellular deformation. Circ. Res. *64*:1079, 1989.

65. Simpson, R.: Stimulation of hypertrophy of cultured neonatal rat heart cells through an alpha₁- and beta₁-adrenergic receptor interaction. Evidence for independent regulation of growth. Circ. Res. *56*:884, 1985.

66. Watson, P. A., Haneda, T., and Morgan, H. E.: Effect of higher aortic pressure on ribosome formation and cAMP content in rat heart. Am. J. Physiol. *256*:C1257, 1989.

67. Yazaki, Y., and Komuro, I.: Molecular analysis of cardiac hypertrophy due to overload. J. Mol. Cell. Cardiol. *21*(Suppl. III):S29, 1989.

68. Bauters, C., Moalic, J. M., Bercovici, J., et al.: Augmentation de l'expression des oncogenenes c-myc et c-fos en fonction de l'activite mecanique du coeur isole de rat adulte. C. R. Acad. Sci. [III] *306*:597, 1988.

69. Cooper, G., IV, Mercer, W. E., Hoober, J. K., et al.: Load regulation of the properties of adult feline cardiocytes. Role of substrate adhesion. Circ. Res. *58*:692, 1986.

70. Bauters, C., Moalic, J. M., Bercovici, J., et al.: Coronary flow as a determinant of c-myc and c-fos proto-oncogene expression in an isolated adult rat heart. J. Mol. Cell. Cardiol. *20*:97, 1988.

71. Lee, H. R., Henderson, S. A., Reynolds, R., et al.: α₁-Adrenergic stimulation of cardiac gene transcription in neonatal rat myocardial cells. J. Biol. Chem. *263*:7352, 1988.

72. von Harsdorf, R., Lang, R. E., Fullerton, M., and Woodcock, E. A.: Myocardial stretch stimulates phosphatidylinositol turnover. Circ. Res. *65*:494, 1989.

73. Craelius, W., Chen, V., and El-Sherif, N.: Stretch activated ion channels in ventricular myocytes. Biosci. Rep. *8*:407, 1988.

74. Watkins, S. C., Samuel, J. L., Marotte, F., et al.: Microtubules and desmin filaments during onset of heart hypertrophy in rat: A double immunoelectron microscope study. Circ. Res. *60*:327, 1987.

75. Hoh, J.F.Y., McGrath, P. A., and Hale, P. T.: Electrophoretic analysis of multiple forms of rat cardiac myosin: Effects of hypophysectomy and thyroxine replacement. J. Mol. Cell. Cardiol. *10*:1053, 1977.

76. Isumo, S., Nadal-Ginard, B., and Mahdavi, V.: All members of the MHC multigene family respond to thyroid hormone in a highly tissue-specific manner. Science *231*:597, 1986.

77. Lompre, A. M., Nadal-Ginard, B., and Mahdavi, V.: Expression of the cardiac ventricular α- and β-myosin heavy chain genes is developmentally and hormonally regulated. J. Biol. Chem. *259*:6437, 1984.

78. Carter, W. J., Kelly, W. F., Faas, F. H., et al.: Effect of graded doses of tri-iodothyronine on ventricular myosin ATPase activity and isomyosin profile in young and old rats. Biochem. J. *247*:329, 1987.

79. Reaven, E. P., and Reaven, P. D.: Structure and function changes in the endocrine pancreas of aging rats with reference to the modulating effects of exercise and caloric restriction. J. Clin. Invest. *68*:75, 1981.

80. Ashok, K., Scheuer, B., and Scheuer, J.: Effects of physical training on cardiac myosin ATPase activity. Am. J. Physiol. *228*:1178, 1975.

81. Dillmann, W. H.: Influence of thyroid hormone administration on myosin ATPase activity and myosin isoenzyme distribution in the heart of diabetic rats. Metabolism *31*:199, 1982.

82. Malhotra, A., Penpargkul, S., Fein, F., et al.: The effect of streptozotocin-induced diabetes in rats on cardiac contractile proteins. Circ. Res. *49*:1243, 1981.

83. Ganguly, P. K., Pierce, G. N., Dhalla, K. S., and Dhalla, N. S.: Defective sarcoplasmic reticulum calcium transport in diabetic cardiomyopathy. Am. J. Physiol. *244*:E528, 1983.

84. Lopaschuk, G. D., Tahiliani, A. G., Vadlamudi, R. V., et al.: Cardiac sarcoplasmic reticulum function in insulin- or carnitine-treated diabetic rats. Am. J. Physiol. *245*:H969, 1983.

85. Penpargkul, S., Fein, F., Sonnenblick, E. H., and Scheuer, J.: Depressed cardiac sarcoplasmic reticulum function from diabetic rats. J. Mol. Cell. Cardiol. *13*:303, 1981.

86. Fein, F. S., Kornstein, L. B., Strobeck, J. E., et al.: Altered myocardial mechanics in diabetic rats. Circ. Res. *47*:911, 1980.

87. Yu, B. P., Masoro, E. J., and McMahan, C. A.: Nutritional influences on aging of Fischer 344 rats. I. Physical, metabolic, and longevity characteristics. J. Gerontol. *40*:657, 1985.

88. Peng, M., and Kang, M.: Circadian rhythms and patterns of running-wheel activity, feeding and drinking behaviors of old rats. Physiol. Behav. *4*:615, 1984.

89. Lakatta, E. G., and Spurgeon, H. A.: Effect of exercise on cardiac muscle performance in aged rats. Fed. Proc. *46*:1844, 1987.

90. Gwathmey, J. K., Slawsky, M. T., Perreault, C. L., et al.: The effect of exercise conditioning on excitation-contraction coupling in aged rats. J. Appl. Physiol. *69*:1366, 1990.

91. Tate, C. A., Taffet, G. E., Hudson, E. K., et al.: Enhanced calcium uptake of cardiac sarcoplasmic reticulum in exercise-trained old rats. Am. J. Physiol. *258*:H431, 1990.

92. Iscaum K. B., Mole, P. A., and Holloszy, J. O.: Effects of exercise on cardiac weight and mitochondria in male and female rats. Am. J. Physiol. *220*:1944, 1971.

93. Starnes, J. W., Beyer, R. E., and Edington, D. W.: Myocardial adaptations to endurance exercise in aged rats. Am. J. Physiol. *245*:H560, 1983.

94. Steinhagen-Thiessen, E., Reznick, A. S., and Ringe, J. D.: Age dependent variations in cardiac and skeletal muscle during short and long term transmill-running of mice. Eur. Heart J. *5*(Suppl. E):27, 1984.

95. Chesky, J. A., LaFollette, S., Travis, M., and Fortado, C.: Effects of physical training on myocardial enzyme activities in aging rats. J. Appl. Physiol. *55*:1349, 1983.

96. Farrar, R. P., Starnes, J. W., Carter, G. D., et al.: Effects of exercise on cardiac myosin isozyme composition during the aging process. J. Appl. Physiol. *64*:880, 1988.

97. Wei, J. Y., Li, Y. X., Lincoln, T., et al.: Chronic exercise training protects aged cardiac muscle against hypoxia. J. Clin. Invest. *83*:778, 1989.

98. Isoyama, S., Wei, J. Y., Izumo, S., et al.: Effect of age on the development of cardiac hypertrophy produced by aortic constriction in the rat. Circ. Res. *61*:337, 1987.

99. Grossman, W., and Wei, J. Y.: Effect of age on myocardial adaptation to volume overload in the rat. J. Clin. Invest. *81*:1850, 1988.

100. Buttrick, P., Malhorta, A., Factor, S., et al.: The effect of aging and hypertension on myosin biochemistry and gene expression in the rat heart. Am. J. Physiol. (in press).

101. Walford, G. D., Spurgeon, H. A., and Lakatta, E. G.: Diminished cardiac hypertrophy and muscle performance in older compared to younger adult rats with chronic atrioventricular block. Circ. Res. 63:502, 1988.

102. Boluyt, M. O., Opiteck, J. A., Esser, K. A., and White, T. P.: Cardiac adaptations to aortic constriction in adult and aged rats. Am. J. Physiol. 257:H643, 1989.

103. Sakai, M., Danziger, R. S., Spurgeon, H. A., and Lakatta, E. G.: Decreased contractile response to norepinephrine with aging. Circulation 76(Suppl. IV):153, 1987.

104. Sakai, M., Danziger, R. S., Staddon, J. M., et al.: Decrease with senescence in the norepinephrine-induced phosphorylation of myofilament proteins in isolated rat cardiac myocytes. J. Mol. Cell. Cardiol. 21:1327, 1989.

105. Dobson, J. G., Jr., Fenton, R. A., and Romano, F. D.: Increased myocardial adenosine production and reduction of beta-adrenergic contractile response in aged hearts. Circ. Res. 66:1381, 1990.

106. Guarnieri, T., Spurgeon, H. A., Froehlick, J. P., et al.: Diminished inotropic response but unaltered toxicity to acetylstrophanthidin in the senescent beagle. Circulation 60:1548, 1979.

CARDIAC FUNCTION IN NORMAL AGING HUMANS

107. Fleg, J. L., and Lakatta, E. G.: Loss of muscle mass is a major determinant of the age-related decline in maximal aerobic capacity [abstr.]. Circulation 72(Suppl. III):464, 1985.

108. Tejada, C., Strong, J. P., Montenegro, M. R., et al.: Distribution of coronary and aortic atherosclerosis by geographic location, race and sex. Lab. Invest. 18:509, 1968.

109. Kennedy, R. O., Andrews, G. R., and Caird, F. I.: Ischemic heart disease in the elderly. Br. Heart J. 39:1121, 1977.

110. Brandfonbrener, M., Landowne, M., and Shock, N. W.: Changes in cardiac output with age. Circulation 12:557, 1955.

111. Strandell, T.: Circulatory studies on healthy old men. Acta Med. Scand. 175:1, 1964.

112. Conway, J., Wheeler, R., and Sannerstedt, R.: Sympathetic nervous activity during exercise in relation to age. Cardiovasc. Res. 5:577, 1971.

113. Rodeheffer, R. J., Gerstenblith, G., Becker, L. C., et al.: Exercise cardiac output is maintained with advancing age in healthy human subjects: Cardiac dilatation and increased stroke volume compensate for a diminished heart rate. Circulation 69:203, 1984.

114. Port, S., Cobb, F. R., Colema, E., and Jones, R. H.: Effect of age on the response of the left ventricular ejection fraction to exercise. N. Engl. J. Med. 303:1133, 1980.

115. Proper, R., and Wall, F.: Left ventricular stroke volume measurements not affected by chronologic aging. Am. Heart J. 83:843, 1972.

116. Gerstenblith G., Frederiksen, J., Yin, F.C.P., et al.: Echocardiographic assessment of a normal adult aging population. Circulation 56:273, 1977.

117. Avolio, A. P., Fa-Quan, D., Wei-Qiang, L., et al.: Effects of aging on arterial distensibility in populations with high and low prevalence of hypertension: Comparison between urban and rural communities in China. Circulation 71:202, 1985.

118. Sjogren, A. L.: Left ventricular wall thickness determined by ultrasound in 100 subjects without heart disease. Chest 60:341, 1971.

119. Gerstenblith, G., Fleg, J. L., Becker, L. C., et al.: Maximum left ventricular filling rate in healthy individuals measured by gated blood pool scans: Effect of age. Circulation 68(Suppl. III):101, 183.

120. Miyatake, K., Okamoto, M., Kinoshita, N., et al.: Augmentation of atrial contribution to left ventricular inflow with aging as assessed by intracardiac Doppler flowmetry. Am. J. Cardiol. 53:586, 1984.

121. Bonow, R. O., Vitale, D. F., Bacharach, S. L., et al.: Effects of aging on asynchronous left ventricular regional function and global ventricular filling in normal human subjects. J. Am. Coll. Cardiol. 11:50, 1988.

122. Nixon, J. V., Hallmark, H., Page, K., et al.: Ventricular performance in human hearts aged 61 to 73 yeas. Am. J. Cardiol. 56:932, 1985.

123. Lima, J.A.C., Weiss, J. L., Guzman, P. A., et al.: Incomplete filling and incoordinate contraction as mechanisms of hypotension during ventricular tachycardia in man. Circulation 68:928, 1983.

124. Dehn, M. M., and Bruce, R. A.: Longitudinal variations in maximal oxygen intake with age and activity. J. Appl. Physiol. 33:805, 1971.

125. Hagberg, J. M., Allen, W. K., Seals, D. R., et al.: A hemodynamic comparison of young and older endurance athletes during exercise. J. Appl. Physiol. 58:2041, 1985.

126. Yin, F.C.P., Raizes, G. S., Guarnieri, T., et al.: Age associated decrease in ventricular response to hemodynamic stress during beta-adrenergic blockade. Br. Heart J. 40:1349, 1978.

127. Yin, F.C.P., Weisfeldt, M. L., and Milnor, W. R.: The role of aortic input impedance in the decreased cardiovascular response to exercise with aging in the dog. J. Clin. Invest. 68:28, 1981.

128. Fleisch, J. H., and Hooker, C. S.: The relationship between age and relaxation of vascular smooth muscle in the rabbit and rat. Circ. Res. 38:243, 1976.

129. Fleg, J. L., Tzankoff, S. P., and Lakatta, E. G.: Age-related augmentation of plasma catecholamines during dynamic exercise in healthy males. J. Appl. Physiol. 59:1033, 1985.

AGING, DISEASE, AND CARDIAC FUNCTION

130. World Health Organization: World Health Statistics Annual. Geneva, 1979.

131. MacDonald, J. B.: Presentation of acute myocardial infarction in the elderly—a review. Age/Ageing 14:196, 1984.

132. Spodick, D. H., and Quarry, V. M.: Prevalence of the fourth heart sound by phonocardiography in the absence of heart disease. Am. Heart J. 87:11, 1974.

133. Slodki, S. J., Hussain, A. T., and Luisada, A. A.: The Q-T interval. III. A study of the second heart sound in old age. J. Am. Geriatr. Soc. 17:673, 1969.

134. Burch, G. E., and DePlaquale, N. P.: Geriatric cardiology. Am. Heart J. 78:700, 1969.

135. Lam, J.Y.T., Chaitman, B. R., Glaenzer, M., et al.: Safety and diagnostic accuracy of dipyridamole-thallium imaging in the elderly. J. Am. Coll. Cardiol. 11:585, 1988.

136. Hypertension Detection and Follow-up Program Cooperative Group: Five-year findings of the Hypertension Detection and Follow-up Program. Mortality by race, sex, and age. J.A.M.A. 242:2572, 1979.

137. European Working Party on High Blood Pressure in the Elderly: Mortality and morbidity results from the European Working Party on High Blood Pressure in the Elderly Trial. Lancet 1:1349, 1985.

138. Jajich, C. L., Ostfeld, A. M., and Freeman, D. H.: Smoking and coronary heart disease mortality in the elderly. J.A.M.A. 252:2831, 1984.

139. Mock, M. B., Holmes, D. R., Vlietstra, R. E., et al.: Percutaneous transluminal coronary angioplasty (PTCA) in the elderly patient: Experience in the National, Heart, Lung and Blood Institute PTCA Registry. Am. J. Cardiol. 53:89C, 1984.

140. Raizner, A. E., Hust, R. G., Lewis, J. M., et al.: Transluminal coronary angioplasty in the elderly. Am. J. Cardiol. 57:29, 1986.

141. Gersh, B. J., Kronmal, R. A., Schaff, H. V., et al.: Long-term (5-year) results of coronary bypass surgery in patients 65 years old and older: A report from the Coronary Artery Surgery Study. Circulation 68(Suppl. II):190, 1983.

142. Roberts, A. J., Woodhall, D. D., Conti, C. R., et al.: Mortality, morbidity, and cost-accounting related to coronary artery bypass graft surgery in the elderly. Ann. Thorac. Surg. 39:426, 1985.

143. Elayda, M. A., Hall, R. J., Gray, A. G., et al.: Coronary revascularization in the elderly patient. J. Am. Coll. Cardiol. 3:1398, 1984.

144. Kunis, R., Greenberg, H., Yeoh, C. B., et al.: Coronary revascularization for recurrent pulmonary edema in elderly patients with ischemic heart disease and preserved ventricular function. N. Engl. J. Med. 313:1207, 1985.

145. Gersh, B. J., Kronmal, R. A., Schaff, H. V., et al.: Comparison of coronary artery bypass surgery and medical therapy in patients 65 years of age or older. N. Engl. J. Med. 313:217, 1985.

146. Letting, C. A., and Silverman, M. E.: Acute myocardial infarction in hospitalized patients over age 70. Am. Heart J. 100:331, 1980.

147. Williams, B. O., Begg, T. B., Semple, T., and McGuinness, J. B.: The elderly in a coronary care unit. Br. Med. J. 2:451, 1976.

148. Zerman, F. D., and Rodstein, M.: Cardiac rupture complicating myocardial infarction in the aged. Arch. Intern. Med. 105:431, 1960.

149. Schuster, E. H., and Bulkley, B. H.: Expansion of transmural myocardial infarction: A pathophysiologic factor in cardiac rupture. Circulation 60:1532, 1979.

150. DeWood, M. A., Spores, J., Notske, R., et al.: Prevalence of total coronary occlusion during the early hours of transmural myocardial infarction. N. Engl. J. Med. 303:897, 1980.

151. Gruppo Italiano per lo studio della streptochinasi nell'infarto miocardico (GISSI): Effectiveness of intravenous thrombolytic therapy in acute myocardial infarction. Lancet 1:397, 1986.

152. Wilcox, R. G., Olsson, C. G., Skene, A. M., et al.: Trial of tissue plasminogen activator for mortality reduction in acute myocardial infarction. Lancet 2:525, 1988.

153. AIMS Trial Study Group: Effect of intravenous APSAC on mortality after acute myocardial infarction: Preliminary report of a placebo-controlled clinical trial. Lancet 1:545, 1988.

154. ISIS-2 (Second International Study of Infarct Survival Collaborative Group): Randomized trial of intravenous streptokinase, oral aspirin, both, or neither among 17 187 cases of suspected acute myocardial infarction: Lancet 2:349, 1988.

155. Guerci, A. D., Gerstenblith, G., Brinker, J. A., et al.: A randomized trial of intravenous tissue plasminogen activator for acute myocardial infarction with subsequent randomization to elective coronary angioplasty. N. Engl. J. Med. 317:1613, 1987.

156. Lie, K. I., Wellens, H. J., van Capelle, F. J., et al.: Lidocaine in the prevention of primary ventricular fibrillation. N. Engl. J. Med. 291:1324, 1974.

157. Jick, H., Sloan, D., and Borda, I. T.: Efficacy and toxicity of heparin in relation to age and sex. N. Engl. J. Med. 279:284, 1968.

158. The Norwegian Multicenter Study Group: Timolol-induced reduction in mortality and reinfarction in patients surviving acute myocardial infarction. N. Engl. J. Med. 304:801, 1981.

159. Sixty Plus Reinfarction Study Research Group: A double-blind trial to assess long-term oral anticoagulant therapy in elderly patients after myocardial infarction. Lancet 2:990, 1980.

160. Weintraub, R. M., Thurer, R. L., Wei, J., and Aroesty, J. M.: Repair of postinfarction ventricular septal defect in the elderly. J. Thorac. Cardiovasc. Surg. 85:191, 1983.

161. Fleg, J. L., and Kennedy, H. L.: Cardiac arrhythmias in a healthy elderly

population: Detection by 24 hour ambulatory electrocardiography. Chest 81:302, 1982.

162. Fleg, J. L., and Lakatta, E. G.: Prevalence and prognosis of exercise-induced nonsustained ventricular tachycardia in apparently healthy volunteers [abstr.]. Am. J. Cardiol. 54:762, 184.

163. Berger, M., Berdoff, R. L., Gallerstein, P. E., and Goldberg, E.: Evaluation of aortic stenosis by continuous wave Doppler ultrasound. J. Am. Coll. Cardiol. 3:150, 1984.

164. Pomerance, A.: Cardiac pathology in the elderly. In Noble, R. J., and Rothbaum, D. A. (eds.): Geriatric Cardiology, Cardiovascular Clinics. Philadelphia, F. A. Davis, 1981, p. 9.

165. Hochberg, M. S., Morrow, A. G., Michaelis, L. L., et al.: Aortic valve replacement in the elderly. Encouraging postoperative clinical and hemodynamic results. Arch. Surg. 112:1475, 1977.

166. Kaplan, O., Yakirevich, V, and Vidne, B. A.: Aortic valve replacement in septuagenarians. Texas Heart Inst. J. 12:295, 1985.

167. Litvack, F., Jakubowski, A. T., Buchbinder, N. A., and Eigler, N.: Lack of sustained clinical improvement in an elderly population after percutaneous aortic valvuloplasty. Am. J. Cardiol. 62:270, 1988.

168. Caird, F. I.: Valvular heart disease. In Caird, F. I., Dall, J.L.C., and Kennedy, R. D. (eds.): Cardiology in Old Age. New York, Plenum Press, 1976, pp. 231–247.

169. Hochberg, M. S., Derkae, W. M., Conkle, D. M., et al.: Mitral valve replacement in elderly patients. Encouraging postoperative clinical and hemodynamic results. J. Cardiovasc. Thorac. Surg. 77:422, 1979.

170. Jamieson, W.R.E., Dooner, J., Munro, A. I., et al.: Cardiac valve replacement in the elderly. A review of 320 consecutive cases. Circulation 64(Suppl. II):177, 1981.

171. Curb, J. D., Borhani, N. O., Schnaper, H., et al.: Detection and treatment of hypertension in older individuals. Am. J. Epidemiol. 121:371, 1985.

172. Management Committee of the Australian Therapeutic Trial in Mild Hypertension: Treatment of mild hypertension in the elderly. Med. J. Aust. 2:398, 1981.

173. Kannel, W. B.: Blood pressure and risk of coronary heart disease: The Framingham Study. Dis. Chest 56:43, 1969.

174. Kannel, W. B., Dawber, T. R., and McGee, N. L.: Perspectives on systolic hypertension. The Framingham Study. Circulation 61:1179, 1980.

175. Pooling Project Research Group: Relationship of blood pressure, serum cholesterol, smoking, relative weight, and ECG abnormalities to incidence of major coronary events. Final report of the Pooling Project. J. Chron. Dis. 31:201, 1978.

176. Kannel, W. B.: Blood pressure and development of cardiovascular disease in the aged. In Caird, F. I., Randall, J.L.C., and Kennedy, R. D. (eds.): Cardiology in Old Age. New York, Plenum Press, 1976.

176a. Amery, A., and de Schaepdryver, A.: The European working party on high blood pressure in the elderly. Am. J. Med. 90(Suppl. 3A):15, 1991.

176b. Freis, E. D., for the Veterans Administration Cooperative Study Group on Antihypertensive Agents: Effects of age on treatment results. Am. J. Med. 90(Suppl. 3A):20S, 1991.

177. Hulley, S. B., Furberg, C. D., Gurland, B., et al.: Systolic Hypertension in the Elderly Program (SHEP): Antihypertensive efficacy of chlorthalidone. Am. J. Cardiol. 56:913, 1985.

178. Joint National Committee on Detection, Evaluation, and Treatment of High Blood Pressure: The 1984 Report of the Joint National Committee on Detection, Evaluation and Treatment of High Blood Pressure. Arch. Intern. Med. 144:1045, 1984.

179. Multiple Risk Factor Intervention Trial Research Group: Baseline resting electrocardiographic abnormalities, antihypertensive treatment and mortality in the Multiple Risk Factor Intervention Trial. Am. J. Cardiol. 55:1, 1985.

180. Buhler, F. R.: Age and cardiovascular response adaptation. Determinants of an antihypertensive treatment concept primarily based on beta-blockers and calcium entry blockers. Hypertension 5:94, 1983.

181. Massie, B. M., Hirsch, A. T., Inouye, E. K., and Tubau, J. F.: Calcium channel blockers as antihypertensive agents. Am. J. Med. 77:(Suppl. 4A):135, 1984.

182. Dunn, F. G., Oigman, W., Ventura, H. O., et al.: Enalapril improves systemic and renal hemodynamics and allows regression of left ventricular mass in essential hypertension. Am. J. Cardiol. 53:105, 1985.

183. Levy, D., Garrison, R. J., Savage, D. D., et al.: Left ventricular mass and incidence of coronary heart disease in an elderly cohort. Ann. Intern. Med. 110:101, 1989.

184. Schulman, S. P., Weiss, J. L., Becker, L. C., et al.: The effects of antihypertensive therapy on left ventricular mass in elderly hypertensive patients. N. Engl. J. Med. 322:1350, 1990.

185. Topol, E. J., Traill, T. A., and Fortuin, N. J.: Hypertensive hypertrophic cardiomyopathy of the elderly. N. Engl. J. Med. 312:277, 1985.

USE OF CARDIOVASCULAR DRUGS IN THE ELDERLY

186. Vestal, R. E., and Dawson, G. W.: Pharmacology and aging. In Finch, C. E., and Schneider, E. L. (eds.): Handbook of the Biology of Aging. 2nd ed. New York, Van Nostrand, 1985, p. 744.

187. Greenblatt, D. J., Sellers, E. M., and Shader, R. I.: Drug disposition in old age. N. Engl. J. Med. 306:1081, 1982.

188. Sjoqvist, F., and Alvan, G.: Aging and drug disposition-metabolism. J. Chron. Dis. 36:31, 1983.

189. Dybkaer, R., Lauritzen, M., and Krakauer, R.: Relative reference values for clinical chemical and haematological quantities in "healthy" elderly people. Acta Med. Scand. 209:1, 1981.

190. Bruce, A., Andersson, M., Arvidsson, B., and Isaksson, B.: Body composition. Prediction of normal body potassium, body water and body fat in adults on the basis of body height, body weight and age. Scand. J. Clin. Lab. Invest. 40:461, 1980.

191. Verbeeck, R. K., Cardinal, J. A., and Wallace, S. M.: Effect of age and sex on the plasma binding of acidic and basic drugs. Eur. J. Clin. Pharmacol. 27:91, 1984.

192. Rowe, J. W., Andres, R., Tobin, J. D., et al.: Age-adjusted standards for creatinine clearance. Ann. Intern. Med. 84:567, 1976.

193. Kerremans, A.L.M., and Gribnau, F.W.J.: Changes in pharmacokinetics and in effect of furosemide in the elderly. Clin. Exp. Hyper. [A] A5:271, 1983.

194. Vestal, R. E., Wood, A.J.J., and Shand, D. G.: Reduced beta-adrenoceptor sensitivity in the elderly. Clin. Pharmacol. Ther. 26:181, 1979.

Medical Management of the Patient Undergoing Cardiac Surgery

by ELLIOTT M. ANTMAN, M.D.

Advances in cardiac surgery have made the operative repair of a variety of cardiac lesions a viable therapeutic option for an increasing number of patients with cardiovascular disease. The care of the patient undergoing cardiac surgery requires the collaboration of surgeons, cardiologists, anesthesiologists, radiologists, and various other professionals. This chapter summarizes the information required by the cardiologist, whose responsibilities include both preoperative evaluation and postoperative care, especially of the medical complications that may develop. The indications for operation are discussed in the chapters on the individual forms of heart disease.

PREOPERATIVE EVALUATION

PATIENT'S KNOWLEDGE BASE. A sensitive and thoughtful review of the indications for the operation and an explanation of the postoperative procedures will have a calming effect that may translate into a reduced need for antihypertensive and anxiolytic agents perioperatively.[1] The preoperative interview also should be used to assess the patient's potential ability to comply with postoperative medical issues such as anticoagulation and follow-up procedures for permanent pacemakers and implanted defibrillators (see Chap. 25).

TABLE 53-1 IMPORTANT ASPECTS OF PHYSICAL EXAMINATION IN PATIENTS SCHEDULED FOR CARDIAC SURGERY

PORTION OF PHYSICAL EXAMINATION	ABNORMAL FINDING	COMMENT
Head, eyes, ears, nose, throat	Dental caries, ENT infection	Risk of endocarditis in valvular surgery
Chest	Prior radical mastectomy	Previous mastectomy (especially left) may compromise thoracic blood supply[2] and therefore contraindicate use of internal mammary artery as conduit because of lack of patency or possible inadequate sternal wound healing.
Cardiovascular	Murmur of aortic regurgitation	Aortic regurgitation may worsen during cardiopulmonary bypass because of a jet from aortic cannulation; left ventricular distention may ensue. Intraaortic balloon pump contraindicated.
Abdomen	Abdominal aorta	Presence of abdominal aortic aneurysm or significant atherosclerosis may contraindicate use of intraaortic balloon pump.
Extremities	1. Peripheral arterial insufficiency 2. Venous varicosities in lower extremities 3. Tinea pedis	1. May prevent use of intraaortic balloon pump. 2. Insufficient venous conduits may be available in lower extremities, necessitating use of arm veins. If this is the case, intravenous lines should not be inserted in the arm veins that will be harvested. For reoperation cases cardiac catheterization should include imaging of the left internal mammary artery; a lesser saphenous venogram also is advisable. 3. Increased risk of lower-extremity cellulitis
Neurological	1. Carotid bruits 2. Preoperative neurological deficit(s)	1. Cerebrovascular accident may occur perioperatively. 2. Neurological status may deteriorate postoperatively because of compromised cerebral perfusion.

TABLE 53-2 PREOPERATIVE LABORATORY EVALUATIONS FOR PATIENTS UNDERGOING CARDIAC SURGERY

PREOPERATIVE LABORATORY TEST	ABNORMAL FINDING	COMMENT
Complete blood count	1. Anemia, especially HCt < 35% 2. WBC > 10,000	1. Anticipate that hemodilution will occur on cardiopulmonary bypass and blood loss will occur intraoperatively. Preoperative RBC transfusions may be needed. In addition, patients with unstable angina, congestive heart failure, aortic stenosis, and left main coronary artery disease should be advised against autologous donation of blood in the preoperative period. 2. Search for possible infection.
Coagulation screen	1. Prolonged bleeding time 2. Elevated PT and/or PTT 3. Thrombocytopenia	All of these laboratory abnormalities suggest that the patient is at risk for bleeding postoperatively and may have excessive chest tube drainage. Corrective measures (e.g., vitamin K, fresh frozen plasma, platelet transfusions) should be considered preoperatively, and surgery may need to be postponed. Hematological consultation may be required if an inherited defect in coagulation (e.g., von Willebrand's factor deficiency) is suspected.
Chemistry profile	1. Elevated BUN/creatinine 2. Potassium < 4.0 mEq/liter 3. Abnormal liver function tests	1. Abnormal renal function that may worsen in perioperative period (caused by nonpulsatile flow on cardiopulmonary bypass and potential low flow postoperatively); this may necessitate temporary or even permanent hemodialysis. 2. Hypokalemia will place the patient at risk of arrhythmias perioperatively and should be corrected before induction of anesthesia. 3. Patient may clear anesthetic agents as well as other cardioactive drugs more slowly. Low albumin level may indicate a state of relative malnutrition that may need to be corrected with nutritional support perioperatively.
Stool hematest	Positive for occult blood	Because heparinization will take place while on cardiopulmonary bypass apparatus, the patient may be at risk for gastrointestinal (GI) bleeding perioperatively. The source of GI heme loss should be investigated preoperatively, if clinical circumstances permit. The potential for bleeding in the future may influence the choice of prosthetic valve inserted.
Pulmonary function	Reduced VC or prolonged FEV_1	Anticipate longer than usual process of weaning from ventilator postoperatively if FEV_1 < 65% VC or FEV_1 < 1.5–2.0 liters. Obtain baseline arterial blood gas analysis on room air to help guide respiratory management postoperatively.
Thyroid function	These tests are not ordered routinely but should be drawn in cases of suspected hypothyroidism or hyperthyroidism, known thyroid dysfunction on replacement therapy, and in patients with atrial fibrillation who have not undergone evaluation of thyroid function.	1. Hypothyroid patients require prolonged period of ventilatory support postoperatively because of slower clearance of anesthetic agents. 2. Hyperthyroid patients have a hypermetabolic state that places them at increased risk of myocardial ischemia, vasomotor instability, and poorly controlled ventricular rate in atrial fibrillation.
Cardiac catheterization	1. Elevated left ventricular end-diastolic pressure and pulmonary capillary wedge pressure 2. Elevated right atrial pressure 3. Elevated pulmonary artery pressure (and pulmonary vascular resistance) 4. Left ventricular mural thrombus	1. These may remain elevated in the early postoperative period and indicate a need for careful attention to maintenance of adequate preload postoperatively. 2. This may reflect tricuspid regurgitation or right ventricular dysfunction from prior infarction. Such patients require vigorous volume expansion postoperatively to maintain an adequate cardiac output. 3. Fixed pulmonary vascular resistance should be suspected when the pulmonary artery diastolic pressure exceeds the mean pulmonary capillary wedge pressure. Vigorous oxygenation and pharmacological support with a pulmonary vasodilator (isoproterenol, prostaglandin E_1) are important in such cases. Patients with a pulmonary artery diastolic pressure equal to the pulmonary capillary wedge pressure usually have a more rapid resolution of pulmonary hypertension postoperatively. 4. Increased risk of stroke perioperatively.

Hct, hematocrit; RBC, red blood cell; PT, prothrombin time; PTT, partial thromboplastin time; BUN, blood urea nitrogen; VC, vital capacity; FEV_1, volume of air expired at 1 second.

Serious language barriers and lack of a family support system, especially in the elderly patient, can turn a technical surgical success into a postoperative medical failure. Enlistment of support from social workers and nurse practitioners may be essential for minimizing such an unfortunate outcome.

GENERAL MEDICAL CONDITION. Except for life-threatening conditions (e.g., proximal aortic dissection, cardiogenic shock caused by ruptured papillary muscle in acute myocar-

dial infarction, penetrating wound of the heart), it behooves the consulting cardiologist to assess the overall medical condition of the patient and advise the surgical team if postponement of the operation seems warranted. When performing the clinical examination (Table 53–1)[2] and reviewing laboratory data (Table 53–2), particular attention should be paid to the patient's potential for developing one or more of the following complications: (1) bleeding while heparinized on cardiopulmonary bypass; (2) deterioration of renal function; (3) development of arrhythmias because of electrolyte imbalance; (4) sepsis because of incompletely treated pulmonary, urinary tract, or dental infections, or dermatologic infections over the sternum or saphenous vein harvest site; (5) the need for prolonged ventilatory support postoperatively because of underlying pulmonary disease and preoperative malnutrition (cardiac cachexia); and (6) development or exacerbation of a neurological deficit because of carotid artery disease or prior stroke.[3] In cases where perioperative intraaortic balloon pump support may be needed, the status of the ileofemoral circulation should be assessed bilaterally. Preoperative cessation of cigarette smoking should be emphasized. If a delay in elective surgery while preoperative infections, electrolyte disorders, or nutritional deficits are rectified is necessary, the cardiology consultant to the patient and the surgical team are responsible for making this determination.

The *protein-calorie malnutrition* associated with cardiac cachexia has been shown to compromise cardiac function, and is associated with a greater risk of respiratory failure, sepsis, and prolonged hospitalization.[4] If the clinical situation

TABLE 53–3   PRINCIPLES OF NUTRITIONAL SUPPORT IN CARDIAC SURGICAL PATIENTS

I. Recognize nutritionally deficient patient: current weight less than 10% of ideal body weight or a history of loss of >10% of ideal body weight; inadequate daily caloric intake (<1000 calories) for ≥1 week, serum albumin ≤2.5

II. Calculate daily caloric requirements
  A. Determine basal energy expenditure (BEE) in kcal/24 hr from the following Harris-Benedict formulae[5] (where W is ideal body weight in kg, H is height in cm, and A is age in years):

$$BEE_{men} = 66 + (13.7 \times W) + (5 \times H) - (6.8 \times A)$$
$$BEE_{women} = 65.5 + (9.6 \times W) + (1.8 \times H) - (4.7 \times A)$$

  B. Adjust for level of activity
    1. Add [0.25 × BEE] for hospitalization and postoperative state.
    2. Do not apply activity "factor" for patients who are at a reduced level of physical activity: on ventilator; comatose
  C. Adjust for stress (e.g., fever)
    1. Add [0.13 × BEE] for each 1° C rise in temperature above normal (use [0.07 × BEE]/1° F).
    2. Septic patients may need as much as 0.25–0.45 × BEE added to their daily caloric intake.
  D. Add additional calories if weight gain is desired (e.g., to treat cardiac cachexia): 1000 kcal/day will result in a weight gain of 2 lb/wk. A diet containing 150 kcal: 1 gm of nitrogen should be used (assuming renal or hepatic failure is absent). (Total calories ÷ 150 = # grams of nitrogen; multiply by 6.25 to determine number of grams of protein).

III. Determine route for nutritional support
  A. *Functioning gastrointestinal tract*
    1. Adequate oral intake: provide calculated calories in a diet that is 15–20% protein, 50–60% carbohydrate, and the remainder as fat.
    2. Inadequate oral intake: use enteral feeding to deliver daily caloric requirement (e.g., Osmolite = 1 cal/cc; Ensure Plus = 1.5 cal/cc). If renal or hepatic failure is present, use modified enteral feeding (e.g., Travesorb Renal or Travesorb Hepatic).
  B. *Nonfunctioning gastrointestinal tract or intolerance of enteral feedings*
    1. Normal renal function and can tolerate at least 2500 ml/day: peripheral parenteral nutrition
    2. Renal dysfunction and in need of fluid restriction: insert sterile central line for parenteral nutrition and prescribe central parenteral nutrition or total parenteral nutrition in consultation with nutritional support service. Prescription may need to be modified daily.

TABLE 53–4   PREOPERATIVE RISK FACTORS FOR ADVERSE OUTCOMES IN PATIENTS UNDERGOING CARDIAC SURGERY

I. Increased morbidity and mortality after CABG[6]
  A. Advanced age[6–8]
  B. Female gender[*9]
  C. Left ventricular dysfunction
  D. Symptomatic congestive heart failure
  E. Critical left main stenosis
  F. Urgent or emergency surgery

II. Increased risk of mediastinal infection[11]**
  A. Obesity
  B. Diabetes mellitus (especially if bilateral internal mammary artery grafting is performed)
  C. Malnutrition (see Table 53–3)
  D. Advanced age
  E. Severe pulmonary disease that is likely to lead to prolonged postoperative ventilatory support
  F. Hospitalization for more than 5 days preoperatively

CABG, coronary artery bypass grafting.

* A recent study casts doubt on the significance of female gender as an *independent* risk factor for coronary artery bypass surgery.[10] Women may be referred for surgery later in the course of their disease and undergo operation when they are older and have more advanced disease than do men. Thus differences in functional status and age may account for prior reports of the adverse impact of female gender.

** Highly correlated with increased length of stay and greater hospital costs related to surgery.

allows, patients diagnosed as having cardiac cachexia should receive 1 to 2 weeks of preoperative nutritional support before undergoing elective cardiac surgery. The general principles of nutritional support in cardiac surgical patients are outlined in Table 53–3.

The risk factors for morbidity and mortality after coronary revascularization surgery and postoperative mediastinal infection are outlined in Table 53–4. Several centers have noted a higher mortality risk profile of patients referred for cardiac surgery over the past few years, including older persons with complex medical issues (e.g., diabetes mellitus, renal dysfunction) and a history of cardiac surgery.[12,13]

HEMODYNAMIC COMPENSATION. An especially important aspect of the preoperative evaluation of the cardiac surgical patient involves estimating the extent of underlying ventricular dysfunction, using preoperative echocardiography, radionuclide ventriculography, and contrast ventriculography. Careful consideration should be given to the possibility, sometimes occult, of right ventricular dysfunction (Table 53–2).[14] The latter should be suspected in patients with preoperative elevation of pulmonary artery systolic pressure (>60 mm Hg), a history of inferoposterior left ventricular infarction (and possibly associated right ventricular infarction), and longstanding tricuspid regurgitation. Patients with right ventricular dysfunction should be placed on maintenance digitalis and receive supplemental oxygen preoperatively to attempt to lower pulmonary vascular resistance and improve right ventricular systolic performance. Intravenous nitrate infusions in the perioperative period also have been shown to reduce pulmonary hypertension and ameliorate right ventricular failure.[15] Patients with mitral regurgitation and severe heart failure should undergo preoperative afterload reduction with such agents as oral angiotensin converting enzyme (ACE) inhibitors and intravenous sodium nitroprusside to a systolic pressure of about 90 to 100 mm Hg.

RISK OF MYOCARDIAL ISCHEMIA. Many patients with active unstable angina pectoris or critical coronary artery disease (e.g., significant left main coronary artery stenosis or severe three-vessel coronary artery disease), especially if it is associated with left ventricular dysfunction and/or mitral regurgitation, are in a tenuous hemodynamic balance as they proceed to the operating room. Delays while awaiting surgery and the time between the induction of anesthesia and the institution of cardiopulmonary bypass are high-risk periods during which a vicious spiral of myocardial ischemia and low-output syndrome can rapidly develop. Such patients should be protected by an intraaortic balloon pump inserted preoperatively and an infusion of nitroglycerin intraoperatively.[16]

ANESTHESIA FOR CARDIAC SURGERY. The details of the practice of cardiac anesthesia are beyond the scope of this chapter and are available in other sources.[17] As regards the preoperative evaluation, an important consideration relates to the form of anesthesia that may be used in cardiac surgical procedures today. Intravenous morphine in a dose of 1 to 3 mg/kg has been used in association with the inhaled anesthetic nitrous oxide. Although morphine has the advantage of being free of any significant myocardial depression, it does cause vasodilatation (by means of histamine release) and reduces preload and afterload.[18] High-dose synthetic narcotics, such as fentanyl and sufentanil, that do not cause vasodilatation have replaced morphine in many centers. The newer, inhaled anesthetics—enflurane and isoflurane—that have replaced nitrous oxide, still have the potential to cause vasodilatation. Patients with critical aortic stenosis, critical mitral stenosis, and large right-to-left shunts may experience a dramatic reduction in cardiac output as ventricular stroke volume falls with a reduction in preload. Preoperative volume expansion and even administration of vasopressor agents may be necessary to avoid this problem.

STATUS OF CARDIAC RHYTHM. Although supraventricular arrhythmias after cardiac surgery are seldom life-threatening, they frequently jeopardize hemodynamic stability and provoke disturbing symptoms. It is a common preoperative practice in many institutions to administer digitalis prophylactically to patients undergoing cardiac surgery, not only for inotropic support, but also for "control" of the ventricular rate if atrial fibrillation should occur postoperatively.[19,20] The support for this practice is less than compelling. Although the prophylactic use of digoxin has been reported to be "beneficial" by some,[20-22] this is by no means a consistent observation.[19,23] There is little reason to believe that digoxin prevents the development of atrial fibrillation, and indeed, clinical trials do not clearly substantiate either a lower incidence of atrial fibrillation[19] or a slower ventricular rate in atrial fibrillation in digoxin-treated patients.[20] *Furthermore, hypoxia, hypokalemia, and elevated catecholamine levels are common postoperatively, and these may predispose the patient to digoxin toxicity.*[24] Because many patients undergoing cardiac surgery are over age 60, there is likely to be a slower than normal clearance of digoxin, which contributes to the risk of digitalis intoxication.

Attention also has focused on the prophylactic use of beta-adrenoceptor blocking agents.[25] This stems from a number of considerations: (1) there is evidence that a rebound phenomenon after withdrawal of such agents at the time of surgery may contribute to the appearance of arrhythmias in the postoperative period[26]; (2) there is a heightened level of sympathetic nervous system tone in the postoperative period, and this may provoke supraventricular arrhythmias[27]; (3) the therapeutic index for digitalis glycosides is narrow. Clinical trials with several beta blockers have shown a statistically significant reduction not only in the frequency of supraventricular arrhythmias, but also in the severity (duration, speed of ventricular response) of the arrhythmia when it does occur.[23,25-28] In the absence of an ejection fraction less than 30 per cent, severe bronchospastic lung disease, or bradyarrhythmias, we advocate the use of prophylactic beta blockers in patients undergoing coronary artery bypass grafting.[28a]

Insufficient data are available to provide definitive recommendations for prophylaxis against atrial fibrillation in patients undergoing valve surgery. We individualize our recommendations for prophylaxis in such cases, and usually do not start beta blockers in patients who have not been on them chronically preoperatively. Young patients (<40 years) undergoing isolated repair of an atrial septal defect or patent ductus arteriosus need not receive prophylactic beta blockers preoperatively, since they are likely to tolerate a postoperative supraventricular arrhythmia during the time it takes to initiate measures to slow the ventricular rate or terminate the arrhythmia. Suggested doses of beta-adrenoceptor blockers for prophylaxis against atrial fibrillation are as follows: propranolol, 10 to 40 mg every 6 hours; metoprolol, 50 mg every 6 to 12 hours. For patients with depressed left ventricular function who cannot tolerate the negative inotropic effects of beta blockers, digoxin (0.25 to 0.375 mg/day) remains a suitable choice for a prophylactic agent.

Although oral verapamil (40 to 120 mg every 8 hours) also may be considered for prophylaxis against supraventricular arrhythmias, its use for that purpose is less well studied.[29] More commonly, intravenous verapamil is used for the acute postoperative management of supraventricular arrhythmias that may occur despite prophylaxis with other drugs.[30]

With the exception of amiodarone, antiarrhythmic drugs that have been prescribed for hemodynamically compromising ventricular tachyarrhythmias should be continued up to the time of operation because of the risk of "break through" of a potentially lethal ventricular arrhythmia in the preoperative period. Few data support the *initiation* of membrane-active agents such as quinidine and procainamide for prophylaxis against supraventricular arrhythmias; there may even be the potential for harm when such agents are used in the patient with ischemic heart disease.[31] Antiarrhythmic agents that have previously been prescribed for troublesome supraventricular arrhythmias or life-threatening ventricular arrhythmias should be continued up to the time of operation. A possible exception to this is amiodarone, since that agent has been associated with increased difficulty weaning from cardiopulmonary bypass, low cardiac output postoperatively, and a higher risk of hypoxia and bleeding postoperatively.[32,33] The necessity of continuing amiodarone preoperatively should be carefully reviewed. Patients with a documented history of resuscitation from sudden cardiac death should continue to receive amiodarone. In cases where amiodarone was prescribed for a less overtly life-threatening arrhythmia (e.g., atrial fibrillation), we prefer to discontinue the drug if surgery is being performed on an elective basis. Unfortunately adipose tissue stores of amiodarone are extensive with long-term (>1 month) treatment,[34] and electrophysiological effects have been reported for up to 1 year after discontinuation of the medication. No guidelines have been established for a minimum period of withdrawal of amiodarone preoperatively to reduce the perioperative risks noted above, but we advocate at least a 3-month period off the drug before subjecting the patient to elective cardiopulmonary bypass.

BRADYARRHYTHMIAS AND ATRIOVENTRICULAR AND INTRAVENTRICULAR BLOCK. Patients with high-grade (third-degree or type II second-degree) atrioventricular block and hemodynamic compromise (systolic pressure <90 mm Hg) are at high risk for general anesthesia unless a temporary transvenous pacemaker wire is inserted preoperatively.

The specifications (model, mode, and settings) of a permanent pacemaker system and, if possible, a statement as to the pacemaker dependency of the patient should be noted in the medical record. The possibility of postoperative malfunction of the permanent pacing system should be anticipated because of the effects of anesthesia, electrocautery, and surgical manipulation of the leads (e.g., during caval cannulation).[35,36] It is our practice to have the appropriate pacemaker programming equipment available postoperatively, since many problems (e.g., reversion to the VOO mode [p. 746] because of electromagnetic interference from the electrocautery apparatus) can be quickly resolved by interrogation of the generator and reprogramming in the recovery area.

In patients with left bundle branch block preoperatively who are about to undergo aortic or mitral valve replacement, there is an increased risk of permanent complete heart block postoperatively. The surgical team should be alerted to the need for placement of permanent epicardial leads intraoperatively, or plans should be made for implantation of a permanent transvenous pacing system in the early postoperative period if complete heart block develops. In addition to the rhythm considerations noted above, patients with left bundle branch block should be thoroughly evaluated for evidence of uncorrected congestive heart failure, since left bundle branch block often is a "marker" of poor ventricular function. Optimization of hemodynamics with digitalization, diuresis (to the point of clear lung fields), and afterload reduction (to a systolic blood pressure of 100 mm Hg) should be undertaken before the patient is taken to the operating room.

DRUG THERAPY. With the exception of oral anticoagulation with warfarin compounds, most medications can and should be continued up to the time of surgery. Although some cardiac surgeons are reluctant to operate on patients who have received aspirin within the preceding 2 weeks because of the risk of postoperative bleeding,[37] this must be weighed against the accumulated data documenting a greater rate of vein graft patency when an antiplatelet agent is administered preoperatively.[38,38a] Although there may be an increased requirement for postoperative transfusions in the aspirin-treated patient,[39] preoperative donations of autologous red cells,[40] cell-saver techniques, and autotransfusions of shed blood intraoperatively and postoperatively[41,42] should help to minimize the need for and potential hazards of homologous blood transfusions. There are no convincing data to indicate that other antiplatelet agents offer sufficient beneficial effects in addition to aspirin to advocate their routine prophylactic use preoperatively.[43] Warfarin therapy should be stopped 2 days preoperatively and, if necessary, treatment with heparin or low molecular weight dextran initiated. The heparin infusion can be terminated 4 to 6 hours before surgery, but in coronary artery disease patients we prefer that it be continued into the operating room in those cases where one is concerned about unstable ischemic symptoms developing (e.g., catheterization-documented intracoronary thrombus in a patient with unstable angina).

Calcium antagonists previously prescribed for control of ischemic heart disease should be continued up to the time of operation to reduce the chance of myocardial ischemia and rebound coronary vasospasm from withdrawal of the drug.[44-46] In the case of diltiazem and verapamil, the dose may need to be reduced, since these agents may provoke bradycardia and a low-output syndrome postoperatively, especially if a beta blocker or amiodarone is given concurrently or the patient is elderly. Profound atropine- and isoproterenol-resistant bradyarrhythmias may occur postoperatively in patients on these calcium antagonists, particularly when the patient has not yet recovered from the hypothermia that is imposed intraoperatively; temporary dual-chamber pacing support should be available to manage such patients.

INTRAOPERATIVE MANAGEMENT

The technical aspects of intraoperative management of the cardiac surgical patient are obviously of great importance but are beyond the scope of this chapter. The reader is referred to excellent sources currently available.[47] Table 53–5 provides a summary of the general sequence of cardiac surgical procedures, and Figures 53–1 and 53–2 provide examples of pump oxygenators and the usual monitoring devices in place when the patient returns from the operating room.

POSTOPERATIVE MANAGEMENT

FLUID, ELECTROLYTE, AND ACID–BASE BALANCE. After extracorporeal circulation there is an increase in extracellular fluid and total exchangeable sodium, along with a decrease in exchangeable potassium. The cumulative experience in many centers has led to the following basic principles of management:

1. For the first 48 hours after operation, free water is limited to about 1000 ml/day and intravenous fluids are in the form of

TABLE 53–5   GENERAL SEQUENCE OF ELECTIVE CARDIAC OPERATIONS

1. Preoperative medications (anxiolytic and narcotic) administered on call to operating room
2. Insertion/positioning of the following devices:
   a. Arterial line (usually radial artery)
   b. Central venous pressure or pulmonary artery catheter
   c. Urinary catheter
   d. ECG electrodes for oscilloscopic monitoring
   e. Grounding plate for electrocautery apparatus (over buttock)
3. Induction of anesthesia and endotracheal intubation
4. Skin preparation and draping of patient
5. Median sternotomy (with simultaneous harvesting of greater saphenous vein if coronary revascularization is to be performed.)
6. Mobilization of internal mammary artery (usually left) if coronary revascularization is to be performed.
7. Heparinization
8. Cannulation for cardiopulmonary bypass usually by one of the following routes:
   Venous: Right atrium, superior/inferior vena cava, femoral
   Arterial: ascending aorta; femoral artery
9. Initiation of cardiopulmonary bypass
10. Cross-clamping of aorta
11. Myocardial protection: topical cooling, cold potassium cardioplegia solution injected by cannulae in root of aorta, systemic cooling by way of cardiopulmonary bypass apparatus
12. Operative procedure*
13. Weaning from extracorporeal circulation: rewarming by means of cardiopulmonary bypass apparatus, evacuation of air from left ventricle and aorta if heart has been entered. Discontinuation of bypass occurs by means of a gradual reduction of venous return and incremental volume loading of the heart. Reversal of anticoagulation by protamine with guidance by activated clotting time results intraoperatively. Removal of bypass cannulae.
14. Placement of the following devices:
   a. Atrial, ventricular, and ground (subcutaneous) pacing electrodes
   b. Additional monitoring lines: right atrial, left atrial catheters (variable)
   c. Anterior and posterior mediastinal chest tubes; pleural tube if needed
15. Wire closure of sternum and skin closure
16. Transportation to recovery facility by team consisting of surgeon, anesthesiologist, and nurse.

* The precise sequence of operative procedures such as valve replacement, aneurysm resection, and coronary revascularization is variable. Coronary revascularization usually is accomplished according to the following scheme: Distal venous anastomoses are performed (frequently followed by supplemental injection of cardioplegia solution down graft). Distal end of internal mammary artery is directly anastomosed to target coronary vessel. Aortic cross-clamp is removed. Proximal venous anastomoses to ascending aorta are performed. (The precise sequence is variable with some surgeons preferring to perform the proximal and distal venous anastomoses first followed by internal mammary anastomosis.)

5 per cent glucose in water. Sodium replacement varies with volume needs.

2. Serum potassium levels can fluctuate dramatically, and therefore frequent measurement of serum potassium is indicated, especially in diabetics.[48] We attempt to maintain the serum potassium in the range of 4.5 ± 0.5 mEq/liter to minimize the chance of cardiac arrhythmias.

3. Serum glucose levels are frequently elevated (250–400 mg/dl), resulting from glucose-containing intravenous solutions and surgically induced increases in cortisol and catecholamine levels. In nondiabetic patients insulin therapy usually is not required, whereas it is routinely used in insulin-requiring diabetic patients to avoid uncontrolled hyperglycemia.

4. Mild metabolic acidosis or metabolic alkalosis may be present for the first 24 hours postoperatively, particularly during rewarming. These acid–base abnormalities usually do

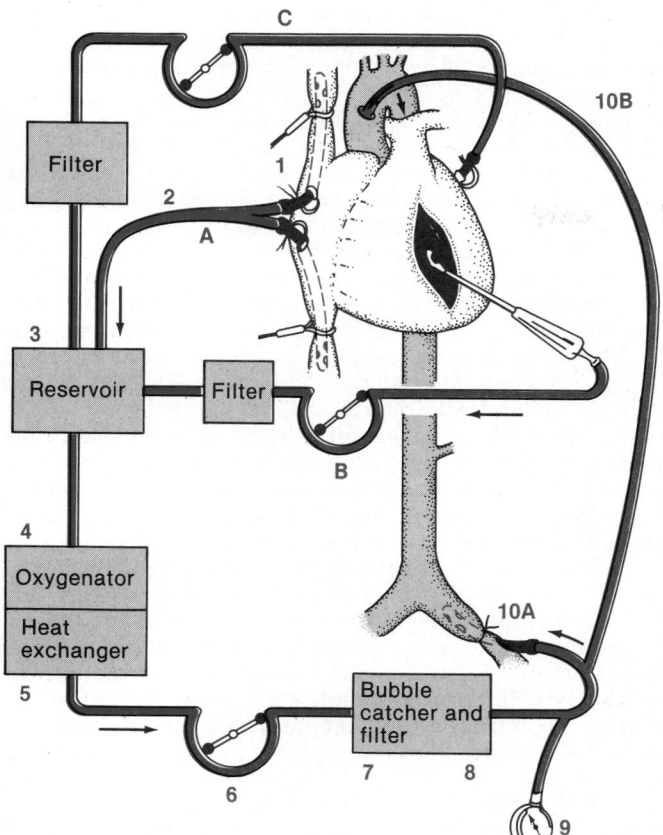

FIGURE 53–1. Schematic diagram of a typical cardiopulmonary bypass circuit. Blood is drained by gravity from the venae cavae (1) through venous cannula (2) into a venous reservoir (3). Blood from surgical field suction and from a ventricular vent (if used during operation) is pumped (*B, C*) into a cardiotomy reservoir (not shown) and then drained into a venous reservoir (3). Venous blood is oxygenated (4), temperature adjusted (5), raised to arterial pressure (6), filtered (7–8), and returned to the patient by way of a cannula either in the aorta (10*B*) or femoral artery (10*A*). Arterial line pressure is monitored (9). (Modified from Nose, Y.: The Oxygenator. Vol. II. St. Louis, C. V. Mosby, 1973.)

not require correction in the absence of preoperative renal dysfunction or acute renal failure developing postoperatively.

5. Serum total calcium, phosphorus, and magnesium levels are frequently depressed for about 24 to 48 hours in the normally convalescing patient, owing in part to the effects of hemodilution. These electrolyte abnormalities usually are self-correcting, and replacement therapy usually is not required. A possible exception is hypomagnesemia because of recent data suggesting a relation between hypomagnesemia and the development of cardiac arrhythmias.[49]

RESPIRATORY MANAGEMENT

EFFECTS OF ANESTHESIA, STERNOTOMY, AND CARDIOPULMONARY BYPASS ON PULMONARY FUNCTION. Four broad areas should be considered, as outlined in Table 53–6. Almost all patients experience alveolar dysfunction after open-heart surgery because of right-to-left intrapulmonary shunting of blood from various intrinsic alveolar abnormalities (e.g., atelectasis, edema, infection) and pulmonary vascular events (e.g., extravasation of fluid, inhibition of hypoxia-induced vasoconstriction). Central respiratory drive and respiratory muscle function are depressed postoperatively because of a combination of pharmacological effects and mechanical derangements of thoracic function. Patients with preexisting pulmonary disease may experience a more profound depression of respiratory function, necessitating vigorous pulmonary toilette and an extended period of ventilatory support.

VENTILATORS

Principles. It is standard practice to use a volume-controlled mechanical ventilator for pulmonary support (positive-pressure delivery of warmed, humidified gas) during the early postoperative period until the effects of anesthetic agents have dissipated. Although most patients receive between 6 and 18 hours of ventilatory support, several studies have suggested that early extubation (<6 hours) is possible if low-dose synthetic narcotics (e.g., fentanyl) and inhaled anesthetic agents are used, muscle relaxants are reversed, the total cardiopulmonary bypass time is less than 100 minutes, and the patient is hemodynamically stable and mentally alert and has a vital capacity equal to or greater than 10 cc/kg.[53]

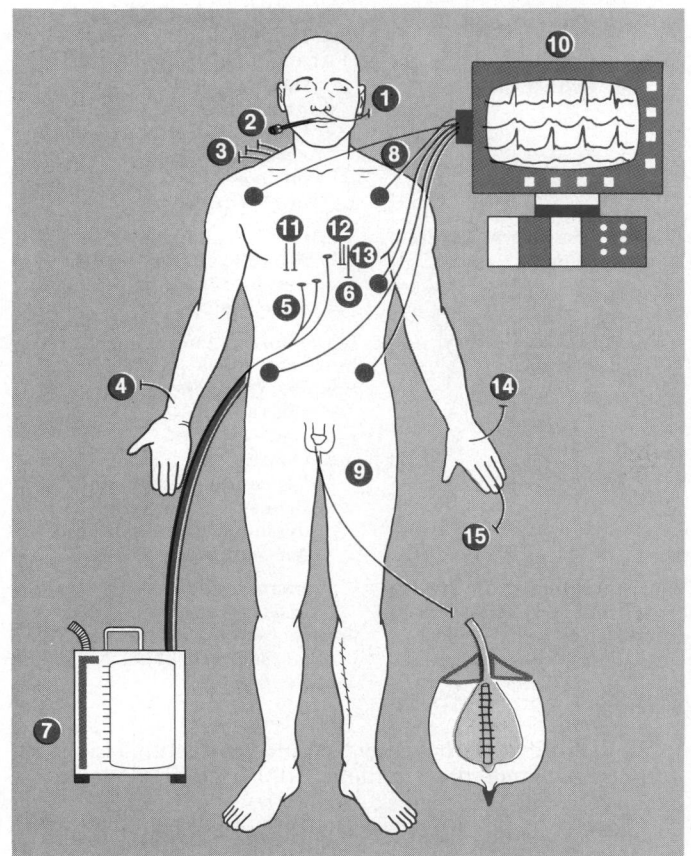

FIGURE 53–2. Schematic diagram of the various devices commonly used after cardiac surgery. (1) Nasogastric tube. (2) Endotracheal tube. (3) Central venous access catheter. This may have multiple ports for the simultaneous measurement of central venous pressure, pulmonary arterial pressure, and pulmonary capillary wedge pressure. Through a sheath introducer a triple-lumen catheter for drug administration and hyperalimentation also may be inserted. (4) Radial arterial pressure monitoring line. (5) Mediastinal chest tubes. One tube is positioned in the anterior mediastinum and the other in the posterior mediastinum. (6) Left pleural chest tube (the left pleural space having been entered during mobilization of the left internal mammary artery for bypass surgery). (7) Chest tube drainage apparatus. (8) Multiple-lead electrocardiograph cable. (9) Urinary drainage catheter. (10) Oscilloscopic monitor capable of the simultaneous recording of multiple electrocardiographic leads and pressures (systemic arterial, pulmonary arterial, central venous). Many contemporary monitoring systems provide modules for calculation of cardiac output by the thermodilution method, automated temperature, and end tidal-CO_2 pressure measurements, and on-line help screens for calculations of the infusion rate of various medications and important hemodynamic variables, such as systemic and pulmonary vascular resistance. (11) Right atrial pacing wires. (12) Right ventricular pacing wires. (13) Subcutaneous "ground" (indifferent) pacing wire. The median sternotomy has been secured with stainless steel wires (not shown). The skins wounds from the median sternotomy and saphenous vein harvest site (left leg in this diagram) are typically covered with dry sterile dressings for the first several days postoperatively. (14) Peripheral intravenous line. (15) Pulse oximeter monitoring line. (Diagram courtesy of Cheryl Warrick-Brooks, R. N., Brigham and Women's Hospital, Boston.)

TABLE 53-6   ABNORMALITIES OF RESPIRATORY FUNCTION AFTER CARDIAC SURGERY

EFFECTS OF ANESTHESIA, THORACIC SURGERY, AND CARDIOPULMONARY BYPASS ON PULMONARY FUNCTION	POTENTIAL CAUSES
Alveolar dysfunction (e.g., widened alveolar-arterial oxygen gradient because of right-to-left intrapulmonary shunting)	a. Scattered regions of atelectasis with preserved perfusion[50] b. Pulmonary edema (e.g., cardiogenic, noncardiogenic "post pump" alveolar capillary leak)[51] c. Infection d. Inhibition of hypoxic pulmonary vasoconstriction by anesthetic agents[52] e. Exacerbation of ventilation/perfusion mismatch by vasodilating agents used postoperatively (e.g., nitroprusside)
Decreased central respiratory drive	a. General anesthetics b. Narcotic analgesics c. Cerebral insult in perioperative period
Decreased respiratory muscle function	a. Thoracic pain (incision, chest tubes) b. Persistent effects of muscle relaxants c. Age d. Obesity e. Depressed cardiac function f. Primary diaphragmatic dysfunction (e.g., phrenic nerve injury)
Exacerbation of underlying chronic pulmonary disease	a. Increase in airway resistance b. Increased secretions and worsening bronchitis c. Pneumonia

While intubated, the patient should be breathing in the intermittent mandatory ventilation (IMV) mode, and arterial blood gases should be checked every hour for the first 6 hours to ensure adequate oxygenation. Positive end-expiratory pressure (PEEP) often is used to minimize the number of collapsed alveolar segments. PEEP should be used cautiously in patients with obstructive pulmonary disease (risk of pneumothorax from air trapping and barotrauma), and it is contraindicated in patients who have undergone operative procedures in which elevation of the right atrial pressure would be undesirable (e.g., interatrial transposition of venous return, Fontan procedure, superior vena caval–right atrial anastomosis [p. 939]). Initiation of PEEP may not be tolerated in patients with relative hypovolemia and inadequate preload (p. 378).

Guidelines for Weaning. Suggested guidelines for identifying the patient who is ready to be weaned from the ventilator are shown in Table 53–7. The IMV setting is progressively reduced to about 2 to 4 breaths per minute, and then the patient may be given a brief trial of T-tube ventilation (with or without continuous positive airway pressure) before extubation occurs. In certain situations extubation should not take place even if the patient "qualifies" on the basis of pulmonary criteria. These situations include hemodynamic instability, malignant ventricular arrhythmias, and postoperative bleeding that may require reoperation.

SPECIAL PROBLEMS

An increased alveolar-arterial (A-a) gradient postoperatively is a serious problem that demands a thorough evaluation. The ventilator settings should be checked, and a chest

radiograph obtained to ascertain the position of the tip of the endotracheal tube (e.g., exclude intubation of the right mainstem bronchus) and to rule out pneumothorax, lobar atelectasis or pneumonia, or a large pleural effusion. Hemodynamic monitoring by means of a pulmonary artery catheter can cause pulmonary hemorrhage because of overinflation of the balloon, and bronchoscopy may need to be performed to diagnose and manage the problem (e.g., occlusion of the bronchus draining the bleeding segment of lung).

PULMONARY EDEMA (see also Chap. 20). The most common cause of pulmonary edema postoperatively is elevated pulmonary venous pressure arising from left ventricular dysfunction and/or a valvular lesion (e.g., mitral regurgitation). Such patients require aggressive diuresis and vasodilator and inotropic support. Mechanical ventilation with PEEP is used until the patient's ventricular function improves.

In a minority of patients pulmonary edema is due to the adult respiratory distress syndrome (ARDS). In its most extreme form, this disorder is associated with a generalized whole-body *postpump syndrome*, characterized by increased capillary permeability, interstitial edema, fever, leukocytosis, renal dysfunction, and hemodynamic collapse. Although the inciting cause of ARDS in some patients may be sepsis, transfusion reactions, or anaphylaxis, in most cases it is the adverse consequences of exposure of the blood to foreign surfaces during prolonged cardiopulmonary bypass. Included among these are platelet clumping and embolization, protein denaturation, liberation of free fat by lipoproteins, and activation of the coagulation cascade, fibrinolytic system, complement system (by way of C3a and C5a), and the kallikrein-bradykinin system. Generation of the anaphylatoxins C3a and C5a mediates leukocyte chemotaxis, aggregation, and enzyme release.[51,54] Pulmonary sequestration of activated leukocytes and platelets occurs with attendant damage to the pulmonary endothelium.[55] There is a direct relation between the duration of cardiopulmonary bypass and the development of the derangements of pulmonary and vascular integrity noted above.[56] Management of ARDS includes mechanical ventilation with PEEP (often for extended periods), minimization of the pulmonary capillary wedge pressure without compromising cardiac output, and nutritional support as needed (Table 53–3).

UNDERLYING CHRONIC LUNG DISEASE. General surgical preparation of patients with obstructive lung disease, including antibiotics, bronchodilators, and cessation of cigarette smoking, has been reported to prevent or diminish respiratory failure from postoperative atelectasis and pneumonia.[57] Inhaled bronchodilators should be continued postoperatively

TABLE 53-7   CRITERIA FOR SUCCESSFUL WEANING FROM VENTILATORY SUPPORT*

Tests of mechanical capability
A. Vital capacity $> 10-15$ cc/kg body weight
B. Forced expiratory volume in 1 sec > 10 cc/kg body weight
C. Peak inspiratory pressure > -20 to -30 cm H_2O
D. Resting minute ventilation < 10 liters/min (can be doubled with maximal voluntary ventilation)
E. Spontaneous respiratory rate under 25 on intermittent mandatory ventilation (IMV) of 6 while resting comfortably, and no apparent increase in work of breathing

Tests of oxygenation capability
A. Alveolar-arterial gradient on 100% O_2 $< 300-500$ torr
B. Arterial P_{O_2} > 80 torr in the absence of intracardiac right-to-left shunting when the FIO_2 is ≤ 0.5
C. Arterial P_{CO_2} < 45 and pH > 7.37
D. Shunt fraction (Q_s/Q_t) $< 10-20\%$
E. Dead space/tidal Volume (V_d/V_t) $< 0.55-0.60$

* Modified from Snow, J. C.: Respiration and respiratory care. *In* Snow, J. C. (ed.): Manual of Anesthesia. Boston, Little, Brown, 1977, pp. 317–331; and Kirklin, J. K., Daggett, W. M., and Lappas, D. G.: Postoperative care following cardiac surgery. *In* Johnson, R. A., Haber, E., and Austen, W. G.: The Practice of Cardiology. The Medical and Surgical Cardiac Units at the Massachusetts General Hospital. Boston, Little, Brown, 1980, pp. 110–113.

and supplemented with intravenous theophylline (0.4 mg/kg/hr to obtain plasma levels of 10 to 20 μg/ml).[58] Plasma levels of theophylline should be monitored at least once every 24 hours in the intensive care unit to minimize the chance of toxicity manifested by agitation, arrhythmias, and grand mal seizures.[59] Particularly refractory patients may require a short course of corticosteroids (e.g., methylprednisolone, 0.5 mg/kg every 6 hours for 3 days) to be weaned from the ventilator.[60]

Patients with chronic obstructive pulmonary disease should be weaned from the ventilator slowly. It is helpful to maintain the arterial carbon dioxide tension close to the patient's baseline level to ensure an adequate respiratory drive.[61]

DIAPHRAGMATIC FAILURE. Diaphragmatic dysfunction after cardiac surgical procedures usually occurs as a result of injury to the phrenic nerve(s). An elevated hemidiaphragm may be seen on postoperative roentgenograms in 25 per cent of patients who undergo myocardial preservation, including a topical ice slush and harvesting of an internal mammary artery.[62] Of note, an elevated hemidiaphragm usually is not associated with increased postoperative morbidity or mortality; recovery of the hemidiaphragm to normal position occurs in 80 per cent of patients at 1 year and nearly all patients by 2 years postoperatively. Less than 1 per cent of patients develop clinically important diaphragmatic dysfunction after cardiac surgery because of unilateral or bilateral phrenic nerve injury. Evidence of diaphragmatic failure includes the inability to wean the patient from the ventilator, a vital capacity less than 500 cc, and paradoxical movement of the diaphragm on fluoroscopy or ultrasonography. Because it may take up to 6 weeks for an injured phrenic nerve to recover function, management includes a more prolonged period of mechanical ventilation and, for some patients, transition to a rocking bed.[63] In cases of permanent unilateral phrenic nerve damage, plication of the diaphragm may help to improve respiratory function.[64]

PROLONGED VENTILATORY INSUFFICIENCY. Patients who fail to wean from the ventilator within 48 hours require special medical attention. To maximize the efficiency of mechanical ventilation, such patients should be sedated and consideration given to neuromuscular blockade if the patient is not breathing synchronously with the respirator. Because of the risk of stress-induced gastritis, an H_2-receptor blocker (e.g., ranitidine, 50 mg intravenously every 8 to 12 hours) is administered. To maintain hemodynamic stability, such patients frequently receive large volumes of intravenous fluids; packed red blood cells should be used to maintain an adequate oxygen-carrying capacity. Nutritional support in the form of tube feedings (preferably as a continuous infusion with the patient positioned in the right lateral decubitus position) or parenteral feedings is critical to provide adequate metabolic needs and prevent catabolism of skeletal muscles (e.g., respiratory muscles) (Table 53-3).

If the patient remains intubated beyond 10 to 14 days, the risks of tracheal stenosis, vocal cord damage, retropharyngeal abscess formation, and tracheoesophageal fistula increase. High-compliance, low-pressure cuffs on endotracheal tubes have reduced the risk of such complications, and permit patients to remain intubated continuously for up to 20 or even 30 days, provided the cuff pressures are maintained below 20 mm Hg and meticulous respiratory care technique is used. Placement of a tracheostomy tube is not a trivial decision, since it can be associated with a number of complications that may offset the advantages of improved endotracheal suctioning and reduced risk of upper airway damage, but tracheostomy usually is desirable if it is clear that the patient will remain intubated beyond 3 weeks.

Finally, patients who fail to maintain adequate oxygenation despite adequate sedation, neuromuscular blockade, large tidal volumes, and PEEP, or who develop marked depression of cardiac output, may be candidates for high-frequency jet ventilation.[65] This mode of ventilatory support provides small tidal volumes at high respiratory rates (e.g., 60 breaths per minute) and produces minimal adverse effects on cardiovascular function. In rare cases extracorporeal membrane oxygenators have been used in patients with severe compromise of diffusing capacity caused by ARDS; the mortality remains high in such cases.

HYPERTENSION

Postoperative hypertension has been defined variably in the literature,[66,67] but we consider it to be present if the systolic pressure exceeds 140 mm Hg.[68] The incidence of postoperative hypertension ranges from 40 to 60 per cent of patients.[69] It occurs more commonly in patients with a preoperative history of hypertension, prior maintenance therapy with a beta blocker, and well-preserved left ventricular function.[70] Postoperative hypertension is especially frequent after coronary artery bypass grafting and surgical relief of left ventricular outflow tract obstruction (e.g., aortic valve replacement, correction of coarctation of the aorta).[71]

The mechanisms of postoperative hypertension probably vary from patient to patient, but usually include (1) a "rebound" effect from withdrawal of beta blockade administered preoperatively[26]; (2) excessive sympathetic nervous system activity with elevations of circulating catecholamine levels (especially norepinephrine)[69,70]; (3) pressor reflexes originating in the heart, great vessels, or coronary arteries[72]; and (4) following correction of aortic coarctation, a drop in the aortic pressure proximal to the site of the prior coarctation with resultant stimulation of aortic and carotid baroreceptors by apparent "hypotension." The renin-angiotensin system is stimulated and peripheral resistance is increased. The sudden exposure of vascular beds downstream to the coarctation to "undamped" aortic pressure also has been reported to cause mesenteric arteritis.

The adverse consequences of elevated systemic pressure include an increased risk of postoperative bleeding, suture line disruption, and aortic dissection[73]; elevated left ventricular afterload and consequent reduction of left ventricular output; injury to aortocoronary bypass grafts[74]; and postoperative stroke.

Although a variety of agents may be used for treating acute postoperative hypertension, we prefer those that are rapidly acting and titratable and have a short half-life. Such drugs include sodium nitroprusside (0.5 to 2.0 μg/kg/min),[75] esmolol (50 to 250 μg/kg/min),[76] labetalol (1 to 2 mg/min),[77] and nitroglycerin (25 to 300 μg/min).[66] Many centers are starting to use closed-loop systems designed to titrate the intravenous infusion rate of a drug to a preset pressure level that is constantly being monitored invasively.[78] The need for transition to oral antihypertensive therapy is assessed on an individual basis; chronic treatment usually is required only in the patient with a preoperative history of hypertension.

PERIOPERATIVE MYOCARDIAL INFARCTION

Despite modern intraoperative myocardial protection and improvements in surgical techniques, some degree of ischemia occurs nearly uniformly during coronary artery bypass surgery.[79] Only a minority of patients (5 to 15 per cent of patients undergoing coronary artery bypass graft surgery), however, actually experience a *perioperative myocardial infarction*.[80,81] The potential causes of myocardial ischemia and infarction in the perioperative period include incomplete revascularization; diffuse atherosclerotic disease of the distal coronary arteries; spasm, embolism, or thrombosis of the native coronary vessels or bypass grafts[82-85]; technical problems with graft anastomoses; inadequate myocardial preservation intraoperatively; increased myocardial oxygen needs, as in left ventricular hypertrophy; and hemodynamic derangements in the postoperative period (e.g., hypotension, hypertension, tachycardia). Although initially one might suspect that perioperative myocardial infarction results from occlu-

TABLE 53-8   DIAGNOSIS OF MYOCARDIAL INFARCTION AFTER CARDIAC SURGERY

DIAGNOSTIC FINDING	COMMENT
Symptoms	
Early (<48 hr postop)	Not reliable because of residual effects of anesthesia and postoperative analgesics
Late (>48 hr postop)	Potentially reliable but may be confused with incisional pain and pleuritic pain from chest tubes, pericarditis
Electrocardiogram	
New, persistent Q waves	This is the most reliable diagnostic finding but only if the Q waves persist on serial ECG's over several days.
Evolutionary ST-T changes	Supportive data favoring the diagnosis of MI only if a typical evolutionary pattern is observed. Because of the effects of cardiopulmonary bypass, hypothermia, postoperative pericarditis, mediastinal chest tubes, and medications (e.g., digitalis), a variety of nonspecific ST-Tw abnormalities may be seen and should not be relied on for diagnosing a perioperative MI.
Myocardial specific enzymes	
Total CK	Elevated total CK levels postoperatively may arise from multiple sources, including skeletal muscle in the thorax and calf as well as myocardium.
CK-MB	Myocardial-specific CK may be released from ischemia occurring during cardiopulmonary bypass as well as myocardial and aortic incisions made intraoperatively (e.g., right atrium for cannulation of cavae). Because of the nearly universal release of CK-MB, a diagnosis of MI should not be made unless the CK-MB is significantly elevated (e.g., >30 units/liter).
Echocardiogram	A regional wall motion abnormality is a helpful finding, particularly if it can be shown to be a new finding by comparison with a preoperative study. Paradoxical motion of the high anterior portion of the interventricular septum is a common finding postoperatively in the absence of MI, and should not be taken as the sole evidence of new perioperative myocardial necrosis.
Scintigrams	Abnormal technetium-99m stannous pyrophosphate scintigrams are more sensitive and more specific than the development of new Q waves on the ECG and more specific than the presence of CK-MB in the serum for the diagnosis of perioperative MI. It is important to differentiate between blood pool activity and diffuse left ventricular uptake and to differentiate between rib uptake secondary to operative trauma and localized myocardial uptake.

MI, myocardial infarction; CK, creatine kinase.

sion of bypass grafts placed to diseased coronary arteries, autopsy studies have shown that bypass grafts usually are patent in patients dying of a perioperative myocardial infarction.[86] This observation lends support to the concept that a mismatch between myocardial oxygen supply and demand in the operating room accounts for much of the infarction noted postoperatively.

The diagnosis of a myocardial infarction after cardiac surgery is more difficult than at other times because of the nonspecific ST-T wave abnormalities on the electrocardiogram and nearly universal elevation of creatine-kinase (CK) levels postoperatively. A number of diagnostic findings (Table 53-8) must be carefully interpreted and then integrated along the lines of the algorithm shown in Table 53-9.

A 12-lead electrocardiogram should be obtained immediately on the patient's arrival in the intensive care unit after operation and no less frequently than once every 24 hours for the first 3 postoperative days. Measurements of total CK and

CK-MB should be made every 8 hours for the first 24 hours and every 24 hours thereafter for the first 3 postoperative days. If there is clinical suspicion of a perioperative myocardial infarction, the CK measurements are made more frequently (every 8 hours) during the 2nd and 3rd postoperative days and a confirmatory bedside echocardiogram is obtained. It is especially helpful to review new echocardiograms in comparison with the preoperative studies that are almost always available.

The electrocardiogram is the most reliable tool for diagnosing a perioperative myocardial infarction. New and persistent Q waves accompanied by new, persistent, and evolutionary ST-T wave abnormalities are the most helpful criteria. Pathological Q waves owing to perioperative myocardial infarction may appear with an earlier time course (i.e., immediately on arrival from the operating room) than in the nonrevascularized patient; they should be considered diagnostic, however, only if they are seen on serial electrocardiograms once the

TABLE 53-9   ALGORITHM FOR DIAGNOSIS OF PERIOPERATIVE MI AFTER CARDIAC SURGERY

NEW Q's ON ECG	CK-MB >30 IU/LITER	NEW RWMA ON ECHO*	DIAGNOSIS	COMMENT
Yes	Yes	Yes	Definite MI	
Yes	Yes	No	Probable MI	New zone of necrosis not evident on echo. The persistence of new Q waves and abnormally elevated CK-MB suggests that the Q waves are not a "benign" postoperative finding.
Yes	No	Yes	Definite MI	CK-MB peak probably missed because of infrequent sampling.
Yes	No	No	Possible MI	New Q waves may be false-positive finding.
No	Yes	Yes	Probable MI	Non-Q wave MI.
No	Yes	No	MI unlikely	Small non-Q wave MI cannot be entirely excluded.
No	No	Yes	MI unlikely	Removal of "restraining" effect of pericardium may result in new RWMAs, especially in high anterior septal area
No	No	No	No MI	Although small patchy areas of necrosis may be seen histologically, these are not of clinical significance.

* Perioperative echocardiography is not *required* for the diagnosis of a perioperative MI but can provide useful supportive data or aid in the diagnosis in unclear cases, especially if obtained acutely. RWMA, regional wall motion abnormality; MI, myocardial infarction.

early postoperative hypothermia, axis shifts, and any potentially reversible myocardial ischemia have resolved.[87]

Operative variables that have been found to correlate with the development of a perioperative myocardial infarction in patients undergoing coronary bypass grafting include prolonged pump time (>75 minutes) and increased total ischemic time (>50 minutes); although some investigators found that an increased number of grafts also correlated with myocardial infarction, this has not been a uniform finding.[88,89]

Although the unique circumstances of perioperative myocardial infarction (early reperfusion, revascularization of adjacent ischemic zones, potential for early intervention if complications should arise) may lessen the potential adverse impact of myocardial infarction on ventricular function, most patients with a perioperative myocardial infarction have an increased hospital mortality (about 10 per cent) compared with patients undergoing coronary bypass grafting who have not sustained a perioperative myocardial infarction (about 1 per cent).[89,90] Characteristics of patients who are especially at risk of increased short-term mortality after a perioperative myocardial infarction include age over 65 years, unstable angina preoperatively, a myocardial infarction within 1 week before operation, left ventricular aneurysm, intraventricular conduction disturbance (e.g., left bundle branch block), and the need for reoperation for bleeding. About two-thirds of the postoperative mortality is due to pump failure and one-third is due to malignant ventricular tachyarrhythmias.[90] A recent study suggests that perioperative myocardial infarction also affects long-term prognosis, particularly if associated with inadequate revascularization and depressed left ventricular function.[90a]

LOW-OUTPUT SYNDROME AND SHOCK STATES

Sometimes diagnosis of the low-output syndrome and a shock state after cardiac surgery is difficult. Because cold extremities and mottled skin may result from hypothermia postoperatively, these observations lack sufficient specificity. Although reduced systolic pressure is the most striking manifestation of this disorder, a low-output syndrome may be present even if the arterial systolic pressure exceeds 100 mm Hg, since an increased systemic vascular resistance (>1500 dynes-sec-cm^{-5}) may be supporting the peripheral perfusion pressure. It is important to recognize this syndrome, since there is a strong relation between the cardiac index in the early postoperative period and the probability of cardiac death after surgery. Common clinical features of the low-output syndrome and shock states after cardiac surgery include cold extremities, mottled skin, reduced systolic pressure (<90 mm Hg), decreased urine output (<30 ml/hr), low cardiac index (<2.0 liter/min/m^2), low mixed venous oxygen saturation (<50 per cent), and acidosis. One should make careful hemodynamic measurements and integrate them with bedside echocardiographic recordings to confirm the diagnosis of a low-output syndrome and attempt to segregate the findings into one of the patterns (*reduced preload, cardiogenic,* or *septic*) in Table 53–10. Although there is overlap of the hemodynamic findings among these patterns, and coexistence of multiple disorders (e.g., bradycardia and hypovolemia) may blur the distinctions between patterns, they offer a clinically useful approach to the evaluation of the patient with a low-output syndrome. In addition to the specific treatment measures discussed below, a number of general measures are applicable to all patients who are in a shock-like condition after cardiac surgery, including prompt correction of any electrolyte and acid–base disturbances, transfusion to a hematocrit over 30 per cent for improved oxygen-carrying capacity of the blood, and a "low threshold" for mechanical ventilatory support to minimize the work of breathing and thereby reduce total body oxygen needs.

REDUCED PRELOAD

Hypovolemia. Low ventricular filling pressures, a normal systemic vascular resistance, and a reduced cardiac index, coupled with echocardiographic demonstration of small ventricular volumes with preserved systolic function, are indicative of *hypovolemia.* Possible causes of hypovolemia include bleeding, excessive diuresis, the "leaky capillary state" associated with the postpump syndrome, and, less frequently, inadequate vascular volume because of insufficient return of fluids at the conclusion of cardiopulmonary bypass. Rarely, adrenal cortical insufficiency owing to perioperative hemorrhage into the adrenals has been reported as a cause of hypovolemic hypotension after cardiac surgery.

Therapeutic maneuvers include administration of intravenous fluids (normal saline solution, lactated Ringer's solution), transfusion with packed red blood cells if the hemoglobin is less than 10 gm/dl and administration of colloid-type volume expanders. It also is important to discontinue any vasodilators that may have been prescribed during a period when the patient was hypertensive. While waiting for the above measures to take effect, the patient may require a transient infusion of an inotropic pressor agent, usually dopamine (p. 501).

Vasodilatation. Inhibition of sympathetic tone by the effects of anesthetic agents may cause peripheral vasodilatation. In combination with increased venous capacitance that may occur during rewarming, a low-output syndrome may develop owing to a markedly reduced systemic vascular resistance (<1000 dynes-sec-cm^{-5}). This situation is best treated by an infusion of a vasoconstrictor such as epinephrine or norepinephrine in a dose of 1 to 10 μg/min until the systemic vascular resistance returns to a normal level.

CARDIOGENIC SHOCK. When the right ventricular and left ventricular filling pressures are in the normal range and systemic vascular resistance is not reduced, a frequent cause of a cardiac index less than 2 liters/min/m^2 is *bradycardia.* Because cardiac index is the product of stroke volume and heart rate, this abnormality is easily corrected by atrial or atrioventricular pacing at 85 to 100 beats/min.

Left Ventricular Failure. The pattern of predominant *left ventricular failure* is characterized by a disproportionately elevated pulmonary capillary wedge pressure as compared with right atrial pressure, low cardiac index, and normal or elevated systemic vascular resistance. Echocardiography usually reveals a dilated, poorly contractile left ventricle, often exhibiting multiple regional wall motion abnormalities. The differential diagnosis of left ventricular failure after cardiac surgery includes the following conditions (which may coexist in the same patient): preoperative left ventricular dysfunction, inadequate surgical correction of the cardiac lesion (e.g., persistent aortic valve gradient owing to mismatch between the patient's aortic ring and prosthesis, residual left ventricular outflow tract obstruction after repair of idiopathic hypertrophic subaortic stenosis, residual atrial or ventricular septal defect), complication of surgical procedure (e.g., prosthetic valve leak or thrombosis, depression of stroke volume after correction of mitral regurgitation caused by the elevation of afterload), dysrhythmia, depressant effect of pharmacological agent (e.g., antiarrhythmic drug), acid–base or electrolyte disturbance, or myocardial ischemia and/or infarction. Bedside echocardiography usually can help to identify mechanical disorders such as prosthetic valve dysfunction and dysrhythmias, and metabolic abnormalities and toxic drug levels can be readily recognized by electrocardiogram and laboratory measurements.

The objectives of hemodynamic management of patients with *left ventricular failure* postoperatively are to correct hypotension if present, increase forward left ventricular output, and return left and right ventricular filling pressures to the normal range. These parameters are intimately related, and treatment may require careful titration of several intravenous agents for pharmacological support of the failing circulation. Boluses of calcium chloride (0.5 to 1.0 gm) will increase myocardial contractility, but the effect is modest and short-lived. A continuous infusion of dopamine (5 to 10 μg/kg/min) is preferable if the primary goal is to increase systemic arterial

TABLE 53-10 LOW-OUTPUT SYNDROME AND SHOCK STATES AFTER CARDIAC SURGERY

	REDUCED PRELOAD		CARDIOGENIC SHOCK				SEPTIC
Causes	Hypovolemia	Vasodilatation	Bradycardia (Inappropriately slow HR postoperatively)	LV failure	RV failure	Cardiac tamponade	Sepsis
Hemodynamics							
RA	<8	<8	≤10	≥10	>10	≫15	<10
PCW	<15	<15	>15	>20	≤15*	≫15	<15
CI	<2.0	<2.0	<2.0	<2.0	<2.0	<2.0	≥2.0
SVR	>1200	<1000	>1200	>1000	>1000	≫1000	<1000
Other			HR < 60		PCW > 15 if LV failure is present	RA = PCW = PAd (within 5 mm Hg) unless "asymmetric" tamponade occurs due to pericardial clots	Narrow AV O₂ difference
Echocardiogram	Small ventricular chambers with vigorous systolic contraction unless LV dysfunction was present preoperatively	Small ventricular chambers with normal systolic contraction unless LV dysfunction was present preoperatively	Normal-sized ventricular chambers with vigorous systolic contraction, albeit at a slow rate	Dilated LV with reduced systolic performance; regional wall motion abnormalities may reflect old or new myocardial ischemia and/or infarction.	Dilated RA and RV with reduced RV systolic contraction. TR often present on Doppler study. The contractile performance of LV is variable.	Small cardiac chambers with diastolic collapse of RA and RV. Systolic contraction of RV and LV usually normal unless dysfunction was present preoperatively or coexistent LV or RV failure has occurred postoperatively.	Small ventricular chambers with normal or slightly depressed contractile function (myocardial depressant factor)
Management	IV fluids Transfusion if Hgb <10 Inotropes	Vasopressors	Cardiac pacing	Search for correctible lesion, offending agent, or laboratory abnormality Inotropes Vasopressors and vasodilators Mechanical assistance	Supplemental O₂ Pulmonary vasodilators Inotropes Mechanical assistance	Reexploration Supportive measures: IV fluids, inotropes	IV fluids Antibiotics Vasopressors Inotropes

LV, left ventricular; RV, right ventricular; RA, right atrial; PCW, pulmonary capillary wedge; CI, cardiac index; SVR, systemic vascular resistance; TR, tricuspid regurgitation.

pressure and cardiac output.[91] Dobutamine (2 to 5 μg/kg/min) or amrinone (2 to 5 μg/kg/min) also will both augment cardiac output and should be selected if reduction of ventricular filling pressure is desired; systemic arterial pressure usually will be unchanged or may even drop slightly because of the peripheral vasodilatory effects of these drugs.[92] A commonly used combination is dopamine (2 μg/kg/min) to achieve greater renal perfusion in conjunction with dobutamine (2–5 μg/kg/min) for augmentation of cardiac output. If the arterial pressure is equal to or greater than 90 mm Hg, vasodilator therapy with sodium nitroprusside or nitroglycerin will increase forward cardiac output and lower the pulmonary capillary wedge pressure further. In cases where hypotension is profound (e.g., systolic pressure <70 mm Hg), norepineph-

rine, 1 to 10 μg/min, may be necessary to prevent coronary hypoperfusion.[93]

We prefer to use an intraaortic balloon pump (Chap. 19) for mechanical support of the circulation along with pharmacotherapy early in the course of management of postoperative left ventricular failure that does not respond to the initial pharmacological maneuvers already discussed. This has the advantages of avoiding a continuous upward titration of the dose of sympathomimetic inotropic agents and vasoconstrictors associated with downregulation of beta adrenoceptors and diminished perfusion of the renal, mesenteric, and coronary vascular beds. Also, intraaortic balloon counterpulsation will not increase myocardial oxygen demand. The intraaortic balloon pump is particularly helpful if significant mitral regurgitation is present, but is contraindicated in the presence of aortic regurgitation and if an abdominal aortic aneurysm is present. If the patient does not improve despite a combination of intraaortic balloon pumping and pharmacotherapy, and cardiac transplantation is decided on, then a left ventricular assist device as a "bridge" to transplantation may be considered until a donor is located (Chap. 19).

Right Ventricular Failure. The pattern of predominant *right ventricular failure* is characterized by a disproportionate elevation of the right atrial pressure in comparison with the pulmonary capillary wedge pressure. In severe cases of postoperative right ventricular failure, the right atrial pressure may exceed 20 mm Hg while the pulmonary capillary wedge pressure remains equal to or less than 15 mm Hg. When left ventricular failure is present simultaneously, the difference between the right atrial and pulmonary capillary wedge pressures lessens and differentiation from cardiac tamponade becomes difficult. Bedside echocardiography is useful for making a proper diagnosis (Table 53–10).

Postoperatively, predominant right ventricular failure may be seen as a result of one or more of the following conditions: elevated pulmonary vascular resistance (persistently elevated from preoperative elevations of pulmonary artery pressure; postoperative hypoxia, pulmonary embolus, or pneumothorax), primary right ventricular ischemia/infarction,[94] or a mechanical lesion (tricuspid regurgitation, residual shunt flow, right ventriculotomy). *Massive pulmonary embolism* is a rare occurrence after cardiac surgery (Chap. 48). The diagnosis should be suspected when sudden deterioration in oxygenation occurs in association with systemic hypotension and elevation of right atrial pressure. Because thrombolytic therapy usually is contraindicated (because of the risk of bleeding postoperatively), management consists of prompt confirmation of the diagnosis with pulmonary arteriography followed by anticoagulation. Pulmonary emboli that cause less hemodynamic compromise (right atrial pressure <15 mm Hg, arterial pressure >90 mm Hg, cardiac index ≥2 liters/min/m²) can be treated with anticoagulation alone. An inferior vena caval filter should be inserted if venography reveals lower-extremity venous thrombosis and recurrences are detected, or if, after the index event, it is felt that the patient could not survive a recurrent embolus. Because a caval filter will not prevent embolization from right atrial or right ventricular thrombi, an echocardiogram should be performed with consideration of surgical removal of any large mobile, nonsessile right heart thrombi.

Hemodynamic management of predominant right ventricular failure should focus on improvement of right ventricular output to allow adequate filling of the left ventricle. Supplemental oxygen is provided to lower the pulmonary artery pressure. Bradycardia (<60 beats/min) is corrected by atrial or atrioventricular pacing. Isoproterenol (1 to 2 μg/min in the average adult) increases right ventricular contractility and also causes pulmonary vasodilatation. Pulmonary hypertension also may be reduced by prostaglandin E$_1$[95] and intravenous nitroglycerin.[15] Further reduction in right ventricular afterload can be achieved by an infusion of dobutamine to decrease the pulmonary capillary wedge pressure and lower the driving force across the pulmonary vascular circuit. Profound hypotension caused by right ventricular failure that does not respond to the above measures can be treated with an infusion of a pulmonary vasodilator (isoproterenol, phentolamine) directly into the pulmonary artery by way of a Swan-Ganz catheter. Insertion of a counterpulsation balloon catheter directly into the pulmonary artery has been reported, but the survival rate in such cases has been poor.[96] Mechanical support of the failing right ventricle is now being used more frequently (see Chap. 19). Rarely, pulmonary embolectomy may be considered in the presence of refractory failure or shock (p. 1574).

Cardiac Tamponade (see Chap. 45). Postoperative echocardiography has shown that virtually all patients have a pericardial effusion after cardiac surgery.[97] Many such effusions

are asymmetrical, with most of the fluid collecting posteriorly; this is probably because the cut anterior surfaces of the pericardium frequently are left unopposed at the conclusion of the operation, and positioning of the patient supine leaves the posterior mediastinum dependent.[98] Even with mediastinal drains in place, it is possible for a patient to develop cardiac tamponade postoperatively; recognition of this condition requires a high index of suspicion and assessment of hemodynamics at the bedside.[99]

Important clinical features of tamponade, such as diminished heart sounds and pulsus paradoxus, may be obscured by mechanical ventilation. Asymmetrical, loculated accumulation of blood and clots in the mediastinum and pericardial space may cause isolated tamponade of one or two cardiac chambers, producing unusual elevations of diastolic pressures (e.g., right atrial tamponade with elevation of central venous pressure without an increase in right ventricular end-diastolic pressure or pulmonary capillary wedge pressure).[100,101] Bedside two-dimensional echocardiography is extremely helpful for diagnosing pericardial effusions and assessing the hemodynamic significance of fluid collections. Diastolic collapse of the right atrium and right ventricle is an indication of a hemodynamically significant external compressive force, and should prompt urgent treatment. Although pericardiocentesis may be helpful in nonsurgical tamponade, it is unlikely to be successful in evacuating the organized pericardial and mediastinal material that develops after cardiac surgery; subxiphoid drainage and/or emergency sternotomy is preferred. Supportive measures that can be attempted in the interim include volume expansion with intravenous fluids (Plasmanate, whole blood), and inotropic agents (dobutamine).

SEPTIC SHOCK. Low ventricular filling pressures, a markedly reduced systemic vascular resistance, and a normal or unexpectedly high cardiac index in the setting of hypotension and a shock-like state should raise the suspicion of the early stages of *sepsis*. With progression of septic shock, a capillary leak syndrome develops (hypovolemia) and myocardial depression may occur, resulting in a somewhat reduced contractile pattern of the ventricles on echocardiography. Combined therapy with intravenous fluids, antibiotics, and inotropic agents is required to interrupt the vicious cycle of hypotension, acidosis, and diminished coronary perfusion. Most patients who are septic during the first 48 hours after cardiac surgery are infected with a skin organism (incision, monitoring lines) or from seeding the bloodstream from a pulmonary or urinary source. Broad antibiotic coverage with one of the following combinations should be instituted: vancomycin plus an aminoglycoside, or ampicillin plus oxacillin and an aminoglycoside. Because the offending organism is likely to be resistant to the prophylactic antibiotic given preoperatively, it is wise not to include it as one of the empiric antibiotics selected to treat sepsis.

ARRHYTHMIAS

EVALUATION AND TREATMENT. There appear to be two peaks in the incidence of arrhythmias perioperatively: the first occurs in the operating room (most commonly during induction of anesthesia, weaning from cardiopulmonary bypass, rewarming) and the second occurs in the intensive care unit between the 2nd and 5th postoperative days. The electrophysiologic mechanisms underlying perioperative arrhythmias are incompletely understood, but they can probably be ascribed to a combination of the effects of circulating catecholamines, alterations in autonomic nervous system tone, transient electrolyte imbalances, myocardial ischemia or infarction, and mechanical irritation of the heart.

The physician caring for the postoperative cardiac surgical patient is frustrated by the lack of clinical data on which to base treatment decisions. Most of the emphasis in the literature is placed on prophylaxis against supraventricular tachyarrhythmias with digoxin (p. 691) and extrapolation of the early (and now outdated) coronary care unit guidelines for treating "warning" ventricular arrhythmias to the postoperative cardiac surgical patient. The availability of newer antiarrhythmic agents (verapamil, esmolol, adenosine) with efficacy against supraventricular arrhythmias coupled with published reports of the successful use of atrial pacing techniques have begun to provide a more rational approach to *supraventricular arrhythmias.* The management of *ventricular arrhythmias* remains controversial, especially in light of data from the nonsurgical ischemic heart disease population that prophylactic and suppressive antiarrhythmic therapy for the asymptomatic or minimally symptomatic patient may be associated with an increased mortality.[31,102] Studies of the prognostic significance of ventricular arrhythmias after cardiac surgery and the impact of antiarrhythmic therapy on postoperative mortality are virtually nonexistent.

In the absence of more definitive data, clinicians can only cautiously apply the information gleaned from arrhythmia-intervention trials in nonsurgical patients and individualize treatment decisions based on the specifics of the patient's medical history and the circumstances present in the intensive care unit. For example, a patient with depressed left ventricular function and a preoperative history of resuscitation from sudden cardiac death who has just undergone coronary revascularization requires an aggressive approach to prevent recurrent ventricular tachycardia or ventricular fibrillation. Alternatively, a young patient with normal left ventricular function who has undergone closure of an atrial septal defect or mitral valve repair for ruptured chordae tendineae probably does not require suppression of ventricular arrhythmias in the absence of sustained ventricular tachycardia causing hemodynamic compromise.

When evaluating rhythm disturbances after open heart surgery, a number of general principles should be kept in mind. Several factors may predispose to the development of arrhythmias, including ventilatory dysfunction, fever, electrolyte imbalance (hypokalemia,[103] hypomagnesemia,[49] hypocalcemia), anemia, myocardial ischemia or infarction, low cardiac output and reflex increase in sympathetic tone, hypertension, pericardial inflammation, and toxic effects of cardioactive medications (e.g., digitalis toxicity, bradycardia induced by diltiazem). *Every effort should be made to look for and eliminate any of the factors that may be provoking the arrhythmia.*

Although antiarrhythmic drug therapy and direct-current cardioversion are traditional methods for treating postoperative arrhythmias, cardiac pacing techniques have a number of advantages. These include a more rapid onset and offset of action, avoidance of potential drug toxicity—especially proarrhythmia—elimination of the need for anesthesia (required for cardioversion), reduced anxiety for the patient, greater safety in patients receiving digitalis, and, perhaps most important, the ability to repeat the pacing protocol if the arrhythmia should recur, a not infrequent event. In addition to terminating arrhythmias, cardiac pacing can be used to suppress arrhythmias in many patients by atrial, atrioventricular sequential, or ventricular stimulation at a critical rate (e.g., 85–100 beats/min).

Surface Electrocardiogram. In an attempt to improve arrhythmia-detection algorithms, many manufacturers have built cardiac monitors that simultaneously record two to four electrocardiograph leads. It usually is unwise, however, to base a treatment decision on monitor lead rhythm strips, especially if one is attempting to analyze a wide-complex tachycardia. The value of a 12-lead electrocardiogram and simultaneously recorded multiple standard electrocardiograph lead rhythm strips cannot be overemphasized in this regard. Unfortunately a number of the criteria for differentiating supraventricular tachycardia with aberrant conduction from ventricular tachycardia (p. 704) may not be applicable to postoperative patients because of previous or newly acquired infarction patterns, transient conduction defects (seen in 5–15 per cent of patients in the early recovery period), and nonspecific repolarization patterns. Although carotid sinus mas-

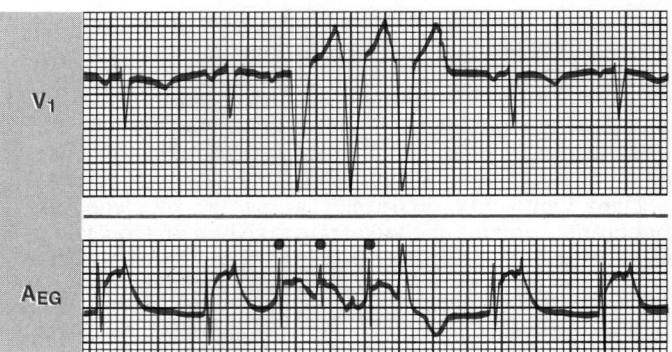

FIGURE 53–3. Simultaneous recordings of electrocardiographic lead V1 and a bipolar atrial electrogram (A_{EG}). The three consecutive beats with wide QRS complexes recorded in the electrocardiogram do not represent ventricular tachycardia, but are due to aberrant ventricular conduction of three premature atrial beats (black dots), as documented in the bipolar atrial electrogram. The appearance of a small ventricular complex after each atrial complex in the bipolar atrial electrogram recording helps to confirm the diagnosis. (From Waldo, A. L., and MacLean, W. A. H.: Diagnosis and Treatment of Cardiac Arrhythmias Following Cardiac Surgery. Mt. Kisco, NY, Futura Publishing Co., 1980.)

sage and specialized electrocardiograph lead recordings to detect atrial activation may be helpful, it is important to take advantage of the additional recording capabilities provided by the atrial and ventricular epicardial electrodes placed at the conclusion of cardiopulmonary bypass (Fig. 53–3).

Epicardial Electrodes. Although many cardiac surgeons place only single atrial and ventricular pacing wires and a subcutaneous wire for the indifferent electrode, it is preferable that two wires be positioned high on the free wall of the

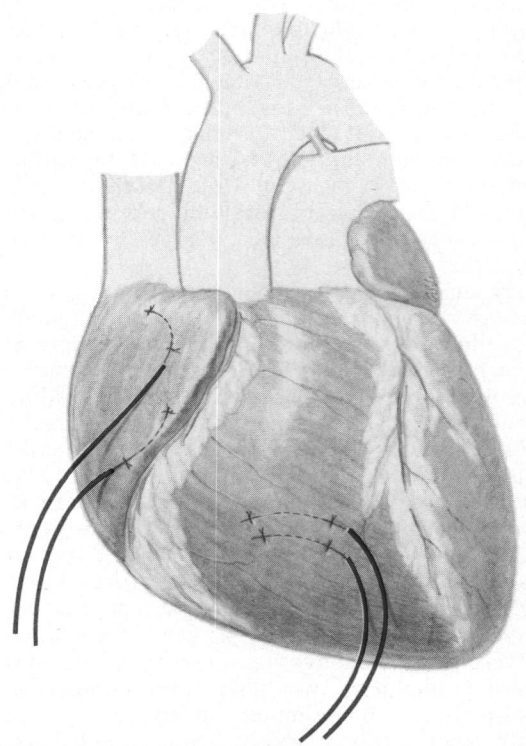

FIGURE 53–4. Placement of atrial and ventricular pacing wires during cardiac surgery. Although two atrial and ventricular electrodes are shown in this diagram (allowing bipolar recording and pacing), some surgeons place only one electrode in each of the sites (restricting recording and pacing to a unipolar configuration). Not shown in this diagram is an indifferent (ground) electrode that is placed in a subcutaneous position. The distal ends of the pacing wires are brought out to the skin through small stab wounds and positioned as shown in Figure 53–2. (From Behrendt, D. M., and Austen, W. G.: Patient Care in Cardiac Surgery. 4th ed. Boston, Little, Brown, 1985.)

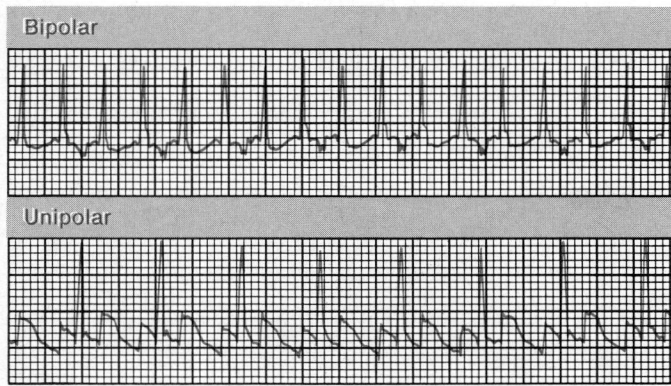

FIGURE 53-5. Simultaneous recording of bipolar and unipolar atrial electrograms utilizing a two-channel electrocardiography machine with the standard right and left arm leads of the electrocardiograph patient cable attached to the two atrial wires and the recording selector set to the standard lead I (bipolar atrial electrogram) and standard lead II (unipolar atrial electrogram) positions. The rhythm disorder is type I (classical) atrial flutter with an atrial rate of 280 beats/min and 2:1 AV conduction. This type of atrial flutter is easily treated with rapid atrial pacing techniques. More rapid forms of atrial flutter (atrial rate 340–430 beats/min) are less responsive to atrial pacing, and have been designated type II flutter. (From Waldo, A. L., and MacLean, W. A. H.: Diagnosis and Treatment of Cardiac Arrhythmias Following Cardiac Surgery. Mt. Kisco, NY, Futura Publishing Co., 1980.)

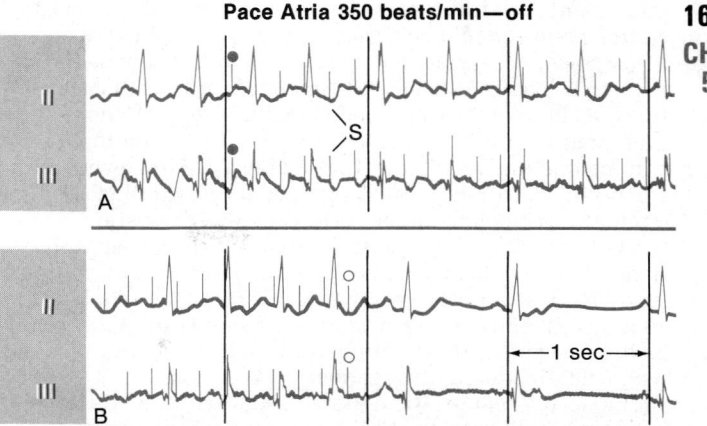

FIGURE 53-6. Recording of electrocardiographic leads II and III in a patient with atrial flutter. Panels A and B are not continuous tracings. The dots in Panel A mark the onset of rapid atrial pacing at 350 beats/min using a pacing stimulator capable of high drive rates. The morphology of the atrial complexes changes dramatically, such that by the end of the trace in Panel A, the atrial complexes are positive in leads II and III. Panel B shows the termination of 30 seconds of atrial pacing at 350 beats/min. The circles represent the last paced atrial beat. With abrupt termination of the rapid atrial pacing, sinus rhythm appears. S = stimulus artifact. Time lines are at 1-second intervals. (From Waldo, A. L., and MacLean, W. A. H.: Diagnosis and Treatment of Cardiac Arrhythmias Following Cardiac Surgery. Mt. Kisco, NY, Futura Publishing Co., 1980.)

right atrium to allow for bipolar atrial recording and pacing. Waldo and MacLean have enumerated the advantages of bipolar pacing, including a smaller stimulus artifact, the ability to record a bipolar atrial electrogram during ventricular pacing, and a reduced likelihood of precipitating undesired atrial arrhythmias if an atrial wire is used as the indifferent electrode during unipolar ventricular pacing.[104] Schematic diagrams showing the suggested intrathoracic positioning of the right atrial wires and recordings of unipolar and bipolar atrial electrocardiograms are shown in Figures 53-4 and 53-5.

SUPRAVENTRICULAR ARRHYTHMIAS

Atrial Premature Depolarizations (see also p. 679). The hemodynamic consequences of atrial premature depolarizations are almost always minor, and one should resist the urge to suppress them with antiarrhythmic drugs. Instead, they should be considered a signal that the patient is possibly hypoxic or that an electrolyte imbalance is present, and a warning that the patient is at risk of developing a more serious arrhythmia, such as atrial fibrillation or atrial flutter. In the absence of such correctable abnormalities, one may want to administer a beta blocker to inhibit the effects of circulating catecholamines and also to slow the ventricular rate if atrial fibrillation should develop. We reserve the practice of "prophylactic" digitalization in response to the emergence of atrial premature depolarizations to those patients with markedly depressed left ventricular function (ejection fraction < 30 per cent) in whom atrial fibrillation would cause serious hemodynamic compromise.

Atrial Flutter (see also p. 679). Control of the ventricular rate in atrial flutter is more difficult than atrial fibrillation because of the limited number of ventricular responses to atrial activation (usually 2:1, 4:1, but rarely an odd-numbered multiple). Because atrial flutter may be difficult to terminate with antiarrhythmic agents, electrical procedures such as direct-current cardioversion and rapid atrial pacing often are used clinically. Cardioversion can be expected to terminate atrial flutter in more than 90 per cent of patients, with an energy of 25 to 50 watt-seconds delivered as a single discharge. Atrial flutter can also be terminated by rapid atrial pacing using the temporary epicardial atrial wires placed at the time of operation. The likelihood of success is increased if one uses sufficiently rapid rates of pacing (up to 140 per cent of the spontaneous atrial rate), a sufficient duration of pacing (10

to 30 seconds), and adequate strength (5 to 20 mA). To achieve the high drive rates required, a special stimulator is utilized.[104] A bipolar pacing mode is preferred, although unipolar pacing can be attempted but with a lower chance of success. Difficulty also may be encountered if the spontaneous atrial rate is particularly rapid (i.e., > 350 beats/min) and when pacing stimuli are delivered at a distance from the focus initiating the arrhythmia. In the latter instance the pacing protocol may be unable to penetrate and depolarize a portion of the reentrant circuit, allowing the flutter mechanism to persist. Examples of the diagnostic usefulness of atrial electrograms and the successful use of rapid atrial pacing for the termination of atrial flutter are shown in Figures 53-6 and 53-7.

Atrial Fibrillation (see also p. 682). Atrial fibrillation is extremely common after cardiac surgery. Transient symptomatic atrial fibrillation occurs in at least 25 to 30 per cent of patients after coronary artery bypass grafting and 60 per cent of patients after valvular surgery, appearing with greatest incidence on the 2nd or 3rd postoperative day.[105,106] Unless he-

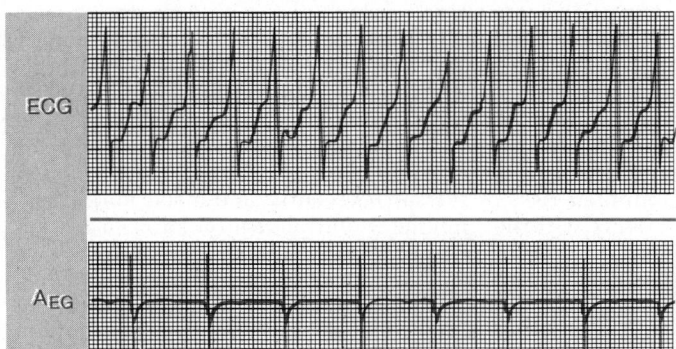

FIGURE 53-7. Monitor electrocardiographic lead recorded simultaneously with bipolar atrial electrogram (A$_{EG}$) during a wide QRS complex tachycardia at 155 beats/min. The A$_{EG}$ demonstrates the presence of sinus rhythm at 90 beats/min. This observation in conjunction with AV dissociation and fusion beats (second and ninth QRS complexes), establishes that the wide QRS complex tachycardia is ventricular in origin. (From Waldo, A. L., and MacLean, W. A. H.: Diagnosis and Treatment of Cardiac Arrhythmias Following Cardiac Surgery. Mt. Kisco, NY, Futura Publishing Co., 1980.)

modynamic collapse is present — in which case direct-current cardioversion should be performed — the treatment of choice in the postoperative patient is to first slow the ventricular rate. Although many textbooks and manuals of patient care continue to list digitalis glycosides as the drugs of choice, the therapeutic index is especially narrow in the postoperative patient, and the likelihood of achieving a desired level of control of the ventricular rate is reduced in the presence of high circulating catecholamine levels. Provided the patient's ventricular function is adequate, acute intravenous administration of beta blockers (e.g., metoprolol, 5 mg, every 5 minutes for up to three doses) or verapamil (e.g., 5-mg bolus every 5 to 10 minutes for three to four doses) is a more desirable option. Esmolol, an ultrashort-acting cardioselective beta blocker, when administered intravenously in a dose of 50 to 250 μg/kg/min, provides the option of rapid onset of a titratable level of beta blockade with a cardioselective agent; in the event of hemodynamic deterioration, the effects of the drug usually are dissipated within 30 minutes after discontinuation of the infusion. In addition, the probability of conversion to sinus rhythm with esmolol appears to be superior to that with other agents, such as verapamil.[107]

Although direct-current cardioversion with an average energy of 100 watt-seconds is likely to restore sinus rhythm, we prefer to control the ventricular rate by pharmacotherapy, and to postpone the cardioversion procedure until 7 to 10 days postoperatively, when the risk of recurrent atrial fibrillation is decreased because pericardial and mediastinal inflammation have resolved somewhat and the level of sympathetic tone has decreased. In the nonsurgical patient the current recommendation is that anticoagulation be initiated for patients who have been in atrial fibrillation for more than 3 days because of the risk of embolism.[108] We usually do not initiate anticoagulation in the early (<2 weeks) postoperative period before cardioversion if the presence of atrial fibrillation is the only indication for antithrombotic therapy. The advantages of intravenous heparin in reducing the risk of embolism from atrial fibrillation must be weighed against the risk of bleeding as a result of recent surgery. Patients in whom sinus rhythm cannot be successfully restored and who are discharged in chronic atrial fibrillation *should* be considered candidates for anticoagulation.[108]

About 48 hours before cardioversion, antiarrhythmic treatment to possibly restore sinus rhythm pharmacologically (albeit successfully in only 5 to 15 per cent of patients) and to suppress recurrences of atrial fibrillation is started in those patients in whom long-term antiarrhythmic therapy is considered appropriate (e.g., preoperative history of atrial fibrillation, depressed left ventricular function, valvular surgery). Because patients are most likely to relapse into atrial fibrillation during the first 2 months after cardioversion, it is wise to administer suppressive antiarrhythmic therapy for at least this period. Permanent suppressive antiarrhythmic therapy often is still necessary in patients with rheumatic heart disease and a preoperative history of atrial fibrillation despite successful aortic or mitral valve surgery, even if sinus rhythm is present during the early postoperative period. Such patients typically have scarring of enlarged atria that places them at continued risk for intraatrial reentry and atrial fibrillation. Patients with nonrheumatic mitral regurgitation (e.g., ruptured chordae tendineae) who have undergone mitral valve repair or replacement may be observed off antiarrhythmic therapy post cardioversion, despite a preoperative history of atrial fibrillation, since relief of the hemodynamic burden may decrease their propensity to atrial premature depolarizations and atrial fibrillation.

Patients with atrial fibrillation postoperatively are at risk for systemic embolization, but the risk varies with the pattern (chronic > paroxysmal) and underlying cardiovascular pathology (valvular heart disease, dilated or hypertrophic cardiomyopathy, and congestive heart failure > nonvalvular heart disease > lone atrial fibrillator).[108] For patients with persistent atrial fibrillation and mitral valve disease, dilated car-

diomyopathy, or a history of systemic embolism, we advocate chronic warfarin therapy designed to achieve a prothrombin time ratio of 1.5 times control.

Paroxysmal Supraventricular Tachycardia (see p. 1715). The reentrant forms of paroxysmal supraventricular tachycardia (PSVT) — atrioventricular nodal reentry tachycardia and atrioventricular reentry tachycardia — occur less frequently in the postoperative patient than atrial fibrillation or atrial flutter, but fortunately retain their responsiveness to vagal maneuvers and pharmacotherapy to inhibit atrioventricular nodal conduction. The antiarrhythmic agent adenosine (p. 650), an endogenous nucleoside, has a number of features making it the drug of choice for treating PSVT in the postoperative patient.[109] A rapid (2 seconds) intravenous bolus of 6 mg will terminate about 60 per cent of episodes of PSVT within 20 seconds; a subsequent bolus of 12 mg administered 1 to 2 minutes later will terminate PSVT in virtually all those cases that failed to respond to the lower dose. Because adenosine is rapidly transported into the cell or degraded enzymatically to inosine, the physiological effects of adenosine are dissipated by 5 minutes. Untoward reactions such as flushing and hypotension are mild and short-lived.

PSVT also may be diagnosed by atrial recordings, and terminated by burst atrial pacing or randomly delivered atrial or ventricular premature depolarizations that invade the reentrant circuit and interrupt the arrhythmia. The automatic form of PSVT (i.e., ectopic automatic atrial tachycardia) is sufficiently unusual postoperatively that its presence should strongly raise the suspicion of digitalis toxicity.

VENTRICULAR ARRHYTHMIAS

Ventricular Premature Depolarizations (see p. 701). Isolated ventricular premature depolarizations (VPDs) commonly occur after cardiac surgery. There may be an increase in the density of VPDs in patients with a preoperative history of VPDs, or they may appear de novo in patients with no history of ventricular arrhythmias. Although there may be a fall in arterial pressure associated with isolated VPDs, this usually is extremely brief and of no significant hemodynamic consequence to the patient unless prolonged periods of bigeminy occur. The emergence of frequent VPDs should trigger a search for any potentially correctable factors. Such a search would include measurement of serum electrolyte levels (potassium, calcium, magnesium), hematocrit, and blood pressure; assessment of the level of oxygenation; estimation of volume status (central venous pressure, pulmonary capillary wedge pressure, urine output); and screening for possible toxic levels of cardioactive agents (digitalis, theophylline).

It is a common, but not uniform practice in most surgical centers to initiate intravenous lidocaine or procainamide to suppress VPDs as prophylaxis against more serious ventricular arrhythmias. These variations in practice reflect the confusion regarding the prognostic significance of VPDs in the postoperative setting. The benefits of prophylactic antiarrhythmic therapy postoperatively have never been adequately addressed in a randomized clinical trial. Because ventricular fibrillation in the early postoperative period is an infrequent event, and probably most often is the result of transitory electrolyte disturbances and/or myocardial ischemia, aggressive correction of electrolyte deficits and antiischemic therapy with intravenous nitroglycerin and beta blockers alone may be effective for preventing ventricular fibrillation without exposing the patient to the potential hazards of antiarrhythmic therapy (myocardial depression, torsades de pointes).

We advocate a conservative approach focusing on prompt detection and correction of provocative factors, liberal use of beta blockers in patients with an ejection fraction greater than 30 per cent, overdrive atrial or atrioventricular sequential pacing between 85 and 100 beats/min, and restriction of suppressive antiarrhythmic therapy to patients with a preoperative history of serious ventricular tachyarrhythmias. If the decision is made to suppress VPDs in patients without a history of symptomatic ventricular arrhythmias, the treatment period should be brief (6 to 24 hours) and the patient should not be automatically converted to an oral antiarrhythmic drug regimen without careful reconsideration of the indications for treatment.

Ventricular Tachycardia (see p. 703). Many of the same arguments cited above for isolated VPDs can be applied for paroxysms of nonsustained ventricular tachycardia (VT). No definitive guidelines are available, but we believe that episodes of VT lasting for 15 to 30 seconds or more in the absence of correctable factors and attempts at overdrive atrial or atrioventricular sequential pacing are an indication for antiarrhythmic therapy, especially if the episodes are associated with hemodynamic compromise. Sustained VT is a serious emergency that should be handled with an orderly approach. If the clinical situation permits, a 12-lead electrocardiogram should be obtained for future reference and confirmation of the diagnosis; simultaneous recording of surface electrocardiographic leads with electrograms from the epicardial wires may be helpful in establishing the mechanism of a wide complex tachycardia (Fig. 53–7). Acute attempts at conversion of the tachycardia include the following maneuvers in the sequence listed: thumpversion, burst ventricular pacing (see p. 705), and boluses of antiarrhythmic agents (lidocaine, 100 mg; procainamide, up to 500 to 1000 mg over 20 minutes; or bretylium, 500 to 1000 mg over 5 to 10 minutes). In urgent circumstances synchronized direct-current cardioversion with a low-energy shock (5 to 50 watt-seconds) may be used. Unsynchronized shocks of 100 to 200 watt-seconds should be used if the tachycardia rate is greater than 160 beats/min and/or has a sinusoidal waveform on the electrocardiogram. After conversion a search for correctable disorders should be undertaken, and if none is found a continuous infusion of lidocaine (2 mg/min), procainamide (2 mg/min), or bretylium (1 to 2 mg/min) is started.

Ventricular Fibrillation (see p. 709). As in the nonsurgical patient, ventricular fibrillation (VF) must be promptly treated with an unsynchronized direct-current shock. Extrapolating from experience in the electrophysiology laboratory, where VF frequently is provoked iatrogenically, it often can be reverted with shocks of 50 to 200 watt-seconds, provided the intervention is performed in less than 1 minute. It should be possible to defibrillate postoperative patients in the intensive care unit expeditiously; therefore, the higher energies (360 to 400 watt-seconds) used in the "field" probably are unnecessary—at least initially. The development of VF should raise the suspicion of a perioperative myocardial infarction. VF may occur in the early postoperative period without any evidence of myocardial necrosis and with electrolyte and drug levels "in the normal range." In such cases reperfusion of previously ischemic zones or transmembrane shifts of electrolytes probably have occurred, and would not be detected by available laboratory measurements. The majority of such patients are not subject to recurrent ventricular tachyarrhythmias, and their prognosis is determined more by overall left ventricular function than by electrical instability.

ATRIOVENTRICULAR JUNCTIONAL RHYTHMS. Nonparoxysmal atrioventricular junctional rhythms (rate >45 beats/min) occur not infrequently after mitral or aortic valve surgery. Trauma and tissue swelling from surgical debridement and suture placement are believed to be the provocative mechanisms. It typically is transient (≤48 hours), and easily treated with atrial or atrioventricular sequential pacing at a rate above that of the intrinsic junctional mechanism.

BRADYARRHYTHMIAS (see pp. 1240–1244) Sinus bradycardia or sinus arrest with emergence of a slow atrioventricular junction escape rhythm may be seen postoperatively when one or more of the following factors are present: advanced age, hypothermia, as a consequence of drug effects (diltiazem, beta blocker, digitalis, procainamide), preoperative sinus node dysfunction, intraoperative trauma to the sinus node, and postoperative elevation of vagal tone. In addition to modifying the dose or discontinuing offending drugs (such as those noted above), atrial pacing at 85 to 100 beats/min should be initiated to maintain an adequate cardiac output and urine flow. Checks of the intrinsic heart rate every 6 hours during the first 24 to 48 hours will indicate when pacing may be discontinued.

Although up to 15 per cent of patients may develop a new conduction defect after cardiac surgery,[110] the majority usually are transient, related to cardioplegia,[111] hypothermia, perioperative electrolyte shifts, or surgical trauma during valve repair or replacement, or closure of septal defects. In the absence of a low cardiac output syndrome related to bradycardia, the development of a new fascicular block or bundle branch alone is not necessarily an indication for initiation of temporary pacing (although it is a common practice in many centers to attach the epicardial wires to an external generator that is either turned off or programmed in the VVI mode with a low escape rate, in the unlikely event that complete heart block occurs). As with nonsurgically related conduction defects, the prognosis of patients with postoperative conduction defects is closely related to the underlying ventricular function. When other factors affecting long-term prognosis (age, left ventricular function, details of graft anatomy) are considered, the presence of a new postoperative bundle branch block or nonspecific intraventricular conduction delay does not clearly have an adverse impact on mortality or cardiovascular-related events over the long term.[111a]

The decision to insert a permanent pacemaker after cardiac surgery should be based on the hemodynamic consequences of bradycardia in the individual patient rather than on a specific heart rate. Most new conduction defects resolve by the 3rd postoperative day, but some persist for as long as 2 weeks. Although we are willing to observe a younger patient (<65 years) with a temporary pacing system for up to 2 weeks postoperatively to see if a conduction defect will resolve, we have a low threshold for implanting a permanent pacemaker if antiarrhythmic therapy or beta blocker treatment is contemplated, since these pharmacologic measures might "stress" a diseased conduction system. We advocate early insertion of a permanent pacemaker in elderly patients with symptomatic bradycardia, since the recuperative process is facilitated, the period of relative immobilization and electrocardiographic monitoring is minimized, and hospital stay is shortened.[112]

CARDIOVERSION (see p. 651). Direct-current cardioversion should be used in the postsurgical patient with the following additional considerations. The recent cardiotomy with resultant pericardial and mediastinal inflammation, presence of chest tubes and/or pleural effusions, and elevated catecholamine levels after surgery may all contribute to higher energy requirements for reversion of arrhythmias such as atrial fibrillation than are commonly required in patients who have not recently undergone cardiac surgery. To achieve the maximum transcardiac spread of current after a median sternotomy, the anterior paddle should be placed to the right of the sternum between the third and sixth intercostal spaces, and the other paddle should be positioned in the fourth to sixth intercostal space as far in the left axilla as possible or in a posterior location under the tip of the left scapula. Firm pressure is applied to the paddles to maintain contact with the chest wall as the discharge buttons are depressed.

HEMOSTATIC DISTURBANCES (See Chap. 58)

All patients who undergo cardiopulmonary bypass develop a multifactorial derangement of the hemostatic system. These abnormalities are caused by exposure of the blood to artificial surfaces, hemodilution, and the effects of heparin (Table 53–11). Platelet dysfunction is the most significant hemostatic abnormality that occurs after cardiopulmonary bypass, although diminution of coagulation factor levels may assume greater significance in patients with preoperative deficiencies of hemostasis. Administration of the following drugs before surgery may predispose the patient to excessive bleeding: aspirin, nonsteroidal antiinflammatory agents, thrombolytic agents,[119] certain antibiotics (carbenicillin, ticarcillin, moxalactam, cefamandole, third-generation cephalosporins), dex-

TABLE 53–11 HEMOSTATIC DISTURBANCES AFTER CARDIOPULMONARY BYPASS

ABNORMALITY	CAUSE
Exposure of blood to artificial surfaces	

1. Platelet dysfunction
  a. Prolonged bleeding time
  b. Decreased adhesiveness
	1. Depletion of platelet α-granules, reduced membrane binding of fibrinogen and α-adrenergic agonists, and increased plasma levels of platelet factor 4 and β-thromboglobulin[113,114]

2. Complement activation	2. C3a and C5a are generated and increase microvascular permeability. C5b–9 complexes are deposited on red cells and platelets, causing hemolysis and platelet activation.[115,116]
Hemodilution	
1. Thrombocytopenia	1. Priming of extracorporeal bypass circuit with crystalloid solutions. Heparin-mediated immune thrombocytopenia may occur in about 5% of patients.[117]
2. Coagulation factor depletion	2. Most coagulation factor levels are reduced by hemodilution by about 50%; factor V is reduced to 20–30% of normal and factor VIII is relatively unaffected. Factor levels usually return to normal within 12 hours after completion of cardiopulmonary bypass. Although plasminogen and fibrinogen levels are decreased by about 50%, fibrin degradation products usually do not appear in the plasma during bypass.[113]
Heparinization*	Thrombus formation is inhibited and excessive bleeding is avoided intraoperatively by maintaining the activated clotting time between 400 and 480 seconds.

* Heparin effects are reversed with protamine sulfate. Vascular collapse has been reported in some patients during protamine treatment.[118]

tran, amrinone, quinidine, cytotoxic agents, gold, phenylbutazone, and fish oils.[120,121] In some institutions, for patients who are undergoing a reoperation or are polycythemic (p. 1749), when the risk of early postoperative bleeding is increased, 2 units of fresh frozen plasma are administered prophylactically after cardiopulmonary bypass.

The most obvious evidence of bleeding in the postoperative cardiac surgical patient is by means of chest tube drainage. "Acceptable" rates of bleeding vary slightly among institutions but usually are less than 100 ml/hr. In our institution, guidelines for returning to the operating room because of excessive bleeding include more than 500 ml/hr for 1 hour, more than 300 ml/hr for 3 hours, and 200 to 300 ml/hr for 5 hours. These guidelines may be tempered by correctable extenuating circumstances, such as uncontrolled hypertension postoperatively, failure to achieve normothermia, or an abnormal coagulation status that is being corrected. Emergency

medical maneuvers that can be attempted after sending coagulation studies to the laboratory include the use of PEEP up to 10 cm H_2O for mediastinal tamponade; empirical "correction" of putative platelet dysfunction with desmopressin acetate (DDAVP, a synthetic analog of arginine vasopressin that increases plasma levels of von Willebrand factor), 0.3 μg/kg, infused over 15 to 30 minutes[122,123]; and empirical administration of a small dose of protamine sulfate, 25 to 50 mg, since heparin may be liberated from the patient's fat stores as rewarming occurs.

Once the coagulation profile returns, additional therapy in the form of platelet transfusions for a platelet count less than 100,000/mm³ and fresh frozen plasma to correct an elevated prothrombin time can be prescribed. When monitoring bleeding from a chest tube, it is important to be alert to a sudden cessation of hemorrhage. This may indicate that the chest tubes have clotted and the fluid is now draining into the mediastinum or the pleural spaces. Serial chest radiographs may be helpful while observing a patient during a bleeding episode. With correct medical management, only about 5 per cent of patients need to return to the operating room for control of bleeding; this should be accomplished within 3 to 4 hours of the original surgery, before hemodynamic destabilization occurs and large volumes of blood products are administered.

ANTITHROMBOTIC THERAPY IN PATIENTS WITH PROSTHETIC HEART VALVES (see p. 1062). Patients who have undergone implantation of a prosthetic heart valve are exposed to a lifelong risk of thromboembolism. The degree of risk varies with the type of valve implanted (mechanical > bioprosthetic), valve location (mitral > aortic), the presence of atrial fibrillation, the size of the left atrium, a history of thromboembolism or the presence of left atrial thrombi at the time of operation, and the adequacy of anticoagulation. For mechanical prosthetic heart valves it is strongly recommended that all patients receive lifelong warfarin therapy designed to prolong the prothrombin time to 1.5 times control (p. 1777).[43,124] Patients with bioprosthetic valves appear to be at greatest risk of thromboembolism in the first 3 months after valve implantation. For patients in sinus rhythm who have a bioprosthetic valve placed in the mitral position, we prescribe warfarin for 3 months, designed to prolong the prothrombin time to 1.3 to 1.5 times control; if atrial fibrillation persists, warfarin is continued permanently. We usually do not anticoagulate patients with bioprosthetic valves inserted in the aortic position, provided the patient is in sinus rhythm.

INFECTION

Despite its nonspecific nature, fever is the most common initial clinical sign of a postoperative infection.[125] It should be emphasized, however, that patients who experience a normal course of convalescence continue to show an elevated temperature for up to 6 days postoperatively (Fig. 53–8).[126] In the absence of infection such early fevers are believed to be caused by alterations in blood components after cardiopulmonary bypass. In addition to infectious causes, fevers that occur beyond 6 days may be due to drug reactions, phlebitis at the site of intravenous lines, atelectasis, pulmonary emboli, or the postpericardiotomy syndrome.

WOUND

Leg. Infections of the leg wound typically present with fever, induration, pain, erythema, local warmth, and drainage from the suture line. The usual infectious agents include staphylococcus, streptococcus, and aerobic gram-negative bacilli. Wound aspiration and Gram's stain should be used to guide antibiotic treatment. More advanced cases require wound debridement and open drainage. Recurrent bacterial cellulitis in the leg used for saphenous vein harvest may be a recalcitrant problem that appears months to years after operation.[127] Antibiotic courses directed against staphylococcus and streptococcus species for each individual occurrence may be insufficient, and a long-term course of antibiotic therapy may be needed. It is important to search for evidence of super-

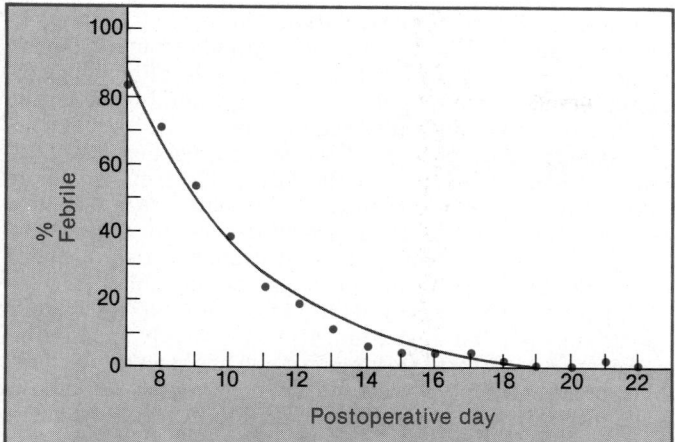

FIGURE 53–8. The decay of fever in a group of 118 retrospectively identified patients with unexplained postoperative fever after postoperative day 6. The percentage of patients that remain febrile is plotted as a function of postoperative day beyond postoperative day 6. A patient is considered febrile if any temperature determination for a given day is equal to or greater than 37.8° C. The percentage of patients febrile on postoperative day 7 is 83 per cent rather than 100 per cent because in 17 per cent of patients fever developed after postoperative day 7. (From Livelli, F. D., Johnson, R. A., McEnany, M. T., et al.: Unexplained in-hospital fever following cardiac surgery. Natural history, relationship to postpericardiotomy syndrome, and a prospective study of therapy with indomethacin versus placebo. Circulation 57:968, 1978, by permission of the American Heart Association, Inc.)

ficial fungal infections in the affected leg, since persistent tinea pedis infection has been reported to cause recurrent lower-extremity cellulitis.[128] If a fungal infection is identified, treatment with topical miconazole or clotrimazole should be given in addition to antibacterial therapy. Persistent fungal infections (owing to breaks in integrity of the dermal barrier) should be treated with either oral ketoconazole or griseofulvin.

Mediastinitis. Mediastinitis and sternal osteomyelitis are among the most serious complications of a median sternotomy.[129] If one excludes operations that occur after thoracic trauma, it is estimated that mediastinitis occurs in about 2 per cent of patients who undergo median sternotomy.[130]

Most cases present within 2 weeks after sternotomy. Important diagnostic features of patients who develop mediastinitis early after cardiac surgery include persistent fever in excess of 101° F beyond the 4th postoperative day, a systemic toxic condition, leukocytosis, bacteremia, and a purulent discharge from the sternal wound. Wound erythema, abnormal sternal tenderness or instability, and mediastinal widening may all be absent or clinically unapparent early in the development of mediastinitis. Recognition of mediastinitis requires a high index of suspicion and a vigorous, repetitive search for evidence of sternal wound drainage in patients who are persistently febrile late into the 1st week after surgery and in whom there is no other obvious focus of infection, such as pneumonia or urinary tract infection. The diagnosis can be confirmed by needle aspiration from the subxiphoid approach followed by Gram's stain and culture.

In addition to the preoperative risk factors noted in Table 53–4, there are a number of intraoperative and postoperative risk factors for the development of mediastinitis. These include prolonged cardiopulmonary bypass time, excessive postoperative bleeding with reexploration for control of hemorrhage, and diminished cardiac output in the postoperative period. There is an increase in the development of mediastinitis when both internal mammary arteries are mobilized bilaterally for use as bypass conduits.[131] For that reason many surgeons prefer to utilize only the left internal mammary artery, particularly in elderly diabetic patients who may already be predisposed to delayed sternal wound healing. The spectrum of microorganisms that cause mediastinitis includes *Staphylo-*

coccus (*aureus* and *epidermidis*) in about 50 per cent of patients and a variety of gram-negative bacilli in about 40 per cent of cases.[132] Mixed infections and fungal infections are rare. The organism isolated frequently is resistant to the prophylactic antibiotic used preoperatively, especially if the isolate includes a gram-negative bacillus or a β-lactamase–producing S. aureus.[133]

Definitive diagnosis of a sternal wound infection requires exploration of the wound and culture of suspicious areas. Specialized radiological techniques such as CT and MRI scanning also have been reported to be helpful in localizing the sites of infection. Although both closed and open methods of treatment of mediastinitis have been reported, most authorities comment on the need for experienced surgical judgment if the closed approach (debridement, reclosure, and antibiotic irrigation) is utilized. The open approach is more frequently used for chronic or extensive infections, and often entails removal of involved bony or cartilaginous structures. Although previously the wound was allowed to heal by secondary intention, current strategy involves formation of a myocutaneous flap over the sternal area. The patient is treated with nutritional (Table 53–3) and respiratory support as needed. With both the closed and open method intravenous antibiotics and sternal antibiotic irrigation are continued for at least 10 to 14 days[134]; 4 to 6 weeks of treatment may be needed in cases of documented sternal osteomyelitis.

The reported mortality associated with mediastinitis varies greatly and appears to be related to the delay in initiation of treatment; patients diagnosed and treated aggressively within 1 month of surgery have a mortality of about 10 per cent, whereas those treated later have a mortality of about 25 per cent.[132,134,135] Surprisingly, the presence of a mediastinal infection does not appear to reduce the likelihood of patency of coronary artery bypass grafts.[136]

INFECTIVE ENDOCARDITIS (see Chap. 35). It has been convincingly shown that perioperative antibiotic prophylaxis is of benefit in patients undergoing cardiac surgery.[137] Although the antibiotic regimen varies, in part related to local differences in microbiological flora and personal preference, it is directed against gram-positive cocci (the most frequent causative pathogen in infections after cardiac surgery) and usually contains a cephalosporin. The regimen utilized in our institution consists of 1 gm of cefazolin intravenously 30 minutes before the skin incision and then repeated at 8-hour intervals for 48 hours after operation.

Cardiac surgery does not appear to increase the risk of endocarditis in patients with abnormal native valves that are not repaired or replaced during the operative procedure, in patients with intracardiac shunts, or in patients with intravascular devices (e.g., permanent pacemaker wires or renal dialysis shunts).[138] Assuming no infection is present preoperatively, such patients need only receive the standard antibiotic prophylaxis regimen in force at the institution in which the surgery is being performed.

Prosthetic Valve Endocarditis (see p. 1081). Prosthetic valve endocarditis is a rare complication of cardiac surgery, estimated to occur in only 2 to 4 per cent of patients; about half of the cases are classified as "early" (<60 days from the date of operation) and half as "late" (>60 days from the date of operation).[139–141] The pooled data from several series indicate that the organism responsible for early prosthetic valve endocarditis includes a *Staphylococcus* species in about 50 per cent of cases.[139,141] The remainder of early cases of prosthetic valve endocarditis are caused by gram-negative bacilli, diphtheroids, and fungi. The microbiological spectrum of late prosthetic valve endocarditis is more characteristic of that seen with native valve endocarditis. Only 30 per cent of cases are due to either S. epidermidis or S. aureus, and slightly more than one-third are caused by Streptococcus species (group D streptococci and Streptococcus pneumoniae). The nature of the pathology in prosthetic valve endocarditis varies, depending on the type of prosthesis.[141] Mechanical valves typically show a ring abscess or myocardial abscess, whereas porcine heterografts more commonly develop valvar stenosis or regurgitation as a result of the endocarditis.

Features of prosthetic valve endocarditis that have been associated with increased mortality include invasive infection (i.e., extension into the myocardium), congestive heart failure resulting from dysfunction of the prosthesis, and the presence of antibiotic-resistant, virulent microorganisms or a fungal organism.[141] Appropriate antibiotic therapy for prosthetic valve endocarditis is discussed in Chap. 35. The following clinical characteristics indicate the need for early operative intervention[141,142]: (1) moderate to severe congestive heart failure caused by prosthetic valve dysfunction (incompetence or stenosis); (2) signs of extension of the infection into the perivalvular tissue or formation of a myocardial abscess (new electrocardiographic conduction abnormalities, pericarditis, valve dehiscence, persistent unexplained fever beyond 10 days of antibiotic treatment); (3) infection caused by aggressive, invasive organisms or those that are difficult to eradicate (fungi, S. aureus, some cases of S. epidermidis); (4) persistently positive blood cultures despite appropriate antibiotic therapy; (5) relapse of the clinical syndrome of endocarditis after appropriate antibiotic therapy; and (6) recurrent systemic emboli.

VIRAL. Viral infections that occur after cardiac surgery are almost exclusively the result of infectious complications of transfusion therapy, and usually result in hepatitis. The incidence of viral infections after cardiac operations is decreasing as a result of a reduction in the number of transfusions of blood bank products (e.g., cell-saver techniques and preoperative autologous blood donations) and improved screening techniques in contemporary blood bank practice. The two most common transfusion-related viral infections after cardiac surgery are cytomegalovirus (CMV) infection and non-A, non-B hepatitis (currently referred to as hepatitis C). CMV infection is a febrile syndrome that typically presents 1 month postoperatively. It is characterized by high-spiking fevers, abnormalities of liver function tests, and arthralgias. A self-limited illness, it is best treated with antipyretics and supportive fluid therapy.

Hepatitis C is caused by an RNA virus, and is characterized by a protracted course with fluctuating transaminase levels.[143] About 50 per cent of patients respond to a course of interferon therapy with a reduction in transaminase levels; half of the responders relapse over the long term.[144,145] It is hoped that the incidence of hepatitis C will decrease with improvements in blood bank screening procedures for hepatitis C as are currently in place for hepatitis A and hepatitis B.

FUNGAL. Fungal infections that involve the heart are rare. They typically are seen in cases of fungemia and usually are fatal. Although the problem of fungemia is well described in the immunocompromised host (e.g., heart transplant recipient), in an autopsy study of 60 patients with fungal infections of the heart 25 per cent of cases occurred in association with conventional valvular surgery.[146] About half of fungal infections of the heart are confined to the endocardium, and half involve both the endocardium and the myocardium. Extracardiac involvement is common, with spread of the infection to the lungs, cerebrospinal fluid, urine, and skin. The most commonly encountered organisms, in descending order of frequency, are Candida, Aspergillus, and Cryptococcus species. Patients who appear at particular risk of fungal involvement of the heart are those who have received corticosteroids and long courses of antibiotic treatment postoperatively.

PERIPHERAL VASCULAR COMPLICATIONS

Most adult patients who undergo cardiac surgery—especially coronary revascularization—have atherosclerosis of the peripheral vasculature (e.g., ileofemoral system), and may experience lower-extremity ischemia after surgery because of low flow in the perioperative period with in situ thrombosis, embolism from the heart or aorta, or vascular compromise from an intraaortic balloon pump catheter. Man-

agement consists of anticoagulation and removal of indwelling catheters, if clinically feasible. Thrombectomy and even revascularization surgery of the lower extremities (e.g., femorofemoral, femoropopliteal, or axillofemoral bypass) may be required to salvage threatened limbs.

When aggressive preventive measures are not used, asymptomatic deep venous thrombosis of the calf can evolve before hospital discharge in one-third to one-half of patients who receive saphenous vein bypass grafts. Rarely, this causes massive pulmonary embolism. The best strategy is rigorous perioperative prophylaxis against venous thromboembolism in all such patients. The efficacy of "minidose heparin" (5000 units subcutaneously initiated 2 hours preoperatively and continued every 8 to 12 hours postoperatively) has been established. The potential benefit of prevention of deep venous thrombosis with intermittent pneumatic compression devices is under investigation.

OTHER COMPLICATIONS

PERICARDITIS (see Chap. 45). Pericardial friction rubs frequently are audible in the early postoperative period, and probably are the result of mechanical irritation from the mediastinal chest tubes. They usually disappear by the 2nd or 3rd postoperative day and are asymptomatic because of the narcotic analgesics prescribed at that stage of recovery. Although some patients develop pericardial rubs toward the end of the 1st postoperative week, these usually are benign, do not indicate a need for prolongation of hospitalization, and do not require treatment. A separate clinical syndrome that appears late in the 1st postoperative month is the *postpericardiotomy syndrome* (p. 227).[147] The relation between the postpericardiotomy syndrome and chronic constrictive pericarditis is not firmly established, but a number of case reports of patients with *postoperative constrictive pericarditis*[148] include patients with a history of postpericardiotomy syndrome.

RENAL FAILURE (see Chap. 62). All patients who undergo cardiac surgery experience a reduction in renal blood flow and glomerular filtration rate (GFR) as a consequence of both anesthesia and cardiopulmonary bypass. Risk factors for the development of persistent renal failure after cardiac surgery include a preoperative history of renal dysfunction or left ventricular dysfunction, prolonged bypass time (>180 minutes), prolonged aortic cross-clamping (>40 minutes), perioperative hypotension, advanced age (>70 years), and the development postoperatively of medical complications.[149–151] Most cases of acute renal failure after cardiac surgery result from renal ischemia that lowers the GFR directly (prerenal disease) or, if severe or prolonged, can induce acute tubular necrosis. Possible additional contributory factors include sepsis, nephrotoxic drugs, radiocontrast material injections, cholesterol plaque embolization to the renal circulation, increased urine free hemoglobin levels from hemolysis while on cardiopulmonary bypass, and the effects of angiotensin converting enzyme (ACE) inhibitors on glomerular capillary pressure.[150] The detrimental effects of ACE inhibitors are most likely to occur when renal perfusion pressure is low because of renal artery stenosis or systemic hypotension caused by cardiac failure.

Urine output is variable in patients with postoperative acute renal failure. Anuria is uncommon and, if present, should raise the suspicion of urinary tract obstruction (e.g., occluded Foley catheter). More commonly patients are either oliguric (<400 ml/day) or nonoliguric. Oliguric acute renal failure occurs less frequently than nonoliguric renal failure, usually reflects more severe renal injury, and is associated with a greater probability of requiring dialysis during the acute phase.[152,153]

Important diagnostic studies in all patients with acute renal failure include a urinalysis, and estimation of pulmonary capillary wedge pressure and cardiac output by means of pulmonary artery catheterization. Prerenal azotemia should be suspected if the urine sodium level is less than 20 mEq/liter, the fractional excretion of sodium is less than 1 per cent, and the urine osmolality level is greater than 500 mOsm/liter. Acute tubular necrosis should be suspected if the urine sodium level is greater than 40 mEq/liter, the fractional excretion of sodium is greater than 2 per cent, and the urine osmolality level is less than 350 mOsm/liter.

TREATMENT. Essential elements of treatment for both prerenal azotemia and acute tubular necrosis include optimization of intravascular fluid volume and cardiac output. The latter is best accomplished with vasodilators and inotropic agents (p. 1871) rather than with vasopressors, to avoid further reductions in renal blood flow. Experimental studies suggest that several modalities may protect against the development of progressive renal failure in models of acute renal ischemic injury (e.g., renal artery clamping that simulates the effects of suprarenal aortic cross-clamping while on cardiopulmonary bypass). Mannitol (which washes out obstructing casts), a loop diuretic (which decreases energy requirements in the

TABLE 53–12 GASTROINTESTINAL COMPLICATIONS AFTER CARDIAC SURGERY

COMPLICATION	COMMON CAUSES	EVALUATION	TREATMENT	COMMENT
Hyperbilirubinemia				
Early (1–10 days)	"Shock liver" syndrome[162]	Check full chemistry profile	Maximize cardiac output, BP, and oxygenation	Markedly elevated enzyme levels are seen early after onset of shock state
	Hemolysis on cardiopulmonary bypass[163]	↑ Plasma free hemoglobin	Observe	Isolated elevation of direct and indirect bilirubin without enzyme elevation
	Right heart failure[162]	Chest x-ray, hemodynamic monitoring	Digitalis, diuretics, oxygen, consider isoproterenol infusion	Elevated direct bilirubin and alkaline phosphatase but without enzyme elevation
Late (10–90 days)	Infection (cytomegalovirus, hepatitis C)[164]	Viral serology	Observe	Consider interferon for hepatitis C
	Cholecystitis	Ultrasound, biliary isotopic scan (e.g., HIDA, PIPIDA)	General surgical consultation	May require ERCP, cholecystectomy, cholecystotomy
Gastroduodenal disease[160]				
Hemorrhage	Stress gastritis	Nasogastric aspirate (pH and Hematest), CBC	Nasogastric tube, antacids, H$_2$-receptor antagonists, transfusions	Because of the increased risk of developing this complication, it is important to provide prophylactic treatment (antacids, H$_2$-receptor antagonists) to patients with COPD and postoperative hypotension, bleeding, or reoperation.[165] Early endoscopy and consideration of surgical intervention are strongly advised if supportive medical care is unsuccessful.
	Peptic ulcer disease	Nasogastric aspirate (pH and Hematest), CBC	Nasogastric tube, antacids, H$_2$-receptor antagonists, transfusions	Early endoscopy and consideration of surgical intervention are strongly advised if supportive medical care is unsuccessful.
Mesenteric ischemia[166]	Combination of low cardiac output, embolization of atherosclerotic debris or thrombi, and vascular dissection by intraaortic balloon pump	High index of suspicion and early surgical consultation	Early laparotomy with resection of affected bowel and embolectomy when possible	Mortality rate remains high.
Pancreatitis	Hypotension, thromboembolism of vascular supply, splanchnic vasoconstriction	Serum amylase measurements serially, abdominal ultrasonogram	Nasogastric suction and fluid support	Hyperamylasemia is common after cardiac surgery, but clinical pancreatitis is rare.[167] Severe, fulminating acute pancreatitis in postcardiac surgical patients has a poor prognosis despite aggressive surgical treatment.[168]
Miscellaneous				
Intraabdominal bleeding	Trauma (intraop, chest tubes)	Abdominal lavage	General surgical consultation	
	Preexisting lesion (e.g., hamartoma)			
Lower gastrointestinal tract bleed	Colonic pathology (e.g., polyp)	Plain film of abdomen, colonoscopy		
Ileus	Narcotics	Plain film of abdomen	Nasogastric suction	
	Adhesions			

CBC, complete blood count; COPD, chronic obstructive pulmonary disease; ERCP, endoscopic retrograde cholangiopancreatography.

thick ascending limb of the loop of Henle, thereby decreasing ischemic injury), and the combination of dopamine and atrial natriuretic peptide (but neither alone) have all been effective.[154] There are, however, no good clinical trials to confirm the efficacy of these interventions. Several uncontrolled observations suggest that those patients who appear to be protected by a loop diuretic, mannitol, or dopamine were all treated within 12 to 24 hours of the onset of renal dysfunction.[155,156]

It is prudent to undertake a trial of furosemide and mannitol (only if the patient can tolerate the volume load of the latter) within the first 12 to 24 hours after the development of oliguria. The aim of such therapy is to increase urine output. Because of the renal vasodilating effects of dopamine (3 μg/kg/min), patients with both oliguric and nonoliguric renal failure may experience an increase in urine output.[150] There is, however, no evidence that dopamine alone given in this setting is helpful for recruiting salvageable, but nonfunctioning nephrons.[157]

If oliguria persists beyond 12 hours, a number of supportive measures must be activated, including careful attention to electrolyte balance, specifically avoiding hyperkalemia; excessive free water administration that might lead to hyponatremia; correction of acidosis (adding bicarbonate to daily fluids); and adjustment of medication dosages for delayed excretion if the drug is cleared by renal mechanisms.[154] There seems little benefit to instituting dialysis prophylactically for a given level of blood urea nitrogen or creatinine. Rather, dialysis should be carried out for pericarditis, refractory hyperkalemia, uremic encephalopathy, or colitis. Continuous arteriovenous hemofiltration is a simpler modality that can be used to remove excess fluid.

Finally, the patient with chronic renal failure who undergoes surgery is at increased risk of exacerbation of renal dysfunction perioperatively. This may require temporary or even permanent hemodialysis, and these eventualities should be addressed with the patient and the cardiac surgical team preoperatively. Surgery can be safely performed in patients who are already on hemodialysis, but careful coordination of the surgical and dialysis schedules is essential to minimize postoperative problems with fluid and electrolyte management.[158,159] Ultrafiltration can be performed while on cardiopulmonary bypass, to help minimize the intraoperative fluid load received by the patient.

GASTROINTESTINAL COMPLICATIONS (Table 53–12). Serious gastrointestinal complications after cardiac surgery are rare (occurring in about 1 per cent of patients), and usually can be handled by a conservative approach. Only about 0.5 per cent of patients who undergo cardiac surgery require a general surgical operation for a gastrointestinal complication.[160] Patients with circulatory compromise and those who require intraaortic balloon pump support are more likely to develop gastrointestinal complications.[160,161] Despite their relative rarity, gastrointestinal complications are associated with a significant mortality (approaching 40 per cent in some series), highlighting the need for careful monitoring and repeated physical examination in high-risk patients.[160] Most complications occur within 7 days of surgery.

NEUROLOGICAL. Neurologic complications after cardiac surgery are quite common, particularly in the elderly, if one is attentive to the subtle cognitive (short-term memory loss, lack of concentration) and psychological (depression, increased sense of dependency) changes seen early after operation.[169,170] A positive and supportive attitude on the part of the staff and enlistment of the aid of family members help to minimize these problems. Although many patients return to their preoperative state by 4 to 6 weeks after surgery,[171] about 10 per cent will continue to show deterioration of their neuropsychological function over the next 6 months, especially if they are over age 65.[172] More serious neurological complications, such as stroke (Table 53–13), occur in 1 to 5 per cent of patients, but may be seen in as many as 10 per cent of patients over age 65.

Symptomatic visual defects may be seen after cardiac surgery, and result from retinal emboli, occipital lobe infarction, or anterior ischemic optic neuropathy.[176] Risk factors for cerebrovascular accident (CVA) or transient ischemic attack (TIA) after cardiac surgery include preoperative carotid bruit,[177] previous CVA or TIA,[174] postoperative atrial fibrillation,[174] prolonged cardiopulmonary bypass (>2 hours),[177] and preoperative left ventricular mural thrombus.[175] Patients with *symptomatic* carotid bruits should undergo combined carotid endarterectomy along with their cardiac procedure. However, despite the recognition of a carotid stenosis greater than 50 per cent as a risk factor for perioperative CVA, no clinical trial has convincingly shown a benefit of preoperative or simultaneous carotid endarterectomy (which is inherently associated with a 3 to 4 per cent risk of cerebral ischemia) in reducing the incidence of CVA or TIA after cardiac surgical procedures.[178,179]

Neuropathies in the upper extremities have been reported after cardiac operations. The pattern of injury involving predominantly the ulnar nerve and medial antebrachial cutaneous nerve suggests that the lesion involves a brachial plexus compression or traction injury.[180] The average duration of symptoms after such an injury is 2 months, but some patients show a slower time course of improvement extending over 6 to 12 months.

CHYLOTHORAX, CHYLOPERICARDIUM. These are rare postcardiac

TABLE 53–13 POSSIBLE CAUSES OF STROKE AFTER CARDIAC SURGERY

Embolism
  Debridement or replacement of calcified aortic valve
  Dislodgment of atherosclerotic plaque during cannulation of aorta
  Introduction of air into the arterial circulation intraoperatively[173]
  Dislodgment of atherosclerotic plaque from carotid artery stenosis by means of "jet effect" from aortic inflow cannula
  Arrhythmia (e.g., atrial fibrillation)[174]
  Thrombosis of mechanical prosthetic valve
  Dissection of aorta during cannulation
  Left ventricular thrombus[175]
  Dislodgment of fragment of left atrial myxoma
  Endocarditis
  Microaggregate formation on cardiopulmonary bypass[173]
Hemorrhage
  Anticoagulation perioperatively
  Hypertension
Hypotension
  Hypoperfusion of cerebral circulation while on cardiopulmonary bypass
  Hypoperfusion of cerebral circulation during period of postoperative shock

surgical complications in adults, occurring in less than 0.5 per cent of cases. Treatment of chylothorax consists of prolonged chest tube drainage and dietary support with medium-chain triglycerides. Refractory cases of chylothorax have been successfully treated by the creation of a pleuroperitoneal shunt.[181] Chylopericardium may cause cardiac tamponade (p. 1479), and is treated by creation of a pericardial window into the pleural space and management as above for chylothorax. Persistent chyle leaks may necessitate thoracic duct ligation.

REHABILITATION AND PREPARATION FOR DISCHARGE
(See Chap. 42)

A coordinated, multidisciplinary cardiac exercise program is essential to overcome the physical deconditioning and psychosocial upheaval associated with cardiac surgery. Emphasis should be placed on early mobilization and progressively more patient self-care, including in the intensive care unit during the first 48 hours postoperatively. After transfer out of the intensive care unit, the patient should be encouraged to engage in low-intensity (2 to 3 METS) isotonic activities such as walking and range-of-motion exercises. The nursing staff should monitor the patient's progress, being alert to any undue acceleration of the heart rate (>120 beats/min) or hemodynamically compromising arrhythmias. Patients also should participate in an education program focusing on instructions regarding postoperative medications and plans for returning to work (by about 6 to 8 weeks). Despite the extensive publicity surrounding coronary bypass surgery and the efforts of many personnel in institutions in which such operations are performed, there is a disappointing rate of return to work reported in several series, even allowing for the advanced age of many patients who undergo coronary artery bypass grafting.[182–184] Innovative strategies are needed to encourage patients to return to work, and society to accept postcardiac surgical patients back into the work force.[185]

REFERENCES

PREOPERATIVE EVALUATION

1. Anderson, E. A.: Preoperative preparation for cardiac surgery facilitates recovery, reduces psychological distress, and reduces the incidence of acute postoperative hypertension. J. Consult. Clin. Psychol. 55:513, 1987.
2. Hanet, C., Marchand, E., and Keyeux, A.: Left internal mammary artery occlusion after mastectomy and radiotherapy. Am. J. Cardiol. 65:1044, 1990.
3. Kuan, P., Bernstein, S. B., Ellesstad, M. H., et al.: Coronary artery bypass surgery morbidity. J. Am. Coll. Cardiol. 3:1391, 1984.
4. Rich, M. W., Kelller, A. J., Schechtman, K. B., et al.: Increased complica-

tions and prolonged hospital stay in elderly cardiac surgical patients with low serum albumin. Am. J. Cardiol. 63:714, 1989.

5. Jeejeebhoy, K. N.: Nutrition in critical illness. In Shoemaker, W. C., Ayres, S., Grenovik, A., et al. (eds.): Textbook of Critical Care. Philadelphia, W. B. Saunders, 1989, p. 1093.

6. Gersh, B. J., Kronman, R. A., Frye, R. L., et al.: Coronary arteriography and coronary artery bypass surgery: Morbidity and mortality in patients age 65 years and older. Circulation 67:483, 1983.

7. Naunheim, K. S., Kern, M. J., McBride, L. R., et al.: Coronary artery bypass surgery in patients aged 80 years and older. Am. J. Cardiol. 59:804, 1987.

8. Birnbaum, P. L., Weisel, R. D., Ivanov, J., et al.: The changing pattern of coronary bypass surgery (CABG). Circulation 78(Supp II):II-476, 1988.

9. Loop, F. D., Golding, L. R., MacMillan, J. P., et al.: Coronary artery surgery in women compared with men: Analysis of risks and long term results. J. Am. Coll. Cardiol. 1:383, 1983.

10. Khan, S. S., Nessim, S., Gray R., et al.: Increased mortality of women in coronary artery bypass surgery: Evidence for referral bias. Ann. Intern. Med. 112:561, 1990.

11. Loop, F. D., Lytle, B. W., Cosgrove, D. M., et al.: Sternal wound complications after isolated coronary artery bypass grafting: Early and late mortality, morbidity, and cost of care. Ann. Thorac. Surg. 49:179, 1990.

12. McGrath, L. B., Laub, G. W., Graf, D., and Gonzalez-Lavin, L.: Hospital death on a cardiac surgical service: Negative influence of changing practice patterns. Ann. Thorac. Surg. 49:410, 1990.

13. Weintraub, W. S., Jones, E. L., Craver, J., et al.: Determinants of prolonged length of hospital stay after coronary artery bypass surgery. Circulation 80:276, 1989.

14. Boldt, J., Kling, D., Hempelmann, G.: Right ventricular function and cardiac surgery. Intensive Care Med. 14:496, 1988.

15. Parsons, R. S., Mohandas, K., and Riaz, N.: The effects of an intravenous infusion of isosorbide dinitrate during open heart surgery. Eur. Heart J. 9(Suppl A): 195, 1988.

16. Coriat, P., Daloz, M., Bousseau, D., et al.: Prevention of intraoperative myocardial ischemia during noncardiac surgery with intravenous nitroglycerin. Anesthesiology 61:193, 1984.

17. Hensley, F. A., and Martin, D. E.: The Practice of Cardiac Anesthesia. Boston, Little, Brown, 1990.

18. Knight, P. R., Kroll, D. A., Nahrwald, M. L., et al.: Comparison of cardiovascular responses to anesthesia and operation when intravenous lidocaine or morphine sulfate is used as adjunct to diazepam-nitrous oxide for cardiac surgery. Anesth. Analg. 59:130, 1980.

19. Tyras, D. H., Stothert, J. C. Jr., Kaiser, G. C., et al.: Supraventricular tachyarrhythmias after myocardial revascularization: A randomized trial of prophylactic digitalization. J. Thorac. Cardiovasc. Surg. 77:310, 1979.

20. Csicsko, J. F., Schatzlein, M. H., and King, R. D.: Immediate postoperative digitalization in the prophylaxis of supraventricular arrhythmias following coronary artery bypass. J. Thorac. Cardiovasc. Surg. 81:419, 1981.

21. Johnson, L. W., Dickstein, R. A., Fruehan, C. T., et al.: Prophylactic digitalization for coronary artery bypass. Circulation 53:819, 1976.

22. Chee, T. P., Prakash, N. S., Desser, K. B., and Benchimol, A.: Postoperative supraventricular arrhythmias and the role of prophylactic digoxin in cardiac surgery. Am. Heart J. 104:974, 1982.

23. Ormerod, O. J., McGregor, C. G., Stone, D. L., et al.: Arrhythmias after coronary bypass surgery. Br. Heart J. 51:618, 1984.

24. Selzer, A., Kelly, J. J. Jr., Gerbode, F., et al.: Case against routine use of digitalis in patients undergoing cardiac surgery. J.A.M.A. 195:549, 1966.

25. Lauer, M. S., Eagle, K. A., Buckley, M. J., and DeSanctis, R. W.: Atrial fibrillation following coronary artery bypass surgery. Prog. Cardiovasc. Dis. 31:367, 1989.

26. Oka, Y., Frishman, W., Becker, R. N., et al.: Clinical pharmacology of the new beta adrenergic blocking drugs. 10. Beta adrenoceptor blockade and coronary artery surgery. Am. Heart J. 99:255, 1980.

27. Hammon, J. W. Jr., Wood, A. J., Prager, R. L., et al.: Perioperative beta blockade with propranolol: Reduction in myocardial oxygen demands and incidence of atrial and ventricular arrhythmias. Ann. Thorac. Surg. 38:363, 1984.

28. White, H. D., Antman, E. M., Glynn, M. A., et al.: Efficacy and safety of timolol for prevention of supraventricular tachyarrhythmias after coronary artery bypass surgery. Circulation 70:479, 1984.

28a. Andrews, T. C., Reimold, S. C., Berlin, J. A., and Antman, E. M.: Prevention of supraventricular arrhythmias after coronary artery bypass surgery: A meta-analysis. Circulation 82 (Suppl. III):296, 1990.

29. Davison, R., Hartz, R., Kaplan, K., et al.: Prophylaxis of supraventricular tachyarrhythmia after coronary bypass surgery with oral verapamil: A randomized, double-blind trial. Ann. Thorac. Surg. 39:336, 1985.

30. Gray, R., Conklin, C., Sethna, D., et al.: The role of intravenous verapamil in supraventricular tachyarrhythmias after open-heart surgery. Am. Heart J. 104:799, 1982.

31. Cardiac Arrhythmia Suppression Trial (CAST) Investigators: Preliminary Report: Effect of encainide and flecainide on mortality in a randomized trial of arrhythmia suppression after myocardial infarction. N. Engl. J. Med. 321:406, 1989.

32. Nalos, P. C., Kass, R. M., Gang, E. S., et al.: Life-threatening postoperative pulmonary complications in patients with previous amiodarone pulmonary toxicity undergoing cardiothoracic operations. J. Thorac. Cardiovasc. Surg. 93:904, 1987.

33. Kupferschmid, J. P., Rosengart, T. K., McIntosh, C. L., et al.: Amiodarone-induced complications after cardiac operation for obstructive hypertrophic cardiomyopathy. Ann. Thorac. Surg. 48:359, 1989.

34. Barbieri, E., Conti, F., Zampieri, P., et al.: Amiodarone and desethylamiodarone distribution in the atrium and adipose tissue of patients undergoing short- and long-term treatment with amiodarone. J. Am. Coll. Cardiol. 8:210, 1986.

35. Lamas, G. A., Rebecca, G. S., Braunwald, N. S., and Antman, E. M.: Pacemaker malfunction after nitrous oxide anesthesia. Am. J. Cardiol. 56:995, 1985.

36. Lamas, G. A., Antman, E. M., Gold, J., et al.: Pacemaker back-up mode reversion and injury during cardiac surgery. Ann. Thorac. Surg. 41:155, 1986.

37. Forraris, V., Ferraris, S. P., Lough, F. C., et al.: Preoperative aspirin ingestion increases operative blood loss after coronary artery bypass grafting. Ann. Thorac. Surg. 45:71, 1988.

38. Henderson, W. G., Goldman, S., Copeland, J. G., et al.: Antiplatelet or anticoagulant therapy after coronary artery bypass surgery: A meta-analysis of clinical trials. Ann. Intern. Med. 111:743, 1989.

38a. Buring, J. E., Hennekens, C. H.: Antiplatelet therapy to prevent coronary artery bypass graft occlusion. Circulation 82:1046, 1990.

39. Sethi, G. K., Copeland, J. G., Goldman, S., et al.: Implications of preoperative administration of aspirin in patients undergoing coronary artery bypass grafting. J. Am. Coll. Cardiol. 15:15, 1990.

40. Owings, D. V., Kruskall, M. S., Thurer, R. L., and Donovan, L. M.: Autologous blood donations prior to elective cardiac surgery. Safety and effect on subsequent blood use. J.A.M.A. 262:1963, 1989.

41. Giordano, G. F., Goldman, D. S., Mammana, R. B., et al.: Intraoperative autotransfusion in cardiac operations. Effect on intraoperative and postoperative transfusion requirements. J. Thorac. Cardiovasc. Surg. 96:382, 1988.

42. Dietrich, W., Barankay, A., Dilthey, G., and Richter, J. A.: Autotransfusion and hemoseparation in cardiac surgery. What can be saved in cardiac reoperations and operations of thoracic aortic aneurysms? Thorac. Cardiovasc. Surg. 37:84, 1989.

43. Stein, B., Fuster, V., Halperin, J. L., and Chesebro, J. H.: Antithrombotic therapy in cardiovascular disease. An emerging approach based on pathogenesis and risk. Circulation 80:1501, 1989.

44. Subramanian, V. B., Bowles, M. J., Khurmi, N. S., et al.: Calcium antagonist withdrawal syndrome: Objective demonstration with frequency-modulated ambulatory ST-segment monitoring. Br. Med. J. 286:520, 1983.

45. Gottlieb, S. O., and Gerstenblith, G.: Safety of acute calcium antagonist withdrawal: Studies in patients with unstable angina withdrawn from nifedipine. Am. J. Cardiol. 55:27E, 1985.

46. Mehta, J., and Lopez, L. M.: Calcium-blocker withdrawal phenomenon: Increase in affinity of alpha 2 adrenoceptors for agonist as a potential mechanism. Am. J. Cardiol. 58:242, 1986.

INTRAOPERATIVE EVALUATION

47. Kirklin, J. W., and Barratt-Boyes, B. G.: Cardiac Surgery. New York, John Wiley & Sons, 1986.

POSTOPERATIVE EVALUATION

48. Weber, D. O., and Yarnoz, M. D.: Hyperkalemia complicating cardiopulmonary bypass: Analysis of risk factors. Ann. Thorac. Surg. 34:439, 1982.

49. Keren, A., and Tzivoni, D.: Magnesium therapy in ventricular arrhythmias. Pace 13:937, 1990.

50. Osborn, J. J., Popper, R. M., Kerth, W. J., et al.: Respiratory insufficiency following open heart surgery. Ann. Surg. 156:638, 1962.

51. Chenoweth, D. E., Cooper, S. W., Hugli, T. E., et al.: Complement activation during cardiopulmonary bypass: Evidence for generation of C3a and C5a anaphylatoxins. N. Engl. J. Med. 304:497, 1981.

52. Benumof, J. L., and Wahrenbrock, E. A.: Local effects of anesthetics on regional hypoxic pulmonary vasoconstriction. Anesthesiology 43:525, 1975.

53. Quasha, A. C., Loeber, N., Feeley, T. W., et al.: Postoperative respiratory care: A controlled trial of early and late extubation following coronary artery bypass grafting. Anesthesiology 52:135, 1980.

54. Fountain, S. W., Martin, B. A., and Musclow, C. E.: Pulmonary leukostasis and its relationship to pulmonary dysfunction in sheep and rabbits. Circ. Res. 46:175, 1980.

55. Jorgensen, L., Hoving, T., Rowsell, H. C., et al.: Adenosine diphosphate-involved platelet aggregation and vascular injury in swine and rabbit. Am. J. Pathol. 61:161, 1970.

56. Edmunds, L. H. Jr., and Alexander, J. A.: Effect of cardiopulmonary bypass on the lungs. In Fishman, A. (ed.): Pulmonary Disease and Disorders. New York, McGraw-Hill, 1980, p. 1728.

57. Stein, M., and Cassara, E. L.: Preoperative pulmonary evaluation and therapy for surgery patients. J.A.M.A. 211:787, 1970.

58. Aubier, M., and Roussos, S.: Effect of theophylline on respiratory muscle function. Chest 88:915, 1985.

59. Weinberger, M., Hendeles, L., and Ahrens, R.: Pharmacologic management of reversible obstructive airways disease: Symposium on chronic lung obstructive airways disease. Med. Clin. North Am. 65:579, 1980.

60. Albert, R. K., Martin, T. R., and Lewis, S. W.: Controlled clinical trial of methylprednisolone in patients with chronic bronchitis and acute respiratory insufficiency. Ann. Intern. Med. 92:753, 1980.

61. Morgenroth, M. L., Morganroth, J. L., Nett, L. M., et al.: Criteria for wean-

ing from prolonged mechanical ventilation. Arch. Intern. Med. 144:1012, 1984.

62. Curtis, J. J., Weerachai, N., Walls, J. T., et al.: Elevated hemidiaphragm after cardiac operations: Incidence, prognosis, and relationship to the use of topical ice slush. Ann. Thorac. Surg. 48:764, 1989.

63. Abd, G. A., Braun, N. M. T., Baskin, M. I., et al.: Diaphragmatic dysfunction after open heart surgery: Treatment with a rocking bed. Ann. Intern. Med. 111:881, 1989.

64. Graham, D. R., Kaplan, D., Evans, C. C., et al.: Diaphragmatic plication for unilateral diaphragmatic paralysis: A 10-year experience. Ann. Thorac. Surg. 49:248, 1990.

65. Carlin, G. C., Howland, W. S., Ray, C., et al.: High frequency jet ventilation. A prospective randomized evaluation. Chest 84:551, 1983.

66. Flaherty, J. T., Magee, P. A., Gardner, T. L., et al.: Comparison of intravenous nitroglycerin and sodium nitroprusside for treatment of acute hypertension developing after coronary artery bypass surgery. Circulation 65:1072, 1982.

67. Fremes, S. E., Weisel, R. D., Baird, R. J., et al.: Effects of postoperative hypertension and its treatment. J. Thorac. Cardiovasc. Surg. 86:47, 1983.

68. Gray, R. J., Bateman, T. M., Czer, L. S., et al.: Use of esmolol in hypertension after cardiac surgery. Am. J. Cardiol. 56:SGF, 1985.

69. Estafanous, F. G., and Tarazi, R. C.: Systemic arterial hypertension associated with cardiac surgery. Am. J. Cardiol. 46:685, 1980.

70. Cooper, T. J., Clutton Brock, T. H., Jones, S. N., et al.: Factors relating to the development of hypertension after cardiopulmonary bypass. Br. Heart J. 54:91, 1985.

71. Rocchini, A. P., Rosenthal, A., Barger, A. C., et al.: Pathogenesis of paradoxical hypertension after coarctation resection. Circulation 54:382, 1976.

72. James, T. N., Hageman, G. R., and Urthaler, F.: Anatomic and physiologic considerations of a cardiogenic hypertensive reflex. Am. J. Cardiol. 44:852, 1979.

73. Kirklin, J. W., and Barratt-Boyes, B. G.: Postoperative care. In Kirklin, J. W., and Barratt-Boyes, B. G. (eds.): Cardiac Surgery. New York, John Wiley & Sons, 1986, p. 139.

74. Brody, W. R., Kosek, J. C., and Angell, W. W.: Changes in vein grafts following aorto-coronary bypass induced by pressure and ischemia. J. Thorac. Cardiovasc. Surg. 46:847, 1972.

75. Kaplan, J. A., Finlayson, D. C., and Woodward, S.: Vasodilator therapy after cardiac surgery: A review of the efficacy and toxicity of nitroglycerin and nitroprusside. Can. Anaesth. Soc. J. 27:254, 1980.

76. Gray, R. J., Bateman, T. M., Czer, L. S., et al.: Comparison of esmolol and nitroprusside for acute post-cardiac surgical hypertension. Am. J. Cardiol. 59:887, 1987.

77. Gabrielson, G., Lingham, R., Dimich, I., et al: Comparative study of labetalol and hydralazine in the treatment of postoperative hypertension. Anesth. Analg. 66:S63, 1987.

78. Cosgrove, D. M., Petre, J. H., Waller, J. L., et al.: Automated control of postoperative hypertension: A prospective, randomized multicenter study. Ann. Thorac. Surg. 47:678, 1989.

79. Gray, R. J., Harris, W. S., Shah, P. K., et al.: Coronary sinus blood flow and sampling for detection of unrecognized myocardial ischemia and injury. Circulation 56(Suppl 2):58, 1977.

80. Slogoff, S., and Keats, A. S.: Does perioperative myocardial ischemia lead to postoperative myocardial infarction? Anesthesiology 62:107, 1985.

81. London, M. J., Hollenberg, M., Wong, M. G., et al.: Intraoperative myocardial ischemia: Localization by continuous 12-lead electrocardiography. Anesthesiology 69:232, 1988.

82. Lemmer, J. H. Jr., and Krish, M. M.: Coronary artery spasm following coronary artery surgery. Ann. Thorac. Surg. 46:108, 1988.

83. Lawrence, G. H., McKay, H. A., and Sherensky, R. T.: Effective measures in the prevention of intraoperative aeroembolus. J. Thorac. Cardiovasc. Surg. 62:731, 1971.

84. Keon, W. J., Heggtveit, H. A., and Leduc, J.: Perioperative myocardial infarction caused by atheroembolism. J. Thorac. Cardiovasc. Surg. 84:849, 1982.

85. Obarski, T. P., Loop, F. D., Cosgrove, D. M., et al.: Frequency of acute myocardial infarction in valve repairs versus valve replacement for pure mitral regurgitation. Am. J. Cardiol. 65:887, 1990.

86. Bulkley, B. H., and Hutchins, G. M.: Myocardial consequences of coronary artery bypass graft surgery. The paradox of necrosis in areas of revascularization. Circulation 56:906, 1977.

87. Albert, D. E., Califf, R. M., LeCocq, D. A., et al.: Comparative rates of resolution of QRS changes after operative and nonoperative acute myocardial infarcts. Am. J. Cardiol. 51:378, 1983.

88. Gray, R. J., Matloff, J. M., Conklin, C. M., et al.: Perioperative myocardial infarction: Late clinical course after coronary artery bypass surgery. Circulation 66:1185, 1982.

89. Chaitman, B. R., Alderman, E. L., Sheffield, L. T., et al.: Use of survival analysis to determine the clinical significance of new Q waves after coronary bypass surgery. Circulation 67:302, 1983.

90. Bateman, T. M., Matloff, J. M., and Gray, R. J.: Myocardial infarction during coronary artery bypass surgery—benign event or prognostic omen? Int. J. Cardiol. 6:259, 1984.

90a. Force, T., Hibberd, P., Weeks, G., et al.: Perioperative myocardial infarction after coronary artery bypass surgery. Circulation 82:903, 1990.

91. Salomon, N. W., Plachetka, J. R., and Copeland, J. G.: Comparison of dopamine and dobutamine following coronary artery bypass grafting. Ann. Thorac. Surg. 33:48, 1982.

92. Makabali, C., Weil, M. H., and Henning, R. J.: Dobutamine and other

93. Gray, R., Shah, P. K., Singh, B., et al.: Low cardiac output states after open heart surgery. Chest 80:16, 1981.

94. Bastien, O., Durand, P. G., George, M., et al.: Evolution of right ventricular performance after CABG. Intensive Care Med. 14:499, 1988.

95. D'Ambra, M. N., LaRaia, P. J., Philbin, D. M., et al.: Prostaglandin E₁: A new therapy for refractory right heart failure and pulmonary hypertension after mitral valve replacement. J. Thorac. Cardiovasc. Surg. 89:567, 1985.

96. Miller, D. C., Moreno-Cabral, R. J., Stinson, E. B., et al.: Pulmonary artery balloon counterpulsation for acute right ventricular failure. J. Thorac. Cardiovasc. Surg. 80:760, 1980.

97. Weitzman, L. B., Tinker, P. W., Kronzon, I., et al.: The incidence and natural history of pericardial effusion after cardiac surgery. Circulation 69:506, 1984.

98. D'Cruz, I. A., Kensey, K., Campbell, C., et al.: Two-dimensional echocardiography in cardiac tamponade occurring after cardiac surgery. Circulation 5:1250, 1985.

99. Weeks, K. R., Chatterjee, K., Block, S., et al.: Bedside hemodynamic monitoring—its value in the diagnosis of tamponade complicating cardiac surgery. J. Thorac. Cardiovasc. Surg. 71:259, 1976.

100. Jones, M. R., Vine, D. L., Attas, M., et al.: Late isolated left ventricular tamponade: Clinical, hemodynamic and echocardiographic manifestations of a previously unreported postoperative complication. J. Thorac. Cardiovasc. Surg. 77:142, 1979.

101. Bateman, T., Gray, R., Chaux, A., et al.: Right atrial tamponade caused by hematoma complicating coronary artery bypass graft surgery: Clinical hemodynamic and scintigraphic correlates. J. Thorac. Cardiovasc. Surg. 84:413, 1982.

102. MacMahon, S., Collins, R., Peto, R., et al.: Effects of prophylactic lidocaine in suspected acute myocardial infarction. An overview of results from the randomized, controlled trials. J.A.M.A. 260:1910, 1988.

103. Rao, G., Ford, W. B., Zikria, E. A., et al.: Prevention of arrhythmias after direct myocardial revascularization surgery. Vasc. Surg. 8:82, 1974.

104. Waldo, A. L., and MacLean, W. A.: Treatment of cardiac arrhythmias with emphasis on cardiac pacing. In Diagnosis and Treatment of Cardiac Arrhythmias Following Open Heart Surgery: Emphasis on the Use of Atrial and Ventricular Epicardial Wire Electrodes. Mount Kisco, Futura, 1980, p. 115.

105. Douglas, P., Hirshfield, J. W., and Edmunds, L. H.: Clinical correlates of postoperative atrial fibrillation. Circulation 70(Suppl II):165, 1984.

106. Fuller, J. A., Adams, G. G., and Buxton, B.: Atrial fibrillation after coronary artery bypass grafting. Is it a disorder of the elderly? J. Thorac. Cardiovasc. Surg. 97:821, 1989.

107. Platia, E. V., Fitzpatrick, P., Wallis, D., et al.: Esmolol vs verapamil for the treatment of recent-onset atrial fibrillation/flutter. J. Am. Coll. Cardiol. 11:170A, 1988.

108. Dunn, M. I., Alexander, J. K., deSilva, R., and Hildner, F.: Antithrombotic therapy in atrial fibrillation. Chest 95(Suppl):119S, 1989.

109. Dimarco, J. P., Miles, W., Akhtar, M., et al.: Adenosine for paroxysmal supraventricular tachycardia: Dose ranging and comparison with verapamil. Assessment in placebo-controlled multicenter trials. Ann. Intern. Med. 113:104, 1990.

110. Wexelman, W., Lichstein, E., Cunningham, J. N., et al.: Etiology and clinical significance of new fascicular conduction defects following coronary bypass surgery. Am. Heart J. 111:923, 1986.

111. Gundry, S, R., Sequeira, A., Coughlin, T. R., and McLaughlin, J. S.: Postoperative conduction disturbances: A comparison of blood and crystalloid cardioplegia. Ann. Thorac. Surg. 47:384, 1989.

111a. Tuzcu, E. M., Emre, A., Goormastic, M., et al.: Incidence and prognostic significance of intraventricular conduction abnormalities after coronary bypass surgery. J. Am. Coll. Cardiol. 16:607, 1990.

112. Tsai, T., and Matloff, J. M.: Cardiac surgery in the elderly. In Gray, R., and Matloff, J. (eds.): Medical Management of the Cardiac Surgical Patient. Baltimore, Williams & Wilkins, 1990, p. 27.

113. Harker, L. A.: Bleeding after cardiopulmonary bypass. N. Engl. J. Med. 314:1146, 1986.

114. Mammen, E. F., Koets, M. H., Washington, B. C., et al.: Hemostasis changes during cardiopulmonary bypass surgery. Semin. Thromb. Hemost. 11:281, 1985.

115. Kirklin, J. K., Westaby, S., Blackstone, E. H., et al.: Complement and the damaging effects of cardiopulmonary bypass. J. Thorac. Cardiovasc. Surg. 86:845, 1983.

116. Salama, A., Hugo, F., Heinrich, D., et al.: Deposition of terminal C5b-9 complement complexes on erythrocytes and leukocytes during cardiopulmonary bypass. N. Engl. J. Med. 318:408, 1988.

117. Cines, D. B., Tomaski, A., and Tannenbaum, S.: Immune endothelial-cell injury in heparin-associated thrombocytopenia. N. Engl. J. Med. 316:581, 1987.

118. Horrow, J. C.: Protamine allergy. J. Cardiothorac. Anesth. 2:225, 1988.

119. Sane, D. C., Califf, R. M., Topol, E. J., et al.: Bleeding during thrombolytic therapy for acute myocardial infarction: Mechanisms and management. Ann. Intern. Med. 111:1010, 1989.

120. Schrier, S. L.: Disorders of hemostasis and coagulation. In Rubenstein, E., and Federman, D. D. (eds.): Scientific American Medicine. New York, Scientific American, 1988 (5 Hematology), p. 1.

121. Sattler, F. R., Weitekamp, M. R., and Ballard, J. O.: Potential for bleeding with the new beta-lactam antibiotics. Ann. Intern. Med. 105:924, 1986.

122. Czer, L. S., Bateman, T. M., Gray, R. J., et al.: Treatment of severe platelet dysfunction and hemorrhage after cardiopulmonary bypass: Reduction

in blood product usage with desmopressin. J. Am. Coll. Cardiol. 9:1139, 1987.

123. Salzman, E. W., Weinstein, M. J., Weintraub, R. M., et al.: Treatment with desmopressin acetate to reduce blood loss after cardiac surgery: A double-blind randomized trial. N. Engl. J. Med. 314:1402, 1986.

124. Saour, J. N., Sieck, J. O., Mamo, L. A. R., and Gallus, A. S.: Trial of different intensities of anticoagulation in patients with prosthetic heart valves. N. Engl. J. Med. 322:428, 1990.

125. Verkkala, V., Valtonen, V., Jarvinen, A., and Tolppanen, E. M.: Fever, leukocytosis and C-reactive protein after open-heart surgery and their value in the diagnosis of postoperative infections. Thorac. Cardiovasc. Surg. 35:78, 1987.

126. Livelli, F. D., Johnson, R. A., McEnany, M. T., et al.: Unexplained in-hospital fever following cardiac surgery. Natural history, relationship to postpericardiotomy syndrome, and a prospective study of therapy with indomethacin versus placebo. Circulation 57:968, 1978.

127. Baddour, L. M., and Bisno, A. L. Recurrent cellulitis after saphenous venectomy for coronary bypass surgery. Ann. Intern. Med. 97:493, 1982.

128. Greenberg, J., DeSanctis, R. W., and Mills, R. M., Jr.: Vein-donor-leg cellulitis after coronary artery bypass surgery. Ann. Intern. Med. 97:565, 1982.

129. Spencer, F. C., and Grossi, E. A.: Mediastinitis after cardiac operations. Ann. Thorac. Surg. 49:506, 1990.

130. Demmy, T. L., Park, S. B., Liebler, G. A., et al.: Recent experience with major sternal wound complications. Ann. Thorac. Surg. 49:458, 1990.

131. Kouchoukos, N. T., Wareing, T. H., Murphy, S. F., et al.: Risks of bilateral internal mammary artery bypass grafting. Ann. Thorac. Surg. 49:210, 1990.

132. Bor, D. H., Rose, R. M., Modlin, J. F., et al.: Mediastinitis after cardiovascular surgery. Rev. Infect. Dis. 5:885, 1983.

133. Kernodle, D. S., Classen, D. C., Burke, J. P., and Kaiser, A. B.: Failure of cephalosporins to prevent *Staphylococcus aureus* surgical wound infections. J.A.M.A. 263:961, 1990.

134. Culliford, A. T., Cunningham, J. W., Zeaff, R. N., et al.: Sternal and costochondral infections following open heart surgery. J. Thorac. Cardiovasc. Surg. 72:714, 1976.

135. Engelman, R. M., Williams, C. D., Gouge, T. H., et al.: Mediastinitis following open-heart surgery. Am. J. Surg. 107:772, 1973.

136. Macmanus, Q., and Okies, J. E.: Mediastinal wound infection and aortocoronary graft patency. Am. J. Surg. 132:558, 1976.

137. Platt, R., Munoz, A., Stell, J., et al.: Antibiotic prophylaxis for cardiovascular surgery. Efficacy with coronary artery bypass. Ann. Intern. Med. 101:770, 1984.

138. Keys, T. F.: Antimicrobial prophylaxis for patients with congenital or valvular heart disease. Mayo Clin. Proc. 57:171, 1982.

139. Wilson, W. R., Danielson, G. K., Giuliani, E. R., and Geraci, J. E.: Prosthetic valve endocarditis. Mayo Clin. Proc. 57:155, 1982.

140. Ivert, T. S. A., Dismukes, W. E., Cobbs, C. G., et al.: Prosthetic valve endocarditis. Circulation 69:223, 1984.

141. Cowgill, L. D., Addonizio, V. P., Hopeman, A. G., and Harken, A. H.: A practical approach to prosthetic valve endocarditis. Ann. Thorac. Surg. 43:450, 1987.

142. Dinubile, M. J.: Surgery in active endocarditis. Ann. Intern. Med. 96:650, 1982.

143. Alter, H. J., Purcell, R. H., Shih, J. W., et al.: Detection of antibody to hepatitis C virus in prospectively followed transfusion recipients with acute and chronic non-A, non-B hepatitis. N. Engl. J. Med. 321:1494, 1989.

144. Davis, G. L., Balart, L. A., Schiff, E. R., et al.: Treatment of chronic hepatitis C with recombinant interferon alfa. A multicenter randomized, controlled trial. N. Engl. J. Med. 321:1501, 1989.

145. DiBisceglie, A. M., Martin, P., Kassiandes, C., et al.: Recombinant interferon ALFA therapy for chronic hepatitis C. N. Engl. J. Med. 321:1506, 1989.

146. Atkinson, J. B., Connor, D. H., Robinowitz, M., et al.: Cardiac fungal infections: Review of autopsy findings in 60 patients. Human Pathol. 15:935, 1984.

147. Miller, R. H., Horneffer, P. J., Gardner, T. J., et al.: The epidemiology of the postpericardiotomy syndrome: A common complication of cardiac surgery. Am. Heart J. 116:1323, 1988.

148. Ng, A. S., Dorosti, K., and Sheldon, W. C.: Constrictive pericarditis following cardiac surgery—Cleveland Clinic experience: Report of 12 cases and review. Cleve. Clin. Q. 51:39, 1984.

149. Abel, R. M., Buckley, M. J., Austen, W. G., et al.: Etiology, incidence, and prognosis of renal failure following cardiac operations. Results of a prospective analysis of 500 consecutive patients. J. Thorac. Cardiovasc. Surg. 71:323, 1976.

150. Bhat, J. G., Gluck, M. C., Lowenstein, J., and Baldwin, D. S.: Renal failure after open heart surgery. Ann. Intern. Med. 84:677, 1976.

151. Alfieri, A., and Kotler, M. N.: Noncardiac complications of open-heart surgery. Am. Heart J. 119:149, 1990.

152. Gailiunas, P., Chawla, R., Lazarus, J. M., et al.: Acute renal failure following cardiac operations. J. Thorac. Cardiovasc. Surg. 79:241, 1980.

153. Lange, H. W., Aeppli, D. M., and Brown, D. C.: Survival of patients with acute renal failure requiring dialysis after open-heart surgery: Early prognostic indicators. Am. Heart J. 113:1138, 1987.

154. Rose, B. D.: Acute renal failure—prerenal disease versus acute tubular necrosis. *In* Rose, B. D. (ed): Pathophysiology of Renal Disease. New York, McGraw-Hill, 1987, p. 63.

155. Luke, R. G., Briggs, J. D., Allison, M. E. M., and Kennedy, A. C.: Factors determining response to mannitol in acute renal failure. Am. J. Med. Sci. 259:168, 1970.

156. Graziani, G. A., Cantaluppi, S., Casati, A., et al.: Dopamine and furosemide in oliguric acute renal failure. Nephron 37:39, 1984.

157. Conger, J. D., Falk, S. A., Yuan, B. H., and Schrier, R. W.: Atrial natriuretic peptide and dopamine in a rat model of ischemic acute renal failure. Kidney Int. 35:1126, 1989.

158. Francis, G. S., Sharma, B., Collins, A. J., et al.: Coronary-artery surgery in patients with end-stage renal disease. Ann. Intern. Med. 92:499, 1980.

159. Opsahl, J. A., Husebye, D. G., Helseth, H. K., et al.: Coronary artery bypass surgery in patients on maintenance dialysis: Long-term survival. Am. J. Kidney Dis. 12:271, 1988.

160. Aranha, G. V., Pickleman, J., Pifarre, R., et al.: The reasons for gastrointestinal consultation after cardiac surgery. Am. Surg. 50:301, 1984.

161. Moneta, G. L., Misbach, G. A., and Ivey, T. D.: Hypoperfusion as a possible factor in the development of gastrointestinal complications after cardiac surgery. Am. J. Surg. 149:648, 1985.

162. Kumon, K., Kaznihiko, T., Takahiko, H., et al.: Organ failure due to low cardiac output syndrome following open heart surgery. Jpn. Circ. J. 50:329, 1986.

163. Kleptko, W.: Jaundice after open-heart surgery: A prospective study. Thorax 40:80, 1985.

164. Tremolada, F., Loreggian, M., Antona, C., et al.: Blood transmitted and clotting factor transmitted non-A, non-B hepatitis. J. Clin. Gastroenterol. 10:413, 1988.

165. Heikkinen, L., and Alz Kulju, K.: Abdominal complications following cardiopulmonary bypass in open-heart surgery. Scand. J. Thorac. Cardiovasc. Surg. 21:1, 1987.

166. Wallwork, J.: The acute abdomen following cardiopulmonary bypass surgery. Br. J. Surg. 67:410, 1980.

167. Svensson, L. G., Decker, G., and Kinsley, R. B.: A prospective study of hyperamylasemia and pancreatitis after cardiopulmonary bypass. Ann. Thorac. Surg. 39:409, 1985.

168. Rose, D. M., Ranson, J. H., Cunningham, J. N. Jr., and Spencer, F. C.: Patterns of severe pancreatic injury following cardiopulmonary bypass. Ann. Surg. 199:168, 1984.

169. Heller, S. S., Frank, K. A., Kornfield, D. S., et al.: Psychological outcome following open-heart surgery. Arch. Intern. Med. 134:908, 1974.

170. Adrian, J., Brankshaw, D. P., Tiller, J. W., et al.: Affective, cognitive and subjective changes in patients undergoing cardiac surgery—a preliminary report. Anaesth. Intensive Care 16:144, 1988.

171. Fish, K. J., Helms, K. N., Sarnquist, F. H., et al.: A prospective randomized study of the effects of prostacyclin on neuropsychological dysfunction after coronary artery surgery. J. Thorac. Cardiovasc. Surg. 93:609, 1987.

172. Townes, B. D., Bashein, G., Hornbein, T. F., et al.: Neurobehavioral outcomes in cardiac operations. J. Thorac. Cardiovasc. Surg. 98:774, 1989.

173. Furian, A. J., and Brener, A. C.: Central nervous system complications of open heart surgery. Stroke 15:912, 1984.

174. Taylor, G. J., Malik, S. A., Colliver, J. A., et al.: Usefulness of atrial fibrillation as a predictor of stroke after isolated coronary artery bypass grafting. Am. J. Cardiol. 60:905, 1987.

175. Breuer, A. C., Franco, I., Marzewski, D., et al.: Left ventricular thrombi seen by ventriculography are a significant risk factor for stroke in open heart surgery. Ann. Neurol. 10:103, 1981.

176. Shahian, D. M., and Speert, P. K.: Symptomatic visual deficits after open heart surgery. Ann. Thorac. Surg. 48:275, 1989.

177. Reed, G. L., Singer, D. E., and Pilard, E. H.: Stroke following coronary artery bypass surgery. A case control estimate of the risk of carotid bruits. N. Engl. J. Med. 319:1246, 1988.

178. Hertzer, N. R., Loop, F. D., Taylor, P. C., et al.: Staged and combined surgical approach to simultaneous carotid and coronary vascular disease. Surgery 84:803, 1978.

179. Mehigan, J. T., Buch, W. S., Pipkin, R. D., et al.: A planned approach to co-existent cerebrovascular disease in coronary artery bypass candidates. Ann. Surg. 112:1403, 1977.

180. Seyfer, A. E., Grammer, N. Y., Bogumill, G. P., et al.: Upper extremity neuropathies after cardiac surgery. J. Hand Surg. [Am.] 10:16, 1985.

181. Murphy, M. C., Newman, B. M., and Rodgers, B. M.: Pleuroperitoneal shunts in the management of persistent chylothorax. Ann. Thorac. Surg. 48:195, 1989.

182. Gutmann, M. C., Knapp, D. N., Pollock, M. L., et al.: Coronary artery bypass patients and work status. Circulation 66:33, 1982.

183. Oberman, A., Wayne, J. B., Kouchoukos, N. T., et al.: Employment status after coronary artery bypass surgery. Circulation 65:115, 1982.

184. CASS Principal Investigators and Their Associates. Coronary Artery Surgery Study (CASS): A randomized trial of coronary artery bypass surgery. Quality of life in patients randomly assigned to treatment groups. Circulation 68:951, 1983.

185. Boulay, F. M., David, P. P., and Bourassa, M. G.: Strategies for improving the work status of patients after coronary artery bypass surgery. Circulation 66:43, 1982.

Cost-Effective Strategies in Cardiology
by LEE GOLDMAN, M.D.

The availability of an increasing number of diagnostic and therapeutic technologies, coupled with concerns over the rising costs of health care, has generated increasing interest in determining the costs and effectiveness of cardiologic care. Cost-effectiveness analysis, which initially had been used principally by economists and policymakers, is a potentially useful technique for evaluating how best to diagnose, prevent, and treat medical illnesses. Such analyses highlight the important issues that should guide the physician–decision maker. They can help in identification of gaps in knowledge and establishment of priorities for research to be carried out by clinical investigators. To appreciate the implications of the emerging literature on cost-effectiveness in cardiology, it is important to understand the basic concepts that underlie formal cost-effectiveness analysis.

QUANTITATIVE ANALYSES OF COSTS AND EFFECTIVENESS

Analysts commonly distinguish between *cost-benefit analysis*, in which both costs and benefits are expressed in the same units (such as dollars), and *cost-effectiveness analysis*, in which the costs are commonly expressed in monetary terms while the effectiveness is expressed in terms of the health benefit.[1] The health benefit commonly is measured in units such as the number of lives that are saved, the years of life gained, the quality-adjusted years of life saved,[1-3] the days of disability avoided, or other suitable measurements.

SENSITIVITY ANALYSIS. Cost-effectiveness analyses are critically dependent on the accuracy of the assumptions on which they are based. Therefore, the analysis should include a "sensitivity analysis," in which the calculations are repeated with varying assumptions to determine whether the conclusions are altered.[1,2] It is vital to determine whether the final conclusions are critically dependent on a tenuous estimate by determining whether reasonable variations in important assumptions make major differences in the results of the analysis.

For example, in an analysis of the cost-effectiveness of admitting patients with chest pain and possible uncomplicated acute myocardial infarction in the absence of ST-segment elevation to a full-fledged coronary care unit as opposed to a nonintensive care unit bed with telemetry monitoring, it would be critical to estimate the relative difference, if any, in the rate of successful resuscitation from primary ventricular fibrillation in the two settings. The larger the estimated difference, the more cost-effective the coronary care unit would appear. If the two settings were assumed to be equally effec-

tive, the additional cost of the coronary care unit would not yield additional effectiveness for this purpose. Because there are no randomized controlled data to address this issue, any analysis of the relative cost-effectiveness of care of patients with possible myocardial infarction in these two settings depends on the estimates that are made. When a sensitivity analysis was performed, the nonintensive care bed with telemetry monitoring remained the more cost-effective option for patients whose probability of acute myocardial infarction was 10 per cent or less, even if it was assumed that the rate of successful resuscitation from primary ventricular fibrillation in this setting was no better than the success rate among patients seen by trained ambulance personnel within 5 minutes after onset of ventricular fibrillation in the out-of-hospital setting.[4]

THE CLINICAL DECISION TREE. Some cost-effectiveness analyses address difficult clinical problems for which no clear agreement exists, often because available data are not adequate even for the experienced clinician. In such situations, cost-effectiveness analysis may not yield clear answers, usually because the relative differences between competing strategies are small. For example, it may be difficult to decide whether or not to implant a permanent pacemaker in an elderly patient who has symptoms that are suggestive of a pacemaker-responsive arrhythmia but in whom the relation between arrhythmia and symptoms has not been proved. The therapeutic options can be displayed using a decision tree (Fig. 54–1) that explicitly outlines the various possibilities.[5] In this decision analysis, estimates about the relative cost-effectiveness of various therapeutic strategies would depend on the patient's subjective assessment of the quality of life under different scenarios, including persistent symptoms and no pacemaker, persistent symptoms despite a pacemaker, and the pacemaker without symptoms. Because small changes in the assessment of quality of life under these different circumstances would alter the preferred strategy, this particular analysis could not provide a definitive solution for all cases involving this therapeutic dilemma. Nevertheless, this analysis demonstrated that empiric pacing was an attractive option in an elderly patient with unexplained syncope even when there was only about a 25 per cent chance that the syncope was caused by a pacemaker-responsive arrhythmia.

The goal of cost-effectiveness analysis is not to find the greatest possible benefit for the lowest possible cost, because it is not possible to achieve both simultaneously.[2,3,6] Instead, it is necessary either to determine the resources that are available and then find the greatest possible effectiveness that can be purchased for those resources, or to determine the desired effectiveness and then find the lowest cost to achieve it. In either case, it is important to have a preconceived idea of the

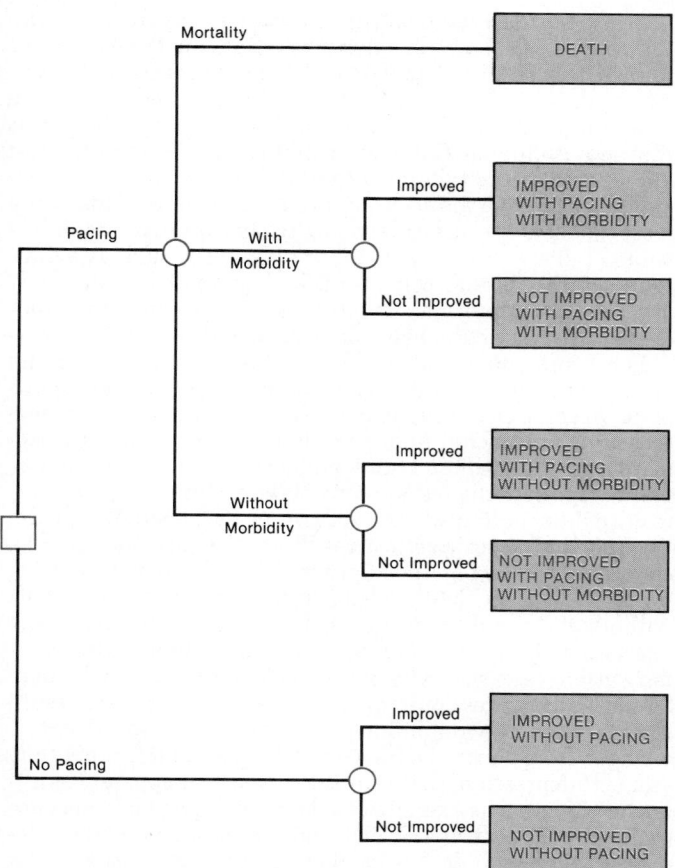

FIGURE 54–1. Decision tree for whether or not to perform empiric pacing in the elderly patient with syncope that may or may not be caused by a pacemaker-responsive arrhythmia. Branches of this decision tree explicitly detail the potential outcomes from the various options. The squares denote the outcomes of decisions that the physician must make, while the circles denote events over which the physician has no control, i.e., occur "by chance." In constructing the decision tree, physicians would use either their own judgment or probabilities derived from the literature to estimate the likelihood of each of the events that can occur at a "chance" node. The sum of the probabilities of these chance events is always 100 per cent. In a cost-effectiveness analysis, each of the potential outcomes, as displayed in the rectangles in the right column, would be assigned a cost and a "utility." The utility would denote how highly the outcome is valued compared to perfect health, which traditionally has a value of 1.0, versus death, which traditionally has a value of 0. Cost-effectiveness calculations would compute the average expected costs and utilities for each of the various options that might be chosen by the physician, in this case the "pacing" and "no pacing" options that emanate from the initial square node. (From Kwoh, C. K., Beck, J R., and Pauker, S. G.: Repeated syncope with negative diagnostic evaluation. Med. Decis. Making 4:351, 1984.)

desirable or acceptable relative ratio of cost to effectiveness. Although cost-effectiveness analyses determine the ratio of cost to effectiveness, two strategies with the same ratio may have quite different absolute costs and absolute effectiveness. For example, a program that saves 100 lives for $10,000 has the same cost-effectiveness ratio as one that saves 10,000 lives for $1,000,000, but the two programs' absolute costs and absolute effectivenesses vary 100-fold. In cost-effectiveness analyses, any potentially new strategy usually is compared with the current, or baseline, strategy by calculating the *incremental cost:incremental effectiveness* ratio.[1–3,6,7]

CALCULATION OF COSTS

In determining costs, several types must be considered.[7,8] *Operating costs* may include both direct costs such as salaries and indirect costs such as overhead, including utilities and

maintenance. Costs also can be categorized as fixed versus variable costs. For example, the first 100 cardiac scans carried out in an imaging center may cost $100,000 for an average cost of $1000 per scan because of the high capital costs of the equipment. If the laboratory were to "increase its output," the incremental cost for the next 100 scans would be much less than the cost for the first 100 scans because the capital costs of the equipment would be nearly the same regardless of whether 100 scans or 200 scans were performed. Thus one could distinguish between the incremental cost of performing the second 100 scans versus the average cost of all 200 scans. In many medical analyses, true costs are not available, and charges are used in the calculation of "cost" effectiveness. Because charges often are the same regardless of volume, they usually do not consider fully the important differences between average and incremental costs.

In calculating net health care costs, a useful approach is shown in Table 54–1. Unfortunately many cost-effectiveness analyses have concentrated only on direct medical costs, without fully taking into account the other terms in the equation.

DISCOUNTING. In virtually all cost analyses, it is important to consider the time frame when costs and effects will be achieved. Because current dollars or benefits are more highly valued than a promise of future dollars or health benefits, a cost or benefit achieved immediately is more highly valued than one that is achieved later.[1] For example, one would be more willing to spend $10,000 today to prevent a death that otherwise would occur tomorrow than to spend $10,000 today to prevent a death that otherwise would occur in 10 years, even if there were no inflation and if there were no interest to be earned on the dollars. There is a preference to achieve an immediate benefit for several reasons. First, other events may intercede so that the projected future death may not occur or might be avoided as a consequence of newly available options that cost less than $10,000. Second, another illness could terminate life during the intervening period. Also, the $10,000 might be spent during the intervening 10 years in ways that are deemed more valuable. Furthermore, there is always a lingering doubt that the money spent now will not actually achieve the desired effect 10 years hence. This principle, by which the promise of future events is less valued than known immediate events, is termed "discounting," and is independent of monetary inflation. It is common practice to "discount" both future costs and future benefits by about 5 per cent per year.

In discussions of cost and effectiveness, several common misconceptions occur.[6] Cost-effective should not be equated with cost-saving because one often must spend to achieve a real benefit. Although a strategy that saves money *and* achieves an equal or better outcome is obviously cost-effective, a program is also cost-effective if it yields an additional benefit that is worth the additional cost. The definition of "worth the cost" may be a somewhat arbitrary value judgment because it is difficult to place a monetary value on years of life and productivity. In many analyses, the approximately

TABLE 54–1 CALCULATION OF NET HEALTH CARE COSTS FOR A PROGRAM

Net costs = direct medical costs*
  + health care costs associated with the adverse effects of treatment
  − savings of health care, rehabilitation, and custodial costs owing to prevention or alleviation of disease
  + costs of treating disease that would not have occurred if the patient had not lived longer as a result of the original treatment

* Costs of hospitalization, physician time, medications, laboratory services, and other ancillary services.
See reference 2 for more details.

$30,000 to $35,000 per year cost in 1990 dollars of renal dialysis,[9,10] a program that the United States has decided to support with tax dollars, has been used as the benchmark for the amount of cost that the public appears willing to bear to prolong useful life by 1 year.

Although physicians must be aware of the relative cost-effectiveness of various diagnostic and therapeutic options if they are to make optimal choices for their patients, decisions about the number of dollars that *should* be spent to achieve specific health care benefits will ultimately be determined by society. Physicians have a critical role to play in developing appropriate data on cost-effectiveness issues, but the individual physician's primary responsibility is to the patient, within the confines of the economic limitations that may be imposed on both the physician and the patient by society.

One example of societal constraints on medical care expenditures is the diagnosis-related groups (DRG) system of prospective reimbursement. By defining in advance the number of dollars that a hospital will be reimbursed for the care of certain types of patients, the physician, the hospital, and the patient may all become more concerned with issues of cost-effectiveness. In an analogous manner, capitation systems, in which physicians are prepaid a fixed sum to assume the care of a patient, place an increased emphasis on the determination of cost-effective strategies.

DIAGNOSTIC TESTING

Modern cardiology includes an impressive armamentarium of diagnostic tests. Good clinical judgment requires that the physician choose tests in a cost-effective manner, in which the tests individually or sequentially may lead to improved diagnosis and management. The cost-effective use of diagnostic tests requires the physician to proceed logically through evaluation of the patient, selection of diagnostic tests, integration of the test with clinical data, and formulation of management strategies.[11,12] Each of these steps must be carefully considered for the proper utilization of diagnostic testing.

THE ESTIMATION OF CLINICAL PROBABILITIES. Regardless of the condition in question, the physician must utilize data from the medical history and physical examination to estimate the likelihood of its presence. For example, in evaluating the patient with chest pain, the physician may consider the patient's age and sex, as well as the typicality of the discomfort for angina pectoris.[12-16] The symptom may be categorized as typical angina pectoris, atypical angina pectoris, or nonanginal chest discomfort on the basis of its character, location, provocation, and response to rest or nitroglycerin (p. 1293). Similarly, in estimating the probability of the presence of hemodynamically significant aortic stenosis in an adult with a systolic murmur, one would consider factors such as the intensity, location, and radiation of the murmur, the volume and rate of upstroke of the carotid arterial pulse, and the second heart sound (p. 1038).[17] Although these estimates of clinical probabilities can be based on the judgment of an experienced physician, in some circumstances, the physician can be aided by accumulated data from large series of patients in whom the clinical probability of conditions such as significant coronary artery disease[16] or acute myocardial infarction or unstable angina pectoris[18,19] have been determined.

ORDERING A DIAGNOSTIC TEST. When considering a test that may be ordered, the physician must determine whether the test is efficacious and sufficiently accurate for indications for which it is being considered, that no other test with acceptable efficacy is less hazardous or less expensive, and that this is the most appropriate time for ordering the test.[11,19,20] In one such study carried out in 1977, soon after cardiac nuclear medicine scans became clinically available, 35 per cent were found *not* to have been ordered appropriately.[19] By comparison, the rate of inappropriate ordering for M-mode echocardiograms, which had been routinely available for some time and were presumably well understood by physicians, was only 14 per cent.[20]

Tests may be ordered for such indications as to plan or monitor therapy, to establish a diagnosis, to define the extent of a known disease, to estimate prognosis, or to reassure the physician or the patient.[19-21] Although each of these indications can be a legitimate reason for ordering a diagnostic test, test results that may influence therapeutic action usually are the most valued and are certainly the most cost-effective.

When assessing the accuracy of a test, one must understand terms such as sensitivity, specificity, and positive predictive value (Table 6-2, p. 168).[1,2,11] For some tests, such as a thallium scintiscan, the result is often dichotomized into "normal" versus "abnormal," even though it is understood that the precise distinction between normal and abnormal may be difficult and somewhat arbitrary. Other tests, such as the ejection fraction, commonly are reported on a continuous scale. In some circumstances, such as with the exercise electrocardiogram, a continuous result (e.g., the extent of ST-segment depression) often is dichotomized into normal or abnormal to facilitate the test's interpretation. When a continuous result is dichotomized, an increase in its sensitivity, or the likelihood of a positive test result among patients with the condition, can be obtained only at the expense of decreasing specificity, or the likelihood of a normal test result in patients without the condition.[22] For example, the sensitivity of the exercise electrocardiogram for detecting patients with coronary artery disease can be increased by reducing the depth of ST-segment depression required for a "positive" test result. However, as the definition of a "positive" test result is changed from 2 mm of ST-segment depression to 1 mm of ST-segment depression, the resulting increase in apparent sensitivity will be at the expense of a decreased specificity because patients who have between 1 and 2 mm of ST-segment depression and who do not have coronary artery disease now will be misclassified.

In an era of cost consciousness, the physician often must be asked to decide between two tests that may offer similar types of information. For example, a radionuclide ventriculogram may provide a more accurate assessment of the left ventricular ejection fraction than a two-dimensional echocardiogram, but the latter frequently provides a sufficiently accurate estimate of left ventricular function to obviate the need for the more expensive radionuclide study.

The choice of tests also may depend on the timing of clinical events. For example, a technetium pyrophosphate scan can diagnose a transmural myocardial infarction (p. 315) accurately, but it is unnecessary to order such a test in patients who arrive early enough after the onset of symptoms for enzymes such as creatine kinase isoenzymes to be diagnostic. Technetium pyrophosphate scans can potentially be helpful in patients who arrive long enough after the onset of symptoms so that creatine kinase levels would have returned to normal, but even in such patients, lactic dehydrogenase (LDH) isoenzyme levels appear to be at least as accurate and far less expensive.[23,24]

Thus technetium pyrophosphate scans usually are helpful diagnostically only in patients who arrive long enough after the acute event for creatine kinase isoenzymes to be unhelpful and who have other conditions, such as hemolysis or renal infarction, that make LDH isoenzyme tests unreliable.

INTEGRATING THE TEST RESULT WITH CLINICAL DATA. To use diagnostic tests efficiently, the physician should decide the threshold probability above or below which the future diagnostic or management strategy would be altered.[25,26] For example, consider that a patient has recurrent chest pain, and on the basis of history and physical examination, the physician estimates that there is a 50 per cent probability that it is caused by coronary artery disease. The physician also knows that coronary arteriography would be required to decide whether coronary artery bypass grafting or percutaneous transluminal coronary angioplasty should be carried out if coronary artery disease were present. For cost-effective test ordering, the physician then must estimate how unlikely coronary artery disease would have to be for this

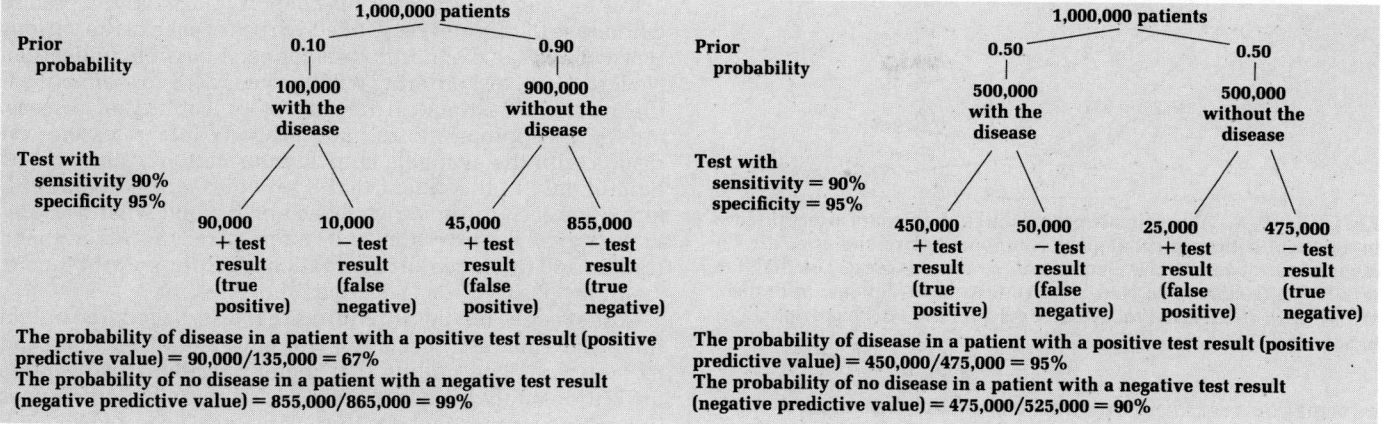

TABLE 54–2 HOW THE POSITIVE AND NEGATIVE PREDICTIVE VALUES OF THE SAME TEST VARY DEPENDING ON THE PRIOR PROBABILITY OF DISEASE

INTERPRETATION OF THE TEST RESULT WHEN 10% OF THE PATIENTS BEING TESTED HAVE THE DISEASE (PRIOR PROBABILITY = 10%)	INTERPRETATION OF THE TEST RESULT WHEN 50% OF THE PATIENTS BEING TESTED HAVE THE DISEASE (PRIOR PROBABILITY = 50%)
1,000,000 patients	1,000,000 patients
Prior probability 0.10 / 0.90	Prior probability 0.50 / 0.50
100,000 with the disease / 900,000 without the disease	500,000 with the disease / 500,000 without the disease
Test with sensitivity 90% specificity 95%	Test with sensitivity = 90% specificity = 95%
90,000 + test result (true positive) 10,000 − test result (false negative) 45,000 + test result (false positive) 855,000 − test result (true negative)	450,000 + test result (true positive) 50,000 − test result (false negative) 25,000 + test result (false positive) 475,000 − test result (true negative)
The probability of disease in a patient with a positive test result (positive predictive value) = 90,000/135,000 = 67% The probability of no disease in a patient with a negative test result (negative predictive value) = 855,000/865,000 = 99%	The probability of disease in a patient with a positive test result (positive predictive value) = 450,000/475,000 = 95% The probability of no disease in a patient with a negative test result (negative predictive value) = 475,000/525,000 = 90%

From Goldman, L.: Quantitative aspects of clinical reasoning. In Wilson, J. D., et al. (eds.): Harrison's Principles of Internal Medicine 12th ed. New York, McGraw-Hill Book Company, 1991, p. 7.

strategy to be altered. If the physician would proceed with catheterization provided that the probability of coronary artery disease were as low as 10 per cent (or higher), then a test such as an exercise radionuclide ventriculogram, whose negative result might reduce the probability of coronary artery disease to 30 per cent, would not be helpful in decision-making.

Threshold Approach. This concept has been called the "threshold approach" to test utilization and decision-making.[26] In essence, it emphasizes that a test is potentially helpful only if its result would change the pretest probability of disease to a degree that could be sufficient to alter the approach to the patient. If it is highly unlikely that the available diagnostic test could move the probability of disease across such a threshold, the test would not be cost-effective and ordinarily would not be ordered. In some situations, the diagnostic threshold may be redefined because of the special characteristics of the patient at hand. For example, it would be considered important to rule out significant coronary artery disease in an otherwise healthy airline pilot who has atypical chest pain. In this situation, the combination of a normal exercise electrocardiogram and a normal exercise thallium scintiscan would make the presence of coronary disease unlikely. If it were argued that the airline pilot's occupational responsibilities would require even a greater degree of certainty, it would be preferable to proceed directly to the test that usually is considered the benchmark, in this case, coronary arteriography, if it were necessary to be as certain as possible that coronary disease was not present.

BAYES' THEOREM (see also p. 169). One way to understand the concepts of prior probability, thresholds, and the impact of diagnostic tests is through Bayes' theorem.[1,11] When the prior probability (prevalence) of the disease is known in patients who are similar to the patient under consideration, and when the sensitivity and specificity of the test to be ordered are known, the post-test probability that the disease is present can be calculated (Table 54–2). Table 54–2 emphasizes how the physician must consider both the prior (pretest) probability that the patient has a disease and the test result in estimating the post-test probability. For example, if a test has a sensitivity of 90 per cent and a specificity of 95 per cent, a patient whose prior probability of disease was 10 per cent and who has a positive test result would have a 67 per cent probability of disease after the test. By comparison, the same test result in a patient whose prior probability was 50 per cent would yield a post-test probability of 95 per cent.

A test is potentially useful if it changes the probability of

disease sufficiently to cross the threshold for decision-making. Unfortunately, available data do not always provide precise guidelines for establishing such appropriate thresholds for diagnostic decision-making. Nevertheless, common clinical judgment is often a sufficient guide. For example, using pooled data from the literature, the effects of exercise electrocardiography and exercise thallium testing can be estimated for a patient with typical angina pectoris (Fig. 54–2), a patient with atypical angina (Fig. 54–3), and a patient with presumably nonanginal chest pain (Fig. 54–4). These estimated probabilities correspond well to the actual probability of disease in patients who have been evaluated.[27]

NONINVASIVE TESTING IN PATIENTS WITH POSSIBLE ANGINA PECTORIS (see also p. 1298). The patient with symptoms typical for angina pectoris already has a high probability of coronary artery disease on the basis of the history alone (80 to 85 per cent); the probability becomes even higher (95 per cent) if the exercise electrocardiogram is positive and becomes overwhelming (99 per cent) after a confirmatory exercise thallium scan. For diagnosing the presence or absence of coronary disease, however, the exercise thallium scan adds little to the results of the exercise test. Although the exercise thallium test may have some additional prognostic value,[28,29] in most situations, the results of the exercise thallium test would be unlikely to add substantial independent

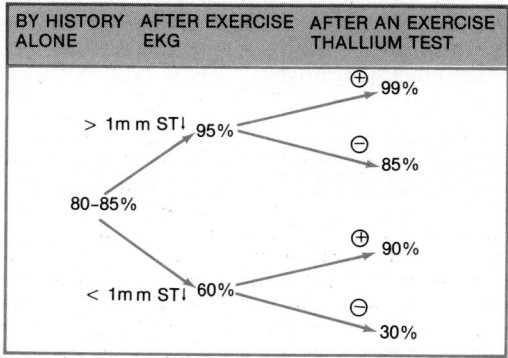

FIGURE 54–2. Approximate probabilities of coronary artery disease in a patient with typical angina pectoris before and after the sequential use of an exercise electrocardiogram and an exercise thallium test. (From Goldman, L.: Non-invasive tests in cardiology. In Branch, W., Jr. [ed.]: The Office Practice of Medicine. 2nd ed. Philadelphia, W. B. Saunders Company, 1987.)

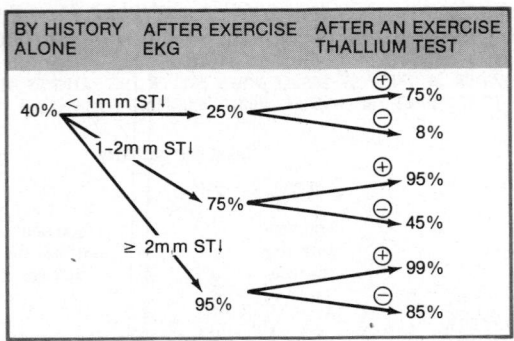

FIGURE 54–3. Approximate probabilities of coronary artery disease in a patient with atypical anginal symptoms before and after the sequential use of an exercise electrocardiogram and an exercise thallium test. (From Goldman, L.: Non-invasive tests in cardiology. *In* Branch, W., Jr. [ed.]: The Office Practice of Medicine. 2nd ed. Philadelphia, W. B. Saunders Company, 1987.)

information regarding the diagnosis of the presence of coronary artery disease. If the exercise electrocardiogram and exercise thallium test give conflicting information, the probability of coronary artery disease in the patient with typical angina pectoris remains similar to what it was before either test was obtained (80 to 90 per cent). If both tests are negative, the patient with typical angina pectoris still has a reasonable probability of having significant coronary artery disease (30 per cent). Thus even two negative tests have not "ruled out" coronary artery disease in a patient with typical angina to an extent to which one could simply reassure the patient, even though they imply a favorable prognosis if coronary artery disease should be present.[28,29] Thus, if one were trying to rule out coronary artery disease in a patient with typical angina pectoris, coronary arteriography still would be required.[12,30]

In the patient with atypical angina (Fig. 54–3), positive results on both exercise electrocardiography and exercise thallium testing would raise the probability of coronary artery disease from 40 to 95 to 99 per cent. Conversely, negative results on both tests would lower the probability of coronary artery disease substantially (to 8 per cent), perhaps to a low enough level that one would not feel compelled to obtain coronary arteriography except in unusual circumstances. If the two tests give conflicting results, the probability of the disease has not been altered appreciably by the two tests.

In asymptomatic healthy people, a resting electrocardiogram appears to have little value as a screening test.[3] Similarly, screening exercise tests have too small a yield to justify their use in healthy people.[32] If, however, an asymptomatic subject who is in the age range in which coronary disease usually occurs has a strongly positive exercise electrocardiogram, the probability of coronary disease is increased substantially (from about 5 to about 50 per cent), and a subsequent negative exercise thallium test is not sufficiently reassuring to eliminate the possibility of coronary disease. Thus one cannot simply use the negative exercise thallium scan to "prove" that the exercise electrocardiogram was a false-positive result.

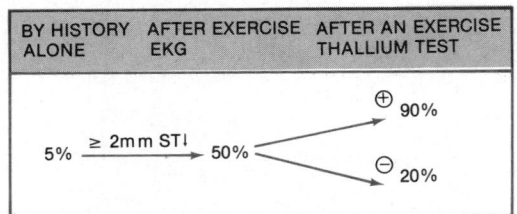

FIGURE 54–4. Approximate probabilities of coronary artery disease in an asymptomatic subject in the coronary artery disease age range before and after the sequential use of an exercise electrocardiogram and an exercise thallium test. (From Goldman, L.: Non-invasive tests in cardiology. *In* Branch, W., Jr. [ed.]: The Office Practice of Medicine. 2nd ed. Philadelphia, W. B. Saunders Company, 1987.)

Coronary arteriography will be required to determine whether the exercise electrocardiogram was a true or false-positive result, and this frequent need to proceed to invasive testing greatly increases the cost of any program that uses screening exercise electrocardiography.

It is beyond the scope of this chapter to discuss the precise guidelines for the most cost-effective use of each of the various types of cardiac diagnostic tests for each possible indication. Nevertheless, test ordering will become more cost-effective if the physician estimates the pretest probability of disease, orders the appropriate test, and properly integrates the test results with the available clinical information. A test will be helpful only to the extent that it provides nonredundant information (i.e., information above and beyond what was previously available).[11,33] It must be emphasized, however, that a test can add incremental information regardless of whether its result is "positive" or "negative."[34]

Cost-effective medicine requires that tests be ordered only if their incremental information will have a positive impact on patient care. The finding that major variations in resource utilization often do not correlate with discernible differences in health outcome suggests that many tests do not meet such criteria.[35] Substantial financial savings can be realized by reducing the utilization of low- or moderate-cost tests as well as by reducing the utilization of expensive procedures.[36–38]

PREVENTION AND TREATMENT

The current and projected future costs of heart disease are substantial. The rate of death from coronary heart disease has been declining in the United States since the late 1960's,[39,40] but the increase in the total population and especially its age portends a rise in the total absolute number of cases of coronary heart disease unless there are major declines in risk factors.[41] Furthermore, the high cost of medical care for prevalent cases of coronary heart disease indicates that coronary disease will remain a major cost for the American public.[41,42]

Among the various preventive and therapeutic modalities in cardiology, some have been studied by means of formal cost-effectiveness analysis, whereas others have been studied in a more qualitative manner. In evaluating the cost-effectiveness of any program, it must be compared with a baseline or standard current approach. In the following sections, selected data on the costs and effectiveness of several modalities for the diagnosis, prevention, and treatment of heart disease are considered.

DETECTION AND TREATMENT OF HYPERLIPIDEMIA
(See also Chap. 37)

Substantial data indicate that the serum cholesterol level is significantly correlated with the risk of coronary artery disease (p. 1116), and after controlling for the cholesterol level, the triglyceride level is not an important independent predictor.[43–45] The high-density lipoprotein cholesterol fraction (p. 1128) appears to be even more important than the low-density lipoprotein fraction for prediction.[44] For primary care settings, the most prudent screening technique is to obtain a total serum cholesterol level. If it is elevated, fasting levels of total cholesterol, high-density lipoprotein cholesterol, and triglycerides can be obtained to define risk more precisely and to determine the hyperlipidemia pattern to guide future dietary and perhaps drug therapy (Chap. 37).[46]

The relation between the intake of dietary fats and the serum cholesterol level is well established.[47,48] There is evidence that increased dietary fat intake is correlated with the progression of coronary atherosclerosis and with long-term coronary mortality,[49,50] whereas reduced intake can retard the progression of atherosclerosis.[51–53] The Lipid Research Clinics Coronary Primary Prevention Trial[54,55] demonstrated that treatment with cholestyramine resulted in a 13.4 per cent reduction in the serum cholesterol level in the group randomized to treatment, whereas cholesterol levels declined by only 4.9 per cent in the randomized control group. The risk of coronary heart disease death was 24 per cent lower and the risk of myocardial infarction was 19 per cent lower in the treated group than in the control group, and the reductions in events were almost exactly what would be predicted on the basis of the reductions in serum cholesterol levels and the known association between cholesterol and event rates.[56]

The Helsinki Heart Study, which used gemfibrozil, demonstrated that the risk of coronary heart disease was lowered because of both a reduction in low-density lipoprotein cholesterol and an increase in high-density lipoprotein cholesterol.[57] In patients treated with niacin in the Coronary Drug Project, a benefit also was found.[58]

Because of the high prevalence of an elevated serum cholesterol level, issues relating to screening and to treatment, with either diet or medications, have major public health implications.[59] One analysis indicated that a 10 mg/dl population-wide reduction in serum cholesterol level in men would yield the same benefit that could be realized by identifying and treating all individual men with serum cholesterol levels above 250 mg/dl and lowering them to 250 mg/dl.[60] This analysis suggested that it would be inadvisable to rely just on a cholesterol reduction program targeted to patients with hypercholesterolemia to reduce national coronary heart disease. Community-based programs in North Karelia, Finland, and in California have achieved about a 3 to 4 per cent net reduction in serum cholesterol levels.[61-66] It is not currently possible to assess the cost-effectiveness of such efforts on a broader regional or national scale.

Although cholesterol-reduction programs targeted to patients with hypercholesterolemia are probably not sufficient for addressing a risk factor such as cholesterol, for which the risk of coronary heart disease is graded and continuous,[43] it is more practical to estimate cost-effectiveness of cholesterol reduction in high-risk groups. Berwick et al.[57] estimated that screening and dietary intervention programs for hypercholesterolemia in the pediatric population would cost about $33,000 (in 1990 dollars) for 10-year-old boys and $29,000 for 10-year-old girls per year of life gained. If the screening was limited to children with a known family history, the cost would be about $21,000 for boys and $24,000 for girls per year of life saved, whereas for children without a family history, the figures would be about $39,000 for boys and $31,000 for girls. Thus, in this example, a "targeted" program, which is limited to children who are at higher risk because of a known family history, would be more cost-effective than a nontargeted program.

In an analysis of the use of screening serum cholesterol levels in asymptomatic adults, it was estimated that screening should be performed about every 5 years in low-risk asymptomatic men and more frequently in high-risk asymptomatic men but was optional in women and in the elderly.[68] Various consensus groups have not currently reached agreement with one another about screening and treatment guidelines in asymptomatic adults.[46,69-73]

Analyses of medication therapy have raised serious questions about the affordability of cholesterol-lowering medications, except in some very high risk groups. As calculated by Weinstein and Stason, the cost per year of life gained for cholestyramine among men aged 45 to 50 years with cholesterol levels above 265 mg/dl would be about $180,000 in 1991 dollars, given a 5 per cent per year discount rate.[73]

Another analysis found that cholestyramine had a cost-effectiveness ratio below about $45,000 per year of life saved only in very selected types of patients, such as those with cholesterol levels of 315 mg/dl or higher in whom treatment was begun between ages 35 and 50 and continued through age 55, or people who smoked, were hypertensive, had diabetes, and in whom new treatment was begun between ages 35 and 49 and continued through age 70.[74] Kinosian and Eisenberg

reported that colestipol and cholestyramine, even when used in the less expensive bulk form, cost under $50,000 per year of life saved only when used in relatively high-risk, middle-aged males.[75] Other authors have suggested that cholestyramine is even less cost-effective.[76] In another analysis, in which it was assumed that the relative benefits of cholesterol reduction for secondary prevention in patients who already have coronary heart disease were similar to the benefits of cholesterol reduction for primary prevention,[54,55] secondary prevention was very cost-effective or even cost-saving.[77] Primary prevention with lovastatin was relatively cost-effective only in isolated subgroups, such as people between ages 45 and 74 who had two or more additional risk factors (hypertension, cigarette smoking, or obesity) and whose cholesterol levels were markedly elevated, usually above 300 mg/dl.

In summary, the high prevalence of hypercholesterolemia implies that populationwide interventions, such as dietary changes, will be required if there is to be a major reduction in national coronary heart disease rates. Screening and targeted diet therapy are indicated in high-risk pediatric and adult populations. Medications may be cost-effective in high-risk primary prevention situations and are likely to be very cost-effective and perhaps even cost-saving when used for secondary prevention in people who have existing coronary heart disease, assuming that the benefits to be realized by secondary prevention are truly analogous to those that have been reported for primary prevention.[79-82]

DETECTION AND TREATMENT OF HYPERTENSION
(See also Chaps. 28 and 29)

Most epidemiological data emphasize that the systolic blood pressure is an independent significant predictor of coronary heart disease but that the diastolic blood pressure is not (after controlling for the systolic blood pressure).[56] Nevertheless, it has been common practice to define the threshold for treating hypertension on the basis of the diastolic blood pressure, and virtually all treatment trials use definitions that are based on the diastolic blood pressure level.

About 20 per cent of adults in the United States have diastolic blood pressures above 95 mm Hg, and about another 10 per cent have blood pressures of 90 to 94 mm Hg.[83] There is virtually unanimous agreement that treatment of people whose diastolic blood pressure exceeds about 105 mm Hg will reduce mortality, although the main benefit in the Veterans Administration Trials was to prevent death from conditions other than coronary heart disease.[84-86] Of course, by preventing death from strokes, congestive heart failure, and renal failure, the treatment of hypertension permits more people to survive and potentially to develop coronary heart disease.

Numerous trials have evaluated the benefit of drug treatment for mild hypertension.[87] Many medications that are used to treat hypertension may raise the serum cholesterol and glucose concentrations, thereby theoretically offsetting some of their blood pressure–lowering benefits. Data suggest that the modest elevations in serum cholesterol levels and the occasional precipitation of hyperglycemia are outweighed by the predicted benefit obtained by blood pressure reduction, thus supporting the value of antihypertensive therapy.[87,88] Of course, it would be even more desirable to treat hypertension without raising serum cholesterol or blood sugar.

The Australian National Blood Pressure Study[89] demonstrated that treatment of people with diastolic blood pressure of 95 to 109 mm Hg reduced cardiovascular mortality significantly, and the reduction in incidence of coronary heart disease events was similar to what would be predicted, given the reductions in blood pressure levels using projections from the Framingham equations.[88] The Hypertension Detection and Follow-up Program[90-92a] showed a significant 20 per cent reduction in mortality in the stepped-care group. When data from all the randomized trials of the treatment of mild to moderate hypertension are pooled, there appears to be about a 10 per cent reduction in myocardial infarction in the treated

TABLE 54–3 APPROXIMATE COST PER QUALITY-ADJUSTED YEAR OF LIFE GAINED BY SCREENING AND/OR TREATMENT OF HYPERTENSION (1991 DOLLARS) GIVEN EXPECTED COMPLIANCE

Treat if diastolic blood pressure 105 mm Hg or greater	$20,000
Treat if diastolic blood pressure 95–104 mm Hg	$40,200
Screen for hypertension, treat if blood pressure 95 mm Hg or greater	$41,000

See references 95 and 207.

patients.[87] Treatment is predicted to have the greatest absolute benefit in patients with higher blood pressures[88] and in patients with other risk factors for coronary disease. There is uncertainty as to whether diuretic therapy for hypertensive men with resting electrocardiographic abnormalities would actually increase mortality (p. 852).[93,94]

One recent analysis concluded that screening to detect and treat hypertension was relatively cost-effective for men and women of all ages (Table 54–3).[95] The marginal cost per quality-adjusted year of life gained ranged from about $8000 for men aged 60 to about $29,000 for men aged 20. For women, the cost ranged from about $12,000 at age 60 to about $44,000 at age 20. The results of the analysis were affected relatively little when the authors varied many of the assumptions inherent in their analysis, except that the results were dependent on the cost of medication.

Weinstein and Stason used data from the Framingham Heart Study to calculate the cost-effectiveness of the treatment of mild hypertension.[96] They concluded that the reduction in direct medical care costs for stroke and coronary heart disease would offset about 22 per cent of the cost of treating moderate to severe diastolic hypertension (105 mm Hg and above) and about 15 per cent of the cost for treating mild hypertension (95 to 104 mm Hg), an estimate similar to those made by Stokes and Carmichael.[97] These cost-effectiveness estimates also are similar to those of Littenberg et al.,[95] who found that a program that would screen for hypertension and treat if the diastolic blood pressure was 95 mm Hg or greater would cost about $41,000 per quality-adjusted year of life gained. Treatment programs aimed at people with diastolic blood pressures of 105 mm Hg or greater would be more cost-effective: the cost would be only about $20,000 per year of life gained.

Edelson et al. reported that the cost of primary prevention to treat people 35 to 60 years of age with diastolic blood pressures of 95 mm Hg or greater and no known coronary heart disease was about $11,000 per year of life saved for propranolol and about $16,000 for hydrochlorothiazide.[98] Once again, however, cost-effectiveness was dependent on the cost of the medication and the costs per year of life saved were not estimated to be as favorable for the newer, more expensive medications.

Thus several analyses indicate that screening and treating people with hypertension is reasonably cost-effective and is in the range of the inflation-adjusted annual cost of hemodialysis for chronic renal failure.[9,11] Although hypertension detection and treatment is most cost-effective when it is performed by the patients' own physicians as part of routine medical care,[95,99] worksite programs for the detection and treatment of hypertension can more than pay for themselves by reducing direct medical costs and absenteeism.[100]

CIGARETTE SMOKING

Cigarette smoking is an independently significant correlate of the risk of developing coronary heart disease (p. 1146) and also is a major risk factor for several types of cancer. Many of these risks appear to be reversed after smokers stop smoking. Oster et al. used data from the American Cancer Society and from other sources to estimate the increase in life expectancy that could be realized by smoking cessation (Table 54–4).[101,102]

Although it is not possible to design a trial in which patients are randomized to continue smoking or to guarantee smoking cessation, substantial data confirm that discontinuing smoking improves prognosis. For example, in the Multiple-Risk Factor Intervention Trial,[93] the enrollees who discontinued smoking had a 48 per cent reduction in coronary deaths compared with those who continued smoking, and other data confirm that quitters have lower risks than persistent smokers.[103–107]

There are a variety of interventions to reduce smoking. On average, about 5 per cent of smokers will discontinue the habit for 1 year after receiving a physician's advice, although the rate of quitting will be higher in more highly motivated cohorts.[108–112] Nicotine gum or transdermal patches may increase the 1-year likelihood of smoking cessation by 30 to 100 per cent, suggesting that the cost of a physician's advice plus the availability of nicotine gum per year of life saved will range from about $5700 to $9200 in men aged 35 to 69 and from about $9800 to $13,000 in women aged 35 to 69 in 1990 dollars.[101,113–121] Clonidine has been unsuccessful in the primary care setting.[122]

Group counseling can increase rates of quitting.[121,123] Public programs also are effective, with television advertisements against smoking among the most cost-effective.[124,125] Physicians should not be discouraged by the relatively low rate of quitting that occurs immediately after their advice, since this advice is among the most cost-effective of all the interventions and may be a necessary psychological prelude to the patient's response to subsequent interventions.[126]

OBESITY

In long-term follow-up of the Framingham cohort, obesity emerged as an independently significant risk factor for the development of coronary artery disease (p. 1150). Unfortunately, it is extremely difficult for most adults to lose weight and to maintain the weight loss over the long term. Programs in schools or at the worksite commonly can help to achieve weight losses of 2 to 5 kg at costs that are about $10 to $30 per kilogram lost, which would be highly cost-effective.[128,129] Lay organizations such as Weight Watchers also can aid in producing similar losses at similar costs and are clearly cost-effective despite the high attrition rate.[130] More intensive weight-loss programs for motivated people may still be very cost-effective for those people for whom simpler measures are ineffective.[130] Although physicians may become discouraged over the inability of their patients to lose weight, the usual effects of these other programs are not substantially greater than what may be achieved simply by a physician's advice. Furthermore, it often

TABLE 54–4 INCREASE IN LIFE EXPECTANCY DUE TO SMOKING CESSATION, BY SEX AND AGE AT QUITTING

AGE AT QUITTING*	UNDISCOUNTED INCREASE IN YEARS OF LIFE EXPECTANCY DUE TO SMOKING CESSATION	
	Men	Women
35–39	5.08	3.18
40–44	4.60	2.94
45–49	4.00	2.64
50–54	3.32	2.28
55–59	2.60	1.85
60–64	1.90	1.40
65–69	1.32	0.97

* Median age used for purposes of calculation.

Adapted from Oster, G., Huse, D. M., Delea, T. E., and Colditz, G. A.: Cost effectiveness of nicotine gum as an adjunct to the physician's advice against cigarette smoking. JAMA 256:131, 1986. Copyright 1986, American Medical Association.

is a physician's advice that influences patients to try other interventions that might not be considered if the physician had not identified overweight as a medical problem.

PHYSICAL ACTIVITY

Substantial data indicate that physical activity reduces coronary heart disease and all-cause mortality, partly because of its beneficial effects on other risk factors but apparently partly independently.[131-137] Unfortunately, it has been reported that less than 10 per cent of physicians recommend exercise for their patients.[138] Many patients, however, both want and expect their physicians to make recommendations regarding physical activity,[138] and in one survey, about 25 per cent of active people ascribed their activity in large part to the advice of a physician.[139]

Worksite exercise programs also are potentially cost-effective independent of their possible effect on the development of clinical coronary artery disease. In one study, employees in the experimental exercise program group missed fewer days of work, were more likely to remain employed, and had fewer hospital days and fewer medical claims, thus resulting in substantial health care savings.[140,141] In fact, some employers have decided to pay their employees directly for participating in exercise programs, such as jogging. Unlike antismoking campaigns, media campaigns advocating exercise seem to encourage people to seek out other programs in the community but not to lead to direct changes in behavior by themselves.[139,142] Thus it appears that a physician's encouragement of increased physical activity, especially if combined with direct guidance on how to implement the suggestion, can lead to major changes in health behavior. Although it is difficult to determine the exact degree of effectiveness to be gained for the cost, there are substantial data linking physical activity to other cardiovascular risk factors and apparently independently to cardiovascular and all-cause mortality.[132-137] These data suggest that efforts to increase physical activity have the potential for being highly cost-effective.

Cardiac rehabilitation in patients who have suffered a myocardial infarction (Chap. 39) appears to lower by about 20 per cent the subsequent rates of reinfarction, cardiovascular mortality, and total mortality.[143] These programs improve the functional and symptomatic status of patients, and the exercise programs themselves are associated with a very small risk of major adverse events.[144-146] Such programs also can help patients return to work earlier after uncomplicated myocardial infarction,[147] and, as a result, can both reduce costs of medical care and increase productivity.[148] Thus the combination of cardiac rehabilitation services and occupational work evaluations appears to be very cost-effective for the post–myocardial infarction patient.

PREVENTION OF INFECTIVE ENDOCARDITIS IN VALVULAR HEART DISEASE
(See also p. 1097)

By extrapolation from cost-effectiveness analyses, penicillin prophylaxis to prevent bacterial endocarditis in patients with rheumatic valvular heart disease appears to have a cost-effectiveness of about $13,000 per year of life gained.[149,150] In patients with prosthetic heart valves, in whom the risk of endocarditis is higher, the cost-effectiveness is likely to be even more favorable. By comparison, two detailed cost-effectiveness analyses indicate that penicillin prophylaxis before dental work to prevent bacterial endocarditis is not cost-effective for patients with mitral valve prolapse[149,150] (p. 1035). Using the most likely assumptions, people are as likely to die of penicillin reactions as they are to die of endocarditis, and even given the most optimistic assumptions, it is estimated that routine penicillin prophylaxis for dental procedures in patients with mitral valve prolapse would cost more than a million dollars to save a year of life. In most studies of mitral

valve prolapse, the risk of endocarditis is substantially higher in patients with murmurs of mitral regurgitation. Although the cost-effectiveness in this subpopulation of patients with mitral valve prolapse is unclear, the use of prophylactic antibiotics in the presence of a murmur of mitral valve prolapse is often recommended.[151,152]

PREHOSPITAL EMERGENCY SERVICES
(See also Chap. 26)

Prehospital emergency services range from basic life support to advanced life support services. Advanced life support programs, which include interventions such as defibrillation, endotracheal intubation, and intravenous or intramuscular medications, have been instituted throughout much of the United States.[153] Because about 60 per cent of patients whose death certificates list the cause of death as myocardial infarction die outside of the hospital, advances in prehospital emergency services, such as better training in the community or dispatcher-assisted instruction, could have a substantial impact on survival.[154]

Prehospital emergency care appears to be extremely successful in patients who have ventricular fibrillation and who are seen very soon after cardiac arrest (p. 773). For example, in pooled data, about two-thirds of patients who are seen within 5 minutes of a ventricular fibrillation arrest survive to leave the hospital.[155] Unfortunately, many arrests are not caused by ventricular fibrillation, and even the most successful prehospital emergency services often cannot deliver care within 5 minutes. Thus only about 15 to 20 per cent of prehospital cardiac arrest patients commonly survive to leave the hospital in even the best programs.[156,157] These higher rates are achieved principally through advanced life support programs utilizing paramedics, which appear to increase the likelihood of reaching the hospital alive from about 19 to 34 per cent and the likelihood of being discharged alive from the hospital from 7 to 17 per cent.[153] However, the prognosis after hospital discharge of patients who were resuscitated from prehospital arrest is only about 75 per cent as high as age- and sex-matched comparison groups who have survived myocardial infarction without prehospital arrest, and it is only about 60 per cent as high as for age- and sex-adjusted members of the general population.[156]

The cost-effectiveness of prehospital emergency programs is difficult to estimate. One analysis estimated that a mobile coronary care unit has an incremental cost of about $25,000 (in 1991 dollars) per life saved above and beyond the cost of the ambulance system itself.[157] Another analysis estimated that the incremental cost-effectiveness of a mobile coronary care unit was about $100,000 (in 1991 dollars) per life saved and $50,000 (in 1991 dollars) per year of life saved, but this analysis included only the incremental costs of the mobile coronary care unit program and not the costs of the existing emergency medical technician and community training program to which it was added.[158]

Analyses of the cost-effectiveness of prehospital emergency services depend on assumptions about the mean response time and the patients' prognoses, both in terms of life expectancy and in terms of quality of life and neurological impairment. For example, the longer the response time, the more likely it is that survivors of prehospital cardiac arrest will have neurological impairment. If the years of life expectancy that are gained are compromised by such neurological impairment, then the *quality* of those years of life will not be the same as the quality of the years of life that might be gained from preventive measures that delay the onset of disease. Thus, when the calculation of cost-effectiveness is adjusted for the years of life that are gained without major neurological impairment, the apparent benefit of prehospital resuscitation may be reduced. Furthermore, patients whose lives are saved by prehospital emergency services are likely to require careful medical follow-up, sometimes including expensive interventions such as coronary bypass grafting. Most studies have not clearly considered the fact that the survivors of out-of-hospital cardiac arrest will have costs other than those included in the first term of the equation in Table 54–1, such as the costs for rehabilitative and custodial care and the costs for additional diagnosis and therapy of the substantial coronary disease that may have precipitated the arrest. If these costs are taken into account, the relative cost-effectiveness of prehospital emergency services programs would be less appealing than the preceding estimates.

CORONARY CARE UNITS

(See also Chap. 39)

Coronary care units were originally designed to provide the ready availability of resuscitative services to patients with obvious acute myocardial infarction (p. 1223). The mission of these units subsequently has been substantially broadened: patients are now admitted to rule out a myocardial infarction if there is a reasonable suspicion that one may have occurred. The interventions in these units now include prevention of arrhythmias, medical and surgical treatment of acute ischemia, treatment of severe pump failure, and procedures designed to prevent or to limit the size of the acute myocardial infarction. It is difficult, if not impossible, to disentangle each of these potential aspects of coronary care units.

HOME CARE VS. CORONARY CARE. Two trials in Great Britain showed no significant difference in the survival of patients who were admitted to coronary care units compared with randomized controls who were treated at home.[159,160] These studies were too small, however, to detect the expected difference in mortality.[161] Furthermore, patients were eligible for randomization only after prolonged home observation, during which time high-risk patients were excluded and a substantial proportion of patients were actually resuscitated. Thus these studies do not appear to apply to unselected patients coming to American hospitals. In fact, available data suggest that patients who are mistakenly discharged from the emergency room appear to have a significantly higher mortality with their acute myocardial infarctions than patients who are correctly admitted.[162]

REDUCTION OF MORTALITY IN THE CCU. If one assumes that the risk of primary ventricular fibrillation in an acute myocardial infarction is about 4.5 per cent and that the likelihood of successful resuscitation and hospital survival is about 88 per cent in coronary care units, the availability of defibrillation and resuscitation would result in about a 4-percentage-point decline in the in-hospital mortality from acute myocardial infarction compared with the pre–coronary care unit era when defibrillation could not be carried out promptly on a regular nursing unit.[163] Data from the Minnesota area document a positive effect of about this magnitude.[164]

Between the initial development of defibrillation and resuscitation and the subsequent advent of thrombolysis, a variety of intensive care interventions such as intra-aortic balloon counterpulsation, intravenous afterload reduction, and intravenous inotropic agents were used in the care of patients with acute myocardial infarction. Although these interventions certainly saved individual lives, their precise impact on overall mortality rates is less certain.[165,166]

More recently intravenous thrombolysis has been shown to have a statistically significant and clinically important impact on mortality in patients with acute myocardial infarction (p. 1230).[167–172] Depending on the criteria for eligibility for thrombolysis, as few as 15 per cent of patients with acute myocardial infarctions may receive such therapy.[173] The use of prehospital thrombolysis, as well as interventions to speed the access to thrombolysis, could greatly increase the impact of thrombolytic therapy.[174]

Although thrombolytic therapy in the management of acute myocardial infarction has been rapidly adopted,[175] there is still not a broad consensus about which thrombolytic agent is best[176] or about the role of adjunctive aspirin and heparin.[177]

The role of subsequent percutaneous transluminal coronary angioplasty also is evolving, with emerging evidence that a conservative strategy of reserving angioplasty for patients with specific clinical indications is as efficacious as routine angioplasty.[178]

Issues related to the choice of thrombolytic agent and the use of angioplasty are critical to the determination of the cost-effectiveness of reperfusion therapy. The cost of thrombolysis per 1-year survivor was estimated to range from about $35,000 for a large myocardial infarction to $200,000 for a moderate-sized myocardial infarction, and $800,000 for a small myocardial infarction when intravenous thrombolysis was followed by catheterization only when the patient was symptomatic or had a positive exercise tolerance test.[179] The cost *per year of life saved* is uncertain, since long-term survival data are still emerging. Another cost-effectiveness analysis also emphasized the importance of the costs of medications and of the additional procedures that are generated in patients who receive thrombolytic therapy.[180]

Another important group to consider are patients who are admitted to the coronary care unit for suspected or "rule-out" myocardial infarction. Coronary care unit admission can be applied selectively only to patients whose probability of myocardial infarction is sufficiently high for it to be cost-effective.[4] Thus, if the probability of myocardial infarction is only 5 per cent, the incremental cost per year of life saved by admission to the coronary care unit compared with an intermediate care unit is about $260,000 (in 1991 dollars); and the cost will fall to about $60,000 (in 1991 dollars) per year of life saved if the potential for acute myocardial infarction is 20 per cent. These estimates suggest that it may be worthwhile for physicians to estimate the probability of acute myocardial infarction from clinical data or from more sophisticated calculations.[17,18] One study indicates that the intermediate-care option, which would be analogous to many "stepdown" units in which electrocardiographic monitoring and resuscitative facilities are available but in which patients do not receive intensive care nursing, is safe for patients who are admitted to rule out a myocardial infarction and in whom this diagnosis is confirmed.[181]

LENGTH OF STAY. The coronary care unit also can be made more cost-effective by limiting the length of stay. Data indicate that, except in patients who have recurrent ischemic pain, 24 hours is nearly always sufficient to determine whether or not a myocardial infarction has occurred.[182] Similar protocols using the electrocardiogram, the history, and serum enzyme levels substantiate that 24 hours is often a sufficient length of stay.[183] If coronary care units were used in this more cost-effective manner, the relative cost-effectiveness for patients with symptoms indicative of but not diagnostic of an acute myocardial infarction would be improved, since the original calculations noted above assumed a longer average length of stay.

When faced with a shortage of coronary care unit beds, physicians can identify correctly which patients are most in need.[184] It is likely that coronary care units can become substantially more cost-effective by limiting admission to patients whose probability of acute myocardial infarction is at about 20 per cent or higher or in whom serious complications are more likely and by shortening the average length of stay for patients who do not have documented myocardial infarctions or complications. Intermediate care (or "stepdown") unit admission appears to be quite cost-effective and safe for patients whose probability of acute myocardial infarction is too high for discharge to be appropriate but not high enough for coronary care unit admission to be worthwhile.

MEDICAL THERAPY OF CORONARY ARTERY DISEASE

(See also Chap. 40)

Although the natural history of patients with medically treated coronary artery disease appears to be improving, it is difficult to measure the impact of specific aspects of the medical treatment. The best-studied intervention is the use of "prophylactic" beta-adrenoceptor antagonists in survivors of a recent myocardial infarction. Numerous studies have shown a substantial benefit from routine use of beta-adrenoceptor antagonists in patients who are ready for discharge after an acute myocardial infarction (p. 1265).[185-189] Several studies indicate that the relative reduction in mortality in years 2 and 3 is similar to the 25 to 30 per cent reduction found in year 1.[185,186,189,191-194] In the fourth, fifth, and sixth years, the benefit appears to be smaller, closer to 8 to 9 per cent.[195] Based on the costs of the medications, and the likely benefits in patients with various risks of short- and long-term complications, cost-effectiveness analysis indicates that the cost of beta-adrenoceptor antagonist therapy to save 1 year of life is about $4700 (in 1991 dollars) in patients at high risk for complications, about $7400 for medium-risk patients, and about $27,000 for low-risk patients. Altering the patients' age from 45 to 65 years had little effect on the analysis. These calculations suggest that beta-adrenoceptor antagonist therapy in the post–myocardial infarction patient is extremely cost-effective in high- and medium-risk patients and is still rather cost-effective even in low-risk patients.[196] It is not possible, as of this writing, to make analogous calculations in patients with angina who have not recently survived a myocardial infarction.

CORONARY ARTERY BYPASS GRAFTING

(See also p. 1320)

Coronary artery bypass grafting prolongs the life of patients with left main coronary artery disease and of patients with three-vessel disease and left ventricular dysfunction.[197-199] Data on patients with less severe degrees of disease are conflicting, with the European trial being the only major randomized study that showed a significant advantage for surgery among patients with two-vessel disease that included the left anterior descending artery.[200,201] The benefit of operation diminishes after about 7 years,[201] presumably because of late graft failure, which appears to be less common with internal mammary grafts than with vein grafts.[202]

In patients with marked symptoms, coronary artery bypass grafting is efficacious in improving symptomatic status. Several studies, however, indicate that coronary artery bypass grafting does not, in general, improve work status[203-205] even though it improves quality of life.[203,206] Weinstein and Stason estimated that the net cost of coronary bypass grafting is about $25,000 to $29,000 (in 1991 dollars).[207] Data also indicate that the initial investment in coronary artery bypass surgery is not offset by lower subsequent treatment costs.[208] The costs vary, depending on postoperative length of stay, which appears to be partly related to predetermined protocol and largely related to postoperative complications.[209,210] Interestingly, professional fees for coronary bypass grafting have not fallen, even as the procedure has become quicker and more routine.[211]

Weinstein and Stason also have performed the most extensive cost-effectiveness analysis of coronary artery bypass grafting in patients with various symptomatic states and extents of disease (Table 54–5).[207] These calculations suggest that in patients with three-vessel disease or left main coronary artery disease, or in patients with two-vessel disease and severe angina, the cost per year of life gained from coronary bypass grafting compares favorably with the cost per year of life gained from renal dialysis in patients with chronic renal failure. It also has been estimated that coronary bypass grafting compares favorably with valve replacement for aortic stenosis and implantation of a pacemaker for heart block in terms of its cost-effectiveness, and that it is more cost-effective than heart transplantation or the treatment of end-stage renal failure and is probably somewhat less cost-effective than hip replacement for disabling arthritis.[212] Of course, patient selec-

TABLE 54–5 ESTIMATED APPROXIMATE COST PER GAIN IN ONE QUALITY-ADJUSTED YEAR OF LIFE FOR CORONARY ARTERY BYPASS GRAFTING (SEE REFERENCE 207; CALCULATIONS ARE UPDATED TO 1991 DOLLARS)

	ONE-VESSEL DISEASE	TWO-VESSEL DISEASE	THREE-VESSEL DISEASE	LEFT MAIN DISEASE
Very mild angina	*	86,000	14,000	6300
Mild angina	850,000	55,000	13,500	6600
Severe angina	55,000	32,000	13,000	7000

* Quality-adjusted life expectancy is reduced.

tion is paramount to maximizing cost-effectiveness, and sometimes a second opinion is helpful in this regard.[213]

PERCUTANEOUS TRANSLUMINAL CORONARY ANGIOPLASTY

(See also Chap. 41)

The initial charges for percutaneous transluminal coronary angioplasty (PTCA) have been reported to be about 60 per cent as high as for coronary artery bypass grafting,[214-216] but this estimate included the substantial cost of the availability of standby surgery.[217] The true costs of a treatment strategy, including PTCA, must consider the immediate failure rate, the possible need for urgent coronary artery bypass grafting, and the likelihood of restenosis and its subsequent treatment. If the PTCA can be performed at a time of day when an operating suite and team normally would be "between cases," without causing them to be idle during a period when they would otherwise be in full use, the actual cost of the availability of standby surgery would be minimal and angioplasty becomes more cost-effective.

Even given the full costs of surgical standby, the expenditures for patients undergoing PTCA were significantly lower at 1 year than those of patients treated with coronary artery bypass grafting.[214] Because this study reported a 30 per cent immediate failure rate and a 22 per cent restenosis rate at 1 year, the cost-effectiveness of PTCA is even better now that immediate success rates usually are higher.

SUMMARY

The gratifying reduction in mortality from ischemic heart disease usually is regarded as testimony to the effectiveness of a variety of primary and secondary preventive and therapeutic measures.[218-220] It will be necessary, however, for current and future interventions to be carefully analyzed, so that the benefit of medical care to reduce cardiovascular morbidity and mortality can be maximized within the constraints of the resources that will be available.

Physicians should not view the current emphasis on cost-effective care as contradictory to excellent care. Patients should not be treated as numbers, and optimal medical care cannot be routinely derived from equations. The physician's principal responsibility is to render the best possible medical care to the patient as an individual. An understanding of the principles of cost-effectiveness should allow the physician to improve the choice of diagnostic and therapeutic strategies, and it should assist the physician's ability to determine strategies that are optimal in the aggregate and to adopt or adapt them for the person at hand. In such a context, more cost-effective care implies better care for the individual patient as well as the conservation of resources to improve care for the population as a whole.

REFERENCES

QUANTITATIVE ANALYSES OF COSTS AND EFFECTIVENESS

1. Weinstein, M. C., and Fineberg, H. V.: Clinical Decision Analysis. Philadelphia, W. B. Saunders Company, 1980.
2. Weinstein, M. C., and Stason, W. B.: Foundations of cost-effectiveness analysis for health and medical practices. N. Engl. J. Med. 296:716, 1977.
3. Sox, H. C., Blatt, M. A., Higgins, M. C., and Marton, K. I.: Cost-effectiveness analysis and cost-benefit analysis. Med. Decis. Making 317: 1988.
4. Fineberg, H., Scadden, D., and Goldman, L.: Management of patients with a low probability of acute myocardial infarction: Cost-effectiveness of alternatives to coronary care unit admission. N. Engl. J. Med. 310:1301, 1984.
5. Kwoh, C. K., Beck, J. R., and Pauker, S. G.: Repeated syncope with negative diagnostic evaluation. To pace or not to pace? Med. Decis. Making 4:351, 1984.
6. Doubilet, P., Weinstein, M. D., and McNeil, B. J.: Use and misuse of the term "cost effective" in medicine (Editorial). N. Engl. J. Med. 314:253, 1986.
7. Eisenberg, J. M.: Clinical economics: A guide to the economic analysis of clinical practices. JAMA 262:2879, 1989.
8. Drummond, M., Stoddart, G., LaBelle, R., and Cushman, R.: Health economics: An introduction for clinicians. Ann. Intern. Med. 107:88, 1987.
9. Roberts, S. D., Maxwell, D. R., and Gross, T. L.: Cost-effective care of end-stage renal disease: A billion-dollar question. Ann. Intern. Med. 92:243, 1980.
10. Goldman, L. Cost-awareness in medicine. In Wilson, J. D., et al. (eds.): Harrison's Principles of Internal Medicine. 12th ed. New York, McGraw-Hill Book Co. 1991, p. 11.

DIAGNOSTIC TESTING

11. Goldman, L.: Quantitative aspects of clinical reasoning. In Wilson, J. D., et al. (eds.): Harrison's Principles of Internal Medicine. 12th ed. New York, McGraw-Hill Book Co., 1991, pp. 5–11.
12. Goldman, L.: Noninvasive tests in cardiology. In Branch, W., Jr. (ed.): The Office Practice of Medicine. 2nd ed. Philadelphia, W. B. Saunders Company, 1987, p 55.
13. Rifkin, R. D., and Hood, W. B.: Bayesian analysis of electrocardiographic exercise stress testing. N. Engl. J. Med. 297:681, 1977.
14. Diamond, G. A., Staniloff, H. M., Forrester, J. S., et al.: Computer-assisted diagnosis in the noninvasive evaluation of patients with suspected coronary artery disease. J. Am. Coll. Cardiol. 1:444, 1983.
15. Goldman, L., Cook, E. F., Mitchell, N., et al.: Incremental value of the exercise test for diagnosing the presence or absence of coronary artery disease. Circulation 66:945, 1982.
16. Weiner, D. A., Ryan, T. J., McCabe, C. H., et al.: Exercise stress testing: Correlations among history of angina, ST-segment response and prevalence of coronary-artery disease in the coronary artery surgery study (CASS). N. Engl. J. Med. 300:230, 1979.
17. Hoagland, P. M., Cook, E. F., Wynne, J., and Goldman, L.: Value of noninvasive testing in adults with suspected aortic stenosis. Am. J. Med. 80:1041, 1986.
18. Goldman, L., Cook, E. F., Brand, D. A., et al.: A computer protocol to predict myocardial infarction in emergency department patients with chest pain. N. Engl. J. Med. 318:797, 1988.
19. Goldman, L., Feinstein, A. R., Batsford, W. P., et al.: Ordering patterns and clinical impact of cardiovascular nuclear medicine procedures. Circulation 62:680, 1980.
20. Goldman, L., Cohn, P. F., Mudge, G. H. Jr. et al.: Clinical utility and management impact of M-mode echocadiography. Am. J. Med. 75:49, 1983.
21. Sox, H. C., Margulies, I., and Sox, C. H.: Psychologically mediated effects of diagnostic tests. Ann. Intern. Med. 95:680, 1981.
22. McNeil, B. J., Keeler, E., and Adelstein, S. J.: Primer on certain elements of medical decision-making. N. Engl. J. Med. 293:211, 1975.
23. Lee, T. H., and Goldman, L.: Serum enzyme assays in the diagnosis of acute myocardial infarction. Recommendations based on a quantitative analysis. Ann. Intern. Med. 105:221, 1986.
24. Vasudevan, G., Mercer, D. W., and Varat, M. A.: Lactic dehydrogenase isoenzyme determination in the diagnosis of acute myocardial infarction. Circulation 57:1055, 1978.
25. Pauker, S. G., and Kassirer, J. P.: Therapeutic decision-making: A cost-benefit analysis. N. Engl. J. Med. 293:229, 1975.
26. Pauker, S. G., and Kassirer, J. P.: The threshold approach to clinical decision-making. N. Engl. J. Med. 302:1109, 1980.
27. Weintraub, W. S., Madeira, S. W., Bodenheimer, M. M., et al.: Critical analysis of the application of Bayes' theorem to sequential testing in the noninvasive diagnosis of coronary artery disease. Am. J. Cardiol. 54:43, 1984.
28. Pamelia, F. X., Gibson, R. S., Watson, D. D., et al.: Prognosis with chest pain and normal thallium-201 exercise scintigrams. Am. J. Cardiol. 55:920, 1985.
29. Gordon, D. J., Ekelund, L., Karon, J. M., et al.: Predictive value of the exercise tolerance test for mortality in North American men: The Lipid Research Clinics Mortality Follow-up Study. Circulation 74:252, 1986.
30. Patterson, R. E., Eng, C., Horowitz, S. F., et al.: Bayesian comparison of cost-effectiveness of different clinical approaches to diagnose coronary artery disease. J. Am Coll. Cardiol. 4:278, 1984.

31. Sox, H. C., Garber, A. M., and Littenberg, B.: The resting electrocardiogram as a screening test: A clinical analysis. Ann. Intern. Med. 111:489, 1989.
32. Sox, H. C., Littenberg, B., and Garber, A. M.: The role of exercise testing in screening for coronary artery disease. Ann. Intern. Med. 110:456, 1989.
33. Harrell, F. E., Califf, R. M., Pryor, D. B., et al.: Evaluating the yield of medical tests. JAMA 247:2543, 1982.
34. Gorry, G. A., Pauker, S. G., and Schwartz, W. B.: The diagnostic importance of the normal finding. N. Engl. J. Med. 298:486, 1978.
35. Wennberg, J. E., Freeman, J. L., and Culp, W. J.: Are hospital services rationed in New Haven or over-utilised in Boston? Lancet 1:1185, 1987.
36. Fineberg, H. V., and Hiatt, H. H.: Evaluation of medical practices. The case for technology assessment. N. Engl. J. Med. 301:1086, 1979.
37. Moloney, T. W., and Rogers, D. E.: Medical technology—a different view of the contentious debate over costs. N. Engl. J. Med. 301:1413, 1979.
38. Griner, P. F., and the Medical House Staff, Strong Memorial Hospital, Rochester, New York: Use of laboratory tests in a teaching hospital: Long-term trends. Reductions in use and relative cost. Ann. Intern. Med. 90:243, 1979.

PREVENTION AND TREATMENT

39. Goldman, L., and Cook, E. F.: The decline in ischemic heart disease mortality rates: An analysis of the comparative effects of medical interventions and changes in lifestyle. Ann. Intern. Med. 101:825, 1984.
40. Sempos, C., Cooper, R., Kovar, M. G., and McMillen, M.: Divergence of the recent trends in coronary mortality for the four major race-sex groups in the United States. Am. J. Public Health 78:1422, 1988.
41. Weinstein, M. C., Coxson, P. G., Williams, L. W., et al.: Forecasting coronary heart disease incidence, mortality, and cost: The coronary heart disease policy model. Am. J. Public Health 77:1417, 1987.
42. Wittels, E. H., Hay, J. W., and Gotto, A. M.: Medical costs of coronary artery disease in the United States. Am. J. Cardiol. 65:432, 1990.
43. Stamler, J., Wentworth, D., and Neaton, J. D.: Is relationship between serum cholesterol and risk of premature death from coronary heart disease continuous and graded? Findings in 356,222 primary screenees of the Multiple-Risk Factor Intervention Trial (MRFIT). JAMA 256:2823, 1986.
44. Kannel, W. B., Castelli, W. P., and Gordon, T.: Cholesterol in the prediction of atherosclerotic disease. New perspectives based on the Framingham Study. Ann. Intern. Med. 90:85, 1979.
45. NIH Consensus Conference: The treatment of hypertriglyceridemia. JAMA 251:1196, 1984.
46. Expert Panel: Report of the national cholesterol education program. Expert panel on detection, evaluation, and treatment of high blood cholesterol in adults. Arch. Intern. Med. 148:36, 1988.
47. Keys, A., Anderson, J. T., and Grande, F.: Serum cholesterol response to changes in diet. IV. Particular saturated fatty acids in the diet. Metabolism 14:776, 1965.
48. Hegsted, D. M., McGandy, R. B., Myers, M. L., and Stare, F. J.: Quantitative effects of dietary fat on serum cholesterol in man. Am. J. Clin. Nutr. 17:281, 1965.
49. Arntzenius, A. C., Kromhout, D., Barth, J. D., et al.: Diet, lipoproteins, and the progression of coronary atherosclerosis. The Leiden Intervention Trial. N. Engl. J. Med. 312:805, 1985.
50. Kushi, L. H., Lew, R. A., Stare, F. J., et al.: Diet and 20-year mortality from coronary heart disease. The Ireland-Boston Diet-Heart Study. N. Engl. J. Med. 312:811, 1985.
51. Blankenhorn, D. H., Alaupovic, P., Wickham, E., et al.: Prediction of angiographic change in native human coronary arteries and aortocoronary bypass grafts: Lipid and non-lipid factors. Circulation 81:470, 1990.
52. Blankenhorn, D. H., Johnson, R. L., Mack, W. J., et al.: The influence of diet on the appearance of new lesions in human coronary arteries. JAMA 263:1646, 1990.
53. Blankenhorn, D. H., Nessim, S. A., Johnson, R. L., et al.: Beneficial effects of combined colestipol niacin therapy in coronary atherosclerosis and coronary venous bypass grafts. JAMA 257:3233, 1987.
54. The Lipid Research Clinics Program: The Lipid Research Clinics Coronary Primary Prevention Trial results. I. Reduction in incidence of coronary heart disease. JAMA 251:351, 1984.
55. The Lipid Research Clinics Program: The Lipid Research Clinics Coronary Primary Prevention Trial results. II. The relationship of reduction in incidence of coronary heart disease to cholesterol lowering. JAMA 251:365, 1984.
56. Kannel, W. B., and Gordon, T. (eds.): The Framingham Study: An Epidemiologic Investigation of Cardiovascular Disease. Sections 1–32. Washington, D.C., U.S. Government Printing Office, 1970–1977.
57. Frick, M. H., Elo, O., Haapa, K., et al.: Helsinki Heart Study: Primary-prevention trial with gemfibrozil in middle-aged men with dyslipidemia. N. Engl. J. Med. 317:1237, 1987.
58. Canner, P. L., Berge, K. G., Wenger, N. K., et al.: Fifteen year mortality in coronary drug project patients; long-term benefits with niacin. J. Am. Coll. Cardiol. 8:1245, 1986.
59. Sempos, C., Fulwood, R., Haines, C., et al.: The prevalence of high blood cholesterol levels among adults in the United States. JAMA 262:45, 1989.
60. Goldman, L., Weinstein, M. C., and Williams, L. W.: Relative impact of targeted versus populationwide cholesterol interventions on the incidence of coronary heart disease. Circulation 80:254, 1989.
61. Pusko, P., Tuomilehto, J., Salonen, J., et al.: Changes in coronary risk

factors during comprehensive five-year community programme to control cardiovascular diseases (North Karelia project). Br. Med. J. 2:1173, 1979.

62. Puska, P., Salonen, J. T., Nissinen, A., et al.: Change in risk factors for coronary heart disease during 10 years of a community intervention programme (North Karelia project). Br. Med. J. 287:1840, 1983.

63. Puska, P., Neittaanmaki, L., and Tuomilehto, J.: A survey of local health personnel and decision makers concerning the North Karelia project: A community program for control of cardiovascular diseases. Prev. Med. 10:564, 1981.

64. Salonen, J. T., Heinonen, O. P., Kottke, T. E., and Puska, P.: Change in health behaviour in relation to estimated coronary heart disease risk during a community-based cardiovascular disease prevention programme. Int. J. Epidemiol. 10:343, 1981.

65. Salonen, J. T., Puska, P., Kottke, T. E., et al.: Decline in mortality from coronary heart disease in Finland from 1969 to 1979. Br. Med. J. 286:1857, 1983.

66. Fortmann, S. P., Williams, P. T., Hulley, S. B., et al.: Effect of health education on dietary behavior: The Stanford Three Community Study. Am. J. Clin. Nutr. 34:2030, 1981.

67. Berwick, D. M., Cretin, S., and Keeler, E.: Cholesterol, Children, and Heart Disease: An Analysis of Alternatives. New York, Oxford University Press, 1980.

68. Garber, A. M., Sox, H. C., and Littenberg, B.: Screening asymptomatic adults for cardiac risk factors: The serum cholesterol level. Ann. Intern. Med. 110:622, 1989.

69. Basinski, A., Frank, J. W., Naylor, C. D., and Rachlis, M. M.: Detection and Management of Asymptomatic Hypercholesterolemia. A Policy Document by the Toronto Working Group on Cholesterol Policy. Toronto, Ontario Ministry of Health, 1989.

70. The British Cardiac Society Working Group on Coronary Heart Disease Prevention. Lancet 1:377, 1987.

71. Study Group, European Atherosclerosis Society: Strategies for the prevention of coronary heart disease: A policy statement of the European Atherosclerosis Society. Eur. Heart J. 8:77, 1987.

72. Assmann, G.: At what levels of total low- or high-density lipoprotein cholesterol should diet/drug therapy be initiated? European guidelines. Am. J. Cardiol. 65:11F, 1990.

73. Weinstein, M. C., and Stason, W. B.: Cost-effectiveness of interventions to prevent or treat coronary heart disease. Ann. Rev. Public Health 6:41, 1985.

74. Oster, G., and Epstein, A. M.: Cost-effectiveness of antihyperlipemic therapy in the prevention of coronary heart disease: The case of cholestyramine. JAMA 248:2381, 1987.

75. Kinosian, B. P., and Eisenberg, J. M.: Cutting into cholesterol: Cost-effective alternatives for treating hypercholesterolemia. JAMA 259:2249, 1988.

76. Himmelstein, D., and Woolhandler, S.: Free care, cholestyramine, and health policy. N. Engl. J. Med. 311:1511, 1984.

77. Goldman, L. G., Edelson, J. T., Tosteson, A. A., et al.: Projected cost-effectiveness of lovastatin for cholesterol reduction. Clin. Res. 36:337A, 1988.

78. Research Committee to the Medical Research Council: Controlled trial of soya-bean oil in myocardial infarction. Lancet 2:693, 1968.

79. Leren, P.: The Oslo Diet Heart Study: Eleven-year report. Circulation 42:35, 1970.

80. Group of Physicians of the Newcastle-Upon-Tyne Region: Trial of clofibrate in the treatment of ischaemic heart disease. Br. Med. J. 4:767, 1971.

81. Coronary Drug Project Group: Clofibrate and niacin in coronary heart disease. JAMA 231:360, 1975.

82. Research Committee of the Scottish Society of Physicians: Ischaemic heart disease: A secondary prevention trial using clofibrate. Br. Med. J. 4:775, 1971.

83. National Center for Health Statistics, U.S. Public Health Service: National Health and Nutrition Examination Survey 1976–1980. Public Use Data Tape. Hyattsville, MD, U.S. Department of Health and Human Services, 1982.

84. Veterans Administration Cooperative Study Group on Antihypertensive Agents: Effects of treatment on morbidity in hypertension. Part 1. JAMA 202:1028, 1967.

85. Veterans Administration Cooperative Study Group on Antihypertensive Agents: Effects of treatment on morbidity in hypertension. Part 2. JAMA 213:1143, 1970.

86. Veterans Administration Cooperative Study Group on Antihypertensive Agents: Effects of treatment on morbidity in hypertension. Part 3. Circulation 45:991, 1972.

87. Hebert, P. R., Fiebach, N. H., Eberlein, K. A., et al.: The community based randomized trials of pharmacologic treatment of mild-to-moderate hypertension. Am. J. Epidemiol. 127:581, 1988.

88. Shea, S., Cook, E. F., Kannel, W. B., and Goldman, L.: Treatment of hypertension and its effect on cardiovascular risk factors: Data from the Framingham Heart Study. Circulation 71:22, 1985.

89. Australian National Blood Pressure Management Committee: The Australian therapeutic trial in mild hypertension. Lancet 1:1261, 1980

90. Hypertension Detection and Follow-up Program Cooperative Group: Five-year findings of the Hypertension Detection and Follow-up Program: I. Reduction in mortality of persons with high blood pressure, including mild hypertension. JAMA 242:2562, 1979.

91. Hypertension Detection and Follow-up Program Cooperative Group: Five-year findings of the Hypertension Detection and Follow-up Program: III. Reduction in stroke incidence among persons with high blood pressure. JAMA 247:633, 1982.

92. Hypertension Detection and Follow-up Program Cooperative Group: The effect of treatment on mortality in "mild" hypertension: Results of the Hypertension Detection and Follow-up Program. N. Engl. J. Med. 307:976, 1982.

92a. Hypertension Detection and Follow-up Program Cooperative Group: Effect of stepped care treatment on the incidence of myocardial infarction and angina pectoris: Five-year findings of the Hypertension Detection and Follow-up Program. Hypertension 6 (Suppl I):198, 1984.

93. Multiple-Risk Factor Intervention Trial Research Group: Multiple-Risk Factor Intervention Trial: Risk factor changes and mortality results. JAMA 248:1465, 1982.

94. The Hypertension Detection and Follow-up Program Cooperative Research Group: The effect of antihypertensive drug treatment on mortality in the presence of resting electrocardiographic abnormalities at baseline: The HDFP experience. Circulation 70:996, 1984.

95. Littenberg, B., Garber, A. M., and Sox, H. C.: Screening for hypertension. Ann. Intern. Med. 112:192, 1990.

96. Weinstein, M. C., and Stason, W. B.: Hypertension: A Policy Perspective. Cambridge, Mass., Harvard University Press, 1976.

97. Stokes, J., III, and Carmichael, D. C.: A Cost-Benefit Analysis of Model Hypertension Control. Bethesda, National Heart, Lung and Blood Institute, 1975.

98. Edelson, J. T., Weinstein, M. C., Tosteson, A. N. A., et al.: Long-term cost-effectiveness of various initial monotherapies for mild to moderate hypertension. JAMA 263:408, 1990.

99. Three-Community Hypertension Control Program. V. Cost-effectiveness of intervention. Mayo Clin. Proc. 56:11, 1981.

100. Hannan, E. L., and Graham, J. K.: A cost-benefit study of hypertension screening and treatment program at the work setting. Inquiry 15:345, 1978.

101. Oster, G., Huse, D. M., Delea, T. E., and Colditz, G. A.: Cost effectiveness of nicotine gum as an adjunct to physician's advice against cigarette smoking. JAMA 256:1315, 1986.

102. Doll, R., and Peto, R.: Mortality in relation to smoking: Twenty years observation of male British doctors. Br. Med. J. 2:1525, 1976.

103. Friedman, G. D., Petitti, D. B., Bawol, R. D., and Siegelaub, A. B.: Mortality in cigarette smokers and quitters. Effect of base-line differences. N. Engl. J. Med. 304:1407, 1981.

104. Rosenberg, L., Kaufman, D. W., Helmrich, S. P., and Shapiro, S.: The risk of myocardial infarction after quitting smoking in men under 55 years of age. N. Engl. J. Med. 313:1511, 1985.

105. Vietstra, R. E., Kronmal, R. A., Oberman, A., et al.: Effect of cigarette smoking on survival of patients with angiographically documented coronary artery disease. JAMA 255:1023, 1986.

106. Hermanson, B., Omenn, G. S., Kronmal, R. A., and Gersh, B. J.: Beneficial six-year outcome of smoking cessation in older men and women with coronary artery disease. N. Engl. J. Med. 319:1365, 1988.

107. Rosenberg, L., Palmer, J. R., and Shapiro, S.: Decline in the risk of myocardial infarctions among women who stop smoking. N. Engl. J. Med. 322:213, 1990.

108. Russell, M. A., Wilson, C., Taylor, C., and Baker, C. D.: Effect of practitioners' advice against smoking. Br. Med. J. 2:231, 1979.

109. Jamrozik, K., Vessey, M., Fowler, G., et al.: Controlled trial of three different antismoking interventions in general practice. Br. Med. J. 288:1499, 1984.

110. Stewart, P. J., and Rosser, W. W.: The impact of routine advice on smoking cessation from family physicians. Can. Med. Assoc. J. 126:1051, 1982.

111. Cohen, S. J., Stookey, G. K., Katz, B. P., et al.: Encouraging primary care physicians to help smokers quit. Ann. Intern. Med. 110:648, 1989.

112. Cummings, S. T., Coates, T. J., Richard, R. J., et al.: Training physicians in counseling and smoking cessation: A randomized trial of the "Quit for Life" program. Ann. Intern. Med. 110:640, 1989.

113. Hjalmarson, A. L.: Effect of nicotine chewing gum in smoking cessation. A randomized, placebo-controlled, double-blind study. JAMA 252: 2835, 1984.

114. Jarvik, M. E., and Schneider, N. G.: Degree of addiction and effectiveness of nicotine gum therapy for smoking. Am. J. Psychiatry 141:790, 1984.

115. Schneider, N. G., Jarvik, M. E., Forsythe, A. B., et al.: Nicotine gum in smoking cessation: A placebo-controlled, double-blind trial. Addict. Behav. 8:253, 1983.

116. British Thoracic Society: Comparison of four methods of smoking withdrawal in patients with smoking-related diseases. Br. Med. J. 286:595, 1983.

117. Hughes, J. R., Gust, S. W., Keenan, R. M., et al.: Nicotine vs placebo gum in general medical practice. JAMA 261:1300, 1989.

118. Hajek, P., Jackson, P., and Belcher, M.: Long-term use of nicotine chewing gum: Occurrence, determinants, and effect on weight gain. JAMA 260:1593, 1988.

119. Fortmann, S. P., Killen, J. D., Telch, M. J., and Newman, B.: Minimal contact treatment for smoking cessation. A placebo controlled trial of nicotine polacrilex and self-directed relapse prevention: Initial results of the Stanford Stop Smoking Project. JAMA 260:1575, 1988.

120. Abelin, T., Muller, P., Buehler, A., et al.: Controlled trial of transdermal nicotine patch in tobacco withdrawal. Lancet 1:7, 1989.

121. Tonnesen, P., Fryd, V., Hansen, M., et al.: Effect of nicotine chewing gum in combination with group counseling on the cessation of smoking. N. Engl. J. Med. 318:15, 1988.

122. Franks, P., Harp, J., and Bell, B.: Randomized, controlled trial of clonidine for smoking cessation in a primary care setting. JAMA 262:3011, 1989.

123. Lando, H. A., McGovern, P. G., Barrios, F. X., and Etringer, B. D.: Comparative evaluation of American Cancer Society and American Lung Association smoking cessation clinics. Am. J. Public Health 80:554, 1990.

124. Danaher, B. G., Berkanovic, E., and Gerger, B.: Mass media–based health behavior change: Televised smoking cessation program. Addict. Behav. 9:245, 1984.

125. Pierce, J. P., Macaskill, P., and Hill, D.: Long-term effectiveness of mass media led antismoking campaigns in Australia. Am. J. Public Health 80:565, 1990.

126. Health and Public Policy Committee, American College of Physicians: Methods for stopping cigarette smoking. Ann. Intern. Med. 105:281, 1986.

127. Hubert, H. B., Feinleib, M., McNamara, P. M., and Castelli, W. P.: Obesity as an independent risk factor for cardiovascular disease: A 26-year follow-up of participants in the Framingham Heart Study. Circulation 67:968, 1983.

128. Brownell, K. D., and Kaye, F. S.: A school-based behavior modification, nutrition, education, and physical activity program for obese children. Am. J. Clin. Nutr. 35:277, 1982.

129. Brownell, K. D., Stunkard, A. J., and McKeon, P. E.: Weight reduction at the worksite: A promise partially fulfilled. Am. J. Psychiatry 142:47, 1985.

130. Stunkard, A. J.: The current status of treatment for obesity in adults. In Stunkard, A. J., and Stellar, E. (eds.): Eating and Its Disorders. New York, Raven Press, 1984.

131. Gibbons, L. W., Blair, S. N., Cooper, K. H., and Smith, M.: Association between coronary heart disease risk factors and physical fitness in healthy adult women. Circulation 67:977, 1983.

132. Brand, R. J., Paffenbarger, R. S. Jr., Sholtz, R. I., and Kampert, J. B.: Work activity and fatal heart attacks studied by multiple logistic risk analysis. Am. J. Epidemiol. 110:52, 1979.

133. Paffenbarger, R. S., Hyde, R. T., Wing, A. L., and Hsieh, C. C.: Physical activity, all-cause mortality, and longevity of college alumni. N. Engl. J. Med. 314:605, 1986.

134. Blair, S. N., Kohl, H. W., Paffenbarger, R. S., et al.: Physical fitness and all-cause mortality: A prospective study of healthy men and women. JAMA 262:2395, 1989.

135. Leon, A. S., Connett, J., Jacobs, D. R., and Rauramaa, R.: Leisure-time physical activity levels and risk of coronary heart disease and death. The multiple risk factor intervention trial. JAMA 258:2388, 1987.

136. Slattery, M. L., Jacobs, D. R., and Nichaman, M. Z.: Leisure time physical activity and coronary heart disease death. The US Railroad Study. Circulation 79:304, 1989.

137. Ekelund, L. G., Haskell, W. L., Johnson, J. L., et al.: Physical fitness as a predictor of cardiovascular mortality in asymptomatic North American men. N. Engl. J. Med. 310:1379, 1988.

138. Iverson, D. C., Fielding, J. E., Crow, R. S., and Christenson, G. M.: The promotion of physical activity in the United States population: The status of programs in medical, worksite, community, and school settings. Public Health Reports 100:212, 1985.

139. Gilmore, A.: Canada fitness survey finds fitness means health. Can. Med. Assoc. J. 129:181, 1983.

140. Cox, M., Shepard, R. J., and Corey, P.: Influence of an employee fitness programme upon fitness, productivity, and absenteeism. Ergonomics 24:795, 1981.

141. Shepard, R. J., Corey, P., Renzland, P., and Cox, M.: The influence of an employee fitness and lifestyle modification upon medical care costs. Can. J. Public Health 73:259, 1982.

142. Oldridge, N. B.: Adherence to adult exercise fitness programs. In Matarazzo, J. D., Miller, N. E., Herd, J. A., and Weiss, S. M. (eds.): Behavioral Health: A Handbook of Health Enhancement and Disease Prevention. New York, John Wiley and Sons, 1984, pp. 467–487.

143. O'Connor, G. T., Buring, J. E., Yusuf, S., et al.: An overview of randomized trials of rehabilitation with exercise after myocardial infarction. Circulation 80:234, 1989.

144. AMA-Council on Scientific Affairs. Physician-supervised exercise programs in rehabilitation of patients with coronary heart disease. JAMA 245:1463, 1981.

145. Greenland, P., and Chu, J. S.: Efficacy of cardiac rehabilitation services. With emphasis on patients after myocardial infarction. Ann. Intern. Med. 109:650, 1988.

146. U.S. Department of Health and Human Services: Health Technology Assessment Reports, 1987. Cardiac Rehabilitation Services DHHS Publication No. (PHS) 88-3427. Rockville, Md.: National Center for Health Services Research and Health Care Technology Assessment.

147. Dennis, C. A., Houston-Miller, N., Schwartz, R. G., et al.: Early return to work after uncomplicated myocardial infarction: Results of a randomized trial. JAMA 260:214, 1988.

148. Picard, M. H., Dennis, C., Schwartz, R. G., et al.: Cost-benefit analysis of early return to work after uncomplicated acute myocardial infarction. Am. J. Cardiol. 63:1308, 1989.

149. Bor, D. H., and Himmelstein, D. U.: Endocarditis prophylaxis for patients with mitral valve prolapse. A quantitative analysis. Am. J. Med. 76:711, 1984.

150. Clemens, J. D., and Ransohoff, D. F.: A quantitative assessment of predental antibiotic prophylaxis for patients with mitral valve prolapse. J. Chron. Dis. 37:531, 1984.

151. Clemens, J. D., Horwitz, R. I., Jaffe, C. C., et al.: A controlled evaluation of the risk of bacterial endocarditis in persons with mitral valve prolapse. N. Engl. J. Med. 307:776, 1982.

152. Mills, P., Rose, J., Hollingsworth, J., et al.: Long-term prognosis of mitral valve prolapse. N. Engl. J. Med. 297:13, 1977.

153. Eisenberg, M. S., Bergner, L., and Hallstrom, A.: Out-of-hospital cardiac arrest: Improved survival with paramedic services. Lancet 1:812, 1980.

154. Kellerman, A. L., Hackman, H. B., and Somes, G.: Dispatcher-assisted cardiopulmonary resuscitation—validation of efficacy. Circulation 80:1231, 1989.

155. Crampton, R. S., Aldrich, R. F., Gascho, J. A., et al.: Reduction of prehospital, ambulance, and community coronary death rates by the community-wide emergency cardiac care system. Am. J. Med. 58:151, 1975.

156. Eisenberg, M. S., Hallstrom, A., and Bergner, L.: Long-term survival after out-of-hospital arrest. N. Engl. J. Med. 306:1340, 1982.

157. Cummins, R. O., and Eisenberg, M. S.: Prehospital cardiopulmonary resuscitation: Is it effective? JAMA 253:2408, 1985.

158. Urban, N., Bergner, L., and Eisenberg, M. S.: The costs of a suburban paramedic program in reducing deaths due to cardiac arrest. Med. Care 19:379, 1981.

159. Hill, J. D., Hampton, J. R., and Mitchell, J. R. A.: A randomized trial of home-versus-hospital management for patients with suspected myocardial infarction. Lancet 1:837, 1978.

160. Mather, H. G., Morgan, D. C., Pearson, N. G., et al.: Myocardial infarction: A comparison between home and hospital care for patients. Br. Med. J. 1:925, 1976.

161. Goldman, L.: Coronary care units: A perspective on their epidemiologic impact. Int. J. Cardiol. 2:284, 1982.

162. Lee, T. H., Rouan, G., Weisberg, M. C., et al: Clinical characteristics and natural history of patients with acute myocardial infarction sent home from the emergency room. Am. J. Cardiol. 60:219, 1987.

163. Goldman, L., and Batsford, W. P.: Risk-benefit stratification as a guide to lidocaine prophylaxis of primary ventricular fibrillation in acute myocardial infarction: An analytic review. Yale J. Biol. Med. 52:455, 1979.

164. Gillum, R. F., Folsom, A., Leupker, R. V., et al.: Sudden death and acute myocardial infarction in a metropolitan area, 1970-1980: The Minnesota Heart Survey. N. Engl. J. Med. 309:1353, 1983.

165. Goldman, L., Cook, F., Hashimoto, B., et al.: Evidence that hospital care for acute myocardial infarction has not contributed to the decline in coronary mortality between 1973–1974 and 1978–1979. Circulation 65:936, 1982.

166. Pell, S., and Fayerweather, M. P. H.: Trends in the incidence of myocardial infarction and in associated mortality and morbidity in a large employed population, 1957–1983. N. Engl. J. Med. 312:1005, 1985.

167. Kennedy, J. W., Martin, G. V., Davis, K. B., et al.: The Western Washington intravenous streptokinase in acute myocardial infarction randomized trial. Circulation 77:345, 1988.

168. ISIS-2 (Second International Study of Infarct Survival) Collaborative Group: Randomised trial of intravenous streptokinase, oral aspirin, both, or neither among 17,187 cases of suspected acute myocardial infarction: ISIS-2. Lancet 2:349, 1988.

169. AIMS Trial Study Group: Long-term effects of intravenous anistreplase in acute myocardial infarction: Final report of the AIMS study. Lancet 1:427, 1990.

170. Mauri, F., Gasparini, M., Barbonaglia, L., et al.: Prognostic significance of the extent of myocardial injury in acute myocardial infarction treated by streptokinase (the GISSI Trial). Am. J. Cardiol. 63:1291, 1989.

171. Dalen, J. E., Gore, J. M., Braunwald, E., et al.: Six- and twelve-month follow-up of the phase I thrombolysis in myocardial infarction (TIMI) trial. Am. J. Cardiol. 62:179, 1988.

172. White, H. D., Rivers, J. T., Maslowski, A. H., et al.: Effect of intravenous streptokinase as compared with that of tissue plasminogen activator on left ventricular function after first myocardial infarction. N. Engl. J. Med. 320:817, 1989.

173. Lee, T. H., Weisberg, M. C., Brand, D. A., et al.: Candidates for thrombolysis among emergency room patients with acute chest pain. Ann. Intern. Med. 110:957, 1989.

174. Maynard, C., Althouse, R., Olsufka, M., et al.: Early versus late hospital arrival for acute myocardial infarction in the western Washington thrombolytic therapy trials. Am. J. Cardiol. 63:1296, 1989.

175. Hlatky, M. A., Cotugno, H., O'Connor, C., et al.: Adoption of thrombolytic therapy in the management of acute myocardial infarction. Am. J. Cardiol. 61:510, 1988.

176. Collen, D.: Coronary thrombolysis: Streptokinase or recombinant tissue-type plasminogen activator? Ann. Intern. Med. 112:529, 1990.

177. Braunwald, E.: Thrombolytic reperfusion of acute myocardial infarction: Resolved and unresolved issues. J. Am. Coll. Cardiol. 12:85A, 1988.

178. The TIMI Study Group: Comparison of invasive and conservative strategies after treatment with intravenous tissue plasminogen activator in acute myocardial infarction: Results of the Thrombolysis in Myocardial Infarction (TIMI) Phase II Trial. N. Engl. J. Med. 320:618, 1989.

179. Laffel, G. L., Fineberg, H. V., and Braunwald, E.: A cost-effectiveness model for coronary thrombolysis/reperfusion therapy. J. Am. Coll. Cardiol. 10:79B, 1987.

180. Steinberg, E. P., Topol, E. J., Sakin, J. W., et al.: Cost and procedure implications of thrombolytic therapy for acute myocardial infarction. J. Am. Coll. Cardiol. 23:58A, 1988.

181. Feibach, N. H., Cook, E. F., Lee, T. H., et al.: Outcomes in patients with myocardial infarction who are initially admitted to stepdown units: Data from the Multicenter Chest Pain Study. Am. J. Med. 89:15, 1990.

182. Lee, T. H., Rouan, G. W., Weisberg, M. C., et al.: Sensitivity of routine clinical criteria for diagnosing myocardial infarction within 24 hours of hospitalization. Ann. Intern. Med. 106:181, 1987.

183. Mulley, A. G., Thibault, G. E., Hughes, R. A., et al.: The course of patients with suspected myocardial infarction: The identification of low-risk patients for early transfer from intensive care. N. Engl. J. Med. *302*:943, 1980.

184. Singer, D. E., Carr, P. L., Mulley, A. G., and Thibault, G. E.: Rationing intensive care—physician responses to a resource shortage. N. Engl. J. Med. *309*:1155, 1983.

185. Beta-Blocker Heart Attack Trial Research Group: A randomized trial of propranolol in patients with acute myocardial infarction. I. Mortality results. J.A.M.A. *247*:1707, 1982.

186. Norwegian Multicenter Study Group: Timolol-induced reduction in mortality and reinfarction in patients surviving acute myocardial infarction. N. Engl. J. Med. *304*:801, 1981.

187. Hansteen, V., Moinichen, E., Lorensten, E., et al.: One year's treatment with propranolol after myocardial infarction: Preliminary report of Norwegian Multicentre Trial. Br. Med. J. *284*:155, 1982.

188. Multicentre International Study: Improvement in prognosis of myocardial infarction by long-term beta-adrenoreceptor blockade using practolol. Br. Med. J. *3*:735, 1975.

189. Multicentre International Study: Reduction in mortality after myocardial infarction with long-term beta-adrenoceptor blockade. Br. Med. J. *2*:419, 1977.

190. Yusuf, S., Peto, R., Lewis, J., et al.: Beta blockade during and after myocardial infarction: An overview of the randomized trials. Prog. Cardiovasc. Dis. *27*:335, 1985.

191. Alhmark, G., and Saetre, H.: Long-term treatment with beta blockers after myocardial infarction. Eur. J. Clin. Pharmacol. *10*:77, 1976.

192. Australian and Swedish Pindolol Study Group: The effect of pindolol on the two years mortality after complicated myocardial infarction. Eur. Heart J. *4*:367, 1983.

193. Rehnqvist, N., and Olsson, G.: Influence on ventricular arrhythmias by chronic postinfarction treatment with metoprolol. Circulation *68*:III-369, 1983.

194. Wilhelmsson, C., Vedin, J. A., Wilhelmsen, L., et al.: Reduction of sudden deaths after myocardial infarction by treatment with alprenolol. Preliminary results. Lancet *2*:1157, 1974.

195. Pedersen, T. R., and the Norwegian Multicenter Study Group: Six-year follow-up of the Norwegian Multicenter Study on timolol after acute myocardial infarction. N. Engl. J. Med. *313*:1055, 1985.

196. Goldman, L., Sia, S.T.B., Cook, E. F., et al.: Cost-effectiveness of routine long-term beta-adrenergic antagonist therapy following acute myocardial infarction. N. Engl. J. Med. *319*:152, 1988.

197. Takaro, T., Hultgren, H. N., Lipton, M. J., et al.: The VA cooperative randomized study of surgery for coronary arterial occlusive disease. II. Subgroup with significant left main lesions. Circulation *54*(Suppl. III):107, 1976.

198. The Veterans Administration Coronary Artery Bypass Surgery Cooperative Study Group: Eleven-year survival in the Veterans Administration randomized trial of coronary artery bypass surgery for stable angina. N. Engl. J. Med. *311*:1333, 1984.

199. Passamani, E., Davis, K. B., Gillispie, M. J., et al.: A randomized trial of coronary artery bypass surgery. Survival of patients with a low ejection fraction. N. Engl. J. Med. *312*:1665, 1985.

200. European Coronary Surgery Study Group: Prospective randomized study of coronary artery bypass surgery in stable angina pectoris: A progress report on survival. Circulation *65*(Suppl. II):67, 1982.

201. Varnauskas, E., and the European Coronary Surgery Study Group: Twelve-year follow-up of survival in the randomized European coronary surgery study. N. Engl. J. Med. *319*:332, 1988.

202. Cameron, A., Kemp, H. G., and Green, G. E.: Bypass surgery with the internal mammary artery graft: 15 year follow-up. Circulation *74*(Suppl. III):30, 1986.

203. CASS Principal Investigators and their Associates: A randomized trial of coronary artery bypass surgery: Quality of life in patients randomly assigned to treatment groups. Circulation *68*:951, 1983.

204. Charles, E. C., Wayne, J. B., Oberman, A., et al.: Costs and benefits associated with treatment for coronary artery disease. Circulation *66*(Suppl. III):87, 1982.

205. Varnauskas, E., and the European Coronary Surgery Study Group: Survival, myocardial infarction, and employment status in a prospective randomized study of coronary bypass surgery. Circulation *72*(Suppl. V):90, 1985.

206. Kornfeld, D. S., Heller, S. S., Frank, K. A., et al.: Psychological and behavioral responses after coronary artery bypass surgery. Circulation *66*(Suppl. III):24, 1982.

207. Weinstein, M. C., and Stason, W. B.: Cost-effectiveness of coronary artery bypass surgery. Circulation *66*(Suppl. III):56, 1982.

208. Hemenway, D., Sherman, H., Mudge, G. H. Jr., et al.: Comparative costs versus symptomatic and employment benefits of medical versus surgical treatment of stable angina pectoris. Med. Care *23*:133, 1985.

209. Weintraub, W. S., Jones, E. L., Craver, J., et al.: Determinants of prolonged length of hospital stay after coronary bypass surgery. Circulation *80*:276, 1989.

210. Taylor, G. J., Mikell, F. L., Moses, H. W., et al.: Determinants of hospital charges for coronary artery bypass surgery: The economic consequences of postoperative complications. Am. J. Cardiol. *65*:309, 1990.

211. Cromwell, J., Mitchell, J. B., and Stason, W. B.: Learning by doing in CABG surgery. Med. Care *28*:6, 1990.

212. Williams, A.: Economics of coronary artery bypass grafting. Br. Med. J. *291*:326, 1985.

213. Graboys, T. B., Headley, A., Lown, B., et al.: Results of a second opinion program for coronary artery bypass graft surgery. JAMA *258*:1611, 1987.

214. Reeder, G. S., Krishan, I., Nobrega, F. T., et al.: Is percutaneous coronary angioplasty less expensive than bypass surgery? N. Engl. J. Med. *311*:1157, 1984.

215. Jang, G. C., Block, P. C., Cowley, M. J., et al.: Relative cost of coronary angioplasty and bypass surgery in a one-vessel disease model. Am. J. Cardiol. *53*:52C, 1984.

216. Kelly, M. E., Taylor, G. J., Moses, H. W., et al.: Comparative cost of myocardial revascularization: Percutaneous transluminal angioplasty and coronary artery bypass surgery. J. Am. Coll. Cardiol. *5*:16, 1985.

217. Wilson, J. M., Dunn, E. J., Wright, C. B., et al.: The cost of simultaneous surgical standby for percutaneous transluminal coronary angioplasty. J. Thorac. Cardiovasc. Surg. *91*:362, 1986.

218. Goldman, L., and Cook, E. F.: The decline in ischemic heart disease mortality rates. An analysis of the comparative effects of medical interventions and changes in lifestyle. Ann. Intern. Med. *101*:825, 1984.

219. Sytkowski, P. A., Kannel, W. B., and D'Agostino, R. B.: Changes in risk factors and the decline in mortality from cardiovascular disease: The Framingham Heart Study. N. Engl. J. Med. *322*:1635, 1990.

220. Cohn, B. A., Kaplan, G. A., and Cohen, R. D.: Did early detection and treatment contribute to the decline in ischemic heart disease mortality? Prospective evidence from the Alameda County Study. Am. J. Epidemiol. *127*:1143, 1988.

221. Kaplan, G. A., Cohen, B. A., Cohen, R. D., and Guralnik, J.: The decline in ischemic heart disease mortality: Prospective evidence from the Alameda County Study. Am. J. Epidemiol. *127*:1131, 1988.

PART V

HEART DISEASE AND DISORDERS OF OTHER ORGAN SYSTEMS

55

General Anesthesia and Noncardiac Surgery in Patients With Heart Disease

by LEE GOLDMAN, M.D., and EUGENE BRAUNWALD, M.D.

The cardiovascular system of patients undergoing general anesthesia and noncardiac surgical procedures is subject to multiple stresses owing to depression of myocardial contractility and respiration as well as fluctuations in temperature, arterial pressure, ventricular filling pressures, blood volume, and activity of the autonomic nervous system. Complications of anesthesia and operation, such as hemorrhage, infection, fever, pulmonary embolism, and myocardial infarction, impose additional burdens on the cardiovascular system. The patient with cardiac disease who is compensated preoperatively may be unable to meet these increased demands during the perioperative period, in which case arrhythmias, myocardial ischemia, and/or heart failure may develop.[1,2] As a consequence, a substantial proportion of all deaths in most series of noncardiac operations results from cardiovascular complications.

Because both the frequency and the seriousness of cardiovascular complications of general anesthesia and operation are considerably increased in the patient with known cardiovascular disease, the magnitude of these risks must be appreciated to decide on the advisability of noncardiac surgery in the cardiac patient. In addition, both the life expectancy and the quality of life of the patient must be taken into account. For instance, a noncardiac surgical procedure with a high risk, directed to correct a disorder which is not life threatening, may be difficult to justify if the patient's cardiac condition precludes a survival period sufficient to allow the patient to reap the benefits of the operation. Obviously the dangers and disability of the disease for which an operation is being proposed must also be balanced against the risk of the operation itself.

ANESTHESIA

Changes in cardiovascular function during general anesthesia are due to many factors, including direct effects of the anesthetic agent(s) and indirect effects mediated primarily through the autonomic nervous system. In addition, if respiration is inadequately maintained, the resulting hypoxemia, hypercarbia, and acidosis may further depress myocardial contractility and increase cardiac irritability. The interplay of these several variables may produce changes in arterial and central venous pressures, cardiac output, and rate and rhythm. To minimize the risk of operation in the patient with a compromised cardiovascular system, it is essential to minimize these changes.[3]

The choice of the anesthetic approach and the specific anesthetic agents to be used should be made by a qualified anesthesiologist, commonly after careful evaluation of the patient's medical and cardiac condition and often after consultation with the surgeon and the internist or cardiologist. Different anesthesiologists may have preferences for different anesthetic techniques, and the anesthesiological literature clearly indicates that there is little, if any, correlation between the anesthetic route or agents and the likelihood of major clinical complications. Thus, it is the skill and experience of the anesthesiologist, including the ability to monitor hemodynamics and respond quickly, that are far more important than the specific agent that is used. While the cardiological consultant should not expect to dictate the anesthetic approach, the quality of the consultation will be improved if the consultant appreciates the clinical pharmacology of the anesthetic agents and the effects of intubation and extubation.

GENERAL ANESTHESIA

The induction of anesthesia is usually accomplished with intravenous anesthetics. With the exception of ketamine, the agents used for the induction of anesthesia commonly lower systemic arterial pressure by about 20 to 30 per cent in healthy patients, but sometimes by a greater amount in hypertensive patients.[4] During laryngoscopy and tracheal intubation, blood pressure commonly increases by 20 to 30 mm Hg, but it may increase even more in the hypertensive patient,[4] in whom these changes in blood pressure may be associated with electrocardiographic evidence of myocardial ischemia.[5,6] Much of this hypertensive response can be avoided by adequate topical anesthesia of the upper airways, larynx, and trachea, or by blind nasal intubation because the hypertension appears to be caused by the laryngoscopy rather than by the passage of a tube into the trachea.

INHALATION AGENTS. These agents enter the bloodstream by way of the alveoli and are excreted across the alveoli essentially unchanged. In most major operations a combination of inhalation agents and/or intravenous anesthetics is used.[3,7]

Nitrous oxide usually causes a modest decrease of about 15 per cent in cardiac output but usually does not cause substantial hypotension because of reflex vasoconstriction (Table 55–1). Unfortunately, in many patients it is impossible to achieve full anesthesia with concentrations of nitrous oxide that also permit adequate oxygenation.

Halothane and related agents also cause a reduction in myocardial contractility,[8] but unlike nitrous oxide, they are not associated with substantial reflex vasoconstriction. Thus, when halothane is added to nitrous oxide, there are often further reductions in arterial pressure because of reductions in cardiac output without concomitant vasoconstriction.[5] Halothane also appears to sensitize the myocardium to catecholamines, sometimes resulting in arrhythmias. *Enflurane* has properties similar to halothane but appears to result in less sensitization to catecholamines. *Isoflurane* appears to have less of a negative inotropic effect than halothane or enflurane, but it can be associated with marked decreases in systemic vascular resistance, and hence a fall in systemic blood pressure.

INTRAVENOUS ANESTHETICS. Among the narcotic analgesics, *morphine* is generally well tolerated, although it does cause venodilation, thereby decreasing preload and cardiac output. *Fentanyl* is less likely to cause as much hypotension or vasodilation as morphine, and it has a shorter duration of action. Like morphine, it tends not to have major effects on myocardial contractility, but it is more likely than morphine to cause bradycardia. *Sufentanil* and *alfentanil* have cardiovascular effects that are generally similar to those of fentanyl.

Short-acting barbiturates, especially *thiopental*, often cause a fall in blood pressure because of depressive actions on myocardial contractility and sympathetic tone. In patients who have severe hypovolemia or severe cardiac dysfunction, serious reductions in cardiac output can occasionally occur after a small dose of thiopental.

Benzodiazepines can achieve adequate sedation with only mild cardiovascular depression. However, occasionally patients may become apneic or hypotensive after small doses. *Droperidol* causes vasodilation because of its alpha-adrenergic blocking action and its effect on the central nervous system.

Ketamine is unlike other commonly used intravenous anesthetics in that it does not cause cardiovascular depression. Although it may cause minimal direct myocardial depressant activity, this is commonly counterbalanced by an increase in circulating catecholamines.

MUSCLE RELAXANTS. Drugs used for muscle relaxation also may have cardiovascular effects. *Succinylcholine* can cause bradycardia, which can be reversed or prevented by the administration of atropine. In patients anesthetized with halothane, *pancuronium* and *gallamine* cause an increase in heart rate, arterial pressure, and cardiac output, while *tubocurarine* and *metocurine* result in a fall in mean arterial pressure with mild elevations in heart rate and little, if any, change in cardiac output. *Vecuronium* has essentially no cardiovascular side effects.

SPINAL AND EPIDURAL ANESTHESIA

Spinal and epidural anesthesia cause sympathetic denervation, which produces peripheral arteriodilation and venodilation. Systemic vascular resistance may be reduced by 10 to 15 per cent. Venodilation may cause a marked reduction in right ventricular preload as a consequence of sympathetic denervation. Under these circumstances, right ventricular preload depends critically on the effects of gravity on the patient's position, and on the total blood volume (Fig. 13–35, p. 378).

REGIONAL AND LOCAL ANESTHESIA. Regional and local anesthesia cause cardiovascular effects only to the extent that the agents are absorbed into the bloodstream or where there is sympathetic blockade accompanying the local sensory block. A major concern with local or regional anesthesia is whether the technique is adequate for the planned procedure; the cardiological consultant should not underestimate the cardiovascular consequences of inadequate anesthesia.

TABLE 55–1 CARDIOVASCULAR CHANGES WITH NITROUS OXIDE AND AFTER ITS ADDITION TO PREEXISTING GENERAL ANESTHETICS

	EFFECT			
MEASUREMENT	NITROUS OXIDE	NITROUS OXIDE–HALOTHANE	NITROUS OXIDE–ENFLURANE	NITROUS OXIDE–MORPHINE
Blood pressure	None	Increased	None	None
Heart rate	Decreased	None	Decreased	Decreased
Cardiac output	Decreased	None	Increased	Decreased
Systemic vascular resistance	Increased	Increased	None	Increased
Central venous pressure	Increased	Increased	None	Increased

From Tarhan, S. (ed.): Cardiovascular Anesthesia and Postoperative Care. Chicago, Year Book Medical Publishers, 1982. Copyright © 1982 by Year Book Medical Publishers, Inc., Chicago.

One study of 53 patients suggested that epidural anesthesia and postoperative analgesia were preferable to standard general anesthesia for high-risk surgical patients.[9] At the present time, however, the potential benefit of regional anesthesia compared to general anesthesia is uncertain,[10-12] in part because the decline in systemic blood pressure from regional anesthesia can cause transient myocardial ischemia.[13] Postoperative epidural analgesia can attenuate sympathetic nervous system hyperactivity, reduce the need for parenteral analgesia, and may be of benefit for patients with coronary artery disease.[14,15]

INTRAOPERATIVE HEMODYNAMICS AND ARRHYTHMIAS

During the operative procedure, it is not uncommon for systolic blood pressure to fall into the range of 95 to 105 mm Hg. Such blood pressure reductions are often brief and may respond to a lightening of the anesthesia or, in 20 to 30 per cent of patients, either to a brisk fluid challenge or the use of intravenous sympathomimetic agents. Any severe reduction in arterial pressure in patients with ischemic heart disease can reduce coronary flow and precipitate myocardial ischemia. In general, such reductions in blood pressure are not associated with major cardiac complications, such as myocardial infarction, unless they are marked and sustained. For example, increased complication rates have been reported for reductions in systolic arterial pressures that exceed approximately 33 per cent of the preoperative blood pressure and that persist for 10 or more minutes, or are more than 50 per cent below the preoperative blood pressure, or for mean arterial pressure reductions of 20 mm Hg or greater for 60 or more minutes, or for 20-mm Hg increases in mean arterial pressure sustained for 15 or more minutes.[16-19] Fluids that are administered to maintain intraoperative blood pressure can potentially cause postoperative fluid overload.

The risk of unplanned intraoperative hypotension is at least as great with spinal or epidural anesthesia as with general anesthesia.[20] However, because spinal and epidural anesthesia are not direct myocardial depressants, they may be advantageous in patients with severe myocardial dysfunction; but even in those circumstances, well-balanced general anesthesia, sometimes including ketamine, has been used successfully.

Transient bradycardias, such as sinus bradycardia and junctional rhythm, may occur during periods of vagal stimulation. These bradyarrhythmias commonly respond to a lightening of the anesthesia or to the administration of atropine or beta$_1$-adrenoceptor agonists such as isoproterenol or epinephrine. Tachyarrhythmias may result from hypovolemia or vasodilation as well as from sensitization of the myocardium to catecholamines that are circulating and/or released by sympathetic nerve endings in the heart. Tachycardia is poorly tolerated by patients with mitral stenosis (p. 1007) and may cause myocardial ischemia in patients with coronary artery disease. Therapy with specific antiarrhythmic medications is usually indicated only when the arrhythmia causes circulatory compromise and does not respond to changes in the depth of anesthesia or to attention to problems such as hypoxemia, hypovolemia, hypotension, or the potentially precipitating surgical manipulation.

Positive-pressure ventilation during general anesthesia reduces the return of blood to the right side of the heart and tends to reduce ventricular preload. Fluid that is administered during positive-pressure ventilation will not increase preload to the extent that it would in the patient who is ventilating spontaneously. When the positive-pressure ventilation of general anesthesia ceases, ventricular preload increases, often abruptly, and hypertension or pulmonary congestion may result. Analogous physiological changes can occur with the cessation of spinal or epidural anesthesia because the venodilation caused by these agents also reduces right ventricular preload.

MONITORING. In patients with severe underlying heart disease undergoing noncardiac surgery, it is mandatory to monitor cardiac function during anesthesia,[21] including cardiac rate and rhythm and directly recorded arterial blood pressure. A radial artery line permits not only monitoring of intraarterial pressure but also frequent sampling for determination of blood gases. In the presence of peripheral vasoconstriction, indirect (cuff) blood pressure measurements may greatly underestimate true arterial pressure. Monitoring of the pulmonary artery (or, preferably, pulmonary artery wedge) pressure and cardiac output is often desirable in patients who are critically ill, who have marginal cardiovascular reserve, who are to undergo prolonged operative procedures in which major blood losses might occur, and in whom hypotensive anesthesia is to be used. Both pulmonary artery wedge pressure and cardiac output can be measured with the aid of a multiple-lumen balloon flotation catheter (Swan-Ganz) and the thermodilution method (Chap. 7). For detection of intraoperative myocardial ischemia, transesophageal echocardiography is about as accurate as 12-lead electrocardiography, and both are preferable to the monitoring of only one or two electrocardiographic leads.[22] Pulmonary capillary wedge pressure is a poor marker of ischemia, but the pulmonary capillary wedge pressure remains the best index of fluid balance.[23] In seriously ill patients, urine output should be monitored with a Foley catheter.

THE OPERATION

Just as consultant cardiologists must understand the pharmacological effects of anesthesia, they must also recognize the physiological effects of surgery, including the direct consequences of the operation and the expected responses to postoperative recuperation.

NATURE OF THE OPERATION. Although ophthalmological surgery[24] and transurethral prostatic resection[25] are almost always safe, even in patients with a history of serious cardiac disease, general surgical mortality is often 25 to 50 per cent higher in patients with underlying cardiovascular conditions than in patients with normal cardiac function.[17,20,26-29] Among noncardiac surgical procedures, the highest cardiovascular complication rates are commonly associated with abdominal aortic aneurysm surgery,[26,30] which causes substantial myocardial stress because of aortic cross-clamping and major shifts in fluid and electrolytes. The risk of cardiac complications is also higher in other major abdominal and thoracic procedures than in procedures on the extremities, in large part because of the more difficult postoperative course. Patients who undergo operation for aortic aneurysm, carotid arterial disease, or peripheral vascular disease often have substantial coronary artery disease as well, and the extent of the latter may be underestimated because of the limitations caused by the peripheral arterial disease.

DURATION. The risk of cardiovascular mortality and morbidity is generally correlated with the duration of anesthesia, but this is principally because the longest operations are more often on the aorta or in the abdomen or chest than on the extremities. In most series[20,28,29] the risk of major cardiovascular complications did not correlate with the duration of surgery after controlling for the type of surgery. However, if the operation is prolonged because of intraoperative complications, it would be expected that the risk of postoperative cardiovascular complications might increase, especially among patients with a prior myocardial infarction[17] or in situations in which the operation takes longer than 5 hours.[20]

EMERGENCY OPERATION. When an operation is carried out under emergency conditions, it is associated with greatly increased mortality in patients with cardiovascular disease. The risk of postoperative cardiac complications, including postoperative myocardial infarction or cardiac death, is increased anywhere from 2.5- to 4-fold in emergency compared with elective surgery.[20,26,28,29] Part of this increased risk is because patients undergoing emergency operations may often have poorly controlled or unappreciated general medical problems, such as fluid and electrolyte imbalance or hepatic dysfunction.[26,28] However, emergency surgery appears to be an important correlate of postoperative complications, even after controlling for the underlying medical disease.[26,28,31]

The application of invasive hemodynamic monitoring to noncardiac surgical procedures in patients with underlying heart disease may reduce the risk of intraoperative and postoperative cardiovascular complications. Thus the risk of a new infarction was reduced from 7.7 to 1.9 per cent when patients with a history of infarction were aggressively monitored during the period from 1977 to 1982 compared with when minimal invasive monitoring was used in the period from 1973 to 1976.[32] Although this nonrandomized study did not control for other secular changes in medical care, it should not be surprising that the application of cardiovascular anesthesiological techniques to noncardiac surgery would have a beneficial effect. Thus, in patients who have suffered a myocardial infarction within the past 3 months, who have angina that is more severe than Canadian Class II (p. 11, 12), who have severe heart failure, or who are at high risk based on indices such as the multifactorial index of cardiac risk in noncardiac surgery[26,28,33-35] (p. 1717), available data support the use of intraarterial and pulmonary artery catheters for careful hemodynamic monitoring. In general, arterial and pulmonary artery pressure should not be allowed to fluctuate by more than 20 per cent of the preinduction values for longer than 5 minutes. For patients with a recent myocardial infarction or severe angina, careful monitoring should usually extend into the postoperative period, usually for at least 24 hours.[32]

INFLUENCE OF UNDERLYING CARDIOVASCULAR DISEASE

ISCHEMIC HEART DISEASE

ASSESSMENT OF RISK

Clinical. Ischemic heart disease is a major determinant of perioperative morbidity and mortality. The incidence of perioperative myocardial infarction is increased 10- to 50-fold in patients who have previously suffered infarcts compared with patients who do not have a clinical history of coronary disease.

During the 1970's, several studies reported about a 30 per cent risk of reinfarction or cardiac death when patients were operated on within 3 months of the previous myocardial infarction, about a 15 per cent risk when the operation was performed 3 to 6 months after a prior infarction, and about a 5 per cent risk when the operation was performed more than 6 months after the infarction.[9,20] However, recent data suggest that the application of invasive hemodynamic monitoring and careful regulation of oxygenation, electrolytes, volume status, and the hematocrit have markedly reduced the complication rate. For example, Wells and Kaplan[36] reported no reinfarctions in 48 patients who were operated on within 3 months after a myocardial infarction, while Rao et al.[32] reported only a 6 per cent reinfarction rate within 3 months after preoperative myocardial infarction and only a 2 per cent reinfarction rate between 3 and 6 months after a myocardial infarction.

Obviously, truly life-saving procedures must be performed almost regardless of the cardiac risk, and purely elective surgery should commonly be delayed for 6 months after infarction, when the cardiovascular risks will have returned to a stable, long-term baseline risk. The more difficult issue is in patients in whom the operation is not truly emergent but is also not purely elective, for example, a patient with severe symptomatic peripheral vascular disease or a patient with a potentially resectable malignant tumor. In such situations one would like to delay operation sufficiently long for cardiac risk to be reduced but not wait a full 6 months. Because full healing of a myocardial infarction usually takes about 4 to 6 weeks, one rational approach is to evaluate the patient with postmyocardial infarction prognostic studies, such as a submaximal exercise tolerance test,[37] and to use the patient's clinical and cardiological conditions as the guide for surgery sometime between 4 weeks and 3 months after the infarction.

A recent preoperative myocardial infarction will increase a patient's relative risk of reinfarction with operation, but the absolute risk depends on a variety of factors in addition to the timing of the infarction. In general, one should be influenced less by whether or not a preoperative myocardial infarction was associated with the development of new Q waves than by the state of left ventricular function and the severity of preoperative angina. Thus, patients who have good exercise tolerance and left ventricular function after infarction and who can resume normal activity levels within 4 to 6 weeks after infarction should be able to undergo operation with relatively small absolute risks, even if their relative risk might be slightly lower if one could wait the full 6 months. By comparison, risks are likely to be substantially higher in patients who have postinfarction angina, large reversible defects on thallium scintigraphy, reduced left ventricular function, marked ST-segment depression with exercise, or other evidence of easily provokable ischemia (p. 1270).

When the patient with angina pectoris is evaluated, the patient's current (preoperative) exercise tolerance should be ascertained and an assessment made as to whether the anginal pattern is stable or unstable (p. 1293). Patients who are Class II by the criteria of the Canadian Cardiovascular Society[38] or the Specific Activity Scale[39,40] can carry objects such as two grocery bags or a young child up a flight of stairs without stopping and without appreciable symptoms. In such patients most surgical procedures are generally well tolerated. Physicians should avoid relying on the *frequency* of angina because patients who voluntarily reduce their activity level may also greatly reduce their symptoms.[40] This phenomenon is especially true in patients whose surgical conditions, such as orthopedic disorders or peripheral vascular disease, limit ambulation.

Laboratory. *Exercise treadmill testing* is an objective means for assessing exercise tolerance and is especially beneficial if the history is unreliable. Unfortunately, the limited sensitivity and specificity of standard electrocardiographic exercise tolerance testing limit the use of this test for diagnosing coronary artery disease (see Chap. 6). In two studies of vascular surgery patients,[41,42] postoperative cardiac complications were significantly less in patients who exercised to higher heart rates and cardiac workloads. The prognostic value of limited exercise tolerance has also been reported in persons over age 65[43,44] in whom the inability to perform 2 minutes of bicycle exercise in a supine position and to raise the heart rate above 99 beats per minute was an independent important predictor of cardiac complications in noncardiac surgery. Of note was that poor exercise capacity was an independent predictor of cardiac complications, but electrocardiographic changes with exercise were not. Although some investigators have used radionuclide ventriculography to predict risk,[45] in other studies data from resting and exercise radionuclide ventriculography did not add important independent information for predicting perioperative cardiac risk.[43,46-48]

In patients who are unable to exercise because of noncardiac disability (e.g., intermittent claudication or orthopedic abnormalities), ambulatory ischemia monitoring and dipyridamole thallium imaging can be used to assess perioperative risk. In one study of vascular surgery patients with normal resting electrocardiograms, the presence of ischemia on ambulatory electrocardiographic monitoring identified more than 90 per cent of patients who had major postoperative cardiac ischemic events.[49] More than one-third of the patients with preoperative ambulatory ischemia had major events. In this study[49] and another report,[50] ambulatory ischemia was a statistically significant independent correlate of major postoperative ischemic events, but asymptomatic postoperative ischemia appears to be an even better predictor of clinical postoperative ischemic events.[50a-c]

Dipyridamole thallium imaging has also been successful in identifying high-risk patients among selected subgroups undergoing vascular surgery, and it is especially appealing for patients who have abnormal resting electrocardiograms or are taking medications such as digoxin that make electrocardiographic monitoring unreliable for the detection of ischemia.[51-55] In one study,[51] all eight postoperative ischemic events, including three myocardial infarctions, occurred in patients who had transient thallium defects precipitated by dipyridamole; there were no such events in 32 patients who had no fixed defects. Among the 16 patients with dipyridamole thallium defects, there were three myocardial infarctions and five additional patients who developed episodes of angina with ST-segment depression postoperatively. In one series, however, dipyridamole thallium imaging was not correlated with the risk of postoperative ischemic events.[56]

The utility of both ambulatory ischemia monitoring and dypyridamole thallium imaging can be improved when these techniques are used in appropriate patient subsets. For example, in patients who do not have Q waves on their electrocardiograms, are less than 70 years of age, and who do not have a history of angina, ventricular ectopic activity requiring treatment, or diabetes mellitus requiring treatment the risk of major postoperative events appears to be sufficiently low that neither technique should be used as a screening test.[49,53]

Patients who have undergone successful coronary revascularization can undergo major noncardiac surgical procedures with a low mortality rate,[21,57] except perhaps in the first 30 days postoperatively. In some circumstances both the coronary artery bypass operation and the noncardiac operation can be performed during the course of the same procedure. It must be remembered, however, that the operative mortality rate for major noncardiac surgery in patients with stable angina and good exercise tolerance is relatively low, usually in the range of 2 per cent. No randomized controlled trials are available to assess the value of coronary artery bypass grafting preoperatively in patients with stable angina pectoris who are about to undergo noncardiac surgery. An analysis of patients in the Coronary Artery Surgery Study registry[57] showed that total operative mortality was 2.4 per cent in 458 patients who had significant coronary artery disease and underwent noncardiac operations without prior coronary artery bypass grafting. By comparison, operative mortality was 0.9 per cent among 399 patients who had had a coronary artery bypass grafting procedure performed before noncardiac surgery. The mortality was higher in patients who had more severe left ventricular dysfunction or dyspnea on exertion and in patients who used nitrates, were older, and had diabetes. The risk of myocardial infarction, however, was not significantly different between the patients with and without preoperative coronary artery bypass grafting. Furthermore, if one considers the mortality associated with coronary artery bypass grafting, which was 1.4 per cent in the Coronary Artery Surgery Study, the overall mortality from combined coronary artery bypass grafting and noncardiac surgery (2.3 per cent) would be as high as for the noncardiac surgery done in the non-bypassed group (2.4 per cent). Thus the data do not argue in favor of prophylactic coronary artery bypass grafting for patients whose symptoms would not otherwise warrant revascularization, who have stable angina with good exercise tolerance, and who do not have other factors that define a high-risk status (see below).

A practical approach to the patient with known or suspected ischemic heart disease should utilize information from the history as well as diagnostic tests.[58-60] If the patient's history indicates reliably that Class I or Class II activities[38,40,61] can be performed, the patient will commonly be raising the double product (the heart rate multiplied by the systolic blood pressure) above the range to be expected with general anesthesia and surgery, and hence should be able to withstand the stress of the procedure. If the history is unreliable, exercise testing to assess physical function[41-44] will aid in risk assessment. If the patient is unable to exercise because of noncar-

diac conditions, ambulatory ischemia monitoring (in a patient with a normal resting electrocardiogram who is not receiving medication such as digoxin) or dypyridamole thallium imaging should be used unless the patient has no historical risk factors.[49,53]

Patients who can exercise to Class I or II levels, or who have normal ambulatory ischemia monitoring or normal dipyridamole thallium imaging, can undergo most operations with acceptable risk. Patients who cannot perform Class I or II activities or who have positive ambulatory ischemia monitoring or dypyridamole thallium images should have their medical regimens intensified, if possible, and then have repeat testing. If tests remain positive or physical functioning remains limited after optimization of medical management, coronary arteriography will usually be indicated prior to elective surgery to determine whether coronary revascularization, with either percutaneous transluminal coronary angioplasty or coronary bypass surgery, would be feasible. The decision to proceed with revascularization depends more on the functional limitations that result from the coronary lesions than on their anatomical severity. Although the latter is important for long-term prognosis, the former is probably the most relevant correlate of perioperative risk.

COMBINED CAROTID AND CORONARY ARTERY SURGERY. There is some controversy as to the indications for combined coronary revascularization and carotid endarterectomy in patients with coexisting coronary and carotid stenoses. It has been shown experimentally that carotid perfusion is maintained or increased during cardiopulmonary bypass,[62] thus suggesting that nonpulsatile cardiopulmonary bypass per se is unlikely to cause a stroke due to hypoperfusion. Most strokes that occur during coronary revascularization appear to be embolic in origin.[63] Combined coronary and carotid surgery can be performed at an acceptable risk,[64,65] but we recommend combined surgery only when there is severe bilateral or currently symptomatic carotid disease associated with unstable angina, left main coronary disease, or very symptomatic three-vessel coronary disease. If the coronary disease is stable and relatively mild but the carotid disease is symptomatic, the carotid surgery should be performed first and the coronary revascularization at a later date. If the carotid disease is and has always been asymptomatic and is not bilateral and severe, coronary revascularization can be performed without a proven need for prophylactic carotid surgery.[63,64]

USE OF BETA BLOCKERS AND CALCIUM ANTAGONISTS. Although some concern has been expressed about the use of general anesthesia in patients receiving beta-adrenoceptor blocking agents and calcium antagonists, there are no clinical data to indicate that such medications should routinely be discontinued preoperatively. For beta-adrenoceptor blocking agents, early concerns[66] about the safety of propranolol have been contradicted by substantial subsequent data demonstrating the safety of their use[67] and the dangers of discontinuing beta-adrenoceptor blocking agents preoperatively.[68] Propranolol appears to reduce the risk of severe hypertensive episodes and ischemic electrocardiographic responses to the stresses of intubation, anesthesia, and surgery.[69,70] In patients who rely on beta-adrenoceptor blocking agents for the control of severe angina, the medication should be continued up to and including the morning of operation with a small sip of water.[68] Postoperatively, the medication can be resumed orally or sometimes given through a nasogastric tube. However, intravenous propranolol, metoprolol, or esmolol should be used in patients with a prior history of severe angina that required beta-adrenoceptor blocking agents for its control or in patients who have evidence of postoperative myocardial ischemia or otherwise unexplained hypertension or tachycardia.

Propranolol can be given as a 1-mg intravenous bolus, which is repeated up to a total loading dose of 10 mg and followed by 1 mg intravenously every 20 to 60 minutes. The second option is a 5- to 10-mg loading dose given slowly over 60 minutes, followed by a continuous intravenous infusion of

0.01 to 0.05 mg/min.[71,72] Esmolol, an ultra-short-acting beta-adrenoceptor blocker, can be used in doses ranging from 100 to 300 μg/kg/min after a 500 μg/kg/min loading dose.[73] If the patient suffers side effects attributable to administration of a beta-adrenoceptor blocker, treatment should be instituted with isoproterenol or dobutamine, or with glucagon, if the others are not effective.

Nifedipine can be given sublingually, and nitrates can be given sublingually, topically, or intravenously, to aid in the management of the early postoperative patient with angina, but neither of these agents substitutes for beta-adrenoceptor blockers in patients who have relied on the latter for the control of their ischemic heart disease.

HYPERTENSION

Several studies have documented that patients with hypertension have higher risks of suffering major cardiac complications during or shortly after noncardiac operation than do patients who have always been normotensive. However, most, if not all, of this increased risk is because of the ischemic heart disease, left ventricular dysfunction, renal failure, or other abnormalities that often occur in patients with hypertension. Thus, in patients with mild to moderate hypertension, diastolic pressures below 100 mm Hg, and no evidence of serious end-organ damage, general anesthesia and major noncardiac surgery are generally well tolerated.[18] Halothane anesthesia may be more likely than other anesthetic agents to induce intraoperative hypotension in patients with a history of hypertension,[18] and hypertensive patients are at higher risk for labile blood pressures and for hypertensive episodes during surgery and especially just after extubation.

Although uncontrolled early studies suggested that the continuation of any hypertensive agents might increase the risk of perioperative hypotension, substantial subsequent data from more careful studies indicate that patients whose hypertension is well controlled will do at least as well, if not better, if their medications are, in fact, continued up to the time of operation.[5,18,74] Thus, although it is not mandatory to delay noncardiac operation for the weeks or months that may be required to achieve ideal blood pressure control in the stable patient with mild to moderate hypertension who has no complications of the hypertension, there is also no apparent benefit, and some potential harm, from discontinuing successful antihypertensive therapy before surgery.

Thiazide and other diuretics cause some degree of chronic volume depletion,[75] and patients receiving these drugs may require more fluid administration early during the operative procedure. Guanethidine causes depletion of norepinephrine at adrenergic nerve endings, and when hypotension develops in patients receiving these drugs and they require adrenergic agonists, direct-acting agents such as norepinephrine, methoxamine, or phenylephrine should be used rather than indirect-acting agents such as ephedrine. If severe perioperative hypertension develops in a patient who has previously been receiving clonidine, and if the clonidine cannot be given orally, it can be administered intramuscularly in doses about one-half as large as the patient's usual daily dose or it can be administered topically,[76] or the patient can be treated with sublingual captopril, with methyldopa, or with a beta blocker. Although it may be desirable to use propranolol, metoprolol, or esmolol intravenously in patients who rely on beta-adrenoceptor blockers for the control of ischemic heart disease, it is less often necessary to use such agents intravenously in patients who take these medications for their antihypertensive effects. Commonly, intravenous labetolol[77] or nitroprusside can be used for acute episodes of hypertension and methyldopa for nonacute situations.

Patients with valvular heart disease undergoing anesthesia and noncardiac operation are subject to many potential hazards: heart failure, infection, tachycardia, and embolization. As might be expected, patients with no or only mild limitation of activity (i.e., those in Class I or II[38-40]) tolerate operation well[78] and probably require little more than careful perioperative care and prophylaxis for infective endocarditis (p. 1097). Those with more serious impairment of cardiac reserve (i.e., those in Class III or IV) tolerate major noncardiac operations poorly, and their prognosis for surviving major surgery is distinctly worse,[20,29] although as is the case for patients with rheumatic heart disease who face the stress of pregnancy (p. 1796), the risk of operation depends on the functional state of the heart. Patients with symptomatic critical aortic[28] or mitral stenosis are especially prone to sudden death or acute pulmonary edema during the perioperative period; this may occur if demands on cardiac output are suddenly increased or if atrial fibrillation and a rapid ventricular rate are precipitated by anesthesia or operation. Every effort should be made to treat heart failure preoperatively. Patients with severe stenotic or regurgitant valve disease should undergo corrective valvular surgery before an elective operation, while those who require an emergency noncardiac operation may benefit from intraoperative hemodynamic monitoring, afterload reduction, and preload augmentation.[79] In some patients with mitral or aortic stenosis, balloon valvuloplasty (p. 1376) may offer relief of severe obstruction at a low risk when it might not be desirable to carry out valve replacement.[80]

HYPERTROPHIC CARDIOMYOPATHY. Patients with hypertrophic cardiomyopathy are intolerant of hypovolemia, which may lead to both a reduction in the elevated preload necessary to maintain cardiac output and an increase in the obstruction to left ventricular outflow (p. 1404). With careful perioperative, intraoperative, and postoperative care, however, the risk of major cardiac complications in such patients is small. In one series of 56 operations in patients with hypertrophic cardiomyopathy, there were no deaths and the only major complication was a myocardial infarction with congestive heart failure in a patient who also had underlying coronary artery disease. Intraoperative or postoperative hypotension requiring vasoconstrictors occurred in less than 10 per cent of patients.[81] It has been suggested that spinal anesthesia may be relatively contraindicated in patients with hypertrophic obstructive cardiomyopathy because of its tendency to reduce systemic vascular resistance and increase venous pooling and thereby increase the severity of obstruction to outflow.[81] Hemodynamic monitoring is not routinely required but may be helpful when these patients undergo major aortic, abdominal, or thoracic procedures.

PROSTHETIC HEART VALVES. Most patients with mechanical prosthetic heart valves receive anticoagulants on a long-term basis to prevent thromboembolic complications (p. 1062). If these medications are continued through the period of noncardiac operation, hemostasis, hematoma formation, and persistent postoperative bleeding may ensue. Anticoagulants can be temporarily discontinued during the perioperative period with minimal risk of thrombosis. In one study,[82] no thromboembolic complications occurred in 159 patients with prosthetic valves undergoing 180 noncardiac operations when warfarin was discontinued an average of 2.9 days preoperatively and resumed 2.7 days postoperatively.[82] Using a similar approach, Katholi et al. did not observe thromboembolic complications in 25 noncardiac operations on patients with prosthetic aortic valves[83]; however, two such complications occurred in the 10 patients with mitral valve prostheses when anticoagulants were discontinued for noncardiac operations, although these patients had Kay-Shiley caged-disc valves, which are associated with a somewhat higher risk of thromboembolic complications. Because there is a distinct risk of hemorrhagic complications in patients whose anticoagulants have been discontinued for only 2 or 3 days,[82] prothrombin time should be restored to within 20 per cent of normal before one proceeds with the noncardiac surgery.[84] Low molecular weight dextran can be used in the postoperative period to minimize thrombotic complications during the 2 to 3 days when the risk of hemorrhagic complications from resuming anticoagulation is relatively higher. In patients with prostheses that are at high risk for thrombosis, such as caged-disc valves, we recommend discontinuing warfarin, allowing the prothrombin time to come to within about 2 to 3 seconds of normal, using intravenous heparin until about 6 hours before the operation, restarting the heparin about 36 to 48 hours after surgery, and switching to warfarin about 2 to 5 days later. Recent analyses indicate that these various anticoagulation regimens are cost-effective provided that they do not result in lengthening the hospitalization.[85] Even one day of additional hospitalization is relatively costly, and the daily risk of thromboembolic complications is low. Thus, perioperative anticoagulation management should focus on regimens that provide reasonable protection from thromboembolic disease but that permit the patient to be discharged when the surgical condition itself permits.[85]

ENDOCARDITIS PROPHYLAXIS. Patients with valvular heart disease and those with prosthetic heart valves should receive prophylactic antibiotics for surgical procedures likely to be complicated by bacteremias.[86,87] These include incision and drainage of an infected site; oral, lower gastrointestinal, and gallbladder surgery; and genitourinary procedures. Penicillin can be used before operation involving the upper respiratory tract, with erythromycin or vancomycin an acceptable alternative for patients with a penicillin allergy. For gastrointestinal and genitourinary surgery, which can be complicated by either enterococci or gram-negative bacteremia, gentamicin or streptomycin is required in addition to penicillin. (Suggested doses are given on p. 1099).

The value of antibiotic prophylaxis before noncardiac operation in patients with *mitral valve prolapse* is controversial (p. 1035). Most studies indicate that patients with this condition who have murmurs of mitral regurgitation are at substantially higher risk than patients who do not have murmurs,[88] and cost-effectiveness analyses argue *against* routine antibiotic prophylaxis in patients without a murmur.[89,90] At the present time a reasonable compromise is to use antibiotic prophylaxis before surgery in patients with mitral valve prolapse who have clinical evidence of mitral regurgitation.

CONGENITAL HEART DISEASE

Depending on the nature of the malformation, the patient with congenital heart disease may be subject to one or more potentially serious complications, such as infection, bleeding, hypoxemia, and paradoxical embolization during general anesthesia and operation. As is the case for patients with valvular heart disease, patients with congenital heart disease who are to undergo a surgical procedure require prophylaxis to prevent infective endocarditis (p. 1098). Patients with cyanotic congenital heart disease and secondary polycythemia are at increased risk of intraoperative and postoperative hemorrhage as a consequence of coagulation defects and thrombocytopenia (p. 894); this risk can be reduced with careful preoperative phlebotomy, usually to a hematocrit of 50 to 55 per cent.[91]

Patients with cyanotic congenital heart disease tolerate systemic hypotension poorly, since this increases the right-to-left shunt and the severity of hypoxemia. In one large series, induction was commonly accomplished using ketamine or fentanyl to avoid hypotension, and anesthesia was maintained with morphine and nitrous oxide or with large doses of fentanyl with or without nitrous oxide. Halothane in very low concentrations can be used in patients with less severe degrees of cyanosis.[92] With use of careful anesthetic techniques, the risk of major anesthetic complications is extremely low

even in very ill and cyanotic patients. However, spinal anesthesia, which causes peripheral arterial vasodilatation and reduces venous return, can have deleterious hemodynamic effects in patients with cyanotic congenital heart disease. Occasionally, infusion of a vasoconstrictor such as phenylephrine may be required to raise systemic vascular resistance and thereby decrease the magnitude of the right-to-left shunt. Because patients with right-to-left shunts are subject to the risk of paradoxical emboli, including air emboli, meticulous techniques with regard to intravenous solutions and injections are mandatory to prevent such complications.

CONGESTIVE HEART FAILURE

Congestive heart failure is a major determinant of perioperative risk, irrespective of the nature of the underlying cardiac disorder. Mortality with noncardiac surgery increases with worsening cardiac class[20,29] and with the presence of pulmonary congestion,[20] especially when a third heart sound is noted.[28] Because the perioperative mortality rate appears to depend more on the patient's condition at the time of operation than on the most severe depression of cardiovascular status the patient has ever experienced, it is clearly advisable to treat the congestive heart failure before the contemplated major elective noncardiac surgery. However, because such a therapeutic regimen almost always includes a diuretic, both hypovolemia and hypokalemia are potential problems for patients treated just before operation. It is therefore desirable, if possible, to stabilize the patient's condition by treating heart failure for approximately 1 week rather than for only 1 or 2 days before the contemplated operation. Also, great care should be taken to avoid dehydration because hypovolemic patients may be especially likely to experience marked hypotension during the early phases of anesthesia. Perioperative cardiogenic pulmonary edema will develop in about 2 per cent of patients over age 40 undergoing major noncardiac surgery without prior congestive heart failure, in about 6 per cent of patients whose heart failure is well controlled, and in about 16 per cent of patients whose heart failure persists on physical examination or chest radiograph before surgery.[20]

Although digitalis can counteract the myocardial depressant actions of many general anesthetic agents,[93] the value of digitalis in patients with congestive heart failure appears to be limited to certain subsets of patients, especially those who have a third heart sound.[94] Digitalis is one of the most common causes of iatrogenic complications in hospitalized patients, and it may be associated with a higher risk of intraoperative bradyarrhythmias.[20] Therefore, preoperative digitalization is *not* recommended except in patients whose congestive heart failure is sufficiently severe that they would normally meet the criteria for long-term digitalization (p. 479).

ARRHYTHMIAS

Arrhythmias may be a manifestation of underlying heart disease, and hence are frequently markers for the likelihood of perioperative cardiac complications. For example, the frequency of ventricular premature contractions correlates with left ventricular dysfunction and the severity of coronary artery disease,[95,96] and thus frequent ventricular premature contractions in patients with coronary artery disease represent a risk factor for the development of cardiac complications.[28] Because patients who have ventricular premature contractions but no evidence of underlying heart disease on detailed examination have an apparently normal cardiac prognosis,[97] ventricular premature contractions in the *absence* of underlying heart disease should not be considered a risk factor for cardiac complications with noncardiac surgery. Atrial arrhythmias are often a manifestation of atrial enlargement, and a supraventricular rhythm other than sinus appears to be a risk factor for the development of perioperative complications.[28]

Although it would be ideal for arrhythmias to be well controlled preoperatively, the risks associated with arrhythmias appear to be related more to the underlying cardiac disease than to the arrhythmias per se. Therefore, there currently is no evidence that asymptomatic ventricular premature contractions require aggressive preoperative control or prophylactic intraoperative suppression. Similarly, in the patient with well-controlled atrial fibrillation, cardioversion need not be carried out specifically because of planned noncardiac surgery if such a management option would not otherwise be appropriate.

Patients who are most at risk for the development of postoperative supraventricular tachyarrhythmias include elderly patients undergoing pulmonary surgery, patients with subcritical valvular stenoses, and patients with prior histories of supraventricular tachyarrhythmias. Although data are less than decisive, there is a suggestion that digitalis may reduce the risk of the development of postoperative supraventricular tachycardia in such patients,[98] and that the rate of the supraventricular tachycardia will be slower in the digitalized patient.[20] Thus, we generally recommend prophylactic preoperative digitalization in elderly patients undergoing major pulmonary surgery, patients with subcritical valvular stenoses, and patients with a prior history of symptomatic supraventricular tachycardias, except if the latter are already taking other medications for the control of such arrhythmias. Verapamil may also be useful in these settings, but its negative inotropic effects make it theoretically less appealing than digitalis for many patients.

CONDUCTION DEFECTS. The patient with *complete heart block* (p. 710) must respond to the demands for an increased cardiac output by augmenting stroke volume, but this compensatory response is prevented in many patients by a concurrent impairment of cardiac contractility. In addition, most anesthetic agents depress myocardial contractility and/or produce peripheral vasodilatation. Furthermore, anesthesia may cause further depression of the automaticity, and therefore the ventricular rate, of the patient with heart block. Thus patients with untreated complete heart block may be unable to meet the increased demands placed on the cardiovascular system by anesthesia and operation, and a permanent or temporary pacemaker should be inserted before general anesthesia, even in asymptomatic patients (Chap. 26).

Another problem is presented by the patient with *chronic bifascicular block* (p. 131).[20,99] A significant fraction of patients developing this abnormality in the course of an acute myocardial infarction progress to complete heart block, often accompanied by sudden severe hemodynamic compromise (p. 1241). In several series, progression from bifascicular to complete heart block has not been documented during the perioperative period in patients without a previous history of third-degree heart block. Therefore, we do *not* recommend prophylactic pacemaker placement for such patients or for patients with first-degree atrioventricular (AV) block or type I second-degree AV block (Wenckebach), although a pacemaker should always be available in the operating room for emergency placement. However, in patients who have bifascicular block, and either type II second-degree AV block or a history of unexplained syncope or transient third-degree AV block, the risk of development of complete heart block is much higher, and a temporary pacemaker should be inserted preoperatively.

THE PATIENT WITH A PERMANENT PACEMAKER. When a patient with a permanent pacemaker in situ is about to undergo operation, the device should be carefully evaluated to insure that it is functioning properly preoperatively (Chap. 26). Demand pacemakers are sensitive to electromagnetic interference, such as that produced by the electrocautery, which may result in failure to pace. The danger of this potentially hazardous interaction can be reduced by placing the indifferent plate of the cautery unit as far as possible from the lead and pulse generator, and the electrocautery should be used in brief bursts rather than continuously. Also, a magnet should be available in the operating room to convert the pacemaker from the demand to the fixed-rate mode. Because the cautery may also interfere with the electrocardiographic monitor and render it temporarily uninterpretable, arterial pressure should be monitored directly when the cautery is being used on patients with permanent pacemakers.

In general, a prophylactic *temporary pacemaker* should be inserted before noncardiac operations only if the patient meets the indications for permanent pacemaker insertion[100] (see also p. 728) and the operation should not be delayed for the time required for a permanent pacemaker insertion, or if the operative course is likely to be complicated by transient bacteremia. In such situations a temporary pacemaker should be placed initially, and the permanent pacemaker can be inserted after the operation. The occasional exception is the patient who has a severe bradycardiac response to vagal stimuli and who might be difficult to manage during a major operation without a pacemaker.

GENERAL MEDICAL PROBLEMS

Patients with heart disease whose general medical status is complicated by renal insufficiency, hepatic abnormalities, hypoxemia, or electrolyte abnormalities have a higher risk of cardiac complications, presumably because these nonmedical conditions exacerbate the stress placed on the heart by the operation.[20,26,28] Morbidity is also higher in markedly obese patients[101] because obesity is often associated with abnormal cardiorespiratory function, metabolic function, and hemostasis. Every effort should be made to correct any of these noncardiac problems before operations, and the potential long-term benefits of surgery must also be interpreted in light of the patient's general prognosis.

POSTOPERATIVE COMPLICATIONS

MYOCARDIAL INFARCTION. Transient intraoperative ischemia does not appear to be a major correlate of postoperative ischemic events in patients undergoing noncardiac surgery,[102] but most clinical postoperative ischemic events are preceded by asymptomatic episodes of postoperative ischemia that can be detected by ambulatory ischemic monitoring.[102,103] Although series from before 1980 showed a peak in the risk of myocardial infarction on about the third postoperative day,[104] more recent series show that a combination of frequent electrocardiograms and cardiac enzymes detects many non-Q-wave infarctions in the first 24 hours postoperatively.[49,105,106] Although care must be taken in interpreting cardiac enzymes in the perioperative period,[107] it may be that supply-demand imbalances cause an early peak in non-Q-wave postoperative infarctions, while the hypercoagulable postoperative state leads to a later (3 to 5 days postoperatively) peak in Q-wave infarctions. For both types of infarction, postoperative stresses include general surgical complications, hypoxia and other pulmonary complications, fluid and electrolyte abnormalities, and the stresses of modern postoperative ambulation protocols. Substantial data indicate that prophylactic anticoagulation with low-dose heparin will reduce the risk of postoperative thromboembolic complications,[108] and such therapy is routinely indicated in most cardiac patients who undergo noncardiac operations. In fact, such anticoagulation regimens may permit a more gradual postoperative ambulation protocol in cardiac patients, and hence possibly lower the incidence of postoperative myocardial infarction.

Myocardial infarction occurring in the perioperative period is often painless. Obviously, then, the incidence of perioperative infarction will be underestimated if electrocardiograms and serial estimations of serum creatine kinase isoenzyme

(MB fraction) are not obtained routinely during the postoperative period in high-risk patients.[105]

HYPERTENSION. Postoperative hypertension is most likely to occur soon after the cessation of positive-pressure ventilation or in the recovery room, and it is more common after carotid endarterectomy and major abdominal vascular procedures.[18]

Common precipitants include fluid overload after cessation of positive-pressure ventilation, hypoxemia, anxiety, and pain.[109] The principal therapeutic approaches should therefore concentrate on assuring adequate oxygenation, pain control, and fluid control. In general, supplemental oxygen, morphine, and diuretics are the mainstays of the treatment of postoperative hypertension. Nitroprusside (p. 869) and labetalol[77] (p. 866) are the preferred medications for more severe hypertension. Intravenous hydralazine in small doses is effective for treating postoperative hypertension, but it has the potential of precipitating supraventricular tachyarrhythmias. Methyldopa will not be helpful in the emergency situation, but it may be an important part of the overall regimen because it will have its onset of effect about 4 hours after administration, at a time when one would like to be able to discontinue more vigorous intravenous antihypertensive regimens.

CONGESTIVE HEART FAILURE. Although postoperative heart failure may be precipitated by myocardial infarction or ischemia, a substantial proportion of the cases are directly caused by excess fluid administration. Heart failure tends to occur soon after cessation of positive-pressure ventilation and again at about 24 to 48 hours after operation, when the fluid that was given in the perioperative period is mobilized from the extravascular sites. Diuretics, often given intravenously, and rarely supplemented by digitalis glycosides, are usually sufficient therapy for postoperative congestive heart failure.

POSTOPERATIVE ARRHYTHMIAS. Arrhythmias are common after operation and are often a manifestation of a noncardiac complication, such as bleeding, infection, or an acid-base or electrolyte imbalance occurring in a patient with heart disease. Management of such arrhythmias often requires recognition and correction of extracardiac factors.

In one study of 916 patients with sinus rhythm throughout the course of major noncardiac surgery, 35 patients (4 per cent) developed new supraventricular tachyarrhythmias postoperatively.[110] Of these 35 patients, 46 per cent had acute cardiac conditions, 31 per cent had major infections, 29 per cent had preexisting hypotension, 26 per cent had anemia, 23 per cent had metabolic derangements, 23 per cent had received new parenteral drugs that could be implicated, and 20 per cent were hypoxic. Forty per cent of the patients required no new therapy with cardiac medications, and only two patients required electrical cardioversion; the arrhythmias of all treated patients reverted to sinus rhythm. No deaths were related to the supraventricular tachyarrhythmias per se, but a substantial proportion of the patients in whom these arrhythmias occurred died as a result of the concurrent medical problems. Thus, a new postoperative supraventricular tachyarrhythmia should prompt a search for remediable medical problems. Direct antiarrhythmic therapy is often unnecessary and is usually secondary in importance to correction of the underlying cause of the arrhythmia.

Sinus tachycardia is the most common rhythm disturbance in the postoperative patient. Multiple noncardiac etiologic factors have been identified, including pain, hypovolemia, hypervolemia, fever, anemia, hypoxemia, pulmonary emboli, anxiety, infection, hypotension, and electrolyte abnormalities (especially hypokalemia). These noncardiac factors are much more common causes of sinus tachycardia in the postoperative cardiac patient than is either myocardial infarction or heart failure. Sinus tachycardia not caused by congestive heart failure will not slow with cardiac glycosides. The therapeutic:toxic ratio of these drugs is actually reduced by most of the above-mentioned noncardiac causes of sinus tachycardia, and therefore digitalis glycosides are not considered appropri-

ate for postoperative patients unless the sinus tachycardia is caused by impaired cardiac function.

Atrial fibrillation is also a common postoperative arrhythmia. Atrial dilatation, which lowers the threshold for development of this arrhythmia, may result from heart failure, mitral valve disease, and/or hypervolemia. Noncardiac precipitants include pneumonia, atelectasis, and pulmonary emboli. Initially, the postoperative patient with atrial fibrillation should be treated with a digitalis glycoside or verapamil; in addition, a beta-adrenoceptor blocker can be used to help gain rapid control of the ventricular rate. Cardioversion is usually delayed until the precipitating factors have been eliminated, since in the patient who has cardioversion before clearing of the atelectasis or pneumonia there is frequently reversion to atrial fibrillation, while in the patient whose pulmonary problem or congestive heart failure is adequately treated there is often spontaneous reversion to sinus rhythm.

Atrial flutter is often poorly tolerated because of the rapid ventricular rate and the difficult pharmacological management. Cardioversion is usually the treatment of choice, along with quinidine or procainamide administered to prevent recurrence (p. 681).

IMPLICATIONS OF POSTOPERATIVE COMPLICATIONS FOR LONG-TERM MANAGEMENT. When a patient develops a perioperative myocardial infarction, the evaluation and the recuperative process generally should be analogous to when a myocardial infarction occurs in other patients (see Chap. 39). Because postoperative congestive heart failure is commonly precipitated by iatrogenic fluid overload, the patient commonly will not need long-term therapy for congestive heart failure. Similarly, perioperative arrhythmias are often precipitated by specific stimuli, and the patient with a postoperative arrhythmia should not automatically be consigned to long-term antiarrhythmic therapy. In patients who develop either postoperative congestive heart failure or arrhythmias, it is often appropriate to discontinue new cardiac therapies several days before discharge and observe the patient to see whether long-term therapy is indicated.

THE ROLE OF THE MEDICAL CONSULTANT

The physician called on to evaluate the status of a patient with suspected or overt cardiac disease before elective or emergency noncardiac surgery must first determine whether cardiovascular disease is present and, if it is, must identify those factors that may increase the risk of operation. It may be necessary to invest considerable time and effort to prepare the patient for operation. In addition, the patient must be followed carefully after operation to detect and manage the cardiac problems that frequently complicate the postoperative period.

ESTIMATION OF RISK

A few patients have such compelling reasons for operation (e.g., rupturing aortic aneurysm, perforated or necrotic bowel, life-threatening hemorrhage, or some forms of intestinal obstruction) that estimation of operative risk is an academic exercise, since failure to operate almost certainly will result in the patient's death. Often, however, the timing or even the performance of an operation is elective, and under these circumstances estimation of risk is an important aspect of the medical consultant's role. Certain cardiovascular problems, such as recent myocardial infarction (less than 1 month), inadequately treated congestive heart failure, and severe mitral or aortic stenosis, are *absolute contraindications* to *elective* surgery. *Relative contraindications*, which commonly require further clinical or laboratory evaluation or treatment before elective surgery, include more remote myocardial infarction (1 month to 6 months previously), angina pectoris, mild heart failure, cyanotic congenital heart disease with severe polycythemia, and a coagulation abnormality. Several other problems should be recognized and treated before operation: ane-

TABLE 55-2 COMPUTATION OF THE CARDIAC RISK INDEX

CRITERIA	POINTS
1 History	
(a) Age > 70 yr	5
(b) MI in previous 6 mo	10
2 Physical examination	
(a) S₃ gallop or JVD	11
(b) Important VAS	3
3 Electrocardiogram	
(a) Rhythm other than sinus or PACs on last preoperative ECG	7
(b) > 5 PVCs/min documented at any time before operation	7
4 General status	
PO₂ < 60 or PCO₂ > 50 mm Hg, K < 3.0 or HCO₃ < 20 mEq/liter, BUN > 50 or Cr > 3.0 mg/dl, abnormal SGOT, signs of chronic liver disease, or patient bedridden from noncardiac causes	3
5 Operation	
(a) Intraperitoneal, intrathoracic, or aortic operation	3
(b) Emergency operation	4
Total possible	**53 points**

To calculate a patient's score, the number of points from all factors he or she possesses are summed. MI, myocardial infarction; JVD, jugular vein distention; VAS, valvular aortic stenosis; PACs, premature atrial contractions; ECG, electrocardiogram; PVCs, premature ventricular contractions; PO₂, partial pressure of oxygen; PCO₂, partial pressure of carbon dioxide; K, potassium; HCO₃, bicarbonate; BUN, blood urea nitrogen; Cr, creatinine; and SGOT, serum glutamic oxalacetic transaminase.

Reprinted by permission from Goldman, L., et al.: Multifactorial index of cardiac risk in noncardiac surgical procedures. N. Engl. J. Med. 297:845, 1977.

FIGURE 55-1. Cardiac complications in patients over age 65 having intraperitoneal or intrathoracic surgery.[43,44] *Ability to exercise = ability to pedal a supine bicycle for at least 2 minutes to a heart rate of ≥100; †Goldman indicator = factor on cardiac risk index[28] other than age or type of operation. (Data from Gerson, M.C., et al.: Prediction of cardiac and pulmonary complications related to elective abdominal and noncardiac thoracic surgery in geriatric patients. Am. J. Med. 88:101, 1990.)

mia, hypovolemia, polycythemia, pulmonary disease causing hypoxemia, adrenal hyporesponsiveness secondary to long-term administration of adrenal steroids, hypertension, electrolyte abnormalities, as well as the entire gamut of cardiac arrhythmias. Considerable judgment must be exercised when one or more of the above-mentioned problems are present and when a patient requires prompt surgical treatment but the situation is not a true emergency, as for neoplastic disease.

To identify those preoperative factors associated with the development of cardiac complications after major noncardiac operation in patients over 40 years of age, one analysis[20] identified nine independently significant correlates of life-threatening and fatal cardiac complications. When these factors were weighted based on their relative significance as predictors of cardiac outcome, a multifactorial index was developed

for predicting perioperative risk (Table 55-2). Notably, *unimportant* factors included smoking, glucose intolerance, hyperlipidemia, hypertension, peripheral atherosclerotic vascular disease, stable Class I or II angina, and remote myocardial infarction.

The value of the information in this index has been confirmed in two large prospective series of general surgical patients[33,34] (Table 55-3) and in several other studies.[21,43,105,111-113] In one series,[34] risk stratification was equally good when several minor modifications were made in point assignment and when a prior history of Class III or IV angina, unstable angina, and pulmonary edema was included in the index.

However, because the index was derived from unselected general surgical patients above age 40, it appears to underestimate risk by about 40 per cent in patients who undergo resection of an abdominal aortic aneurysm,[30] and it also underestimates risk in patients who are selected on the basis of any high-risk status. One way to take into account the fact that some patients have higher baseline risks is to know the baseline probability of cardiac complications for specific types of patients or types of surgery and then to modify these "pretest" probabilities on the basis of the patient's cardiac condition.[34,113-115] As shown in Table 55-4, this can be a useful approach to estimating the risk of major cardiac complications. Even at its best, however, any index for predicting cardiac complications should be viewed as an aid and not as a crutch; it should supplement, not substitute for, clinical judgment.

TABLE 55-3 MAJOR COMPLICATION* RATES IN FOUR STUDIES THAT HAVE ANALYZED THE MULTIFACTORIAL CARDIAC RISK INDEX[18]

TYPE OF PATIENTS	GOLDMAN ET AL[28] UNSELECTED NONCARDIAC SURGERY ≥ 40 y.o.	ZELDIN[33] UNSELECTED NONCARDIAC SURGERY ≥ 40 y.o.	DETSKY ET AL.[34]† PREOPERATIVE MEDICAL CONSULTATIONS	JEFFREY ET AL[30]‡ ABDOMINAL AORTIC ANEURYSM SURGERY	POOLED	POOLED LIKELIHOOD RATIO (Sensitivity/ 1-specificity)
Overall complication rate	58/1001 (6%)	35/1140 (3%)	27/268 (10%)	11/99 (11%)	131/2508 (5.2%)	
Complication rate by class						
Class I (0-5 points)†	5/537 (1%)	4/590 (1%)	8/134 (6%)	4/56 (7%)	21/1317 (1.6%)	.29
Class II (6-12 points)	21/316 (7%)	13/453 (3%)	6/85 (7%)	4/35 (11%)	44/889 (5%)	.94
Class III (13-25 points)	18/130 (14%)	11/74 (15%)	9/45 (20%)	3/8 (38%)	41/257 (16%)	3.4
Class IV (≥ 26 points)	14/18 (78%)	7/23 (30%)	4/4 (100%)	0	25/45 (56%)	22.7

* Documented myocardial infarction, cardiogenic pulmonary edema, ventricular tachycardia, or cardiac death.
† Actual unpublished numbers provided by Dr. Detsky.
‡ See Table 55-2 for calculation of point total.
From Goldman, L.: Multifactorial index of cardiac risk in noncardiac surgery: Ten-year status report. J. Cardiothorac. Anesth. 1:237, 1987.

TABLE 55-4   ESTIMATION OF PROBABILITY OF CARDIAC COMPLICATIONS

TYPE OF PATIENT	APPROX-IMATE BASELINE RISK (%)	APPROXIMATE RISK AS ADJUSTED USING MULTIFACTORIAL INDEX (%)[18*]			
		CLASS I	CLASS II	CLASS III	CLASS IV
Minor surgery	1	0.3	1	3	19
Unselected consecutive patients over age 40 who have major noncardiac surgery	4	1.2	4	12	48
Patients who have abdominal aortic aneurysm surgery or who are over age 40 and have medical consultations before major noncardiac surgery	10	3	10	30	75

*Calculated by multiplying the prior odds of complications by the likelihood ratio for each class; see Table 55-3.

From Goldman, L.: Multifactorial index of cardiac risk in noncardiac surgery: Ten-year status report. J. Cardiothorac. Anesth. 1:237, 1987.

PREPARATION OF THE PATIENT FOR ANESTHESIA AND OPERATION

Careful preparation of the cardiac patient for operation may diminish the frequency and seriousness of intraoperative and postoperative complications. The medical consultant should, after appropriate discussion with the surgeon, be prepared to urge postponement or cancellation of an elective operation or to insist on sufficient time to institute any measures that are necessary to minimize risk. The consultant should attempt to be brief and to the point, and to provide a limited number of explicit, relevant suggestions.[116-118] The cardiological consultant should work closely with the anesthesiologist and the surgeon so that their talents may be combined to maximize the likelihood of a favorable outcome.

REFERENCES

ANESTHESIA

1. Breslow, M. J., Miller, C. F., and Rogers, M. (eds.): Perioperative Management. St. Louis, C. V. Mosby Co., 1990.
2. Mangano, D. T. (ed.): Perioperative Cardiac Assessment. Philadelphia, J. B. Lippincott Co., 1990.
3. Kaplan J. A. (ed.): Cardiac Anesthesia. Ed. 2. Orlando, Grune & Stratton, 1987.
4. Prys-Roberts, C., and Meloche, R.: Management of anesthesia in patients with hypertension or ischemic heart disease. Int. Anesthesiol. Clin. 18:181, 1980.
5. Prys-Roberts, C., Meloche, R., and Foex, P.: Studies of anesthesia in relation to hypertension: I. Cardiovascular responses of treated and untreated patients. Br. J. Anaesth. 43:1112, 1971.
6. Prys-Roberts, C., Foex, P., Greene, L. T., and Waterhouse, T. D.: Studies of anesthesia in relation to hypertension: IV. The effects of artificial ventilation on the circulation and pulmonary gas exchanges. Br. J. Anaesth. 44:335, 1972.
7. Tarhan, S. (ed.): Cardiovascular Anesthesia and Postoperative Care. Chicago, Year Book Medical Publishers, 1982.
8. Rusy, B. F., and Komai, H.: Anesthetic depression of myocardial contractility: A review of possible mechanisms. Anesthesiology 67:745, 1987.
9. Yeager, M. P., Glass, D. D., Neff, R. K., and Brinck-Johnsen, T.: Epidural anesthesia and analgesia in high-risk surgical patients. Anesthesiology 66:729, 1987.
10. Scott, N. B., and Kehlet, H.: Regional anaesthesia and surgical morbidity. Br. J. Surg. 75:299, 1988.
11. Yeager, M. P.: Regional anesthesia for the patient with heart disease. Pro:

12. Beattie, C.: Con: Regional anesthesia is not preferable to general anesthesia for the patient with heart disease. J. Cardiothorac. Anesth. 3:797, 1989.
13. Saada, M., Duval, A. M., Bonnet, F., et al.: Abnormalities in myocardial segmental wall motion during lumbar epidural anesthesia. Anesthesiology 71:26, 1989.
14. Breslow, M. J., Jordan, D. A., Christopherson, R., et al.: Epidural morphine decreases postoperative hypertension by attenuating sympathetic nervous system hyperactivity. JAMA 261:3577, 1989.
15. Diebel, L. N., Lange, P. M., Schenider, F., et al.: Cardiopulmonary complications after major surgery: A role for epidural analgesia? Surgery 102:660, 1987.
16. Mauney, R. M., Jr., Ebert, P. A., and Sabiston, D. C., Jr.: Postoperative myocardial infarction: A study of predisposing factors, diagnosis and mortality in a high risk group of surgical patients. Ann. Surg. 172:497, 1970.
17. Steen, P.A., Tinker, J. H., and Tarhan, S.: Myocardial reinfarction after anesthesia and surgery. JAMA 239:2566, 1978.
18. Goldman, L., and Caldera, D. L.: Risks of general anesthesia and elective surgery in the hypertensive patient. Anesthesiology 50:285, 1979.
19. Charlson, M. E., MacKenzie, C. R., Gold, J. P., et al.: The preoperative and intraoperative hemodynamic predictors of postoperative myocardial infarction or ischemia in patients undergoing noncardiac surgery. Ann. Surg. 210:637, 1989.
20. Goldman L., Caldera, D. L., Southwick, F. S., et al.: Cardiac risk factors and complications in non-cardiac surgery. Medicine 57:357, 1978.
21. Kaplan J. A., and Dunbar, R. W.: Anesthesia for noncardiac surgery in patients with cardiac disease. In Kaplan, J. A. (ed.): Cardiac Anesthesia. Orlando, Grune & Stratton, 1979, p. 377.
22. Smith, J. S., Cahalan, M. K., Benefiel, D. J., et al.: Intraoperative detection of myocardial ischemia in high risk patients: Electrocardiography versus two-dimensional echocardiography. Circulation 72:1015, 1985.
23. Van Daele, M. E. R. M., Sutherland, G. R., Mitchell, M. M., et al.: Do changes in pulmonary capillary wedge pressure adequately reflect myocardial ischemia during anesthesia? Circulation 81:865, 1990.

THE OPERATION

24. Backer, C. L., Tinker, J. H., Robertson, D. M., and Vliestra, R. E.: Myocardial reinfarction following local anesthesia for ophthalmic surgery. Anest. Analg. 59:257, 1980.
25. Erlik, D., Valero, A., Birkhan, J., and Gersh, I.: Prostatic surgery and the cardiovascular patient. Br. J. Urol. 40:53, 1968.
26. Larsen, S. F., Olesen, K. H., Jacobsen, E., et al.: Prediction of cardiac risk in non-cardiac surgery. Eur. Heart J. 8:179, 1987.
27. Knorring, J.: Postoperative myocardial infarction: A prospective study in a high-risk group of surgical patients. Surgery 90:55, 1981.
28. Goldman, L., Caldera, D. L., Nussbaum, R. R., et al.: Multifactorial index of cardiac risk in noncardiac surgical procedures. N. Engl. J. Med. 297:845, 1977.
29. Skinner, J. R., and Pearce, M. L.: Surgical risk in the cardiac patient. J. Chronic Dis. 17:57, 1964.
30. Jeffrey, C. C., Kunsman, J., Cullen, D. J., and Brewster, D. C.: A prospective evaluation of cardiac risk index. Anesthesiology 58:462, 1983.
31. Lewin, I., Lerner, A. G., Green, S. H., et al.: Physical class and physiological status in the prediction of operative mortality in the aged sick. Ann. Surg. 174:217, 1971.
32. Rao, T. L. K., Jacobs, K. H., and El-Etr, A. A.: Reinfarction following anesthesia in patients with myocardial infarction. Anesthesiology 59:499, 1983.

INFLUENCE OF UNDERLYING CARDIOVASCULAR DISEASE

33. Zeldin, R. A.: Assessing cardiac risk in patients who undergo noncardiac surgical procedures. Can. J. Surg. 27:402, 1984.
34. Detsky, A. S., Abrams, H. B., McLaughlin, J. R., et al.: Predicting cardiac complications in patients undergoing non-cardiac surgery. J. Gen. Intern. Med. 1:211, 1986.
35. Shah, K., Kleinman, B., Rao, T., et al.: Reduction in mortality from cardiac causes in Goldman class IV patients. J. Cardiothorac. Anesth. 2:789, 1988.
36. Wells, P. H., and Kaplan, J. A.: Optimal management of patients with ischemic heart disease for noncardiac surgery by complementary anesthesiologist and cardiologist interaction. Am. Heart J. 102:1029, 1981.
37. DeBusk, R. F., Blomqvist, C. G., Kouchoukos, N. T., et al.: Identification and treatment of low-risk patients after acute myocardial infarction and coronary-artery bypass graft surgery. N. Engl. J. Med. 314:161, 1983.
38. Campeau, L.: Grading of angina pectoris. Circulation 54:522, 1975.
39. Goldman, L., Hashimoto, B., Cook, E. F., and Loscalzo, A.: Comparative reproducibility and validity of systems for assessing cardiovascular functional class: Advantages of a new Specific Activity Scale. Circulation 64:1227, 1981.
40. Goldman, L., Cook, E. F., Mitchell, N., et al.: Pitfalls in the serial assessment of cardiac functional class. J. Chronic Dis. 35:763, 1982.
41. McPhail, N., Calvin, J. E., Shariatmadar, A., et al.: The use of preoperative exercise testing to predict cardiac complications after arterial reconstruction. J. Vasc. Surg. 7:60, 1988.

42. Cutler, B. S., Wheeler, H. B., Paraskos, J. A., and Cardullo, P. A.: Applicability and interpretation of electrocardiographic stress testing in patients with peripheral vascular disease. Am. J. Surg. 141:501, 1981.

43. Gerson, M. C., Hurst, J. M., Hertzberg, V. S., et al.: Cardiac prognosis in noncardiac geriatric surgery. Ann. Intern. Med. 103:832, 1985.

44. Gerson, M. C., Hurst, J. M., Hertzberg, V. S., et al.: Prediction of cardiac and pulmonary complications related to elective abdominal and noncardiac thoracic surgery in geriatric patients. Am. J. Med. 88:101, 1990.

45. Pasternack, P. F., Imparato, A. M., Riles, T. S., et al.: The value of the radionuclide angiogram in the prediction of perioperative myocardial infarction in patients undergoing lower extremity revascularization procedures. Circulation 72 (Suppl. 2):13, 1985.

46. Franco, C. D., Goldsmith, J., Veith, F. J., et al.: Resting gated pool ejection fraction: A poor predictor of perioperative myocardial infarction in patients undergoing vascular surgery for infrainguinal bypass grafting. J. Vasc. Surg. 10:656, 1989.

47. McCann, R. L., and Wolfe, W. G.: Resection of abdominal aortic aneurysm in patients with low ejection fractions. J. Vasc. Surg. 10:240, 1989.

48. Kazmers, A., Cerqueira, M. D., and Zierler, R. E.: The role of preoperative radionuclide ejection fraction in direct abdominal aortic aneurysm repair. J. Vasc. Surg. 8:128, 1988.

49. Raby, K. E., Goldman, L., Creager, M. A., et al.: Correlation between preoperative ischemia and major cardiac events after peripheral vascular surgery. N. Engl. J. Med. 321:1296, 1989.

50. Pasternack, P. F., Grossi, E. A., Baumann, F. G., et al.: The value of silent myocardial ischemia monitoring in the prediction of perioperative myocardial infarction in patients undergoing peripheral vascular surgery. J. Vasc. Surg. 10:617, 1989.

50a. Mangano, D. T., Browner, W. S., Hollenberg, M., et al.: Association of perioperative myocardial ischemia with cardiac morbidity and mortality in men undergoing noncardiac surgery. N. Engl. J. Med. 323:1781, 1990.

50b. Mangano, D. T., Hollenberg, M., Fegert, G., et al.: Perioperative myocardial ischemia in patients undergoing noncardiac surgery—I. Incidence and severity during the 4 day perioperative period. J. Am. Coll. Cardiol. 17:843, 1991.

50c. Mangano, D. T., Wong, M. G., London, M. J., et al.: Perioperative myocardial ischemia in patients undergoing noncardiac surgery—II. Incidence and severity during the first week after surgery. J. Am. Coll. Cardiol. 17:851, 1991.

51. Boucher, C. A., Brewster, D. C., Darling, R. C., et al.: Determination of cardiac risk by dipyridamole-thallium imaging before peripheral vascular surgery. N. Engl. J. Med. 312:389, 1985.

52. Leppo, J., Plaja, J., Gionet, M., et al.: Noninvasive evaluation of cardiac risk before elective vascular surgery. J. Am. Coll. Cardiol. 9:269, 1987.

53. Eagle, K. A., Coley, C. M., Newell, J. B., et al.: Combining clinical and thallium data optimizes preoperative assessment of cardiac risk before major vascular surgery. Ann. Intern. Med. 110:859, 1989.

54. Lette, J., Waters, D., Lapointe, J. et al.: Usefulness of the severity and extent of reversible perfusion defects during thallium-dipyridamole imaging for cardiac risk assessment before noncardiac surgery. Am. J. Cardiol. 64:276, 1989.

55. McPhail, N. V., Ruddy, T. D., Calvin, J. E., et al.: A comparison of dipyridamole-thallium imaging and exercise testing in the prediction of postoperative cardiac complications in patients requiring arterial reconstruction. J. Vasc. Surg. 10:51, 1989.

56. Marwick, T. H., and Underwood, D. A.: Dipyridamole thallium imaging may not be a reliable screening test for coronary artery disease in patients undergoing vascular surgery. Clin. Cardiol. 13:14, 1990.

57. Foster, E. D., Davis, K. B., Carpenter, J. A., et al.: Risk of noncardiac operation in patients with defined coronary disease: The Coronary Artery Surgery Study (CASS) registry experience. Ann. Thorac. Surg. 41:42, 1986.

58. Weitz, H. H., and Goldman, L.: Noncardiac surgery in the patient with heart disease. Med. Clin. North Am. 71:413, 1987.

59. Freeman, W. K., Gibbons, R. J., and Shub, C.: Preoperative assessment of cardiac patients undergoing noncardiac surgical procedures. Mayo Clin. Proc. 64:1105, 1989.

60. Deron, S. J., and Kotler, M. N.: Noncardiac surgery in the cardiac patient. Am. Heart J. 116:831, 1988.

61. McPhail, N., Menkis, A., Shariatmader, A., et al.: Statistical prediction of cardiac risk in patients who undergo vascular surgery. Can. J. Surg. 28:404, 1985.

62. Lunder, T., Lindegaard, K. F., Froysaker, T., et al.: Cerebral perfusion during nonpulsatile cardiopulmonary bypass. Ann. Thorac. Surg. 40:144, 1985.

63. Jones, E. L., Craver, J. M., Michalik, R. A., et al.: Combined carotid and coronary operations: When are they necessary? J. Thorac. Cardiovasc. Surg. 87:7, 1984.

64. Hertzer, N. R., Loop, F. D., Beven, E. G., et al.: Surgical staging for simultaneous coronary and carotid disease: A study including prospective randomization. J. Vasc. Surg. 9:455, 1989.

65. Matar, A. F.: Concomitant coronary and cerebral revascularization under cardiopulmonary bypass. Ann. Thorac. Surg. 41:181, 1986.

66. Viljoen, J. F., Estafanous, G., and Kellner, G. A.: Propranolol and cardiac surgery. J. Thorac. Cardiovasc. Surg. 64:826, 1972.

67. Should propranolol be stopped before surgery? Med. Lett. 18:41, 1976.

68. Goldman, L.: Noncardiac surgery in patients receiving propranolol. Case reports and a recommended approach. Arch. Intern. Med. 141:193, 1981.

69. Prys-Roberts, C., Foex, P., and Roberts, J. G.: Studies of anaesthesia in relation to hypertension. Br. J. Anaesth. 45:671, 1973.

70. Prys-Roberts, C.: Hemodynamic effects of anesthesia and surgery in renal hypertensive patients receiving large does of beta-receptor antagonists. Anesthesiology 51 (Suppl.):122, 1979.

71. Woolsey, R. L., and Shand, D. G.: Pharmacokinetics of antiarrhythmic drugs. Am. J. Cardiol. 41:986, 1978.

72. Smulyan, H., Weinberg, S. E., and Howanitz, P. J.: Continuous propranolol infusion following abdominal surgery. JAMA 247:2539, 1982.

73. Reves, J. G., and Flezzani, P.: Perioperative use of esmolol. Am. J. Cardiol. 56:57F, 1985.

74. Prys-Roberts, C.: Hypertension and anesthesia—fifty years on. Anesthesiology 50:281, 1979.

75. Tarazi, R. C., Dustan, H. P., and Frohlich, E. D.: Long-term thiazide therapy in essential hypertension. Evidence for persistent alteration in plasma volume and renin activity. Circulation 41:709, 1970.

76. Bruce, D. L., Croley, T. F., and Lee, J. S.: Preoperative clonidine withdrawal syndrome. Anesthesiology 51:90, 1979.

77. Orlowski, J. P., Vidt, D. G., Walker, S., and Haluska, J. F.: The hemodynamic effects of intravenous labetalol for postoperative hypertension. Cleve. Clin. J. Med. 56:29, 1989.

78. O'Keefe, J. H., Shub, C., and Rettke, S. R.: Risk of noncardiac surgical procedures in patients with aortic stenosis. Mayo Clin. Proc. 64:400, 1989.

79. Stone, J. G., Hoar, P. F., Calabro, J. R., et al.: Afterload reduction and preload augmentation improve the anesthetic management of patients with cardiac failure and valvular regurgitation. Anesth. Analg. 59:737, 1980.

80. Hayes, S. N., Holmes, D. R., Jr., Nishimura, R. A., and Reeder, G. S.: Palliative percutaneous aortic balloon valvuloplasty before noncardiac operations and invasive diagnostic procedures. Mayo Clin. Proc. 64:753, 1989.

81. Thompson, R. C., Liberthson, R. R., and Lowenstein, E.: Perioperative anesthetic risk of noncardiac surgery in hypertrophic obstructive cardiomyopathy. JAMA 254:2419, 1985.

82. Tinker, J. H., and Tarhan, S.: Discontinuing anticoagulant therapy in surgical patients with cardiac valve prostheses. JAMA 239:738, 1978.

83. Katholi, R. E., Nolan, S. P., and McGuire, L. B.: Living with prosthetic heart valve. Subsequent noncardiac operations and the risk of thromboembolism or hemorrhage. Am. Heart J. 92:162, 1976.

84. Tinker, J. H., Noback, C. R., Vliestra, R. E., and Frye, R. L.: Management of patients with heart disease for noncardiac surgery. JAMA 246:1348, 1981.

85. Eckman, M. H., Beshansky, J. R., Durand-Zaleski, I., et al.: Anticoagulation for noncardiac procedures in patients with prosthetic heart valves. JAMA 263:1513, 1990.

86. Simmons, N. A.: Antibiotic prophylaxis of infective endocarditis. Lancet 335:88, 1990.

87. Millard, H. D., Sanders, W. E., Schwartz, R. H., and Watanakunakorn, C.: Prevention of bacterial endocarditis. A statement for health professionals by the Committee on Rheumatic Fever and Infective Endocarditis of the Council on Cardiovascular Disease in the Young. Circulation 70:1123A, 1984.

88. Clemens, J. D., Horwitz, R. I., Jaffe, C. C., et al.: A controlled evaluation of the risk of bacterial endocarditis in persons with mitral-valve prolapse. N. Engl. J. Med. 307:776, 1982.

89. Bor, D. H., and Himmelstein, D. U.: Endocarditis prophylaxis for patients with mitral valve prolapse. Am. J. Med. 76:711, 1984.

90. Clemens, J. D., and Ransohoff, D. F.: A quantitative assessment of predental antibiotic prophylaxis for patients with mitral valve prolapse. J. Chronic Dis. 37:531, 1984.

91. Sommerville, J., McDonald, L., and Edgill, M.: Postoperative haemorrhage and related abnormalities of blood coagulation in cyanotic congenital heart disease. Br. Heart J. 27:440, 1965.

92. Hickey, P.R., Hansen, D. D., Norwood, W. I., and Castaneda, A. R.: Anesthetic complications in surgery for congenital heart disease. Anesth. Analg. 63:657, 1984.

93. Goldberg, A. H., Maling, H. M., and Gaffney, T. E.: The value of prophylactic digitalization in halothane anesthesia. Anesthesiology 23:207, 1962.

94. Lee, D. C., Johnson, R. A., Bingham, J. B., et al.: Heart failure in outpatients. A randomized trial of digoxin versus placebo. N. Engl. J. Med. 306:699, 1982.

95. Schulze, R. A., Jr., Rouleau, J., Rigo, P., et al.: Ventricular arrhythmias in the late hospital phase of acute myocardial infarction: Relation to left ventricular function detected by gated cardiac blood pool scanning. Circulation 52:1006, 1975.

96. Schulze, R. A., Jr., Strauss, H. W., and Pitt, B.: Sudden death in the year following myocardial infarction: Relation to ventricular premature contractions in the late hospital phase and left ventricular ejection fraction. Am. J. Med. 62:192, 1977.

97. Kennedy, H. L., Whitlock, J. A., Sprague, M. K., et al.: Long-term follow-up of asymptomatic healthy subjects with frequent and complex ventricular ectopy. N. Engl. J. Med. 312:193, 1985.

98. Bergh, N. P., Dottori, O., and Malmberg, R.: Prophylactic digitalis in thoracic surgery. Scand. J. Resp. Dis. 48:197, 1967.

99. Pastore, J. O., Yurchak, P. M., Janis, K. M., et al.: The risk of advanced heart block in surgical patients with right bundle branch block and left axis deviation. Circulation 57:677, 1978.

100. Frye, R. L., Collins, J. J., DeSanctis, R. W., et al.: Guidelines for permanent cardiac pacemaker implantation, May 1984. A report of the Joint Amer-

ican College of Cardiology/American Heart Association Task Force on Assessment of Cardiovascular Procedures (Subcommittee on Pacemaker Implantation). J. Am. Coll. Cardiol. 4:434, 1984.

101. Pasulka, P. S., Bistrian, B. R., Benotti, P. N., and Blackburn, G. L.: The risks of surgery in obese patients. Ann. Intern. Med. 104:540, 1986.

POSTOPERATIVE COMPLICATIONS

102. Raby, K. E., Goldman, L., Creager, M. E., and Selwyn, A. P.: Detection of intraoperative and postoperative myocardial ischemia in peripheral vascular surgery (abstract). Circulation 78:(Suppl. 2):333, 1988.

103. Ouyang, P., Gerstenblith, G., Furman, W. R., et al.: Frequency and significance of early postoperative silent myocardial ischemia in patients having peripheral vascular surgery. Am. J. Cardiol. 64:1113, 1989.

104. Salem, D. N., Homans, D. C., and Isner, J. M.: Management of cardiac disease in the general surgical patient. In Harvey, W. P. (ed.): Current Problems in Cardiology. Vol. 5. Chicago, Year Book Medical Publishers, 1980.

105. Charlson, M. E., MacKenzie, C. R., Ales, K. L., et al.: Surveillance for postoperative myocardial infarction after noncardiac operations. Surg. Gynecol. Obstet. 167:407, 1988.

106. Charlson, M. E., MacKenzie, C. R., Ales, K. L., et al.: The post-operative electrocardiogram and creatine kinase: Implications for diagnosis of myocardial infarction after non-cardiac surgery. J. Clin. Epidemiol. 42:25, 1989.

107. Lee, T. H., and Goldman, L.: Serum enzyme assays in the diagnosis of acute myocardial infarction. Recommendations based on a quantitative analysis. Ann. Intern. Med. 105:221, 1986.

108. Oster, G., Tuden, R. L., and Colditz, G. A.: Prevention of venous thromboembolism after general surgery. Cost-effectiveness analysis of alternative approaches to prophylaxis. Am. J. Med. 82:889, 1987.

109. Goldman, L.: Anesthesia and surgery in the hypertensive patient. In Amery, A. (ed.): Hypertensive Cardiovascular Disease: Pathophysiology and Treatment. The Hague, Martinus Nijhoff Publishing, 1982, p. 916.

110. Goldman, L.: Supraventricular tachyarrhythmias in hospitalized adults after surgery. Chest 73:450, 1978.

THE ROLE OF THE MEDICAL CONSULTATION

111. Weathers, L. W., and Paine R.: The risk of surgery in cardiac patients. Intern. Med. 2:57, 1981.

112. Perry, M. O., and Calcagno, D.: Abdominal aortic aneurysm surgery: The basic evaluation of cardiac risk. Ann. Surg. 208:738, 1988.

113. Rivers, S. P., Scher, L. A., Gupta, S. K., and Veith, F. J.: Safety of peripheral vascular surgery after recent acute myocardial infarction. J. Vasc. Surg. 11:70, 1990.

114. Detsky, A. S., Abrams, H. B., Forbath, N., et al.: Cardiac assessment for patients undergoing noncardiac surgery. A multifactorial clinical risk index. Arch. Intern. Med. 146:2131, 1986.

115. Goldman, L.: Multifactorial index of cardiac risk in noncardiac surgery: Ten-year status report. J. Cardiothorac. Anesth. 1:237, 1987.

116. Lee, T., Pappius, E. M., and Goldman, L.: Impact of inter-physician communication on the effectiveness of medical consultations. Am. J. Med. 74:106, 1983.

117. Horwitz, R. I., Henes, C. G., and Horwitz, S. M.: Strategies for improving the diagnostic and management efficacy of medical consultations. J. Chronic Dis. 36:213, 1983.

118. Lee, T. H., and Goldman, L.: Role of consultant. In Breslow, M. J., Mullen, C. F., and Rogers, M. (eds.): Perioperative Management. St. Louis, C. V. Mosby Co., 1990.

Rheumatic Fever and Other Rheumatic Diseases of the Heart

by GENE H. STOLLERMAN, M.D.

Two groups of diseases that affect connective tissues are the so-called rheumatic diseases and the heritable disorders of connective tissues. The *rheumatic diseases* have many clinical features in common and are often classified together because they produce acute or chronic arthritis, or both, associated with a variety of systemic inflammatory manifestations. Pathologically, they are characterized by diffuse vascular lesions with varying degrees of exudation and fibrosis, and some seem to be associated with hyperimmune phenomena. In some of the syndromes the etiology has been established as complications of well-recognized infections; however, several of the rheumatic diseases remain obscure in regard to both etiology and pathogenesis. They all involve the heart differently and to varying degrees, as would be expected considering the variety of connective tissue structures that make up the heart's "skeleton"—its valve rings, valves, septa, and pericardial sac and the myocardial interstitium, through which courses its rich blood supply.

The *heritable disorders of connective tissue* are rare, genetically determined biochemical lesions of collagen, elastic tissue, or the mucopolysaccharides. In all, structural lesions are produced when cardiac action stresses the defective cardiac skeleton. These conditions are presented in Chapter 51.

Rheumatic Fever

Rheumatic fever (RF) is frequently classified as a connective tissue disease because its anatomical hallmark is damage to collagen fibrils and to the ground substance of connective tissue (especially in the heart). Of major clinical importance is the presence of potentially lethal myocarditis during the acute attack or, more commonly, the fibrosis of the heart valves, which leads to the crippling hemodynamics of chronic rheumatic heart disease. Its uniqueness from other rheumatic diseases is that it is specifically a delayed nonsuppurative sequel of pharyngeal infection with group A streptococci.

EPIDEMIOLOGY

The relation between the epidemiology of RF and that of streptococcal infection has been reviewed extensively.[1] The current confusion concerning the epidemiology of RF stems from the dramatic decline in incidence and prevalence of the disease despite the fact that group A streptococcal pharyngitis still appears to be common among populations in which RF has become rare.[2] In recent years, focal outbreaks of RF in military and civilian populations in the United States have been found to correlate with the reappearance of virulent, encapsulated, M protein–rich strains belonging to M-serotypes previously noted to be associated with epidemic rheumatic fever, and thus referred to as "rheumatogenic" group A streptococci.[3]

THE CHANGING PATTERN OF RHEUMATIC FEVER
(Fig. 56–1)

Reasons for the spectacular decline in RF in the 60's, 70's, and early 80's are undoubtedly multiple. Certainly antibiotics for the treatment and prevention of streptococcal infection have been a factor, as demonstrated particularly in military populations.[4,5] However, the incidence and death rate from the disease were decreasing before the introduction of antibiotics. Changes in the virulence and serotypes of group A streptococci have been most noteworthy[3] (see below). Improved social conditions, such as better housing and slum clearance, have contributed to the decline, since crowding because of inadequate housing is probably the chief reason for the magnified risk of streptococcal infection and acute rheumatic fever (ARF) in certain ethnic and disadvantaged populations. Improvement in the delivery of health care in defined populations may also be significant.[6]

Notwithstanding its decline, rheumatic heart disease still

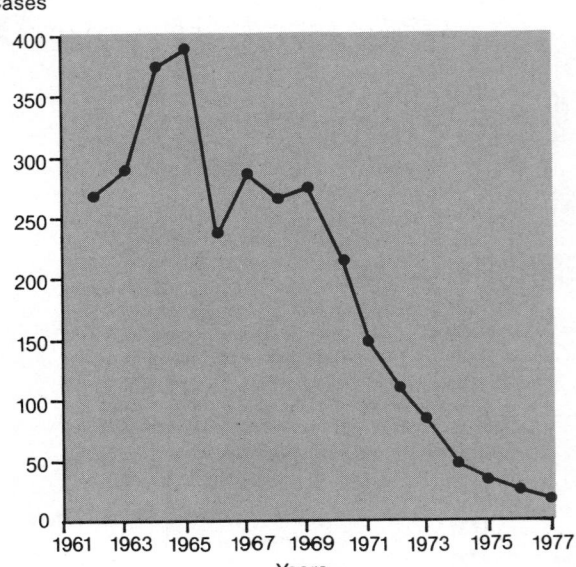

FIGURE 56-1. Acute rheumatic fever attacks reported from 1962 to 1977 to the rheumatic fever registry of the Chicago Department of Health. (From Stollerman, G. H.: Global changes in group A streptococcal diseases and strategies for their prevention. Adv. Intern. Med. 27:373, 1982.)

constitutes the leading cause of death from heart disease in the 5- to 24-year-old age group in many parts of the world and continues to be a serious public health problem, particularly in the slums of the industrializing nations of the Third World.[6-8] The surprising reappearance of outbreaks of RF associated with concomitant reappearance of highly virulent group A streptococcal strains (Fig. 56-2) has made the need for intensified treatment and prevention of streptococcal pharyngeal infection compelling, especially in individuals with rheumatic heart disease (see below, "Prevention").

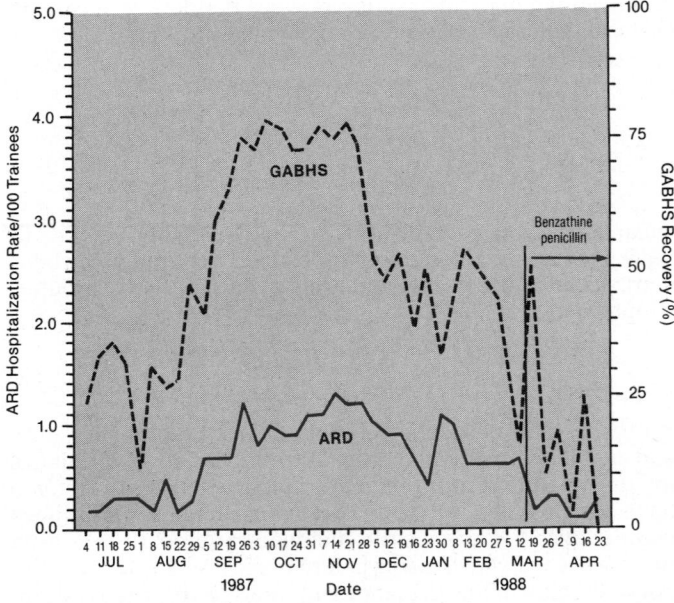

FIGURE 56-2. Hospitalization for acute respiratory disease (ARD, left ordinate) and present recovery of group A streptococci (GABHS, upper curve, right ordinates) among army trainees at Fort Leonard Wood, Missouri, plotted for July 1987 to April 1988. Thirteen cases of ARF were diagnosed between October 1987 and February 1988. No new cases had been reported since the second week of March when benzathine penicillin G was given once to all nonallergic soldiers and thereafter to all new trainees on arrival at the base (From Centers for Disease Control: Acute rheumatic fever among army trainees—Ft Leonard Wood, MO, 1987-1988. MMWR 37:519, 1988.)

FACTORS IN THE ATTACK RATE OF RHEUMATIC FEVER

QUANTITATIVE FACTORS. One factor is the severity of the antecedent pharyngeal streptococcal infection. The clearest relationship of group A streptococcal infection to RF is found in military populations subject to epidemic streptococcal sore throat. In patients with frank, exudative streptococcal pharyngitis caused by rheumatogenic strains of virulent group A streptococci, RF followed at a fairly predictable attack rate (approximately 3 per cent) regardless of the age, race, or ethnic group studied and regardless of the year or season in which the study was made.[4] The major variables which seem to be related to this attack rate in such studies are the magnitude of the immune response to the antecedent streptococcal infection[9] and the duration of convalescent carriage of the organism.[10] Weak antistreptolysin O (ASO) responses are associated with ARF attack rates considerably less than 1 per cent, whereas strong responses are associated with rates well in excess of 5 per cent. If the infecting organism in the pharynx was not eradicated during convalescence, treatment of streptococcal pharyngitis failed to reduce the attack rate of rheumatic fever.

In contrast to the military studies, reports from civilian medical practice indicate that RF occurs less frequently or not at all following endemic, sporadic streptococcal disease.[3,11-14]

VARIATION IN GROUP A STREPTOCOCCAL INFECTIONS. Variations in the rheumatogenicity of group A streptococcal strains are a factor influencing the attack rate of RF.[3] In several laboratories where regular serotyping of group A streptococci isolated from pharyngeal infections is performed with available antisera prepared against known M-protein serotypes, the frequency of identification of such strains has decreased. Furthermore, the prevalence of several of the virulent M types notorious for causing epidemic RF (e.g., types 5, 14, and 24) has apparently declined, and attention has shifted to the study of "new" M types among both pharyngeal strains and "skin" strains.[2,15] The issue of whether there are "nonrheumatogenic group A streptococci"[16] has been sharpened by the clear demonstration that group A streptococcal pyoderma, with or without complicating acute glomerulonephritis (AGN), does not cause ARF.[17] These skin infections are nonrheumatogenic. Since the pharyngeal route of infection is now an accepted requirement for the pathogenesis of ARF[18] (see below), the question of whether such pyoderma strains can cause RF when they produce pharyngitis is of particular interest. Studies in the southwestern United States have clearly shown seasonal epidemiological separation of ARF and AGN.[19] A study of the streptococcal strains in an island population such as Trinidad shows a clear distinction between the serotypes associated with AGN and those associated with ARF.[20,21] In the past, several studies suggested that RF was associated with infections due to virulent encapsulated ("mucoid") strains capable of causing strong type-specific immune responses to M protein and other streptococcal antigens. Such strains belong to the classic M serotypes known to cause ARF.[22,23] The reappearance of severe epidemic rheumatic fever associated with the reappearance of these virulent strains has greatly strengthened the concept of rheumatogenic strains of group A streptococci.[3] Thus, qualitative and quantitative changes in streptococcal pharyngitis have affected greatly the epidemiology of rheumatic fever in various parts of the world.

GEOGRAPHY AND CLIMATE. The relationship of RF to the intensity and severity of streptococcal disease is the same in the tropics as in the temperate climates.[24] In *prospective* studies in which all patients suspected of having ARF were admitted and recurrent attacks were excluded, the frequency of the clinical manifestations of rheumatic fever is the same as in the studies in the United States.[25,26]

Host Factors

AGE, SEX, AND RACE. Like streptococcal sore throat, ARF occurs most commonly in the young school-age child, median age between 9 and 11 years, and very rarely in early infancy. It is estimated that 40 per cent of streptococcal infections in pediatric populations occur in children 2 to 6 years of age, suggesting that repeated streptococcal infections and early sensitization of the host are prerequisite to the development of RF. No true differences in sex, race, or ethnic group susceptibility have been established. Crowded living conditions account for whatever apparent increased susceptibility has been reported.

ACQUIRED SUSCEPTIBILITY. Because ARF develops in only a relatively small percentage of patients following even the most virulent bouts of streptococcal pharyngitis, the question of host predisposition is often raised. Once RF is acquired, its activation following subsequent streptococcal infection is many times greater in rheumatic subjects than in the general population. The recurrence rate per infection, which is as high as 50 per cent during the first year after the initial attack, decreases sharply until 4 to 5 years after the attack.[27,28] It then levels off at approximately 10 per cent and does not seem to fall much lower.[29] Although the persistently high attack rate in individuals having had RF suggests genetic predisposition (see below), the diminishing recurrence rate per infection also suggests loss of acquired hyperreactivity. An alternative explanation may be acquired sensitization in a genetically predisposed host that persists throughout life.

GENETIC FACTORS. Many investigators have sought genetic markers for rheumatic hosts without more than suggestive results.[30] Only a few adequate studies in identical twins have been made and these have shown a relatively low concordance of RF (less than 20 per cent), actually considerably lower than the concordance found in identical twins with other infectious diseases such as tuberculosis or poliomyelitis.[1,30] No clear correlation of conventional HLA genotypes with rheumatic fever has yet been shown. In contrast, non-HLA B cell alloantigens have been found to be expressed more frequently in rheumatic fever probands than in their unaffected siblings and parents.[31-33] Thus, these B cell alloantigens are not unique to the rheumatic hosts but may be more expressible in them if they are stimulated by putative rheumatogenic antigens of group A streptococci (see below). The uniqueness of the group A streptococcus in initiating a cardiodestructive disease in a limited segment of the human species, regardless of race or ethnic group, continues to make the quest for a unique host response to a specific streptococcal antigen a persisting challenge, particularly for investigators interested in autoimmunity.[34]

ETIOLOGY

The lines of evidence establishing the group A streptococcus as the sole agent causing initial and recurrent attacks of RF (described below) are of necessity indirect, because group A streptococci cannot be recovered from the lesions of RF and no satisfactory experimental model of the disease has been demonstrated.

CLINICAL EVIDENCE. Although the frequency with which septic sore throat preceded ARF has been recognized for over 100 years, inconsistencies in this relationship have been pointed out repeatedly.[1] Almost one-third of patients with ARF deny the occurrence of antecedent sore throat. Throat and blood cultures in such patients show that the former is frequently negative and the latter virtually always sterile at the onset of the rheumatic attack. Recurrences of RF appeared even more mysterious when antecedent streptococcal sore throat was unrecognized and particularly when the chronicity of a rheumatic attack and the hemodynamic complications of rheumatic heart disease made it difficult to distinguish continued versus reactivated rheumatic carditis. On clinical grounds alone, therefore, it is difficult to establish the group A streptococcus as the *sole* etiological agent.

EPIDEMIOLOGICAL EVIDENCE. Such factors as latitude, altitude, crowding, dampness, economic factors, and age all affect the incidence of RF because they are related to the incidence and severity of streptococcal infections in general (see above). Careful epidemiological studies over a period of 20 years show a clear sequential relationship between outbreaks of streptococcal pharyngitis and RF.

IMMUNOLOGICAL EVIDENCE. Initial (primary) or recurrent (secondary) RF does not occur without a streptococcal antibody response.[35] Furthermore, the magnitude of the antibody response is a major variable determining the attack rate (but not the severity or duration) of RF following streptococcal pharyngitis.[9] This is true for both primary and secondary attacks.[27] Indeed, the streptococcal immune response is an important criterion for the diagnosis of RF (see below).

PROPHYLACTIC EVIDENCE. The final and perhaps most convincing evidence is the prevention of both initial and recurrent attacks of RF by, in the former case, penicillin therapy and, in the latter, continuous chemoprophylaxis against streptococcal infections. Completely effective prophylaxis of streptococcal infections in rheumatic subjects allows us to conclude that RF cannot be reactivated by any other infection, illness, or trauma.[27,35]

PATHOGENESIS

Despite the elusiveness of the pathogenesis of RF, there are a few well-established requirements for the development of this postinfectious sequel: (1) the presence of the group A streptococcus, (2) a streptococcal antibody response indicative of actual recent infection, (3) persistence of the organism in the pharynx for a sufficient period, and (4) location of the infection in the throat.

THE ROLE OF TOXINS. Despite the popularity of the concepts of hyperimmunity and autoimmunity in the pathogenesis of RF (see below), none of the antibodies described to date, including those reactive with the heart, has been shown to be cytotoxic. A direct toxic effect, therefore, of some streptococcal product, particularly on the heart, has not yet been ruled out as a pathogenetic mechanism.[1]

IMMUNOLOGICAL THEORIES

The most popular pathogenic theory is that RF results from some type of hyperimmune reaction due either to bacterial allergy or autoimmunity. This view is supported by strong evidence, since RF patients are, in general, the population most intensively hyperimmune to all streptococcal products.

The mean antibody titer to virtually every streptococcal antigen that has been studied is increased in patients during the acute stage of RF.[1] Yet no single humoral mechanism of tissue injury has been defined. Complement levels are increased rather than decreased, and autoantibodies associated with immune complex disease (e.g., rheumatoid factor, anti-DNA, and others) are not present. Although low-grade microscopic hematuria may occur, frank lesions of glomerulonephritis are absent. Careful studies have identified circulating immune complexes, but they are of small size and not high titer and quickly disappear after the acute stage of polyarthritis.[36]

AUTOIMMUNITY. Modern theories of the possible autoimmune pathogenetic mechanisms of RF have been extensively reviewed.[34,37] It has been known for many years that the serum of some patients with ARF contains autoantibodies to heart tissues, and numerous reports using a variety of techniques, mostly immunofluorescence, have confirmed this finding.[38-40] Antiheart antibodies are gamma globulins with specificity for cardiac components reacting primarily with the sarcolemma. Their binding is also associated with deposition of large amounts of complement component C3.

CROSS-REACTIVE ANTIBODIES AND AUTOIMMUNITY. In the early 1960's Kaplan and his associates demonstrated that rabbit antisera against certain group A streptococci react with human heart preparations in the immunofluorescent test.[40,41] Since then, many additional immunological cross reactions have been described between streptococci and human tissues[42-47] (Fig. 56–3). The immunological details of these reactions and their possible relation to the pathogenesis of RF[1,34,37] are summarized below.

Group A streptococci have a number of structural components that are related to mammalian tissues.[1] The hyaluronate capsule of the organism, for example, is identical with human hyaluronate. Antibodies to the group A cell wall polysaccharide cross-react with glycoproteins of heart valves.[43] Membrane antigens of group A streptococci cross-react with sarcolemma and smooth muscle of endocardial and myocardial arteries.[42]

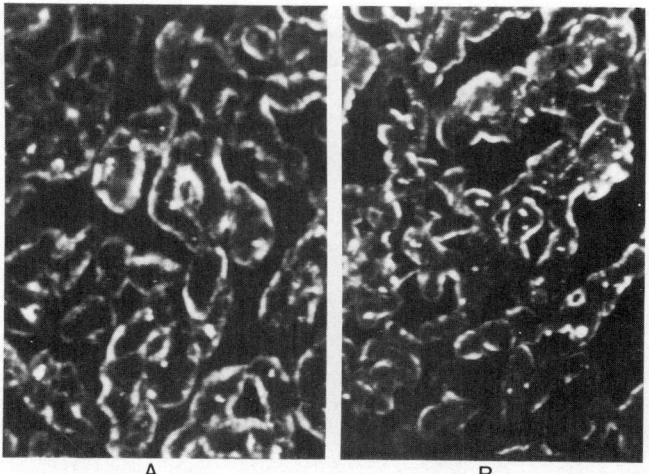

FIGURE 56–3. Immunofluorescent staining patterns of cryostat sections of heart tissue stained with sera containing heart-reactive antibody. *A,* The pattern obtained with a serum sample from a patient with acute rheumatic fever. *B,* The pattern seen with serum from a rabbit immunized with group A streptococcal membranes. (From Zabriskie, J. B.: Rheumatic fever. The interplay between host, genetics, and microbe. Circulation 71:1077, 1985, by permission of the American Heart Association, Inc.)

Antibodies that are of specific interest for their potential relationship to autoimmune injury of the heart are those absorbable by streptococcal products. A sustained rise in titer of antibodies that cross-react with the cardiac tissue often precedes an attack of RF, but such antibodies do not correlate clearly with the presence or severity of rheumatic carditis, and they have not been shown to be cytotoxic. Antibody to the streptococcal group A polysaccharide has received particular attention because of prolonged persistence of elevated levels in the serum of patients with rheumatic mitral valvular disease in contrast with its more rapid decline in patients with RF without cardiac involvement and in patients with transient mitral insufficiency, including those with mitral valve prolapse.[44,45] Antibodies reactive with cytoplasm of neurons in the subthalamic and caudate nuclei have been found more frequently in rheumatic patients with Sydenham's chorea than in those rheumatic patients without this manifestation.[46] Most recently, delineation of the molecular structure of several streptococcal M proteins has led to the demonstration of epitopes of these serotypes cross-reactive with myosin.[47-50] The tertiary structure of streptococcal coil[50] and to be similar to other coiled proteins in human tissues which include not only myosin but keratin and other connective tissue structures.[47-49] Moreover, the M protein in rheumatogenic strains has been shown to be a very large molecule[51] containing not only the type-specific epitopes that make it capable of producing protective opsonic antibodies but also containing moieties that are powerful blastogens for

human T lymphocytes. These moieties are so-called "superantigens" that may stimulate subsets of T cells with specificity for self-antigens (e.g., cardiac tissues) above a threshold of tolerance needed to permit an autoimmune response.[52]

Little doubt remains that streptococcal antigens of various kinds are shared with human myocardium, but it has not yet been shown that they are actually responsible for tissue injury in certain hosts and are thus related to the pathogenesis of rheumatic fever.[33]

PATHOLOGY

There is often considerable disparity between the severity of the clinical manifestations of RF and the extent of the morbid anatomical changes it produces. Sydenham's chorea, cardiac atrioventricular conduction blocks, and erythema marginatum all appear to be related more to functional disturbances than to visible lesions. In contrast, the persistent focal inflammatory lesions of the myocardium, such as the Aschoff nodule, do not always correlate with clinical manifestations of active carditis and have led to differences of opinion between pathologists and clinicians with regard to the definition of rheumatic activity. In general, however, the acute phase of RF is characterized by diffuse exudative and proliferative inflammatory reactions in the heart, joints, and skin. Small blood vessels and arterioles are commonly involved, but unlike the arteritis of some other connective tissue diseases, thrombotic lesions are not seen.

The term *fibrinoid degeneration* describes the basic structural changes

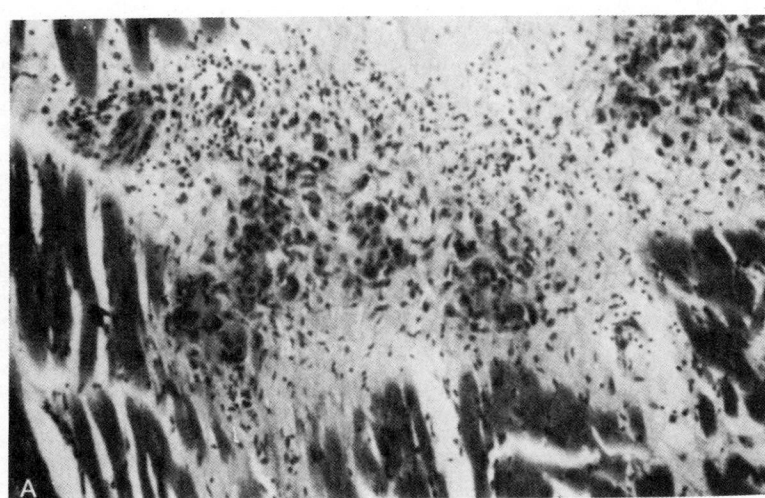
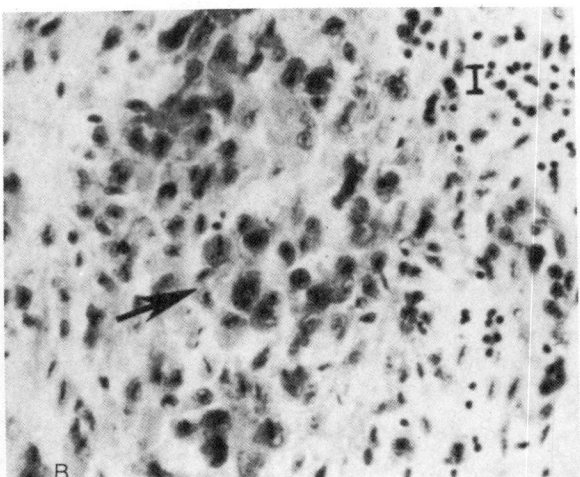
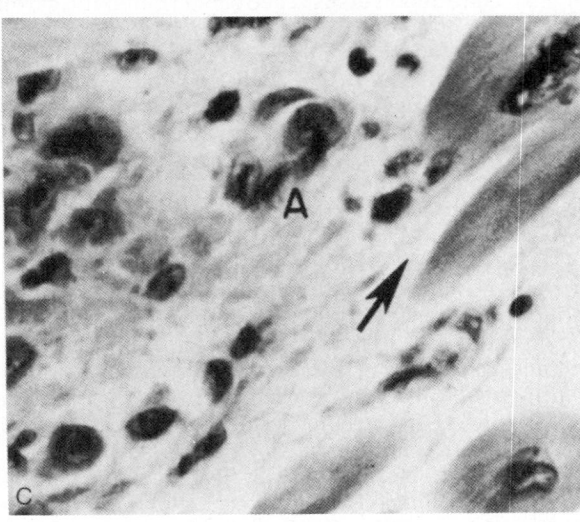

FIGURE 56-4. *A,* Multiple Aschoff lesions in the left ventricle, showing confluence of large monocyte macrophage-appearing cells surrounded by cell infiltrate and dissolution of adjacent myocardial muscle with fibrous tissue replacement. *B,* Higher-power view showing large mononuclear cells *(arrow)* and interstitial lymphocytes (I). *C,* High-power view. (From Husby, G., et al.: Immunofluorescent studies of florid rheumatic Aschoff lesions. Arthritis Rheum. *29:*207, 1986.)

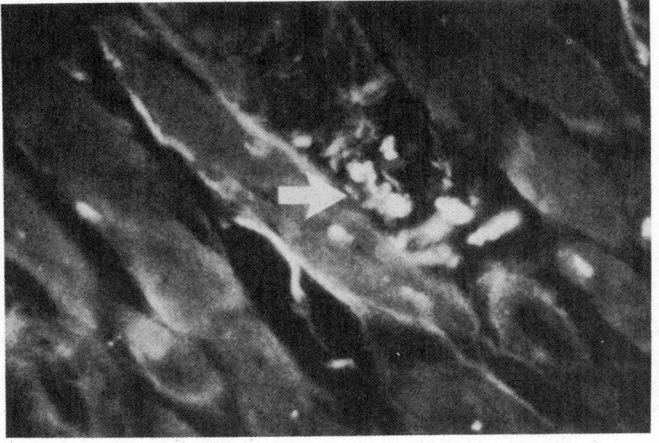

FIGURE 56-5. Postmortem myocardial specimen from a 20-year-old patient with severe rheumatic carditis. Immunofluorescent staining shows many large monocytoid cells that appear to have ingested myosin *(arrow).* (From Husby, G., et al.: Immunofluorescent studies of florid rheumatic Aschoff lesions. Arthritis Rheum. *29:*207, 1986.)

in the collagen of connective tissues. The fibrinoid substance resembles and stains like fibrin and is a feature of the earliest phase of the myocardial lesions. The collagen fibers in these mucoid areas become swollen and eosinophilic, forming a meshwork of rigid, waxlike fibers. This exudative-degenerative phase lasts for 2 to 3 weeks, following which the most characteristic lesion of RF develops — the myocardial *Aschoff nodule*. The proliferative and healing phase then follows and may persist for many months or even years (Figs. 56–4 and 56–5).

Ironically, the only lesion pathognomonic of RF is vague with regard to its origin, functional impact on the heart, and relation to the course and severity of the rheumatic attack.[54] Aschoff nodules do not seem to account for the acute dilatation of the heart in first attacks of severe carditis. The persistence of Aschoff nodules for many years after a rheumatic attack has been well recognized by pathologists. Biopsies of the left atrial appendage obtained during mitral valve surgery for mitral stenosis have shown persistence of Aschoff nodules in patients who no longer have clinical or laboratory evidence of rheumatic activity[55–57] and who have no recent evidence of streptococcal infection.[58] The persistence of Aschoff nodules seems to be correlated, however, with progressive fibrosis and stenosis of the mitral valve. One series[56,57] showed such lesions in 21 per cent of 191 surgically excised left atrial appendages in patients with mitral stenosis. In the same series, of 91 patients with pure mitral regurgitation, Aschoff nodules were present in the left atrial appendage of only one patient.

CARDIAC LESIONS

On gross inspection of the heart, a pancarditis is almost always evident, with fresh exudative pericardial lesions, dilatation of the heart, and verrucous endocardial lesions on the valves.[59]

PERICARDITIS (see also p. 1501). Both layers of the pericardium are thickened and covered with a fibrinous exudate, and serosanguineous pericardial fluid may be present. With healing, fibrosis and adhesions develop which partially or completely obliterate the pericardial sac, but constrictive pericarditis does *not* occur.

MYOCARDITIS. In addition to the Aschoff bodies, a diffuse cellular infiltrate is present in interstitial tissues. The cells are usually lymphocytes, but polymorphonuclear leukocytes, histiocytes, and eosinophils may also be present. Exudate may be associated with damaged muscle. This interstitial myocarditis may be more important than the nodular Aschoff bodies in producing heart failure. Myocardial fibers are also damaged, and the greatest damage occurs in the vicinity of Aschoff nodules and around blood vessels.[60,61] Macrophages containing cardiac myosin have been identified in Aschoff nodules by immunofluorescent studies of florid acute myocarditis (Fig. 56–5).[61]

THE CONDUCTION SYSTEM. Despite the high frequency of prolonged atrial ventricular conduction in ARF, visible changes in the bundle of His are seen in the minority of autopsy cases of ARF. The evanescence of heart block and its easy reversibility in most cases by the administration of atropine fit the concept that a pathophysiological defect rather than an anatomical lesion is responsible for this conduction defect.

ENDOCARDITIS. The verrucous lesions at the valve edge appear as a mass of eosinophilic material staining as fibrin. At the base and edges of the valve, the cells line up in palisades at right angles to the base and often have elongated Aschoff-like nuclei. As the lesions progress, granulation tissue develops and vascularization and progressive fibrosis take place. The changes involve the annulus as well as the cusps and chordae tendineae, which, as a result of scarring, thicken and shorten.

RHEUMATIC VALVULAR DEFORMITIES

(See also Chap. 34)

MITRAL REGURGITATION. Incompetence or regurgitation may result from shortening of one or both cusps, from shortening and fusing of chordae and papillary muscles, or from dilatation of the valve ring. By far, the most common clinically apparent lesion of rheumatic heart disease is mitral regurgitation, and such lesions often occur subclinically when extracardiac symptoms of ARF are absent. Dilatation of the valve ring occurs in active carditis more frequently as a result of acute dilatation of the left ventricle. Marked mitral regurgitation also occurs, however, without acute left ventricular dilatation when the valve cusps and the musculotendinous structures are severely swollen and disorganized by the rheumatic process without coexisting severe myocarditis.

MITRAL STENOSIS. This lesion occurs with varying degrees of mitral regurgitation. When stenosis is severe, regurgitation may be relatively unimportant, and the main hemodynamic problem is obstruction to blood flow during diastole. The gross changes in the mitral valve are variable. The cusps may fuse, leaving an ovoid opening, but the cusps themselves may remain thin and pliable. In other instances the cusps become thick, rigid, or even calcified. A "funnel-shaped valve" with its opening at the apex may result when fusion of the cusps occurs with shortening and thickening of the chordae tendineae and papillary muscles.

AORTIC VALVE DEFORMITIES. The most common aortic lesion is a combination of stenosis and regurgitation. Pure aortic stenosis is relatively uncommon, but a minimal degree of aortic regurgitation occurs frequently in mild rheumatic involvement. In most cases of symptomatic rheumatic aortic disease, both stenosis and regurgitation occur, but one or the other may be functionally predominant. Deformity of the valve results from fusion of the cusps at the commissures, rigidity and shortening of the cusps alone, or combinations of both processes with calcification superimposed (Fig. 56–6).

TRICUSPID VALVE DEFORMITIES. These almost always exist in association with mitral and aortic lesions and occur in approximately 10 per cent of patients with chronic rheumatic heart disease.[59]

PULMONARY VALVE DEFORMITIES. Pulmonary valve deformities are rarest of all. When they occur, stenosis is more usual than is incompetence. The pathological changes in the pulmonary valve are similar to those in the aortic valve.

PROGRESSIVE PATHOLOGICAL CHANGES IN HEALED RHEUMATIC HEART DISEASE. There are manifestations of progressive changes and continued inflammation that seem unrelated to the original rheumatic process. Disruption of red blood cells ("cardiac hemolytic anemia") can result from valvular defects; platelet turnover and destruction have recently been proved to be excessive in rheumatic heart disease[62]; and resultant thrombosis and fibrosis can occur along with calcification. Recurrent congestive heart failure may cause fatty changes in the myocardium and progressive fibrosis. The endocardium, especially the left atrium in mitral valvular deformity, is prone to develop organized thrombi, to stretch and dilate progressively, and to develop chronic inflammatory changes that are not exudative or clearly due to the rheumatic process at all.

EXTRACARDIAC LESIONS

JOINTS. Swelling and edema of the articular and periarticular structures with serous effusion into the joint space occur without erosion of the joint surface or pannus formation. The synovial membrane is reddened and thickened and covered with fibrinous exudate. Histologically there is marked edema, engorgement and dilation of blood vessels, and diffuse and focal infiltrates of lymphocytes and polymorphonuclear leukocytes, the latter more numerous initially. Later, focal fibrinoid lesions with histiocytic granulomas may appear, but these lesions heal also without residua.

SUBCUTANEOUS NODULES. A central zone of fibrinoid necrotic material is surrounded by histiocytes and fibroblasts, and lymphocytes and polymorphonuclear leukocytes collect around small vessels. The structure resembles Aschoff bodies and may heal very rapidly, leaving no apparent scars.

CHOREA. Considerable confusion exists concerning the pathology of Sydenham's chorea because (1) few patients die of "pure" chorea, (2) those who die of severe carditis may have inflammatory lesions of the central nervous system without chorea,[63] (3) no single site is consistently involved, (4) Aschoff bodies are not found in the brain,[64,65] and (5) it has not been possible to correlate clinical findings with pathological changes. Changes found in the central nervous system include arteritis, cellular degeneration, perivascular round cell infiltration, and occasional petechial hemorrhages, but on the whole these are not impressive and are scattered throughout the cortex, cerebellum, and basal ganglia.[66,67]

RHEUMATIC PNEUMONITIS. Because this finding usually occurs with severe carditis only, there has been argument about whether the pulmonary lesion is a form of the acute respiratory distress syndrome secondary to heart failure or part of the rheumatic process itself. It has been described, however, in the absence of heart failure.[68]

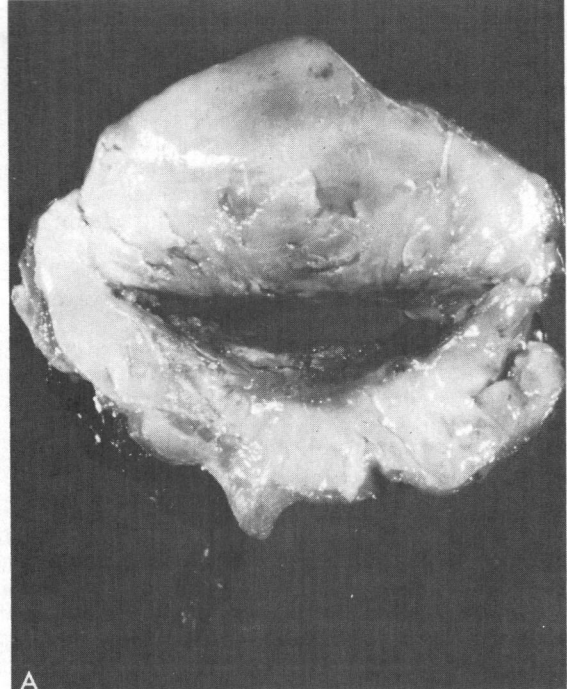

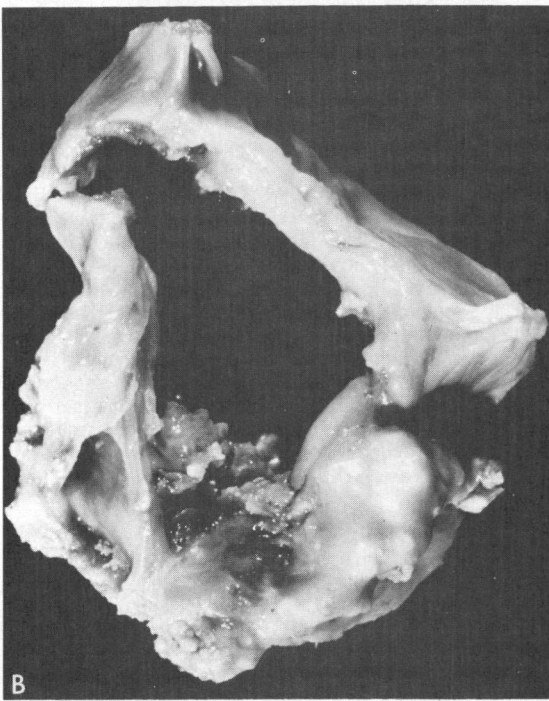

FIGURE 56–6. Excised rheumatic valve. *A,* "Fishmouth" mitral valve. *B,* Aortic valve fixed in open position. (Courtesy of James W. Pate, M.D. From Stollerman, G. H.: Rheumatic Fever and Streptococcal Infection. New York, by permission of Grune and Stratton, 1975.)

CLINICAL MANIFESTATIONS

The signs and symptoms of ARF vary greatly and are determined by the systems involved, the severity of the lesions and when they appear in the course of the disease, and the stage of the disease when the patient is first observed by the physician. Certain manifestations that follow streptococcal infections (with a frequency far exceeding chance) occur simultaneously, in close succession, or singly. They have been called *major manifestations* and consist of carditis, arthritis, chorea, subcutaneous nodules, and erythema marginatum. The word "major" refers to their importance as diagnostic criteria and not to their importance in the severity of the process or its activity, or to the prognosis.

Minor manifestations of ARF are frequently present and helpful in recognizing the disease. They are too nonspecific, however, to be of major importance in diagnosis. Minor manifestations include such findings as fever, arthralgia, acute phase reactants in the blood, heart block, and a history of previous ARF or rheumatic heart disease.

ANTECEDENT STREPTOCOCCAL INFECTION. Clinical evidence for an antecedent streptococcal infection may not be apparent. As many as one-third of patients do not remember having had any illness in the preceding month (see above). Furthermore, in patients with previous RF who were followed prospectively for recurrences, asymptomatic streptococcal infections accounted for 54[27] to 70 per cent[29] of recurrences of RF. The average interval between onset of symptoms of pharyngitis and the symptoms of RF (the latent period) was 18.6 days in one prospective study,[69] but may be as short as 1 week or as long as 5 weeks. The latent period is no shorter in patients with previous RF than in those without.

ARTHRITIS. The manifestation occurs in about three-fourths of patients during the acute stage of the disease. In general, joint involvement becomes more common with increasing age of the patient, a trend related to the concomitant decrease in the incidence of carditis and chorea.[70,71] The arthritis of RF usually involves the large joints, particularly the knees, ankles, elbows, and wrists. Almost any joint, however, may be affected. In the classic attack, several joints are involved in quick succession, each for a brief time, resulting in the typical picture of migratory polyarthritis. Each joint remains inflamed for usually no more than a week before the inflammation begins to subside, and the inflammation usually abates spontaneously in 2 or 3 weeks.[72-74] Acute polyarthritis rarely occurs more than 35 days after the onset of the streptococcal infection, and *for that reason, it is almost always associated with a rising or peak titer of streptococcal antibodies.* This fact aids in identifying an isolated bout of polyarthritis as rheumatic or in *excluding* RF as a cause for a given bout of polyarthritis when streptococcal antibodies are not increased.

CARDITIS

VARIATIONS IN ONSET AND COURSE. The most important manifestation of ARF is carditis, which, in its most severe form, causes death from acute cardiac failure. Much more commonly, however, carditis is less intense, and the predominant effect is scarring of the heart valves. In contrast to the seriousness of its prognosis, rheumatic carditis most often causes no symptoms of its own and is usually diagnosed in the course of the examination of a patient with arthritis or chorea, which directs the physician's attention to the heart, where murmurs are detected. Carditis, therefore, does not come to medical attention if other symptoms of rheumatic fever are absent or if the carditis is not severe enough to cause heart failure, prolonged or severe fever, or the pain of pericarditis. Patients with undiagnosed carditis may later prove to have rheumatic heart disease and usually give no history of a previous rheumatic attack.

Murmurs indicative of carditis are usually present during the first week of the illness in about three-fourths of all patients in whom carditis is eventually diagnosed.[75] By the second or third week, murmurs become evident in 85 per cent of those in whom they will eventually develop.

Acute heart failure in a young patient who has had rheumatic heart disease previously but who has been well compensated *should always be suspected as a recurrence of acute rheumatic carditis.* Young hearts with rheumatic disease rarely fail abruptly because of hemodynamic handicaps alone except when the latter are severe and protracted. On the other hand, it is often not possible to detect carditis during mild rheumatic recurrences in patients with old rheumatic valvular lesions. Like most episodes of carditis, heart failure or signs of pericarditis will be absent, and the diagnosis of a recurrence will depend on other major and minor criteria in cases in which changing heart murmurs (the most common sign of carditis in first rheumatic attacks) are undetectable.

CLINICAL SIGNS AND CRITERIA. The four major criteria for the clinical diagnosis of rheumatic carditis are (1) an organic heart murmur or murmurs not previously present, (2) enlargement of the heart, (3) congestive heart failure, and (4) pericardial friction rubs or signs of effusion. If any one of these is unequivocal in a patient with active RF, the diagnosis of carditis is justified.

MURMURS OF ACUTE RHEUMATIC CARDITIS. Organic murmurs are almost invariably present. They may not be heard when the heart rate is too rapid, when cardiac output is very low in severe congestive heart failure, when they are obscured by a loud pericardial rub, or, rarely, when there is marked pericardial effusion. Otherwise, the signs of endocarditis are always associated with those of involvement of other layers of the heart, although the latter may not be clinically apparent.

Apical Systolic Murmur. The mitral valve is the most common site of rheumatic inflammation—about three times as frequently involved as the aortic valve. Inflammation ("valvulitis") causing edema, thickening, and verrucae leads to mitral regurgitation early in the course of the disease and often with mild cardiac involvement. The systolic murmur is heard best at the apex, usually grade 3 or more on a scale of 6 in intensity, and, most important, it has a high-pitched blowing quality.

Apical Mid-diastolic Murmur (Carey-Coombs Murmur). This murmur begins directly after the onset of the third heart sound and ends before the first heart sound. The mid-diastolic murmur is often transient, low pitched, and easily missed. The presence of this murmur makes the diagnosis of "mitral valvulitis" more definite, confirms the significance of the apical systolic murmur, and adds to the seriousness of the prognosis for permanent valve injury.

Aortic Diastolic Murmur. This murmur may appear early in the course of the disease as an expression of aortic valvulitis and may occur alone or with mitral valvulitis. The aortic diastolic blow may be audible only intermittently, depending, again, on cardiac output. The murmur is a soft, high-pitched, decrescendo blow heard immediately after the second heart sound. A diastolic cooing or crying "sea gull" murmur is rarely heard, but can be present evanescently in the aortic valvulitis of acute carditis.

CARDIAC ENLARGEMENT AND FAILURE. The most reliable clinical expression of rheumatic myocarditis from the standpoint of diagnosis and prognosis is *dilatation*, particularly of the left atrium and ventricle. In two careful cooperative studies designed to evaluate treatment of rheumatic carditis, cardiomegaly occurred in a little more than half the children who developed carditis.[72,76,77]

Congestive heart failure is the least common but most serious manifestation of rheumatic carditis. It is reported in 5 to 10 per cent of first attacks of rheumatic carditis. It is more common, however, to encounter severe and fatal heart failure as a manifestation of a *rheumatic recurrence* than of a primary attack.

PERICARDITIS. Pericarditis occurs in approximately 5 to 10 per cent of most large series of ARF.[72,75] Occasionally, pericardial reaction and effusion will be more striking and prominent than the degree of myocarditis. In such cases the regression in apparent heart size and the rate of healing of the attack can be rapid. Conversely, the pericarditis may be a relatively minor aspect of a profound case of heart failure due to severe myocarditis. One rarely sees tamponade without severe heart failure as well.

ARRHYTHMIAS. Delayed atrioventricular (AV) conduction, as reflected in prolongation of the P-R interval, occurs with a frequency similar to that of the polyarthritis of ARF, whether or not clear evidence of carditis is present. The prolongation of AV conduction is easily reversed with atropine,[78]

suggesting that this feature is usually due to functional effects of the disease on AV conduction rather than to direct inflammation and fibrosis of the conduction system. Prolongation of AV conduction may lead to second-degree and, rarely, even third-degree block.[79] The latter is usually of brief duration and reverts spontaneously. Interference and dissociation phenomena are also characteristic of occasional nodal rhythms.

EXTRACARDIAC MANIFESTATIONS

SUBCUTANEOUS NODULES. These are a major manifestation of ARF.[80] However, they are not pathognomonic of RF, since they occur in rheumatoid arthritis and systemic lupus erythematosus as well. They rarely occur as an isolated manifestation and are associated most often with severe carditis, appearing usually several weeks after its onset.[81]

Nodules are round, firm, painless subcutaneous lesions varying in size from approximately 0.5 to 2.0 cm. The skin over them is freely movable and not inflamed. They are located over bony surfaces or prominences and over tendons, particularly the extensor of the fingers and toes and flexors of the wrists and ankles. They occur in crops and vary in number from one to usually three or four dozen; when numerous, they tend to be symmetrical. Nodules are evanescent, disappearing sometimes within several days but usually lasting a week or two and rarely more than a month. They tend, therefore, to be much smaller and less persistent than rheumatoid nodules.

ERYTHEMA MARGINATUM. This is a less common feature of RF, but is so characteristic that it has taken its rightful place among the five major diagnostic manifestations of the disease. However, it cannot be considered pathognomonic of ARF because it has been reported in sepsis, particularly staphylococcal, in drug reactions, in patients with glomerulonephritis, and in children in whom no etiological factor can be identified.

Erythema marginatum appears as a bright-pink "smoke ring" spreading serpiginously through pale skin. It is nonpruritic, nonpainful, and neither indurated nor raised. It blanches completely on pressure and is evanescent. The individual lesions usually appear on the trunk and the proximal parts of the extremities but not on the face; they rarely extend distally beyond the elbows or knees. Erythema marginatum may recur intermittently for months, uninfluenced by antirheumatic agents, and when all other signs of rheumatic activity are gone, one can allow the patient to begin to ambulate without fear of a relapse.

CHOREA (SYDENHAM'S CHOREA, ST. VITUS' DANCE). This neurological disorder, characterized by involuntary, purposeless, rapid movements, muscular weakness, and emotional lability, may be associated with other manifestations of ARF, but it also may appear as the sole expression of the disease—so-called pure chorea. After puberty it is present exclusively in women, and even in them it declines rapidly after adolescence. Chorea has decreased strikingly in frequency compared with arthritis and carditis. In a recent outbreak of rheumatic fever in children in Utah, however, the frequency of chorea in the acute attack was as high as that described in the United States several decades ago—approximately 25 per cent of cases.[82]

The movements of chorea are abrupt and erratic, not rhythmic or repetitive. In even the most violent attacks, all choreiform movements disappear during sleep and are less violent during rest and sedation.[1]

Chorea may last from 1 week to more than 2 years, but usually about 8 to 15 weeks, with a mean of 13.7. Chorea is never seen simultaneously with arthritis, but often coexists with carditis. When chorea appears alone, however, the other minor clinical and laboratory signs of ARF may be entirely absent. The erythrocyte sedimentation rate and C-reactive protein may be normal. Even more confusing, in such cases the ASO and other streptococcal antibody titers may not be increased because chorea appears only after a relatively long latent period (as long as 1 to 6 months) following the antecedent streptococcal infection, and after the longest latent period, both the acute phase reactants and the streptococcal antibody titers may have returned to normal.[83,84]

FEVER. Some degree of fever accompanies almost all rheumatic attacks at their onset. Temperature usually ranges from 101° to 104°F (38.4° to 40°C), is rarely higher, and has no characteristic pattern. In the usual attack, fever decreases in approximately a week without antipyretic treatment and may become low grade for another week or two. It rarely lasts for more than several weeks. When antirheumatic agents are used, however, a "rebound" of fever may occur after 4 to 6 weeks of treatment, but it usually subsides spontaneously within a few days except in unusually persistent attacks.

ABDOMINAL PAIN. The abdominal pain of RF, which occurs in fewer than 5 per cent of patients with ARF, resembles that seen in other conditions in which acute microvascular mesenteric disease occurs, such as sickle cell crises, sepsis, endotoxin or anaphylactic shock, transfusion reactions, and anaphylactoid purpura.

EPISTAXIS. In the past, the incidence of epistaxis was reported from as high as 48 per cent in the early 1930's to a low of 4 to 9 per cent in the late 1950's,[70] and perhaps it is even less frequent now.

LABORATORY FINDINGS

Although there are no pathognomonic tests for RF, laboratory findings are helpful in two major ways: (1) in establishing the antecedent streptococcal infection and (2) in documenting the presence or persistence of an inflammatory process.

ANTECEDENT STREPTOCOCCAL INFECTION. The diagnosis of recent streptococcal infection can be made only tentatively by throat culture but definitely by antibody determinations. Throat cultures are usually negative by the time RF appears. When they are positive, one still cannot be certain whether the organism isolated represents convalescent carriage of the antecedent infection or an intercurrent acquisition of a different strain. Streptococcal antibodies are therefore more useful because they reach a peak titer shortly after the onset of ARF and indicate true infection rather than transient carriage.

ANTIBODIES. The specific antibodies used to diagnose streptococcal infections are primarily antistreptolysin O and anti-DNAase B. Antistreptolysin O has been the most extensively used test and is generally available in hospitals in the United States.

ASO titers vary with age, geographical area, and other factors influencing the frequency of streptococcal infection. Titers of 200 to 300 units/ml are common in healthy children 6 to 14 years of age who live in crowded cities in the temperate zone of the United States.

The chance of detecting a significant antibody response is greatest 2 to 3 weeks after the onset of ARF, which is usually 4 to 5 weeks after the antecedent streptococcal infection. Thereafter, antibody titers fall off rapidly in the next few months, and after 6 months the decline levels off slowly. For this reason, evidence of increased streptococcal antibodies should be present in all patients at the onset of the rheumatic attack if such onset is well defined. Acute polyarthritis always occurs within a latent period of no more than 4 to 5 weeks after the antecedent streptococcal infection and therefore at or near the peak of the antibody response.

Anti-DNAase B, together with the ASO, has become most generally recommended for diagnosis, with antihyaluronidase a third choice.[85]

ACUTE PHASE REACTANTS. Acute phase reactants include leukocyte counts, erythrocyte sedimentation rate (ESR), C-reactive protein (CRP),[86] serum mucoprotein, serum hexosamine, serum protein electrophoresis, and several others. The two tests that have gained widest use are the CRP and the ESR. These tests are, of course, not specific for RF, but they are almost always abnormal during the active rheumatic process if it is not suppressed by antirheumatic drugs.

ANEMIA. The anemia of RF is the normocytic normochromic anemia of chronic inflammation and is of mild to moderate degree. Suppression of inflammation usually corrects the anemia partially or completely, and corticosteroids are particularly potent in this regard. Anemia is a good index of the severity and chronicity of RF.

ELECTROCARDIOGRAPHIC FINDINGS. The electrocardiogram in RF has no characteristic pattern, and the diagnosis of rheumatic carditis should never be made on the basis of ECG changes alone. Too often the diagnosis of carditis has been made incorrectly when a doubtful systolic murmur has been associated with a prolonged P-R interval or nonspecific ST-T changes. Neither the course of the acute rheumatic attack nor the subsequent development of valvular or myocardial damage can be predicted from the electrocardiographic changes.[74,87] Patients with ECG changes but with no other signs of carditis recover completely without the stigmata of rheumatic heart disease.[88]

DIAGNOSIS

JONES CRITERIA. When T. Duckett Jones formulated his criteria for the diagnosis of ARF in 1944,[89] there was immediate recognition of their value and considerable agreement about their use. These criteria were adopted in modified form in 1955 by the American Heart Association's Council on Rheumatic Fever and Congenital Heart Disease and were further revised by the same Council's committee in 1965.[90] The current criteria (Table 56–1) emphasize the importance of establishing the presence of the antecedent streptococcal infection by demonstration of increased streptococcal antibodies. If supported by such evidence, two major (or one major and two minor) manifestations indicate a high probability of ARF. However, because virtually all patients with Sydenham's chorea are rheumatic subjects, the diagnosis can be made even when chorea is the sole manifestation. Because of the numerous causes of polyarthritis, the diagnosis of RF is weakest when this manifestation appears alone, and particularly in the adolescent or adult population in which other arthritides are common.

CARDITIS

Functional ("Innocent") Murmurs. When functional or organic murmurs are typical, there is little problem for the experienced physician. At times, however, a nondescript murmur, especially in an obese or heavy-chested person, may defy sharp distinctions, and repeated examinations and other studies may be required. Such murmurs are often classified as "doubtful" or "questionable" when no other decision can be made.

Myocarditis. In its severe and chronic form, myocarditis due to other diseases may be impossible to distinguish from chronic rheumatic carditis if the heart is dilated and mitral regurgitation is prominent. This situation occurs when patients with ARF have heart failure with no associated extracardiac manifestations to provide clues. In rheumatic carditis, as the patient recovers cardiac compensation, the valvular lesions persist, and the murmurs become, if anything, louder.

Pericarditis. Rheumatic carditis does not produce an isolated pericarditis. At the onset of RF, however, pericarditis may appear before valvulitis and myocarditis are evident. Although many causes of pericarditis can be listed (Chap. 45), primary viral pericarditis most often enters the differential diagnosis in children.

COURSE AND PROGNOSIS

The clinical course of RF can be quite variable, but in general there is a characteristic sequence of the major manifestations and usually a predictable duration. The latent period between streptococcal infection and the onset of ARF is shortest in arthritis and erythema marginatum and longest in chorea, with that of carditis and subcutaneous nodules in be-

TABLE 56–1 JONES CRITERIA (REVISED)

MAJOR MANIFESTATIONS	MINOR MANIFESTATIONS
Carditis	Fever
Polyarthritis	Arthralgia
Chorea	Previous rheumatic fever or
Erythema marginatum	rheumatic heart disease
Subcutaneous nodules	Elevated ESR or positive CRP
	Prolonged P-R interval
Plus supporting evidence of preceding streptococcal infection: history of recent scarlet fever; positive throat culture for group A streptococcus; increased ASO titer or other streptococcal antibodies.	

From Jones Criteria (revised) for guidance in the diagnosis of rheumatic fever. Circulation 32:664, 1965, by permission of the American Heart Association, Inc.

tween. The usual duration of a rheumatic attack is rarely longer than 3 months. When severe carditis is present, clinical rheumatic activity may continue for 6 months or more. In fewer than 5 per cent of patients, ARF may remain active for more than 6 months.[91] These cases are classified as "chronic" rheumatic fever.

CARDITIS. Of the patients in whom carditis develops, murmurs occur during the first week of illness in 76 per cent. In 93 per cent of patients there is evidence of carditis in the first 3 months. Age of onset and severity of carditis influence its chronicity. Before the age of 3 years, 92 per cent of patients in one study[92] and 90 per cent in another[93] had carditis. The incidence of carditis decreased to 50 per cent in the 3- to 6-year age group and to 32 per cent in the 14- to 17-year age group[70] in first attacks. Carditis occurs occasionally after the age of 25 in what are apparently first attacks of ARF. When carditis is mild or evidence for it is borderline, it usually disappears rapidly. Severe carditis prolongs the attack. When severe carditis subsides, low-grade fever and tachycardia often continue, cardiac enlargement usually persists, and new murmurs may appear. Congestive heart failure may occur at any time while carditis is still active.

PROGNOSIS. RF does not recur when streptococcal disease is prevented. The prognosis is excellent for the rheumatic subject who escapes carditis during an initial attack of RF. In one 5-year follow-up, rheumatic heart disease did not develop when the acute attack was not accompanied by the appearance of organic heart murmurs.[87] In the United Kingdom–United States Cooperative Study on the treatment of RF,[73,74] similar patients without carditis (defined as the absence of organic murmurs) during the acute attack showed virtually no evidence of late or insidious development of rheumatic heart disease. The percentage of this group of patients with "no carditis" who subsequently had normal hearts was 96 at 5 years and 94 at 10 years. The prognoses become poorer with the increasing severity of initial carditis, so that the percentage of those with congestive heart failure during the acute attack showing complete healing was 30 at 5 years and 40 at 10 years. It is apparent that the healing rate of rheumatic carditis is remarkably high if recurrences are prevented.

Prospective cooperative studies[74] have shown, at 5 years, that the frequency of mitral stenosis was equally distributed between the sexes and was related to the severity of the initial attack of carditis. In fact, a large percentage of the deaths within 5 years was due to such severe mitral valvular deformity. The analysis at 10 years, however, showed the emergence of another group—those whose initial mitral lesion had been relatively mild and who showed slow, progressive obstruction without evidence of recurrent RF or streptococcal disease. This group consisted of predominantly female subjects. It is apparent, therefore, that host factors, as yet undefined, influence the course of valvular sclerosis once mitral deformity has occurred and that progression of rheumatic heart disease may be related to more than the rheumatic inflammation itself. In addition, the tendency of stenotic mitral valves that have been fractured or incised surgically to restenose without evidence of recurrent or active RF is quite apparent in several long-term follow-up studies.[94]

Recurrences. First attacks of RF in the general population following epidemic streptococcal pharyngitis due to rheumatogenic strains average 3 per cent, whereas such infections in patients with a history of recent RF may produce a secondary attack rate as high as 65 per cent.[27] In the Irvington House study,[95] rheumatic attack rate per infection (R/I) in children decreased from 23 to 11 per cent between the first and fifth year after a rheumatic attack.[28] In adults with rheumatic heart disease, this rate was 4.8 per cent 10 or more years after the last attack.[29] Recurrence rates decline, therefore, with the length of time elapsed since the last attack.

A second factor that clearly increases the chance that a streptococcal infection will be followed by a rheumatic attack is the presence of residual rheumatic heart disease. In the Irvington House studies, the recurrence rate in children with

rheumatic heart disease and cardiomegaly was 43 per cent; in patients with rheumatic heart disease and no cardiomegaly, 27 per cent; and in patients without apparent residual heart disease, 10 per cent.[28]

A third factor influencing the R/I is the magnitude of the immune response to the antecedent streptococcal disease as reflected in the increase of ASO titer. The decline in first attacks of ARF is also associated with a decline in rheumatic recurrences, and both may be due to the disappearance of rheumatogenic strains of group A streptococci.[3] In the absence of such strains in a rheumatic population, even those subjects with rheumatic heart disease who develop intercurrent streptococcal infections associated with a rise in antistreptococcal antibodies do not have reactivated rheumatic fever.[96]

THE CHANGING NATURAL HISTORY OF RHEUMATIC HEART DISEASE. The current longevity of patients in the United States with inactive rheumatic heart disease can be projected from a subgroup of such patients followed prospectively for more than 30 years as part of the Framingham Study.[97] As expected, compared with a cohort control group, there was a relatively sharp decline in survival during the first half of the study, reflecting, no doubt, hemodynamic changes in the more severely involved hearts, because rheumatic recurrences were extremely rare. Nonetheless, a large proportion of patients with rheumatic heart disease survived. After 36 years of follow-up, in males the percentage surviving in the rheumatic heart disease group was only slightly below 40, compared with somewhat more than 40 per cent in their cohorts without rheumatic heart disease. Among the women the discrepancy in survival between the patients with rheumatic heart disease and their cohorts was greater.[96] The reservoir of relatively benign rheumatic valvular disease in the elderly population has been well recognized by clinicians for many years, but because of the sharp decline in new cases of rheumatic fever, rheumatic heart disease in the United States is becoming a "geriatric" disease. This phenomenon also contributes to the increasing mean age of patients with infective endocarditis.

TREATMENT

GENERAL MANAGEMENT. In any given case of RF, general management depends upon the manifestations and severity of the attack. Patients should remain in bed for the duration of the acute and febrile portion of the illness until clinical and laboratory evidence of inflammation abates.

The administration of antiinflammatory or suppressive therapy should ordinarily be delayed until the disease process is clearly expressed in order to establish the diagnosis. Aspirin or corticosteroids administered prematurely to a patient with arthralgia or early monoarticular arthritis and fever may mask the disease process and cause diagnostic confusion. Furthermore, in isolated polyarthritis a trial of penicillin therapy is often essential to eliminate the diagnosis of septic arthritis, especially gonococcemia, and the therapeutic response to the antibiotic must be carefully evaluated.

Once the diagnosis is established, treatment can begin, usually with a *course of penicillin* adequate to eradicate residual group A streptococci. Massive penicillin treatment has been used by some investigators in an attempt to alter the frequency of cardiac damage, but without success.[98] The usual course of penicillin consists of a single injection of 1.2 million units of benzathine penicillin intramuscularly, or 600,000 units of procaine penicillin intramuscularly, daily for 10 days. This is followed by continuous (secondary) prophylaxis (see below).

ANTIRHEUMATIC THERAPY. The selection of an antirheumatic agent is not critical to the outcome of most attacks of RF.[72-77] Corticosteroids and salicylates can be regarded as valuable symptomatic and supportive therapy, but they are not curative and may actually prolong the course of the disease. However, both steroids and salicylates control the toxic manifestations of the disease; contribute to the comfort of the

CHAP
56

patient; and combat anemia, anorexia, and other constitutional symptoms. In severe rheumatic carditis associated with heart failure, such nonspecific antiinflammatory effects may reduce the burden on the heart and occasionally such supportive therapy may tilt the balance in favor of the survival of a critically ill patient.

Patients with mild arthritis or arthralgia and no carditis may be treated with analgesics only, such as codeine, as needed. Two goals will be thus accomplished: First, the diagnosis may be made more certain by the appearance of definite arthritis in some of the initially questionable cases; and second, the duration of hospitalization or of close observation at home will be decreased because many of the patients will get well in 2 or 3 weeks; moreover, one will not have to worry about, and deal with, post-therapeutic rebounds.

Most current general policy is to administer salicylates when no clear evidence of carditis exists. If signs and symptoms are not adequately suppressed by salicylates, corticosteroids should be substituted. Patients with mild carditis are often given corticosteroids, but without the conviction that these are superior to salicylates. Those with severe carditis are usually treated promptly with corticosteroids, particularly if heart failure is evident, and with the precaution of adequate doses of diuretics and restriction of salt intake to combat sodium retention.

Since neither corticosteroids nor salicylates shorten the course of RF, the duration of therapy must be estimated according to the expected course of the attack. It is important to reduce the dose of corticosteroids gradually over a period of about 2 weeks and to recognize that abrupt cessation of treatment leaves the patient in a state of temporary adrenal insufficiency resulting from suppression of endogenous adrenocortical activity during prolonged hormone therapy.

When treatment of ARF is initiated with salicylates, a dose of 6 to 9 gm/day of acetylsalicylic acid is administered to patients weighing 70 kg or more, and proportionately smaller doses are given to patients weighing less. This is administered in divided doses every 4 hours. The initial doses of acetylsalicylic acid should be continued until a satisfactory clinical response is obtained, that is, until there is complete relief of symptoms and signs of arthritis and the temperature has returned to a normal range. Thereafter the dosage may be reduced to two-thirds the initial value and may be maintained until all laboratory manifestations of inflammatory disease have returned to normal. For the remainder of the course of therapy, the dosage may be reduced to half the initial daily dose. Should clinical or laboratory evidence of relapse occur when doses are reduced, it is advisable to return to the previous higher dosage that suppressed the process.

An initial dose of prednisone of 40 to 60 mg/day for adults and children alike may be started and varied according to the patient's response. With other analogs, such as triamcinolone and dexamethasone, the dosage is based on their potency relative to prednisone.

REBOUNDS OF RHEUMATIC ACTIVITY. Clinical or laboratory evidence of rheumatic activity may reappear when suppressive antirheumatic therapy is discontinued. Such reactivation has been termed a *rebound* and should clearly be distinguished from a recurrence. Spontaneous rebounds do not occur more than 5 weeks after complete cessation of all antirheumatic therapy; by far the majority occur within 2 weeks, but most occur within a few days or while dosage is being reduced. Mild rebounds subside spontaneously within a week or two and do not require medication.

TREATMENT OF CHOREA. This is nonspecific and consists of tranquilization and sedation. For complete details the reader is referred elsewhere.[1,99]

PREVENTION

The most effective preventive measures against RF are probably socioeconomic. The almost total absence of the disease in the affluent sections of the cities of the western world suggests that spacious housing and noncrowding are at least as important as good diagnosis and treatment of streptococcal sore throat in the prevention of rheumatic attacks. Nevertheless, the natural history of RF can be dramatically altered in several ways by the use of antimicrobials. Mass penicillin prophylaxis can halt epidemics of streptococcal sore throat. Adequate penicillin treatment of acute streptococcal sore throat will abort an initial attack and, less often, rheumatic recurrences. Continuous administration of sulfadiazine or penicillin will prevent recurrent attacks in rheumatic subjects. The resurgence of localized outbreaks of ARF in the United States in recent years[1,81,100-103] has been blamed, in part, upon less faithful adherence to conventional recommendations for rigorous penicillin regimens known to be highly effective in the prevention of primary and secondary rheumatic attacks by pharyngeal infections caused by rheumatogenic strains of group A streptococci. The disappearance of such strains in many populations has caused uncertainty as to how faithfully the recommended penicillin regimens should be applied. The regimens recommended below are those known to be effective when rheumatic fever exists in the population.

SECONDARY PROPHYLAXIS. The term secondary prophylaxis is used to describe protection against rheumatic recurrences by means of continuous chemoprophylaxis. After a diagnosis of RF is established, residual streptococci, which may or may not be detectable on throat cultures, should be eradicated by a therapeutic course of penicillin as described below for primary prevention. The most effective form of continuous prophylaxis is a single monthly intramuscular injection of 1.2 million units of benzathine penicillin G.[104,106] An attack rate of less than 1 recurrence per 250 patient-years was documented in patients using this form of prophylaxis in the extensive studies reported by the Irvington House group.[104,105] Although the reaction rate is somewhat higher for all injectable forms of penicillin, regardless of kind, than with oral penicillin, reactions are very rare after the first months of prophylaxis. Monthly injections of benzathine penicillin G are undoubtedly the preferred form of prophylaxis in populations in which RF continues to appear, or, indeed, is on the increase. In affluent societies, however, and in countries in which RF has become rare, it is unlikely that this form of prophylaxis will be employed except when major risk factors of recurrences coexist.[106]

Oral prophylaxis is less reliable than repository penicillin prophylaxis. In the Irvington House studies, a recurrence rate of almost 1 per 25 patient-years (10 times that of intramuscular benzathine penicillin G) was observed in patients receiving oral medication.[105] The recommended dosages for oral sulfadiazine prophylaxis are 0.5 gm once daily for patients weighing less than 27 kg (60 lb) and 1 gm once a day for patients weighing more than 27 kg. For oral penicillin prophylaxis, the recommended dose is 200,000 to 250,000 units daily of penicillin G or 125 to 250 mg of penicillin V twice a day.[106] Even when oral penicillin is administered twice daily, no superiority over sulfadiazine has been demonstrated.

Strains of streptococci resistant to sulfonamide have appeared with mass sulfonamide prophylaxis in military populations, but have not been a problem in secondary prophylaxis of rheumatic subjects. Reaction rates are low with both oral medications and are rare after the first months of prophylaxis. For the rare patient who is sensitive to both sulfadiazine and penicillin, oral erythromycin may be substituted in a dose of 250 mg twice daily.

It has been difficult to establish a general recommendation concerning the duration of prophylaxis because of the number of variables that influence the attack rate of recurrences following streptococcal infections (see Course and Prognosis, above). Although risks of recurrences decline with age and with increased interval from the last rheumatic attack, a relatively high recurrence rate per infection persists for a very long time—5 to 10 years or more. Exceptions to instituting or maintaining prophylaxis should be made only after assessing the risk of high exposure to rheumatogenic streptococcal infection. Patients with significant degrees of rheumatic heart disease or with a history of repeated recurrences (including chorea) or those having had a recent attack require most careful consideration before discontinuation of prophylaxis.

PRIMARY PROPHYLAXIS. The term *primary prophylaxis* is applied to the prevention of first attacks of RF by treatment of the preceding streptococcal pharyngitis. The appearance of RF in a community signals the presence of rheumatogenic streptococci, whose spread must be interrupted by use of penicillin regimens that eradicate pharyngeal carriage or cause attenuation of surviving strains, which then are harmlessly carried. In military populations with a high frequency of severe streptococcal pharyngitis, penicillin therapy reduced the attack rate of RF from 3.0 to 0.3 per cent.[107] The application of primary prevention to civilian populations, particularly children with sporadic or endemic streptococcal infections, has been more difficult because of the problem of differentiating viral pharyngitis in carriers of group A streptococci from current streptococcal infection and because prevalent streptococcal strains may no longer be rheumatogenic. Throat cultures, when negative, are helpful, however, in eliminating the need for intensive penicillin therapy in patients with nonstreptococcal infection.

Effective therapy demands eradication of the infecting organism, which requires 10 days of consistent treatment if penicillin is administered orally.

Many patients fail to extend such treatment beyond the first few days if acute symptoms of streptococcal pharyngitis subside. A single intramuscular injection of benzathine penicillin G (600,000 units in children under 27 kg [60 lb] and 1.2 million units in those over 27 kg) is the treatment of choice when the risk of RF still exists. Oral penicillin is now usually preferred for the treatment of streptococcal infections in populations in which the risk of RF is very low. The dose of penicillin G is 200,000 to 250,000 units three to four times daily. Penicillin V in doses of 250 mg t.i.d. may be substituted. Treatment is still recommended for a full 10 days.[102] For those sensitive to penicillin, erythromycin (250 mg two to four times a day or 40 mg/kg per day in younger children) may be substituted.

Mass Antibiotic Prophylaxis. This type of prophylaxis is effective in populations in which rheumatogenic streptococcal pharyngeal infections are epidemic.[108] This approach may be indicated occasionally in civilian or institutional epidemics, especially if cases of RF occur within a few weeks. Mass intramuscular administration of 1.2 million units of benzathine penicillin G to all members of the affected population has been extremely effective.[5]

IMMUNIZATION WITH STREPTOCOCCAL VACCINES. Although no vaccine is currently available for general distribution, considerable progress has been made on the purification and immunology of streptococcal M proteins and holds promise for future streptococcal vaccine development.[109-111]

Other Rheumatic Diseases Affecting the Heart and Circulation

SERONEGATIVE SPONDYLOARTHROPATHIES

COMMON CLINICAL FEATURES AND NOSOLOGY. A group of rheumatological syndromes has been classified under the heading of seronegative spondyloarthropathies because they have clinical features in common and some pathological lesions, including those of the heart, that are identical.[112-114] They are distinguished from rheumatoid arthritis by the *absence of the characteristic serological changes of the latter* (e.g., increased rheumatoid factor); by the predilection of the arthritis for the sacroiliac, lumbosacral, and apophyseal joints of the spine; by the predominance in men over women; by the predilection for involvement of the entheses (insertions of ligaments and capsules into bone); and by the extraarticular manifestations of iritis and aortic regurgitation due to a characteristic lesion at the root of the aorta. The spondyloarthropathies are also distinguished by association with haplotype HLA-B27. The group of syndromes includes ankylosing spondylitis, Reiter's disease, psoriatic arthritis, and the intestinal arthropathies. Two of the major syndromes, ankylosing spondylitis and Reiter's disease, have been associated with dysentery and urethritis. Although the causative agents are usually not apparent, dysentery due to specific bacteria (*Yersinia enterocolitica, Shigella, Salmonella,* and *Campylobacter*) has produced most of the features of these syndromes.[115] Urethritis due to *Chlamydia trachomatis* has also been implicated as one of the causes of Reiter's disease,[116] but in most cases the etiological agent has not been identified.

HISTOCOMPATIBILITY ANTIGEN B27. The concept of a genetically determined aberrant host response to a variety of infectious agents that can invade the bowel or genitourinary tract has emerged from the demonstration of the striking association of the seronegative spondyloarthropathies with the histocompatibility antigen HLA-B27.[112-114] This membrane antigen occurs with a frequency of approximately 4 to 8 per cent in the normal population, whereas over 90 per cent of patients with either ankylosing spondylitis or Reiter's disease with spondyloarthropathy are B27-positive. When spondyloarthropathy complicates inflammatory bowel disease, the association with B27 is greater than 80 per cent, and 50 per cent of psoriatic patients with spondylitis are B27-positive. So far, 50 per cent of patients with anterior uveitis have this antigen. When an outbreak of a specific form of dysentery has

permitted careful prospective studies, patients with the B27 antigen have had a much greater tendency to develop any form of arthritis than those lacking this antigen. The more specific features of the syndrome such as spondyloarthropathy, iritis, and cardiac involvement have been confined primarily to those who are B27-positive.

ANKYLOSING SPONDYLITIS

CARDIAC PATHOLOGY. The incidence of cardiovascular involvement varies from 3.5 per cent of cases with a 15-year history to 10 per cent with up to 30 years of disease. Several excellent prospective studies have documented the form of cardiac and aortic disease peculiar to ankylosing spondylitis, consisting of the following: dilatation of the aortic valve ring; fibrous thickening, scarring, and variable focal inflammatory lesions of the aortic valve cusps, which sag into the ventricular cavity; dilatation of the sinuses of Valsalva;

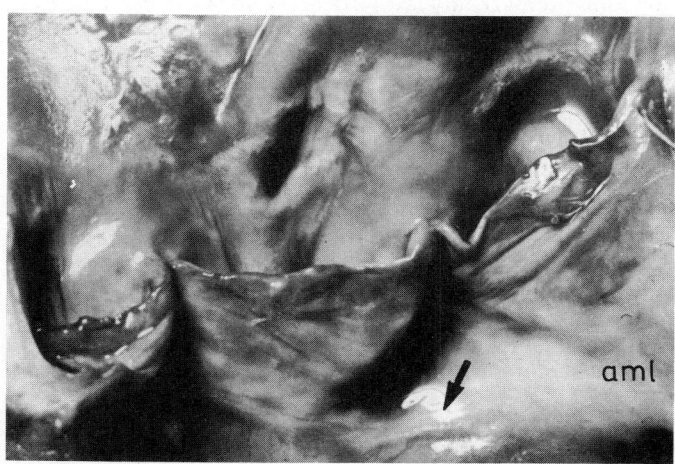

FIGURE 56–7. The aortic valve and sinus of Valsalva cut open in a patient with ankylosing spondylitis who was HLA-B27-positive. The base of the cusps is thickened. The orifice of the right coronary artery is distorted. Aortic regurgitation had been present during life. aml = anterior mitral leaflet. (From Bergfeldt, L.: HLA-B-27—associated heart disease. Am. J. Med. 77:961, 1984.)

focal degenerative changes of elastic and muscle fibers of the aortic media; and patchy inflammatory lesions in all layers of the aorta, predominantly in the region adjacent to the aortic valve ring[117-119] (Fig. 56-7). The lesions resemble those of syphilis except that in ankylosing spondylitis they remain close to the valve ring and do not affect the rest of the aorta. In addition, the basal rather than distal portion of the aortic cusps is thickened in ankylosing spondylitis and the dense adventitial scarring extends into the endocardium in the immediate subaortic region. This extension may involve the base of the anterior mitral leaflet and the upper portion of the ventricular septum. In view of the enthesopathical lesions that characterize the pathology of this condition, patients may present with insertional tendinitis at any site, and the heart valve lesions may reflect this connective tissue localization.

Aortic regurgitation results from thickening and shortening of the cusps and from their displacement caudally by the mass of fibrous tissue behind the commissures, the subaortic ridge or bump, and by dilatation of the aortic valve root consequent to the destruction of elastic tissue (Figs. 56-7 and 56-8). Mitral regurgitation is infrequent and usually insignificant but can result from dilatation of the left ventricle from mitral valve prolapse, an extension of the subaortic bump[120] and from fibrous thickening of the basal portion of the anterior mitral leaflet. The frequent heart block and conduction defects of ankylosing spondylitis are due to the extension of fibrosis into the muscular septum and destruction of the bundle of His and proximal bundle branches.[122-124]

The lesions of the myocardium are rather nonspecific, consisting of fibrosis, perivascular lymphocytic infiltration, and increased mucinous ground substance. Cardiac enlargement without any apparent cause and hypertrophy and dilatation of the left ventricle are often described.[125]

Chronic fibrous obliteration of the pericardial cavity has been found at autopsy, but pericarditis is not a prominent clinical feature of the disease. Pericardial rubs and chest pain have been described, however, during more severe, acute, toxic episodes when there is active peripheral polyarthritis and in association with presumably early phases of the disease, especially in association with early Reiter's syndrome or dysentery with polyarthritis.

CLINICAL CARDIAC FEATURES. In many patients there is evidence of active carditis before aortic regurgitation appears. Precordial pain, pericardial friction rubs, marked tachycardia, cardiac enlargement not explained by hypertension, or other recognizable forms of heart disease and varying P-R intervals greater than 0.24 sec are frequently described, usually when patients have active peripheral arthritis and/or spondylitis with fever and increased erythrocyte sedimentation rates. Remarkably few critical studies have been made of myocardial function in patients with ankylosing spondylitis before evidence of aortic regurgitation draws attention to cardiac involvement, but it is clear that cardiomyopathy may precede valvular involvement.[125] Indeed, the high cardiovascular morbidity and mortality in these diseases may be due to myocardial abnormalities in the absence of valve disease.[125] The usual cardiac features of ankylosing spondylitis are the gradual evolution of aortic regurgitation and varying degrees of AV block. The prevalence of the valve lesion is related to the duration of spondylitis and peripheral joint involvement, reaching an incidence in one series of 10 per cent in those with spondylitis for 30 years or more and of 18 per cent if peripheral joint involvement was also present. The incidence of AV block in each of the above groups was 8.5 and 15.5 per cent, respectively.[117]

In one long follow-up of 97 patients with ankylosing spondylitis, of whom 14 had cardiovascular lesions, aortic regurgitation occurred in 10 patients. Mitral regurgitation and AV block appeared as isolated findings in 1 and 3 patients, respectively. Nine of the 14 patients had peripheral arthritis, and 3 had iritis.[118] Anterior uveitis and extraspinal disease may also precede the articular lesions of ankylosing spondylitis by months or years. Hence the discovery of isolated aortic regur-

gitation in young or middle-aged men requires that ankylosing spondylitis be considered in the differential diagnosis. In addition, the aortic regurgitation of ankylosing spondylitis is now well documented to occur in so-called secondary forms of the disease such as spondylitis associated with psoriasis, regional enteritis,[118] ulcerative colitis,[126] and Reiter's disease.[127]

Aortic valve replacement (p. 1052) has been performed successfully in several centers, and patients with ankylosing spondylitis may be suitable candidates when such a procedure is indicated. Cardiac pacemakers have been implanted for AV block.

REITER'S DISEASE

Cardiac involvement in the acute stages of Reiter's disease has been described frequently and consists most commonly of acute pericarditis, apical systolic murmurs, gallops, and cardiac conduction abnormalities, particularly AV block. These changes disappear rapidly, and long-term follow-up of large series reveals only an occasional case of cardiac failure or third-degree AV block.[128] This acute form of Reiter's disease usually features nonspecific urethritis, nonsuppurative migratory polyarthritis, conjunctivitis, circinate balanitis, and keratoderma blennorrhagica. Initial attacks usually subside spontaneously, but second attacks occur in about 15 per cent of cases, and chronic manifestations (almost always in B27-positive individuals[114]) may then ensue, with recurrent anterior uveitis, painful mutilating deformities of the feet, sacroiliitis, spondylitis, AV block, and an aortic valve lesion leading to aortic and occasionally to mitral regurgitation.

Postmortem studies of the aortic valves have shown the cusps to be thickened, with rolled edges, and the aorta to incur changes similar if not identical to the lesions described in AS.[129,130]

The development of Reiter's disease in patients with *Yersinia arthritis* or associated with various other dysentery-producing bacteria has emphasized the role of the B27 antigen in the frequency of expression of various clinical features of the syndrome, including its cardiac manifestations.[131-133] Of 19 patients with Reiter's syndrome observed at one institution, all 5 who had conduction abnormalities were B27-positive.[134]

RELAPSING POLYCHONDRITIS

This relatively poorly known condition is a rheumatic vasculitis characterized by recurrent inflammation of cartilage and most commonly auricular and nasal and seronegative arthritis. Both mitral and aortic regurgitation, sometimes severe enough to require valve replalcement, have been reported,[135-137] as have aneurysms of the aorta and its major branches.

RHEUMATOID ARTHRITIS

PATHOLOGY. The heart is frequently involved in the inflammatory process of rheumatoid arthritis (RA), yet its function is seldom compromised by the lesions produced.[135,136] The exudative type of rheumatoid inflammation affects the pericardial surfaces, producing a fibrinous pericarditis that is usually low grade and subclinical. Pericardial inflammation becomes symptomatic and clinically significant in its more florid form and may even be the presenting complaint.

The most characteristic pathological lesion of RA, the nodular granuloma, involves the myocardium, endocardium, and valves of the heart.[140,141] The extent of this kind of involvement is generally proportionate to the severity of the disease and is almost always associated with diffusely distributed rheumatoid nodules, subcutaneously and elsewhere. These granulomas rarely compromise the function of the myocardium, however, nor do they often affect the function of the heart valves unless they become large and numerous enough to distort them (Fig. 56-8).

Diffuse arteritis, when present, affects small vessels, causing round cell infiltration, edema, fibrosis, and proliferation of the intima. Such involvement of the pericardial vessels may be extensive when it reflects an intense systemic form of RA, and the disease may begin in the pericardium before the joints become involved. Coronary arteritis is often observed at necropsy in severe RA, but it very rarely results in clinically apparent myocardial ischemia.

Clinical Features

PERICARDITIS (see also p. 1501). The frequency of rheumatoid pericarditis in necropsy studies ranges from 11 to 50 per cent, with an overall estimate of about 30 per cent.[142] Clinically, the diagnosis of pericarditis is made in about 2 per cent of cases in the adult form and in about 6 per cent in the juvenile form of RA. In careful studies of the more severe forms of the disease which require hospital admission, approximately 10 per cent of patients with rheumatoid arthritis have clinical

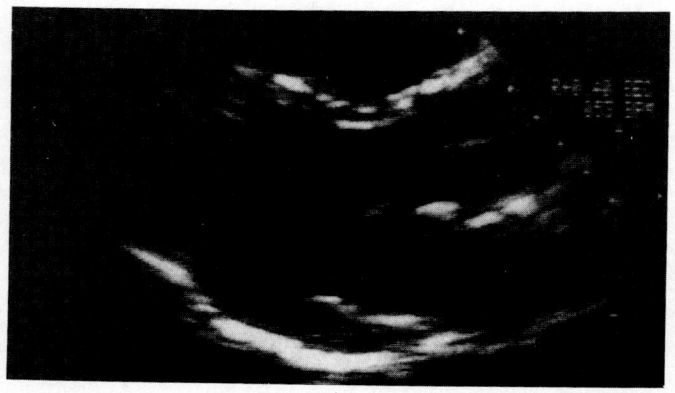
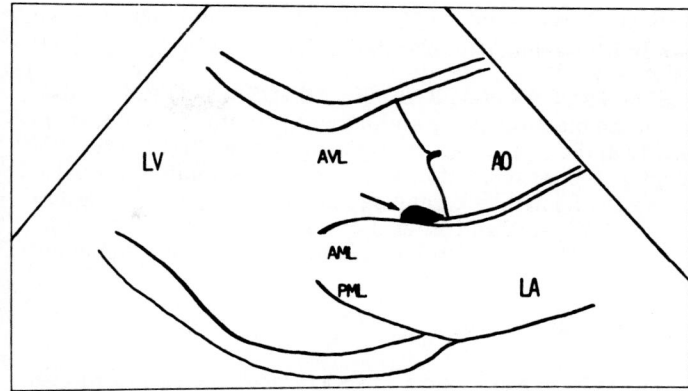

FIGURE 56-8. Long-axis view in a patient with ankylosing spondylitis. Subaortic thickening (*arrow*) is present, and there is an increase in aortic diameter and thickening of the aortic walls and aortic root echodensity. AML = anterior mitral leaflet; AO = aortic root; AVL = aortic valve leaflets; LA = left atrium; LV = left ventricle; PML = posterior mitral leaflet. (From Labresh, K. A., et al.: Two-dimensional echocardiographic detection of preclinical aortic root abnormalities in rheumatoid variant diseases. Am. J. Med. *78*:908, 1985.)

evidence of rheumatoid pericarditis during the lifetime course of their disease. Part of the disparity between clinical and autopsy findings is due to the fact that the chest pain may be overshadowed by arthritic pains and may be masked by antirheumatic agents or mistaken for arthritic pain in neighboring joints.

The pathophysiology of the acute fibrinous pericarditis of RA is not clear, but in severe cases the pericardial fluid, like synovial fluid, shows decreased hemolytic complement (CH$_{50}$) and C3 levels. Immunofluorescence staining of the pericardium shows plasma cell infiltration and deposits of IgG, IgM, IgA, or C3 in the pericardial vessels.[143] Moreover, the polymorphonuclear leukocytes in the pericardial fluid may show cytoplasmic inclusions which stain for IgM, indicative of ingested immune complexes such as are also seen in the polymorphonuclear cells of synovial fluid in the same patients. These findings are associated with extremely low levels of glucose, indicative of active phagocytosis, as observed in pleural and synovial rheumatoid fluids. About half the patients with overt rheumatoid pericarditis also have rheumatoid pleural and lung lesions.

In reports of patients with rheumatoid arthritis studied by echocardiography, pericardial effusion was demonstrated in 30 per cent of all patients studied and in 50 per cent of those with subcutaneous nodules.[135,144] This incidence is as high as the reported frequency of postmortem findings of rheumatoid pericarditis.

Pericarditis may appear without relation to the duration of rheumatoid arthritis[145] and sometimes may even be the harbinger of the onset of a severe form of the disease. It occurs most often in middle-aged men in whom arthritis was of acute onset. Most often, the clinical course is benign, and symptoms and signs will respond to moderate amounts of prednisone. Occasionally, however, the disease may be more protracted and severe, leading to hemopericardium,[146] cardiac tamponade,[147] and constrictive pericarditis.[145,148]

In its florid form the disease has the usual symptoms and signs of pericarditis, and when persistent, it imitates closely tuberculous pericarditis, from which it must be carefully differentiated. Although some fatal cases have been described in which a true pancarditis was present,[149] such cases are exceptional, and even severe rheumatoid pericarditis usually spares myocardial and endocardial function.

Treatment of rheumatoid pericarditis is the same as that for the arthritic disease. Although corticosteroids tend to be used more liberally in pericarditis to suppress inflammation, there is no evidence that such suppression will prevent adhesive or constrictive pericarditis.

RHEUMATOID MYOCARDITIS. Except for rare cases of myocarditis with diffuse granulomas or amyloid infiltration of the myocardium associated with very severe rheumatoid arthritis, myocarditis is mostly nonspecific and subclinical in

the great majority of patients. The histological lesions may be focal or generalized infiltrations of lymphocytes, plasma cells, palisading histiocytes, and fibroblasts.[140] The incidence of myocarditis in autopsies of rheumatoid arthritis patients is reported as 19 per cent. Most of such cases are associated with severe arthritis, vasculitis, and endocarditis or pericarditis.

Although left ventricular function may be compromised by a variety of pathological processes in severe rheumatoid arthritis, the typical case is remarkable for its characteristic sparing of the myocardial musculature despite extensive involvement of the fibrous structures of the heart. Nevertheless, when there are unusually severe systemic manifestations of rheumatoid arthritis, rheumatoid pancarditis with congestive heart failure has been well described and confirmed by necropsy. Such patients exhibit the whole spectrum of rheumatoid inflammation of the heart.[149]

CORONARY ARTERY DISEASE. Clinicopathological correlation suggests that the nature of the coronary artery disease analyzed in some studies of patients with rheumatoid arthritis is probably rheumatoid rather than arteriosclerotic. Coronary arteritis is observed in about 20 per cent of patients with rheumatoid arthritis at autopsy. This arteritis is probably a manifestation of generalized vasculitis often seen in rheumatoid arthritis. Inflammation with edema of the intima of the artery may lead to severe narrowing or occlusion of its lumen, to necrosis, and to angina or infarction.[150] Nevertheless, myocardial necrosis secondary to this form of arteritis is rare.

Rheumatoid vasculitis of the pulmonary arteries causing severe pulmonary hypertension and right heart failure has been reported.[151]

VALVULAR AND ENDOCARDIAL LESIONS. As in myocarditis, the histological picture of the valves and adjacent endocardial areas of patients with rheumatoid arthritis shows nonspecific inflammation with fibrotic and sclerotic changes and infiltrations of histiocytes, plasma cells, lymphocytes, and occasional eosinophils.[140] The most characteristic lesions, however, are granulomas resembling rheumatoid nodules. Usually these do not interfere with valvular function unless they reach large enough proportions to produce frank valvular regurgitation by destroying the base of the valve and its cusps. Such regurgitation may be of sufficient magnitude and rapidity of onset to cause severe cardiac decompensation and death unless valve replacement is undertaken in a timely manner[152] (Chap. 34).

All valves may be involved, but the descending order of frequency is similar to that in rheumatic fever, i.e., mitral, aortic, tricuspid, and pulmonary. Echocardiographic studies have shown a significant slowing of mitral valve movement in patients with rheumatoid arthritis correlating with the duration of the disease and the extent of the formation of subcutaneous nodules.[144] In a few well-described cases, however, mitral and aortic valvular deformity with marked regurgitation due to rheumatoid nodules was the characteristic pathological picture.[149]

ELECTROCARDIOGRAPHIC ABNORMALITIES. Studies of the electrocardiogram in patients with rheumatoid arthritis and in matched controls show that first degree AV block is the most significant finding in rheumatoid arthritis. Complete heart block causing Adams-Stokes syndrome has been described,[152] and other abnormalities include left bundle branch block, atrial fibrillation, and atrial and ventricular ectopic beats.

JUVENILE RHEUMATOID ARTHRITIS (STILL's DISEASE)

This syndrome, one of the more common chronic illnesses of childhood, may also have its onset in adults and is particularly noteworthy for involvement of the serosal surfaces, producing pleuritis and pericarditis as well as arthritis, and is featured by a characteristic rash.[154] Pericarditis can be diagnosed clinically in approximately 7 per cent of children with juvenile rheumatoid arthritis. As in rheumatoid arthritis, postmortem examinations show a much higher incidence of pericarditis, and echocardiography is needed to reveal its clinical frequency.[155] Pericardial tamponade has been reported in both children and adults with this syndrome, but it is very rare. Myocarditis is less common than pericarditis, but may produce cardiac enlargement and heart failure, especially in adult Still's disease.[156-158] Valvular heart disease is rare, but severe aortic regurgitation requiring valve replacement has been described in a young adult.[147]

SYSTEMIC LUPUS ERYTHEMATOSUS

PATHOLOGICAL FEATURES. The hallmark of this disease is the presence of a number of antibodies to nuclear components, the antinuclear antibodies (ANA), as well as antibodies against phospholipids that may participate in the pathogenesis of SLE by forming antigen-antibody-complement complexes that are found in many of the lesions. These and other hyperimmune phenomena explain many of the protean clinical manifestations of SLE. Although anti-heart antibodies have been described in the sera of patients with SLE, they bear no clear relationship to the frequency and severity of cardiac lesions and may be a result rather than a cause of cardiac inflammation, presumably owing to release of myocardial antigens into the circulation.[160] Other etiological ad pathogenetic processes associated with autoimmunity have been extensively reviewed.

Cardiac Abnormalities

Because the basic anatomical lesion of SLE is a diffuse microvasculitis (Fig. 56–9)[161,162] the heart is almost always found to be involved at autopsy.[163] The clinical manifestations, however, are usually overshadowed by the symptoms and signs related to involvement of other organs, and attention is drawn to the heart only when the lesions of pericarditis, myocarditis, or endocarditis are florid. Clinical evidence of cardiac abnormalities has been observed, however, in as many as 50 to 60 per cent of cases in two large series.[164,165] As diagnostic methods become more sophisticated, detection of cardiac involvement during life begins to approach that found at necropsy (see below).

PERICARDITIS. This is found in approximately two-thirds to three-fourths of autopsies and is the most common cardiac lesion of SLE (p. 1501). The acute pericardial inflammation may extend into the sinoatrial and AV nodes, with destruction of conducting fibers.[166,167] Pericardial fluid may be clear or sanguineous and has a high protein content. Effusions may be voluminous and occasionally cause tamponade.[168] Histologically, the pericardium shows fibrinoid degeneration, edema, and necrosis of connective tissue when the process is acute, and various stages of fibrosis with the formation of adhesions are found during the healing or chronic phase. Constrictive pericarditis occurs only rarely;[169] however, pericardial tamponade and constrictive pericarditis both have been reported in cases of procainamide-induced lupus erythematosus.[170,171] Pericarditis, which is frequently detected in lupus patients by echocardiography,[172,173] like arthritis, tends to be episodic and to heal well in remissions rather than to become chronic and sclerosing.

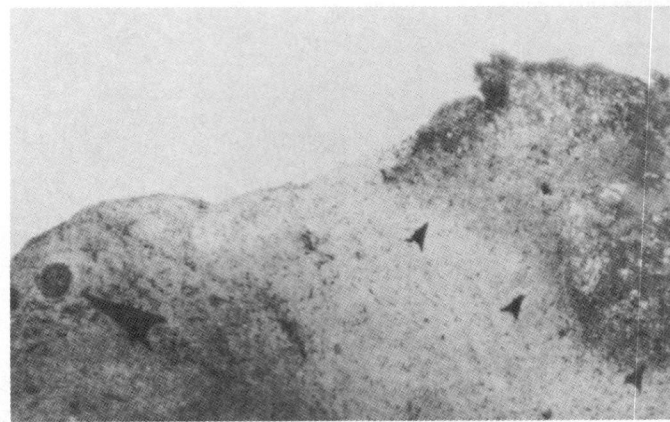

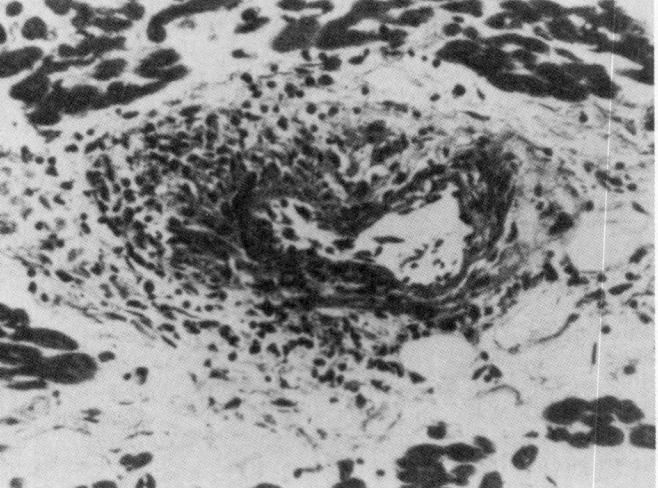

FIGURE 56–9. *Top,* Vasculopathy (large arrow) and necrosis (small arrows) of mitral valve in SLE (original magnification 40×). *Bottom,* Vasculitis of sinus node artery in SLE (original magnification 100×). (From Straaton, K. V., Chatham, W. W., Reveille, J. D., et al.: Clinically significant valvular heart disease in systemic lupus erythematosus. Am. J. Med. *85:*645, 1988.)

MYOCARDITIS. Subclinical myocarditis manifested as left ventricular dysfunction on echocardiography is common.[172-174] Its severity is proportionate to the severity of the systemic disease process. The lesions observed at autopsy and endomyocardial biopsy[175] consist of fibrinoid necrosis involving interstitial tissues and blood vessels, and only rarely are the cardiac myofibrils destroyed. Small vessel changes include an arteriopathy of vessels 0.1 to 1.0 mm in diameter. The abnormal vessels are located in the conduction system of patients selected for study because of the presence of arrhythmias. Segmental arteritis and periarteritis with some occlusions of the arterial lumen and small areas of fibrosis distal to the obstruction are found. Involvement of the AV as well as the sinoatrial node in the inflammatory process of SLE has been shown at autopsy. Rare cases of myocardial infarction, presumably due to arteritis of larger coronary vessels, have been reported.[178]

ENDOCARDITIS. This is the most characteristic cardiac lesion of SLE.[166,179] The Libman-Sacks verrucous valvular lesions are wartlike, varying from pinhead size to 3 to 4 mm. The lesions may be discrete or in clumps and are composed of degenerating valve tissue apparently extruded beyond the endothelium and accompanied by some fibrosis of the underlying leaflet. The lesions usually contain granular, basophilic masses of cellular debris, the characteristic so-called hematoxylin bodies composed of basophilic fragments in the cytoplasm of cells. They may be found anywhere on the endocardial surface of the heart, but are most common in the angles of the AV valves and on the underside of the base of the mitral valve. They may also extend onto the chordae tendineae or papillary muscles. Generalized involvement of the entire thickness of the heart valves with inflammatory and fibrous changes may also occur. Aortic valve involvement is rare, but has been well described.[180] Despite the frequency and extent of the endocardial lesions of SLE, they profoundly affect the function of the valves in only a minority of cases and, unlike rheumatic fever, do not produce serious regurgitation during the acute phase of the disease. Only rarely do they lead to marked scarring and deformity during healing, requiring valve replacement. The subclinical nature of the valvular lesions has been demonstrated by prospective clinical and echocardiographic studies (Fig. 56–10).[172,173]

Clinical Features

Although autopsy shows that at least two-thirds of patients have pericarditis at some time during the course of SLE, only one-third have recognizable symptoms and signs during life.[164,165] Typical pericardial pain may occur, but often the friction rubs, characteristic electrocardiographic changes, or enlargement of the cardiac silhouette on chest x-ray due to pericardial effusion may be found in the absence of symptoms, and therefore evidence of pericarditis should always be suspected and sought by clinical means and at intervals by echocardiography in *all* patients with SLE, even in those without clinical manifestations. Cardiac tamponade is rare but can occur,[168] requiring repeated aspirations of fluid. Systolic and diastolic murmurs at the mitral area, and less often at the aortic area, seem to come and go during the course of acute exacerbations of the disease and are presumably due to Libman-Sacks endocarditis. However, at autopsy the presence of these lesions is not always confirmed, and other factors such as anemia, tachycardia, fever, myocarditis, transient papillary muscle dysfunction, and the adventitious sounds of pleuropericarditis must be considered. Hemodynamically significant and permanent valvular regurgitation from lupus carditis is rare, but such cases have been reported and have even required valve replacement.[181–183]

Although myocardial dysfunction may be present, overt congestive heart failure due primarily to SLE is uncommon[184] except when associated with hypertension secondary to renal disease. Heart failure may be mistakenly diagnosed in the presence of edema due to renal disease or pericardial effusion or both. Clinically apparent myocarditis, like that of rheumatic fever, producing tachycardia, gallop rhythm, and cardiac dilatation, is usually a feature of very toxic cases of SLE when high fever and other multisystem manifestations of acute vasculitis are present. Arrhythmias are also relatively uncommon and consist of atrial flutter and fibrillation with varying degrees of AV block.[184] The latter may be associated with myocarditis and circulating antibodies to nuclear ribonucleoprotein.[185] Attention has been called to the development of congenital complete heart block, a lupus-like syndrome, and pericarditis in infants born to mothers with active SLE.[188,189] The observation suggests that transplacental transfer of abnormal antibodies may be of pathogenetic importance in these cases. During examination of a pregnant woman with SLE, fetal bradycardia should be recognized as a possible complication of lupus rather than fetal distress from other causes. The maternal antibodies that damage the fetal conduction system appear to be approximately 50 kD and to the SSA/Ro-55b/La system.[186]

Echocardiography may be useful in SLE for demonstrating pericardial involvement and for evaluating valve function in the presence of various murmurs.[176] Extensive hemodynamic studies carried out on patients who had had SLE for 2½ to 7 years prior to heart catheterization and who had no obvious clinical findings of cardiac involvement nonetheless showed considerable evidence of impairment of myocardial function.[190] Myocardial involvement has also been detected by magnetic resonance imaging.[191] More sophisticated studies will be necessary to sort out the complex factors that may compromise myocardial function in a disease that can affect all layers of the heart and the coronary vascular bed as well.[192]

TREATMENT. To the extent that their antiinflammatory effect can control active myocarditis, corticosteroids may be necessary to manage severe cardiac involvement in SLE. Control of hypertension is also helpful in the treatment and prevention of congestive heart failure. There is no evidence that corticosteroid treatment can prevent the rare cases of constrictive pericarditis or valvular deformity. Although the inflammatory reaction may be dramatically suppressed, the basic disease process and tissue injury are not altered by corticosteroid therapy, which is at most supportive and sometimes causes problems (hypertension and fluid retention). Immunosuppressive therapy is usually reserved for the most severe, corticosteroid-resistant forms of the disease and especially for renal involvement. Death from the cardiac disease of SLE compared with other causes of fatality in this disease is rare, so that cardiac manifestations usually do not determine the choice of antiinflammatory therapy.

Among the antibodies found in high concentrations in patients with SLE are a variety of antiphospholipid antibodies, which include the lupus "anticoagulant," the antibodies responsible for a positive VDRL, and more specific anti-phospholipid antibodies such as the anticardiolipin antibody. Elevated levels of these antiphospholipid antibodies are associated with a syndrome consisting of recurrent venous and/or arterial thromboses, placental thrombosis leading to abortion, thrombocytopenia, and cutaneous vascular abnormalities such as livedo reticularis.[193,194] Occasionally, this clinical complex occurs in patients without lupus.[196] High levels of anticardiolipin antibodies have been found in patients with SLE to be highly associated with cardiac abnormalities, especially valvular heart disease.[196–198]

POLYARTERITIS NODOSA

As noted above, necrotizing inflammation of blood vessels is a common finding in immune complex diseases of known and unknown etiology; however, because the origin and nature of the offending agent are unknown in most instances the vasculitides continue to be classified on the basis of their histological and clinical features. These depend largely upon the size of the involved blood vessels, their anatomical sites, the stage of the inflammation, and the characteristics of the lesions.

The clinical features of most cases fit into one of the following five major categories: polyarteritis nodosa (PAN; also termed periarteritis nodosa),

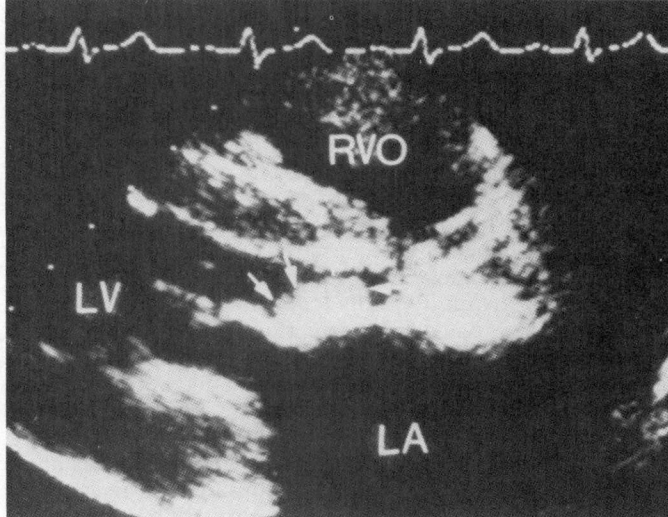

FIGURE 56–10. Parasternal long-axis view of the heart from a patient with systemic lupus erythematosus and high levels of anticardiolipin antibodies. A massive vegetation on ventricular surface of the anterior mitral leaflet (*arrows*) not interfering with the valve mobility, is clearly visualized. LA = left atrium, LV = left ventricle, RVO = right ventricular outflow. (From Nihoyannopoulos, N., et al.: Cardiac abnormalities in systemic lupus erythematosus: Association with raised anticardiolipin antibodies. Circulation *82:*369, 1990, by permission of the American Heart Association.)

allergic granulomatosis, Wegener's granulomatosis, hypersensitivity vasculitis, and giant cell arteritis.

PATHOLOGICAL FEATURES. The muscular arteries, adjacent veins, and occasionally arterioles and venules (but not the capillaries) are involved in a necrotizing inflammation. Segments of vessels, at times only part of the circumference being affected, are involved in the lesions, especially at the bifurcation of arteries. Small aneurysms may form and rupture. In the acute stage of inflammation the lesions contain predominantly polymorphonuclear leukocytes whereas in chronic lesions mononuclear cell infiltration and partial healing are apparent. However, both phases may be present at once, suggesting repeated or continuous insults.

The lesions are commonly found in the coronary arteries as well as kidneys, muscles, and vasa nervorum, but the lungs are usually spared. *Myocardial infarction* is therefore relatively common, and this leads to patchy myocardial fibrosis and left ventricular enlargement. The latter is also secondary to hypertension, frequently present owing to renal involvement. Hemorrhage into the pericardial sac with tamponade and death, inflammatory pericarditis, and uremic pericarditis are causes of pericardial involvement. Endocardial or valvular lesions do not occur unless the papillary muscle is injured by ischemia.

CLINICAL FEATURES. PAN may occur at any age, produces fever and multisystem involvement, and may persist for months or years. Pericarditis may be clinically evident, frequently associated with pleuritis, but is not a prominent feature of the disease. Chest pain due to true angina pectoris is also relatively rare[199] despite the occurrence of myocardial infarction. In one series of 41 cases of PAN and myocardial infarction, only three were diagnosed clinically.[200] The most common form of heart involvement is congestive failure and hypertension due to renal disease, which causes most deaths. Cardiac arrhythmias, most often atrial flutter and fibrillation, can occur. Death from ruptured aneurysms, particularly gastrointestinal bleeding, is not uncommon.

COURSE AND TREATMENT. The prognosis of PAN is grave; one-half to two-thirds of patients died within a year when series comprised hospitalized cases. Treatment with corticosteroids is frequently followed by temporary improvement with doses of 40 to 60 mg of prednisone or prednisolone per day. Five-year survival of untreated patients is estimated at 13 per cent. Studies with immunosuppressive drugs have been encouraging in apparently prolonging the course in some cases, but adequate controlled studies have not been made.[202]

Other Forms of Diffuse Vasculitis

ALLERGIC GRANULOMATOSIS (CHURG-STRAUSS VASCULITIS, HYPEREOSINOPHILIC SYNDROME)

This disease involves the vessels of the heart in the same way as PAN, but eosinophils tend to be more abundant in the lesions, and granulomatous collections of epithelioid and giant cells are formed, accounting for the name of the condition.[202] Pulmonary involvement, especially asthma, dominates the clinical picture, and patients tend to have a history of respiratory infection and fever, often with a striking peripheral eosinophilia. The heart, however, may be a primary target organ. Pericarditis, occasionally constrictive, myocarditis with acute heart failure, and myocardial infarction have been reported, as well as endomyocardial fibrosis in some variants of the syndrome.[203]

WEGENER'S GRANULOMATOSIS

This syndrome is distinguished by necrotizing granulomas of the upper respiratory tract, especially the destructive lesions of the nasopharynx and paranasal sinuses, middle ear, and bronchial tree. Necrotizing inflammation extends into the smaller pulmonary vessels of the lungs and other organs, particularly the kidneys. Pericardial and myocardial involvement is not uncommon, but the clinical picture is dominated by respiratory and renal involvement, without which the diagnosis cannot be made. The special feature of treatment is the encouraging response of this particular syndrome to cyclophosphamide therapy, resulting in dramatic remissions, often complete, and in prolonged survival.[202,204] Although cardiac complications are considered unusual in Wegener's granulomatosis, they have been found in 12 per cent of some recent series[204] and in sporadic case reports that include constrictive pericarditis, high-grade AV block, supraventricular tachycardia, as well as complications secondary to involvement of the coronary arteries.[205,206]

HYPERSENSITIVITY VASCULITIS (LEUKOCYTOBLASTIC VASCULITIS)

Hypersensitivity vasculitis is also called small-vessel vasculitis or angiitis and is characterized by involvement of arterioles, venules, and capillaries only. Antigen-antibody complexes present in the lesions all tend to be of the same age. It is difficult to tell at the inception of the disease

whether it is part of a larger syndrome, such as SLE, subacute infective endocarditis, mixed cryoglobulinemia, Henoch-Schönlein purpura, or a drug reaction except by the course and distinguishing features of the other syndromes. Hypersensitivity vasculitis is the most common form of immune complex disease. Muscular and large arteries are spared, so that the tissue lesions are due to microinfarcts and hemorrhagic and exudative reactions at the capillary level rather than to thrombosis of large vessels with resulting ischemia and necrosis. The most common cardiac finding is pericarditis, but such involvement occurs along with that of many other organs, skin, mucous membranes, joints, and so on.

GIANT CELL ARTERITIS[202-208]

Giant cell arteritis, also called cranial or temporal arteritis, affects predominantly older individuals. Large or medium-sized arteries, including the superficial temporal artery, are involved without small-vessel or capillary lesions. The lesions are usually cellular and granulomatous and contain multinucleated giant cells. Involvement of the arteries is spotty and segmented and tends to produce thrombosis at the site of involvement. The aorta is often involved and aneurysms and dissection can result (p. 1547). External and internal carotids and vertebral arteries can be affected, and thrombosis of the ophthalmic or central retinal artery leads to blindness. Thrombosis of the coronary, iliac, femoral, or mesenteric arteries produces ischemia and infarctions. Aortic regurgitation is a rare but well-documented complication.[209]

BEHÇET'S SYNDROME

This diffuse vasculitis causes recurrent genital and oral ulcerations and uveitis.[210] Cardiac manifestations occur in about 5 per cent of patients and include pericarditis, aortic and mitral regurgitation, and endomyocardial fibrosis involving the right side of the heart.[211]

PROGRESSIVE SYSTEMIC SCLEROSIS (DIFFUSE SCLERODERMA)

Progressive systemic sclerosis (PSS) is an insidious, chronic, fibrosing condition that presents as progressive tightening and thickening of the skin (scleroderma), developing over a period of many years. Raynaud's phenomenon occurs at some time in almost all patients. Visceral involvement may occur at any time during the course of the disease, affecting the gastrointestinal tract, lungs, heart or kidney. Much attention has been given to the classification of various subgroups of this syndrome that include patients with diffuse scleroderma, those without diffuse skin changes but with other shared features, such as calcinosis, Raynaud's phenomenon, esophageal dysfunction, sclerodactyly, and telangiectasia (the CREST syndrome), and those with features overlapping polymyositis or systemic lupus erythematosus or both.[212-214]

Pathological Features and Pathogenesis

In contrast to the acute exudative forms of vasculitis associated with the necrotizing lesions described above, PSS seems to be a disease at the opposite end of the inflammatory scale, in which very slow scarring and fibrosis result from gradual obliteration of small vessels. It is difficult to classify PSS pathophysiologically because the cause of the extensive fibrosis is not known, but the importance of small artery spasm and the possibility of its reversal by arterial vasodilators has received considerable attention.[215-225] Pulmonary hypertension has been at least temporarily reduced with such vasodilators as captopril,[221] nifedipine,[223] and verapamil,[224] as have attacks of Raynaud's phenomenon. Left ventricular regional wall motion abnormalities have been demonstrated during cold exposure in 9 of 16 patients with Raynaud's phenomenon and PSS or the CREST syndrome, and in most of these cases treatment with nifedipine blunted the severity of the abnormal ventricular response.[225] Short-term improvement in myocardial perfusion with nifedipine, demonstrated by thallium-201 single-photon-emission computed tomography, was observed in a study of 29 patients with diffuse scleroderma and Raynaud's phenomenon.[217]

Hereditary factors have not been identified. Qualitative abnormalities of collagen are not documented. The disease apparently results from injury or spasm at the level of very small arteries, 150 to 500 μm in diameter, and capillaries are gradually obliterated.[215] Early in the course of lesions, mononuclear cell infiltrates occur around small arteries and in the interstitium. The basement membrane of the capillaries appears thickened. Fibroblastic proliferation and overproduction of collagen result from the low-grade inflammatory process. Narrowing and obliteration of small arteries result in decreased vascularization of the skin, skeletal muscles, lung, and heart, followed by fibrosis. The interlobular arteries of the kidney are involved by intensive intimal proliferation, which causes rapid renal failure, often with severe hypertension.

CARDIAC LESIONS. The importance of primary cardiac involvement in the natural history of the disease has been repeatedly emphasized,[213-221] but only with the advent of noninvasive cardiac evaluation methods of thallium-201 scintigraphy, rest and exercise radionuclide ventriculography, continuous 24-hour Holter ECG monitoring, two-dimensional echocardiography, and pulmonary-function testing has the full picture of the frequency and extent of cardiac dysfunction become apparent.[215-221] Thallium scintigraphy may show fixed defects, but even more common are cold-induced reversible defects[226] compatible with severe coronary vasospasm. Defective perfusion of organs by spastic small arteries may account for the general observation that functional disability of the myocardium and lungs exceeds anatomical changes.[216-225] Heart involvement is a frequent cause of death and second only to involvement of the kidneys as a factor shortening the survival of patients with this disease. Confusion concerning the question of primary involvement of the heart by the sclerosing process has been caused by the frequency of cor pulmonale resulting from pulmonary involvement of PSS and severe hypertension and hypertensive heart disease resulting from the renal involvement. In one study of patients with systemic sclerosis, ambulatory electrocardiography revealed ventricular ectopy in 67 per cent of patients, with more serious ventricular arrhythmias in 25 per cent.[227] These arrhythmias tend to be more severe in patients with other evidence of cardiac disease and are an independent risk factor for death.

"Scleroderma heart" is primarily a myocardial disease, and the heart's small vessels are all vulnerable to the sclerosing process. Atherosclerosis of the major coronary arteries occurs to the same degree in patients with PSS as in age- and sex-matched controls. PSS patients, however, have much more intimal sclerosis of the small coronary arteries than do controls, and such involvement may lead to ischemia, small infarctions, and fibrosis. The combination of vascular insufficiency and fibrosis produces a cardiomyopathy with congestive heart failure and conduction system abnormalities.[215-221] Acute and chronic pericarditis, even in the absence of uremia, is common but usually asymptomatic. At times the resulting effusion can be large enough to cause tamponade,[228] although this degree of effusion is rare. Pericardial fluid, when obtainable, has the features of an exudate but lacks evidence of autoantibodies, immune complexes, or complement depletion, such as that seen in rheumatoid arthritis or SLE.[229] Endocardial involvement is rare, and the deformities of mitral and aortic valves that have been reported probably have little hemodynamic significance.

Clinical Features

The primary clinical manifestations of scleroderma heart disease are those of pericarditis (see also p. 1502) and congestive heart failure. In one series, pericarditis patients had a 7-year cumulative survival rate of 33 per cent, whereas none of the PSS patients with heart failure survived for 7 years.[230] Men have significantly worse survival rates than women, as do blacks and older patients. Although cardiac symptoms may appear months or even years before the skin is involved, as a rule overt heart disease is not a prominent part of the clinical picture of PSS until late in its course, when myocardial involvement and resultant heart failure indicate a grim prognosis. The relative risk of death for a PSS patient with an S_3 gallop indicative of myocardial disease was reported to be many times that for a patient without an S_3 gallop.[231] Pericarditis, however, may be intermittently symptomatic for long periods.

When dyspnea with exertion or at rest occurs in the patient with PSS, primary myocardial failure must be distinguished from myocardial failure secondary to hypertension from renal disease and pulmonary insufficiency from pulmonary fibrosis due to PSS. Cardiac murmurs are not usually due to valvular deformity but to cardiac dilatation and to anemia or to papillary weakness. Chest pain simulating ischemic heart disease as well as typical pericardial pain may occur.

The *roentgenogram of the chest* may reveal cardiac enlargement from pericardial effusion, cardiomyopathy, or hypertension. The electrocardiographic findings are also nonspecific and may, indeed, be normal when the heart is seriously involved. All degrees of AV conduction blocks, right and left ventricular hypertrophy, and all varieties of arrhythmias have been described,[227] but conduction defects are found most often in patients with the primary cardiomyopathy of PSS.[218-221]

Echocardiographic studies reveal patterns consistent with a congestive cardiomyopathy or a restrictive cardiomyopathy, and pericardial effusion can be demonstrated often when not suspected clinically.

TREATMENT. The value of corticosteroids is limited to improvement of the early edematous phase of the disease, but this effect on the heart has not been systematically evaluated and probably will not influence the eventual course of the disease.

As noted above, the most interesting and encouraging recent therapeutic development is the demonstration of improved perfusion of the heart, lungs, and, in the case of Raynaud's phenomenon, the hands, of patients with PSS or the CREST syndrome by the administration of calcium channel blockers such as nifedipine[217,223] and verapamil[225] and other vasodilators such as captopril.[222,232] The possible benefits of long-term therapy with these agents remain to be defined.

POLYMYOSITIS AND DERMATOMYOSITIS

Polymyositis is a diffuse inflammatory disease of unknown cause affecting primarily proximal striated muscles and various connective tissues of the body, especially skin and joints.[233] When the disease also involves the skin, it is called *dermatomyositis*. Polymyositis may be due to a pathological process common to several etiologies because it is seen in association with a variety of syndromes. It is grouped with the connective tissue or rheumatic diseases because of its overlapping clinical and laboratory features, especially when it is associated with rheumatoid arthritis and PSS but also with SLE or polyarteritis. Involvement of the heart in polymyositis has just begun to be fully appreciated in the past decade and was mentioned in earlier publications only as a rare finding, if at all.

Pathological Features

Polymyositis is either increasing in incidence and/or is being more frequently diagnosed, and it is now well recognized as one of the most common myopathies. The principal changes in muscle tissue consist of widespread destruction of muscle fibers with phagocytosis of destroyed cells. There may be focal infiltrates of inflammatory cells, such as lymphocytes, mononuclear leukocytes, plasma cells, and, only rarely, neutrophilic leukocytes. Regeneration of destroyed muscle in the form of proliferating sarcolemmal nuclei, basophilic sarcoplasm, and new myofibrils is a prominent feature. Residual muscle fibers may be small. In any given biopsy specimen, either degeneration of muscle fibers or infiltrations of inflammatory cells may predominate. In electron microscopic studies, the most significant changes, in addition to those in muscle fibers, are found in the endothelium and basement

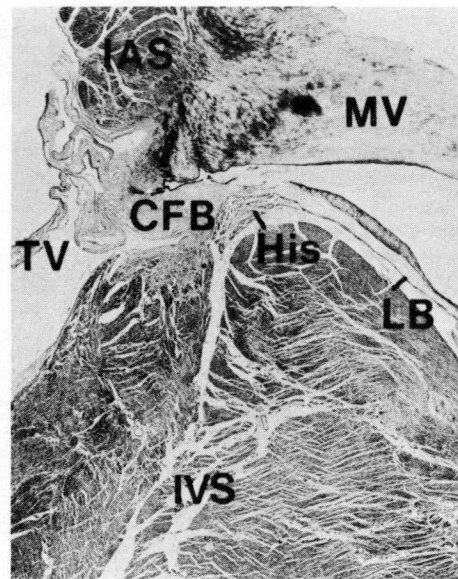
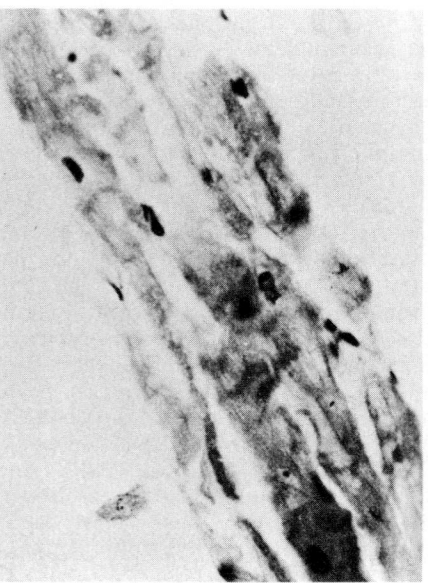

FIGURE 56–11. Cardiac conduction system in a 53-year-old woman with polymyositis-dermatomyositis left bundle branch block. *Left,* the left bundle (LB) and distal portion of the His bundle (His). The interatrial septum (IAS) is at the top and the interventricular septum (IVS) below. The mitral (MV) and tricuspid (TV) valves are attached to the central fibrous body (CFB). *Right,* contraction band necrosis of the left bundle. The myocytes of the bundle show irregular coarse transverse condensations of sarcoplasm and their nuclei are pyknotic. (From Haupt, H. M., and Hutchins, G. M.: The heart and conduction system in polymyositis-dermatomyositis: A clinicopathologic study of 16 autopsied patients. Am. J. Cardiol. *50*:998, 1982.)

membrane of capillaries and small arterioles, much like those described in scleroderma and SLE. Inclusions in the cytoplasm of endothelial cells that are identical to those found in SLE and scleroderma have been described.[234]

CARDIAC PATHOLOGY.[235-239] The cardiac lesions involve the conducting system predominantly but also can produce an extensive cardiomyopathy and pericarditis. The latter may appear far more often than would be suspected on clinical grounds. The cardiac valves and coronary arteries are spared except in overlap syndromes. The sinoatrial node shows conspicuous fibrosis, swelling and degeneration of collagen, and focal or complete replacement. The fibrosis extends into the adjacent myocardium of the right atrium. The AV node, bundle of His, and both bundle branches all may be involved in the degenerative and fibrotic processes (Fig. 56–11). Cardiac muscle fibers in the atria and ventricles are replaced in scattered areas by fibrosis, and, in some cases, the pattern of focal myocardial necrosis and inflammation is the same as that seen in skeletal muscle. Pericarditis is described more often clinically than pathologically.

CLINICAL FEATURES. Almost all authors comment on the rarity of cardiovascular manifestations in polymyositis, and, indeed, the best reported studies of survivorship do not relate death to cardiac causes but rather to pneumonitis, which is relatively common from aspiration secondary to respiratory muscle weakness and dysphagia. However, more careful studies of the heart for subtle signs of involvement in polymyositis patients without cardiac symptoms and signs[238,239] and careful review of autopsied patients with polymyositis-dermatomyositis syndromes[237] show a much higher frequency of cardiac involvement in polymyositis than was previously appreciated. When standard 12-lead electrocardiograms are analyzed systematically, arrhythmias may be quite frequent.[239] These usually consist of supraventricular tachycardia, but ventricular tachycardia and advanced heart block associated with syncope or cardiac arrest have also been observed. Deaths have been attributed directly to myocardial failure or arrhythmias or both in some cases, and cardiac muscle histology has been found to be abnormal on autopsy. Sudden death is not unusual, especially in patients with documented heart block.[239] Constrictive pericarditis has been reported.[235]

TREATMENT. Corticosteroids and immunosuppressive drugs may be of benefit in the treatment of polyositis-dermatomyositis, but only a controlled prospective study can settle this issue. The course of the disease, including myocardial involvement, may not be truly modified by corticosteroids, but the complications of muscle weakness, especially of the respiratory and deglutitional muscles, which lead to pulmonary disease and death, might be diminished by the frequent improvement of muscle strength observed after this treatment.

In the absence of malignancy, survival statistics are favorable for all groups (87 to 91 per cent) in several studies. The leading causes of death, which in one series were metastatic malignant disease (24 per cent), sepsis (19 per cent), profound muscular weakness (9.5 per cent), and cardiovascular and cerebrovascular disorders (unspecified percentage), suggest that at least some of these may be modified by supportive therapy and management to improve the prognosis.

MIXED CONNECTIVE TISSUE DISEASE

As its name implies, this condition is characterized by overlapping features and combinations of rheumatoid arthritis, progressive systemic stenosis, polymyositis, and systemic lupus erythematosus. Patients have high titers of circulating antibodies to nuclear ribonucleoprotein.[240] Cardiac involvement includes pericardial effusion and thickening as well as valvular, usually mitral, regurgitation.[241]

REFERENCES

REUMATIC FEVER

1. Stollerman, G. H.: Rheumatic Fever and Streptococcal Infection. New York, Grune and Stratton, 1975.
2. Bisno, A. L.: The rise and fall of rheumatic fever. J.A.M.A. 254:538, 1985.
3. Stollerman G. H.: Rheumatogenic group A streptococci and the return of rheumatic fever. Adv. Intern. Med. 35:1, 1990.
4. Ramelkamp, C. H., Denny, F. W., and Wannamaker, L. W.: Studies on the epidemiology of rheumatic fever in the armed services. In Thomas, L. (ed.): Rheumatic Fever. Minneapolis, University of Minnesota Press, 1952, pp. 72–89.
5. Frank, P. F., Stollerman, G. H., and Miller, L. F.: Protection of a military population from rheumatic fever. J.A.M.A. 193:775, 1965.
6. Gordis, L.: The virtual disappearance of rheumatic fever in the United States; lessons in the rise and fall of disease. Circulation 72:1155, 1985.
7. Markowitz, M.: The decline of rheumatic fever, role of medical intervention. J. Pediatr. 106:545, 1985.
8. Argarwal, B. L.: Rheumatic heart disease unabated in developing countries. Lancet 2:910, 1981.
9. Stetson, C. A.: The relation of antibody response to rheumatic fever. In McCarty, M. (ed.): Streptococcal Infections. New York, Columbia University Press, 1954, pp. 208–218.
10. Rammelkamp, C. H., Jr.: The Lewis A. Conner Memorial Lecture. Rheumatic heart disease—A challenge. Circulation 17:842, 1958.
11. Siegel, A. C., Johnson, E. E., and Stollerman, G. H.: Controlled studies of streptococcal pharyngitis in a pediatric population: I. Factors related to the attack rate of rheumatic fever. N. Engl. J. Med. 265:559, 1961.
12. Stollerman, G. H.: Factors determining the attack rate of rheumatic fever. J.A.M.A. 177:823, 1961.
13. Stollerman, G. H., Siegel, A. C., and Johnson, E. E.: Variable epidemiology of streptococcal disease and the changing patterns of rheumatic fever. Mod. Concepts Cardiovasc. Dis. 34:45, 1965.
14. Kaplan, E. L., Top, F. H., Dudding, B. A., and Wannamaker, L. W.: Diagnosis of streptococcal pharyngitis: Differentiation of active infection from the carrier state in the symptomatic child. J. Infect. Dis. 123:490, 1971.
15. Top, F. H., Wannamaker, L. W., Maxted, W. R., and Anthony, G. V.: M antigens among group A streptococci isolated from skin lesions. J. Exp. Med. 126:667, 1967.
16. Stollerman, G. H.: Nephritogenic and rheumatogenic group A streptococci. J. Infect. Dis. 120:258, 1969.
17. Wannamaker, L. W.: Medical progress. Differences between streptococcal infections of the throat and of the skin. N. Engl. J. Med. 282:23 and 78, 1970.
18. Wannamaker, L. W.: The chain that links the heart to the throat. Circulation 48:9, 1973.
19. Bisno, A. L., Pearce, I. A., Wall, H. P., et al.: Contrasting epidemiology of acute rheumatic fever and acute glomerulonephritis. Nature of the antecedent streptococcal infection. N. Engl. J. Med. 283:561, 1970.
20. Poon-King, T., Mohammed, I., Cox, R., et al.: Recurrent epidemic nephritis in South Trinidad. N. Engl. J. Med. 277:728, 1967.
21. Potter, E. V., Svartman, M., Poon-King, T., and Earle, D. P.: The families of patients with acute rheumatic fever or glomerulonephritis in Trinidad. Am. J. Epidemiol. 106:130, 1977.
22. Widdowson, J. P., Maxted, W. R., Notley, C. M., and Pinney, A. M.: The antibody responses in man to infection with different serotypes of group A streptococci. J. Med. Microbiol. 7:483, 1974.

23. Bisno, A. L.: The concept of rheumatogenic and nonrheumatogenic group A streptococci. *In* McCarty, M., and Zabriskie, J. B. (eds.): Streptococcal Diseases and the Immune Response. New York, Academic Press, 1980, p. 789.
24. Stollerman, G. H.: The streptococcus, rheumatic fever and rheumatic heart disease. *In* Shaper, A. G., Hutt, M. S. R., and Fejfar, Z. (eds.): Cardiovascular Disease in the Tropics. London, British Medical Associates, 1974.
25. Sanyal, S. K., Berry, A. M., Duggal, S., et al.: Sequelae of the initial attack of rheumatic fever in children from North India. Circulation *65*:375, 1982.
26. Sanyal, S. K., Thapar, M. K., Ahmed, S. H., et al.: The initial attack of acute rheumatic fever during childhood in North India. A prospective study of the clinical profile. Circulation *49*:7, 1974.
27. Taranta, A.: Rheumatic fever in children and adolescents. A long-term epidemiologic study of subsequent prophylaxis, streptococcal infections, and clinical sequelae: IV. Relation of the rheumatic fever recurrence rate per streptococcal infection to the titers of streptococcal antibodies. Ann. Intern. Med. *60*(Suppl. 5):47, 1964.
28. Taranta, A., Kleinberg, E., Feinstein, A. R., et al.: Rheumatic fever in children and adolescents. A long-term epidemiologic study of subsequent prophylaxis, streptococcal infections, and clinical sequelae: V. Relation of the rheumatic fever recurrence rate per streptococcal infection to pre-existing clinical features of the patients. Ann. Intern. Med. *60*(Suppl. 5):58, 1964.
29. Johnson, E. E., Stollerman, G. H., and Grossman, B. J.: Rheumatic recurrences in patients not receiving continuous prophylaxis. J.A.M.A. *190*:74, 1964.
30. Taranta, A.: Rheumatic fever made difficult. A critical review of pathogenetic theories. Paediatrician *5*:74, 1976.
31. Pattarroyo, M. E., Winchester, R., Vejerano, A., et al.: Association of B-cell alloantigen with susceptibility to rheumatic fever. Nature *278*:173, 1979.
32. Zabriskie, J. B., Lavenchy, D., Williams, R. C., Jr., et al.: Rheumatic fever associated B cell alloantigen as identified by monoclonal antibodies. Arthritis Rheum. *28*:1047, 1985.
33. Khanna, A. K., Buskirk, D. R., Williams, R. C., Jr., et al.: Presence of a non-HLA B cell antigen in rheumatic fever patients and their families as defined by a monoclonal antibody. J. Clin. Invest. *83*:1710, 1989.
34. Stollerman, G. H.: Streptococci and Rheumatic Heart Disease. *In* De Vries, RRP, Cohen, I. R., and van Rood, J. J. (eds.): The Role of Microorganisms in noninfectious diseases. London, Springer-Verlag, 1990, pp. 9–20.
35. Stollerman, G. H.: The epidemiology of primary and secondary rheumatic fever. *In* Uhr, J. W. (ed): The Streptococcus, Rheumatic Fever and Glomerulonephritis. Baltimore, Williams and Wilkins, 1964, pp. 331–337.
36. Yoshimoya, S., and Pope, R. M.: Detection of immune complexes in acute rheumatic fever and their relationship to HLA-B5. J. Clin. Invest. *65*:136, 1980.
37. Stollerman, G. H.: Autoimmunity and rheumatic fever. *In* Cohen, I. R. (ed.): Perspectives in Autoimmunity. Boca Raton, Fl., CRC Press, 1986.
38. Kaplan, M. H., Meyeserian, M., and Kishner, I.: Immunologic studies of heart tissue: IV. Serologic reactions with human heart tissue as revealed by immunofluorescent methods. Isoimmune, Wassermann, and auto-immune reactions. J. Exp. Med. *113*:17, 1961.
39. Hess, E. V., Fink, C. W., Taranta, A., and Ziff, M.: Heart muscle antibodies in rheumatic fever and other diseases. J. Clin. Invest. *43*:886, 1964.
40. Kaplan, M. H.: Immunologic relation of streptococcal and tissue antigens. I. Properties of an antigen in certain strains of group A streptococci exhibiting an immunologic cross-reaction with human heart tissue. J. Immunol. *90*:595, 1963.
41. Kaplan, M. H., and Suchy, M. L.: Immunologic relation of streptococcal and tissue antigens. II. Cross reactions of antisera to mammalian heart tissue with a cell wall constituent of certain strains of group A streptococci. J. Exp. Med. *119*:643, 1964.
42. Zabriskie, J. B., and Freimer, E. H.: An immunological relationship between the group A streptococcus and mammalian muscle. J. Exp. Med. *124*:661, 1966.
43. Goldstein, I., Halpern, B., and Robert, L.: Immunological relationship between streptococcus A polysaccharide and the structural glycoproteins of heart valves. Nature *213*:44, 1967.
44. Dudding, B. A., and Ayoub, E. M.: Persistence of streptococcal group A antibody in patients with rheumatic valvular disease. J. Exp. Med. *129*:1081, 1968.
45. Appleton, R. S., Victoria, B. C., Tamer, D., and Ayoub, E. M.: Specificity of persistence of antibody to the streptococcal group A carbohydrate in rheumatic valvular heart disease. J. Lab. Clin. Med. *105*:114, 1985.
46. Husby, G., van de Rijn, I., Zabriskie, J. B., et al.: Antibodies reacting with cytoplasm of subthalamic and caudate nuclei neurons in chorea and acute rheumatic fever. J. Exp. Med. *144*:1094, 1976.
47. Dale, J. B., and Beachey, E. H.: Epitopes of streptococcal M proteins shared with cardiac myosin. J. Exp. Med. *162*:583, 1985.
48. Cunningham, M. W., and Swerlick, R. A.: Polyspecificity of antistreptococcal murine monoclonal antibodies and their implications in autoimmunity. J. Exp. Med. *164*:998, 1987.
49. Bronze, M. S., Beachey, E. H., and Dale, J. B.: Protective and heart cross-reactive epitopes within the NH2 terminus of type 19 streptococcal M protein. J. Exp. Med. *167*:1849, 1988.
50. Manjula, B. N., Trus, B. L., and Fischetti, V. A.: Presence of two distinct regions in the coiled-coil structure of the streptococcal pep M5 protein: relationship to mammalian coiled-coil proteins and implications to its biological properties. Proc. Natl. Acad. Sci. *82*:1064, 1985.
51. Bessen, D., Jones, K. F., and Fischetti, V. A.: Evidence for two distinct classes of streptococcal M protein and their relationship to rheumatic fever. J. Exp. Med. *169*:269, 1989.
52. Tomai, M., Kotb, M., Majundar, G., and Beachey E. H.: Superantigenicity of streptococcal M protein. J. Exp. Med. *172*:359, 1990.
53. Murphy, G. E.: Nature of rheumatic heart disease with special reference to myocardial disease and heart failure. Medicine *39*:289, 1960.
54. Aschoff, L.: The rheumatic nodules in the heart. Ann. Rheum. Dis. *1*:161, 1939.
55. Kuschner, M., Ferrer, M. I., Harvey, R. M., and Wylie, R. H.: Rheumatic carditis in surgically removed appendages. Am. Heart J. *43*:286, 1952.
56. Virmani, R., and Roberts, W. C.: Aschoff bodies in operatively excised atrial appendages and in papillary muscles. Frequency and clinical significance. Circulation *55*:559, 1977.
57. Roberts, W. C., and Virmani, R.: Aschoff bodies at necropsy in valvular heart disease. Evidence from an analysis of 543 patients over 14 years of age that rheumatic heart disease, at least anatomically, is a disease of the mitral valve. Circulation *57*:803, 1978.
58. Stollerman, G. H., Lynch, W. F., Dolman, M. A., et al.: Immunologic evidence of streptococcal infection in patients undergoing mitral commissurotomy. Circulation *15*:267, 1957.
59. Lanningan, R.: Cardiac Pathology. London, Butterworth and Co., 1966.
60. Becker, C. G., and Murphy, G. E.: On the pathology of rheumatic heart disease. *In* Read, S. E., and Zabriskie, J. B. (eds.): Streptococcal Diseases and the Immune Response, New York, Academic Press, 1980, p. 23.
61. Husby, G. H., Arora, R., Williams, R. C., et al.: Immunofluorescent studies of florid rheumatic Aschoff lesions. Arthritis Rheum. *29*:207, 1986.
62. Steele, P. P., Weily, H. S., Davies, H., and Genton, E.: Platelet survival in patients with rheumatic heart disease. N. Engl. J. Med. *290*:537, 1974.
63. Winkelman, N. W., and Eckel, J. L.: The brain in acute rheumatic fever. Nonsuppurative meningoencephalitis rheumatica. Arch. Neurol. Psychiatr. *28*:844, 1932.
64. Neubuerger, K. T.: The brain in rheumatic fever. Dis. Nerv. System *8*:259, 1947.
65. Costero, I.: Cerebral lesions responsible for death of patients with active rheumatic fever. Arch. Neurol. Psychiatr. *62*:48, 1949.
66. Buchanan, D. N.: Pathologic changes in chorea. Am. J. Dis. Child. *62*:443, 1941.
67. Kernohan, J. W., Woltman, H. W., and Barnes, A. R.: Involvement of the nervous system associated with endocarditis. Neuropsychiatric and neuropathologic observations in 42 cases of fatal outcome. Arch. Neurol. Psychiatr. *42*:789, 1939.
68. Raz, I., Fisher, J., Israel, A., et al.: An unusual case of rheumatic pneumonia. Arch. Intern. Med. *145*:1130, 1985.
69. Rammelkamp, C. H., Jr., and Stolzer, B. L.: The latent period before the onset of acute rheumatic fever. Yale J. Biol. Med. *34*:386, 1961.
70. Feinstein, A. R., and Spagnuolo, M.: The clinical patterns of acute rheumatic fever: A reappraisal. Medicine *41*:279, 1962.
71. Ben-Dov, I., and Berry, E.: Acute rheumatic fever in adults over the age of 45 years: An analysis of 23 patients together with a review of the literature. Semin. Arthritis Rheum. *10*:10, 1980.
72. United Kingdom and United States Joint Report on Rheumatic Fever: The treatment of acute rheumatic fever in children. A cooperative clinical trial of ACTH, cortisone and aspirin. Circulation *11*:343, 1955.
73. United Kingdom and United States Joint Report on Rheumatic Heart Disease: The evolution of rheumatic heart disease in children. Five-year report of a cooperative clinical trial of ACTH, cortisone and aspirin. Circulation *22*:503, 1960.
74. United Kingdom and United States Joint Report on Rheumatic Heart Disease: The natural history of rheumatic fever and rheumatic heart disease. Ten-year report of a cooperative clinical trial of ACTH, cortisone and aspirin. Circulation *32*:457, 1965.
75. Massell, B. V., Fyler, D. C., and Roy, S. B.: The clinical picture of rheumatic fever. Diagnosis, immediate prognosis, course and therapeutic implications. Am. J. Cardiol. *1*:436, 1958.
76. Combined Rheumatic Fever Study Group, 1960: A comparison of the effect of prednisone and acetylsalicylic acid on the incidence of residual rheumatic heart disease. N. Engl. J. Med. *262*:895, 1960.
77. Combined Rheumatic Fever Study Group, 1965: A comparison of the short-term, intensive prednisone and acetylsalicylic acid therapy in the treatment of acute rheumatic fever. N. Engl. J. Med. *272*:63, 1965.
78. Robinson, R. W.: Effect of atropine upon the prolongation of the P-R interval found in acute rheumatic fever and certain vagotonic persons. Am. Heart J. *29*:378, 1945.
79. Lenox, C. C., Zuberbuhler, J. R., Park, S. C., et al.: Arrhythmias and Stokes-Adams attacks in acute rheumatic fever. Pediatrics *61*:599, 1979.
80. Meynet, P.: Rheumatisme articulaire subaigu avec production de tumeurs multiples dans les tissus fibreux periarticulaires et sur le périoste d'un grand numbre d'os. Lyons Med. *19*:495, 1875.
81. Baldwin, J. S., Kerr, J. M., Kuttner, A. G., and Loyle, E. F.: Observations on rheumatic nodules over a 30-year period. J. Pediatr. *56*:465, 1960.
82. Veasy, L. G., Wiedmeier, S. E., Garth, S. O., et al.: Resurgence of acute rheumatic fever in the intermountain area of the United States. N. Engl. J. Med. *316*:421, 1987.
83. Taranta, A., and Stollerman, G. H.: The relationship of Sydenham's chorea to infection with group A streptococci Am. J. Med. *20*:170, 1956.
84. Bland, E. F.: Chorea as a manifestation of rheumatic fever. A long-term perspective. Trans Am. Clin. Climatol. Assoc. *73*:209, 1961.
85. Whitnack, E., and Stollerman, G. H.: Antistreptococcal antibodies in the diagnosis of rheumatic fever: *In* Cohen, A. S., (ed.): Laboratory Diagnostic Procedures in Rheumatic Diseases, 3rd Ed. Boston, Little, Brown and Co., 1985, pp. 273–292.
86. Gewurz, H., Mold, C., Siegel, J., and Fiedel, B.: C-reactive protein and the acute phase response. Adv. Intern. Med. *27*:345, 1982.
87. Feinstein, A. R., and DiMassa, R.: Prognostic significance of valvular involvement in acute rheumatic fever. N. Engl. J. Med. *260*:1001, 1959.
88. Feinstein, A. R., Wood, H. F., Spagnuolo, M., et al.: Rheumatic fever in children and adolescents: VII. Cardiac changes and sequelae. Ann. Intern. Med. *60*(Suppl. 5):87, 1964.
89. Jones, T. D.: The diagnosis of rheumatic fever. J.A.M.A. *126*:481, 1944.
90. Jones Criteria (revised) for guidance in the diagnosis of rheumatic fever. Circulation *32*:664, 1965.
91. Taranta, A., Spagnuolo, M., and Feinstein, A. R.: "Chronic" rheumatic fever. Ann. Intern. Med. *56*:367, 1962.
92. McIntosch, R., and Wood, C. L.: Rheumatic infections occurring in the first three years of life. Am. J. Dis. Child. *49*:835, 1935.
93. Rosenthal, A., Czoniczer, G., and Massell, B. F.: Rheumatic fever under three years of age. A report of ten cases. Pediatrics *41*:612, 1968.
94. Ellis, L. B.: Recurrent mitral stenosis. Mod. Concepts Cardiovasc. Dis. *33*:851, 1964.
95. Wood, H. F., Simpson, R., Feinstein, A. R., et al.: Rheumatic fever in children and adolescents. I. Description of the investigative techniques and of the population studied. Ann. Intern. Med. *60*(Suppl. 5):6, 1964.
96. Bisno, A. L., Pearce, I. A., and Stollerman, G. H.: Streptococcal infections that fail to cause recurrences of rheumatic fever. J. Infect. Dis. *136*:278, 1977.
97. Goetzler, R., Stokes, J., III, and Anderson, K.: Prognosis of subjects in the Framingham Study with rheumatic heart disease. J. Am. Geriatr. Soc. *33*:693, 1985.
98. Vaisman, S., Guasch, J., Vignau, A., et al.: The failure of penicillin to alter acute rheumatic valvulitis. J.A.M.A. *194*:1284, 1965.
99. Lockman, L. A.: Movement disorders. *In* Swaiman, K., and Wright, F. (eds.): Practice of Pediatric Neurology. St. Louis, C. V. Mosby Co., 1975.
100. Centers for Disease Control: Acute rheumatic fever—Utah. M.M.W.R. *36*:108, 1987.
101. Centers for Disease Control: Acute rheumatic fever in a Navy training center—San Diego, California. M.M.W.R. *37*:101, 1988.
102. Centers for Disease Control: Acute rheumatic fever among Army trainees—Ft. Leonard Wood, MO 1987–1988. M.M.W.R. *37*:519, 1988.
103. Kaplan, E. L., Johnson, D. R., and Cleary, P. P.: Group A streptococcal serotypes isolated from patients and sibling contacts during the resurgence of rheumatic fever in the United States in the mid-1980's. J. Infect. Dis. *159*:101, 1989.
104. Stollerman, G. H., Rusoff, J. H., and Hirschfeld, I.: Prophylaxis against group A streptococci in rheumatic fever. The use of single monthly injections of benzathine penicillin G. N. Engl. J. Med. *252*:787, 1955.
105. Albam, B., Epstein, J. A., Feinstein, A. R., et al.: Rheumatic fever in children and adolescents. A long-term epidemiologic study of subsequent prophylaxis, streptococcal infections, and clinical sequelae. Ann. Intern. Med. *60*(Suppl. 5): No. 2, Part II, 1964.
106. American Heart Association, Committee on Rheumatic Fever and Bacterial Endocarditis: Prevention of rheumatic fever. Circulation *78*:1082, 1988.
107. Wannamaker, L. W., Rammelkamp, C. H., Jr., Denny, F. W., et al.: Prophylaxis of acute rheumatic fever by treatment of the preceding streptococcal infection with various amounts of depot penicillin. Am. J. Med. *10*:673, 1951.
108. Wannamaker, L. W., Denny, F. W., Perry, W. D., et al.: The effect of penicillin prophy-

laxis on streptococcal disease rates and the carrier state. N. Engl. J. Med. *249*:1, 1953.

109. Dale, J. B., and Beachey, E. H.:Localization of protective epitopes of the amino terminus of type 5 streptococcal M protein. J. Exp. Med. *163*:1191, 1986.
110. Beachey, E. H., Stollerman, G. H., Johnson, R. H., et al.: Human immune response to immunization with a structurally defined polypeptide fragment of streptococcal M protein. J. Exp. Med. *150*:862, 1979.
111. Beachey, E. H., Grus-Masse, H., Tarter, A., et al.:Opsonic antibodies evoked by hybrid peptide copies of types 5 and 24 streptococcal M proteins synthesized in tandem. J. Exp. Med. *163*:1451, 1986.
112. Bluestone, R., and Pearson, C. M.: Ankylosing spondylitis and Reiter's syndrome: The interrelationships and association with HLA B27. Adv. Intern. Med. *22*:1, 1977.
113. Khan, M. A., and Khan, M. K.: Diagnostic value of HLA-B27 testing in ankylosing spondylitis and Reiter's syndrome. Ann. Intern. Med.*96*:70, 1982.
114. Calin, A. (ed.): Spondyloarthropathies. Orlando, Fl., Grune and Stratton, 1984.
115. Laitinen, O., Leirisalo, M., and Skylv, G.: Relation between HLA-B27 and clinical features in patients with Yersinia arthritis. Athritis Rheum. *20*:1121, 1977.
116. Schachter, J.: Can chlamydial infections cause rheumatic disease? *In* Dumonde, D. C. (ed.): Infection and Immunology in Rheumatic Diseases. Oxford, Blackwell Scientific Publications, 1976, pp. 151–157.

ANKYLOSING SPONDYLITIS

117. Alves, M. G., Espirito-Santo, J., Queiroz, M. V., et al.: Cardiac alterations in ankylosing spondylitis. Angiology *39*:567, 1988.
118. Thomas, D., Hill, W., Geddes, R., et al.: Early detection of aortic dilatation in ankylosing spondylitis using echocardiography. Aust. N.Z. J. Med. *12*:10, 1982.
119. LaBresh, K. A., Lally, E. V., Sharma, S. C., and Ho, G.: Two-dimensional echocardiographic detection of preclinical aortic root abnormalities in rheumatoid variant diseases. Am. J. Med. *78*:908, 1985.
120. Shah, A.: Echocardiographic features of mitral regurgitation due to ankylosing spondylitis. Am. J. Med. *82*:353, 1987.
121. Roberts, W. C., Hollingsworth, J. F., Bulkley, B. H., et al.: Combined mitral and aortic regurgitation in ankylosing spondylitis. Angiographic and anatomic features. Am. J. Med. *56*:237, 1974.
122. Nitter-Hauge, S., and Otterstad, J. E.: Characteristics of atrioventricular conduction disturbances in ankylosing spondylitis. Acta Med. Scand. *210*:197, 200, 1981.
123. Bergfeld, E. L.: HLA-B27-associated rheumatic diseases with severe cardiac bradyarrhythmias. Clinical features in 223 men with permanent pacemakers. Am. J. Med. *75*:210, 1983.
124. Bulkley, B. H., and Roberts, W. C.: Ankylosing spondylitis and aortic regurgitation. Description of the characteristic cardiovascular lesion from study of eight necropsy patients. Circulation *48*:1014, 1973.
125. Ribiero, P., Morley, L. M., Shapiro, R. A., et al.: Left ventricular function in patients with ankylosing spondylitis and Reiter's disease. Eur. Heart J. *5*:419, 1984.
126. Cowan, G. O.: Aortic incompetence associated with ulcerative colitis and ankylosing spondylitis. Proc. Roy. Soc. Med. *63*:4, 1970.

REITER'S DISEASE

127. Good, A. E.: Reiter's disease: A review with special attention to cardiovascular and neurologic sequelae. Semin. Arthr. Rheum. *3*:253, 1974.
128. Sairanen, E., Paronen, I., and Mahonen, H.: Reiter's syndrome: A follow-up study. Acta Med. Scand. *185*:57, 1969.
129. Paulus, H. E., Pearson, C. M., and Pitts, W., Jr.: Aortic insufficiency in five patients with Reiter's syndrome: A detailed clinical pathological study. Am. J. Med. *53*:464, 1972.
130. Collins, P.: Aortic incompetence and active myocarditis in Reiter's disease. Br. J. Vener. Dis. *48*:300, 1972.
131. Ahvonen, P., Hiisi-Brummer, L., and Aho, K.: Electrocardiographic abnormalities and arthritis in patients with *Yersinia enterocolitica* infection. Ann. Clin. Res. *3*:69, 1971.
132. Aho, K., Ahvonen, P., and Lassus, A.: HLA B27 in reactive arthritis. A study of Yersinia arthritis and Reiter's disease. Arthritis Rheum. *17*:521, 1974.
133. Hakansson, U., Eitrem, R., Löw, B., and Winblad, S. W.: HLA-antigen B27 in cases with joint affects in an outbreak in salmonellosis. Scand. J. Infect. Dis. *8*:245, 1976.
134. Ruppert, G. B., Lindsay, J., and Barth, W. F.: Cardiac conduction abnormalities in Reiter's syndrome. Am. J. Med. *73*:335, 1982.
135. Mody, G. M., Stevens, J. E., and Meyers, O. L.: The heart in rheumatoid arthritis—a clinical and echocardiographic study. Q. J. Med. *65*:921, 1987.
136. Esdaile, J., Hawkins, D., Gold, P., et al.: Vascular involvement in relapsing polychondritis. CMA J. *116*:1019, 1977.
137. Balsa-Criado, A., Garcia-Fernandez, F., and Roldan, I.: Cardiac involvement in relapsing polychondritis. Int. J. Cardiol. *14*:381, 1987.
138. Mutru, O., Laakso, M., Isomaki, H., and Koota, K.: Cardiovascular mortality in patients with rheumatoid arthritis. Cardiology *76*:71, 1989.
139. VanDecker, W., and Panidis, I. P.: Relapsing polychondritis and cardiac valvular involvement. Ann. Intern. Med. *109*:340, 1988.

RHEUMATOID ARTHRITIS

140. Lanningan, R.: Cardiac Pathology. London, Butterworth and Co., 1966.
141. Bonfiglio, T., and Ativater, E. C.: Heart disease in patients with seropositive rheumatoid arthritis. A controlled autopsy study and review. Arch. Intern. Med. *124*:714, 1969.
142. Khan, A. H., and Spodick, D. H.: Rheumatoid heart disease. Semin. Arthritis Rheum. *1*:327, 1972.
143. Butman, S., Espinoza, L. R., Del Carpio, J., and Osterland, C. K.: Rheumatoid pericarditis. Rapid deterioration with evidence of local vasculitis. J.A.M.A. *238*:2394, 1977.
144. MacDonald, W. J., Jr., Crawford, M. H., Klippel, J. H., et al.: Echocardiographic assessment of cardiac structure and function in patients with rheumatoid arthritis. Am. J. Med. *63*:890. 1977.
145. Kelly, C. A., Bourke, J. P., Malcolm, A., and Griffiths, I. D.: Chronic pericardial disease in patients with rheumatoid arthritis: A longitudinal study. Q. J. Med. *75*:461, 1990.
146. Stables, R. H., Campbell, S., and Ormerod, O.J.M.: Haemopericardium in rheumatoid arthritis. Int. J. Cardiol. *23*:268, 1989.
147. Breut, C., Drouelle, S., Lognone, T., et al.: Complications des pericardites rhumatoides: Constriction et tamponnade. Presse Med. *18*:1151, 1989.
148. Thould, A. K.: Constrictive pericarditis in rheumatoid arthritis. Ann. Rheum. Dis. *45*:89, 1986.
149. Roberts, W. C., Kehoe, J. A., and Carpenter, D. F.: Cardiac valvular lesions in rheumatoid arthritis. Arch. Intern. Med. *122*:141, 1968.
150. Morris, P. B., Imber, M. J., Heinsimer, J. A., et al.: Rheumatoid arthritis and coronary arteritis. Am. J. Cardiol. *57*:689, 1986.
151. Young, I. D., Ford, S. E., and Ford, P. M.: The association of pulmonary hypertension with rheumatoid arthritis. J. Rheumatol. *16*:1266, 1989.
152. Linch, D. C., GIllmer, D. J., Whimster, W. F., and Keates, J.R.W.: Rheumatoid aortic valve prolapse requiring emergency valve replacement. Br. Heart J. *43*:237, 1980.
153. Ahern, M., Lever, J. W., and Cash, J.: Complete heart block in rheumatoid arthritis. Ann. Rheum. Dis. *42*:389, 1983.
154. Cassidy, J. T.: Juvenile rheumatoid arthritis. *In Kelly*, W. N., Harris, E. D., Ruddy, S., and Sledge, C. B. (eds.): Textbook of Rheumatology, 2nd ed. Philadelphia, W. B. Saunders Company, 1985.
155. Bernstein, B.: Pericarditis in juvenile rheumatoid arthritis. Arthritis Rheum. *20*:241, 1977.
156. Bank, L., Marboe, C. C., Redberg, R. F., and Jacob, J.: Myocarditis in adult Still's disease. Arthritis Rheum. *28*:452, 1985.
157. Bank, I., Marboe, C. C., Redberg, R. F., and Jacobs, J.: Myocarditis in adult Still's disease. Arthritis Rheum. *28*:452, 1985.
158. Sachs, R. N., Talvard, O., and Lanfranchi, J.: Myocarditis in adult Still's disease. Int. J. Cardiol. *27*:377, 1990.
159. Kramer, P. H., Imboden, J. B., Waldman, F. M., et al.: Severe aortic insufficiency in juvenile chronic arthritis. Am. J. Med. *74*:1088, 1983.
160. Hah, B. H.: Systemic lupus erythematosus. *In* Wilson, J. D., et al. (eds.): Harrison's Principles of Internal Medicine. 12th ed. New York, McGraw-Hill, 1991, pp. 1432–1437.
161. Klemperer, P., Pollack, A., and Baehr, G.: Pathology of disseminated lupus erythematosus. Arch. Pathol. *32*:569, 1941.
162. Liberthson, R. R., Homcy, C., Fallon, J. T., et al.: Systemic lupus erythematosus and heart disease. Primary Cardiol. *9*:77, 1983.
163. Gross, L.: Cardiac lesions in Libman-Sacks disease with consideration of its relationship to acute diffuse lupus erythematosus. Am. J. Pathol. *16*:375, 1940.
164. Harvey, A. M., Shulman, L. E., Tumulty, P. A., et al.: Systemic lupus erythematosus: A review of the literature and clinical analyses of 138 cases. Medicine *33*:291, 1954.
165. Hejtmancik, M. R., Wright, J. C., Quint, R., and Jennings, F.: The cardiovascular manifestations of systemic lupus erythematosus. Am. Heart J. *68*:119, 1964.
166. Bulkley, B. H., and Roberts, W. C.: The heart in systemic lupus erythematosus and the changes induced in it by corticosteroid therapy: A study of 36 necropsy patients. Am. J. Med. *58*:243, 1975.
167. Bharati, S., de la Fuente, D. J., Kallen, R. J., et al.: Conduction system in lupus erythematosus with atrioventricular block. Am. J. Cardiol. *35*:299, 1975.
168. Porcel, J. M., Selva, A., Tornos, M. P., et al.: Resolution of cardiac tamponade in systemic lupus erythematosus with indomethacin. Chest *96*:1193, 1989.
169. Wolf, R. E., King, J. W., and Brown, T. A.: Antimyosin antibodies and constrictive pericarditis in lupus erythematosus. J. Rheumatol. *15*:1284, 1988.
170. Sunder, S. K., and Shah, A.: Constrictive pericarditis in procainamide-induced lupus erythematosus syndrome. Am. J. Cardiol. *36*:960, 1975.
171. Ghose, M. K.: Pericardial tamponade. A presenting manifestation of procainamide-induced lupus erythematosus. Am. J. Med. *58*:581, 1975.
172. Enomoto, K., Kaji, Y., Mayumi, T., et al.: Frequency of valvular regurgitation by color Doppler echocardiography in systemic lupus erythematosus. Am. J. Cardiol. *67*:209, 1991.
173. Leung, W-H., Wong, K-L., Lau, C-P., et al.: Cardiac abnormalities in systemic lupus erythematosus: A prospective M-mode, cross-sectional and Doppler echocardiographic study. Int. J. Cardiol. *27*:367, 1990.
174. Murai, K., Oku, H., Takeuchi, K., et al.: Alterations in myocardial systolic and diastolic function in patients with active systemic lupus erythematosus. Am. Heart J. *113*:966, 1987.
175. Salomone, E., Tamburino, C., Bruno, G., et al.: The role of endomyocardial biopsy in the diagnosis of cardiac involvement in systemic lupus erythematosus. Heart Vessels *5*:52, 1989.
176. Elkayam, U., Weiss, S., and Laniado, S.: Pericardial effusion and mitral valve involvement in systemic lupus erythematosus: Echocardiographic study. Ann. Rheum. Dis. *36*:349, 1977.
177. Doherty, N. E., and Siegel, R. J.: Cardiovascular manifestations of systemic lupus erythematosus. Am. Heart J. *110*:1257, 1985.
178. Takatsu, Y., Hattori, R., Sakuguchi, K., et al.: Acute myocardial infarction associated with systemic lupus erythematosus. Chest *88*:147, 1985.
179. Libman, E., and Sacks, B.: A hitherto undescribed form of valvular and mitral endocarditis. Arch. Intern. Med. *33*:701, 1924.
180. Rawsthorne, L., Ptacin, M. J., Choi, H., et al.: Lupus valvulitis necessitating double valve replacement. Arthritis Rheum. *24*:561, 1981.
181. Dajee, H., Hurley, E. J., and Szarnicki, R. J.: Cardiac valve replacement in systemic lupus erythematosus. A review. J. Thorac. Cardiovasc. Surg. *85*:718, 1983
182. Straaton, K. V., Chatham, W. W., Reveille, J. D., et al.: Clinically significant valvular heart disease in systemic lupus erythematosus. Am. J. Med. *85*:645, 1988.
183. Galve, E., Candell-Riera, J., Pigrau, C., et al.: Prevalence, morphologic types, and evolution of cardiac valvular disease in systemic lupus erythematosus. N. Engl. J. Med. *319*:817, 1988.
184. Maier, W. P., Ramirez, H. E., and Miller, S. B.: Complete heart block as the initial manifestation of systemic lupus erythematosus. Arch. Intern. Med. *147*:170, 1987.
185. Gur, H., Keren, G., Averbuch, M., and Levo, Y.: Severe lupus congestive cardiomyopathy complicated by an intracavitary thrombus: A clinical and echocardiographic followup. J. Rheumatol. *15*:1278, 1988.
186. Bilazarian, S. D., Taylor, A. J., Brezinski, D., et al.: High-grade atrioventricular heart block in an adult with systemic lupus erythematosus: The association of nuclear RNP (U1 RNP) antibodies, a case report, and review of the literature. Arthritis Rheum. *32*:1170, 1989.
187. Buyon, J. P., Ben-Chetrit, E., Karp, S., et al.: Acquired congenital heart block: Pattern of maternal antibody response to biochemically defined antigens of the SSA/Ro-SSB/La system in neonatal lupus. J. Clin. Invest. *84*:627, 1989.
188. Scott, J. S., Maddison, P. J., Taylor, P. V., et al.: Connective-tissue disease, antibodies to ribonucleoprotein and congenital heart block. N. Engl. J. Med. *309*:209, 1983.
189. Litsey, S. E., Noonan, J. A., Connor, W. N., et al.: Maternal connective tissue disease and congenital heart block. N. Engl. J. Med. *312*:98, 1985.
190. Strauer, B. E., Brune, I., Schenk, H., et al.: Lupus cardiomyopathy: Cardiac mechanics, hemodynamics, and coronary blood flow in uncomplicated systemic lupus erythematosus. Am. Heart J. *92*:715, 1976.
191. Been, M., Thomson, B. J., Smith, M. A., et al.: Myocardial involvement in systemic lupus erythematosus detected by magnetic resonance imaging. Eur. Heart J. *9*:1250, 1988.
192. Homcy, C. J., Liberthson, R. R., Fallon, J. T., et al.: Ischemic heart disease in systemic lupus erythematosus in the young patient: Report of six cases. Am. J. Cardiol. *49*:478, 1982.
193. Hughes, G.R.V., Harris, N. N., and Gharavi, A. E.: The anticardiolipin syndrome. J. Rheum. *13*:486, 1986.
194. Sontheimer, R. D.: The anticardiolipin syndrome: A new way to slice an old pie, or a new pie to slice? Arch. Dermatol. *123*:590, 1987.
195. O'Rourke, R. A.: Antiphospholipid antibodies: A marker of lupus carditis? Circulation *82*:636, 1990.

196. Nihoyannopoulos, P., Gomez, P. M., Joshi, J., et al.: Cardiac abnormalities in systemic lupus erythematosus. Circulation 82:369, 1990.
197. Khamashta, M. A., Cervera, R., Asherson, R. A., et al.: Association of antibodies against phospholipids with heart valve disease in systemic lupus erythematosus. Lancet 335:1541, 1990.
198. Chartash, E. K., Lans, D. M., Paget, S. A., et al.: Aortic insufficiency and mitral regurgitation in patients with systemic lupus erythematosus and the antiphospholipid syndrome. Am. J. Med. 86:407, 1989.

POLYARTERITIS NODOSA

199. Zeek, P. M.: Periarteritis nodosa and other forms of necrotizing angiitis. N. Engl. J. Med. 148:764, 1953.
200. Schrader, M. L., Hockman, J. S., and Bulkley, B. H.: The heart in polyarteritis nodosa: A clinicopathologic study. Am. Heart J. 109:1353, 1985.
201. Frayha, R. A.: Trichinosis-related polyarteritis nodosa. Am. J. Med. 71:307, 1981.
202. Cupps, T. R., and Fauci, A. S.: The vasculitis syndromes. Adv. Intern. Med. 27:315, 1982.
203. Lonham, J. G., Elkon, K. B., Pusey, C. D., and Hughes, G.R.V.: Systemic vasculitis with asthma and eosinophilia: A clinical approach to the Churg-Strauss syndrome. Medicine 63:65, 1984.
204. Fauci, A. S., Haynes, B. F., Katz, P., and Wolff, S. M.: Wegener's granulomatosis: Prospective clinical and therapeutic experience with 85 patients for 21 years. Ann. Intern. Med. 98:76, 1983.
205. Forstot, J. Z., Overlie, P. A., Neufeld, G. K., et al.: Cardiac complications of Wegener granulomatosis: A case report of complete heart block and review of the literature. Semin. Arthritis Rheum. 10:148, 1980.
206. Schiavone, W. A., Ahmad, M., and Ockner, S. A.: Unusual cardiac manifestations of Wegener's granulomatosis. Chest 88:5, 1985.
207. Sams, W. M., Jr., Claman, H. N., and Kohler, P. F.: Human necrotizing vasculitis: Immunoglobulins and complement in vessel walls of cutaneous lesions and normal skin. J. Invest. Derm. 64:441, 1975.
208. Huston, K. A., and Hunder, G. G.: Giant cell (cranial) arteritis: A clinical review. Am. Heart J. 100:99, 1980.
209. Klinkhoff, A. V., Reid, G. D., and Moscovich, M.: Aortic regurgitation in giant cell arteritis. Arthritis Rheum. 28:582, 1985.
210. Moutsopoulos, H. M.: Behçet's syndrome. In Wilson, J. D., et al. (eds.): Harrison's Principles of Internal Medicine. 12th ed. New York, McGraw-Hill, 1991, pp. 1455–56.
211. Bletry, O., Monhattane, A., Wechsler, B., et al.: Atteinte cardiaque de la maladie de Behçet: Douze observations. Presse Med. 17:2388, 1988.

PROGRESSIVE SYSTEMIC SCLEROSIS

212. Masi, A. T., and Rodnan, G. P.: Preliminary criteria for the classification of systemic sclerosis (scleroderma). Bull. Rheum. Dis. 31:1, 1981.
213. Botstein, G. R., and LeRoy, E. C.: Primary heart disease in systemic sclerosis (scleroderma): Advances in clinical and pathologic features, pathogenesis, and new therapeutic approaches. Am. Heart J. 102:913, 1981.
214. Weiss, S., Stead, E., Warren, J., and Bailey, O.: Scleroderma heart disease. Arch. Intern. Med. 71:749, 1943.
215. LeRoy, E. C.: The heart in systemic sclerosis. N. Engl. J. Med. 310:188, 1984.
216. Follansbee, W. P., Curtiss, E. I., Medsger, T. A., Jr., et al.: Physiologic abnormalities of cardiac function in progressive systemic sclerosis with diffuse scleroderma. N. Engl. J. Med. 310:142, 1984.
217. Kahan, A., Devaux, J. Y., Amor, B., et al.: Nifedipine and thallium-201 myocardial perfusion in progressive systemic sclerosis. N. Engl. J. Med. 314:1397, 1986.
218. Roberts, N. K., Cabeen, W. R., Jr., Moss, J., et al.: The prevalence of conduction defects and cardiac arrhythmias in progressive systemic sclerosis. Ann. Intern. Med. 94:38, 1981.
219. Ferri, C., Bernini, L., Gongiorni, M. G., et al.: Noninvasive evaluation of cardiac dysrhythmias and their relationship with multisystemic symptoms in progressive systemic sclerosis patients. Arthritis Rheum. 28:1259, 1985.
220. Follansbee, W. P., Curtiss, E. I., Rahko, P.S., et al.: The electrocardiogram in systemic sclerosis (scleroderma). Am. J. Med. 79:183, 1985.
221. Kahan, A., Nitenberg, A., Foult, J. M., et al.: Decreased coronary reserve in primary scleroderma myocardial disease. Arthritis Rheum. 28:637, 1985.
222. Niarchose, A. P., Whitman, H. H., Goldstein, J. E., and Laragh, J. H.: Hemodynamic effects of captopril in pulmonary hypertension of collagen vascular disease. Am. Heart J. 104:834, 1982.
223. Ocken, S., Reinitz, E., and Strom, J.: Nifedipine treatment for pulmonary hypertension in a patient with systemic sclerosis. Arthritis Rheum. 26:794, 1983.
223a. Morgan, J.M., Griffiths, M., duBois, R. M., and Evans, T. W.: Hypoxic pulmonary vasoconstriction in systemic sclerosis and primary pulmonary hypertension. Chest 99:551, 1991.
224. O'Brien, J. T., Hill, J. A., and Pepine, C. J.: Sustained benefit of verapamil in pulmonary hypertension with progressive systemic sclerosis. Am. Heart J. 109:380, 1985.
225. Ellis, W. W., Baer, A. N., Robertson, R. M., et al.: Left ventricular dysfunction induced by cold exposure in patients with systemic sclerosis. Am. J. Med. 80:385, 1986.
226. Gustafsson, R., Mannting, F., Kazzam, E., et al.: Cold-induced reversible myocardial ischaemia in systemic sclerosis. Lancet August 26, 1989, pp. 475–479.
227. Kostis, J. B., Seibold, J. R., Turkevich, D., et al.: Prognostic importance of cardiac arrhythmias in systemic sclerosis. Am. J. Med. 84:1007, 1988.
228. McWhorter, J. E., and LeRoy, E. C.: Pericardial disease in scleroderma (systemic sclerosis). Am. J. Med. 57:566, 1974.
229. Gladman, D. D., Gordon, D. A., Urowitz, M. B., and Levy, H. L.: Pericardial fluid analysis in scleroderma (systemic sclerosis). Am. J. Med. 60:1064, 1976.
230. Medsger, T. A., Jr., and Masi, A. T.: Survival with scleroderma. II. A life-table analysis of clinical and demographic factors in 358 male U.S. veteran patients. J. Chron. Dis. 26:647, 1973.
231. Wynn, J., Fineberg, N., Matzer, L., et al.: Prediction of survival in progressive systemic sclerosis by multivariate analysis of clinical features. Am. Heart J. 110:123, 1985.
232. Whitman, H. H., Case, D. B., Laragh, J. H., et al.: Variable response to oral angiotensin-converting enzyme blockade in hypertensive scleroderma patients. Arthritis Rheum. 25:241, 1982.
233. Bohan, A., Peter, J. B., Bowman, R. L., and Pearson, C. M.: A computer assisted analysis of 153 patients with polymyositis and dermatomyositis. Medicine 56:255, 1977.
234. Norton, W. L., Velayos, E., and Robison, L.: Endothelial inclusions in dermatomyositis. Ann. Rheum. Dis. 29:67, 1970.
235. Tamir, R., Pick, A. J., and Theodor, E.: Constrictive pericarditis complicating dermatomyositis. Ann. Rheum. Dis. 47:961, 1988.
236. Oka, M., and Raasakka, T.: Cardiac involvement in polymyositis. Scand. J. Rheumatol. 7:203, 1978.
237. Haupt, H. M., and Hutchins, G. M.: The heart and conduction system in polymyositis-dermatomyositis: A clinicopathologic study of 16 autopsied patients. Am. J. Cardiol. 50:998, 1982.
238. Raju, N.V.R., Hart, N., Maloney, J., et al.: Cardiac involvement in polymyositis: A case report and review of the literature. Cleve. Clin. Q. 51:89, 1984.
239. Stern, R., Godbold, J. H., Chess, Q., and Kogan, L. J.: ECG abnormalities in polymyositis. Arch. Intern. Med. 144:2185, 1984.
240. Sharp, G. C.: Mixed connective tissue diseases. In Wilson, J. D., et al. (eds.): Harrison's Principles of Internal Medicine. 12th ed. New York, McGraw-Hill, 1991, pp. 1448–1449.
241. Leung, W-H., Wong, K-L., Lau, C-P., et al.: Echocardiographic identification of mitral valvular abnormalities in patients with mixed connective tissue disease. J. Rheumatol. 17:485, 1990.

Hematological-Oncological Disorders and Heart Disease

by DAVID S. ROSENTHAL, M.D., and EUGENE BRAUNWALD, M.D.

The increased frequency of cardiovascular abnormalities in patients with hematological and neoplastic disorders and, conversely, of blood disorders in patients being treated for a variety of cardiovascular diseases has led to greater interaction between cardiologists and hematologist-oncologists. Blood dyscrasias often complicate the use of cardiac medications and prosthetic heart valves and cardiovascular surgery.

Hematologist-oncologists must often consult cardiologists regarding clinical problems that range from interpreting abnormal physical findings and electrocardiographic and echocardiographic changes in their patients to obtaining advice about how to treat heart failure, pericardial effusion, or other cardiac complications common among patients with anemia and hematological malignant diseases.

Anemia and Cardiovascular Disorders

(See also p. 458)

Anemia is one of the most common causes of increased cardiac output and when extremely severe sometimes results in heart failure due to a high-output state in the absence of heart disease. As discussed in Chapter 16, tissue hypoxia combined with reduced blood viscosity leads to a reduction in systemic vascular resistance, which is associated with an increase in cardiac output.[1-3] Acutely induced anemia lowers coronary vascular resistance, whereas chronic anemia enhances formation of intercoronary collaterals and causes increases in preload and reduction of afterload.[4] When the normal hemoglobin concentration is restored, all signs and symptoms of cardiovascular disease usually disappear. The gradual development of severe anemia may lead to cardiac hypertrophy, by causing vasodilation, which increases venous return (and thereby preload) and reduces peripheral resistance (and thereby afterload). Left ventricular end-diastolic volume is increased in patients with chronic anemia, and afterload reduction, as reflected in left ventricular end-systolic stress, has been demonstrated. Such changes may favor maintaining a sufficiently high stroke volume.[5] Another mechanism of enhanced left ventricular function in chronic anemia has been attributed to increased levels of catecholamine and noncatecholamine inotropic factors in plasma.[6,7] For example, papillary muscles placed in serum obtained from patients with chronic anemia exhibit increased contractility.[7]

CARDIAC SYMPTOMS OF ANEMIA. The severity of reduction of cardiac reserve, of fatigue, exertional dyspnea, and edema depend on the severity of the anemia and the presence of an underlying cardiovascular disorder such as myocardial, coronary arterial, or valvular heart disease. Severely anemic patients without heart disease have few if any cardiac symptoms. When hemoglobin values decline below 9 gm/dl, rest-

ing cardiac output increases[1,8-10] Symptoms also depend on the rapidity with which the anemia develops, as well as the physical activity of the patient. For example, if the anemia develops gradually in a normal person, patients with hemoglobin levels as low as 7 gm/dl may be able to carry out all but the most strenuous activities, whereas in the presence of coronary artery disease, anemia lowers the threshold for development of angina pectoris, so that patients with mild anemia may develop intensified angina.

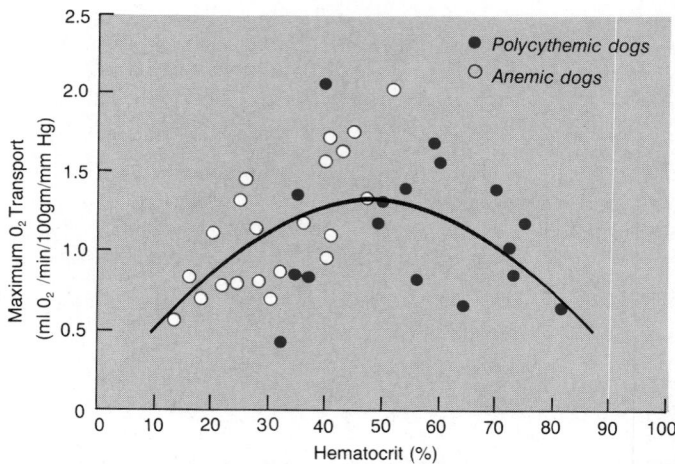

FIGURE 57-1. Maximum oxygen transport adjusted per unit perfusion pressure is shown as a function of hematocrit in anemic and polycythemic dogs. (From Baer, R. W., et al.: Maximum myocardial oxygen transport during anemia and polycythemia in dogs. Am. J. Physiol. *252*:H1086, 1987.)

Although uncommon, congestive heart failure with pulmonary edema can occur solely on the basis of very severe anemia (Hb < 4 gm/dl) even in the absence of underlying heart disease. It may be difficult to distinguish congestive heart failure secondary to chronic anemia from that related to myocardial iron infiltration secondary to transfusion-related hemosiderosis (p. 1747). However, the symptoms of reduced cardiac reserve secondary to anemia alone are usually relieved when the anemia is corrected and a normal red cell mass has been restored.

Electrocardiographic findings are not uncommon as the anemia progresses. With hemoglobin levels below 7 gm/dl, T-wave depression and inversion may be found, simulating myocardial disease. With transfusions, these findings usually return to normal.

Studies in anesthetized dogs have shown that maximal myocardial oxygen delivery far exceeds the supply at all levels of hematocrit. When one is plotting maximum oxygen transport against hematocrit, an "inverted U-shaped" relationship results (Fig. 57–1.)[11] In otherwise normal subjects, the gradual occurrence of severe anemia rarely if ever results in myocardial hypoxia, because of several compensatory mechanisms, including oxygen dissociation, 2,3-diphosphoglycerate (2,3-DPG) levels in red cells, and its effect on the hemoglobin-oxygen dissociation curve, as described below.

OXYGEN DISSOCIATION AND LEVELS OF 2,3-DIPHOSPHOGLYCERATE IN RED CELLS

To account for the circulatory adaptation that occurs in chronic anemia, it is important to appreciate that factors other than hemoglobin concentration and blood flow play a role in the quantity of oxygen delivered to tissues. These factors include tissue oxygen tension and the position of the hemoglobin-oxygen (Hb-O_2) dissociation curve. Normally, 1 gm of hemoglobin binds 1.34 ml of O_2. With a hemoglobin concentration of 15 gm/dl, 100 ml of arterial blood contains 20 ml of O_2. As can be calculated from the Hb-O_2 dissociation curve (Fig. 57–2), 100 ml of mixed venous blood having a PO_2 of 40 mm Hg will contain 15.5 ml of O_2. The difference (i.e., 4.5 ml of O_2 per 100 ml of arterial blood) would be available for delivery to tissues.

SHIFTS OF THE HEMOGLOBIN-OXYGEN DISSOCIATION CURVE. In most patients with anemia, the Hb-O_2 dissociation curve shifts to the right, and more oxygen is released from hemoglobin as the PO_2 declines. The red cell concentrations of 2,3-diphosphoglycerate (2,3-DPG), which are known to vary in a number of disease states,[10] profoundly affect the binding and release of O_2 by hemoglobin. Deoxygenated hemoglobin, which is more alkaline than oxyhemoglobin, stimulates the production of 2,3-DPG, a byproduct of glycolysis. As a consequence, the intraerythro-

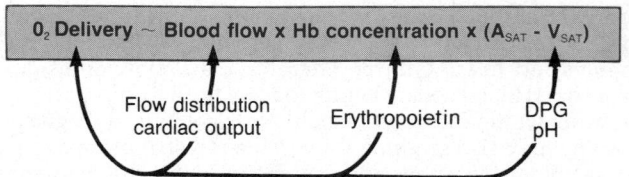

FIGURE 57–3. Oxygen delivered to an organ or tissue is directly proportional to blood flow, hemoglobin concentration, and the difference in oxygen saturation between arterial and venous blood. Patients with various types of hypoxia may compensate in the following ways: (1) Blood flow distribution may be altered to maintain oxygenation of vital organs, with an increase in total cardiac output when hypoxia is severe. (2) Increased erythropoietin production may stimulate erythropoiesis. (3) Oxygen unloading may be enhanced by a shift to the right in the oxygen dissociation curve, mediated by an increase in red cell 2,3-DPG. (From Bunn, H. F.: Pathophysiology of the anemias. In Wilson, J. E. et al. (eds.): Harrison's Principles of Internal Medicine. 12th ed. New York, McGraw-Hill Book Co., 1990, p.1517.)

cytic ratio of deoxyhemoglobin to oxyhemoglobin serves as a critical regulator of 2,3-DPG concentration. For example, the decreased oxygen affinity present in chronic anemia can be accounted for by this increase in red cell 2,3-DPG. At a normal arterial PO_2, arterial oxygen saturation remains high despite the reduction in oxygen affinity. However, at the lower PO_2 in the venous blood, elevated 2,3-DPG displaces the Hb-O_2 dissociation curve to the right, enabling greater release of oxygen from the cells at any level of PO_2. Oski et al. have calculated that decreased oxygen affinity mediated by increased red cell 2,3-DPG may compensate for up to half the oxygen deficit in anemia.[12] High levels of 2,3-DPG have also been found in subjects exposed to altitude[13] and in patients with pulmonary disease.[14]

The position of the Hb-O_2 dissociation curve can be expressed by the value of P_{50}, i.e., the partial pressure of O_2 at which hemoglobin is 50 per cent saturated. A reduction of the oxygen affinity of hemoglobin, i.e., a shift of the dissociation curve to the right, is reflected in an elevation of P_{50}. With a P_{50} of 34 mm Hg (instead of the normal P_{50} of 26.5 mm Hg), 3.3 ml of O_2 is unloaded per 100 ml of blood. As a consequence, an anemic individual with a 50 per cent reduction in red cell mass would suffer only a 27 per cent reduction in oxygen unloading (Fig. 57–2).

RESPONSE TO HYPOXIA. Figure 57–3 summarizes the factors responsible for oxygenation in response to hypoxia. O_2 delivery to the metabolizing tissues depends directly on three principal factors: (1) blood flow; (2) hemoglobin concentration (i.e., the O_2-carrying capacity of the blood); and (3) the O_2 unloaded per unit of blood, as represented by the difference between arterial and venous blood oxygen saturations. Each of these three factors varies independently. Blood flow to any tissue is a function of total cardiac output and its fractional distribution. The red cell mass is regulated by erythropoietin in response to tissue oxygenation. The position of the Hb-O_2 dissociation curve is determined primarily by red cell 2,3-DPG levels and blood pH. Chronic anemia is usually well tolerated when these compensatory mechanisms operate effectively, i.e., with an increased cardiac output, redistribution of blood flow, and decreased O_2 affinity.

CARDIAC EXAMINATION. The cardiac enlargement that develops with severe, chronic anemia usually results from dilatation and eccentric hypertrophy with a normal ratio of wall thickness to cavity diameter, as occurs in other forms of volume overload (see Fig. 14–8, p. 400). The precordium is usually hyperactive, not unlike that in mitral regurgitation (Fig. 2–16, p. 27). Third and fourth heart sounds are frequently present, and a midsystolic murmur, maximal at the left sternal border, is usually audible.[15,16] The murmur is probably secondary to the combined effects of increased velocity of blood flow across the pulmonic and aortic valve orifices and reduced blood viscosity. Less frequently, an early, midsystolic rumbling murmur may be heard at the apex or along the left sternal border. This diastolic murmur is probably related to the increase in blood flow across the mitral or tricuspid valves and may be difficult to distinguish from the murmurs of mitral or tricuspid stenosis, although the murmur follows a third heart sound rather than an opening snap. Accurate diagnosis may require echocardiography as well as reexamination after correction of the anemia.

In patients with chronic anemia whose hearts are compensated at a reduced concentration of hemoglobin, blood volume expansion achieved by the transfusion of whole blood may be

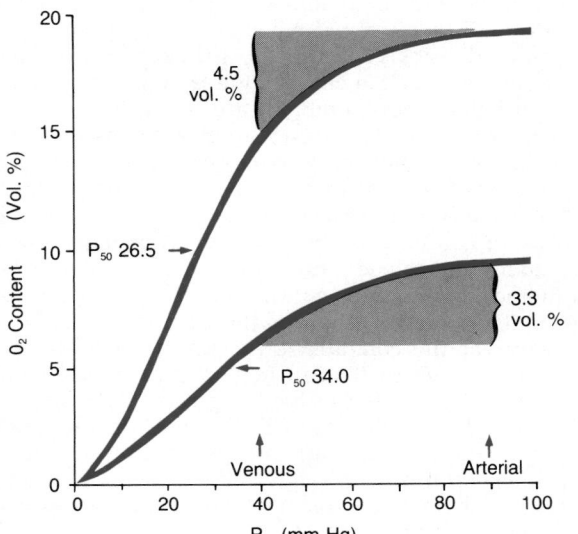

FIGURE 57–2. Enhancement of oxygen unloading by decreased red cell oxygen affinity in anemia with an increase in P_{50} from 26.5 to 34.0. (From Klocke, R. A.: Oxygen transport and 2,3-diphosphoglycerate. Chest 62:7951, 1972.)

poorly tolerated. Expanding the blood volume and augmenting left ventricular filling pressure will risk precipitating or aggravating heart failure. Therefore, the slow infusion of packed red blood cells accompanied by the administration of a diuretic would be more useful. Intravenous nitroglycerin therapy may also produce a favorable redistribution of circulating blood volume and antagonize the hemodynamic changes caused by transfusion.[17]

CARDIAC DISORDERS ASSOCIATED WITH HEMOLYTIC ANEMIA

Cardiomegaly, congestive heart failure, and sudden death have been reported frequently in patients with chronic hemolytic anemias such as sickle cell disease and thalassemia. In addition, hemolysis secondary to cardiac disease may cause acute symptoms. Hemolytic anemias are usually characterized by marked reticulocytosis and erythroid hyperplasia of the bone marrow. Indirect hyperbilirubinemia, increased serum lactic dehydrogenase, and reduced haptoglobin are also common findings. If lysis of red cells occurs within the circulation (intravascular hemolytic anemia), hemoglobinemia and hemoglobinuria may occur and will reflect the severity of hemolysis. Specific laboratory investigations will identify the type of hemolytic anemia, examples being a positive antiglobulin (or Coombs) test in immunohemolytic anemia, increased red cell osmotic fragility in hereditary spherocytosis, and abnormal hemoglobin electrophoresis in sickle cell anemia and the thalassemic syndromes. Acquired hemolytic anemias may occur precipitously, and the resulting symptoms may resemble those of acute blood loss with peripheral vasoconstriction, hypotension, tachycardia, fatigue, lightheadedness, and dyspnea on exertion.

HEMOGLOBINOPATHIES

Sickle Cell Disease

Sickle hemoglobin results from a mutation in the codon for the sixth amino acid of the beta globin chain from glutamic acid to valine (alpha-2, beta-2$^{6glu \rightarrow val}$). Eight to 10 per cent of black Americans are heterozygous for this trait. In certain regions of central Africa, the gene frequency is as high as 20 per cent, and it is likely that the high frequency of hemoglobin S in these areas is associated with resistance to or protection against falciparum malaria. With decreased oxygen tension, red cells containing hemoglobin S acquire an elongated crescent (sickle) shape. Electron microscopy demonstrates bundles of fibers running parallel to the long axis of the cells.[18] If sickle cells are reoxygenated within a short time, their normal red shape can be restored. However, as red cells remain sickled in vivo, their membranes become damaged and rigid, resulting eventually in irreversibly sickled cells that have a shortened survival and may block small blood vessels. The continuous formation and destruction of irreversibly sickled cells contribute to the symptoms of sickle cell disease. Factors that decrease oxygen affinity, such as acidosis and increased red cell 2,3-DPG levels, lead to the deoxygenation of hemoglobin and promote the formation of sickled cells.

Persons who are heterozygous for sickle cell disease are not anemic and rarely have symptoms except at high altitudes or as a result of marked hypoxia. In contrast, the signs and symptoms in patients homozygous for sickle cell anemia (SS) begin at about 6 months of age, when the conversion from fetal to adult hemoglobin production is completed.

The cardiopulmonary system is frequently involved in sickle cell anemia.[19-27] As in other chronic anemias, both cardiac output and oxygen extraction by tissues are increased, and the reduced oxygen content of these red cells leads to further sickling. In addition, for any given value of hematocrit, the elevation of cardiac output and the auscultatory findings associated with anemia are greater in sickle cell anemia[24] compared with other anemias. A normal left ventricle is able to tolerate the volume overload of chronic, moderately severe anemia for indefinite periods with no deterioration in functional capacity.[25] The increased preload and decreased afterload characteristic of chronic anemia (Fig. 57-4) compensate

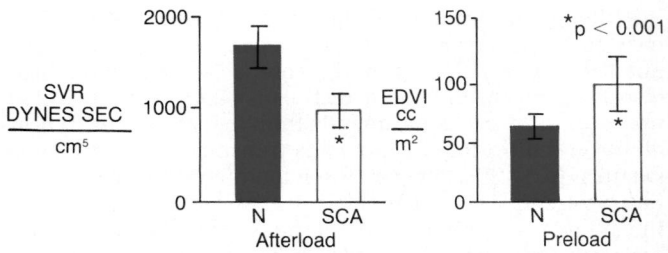

FIGURE 57-4. Loading conditions in 11 patients with sickle cell anemia (SCA) and 11 normal subjects (N). *Left,* Afterload, as indicated by systemic vascular resistance (SVR), was significantly decreased in patients with SCA. *Right,* Preload, as indicated by end-diastolic volume index (EDVI), was significantly increased in patients with SCA. (From Dennenberg, B. S., et al.: Cardiac function in sickle cell anemia. Am. J. Cardiol. *51*:1675, 1983.)

for any left ventricular dysfunction and maintain a normal ejection fraction and high cardiac output in sickle cell anemia.[26] When cardiac decompensation occurs in patients with sickle cell anemia, it is usually the result of other coexisting complications of the SS disease or the presence of underlying cardiovascular abnormalities. Deaths secondary to congestive heart failure occurring in children and young adults with sickle cell anemia are usually precipitated by chronic renal failure, pulmonary thrombosis, or infections.[27,28]

Acute myocardial infarction is a rare complication of sickle cell disease and has been confirmed at postmortem examination in a few patients without significant coronary atherosclerosis.[29-31] More O_2 is extracted by the myocardium than by any other tissue, and transmural infarction due to in situ thrombosis by sickled cells is rare. However, infarction of the papillary muscles of the heart does occur. This should not be surprising, since the papillary muscles are at the terminal portion of the coronary circulation, where collateral vessels are scant and hypoxia is marked.

Pulmonary infarction, a common complication of sickle cell anemia, is probably due to thrombosis in situ rather than to embolization.[32] Although infrequent, fat and bone marrow emboli to the lungs have been reported, the latter resulting from necrosis caused by sickling within the marrow sinusoids. Patients with sickle cell anemia are unusually susceptible to infection. In addition, damage to the lung caused by repeated vascular insults creates a suitable milieu for bacterial growth; as a consequence, pneumonia is a frequent and serious complication. Mortality and morbidity are high in the setting of pneumonia and hypoxia, so that treatment of these complications must be immediate and vigorous. However, it may be difficult to differentiate pulmonary infection from infarction in patients with sickle cell anemia. Although impaired pulmonary function in sickle cell anemia is common, pulmonary hypertension and cor pulmonale are rarely encountered.[24]

In almost all patients with sickle cell anemia the heart ultimately becomes enlarged, and at autopsy strikingly high heart weights are noted in a majority of patients despite the absence of other causes of cardiomegaly such as hypertension, atherosclerosis, or coronary artery disease.[33] In patients who have received multiple blood transfusions, myocardial iron deposition (hemosiderosis) may contribute both to the cardiac enlargement and to the associated impairment of cardiac function. However, this complication occurs much less frequently in sickle cell anemia than in homozygous thalassemia (see below). Histological studies have suggested that the increase in heart weight is secondary to fibrosis, presumably caused by the combination of anemia and papillary muscle infarction. With time, children with sickle cell disease exhibit progressive cardiac chamber enlargement with a progressive increase in left ventricular mass.[34]

There are no specific electrocardiographic changes in sickle cell anemia. However, almost 80 per cent of patients with sickle cell anemia have an abnormal electrocardiogram. These abnormalities include left ventricular hypertrophy and first-degree atrioventricular (AV) block as well as nonspecific ST-segment and T-wave changes and abnormal septal Q waves; this last finding is believed to be secondary to excessive septal thickness.[20,35,36] Arrhythmias rarely occur with sickle cell anemia, although continuous electrocardiographic monitoring during painful crises has revealed both atrial and ventricular arrhythmias in the majority of patients.[36] Echocardiographic measurements in patients with cardiac symptoms are useful in documenting both cardiac hyperactivity and depressed left ventricular performance.[20] Radiological studies may be entirely normal. With exercise, cardiac dysfunction may be manifested by an abnormal ejection fraction response, abnormalities of wall motion, and slowed left ventricular filling.[37-40] M-mode echocardiographic studies demonstrated an incidence of mitral valve prolapse in 25 per cent of SS patients,[21,41] far in excess of that expected. More recent two-dimensional echo and Doppler ultrasonography performed in adult patients with SS disease demonstrated a 22 per cent incidence of diastolic murmurs but no instances of myxomatous valvular degeneration or mitral valve prolapse.[21]

Thalassemic Syndromes

The thalassemias are a group of inherited disorders caused by an imbalance in the synthesis of hemoglobin chains rather than by a single amino acid substitution, as in sickle cell disease. The two principal types are referred to as α-thalassemia, in which α-chain synthesis is absent or reduced (a condition found mainly in Asians), and β-thalassemia, in which β-chain synthesis is absent or reduced. The homozygous form of β-thalassemia is also referred to as Cooley's or Mediterranean anemia and is common in persons of Greek and Italian descent. Heterozygous α- and β-thalassemias are also common in American blacks, particularly in association with sickle cell trait. These inherited autosomal dominant defects have been linked to molecular lesions that interfere with the synthesis of globin subunits. The net result in both types of thalassemia is decreased production of hemoglobin A (Hb A) and therefore hemoglobin-deficient red cells that are both microcytic and hypochromic. In addition, the red cells are target shaped and demonstrate basophillic stippling.

The diagnosis of β-thalassemia is confirmed by quantitative hemoglobin electrophoresis in which levels of Hb A are decreased or absent and levels of Hb A_2 and fetal hemoglobin (Hb F) are increased. The anemia in homozygous β-thalassemia results from a combination of hemolysis and ineffective erythropoiesis. Children have a characteristic "chipmunk" appearance owing to marked hyperplasia of the marrow in the facial bones and massive hepatosplenomegaly owing to extramedullary hematopoiesis. Occasionally, the expanding marrow extrudes from the ribs, sternum, and vertebrae, forming a mass resembling a lymphoma on chest roentgenogram.

CARDIAC ABNORMALITIES IN THALASSEMIA. Cardiac complications are the major cause of death in patients with thalassemia.[42] As with sickle cell disease, these events may be due in part to chronic anemia. In addition, cardiac siderosis is a frequent problem in thalassemia, unlike the situation in sickle cell anemia or many other chronic anemias.[43,44] Iron overload results from a combination of extravascular hemolysis, frequent transfusions, and an inappropriate increase in intestinal iron absorption. Consequently, heart failure and arrhythmias are the common causes of death in children with this condition.[43] Although anemia per se undoubtedly contributes to cardiomegaly, iron overload of the heart is the most likely cause of myocardial damage.[45-47]

Prior to the era of hypertransfusion and chelation therapy, patients with transfusion-dependent, chronic, severe refractory thalassemia regularly manifested serious cardiac involvement, usually by the second decade of life. Although most died within months of the development of congestive heart failure, occasional patients died suddenly, presumably secondary to an arrhythmia. Intensive treatment of heart failure and antiarrhythmic therapy do not appear to change the natural history. At postmortem examination, widespread iron deposition characteristic of hemochromatosis is found in all viscera, including the heart, which is hypertrophied and sometimes twice its normal weight; it is often a deep brown, with large quantities of iron in myocardial cells, demonstrated by staining with Prussian blue dye. The sinoatrial node is

usually spared, but the AV node is frequently involved. Apparently cardiac dysfunction depends on the quantity of iron deposited in the ventricles, and it has been suggested that myocardial damage results from iron-induced release of acid hydrolases from lysosomes.[14]

Pericarditis occurs in about half of all patients with thalassemia and is often recurrent and associated with fever, precordial pain, and electrocardiographic changes characteristic of acute pericarditis (p. 1469). Pericardial effusion is common; in rare cases, creation of a pericardial window is necessary to relieve tamponade or a recurrent effusion.

The *electrocardiogram* often shows left ventricular hypertrophy, nonspecific ST-segment and T-wave abnormalities, supraventricular or ventricular premature contractions, and first- or second-degree AV block. The His bundle electrogram may show prolongation of the P-R interval, signifying abnormal conduction through the AV node. The chest roentgenogram may show slight to moderate cardiac enlargement, and *echocardiographic* assessment may disclose increased left ventricular end-diastolic, left atrial, and aortic root dimensions as well as a thickened left ventricular wall[44] and diastolic abnormalities.[44a] At cardiac catheterization, the usual findings comprise a normal or elevated cardiac index with moderate elevations in left ventricular end-diastolic pressure and volume and end-systolic volume with a reduced ejection fraction.

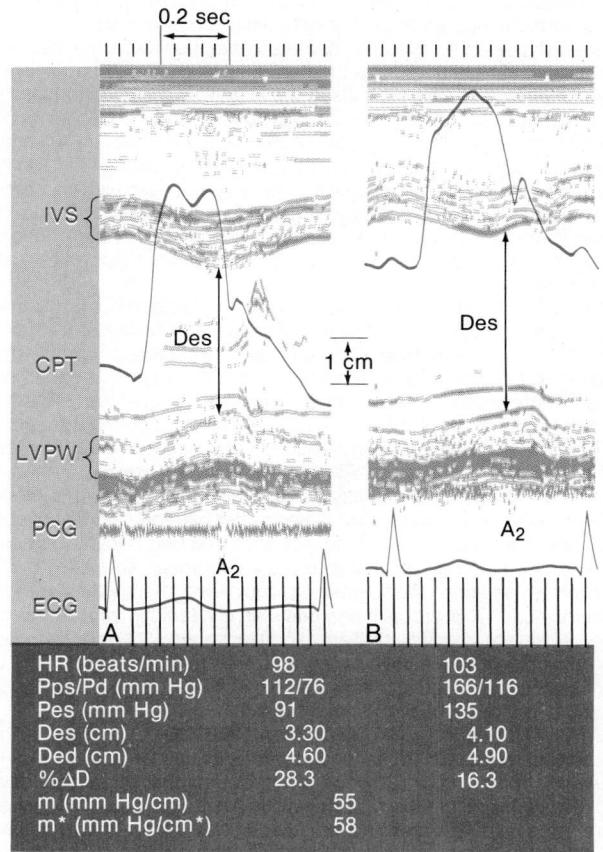

FIGURE 57–5. Recordings from a 16-year-old patient with thalassemia major during baseline conditions (*A*) and at peak methoxamine effect (*B*). Both the actual and corrected slope values (m and m*) were abnormal despite normal resting fractional shortening (%ΔD). The 44-mm Hg increase in end-systolic pressure (Pes) resulted in a 0.80-cm increase in end-systolic dimension (Des). For the control population, a comparable change in Pes resulted in a 0.40 ± 0.05-cm increase in Des. IVS = interventricular septum; LVPW = left ventricular posterior wall; A_2 = aortic component of the second heart sound; HR = heart rate; Pps = peak systolic pressure; Pd = aortic diastolic pressure; %ΔD = per cent fractional shortening; m = slope; m* = corrected slope. (From Borow, K. M., et al.: The left ventricular end-systolic pressure-dimensions relation in patients with thalassemia major. A new noninvasive method for assessing contractile state. Circulation 66:980, 1982, by permission of the American Heart Association, Inc.)

There has been considerable interest in defining abnormalities of cardiac performance noninvasively in asymptomatic patients. Valdes-Cruz et al. have reported that in asymptomatic children with thalassemia major[48] the left ventricular posterior wall thinned more slowly than normal during diastole. Utilizing the relationship between ventricular fractional shortening and end-systolic pressure (p. 431), Borow et al. identified preclinical left ventricular dysfunction (Fig. 57–5),[49] an approach that may be useful in the serial assessment of left ventricular contractility in response to chelation therapy.

Management. Supportive therapy consisting primarily of an adequate transfusion program (and even hypertransfusions), splenectomy, and early treatment of infections has prolonged the life of many patients with thalassemia.[51] Roentgenographic evidence of cardiomegaly in children often regresses when hemoglobin is maintained above 10 gm/dl. Indeed, in one study, in four of seven patients with significant cardiomegaly, heart size returned to normal 1 week after multiple transfusions restored hemoglobin to near-normal levels. The use of chelating agents for both treatment and prevention of iron overload and left ventricular systolic function is necessary and is discussed on page 1749).

HEMOLYTIC ANEMIA IN PATIENTS WITH VALVULAR HEART DISEASE

In 1964, Dameshek described an interesting patient with aortic, mitral, and tricuspid stenosis and mitral regurgitation who had hemolytic anemia with distorted and fragmented red cells, including helmet cells, burr cells, and schistocytes.[52] At autopsy, numerous calcified excrescences were present on the mitral valve and the free margins of the aortic valve. The presence of excess iron deposits in the kidney suggested intravascular hemolysis, but it could not be established whether the cardiac abnormalities were the cause. Subsequently, shortened red cell survival was demonstrated in other patients with aortic valve disease, some of whom had anemia.[53] In patients with rheumatic aortic valve disease with mild hemolytic anemia, red cell survival may be significantly reduced during periods of exercise.[54] Although this form of hemolytic anemia is probably uncommon, it should be considered in patients with valvular heart disease and unexplained anemia.

HEMOLYTIC ANEMIA DURING CARDIAC SURGERY. In the past, hemolysis frequently occurred as a consequence of extracorporeal circulation. When the blood of many donors must be transfused or is mixed in a pump-oxygenator, as may occasionally be the case in patients undergoing cardiac surgery, the question arises whether the samples should be crossmatched with each other as well as with the patient. The plasma of one donor may contain a potent antibody that might interact with cells from a donor who has the antigen specific for that antibody. Although infrequent, this phenomenon may explain some cases of mild-to-moderate hemolysis and hemoglobinemia seen after cardiopulmonary bypass.

With the use of earlier heart-lung machines, red cells became damaged as they passed through the pump-oxygenator, presumably as a result of shear forces, leading to slight hemolysis and causing hemoglobinemia and hemoglobinuria. This problem has been largely avoided with newer machines, which also require little if any blood for priming. As a consequence, hemolytic complications have become far less frequent. In addition, the use of autologous blood and aspirated blood filtered for reuse during the operation has been helpful in this regard.

HEMOLYTIC ANEMIA AFTER CARDIAC SURGERY. In 1954, following surgical implantation of Hufnagel valves in the descending aorta for the treatment of aortic regurgitation, a significant number of patients developed anemia,[55] presumably on a hemolytic basis. The potentially serious nature of the hemolytic anemia associated with an intracardiac prosthesis was not really appreciated until chronic and severe hemolytic anemia characterized by microangiopathic red cell changes (consisting of fragmented red cells, burr cells, and schistocytes) was noted after a Teflon patch repair of an ostium primum atrial septal defect (Fig. 57–6).[56] Chromium-51 red cell survival studies confirmed that the half-life of not only autologous red cells but also of donor cells was shortened, indicating a defect extrinsic to the red cell. In keeping with intravascular hemolysis, high concentrations of hemoglobin in the plasma and urine were noted along with hemosiderinuria. At reoperation a jet of blood was found regurgitating through a cleft in the mitral valve that had been impinging on the prosthetic interatrial Teflon patch. Part of the septum had become denuded of endothelium and had formed a small cul-de-sac in contact with the jet of blood. With repair of the cul-de-sac and reendothelialization of the area, hemolysis ceased. Torn cusps of porcine mitral valve or dehiscence of an implanted mitral ring can also cause the sudden onset of a hemolytic anemia.[57,58]

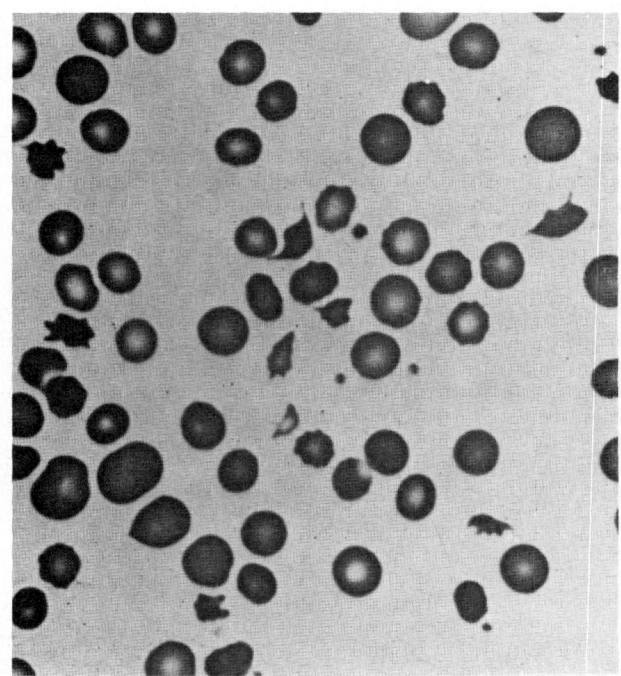

FIGURE 57–6. Peripheral blood smear from patient with microangiopathic hemolytic anemia secondary to abnormal prosthetic heart valve (×1000).

Microangiopathic Hemolytic Anemia

This condition has now been reported in association with many cardiac defects (Table 57–1). Its incidence after valve surgery depends on many variables, including the specific operation, the surgical technique, and the tests used to determine hemolysis, and varies widely.[59] In many instances, diurnal variations occur, with greater intravascular hemolysis during physical activity.[60]

CLINICAL PRESENTATION. With newer surgical techniques and prosthetic valves, the incidence of microangiopathic hemolytic anemia appears to be declining.[61] Symptoms and signs may develop suddenly or gradually, usually with no associated splenomegaly. Rarely, a vicious circle develops in a

TABLE 57–1 CAUSES OF MACROVASCULAR HEMOLYTIC ANEMIA

I. **Abnormalities of heart and large vessels**
  A. **Without surgery**
    1. **Aortic stenosis**
    2. **Ruptured sinus of Valsalva**
    3. **Ruptured chordae tendineae**
    4. **Coarctation of aorta**
    5. **Aortic aneurysm**
  B. **Following surgery**
    1. **"Patching" operations**
      a. **Ostium primum repair, especially if mitral regurgitation present**
      b. **Aortic aneurysm repair (aortofemoral bypass)**
      c. **Hemodialysis shunt**
    2. **Valvular replacement**
      a. **Uncomplicated**
        (1) **Outflow too small**
        (2) **Large area of exposed plastic**
        (3) **Cloth-covered struts**
        (4) **Two or more valves replaced**
        (5) **Xenograft**
      b. **Complicated**
        (1) **Ball variance**
        (2) **Regurgitation around seating of valve**
        (3) **Rupture of cloth-covered strut**

From Ersley, A. J.: Traumatic cardiac hemolytic anemia. *In* Williams, W. J. et al. (eds.): Hematology. 4th ed. New York, McGraw-Hill Book Co., 1990, p. 656.

patient with a perivalvular leak: the resultant shear stress produces hemolytic anemia, increasing stroke volume and shear stress, and in turn intensifying the anemia. While it is agreed that direct mechanical trauma to the red cells is the cause of hemolysis, the relative contributions of valve closure, denuded endothelium, turbulence, and the development of antierythrocyte autoantibodies are still not clear and probably vary among patients. In some instances, the hemolytic anemia observed in the early postoperative period is probably due simply to multiple intraoperative transfusions or to the lymphocyte-splenomegaly syndrome (post–pump-oxygenator syndrome) associated with cytomegaloviral infection.

CAUSE. Excessive blood turbulence is the most common feature of all hemolytic anemias due to valvular disease and cardiac surgery. For example, after insertion of a prosthetic valve, perivalvular regurgitation will increase the stroke volume and therefore the turbulence of flow through the narrowed orifice. Experiments in vitro have demonstrated that shearing stresses in excess of 3000 dynes/cm^2 can easily cause

hemolysis and that such degrees of stress may readily develop with perivalvular leaks, causing regurgitation from the aorta to the left ventricle,[62] as well as in situations in which the lumen of the aortic valve prosthesis is small relative to the stroke volume or when the ball is large relative to the diameter of the aorta. Although much less common, similar phenomena can occur with prosthetic mitral valves.[57,58] Rarely, chronic intravascular hemolytic anemia may occur in the presence of hypertrophic cardiomyopathy, probably secondary to abnormal turbulence due to the primary underlying cardiac disease.[63] This rare condition may be managed by reducing the outflow gradient by beta-adrenoceptor blocker or calcium antagonist therapy, or by operation (p. 1412).

Definitive treatment of the hemolytic syndrome secondary to turbulence consists of surgical repair of the cardiac abnormality, i.e., either replacement or correction of the prosthesis or correction of the perivalvular leak. If a patient is not readily operable, rest should alleviate the condition, and iron and folate replacement may be helpful.

Hemochromatosis and Hemosiderosis

(See also p. 1419)

A number of disease states are characterized by excessive iron stores in the body (Table 57–2). The deposition of a significant amount of iron in the myocardium, liver, and pancreas may lead to varying degrees of dysfunction of these organs.[64] Insofar as the heart is concerned, myocardial deposits of iron may lead to congestive heart failure, conduction disturbances, and arrhythmias. Significant siderosis is most often encountered in patients with idiopathic hemochromatosis or in anemic patients with large and longstanding transfusion requirements.

IDIOPATHIC HEMOCHROMATOSIS. In this condition, inappropriately large quantities of iron are absorbed from the gastrointestinal tract. This inherited disorder, with a variable clinical expression, develops slowly and depends in part upon environmental factors, such as the magnitude of dietary iron intake, alcohol intake, and the severity of any underlying liver disease. HLA subtyping associated with HLA-A3, HLA-B14, and HLA-B7 antigens has suggested a recessive mode of transmission, has linked the disease to chromosome 6, and has helped to distinguish idiopathic hemochromatosis from iron overload secondary to liver disease.[65]

Clinical manifestations of hemochromatosis occur more frequently in men than in women, and the disease rarely becomes manifest before age 20 years, reaching its peak in the fifth decade. Diabetes is the most common initial manifestation, occurring in half of the patients. The classic clinical presentation includes increased pigmentation of the skin, hepatomegaly, and cardiac dysfunction. Loss of libido and other endocrinopathies, such as hypopituitarism, may also become apparent. Cellular damage results from iron-induced release of lysosomal acid hydrolases.[66]

The incidence of cardiac symptoms increases with time.[66,67] Dyspnea, edema, and ascites are noted early in the course in 15 to 20 per cent of the patients, but eventually about one-third develop symptoms referable to the heart, and approximately the same fraction of patients eventually die of cardiac failure.[67] Arrhythmias are common and include paroxysmal atrial tachycardia and flutter, chronic atrial fibrillation, and frequent premature ventricular contractions; varying degrees of AV block have also been noted. Of all men with second and third degree heart block requiring pacemaker insertion, idiopathic hemochromatosis[68] is retrospectively diagnosed in a significant percentage. Heart block and arrhythmias are often associated with iron deposits in the AV node[69] and supraventricular arrhythmias with deposits in the atria. Low-voltage and nonspecific T-wave changes are also frequently present.

Radiographic studies in symptomatic patients usually reveal a globular heart with biventricular enlargement and weak pulsations. Some patients may have elevated right ventricular and right atrial pressures[70] consequent to the restrictive cardiomyopathy secondary to iron deposition in the myocardium as well as involvement of the pericardium itself.[71]

TRANSFUSIONAL HEMOSIDEROSIS. Iron overload may become a clinical problem in patients with severe chronic anemia who survive long enough to accumulate toxic quantities of iron from transfused blood. For example, patients with thalassemia, other serious chronic refractory anemias, myeloid metaplasia, pure red cell aplasia, and aplastic anemia may accumulate 50 gm of iron from transfusions, resulting in a variety of clinical problems similar to those encountered in idiopathic hemochromatosis. Indeed, children with β-thalassemia major maintained on hypertransfusion programs, while spared the cardiac consequences of severe anemia, generally die of heart failure in the second decade as a consequence of myocardial siderosis.[43] In adults with chronic anemias, cardiac iron deposition secondary to transfusional hemosiderosis may contribute to cardiovascular disability, which is often inappropriately attributed solely to high-output heart failure. Undoubtedly, the combination of impaired cardiac function

---

TABLE 57–2   CAUSES OF IRON OVERLOAD

GENETIC

Hereditary hemochromatosis
Thalassemia major
Hereditary sideroblastic anemia
Certain hereditary hemolytic anemias
  Pyruvate kinase deficiency
  Glucose-6-phosphate dehydrogenase deficiency
  Congenital dyserythropoietic anemia
Neonatal hemochromatosis
Congenital atransferrinemia

ACQUIRED

Chronic ingestion of medicinal iron
Transfusional iron overload
Acquired sideroblastic anemia
Porphyria cutanea tarda
African nutritional hemochromatosis
Shunt siderosis

From Fairbanks, V. F., and Baldus, W. P.: Production of erythrocytes. *In* Williams, W. J. et al. (eds.): Hematology. 4th ed. New York, McGraw-Hill Book Co., 1990, p. 752.

secondary to iron deposition and the increased burden on the heart imposed by the persistent, incompletely treated anemia is responsible.

Pathological Findings. In a review of 135 hearts studied at autopsy, including four from patients with hemochromatosis and 131 from patients with chronic anemia requiring repeated transfusions, 19 were found to have iron deposits.[72] Grossly visible iron deposits in the heart were always associated with a prior history of cardiac dysfunction and usually of chronic heart failure. Deposits were usually most extensive in idiopathic hemochromatosis and in patients who received more than 100 units of blood without evidence of blood loss. In patients with cardiac hemosiderosis, histological examination revealed that the ventricular free wall and septum contained heavier deposits than did the atrial wall (Fig. 57–7). The quantity of iron in the various layers of the ventricular myocardium is variable, with the epicardium and papillary muscles containing the most iron, the subendocardium containing intermediate amounts, and the midmyocardium and conduction tissue containing the least.

Diagnosis. It is often difficult to determine whether myocardial dysfunction results from the chronic anemia or hemosiderosis. Two techniques are useful: with the use of atomic absorption spectrophotometry, the exact concentrations of iron can be determined in various body organs or tissues. Iron-stained endomyocardial biopsy specimens can confirm hemochromatosis as a cause of cardiac dysfunction.[73] Rarely is iron deposition limited to the heart in these conditions. Since the liver is easily accessible by biopsy and its iron concentration is closely related to that in the myocardium, liver biopsy is a convenient way of confirming a diagnosis of myocardial siderosis. In some patients, echocardiography may detect

early left ventricular dysfunction prior to the development of symptoms.[44,74,75] In a group of patients with severe β-thalassemia or transfusion-dependent anemias without clinical cardiac symptoms, left ventricular dysfunction measured by radionuclide angiography was demonstrated during exercise but not at rest.[74] Noninvasive assessment of the left ventricular end-systolic pressure-dimension relation (using a methoxamine challenge) can identify preclinical left ventricular dysfunction not evident on resting or dynamic exercise studies and not due to chronic anemia per se. This technique is a sensitive means of monitoring therapeutic response or iron overload diseases to prevent cardiac complications.[76,77]

Management. Since the majority of patients with myocardial siderosis ultimately die of irreversible cardiac failure and arrhythmias, reversal of the iron overload should be attempted. In patients with idiopathic hemochromatosis, it is possible to mobilize iron stores by repeated phlebotomies, which is the preferred mode of therapy.[75,77–79] Decreases in hepatic iron stores and fibrosis, improvement of liver function, amelioration of diabetes, and reversal of cardiomyopathy have all occurred with such treatment. Since the average patient with idiopathic hemochromatosis has 20 to 40 gm of stored iron, weekly to bimonthly phlebotomies usually have to be continued for 2 to 3 years. Initially the hematocrit will drop but will then return toward normal despite repeated phlebotomies. Removal of excess body iron by phlebotomy has been possible in patients with hematocrits as low as 30 per cent.

The distribution of iron in the tissues differs somewhat between individuals with idiopathic hemochromatosis and those with transfusion siderosis, who have relatively more iron stored in the reticuloendothelial cells. However, repeated

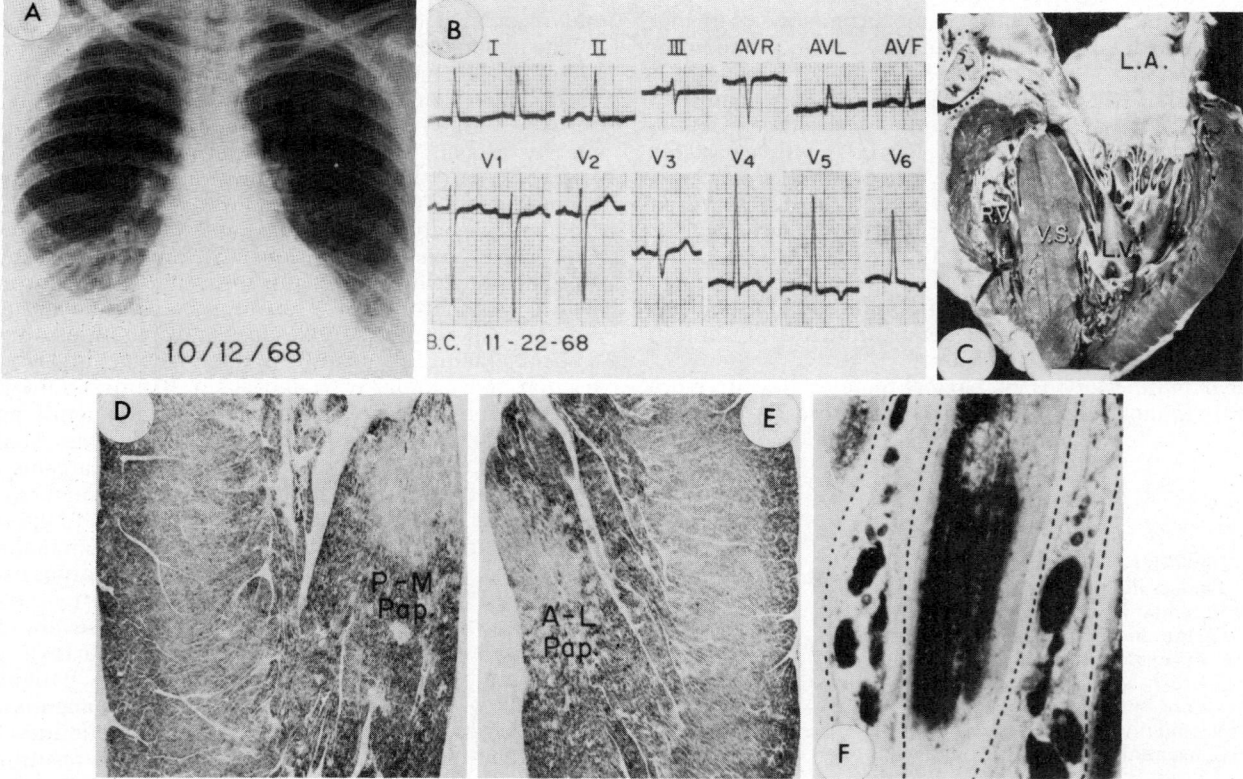

FIGURE 57–7. Observations in a 42-year-old woman with sickle cell anemia who developed congestive heart failure after cumulative transfusions of 260 units of blood. By the time of death, she had received a total of 359 units of blood (90 gm iron). *A*, Chest roentgenogram 2 weeks prior to death, showing cardiomegaly. *B*, Ischemic ST-segment and T-wave changes can be seen on the electrocardiogram. *C*, At autopsy the walls of the right (R.V.) and left (L.V.) ventricles and left atrium (L.A.) and the atrial and ventricular (V.S.) septa were rusty brown, owing to extensive iron deposits. The right atrial wall (partially enclosed by dotted line), in contrast, was tan; only minute particles of iron were present on microscopic examination. *D* and *E*, Large areas of replacement fibrosis (pale areas) were present in both left ventricular papillary muscles. *F*, Severely degenerated myocardial fibers (enclosed by dotted lines) that also contained iron deposits were often found adjacent to viable myocardial fibers. (Prussian blue stains.) (From Buja, L. M., and Roberts, W. C.: Iron in the heart. Am. J. Med. **51**:209, 1971.)

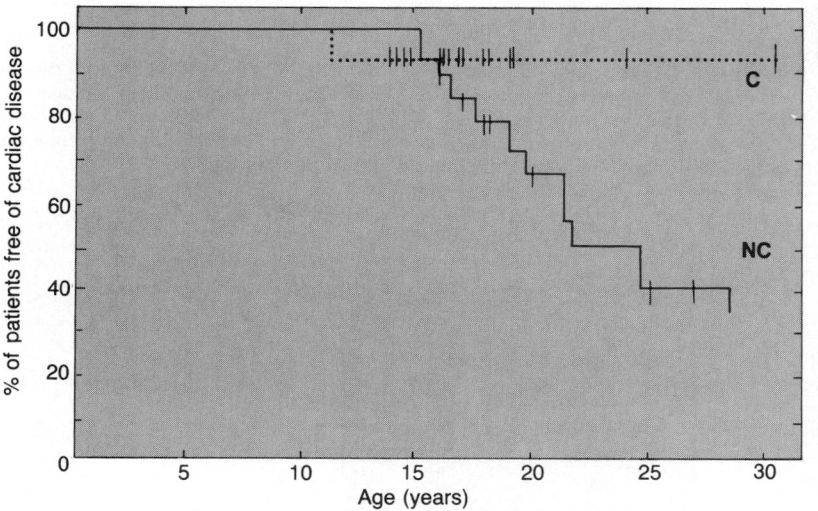

FIGURE 57–8. Life-table depiction of survival free of cardiac disease in patients with thalassemia major treated with desferrioxamine. Dotted line represents the compliant group (C) and solid line represents the current ages of patients still free of cardiac disease. (Reprinted by permission from Wolfe, L., et al.: Prevention of cardiac disease by subcutaneous desferrioxamine in patients with thalassemia major. N. Engl. J. Med. *312*:1600, 1985.)

transfusions in the latter result in a pattern of organ dysfunction similar to that in idiopathic hemochromatosis.[80] Phlebotomy is, of course, not a therapeutic alternative in the management of iron overload due to chronic blood transfusion therapy for anemia or in some patients with idiopathic hemochromatosis and chronic anemia. Rather, chelation therapy is the only approach available for removing iron in these anemic patients.[67-69,81-88]

Deferoxamine is the most widely studied iron chelator. This hydroxamic acid compound has a very high affinity for trivalent iron. It must be administered parenterally, and most of the chelated iron will be excreted in the urine within 4 hours of the injection. Initial studies with intramuscular deferoxamine were unsuccessful in achieving sustained negative iron balance. The addition of oral ascorbic acid doubles iron excretion[81]; when ascorbic acid loading was combined with the continuous, subcutaneous administration of deferoxamine, a negative iron balance was achieved in children with thalassemia.[89] However, ascorbate supplementation in patients with iron overload may be hazardous. Clinical cardiotoxicity manifested by fatal congestive heart failure and arrhythmias has been reported in patients treated simultaneously with deferoxamine and ascorbic acid. Not only does ascorbate make more cellular iron available for chelation, but it also liberates free intracellular iron, which can generate membrane-damaging free oxygen radicals.[90] The adverse effect of ascorbate may be prevented by using this agent *after* the patient has been started on chelation therapy.[91]

Long-term deferoxamine iron chelation therapy is effective not only in delaying but in reversing organ damage caused by transfusional iron overload.[84,86,87] Early and regular treatment with iron chelation appears to protect children with thalassemia major from developing cardiac disease induced by iron overload[85] (Fig. 57–8). An orally active chelator of iron may be just as effective and more easily administered.[91a]

Disorders Associated with Increased Blood Viscosity

As discussed on p. 1743, delivery of oxygen to an organ or tissue is directly proportional to blood flow, hemoglobin concentration, and the difference in oxygen saturation between arterial and venous blood (Fig. 57–3). In anemic patients, an increase in blood flow, due in part to reduced blood viscosity, and enhanced oxygen delivery through elevated levels of red cell 2,3-DPG compensate for the reduced hemoglobin levels. In contrast, conditions associated with increased viscosity cause an increase in resistance to flow and a reduction in blood flow. Disorders with increased viscosity and abnormal blood rheology include the erythrocytoses, such as polycythemia vera, and disease states associated with hypergammaglobulinemia, such as multiple myeloma and cryoglobulinemia.

POLYCYTHEMIA

Polycythemia is characterized by an increase in red cells, as determined by hematocrit, hemoglobin, and/or red blood cell count.[92] However, the terms *polycythemia* and its synonym *erythrocytosis* do not refer to a specific disease entity but to a variety of conditions. *Absolute* polycythemias refer to conditions in which there is an absolute increase in red cell mass (as measured by ^{51}Cr labeling or other dilution techniques). The absolute erythrocytoses are subclassified as primary or secondary, depending whether the elevation in red cell mass is autonomous (primary) or under hormonal (erythropoietin) control. *Primary* polycythemia, i.e., polycythemia vera, is part of the spectrum of myeloproliferative disorders. *Secondary*

polycythemia is further classified into those disorders which cause an appropriate increase in erythropoietin secretion (e.g., disorders associated with hypoxemia, such as cyanotic forms of congenital heart disease and pulmonary disease) and those which cause an inappropriate increase in erythropoietin production, as occurs with tumors and a variety of renal diseases. In the *relative* polycythemias, red cell mass is normal but plasma volume is decreased, causing hematocrit, hemoglobin, and red cell values to be elevated.

Although the symptoms of secondary polycythemia depend on the underlying disease state, they are also usually a consequence of increased blood volume and viscosity; the latter increases exponentially with increased hematocrit.[93] When flow rate through a capillary tube is determined at various levels of hematocrit, flow decreases as an essentially linear function of hematocrit (Fig. 57–9). The product of flow rate and arterial oxygen content provides a relative measure of the rate of oxygen transport through a single blood vessel; optimal hematocrit is just below 40 per cent. Delivery of oxygen to the body depends on the product of total blood flow and the oxygen content of arterial blood, which tends to be high in polycythemia vera, in which blood volume, cardiac output, and arterial blood oxygen content are all increased, despite the increase in viscosity (Fig. 57–10). Although the increases in oxygen content, blood volume, and cardiac output in polycythemia vera are not required for adequate tissue oxygenation, in the polycythemias secondary to hypoxemia the increases in blood oxygen content and cardiac output represent an attempt to improve oxygen delivery.

FIGURE 57-9. Viscosity of heparinized normal blood related to hematocrit. Viscosity was measured with an Ostwald viscosimeter at 37° C and expressed in relation to viscosity of water. Oxygen transport was calculated from the product of hematocrit and 1/viscosity and is recorded in arbitrary units. (From Williams, W. J. [ed.]: Hematology, 2nd ed. New York, McGraw-Hill Book Co., 1977, p. 256.)

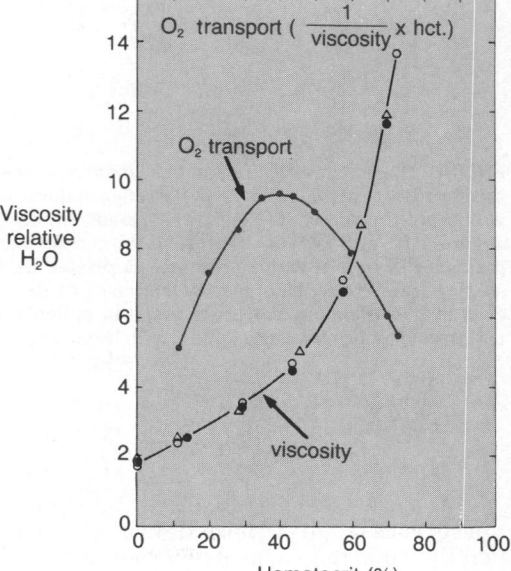

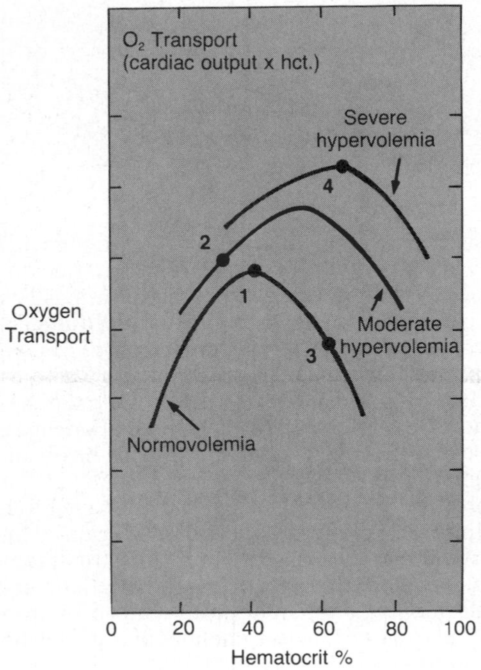

FIGURE 57-10. Oxygen transport at various hematocrit levels in normovolemic, mildly hypervolemic, and severely hypervolemic individuals. The oxygen transport is estimated by multiplying hematocrit by cardiac output. As can be seen in 1, the optimal oxygen transport for the normovolemic subjects is at a hematocrit of about 45 percent with a progressive rise in the optimal hematocrit as the blood volume increases. A suboptimal hematocrit in a hypervolemic person (anemia of pregnancy), as in 2, may be associated with a higher oxygen transport than that of a normovolemic person with normal hematocrit. However, a high hematocrit without increase in blood volume (3) may be associated with an absolute reduction in oxygen transport and tissue hypoxia. Only high hematocrit coupled with high blood volume (4) enhances oxygen transport to the tissues. (From Erslev, A. J.: Clinical manifestations and classification of erythrocyte disorders. *In* Williams, W. J., et al. (eds.): Hematology. 4th ed. New York, McGraw-Hill Book Co., 1990, p. 428.)

POLYCYTHEMIA VERA

Although the pathogenesis of polycythemia vera is not understood, this condition has been classified as a myeloproliferative disorder.[94] All hematopoietic cells are monoclonal based on assays of glucose-6-phosphate dehydrogenase (G-6-PD) isoenzymes,[95] an enzymatic marker that has been used as evidence of the clonal origin of tumors. In black patients heterozygous for G-6-PD, normal tissues possess both isoenzymes A (phenotype: Gd-A) and B (phenotype: Gd-B); if only one isoenzyme is present in the neoplastic cells of such a patient, a clonal origin of the neoplasm or, in this case, the disease polycythemia vera is likely. Thus, erythropoietin is not the stimulus for increased red cell production; indeed, erythropoietin concentrations may be low in this condition.

If erythrocytosis is accompanied by an increased red cell mass, arterial oxygen saturation more than 92 per cent, and splenomegaly, the diagnosis of polycythemia vera is confirmed. In the absence of splenomegaly, any two of the following laboratory findings will satisfy the diagnostic criteria: thrombocytosis, leukocytosis (in the absence of infection), elevated leukocyte alkaline phosphatase activity, or a combination of elevated serum vitamin B_{12} concentration and unsaturated B_{12}-binding capacity.[96]

CLINICAL MANIFESTATIONS. Symptoms are divided into those secondary to the increased red cell mass and increased blood volume, including headache, plethora, pruritus, dyspnea, and bleeding; those due to increased blood viscosity, including paresthesias and thrombosis; and those due to hypermetabolism, including weight loss despite a good appetite and night sweats. Angina pectoris, intermittent claudication, and arterial hypertension occur frequently.

It seems paradoxical that both bleeding and thrombosis can be complications of this disease; however, each occurs in 33 to 50 per cent of patients, and they are the major causes of morbidity and mortality. Bleeding is caused by the distention of veins and capillaries due to the increased blood volume, defective platelet function, or both. Thrombosis has been thought to be related to increased blood viscosity, thrombocytosis, and abnormally increased aggregation of platelets. Thrombotic sites include coronary and cerebral arteries as well as those in the extremities. Less frequently, thrombosis may involve the mesenteric and portal veins. Surgical morbidity is high in patients with polycythemia vera who are inade-

quately treated, and anesthesia and the stress of operation increase further the risk of hemorrhagic and thrombotic events during the immediate postoperative period.

TREATMENT. Therapy is aimed primarily at decreasing the potential for both hemorrhage and thrombosis. Ideally, this consists of phlebotomy alone. If control of thrombocytosis is necessary, hydroxyurea appears to be the most efficacious agent.[96]

MECHANISMS OF SYMPTOMS. The clinical severity of polycythemia is usually related to the degree of hypervolemia and increased viscosity.[93,94] Myocardial oxygen transport is not impaired with high hematocrit values.[11] In older patients with underlying atherosclerotic vascular disease, cardiac output tends not to be elevated, and as a consequence of the increased viscosity without increased flow, the incidence of ischemic episodes may be higher. In vitro studies suggest that white blood cells can contribute significantly to blood viscosity[97]; since leukocytosis is characteristic of polycythemia vera, white cells undoubtedly play a role in the increased viscosity seen in this disease.

Cerebral blood flow is significantly reduced and is associated with cerebral symptoms in about half the patients with hematocrit values averaging 53.6 per cent, confirming the relationship between cerebrovascular insufficiency and blood viscosity.[98] When hematocrit is lowered to approximately 45 per cent, viscosity declines by 30 per cent and cerebral blood flow increases substantially. With hematocrit values ranging from 46 to 52 per cent, cerebral blood flow is still less than normal, suggesting that even slight increases in red cell mass may interfere with cerebral perfusion. These results imply that patients with polycythemia vera should undergo phlebotomy until hematocrit levels reach the low 40's rather than the previously recommended level of about 47 per cent.

SECONDARY POLYCYTHEMIAS

The secondary polycythemias may be divided into two subgroups: (1) those in which the increased red cell mass compensates for a reduction in oxygen transport with appropriate stimulation by erythropoietin and (2) those in which erythrocytosis is associated with an inappropriate increase in erythropoietin production. It has been suggested that any hypoxic stimulus will cause production of the enzyme erythrogenin in the kidney, which generates erythropoietin by acting enzymatically on a proposed plasma protein substrate, possibly of hepatic origin (Fig. 57-11). If an individual living at sea level is transported to a high altitude, hemoglobin concentrations will rise[99] accompanied by an increase in erythropoietin. Similarly, with severe degrees of chronic hypoxemia in chronic obstructive pulmonary disease, an arterial PO_2 less than 60 mm Hg usually leads to an increase in red cell mass. Although in some instances hemoglobin has been reported to be as high as 24 gm/dl and the hematocrit as high as 75 per cent, in most patients with chronic pulmonary disease these values do not exceed 17 gm/dl and 57 per cent, respectively.[100] In cyanotic congenital heart disease, red cell mass increases as resting arterial oxygen saturation falls (p. 895). Hematocrits as high as 86 per cent may be seen with red blood cell masses almost three times normal.[101] Although plasma volume may be diminished, total blood volume remains significantly elevated because of the striking increase in red cell mass. The most common congenital malformations producing these elevations include tetralogy of Fallot, transposition of the great arteries, and persistent truncus arteriosus (see Chap. 31).

CLINICAL MANIFESTATIONS. Signs and symptoms of hyperviscosity generally occur as hematocrit exceeds 60 per cent; cardiac function may be compromised because of the combination of hypervolemia and the constant volume load and augmented vascular resistance secondary to the increased viscosity of the blood. Ruddy cyanosis, headache, dizziness, roaring in the ears, thrombotic episodes, and bleeding are the major clinical findings and may be treated with phlebotomy.[102] Careful monitoring of arterial pressure, heart rate, and general condition is necessary during phlebotomy, and the acute reduction in blood volume may have to be avoided by the simultaneous administration of plasma expanders.[103] After isovolemic phlebotomy to reduce the hematocrit from the 70's to the 60's, cardiac output rises, and despite the fall in arterial oxygen content, systemic oxygen transport usually increases. These favorable changes are attributed to the reduced blood viscosity and vascular resistance. Although the erythrocytosis is a homeostatic mechanism compensating for the chronic arterial hypoxemia, greatly increased hematocrits are generally undesirable. Studies by Erslev and Caro suggest that secondary polycythemia is not necessarily a boon but could be a burden, and that secondary erythrocytosis cannot always be considered optimal for overall oxygen transport.[104] Secondary polycythemia due to cyanotic congenital heart disease has been reported to cause myocardial infarction without manifestations of coronary atherosclerosis.[105,106]

MANAGEMENT. Phlebotomy, or preferably erythropheresis, in secondary polycythemia reduces blood viscosity, increases systemic oxygen transport without lowering peripheral oxygen consumption, and simultaneously increases effective renal plasma flow.[107,108] The optimal hematocrit for patients with cyanotic congenital heart disease and other chronically hypoxemic states is poorly defined and presents an interesting and perplexing dilemma. The clinical presentation of the patient must be carefully considered. Cerebral blood flow is reduced in secondary erythrocytosis as well as in polycythemia vera and improves with phlebotomy.[109,110] As might be expected from the decreased oxygen transport associated with right-to-left shunts, P_{50} and red cell 2,3-DPG are increased, but the relationship between decreased arterial PO_2 and the rise in P_{50} and red cell 2,3-DPG varies greatly.[111] Successful surgical correction of the cardiac defect will result in normal saturation and obviate the adaptive mechanism, and hematocrit and blood volume will return to normal.

HEMOGLOBIN VARIANTS WITH INCREASED AFFINITY FOR OXYGEN. In 1966, it was first recognized that a hemoglobin variant with increased oxygen affinity could be associated with erythrocytosis.[112] These variants, which generally have amino acid substitutions at structural sites crucial to hemoglobin function and individually are quite rare, now number over 40. They are transmitted in an autosomal dominant fashion and cause a shift in the oxygen dissociation curve to the left with reduced levels of P_{50}. The shift to the left of the Hb-O_2 dissociation curve results in a marked reduction in oxygen extraction by the tissues. Increased hemoglobin concentration and blood flow are available compensatory mechanisms to maintain oxygen delivery (Fig. 57–3). However, the primary response appears to be erythrocytosis mediated by increases in erythropoietin.[113–115] The cardiac output is usually normal. Polycythemia constitutes the primary adjustment for oxygen delivery in patients with these hemoglobin variants, who have no increased incidence of myocardial ischemia or other forms of organ hypoxia.

OTHER CAUSES. True erythrocytosis without demonstrable cause, other than excessive cigar and cigarette smoking, has also been noted in a significant number of individuals.[116] All had elevated levels of carboxyhemoglobin with shifts of the Hb-O_2 dissociation curve to the left, stimulating erythropoiesis. In most cases of polycythemia secondary to inappropriate erythropoietin production, such as tumors, renal cysts, and hydronephrosis, the red cell mass, although increased, does not generally cause symptoms of hyperviscosity.

RELATIVE POLYCYTHEMIA. This is a distinct and commonly encountered entity that is also referred to as spurious polycythemia, *Gaisböck syndrome*, and *stress erythrocytosis*. It is not a primary disease process and may be merely a physiological state in which the plasma volume is slightly reduced and the red cell mass is slightly increased. Hematocrit rarely exceeds 60 per cent, and other blood constituents are normal. This disorder can be distinguished from polycythemia vera by measuring the red cell mass, which by definition is normal in relative polycythemia and increased in polycythemia vera. Patients are often hypertensive, prone to thromboembolic complications,[117] and obese; however, these complications appear to be unrelated to the hematological changes, so that reducing the red cell mass by phlebotomy, radiation therapy, or chemotherapy is not appropriate. When present, hypertension and thromboembolic complications should be treated in the usual manner.

THROMBOCYTOSIS

Occasionally thrombocytosis value may be seen alone as a manifestation of a myeloproliferative disorder without an increased hematocrit.[118–123] Essential thrombocytosis has been associated in several instances of sudden catastrophic events such as massive arterial thrombosis in the cerebral and coronary arteries, occurring even in young adults without underlying atherosclerosis.[118–122] Such complications rarely occur in the thrombocytosis secondary to nonmyeloproliferative states such as iron deficiency or postsplenectomy states unless coexistent with severe anemia.[123] Rheological changes in the blood have been found to be associated with myocardial infarction, but it is not clear whether these changes are secondary to infarction or whether they play an initiating role.[124–126] Changes in blood viscosity, plasma viscosity, and red cell filterability occur in patients with myocardial infarction or unstable angina and may play an important role in its pathogenesis. Although these changes may not contribute to disease in many other parts of the body, they may be significant in the coronary microcirculation.

FIGURE 57–11. Feedback circuit linking an oxygen sensor in the kidney with erythroid progenitor cells in the bone marrow. The circuit is moved in one direction by red cells containing oxygen and in the opposite direction by erythropoietin. Oxygen sensing and erythropoietin production may also take place in the liver and in some macrophages. The target for erythropoietin is primarily the erythropoietin-dependent progenitor cells (CFU-E), with milder actions on the burst-forming progenitor cells (BFU-E) and the precursor cells. (From Erslev, A. J.: Production of erythrocytes. *In* Williams, W. J., et al. (eds.): Hematology. 4th ed, New York, McGraw-Hill Book Co., 1990, p. 395.)

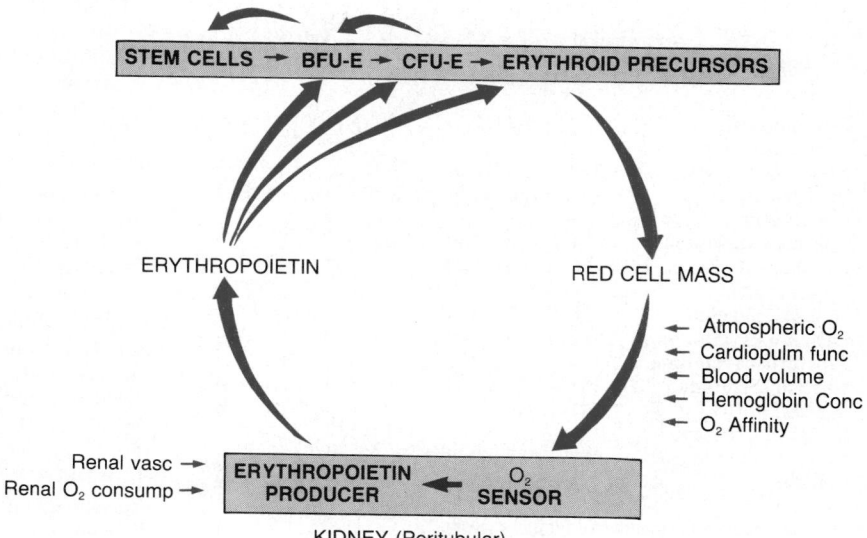

STEM CELLS → BFU-E → CFU-E → ERYTHROID PRECURSORS

ERYTHROPOIETIN

RED CELL MASS

← Atmospheric O_2
← Cardiopulm func
← Blood volume
← Hemoglobin Conc
← O_2 Affinity

Renal vasc →
Renal O_2 consump →

ERYTHROPOIETIN PRODUCER ← O_2 SENSOR

KIDNEY (Peritubular)
Liver (Kupffer cells?)
Macrophages?

INCIDENCE. Primary tumors of the heart which are discussed in Chap. 44, are rare, occurring in less than 0.1 per cent of autopsies. Here we deal with tumors metastatic to the pericardium or heart, which are far more common, ranging from 1.5 to 20.6 per cent (average 6 per cent) of autopsies on patients with malignant diseases, and actually appear to be increasing in incidence.[127] Prolonged survival of cancer patients may be the reason for this higher incidence. Usually the metastases involve the pericardium and myocardium, with the valves or endocardium rarely affected, and the right side of the heart appears to be affected more frequently than the left.[128] Solitary metastases to the heart are rare. Although metastatic nodules in the heart are generally multiple (Fig. 57–12), they may become diffuse and lead to the manifestations of restrictive cardiomyopathy (p. 1415). The mode of spread to the heart may be by direct extension, as occurs in lung cancer; via the hematogenous route, as in malignant melanoma; or through lymphatic channels, as in lymphoma.

The most common primary tumor producing cardiac metastases is carcinoma of the bronchus (Fig. 57–12), with carcinoma of the breast, malignant melanoma, lymphomas, and leukemias next in order of frequency (Table 57–3).[128,129] At autopsy, 15 to 35 per cent of patients dying with primary lung cancer show cardiac involvement, while over 60 per cent of patients with melanoma have cardiac metastases.[130] Hematological malignant tumors, especially lymphomas, have been reported to account for 15 per cent of all cardiac and pericardial metastases,[131] and about 15 per cent of patients dying of malignant lymphomas show metastases to the heart. Metastatic cardiac lesions secondary to mesothelioma and sarcoma, as well as melanoma and breast cancer, are all increasing in number.

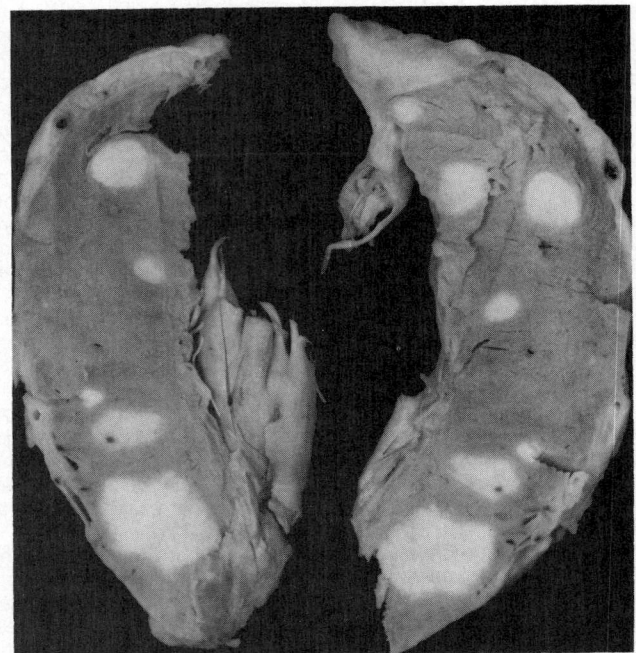

FIGURE 57–12. Sections of left ventricle showing metastatic nodules in the myocardium. Primary tumor was in a bronchus. (From Edwards, J. E.: Effects of malignant noncardiac tumors upon the cardiovascular system. *In* Brest, A. N. [ed.]: Cardiovascular Clinics, Vol. 4. Philadelphia, F. A. Davis, 1972, p. 282.)

CLINICAL MANIFESTATIONS

Many metastatic cardiac lesions are clinically silent and are found only at necropsy. For example, despite massive heart involvement with melanoma ("charcoal heart"), sometimes there is surprisingly little evidence of cardiac dysfunction.[132] Specific clinical manifestations of cardiac involvement by cancer may be divided into those due to pericardial, myocardial, or endocardial involvement; cardiac compression by extracardiac tumors[133]; indirect consequences of tumor complications of circulating mediators; embolization in patients in a hypercoagulable state; or the effects of specific tumor therapy, such as chemotherapy and radiation therapy (Table 57–4).[128,129] The most common clinical manifestations result from pericardial effusion with tamponade, tachyarrhythmias, AV block,[134] or congestive heart failure.[133] Metastatic cardiac disease is rarely the presenting symptom of a tumor. The mode of spread may be by direct extension via the hematogenous route or through lymphatic channels. Routine chest radiographs, computed chest tomography, magnetic resonance imaging, echocardiography, and/or radionuclide imaging with gallium or thallium are often helpful in diagnosis.[135–138] Osteogenic sarcoma, which may metastasize to the heart, is unique because the metastases contain bone and may be radiographically visible.[139]

PERICARDIAL INVOLVEMENT (see also p. 1415). Ten to 25 per cent of all patients with cancer have pericardial involvement at autopsy, with slightly more than half being due to tumor, the rest due to therapy or other causes.[140] Signs and symptoms of pericarditis with pericardial effusion and cardiac tamponade are particularly common in patients with carcinoma of the lung and breast as well as in Hodgkin's disease, non-Hodgkin's lymphoma,[141] and the leukemias,[142] particularly acute myelogenous, lymphoblastic leukemia and the blast crisis of chronic myelogenous leukemia. Pericardial involvement is usually diagnosed ante mortem because of the resultant symptomatology and radiographic and echocardiographic evidence. Clinically, this takes the form of either cardiac tamponade or adhesive pericarditis, associated with extensive nodular tumor infiltration of the pericardium.[143–147] The finding of chylous pericardial effusion is usually characteristic of lymphoma.[148] Echocardiography is a key tool in the diagnosis of neoplastic involvement of the pericardium[119,120,136,149] (Fig. 57–13) (see also Fig. 4–102, p. 103 and Fig. 45–27, p. 1506). Pericardiocentesis may be necessary to differentiate tumor from radiation effects.[150] Computed tomography and magnetic resonance imaging are also helpful in detecting pericardial tumors.

TABLE 57–3 METASTATIC CARDIAC DISEASE

TUMOR TYPE	TOTAL NO.	Heart	Pericardial	Both
Bronchogenic carcinoma	402	43 (10.2)	66 (15.7)	23 (5.4)
Breast carcinoma	289	24 (8.3)	34 (11.8)	3 (1.4)
Malignant melanoma	59	20 (34.0)	14 (23.7)	12 (20.4)
Colonic carcinoma	214	2 (0.9)	6 (2.8)	0
Esophageal carcinoma	65	5 (7.7)	5 (7.7)	2 (3.6)
Hypernephroma	95	5 (5.3)	0	0
Ovarian carcinoma	115	6 (5.7)	8 (7.0)	3 (2.6)
Prostatic carcinoma	186	5 (2.7)	2 (1.0)	0
Gastric carcinoma	308	11 (3.6)	10 (3.2)	3 (0.9)
Sarcoma*	207	19 (9.2)	19 (9.2)	8 (3.9)
Hodgkin's disease	75	—	11 (14.6)	—
Acute leukemia	420	227 (53.9)	95 (22.4)	—
Total	2,435	367 (15.1)	270 (11.1)	54 (2.2)

* Reticulum cell sarcoma and lymphosarcoma.
Note: Numbers in parentheses represent percentages.
From Applefeld, M. M., and Pollock, S. H.: Cardiac disease in patients who have malignancies. Curr. Probl. Cardiol. 4(6):5, 1980.

TABLE 57-4 CLINICAL MANIFESTATIONS OF CARDIAC INVOLVEMENT IN MALIGNANT DISEASE

Pericardial involvement
   Pericarditis
   Cardiac tamponade
Superior vena caval syndrome
Arrhythmias
   Supraventricular tachycardia
   Carotid sinus syncope
   Atrioventricular block
Cardiomegaly and congestive heart failure
Unexplained heart murmur
Unexplained hypotension
Noninfective (marantic) endocarditis

Pericardial tumor or fibrosis secondary to radiation therapy may mimic chronic constrictive pericarditis or chronic effusive pericardial disease and cause problems in differential diagnosis (p. 1499). In patients with carcinoma of the lung, Hodgkin's disease, and non-Hodgkin's lymphoma, who commonly undergo irradiation of the thorax, radiation-induced pericarditis is common, and it was believed that this condition could be differentiated from tumor involvement because it occurred usually within a year of such therapy. However, it has become clear that radiation-induced pericarditis may occur as late as 8 years after therapy.[151]

MYOCARDIAL METASTASES. Direct myocardial or endocardial involvement by tumor such as lung cancer, lymphoma, or melanoma may result in arrhythmias, congestive heart failure, ventricular outflow tract obstruction, and peripheral emboli.[131,152] Cardiac metastases can be detected on two-dimensional echocardiography (Figs. 57-12 and 57-14),[136] computed tomography, and magnetic resonance imaging (Fig. 11-36, p. 330).[136,153,154]

VENA CAVAL OBSTRUCTION. The superior vena caval syndrome, resulting from obstruction of this vessel by tumor, is also a recognized complication in patients with carcinoma of the lung and malignant lymphoma.[155] Enlarged mediastinal nodes or the primary tumor itself may impinge upon or even occlude the superior vena cava, causing dyspnea, distention of the neck veins, edema of the face and arms, proptosis, headache, and syncope. Because of the potential life-threatening nature of these problems, local irradiation may have to be initiated prior to any diagnostic procedure. Similar enlargement of nodes or tumor may cause obstruction of the inferior vena cava, with massive leg edema, congestive hepatomegaly, and hypotension.[156]

CARDIAC AMYLOIDOSIS (see also p. 1416). The heart is involved in the majority of cases of primary amyloidosis and also in many instances of amyloidosis secondary to multiple myeloma. Symptoms often include congestive heart failure, hypotension, arrhythmias, and conduction disturbances.[157,158] Echocardiographic examination, contrast tomography, and endomyocardial biopsy have made it easier to confirm this

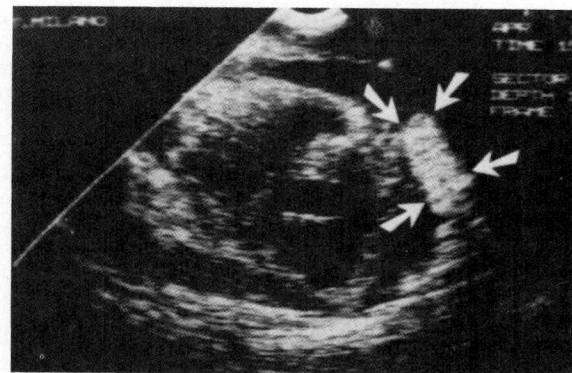
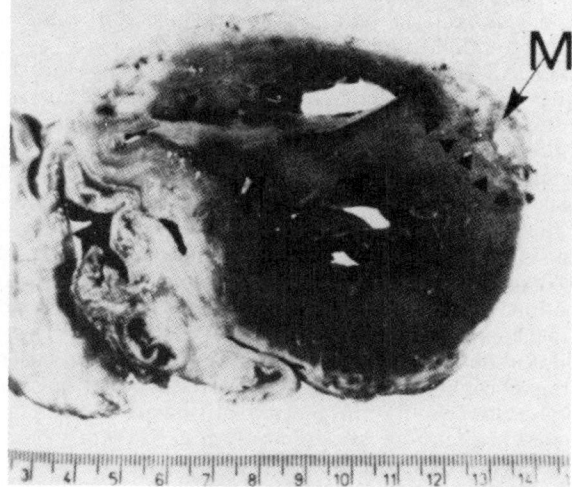

FIGURE 57-14. *Top,* Echocardiogram in parasternal short-axis view. A large echogenic mass (arrows) infiltrates the left lateral ventricular wall and the septum. *Bottom,* Postmortem specimen (cross section). The neoplastic mass (M) infiltrates the epicardium and the subepicardial myocardium (arrowheads). (From Lestuzzi, C., et al.: Secondary neoplastic infiltration of the myocardium diagnosed by two-dimensional echocardiography in seven cases with anatomic confirmation. J. Am. Coll. Cardiol. 9:439, 1987.)

diagnosis. A low myocardial density on contrast-aided tomography, diffuse myocardial thickening, and diffuse hypokinetic wall motion may be the result of cardiac amyloidosis and may simulate hypertrophic cardiomyopathy. Endomyocardial biopsy may be necessary to confirm the diagnosis.[159-161]

ELECTROCARDIOGRAPHIC AND ROENTGENOGRAPHIC FINDINGS. Arrhythmias and a wide variety of electrocardiographic changes are common in patients with metastatic disease. Although they may certainly be caused by tumor involvement of the heart, they are more often due to concomitant factors, such as altered electrolyte concentrations, anemia, and hypoxia. Nonspecific ST-segment and T-wave changes, low voltage, and sinus tachycardia are frequent electrocardiographic abnormalities and cannot be considered diagnostic.[162] Clinically it may be difficult to determine whether any such abnormality is attributable to cardiac metastases or is due to an associated cardiac problem, irradiation, or the cardiotoxic effects of drugs. Atrial arrhythmias, such as fibrillation and flutter, may occur secondary to either neoplastic involvement of autonomic fibers supplying the atria or tumor invasion of the coronary arteries perfusing the atria, with resulting atrial infarction, or to neoplastic infiltration of the atrial myocardium or sinus node. Similarly, electrocardiographic changes of acute myocardial infarction can be produced by tumor infiltration or hemorrhage into the ventricle or occlusion of one of the coronary arteries. Occasionally, the exact area of tumor involvement may be pinpointed based on the acute electrocardiographic changes.[163] Involvement of the

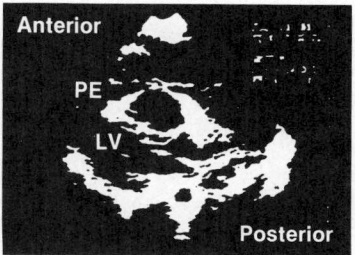
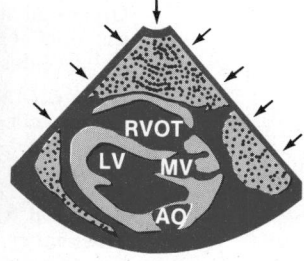

FIGURE 57-13. Two-dimensional, parasternal, long-axis view *(left)* with schematic diagram *(right)* in lymphoblastic lymphoma involving the pericardium. Note a small amount of pericardial effusion (PE) and extensive thickening of the pericardium encasing the heart (arrowheads in right panel). AO = aorta; LV = left ventricle; MV = mitral valve; RVOT = right ventricular outflow tract. (From Kutalek, S. P., et al.: Metastatic tumors of the heart detected by two-dimensional echocardiography. Am. Heart J. *109:*343, 1985.)

AV node is a rare cause of complete heart block but may be the presenting symptom of the tumor.[164] In addition, tumor involvement of cervical lymph nodes without mediastinal involvement has been associated with carotid sinus syncope.[165]

Roentgenographic evidence of cardiac enlargement and the development of congestive heart failure may be the only clinical signs of malignant involvement of the heart. New systolic murmurs may occur with intraluminal invasion or external compression of the carotid or pulmonary arteries by the tumor. In addition to coincidental atherosclerosis, coronary artery disease in cancer patients can be caused by tumor emboli, extrinsic compression of the coronary arteries or ostia, or thromboemboli brought about by tumor-associated coagulation disorders.

If myocardial metastases are suspected from clinical or electrocardiographic data, a two-dimensional echocardiogram is often helpful diagnostically.

MYOCARDIAL INFARCTION. In a necropsy study of 816 patients with solid tumors, 33 (4 per cent) died of myocardial infarction.[166] Patients with carcinoma of the lung, malignant lymphoma, and leukemia are most commonly afflicted; less frequently affected were patients with cancer of the breast and gastrointestinal tract and malignant melanoma.[167] In general, the etiology of coronary artery disease in patients with cancer is most likely coincidental spontaneous atherosclerosis.[168] The most common cause of tumor-related myocardial infarction is extrinsic compression of a coronary artery, occurring in 60 per cent of cases, whereas tumor emboli are responsible for about 35 per cent.[167,169] Widespread thromboses, including coronary artery thromboses due to disseminated intravascular coagulation, occasionally occur in patients with metastatic tumors, most commonly mucin-secreting adenocarcinomas. Approximately half of all patients with acute myocardial infarction secondary to malignant disease had a history of typical chest pain prior to death. An acute myocardial infarction in a patient with advanced malignant disease is a particularly poor prognostic sign, since more than two-thirds of such patients die within 3 weeks of the event.

VALVULAR EFFECTS: NONBACTERIAL THROMBOTIC ENDOCARDITIS (NBTE). Metastatic tumors may affect cardiac valves in a variety of ways, including direct invasion of valves, interference with valvular function by compression, valvular dysfunction secondary to malignant carcinoid (p. 1424), but most commonly by NBTE.[170-172] Although the pathogenesis is unclear, this condition is associated with adenocarcinomas—especially of the pancreas and lung—as well as hematological malignant disease and lymphomas.[173] It has been suggested that immune complexes elicited by the underlying malignant process play a role in the formation of thrombi.[174] Other causes of NBTE include disseminated intravascular coagulation and nonneoplastic causes of debilitation and cachexia.[173] The fibrin matrix is attached to, but does not destroy, valve leaflets that may be normal or show degenerative changes.[171,172] NBTE involves principally the aortic and mitral valves equally. (The pulmonic valve may be involved in patients with catheters in place for long periods in the right heart and pulmonary artery.[175])

Patients may have clinical evidence of arterial embolization and microembolic events resembling those of infective endocarditis (p. 1083), and changing murmurs, often without fever or leukocytosis (unless an unrelated infection is present). The most serious complications are cerebral emboli with neurological sequelae. Rarely coronary embolization may occur, causing myocardial infarction.

The diagnosis is aided immensely by two-dimensional echocardiography. Antiplatelet therapy with aspirin or anticoagulants has been employed to prevent recurrent embolization, but its effectiveness has yet to be demonstrated.

ENDOCARDIAL INVOLVEMENT. There is a high correlation between eosinophilia in the bone marrow and peripheral blood and the occurrence of endomyocardial fibrosis,[176] which may cause restrictive cardiomyopathy (p. 1415). Ever since Loeffler described the entity "endocarditis parietalis fibroplastica" with eosinophilia, this association has been of interest but remains unexplained. In some patients, the cardiac manifestations predominate, most commonly cardiomegaly, congestive heart failure, arrhythmias, and heart murmurs, whereas in others, all or most of the clinical manifestations are secondary to the *eosinophilic leukemia*. Pathologically, these syndromes are characterized by local or widespread eosinophilic infiltrates with fibrous scarring and thickening of the endocardium, including the atrioventricular valves. In many patients, the course is chronic and insidious, but death is usually the direct result of cardiac involvement.

CARDIAC EFFECTS OF RADIATION THERAPY AND CHEMOTHERAPY

With the advent of intensive radiation therapy and aggressive chemotherapy, cardiac toxicity of antitumor treatment has increased greatly. Formerly, the heart was considered one of the most radioresistant organs and seemed to be spared most of the side effects of chemotherapy. However, radiation can cause myocardial damage.[177] The incidence of cardiovascular complications has risen sharply with the use of curative forms of radiation therapy for Hodgkin's disease and non-Hodgkin's lymphoma involving the mediastinum and the addition of one of the most potent classes of chemotherapeutic agents, the anthracyclines. The addition of growth factors and cytokines such as interferon and interleukin-2 to the armamentarium of the therapist has also brought on unexpected cardiac complications.

RADIATION THERAPY

Therapeutic radiation can cause heart damage by injuring various structures either acutely or chronically (Table 57–5). Most commonly affected is the pericardium, with less damage to the myocardium, endocardium, and papillary muscles, and the least damage to the heart valves and coronary arteries

TABLE 57–5 EFFECT OF RADIATION ON THE HEART

EARLY CHANGES
Cytoplasmic damage
Capillary injury
DNA damage
Local chemical reactions
von Willebrand factor release
Platelet and fibrin deposition
Acute inflammatory reaction
Increased vascular permeability
Protein damage
Transient pericardial effusion
INTERMEDIATE CHANGES
Cellular immune response
Vascular compromise
Attempts at repair
Organized fibrin formation
Endothelial proliferation
Collagen deposition
LATE CHANGES
Compromised vascular supply
Cell death
Fibroblastic proliferation
Altered cell morphology
Enhanced atherosclerosis
Thickening of pericardium
Loss of adventitial tissue
Pericardial effusion
Endocardial thickening
Valvular heart disease
Arrhythmias

From Niemtzow, R. C., and Reynolds, R. D.: Radiation therapy and the heart. *In* Kapoor, A. S. (ed.): Cancer and the Heart. New York, Springer-Verlag, 1986, p. 240.

TABLE 57-6 CLASSIFICATION OF RADIATION-RELATED CARDIAC DISEASE

1. **Acute pericarditis (caused by necrosis of tumor adjacent to the heart)**

2. **Delayed pericarditis**
   a. **Acute radiation-induced pericarditis, without effusion**
   b. **Acute radiation-induced pericarditis, with effusion, with/without cardiac tamponade**
   c. **Chronic effusive pericarditis**
   d. **Effusive constrictive pericarditis**
   e. **Chronic pericardial constriction**
   f. **Occult constrictive pericarditis**

3. **Myocardial fibrosis**

4. **Occlusive coronary artery disease**

5. **Conduction abnormalities**

6. **Valvular regurgitation or stenosis**

(Table 57-6).[178,178a] Severe pericardial damage with pericarditis,[179-181] acute myocardial infarction,[151,182-186] valvular disease,[187-190] cardiomyopathy,[191] and arrhythmias[192] are the most frequently observed complications.

PERICARDIAL EFFECTS (see also p. 1499). Radiation-induced pericardial abnormalities can be divided into early, intermediate, and late changes (Table 57-5).[178,193,194] The most common acute cardiovascular complication of radiation therapy is pericarditis.[180] Acute pericarditis occurs in 10 to 15 per cent of patients with Hodgkin's disease who receive over 4000 rads to the mediastinum.[181] These episodes are characterized by fever, pleuritic pain, pericardial friction rub, and electrocardiographic and echocardiographic changes typical of this condition (p. 1500). The time from completion of radiotherapy to the clinical onset of pericarditis ranges from 0 to 85 months, with the peak incidence occurring between 5 and 9 months. Echocardiography demonstrates a pericardial effusion in almost all patients with clinical evidence of pericarditis.[195] With long follow-up of patients cured of their underlying neoplastic disease, the clinical manifestations of pericarditis may not develop for 8 to 10 years.[151,193,194] The incidence of pericarditis appears to be a function of the fractional and total dose of radiation to the pericardium and the quantity of the heart irradiated. When the entire dose of radiation is delivered through an anterior port, the incidence of pericarditis is increased. However, when chest irradiation is delivered in divided doses to anterior and posterior ports and with a subcarinal shield, the incidence of pericarditis has decreased to 2.5 per cent, without increasing the risk of relapse of Hodgkin's disease.[196] If the entire heart receives therapeutic doses of radiation, up to 50 per cent of patients may develop pericardial complications.[197] As a consequence whole-heart irradiation has been replaced with chemotherapy for many patients with large mediastinal masses.

It has been suggested that routine follow-up during the first year after radiation of the mediastinum should consist of frequent echocardiography and chest roentgenography. If any evidence of increased cardiac diameter is noted, or if clinical manifestations suggestive of pericarditis or pericardial effusion develop and there is no reason to suspect another cause of pericarditis, patients may be treated symptomatically but occasionally may require pericardiocentesis and/or pericardiectomy.[150,151]

MYOCARDIAL AND ENDOCARDIAL EFFECTS. Echocardiographic studies carried out before and within 6 months after conventional irradiation therapy in women with breast cancer revealed an asymptomatic decrease of the fractional systolic shortening of the left ventricular minor-axis diameter and of the systolic blood pressure/end-systolic diameter ratio. These changes, which reflect slight transient depression of left ventricular function, occurred within the first 6 months after postoperative radiation and disappeared by 6 months.[198]

Radiation-induced endocardial fibrosis may cause manifestations of restrictive cardiomyopathy[191,199] (p. 1415) and a variety of nonspecific electrocardiographic changes[200] as well as varying degrees of AV block.[192] Mitral regurgitation may develop secondary to radiation-induced papillary muscle dysfunction and aortic regurgitation as a consequence of endocardial valvular thickening.[187,189] The onset of new murmurs occurring after radiation therapy should alert the physician to these possibilities. In an autopsy study of the cardiac effects of radiation exposure, three-fourths of the patients exposed to more than 3500 rads, with a field resulting in a large exposure of the anterior thorax, developed interstitial myocardial fibrosis, with more extensive involvement of the right than the left ventricle. Functional abnormalities demonstrated on echocardiography and radionuclide angiocardiography may occur 5 to 15 years after radiation but, as with pericarditis, should become less frequent with new techniques of radiotherapy.[179]

CORONARY AND CAROTID ARTERIAL EFFECTS. Since the report in 1967 of a 15-year-old boy suffering a fatal myocardial infarction 16 months after receiving 4000 rads to the heart for Hodgkin's disease, a number of similar occurrences have been reported.[151,182-186,201-203] Supportive evidence for radiation-induced coronary artery disease includes (1) its occurrence in subjects who are very young with no predisposing factors and disease limited to coronary vessels within the path of the radiation beam, (2) the lack of atherosclerosis in arteries not exposed to irradiation, (3) reports of occlusive lesions in other arteries such as the carotid artery after irradiation,[204] (4) the presence of distinctive pathological changes, and (5) the production of similar lesions in experimental models.

Occlusive coronary and carotid artery disease following irradiation generally occurs 6 to 12 years after exposure. In rabbits, 2500 rads has produced coronary atherosclerosis similar to that in humans.[205] However, rabbits do not develop radiation-induced atherosclerosis unless they also receive a diet high in lipids and cholesterol, which by itself is insufficient to produce the atherosclerotic lesion. Coronary artery lesions presumably induced by radiotherapy in patients appear to be distinct pathologically and to contain severe medial and adventitial fibrosis in continuity with overlying epicardial fibrous tissue and a marked paucity of lipid in the intimal lesions.[206] In affected young patients examined at autopsy, the proximal portions of the arteries are significantly more narrowed than the distal portions. In addition, there is significant loss of smooth muscle cells from the media.[206]

Radiation-induced coronary artery or carotid artery obstruction or occlusion may require surgical treatment. Because of the relatively low incidence of this complication and the concern that lowering the dose of radiation might preclude effective treatment of the neoplastic process, no systematic attempts have been made to try to prevent this complication other than considering chemotherapeutic alternatives if whole-heart irradiation is otherwise deemed necessary for curative purposes. It is anticipated that with changes in radiotherapeutic techniques and available curative chemotherapy, the incidence of all forms of radiation-induced heart disease will continue to decline.

CHEMOTHERAPY

Since the late 1960's there have been major advances in the management of a variety of neoplastic disorders using combination chemotherapy. Therapies have become more aggressive and new agents have been introduced, resulting in significant responses and longer survival. Unfortunately, concomitant with this increased response rate has been an increase in toxicity. Although most complications due to drugs are limited to rapidly proliferating tissues such as the bone marrow and gastrointestinal tract, cardiotoxicity, both early and late, has been recognized with increasing frequency (Table 57-7).[207-210]

TABLE 57-7 MAJOR CARDIOVASCULAR COMPLICATIONS OF CHEMOTHERAPEUTIC AGENTS

AGENT	CARDIAC TOXICITY
Amsacrine	Arrhythmia, cardiomyopathy
Busulfan	Pulmonary fibrosis
	Pulmonary hypertension
	Endocardial fibrosis
Cisplatin	ECG changes, vaso-occlusion
Cyclophosphamide	Cardiac necrosis, cardiomyopathy
Cytosine arabinoside	Congestive heart failure
	Pericarditis
Diethylstilbestrol	Cardiovascular deaths
Doxorubicin	ECG changes, cardiomyopathy
Etoposide	Myocardial infarction
5-Fluorouracil	Vaso-occlusion, myocarditis
Methotrexate	ECG changes
Mitomycin	Myocardial damage
Mitoxantrone	Cardiomyopathy
Vincristine	Hypotension

For many years, the only notable cardiopulmonary complications of chemotherapy for neoplastic disease were orthostatic hypotension and the rare myocardial infarctions that occurred in the course of therapy with vincristine, a periwinkle alkaloid, and the interstitial lung disease and mild pulmonary hypertension secondary to pulmonary fibrosis created by bleomycin or busulfan.[211] However, with the use of higher doses of conventional therapy for curative intent and the addition of the anthracycline group of drugs (doxorubicin, daunorubicin), the incidence of cardiac toxicity as a consequence of chemotherapy for neoplastic disease has increased greatly.

ANTHRACYCLINE CARDIOTOXICITY. Doxorubicin is a glycoside antibiotic (Fig. 57-15). Its potent antitumor effect is attributed to its ability to inhibit nucleic acid synthesis by binding to both strands of the DNA helix, intercalating between base pairs, and thereby inhibiting the normal function of DNA and RNA polymerases. Doxorubicin has received more attention than the related compound daunorubicin because of its wider spectrum of antitumor activity in solid tumors and hematological malignant disease.[212] Complete remissions in 30 to 40 per cent of patients with Hodgkin's disease and non-Hodgkin's lymphoma and all types of acute leukemia have been reported with doxorubicin treatment alone. However, its effectiveness is enhanced when it is combined with other chemotherapeutic agents. Remission rates of 60 to 80 per cent have been attained in adults with acute leukemia when doxorubicin was used in combination with cytosine arabinoside and in patients with lymphomas when it was combined with bleomycin, cyclophosphamide, vincristine, and corticosteroids.[212] Although the majority of toxic manifestations produced by these drugs, including alopecia, gastrointestinal distress, myelosuppression, and mucositis, had been predicted on the basis of animal studies, the occurrence of cardiac toxicity and the interactions with radiation therapy were unexpected. Anthracycline cardiotoxicity can be divided into early and late (Table 57-8).

TABLE 57-8 DOXORUBICIN CARDIAC TOXICITY

EARLY OR ACUTE
Arrhythmias
ECG changes
Left ventricular dysfunction
Pericarditis-myocarditis syndrome
Myocardial infarction
Sudden death

LATE OR CHRONIC
Cardiomyopathy
Sinus tachycardia
Pericardial effusion
Left ventricular dysfunction
Low-output heart failure

Modified from Kapoor, A. S.: Doxorubicin toxicity. In Kapoor, A. S. (ed.): Cancer and the Heart. New York, Springer-Verlag, 1986, p. 228.

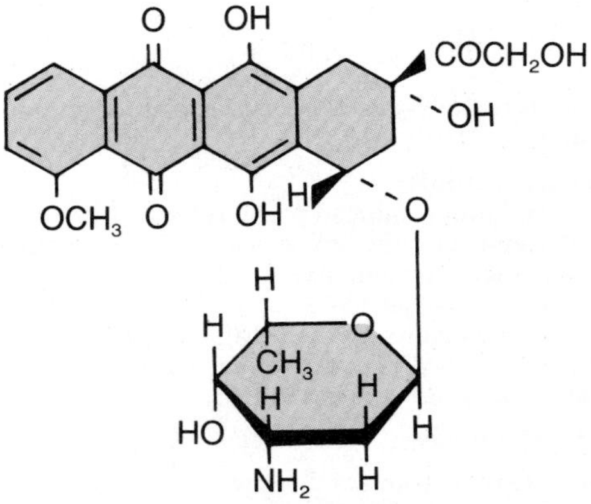

FIGURE 57-15. Structure of doxorubicin.

Early or Acute Cardiotoxicity. This includes arrhythmias, electrocardiographic abnormalities, left ventricular dysfunction, a pericarditis-myocarditis syndrome, and rarely sudden death and myocardial infarction. Arrhythmias, which include supraventricular tachyarrhythmias and premature atrial and ventricular contractions, and abnormalities of conduction such as left axis deviation, decreased QRS voltage, and a variety of nonspecific ST-segment and T-wave abnormalities occur in approximately 11 per cent of patients (range 0 to 41.2 per cent).[213,214] These electrocardiographic changes are usually transient, may occur even at low doses of the anthracycline, and are usually seen within several days after administration of the drug.

The pericarditis-myocarditis syndrome and acute left ventricular dysfunction are rare events. The latter may occur in patients with marginal cardiac reserve, while the acute pericarditis-myocarditis syndrome has been seen in patients with no previous cardiac history.[215] Sudden death may occur as a result of an arrhythmia, myocardial infarction, or acute left ventricular dysfunction.[216]

Late or Chronic Cardiotoxicity. This is primarily due to the development of a dose-dependent degenerative cardiomyopathy.[217] The clinical manifestations consist of sinus tachycardia, tachypnea, cardiomegaly, peripheral and pulmonary edema, hepatomegaly, venous congestion, and pleural effusion. Cardiomyopathy is usually secondary to a cumulative effect of the drug, occurring with increasing frequency at higher doses. Most commonly, congestive heart failure occurs from 9 to 192 days, with a median of 34 days, after the administration of the last dose. It is usually refractory to therapy; when it is severe, as in patients with marked dyspnea and with evidence of heart failure within 4 weeks of the last dose of doxorubicin, survival is short, usually less than 2 weeks.[217,218] The majority of patients with less severe symptoms may be treatable with digitalis and diuretics, but the incidence of cardiac death is high (Fig. 57-16).[217] With long-term follow-up of cancer survivors, there are many reports of congestive heart failure developing 6 to 10 years after doxorubicin therapy. Although in some cases the occurrence may be associated with other risk factors for heart failure, the development of symptoms in childhood survivors suggests a direct relationship with previous anthracycline therapy.[219-221]

Pathological Examination. In chronic anthracycline toxicity, the heart is enlarged, pale, and flabby, with dilated ventricles. Mural thrombi are occasionally found, but the coronary arteries and cardiac valves appear normal. Light microscopy reveals a severe cardiomyopathy with fewer myocardial cells, which show degenerative changes. Electron microscopy shows extensive depletion of myofibrillar bundles, myofibrillar lysis, and distortion and disruption of the Z lines; the mitochondria are swollen with disrupted cristae and inclusion bodies[214,218] (Fig. 57-17). There may be almost complete loss of contractile elements.[222] Routine autopsy studies on patients who had received anthracycline chemotherapy have revealed that clinical evidence of toxicity may be

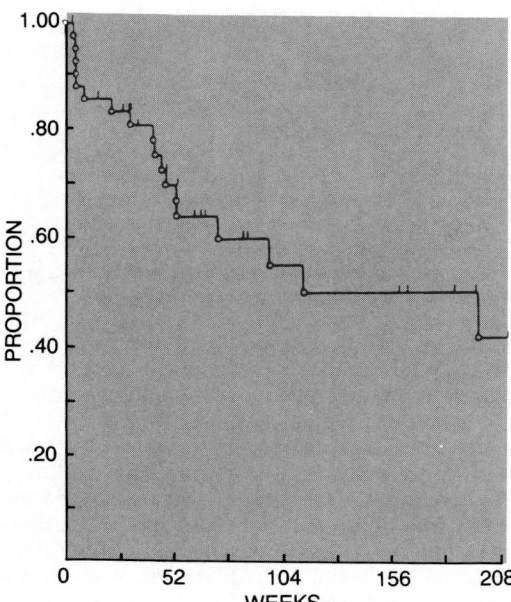

FIGURE 57–16. Actuarial survival plotted for all patients with doxorubicin-induced congestive heart failure. Eighteen patients died of congestive heart failure, 1 died from tumor, and 25 were alive. (From Haq, M. M., et al.: Doxorubicin-induced congestive heart failure in adults. Cancer 56:1361, 1985.)

culture model has been adapted to study the toxic mechanism.[235,236] Tumor cells and myocardial cells cultured in media containing anthracycline are similarly damaged.[237] Drug-exposed cells have decreased alpha-actin synthesis, which morphologically correlates with the disruption of the thin filaments and the Z lines and relates to poor contractility.[235]

Early Detection. Because of the importance of these drugs in cancer chemotherapy and the high incidence of serious cardiac toxicity, several approaches have been suggested for early detection of this complication and for predicting susceptibility.[238–241] Noninvasive studies include serial follow-up of systolic time intervals, in particular the pre-ejection period/left ventricular ejection time (PEP/LVET) ratio, and radionuclide angiogram (p. 297). The PEP/LVET ratio was at first thought to be a sensitive parameter for monitoring toxicity; however, this has not been confirmed on further study and, in fact, has been criticized, since false-positive changes may have been responsible for the inappropriate withholding of potentially life-saving doxorubicin therapy.[242] Radionuclide angiography appears to provide a sensitive and reproducible measurement of left ventricular dysfunction due to

present without histological signs; conversely, histological signs of drug toxicity may be seen in the absence of a history of clinical manifestations.[223]

Incidence. The incidence of cardiomyopathy with doxorubicin is 1.7 per cent and with daunorubicin 4.4 per cent. It is fatal in over half the cases.[213] With anthracycline, there is a clear dose-related incidence of cardiomyopathy. None of 764 patients who received a cumulative dose of less than 500 mg/m² showed cardiomyopathy, but a progressive increase in the frequency of this complication was noted with higher doses (Table 57–9).[218] It is therefore recommended that cumulative doses of doxorubicin be held to less than 450 to 500 mg/m² and 500 to 600 mg/m² for daunorubicin. However, cardiomyopathy is being reported with increasing frequency with doxorubicin doses below 450 mg/m².[214,218,224] It has been suggested that use of these agents in combination with other modalities of therapy, such as radiation or cyclophosphamide, may be synergistic in the pathogenesis of the cardiomyopathy in some patients, since both radiation and cyclophosphamide alone have been described as potentially cardiotoxic.[206,244–227]

Mechanism. No mechanism for doxorubicin cardiotoxicity has been established, although numerous proposals have been put forward.[228,228a,229] For example, lipid peroxidation may be caused by the binding of DNA by the drug, specifically bound to spectrin, actin, or cardiolipin.[230] Doxorubicin inhibits ATP production, interferes with the sarcolemmal sodium-potassium pump, inhibits oxidative phosphorylation, may provoke an autoimmune response, binds to DNA precursors, interferes with mitochondrial respiration by inhibiting coenzyme Q, and causes myocardial necrosis by allowing the buildup of myocardial calcium.[231–234] A rat myocardial cell

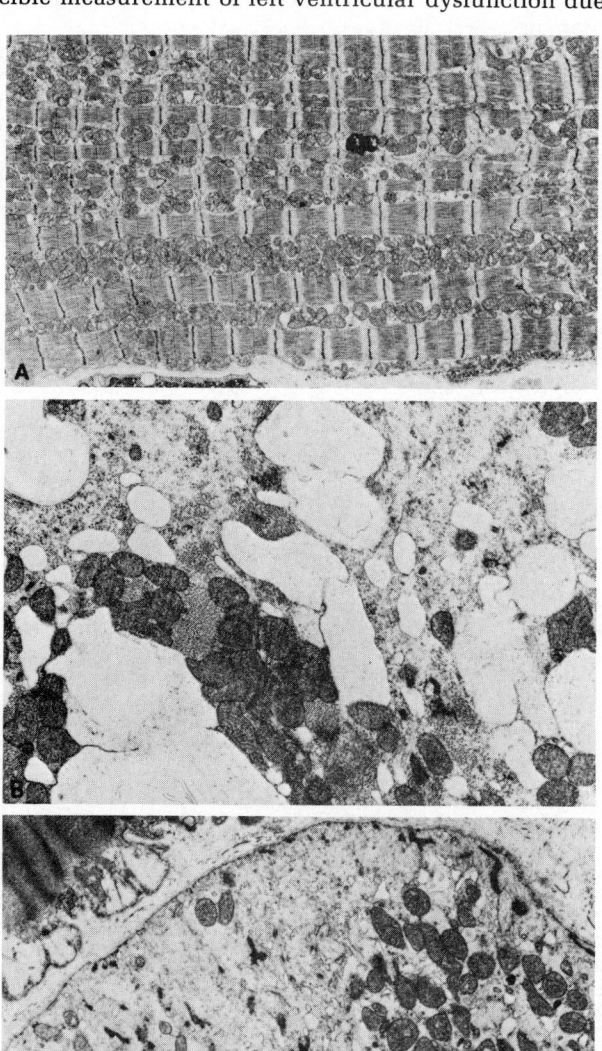

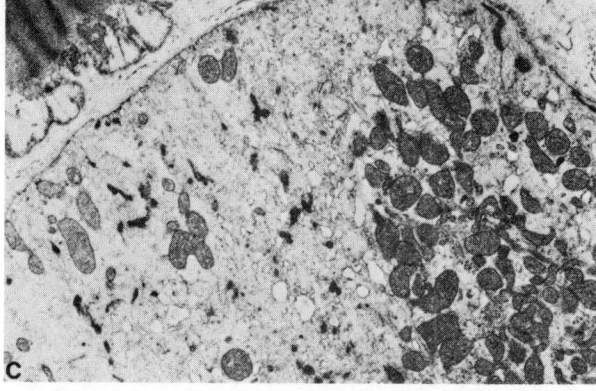

FIGURE 57–17. Electron microscopic images of cardiac biopsy specimens. A, Normal cardiac muscle fiber (grade O). B, Vacuolation. C, Myofibrillar dropout (×3,575). (From Ali, M. D., and Ewer, M. S.: Cancer and the Cardiopulmonary System. New York, Raven Press, 1984, pp. 62 and 63.)

TABLE 57–9   CORRELATION OF CARDIOMYOPATHY (CMY) AND THE TOTAL DOSE OF DOXORUBICIN IN ADULTS

TOTAL DOSE (mg/m²)	PATIENTS AT RISK	PATIENTS WITH CMY	FREQUENCY (%)
<450	738	0	0
451 to 500	26	0	0
501 to 550	32	3	9
551 to 600	15	3	20
>600	37	15	41
1 Total			
>550	52	18	35
Total <550	796	3	0.4

doxorubicin cardiotoxicity.[240,241,243] Sequential studies demonstrate the frequent presence of subclinical left ventricular abnormalities. However, the increased incidence of abnormal results may not be clinically significant if the studies are performed after exercise. Since left ventricular diastolic function can occur before systolic dysfunction, both measurements may be necessary.[241,243,244]

Endomyocardial biopsy appears to be more diagnostic of toxicity than are any of the noninvasive evaluations. In the hands of trained personnel, this technique may be considered a safe procedure[245] (p. 199). Administration of doxorubicin was associated with a dose-related increase in the degree of myocyte damage; drug-associated degenerative changes were identified in 27 of 129 patients at doses greater than or equal to 240 mg/m². Simultaneous studies using endomyocardial biopsy and radionuclide angiography demonstrate good correlation; while the noninvasive studies reveal an accelerating decrease in myocardial function with drug levels exceeding 400 mg/m², biopsy studies show a fairly constant progression of myocardial damage as a function of cumulative dose.[246] These findings suggest that compensatory mechanisms are available to maintain myocardial function despite pathological damage.

It is helpful to grade the hemodynamic abnormalities that occur in patients undergoing doxorubicin chemotherapy[247,248] (Table 57–10). Cardiac monitoring has demonstrated a reduction in the severity and mortality of doxorubicin-associated cardiac failure. Unfortunately, endomyocardial biopsy is invasive and moderately expensive. It has been suggested that different strategies be devised for patients at high risk for car-

TABLE 57–11 RISK FACTORS FOR DEVELOPMENT OF DOXORUBICIN CARDIOTOXICITY

Cumulative dose (> 550 mg/m²)
Age extremes
Prior history of cardiac disease
Hypertension
Coronary artery disease
Valvular disorders
Metastatic pericardial or myocardial disease
Prior mediastinal irradiation
Coexistent chemotherapy with alkylating agents
Hypoxic

diotoxicity. Risk factors for the development of drug cardiotoxicity are shown in Table 57–11.[222,224,249–252]

On the basis of large retrospective analyses of high-risk and normal-risk individuals treated with anthracyclines, guidelines have been recommended as to when to discontinue the drug without any acute or late consequences. Guidelines include radionuclide angiocardiography alone[253] (Table 57–12) or radionuclide studies plus the histopathological findings of an endomyocardial biopsy[222] (Table 57–13).

Prevention. The best management of anthracycline cardiac toxicity is prevention by limiting dosage. However, several possibilities for preventing doxorubicin-induced cardiotoxicity have been suggested. The use of free-radical scavengers (vitamin E),[231] ICRF-187 (a bispiperazine[232–234]), sulfhydryl compounds,[254] coenzyme Q10 (a mitochondrial quinone),[255] cardiac glycosides,[256] calcium-channel antagonists,[257] doxorubicin bound to liposomes,[258,259] and histaminergic and adrenergic blockade have all been reported to lessen cardiac toxicity; prospective studies to determine the efficacy of these interventions are now in progress. Lowering the peak blood levels of the drug appears to offer the best means of reducing cardiac toxicity. In a controlled study monitoring cardiac toxicity by both noninvasive techniques and endomyocardial biopsy, drug-related damage was significantly reduced but not eliminated when the drug was administered by prolonged continuous intravenous infusion rather than by bolus injection; the reduction in toxicity clearly appears to be related to reduced peak plasma levels.[260–262] Similarly, lower dosages given more frequently reduce peak plasma levels and seem to lower the incidence of cardiac toxicity.[263] Antitumor activity does not appear to be compromised by altering the technique of administration in these ways.[260]

Another approach to this problem has been the develop-

TABLE 57–10 HEMODYNAMIC GRADING OF PATIENTS UNDERGOING DOXORUBICIN CHEMOTHERAPY

GRADE	HEMODYNAMIC FINDINGS
0 Normal	Mean RA <7 mm Hg RVEDP <8 mm Hg LVEDP/Mean PAW <12 mm Hg Cardiac index >2.5 L/min/m² Exercise factor >5.0
1 Mildly abnormal	Any of the following: Mean RA = 7 to 10 mm Hg RVEDP = 8 to 12 mm Hg at rest with increase on exercise = 5 to 9 mm Hg LVEDP/Mean PAW = 12 to 15 mm Hg at rest with increase on exercise = 5 to 11 mm Hg Cardiac index = 2.2 to 2.5 L/min/m² Exercise factor = 4.0 to 5.0
2 Moderately abnormal	Any of the following: Two or more grade 1 features Mean RA = 10 to 15 mm Hg RVEDP = 12 to 17 mm Hg at rest with increase on exercise ≥9 mm Hg Cardiac index = 1.8 to 2.2 L/min/m² Exercise factor <4.0
3 Severely abnormal	Any of the following: Two or more grade 2 features Mean RA ≥16 mm Hg RVEDP ≥19 mm Hg LVEDP/Mean PAW ≥20 mm Hg Cardiac index <1.8 L/min/m²

RA = right atrium; RVEDP and LVEDP = right and left end-diastolic pressure, respectively; PAW = pulmonary artery wedge pressure. Abnormal cardiac index is accompanied by elevated AV oxygen content difference (>5 vol%). Exercise factor = increase in cardiac output (ml/min)/increase in total body oxygen consumption.

From Bristow, M. R., et al.: Efficacy and the cost of cardiac monitoring in patients receiving doxorubicin. Cancer 50:32, 1982.

TABLE 57–12 GUIDELINES FOR MONITORING PATIENTS RECEIVING DOXORUBICIN

Perform baseline radionuclide angiocardiography at rest for calculation of left ventricular ejection fraction (LVEF) prior to administration of 100 mg/m² doxorubicin. Subsequent studies are performed at least 3 wk. after the indicated total cumulative doses have been given, before consideration of the next dose

PATIENTS WITH NORMAL BASELINE LVEF (≥50%)
Perform the second study after 250 to 300 mg/m².
Repeat study after 400 mg/m² in patients with known heart disease, radiation exposure, abnormal ECG results, or cyclophosphamide therapy, or after 450 mg/m² in the absence of any of these risk factors.
Perform sequential studies thereafter prior to each dose.
Discontinue doxorubicin therapy once functional criteria for cardiotoxicity develop, i.e., absolute decrease in LVEF ≥10% (EF units) associated with a decline to a level ≤50% (EF units).

PATIENTS WITH ABNORMAL BASELINE LVEF (<50%)
Doxorubicin therapy should not be initiated with baseline LVEF ≤30%.
In patients with LVEF >30% and <50%, sequential studies should be obtained prior to each dose.
Discontinue doxorubicin with cardiotoxicity: absolute decrease in LVEF ≥10% (EF units) and/or final LVEF ≤30%.

TABLE 57–13 SEMIQUANTITATIVE SCALE OF BIOPSY-DETERMINED ANTHRACYCLINE MYOCARDIAL DAMAGE

BIOPSY GRADE	HISTOPATHOLOGICAL FEATURES
0	No detectable change from normal
1	Scant number of cells (≤5%) showing distended sarcoplasmic reticulum and/or early myofibrillar loss
1.5	Small numbers of cells (5 to 15%), some showing definite cytoplasmic vacuolization and/or myofibrillar loss
2	Groups of cells (16 to 25%), some showing definite cytoplasmic vacuolization and/or myofibrillar loss. Biopsy grades up to 2 carry <10% risk of heart failure with 100 mg/m² incremental dose of doxorubicin
2.5	Groups of cells (26 to 35%), some showing definite cytoplasmic vacuolization and/or marked myofibrillar loss. Biopsy grade of 2.5 carries a 10 to 25% risk of heart failure with 100 mg/m² incremental dose of doxorubicin
3	Diffuse cell injury (>35%) showing advanced loss of organelles, total loss of myofibrils, and mitochondrial and nuclear degeneration. Biopsy grade 3 is associated with >25% risk of heart failure if more doxorubicin is given

From Fowles, R. E.: Cardiac catheterization and endomyocardial biopsy. *In* Kapoor, A. S. (ed.): Cancer and the Heart. New York, Springer-Verlag, 1986, p. 48.

ment of anthracycline analogs that retain their antitumor effect but do not cause cardiac toxicity. However, most agents that have been studied, such as epirubicin, 4-demethyl-6-demethyl-doxorubicin, rubidazone, and aclacinomycin, continue to show toxicity, either clinically or in animal models.[264,264a] To date, more than 16 such analogs have been described. The 4'-substituted derivatives, i.e., 4'-epi-adriamycin (epirubicin), 4'-deoxydoxorubicin, 4'-deoxy-u'-iodo-doxorubicin (idarubicin), and other analogs have been associated with decreased histological abnormalities in animal models but turn out to have decreased antitumor effect.[265-270]

CHEMOTHERAPY AND VASO-OCCLUSION. Vaso-occlusive complications, including acute myocardial infarction, often occur in patients with malignant tumors. There is increasing suspicion that chemotherapeutic agents such as 5-fluorouracil[271-274] may be the sole precipitating factor in a small but significant percentage of cases. Ischemic coronary complications have also been reported after treatment with cisplatinum,[275,276] bleomycin,[277] and vinca alkaloids,[278-280] such as vincristine, vinblastine, and VP-16-213 (etoposide). Acute endothelial injury, vasospasm and/or autonomic dysfunction, hypomagnesemia, autoimmune response, increases in platelet aggregability and a synergistic effect of irradiation to the heart are all possible mechanisms.

CYCLOPHOSPHAMIDE. As noted in Table 57–7, cardiomyopathies have been reported secondary to high doses of intravenous cyclophosphamide.[227,267-269] In contrast to doxorubicin, the cardiotoxicity of cyclophosphamide is acute and not due to cumulative doses. It causes reductions in ECG voltage and systolic function and an increase in myocardial mass, presumably secondary to edema. Cyclophosphamide may also cause acute pericarditis. A prior history of heart failure and a pretreatment ejection fraction less than 50 per cent correlate with clinical cardiotoxicity. Although mortality is appreciable, survivors exhibit no residual cardiac abnormalities.[281] Ifosfamide, an active compound related to cyclophosphamide, may also cause cardiac side effects in the form of supraventricular arrhythmias and ST-T wave changes.[282]

OTHER ANTINEOPLASTIC AGENTS. *Amsacrine* (AMSA) has been associated with acute cardiac arrhythmias and cardiomyopathy. Although AMSA-related cardiac events are frequent, they are less common than those due to doxorubicin. Manifestations of toxicity include ECG abnormalities, sudden death, and congestive heart failure. Hypokalemia appears to be a risk factor for the development of severe arrhythmias with this agent.[250,283-285] The anthraquinones, mitoxantrone and nonvantrone, are a new group of antineoplastic agents with significant clinical activity.[286] They have been shown to produce favorable results in leukemias as well as in advanced breast cancer. Deterioration in ejection fraction and congestive heart failure have been reported.[287-289] The anthraquinones are being compared in a randomized fashion with the anthracyclines in terms of both therapeutic efficacy and incidence of cardiac toxicity.[290]

5-Fluorouracil has been reported to cause angina pectoris and other manifestations of myocardial ischemia, presumably secondary to coronary vasospasm.[291,291a] Supportive therapy given to cancer patients may also be cardiotoxic when combined with chemotherapeutic agents. Lithium, which is occasionally used to increase the white blood cell count so that more therapy can be given, has been associated with sudden death in patients who are simultaneously receiving combination chemotherapy that includes an anthracycline agent.[250] In addition, antiemetic drugs such as domperidone have been associated with cardiac arrhythmias and cardiac arrest in several patients receiving antineoplastic agents.[292,293] As new antineoplastic agents are brought to trial, lessons learned in the evaluation of cardiac toxicity with doxorubicin are likely to prove helpful.

Bone marrow transplantation, either allogeneic or autolo-

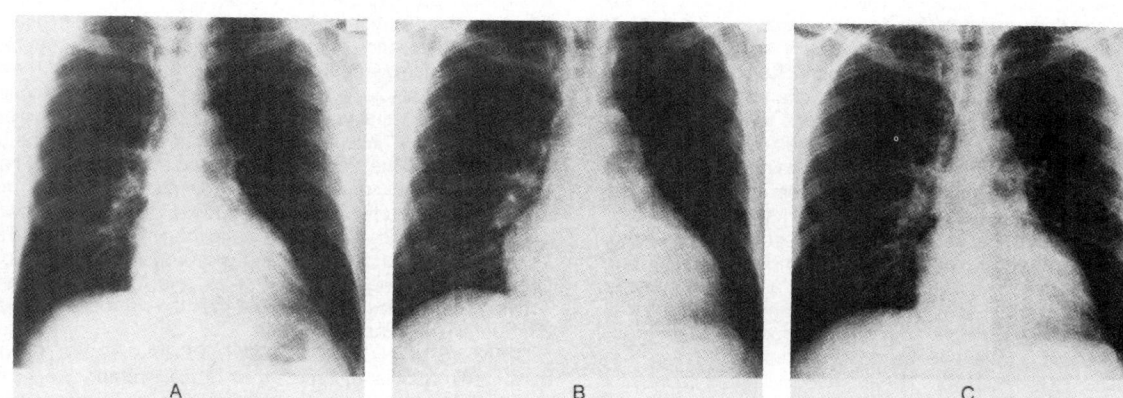

FIGURE 57–18. *A* shows a base-line chest radiograph before treatment, *B* the development of congestive cardiomyopathy during interferon alpha therapy, and *C* its subsequent resolution after the drug was discontinued. The increased cardiac silhouette was shown on echocardiography to be due to left ventricular enlargement and a moderate pericardial effusion.

gous, involves the combination of large doses of whole-body irradiation therapy with high-dose chemotherapy. Cardiac complications are frequent during these transplant procedures and may be an important factor in limiting the success rate.[294] Fatal cardiomyopathies, pericarditis, and significant arrhythmias are not infrequent. High-dose cyclophosphamide and cytosine arabinoside are commonly associated with cardiotoxicity. In addition, the effect of whole-heart irradiation in conjunction with anthracycline drugs and cyclophosphamide appears to be additive.

Hematopoietic growth factors and cytokines are leukocyte/lymphocyte-derived glycoproteins that are antiviral, immunomodulating, and antiproliferative as well as cell-specific stimulative. The glycoproteins of the interferon and interleukin family have become potential agents in treating many refractory cancers. Interferon alpha is effective against hairy cell leukemia, chronic myelogenous leukemia, and condyloma acuminatum and also is approved for use in treating Kaposi's sarcoma. In high doses, interferon can cause a severe congestive cardiomyopathy with severe myocardial dysfunc-

tion, usually reversible with discontinuation of the agents (Fig. 57–18).[295,296]

Recombinant interleukin-2 (rIl-2) used in association with lymphokine-activated killer (LAK) cells can cause significant tumor destruction in renal cell cancer and malignant melanoma. Eight to thirty per cent of the patients experience myocardial ischemia during or immediately after this infusional therapy. Most affected patients had no or minimal cardiac risk factors, and several cardiac deaths have been directly related to the therapy.[297–301] Despite vasopressor support during the therapy, there has been evidence of reduced left ventricular stroke work and decreased cardiac contractility.[300] Although radionuclide ventriculography and echocardiography may suggest a localized wall motion disorder, no coronary arterial abnormalities have been reported, raising the question of toxic myocarditis or a peripheral vascular effect and not endovascular injury.[301,302] Patients need to be closely monitored while receiving these experimental therapies and the infusions immediately discontinued when any clinical cardiac or electrocardiographic abnormality occurs.

Hematological Abnormalities Related to Cardiac Drugs

Blood dyscrasias are frequent complications of drugs used to treat cardiac disorders. The development of unexplained anemia, leukopenia or thrombocytopenia in a patient receiving a diuretic, antihypertensive, or antiarrhythmic agent should immediately raise the suspicion that a drug used in the treatment of cardiac disease might be responsible.

Many different types of blood dyscrasias occur secondary to drug ingestion. The anemias may be of the aplastic, hemolytic, megaloblastic, or sideroblastic type; other disorders may include granulocytopenia and agranulocytosis, thrombocytopenia, thrombocytosis, defects of platelet function, and a variety of miscellaneous disorders (Table 57–14). Underlying mechanisms include suppression of one or more of the three cellular elements in the bone marrow as well as a variety of immune phenomena with increased peripheral destruction of the formed elements. The drug effect may be dose related or idiosyncratic.

APLASTIC ANEMIA. Many chemical agents are capable of suppressing marrow function and producing hypoplasia or aplasia. Chloramphenicol, benzene, cytostatic agents used in the treatment of malignant disease, and phenylbutazone are the drugs most commonly implicated. Less frequently involved, and perhaps less well documented, are antibiotics such as sulfonamides, hypoglycemic agents, and insecticides. Among drugs used to treat cardiovascular disease, the antiarrhythmic agent phenytoin (p. 641), the diuretic agent acetazolamide, and the angiotensin-converting enzyme inhibitor captopril[303] (p. 867) have been reported, on rare occasion, to lead to such reactions. The onset of aplastic anemia is usually insidious, and the symptoms are directly related to the degree of pancytopenia. If the causative agent is immediately discontinued upon detection of the blood dyscrasia, the latter can often be reversed.

MEGALOBLASTIC ANEMIA. A pancytopenia characterized by macrocytic red cells due to impairment of DNA synthesis may be caused by vitamin B_{12} or folate deficiency or by purine and pyrimidine inhibitors. Most commonly, drugs cause megaloblastic anemia by impairing the absorption of folic acid or acting as folate antagonists. Phenytoin (p. 632), oral contraceptives, and a variety of other drugs can impair folate absorption by interfering with the liver conjugases needed to break down the polyglutamate structure of naturally occurring folates to the monoglutamate form appropriate for absorption by the gastrointestinal tract. Triamterene, a potassium-sparing diuretic (p. 474), is a pteridine analog that exhibits antifolate activity, similar to aminopterin, in vitro. Its propensity to produce a megaloblastic anemia appears to be dose related.

IMMUNOHEMOLYTIC ANEMIAS. There are four different causes for the development of a positive direct Coombs or antiglobulin test, two of which involve cardiac medications: the first mechanism, which is uncommon, involves some drugs that bind to plasma protein and thereby become antigenic, including quinidine and the sulfonamides. The resultant antigen-antibody complex may deposit on the red cell surface and cause

agglutinability by anticomplement sera. Hemolysis may be severe, but rapid improvement follows withdrawal of the drug.

The second type of reaction that results in a positive Coombs' test involves the antihypertensive drug alpha-methyldopa[304] (p. 863). The mechanism of antibody formation is unknown, but presumably antibody induced by alpha-methyldopa has an affinity for the Rh locus of the red cell, similar to that of IgG antibodies in idiopathic immunohemolytic anemia. The frequency of positive results on Coombs' test varies from 11 per cent for patients who are receiving 0.75 gm per day for over 3 months to 40 per cent for those receiving 2 gm per day for the same time. Fortunately, the affinity of the alpha-methyldopa antibody for red cells is low, and fewer than 1 per cent of patients whose antiglobulin test is positive will manifest significant hemolytic anemia. Nonetheless, alpha-methyldopa surpasses all other drugs in causing immunohemolytic anemia. On withdrawal of the drug, hemolysis improves within 1 or 2 weeks, with full recovery in 1 month, although the positive Coombs' test may persist for 6 to 24 months. A positive Coombs' test without hemolysis is not an indication to discontinue alpha-methyldopa if its administration is otherwise indicated in the treatment of hypertension.

The other two mechanisms of drug-related positive antiglobulin reactions do not involve cardiovascular drugs. The third is represented by penicillin, in which the drug binds to the red cell membranes, creating a cell-drug complex and antigenic stimulation of an IgG antibody. The fourth mechanism involves cephalothin, which is bound to the red cell membrane; normal serum proteins adhere nonspecifically to red cell membranes.

GRANULOCYTOPENIA AND AGRANULOCYTOSIS. A reduction in circulating neutrophils is the most toxic hematological effect of drugs. It may be secondary to depression of the marrow, or it may be an immune mechanism causing peripheral destruction. When there is immune suppression, examination of the marrow reveals active myeloid precursors, whereas the absence of myeloid elements suggests suppression of synthesis. The marrow-depressive effect is dose related.[305] Anticoagulants such as phenindione, antiarrhythmics such as procainamide and tocainide,[306–308] antihypertensives such as captopril, and diuretics such as the thiazides have all been reported to produce granulocytopenia. Procainamide is the most dangerous and most frequently implicated cardiac drug in granulocytopenia.[309] Presenting symptoms may include a sore throat, ulcerations of mucous membranes, fever, malaise, fatigue, and weakness. Discontinuation of the drug may be followed by a rebound in the white blood cell count and occasionally a leukemoid picture. Because laboratory tests are not conclusive for white cell antibodies, an accurate definition of the immune mechanism responsible for white cell destruction remains unclear.

DRUG-INDUCED THROMBOCYTOPENIA. Many of the drugs used to treat cardiovascular disorders may cause thrombocytopenia, either by a direct effect on the bone marrow or by inducing formation of drug-specific antibody.[310] For example, the thiazide diuretics (p. 860) directly suppress megakaryocyte production. Thiazide-induced thrombocytopenia is usually mild, with the platelet count rarely falling below $50,000/\mu l$. This condition is unique, since it persists for 6 to 8 weeks after drug withdrawal.

TABLE 57–14 BLOOD DYSCRASIAS ASSOCIATED WITH CARDIAC MEDICATIONS

	ANEMIA			NEUTROPENIA	THROMBOCYTOPENIA	OTHER
	Aplastic	Megaloblastic	Hemolytic			
Antiarrhythmics						
Digitoxin	–	–	–	–	+	L
Phenytoin	+	+	–	+	+	L,P
Procainamide	–	–	–	+(A)	–	–
Propranolol	–	–	–	+	–	–
Quinidine	–	–	+	+	+	–
Tocainide	+	–	–	+(A)	–	–
Moricizine	–	–	–	–	+	–
Propafenone	–	–	–	+(A)	–	–
Anticoagulants						
Heparin	+*	–	–	–	+	–
Phenindione	–	–	–	+	–	–
Antihypertensives						
Captopril	+	–	–	+	+	–
Glutethimide	+*	–	–.	–	–	P
Hydralazine	–	–	–	–	+	L
Methyldopa	–	–	+	+	+	P
Reserpine	–	–	–	–	+	–
Diuretics						
Acetazolamide	+	–	–	+	+	–
Chlorothiazide	–	–	–	+	+	–
Chlorthalidone	–	–	–	+	+	–
Diazoxide	–	–	–	–	+	–
Ethacrynic acid	–	–	–	+	–	–
Hydrochlorothiazide	–	–	–	+	–	–
Mercurials	–	–	–	+	+	–
Spironolactone	–	–	–	+	+	–
Triamterene	–	+	–	–	–	–
Coronary dilators						
Amyl nitrite	–	–	–	–	–	M
Nitroglycerin	–	–	–	–	–	M
Other						
Amrinone	–	–	–	–	+	–

* Pure red cell aplasia.
L = lupus-like syndrome; P = porphyria; A = agranulocytosis; M = methemoglobinemia.

Thrombocytopenia caused by amrinone, a positive inotropic agent with vasodilator properties (p. 503), is less well studied but is clearly related to the total dose of drug administered and to peripheral destruction of platelets.[311] Other common agents like alcohol and some estrogen preparations may cause thrombocytopenia by a direct depressant effect on the bone marrow. Shortened platelet survival secondary to antibody or complement binding to platelets can cause severe thrombocytopenia and life-threatening hemorrhage. The onset is abrupt and is not related to the dose of medication or the duration of its use. In most cases of immunological thrombocytopenia, the offending agent induces a specific antibody. The resulting drug-antibody complex then binds to the platelet, thereby shortening its survival. Quinidine, one of the first cardiac drugs to produce this response, has been well studied as a cause of thrombocytopenia. The defect can be transferred to a normal individual by administering serum from a patient with quinidine-induced thrombocytopenia, followed by a quinidine challenge to the normal subject.[312] A similar defect can be caused by antibodies to quinine, including the small quantities present in tonic drinks. Acetaminophen (a common analgesic given to cardiac patients), acetazolamide, digitoxin, phenytoin, ethacrynic acid, alpha-methyldopa, and spironolactone have all been implicated in various cases of suspected drug-induced thrombocytopenia, although the mechanism has not always been well defined.

Although in vitro laboratory tests for drug-dependent platelet antibody are available, the results do not always correlate with clinical events. The best proof of drug-induced thrombocytopenia is prompt recovery of the platelet count after drug withdrawal followed by a second episode of thrombocytopenia upon readministration of the suspected drug. (Because of this potential hazard, the drug challenge is not advised.) If serious hemorrhage persists after the drug is withdrawn, treatment with 1 mg/kg prednisone or its equivalent may be necessary. Corticosteroids may hasten the return of a normal platelet count and may also protect capillaries and small vessels even without altering the platelet count. Platelet transfusions are not usually helpful but can be tried in desparate situations in which hemorrhage is life threatening. They are most useful if thrombocy-topenia persists well after the drug-antibody complex has been cleared. In this situation, a gratifying elevation in platelet count sometimes occurs.

Heparin. Treatment with this drug is one of the most important causes of thrombocytopenia in cardiac patients (p. 1780). The incidence varies from 5 to 25 per cent among patients receiving heparin; it is more common in those given heparin derived from beef lung and has been associated with all modes and doses of heparin administration.[313] Heparin has a direct platelet-aggregating effect that may contribute to thrombocytopenia. This property is most marked in those fractions with the highest molecular weight and the lowest affinity for antithrombin. There is an increase in platelet-associated immunoglobulin in many of the cases, suggesting an immune etiology. However, the nature of the offending antigen in heparin and its relationship to the biologically active heparin fractions remain unclear. In addition, some patients with heparin-induced thrombocytopenia develop paradoxical thrombosis and disseminated intravascular coagulation. The development of thromboembolism in association with thrombocytopenia is unique to heparin.

OTHER HEMATOLOGICAL ABNORMALITIES CAUSED BY CARDIAC DRUGS. Amyl nitrite, sodium nitrite, and nitroglycerin can oxidize hemoglobin to methemoglobin, which cannot effectively carry oxygen. The patient with methemoglobinemia appears cyanotic but has a normal arterial PO_2, and oxygen therapy will not improve the pallor. Although symptomatic methemoglobinemia may occur in adults, most cases are seen in children who accidentally ingest medications prescribed for adults. Occasionally, adults with mild congenital methemoglobinemia will become markedly symptomatic when exposed to small doses of these same medications. With the increasing use of intravenous nitroglycerin, this complication may become more frequent.[314] If venous blood is chocolate brown and this color persists after the blood is shaken in air, the diagnosis of methemoglobinemia is almost certain. The diagnosis is confirmed by the addition of a few drops of 10 per cent potassium cyanide, which results in the rapid production of the bright red cyanmethemoglobin. Symptoms are nonspecific and consist of dyspnea, headache, fatigue, and dizziness. They are usually self-limited if the responsible drugs are discontinued, since normal red cells can enzymatically reduce the methemoglobin. In severe cases or in patients with enzyme defects, methylene blue may be administered to stimulate reduction of the methemoglobin.

Other medications may interfere with oxygen delivery to tissues. For example, sodium nitroprusside used to treat hypertensive emergencies and to reduce afterload in the management of heart failure may cause fatigue, nausea, abnormal behavior, and muscle spasm as the agent reacts with oxyhemoglobin, producing cyanmethemoglobin and free cyanide ions.[315]

Hydralazine (p. 1051), procainamide (p. 630), and rarely phenytoin (p. 641) can cause a lupus erythematosus-like syndrome, with urticaria, erythema multiforme, photosensitivity, delirium, and immune-mediated blood cell destruction.[316] Although patients with drug-induced lupus have positive antinuclear antibody tests and many of the clinical manifestations of the systemic form, renal function is not usually impaired, and all these manifestations usually remit within several months if the drugs are discontinued. The syndrome is of particular importance in cardiac patients, since the onset of chest pain, pleurisy, or pericardial effusion in the patient with heart disease could lead to an erroneous diagnosis unless drug-induced lupus is suspected.

REFERENCES

ANEMIA AND CARDIOVASCULAR DISORDERS

1. Graettinger, J. S., Parsons, R. L., and Campbell, J. A.: A correlation of clinical and hemodynamic studies in patients with mild and severe anemia with and without congestive heart failure. Ann. Intern. Med. 58:617, 1963.
2. Ali, M. K., and Ewer, M. S.: Cancer and the cardiopulmonary system. New York, Raven Press, 1984, p. 242.
3. Datta, B. N., and Silver, M. D.: Cardiomegaly in chronic anemia in rats; an experimental study including ultrastructural, histometric and stereological observations. Lab. Invest. 2:503, 1975.
4. Eckstein, R. W.: Development of interarterial coronary anastomoses by chronic anemia. Disappearance following correction of anemia. Circ. Res. 3:306, 1955.
5. Reichek, N., Wilson, J., Sutton, M. S., et al.: Noninvasive determination of left ventricular end systolic stress: Validation of the method and initial application. Circulation 65:99, 1982.
6. Rossi, M. A., Carillo, S. V., and Oliveria, J.S.M.: The effect of iron deficiency anemia in the rat on catecholamine levels and heart morphology. Cardiovasc. Res. 15:313, 1981.
7. Florenzano, F., Diaz, G., Regonesi, C., and Escobar, E.: Left ventricular function in chronic anemia: Evidence of noncatecholamine positive inotropic factor in the serum. Am. J. Cardiol. 54:638, 1984.
8. Duke, M., and Abelmann, W. H.: The hemodynamic response to chronic anemia. Circulation 39:503, 1969.
9. Varat, M. A., Adolph, R. J., and Fowler, N. O.: Cardiovascular effects of anemia. Am. Heart J. 83:415, 1972.
10. Torrance, J. D., Jacobs, P., Restrepo, A., et al.: Intraerythrocyte adaptation to anemia. N. Engl. J. Med. 283:165, 1970.
11. Baer, R. W., Vlahakes, G. J., Uhlig, P. N., and Hoffman, I. E.: Maximum myocardial oxygen transport during anemia and polycythemia in dogs. Am. J. Physiol. 252:H1086, 1987.
12. Oski, F. A., Marshall, B. D., Cohen, P. J., et al.: Exercise with anemia. The role of the left or right shifted oxygen-hemoglobin equilibrium curve. Ann. Intern. Med. 74:44, 1971.
13. Lenfant, C., Torrance, J., English, E., et al.: Effect of altitude on the oxygen binding by hemoglobin and on organic phosphate levels. J. Clin. Invest. 47:2652, 1968.
14. Oski, F. A., Gottlieb, A. J., Delivoria-Papadopoulos, M., and Miller, W. W.: Red-cell 2,3-diphosphoglycerate levels in subjects with chronic hypoxemia. N. Engl. J. Med. 280:1165, 1969.
15. Hunter, A.: The heart in anemia. Q. J. Med. 15:107, 1946.
16. Harris, T. N., Friedman, S., Tuncali, M. T., and Hallidie-Smith, K. A.: Comparison of innocent murmur of childhood with cardiac murmurs in high output states. Pediatrics 33:341, 1964.
17. Varriale, P., Kwa, R. P., and Vyas, P.: Intravenous nitroglycerin in transfusion therapy for severe anemia. Association with congestive heart failure. Arch. Intern. Med. 144:401, 1984.
18. Bunn, H. F.: Disorders of hemoglobin. In Wilson, J., and Braunwald E. et al. (eds.): Harrison's Principles of Internal Medicine, 12th ed. New York, McGraw-Hill, 1991, pp. 1543–1552.
19. Denenberg, B. S., Criner, G., Jones, R., and Spann, J. F.: Cardiac function in sickle cell anemia. Am. J. Cardiol. 51:1674, 1983.
20. Falk, R. H., and Hood, W. B.: The heart in sickle cell anemia. Arch. Intern. Med. 142:1680, 1982.
21. Simmons, B. E., Santhanam, V., Castaner, A., et al.: Sickle cell heart disease. Two dimensional echo and doppler ultrasonographic findings in the hearts of adult patients with sickle cell anemia. Arch. Intern. Med. 148:1526, 1988.
22. Miller, G. J., Serjeant, G. R., Sivapragasam, S., and Petch, M.: Cardiopulmonary responses and gas exchange during exercise in adults with homozygous sickle cell disease. Clin. Sci. 44:113, 1973.
23. Sharache, S., Scott, J. C., and Sharache, P.: "Acute chest syndrome" in adults with sickle cell disease: Microbiology, treatment and prevention. Arch. Intern. Med. 139:67, 1979.
24. Shubin, H., Kaufmann, R., Shapiro, M., and Levinson, D. C.: Cardiovascular findings in children with sickle cell anemia. Am. J. Cardiol. 6:875, 1960.
25. Gaffney, J. W., Bierman, F. Z., Donnelly, C. M., et al.: Cardiovascular adaptation to transfusion/chelation therapy of homozygote sickle cell anemia. Am. J. Cardiol. 62:121, 1988.
26. Estrade, G., Pointrineau, D., Bernasconi, F., et al.: Left ventricular function and sickle-cell anemia. Echocardiographic Study. Arch. Mal. Coeur 82:1975, 1989.
27. Perrine, R. P., Pembrey, M. E., John, P., et al.: Natural history of sickle cell anemia in Saudi Arabs: A study of 270 subjects. Ann. Intern. Med. 88:1, 1978.
28. Gerry, J. L., Bulkley, B. H., and Hutchins, G. M.: Clinicopathologic analysis of cardiac dysfunction in 52 patients with sickle cell anemia. Am. J. Cardiol. 42:211, 1978.
29. Barrett, O., Saunders, D. E., McFarlend, D. E., and Humphries, J. O.: Myocardial infarction in sickle cell disease. Am. J. Hematol. 16:139, 1984.
30. Martin, C. R., Cobb, C., Tatter, D., et al.: Acute myocardial infarction in sickle cell anemia. Arch. Intern. Med. 143:830, 1983.
31. McCormick, W. F.: Massive nonatherosclerotic myocardial infarction in sickle cell anemia. Am. J. Forensic Med. Pathol. 9:151, 1988.
32. Rubler, S., and Fleischer, R. A.: Sickle cell states and cardiomyopathy. Sudden death due to pulmonary thrombosis and infarction. Am. J. Cardiol. 19:867, 1967.
33. Burnheimer, J., and Haywood, L. J.: Prevalence of hemoglobinopathies in patients with ischemic heart disease. J. Natl. Med. Assoc. 68:312, 1976.
34. Balfour, I. C., Covitz, W., Davis, H., et al.: Cardiac size and function in children with sickle cell anemia. Am. Heart J. 108:345, 1984.
35. Lippman, S. M., Niemann, J. T., Thigpen, T., et al.: Abnormal septal Q waves in sickle cell disease. Prevalence and causative factors. Chest 88:543, 1985.
36. Maisel, A., Friedman, H., Flint, L., et al.: Continuous electrocardiographic monitoring in patients with sickle cell anemia during pain crisis. Clin. Cardiol. 6:339, 1983.
37. Covitz, W., Eubig, C., Balfour, I. C., et al.: Exercise-induced cardiac dysfunction in sickle cell anemia. Radionuclide study. Am. J. Cardiol. 51:570, 1983.
38. Manno, B. V., Burka, E. R., Hakki, A., et al.: Biventricular function in sickle cell anemia: Radionuclide angiographic and thallium-201 scintigraphic evaluation. Am. J. Cardiol. 52:584, 1983.
39. Willens, H. J., Lawrence, C., Frishman, W. H., and Strom, J. A.: A noninvasive comparison of left ventricular performance in sickle cell anemia and chronic aortic regurgitation. Clin. Cardiol. 6:542, 1983.
40. Alpert, B. S., Dover, E. V., Strong, W. B., and Covits, W.: Longitudinal exercise hemodynamics in children with sickle cell anemia. Am. J. Dis. Child. 138:1021, 1984.
41. Lippman, S. M., Ginzton, L. E., Thigpen, T., et al.: Mitral valve prolapse in sickle cell disease: Presumptive evidence for a linked connective tissue disorder. Arch. Intern. Med. 145:435, 1985.
42. Sanakul, D., Thakerngpol, K., and Pacharee, P.: Cardiac pathology in 76 thalessemic patients. Birth Defects 23:177, 1988.
43. Ohene-Frempong, K., and Schwartz, E.: Clinical features of thalassemia. Pediatr. Clin. North Am. 27:403, 1980.
44. Ehlers L. H., Levin, A. R., Klein, A. A., et al.: The cardiac manifestations of thalassemia major: Natural history, noninvasive cardiac diagnostic studies, and results of cardiac catheterization. In Engle, M. A. (ed.): Pediatric Cardiovascular Disease. Cardiovascular Clinics II. Philadelphia, F. A. Davis Co., 1981, pp. 171–186.
44a. Spirito, P., Lupi, G., Melevendi, C., and Vecchio, C.: Restrictive diastolic abnormalities identified by Doppler echocardiography in patients with thalassemia major. Circulation 82:88, 1990.
45. Sapoznikov, D., Lewis, N., Rachmilewitz, E. A., et al.: Left ventricular filling and emptying patterns in anemia due to beta-thalassemia. A computer-assisted echocardiographic study. Cardiology 69:276, 1982.
46. Sapoznikov, D., Lewis, N., Degan, I., et al.: Studies of left ventricular function in anemia due to beta-thalassemia. Isr. J. Med. Sci. 18:928, 1982.
47. Lau, K. C., Li, A.M.C., Hui, P. W., and Yeung, C. Y.: Left ventricular function in β thalassemia major. Arch. Dis. Child. 64:1046, 1989.
48. Valdes-Cruz, L. M., Reinecke, C., Rutkowski, M., et al.:Preclinical abnormal segmental cardiac manifestations of thalassemia major in children on transfusion-chelation therapy: Echographic alterations of left ventricular posterior wall contractions and relaxation patterns. Am. Heart J. 103:505, 1982.
49. Borow, K. M., Propper, R., Bierman, F. Z., et al.: The left ventricular end-systolic pressure-dimensions relation in patients with thalassemia major. A new noninvasive method for assessing contractile state. Circulation 66:980, 1982.
50. Canale, C., Terrachini, V., Vallebena, A., et al.: Thalassemic cardiomyopathy: Echocardiographic difference between major and intermediate thalassemia at rest and during isometric effort: Yearly follow-up. Clin. Cardiol. 11:563, 1988.
51. Yee, H., Mra, R., and Nyunt, K. M.: Cardiac abnormalities in the thalassemia syndromes. Southeast Asian J. Trop. Med. Public Health 15:414, 1984.
52. Dameshek, W., and Roth, S. I.: Case Records of the Massachusetts General Hospital—Weekly Clinicopathological exercises. Case 52. N. Engl. J. Med. 271:898, 1964.
53. Westring, D. W.: Aortic valve disease and hemolytic anemia. Ann. Intern. Med. 65:203, 1966.

54. Miller, D. S., Mengel, C. E., Kremer, W. B., et al.: Intravascular hemolysis in a patient with valvular heart disease. Ann. Intern. Med. 65:210, 1966.
55. Rose, J. C., Hufnagel, C. A., Freis, C. D., et al.: The hemodynamic alterations produced by a plastic valvular prosthesis for severe aortic insufficiency in man. J. Lab. Clin. Med. 33:891, 1954.
56. Sayed, H. M., Dacie, J. V., Handley, D. A., et al.: Hemolytic anemia of mechanical origin after open-heart surgery. Thorax 16:356, 1961.
57. Sonaer, D. H., Cheng, T. O., and Aaron, B. L.: Hemolytic anemia and acute mitral regurgitation caused by a torn cusp of a porcine mitral prosthetic valve 7 years after its implantation. Am. Heart J. 113:404, 1987.
58. Mok, P., Lieberman, E. H., Lilly, L. S., et al. Severe hemolytic anemia following mitral valve repair. Am. Heart J. 117:1171, 1989.
59. Dacie, J. V.: The Hemolytic Anemias. Part III. 2nd ed. New York, Grune and Stratton, 1967, p. 957.
60. Sears, A. D., and Crosby, W. H.: Intravascular hemolysis due to intracardiac prosthetic devices. Diurnal variations related to activity. Am. J. Med. 39:341, 1965.
61. DiSosa, V. J., Collins, J. J., Jr., and Cohn, C. H.: Hematological complications with the St. Jude valve and reduced-dose coumadin. Ann. Thorac. Surg. 48:280, 1989.
62. Nevaril, C. G., Lynch, E. C., Alfrey, C. P., Jr., and Hellums, J.: Erythrocyte damage and destruction induced by shearing stress. J. Lab. Clin. Med. 71:784, 1986.
63. Zezulka, A., Schapiro, L., and Sind, S.: Chronic haemolytic anemia in hypertrophic cardiomyopathy. Br. Heart J. 52:474, 1984.

HEMOCHROMATOSIS AND HEMOSIDEROSIS

64. Schafer, A. I.: Iron overload. In Fairbanks, V. F. (ed.): Current Hematology. New York, John Wiley and Sons, 1981, pp. 191–218.
65. Edwards, C. Q., Dadone, M. M., Skolnick, M. H., and Kushner, J. P.: Hereditary hemochromatosis. Clin. Hematol. 11:411, 1982.
66. Swan, W.G.A., and Dewar, H. A.: The heart in hemochromatosis. Br. Heart J. 14:117, 1952.
67. Finch, S. C., and Finch, C. A.: Idiopathic hemochromatosis, an iron storage disease. Medicine 34:381, 1955.
68. Rosenqvist, M., and Hultcrantz R.: Prevalence of haemochromatosis among men with clinically significant bradyarrhythmias. Eur. Heart J. 10:473, 1989.
69. James, T. N.: Pathology of the cardiac conduction system in hemochromatosis. N. Engl. J. Med. 271:92, 1964.
70. Wasserman, A. J., Richardson, D. W., Baird, C. L., and Wyso, E. M.: Cardiac hemochromatosis simulating constrictive pericarditis. Am. J. Med. 32:316, 1962.
71. Cutler, H. J., Isner, J. M., Bracey, A. W., et al.: Hemochromatosis heart disease: An unemphasized cause of potentially reversible restrictive cardiomyopathy. Am. Heart J. 69:923, 1980.
72. Buja, L. M., and Roberts, W. C.: Iron in the heart. Etiology and clinical significance. Am. J. Med. 51:209, 1971.
73. Olson, L. J., Edwards, W. D., Holmes, D. R., et al.: Endomyocardial biopsy in hemochromatosis: Clinicopathologic correlates in six cases. J. Am. Coll. Cardiol. 13:116, 1989.
74. Leon, M. D., Borer, J. S., Bacharach, S. L., et al.: Detection of early cardiac dysfunction in patients with severe beta-thalassemia and chronic iron overload. N. Engl. J. Med. 301:1143, 1979.
75. Candell-Riera, J., Permanger-Miralda, G., and Soler-Soler, J.: Cardiac hemochromatosis. Primary Cardiol. 12 (October):123, 1986.
76. Grisaru, D., Goldfarb, A. W., Gotsman, M. S., et al.: Deferoxamine improves left ventricular function in β-thalassemia. Arch. Intern. Med. 146:2344, 1986.
77. Rivers, J., Garrahy, P., Robinson, W., and Murphy, A.: Reversible cardiac dysfunction in hemochromatosis. Am. Heart J. 113:216, 1987.
78. Easley, R. M., Schreiner, B. F., and Yu, P. N.: Reversible cardiomyopathy associated with hemochromatosis. N. Engl. J. Med. 287:866, 1972.
79. Skinner, C., and Kenmore, C. F.: Haemochromatosis presenting as congestive cardiomyopathy and responding to venesection. Br. Heart J. 35:466, 1973.
80. Schafer, A. I., Cheron, R. G., Dluhy, R., et al.: Clinical consequences of acquired tranfusional iron overload in adults. N. Engl. J. Med. 304:319, 1981.
81. Schafer, A. I.: Treatment of iron overload with parenteral deferoxamines. In Isselbacher, K. J. et al. (eds.): Update III to Harrison's Principles of Internal Medicine. New York, McGraw-Hill Book Co., 1982, pp. 157–166.
82. Wolfe, L., Olivieri, N., Sallan, D., et al.: Prevention of cardiac disease by subcutaneous deferoxamine in patients with thalassemia major. N. Engl. J. Med. 312:1600, 1985.
83. Schafer, A. I., Rabinowe, S., LeBoff, M. S., et al.: Long term efficacy of deferoxamine iron chelation therapy in adults with acquired transfusional overload. Arch. Intern. Med. 145:1217, 1985.
84. Rahko, P. S., Salerni, R., and Uretsky, B. F.: Successful reversal by chelation therapy of congestive cardiomyopathy due to iron overload. J. Am. Coll. Cardiol. 8:436, 1986.
85. Maurer, H. S., Lloyd-Still, J. D., Ingrisano, C., et al.: A prospective evaluation of iron chelation therapy in children with severe beta-thalassemia. A six year study. Am. J. Dis. Child. 142:287, 1988.
86. Freeman, A. P., Giles, R. W., Berdoukas, V. A., et al.: Sustained normalization of cardiac function by chelation therapy in thalassaemia major. Clin. Lab. Haematol. 11:299, 1989.
87. Cohen, A. R., Mizanin, J., and Schwartz, E.: Rapid removal of excessive iron with daily, high-dose intravenous chelation therapy. J. Pediatr. 115:151, 1989.
88. Freeman, A. P., Giles, R. W., Berdoukas, V. A., et al.: Sustained normalization of cardiac function by chelation therapy in thalassaemia major. Clin. Lab. Haematol. 11:299, 1989.
89. Cohen, A., and Schwartz, E.: Iron chelation therapy with deferoxamine in Cooley anemia. J. Pediatr. 92:643, 1978.
90. Nienhuis, A. W.: Vitamin C and iron. N. Engl. J. Med. 304:170, 1981.
91. Bridges, K. R., and Hoffman, K. E.: The effects of ascorbic acid on the intracellular metabolism of iron and ferritin. J. Biol. Chem. 261:14273, 1986.
91a. Kontoghiorges, G. T., Aldouri, M. A., Sheppard, L., and Hoffbrand, A. V.: 1, 2-Dimethyl-3-hydroxypyrid-4-one, an orally active chelator for treatment of iron overload. Lancet 1:1294, 1987.

DISORDERS ASSOCIATED WITH ABNORMAL BLOOD FLOW DISTRIBUTION OR INCREASED VISCOSITY

92. Braunwald, E.: Cyanosis, hypoxia, and polycythemia. In Braunwald, E., et al. (eds.): Harrison's Principles of Internal Medicine, 11th ed. New York, McGraw-Hill Book Co., 1987, pp. 145–149.
93. Castle, W. B., and Jandl, J. H.: Blood viscosity and blood volume: Opposing influences upon oxygen transport in polycythemia. Semin. Hematol. 3:193, 1966.
94. Adamson, J. W.: The myeloproliferative disease. In Braunwald, E., et al. (eds.): Harrison's Principles of Internal Medicine, 11th ed. New York, McGraw-Hill, 1987, pp. 1527–1533.
95. Adamson, J. W., and Fialkow, P. J.: Polycythemia vera: Stem cell and probable clinical origin of the disease. N. Engl. J. Med. 245:913, 1976.
96. Berlin, N. I. (ed.). Polycythemia vera: An update. Semin. Hematol. 23:131, 1986.
97. Dintenfass, L.: Viscosity of the packed red and white blood cells. Exp. Molec. Pathol. 4:597, 1965.
98. Thomas, D. J., Marshall, J., Russell, R. W., et al.: Effect of hematocrit on cerebral blood flow in man. Lancet 2:941, 1977.
99. Torrance, J. D., Lenfant, C., and Cruz, J.: Oxygen transport mechanisms in residents at high altitude. Respir. Physiol. 11:1, 1970.
100. Balcerzak, S. P., and Bromberg, P. A.: Secondary polycythemia. Semin. Hematol. 12:353, 1976.
101. Rosenthal, A., Button, L. N., and Nathan, D. G.: Blood volume changes in cyanotic congenital heart disease. Am. J. Cardiol. 29:162, 1971.
102. Golde, D. W., Hocking, W. G., Koeffler, H. P., and Adamson, J. W.: Polycythemia: Mechanism and management. Ann. Intern. Med. 95:71, 1981.
103. Rosenthal, A., Nathan, D. G., Marty, A. T., et al.: Acute hemodynamic effects of red cell production in polycythemia of cyanotic congenital heart disease. Circulation 42:197, 1970.
104. Erslev, A. J., and Caro, J.: Secondary polycythemia: A boon or a burden? Blood Cells 10:177, 1984.
105. Yeager, S. B., and Freed, M. D.: Myocardial infarction as a manifestation of polycythemia in cyanotic heart disease. Am. J. Cardiol. 53:952, 1984.
106. Grant, P., Patel, P., and Singh, S.: Acute myocardial infarction secondary to polycythemia in a case of cyanotic congenital heart disease. Int. J. Cardiol. 9:108, 1985.
107. Wallis, P. J., Skehan, J. D., Newland, A. C., et al.: Effects of erythropheresis on pulmonary hemodynamics and oxygen transport in patients with secondary polycythemia and cor pulmonale. Clin. Sci. 70:91, 1986.
108. Wallis, P. J., Cunningham, J., Few, J. D., et al.: Effects of packed cell volume reduction on renal hemodynamics and the renin angiotensin aldosterone system in patients with secondary polycythemia and hypoxic cor pulmonale. Clin. Sci. 70:81, 1986.
109. Willison, J. R., Thomas, D. J., and duBoulay, G. H., et al.: Effect of high hematocrit on alertness. Lancet 1:846, 1980.
110. York, E. L., Junes, R. L., Menon, D., and Sproule, B. J.: Effects of secondary polycythemia on cerebral blood flow in chronic obstructive pulmonary disease. Am. Rev. Respir. Dis. 121:813, 1980.
111. Rosenthal, A., Mentzer, W. C., and Eisenstein, E. B.: The role of red blood cell organic phosphates in adaptation to congenital heart disease. Pediatrics 47:537, 1971.
112. Charache, S., Weatherall, D. J., and Clegg, J. B.: Polycythemia associated with hemoglobinopathy. J. Clin. Invest. 45:813, 1966.
113. Adamson, J. W., and Finch, C. A.: Erythropoietin and the polycythemias. Ann. N. Y. Acad. Sci. 149:560, 1968.
114. Bromberg, P. A., Padilla, F., Boy, J. T., and Balcerzak, S. P.: Effect of a new hemoglobin (Hb Little Rock) on the physiology of oxygen delivery. J. Lab. Clin. Med. 78:837, 1971.
115. Charache, S., Achuff, S., Winslow, R., et al.: Variability of the homeostatic response to P50. Blood 52:1156, 1978.
116. Smith, J., and Landow, S. A.: Smoker's polycythemia. N. Engl. J. Med. 298:6, 1978.
117. Weinreb, N. J., and Shih, C. F.: Spurious polycythemia. Semin. Hematol. 12:397, 1975.
118. Saffitz, J. E., Phillips, E. R., Temesy-Armos, P. N., and Roberts, W. C.: Thrombocytosis and fetal coronary heart disease. Am. J. Cardiol. 52:651, 1983.
119. Pick, R. A., Glover, M. U., Nanfro, J. J., et al.: Acute myocardial infarction with essential thrombocythemia in a young man. Am. Heart J. 106:406, 1983.
120. Hanger, K. H., Kilgore, J., and James, E.: Essential thrombocythemia and coronary artery disease. Chest. 86:933, 1984.

121. Virmani, R., Popuvsky, M. A., and Roberts, W. C.: Thrombolysis, coronary thrombosis and acute myocardial infarction. Am. J. Med. 67:498, 1979.

122. Mitus, A. J., Barbui, R., Shulman, L. N., et al.: Hemostatic complications in young patients with essential thrombocythemia. Am. J. Med. 88:371, 1990.

123. Knizley, H., Jr., and Noyes, W. D.: Iron deficiency anemia, papilledema, thrombocytosis and transient hemiparesis. Arch. Intern. Med. 129:480, 1972.

124. Karwinski, B., and Svendsen, E.: Trends in cardiac metastasis. Acta Pathol Microbiol Immunol Scand 97:1018, 1989.

124a. Fuchs, J., Weinberger, I., Rotenberg, Z., et al.: Plasma viscosity in ischemic heart disease. Am. Heart J. 108:435, 1984.

125. Zannad, F., Stoltz, J. F., Laprevote-Heully, M. C., et al.: Hemorrhagic disorders in the threatened myocardial infarct syndrome. Arch. Mal. Coeur. 78:1237, 1985.

126. Strano, A., Avellone, G., Novo, S., et al.: Evaluation of blood viscosity and erythrocyte filterability in chronic ischemic heart disease. Ric. Clin. Lab. 1:179, 1985.

CARDIAC MANIFESTATIONS OF NEOPLASTIC DISEASE

127. Israeli, A., Rein, A.J.J.T., Kriski, M., et al.: Right ventricular outflow tract obstruction due to extracardiac tumors: A report of three cases diagnosed and followed up by echocardiographic studies. 149:2105, 1989.

128. Kapoor, A. S.: Clinical manifestations of neoplasia of the heart. In Kapoor, A. S. (ed.): Cancer and the Heart. New York, Springer-Verlag, 1986, pp. 21–25.

129. Schoen, F. J., Berger, B. M., and Guerina, N. G.: Cardiac effects of noncardiac neoplasms. Cardiol. Clin. 2:657, 1984.

130. Roberts, W. C., Glancy, D. L., and DeVita, V. T.: Heart in malignant lymphoma. A study of 196 autopsy cases. Am. J. Cardiol. 22:85, 1968.

131. Petersen, C. D., Robinson, Q. A., and Kurnich, J. E.: Involvement of the heart and pericardium in the malignant lymphomas. Am. J. Med. Sci. 272:161, 1976.

132. Waller, B. F., Gottdiener, J. S., Virmni, R., and Roberts, W. C.: Structure-function correlations in cardiovascular and pulmonary diseases. The charcoal heart. Chest 77:671, 1980.

133. McBride, W., Jackman, J. D., Gammon, R. S., and Willerson, J. T.: High output cardiac failure in patients with multiple myeloma. N. Engl. J. Med. 319:1651, 1988.

134. Almange, C., Lebrestec, T., Louvet, M., et al.: Bloc auriculo-ventriculaire complet par metastase cardiaque: A propos dune observation. Sem. Hop. Paris 54:1419, 1978.

135. McDonnell, P. J., Becker, L. C., and Bulkley, B. H.: Thallium imaging in cardiac lymphoma. Am. Heart J. 101:809, 1981.

136. Kutalek, S. P., Panidis, I. P., Kotler, M., et al.: Metastatic tumors of the heart detected by two-dimensional echocardiography. Am. Heart J. 109:343, 1985.

137. Moncada, R., and Posnik, H.: Computed tomograph of neoplastic disease in the pericardium. In Kapoor, A. S.: Cancer and the Heart. New York, Springer-Verlag. 1986, pp. 26–41.

138. Goldman, A. P., Kotler, M. N., and Perry, W. R.: Arterial tumors. In Kapoor, A. S. (ed.): Cancer and the Heart. New York, Springer-Verlag, 1986, pp. 82–109.

139. Seibert, K. A., Rettenmier, C. W., Waller, B. F., et al.: Osteogenic sarcoma metastatic to the heart. Am. J. Med. 73:136, 1982.

140. Kralstein, J., and Frishman, W.: Malignant pericardial disease: Diagnosis and treatment. Am. Heart J. 113:785, 1987.

141. Lloyd, E. A., and Curcio, C. A.: Lymphoma of the heart as an unusual cause of pericardial effusion. S. Afr. Med. J. 58:937, 1980.

142. Haedersdal, C., Hasselbach, H., Devantier, A., and Saunamak, K.: Pericardial hematopoiesis with tamponade in myelofibrosus. Scand. J. Haematol. 34:270, 1985.

143. Hancock, E. W.: Pericardial disease in patients with neoplasm. In Reddy, R. S., Leon, D. F., and Shaver, J. A. (eds.): Pericardial Disease. New York, Raven Press, 1981, p. 327.

144. Ramarkrishnan, S., Marshall, A. J., Richard, J. G., and Tyrell, C. J.: Pericardiocentesis and systemic cytotoxic chemotherapy in the management of cardiac tamponade secondary to disseminated breast carcinoma. Br. Heart J. 60:162, 1988.

145. Leung, W., Tai, Y., Lau, C., et al.: Cardiac tamponade complicating leukaemia: Immediate chemotherapy or pericardiocentesis? Postgrad. Med. J. 65:773, 1989.

146. Press, O. W., and Livingston, R.: Management of malignant pericardial effusion and tamponade. JAMA 256:2301, 1987.

147. Rudoff, J., Perey, R., Benrubi, G., and Ostrewski, M. L.: Recurrent squamous cell carcinoma of the cervix presenting as cardiac tamponade. Case report and subject review. Gynecol. Oncol. 34:226, 1989.

148. Barton, J. C., and Durant, J. R.: Isolated chylopericardium associated with lymphoma. South. Med. J. 73:1551, 1980.

149. Buck, M., Ingle, J. N., Giuliani, E. R., et al.: Pericardial effusion in women with breast cancer. Cancer 60:263, 1987.

150. Posner, M. R., Cohen, G. I., and Skarin, A. T.: Pericardial disease in patients with cancer. The differentiation of malignant from idiopathic and radiation-induced pericarditis. Am. J. Med. 71:407, 1981.

151. Applefeld, M. M., Spicer, K. M., Slawson, R. G., et al.: The long-term cardiac effects of radiotherapy in patients treated for Hodgkin's disease. Cancer Treat. Rep. 66:1003, 1982.

152. Gouldesbrough, D. R., and Carder, P. J.: Rapidly progressive cardiac fail-

ure due to lymphomatous infiltration of the myocardium. Postgrad. Med. J. 65:668, 1989.

153. Lestuzzi, C., Biasi, S., Nicolosi, G. L., et al.: Secondary neoplastic infiltration of the myocardium diagnosed by two-dimensional echocardiography in seven cases with anatomic confirmation. J. Am. Coll. Cardiol. 9:439, 1987.

154. Wig, I. L., Mehva, S., Azueta, V., and Rosner, F.: Cardiac metastasis from adenocarcinoma of the lung. Echocardiographic pathologic correlation. Am. J. Med. 80:108, 1986.

155. Perez, C. A., Presant, C. A., and Amburg, A. L.: Management of superior vena caval syndrome. Semin. Oncol. 5:123, 1978.

156. Lopez, M. I., and Vincent, R. J.: Malignant superior vena cava syndrome. In Kapoor, A. S. (ed.): Cancer and the Heart. New York, Springer-Verlag, 1986, p. 206.

157. Wahlin, A., Olofsson, B., Eriksson, A., and Backman, C.: Myeloma-associated cardiac amyloidosis. Acta Med. Scand. 215:189, 1984.

158. Alpert, M. A.: Cardiac amyloidosis. In Kapoor, A. S. (ed.): Cancer and the Heart. New York, Springer-Verlag, 1986, p. 162.

159. Sedlis, S. P., Saffitz, J. E., Schwob, V. S., and Jaffe, A. S.: Cardiac amyloidosis simulating hypertrophic cardiomyopathy. Am. J. Cardiol. 53:969, 1984.

160. Laurent, M., Taulet, R., Ramee, M. P., et al.: Light-chain disease with terminal myocardiopathy. Arch. Mal. Coeur 78:943, 1985.

161. Ursell, P. C., and Fenogolio, J. J.: Spectrum of cardiac disease diagnosed by endomyocardial biopsy. Pathol. Annu. 19:197, 1984.

162. Koiwaya, Y., Nakamura, M., and Yamamoto, K.: Progressive ECG alterations in metastatic cardiac mural tumor. Am. Heart J. 105:339, 1983.

163. Hartman, R. B., Clark, P. I., and Schulman, P.: Pronounced and prolonged ST segment elevation. A pathognomonic sign of tumor invasion of the heart. Arch. Intern. Med. 142:1917, 1982.

164. Cole, T. O., Attah, E. B., and Onyemelukwe, G. C.: Burkitt's lymphoma presenting with heart block. Br. Heart J. 37:94, 1975.

165. Ballentyne, F., VanderArk, C. R., and Holick, M.: Carotid sinus syncope and cervical lymphoma. Wis. Med. J. 74:91, 1975.

166. Inagaki, R., Rodriguez, M., and Brody, G. P.: Causes of death in cancer patients. Cancer 33:568, 1974.

167. Kopelson, G., and Herwig, K. J.: The etiologies of coronary artery disease in cancer patients. Int. J. Radiat. Oncol. Biol. Phys. 4:895, 1978.

168. Stewart, J. R., and Fajardo, L. F.: Cancer and coronary artery disease. Int. J. Radiat. Oncol. Biol. Phys. 4:915, 1978.

169. Ackerman, D. M., Hyma, B. A., and Edwards, W. D.: Malignant neoplastic emboli to the coronary arteries. Report of two cases and review of the literature. Hum. Pathol. 18:955, 1987.

170. Parker, B. M.: Valvular involvement in cancer. In Kapoor, A. S. (ed.): Cancer and the Heart. New York, Springer-Verlag, 1986, p. 64.

171. MacDonald, R. A., Robbins, S. L.: The significance of nonbacterial thrombotic endocarditis: An autopsy and clinical study of 78 cases. Ann. Intern. Med. 46:255, 1957.

172. Chino, F., Kodama, A., Otake, M., and Dock, D. S.: Nonbacterial thrombotic endocarditis in a Japanese autopsy sample. A review of eighty cases. Am. Heart J. 90:190, 1975.

173. Gonzalez Quintela, A., Candela, M. J., Vidal, C., et al.: Nonbacterial thrombotic endocarditis in cancer patients. Acta Cardiologica XLVI:1, 1991.

174. Lehto, V. P., Stenman, S., and Somer, T.: Immunohistological studies on valvular vegetations in nonbacterial thrombotic endocarditis. Arch. Pathol. Microbiol. Scand. 90:207, 1982.

175. Lange, H. W., Galliani, C. A., and Edwards, J. E.: Local complications associated with indwelling Swan-Ganz catheters: Autopsy study of 36 cases. Am. J. Cardiol. 52:1108, 1983.

176. Yam, L. T., Li, C. Y., Necheles, T. F., and Katayama, I.: Pseudoeosinophilic, eosinophilic endocarditis and eosinophilic leukemia. Am. J. Med. 53:193, 1972.

177. Cilliers, G. D., Harper, I. S., and Lochner, A.: Radiation-induced changes in the ultrastructure and mechanical function of the rat heart. Radiotherapy Oncol. 16:311, 1989.

178. Niemtzow, R. C., and Reynolds, R. D.: Radiation therapy and the heart. In Kapoor, A. S. (ed.): Cancer and the Heart. New York, Springer-Verlag, 1986, pp. 232–237.

178a. Geist, B. J., Lauk, S., Bornhausen, M., and Trott, K-R.: Physiologic consequences of local heart irradiation in rats. Int. J. Radiat. Oncol. Biol. Phys. 18:1107, 1990.

179. Gottdeiner, J. S., Katin, M. J., Borer, J. S., et al.: Late cardiac effects of therapeutic mediastinal irradiation: Assessment by echocardiography and radionuclide angiography. N. Engl. J. Med. 308:569, 1983.

180. Applefeld, M. M., and Wiernik, P. H.: Cardiac disease after radiation therapy for Hodgkin's disease. Analysis of 48 patients. Am. J. Cardiol. 51:1679, 1983.

181. Taymor-Luria, H., Kohn, K., and Pasternak, R. C.: Radiation heart disease. J. Cardiovasc. Med. 8:113, 1983.

182. Iqbal, S. M. Hanson, E. L., and Gensini, G. G.: Bypass graft for coronary arterial stenosis following radiation therapy. Chest 71:664, 1977.

183. Miller, D. D., Waters, D. D., Dangoisse, V., and David, P. R.: Symptomatic coronary artery spasm following radiotherapy for Hodgkin's disease. Chest 83:284, 1983.

184. Stegaru-Hellring, B., Keller, H., Bode, H. et al.: Ostium stenosis of both coronary arteries and latent hypothyroidism as sequelae of radiotherapy in Hodgkin's disease. Z. Kardiol. 74:485, 1985.

185. Simon, E. B., Ling, J., Mendizabal, R. C., and Midawell, J.: Radiation-induced coronary artery disease. Am. Heart J. 108:1031, 1984.

186. Tracy, G. P., Brown, D. E., Johnson, L. W., and Gottlieb, A. J.: Radiation-induced coronary artery disease. JAMA 228:1660, 1974.

187. Shashaty, G. G.: Aortic insufficiency following mediastinal radiation for Hodgkin's disease. Am. J. Med. Sci. 287:46, 1984.

188. Warda, M., Kahn, A., Massumi, A., et al.: Radiation-induced valvular dysfunction. J. Am. Coll. Cardiol. 2:180, 1983.

189. Detrano, R. C., Yiannikas, J., and Salcedo, E. E.: Two-dimensional echocardiographic assessment of radiation-induced valvular heart disease. Am. Heart J. 107:584, 1984.

190. Rummeny, E., Hausen, W., Lorbacher, P., and Willems, D.: Acquired infundibular pulmonary stenosis. Possible late complication following radiotherapy of Hodgkin's disease. Z. Kardiol. 73:641, 1984.

191. Gomez, G. A., Park, J. J., Panahoh, A. M., et al.: Heart size and function after radiation therapy to the mediastinum in patients with Hodgkin's disease. Cancer Treat. Rep. 67:1099, 1983.

192. Cohen, I. S., Bharati, S., Glass, J., and Lev, M.: Radiotherapy as a cause of complete atrioventricular block in Hodgkin's disease. Arch. Intern. Med. 141:676, 1981.

193. Loeffler, J. S., Mauch, P., and Hellman, S.: Late effects of radiation therapy in the treatment of Hodgkin's disease. In Lacher, M. J., and Redman, J. R. (eds.): Hodgkin's Disease: The Consequences of Survival. Philadelphia, Lea and Febiger, 1990, pp. 27–46.

194. Gerling, G., Gottdiener, J., and Burer, J. S.: Cardiovascular complications of the treatment of Hodgkin's disease. In Lacher, M. J., and Redman, J. R. (eds.): Hodgkin's Disease: The Consequences of Survival. Philadelphia, Lea and Febiger, 1990, pp. 267–295.

195. Akaike, A., Cogure, R., Oyama, K., and Oda, M.: Damage to the heart from tumor irradiation in the thorax: An echocardiographic study. Radiology 25:430, 1985.

196. Green, D., Gingell, R. L., Pearce, J., et al.: The effect of mediastinal irradiation on cardiac function of patients treated during childhood and adolescence for heart disease. J. Clin. Oncol. 5:239, 1987.

197. Carmel, R. J., and Kaplan, H. S.: Mantle irradiation in Hodgkin's disease. Cancer 37:2813, 1976.

198. Ikaheimo, M. J., Niemela, K. O., Linnaluoto, M. M., et al.: Early cardiac changes related to radiation therapy. Am. J. Cardiol. 56:943, 1985.

199. O'Donnell, L. O., O'Neill, T., Toner, M., et al.: Myocardial hypertrophy, fibrosis and infarction following exposure of the heart to radiation for Hodgkin's disease. Postgrad. Med. J. 62:1055, 1986.

200. Strender, L. E., Lindhal, J., and Larsson, L. E.: Incidence of heart disease and functional significance of changes in the electrocardiogram 10 years after radiotherapy for breast cancer. Cancer 57:929, 1986.

201. Lederman, G. S., Sheldon, T. A., Chaffey, J. T., et al.: Cardiac disease after mediastinal irradiation for seminoma. Cancer 60:772, 1987.

202. Radwanen, B. A., Geringer, R., Goldmann, A. M., et al.: Left main coronary artery stenosis following mediastinal irradiation. Am. J. Med. 82:1017, 1987.

203. Joesuu, H.: Acute myocardial infarction after heart irradiation in young patients with Hodgkin's disease. Chest 95:388, 1989.

204. Silverberg, G. O., Britt, R. H., and Goffinet, D. R.: Radiation induced carotid artery disease. Cancer 41:130, 1978.

205. Amromin, G. G., Gildenhorn, H. C., and Solomon, R. D.: The synergism of x-irradiation and cholesterol-fat feeding on the development of coronary artery lesions. J. Atheroscler. Res. 4:325, 1975.

206. Brosius, F. C., Waller, B. F., and Roberts, W. C.: Radiation heart disease: Analysis of 16 young (aged 15 to 33 years) necropsy patients who received over 3500 rads to the heart. Am. J. Med. 7:519, 1981.

207. Kantrowitz, N. E., and Bristow, M. R.: Cardiotoxicity of antitumor agents. Prog. Cardiovasc. Dis. 27:195, 1984.

208. Sunnenberg, D., and Kramer, B.: Long-term effects of cancer chemotherapy. Compr. Ther. 11:58, 1985.

209. Perry, M. C.: Effects of chemotherapy on the heart. In Kapoor, A. S. (ed.): Cancer and the Heart. New York, Springer-Verlag, 1986, p. 223.

210. Lancaster, L. D., and Ewy, G. A.: Cardiac consequences of malignancy and their treatment. Adv. Intern. Med. 30:275, 1984.

211. Schoenberger, C. I., and Crystal R.: Drug-induced lung disease. In Isselbacher, K. J. (ed.): Update IV to Harrison's Principles of Internal Medicine. New York, McGraw-Hill Book Co., 1982, pp. 49–74.

212. Young, R. C., Oxols, R. F., and Myers, C. E.: The anthracycline antineoplastic drugs. N. Engl. J. Med. 305:139, 1981.

213. Lena, L., and Page, J. A.: Cardiotoxicity of Adriamycin and related anthracyclines. Cancer Treat. Rev. 3:111, 1976.

214. Ali, M. K., Soto, P. A., Maroongroge, D., et al.: Electrocardiographic changes after Adriamycin chemotherapy. Cancer 43:465, 1979.

215. Bristow, M. R., Billingham, M. E., Mason, J. W., and Daniels, J. R.: Clinical spectrum of anthracycline antibiotic cardiotoxicity. Cancer Treat. rep. 62:873, 1978.

216. Wortman, J. E., Lucas, V. S., Jr., Schuster, E., et al.: Sudden death during doxorubicin administration. Cancer 44:1588, 1979.

217. Lipshultz, S. E., Colan, S. D., Gelber, R. D., et al.: Late cardiac effects of doxorubicin therapy for acute lymphoblastic leukemia in childhood. N. Engl. J. Med. 324:808, 1991.

218. Greene, H. L., Reich, S. D., and Dalen, J. E.: How to minimize doxorubicin toxicity. J. Cardiovasc. Med. 7:306, 1982.

219. Freter, C. E., Leet, C., Billingham, M. E., et al.: Doxorubicin cardiac toxicity manifesting seven years after treatment. Am. J. Med. 80:483, 1986.

220. Steinherz, L. J., and Steinherz, P.: Cardiac failure more than six years post anthrcyclines. Am. J. Cardiol. 52:505, 1988.

221. Goorin, A. M., Chauvenet, A. R., Perez-, Perez-Atayde, A. R. Gruz J, et al.: Initial congestive heart failure, six to ten years after doxorubicin chemotherapy for childhood cancer. J. Pediatr. 116:144, 1990.

222. Porembka, D. T., Lowder, J. N., Orlowski, J. P., et al.: Etiology and management of doxorubicin cardiotoxicity. Crit. Care Med. 17:569, 1989.

223. Isner, J. M., Ferrans, V. J., Cohen, S. R., et al.: Clinical and morphological cardiac findings after anthracycline chemotherapy. Analysis of 64 patients studied at necroscopy. Am. J. Cardiol. 51:1167, 1983.

224. Merrill, J., Greco, F. A., Zimbler, H., et al.: Adriamycin and radiation: Synergistic cardiotoxicity. Ann. Intern. Med. 82:122, 1975.

225. Fajardo, L. F., and Stewart, J. F.: Pathogenesis or radiation-induced myocardial fibrosis. Lab. Invest. 29:244, 1973.

226. O'Connell, T. X., and Berenbaum, M. D.: Cardiac and pulmonary effects of high doses of cyclophosphamide and isophosphamide. Cancer Res. 34:1586, 1974.

227. Mills, B. A., and Roberts, R. W.: Cyclophosphamide-induced cardiomyopathy. A report of two cases and a review of the English literature. Cancer 43:2223, 1979.

228. Severs, N. J., Twist, V. W., and Powell, T.: Acute effects of Adriamycin on the macromolecular organization of the cardiac muscle cell plasma membrane. Cardioscience 2:35, 1991.

228a. Lewis, W., and Gonzalez, B.: Actin isoform mRNA alterations induced by doxorubicin in cultured heart cells. Lab. Invest. 62:69, 1990.

229. Papoian, T., and Lewis, W.: Adriamycin cardiotoxicity in vivo. Am. J. Pathol. 136:1201, 1990.

230. Lewis, W., Kleinerman, J., and Poszkin, S.: Interaction of Adriamycin in vitro with cardiac myofibrillar proteins. Circ. Res. 50:547, 1982.

231. Milei, J., Bovevis, A., Llesoy, S., et al.: Amelioration of Adriamycin-induced cardiotoxicity in rabbits by prenylamine and vitamin A + E. Am. Heart J. 111:95, 1986.

232. Speyer, M., et al.: Protective effect of ICRF against doxorubicin-induced cardiotoxicity in advanced breast cancer. N. Engl. J. Med. 319:745, 1988.

233. Villani, F., Galimberti, M., Monti, E., et al.: Effect of ICRF-187 pretreatment against doxorubicin-induced delayed cardiotoxicity in the rat. Toxicol. Appl. Pharmacol. 102:292, 1990.

234. Kajagopalan, S., Puliti, P. M., Sinha, B. K., et al.: Adriamycin-induced free radical formation in the perfused rat heart: Implications of cardiotoxicity. Cancer Res. 48:4766, 1988.

235. Lewis, W., Perillo, N. L., and Gonzales, B.: α-Actin synthesis changes in cultural cardiac myocytes: Relationship to anthracycline structure. J. Lab. Clin. Med. 112:43, 1988.

236. Dorr, R. T., Bozak, K. A., Shipp, N. G., et al.: In vitro rat, myocyte cardiotoxicity model for antitumor antibiotics using adenosine triphosphate/protein ratios. Cancer Res. 48:5222, 1988.

237. Singh, Y., Ulrich, L., Katz, D., et al.: Structural requirements for anthracycline-induced cardiotoxicity and antitumor effects. Toxicol. Appl. Pharmacol. 100:9, 1989.

238. Binacaniello, T., Myer, R. A., Wong, K. Y., et al.: Doxorubicin cardiotoxicity in children. J. Pediatr. 97:45, 1980.

239. Danesi, R., Del Tacca, M., Bernardini, N., et al.: Evaluation of the JT and corrected JT intervals as a new ECG method for monitoring doxorubicin cardiotoxicity in the dog. J. Pharmacol Meth. 21:317, 1989.

240. Boujon, B., Lechat, P., Mantz, J., et al.: Echocardiographic detection of adriamycin cardiotoxicity. Study of the relationship between the shortening fraction-constraint and the systolic shortening fraction-diameter of the left ventricle. Arch. Mal. Coeur 82:167, 1989.

241. Merchandise, B., Schroeder, E., Bosly, A., et al.: Early detection of doxorubicin cardiotoxicity: Interest of Doppler echocardiographic analysis of left ventricular filling dynamics. Am. Heart J. 118:92, 1989.

242. Applefeld, M. M., and Pollock, S. H.: Cardiac disease in patients who have malignancies. Curr. Probl. Cardiol. 4:1, 1980.

243. Hausdorf, G., Morf, G., Beron, G., et al.: Long-term doxorubicin cardiotoxicity in childhood: Noninvasive evaluation of the contractile state and diastolic filling. Br. Heart J. 60:309, 1988.

244. Lee, B. H., Goodenday, L. S., Muswick, G. J., et al.: Alterations in left ventricular diastolic function with doxorubicin therapy. J. Am. Coll. Cardiol. 9:184, 1987.

245. Bristow, M. R., Mason, J. W., Billingham, M. E., and Daniels, J. R.: Doxorubicin cardiomyopathy. Evaluation by phonocardiography, endomyocardial biopsy, and cardiac catheterization. Ann. Intern. Med. 88:168, 1978.

246. Bristow, M. R., Mason, J. W., Billingham, M. E., and Daniels, J. R.: Dose effect and structure-function relationships in doxorubicin cardiomyopathy. Am. Heart J. 102:709, 1981.

247. Fowles, R. E.: Cardiac catheterization and endomyocardial biopsy. In Kapoor, A. S. (ed.): Cancer and the Heart. Springer-Verlag, New York, 1986, pp. 42–50.

248. Bristow, M. R., Lopez, M. R., Mason, J. W., et al.: Efficacy and the cost of cardiac monitoring in patients receiving doxorubicin. Cancer 50:32, 1982.

249. Von Hoff, D. D., Layard, M. W., Basa, P., et al.: Risk factors for doxorubicin-induced congestive heart failure. Ann. Intern. Med. 91:710, 1979.

250. Weiss, R. B., Grillo-Lopez, A. J., Marsoni, S., et al.: Amsacrine associated cardiotoxicity: An analysis of 82 cases. J. Clin. Oncol. 4:918, 1986.

251. Lyman, G. H., Williams, C. C., Dinwoodie, W. R., and Schocken, D. D.: Sudden death in cancer patients receiving lithium. J. Clin. Oncol. 2:1270, 1984.

252. Bradamante, S., Monti, E., Paracchini, L., and Perletti, G.: Hypoxia as a risk factor for doxorubicin-induced cardiotoxicity: A NMR evaluation. Biochem. Biophys. Res. Commun. 163:682, 1989.

253. Schwartz, R. G., McKenzie, W. B., Alexander, J., et al.: Congestive heart failure and left ventricular dysfunction complicating doxorubicin therapy. Seven-year experience using serial radionuclide angiocardiography. Am. J. Med. 82:1109, 1987.

254. Doroshow, H. J., Locker, G. Y., Ifrim, I., and Myers, C. E.: Prevention of doxorubicin cardiac toxicity in the mouse by N-acetylcysteine. J. Clin. Invest. 68:1053, 1981.

255. Cortes, E. P., Gupta, M., Chew, C., et al.: Adriamycin cardiotoxicity: Early detection by systolic time interval and possible prevention by coenzyme Q. Cancer Treat. Rep. 62:887, 1978.

256. Somberg, J., Cagin, N., Levitt, L. B., et al.: Blockade of tissue uptake of the antineoplastic agent doxorubicin. J. Pharmacol. Exp. Ther. 204:226, 1978.

257. Milei, J., Marantz, A., Ale, J., et al.: Prevention of adriamycin-induced cardiotoxicity by prenylamine: A pitot double blind study. Cancer Drug Delivery 4:129, 1987.

258. Bellelli, A., Giomini, M., Giuliani, A. M., et al.: Antitumor effect and cardiotoxicity of a doxorubicin-lecithin association. Anti Cancer Res. 8:177, 1988.

259. Storm, G., Hoesel, Q. G., deGroot, G., et al.: A comparative study on the antitumor effect, cardiotoxicity and nephrotoxicity of doxorubicin given as a bolus continuous infusion or entrapped in liposomes in the Lou/M WSI rat. Cancer Chemother. Pharmacol. 24:341, 1989.

260. Legla, S. S., Benjamin, R. S., MacKay, B., et al.: Reduction of doxorubicin cardiotoxicity by prolonged continuous intravenous infusion. Ann. Intern. Med. 96:133, 1982.

261. Anders, R. J., Shanes, J. G., and Zeller, F. P.: Lower incidence of doxorubicin cardiomyopathy by one-a-week low-dose administration. Am. Heart J. 111:755, 1986.

262. Shapira, J., Gotfried, M., Lishner, M., et al.: Reduced cardiotoxicity of doxorubicin by a 6-hour infusion infusion regimen. A prospective randomized evaluation. Cancer 65:870, 1990.

263. Valdirieso, M., Burgess, M. A., Awer, M. S., et al.: Increased therapeutic index of weekly doxorubicin in the therapy of non small cell lung cancer: A prospective randomized study. J. Clin. Oncol. 2:207, 1984.

264. Taylor, A. L., Applefeld, M. N., Wiernik, P. H., et al.: Acute anthracycline cardiotoxicity. Comparative morphologic study of three analogues. Cancer 53:1660, 1984.

264a. Nielsen, D., Jensen, J. B., Dombernowsky, P., et al.: Epirubicin cardiotoxicity: A study of 135 patients with advanced breast cancer. J. Clin. Oncol. 8:1806, 1990.

265. Leitner, S. P., Casper, E. S., Hakes, T. B., et al.: A phase II trial of 4'-deoxy-doxorubicin in patients with advanced breast cancer. Cancer Treat. Rep. 69:1319, 1985.

266. Bramhilla, C., Rossi, A., Bonfonta, B., et al.: Phase II study of doxorubicin versus epirubicin in advanced breast cancer. Cancer Treat. Rep. 70:261, 1986.

267. Baello, E. B., Ensberg, M. E., Fergoson, D. W., et al.: Effect of high dose cyclophosphamide and total-body irradiation on left ventricular function in adult patients with leukemia undergoing allogeneic bone marrow transplantation. Cancer Treat. Rep. 70:1187, 1986.

268. Goldberg, M. A., Antin, J. H., Guinan, E. C., and Rappeport, J. M.: Cyclophosphamide cardiotoxicity. An analysis of dosing as a risk factor. Blood 68:1114, 1986.

269. Braverman, A. C., Antin, J. H., Plappert, M. T., et al.: Cyclophosphamide cardiotoxicity: A prospective evaluation of new dosing regimens. (Submitted for publication.)

270. Lopez, M., Contegiacomp, A., Vici, P., et al.: A prospective, randomized trial of doxorubicin versus idarubicin in the treatment of advanced breast cancer. Cancer 64:2431, 1989.

271. Baker, W. P., Dainer, P., Lester, W. M., et al.: Ischemic chest pain after 5-fluorouracil therapy for cancer. Am. J. Cardiol. 57:497, 1986.

272. Freeman, N. J., and Costanza, M. E.: 5-Fluorouracil-associated cardiotoxicity. Cancer 61:36, 1988.

273. Cristofini, P., Desnos, M., Guenot, O., et al.: Cardiotoxicity of 5-fluorouracil: Coronary spasm? Apropos of two cases with normal coronarography. Ann. Med. Interne 140:9, 1989.

274. Ensley, J. F., Patel, B., Kloner, R., et al.: The clinical syndrome of 5-fluorouracil cardiotoxicity. Invest. New Drugs 7:101, 1989.

275. Doll, D. C., List, A. F., Greco, F. A., et al.: Acute ventricular ischemic events after cisplatin-based combination chemotherapy for germ-cell tumors of the testis. Ann. Intern. Med. 105:48, 1986.

276. Anjo, A., Dantchev, D., and Mathe, G.: Notes on the cardiotoxicity of platinum complexes in ultrastructural study. Biomed. Pharmacother. 43:265, 1989.

277. Burkhardt, A., Haltje, W. J., and Gebbens, J. O.: Vascular lesions following perfusion with bleumycin: Electron-microscopic observations. Virchows Arch. Pathol. Anat. 372:227, 1976.

278. Mandel, E. M., Lewinski, U., and Djaldetti, M.: Vincristine-induced myocardial infarction. Cancer 30:1979, 1975.

279. Lejonc, J. L., Vernant, J. P., Macquin, J., and Castaigne, A.: Successful removal of aluminum from patient with dialysis encephalopathy. Lancet 2:692, 1980.

280. Aisner, J., VanEcho, D. A., Whitacre, M., and Wiernik, P. H.: A phase-I trial of continuous infusion VP-16-213 (etoposide). Cancer Chemother. Pharmacol. 7:157, 1982.

281. Gottdiener, J. S., Applebaum, F. R., Ferrans, V. J., et al.: Cardiotoxicity associated with high dose cyclophosphamide therapy. Arch. Intern. Med. 141:758, 1981.

282. Kandylis, K., Vassilomanolakis, M., Tsoussis, S., and Efremidis, A. P.: Ifosfamide cardiotoxicity in humans. Cancer Chemother. Pharmacol. 24:395, 1989.

283. Steinherz, L. J., Steinherz, P. G., Mangiacasale, D., et al.: Cardiac abnormalities after AMSA administration. Cancer Treat. Rep. 66:483, 1982.

284. Lindpainter, K., Lindpainter, L. S., Wentworth, M., and Burns, C. P.: Acute myocardial necrosis during administration of amsacrine. Cancer 57:1284, 1986.

285. Weiss, R. B., Grillo-Lopez, A. J., Marsoni, S., et al.: Amsacrine-associated cardiotoxicity: An analysis of 82 cases. J. Clin. Oncol. 4:919, 928, 1986.

286. Shenkenberg, T. D., and VonHoff, D. D.: Mitoxantrone: A new anticancer drug with significant clinical activity. Ann. Intern. Med. 105:67, 1986.

287. Colman, R. E., Maisey, M. N., Knight, R. K., and Rubens, R. D.: Mitoxantrone in advanced breast cancer: A phase II study with special attention to cardiotoxicity. Eur. J. Cancer Clin. Oncol. 20:771, 1984.

288. Pratt, C. G., Vietti, T. J., Etcubanas, E., et al.: Nonvantrone for childhood malignant solid tumors. A pediatric oncology group phase II study. Invest. New Drugs 4:43, 1986.

289. Landys, K., Bergstom, S., Andersson, T., and Noppa, H.: Mitoxantrone as a first line treatment of advanced breast cancer. Invest. New Drugs 3:133, 1985.

290. Allegra, J. C., Woodcock, T., Woolf, S., et al.: A randomized trial comparing mitoxantrone with doxorubicin in patients with stage IV breast cancer. Invest. New Drugs 3:153, 1985.

291. Baker, W. P., Dainer, P., Lester, W. M., et al.: Ischemic chest pain after 5-fluorouracil therapy for cancer. Am. J. Cardiol. 57:497, 1986.

291a. May, D., Wandl, U., Becher, R., et al.: Kardiale nebenwirkungen von 5-fluorouracil. Dtsch. Med. Wochenschr. 115:618, 1990.

292. Cameron, H. A., Reyntjens, A. J., and Lake-Bakaar, G.: Cardiac arrest after treatment with intravenous domperidone. Br. Med. J. (Clin. Res.) 290:160, 1985.

293. Osborne, A. J., Slevin, N. L., Hunter, L. W., and Hamer, J.: Cardiac arrhythmias during cytotoxic chemotherapy: Role of domperidone. Hum. Toxicol. 4:617, 1985.

294. Cazin, V., Gorin, C., Laport, J. P., et al.: Cardiac complications after bone marrow transplantation. A report on a series of 63 consecutive transplantations. Cancer 57:2061, 1986.

295. Cohen, M. C., Huberman, M. S., and Nesto, R. W.: Recombinant alpha-2 interferon-related cardiomyopathy. Am. J. Med. 85:549, 1988.

296. Deyton, L. R., Walker, R. E., Kovacs, J. A., et al.: Reversible cardiac dysfunction associated with interferon alpha therapy in AIDS patients with Kaposi's sarcoma. N. Engl. J. Med. 321:1246, 1989.

297. Nora, R., Abrams, J., and Silverman, H. J.: Infarction in patients receiving high dose recombinant interleukin-2 (rll-2). Proc. Am. Soc. Clin. Cardiol. 6:245, 1987.

298. Margolin, K., Jaffe, H. S., Hawkins, M., et al.: Toxicity of interleukin-2 and lymphokine-activated killer cell therapy. Proc. Am. Soc. Clin. Oncol. 6:251, 1987.

299. Rosenberg, S. A., Lotze, M. T., Muul, L. M., et al.: A progress report on the treatment of 157 patients with advanced cancer using lymphokine-activated hilar cells and interleukin-2 or high dose interleukin-2 alone. N. Engl. J. Med. 316:889, 1987.

300. Nora, R., Abrams, J. S., Tait, N. S., et al.: Myocardial toxic effects during recombinant interleukin-2 therapy. J. Natl. Cancer Inst. 81:59, 1989.

301. Osanto, S., Cluitman, F. H. M., Franks, C. R., et al.: Myocardial injury after interleukin-2 therapy. Lancet 2:48, 1988.

302. Dorr, R. T., and Shipp, N. G.: Effect of interferon, interleukin-2, and tumor necrosis factor in myocardial cell viability and doxorubicin cardiotoxicity in vitro. Immunpharmacology 18:31, 1989.

HEMATOLOGICAL ABNORMALITIES RELATED TO CARDIAC DRUGS

303. Gavras, F., Graff, L. G., Rose, B. D., et al.: Fatal pancytopenia associated with the use of captopril. Ann. Intern. Med. 94:58, 1981.

304. Lundh, B., and Hasselgren, K. H.: Hematological side effects from antihypertensive drugs. Acta Med. Scand. (Suppl.) 628:73, 1979.

305. Erslev, A. J. Aplastic anemia. In Williams, W. J. (ed.): Hematology, 3rd. ed. New York, McGraw-Hill Book Co., 1983, pp. 155–158.

306. Volosin, K., Greenberg, R. M., and Grenspon, A. J.: Tocainide-associated agranulocytosis. Am. Heart J. 109:1392, 1985.

307. Soff, G. A., and Kadin, M. E.: Tocainide-induced reversible agranulocytosis and anemia. Arch. Intern. Med. 147:598, 1987.

308. Morrill, G. B., and Gibson, S. M.: Tocainide-induced aplastic anemia (letter). Drug Intell. Clin. Pharm. 23:90, 1989.

309. Finch, S. C.: Neutropenia. In Williams, W. J. (ed.): Hematology. New York, McGraw-Hill, 1983, pp. 777–786.

310. Hackett, T., Kelton, J. G., and Powers, P.: Drug-induced platelet destruction. Semin. Thromb. Hemostas. 8:116, 1982.

311. Ansell, J., McCue, J., Tiarks, C., et al.: Amrinone-induced thrombocytopenia. Blood 58(Suppl. 1):187a, 1981.

312. Packman, C. H., and Leddy, J. P.: Drug-related immunologic injury of erythrocytes. In Williams, W. J. (ed.): Hematology. New York, McGraw-Hill Book Co., 1983, pp. 647–650.

313. Bell, W. R., and Royall, R. M.: Heparin-associated thrombocytopenia: A comparison of three heparin preparations. N. Engl. J. Med. 303:902, 1980.

314. Gibson, G. R., Hunter, J. B., Raabe, D. S., et al.: Methemoalbuminemia produced by high-dose intravenous nitroglycerin. Ann. Intern. Med. 96:615, 1982.

315. Vesey, C. J., and Cole, P. V.: Blood cyanide and thiocyanate concentrations produced by long-term therapy with sodium nitroprusside. Br. J. Anaesth. 57:148, 1985.

316. Weisbart, R. H., Yee, W. S., Colburn, K. K., et al.: Antiguanosine antibodies: A new marker for procainamide-induced systemic lupus erythematosus. Ann. Intern. Med. 104:310, 1986.

Hemostasis, Thrombosis, Fibrinolysis, and Cardiovascular Disease

by ROBERT I. HANDIN, M.D., and JOSEPH LOSCALZO, M.D., Ph.D.

Thrombosis and embolism either contribute to the pathogenesis of many cardiovascular disorders or complicate their clinical course. After some initial skepticism, several decades of laboratory and clinical research have established a role for platelets and coagulation proteins in the pathogenesis of atherosclerosis (see Chap. 36). The coagulation system plays a role in the clinically silent evolution and progression of atheroma, and in the events that follow plaque rupture and activation which produce clinical symptoms. This close pathogenic relation has led some authors to refer to the overall process as "atherothrombosis."[1] Not only do many acute cardiovascular events, such as myocardial infarction and stroke, arise from thrombotic occlusion of atherosclerotic arteries, but also patients with preexisting chronic disorders such as congestive heart failure, cardiomyopathy, and valvular or congenital heart disease are at increased risk of venous or arterial thromboembolism. As a result of these clinical and experimental observations, anticoagulant, antiplatelet, and, most recently, fibrinolytic agents have become increasingly important therapeutic tools for the cardiologist.

In this chapter the pathophysiology of normal hemostasis is reviewed, and those disorders are described that cause failure of hemostasis with hemorrhage as well as those that increase the risk of thrombosis. The inherited prethrombotic or hypercoagulable states, including fibrinolytic disorders, are used to illustrate more general mechanisms of venous and arterial thromboembolism in patients with cardiovascular disorders. Finally, methods for preventing and treating thromboembolism associated with cardiovascular diseases are discussed, including new options for clot dissolution—an area in which rapid and impressive strides have been made over the past few years.

HEMOSTASIS

Unactivated *platelets* circulate as individual, smooth-surfaced discs that do not interact with other cells in the blood or with the endothelial cells that line the blood vessels. Platelets will adhere, however, to subendothelium that has been exposed as a result of vascular injury or to any foreign or prosthetic material in contact with blood. Adherent, activated platelets generate potent mediators that cause vasoconstriction and leukocyte chemotaxis. The platelets then degranulate, releasing materials that attract platelets, forming a multicellular aggregate or hemostatic plug on the adherent monolayer. These events, collectively referred to as *primary hemostasis*, are the first line of defense against hemorrhage after vascular injury. They are particularly important in capillaries and small arterioles where shear forces are high and the formation of a platelet plug is critical for effective hemostasis.

The *plasma coagulation system*, or secondary hemostatic system, is simultaneously activated in response to vascular injury and, within several minutes, generates insoluble fibrin strands that interdigitate with and strengthen the primary platelet plug. Fibrin is produced by the action of thrombin on fibrinogen. Thrombin is generated by a series of linked proteolytic reactions that take place on phospholipid-rich cell surfaces and are regulated by plasma cofactors and calcium, which accelerate coagulation, and by a series of naturally occurring inhibitors, or anticoagulants. Although platelet activation and fibrin production are described as separate processes, they actually are closely linked and interdependent. For example, the surface of the activated platelet provides the optimal locus for several critical coagulation reactions and accelerates them several hundredfold. Conversely, thrombin generated during plasma coagulation also is a potent agonist, and stimulates platelet secretion and aggregation. The endothelial cells that line the blood vessels also bind coagulation proteins, accelerate their interactions, and secrete both inhibitory and procoagulant molecules.

Although the hemostatic system has evolved to minimize blood loss from injured vessels, there is little difference between the physiological process of normal hemostasis and the pathological events that lead to thrombosis and embolism. Because of this similarity, thrombosis has been described as hemostasis occurring in the wrong place or at the wrong time. Although both inherited and acquired disorders may predispose a patient to thrombosis, in many cases the triggering event is simply the interaction of normal blood components with an abnormal surface such as a diseased or atherosclerotic vessel, a prosthetic cardiac valve, or a vascular graft. Furthermore, bleeding caused by failure of a component in the hemostatic system is similar to the purposeful or therapeutic failure of hemostasis induced by anticoagulant agents used to prevent recurrent thromboembolism. Most of the available anticoagulant drugs are not selective and have a relatively poor therapeutic index. Thus, the dose of drug needed to produce the desired antithrombotic effect also may cause undesirable hemorrhage. Finally, because pathological thrombi may coexist with physiological and vital hemostatic plugs, even the more selective drugs, such as the relatively fibrin-specific plasminogen activators, cannot discriminate between fibrin within pathological thrombi and that within physiological hemostatic plugs.

PLATELETS IN COAGULATION

PLATELET ADHESION TO THE VESSEL WALL. Platelet adhesion, the initial event in both normal hemostasis and thrombosis, is a complex process that involves constituents of the vascular subendothelium, receptor sites on the platelet membrane, and plasma glycoproteins (Fig. 58–1). In normal hemostasis, platelets adhere to exposed subendothelial collagen after the traumatic removal of endothelial cells that normally line the blood vessel. In addition, thrombus formation may be initiated by the adhesion of platelets to damaged endothelial cells or denuded atherosclerotic plaques. Although several candidates have been proposed as the platelet collagen receptor, the collagen-binding site is probably located on the platelet glycoprotein Ia/IIa complex.[2,3] The initial bond between the platelet and the vessel wall is strengthened by the interaction of several adhesive glycoproteins.

Fibronectin. This 440,000-dalton dimeric protein binds to collagen and to platelets through receptor sites on the platelet glycoprotein IIb/IIIa (GpIIb/IIIa) complex.[4,5] Fibronectin binding facilitates both initial platelet attachment to the vessel wall and subsequent spreading over the subendothelial surface.[6]

von Willebrand's Factor (vWF). This protein circulates as a heterogeneous series of high molecular weight multimers and also binds to collagen[7] and to two separate platelet receptor sites. The best defined receptor site for vWF is on the platelet glycoprotein Ib/IV complex.[8] Binding to this site is critically important for normal platelet adhesion. vWF binding to a second platelet receptor site on glycoproteins IIb/IIIa may facilitate both adhesion and platelet-platelet cohesion or aggregate formation.[9] This factor plays a critical role in hemostasis, since it stabilizes the attachment of platelets to the vessel wall under conditions of high shear stress.[10,11] Neither the initial collagen-GpIa/IIa interaction nor the secondary interposition of fibronectin between platelets and collagen is sufficient to sustain platelet adhesion in the face of the high shear stresses encountered with normal blood flow. This unique property of vWF is clinically important, since bleeding and abnormal platelet function are found in patients with a mild or moderate deficiency in vWF despite normal interactions between the platelet membrane and subendothelial collagen and normal binding of fibronectin to the platelet and vessel wall.

PLATELET ACTIVATION AND SECRETION

Platelet activation follows the adhesion of platelets to vascular subendothelium, or the binding of soluble agonists to platelet membrane receptors, and culminates in granule release and the formation of a platelet aggregate or hemostatic plug. Platelets have specific binding sites for adenosine diphosphate (ADP), thrombin, serotonin, and alpha$_2$-adrenergic agonists.[12] As shown in Figure 58–2, occupancy of these receptors by the appropriate agonists activates two intracellular enzymes, protein kinase A [the cyclic adenosine monophosphate (AMP)–dependent protein kinase] and protein kinase C, which then catalyze the phosphorylation of critical regulatory proteins within the platelet. Protein kinase A activity is regulated by the level of intracellular cyclic AMP and protein kinase C by diacylglycerol (DAG), a product of phospholipid hydrolysis. Inhibition of platelet adenylate cyclase activity activates protein kinase A, which then phosphorylates myosin light chain and enhances the contractile activity of platelet actomyosin. In contrast, the major substrate for protein kinase C is a 47,000-dalton protein that may serve as a feedback inhibitor of platelet activation, as described below. Although the specific target proteins may differ slightly, the sequence of reactions resembles that seen after the activation of beta-adrenoceptors in heart muscle (p. 363).

MECHANISMS OF ACTIVATION. Although there are two separate signal transduction pathways, mediated by protein kinases A and C within the platelet, their relative contributions to platelet activation are still being debated. Agonists like epinephrine clearly inhibit adenylate cyclase activity in platelet membrane fractions; however, incubating intact platelets with epinephrine does not reduce intraplatelet cyclic AMP to below basal levels, suggesting that cyclic AMP levels do not regulate platelet signal transduction and activation.[13] Alternatively, because cyclic AMP is compartmentalized within the platelet, regulation of cyclic AMP content within a specific compartment may be an important mechanism for signal transduction by certain agonists. The bulk of recent evidence suggests that the adenylate cyclase–cyclic AMP system provides a mechanism to *inhibit* platelet activation. In fact, many agents that stimulate platelet adenylate cyclase activity and raise intraplatelet cyclic AMP levels, such as prostaglandins E$_1$, D$_2$, and I$_2$, are potent platelet inhibitors.[14,15]

Transduction of the signal initiated by platelet agonist binding to membrane receptors is more likely to be mediated by the intracellular enzyme phospholipase C, which hydrolyzes a trace membrane phospholipid, phosphatidylinositol 4,5-bisphosphate (PIP$_2$), yielding inositol 1,4,5,-trisphosphate (IP$_3$) and DAG.[16,17] Although the role of cyclic AMP in platelet activation may be unclear, the two products of PIP$_2$ hydrolysis are clearly important mediators of platelet signal transduction. IP$_3$ acts as a calcium ionophore, transiently raising intraplatelet calcium levels, while DAG activates protein kinase C, which then phosphorylates several intracellular proteins.[18,19] One prominent substrate is a 47,000-dalton protein present in platelets and leukocytes called *plekstrin*.[20] The function of this phosphoprotein is unknown. There also is pharmacological evidence that IP$_3$ and DAG themselves mediate signal transduction directly. The ability of a calcium ionophore to initiate platelet signal transduction has been well established. Furthermore, incubation of platelets with DAG analogs like oleylacylglycerol, which cross the platelet membrane, can mimic the effect of endogenous DAG.[21] Likewise, incubation of platelets with phorbolmyristate acetate, an agent that directly activates protein kinase C, eliminates the requirement for phospholipid hydrolysis and DAG generation for platelet activation.[22]

ROLE OF ARACHIDONIC ACID AND PROSTAGLANDINS

Arachidonic acid (5,8,11,14-eicosatetraenoic acid), a 20-carbon polyunsaturated fatty acid derived from dietary linoleic acid, is the precursor of the prostaglandins, leukotrienes, and thromboxane — eicosanoid mediators generated by activated platelets, leukocytes, and endothelial cells.[23,24] Arachidonate is taken up by the platelet from plasma and is esterified into platelet phospholipids. As outlined in Figures 58–2 and 58–3, the combined action of phospholipase C and diglyceride lipase on phosphatidylinositol rapidly releases arachidonic acid early in platelet acti-

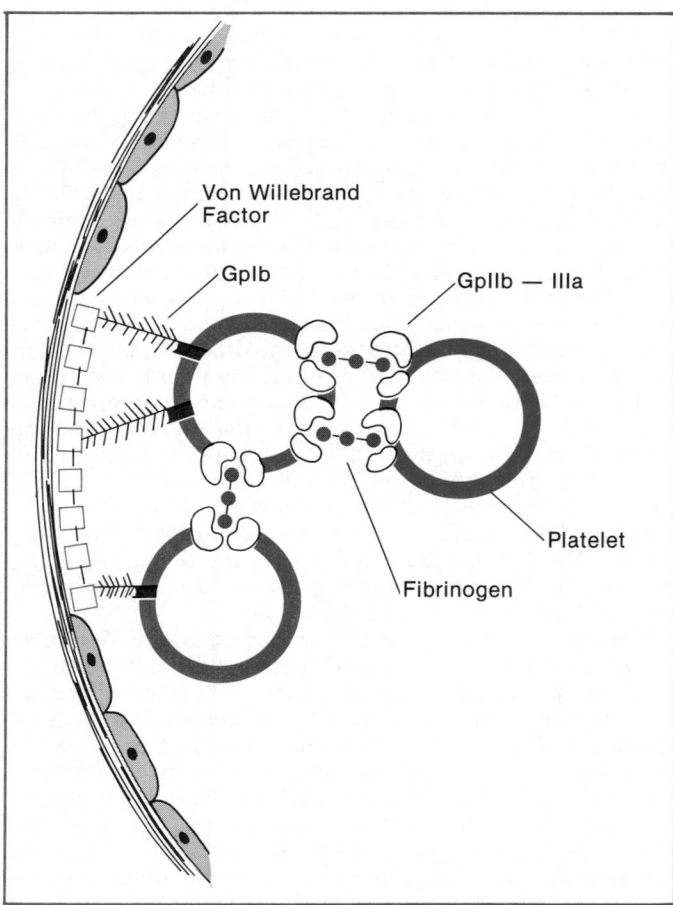

FIGURE 58–1. Molecular mechanisms of platelet attachment to vascular subendothelium (platelet adhesion) and of platelet-platelet interactions (platelet aggregation) in a cross-sectional view of a blood vessel. von Willebrand's multimers attach to exposed vascular subendothelial collagen and to a platelet membrane receptor site on glycoprotein Ib (GpIb). This is the initial interaction in hemostasis and stabilizes platelets so that they remain attached despite the high shear forces generated by flowing blood. Receptor sites on platelet membrane glycoproteins IIb and IIIa (GpIIb–IIIa) then become available to bind fibrinogen. The fibrinogen molecule links platelets together to form the hemostatic plug.

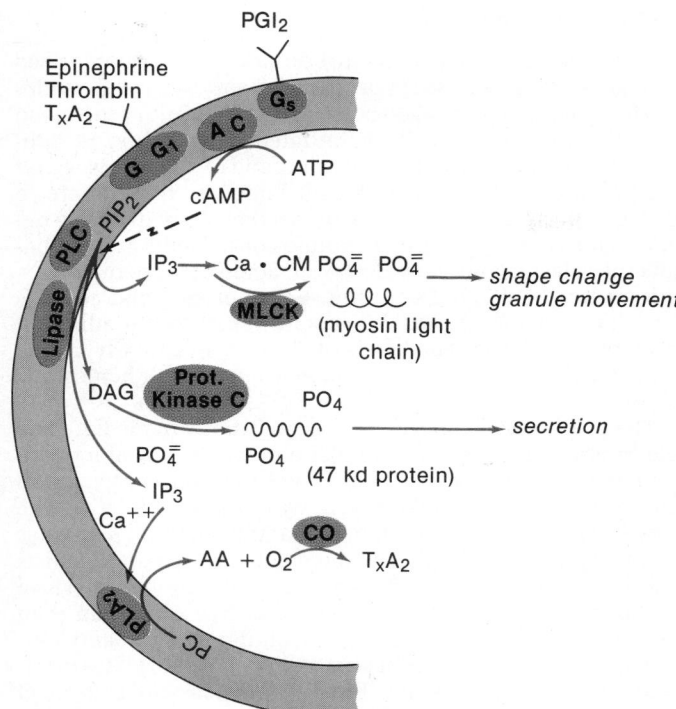

FIGURE 58–2. Biochemical pathways for stimulus-response coupling in the platelet. Platelets contain receptors that bind various agonists, including epinephrine, thrombin, and thromboxane A_2 (TxA_2) and the antagonist prostaglandin I_2 (PGI_2). Receptors for agonists and antagonists are coupled to two enzymes, adenylate cyclase (AC) and phospholipase C (PLC), by means of guanine nucleotide binding (G) proteins. Coupling to AC occurs by way of separate G_i (inhibitory) and G_s (stimulatory) proteins. It is not yet known whether coupling of receptors to PLC is by the same or a different set of G proteins. Activation of AC by PGI_2 raises intracellular cyclic AMP (cAMP) and inhibits platelet function, whereas inhibition of AC facilitates platelet activation by an incompletely worked-out set of reactions. PLC hydrolyzes the membrane phospholipid phosphatidylinositol bisphosphate (PIP$_2$) to yield diacylglycerol (DAG) and inositol triphosphate (IP$_3$). IP$_3$ functions as a calcium ionophore and transiently increases intracellular ionized calcium (Ca), which facilitates several important intraplatelet reactions. In one, Ca bound to calmodulin (CM) activates myosin light chain kinase (MLCK), which then phosphorylates the light chain of platelet myosin. The phosphorylated light chain participates in contractile force generation within the platelet, which causes shape change and granule movement. DAG activates protein kinase C, which, in turn, phosphorylates several other intracellular proteins that regulate secretion. Two mechanisms hydrolyze arachidonic acid (AA) from membrane phospholipids. First, DAG generated by PLC is the substrate for an intramembrane diglyceride lipase. Second, the IP$_3$-induced calcium flux activates a second enzyme, phospholipase A_2 (PLA_2), which hydrolyzes AA from phosphatidylcholine (PC). AA is then oxygenated by the enzyme cyclo-oxygenase (CO) and subsequently converted to TxA_2, a potent platelet agonist and vasoconstrictor. TxA_2 then stimulates additional platelet activation by way of the previously described pathways. Aspirin and nonsteroidal antiinflammatory agents act as antiplatelet agents by irreversibly acetylating CO and preventing TxA_2 generation.

vation.[25] Additional arachidonate subsequently is liberated from phosphatidylcholine by a phospholipase A_2 enzyme.[26] Released arachidonate is rapidly oxygenated by cyclo-oxygenase or lipoxygenase enzymes in platelets, leukocytes, and endothelial cells to yield various prostanoid and eicosanoid mediators.

THROMBOXANE A_2 (TxA_2). This potent vasoconstrictor and platelet agonist is the most important platelet eicosanoid mediator.[24] The generation of TxA_2 by activated platelets may explain the vasoconstriction and vessel retraction that accompany vascular injury and may contribute to the vasospasm observed in partially occluded atherosclerotic coronary and cerebral vessels. Inhibition of TxA_2 synthesis by agents like aspirin may explain their beneficial antithrombotic effect.[23] The principal platelet lipoxygenase product, 12-hydroxyeicosatetraenoic acid (12-HETE), has no direct role in hemostasis but may serve as a chemotactic agent for neutrophils and contribute to the inflammatory response.[27]

PROSTACYCLIN (PGI_2). The endothelial cell converts arachidonic acid into PGI_2, a labile cyclic prostaglandin.[28] In contrast to TxA_2, PGI_2 is a potent vasodilator that inhibits platelet aggregation and secretion by activating platelet adenylate cyclase and elevating intraplatelet cyclic AMP. Thrombin, calcium ionophore, bradykinin, serotonin, platelet-derived growth factor, and mechanical injury can all induce the synthesis of PGI_2 by endothelial cells. Although it is tempting to postulate that a balance between TxA_2 and PGI_2 synthesis by their respective cells regulates platelet vessel wall interactions and vessel tone, it is difficult to test this hypothesis, since both eicosanoids have very short half-lives, are produced in small quantities, and function locally within the microcirculation. Whole-body turnover studies that assess the excretion of thromboxane and prostacyclin metabolites in urine by gas chromatography and mass spectrometry demonstrate that the production of both eicosanoids is increased in thrombotic states and vascular disease.[29,30]

THE LEUKOTRIENES AND LIPOXINS. A relatively new class of eicosanoid mediators, the leukotrienes, play an important role in inflammation (Fig. 58–3).[31] The major derivative of arachidonic acid in polymorphonuclear leukocytes is 5-hydroxyeicosatetraenoic acid (5-HETE), which is converted to leukotriene A_4 (LTA_4). LTA_4 is then converted to LTB_4 by the addition of a 12-OH group. LTA_4 also is converted to leukotrienes C_4, D_4, and E_4 by the addition and subsequent metabolism of glutathione. The mediator responsible for acute anaphylaxis, formerly called the slow reacting substance of anaphylaxis, or SRS-A, is actually a mixture of the peptidolipid leukotrienes C_4, D_4, and E_4, which are potent bronchoconstrictors and vasoconstrictors. These leukotrienes also may be important in hemostasis, since they constrict the microvasculature and coronary arteries. The lipoxins are conjugated tetraene derivatives of arachidonic acid.[32] They tend to oppose the actions of leukotrienes. Because leukotrienes and lipoxins are products of lipoxygenase reactions, their biosynthesis is not inhibited by cyclo-oxygenase inhibitors such as aspirin.

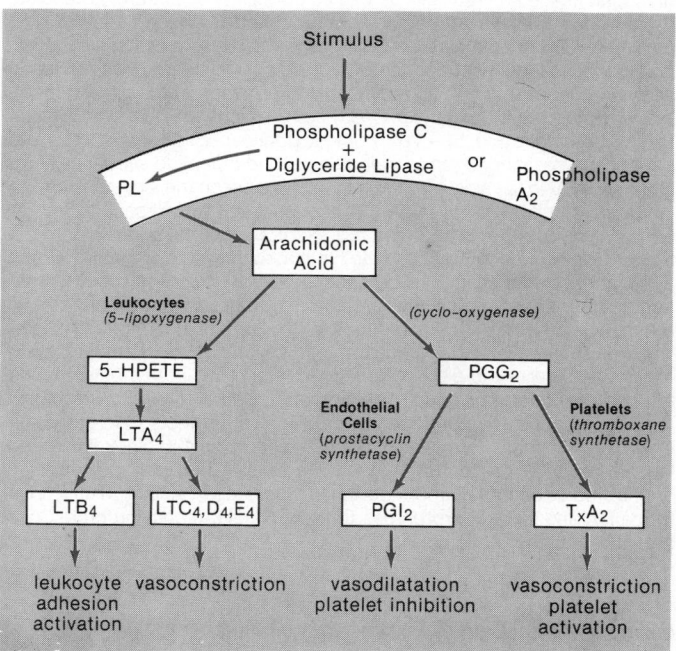

FIGURE 58–3. Liberation of arachidonic acid from membrane phospholipids and its subsequent conversion into biologically active mediators in leukocytes, platelets, and endothelial cells. Arachidonic acid is liberated from membrane phospholipids after cellular activation by the combined effects of the enzymes phospholipase C and diglyceride lipase or by the action of a phospholipase A_2 enzyme. In leukocytes, arachidonic acid is converted to an unstable intermediate, 5-hydroperoxyeicosatetraenoic acid (5-HPETE), by a 5-lipoxygenase enzyme. 5-HPETE is then converted into the leukotrienes (LT). Leukotriene B_4 (LTB_4) stimulates leukocyte adhesion to endothelial cells; leukotrienes C_4, D_4, and E_4 are potent vasoconstrictors. In platelets and endothelial cells the principal pathway for arachidonic acid metabolism is by way of cyclo-oxygenase, which forms the unstable intermediate prostaglandin G_2 (PGG_2). It is then converted to prostaglandin I_2 (PGI_2, or prostacyclin) by means of prostacyclin synthetase within endothelial cells. Prostacyclin, a labile compound, is a potent vasodilator that inhibits platelet activation. Within the platelet, PGG_2 is converted to thromboxane A_2 (TxA_2), another labile compound that is a potent vasoconstrictor and platelet agonist. Aspirin and other nonsteroidal antiinflammatory agents interfere with hemostasis by inhibiting the enzyme cyclooxygenase. They have no effect on leukotriene biosynthesis.

There also is active transcellular metabolism of eicosanoids. For example, two of the prostaglandin endoperoxide precursors, PGG_2 and PGH_2, can leave the platelet and enter the endothelial cell to be converted to PGI_2. Thus, a byproduct of platelet activation is transformed into a platelet inhibitor and acts as a feedback regulator, a phenomenon referred to as the "endoperoxide steal."[33,34] There also is evidence that unmetabolized arachidonic acid derived from aspirin-treated platelets may be converted into the vasoactive leukotrienes by polymorphonuclear leukocytes.

GRANULE SECRETION OR RELEASE

Platelets contain two classes of secretory granules, which are most readily classified by their density on electron micrographs. The most electron-dense (delta) granules contain adenine nucleotides (ADP and ATP), calcium, and serotonin, whereas the least electron-dense alpha granules contain enzymes, adhesive and coagulation proteins, and growth factors.[35] After platelet activation, both granule classes release their contents into the vicinity of the platelet plug, where they diffuse into plasma and into the vessel wall.[36] Platelet-derived growth factor and transforming growth factor beta (TGF-beta), which are both released by activated platelets, stimulate smooth muscle cell and fibroblast migration and proliferation.[37] This may be of importance both in wound healing and in the pathogenesis of atherosclerosis. TGF-beta also may inhibit the migration and proliferation of endothelial cells. Other secreted molecules enhance vascular permeability, bind glycosaminoglycans, and induce the chemotaxis of leukocytes to sites of vascular injury.[38]

PLATELET AGGREGATION

Fibrinogen is an essential cofactor for platelet aggregation. Although platelets circulate in a milieu rich in fibrinogen, they do not bind to it but remain as single, disc-shaped particles. Contact with ADP, derived from damaged tissue and red cells as well as from platelet secretory granules, initiates both platelet aggregate formation and fibrinogen binding. The binding of ADP to a platelet receptor induces platelets to become spherical and to extend large pseudopods. A protein, aggregin, has been proposed as the ADP receptor.[39] In addition, the conformation of the platelet membrane glycoprotein IIb/IIIa (GpIIb/IIIa) complex changes, so that it binds plasma fibrinogen (Fig. 58–1).[40] A unique dodecapeptide sequence on the gamma chain of fibrinogen as well as a second tripeptide sequence (Arg-Gly-Asp-RGD in the single letter amino acid code) on the alpha chain each binds to the platelet.[41,42] The RGD sequence is also present in 8 other adhesive glycoproteins and may represent a universal adhesive protein recognition sequence. Because the fibrinogen molecule contains pairs of alpha and gamma chain binding sites, it can link platelets together into aggregates. Patients with the rare platelet defect *thrombasthenia* have reduced or absent GpIIb/IIIa, reduced fibrinogen binding, markedly diminished or absent platelet aggregation, and severe bleeding, underscoring the importance of the platelet-fibrinogen interaction in hemostasis. The infusion of monoclonal antibodies directed against GpIIb/IIIa, which prevent aggregation and fibrinogen binding in vivo, protects laboratory animals from thrombus formation.[43] Synthetic peptides that block fibrinogen binding to platelet receptors may have a similar antithrombotic effect.[44] These studies document the importance of fibrinogen binding in thrombus formation and provide prototypes for new platelet-modifying drugs with potential antithrombotic activity.

Endothelial Inhibition of Platelet Aggregation

Under normal circumstances, the vascular endothelium presents an antithrombotic surface which inhibits platelet activation. Factors produced by the endothelial cell that are inhibitory include prostacyclin, endothelium-derived relaxing factor (EDRF), tissue-type plasminogen activator (t-PA), and an endothelial surface ADPase. Prostacyclin activates adenylate cyclase and increases intraplatelet cyclic AMP, and EDRF, one form of which is nitric oxide or an S-nitrosothiol derivative, activates platelet guanylate cyclase,[45,46] raising intraplatelet levels of cyclic GMP. Both antagonists inhibit platelet activation, prevent intraplatelet calcium flux, and reduce surface fibrinogen binding.[47] t-PA released from the endothelial cell binds to the platelet surface and activates platelet-bound plasminogen.[48-50] Finally, an endothelial surface ADPase may hydrolyze ADP released from damaged tissue or other platelets. These four independent endothelial-dependent reactions can be synergistic and effectively inhibit platelet plug formation and maintain blood fluidity,[51] and endothelial removal, injury, or dysfunction can enhance platelet plug formation.

Summary of the Role of Platelets

The sequence of reactions just described and summarized in Figure 58–4 represents primary hemostasis and provides the first line of defense against blood loss after injury to a blood vessel. Hemostasis usually is initiated when injury is sufficient to remove the endothelial lining and expose the vascular subendothelium to flowing blood. Platelets then adhere to collagen fibrils in the vessel wall, become activated, and degranulate, thereby releasing granule constituents and mediators into plasma and the vessel wall. Some of these materials, principally ADP and TxA_2, diffuse into plasma and activate circulating platelets, which become linked to the adherent platelet monolayer. The layers of platelets eventually fill the lumen of the vessel, forming a platelet aggregate or hemostatic plug.

The processes of adhesion and aggregation are mediated by the interaction of specific platelet membrane receptors with components of the vessel wall or with plasma proteins like fibronectin, vWF, and fibrinogen, which link platelets to the vessel wall and to one another. Signal transduction pathways in the platelet are complex, and regulated by specific agonists that bind to platelet receptors and activate the hydrolysis of phosphatidylinositol. These products of hydrolysis can then induce transient increases in intracellular calcium and activate an intracellular protein kinase that phosphorylates intraplatelet regulatory proteins. Finally, the eicosanoids derived from arachidonic acid in platelets, leukocytes, and endothelial cells provide short-acting biological mediators that can optimize the degree of platelet activation and vasoconstriction during local hemostasis. The plasma coagulation, or secondary hemostatic, system then generates fibrin strands that are interposed into the platelet plug to provide a stronger and more permanent hemostatic plug.

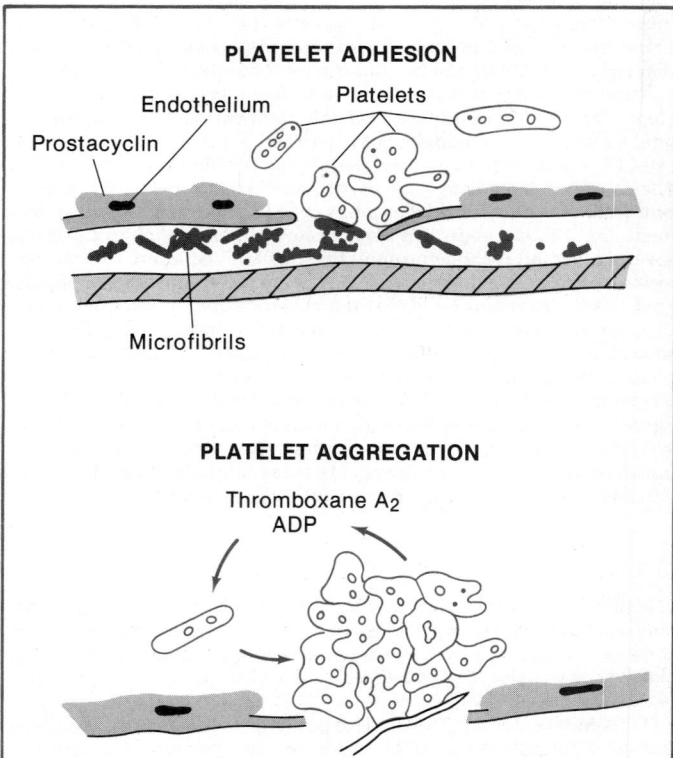

FIGURE 58–4. Overview of primary hemostasis. The initial event is adhesion of platelets to areas of the vessel wall in which the subendothelium has been exposed by endothelial cell disruption or injury. After adhesion, platelets become activated and, under the influence of mediators like ADP and thromboxane A_2, recruit additional circulating platelets to bind to the adherent monolayer and form a platelet aggregate.

FIBRIN GENERATION AND CLOT FORMATION

Blood coagulation is initiated by the interaction of flowing blood with vascular subendothelium or tissue thromboplastin (tissue factor) exposed on cell surfaces after cellular injury. Although the blood coagulation reactions often are referred to as the "fluid phase" of hemostasis, the reactions actually occur on vascular subendothelium or negatively charged, phospholipid-rich surfaces, such as the plasma membrane of suitably activated platelets or endothelial cells. The adsorption of coagulation proteins onto these surfaces increases their concentration, effectively increasing reaction rates and localizing their activity. As shown in Figure 58–5, the interactions among the procoagulants can be conveniently grouped into a series of surface-bound enzyme–cofactor complexes. Several of the coagulation proteins, including factors II, VII, IX, and X, are bound to surfaces by means of bridges formed between calcium, the negatively charged cell surface, and digamma-carboxyglutamic acid (Gla) residues on the proteins.[52] Other proteins are bound by electrostatic or hydrophobic interactions. After adsorption and complex formation, precursor proteins, or zymogens, are converted to active enzymes by limited proteolysis. Reaction rates are controlled by high molecular weight protein cofactors like factors V and VIII that markedly accelerate proteolysis. In each case, the cleavage of one or more relatively small peptides from the parent molecule converts it to an active protease, which then acts on another zymogen in the coagulation cascade.

INTRINSIC COAGULATION PATHWAY. The intrinsic, or contact activation, pathway of coagulation is initiated by the formation of a complex among three plasma proteins—Hageman factor (factor XII), high molecular weight kininogen (HMWK), and prekallikrein (PK) (Fig. 58–6A). HMWK and PK circulate in plasma as a noncovalent complex. This complex,

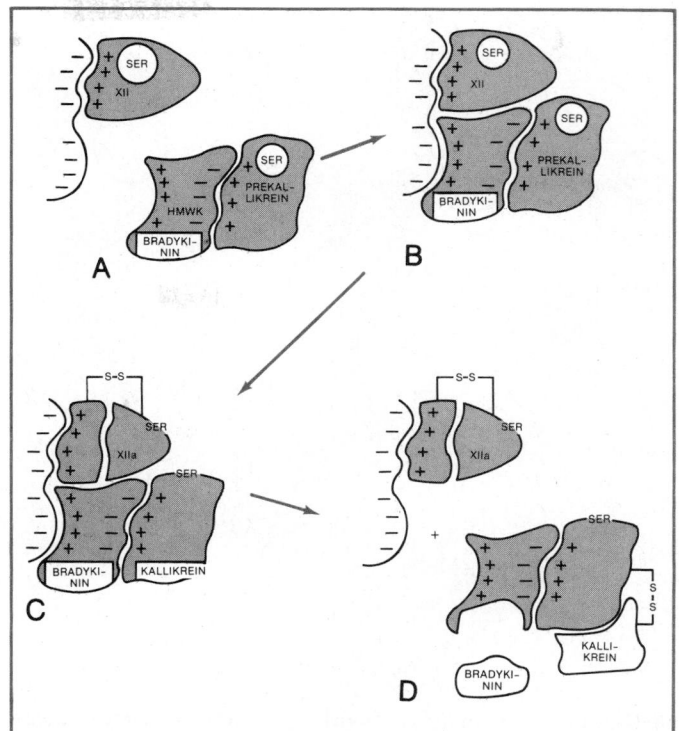

FIGURE 58–6. Reactions comprising the contact activation or intrinsic pathway of coagulation. *A* and *B*, High molecular weight kininogen (HMWK) and prekallikrein (PK), which circulate as a noncovalent complex, attach to a surface such as the vascular subendothelium along with Hageman factor (factor XII). *C, D,* This converts PK to the active serine protease kallikrein, which then converts factor XII to its active form, XIIa, and also liberates bradykinin from HMWK. The subsequent reaction (not shown in the figure) is between surface-bound XIIa and factor XI, which initiates coagulation. (From Verstraete, M., and Vermylen, J.: Thrombosis. Oxford, Pergamon Press, 1984, p. 27.)

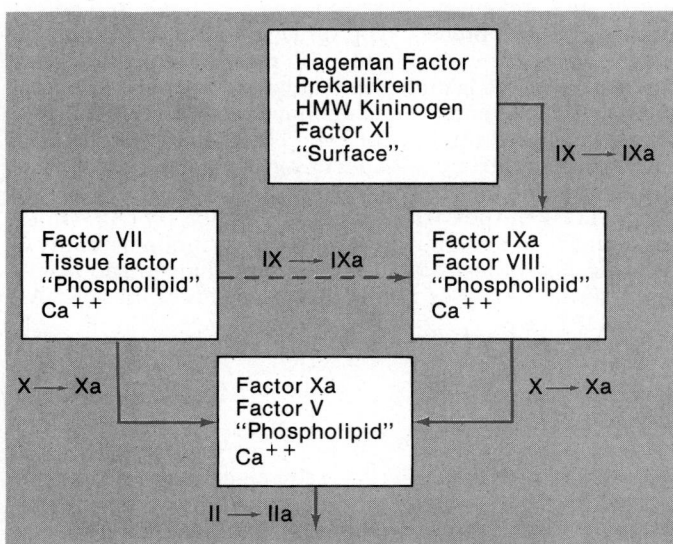

FIGURE 58–5. Major enzyme complexes of the coagulation cascade. The intrinsic, or contact activation, pathway is represented by the box at the top containing Hageman factor, prekallikrein, high molecular weight (HMW) kininogen, and factor XI and the initiating stimulus contact of blood with a "surface." The result of these interactions is formation of an enzyme, factor XIa, that converts factor IX to IXa. In the second reaction, factor IXa along with factor VIII, a source of phospholipid, and calcium assemble to convert factor X to Xa. In the extrinsic, or tissue factor–dependent, pathway, tissue factor and factor VII along with phospholipid and calcium can either directly activate factor X to Xa or activate IX. In the final reaction, factor Xa and factor V along with phospholipid and calcium convert factor II (prothrombin) to IIa (thrombin). Because both initiating pathways can activate factors IX and X, there is no need to make a distinction between intrinsic and extrinsic activation of the coagulation system. (From Mann, K. G., and Fass, D. N.: The molecular biology of blood coagulation. *In* Fairbanks, V. F. [ed.]: Current Hematology. Vol 2. New York, John Wiley & Sons, 1983, p. 347.)

when adsorbed onto a suitable surface, binds factor XII and slowly converts some of it to an active enzymatic form called factor XIIa (Fig. 58–6B). Factor XIIa then converts a second component of the complex, PK, to kallikrein (Fig. 58–6C). The resulting protease, kallikrein, both liberates the vasoactive peptide bradykinin from the third member of the complex, HMWK, and accelerates the conversion of factor XII to XIIa (Fig. 58–6D). In a subsequent reaction, factor XI is attached to this trimolecular complex and converted to its active form, XIa, by the proteolytic action of surface-bound XIIa.

EXTRINSIC COAGULATION PATHWAY. Tissue factor, a ubiquitous cellular lipoprotein, initiates the extrinsic coagulation pathway by forming a calcium-dependent complex with another protein, factor VII, a member of a group of Gla-containing coagulation proteins synthesized in the liver. After complex formation, factor VII develops proteolytic activity (VIIa), which converts factor X to its active form, Xa. The term extrinsic coagulation pathway was derived from an earlier observation that vesicles rich in tissue factor may be released into the blood from damaged tissues or cells. It is now known that endothelial cells still attached to subendothelium, along with circulating leukocytes, may express tissue factor activity and accelerate coagulation reactions after activation by agents like interleukin-1 or bacterial endotoxin.

COMMON PATHWAY. Factor X is activated by products generated by the contact activation or Hageman factor–dependent pathway as well as by the tissue factor–VII complex (Fig. 58–7). Factor XIa first converts factor IX to IXa. Factor X is then activated by IXa, in conjunction with factor VIII, by the formation of a calcium- and lipid-dependent macromolecular complex. Factor VIII has little biological activity until it is converted to VIIIa by traces of thrombin. Formation

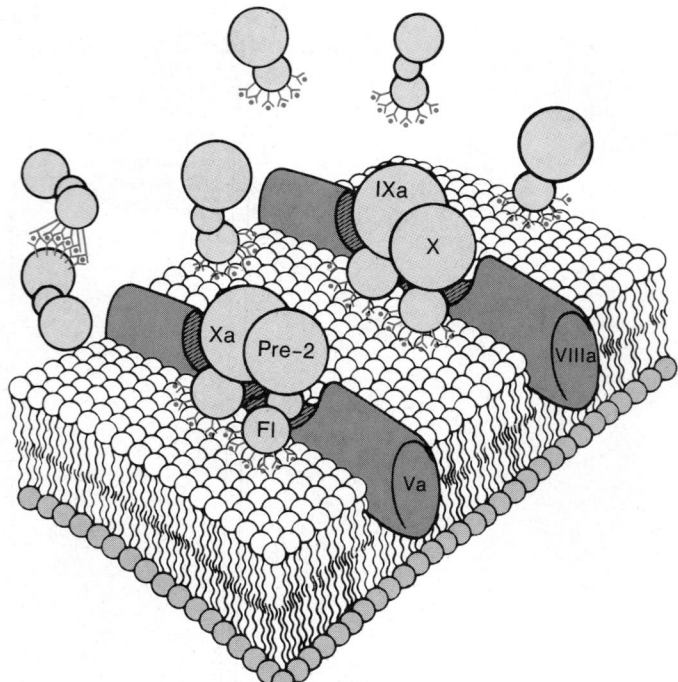

FIGURE 58-7. Hypothetical model of the prothrombinase complex and the complex responsible for factor X activation. Factors Va and VIIIa attach to a model cell membrane by hydrophobic interactions and also develop binding sites for specific coagulation factors. Factors IXa and X bind to factor VIIIa and to the membrane. Binding is partially mediated by gammacarboxyglutamic acid (Gla) residues and calcium. After its activation, factor Xa becomes part of a second adjacent complex with factor Va and prothrombin (depicted here as Pre-2). Again, Xa and prothrombin interact with the cell membrane by means of Gla residues and calcium. Thrombin is then liberated from the surface to participate in additional coagulation reactions. (From Mann, K. G., et al.: The role of factor V in the assembly of the prothrombinase complex. In Walz, D. A., and McCoy L. E. [eds.]: Annals of the New York Academy of Sciences. New York, 1981, p. 378.)

of the IXa–X–VIIIa complex occurs on a cell surface, probably on activated endothelial cells or platelets. In addition to activating factor X, the tissue factor–VIIa complex also may activate factor IX. This alternative pathway provides a link between the contact activation and tissue factor–dependent pathways of coagulation, and its existence may help to explain why patients with severe factor VIII or IX deficiency who have a normal tissue factor–dependent mechanism still have defective hemostasis.

Factor Xa then converts prothrombin to thrombin in conjunction with factor Va, calcium, and phospholipid (Fig. 58-7). Prothrombin conversion, which also takes place on activated platelet or endothelial surfaces, requires the assembly of a macromolecular complex among factor Va, Xa, and prothrombin. Thrombin, the product of this reaction, is a potent and versatile protease that has multiple actions in hemostasis, which include activating factors V, VIII, and XIII and binding to and activating platelets and endothelial cells. A most important function is the cleavage of peptides from the A and B chains of fibrinogen to form fibrin of thrombin monomers that subsequently polymerize into large fibrillar polymers (Fig. 58-8). Fibrin polymerization, the basis for the familiar clotting reaction, markedly changes plasma viscosity and converts blood from a sol to a gel. Polymers are initially held together by weak noncovalent bonds that are readily dissociated. They subsequently are cross-linked by a plasma transglutaminase, factor XIIIa, providing optimal mechanical stability.

LIMITING REACTIONS—THE NATURAL ANTICOAGULANTS

During normal hemostasis, only a small quantity of the coagulation protein in plasma is converted into an active protease or cofactor. The rate and extent of serine protease generation are carefully regulated by a group of inhibitor proteins that function as natural anticoagulants (Fig. 58-8). Such tight regulation is critical, since there is enough prothrombin in a single milliliter of blood, if converted to thrombin, to clot the entire volume of blood within 15 seconds. The natural anticoagulants permit coagulation to proceed locally, in response to injury, and prevent it from becoming a systemic and potentially dangerous process. The three most important natural anticoagulants are antithrombin III, protein C, and protein S. Their importance is underscored by the observation that patients with deficiency or dysfunction of any of the three proteins have a prethrombotic or hypercoagulable disorder characterized by recurrent episodes of venous and, rarely, arterial thrombosis and embolism.

ANTITHROMBIN III. This 60,000-dalton protein, which is a member of the serpin or serine protease inhibitor family of proteins, is synthesized in the liver and binds to and inactivates serine proteases within the coagulation cascade. Al-

FIGURE 58-8. Overview of the entire coagulation cascade, including the limiting reactions of the natural anticoagulants. There are two major activation pathways: the intrinsic pathway, which involves factors XII, IX, and VIII, and the extrinsic, or tissue factor, system, which involves tissue factor and factor VII. Both pathways result in the conversion of inactive factor X to its active form, Xa. In the third, or common, pathway Xa converts prothrombin to thrombin in a reaction that is accelerated by factor Va. Thrombin then converts fibrinogen to fibrin monomers, which polymerize and are cross-linked by factor XIIIa, a plasma transglutaminase. The interaction of factors VIIIa, IXa, and X; the interaction of the tissue factor–VII complex with factor X; and the conversion of prothrombin to thrombin are all reactions that require phospholipid (PL) and calcium. Two major anticoagulant systems limit coagulation reactions. Antithrombin binds to

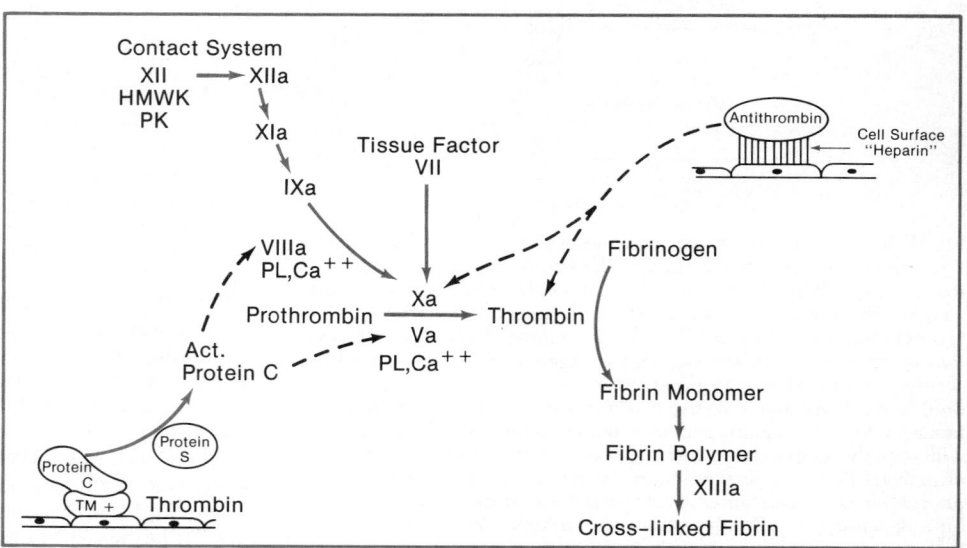

thrombin, factor Xa, and other coagulation serine proteases except factor VII in a reaction that is accelerated by exogenous heparin or heparin-like molecules on endothelial cells. Protein C is activated by thrombin after it is bound to the endothelial cell protein thrombomodulin. Activated protein C and protein S inactivate the two coagulation cofactors VIIIa and Va, which also limits thrombin generation. (From Handin, R. I.: Bleeding and thrombosis. In Wilson, J., et al. [eds.]: Harrison's Principles of Internal Medicine. 12th ed. New York, McGraw-Hill Book Co., 1991, p. 350.)

though named for its interaction with thrombin, it also inactivates factors XIIa, XIa, Xa, and IXa by binding to a serine residue at the active site of these proteases.[53] The kinetics of the interaction vary for the different proteases but, in each case, can be accelerated many times by the addition of heparin. Heparin binds to a site on antithrombin III that is separate from the region that binds proteases, and acts as an "allosteric" regulator. After the formation of a protease–antithrombin complex, heparin is released and can bind to additional antithrombin molecules. In this way its function is analogous to that of an enzyme or catalyst. The "catalytic" acceleration of antithrombin activity by heparin, referred to as its heparin cofactor activity, accounts for the entire anticoagulant action of heparin in plasma. During normal hemostasis, antithrombin is activated by binding to heparin-like glycosaminoglycans (heparans) present on the surface of endothelial cells.

PROTEINS C AND S. The second regulatory system involves protein C, protein S, and an endothelial membrane protein, *thrombomodulin*.[54–56] When bound to thrombomodulin, protein C is converted to an active serine protease by thrombin. Activated protein C then inhibits coagulation by inactivating factors Va and VIIIa. Protein S increases the rate of proteolysis of factors Va and VIIIa by activated protein C. Activated protein C can be inhibited by another serpin plasminogen activator inhibitor 1 (PAI-1). This interaction limits access of activated protein C to Va and VIIIa.[57,58]

RHEOLOGY AND THROMBOSIS

Any discussion of hemostasis should include the effects of blood flow and vascular geometry on thrombus formation.[59] Stress, in rheological terms, is the force per unit area generated during blood flow. When this force is applied at right angles to a surface, it is referred to as "normal" stress, and when applied parallel to a surface, as tangential stress or "shear." Figure 58–9 shows a longitudinal cross section of a blood vessel, with h representing wall thickness and r the inner radius. The parabola represents the range of velocities, V, at which laminar "plates" of blood travel along the longitudinal axis of the vessel at varying distances (y) from its center. Normal or circumferential stress (S_c) can be defined mathematically as

$$S_c = Px\eta/h, \qquad (1)$$

where P is the distending luminal pressure. In this idealized system of laminar, nonturbulent flow through a vessel of uniform diameter, the shear or tangential stress is

$$S_t = n\eta/Y = P\,Y/2, \qquad (2)$$

where η is blood viscosity and P the pressure gradient per unit length of vessel. Finally, the velocity of any laminar plate can be related to the radius of the vessel, the pressure generated, blood viscosity, and vessel length, L, as follows:

$$\eta \times \pi Pr^4/8\,\eta L \qquad (3)$$

From Equation 3 one can determine that velocity is maximal at the center of the vessel as it is proportional to the fourth power of the radius and falls off to nearly zero at the vessel wall. In addition, this equation predicts that the greater the viscosity of the blood, the lower its velocity. In addition, from Equation 2, it is clear that an increase in viscosity (η) will increase shear stress. These concepts have some practical applications. First, because plasma proteins, erythrocytes, and platelets require some minimal time to interact with one another and with subendothelial surfaces,

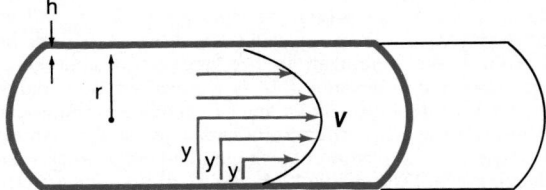

FIGURE 58–9. Biophysical variables that affect blood shear and rheology in a model cross section of a blood vessel. h = thickness of the vessel wall; r = radius of the vessel. Blood travels at different velocities (V), depending on its distance (Y) from the vessel wall. These parameters along with measurements of blood viscosity and blood pressure can be used to calculate shear stress on the vessel wall and blood flow.

conditions of high viscosity and low velocity favor platelet adhesion and thrombus formation. In fact, in the venous circulation, where velocity is low, relatively minor variations in flow, when coupled with minor degrees of injury to venous endothelium, may induce thrombus formation. Venous clots also take on their typical red appearance because of the large numbers of trapped red cells and amount of fibrin that accumulate under conditions of low flow. In the more rapid arterial circulation, platelet-platelet interactions predominate, there is insufficient time for fibrin formation and red cell trapping, and thrombi appear white. Adequate quantities of vWF multimers also are critical to stabilize adhesion of platelets to the vessel wall under conditions of high flow and shear stress. A modest reduction in this protein may lead to impaired hemostasis and clinical bleeding.

Rheology also influences the location of vascular disease, which occurs more frequently at bifurcations. Velocity is reduced as the "plates" of flowing blood are divided. This prolongs the residence time of platelets at the vessel surface and may enhance their deposition onto subendothelium when the bifurcation site is injured. Turbulence, which may occur in a stenotic vessel, adds another variable to the analysis by producing non-Newtonian flow. This also increases the residence time of proteins and platelets, reduces velocity, enhances local viscosity, and promotes platelet and fibrin deposition near flow vortices.

Finally, rheological principles have been applied to the design of therapeutic agents. Improving blood flow and reducing blood viscosity should reduce thrombus formation. There is evidence that cerebral blood flow can be dramatically increased by a slight reduction in the hematocrit.[60] Volume expanders like dextran, which have minimal effects on coagulation reactions, may act as antithrombotic agents by improving flow and reducing viscosity.[61] It also has been suggested that defibrination with agents like *ancrod* or the defibrination that accompanies systemic fibrinolytic therapy may be beneficial, in part, because it markedly reduces blood viscosity and improves blood flow.

CLOT DISSOLUTION — THE FIBRINOLYTIC SYSTEM

The fibrinolytic system, which dissolves fibrin-thrombi and restores blood flow within obstructed blood vessels, is a critically important component of the normal hemostatic system. Orderly, localized clot lysis is achieved by the concerted actions of a complex system that includes proteolytic enzymes, specific activators, and inhibitors of both the proteases and their activators. Although there are several enzymes like leukocyte elastase, which can digest fibrin, the major protease of the fibrinolytic system is *plasmin*. Three principal activators convert the precursor zymogen plasminogen to its active form, plasmin; these are activated Hageman factor fragments, urokinase-type plasminogen activators (UKs), and t-PA. Both the rate and the extent of fibrinolysis are regulated by a circulating inhibitor of plasmin, the alpha$_2$-plasmin inhibitor, a serpin, and endothelial cell–derived inhibitors of the principal activators, the plasminogen activator inhibitors types 1 and 2 (PAI-1 and PAI-2). The fibrinolytic process usually is localized to fibrin clots because plasminogen is selectively incorporated into fibrin thrombi at the time of thrombus formation. In addition, the two endogenous activators UK and t-PA are derived from stimulated endothelial cells at the site of thrombus formation and diffuse into the adjacent thrombus.

PLASMINOGEN

This 92,000-dalton plasma glycoprotein contains 790 amino acids, including 48 cysteines that form 24 intramolecular disulfide bonds, leaving no free sulfhydryl groups. Although the tissue of origin is still debated, plasminogen synthesis has been described in both liver and kidney, and plasminogen is present in eosinophilic leukocytes. The plasma concentration is approximately 21 mg/dl and does not vary greatly during normal blood coagulation. As shown in Figure 58–10, the parent molecule (Glu-plasminogen) has a glutamic acid at its amino terminus. Variable amounts of Glu-plasminogen are converted to Lys-plasminogen by the cleavage of an 8000-dalton polypeptide. Both Glu- and Lys-plasminogen are converted to plasmin by the scission of a single Arg-Val bond,

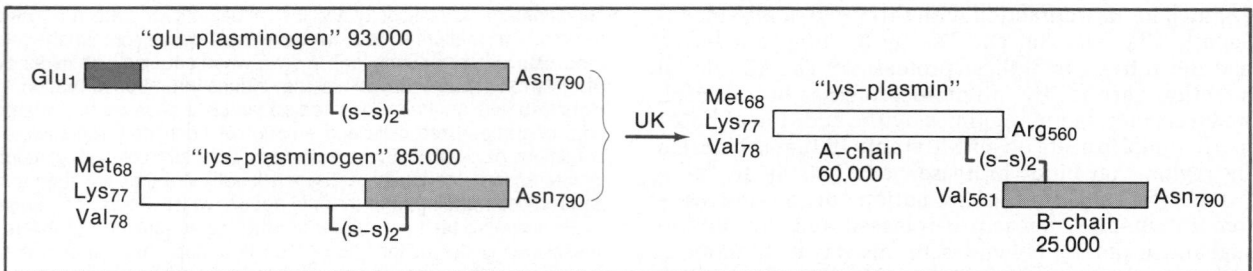

FIGURE 58-10. Molecular forms of plasminogen in plasma. The native molecule has 790 amino acids and a molecular weight of 93,000 daltons, with a glutamic acid as the initial or amino terminal amino acid residue (Glu-plasminogen). In plasma an 8000-dalton preactivation peptide is cleaved from Glu-plasminogen to produce a somewhat smaller form of plasminogen, with lysine as the amino terminal amino acid (Lys-plasminogen). Both Glu- and Lys-plasminogen circulate in plasma and can be converted to plasmin.

This requires two steps for Glu-plasminogen, cleavage of the 8000-dalton peptide, and scission of an internal peptide bond. Lys-plasminogen is activated by the internal bond scission alone. Plasmin is a two-chain molecule linked by disulfide bonds that has proteolytic activity against fibrinogen and fibrin as well as a number of other blood and cellular substrates. (Modified from Verstraete, M., and Vermylen, J.: Thrombosis. London, Pergamon Press, 1984, p. 46.)

through which the single-chain precursor is converted into a disulfide-linked, two-chain protease. Plasmin is a potent protease with broad reactivity. In addition to fibrin, it can digest fibrinogen, coagulation factors V and VIII, and platelet membrane glycoprotein Ib.

The complete covalent structure of plasminogen has been determined by direct protein sequencing and has been deduced from sequencing of plasminogen cDNA. As summarized in Figure 58-11, there are important structural similarities between plasminogen and the various plasminogen activators. Within the plasminogen molecule are five repeated regions of sequence homology that begin at the amino terminus of the molecule. These homologous repeats form looped structures held together by disulfide bonds and referred to as "kringles." (Kringles are a Danish breakfast pastry with a similar twisted, pretzel-like shape.) Plasminogen binds to fibrin through lysine binding sites located on the five nodular "kringle" domains, shown in Figure 58-11 as K_1 through K_5. These noncovalent interactions permit plasminogen to become con-

centrated within fibrin-rich thrombi for more effective and localized fibrinolysis.[62]

ENDOGENOUS PLASMINOGEN ACTIVATORS

(See also p. 1785)

As already mentioned, three endogenous plasminogen activators have now been identified.[63] They can be distinguished by their mechanism of plasminogen activation and the ability of fibrin to enhance their activity. Hageman factor (factor XII) fragments, generated during the early phase of coagulation, are relatively weak plasminogen activators (Fig. 58-6). Their activity is not enhanced by the adsorption of plasminogen to fibrin.

Tissue-type Plasminogen Activator

The major physiological activator is t-PA, a 70,000-dalton protein synthesized predominantly in endothelial cells. Be-

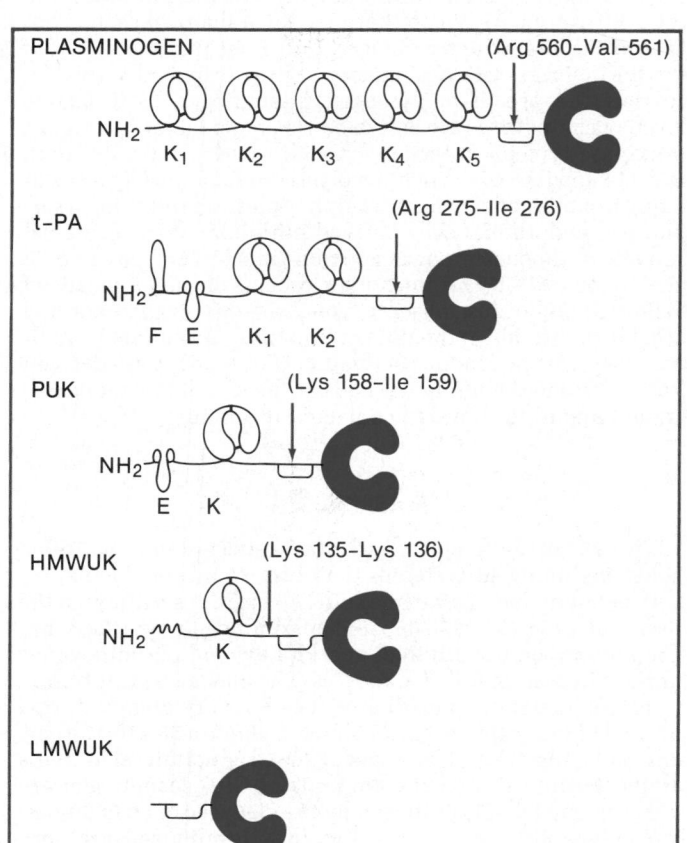

FIGURE 58-11. Structural homologies between plasminogen and the major activators of the fibrinolytic system. Plasminogen, tissue plasminogen activator (t-PA), pro-urokinase (PUK), and the high molecular weight form of urokinase (HMWUK) all contain "pretzel-like" kringle domains which are held together by disulfide bonds. In addition, t-PA contains a finger-like projection (F) at its amino (NH_2) terminus, also held together by disulfide bonds, which is homologous to a finger structure first recognized in the adhesive glycoprotein fibronectin. t-PA and PUK also contain a second slightly differently shaped projection (E) first noted in another molecule, the epidermal growth factor, and now recognized in many other proteins. The large "C"-shaped region on the right-hand end of each molecule represents the proteolytically active region. The K domains numbered 1 through 5 on various molecules and the F domains are the sites on each molecule which interact with fibrin and confer fibrin "specificity." The varying numbers of K domains, in combination with the F domains, confer differing affinities for fibrin. The arrows indicate sites in each of the proteins that are cleaved by proteolytic enzymes. Plasminogen is a single-chain zymogen or precursor which has no proteolytic activity. The scission of the peptide bond between arginine 560 and valine 561 converts it to a two-chain molecule, plasmin, which can proteolyze fibrinogen, fibrin, and various other substrates. As shown in Figure 58-10, a second peptide bond is cleaved from Glu-plasminogen to produce Lys-plasminogen. Both forms are converted to plasmin. t-PA is synthesized as a single-chain form which has proteolytic activity and can activate plasminogen. It is quickly converted to a two-chain form with somewhat enhanced proteolytic activity, by the scission of a single bond between arginine 275 and isoleucine 276. PUK, unlike t-PA, has no proteolytic activity until the bond between lysine 158 and isoleucine 158 is clipped, converting it to a two-chain protease. Both HMWUK and LMWUK circulate as two-chain active proteases. Scission of a bond between lysines 135 and 136 removes the single K domain but does not appreciably alter the specificity or biological activity of UK, which has no fibrin specificity.

cause there are only trace quantities of this protein in normal plasma, it had been difficult to purify and characterize t-PA until the cDNA-encoding t-PA was cloned and the recombinant molecule expressed in heterologous cells (Fig. 58–12).[64] As shown in Figures 58–11 and 58–12, t-PA is synthesized as a single-chain molecule, which is readily converted to a two-chain form by the proteolytic cleavage of a single plasmin-sensitive site. Unlike most other serine proteases, both the single-chain and the two-chain forms have proteolytic activity. t-PA is a relatively selective or fibrin-specific activator, since it converts plasminogen to plasmin two to three orders of magnitude more efficiently in vitro in the presence of fibrin than in plasma free of fibrin. Based on preliminary clinical studies, a similar degree of specificity may not be achieved in vivo. As shown in Figure 58–11, the A chain of t-PA, which is derived from the NH$_2$ terminal portion of single-chain t-PA, has a molecular weight of 40,000 daltons and contains two "kringle" domains (K$_1$ and K$_2$ in Fig. 58–11), a fibronectin-like "finger" domain, and an epidermal growth factor domain (EGF). The fibronectin-like finger domain is indicated in Figure 58–11 as F and the EGF homolog as E. The K$_2$ and F domains of t-PA both interact with fibrin. The smaller (30,000-dalton) B chain of t-PA contains the proteolytic site that converts plasminogen to plasmin. The B chain is homologous to the active site of other serine proteases like elastase, urokinase, trypsin, and plasmin.

Urokinase-type Plasminogen Activators

Endothelial and renal tubular epithelial cells synthesize urokinase-type plasminogen activators (u-PAs) in addition to t-PA. The u-PAs are immunologically distinct from t-PA,[54] but convert plasminogen to plasmin by hydrolyzing the same Arg-Val bond as t-PA. They are derived from a parent single-chain molecule, single-chain u-PA, or scu-PA (also called pro-urokinase or PUK). scu-PA has a molecular weight of 54,000 daltons and only minimal proteolytic activity in the absence of fibrin. scu-PA is quantitatively converted to the high molecular weight two-chain form (HMW-tc-UK), which has full proteolytic activity.[65,66] The ability to activate plasminogen is somewhat enhanced by the presence of fibrin. HMW-tc-UK is converted to a lower molecular weight species of 33,000 daltons (LMW-tc-UK) that is not fibrin-specific, but is proteolytically active. scu-PA and HMW-tc-UK have a single kringle domain (K), like t-PA, although its role in conferring fibrin specificity has not been established. Fibrin selectivity may be conferred by an increased affinity for plasminogen bound to internal lysine sites on fibrin that are exposed by partial clot lysis.[55] Because scu-PA has only minimal proteolytic activity, the mechanism by which it activates plasminogen in a relatively fibrin-specific manner is not fully understood. One possible explanation is that t-PA secreted from endothelial cells in the vicinity of a thrombus generates small quantities of plasmin which, in turn, rapidly converts scu-PA to HMW-tc-UK, and thereby activates additional plasminogen.

Endogenous Inhibitors of Fibrinolysis

PLASMINOGEN ACTIVATOR INHIBITORS. Activity of the endogenous fibrinolytic system is carefully regulated. Endothelial cells and platelets both secrete a plasminogen activator inhibitor (PAI-1) that irreversibly inactivates t-PA and UK[67] monocytes, and placental cells also secrete a second species, PAI-2, that is a more selective inhibitor of u-PA than of

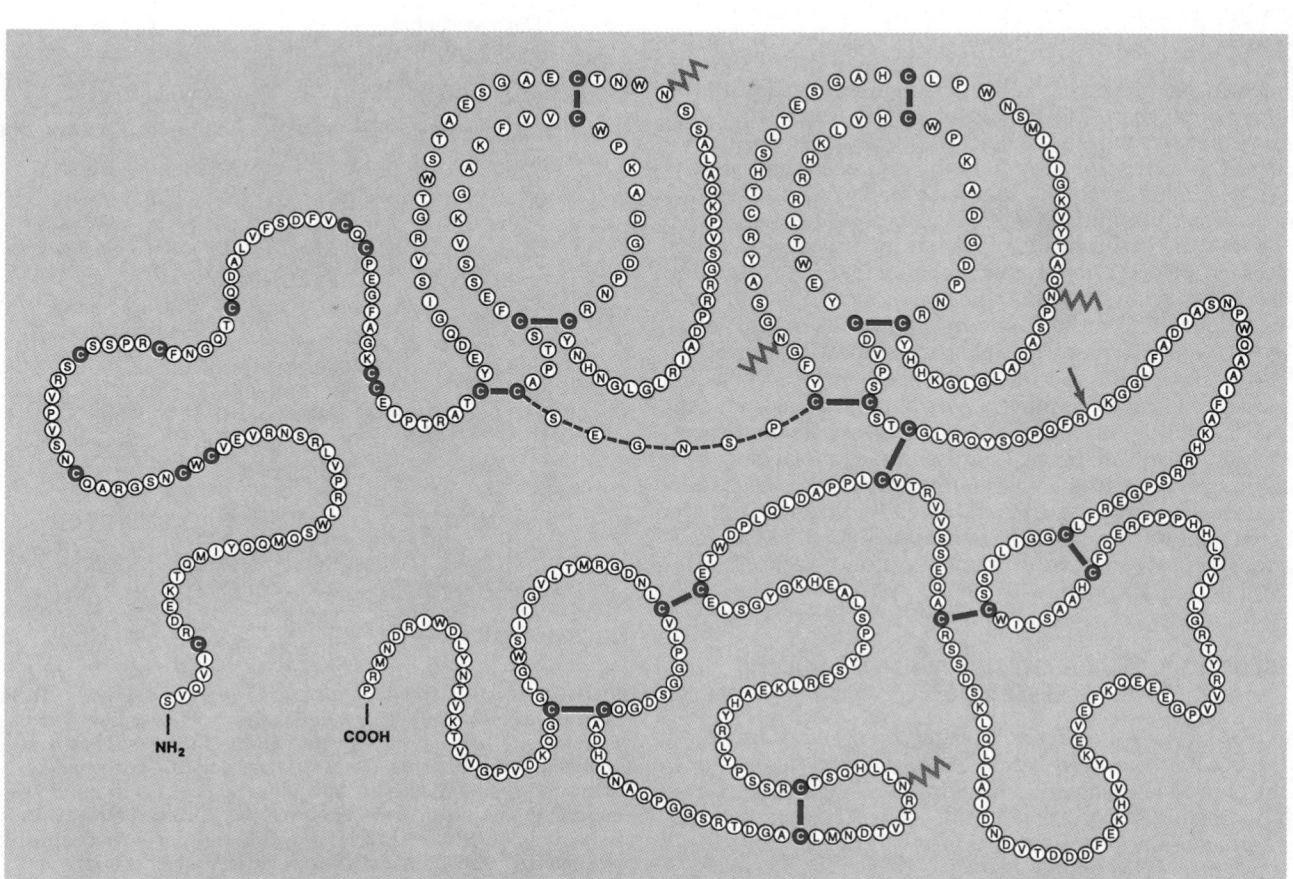

FIGURE 58–12. Structure of tissue plasminogen activator deduced from cDNA cloning and sequencing. The one-letter abbreviations for amino acid residues are used. Solid bars mark sites for potential disulfide bonds between cysteine residues, and zigzag lines mark attachment sites for N-linked carbohydrate. The arrow marks the position of the bond scission, which converts one-chain t-PA to the two-chain form. Finally, the broken line indicates the short stretch of six amino acids that connects the two kringle domains. (From Pennica, D., et al.: Cloning and expression of human tissue-type plasminogen activator cDNA in E. coli. Nature 301:214, 1983.)

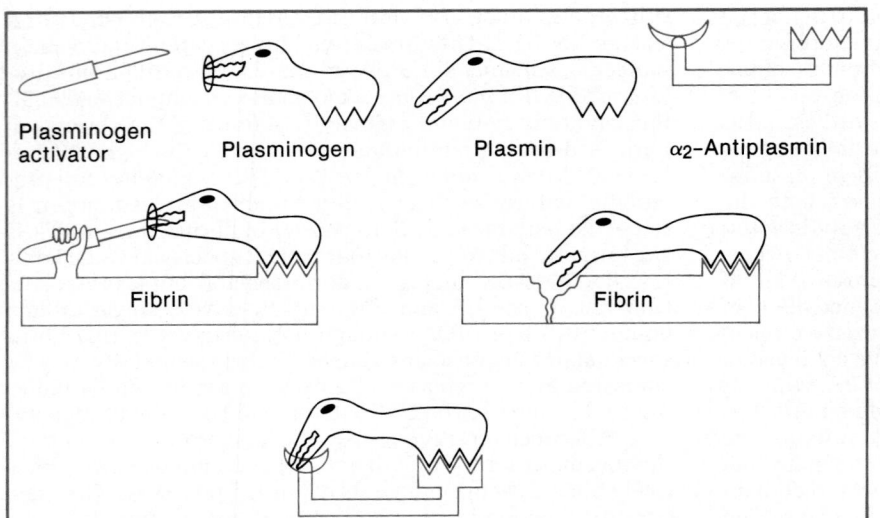

FIGURE 58-13. Schematic view of the interactions among a plasminogen activator (such as tissue plasminogen activator, which binds to fibrin), a fibrin clot, and the alpha$_2$-plasmin inhibitor. The plasminogen activator both binds to fibrin and converts fibrin-bound plasminogen to the active protease plasmin. Plasmin then digests the fibrin clot. Alpha$_2$-plasmin inhibitor binds to and inhibits free plasmin but cannot neutralize plasmin when it is bound to the fibrin clot, since it must bind to both the protease active site and the fibrin-binding site. This mechanism helps to limit fibrinolysis to areas of fibrin clot formation and prevents plasmin from entering the circulation. (From Verstraete, M., and Vermylen, J.: Thrombosis. London, Pergamon Press, 1984, p. 43.)

t-PA. The PAIs are structurally homologous to other serpins such as alpha$_1$-antitrypsin and antithrombin III.

ALPHA$_2$-PLASMIN INHIBITOR. As shown in Figure 58-13, another molecule circulating in plasma, alpha$_2$-plasmin inhibitor (α_2PI), rapidly neutralizes free plasmin.[68] However, the lysine-binding "kringle" domains as well as the active-site serine of plasmin must be available for binding and neutralization by α_2PI. Thus, when it is bound to fibrin, plasmin is protected from the neutralizing effect of α_2PI. This helps to sustain the fibrinolytic activity of plasmin within a thrombus and minimizes systemic fibrinolysis, since α_2PI rapidly neutralizes any release of "free" plasmin. α_2PI also may inhibit fibrinolysis by competing for lysine-binding sites on fibrinogen.

The fibrin clot plays a key role in the regulation of fibrinolysis. Fibrin binds plasminogen, enriching this key fibrinolytic enzyme precursor within the clot. The presence of fibrin also enhances the activity of t-PA and inhibits the activity of α_2PI and PAI-1. Finally, products generated during fibrin clot formation, such as thrombin, enhance the local release of t-PA as well as its principal inhibitor PAI-1 from endothelial cells. The surface of endothelial and mononuclear cells and the platelet also provide sites for enhanced or more efficient conversion of plasminogen to plasmin. These cells express specific surface receptors for plasminogen and for t-PA, as well as u-PA. Binding to these receptors enhances plasminogen activation. This cell surface property may help to maintain blood fluidity, facilitate production of inflammatory mediators on the mononuclear cell surface, and enhance clot lysis after tissue injury. Unregulated systemic fibrinolysis is a rare event, and occurs only in patients with disseminated intravascular coagulation, those with advanced liver disease, and those receiving systemic infusions of fibrinolytic activators to lyse pathological thrombi.

SUMMARY OF COAGULATION AND FIBRINOLYTIC REACTIONS

The plasma coagulation and fibrinolytic systems are complicated because they involve the closely linked interactions of multiple serine proteases. In addition, the reactions are carefully regulated by plasma and cell surface activators, plasma cofactors, and a series of naturally occurring anticoagulants or fibrinolytic inhibitors.

The major coagulation reactions are summarized in Figure 58-8 and the fibrinolytic pathway in Figure 58-14. Two major stimuli initiate coagulation—contact of blood with vascular subendothelium and liberation of tissue thromboplastin or tissue factor. The net result of activation of these two pathways is the generation of thrombin, a potent protease that converts fibrinogen to fibrin. Fibrin then polymerizes and is cross-linked to form a stable clot. There are two critical plasma cofactors—factors Va and VIIIa—that regulate the rates of factor Xa generation by the contact or intrinsic pathway and the rate of thrombin generation from Xa produced by either the extrinsic or the intrinsic pathway. The most impor-

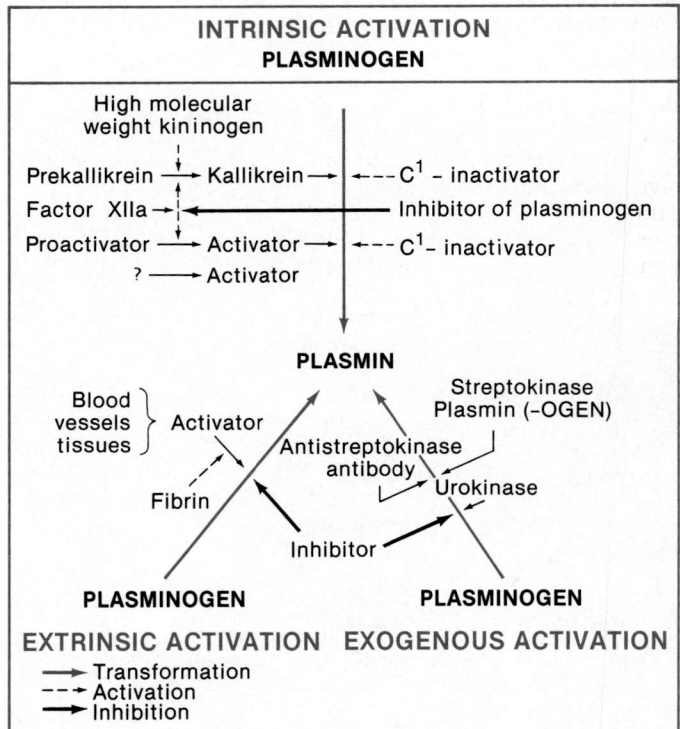

FIGURE 58-14. Overview of the fibrinolytic pathways. There are three principal pathways for the conversion of plasminogen to plasmin. The intrinsic pathway is activated during the early phases of blood coagulation by Hageman factor fragments. This is a relatively weak activation system of questionable physiological significance. The most important physiological mechanism is the extrinsic pathway. Endothelial cells in blood vessels release two fibrin-specific activators, tissue plasminogen activator and pro-urokinase, which rapidly and effectively convert plasminogen to plasmin. Finally, several potential exogenous activators are used in fibrinolytic therapy. The bacterial protein streptokinase and the urinary product urokinase are two standard nonspecific activators. In addition, the two physiological and fibrin-specific activators, tissue plasminogen activator and prourokinase, are now available and being used in clinical trials. (From Verstraete, M., and Vermylen, J.: Thrombosis. London, Pergamon Press, 1984, p. 41.)

tant naturally occurring anticoagulants are antithrombin III, which is activated by cell surface heparin-like molecules (heparans) and rapidly neutralizes coagulation proteases, and protein C, which is activated by thrombin and cell surface thrombomodulin. Along with protein S, activated protein C inactivates factors Va and VIIIa.

The fibrinolytic system may be activated by two endogenous substances: t-PA and the u-PAs. In each case activation is accomplished by converting plasminogen to plasmin directly. Plasmin then digests fibrin thrombi. The rate of plasminogen activation by t-PA, scu-PA, or HMW-tc-UK is enhanced by the presence of fibrin and permits the activation process to be localized to areas that contain fibrin thrombi. t-PA and scu-PA are secreted from endothelial cells after the generation of thrombin. Fibrinolytic activity is regulated at two levels. First, there is endothelial PAI (PAI-1), which may bind to any free plasminogen activator. In addition, there is another serpin, α_2PI, which binds to any free plasmin and rapidly neutralizes its proteolytic activity. In normal hemostasis, fibrinolysis is activated shortly after thrombus formation to restore vessel patency and reestablish normal blood flow rapidly.

EVALUATION OF HEMOSTASIS IN CARDIOVASCULAR PATIENTS

Many patients with cardiovascular disorders require corrective surgery or invasive diagnostic and therapeutic procedures such as cardiac catheterization, coronary angiography, or transluminal angioplasty. Although special precautions usually are not necessary, a specific evaluation of the hemostatic system may be necessary in three clinical situations. First, some patients may have a suspected or poorly documented hemorrhagic disorder that may have produced only minimal symptoms but might cause excess bleeding after an invasive diagnostic or surgical procedure. For example, many patients with mild von Willebrand's disease have little or no spontaneous bleeding but may bleed profusely after an operation. Second, the antiplatelet or anticoagulant medications administered to cardiac patients increase their risk of hemorrhage. This problem is especially serious when patients are to undergo invasive cardiovascular or surgical procedures, since they may have few bleeding symptoms before surgery. Finally, although most cardiovascular disorders do not increase the risk of hemorrhage, certain types of cardiac disease perturb hemostasis and cause bleeding.

Although it may be tempting to order a battery of screening laboratory tests on all cardiac patients with a suspected hemorrhagic disorder, the most useful part of the evaluation is still a careful history. For example, a past history of excessive bleeding after dental extractions or tonsillectomy, bleeding after minor trauma, recurrent epistaxis, abnormal menses, or recurrent joint or muscle bleeding without antecedent trauma all suggest an inherited coagulation disorder. Many, but not all, patients also have a family history of bleeding. Finally, a careful drug history is essential, since many commonly used drugs, including aspirin and other nonsteroidal antiinflammatory agents, may cause platelet dysfunction and clinical bleeding.

Patients with deficits in platelet number or function usually bleed into the skin and mucous membranes and may present with epistaxis, gastrointestinal bleeding, or abnormal menses. Bleeding develops immediately after surgery or trauma and may respond to local pressure or packing. The most common platelet disorders are (1) thrombocytopenia, (2) platelet dysfunction secondary to ingestion of medications such as aspirin, and (3) von Willebrand's disease. Platelet function is readily evaluated by a platelet count and bleeding time. Current techniques for measuring bleeding time are reproducible and sensitive and can detect even mild platelet dysfunction. In most laboratories, the average bleeding time is 5 ± 2 (S.D.)

min, so that a value greater than 10 min probably indicates impaired primary hemostasis.

In contrast, in patients with plasma coagulation defects, musculoskeletal and soft tissue bleeding occurs hours or days after surgery or trauma, and usually requires specific replacement therapy. The most common inherited abnormalities are the hemophilias—specifically, deficiencies in the activity of factors VIII and IX, which are sex-linked recessive disorders that cause recurrent hemorrhage and joint deformity. The most common acquired defects are those associated with (1) vitamin K deficiency, (2) liver disease, and (3) disseminated intravascular coagulation (DIC).

The integrity of the plasma coagulation system is readily assessed with a group of simple laboratory tests—the partial thromboplastin time (PTT), prothrombin time (PT), and, in some cases, thrombin time (TT) or fibrinogen level. In rare cases additional assays of clot solubility and fibrin cross-linking may be useful. The PTT exclusively measures the activity of coagulation factors in the intrinsic or contact activation pathway, which include Hageman factor (factor XII), high molecular weight kininogen, prekallikrein, and factors XI, IX, and VIII (Fig. 58–8). The PT, which is used to assay the extrinsic or tissue factor–dependent pathway of coagulation, exclusively measures factor VII. The PT and PTT both assess the integrity of factors in the common pathway, which include factors X and V, prothrombin, and fibrinogen. When a patient has an isolated increase in either the PT or the PTT, the group of factors that are potentially defective can be readily pinpointed. When both PT and PTT are prolonged, fibrinogen level or function also should be assessed, since either reduced or dysfunctional fibrinogen or a common pathway defect involving factor X or V or prothrombin will prolong both tests. Defective fibrin cross-linking and abnormal clot solubility are extremely rare and should be suspected only when a patient has a severe bleeding disorder with a normal PT and PTT.

THROMBOCYTOPENIA

The platelet count normally ranges between 150,000 and 450,000/μl. Low counts may be due to decreased marrow production, accelerated peripheral destruction, or platelet sequestration in an enlarged spleen. The most common causes of decreased production are exposure to marrow toxins, including chemotherapeutic agents, binge consumption of alcohol, and thiazide diuretics. Accelerated destruction can occur from platelet interaction with a prosthetic valve, Dacron vascular grafts or intracardiac patches, or activation of the coagulation system and platelet entrapment in fibrin thrombi. This is particularly prominent in patients with DIC but also occurs in disorders like thrombotic thrombocytopenic purpura and the hemolytic uremic syndrome. Finally, destruction may result from the interaction of antibodies or immune complexes with the platelet surface. Antibodies may arise in response to viral infections or the administration of drugs like quinidine, procainamide, or heparin.

PLATELET DYSFUNCTION

The most common cause of platelet dysfunction is the ingestion of aspirin and related nonsteroidal antiinflammatory agents. Patients usually have a mildly prolonged bleeding time, although in some susceptible individuals bleeding time may be as long as 20 to 30 minutes. This is accompanied by reduced platelet aggregation in response to agents like collagen, ADP, or epinephrine. Aspirin and the nonsteroidal antiinflammatory drugs inhibit platelet synthesis of TxA_2 and other eicosanoids by inhibiting platelet cyclo-oxygenase. Aspirin irreversibly acetylates cyclo-oxygenase; because the platelets cannot synthesize new enzyme, hemostasis is impaired for 5 to 7 days after a single dose of aspirin. The other common nonsteroidal compounds like indomethacin and ibuprofen are competitive inhibitors of cyclo-oxygenase, and induce transient and dose-dependent inhibition of the enzyme. Administration of other drugs, including large doses of penicillin G or semisynthetic penicillins, also may impair platelet function. In addition, certain metabolic disturbances, including uremia, may impair platelet adhesion, release, and aggregation.

VON WILLEBRAND'S DISEASE

The most common inherited defect of primary hemostasis is von Willebrand's disease, which affects as many as 1 in 800 to 1000 persons in the general population.[69] Patients almost always have a prolonged bleeding time; normal platelet aggregation with ADP, epinephrine, and collagen;

and variable defects in vWF concentration and function. In the most common form, type I, vWF content is modestly reduced to less than 50 per cent of normal. There is a parallel reduction in biological activity, as measured by ristocetin-dependent platelet agglutination, and in factor VIII activity, since vWF serves as the intravascular carrier for this factor. Less commonly, patients have variant syndromes (type II) characterized by a severe reduction in vWF activity despite a normal quantity of circulating protein. Patients with von Willebrand variants have a selective loss of the largest and most hemostatically effective multimers.[70] In type IIa disease, this is due to the rapid proteolysis and catabolism of genetically altered forms of vWF after normal synthesis. In type IIb disease, the large multimers spontaneously bind to circulating platelets, causing intravascular aggregation and mild thrombocytopenia. Rarely, patients will present with type III disease, in which there is an almost total absence of antigen or activity. These patients probably have homozygous or doubly heterozygous forms of von Willebrand's disease. No patient with von Willebrand's disease should receive antiplatelet agents, and all patients require treatment before surgery or cardiac catheterization with either cryoprecipitate, which replaces vWF, or 1-deamino-8-D-arginine vasopressin (DDAVP), which can transiently raise vWF levels and improve hemostasis in type I patients.[71]

HEMOPHILIA AND RELATED COAGULATION DEFECTS

Deficiencies in factors VIII and IX are the two most common inherited coagulation disorders. They are both X-linked recessive traits and cause recurrent musculoskeletal bleeding and hemarthroses in male patients. There is a close relation between factor level and clinical severity. Patients with levels of less than 1 per cent have severe disease and bleed frequently, even after minimal trauma; those with 1 to 5 per cent have more moderate disease; and those with greater than 5 per cent activity have mild disease with infrequent bleeding. Patients with factor VIII or IX levels above 15 to 20 per cent may be especially difficult to diagnose, since bleeding may occur only after major trauma or surgery. The third most common disorder is factor XI deficiency, an autosomal recessive trait frequently found among Ashkenazi Jews. Hemarthroses are uncommon, and many patients present with postoperative bleeding. There is little correlation between factor XI activity or antigenic level and clinical severity. All these disorders cause an increase in PTT with no change in PT. It is of interest that in patients with deficiencies in factors XII, HMWK, and PK, PTT is markedly prolonged but bleeding does not occur. Patients with true hemorrhagic disorders are treated with plasma fractions (VIII and IX deficiency) or fresh frozen plasma (XI deficiency), whereas those with laboratory abnormalities of no clinical significance (XII, HMWK, and PK deficiency) do not require therapy.

VITAMIN K DEFICIENCY AND LIVER DISEASE

Patients with biliary obstruction, liver disease, or inadequate food intake and those receiving broad-spectrum antibiotics may rapidly become deficient in vitamin K. The earliest manifestation of vitamin K deficiency is prolongation of the PT due to a fall in the factor VII level. Later, as the other prothrombin complex proteins with a longer half-life decline, the PTT also becomes prolonged. Patients should rapidly be treated with parenteral vitamin K, which can reverse the hemostatic defect in 8 to 10 hours. More rapid correction can be achieved with infusion of fresh frozen plasma. In contrast, patients with liver disease have a more complex coagulation defect, with a combination of vitamin K deficiency, impaired production of multiple coagulation factors, including fibrinogen, production of abnormal clotting proteins, systemic fibrinolysis, intravascular coagulation, and thrombocytopenia secondary to splenomegaly and platelet sequestration. These patients do not tolerate therapy with prothrombin complex concentrates, many of which contain trace quantities of activated coagulation factors, since they cannot clear activated coagulation proteins effectively. Inadvertent infusion has caused fatal thromboembolism. The best therapy for these patients is a combination of vitamin K, platelet concentrates, and fresh frozen plasma.

DISSEMINATED INTRAVASCULAR COAGULATION (DIC)

DIC begins as a thrombotic disorder with the rapid generation of thrombin, extensive fibrin deposition in the microvasculature, and intense secondary fibrinolysis. In some patients this leads to thrombosis of peripheral vessels and tissue damage. If untreated, there is progressive depletion of coagulation proteins and platelets, and diffuse hemorrhage. Various pathological events trigger DIC, including tissue damage from extreme heat, cold, or trauma; malignant tumors; bacterial or viral infections; extensive vascular malformations (Kasabach-Merritt syndrome); and obstetrical mishaps such as abruptio placentae. Treatment of DIC should focus on identifying and removing the triggering mechanism. Plasma and platelet transfusions are indicated to stop diffuse bleeding, and heparin is used to treat patients with microvascular thrombosis. Occasionally heparin also is administered to patients with intractable bleeding despite adequate plasma and platelet replacement.

CARDIAC DISORDERS WITH HEMOSTATIC DEFECTS

As previously mentioned, certain cardiovascular disorders may impair hemostasis. For example, patients with chronic right-sided heart failure may develop liver dysfunction and cardiac cirrhosis. This results in impaired vitamin K absorption, impaired production of the prothrombin complex proteins, and thrombocytopenia from splenomegaly and platelet sequestration. Patients with severe cyanotic congenital heart disease, who have a markedly expanded red cell volume and increased whole blood viscosity, may develop a DIC-like syndrome characterized by thrombocytopenia, shortened platelet survival, and increased consumption of fibrinogen and other coagulation proteins. The factors which trigger DIC in this setting are unknown, although reduced blood flow and increased viscosity because of the marked increase in red cell mass are implicated. The coagulation abnormalities are corrected by red cell removal and plasma replacement.[72] Patients with acute bacterial endocarditis may develop subclinical DIC, which may be exacerbated by insertion of a prosthetic valve. Patients undergoing cardiopulmonary bypass may develop a complex platelet disorder that can cause postoperative bleeding. Platelet dysfunction is due to platelet activation and secretion during bypass and plasmin-mediated proteolysis of glycoproteins Ib/IX and IIb/IIIa.[73]

EVALUATION OF THROMBOTIC AND PRETHROMBOTIC PATIENTS

Although the clinical and laboratory evaluation of hemorrhagic disorders has become straightforward, there are, as yet, no clinically useful laboratory tests that detect either subclinical thrombosis or the prethrombotic state. Several tests have been devised to measure platelet activation in patients with thrombosis and vascular disease. First, intravascular platelet survival, as measured by the infusion of autologous radiolabeled platelets, is shortened in patients with arterial vascular disease as well as in patients with vascular grafts, arteriovenous shunts, and prosthetic cardiac valves.[74] There also is evidence that this shortened survival may be corrected by the administration of antiplatelet agents.[75] The plasma content of platelet alpha granule proteins such as platelet factor 4 (PF-4) and β-thromboglobulin (β-TG) is increased in patients with thrombosis or embolism but usually is not elevated in patients with prethrombotic disorder.[76,77] These radioimmunoassays are difficult to standardize, since their interpretation depends on the ability to totally suppress the secretion of platelet proteins during blood collection. In addition, extraneous metabolic factors that do not affect platelet activation and release may affect plasma measurements. PF-4 has a very short intravascular half-life, since it has a high affinity for glycosaminoglycans and binds to heparans on the surface of endothelial cells. The administration of heparin is accompanied by a transient rise in plasma PF-4 as the endothelial cell surface pool of PF-4 binds to intravascular heparin.[78] In contrast, β-TG, which does not bind to the endothelial cell, is cleared exclusively by a renal mechanism. Thus, the plasma β-TG level is inversely related to creatinine clearance and increases with serum creatinine independent of platelet activation.[79] Measuring β-TG levels to monitor platelet activation may therefore prove inaccurate in patients with renal insufficiency.[80]

Laboratory tests that detect coagulation system activation rather than platelet activation, although equally cumbersome, may be more useful. The pioneering studies of Nossel and colleagues demonstrated an increase in fibrinopeptide A (FPA), one of the peptides cleaved from fibrinogen by thrombin, in patients with deep venous thrombosis and pulmonary embolism.[81] The elevated FPA level returns to normal after the administration of heparin. More recent studies have used radioimmunoassays for a prothrombin activation fragment and for circulating thrombin–antithrombin complexes.[82] Both products are elevated in patients with thromboembolism. The ambient levels of prothrombin fragment and thrombin–antithrombin complex also are elevated in elderly patients with vascular disease and in patients with inherited prethrombotic disorders like antithrombin III or protein C deficiency. The protein elevations in these patients can be suppressed by the administration of warfarin-type anticoagulants. These studies provide the first definitive evidence for activation of the coagulation system in patients with inherited or acquired prethrombotic disorders as well as in patients with asymptomatic vascular disease. However, despite these promising results, neither of the tests is yet available in routine clinical laboratories, since they require specialized reagents and meticulous venipuncture technique.

PRETHROMBOTIC OR HYPERCOAGULABLE DISORDERS

There are no clearly identified disorders in which well-documented abnormalities in platelet function can be linked to arterial or venous thrombosis. Certain patients with myeloproliferative disorders and patients with Types I and II diabetes mellitus are said to have "hyperactive" platelets based on standard platelet aggregation assays.[83] In addition, there is evidence that lipid abnormalities such as those seen in familial hypercholesterolemia may increase platelet membrane cholesterol content, decrease membrane fluidity, and enhance platelet reactivity to agonists in vitro.[84] Patients with homozygous homocystinuria clearly have an increased incidence of cerebrovascular thrombosis and develop premature atherosclerosis.[85] In some studies intravascular platelet survival also was shown to be reduced in patients with homocystinuria.[86] These patients are readily recognized because they may have a "marfanoid" body habitus (resembling the Marfan syndrome), ectopia lentis, and mild mental retardation. In laboratory animals, infusion of homocysteine induces similar arterial lesions, which are accompanied by patchy desquamation of endothelial cells. Platelets then adhere to exposed subendothelium and induce smooth muscle cell proliferation and vascular lesions. There also is evidence that environmental changes can enhance platelet reactivity. One group has reported that the circadian variation in incidence of myocardial infarction is accompanied by a diurnal variation in platelet aggregation in vitro.[87]

DEFICIENCY OR DYSFUNCTION OF THE NATURAL ANTICOAGULANTS

The most thoroughly characterized of the prethrombotic or hypercoagulable disorders are those caused by inherited deficiency or dysfunction of one of three natural anticoagulants: antithrombin III, protein C, or protein S.[88-90] The true incidence of these disorders in the general population is not clear, although preliminary surveys of antithrombin III levels have suggested an incidence of antithrombin III deficiency as high as 1 in 2000 persons. When the clinical experience of large centers that treat venous thromboembolism is reviewed, the congenital disorders identified to date account for no more than 20 per cent of patients with recurrent venous thromboembolism and fewer than 5 per cent of all patients with deep venous thrombosis.

CLINICAL MANIFESTATIONS. Patients with a congenital deficiency of any one of the natural anticoagulants present with remarkably similar histories of familial, recurrent venous thrombosis and pulmonary embolism. Rarely, these patients also have arterial thrombosis. Thromboembolic events are uncommon in infancy and childhood. The incidence of venous thrombosis and pulmonary embolism increases during each ensuing decade, and 90 per cent of patients will have had a thromboembolic episode by the third decade of life. Each of the three abnormalities usually is in-

herited as an autosomal dominant trait, although a few patients with homozygous protein C deficiency have now been identified. These rare patients become symptomatic shortly after birth and develop neonatal purpura fulminans and DIC.[91] Patients with the heterozygous or autosomal dominant forms of antithrombin III, protein C, or protein S deficiency have only a modestly decreased level of circulating protein. In fact, in many cases, values are just below the normal range. This is quite different from the majority of the X-linked or autosomal recessive coagulation protein disorders, in which patients are not symptomatic until levels are well below normal. Thus, it is important to pay attention to modest deficiencies in the natural anticoagulants.

To date, most patients with antithrombin III deficiency have had a modest reduction in antithrombin level, and no cases of homozygous antithrombin deficiency have been reported. However, families have been identified who have dysfunctional antithrombin molecules. In these cases, the plasma antithrombin level is normal based on immunoassay even though the dysfunctional molecule may not neutralize thrombin effectively or may not bind or become activated by heparin.[92] Effective screening of patients with suspected antithrombin deficiency must include both an immunoassay for total content of the protein and functional assays that measure both the thrombin-neutralizing and heparin cofactor activities of the protein. Families with protein C and S deficiency have shown either a reduction in protein or dysfunctional molecules. Accurate immunoassays for protein C and S are readily available. Functional assay of proteins is complicated by the partitioning of protein S into two compartments—free (active) and bound to C4 binding protein (inactive).

MANAGEMENT. Any patients with symptomatic thromboembolism should be treated acutely with heparin and then placed on an oral anticoagulant. To prevent recurrent thromboembolism, which may be fatal, patients should remain on anticoagulants for life. The only group who may not respond to acute heparin therapy are those rare patients with antithrombin variants that are not activated by heparin. In these cases, patients also should receive infusions of plasma or antithrombin concentrates to provide a source of normal antithrombin. Treatment of protein C and S deficiencies poses a special problem, since administration of warfarin to these patients may further depress protein C and S levels and increase the risk of thrombosis. This is thought to be the mechanism underlying hemorrhagic skin necrosis, a rare complication of warfarin therapy.[93] In several retrospective surveys, all identified cases have had protein C deficiency. Patients with either abnormality who require anticoagulant therapy should receive plasma infusions to raise the protein C or S level or should continue anticoagulation with heparin during the first week of warfarin administration.

It is important to carry out thorough family studies and identify all the affected members of a kindred who are deficient in the natural anticoagulants. Asymptomatic family members, particularly those under the age of 30, need not be placed on oral anticoagulants; however, they should receive prophylactic plasma or antithrombin concentrate replacement and perhaps heparin therapy during any period of prolonged immobility owing to a fracture, trauma, or surgery.

OTHER CAUSES OF VENOUS AND ARTERIAL THROMBOSIS

The inherited prethrombotic disorders account for a small but important fraction of patients with thromboembolism. They also provide interesting model systems in which the relation betweeen a discrete molecular defect and thrombosis can be accurately correlated. In the majority of patients, however, the etiology or pathophysiology remains unclear. Nonetheless, certain acquired disorders or physiological states predispose patients to the development of venous thrombosis. Immobilization, especially when coupled with trauma or surgery, may precipitate deep venous thrombosis. In most patients, the thrombi are small and limited to the calf veins. Proximal extension to the femoral system greatly increases the risk of pulmonary embolism.[94] Calf vein thrombi can be detected by venography as well as by Doppler flow and impedance plethysmographic measurements. Patients with certain primary or metastatic malignancies, particularly those with cancer arising in the pancreas, stomach, and kidney, as well as patients with chronic congestive heart failure or women who take oral contraceptives, are at increased risk for venous thrombosis and embolism. The association of malignancy and thromboembolism has been referred to as *Trousseau's syndrome*, and occasionally the thromboembolic complications may present well before the tumor can be diagnosed. In most of these cases, the pathological mechanism is unclear. A combination of tissue factor generation from tumor or damaged tissue and venous stasis may explain many cases of thrombosis in surgical and cancer patients. Oral contraceptive use also lowers antithrombin III levels and may place some patients in the symptomatic range.[95]

Arterial thrombosis seldom occurs de novo in a normal, uninjured vessel, and usually develops in a stenotic or atherosclerotic artery. One of the best clinical examples of arterial thromboembolism is the transient ischemic attack (TIA) syndrome. In this condition, platelet thrombi form on ulcerated atherosclerotic carotid vessel plaques. After the thrombus reaches a critical size, fragments break off and embolize to the distal cerebral or retinal circulation. In most patients, the distal emboli will break up, so that blood flow is restored to normal and visual impairment or neurological symptoms disappear. Occasionally, emboli can cause permanent neurological dysfunction and produce a completed stroke or cerebrovascular accident (CVA). Patients may have repeated TIAs without suffering a CVA and can be effectively treated with antiplatelet agents that prevent or reduce platelet plug formation on the ulcerated carotid plaque.

Firm evidence has emerged supporting a similar mechanism underlying transient or permanent obstruction of coronary arteries.[96] In fact, it is now clear that the majority of transmural myocardial infarcts are due to coronary thrombosis after the fracture or disruption of an atherosclerotic coronary arterial plaque, producing a surface which activates coagulation reactions. In addition, many patients with unstable angina (p. 1334), like those with TIAs, may have repeated bouts of thrombosis and embolism causing their cardiac instability and chest pain. In addition, their symptoms may abate with antiplatelet therapy, which also may reduce the risk of subsequent myocardial infarction (p. 1340). In addition to forming thrombi in diseased coronary arteries, cardiac patients may develop intracavitary or intracardiac thrombi. For example, patients who have had a transmural myocardial infarction may have residual endocardial scarring or hypokinesis. The damaged endocardium may provide a site for development of a mural thrombus, which may then break up and produce systemic emboli. Similarly, in patients with mitral stenosis, left atrial enlargement, and atrial fibrillation, thrombi often develop in the left atrium or on the mitral valve and can embolize into the systemic circulation. Patients with prosthetic cardiac valves also are at risk for systemic embolization. Although these intracavitary cardiac thrombi are "arterial," they form in areas of low blood flow and are rich in fibrin. In this respect, they more closely resemble the fibrin and red cell–rich thrombi that form in the venous circulation. Thus, effective treatment of intracavitary thrombi requires anticoagulants such as heparin or warfarin or a combination of anticoagulants and antiplatelet drugs.

DISORDERS OF FIBRINOLYSIS

Until recently, the study of potential disorders of the fibrinolytic system and their relation to thromboembolism has been hampered by a lack of precise assays for components of the system. Now, with the molecular cloning of t-PA, scu-PA,

and the fibrinolytic inhibitors PAI-1 and -2, it is possible to analyze fibrinolysis with more precision. In fact, several congenital or acquired abnormalities of the fibrinolytic system have been described that may increase the risk of thrombosis. Both a decreased concentration of plasminogen and abnormal plasminogen molecules have been associated with recurrent thrombosis.[97] Production of abnormal fibrinogen molecules (dysfibrinogenemias) usually causes bleeding; however, in certain dysfibrinogenemias, fibrin thrombi are formed that are unusually resistant to the action of plasmin and can predispose patients to thrombosis.[98] In addition, reduced fibrinolytic activity has been described in patients with CVAs,[99] recurrent venous thrombosis,[100] and mesenteric venous thrombosis.[101] In one case, defective release of t-PA from endothelial cells has been postulated as the cause of the fibrinolytic defect and recurrent venous thrombosis.[102] In a provocative report, elevated levels of PAI-1 have been noted in the plasma of young patients who survive myocardial infarction.[103] This raises the interesting possibility that coronary thrombosis might be due to a failure to lyse intracoronary thrombi owing to rapid neutralization of t-PA.

LIPOPROTEIN (a) (see also Fig. 37–3, p. 1129). A unique lipoprotein particle, lipoprotein (a), also impairs fibrin enhancement of plasminogen activation by t-PA and impairs the binding of t-PA to endothelial cells.[104] This lipoprotein is composed of low-density lipoprotein linked by a disulfide bridge(s) to a unique apolipoprotein, apo(a).[105] Apo(a) is 80 to 90 per cent homologous to plasminogen and contains a serine protease active site, a single kringle 5–like domain, and 37 copies of a kringle 4–like domain. Because of a crucial substitution of serine for arginine at the active site in the homolog, protease activity cannot be generated. The molecule is of particular interest, since elevated levels are highly predictive of atherosclerotic coronary disease. In addition, the lipoprotein colocalizes with fibrin in atheroma, where it may impair fibrinolysis. Thus, lipoprotein (a) may provide a link between the pathological processes of thrombosis and atherosclerosis.

Finally, there is one fibrinolytic abnormality that can cause bleeding rather than thrombosis. Absence of α_2PI, the principal plasmin inhibitor, permits excessively rapid fibrinolysis of hemostatic plugs and recurrent hemorrhage.[106] In summary, it is now clear that inherited molecular defects in the fibrinolytic system, like the inherited defects in the natural anticoagulants, may be added to the growing list of disorders that predispose patients to both arterial and venous thromboembolism.

ANTICOAGULANT THERAPY FOR CARDIOVASCULAR DISORDERS

HEPARIN

Heparin is clearly the most effective anticoagulant agent available for the treatment of thromboembolic disorders. Since the pioneering studies by Barrett and Jordan that demonstrated the efficacy of parenteral heparin in patients with pulmonary embolism, it has become the standard therapy for acute venous and arterial thrombosis and embolism.[107] Heparin activity resides in a heterogeneous series of sulfated glycosaminoglycans that function as anticoagulants by binding to and activating antithrombin III.[108] For pharmaceutical applications, heparin is extracted from porcine intestinal mucosa. There is now abundant evidence that heparin-like molecules also are present on endothelial cells throughout the vascular tree, where they regulate the rate of normal coagulation reactions and help to maintain blood fluidity.[109] Commercial heparin preparations are heterogeneous with respect to both the molecular size and the biological activity of the glycosaminoglycans. In fact, only a small fraction of the molecules in commercial heparin (usually about 20 per cent) have anticoagulant activity.

MECHANISM OF ACTION. Heparin can be conveniently fractionated on the basis of its molecular size and antithrombin affinity. Those heparin species with a low affinity for antithrombin—and therefore little or no anticoagulant activity—may have other biological properties of potential importance. For example, such species inhibit the proliferation of vascular smooth muscle cells in culture and prevent smooth muscle cell migration and proliferation within the arterial wall after experimental injury.[110] In the future, this antiproliferative property of heparin could be exploited to produce agents that inhibit atherogenesis. These low-affinity, high molecular weight forms of heparin also bind to and agglutinate platelets and may be the cause of heparin-induced thrombocytopenia. Heparin size also affects the kinetics of substrate neutralization by antithrombin III. For example, high and low molecular weight species neutralize factor Xa equally well. However, the high molecular weight species are more effective in facilitating the neutralization of thrombin by antithrombin III. This difference could be of importance as various heparin fractions are utilized clinically as antithrombotic agents.

Heparin is administered continuously by intravenous pump, by intermittent intravenous infusion, or subcutaneously. It is metabolized within the liver by the enzyme heparinase and excreted unchanged by the kidney. This explains the increased sensitivity and erratic metabolism of heparin by some patients with renal or hepatic disease. The dose and route of administration vary with the clinical situation and the therapeutic goal. As shown in Figure 58–15, varying methods of heparin administration have a marked effect on plasma heparin level and on the magnitude and duration of impaired hemostasis. Administration of a bolus of heparin followed by a continuous infusion of the drug will maintain heparin levels within the "therapeutic" range with minimal oscillation. Intermittent bolus infusion causes a more dramatic increase and subsequent fall in heparin level. After subcutaneous heparin, levels are not as high but are more sustained. The standard heparin regimens are summarized in Table 58–1.

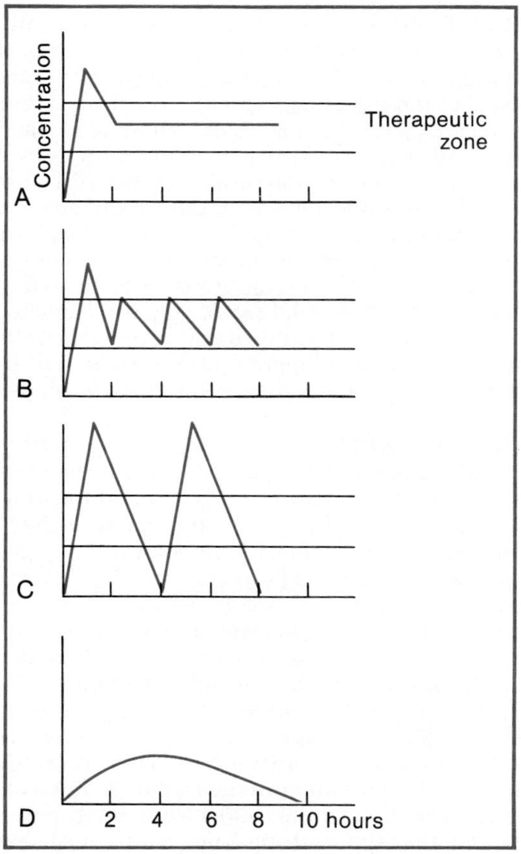

FIGURE 58–15. Concentration of heparin in blood after various routes of administration. *A,* Effect of a heparin bolus followed by a continuous intravenous infusion, the most common method of heparin administration for patients with acute thromboembolism. *B* and *C,* Effects of intermittent intravenous infusions. With this route, heparin levels oscillate widely and frequently are outside the broadly defined "therapeutic zone." This may increase the risk of bleeding and increase the rate of rethrombosis. *D,* Effects of subcutaneous injection, the route used for prophylactic "low-dose" heparin, in which there is a low but sustained level of heparin in the blood. (From Verstraete, M., and Vermylen, J.: Thrombosis. London, Pergamon Press, Copyright 1984, p. 85.)

TABLE 58–1 CLINICAL USE OF HEPARIN

INDICATION	DOSE (USP UNITS)	FREQUENCY	ROUTE
Prophylaxis in elective general surgery	5000	q12h	SC
Prophylaxis in congestive heart failure, cardiomyopathy, myocardial infarction	10,000	q12h	SC
Venous thromboembolism	5000 (bolus)	1000/hr	IV
Massive pulmonary embolism*	20,000 (bolus)	2000/hr	IV

* Reported to be effective in small studies; no randomized trials. Fibrinolytic therapy is a better alternative. SC = subcutaneous; IV = intravenous.

INDICATIONS. The most frequent indications for heparin in cardiac patients are (1) to prevent proximal extension of deep venous thrombosis or the recurrence of pulmonary embolism (p. 1568); (2) to prevent the recurrence of cerebral or other systemic embolism from intracardiac sources in the left atrium, left ventricle, or mitral valve; (3) to preclude development of deep venous thrombosis or pulmonary embolism in high-risk patients, such as those who are immobilized or have congestive heart failure, acute myocardial infarction, or cardiomyopathy or those who are undergoing abdominal surgery; and (4) as long-term therapy for the occasional patient who has recurrent thrombosis or embolism on warfarin or who cannot receive warfarin therapy.

METHOD OF ADMINISTRATION. When full-dose heparin is required, the usual procedure is to administer 5000 USP units of heparin rapidly intravenously followed by a continuous infusion of approximately 1000 USP units per hour. The dose of heparin is adjusted to prolong the PTT to 1.5 times the patient's PTT before instituting heparin therapy. Alternatively, patients may be given an intermittent intravenous infusion of 5000 units four to six times daily. There is good evidence that the risk of bleeding is less with continuous infusion and careful monitoring of the PTT. A less desirable third alternative is to administer 5000 units every 4 to 6 hours by subcutaneous injection. The administration of full-dose heparin is continued for 5 to 7 days, with close monitoring of the PTT and hematocrit along with examination of the stool for occult blood and periodic urinalysis for hematuria. Even with careful control, 10 to 20 per cent of patients experience some bleeding and 1 to 5 per cent have a major hemorrhage. Patients usually are begun on an oral anticoagulant such as warfarin within the first 3 to 5 days of heparinization, although heparin is continued while the dose of warfarin is adjusted.

Low-Dose Heparin. The rationale for low-dose heparin to prevent initial thrombus formation has evolved from extensive clinical studies conducted by Kakkar and colleagues.[111] Their studies demonstrated a clear reduction in both the incidence of and mortality from pulmonary embolism in a large cohort of middle-aged men undergoing major abdominal surgery. Because the incidence of fatal pulmonary embolism also was low in the control group, a multicenter study that enrolled more than 4000 patients was required to prove efficacy. The recommended regimen is 5000 USP units of heparin subcutaneously every 8 to 12 hours beginning 2 hours before surgery. This regimen reduced the rate of deep venous thrombosis by 60 per cent and the risk of fatal pulmonary embolus by 71 per cent in the Kakkar studies. A recent study has shown that the efficacy of low-dose heparin can be improved by monitoring the PTT for minor but reproducible prolongations.[112]

Theoretically, a low-dose heparin regimen should be successful in other surgical and medical settings in which the risk of venous thrombosis and embolism is high. Patients with acute myocardial infarction as well as hospitalized patients with chronic congestive heart failure and low output states, including those with cardiomyopathy, might benefit from prophylactic heparin administration. The regimen does not prevent venous thrombosis and embolism in gynecological patients undergoing pelvic surgery or in orthopedic patients undergoing open reduction and nailing of hip fractures. In addition, in patients who require ophthalmological or neurosurgical procedures, the risk of bleeding, even with low-dose heparin, is prohibitive, and the medication should not be given. Thus, despite careful clinical trials, the use of prophylactic heparin has not become widespread. The trend toward early mobilization of patients after major surgery may have lowered the incidence of venous thrombosis and embolism in the absence of heparin and may limit physician enthusiasm for this regimen.

COMPLICATIONS. The major complication of heparin therapy is hemorrhage caused by interruption of normal hemostasis. Patients may bleed from surgical wounds or catheterization sites or around indwelling vascular catheters and tubes. Patients also may develop gastrointestinal, genitourinary, or retroperitoneal bleeding. Age of the patient, dose and route of administration, presence of pathological lesions in the gastrointestinal or genitourinary tract, and concomitant administration of medications that impair platelet function all affect the incidence and severity of bleeding. Heparin also causes thrombocytopenia in as many as 20 per cent of recipients.[113] More rarely, heparin may provoke intravascular platelet agglutination and paradoxical thrombosis.[114] The antiplatelet effect of heparin is more pronounced with beef lung heparin preparations and, as previously described, is largely caused by the heparin species having low antithrombin affinity and high molecular weight. Because of this adverse effect, beef lung heparin is no longer manufactured. Heparin administration also may induce osteoporosis, although substantial bone loss is not apparent until the 6th to 8th week of therapy.[115] Fortunately, this exceeds the usual duration of heparin therapy for acute thrombosis, but it can become a problem in the occasional patient who requires prolonged intravenous heparin for recurrent thromboembolism.

To reduce complications and improve efficacy, heparin species of low molecular weight and high antithrombin affinity have been prepared by the fractionation of commercial heparin and currently are being tested clinically and in experimental models.[108] Although low molecular weight heparin fractions are effective antithrombotic agents, they are more expensive to produce than standard heparin. Because they are less likely to cause thrombocytopenia, they are the agents of choice in patients with a history of heparin-associated thrombocytopenia who require heparin therapy.

CHRONIC ORAL ANTICOAGULATION

The oral anticoagulants, which are all derivatives of the parent compound warfarin, are the agents of choice for preventing the recurrence of thrombosis and embolism after an initial course of therapy with heparin. The most frequent *indications* for therapy are patients with (1) established deep venous thrombosis and pulmonary embolism, (2) cerebral embolism, (3) atrial fibrillation[116] or mitral stenosis with a history of embolism, (4) prosthetic cardiac valves, and (5) an inherited prethrombotic disorder. The duration of therapy varies. Most patients with a single episode of thromboembolism receive treatment for 3 to 6 months. There is evidence that 90 per cent of patients with deep venous thrombosis will relapse if they do not receive oral anticoagulant therapy and that the risk decreases markedly by 3 months and plateaus by the 6th month. Patients with a noncorrectable cardiac disorder or an inherited prethrombotic state may require prolonged or even lifelong oral anticoagulation. Prophylactic anticoagulation has been proposed for patients (1) with atrial fibrillation who are to undergo cardioversion, (2) with chronic congestive heart failure or low output states such as cardiomyopathy, and (3)

who have undergone hip surgery to prevent perioperative thrombosis.

Warfarin-Type Drugs

These are vitamin K antagonists, which prevent the reduction of vitamin K to its active epoxide form by blocking an intrahepatic epoxide reductase. This, in turn, prevents the formation of Gla residues on prothrombin and factors VII, IX, and X as well as on the proteins C and S. The net effect of warfarin administration is to reduce coagulation factor activity and prolong the PT and PTT. The reduction in coagulation factor activity is directly related to the half-life of each plasma factor. Factor VII, which has the shortest half-life, decreases first, followed by proteins C and S, factors IX and X, and prothrombin. Although therapy with warfarin derivatives usually is evaluated by the degree to which the PT is prolonged, prevention of thrombosis requires a reduction in factors IX and X, which are not measured by the PT. Paradoxically, a profound reduction in factor VII, which prolongs the PT, may not protect a patient from recurrent thrombosis but may increase the risk of bleeding. Although warfarin therapy decreases the activity of both procoagulant and anticoagulant molecules, the net effect is to impair coagulation and reduce the rate of thrombus formation. In patients with congenital protein C or S deficiency, who already have low levels of these proteins, the net balance may shift toward thrombus formation, since protein C and S may have fallen to dangerously low levels while the procoagulant proteins are still elevated. This may predispose patients to a rare thrombotic event, hemorrhagic skin necrosis.

PHARMACOKINETICS. The warfarin derivatives are readily absorbed in the stomach and jejunum and, after absorption, are bound to albumin and become distributed in the intravascular and interstitial spaces. Free drug is then taken up by hepatocytes, where it blocks vitamin K metabolism. Warfarin, like many other drugs, is inactivated by hepatic microsomal enzymes, and the resulting metabolites are either excreted into the bowel by way of the enterohepatic circulation or filtered and excreted by the kidneys. The plasma half-life of the different warfarin derivatives varies considerably. In addition, each of the derivatives is optically active and is produced as a racemic mixture of D and L isomers. The D isomers have a longer half-life, so that varying the ratio of D to L isomers also could influence intravascular half-life. The most frequently used derivative, sodium warfarin, has a half-life of 42 hours.

METHOD OF ADMINISTRATION. Oral anticoagulant therapy with an agent like warfarin is initiated by administering 10 to 15 mg/day of the drug for 3 days to the average-sized adult. The daily dose is then adjusted to maintain the PT at 1.5 to 2.0 times the control value. It is important to recognize that laboratory reagents used to measure the PT are not standardized, so that the patient's PT before therapy should be used as a guideline. Ideally, all measurements should be made in the same laboratory with the same reagents, since the correlation between prolongation of the PT and reduction in activity of the prothrombin complex proteins II, VII, IX, and X varies among PT reagents. One approach, used in Great Britain, has been to supply a reference thromboplastin to each clinical laboratory. Each laboratory can then calibrate its local thromboplastin reagent against the British National thromboplastin standard. Another approach has been to introduce new assays that measure the prothrombin complex proteins but do not rely on the PT reagent. In one study, a conformation-specific antibody that recognized the biologically inactive Gla-deficient prothrombin molecules produced by warfarin therapy was used to assess therapeutic efficacy and was slightly superior to the conventional PT-based test.[117]

DRUG INTERACTIONS. The pharmacology of warfarin is complex. It is well recognized that the anticoagulant effect of warfarin derivatives is dramatically affected by the simultaneous administration of other drugs that may enhance or reduce their activity.[118] The biological effect of a given dose also depends on the rapidity of its uptake by the liver, the integrity and vitamin K stores of the hepatocyte, and the activity of hepatic microsomal degrading enzymes. As shown in Table 58–2, some drugs commonly prescribed for patients with heart disease such as quinidine, cimetidine, and clofibrate may enhance warfarin activity. These drugs compete for albumin-binding sites, displace warfarin from the blood, and increase its rate of delivery to the liver. Conversely, drugs such as glutethimide and other common sedatives reduce the potency of a given warfarin dose by increasing liver microsomal enzyme activity and enhancing drug catabolism. In addition, some drugs like antacids and cholestyramine may impair intestinal absorption of the drug and reduce the activity of a given dose.

In addition to these well-documented drug interactions, metabolic abnormalities that alter hepatic or renal function or that lower albumin levels or vitamin K stores can make patients more sensitive to a given dose of warfarin. Conversely, ingestion of foods rich in vitamin K or the presence of a hypometabolic state such as hypothyroidism may require administration of a larger than usual dose of warfarin. In patients with fever, sepsis, or hyperthyroidism, catabolism of the vitamin K–dependent coagulation factors may have increased, so they require less warfarin for an equivalent anticoagulant effect. In addition to these effects on drug absorption and metabolism, the concomitant administration of drugs that impair platelet function, like aspirin, may cause hemorrhage without altering the PT or warfarin level.

COMPLICATIONS. Hemorrhagic complications occur in 7 to 10 per cent of patients who are anticoagulated for more than 4 months.[119] Death from hemorrhage occurs in approximately 1 per cent of patients who receive warfarin for a similar duration. The frequency of bleeding increases with anticoagulant dose and the degree to which the PT is prolonged, but it also is affected by the patient's age and associated medical conditions. For example, in one large study, bleeding occurred during 7 of 1000 days of warfarin treatment when the residual PT activity was between 10 and 29 per cent of normal. This is equivalent to a PT of 18 to 20 seconds. The rate of hemorrhage increased to 85 per 1000 days of treatment when residual PT activity was less than 10 per cent (PT above 20 seconds).[120]

TABLE 58–2 FACTORS INFLUENCING THE DOSE OF COUMARIN NEEDED FOR A CONSTANT ANTICOAGULANT EFFECT

METABOLIC AND DIETARY FACTORS

Decrease dose:	Increase dose:
Decreased oral intake and vitamin K stores (surgery, antibiotics)	Increased vitamin K intake (liver, cauliflower, green vegetables like broccoli, spinach, green beans)
Liver disease	Hypometabolism (hypothyroidism)
Renal disease leading to hypoalbuminemia	Hereditary resistance
Malignancy, sepsis	
Diarrhea, malabsorption syndromes	
Hypermetabolism (hyperthyroidism, fever)	

DRUG INTERACTIONS

Decrease dose:	Increase dose:
Antibiotics	Vitamin K
Cimetidine	Antacids
Anabolic steroids	Cholestyramine
D-Thyroxine	Barbiturates
Clofibrate	Griseofulvin
Sulfinpyrazone	Rifampin
Phenylbutazone	Antihistamines
Quinidine	
Alpha-methyldopa	

Modified from Chesebro, J., et al.: Antithrombotic therapy in valvular heart disease. By permission of The American College of Cardiology. J. Am. Coll. Cardiol. 8:52B, 1986.

Because of this unacceptably high rate of hemorrhage, modified regimens have been introduced that use less intense anticoagulation.[121] In these regimens, the warfarin dose is adjusted so that the PT is prolonged to no more than 1.5 times the control value. In one study of "low-dose" warfarin, the frequency of bleeding was markedly reduced when compared with standard therapy (4 vs. 22 per cent), whereas the frequency of recurrent venous thromboembolism remained at 2 per cent in both groups.[122]

RECOMMENDATIONS. It is hard to develop a general set of recommendations regarding the duration and intensity of anticoagulation with warfarin-type drugs. Based on the available evidence, however, the authors recommend that patients who receive prophylactic anticoagulation, such as those with prosthetic cardiac valves, chronic atrial fibrillation or mitral stenosis, cardiomyopathy, or chronic congestive heart failure, or those undergoing hip surgery, receive sufficient warfarin to prolong the PT to 1.5 times the control value. Patients given warfarin after an episode of deep venous thrombosis or pulmonary embolism, who are at high risk for recurrent thromboembolism, or patients with a mechanical cardiac valve, should probably receive a slightly higher dose of warfarin to keep the PT prolonged to 1.5 to 2.0 times the control value. Additional clinical studies coupled with the introduction of more reliable assays to monitor biological effects should make warfarin therapy safer and more effective and will allow the dose to be adjusted to the needs of the individual patient.

ANTIPLATELET DRUG THERAPY IN CARDIOVASCULAR DISEASE

Agents that modify platelet function have now been administered to patients with a wide range of cardiovascular disorders. These drugs have been given to patients with unstable angina, at high risk for arrhythmia and sudden death, with prosthetic cardiac valves or saphenous vein bypass grafts, or undergoing percutaneous transluminal angioplasty as well as to those with a history of acute myocardial infarction, stroke, or transient ischemic attacks. In each of these clinical situations there is evidence for platelet participation in the pathophysiology of the clinical disorder and there are some reports of clinical efficacy.[123,124]

Four fundamental problems have made evaluation of antiplatelet therapy difficult: (1) a lack of firm guidelines regarding disorders or clinical events that might potentially benefit from such therapy; (2) the variable quality of clinical trials on which therapeutic decisions must be based; (3) a lack of correlation between in vitro inhibition of platelet function and a clinical antithrombotic effect; and (4) the inability of available drugs to inhibit platelet participation in thrombus formation completely. The ideal antiplatelet drug, which is not yet available, should substantially reduce arterial thrombosis and embolism without causing undue bleeding or other undesirable side effects. This last limitation of antiplatelet therapy may be most important, since an ideal procedure for patient selection and a perfectly organized clinical trial are of limited value if the agent to be tested has minimal or no efficacy.

PHARMACOLOGY OF ANTIPLATELET DRUGS

CYCLO-OXYGENASE INHIBITORS. The most widely studied antiplatelet agents interfere with platelet signal transduction and stimulus-response coupling. One group of drugs, which includes aspirin and other nonsteroidal antiinflammatory agents such as indomethacin, sulfinpyrazone, and ibuprofen, inhibits platelet cyclo-oxygenase. Aspirin is unique in that it is the only drug that irreversibly inhibits cyclo-oxygenase. Because the platelet cannot synthesize any new enzyme, the antiplatelet effect of a single dose of aspirin can persist for 5 to 7 days. In contrast, other tissues rapidly recover from aspirin inhibition by synthesizing new cyclo-oxygenase. Thus endothelial cells regain their capacity to synthesize prostacyclin within a few hours of aspirin administration.[125] The concept of using low doses of aspirin to selectively inhibit platelet function has gained considerable popularity. In fact, it is possible to inhibit platelet thromboxane production effectively with as little as 20 to 100 mg aspirin per day.[126] There is, as yet, no convincing clinical evidence that low-dose aspirin is more effective than the conventional daily doses of 625 to 1250 mg or that these higher doses are harmful. The antiplatelet effect of the competitive inhibitors is much less dramatic than that of aspirin when measured by in vitro laboratory tests as well as by clinical studies assessing thrombus formation in vivo, and they are not frequently used in clinical trials.

DIPYRIDAMOLE. This agent (Persantine) inhibits platelet phosphodiesterase activity and raises platelet cyclic AMP levels in vitro, although the usual doses do not alter in vitro tests of platelet function or prolong the bleeding time in patients. Like aspirin, dipyridamole has undergone extensive clinical testing[127] but has limited clinical efficacy.[128]

OTHER ANTIPLATELET AGENTS. In addition to aspirin and dipyridamole, a number of new antiplatelet agents have been introduced that have more selective effects on arachidonic acid metabolism or affect other steps in the platelet activation process. Several *thromboxane synthetase inhibitors* have been designed to circumvent the fact that aspirin inhibits both thromboxane and prostacyclin synthesis. Unfortunately drugs in this class, such as *dazoxiben,* increase the concentration of the prostaglandin endoperoxide precursors of TxA_2 to levels that can activate the platelets.[129] Several *thromboxane receptor antagonists* that are active in vitro may soon become available for clinical testing, possibly in conjunction with the thromboxane synthetase inhibitors.[130] *Inhibitory prostaglandins* (e.g., PGD_2) or stable synthetic analogs of prostacyclin, prostaglandin-like BW 245C, or carbacyclin have been administered to normal volunteers and to a small number of patients with occlusive vascular disease or fulminant thrombotic thrombocytopenic purpura.[131,132] Although some beneficial effects were noted, the potent hypotensive effects of these compounds may limit their utility for in vivo studies. Inhibitory prostaglandins have been used to prevent the interaction of platelets with artificial surfaces during ex vivo perfusion and may be of value during hemodialysis and cardiopulmonary bypass.[133]

Ticlopidine is a novel platelet inhibitor with a poorly defined mechanism of action. It has the unique property of having little effect on platelets after direct addition in vitro, although it markedly prolongs the bleeding time and platelet response to aggregating agents after administration to patients. It is thought to alter membrane reactivity to multiple agonists and currently is under study in several multicenter trials.[134] Other agents currently under study are inhibitors of platelet-activating factor (1-alkyl-2-acetyl-sn-glycero-3-phosphorylcholine), a lipid mediator generated from leukocytes during allergic and immunological reactions, that aggregates platelets.[135] In addition, peptides that inhibit fibrinogen binding to platelets and monoclonal antibodies to platelet surface glycoproteins may block platelet aggregation and are being tested in laboratory animals as well as in clinical trials.[136] Several well-known cardiovascular drugs such as nitroglycerin[137] and the calcium channel antagonists[138] may have antiplatelet effects, although their possible utility as antithrombotic agents has only recently been the subject of clinical investigation.

ANTIPLATELET AGENTS IN TREATMENT OF MYOCARDIAL ISCHEMIA AND INFARCTION

It is now well accepted that a majority of acute transmural myocardial infarctions are caused by thrombotic occlusion of a diseased coronary artery.[139] The occluding thrombus, which forms on an ulcerated or ruptured atherosclerotic plaque, can be demonstrated in 90 per cent of patients by means of prompt angiography. Although platelets may initiate thrombus formation, fibrin deposition occurs secondarily. These fibrin-rich thrombi are effectively removed by the administration of fibrinolytic agents that restore vascular patency. Platelets also are implicated in the pathogenesis of coronary arterial vasospasm, which may cause transient ischemia and angina pectoris or, less frequently, myocardial infarction. Activated platelets produce TxA_2, a potent vasoconstrictor that may produce or enhance vasospasm. The concentration of the stable metabolite TxB_2 is elevated in coronary sinus blood obtained during pacing or exercise-induced angina and in blood obtained soon after spontaneous anginal episodes.[140] It also is

elevated in patients with variant anginal syndromes who have pain at rest and ST-segment elevation, as well as in those with the clinical syndrome of unstable angina.

UNSTABLE ANGINA (see also p. 1340). Three large randomized placebo-controlled double-blind trials of aspirin in patients with unstable angina have yielded impressive positive results.[141-143] In the first study, the Veterans Administration Cooperative Trial, 1266 men with unstable angina were given 324 mg of aspirin daily, with a 51 per cent decrease in the number of subsequent infarctions and an identical reduction in mortality. A second, Canadian cooperative trial confirmed these results, reporting a 55 per cent reduction in myocardial infarction and a 43 per cent reduction in mortality. In the Theroux study,[143] the number of patients given aspirin who progressed to infarction was reduced by 75 per cent compared with those given placebo. In contrast, there is no evidence that aspirin or any other antiplatelet agents affect the frequency of, duration of, or precipitating events that cause spontaneous or exercise-induced angina pectoris, despite clear evidence for platelet activation in these patients. This striking difference in aspirin's efficacy in various forms of myocardial ischemia as well as the marginal results in most other patients with stable coronary artery disease highlights the problems facing investigators who design clinical trials as well as physicians who must recommend appropriate treatment for their patients. Aspirin currently can be unequivocally recommended only for patients with unstable angina. The differing efficacy may relate to differences in the pathophysiology of unstable angina as compared with chronic angina.

MYOCARDIAL INFARCTION (see also p. 1266). Over the past 12 years there have been several randomized double-blind trials of antiplatelet therapy for the secondary prevention of myocardial infarction.[123] The results are summarized in Table 58-3. Five trials utilized aspirin alone, two had a combination of aspirin and dipyridamole (Persantine), and two used sulfinpyrazone (Anturane). The doses of aspirin varied from 160 to 1500 mg/day, and the studies enrolled 600 to 17,000 patients, predominantly men, who had a well-documented myocardial infarct. Although aspirin therapy was reported to reduce mortality from subsequent infarcts by from 17 to 30 per cent in various studies, none of these trends reached statistical significance. In the second International Study of Infarct Survival, one finds the strongest evidence for the use of aspirin. More than 17,000 patients were randomized to receive either aspirin or streptokinase, both drugs, or placebo. Mortality 5 weeks post infarct was reduced 23 per cent with aspirin, 25 per cent with streptokinase, and 42 per cent with both drugs—all statistically significant reductions.[144]

The first sulfinpyrazone trial reported a striking reduction in sudden death and mortality during the first 6 months of therapy, and the second trial reported a reduction in reinfarction rate. These studies have been criticized, however, on technical grounds relating to the method of patient exclusion and the time of enrollment of subjects.

One investigator has suggested that the lack of statistical significance in many of the aspirin studies may be an insurmountable problem, given the relatively small numbers of patients enrolled in each of these secondary prevention trials. However, when data from all the aspirin trials are pooled to increase the number of evaluable patients, a statistically significant reduction in mortality can be demonstrated. The use of this statistical technique, meta analysis, is subject to the criticism that the study populations may be dissimilar.

The benefits of antiplatelet agents in the primary prevention of cardiovascular disease have been documented in the U.S. Physicians' Health Study.[145] In this study 22,071 male physicians, half of whom received 325 mg of aspirin every other day, were followed for 4.8 years. Aspirin use reduced the incidence of myocardial infarction by 44 per cent, from 0.4 to 0.25 per cent per year, but did not reduce cardiovascular mortality. In the British primary prevention trial, 5139 male physicians, 66 per cent of whom received 500 mg aspirin daily,

TABLE 58–3 ANTIPLATELET THERAPY IN SECONDARY PREVENTION OF MYOCARDIAL INFARCTION

STUDY	DRUGS (DOSAGE)	PATIENTS (DURATION)	OUTCOME*
Elwood et al., 1974	ASA (300 mg/day)	1239 (30 mo)	Mortality ↓ 25%
CDP, 1976	ASA (1 gm/day)	1529 (24 mo)	Mortality ↓ 30%
Breddin et al., 1977	ASA (1.5 gm/day)	946 (24 mo)	No change
Elwood and Sweetman, 1979	ASA (900 mg/day)	1682 (12 mo)	Mortality ↓ 17%
AMIS, 1980	ASA (1 gm/day)	4524 (36 mo)	No change
ART, 1980	Sulfinpyrazone (800 mg/day)	1558 (16 mo)	Reinfarction ↓ 57%
ARIS, 1982	Sulfinpyrazone (800 mg/day)	727 (9 mo)	Reinfarction ↓ 56%
PARIS I, 1980	ASA (1 gm/day) Dipyridamole (225 mg/day)	2206 (36 mo)	Reinfarction ↓ 50%
PARIS II, 1986	Same as PARIS I	3128 (24 mo)	30% ↓ reinf. at 1 yr; 24% ↓ reinf. at 2 yr

All studies cited in Harker, L.A.: Circulation 23:206, 1986 except PARIS II, which is in Klimt, C.R., et al.: J. Am. Coll. Cardiol. 7:251, 1986.

* The reduction in reinfarctions in PARIS II was statistically significant at one and two years. Although trends are given, reductions in mortality were not statistically significant.

Abbreviations: CDP = Coronary Drug Project; AMIS = Acute Myocardial Infarction Study; ART = Anturane Reinfarction Trial; ARIS = Anturane Reinfarction Study; PARIS = Persantine-Aspirin Reinfarction Study; ASA = aspirin.

were followed for 6 years.[146] In contrast to the much larger U.S. trial, no significant difference in myocardial infarction or cardiovascular death was noted in the two groups. In both studies, a slight increase in the incidence of severe or disabling stroke was observed in the men who received aspirin.

ANTIPLATELET THERAPY AFTER CORONARY BYPASS GRAFTING OR PROSTHETIC VALVE INSERTION. The efficacy of antiplatelet therapy for patients who undergo coronary bypass grafting has been extensively studied.[147,148] (Although the majority of the studies have demonstrated a beneficial effect of platelet-modifying drugs, differences in dosage regimens, timing of the onset of therapy, and surgical technique, which may affect the incidence of graft occlusion in placebo groups, complicate interpretation of the data.) Although several early studies utilizing aspirin were begun shortly after surgery improved graft patency, the most dramatic results are those of Chesebro et al., who used a combination of ASA and dipyridamole.[148a] Dipyridamole was begun before surgery and continued by gastric lavage throughout the perioperative period. In addition, they began patients on

aspirin within 24 hours of surgery. Their results, which are summarized in Figure 58–16, show a marked improvement in graft patency both 1 month and 1 year after surgery in patients who received the prescribed antiplatelet therapy. To date, all studies support the use of antiplatelet therapy for at least the first year after coronary bypass grafting. Although perioperative regimens that involve aspirin improve graft patency, the incidence of postoperative bleeding and the need for reoperation also increase. A prospective trial currently is under way to address this important issue.

Some of the earliest studies of antiplatelet drug efficacy involved patients with prosthetic cardiac valves who had cerebral embolic episodes while receiving warfarin.[149] At least six separate studies have demonstrated a beneficial effect of antiplatelet drugs when used with conventional warfarin-type anticoagulants. The regimens have used aspirin alone, aspirin and dipyridamole, and dipyridamole alone. Although all three regimens have been effective, the combination of aspirin and warfarin causes gastrointestinal bleeding. The type of valve and its position in the heart also affected study outcome. The highest incidence of thromboembolism is seen with older types of prostheses in the mitral position. The increasing use of less thrombogenic porcine homograft or "bioprosthetic" valves has lowered the incidence of thromboembolism. Current recommendations are to use warfarin and, if embolism should occur, 400 mg/day of dipyridamole in patients who receive prosthetic valves. Patients who receive bioprosthetic valves should be treated with anticoagulants for 3 months after valve replacement and then should require no further anticoagulant therapy unless they continue to have atrial fibrillation or their valve is placed in the mitral position.

THROMBOLYTIC THERAPY

(See also pp. 1176, 1190, and 1230)

As discussed earlier, there are two general classes of plasminogen activators: the endogenous agents that are derived from human sources—t-PA and the u-PAs—and the exogenous agents that are derived from nonhuman sources—streptokinase (SK) and its anisoylated derivative complexed to plasminogen (APSAC). These agents differ in their mechanism of action, pharmacokinetics, degree of fibrin selectivity, and side effects.

STREPTOKINASE AND ANISOYLATED PLASMINOGEN–STREPTOKINASE COMPLEX

SK, a 47,000-dalton single-chain protein produced by β-hemolytic streptococci, is the oldest available plasminogen activator. It does not enzymatically activate plasminogen but forms a stoichiometric complex with the proenzyme, thereby

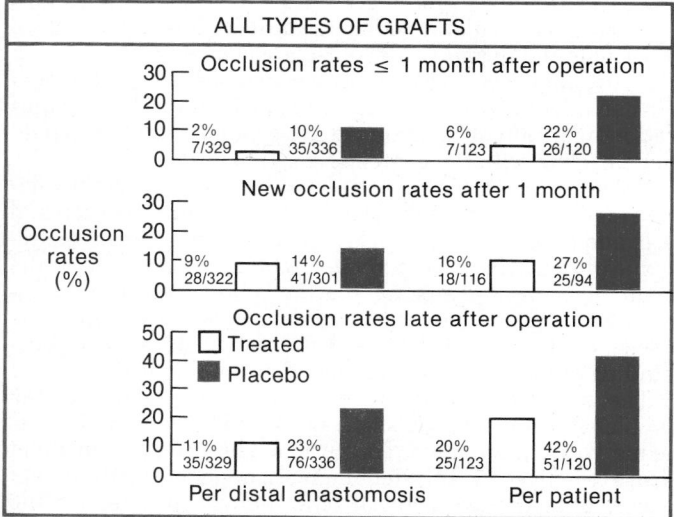

FIGURE 58–16. Occlusion rates of saphenous vein grafts to the coronary artery after treatment with a combination of aspirin (625 mg/day) and dipyridamole (500 mg t.i.d.) beginning at the time of surgery. Rates are expressed per distal anastomosis and per patient. Occlusion is shown 1 month after surgery and as new events beyond 1 month. Data include only patients who underwent angiography 1 month and 1 year after surgery. Below each percentage of occlusion is the total number of anastomoses or patients. (Reprinted by permission from Chesebro, J. H., et al.: Effect of dipyridamole and aspirin on late vein-graft patency after coronary bypass operations. N. Engl. J. Med. 310:211, 1984.)

leading to a conformational change that confers plasmin-like activity on the bimolecular species.[150] This complex then converts uncomplexed plasminogen molecules to plasmin, which initiates fibrinolysis. APSAC is an inactive derivative produced by acylation of the plasminogen active site. This molecular complex does not interact with plasminogen until spontaneous deacylation occurs in plasma.[151] APSAC is not inhibited by α_2PI.

SK and APSAC have been used in a number of clinical settings and can effectively lyse thrombi. They do, however, produce a number of side effects, including febrile reactions, urticarial skin lesions, angioedema, bronchospasm, and hypotension. Serum sickness–like reactions have been reported 7 days after the completion of therapy owing to the formation of immune complexes. In addition, the presence of neutralizing antibodies can make dosage calculations unpredictable. Antibodies induce platelet aggregates in as many as 15 per cent of patients who receive the drug.[152] Clots in these patients, paradoxically, may propagate rather than lyse. Given the allergic potential of SK and APSAC, some investigators believe that patients should be pretreated with diphenhydramine and hydrocortisone, although this approach is infrequently taken in practice.

SK has a plasma half-life of 30 minutes, whereas APSAC has a longer half-life of 70 minutes. For the therapy of acute myocardial infarction, a dose of 1.5 million units of SK is infused over 1 hour, whereas APSAC is administered as an intravenous bolus (30 units over 5 minutes). Therapeutic regimens for deep venous thrombosis and pulmonary embolism commonly call for prolonged infusions of SK over 24 to 72 hours. These lengthy infusions increase the incidence of hemorrhagic complications.

UROKINASE-TYPE PLASMINOGEN ACTIVATORS

As discussed earlier (p. 1775), the u-PAs are synthesized by endothelial cells and renal tubular epithelial cells as a single-chain species (scu-PA or PUK) with minimal endogenous plasminogen activator activity.[153] This proenzyme is converted to a fully active high molecular weight two-chain form and to a smaller form, the conventional UK species used clinically in North America. Low molecular weight two-chain UK (LMW-tc-UK) has a plasma half-life of 10 minutes, whereas scu-PA has an initial plasma half-life of 5 minutes and a terminal half-life of 6 to 7 hours in rabbits and dogs.[154] LMW-tc-UK has been used to treat deep venous thrombosis and also is approved for intracoronary administration in acute myocardial infarction. Because they are of human origin, allergic reactions are rare with this group of activators.

TISSUE-TYPE PLASMINOGEN ACTIVATOR

t-PA also is secreted by the endothelial cell as a single-chain polypeptide with significant plasminogen activator activity.[155] It is converted to a two-chain species which predominates in plasma. t-PA is a relatively unique plasminogen activator, as it is more than 300-fold more efficient at activating plasminogen in the presence of fibrin. Two-chain t-PA is somewhat less fibrin-selective.[156] Fibrin-binding site requires the second kringle domain of t-PA, a triple-looped structure containing lysine residues present in a number of coagulation proteins, and the fibronectin finger-like domain.[157]

Traditionally, a continuous infusion of 100 mg of t-PA is administered over 3 hours to patients with acute myocardial infarction. Newer regimens which use t-PA administered as a bolus may be even more efficacious[158] and may become the preferred treatment mode. t-PA also has been approved for the treatment of pulmonary embolism (p. 1571). Although not yet approved for use in these disorders, in clinical trials t-PA also is effective in the treatment of deep venous thrombosis and peripheral arterial occlusion as well as thrombotic cerebrovascular occlusion.[159-162] Single-chain t-PA has an initial

plasma half-life of 4 minutes and a terminal half-life of approximately 46 minutes.[163] Two weeks after treatment with t-PA one group of investigators failed to detect antibodies in patient plasma.[164]

Indications and Contraindications for Thrombolytic Therapy

There is a general consensus that this form of therapy is indicated in patients with acute myocardial infarction, extensive deep venous thrombosis, major pulmonary embolism with hypotension and/or severe hypoxia, and acute peripheral arterial occlusion. Thrombolytic therapy also has been effective in restoring the patency of indwelling vascular catheters and arteriovenous shunts, as well as in treating patients with axillary vein thrombosis, a condition that is not effectively treated with conventional anticoagulants. General contraindications for use of these agents include a history of abnormal bleeding (particularly from the gastrointestinal or genitourinary tract), uncontrolled hypertension, central nervous system disease, conditions such as peptic ulcer or gastrointestinal neoplasm that potentially can be associated with bleeding, and recent major surgery or organ biopsy.

Limitations of Thrombolytic Therapy

Although thrombolytic therapy usually can restore vessel patency and may be of considerable benefit to selected patients, it is sometimes difficult to demonstrate that pharmacological clot lysis improves clinical outcome. For example, studies of thrombolytic therapy in patients with deep venous thrombosis have not demonstrated any significant reduction in the incidence of postphlebitic complications in treated patients. The often-cited urokinase in pulmonary embolism trial clearly demonstrated superior resolution and lung perfusion in patients treated with urokinase.[165] Until recently,[166] however, this benefit had been shown to correlate with improved long-term outcome.

The appropriate approach to patients with acute coronary thrombosis (see also p. 1230) presents a particularly vexing problem, and highlights the three major shortcomings of thrombolytic therapy for arterial disorders. First, it is clear that treating patients with acute myocardial infarction opens occluded vessels in a timely manner in most patients (70 to 80 per cent), improves mortality rates (at 5 weeks), and leads to improved ventricular function, regardless of the agent chosen. All agents and regimens, however, are plagued by (1) delay in time to patency or, in some cases, resistance to lysis; (2) reocclusion rates of 10 to 20 per cent; and (3) hemorrhagic complications that cannot be predicted in a given patient and that do not correlate with the degree of systemic lysis.

Delays in lysis have been explained on the basis of the relative platelet content of the clot, its degree of organization and age, and a cell surface or plasma plasminogen "steal" of systemically administered activator which might decrease the availability of activator for the thrombus itself. Newer approaches to the administration of the activators as well as the design of mutants with longer half-lives or different surface-binding properties may overcome these problems.

The problem of reocclusion is intimately related to the problem of hemorrhage, since agents that intensify the systemic lytic state reduce reocclusion. The use of antiplatelet drugs to temper the transient increase in platelet activity that occurs after the initiation of lytic therapy may reduce the magnitude of this problem. The simultaneous administration of agents that reverse the bleeding tendency caused by plasminogen activators, like recombinant PAI-1 or DDAVP, may attenuate the hemorrhagic complications.[167]

Management of Patients Receiving Thrombolytic Agents

All candidates for thrombolytic therapy should have screening tests of hemostasis, including a platelet count, PT, and PTT, as well as a bleeding time. The bleeding time correlates fairly well with the likelihood of a hemorrhagic complication. During fibrinolytic therapy, surgical and invasive cardiovascular procedures should be avoided whenever possible. Intramuscular injections also should be avoided. In patients undergoing coronary thrombolysis it is common practice to administer aspirin before infusion of the thrombolytic. Approximately 2 to 4 hours after the completion of treatment, heparin is initiated, and continued for 24 to 72 hours. There is no need to routinely measure fibrinogen, fibrin degradation products, plasminogen consumption, or α_2PI consumption, since changes in these parameters predict neither efficacy nor complications arising from therapy.

Bleeding that develops during thrombolytic therapy is best managed by applying direct pressure whenever possible, discontinuing the thrombolytic agent, reversing heparin with protamine, and transfusing the patient with fresh frozen plasma and packed erythrocytes. In extreme cases ϵ-aminocaproic acid (Amicar) may be administered.

REFERENCES

HEMOSTASIS

1. Loscalzo, J.: Lipoprotein a—a unique risk factor for atherothrombotic disease. Arteriosclerosis 10:672, 1990.
2. Nieuwenhuis, H. K., Akkerman, J.W.M., Houdjik, W.P.M., and Sixma, J. J.: Human blood platelets showing no response to collagen fail to express glycoprotein Ia. Nature 318:470, 1985.
3. Santoro, S. A.: Identification of a 160,000-dalton platelet membrane protein that mediates the initial divalent cation-dependent adhesion of platelets to collagen. Cell 46:913, 1986.
4. Yamada, K. M., and Olden, K.: Fibronectins—adhesive glycoproteins of cell surface and blood. Nature 275:179, 1978.
5. Plow, E. F., and Ginsberg, M. H.: Specific and saturable binding of plasma fibronectin to thrombin-stimulated human platelets. J. Biol. Chem. 256:9477, 1981.
6. Haverstick, D. M., Coawa, J. F., Yamada, K. M., and Santoro, S. A.: Inhibition of platelet adhesion to fibronectin, fibrinogen, and von Willebrand factor substrates by a synthetic tetrapeptide derived from the cell binding domain of fibronectin. Blood 66:946, 1985.
7. Bockenstedt, P., McDonagh, J., and Handin, R. I.: The binding and covalent crosslinking of purified von Willebrand's factor to native monomeric collagen. J. Clin. Invest. 77:743, 1986.
8. Michelson, A. D., Loscalzo, J., Melnick, B., et al.: Partial characterization of a binding site for von Willebrand factor on glycocalicin. Blood 67:19, 1986.
9. Ruggeri, Z. M., DeMarco, L., Gatti, L., et al.: Platelets have more than one binding site for von Willebrand factor. J. Clin. Invest. 72:1, 1983.
10. Baumgartner, H. R., Tschopp, T. B., and Weiss, H. J.: Platelet interaction with collagen fibrils in flowing blood. II. Impaired adhesion and aggregation in bleeding disorders. Thromb. Haemost. 37:17, 1977.
11. Houdjik, W.P.M., Sakariassen, K. S., Nievelstein, P.F.E.M., and Sixma, J. J.: Role of factor VIII–von Willebrand factor and fibronectin in the interaction of platelets in flowing blood with monomeric and fibrillar human collagen types I and III. J. Clin. Invest. 75:531, 1985.
12. Shattil, S. J.: Platelets and their membranes in hemostasis: Physiology and pathophysiology. Ann. Intern. Med. 94:108, 1981.
13. Cooper, B., Handin, R. I., Young, L. H., and Alexander, R. W.: Agonist regulation of the human platelet alpha-adrenergic receptor. Nature 274:703, 1978.
14. Schafer, A. I., Cooper, B., O'Hara, D., and Handin, R. I.: Identification of platelet receptors for prostaglandins I_2 and D_2. J. Biol. Chem. 254:2914, 1979.
15. Moncada, S., and Vane, J. R.: Arachidonic acid metabolites and the interactions between platelets and blood vessel walls. N. Engl. J. Med. 300:1142, 1979.
16. Berridge, M. J.: Inositol triphosphate and diacylglycerol as second messengers. Biochem. J. 220:345, 1984.
17. Majerus, P. W., Connolly, T. M., Deckman, H. et al.: The metabolism of phosphoinositide-derived messenger molecules. Science 234:1519, 1986.
18. Berridge, M. J., and Irvine, R. F.: Inositol triphosphate: A novel second messenger in cellular signal transduction. Nature 312:315, 1984.
19. Nishizuka, Y.: The role of protein kinase C in cell surface signal transduction and tumour promotion. Nature 308:693, 1984.
20. Tyers, M., Rachubirski, R. A., Stewart, M. I., et al.: Molecular cloning and expression of the major protein kinase L substrate of platelets. Nature 2:470, 1988.
21. Chaffoy de Courcelles, D., Roevens, P., and Van Belle, H.: 1-Oleoyl-2-acetyl-glycerol (OAG) stimulates the formation of phosphatidylinositol-4-phosphate in intact human platelets. Biochem. Biophys. Res. Commun. 123:589, 1984.
22. Halenda, S. P., Zavoico, G. B., and Feinstein, M. B.: Phorbol esters and

oleoyl acetyl glycerol enhance release of arachidonic acid in platelets stimulated by Ca^{2+} ionophore A23187. J. Biol. Chem. 260:12484, 1985.
23. Majerus, P. W.: Arachidonate metabolism in vascular disorders. J. Clin. Invest. 72:1521, 1986.
24. Hamberg, M., Svensson, J., and Samuelsson, B.: Thromboxanes: A new group of biologically active compounds derived from prostaglandin endoperoxides. Proc. Natl. Acad. Sci. U.S.A. 72:2994, 1975.
25. Rittenhouse, S. E.: Activation of phospholipase C in human platelets. In Hayaishi, O. (ed.): Advances in Thromboxane and Prostaglandin Research. Vol. 15. New York, Raven Press, 1985, pp. 113–114.
26. Rittenhouse-Simmons, S., and Deykin, D.: The mobilization of arachidonic acid in platelets exposed to thrombin or ionophore A23187. J. Clin. Invest. 60:495, 1977.
27. Turner, J. R., and Tainer, J. A.: Biogenesis of chemotactic molecules by the arachidonate lipoxygenase system of platelets. Nature 257:680, 1975.
28. Gerrard, J. M., and White, J. G.: Prostaglandins and thromboxanes: "Middlemen" modulating platelet function in hemostasis and thrombosis. In Spaet, T. H. (ed.): Progress in Hemostasis and Thrombosis. Vol. 4. New York, Grune and Stratton, 1982, pp. 87–126.
29. Fitzgerald, G. A., Oates, J. A., Hawiger, J., et al.: Endogenous synthesis of prostacyclin and thromboxane and platelet function during aspirin administration in man. J. Clin. Invest. 71:767, 1983.
30. Fitzgerald, G. A., Smith, G. K., Pedersen, A. K., and Brash, A. R.: Increased prostacyclin biosynthesis in patients with severe atherosclerosis and platelet activation. N. Engl. J. Med. 310:1065, 1984.
31. Samuelsson, B.: Leukotrienes: Mediators of immediate hypersensitivity and inflammation. Science 220:568, 1983.
32. Samuelsson, B., Dahlen, S-E., Lindgren, J. A., et al.: Leukotrienes and lipoxins: Structures, biosynthesis and biological effects. Science 237:1171, 1987.
33. Marcus, A. J., Weksler, B. B., Jaffe, E. A., and Broekman, M. J.: Synthesis of prostacyclin from platelet-derived endoperoxides by cultured human endothelial cells. J. Clin. Invest. 66:979, 1980.
34. Schafer, A. I., Crawford, D. D., and Gimbrone, M. A.: Unidirectional transfer of prostaglandin endoperoxides between platelets and endothelial cells. J. Clin. Invest. 73:1105, 1984.
35. White, J. G.: Electron microscopic studies of platelet secretion. In Spaet, T. H. (ed.): Progress in Hemostasis and Thrombosis. Vol. 2. New York, Grune and Stratton, 1974, pp. 49–98.
36. Goldberg, I. D., Stemerman, M. B., and Handin, R. I.: Vascular permeation of platelet factor four following endothelial injury. Science 209:611, 1980.
37. Sporn, M. B., Roberts, A. B., Wakefield, L. M., and Assoian, R. K.: Transforming growth factor-beta: Biological function and chemical structure. Science 233:532, 1986.
38. Deuel, T. F., and Huang, J. S.: Platelet-derived growth factor. Structure, function, and roles in normal and transformed cells. J. Clin. Invest. 74:664, 1984.
39. Colman, R. W.: Aggregin—a platelet ADP receptor that mediates activation. FASEB J. 4:1425, 1990.
40. Bennett, J. S., Vilaire, G., and Cines, D. B.: Identification of the fibrinogen receptor on human platelets by photoaffinity labeling. J. Biol. Chem. 257:8049, 1982.
41. Kloczewiak, M., Timmons, S., Lukas, T. J., and Hawiger, J.: Platelet receptor recognition site on human fibrinogen: Synthesis and structure-function relationship of peptides corresponding to the carboxy terminal segment of the gamma chain. Biochemistry 23:1767, 1984.
42. Plow, E. F., Srouji, A. H., Meyer, D., et al.: Evidence that three adhesive proteins interact with a common recognition site on activated platelets. J. Biol. Chem. 259:5388, 1984.
43. Coller, B. S., Folts, J. D., Scudder, L. E., and Smith, S. R.: Antithrombotic effect of a monoclonal antibody to the platelet glycoprotein IIb/IIIa receptor in an experimental animal model. Blood 68:783, 1986.
44. Ruggeri, Z. M., Houghten, R. A., Russel, S. R., and Zimmerman, T. S.: Inhibition of platelet function with synthetic peptides designed to be high affinity antagonists of fibrinogen binding to platelets. Proc. Natl. Acad. Sci. U.S.A. 83:5708, 1986.
45. Azuma, H., Ishikawa, M., and Sezizaki, S.: Endothelium-dependent inhibition of platelet aggregation. Br. J. Pharmacol. 88:411, 1986.
46. Stamler, J., Mendelsohn, M. E., Amarante, P., et al.: N-acetylcysteine potentiates platelet inhibition by endothelium-drived relaxing factor. Circ. Res. 65:789, 1989.
47. Mendelsohn, M. E., and Loscalzo, J.: The effect of S-nitrosothiols on fibrinogen binding to human platelets. Blood 74:4030, 1989.
48. Vaughan, D. E., Mendelsohn, M. E., Dalllerck, P. J., et al.: Characterization of the binding of human tissue-type plasminogen activator to platelets. J. Biol. Chem. 264:15869, 1989.
49. Loscalzo, J., and Vaughan, D. E.: Human tissue-type plasminogen activator facilitates platelet disaggregation. J. Clin. Invest. 79:12749, 1987.
50. Stamler, J. S., Vaughan, D. E., and Loscalzo, J.: Synergistic disaggregation of platelets by tissue-type plasminogen activator, prostaglandin E_1 and nitroglycerin. Circ. Res. 65:756, 1989.
51. Marcus, A. J.: Thrombosis and inflammation as multicellular processes. Blood 76:1903, 1990.
52. Mann, K. G., Nesheim, M. E., Church, W. R., et al.: Surface-dependent reactions of the vitamin K–dependent enzyme complexes. Blood 76:1, 1990.
53. Rosenberg, R. D., and Rosenberg, J. S.: Natural anticoagulant mechanisms. J. Clin. Invest. 74:1, 1984.
54. Clouse, L. H., and Comp, P.: The regulation of hemostasis: The protein C system. N. Engl. J. Med. 314:1298, 1986.

55. Esmon, N. L., Owen, W. G., and Esmon, C. T.: Isolation of a membrane-bound cofactor for thrombin-catalyzed activation of protein C. J. Biol. Chem. 257:859, 1982.

56. Walker, F. J.: Regulation of activated protein C by a new protein: A possible function for protein S. J. Biol. Chem. 255:5521, 1980.

57. De Fouw, N. J., von Hirsbergh, V.W.M., de Jong, W. F., et al.: The interaction of activated protein C and thrombin with the plasminogen activator inhibitor release from human endothelial cells. Thromb. Haemost. 57:176, 1987.

58. Fay, W. P., and Owen, W. G.: Platelet plasminogen activator inhibitor: Purification and characterization of interaction with plasminogen activators and activated protein C. Biochemistry 28:5773, 1989.

59. Chien, S.: Transport across arterial endothelium. In Spaet, T. H. (ed.): Progress in Hemostasis and Thrombosis. Vol. 4. New York, Grune and Stratton, 1978, pp. 1–36.

60. Thomas, D. J.: The influence of blood viscosity on cerebral blood flow and symptoms. In Greenhalsh, R. M., and Rose, F. L. (eds.): Progress in Stroke Research. Kent, England, Pitman Medical Publishing Company, 1979, pp. 47–55.

61. Segal, A.: The Clinical Use of Dextran Solutions. New York, Grune and Stratton, 1964.

CLOT DISSOLUTION—THE FIBRINOLYTIC SYSTEM

62. Adams, L. M., Fretto, L. J., and McKee, P. A.: The binding of human plasminogen to fibrin and fibrinogen J. Biol. Chem. 258:4249, 1983.

63. Collen, D., and Lijnen, H. R.: The fibrinolytic system in man: An overview. In Collen, D., Lijnen, H. R., and Verstraete, M. (eds.): Thrombolysis: Biological and Therapeutic Properties of New Thrombolytic Agents. New York, Churchill Livingstone, 1985, pp. 1–14.

64. Pennica, D., Holmes, W. E., Kohr, W. J., et al.: Cloning and expression of human tissue-type plasminogen activator. Nature 301:214, 1983.

65. Steffens, G. J., Günzler, W. A., Otting, F., et al.: The complete amino acid sequence of low molecular mass urokinase from human urine. Physiol. Chem. 363:1043, 1982.

66. Pannell, R., Block, J., and Gurewich, V.: Complementary modes of action of tissue-type plasminogen activator and pro-urokinase by which their synergistic effects on clot lysis may be explained. J. Clin. Invest. 81:853, 1988.

67. Ginsburg, D., Zeheb, R., Yang, A. Y., et al.: cDNA cloning of human plasminogen activator-inhibitor from endothelial cells. J. Clin. Invest. 78:1673, 1986.

68. Moroi, M., and Aoki, N.: Isolation and characterization of alpha$_2$-plasmin inhibitor from human plasma. A novel proteinase inhibitor which inhibits activator-induced lysis. J. Biol. Chem. 251:5956, 1976.

EVALUATION OF HEMOSTASIS IN CARDIOVASCULAR PATIENTS

69. Meyer, D., and Zimmerman, T. S.: von Willebrand's disease. In Colman, R. W., Hirsh, J., Marder, V. J., and Salzman, E. W. (eds.): Hemostasis and Thrombosis. Philadelphia, J. B. Lippincott, 1982, pp. 64–74.

70. Ruggeri, Z. M., and Zimmerman, T. S.: Variant von Willebrand's disease. Characterization of two subtypes by analysis of multimeric composition of factor VIII/von Willebrand factor in plasma and platelets. J. Clin. Invest. 63:1318, 1980.

71. Mannucci, P. M., Canciani, M. T., Rota, L., and Donovan, B. S.: Response of factor VIII/von Willebrand factor to DDAVP in healthy volunteers and in patients with von Willebrand's disease. Br. J. Haematol. 47:283, 1981.

72. Milan, J. D., Austin, S. F., Nihill, M. R., et al.: Use of sufficient hemodilution to prevent coagulopathies following surgical correction of cyanotic heart disease. J. Thorac. Cardiovasc. Surg. 89:623, 1985.

73. Michelson, A.: Pathomechanism of defective hemostasis during and after extracorporeal circulation: The role of platelets. In Hetzer, R. (ed.): Blood Use in Cardiac Surgery. Darmstadt, Steinkopff (in press).

74. Abrahamsen, A. F.: Platelet survival studies in man with special reference to thrombosis and atherosclerosis. Scand. J. Haematol. 3(Suppl.):1, 1968.

75. Harker, L. A., and Slichter, S. J.: Studies of platelet and fibrinogen kinetics in patients with prosthetic heart valves. N. Engl. J. Med. 283:1302, 1970.

76. Handin, R. I., McDonough, M., and Lesch, M.: Elevation of platelet factor 4 in acute myocardial infarction: Measurement by radioimmunoassay. J. Lab. Clin. Med. 91:340, 1978.

77. Kaplan, K. L., Nossel, H. L., Drillings, M., and Lasznik, G.: Radioimmunoassay of platelet factor 4 and B-thromboglobulin: Development and application to studies of platelet release in relation to fibrinopeptide A generation. Br. J. Haematol. 39:129, 1978.

78. Dawes, J., Smith, R. C., and Pepper, D. S.: The release, distribution and clearance of human B-thromboglobulin and platelet factor 4. Thromb. Haemost. 37:73, 1977.

79. Guzzo, J., Niewiarowski, S., Musial, J., et al.: Secreted platelet proteins with antiheparin and mitogenic activities in chronic renal failure. J. Lab. Clin. Med. 96:102, 1980.

80. Ludlam, C. A., and Cash, J. D.: Studies on the liberation of B-thromboglobulin from human platelets in vitro. Br. J. Haematol. 33:2339, 1976.

81. Yudelman, I., Nossel, H. L., and Kaplan, K. L.: Fibrinopeptide A levels in symptomatic thromboembolism. Blood 51:1189, 1978.

82. Bauer, K. A., Goodman, T. L., Kass, B. L., and Rosenberg, R. D.: Elevated factor Xa activity in the blood of asymptomatic patients with congenital antithrombin deficiency. J. Clin. Invest. 76:826, 1985.

83. Halushka, P. V., Lurie, D., and Colwell, J. A.: Increased synthesis of prostaglandin E–like material by platelets from patients with diabetes mellitus. N. Engl. J. Med. 297:1306, 1977.

84. Carvalho, A., Colman, R. W., and Lees, R. S.: Platelet function in hyperbetalipoproteinemia. N. Engl. J. Med. 290:434, 1974.

85. Gerritsen, T., and Waisman, H. A.: Homocystinuria. Cystathionine synthase deficiency. In Stanbury, J. B., et al. (eds.): The Metabolic Basis of Inherited Disease. 3rd ed. New York, McGraw-Hill Book Co., 1972, pp. 404–412.

86. Harker, L. A., Slichter, S. J., and Scott, C. R.: Homocystinemia. Vascular injury and arterial thrombosis. N. Engl. J. Med. 291:537, 1974.

87. Tofler, G. H., Brezinski, D., Schafer, A. I., et al.: Concurrent morning increase in platelet aggregability and the risk of myocardial infarction and sudden cardiac death. N. Engl. J. Med. 316:1514, 1987.

88. Winter, J. H., Fenech, A., Ridley, W., et al.: Familial antithrombin III deficiency. Q. J. Med. 51:373, 1982.

89. Broekmans, A. W., Veltkamp, J. J., and Bertina, R. M.: Congenital protein C deficiency and venous thromboembolism: A study of three Dutch families. N. Engl. J. Med. 309:340, 1983.

90. Comp, P. C., Nixon, R. R., Cooper, M. R., and Esmon, C. T.: Familial protein S deficiency is associated with recurrent thrombosis. J. Clin. Invest. 74:2082, 1984.

91. Seligson, U., Berger, A., Abend, M., et al.: Homozygous protein C deficiency manifested by massive venous thrombosis in the newborn. N. Engl. J. Med. 310:559, 1984.

92. Bauer, K. A., Ashenhurst, J. B., Chediak, J., and Rosenberg, R. D.: Antithrombin "Chicago": A functionally abnormal molecule with increased heparin affinity causing thrombophilia. Blood 57:1242, 1981.

93. McGehee, W. G., Klotz, T. A., Epstein, D. J., and Rapaport, S. I.: Coumarin necrosis associated with hereditary protein C deficiency. Ann. Intern. Med. 101:59, 1984.

94. Moser, K. M., and LeMoine, J. R.: Is embolic risk conditioned by location of deep venous thrombosis? Ann. Intern. Med. 94:855, 1981.

95. Sagar, S., Thomas, D. P., Stamatakis, J. D., and Kakkar, V. V.: Oral contraceptives, antithrombin-III activity, and post-operative deep-vein thrombosis. Lancet 1:509, 1976.

96. Rentrop, P., Blanke, H., Karsch, K. R., et al.: Selective intracoronary thrombolysis in acute myocardial infarction and unstable angina pectoris. Circulation 63:307, 1981.

97. Aoki, N., Moroi, M., Sakata, Y., and Yoshida, N.: Abnormal plasminogen. A hereditary molecular abnormality found in a patient with recurrent thrombosis. J. Clin. Invest. 61:1186, 1978.

98. Carrell, N., Gabriel, D. A., Blatt, P. M., et al.: Hereditary dysfibrinogenemia in a patient with thrombotic disease. Blood 62:439, 1983.

99. Mettinger, K. L., Nyman, D., Kjellin, K. G., et al.: Factor VIII related antigen, antithrombin III, spontaneous platelet aggregation, and plasminogen activator in ischemic cerebrovascular disease. J. Neurosci. 41:31, 1979.

100. Isacson, S., and Nilsson, I. M.: Defective fibrinolysis in blood and vein walls in recurrent "idiopathic" venous thrombosis. Chir. Scand. 138:313, 1972.

101. Boyko, O. B., and Pizzo, S. V.: Mesenteric vein thrombosis and vascular plasminogen activator. Arch. Pathol. Lab. Med. 107:541, 1983.

102. Latham, B., Kafoy, G. A., Barrett, O., Jr., et al.: Deficient tissue plasminogen activator release with recurrent deep vein thrombosis. Am. J. Med. 88:199, 1990.

103. Hamsten, A., Wiman, B., deFaire, U., and Blomback, M.: Increased plasma levels of a rapid inhibitor of tissue plasminogen activator in young survivors of myocardial infarction. N. Engl. J. Med. 313:1551, 1985.

104. Loscalzo, J., Weinfeld, M., Fless, G., and Scanu, A. M.: Lipoprotein (a), fibrin binding and plasminogen activation. Arteriosclerosis 10:240, 1990.

105. Scanu, A. M., and Fless, G. M.: Lipoprotein (a). Heterogeneity and biological relevance. J. Clin. Invest. 85:1709, 1990.

106. Aoki, N., Saito, H., Kamya, T., et al.: Congenital deficiency of alpha$_2$ plasmin inhibitor associated with severe hemorrhagic tendency. J. Clin. Invest. 63:877, 1979.

ANTICOAGULANT THERAPY FOR CARDIOVASCULAR DISORDERS

107. Barrett, D. W., and Jordan, S. C.: Anticoagulant drugs in the treatment of pulmonary embolism. A controlled clinical trial. Lancet 1:1309, 1960.

108. Rosenberg, R. D.: The heparin-antithrombin system. In Colman, R. W., Hirsh, J., Marder, V. J., and Salzman, E. W. (eds.): Hemostasis and Thrombosis: Basic Principles and Clinical Practice. Philadelphia, J. B. Lippincott, 1982, p. 962.

109. Marcum, J. A., McKenney, J. R., and Rosenberg, R. D.: Acceleration of thrombin-antithrombin complex formation in rat hindquarters via heparin-like molecules bound to the endothelium. J. Clin. Invest. 74:341, 1984.

110. Castellot, J. J., Beeler, D. L., Rosenberg, R. D., and Karnovsky, M. J.: Structural determinants of the capacity of heparin to inhibit the proliferation of vascular smooth muscle cells. J. Cell. Physiol. 120:315, 1984.

111. Kakkar, V. V., Corrigan, T., and Spindler, J.: Efficacy of low doses of heparin in prevention of deep-vein thrombosis after major surgery: A double blind, randomized trial. Lancet 2:101, 1972.

112. Turpie, A. G., Robinson, J. G., Doyle, D. J., et al.: Comparison of high-dose with low-dose subcutaneous heparin to prevent left ventricular mural thrombosis in patients with acute transmural anterior myocardial infarction. N. Engl. J. Med. 320:352, 1989.

113. Bell, W. R., and Royall, R. M.: Heparin-induced thrombocytopenia. A comparison of three heparin preparations. N. Engl. J. Med. *303*:902, 1980.

114. Ansell, J., and Deykin, D.: Heparin-induced thrombocytopenia and recurrent thromboembolism. Am. J. Haematol. *8*:235, 1980.

115. Jaffe, M. D., and Willis, P. W.: Multiple fractures associated with heparin therapy. J.A.M.A. *193*:158, 1965.

116. Petersen, P., Roysen, G., Godtfredsen, J., et al.: Placebo-controlled randomized trial of warfarin and aspirin for prevention of thromboembolic complications in chronic atrial fibrillation. Lancet *1*:175, 1989.

117. Furie, B., Liebman, H. A., Blanchard, R. A., et al.: Comparison of native prothrombin antigen and the prothrombin time for monitoring oral anticoagulant therapy. Blood *64*:445, 1984.

118. O'Reilly, R. A.: Vitamin K antagonists. *In* Colman, R. W., Hirsh, J., Marder, V. J., and Salzman, E. W. (eds.): Hemostasis and Thrombosis: Basic Principles and Clinical Practice. Philadelphia, J. B. Lippincott, 1982, p. 955.

119. Deykin, D.: Warfarin therapy. N. Engl. J. Med. *283*:691–694 and 801–803, 1970.

120. Husted, S., and Andreasen, F.: Problems encountered in long-term treatment with anticoagulants. Acta Med. Scand. *200*:379, 1976.

121. Hull, R., Delmore, T., Carter, C., et al.: Adjusted subcutaneous heparin versus warfarin sodium in the treatment of venous thrombosis. N. Engl. J. Med. *306*:189, 1982.

122. Hirsh, J., Deykin, D., and Poller, L.: "Therapeutic range" for oral anticoagulant therapy. Chest *82*(Suppl. 2):11S, 1986.

ANTIPLATELET DRUG THERAPY IN CARDIOVASCULAR DISEASE

123. Stein, B., Fuster, V., Israel, D. H., et al.: Platelet inhibitor agents in cardiovascular disease—an update. J. Am. Coll. Cardiol. *14*:813, 1986.

124. Antiplatelet Trialists' Collaboration: Secondary prevention of vascular disease by prolonged antiplatelet treatment. Br. Med. J. *296*:320, 1988.

125. Jaffe, E. A., and Weksler, B. B.: Recovery of endothelial cell prostacyclin production after inhibition by low doses of aspirin. J. Clin. Invest. *63*:532, 1979.

126. FitzGerald, G. A., Brash, A. R., Oates, J. A., and Pedersen, A. K.: Endogenous prostacyclin biosynthesis and platelet function during selective inhibition of thromboxane synthase in man. J. Clin. Invest. *71*:1336, 1983.

127. Hanson, S. R., Harker, L. A., and Bjornsson, T. D.: Effects of platelet-modifying drugs on arterial thromboembolism in baboons: Aspirin potentiates the antithrombotic actions of dipyridamole and sulfinpyrazone by mechanism(s) independent of platelet cyclooxygenase inhibition. J. Clin. Invest. *75*:1591, 1985.

128. FitzGerald, G. A.: Dipyridamole. N. Engl. J. Med. *316*:1247, 1987.

129. Lewis, P., and Taylor, H. M.: Dazoxiben—Clinical prospects for a thromboxane synthase inhibitor. Br. J. Clin. Pharmacol. *15*:1S, 1983.

130. Brittain, R. T., Boutal, L., Carter, M. C., et al.: AH23848: A thromboxane receptor blocking drug that can clarify the pathophysiologic role of thromboxane A₂. Circulation *72*:1208, 1985.

131. Kelton, J. G., and Blajchman, M. A.: Prostaglandin I₂ (prostacyclin). Can. Med. Assoc. J. *122*:175, 1980.

132. FitzGerald, G. A., Maas, R. L., Stein, R., et al.: Intravenous prostacyclin in thrombotic thrombocytopenic purpura. Ann. Intern. Med. *95*:319, 1981.

133. Zussman, R., Rubin, R. H., Cato, A. E., et al.: Hemodialysis using prostacyclin instead of heparin as the sole antithrombotic agent. N. Engl. J. Med. *304*:934, 1981.

134. Haes, W. K., and Kamm, B.: The North American Ticlopidine Aspirin Stroke Study: Structure, stratification, variables and patient characteristics. Ticlopidine: quo vadis? Agents Actions *15*(Suppl.):273, 1984.

135. Voelkel, N. F., Chang, S. W., Pfeffer, K. D., et al.: PAF antagonists: Different effects on platelets, neutrophils, guinea pig ileum and PAF-induced vasodilation in isolated rat lung. Prostaglandins *32*:359, 1986.

136. Gold, H. K., Coller, B. S., Yasuda, T., et al: Rapid and sustained coronary artery recanalization with combined bolus injection of recombinant tissue-type plasminogen activator and monoclonal antiplatelet GpIIb/IIIa antibody in a canine preparation. Circulation *77*:670, 1988.

137. Schror, K., Ahland, B., Darius, H., and Weiss, P.: Stimulation of vascular PGI₂ by organic nitrates and its significance for the antianginal effect. Scand. J. Lab. Clin. Invest. *173*(Suppl.):33, 1984.

138. Pumphrey, C. W., Fuster, V., Dewarjee, M. K., et al.: Comparison of the antithrombotic action of calcium antagonist drugs with dipyridamole in dogs. Am. J. Cardiol. *51*:591, 1983.

139. DeWood, M. A., Stifter, W. F., Simpson, C. S., et al.: Coronary arteriographic findings soon after non-Q-wave myocardial infarction. N. Engl. J. Med. *315*:417, 1986.

140. Mehta, J., Mehta, P., Feldman, R. J., and Horalek, C.: Thromboxane release in coronary artery disease: Spontaneous angina versus pacing-induced angina. Am. Heart J. *107*:286, 1984.

141. Lewis, H. D., David, J. W., Archibald, D. G., et al.: Protective effects of aspirin against acute myocardial infarction and death in men with unstable angina. N. Engl. J. Med. *309*:396, 1983.

142. Cairns, J., Gent, M., Singer, J., et al.: Aspirin, sulfinpyrazone or both in unstable angina. Results of a Canadian multicenter trial. N. Engl. J. Med. *313*:1369, 1985.

143. Theroux, P., Ouimet, H., McCano, J., et al.: Aspirin, Heparin or both to treat acute unstable angina. N. Engl. J. Med. *319*:1105, 1988.

144. ISIS-2 Collaborative Group: Randomized trial of intravenous streptokinase and aspirin both or neither among 17, 187 cases of suspected acute myocardial infarction. Lancet *2*:348, 1988.

145. The Steering Committee of the Physicians' Health Study Research Group: Final report of the aspirin component of the ongoing physicians' health study. N. Engl. J. Med. *321*:129, 1989.

146. Peto, R., Gray, R., Collins, R., et al.: A randomized trial of the effects of prophylactic daily aspirin among male British doctors. Br. Med. J. *296*:313, 1988.

147. Sethi, G., Copeland, J. G., Goldman, S., et al.: Implications of preoperative administration of aspirin to patients undergoing coronary bypass grafting. J. Am. Coll. Cardiol. *15*:15, 1990.

148. Goldman, S., Copeland, J., Moritz, T., et al.: Improvement in early saphenous vein graft patency after coronary artery bypass surgery with antiplatelet therapy: Results of a Veterans Administration Cooperative Study. Circulation *77*:1324, 1988.

148a. Chesebro, J. H., Fuster, V., Elveback, L. R., et al.: Effect of dipyridamole and aspirin on late vein–graft patency after coronary bypass operations. N. Engl. J. Med. *310*:209, 1984.

149. Goldman, S., Copeland, J., Moeritz, T., et al.: Saphenous vein graft patency one year after coronary artery bypass surgery and effects of antiplatelet therapy: Results of a Veterans Administration Cooperative Study. Circulation *80*:1190, 1989.

THROMBOLYTIC THERAPY

150. Reddy, K.N.N.: Mechanism of activation of human plasminogen by streptokinase. *In* Kline, D. L., and Reddy, K. N. (eds.): Fibrinolysis. Boca Raton, CRC Press, 1980, p. 71.

151. Anderson, J. L.: Development and evaluation of anisoylated plasminogen-streptokinase activator complex (APSAC) as a second generation thrombolytic agent. J. Am. Coll. Cardiol. *10*:228, 1987.

152. Vaughan, D. E., Kirshenbaum, J., and Loscalzo, J.: Streptokinase-induced, antibody-mediated platelet aggregation: A potential cause of clot propagation in vitro. J. Am. Coll. Cardiol. *11*:1343, 1988.

153. Hussain, S. S., Gurewich, V., and Lipinski, B.: Purification and partial characterization of a single chain high molecular weight form of urokinase from human urine. Arch. Biochem. Biophys. *220*:31, 1983.

154. Gurewich, V., Pannell, R., Louie, S., et al.: Effective and fibrin-specific clot lysis by a zymogen precursor form of urokinase (pro-urokinase). J. Clin. Invest. *73*:1731, 1984.

155. Rijken, D. C., and Collen, D. C.: Purification and characterization of the plasminogen activator secreted by human melanoma cells in culture. J. Biol. Chem. *257*:7035, 1981.

156. Loscalzo, J.: A structural and kinetic comparison of recombinant human single-chain and two-chain tissue plasminogen activator. J. Clin. Invest. *82*:1391, 1988.

157. vanZonnenveld, A. J., Veerman, H., and Pannekoek, H.: Autonomous functions of structural domains on human tissue-type plasminogen activator. Proc. Natl. Acad Sci. U.S.A. *83*:4670, 1986.

158. Neuhaus, K. L., Feuerer, W., Jeep-Tebbe, S., et al.: Improved thrombolysis with a modified dose regimen of recombinant tissue-type plasminogen activator. J. Am. Coll. Cardiol. *14*:1566, 1989.

159. Goldhaber, S. Z., Vaughan, D. E., Markis, J. E., et al.: Acute pulmonary embolism treated with tissue plasminogen activator. Lancet *2*:886, 1986.

160. Goldhaber, S. Z., Meyerowitz, M. F., Green, D., et al.: Randomized controlled trial of tissue plasminogen activator in proximal deep venous thrombosis. Am. J. Med. *88*:235, 1990.

161. Graor, R. A., Risius, B., Young, J. R., et al.: Peripheral artery and bypass graft thrombolysis with recombinant tissue-type plasminogen activator. J. Vasc. Surg. *3*:115, 1986.

162. DelZoppo, G. J.: Investigational use of t-PA in acute stroke. Ann. Emerg. Med. *17*:1196, 1988.

163. Garabedian, H. D., Gold, H. K., Leinbach, R. C., et al.: Comparative properties of two clinical preparations of recombinant human tissue-type plasminogen activator in patients with acute myocardial infarction. J. Am. Coll. Cardiol. *9*:599, 1987.

164. Jang, I. K., van Haecke, J., and de Geest, H.: Coronary thrombolysis with recombinant tissue-type plasminogen activator: Patency rate and regional wall motion after three months. J. Am. Coll. Cardiol. *8*:15, 1986.

165. The Urokinase Pulmonary Embolism Trial: A national cooperative study. Circulation *47*:II-1, 1973.

166. Sharma, G.V.R.K., and Sasahara, A. A.: Long-term benefits of treatment of pulmonary embolism with thrombolytic therapy. J. Am. Coll. Cardiol. (in press).

167. Loscalzo, J.: Shortcomings of thrombolytic therapy. J. Myocard. Isch. *2*:48, 1990.

Pregnancy and Cardiovascular Disease

by URI ELKAYAM, M.D.

CARDIOVASCULAR PHYSIOLOGY DURING PREGNANCY AND THE PUERPERIUM

Pregnancy and the peripartum period are associated with substantial cardiocirculatory changes. In the woman with heart disease, these changes can lead to rapid clinical deterioration and result in greater morbidity and possibly death.[1] Therefore, the management of these disorders in the pregnant patient requires an understanding of cardiovascular physiology during gestation, labor, delivery, and the puerperium. Hemodynamic changes occurring during pregnancy are summarized in Table 59–1.

BLOOD VOLUME. Blood volume increases substantially during pregnancy, starting as early as the sixth week of gestation and rising rapidly until midpregnancy, when the volume continues to rise, but at a much slower rate.[1a] Although the degree of volume expansion varies considerably in the individual patient (20 to 100 per cent), the augmentation averages 50 per cent of the volume in the nonpregnant state.[2] This increase is reported to correlate with fetal weight, placental mass, weight of the products of conception, neonatal weight, and maternal weight. A higher increment in blood volume is reported in multigravidas and in women with multiple pregnancies.[1]

Because the increase in blood volume is more rapid than the increase in red blood cell mass (Fig. 59–1), hemoglobin concentration falls during pregnancy, causing the "physiological anemia of pregnancy."[3] Hematocrit and hemoglobin levels are frequently as low as 33 to 38 per cent and 11 to 12 gm/100 ml, respectively.[1] Changes in blood volume during pregnancy may be attributable to estrogen-mediated stimulation of renin,[4] which then promotes aldosterone secretion and hypervolemia as a result of sodium and water retention.[3,5] (Fig. 59–2). Chorionic somatomammotropin, a hormone-like substance in the placenta, may also be a factor.[3]

CARDIAC OUTPUT, STROKE VOLUME, AND HEART RATE. Augmentation of blood volume alters stroke volume and cardiac output (Table 59–1). Cardiac output during pregnancy is estimated to exceed the output during the nonpregnant state by 30 to 50 per cent.[1,3,6] It begins to rise around the fifth week and peaks between the middle of the second and the third trimesters. After that time, cardiac output seems to be maintained at the same level. Changes in body position can induce substantial changes in cardiac output with levels rising in the lateral position and declining in the supine position, owing to caval compression by the gravid uterus and thus decreased venous return to the heart. The increase in cardiac output early in pregnancy can be attributed predominantly to the augmentation in stroke volume; during the third trimester, the increase is largely due to an accelerated heart rate,

while stroke volume declines toward prepregnancy values as a result of caval compression.

Heart rate also increases, peaking during the third trimester. The average rise in heart rate is 10 to 20 beats per minute.[6] Although the rate may on occasion be markedly faster, it may decrease slightly in the lateral position compared with the supine position.[7]

BLOOD PRESSURE AND SYSTEMIC VASCULAR RESISTANCE. Systemic arterial pressure begins to fall during the first trimester, reaches a nadir in midpregnancy, and returns toward pregestational levels before term.[1] Since the fall in diastolic blood pressure is substantially greater than the fall in systolic pressure, the pulse pressure widens.[1,8] The reduction in blood pressure results from a decline in systemic vascular resistance due to vasodilation, probably mediated by gestational hormonal activity,[9] increased levels of circulating prostaglandins,[10] increased heat production by the developing fetus, and the creation of low-resistance circulation in the pregnant uterus.[11] A phenomenon unique to pregnancy and described as the supine hypotensive syndrome of pregnancy or the uterocaval syndrome presents with significant decreases in heart rate and blood pressure and occurs in up to 11 per cent of pregnant women.[1–7] These hemodynamic changes are associated with weakness, lightheadedness, nausea, dizziness, and even syncope and are explained by acute occlusion of the inferior vena cava by the enlarged uterus. When the

TABLE 59–1 HEMODYNAMIC CHANGES DURING NORMAL PREGNANCY

PARAMETER	1ST TRIMESTER	2ND TRIMESTER	3RD TRIMESTER
Blood volume	↑	↑↑	↑↑↑
Cardiac output	↑	↑↑ to ↑↑↑	↑↑↑ to ↑↑
Stroke volume	↑	↑↑↑	↑, ↔, or ↓
Heart rate	↑	↑↑	↑↑↑
Systolic blood pressure	↔	↓	↔
Diastolic blood pressure	↓	↓↓	↓
Pulse pressure	↑	↑↑	↔
Systemic vascular resistance	↓	↓↓↓	↓↓

↔ = no change compared to nonpregnant level; ↑ = small increase; ↑↑ = moderate increase; ↑↑↑ = large increase; ↓ = small decrease; ↓↓ = moderate decrease; ↓↓↓ = large decrease

Modified from Elkayam, U., and Gleicher, N.: Hemodynamics and cardiac function during normal pregnancy and the puerperium. In Elkayam, U., and Gleicher, N. (eds.): Cardiac Problems in Pregnancy: Diagnosis and Management of Maternal and Fetal Disease. 2nd ed. New York, Alan R. Liss, Inc., 1990, p. 5.

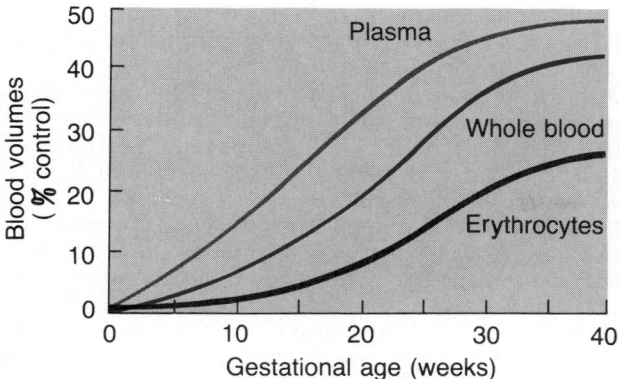

FIGURE 59–1. Alterations in plasma volume, blood volume, and erythrocyte mass during pregnancy. Predominance of increase in plasma volume results in the "physiological anemia of pregnancy." (From Longo, L. O.: Maternal blood volume and cardiac output during pregnancy: A hypothesis of endocrinologic control. Am. J. Physiol. 245:R720, 1983.)

supine position is abandoned, these hemodynamic effects and symptoms usually are promptly relieved.

HEMODYNAMIC CHANGES DURING LABOR AND DELIVERY. Anxiety, pain, and uterine contractions all alter hemodynamics substantially during labor and delivery. Cardiac output increases by up to 50 per cent during contractions, mainly owing to changes in stroke volume,[12] and total cardiac output is higher in the lateral position than in the supine position.[13] The effect of uterine contractions on the heart rate varies[12] and may be influenced by the woman's position during labor and the form of sedation used. Both systolic and diastolic blood pressures increase markedly during contractions, with greater augmentation during the second stage.[1,12]

Hemodynamic changes during labor are associated with a threefold increase in oxygen consumption and are greatly influenced by the form of anesthesia or analgesia used.[1,14,15] In general, reducing the pain and apprehension associated with local and caudal anesthesia will limit the rise in cardiac output; however, these forms of anesthesia will not prevent the increase in cardiac output related to uterine contractions.

HEMODYNAMIC EFFECTS OF CESAREAN SECTION. To avoid the hemodynamic changes associated with vaginal delivery, cesarean section is frequently recommended for women with cardiovascular disease. However, this form of delivery can also be associated with considerable hemodynamic fluctuation related largely to intubation, the form of anesthesia, the anesthetic and analgesic agent(s), the extent of blood loss during the procedure, abdominal surgery, the relief of caval compression, extubation, and postoperative awakening.[14,15]

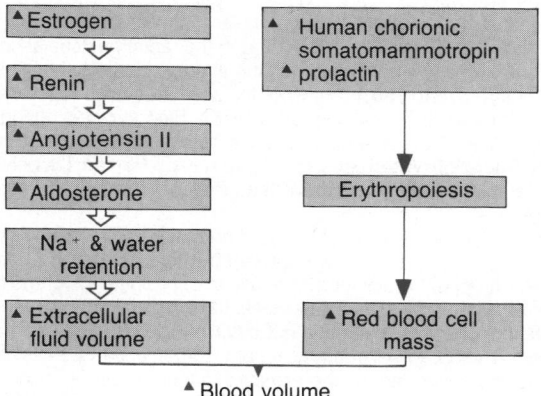

FIGURE 59–2. Potential mechanisms of hypervolemia of pregnancy. (From Elkayam, U., and Gleicher, N.: Hemodynamics and cardiac function during normal pregnancy and the puerperium. In Elkayam, U., and Gleicher, N. [eds.]: Cardiac Problems in Pregnancy: Diagnosis and Management of Maternal and Fetal Disease. 2nd ed. New York, Alan R. Liss, Inc., 1990, p. 5.)

HEMODYNAMIC CHANGES POST PARTUM. Clinical status often deteriorates in the immediate postpartum period when venous return increases after the fetus is removed and caval compression has been relieved.[1] In addition, blood shifting from the contracting, emptied uterus into the systemic circulation (autotransfusion) increases the preload. This change in effective blood volume occurs despite blood loss associated with delivery and leads to a substantial rise in stroke volume and cardiac output immediately after delivery. Within the first hour, however, the reduction in heart rate decreases cardiac output, which falls to prepregnancy levels 24 hours post partum as stroke volume normalizes.[12]

HEMODYNAMIC RESPONSE TO EXERCISE. Exercise-mediated increases in cardiac output are limited during gestation; in the third trimester output during exercise may be more than 20 per cent lower than it is in nonpregnant women.[16] This attenuated rise in cardiac output is due to the lower responses of heart rate and stroke volume; the latter is probably the result of a reduction in venous return during pregnancy.[17] In normal women during the third trimester, uterine blood flow is reduced 25 per cent during mild exercise.[18] Such reductions may be associated with fetal hypoxia, manifested by brief episodes of fetal bradycardia.[18,19] Strenuous physical activity may be associated with fetal compromise and is therefore not recommended during pregnancy.[18]

CARDIAC EVALUATION DURING PREGNANCY

The evaluation of cardiac disease in pregnancy may be complicated by the normal anatomical and functional changes of the cardiovascular system during gestation. Such changes may result in signs and symptoms that can either simulate or obscure heart disease.[20] In addition, the diagnostic approach to cardiac disease in pregnancy is influenced by the potential risk to the fetus posed by certain diagnostic methods.

HISTORY AND PHYSICAL EXAMINATION
(Table 59–2)

Normal pregnancy is often accompanied by symptoms of fatigue, decreased exercise capacity, dyspnea, lightheadedness, and, rarely, syncope.[20] Respirations are often shallow and rapid and may be erroneously interpreted as dyspnea. In addition, distention of the jugular veins due to increased blood volume and the leg edema often observed in late pregnancy could lead to an inappropriate diagnosis of heart failure or overestimation of its severity. Systemic arterial pulses are full and collapsing and are similar to those palpated in patients with aortic regurgitation or hyperthyroidism. A left ventricular impulse is easily detected in most women in late pregnancy; usually it is hyperactive, brisk, and unsustained and may be displaced to the left. The quality of the impulse may simulate a volume overload state such as that seen in aortic or mitral valve regurgitation. The pulmonary trunk, right ventricle, and pulmonic valve closure are often palpable, and this group of findings may lead to the misdiagnosis of pulmonary hypertension.

CARDIAC AUSCULTATION. Especially after the first trimester, auscultation often reveals an increased first heart sound (S_1) with exaggerated splitting[21] that may be misinterpreted as S_4 or as a systolic click. The physiological increase in the amplitude of the second element of S_1 during inspiration should help differentiate it from an abnormal auscultatory event. S_2 is often increased in late pregnancy and may exhibit expiratory splitting when the patient is examined in the lateral position. These changes in S_2 may be interpreted as signs of pulmonary hypertension (loud S_2) or atrial septal defect (fixed splitting of S_2). Although S_3 and S_4 have been reported to be extremely frequent during gestation,[21] in the author's experience, auscultation of these sounds is actually uncommon in normal pregnancy, and their presence warrants further investigation to detect possible underlying disease.

TABLE 59-2 CARDIAC SYMPTOMS AND FINDINGS DURING NORMAL PREGNANCY

SYMPTOMS
Decreased exercise capacity
Tiredness
Dyspnea
Orthopnea
Lightheadedness
Syncope

PHYSICAL FINDINGS
Inspection
  Hyperventilation
  Peripheral edema
  Distended neck veins with prominent A and V waves and
    brisk x and y descents
  Capillary pulsation
Precordial palpation
  Brisk, diffuse, and displaced left ventricular impulse
  Palpable right ventricular impulse
  Palpable pulmonary trunk impulse
Auscultation
  Pulmonary basilar rales
  Increased S₁ with exaggerated splitting
  Persistent splitting of S₂
  Early and midsystolic ejection-type murmurs at the lower
    left sternal edge and/or over the pulmonary area
  Continuous murmurs (cervical venous hum, mammary
    souffle)
  Diastolic murmurs

ELECTROCARDIOGRAM
QRS-axis deviation
ST-segment and T-wave changes
Small Q wave and inverted P wave in lead III (abolished by
  inspiration)
Increased R-wave amplitude in lead V₂
Frequent sinus tachycardia
Increased incidence of arrhythmias

CHEST X-RAY
Straightening of the left upper cardiac border
Horizontal position of the heart
Increased lung marking
Small pleural effusion early post partum

ECHO-DOPPLER
Increased left and right ventricular dimensions
Unchanged or slightly improved left ventricular systolic func-
  tion
Enlargement of the ventricular dimensions
Mild increase in left and right atrial size
Small pericardial effusion
Increased diameter of tricuspid annulus
Functional tricuspid and pulmonary insufficiency

Modified from Elkayam, U., and Gleicher, N.: Changes in cardiac findings during normal pregnancy. In Elkayam, U., and Gleicher, N. (eds.): Cardiac Problems in Pregnancy: Diagnosis and Management of Maternal and Fetal Disease. 2nd ed. New York, Alan R. Liss, Inc., 1990, p. 31.

Innocent Systolic Murmurs. These can be heard in most pregnant women[20,21] and are the result of the hyperkinetic circulation of pregnancy. They are heard best at the lower left sternal edge and over the pulmonic area radiating to the suprasternal notch and to the left and, at times, also to the right side of the neck. The murmurs often sound like those associated with atrial septal defect or stenosis of one of the semilunar valves. Two benign continuous murmurs that can be heard frequently during gestation are the cervical venous hum and the mammary souffle. The venous hum is usually heard maximally over the right supraclavicular fossa but can radiate to the contralateral area and sometimes to the area below the clavicle.[22] The mammary souffle, which is heard mostly over the breast late in gestation or in the lactating woman post partum, is caused by increased flow in the mammary vessels and can be either systolic or continuous. Characteristically, the murmur decreases or vanishes when pressure is applied to the stethoscope or when the patient moves into the upright position.[23] The continuous murmurs may be incorrectly attributed to patent ductus arteriosus or arteriovenous fistulas. In addition, these murmurs can be misinterpreted as systolic and/or diastolic murmurs, leading to erroneous diagnosis.

A soft, medium- to high-pitched diastolic murmur has been reported in normal pregnant women.[21] However, in the author's experience, such a finding is infrequent in the healthy pregnant woman and therefore requires a careful diagnostic work-up to rule out organic disease.

Increases in blood volume and flow across the various cardiac valves may augment systolic murmurs of aortic or pulmonic stenosis and the diastolic murmur of mitral stenosis. In contrast, the murmurs associated with mitral or aortic regurgitation may decrease in intensity secondary to a reduction in systemic vascular resistance during pregnancy.[24] The physiological increase in blood volume with gestation may also affect auscultatory findings in other volume-dependent abnormalities, such as mitral valve prolapse and obstructive hypertrophic cardiomyopathy; the change in volume may abolish the systolic click and murmur commonly heard in patients with mitral valve prolapse[25] and may decrease the systolic murmur typical of hypertrophic cardiomyopathy.[26,27]

FUNCTIONAL CLASSIFICATION

Functional classification, as recommended by the New York Heart Association, attempts to define a cardiac patient's status according to symptoms at different levels of activity.[28] Traditionally, this classification has also been used to assess the severity of cardiac disease and prognosis during pregnancy.[29] In general, pregnancy is considered safe for cardiac patients in Classes I and II (prior to pregnancy). For Class III patients, special attention during pregnancy and early admission before delivery are recommended. Pregnancy is generally contraindicated for patients in Class IV. Although the functional classification has been widely accepted, it is important to note that this method (which relies on signs and subjective symptoms) may be inaccurate and misleading owing to the major anatomical and functional changes in the cardiovascular system that take place during pregnancy. It is therefore imperative to use additional diagnostic tools to obtain objective and reliable information about cardiac status.

LABORATORY EXAMINATIONS

ELECTROCARDIOGRAPHY (Table 59-2). In normal pregnancy, the QRS axis shifts to either the left or the right.[20] Transient ST-segment depressions and T-wave changes are common. A small Q wave and an inverted P wave in lead III that vary with respiration[20] as well as a greater R-wave amplitude in lead V₂ are often present.[30] The pregnant woman's increased susceptibility to arrhythmias[31] can also be apparent in the frequent finding of sinus tachycardia and atrial and/or ventricular premature beats. Arrhythmias with a high incidence during labor and delivery include atrial and ventricular premature beats, sinus arrhythmia, sinus tachycardia, sinus bradycardia, wandering atrial pacemaker, sinus arrest with nodal escape rhythm, and supraventricular tachycardia.[32]

CHEST X-RAY (Table 59-2). Although the radiation dose associated with a routine chest x-ray is minimal (the average dose to the skin in the primary beam is 70 to 150 mrad, while the estimated dose to the uterus is 0.2 to 43.0 mrad),[33,34] this diagnostic test is best avoided during pregnancy because of the potential for adverse biological effects from any amount of radiation. When chest radiography is performed, the pelvic area should be shielded by a protective lead material from accidental direct exposure.

Since changes seen on chest x-rays in normal pregnancy may simulate cardiac disease, they should be interpreted with caution.[20,35] Straightening of the left upper cardiac border because of prominence of the pulmonary conus is often seen and may mimic the left atrial enlargement commonly associated with rheumatic mitral valve disease. The heart seems enlarged on radiography in many pregnant women because of its horizontal positioning secondary to the elevated diaphragm. In addition, an increase in lung markings may simulate the flow redistribution seen with increased pulmonary venous pressure due to left ventricular failure or mitral valve disease. Pleural effusion early post partum has been a frequent finding[36,37]; the effusion is usually small and resorbs 1 to 2 weeks after delivery.

DOPPLER ECHOCARDIOGRAPHY (Table 59-2). Despite concern regarding the use of ultrasound during pregnancy, no hazard has been

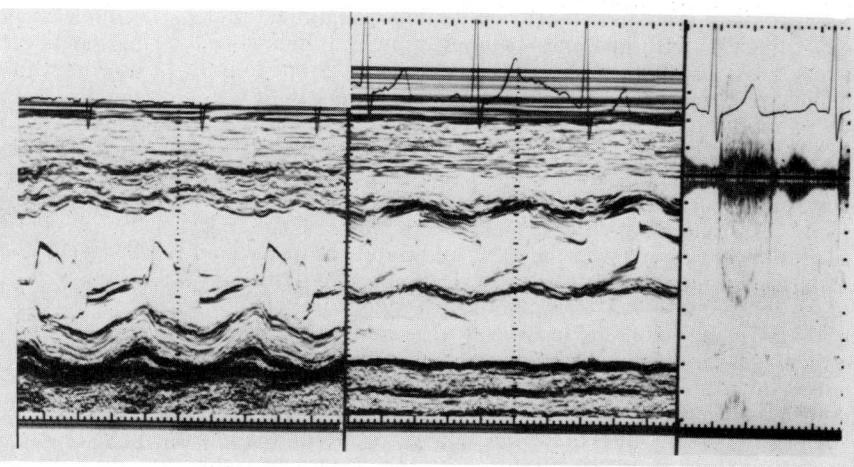

FIGURE 59–3. M-mode echocardiogram at the level of the mitral valve *(left panel)* and the aortic valve *(middle panel)* and Doppler aortic blood flow study *(right panel)* in a 27-year-old woman with congenital bicuspid valve and aortic stenosis at 32 weeks' gestation. The patient had symptoms of fatigue and shortness of breath. Peak instantaneous pressure gradient across the aortic valve by the Doppler technique was 81 mm Hg. The patient had successful pregnancy, labor, and delivery of a normal baby. Small pericardial effusion seen on the left is a common benign finding in pregnancy.

identified in humans, so that both maternal and fetal echocardiography may be considered safe.[38] Normal gestational changes in the cardiovascular system are reflected echocardiographically and should be taken into consideration. When the patient is examined in the left lateral position, an increase in left and right ventricular end-diastolic dimensions is to be expected as a result of volume overload.[39,40] These changes progress with the pregnancy but return to baseline dimensions post partum. Left ventricular systolic dimension and function are either unchanged or increased during pregnancy, and the left and right atria may increase slightly in size.

Pericardial effusion, usually minimal, has been noted in 40 per cent of normal pregnant women late in pregnancy (Fig. 59–3).[41,42] Recent studies have demonstrated mild tricuspid and pulmonary regurgitation, mainly near term,[40,43] that seem related to right-sided chamber enlargement and dilatation of the valve annulus. These findings do not appear to be important clinically but need to be considered when one is interpreting Doppler echocardiograms obtained during pregnancy.

STRESS TESTING. An exercise test using bicycle ergometry or a treadmill may be carried out during pregnancy to help establish the diagnosis of ischemic heart disease and to assess functional capacity and cardiac reserve. The safety of such testing in pregnancy has not been fully established. Since fetal bradycardia has been reported with maximal but not with submaximal exercise,[44] a low-level exercise protocol with fetal monitoring is recommended when stress testing is indicated.[45]

PULMONARY ARTERY FLOTATION CATHETERIZATION. Hemodynamic monitoring with the aid of a pulmonary artery catheter can be of great help in managing patients at high risk during pregnancy, labor, delivery, and the postpartum period. The ability to insert and position the flotation catheter under pressure monitoring without the need for fluoroscopy makes it particularly attractive for use during pregnancy.[46] Hemodynamic monitoring can provide useful diagnostic and prognostic information and should be used without hesitation at any time during pregnancy if a noninvasive cardiac work-up does not provide conclusive information.

Hemodynamic monitoring is recommended throughout labor and delivery for any patient with symptomatic cardiac disease during pregnancy or with the potential for deterioration due to valvular, vascular, myocardial, or ischemic heart disease. Since significant circulatory changes that may lead to hemodynamic deterioration occur in the early postpartum period,[1] hemodynamic monitoring should be continued for 24 hours after delivery to assure stability.

CARDIAC CATHETERIZATION. When cardiac decompensation occurs during pregnancy, particularly if cardiac surgery or balloon valvulo-

plasty is being considered, cardiac catheterization may be required. Although this technique provides high-quality images, it is associated with a relatively high dose of radiation. The median dose to the skin is 47 rads per examination with 10 to 15 per cent exposure to an unshielded abdomen and approximately 500 mrad estimated dose to the conceptus, even with an appropriate pelvic shield.[33,34]

The potentially deleterious effect of ionizing radiation is linearly proportional to the absorbed dose and is present at all times after fertilization. The type and likelihood of this effect vary with the stage of fetal development and the dose of radiation. An increase in the incidence of fetal malformation appears to be highly unlikely with doses below 5 rads, even when these are delivered at a time when the induction of any specific type of maldevelopment is critical.[47] In general, radiation exposure during the first week of pregnancy may result in absorption or resorption of the preimplanted blastocyst, whereas the risk of teratogenic effects predominates during the second to sixth weeks of gestation. Developing brain cells can be affected by radiation during the seventh to fifteenth weeks, which may lead to alterations in neurological function or behavior. In addition, irradiation at any time during the entire pregnancy may increase the risk for childhood cancer[48]; this risk seems to be higher with exposure during the first trimester.

Therefore, because of its risk to the fetus, cardiac catheterization during gestation should be performed only if information cannot be obtained by alternative noninvasive methods. The procedure should involve the brachial rather than the femoral approach to minimize radiation to the pelvic and abdominal areas, which should be appropriately shielded, and x-ray exposure should be kept to a minimum. To minimize the use of ionizing radiation, techniques such as contrast[49] and Doppler echocardiography with cardiac catheterization should be combined for a complete evaluation.

RADIONUCLIDE IMAGING. A potential limitation of these techniques during pregnancy is radiation exposure to the fetus. The dose estimated to reach the fetus with the radiopharmaceuticals generally used for cardiac imaging is equal to or less than 800 mrad.[50] However, calculations of the dose to the conceptus are only approximations and can vary from person to person owing to differences in the uptake of radionuclides by maternal organs, metabolism, and placental uptake and transfer. Because of these uncertainties and the potential risk, *use of radionuclide imaging should be avoided if possible during gestation and in particular during the first trimester.* In addition, such imaging should be performed only when the information desired cannot be obtained by other, noninvasive techniques, such as two-dimensional and Doppler echocardiography.

Cardiovascular Diseases and Pregnancy

CONGENITAL HEART DISEASE (CHD)
(See also Chap. 32)

PRECONCEPTION COUNSELING. The management of patients with CHD should begin before conception. An accurate diagnostic and functional evaluation is supplemented by counseling of both the patient and her family regarding potential maternal and fetal risks of pregnancy, expected maternal morbidity, and, when appropriate, long-term survival as well as the risk that the offspring will inherit CHD. In addition, guidance concerning anticoagulation and prophylactic antibiotics, if needed, should be provided.[51]

MATERNAL AND FETAL OUTCOME. Maternal outcome is determined by the nature of the disease, surgical repair, the presence of cyanosis, and functional capacity.[52,53] Whittemore et al.[53,54] reported no maternal deaths in 237 women with CHD involving 488 pregnancies. Congestive heart failure, arrhythmias, and hypertension are commonly seen in patients with impaired functional status and with cyanosis.[52,53] Other reported complications in patients with CHD during pregnancy include angina and infective endocarditis.

Maternal functional capacity and the presence of cyanosis also determine fetal outcome. Fetal wastage was reported in 45 per cent of cyanotic mothers, compared with 20 per cent of acyanotic mothers with CHD.[53] Low birth weight for gestational age and prematurity are common in cyanotic mothers and correlate with maternal hemoglobin and hematocrit levels.[54] Risk of substantial cardiac and noncardiac congenital defects is increased for the offspring of mothers with CHD with a reported incidence of CHD of about 10 per cent (3.4 to 16.1 per cent).[53-55] In addition, there are a greater number of noncardiac abnormalities as well as mental and physical impairments in children born to mothers with CHD.[53]

LABOR AND DELIVERY. Cesarean section is not indicated in most patients with CHD[53-55] and should be performed primarily for obstetrical reasons or in response to deteriorating maternal status. Oxygen should be given to hypoxemic mothers during labor and delivery, and hemodynamic as well as blood gas monitoring is recommended in patients with impaired functional capacity, cardiac dysfunction, pulmonary hypertension, and cyanotic malformations.[46]

ANTIBIOTIC PROPHYLAXIS. Official recommendations for antibiotic prophylaxis proposed by the American Heart Association (p. 1806) do not include patients with CHD who are undergoing uncomplicated vaginal delivery unless they have a prosthetic heart valve or a surgically constructed systemic-to-pulmonary shunt.[56] Despite these recommendations, the use of antibiotic prophylaxis is not uncommon in many hospitals for patients with CHD, with the exception of those with an isolated secundum type of atrial septal defect and those who underwent ligation and division of a patent ductus arteriosus more than 6 months earlier. The risk for endocarditis may be increased after manual removal of the placenta, so that antibiotic prophylaxis is recommended for this procedure in patients with CHD.[55]

Atrial Septal Defect (ASD) (see also p. 977)

This common type of maternal CHD is frequently discovered during pregnancy when the murmur is first elicited. This condition is usually well tolerated in pregnancy, even among patients with large left-to-right shunts. Pulmonary hypertension rarely occurs until the fourth decade of life, and the same is true for atrial arrhythmias, which are uncommon before age 40. Because endocarditis is rare, antibiotic prophylaxis is not indicated in patients with secundum-type ASD. Recommendations concerning pregnancy in such patients should be made on an individual basis, account being taken of the functional status and the level of pulmonary artery pressure.

Ventricular Septal Defect (VSD) (see also p. 971)

Women with isolated VSD usually tolerate pregnancy well, although congestive heart failure and arrhythmias have been reported in patients with uncorrected lesions.[46] The risk posed by pregnancy after closure of an uncomplicated VSD should not differ from that in patients without heart disease. The incidence of CHD was found to be as high as 22 per cent among live-born offspring in one report, with a recurrence of VSD in 50 per cent of this group.[53] Marked reduction in blood pressure during or after delivery as a result of blood loss or anesthesia may lead to shunt reversal in patients with pulmonary hypertension. The use of vasopressors and volume replacement to stabilize blood pressure promptly should prevent further complications.

Patent Ductus Arteriosus (PDA) (see also p. 977)

This common congenital defect occurs predominantly in women (2:1 female/male ratio). With early diagnosis and surgical correction in early childhood, a patent ductus has become a rare finding in pregnancy.[57] Although maternal outcome in patients with PDA is usually favorable,[58] some patients deteriorate clinically because of congestive heart failure.[55] Although early reports cited a maternal mortality rate of approximately 5 per cent, more recent experience has revealed no maternal deaths among a large number of patients with PDA.[52,53,57] The occasional patient with heart failure should be treated with bed rest, diuretics, and digitalis. Al-

though surgical intervention or catheter-induced closure during pregnancy may be successful,[58] these procedures should be reserved for patients with heart failure unresponsive to medical therapy. In the early postpartum period, shunt reversal may occur in women with pulmonary hypertension who develop systemic hypotension, so that any decrease in systemic blood pressure should be immediately corrected by means of volume replacement or vasopressor agents.

Congenital Aortic Valve Disease (see also p. 978)

A bicuspid aortic valve is the most common type of CHD, occurring in 1 per cent to 2 per cent of the population. This defect may lead to significant aortic stenosis in women of childbearing age. Obstruction of left ventricular outflow can also result from unicuspid or tricuspid valves or supravalvular and subvalvular obstruction. Aortic stenosis, especially if mild, can easily be missed on physical examination, since its murmur may be attributed to the flow-related systolic murmur commonly heard in the normal pregnant woman. The presence of a sustained left ventricular impulse, aortic ejection sound, and S_4 should raise the level of suspicion.

Although data concerning pregnancy in women with surgically uncorrected aortic stenosis are limited, they indicate the potential for clinical deterioration, due to the development of heart failure, hypertension, and angina, and even for death during pregnancy and the peripartum period.[52,53,59] Whittemore et al.[53] reported a high incidence (20 per cent) of cardiac defects in live-born infants of mothers with left heart obstruction.

The author's experience with several patients with moderate to severe aortic stenosis indicates that with early diagnosis and appropriate care, including hemodynamic monitoring during labor and delivery and appropriate anesthesia, the outcome will be favorable in most cases (Fig. 59-3).[55] Patients with severe aortic stenosis (aortic valve area $< 1.0\ cm^2$) should be advised against pregnancy or should agree to an early abortion so that the valve can be corrected surgically. When clinical deterioration after the 22nd week of gestation does not respond to medical therapy, surgical intervention is indicated.

Percutaneous balloon valvuloplasty (p. 1377) has been performed successfully in pregnant women with aortic stenosis.[60] Although this procedure obviates the general anesthesia and cardiopulmonary bypass required for surgery, it is associated with significant and often unpredictable radiation exposure and hemodynamic fluctuations that may lead to immediate and late fetal complications.[33,34,37] In addition, significant restenosis may occur within 6 months of the procedure. For all of these reasons, percutaneous balloon valvuloplasty should be considered only in patients with severe symptoms not manageable with drug therapy and should be performed as late as possible during gestation.

Coarctation of the Aorta (see also p. 967)

Uncorrected coarctation of the aorta is found less commonly during pregnancy, since surgical correction is usually performed prior to the childbearing age.[57] In uncomplicated coarctation, pregnancy is usually safe for the mother; however, fetal development may be impaired since uteroplacental blood flow is decreased owing to the aortic obstruction. In a review of reports published since 1958, Metcalfe et al.[58] found 13 cases of maternal death among 230 women with aortic coarctation involving 565 pregnancies. Whittemore et al.[53] found no deaths, but reported complications such as hypertension, congestive heart failure, and angina. Aortic dissection and rupture have also been associated with coarctation of the aorta during pregnancy.[61] In addition, a higher incidence of CHD has been shown in infants of mothers with surgically uncorrected coarctation compared with mothers whose coarctation had been corrected.[53] For all of these reasons, it seems advisable to correct aortic coarctation prior to pregnancy.

Treatment to reduce the incidence of aortic rupture and

cerebral aneurysms during pregnancy consists of limiting physical activity and controlling blood pressure. Excessive reduction of blood pressure, however, may compromise uteroplacental blood flow and should be avoided. Surgical correction of coarctation has been performed successfully during pregnancy[62] and may be indicated in patients with uncontrollable, severely elevated systolic blood pressure or severe heart failure refractory to medical therapy. Contrary to earlier opinion, most pregnancy-related aortic ruptures and dissections in patients with coarctation of the aorta occur prior to labor and delivery.[62]

Pulmonic Stenosis (see also p. 1059)

Over 175 pregnancies in women with pulmonic stenosis have been reported since 1960.[55,57] Although complications such as congestive heart failure have been described, recent reports suggest that the incidence of heart failure is low, and most pregnant women seem to tolerate the additional hemodynamic load.[51,63] In the rare instance of persistent heart failure despite appropriate drug therapy, surgical valvotomy should be considered. Percutaneous balloon valvuloplasty of the pulmonic valve during pregnancy has not been reported. Although this procedure may be attractive since it obviates surgery, it is not free of side effects and may be associated with considerable radiation exposure and acute hemodynamic changes, possibly harming the fetus.

Tetralogy of Fallot (see also p. 971)

Tetralogy of Fallot is the most common type of cyanotic CHD in adults. As a result of palliative or definitive surgical repair in most children with this defect, more patients are reaching childbearing age.[64]

Hemodynamic changes associated with pregnancy may become severe and cause clinical deterioration in women with tetralogy of Fallot. Increases in blood volume and venous return to the right atrium raise right ventricular pressure, and the fall in peripheral vascular resistance can cause or exacerbate a right-to-left shunt and cyanosis.

Maternal hematocrit above 60 per cent, arterial oxygen saturation below 80 per cent, right ventricular hypertension, and syncopal episodes are poor prognostic signs. Close monitoring of hemodynamic parameters and blood gases during labor and delivery is recommended for cyanotic or symptomatic patients. Palliative or corrective surgery will reduce the risks posed by pregnancy. Although reports of pregnancies in 37 women with corrected tetralogy of Fallot described no maternal deaths,[53] worsening of the clinical condition necessitating interruption of the pregnancy is not uncommon. Cardiac defects were reported by Whittemore in 15 and 17 per cent of infants born, respectively, to cyanotic and acyanotic mothers with tetralogy of Fallot.[53] In contrast, an incidence of only 3 per cent has been reported by other authors.[58]

Since maternal and fetal outcomes seem to be markedly improved in women whose defects have been surgically repaired, this procedure should be performed prior to conception. Patients who have undergone only palliative procedures or who have significant residual defects after repair are still at higher risk during pregnancy. Although mortality associated with complete repair is slightly increased in older patients who have previously undergone a palliative procedure,[64,65] surgical repair is recommended *prior* to pregnancy in patients in the absence of contraindications. Since revision of an incompletely repaired defect is recommended in patients with residual VSD when the pulmonary/systemic flow ratio is greater than 1.5:1, in those with right ventricular outflow obstruction (right ventricular systolic pressure > 60 mm Hg), and in those with right ventricular failure due to pulmonic regurgitation,[64] such revision should be performed prior to conception in a woman who plans to conceive.

Inhalation analgesia and paracervical or pudendal block have been recommended for labor and vaginal delivery.[66] Epidural block could result in systemic hypotension and shunt

reversal and should therefore be used with great care. To minimize potential hemodynamic problems, a segmental epidural block for the first stage of labor with pudendal or caudal block for the second stage has been recommended along with opiates to decrease the concentration of anesthetics injected epidurally.

EBSTEIN'S ANOMALY (see also p. 970). Most patients with Ebstein's anomaly survive to childbearing age. Long-term prognosis depends on the severity of tricuspid regurgitation, the presence of right ventricular failure, cyanosis due to shunting from right to left through a patent foramen ovale, and the performance and adequacy of surgical intervention. Several successful pregnancies have been reported in patients with Ebstein's anomaly.[55] At the same time, pregnancy may be complicated by right ventricular failure, infective endocarditis, and paradoxical embolism. The incidence of maternal and fetal complications is increased among cyanotic patients.[53,54] The approach to labor and delivery in symptomatic or cyanotic patients with Ebstein's anomaly includes antibiotic prophylaxis, hemodynamic monitoring, oxygen administration, and efforts to prevent a drop in systemic blood pressure in response to peripheral vasodilation or blood loss.

COMPLEX CYANOTIC CHD. The more widespread use of palliative and corrective surgical procedures for complex cyanotic congenital cardiac anomalies has allowed more of these women to reach childbearing age.[55] Although successful pregnancies have been reported in patients with tricuspid atresia,[67] corrected and uncorrected transposition of the great vessels,[68,69] truncus arteriosus,[55] and a single ventricle,[68,70] pregnancy is risky in these patients and cannot be recommended. A high incidence of hemodynamic and functional deterioration with increased maternal morbidity and even mortality may occur.[52,53,71,72] In addition, a high incidence of fetal wastage, premature deliveries, and both cardiac and noncardiac congenital malformations should be anticipated, as well as small-for-gestational-age newborns.[52,53,70,72]

Patients should be informed prior to conception about expected maternal and fetal complications. When the potential mother is believed to be at risk, pregnancy should be discouraged prior to conception or should be interrupted early if it has already begun. If the patient wishes to continue the pregnancy, the hemodynamic load should be reduced by restricting physical activity, and the patient should be closely observed for early detection and management of heart failure and/or arrhythmias. Antibiotic prophylaxis and oxygen therapy are recommended for delivery, and hemodynamic and blood gas monitoring are essential to assure stability. Although vaginal delivery appears to be tolerated by most women, attempts should be made to shorten the second stage by the use of forceps or vacuum extraction.

In providing anesthesia or analgesia for labor and vaginal delivery, the physician should try to avoid increasing the right-to-left shunt. For that reason, regional anesthetic techniques should be avoided; systemic medication, inhalation analgesia, nerve blocks, and intrathecal morphine have been recommended.[66,73]

EISENMENGER'S SYNDROME (see also p. 971). In an extensive review of the literature published in 1979, Gleicher et al.[74] described the outcome of 70 pregnancies among 44 patients with documented Eisenmenger's syndrome and reported a maternal mortality rate of 52 per cent. A more recent review of 24 women with this syndrome revealed a mortality rate of 38 per cent.[55] Recently, more emphasis has been placed on reporting successful rather than unsuccessful pregnancy outcomes in patients with Eisenmenger's syndrome.

Eisenmenger's syndrome is also associated with a poor fetal outcome. Only 26 per cent of all pregnancies reported by Gleicher et al. reached term.[74] In addition, more than 55 per cent of the live-born infants were premature, 30 per cent had intrauterine growth retardation, and perinatal death occurred in 28 per cent.

Because of the high maternal mortality associated with Eisenmenger's syndrome, patients should be advised against pregnancy, and early abortion should be recommended for patients who are already pregnant. Management of a pregnant patient with Eisenmenger's syndrome who decides to proceed to term must include both close medical follow-up to detect deterioration early and restriction of physical activity to minimize the hemodynamic burden. Because of the increased incidence of thromboembolic events—which are often the cause of death in such patients—anticoagulant therapy seems indicated for at least the last 8 to 10 weeks of gestation and for 4 weeks post partum. Since premature delivery is common, these women should be hospitalized if there is any sign of premature uterine activity. For this reason and to assure restriction of activity and close follow-up, early elective hospitalization is recommended. Spontaneous labor is preferred to induction and should lower the chance of prematurity or the need for cesarean section. Hemodynamic, electrocardiographic, and blood gas monitoring are essential during labor and delivery to ensure the early detection and correction of problems; high concentrations of oxygen may be helpful.[75] Most patients in stable condition will tolerate vaginal delivery; however, an attempt should be made to shorten the second stage of labor by the use of forceps or vacuum extraction.

Since epidural anesthesia may lead to peripheral vasodilation and increased shunting from right to left, local anesthetics should be titrated carefully to achieve the epidural block.[66] Delivery has been successful with lumbar epidural block for the first stage of labor and caudal block for delivery; other authors have preferred the use of systemic medication, inhalation analgesia, and paracervical or pudendal block.[66,76] For cesarean section, general anesthesia with a drug having a minimal negative inotropic effect is recommended.[66,76] In addition, segmental epidural anesthesia has been used successfully for cesarean section in patients with Eisenmenger's syndrome.[66,77]

RHEUMATIC HEART DISEASE

Although the incidence of rheumatic heart disease is declining in the United States,[78] it continues to be prevalent in many parts of the world[79] and still frequently complicates pregnancy.[57]

ACUTE RHEUMATIC FEVER
(See also Chap. 56)

This disease occurs most commonly in children, before puberty, and may recur during pregnancy. Acute rheumatic fever associated with carditis and congestive heart failure may be fatal in the pregnant woman.[80] The incidence of Sydenham's chorea, like acute rheumatic fever itself, has been reported to be increased in pregnancy (chorea gravidarum). Chorea gravidarum has been reported to cause preterm labor and fetal and maternal death. Because of the problems faced by women with recurrent rheumatic fever during pregnancy, it is prudent to continue antibiotic prophylaxis against streptococcal infection in the pregnant patient with a history of this condition.[56] The recommended antibiotic regimen is discussed in detail on p. 1729.

CHRONIC RHEUMATIC VALVULAR DISEASE
(See also Chap. 34)

Significant valve deformities due to rheumatic valvular disease may increase morbidity and even mortality during gestation and the peripartum period. Although patients with chronic rheumatic valvular disease should be managed individually according to the location and severity of the lesion, certain general guidelines apply to the care of all patients. These include rheumatic fever prophylaxis, restriction of physical activity, antibiotic prophylaxis for bacterial endocarditis, and hemodynamic monitoring during labor and delivery.

To reduce the cardiovascular load and prevent hemodynamic and symptomatic worsening, physical activity should be restricted for symptomatic patients. All those with chronic rheumatic heart disease should be treated prophylactically with antibiotics to prevent streptococcal infection and recurrence. Although antibiotic prophylaxis during labor and delivery has not been uniformly recommended,[56] it is commonly used for vaginal and abdominal deliveries.[80]

Hemodynamic monitoring is strongly recommended from the onset of labor to 24 hours post partum in any patient who experiences symptoms of heart failure during pregnancy and for those with severe valvular disease, left ventricular dysfunction, or pulmonary hypertension.[46]

Mitral Valve Disease

MITRAL STENOSIS (see also p. 1007). This condition is The most common rheumatic valvular lesion in pregnancy.[57] The status of patients with mitral stenosis may deteriorate significantly during gestation. Although mitral stenosis is often accompanied by some degree of mitral regurgitation, hemodynamic problems are related predominantly to flow obstruction. The pressure gradient across the narrowed mitral valve may increase greatly as left ventricular diastolic filling

time decreases secondary to the physiological increase in heart rate and the increased cardiac output of pregnancy.[1] Increased left atrial pressure and the arrhythmogenic effect of pregnancy[31] may result in atrial flutter or fibrillation, substantially accelerating the ventricular rate and further elevating left atrial pressure. In addition to the decreased serum colloid osmotic pressure—often a result of peripartum intravenous fluid administration—these changes predispose to pulmonary edema during the peripartum period.

The therapeutic approach to patients with significant mitral stenosis is designed to reduce the heart rate and decrease blood volume. Both heart rate and symptoms can be controlled effectively by restricting physical activity and administering beta-adrenergic receptor blockers. In patients with atrial fibrillation, digoxin may control further the ventricular rate. Blood volume can be decreased through the restriction of salt intake and the use of oral diuretics; the aggressive use of diuretic agents should be avoided to prevent hypovolemia, which may reduce uteroplacental perfusion (p. 1014).

Vaginal delivery can be allowed in most patients with mitral stenosis. In symptomatic patients or those with moderate or severe stenosis (mitral valve area < 1.5 cm^2), hemodynamic monitoring is recommended during labor, delivery, and the puerperium. By inserting a pulmonary artery catheter at the start of labor, one can optimize hemodynamic status by means of intravenous diuretics, digoxin (in case of atrial fibrillation), beta blockers, or nitroglycerin and prevent a rise in left atrial pressure during labor and delivery.[81] With delivery and thus relief of venocaval obstruction due to the gravid uterus, there is an immediate increase in venous return, and one sees a substantial increase in pulmonary artery wedge pressure (Fig. 59–4).[82] For this reason, hemodynamic monitoring should be continued for at least 24 hours post partum.[46]

Epidural anesthesia is the most appropriate form of analgesia in patients with mitral stenosis[66,81,83] and is often associated with a significant fall in pulmonary arterial and left atrial pressures due to systemic vasodilation. By the same mechanism, systemic hypotension may occur and can be prevented by fluid replacement. With this approach, the great majority of patients with mitral stenosis, even if it is severe, can be delivered with few complications.

Mitral Valvuloplasty. Surgical (p. 1016) or percutaneous balloon mitral valvuloplasty (p. 1376) or mitral valve replacement (p. 1027) has been performed in severely symptomatic patients with mitral stenosis during pregnancy.[57,84–86] Becker[86] described 101 cases of closed surgical mitral commissurotomy during pregnancy in which there were no maternal deaths and the fetus survived in 98 of the cases. The same author reported similar favorable results in 23 cases of open

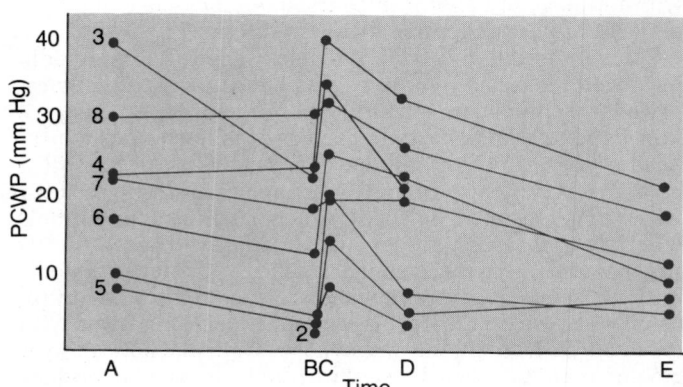

FIGURE 59–4. Intrapartum alterations in pulmonary capillary wedge pressure (PCWP) in eight patients with mitral stenosis. _A_, First-stage labor; _B_, Second-stage labor 15 to 30 minutes before delivery; _C_, 5 to 15 minutes post partum; _D_, 4 to 6 hours post partum; _E_, 18 to 24 hours post partum. (From Clark, S. C., et al.: Labor and delivery in the presence of mitral stenosis: Central hemodynamic observations. Am. J. Obstet. Gynecol. _152_:984, 1985.)

mitral commissurotomy. Mitral valve replacement in 19 cases resulted in a single maternal death due to hepatitis, occurring 7 weeks after surgery; fetal death in four cases; and cerebral palsy in one infant, thought to be due to heparin management. Recently, successful percutaneous mitral balloon valvuloplasty has been reported in two cases during pregnancy and has been recommended for palliation of symptoms.[85,87] Although repair or replacement of the valve may be indicated in some patients with severe mitral stenosis, these procedures are not free of risk and can result in fetal loss (surgery) and irradiation (balloon valvuloplasty). For this reason, they should be recommended only for women who fail to respond to adequate medical therapy.

The author's experience with patients with critical mitral stenosis (mitral valve area < 1.0 cm²) indicates that careful medical therapy, with particular emphasis on lowering the heart rate, should allow successful completion of pregnancy in the great majority without the need for valve correction or replacement. When a surgical procedure seems indicated, closed mitral valvotomy will avoid the fetal complications that may be associated with the use of extracorporeal circulation and is therefore preferable to the open technique.[86,88] However, this procedure should be recommended only in centers where it is performed routinely. Although percutaneous balloon valvuloplasty is an attractive alternative to surgery, it is limited by the high radiation exposure and hemodynamic fluctuations attending this procedure. When valve replacement is indicated, selection of the type of prosthesis should be based on its hemodynamic profile and durability and the need for anticoagulation (p. 1015).

MITRAL REGURGITATION. This lesion is usually well tolerated in pregnancy,[46] presumably because of the unloading resulting from the physiological fall in systemic vascular resistance. In symptomatic patients, drug therapy with diuretics is indicated, and digoxin may be useful in those with impaired left ventricular systolic function. Since hydralazine has been shown to be safe for use during pregnancy,[89] its use should be considered as a means of reducing left ventricular afterload and mitral regurgitation and preventing the hemodynamic worsening associated with isometric exercise during labor.[90]

Aortic Valve Disease

Aortic valve involvement occurs in conjunction with mitral valve disease in approximately 10 per cent of pregnant patients with rheumatic valvular disease.[91]

AORTIC STENOSIS (see also p. 1035). Rheumatic aortic valve stenosis is uncommon in pregnancy. However, a severe form of this deformity presents significant risk to the mother. Reported clinical experience with aortic stenosis is limited, with information based mostly on anecdotal reports. A survey of the literature by Arias and Pineda[59] revealed a maternal mortality rate of 17 per cent and high rates of therapeutic abortion and fetal mortality among 23 patients with aortic stenosis. These data illustrate the potential hazard posed by this lesion in pregnancy. Nevertheless, recent improvements in diagnostic capabilities, hemodynamic monitoring, and fetal monitoring have increased maternal and fetal safety for pregnant women with aortic stenosis.[46] Management of patients with rheumatic aortic stenosis is similar to that for congenital aortic stenosis (p. 1035).

AORTIC REGURGITATION (see also p. 1043). This lesion is more common during pregnancy than is aortic stenosis.[57,80,91] Similar to mitral regurgitation, aortic regurgitation is also tolerated well during pregnancy, probably because systemic vascular resistance is reduced and heart rate and thus diastolic time are increased. In symptomatic patients, diuretics, digoxin, and hydralazine for afterload reduction can be safely used during pregnancy. Since hydralazine has been shown to prevent an increase in pulmonary artery wedge pressure during isometric exercise,[92] it can be administered intravenously in increments of 2.5 to 5.0 mg during labor with the aid of hemodynamic monitoring to prevent the hemody-

namic changes associated with the Valsalva maneuver during labor.

MITRAL VALVE PROLAPSE (MVP) (see also p. 1029). As diagnosed by M-mode echocardiography, MVP has been reported in approximately 15 per cent of women of childbearing age.[93] However, when the diagnosis was based on two-dimensional echocardiographic criteria, the incidence was reported to be only about 2 per cent.[94] In a review of heart disease in pregnancy, MVP was found in only two of 145 pregnant women, and Rayburn et al. reported that MVP was clinically suspected in 1.2 per cent of women examined in prenatal clinics.[95] A combined experience involving 128 pregnant women showed that MVP has no effect on maternal or fetal outcome.[86,97]

Pregnancy has been reported to reduce the incidence of prolapse-related auscultatory and echocardiographic changes that result from an increase in left ventricular end-diastolic volume.[25,95] For the few patients with chest pain or cardiac arrhythmias, the emphasis should be on reassurance and attempts to avoid the use of medications. Beta-adrenergic blocking agents are recommended if symptomatic arrhythmias or chest pain persists, with periodic reassessment of the need to continue drug therapy. Patients with MVP, especially those with a thickened mitral valve and regurgitation, are at increased risk for infective endocarditis. Although antibiotic prophylaxis for uncomplicated vaginal delivery has not been uniformly recommended,[56] the development of bacteremia during vaginal delivery and cesarean section cannot always be predicted,[80] so that some authors have recommended prophylaxis for labor and delivery in patients with MVP accompanied by valve thickening and/or regurgitation.[96]

THE MARFAN SYNDROME
(See also p. 1641)

A review of the literature revealed a high incidence of aortic dissection and death (mostly occurring during the peripartum period) among 32 pregnant patients with the Marfan syndrome. Most of these women had preexisting cardiovascular problems, including aortic dilatation, aortic regurgitation, aortic coarctation, hypertension, cardiomegaly, and patent ductus arteriosus.[98] In addition, the incidence of spontaneous abortion was increased, suggesting their susceptibility to recurrent abortions. In contrast, a retrospective analysis of 105 unselected pregnancies among 26 women with this syndrome revealed only one death from endocarditis in a patient with severe mitral regurgitation.[99] Similarly, no cardiovascular complications were reported among 10 women with this condition and an aortic diameter of less than 45 mm involving 12 term pregnancies.[100] These findings suggest that anecdotal reports in the literature represent a selected group of patients at high risk in which pregnancy-related complications in women with the Marfan syndrome are overrepresented.

The management of pregnant women with the Marfan syndrome should include preconception counseling to discuss potential maternal and fetal risks, including the 50 per cent chance that this syndrome will be inherited.[99] Based on available information, women with significant cardiac involvement, including asymptomatic dilatation of the aorta, should be advised against conception or, if they are already pregnant, to agree to early abortion. In contrast, the risk is significantly lower in patients with no cardiac complications and a normal aortic diameter. Still, a favorable outcome is not guaranteed, and aortic dissection can occur, albeit infrequently, in patients without aortic dilatation.[100] During pregnancy, physical activity should be limited. Beta blockers, which have been shown to reduce the rate of aortic dilatation and the risk of complications in patients with the Marfan syndrome, should be administered.[101]

In women with aortic dilatation or other cardiac complications, abdominal delivery by cesarean section may be preferred to prevent the potential deleterious effect of bearing down.

CARDIOMYOPATHIES

HYPERTROPHIC CARDIOMYOPATHY

(See also p. 1404)

A review of 82 pregnancies among 35 patients with hypertrophic cardiomyopathy (HC) revealed a favorable outcome in most cases; however, the development or worsening of cardiac symptoms was common.[26] Congestive heart failure was first diagnosed or became worse in 21 per cent of patients, and a few patients experienced chest pain, palpitations, dizzy spells, and syncope. Two patients had ventricular arrhythmias, which proved fatal in one.[102] Fetal outcome does not seem to be affected by maternal HC; however, the risk of inheriting this condition may be as high as 50 per cent in familial cases and less in sporadic cases.[26]

Diagnosis of HC may be missed during pregnancy, since the systolic murmurs associated with obstructive HC may be attributed to the innocent heart murmurs frequently heard in pregnancy. The presence of left ventricular hypertrophy, an S_4, a systolic thrill along the lower left sternal border and apex, and a more intense murmur in the upright position or during the strain phase of the Valsalva maneuver warrants further evaluation using echocardiography, the key definitive diagnostic test for HC.[103]

The therapeutic approach to the pregnant patient with HC depends on the presence of symptoms and left ventricular outflow obstruction. No treatment is indicated in the asymptomatic patient without resting or provocable left ventricular obstruction. In the symptomatic patient with obstructive HC, blood loss during delivery, vasodilation, and sympathetic stimulation during anesthesia must be avoided. Indications for drug therapy include symptoms and the presence of arrhythmias. Symptoms associated with elevated left ventricular filling pressures should be treated with beta-adrenergic blocking agents, with diuretics added if beta blockers alone are not sufficient. While calcium antagonists appear to be useful in nonpregnant patients,[104] the fetal effect of administration of these drugs has not been established.[105]

Although pregnancy per se does not seem to increase the risk for sudden death in patients with HC, such events are most commonly seen during the childbearing years.[106] The presence of ventricular arrhythmias — an important prognostic sign — should be sought on Holter monitoring, and complex ventricular arrhythmias should be treated with drugs that will not harm the fetus, such as quinidine, procainamide, and beta blockers (if effective). The safety of amiodarone during pregnancy, shown to prevent sudden death in nonpregnant patients with HC, has not been established.[105] Amiodarone should therefore be used only in patients with life-threatening arrhythmias that do not respond to other drugs.[107] Supraventricular arrhythmias, especially atrial fibrillation, should be treated with Class 1A antiarrhythmic drugs (p. 634) during pregnancy. Electrical cardioversion can be used when patients with symptomatic atrial fibrillation do not respond to medical therapy.[108] Since digoxin may have unfavorable hemodynamic effects in obstructive HC and the long-term safety of calcium antagonists is unknown, beta blockers are the drugs of choice for controlling heart rate in patients with resistant atrial fibrillation.

Vaginal delivery has been shown to be safe in women with HC. In those with symptoms or outflow obstruction, the second stage of labor may be shortened by the use of forceps.[26,104] The use of prostaglandins to effect uterine contractions may be unfavorable owing to their vasodilatory effect, whereas oxytocin seems to be tolerated well.[102] Since beta-sympathomimetic tocolytic agents may aggravate left ventricular outflow tract obstruction, magnesium sulfate is preferred.[102] Similarly, spinal and epidural anesthetics should be avoided in obstructive HC because of their vasodilatory effect,[109] and excessive blood loss should be avoided or replaced promptly with intravenous fluid or blood.[26]

Because the risk for infective endocarditis is increased in HC, especially the obstructive form, antibiotic prophylaxis should be considered for labor and delivery.

PERIPARTUM CARDIOMYOPATHY

(See also p. 1398)

This form of dilated cardiomyopathy has signs and symptoms of heart failure due to left ventricular systolic dysfunction that become manifest for the first time in the peripartum period. Rarely for the most part, symptoms occur during the last month of gestation or immediately post partum, although occasional cases may appear at any time during the last 3 months of pregnancy or the first 6 months post partum (Fig. 59–5).[110] Any other causes of left ventricular dilatation and systolic dysfunction must be excluded to establish the diagnosis of peripartum cardiomyopathy (PPCM).[111] The reported incidence of the disease in the United States varies from one in 1300 to one in 15,000, with a higher incidence (one in 100) in certain parts of Africa.[112]

Patients usually have symptoms of congestive heart failure, chest pain, palpitations, and occasionally peripheral or pulmonary embolization.[110-113,113a] Physical examination often reveals an enlarged heart and an S_3, and murmurs of mitral and tricuspid regurgitation are not uncommon.[110,112,114] The electrocardiogram may show left ventricular hypertrophy, ST-T changes, conduction abnormalities, and arrhythmias. Chest x-ray may reveal cardiomegaly, pulmonary venous congestion with interstitial or alveolar edema, and occasionally pleural effusion. On Doppler echocardiography, all four chambers are enlarged, with marked reduction in left ventricular systolic function. Small-to-moderate pericardial effusion may be found; mitral, tricuspid, and pulmonic regurgitation may be evident. Hemodynamic changes are indistinguishable from those other forms of dilated cardiomyopathy.[114] A few patients with high-output heart failure have been reported.[113a]

The incidence of PPCM is greater in women with twin pregnancies and in women who are multiparous, over 30 years of age, and black.[110-112] Although the etiology of PPCM is still unknown, the unique nature of this syndrome is suggested by its occurrence at a relatively young age compared with other forms of dilated cardiomyopathy, the recovery of cardiac size and function in a large number of patients, and its relation to pregnancy. It has been postulated that PPCM may be due to myocarditis, nutritional deficiency, small-vessel coronary artery abnormalities, hormonal effects, toxemia, or the maternal immunological response to fetal antigen.[110,112,114] Recently, the use of endomyocardial biopsy in patients with PPCM has revealed a greater incidence of myocarditis[115] compared with other forms of dilated cardiomyopathy. Although biopsy results were normal for myocarditis in some investigations,[116,117] the incidence of this condition in other reports ranged from 29 per cent to 100 per cent.[110,114,115] These findings may suggest an etiological role for myocarditis in patients with PPCM.

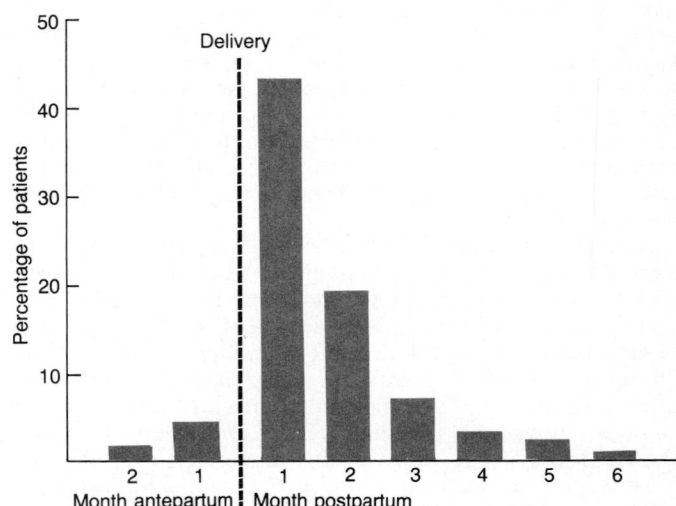

FIGURE 59–5. Onset of peripartum cardiomyopathy in relation to time of delivery in 347 patients. (From Homans, D. C.: Peripartum cardiomyopathy. N. Engl. J. Med. *312*:1432, 1985.)

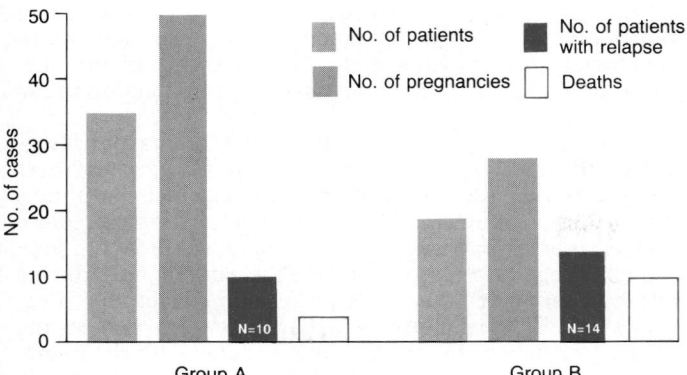

FIGURE 59-6. Incidence of relapse and death in subsequent pregnancies in patients with peripartum cardiomyopathy (PPCM). Group A, patients with PPCM demonstrating clinical improvement with normalization of heart size on chest X-ray or left ventricular size and function by echocardiography. Group B, patients with PPCM with persistent cardiomyopathy and/or left ventricular dysfunction. N, number. Data are derived from previous reports of 54 patients (references 111, 125–132).

The clinical course of PPCM varies. Approximately 50 per cent of patients show complete or near-complete recovery of cardiac function and clinical status within the first 6 months post partum; the other 50 per cent demonstrate either continuous clinical deterioration, leading to early death, or persistent left ventricular dysfunction and chronic heart failure, with high morbidity and mortality.[110–112, 117]

Acute heart failure should be treated vigorously with oxygen, diuretics, inotropic support with digitalis, and vasodilator agents. The use of hydralazine as an afterload-reducing agent is safe during pregnancy.[90] Experience with organic nitrates is limited, although hypotension secondary to an excessive dose has been associated with fetal bradycardia.[118] Nitroprusside has been used successfully during pregnancy, but experiments in animals have shown the potential for fetal toxicity.[105] Angiotensin-converting enzyme inhibitors have had deleterious effects on blood pressure control and renal function in the fetus[119] and are therefore *not* recommended for antepartum therapy. Because of the increased incidence of thromboembolic events in PPCM, anticoagulant therapy is recommended. Since the disease may be reversible, the temporary use of an intraaortic balloon pump may help stabilize the patient's condition pending improvement.[120]

Recent data have provided circumstantial evidence of the potential benefits of immunosuppression in patients with PPCM.[115,121] Midei et al.[115] recently reported both objective and subjective improvement in nine of ten patients with PPCM who had biopsy evidence of myocarditis. However, significant clinical improvement as well as the rapid improvement of left ventricular function was also reported in patients with PPCM given supportive therapy alone.[116,117] Since information about the effect of immunosuppressive therapy in PPCM is insufficient,[122] no recommendation can be made at the present time. However, such treatment seems reasonable in patients with acute clinical deterioration who do not respond to conventional therapy. Because of the high mortality and morbidity among patients who do not recover early, such patients should also be considered for cardiac transplantation.[117,123,124]

Subsequent pregnancies in women with PPCM are often associated with relapses and a high risk for maternal mortality. Although the likelihood of such relapse is greater in patients with persistently abnormal heart size and/or function, it has also been reported in women in whom left ventricular function is restored after the first episode[111,125–132] (Fig. 59–6). For these reasons, subsequent pregnancies should be discouraged in patients with PPCM who have persistent cardiac dysfunction; women in whom cardiac function is recovered after one episode of PPCM should be informed about the increased risk that attends later pregnancies.

PATHOGENESIS. Coronary artery disease (CAD) is rare among women of childbearing age, and the incidence of peripartum acute myocardial infarction (AMI) is estimated to be less than one in 10,000 pregnancies.[133]

Risk factors for CAD in women under age 50 include high levels of total plasma cholesterol, low levels of high-density lipoproteins, cigarette smoking, diabetes mellitus, hypertension, a family history of CAD, toxemia of pregnancy, and the use of oral contraceptives.[134,135] The combination of heavy smoking and concurrent use of oral contraceptives has been shown to be a powerful predictor of AMI.[136] In addition, an increased risk has been related to the age of the mother at the time of delivery of the first child (below the age of 20)[137] and to a lifelong irregular pattern of menstruation.[138]

Several mechanisms have been proposed to explain the relationship between oral contraceptives and AMI (see also p. 1153). For example, these drugs may trigger clot formation and embolization, as suggested by the increased incidence of venous thrombosis, pulmonary embolism, and cerebral thromboembolism.[133] In addition, oral contraceptives may raise serum levels of triglycerides, total cholesterol, and low-density lipoprotein; lower the level of high-density lipoprotein; increase the incidence of hypertension; and precipitate the ulceration of atherosclerotic plaques.[133] To reduce the risk for AMI, oral contraceptives should be avoided or formulations with lower effective doses of estrogen should be used in women over age 35, cigarette smokers, and those who develop hypertension while using this form of birth control.

Peripartum AMI is often associated with normal coronary angiographic findings[138]; this suggests a decrease in coronary perfusion, possibly due to spasm or in situ thrombosis, as a relatively common etiological factor in this patient population.[133,139,140] Although the cause of spasm is not clear, it has often been associated with pregnancy-induced hypertension and in some instances with the use of ergot derivatives to suppress lactation.[139] Coronary arterial dissection that occurs immediately post partum is another relatively common cause of peripartum AMI.[141,142] Advanced maternal age and parity may predispose to the development of coronary arterial dissection, and nearly all reported cases have involved the left anterior descending coronary artery.[141] Another potential cause of AMI during pregnancy has been collagen vascular disease.[143]

DIAGNOSIS. The diagnostic approach to ischemic myocardial disease in pregnancy is influenced to some extent by whether a diagnostic procedure could harm the fetus. No information is available regarding the safety of exercise testing during pregnancy. Because fetal bradycardia has been reported during maximal exercise in normal women,[44] a submaximal exercise protocol with fetal monitoring is recommended to evaluate ischemic myocardial disease during pregnancy.[45] Radionuclide myocardial perfusion scans and radionuclide ventriculography expose the fetus to radiation and should be used only when the potential benefits seem to outweigh fetal risk.[45] For similar reasons, cardiac catheterization involving fluoroscopy and cineangiography should be used only when relevant information cannot be obtained by other, noninvasive methods.[45]

MANAGEMENT. Fetal safety should also influence the therapeutic approach to ischemic heart disease during pregnancy. Since the safety of long-term therapy with organic nitrates and calcium antagonists in pregnancy has not been established, beta blockers appear to be the most appropriate choice for the treatment of ischemia during gestation. Coronary reperfusion by means of percutaneous transluminal coronary angioplasty or coronary artery bypass graft surgery has been reported to be successful during pregnancy,[144,145] although experience is still limited. Such procedures should be avoided during the first trimester, if possible, owing to the potential deleterious effects on the fetus of both ionizing radiation and cardiopulmonary bypass.[133]

Myocardial infarction is associated with high maternal mortality, especially when it occurs during the third trimester and labor,[146] and is probably related to a delay in diagnosis due to a low level of suspicion as well as the normal increase in cardiovascular work and myocardial oxygen consumption during gestation. Intrapartum management should focus on reducing cardiovascular stress during pregnancy and the peripartum period. Pulmonary artery catheterization with monitoring of pressure and cardiac output can help in the early detection and correction of hemodynamic abnormalities during labor and delivery. During labor, adequate analgesia and supplemental oxygen should be given, and if desired, cardiac output can be increased by placing the patient in the left lateral decubitus position. Labor in the supine position may decrease venous return and thus reduce right and left ventricular filling pressures. Low forceps can be used to shorten the second stage of labor. Although elective cesarean section is not indicated in every case, it should be used in patients with active ischemia or hemodynamic instability despite adequate medical therapy. Epidural anesthesia can reduce hemodynamic fluctuations during labor and is associated with left ventricular unloading due to vasodilation. If general anesthesia is indicated, *halothane should be avoided* in patients with depressed left ventricular systolic function.[66] In addition, atropine and ketamine should be used with caution to prevent tachycardia. Continued hemodynamic monitoring is advisable for 24 hours post partum to prevent hemodynamic worsening associated with the postpartum hemodynamic changes described earlier.[1]

CARDIAC ARRHYTHMIAS

Although the exact prevalence of arrhythmia during pregnancy is not known, anecdotal reports and clinical experience suggest a gestational arrhythmogenic effect, in women both with and without organic heart disease.[31] Palpitations, dizziness, and syncope are relatively common symptoms during pregnancy. Recently, 24-hour Holter monitoring was employed in 86 women referred for such symptoms and found multiple ventricular premature beats, atrial premature beats,

or both in 18 per cent of the patients; no supraventricular or ventricular tachycardia was noted.[147] The presence of multiple premature beats was not associated with any adverse maternal or fetal effect, and there was marked reduction in the number of premature beats post partum.

Early studies reported an incidence of supraventricular tachycardia (SVT) during pregnancy of 1.5 per cent to 3.0 per cent in women with heart disease. However, since continuous electrocardiographic monitoring was not performed, these studies probably underestimated the incidence of SVT in such patients. Reports of paroxysmal SVT occurring only during gestation support the arrhythmogenic effect of pregnancy.[31,148,149] Atrial flutter and fibrillation are rare during normal pregnancy and are usually associated with rheumatic mitral valve disease. Ventricular tachycardia or fibrillation is also rare in pregnancy and is usually associated with structural heart disease,[150] although sustained symptomatic ventricular tachycardia in otherwise healthy pregnant women has been described in a few cases.[151]

Among pregnant women who were otherwise healthy, Copeland and Stern[152] reported type I (Wenckebach) second degree atrioventricular (AV) block on six of 26,000 electrocardiograms. However, similar findings were noted for nonpregnant women.[153] Complete heart block has been described during pregnancy; although usually congenital, it can be acquired[154] as a result of myocarditis, congenital heart disease, acute myocardial infarction, or infective endocarditis. Symptomatic patients have been treated with pacemakers, and numerous pregnancies have been reported in patients after a pacemaker has been implanted.[155] A rate-adaptive pacemaker (p. 742) seems to be indicated in women of childbearing age. Reports of skin irritation and ulceration at the implant site due to enlargement of the breast and abdomen during pregnancy have led to placement of the battery under the breast in such women.[108]

Figure 59–7 shows an approach to management of patients with arrhythmias. A complete evaluation is indicated to rule out a cardiac cause as well as electrolyte imbalance, thyroid disease, and arrhythmogenic effects due to drugs, alcohol, caffeine, and cigarette smoking. The identified cause should be treated and antiarrhythmic drug therapy initiated only if the

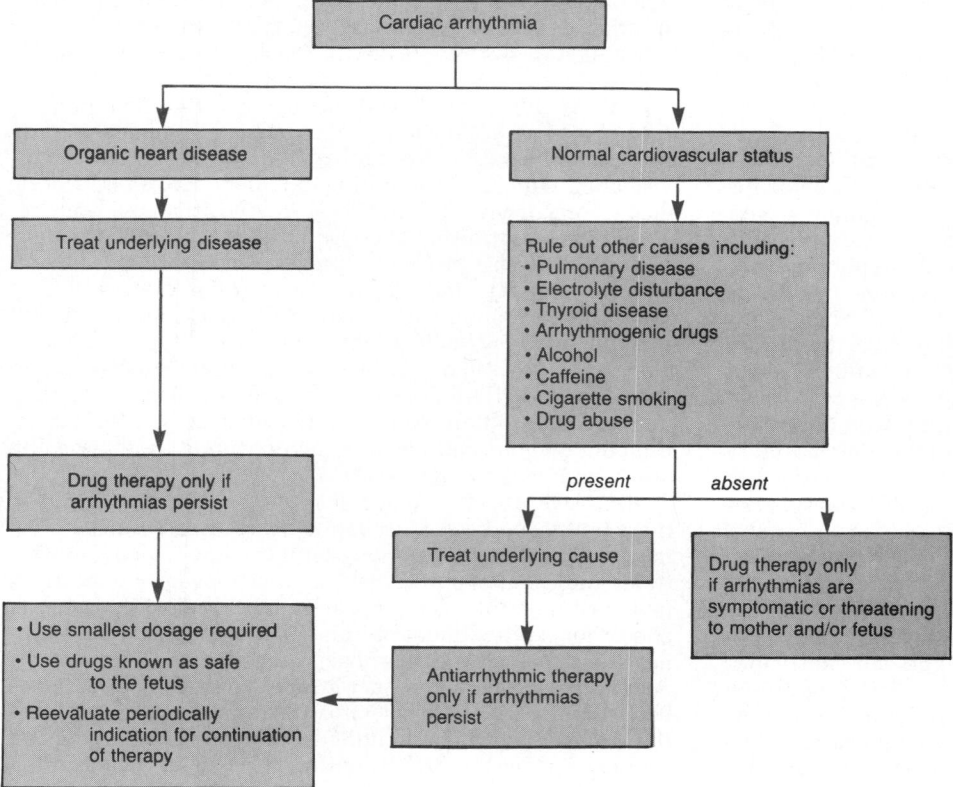

FIGURE 59–7. Management of cardiac arrhythmias during pregnancy. (From Rotmensch, H. H., et al.: Management of cardiac arrhythmias during pregnancy: Current concepts. Drugs 33:623, 1987.)

arrhythmia persists and is symptomatic or threatens the mother and/or fetus. When drug therapy seems necessary, drugs known to be safe for the fetus (p. 1803) should be used at the smallest dose required to achieve effect and/or therapeutic blood levels, and the indication(s) for continuous drug therapy should be reevaluated periodically.[107]

OTHER CARDIOVASCULAR DISEASES

Aortic Dissection (see also p. 1535)

Although aortic dissection occurs two to three times more frequently in males than in females, a predisposition to this condition during gestation has been suggested.[141,156] Over the last 50 years, approximately 200 cases of aortic dissection in association with pregnancy have been reported.[141] The incidence is increased among women over age 30, multiparous women, and patients with coarctation of the aorta and Marfan syndrome (see p. 1641).[157] Pregnancy-related aortic dissection seems to occur most often during the third trimester and peripartum period.[141]

The diagnostic approach to the pregnant patient suspected of having aortic dissection is similar to that for the nonpregnant patient. Since contrast aortography is often required to establish the diagnosis, an attempt should be made to minimize the radiation dose, and the fetus should be appropriately shielded. The use of transesophageal echocardiography has provided a powerful tool for diagnosing aortic dissection in pregnancy (p. 1538).[158] This method is preferable to computed tomography (CT), which involves radiation exposure, and to magnetic resonance imaging, the safety of which during gestation has not yet been established.

The combination of nitroprusside and propranolol is currently recommended to control hypertension in patients with aortic dissection. Since nitroprusside may result in fetal toxicity (see p. 1804) it should be used only in patients refractory to other drugs. Hydralazine, either intravenously or orally, is the drug of choice for blood pressure reduction in pregnant women with aortic dissection. To avoid the pressure elevation associated with labor and vaginal delivery in women with aortic dissection, abdominal delivery by cesarean section under epidural anesthesia is recommended.[141]

Takayasu's Arteritis (see also p. 1544)

A review of the literature revealed 116 pregnancies in 89 women with Takayasu's disease.[141,159-162] Cerebral hemorrhage, heart failure, and even death have been reported in pregnant patients with Takayasu's arteritis.[159,162] In addition, systolic blood pressure was markedly elevated during uterine contractions in some patients.[159] Low birth weights were noted when the disease was complicated by retinopathy, hypertension, aortic regurgitation, or arterial aneurysms. The management of pregnant patients with Takayasu's arteritis includes treatment of hypertension to prevent complications such as congestive heart failure and cerebral hemorrhage. However, to avoid compromising uteroplacental blood flow, blood pressure should not be reduced excessively in patients with aortic narrowing. Adrenal glucocorticoids have been used in some cases of Takayasu's arteritis during pregnancy[159,161]; however, since pregnancy does not seem to change the inflammatory activity of this disorder, glucocorticoids should be reserved for patients who become pregnant during the acute phase of the disease. Prophylactic antibiotics may be given for labor and delivery in patients with aortic regurgitation and vascular stenoses.

Vaginal delivery is likely to be tolerated in the majority of patients with Takayasu's arteritis. Abdominal delivery may be considered for those with severe systemic hypertension and heart failure that does not respond to medical therapy. Vacuum extraction or forceps can be used to shorten the second stage of labor in patients with a marked increase in blood pressure during uterine contractions. In patients with substantial aortic narrowing, epidural anesthesia may markedly reduce blood pressure distal to the narrowing and compromise placental perfusion.

The use of oral contraceptives may accelerate the progression of Takayasu's arteritis[163] and should therefore be avoided in patients with this condition.

Primary Pulmonary Hypertension (PPH) (see also p. 806)

PPH is one of the few cardiovascular conditions in which pregnancy may be associated with a high maternal mortality rate. A review of the literature as well as of our own experience has revealed that 15 of 37 patients with PPH (41 per cent) died during pregnancy or in the early postpartum period.[164,165] Clinical deterioration or death during pregnancy cannot always be predicted on the basis of the patient's preconception clinical status. Symptomatic deterioration usually occurs in the second trimester and is manifested by fatigue, dyspnea, syncope, chest pain, and right ventricular failure. Death occurs most often during late gestation or in the early postpartum period. Since hemodynamic or electrocardiographic information has not been available, the exact cause of death in patients with PPH is not clear. However, right ventricular ischemia and failure due to an increased hemodynamic load that leads to cardiac arrhythmias and pulmonary embolism are likely mechanisms. In addition to high maternal risk, the incidence of spontaneous abortions and of neonatal deaths due to congenital heart disease is high.[164]

Because of the potentially deleterious effect of pregnancy on both mothers with PPH and their fetuses, pregnancy seems contraindicated in these patients. Since an etiological link between pulmonary hypertension and oral contraceptives has been suggested,[166] this form of birth control is not recommended for women with PPH. Tubal ligation should provide maximum protection against the undesired risks of pregnancy; however, this procedure should be carried out under local or epidural anesthesia and in conjunction with hemodynamic as well as electrocardiographic monitoring. Early abortion is indicated in patients who become pregnant. If the patient elects to continue the pregnancy, physical exertion should be restricted to reduce the circulatory load. In addition, elective early hospitalization is recommended to ensure limited activity and close follow-up. The incidence of premature deliveries is increased in patients with PPH and should be anticipated.

Because of the beneficial effect of anticoagulation in patients with PPH[167] and the increased incidence of thromboembolism during pregnancy, such therapy is recommended throughout gestation and at least during the early postpartum phase. Hemodynamic monitoring and blood gas measurements should be performed regularly during labor and delivery. Oxygen should be provided to prevent hypoxemia, and every effort should be made to prevent or immediately replace blood lost during delivery.[164]

Segmental epidural anesthesia and intrathecal morphine have been successful in relieving pain in these patients.[168,169] Because right ventricular dysfunction is likely, anesthetics having a negative inotropic effect should be avoided in patients with PPH. Most patients can tolerate vaginal delivery, and spontaneous labor is preferable to induction. Continued hemodynamic monitoring for 24 to 48 hours after delivery and a hospital stay of 10 to 14 days are recommended to prevent the complications commonly seen post partum.

CARDIAC SURGERY DURING PREGNANCY

Since heart disease that requires surgery is usually diagnosed and treated prior to pregnancy, cardiac surgery during gestation is uncommon. In general, cardiac surgery in the pregnant woman is not associated with increased maternal risk but may lead to fetal wastage.[86,170] Although many cardiac operations during gestation have been reported in the last 40 years, little information is available regarding the effects of anesthesia and the procedure, especially cardiopulmonary bypass, on the uteroplacental circulation and fetal outcome.[170] Therefore, surgery should be recommended only for patients who do not respond to medical therapy, and procedures not requiring cardiopulmonary bypass are preferred.[88,171] To minimize the risk of teratogenicity, surgery should be avoided during the first trimester.[170] Since heart surgery is indicated when medical therapy has not led to satisfactory improvement, many of these patients will be hemodynamically unstable and will require hemodynamic monitoring for stabilization and careful anesthetic technique. Anesthetic agents should be selected on the basis of their hemodynamic effects and fetal safety.[66] When the patient is at or near term, abdominal delivery by cesarean section can be performed at the same time as cardiac surgery, once fetal maturity has been confirmed.[172] Fetal monitoring is essential for early detection of the fetal bradycardia commonly seen in surgery involving cardiopulmonary bypass. This finding most likely indicates fetal distress due to a decrease in placental blood flow, so that bradycardiac episodes can frequently be managed by increasing the flow rate.[173,174]

PREGNANCY IN PATIENTS WITH VALVE PROSTHESES
(See also p. 1061)

The risk of pregnancy in women with a valve prosthesis is multifactorial and should be assessed and discussed with the patient and her family before conception. Potential problems may be related to an increased hemodynamic load, the hypercoagulable state of pregnancy with the increased likelihood of thromboembolic events, and risk to the fetus due to anticoagulants (p. 1805) and other cardiovascular drugs. In addition, the expected limitation in maternal functional capacity as well as postpartum morbidity and mortality should be taken into consideration. Most patients with an adequately functioning mechanical prosthesis, including those with two and three prosthetic valves, can tolerate the hemodynamic load of pregnancy. This fact was well demonstrated by Salazar et al.,[175] who reported favorable outcomes in 223 pregnancies in women with prosthetic heart valves. Although functional classification was not reported, 60 per cent of these patients required digitalis and diuretics, and 30 per cent were in atrial fibrillation, indicating advanced disease in many cases. In questionable cases, exercise testing prior to conception may be used to predict whether a patient with a prosthetic heart valve can tolerate the increased hemodynamic load of pregnancy.[29]

Significant changes in the levels of coagulation factors increase the risk for thrombosis during gestation.[176] Although thrombosis of prosthetic valves during pregnancy has been reported in isolated cases despite anticoagulation,[177-180] the anticoagulant regimen used was inadequate in most of these cases. In the combined experience of Salazar et al.[175,177] involving women with mechanical valves treated with anticoagulation during pregnancy, thromboembolic events occurred in 6 of 165 patients with mitral prostheses (3.6 per cent) and in none of 37 patients with aortic prostheses.[181] Considering the fact that a fixed dose of heparin (5000 units every 12 hours) rather than adjusted dose was used in some of these patients, the incidence of thromboembolic events in patients with prosthetic heart valves who are adequately treated with anticoagulants during pregnancy is probably comparable to that in the nongravid population.[182] (The approach to and hazards of an-

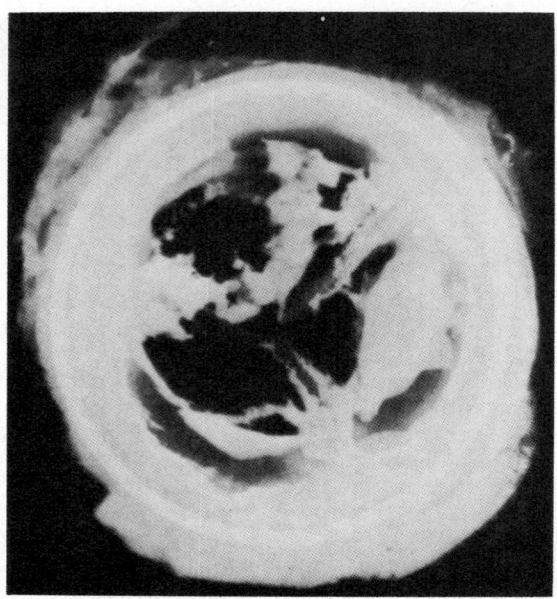

FIGURE 59-8. X-ray examination of a calcified mitral porcine bioprosthesis. This valve was recovered at reoperation, performed shortly after delivery, for severe prosthetic stenosis. (From Bortolotti, U., et al.: Pregnancy in patients with porcine valve bioprostheses. Am. J. Cardiol. *50*:1051, 1982.)

ticoagulation therapy during pregnancy are described on p. 1805.)

The selection of a prosthetic valve for pregnant patients or women of childbearing age should be individualized (p. 1065). Since it is desirable to avoid anticoagulation during pregnancy, the use of tissue valves is often recommended.[175,183,184] However, the long-term durability of these valves is limited, and frequently reoperation is required, with its related morbidity and mortality. In addition, tissue valves deteriorate more rapidly in young patients, and the incidence of calcification appears to be increased during pregnancy (Fig. 59-8).[185] A mechanical valve is recommended for patients who are willing to follow a strict regimen of anticoagulation and for those who require anticoagulation therapy for other conditions such as thrombophlebitis, atrial fibrillation, rheumatic mitral valve disease with an enlarged left atrial diameter, intracardiac thrombus, or a history of pulmonary embolism.

A review of the literature has suggested that fetal complications significantly increase with anticoagulation.[186] However, more recent prospective studies have demonstrated a normal fetal outcome when an adjusted dose of heparin is given throughout pregnancy, or at least during the first trimester.[175,177,187] Similar results have been reported with the use of oral Coumadin during pregnancy.[188]

In summary, the cumulative experience involving over 450 pregnancies reported by numerous groups from different parts of the world has demonstrated that asymptomatic or mildly symptomatic women with prosthetic heart valves can tolerate the hemodynamic load of pregnancy without difficulties. The incidence of thromboembolic events during pregnancy in women treated with anticoagulation is comparable to that in the nonpregnant population[181,182] and can be further reduced by the careful adjustment and monitoring of therapy during gestation.[187] Thus, pregnancy is not absolutely contraindicated in women with prosthetic heart valves, including mechanical prostheses.[175]

(Table 59–3)

Because of their potentially unfavorable effects on the developing fetus, all drugs should be avoided, if possible, during pregnancy. When drugs are needed, however, risk/benefit ratio must be evaluated carefully, and the smallest effective dose should be used. Another source of concern is the transfer of drugs into breast milk and subsequently to the neonates during lactation. Generally, only 1 per cent to 2 per cent of the maternal dose appears in breast milk.[189] Most data regarding drug excretion in human milk are anecdotal, and except for some drugs that are clearly contraindicated, there is not enough information to allow or prohibit breast-feeding in mothers receiving medications. Because the mechanisms involved in drug excretion into breast milk are complex, the various models and formulas used to estimate plasma/milk ratios are of limited clinical value. Therefore, close monitoring of the infant's ingested dose and plasma levels, as well as close observation for adverse effects or toxicity, is necessary to ensure safety.

Cardiac Glycosides (see also p. 479)

Recommendations for the gestational use of cardiac glycosides are based on their extensive use in maternal congestive heart failure and supraventricular arrhythmias.[190] During the past decade, digoxin alone or combined with a second drug, such as verapamil[191] or quinidine,[192] has been employed with increasing frequency to treat fetal supraventricular tachycardia and congestive heart failure.[191-193] Digoxin's volume of distribution is markedly increased during pregnancy. Since the drug is only 20 per cent to 25 per cent bound to proteins, its concentration is not greatly affected by the decrease in albumin levels during gestation. Transplacental passage of digoxin has been extensively documented, and the fetomaternal serum digoxin concentration ratio has been shown to range from 0.5 to 1.0.[190]

Pregnancy, especially when complicated by hypertension, is associated with increased levels of digoxin-like substances.[194,195] This phenomenon can interfere with digoxin radioimmunoassay and may cause errors of up to 2 μg/ml.[190,194,195]

To date, few adverse effects have been observed in fetuses of mothers who have undergone long-term treatment with digoxin. Low birth weight has been reported and has been postulated to be secondary to the effect of digoxin on amino acid transport through the placenta, with consequent growth retardation.[105] However, since the duration of pregnancy has been noted to be shorter in mothers with long-term digoxin therapy, it is possible that the reported low birth weight has been due to prematurity rather than intrauterine growth retardation.[105]

Despite these concerns, the gestational use of digoxin is considered safe, and to date there are no reports of teratogenesis in humans.[105,190] Caution is advised in digitalis administration, however, since overdose can be detrimental to the mother and may be lethal to the fetus.[105]

EFFECTS ON THE FETUS. Digoxin is excreted in breast milk and the milk/plasma ratio ranged from 0.59 to 0.90.[189] The total amount of digoxin ingested daily by the infant has been estimated to be approximately 1/100 of the pediatric recommended dose. No apparent clinical effects have been demonstrated in newborns, so that digoxin therapy of the mother should not affect breast-feeding decisions.[189]

Antiarrhythmics (see also Chap. 23)

QUINIDINE (see also p. 633). There is substantial clinical experience with the use of quinidine for the treatment of maternal arrhythmias.[105,108] One report has demonstrated successful treatment of fetal supraventricular tachycardia with quinidine and digoxin.[192] Since the drug is 60 per cent to 80 per cent bound to protein, the unbound fraction may increase owing to the hypoalbuminemia of pregnancy. Transplacental passage of quinidine has been demonstrated with a fetomaternal serum concentration ratio ranging from 0.25 to 0.8.[105]

Effects on the Fetus. Fetal thrombocytopenia has been associated with quinidine treatment, and minimal oxytocic activity has been reported mostly during development of spontaneous uterine contractions. Toxic doses of quinidine, however, may cause premature labor, abortion, or damage to the fetal eighth cranial nerve.[105,108] Although these side effects are of concern, they are rare, and the drug is considered safe for the treatment of both maternal and fetal arrhythmias. Quinidine is secreted in breast milk, with a milk/plasma ratio of 0.71.[189] The calculated total dose of quinidine likely to be ingested by the infant is far below the recommended therapeutic daily pediatric dose.

PROCAINAMIDE (see also p. 636). Information regarding the use of procainamide in pregnancy is limited. Transplacental transfer of procainamide is well documented by its use in the treatment of fetal supraventricular tachycardia.[196] Fetomaternal drug level ratios have been found to be 0.28 and 1.32 in two different patients.[105] At present, no information is available concerning procainamide pharmacokinetics in the maternofetal unit. No teratogenic effects have been reported; however, because of the limited experience with procainamide, quinidine should be used as the drug of choice during pregnancy.

Translactal passage of procainamide was reported, with a milk/plasma ratio of 4.3 ± 2.4 for procainamide and 3.8 ± 1.8 for N-acetylprocainamide (NAPA).[197] Although the high ratio may indicate accumulation in the milk, the amount of both procainamide and NAPA ingested daily by the infant is not expected to produce significant plasma levels.[189]

DISOPYRAMIDE (see also p. 638). Reports regarding disopyramide treatment in pregnancy are limited to only a few patients treated for ventricular and supraventricular arrhythmias.[105,108,198] No teratogenic effects have been reported; however, the use of disopyramide for refractory supraventricular tachycardia in a pregnant patient with mitral valve prolapse triggered uterine contractions that abated upon withdrawal of the drug.[105]

Disopyramide is secreted in breast milk in concentrations similar to those in plasma. The estimated dose likely to be ingested by the infant is less than 2 mg/kg/day.[189] Although no adverse effects were noted in such infants,[199] until further investigation provides sufficient information re-

TABLE 59–3 SAFETY AND ADVERSE EFFECTS OF CARDIOVASCULAR DRUGS DURING PREGNANCY

DRUG	POTENTIAL FETAL ADVERSE EFFECTS	SAFETY
Digoxin	Low birth weight	Safe
Quinidine	Toxic dose may induce premature labor and damage to the fetal eighth cranial nerve.	Safe
Procainamide	None reported	*
Disopyramide	May initiate uterine contractions	*
Lidocaine	In high blood levels and fetal acidosis may cause central nervous system depression	Safe
Mexiletine	None reported	*
Admiodarone	Fetal hypothyroidism	*
Calcium antagonists	None reported	*
Beta-adrenergic blocking agents	Intrauterine growth retardation, apnea at birth, bradycardia, hypoglycemia, hyperbilirubinemia. Beta₂ blockade may initiate uterine contractions.	Safe
Sodium nitroprusside	Potential thiocyanate toxicity with high dose, fetal mortality in animal studies	Potentially unsafe
Organic nitrates	Fetal heart rate deceleration and bradycardia	*
ACE inhibitors (captopril and enalapril)	Skull ossification defect, premature deliveries, low birth weight, oligohydramnios, neonatal anuria, and renal failure	Unsafe
Diuretic agents	Impairment of uterine blood flow, thrombocytopenia, jaundice, hyponatremia, bradycardia	Potentially unsafe

* To date, only limited information is available and safety during pregnancy cannot be established.

garding its safety, use of disopyramide should be limited to patients with arrhythmias refractory to treatment with more established drugs.

LIDOCAINE (see also p. 639). This drug has been used during pregnancy mainly for epidural or local anesthesia; occasional reports describe its use as an antiarrhythmic agent.[105,108,200] Lidocaine crosses the placenta and can be detected rapidly in the umbilical cord after maternal administration. The fetomaternal plasma concentration ratio is 0.5 to 0.7.[105,189] Elevated lidocaine levels have been associated with infant central nervous system depression and apnea, hypotonia, dilated pupils, and seizures. Bradycardia has also been described. These side effects were reversible with appropriate treatment. As a weak base, lidocaine may be trapped by an acidic environment. For this reason, fetal acidosis may be associated with increased blood levels of the drug and the likelihood of toxicity. Lidocaine use during pregnancy has *not* been associated with teratogenic effects.

In *summary*, the available data indicate that lidocaine is safe for use during pregnancy as long as blood levels are closely monitored. Caution should be exercised in cases with fetal distress when fetal acidosis is likely. To prevent toxicity, maternal lidocaine levels should be maintained below 4 μg/ml.[105]

MEXILETINE (see also p. 640). A limited number of pregnant women have been reported to have been treated for cardiac arrhythmias with mexiletine at doses between 600 and 800 mg/day.[105,201,202] This drug appears to cross the placenta freely, and the fetomaternal ratio ranges from 0.7 to 1.0. Fetal bradycardia, infants small for gestational age, low Apgar score, and neonatal hypoglycemia have all been reported in cases of maternal treatment with mexiletine.[105] Despite these concerns, no teratogenic or long-term adverse effects have been reported. Mexiletine is secreted in breast milk and was found in higher concentrations in breast milk than in maternal plasma (the milk/plasma ratio varied between 0.8 and 1.9)[105,189]; however, the calculated daily quantity ingested by the infant appears to be below the therapeutic range, and drug levels were undetectable in infants' blood. Owing to very limited information and reported untoward effects, mexiletine cannot be recommended for use during gestation until its safety is further investigated.

AMIODARONE (see also p. 646). The use of amiodarone during pregnancy for the treatment of maternal and fetal arrhythmias has been reported in several cases.[105,189,203-205] Transplacental transfer of amiodarone and its metabolite desethylamiodarone has been reported to be 10 to 25 per cent.[105]

Although fetal outcome has been favorable in most cases, side effects, including congenital hypothyroidism with goiter, premature birth, hypotonia, bradycardia, and large anterior and posterior fontanelles, have been reported,[105,204-206] casting doubts on amiodarone's safety during pregnancy. Pending further studies, amiodarone should be used only in refractory cases of maternal or fetal tachyarrhythmias. Close monitoring of maternal and neonatal thyroid size and function is important for early detection of abnormalities.

Amiodarone is secreted in breast milk in quantities significant enough to be detected in the infant's blood.[105,189] The effect of long-term amiodarone exposure in infants is unknown; however, because of the well-known potential side effects of this drug, breast-feeding is *not* recommended in women being treated with amiodarone.[105]

Calcium Channel Antagonists (see also p. 867)

VERAPAMIL (see also p. 648). This drug has been used in pregnancy for various indications, including maternal and fetal supraventricular arrhythmias, premature labor, severe preeclampsia, and severe gestational proteinuric hypertension.[105,207,208]

Transplacental passage of verapamil forms the basis for in utero treatment of fetal tachycardias, which is often successful with this drug alone or combined with digoxin.[191,208] Although dysfunctional labor or postpartum hemorrhage attributable to verapamil has not been reported, discontinuation of the drug at the onset of labor has been recommended. More data are required to establish the safety of long-term therapy during pregnancy. Verapamil is excreted in breast milk[105,209]; its concentration ranges from 23 to 94 per cent of maternal blood level. The estimated total amount of verapamil secreted in milk is less than 0.01 to 0.04 per cent of the administered dose, and no pharmacological effects have been observed in neonates.

NIFEDIPINE (see also p. 867). Limited use of nifedipine in pregnancy as a tocolytic agent[210] and for the acute treatment of hypertensive emergencies[211] and chronic essential hypertension has also been reported.[212] The drug was reported to lower blood pressure without any apparent reduction in uteroplacental blood flow.[213] Constantine et al.[212] combined nifedipine with beta blockers for long-term treatment of hypertensive patients who were pregnant and found a high rate of cesarean section, abnormal antenatal cardiotocograph, premature delivery, and small-for-date infants. For these reasons and until further information is available regarding the safety of nifedipine in pregnancy, long-term use of this agent during gestation cannot be recommended.

Beta-Adrenoceptor Blocking Agents (see also p. 644)

PROPRANOLOL (see also p. 644). This drug has been used in pregnancy for the treatment of cardiac arrhythmias, hypertrophic cardiomyopathy, and hyperthyroidism.[105,108] Propranolol readily crosses the placenta; at delivery, fetal serum concentrations are equal to or lower than maternal concentrations. Because of decreased hepatic metabolism and altered protein binding, serum concentration and half-life may be increased in the neonate during the first 10 days of life. Several adverse effects on the fetus and neonate have been reported, including intrauterine growth retardation, delayed onset of respiration in the newborn, bradycardia, hypoglycemia, and hyperbilirubinemia.[105] Although increasing experience with the use of propranolol in pregnancy has demonstrated the rarity of these side effects, they should be anticipated by the clinician. Since blockade of myometrial beta$_2$-adrenergic receptors with propranolol may stimulate uterine contractions, selective beta$_1$-receptor blockers may be preferable for use during gestation.

Propranolol is excreted in breast milk, with a milk/plasma ratio of approximately 0.5 to 1.0.[105,189] No adverse effects were observed in infants breast-fed by mothers treated with propranolol. However, careful observation of such infants is recommended, since propranolol may accumulate owing to the immature hepatic microsomal enzyme system of the neonate.

METOPROLOL. This drug has been used alone or in combination with hydralazine to treat hypertensive pregnant patients without causing teratogenic or major side effects.[214] Metoprolol is secreted in breast milk[189]; however, the daily quantity ingested by the neonate is very small. Unless hepatic function in the newborn is markedly impaired, breast-feeding is probably safe.

ATENOLOL. Several studies have reported the use of atenolol in the treatment of hypertension during gestation.[105] Transplacental transfer of atenolol has been well documented with a fetomaternal ratio of 1.0.[105,189] Although available data indicate that the safety of atenolol is similar to that of other beta blockers, low birth weight has been reported in association with its use during pregnancy.[105] Atenolol is secreted in breast milk. No adverse effects have been noted in babies exposed to breast milk of women treated with atenolol, so that breast-feeding need not be discontinued.

LABETALOL (see also p. 866). This drug is an antihypertensive agent with selective alpha$_1$ nonselective beta-adrenergic blocking activity and low beta-agonist activity. Labetalol crosses the placenta, and the fetomaternal ratio is 0.5.[189,215] Its clearance and volume of distribution are not altered during pregnancy. A number of favorable reports have described the efficacy and safety of labetalol in the treatment of hypertensive pregnancies.[105,215,216] Despite significant reduction in blood pressure, uterine blood flow has not been affected.[216] Labetalol is secreted in breast milk, and no adverse effects have been noted in neonates.[217]

Sodium Nitroprusside

During pregnancy, nitroprusside (NP) has been used to control blood pressure and heart failure in patients with intracranial aneurysm, surgery, or severe gestational hypertension.[105,218,219] Data concerning the effect of NP on uterine blood flow are conflicting. The drug has been demonstrated to cross the placenta, both in animals and in humans. In pregnant ewes, maternal and fetal levels achieved equilibrium within 20 minutes. A large dose of NP in animals resulted in significant accumulation of maternal and fetal cyanide and fetal death.[218] In the limited number of patients treated with NP during pregnancy, no unfavorable drug-related effect on the fetus was noticed.[105,218] Therefore, NP is a very effective but potentially toxic drug. It has been employed in pregnancy mostly in gravely ill patients, and the data available are small. Until further studies clarify its pharmacodynamics, kinetics, and safety during pregnancy, caution is recommended.

Organic Nitrates

Intravenous nitroglycerin has been used effectively and safely to control severe pregnancy-induced hypertension.[89,118] In one report, however, the reduction of blood pressure with nitroglycerin was associated with fetal heart rate deceleration and bradycardia in a few patients and attenuation of spontaneous beat-to-beat variability, probably owing to loss of cerebral autoregulation and increased intracranial pressure. It appears, therefore, that treatment with nitrates may not be free from side effects. Further studies are needed to clarify the effects of these drugs on uterine blood flow and fetal safety before they can be recommended for use during pregnancy.

Angiotensin-Converting Enzyme (ACE) Inhibitors
(see also p. 867)

Both captopril and enalapril have been used in the treatment of hypertension in pregnancy.[220,221] Passage of captopril from the mother to the fetus has been reported in two patients with maternal/fetal plasma concentration quotients of 3.4 and 1.0.[220] In animals, exposure to ACE inhibitors during pregnancy has been reported to produce prolonged fetal hypotension and death.[221] Although there are no reports of direct teratogenicity, two cases have been reported of a rare skull ossification defect in fetuses born to mothers treated with ACE inhibitors.[222] In addition, increased risk of early delivery, low birth weight, severe oligohydramnios, and/or neonatal anuria and renal failure that may be fatal has been reported.[218,222] Despite the limited and anecdotal nature of the available information, the published data indicate a potential risk and suggest that, for the time being, ACE inhibitors should not be used during gestation.[89]

Diuretic Agents

Diuretics have been used in pregnancy for the management of hypertension, heart failure, fluid retention, and prophylactically to prevent preeclampsia.[89,218] Because of the benign nature of dependent edema in pregnancy and the potential impairment of uterine blood flow and placental perfusion due to decreased blood volume, diuretics are not recommended for dependent edema. The prophylactic use of diuretics has not been proved effective in patients with preeclampsia; moreover, further volume restriction with these drugs may be deleterious.[89] Although diuretic therapy during pregnancy in patients with chronic hypertension is controversial, the continuation of diuretic therapy initiated prior to conception does not seem unfavorable. However, because of the potential for a decrease in placental perfusion, initiating diuretics during pregnancy is not recommended. Recent data have shown, however, that thiazide diuretics are safe and effective when used in combination with methyldopa.[223] Placental transfer of both hydrochlorothiazide and furosemide[224,225] has been documented, with similar maternal and fetal serum levels. Although no teratogenic effects have been described, case reports of neonatal thrombocytopenia, jaundice, hyponatremia, and bradycardia have been reported with the use of thiazides.[218]

In *summary*, because of the potential fetal adverse effects, the use of diuretics in pregnancy should be limited to the treatment of heart failure and selected cases of hypertension. The *routine* use of these drugs for the treatment of hypertension or dependent edema is *not* recommended.

Anticoagulant Therapy

Anticoagulants may be necessary to prevent or control the following cardiovascular conditions during pregnancy: venous thrombophlebitis, pulmonary embolism, rheumatic mitral valve disease, prosthetic heart valves, peripartum cardiomyopathy, primary pulmonary hypertension, and Eisenmenger's syndrome.[176]

Because of its large molecular size, heparin does not cross the placenta and is the drug of choice during pregnancy. In a review of anticoagulation during pregnancy, Hall et al.[186] reported a high incidence of maternal and fetal complications associated with heparin; however, other prospective studies have demonstrated a favorable outcome with heparin therapy.[175,177,187]

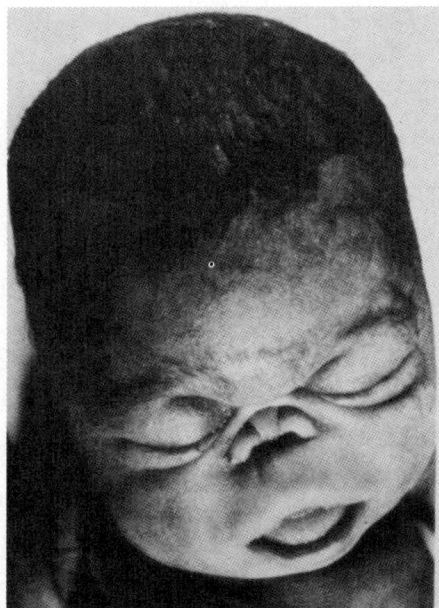

FIGURE 59–9. Severe nasal deformity in a newborn from a mother with aortic valve prosthesis taking Coumadin throughout pregnancy. (From Becker, M. H., et al.: Chondrodysplasia punctata. Is maternal warfarin therapy a factor? Am. J. Dis. Child. *129*:356, 1975.)

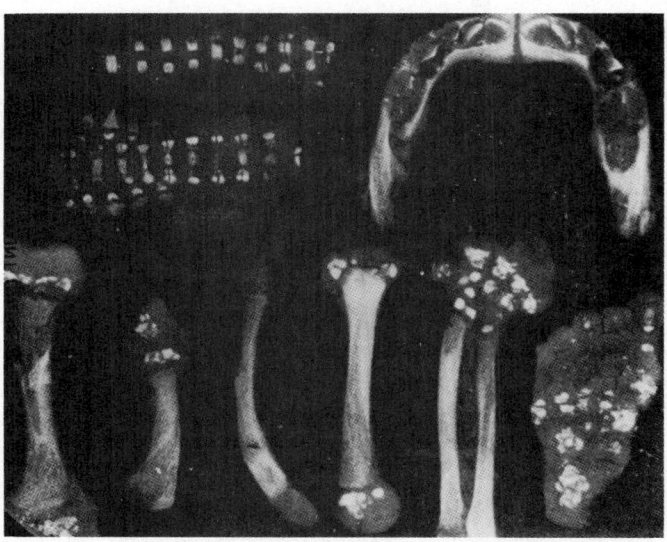

FIGURE 59–10. Roentgenograph of dissected skeleton showing stippling in cartilaginous portions of skeleton. Same case as Figure 59–9. (From Becker, M. H., et al.: Chondrodysplasia punctata. Is maternal warfarin therapy a factor? Am. J. Dis. Child. *129*:356, 1975.)

The use of Coumadin during pregnancy is associated with substantial teratogenic risk, including a high incidence of fetal wastage due to spontaneous abortion and stillbirths[176,179,226]; central nervous system disease such as optic nerve atrophy and blindness, mental retardation, microcephaly, and spasticity; and even death secondary to intracranial hemorrhage.[176,226] Use of this drug during the first trimester has been associated with "coumarin embryopathy" in 5 to 30 per cent of newborns.[176,177,226] This syndrome includes nasal bone hypoplasia (Fig. 59–9) and epiphyseal stippling (chondrodysplasia punctata[227]; Fig. 59–10). Labor and delivery while the patient is taking Coumadin places both the mother and fetus at risk of hemorrhage. Because the drug(s)' half-life is longer in the fetus, the effect of Coumadin may persist for 7 to 10 days after its administration has been discontinued. Our recommended strategy for peripartum anticoagulation therapy is shown in Figure 59–11.

Patients of childbearing age who are taking anticoagulants on a long-term basis should be advised prior to conception regarding the maternal and fetal risks of these agents. If pregnancy is planned, oral anticoagulants should be discontinued and subcutaneous heparin started. To avoid prolonged treatment with heparin prior to conception, the fertility of both parents should be investigated before heparin administration is begun. In cases of conception during Coumadin therapy, heparin should be substituted. A brief period of hospitalization is advisable to establish the required heparin dose and assure continuity of effective anticoagulation.

Self-injection of an adjusted dose of heparin subcutaneously is the recommended approach for the duration of pregnancy. Because of interpatient dose variability and changes in the dose requirement as pregnancy progresses,[176,187] a fixed dose of heparin may not prevent thromboembolic events and cannot be recommended.[228,229] Heparin is administered into the lower abdominal subcutaneous tissue at 12-hour intervals, with dose adjustment to prolong the activated partial thromboplastin time to 1.5 to 2.0 times normal. To reduce pain, concentrated heparin (20,000 units/ml) should be used.[176]

Complications related to long-term heparin therapy may occur and include sterile abscesses and hematomas in the abdominal wall, thrombocytopenia, and osteoporosis.[176,230,231] To reduce the risk of bleeding at delivery, subcutaneous heparin should be replaced in the hospital with intravenous heparin at 38 weeks' gestation. If heparin is needed, it can be substituted with oral Coumadin, adjusted to increase protime 1.5 to 2.0 times normal value, at the end of the first trimester.[177] Heparin and Coumadin should be given concomitantly for 4 days before heparin is stopped.[232]

Heparin should be discontinued at the onset of labor to allow clotting time to normalize prior to delivery. It has been recommended that heparin be continued into early labor when longer labor is anticipated, such as for primigravidas.[233] Since anticoagulation is reinstituted soon after delivery in patients who require this form of therapy, epidural anesthesia may increase the risk of bleeding into the epidural and subarachnoid space.[233] Pudendal anesthesia may also be associated with increased risk of bleeding complications in patients who have had anticoagulative therapy, since pudendal blood vessels are commonly punctured. Hemostatic stitches should be used to avoid bleeding in patients undergoing episiotomy, and uterine contraction should be stimulated by massage and Pitocin or ergot derivatives. Intravenous heparin can be resumed after delivery once he-

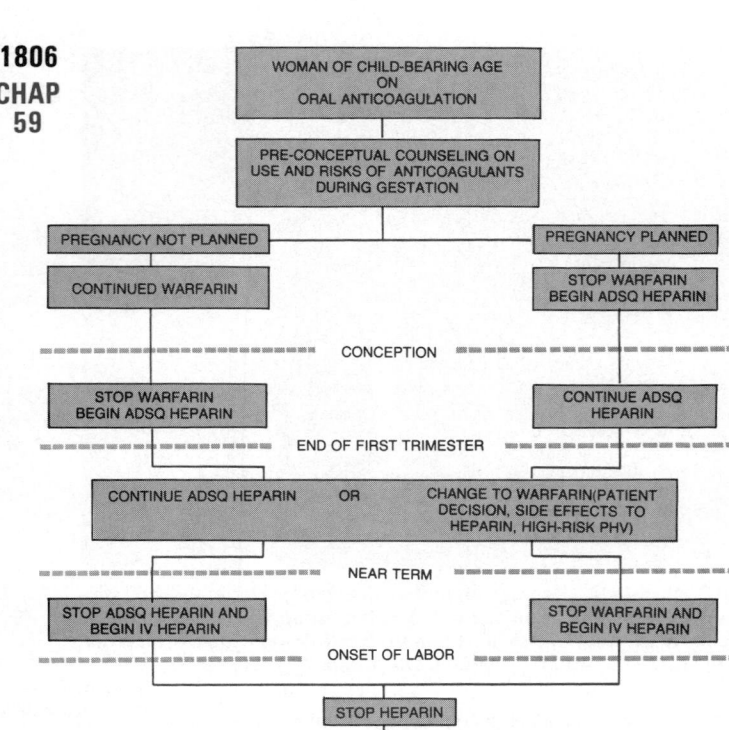

FIGURE 59–11. Recommended strategy for peripartum anticoagulation therapy. ADSQ, adjusted dose subcutaneous; H, hours; IV, intravenous; PHV = prosthetic heart valve. (From McGehee, W.: Anticoagulation in pregnancy. In Elkayam, U., and Gleicher, N. [eds.]: Cardiac Problems in Pregnancy: Diagnosis and Management of Maternal and Fetal Disease. 2nd ed. New York, Alan R. Liss, Inc., 1990, p. 397.)

mostasis is deemed adequate, and oral anticoagulation can be started 24 hours post partum after bleeding and hemorrhage have been ruled out.[176,233] Oral anticoagulation can be safely used after delivery, even in lactating women.[176]

Prophylactic Antibiotics

Antibiotic prophylaxis is indicated to prevent recurrent acute rheumatic fever in patients with a history of this disease and to prevent bacterial endocarditis in patients with certain types of underlying heart disease.

The recommended regimen for the prevention of rheumatic fever is the same as in the nongravid state (p. 1729) and includes 1.2 million units of benzathine penicillin G intramuscularly every 4 weeks, 250,000 units of oral penicillin V twice a day, or 1 gm/day of sulfadiazine.[234] Because of predisposition to kernicterus with the use of sulfadiazine, these drugs are not recommended during the third trimester of pregnancy and in women with a previous history of children with neonatal jaundice or blood-group incompatibility.[235]

Similar to the nongravid state, antibiotic prophylaxis for infective endocarditis is indicated during gestation in patients with prosthetic heart valves, congenital heart disease, rheumatic valvular disease, obstructive hypertrophic cardiomyopathy, and mitral valve prolapse with thickened mitral valve and mitral insufficiency who are undergoing procedures likely to result in bacteremia.[56] Since the incidence of bacteremia associated with uncomplicated vaginal delivery has been reported to be low (0 to 5 per cent),[236] the indication for antibiotic prophylaxis is questionable.[234]

The Committee on Bacterial Endocarditis, formed by the American Heart Association, has recommended routine prophylaxis for anticipated normal delivery only in patients with prosthetic heart valves.[56] Despite these recommendations, and since complications and bacteremia are not always predictable, we routinely administer prophylactic antibiotics to all patients susceptible to bacterial endocarditis. The antibiotic regimen recommended for delivery is 2 gm of ampicillin intramuscularly or intravenously, plus 1.5 mg/kg of gentamicin (maximum of 80 mg) intramuscularly or intravenously 30 minutes to 1 hour before the procedure. A second dose may be given 8 hours later. In patients allergic to penicillin, 1 gm of vancomycin is given intravenously, slowly over 1 hour, plus 1.5 mg/kg of gentamicin (to a maximum of 80 mg) intramuscularly or intravenously 1 hour before the procedure. This may be repeated 8 to 12 hours later.[56,234]

REFERENCES

CARDIOVASCULAR PHYSIOLOGY DURING PREGNANCY AND THE PUERPERIUM

1. Oakley, C. M.: Cardiovascular disease in pregnancy. Can. J. Cardiol. 6:(Suppl B):33B, 1990.
1a. Elkayam, U., and Gleicher, N.: Hemodynamics and cardiac function during normal pregnancy and the puerperium. In Elkayam, U., and Gleicher, N. (eds.): Cardiac Problems in Pregnancy: Diagnosis and Management of Maternal and Fetal Disease, 2nd ed. New York, Alan R. Liss Inc., 1990, p. 5.
2. Ueland, K.: Maternal cardiovascular dynamics: VII. Intrapartum blood volume changes. Am. J Obstet. Gynecol. 126:671, 1976.
3. Longo, L. D.: Maternal blood volume and cardiac output during pregnancy: A hypothesis of endocrinologic control. Am. J. Physiol. 245:R720, 1983.
4. Hsueh, W. A., Luetscher, J. A., Carlson, E. J., et al.: Changes in active and inactive renin throughout pregnancy. J. Clin. Endocrinol. Metab. 54:1010, 1982.
5. Cheek, D. B., Petrucco, O. M., Gillespie, A., et al.: Muscle cell growth and the distribution of water and electrolyte in human pregnancy. Early Hum. Dev. 11:293, 1985.
6. Robson, S. C., Hunter, S., Boys, R. J., et al.: Serial study of factors influencing changes in cardiac output during human pregnancy. Am. J. Physiol. 256:H1060, 1989.
7. Kjeldsen, J.: Hemodynamic investigations during labor and delivery. Acta Obstet. Gynecol. Scand. 89(Suppl.):20, 1979.
8. Katz, R., Karliner, J. S., and Resnik, K. R.: Effects of a natural volume overload state (pregnancy) on left ventricular performance in normal human subjects. Circulation 58:434, 1978.
9. Bryant, E. E., Douglas, B. H., and Ashburn, A. D.: Circulatory changes following prolactin administration. Am. J. Obstet. Gynecol. 115:53, 1973.
10. Gerber, J. G., Payne, N. A., Murphy, R. R., et al.: Prostacyclin produced by the pregnant uterus in the dog may act as a circulating vasodepressor substance. J. Clin. Invest. 67:632, 1981.
11. Metcalfe, J., and Ueland, K.: Maternal cardiovascular adjustment to pregnancy. Prog. Cardiovasc. Dis. 16:363, 1974.
12. Robson, S. C., Dunlop, W., Boys, R. J., et al.: Cardiac output during labour. Br. Med. J. 295:1169, 1987.
13. Ueland, K., and Hansen, J. M.: Maternal cardiovascular dynamics: II. Posture and uterine contractions. Am. J. Obstet. Gynecol. 103:1, 1969.
14. Ueland, K.: Cardiovascular physiology of the normal pregnancy. In Gleicher, U., Elkayam, U., Galbraith, R. M., et al. (eds.): Principles of Medical Therapy in Pregnancy. New York, Plenum, 1985, p. 643.
15. Ueland, K., and Hansen, J. M.: Maternal cardiovascular dynamic: III. Labor and delivery under local and caudal analgesia. Am. J. Obstet. Gynecol. 103:8, 1969.
16. Artal, R., Khodiguian, N., Rutherford, S., et al.: Cardiopulmonary and metabolic responses to bicycle ergometry in pregnancy. In Proceedings of the Society for Gynecologic Investigation, 1987, p. 48.
17. Morton, M. J., and Metcalfe, J.: Changes in maternal hemodynamics during pregnancy. In Artal, R., and Wiswell, R. (eds.): Exercise in Pregnancy. Baltimore, Williams and Wilkins, 1986.
18. Artal, R.: Cardiopulmonary responses to exercise in pregnancy. In Elkayam, U., and Gleicher, N. (eds.): Cardiac Problems in Pregnancy: Diagnosis and Management of Maternal and Fetal Disease, 2nd ed. New York, Alan R. Liss, Inc., 1990, p. 25.
19. Artal, R., Romem, Y., Paul, R. H., et al.: Fetal bradycardia induced by maternal exercise. Lancet 2:258, 1984.

CARDIAC EVALUATION DURING PREGNANCY

20. Elkayam, U., and Gleicher, N.: Changes in cardiac findings during normal pregnancy: Cardiovascular physiology of pregnancy: In Elkayam, U., and Gleicher, N. (eds.): Cardiac Problems in Pregnancy: Diagnosis and Management of Maternal and Fetal Disease. 2nd ed. New York, Alan R. Liss, Inc., 1990, p. 31.
21. Cutforth, R., and MacDonald, C. B.: Heart sounds and murmurs in pregnancy. Am. Heart J. 71:741, 1966.
22. Perloff, J. K.: Normal or innocent murmurs. In Perloff, J. K. (ed.): The Clinical Recognition of Congenital Heart Disease. 3rd ed. Philadelphia, W. B. Saunders Company, 1987, p. 8.
23. Tabaznik, B., Randall, T. W., and Hersch, C.: The mammary souffle of pregnancy and lactation. Circulation 22:1069, 1960.
24. Marcus, F. L., Ewy, G. A., O'Rourke, R. A., et al.: The effect of pregnancy on the murmurs of mitral and aortic regurgitation. Circulation 41:795, 1970.
25. Haas, J. M.: The effect of pregnancy on the midsystolic click and murmur of the prolapsing posterior leaflet of the mitral valve. Am. Heart J. 92:407, 1976.
26. Kumar, A., and Elkayam, U.: Hypertrophic cardiomyopathy in pregnancy: In Elkayam, U., and Gleicher, N. (eds.): Cardiac Problems in Pregnancy: Diagnosis and Management of Maternal and Fetal Disease. 2nd ed. New York, Alan R. Liss, Inc., 1990, p. 129.
27. Perloff, J. K.: Pregnancy and cardiovascular disease. In Braunwald, E. (ed.): Heart Disease. 2nd ed. Philadelphia, W. B. Saunders Company, 1984, p. 1763.
28. Criteria Committee of the New York Heart Association: Nomenclature and Criteria for Diagnosis of Diseases of the Heart and Great Vessels. 6th ed. Boston, Little, Brown and Co., 1964, p. 1.
29. Elkayam, U., and Gleicher, N.: Cardiac problems in pregnancy: I. Mater-

nal aspects: The approach to the pregnant patient with heart disease. JAMA 251:2838, 1984.

30. Elkayam, U.: Unpublished data.

31. Hong, R. A., and Bhandari, A. K.: Cardiac arrhythmias and pregnancy. In Elkayam, U., and Gleicher, N. (eds.): Cardiac Problems in Pregnancy: Diagnosis and Management of Maternal and Fetal Disease. 2nd ed. New York, Alan R. Liss, Inc., 1990, p. 167.

32. Upshaw, C. B., Jr.: A study of maternal electrocardiograms recorded during labor and delivery. Am. J. Obstet. Gynecol. 107:17, 1970.

33. Department of Health Services: Syllabus on Diagnostic X-ray Radiation Protection for Certified X-ray Supervisors and Operators. Sacramento, Calif., Department of Health Services, 1982, p. 71.

34. Wagner, C. K., Lester, R. G., and Saldana L. R.: Exposure of the pregnant patient to diagnostic radiation. A Guide to Medical Management. Philadelphia, J. B. Lippincott Co., 1985, p. 52.

35. Turner, A. F.: The chest radiograph in pregnancy. Clin. Obstet. Gynecol. 183:65, 1975.

36. Hughson, W. G., Friedman, P. J., Feigin, D. S., et al.: Postpartum pleural effusion: A common radiologic finding. Ann. Intern. Med. 97:856, 1982.

37. Austin, J.H.M.: Postpartum pleural effusions. Ann. Intern. Med. 98:555, 1983.

38. Bioeffects Committee of the American Institute of Ultrasound in Medicine. J. Ultrasound Med. Biol. 2:R14, 1983.

39. Katz, R., Karliner, J. S., and Resnik, R.: Effects of a natural volume overload state (pregnancy) on left ventricular performance in normal human subjects. Circulation 58:434, 1978.

40. Limacher, M. C., Ware, J. A., O'Meara, M. E., et al.: Tricuspid regurgitation during pregnancy. Am. J. Cardiol. 55:1059, 1985.

41. Haiat, R., and Halphen, C.: Silent pericardial effusion in late pregnancy: A new entity. Cardiovasc. Intervent. Radiol. 7:267, 1984.

42. Enein, M., Aziz, A., Zima, A., et al.: Echocardiography of the pericardium in pregnancy. Obstet. Gynecol. 69:851, 1987.

43. Campos, O., Martinez, E., Andrade, J. L., et al.: Detection of right-sided valve regurgitation during normal pregnancy by Doppler echocardiography. J. Am. Coll. Cardiol. 15:139A, 1990.

44. Carpenter, M. W., Sady, S. P., Hoegsberg, B., et al.: Fetal heart rate response to maternal exertion. JAMA 259:3006, 1988.

45. Elkayam, U., and Gleicher, N.: Diagnostic approaches to maternal heart disease. In Elkayam, U., and Gleicher, N. (eds.): Cardiac Problems in Pregnancy. 2nd ed. New York, Alan R. Liss, Inc., 1990, p. 41.

46. Lee, W., Shah, P. K., Amin, D. K., et al.: Hemodynamic monitoring of cardiac patients during pregnancy. In Elkayam, U., and Gleicher, N. (eds.): Cardiac Problems in Pregnancy: Diagnosis and Management of Maternal and Fetal Disease. 2nd ed. New York, Alan R. Liss, Inc., 1990, p. 47.

47. Medical Radiation Exposure of Pregnant and Potentially Pregnant Women: Recommendations of the National Council on Radiation Protection and Measurements. Washington, National Council on Radiation Protection and Measurements, 1977, p. 13.

48. Bithell, J. F., and Stewart, A. M.: Pre-natal irradiation and childhood malignancy: A review of British data from the Oxford survey. Br. J. Cancer 31:271, 1975.

49. Elkayam, U., Kawanishi, D., Reid, C. L., et al.: Contrast echocardiography to reduce ionizing radiation associated with cardiac catheterization during pregnancy. Am. J. Cardiol. 52:213, 1983.

50. Kereiakes, J. J., and Rosenstein, M.: Handbook of Radiation Doses of Nuclear Medicine and Diagnostic X-ray. Boca Raton, Fl, CR Press, 1980, p. 170.

CARDIOVASCULAR DISEASES AND PREGNANCY

51. Canobbio, M. M.: Counseling the adult with congenital heart disease. In Roberts W. C. (ed.): Adult Congenital Heart Disease. Philadelphia, F. A. Davis Co., 1987, p. 733.

52. Shime, J., Mocarski, E.J.M., Hastings, D., Webb, G. D., and McLaughlin, P. R.: Congenital heart disease in pregnancy: Short- and long-term implications. Am. J. Obstet. Gynecol. 156:313, 1987.

53. Whittemore, R., Hobbins, J. C., and Engle, M. A.: Pregnancy and its outcome in women with and without surgical treatment of congenital heart disease. Am. J. Cardiol. 50:641, 1982.

54. Whittemore, R.: Congenital heart disease: Its impact on pregnancy. Hosp. Pract. 18:65, 1983.

55. Elkayam, U., Cobb, T., and Gleicher, N.: Congenital heart disease and pregnancy. In Elkayam, U., and Gleicher, N. (eds.): Cardiac Problems in Pregnancy. 2nd ed. New York, Alan R. Liss, Inc., 1990, p. 73.

56. Shulman, S. T., Amren, D. P., Bisno, A. L., et al.: Prevention of bacterial endocarditis. Circulation 70:1123A, 1984.

57. McFaul, P. B., Dorman, J. C., Lamki, H., et al.: Pregnancy complicated by maternal heart disease. A review of 519 women. Br. J. Obstet. Gynecol. 95:861, 1988.

58. Metcalfe, J., McAnulty, J. H., and Ueland, K.: Heart Disease and Pregnancy, Physiology and Management. Boston, Little, Brown and Co., 1986, p. 223.

59. Arias, F., and Pineda, J.: Aortic stenosis and pregnancy. J. Reprod. Med. 4:229, 1978.

60. Angel, J. L., Chapman, C., Knappel, R. A., et al.: Percutaneous balloon aortic valvuloplasty in pregnancy. Obstet. Gynecol. 72:438, 1988.

61. Wachtel, H. L., and Czarnecki, S. W.: Coarctation of the aorta and pregnancy. Am. Heart J. 72:251, 1966.

62. Barash, P. G., Hobbins, J. C., Hook, R., et al.: Management of coarctation of the aorta during pregnancy. J. Thorac. Cardiovasc. Surg. 69:781, 1975.

63. Togo, T., Sugishita, Y., Tamura, T., et al.: Uneventful pregnancy and delivery in a case of multiple peripheral pulmonary stenosis. Acta Cardiol. 18:143, 1983.

64. Garson, H., McNamara, D. G., and Cooley, D. A.: Tetralogy of Fallot in adults. In Roberts, W. C. (ed.): Congenital Heart Disease in Adults. Philadelphia, F. A. Davis Co., 1987, p. 493.

65. Zitnik, R. S., Bradenburg, R. O., Sheldon, R., et al.: Pregnancy and open heart surgery. Circulation 39(Suppl. I):257, 1969.

66. Geller, E., Rudick, V., and Niv, D.: Analgesia and anesthesia during pregnancy. In Elkayam, E., and Gleicher, N. (eds.): Cardiac Problems in Pregnancy: Diagnosis and Management of Maternal and Fetal Disease. 2nd ed. New York, Alan R. Liss, Inc., 1990, p. 283.

67. Hatjis, C. G., Gibson, M., Capeless, E. L., et al.: Pregnancy in a patient with tricuspid atresia. Am. J. Obstet. Gynecol. 145:114, 1983.

68. Baumann, H., Schneider, H., Drack, G., et al.: Pregnancy and delivery by cesarean section in a patient with transposition of the great arteries and single ventricle. Case report. Br. J. Obstet. Gynaecol. 94:704, 1987.

69. Neukermans, K., Sullivan, T. J., Pitlick, P. T.: Successful pregnancy after the Mustard operation for transposition of the great arteries. Am. J. Cardiol. 62:838, 1988.

70. Ahmed, S., Hawes, D., Dooley, S., et al.: Intrathecal morphine in a patient with a single ventricle. Anesthesiology 54:515, 1981.

71. Simon, D. L., and Lustberg, A.: A case of truncus arteriosus communis compatible with full-term pregnancy. Am. Heart J. 42:617, 1951.

72. Mandel, A., and Hirsch, V.: Cor triloculare biatriatum: Report of a case with survival to the age of 29 years. Am. Heart J. 66:104, 1963.

73. Copel, J. A., Harrison, D., Whittemore, R., et al.: Intrathecal morphine analgesia for vaginal delivery in a woman with a single ventricle. A case report. J. Reprod. Med. 31:274, 1986.

74. Gleicher, N., Midwall, J., Hochberger, D., et al.: Eisenmenger's syndrome and pregnancy. Obstet. Gynecol. Surv. 34:721, 1979.

75. Midwall, J., Jaffin, H., Herman, M. V., et al.: Shunt flow and pulmonary hemodynamics during labor and delivery in the Eisenmenger's syndrome. Am. J. Cardiol. 42:299, 1978.

76. Mangano, D. T.: Anesthesia for the pregnant cardiac patient. In Shnider, S. M., and Levinson, G. (eds.): Anesthesia for Obstetrics. Baltimore, Williams and Wilkins, 1986, p. 345.

77. Rosenberg, B., Simon, K., Peretz, B. A., et al.: Eisenmenger's syndrome in pregnancy. Controlled segmental epidural block for cesarean section. Reg. Anaesth. 7:131, 1984.

78. Gordis, L.: The virtual disappearance of rheumatic fever in the United States: Lessons in the rise and fall of disease. Circulation 72:1155, 1985.

79. Argarwal, B. L.: Rheumatic heart disease unabated in developing countries. Lancet 2:910, 1981.

80. Ueland, K.: Rheumatic heart disease and pregnancy. In Elkayam, U., and Gleicher, N. (eds.): Cardiac Problems in Pregnancy. 2nd ed. New York, Alan R. Liss, Inc., 1990, p. 99.

81. Jacobi, P., Adler, Z., Zimmer, E. Z., et al.: Effect of uterine contractions on left atrial pressure in pregnant woman with mitral stenosis. Br. J. Med. 298:27, 1989.

82. Clark, S. L., Phelan, J. P., Greenspoon, J., et al.: Labor and delivery in the presence of mitral stenosis: Central hemodynamic observations. Am. J. Obstet. Gynecol. 152:984, 1985.

83. Hemmings, G. T., Whalley, D. G., O'Connor, P. H., et al.: Invasive monitoring and anesthetic management of a patient with mitral stenosis. Can. Anaesth. Soc. J. 34:182, 1987.

84. Bernal, J. M., and Miralles, P. J.: Cardiac surgery with cardiopulmonary bypass during pregnancy. Obstet. Gynecol. Surv. 41:1, 1986.

85. Palacios, I. F., Block, P. C., Wilkins, G. T., et al.: Percutaneous mitral balloon valvotomy during pregnancy in a patient with severe mitral stenosis. Cathet. Cardiovasc. Diagn. 15:109, 1988.

86. Becker, R. M.: Intracardiac surgery in pregnant women. Ann. Thorac. Surg. 36:453, 1983.

87. Safian, R. D., Berman, A. D., Sachs, B., et al.: Percutaneous balloon mitral valvuloplasty in a pregnant woman with mitral stenosis. Cathet. Cardiovasc. Diagn. 15:103, 1988.

88. Goon, M. S., Raman, S., and Sinnathuray, T. A.: Closed mitral valvotomy in pregnancy—A Malaysian experience. Aust. N. Z. J. Obstet. Gynaecol. 27:173, 1987.

89. Myers, S. A.: Antihypertensive drug use during pregnancy. In Elkayam, U., and Gleicher, N. (eds.): Cardiac Problems in Pregnancy: Diagnosis and Management of Maternal and Fetal Disease. 2nd ed. New York, Alan R. Liss, Inc., 1990, p. 381.

90. Roth, A., Rahimtoola, S., and Elkayam, U.: Enhancement of hemodynamic effects of hydralazine with nitroglycerin in patients with chronic mitral regurgitation. Circulation 76(Suppl. IV):89, 1987.

91. Panja, M., Nutra, K., Kar, A. K., et al.: A clinical profile of heart disease in pregnancy. Indian Heart J. 38:392, 1986.

92. Elkayam, U., McKay, C. R., Weber, L., et al.: Favorable effects of hydralazine on the hemodynamic response to isometric exercise in chronic severe aortic regurgitation. Am. J. Cardiol. 53:1604, 1984.

93. Savage, D. D., Garrison, R. J., Devereux, R. B., et al.: Mitral valve prolapse in the general population: I. Epidemiology features: The Framingham Study. Am. Heart J. 106:571, 1983.

94. Wann, L. S., Grove, J. R., Hess, T. R., et al.: Prevalence of mitral prolapse by two-dimensional echocardiography in healthy young women. Br. Heart J. 49:334, 1983.

95. Rayburn, W. F., LeMire, M. S., Bird, J. L., et al.: Mitral valve prolapse: Echocardiographic changes during pregnancy. J. Reprod. Med. 32:185, 1987.

96. Rayburn, W. F.: Mitral valve prolapse and pregnancy. In Elkayam, U., and Gleicher, N. (eds.): Cardiac Problems in Pregnancy. 2nd ed. New York, Alan R. Liss, Inc., 1990, p. 181.

97. Tank, L.C.H., Chan, S.Y.W., Wong, V.C.W., et al.: Pregnancy in patients with mitral valve prolapse. Int. J. Gynaecol. Obstet. 23:217, 1985.

98. Pyeritz, R. E.: Maternal and fetal complications of pregnancy in the Marfan syndrome. Am. J. Med. 71:784, 1981.

99. Pyeritz, R. E.: The Marfan syndrome. Am. Fam. Physician 34:83, 1986.

100. Rosenblum, N. G., Grossman, A. R., Mennuti, M. T., et al.: Failure of serial echocardiographic studies to predict aortic dissection in pregnant patient with Marfan's syndrome. Am. J. Obstet. Gynecol. 146:470, 1983.

101. Pyeritz, R. E.: Propranolol retards aortic root dilatation in the Marfan syndrome. Circulation 68(Suppl. III):365, 1983.

102. Shah, D. M., and Sunderji, S. G.: Hypertrophic cardiomyopathy and pregnancy: Report of the maternal mortality and review of the literature. Obstet. Gynecol. Surv. 40:444, 1985.

103. Maron, B. J., Bonow, R. D., Cannon, R. O., et al.: Hypertrophic cardiomyopathy. Interrelations of clinical manifestations, pathophysiology and therapy. N. Engl. J. Med. 316:844, 1987.

104. Rosing, D. R., Idanpaan-Heikkila, U., Maron, B. J., et al.: Use of calcium-channel blocking drugs in hypertrophic cardiomyopathy. Am. J. Cardiol. 55:185B, 1985.

105. Widerhorn, J., Rubin, J. N., Frishman, W. H., et al.: Cardiovascular drugs in pregnancy. Cardiol. Clin. 5:651, 1987.

106. McKenna, W. J., Deanfield, J. F., Faruqui, A. M., et al.: Prognosis in hypertrophic cardiomyopathy: Role of age and clinical, electrocardiographic, and hemodynamic features. Am. J. Cardiol. 47:532, 1981.

107. Rotmensch, H. H., Rotmensch, S., and Elkayam, U.: Management of cardiac arrhythmia during pregnancy; Current concepts. Drugs 33:623, 1987.

108. Rotmensch, H. H., Pines, A., and Donchin, Y.: Antiarrhythmic drugs in pregnancy. In Elkayam, U., and Gleicher, N. (eds.): Cardiac Problems in Pregnancy. 2nd ed. New York, Alan R. Liss, Inc., 1990, p. 361.

109. Boccio, R. V., Chung, J. H., and Harrison, D. M.: Anesthetic management of cesarean section in a patient with idiopathic hypertrophic subaortic-stenosis. Anesthesiology 65:663, 1986.

110. Homans, D. C.: Peripartum cardiomyopathy. N. Engl. J. Med. 312:1432, 1985.

111. Demakis, J. G., Rahimtoola, S. H., Sutton, E. C., et al.: Natural course of peripartum cardiomyopathy. Circulation 44:1053, 1971.

112. Ribner, H. S., and Silverman, R. I.: Peripartal cardiomyopathy. In Elkayam, U., and Gleicher, N. (eds.): Cardiac Problems in Pregnancy: Diagnosis and Management of Maternal and Fetal Disease. 2nd ed. New York, Alan R. Liss, Inc., 1990, p. 115.

113. McAdams, S. A., and Maguire, F. E.: Unusual manifestations of peripartal cardiac disease. Crit. Care Med. 14:910, 1986.

113a. Marin-Neto, J. A., Maciel, B. C., Teran Urbanetz, L. L., et al: High output failure in patients with peripartum cardiomyopathy: A comparative study with dilated cardiomyopathy. Am. Heart J. 121:134, 1990.

114. O'Connell, J. B., Rosa Costanzo-Nordin, M., Subramanian, R., et al.: Peripartum cardiomyopathy: Clinical, hemodynamic, histologic and prognostic characteristics. J. Am. Coll. Cardiol. 8:52, 1986.

115. Midei, M. C., DeMent, S. H., Feldman, A. M., et al.: Peripartum myocarditis and cardiomyopathy. Circulation 81:922, 1990.

116. Cole, P., Cook, F., Plappert, T., et al.: Longitudinal changes in left ventricular architecture and function in peripartum cardiomyopathy. Am. J. Cardiol. 60:871, 1987.

117. Carvalho, A., Brandao, A., Martinez, E. E., et al.: Prognosis in peripartum cardiomyopathy. Am. J. Cardiol. 64:540, 1989.

118. Cotton, D. B., Longmire, S., Jones, M. M., et al.: Cardiovascular alterations in severe pregnancy-induced hypertension: Effects of intravenous nitroglycerin coupled with blood volume expansion. Am. J. Obstet. Gynecol. 154:1053, 1986.

119. Rosa, F. W., Bosco, L. A., Graham, C. F., et al.: Neonatal anuria with maternal angiotensin-converting enzyme inhibitors. Obstet. Gynecol. 74:371, 1989.

120. Brantigan, C. O., Grow, J. B., and Schoonmaker, F. W.: Extended use of intra-aortic balloon pumping in peripartum cardiomyopathy. Ann. Surg. 183:1, 1976.

121. Melvin, R. R., Richardson, P. J., Olesen, E.G.J., et al.: Peripartum cardiomyopathy due to myocarditis. N. Engl. J. Med. 307:731, 1982.

122. Mason, J. W., and O'Connell, J. B.: A model of myocarditis in humans. Circulation 81:1154, 1990.

123. Hovsepian, P. G., Ganzel, B., Sohi, G. S., et al.: Peripartum cardiomyopathy treated with a left ventricular assist device as a bridge to cardiac transplantation. South. Med. J. 82:527, 1989.

124. Aravot, D. J., Banner, N. R., Dhalla, N., et al.: Heart transplantation for peripartum cardiomyopathy. Lancet 2:1024, 1987.

125. Meadows, W. R.: Idiopathic myocardial failure in the last trimester of pregnancy and the puerperium. Circulation 15:903, 1957.

126. Seffel, H., and Susser, M.: Maternal and myocardial failure in African women. Br. Heart J. 23:43, 1961.

127. Willmer, G.: Postpartal heart disease. South. Med. J. 56:803, 1963.

128. Walsh, J., and Burch, G.: Idiopathic cardiomyopathy of the puerperium (postpartal heart disease). Circulation 32:19, 1965.

129. Stuart, K. L.: Cardiomyopathy of pregnancy and the puerperium. Q. J. Med. 37:463, 1968.

130. Brockington, I. F.: Postpartum hypertensive heart failure. Am. J. Cardiol. 27:650, 1971.

131. Lee, W., and Cotton, D. B.: Peripartum cardiomyopathy: Current concepts and clinical management. Clin. Obstet. Gynecol. 32:54, 1989.

132. St. John Sutton, M., Cole, P., Saltzman, D., et al.: Risks of cardiac dysfunction in peripartum cardiomyopathy (PPCM) with subsequent pregnancy. Circulation 80:II-320, 1989.

133. Goldman, M. E., and Meller, J.: Coronary artery disease in pregnancy. In Elkayam, U., and Gleicher, N. (eds.): Cardiac Problems in Pregnancy. 2nd ed. New York, Alan R. Liss, Inc., 1990, p. 153.

134. Sullivan, J. M., and Ramanathan, K. B.: Management of medical problems in the pregnancy—severe cardiac disease. N. Engl. J. Med. 313:304, 1985.

135. La Vecchia, C., Franceschi, S., Decarli, A., et al.: Risk factors for myocardial infarction in young women. Am. J. Epidemiol. 125:832, 1987.

136. Croft, P., and Hannaford, P. C.: Risk factors for acute myocardial infarction in women: Evidence from the Royal College of General Practitioners' Oral Contraception Study. Br. Med. J. 298:165, 1989.

137. La Vecchia, C., Decarli, A., Franceschi, S., et al.: Menstrual and reproductive factors and the risk of myocardial infarction in women under fifty-five years of age. Am. J. Obstet. Gynecol. 157:1108, 1987.

138. Raymond, R., Lynch, J., Underwood, D., et al.: Myocardial infarction and normal coronary arteriography: A 10-year clinical and risk analysis of 74 infants. J. Am. Coll. Cardiol. 11:471, 1988.

139. Ruch, A., and Duhring, J. L.: Postpartum myocardial infarction in a patient receiving bromocriptine. Obstet. Gynecol. 74:448, 1989.

140. Sonel, A., Erol, C., Oral, D., et al.: Acute myocardial infarction and normal coronary arteries in a pregnant woman. Cardiology 75:218, 1988.

141. Elkayam, U., Rose, J., and Jamison, M.: Vascular aneurysms and dissections during pregnancy: In Elkayam, U., and Gleicher, N. (eds.): Cardiac Problems in Pregnancy. 2nd ed. New York, Alan R. Liss, Inc., 1990, p. 215.

142. Movsesian, M. A., and Wray, R. B.: Postpartum myocardial infarction. Br. Heart J. 62:154, 1989.

143. Rallings, P., Exner, T., and Abraham, R.: Coronary artery vasculitis and myocardial infarction associated with antiphospholipid antibodies in a pregnant woman. Aust. N. Z. J. Med. 19:347, 1989.

144. Madjan, J. F., Walinsky, P., Cowchuck, J. F., et al.: Coronary bypass surgery during pregnancy. Am. J. Cardiol. 52:1145, 1983.

145. Cowan, N. C., de Belder, M. A., and Rothman, M. T.: Coronary angioplasty in pregnancy. Br. Heart J. 59:588, 1988.

146. Hankins, G.D.V., Wendel, G. D., Jr., Leveno, K. J., et al.: Myocardial infarction during pregnancy: A review. Obstet. Gynecol. 65:139, 1985.

147. Elkayam U: Unpublished data.

148. Szekely, P., and Snaith, L.: Paroxysmal tachycardia in pregnancy. Br. Heart J. 15:195, 1953.

149. Gleicher, N., Meller, J., Sandler, R. Z., et al.: Wolff-Parkinson-White syndrome in pregnancy. Obstet. Gynecol. 58:748, 1981.

150. O'Donnell, M., Meecham, J., Tosson, S. R., et al.: Ventricular fibrillation and reinfarction in pregnancy. Postgrad. Med. J. 63:1095, 1987.

151. Brodsky, M. A., Sato, D. A., Oster, P. D., et al.: Paroxysmal ventricular tachycardia with syncope during pregnancy. Am. J. Cardiol. 58:563, 1986.

152. Copeland, G. D., and Stern, T. N.: Wenckebach periods in pregnancy and puerperium. Am. Heart J. 56:291, 1958.

153. Sobotka, P. A., Mayer, J. H., Bauernfeind, R. A., et al.: Arrhythmias documented by 24-hr continuous ambulatory electrocardiographic monitoring in young women without apparent heart disease. Am. Heart J. 101:753, 1981.

154. Schonbaum, M., Rowland, W., and Quiroz, A. C.: Complete heart block in pregnancy. Successful use of an intravenous pacemaker in 2 patients during labor. Obstet. Gynecol. 27:243, 1966.

155. Jaffe, R., Gruber, A., Fejgin, M., et al.: Pregnancy with an artificial pacemaker. Obstet. Gynecol. Surv. 42:137, 1987.

156. Barrett, J. M., Van Hooydonk, J. E., and Boehm, F. H.: Pregnancy related rupture of arterial aneurysms. Obstet. Gynecol. Surv. 37:557, 1982.

157. Konishi, Y., Tatsuta, N., Kumada, K., et al.: Dissecting aneurysms during pregnancy and the puerperium. Jpn. Circ. J. 44:726, 1980.

158. Chandrasekaran, K., and Currie, P. J.: Transesophageal echocardiography in aortic dissection. J. Invasive Cardiol. 1:328, 1989.

159. Ishikawa, K., and Matsuura, S.: Occlusive thromboaortopathy (Takayasu's disease) and pregnancy: Clinical course and management of 33 pregnancies and deliveries. Am. J. Cardiol. 50:1293, 1982.

160. Wong, V.C.W., Wang, R.Y.E., and Tse, T. F.: Pregnancy and Takayasu's arteritis. Am. J. Med. 75:597, 1983.

161. Sise, M. J., Couniham, C. M., Shackford, S. R., et al.: The clinical spectrum of Takayasu's arteritis. Surgery 104:905, 1988.

162. Winn, H. N., Setaro, J. F., Mazor, M., et al.: Severe Takayasu's arteritis in pregnancy: The role of central hemodynamic monitoring. Am. J. Obstet. Gynecol. 159:1135, 1988.

163. Ask-Upmark, E.: Case of Takayasu's syndrome accelerated (initiated?) by oral contraceptives. Acta Med. Scand. 185:119, 1969.

164. Elkayam, U., and Gleicher, N.: Primary pulmonary hypertension and pregnancy. In Elkayam, U., and Gleicher, N., (eds.): Cardiac Problems in Pregnancy. 2nd ed. New York, Alan R. Liss, Inc., p. 189, 1990.

165. Takenchi, T., Nishii, O., Okamura, T., et al.: Primary pulmonary hypertension in pregnancy. Int. J. Gynaecol. Obstet. 26:145, 1988.

166. Rich, S., Dantzker, D. R., Ayres, S. M., et al.: Primary pulmonary hypertension: A national prospective study. Ann. Intern. Med. 107:216, 1987.

167. Fuster, V., Steele, P. M., Edwards, W. D., et al.: Primary pulmonary hypertension: Natural history and the importance of thrombosis. Circulation 70:580, 1984.

168. Nelson, D. M., Main, E., Crafford, W., et al.: Peripartum heart failure due to primary pulmonary hypertension. Obstet. Gynecol. 62:59S, 1983.

169. Abboud, T. K., Raya, J., Noueihed, R., et al.: Intrathecal morphine for relief of labor pain in a parturient with severe pulmonary hypertension. Anesthesiology 59:477, 1983.

170. Gazzaniga, A.: Cardiac surgery during pregnancy. In Elkayam, U., and Gleicher, N. (eds.): Cardiac Problems in Pregnancy. 2nd ed. New York, Alan R. Liss, Inc., 1990, p. 259.

171. El-Maraghy, M., Abon Senna, I., El-Tehewy, F., et al.: Mitral valvotomy in pregnancy. Am. J. Obstet. Gynecol. 145:708, 1983.

172. Martin, M. C., Pernall, M. L., Borhszak, A. N., et al.: Cesarean section while on cardiac bypass. Report of a case. Obstet. Gynecol. 6:41S, 1981.

173. Levy, D. L., Warriner, R. A., Burgess, G. E.: Fetal response to cardiopulmonary bypass. Obstet. Gynecol. 56:112, 1980.

174. Eilen, B., Kaiser, I., Becker, R., et al.: Aortic valve replacement in the third trimester of pregnancy. Obstet. Gynecol. 57:119, 1981.

175. Salazar, E., Zajarias, A., Gutierrez, N., et al.: The problem of cardiac valve prosthesis, anticoagulants and pregnancy. Circulation 70(Suppl. 1):169, 1984.

176. McGehee, W.: Anticoagulation in pregnancy. In Elkayam, U., and Gleicher, N. (eds.): Cardiac Problems in Pregnancy. 2nd ed. New York, Alan R. Liss, Inc., 1990, p. 397.

177. Iturbe-Alessio, I., Del Carmen Fonseca, M., Mutchinik O., et al.: Risks of anticoagulant therapy in pregnant women with artificial heart valve. N. Engl. J. Med. 315:1390, 1986.

178. Donzeau, G. P., Nguyen, A., Touchot, B., et al.: Acute thrombosis of a St. Jude medical aortic prosthesis in a pregnant woman. Thorac. Cardiovasc. Surg. 33:248, 1985.

179. Shemin, R. J., Phillippe, M., and Dzau, V.: Acute thrombosis of a composite ascending aortic conduit containing a Björk-Shiley valve during pregnancy. Successful emergency cesarean section and operative repair. Clin. Cardiol. 9:299, 1986.

180. Gonzaelz-Santos, M. L., Horno, R., and Garcia-Dorado, D.: Thrombosis of a mechanical valve prosthesis late in pregnancy. Thorac. Cardiovasc. Surg. 34:335, 1986.

181. Elkayam, U., and Gleicher, N.: Anticoagulation in pregnant women with artificial heart valves. N. Engl. J. Med. 316:1663, 1987.

182. Norris, D. C.: Management of patients with prosthetic heart valves. Curr. Probl. Cardiol. 7:1, 1982.

183. Guidozzi, F.: Pregnancy in patients with prosthetic cardiac valves. S. Afr. Med. J. 64:961, 1984.

184. Cohn, L. H.: Anticoagulation in pregnant women with artificial heart valves. N. Engl. J. Med. 316:1662, 1987.

185. Deviri, E., Yechezkel, M., Levinsky, C., et al.: Calcification of a porcine valve xenograft during pregnancy: A case report and review of the literature. Thorac. Cardiovasc. Surg. 32:266, 1984.

186. Hall, J., Pauli, R. M., and Wilson, K. M.: Maternal and fetal sequelae of anticoagulation during pregnancy. Am. J. Med. 68:122, 1980.

187. Lee, P. K., Wang, R.Y.C., Chow, J.S.F., et al.: Combined use of warfarin and adjusted subcutaneous heparin during pregnancy in patients with an artificial heart valve. J. Am. Coll. Cardiol. 8:221, 1986.

188. Oakley, C.: Valve prosthesis and pregnancy. Br. Heart J. 58:303, 1987.

CARDIOVASCULAR DRUGS IN PREGNANCY

189. Mitani, G. M., Steinberg, I., Lien, E., et al.: The pharmacokinetics of antiarrhythmic agents in pregnancy and lactation. Clin. Pharmacokinet. 12:253, 1987.

190. Mitani, G. M., Harrison, E. C., Steinberg, I., et al.: Digitalis glycosides in pregnancy. In Elkayam, U., and Gleicher, N. (eds.): Cardiac Problems in Pregnancy. 2nd ed. New York, Alan R. Liss, Inc., 1990, p. 417.

191. Lilja, H., Karlsson, K., Lindecranz, K., et al.: Treatment of intrauterine supraventricular tachycardia with digoxin and verapamil. J. Perinat. Med. 12:151, 1984.

192. Spinnato, J. A., Shaver, D. C., Flinn, G. S., et al.: Fetal supraventricular tachycardia: In utero therapy with digoxin and quinidine. Obstet. Gynecol. 64:730, 1984.

193. Gleicher, N., and Elkayam, U.: Intrauterine therapy of rhythm and rate disorders and heart failure. In Elkayam, U., and Gleicher, N. (eds.): Cardiac Problems in Pregnancy. 2nd ed. New York, Alan R. Liss, Inc., 1990, p. 749.

194. Valdes, A., Jr.: Endogenous digoxin-like immunoreactive factors: Impact on digoxin measurements and potential physiologic implications. Clin. Chem. 31:1525, 1985.

195. Fievet, P., Gregoire, I., Fournier, A., et al.: Ouabain-like natriuretic factor and atrial natriuretic factor in pregnancy. Kidney Int. 34(Suppl. 25):A-89, 1988.

196. Given, B. D., Phillippe, M., Sanders, S. P., et al.: Procainamide cardioversion of fetal supraventricular tachyarrhythmia. Am. J. Cardiol. 53:1460, 1984.

197. Pittard, W. B., II, and Glazier, H.: Procainamide excretion in human milk. J. Pediatr. 102:631, 1984.

198. Ellsworth, A. J., Horn, J. R., Raisys, V. A., et al.: Disopyramide and N-monodesalkyl disopyramide in serum and breast milk. Drug Intell. Clin. Pharmacy 23:56, 1989.

199. Hopper, K., Neuvonen, P. J., and Korte, T.: Disopyramide and breast feeding. Br. J. Clin. Pharmacol. 21:553, 1986.

200. Juneja, M. M., Ackerman, W. E., Kaczorowski, D. M., et al.: Continuous epidural lidocaine infusion in the parturient with paroxysmal ventricular tachycardia. Anesthesiology 71:549, 1989.

201. Lownes, H. E., and Ives, T. J.: Mexiletine use in pregnancy and lactation. Am. J. Obstet. Gynecol. 157:446, 1987.

202. Gregg, A. R., and Tomich, P. G.: Mexiletine use in pregnancy. J. Perinat. 8:33, 1988.

203. Foster, C. J., and Love, H. G.: Amiodarone in pregnancy: Case report and review of literature. Int. J. Cardiol. 20:307, 1988.

204. DeWolf, D., De Schlepper, H., Verhaaren, H., et al.: Congenital hypothyroid goiter and amiodarone. Acta Paediatr. Scand. 77:616, 1988.

205. Arnoux, P., Seyral, P., Llurens, M., et al.: Amiodarone and digoxin for refractory fetal tachycardia. Am. J. Cardiol. 59:166, 1987.

206. Laurent, M., Betremieux, P., Biron, Y., et al.: Neonatal hypothyroidism after treatment by amiodarone during pregnancy. Am. J. Cardiol. 60:142, 1987.

207. Belfort, M. A., and Moore, P. J.: Verapamil in the treatment of severe postpartum hypertension. S. Afr. Med. J. 74:265, 1988.

208. Maxwell, D. J., Crawford, D. C., Curry, P.V.M., et al.: Obstetric importance: Diagnosis and management of fetal tachycardia. Br. Heart J. 297:107, 1988.

209. Miller, M. R., Withers, R., Bhamra, R., et al.: Verapamil and breast feeding. Eur. J. Pharmacol. 301:125, 1986.

210. Read, M. D., and Wellby, D. E.: The use of calcium antagonist (nifedipine) to suppress preterm labor. Br. J. Obstet. Gynecol. 93:933, 1986.

211. Seabe, S. J., Moodley, J., and Becker, P.: Nifedipine in acute hypertensive emergencies in pregnancy. S. Aft. Med. J. 76:248, 1989.

212. Constantine, G., Beevers, D. G., Reynolds, A. L., et al.: Nifedipine as a second line antihypertensive drug in pregnancy. Br. J. Obstet. Gynecol. 94:1136, 1987.

213. Lindow, S. W., Davey, N., Davy, D. A., et al.: The effect of sublingual nifedipine on uteroplacental blood flow in hypertensive pregnancy. Br. J. Obstet. Gynecol. 95:1276, 1988.

214. Högstedt, S., Lindebey, S., Axelsson, O., et al.: A prospective controlled trial of metroprolol-hydralazine treatment in hypertension during pregnancy. Acta Obstet. Gynecol. Scand. 64:505, 1985.

215. Plokin, P. F., Breart, G., Maillard, F., et al.: Comparison of antihypertensive efficacy and prenatal safety of labetalol and methyldopa in the treatment of hypertension in pregnancy: A randomized controlled trial. Br. J. Obstet. Gynaecol. 95:868, 1988.

216. Jouppila, P., Kirkinen, P., Koivula, A., et al.: Labetalol does not alter the placental and fetal blood flow or maternal prostanoids in pre-eclampsia. Br. J. Obstet. Gynaecol. 93:543, 1986.

217. Lunrel, N. O., Kulas, J., Rane, A.: Transfer of labetalol into amniotic fluid and breast milk in lactating women. Eur. J. Clin. Pharmacol. 28:597, 1985.

218. Dicke, J. M.: Cardiovascular drugs in pregnancy. In Gleicher, N., Elkayam, U., Galbraith, R. M., et al. (eds.): Principles of Medical Therapy in Pregnancy. New York, Plenum, 1985, p. 646.

219. Shoemaker, C. T., and Meyers, M.: Sodium nitroprusside for control of severe hypertensive disease of pregnancy: A case report and discussion of potential toxicity. Am. J. Obstet. Gynecol. 149:171, 1984.

220. Boutroy, M. J.: Fetal effects of maternally administered clonidine and angiotensin-converting enzyme inhibitors. Dev. Pharmacol. Ther. 13:199, 1989.

221. Rosa, F. W., Bosco, L. A., Graham, C. F., et al.: Neonatal anuria with maternal angiotensin converting enzyme inhibition. Obstet. Gynecol. 74:371, 1989.

222. Are ACE inhibitors safe in pregnancy? Lancet 2:482, 1989.

223. Ferris, T. F.: Toxemia and hypertension. In Burrow, G. N., and Ferris, T. F. (eds.): Medical Complications During Pregnancy. Philadelphia, W. B. Saunders Company, 1982, p. 1.

224. Garnet, J. D.: Placental transfer of chlorothiazide. Obstet. Gynecol. 21:123, 1963.

225. Riva, E., Farina, P., Tognoni, G., et al.: Pharmacokinetics of furosemide in gestosis of pregnancy. Eur. J. Clin. Pharmacol. 14:361, 1978.

226. Sareli, P., England, M. J., Berk, H. R., et al.: Maternal and fetal sequelae of anticoagulation during pregnancy in patients with mechanical heart valve prosthesis. Am. J. Cardiol. 63:1462, 1989.

227. Becker, M. H., Genieser, N. B., Finegold, M., et al.: Chondrodysplasia punctata: Is maternal warfarin therapy a factor? Am. J. Dis. Child. 129:356, 1975.

228. Matorras, R., Reque, J. A., Usandizaga, J. A., et al.: Prosthetic heart valve and pregnancy. A study of 59 cases. Gynecol. Obstet. Invest. 19:21, 1985.

229. Wang, R.Y.C., Lee, P. K., Chow, J.S.F., et al.: Efficacy of low dose subcutaneously administered heparin in the treatment of pregnant women with artificial heart valves. Med. J. Aust. 2:126, 1983.

230. Hatjis, C. G.: Heparin-induced thrombocytopenia in pregnancy. A case report. J. Reprod. Med. 29:337, 1984.

231. DeSwiet, M., Dorrington, W., Fidler, J., et al.: Prolonged heparin therapy in pregnancy causes bone demineralization. Br. J. Obstet. Gynaecol. 90:1129, 1983.

232. Hirsh, J.: Mechanism of action and monitoring of anticoagulants. Semin. Thromb. Hemostas. 12:1, 1986.

233. Noller, K. L.: Cardiac surgery and pregnancy. In Gleicher, N., Elkayam, U., and Galbraith, R. M. (eds.): Principles of Medical Therapy in Pregnancy. New York, Plenum, 1985, p. 713.

234. Cesario, T. C.: Antibiotic therapy in pregnancy. In Elkayam, U., Gleicher, N. (eds.): Cardiac Problems in Pregnancy. 2nd ed. New York, Alan R. Liss, Inc., 1990, p. 437.

235. McCans, J., and Wenger, N.: Problems in management of the pregnant patient with rheumatic heart disease and valve prosthesis. South. Med. J. 69:1007, 1976.

236. Sugrue, D., Blake, S., Troy, P., et al.: Antibiotic prophylaxis against infective endocarditis after normal delivery. Is it necessary? Br. Heart J. 5:44, 1980.

Neurological Disorders and Heart Disease

by JOSEPH K. PERLOFF, M.D.

Cardiovascular disorders occur as consequences of diseases of the nervous system, and disorders of the nervous system occur secondary to diseases of the heart and circulation. This chapter deals with the varied and complex interplay between cardiology and neurology and focuses on six general topics: (1) major heredofamilial neuromyopathic disorders in which cardiac disease is an inherent part; (2) less common neuromyopathic disorders that are sometimes associated with diseases of the heart; (3) acute cerebral disorders accompanied by cardiovascular abnormalities; (4) cardiac complications of drugs used in treating neuromuscular diseases; (5) neurological complications of therapy for cardiovascular diseases; and (6) cardiac denervation. Cardiac causes of syncope are discussed in Chapter 30. Neurological complications associated with congenital and acquired heart disease are discussed in the chapters dealing specifically with those disorders.

MAJOR HEREDOFAMILIAL NEUROMYOPATHIC DISORDERS

Cardiac involvement is an inherent part of three major categories of heredofamilial neuromyopathic disorders: the progressive muscular dystrophies, myotonic muscular dystrophy, and Friedreich's ataxia.[1-4] The majority of non-myotonic progressive muscular dystrophies are classified as:

1. X-linked progressive muscular dystrophies
   a. Early-onset, rapidly progressive (classic Duchenne dystrophy)
   b. Late-onset, slowly progressive (Becker muscular dystrophy)
2. Limb-girdle dystrophy of Erb
3. Facioscapulohumeral dystrophy of Landouzy-Dejerine

PROGRESSIVE MUSCULAR DYSTROPHIES

Early-Onset, Rapidly Progressive X-Linked (Duchenne) Dystrophy

Classic Duchenne muscular dystrophy is a sex-linked recessive disorder, transmitted by the mother to one-half of her sons as overt disease and to one-half of her daughters as a carrier state.[5,6] The average incidence of Duchenne dystrophy in the general population is around 1 in 5000 male births, but it is believed that the true incidence is as high as 1 in 3000 male births.[7] Assuming that the mutation rate is equal in the two sexes, one-third of cases represent new mutations in either the patient or his mother.[8] Duchenne muscular dystrophy is caused by a defective gene located on the X chromosome. *Dystrophin*, the high-molecular-weight protein product of the gene, is localized to the sarcolemmal membrane of normal skeletal muscle but is absent from skeletal muscle of patients with Duchenne dystrophy.[9] The rare but well-documented cases of clinical Duchenne dystrophy in females have been attributed to X translocation of a single mutant gene at band Xp21 of the X-chromosome short arm.[7,10] The normal X is inactivated, so the mutant X-linked recessive gene expresses itself. Creatine kinase has had important but limited use in the detection of carrier females, but quantification of dystrophin on skeletal muscle biopsies has been a major step forward in carrier identification.[9]

Overt clinical manifestations usually begin in the second year of life, although there is histological and enzymatic evidence that the disease exists from birth.[5] The clumsy, waddling gait and frequent falls often go unnoticed in a child just learning to walk, and the boy's difficulty in rising from the floor by "climbing up" himself (Gowers' sign) tends to be initially ignored by parents and physicians. Because of the seemingly good muscle development and early pseudohypertrophy of the calves (Fig. 60–1), reduced strength is not ascribed to an abnormality of skeletal muscle. Lumbar lordosis, hyperextension of the knees, and shortening of the Achilles tendons contribute to a precarious balance on the toes (Fig. 60–1). Kyphoscoliosis becomes marked, and in terminal stages of the disease the boy sits in a wheelchair, twisted like a pretzel, with his head lolling unsupported because of inadequate neck muscles. Dystrophy of thoracic muscles and diaphragm together with kyphoscoliosis compromises coughing and breathing. Patients are likely to succumb to pulmonary infection in the second decade, although cardiac disease is an important and sometimes dramatic cause of death. Rapidly progressive preterminal heart failure may follow years of circulatory stability during which the chief, if not only, suspicion of cardiac involvement is an abnormal electrocardiogram (Fig. 60–2). Pulmonary emboli have been reported in patients with end-stage Duchenne dystrophy, and systemic emboli can originate in the left ventricle.[11,12]

Physical and radiological examinations of the heart disclose thoracic deformities and the high diaphragm of diaphragmatic dystrophy. A reduction in anteroposterior chest dimension is often striking and is commonly responsible for a systolic im-

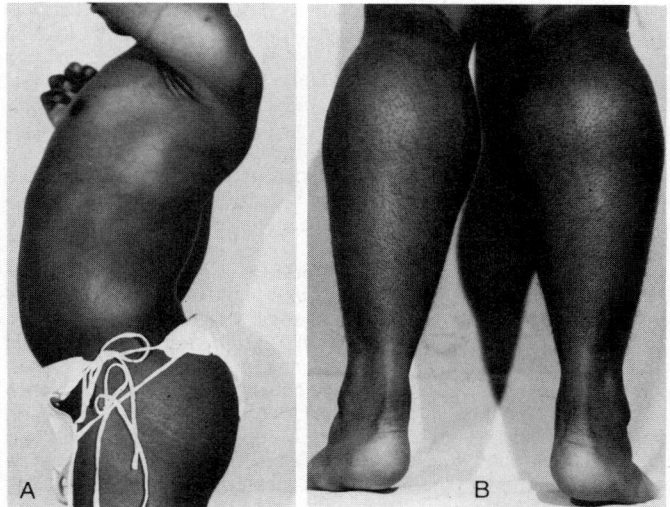

FIGURE 60–1. Classic X-linked Duchenne muscular dystrophy. *A,* Exaggerated lumbar lordosis. *B,* Calf pseudohypertrophy and shortening of the Achilles tendons.

pulse at the left sternal edge, a grade 1–3/6 short impure midsystolic murmur in the second left interspace, and a loud pulmonic component of the second heart sound. These signs should *not* be taken as evidence of pulmonary hypertension, which if present at all, occurs in the terminal stage of the disease with respiratory failure.[13] An increase in transverse heart size on x-ray examination is more often than not caused by the narrow anteroposterior chest dimension and high diaphragm rather than by ventricular dilatation.[1] The murmur of mitral regurgitation has a relatively firm anatomical basis, namely, dystrophic involvement of the posterior papillary muscle and contiguous posterobasal left ventricular wall.[14,15]

ELECTROCARDIOGRAPHY. Twenty-four-hour electrocardiographic recordings show that the most common rhythm disturbance is inappropriate sinus tachycardia,[16,17] which may be labile and gradual or abrupt in onset. The cause(s) of the rate acceleration or of relatively frequent sinus arrhythmias is(are) unknown but may involve abnormal autonomic regulation.[16,18] Alternatively, "dystrophic" disease of the sinoatrial node may prove to be the substrate not only for abnor-

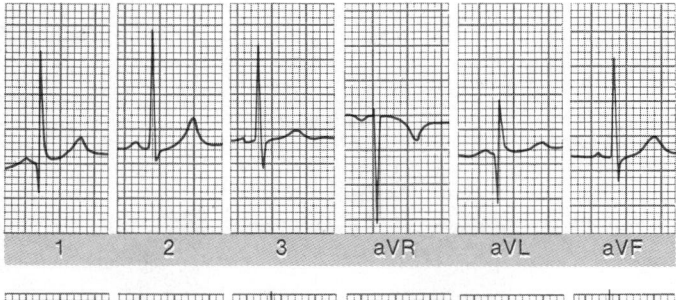

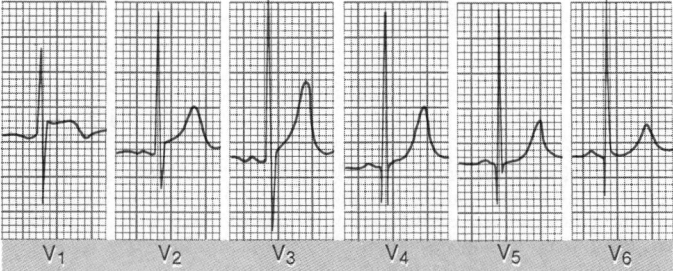

FIGURE 60–2. Electrocardiogram from a 10-year-old boy with classic Duchenne muscular dystrophy. The P-R interval is short (100 msec in lead 2). The QRS complex is typical of Duchenne dystrophy, showing an anterior shift in the right precordial leads and deep but narrow Q waves in leads I, aVl, and V$_{4-6}$. (From Perloff, J. K.: Cardiac rhythm and conduction in Duchenne's muscular dystrophy. Reprinted by permission of the American College of Cardiology. J. Am. Coll. Cardiol. 3:1263, 1984.)

mal sinus node automaticity but also for sinus node reentry and labile sinus tachycardia, especially the abrupt-onset type.[16] Intraatrial or interatrial conduction abnormalities are not uncommon. An abnormal P-terminal force in lead V$_1$ in the presence of normal left atrial size on the echocardiogram implies an intrinsic disorder of left atrial or interatrial conduction.[17] It is unclear whether the conduction disorder sets the stage for unstable atrial rhythms (see below).

In approximately 50 per cent of patients, atrioventricular (AV) conduction, as judged by the P-R interval, is either definitely or marginally accelerated without delta waves (Fig. 60–2).[16] Short P-R intervals may represent atriofascicular bypass tracts or accelerated conduction within the AV node (p. 696).[16] Paroxysmal rapid heart action via bypass tracts is, however, unknown in Duchenne dystrophy, and atrial flutter, a common preterminal arrhythmia, has not been reported with 1:1 AV conduction.[16,19,20] Proximal infranodal conduction abnormalities sometimes take the form of a rightward QRS axis that implies left posterior fascicular block.[16] Significant electrical ventricular instability seldom occurs despite regional left ventricular dystrophy. Multiform ventricular premature complexes, couplets, and episodes of ventricular tachycardia are uncommon but not unknown, especially as the disease advances.[16] Death is occasionally sudden.

Disorders of atrial rhythm are more common than are disturbances of ventricular rhythm, even though involvement of atrial myocardium is relatively scant.[14,15,20,21] These observations suggest that ectopic atrial rhythms are prompted by abnormalities of specialized conduction tissues. A similar speculation applies to the observed or reported disorders of infranodal conduction.[16]

The standard scalar electrocardiogram is the simplest and most reliable tool for detecting cardiac involvement in Duchenne dystrophy (Fig. 60–2).[1,15,22,23] Abnormal electrocardiograms are present even in early childhood.[23,24] Tall right precordial R waves and increased R/S amplitude ratios together with deep Q waves in leads 1, aV$_1$, and V$_{5,6}$ are characteristic of the classic rapidly progressive pseudohypertrophic X-linked dystrophy of Duchenne (Fig. 60–2).[15,17,20,25] A reduction in or a loss of electromotive force caused by myocardial dystrophy in the posterobasal left ventricular wall (anterior shift of the QRS) and contiguous lateral wall (deep Q waves in leads 1, aV$_1$, and V$_{5,6}$) is believed to be responsible for the characteristic electrocardiogram.[1,15,17] Necropsy studies have disclosed that these regions are the initial and most extensive sites of myocardial fibrosis (Fig. 60–3),[15,17,20] which is preceded by ultrastructural (subcellular) abnormalities.[17] Electron microscopic examination of right ventricular endomyocardial biopsy specimens has identified abnormalities of mitochondria, C bands, sarcoplasmic reticulum, and nuclei.[26] Primary posterobasal involvement spreads to the epicardial third of the contiguous lateral left ventricular free wall, with progressive transmural fibrous replacement.[17,21] There is relative sparing of the ventricular septum and comparatively little involvement of right ventricular and atrial myocardia.[15,17,21] Based on these observations, Duchenne dystrophy emerges as a unique form of heart disease characterized by a genetically determined predilection for specific regions of the heart — the posterobasal and lateral left ventricular walls.[1,15,17,25] Interestingly, relatively specific electrocardiographic and histopathological abnormalities have been reported in dystrophic hamsters with cardiomyopathy.[27]

HISTOLOGICAL FINDINGS. Light microscopy has disclosed fatty infiltration and mild fibrosis in the sinus and AV nodes, although there is little or no evidence of degeneration of the conduction fibers themselves in either of these nodes or in the His bundle.[28] However, the peripheral conduction system (Purkinje fibers) shows significant degeneration (eosinophilic, necrotic, and vascular changes with fibrosis).[28] In two light microscopic studies, fibers in the sinus node, His bundle, and proximal bundle branch were normal.[15,29] Ultrastructural data on specialized cardiac tissues are scanty and inconclusive.[17] The small intramural coronary arteries are sometimes

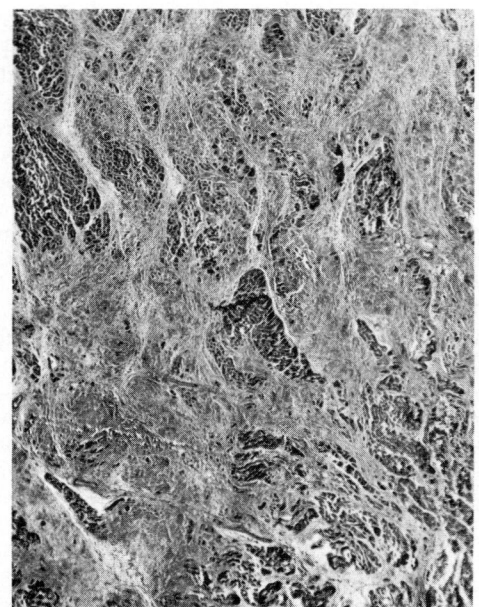

FIGURE 60-3. Photomicrograph from an 18-year-old boy who died of classic Duchenne progressive muscular dystrophy. The posterobasal left ventricular wall is extensively scarred (hematoxylin and eosin stains). (From Perloff, J. K., et al.: The distinctive electrocardiogram of Duchenne's muscular dystrophy. Am. J. Med. 42:179, 1967.)

thick walled, with varying degrees of luminal narrowing.[15,21,29] The arteriopathy occasionally involves sinus nodal and AV nodal arteries,[15,20,29] but an association between the small-vessel coronary arteriopathy and abnormalities of rhythm and conduction remains speculative.

Mitral regurgitation may occur in Duchenne dystrophy. The cause is papillary muscle dysfunction (dystrophic involvement of the posterolateral papillary muscle and contiguous left ventricular wall) rather than an abnormality of leaflets, chordae tendineae, and annulus.[14]

Malignant hyperthermia and cardiac arrest have occurred during anesthesia in a number of children with Duchenne muscular dystrophy after use of halothane, suxamethonium, isoflurane, and succinylcholine.[30,31]

POSITRON EMISSION TOMOGRAPHY (see also p. 302)

Investigators have sought to ascertain whether regional metabolic, perfusion, or wall-motion abnormalities were present during life in patients with Duchenne dystrophy.[2,32] To determine whether segmental abnormalities of the left ventricular wall were present in living subjects, noninvasive methods, including positron-emission tomography (see p. 304) using radioactive tracers for metabolism, supplemented by thallium-201 perfusion scans, gated equilibrium radionuclide angiography, and two-dimensional echocardiography, were employed.[2,32] Accelerated exogenous glucose (^{18}F fluorodeoxyglucose) utilization in the posterobasal and contiguous lateral left ventricular walls (Fig. 60-4) provided evidence of a regional myocardial metabolic abnormality[2] (p. 536). [13]NH₃ activity was reduced in segments in which uptake of exogenous glucose was accelerated (Fig. 60-4). These sites corresponded to those of primary dystrophic replacement found at necropsy.[15,17,20]

The observed regional increases in ^{18}F fluorodeoxyglucose concentrations are believed to indicate a segmental alteration in membrane permeability, an increase in the rate of phosphorylation due to the abnormality in adenyl cyclase identified in skeletal muscle,[33,34] or a compensatory increase in glycolysis in response to a decline in fatty acid oxidation.[2] Regional decreases in [13]NH₃ activity in Duchenne dystrophy (Fig. 60-4) are believed to reflect a metabolic abnormality, a regional decrease in flow, or both of these causes.[2]

EARLY FINDINGS. Early in the natural history (i.e., in very young patients), segmental reductions in [13]NH₃ probably reflect altered regional myocardial metabolic uptake and trapping of the isotope.[2] If these alterations in the myocardium are analogous to those in skeletal muscle in Duchenne dystrophy, a longer diffusion distance of an altered ionic milieu could decrease the extraction fractions of [13]NH₃.[2] Regional depletion of the pool of glutamic acid, which binds the tracer in tissue, might also contribute to a segmental reduction in [13]NH₃.[2]

LATE FINDINGS. Regional perfusion defects sometimes occur in older patients with Duchenne dystrophy, as demonstrated by thallium scintigraphy. In these late stages of the disease, decreased perfusion might contribute to segmental reductions in [13]NH₃ activity.[2] It is likely that the mechanism(s) governing a regional reduction in myocardial blood flow relate(s) to a decrease in the number of myofibers per unit mass (fibrous replacement) and/or to an increase in the number of intrinsically injured but viable posterobasal and lateral left ventricular myocardial cells that require less oxygen and, accordingly, less flow.[2] Necropsy studies (light microscopy) identified no luminal narrowing of extramural or intramural coronary arteries in the involved segments.[15]

MECHANISM OF ABNORMAL POSITRON-EMISSION TOMOGRAPHY FINDINGS. It has been hypothesized that the regional myocardial abnormalities of ^{18}F fluorodeoxyglucose and [13]NH₃ activity represent secondary metabolic alterations initiated by the basic defect in cardiac plasma cell membrane[2] represented in skeletal muscle by absence from the sarcolemmal membrane of dystrophin, the protein product of the Duchenne muscular dystrophy gene (see earlier).[9] Current evidence—both ultrastructural and biochemical—supports the proposition that the fundamental structural and biochemical abnormalities in Duchenne dystrophy reside in plasma cell membranes, not only in those of striated (skeletal and cardiac) muscle fibers but also in those of red blood cells and probably also of fibroblasts.[35-38]

If a reduction in or loss of posterolateral left ventricular electrical forces is the cause of the distinctive electrocardiogram in Duchenne dystrophy,[1,15,17] this loss of forces does not require transmural replacement of

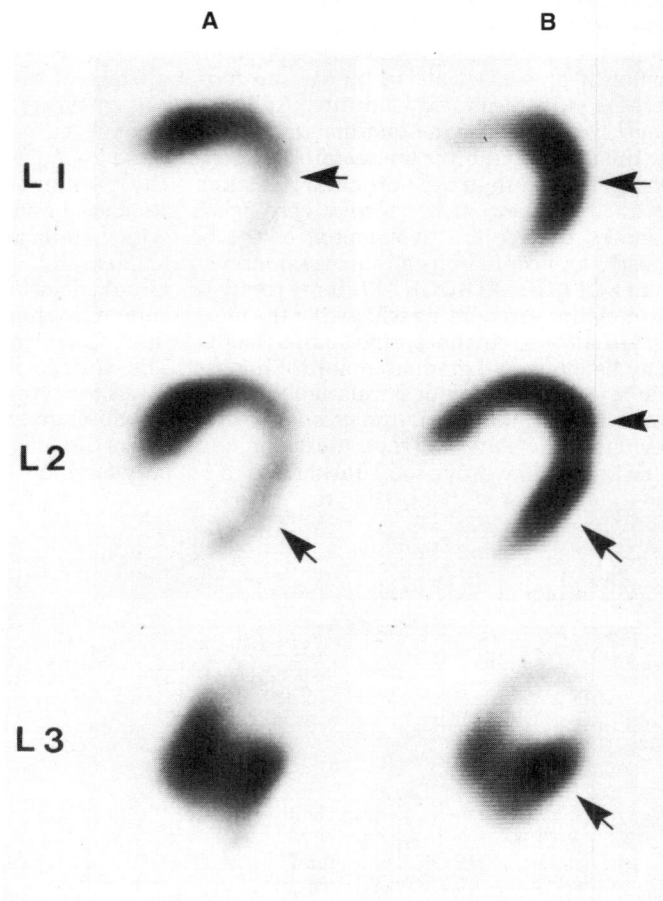

FIGURE 60-4. Regional myocardial uptake of [13]NH₃ (*A*) and ^{18}F fluorodeoxyglucose (*B*) visualized in three contiguous positron CT images of left ventricular myocardium in a 24-year-old man with classic Duchenne dystrophy. There is a segmental decrease in [13]NH₃ activity in the posterolateral wall (arrows) with a discordant increase in ^{18}F fluorodeoxyglucose concentration in the same region (arrows). This patient had a moderate posterolateral thallium-201 defect, posterolateral akinesis on technetium-99m radionuclide imaging, and a left ventricular ejection fraction of 46 per cent. (From Perloff, J. K., et al.: Alterations in regional myocardial metabolism, perfusion and wall motion in Duchenne muscular dystrophy studied by radionuclide imaging. Circulation 69:33, 1984, by permission of The American Heart Association, Inc.)

myocardium by inert connective tissue. Increased ^{18}F fluorodeoxyglucose concentrations in these areas together with normal regional wall motion are consistent with the presence of abnormal but viable (metabolically active) contracting myofibers or the preservation of a sufficient population of normal myofibers.[2]

RELEASE OF MUSCLE ENZYMES

Skeletal muscle enzymes are copiously released into the plasma in Duchenne dystrophy. It was hoped that distinctive profiles of an isozyme, such as MB creatine phosphokinase (CPK), might be used to identify active myocardial dystrophy, but the isozyme originates in dystrophic skeletal muscle and not in cardiac muscle, thus compromising the specificity of the determination.[39,40] CPK quantification is a useful but limited means of identifying carrier females in families with Duchenne dystrophy.[41,42] However, dystrophin quantification in skeletal muscle biopsies has been the major step forward in diagnosing carrier females[9] who sometimes manifest occult or overt muscle weakness and mild calf pseudohypertrophy[41,43] in addition to electrocardiographic evidence of cardiac involvement.[41,42,44–46] Electrocardiograms in carrier females differ significantly from those of normal adult women, with R/S ratios larger in leads V_{1-2} in the carrier group.[42,44] Cardiac involvement in female carriers is occasionally expressed overtly as dilated cardiomyopathy.[44,46]

Late-Onset, Slowly Progressive X-Linked (Becker) Dystrophy

A type of X-linked recessive muscular dystrophy that resembles Duchenne dystrophy was first described by Becker.[5,6,47–49] Becker dystrophy can now be distinguished from Duchenne dystrophy by dystrophin assays of skeletal muscle biopsies. In Becker dystrophy, the protein product of the gene is present but abnormal in molecular weight, while in Duchenne dystrophy the protein product is absent or scanty but of normal molecular weight.[9] The Becker and Duchenne muscular dystrophy genes are on separate but close regions of the short arm of the X chromosome.

Becker dystrophy is later in onset and slower in progression than Duchenne dystrophy, with most patients remaining ambulant into adulthood[5] (Fig. 60–5). Becker dystrophy has been called benign sex-linked muscular dystrophy,[48] a designation more appropriate for the skeletal muscle disease than for the heart disease.[1,50] Skeletal muscle impairment is sometimes relatively mild and slowly progressive, while the cardiomyopathy is severe and rapidly progressive.[51–53]

Because the diagnosis of Becker dystrophy was less than secure before the advent of dystrophin assays, some reports of

the incidence and type of associated heart disease are open to question. There is evidence, however, that the frequency of cardiac involvement increases after adolescence, and patients who reach adulthood not only have cardiomyopathy but may succumb to it[51,54] (Fig. 60–6). The type of cardiac disease differs substantially from that of Duchenne dystrophy.[51–53,55] All four chambers are involved, with dilatation and failure of the ventricles (Fig. 60–6) in addition to abnormalities of the His bundle and of infranodal conduction that express themselves as fascicular block and complete heart block (Fig. 60–6).

LIMB-GIRDLE DYSTROPHY OF ERB

The heterogeneous collection of conditions designated limb-girdle dystrophy is perhaps the most poorly defined group within the major muscular dystrophies.[5] There is variation in the mode of inheritance, the age of onset, and progression of the illness, as well as in the distribution of muscle weakness. If there is a dominant theme, it is represented by the combination of onset in late childhood or adolescence with difficulty walking; the pelvic girdle is chiefly affected, the upper limbs and shoulder girdle less so, and the face spared. Because of disproportionate pelvic involvement, the patient is often confined to a wheelchair even though skeletal deformities are infrequent.[5] Calf pseudohypertrophy occurs but is relatively late in onset and mild to moderate in degree. Because limb-girdle dystrophy has been poorly defined, conclusions regarding the type and prevalence of heart disease cannot be drawn with confidence. Disorders of cardiac muscle (cardiomyopathy) and of the cardiac conduction system have been reported.[56,57]

FACIOSCAPULOHUMERAL DYSTROPHY (LANDOUZY-DEJERINE)

Facioscapulohumeral dystrophy is inherited as an autosomal dominant with strong penetrance and an incidence estimated at three to ten cases per million population.[5] The disease typically becomes overt at the end of the first decade or the beginning of the second. Facial weakness may be signaled initially by no more than inability to whistle or drink through a straw. More distinctive and troublesome is inability to close the eyes, even during sleep. The face ultimately becomes smooth and the forehead unlined; loss of the normal upward curvature of the lower lip creates a pouting appearance, and the only marks on an otherwise expressionless face are the dimples on either side of the angles of the mouth (Fig. 60–7). Concurrently, the muscles of the arms and shoulders (scapulohumeral) are involved, and winging of the scapulae becomes apparent (Fig. 60–7). Infrequently, the disease expresses itself in infancy and runs a rapid course that leads to death in adolescence.[58] Asymptomatic or minimally affected parents may have severely affected offspring with the infantile form of the disease.[58]

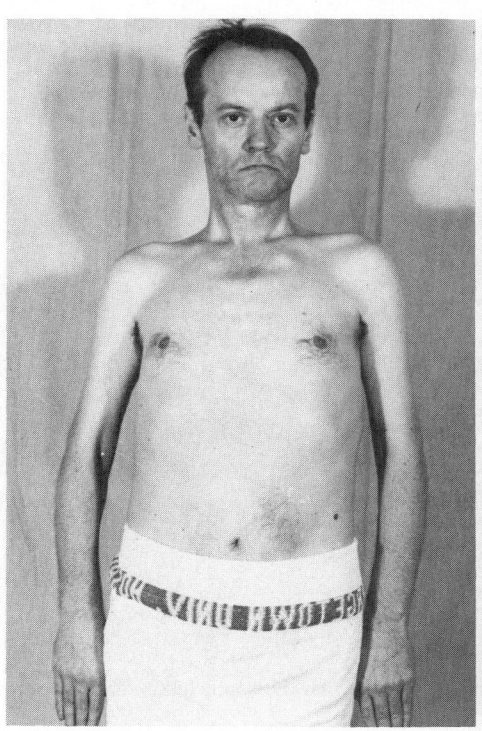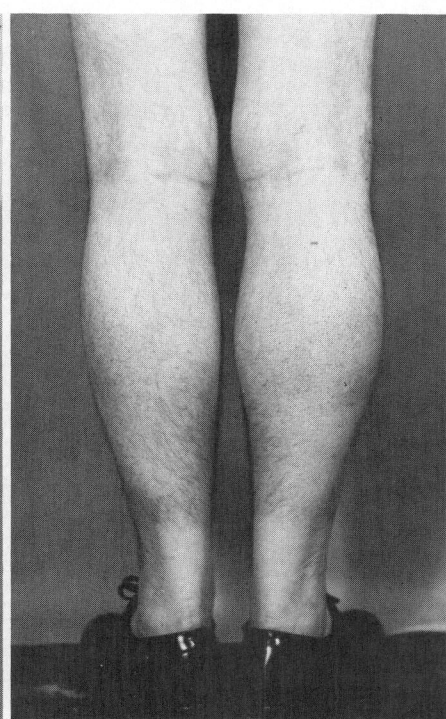

FIGURE 60–5. A 40-year-old man believed to have late-onset, slowly progressive Becker dystrophy. He died because of cardiomyopathy and complete heart block. Dystrophy of shoulder girdle, arms, pelvic girdle, and proximal leg muscle is seen, with mild asymmetrical pseudohypertrophy of the calves. (From Perloff, J. K., et al.: The cardiomyopathy of progressive muscular dystrophy. Circulation 33:625, 1966, by permission of The American Heart Association, Inc.)

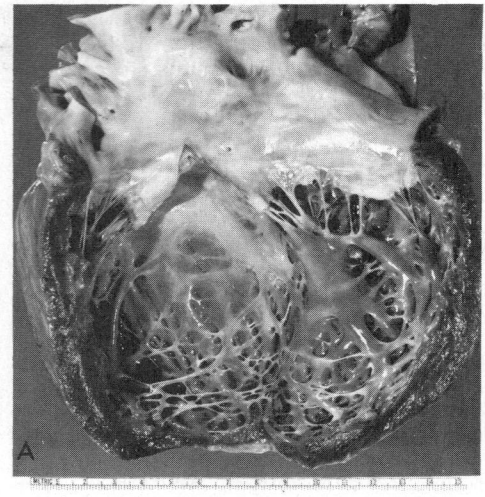

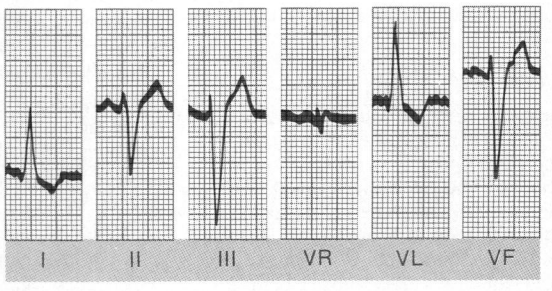

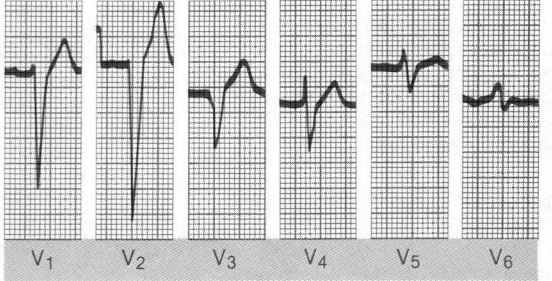

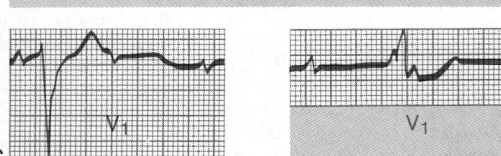

FIGURE 60-6. Gross and microscopic cardiac pathological specimens and the electrocardiogram from a 45-year-old man with late-onset, slowly progressive Becker muscular dystrophy. A, Dilated, flabby left ventricle with focal endocardial thickening. The left atrium is also dilated. B, Microscopic section from the left ventricle shows marked confluent scarring with variations in fiber size; there was no significant coronary artery disease. C, Electrocardiogram recorded at age 40 years. The 12-lead tracing shows left-axis deviation, a QRS of 0.14 sec, small Q waves in leads I and aVl and loss of R-wave amplitude in leads V₂ and V₃. The lower tracings, taken 4 years later (a year before death), show complete heart block with a variable QRS configuration. (From Perloff, J. K., et al.: The cardiomyopathy of progressive muscular dystrophy. Circulation 33:625, 1966, by permission of The American Heart Association, Inc.)

CARDIAC FINDINGS. The type of cardiac abnormality previously ascribed to facioscapulohumeral dystrophy (adult form) was a unique variety of heart disease — permanent atrial paralysis. However, the cases reported as facioscapulohumeral dystrophy[59-61] are now believed to have been phenotypically similar to Emery-Dreifuss dystrophy (see below).[62] The first secure evidence of cardiac involvement in facioscapulohumeral dystrophy was reported only recently in a prospective investigation of the electrophysiological properties of the atria and AV node and infranodal conduction in 30 rigorously documented cases.[62] The involvement was not represented by atrial paralysis but by a relatively high susceptibility to induced atrial flutter or fibrillation during electrophysiological study, together with less frequent evidence of abnormal sinus node function and abnormal AV nodal or infranodal conduction.[62] It was hypothesized that the genetic marker for facioscapulohumeral dystrophy resulted in a form of cardiac involvement analogous to but much more benign than that in phenotypically similar but genetically distinct Emery-Dreifuss dystrophy and its variants.[62]

EMERY-DREIFUSS MUSCULAR DYSTROPHY

Emery-Dreifuss dystrophy has been separated from facioscapulohumeral dystrophy, which it superficially resembles.[63-65] Scapulohumeral

and scapuloperoneal muscular dystrophy are believed to be genetic variants of the Emery-Dreifuss form.[66-69] Emery-Dreifuss dystrophy is an X-linked disorder characterized by slowly progressive muscle wasting and weakness with a humeral-peroneal distribution and early contractures of the elbows, Achilles tendons, and postcervical muscles. Permanent paralysis of the atria (atrial standstill) is the unusual if not unique form of electrophysiological heart disease that occurs in Emery-Dreifuss dystrophy; partial or permanent atrial standstill has also been reported as an isolated disorder in adults, rarely in children, and occasionally in families.[70-74] Criteria for the diagnosis of atrial paralysis include absence of P waves on scalar, esophageal, and intracardiac electrocardiograms; lack of response to direct (intracardiac) electrical or mechanical stimulation of the atria; absence of a waves in the jugular venous and right atrial pressure pulses; a supraventricular QRS; and immobility of the atria on fluoroscopy or on two-dimensional echocardiography.[72] The entire atrial myocardium ultimately becomes inexcitable, but prior to this stage, atrial standstill appears to be regional, with certain focal areas that are inert while others are subject to enhanced atrial electrical activity (atrial tachycardia or flutter).[71,73,74] Permanent atrial paralysis, atrial fibrillation, and atrial flutter are features of Emery-Dreifuss dystrophy, but the greatest threats are abnormalities of infranodal conduction with slow junctional

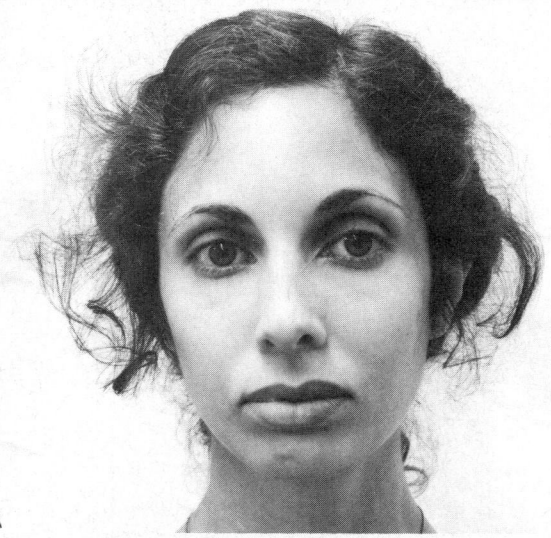

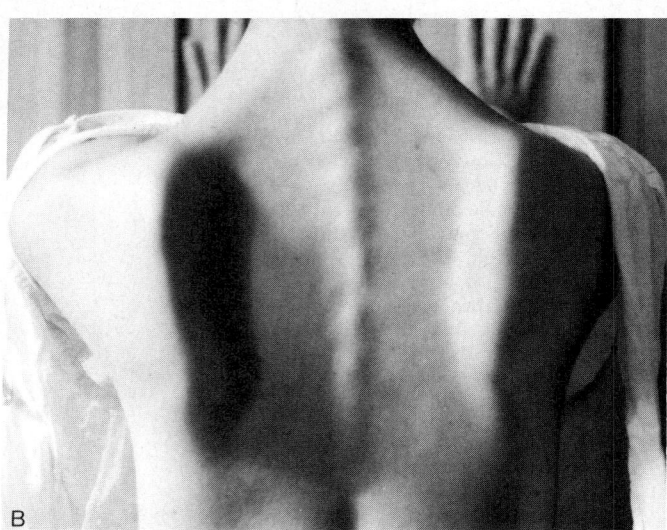

FIGURE 60-7. Facioscapulohumeral muscular dystrophy in 32-year-old woman. A, The face is in repose (myopathic). B, Typical winging of the scapulae.

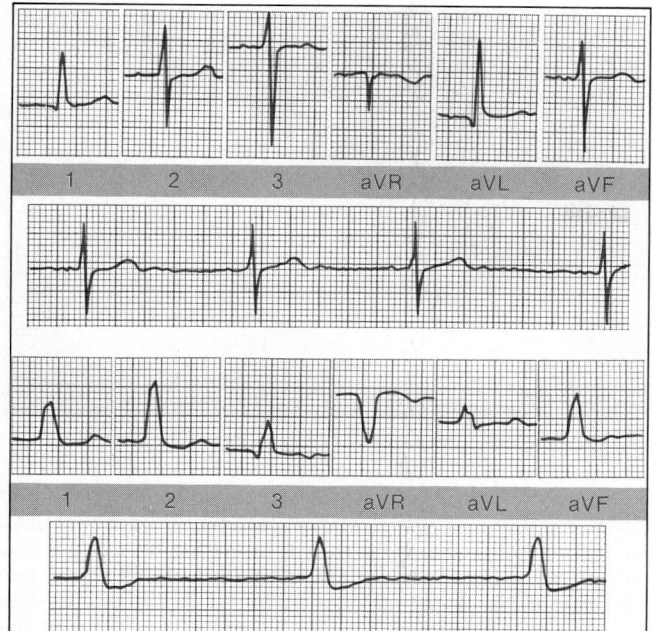

FIGURE 60-8. Limb leads and rhythm strips from two patients, a 16-year-old son (*upper*) and his 38-year-old father (*lower*) with Emery-Dreifuss muscular dystrophy. The son's tracing shows left anterior fascicular block. The P waves are low voltage and bifid, and the rate is bradycardiac. The father's tracing shows complete left bundle branch block. There is fine atrial fibrillation with a slow ventricular response. A pacemaker was inserted a month later.

rhythms or complete AV block[64,67,75,76,79-82] (Fig. 60-8). A permanent pacemaker is often required. It is the cardiac involvement, not the systemic neuromuscular disease, that places the patient at risk. In addition to the defects in rhythm and conduction in Emery-Dreifuss dystrophy and its genetic variants, myocardial fibrosis has been described at necropsy[78] and on myocardial biopsy.[67]

MYOTONIC MUSCULAR DYSTROPHY

Myotonic muscular dystrophy (Steinert's disease) is a multisystem disorder inherited as an autosomal dominant (locus on chromosome 19) with an estimated incidence between three and five per 100,000 population, making it a relatively common neuromuscular disease.[83,84] A consistent and early feature is weakness of the flexor muscles of the neck; atrophy of the sternocleidomastoid muscles often progresses to virtual disappearance. The phenotype of the adult with myotonic dystrophy is characteristic.[5,83] The presence of myotonia (delayed relaxation after contraction) is provoked by voluntary, mechanical, or electrical stimulation of muscles of the hands, forearms, tongue, and jaw. Myotonic responses are best elicited by tapping the thenar eminence (percussion myotonia),

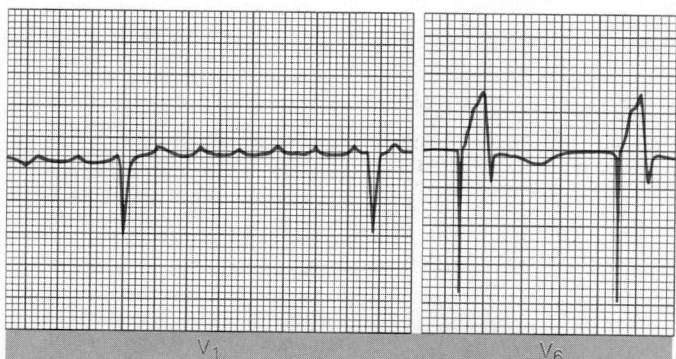

FIGURE 60-9. Rhythm strip from a 34-year-old man with myotonic muscular dystrophy. Lead V_1 shows atrial flutter, with high degree heart block. A syncopal episode prompted insertion of a right ventricular pacemaker (lead V_6).

especially after patients rapidly open and close their fists. Myotonic dystrophy is a systemic disease with important non-myotonic/nonmyopathic features, including cataracts, testicular atrophy, premature baldness, mental deterioration, and involvement of smooth muscle (esophagus, colon, uterus).[83]

Clinically important cardiac manifestations generally reside in specialized tissues rather than in myocardium.[3,85-87] Involvement is relatively specific, primarily assigned to the His-Purkinje system. At necropsy the most frequent histopathological lesions of the cardiac conduction system are fibrosis, fatty infiltration, and atrophy involving the sinus node, AV node, His bundle, and bundle branches.[88] Involvement of cardiac muscle, generally occult, takes the form of dystrophy rather than myotonia and is not selective, appearing with approximately equal distribution in all four chambers.[3] Myocardial dystrophy may be responsible for atrial and ventricular arrhythmias, including sinus bradycardia, premature atrial beats, atrial flutter (Fig. 60-9), atrial fibrillation, premature ventricular beats, and ventricular tachycardia.[89-91] Preferential selection of the His-Purkinje system (80 per cent of patients) is reflected in intraventricular conduction defects, prolongation of the H-V interval and of the effective refractory period of the right bundle branch, the development of right bundle branch block, or some other abnormal response to atrial pacing or extrastimuli.[3] The most common electrocardiographic abnormalities—prolongation of the P-R interval, left anterior fascicular block, increased QRS duration—reflect the His-Purkinje disease that can progress rapidly, although neither the scalar electrocardiogram nor a single H-V interval predicts the rate of progression.[92] His-Purkinje disease can culminate in fatal Stokes-Adams episodes unless anticipated and treated by pacemaker insertion[90,93,94] (Fig. 60-9). Although sudden death caused by AV block is relatively rare, it is the most grave cardiac threat in myotonic dystrophy. Ventricular tachycardia has also been held responsible for sudden death.[87,91]

The myocardium is seldom involved extensively enough to cause clinically overt signs or symptoms.[3] Fewer than 10 per cent of patients have clinical evidence of heart failure.[88] The electrocardiogram is a sensitive determinant of involvement of specialized cardiac tissues but not of myocardium. Nevertheless, abnormal Q waves with normal coronary arteries indicate regional myocardial dystrophy (Fig. 60-10). Findings on light microscopic examination of the myocardium vary from few or no changes to focal or diffuse fatty infiltration and fibrosis in all four cardiac chambers.[90,95-97] Apart from abnor-

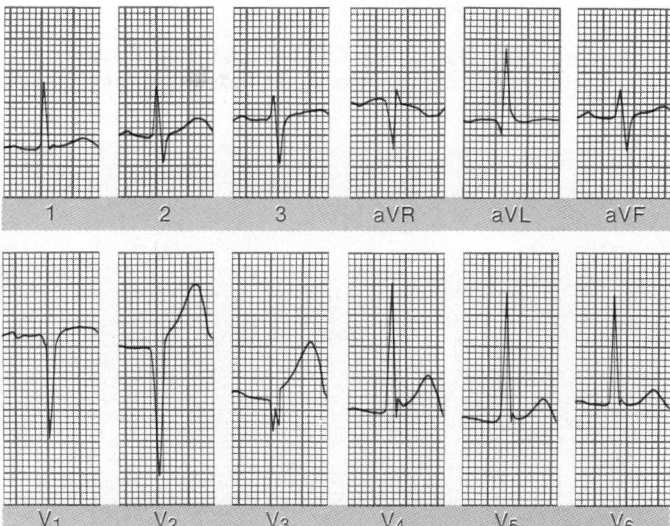

FIGURE 60-10. Electrocardiogram from a 38-year-old man with myotonic muscular dystrophy. Prominent QS deformities are present in leads V_{1-3}. The P-R interval is 0.21 sec and the frontal plane QRS axis is horizontal. (From Perloff, J. K., et al.: Cardiac involvement in myotonic muscular dystrophy [Steinert's disease]: A prospective study of 25 patients. Am. J. Cardiol. *54*:1074, 1984.)

malities of initial forces in the electrocardiogram, occult clinical involvement of the myocardium can be assessed by radionuclide angiography during exercise.[3,98]

Myotonia in skeletal muscle reflects the inability of the muscle cell membrane to reestablish its resting membrane potential quickly after contraction. Whether significant myotonia occurs in cardiac muscle is unproven. Should that be the case, the physiological derangement would, in all probability, be a relatively mild abnormality of diastolic relaxation. There is recent evidence that this, in fact, may be so.[99]

Myotonic dystrophy is genetically transmitted, with complete expression of the gene toward striated muscle tissue, whether skeletal or cardiac.[3] Because specialized cardiac tissues and myocardium have close embryological origins, it is not surprising that the genetic marker affects both. Cardiac involvement is therefore an integral part of myotonic dystrophy with the genetic marker targeting the infranodal conduction system, the sinus node to a lesser extent, and still less specifically the myocardium.[3,100]

An important variation from the above pattern is seen in the offspring of mothers with myotonic dystrophy.[83] The disorder in infants expresses itself as hypotonia and facial paralysis with no evidence of myotonia, at least initially. Respiratory distress is largely responsible for neonatal death from congenital myotonic dystrophy.[83] Affected children have characteristic facies with the upper lip forming a cupid's bow. Studies on cardiac involvement are limited but have reportedly disclosed atrioventricular and intraventricular conduction defects, less commonly reduced left ventricular systolic function.[101] Apart from genetic transmission from the mother (cytoplasmic inheritance), pregnancy is hazardous to the gravida with myotonic dystrophy.[83]

Myotonia congenita (Thomsen's disease) and *paramyotonia congenita* must be distinguished from myotonic muscular dystrophy.[83] Thomsen's disease is characterized by myotonia but not dystrophy. In fact, the skeletal muscles are well developed, even hypertrophied.[5,83] Because the natural history of Thomsen's disease is benign, longevity permits secure conclusions regarding cardiac involvement, which is conspicuously absent. In a single case, cardiac conduction abnormalities similar to those found in myotonic dystrophy were reported.[102] Paramyotonia congenita is an uncommon to rare autosomal dominant disorder characterized by prolonged myotonic reaction to cold.[5,103,104] Dystrophy of skeletal muscle is absent, and cardiac involvement is unknown.

FRIEDREICH'S ATAXIA

The hereditary ataxias are divided into (1) the hereditary spinocerebellar ataxia of Friedreich, (2) hereditary ataxia

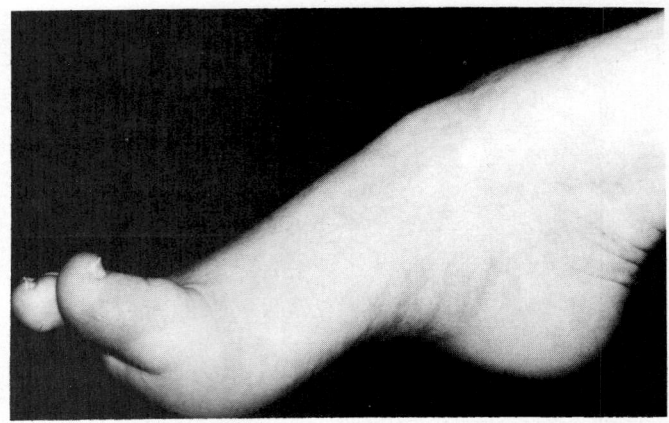

FIGURE 60–11. Pes cavus with hammer toe (Friedreich's foot).

with muscular atrophy (Roussy-Lévy syndrome), (3) hereditary spinocerebellar ataxia, and (4) olivopontocerebellar atrophy.[105] Despite a century of lively interest, Friedreich's ataxia has resisted precise clinical and biochemical definition, and there is still disagreement about where this spinocerebellar degenerative disease fits into the complex framework of the hereditary ataxias.[105-107] It is important to underscore, however, that the disorder is essentially neurological rather than myopathic.[105-107] Friedreich's ataxia is inherited as an autosomal recessive trait and is characterized by ataxia of the limbs and trunk, absence of tendon reflexes, extensor plantar responses, and loss of proprioceptive sensations in the limbs.[107] There are no remissions; instead, ataxia of gait and muscle weakness progress relentlessly, affecting first the lower limbs and then all four extremities. Pes cavus (Friedreich's foot) (Fig. 60–11) and kyphoscoliosis develop within a few years of onset.

When strict neurological and genetic criteria were used to identify a clinically homogeneous group of patients with Friedreich's ataxia, the incidence of cardiac involvement exceeded 90 per cent.[4,108-114] Severe ataxia occurs long before overt heart disease, and there is no relationship between the degrees of neurological and cardiac involvement.[4] Nevertheless, cardiac disease is often the cause of death.[4,115] There is reason to believe that phenotypically identical Friedreich patients are not genetically homogeneous, so the cardiac expressions might be expected to vary. This, in fact, proved to be the case in a prospective study of 75 patients.[4] Cardiac involvement, usually occult and asymptomatic, is the rule.[115,116] Scalar electrocardiography and echocardiography detected one or more abnormalities in 95 per cent of study patients.[4]

HYPERTROPHIC CARDIOMYOPATHY. The most com-

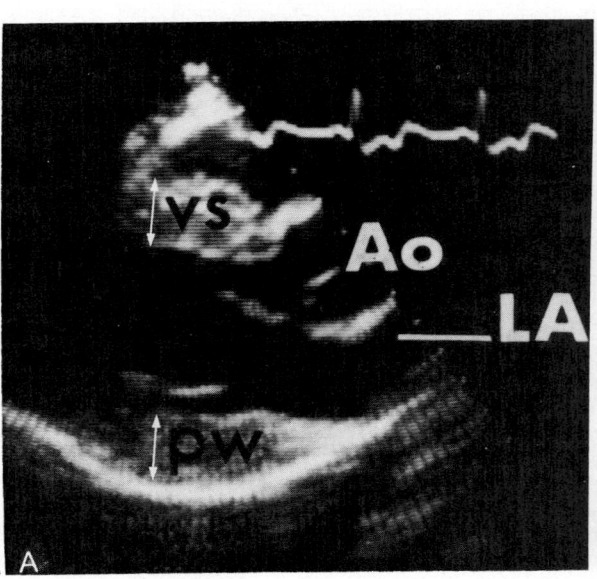
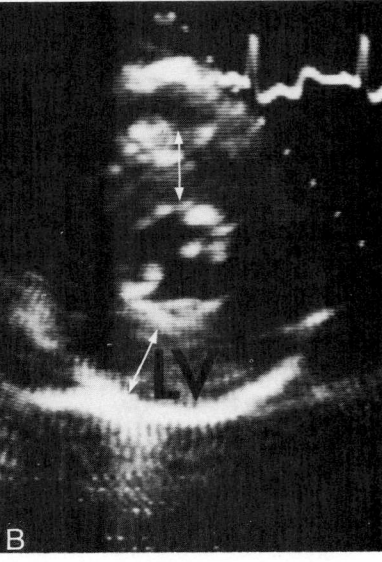

FIGURE 60–12. Two-dimensional echocardiographic parasternal long-axis view (*A*) and short-axis view (*B*) in a 16-year-old boy with Friedreich's ataxia and concentric left ventricular hypertrophy. When he was 13 years of age, the echocardiogram was normal. Ao = aorta; LA = left atrium; LV = left ventricle; PW = posterior wall; VS = ventricular septum. (From Child, J. S., et al.: Cardiac involvement in Friedreich's ataxia. Reprinted by permission of the American College of Cardiology. J. Am. Coll. Cardiol. 7:1370, 1986.)

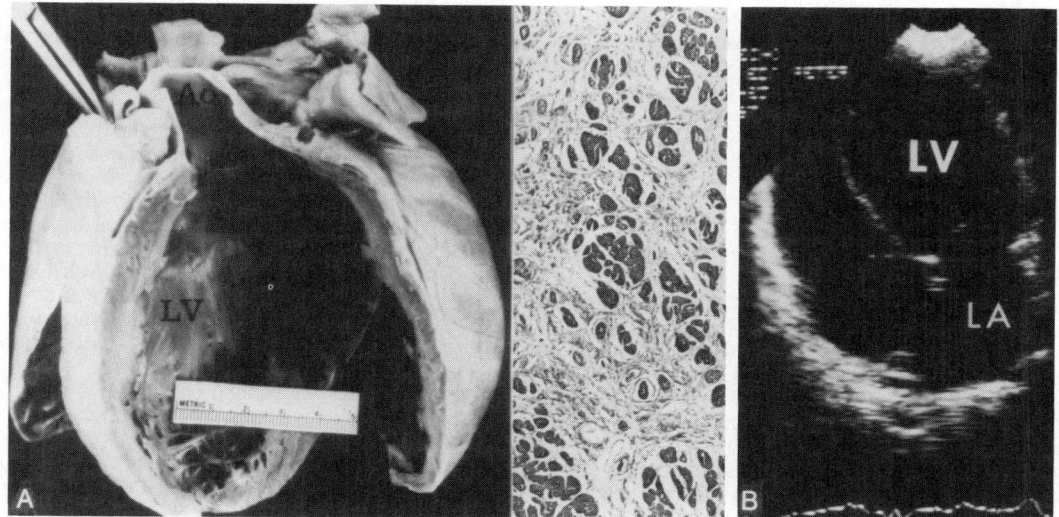

FIGURE 60-13. *A*, Gross and histological specimens from a 17-year-old boy with Friedreich's ataxia whose echocardiogram progressed from normal at age 13 years to a minimally dilated, hypocontractile left ventricle 3 to 4 years later. The gross specimen shows a mildly dilated left ventricle with normal wall thickness; the walls were flabby. The microscopic section from the left ventricular free wall shows marked connective tissue replacement. Although specifically sought, small-vessel coronary artery disease was not identified. *B*, Two-dimensional echocardiogram (apical window) showing the mildly dilated, thin-walled left ventricle (LV). LA = left atrium. (From Child, J. S., et al.: Cardiac involvement in Friedreich's ataxia. Reprinted by permission of the American College of Cardiology. J. Am. Coll. Cardiol. 7:1370, 1986.)

mon echocardiographic finding has been concentric (symmetrical) left ventricular hypertrophy (Fig. 60-12); asymmetrical septal thickening occurs, but less frequently.[110,112,117-119] Left ventricular outflow gradients have been reported in some cases with disproportionate septal thickness[112] but not in others.[110] Importantly, septal cellular disarray—the histological hallmark of genetic hypertrophic cardiomyopathy (p. 1636)—has been absent or only focal in necropsy studies of Friedreich's ataxia.[108,111,120,121] This observation may, in part, explain why the potentially malignant ventricular arrhythmias common in genetic hypertrophic cardiomyopathy are essentially unknown in Friedreich's ataxia.[122] In the hypertrophic cardiomyopathy of Friedreich's ataxia, systolic ventricular function is normal, not supernormal, and diastolic function is not deranged as in genetic hypertrophic cardiomyopathy.[123,124]

DILATED CARDIOMYOPATHY. A second and much less common form of cardiac involvement in Friedreich's ataxia is dilated cardiomyopathy that may initially express itself as global hypokinesis with normal left ventricular internal dimensions (Fig. 60-13).[4,119] There is one report of dilated cardiomyopathy, chiefly involving the right ventricle, with ventricular tachyarrhythmias.[125] In contrast to the favorable prognosis of Friedreich's ataxia with hypertrophic cardiomyopathy, the outlook is poor in dilated cardiomyopathy patients who experience relentless, progressive cardiac deterioration.[4,119] There is convincing evidence that the dilated form of cardiomyopathy in Friedreich's ataxia is distinct from the hypertrophic form (i.e., not a transition) and represents a fundamentally different type of cardiac involvement designated dystrophic.[4] This view is supported by the flabby myocardium with normal wall thickness in necropsy cases that exhibited premortem progression on echocardiography from normal to dilated globally hypofunctional left ventricles with normal wall thickness (Fig. 60-13).[4] The initial force deformities on electrocardiograms and vectorcardiograms (Fig. 60-14)[4,113] are believed to represent areas of regional ventricular myocardial dystrophy which, if sufficiently widespread, might result in depressed systolic function.[4] Atrial arrhythmias (flutter, fibrillation) and ventricular arrhythmias are features of the dilated cardiomyopathy of Friedreich's ataxia.[4,125] Disease of the coronary arteries, especially small intramural coronary arteries, has been reported in Friedreich's ataxia,[121] but a relationship between the coronary arteriopathy and regional wall abnormalities is doubtful.

In summary, there appear to be two distinct types of cardiac involvement in Friedreich's ataxia: (1) hypertrophic cardiomyopathy, represented by symmetrical (less commonly asymmetrical) left ventricular hypertrophy with normal cavity size and ventricular function, and (2) relatively uncommon dilated cardiomyopathy, represented by depressed systolic function with normal or increased ventricular cavity size. Whether the frequently observed initial force abnormalities on the scalar electrocardiogram represent regional "dystrophic" disease that anticipates dilated cardiomyopathy remains to be proven.

Why a nonmyopathic spinocerebellar corticospinal disorder is accompanied by two widely disparate types of cardiac disease is unknown. An important implication is that phenotypically indistinguishable patients are genetically different.[126,127] The relationship between the spinocerebellar-corticospinal disorder and an increase in ventricular

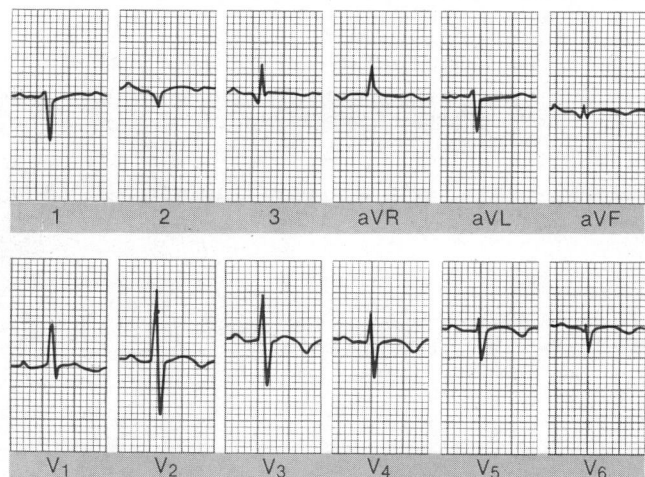

FIGURE 60-14. Electrocardiogram in a 28-year-old man with Friedreich's ataxia. The QRS shows marked right-axis deviation. There are 40-msec Q waves in leads 2, 3, and aVl. A prominent 60-msec R wave appears in lead V_1. A vectorcardiogram and echocardiogram showed no evidence of right ventricular hypertrophy. The ECG pattern reflects loss of inferior and posterior electrical forces without a corresponding regional wall motion abnormality on echocardiography. (From Child, J. S., et al.: Cardiac involvement in Friedreich's ataxia. Reprinted by permission of the American College of Cardiology. J. Am. Coll. Cardiol. 7:1370, 1986.)

mass—hypertrophic cardiomyopathy—is also an enigma. A unifying thread may be the "catecholamine hypothesis," which has been a focus of interest in the pathogenesis of genetic hypertrophic cardiomyopathy.[128] Plasma catecholamine levels are reportedly increased in patients with Friedreich's ataxia.[129,130]

LESS COMMON NEUROMYOPATHIC DISEASES SOMETIMES ASSOCIATED WITH HEART DISEASE

PERONEAL MUSCULAR ATROPHY (CHARCOT-MARIE-TOOTH SYNDROME). Peroneal muscular atrophy includes several genetic disorders (the hereditary motor and sensory neuromyopathies) characterized by distal weakness of the legs with predilection for muscles innervated by the peroneal nerves, particularly the everters of the foot and occasionally intrinsic muscles of the hands.[131] Peroneal muscular atrophy is an autosomal dominant disorder; one form begins during the first 20 years of life, while the other form begins later, with initial symptoms appearing in early life or not until middle age. Cardiac involvement is not a feature of peroneal muscular atrophy.[114,132,133] Arrhythmias, conduction abnormalities, and dilated heart failure have been sporadically reported in patients with peroneal muscular atrophy,[134-138] but are believed to be chance associations.[133]

MYOTUBULAR MYOPATHY (CENTRONUCLEAR MYOPATHY). Centronuclear myopathy typically exhibits internal nuclei, i.e., structures resembling fetal myotubes (rows of nuclei separated by spaces).[139-140] The disorder is characterized clinically by slow but progressive wasting and weakness of skeletal muscle beginning at birth. Ptosis is the rule, and patients are hyporeflexic or areflexic. Few examples are available for study, but presumptive evidence indicates that myotubular myopathy can be associated with extensive myocardial fibrosis, cardiac dilatation, and early death.[139] In an illustration in one report on skeletal muscle in "idiopathic cardiomyopathy," numerous internal nuclei could be seen.[141] Centronuclear myopathy had apparently presented as cardiomyopathy before the neuromuscular disease was identified.

KEARNS-SAYRE SYNDROME (PROGRESSIVE EXTERNAL OPHTHALMOPLEGIA WITH PIGMENTARY RETINOPATHY). Kearns-Sayre syndrome is a mitochondrial myopathy characterized by progressive external ophthalmoplegia (Fig. 60–15), pigmentary retinopathy, and *heart block*.[142-144] Morphological alterations in skeletal muscle are identified in the trichrome stain as ragged red fibers.[142] Cardiac involvement primarily afflicts the specialized conduction pathways.[145,146] Clinically overt myocardial disease is the exception, despite the fact that ultrastructural abnormalities, especially of mitochondria, are well established.[147-149] Occasional patients exhibit dilated cardiomyopathy with progressive heart failure.[147-149] Patients are chiefly at risk because of the abnormalities of the specialized conduction pathways. Two derangements in cardiac conduction coexist: (1) gradually progressive impairment of infranodal conduction (left anterior hemiblock, right bundle branch block, complete heart block) (Fig. 60–16A) and (2) concomitant enhancement of AV nodal conduction.[145,150] The morphological basis for impaired infranodal conduction

lies in the extensive changes in distal portions of the bundle of His extending to the origins of the bundle branches.[150] Evidence of enhanced AV nodal conduction has been identified by His bundle electrocardiography[145] (Fig. 60–16B). A short or relatively short P-R interval should not be used to weigh against the risk inherent in trifascicular disease in patients with Kearns-Sayre syndrome, right bundle branch block, and left anterior hemiblock.[145] Pacemaker implantation is often necessary.

GUILLAIN-BARRÉ SYNDROME. This syndrome is the most common of the acquired demyelinative neuropathies.[151] The incidence gradually increases with age, but the disease may occur at any age, and both sexes are equally affected. The syndrome often appears days to weeks after a viral respiratory or gastrointestinal infection, with neurological symptoms comprising symmetrical weakness of the limbs often accompanied by paresthesias. The incidence of the acute polyneuropathy is higher in patients with Hodgkin's disease, and the disorder may be precipitated by pregnancy, general surgery, or vaccinations. Myocardial infarction was believed to be the precipitating cause in two cases.[152] Important and characteristic features of the syndrome are flaccid motor paralysis with a distinctive tendency to ascend (Landry's ascending paralysis) and elevation of the cerebrospinal protein concentration without an increase in the number of white blood cells. Involvement of thoracic muscles often requires assisted ventilation. Despite respiratory support, the Guillain-Barré syndrome is fatal in approximately 20 per cent of children with significant involvement of trunk muscles and associated pulmonary insufficiency.[153]

Cardiac Findings. When sudden death occurs, postmortem studies have shed little or no light on the cause. There is substantial evidence, however, that deaths are often if not invariably related to cardiac arrhythmias.[153-155] Bradyarrhythmias (sinus arrest, complete heart block) and tachyarrhythmias (supraventricular and ventricular) as well as premature atrial and ventricular beats are relatively frequent occurrences and may be increased by the use of a respirator.[154] Occasionally, patients exhibit autonomic dysfunction, especially sympathetic hyperactivity, reflected in orthostatic hypotension, transient hypertension, wide fluctuations in blood pressure and in heart rate, and variations in the R-R interval.[156-158] Pacemaker support has been required because of recurrent asystole.[154] In one patient, tracheal aspiration produced an idioventricular rhythm of 40 beats per minute that reverted to sinus rhythm when aspiration ceased.[153] Cardiac monitoring is advisable, especially when the Guillain-Barré syndrome is sufficiently severe to warrant assisted ventilation.[153] ECG occasionally shows widespread deep T-wave inversions.[158]

NEMALINE MYOPATHY. This condition is characterized by myriads of small, rodlike particles in striated muscle.[159-160,160a] Inheritance is either autosomal dominant or recessive, with occasional sporadic cases. The most common clinical manifestation is hypotonia with diffuse weakness of limbs and trunk beginning at an early age. Children are often dysmorphic with an elongated, narrow face, high arched palate, and slender musculature.[5] Alternatively, symptoms begin in adolescence or adult life and are characterized by scapuloperoneal weakness and footdrop.[161] Nemaline myopathy is only rarely associated with cardiac involvement, but nemaline rods in the myocardium and in the cardiac conduction tissues have been held responsible for cardiac dilatation and conduction defects.[162,163]

MYASTHENIA GRAVIS. This is a "neuroimmunological" disease caused by a disorder of neuromuscular transmission due to antibodies to

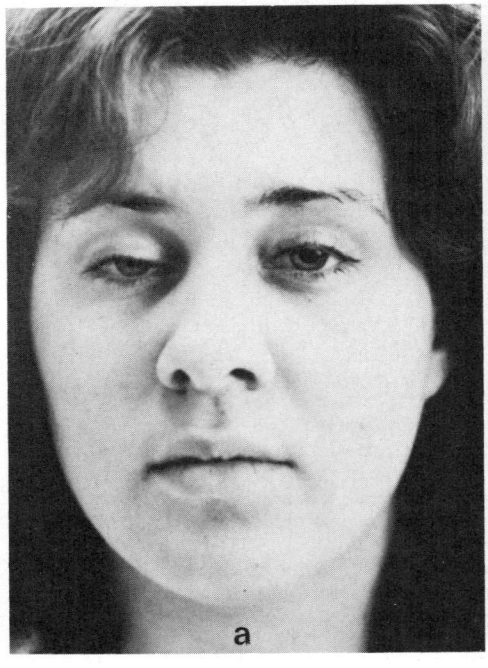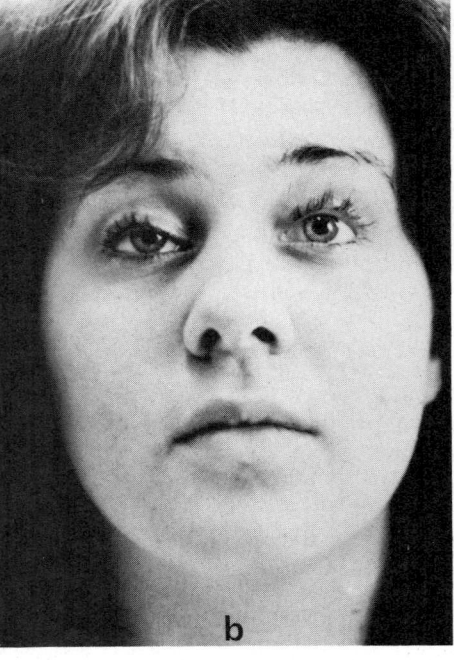

a   b

FIGURE 60–15. An 18-year-old girl with Kearns-Sayre syndrome and bilateral asymmetrical ptosis. Within 24 months, her electrocardiogram changed from normal to bifascicular block (complete right bundle branch block and left anterior fascicular block). *A,* The asymmetrical ptosis when the patient looks straight ahead. *B,* Ptosis of the right lid persists when the patient looks up. She also had atypical pigmentary retinopathy.

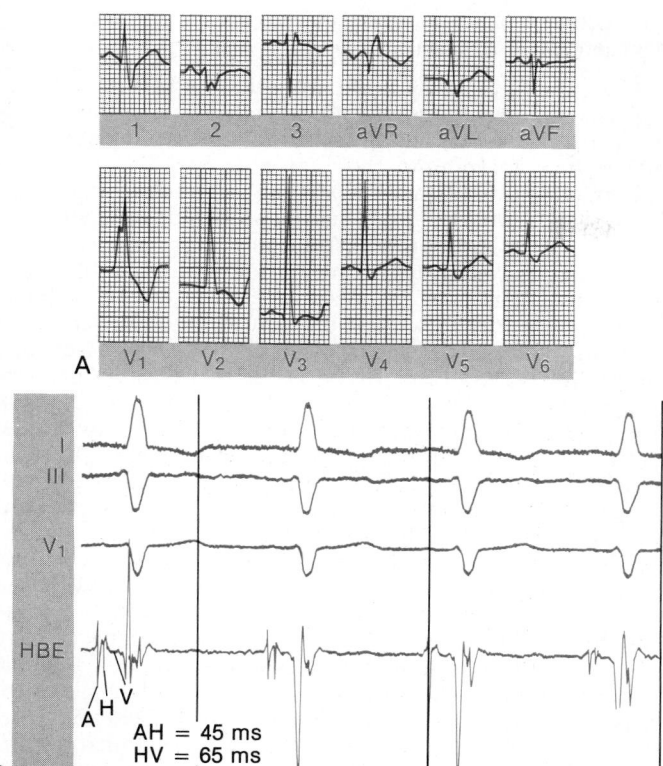

FIGURE 60–16. *A*, Electrocardiogram from a 13-year-old boy with Kearns-Sayre syndrome. There is a short P-R interval (110 msec), left anterior hemiblock, and complete right bundle branch block. *B*, Leads I, III, and V₁ with His bundle electrogram (HBE) in a 21-year-old woman with Kearns-Sayre syndrome. Time lines are at 1-sec intervals. The A-H interval is 45 msec (short) and the H-V interval is 65 msec (prolonged). (From Roberts, N. K., et al.: Cardiac conduction in Kearns-Sayre syndrome. Am. J. Cardiol. *44:*1396, 1979.)

acetylcholine receptors.[164,165] The abnormality may become manifest at any age but is most common in the second to fourth decades. Overt pathological evidence of myasthenia gravis is primarily in the thymus, which shows lymphoid hyperplasia and numerous lymphoid follicles with germinal centers in the medulla. Ocular muscles are affected first, and weakness characteristically fluctuates during the course of a single day, sometimes within minutes. The association of myocardial disease with thymoma, especially malignant thymoma, is generally accepted, whereas the association of myasthenia gravis with heart disease is less clear despite a considerable body of suggestive evidence.[166] Specific cardiac involvement is unproven even though clinical, electrocardiographic, and vectorcardiographic data implicate the myocardium.[166]

Early in this century quinine was used as a provocative diagnostic test for myasthenia gravis. Quinidine and procainamide, like quinine, have anticholinergic properties that depress neuromuscular conduction.[167] These antiarrhythmic agents can unmask previously unsuspected myasthenia gravis and can exacerbate symptoms in previously well controlled patients.[167,168] Accordingly, quinidine and procainamide should be avoided in this disorder.

McARDLE SYNDROME. This metabolic myopathy (muscle phosphorylase deficiency) results in inadequate skeletal muscle glycolysis.[169] The disease is characterized by exercise-induced muscle cramps. The electrocardiogram occasionally reveals sinus bradycardia, increased QRS voltage, and prolongation of the P-R interval, but the most common feature is a rapid acceleration of heart rate and respiratory rate with the beginning of exercise.[5,169] McArdle syndrome differs from the metabolic mitochondrial myopathy of skeletal and cardiac muscle with exercise-induced lactic acidemia and storage of glycogen and lipid.[170]

KUGELBERG-WELANDER SYNDROME. Proximal spinal muscular atrophies are autosomal recessive.[171] The childhood form is subdivided into three groups: the acute Werdnig-Hoffmann, the intermediate Werdnig-Hoffmann, and the Kugelberg-Welander.[171] The last variety of spinal muscular atrophy is characterized by onset in childhood or adolescence, atrophy and weakness principally of proximal limb muscles, slowly progressive clinical course, development of fasciculations, and evidence of neurogenic changes in the electromyogram and on muscle biopsy. There have been a few reports of cardiac involvement in the Kugelberg-Welander syndrome, including atrial fibrillation, atrial standstill, conduction defects (H-V prolongation, complete AV block), and dilated heart failure.[172]

POLIOMYELITIS. Cardiac involvement is believed to occur only rarely in childhood poliomyelitis but may simply be clinically occult.[173,174] In adults, the infrequency of symptomatic involvement of the heart contrasts with a relatively high incidence of electrocardiographic abnormalities, especially of rhythm and conduction.[173,174] Disturbances of rhythm take the form of premature beats (atrial and ventricular) and atrial fibrillation or flutter; disturbances in conduction are manifested by impaired AV conduction (first, second, and third degree heart block) and abnormalities of infranodal conduction (left-axis deviation and bundle branch block).[173,174] Respiratory failure can provoke hypoxemia-induced pulmonary hypertension[175] and multifocal atrial tachycardia.

At necropsy, the sinoatrial node, distal His bundle, and left and right bundle branches show infiltration, degeneration, and fibrous replacement that wholly or in part account for the conduction defects.[173,174] Pathological changes in the myocardium tend to be similar to those in skeletal muscle, including diffuse mononuclear cell infiltration and myofibril degeneration, regeneration, and fibrosis.

PERIODIC PARALYSIS. Periodic paralysis is characterized by recurrences of flaccid weakness accompanied by either abnormally high or abnormally low levels of serum potassium.[176,177] *Hypokalemic attacks* typically begin in late childhood or adolescence, usually occur at night, tend to be severe, and last a day or longer.[177] *Hyperkalemic attacks* have their onset at a younger age. Episodes occur more frequently than with hypokalemia but tend to be milder and shorter in duration (minutes or hours). Many features are common to both varieties of periodic paralysis, including familial recurrence (autosomal dominant inheritance), heightened susceptibility immediately after cessation of strenuous exercise, termination of incipent attacks by *mild* exercise, onset of weakness in the lower extremities with progression to the arms but not to the respiratory muscles, intensification by cold, and persistent weakness between attacks even though potassium levels may be normal.[176,178] During hyperkalemia, the electrocardiogram exhibits peaked T waves, and during hypokalemia there are low-voltage T waves and digitalis sensitivity.

More important are the cardiac arrhythmias that accompany periodic paralysis, including ventricular ectopic beats, ventricular bigeminy, and fusion beats producing multiform complexes.[177-179] Of particular interest is bidirectional tachycardia that is believed to originate in the left ventricle, that is refractory to antiarrhythmic therapy, that occurs independent of attacks of muscle weakness, that exhibits no correlation with serum electrolyte concentrations, and that is regularly converted to sinus rhythm by mild exercise.[180,181] Hypokalemic episodes are best treated with oral potassium chloride, and hyperkalemic episodes, with glucose and insulin, but it should be pointed out that administration of potassium does not necessarily suppress the ventricular electrical instability during hypokalemic attacks.[179]

ALCOHOLIC CARDIOMYOPATHY (see also p. 1819). Dilated cardiomyopathy associated with long-term ingestion of large amounts of ethyl alcohol may be accompanied by clinically occult skeletal myopathy.[182-184] The teratogenic potential of alcohol, exemplified by the fetal alcohol syndrome, afflicts the central nervous system but not the fetal myocardium, although congenital malformations of the heart are not uncommon in the offspring of alcoholic mothers.[185]

ACUTE CEREBRAL DISORDERS ACCOMPANIED BY CARDIOVASCULAR ABNORMALITIES

Acute cerebral injury can provoke cardiovascular abnormalities, and abnormalities of the heart can set the stage for acute cerebral injury. A connection between certain acute cerebral events—subarachnoid hemorrhage, intracranial hemorrhage, space-occupying lesions—and overt cardiovascular abnormalities has been recognized for nearly a century, and a relationship between head trauma and cardiac abnormalities was proposed 50 years ago.[186] The cardiac abnormalities that were emphasized in these settings were disturbances in rhythm and conduction and abnormalities of repolarization. *Neurogenic pulmonary edema* (p. 559) has been reported with a variety of disorders of the central nervous system[187,188] and with brain stem hemorrhage.[189] A rise in systemic blood pressure in response to cerebral injury[190] was known to Harvey Cushing at the turn of the century (the *Cushing pressor response*),[191] and experimentally induced intense cerebral compression in rats evokes a marked increase in systemic vascular resistance, a profound decrease in cardiac output, pulmonary venous congestion, and hemorrhagic pulmonary edema.[187] Interest has also focused on the importance of damage to the myocardium in response to cerebral injury, especially severe brain injury caused by craniocerebral trauma.[192-197]

ARRHYTHMIAS, CONDUCTION DEFECTS, AND REPOLARIZATION ABNORMALITIES. Approximately 90 per cent of patients with *acute cerebral accidents*—most notably spontaneous cerebral or subarachnoid hemorrhage or acute cerebral trauma—exhibit electrocardiographic abnormalities that consist chiefly of disturbances of cardiac rhythm and repolarization.[189,195,196,198-207] Disturbances in cardiac rhythm include sinus bradycardia (sometimes profound), sinus tachycardia, atrial arrhythmias (ectopic beats, fibrillation, flutter, or supraventricular tachycardia), junctional rhythms, and ventricular arrhythmias (ectopic beats, ventricular tachycardia, or fibrillation).[199,208,209] Conduction disturbances include first, second, or third degree AV block.[196] Repolarization abnormalities closely resemble those of ischemic heart disease and consist mainly of abnormal ST segments and T waves in addition to prominent U waves, and a prolonged Q-T interval.[189,202,210] ST segments may be dramatically elevated and T waves dramatically inverted (Fig. 60-17).

MYOCARDIAL INJURY. There is substantial evidence that the "catecholamine storm"—copious release of norepinephrine at cardiac beta$_1$-receptor sites—is responsible for myocardial damage, reflected in an increase in serum cardiac enzymes (CK MB), in left ventricular wall motion abnormalities,[197] in evidence of myofibrillar degeneration on light microscopy, and in subendocardial injury.[190,194,205] Potentially additive effects of glucocorticoids combined with catecholamines have been emphasized in the genesis of stress myocardial injury.[199] The myocardial damage associated with acute cerebral injury puts patients at additional risk (see above). It is important to emphasize that the major sources of donor hearts for cardiac and for heart and lung transplantation are motor vehicle accident or gunshot wound victims who have suffered massive cerebral injury and, in all probability, have varying degrees of catecholamine- and stress-induced myocardial and lung injury.[195,209]

NEUROGENIC PULMONARY EDEMA AND CARDIOPULMONARY ARREST. Cerebrogenic hemorrhagic pulmonary edema has been experimentally induced by cranial compression in rats,[187] and neurogenic pulmonary edema sometimes accompanies acute cerebral injury in patients[187-189] (p. 559). Myocardial damage may aggravate the pulmonary edema but is not necessary for its genesis. Respiratory arrest without circulatory collapse is more common than cardiac arrest in patients with acute cerebral injury.[211] Cardiac arrest per se is likely to be triggered by disturbances in ventricular rhythm (see above). Cerebrogenic cardiac arrhythmias and neurogenic pulmonary edema have been reported following generalized tonic-clonic epileptic seizures without acute cerebral injury.[212,213] Acute injury to the cervical spinal cord without cerebral damage is frequently accompanied by disturbances in cardiac rhythm and conduction and occasionally by sudden death.[214] Bradyarrhythmias are most prevalent, but supraventricular and ventricular tachyarrhythmias and AV block also occur, in addition to marked hypotension. The cardiac abnormalities are believed to arise from acute autonomic imbalance imposed on the heart by the cervical cord injury.[214]

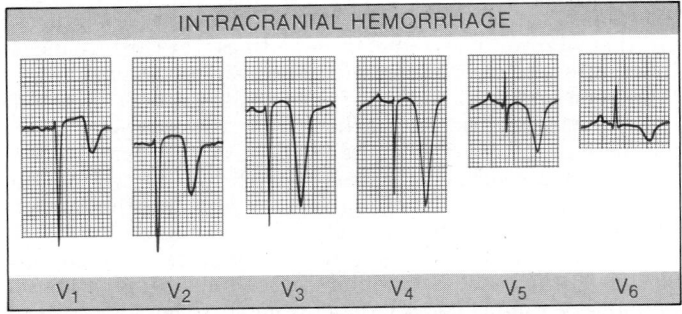

INTRACRANIAL HEMORRHAGE

V$_1$ V$_2$ V$_3$ V$_4$ V$_5$ V$_6$

FIGURE 60-17. Deep, symmetrical T-wave inversions in precordial leads of a patient with a cerebral hemorrhage. (Courtesy of John H. Phillips, M.D., Tulane Medical Center, New Orleans, Louisiana.)

Coexistence of Cerebrovascular Disease and Coronary Heart Disease

The preceding section pointed out that acute cerebrovascular accidents in patients with normal hearts (i.e., without coronary artery disease) often result in electrocardiographic abnormalities resembling those of myocardial ischemia or infarction with release of CK MB; however, in older patients, these electrocardiographic abnormalities and isoenzyme elevations may in fact represent an accompanying acute myocardial ischemic event caused by coexisting atherosclerotic coronary artery disease.[215,216] Because ST-segment elevations, deep T-wave inversions, and an increase in CK MB occur in patients with cerebrovascular accidents *without* ischemic heart disease, one cannot rely on these criteria to diagnose ischemic injury due to coronary artery obstruction. Accordingly, earlier estimates of the incidence of acute myocardial infarction in such patients[217] must be reevaluated.[218] Differential diagnosis is important, because mortality is relatively high in patients with coexisting acute cerebrovascular accident and acute myocardial infarction.[210]

DIAGNOSIS. Patients with clinically overt atherosclerotic coronary artery disease should be examined for occult carotid artery disease, and those with overt carotid artery disease should be assessed for occult atherosclerotic coronary artery disease. Cervical arterial murmurs were found in 4.4 to 12.6 per cent of persons 45 years of age and older with no history of stroke, transient cerebral ischemia, or overt ischemic heart disease.[219-221] The prevalence of these asymptomatic murmurs increased with age and was higher among women and among patients with systemic hypertension. In a prospective study of 735 unselected patients over age 55 years who were scheduled for elective surgery, 14 per cent had cervical arterial murmurs.[222] Pooled data on 2205 patients undergoing elective surgery disclosed cervical arterial murmurs in 15 per cent but no difference in stroke distribution between patients with and without carotid murmurs.[222] It was concluded that strokes in patients undergoing operations other than coronary artery bypass are so rare that further evaluation seems unnecessary. Still, it is important to distinguish between hemodynamically mild carotid stenosis with an exceedingly low risk of stroke and hemodynamically significant lesions in which the risk of even nonfatal cerebral infarction is appreciable.[221,223,224]

The need to identify hemodynamically significant carotid artery obstruction—either symptomatic or asymptomatic—was underscored in the Framingham Study, in which attention was called to the relative frequency of cerebral infarction in vascular territories different from that predicted based on an asymptomatic carotid artery murmur.[225] Ruptured aneurysm, embolism from the heart, and lacunar infarction were the mechanisms of stroke in nearly half the cases (see later).

The *physical examination* serves to detect carotid artery murmurs but does not accurately determine the severity of carotid obstruction. Of the currently available noninvasive neurovascular tests that reliably assess carotid artery disease, the first choice is ultrasonic duplex scanning that combines B-mode imaging to visualize specific arterial segments with the pulsed Doppler technique to determine the physiological significance of the obstruction.[226,227]

MANAGEMENT. Expert opinion regarding carotid endarterectomy for prevention of stroke has varied widely.[224] Given relatively secure information regarding the carotid and coronary circulations, however, judgments concerning management before coronary revascularization can be based on the following suppositions[221,224,228-230]: (1) in patients with symptomatic carotid artery murmurs (prior stroke or transient ischemic attacks) and hemodynamically significant carotid artery obstruction (especially bilateral) in whom myocardial revascularization *cannot* safely be deferred (left main coronary obstruction, unstable angina pectoris, severe multivessel disease), *combined* carotid endarterectomy and coronary bypass grafting are recommended: (2) in patients with symptomatic carotid artery murmurs and hemodynamically significant carotid obstruction in whom myocardial revascularization *can* safely be deferred, carotid endarterectomy should be carried out first, followed at a later date by coronary revascularization: (3) in patients with asymptomatic carotid artery murmurs and obstruction that is considered hemodynamically insignificant, myocardial revascularization alone can proceed as clinically indicated; (4) less clear is the management of patients with asymptomatic carotid artery murmurs and hemodynamically significant carotid obstruction.[221,224] It has been argued that elective myocardial revascularization can be performed either alone or, if clinically urgent (as already defined), combined with carotid endarterectomy.[228]

An important corollary to these observations is the incidence of neurological complications unassociated with carotid artery obstruction in patients undergoing coronary artery bypass grafting.[228,230–233] These complications are in addition to and distinct from those accompanying open-heart surgery per se.[234,325] Major central nervous system events are associated with coronary bypass operations in 1 to 2 per cent of cases.[230,232,233] The majority of cerebral events complicating coronary bypass grafting are believed to be related to embolization of atheromatous material from the ascending aorta or embolization from a postinfarction left ventricular mural thrombus.[230,233]

Cardiogenic Brain Embolism

Aggregate clinical data on cardiac sources of embolic stroke (the Cerebral Embolism Task Force) emphasize "nonvalvular" atrial fibrillation, ischemic heart disease (acute myocardial infarction, ventricular aneurysm), rheumatic heart disease (mitral stenosis), and prosthetic cardiac valves.[236] Important but less common sources include nonischemic dilated cardiomyopathy, infective endocarditis, nonbacterial thrombotic endocarditis, mitral valve prolapse, mitral annular calcification, calcific aortic stenosis, left atrial myxoma, atrial septal aneurysm, and paradoxical embolization especially but not necessarily with congenital heart disease.[236] Nonvalvular atrial fibrillation encompasses a wide spectrum, from "lone atrial fibrillation" without other clinical evidence of heart disease to ventricular dilatation with congestive heart failure. Nonvalvular atrial fibrillation is the most common cardiac disorder believed to be associated with cerebral embolic events, accounting for almost one-half of cardiogenic embolic strokes.[236] Although some studies report a low stroke incidence in patients with lone atrial fibrillation,[237] other studies conclude that atrial fibrillation unassociated with structural heart disease predisposes to cerebral embolism.[238] Preliminary results indicate that aspirin or Coumadin (given separately) is effective in preventing systemic embolism and ischemic stroke and is comparatively safe in patients with nonvalvular atrial fibrillation. The absolute reduction in risk according to the Stroke Prevention in Atrial Fibrillation Study Group[238] was 6.8 per cent per year, exceeding the incremental risk of clinically important hemorrhage (<1 per cent per year). When that report was compiled, it was not possible to establish an advantage of either warfarin or aspirin over the other.

Focal neurological signs are occasionally seen in patients with *mitral valve prolapse* (p. 1029) and are believed to be embolic (platelet fibrin aggregates).[239–240] *Left atrial myxomas* (p. 1452) result in peripheral emboli in about 45 per cent of cases, and the brain is affected in one-half of these. Occasionally, patients with left atrial myxoma are initially seen by neurologists because of predominantly or exclusively neurological manifestations.[241] *Left ventricular mural thrombi* set the stage for cerebral emboli, most commonly in patients with myocardial infarction because of the prevalence of ischemic heart disease, but left ventricular mural thrombi in patients with dilated cardiomyopathy are much more likely to give rise to cerebral emboli than are mural thrombi associated with myocardial infarction.[182] Infants with endocardial fibroelastosis of the dilated type also suffer strokes caused by emboli from left ventricular endocardial thrombi.[242] *Infective endocarditis* (p. 1078) on native or prosthetic cardiac valves gives rise to neurological complications, including stroke, toxic

confusion, and meningitis. Rupture of a mycotic aneurysm is a catastrophic event associated with 80 per cent mortality.[243–245] Septic cerebral emboli may give rise to acute intracranial hemorrhage or cerebral abscess after a misleading interval of quiescence.

Bland emboli from *marantic endocarditis* (p. 1551), especially on the aortic valve, are believed to be more common than clinically recognized.[246] The use of anticoagulants coupled with improved rigid prostheses has decreased the incidence of cerebral emboli after *left cardiac valve replacement*. Drug abuse not only causes infective endocarditis but, depending on the drug and vehicle (embolism of foreign matter), may be associated with intracranial or subarachnoid hemorrhage, cerebral emboli, and ischemic stroke.[247]

Paradoxical emboli reach the brain when peripheral venous blood enters the systemic arterial circulation via right-to-left shunts of cyanotic congenital heart disease.[242,248] An important variation on this theme is what are believed to be paradoxical emboli in acyanotic patients with interatrial communications (ostium secundum atrial septal defect or patent foramen ovale).[248–250] Especially vulnerable are pregnant women with an ostium secundum atrial septal defect; inferior caval to left atrial streaming provides a pathway into the left atrium.[251] Recent interest has focused on younger adults with embolic stroke ascribed to paradoxical emboli through a patent foramen ovale[249] (Fig. 60–18). Evidence in this regard has been considered sufficient to warrant sealing the patent foramen using interventional catheterization techniques. Atrial septal aneurysm, an uncommon localized malformation of the interatrial septum, protrudes into the right or left atrium and is a potential occult source of cerebral embolism[252] (Fig. 60–19).

Focal discrete neurological deficits are well-known sequelae of cerebral emboli; less well known are the diffuse cerebral symptoms believed to result from recurrences of multiple small corticoemboli that cause agitated confusion, dulled sensorium, and seizures.[253]

CYANOTIC CONGENITAL HEART DISEASE WITH NEUROLOGICAL MANIFESTATIONS

Brain damage, mental retardation, venous sinus thromboses, paradoxical cerebroembolism (see earlier), and brain abscess constitute a formidable list of central nervous system complications in cyanotic congenital heart disease.[242,254] Cyanotic spells of tetralogy of Fallot may culminate in syncope, seizures, and rarely in hemiplegia[255] (p. 935). The erythrocytosis of cyanotic congenital heart disease is a risk of stroke chiefly in infants under 2 years of age with iron deficiency, but the risk of stroke is low in cyanotic adults, whether the erythrocytosis is compensated (normochromic) or decompensated (hypochromic) and irrespective of hematocrit level.[254]

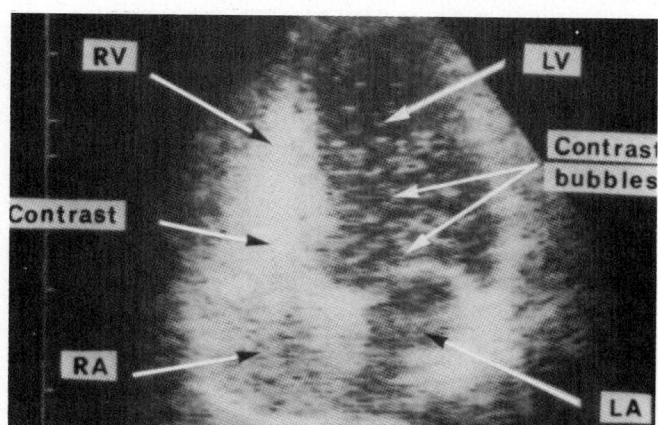

FIGURE 60–18. **Two-dimensional contrast echocardiograms (apical four-chamber view) in a patient with a patent foramen ovale.** Isotonic saline containing microbubbles was injected into a peripheral vein. Contrast material fills the right atrium (RA) and right ventricle (RV) and appears in the left atrium (LA) and left ventricle (LV) through a patent foramen ovale. (From Lechat, P., et al.: Prevalence of patent foramen ovale in patients with stroke. N. Engl. J. Med. *318:*1148, 1988.) Relabeled for clarity.

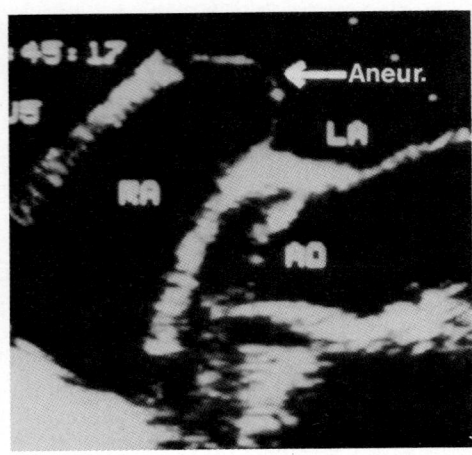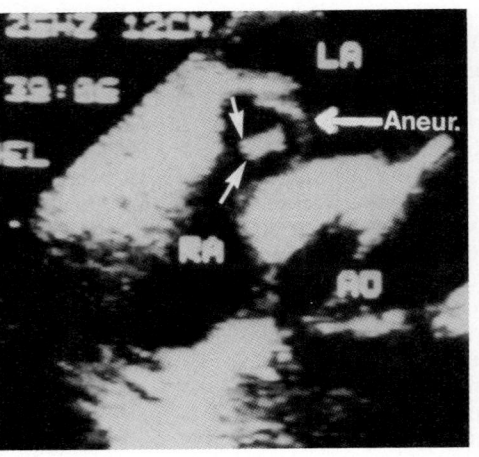

FIGURE 60–19. *Left panel,* Early systolic frame of a thin atrial septal aneurysm (Aneur.) on transesophageal echocardiogram. LA = left atrium; Ao = aorta. *Right panel,* A mobile thrombus (paired arrows) on the right atrial side of an atrial septal aneurysm. (From Schneider, B., Hannath, P., Vogel, P., and Meinertz, T.: Improved morphologic characterization of atrial septal aneurysm by transesophageal echocardiography: Relation to cerebrovascular events. Reprinted by permission of the American College of Cardiology. J. Am. Coll. Cardiol. *16*:1000, 1990.) Relabeled for clarity.

NEUROLOGICAL COMPLICATIONS AFTER CARDIAC ARREST

Broadly speaking, neurological outcomes cover a broad spectrum, ranging from complete recovery to the vegetative state.[256–258] A reversible "metabolic encephalopathy" occurs in patients with brief episodes of systemic circulatory arrest and mild degrees of cerebral hypoxia. Recovery is rapid and complete. In contrast, patients with severe cerebral hypoxia suffer structural damage to specific areas of the brain, as if they had had a stroke, and on awakening manifest permanent focal or multifocal motor, sensory, and intellectual deficits.[256–258] Still other patients with more widespread brain injury remain hospitalized in a state of wakefulness without awareness (vegetative state) or die a neurological death (brain death). Of patients discharged from a hospital, serious neurological deficits are seen in only about 10 per cent because severe postarrest neurological complications frequently lead to death.[257] Preexisting neurological deficits bode ill in survivors of cardiopulmonary resuscitation. Early return to consciousness, and return of cranial nerve function and electroencephalographic function imply a better cerebral prognosis, but do not guarantee a good overall outcome.[257] Delayed electroencephalographic return signifies a poor neurological prognosis.

CARDIAC COMPLICATIONS OF DRUGS USED IN TREATING NEUROMUSCULAR DISEASE

Neuromuscular and cardiovascular diseases may be related to cardiac complications of certain drugs used by the neurologist.

Methysergide prescribed for migraine headache is occasionally accompanied by inflammatory retroperitoneal fibrosis and by a similar fibrotic disease of pleura, systemic arteries, cardiac valves, endocardium, and pericardium.[259–261] Methysergide-induced lesions do little or no damage to underlying cardiac structures, but instead a layer of fresh collagen is deposited on the surfaces of otherwise unharmed cardiac tissue.[260] The aortic valve lesion induced by methysergide causes both stenosis and regurgitation, while the mitral lesion generally causes regurgitation. If the drug is continued, the valvular abnormalities generally progress; however, in some patients, regression or complete disappearance (at least of the cardiac murmurs) has followed discontinuation of methysergide.[260]

In *Parkinson's disease,* neurons are selectively destroyed and cannot release the neurotransmitter dopamine.[262] Accordingly, levodopa (L-dopa), the precursor of dopamine, is used in treatment. A relatively large dose is required for a therapeutic response because only a small percentage of oral L-dopa penetrates the blood-brain barrier. Such doses are seldom tolerated without side effects. L-dopa provokes hypotension (supine and postural) as well as ventricular ectopic beats.[262] The drug must therefore be used cautiously in patients with cerebral ischemia, angina pectoris, recent myocardial infarction, or cardiac arrhythmias, even though after weeks (sometimes months) of use, tolerance improves and side effects diminish. The cardiovascular effects are mediated by the action of L-dopa on the central and peripheral nervous systems.

Bromocriptine, an ergot derivative, stimulates dopamine-sensitive receptors and is also useful in parkinsonism.[262] In high doses, the drug may cause a significant postural fall in blood pressure, and the hypotensive effect may persist for as long as 6 weeks. Rarely, severe hypotension, both supine and erect, occurs after the initial dose of bromocriptine.

Cyclosporine neurotoxicity is only one of the neuropathological concerns accompanying cardiac transplantation.[263] Cyclosporine may produce a wide range of neurological disorders, including coma, encephalopathy, cortical blindness, tremor, ataxia, peripheral neuropathy, and paraparesis.[263] There is no necessary correlation between blood levels and neurotoxic effects of the drug. However, while withdrawal of cyclosporine or reduction in dose generally results in resolution of the signs and symptoms, cases of fatal convulsions and coma have been reported.[263] Perioperative neurological complications of cardiac transplantation (first 2 weeks) include cerebrovascular disorders, encephalopathy, acute psychosis, and mononeuropathy.[264,265] Late neurological complications are related primarily to the use of chronic immunosuppressive therapy (see above), with cerebrovascular disorders becoming less frequent.[264,265]

NEUROLOGICAL COMPLICATIONS OF THERAPY FOR CARDIOVASCULAR DISEASE

Certain therapies for cardiovascular disease can result in serious neurological sequelae, such as those that are sequelae of cardiac arrest and resuscitation (see above). Systemic emboli related to cardioversion for chronic atrial fibrillation occur either at the time of reversion to sinus rhythm or on recurrence of atrial fibrillation. If an anticoagulant is administered for prophylaxis, it must not only precede cardioversion but must be maintained until stable sinus rhythm seems assured.[266]

Several commonly used cardiac drugs have important, although relatively rare, central or peripheral nervous system effects. The adverse responses to quinidine and procainamide in patients with myasthenia gravis were mentioned already (p. 1819). *Lidocaine neurotoxicity* (p. 640) includes drowsiness, dizziness, dysarthria, blurred vision, muscular fasciculations, and occasionally convulsions.[267] Beta-adrenoceptor blockers (p. 1309), in addition to causing drowsiness and lightheadedness, sometimes result in mental depression. Even digitalis glycosides are not exempt from neurotoxic effects[268] (p. 490). William Withering reported that, "The Foxglove when given in very large and quickly repeated doses occasions giddiness, confused vision, objects appearing green or yellow . . . cold sweats, convulsions, syncope, death."[269]

CARDIAC DENERVATION

The most common cause of cardiac denervation is transplantation of the heart (Chap. 18). Less well known is the remarkable denervation of the heart's intrinsic nervous system that occurs in Chagas heart disease (p. 1432).[270,271] Chagasic dysautonomia is associated with pathological changes in the cardiovascular, digestive, and autonomic nervous systems.[271] The cardioneuropathy is characterized by bradycardia, absence of postural reflexes, arterial hypotension, and an abnormal hyperventilation response.[271] The increased capacity of the coronary arteries (judged at necropsy by the volume of barium sulfate – gelatin mass taken up by the coronary arterial bed relative to heart weight) has been attributed to relative sympathetic overdrive in this disease.[270]

REFERENCES

MAJOR HEREDOFAMILIAL NEUROMYOPATHIC DISORDERS

1. Perloff, J. K., deLeon, A. C., and O'Doherty, D.: The cardiomyopathy of progressive muscular dystrophy. Circulation 33:625, 1966.
2. Perloff, J. K., Henze, E., and Schelbert, H. R.: Alterations in regional myocardial metabolism, perfusion and wall motion in Duchenne muscular dystrophy studied by radionuclide imaging. Circulation 69:33, 1984.
3. Perloff, J. K., Stevenson, W. G., Roberts, N. K., et al.: Cardiac involvement in myotonic muscular dystrophy (Steinert's disease): A prospective study of 25 patients. Am. J. Cardiol. 54:1074, 1984.
4. Child, J. S., Perloff, J. K., Bach, P. M., et al.: Cardiac involvement in Friedreich's ataxia. J. Am. Coll. Cardiol. 7:1370, 1986.
5. Brooke, M. H.: A Clinician's View of Neuromuscular Disease. 2nd ed. Baltimore, Williams and Wilkins Co., 1986.
6. Kunkel, L. M.: Analysis of deletions in DNA from patients with Becker and Duchenne muscular dystrophy. Nature 322:73, 1986.
7. Boyd, Y., Buckle, V., Holt, S., et al.: Muscular dystrophy in girls with X; autosome translocations. J. Med. Genet. 23:484, 1986.
8. Roses, A. D.: Progressive muscular dystrophies. In Rowland, L. P. (ed.): Merritt's Textbook of Neurology. 7th ed. Philadelphia, Lea & Febiger, 1984.
9. Ervasti, J. M., Ohlendieck, K., Kahl, S. D., et al.: Deficiency of a glycoprotein component of the dystrophin complex in dystrophic muscle. Nature 345:315, 1990.
10. Boyd, Y., and Buckle, V. J.: Cytogenetic heterogeneity of translocations associated with Duchenne muscular dystrophy. Clin. Genet. 29:108, 1986.
11. Riggs, T.: Cardiomyopathy and pulmonary emboli in terminal Duchenne's muscular dystrophy. Am. Heart J. 119:690, 1990.
12. Gaffney, J. F., Kingston, W. J., Metlay, L. A., and Gramiak, R.: Left ventricular thrombus and systemic emboli complicating the cardiomyopathy of Duchenne's muscular dystrophy. Arch. Neurol. 46:1249, 1989.
13. Yotsukura, M., Miyagawa, M., Tsuya, T., et al.: Pulmonary hypertension in progressive muscular dystrophy of the Duchenne type. Jpn. Circ. J. 52:321, 1988.
14. Sanyal, S. K., Johnson, W. W., Dische, M. R., et al.: Dystrophic degeneration of papillary muscle and ventricular myocardium. A basis for mitral valve prolapse in Duchenne's muscular dystrophy. Circulation 62:430, 1980.
15. Perloff, J. K., Roberts, W. C., deLeon, A. C., and O'Doherty, D.: The distinctive electrocardiogram of Duchenne's progressive muscular dystrophy. Am. J. Med. 42:179, 1967.
16. Perloff, J. K.: Cardiac rhythm and conduction in Duchenne's muscular dystrophy. J. Am. Coll. Cardiol. 3:1263, 1984.
17. Sanyal, S. K., Johnson, W. W., Thapar, M. K., and Pitner, S. E.: An ultrastructural basis for the electrocardiographic alterations associated with Duchenne's progressive muscular dystrophy. Circulation 57:1122, 1978.
18. Miller, G., D'Orsogna, L., and O'Shea, J. P.: Autonomic function and the sinus tachycardia of Duchenne muscular dystrophy. Brain Dev. 11:247, 1989.
19. Zalman, F., Perloff, J. K., Durant, N. N., and Campion, D. S.: Acute respiratory failure following intravenous verapamil in Duchenne's muscular dystrophy. Am. Heart J. 105:510, 1983.
20. Rubler, S., Perloff, J. K., and Roberts, W. C.: Clinical Pathological Conference—Duchenne's muscular dystrophy. Am. Heart J. 94:776, 1977.
21. Frankel, K. A., and Rosser, R. J.: The pathology of the heart in progressive muscular dystrophy. Hum. Pathol. 7:375, 1976.
22. Skyring, A., and McKusick, V. A.: Clinical, genetic and electrocardiographic studies in childhood muscular dystrophy. Am. J. Med. Sci. 242:54, 1961.
23. Slucka, C.: The electrocardiogram in Duchenne's progressive muscular dystrophy. Circulation 38:933, 1968.
24. Fitch, C. W., and Ainger, L. E.: The Frank vectorcardiogram and the electrocardiogram in Duchenne muscular dystrophy. Circulation 35:1124, 1967.
25. Ronan, J. A., Perloff, J. K., Bowen, P. J., and Mann, O.: The vectorcardiogram in Duchenne's progressive muscular dystrophy. Am. Heart J. 84:588, 1972.
26. Wakai, S., Minami, R., Kameda, K., et al.: Electron microscopic study of the biopsied cardiac muscle in Duchenne muscular dystrophy. J. Neurol. Sci. 84:167, 1988.
27. Bhattacharya, S. K., Crawford, A. J., and Pate, J. W.: Electrocardiographic, biochemical, and morphologic abnormalities in dystrophic hamsters with cardiomyopathy. Muscle Nerve 10:168, 1987.

28. Nomura, H., and Hizawa, K.: Histopathological study of the conduction system of the heart in Duchenne progressive muscular dystrophy. Acta Pathol. 32:1027, 1982.
29. James, T. N.: Observations on the cardiovascular involvement, including the cardiac conduction system, in progressive muscular dystrophy. Am. Heart J. 63:48, 1962.
30. Chalkiadis, G. A., and Branch, K. G.: Cardiac arrest after isoflurane anaesthesia in a patient with Duchenne's muscular dystrophy. Anaesthesia 45:22, 1990.
31. Sethna, N. F., and Rockoff, M. A.: Cardiac arrest following inhalation induction of anaesthesia in a child with Duchenne's muscular dystrophy. Can. Anaesthes. Soc. J. 33:799, 1986.
32. Schelbert, H. R., Benson, L., Schwaiger, M., and Perloff, J. K.: Positron emission tomography. In Friedman, W. F., and Higgins, C. B. (eds.): Pediatric Cardiac Imaging, Cardiology Clinics. Philadelphia, W. B. Saunders Company, 1983.
33. Mawatari, S., Miranda, A., and Rowland, L. P.: Adenyl cyclase abnormality in Duchenne muscular dystrophy: Muscle cells in culture. Neurology 67:1016, 1976.
34. Wilner, J. H., Cerri, C., and Wood, D. S.: Adenyl cyclase in human genetic myopathies. In Schotland, D. L. (ed.): Disorders of the Motor Unit. New York, John Wiley and Sons, 1982, p. 431.
35. Carpenter, S., and Karpati, G.: Duchenne muscular dystrophy. Plasma membrane loss initiates muscle cell necrosis unless it is repaired. Brain 102:147, 1979.
36. Mokri, B., and Engel, A. G.: Duchenne dystrophy: Electronmicroscopic findings pointing to a basic or early abnormality in the plasma membrane of the muscle fiber. Neurology 25:1111, 1975.
37. Bonilla, E., Schotland, D. L., and Yakayama, Y.: Duchenne dystrophy: Focal alterations in the distribution of concanavalin A binding sites at the muscle cell surface. Ann. Neurol. 4:117, 1978.
38. Roses, A. D., Harwig, G. B., Mabry, M., et al.: Red blood cell and fibroblast membranes in Duchenne and myotonic muscular dystrophy. Muscle Nerve 3:36, 1980.
39. Pennington, R.J.T.: Serum enzymes. In Rowland, L. P. (ed.): Pathogenesis of Human Muscular Dystrophies. Amsterdam-Oxford, Excerpta Medica, 1977, p. 341.
40. Sutton, T. M., O'Brien, J. F., Kleinberg, F., et al.: Serum levels of creatine phosphokinase and its isoenzymes in normal and stressed neonates. Mayo Clin. Proc. 56:150, 1981.
41. Yoshioka, M.: Clinically manifesting carriers in Duchenne muscular dystrophy. Clin. Genet. 20:6, 1981.
42. Lane, R.J.M., Gardner-Medwin, D., and Roses, A. D.: Electrocardiographic abnormalities in carriers of Duchenne muscular dystrophy. Neurology 30:497, 1980.
43. Fowler, W. M., Gardner, G. W., Taylor, R. G., et al.: Quantitative measurements in female siblings and mothers of boys with Duchenne dystrophy. Arch. Phys. Med. Rehab. 50:301, 1969.
44. Mann, O., deLeon, A. C., Perloff, J. K., et al.: Duchenne's muscular dystrophy: The electrocardiogram in female relatives. Am. J. Med. Sci. 255:376, 1968.
45. Paillonry, M., Citron, B., Hersch, B., et al.: Electrocardiograms of women carriers of Duchenne-type muscular dystrophy. Ann. Cardiol. Angiol. 31:47, 1982.
46. Wiegand, V., Rahlf, G., Meinck, M., and Kreuzer, H.: Cardiomyopathy in female carriers of the Duchenne gene. Z. Kardiol. 73:188, 1984.
47. Becker, P. E.: Two new families of benign sex-linked recessive muscular dystrophy. Rev. Can. Biol. 21:551, 1962.
48. Markand, O. N., North, R. R., D'Agostino, A. N., and Daly, D. D.: Benign sex-linked muscular dystrophy. Neurology 19:617, 1969.
49. Borgeat, A., Goy, J. J., and Sigwart, U.: Acute pulmonary edema as the inaugural symptom of Becker's muscular dystrophy in a 19-year-old patient. Clin. Cardiol 10:127, 1987.
50. Vrints, C., Mercelis, R., Vanagt, E., et al.: Cardiac manifestations of Becker-type muscular dystrophy. Acta Cardiol. 38:479, 1983.
51. Yazawa, M., Ikeda, S., Owa, M., et al.: A family of Becker's progressive muscular dystrophy with severe cardiomyopathy. Eur. Neurol. 27:13, 1987.
52. Lazzeroni, E., Favaro, L., and Botti, G.: Dilated cardiomyopathy with regional myocardial hypoperfusion in Becker's muscular dystrophy. Int. J Cardiol. 22:126, 1989.
53. Casazza, F., Brambilla, G., Salvato, A., et al.: Cardiac transplantation in Becker muscular dystrophy. J. Neurol. 235:496, 1988.
54. Nigro, G., Comi, L. I., Limonselli, F. M., et al.: Prospective study of X-linked progressive muscular dystrophy in Campania. Muscle Nerve 6:253, 1983.
55. Levin, R. N., and Narahara, K. A.: Right axis deviation and anterior wall thallium-201 defect in Becker's muscular dystrophy. Am. J. Cardiol. 56:203, 1985.
56. Kawashima, S., Ulno, M., Kondo, T., et al.: Marked cardiac involvement in limb girdle muscular dystrophy. Am. J. Med. Sci. 299:411, 1990.
57. Hoshio, A., Kotake, H., Saitoh, M., et al.: Cardiac involvement in a patient with limb-girdle muscular dystrophy. Heart and Lung 16:439, 1987.
58. Bailey, R. O., Marzulo, D. C., and Hans, M. B.: Infantile facioscapulohumeral muscular dystrophy: new observations. Acta Neurol. Scand. 74:51, 1986.
59. Bloomfield, D. A., and Sinclair-Smith, B. C.: Persistent atrial standstill. Am. J. Med. 39:335, 1965.
60. Caponnetto, S., Patorini, C., and Tirelli, G.: Persistent atrial standstill in a patient affected with facioscapulohumeral dystrophy. Cardiologia 53:341, 1968.
61. Baldwin, A. J., Talley, R. C., Johnson, C., and Nutter, O.: Permanent paral-

ysis of the atrium in a patient with facioscapulohumeral muscular dystrophy. Am. J. Cardiol. 31:649, 1973.

62. Stevenson, W. G., Perloff, J. K., Weiss, J. N., and Anderson, T. L.: Facioscapulohumeral muscular dystrophy: Evidence for selective, genetic electrophysiologic cardiac involvement. J. Am. Coll. Cardiol. 15:292, 1990.

63. Emery, A.E.H., and Dreifuss, F. E.: Unusual type of benign X-linked muscular dystrophy. J. Neurol. Neurosurg. Psychiatry 29:338, 1966.

64. Emery, A.E.H.: X-linked muscular dystrophy with early contractures and cardiomyopathy (Emery-Dreifuss type). Clin. Genet. 32:360, 1987.

65. Hopkins, L. C., Jackson, J. A., and Elsas, L. J.: Emery-Dreifuss humeroperoneal muscular dystrophy: An X-linked myopathy with unusual contractures and bradycardia. Ann. Neurol. 10:230, 1981.

66. Fenichel, G. M., Sul, Y. C., Kilroy, A. W., and Blouin, R.: An autosomal-dominant dystrophy with humeropelvic distribution and cardiomyopathy. Neurology 32:1399, 1982.

67. Takamoto, K., Hirose, K., and Nonaka, I.: A genetic variant of Emery-Dreifuss disease. Arch. Neurol. 41:1292, 1984.

68. Tanaka, K., Yoshimura, T., Muratani, H., et al.: Familial myopathy with scapulohumeral distribution, rigid spine, cardiomyopathy and mitochondrial abnormality. J. Neurol. 236:52, 1989.

69. Bergia, B., Sybers, H. D., and Butler, I. J.: Familial lethal cardiomyopathy with mental retardation and scapuloperoneal muscular dystrophy. J. Neurol. 49:1423, 1986.

70. Woolliscroft, J., and Tuna, N.: Permanent atrial standstill: The clinical spectrum. Am. J. Med. 49:2037, 1982.

71. Ward, D. E., Ho, S. Y., and Shinebourne, E. A.: Familial atrial standstill and inexcitability in childhood. Am. J. Cardiol. 53:965, 1984.

72. Disertori, M., Guarnerio, M., Vergara, G., et al.: Familial endemic persistent atrial standstill in a small mountain community. Eur. Heart J. 4:354, 1983.

73. Levy, S., Pouget, B., Bemurat, M., et al.: Partial atrial electrical standstill: Report of three cases and review of clinical and electrophysiological features. Eur. Heart J. 1:107, 1980.

74. Effendy, F. N., Bolognesi, R., Bianchi, G., and Visioli, O.: Alternation of partial and total atrial standstill. J. Electrocardiol. 12:121, 1979.

75. Miller, R. G., Layzer, R. B., Mellenthin, M. A., et al.: Emery-Dreifuss muscular dystrophy with autosomal dominant transmission. Neurology 35:1230, 1985.

76. Rowland, L. P., Fetell, M., Alarte, M., et al.: Emery-Dreifuss muscular dystrophy. Ann. Neurol. 5:111, 1979.

77. Fenichel, G. M., Sul, Y. C., Kilroy, A. W., and Blouin, R.: An autosomal dominant dystrophy with humeropelvic distribution and cardiomyopathy. Neurology 32:1399, 1982.

78. Hopkins, L. C., Jackson, J. H., and Elsas, L. J.: Emery-Dreifuss humeroperoneal muscular dystrophy: An X-linked myopathy with unusual contractures and bradycardia. Ann. Neurol. 10:230, 1981.

79. Dickey, P. P., Ziter, F. A., and Smith, R. A.: Emery-Dreifuss muscular dystrophy. J. Pediatr. 104:555, 1984.

80. Oswald, A. H., Goldblatt, J., Horak, A. R., and Beighton, P.: Lethal cardiac conduction defects in Emery-Dreifuss muscular dystrophy. S. Afr. Med. J. 72:567, 1987.

81. Wyse, D. G., Nath, F. C., and Brownell, A.K.W.: Benign X-linked (Emery-Dreifuss) muscular dystrophy is not benign. PACE 10:533, 1987.

82. Yoshioka, M., Saida, K., Itagaki, Y., and Kamiya, T.: Follow up study of cardiac involvement in Emery-Dreifuss muscular dystrophy. Arch. Dis. Child. 64:713, 1989.

83. Harper, P. S.: Myotonic Dystrophy. 2nd ed. Philadelphia, W. B. Saunders Company, 1989.

84. Wieringa, B., Brunner, H., Hulsebos, T., et al.: Genetic and physical demarcation of the locus for dystrophia myotonica. Adv. Neurol. 48:47, 1988.

85. Bharati, S., Bump, F. T., Bauernfeind, R., and Lev, M.: Dystrophica myotonia. Correlative electrocardiographic, electrophysiologic and conduction system study. Chest 86:444, 1984.

86. Moorman, J. R., Coleman, R. E., Packer, D. L., et al.: Cardiac involvement in myotonic muscular dystrophy. Medicine 64:371, 1985.

87. Hiromasa, S., Ikeda, T., Kubota, K., et al.: Ventricular tachycardia and sudden death in myotonic dystrophy. Am. Heart J. 115:914, 1988.

88. Nguyen, H. H., Wolfe, J. T., III, Holmes, D. R., Jr., and Edwards, W. D.: Pathology of the cardiac conduction system in myotonic dystrophy: A study of 12 cases. J. Am. Coll. Cardiol. 11:662, 1988.

89. Hiromasa, S., Ikeda, T., Kubota, K., et al.: A family with myotonic dystrophy associated with diffuse cardiac conduction disturbances as demonstrated by His bundle electrocardiography. Am. Heart J. 111:85, 1986.

90. Olofsson, B., Forsberg, H., Andersson, S., et al.: Electrocardiographic findings in myotonic dystrophy. Br. Heart J. 59:47, 1988.

91. Grigg, L. E., Chan, W., Mond, H. G., et al.: Ventricular tachycardia and sudden death in myotonic dystrophy: Clinical, electrophysiologic and pathologic features. Am. J. Cardiol. 6:254, 1985.

92. Prystowsky, E. N., Pritchett, E.L.C., Roses, A. D., and Gallagher, J. J.: The natural history of conduction system disease in myotonic muscular dystrophy as determined by serial electrophysiologic studies. Circulation 60:1360, 1979.

93. Uemura, N., Tanaka, H., Niimura, T., et al.: Electrophysiological and histological abnormalities of the heart in myotonic dystrophy. Am. Heart J. 86:616, 1973.

94. Petkovich, N. J., Dunn, M., and Reed, W.: Myotonia dystrophica with AV dissociation and Stokes-Adams attacks. Am. Heart J. 68:391, 1964.

95. Motta, J., Guilleminault, C., Bilingham, M., et al.: Cardiac abnormalities in myotonic dystrophy: Electrophysiologic and histopathologic studies. Am. J. Med. 67:467, 1979.

96. Ludatscher, R. M., Kerner, H., Amikam, S., and Gellei, B.: Myotonia dystrophica with heart involvement: An electron microscopic study of skeletal, cardiac, and smooth muscle. J. Clin. Pathol. 31:1057, 1978.

97. Tanaka, N., Tanaka, H., Takeda, M., et al.: Cardiomyopathy in myotonic dystrophy: A light and electron microscopic study of the myocardium. Jpn. Heart J. 14:202, 1973.

98. Hartwig, G. R., Ran, K. R., Radoff, F. M., et al.: Radionuclide angiocardiographic analysis of myocardial function in myotonic muscular dystrophy. Neurology 33:657, 1983.

99. Child, J. S., and Perloff, J. K.: Diastolic properties of the left ventricle in myotonic muscular dystrophy (Steinert's disease). To be published.

100. Hiromasa, S., Ikeda, T., Kubota, K., et al.: A family with myotonic dystrophy associated with diffuse cardiac conduction disturbances as demonstrated by His bundle electrocardiography. Am. Heart J. 111:85, 1986.

101. Forsberg, H., Olofsson, B., Eriksson, A., and Andersson, S.: Cardiac involvement in congenital myotonic dystrophy. Br. Heart J. 63:119, 1990.

102. Anderson, M.: Probable Thomsen's disease with cardiac involvement. J. Neurol. 214:301, 1977.

103. Subramony, S. H., Malhotra, C.P., and Mishra, S. K.: Distinguishing paramyotonia congenita and myotonia congenita by electromyography. Muscle Nerve 6:374, 1983.

104. Streib, F. W., Sun, S. F., and Hanson, M.: Paramyotonia congenita: Clinical and electrophysiologic studies. Electromyogr. Clin. Neurophysiol. 23:315, 1983.

105. Rosenberg, R. N.: Hereditary ataxias. In Rowland, L. P. (ed.): Merritt's Textbook of Neurology. Philadelphia, Lea & Febiger, 1984, p. 499.

106. Barbeau, H.: Friedreich's ataxia 1980. Our overview of the pathophysiology. J. Can. Sci. Neurol. 7:455, 1980.

107. Harding, A. E.: Friedreich's ataxia: A clinical and genetic study of 90 families with an analysis of early diagnostic criteria and intrafamilial clustering of clinical features. Brain 104:589, 1981.

108. Brumback, R. A., Panner, B. J., and Kingston, W. J.: The heart in Friedreich's ataxia. Arch. Neurol. 43:189, 1986.

109. Grenadier, E., Goldberg, S. J., Stern, L. Z., and Feldman, J.: M-mode and two-dimensional echocardiographic examination of patients with Friedreich's ataxia. J. Cardiovasc. Ultrasonog. 3:5, 1984.

110. Gottdiener, J. S., Hawley, R. J., Maron, B. J., et al.: Characteristics of the cardiac hypertrophy in Friedreich's ataxia. Am. Heart J. 103:525, 1982.

111. Barbeau, A.: Pathophysiology of Friedreich's ataxia. In Matthews, W. B., and Glaser, G. H. (eds.): Recent Advances in Clinical Neurology, No. 3. Edinburgh, Churchill Livingstone, 1982, p. 129.

112. Pasternac, A., Drol, R., Petitclerc, R., et al.: Hypertrophic cardiomyopathy in Friedreich's ataxia: Symmetric or asymmetric? J. Can. Sci. Neurol. 7:379, 1980.

113. Harding, A. E., and Hewer, R. L.: The heart disease of Friedreich's ataxia: A clinical and electrocardiographic study of 115 patients, with an analysis of serial electrocardiographic changes in 30 cases. Q. J. Med. 28:489, 1983.

114. Zimmermann, M., Gabathuler, J., Adamec, R., and Pinget, L.: Unusual manifestations of heart involvement in Friedreich's ataxia. Am. Heart J. 111:184, 1986.

115. Hawley, R. J., and Gottdiener, J. S.: Five-year follow-up of Friedreich's ataxia cardiomyopathy. Arch. Intern. Med. 146:483, 1986.

116. Unverferth, D. V., Schmidt, W. R., Baker, P. B., and Wooley, C. F.: Morphologic and functional characteristics of the heart in Friedreich's ataxia. Am. J. Med. 82:5, 1987.

117. Pentland, B., and Fox, K.A.A.: The heart in Friedreich's ataxia. J. Neurol. Neurosurg. Psychiatry 46:1138, 1983.

118. Hawley, R. J., and Gottdiener, J. S.: Five-year follow-up of Friedreich's ataxia cardiomyopathy. Arch. Intern. Med. 146:483, 1986.

119. Alboliras, E. T., Shub, C., Gomez, M. R., et al.: Spectrum of cardiac involvement in Friedreich's ataxia: Clinical, electrocardiographic and echocardiographic observations. Am. J. Cardiol. 58:518, 1986.

120. Pentland, B., and Fox, K.A.A.: The heart in Friedreich's ataxia. J. Neurol. Neurosurg. Psychiatry 46:1138, 1983.

121. James, T. N., Cobbs, B. W., Coghlan, H. C., et al.: Coronary disease, cardioneuropathy, and conduction system abnormalities in the cardiomyopathy of Friedreich's ataxia. Br. Heart J. 57:446, 1987.

122. Spach, N. S., and Kootsey, J. M.: The nature of electrical propagation in cardiac muscle. Am. J. Physiol. 244:H3, 1983.

123. Palagi, B., Picozzi, R., Casazza, F., et al.: Biventricular function in Friedreich's ataxia: A radionuclide angiographic study. Br. Heart J. 59:692, 1988.

124. Giunta, A., Maione, S., Biagini, R., et al.: Noninvasive assessment of systolic and diastolic function in 50 patients with Friedreich's ataxia. Cardiology 75:321, 1988.

125. Zimmermann, M., Gabathuler, J., Adamec, R., and Pinget, L.: Unusual manifestations of heart involvement in Friedreich's ataxia. Am. Heart J. 111:184, 1986.

126. Rowland, L. P.: Molecular genetics, pseudogenetics and clinical neurology. Neurology 33:179, 1983.

127. Rosenberg, R. N.: Biochemical genetics of neurologic disease. N. Engl. J. Med. 305:1181, 1981.

128. Perloff, J. K.: Pathogenesis of hypertrophic cardiomyopathy. In Goodwin, J. F. (ed.): Heart Muscle DIsease. Lancaster, MTP Press Ltd., 1985.

129. Pasternac, A., Wagniart, P., Olivenstein, R., et al.: Increased plasma catecholamines in patients with Friedreich's ataxia. J. Can. Sci. Neurol. 9:195, 1982.

130. Merkel, A. D., and Barbeau, A.: Plasma catecholamines in Friedreich's ataxia assayed using high performance liquid chromatography with electrochemical detection. J. Can. Sci. Neurol. 9:205, 1982.

LESS COMMON NEUROMYOPATHIC DISEASES SOMETIMES ASSOCIATED WITH HEART DISEASE

131. Pleasure, D. E., and Schotland, D. L.: Hereditary neuropathies. *In* Rowland, L. P. (ed.): Merritt's Textbook of Neurology. Philadelphia, Lea & Febiger, 1984.

132. Isner, J. M., Hawley, R. J., Weintraub, A. B., and Engel, W. K.: Cardiac findings in Charcot-Marie-Tooth disease. Arch. Intern. Med. *139*:1161, 1979.

133. Dyck, P. J., Swanson, C. J., Nishimura, R. A., et al.: Cardiomyopathy in patients with hereditary motor and sensory neuropathy. Mayo Clin. Proc. *62*:672, 1987.

134. Leak, D.: Paroxysmal atrial flutter in peroneal muscular atrophy. Br. Heart J. *23*:326, 1961.

135. Littler, W. A.: Heart block and peroneal muscular atrophy. Q. J. Med. *39*:431, 1970.

136. Kaj, J. M., Littler, W. A., and Meade, J. B.: Ultrastructure of the myocardium in familial heart block and peroneal muscular atrophy. Br. Heart J. *34*:1081, 1972.

137. Lowry, P. I., and Littler, W. A.: Peroneal muscular atrophy associated with cardiac conduction tissue disease. Postgrad. Med. J. *59*:530, 1983.

138. Martin-Du Pan, R. C., Juse, C., and Perrenoud, J. J.: Congestive cardiomyopathy and pyruvate elevation in a case of Charcot-Marie-Tooth disease. Schweiz. med. Wochenschr. *5*:114, 1984.

139. Spiro, A. J., Shy, G. M., and Gonatas, N. K.: Myotubular myopathy. Arch. Neurol. *14*:1, 1966.

140. Verhiest, W., Brucher, J. M., Goddeeris, P., et al.: Familial centronuclear myopathy associated with cardiomyopathy. Br. Heart J. *38*:504, 1976.

141. Shafiq, S. A., Sande, M. A., Carruthers, R. R., et al.: Skeletal muscle in idiopathic cardiomyopathy. J. Neurol. Sci. *15*:303, 1972.

142. Berenberg, R. A., Pellock, J. M., DiMauro, S., et al.: Lumping or splitting? "Ophthalmoplegia-plus" or Kearns-Sayre syndrome? Ann. Neurol. *1*:37, 1977.

143. Lowes, M.: Chronic progressive external ophthalmoplegia, pigmentary retinopathy and heart block (Kearns-Sayre syndrome). Acta Ophthalmol. *53*:610, 1975.

144. Charles, R., Holt, S., Kay, J. M., et al.: Myocardial ultrastructure and the development of atrioventricular block in Kearns-Sayre syndrome. Circulation *63*:214, 1981.

145. Roberts, N. K., Perloff, J. K., and Kark, P.: Cardiac conduction in Kearns-Sayre syndrome. Am. J. Cardiol. *44*:1396, 1979.

146. Schwartzkopff, B., Frenzel, H., Losse, B., et al.: Heart involvement in progressive external ophthalmoplegia (Kearns-Sayre syndrome): Electrophysiologic, hemodynamic and morphologic findings. Z. Kardiol. *75*:161, 1986.

147. Schwartzkopff, B., Frenzel, H., Breithardt, G., et al.: Ultrastructural findings in endomyocardial biopsy of patients with Kearns-Sayre syndrome. J. Am. Coll. Cardiol. *12*:1522, 1988.

148. Channer, K. S., Channer, J. L., Campbell, M. J., and Rees, J. R.: Cardiomyopathy in the Kearns-Sayre syndrome. Br. Heart J. *59*:486, 1988.

149. Kenny, D., and Wetherbee, J.: Kearns-Sayre syndrome in the elderly: Mitochondrial myopathy with advanced heart block. Am. Heart J. *120*:440, 1990.

150. Clark, D. S., Myerburg, R. J., Morales, R. R., et al.: Heart block and Kearns-Sayre: Electrophysiologic-pathologic correlation. Chest *68*:727, 1975.

151. Pleasure, D. E., and Schotland, D. L.: Acquired neuropathies. *In* Rowland, L. P. (ed.): Merritt's Textbook of Neurology. 7th ed. Philadelphia, Lea & Febiger, 1984.

152. McDonagh, A.J.G., and Dawson, J.: Guillain-Barré syndrome after myocardial infarction. Br. Med. J. *294*:613, 1987.

153. Emmons, P. R., Blume, W. T., and DuShane, J. W.: Cardiac monitoring and demand pacemaker in Guillain-Barré syndrome. Arch. Neurol. *32*:59, 1975.

154. Greenland, P., and Griggs, R. C.: Arrhythmic complications in the Guillain-Barré syndrome. Arch. Intern. Med. *140*:1053, 1980.

155. Narayam, D., Huang, M. T., and Matthew, P. K.: Bradycardia and asystole requiring pacemaker in Guillain-Barré syndrome. Am. Heart J. *108*:426, 1984.

156. Fagius, J., and Wallin, B. G.: Microneurographic evidence of excessive sympathetic outflow in the Guillain-Barré syndrome. Brain *106*:589, 1983.

157. Persson, A., and Solders, G.: R-R variations in Guillain-Barré syndrome: A test of autonomic dysfunction. Acta Neurol. Scand. *67*:294, 1983.

158. Palferman, T. G., Wright, I., Doyle, D. V., and Amiel, S.: Electrocardiographic abnormalities and autonomic dysfunction in Guillain-Barré syndrome. Br. Med. J. *284*:1231, 1982.

159. Shy, G. M., Engel, W. K., Somers, J. E., and Wanko, T.: Nemaline myopathy; a new congenital myopathy. Brain *86*:793, 1963.

160. Conen, P. E., Murphy, G. E., and Donohue, W. L.: Light and electron microscopic studies of "myogranules" in a child with hypotonia and muscle weakness. Can. Med. Assoc. J. *89*:983, 1963.

160a. Ishibashi-Veda, H., Imakita, M., Yutani, C., et al.: Congenital nemaline myopathy with dilated cardiomyopathy: An autopsy study. Hum. Pathol. *21*:77, 1990.

161. Kinoshita, M., and Satoyoshi, E.: Type I fiber atrophy and nemaline bodies. Arch. Neurol. *31*:423, 1974.

162. Meier, C., Gertsch, M., Zimmerman, A., et al.: Nemaline myopathy presenting as cardiomyopathy. N. Engl. J. Med. *308*:1536, 1983.

163. Meier, C., Voellmy, W., Gertsch, M., et al.: Nemaline myopathy appearing in adults as cardiomyopathy: A clinicopathologic study. Arch. Neurol. *41*:443, 1984.

164. Penn, A. S., and Rowland, L. P.: Neuromuscular junction. *In* Rowland, L.

165. Barnes, D. M.: Nervous and immune system disorders linked in a variety of diseases. Science *232*:160, 1985.

166. Gibson, T. C.: The heart in myasthenia gravis. Am. Heart J. *90*:389, 1975.

167. Kornfeld, P., Horowitz, S. H., Genkins, G., and Papatestas, A.: Myasthenia gravis unmasked by antiarrhythmic agents. Mt. Sinai J. Med. *43*:10, 1976.

168. Niakan, E., Bertorini, T. E., Acchiardo, S. R., and Werner, M. F.: Procainamide-induced myasthenia-like weakness in a patient with peripheral neuropathy. Arch. Neurol. *38*:378, 1981.

169. Ratinov, G., Baker, W. P., and Swaiman, K. F.: McArdle's syndrome with previously unreported electrocardiographic and serum enzyme abnormalities. Ann. Intern. Med. *62*:328, 1965.

170. Sengers, R.C.A., ter Haar, B.G.A., Trijhels, J.M.F., et al.: Congenital cataract and mitochondrial myopathy of skeletal and heart muscle associated with lactic acidosis after exercise. J. Pediatr. *86*:873, 1975.

171. Melki, J., Abdelhak, S., Sheth, P., et al.: Gene for chronic proximal spinal muscular atrophies maps to chromosome 5q. Nature *344*:767, 1990.

172. Kimura, S., Yokota, H., Tateda, K., et al.: A case of the Kugelberg-Welander syndrome complicated with cardiac lesions. Jpn. Heart J. *21*:417, 1980.

173. Gottdiener, J. S., Sherber, H. S., Hawley, R. J., and Engel, W. K.: Cardiac manifestations in polymyositis. Am. J. Cardiol. *41*:1141, 1978.

174. Singsen, B., Goldreyer, B., Stanton, R., and Hanson, V.: Childhood polymyositis with cardiac conduction defects. Am. J. Dis. Child. *131*:72, 1976.

175. Farber, H. W., and Make, B.: Physiologic closure of a symptomatic patent foramen ovale with oxygen therapy. Am. Rev. Resp. Dis. *131*:181, 1985.

176. Lisak, R. P., Lebeau, J., Tucker, S. H., and Rowland, L. P.: Hyperkalemic periodic paralysis and cardiac arrhythmias. Neurology *22*:810, 1972.

177. Buruma, O. J., Schipperheyn, J. J., and Bots, G. T.: Heart muscle disease in familial hypokalemic periodic paralysis. Circulation *64*:12, 1981.

178. Klein, R., Ganelin, R., Marks, J. F., et al.: Periodic paralysis with cardiac arrhythmia. J. Pediatr. *62*:371, 1963.

179. Kastor, J. A., and Goldreyer, B. N.: Ventricular origin of bidirectional tachycardia. Circulation *48*:897, 1973.

180. Karpawich, P. P., Hart, Z. H., Perry, B. L., et al.: Childhood periodic paralysis with dysrhythmias: Electrophysiologic and histopathologic evaluation. Am. Heart J. *114*:186, 1987.

181. Fukuda, K., Ogawa, S., Yokozuka, H., et al.: Long-standing bidirectional tachycardia in a patient with hypokalemic periodic paralysis. J. Electrocardiol. *21*:71, 1988.

182. Perloff, J. K. (ed.): The Cardiomyopathies. Philadelphia, W. B. Saunders Company, 1988.

183. Meyer, J. G., and Urban, K.: Electrolyte changes and acid-base balance after alcohol withdrawal. With special reference to rum fits and magnesium depletion. J. Neurol. *215*:135, 1977.

184. Rubin, E.: Alcoholic myopathy in heart and skeletal muscle. N. Engl. J. Med. *301*:28, 1979.

185. Clarren, S. K., and Smith, D. W.: The fetal alcohol syndrome. N. Engl. J. Med. *298*:1063, 1978.

ACUTE CEREBRAL DISORDERS ACCOMPANIED BY CARDIOVASCULAR ABNORMALITIES

186. Bramwell, C.: Can head injury cause auricular fibrillation? Lancet *1*:8, 1934.

187. Chen, H. I., Liao, J. F., and Ho, S. T.: Centrogenic pulmonary hemorrhagic edema induced by cerebral compression in rats. Circ. Res. *47*:366, 1980.

188. Schell, A. R., Shenoy, M. M., Friedman, S. A., and Patel, A. R.: Pulmonary edema associated with subarachnoid hemorrhage. Arch. Intern. Med. *147*:591, 1987.

189. Yamour, B. J., Sridharan, M. R., Rice, J. F., and Flowers, N. C.: Electrocardiographic changes in cerebrovascular hemorrhage. Am. Heart J. *99*:294, 1980.

190. Robertson, C. S., Clifton, G. L., Taylor, A. A., and Grossman, R. G.: Treatment of hypertension associated with head injury. J. Neurosurg. *59*:455, 1983.

191. Cushing, H.: Concerning a definite regulatory mechanism of the vasomotor center which controls blood pressure during cerebral compression. Bull. Johns Hopkins Hosp. *12*:390, 1901.

192. Sciarra, D.: Head injury. *In* Rowland, L. P. (ed.): Merritt's Textbook of Neurology. 7th ed. Philadelphia, Lea & Febiger, 1984, p. 277.

193. Hackenberry, L. E., Miner, M. E., Rea, G. L., et al.: Biochemical evidence of myocardial injury after severe head trauma. Crit. Care Med. *10*:641, 1982.

194. Clifton, G. L., Robertson, C. S., Kyper, K., et al.: Cerebrovascular response to severe head injury. J. Neurosurg. *59*:447, 1983.

195. McLeod, A. A., Neil-Dwyer, G., Meyer, C.H.A., et al.: Cardiac sequelae of acute head injury. Br. Heart J. *47*:221, 1982.

196. Tobias, S. L., Bookatz, B. J., and Diamond, T. H.: Myocardial damage and electrocardiographic changes in acute cerebrovascular hemorrhage: A report of three cases and review. Heart Lung *16*:521, 1987.

197. Pollick, C., Cujec, B., Parker, S., and Tator, C.: Left ventricular wall motion abnormalities in subarachnoid hemorrhage: An echocardiographic study. J. Am. Coll. Cardiol. *12*:600, 1988.

198. Baur, H. R., Gobel, F. L., and Pierach, C. A.: Electrocardiographic changes after cervical laminectomy. Int. J. Cardiol. *1*:37, 1981.

199. Samuels, M. A.: Electrocardiographic manifestations of neurologic disease. Semin. Neurol. *4*:453, 1984.

200. Carruth, J. E., and Silverman, M. E.: *Torsades de pointes* atypical ventricular tachycardia complicating subarachnoid hemorrhage. Chest 78:886, 1980.

201. Mikolich, J. R., Jacobs, W. C., and Fletcher, G. F.: Cardiac arrhythmias in patients with acute cerebrovascular accidents. J.A.M.A. 246:1314, 1981.

202. Goldberger, A. L.: Recognition of ECG pseudoinfarct patterns. Mod. Concepts Cardiovasc. Dis. 49:13, 1980.

203. Taylor, A. L., and Fozzard, H. A.: Ventricular arrhythmias associated with CNS disease. Arch. Intern. Med. 142:232, 1982.

204. Gould, L., Reddy, R. C., Kollali, M., et al.: Electrocardiographic normalization after cerebral vascular accident. J. Electrocardiol. 14:191, 1981.

205. Myers, M. G., Norris, J. W., Hachinski, V. C., et al.: Cardiac sequelae of acute stroke. Stroke 13:838, 1982.

206. Stober, T., Anstätt, T., Sen, S., et al.: Cardiac arrhythmias in subarachnoid haemorrhage. Acta Neurochir. 93:37, 1988.

207. Rudehill, A., Olsson, G. L., Sundqvist, K., and Gordon, E.: ECG abnormalities in patients with subarachnoid haemorrhage and intracranial tumours. J. Neurol. Neurosurg. Psychiatry 50:1375, 1987.

208. Melin, J., and Fogelhohm, R.: Electrocardiographic findings in subarachnoid hemorrhage. Acta Med. Scand. 213:5, 1983.

209. Brunninkhuis, L.G.H.: Electrocardiographic abnormalities suggesting myocardial infarction in a patient with severe cranial trauma. PACE 6:1336, 1983.

210. Gascon, P., Ley, T. J., Toltzis, R. J., and Bonow, R. O.: Spontaneous subarachnoid hemorrhage simulating acute transmural myocardial infarction. Am. Heart J. 105:511, 1983.

211. Tabbaa, M. A., Ramirez-Lassepas, M., and Snyder, B. D.: Aneurysmal subarachnoid hemorrhage presenting as cardiorespiratory arrest. Arch. Intern. Med. 147:1661, 1987.

212. Fredberg, U., Bøtker, H. E., and Rømer, F. K.: Acute neurogenic pulmonary oedema following generalized tonic clonic seizure. A case report and a review of the literature. Eur. Heart J. 9:933, 1988.

213. Oppenheimer, S. M., Cechetto, D. F., and Hachinski, V. C.: Cerebrogenic cardiac arrhythmias. Arch. Neurol. 47:513, 1990.

214. Lehmann, K. G., Lane, J. G., Piepmeier, J. M., and Batsford, W. P.: Cardiovascular abnormalities accompanying acute spinal cord injury in humans: Incidence, time course and severity. J. Am. Coll. Cardiol. 10:46, 1987.

215. Miah, K., von Arbin, M., Britton, M., et al.: Prognosis in acute stroke with special reference to some cardiac factors. J. Chronic Dis. 36:279, 1983.

216. Komrad, M. S., Coffey, C. E., Coffey, K. S., et al.: Myocardial infarction and stroke. Neurology 34:1403, 1984.

217. Chin, P. L., Kaminski, J., and Rout, N.: Myocardial infarction coincident with cerebrovascular accidents in the elderly. Age Ageing 6:29, 1977.

218. Gillum, R. F., Fortmann, S. P., Prineas, R. J., and Kottke, T. E.: International diagnostic criteria for acute myocardial infarction and acute stroke. Am. Heart J. 108:150, 1984.

219. Sandok, B. A., Whisnant, J. P., Furlan, A. J., and Mickell, J. L.: Carotid arterial bruits. Mayo Clin. Proc. 57:227, 1982.

220. Heyman, A., Wilkinson, W. E., Heyden, S., et al.: Risk of stroke in asymptomatic persons with cervical arterial bruits. N. Engl. J. Med. 302:838, 1980.

221. Sundt, T. M., Jr., Whisnant, J. P., Houser, O. W., and Fode, N. C.: Prospective study of the effectiveness and durability of carotid endarterectomy. Mayo Clin. Proc. 65:625, 1990.

222. Roper, A. H., Wechsler, L. R., and Wilson, L. S.: Carotid bruit and the risk of stroke in elective surgery. N. Engl. J. Med. 307:1388, 1982.

223. Busuttil, R. W., Baker, J. D., Davidson, R. K., and Machleder, H. I.: Carotid arterial stenosis: Hemodynamic significance and clinical course. J.A.M.A. 245:1438, 1981.

224. Matchar, D. B.: Decision making in the face of uncertainty: The case of carotid endarterectomy. Mayo Clin. Proc. 65:756, 1990.

225. Wolf, P. A., Kannel, W. B., Sorlie, P., and McNamara, P.: Asymptomatic carotid bruit and risk of stroke. J.A.M.A. 245:1442, 1981.

226. Langlois, Y., Roederer, G. O., Chan, A., et al.: Evaluating carotid arterial disease. Ultrasound Med. Biol. 9:51, 1983.

227. Cebul, R. D., and Ginsberg, M. D.: Noninvasive neurovascular tests for carotid artery disease. Ann. Intern. Med. 97:867, 1982.

228. Jones, E. L., Craver, J. M., Michalik, R. A., et al.: Combined carotid and coronary operations: When are they necessary? J. Thorac. Cardiovasc. Surg. 87:7, 1984.

229. Rice, P. L., Pifarre, R., Sullivan, H. J., et al.: Experience with simultaneous myocardial revascularization and carotid endarterectomy. J. Thorac. Cardiovasc. Surg. 79:922, 1980.

230. Breslau, P. J., Fell, G., Ivey, T. D., et al.: Carotid arterial disease in patients undergoing coronary artery bypass operations. J. Thorac. Cardiovasc. Surg. 82:765, 1981.

231. Breuer, A. C., Hanson, M. R., Furlan, A. J., et al.: Central nervous system complications of myocardial revascularization. A prospective analysis of 400 patients. Stroke 11:136, 1980.

232. Gonzalez-Scarano, F., and Hurtig, H. I.: Neurologic complications of coronary artery bypass grafting: Case-control study. Neurology 31:1032, 1981.

233. Bojar, R. M., Najafi, H., De Laria, G. A., et al.: Neurological complications of coronary revascularization. Ann. Thorac. Surg. 36:427, 1983.

234. Sotaniemi, K. A.: Brain damage and neurological outcome after open heart surgery. J. Neurol. Neurosurg. Psychiatry 43:127, 1980.

235. Ferry, P. C.: Neurologic sequelae of cardiac surgery in children. Am. J. Dis. Child. 141:309, 1987.

236. Cerebral Embolism Task Force: Cardiogenic brain embolism. Arch. Neurol. 43:71, 1986.

237. Kopecky, S. L., Gersh, B. J., McGoon, M. D., et al.: The natural history of lone atrial fibrillation. N. Engl. J. Med. 317:669, 1987.

238. Stroke Prevention in Atrial Fibrillation Study Group Investigators: Preliminary report of the stroke prevention in atrial fibrillation study. N. Engl. J. Med. 322:863, 1990.

239. Perloff, J. K., and Child, J. S.: Clinical and epidemiological issues in mitral valve prolapse. Am. Heart J. 113:1324, 1987.

240. Wolf, P. A., and Sila, C. A.: Cerebral ischemia with mitral valve prolapse. Am. Heart J. 113:1308, 1987.

241. Yufe, R., Karpati, G., and Carpenter, S.: Cardiac myxoma: A diagnostic challenge for the neurologist. Neurology 26:1060, 1976.

242. Perloff, J. K.: The Clinical Recognition of Congenital Heart Disease. 3rd ed. Philadelphia, W. B. Saunders Company, 1987.

243. Salgado, A. V., Furlan, A. J., and Keys, T. F.: Mycotic aneurysm, subarachnoid hemorrhage, and indications for cerebral angiography in infective endocarditis. Stroke 18:1057, 1987.

244. Salgado, A. V., Furlan, A. J., Keys, T. F., et al.: Neurologic complications of endocarditis: A 12-year experience. Neurology 39:173, 1989.

245. Grandsden, W. R., Eykyn, S. J., and Leach, R. M.: Neurological presentations of native valve endocarditis. Q. J. Med. 73:1135, 1989.

246. Baron, K. D., Siqueira, E., and Hirano, A.: Cerebral embolism caused by nonbacterial thrombotic endocarditis. Neurology 10:391, 1960.

247. Caplan, L. R., Hier, D. B., and Banks, G.: Stroke and drug abuse. Curr. Concepts Cerebrovasc. Dis. 17:9, 1982.

248. Biller, J., Johnson, M. R., Adams, H. P., Jr., et al.: Further observations on cerebral or retinal ischemia in patients with right-left intracardiac shunts. Arch. Neurol. 44:740, 1987.

249. Lechat, P., Mas, J. L., Lascault, G., et al.: Prevalence of patent foramen ovale in patients with stroke. N. Engl. J. Med. 318:1148, 1988.

250. Harvey, J. R., Teague, S. M., Anderson, J. L., et al.: Clinically silent atrial septal defects with evidence for cerebral embolization. Ann. Intern. Med. 105:695, 1986.

251. Pitkin, R. M., Perloff, J. K., Koos, B. J., and Beall, M. H.: Pregnancy and congenital heart disease. Ann. Intern. Med. 112:445, 1990.

252. Schneider, B., Hanrath, P., Vogel, P., and Meinertz, T.: Improved morphologic characterization of atrial septal aneurysm by transesophageal echocardiography: Relation to cerebrovascular events. J. Am. Coll. Cardiol. 16:1000, 1990.

253. Dodge, R. P., Richardson, E. P., and Victor, M.: Recurrent convulsive seizures as a sequel to cerebral infarction. Brain 77:610, 1959.

254. Perloff, J. K., Rosove, M. H., Child, J. S., and Wright, G. B.: Adults with cyanotic congenital heart disease: Hematologic management. Ann. Intern. Med. 109:406, 1988.

255. Daniels, S. R., Bates, S. R., and Kaplan, S.: EEG monitoring during paroxysmal hyperpnea of tetralogy of Fallot: An epileptic or hypoxic phenomenon? J. Child Neurol. 2:98, 1987.

256. Longstreth, W. T., Inui, T. S., Cobb, L. A., and Copass, M. K.: Neurologic recovery after out-of-hospital cardiac arrest. Ann. Intern. Med. 98:588, 1983.

257. Bircher, N. G.: Neurologic management following cardiac arrest. Neurol. Crit. Care 5:773, 1989.

CARDIAC COMPLICATIONS OF DRUGS USED IN TREATING NEUROMUSCULAR DISEASE

258. Bircher, N. G.: Brain resuscitation. Resuscitation 18:S1, 1989.

259. Orlando, R. C., Moyer, P., and Barnett, T. B.: Methysergide therapy and constrictive pericarditis. Ann. Intern. Med. 88:213, 1978.

260. Bana, D. S., MacNeal, P. S., LeCompte, P. M., et al.: Cardiac murmurs and endocardial fibrosis associated with methysergide therapy. Am. Heart J. 88:640, 1974.

261. Dorne, H. L., and Satin, R.: Methysergide-induced lower extremity arterial insufficiency. J. Can. Assoc. Radiol. 37:210, 1986.

262. Yahr, M. D.: Parkinsonism. In Rowland, L. P. (ed.): Merritt's Textbook of Neurology. 7th ed. Philadelphia, Lea & Febiger, 1984, p. 526.

263. Lane, R.J.M., Roche, S. W., Leung, A.A.W., et al.: Cyclosporin neurotoxicity in cardiac transplant recipients. J. Neurol. Neurosurg. Psychiatry 51:1434, 1988.

264. Hotson, J. R., and Enzmann, D. R.: Neurologic complications of cardiac transplantation. Neurol. Clin. 6:349, 1988.

265. Ang, L. C., Gillett, J. M., and Kaufmann, J.C.E.: Neuropathology of heart transplantation. Can. J. Neurol. Sci. 16:291, 1989.

266. Francis, D. A., Heron, J. R., and Clarke, M.: Ambulatory electrocardiographic monitoring in patients with transient focal cerebral ischaemia. J. Neurol. Neurosurg. Psychiatry 47:256, 1984.

267. Benorvitz, N. L.: Clinical applications of the pharmacokinetics of lidocaine. Cardiovasc. Clin. 6:77, 1974.

268. Weidler, D. J., Jallad, N. S., Keener, D. B., et al.: The effects of acute focal cerebral ischemia on digoxin toxicity and pharmacokinetics. Pharmacology 20:188, 1980.

269. Withering, W.: An account of the Foxglove. In Willius, F. A., and Keys, T. E.: Classics of Cardiology. Vol. 1. Malabar, Fla., Robert E. Krieger Publishing Co., 1983, p. 244.

270. Oliveira, J.S.M., dos Santos, J.C.M., Muccillo, G., and Ferreira, A. L.: Increased capacity of the coronary arteries in chronic Chagas' heart disease: Further support for the neurogenic pathogenetic concept. Am. Heart J. 109:304, 1985.

271. Iosa, D., DeQuattro, V., Lee, D. D., et al.: Plasma norepinephrine in Chagas' cardioneuromyopathy: A marker of progressive dysautonomia. Am. Heart J. 117:882, 1989.

Endocrine and Nutritional Disorders and Heart Disease

by GORDON H. WILLIAMS, M.D., and EUGENE BRAUNWALD, M.D.

In 1835, Robert Graves described "three cases of violent and long-continued palpitation in females" with thyrotoxicosis.[1] Twenty years later, Thomas Addison reported that patients with disease of the "suprarenal capsules" had a "pulse, small and feeble . . . excessively soft and compressible." As the disease progressed, "the body wastes . . . the pulse becomes smaller and weaker, and . . . the patient at length gradually sinks and expires."[2] Thus, since the mid-19th century, it has been known that deranged hormonal secretion can significantly alter cardiovascular function. The purpose of this chapter is to summarize the more important cardiovascular manifestations of endocrine and nutritional diseases.

ACROMEGALY

The anterior pituitary gland secretes at least seven polypeptide hormones. Four (ACTH and related peptides, FSH, LH, and TSH) primarily produce their biological effect indirectly by altering hormonal secretion from a specific target gland (adrenal cortex, gonad, or thyroid). Thus, the pathophysiological manifestations of a derangement in their secretion are the same as those of their target organs and will be discussed later. There are no cardiovascular manifestations of altered prolactin secretion or growth hormone deficiency; however, acromegaly (growth hormone excess) is associated with a number of clinical signs and symptoms related to the cardiovascular system.

ACTIONS OF GROWTH HORMONE. Growth hormone is only one of a family of peptides whose overall function is to regulate growth of the organism.[3,4] Two hormones secreted by the hypothalamus (somatotropin-releasing hormone and somatostatin) regulate the release of growth hormone from the anterior pituitary.[5,6] After growth hormone is released into the circulation, it stimulates the production of insulin-like growth factors (IGF-I and IGF-II).[7] These growth factors are primarily made under the influence of growth hormone in the liver. They are homologs of the proinsulin molecule and therefore have biological effects that are qualitatively similar to those of insulin. It is uncertain whether either or both can be produced in the absence of growth hormone, although presently available data suggest that at least IGF-II, the weaker growth-promoting hormone, may not require growth hormone for synthesis. Thus, it is likely that IGF-I (somatomedin C) may be the major final mediator of growth hormone's biological effects.[3,4] It feeds back on the pituitary, modifying mRNA levels in the pituitary and growth hormone secretion.[8] In this chapter, by convention the term *growth hormone effects* is used, although most of these effects are probably mediated by the insulin-like growth factors, particularly somatomedin C.

Growth hormone effects influence many metabolic processes, but the net effect is anabolic. Thus, when growth hormone is administered to a growth hormone–deficient individual, positive nitrogen balance, with retention of calcium, sodium, potassium, magnesium, and chloride, is manifest within days.[3,4] While many facets of nitrogen metabolism following administration of growth hormone have been studied, its primary effect has not been assessed definitively. Growth hormone increases the synthesis of both transfer and messenger RNA.[9] It reduces the breakdown of amino acids to urea and increases the transport of amino acids into skeletal and cardiac muscle, thus augmenting the substrate available for protein synthesis.[10] However, direct measurement of intracellular amino acid content has not documented the increase expected if these actions were the only ones responsible for the increased protein synthesis.

Growth hormone also induces changes in both fat and carbohydrate metabolism.[3] When administered for a short time, it increases the uptake and utilization of glucose by fat cells, thus increasing lipogenesis. However, when administered over a long period, it promotes lipolysis, thus increasing plasma free fatty acid levels and their oxidation and promoting ketogenesis, particularly in diabetic patients or animals. Growth hormone reduces glucose uptake by fat and muscle cells, increases gluconeogenesis, and increases peripheral resistance to insulin; as a consequence, plasma glucose levels rise. Because of this reduced tissue uptake of glucose and the increased blood levels of free fatty acids and ketones, those tissues, like the myocardium, that are able to use these latter compounds as energy substrates do so. Growth hormone also increases the synthesis and/or accumulation of sulfated mucopolysaccharides in connective tissue.

EFFECT OF GROWTH HORMONE AND SOMATOSTATIN ON THE HEART. Short-term administration of growth hormone to normal subjects, which produces changes in growth hormone levels similar to those observed in patients with mild acromegaly, increases heart rate and myocardial contractility, the latter reflected in fractional shortening of the left ventricle and mean circumferential shortening of velocity, determined by echocardiography.[11] There is no effect on mean arterial blood pressure. *Somatostatin* has an effect on the heart beyond that induced by its effect on growth hormone secretion. Infusion of somatostatin causes bradycardia and a fall in cardiac output. Furthermore, in some cases of supraventricular arrhythmias somatostatin administration restores sinus rhythm.[12] Finally, cardiac nerves have been shown to contain somatostatin, suggesting that this hormone may be an important physiological regulator of cardiac conduction.[13]

CLINICAL AND BIOCHEMICAL MANIFESTATIONS. Acromegaly is almost invariably the result of a growth hormone – producing chromophobic or eosinophilic pituitary adenoma, although rarely it may be secondary to ectopic production of growth hormone or somatotropin-releasing hormone.[14] Characteristically, the disease is a slowly progressive one with signs and symptoms often predating diagnosis by more than 10 years. The striking physical findings (broad, spadelike hands and feet) are the result of growth hormone's effect on bone, muscle, and connective tissue. Osteoarthritis is common, as are organomegaly, hypertrichosis, hyperhidrosis, and modest weight gain.[15]

A derangement in carbohydrate metabolism is the most common metabolic consequence of chronic overproduction of growth hormone. Impaired glucose tolerance is found in half the patients, and hyperinsulinism is present in nearly all; thus a state of insulin resistance exists. However, clinical diabetes mellitus is present in only 10 per cent of patients, which suggests that only those who are predisposed and have limited insulin reserve actually develop overt disease.[16] The insulin-resistant state also may contribute to other features of the disease, e.g., the hypertension. While it might be anticipated that hyperlipidemia would be common in acromegaly, it is in fact infrequently observed except in patients with clinical diabetes mellitus.[3,4,16] Even in these patients, it is probably secondary to the decreased secretion of insulin rather than to the increased secretion of growth hormone.

CARDIOVASCULAR MANIFESTATIONS

The cardiac manifestations of acromegaly include cardiac enlargement that is greater than would be anticipated for the generalized organomegaly. In addition, the frequency of a number of other cardiovascular disorders is increased in acromegaly: hypertension, premature coronary artery disease, congestive heart failure, and cardic arrhythmias, particularly frequent ventricular premature beats and intraventricular conduction defects.[17,18] Indeed, because of the frequent occurrence of congestive heart failure and cardic arrhythmias in patients who otherwise have no predisposing factors (e.g., no hypertension or arteriosclerosis), it has been suggested that a specific acromegalic cardiomyopathy exists[19] (see below).

CARDIOMEGALY. Nearly all patients with acromegaly have cardiomegaly (Fig. 61–1), particularly after the fifth decade.[20,21] Echocardiographic assessment suggests that frequently there is an increase in cardiac mass, particularly asymmetrical septal hypertrophy, and in a sizable minority left ventricular dilatation and a reduced ejection fraction.[21] Although the cardiomegaly may be related to the generalized

effect of growth hormone on protein synthesis, some data suggest that other factors may also be important. For example, enlargement of the heart is often greater than that of other organs. Furthermore, there is no direct relationship between the degree of cardiomegaly and the level of circulating growth hormone.[17] While there is a correlation between the duration of acromegaly and the severity of cardiac hypertrophy,[19] other factors which may be important in the genesis of cardiomegaly include hypertension and atherosclerosis, both of which occur with increased frequency in acromegaly. Focal cardiac interstitial fibrosis and a myocarditis with lymphocytic infiltrate also have been reported in the majority of cases.[19,22] The former is probably due to the effect of growth hormone on collagen synthesis. Additionally, small-vessel disease of the myocardium occasionally may be present.[19] The resultant dysfunction in cardiac contraction secondary to any of these pathological changes could also contribute to the cardiac hypertrophy. Finally, the cardiomyopathy characteristic of acromegaly may also contribute to the cardiomegaly.

HYPERTENSION. This is the most common cardiovascular manifestation of acromegaly, occurring in 15 to 50 per cent of patients if individuals with hypopituitarism are excluded. Hypertensive acromegalic patients tend to be older and to have had their acromegaly longer than nonhypertensive acromegalic patients. The underlying pathophysiology is uncertain. However, the hypertension usually is mild, uncomplicated, and readily responsive to drugs.[17] Most investigators either have searched for factors other than growth hormone that could cause hypertension or have attempted to determine how growth hormone itself may produce hypertension. In many respects, in patients with acromegaly there appears to be volume expansion; the presence of an increase in glomerular filtration rate, renal plasma flow, extracellular fluid volume and sodium space, and reduction in plasma renin activity all support this hypothesis.[4,23] Indeed, there is a striking increase in total exchangeable sodium in active acromegaly that is reduced following treatment. Thus, several studies have assessed the secretion of aldosterone in acromegaly; while increased secretion has been reported, this is an uncommon finding.[23] What does appear to occur frequently in acromegalics, however, is a change in tissue responsiveness to angiotensin II. Thus, with a sodium-restricted intake the response of aldosterone production to angiotensin II is decreased, but the vasoconstrictor response is increased when compared to normal subjects. This abnormality is present in both hypertensive and normotensive acromegalics.[24] Whether this is related to the pathogenesis of the elevated arterial pressure or is simply a reflection of an expanded extracellular fluid volume is unclear.

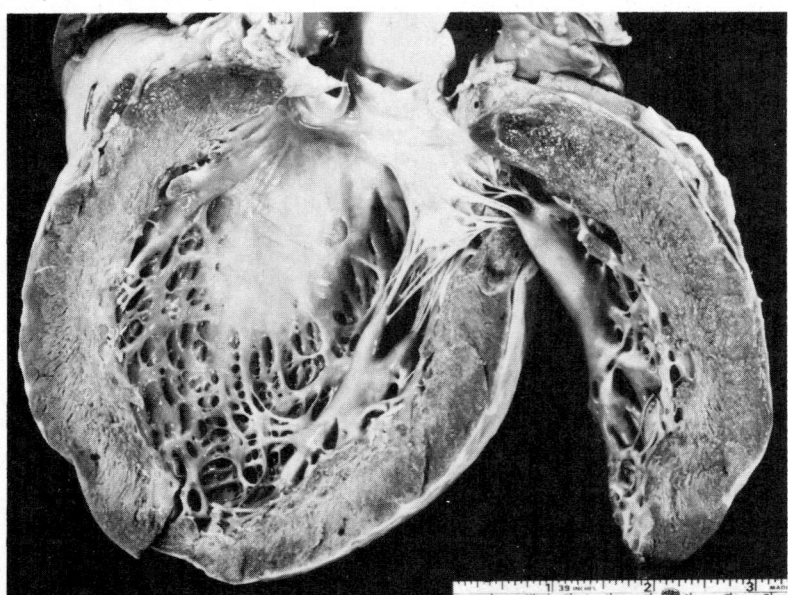

FIGURE 61–1. Opened left ventricle of the heart, showing the marked dilatation and hypertrophy, with fibrosis in the left septal endocardium. (From Rossi, L., et al.: Dysrhythmias and sudden death in acromegalic heart disease. A clinicopathologic study. Chest 72:496, 1977.)

A number of studies have suggested that growth hormone itself may be responsible for the hypertension. Thus, pituitary irradiation or hypophysectomy significantly reduces arterial pressure in hypertensive acromegalic patients, even when full glucocorticoid replacement is carried out, unless growth hormone levels are not normalized.[18,24] Indeed, the apparent volume expansion may be directly related to the elevated growth hormone levels, since administration of growth hormone can produce retention of sodium, expansion of extracellular fluid volume, and abnormalities in white blood cell sodium transport.[25,26] It has been proposed that the pathophysiology of the hypertension in acromegaly may be similar to that in essential hypertension. In both conditions, there may be initial elevation of cardiac output secondary to expansion of extracellular fluid volume (Chap. 28). This could elevate arterial pressure and lead ultimately to changes in the peripheral vasculature producing fixed hypertension.

ATHEROSCLEROSIS. In view of the alterations in carbohydrate and lipid metabolism caused by growth hormone (see above) as well as the high incidence of hypertension, it is not surprising that premature atherosclerosis occurs in patients with acromegaly. What is uncertain is its frequency.[19] Coronary atherosclerosis could also contribute to the cardiomegaly observed in these patients.

ACROMEGALIC CARDIOMYOPATHY. Some patients with acromegaly without evidence of hypertension or atherosclerosis have significant cardiac dysfunction.[19] They primarily have cardiomegaly, congestive heart failure, and/or cardiac dysrhythmias[22]; the congestive heart failure is particularly resistant to conventional therapy. It has been suggested that these are manifestations of an acromegalic cardiomyopathy which is related to the higher collagen content per gram of heart than in normal myocardium.[19] Histological observations show cellular hypertrophy, patchy fibrosis, and myofibrillar degeneration (Fig. 61–2). Sudden death has been associated with inflammatory and degenerative damage to the sinoatrial perinodal nerve plexus and degeneration of the AV node.[22]

It is not clear whether acromegalic cardiomyopathy is a specific entity. The evidence favoring this view, though indirect, comes from five types of observations: (1) Nearly 50 per cent of acromegalic patients have electrocardiographic abnormalities.[27] The most common findings are ST-segment depression with or without T-wave abnormalities, patterns consistent with left ventricular hypertrophy, intraventricular conduction disturbances—specifically, bundle branch block

—and, infrequently, supraventricular or ventricular ectopic rhythms. While hypertension or signs of atherosclerosis are present in many, 10 to 20 per cent of patients with acromegaly and electrocardiographic changes have no evidence of these conditions. (2) Ten to twenty per cent of acromegalics have overt congestive heart failure. In perhaps a fourth of these there is no known predisposing cause. (3) The majority of patients with acromegaly but without hypertension or atherosclerosis have subclinical evidence for cardiac, particularly diastolic, dysfunction.[28,29] (4) Approximately half of all patients with acromegaly, including patients without hypertension, have echocardiographic evidence of left ventricular hypertrophy.[30,31] These patients have growth hormone levels that are significantly higher than those of patients without left ventricular hypertrophy. Half of the patients with left ventricular hypertrophy exhibit asymmetrical septal hypertrophy, and these patients have a significantly greater percentage of internal dimensional shortening during systole than either the patients with concentric hypertrophy or those without left ventricular hypertrophy. (5) In one series of 256 acromegalic patients, 10 had cardiac abnormalities that could not be explained by diabetes, valvular disease, thyroid disease, angina, or myocardial ischemia. In six of these 10 patients, biochemical cure was achieved with surgery, but cardiac function did not improve appreciably. In one of these, who died, there was histological evidence of myocarditis. Of those patients in whom acromegaly remained active, three died; in one, postmortem examination revealed interstitial cardiac fibrosis.

DIAGNOSIS AND TREATMENT

The *diagnosis* of acromegaly is established by documenting the nonsuppressibility of serum growth hormone levels following glucose loading.[4] In most laboratories, growth hormone concentrations in normal subjects are less than 2 ng/ml 120 minutes after the oral administration of 100 gm of glucose. It is also important to evaluate the integrity of the other pituitary hormones, and, in hypertensive patients, to rule out an associated pheochromocytoma or aldosteronoma. The presence of sinus tachycardia or atrial fibrillation in a patient with acromegaly warrants a careful search for coexisting hyperthyroidism.

Surgery and irradiation remain the mainstays of treatment. The surgical approach is more often transsphenoidal rather than transfrontal; heavy particle (proton beam) instead of conventional irradiation is often used.[32] Because of the delayed reduction in growth hormone levels with the latter method, progression of cardiovascular disease in acromegalics continues even though growth hormone levels are falling. In a 10-year follow-up of 11 acromegalic patients, myocardial infarction, dysrhythmias, hypertension,

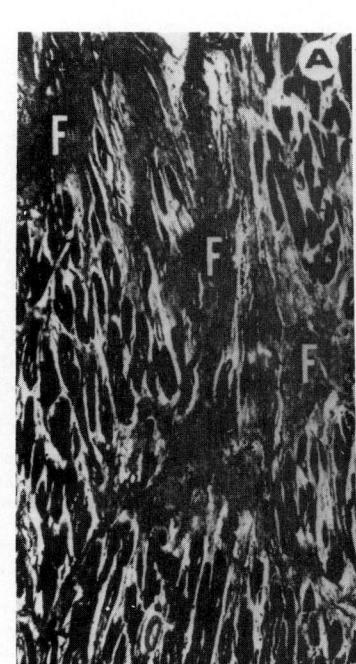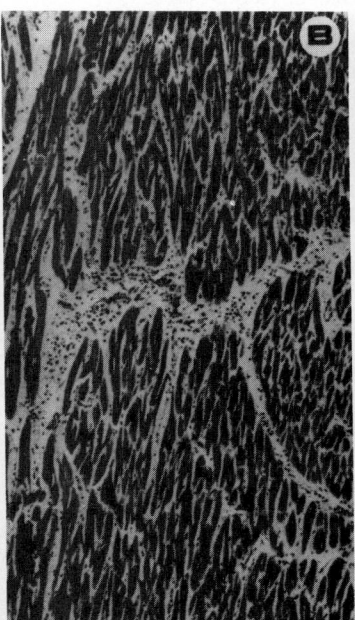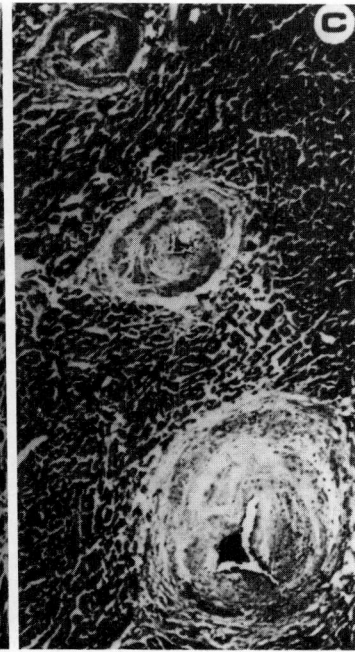

FIGURE 61–2. Histopathological features of acromegalic heart disease. *A*, Nonspecific myocardial hypertrophy and interstitial fibrosis (F). *B*, Myocarditis with predominantly lymphomononuclear cell infiltrate. *C*, Small-vessel disease (proliferative fibrous wall thickening) or intramural coronary artery branches. (Reproduced with permission from Lie, J. T.: Acromegaly and heart disease. Primary Cardiol. *7*:53, 1981. Copyright PW Communications, Inc.)

major artery disease, and heart failure all increased significantly even though the growth hormone levels were falling.[18] The secretion of growth hormone can be suppressed in some acromegalics with the dopamine agonist bromocriptine, and somatostatin.[33,34] Whether these agents have any effect on tumor growth, however, is unclear.

Acromegalic patients with cardiovascular abnormalities usually respond to conventional therapeutic measures for hypertension, heart failure, and arrhythmias. Two caveats: (1) those with hypertension appear to be particularly responsive to volume-depleting maneuvers, i.e., diuretics and sodium restriction, perhaps even more so than patients with essential hypertension; (2) on the other hand, some patients with congestive heart failure, primarily those *without* underlying hypertensive heart disease (i.e., those who are considered to have acromegalic cardiomyopathy), appear to be particularly resistant to therapy.

THYROID DISEASE

Thyroid hormone has a profound effect on a number of metabolic processes in virtually all tissues, with the heart being particularly sensitive to its effects. Therefore, it is not surprising that thyroid dysfunction can produce dramatic cardiovascular effects, often mimicking primary cardiac disease.

ACTION OF THYROID HORMONE. Two biologically active hormones are secreted by the thyroid: thyroxine (T4) and triiodothyronine (T3). Most studies support the hypothesis that T3 is the final mediator and that T4 is a prohormone, primarily because of the universal presence of T3 but not T4 nuclear receptors in tissues responsive to thyroid hormone, specifically the heart.[35–39]

Even though the mechanism of action of thyroid hormone has been intensively investigated over the past three decades, uncertainty still exists about its principal effects. The preponderance of evidence now suggests that the major site of initiation of action of thyroid hormone is on the cell nucleus.[36] It has been observed that thyroid hormone is specifically bound to a chromatin-bound nonhistone nucleoprotein in the nucleus. As a result of this binding, alterations occur in protein synthesis, leading to many of the biochemical and metabolic effects observed with T4 administration.[37,38] According to this hypothesis, the increased oxygen consumption results not from a direct interaction between thyroid hormone and mitochondria, an older hypothesis, but rather indirectly via an increase in mitochondrial protein synthesis secondary to the effect of the thyroid hormone on the nucleus. Support for this hypothesis comes from several sources: (1) specific binding of T3 and, much less strongly, of T4 to nuclear receptor sites has been documented[39]; (2) those tissues sensitive to thyroid hormone have nuclear binding sites[36]; (3) the addition of thyroid hormone in vitro produces an increase in O_2 consumption only after a significant time lag; (4) an early metabolic effect of T4 is an increased rate of incorporation of a labeled precursor into nuclear RNA[40]; (5) inhibitors of protein synthesis prevent many, if not most, of thyroid hormone's effects[41]; and (6) treatment of hypothyroid animals with T3 causes increases in in vivo synthesis of specific messenger RNA's in several tissues, including the heart.[42]

Effect on Na^+, K^+-ATPase. Guernsey and Edelman have extended this hypothesis one step further.[43] They postulated that not only does thyroid hormone enhance protein synthesis, but it specifically increases the activity of Na^+, K^+-ATPase. Thus, the augmented hydrolysis of ATP at the site of the sodium pump in the sarcolemma stimulates cellular (mitochondrial) oxygen consumption. Support for this hypothesis includes the observations that (1) hypothyroid rats treated with T3 exhibit a reduction in active sodium transport in crude homogenates and membrane-rich fractions and a decrease in intracellular Na^+/K^+ ratio in liver, diaphragm, and kidney, and (2) the number of renal Na^+ pump sites and the incorporation of radiolabeled methionine into renal cortical Na^+, K^+-ATPase are both increased, suggesting an increase in protein synthesis as the primary event. Some reports, however, have suggested that the effect of thyroid hormone on cellular respiration cannot be entirely secondary to a change in the activity of this enzyme[44,45] and that thyroid hormone also affects other cellular processes, e.g., the transport of glucose and calcium, particularly in the heart.[46–48]

RELATION BETWEEN THE THYROID AND THE SYMPATHETIC NERVOUS SYSTEM

While the effects of thyroid hormone on the heart are varied and complex, it has been proposed that some of them are indirect, being secondary

to changes in the activity of the sympathetic nervous system (Table 61–1). For example, many of the cardiovascular effects of hyperthyroidism, i.e., tachycardia, systolic hypertension, increased cardiac output, and myocardial contractility, can be abolished or reduced by blocking the activity of the sympathetic nervous system.[49] It has been proposed that thyroid hormone may alter the relationship between the sympathetic nervous and cardiovascular systems, either by increasing the activity of the sympathoadrenal system or by enhancing the response of cardiac tissue to normal sympathetic stimulation.[50] Also, it has been suggested that sympathetic stimuli merely exert a direct additive effect on cardiovascular function above that produced by thyroid hormone. On the other hand, there is also evidence that hyperthyroidism reduces the sensitivity of cardiac tissue to sympathetic stimuli.[51]

Thus the results of experiments on the relationship between the sympathoadrenal system and hyperthyroidism have evoked considerable controversy. The plasma and urine levels of norepinephrine, epinephrine, dopamine, and beta-hydroxylase are either low or normal in hyperthyroidism and either normal or elevated in hypothyroidism.[52] These data suggest that the sympathomimetic features of hyperthyroidism cannot be due simply to an overall increase in adrenergic activity but rather are due to a change in the affinity of catecholamines for their receptors or to a modification of a postreceptor mechanism. Previously such changes were difficult to document, primarily because thyroid hormone appears to have different effects on adrenoceptors in different tissues. For example, the effect of thyroid hormone in the rat liver is different from that in the rat heart. Thyroid hormones reduce beta-adrenoceptor number in the rat liver, and hypothyroid animals show an increase in these receptors.[53,54] In contrast, in the rat heart, which has been the organ most extensively studied, administration of thyroid hormone causes both an increase in the number of receptors and their affinity for their ligand, while hypothyroidism induces the opposite effect.[50,55,56]

These changes in receptor number and affinity lead to appropriate changes in sensitivity of the myocardium to beta-adrenoceptor agonists. For example, stimulation of adenylate cyclase activity by isoproterenol is increased in hyperthyroidism and reduced in hypothyroidism. Finally, there are also changes in the force of contraction with increased sensitivity of the ventricular muscle to isoproterenol-induced contraction in hyperthyroidism and reduction in hypothyroidism.[50] That this effect is specific is shown by an unaltered change in calcium-stimulated contractility in hypo-

TABLE 61–1   CLINICAL FEATURES OF HYPERTHYROIDISM

DIRECT THYROID HORMONE EFFECT†	BETA-ADRENERGIC-LIKE EFFECT†
Resting heart rate > 90/min (90%)	Resting heart rate > 90/min (90%)
Palpitations (85%)	Palpitations (85%)
Atrial fibrillation (10%)	Exertional dyspnea (80%)
Pedal edema (30%)	Increased pulse pressure (systolic hypertension)
Increased oxygen consumption (basal metabolism)	Active apical impulse
Weight loss	Loud first heart sound and pulmonic component of second heart sound
Skeletal muscle myopathy	
Increased bone turnover (occasional osteoporosis or hypercalcemia)	Midsystolic murmur, usually basal
Fair skin	Third heart sound (occasional)
Fine brittle hair	Means-Lerman scratch (rate)‡
Brittle nails	Tremor
Oligomenorrhea or amenorrhea	Brisk reflexes
Increased bowel frequency	Increased perspiration
	Heat intolerance
	Insomnia
	Anxiety
	Stare, lid lag§

The numbers in parentheses are approximate prevalences of the findings, compiled from several large series. Goiter is almost always present, though in elderly patients the thyroid enlargement may be minimal or absent.

† Both types of effects contribute to the tachycardia and palpitations.

‡ A systolic scratch or click in the second left intercostal space that is probably generated by the pleura and pericardium rubbing together.

§ These reflect upper-lid retraction. Infiltrative ophthalmopathy with exophthalmos is found only when Graves' disease is the cause of the hyperthyroidism and is not related to the hyperthyroid state per se.

Reproduced with permission from Kaplan, M. M.: The thyroid and the heart: How do they interact? J. Cardiovasc. Med. 7:893, 1982.

thyroid animals.[55] These effects were also observed in vivo in dogs in which propranolol-induced reductions of heart rate and myocardial contractility were greater in hyperthyroid than in euthyroid animals.[57]

Further support comes from the study by Guarnieri et al., who showed that hyperthyroid rats have enhanced activation of protein kinase and contractile response following administration of a threshold dose of the beta-adrenoceptor agonist isoproterenol.[58] In the aforementioned study in conscious hyperthyroid dogs,[57] however, we found no alteration in the sensitivity of the inotropic response to isoproterenol and norepinephrine.

Circulating blood elements have also provided additional evidence in support of the concept that thyroid hormone "up-regulates" beta-adrenoceptors. When patients are used as their own control, both the number of beta-adrenoceptors and the sensitivity of adenylate cyclase to isoproterenol stimulation in mononuclear cells are increased by thyroid hormone.[59] Additionally, in circulating reticulocytes of hypothyroid animals, the number of receptors is decreased.[60]

While there is compelling evidence for changes in the receptor number and affinity induced by thyroid hormone, it is unclear whether thyroid hormone also has additional effects by which it could alter sensitivity to adrenergic stimuli. There are no data regarding the effect of thyroid hormone on cardiac nucleotide regulatory (G) protein (Fig. 13–12, p. 380), although the presence of hypothyroidism does reduce the concentration of N protein in erythrocyte membranes.[60] On the other hand, no change in N-protein concentration has been observed in adipose tissue.[61] Yet in adipose tissue, hypothyroidism does reduce the lipolytic response to catecholamines.[62] Thus, in this tissue, in which there is no alteration in the number of beta-adrenoceptors, the mechanism underlying the hypothyroid-induced alteration in tissue effect is unclear, but probably occurs downstream from the interaction of the agonist with its receptor.

EFFECT OF THYROID HORMONE ON THE HEART

There is abundant evidence that thyroid hormone may alter cardiac function directly. Thus the addition of thyroid to fragments of chick embryonic heart increases the frequency of beating of the cells.[63] Additionally, the increased heart rate and myocardial contractility observed in experimental hyperthyroidism are not completely reversed by either sympathetic or parasympathetic blockade.[51,57] Finally, T4 enhances the rate of contraction of cardiac muscle even in the presence of adrenergic blockade.[64] Right ventricular papillary muscles isolated from cats rendered hyperthyroid exhibited augmented myocardial contractility, as reflected in an upward shift of the myocardial force-velocity curve,[51] with a greatly increased velocity of myocardial fiber shortening, a reduced time to peak tension during isometric contraction, and an augmented peak tension development (Fig. 61–3). Single ventricular myocytes isolated from hyperthyroid rats exhibited a marked augmentation of twitch velocity and abbreviated both the time required for contraction and relaxation.[64a] Prior catecholamine depletion by pretreatment of the hyperthyroid cats with reserpine did not alter this inotropic effect of hyperthyroidism, providing further evidence for a direct cardiac effect.[51] This hypothesis has been assessed in the intact conscious calf. The results suggest that the major actions of T4 on the left ventricle are (1) a direct positive inotropic effect and (2) an increase in the size of the ventricular cavity without a change in the end-diastolic pressure or length of the sarcomere in diastole, although hypothyroidism does not necessarily impair pump function.[65,66]

The available data suggest that the direct effect of thyroid hormone on the heart is mediated via a change in protein synthesis.[67,68] Thyroid hormone increases the activity of the sodium pump in myocardial cells as it does in other tissues. Philipson and Edelman have documented that the activity of both the Na^+, K^+-ATPase and K^+-dependent p-nitrophenyl phosphatase in the heart is increased by more than 50 per cent when T3 is administered to hypothyroid rats.[69] The hearts of euthyroid rabbits rendered hyperthyroid exhibited a doubling of myofibrillar ATPase activity.[70] Reverse T3 (a biologically inactive analog) has no effect. Curfman et al. have suggested that this increased activity is the result of an increase in the number of functional enzyme complexes.[71] There is evidence that thyroid hormone both increases the synthesis of myosin and alters its structure, increasing its con-

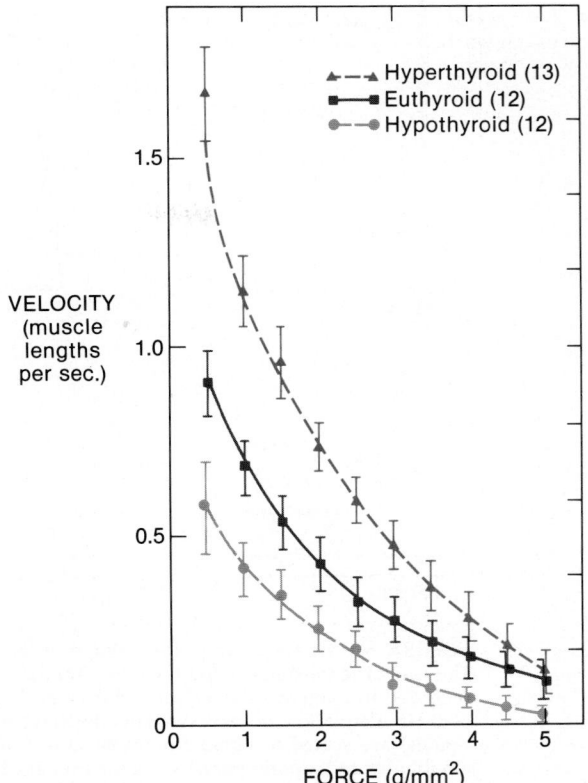

FIGURE 61–3. The average force-velocity relationship for papillary muscles from hyperthyroid, euthyroid, and hypothyroid cats. Initial velocity of shortening is normalized in terms of muscle lengths per second; load, corrected for cross-sectional area of individual muscles, is expressed in gm/mm². Brackets represent ± SEM. (From Buccino, R. A., et al.: Influence of the thyroid state on the intrinsic contractile properties and the energy stores of the myocardium. J. Clin. Invest. 46:1669, 1967.)

tractile properties, particularly by increasing the more mobile myosin isoenzyme (V_1) as determined by polyacrylamide gel electrophoresis, which is composed of two alpha myosin heavy chains (alpha MHC).[68,72] The mRNA for alpha MHC is substantially increased when hypothyroid rats are given T3, while the beta MHC mRNA, which primarily forms the slower V_3 myosin isoform, is substantially reduced.[68] Thus, the heart appears to respond to thyrotoxicosis by enhancing synthesis of a myosin isoenzyme with a fast ATPase activity.[68,70-73] In addition, α-actin mRNA is increased transiently in hyperthyroidism.[68] The augmented myosin ATPase activity of the hyperthyroid heart appears to contribute to the enhanced contractile response of the hyperthyroid heart, since the activity level of this enzyme is thought to regulate the rate of turnover of actin-myosin cross-bridge links in cardiac muscle. Hypothyroidism induces the opposite effects.[73,74] Goto et al. demonstrated in the hyperthyroid rabbit heart that the increase in myosin isoform V_1/V_3 is associated with decreased contractile efficiency and increased energy costs of excitation-contraction coupling.[75]

Thyroid hormone's effect on cardiac contractility also appears to be mediated in part by changes in intracellular calcium handling. Thyroid hormone increases the number of slow calcium channels, which augments transsarcolemmal calcium influx in cultured ventricular cells.[47] In ferret ventricular muscle, hypothyroidism reduces peak tension and prolongs the duration of contraction in association with changes in cytosolic calcium that are decreased and prolonged in relation to ventricular muscle obtained from euthyroid animals (Fig. 61–4). Hyperthyroidism produces the opposite changes. Thus, alteration in intracellular calcium handling, specifically related to recycling of calcium by the sarcoplasmic reticulum, may account for the thyroid-induced changes in myocardial contractile function.[48,76] Finally, the effect of

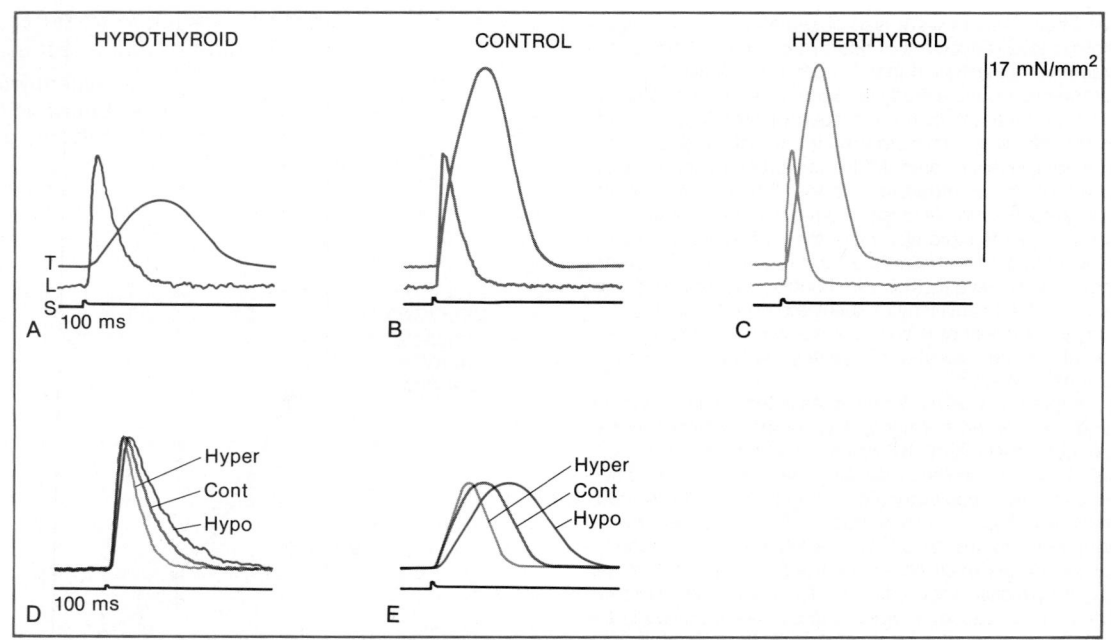

FIGURE 61–4. The thyroid state influences the time course of the isometric contraction and the Ca^{++} transient. The isometric tension (T) and the aequorin light signal, reflecting intracytoplasmic [Ca]$^{++}$ (see p. 357) (L), were recorded from myocardium obtained from a hypothyroid (*A*), euthyroid (*B*), and hyperthyroid (*C*) ferret at 30°C; 0.33 Hz stimulation. I is expressed in milliNewtons/m² muscle cross-sectional area. The Ca^{++} transients (aequorin signals) are scaled to equal amplitudes and superimposed in *D*. In *E*, the tensions have been scaled to equal amplitudes and superimposed. The time from the beginning of the stimulus sweep (S) to the stimulus represents 100 msecs. (From MacKinnon, R., et al.: Modulation by the thyroid state of intracellular calcium and contractility in ferret ventricular muscle. Circ. Res. *63*:1084, 1988. Used with permission from the American Heart Association.)

thyroxine on myosin isoenzyme appears to be localized primarily to the ventricles with atrial isoenzymes relatively unaltered by changes in thyroid hormone.[72] Klein and Hong, using heterotopic cardiac isografts, have suggested that thyroid's effect on protein synthesis in the heart is, for the most part, secondary to changes in cardiac work rather than a direct effect of thyroid hormone. Indeed, they suggested that even the changes in myosin isoenzyme may in part be secondary to changes in workload, although it is clear that thyroid hormone can induce a separate direct effect.[77,78]

The tachycardia observed in hyperthyroidism appears to be due to a combination of an increased rate of diastolic depolarization and a decreased duration of the action potential in the sinoatrial node cells.[79] The propensity for the development of atrial fibrillation may be due to the shortened refractory period of atrial cells.[80]

HYPERTHYROIDISM

Hyperthyroidism is the clinical state resulting from the excess production of T3, thyroxine (T4), or both. The most common cause is a diffuse toxic goiter (Graves' disease). Although the etiology of this condition is still unknown, the hyperproduction of T4 and T3 is thought to result from circulating IgG autoantibodies that bind to the thyrotropin receptor on the thyroid gland. The second most common form of hyperthyroidism is nodular toxic goiter, a condition in which localized areas of the gland function excessively and autonomously. Less common causes include a single toxic adenoma, ingestion of excessive amounts of thyroid hormone, and subacute thyroiditis, in which there may be a self-limit phase of hyperthyroidism. Rarely, hyperthyroidism may also occur as a result of the production of thyroid hormone by a thyroid carcinoma or production of a thyrotropic substance (probably HCG) by a hydatidiform mole or choriocarcinoma.[81]

Hyperthyroidism is a relatively common disease, occurring four to eight times more commonly in women than in men, with a peak incidence in the third and fourth decades. The commonly associated signs and symptoms (Table 61–1) include fatigue, hyperactivity, insomnia, heat intolerance, palpitations, dyspnea, increased appetite with weight loss, nocturia, diarrhea, oligomenorrhea, muscle weakness, tremor, emotional lability, increased heart rate, systolic hypertension, hyperthermia, warm moist skin,

lid lag, stare, and brisk reflexes. In the vast majority of cases a goiter can be palpated. Hyperthyroidism in childhood occurs most frequently just before or during adolescence. It is usually associated with a diffuse goiter. The most common early manifestations in juvenile hyperthyroid patients are excessive movements and emotional lability.

T3 levels are invariably elevated, and serum T4 levels are usually increased as well. In addition to the signs and symptoms directly related to increased production of thyroid hormone, patients with Graves' disease often have exophthalmos and occasionally circumscribed areas of thickening of the skin, particularly of the lower extremities; presumably these are related to the immunological aspects of the disease.

Particularly in older patients, the typical clinical picture is occasionally absent. In these individuals with so-called *apathetic hyperthyroidism,* few clinical manifestations are apparent except for cardiovascular dysfunction. Thus, cardiac arrhythmias and heart failure resistant to conventional forms of therapy are common.

CARDIOVASCULAR MANIFESTATIONS. The heart is among the most responsive organs in thyroid disease, and cardiovascular signs and symptoms are therefore important clinical features of hyperthyroidism.[81,82] Palpitations, dyspnea, tachycardia, and systolic hypertension are common findings. Diastolic hypertension can also occur. Typically, there is a hyperactive precordium with a loud first heart sound, an accentuated pulmonic component of the second heart sound, and a third heart sound; occasionally, a systolic ejection click is heard. Midsystolic murmurs along the left sternal border are common, and a systolic scratch, the so-called Means-Lerman scratch, is occasionally heard in the second left intercostal space during expiration. It is presumed to be secondary to the rubbing together of normal pleural and pericardial surfaces by the hyperdynamic heart.

As would be anticipated, and as described on page 458, cardiac and stroke volume index, mean systolic ejection rate, velocity and extent of wall shortening (Fig. 61–5), and coronary blood flow[83] are all increased, the systolic ejection period and preejection period are abbreviated, the pulse pressure is widened, and systemic vascular resistance is reduced in hyperthyroidism.[84] The changes in left ventricular performance

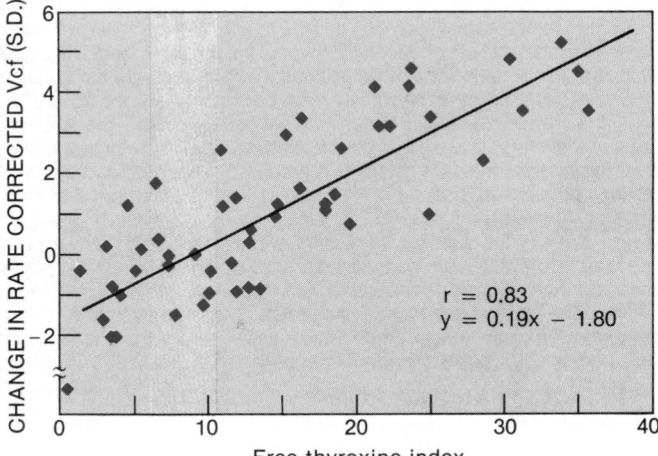

FIGURE 61–5. Rate-corrected velocity of shortening (V_{cf}) in SD units from the normal mean regression line obtained from 11 patients at varying levels of the free thyroxine index. There is a strong positive correlation between the level of thyroid hormone and the change in contractile state. The shaded area represents the normal range for serum free thyroxine index. (From Feldman, T., et al.: Myocardial mechanics in hyperthyroidism: Importance of left ventricular loading conditions, heart rate and contractile state. By permission of the American College of Cardiology. J. Am. Coll. Cardiol. 7:972, 1986.)

induced by thyroid hormone appear to be secondary to augmented contractility rather than to reduction in afterload or change in heart rate.[85] If the hyperthyroidism is relatively mild, many of the indices of left ventricular function are normal, with exercise needed to bring out abnormalities.[86,87] It has been suggested that many of the changes in cardiac function are secondary to the increased metabolic demands of peripheral tissue. However, the increase in cardiac output is greater than would be predicted on the basis of the increased total body oxygen consumption, supporting the view that thyroid hormone exerts a direct cardiac stimulant action independent of its effect on general tissue metabolism. Furthermore, normalization of myocardial contractile response to exercise may not occur until several months after normalization of thyroid function.[88]

Roentgenographic and electrocardiographic changes are common but are nonspecific in hyperthyroidism.[81] Thus the left ventricle, the aorta, and the pulmonary artery are prominent, and, in some cases, there is generalized cardiac enlargement, which may be accompanied by signs and symptoms of heart failure. In patients with sinus rhythm, the magnitude of the tachycardia, in general, parallels the severity of the disease. Sinus tachycardia, i.e., a rate exceeding 100 beats/min, is present in 40 per cent of patients with hyperthyroidism, occurring most frequently in the younger age groups, and often at night.[89] Fifteen to twenty-five per cent of patients with hyperthyroidism have persistent atrial fibrillation, which is often heralded by one or more transient episodes of this arrhythmia.[90,91] There is shortening of the A-V conduction time and functional refractory period, resulting in an increased frequency at which the A-V conduction system transmits rapid atrial impulses.[91] Intraatrial conduction disturbances, manifested by prolongation or notching of the P wave and prolongation of the P-R interval in the absence of treatment with digitalis, occur in 15 per cent and 5 per cent of patients with hyperthyroidism, respectively. Occasionally, second- or third-degree heart block may result.[82] The cause of the A-V conduction disturbance is not clear, since animal experiments have shown that the functional refractory period of the A-V conduction system and the conduction time were shortened in dogs with hyperthyroidism and prolonged in dogs with hypothyroidism.[92] Intraventricular conduction disturbances, most commonly right bundle branch block, occur in about 15 per cent of patients with hyperthyroidism without associated heart disease of other etiology.[82] Paroxysmal supraventricular

tachycardia and flutter are rare in hyperthyroidism. Finally, occult thyrotoxicosis may underlie either chronic or paroxysmal isolated atrial fibrillation. Ciaccheri et al. reported a frequency of thyrotoxicosis of 12.5 per cent in 40 consecutive patients with isolated atrial fibrillation.[91]

Both angina pectoris and congestive heart failure occur in patients with hyperthyroidism, and for many years it was assumed that these were seen only in the presence of underlying cardiovascular disease. Support for this position came primarily from the absence of these symptoms in young persons with significant hyperthyroidism. More recently, however, four lines of evidence have suggested otherwise: (1) Congestive heart failure has been produced in experimental animals by simply administering T4. (2) Children with thyrotoxicosis without underlying cardiac disease may develop congestive heart failure.[93] (3) Angina has been reported in a patient with normal coronary arteries, presumably secondary to thyroid-induced coronary artery spasm.[94] (4) Abnormal left ventricular function observed during exercise in hyperthyroid subjects is not reversed by beta blockade but is reversed by treating the hyperthyroidism.[95] Thus, when it is severe enough, thyrotoxicosis can overtax even the normal heart, although, in most instances, the development of clinical manifestations of heart failure and myocardial ischemia in patients with hyperthyroidism signifies the presence of underlying cardiac or coronary vascular disease. There is also increased frequency of hyperthyroidism in patients with familial hypertrophic cardiomyopathy. In one kindred, 3 of 17 members with hypertrophic cardiomyopathy also had hyperthyroidism.[96] Finally, hyperthyroidism has been associated with mitral valve prolapse in more than a third of cases.[97,98]

TREATMENT OF CARDIOVASCULAR DISEASE IN HYPERTHYROIDISM. Hyperthyroid patients with cardiovascular disease are particularly resistant to therapy. For example, it has been well documented that both congestive heart failure and cardiac arrhythmias are resistant to conventional doses of the cardiac glycosides. While the specific mechanisms underlying these altered responses remain obscure, they may be related to both systemic and local effects.[81,99] First, serum levels of cardiac glycosides are diminished in hyperthyroidism, not because there is an augmentation of its metabolism but because there is an increase in its volume of distribution. Second, experimental hyperthyroidism reduces the enhancement of the myocardial contractile force and the prolongation of the atrioventricular nodal refractory period produced by these agents.[99] Because of this decreased sensitivity to cardiac glycosides, toxicity may develop at a dose that has relatively little therapeutic effect.

DIAGNOSIS AND THERAPY OF HYPERTHYROIDISM

The diagnosis is made on the basis of elevated levels of thyroid hormone in the blood. Because only serum T3 is increased in some individuals, it is important to obtain serum levels of *both* T3 and T4 and an index of the thyroid-binding capacity of the patient's serum (resin thyroxine uptake). In most laboratories hyperthyroidism is confirmed when the levels of serum T4 are greater than 10.5 μg/dl or T3 levels are greater than 180 ng/dl with normal resin thyroxine uptakes. Occasionally, patients will have hyperthyroidism with both T3 and T4 within the normal range. If suspected, confirmation may be obtained by measuring the TSH (thyroid-stimulating hormone) basally (if a supersensitive assay is used) or in response to TRH (thyrotropin-releasing hormone), which should be blunted in hyperthyroidism. However, caution needs to be exercised in using the TRH test, since false-positive results are common.[81]

The definitive treatment of hyperthyroidism is surgical removal of the gland or irradiation using radioactive iodide. In severely ill patients, particularly those with thyroid storm or significant cardiovascular symptoms or both, neither of these therapies is appropriate. Thus, medical therapy is directed at reducing both the production and biological effect of thyroid hormone. Since many of the cardiovascular symptoms of thyrotoxicosis are related to increased beta-adrenoceptor activity, treatment with beta-adrenoceptor blocking agents has been useful.[100] Tachycardia, palpitations, tremor, restlessness, muscle weakness, and heat intolerance are reversed by these agents, which offer the additional benefit of inhibiting the conversion of T4 to the biologically active T3 in peripheral tissues.

Prompt treatment of the hyperthyroid state can significantly reduce, if not eliminate, the associated cardiovascular symptoms. About half of patients with concurrent onset of hyperthyroidism and angina pectoris experience complete remission of symptoms after treatment of hyperthyroidism.[101] Furthermore, in 62 per cent of 163 thyrotoxic patients with atrial fibrillation sustained for 1 week or longer, spontaneous reversion to sinus rhythm was found when they became euthyroid.[102] Arterial embolization is not common in patients with thyrotoxicosis and atrial fibrillation, but it does occur. In one series, 8 per cent of 262 patients with both conditions had embolization.[103] Thus it is important to determine quickly whether hyperthyroidism is present in patients with cardiovascular disease, since treatment often results in dramatic improvement. In elderly patients with apathetic hyperthyroidism, cardiovascular manifestations, specifically atrial fibrillation and/or congestive heart failure, predominate, and therefore evaluation of thyroid function in such patients is particularly important. However, it should be noted that these individuals are particularly resistant to cardiac glycosides.

Beta blockers (p. 505) can be administered orally or intravenously, but since these drugs interfere with the effects of sympathetic stimulation on the heart, they must be used with caution in patients with congestive heart failure. However, if the heart failure is in part related to the tachycardia, beta blockade may be beneficial. These agents can be administered in small doses while the patient is under close observation and being treated with digitalis and diuretics and reduction in physical activity. Beta-blocking drugs and cardiac glycosides act synergistically to slow ventricular rate in atrial fibrillation by increasing the refractoriness of the A-V conduction system. Thus, the combination may produce benefit that would require toxic doses of either agent used alone. Beta-adrenoceptor blockade improves many peripheral manifestations of thyrotoxicosis.[81]

While beta-adrenoceptor blockade can produce significant improvement of the cardiovascular status in patients with hyperthyroidism, correction of the basic metabolic defect requires specific therapy directed at reducing the production of thyroid hormone.[81] The most useful agents are the thionamides, such as propylthiouracil. These drugs should be administered concurrently with a beta-blocking agent to reduce the total production of thyroid hormone, as well as to block its effect. The usual starting dosage of propylthiouracil is 300 to 800 mg in divided doses daily; it not only reduces thyroid hormone production but also has the advantage of reducing the peripheral conversion of T4 into T3. Usual maintenance doses range from 50 to 300 mg. The thionamides are not without risk, since between 1 and 5 per cent of patients have significant side effects — usually gastrointestinal disturbances or a suppression of the bone marrow; infrequently, a generalized vasculitis has been reported.

Iodine, most commonly administered in the form of 2 drops of saturated solution of potassium iodide three times daily, inhibits the release of thyroid hormones from the thyrotoxic gland, and its beneficial effects occur rapidly, indeed, more rapidly than those of agents that inhibit the synthesis of the hormone. It is therefore useful in the rapid amelioration of the hyperthyroid state in patients with thyroid heart disease. It may also be utilized along with antithyroid agents to control thyrotoxicosis following ^{131}I treatment until the radioactive iodide has had time to take effect. Most hyperthyroid patients, however, escape from the effects of iodide after 10 to 14 days.

Ipodate, an agent for oral cholecystography, has been reported to be beneficial in the treatment of early hyperthyroidism, particularly in the early treatment of cardiac manifestations of thyrotoxicosis.[104]

HYPOTHYROIDISM

Hypothyroidism results from reduced secretion of both T4 and T3, occurring in most cases as a consequence of destruction of the thyroid gland itself, usually by an inflammatory process. In some cases, it is secondary to decreased secretion of TSH, due to either pituitary or hypothalamic disease. In secondary hypothyroidism, the signs and symptoms associated with deficiency of other pituitary hormones are also usually present. The incidence of hypothyroidism peaks between the ages of 30 and 60 years and is twice as common in women as in men. The following signs and symptoms are common: cold intolerance, dryness of the skin, weakness, impairment of memory, personality changes, shortness of breath, constipation, hoarseness, menorrhagia and other forms of menstrual dysfunction, and, occasionally, heart failure. In addition, in the more severe forms of the disease, there is facial puffiness, particularly around the eyes, a characteristic nonpitting form of edema (myxedema) of the lower extremities, slow speech, decreased hearing, and a yellow hue to the skin due to decreased conversion of carotene into vitamin A. These signs and symptoms may be present for years before treatment is initiated, particularly in patients in whom the disease has developed gradually.

EFFECTS OF AMIODARONE ON THYROID FUNCTION. The antiarrhythmic agent amiodarone (p. 646) has three effects on thyroid function. Its first effect is to antagonize thyroid hormone action on pituitary cells by binding to the intranuclear thyroid hormone receptor, and it thereby inhibits T3-induced changes in mRNA levels and TSH response to TRH.[105,106] Its second effect is to inhibit peripheral conversion of T4 to T3. Thus, in nearly all patients who receive long-term treatment with this drug, there is reduction in serum T3 levels and a transient rise in TSH. Within a few days to weeks this causes an increase in serum T4 levels and a return of serum TSH to normal. Clinically and metabolically, these patients are euthyroid even though their T4 levels are elevated.[107] Amiodarone's third effect is due to its high iodide content (35 per cent by weight). Thus, when it is metabolized there is a massive increase in the available inorganic iodide, resulting in acute inhibition of thyroid organification (Fig. 61–6). Depending upon the state of iodine intake before its administration, patients may develop either hypothyroidism (common in the United States) or thyrotoxicosis (more common in Europe).[107-109] As would be anticipated, amiodarone administration in experimental animals produces changes in serum lipids and lipoprotein lipase levels similar to those found in hypothyroidism.[110]

In addition to the more direct effects of amiodarone on thyroid function, in susceptible individuals this agent can also induce a marked increase in Ia-positive T cells (an abnormality found in patients with spontaneous Graves' disease). These T-cell abnormalities disappear after discontinuation of the amiodarone. Thus, amiodarone may induce T-cell abnormalities leading to an autoimmune state.[111] Because of amiodarone's long half-life, the biochemical and clinical abnormalities can persist for months after it is stopped.

CARDIOVASCULAR MANIFESTATIONS. The heart in overt myxedema is often pale, flabby, and grossly dilated. Histological examination discloses myofibrillar swelling, loss of striations, and interstitial fibrosis. With the development of methods that reliably and easily measure the circulating levels of thyroid hormone, the diagnosis of hypothyroidism is being made with increasing frequency at an earlier stage of the disease. Treatment is therefore also initiated earlier, resulting in a reduction in the incidence of cardiovascular signs and symptoms. Thus, the classic findings of cardiac enlargement, cardiac dilatation, significant bradycardia, weak arterial pulses, hypotension, distant heart sounds, low electrocardiographic voltages, nonpitting facial and peripheral edema, and evidence of congestive heart failure, such as ascites, orthopnea, and paroxysmal dyspnea, are now seen only infrequently. However, exertional dyspnea and easy fatigability continue to be common complaints.

Myxedema is associated with increased capillary permeability and subsequent leakage of protein into the interstitial space, resulting in pericardial effusion, a common clinical finding in overt myxedema, occurring in about one-third of all patients (p. 1505). Rarely, it or the presenting symptom is complicated by cardiac tamponade.[112] Cardiomegaly on chest radiograph and low voltage in the electrocardiogram are not reliable indicators of pericardial effusion; echocardiography is

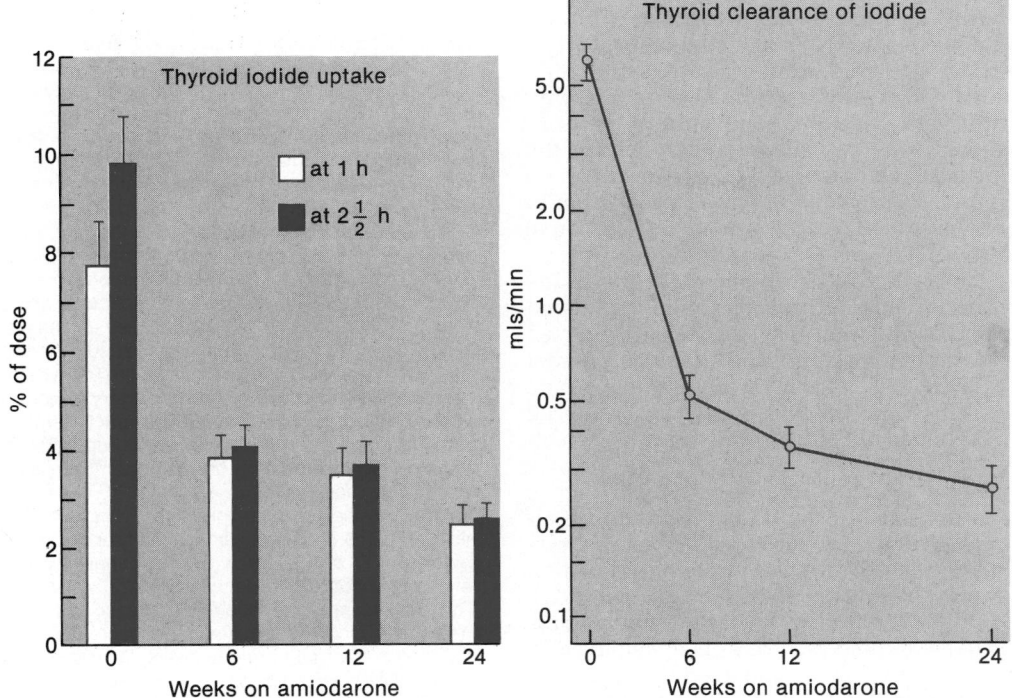

FIGURE 61-6. Effect of amiodarone on mean (±SEM) thyroid iodide uptake (*left*) and thyroid iodide clearance (*right*) in 15 euthyroid patients. (Note that the ordinate of the right panel is plotted on a log scale.) (From Rao, R. H., McCready, V. R., and Spathis, G. S.: Iodine kinetic studies during amiodarone treatment. J. Clin. Endocrinol. Metab. 62:563, 1986) © by The Endocrine Society, 1986.

the most useful method of establishing the diagnosis (p. 102). The effusions disappear with thyroid replacement therapy.[113]

The electrocardiographic changes observed in patients with hypothyroidism other than sinus bradycardia include prolongation of the Q-T interval, but since the T-wave amplitude is low, precise measurement of this interval is often impossible.[27] The P-wave amplitude is usually very low, and in some cases this wave is not even discernible. Sinus tachycardia is very rare, whereas bradycardia is common. It is possible that hypothermia may contribute to reentrant ventricular arrhythmias by slowing the heart rate and increasing the duration of the QRS and the Q-T intervals, which can rarely lead to severe ventricular tachyarrhythmias.[27,114] The incidence of atrioventricular and intraventricular conduction disturbances is about three times greater in patients with myxedema than in the general population.[25] Other electrocardiographic changes are those associated with pericardial effusion.[113] Thus, flattening or inversion of the T waves and low P-, QRS-, and T-wave amplitudes are commonly observed in patients with pericardial effusion. In most cases these revert to normal with the removal of the fluid. In some cases, however, the electrocardiographic changes persist even though the pericardial fluid is removed, which suggests that the lack of thyroid hormone may produce a primary myocardial abnormality suggestive of a cardiomyopathy.[115] Incomplete or complete right bundle branch block has been observed, but other forms of arrhythmias are uncommon.

There is increased frequency of hypertension in patients with hypothyroidism, although not in severe myxedema.[116] In one study of 477 patients, 15 per cent of hypothyroid subjects had a blood pressure greater than 160/95, compared to 5.5 per cent in age-matched euthyroid subjects. Replacement of thyroid hormone resulted in substantial reduction in blood pressure in the hypertensive patients.[117] In a study of 688 consecutive hypertensive patients, hypothyroidism was found in 25 (3.5 per cent). In nearly one-third of this subgroup, treatment of the hypothyroidism lowered the blood pressure to within the normal range.[116] Thus, individuals with mild to moderate hypothyroidism have an increased possibility of developing hypertension, particularly diastolic hypertension, while indi-

viduals with severe hypothyroidism are more likely to have normal or slightly low blood pressures.[116,117]

Cardiovascular manifestations of congenital hypothyroidism are similar except for the rarity of pericardial effusion. Thus the size of the left ventricle, its capacity, and the posterior wall thickness are all less in the hypothyroid infant. Since heart rate is also lower, cardiac output is reduced. There is also a prolongation of the preejection period of the left ventricle.[118]

MYOCARDIAL EFFECTS. Hypothyroid patients have reduced cardiac output, stroke volume, and blood and plasma volumes.[119,120] Circulation time is prolonged, but right and left heart filling pressures are usually within normal limits unless they are elevated by the pericardial effusion. There is a redistribution of blood flow with mild reductions in cerebral and renal flow and significant reductions in cutaneous flow. A delay in the relaxation of skeletal muscle is a well-known finding in hypothyroidism; measurements of isovolumetric relaxation time, by a combination of apex cardiography and phonocardiography, have revealed a prolongation of this interval with an abbreviation to normal during T4 replacement.[121] In addition, there is lengthening of the preejection period and an increased ratio of the preejection period to the left ventricular ejection time (PEP/LVET); these changes are the opposite of those observed in hyperthyroidism.[122]

Cardiac muscle isolated from cats with experimentally produced hypothyroidism exhibited reduced contractility, characterized by a depression of the myocardial force-velocity curve, a reduction of the rate of tension development, and a prolongation of the contractile response (Figs. 61–3 and 61–4).

There is little evidence from either experimental or clinical studies that congestive heart failure is common in myxedema or that it occurs in the absence of other cardiac disease.[123] Presumably the depressed myocardial contractility is sufficient to sustain the reduced workload placed on the heart in hypothyroidism. However, it may be difficult to distinguish between the heart in myxedema and heart failure. Dyspnea, edema, effusions, cardiomegaly, and T-wave changes occur in both conditions. In left heart failure, pulmonary arterial pressure is usually elevated during exercise, cardiac output fails to rise normally, and the Valsalva response is normal, while the opposite occurs in myxedema.[123] The hemodynamic changes in myxedema respond to thyroid hormone administration.

Cardiac catecholamine levels are not reduced in hypothyroidism. Neither the sensitivity of the mechanical performance of the heart to sympathetic nerve stimulation nor the response of the cardiac adenylate cyclase to norepinephrine is altered in hypothyroidism. However, there is a reduction in the total number of myocardial beta receptors.[55] In addition to the effects of hypothyroidism on the beta receptor there also is evidence that the lack of thyroid hormone may modify the contractile process itself. Thus, both isoproterenol-stimulated contractility and the accumulation of cyclic AMP are reduced in hearts obtained from hypothyroid rats.[124] In experimental hypothyroidism, calcium in isolated myocardial sarcoplasmic reticulum particles is reduced, which may explain the altered contractile state.[75] As already noted, thyroid hormone can affect the quantity and function of myosin ATPase activity through a change in protein synthesis. The activity of cardiac myosin ATPase and the rate of calcium uptake and the calcium-dependent ATP hydrolysis by isolated myocardial sarcoplasmic reticulum in the excitation-contraction-relaxation process[74] are reduced in hypothyroidism.

ATHEROSCLEROSIS. It has been suggested that patients with hypothyroidism are at increased risk of developing atherosclerosis, since this disease is accompanied by significant changes in lipid metabolism. Thus, hypercholesterolemia and hypertriglyceridemia, which are associated with the development of premature coronary artery disease, are found in patients with hypothyroidism. Support for this hypothesis has come from several sources, including the documentation that coronary atherosclerosis occurs with twice the frequency in patients with myxedema than in age- and sex-matched controls and that the development of atherosclerosis in cholesterol-fed animals is enhanced by the presence of hypothyroidism and reduced when thyroid hormone is administered.[125] Additionally, hypothyroidism has a deleterious effect on dogs in which a myocardial infarction has been induced. Infarct size was increased, dysrhythmias were more severe, and abnormalities in the microvasculature were present.[126] Yet myocardial infarction and angina pectoris are relatively uncommon occurrences in patients with hypothyroidism. The latter was present in only 7 per cent of a group of patients with hypothyroidism.[127] This low frequency of cardiac complications from atherosclerosis may simply reflect the decreased metabolic demand on the myocardium in hypothyroidism. A definitive study which examines the frequency of atherosclerosis in euthyroid individuals and persons who are now euthyroid but had once been myxedematous has not been reported. However, in one series of treated hypothyroid patients, angina pectoris improved more frequently than it became worse,[127] suggesting that the development of lipid abnormalities may not have the same implications in hypothyroid as in euthyroid individuals.

Other Metabolic Changes in Hypothyroidism

The evaluation of patients with myxedema and chest pain is complicated by the known effects of hypothyroidism on serum enzyme concentrations commonly used to assess myocardial damage. Thus, creatine kinase (CK), lactic dehydrogenase (LDH), and serum glutamic-oxaloacetic transaminase (SGOT) may be moderately or significantly increased in hypothyroidism.[128] The mechanism for the increase in enzymes is uncertain, but it may be related to mild cardiac or skeletal muscle damage with release of enzymes or decreased clearance of normal enzyme concentrations.

DIAGNOSIS AND TREATMENT OF HYPOTHYROIDISM

Caution must be exercised in treating hypothyroid patients who are elderly and who may have underlying heart disease, to avoid precipitating myocardial infarction or severe congestive heart failure; a slow replacement program is indicated in these individuals.

Some have suggested using T3 rather than T4 to treat patients with myxedema; since it has a shorter half-life, if toxic effects develop they will be dissipated more quickly. However, because it has a quicker onset of action, T3 also induces complications more rapidly. Thus, it appears to us more desirable to treat myxedema with T4, usually beginning with a dose as small as 0.0125 mg daily and doubling this every 14 days until a dosage of 0.1 to 0.125 mg is reached. During this process the patient's cardiovascular status is monitored frequently, and, if untoward events occur, the dose is reduced or maintained constant. The measurement of serum TSH levels provides a useful biochemical marker of adequacy of the replacement therapy.

The treatment of congestive heart failure is particularly difficult in patients with myxedema, both because of the effect of thyroid hormone on the heart and because the heart's response to cardiac glycosides is altered.[99] Patients with severe angina pectoris and untreated myxedema pose a difficult clinical dilemma because angina may be exacerbated by thyroid hormone replacement, and the usual medical management of angina with propranolol may induce severe bradycardia. Coronary arteriography often shows severe coronary artery disease in these patients, and an excellent surgical team can perform successful coronary revascularization with minimal thyroid replacement. Full thyroid replacement can then be safely achieved during the postoperative period, without the recurrence of angina.[129]

An increasingly common problem in ill patients is the so-called euthyroid sick syndrome.[130] This occurs in acutely or chronically ill patients who have low serum T4 and T3 levels yet do not have hypothyroidism. The low T3 levels are secondary to decreased extrathyroidal conversion of T4 to T3. The low T4's are often due to a decrease in the concentration of thyroxine-binding globulin, resulting in a decrease in total but only minimal changes in the free hormone levels. In very severe illness, there can be central (CNS) suppression of TSH release and an induced secondary hypothyroid state. Prolonged dopamine infusions can produce this situation also, by direct suppression of TSH secretion. In the euthyroid sick syndrome the serum TSH usually will be normal, whereas in hypothyroidism TSH will be increased, thus providing a biochemical mechanism for distinguishing them.[130,131] T4 therapy is not of benefit in these patients.[132]

DISEASES OF THE ADRENAL CORTEX

Since Addison's description in 1849 of adrenal insufficiency,[2] it has been appreciated that steroids secreted by the adrenal cortex exert a significant effect on the cardiovascular system, primarily by altering blood pressure. Adrenal insufficiency is characterized by significant hypotension, while excessive production of adrenal steroids is often accompanied by hypertension.

Three classes of steroids are secreted by the adrenal cortex: glucocorticoids, e.g., cortisol; mineralocorticoids, e.g., aldosterone; and androgens, e.g., dehydroepiandrosterone. In this section, the physiology and pathophysiology of glucocorticoid and mineralocorticoid secretion will be addressed.

HORMONE ACTIONS

CORTISOL. The primary glucocorticoid, cortisol, is synthesized from cholesterol in the inner layers of the adrenal cortex by a series of enzymatic transformations. After release into the circulation, it is bound to a high-affinity, low-capacity globulin, transcortin. Thus, most of the circulating cortisol is biologically inactive. The daily secretion rate of cortisol ranges from 15 to 30 mg with a pronounced diurnal cycle. Its average plasma concentration is 15 μg/dl in the morning, falling to 5 μg/dl by early evening.[133] The fundamental mechanism of action of the glucocorticoids is similar to that of other steroid hormones. They enter a target tissue by diffusion and combine with a specific high-affinity cytoplasmic receptor protein. The receptor-cortisol complex is then transferred to specific acceptor sites on nuclear chromatin tissue (promoter region) where it produces an increase in RNA and later protein synthesis.

The division of adrenal steroids into glucocorticoids and mineralocorticoids is somewhat arbitrary in that most glucocorticoids have some mineralocorticoid-like properties and vice versa. The major action of glucocorticoids is to promote gluconeogenesis, and, in that respect, they are both catabolic and antiinsulin. They mobilize amino acid precursors from peripheral supporting structures, such as bone, skin, muscle, and connective tissue, and inhibit protein synthesis and amino acid uptake in these same tissues. Gluconeogenesis is also indirectly enhanced by an increase in glucagon secretion secondary to the glucocorticoid-induced hyperaminoacidemia.

Glucocorticoids also have antiinflammatory properties related to their effects on both the microvasculature and the lymphatic system. They maintain normal vascular responsiveness to circulating vasoconstrictors, such as norepinephrine, and have a major effect on both the distribution and excretion of body water. For example, patients with Addison's disease cannot effectively excrete a water load. Finally, glucocorticoids can alter calcium absorption from the gastrointestinal tract by interfering with the activation of vitamin D in the liver and/or blocking its effect on the gastrointestinal tract.[133]

CONTROL OF CORTISOL SECRETION. This is primarily under the control of a negative feedback loop involving the adrenal cortex and the pituitary gland. Thus, as cortisol concentrations fall, ACTH secretion from the pituitary increases, stimulating the adrenal cortex to produce more cortisol and vice versa. The hypothalamus also interacts with this system by releasing corticotropin-releasing hormone, thus modifying ACTH release and the response of the pituitary to the inhibitory effect of cortisol. In addition to this primary negative feedback loop, there is an intrinsic diurnal rhythm in the release of both ACTH and cortisol, probably mediated by changes in the release of corticotropin-releasing hormone from the hypothalamus.

ALDOSTERONE. The major mineralocorticoid produced by the human adrenal gland is aldosterone. It is also synthesized from cholesterol but almost exclusively in the outer layer (glomerulosa) of the adrenal cortex. Aldosterone has two important functions: (1) it is a major regulator of extracellular fluid volume by its effect on sodium retention, and (2) it is a major determinant of potassium metabolism. Aldosterone acts predominantly on the distal convoluted tubule and/or collecting duct of the kidney where it promotes the reabsorption of sodium. Potassium then diffuses into the lumen of the tubules because of the change in electrochemical gradient produced by the active reabsorption of the positively charged sodium ion. Hydrogen ion may also be more freely excreted because of this change in the electrochemical gradient. While aldosterone also acts on salivary and sweat glands and on the endothelial cells of the gastrointestinal tract, these have little impact on total body sodium and potassium homeostasis.

There are three well-defined control mechanisms for aldosterone release.[133,134]

1. The renin-angiotensin system is the major system for the control of extracellular fluid volume by regulating aldosterone secretion. Aldosterone is linked in a negative feedback loop with the renin-angiotensin system. Thus, during periods registered as volume deficiency there is increased release of the enzyme renin from the juxtaglomerular cells of the kidney. Renin then increases the production of angiotensin I from its substrate. Angiotensin I is rapidly converted into the biologically active angiotensin II, which increases aldosterone secretion. Angiotensin II also produces vasoconstriction, thereby raising blood pressure and reducing blood flow to a variety of tissues, especially the kidney.

2. Potassium ion also regulates aldosterone secretion independent of the renin-angiotensin system; elevation of potassium concentration increases aldosterone secretion and vice versa. The adrenal cortex is very sensitive to changes in potassium concentration with as little as a 0.1 mEq/liter increment producing significant changes in the plasma aldosterone levels.

3. ACTH also has been documented to affect aldosterone secretion profoundly. However, because the control of aldosterone release is not appreciably altered in patients who have been on a long-term regimen of steroid therapy, ACTH probably has a smaller role than the other two factors in maintaining normal aldosterone secretion.

In addition to these major stimuli controlling aldosterone secretion, salt-losing hormones such as atrial natriuretic peptide (p. 1858) and dopamine inhibit aldosterone secretion, particularly in response to angiotensin II.[134] Finally, the prior dietary intake of both sodium and potassium alters the magnitude of the aldosterone response to acute stimulation, sodium restriction, and potassium loading, both enhancing the response of the adrenal, perhaps by modifying the local (adrenal) renin-angiotensin system.[133,134]

Diseases of the adrenal cortex, therefore, primarily affect the cardiovascular system via changes in blood pressure or volume homeostasis. Three specific conditions will be discussed next: glucocorticoid excess (Cushing's syndrome), mineralocorticoid excess (primary aldosteronism), and adrenal insufficiency (Addison's disease).

CUSHING'S SYNDROME

(see also p. 839)

In 1932 Harvey Cushing reported a syndrome characterized by truncal obesity, hypertension, fatigue, weakness, amenorrhea, hirsutism, purple abdominal striae, glucosuria, edema, and osteoporosis.[135] Since his original description, a number of specific causes for this syndrome have been described. However, the majority are secondary to bilateral adrenal hyperplasia, with the predominant feature being excess production of glucocorticoids and androgens.[136] Some cases are due to ACTH-producing tumors, of either the pituitary gland (Cushing's disease) or nonendocrine tissue (ectopic ACTH production). Fifteen to twenty per cent of the cases are due to primary adrenal neoplasia, either adenoma or carcinoma. Three

times as many women as men are afflicted, and the onset is usually in the third or fourth decade of life. Most patients have the typical body habitus: central obesity and slender extremities with proximal muscle weakness. Hypertension is present in 80 to 90 per cent of patients, and diabetes occurs in 20 per cent, probably in those individuals with a predisposition.[133,136] Evidence of androgen excess may also be present, including hirsutism, amenorrhea, clitoromegaly, and, in some cases, deepening of the voice. The majority of patients also have significant emotional changes ranging from lability of mood to severe depression, confusion, or even frank psychosis.

Laboratory tests disclose evidence of excess production of both glucocorticoids and androgens in the majority of cases. Thus, urinary metabolites of these steroids, 17-ketosteroids and 17-hydroxysteroids, are characteristically increased. Most patients show some evidence of glycosuria or hyperglycemia. There is usually generalized osteoporosis, most marked in the spine and pelvis; polycythemia is frequently encountered. In severe cases, hypokalemia, a mineralocorticoid manifestation, may also occur.

CARDIOVASCULAR MANIFESTATIONS. Prior to the development of effective treatment for Cushing's syndrome, accelerated atherosclerosis was a common finding. Early death usually occurred from myocardial infarction, congestive heart failure, or stroke. While the pathophysiology of the accelerated atherosclerosis is not clear, the hypertensive process probably contributes. However, it is unlikely to be the sole reason, since the hypertension of patients with primary aldosteronism may be as significant, and yet atherosclerosis is unusual. Some of the atherosclerotic changes may be mediated by the lipid-mobilizing effect of cortisol. Chronic excess production of cortisol leads to hyperlipidemia and hypercholesterolemia, both of which may promote the development of atherosclerosis.[137]

The pathophysiology of the hypertension in Cushing's syndrome has been much debated. Early studies suggested that it was secondary to volume expansion due to cortisol's mineralocorticoid properties. However, recent studies have not supported this hypothesis. Alternative hypotheses include glucocorticoid potentiation of response of vascular smooth muscle to vasoconstrictive agents and ACTH- or cortisol-induced increases in renin substrate.[137] The latter thesis suggests that the increased blood pressure is secondary to increased generation of angiotensin II. Thus, the pathophysiology of the hypertension may be multifactorial, being related to volume expansion, increased production of vasoactive agents, e.g., angiotensin II, and increased sensitivity of vascular smooth muscle to vasoactive agents.

The hemodynamic, electrocardiographic, and roentgenographic studies of patients with Cushing's syndrome have revealed no specific abnormalities except those that are, in general, associated with either hypertension or hypokalemia. The P-R intervals tend to be shorter than normal.

Over the past several years, a new familial syndrome has been described: Cushing's syndrome and cardiac myxoma occurring in the same individual (p. 1454). In addition to having these two conditions, 80 per cent of the patients have a cutaneous abnormality. In most it is a pigmented lesion; in some it is a subcutaneous myxoma. Histologically the adrenal glands show nodular hyperplasia.[138]

DIAGNOSIS AND TREATMENT. The diagnosis of Cushing's syndrome is established by the lack of appropriate suppression of cortisol secretion by dexamethasone. The best screening test is the administration of 1 mg of dexamethasone at bedtime with measurement of plasma cortisol between 7 and 10 the next morning.[133] In normal subjects cortisol levels will be less than 5 μg/dl. Some patients, particularly the obese, may have false-positive responses, but false-negative responses occur only rarely. The definitive diagnosis of Cushing's syndrome is made by administration of 0.5 mg of dexamethasone every 6 hours for 2 days with measurement either of plasma cortisol levels at the end of the second day (normal < 5 μg/dl) or of the 24-hour 17-OH excretory rate on the second day of dexamethasone suppression (normal < 3 mg/24 hours).[137,139]

Therapy of Cushing's syndrome is usually directed at the

specific cause. Thus, patients with adrenal carcinoma or adenoma or an ACTH-producing pituitary tumor are treated surgically. In some cases, patients with adrenal carcinoma have nonresectable lesions, and therefore surgery is combined with chemotherapy. The treatment of patients with bilateral hyperplasia without an evident ACTH-producing tumor is controversial, since the cause is often unknown. In some centers, bilateral adrenalectomy is the treatment of choice, while in others, therapy directed at the pituitary (either surgery or irradiation) is used.[140,141]

The treatment of the *cardiovascular abnormalities* associated with Cushing's syndrome is directed at lowering blood pressure and correcting the hypokalemia if present. Caution should be exercised in treating the hypertension with potassium-losing diuretics because of the tendency for these patients to develop hypokalemia. Thus, potassium-sparing diuretics or potassium supplements are often required. Hypertension in patients with Cushing's syndrome should be treated with agents that block the action or production of renin, such as beta blockers or converting-enzyme inhibitors. As in all clinical conditions in which hypokalemia may be present, cardiac glycosides should be used with caution in patients with Cushing's syndrome.

HYPERALDOSTERONISM
(See also p. 838)

CLINICAL AND BIOCHEMICAL MANIFESTATIONS. Aldosteronism is a syndrome associated with hypersecretion of aldosterone. Primary aldosteronism signifies that the stimulus for the excess aldosterone production resides within the adrenal. In secondary aldosteronism, the stimulus is of extraadrenal origin. These two conditions have similar effects on potassium metabolism.

In patients with primary aldosteronism, which most commonly is due to an aldosterone-producing adrenal adenoma, hypertension, hypokalemia, and metabolic alkalosis are common.[133,142] Polyuria may exist because of the hypokalemia, and glucose intolerance is increased in frequency. Muscle cramps due to the hypokalemia may be present, but little else distinguishes this from other forms of hypertension. Laboratory studies confirm the presence of hypokalemic alkalosis with a low specific gravity of urine and normal levels of adrenal glucocorticoids. The incidence of primary aldosteronism is between 0.5 and 2 per cent of the hypertensive population and it occurs twice as frequently in females as in males, with an initial presentation usually between the ages of 30 and 50 years.[133]

CARDIOVASCULAR MANIFESTATIONS. Many of the cardiovascular effects of aldosteronism are nonspecific, being related to aldosterone's effect on atrial pressure and potassium balance. Thus, T-wave flattening or U-wave prominence on the electrocardiogram (p. 150) and the presence of premature ventricular contractions and other arrhythmias due to hypokalemia are observed.[27] Evidence of left ventricular hypertrophy, either on the electrocardiogram or on the chest roentgenogram, may also be present in patients with longstanding hypertension and hyperaldosteronism. Malignant hypertension and changes in renal function secondary to severe hypertensive angiopathy are infrequent.

DIAGNOSIS AND TREATMENT. The diagnosis of primary aldosteronism is made by the presence of diastolic hypertension without edema, hypersecretion of aldosterone that fails to suppress appropriately during volume expansion, hyposecretion of renin, and hypokalemia with inappropriate urinary potassium loss during salt loading. The state of the renin-angiotensin system is often used to distinguish primary aldosteronism from other conditions that produce hypertension and hypokalemia. For example, hypertension and hypokalemia may be part of the clinical picture of secondary aldosteronism that accompanies malignant or accelerated hypertension or is associated with renal artery stenosis. Secondary aldosteronism can be readily distinguished from primary aldosteronism by the plasma renin activity, which is increased in the former and reduced in the latter. However, the combination of hypertension and a low plasma renin activity does not necessarily mean primary aldosteronism. Be-

tween 15 and 30 per cent of patients with essential hypertension have low renin levels, so-called low-renin essential hypertension.[142] The possibility of excess mineralocorticoid secretion has been extensively evaluated in these patients; however, no definitive evidence for such exists (Chap. 28).

The principal treatment for primary aldosteronism is surgical removal of the aldosterone-producing adenoma. In some cases, this is not possible because of the excessive risk imposed by the general physical status of the patient; then, spironolactone, which pharmacologically blocks the effects of aldosterone, is used long term. This form of therapy may be of limited benefit in males, since compliance is reduced by the undesirable side effects of gynecomastia and impotency, particularly when doses greater than 200 mg per day are required.[143]

Although congestive heart failure occurs infrequently in patients with primary aldosteronism, treatment of patients with this condition with cardiac glycosides must be cautious because of the hypokalemia.

In some patients, primary aldosteronism is due not to a solitary adenoma but to bilateral hyperplasia.[142] While the clinical characteristics of these two conditions are similar, their responses to surgery are different. In both cases hypokalemia is corrected, but patients with bilateral hyperplasia often do not exhibit reduction in arterial pressure. Patients with bilateral hyperplasia are best treated with spironolactone and other antihypertensive agents. Thus, preoperative distinction between bilateral hyperplasia and an adrenal adenoma, using adrenal venography or adrenal scanning, is important.

ADRENAL INSUFFICIENCY

Hypofunction of the adrenal cortex includes all conditions in which the level of secretion of adrenal steroids is less than the needs of the body. There are two major categories: those associated with primary damage to the adrenal cortex and those associated with secondary failure due to the lack of a stimulator such as ACTH. Clinically, patients with adrenal insufficiency can be divided into four types:[133] (1) the most common, primary insufficiency (Addison's disease); (2) secondary insufficiency due to a lack of ACTH; (3) selective hypoaldosteronism; and (4) enzyme deficiency (congenital adrenal hyperplasia).

CLINICAL AND BIOCHEMICAL MANIFESTATIONS. Addison's disease may occur at any age and affects both sexes equally. It is commonly due to a destructive process involving both adrenal glands; this process is sometimes infectious, but most often it is autoimmune.[144] Nearly all patients with primary adrenal insufficiency have weakness, increased skin pigmentation, significant weight loss, anorexia, nausea, vomiting, and hypotension, particularly postural. A significant minority also complain of abdominal pain, salt craving, and diarrhea or constipation. In mild forms, baseline laboratory studies are usually within normal limits. However, as the disease progresses, there is a gradual reduction in serum levels of sodium, chloride, and bicarbonate and an increase in potassium levels. The hyponatremia is due to extravascular loss of sodium, both into the urine (because of aldosterone deficiency) and into the intracellular compartment. The hyperkalemia is due both to the deficiency of aldosterone and to the impaired glomerular filtration rate and acidosis present in these patients. Other nonspecific findings include a reduction in basal metabolic rate with normal thyroid function and a normocytic anemia with relative lymphocytosis. While Addison's disease is often thought of as a common cause of significant eosinophilia, this is observed only occasionally.

CARDIOVASCULAR MANIFESTATIONS. The most common cardiovascular finding in adrenal insufficiency is arterial hypotension. In severe cases the pressure may be in the range of 80/50 mm Hg, with postural accentuation. Indeed, syncope occurs in a significant percentage of patients. In severe cases, heart size and peripheral pulses decrease. The electrocardiogram is abnormal in the majority of patients with Addison's disease.[27] The most common abnormalities are low or inverted T waves, sinus bradycardia, prolonged Q-T$_c$ interval, and low voltage. Conduction defects also occur, with first-degree block present in 20 per cent of patients. Changes secondary to the hyperkalemia are not common even though the serum potassium levels may be elevated. It is of interest that the electrocardiographic abnormalities, other than those secondary to hyperkalemia, do not respond to mineralocorticoids but require glucocorticoid replacement. Cardiac failure in prolonged adrenocortical insufficiency has also been reported rarely, secondary to a high-output state.[145,146]

DIAGNOSIS AND TREATMENT. Decreased response of the adrenal cortex to ACTH establishes the diagnosis of Addison's disease. The best screening test is the administration of synthetic ACTH (cosyntropin), 0.25 mg intramuscularly or intravenously, with measurement of plasma cortisol levels 30 to 60 minutes later. Cortisol levels double or increase by 10 μg/dl in normal subjects. Definitive evaluation is by prolonged (usually 24-hour) infusion of ACTH with assessment of either plasma cortisol or excretion of cortisol or both.[133]

It is possible to differentiate primary adrenal insufficiency from secondary adrenal insufficiency, isolated hypoaldosteronism, or congenital adrenal hyperplasia because one of the adrenal hormonal functions is normal in each of the latter three conditions. Thus in secondary adrenal insufficiency due to ACTH deficiency, aldosterone secretion is normal and the biochemical effects of mineralocorticoid deficiency, i.e., hyperkalemia, are not present. In isolated hypoaldosteronism, glucocorticoid function is normal. Female patients with congenital adrenal hyperplasia have evidence of androgen excess, such as virilization and hirsutism, and hypertension may also be present with a deficiency of 11-hydroxylase[147] (p. 841).

An increasingly common form of hypoaldosteronism is that associated with *hyporeninism*. Most commonly this syndrome is observed in older diabetic patients with a mild degree of renal impairment and hypertension; acidosis is also common. Usually these patients present with unexplained hyperkalemia. The cause is unknown, but may be secondary to damage to the juxtaglomerular apparatus and/or reduced conversion of a renin precursor into the active enzyme.[148] This clinical syndrome is particularly important in terms of cardiovascular diseases. Furthermore, commonly used drugs (beta blockers and calcium antagonists) can exacerbate this condition by further compromising aldosterone release.[149]

The treatment of adrenal insufficiency is accomplished by replacement of the deficient steroid. In adults with primary or secondary insufficiency, hydrocortisone, 20 to 30 mg daily, is administered in divided doses, usually two-thirds in the morning and one-third in midafternoon. In those patients with associated aldosterone deficiency, 9-α-fluorohydrocortisone, 0.05 to 0.10 mg daily, is given. During periods of significant stress (surgery, infection, or trauma), the dose of glucocorticoids should be increased. However, caution needs to be exercised in patients with myocardial infarction, as high-dose steroids could promote early infarct expansion.[150] Occasionally, acute adrenal insufficiency in patients who previously had apparently normal adrenal function is precipitated by the stress of cardiac surgery.[151]

PHEOCHROMOCYTOMA

(See also p. 840)

In 1859, Oliver and Shafer demonstrated that adrenal extract raised blood pressure when injected into experimental animals. In 1901, one active ingredient, epinephrine, was isolated and characterized, and in 1922 a syndrome of paroxysmal hypertension associated with an adrenal medullary tumor, pheochromocytoma, was reported.

EFFECTS OF CATECHOLAMINES ON THE CARDIOVASCULAR SYSTEM

The adrenal medulla and sympathetic nervous system are linked morphologically, biochemically, and physiologically and are often referred to as the sympathoadrenal system.[152] The sympathoadrenal system differs from other endocrine systems in several respects, including the fact that plasma levels of the secretory product, catecholamines, are not regulated by a direct feedback mechanism. Instead, catecholamine secretion is the efferent branch of a reflex arc involving centers in the brain stem, the hypothalamus, and perhaps the cerebral cortex as well. The human adrenal medulla contains about 1 mg of catecholamine per gram of tissue, approximately 85 per cent of which is epinephrine. The strategic location of the adrenal medullary cells within the cortex is associated with their capacity to form epinephrine, since high-dose glucocorticoids induce the formation of phenylethanolamine-*N*-methyltransferase, the enzyme needed to convert norepinephrine into epinephrine.[153]

In addition to their important effects on the cardiovascular system, catecholamines also have significant metabolic effects, stimulating glycogenolysis and gluconeogenesis, that is, increasing the production of glucose from glycogen and amino acid precursors and stimulating lipolysis,

thereby mobilizing free fatty acids and inhibiting secretion of insulin. The absence of the adrenal medulla does not produce definable disease in humans. However, the presence of a hormonally active adrenal medullary tumor produces a number of significant findings.

CLINICAL AND BIOCHEMICAL MANIFESTATIONS. A pheochromocytoma is a catecholamine-producing tumor derived from chromaffin cells. Those arising from extraadrenal chromaffin cells are called nonadrenal pheochromocytomas or paraganglionomas. Probably less than 0.1 per cent of patients with hypertension have a pheochromocytoma. Despite the fact that it is an uncommon disease, pheochromocytomas generate a great deal of interest, largely because the morbidity and mortality associated with these tumors are significant, with detection often resulting in cure. Pheochromocytomas are highly vascular tumors; less than 10 per cent are malignant as indicated by local invasion or metastasis, but, as with other endocrine tumors, malignancy cannot always be determined by microscopic appearance alone.

While the vast majority of tumors occur sporadically, approximately 5 per cent are inherited as an autosomal trait, by which they are often part of a pluriglandular neoplastic syndrome,[152] which, in addition to pheochromocytoma, may consist of medullary carcinoma of the thyroid, parathyroidadenoma, and retinal or cerebellar hemangioblastomas. Most pheochromocytomas are solitary adrenal tumors, with 10 per cent being bilateral and 10 per cent nonadrenal. However, in the familial form of pheochromocytoma nearly half the patients have bilateral adrenal tumors.

The features that suggest pheochromocytoma in hypertensive patients are (1) paroxysmal attacks of any kind, (2) headaches, (3) excessive sweating, (4) signs of hypermetabolism, (5) orthostatic hypotension, and (6) unusual blood pressure elevations due to trauma or operation.[152] Many of the features are similar to those of hyperthyroidism. While paroxysmal attacks are the hallmark of pheochromocytoma, more than half the patients have fixed hypertension and nearly 10 per cent are normotensive.

CARDIOVASCULAR MANIFESTATIONS. Hypertension is the major cardiovascular manifestation of pheochromocytoma. Its lability sometimes distinguishes it from other forms of hypertension; however, only clinical awareness of the entity and specific laboratory testing permit establishment of the proper diagnosis. The lability of blood pressure in patients with pheochromocytoma has been suggested to be due not only to episodic discharge of catecholamines but also to a reduction in plasma volume, as well as to impaired sympathetic reflexes. A number of observations suggest that chronic volume depletion is present.[154] For example, alpha-adrenoceptor blockade or removal of the tumor produces severe hypotension, which is correctable by volume expansion.[155] Cardiac output has been reported to be normal, whereas heart rate is increased, and orthostatic hypotension is accompanied by decreased stroke volume and inadequate adjustments in peripheral resistance indicative of impaired peripheral vascular reflexes.[154] An occasional patient will have markedly elevated central aortic pressure and severe systemic hypotension due to severe arterial vasoconstriction. Patients with pheochromocytoma may also have acute pulmonary edema.[155a]

The electrocardiogram is abnormal in as many as 75 per cent of patients with pheochromocytoma.[27] The changes consist of T-wave inversion, left ventricular hypertrophy, sinus tachycardia, and, in some cases, other alterations in rhythm, such as frequent supraventricular ectopic beats or paroxysmal supraventricular tachycardia.[156] An occasional patient will have a short P-R interval and a narrow QRS complex, suggesting that catecholamines are modifying the A-V conduction system. When arterial pressure increases markedly, changes suggestive of myocardial damage, including transient ST-segment elevations, marked diffuse T-wave inversions, and depression of ST segments, are present. These changes are usually transient, and the electrocardiographic pattern reverts to normal after removal of the tumor or pharmacological blockade.[152,155,157] Some of the electrocardiographic abnormalities are presumably due to hypertensive heart disease or myocardial ischemia. However, a specific catecholamine-induced myocarditis[158] and/or cardiomyopathy[159-161] has also been suggested.

The echocardiogram often shows left ventricular hypertrophy with normal left ventricular function.[162] During a hypertensive crisis it may show systolic anterior involvement of the anterior mitral leaflet, paradoxical septal motion, and proximal exclusion of the posterior wall.[163]

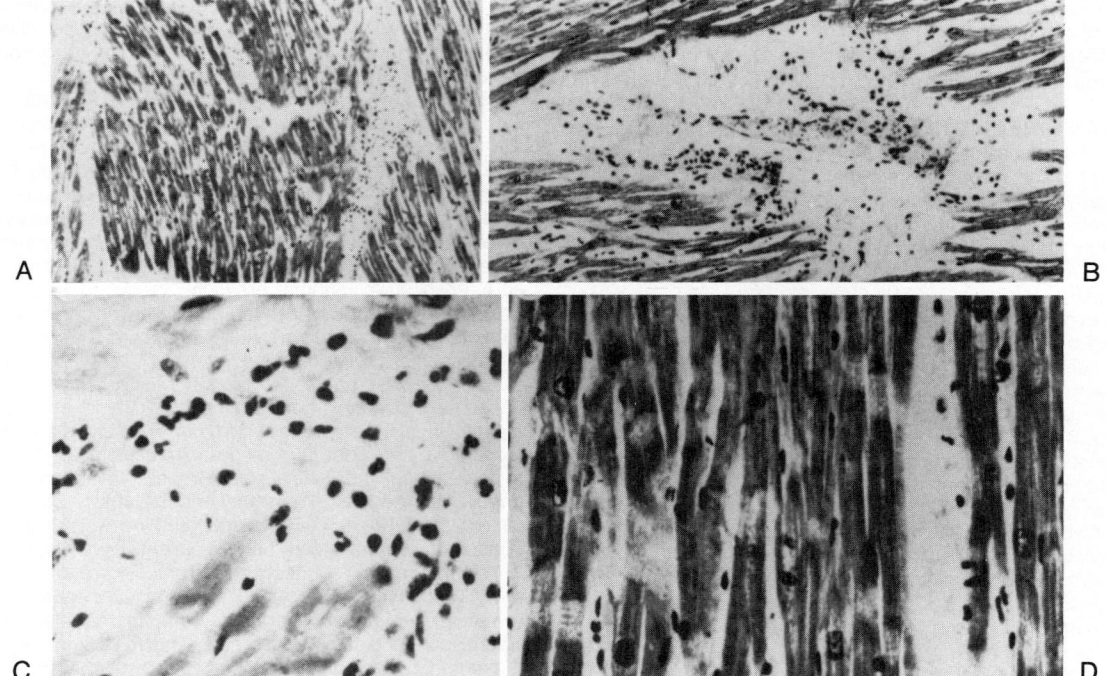

FIGURE 61-7. Left ventricular myocardium with acute myocarditis and contraction band necrosis in a patient with pheochromocytoma dying of catecholamine crisis. *A,* Diffuse infiltration by inflammatory cells through myocardium. *B,* Perivascular inflammation. *C,* Close-up of the inflammatory infiltrate. *D,* Contraction-band necrosis of myocytes. H&E; original magnification ×20 (*A*), ×45 (*B*), ×540 (*C*), ×330 (*D*). (From McManus, B. M., et al.: Fatal catecholamine crisis in pheochromocytoma: Curable cause of cardiac arrest. *Am. Heart J. 102*:930, 1981.)

Myocarditis. Pathologically, the myocarditis consists of focal necrosis with infiltration of inflammatory cells, perivascular inflammation, and contraction band necrosis[164] (Fig. 61-7), finally resulting in fibrosis. In some studies, 50 per cent of patients who died from pheochromocytoma had myocarditis,[155] usually accompanied by left ventricular failure and pulmonary edema. Although coronary atherosclerosis is usually present, medial thickening is the most characteristic lesion of the coronary arteries. When norepinephrine is infused into the rabbit, there is sustained coronary vasoconstriction that within 48 hours leads to histologically documented myocardial damage.[165] Occasionally, patients with pheochromocytoma have manifestations of cardiomyopathy which may be reversed when the tumor is removed[159-161] (Fig. 61-8). Finally, the myositis is not necessarily limited to the myocardium, as it also may occur in skeletal muscle.[166]

DIAGNOSIS AND TREATMENT. The diagnosis of pheochromocytoma is established by documenting increased urinary or plasma levels of catecholamines or one of their metabolites.[152,155] Three tests are commonly employed: (1) total catecholamines, (2) vanillylmandelic acid (VMA), and (3) metanephrine. The last two are metabolites of catecholamine and were first used to screen for pheochromocytoma because they are present in greater quantities. When reliably performed, these tests are probably equivalent in accuracy. The probability of a pheochromocytoma being present in a hypertensive patient with a single normal urine level is less than 5 per cent. It is most desirable to measure both the catecholamines and one of the two metabolites, preferably metanephrine, in screening for pheochromocytoma. If the blood pressure fluctuates, it is particularly important to collect the urine at a time the pressure is elevated. Specific pharmacological tests to screen for pheochromocytoma are of limited benefit, usually hazardous, and therefore warranted only in unusual circumstances. Clonidine has been proposed as a useful definitive test for pheochromocytoma, although it is necessary only in unusual cases. Catecholamine levels are suppressed in normal subjects via stimulation of central alpha-adrenoceptors; following clonidine administration in patients with pheochromocytoma they are not.[152] Unfortunately, profound and prolonged hypotension has been reported in some patients during the course of this test.

Once the diagnosis of pheochromocytoma is established, specific pharmacological blockade should be initiated.[152,155] Administration of phenoxybenzamine hydrochloride should be begun, with the initial dosage 10 mg every 12 hours; the dose is then gradually increased every 2 to 3 days until the arterial pressure is restored to normal. Alternatively, prazosin may be used. However, it should be noted that alpha-adrenoceptor blockade may induce a decline in arterial pressure accompanied by serious postural hypotension, presumably because of the vasodilatation occurring in the presence of hypovolemia. This hypotensive response can be prevented by adequate sodium intake; if the response is very striking, infusion of saline may be required. Adequate control of arterial pressure is essential prior to any arteriographic procedure, before initiating beta-adrenoceptor blockade, and before operation. Serfas and colleagues have suggested that calcium antagonists may be useful both in treating the hypertension associated with pheochromocytoma and in reducing catecholamine production.[167]

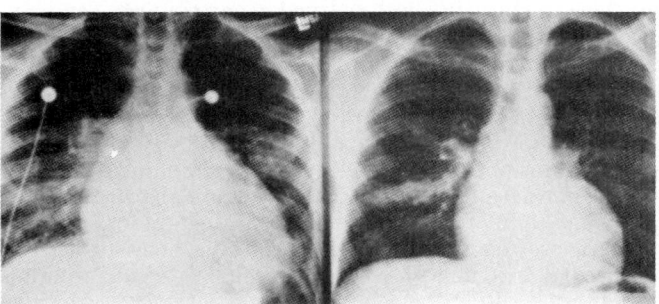

FIGURE 61-8. Pheochromocytoma-induced cardiomyopathy. *Left,* Chest x-ray on admission. Cardiomegaly, right pleural effusion, and signs of congestive heart failure. *Right,* One month after removal of the tumor. No signs of congestion and significant decrease of the heart size. (From Velasquez, G., et al.: Phaeochromocytoma and cardiomyopathy. *Br. J. Radiol. 57*:89, 1984.)

Beta-adrenoceptor blockade is useful in patients with pheochromocytoma who have significant tachycardia, palpitations, and catecholamine-induced arrhythmias. However, beta blockade with a drug affecting beta$_2$ receptors must *not* be initiated prior to inadequate alpha blockade, since severe *hypertension* may occur as a result of unopposed alpha-stimulating activity of the circulating catecholamines.

Definitive treatment is surgical removal of the tumor, usually after localization with computed tomography, arteriography, or scanning using a radioactive iodide derivative of guanethidine as the scanning agent.[155] Scanning may be particularly important in localizing extraadrenal, e.g., thoracic, pheochromocytomas. Although rare, of particular importance to the cardiologist is the presence of a cardiac pheochromocytoma (p. 1457). Precise definition of the anatomical boundaries of this tumor is important preoperatively if surgery is to be successful.[168] In those patients with inoperable lesions, long-term use of the combination of alpha- and beta-adrenoceptor blockers has been helpful. Drugs that inhibit the biosynthesis of catecholamines, such as alpha-methyltyrosine, and generalized chemotherapeutic agents have also been used in patients with malignant pheochromocytoma.[155]

PARATHYROID DISEASE

Disordered parathyroid secretion is associated with two cardiovascular disturbances, cardiac arrhythmias and hypertension. Changes in calcium metabolism as well as a direct effect of parathyroid hormone on the cardiovascular system appear to be responsible.

CLINICAL AND BIOCHEMICAL MANIFESTATIONS. Parathyroid hormone (PTH) is a single-chain polypeptide of 84 amino acids. Its major biological effect is to increase mobilization of calcium into the extracellular fluid from a variety of tissues; this action is linked in a negative feedback loop with serum unbound calcium concentration. Thus, an increase in serum calcium concentration reduces PTH release and vice versa.[169] PTH also increases urinary excretion of phosphate, augments bone resorption, and reduces the urinary excretion of calcium. It also indirectly increases the absorption of calcium from the gastrointestinal tract by increasing the rate of conversion of 25-hydroxyl vitamin D into the biologically active 1,25-dihydroxyvitamin D.[169]

Primary hyperparathyroidism, the excess production of PTH, is usually secondary to a solitary parathyroid adenoma. Occasionally, generalized parathyroid hyperplasia exists, and, infrequently, carcinoma of the parathyroid gland is found. In many cases, hyperparathyroidism is asymptomatic; 10 to 20 per cent of cases are first diagnosed as the result of a routine chemical screening test. *Secondary* hyperparathyroidism is at least equal in frequency to primary hyperparathyroidism. It is most commonly associated with renal disease and chronic hypocalcemia.

The signs and symptoms of primary hyperparathyroidism are related to direct effects of PTH on kidney or bone or those associated with the hypercalcemia. Nearly half the patients have signs and symptoms of renal dysfunction, such as polyuria, nocturia, renal stones, and, in severe cases, nephrocalcinosis and renal failure. In many patients, there are also nonspecific joint and back symptoms, and in unusual circumstances spontaneous fractures occur. Hypercalcemia reduces the excitability of the neuromuscular system, which can lead to such diverse effects as significant myocardial dysfunction and decreased auditory acuity.

Cardiac hypertrophy is found with increased frequency in patients with hyperparathyroidism, even in the absence of hypertension. In one study, five of 18 patients with hypertrophic cardiomyopathy had raised serum PTH levels but normal serum calcium levels. In contrast, left ventricular hypertrophy did not occur in six patients with hypercalcemia alone.[170]

Hypocalcemia is the common biochemical abnormality in both hypoparathyroidism and secondary hyperparathyroidism. Gastrointestinal disturbances and tetany secondary to the hypocalcemia may both occur.

CARDIOVASCULAR MANIFESTATIONS OF PARATHYROID DISEASES
(See also p. 841)

CARDIAC EFFECTS. While most of the effects of parathyroid hormone on the heart are probably secondary to a change in extracellular calcium, PTH also has a direct effect on the

heart, resulting in an increased beating rate of isolated heart cells and a positive inotropic action.[171,172] These effects are probably mediated by PTH binding to specific receptors, leading to increased entry of calcium into cardiac cells, and by the PTH increasing the release of endogenous myocardial norepinephrine. The direct effect of PTH may be deleterious, since it causes necrosis of rat myocytes and may be directly responsible for the increased accumulation of calcium in dystrophic muscles and for the heart damage found in uremia.[171,173] Whether these effects are clinically relevant is uncertain. Gafter and colleagues reported no change in cardiac performance in seven patients with end-stage renal disease who underwent parathyroidectomy for hyperparathyroidism.[174] On the other hand, hypoparathyroidism may cause a dilated cardiomyopathy, presumably secondary to the hypocalcemia. However, since longstanding hypocalcemia does not necessarily produce left ventricular dysfunction,[175] hypomagnesemia and reduced circulating PTH may also be involved.[176] PTH also has a direct effect on vascular smooth muscle, causing vasodilatation. Presently available data suggest that this vasodilating effect is more closely related to the portion of the PTH molecule responsible for its phosphaturic rather than its hypercalcemic effect.[177]

In addition to any direct action of PTH on the heart, hypercalcemia also has an adverse effect. Chronic hypercalcemia from a variety of causes is associated with increased deposition of calcium in the fibrous skeleton of the heart and valvular cusps as well as in coronary arteries and in myocardial fibers[178] (Fig. 61–9). Chronic hypercalcemia also may be a risk factor for accelerated coronary atherosclerosis.[179,180]

The plateau of the action potential of cardiac fibers is prolonged by low and shortened by high extracellular calcium concentrations (Chap. 22). Lengthening of the plateau prolongs the duration of the action potential, whereas shortening of the plateau has the opposite effect. The changes in duration of action potential are accompanied by corresponding changes in the duration of the refractory period, of the ST segment, and of the Q-T interval.[27] Thus the major electrocardiographic change in hypercalcemia is shortening of the Q-T interval. Less frequently, disorders of intraventricular conduction

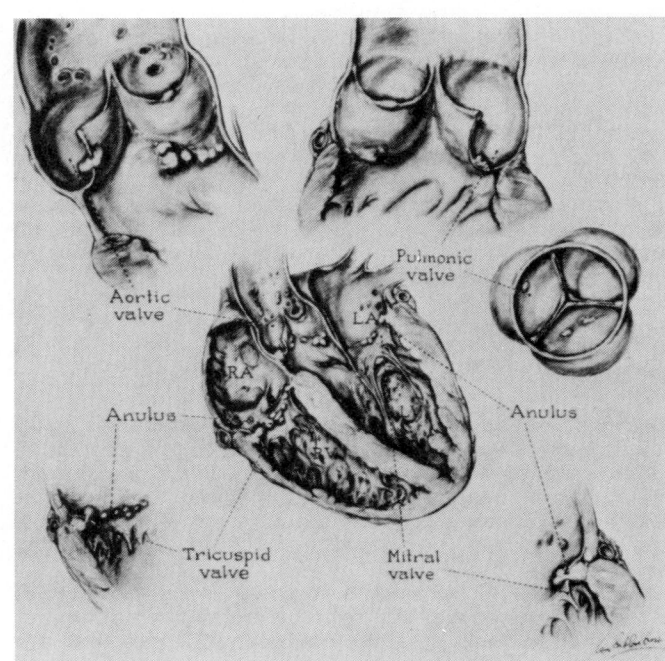

FIGURE 61–9. Heart showing distribution of calcific deposits in the tricuspid and mitral valve annuli and at the bases of both pulmonic and aortic valve cusps in a 43-year-old woman with hypercalcemia secondary to primary hyperparathyroidism. (From Roberts, W. C., and Waller, B. F.: Effect of chronic hypercalcemia on the heart: An analysis of 18 necropsy patients. Am. J. Med. *71*:371, 1981.)

have been reported with shortening of the P-R interval.[27] Complete heart block occurs only rarely.

Hypocalcemia produces the opposite effect on the electrocardiogram with prolongation of the Q-T interval and nonspecific ST- and T-wave changes. Normal contractile function of cardiac muscle requires calcium, and heart failure has been reported in patients with chronic hypocalcemia secondary to hypoparathyroidism.[181]

HYPERTENSION. Hypercalcemic patients detected by routine serum calcium screening techniques have higher arterial pressure than do matched normocalcemic subjects.[182] Yet in patients with hyperparathyroidism, the level of serum calcium is similar in those who are normotensive and those who have hypertension, suggesting that hypercalcemia per se is not the dominant cause for the hypertension. Thus, the pathophysiology of the hypertension is uncertain.[183] For example, hypercalcemia produces nephrocalcinosis, which may lead to renal failure and hypertension. Thus, reversal of hypertension after successful parathyroid surgery is more likely to occur when renal function is normal. Increased serum calcium also increases myocardial contractility, peripheral resistance, and release of or vascular sensitivity to vasoconstrictor agents, such as angiotensin II and norepinephrine. While hypercalcemia can increase cardiac contractility and arterial pressure acutely, it is unlikely that this action produces a significant alteration in cardiac output or performance on a long-term basis in the absence of PTH.[183] Thus an elevation of peripheral resistance is the most likely cause of the hypertension associated with hyperparathyroidism. While the mechanism of hypertension in these patients remains to be elucidated, (1) it may be renin dependent; (2) it is associated with increased circulating PTH, but not necessarily with the level of hypercalcemia; and (3) it is curable surgically in a significant number of patients.[184]

DIAGNOSIS AND TREATMENT

If hypercalcemia is *not* due to primary hyperparathyroidism, circulating concentration of PTH should be suppressed. Thus, an elevated or even a normal concentration of PTH in the presence of hypercalcemia establishes the diagnosis of hyperparathyroidism; many patients with this condition manifest hypercalcemia for the first time after starting thiazide therapy for the associated hypertension. Treatment consists of surgical removal of the parathyroid tumor or hyperplastic glands.

Patients with hypertension should have a determination of serum calcium levels before therapy is begun. If thiazide diuretics are used in treatment, serum calcium levels should be determined every 6 months. If thiazide-induced hypercalcemia occurs, the serum calcium should be determined for 2 to 3 months after discontinuation of the thiazides. Persistence of the hypercalcemia suggests that the patient has primary hyperparathyroidism.[182]

Patients with hypoparathyroidism and hypocalcemia usually are treated with calcium supplementation and vitamin D or one of its metabolites. To minimize the development of nephrolithiasis, serum calcium levels are titrated only to the lower end of the normal range.

DIABETES MELLITUS

Diabetes mellitus is one of the leading public health problems in the industrialized world, and it has a profound effect on the cardiovascular system. Nearly 10 million people are afflicted with this disease in the United States; it is the eighth health-related cause of death. Nearly all the morbidity from diabetes is related to cardiovascular dysfunction— coronary artery disease, hypertension, or renal failure secondary to microvascular disease.

ACTIONS OF INSULIN. Insulin is a double-chain polypeptide derived from proinsulin, which is synthesized in the islet cells of the pancreas. Many stimuli, such as glucose, glucagon, amino acids, catecholamines, and gastrointestinal hormones, can promote insulin secretion, which usually occurs in two phases. The rapid early phase releases preformed insulin stored in granules in the beta cells, while the prolonged late phase results from increased biosynthesis of insulin.[185]

Insulin is an anabolic hormone affecting all metabolic substrates, i.e., carbohydrates, fats, and proteins, as well as nucleic acids. All target tissues for insulin have specific membrane-bound receptors; thus, binding to the receptor is the first step in initiating its metabolic effect. The concept that insulin is the "fed" hormone has been popularized.[185] Thus the ingestion of fuel substrates provokes a rapid rise in the concentration of circulating insulin, which then facilitates the transfer of these substances into their respective depots. According to this theory, in the fasted state insulin levels are low; as a result, there is increased gluconeogenesis by the liver, decreased lipogenesis with lipolysis and fatty acid release from fat tissue, and decreased glucose uptake in cardiac and skeletal muscle. On the other hand, in the fed state insulin levels are high; gluconeogenesis by the liver is reduced; and in cardiac and skeletal muscle glucose and amino acid uptake and protein synthesis are increased. In adipose tissue there is increased glucose and triglyceride uptake, lipogenesis, and absence of release of fatty acids.

In the patient with diabetes, because insulin release is decreased in response to the ingested fuel, there is a delay in the uptake and the disposal of these fuels into their respective depots, which leads to abnormal circulating levels of the substrates. The increased concentrations of lipids in the circulation may be the underlying pathophysiological effect producing a number of the clinical complications of diabetes mellitus.

CLINICAL AND BIOCHEMICAL MANIFESTATIONS. Relatively recently, our understanding of the pathogenesis of diabetes mellitus has been significantly altered. Several lines of evidence suggest that in many instances the insulin-dependent (IDDM) form may be infectious or autoimmune in origin, while in most cases the noninsulin-dependent form (NIDDM) is probably the result of a genetic predisposition.[186]

Most of the signs and symptoms of this disease either are related to the increased levels of blood glucose or are secondary to changes in the cardiovascular system. Thus, the classic presenting symptoms (observed in about 25 per cent of IDDM patients) are polyuria, polydipsia, and polyphagia, all due to the glucosuria. The major pathophysiological consequence of diabetes mellitus is related to changes in the vascular system. The specific target organs include the heart, the eye, the kidney, the autonomic nervous system, and the peripheral vasculature.

CARDIOVASCULAR CHANGES IN DIABETES

PATHOLOGY. The vascular disease associated with diabetes mellitus can be nonspecific (atherosclerosis and arteriosclerosis) or specific (microangiopathic or endothelial proliferative changes of arterioles). The former primarily involves large vessels (especially in the lower extremities), heart, and brain of older patients, while the latter is localized to small vessels and may be seen in patients of all ages. The atherosclerosis tends to be more extensive and more severe than in nondiabetics, resulting in an increased frequency of myocardial infarction and cerebral and peripheral vasculature disease.[187] Indeed, coronary heart disease is the leading cause of death among adult diabetics and accounts for about three times as many deaths among diabetics as among nondiabetics. The incidence of coronary artery disease correlates more closely with the duration of diabetes than with its severity. Of interest is the documentation that diabetics have an increased mortality for noncardiovascular diseases (e.g., cancer) as well.[188] The mechanism(s) responsible for this generalized increased mortality is unclear.

Certainly, diabetes should be considered to be a separate risk factor for coronary heart disease[189-190] (p. 1151). Since each risk factor for vascular disease is thought to add independently (although not equally) to the likelihood for the development of ischemic disease, the diabetic should be considered a high-risk patient in whom all correctable factors should be managed.[191-192] It is logical to approach cigarette smoking and even moderate elevation of blood pressure and plasma lipids more intensively in diabetic than in nondiabetic patients. Contraceptive drugs that suppress ovulation probably should be avoided, since they may contribute to the metabolic abnormalities that underlie their increased risk for vascular disease. The obese diabetic patient should lose weight; this is often accompanied by gratifying improvement of hypertension, hyperglycemia, hyperinsulinemia, and hypertriglyceridemia.

The microangiopathy produces a characteristic thickening of the basement membrane of the capillaries in the retina, conjunctiva, glomerulus, brain, pancreas, and myocardium.[193] In some cases there is also proliferation of the epithelial cells, leading to occlusion of small arterioles similar to that observed in immune arteritis.

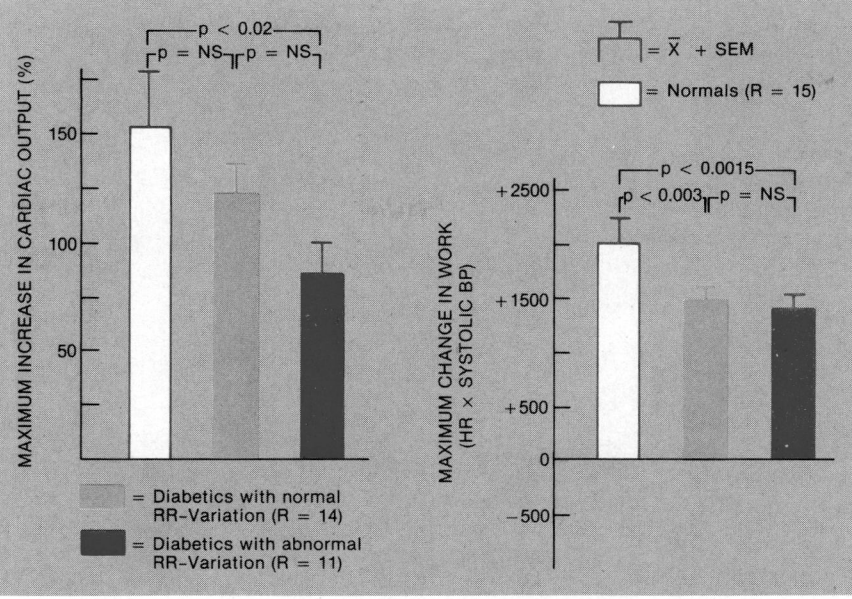

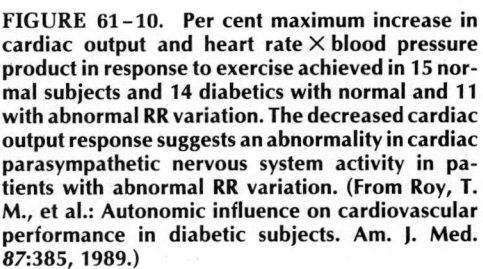

FIGURE 61–10. Per cent maximum increase in cardiac output and heart rate × blood pressure product in response to exercise achieved in 15 normal subjects and 14 diabetics with normal and 11 with abnormal RR variation. The decreased cardiac output response suggests an abnormality in cardiac parasympathetic nervous system activity in patients with abnormal RR variation. (From Roy, T. M., et al.: Autonomic influence on cardiovascular performance in diabetic subjects. Am. J. Med. 87:385, 1989.)

CARDIAC INVOLVEMENT. Not only is the frequency of acute myocardial infarction increased in diabetic patients,[190,191] but also the treatment of the infarct is more complicated than in the nondiabetic patient. Patients with acute myocardial infarction, regardless of the control of their diabetes before hospital admission, exhibit significantly higher mortality and morbidity than do nondiabetics.[189,191,192] Several factors contribute to the increased mortality of diabetic patients with acute myocardial infarction. The size of the infarct tends to be greater in the diabetic than in the nondiabetic; diabetic patients have a greater frequency of both congestive heart failure and shock than do nondiabetics; and the patient is often in a precarious metabolic status compounded by the difficulty of adjusting insulin therapy to prevent ketoacidosis while not precipitating hypoglycemia.[189,192,194]

The occurrence of myocardial infarction has a distinctly adverse effect on carbohydrate and fat metabolism and often leads to stimulation of the sympathetic nervous system and increased catecholamine concentration[195] (p. 1212). Subsequent increases in circulating free fatty acid levels and reductions in glucose tolerance appear to be related to a number of physiological functions—adipose tissue lipolysis, hepatic and muscle glycogenolysis, catecholamine-induced suppression of insulin release, and increased circulating concentrations of growth hormone and cortisol. The net result is that carbohydrate intolerance is common after myocardial infarction, even in nondiabetics. Also, the high concentrations of free fatty acid in the acute phases of myocardial infarction may lead to ventricular arrhythmias.[196] The suppression of insulin release as a consequence of increased catecholamine activity may decrease glucose utilization by a myocardium that may require this fuel for glycolytic activity.[197]

Diabetic patients with acute myocardial infarction differ from nondiabetics in that their pain patterns are more variable, and infarction may actually occur without pain.[198] Also, survival after infarction is more limited than in the nondiabetics, with fatality rates being as high as 25 per cent during the first year after infarction.[189,191,192] Recurrent infarction, heart failure, and dysrhythmias all contribute to this higher death rate.[189–192,194] Administration of beta blockers to diabetics appears to reduce the overall mortality, at least in the immediate postmyocardial infarction period, similar to what has been reported in nondiabetics.[199]

Peripheral somatic neuropathy is a common complication of diabetes mellitus; also, diabetic autonomic neuropathy leading to diarrhea, vomiting, and other gastrointestinal disturbances is well known in this disease. *Cardiac autonomic dysfunction* also exists in many diabetic patients,[200,201] and the anginal threshold is increased, presumably as a consequence

of autonomic and sensory neuropathies.[202a] In two large series it was present in more than a third of the patients and accompanied by depression of left ventricular function. The severity of cardiac dysfunction was directly related to the severity of the cardiac autonomic neuropathy[202,203] (Fig. 61–10). Occasionally it may be present before clinical symptoms of generalized autonomic neuropathy are demonstrable. Furthermore, the neuropathy may involve the sympathetic nervous system and/or the parasympathetic nervous system. Indeed, it may become so severe as to lead to total cardiac denervation. These changes in adrenergic nervous system function result in tachycardia and a fixed, rapid heart rate that barely responds to physiological stimuli, such as the Valsalva maneuver, carotid sinus pressure, or tilting,[204a] or to drugs, such as phenylephrine, atropine, or propranolol. Rarely, these denervated hearts develop arrhythmias.

CONGESTIVE HEART FAILURE. IDDM appears to increase the likelihood of the development of congestive heart failure from all causes. The role of diabetes in congestive heart failure in the Framingham study was analyzed,[192] and the risk of developing heart failure was found to be increased substantially. Even when patients with prior coronary or rheumatic heart disease were excluded, diabetic subjects had a four- to fivefold increased risk of congestive heart failure. Furthermore, this increased risk persisted after age, blood pressure, weight, and cholesterol values, as well as coronary heart disease, were taken into account. On the basis of these findings it appeared that the excessive risk of heart failure in diabetic patients is caused by factors other than accelerated atherogenesis and coronary heart disease. One suggested possibility is a diabetes-induced cardiomyopathy.

Diabetic Cardiomyopathy. There is a substantial increase in the coincidence of diabetes mellitis and cardiomyopathy. The cardiomyopathy occurs in patients who have no evidence of large-vessel disease or abnormalities in myocardial capillary basal lamina documented by endomyocardial biopsies.[205,206] The most common histological abnormalities are interstitial fibrosis (Fig. 61–11) and arteriolar hyalinization (Fig. 61–12). Evidence supporting the presence of cardiomyopathy even in children with diabetes mellitus has been reported. Both systolic and diastolic dysfunction have been observed. The severity of this dysfunction is related to the degree of metabolic control, and there is no clinical evidence of cardiovascular or microvascular disease.[207] Taken together, these studies strongly suggest that in some diabetic patients there is a nonischemic cardiomyopathic process.

ABNORMALITIES OF VENTRICULAR FUNCTION. Several abnormalities of ventricular function, using echocardiographic techniques, have been reported in diabetics. In young

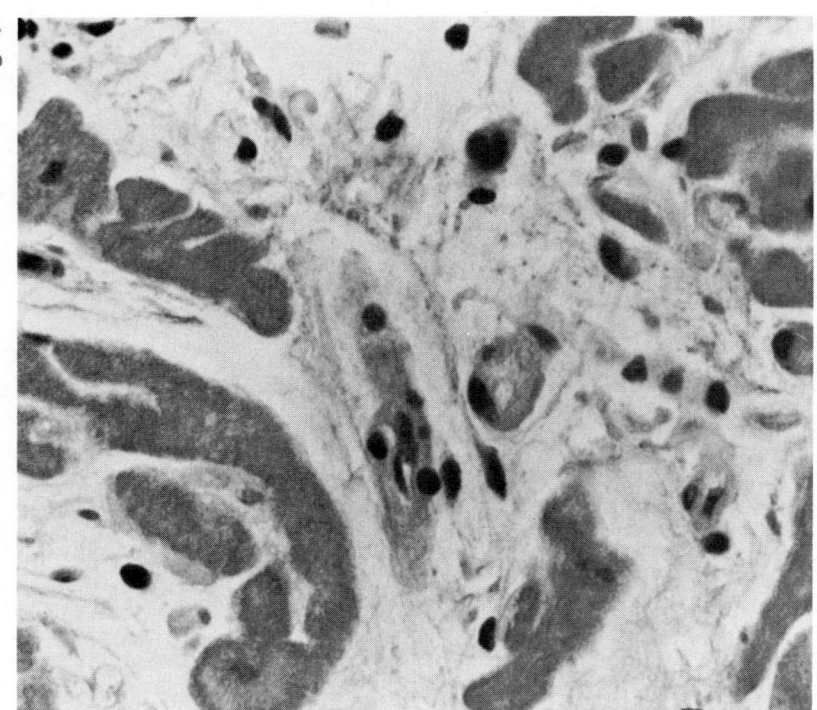

FIGURE 61–11. Myocardium of diabetic patient show-ing atrophied myocytes on right side (compare with more normal fibers on left), increased interstitial fibrous tissue, and thickening of small arteriolar walls. H & E × 300. (From Sutherland, C. G. G., et al.: Endomyocardial biopsy pathology in insulin-dependent diabetic patients with ab-normal ventricular function. Histopathology *14*:596, 1989.)

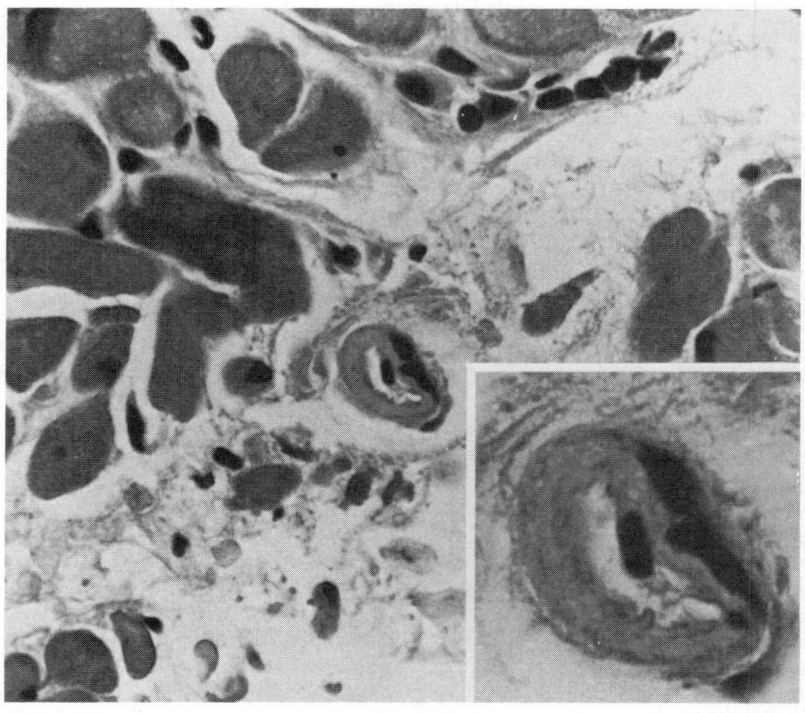

FIGURE 61–12. Hyalinization without luminal narrow-ing of small arteriole in myocardium of diabetic patient. H & E, ×300. Inset, Same arteriole. (H & E, ×750.) (From Sutherland, C.G.G. et al.: Endomyocardial biopsy pathol-ogy in insulin-dependent diabetic patients with abnormal ventricular function. Histopathology *14*:597, 1989.)

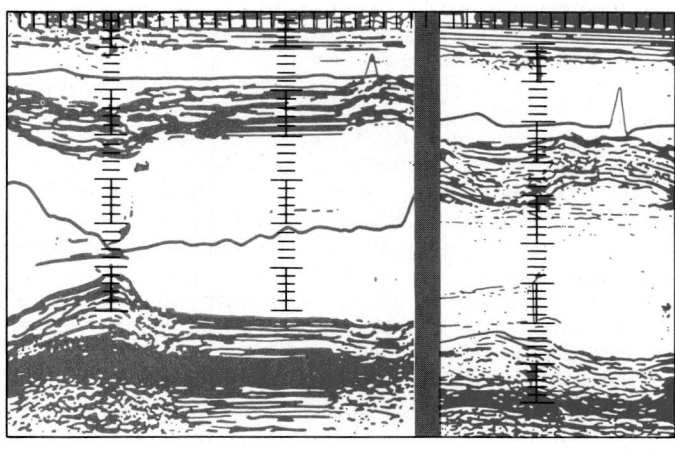

FIGURE 61–13. M-mode echocardiograms from a healthy woman (*left*) and a diabetic woman (*right*). The rate of ventricular filling is much slower in the latter. (From Airaksinen, J., et al.: Impaired left ventricular filling in young female diabetics. An echocardiographic study. Acta Med. Scand. *216*:509, 1984.)

asymptomatic patients, the ratio of early to peak filling velocity is significantly decreased while atrial filling velocity is significantly increased (Fig. 61–13). There is no relationship between the left ventricular diastolic filling abnormalities and evidence of severity of the diabetes, i.e., retinopathy, nephropathy, or peripheral neuropathy.[208] Other reported abnormalities in diabetic subjects include left ventricular asynergy on two-dimensional echocardiograms[208,209]; reduction in the peak diastolic filling rate[210]; an abnormal left ventricular ejection fraction in response to exercise[211,212]; and evidence of diastolic dysfunction, even in normotensive diabetic patients.[213,213a]

Several factors have been reported to contribute to the abnormalities in left ventricular function in diabetics: (1) The role of hypertension with a concomitant increase in left ventricular mass.[214] (2) The potential role of growth hormone. Patients with difficult-to-control diabetes often have increased growth hormone levels. Several investigators have reported that this metabolic abnormality could account for the increased collagen levels present in the left ventricular wall of diabetic humans and animals[215] (Fig. 61–11). Regan et al., however, have reported that in experimental diabetes induced in dogs the collagen accumulation in the myocardium is not related to or dependent on an increase in plasma growth hormone levels.[216] (3) The increased cardiac sorbitol level.[217] (4) The impairment in Ca^{++} handling with hypersensitivity of the myocardium to Ca^{++} secondary to increased sarcolemmal Ca^{++} ATPase activity[218,219] (Fig. 61–14). In a rat model of non-insulin–dependent diabetes mellitus, the abnormalities in myocardial Ca^{++} ATPase activity have also been demonstrated.[220] Further support for this hypothesis comes from the beneficial effect of a calcium antagonist (verapamil), which prevented diabetes-induced myocardial changes in experimental diabetes.[221] (5) Finally, Okumura et al. have suggested that increased 1,2-diacylglycerol levels with resultant activation of protein kinase C may underlie the cardiomyopathy, at least in experimentally induced diabetes.[222] Despite these observations in experimental models, it should be noted that when insulin is administered, the cardiac abnormality is not necessarily corrected. Thus, the relationship between the hyperglycemic state and the abnormalities in myocardial function and metabolism present in experimental diabetes is still unclear.

Pathological Changes. In postmortem studies of 11 diabetic patients, 9 of whom were without significant obstructive disease of the proximal coronary arteries and had died of cardiac failure, all exhibited positive periodic acid–Schiff (PAS) staining material in the interstitium, but none had luminal narrowing of the intramural vessels. Collagen accumulation was present in perivascular loci, between the myofibers, or as replacement fibrosis. Multiple samples of left ventricle and septum revealed abnormally increased deposits of triglyceride and cholesterol.[223] Thus these observations, taken in toto, suggest that a diffuse abnormality, either extravascular or involving the microvasculature, may be the basis for the cardiomyopathic features of diabetes. However, a recent morphological study casts some doubt on small-vessel disease as the producer of cardiac myopathy, because similar findings have been reported in NIDDM subjects. Unsitupa et al., studying 133 patients with NIDDM (Type 2), found a high incidence of impaired left ventricular function already present at the time of initial diagnosis.[224] Hypertension appears to accelerate this process, both in humans and animals, as severe interstitial fibrosis, focal scars, and myocytolytic activity were significantly more frequent in hypertensive diabetics with chronic heart failure examined post mortem than in normotensive diabetics.[225]

Other (nondiabetic) cardiomyopathies may exhibit similar hemodynamic abnormalities; an abnormal rise of ventricular filling pressure without a stroke volume increase in response to afterload increments has also been observed in the preclinical phase of alcoholic cardiomyopathy, in which the interstitium is also altered.[225] More severely altered interstitial

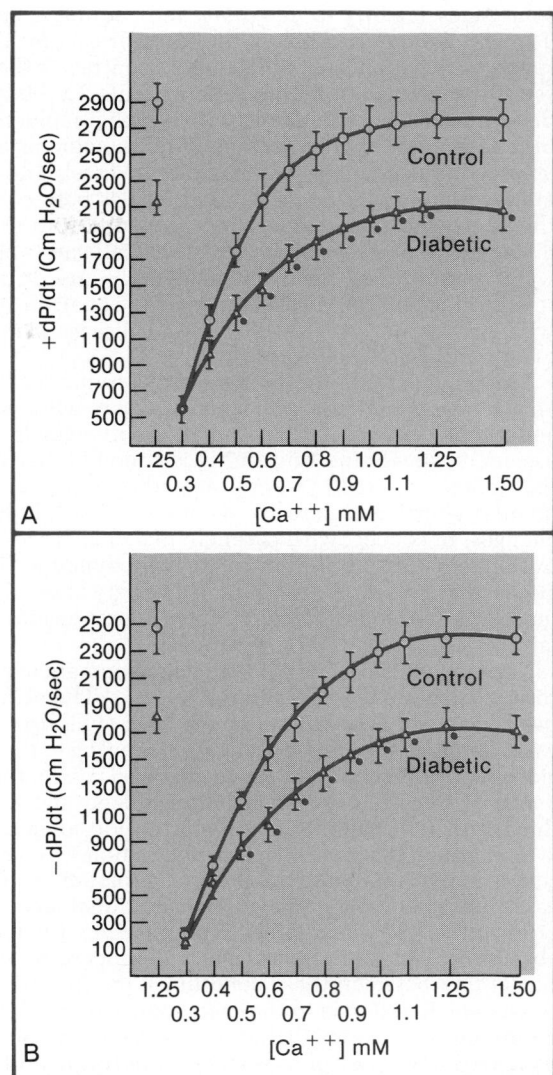

FIGURE 61–14. Effect of non-insulin–dependent diabetes mellitus on myocardial contractility (+ dp/dt, *top*) and relaxation (− dp/dt, *bottom*). Hearts from 12-month-old diabetic rats (triangles) and the age-matched controls (circles) were perfused during the initial 20–minute stabilization period with Krebs-Henseleit buffer containing 11 mM glucose and a calcium concentration of 1.25 mM. At each calcium concentration, + dP/dt (first derivative of left ventricular function, an index of contractility) (*A*) and − dP/dt (an index of relaxation) (*B*) were measured. Each data point represents mean ± SE of five to seven hearts. *Significant difference from control (*P* < 0.05). (From Schaffer, S. W., et al.: Basis for myocardial mechanical defects associated with noninsulin-dependent diabetes. Am. J. Physiol. *256*:E27, 1989.)

changes may be the predominant lesion in the incipient stages of amyloid heart disease.[226]

Diabetes mellitus is associated with another form of cardiomyopathy. Approximately half the infants of diabetic mothers have either radiographic cardiomegaly or clinical features suggesting congestive heart failure[227] (p. 995). The cardiomyopathy in these infants may be transient and secondary to hematological, respiratory, and metabolic problems or a more protracted form of nonobstructive or obstructive hypertrophic cardiomyopathy, which appears to be secondary to maternal hormonal influences and to be reversible.

Electrocardiographic changes are commonly observed in patients with diabetes.[27] While many of the changes are predictable on the basis of the associated hypertension or coronary artery disease, in some there is an unexplained diffuse T-wave abnormality that may be related to the cardiomyopathy.

VASCULAR DISEASE. Peripheral vascular disease is a frequent and significant manifestation of diabetes mellitus, sometimes leading to gangrene and requiring amputation. The smaller arteries below the knee are more likely to be involved in patients with diabetes, in contrast to iliac or femoral artery disease in nondiabetic patients. Cerebral vascular disease is also more frequent, with a greater incidence of cerebral infarction though not cerebral hemorrhage. The increased atherosclerosis of the cerebral vessels and the proliferative changes in the cerebral arterioles both contribute to this increased rate of infarction. In addition to the effect of diabetes on cardiac function, insulin itself can cause salt and water retention by mechanisms still obscure. In most cases this fluid retention is self-limiting. However, in individuals who have underlying cardiovascular disease it may lead to overt cardiac failure.[228]

The renal vasculature is affected in a number of ways: atherosclerosis is common in the larger vessels, with proliferative endothelial changes occurring in small vessels. Capillary basement membrane thickening is common, particularly in the glomerular tuft where a pathognomonic change—nodular glomerulosclerosis—is often found. These vascular changes, in concert with parenchymal changes secondary to pyelonephritis and altered renal hemodynamics (increased glomerular pressure),[229,230] lead to a variety of renal disorders, including the nephrotic syndrome, hypertension, and renal failure.

The mechanism underlying the development of atherosclerosis in diabetes is multifactorial (p. 1151). Hyperinsulinemia itself has been shown to enhance lipid synthesis in arterial walls and may be a major factor contributing to the macroangiopathy.[231] Most studies have reported an increased incidence of hypertension in diabetes. Indeed, more than one-third of diabetic patients have hypertension, an incidence that is higher than that of the general population.[232] The hypertension is in part related to the increased frequency of renal disease. Volume overload may be an additional factor.

Recently the association of hypertension with diabetes and obesity has led some investigators to propose that there is a causal link between these conditions: the link being insulin resistance. Resistance to the metabolic actions of insulin is a prominent feature of NIDDM. It has been suggested that the increased frequency of hypertension in this condition is secondary to selective insulin resistance—the autonomic nervous system and/or the kidney is not insulin-resistant. Elevated levels of insulin acting on the kidney will induce volume retention, while an increased insulin effect on the adrenergic nervous system will increase sympathetic outflow. Either of these can then lead to elevation of blood pressure.[233,234] In the past, the hypertension was assumed to be treated best by diuretics and sodium restriction. This therapy has two substantial drawbacks: (1) diuretics impair glucose homeostasis and (2) they probably accelerate renal deterioration. Because converting-enzyme inhibitors have theoretical advantages both in terms of glucose control and in retarding the deterioration of renal function, they may be the treatment of choice for hypertension in diabetics.[229,235,236]

DIAGNOSIS AND TREATMENT OF DIABETES MELLITUS

It is generally agreed that therapy directed at the control of excessive fatty acid mobilization and oxidation and protein catabolism is essential in diabetes mellitus. On the other hand, disagreement still exists regarding the usefulness of treating asymptomatic hyperglycemia. It has been documented that the synthesis of polyols and basement membrane glycoproteins is increased by hyperglycemia.[193,237] Thus, "tight control" of blood glucose may be important if the long-term complications of diabetes mellitus are to be reduced.

Diet, insulin, and oral hypoglycemic agents have been the mainstays of treatment. However, a controversy has arisen concerning the efficacy of oral hypoglycemic agents, such as the sulfonylureas.[238] While hyperglycemia is better controlled with these agents than it is with diet alone, an increased frequency of myocardial infarction has been reported. Although the interpretation and implications of these findings are controversial, there is some experimental evidence suggesting that sulfonylureas may have an adverse effect on the myocardium. Wu and colleagues have reported increased "stiffness" of the myocardium secondary to interstitial accumulation of PAS-staining material that reduced left ventricular function in dogs treated with tolbutamide.[239]

On the basis of available information, in our judgment patients with diabetes who should use oral hypoglycemic agents, preferably one of the second-generation agents (glyburide or glipizide),[240] are those who are not ketosis prone and whose hyperglycemia cannot be controlled with diet alone. It should also be recognized that beta-adrenoceptor blockers reduce the hyperglycemic reaction to stress, and it is possible that beta-adrenoceptor blocker therapy may require a downward adjustment of insulin dosage, since patients receiving beta blockers may be more susceptible to hypoglycemia, particularly in the elderly.[240] Since many of the symptoms of which the hypoglycemic patient is aware are due to the effects of the epinephrine which is released, both physician and patient must be alert to the possibility that hypoglycemia occurring in the beta blocker–treated diabetic may be relatively asymptomatic. Since certain diuretics, such as the thiazides and furosemide, may result in hypokalemia, and because hypokalemia can inhibit insulin release, these drugs may intensify the glucose intolerance of diabetic patients.

In patients with diabetes mellitus and impairment of left ventricular function, a sudden change in the glucose concentration of extracellular fluid, as occurs with the development of insulin deficiency, may result in the movement of fluid from the intracellular to the extracellular space and the intensification of heart failure. The hyperosmolar state has been shown experimentally to reduce cardiac contractility.[241] This hyperosmolar state responds to the lowering of blood glucose by insulin.[242]

OBESITY

There are two types of obesity: adult onset and lifelong. Adult-onset obesity is extremely common, probably occurring to a varying extent in nearly all individuals in developed countries. Its clinical course consists of normal weight patterns during childhood and adolescence, with a gradual increase in weight beginning between 20 and 40 years of age; it reflects an imbalance between caloric intake and utilization.[243] Much less common is lifelong obesity, characterized by the development of obesity early in childhood, with significant increase in weight during adolescence and, in women, during and after pregnancy. These individuals are usually grossly obese, weighing more than 150 per cent of their ideal weight as adults. The underlying cause of obesity in either condition is unclear.

Hirsch has documented an increase both in the size and the number of adipose cells in individuals with lifelong obesity, while in adult-onset obesity only an increase in cell size occurs.[244] With weight reduction the size of the adipose cells decreases in both conditions; however, the number does not change in either. Whether the increased number of adipose cells in lifelong obesity is determined by genetic or environmental factors is uncertain. However, it has been documented that there is no significant change in the number of adipose cells when obesity develops after late childhood in both experimental animals and humans. On the other hand, some evidence suggests that early infant feeding habits may significantly alter their number.[244] The metabolic consequences of obesity include decreased sensitivity to insulin, with resultant hyperinsulinemia, glucose intolerance, hypercholesterolemia, hypertriglyceridemia, and hyperaminoacidemia.

CARDIOVASCULAR CONSEQUENCES OF SEVERE OBESITY

During the past decade the health risk of obesity has been intensively studied. A conference analyzing data from two national health and nutrition surveys and the Framingham 30-year follow-up study concluded that a significant excess in mortality is evident in individuals with an obesity mass index greater than 27. A value greater than this is present in 34 million adult United States citizens. There is a direct correlation between the levels of blood pressure and cholesterol and the degree of obesity.[245] *Hypertension* is common in the grossly obese,[246] although it must be recognized that indirect measurement of blood pressure frequently leads to overestimation of the arterial pressure by the standard cuff method (p. 20). Nonetheless, direct measurement of arterial pressure frequently shows moderate elevations that can usually be promptly restored to normal by means of weight reduction and salt restriction.

Evidence of circulatory dysfunction in the massively obese, associated with cardiac enlargement during life and at autopsy, was first described by Smith and Willius in 1933.[247] It is now widely appreciated that massive obesity is accompanied by a marked increase in blood volume and cardiac output, which are proportional to the excess of body weight and the duration of obesity[248-250]; the hematocrit is often slightly elevated as well. The increased cardiac output is secondary to increased end-diastolic left ventricular volume[249-250] and stroke volume, since heart rate is normal; the cardiac output rises normally during exercise. Left ventricular filling pressures are at or close to the upper limits of normal in the supine position in the basal state, but increase with passive leg raising, and reach strikingly elevated levels during exercise. These increases in ventricular filling pressure are associated with a high resting central blood volume, which also increases significantly with exertion. A tendency to leftward deviation of the electrical axis correlates significantly with increasing obesity independent of age and blood pressure. However, this association is usually confined to the normal QRS-axis range. Thus, abnormal left-axis deviation is not necessarily a reflection of obesity.[251] The maximum velocity of myocardial fiber shortening and the ratio of stroke work index to left ventricular end-diastolic pressure were reduced, even in relatively young obese persons, without any other evidence of heart disease[248] (Fig. 61–15). Massive edema may occur as a consequence of the elevated ventricular filling pressure, despite elevation of the cardiac output.

Examination of the gross and microscopic anatomy of the heart in patients with marked chronic obesity showed heart weight to be considerably greater than predicted for ideal body weight, with left ventricular dilatation and eccentric hypertrophy and, in a few instances, right ventricular hypertrophy as well[252-253] (Fig. 61–16). Left atrial abnormalities (in-

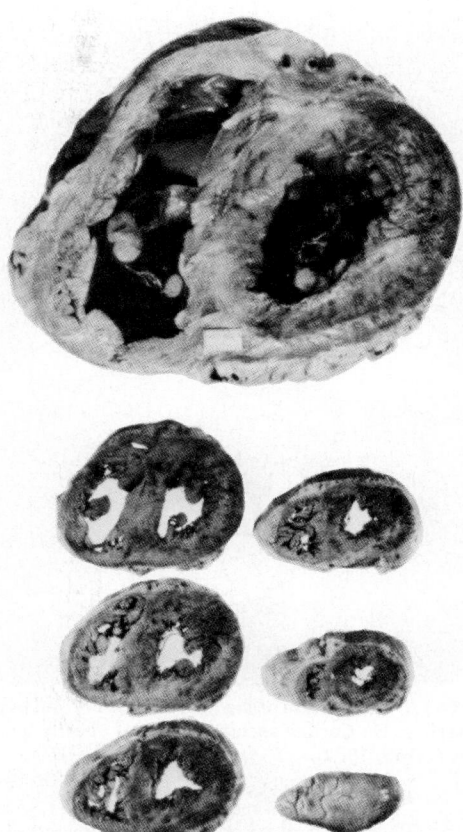

FIGURE 61–16. Cross section of the heart of a 34-year-old man who weighed more than 500 lb. Both ventricular walls are hypertrophied and both cavities are dilated. The heart weight (825 gm) was greatly increased. (From Warnes, C. A., and Roberts, W. C.: The heart in massive [more than 300 pounds or 136 kilograms] obesity: Analysis of 12 patients studied at necropsy. Am. J. Cardiol. *54*:1090, 1984.)

creased size and reduced emptying index) also have been reported.[254] This increase in cardiac weight is not due to excess epicardial fat and fatty infiltration of the myocardium, which were previously considered to be the principal features of the obese heart. However, in at least one study the frequency of atherosclerosis was not increased in persons who were morbidly obese. Obesity-induced cardiac hypertrophy is different from that induced by hypertension. Instead of the concentric left ventricular hypertrophy associated with hypertension, the hypertrophy is eccentric, with chamber dilatation and some wall thickening, as seen in other conditions in which cardiac output is chronically increased (Fig. 61–17). Also, in contrast to the increased afterload associated with systemic hypertension, obesity produces an elevated preload. When hypertension accompanies severe obesity, a combination of concentric and eccentric hypertrophy is present. Obese patients with clinically evident ventricular hypertrophy have an increased propensity to ectopy, in comparison with obese persons without left ventricular hypertrophy or with lean persons.[254] In part, this increased ectopy may be secondary to cardiac autonomic dysfunction.[255] Thus, when these clinical, hemodynamic, and pathological observations are taken together, it appears that manifestations of myocardial dysfunction occur in very obese subjects without evidence of other heart disease and that, in the absence of the obesity hypoventilation syndrome (p. 1593), cor pulmonale is not a presenting feature.

Heart failure in the markedly obese is usually chronic. The pulmonary and systemic congestion with symptoms of dyspnea and edema are, at first, simply related to the reductions in ventricular compliance and elevations of filling pressures. Later, these symptoms are related also to increases in ventricular end-diastolic volume and the reduction of myocardial

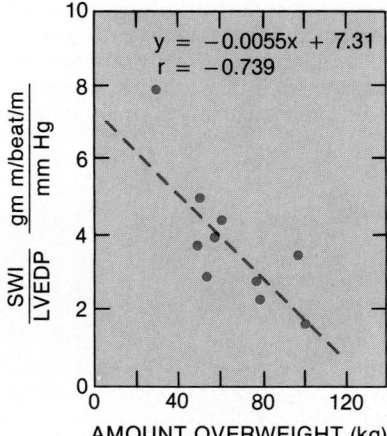

$$y = -0.0055x + 7.31$$
$$r = -0.739$$

FIGURE 61–15. The significant negative correlation between the ratio of the stroke work index (SWI) to the left ventricular end-diastolic pressure (LVEDP) and the amounts of overweight shows that the higher the degree of obesity, the greater the impairment of left ventricular function. (From Divitiis, O., et al.: Obesity and cardiac function. Circulation *64*:477, 1981, by permission of the American Heart Association, Inc.)

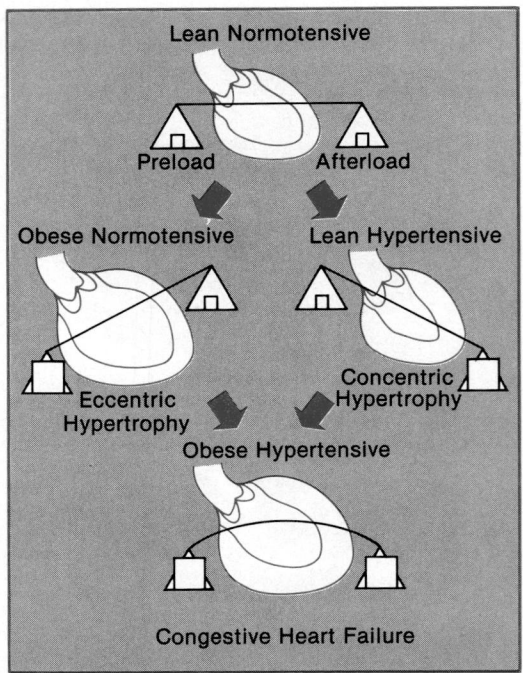

FIGURE 61–17. Adaptation of the heart to obesity and hypertension. (From Masserli, F. H.: Cardiovascular effects of obesity and hypertension. Lancet 1:1165, 1982.)

contractility. Thus, the marked chronic increase in cardiac work, i.e., in cardiac output and arterial pressure, ultimately leads to heart failure.

Fortunately, weight reduction is beneficial in the majority of patients, even those with heart failure. It usually improves the exercise capacity of patients with chronic exogenous obesity and decreases total body oxygen uptake, the cardiothoracic ratio on chest roentgenogram, systemic arterial pressure, blood volume, cardiac output, arteriovenous oxygen difference, and left ventricular filling pressure at rest.[256] MacMahon et al. have documented that weight loss of as little as 8 kg is associated with a significant decrease in left ventricular mass, particularly the thickness of the posterior and central walls.[257] Alpert and colleagues, studying cardiac function in grossly obese individuals, noted a substantial reduction in left ventricular chamber enlargement and an improvement in systemic function with an average weight loss of 55 kg.[258] However, they were unable to show a change in septal or posterior wall thickness, suggesting that some of the beneficial effects of weight loss on cardiac function may occur only if the obesity is mild or of short duration. Supporting this conclusion is the persistence of elevated left ventricular filling pressure with exercise in obese patients following weight reduction.[259]

Treatment of heart failure in these patients consists of maintenance of the reduced body weight, dietary sodium restriction, cardiac glycosides, and diuretics. Often, patients with massive obesity have associated arteriosclerotic coronary artery disease and the salutary results of weight reduction may be particularly striking in them.

TREATMENT

Most cases of adult-onset obesity are the result of imbalance between intake and output. Thus, reduction of intake is the most significant factor in treating this disease. While abnormalities in endocrine function, particularly of the thyroid or adrenal, have often been implicated in the pathophysiology of obesity, this thesis is rarely substantiated by detailed evaluation. The amount and rate of weight loss with a given level of caloric restrictions depend on the degree of energy expenditure. Energy expenditure depends on both the physical activity and mass of the individual. Thus, with a fixed level of

intake and activity, the rate of weight loss decreases as the total weight decreases. There is no evidence that a specific type of diet has any intrinsic benefit except as it is related to its caloric regimen. Thus the claim that high-protein diets are more efficacious is related not to their caloric content but rather to the accompanying ketosis that suppresses appetite.

CARDIAC COMPLICATIONS OF WEIGHT LOSS. Rapid weight loss has been associated with cardiac arrhythmias and sudden death.[260] In some cases, this is probably secondary to inadequate electrolyte supplementation. In others, it may be related to a reduction in myocardial protein and cardiac atrophy, similar to what has been reported in severe malnutrition[261] (Fig. 61–18) (see below). While initially associated with a liquid protein diet, sudden death may occur under any circumstance in which there is rapid weight loss.[262] In nearly all cases, prolongation in the Q-T interval as well as ventricular arrhythmias has been reported, providing strong support for the need for an ECG in any patient undergoing significant rapid weight loss.

MALNUTRITION

Malnutrition, particularly protein-calorie deficiency, is prevalent in many underdeveloped areas of the world. However, in recent years, it has also become a concern in developed countries in those individuals who have chronic diseases, in whom it exists as a result of both anorexia and hypermetabolism. The clinical picture is similar to that of adult kwashiorkor reported from underdeveloped countries, described below.

Protein-calorie malnutrition of childhood refers to syndromes of nutritional deficiency, which range from marasmus to kwashiorkor and which result from a stress like a serious infection superimposed upon an inadequate diet.[263] *Marasmus* is a state of malnutrition in an infant who has been weaned early and fed a diet grossly deficient in calories, protein, and other essential nutrients. *Kwashiorkor* usually occurs in children 1 to 4 years of age and is due to deficiency of protein relative to calories.

CARDIAC CHANGES IN MALNUTRITION. The circulatory status of patients with severe nutritional depletion and electrolyte imbalance is precarious; the cardiac output, systolic pressure, and pulse pressure are abnormally low, and there may be massive, generalized edema; the P-R interval may be shortened (Table 61–2). There is loss of subcutaneous fat and general wasting and atrophy of most organs, including the heart, which is thin-walled, pale, and flabby on gross examination. Histological study reveals atrophy of the muscle fibers, sometimes with interstitial edema. In experimental chronic protein-calorie undernutrition, not only is the heart atrophic, but also left ventricular function may be normal. In the dog there are reductions in left ventricular compliance and contractility, the latter secondary to loss of cardiac tissue, not altered function,[264] whereas in the rat this apparently does not occur, although there is striking atrophy of the heart.[265] The treatment of the dehydrated or severely anemic patient with protein-calorie malnutrition involves correction of hematological, fluid, and electrolyte imbalance and the treat-

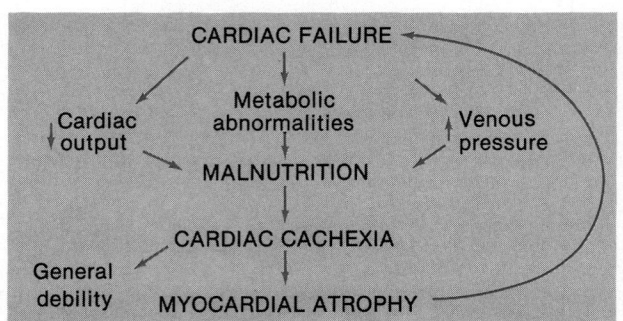

FIGURE 61–18. Possible pathogenesis of cardiac cachexia: Cardiac failure leads to poor nutrition and relative myocardial atrophy. (From Webb, J. G., et al.: Malnutrition and the heart. Can. Med. Assoc. J. 135:755, 1986.)

TABLE 61-2 SPECTRUM OF CARDIAC EFFECTS DUE TO STARVATION AND ANOREXIA NERVOSA

Cellular
Diminished protein synthesis
Activation of calcium-dependent proteinase
Mitochondrial swelling
Decreased glycogen content
Interstitial edema
Myofibrillar atrophy and destruction

Physiological
Decreased contractile force
Decreased cardiac output
Diminished diastolic compliance

Clinical
Bradycardia
Relative hypertension
Nonspecific electrocardiographic changes
Ectopic rhythms
Mitral valve prolapse
Diminished exercise capacity
Heart failure, worsened or precipitated by refeeding

Adapted from Schocken, D. D., Holloway, J. D., and Powers, P. S.: Weight loss and the heart. Effects of anorexia nervosa and starvation. Arch. Intern. Med. 149:878, 1989.

ment of infection. Congestive failure can be avoided if care is taken to avoid overloading with sodium, water, or blood. Digitalis must be given cautiously when these patients are in heart failure because of their sensitivity to glycosides.

In parts of the world where pediatric kwashiorkor is common, there are also cases of adults with similar clinical features. These features include loss of subcutaneous fat and muscle with edema, weakness, depression, anorexia, diarrhea, abdominal distention, hair loss, and thinning of the skin. Classically, plasma albumin and amino acid levels are low, as are serum concentrations of sodium, magnesium, and phosphorus. Urinary excretion of nitrogen is reduced, as is total body potassium. On the other hand, total body and extracellular water and plasma volume are usually increased. The primary pathophysiological event is protein malnutrition. All the clinical signs and symptoms are related to this basic defect.

Anorexia nervosa, a condition more frequently observed in developed countries, produces symptoms similar to those observed in kwashiorkor. Hypomagnesemia with hypocalcemia and hypokalemia frequently occurs in this condition, resulting in heart failure and sometimes sudden death. Cardiac output is low and regional myocardial contraction may be impaired in anorexia nervosa, contributing to the abnormalities in both systolic and diastolic ventricular dysfunction. Congestive heart failure may occur, particularly in the early refeeding phases, probably secondary to an exacerbation of the hypophosphatemia when hyperalimentation and/or oral intake is rich in glucose. Finally, heart rate and blood pressure response to exercise are substantially reduced.[266-269]

MALNUTRITION IN CARDIAC DISEASE

Assessment of protein-calorie nutritional status in cardiac patients has not been extensively evaluated. However, during the last several decades there has been increasing awareness that some patients with cardiovascular disease have clinical features similar to those described above. In these cases, instead of involuntary protein deprivation, anorexia plays a significant role. For example, chronic congestive heart failure leads to cellular hypoxia as well as hypermetabolism. Gastrointestinal hypoxia produces anorexia, which then initiates a vicious cycle. Decreased protein intake produces cardiac atrophy, increased right atrial pressure, tricuspid regurgitation, and increasing congestive heart failure, which produces more cellular hypoxia, greater anorexia, and finally death.[270]

A similar condition has been described in some patients undergoing open-heart surgery for correction of rheumatic

valvular disease. In some malnourished patients the mortality reaches 20 per cent, significantly greater than the 1 to 2 per cent in normally nourished patients undergoing the same procedure. The underlying pathophysiology is uncertain but probably includes (1) decreased cardiac mass, (2) reduction of biosynthetic activity of liver, (3) poor healing due to reduced levels of substrate, and (4) impairment of cell-mediated immunity.[271] As a result, wound healing is retarded, skin ulcers occur, and requirements for artificial ventilation are prolonged. Abel and colleagues have suggested that hyperalimentation in the immediate postoperative period does not significantly alter the increased morbidity.[272] This has led Blackburn et al. to suggest that both preoperative and concurrent nutritional support are necessary.[271] However, definitive studies to distinguish between nutritional status and severity of the cardiovascular disease as the cause for the increased morbidity have not been reported.

Cardiovascular Manifestations of Vitamin Deficiency

(see p. 461)

OTHER VITAMIN DEFICIENCIES. Deficiencies of other vitamins have not led to specifically definable cardiovascular abnormalities, except for the hypocalcemia-accompanied vitamin D deficiency. However, vitamin deficiencies, particularly of the B group and folic acid, have been diagnosed with increasing frequency in patients with cardiovascular disease. For example, nearly a third of infants and children with congenital heart disease have been reported to be deficient in a number of the B vitamins.[273] Folic acid deficiency has been documented in a significant number of patients with congestive heart failure. While the deficient state may simply be related to decreased intake, abnormal intestinal absorption or increased rates of excretion may also contribute.

ALTERATIONS IN GONADAL HORMONE SECRETION

There are no specific cardiovascular abnormalities associated with altered gonadal function except for occasional cardiac structural abnormalities in Kallman's syndrome,[274] a genetic form of hypogonadotropic hypogonadism, and a rare form of cardiomyopathy associated with primary hypogonadism.[275] However, gonadectomy in rats is associated with an impairment of left ventricular filling and left ventricular function, and androgen receptors have been found in the heart.

GONADAL FUNCTION AND CARDIOVASCULAR DISEASE

Middle-aged men are at a higher risk for developing cardiovascular disease than are age-matched women. Because the discrepancy between male and female mortality disappears in older, postmenopausal women, some investigators have suggested that estrogen reduces the rate of development of coronary atherosclerosis (p. 1153). Support for this thesis includes the observation that total cholesterol is lower and HDL cholesterol is higher in postmenopausal women who are taking estrogens than in those who are not.[276] Additionally, the risk ratio of coronary artery disease death varies from 0.3 to 0.7 in postmenopausal estrogen users compared to nonusers.[277-279] Several studies, however, have disputed this thesis. First, it has been documented that the development of coronary artery disease in oophorectomized women is no different from that in age-matched nonoophorectomized women,[280] although the study of Colditz et al. has substantially dampened this objection. The latter reported in 121,700 women that bilateral oophorectomy *increases* the risk of coronary heart disease, which can be prevented by estrogen replacement therapy.[281] Second, widespread use of oral contraceptives, most of which contain estrogen, has proved that estrogen administration is not without cardiovascular risk, since it can increase total cholesterol and beta-lipoprotein (LDL) cholesterol and decrease alpha-lipoprotein (HDL) cholesterol in premenopausal women,[282] although low-dose estrogen therapy, even if combined with a progestational agent, appears to have a beneficial effect on lipid profiles in postmenopausal women.[283,284] Additionally, estrogen administration has been shown to increase the degree of abnormality in postexercise electrocardiograms in those individuals who had abnormal tests prior to estrogen therapy.[285] In summary, in addition to the usual variables (age and smoking), the beneficial effect of estrogen therapy in postmenopausal women is, in part, dependent on (1) whether menopause is induced surgically or is natural; (2) whether low- or normal-dose estrogen is used; and (3) what type of progestational agent, if any, is used. The preponderance of evidence suggests that low-dose estrogen therapy will reduce the risk of cardiovascular disease in the postmenopausal woman.

Hyperestrogenemia in men has been reported to be associated with an increased risk of myocardial infarction.[286] In support of this hypothesis, Wilson and colleagues, using information from the Framingham study, reported an increased risk of cardiovascular morbidity in postmenopausal women taking estrogen.[287] Yet other workers have found no association between estrogen levels and heart disease in men, but have observed an increased frequency of coronary artery disease in patients with lower testosterone levels.[288] Thus, whether estradiol levels are an actual risk factor or an associated finding is unclear.[289] Since, in general, higher levels of estrogen are usually associated with lower levels of testosterone in men, separating effects due to androgens from those due to estrogens is difficult. On the basis of these studies, however, some investigators have suggested that it is not an increased estrogen level but a *decreased* testosterone level that is protective in premenopausal *women*. They base this suggestion on the documented reduction in serum cholesterol levels and the incidence of atherosclerosis in castrated men and the negative correlation between plasma testosterone and HDL cholesterol levels.[290,291] However, the similar frequency of coronary artery disease in postmenopausal women and men of similar age with significantly different testosterone levels is unexplained by this suggestion.

CARDIOVASCULAR EFFECTS OF ORAL CONTRACEPTIVES

Several studies have documented that the use of oral contraceptives may be accompanied by an increased risk of cardiovascular morbidity and mortality in premenopausal females.[282,285,292] Specifically there is increased frequency of diabetes mellitus, hypertension, and thromboembolic disease. While the increased risk is small, caution in the use of oral contraceptive agents by individuals who may be predisposed to the development of these diseases is nevertheless warranted. Fortunately, prior use does not increase risk of subsequent cardiovascular disease.[293]

HYPERTENSION (see also p. 832). The hypertension associated with estrogen administration is probably related to its effect in increasing the production of renin substrate by the liver.[294] It has been clearly documented that oral contraceptives increase the concentration of renin substrate and blood angiotensin II.[295] However, most individuals do not develop clinical hypertension, which suggests that a counterregulatory mechanism(s) is activated, reducing the vascular effect of angiotensin II. Alternatively, blood pressure may increase in all patients, but only the predisposed will develop hypertension. Thus, individuals who have a personal or family history of renal disease are more likely to develop hypertension with estrogen administration.

THROMBOEMBOLIC DISEASE. At least two clearly defined alterations in the clotting system are produced by oral contraceptive agents; either or both could be responsible for the increased frequency of thromboembolic disease.[292] (1) Estrogen enhances the biosynthesis by the liver of a number of the clotting factors. (2) Oral contraceptives increase both the blood viscosity and platelet adhesiveness.

REFERENCES

1. Graves, R. J.: Clinical lectures. London Med. Surg. J. (Part II):7, 516, 1835.
2. Addison, T.: On the Constitutional and Local Effects of Disease of the Suprarenal Capsules. London, Highley, 1855.

ACROMEGALY

3. Frohman, L. A.: Diseases of the anterior pituitary. In Felig, P., et al. (eds.): Endocrinology and Metabolism. 2nd ed. New York, McGraw-Hill Book Co., 1987, p. 247.
4. Faglia, G., Arosio, M., Ambrosi, B.: Recent advances in diagnosis and treatment of acromegaly. In Imura, H. (ed.): The Pituitary Gland. New York, Raven Press, 1985, p. 363.
5. Gomez-Pan, A., and Rodriguez-Arnao, M. D.: Somatostatin and growth hormone releasing factor: Synthesis, location, metabolism and function. J. Clin. Endocrinol. Metab. 12:469, 1983.
6. Frohman, L. A., and Jansson, J.: Growth hormone releasing hormone. Endocr. Rev. 7:223, 1986.
7. Clemmons, D. R., and Van Wyk, J. J.: Somatomedin: Physiological control and effects on cell proliferation. In Baserga, R. (ed.): Handbook of Experimental Pharmacology. Berlin, Springer-Verlag, 1981, p. 161.
8. Yamashita, S., Weiss, M., and Melmed, S.: Insulin-like growth factor I regulates growth hormone secretion and messenger ribonucleic acid levels in human pituitary cells. J. Clin. Endocrinol. Metab. 62:730, 1986.
9. Moore, D. D., Walker, M. D., Diamond, D. J., et al.: Structure, expression, and evolution of growth hormone genes. Recent Prog. Hormone Res. 38:197, 1982.
10. Frelin, C.: The regulation of protein turnover in newborn rat heart cell cultures. J. Biol. Chem. 255:11149, 1980.
11. Thuesen L., Christiansen J. S., Sorensen, J. O. L. et al.: Increased myocardial contractility following growth hormone administration in normal man. Dan. Med. Bull. 35:193, 1988.
12. Greco, A. V., Ghirlanda, G., Barone, C., et al.: Somatostatin in paroxysmal supraventricular and junctional tachycardia. Br. Med. J. 288:28, 1984.
13. Day, S. M., Gu, J., Polak, J. M., and Bloom, S. R.: Somatostatin in the human heart and comparison with guinea pig and rat heart. Br. Heart J. 53:153, 1985.
14. Thorner, M. O., Perryman, R. L., Cronin, M. J., et al.: Somatotroph hyperplasia: Successful treatment of acromegaly by removal of a pancreatic islet tumor secreting a growth hormone-releasing factor. J. Clin. Invest. 70:965, 1982.
15. Melmed, S., Braunstein, G., Chang, R. J., and Becker, D.: Pituitary tumors secreting growth hormone and prolactin. Ann. Intern. Med. 105:238, 1986.
16. Aloia, J. F., Roginsky, M. D., and Field, R. A.: Absence of hyperlipidemia in acromegaly. J. Clin. Endocrinol. 35:921, 1972.
17. McGuffin, W. L., Sherman, B. M., Roth, J. et al.: Acromegaly and cardiovascular disorders. Ann. Intern. Med. 81:11, 1974.
18. Baldwin, A., Cundy, T., Butler, J., and Timmis, A. D.: Progression of cardiovascular disease in acromegalic patients treated by external pituitary irradiation. Acta Endocrinol. 108:26, 1985.
19. Lie, J. T., and Grossman, S. J.: Pathology of the heart in acromegaly: Anatomic findings in 27 autopsied patients. Am. Heart J. 100:41, 1980.
20. Mather, H. M., Boyd, M. J., and Jenkins, J. S.: Heart size and function in acromegaly. Br. Heart J. 41:697, 1979.
21. Csanady, M., Gaspar, L., Hogye, M., et al.: The heart in acromegaly: An echocardiographic study. Int. J. Cardiol. 2:349, 1983.
22. Rossi, L., Thiene, G., Caregaro, L., et al.: Dysrhythmias and sudden death in acromegalic heart disease. A clinicopathologic study. Chest 72:495, 1977.
23. Cain, J. P., Williams, G. H., and Dluhy, R. G.: Plasma renin activity and aldosterone secretion in patients with acromegaly. J. Clin. Endocrinol. 34:73, 1972.
24. Moore, T. J., Thein-Wai, W., Dluhy, R. G., et al.: Abnormal adrenal and vascular responses to angiotensin II and an angiotensin antagonist in acromegaly. J. Clin. Endocrinol. Metab. 51:215, 1980.
25. Souadjian, J. V., and Schirger, A.: Hypertension in acromegaly. Am. J. Med. Sci. 254:629, 1967.
26. Ng, L. L., and Evans, D. J.: Leukocyte sodium transport in acromegaly. Clin. Endocrinol. 26:471, 1987.
27. Surawicz, B., and Mangiardi, M. L.: Electrocardiogram in endocrine and metabolic disorders. In Rios, J. C. (ed.): Clinical Electrocardiographic Correlations. Philadelphia, F. A. Davis Co., 1977, p. 243.
28. Jonas, E. A., Aloia, J. F., and Lane, F. J.: Evidence of subclinical heart muscle dysfunction in acromegaly. Chest 67:190, 1975.
29. Hayward, R. P., Emanuel, R. W., and Navarro, J. D. N.: Acromegalic heart disease: Influence of treatment of the acromegaly on the heart. Q. J. Med. 62:41, 1987.
30. Smallridge, R. C., Rajfer, S., Davis, J., and Schaaf, M.: Acromegaly and the heart. Am. J. Med. 66:22, 1979.
31. Rodrigues, E. A., Caruana, M. P., Lahiri, A., et al.: Subclinical cardiac dysfunction in acromegaly: Evidence for a specific disease of heart muscle. Br. Heart J. 62:185, 1989.
32. Molitch, M. E.: Acromegaly. In Collu, R., Brown, G. M., and Vanloon, G. R. (eds.): Clinical Neuroendocrinology. Boston, Blackwell Scientific Publications, Inc., 1988, p. 189.

33. Vance, M. L., Evans, W. S., and Thorner, M. O.: Bromocriptine. Ann. Intern. Med. *100*:78, 1984.
34. Barkan, A. L., Kelch, R. P., Hopwood, N. J., et al.: Treatment of acromegaly with the long-acting somatostatin analogue SMS 201-995. J. Clin. Endocrinol. Metab. *66*:16, 1988.

THYROID DISEASE

35. Kaplan, M. M.: The thyroid and the heart; how do they interact? J. Cardiovasc. Med. *7*:893, 1982.
36. Oppenheimer, J. H.: The nuclear receptor–triiodothyronine complex: Relationship to thyroid hormone distributions, metabolism, and biological action. *In* Oppenheimer, J. H., and Samuels, H. H. (eds.): Molecular Basis of Thyroid Hormone Action. New York, Academic Press, 1983, p. 1.
37. Ladenson, P. W., Kieffer, J. D., Farwell, A. P., and Ridgway, E. C.: Modulation of myocardial L-triiodothyronine receptors in normal, hypothyroid, and hyperthyroid rats. Metabolism *35*:5, 1986.
38. Jump, D. B., and Oppenheimer, J. H.: Association of thyroid hormone receptors with chromatin. Mol. Cell. Biochem. *55*:159, 1983.
39. Apriletti, J. W., David-Inouye, Y., Baxter, J. D., and Eberhardt, N. L.: Physiochemical characterization of the intranuclear receptor. *In* Oppenheimer, J. H., and Samuels, H. H. (eds.): Molecular Basis of Thyroid Hormone Action. New York, Academic Press, 1983, p. 67.
40. Narayan, P., Liaw, C. W., and Towle, H. C.: Rapid induction of a specific nuclear precursor by thyroid hormone. Proc. Natl. Acad. Sci. USA *81*:4687, 1984.
41. Seelig, S. A., Jump, D. B., Towle, H. C., et al.: Parodoxical effects of cycloheximide on the ultra-rapid induction of two hepatic mRNA sequences by triiodothyronine (T3). Endocrinology *110*:671, 1982.
42. Seelig, S., Liaw, C., Towle, H. C., and Oppenheimer, J. H.: Thyroid hormone attenuates and augments hepatic gene expression at a pretranslational level. Proc. Natl. Acad. Sci. USA *78*:4733, 1981.
43. Guernsey, D. L., and Edelman, I. S.: Regulation of thermogenesis by thyroid hormones. *In* Oppenheimer, J. H., and Samuels, H. H. (eds.): Molecular Basis of Thyroid Hormone Action. New York, Academic Press, 1983, p. 298.
44. Fain, J. N., and Rosenthal, J. W.: Calorigenic action of triiodothyronine on white cells: Effects of ouabain, oligomycin, and cathecholamines. Endocrinology *89*:1205, 1971.
45. Primack, M. P., and Buchanan, J. L.: Control of oxygen consumption in liver slices from normal and T4-treated rats. Endocrinology *95*:619, 1974.
46. Gordon, A., Schwartz, H., and Gross, J.: The stimulation of sugar transport in heart cells grown in a serum-free medium by picomolar concentrations of thyroid hormones: The effects of insulin and hydrocortisone. Endocrinology *118*:52, 1986.
47. Kim, D., Smith, T. W., and Marsh, J. D.: Effect of thyroid hormone on slow calcium channel function in cultured chick ventricular cells. J. Clin. Invest. *80*:88, 1987.
48. MacKinnon, R., Gwathmey, J. K., Allen, P. D., et al.: Modulation by the thyroid state of intracellular calcium and contractility in ferret ventricular muscle. Circ. Res. *63*:1080, 1988.
49. Knight, R. A.: The use of spinal anesthesia to control sympathetic overactivity in hyperthyroidism. Anesthesiology *6*:225, 1945.
50. Hammond, H. K., White, F. C., Buxton, I. L. O., et al.: Increased myocardial beta-receptors and adrenergic responses in hyperthyroid pigs. Am. J. Physiol. *252*:H283, 1987.
51. Buccino, R. A., Spann, J. F., Pool, P. E., and Braunwald, E.: Influence of the thyroid state on the intrinsic contractile properties and the energy stores of the myocardium. J. Clin. Invest. *46*:1669, 1967.
52. Nishizawa, Y., Hamada, N., Fujii, S., et al.: Serum dopamine-beta-hydroxylase activity in thyroid disorders. J. Clin. Endocrinol. Metab. *39*:599, 1974.
53. Malbon, C. C., and Greenberg, M. L.: 3,3′,5′-Triiodothyronine administration in vivo modulates the hormone sensitive adenylate cyclase system of rat hepatocytes. J. Clin. Invest. *69*:414, 1982.
54. Malbon, C. C.: Liver cell adenylate cyclase and β-adrenergic receptors. J. Biol. Chem. *255*:8692, 1980.
55. Brodde, O. E., Schumann, H. J., and Wagner, J.: Decreased responsiveness of the adenylate cyclase system in left atria from hypothyroid rats. Mol. Pharmacol. *17*:180, 1980.
56. Whitsett, J. A., Pollinger, J., and Matz, S.: β-Adrenergic receptors and catecholamine-sensitive adenylate cyclase in developing rat ventricular myocardium: Effect of thyroid status. Pediatr. Res. *16*:463, 1982.
57. Rutherford, J. P., Vatner, S. F., and Braunwald, E.: Adrenergic control of myocardial contractility in conscious hyperthyroid dogs. Am. J. Physiol. *237*:590, 1980.
58. Guarnieri, T., Filburn, C. R., Beard, E. S., and Lakatta, E. G.: Enhanced contractile response and protein kinase activation to threshold levels of β-adrenergic stimulation in hyperthyroid rat heart. J. Clin. Invest. *65*:861, 1980.
59. Andersson, R. G. G., Nilsson, O. R., and Kuo, J. F.: β-Adrenoceptor adenosine 3′,5′-monophosphate system in human leukocytes before and after treatment for hyperthyroidism. J. Clin. Endocrinol. Metab. *56*:42, 1983.
60. Stiles, G. L., Stadel, J. M., De Lean, A., and Lefkowitz, R. J.: Hypothyroidism modulates beta-adrenergic receptor-adenylate cyclase interactions in rat reticulocytes. J. Clin. Invest. *68*:1450, 1981.
61. Malbon, C. C.: The effects of thyroid status on the modulation of fat cell

62. Ling, E., O'Brien, P. J., Salerno, T., et al.: Effects of different thyroid treatments on the biochemical characteristics of rabbit myocardium. Can. J. Cardiol. *4*:301, 1988.
63. Markowitz, C., and Yater, W. M.: Response of explanted cardiac muscle to thyroxine. Am. J. Physiol. *100*:162, 1932.
64. Murayama, M., and Goodkind, M. J.: Effect of thyroid hormone on the frequency-force relationship of atrial myocardium from the guinea pig. Circ. Res. *23*:743, 1968.
64a. Josephson, R. A., Spurgeon, H. A., and Lakatta, E. G.: The hyperthyroid heart: An analysis of systolic and diastolic properties in single rat ventricular myocytes. Circ. Res. *66*:773, 1990.
65. Goldman, S., Olajos, M., Friedman, H., et al.: Left ventricular performance in conscious thyrotoxic calves. Am. J. Physiol. *242*:H113, 1982.
66. McDonough, K. H., Chen, V., and Spitzer, J.: Effect of altered thyroid status on in vitro cardiac performance in rats. Am. J. Physiol. *252*:H788, 1987.
67. Crie, J. S., Wakeland, J. R., Mayhew, B. A., and Wildenthal, K.: Direct anabolic effects of thyroid hormone on isolated mouse heart. Am. J. Physiol. *245*:C328, 1983.
68. Gustafson, T. A., Markham, B. E., and Morkin, E.: Effects of thyroid hormone on alpha-actin and myosin heavy chain gene expression in cardiac and skeletal muscles of the rat: Measurement of mRNA content using synthetic oligonucleotide probes. Circ. Res. *59*:194, 1986.
69. Philipson, K. D., and Edelman, I. S.: Thyroid hormone control of Na⁺,K⁺ATPase and K⁺-dependent phosphatase in rat heart. Am. J. Physiol. *232*:C196, 1977.
70. Litten, R. Z., Martin, B. J., Howe, E. R., et al.: Phosphorylation and adenosine triphosphate activity of myofibrils from thyrotoxic rabbit ears. Circ. Res. *48*:498, 1981.
71. Curfman, G. D., Crowley, T. J., and Smith, T. W.: Thyroid-induced alterations in myocardial sodium- and potassium-activated adenosine triphosphatase, monovalent cation active transport and cardiac glycoside binding. J. Clin. Invest. *59*:586, 1977.
72. Samuel, J. L., Rappaport, L., Syrovy, I., et al.: Differential effect of thyroxine on atrial and ventricular isomyosins in rats. Am. J. Physiol. *250*:H333, 1986.
73. Litten, R. Z., III, Martin, B. J., Low, R. B., and Alpert, N. R.: Altered myosin isozyme patterns from pressure overloaded and thyrotoxic hypertrophied rabbit hearts. Circ. Res. *50*:856, 1982.
74. Holubarsch, C., Goulette, R. P., Litten, R. Z., et al.: The economy of isometric force development, myosin isoenzyme pattern and myofibrillar ATPase activity in normal and hypothyroid rat myocardium. Circ. Res. *56*:78, 1985.
75. Goto, Y., Slinker, B. K., and LeWinter, M. M.: Decreased contractile efficiency and increased nonmechanical energy cost in hyperthyroid rabbit heart: Relation between O₂ consumption and systolic pressure-volume area or force-time integral. Circ. Res. *66*:999, 1990.
76. Poggesi, C., Everets, M., Polla, B., et al.: Influence of thyroid state on mechanical restitution of rat myocardium. Circ. Res. *60*:142, 1987.
77. Klein, I., and Hong, C.: Effects of thyroid hormone on cardiac size and myosin content of the heterotopically transplanted rat heart. J. Clin. Invest. *77*:1694, 1986.
78. Korecky, B., Zak, R., Schwartz, K., et al.: Role of thyroid hormone in regulation of isomyosin composition, contractility, and size of heterotopically isotransplanted rat heart. Circ. Res. *60*:824, 1987.
79. Johnson, P. N., Freedberg, A. S., and Marshall, J. M.: Action of thyroid hormone on the transmembrane potentials from sinoatrial cells and atrial muscle cells in isolated atria of rabbits. Cardiology *58*:273, 1973.
80. Arnsdorf, M. D., and Childers, R. W.: Atrial electrophysiology in experimental hyperthyroidism in rabbits. Circ. Res. *26*:575, 1970.
81. Utiger, R. D.: The thyroid: Physiology, hyperthyroidism, hypothyroidism, and the painful thyroid. *In* Felig, P., et al. (eds.): Endocrinology and Metabolism. 2nd ed. New York, McGraw-Hill Book Co., 1987, p. 389.
82. Skelton, C. L.: The heart and hyperthyroidism. N. Engl. J. Med. *307*:1206, 1982.
83. Talafih, K., Briden, K. L., and Weiss, H. R.: Thyroxine-induced hypertrophy of the rabbit heart. Effect on regional oxygen extraction, flow, and oxygen consumption. Circ. Res. *52*:272, 1983.
84. Friedman, M. J., Okada, R. D., Ewy, G. A., and Hellman, D. J.: Left ventricular systolic and diastolic function in hyperthyroidism. Am. Heart J. *104*:1303, 1982.
85. Feldman, T., Borow, K. M., Sarne, D. H., et al.: Myocardial mechanics in hyperthyroidism: Importance of left ventricular loading conditions, heart rate and contractile state. J. Am. Coll. Cardiol. *7*:967, 1986.
86. Iskandrian, A. S., Rose, L., Hakki, A. H., et al.: Cardiac performance in thyrotoxicosis: Analysis of 10 untreated patients. Am. J. Cardiol. *51*:349, 1983.
87. Maciel, B. C., Gallo, L., Marin-Neto, J., et al.: Autonomic control of heart rate during dynamic exercise in human hyperthyroidism. Clin. Sci. *75*:209, 1988.
88. Forfar, J. C., Matthews, D. M., and Toft, A. D.: Delayed recovery of left ventricular function after antithyroid treatment: Further evidence for reversible abnormalities of contractility in hyperthyroidism. Br. Heart J. *52*:215, 1984.
89. Olshausen, K., Bischoff, S., Kahaly, G., et al.: Cardiac arrhythmias and heart rate in hyperthyroidism. Am. J. Cardiol. *63*:930, 1989.
90. Agner, T., Almdal, T., Thorsteinsson, B., and Agner, E.: A reevaluation of atrial fibrillation in thyrotoxicosis. Dan. Med. Bull. *31*:157, 1984.

β-adrenergic receptor agonist affinity by guanine nucleotides. Mol. Pharmacol. *18*:193, 1980.

1851

CHAP 61

91. Ciaccheri, M., Cecchi, F., Arcangeli, C., et al.: Occult thyrotoxicosis in patients with chronic and paroxysmal isolated atrial fibrillation. Clin. Cardiol. 7:413, 1984.

92. Goel, B. G., Hanson, C. S., and Han, J.: A-V conduction in hyper- and hypothyroid dogs. Am. Heart J. 83:504, 1972.

93. Cavallo, A., Joseph, C. J., and Casta, A.: Cardiac complications in juvenile hyperthyroidism. Am. J. Dis. Child. 138:479, 1984.

94. Featherstone, H. J., and Stewart, D. K.: Angina in thyrotoxicosis: Thyroid-related coronary artery spasm. Arch. Intern. Med. 143:554, 1983.

95. Forfar, J. C., Muir, A. L., Sawers, S. A., and Toft, A. D.: Abnormal left ventricular function in hyperthyroidism: Evidence for a possible reversible cardiomyopathy. N. Engl. J. Med. 307:1165, 1982.

96. Wilson, R., Gibson, T. C., Terrien, C. M., and Levy, A. M.: Hyperthyroidism and familial hypertrophic cardiomyopathy. Arch. Intern. Med. 143:378, 1983.

97. Brauman, A., Algom, M., Gilboa, Y., et al.: Mitral valve prolapse in hyperthyroidism of two different origins. Br. Heart J. 53:374, 1985.

98. Noah, M. S., Sulimani, R. A., Famuyiwa, F. O., et al.: Prolapse of the mitral valve in hyperthyroid patients in Saudi Arabia. Int. J. Cardiol. 19:217, 1988.

99. Morrow, D. H., Gaffney, T. E., and Braunwald, E.: Studies on digitalis: VIII. Effect of autonomic innervation and of myocardial catecholamine stores upon the cardiac action of ouabain. J. Pharmacol. Exp. Ther. 140:236, 1963.

100. Ingbar, S. H.: The role of antiadrenergic agents in the management of thyrotoxicosis. Cardiovasc. Rev. Rep. 2:683, 1981.

101. Sandler, G., and Wilson, G. M.: The nature and prognosis of heart disease in thyrotoxicosis. A review of 150 patients treated with [131]I. Q. J. Med. 28:347, 1959.

102. Nakazawa, H. K., Sakurai, K., Hamada, N., et al.: Management of atrial fibrillation in the postthyrotoxic state. Am. J. Med. 72:903, 1982.

103. Staffurth, J. S., Gibberd, M. C., and Fui, S. T.: Arterial embolism in thyrotoxicosis with atrial fibrillation. Br. Med. J. 2:688, 1977.

104. Chopra, I. J., Huang, T.-S., Hurd, R. E., and Solomon, D. H.: A study of cardiac effects of thyroid hormones: Evidence for amelioration of the effects of thyroxine by sodium ipodate. Endocrinology 114:2039, 1984.

105. Norman, M. F., and Lavin, T. N.: Antagonism of thyroid hormone action by amiodarone in rat pituitary tumor cells. J. Clin. Invest. 83:306, 1989.

106. Lambert, M., Burger, A. G., DeNayer, P., et al.: Decreased TSH response to TRH induced by amiodarone. Acta Endocrinol. 118:449, 1988.

107. Gammage, M. D., and Franklyn, J. A.: Amiodarone and the thyroid. Q. J. Med. 62:83, 1987.

108. Bambini, G., Aghini-Lombardi, F., Rosner, W., et al.: Serum sex hormone–binding globulin in amiodarone-treated patients. Arch. Intern. Med. 147:1781, 1987.

109. Martino, E., Bartalena, L., Mariotti, S., et al.: Radioactive iodine thyroid uptake in patients with amiodarone iodine–induced thyroid dysfunction. Acta Endocrinol. 119:167, 1988.

110. Kasim, S. E., Bagchi, N., Brown, T. R., et al.: Effect of amiodarone on serum lipids, lipoprotein lipase, and hepatic triglyceride lipase. Endocrinology 120:1991, 1987.

111. Rabinowe, S. L., Larsen, P. R., Antman, E. M., et al.: Amiodarone therapy and autoimmune thyroid disease. Am. J. Med. 81:53, 1986.

112. Zimmerman, J., Yahalom, J., and Bar-On, H.: Clinical spectrum of pericardial effusion as the presenting feature of hypothyroidism. Am. Heart J. 106:770, 1983.

113. Khaleeli, A. A., and Memon, N.: Factors affecting resolution of pericardial effusions in primary hypothyroidism: A clinical, biochemical and echocardiographic study. Postgrad. Med. J. 58:1073, 1982.

114. Kumar, A., Bhandari, A. K., and Rahimtoola, S. H.: Torsade de pointes and marked QT prolongation in association with hypothyroidism. Ann. Intern. Med. 106:712, 1987.

115. Shenoy, M. M., and Goldman, J. M.: Hypothyroid cardiomyopathy: Echocardiographic documentation of reversibility. Am. J. Med. Sci. 294:1, 1987.

116. Streeten, D. H. P., Andersen, G. H., Howland, T., et al.: Effects of thyroid function on blood pressure: Recognition of hypothyroid hypertension. Hypertension 11:78, 1988.

117. Saito, I., Kunihiko, I., and Saruta, T.: Hypothyroidism as a cause of hypertension. Hypertension 5:112, 1983.

118. Fouron, J. C., Bourgin, J. H., Letarte, J., et al.: Cardiac dimensions and myocardial function of infants with congenital hypothyroidism: An echocardiographic study. Br. Heart J. 47:584, 1982.

119. Graettinger, J. S., Muenster, J. J., and Checchia, C.: A correlation of clinical and hemodynamic studies in patients with hypothyroidism. J. Clin. Invest. 37:502, 1958.

120. Wieshammer, S., Keck, F. S., Waitzinger, J., et al.: Left ventricular function at rest and during exercise in acute hypothyroidism. Br. Heart J. 60:204, 1988.

121. Vora, J., O'Malley, B. P., Petersen, S., et al.: Reversible abnormalities of myocardial relaxation in hypothyroidism. J. Clin. Endocrinol. Metab. 61:269, 1985.

122. Hillis, W. S., Bremner, W. F., Lawrie, T. D. V., and Thomson, J. A.: Systolic time intervals in thyroid disease. Clin. Endocrinol. 4:617, 1975.

123. McBrion, D. J., and Hindle, W.: Myxoedema and heart failure. Lancet 1:1065, 1963.

124. Levey, G. S., Skelton, C. L., and Epstein, S. E.: Decreased myocardial adenyl cyclase activity in hypothyroidism. J. Clin. Invest. 48:2244, 1969.

125. Steinberg, A. D.: Myxedema and coronary artery disease — a comparative autopsy study. Ann. Intern. Med. 68:338, 1968.

126. Karlsberg, R. P., Friscia, D. A., Aronow, W. S., and Sekhon, S. S.: Deleteri-

ous influence of hypothyroidism on evolving myocardial infarction in conscious dogs. J. Clin. Invest. 67:1024, 1981.

127. Keating, F. R., Parkin, T. W., Selby, J. B., and Dickinson, L. S.: Treatment of heart disease associated with myxedema. Progr. Cardiovasc. Dis. 3:364, 1960.

128. Griffiths, P. D.: Serum enzymes in diseases of the thyroid gland. J. Clin. Pathol. 18:660, 1965.

129. Drucker, D. J., and Burrow, G. N.: Cardiovascular surgery in the hypothyroid patient. Arch. Intern. Med. 145:1585, 1985.

130. Wehmann, R. E., Gregerman, R. I., Burns, W. H., et al.: Suppression of thyrotropin in the low-thyroxine state of severe nonthyroidal illness. N. Engl. J. Med. 312:546, 1985.

131. Hamblin, P. S., Dyer, S. A., Mohr, V. S., et al.: Relationship between thyrotropin and thyroxine changes during recovery from severe hypothyroxinemia of critical illness. J. Clin. Endocrinol. Metab. 62:717, 1986.

132. Brent, G. A., and Hershman, J. M.: Thyroxine therapy in patients with severe nonthyroidal illnesses and low serum thyroxine concentration. J. Clin. Endocrinol. Metab. 63:1, 1986.

DISEASES OF THE ADRENAL CORTEX

133. Williams, G. H., and Dluhy, R. G.: Diseases of the adrenal cortex. In Wilson, J., et al. (eds.): Harrison's Principles of Internal Medicine. 12th ed. New York, McGraw-Hill Book Co., 1991, p. 1713.

134. Quinn, S. J., and Williams, G. H.: Regulation of aldosterone secretion. Annu. Rev. Physiol. 50:409, 1988.

135. Cushing, H.: The basophil adenomas of the pituitary body and their clinical manifestations (pituitary basophilism). Bull. Johns Hopkins Hosp. 50:137, 1932.

136. Liddle, G. W.: Pathogenesis of glucocorticoid disorders. Am. J. Med. 53:638, 1972.

137. Krieger, D. T.: Physiopathology of Cushing's disease. Endocr. Rev. 4:22, 1983.

138. Carney, J. A., Gordon, H., Carpenter, P. C., et al.: The complex of myxomas, spotty pigmentation, and endocrine overactivity. Medicine 64:270, 1985.

139. Sindler, B. H., Griffing, G. T., and Melby, J. C.: The superiority of the metyrapone test vs. the high dose dexamethasone test in the differential diagnosis of Cushing's syndrome. Am. J. Med. 74:657, 1983.

140. Boggan, J. E., Tyrrell, J. B., and Wilson, C. B.: Transsphenoidal microsurgical management of Cushing's disease: Report of 100 cases. J. Neurosurg. 59:195, 1983.

141. Nolan, P. M., Sheeler, L. R., Hahn, J. F., and Hardy, R. W., Jr.: Therapeutic problems with transsphenoidal pituitary surgery for Cushing's disease. Cleve. Clin. Q. 49:199, 1982.

142. Weinberger, M. H.: Primary aldosteronism: Diagnosis and differentiation of subtypes. Ann. Intern. Med. 100:300, 1984.

143. Rose, L. I., Underwood, R. H., Newmark, S. R., et al.: Pathophysiology of spironolactone-induced gynecomastia. Ann. Intern. Med. 87:398, 1977.

144. Rabinowe, S. L., Jackson, R. A., Dluhy, R. G., and Williams, G. H.: Ia-positive T lymphocytes in recently diagnosed idiopathic Addison's disease. Am. J. Med. 77:597, 1984.

145. Knowlton, A. I., and Baer, L.: Cardiac failure in Addison's disease. Am. J. Med. 74:829, 1983.

146. Dorin, R. I., and Kearns, P. J.: High output circulatory failure in acute adrenal insufficiency. Crit. Care Med. 16:296, 1988.

147. New, M. I., and Levine, L. S.: Recent advances in 21-hydroxylase deficiency. Ann. Rev. Med. 35:649, 1984.

148. Schambelan, M., Sebastian, A., and Biglieri, E. G.: Prevalence, pathogenesis and functional significance of aldosterone deficiency in hyperkalemic patients with chronic renal insufficiency. Kidney Int. 17:89, 1980.

149. Lee, T. H., Salomon, D. R., Rayment, C. M., and Antman, E. M.: Hypotension and sinus arrest with exercise-induced hyperkalemia and combined verapamil/propranolol therapy. Am. J. Med. 80:1203, 1986.

150. Mannisi, J. A., Weisman, H. F., Bush, D. E., et al.: Steroid administration after myocardial infarction promotes early infarct expansion. J. Clin. Invest. 79:1431, 1987.

151. Alford, W. C., Meador, C. K., Mihalevich, J., et al.: Acute adrenal insufficiency following cardiac surgical procedures. J. Thorac. Cardiovasc. Surg. 78:489, 1979.

PHEOCHROMOCYTOMA

152. Bravo, E. L., and Gifford, R. W.: Pheochromocytoma: Diagnosis, localization, and management. N. Engl. J. Med. 311:1298, 1984.

153. Wurtman, R. J., and Axelrod, J.: Control of enzymatic synthesis of adrenaline in the adrenal medulla by adrenal cortical steroids. J. Biol. Chem. 241:2301, 1966.

154. Levenson, J. A., Safar, M. E., London, G. M., and Simon, A. C.: Haemodynamics in patients with phaeochromocytoma. Clin. Sci. 58:349, 1980.

155. Landsberg, L., and Young, J. B.: Catecholamines and adrenal medulla. In Wilson, J. D., and Foster, D. W. (eds.): Williams' Textbook of Endocrinology. 7th ed. Philadelphia, W. B. Saunders Company, 1985, p. 891.

155a. Sardesai, S. H., Mourant, A. J., Sivathandon, Y., et al.: Phaeochromocytoma and catecholamine induced cardiomyopathy presenting as heart failure. Br. Heart J. 63:234, 1990.

156. Strenstrom, G., and Swedberg, K.: QRS amplitudes, QT_c intervals and ECG

abnormalities in pheochromocytoma patients before, during and after treatment. Acta Med. Scand. *224*:231, 1988.

157. Haas, G. J., Tzagournis, M., and Boudoulas, H.: Pheochromocytoma: Catecholamine-mediated electrocardiographic changes mimicking ischemia. Am. Heart J. *116*:1363, 1988.

158. Van Vliet, P. D., Burchell, H. B., and Titus, J. L.: Myocarditis associated with pheochromocytoma. N. Engl. J. Med. *274*:1102, 1966.

159. Imperato-McGinley, J., Gautier, T., Ehlers, K., et al.: Reversibility of catecholamine-induced dilated cardiomyopathy in a child with a pheochromocytoma. N. Engl. J. Med. *316*:793, 1987.

160. Scott, I., Parkes, R., and Cameron, D. P.: Pheochromocytoma and cardiomyopathy. Med. J. Aust. *148*:94, 1988.

161. Behrana, A. J., Haselton, P., Leen, C. L. S., et al.: Multiple extra-adrenal paragangliomas associated with catecholamine cardiomyopathy. Eur. Heart J. *10*:182, 1989.

162. Shub, C., Cueto-Garcia, L., Sheps, S. G., et al.: Echocardiographic findings in pheochromocytoma. Am. J. Cardiol. *57*:971, 1986.

163. Cueto, L., Arriaga, J., and Zinser, J.: Echocardiographic changes in pheochromocytoma. Chest *76*:600, 1979.

164. McManus, B. M., Fleury, T. A., and Roberts, W. C.: Fatal catecholamine crisis in pheochromocytoma: Curable form of cardiac arrest. Am. Heart J. *102*:930, 1981.

165. Simons, M., and Downing, S. E.: Coronary vasoconstriction and catecholamine cardiomyopathy. Am. Heart J. *109*:297, 1985.

166. Bhatnagar, D., Carey, P., and Pollard, A.: Focal myositis and elevated creatine kinase levels in a patient with phaeochromocytoma. Postgrad. Med. J. *62*:197, 1986.

167. Serfas, D., Shoback, D. M., and Lorell, B. H.: Phaeochromocytoma and hypertrophic cardiomyopathy: Apparent suppression of symptoms and noradrenaline secretion by calcium-channel blockade. Lancet *2*:711, 1983.

168. David, T. E., Lenkei, S. C., Marquez-Julio, A., et al.: Pheochromocytoma of the heart. Ann. Thorac. Surg. *41*:98, 1986.

PARATHYROID DISEASE

169. Brown, E. M.: Physiology of calcium metabolism. *In* Becker K. L. (eds.): Principles and Practice of Endocrinology and Metabolism. Philadelphia, J. B. Lippincott. Co., 1990, p. 423.

170. Symons, C., Fortune, F., Greenbaum, R. A., and Dandona, P.: Cardiac hypertrophy, hypertrophic cardiomyopathy, and hyperparathyroidism—an association. Br. Heart J. *54*:539, 1985.

171. Bogin, E., Massry, S. G., and Harary, I.: Effect of parathyroid hormone on rat heart cells. J. Clin. Invest. *67*:1215, 1981.

172. Katoh, Y., Klein, K. L., Kaplan, R. A., et al.: Parathyroid hormone has a positive inotropic action in the rat. Endocrinology *109*:2252, 1981.

173. Palmieri, G. M., Nutting, D. F., Bhattacharya, S. K., et al.: Parathyroid ablation in dystrophic hamsters: Effects of Ca content and histology of heart, diaphragm, and rectus femoris. J. Clin. Invest. *68*:646, 1981.

174. Gafter, U., Battler, A., Eldar, M., et al.: Effect of hyperparathyroidism on cardiac function in patients with end-stage renal disease. Nephron *41*:30, 1985.

175. Vered I., Vered, Z., Perez, J. E., et al.: Normal left ventricular performance documented by Doppler echocardiography in patients with long-standing hypocalcemia. Am. J. Med. *86*:413, 1989.

176. Giles, T. D., Iteld, B. J., and Rires, K. L.: The cardiomyopathy of hypoparathyroidism. Chest *79*:225, 1981.

177. Ellison, D. H., and McCarron, D. A.: Structural prerequisites for the hypotensive action of parathyroid hormone. Am. J. Physiol. *246*:F551, 1984.

178. Roberts, W. C., and Waller, B. F.: Effect of chronic hypercalcemia on the heart: An analysis of 18 necropsy patients. Am. J. Med. *71*:371, 1981.

179. Roberts, W. C., and Waller, B. F.: Chronic hypercalcemia as a risk factor for coronary atherosclerosis. Cardiovasc. Rev. Rep. *4*:1275, 1983.

180. Slavich, G. A., Antonucci, F., and Sponza, E.: Primary hyperparathyroidism and angina pectoris. J. Am. Coll. Cardiol. *19*:266, 1988.

181. Csanady, M., Forster, T., and Julesz, J.: Reversible impairment of myocardial function in hypoparathyroidism causing hypocalcaemia. Br. Heart J. *63*:58, 1990.

182. Kleerekoper, M., Rao, D. S., and Frame, B.: Hypercalcemia, hyperparathyroidism and hypertension. Cardiovasc. Med. *3*:1283, 1978.

183. Daniels, J., and Goodman, A. D.: Hypertension and hyperparathyroidism: Inverse relation of sodium phosphate level and blood pressure. Am. J. Med. *75*:17, 1983.

184. Resnick, L. M.: Calcium, parathyroid disease, and hypertension. Cardiovasc. Rev. Rep. *3*:1341, 1982.

DIABETES MELLITUS

185. Halban, P. A., and Weir, G. C.: Islet cell hormones: Production and degradation. *In* Becker, K. L. (ed.): Principles and Practice of Endocrinology and Metabolism. Philadelphia, J. B. Lippincott Co., 1990, p. 1068.

186. Eisenbarth, G. S., and Kahn, C. R.: Etiology and pathogenesis of diabetes mellitus. *In* Becker, K. L. (ed.): Principles and Practice of Endocrinology and Metabolism. Philadelphia, J. B. Lippincott Co., 1990, p. 1074.

187. Waller, B. F., Palumbo, P. J., Lie, J. T., and Roberts, W. C.: Status of the coronary arteries at necropsy in diabetes mellitus with onset after age 30 years: Analysis of 229 diabetic patients with and without clinical evidence of coronary heart disease and comparison of 183 control subjects. Am. J. Med. *69*:498, 1980.

188. Yano, K., Kagan, A., McGee, D., and Rhoads, G. G.: Glucose intolerance and nine-year mortality in Japanese men in Hawaii. Am. J. Med. *72*:71, 1982.

189. Stone, P. H., Muller, J. E., Hartwell, T., et al.: The effect of diabetes mellitus on prognosis and serial left ventricular function after acute myocardial infarction: Contribution of both coronary disease and diastolic left ventricular dysfunction to the adverse prognosis. J. Am. Coll. Cardiol. *14*:49, 1989.

190. Woods, K. L., Samanta, A., and Burden, A. C.: Diabetes mellitus as a risk factor for acute myocardial infarction in Asians and Europeans. Br. Heart J. *62*:118, 1989.

191. Herlitz, J., Malmberg, K., Karlson, B. W., et al.: Mortality and morbidity during a five-year follow-up of diabetics with myocardial infarction. Acta Med. Scand. *224*:31, 1988.

192. Abbott, R. D., Donahue, R. P., Kannel, W. B., et al.: The impact of diabetes on survival following myocardial infarction in men vs women. The Framingham Study. JAMA *260*:3456, 1988.

193. Factor, S. M., Okun, E. M., and Minase, T.: Capillary microaneurysms in the human heart. N. Engl. J. Med. *302*:384, 1980.

194. Savage, M. P., Krolewski, A. S., Kenien, G. G., et al.: Acute myocardial infarction in diabetes mellitus and significance of congestive heart failure as a prognostic factor. Am. J. Cardiol. *62*:665, 1988.

195. Ceremuzynski, L.: Hormonal and metabolic reactions evoked by acute myocardial infarction. Circ. Res. *48*:767, 1981.

196. Flink, E. B., Brick, J. E., and Shane, S. R.: Alterations of long-chain free fatty acid and magnesium concentrations in acute myocardial infarction. Arch. Intern. Med. *141*:441, 1981.

197. Opie, L. H., Tansey, M. J., and Kennelly, B. M.: The heart in diabetes mellitus: II. Acute myocardial infarction and diabetes. S. Afr. Med. J. *56*:256, 1979.

198. Nesto, R. W., Phillips, R. T., Kett, K. G., et al.: Angina and exertional myocardial ischemia in diabetic and nondiabetic patients: Assessment by exercise thallium scintigraphy. Ann. Intern. Med. *108*:170, 1988.

199. Gunderson, T., and Kjekshus, J.: Timolol treatment after myocardial infarction in diabetic patients. Diabetes Care *6*:285, 1983.

200. Roy, T. M., Peterson, H. R., Snider, H. L., et al.: Autonomic influence on cardiovascular performance in diabetic subjects. Am. J. Med. *87*:382, 1989.

201. Sato, N., Hashimoto, H., Takiguchi, Y., et al.: Altered responsiveness to sympathetic nerve stimulation and agonist of isolated left atria of diabetic rats: No evidence for involvement of hypothyroidism. J. Pharmacol. Exp. Ther. *248*:367, 1989.

202. Fernandez-Castaner, M., Figuerola, D., Sorribas, A., et al.: Evaluation des epreuves cardiovasculaires dans le diagnostic des neuropathies diabetiques autonomes. Diabetes Metab. *9*:264, 1983.

202a. Ambepityia, G., Kopelman, P. G., Ingram, D.: Exertional myocardial ischemia in diabetes: A quantitative analysis of anginal perceptual threshold and the influence of autonomic function. J. Am. Coll. Cardiol. *15*:72, 1990.

203. Zola, B., Kahn, J. K., Juni, J. E., and Vinik, A. I.: Abnormal cardiac function in diabetic patients with autonomic neuropathy in the absence of ischemic heart disease. J. Clin. Endocrinol. Metab. *63*:208, 1986.

204. Pfeifer, M. A., Cook, D., Brodsky, J., et al.: Quantitative evaluation of cardiac parasympathetic activity in normal and diabetic man. Diabetes *31*:339, 1982.

204a. Weise, F., Heydenreich, F., Gehrig, W., and Runge, U.: Heart rate variability in diabetic patients during orthostatic load—a spectral analytic approach. Klin. Wochenschr. *68*:26, 1990.

205. Zoneraich, S.: Diabetes and the Heart. Springfield, Ill., Charles C Thomas, Publisher, 1978, p. 303.

206. Sutherland, C. G. G., Fisher, B. M., Frier, B. M., et al.: Endomyocardial biopsy pathology in insulin-dependent diabetic patients with abnormal ventricular function. Histopathology *14*:593, 1989.

207. Hausdorf, G., Rieger, U., and Koepp, P.: Cardiomyopathy in childhood diabetes mellitus: Incidence, time of onset, and relation to metabolic control. Int. J. Cardiol. *19*:225, 1988.

208. Zarich, S. W., Arbuckle, B. E., Cohen, L. R., et al.: Diastolic abnormalities in young asymptomatic diabetic patients assessed by pulsed Doppler echocardiography. J. Am. Coll. Cardiol. *12*:114, 1988.

209. Takenakam K., Sakamoto, T., Amano, K., et al.: Left ventricular filling determined by Doppler echocardiography in diabetes mellitus. Am. J. Cardiol. *61*:1139, 1988.

210. Ruddy, T. D., Shumak, S. L., Liu, P. P., et al.: The relationship of cardiac diastolic dysfunction to concurrent hormonal and metabolic status in Type I diabetes mellitus. J. Clin. Endocrinol. Metab. *66*:113, 1988.

211. Mustonen, J. N., Uusitupa, M. I. J., Tahvanainen, K., et al.: Impaired left ventricular systolic function during exercise in middle-aged insulin-dependent and noninsulin-dependent diabetic subjects without clinically evident cardiovascular disease. Am. J. Cardiol. *62*:1273, 1988.

212. Danielsen, R., Nordrehaug, J. E., and Vik-Mo, H.: Left ventricular function in young long-term Type I (insulin-dependent) diabetic men during exercise assessed by digitized echocardiography. Eur. Heart J. *9*:395, 1988.

213. Bouchard, A., Sanz, N., Botvinick, E. H., et al.: Noninvasive assessment of cardiomyopathy in normotensive diabetic patients between 20 and 50 years old. Am. J. Med. *87*:160, 1989.

213a. Paillole, C., Dahan, M., Paycha, F., et al.: Prevalence and significance of left ventricular filling abnormalities determined by Doppler echocardiography in young Type I (insulin-dependent) diabetic patients. Am. J. Cardiol. *64*:1010, 1989.

214. Danielsen, R.: Factors contributing to left ventricular diastolic dysfunc-

tion in long-term Type I diabetic subjects. Acta Med. Scand. *224*:249, 1988.

215. Ramandaham, S., Rodrigues, B., and McNeill, J. H.: Growth hormone and diabetes-induced cardiomyopathy. J. Lab. Clin. Med. *110*:257, 1987.

216. Regan, T. J., Altszuler, N., Eaddy, C., et al.: Relation of growth hormone and myocardial collagen accumulation in experimental diabetes. J. Lab. Clin. Med. *110*:274, 1987.

217. Nakada, T., and Kwee, I. L.: Sorbitol accumulation in heart: Implication for diabetic cardiomyopathy. Life Sci. *45*:2491, 1989.

218. Schaffer, S. W., Mozaffari, M. S., Artman, M., et al.: Basis for myocardial mechanical defects associated with noninsulin-dependent diabetes. Am. J. Physiol. *256*:E25, 1989.

219. Borda, E., Pascual, J., Wald, M., et al.: Hypersensitivity to calcium associated with an increased sarcolemmal Ca^{++}-ATPase activity in diabetic rat heart. Can. J. Cardiol. *4*:97, 1988.

220. Pierce, G. N., Lockwood, K., and Eckhert, C. D.: Cardiac contractile protein ATPase activity in a diet induced model of noninsulin dependent diabetes mellitus. Can. J. Cardiol. *5*:117, 1989.

221. Afzal, N., Ganguly, P. K., Dhalla, K. S., et al.: Beneficial effects of verapamil in diabetic cardiomyopathy. Diabetes *37*:936, 1988.

222. Okumura, K., Akiyama, N., Hashimoto, H., et al.: Alteration of 1,2-diacylglycerol content in myocardium from diabetic rats. Diabetes *37*:1168, 1988.

223. Sunni, S., Bishop, S. P., Kent, S. P., and Geer, J. C.: Diabetic cardiomyopathy. Arch. Pathol. Lab. Med. *110*:375, 1986.

224. Uusitupa, M., Siitonen, O., Pyorala, K., and Lansimies, E.: Left ventricular function in newly diagnosed noninsulin-dependent (Type 2) diabetes evaluated by systolic time intervals and echocardiography. Acta Med. Scand. *217*:379, 1985.

225. Fein, F. S., Capasso, J. M., Aronson, R. S., et al.: Combined renovascular hypertension and diabetes in rats: A new preparation of congestive cardiomyopathy. Circulation *70*:318, 1984.

226. Regan, T. J., Wu, C. F., Weisse, A. B., et al.: Acute myocardial infarction in toxic cardiomyopathy without coronary obstruction. Circulation *51*:453, 1975.

227. Deorari, A. K., Saxena, A., Singh, M., et al.: Echocardiographic assessment of infants born to diabetic mothers. Arch. Dis. Child. *64*:721, 1989.

228. Sheehan, J. P., Sisam, D. A., and Schumacher, O. P.: Insulin-induced cardiac failure. Am. J. Med. *79*:147, 1985.

229. Zatz, R., Dunn, B. R., Meyer, T. W., et al.: Prevention of diabetic glomerulopathy by pharmacological amelioration of glomerular capillary hypertension. J. Clin. Invest. *77*:1925, 1986.

230. Marre, M., Leblanc, H., Suarez, L., et al.: Converting enzyme inhibition and kidney function in normotensive diabetic patients with persistent microalbuminuria. Br. Med. J. *294*:1448, 1987.

231. Falholt, K., Cutfield, R., Alejandro, R., et al.: The effects of hyperinsulinemia on arterial wall and peripheral muscle metabolism in dogs. Metabolism *34*:1146, 1985.

232. The Working Group on Hypertension in Diabetes: Statement on hypertension in diabetes mellitus. Final report. Arch. Intern. Med. *147*:830, 1987.

233. Ferrannini, E., and DeFronzo, R. A.: The association of hypertension, diabetes, and obesity: A review. J. Nephrol. *1*:3, 1989.

234. Reaven, G. M., and Hoffman, B. B.: Hypertension as a disease of carbohydrate and lipoprotein metabolism. Am. J. Med. *87*:2S, 1989.

235. Williams, G. H.: Converting enzyme inhibitors in the treatment of hypertension. N. Engl. J. Med. *319*:1517, 1988.

236. Houston, M. C.: Treatment of hypertension in diabetes mellitus. Am. Heart J. *118*:819, 1989.

237. Beyer, T. A., and Hutson, N. J.: Introduction: Evidence for the role of the polyol pathway in the pathophysiology of diabetic complications. Metabolism *35*:1, 1986.

238. University Group Diabetes Program: A study of the effects of hypoglycemic agents on vascular complications in patients with adult-onset diabetes: V. Evaluation of phenformin therapy. Diabetes *24* (Suppl. I):65, 1975.

239. Wu, C. F., Haider, B., Ahmed, S. S., et al.: The effects of tolbutamide on the myocardium in experimental diabetes. Circulation *55*:200, 1977.

240. Regan, T. J.: Cardiac disease in the older diabetic: Management considerations. Geriatrics *44*:91, 1989.

241. Bielefeld, D. R., Pace, C. S., and Boshell, B. R.: Hyperosmolarity and cardiac function in chronic diabetic rat heart. Am. J. Physiol. *245*:E568, 1983.

242. Axelrod, L.: Response of congestive heart failure to correction of hyperglycemia in the presence of diabetic nephropathy. N. Engl. J. Med. *293*:1243, 1975.

OBESITY

243. Salan, S.: The obesities. *In* Felig, P., et al. (eds.): Endocrinology and Metabolism. 2nd ed. New York, McGraw-Hill Book Co., 1987, p. 1203.

244. Hirsch, J.: The adipose cell hypothesis. N. Engl. J. Med. *294*:389, 1976.

245. Foster, W. R., and Burton, B. T. (eds.): Health implications of obesity: NIH consensus development conference. Ann. Intern. Med. *103*:979, 1985.

246. Messerli, F. H., Sundgaard-Riise, K., Reisin, E., et al.: Disparate cardiovascular effects of obesity and arterial hypertension. Am. J. Med. *74*:808, 1983.

247. Smith, H. L., and Willius, R. A.: Adiposity of the heart. A clinical and pathological study of one hundred and thirty-six obese patients. Ann. Intern. Med. *52*:911, 1933.

248. De Divitiis, O., Fazio, S., Petitto, M., et al.: Obesity and cardiac function. Circulation *64*:477, 1981.

249. Egan, B., Fitzpatrick, M. A., Juni, J., et al.: Importance of overweight in studies of left ventricular hypertrophy and diastolic function in mild systemic hypertension. Am. J. Cardiol. *64*:752, 1989.

250. Nakajima, T., Fujioka, S., Tokunaga, K., et al.: Correlation of intraabdominal fat accumulation and left ventricular performance in obesity. Am. J. Cardiol. *64*:369, 1989.

251. Zack, P. M., Wiens, R. D., and Kennedy, H. L.: Left-axis deviation and adiposity: The United States health and nutrition examination survey. Am. J. Cardiol. *53*:1129, 1984.

252. Ventura, H. O., Messerli, F. H., Dunn, F. G., and Frohlich, E. D.: Left ventricular hypertrophy in obesity: Discrepancy between echo and electrocardiogram. J. Am. Coll. Cardiol. *1*:682, 1983.

253. Warnes, C. A., and Roberts, W. C.: The heart in massive (more than 300 pounds or 136 kilograms) obesity: Analysis of 12 patients studied at necropsy. Am. J. Cardiol. *54*:1087, 1984.

254. Lavie, C. J., Amodeo, C., Ventura, H. O., et al.: Left atrial abnormalities indicating diastolic ventricular dysfunction in cardiopathy of obesity. Chest *92*:1042, 1987.

255. Rossi, M., Marti, G., Ricordi, L., et al.: Cardiac autonomic dysfunction in obese subjects. Clin. Sci. *76*:567, 1989.

256. Reisin, E., Frohlich, E. D., Messerli, F. H., et al.: Cardiovascular changes after weight reduction in obesity hypertension. Ann. Intern. Med. *98*:315, 1983.

257. MacMahon, S. W., Wilcken, D. E. L., and Macdonald, G. J.: The effect of weight reduction on left ventricular mass: A randomized controlled trial in young, overweight hypertensive patients. N. Engl. J. Med. *314*:334, 1986.

258. Alpert, M. A., Terry, B. E., and Kelly, D. L.: Effect of weight loss on cardiac chamber size, wall thickness and left ventricular function in morbid obesity. Am. J. Cardiol. *55*:783, 1985.

259. Backman, L., Freyschuss, U., Hallberg, D., and Melcher, A.: Reversibility of cardiovascular changes in extreme obesity: Effects of weight reduction through jejunoileostomy. Acta Med. Scand. *205*:367, 1979.

MALNUTRITION

260. Frank, A., Graham, C., and Frank, S.: Fatalities on the liquid protein diet: An analysis of possible causes. Int. J. Obes. *5*:243, 1981.

261. Webb, J. G., Kiess, M. C., and Chan-Yan, C. C.: Malnutrition and the heart. Can. Med. Assoc. J. *135*:753, 1986.

262. Pringle, T. H., Scobie, I. N., Murray, R. G., et al.: Prolongation of the QT interval during therapeutic starvation: A substrate for malignant arrhythmias. Int. J. Obes. *7*:253, 1983.

263. Bergman, J. W., Human, D. G., DeMoor, M. M. A., et al.: Effect of kwashiorkor on the cardiovascular system. Arch. Dis. Child. *63*:1359, 1988.

264. Alden, P. B., Madoff, R. D., Stahl, T. J., et al.: Left ventricular function in malnutrition. Am. J. Physiol. *253*:H380, 1987.

265. Nutter, D. O., Murray, T. G., Heymsfield, S. T., and Fuller, E. O.: The effect of chronic protein-calorie undernutrition in the rat on myocardial function and cardiac function. Circ. Res. *45*:144, 1979.

266. Isner, J. M., Roberts, W. C., Heymsfield, S. B., and Yager, J.: Anorexia nervosa and sudden death. Ann. Intern. Med. *102*:49, 1985.

267. Fonseca, V., Havard, C.W.H.: Electrolyte disturbances and cardiac failure with hypomagnesaemia in anorexia nervosa. Br. Med. J. *291*:1680, 1985.

268. Goldberg, S. J., Comerci, G. D., and Feldman, L.: Cardiac output and regional myocardial contraction in anorexia nervosa. J. Adolesc. Health Care *9*:15, 1988.

269. Schocken, D. D., Holloway, J. D., and Powers, P. S.: Weight loss and the heart. Arch. Intern. Med. *149*:877, 1989.

270. Carr, J. G., Stevenson, L. W., Walden, J. A., et al.: Prevalence and hemodynamic correlates of malnutrition in severe congestive heart failure secondary to ischemic or idiopathic dilated cardiomyopathy. Am. J. Cardiol. *63*:709, 1989.

271. Blackburn, G. L., Gibbons, G. W., Bothe, A., et al.: Nutritional support in cardiac cachexia. J. Thorac. Cardiovasc. Surg. *73*:489, 1977.

272. Abel, R. M., Fischer, J. E., Buckley, M. J., et al.: Malnutrition in cardiac surgical patients. Arch. Surg. *111*:45, 1976.

273. Steier, M., Lopez, R., and Cooperman, J. M.: Riboflavin deficiency in infants and children with heart disease. Am. Heart J. *92*:139, 1976.

ALTERATIONS IN GONADAL HORMONE SECRETION

274. Dimitrovski, C., Plaseski, A., Bogoev, M., and Sadikario, S.: Kallmann's syndrome associated with atrial septal defect. J.A.M.A. *248*:1358, 1982.

275. Warren, S. E., Schnitt, S. J., Bauman, A. J., et al.: Late onset dilated cardiomyopathy in a unique familial syndrome of hypogonadism and metabolic abnormalities. Am. Heart J. *114*:1520, 1987.

276. Wallace, R. B., Hoover, J., Barrett-Conner, E., et al.: Altered plasma lipid and lipoprotein levels associated with oral contraceptive and estrogen use. Lancet *2*:112, 1979.

277. Stampfer, M. J., Willett, W. C., Colditz, G. A., et al.: A prospective study of postmenopausal estrogen therapy and coronary heart disease. N. Engl. J. Med. *313*:1044, 1985.

278. Petitti, D. B., Perlman, J. A., and Sidney, S.: Postmenopausal estrogen use and heart disease. N. Engl. J. Med. *315*:131, 1986.

279. Hillner, B. E., Hollenberg, J. P., and Pauker, S. G.: Postmenopausal estro-

gens in prevention of osteoporosis: Benefit virtually without risk if cardiovascular effects are considered. Am. J. Med. *80*:1115, 1986.

280. Ritterband, A. B., Jaffee, I. A., and Densen, P. M.: Gonadal function and the development of coronary heart disease. Circulation *27*:237, 1963.

281. Colditz, G. A., Willett, W. C., Stamper, M. J., et al.: Menopause and the risk of coronary heart disease in women. N. Engl. J. Med. *316*:1105, 1987.

282. Webber, L. S., Hunter, S. M., Baugh, J. G., et al.: The interaction of cigarette smoking, oral contraceptive use, and cardiovascular risk factor variables in children: The Bogalusa Heart Study. Am. J. Publ. Health *72*:266, 1982.

283. Fletcher, C. D., Farish, E., Dagen, M. M., et al.: The effects of conjugated equine estrogens plus cyclical dydrogesterone on serum lipoproteins and apoproteins in postmenopausal women. Acta Endocrinol. *117*:339, 1988.

284. Wolfe, B. M., and Huff, M. W.: Effects of estrogen and progestin administration on plasma lipoprotein metabolism in postmenopausal women. J. Clin. Invest. *83*:40, 1989.

285. Jaffe, M. D.: Effect of oestrogens on postexercise electrocardiogram. Br. Heart J. *38*:1299, 1976.

286. Luria, M. H.: Estrogen and coronary arterial disease in men. Int. J. Cardiol. *25*:159, 1989.

287. Wilson, P. W. F., Garrison, R. J., and Castelli, W. P.: Postmenopausal estrogen use, cigarette smoking, and cardiovascular morbidity in women over 50: The Framingham Study. N. Engl. J. Med. *313*:1038, 1985.

288. Chute, C. G., Baron, J. A., Plymate, S. R., et al.: Sex hormones and coronary artery disease. Am. J. Med. *83*:853, 1987.

289. Gutin, B., Alejandro, D., Duni, T., et al.: Levels of serum sex hormones and risk factors for coronary heart disease in exercise-trained men. Am. J. Med. *79*:79, 1985.

290. Gutai, J., LaPorte, R., Kuller, L., et al.: Plasma testosterone, high density lipoprotein cholesterol and other lipoprotein fractions. Am. J. Cardiol. *48*:897, 1981.

291. Kiel, D. P., Baron, J. A., Plymate, S. R., et al.: Sex hormones and lipoproteins in men. Am. J. Med. *87*:35, 1989.

292. Merians, D. R., Haskell, W. L., Vranizan, K. M., et al.: Relationship of exercise, oral contraceptive use, and body fat to concentrations of plasma lipids and lipoprotein cholesterol in young women. Am. J. Med. *78*:913, 1985.

293. Stampfer, M. J., Willett, W. C., Colditz, G. A., et al.: A prospective study of past use of oral contraceptive agents and risk of cardiovascular diseases. N. Engl. J. Med. *319*:1313, 1988.

294. Boyd, W. N., Burden, R. P., and Aber, G. M.: Intrarenal vascular changes in patients receiving estrogen-containing compounds—A clinical, histological and angiographic study. Q. J. Med. *44*:415, 1975.

295. Hollenberg, N. K., Williams, G. H., Burger, B., et al.: Renal blood flow and its response to A II: An interaction between oral contraceptive agents, sodium intake and the renin-angiotensin system in healthy young women. Circ. Res. *38*:35, 1976.

Renal Disorders and Heart Disease

by STEPHEN O. PASTAN, M.D., and EUGENE BRAUNWALD, M.D.

Disorders of the heart and of the kidneys are intimately related. On the one hand, some of the principal clinical manifestations of impairment of the heart's performance as a pump are due to renal retention of sodium and water; a number of diseases of the heart, such as infective endocarditis and cardiogenic shock, may result in serious renal disease or dysfunction. On the other hand, renal failure frequently results in hypertension and lipid abnormalities, which often lead to accelerated atherosclerosis, so that coronary artery disease is a common cause of death in patients being treated for chronic renal insufficiency. Also, uremia often causes pericarditis and thereby may lead to cardiac tamponade or constrictive pericarditis; renal failure also can cause secondary hyperparathyroidism, which can produce cardiac calcification and lead to various disturbances of cardiac function.

EFFECTS OF CARDIAC DISEASE ON RENAL FUNCTION

HEART FAILURE

J. P. Peters at Yale is credited with developing the concept that the kidney in heart failure is physiologically similar to the kidney in hypovolemia: because of inadequate cardiac output

---

Editor's note: The pathophysiology of congestive heart failure is described in Chaps. 14 and 16; the use of diuretics in treating heart failure is discussed in Chap. 17; and the alterations in renal function in congestive heart failure are reviewed here.

---

in both states, salt and water are retained in an attempt to restore the effective arterial blood volume—an as yet poorly defined parameter of filling of the arterial tree that is somehow related to the ratio of arterial blood volume to the capacity of the vascular bed.

Total body sodium is uniformly elevated in edematous patients with congestive heart failure.[1] Modulation of the tubular transport of sodium provides the most important mechanism for regulating sodium excretion. The proximal tubule is the primary site of sodium reabsorption in the nephron, with approximately 60 per cent of filtered sodium being reabsorbed isotonically at this site. Current conceptions of the forces governing proximal tubular reabsorption of sodium in the normal state and in heart failure are shown in Figure 62–1. As cardiac output falls, several stimuli—including augmented alpha-adrenergic neural activity, circulating catecholamines, and increased circulating and locally produced angiotensin II—cause renal vasoconstriction, particularly of the efferent arterioles (Figs. 62–2 and 62–3). As a consequence, the glomerular filtration rate declines, but there is a proportionately greater fall in renal blood flow and, therefore, a rise in the filtration fraction (i.e., the ratio of glomerular filtration rate to renal blood flow). This results in an elevated protein concentration in the peritubular capillaries and a decline in the postglomerular capillary hydrostatic pressure; thus, the transcapillary hydraulic pressure gradient falls.[2]

SODIUM RETENTION IN HEART FAILURE. The combination of these events, i.e., the reduction of peritubular capillary hydrostatic pressure and an elevation of peritubular on-

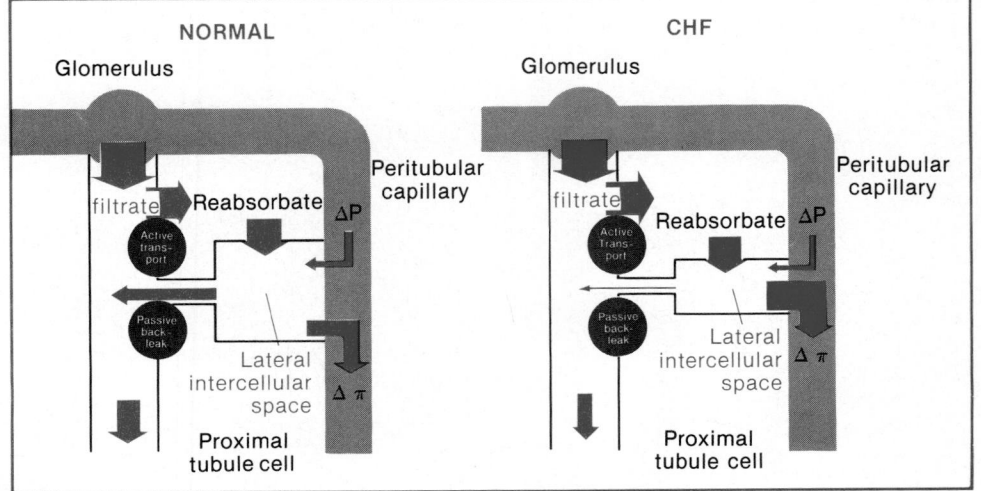

FIGURE 62–1. Peritubular control of proximal tubule fluid reabsorption. Current concept of the role of peritubular capillary physical forces in the regulation of proximal tubule fluid reabsorption in the normal state *(left)* and in congestive heart failure (CHF) *(right)*. ΔP and $\Delta\pi$ are, respectively, the transcapillary hydraulic and oncotic pressure differences operating across the peritubular capillary. The increase in filtration fraction causes $\Delta\pi$ to rise in CHF. The increase in renovascular resistance in CHF is thought to reduce ΔP. Both the increase in $\Delta\pi$ and the fall in ΔP enhance peritubular capillary uptake of proximal reabsorbate and thus increase absolute sodium reabsorption by the proximal tubule. (From Humes, H. D., et al.: The kidney in congestive heart failure. *In* Brenner, B. M., and Stein, J. H. [eds.]: Contemporary Issues in Nephrology. Vol. 1. New York, Churchill Livingstone, 1978, p. 51.)

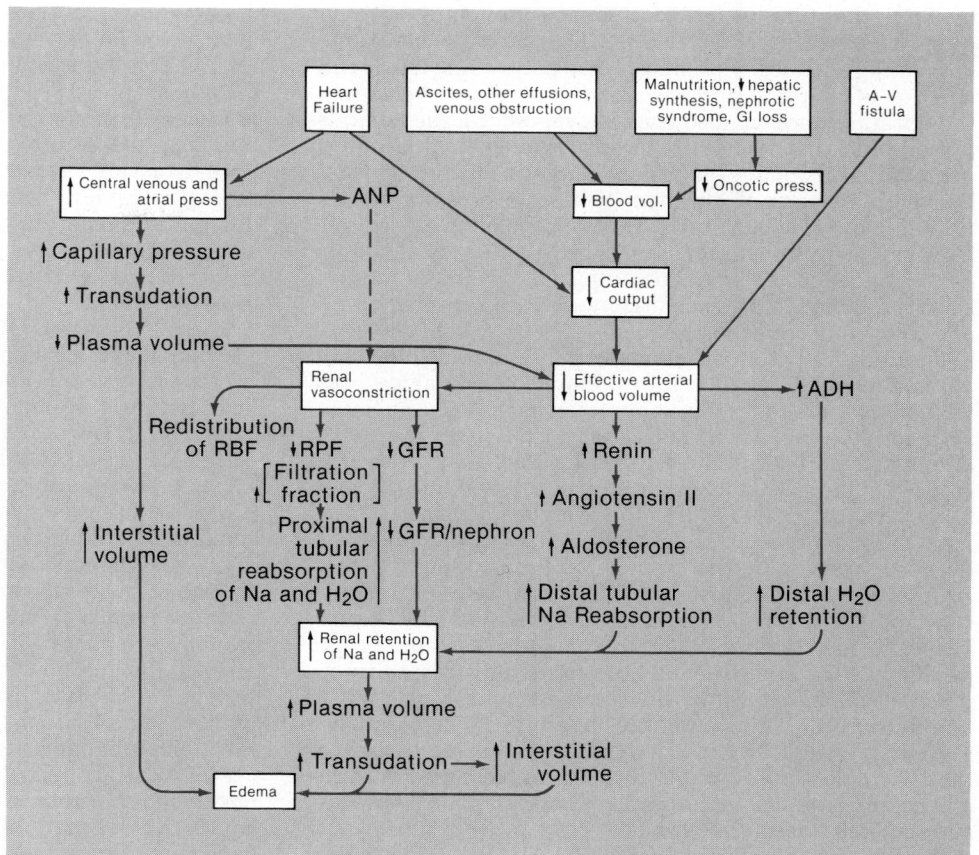

FIGURE 62–2. Major pathophysiological mechanisms leading to salt and water retention and the development of edema. The contribution of heart failure is shown, as well as other major causes. ANP = atrial natriuretic peptide; dotted line indicates inhibition of renal vasoconstriction. (From Braunwald, E.: Edema. *In* Harrison's Principles of Internal Medicine. New York, McGraw-Hill Book Co., 1991, p. 220.)

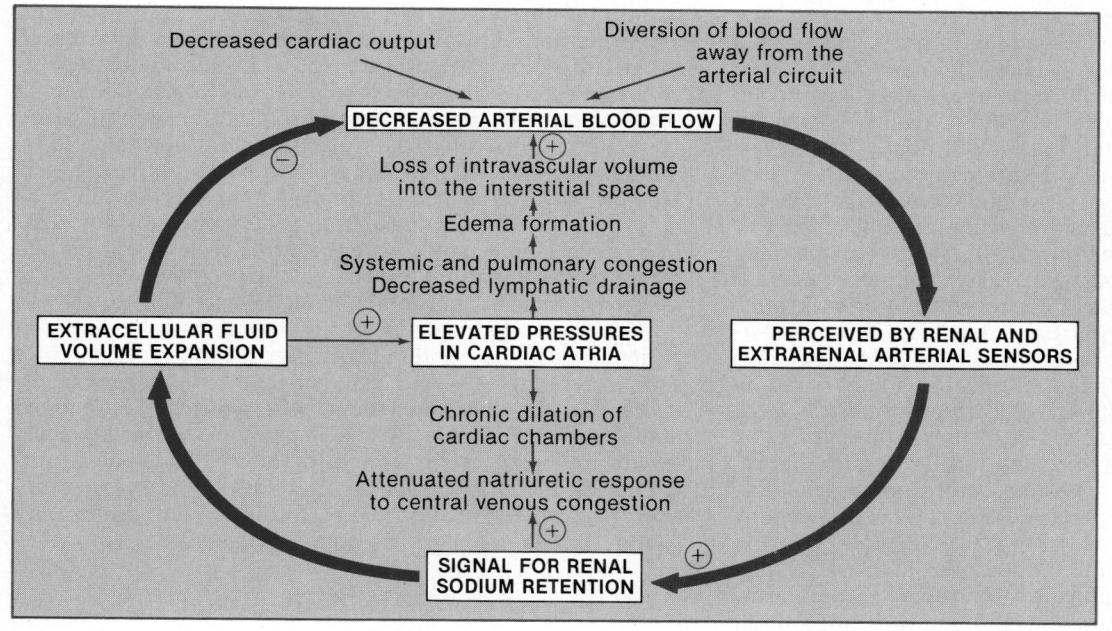

FIGURE 62–3. Sensing mechanisms that initiate and maintain renal sodium retention in congestive heart failure. (Reproduced with permission from Skorecki, K. L., and Brenner, B. M.: Body fluid homeostasis in congestive heart failure and cirrhosis with ascites. Am. J. Med. 72:323, 1982.)

cotic pressure, enhances the peritubular capillary uptake of proximal tubular fluid, and thereby increases the absolute quantity of sodium reabsorbed by the proximal tubule.[3,4] An additional proposed mechanism for sodium retention in heart failure is the redistribution of blood flow from cortical to juxtamedullary nephrons that contain longer loops of Henle and are therefore capable of greater sodium reabsorption.

In addition to the more avid sodium reabsorption in the proximal convoluted tubule, sodium reabsorption also increases in distal nephron sites, including the collecting duct segments. This results from the operation of Starling forces, i.e., a lowering of capillary hydrostatic pressure and an elevation of oncotic pressure, such as those described for the proximal tubule.

The Renin-Angiotensin-Aldosterone System (see also p. 829). In addition, aldosterone, the sodium resorbing activity of which is limited to the terminal segment of the nephron, distal tubule, and collecting duct system, has been recognized as an important factor in sodium retention associated with congestive heart failure. The absolute concentration of circulating aldosterone is increased in some patients with congestive heart failure owing to both the enhanced production of aldosterone stimulated by the renin-angiotensin axis and its diminished metabolism. In acute heart failure, decreased renal perfusion (whether caused by a reduction in total cardiac output or by a decrease in the renal fraction of the cardiac output) activates the juxtaglomerular apparatus to enhance renin release; this in turn augments the generation of angiotensin II, the stimulus for aldosterone secretion and thus for retention of sodium (Fig. 28–13, p. 832). Angiotensin II, both circulating and locally produced, also plays a role in the constriction of efferent arterioles[5] and the resultant elevation in the filtration fraction, discussed above. Indeed, the administration of an angiotensin II–converting enzyme inhibitor in heart failure increases renal blood flow and glomerular filtration with a return of filtration fraction toward normal and usually induces a natriuresis. The impairment in aldosterone biodegradation sometimes seen in heart failure is due to the combination of hepatic congestion as well as reduced splanchnic blood flow secondary to reduced cardiac output and splanchnic vasoconstriction.[6]

The renal retention of sodium expands extracellular fluid volume and tends to return the renin-angiotensin-aldosterone system toward normal. For that reason, circulating angiotensin II and aldosterone concentrations are frequently normal in chronic stable heart failure, although they tend to be high relative to the expanded extracellular fluid volume (Fig. 62–3). In terminal heart failure, however, with further impairment of renal perfusion, renin production is again enhanced, despite expansion of the extracellular fluid volume.

Other Vasoactive Substances. The role of other vasoactive substances, such as prostaglandins, kallikreins, and kinins, has yet to be determined, but they have also been implicated as factors in sodium balance.[7] Intrarenal prostaglandins oppose the actions of angiotensin II on the renal vascular bed. In heart failure the infusion of prostaglandin A_2 may enhance sodium excretion,[8] whereas inhibition of prostaglandin synthesis by means of drugs such as indomethacin may enhance arteriolar resistance, depress the glomerular filtration rate, and increase sodium retention.[9]

WATER RETENTION IN HEART FAILURE. The serum sodium concentration often is reduced in congestive heart failure. With enhanced proximal reabsorption and a decline in glomerular filtration rate, less tubular fluid is delivered to the diluting segments of the nephron.[10] In addition, with a reduction in total renal blood flow, renal medullary blood flow is diminished, which also reduces the nephron's capacity to excrete water. Plasma antidiuretic hormone (ADH) levels are consistently elevated in patients with congestive heart failure, and probably play the dominant role in inducing water retention.[11] The reduced effective arterial blood volume serves as a potent nonosmotic stimulus to enhance the release of ADH. This idea is supported by the observation that the defect in water excretion can be reversed by an antagonist to ADH in rats and dogs with congestive heart failure.[12] Furthermore, water excretion is improved in patients with stage III and stage IV congestive heart failure after afterload reduction with prazosin or captopril. This improvement is associated with a fall in ADH levels, and occurs despite a lowering of blood pressure.[13] This observation further implies that receptors, other than high-pressure baroreceptors, mediate ADH release; these may be ventricular receptors or receptors sensing stroke volume.[11,14]

Heart failure also stimulates the sensation of thirst[15]; angiotensin II, acting centrally, may be responsible for stimulating the thirst mechanism. A number of other nonosmotic stimuli for the release of ADH, such as discomfort, anxiety, beta-adrenoceptor agonists, and central nervous system depressants (including barbiturates and narcotics), are commonly present in congestive heart failure.

PRERENAL AZOTEMIA IN HEART FAILURE. Azotemia is a common finding in severe congestive heart failure.[16] The enhanced water reabsorption in the collecting duct, especially in the presence of inappropriately elevated ADH levels, augments the passive reabsorption of urea. In addition, urea production may be enhanced in some forms of heart failure, especially in acute myocardial infarction; a catabolic state induced by the stress of heart failure may account for the increased urea load. The combination of increased urea production and decreased excretion (secondary to augmented reabsorption) elevates blood urea nitrogen (BUN) levels even before a re-

duction of glomerular filtration rate. However, the principal mechanism for elevation of BUN and serum creatinine levels is reduction of the glomerular filtration rate. As already noted, the latter is preserved by efferent arteriolar constriction in the presence of modest reductions in renal plasma flow, and therefore the serum creatinine level may remain normal until, in severe heart failure, there are marked reductions in renal plasma flow, constriction of afferent arterioles, and reduction of glomerular filtration rate. Thus, an elevation of serum creatinine level usually is a sign of advanced heart failure. It is not uncommon in heart failure for the BUN : creatinine ratio to exceed 10 to 1. In severe heart failure, when glomerular filtration rate declines, the BUN level may exceed 100 mg/dl and the serum creatinine level, 4 mg/dl.

Prerenal azotemia of this degree is a poor prognostic sign in heart failure. Treatment should be directed toward improving cardiac function, as outlined in Chap. 17.

HEART FAILURE IN PATIENTS WITH RENAL DISEASE. The improvement in the therapy of heart failure (Chap. 17) has prolonged the lives of many patients with the combination of cardiac failure and chronic renal disease. In many such patients the intrinsic renal disease is not severe enough to cause salt, water, or nitrogen retention in the presence of a normal cardiac output. However, when heart failure and the attendant alterations in renal hemodynamics described above are superimposed on intrinsic renal disease, serious problems of retention readily occur. Hemodialysis with ultrafiltration or peritoneal dialysis can be effective in the management of this combination of disorders.

POTASSIUM BALANCE IN HEART FAILURE. Mild hypokalemia is a relatively common finding in patients with congestive heart failure, as a consequence of the distal tubular exchange of sodium for potassium and hydrogen under the influence of excess aldosterone. In addition, because all the major diuretics (other than spironolactone, triamterene, and amiloride) inhibit sodium chloride reabsorption proximal to the site of action of aldosterone in the distal tubule, they increase the delivery of sodium to the distal tubule, enhancing the likelihood of the exchange of sodium for hydrogen and potassium. Therefore, the serum potassium level should be monitored in patients with congestive heart failure to ascertain the need for potassium replacement therapy. Because potassium excretion is augmented and accompanied by alkalosis, replacement should be in the form of potassium chloride rather than potassium bicarbonate or gluconate.

In the end stage of chronic congestive heart failure, prerenal azotemia and oliguria may become severe enough to limit the patient's ability to excrete potassium. At this stage, so little sodium is being delivered to the distal tubule, even with diuretic therapy, that its exchange with potassium is reduced and hyperkalemia may develop. In patients with severe heart failure and progressive azotemia and oliguria, potassium-sparing diuretics (spironolactone, amiloride, and triamterene) must be used with caution, if at all, since these agents may hasten the development of hyperkalemia.

ATRIAL NATRIURETIC PEPTIDE

In addition to the aforementioned indirect effects of heart failure on renal function, the atria produce peptides that directly affect renal function.[17] For more than 30 years the atria have been considered important physiological sites of volume regulation.[18,19] Although atrial myocytes have long been known to possess granules characteristic of secretory cells[20] (Fig. 62–4) and the degree of granularity was known to be related to the state of salt balance,[21] it was not until 1981 that DeBold et al. published their landmark experiments showing that infusions of an extract of mammalian atria (but not of the ventricles) induced rapid natriuresis, kaliuresis, and diuresis while lowering systemic arterial pressure.[22] Subsequently, the active material was identified[23] as a family of related *atrial natriuretic peptides* (ANP) that has since been cloned and sequenced.[24] Although ANP has been subjected to intensive ex-

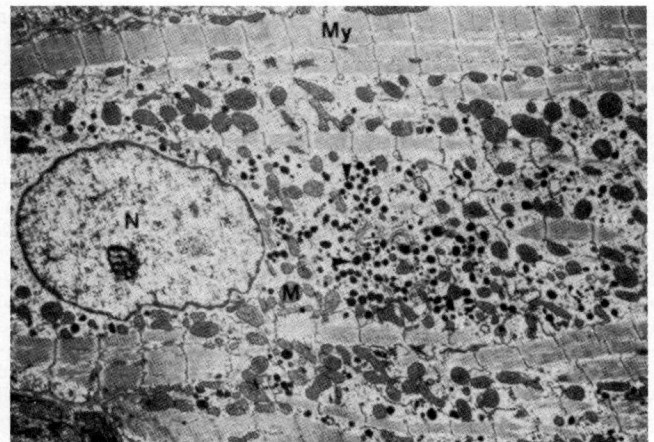

FIGURE 62–4. Electron microscopic view of a rat atrial cardiocyte. N = nucleus; M = mitochondria; My = myofibrils. The central sarcoplasmic core displays morphological features associated with secretory cells that include a large number of storage granules (arrowheads), referred to as specific atrial granules (×3400). (From DeBold, A. J.: Atrial natriuretic factor: A hormone produced by the heart. Science 230:767, 1985. Copyright 1985 by the AAAS. Reproduced by permission of the American Association for the Advancement of Science.)

to 70 picograms/ml of ANP can be measured in normal human plasma.[17] Of interest, messenger RNA for ANP can be detected in ventricular myocardium. Although these levels are only 1 to 2 per cent of atrial levels, ventricular ANP expression rises in the failing heart.[26]

ANP RELEASE. Plasma volume expansion and elevation of left atrial pressure or volume are thought to induce the release of ANP by means of the stretching of myocytes.[27] Release of a natriuretic substance from rat heart-lung preparations in the face of high atrial perfusion pressure[28] as well as elevation of plasma ANP in dogs after atrial distention has been reported.[29] In humans, ANP levels have been found to rise with an increase of salt intake,[30] on assumption of the supine posture,[31] and after water immersion.[32] A rise in plasma ANP after salt and water loading and a fall after furosemide-induced volume depletion have been reported.[33] Patients with congestive heart failure have elevated plasma ANP levels.[30,34] In one study, right atrial and arterial plasma ANP levels correlated with right atrial and pulmonary capillary wedge pressures, respectively.[35] Step-ups in ANP levels across the atria also were demonstrated. ANP levels are elevated in patients with the syndrome of inappropriate antidiuretic hormone secretion, primary hyperaldosteronism, and chronic renal failure with volume overload.[36] Although acute hypertension markedly elevates ANP, levels are normal in patients with essential hypertension.[37] Finally, elevated plasma ANP levels have been described during atrial tachycardia[38] and during atrial pacing[39] and may explain the polyuria sometimes associated with these events. Taken together, these observations support the concept that atrial ANP release is strongly associated with plasma volume status as well as with atrial pressure and/or volume. Of interest, infusions of arginine vasopressin, phenylephrine, angiotensin II, and endothelin also appear to stimulate the release of ANP and increase plasma ANP levels.[40,41]

ANP RECEPTORS. Once released into the circulation, ANP binds to receptors in target tissues that have high affinity and specificity.[42] Receptors have been found in the renal cortex and medulla, aorta, vascular smooth muscle,[43] adrenal zona glomerulosa,[44] and central nervous system.[45] In the kidney and in smooth muscle most ANP receptors serve solely to

perimental investigation, its exact role in circulatory physiology and pathophysiology has yet to be clearly defined. A proposed summary of the actions of ANP as circulating natriuretic hormones is shown in Figure 62–5.

STRUCTURE. Human ANP is synthesized as a 151–amino acid pro-ANP precursor and stored as a 126–amino acid pro-ANP in atrial myocyte granules (Fig. 62–6), in quantities greater on the right side of the heart than on the left. The biologically active circulating molecule consists of a 28–amino acid peptide thought to be cleft from the pro-ANP when it is released. The molecule possesses a 17–amino acid ring formed by a disulfide bridge between two cysteine moieties, which is required for biological activity.[25] Approximately 10

FIGURE 62–5. Summary of the atrial natriuretic peptide (ANP) hormonal system. The 126-amino acid prohormone atriopeptigen, or pro-ANP, is stored in granules in perinuclear atrial cardiocytes. Elevated vascular volume results in the release of atriopeptin (ANP), which acts on the kidney (glomeruli and papilla) to increase glomerular filtration rate (GFR), renal blood flow (RBF), urine volume (UV), and urinary sodium excretion (U_{Na}), and to decrease plasma renin activity. Natriuresis and diuresis also are facilitated by the suppression of aldosterone and of arginine vasopressin (AVP). Diminution of vascular volume provides a negative feedback that suppresses circulating levels of ANP. (Reprinted by permission from Needleman, P., and Greenwald, J. E.: Atriopeptin: A cardiac hormone intimately involved in fluid, electrolyte, and blood pressure homeostasis. N. Engl. J. Med. 314:829, 1986.)

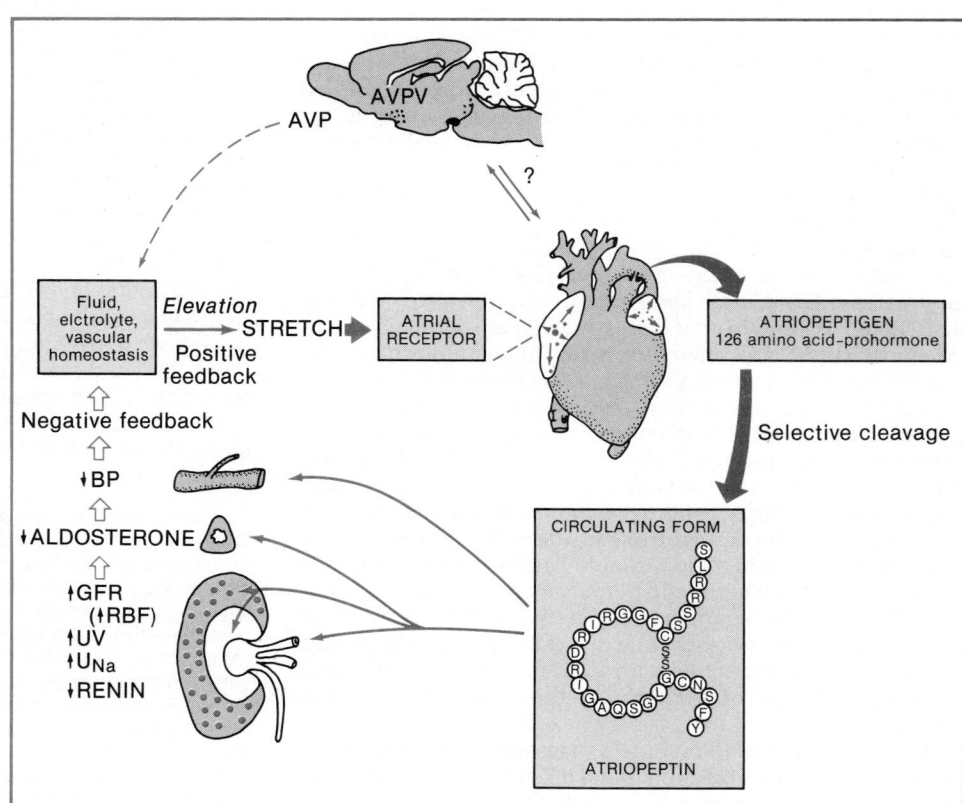

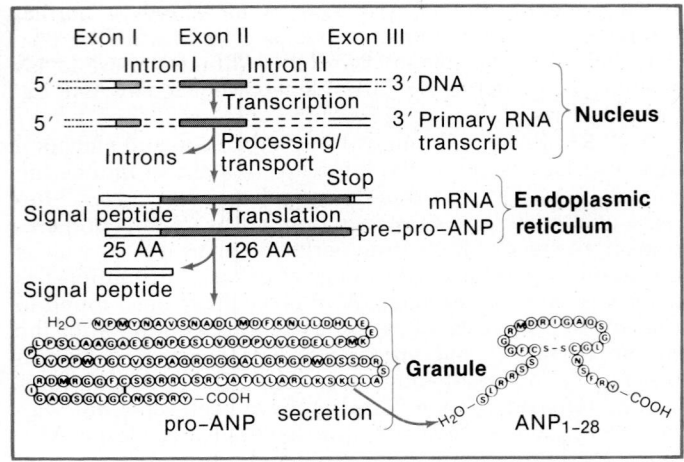

FIGURE 62–6. The biosynthetic pathway, and the sequences of the human pre-pro-ANP gene, pro-ANP, and ANP_{1-28}. ANP_{1-28} is numbered from amino- to carboxyterminus. Specific amino acids in the pro-ANP and ANP sequences are given by single-letter code: alanine = A, arginine = R, asparagine = N, aspartic acid = D, cysteine = C, glutamine = Q, glutamic acid = E, glycine = G, histidine = H, isoleucine = I, leucine = L, lysine = K, methionine = M, phenylalanine = F, proline = P, serine = S, threonine = T, tryptophan = W, tyrosine = Y, valine = V. The pre-pro-ANP gene is present in a single copy on the short arm of chromosome 1. The DNA is transcribed into RNA, and the exon segments are spliced together to form messenger RNA. This is translated to form the initial pro-ANP precursor (pre-pro-ANP). The signal peptide is removed and pro-ANP is stored in atrial myocyte granules. When the peptide is released, the active 28–amino acid fragment is cleaved off and enters the circulation. (From Ballermann, B. J., and Brenner, B. M.: Role of atrial peptides in body fluid homeostasis. Circ. Res. *58:*619, 1986, by permission of the American Heart Association, Inc.)

clear circulating ANP, resulting in its short half-life of about 3 minutes.[46] The biologically active receptor itself is unique, as it both binds ANP and catalyzes the formation of cyclic guanosine monophosphate, which serves as a second messenger for ANP action.[47]

PHYSIOLOGICAL EFFECTS OF ANP. The major direct renal effects of ANP occur in the glomerulus, which has an abundance of receptors,[48] and the inner medullary collecting duct, where sodium uptake is decreased by the inhibition of a membrane sodium channel.[49] Intravenous infusion of ANP in animals and humans results in a brisk natriuresis and diuresis (Fig. 62–7A). An increase in excretion of chloride, potassium, calcium, magnesium, and phosphorus also has been noted.[50,51] Two consistent and dramatic findings have been increases in both glomerular filtration rate and filtration fraction, despite a drop in blood pressure (Fig. 62–7B). In the rat this is associated with constriction of the efferent glomerular arterioles, dilation of afferent arterioles, and an increase in glomerular pressure.[52] Other glomerular effects include an increase in the glomerular capillary ultrafiltration coefficient[52] and inhibition of tubuloglomerular feedback.[53] ANP inhibits renal vasoconstriction, but differing effects of ANP on total renal blood flow have been described, depending on the species studied and on experimental conditions.[50,54] Although changes in the glomerular filtration rate account for the preponderance of the natriuresis in response to ANP, inhibition of distal nephron sodium transport probably contributes as well.[55]

More prolonged effects of ANP on salt balance and hemodynamics may be mediated through changes in the renin-angiotensin-aldosterone system. Renal renin secretion is known to be suppressed by ANP.[56] Aldosterone secretion also is blocked by ANP in vitro and in vivo,[57] as is angiotensin-induced vascular constriction[58] and angiotensin-stimulated aldosterone release. Thus, ANP may play a special role in antagonizing each aspect of the renin-angiotensin-aldosterone axis (Fig. 62–8).

ANP is known to relax smooth muscle, including that found in the renal, coronary, and other vascular beds.[59,59a] However, infusions of ANP into intact animals may increase or decrease vascular resistance, depending on experimental conditions.[50] Thus the fall in blood pressure seen after ANP infusion seems to result mostly from a reduction in cardiac output, which is associated with a decrease in venous return.[60] This hypotensive effect may be augmented by a direct effect of ANP on vascular permeability, resulting in a reversible extravascular fluid shift, and is associated with a rise in hematocrit and total plasma proteins out of proportion to the degree of natriuresis and diuresis.[51]

Other actions of ANP include a suggested role in maintaining sodium balance in chronic renal failure[61] and in mediating the "escape" phenomenon seen with chronic mineralocorti-coid administration.[62] Finally, immunoreactive ANP has been found in the central nervous system and may relate to cardiovascular regulatory functions.[63,64]

Despite the multiplicity of actions of ANP in a variety of tissues, the differences between its physiological and pharmacological effects are not clearly delineated. Although it is certain that ANP will take its place as an important regulatory hormone, further studies are needed to define its role in both normal and pathophysiological conditions, as well as a therapeutic agent.

RENAL MANIFESTATIONS OF CARDIAC DISORDERS

INFECTIVE ENDOCARDITIS (see also Chap. 35). The association between glomerulonephritis and bacterial endocarditis has been appreciated for many years. In 1920, before the availability of antibiotics and when infective endocarditis was uniformly fatal, 11 per cent of patients with this infection ultimately died of renal failure.[65] It was initially thought that the glomerular lesion was secondary to septic embolization to the kidney from infected valvular vegetations, but little firm evidence supports this theory. Instead, the pathogenesis of the renal lesions appears to be more in keeping with the generally accepted pathogenesis of most types of glomerulonephritis.[66] Soluble antigenic components of the infecting organism and antibody directed against these antigens have been demonstrated in the glomeruli. As indicated in Chapter 35, many organisms have been responsible for the infective endocarditis that may be associated with glomerulonephritis. By immunofluorescence, the presence of immune complexes and the third component of complement (C3) can be demonstrated in the glomeruli of patients with endocarditis and glomerulonephritis[66]; early in the course there is a decline in the serum level of C3 and of another component of the complement system, Clq. It now appears that the glomerular lesion of endocarditis results from the deposition of immune complexes along the glomerular basement membrane and in the mesangium.[67]

The most commonly observed abnormality by light microscopy is a focal, proliferative glomerulonephritis, often with focal fibrinoid necrosis. Less commonly, the lesions may be more diffuse, and in some instances extracapillary epithelial proliferation (crescents), such as that seen in rapidly progressive glomerulonephritis, has been observed.[66] Clinically, patients have the typical manifestations of acute or rapidly progressive renal failure, often with hypertension, hematuria, and red cell casts, usually without marked proteinuria and edema. The retention of sodium and water is due to reductions in the glomerular filtration rate and the fractional excretion of sodium. Azotemia usually is progressive, unless rapid bacteriological cure occurs.

Other causes of impaired renal function in patients with infective endocarditis include hypovolemia, congestive heart failure, antibiotic-induced nephrotoxicity, and acute allergic interstitial nephritis secondary to antibiotic therapy.

ANTIBIOTIC TREATMENT IN RENAL FAILURE. Many of the antibiotics used in the treatment of infective endocarditis are excreted by the kidney. These include vancomycin, the penicillins, cephalosporins, and aminoglycosides. It is therefore important to modify the dosage and/or the interval of administration of antibiotics with respect to the degree of renal dysfunction. Because many antibiotics are removed by hemodialysis or peritoneal dialysis, supplementary doses may need to be administered in patients receiving these therapies. Guidelines for antibiotic therapy are presented in Table 62–1. Aminoglycoside and vancomycin levels should be monitored to insure adequate therapeutic dosage and to avoid toxic levels that may contribute to further renal impairment or to ototoxicity. Serum bactericidal titers also may be monitored to assess the adequacy of antibiotic therapy.

The most common cause of endocarditis in dialysis patients is *Staphylococcus aureus*,[68] with *Streptococcus viridans,* enterococci, *Staphylococcus epidermidis,* and gram-negative rods accounting for most of the other cases. Therefore, initial antibiotic therapy should include a penicillinase-resistant penicillin, or vancomycin, and an aminoglycoside, until culture results are available.

ACUTE RENAL FAILURE SECONDARY TO CARDIOGENIC SHOCK (see also p. 574). Prerenal azotemia and, less commonly, acute renal failure (acute tubular necrosis) may occur in association with massive acute myocardial infarction. The mechanism of prerenal azotemia has been discussed above. Acute renal failure occurs when there is a marked, sudden reduction of renal perfusion. The myoglobinuria accompanying excessive myocardial necrosis may play a contributory role. It is critically important to distinguish between prerenal azotemia and acute renal failure, since the former usually responds to measures that improve cardiac output, whereas acute renal failure, once established, is a more serious problem that usually does not respond to extrarenal manipulation. Brief periods of modest hypotension (usually lasting less than an hour) often elicit reversible derange-

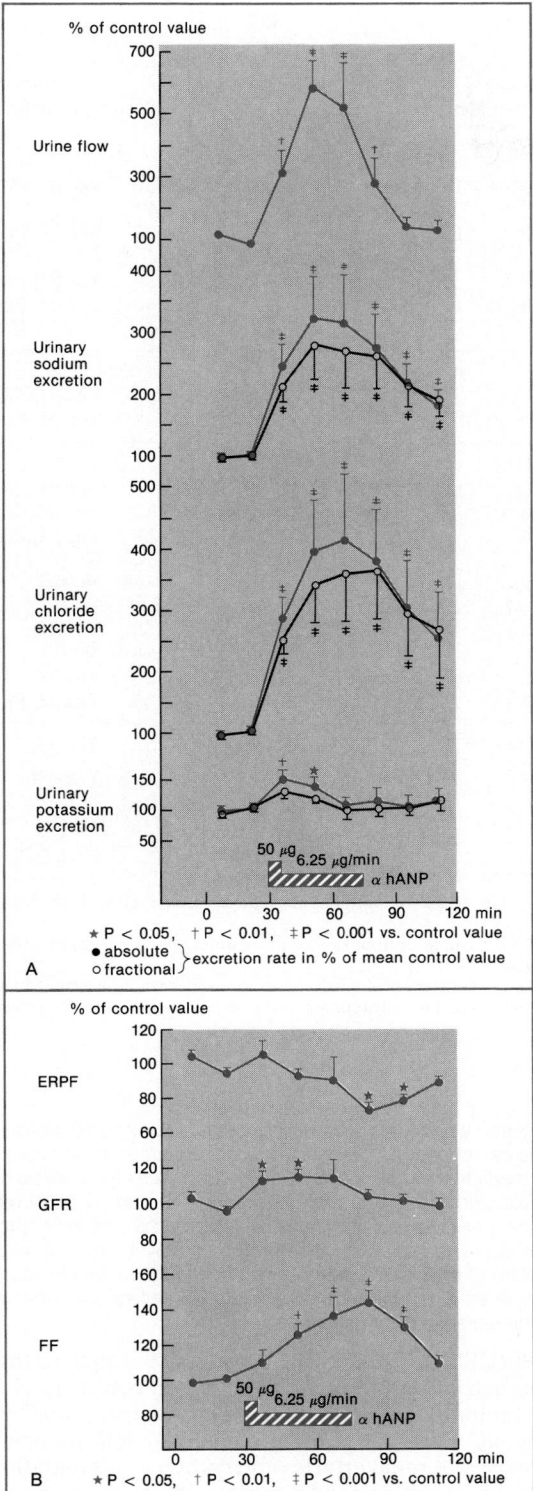

FIGURE 62–7. *A,* Effect of ANP (50 = μg bolus followed by maintenance infusion of 6.25 μ/min) on urine flow and sodium, chloride, and potassium excretion rates in 10 normal subjects (mean ± S.E.M.). The mean of the two control values is taken as 100 per cent. Closed circles are the absolute excretion rates. Open circles are calculated fractional excretion rates (urine/plasma Na, Cl, or K divided by urine/plasma creatinine). *B,* Effect of ANP on ERPF = estimated renal plasma flow; GFR = glomerular filtration rate; FF = filtration fraction. (Reproduced from Weidmann, P., et al.: Blood levels and renal effects of atrial natriuretic peptide in normal man. J. Clin. Invest. *77:*734, 1986, by copyright permission of the American Society for Clinical Investigation.)

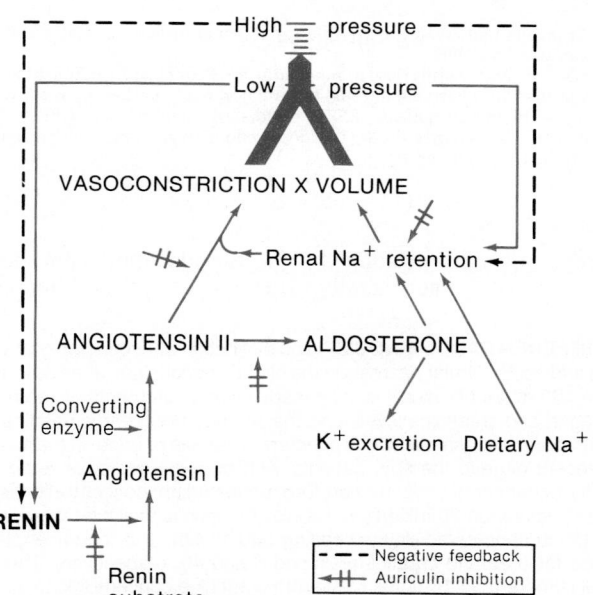

FIGURE 62–8. Atrial natriuretic peptide and the renin-angiotensin-aldosterone system. Renin, secreted in response to reduced renal arterial pressure or a reduction in the sodium supply in the distal tubule, acts to release angiotensin II. Angiotensin II raises blood pressure and stimulates aldosterone secretion, which leads to retention of sodium and water and to improved flow. These pressure and volume effects turn off the renin release. Auriculin opposes the renin system at four points. Within the kidney its natriuretic action opposes aldosterone's action and stops renin secretion. The atrial hormone also opposes the vasoconstrictor action of angiotensin on blood vessels and, at the adrenal cortex, blocks angiotensin's stimulation of aldosterone release. Broken lines = negative feedback; crossed arrows = auriculin inhibition. (Reprinted with permission from Laragh, J. H.: Atrial natriuretic hormone, the renin-aldosterone axis, and blood pressure-electrolyte homeostasis. N. Engl. J. Med. *313:*1330, 1985.)

TABLE 62-1 ANTIBIOTIC THERAPY IN RENAL FAILURE

DRUG	Elimination and Metabolism	Half-life Normal (hr)	Half-life ESRD (hr)	Plasma Protein Binding (%)	Volume of Distribution (liters/kg)	Method	GFR (ml/min) >50	GFR (ml/min) 10-50	GFR (ml/min) <10	Removed by Dialysis
Aminoglycosides[a]										
Amikacin	Renal	2-3	30	<5	0.22-0.29	D	60-90	30-70	20-30	Yes (H, P)
						I	12	12-18	24	
Gentamicin	Renal	2	24-48	<5	0.23-0.26	D	60-90	30-70	20-30	Yes (H, P)[b]
						I	8-12	12	24	
Streptomycin	Renal	2.5	100	35	0.26	I	24	24-72	72-96	Yes (H)
Tobramycin	Renal	2.5	56	<5	0.22-0.25	D	60-90	30-70	20-30	Yes (H, P)
						I	8-12	12	24	
Cephalosporins										
Cefazolin	Renal	1.4-2.2	18-36	80	0.13	I	8	12	24-48	Yes (H), No (P)
Cephalothin	Renal (hepatic)	0.5-0.9	3-18	65	0.26	I	6	6	8-12	Yes (H, P)
Penicillins										
Ampicillin	Renal (hepatic)	0.8-1.5	7-20	8-20	0.17-0.31	I	6	6-12	12-16	Yes (H), No (P)
Azlocillin	Renal (hepatic)	0.8-1.5	5-6	25-30	0.18-0.23	I	4-6	6-8	8	Yes (H), No (P)
Carbenicillin	Renal (hepatic)	1.5	10-20	30-50	0.12-0.20	I	8-12	12-24	24-48	Yes (H), No (P)
Methicillin	Renal (hepatic)	0.5-1.0	4	35-60	0.31	I	4	4-8	8-12	No (H, P)
Nafcillin	Hepatic (renal)	0.5	1.2	80-90	0.31-0.38	D	U	U	U	No (H)
Oxacillin	Renal (hepatic)	0.4	1	85-95	0.12-0.4	D	U	U	U	No (H, P)
Penicillin G[c]	Renal (hepatic)	0.5	6-20	40-60	0.3-0.42	D	U	75	25-50	Yes (H),
						I	6-8	8-12	12-16	No (P)
Piperacillin	Renal (hepatic)	0.8-1.5	3.3-5.1	16-22	0.18-0.30	I	4-6	6-8	8	Yes (H)
Ticarcillin	Renal	1.0-1.5	16	45	0.14-0.21	I	8-12	12-24	24-48	Yes (H, P)
Aztreonam	Renal	1.7-2.9	6-8	50-60	0-20	D	U	50-75	25	Yes (H), No (P)
Imipenem	Renal (hepatic)	1	3.5-4.0	20	0.24-0.27	I	6	8	12	Yes (H)
						D	100	75	50	
Rifampin	Hepatic	2-5	2-5	60-90	0.9	I	U	U	U	No (H)
Vancomycin[d]	Renal	6-8	200-250	10	0.47-0.84	I	24-72	72-240	240	No (H, P)

From Bennett, W. M.: Drug therapy in renal disease. *In* Rubenstein, E., and Federman, D. D. (eds.): Scientific American Medicine. New York, Scientific American, Inc. 1990.

[a] Need usual loading dose in renal failure. [b] Poor clearance from blood to peritoneum in CAPD. [c] Upper limit of 4 to 6 million units/day in severe renal failure. [d] Elimination is variable in renal failure; best guide to therapy is serum level before next dose.

$T_{1/2}$ = biological half-life; ESRD = end-stage renal disease; GFR = glomerular filtration rate; I = interval extension method of dosage adjustment in hours between maintenance doses; D = dose reduction method of dosage adjustment in percentage of usual maintenance dose; H = hemodialysis; P = peritoneal dialysis; U = unchanged.

ments, but more prolonged or profound hypotension lasting for 1 hour or longer usually leads to acute tubular necrosis.

DIFFERENTIAL DIAGNOSIS. The distinction between prerenal azotemia and acute tubular necrosis in the oliguric patient (i.e., urine output less than 400 ml/24 hr) usually can be made by measurements of serum urea nitrogen and creatinine levels and the sodium, urea, and creatinine concentrations and osmolality of a concurrent sample of urine. In the absence of recent diuretic therapy, patients with prerenal azotemia retain their ability to conserve sodium; therefore, urine sodium concentration is low, usually less than 20 mEq/liter. Tubular function is well preserved, as reflected in urine osmolality exceeding 500 mOsm, and the urine:plasma ratios for urea and creatinine exceed 8 and 40, respectively. The BUN level is more than 10 times the serum creatinine concentration.

In acute tubular necrosis, tubular function is impaired and the urine sodium concentration usually exceeds 40 mEq/liter; the impairment of tubular function also is reflected in a urine osmolality less than 350 mOsm; the urine:plasma values for urea and creatinine are below 2 and 20, respectively; and the BUN level exceeds the serum creatinine level by a ratio of less than 10 to 1. The urinary sediment also may be helpful in the differential diagnosis; patients with prerenal azotemia usually have a relatively clear sediment with a few granular or hyaline casts, whereas those with acute tubular necrosis have many tubular cells and casts in the urine.

MANAGEMENT. As in patients with other causes of acute renal failure, the treatment of acute renal failure secondary to myocardial infarction and pump failure consists of controlling fluid intake to levels in accord with urine output and insensible losses, as well as modifying the dosages of medications that are excreted by the kidneys, observing the patient closely for hyperkalemia, and intervening with dialysis for severe hyperkalemia or azotemia. Dialytic therapy, either hemodialysis or peritoneal dialysis, is initiated when serum creatinine levels reach 8 to 10 mg/dl and no reversible component for the renal failure is apparent. In addition, efforts must be made to maintain left ventricular filling pressure at levels that will optimize cardiac output and therefore renal perfusion (18 to 22 mm Hg). Given sufficient time and with no other associated problems, the prognosis for acute renal failure, when appropriately treated, is excellent. When failure of the cardiac pump is severe enough to lead to acute renal failure, myocardial insufficiency rather than the renal failure is the determinant of the patient's poor prognosis.

ATHEROEMBOLIC DISEASE (see also p. 1552). Atheromatous embolization to the kidneys, which results in chronic, fibrotic interstitial disease, is relatively uncommon.[69] It may occur spontaneously but more commonly follows operation on the aorta and renal arteries and catheter manipulation and aortography in patients with severe atheromatous disease of the aorta. Patchy areas of necrosis develop, followed by fibrosis with cholesterol clefts, as well as a foreign body response containing multinucleated giant cells. The disorder may be suspected if there has been some manipulation of the atheromatous aorta preceding the onset of progressive renal insufficiency. Examination of the urine is seldom helpful in confirming the diagnosis; when it is allowed to sediment, fat may be found floating at the top. Careful ophthalmological examination may reveal cholesterol emboli in the retinal arteries. Treatment consists of avoiding further arterial and aortic manipulation, but progressive destruction of renal tissue occurs with subsequent renal insufficiency; the prognosis for improvement of renal function is guarded.

EFFECTS OF RENAL DISEASE ON THE CARDIOVASCULAR SYSTEM

The successful treatment of end-stage renal disease by dialysis and transplantation is widely considered to be one of the major advances of modern medicine. Cardiovascular disease is the principal cause of mortality in dialysis patients, accounting for 30 to 50 per cent of deaths[70] compared with less than 15 per cent of deaths in an age-corrected control population. Heart failure accounts for about 15 per cent of this dialysis-associated mortality, myocardial infarction for about 10 per cent, and pericarditis for about 3 per cent.

CORONARY ATHEROSCLEROSIS

Numerous risk factors for atherosclerosis have been identified in patients with end-stage renal disease.[71] Of these, hypertension is the most important.[72] Uremia itself has been proposed as an independent risk factor,[73] but recently this suggestion has been questioned. It is unclear whether coronary atherosclerosis is unusually prevalent or accelerated in uremic patients when compared with nonuremic patients of comparable age and with similar risk factors.[70,74] The National Cooperative Dialysis Study demonstrated a clear increase in cardiovascular morbid events in patients who received shorter dialysis treatments or who had elevated (time-averaged) BUN concentrations.[75] These observations imply that the adequacy of a dialysis regimen has a significant impact on cardiovascular morbidity.

Coronary bypass surgery has been carried out successfully in patients with renal failure and angina pectoris that is refractory to medical therapy,[76] although postoperative morbidity is increased compared with that of patients without renal disease. Although the short-term results of coronary angioplasty are satisfactory in patients on chronic dialysis, these patients have a high incidence of restenosis, so that coronary bypass surgery is the preferred therapy.[76a] In addition, angina unassociated with coronary atherosclerosis is being increasingly recognized in chronic renal failure, presumably related to the combination of severe hypertension, left ventricular hypertrophy, and anemia.[70] It also has been suggested that reduced coronary artery compliance owing to calcification may restrict coronary vasodilation and limit myocardial oxygen delivery.[74]

HYPERTENSION
(See also p. 833)

Most patients with chronic renal failure that requires dialysis also have hypertension, which is probably the most important risk factor in the development of atherosclerotic cardiovascular disease. Hemodynamic studies in patients with end-stage renal disease have shown an elevated cardiac index and mean arterial pressure but a normal systemic vascular resistance.[70] The elevated cardiac index and normal systemic vascular resistance are related to the anemia; when the anemia is corrected, the cardiac index falls, and both arterial pressure and systemic vascular resistance rise.[77] Many patients with end-stage renal disease who are treated with erythropoietin experience an elevation of blood pressure, related to an increase in peripheral vascular resistance and an increased blood viscosity, when hematocrit rises to more normal levels.[78] This blood pressure elevation may be associated with seizures, and requires initiation of or an increase in blood pressure medication in approximately 25 per cent of patients. Most patients with end-stage renal failure who develop hypertension have so-called volume-dependent hypertension (p. 834). Many studies in patients with end-stage renal failure have shown that arterial pressure is exquisitely dependent on blood volume[79] and that blood pressure control may be achieved by ultrafiltration during dialysis and control of salt and water intake in the interdialytic interval. A minority of patients with chronic renal failure have hypertension that is not volume-related but rather secondary to elevation of plasma renin activity; the hypertension is uncontrollable by lowering blood volume but does respond to bilateral nephrectomy with a consequent reduction in plasma renin activity. Dustan and Page demonstrated the volume-dependent nature of hypertension but also showed that arterial pressure was higher for any given volume when the kidneys were present than after they had been removed.[80] Subsequently a significant correlation between *plasma renin levels* and arterial pressure was demonstrated.[81] The importance of plasma renin also is reflected in observations on patients with renal failure, hypertension, and expanded blood volume who exhibited renin values which, although normal, were higher than expected for the expanded state of their extracellular volume and which therefore may have contributed to the maintenance of hypertension.[82] There also is evidence that local production and action of angiotensin II plays an important part in the hypertension of chronic renal failure.[83]

A third mechanism, which operates in patients whose blood pressure cannot be controlled by either volume reduction or bilateral nephrectomy or explained by elevations in plasma renin activity, may be related to *sympathetically mediated vasoconstriction*. Reduced baroreceptor activity has been demonstrated in patients with chronic renal failure by their response to the inhalation of amyl nitrite and the Valsalva maneuver.[84] Inhalation of amyl nitrite causes peripheral vasodilation, and therefore a fall in blood pressure, which normally results in reflex vasoconstriction and tachycardia. A blunted response in heart rate elevation is taken as evidence of reduced baroreceptor function. Autonomic insufficiency, as evidenced by an inadequate response to the Valsalva maneuver, is said to be present if both bradycardia and arterial pressure overshoot are absent after release of forced expiration against a standard pressure (40 mm Hg) for a set time (12 sec). Many patients with renal insufficiency whose hypertension is caused by sympathetically mediated vasoconstriction exhibit an exaggerated response to the cold pressor test and elevated plasma levels of dopamine beta-hydroxylase as indices of increased adrenergic function but become hypotensive during dialysis.

A fourth mechanism that has been proposed is the *absence of vasodepressor substances* of renal origin, such as the prostaglandins, which may play a role in the genesis of essential hypertension and of renoprival hypertension.[85]

MANAGEMENT. Because volume-dependent hypertension is the most common mechanism in chronic renal disease, the reduction of plasma volume should be the central theme in the management of hypertension in these patients. Before renal function has deteriorated to the point at which dialysis is required, an attempt should be made to reduce plasma volume, but not to the point at which glomerular filtration will decline further; dietary sodium intake should be restricted to the lowest level consistent with a normal sodium balance. Because many patients may have difficulty with this degree of sodium restriction on a long-term basis, and because they may be unable to excrete even this low quantity of sodium, it is often necessary to add diuretics. For most patients with creatinine clearances that exceed 40 ml/min, thiazide diuretics are effective. When the glomerular filtration rate falls below this level, furosemide is required, sometimes in very high doses.

If the arterial pressure remains elevated despite sodium restriction and potent diuretics such as furosemide, antihypertensive agents are required and usually effective. These include calcium channel antagonists, angiotensin converting enzyme (ACE) inhibitors, beta blockers, clonidine, prazosin, hydralazine, and alpha-methyldopa. For the patient whose condition is refractory to these agents, minoxidil may be required. Sympatholytic agents such as guanethidine are not advisable, since they may be associated with particularly profound postural changes in blood pressure in patients with renal failure.

The problem of the control of hypertension is simpler in patients with chronic renal failure who are maintained on intermittent hemodialysis. In addition to dietary restriction of sodium intake, lowering of blood volume by ultrafiltration during hemodialysis may be used. In patients in whom volume reduction does not control blood pressure, pharmacological treatment is indicated, as described above.

Bilateral nephrectomy is seldom used except in those patients who do not respond to antihypertensive drugs, cannot comply with antihypertensive regimens, or experience intolerable side effects with this medication. Although aggressive therapy of hypertension for the patient with renin-mediated malignant hypertension may transiently compromise renal function to the point at which dialysis is required, the increased survival associated with control of the hypertension[86] outweighs the risks attending maintenance hemodialysis.

Hypertension After Renal Transplantation

Hypertension occurs in 30 to 80 per cent of patients during the post-transplant period.[87] Multiple factors have been implicated in its etiology, including acute and chronic rejection, recurrent disease in the transplanted kidney, stenosis of the transplanted renal artery[88], large doses of steroids, and cyclosporin A (CSA).[89] During acute rejection episodes the levels of renin and angiotensin are markedly elevated. In addition, the renin-angiotensin-aldosterone system appears to be of pathogenic importance in the hypertension associated with stenosis of the artery to the transplanted kidney, a complication that occurs in up to 30 per cent of transplant patients who undergo arteriography for refractory hypertension as well as in some patients in whom the diseased native kidneys release renin. CSA-related hypertension is associated with renal vasoconstriction as manifest by decreased renal blood flow, increased renovascular resistance, and decreased glomerular filtration rate, but in humans it is not associated with elevations of renin levels.[89]

MANAGEMENT. To treat hypertension in the posttransplant period the underlying mechanisms of the disorder must be elucidated. Because of activation of the renin-angiotensin-aldosterone system, ACE inhibitors have been found to be effective antihypertensive agents in this setting. Furthermore, ACE inhibitor–induced reversible acute renal insufficiency has been described in patients with functionally significant transplant renal artery stenosis, and its occurrence may serve as a diagnostic test for this entity.[90] In patients with severe refractory hypertension that cannot be ascribed to rejection, angiography and determination of renin activity in venous blood from both the native and the transplanted kidneys are indicated. Surgical revision or angioplasty of a stenosed renal artery or nephrectomy of the native kidney may be in order. Calcium antagonists have been found to counteract some of the adverse effects of CSA on the kidney, and are probably the most effective agents for posttransplant hypertension related to CSA.[91] Also, in some patients, switching from CSA to azathioprine has resulted in noticeable lowering of the blood pressure.[92]

Whereas hypertriglyceridemia is the predominant lipid abnormality in patients with chronic renal failure (see below), hypercholesterolemia Types IIA and B tend to predominate after renal allotransplantation, although in some transplanted patients hypertriglyceridemia persists.[93] The cause of these lipid abnormalities in the posttransplant period is unclear, but they may be related in part to the large doses of glucocorticoids administered to these patients. Furthermore, CSA has been associated with an increased incidence of hypercholesterolemia.[94] In view of the combination of hypertension and lipid abnormalities in a substantial fraction of patients after transplantation, it is not surprising that cardiovascular disease is the most common cause of death greater than 10 years post transplant.[95]

LIPID ABNORMALITIES (see also Chap. 37)

Hypertriglyceridemia with elevations of very low density lipoproteins (VLDL), i.e., Type IV hyperlipoproteinemia (p. 1135), is common in patients with chronic renal failure.[96,96a] There appears to be no relation between the duration of dialysis or the cause of the renal disease and the severity of the hyperlipidemia. A second abnormality in lipid metabolism, *reduced concentration of high-density lipoprotein (HDL) cholesterol,* has also been documented in chronic renal failure,[96,97] a finding of potential importance in view of the strong negative correlation between HDL concentration and the risk of the development of ischemic heart disease. An inverse correlation has been noted between plasma triglyceride and HDL cholesterol levels in both uremic and nonuremic subjects.

MECHANISMS. Several suggestions have been made to explain the elevation of plasma triglycerides in chronic renal failure. The first is that there is increased hepatic synthesis of triglycerides, presumably secondary to increased basal insulin, growth hormone, and glucagon. However, measurements in uremic animals and patients have suggested that the contribution of increased hepatic synthesis is small.[98] A second, more likely possibility[99,100] centers on deficiencies in lipoprotein lipase and hepatic triglyceride lipase known to be necessary for the removal of triglycerides from plasma and their ultimate catabolism; this deficiency also may result from elevated insulin levels, from direct inhibition of these lipases by a nondialyzable factor in uremic serum,[100] or from a deficiency of apoprotein CII in both HDL and VLDL. The reduction of lipoprotein lipase, which is believed to be more important in the generation of hypertriglyceridemia than hepatic lipase, causes a defect in the catabolism of triglyceride-rich lipoproteins, which in turn leads to the accumulation of VLDL[101] and enrichment of intermediate-density lipoproteins and low-density lipoproteins with triglyceride; it also is associated with the appearance of apoprotein B48, an increased concentration of apoprotein AIV, and the presence in LDL of apoproteins C and E (proteins not normally found in LDL). It has been suggested that these abnormal substances may be atherogenic.[100]

Because HDL turnover is diminished in patients with chronic renal failure compared with controls, a decrease in HDL synthesis probably accounts for low HDL levels.[97] In one study HDL cholesterol was significantly reduced in patients with renal failure on chronic hemodialysis (average = 26 mg/dl) compared with normal people (average = 52 mg/dl).[99] This reduction of HDL was due to a reduced protein content in all its subfractions. Apoprotein electrophoresis showed an increase in "arginine-rich" peptide in the VLDL and the HDL fraction and, as noted, a reduction of apoprotein CII, which is transferred to VLDL from HDL and which functions as an activator of the enzyme lipoprotein lipase.[102]

TREATMENT. The standard dietary therapy of patients with type IV hyperlipoproteinemia in the absence of renal failure consists of weight reduction, limitation of alcohol intake, and a reduction in carbohydrate consumption (p. 1140). In patients with chronic renal failure the lipid abnormality usually is not associated with excessive body weight or alcohol consumption, and a reduction in carbohydrate intake is somewhat difficult to achieve, owing to the limitations imposed on the patient's diet by virtue of the reduced protein intake. A reasonable therapeutic approach is to provide caloric replacement through increases in polyunsaturated fat in the diet.[103] With this diet, a significant reduction in plasma triglyceride levels has been observed, both in conservatively treated patients with chronic renal failure and in patients on dialysis.[104]

If conservative measures are unsuccessful, drug therapy may be necessary. *Clofibrate* normally is metabolized by the kidney, and active metabolites can accumulate in patients with severely compromised renal function[105]; patients with renal failure may develop severe myositis in association with the ingestion of the usual doses of this drug.[106] A reduction in total dosage of clofibrate to 1.5 gm per week may lead to a lowering of plasma triglyceride concentration without producing myositis. However, even with this reduced dosage, an increase in serum creatine kinase levels has been reported, presumably as a consequence of damage to skeletal muscle. The metabolism of *gemfibrozil*, another fibric acid derivative, is not dependent on renal function. Modification of the usual dosage of 600 mg twice daily is *not* necessary in patients with renal failure.[106] Although it may be an effective lipid-lowering agent, experience with gemfibrozil in patients with renal dysfunction is small. Neither clofibrate nor gemfibrozil is effectively removed by hemodialysis or peritoneal dialysis. The efficacy and safety of *lovastatin*, an HMG-CoA reductase inhibitor, in patients with chronic renal failure is still being evaluated but appears to be promising. Because less than 10 per cent of the drug is excreted into the urine, it is not necessary to adjust the dosage, which should start at 10 mg twice daily and be slowly increased as needed over a period of months up to a dose of 40 mg twice daily.[106] *Nicotinic acid* also may be used in uremic patients but should be introduced slowly to avoid side effects, starting with a low dose of 100 mg three times daily.

Chronic renal failure can impair cardiac performance by a variety of mechanisms (Table 62–2). It has been found that left ventricular stroke work index, end-diastolic pressure, and size are increased in many patients with end-stage renal disease.[107] Left ventricular hypertrophy also is a frequent finding. In addition, an increase in pulmonary capillary permeability tending to lead to pulmonary edema, even in the absence of elevation of pulmonary capillary wedge pressure, has been reported in renal insufficiency.[108] Impairment of cardiac performance also occurs secondary to ischemic heart disease (see above). The possibility must be considered that dialysis results in the depletion of essential substances; water-soluble vitamins are dialyzable, and it has been suggested that their loss can lead to beriberi heart disease.[109] Therefore, it seems desirable to provide appropriate vitamin supplements for patients on maintenance hemodialysis. Long-term dialysis may deplete other, as yet unidentified, substances necessary for normal cardiac performance, but this has not been established.

The possibility that the uremic state depresses myocardial function is intriguing. As early as 1944, Raab suggested that specific myocardial toxins might be present in uremia.[110] Depression of cardiac function in isolated rat heart preparations perfused with urea, creatinine, guanidinosuccinic acid, and methyl-guanidine—singly and in combination—has been reported.[111] Uremia produces serious disturbances in monovalent cation transport. Red blood cells, leukocytes, lung, and bone from patients with renal insufficiency have an elevated sodium content and a reduction in ouabain-sensitive Na-K–activated adenosinetriphosphatase activity.[112] It is possible that the same fundamental abnormality is responsible for the observed reduction in human skeletal muscle transmembrane potential, which returns toward normal with vigorous hemodialysis.

The observation that cardiac function in patients with renal failure improves after parathyroidectomy has led to the suggestion that parathyroid hormone (PTH) may depress myocardial function.[113] PTH itself stimulates myocardial cell cyclic adenosine monophosphate production, which has been shown to impair energy metabolism, increase cell calcium content, and result in myocardial cell death.[114] Furthermore, abnormally increased myocardial calcium content has been found to correlate with depression of left ventricular ejection fraction in dialysis patients.[115] Thus, PTH-enhanced myocardial calcium uptake may result in myocardial dysfunction. However, data on the cardiosuppressive effects of PTH have been conflicting.[116]

IMPAIRMENT OF VENTRICULAR FUNCTION IN UREMIA. Although the presence of *cardiomyopathy* in uremic patients has been suggested, its existence as a specific entity has been difficult to document in view of the many other possible causes of cardiac dysfunction in such patients.[117] One study involving patients not on dialysis has documented abnormal left ventricular function with exercise early in renal disease that was unrelated to the degree of anemia or the presence of an arteriovenous fistula or of hypertension.[118] This suggests that cardiac performance can become abnormal relatively early in renal failure. Other studies have failed to show an abnormal left ventricular response to exercise in end-stage renal disease patients compared with controls.[118a]

In a study of dialysis patients carefully selected for the absence of coronary disease, valvular abnormalities, diabetes, or hypertension, left ventricular dilatation and hypertrophy were both present.[118b] Furthermore, the ratio of left ventricular radius to left ventricular wall thickness was higher in dialysis patients compared with controls. This observation implies an impaired ability of the uremic myocardium to hypertrophy, resulting in a ventricular mass inadequately adapted to chamber size and pressure.

There is suggestive evidence that uremia-induced myocardial dysfunction may be reversible. Hemodialysis has been found to raise the left ventricular ejection fraction, both

Hypertension	Increased ventricular afterload
Hypervolemia	Increased ventricular preload
Anemia	Increased cardiac work (high-output state)
Lipid abnormalities	Increased atherogenesis
Pericarditis	Restriction of ventricular filling

Ionic alterations
  Hyperkalemia
  Hypocalcemia
  Hypermagnesemia
  Metabolic acidosis
	Negative inotropic effect

Disordered calcium and vitamin D metabolism	(A) Metastatic calcification (cardiac and vascular) (B) ? Vitamin D deficiency cardiomyopathy
Arteriovenous shunt for hemodialysis	Increased cardiac work (high-output state)
Thiamine depletion by dialysis Beriberi (?)	Increased cardiac work (high-output state)
Uremic toxins (?)	Depressed contractility; ? cardiomyopathy

acutely and chronically,[119,120] the greatest improvement occurring in patients with dilated hearts. Reductions in ventricular dilatation and hypertrophy also have been noted with hemodialysis. Some investigators have concluded that an increase in contractile state accounts for the beneficial effects of hemodialysis on cardiac performance.[119,121] In one study comparing different isovolemic dialysis regimens, an increase in ionized plasma calcium was identified as a key factor in this increased contractility.[119] Others suggest that changes in preload and afterload constitute the dominant mechanism.[110,120] It is likely that a combination of these factors is important, depending on the clinical status of the patient and the type of dialysis procedure performed.[121] Left ventricular function also has been found to improve with peritoneal dialysis.[122]

Chronic anemia is another important factor leading to myocardial dysfunction in dialysis patients. Increases in both left ventricular mass index[123] and left ventricular end-diastolic diameter[124] have been found to correlate with the severity of the anemia. Recent studies with recombinant human erythropoietin in hemodialysis patients have shown decreases in

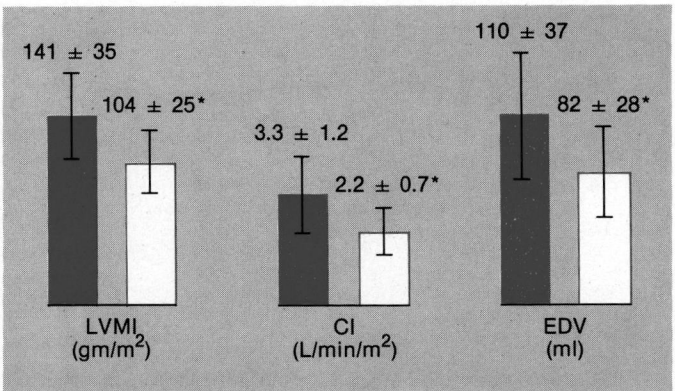

FIGURE 62–9. Echocardiographic changes after kidney transplantation. In 41 patients there were significant decreases in left ventricular mass index (LVMI), cardiac index (CI), and end-diastolic volume (EDV), as measured by echocardiography. Shaded bars = before transplantation; open bars = after transplantation (*p < .05). (From Himmelman, R. B., Landzberg, J. S., Simonson, J. S. et al.: Cardiac consequences of renal transplantation: Changes in left ventricular morphology and function. J. Am. Coll. Cardiol. *12*:915, 1988, by permission of the American College of Cardiology.)

ventricular diameters and improved contractility as hematocrit increases.[125,125a] However, no change in ventricular wall thickness was noted in this short-term study; long-term studies need to be performed to assess the full impact of this hormone on the heart.

After kidney transplantation, serial echocardiograms have documented regression of left ventricular hypertrophy.[126,127] Posttransplant decreases in cardiac index and left ventricular end-diastolic volume also have been found, indicating an improvement over the pretransplant hyperdynamic state (Fig. 62–9). In addition to improvements in lipid profile and blood pressure, these hemodynamic changes may contribute to a decreased cardiac mortality in renal transplant patients.[128] Of interest, no improvement in indices of diastolic function has been noted, which may reflect irreversible myocardial calcification or fibrosis in end-stage renal disease. Finally, dialysis patients with dilated nonischemic cardiomyopathy and class III or IV heart failure have shown symptomatic improvement, as well as increases in ejection fraction, after kidney transplantation.[129] Therefore, patients should not necessarily be denied kidney transplantation, if they are otherwise good transplant candidates.

CARDIOVASCULAR COMPLICATIONS OF HEMODIALYSIS

TECHNICAL CONSIDERATIONS

Hemodialysis is designed to accomplish three objectives. It may (1) remove solutes, (2) alter the electrolyte concentration of the extracellular fluid, and (3) remove as much as 1 liter of extracellular fluid per hour. These three processes should be viewed as being essentially independent of one another, and in the course of a single dialysis it often is desirable to carry out only one or two of these three functions.

HYPOTENSION. A significant fall in blood pressure is a common problem in patients undergoing hemodialysis, occurring in 25 to 50 per cent of dialysis procedures. Many interacting factors appear to be responsible (Fig. 62–10). Ultrafiltration of fluid leads to hypovolemia with a concomitant reduction of venous return and cardiac output. Plasma osmolarity, which falls during dialysis, favors water movement out of the extracellular and into the intracellular space.[130] Autonomic dysfunction, which occurs in up to 50 per cent of dialysis patients,[84] prevents normal compensatory cardioacceleration and an increase in vascular tone. The most common defect seems to reside in the afferent limb of the baroreceptor reflex arc.[84,130] High extracorporeal blood volume, a high blood flow rate, and an underestimation of "dry weight" after dialysis also predispose to hypotension. Drugs that lower blood pressure, such as antihypertensives, some antiarrhythmics, narcotic analgesics, and anxiolytic medications, are commonly prescribed to dialysis patients.

Cardiac disorders that may cause or contribute to hypotension during dialysis include arrhythmias, pericardial effusion with tamponade, cardiomyopathy, and myocardial ischemia. Hypoxemia also should be considered (see below). Finally, acetate, a common dialysate base, has been implicated as a vasodilator and myocardial depressant.[131] Because acetate is metabolized to bicarbonate primarily in muscle cells, it appears to be most poorly tolerated by patients with low muscle mass, typically elderly women. Patients with autonomic insufficiency also may be particularly intolerant of acetate.[132]

The incidence of hypotensive episodes can be reduced by identifying and treating the conditions discussed. Simple measures such as decreasing the size of the dialyzer, removing less fluid during the treatment, or withholding antihypertensive medications before dialysis may be effective. A change in dialysate solution also may be useful. A dialysate sodium concentration that exceeds 135 mEq/liter will reduce the fall in plasma osmolarity and has been shown to improve hemodynamic stability.[133,134] Substituting bicarbonate for acetate as the dialysate base also may be helpful.[131] Finally, sequential ultrafiltration followed by isovolemic dialysis can ameliorate the occurrence of hypotension.[135]

ELECTROLYTE SHIFTS. In adjusting electrolyte concentrations, it is important to appreciate that most dialysates contain 1.5 to 3.0 mEq/liter of potassium and 3.0 to 3.5 mEq/liter of calcium (6 to 7 mg/dl of ionized Ca^{++}). Because most patients commence dialysis with somewhat high serum potassium levels, serum potassium may fall precipitously when dialysis begins, whereas the concentration of ionized calcium rises, setting the stage for digitalis intoxication in digitalized patients (p. 490). This complication is even more likely in cases of digoxin excess, which might come about if the dosage has not been adjusted downward to take into consideration the markedly prolonged half-life of this drug in patients with renal failure (p. 489). A close correlation between the rise in ionized serum calcium and improved myocardial performance has been noted (see above).[119]

ARTERIOVENOUS FISTULAS. To achieve vascular access for dialysis, an arteriovenous fistula must be created. These shunts have a flow rate of 250 to 750 ml/minute, and thereby add to the cardiac workload. As discussed on page 459, in association with the anemia characteristic of chronic renal failure, this may contribute to the development of high-output heart failure.[136] This form of heart failure can be readily controlled if any excess fluid accumulation is prevented by ultrafiltration during dialysis and if the anemia is partially treated by transfusion. It is desirable to use only a single vascular access site at any one time and to limit the size of the anastomosis to the smallest required for successful dialysis. The contribution of the fistula to the heart failure state can be determined by studying the effect of occlusion of the fistula on left ventricular function, as assessed by echocardiography or radionuclide ventriculography.

Infection is a major complication of arteriovenous shunts and may become metastatic. Septic pulmonary emboli and infective endocarditis, most often staphylococcal, have been reported.[68] Because patients on hemodialysis often have functional systolic and occasionally even diastolic murmurs, which may change with the patient's altered hemodynamic

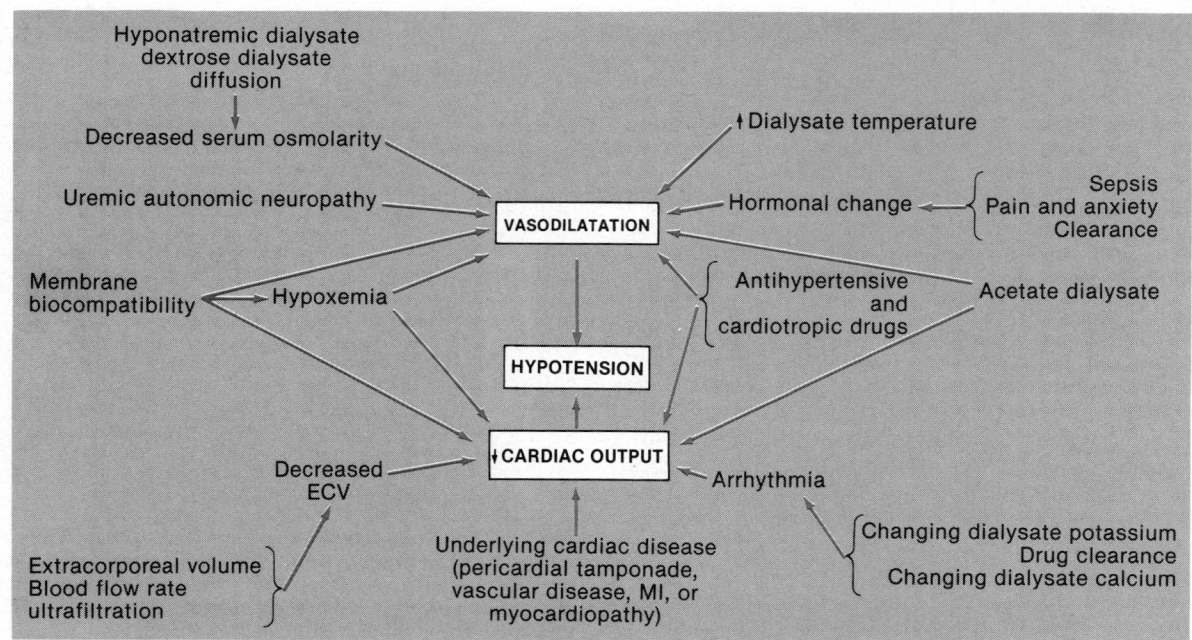

FIGURE 62–10. Major factors leading to dialysis-induced hypotension. (From Hakim, R. M., and Lazarus, J. M.: *Medical aspects of hemodialysis. In* Brenner, B. M., and Rector, F. C. [eds.]: The Kidney. Philadelphia, W. B. Saunders Company, 1986. p. 1820.)

status, the diagnosis of endocarditis may be missed. Therefore, the *early* diagnosis of endocarditis in patients with infected vascular access sites depends on a high index of clinical suspicion and immediate blood cultures. The diagnosis of infective endocarditis may be difficult, since an infected vascular access site without infection of the endocardium can also give rise to positive blood cultures.

HYPOXEMIA. A fall in arterial oxygen tension of 10 to 15 mm Hg frequently occurs within the first 30 minutes of hemodialysis and persists throughout the procedure.[137] This event is undesirable in patients with heart or lung disease, and may lead to serious hypoxemia in patients with even mild arterial desaturation at the commencement of the hemodialysis. Together with the electrolyte changes during hemodialysis referred to above, it may lower the threshold for the development of arrhythmias. Also, the PEP : LVET ratio may increase significantly during dialysis,[138] an increase that correlates significantly with the fall in arterial oxygen tension, suggesting that the latter actually impairs left ventricular function.

The mechanism responsible for the decline in arterial PO_2 during dialysis is in some dispute and is probably multifactorial. It has been reported that activation of complement leads to aggregation of neutrophils in the lungs, which interferes with normal oxygenation.[139] This is particularly observed with cuprophane membranes and not with more biocompatible membranes such as polyacrylonitryl.[140] An additional explanation is that physiological hypoventilation occurs secondary to diffusion of carbon dioxide across the dialyzer. Changing from an acetate- to a bicarbonate-buffered dialysate may prevent this loss of carbon dioxide and lessen the decrease in arterial PO_2.[139]

Of interest, mechanically ventilated patients show a decrease in arterial oxygen tension during dialysis; this indicates that hypoventilation alone cannot account for the observed hypoxemia.[141] Whatever the mechanism, patients with impaired pulmonary function and severe heart disease should be monitored for arterial hypoxemia during the early phase of dialysis and may require inhalation of oxygen during the procedure.

POTASSIUM BALANCE

Life-threatening hyperkalemia may occur in acute oliguric renal failure, in end-stage chronic renal failure, and, rarely, in terminal heart failure (p. 455). The principal detrimental effect of hyperkalemia is in its electrical effect on the heart. The progressive electrocardiographic abnormalities associated with hyperkalemia are shown in Figure 5–51, p. 150. The earliest electrocardiographic sign of hyperkalemia usually is peaking of the T waves, followed progressively by an increase in T-wave amplitude, a widening of the QRS complex, and loss of atrial activity. Finally, with extreme hyperkalemia, a sine wave pattern is noted on the electrocardiogram, followed by cardiac arrest. Unfortunately only a rough correlation exists between the level of serum potassium and the electrocardiographic changes, although in any given patient directional changes in the serum potassium level can be estimated from the electrocardiogram. Even severe hyperkalemia per se produces few, if any, symptoms; occasionally weakness of skeletal muscles or dyspnea presumably secondary to paralysis of respiratory muscles may be noted.

TREATMENT. Severe hyperkalemia is a medical emergency, and its treatment usually can be divided into acute and chronic phases. The most rapid means of counteracting the toxic cardiac effects of potassium is with the administration of intravenous calcium, given in the form of 10 to 20 ml of 10 per cent *calcium chloride* with electrocardiographic monitoring to assure that the signs of hyperkalemia have been reversed. Although administration of calcium chloride is an effective emergency measure, it does not lower the elevated serum potassium concentration.

The second aspect of therapy relies on lowering the serum potassium level. In patients with hyperkalemia and acidosis, *sodium bicarbonate* will reduce the level of serum potassium; the usual dose is 1 to 2 ampules (44 to 88 mEq) administered intravenously. The reduction in [K+] is caused in part by an exchange of hydrogen and potassium ions across cell membranes as well as enhanced secretion of potassium in the distal tubule. Bicarbonate administration lowers serum [K+] in hyperkalemic patients even if the serum pH is not affected, implying a specific effect of the bicarbonate anion itself.[142] The administration of 10 units of regular insulin will result in the redistribution of [K+] from the extracellular to the intracellular space. This should be followed by 50 ml of 50 per cent *glucose* to prevent hypoglycemia. The effects of bicarbonate or glucose and insulin administration can be observed within 15 to 30 minutes and may last for several hours. Although these forms of therapy are useful for rapidly lowering the serum [K+] concentration, they do *not* lower total body potassium stores.

Further treatment of hyperkalemia involves removal of potassium from the body, which can be accomplished by the administration of *cation exchange resins* by enema or orally. The resin most commonly used is sodium polystyrene sulfonate (Kayexalate), 1 gm of which administered orally exchanges approximately 1 mEq of sodium for potassium. The usual dose is 50 gm two or three times daily. When administered orally, it

is desirable to accompany it with an osmotic cathartic to prevent intestinal obstruction as a consequence of inspissation of the resin in the gut.

The most effective means of reducing the body's potassium stores is by means of *dialysis*, either hemodialysis or peritoneal dialysis. However, when using these modalities, one must exercise care not to lower the serum potassium too precipitously, especially in those patients who are receiving cardiac glycosides. This can be accomplished by beginning with a dialysis solution having a potassium concentration of approximately 4 mEq/liter and then progressively lowering it as serum potassium declines.

SECONDARY HYPERPARATHYROIDISM (see also p. 1841)

Ectopic calcification in a variety of tissues, including the heart and arterial bed, is a common manifestation of secondary hyperparathyroidism. This frequent complication of chronic renal failure may involve the sinoatrial and atrioventricular nodes, the intima and media of epicardial coronary arteries, the interventricular septum, the ventricular myocardium, and the valvular annuli and cusps, particularly the mitral annulus and the aortic valve, as shown in Figure 62–11.[143-146] One prospective echocardiographic study identified aortic valve calcification in 28 per cent, and mitral valve calcification in 36 per cent, of 87 maintenance hemodialysis patients.[147] Furthermore, clinically significant valvular stenosis of a tricuspid aortic valve, and less frequently of the mitral valve, may occur. Other clinical and electrocardiographic changes resulting from tissue calcification include varying degrees of atrioventricular block, sinus node dysfunction, supraventricular arrhythmias, infective endocarditis, embolism, mitral regurgitation, and left ventricular failure (see above).[148]

As many as half the patients on maintenance hemodialysis have been reported to have radiological evidence of arterial calcification[149]; calcium deposition usually is in the media, leading to Mönckeberg's sclerosis.[150] Calcium deposition may be associated with almost complete obliteration of the vascu-

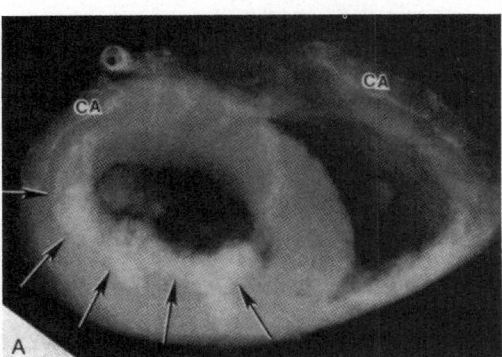

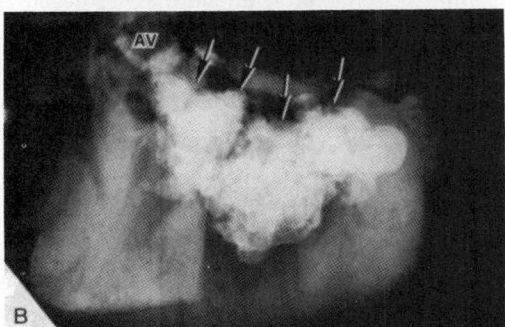

FIGURE 62–11. Postmortem roentgenograms showing severe mitral annular calcification in two patients on hemodialysis. *A*, Superior view of heart showing extensive posterior mitral annular *(arrows)* and coronary arterial (CA) calcification in a patient on dialysis for 14.5 years. *B*, Posteroanterior view of heart revealing extensive calcific deposits in mitral valve apparatus (arrows) and mild calcific deposits in the aortic valve (AV) in a patient on hemodialysis for 7 years. (From Forman, M. B., et al.: Mitral annular calcification in chronic renal failure. Chest **85:**367, 1984.)

lar lumen, and may result in ischemia and, ultimately, gangrene of tissue distal to the involved vessels.[149,150] Case-control studies have shown mitral annular calcification in those dialysis patients with higher ionized calcium, phosphorus, and calcium–phosphorus product levels. These findings suggest that vigorous attempts to normalize calcium–phosphorus metabolism may decrease the incidence of this complication in patients with chronic renal failure.[143,144]

The most effective *treatment* of secondary hyperparathyroidism consists of kidney transplantation or subtotal parathyroidectomy. For patients maintained on dialysis, dietary phospate restriction, calcium supplementation, nonabsorbable aluminum-containing antacids, and oral dihydrotachysterol (a synthetic analog of vitamin D) given in doses of 0.125 to 1.0 mg daily, or 1,25-dihydroxycholecalciferol $(1,25(OH)_2D_3)$ in a dose of 0.25 to 1.0 μg daily also are useful measures.[151,152] Intravenous doses of up to 4.0 μg of $1,25(OH)_2D_3$ after hemodialysis have been shown to markedly suppress PTH levels.[153] Whether this "medical parathyroidectomy" will control secondary hyperparathyroidism over the long term is unknown.

UREMIC PERICARDITIS (see also p. 1496)

Pericarditis is a common complication of both acute and chronic renal failure. Before the era of dialysis the appearance of pericarditis in the uremic patient usually was taken as a sign of terminal renal failure.[154] The incidence of clinically significant pericarditis appears to be declining with the increasing use of early dialysis before progression to advanced uremia. Echocardiography has revealed pericardial effusions in 32 to 56 per cent of patients at the initiation of dialysis, most of which are asymptomatic.[155] The mechanism by which pericarditis and pericardial effusions develop is not clear, but is probably related to the accumulation of uremic toxins, which are responsible for an inflammatory serositis. Volume overload also has been implicated as an important causative factor.[155] The serositis most commonly involves the pericardium but also can involve the pleura.[156] Fibrinous pleuritis, pleural friction rubs,[157] hemorrhagic pleural effusion, and pneumonitis[156] also have been reported to occur in uremia.

A review of published studies reveals that approximately 15 per cent of end-stage renal disease patients develop pericarditis at some time. In renal failure patients, pericarditis carries an average mortality rate of nearly 13 per cent, and in total accounts for about 2.8 per cent of deaths of dialysis patients.[158] Pericarditis that occurs in patients on stable chronic dialysis may be related to inadequate dialysis or to an intercurrent illness, such as a viral infection. In patients with renal failure, pericarditis may be preceded by an otherwise benign respiratory tract infection. Bacterial infection, cytomegalovirus infection, and other conditions such as systemic lupus erythematosus, polyarteritis nodosa, and acute myocardial infarction also have been implicated as causes.[159] In most stable chronic dialysis patients the cause of pericarditis is not certain; the incidence appears to be less in patients on peritoneal dialysis than in those on hemodialysis.

CLINICAL MANIFESTATIONS. The clinical features of uremic pericarditis are summarized in Table 62–3. The diagnosis is made by the same clinical criteria used for other forms of pericarditis, i.e., chest pain usually ameliorated by sitting up and leaning forward, typical echocardiographic changes, increases in heart size on chest roentgenogram, and, with severe pericarditis, evidence of circulatory embarrassment. With echocardiography, small asymptomatic pericardial effusions can be found in approximately one-third of patients on chronic maintenance hemodialysis.[159-161] On electrocardiogram atrial arrhythmias are the most common abnormality, occurring in about 15 per cent of cases. The development of hypotension during dialysis that cannot be readily attributed to changes in intravascular volume is a useful clue to the presence of significant pericardial effusion. A pericardial friction rub is present in almost every patient at some time during

TABLE 62–3   CLINICAL FEATURES OF UREMIC PERICARDITIS

FEATURE	FREQUENCY (%)
Pain	66
Pericardial friction rub	93
Fever	84
Leukocytosis	56
Arrhythmias	23
Hypotension	56
Hepatomegaly	60
Elevated venous pressure	71
Abnormal electrocardiogram	90
Enlarged cardiac silhouette	96

For sources of above data, see Chap. 45.

the course of pericarditis, and should be diligently looked for. However, the diagnosis of pericarditis may be made in error. Many uremic patients develop a systolic ejection murmur, probably related to the high-output state secondary to chronic anemia. Some patients with chronic renal failure and hypertension develop diastolic blowing murmurs resembling those caused by aortic regurgitation, and the combination of these two murmurs may be mistaken for a to-and-fro pericardial friction rub.

Cardiac tamponade, described on page 1473, complicates uremic pericarditis in about 20 per cent of patients[162,163]; it is the major serious complication of pericarditis, and can be lethal. Pericardial fluid usually is exudative and bloody; the heparinization required for hemodialysis may cause serious bleeding into the pericardial cavity in patients with pericarditis. Therefore, it is important to limit the degree of heparinization during hemodialysis as much as possible in the presence of active pericarditis and large effusions. However, systemic heparinization can be used safely in patients with small pericardial effusions without associated physical signs and symptoms of active pericarditis. Chronic constrictive pericarditis is an unusual complication of uremic pericarditis, and has been reported to develop in less than 5 per cent of patients.[162]

TREATMENT. A distinction should be made between "uremic pericarditis" in patients who have not previously been dialyzed, or have initiated dialysis within a few weeks of the episode of pericarditis, and "dialysis pericarditis" in patients on a stable peritoneal or hemodialysis regimen. In a literature review, 50 of 65 reported patients with uremic pericarditis responded to dialysis therapy alone, whereas only 8 of 64 patients with dialysis pericarditis responded to dialysis alone.[158] This difference indicates that uremic toxins are more likely to be responsible for pericardial inflammation in previously undialyzed patients.

Dialysis patients with moderate or large effusions are unlikely to improve with dialysis.[159,163] Elective pericardiocentesis has previously been advocated to drain the pericardial space in such patients, and may be accompanied with the instillation of nonabsorbable corticosteroids into the pericardial cavity.[164] In most centers elective pericardiocentesis is associated with an unacceptable mortality rate approaching 10 per cent,[165] and it is successful in only about 25 per cent of cases.[158] In contrast, surgical drainage is a safe and effective method of draining the pericardial space. Placement of a pericardial window of at least 4 × 4 cm, using the subxiphoid approach, appears to be the safest surgical drainage procedure.[166] The choice of operation should depend on the local experience of the thoracic surgeon, and may include thoracotomy with pericardial window or total pericardiectomy, subxiphoid tube drainage, or pericardiectomy by way of median sternotomy.[167] Oral indomethacin has been suggested as an adjunct to the therapy of pericarditis, but a controlled study has failed to show an effect of this drug on the duration of chest pain, pericardial friction rub, the amount of effusion, or the need for surgery.[163]

It is our practice to treat pericarditis in end-stage renal disease patients with vigorous dialysis if the patient is hemodynamically stable. The size of the effusion should be followed by serial two-dimensional echocardiography. If hemodynamic instability develops, the effusion does not decrease in size, or the effusion enlarges over a period of 1 to 2 weeks, then a subxiphoid pericardial window is placed. In patients already on a stable dialysis regimen who have a moderate or large effusion, immediate elective surgical drainage is strongly considered, as the likelihood of responding to intensive dialysis is small. Emergency pericardiocentesis is reserved for patients with cardiac tamponade, and is closely followed by surgical decompression. Pericardial stripping is the treatment of choice in the rare patient with subacute or chronic constrictive pericarditis.[168]

MANAGEMENT OF PATIENTS WITH CARDIAC DISEASE AND RENAL FAILURE

With the greater availability of dialysis facilities and broader criteria for acceptance of patients into treatment programs for end-stage renal disease, this patient population now encompasses people in whom other diseases may be present, including cardiac disease that may require surgical treatment. Because of the high frequency of coronary artery disease among patients with chronic renal failure and the occasional presence of coexisting valvular heart disease, cardiopulmonary bypass often is a consideration. Patients on maintenance hemodialysis can undergo major operations without excess mortality or morbidity, and several series have been published documenting the ability of patients with renal failure to tolerate open heart surgery, both coronary revascularization and valve replacement.[169] Among patients with end-stage renal disease, cardiac operations may be performed with equal success regardless of whether the renal failure has been treated by dialysis or transplantation.

The major problems associated with operation in patients with chronic renal failure include the development of hyperkalemia, fluid overload, and arrhythmias. With the appropriate use of hemodialysis both before and after operation and careful monitoring of the patient's hemodynamic and electrolyte status, the excess risks have been contained. Although many observers think that patients who have severely impaired renal failure but who do not yet require hemodialysis may undergo cardiac surgery without hemodialysis, others dialyze patients who have a glomerular filtration rate less than 20 per cent of normal on several occasions in the days before and after such operations.

The management of patients with hypertrophic obstructive cardiomyopathy (p. 1404) and chronic renal failure presents a unique problem. It is well established that these patients are particularly sensitive to acute changes in blood volume and to tachyarrhythmias. During hemodialysis, blood volume ordinarily is reduced. Although most patients tolerate this volume depletion without difficulty, many of those with hypertrophic cardiomyopathy develop an acute increase in obstruction to left ventricular outflow. This complication can be avoided by using a dialysis apparatus that requires a low extracorporeal volume and allows precise control of ultrafiltration. In addition, these patients are treated with beta-adrenergic receptor blockers or calcium antagonists and are treated with erythropoietin to maintain a hematocrit in the range of 30 per cent.

MODIFICATION OF COMMON CARDIAC MEDICATIONS IN PATIENTS WITH RENAL FAILURE

Because many drugs (and/or their active metabolites) used in the treatment of heart disease are excreted by the kidney, renal failure affects the pharmacokinetics of many agents, including those commonly used to treat heart disease. Information on the pharmacokinetics of important cardiac medications and dosage adjustments in renal failure are listed in Table 62-4.

CARDIAC GLYCOSIDES (see also p. 479). *Digoxin* is filtered by the glomeruli, and its renal excretion is directly proportional to the glomerular filtration rate. It is not altered by the rate of urine flow and therefore by the administration of diuretics[170]; only very small quantities of digoxin may be secreted by the distal convoluted tubule.[171] The ratio of the clearance of digoxin to endogenous creatinine is 0.8, and the percentage of the body's total stores of digoxin lost per day can be calculated as $14 + 0.2 \times$ creatinine clearance in milliliters per minute. Thus 85 per cent of administered digoxin normally is excreted in the urine, most in unchanged form, and only 10 to 15 per cent is eliminated in the stool through biliary excretion. Normally, 38 per cent of the body's stores of digoxin are either metabolized or excreted per day,[172] whereas in anephric patients only 14 per cent of total body digoxin stores are eliminated per day by way of the biliary tree. Therefore, in the patient with impaired renal function, digoxin elimination is reduced to approximately 37 per cent of normal, and digoxin dosage should be modified accordingly.

In patients with end-stage renal disease who require treatment with digoxin, a loading dose of 0.25 mg and maintenance doses of 0.125 mg every other day are recommended. Digoxin levels are determined 1 week later, and depending on the clinical response, the dose is modified, usually upward, to 0.125 mg orally daily. However, in the emergency setting, when rapid digitalization is required, the *loading* dose of digoxin does not need to be reduced. In contrast to digoxin, the half-life of *digitoxin* is not greatly affected by impaired renal function,[173] and therefore dosage does not need to be altered in patients with renal failure. Because of high tissue and protein binding of both digoxin and digitoxin, little removal occurs with either hemodialysis or peritoneal dialysis.[174] Therefore, these methods are ineffective in the treatment of digitalis overdose in which Fab fragments are the treatment of choice in life-threatening cases.[175]

ANTIARRHYTHMIC DRUGS (see also Chap. 23). The dose of *procainamide* (p. 636) must be modified in patients with end-stage renal disease because this drug normally is eliminated by both renal excretion and hepatic metabolism. Procainamide is readily dialyzable.[176]

Quinidine (p. 634) is metabolized by a variety of tissues, including the liver, mostly to hydroxy derivatives; no specific modification of the dose is necessary in patients with impaired renal function. Quinidine prolongs the half-life of digoxin in patients with renal failure. Therefore, a decrease in digoxin dosage may be required when both drugs are administered.[177] Because quinidine is about 80 per cent protein-bound and is widely distributed in tissue, clearance by dialysis would be expected to be quite poor; indeed, clearance by peritoneal dialysis has been found to be less than 10 ml/min.[178]

The half-life of *lidocaine* (p. 639) is about an hour, and its deactivation largely depends on hepatic metabolism; no dosage modification is necessary in patients with renal failure.[179] It is not removed by hemodialysis.

The liver also is the principal site of inactivation of *phenytoin* (p. 641).[180] Because of the diminished protein-binding of the drug in patients with renal failure, the ranges of therapeutic and toxic levels of total drug are lower than those in patients with normal renal function. Alternatively, free levels of the drug can be measured. No alteration in dosage is necessary in chronic renal failure. As is the case for most antiarrhythmic agents, phenytoin is poorly dialyzed.

Propranolol (p. 644) is used extensively in patients with renal failure for its effects on arterial pressure, angina pectoris, and, less commonly, cardiac arrhythmias. Because it is metabolized primarily by the liver, its half-life is not altered by renal failure.[181] It is largely protein-bound (90 per cent) and has a large volume of distribution[182]; therefore, it is not surprising that it is poorly dialyzed. The long-acting beta blockers *atenolol* and *nadolol* are cleared by the kidney, so that toxic levels may accumulate in patients with renal failure if dosage is not adjusted. They may both be removed by hemodialysis.[183]

Mexiletine (p. 640) is an antiarrhythmic agent which is he-

TABLE 62-4 CARDIOVASCULAR DRUG THERAPY IN RENAL DISEASE

DRUG	Elimination and Metabolism	Half-life Normal (hr)	Half-life ESRD (hr)	Plasma Protein Binding (%)	Volume of Distribution (liters/kg)	Method	GFR (ml/min) >50	GFR (ml/min) 10-50	GFR (ml/min) <10	Removed by Dialysis
Adrenergic modulators and blockers										
Clonidine	Renal	6-23	39-42	20-40	3-6	D	U	U	50-75	No (H)
Guanethidine	Renal (nonrenal)	Biphasic: 48-72 and 96-196[a]	?	0	?	I	24	24	24-36	?
Methyldopa[b]	Renal (hepatic 18%-48%)	Biphasic: 1.4 and 5.8[a]	3-6 and 7-16[a]	<15	0.51	I	6	9-18	12-24	Yes (H, P)
Prazosin	Hepatic (renal)	2-3[c]	?	97	1.2-1.7	D	U	U	U	No (H, P)
Reserpine	Hepatic (GI)	Biphasic: 4.5 and 50-170[a]	87-320	40	?	D	U	U	Avoid	No (H, P)
Angiotensin-converting enzyme inhibitors										
Captopril	Renal (hepatic)	1.9	21-32	25-30	0.7	D	U	U	50	Yes (H)
						I	8-24	24-72	72-108	
Enalapril	Hepatic	24-36	40-60	50-60	?	D	100	75-100	50	Yes (H)
Lisinopril	Renal	12-36	36-48	0-10	1.2-1.4	D	100	75	25-50	Yes (H)
Antiarrhythmic agents[d]										
N-Acetylprocainamide	Renal	6-8	42-70	10	1.5-1.7	I[e]	U	6	12	Yes (H)
						D[e]	U	50	25	
Amiodarone	Hepatic	3-100 Days	U	96	Variable: 1-148	D	U	U	U	No (H)
Bretylium	Renal (non-renal 20%)	6 (PO) 13.6 (IV)	16-32	6	8	D	U	25-50[f]	Avoid[f]	?
Disopyramide	Renal and hepatic	5-8	10-18	5-80	0.8-2.6	I	U	12-24	24-40	No (H)
Encainide	Hepatic	1-3	1-3	71-78	2.7	D	U	50	25	?
Flecainide	Hepatic (renal)	14-20	19-26	50	8-9.5	D	U	U	50-75	No (H)
Lidocaine	Hepatic (renal <20%)	1.2-2.2	1.3-3.0	60-66	1.3-2.2	D	U	U	U	No (H)
Lorcainide	Hepatic	7-13	?	80-85	6-17	D	U	U	U	?
Mexiletine	Hepatic (renal)	8-13	16	75	5.5-6.6	D	U	U	50-75	Yes (H), No (P)
Phenytoin	Hepatic (renal)	24	8	90	0.64	D	U	U	U	No (H)
Procainamide	Renal (hepatic 7%-24%)	2.5-4.9	5.3-5.9	14-23	1.4-2.5	I	4	6-12	8-24	Yes (H)[g]
Quinidine	Hepatic (renal 10%-50%)	5.0-7.2	4-14	70-95	2.0-3.5	I	U	U	U	Yes (H, P)[h]
Tocainide	Hepatic (renal)	11-19	22	10-20	1.6-3.2	D	U	U	50	Yes (H)
Beta blockers										
Acebutolol	Renal (hepatic)	8-9	7	25	1.2	D	U	50[i]	30-50[i]	No (H)
Atenolol	Renal	6-9	15-35	<5	0.7	D	U	50	25[i]	Yes (H), No (P)
						I	24	48	96[i]	
Labetalol	Hepatic	3-8	3-8	50	3-10	D	U	U	U	No (H)
Metoprolol	Hepatic	2.5-4.5	2.5-4.5	12	5-6	D	U	U	U	Yes (H)
Nadolol	Renal	14-24	45	25-30	2	D	U	50	25[i]	Yes (H)
Pindolol	Hepatic (renal)	3-4	3-4	40-57	2	D	U	U	U	?
Propranolol	Hepatic	3.5-6.0	2.3	90-96	3-4	D	U	U	U	No (H)
Sotalol	Renal	5-8	40-50	54	0.7	D	U	30	15-30	Yes (H)
Timolol	Hepatic	3-4	4	10	2-4	D	U	U	U	No (H)
Calcium-channel blockers										
Diltiazem	Hepatic	2-8	2-8	80-86	3-5	D	U	U	U	No (H)
Isradipine	Hepatic	2-5	8.5-14.0	?	1-2	D	U	U	75	?
Nicardipine	Hepatic	1	1	95-98	0.7-0.9	D	U	U	U	No (H)
Nifedipine	Hepatic	4.0-5.5	?	92-98	?	D	U	U	U	No (H)
Nimodipine	Hepatic	1.0-2.8	22	98	0.9-2.3	D	U	U	U	No (H)
Nitrendipine	Hepatic	12	12	98	3-6	D	U	U	U	No (H)
Verapamil	Hepatic	3-7	2.4-4	83-93	3-6	D	U	U	50-75	No (H)
Cardiac glycosides										
Digitoxin	Hepatic (renal)	144-200	210	94	0.6	D	U	U	50-75	No (H, P)
Digoxin	Renal (nonrenal 15%-40%)	36-44	80-120[i]	20-30	5-8	D	U	25-75	10-25	No (H, P)
						I	24	36	48	

DRUG	PHARMACOKINETIC PARAMETERS					ADJUSTMENT FOR RENAL FAILURE				
	Elimination and Metabolism	Half-life		Plasma Protein Binding (%)	Volume of Distribution (liters/kg)	Method	GFR (ml/min)			Removed by Dialysis
		Normal (hr)	*ESRD (hr)*				*>50*	*10-50*	*<10*	
Vasodilators										
Diazoxide	Renal (hepatic)	17-31	>30	>90	0.2-0.3	D	U	U	U	Yes (H, P)
Hydralazine	Hepatic (nonrenal)	2.0-4.5	7-16	87	0.5-0.9	I	8	8	8-16 (fast) 12-24 (slow)	No (H, P)
Minoxidil	Hepatic	2.8-4.2	U	0	2-3	D	U	U	U	Yes (H)
Sodium nitroprusside	Nonrenal	<10 min	<10 min	0	0.20	D	U	U	U^k	Yes (H)^k
Agents used for hyperlipoproteinemia										
Cholestyramine	Not absorbed	—	—	—	—	D	U	U	U	—
Clofibrate	Hepatic (renal)	17	46-110	96	0.14	I^l	6-12	12-18	24-48	No (H)
Colestipol	Not absorbed	—	—	—	—	D	U	U	U	—
Gemfibrozil	Renal (fecal)	1.5	?	Low	?	D	U	50	25	?
Lovastatin	Hepatic	6-8	?	95	?	D	U	U	U	?
Nicotinic acid	Hepatic (renal)	0.5-1.0	?	?	?	GD	U	50	25	?

From Bennett, W. M.: Drug therapy in renal disease. *In* Rubenstein, E., and Federman, D. D. (eds.): Scientific American Medicine. New York, Scientific American, Inc. 1990.

[a] Biexponential pharmacokinetics. [b] Prolonged hypotension due to retention of active metabolites in severe renal failure. [c] $T_{1/2}$ increased to 6-7 hr in congestive heart failure. $T_{1/2}$ may be prolonged in heart disease, or with reduced hepatic blood flow, or both. [c] In practice, a combination of dose and interval adjustment may be necessary. [d] $T_{1/2}$ may be prolonged in heart disease, or with reduced hepatic blood flow, or both. [e] In practice, a combination of dose and interval adjustment may be necessary. [f] No specific data in ESRD. [g] May be able to treat poisoning with hemodialysis. [h] Hemodialysis with low potassium bath may be effective for poisoning. [i] Drug or active metabolite with long $T_{1/2}$ accumulates in ESRD. [j] Volume of distribution and total body clearance decreased in ESRD. [k] Need to monitor thiocyanate levels to keep <10 mg/dL; $t_{1/2}$ for thiocyanate is 1 wk; thiocyanate dialyzable. [l] Daily dose should not exceed 0.5 gm for each gram/dl of serum albumin.

$T_{1/2}$ = biological half-life; ESRD = end-stage renal disease; GFR = glomerular filtration rate; I = Interval extension method of dosage adjustment in hours between maintenance doses; D = dose reduction method of dosage adjustment in per cent of usual maintenance dose; H = hemodialysis; P = peritoneal dialysis; U = unchanged.

patically excreted and does not need dose adjustment with renal failure.[184] It is not removed by peritoneal dialysis, but studies of its removal by hemodialysis have been conflicting. Metabolites of *encainide* (p. 642) are more active than encainide itself and are renally excreted.[185] Thus marked dose reductions of this drug are required and 7 days allowed to pass before steady-state levels are achieved in renal failure patients.[186] *Amiodarone* (p. 646) does not require dosage adjustments in patients with renal disease and is not removed by hemodialysis.[184]

OTHER CARDIOVASCULAR DRUGS. The nitrates and the calcium channel antagonists diltiazem, nifedipine, and verapamil are metabolized by the liver, so that no specific dosage reduction is required in end-stage renal disease.[183]

Acknowledgment

The assistance of Dr. T. Dwight McKinney in the preparation of this chapter is gratefully acknowledged.

REFERENCES

EFFECTS OF CARDIAC DISEASE ON RENAL FUNCTION

1. Birkenfeld, L. W., Liebman, J., O'Meara, M. P., and Edelman, I. S.: Total exchangeable sodium, total exchangeable potassium, and total body water in edematous patients with cirrhosis of the liver and congestive heart failure. J. Clin. Invest. 37:687, 1958.
2. Ichikawa, I., Pfeffer, J. M., Pfeffer, J. A., et al.: Role of angiotensin II in the altered renal function in congestive heart failure. Circ. Res. 55:669, 1984.
3. Skorecki, K. L., and Brenner, B. M.: Body fluid homeostasis in congestive heart failure and cirrhosis with ascites. Am. J. Med. 72:323, 1982.
4. Hostetter, T. H., Pfeffer, J. M., Pfeffer, M. A., Braunwald, E., and Brenner, B. M.: Cardiorenal hemodynamics and sodium excretion in rats with myocardial infarction. Am. J. Physiol. 245:H98, 1983.
5. Francis, G. S.: Neurohumoral mechanisms involved in congestive heart failure. Am. J. Cardiol. 55:15A, 1985.
6. Higgins, C. B., Vatner, S. F., Franklin, D., and Braunwald, E.: Effects of experimentally produced heart failure on the peripheral vascular response to severe exercise in conscious dogs. Circ. Res. 31:186, 1972.
7. Cannon, P. J.: Prostaglandins in congestive heart failure and the effects of nonsteroidal anti-inflammatory drugs. Am. J. Med. 81(Suppl. 2B):123, 1986.
8. DiPerri, T., Forconi, S., Puccetti, F., et al.: Effects of prostaglandin A₁ on renal handling of salt and water in congestive heart failure. J. Cardiovasc. Pharmacol. 2:215, 1980.
9. Raymond, K. H., and Lifschitz, M. D.: Effects of prostaglandins on renal salt and water excretion. Am. J. Med. 80(Suppl. 1A):22, 1986.
10. Berliner, R. W., and Davidson, P. G.: Production of hypertonic urine in the absence of pituitary antidiuretic hormone. J. Clin. Invest. 36:1416, 1957.
11. Schrier, R. W.: Pathogenesis of sodium and water retention in high-output and low-output cardiac failure, nephrotic syndrome, cirrhosis, and pregnancy. N. Engl. J. Med. 319:1065, 1988.
12. Ishikawa, S., Saito, T., Okada, K., et al.: Effect of vasopressin antagonist on water excretion in inferior vena cava constriction. Kidney Int. 30:49, 1986.
13. Bichet, D. G., Korta, S. C., Mettauer, B., et al.: Modulation of plasma and platelet vasopressin by cardiac function in patients with heart failure. Kidney Int. 29:1188, 1986.
14. Hakumeki, M. O., Wang, B. C., Sundet, W. D., et al.: Aortic baroreceptor discharge during nonhypotensive hemorrhage in anesthetized dogs. Am. J. Physiol. 249:H393, 1985.
15. Fitzsimmons, J. T.: Thirst, Physiol. Rev. 52:468, 1972.
16. Badr, K. F., and Ichikawa, I. I.: Pre-renal failure: A deleterious shift from renal compensation to decompensation. N. Engl. J. Med. 319:623, 1988.
17. Cogan, M. G.: Atrial natriuretic peptide. Kidney Int. 37:1148, 1990.
18. Smith, H. W.: Salt and water volume receptors: An exercise in physiologic apologetics. Am. J. Med. 23:623, 1957.
19. Fried, T.: Atrial natriuretic factor: A historic perspective. Am. J. Med. Sci. 294:134, 1987.
20. Jamieson, J. D., and Palade, G. E.: Specific granules in atrial muscle. J. Cell. Biol. 23:151, 1964.
21. DeBold, A. J.: Heart atria granularity: Effects of changes in water-electrolyte balance. Proc. Soc. Exp. Biol. Med. 161:508, 1979.
22. DeBold, A. J., Borenstein, H. B., Veress, A. T., and Sonnenberg, H.: A rapid and potent natriuretic response to intravenous injection of atrial myocardial extract in rats. Life Sci. 28:89, 1981.
23. Genest, J., and Cantin, M.: Atrial natriuretic factor. Circulation 75(Suppl. I):118, 1987.
24. Oikawa, S., Imai, M., Ueno, A., et al.: Cloning and sequence analysis of cDNA encoding a precursor for human atrial natriuretic polypeptide. Nature 309:724, 1984.

25. Baxter, J. D., Lewieki, J. A., and Gardner, D. G.: Atrial natriuretic peptide. Bio/technology 6:529, 1988.

26. Saito, Y., Nakao, R. K., Arai, H., et al.: Augmented expression of atrial natriuretic polypeptide gene in ventricle of failing human heart. J. Clin. Invest. 83:298, 1989.

27. Greenwald, J. E., Apkon, M., Hruska, K. A., et al.: Stretch-induced atriopeptin secretion in the isolated rat myocyte and its negative modulation by calcium. J. Clin. Invest. 83:1061, 1989.

28. Dietz, J. R.: Release of natriuretic factor from rat heart-lung preparations by atrial distention. Am. J. Physiol. 247:R1093, 1984.

29. Goetz, K. L., Wang, B. C., Geer, P. G., et al.: Atrial stretch increases sodium excretion independently of release of atrial peptides. Am. J. Physiol. 250:R946, 1986.

30. Shenker, Y., Sider, R. S., Ostafin, E. A., and Grekin, R. J.: Plasma levels of immunoreactive atrial natriuretic factor in healthy subjects and in patients with edema. J. Clin. Invest. 76:1684, 1984.

31. Yamaji, T., Ishibashi, M., and Takaku, F.: Atrial natriuretic factor in human blood. J. Clin. Invest. 76:1705, 1985.

32. Brenner, B. M., Ballerman, B. J., Gunning, M. E., and Zeidel, M. L.: Diverse biological actions of atrial natriuretic peptide. Physiol. Rev. 70:655, 1990.

33. Kimura, T., Abe, K., Ota, K., et al.: Effects of acute water load, hypertonic saline infusion, and furosemide administration on atrial natriuretic peptide and vasopressin release in humans. J. Clin. Endocrinol. Metab. 62:1003, 1986.

34. Tikkanen, I., Fyhrquist, F., Metsarinne, K., and Leidenius, R.: Plasma atrial natriuretic peptide in cardiac disease and during infusion in healthy volunteers. Lancet 2:66, 1985.

35. Raine, A.E.G., Enre, P., Burgisser, E., et al.: Atrial natriuretic peptide and atrial pressure in patients with congestive heart failure. N. Engl. J. Med. 315:533, 1986.

36. Nicholls, M. G., and Richards, A. M.: Human studies with atrial natriuretic factor. Endocrinol. Metab. Clin. North Am. 16:199, 1987.

37. Genest, J., Larochelle, P., Cusson, J. R., et al.: The atrial natriuretic factor in hypertension. Hypertension 11(Suppl. I):13, 1988.

38. Yamaji, T., Ismibasi, M., Nakaoka, H., et al.: Possible role for atrial natriuretic peptide in polyuria associated with paroxysmal atrial arrhythmias. Lancet 1:1211, 1985.

39. Espiner, E. A., Crozier, I. G., Nicholls, M. G., et al.: Cardiac secretion of atrial natriuretic peptide. Lancet 2:398, 1985.

40. Hu, J. R., Bethinger, U. G., and Lang, R. E.: Endothelin stimulates atrial natriuretic peptide (ANP) release from rat atria. Eur. J. Pharmacol. 158:177, 1988.

41. Manning, P. T., Schwartz, D., Katsube, N. C., et al.: Vasopressin-stimulated release of atriopeptin: Endocrine antagonists in fluid homeostasis. Science 229:395, 1985.

42. Napier, M. A., Vandlen, R. L., Albers-Schonberg, G., et al.: Specific membrane receptors for atrial natriuretic factor in renal and vascular tissue. Proc. Natl. Acad. Sci. USA 81:5946, 1984.

43. Hirata, Y., Tomita, M., Yoshimi, H., and Ikeda, M.: Specific receptors for atrial natriuretic factor (ANF) in cultured vascular smooth muscle cells of rat aorta. Biochem. Biophys. Res. Commun. 125:562, 1984.

44. DeLean, A., Gutkowska, J., NcNicoll, N., et al.: Characterization of specific receptors for atrial natriuretic factor in bovine adrenal zona glomerulosa. Life Sci 35:2311, 1984.

45. Quirion, R., Dalpe, M., DeLean, A., et al.: Atrial natriuretic factor (ANF) binding sites in brain and related structures. Peptides 5:1167, 1984.

46. Fuller, F., Porter, J. G., Arfsien, A. E., et al.: Atrial natriuretic clearance receptor: Complete sequence and functional expression of cDNA clones. J. Biol. Chem. 236H:9395, 1988.

47. Schulz, S., Chinkers, M., and Garbers, D. L.: The guanylate cyclase/receptor family of proteins. FASEB J. 3:2026, 1989.

48. Cogan, M. G.: Renal effects of atrial natriuretic factor. Annu. Rev. Physiol. 52:699, 1990.

49. Light, D. B., Schwiebert, E. M., Karlson, K. H., et al.: Atrial natriuretic peptide inhibits a cation channel in renal inner medullary collecting duct cells. Science 243:383, 1989.

50. Ballermann, B. J., and Brenner, B. M.: Role of atrial peptides in body fluid homeostasis. Circ. Res. 58:619, 1986.

51. Weidmann, P., Hasler, L., Gnadinger, M. P., et al.: Blood levels and renal effects of atrial natriuretic peptides in normal man. J. Clin. Invest. 77:734, 1986.

52. Dunn, B. R., Ichikawa, I., Pfeffer, J. M., et al.: Renal and systemic hemodynamic effects of synthetic atrial natriuretic peptide in the anesthetized rat. Circ. Res. 59:237, 1986.

53. Huang, C. L., and Cogan, M. G.: Atrial natriuretic factor inhibits maximal tubuloglomerular feedback response. Am. J. Physiol. 252:F825, 1987.

54. Pollock, D. M., and Arendshorst, W. J.: Effect of atrial natriuretic factor on renal hemodynamics in the rat. Am. J. Physiol. 251:F795, 1986.

55. Seymore, A. A., Smith, S. G. III, and Mazack, E. K.: Effects of renal perfusion pressure on natriuresis induced by atrial natriuretic factor. Am. J. Physiol. 253:F234, 1987.

56. Henrich, W. L., McAllister, E. A., Smith, P. B., et al.: Guanosine 3',5' cyclic monophosphate as a mediator of inhibition of renin release. Am. J. Physiol. 253:F474, 1988.

57. Laragh, J. H.: Atrial natriuretic hormone, the renin-aldosterone axis, and blood pressure-electrolyte homeostasis. N. Engl. J. Med. 313:1330, 1985.

58. Kleinert, H. D., Maack, T., Atlas, S. A., et al.: Atrial natriuretic factor inhibits angiotensin-, norepinephrine-, and potassium-induced vascular contractility. Hypertension 6(Suppl. 1):1143, 1984.

59. Bolli, P., Muller, F. B., Linder, L., et al.: The vasodilator potency of atrial natriuretic peptide in man. Circulation 75:221, 1987.

59a. Chu, A., Morris, K. G., Kuehl, W. D., et al.: Effects of atrial natriuretic peptide on the coronary arterial vasculature in humans. Circulation 80:1627, 1989.

60. Lappe, R. W., Smits, J.F.M., Todt, J. A., et al.: Failure of atriopeptin II to cause arterial vasodilation in the conscious rat. Circ. Res. 56:606, 1985.

61. Smith, S., Anderson, S., Ballermann, B. J., and Brenner, B. M.: Role of atrial natriuretic peptide in the adaption of sodium excretion with reduced renal mass. J. Clin. Invest. 77:1395, 1986.

62. Ballermann, B. J., Bloch, K. D., Seidman, J. G., and Brenner, B. M.: Atrial natriuretic peptide transcription, secretion, and glomerular receptor activity during mineralocorticoid escape in the rat. J. Clin. Invest. 78:840, 1986.

63. Saper, C. B., Standaert, D. B., Currie, M. G., et al.: Atriopeptin-immunoreactive neurons in the brain: Presence in cardiovascular regulatory areas. Science 227:1047, 1985.

64. Jacobowitz, D. M., Skofitsch, G., Keiser, H. R., et al.: Evidence for the existence of atrial natriuretic factor-containing neurons in the rat brain. Neuroendocrinology 40:92, 1985.

65. Baehr, G., and Laude, H.: Glomerulonephritis as a complication of subacute streptococcus endocarditis. JAMA 75:789, 1920.

66. Neugarten, J., and Baldwin, D. S.: Glomerulonephritis in bacterial endocarditis. Am. J. Med. 77:297, 1984.

67. Bayer, A. S., Theofilopoulos, A. N., Tillman, D. B., et al.: Use of circulating immune complex levels in the serodifferentiation of endocarditis and nonendocarditic septicemias. Am. J. Med. 66:58, 1979.

68. Keane, W. F., and Maddy, M. F.: Host defenses and infectious complications in maintenance hemodialysis patients. In Maher, J. F. (ed.): Replacement of Renal Function by Dialysis. 3rd ed. Dordrect, Kluwer, 1989.

69. Colt, H. G., Begg, R. J., Saporito, J. J., et al.: Cholesterol emboli after cardiac catheterization. Medicine (Baltimore) 67:389, 1988.

EFFECTS OF RENAL DISEASE ON THE CARDIOVASCULAR SYSTEM

70. Rostand, S. G., and Rutsky, E. A.: Ischemic heart disease in chronic renal failure: Management strategies. Semin. Dialysis 2:98, 1989.

71. Hahn, R., Oette, K., Mondorf, H., et al.: Analysis of cardiovascular risk factors in chronic hemodialysis patients with special attention to the hyperlipoproteinemias. Atherosclerosis 48:279, 1983.

72. Vincenti, F., Amand, W. J., Abele, J., et al.: The role of hypertension in hemodialysis-associated atherosclerosis. Am. J. Med. 68:363, 1980.

73. Hopkins, P. N., and Williams, R. R.: A survey of 246 suggested coronary risk factors. Atherosclerosis 40:1, 1981.

74. Rostand, S. G., Kirk, K. A., and Rutsky, E. A.: Dialysis-associated ischemic heart disease: Insights from coronary angiography. Kidney Int. 25:653, 1984.

75. Sreepada Rao, T. K., Roxe, D. M., Laird, N. M., and Santiago, G. C.: Hemodynamic and cardiac correlates of different hemodialysis regimens: The National Cooperative Dialysis Study. Kidney Int. 23(Suppl. 13):S-89, 1983.

76. Deutsch, E., Bernstein, R. C., Addonizion, V. P., et al.: Coronary artery bypass surgery in patients on chronic hemodialysis, a case-control study. Ann. Intern. Med. 110:369, 1989.

76a. Kahn, J. K., Rutherford, B. D., McConahay, D. R., et al.: Short- and long-term outcome of percutaneous transluminal coronary angioplasty in chronic dialysis patients. Am. Heart J. 119:484, 1990.

77. Nonast-Daniel, B., Creutzig, A., Kuhn, K., et al.: Effect of treatment with recombinant erythropoietin on peripheral hemodynamics and oxygenation. Contrib. Nephrol. 66:185, 1988.

78. Eschbach, J. W., Haley, N. R., and Adamson, J. W.: New insights into the treatment of anemia of chronic renal failure with erythropoietin. Semin. Dialysis 3:112, 1990.

79. Heyka, R. J., and Vidt, D. G.: Control of hypertension in patients with chronic renal failure. Cleve. Clin. J. Med. 56:65, 1989.

80. Dustan, H. P., and Page, I. H.: Some factors in renal and renoprival hypertension. J. Lab. Clin. Med. 64:948, 1964.

81. Wilkinson, R., Scott, D. F., Uldall, P. R., et al.: Plasma renin and exchangeable sodium in the hypertension of chronic renal failure. The effect of bilateral nephrectomy. Q. J. Med. 39:377, 1970.

82. Cangiano, J. L., Ramirez-Muxo, O., Ramirez-Gonzalez, R., et al.: Normal renin uremic hypertension. Arch. Intern. Med. 136:17, 1976.

83. Dzau, V.: Significance of the vascular renin-angiotensin pathway. Hypertension 8:553, 1986.

84. Nakashima, Y., Fouad, F. M., Nakamoto, S., et al.: Localization of autonomic nervous system dysfunction in dialysis patients. Am. J. Nephrol. 7:375, 1987.

85. Cinotti, G. A., Mene, P., and Pugliese, F.: Prostaglandins in experimental hypertension. Contrib. Nephrol. 54:9, 1987.

86. Isles, C. G., McLay, A., and Jones, J. M.: Recovery in malignant hypertension presenting as acute renal failure. Q. J. Med. 53:439, 1984.

87. Huysmans, F. T., Hoitsma, A. J., and Koene, R. A.: Factors determining the prevalence of hypertension after renal transplantation. Nephrol. Dial. Transplant. 2:34, 1987.

88. Tilney, N. L., Rocha, A., Strom, T. B., and Kirkman, R. L.: Renal artery stenosis in transplant patients. Ann. Surg. 199:454, 1984.

89. Curtis, J. J., Luke, R. G., Jones, P., et al.: Hypertension in cyclosporine-treated renal transplant recipients is sodium dependent. Am. J. Med. 85:134, 1988.

90. Curtis, J. J., Luke, R. G., Whelchel, J. D., et al.: Inhibition of angiotensin-converting enzyme in renal-transplant recipients with hypertension. N. Engl. J. Med. 308:377, 1983.

91. Steinmuller, D. R.: Refractory hypertension post renal transplantation. Cleve. Clin. J. Med. 56:377, 1989.

92. Chapman, J. R., Marcen, R., Arias, M., et al.: Hypertension after renal transplantation: A comparison of cyclosporine and conventional immunosuppression. Transplantation 43:860, 1987.

93. Kasiske, B. L., and Uman, A. J.: Persistent hyperlipidemia in renal transplant patients. Medicine (Baltimore) 66:309, 1987.

94. Markel, M. S., and Friedman, E. A.: Hyperlipidemia after organ transplantation. Am. J. Med. 87(Suppl. 5N):5N, 1989.

95. Markell, S. S., Brown, C. D., Butt, K.M.H., et al.: Prospective evaluation of changes in lipid profiles in cyclosporine-treated renal transplant patients. Transplant. Proc. 21:1497, 1989.

96. Maschio, G., Oldrizzi, L., Rugiu, C., et al.: Serum lipids in patients with chronic renal failure on long-term, protein-restricted diets. Am. J. Med. 87(Suppl. 5N):5, 1989.

96a. Appel, G. Lipid abnormalities in renal disease. Kidney Int. 39:169, 1991.

97. Fuh, M.M.T., Lee, C-M., Jeng, C-Y., et al.: Effect of chronic renal failure on high-density lipoprotein kinetics. Kidney Int. 37:1295, 1990.

98. Chan, M. K., Varghese, Z., Persaud, J. W., et al.: Hyperlipidemia in patients on maintenance hemo- and peritoneal dialysis: The relative pathogenetic roles of triglyceride production and triglyceride removal. Clin. Nephrol. 17:183, 1982.

99. Rapoport, J., Aviram, M., Chaimovitz, C., and Brook, J. G.: Defective high density lipoprotein composition in patients on chronic hemodialysis. N. Engl. J. Med. 299:1326, 1978.

100. Nestel, P. J., Fidge, N. H., and Tan, M. H.: Increased lipoprotein-remnant formation in chronic renal failure. N. Engl. J. Med. 307:329, 1982.

101. Drueke, T., Lacour, B., Roullet, J. B., and Funcke-Brentano, J. L.: Recent advances in factors that alter lipid metabolism in chronic renal failure. Kidney Int. 24(Suppl. 16):S-134, 1983.

102. Grutzmacher, P., Marz, W., Peschke, B., et al.: Lipoproteins and apolipoproteins during progression of chronic renal disease. Nephron 50:103,1988.

103. Uraemia, lipoproteins and atherosclerosis. Lancet 2:1151, 1981.

104. Sanfelippo, M. L., Swensen, R. S., and Reaven, G. M.: Reduction of plasma triglycerides by diet in subjects with chronic renal failure. Kidney Int. 11:54, 1977.

105. Merk, W., Graben, N., Hartmann, H., et al.: Serum levels of free nonprotein bound clofibrinic acid after single dosing to patients with impaired renal function of various degrees—a multicenter study. Int. J. Clin. Pharmacol. Ther. Toxicol. 25:59, 1987.

106. Guba, E. A., Abel, S. R., and Golper, T. A.: Practical guidelines for drug therapy in dialysis: Lipid lowering agents. Semin. Dialysis 2:186, 1989.

107. Lai, K. N., Barnden, L., and Mathew, T. H.: Effect of renal transplantation on left ventricular function in hemodialysis patients. Clin. Nephrol. 18:74, 1982.

108. Crosbie, W. A., Snowden, S., and Parsons, V.: Changes in lung capillary permeability in renal failure. Br. Med. J. 4:388, 1972.

109. Gotloib, L., and Servadio, C.: A possible case of beriberi heart failure in a chronic hemodialysis patient. Nephron 14:293, 1975.

110. Raab, W.: Cardiotoxic substances in the blood and heart muscle in uremia. J. Lab. Clin. Med. 29:715, 1944.

111. Scheuer, J., and Stezoski, S. W.: The effects of uremic components on cardiac function and metabolism. J. Mol. Cell. Cardiol. 5:287, 1973.

112. Patrick, J., and Jones, N. F.: Cell sodium, potassium and water in uremia and the effects of regular dialysis as studies in the leukocyte. Clin. Sci. Mol. Med. 46:583, 1974.

113. Drüeke, T., Fleury, J., Toure, Y., et al.: Effect of parathyroidectomy on left ventricular function in haemodialysis patients. Lancet 1:112, 1980.

114. Baczynski, R. F., Massry, S. G., Kohan, R., et al.: Effect of parathyroid hormone on myocardial energy metabolism in the rat. Kidney Int. 27:718, 1985.

115. Rostand, S. G. Sanders, C., Kirk, K. A., et al.: Myocardial calcification and cardiac dysfunction in chronic renal failure. Am. J. Med. 85:651, 1988.

116. Gafter, U., Battler, A., Eldar, M., et al.: Effect of hyperparathyroidism on cardiac function in patients with end stage renal disease. Nephron 41:30, 1985.

117. London, G. M., Guerin, A. P., Marchais, S. J., et al.: Cardiomyopathy in end-stage renal disease. Semin. Dialysis 2:102, 1989.

118. Pehrsson, S. K., Jonasson, R., and Lins, L. E.: Cardiac performance in various stages of renal failure. Br. Heart J. 52:667, 1984.

118a. Blake, J. W., Solangi, K. B., Herman, M. V., et al.: Left ventricular response to exercise and autonomic control mechanisms in end-stage renal disease. Arch. Intern. Med. 149:433, 1989.

118b. London, G. M., Fabiani, F., Marchais, S. J., et al.: Uremic cardiomyopathy: An inadequate left ventricular hypertrophy. Kidney Int. 31:973, 1987.

119. Henrich, W. L., Hunt, J. M., and Nixon, J. V.: Increased ionized calcium and left ventricular contractility during hemodialysis. N. Engl. J. Med. 310:19, 1984.

120. Blaustein, A. S., Schmitt, G., Foster, M. C., et al.: Serial effects on left ventricular load and contractility during hemodialysis in patients with concentric hypertrophy. Am. Heart J. 111:340, 1986.

121. Nixon, J. V., Mitchell, J. H., McPhaul, J. J., Jr., and Henrich, W. L.: Effect of hemodialysis on left ventricular function. Dissociation of changes in filling volume and in contractile state. J. Clin. Invest. 71:377, 1983.

122. Leenen, F. H., Smith, D. L., Khanna, R., and Oreopoulos, D. G.: Changes in left ventricular hypertrophy and function in hypertensive patients started on continuous ambulatory peritoneal dialysis. Am. Heart J. 110:102, 1985.

123. Silverberg, J. S., Tahal, D. P., Patton, R., et al.: Role of anemia in the pathogenesis of left ventricular hypertrophy in end-stage renal disease. Am. J. Cardiol. 64:222, 1989.

124. London, G., de Vernejoul, M., Fabiani, F., et al.: Secondary hyperparathyroidism and cardiac hypertrophy in haemodialysis patients. Kidney Int. 32:900, 1987.

125. Low, I., Grutzmacher, P., Bergmann, M., et al.: Echocardiographic findings in patients on maintenance hemodialysis substituted with recombinant human erythropoietin. Clin. Nephrol. 31:26, 1989.

125a. Cannella, G., La Canna, G., Sandrini, M., et al.: Renormalization of cardiac output and of left ventricular size following long-term recombinant human erythropoietin treatment of anemic dialyzed uremic patients. Clin. Nephrol. 34:272, 1990.

126. Himmelman, R. B., Landzberg, J. S., and Simonson, J. S., et al.: Cardiac consequences of renal transplantation: Changes in left ventricular morphology and function. J. Am. Coll. Cardiol. 12:915, 1988.

127. Cueto-Garcia, L., Herrera, J., Arriaga, J., et al.: Echocardiographic changes after successful renal transplantation in young nondiabetic patients. Chest 83:56, 1983.

128. Washer, G. F., Schroter, G.P.J., Starzl, T. E., et al.: Causes of death after kidney transplantation. JAMA 250:49, 1983.

129. Burt, R. K., Gupta-Burt, S., Wadi, W. N., et al.: Reversal of left ventricular dysfunction after renal transplantation. Ann. Intern. Med. 111:635, 1989.

130. Henrich, W. L.: Hemodynamic instability during hemodialysis. Kidney Int. 30:605, 1986.

131. Diamond, S. M., and Henrich, W. L.: Acetate dialysate versus bicarbonate dialysate: A continuing controversy. Am. J. Kidney Dis. 9:3, 1987.

132. Velez, R. L., Woodward, T. D., and Heinrich, W. L.: Acetate and bicarbonate hemodialysis in patients with and without autonomic dysfunction. Kidney Int. 26:59, 1984.

133. Van Stone, J. C., Bauer, J., and Carey, J.: The effects of dialysate sodium concentration on body fluid distribution during hemodialysis. Trans. Am. Soc. Artif. Intern. Organs 26:383, 1980.

134. Henrich, W. L., Woodard, T. D., and McPhaul, J. J., Jr.: The chronic efficacy and safety of high sodium dialysate: Double-blind, crossover study. Am. J. Kidney Dis. 2:349, 1982.

135. Rouby, J. J., Rottembourg, J., Durande, J. P., et al.: Hemodynamic changes induced by regular hemodialysis and sequential ultrafiltration hemodialysis: A comparative study. Kidney Int. 17:801, 1980.

136. Arduson, C. B., Codd, J. R., Graff, R. A., et al.: Cardiac failure in upper extremity arteriovenous dialysis fistulae. Arch. Intern. Med. 136:292, 1976.

137. Aurigemma, N. M., Feldman, N. T., Gottlieb, M. N., et al.: Arterial oxygenation during hemodialysis. N. Engl. J. Med. 297:871, 1977.

138. Thayssen, P., Anderson, K. H., and Pindborg, T.: Noninvasive monitoring of cardiac function during haemodialysis. Scand. J. Urol. Nephrol. 15:313, 1981.

139. Cardoso, M., Vinay, P., Vinet, B., et al.: Hypoxemia during hemodialysis: A critical review of the facts. Am. J. Kidney Dis. 11:281, 1988.

140. Wiegmann, T. B., MacDougall, M. L., and Diederich, D. A.: Dialysis leukopenia, hypoxemia, and anaphylatoxin formation: Effect of membrane, bath, and citrate anticoagulation. Am. J. Kidney Dis. 11:418, 1988.

141. Jones, R. H., Broadfield, J. B., and Parsons, V.: Arterial hypoxaemia during hemodialysis for acute renal failure in mechanically ventilated patients: Observations and mechanisms. Clin. Nephrol. 14:18, 1980.

142. Fraley, D. S., and Adler, S.: Correction of hyperkalemia by bicarbonate despite constant blood pH. Kidney Int. 12:354, 1977.

143. D'Cruz, I. A., Jain, M., Fishman, S., et al.: Calcification of the mitral region in patients with chronic renal failure: 2-D echocardiographic, hormonal and autopsy correlation. J. Am. Coll. Cardiol. 1:625, 1983.

144. Nestico, P. F., DePace, N. L., Kotler, M. N., et al.: Calcium and phosphorus metabolism in dialysis patients with and without mitral anular calcium. Analysis of 30 patients. Am. J. Cardiol. 51:497, 1983.

145. Ferman, M. B., Virmani, R., Robertson, R. M., and Stone, W. J.: Mitral annular calcification in chronic renal failure. Chest 85:367, 1984.

146. Depace, N. L., Rohrer, A. H., Kotler, M. N., et al.: Rapidly progressing, massive mitral annular calcification. Arch. Intern. Med. 141:1663, 1981.

147. Maher, E. R., Yound, G., Smyth-Walsh, B., et al.: Aortic and mitral valve calcification in patients with end-stage renal disease. Lancet 2:875, 1987.

148. Osterberger, L. E., Goldstein, S., Khaja, F., and Lakier, J. B.: Functional mitral stenosis in patients with massive mitral annular calcification. Circulation 64:472, 1981.

149. Rosen, H., Friedman, S. A., Raizner, A. E., and Gerstmann, K.: Azotemic arteriopathy. Am. Heart J. 84:250, 1972.

150. Ejerblad, S., Ericsson, J.L.E., and Eriksson, I.: Arterial lesions of the radial artery in uraemic patients. Acta Chir. Scand. 145:415, 1979.

151. Verberckmoes, R., Bouillon, R., and Krempien, B.: Disappearance of vascular calcifications during treatment of renal osteodystrophy. Ann. Intern. Med. 82:529, 1975.

152. Landsberg, K. F., and Landsberg, D. N.: Vitamin D preparations and their role in renal osteodystrophy. Can. J. Hosp. Pharm. 38:10, 1985.

153. Slatapolsky, E., Weerts, C., Thielan, K., et al.: Marked suppression of secondary hyperparathyroidism by intravenous administration of 1,25-dihydroxycholecalciferal in uremic patients. J. Clin. Invest. 74:2136, 1984.

154. Wacker, W., and Merrill, J. P.: Uremic pericarditis in acute and chronic renal failure. JAMA 156:764, 1954.

155. Frommer, J. P., Young, J. P., and Ayus, J. C.: Asymptomatic pericardial effusion in uremic patients: Effect of long-term dialysis. Nephron 39:296, 1985.

156. Hoops, H. C., and Wissler, R. M.: Uremic pneumonitis. Am. J. Pathol. *31*:361, 1955.

157. Nidus, B. D., Matalon, R., Cantazino, D., and Eisinger, R. P.: Uremic pleuritis—A clinicopathological entity. N. Engl. J. Med. *281*:255, 1969.

158. Ventura, S. C., and Garella, S.: The management of pericardial disease in renal failure. Semin. Dialysis *3*:21, 1990.

159. Luft, F. C., Gilman, J. K., and Weyman, A. E.: Pericarditis in patients with uremia: Clinical and echocardiographic evaluation. Nephron *25*:160, 1980.

160. Lazarus, J. M., Gottlieb, M. N., Lowrie, E. G., et al.: Echocardiographic findings in stable hemodialysis patients. Proc. Clin. Dial. Transplant Forum *6*:53, 1976.

161. Kleiman, J. H., Motta, J., London, E., et al.: Pericardial effusions in patients with end-stage renal disease. Br. Heart J. *40*:190, 1978.

162. Rutsky, E. A., and Rostand, S. G.: Pericarditis in end-stage renal disease: Clinical characteristics and management. Semin. Dialysis *2*:25, 1989.

163. Specter, D., Alfred, H., Siedlecki, M., and Briefel, G.: A controlled study of the effect of indomethacin in uremic pericarditis. Kidney Int. *24*:663, 1983.

164. Quigg, R. J., Idelson, B. A., Yoburn, D. C., et al.: Local steroids in dialysis-associated pericardial effusion. A single intraperitoneal administration of triamcinolone. Arch. Intern. Med. *145*:2249, 1985.

165. Rutsky, E. A., and Rostand, S. G.: Treatment of uremic pericarditis and pericardial effusion. Am. J. Kidney Dis. *10*:2, 1987.

166. Prager, R. L., Wilson, C. H., and Bender, H. W.: The subxiphoid approach to pericardial disease. Ann. Thorac. Surg. *34*:6, 1981.

167. Piehler, J. M., Pluth, J. R., Schaff, H. V., et al.: Surgical management of effusive pericardial disease: Influence of extent of pericardial resection on clinical course. J. Thorac. Cardiovasc. Surg. *90*:506, 1985.

168. Pillay, V.K.G., Sarpel, S. C., and Kurtzman, N. A.: Subacute constrictive uremic pericarditis: Survival after pericardiectomy. JAMA *235*:1351, 1976.

MANAGEMENT OF PATIENTS WITH CARDIAC DISEASE AND RENAL FAILURE

169. Blakeman, B. M., Pifarre, R., Sullivan, H. J., et al.: Cardiac surgery for chronic renal dialysis patients. Chest *95*:509, 1989.

170. Falch, D.: The influence of kidney function, body size and age on plasma concentration and urinary excretion of digoxin. Acta Med. Scand. *194*:251, 1973.

171. Steiness, E.: Renal tubular secretion of digoxin. Circulation *50*:103, 1974.

172. Jelliffe, R. W.: An improved method of digoxin therapy. Ann. Intern. Med. *69*:703, 1968.

173. Rasmussen, K., Jervell, J., Storstein, L., and Gjerdrum, K.: Digitoxin kinetics in patients with impaired renal function. Clin. Pharmacol. Ther. *13*:6, 1972.

174. Ackerman, G. L., Doherty, J. F., and Flanigan, W. J.: Peritoneal dialysis and hemodialysis of tritiated digoxin. Ann. Intern. Med. *67*:718, 1967.

175. Smith, T. W., Butler, V. P., Haber, E., et al.: Treatment of life-threatening digitalis intoxication with digoxin-specific Fab antibody fragments. N. Engl. J. Med. *307*:1357, 1982.

176. Gibson, T. P., Lowenthal, D. T., Nelson, H. A., and Briggs, W. A.: Elimination of procainamide in end-stage renal failure. Clin. Pharmacol. Ther. *17*:321, 1975.

177. Fenster, P. E., Hager, W. D., Perrier, D., et al.: Digoxin-quinidine interaction in patients with chronic renal failure. Circulation *66*:1277, 1982.

178. Hall, K., Meatherall, B., Krahn, J., et al.: Clearance of quinidine during peritoneal dialysis. Am. Heart J. *104*:646, 1982.

179. Thompson, P. D., Melmon, K. L., Richardson, J. A., et al.: Lidocaine pharmacokinetics in advanced heart failure, liver disease and renal failure in humans. Ann. Intern. Med. *78*:499, 1973.

180. Letteri, J. M., Mellk, H., Louis, S., et al.: Diphenylhydantoin metabolism in uremia. N. Engl. J. Med. *285*:648, 1971.

181. Thompson, P. D., Joekes, A. M., and Foulkes, D. M.: Pharmacodynamics of propranolol in renal failure. Br. Med. J. *2*:434, 1972.

182. Shand, D. G., Wed, A.J.J., Vestal, R. E., et al.: Pharmacokinetic and pharmacodynamic factors determining variations in propranolol responsiveness. *In* Braunwald, E. (ed.): Beta-Adrenergic Blockade. New York, Elsevier, 1978, pp. 74–80.

183. Bennett, W. M., Arnoff, G. R., Golper, T. A., et al.: Drug Prescribing in Renal Failure: Dosing Guidelines for Adults. Philadelphia, American College of Physicians, 1987.

184. Epstein, A. E., Kay, G. N., and Plumg, V. J.: Consideration in the diagnosis and treatment of arrhythmias in patients with end-stage renal disease. Semin. Dialysis *2*:31, 1989.

185. Tartini, A., and Kesselbrenner, M.: Encainide-induced encephalopathy in a patient with chronic renal failure. Am. J. Kidney Dis. *15*:178, 1990.

186. Woosley, R. L., Wood, A.J.J., and Roden, D. M.: Encainide. N. Engl. J. Med. *318*:1107, 1988.

Note: Page numbers in *italics* indicate illustrations. Page numbers followed by t indicate tables. **Boldface page numbers** indicate main discussion in the text. **Plate numbers** indicate color plates.